Brief Contents of Volume 2

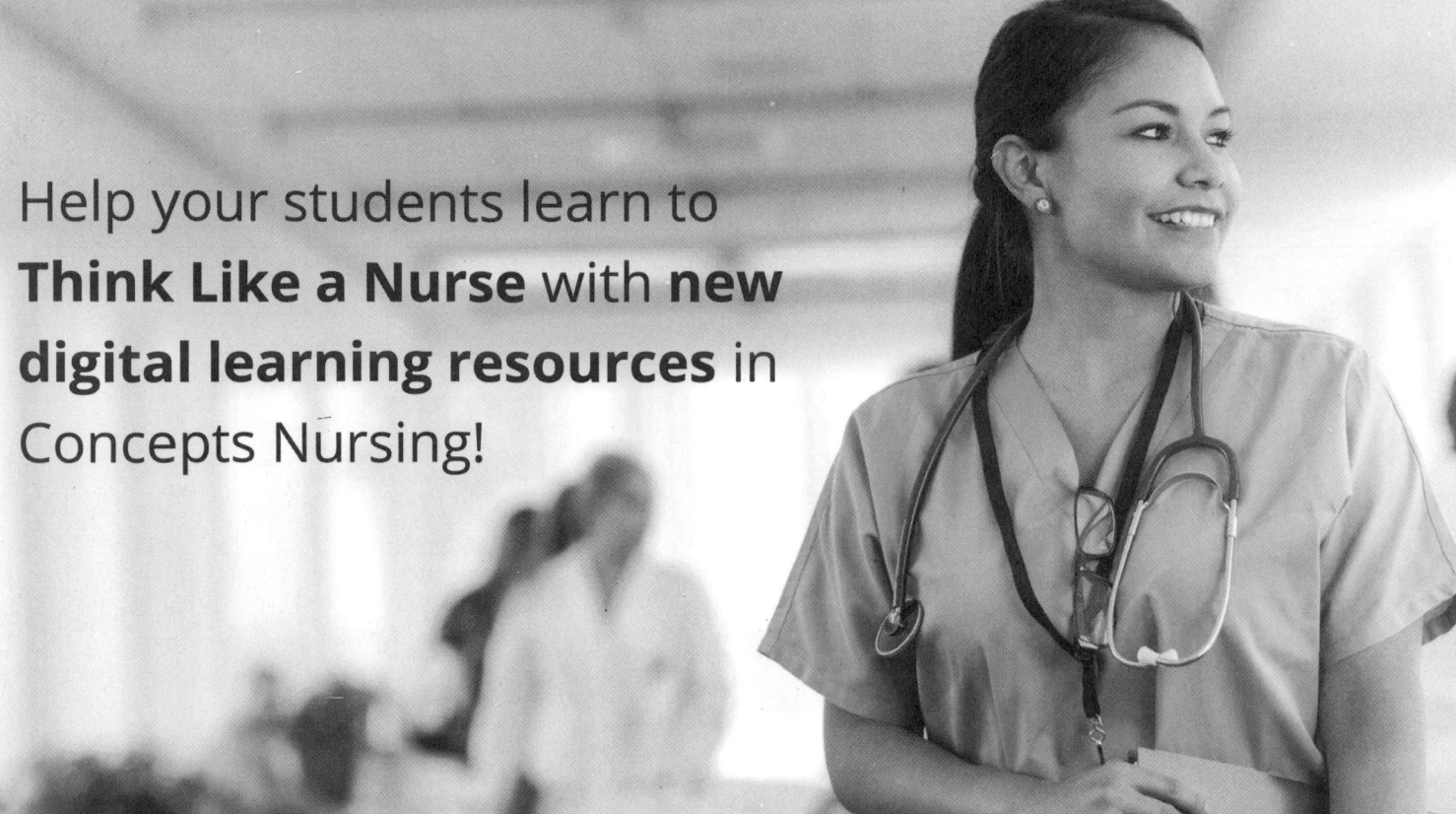

Help your students learn to **Think Like a Nurse** with **new digital learning resources** in Concepts Nursing!

MyLab® Nursing

MyLab Nursing helps students master key concepts, prepare for success on the NCLEX-RN® exam, and develop clinical reasoning skills.

NEW! Adaptive, mobile-enabled Dynamic Study Modules with personalized learning and remediation help students focus their studies and retain information over the long term.

Learn more at pearson.com/mylab/nursing

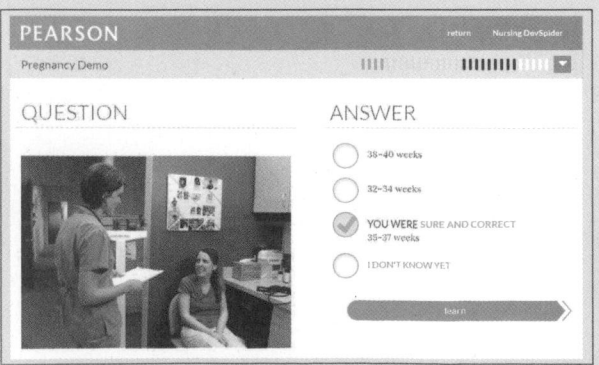

NEW! Concepts Connection in Nursing App

The Concepts Connections in Nursing app helps students make important connections between concepts in nursing and exemplars or alterations. Understanding these key concepts and the connections between them enables students to focus on the critical thinking and decision-making skills necessary for successful clinical practice. Now available on both the Apple App Store and Google Play.

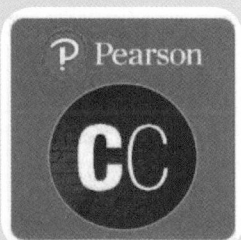

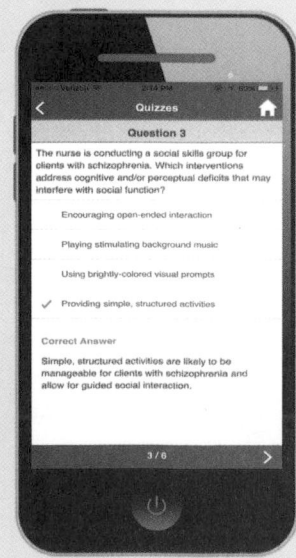

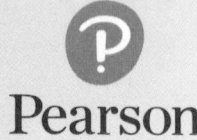

VOLUME 2

NURSING
A Concept-Based Approach to Learning

Third Edition

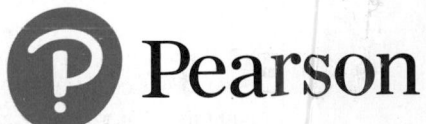

330 Hudson Street, NY, NY 10013

Vice President, Health Science and TED: Julie Levin Alexander
Director of Portfolio Management and Portfolio Manager: Katrin Beacom
Development Editors: Laura S. Horowitz and Adelaide R. McCulloch
Portfolio Management Assistant: Erin Sullivan
Vice President, Content Production and Digital Studio: Paul DeLuca
Managing Producer, Health Science: Melissa Bashe
Content Producer: Bianca Sepulveda
Diversity & Inclusion Specialists: Kendra R. Thomas, JD, and Chuin Phang
Operations Specialist: Maura Zaldivar-Garcia
Creative Director: Blair Brown
Creative Digital Lead: Mary Siener
Director of Digital Production, Digital Studio, Health Science: Amy Peltier
Digital Studio Producer, REVEL and eText 2.0: Jeff Henn
Digital Content Team Lead: Brian Prybella
Digital Content Project Lead: William Johnson
Vice President, Field Marketing: David Gesell
Executive Product Marketing Manager: Christopher Barry
Sr. Field Marketing Manager: Brittany Hammond
Full-Service Project Management and Composition: iEnergizer Aptara®, Ltd.
Project Manager: Kelly Ricci
Inventory Manager: Vatche Demirdjian
Interior Design: Studio Montage
Cover Design: Mary Siener
Cover Art: Studio Montage
Printer/Binder: LSC Communications, Inc.
Cover Printer: Phoenix Color/Hagerstown

Library of Congress Cataloging-in-Publication Data

Title: Nursing: a concept-based approach to learning.
Other titles: Nursing (Pearson)
Description: Third edition. | Boston : Pearson, [2019] | Includes bibliographical references and index.
Identifiers: LCCN 2017043040 | ISBN 9780134616803 (v. 1) | ISBN 0134616804 (v. 1) |
ISBN 9780134616810 (v. 2) | ISBN 0134616812 (v. 2)
Subjects: | MESH: Nursing Care Classification: LCC RT40 | NLM WY 100.1 | DDC 610.73--dc23 LC
record available at https://lccn.loc.gov/2017043040

1 18

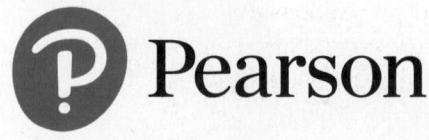

ISBN 13: 978-0-13-461681-0
ISBN 10:   0-13-461681-2

Pearson's Concepts Solution

Nursing: A Concept-Based Approach to Learning is the number one choice for schools of nursing that use a concept-based curriculum. It is the *only* true concept-based learning solution and the *only* concepts curriculum developed from the ground up as a cohesive, comprehensive learning system. The three-volume series, along with MyLab Nursing, provides everything you need to deliver an effective concept-based program that teaches students to think like a nurse and develops practice-ready nurses.

Nursing: A Concept-Based Approach to Learning, Third Edition, represents the cutting edge in nursing education. This uniquely integrated solution provides students with a consistent design of content and assessment that specifically supports a concept-based curriculum. Available as a fully integrated digital experience or in print format, this solution meets the needs of today's nursing student.

Starting with the cover, our goal for the Third Edition is to help students learn the essential knowledge they will need for patient care. The cover, a Möbius strip, represents the relationships among the concepts and how they are all interconnected. By understanding important connections of concepts, students are able to relate topics to broader contexts.

What Makes Pearson's Solution Different?

As demonstrated with the previous two editions of *Nursing: A Concept-Based Approach to Learning,* Pearson's program has successfully met the needs of tens of thousands of students and instructors in concept-based education programs. The Third Edition builds on our commitment to excellence: Every page, every word, every feature has been examined—all to help enhance the learning and teaching process. The result is an integration of content and features that *you,* our customer, have asked for and that you will not find anywhere else.

Pearson's program includes:

- Everything instructors and students need in one package: all concepts, all exemplars, all assessment tools.
- Content designed by instructional designers for conceptual learning that includes learning and enabling objectives for every main section and measurable outcomes for each.
- Content that covers the lifespan from pregnancy and birth, through childhood and adolescence, and into young adulthood and middle and old age.

Why Teach Concept-based Learning?

University and college nursing programs across the United States have begun evaluating how their programs can meet the needs of today's nursing students. The vast array of new knowledge in the "information age" has left nursing students feeling overwhelmed by the quantity of knowledge and skills they must gain in order to become practicing nurses. In light of this, many programs are moving to the model of concept-based learning in an effort to meet the challenges facing nursing students and new nurses today. Aside from creating a streamlined approach in response to content overload/saturation in nursing education, there are a multitude of reasons for nursing programs to consider a concept-based program.

This model provides the impetus for educators to transition away from traditional methods of faculty-centered teaching and passive learning toward active, focused, participative, and collaborative teaching and learning. Pearson's *Nursing: A Concept-Based Approach to Learning,* Third Edition, is designed to assist nursing faculty in providing students with a broader perspective while promoting a deeper understanding of content across the lifespan in a focused, participative, and collaborative learning environment.

What are the benefits of conceptual learning? Some of the often-referenced benefits of conceptual learning in nursing programs are that it:

- Focuses on problems
- Fosters systematic observations
- Fosters understanding of relationships
- Focuses on nursing actions and interprofessional efforts
- Challenges students to be excellent learners.

Organization and Structure of the Third Edition

The basic structure of the Second Edition was retained for the Third Edition. There are:

- Five parts:
  - I: The Biophysical Modules (in the Individual Domain)
  - II: The Psychosocial Modules (in the Individual Domain)
  - III: Reproduction (in the Individual Domain)
  - IV: The Nursing Domain
  - V: The Healthcare Domain
- Fifty-one concepts
- One hundred fifty-eight exemplars

The Concepts were chosen after surveying numerous concept-based curricula and finding the common elements. Some Concepts were added or revised in response to requests by users. The result is a comprehensive set of Concepts that cover the essentials of nursing education.

The Exemplars were chosen based on selected national models and initiatives such as those of the Institute of Medicine, *Healthy People 2020,* The Centers for Disease Control and Prevention, The Joint Commission, the National Institutes of Health, the National Institute of Mental Health, the NCLEX Test Plan, The Centers for Medicare and Medicaid, the Occupational Safety and Health Administration, and Quality and Safety Education for Nurses, among others. Prevalence rates were considered for the biophysical and psychosocial exemplars, with more common disorders prioritized over less common ones. Certain Exemplars were chosen because they lend themselves to teaching across concepts or across the lifespan. In the Third Edition, some Exemplars that focused on a particular stage of the lifespan, such as Diabetes in Children, have been folded into the Lifespan Considerations of another exemplar. Now there are two separate Exemplars on diabetes: one focusing on type 1 diabetes mellitus and the other focusing on type 2 diabetes mellitus. In the Third Edition, nine new/expanded Exemplars have been added:

- Cystic Fibrosis
- Delirium
- Environmental Quality
- Nurse Safety
- Patient Safety
- Sexual Dysfunction
- Traumatic Brain Injury
- Type 1 Diabetes Mellitus
- Type 2 Diabetes Mellitus

For the Third Edition, as shown in the Module Outline and Learning Outcomes listed at the beginning of each module, each main section has a dedicated learning outcome. Our editorial and instructional design teams worked to create consistent, accurate, challenging, achievable, and measurable objective statements based on objective-driven design practices to better engage students, improve performance, increase student gains, and promote deep learning.

Module Outline and Learning Outcomes

The Concept of Acid–Base Balance

Normal Acid–Base Balance

1.1 Analyze the physiology of normal acid–base balance.

Alterations to Acid–Base Balance

1.2 Differentiate alterations in acid–base balance.

Concepts Related to Acid–Base Balance

1.3 Outline the relationship between acid–base balance and other concepts.

Health Promotion

1.4 Explain the promotion of healthy acid–base balance.

Nursing Assessment

1.5 Differentiate common assessment procedures and tests used to examine acid–base balance.

Independent Interventions

1.6 Analyze independent interventions nurses can implement for patients with alterations in acid–base balance.

Collaborative Therapies

1.7 Summarize collaborative therapies used by interprofessional teams for patients with alterations in acid–base balance.

Acid–Base Balance Exemplars

Exemplar 1.A Metabolic Acidosis

1.A Analyze metabolic acidosis as it relates to acid–base balance.

Exemplar 1.B Metabolic Alkalosis

1.B Analyze metabolic alkalosis as it relates to acid–base balance.

Exemplar 1.C Respiratory Acidosis

1.C Analyze respiratory acidosis as it relates to acid–base balance.

Exemplar 1.D Respiratory Alkalosis

1.D Analyze respiratory alkalosis as it relates to acid–base balance.

Structure and Features of the Concepts

The Concepts feature a consistent design throughout the program. This allows students to anticipate the learning they will experience. Special features, which students can use for learning and review, recur in each Concept. The basic structure of the Concepts is shown below with visuals and annotations describing the content. Note that each **red heading** has a corresponding learning outcome.

Normal Presentation ... Each Concept starts with a review of normal, healthy function, including subsections on Physiology Review and Genetic Considerations where appropriate.

Physiology Review

Genetic Considerations

Alterations ... The second section of each Concept focuses on alterations, including subheads on Alterations and Manifestations, Prevalence, and Genetic Considerations and Risk Factors. A standard feature in this section is the Alterations and Therapies table.

Alterations and Manifestations

Prevalence

Genetic Considerations and Risk Factors

Alterations and Therapies
Oxygenation

ALTERATION	DESCRIPTION	MANIFESTATIONS	INTERVENTIONS AND THERAPIES
Hypoxemia	Decreased level of oxygen	▪ Chest wall in-drawing (early manifestation) ▪ Cyanosis (late manifestation)	▪ Identify and treat the underlying cause. ▪ Administer oxygen if O$_2$ saturation level falls below 90%.
Dyspnea	Labored breathing or shortness of breath	▪ Clearly audible, labored breathing; anxiety ▪ Distressed facial expression ▪ Nasal flaring	▪ Identify and treat the underlying cause. ▪ Administer oxygen if O$_2$ saturation level falls below 90%.
Apnea	Absence of breathing	▪ Lack of respiratory effort that can lead to respiratory arrest	▪ Identify and treat the underlying cause. ▪ Administer respiratory stimulants, as appropriate.
Tachypnea	A respiratory rate greater than 20 breaths per minute for children and adults, 60 breaths per minute for an infant	▪ Excessive rapid breathing ▪ Rapid breathing at rest ▪ Shallow breathing	▪ Identify and treat the underlying cause.
Orthopnea	Difficulty breathing when lying down	▪ Dyspnea while lying down	▪ Identify and treat the underlying cause. ▪ Elevate the head, neck, and chest while sleeping.
Pneumothorax	Lung collapse caused by the collection of free air within the pleural space	▪ Chest pain ▪ Shortness of breath	▪ Identify and treat the underlying cause. ▪ Observe the patient. ▪ Use needle decompression or chest tube insertion. ▪ Surgery

Case Studies

Each Concept contains a three-part unfolding case study to help students apply what they are learning to a sample patient.

Case Study » Part 1
Dennis Welborn is a 52-year-old man who visits his primary care physician with complaints of severe pain in his back and abdomen and painful urination with hematuria. As the nurse working at the clinic, you take Mr. Welborn's medical history and make a preliminary assessment. Mr. Welborn is 6'2" tall and weighs 265 pounds. His vital signs include temperature 100.8°F oral, pulse 95 bpm, respirations 22/min, and BP 140/92 mmHg. Mr. Welborn rates his back and abdominal pain as 9 on a scale of 0–10, and his midline abdominal pain level is a 7 when he is urinating. When asked about his diet, Mr. Welborn admits that as a widower, he often eats out with coworkers for lunch and picks up fast food on the way home for his evening meal. He usually drinks three cups of coffee in the morning and diet soda throughout the afternoon and evening. When he gets heartburn, he chews several antacid tablets for relief. An abdominal assessment reveals a distended bladder. Mr. Welborn states he delays urination as long as possible because of the pain. When he does urinate, he has noticed that he has a weak stream and continues to feel the urge to urinate when he has finished. The medical care provider orders lab tests, so a blood

and urine sample are obtained for analysis. Mr. Welborn is transferred to the radiology department to have an abdominal x-ray. The x-ray reveals a large stone (1.2 cm) in Mr. Welborn's proximal right ureter, and the urinalysis indicates the presence of small calcium crystals, RBCs, and bacteria. The blood test also detects high blood calcium levels.

Clinical Reasoning Questions Level I
1. What risk factors does Mr. Welborn have for developing urinary calculi?
2. Other than a distended bladder, what findings might you discover
3. How

Clinical Rea
4. What
5. What
Mr. W
6. Refer
ment

Case Study » Part 3
After 3 days in the hospital, Mr. Welborn is discharged to home. His urinary catheter has been removed, and he states that he can urinate without pain. However, the nephrostomy tube remains in place. In addition, his IV morphine has been discontinued, and he now receives acetaminophen (1000 mg q6h). With initiation and discontinuation of morphine, Mr. Welborn had two bowel movements before discharge.

Clinical Reasoning Questions Level I
1. What methods can you teach Mr. Welborn to help prevent future renal calculi?
2. Describe the patient teaching you will provide Mr. Welborn about caring for his nephrostomy tube.
3. What assessment should be performed on Mr. Welborn before discharge?

Clinical Reasoning Questions Level II
4. What medications might the healthcare provider prescribe for Mr. Welborn upon discharge?
5. What follow-up appointments should you schedule for Mr. Welborn? Why?
6. How would a referral to a nutritionist benefit Mr. Welborn?

Case Study » Part 2
Mr. Welborn's physician consults with a urologist, who suggests that Mr. Welborn be admitted to the hospital for a percutaneous nephrolithotomy. The urologist prescribes intravenous (IV) morphine for pain and schedules the surgery for 8:00 the next morning. The procedure is successful, without complications, and a urinary catheter and nephrostomy tube are put in place during surgery to drain urine. Postoperative pain is again managed with IV morphine, and Mr. Welborn states that his pain is manageable. He is confined to bed until 1 day postsurgery. The day after surgery, Mr. Welborn reports that he did not have his normal morning bowel movement. When he sat on the toilet, he was unable to defecate, and he was afraid to push too hard because of his surgery. He was also unable to have a bowel movement the previous morning because of anxiety about the surgery, and his abdomen is feeling full. Abdominal assessment reveals diminished bowel sounds and dullness to percussion.

Clinical Reasoning Questions Level I
1. What factors may have contributed to Mr. Welborn's constipation?
2. What independent nursing interventions can you implement to help Mr. Welborn eliminate feces?
3. What patient teaching can you provide to help Mr. Welborn prevent constipation in the future?

Clinical Reasoning Questions Level II
4. What effects might Mr. Welborn's constipation have on his urinary problems?
5. What complications may develop as a result of Mr. Welborn's constipation? What assessments should you perform to detect these complications?
6. What side effects of the percutaneous nephrolithotomy may Mr. Welborn experience related to his urinary system?

Concepts Related to
Immunity

CONCEPT	RELATIONSHIP TO IMMUNITY	NURSING IMPLICATIONS
Comfort	Painful conditions, such as swelling and skin reactions, often occur during immune response.	■ Assess related symptoms, such as edema, rash, malaise, loss of appetite, and trouble sleeping. ■ Be alert to topical and latex allergies that could worsen symptoms. ■ *Anticipate:* Additional assessments, comfort measures
Infection	Patients with alterations in immunity can experience acute or chronic infections.	■ Assess area of suspected infection (see Infection Assessment section in the module on Infection). ■ Educate patients regarding the importance of immunizations and encourage their use. ■ Educate patients regarding the importance of avoiding situations that could increase exposure to infection. ■ Practice standard precautions, proper hand hygiene, and aseptic/sterile technique with all procedures. ■ Assess complete blood count (CBC) results; be alert for elevated WBC count.
Inflammation	Movement of fluid and cells to the site of injury or infection causes inflammation during an immune response.	■ Assess for fever, skin warmth and redness, edema, and generalized pain. ■ Be alert for abscess formation, purulent exudate, and increased WBC count. ■ *Anticipate:* Aspirin, antipyretics, cold packs
Managing Care	Patients with alterations in their immune system can greatly benefit from participating in managed care and have more positive health outcomes.	■ Assess the needs of patients to identify actual or potential problems related to care. ■ Advocate for patients in relation to their care needs.

Concepts Related to ... Enhanced for the Third Edition, the Concepts Related to section and feature are designed to help students make linkages between and among different Concepts.

Health Promotion ... New to the Third Edition is a focus on health promotion, one of the foundations of nursing. Many Health Promotion sections include a Patient Teaching feature. Examples of subsections include.

Modifiable Risk Factors

Care in the Community

Patient Teaching
Health Promotion for Cancer Prevention: Modifiable Risk Factors

■ *Discourage smoking or use of other tobacco products.* Emphasize the importance of patients protecting children and themselves from exposure to tobacco smoke. This is one of the most important health decisions an individual can make.

■ *Encourage patients, especially children, to consume a healthy diet.* This should include a minimum of five servings of fruits and vegetables daily as well as whole grains, iron-rich foods, and foods that are rich in vitamin B_{12}. Teach patients to limit their consumption of processed meats; drink alcohol in moderation; and choose fewer high-calorie foods.

■ *Explain the importance of maintaining a healthy weight and being physically active.* Physical activity helps to control weight. Together, these factors may lower the risk for various types of cancer.

■ *Teach patients effective ways to protect themselves from ultraviolet radiation.* Early excessive exposure to sun and one or more severe sunburns during childhood increase the chances of skin cancers developing in adulthood. Patients who work outdoors, athletes, coaches, and others who spend time outside

regularly should use sunscreen daily (SPF 15 or greater), regardless of the climate in which they live. Emphasize the importance of avoiding midday sun, when the sun's rays are strongest. Instruct patients to cover exposed skin and wear a hat with a wide brim. They should avoid tanning beds and sunlamps.

■ *Explain the importance of avoiding risky behaviors.* Practicing risky behaviors such as needle sharing or unsafe sexual contact can increase the risk of developing certain cancers.

■ *Suggest that patients have their homes tested for radon and explore their exposure to harmful chemicals.* Patients may be exposed to hazardous substances in the home or in the workplace.

■ *Stress the importance of getting immunizations, receiving regular medical care, and doing self-examinations.* By protecting against certain viral infections, immunizations can decrease the risk of some cancers. Regular screenings and self-examinations increase the chances of early detection of cancer, allowing for a better chance of successful treatment (Mayo Clinic, 2015a).

Oxygenation Assessment

ASSESSMENT/ METHOD	NORMAL FINDINGS	ABNORMAL FINDINGS	LIFESPAN OR DEVELOPMENTAL CONSIDERATIONS
Nasal Assessment			
Inspect the nose symmetry.	The nose should be midline and symmetrical.	■ Asymmetry indicates trauma or surgery.	■ Nasal flaring in the neonate may be indicative of respiratory compromise.
Inspect nasal cavity using a flashlight.	The septum should fall midline and be intact. The mucosa of the nares should be pink and moist without drainage. Both nares should be patent.	■ Redness and/or swelling is observed. ■ Deviated septum narrows or occludes one naris. ■ Foreign bodies may be found in the nares, especially of infants, toddlers, and preschoolers. ■ Purulent or watery nasal drainage is present. ■ Pale turbinates are seen.	■ Nasal passages of neonates and small children are smaller than those of adults. Ensuring a clear nasal cavity may decrease the risk for respiratory compromise, as neonates and infants are nasal breathers.
Respiratory Rate Assessment			
Count respiratory rate for one full minute, counting one inspiration and one expiration as one breath.	Normal respiratory rate is eupnea (see Table 15–1 for developmental impact on rate).	■ Bradypnea ■ Tachypnea ■ Apnea ■ Cheyne-Stokes respirations	■ A child's respiratory rate is higher than that of an adult's. Rely on both sight and touch to obtain an accurate respiratory rate. Neonates are sporadic breathers so short periods of apnea (less than 15 seconds) are expected.
Assess quality of breathing: determine regularity in timing. Assess depth of inspiration. Observe effort to breathe.	The I:E ratio is normally 1:2. The cycle of inspiration and expiration should be followed by a resting period in which the sensors of the respiratory system will initiate the next cycle. Normal breathing is referred to as eupnea.	■ Shortness of breath ■ Dyspnea ■ Orthopnea	■ Infants and children have softer chest walls and depend more heavily on the diaphragm to breathe. Therefore, they exhibit what is known as "seesaw" breathing, an indicator of severe distress. ■ In older adults, lifestyle choices such as smoking can affect the quality of breathing, as can the development of respiratory diseases.
Inspection of Thoracic Cavity			
Anteroposterior diameter is half the transverse diameter.	Normal ratio is 1:2. (See **Figures 15–5 »** and **15–6 »**.)	■ Anteroposterior equals transverse thoracic diameter measurements, called a barrel chest.	■ Rapid growth early in life, the plateau in young adulthood, and decline in later life can affect normal ratios.

Nursing Assessment ... Restructured for the Third Edition, this section covers everything the new nurse needs to know about assessing patients. It includes information on.

Observation and Patient Interview

Physical Examination

Diagnostic Tests

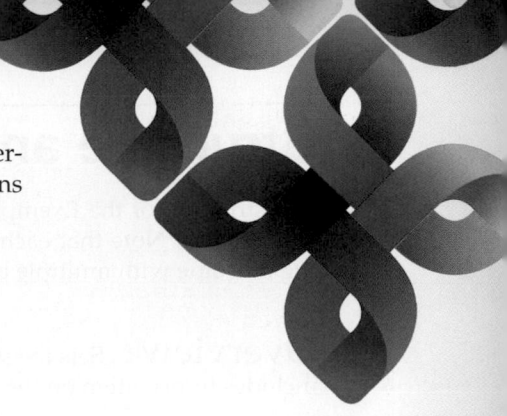

Independent Interventions

Independent Interventions ... Emphasizes interventions that nurses can perform on their own, without an order from the healthcare provider. Examples of subsections include:

Prevent Infection

Promote Safety

Sleep Hygiene

Collaborative Therapies

Collaborative Therapies ... Each Concept includes an overview of relevant therapies that require collaboration with the interprofessional team. A Medications feature covers the most common drugs used to treat alterations. Examples of subsections include.

Surgery

Pharmacologic Therapy

Nonpharmacologic Therapy

Complementary Health Approaches

Medications
Antimicrobial Agents

CLASSIFICATION AND DRUG EXAMPLES	MECHANISMS OF ACTION	NURSING CONSIDERATIONS
Antibiotics ■ Amino-glycosides ■ Macrolides ■ Tetracyclines ■ Cephalosporins ■ Penicillins ■ Sulfonamides ■ Fluoroquinolones *Drug examples:* Cefaclor, erythromycin, penicillin, tobramycin, trimethoprim-sulfamethoxazole	Antibiotics may be used prophylactically to prevent infection or used to treat existing bacterial infection. A specific antibiotic is chosen on the basis of the pathogen causing the infection.	■ Teach patients the importance of taking the entire prescribed amount. ■ Encourage adequate fluid intake. ■ Monitor for signs of allergic reaction. ■ Assess renal and hepatic function and vital signs.
Antifungal *Drug examples:* Amphotericin B, anidulafungin, caspofungin acetate, flucytosine, micafungin, fluconazole, nystatin	These drugs are selective for fungal plasma membranes. They inhibit ergosterol synthesis.	■ Carefully monitor the patient's condition. ■ Use cautiously in patients with renal impairment and severe bone marrow suppression as well as patients who are pregnant. ■ Closely monitor kidney function (intake and output, BUN, creatinine, daily weights). ■ Monitor serum electrolytes.
Antipyretic, Analgesic *Drug example:* Acetaminophen	These drugs relieve pain and reduce fever.	■ Monitor temperature. ■ Assess pain level. ■ Teach proper administration.
Antipyretic, Analgesic, Anti-inflammatory *Drug examples:* Aspirin, ibuprofen	These drugs reduce fever and inflammation, in addition to relieving pain.	■ Monitor temperature. ■ Assess pain level. ■ Teach proper administration.

REVIEW The Concept of ...

REVIEW The Concept of ... As in the Second Edition, each Concept ends with a review that includes linking questions, a list of relevant skills from Volume 3, and a short case study with questions so students can apply their knowledge.

REVIEW The Concept of Elimination

RELATE Link the Concepts

Linking the concept of elimination with the concept of infection:

1. What changes in urinary elimination indicate the presence of a UTI?
2. List the effects viral gastroenteritis has on bowel elimination.

Linking the concept of elimination with the concept of communication:

3. How can therapeutic communication be beneficial when assessing patients with urinary or bowel elimination problems?
4. Describe the importance of accurate documentation when caring for a hospitalized patient with urinary or bowel elimination problems.

READY Go to Volume 3: Clinical Nursing Skills

■ SKILL 1.10	Abdomen: Assessing
■ SKILL 2.25	Rectal Medication: Administering
■ SKILLS 4.1–4.5	Elimination: Assessment—Collecting Specimens
■ SKILLS 4.6–4.16	Elimination: Bladder Interventions
■ SKILLS 4.17–4.23	Elimination: Bowel Interventions
■ SKILLS 4.24–4.27	Elimination: Dialysis
■ SKILL 6.1	Hand Hygiene: Performing

REFER Go to Pearson MyLab Nursing and eText

■ Additional review materials
■ MiniModule: Anatomy and Physiology of Urinary Elimination

REFLECT Apply Your Knowledge

Tony Norwinski is a 7-year-old boy in the second grade. He and his 4-year-old sister, Nyla, live at home with their mother, Diane Norwinski.

Ms. Norwinski is a single parent who works in the cafeteria at the high school. Tony has a problem with wetting the bed occasionally and is too embarrassed to discuss it with anyone. Ms. Norwinski thinks Tony wets the bed because of emotional problems caused by his father leaving them when he was so young. Ms. Norwinski does not want to try anything new to help with the bedwetting because she is afraid it will cause Tony more embarrassment and emotional upset. They try not to talk about the bedwetting because Ms. Norwinski thinks it will make matters worse for Tony and prolong the problem.

Today, both children have an appointment for an annual physical examination with the nurse practitioner prior to starting the new school year. Tony is soft spoken and reserved when questioned about his general heath. Ms. Norwinski is a good historian and offers complete answers about Tony's health history. The nurse notices the odor of urine on Tony's undergarments during the initial assessment. When questioned, Tony looks at his mother and does not answer. Ms. Norwinski looks away and does not answer right away. The nurse remains silent, waiting for a response to the questions.

After a period of silence, Ms. Norwinski reassures Tony and answers the nurse's questions about the odor. Though embarrassed, Tony appears to trust the nurse because he helps his mother explain about the bedwetting.

1. What therapeutic communication techniques could the nurse use to facilitate a full disclosure of the problem?
2. What are some questions the nurse could ask Tony and his mother to obtain the most pertinent information about Tony's situation? What nursing diagnosis would best describe the priority problem?
3. List four other possible nursing diagnoses the nurse may want to incorporate in the plan of care.

Structure and Features of the Exemplars

The structure of the Exemplars is picked up from the Second Edition. Note that each Exemplar has one main learning outcome with multiple enabling objectives.

Overview … Sets the stage for the Exemplar and often includes information on the prevalence of the disorder.

Pathophysiology and Etiology … Describes not only the pathophysiology and etiology of the disorder, but also risk factors and prevention methods.

Pathophysiology

Etiology

Risk Factors

Prevention

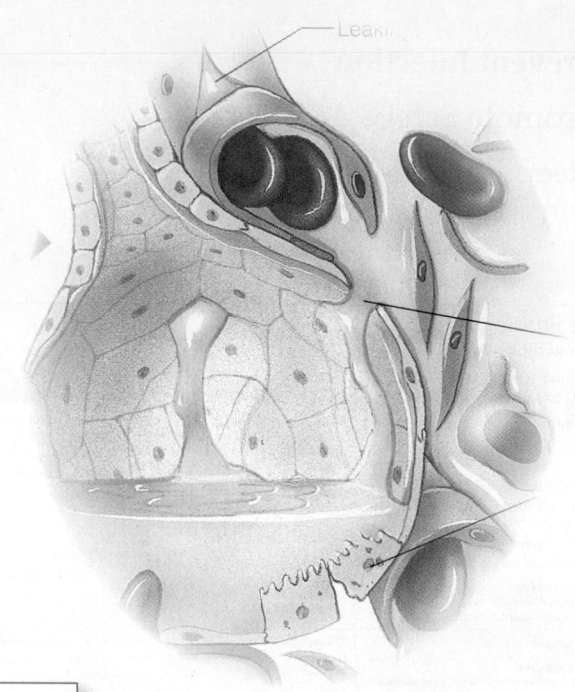

Clinical Manifestations and Therapies
Chronic Obstructive Pulmonary Disease

ETIOLOGY	CLINICAL MANIFESTATIONS	CLINICAL THERAPIES
Bronchitis	<ul><li>Chronic cough with mucus production</li><li>Dyspnea</li><li>Tachycardia</li><li>Narrowed airway passages</li><li>Wheezing</li><li>Air trapping</li></ul>	<ul><li>Smoking cessation</li><li>Bronchodilators</li><li>Corticosteroids</li><li>Fluids to thin secretions</li><li>Elevating the head of the bed</li><li>Low-flow oxygen</li><li>Monitoring of ABGs and oxygen</li><li>Mechanical ventilation if patient cannot meet oxygen demands</li></ul>
Emphysema	<ul><li>Air trapping</li><li>Possible wheezing</li><li>Dyspnea</li><li>Barrel chest</li><li>Pursed-lip breathing</li><li>Posturing</li></ul>	<ul><li>Oxygen administration as needed</li><li>Pursed-lip breathing technique</li><li>Patient education of posture changes to improve ventilation</li><li>Low-flow oxygen</li><li>Monitoring of ABGs and oxygen</li><li>Mechanical ventilation if patient cannot meet oxygen demands</li><li>Nutritional assessment and increased calorie intake</li></ul>
Cardiac dysfunction	<ul><li>Chest pain</li><li>Poor perfusion</li><li>Arrhythmias, particularly premature ventricular contractions</li><li>Hypertension</li><li>Cardiac hypertrophy</li><li>Congestive heart failure</li></ul>	<ul><li>Medications: a. Positive inotropics b. Calcium blockers c. Antiarrhythmic medications d. Diuretics e. Nitrites f. Antihypertensives</li><li>Monitoring of exercise tolerance</li><li>Holter monitoring</li><li>Antiembolism stockings to improve venous return</li><li>Fluid restrictions if cardiac dysfunction not medically managed</li></ul>

Clinical Manifestations … Includes information on clinical manifestations the nurse might see in a patient with the disorder. The Clinical Manifestations and Therapies feature is an excellent tool for review.

Collaboration … Outlines interprofessional interventions and therapies appropriate for patients with the disorder.

Diagnostic Tests

Surgery

Pharmacologic Therapy

Nonpharmacologic Therapy

Complementary Health Approaches

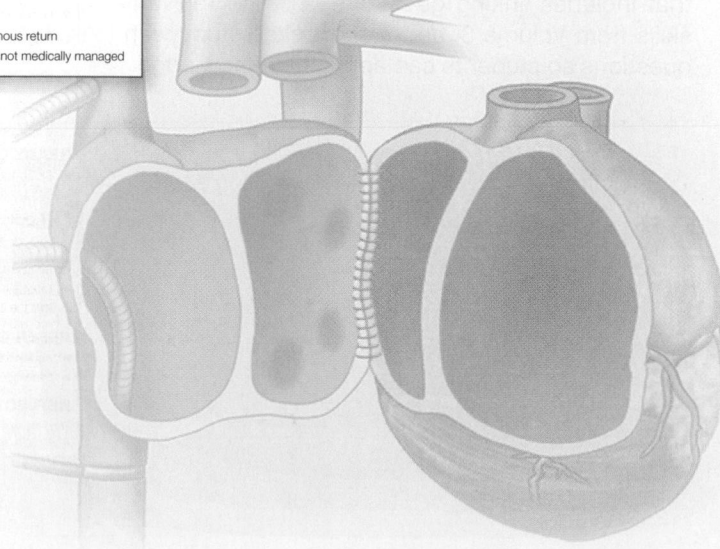

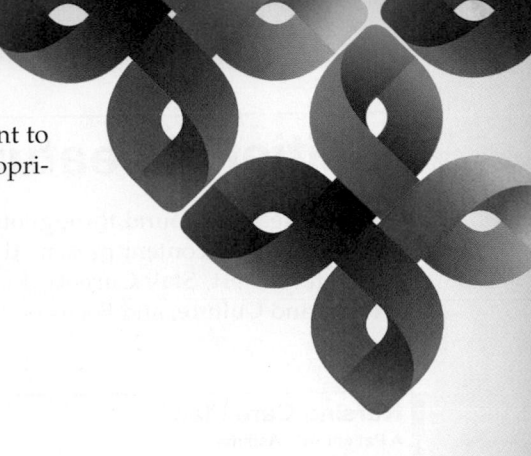

Lifespan Considerations ... New to the Third Edition, all specifics relevant to the lifespan are gathered in one section. Lifespan Considerations are provided as appropriate for both Concepts and Exemplars. Examples of subsections include.

Considerations for Infants

Considerations for Children and Adolescents

Considerations for Pregnant Women

Considerations for Older Adults

Nursing Process ... A detailed look at the nursing process helps students put together all of the content in the exemplar and learn the essentials of providing care to patients with the disorder.

Assessment

Diagnosis

Planning

Implementation

Evaluation

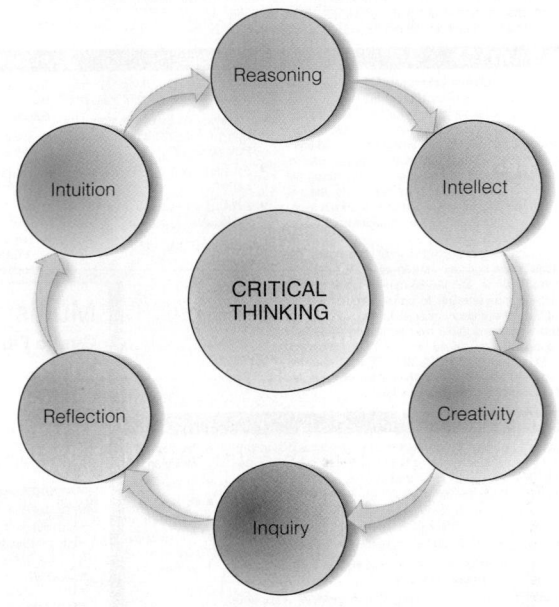

REVIEW Exemplar ... As in the Second Edition, each exemplar ends with a Review that includes linking questions and a short case study with questions to help students apply their knowledge.

REVIEW Benign Prostatic Hyperplasia

RELATE Link the Concepts and Exemplars

Linking the exemplar of BPH with the concept of sexuality:

1. What communication strategies would the nurse use to discuss the impact BPH will have on sexuality without making an older man feel uncomfortable?

2. How can you assess his concerns, fears, and knowledge regarding the impact of BPH on his sexuality?

Linking the exemplar of BPH with the concept of infection:

3. What pathophysiology of BPH could increase the risk of UTIs?

4. What nursing interventions will reduce the risk of UTIs?

READY Go to Volume 3: Clinical Nursing Skills

REFER Go to Pearson MyLab Nursing and eText

■ Additional review materials

REFLECT Apply Your Knowledge

Clifford Allen is a middle manager for a small manufacturing company where he has worked for the last 20 years. Overall, Mr. Allen is in good health, although he has been undergoing treatment recently for BPH. He has a history of depression, for which he does not seek treatment because he fears the social stigma connected to the diagnosis. Mr. Allen has been considering retiring within the next few years so he and his wife can travel, but mostly to escape his stressful work environment. He enjoys bowling and is involved in activities at church. He and his wife go for a walk each evening after supper.

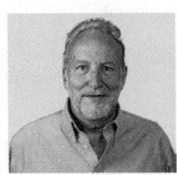

One evening while bowling, he notices that his bladder feels somewhat full. Mr. Allen calls to make an appointment to see his urologist for a follow-up examination. He has been taking finasteride (Proscar) for the last 6 months but does not believe it has been particularly effective. He still has trouble urinating and believes that his symptoms are worse than before he started taking the drug. When he sees the urologist 2 weeks later, he reports that he often feels his bladder is full after voiding, he has difficulty starting his stream of urine, and his stream is weak once started. He gets up frequently at night to void. His score on the AUASI is 28, which has increased from his score of 18 six months ago. The urologist confirms that the medication has not been effective and schedules further tests, including uroflowmetry, check postvoid residual, a PSA blood test, and a urinalysis. Results from the uroflowmetry and postvoid residual test show a significant obstruction of urinary flow. The serum PSA is negative, and the urinalysis is consistent with bladder inflammation. A TURP is recommended in the upcoming weeks.

1. To determine Mr. Allen's understanding of the procedure, what will the nurse want to ask him upon admission to the surgical center?

2. What teaching will the nurse prepare regarding postoperative self-care?

3. Design a nursing plan of care for this patient postoperatively.

Additional Features

Additional features found throughout the program include numbered tables, figures, and boxes that contain content presented in visual formats, and the following highlighted features: Safety Alert, Stay Current, Evidence-Based Practice, Nursing Care Plan, Focus on Diversity and Culture, and Focus on Integrative Health.

Nursing Care Plan
A Patient with Asthma

Sarah Mitchell is a 35-year-old working mother with moderate persistent asthma. Her known triggers are allergies to dust mites, cockroach feces, grass and tree pollens, and some molds. She takes immunotherapy once a week and takes maintenance medications daily. She works as a full-time preschool teacher.

Ms. Mitchell calls her allergist's office asking to be seen because she is having a bad asthma flare. She reports having to use her rescue inhaler every 3–4 hours, that her chest is very tight, and that she is having trouble breathing. She has used her home peak flow meter three times since late yesterday and has been in the yellow zone each time. She did not sleep last night because of her asthma symptoms.

ASSESSMENT	DIAGNOSES	PLANNING
The nurse, Clancy O'Hara, admits Ms. Mitchell when she arrives at the allergist's office. During the health history Ms. Mitchell confirms she is compliant with her medication regimen. She takes a LABA in combination with a low-dose corticosteroid, a daily antihistamine, and montelukast. In checking Ms. Mitchell's medical record, Nurse O'Hara notes that the patient is maintaining her scheduled immunotherapy appointments. Ms. Mitchell reports that she is not aware of any unusual allergy exposure but says that several of her students have a cold this week. On physical examination, Nurse O'Hara notes that Ms. Mitchell's vital signs are as follows: T 37°C (98.6°F); P 96 bpm; R 36/min; BP 128/86 mmHg. Other assessment data include needing to pause frequently while speaking, use of accessory muscles for respirations, and scattered wheezes audible over both lung fields with stethoscope. ABG results are pH 7.32, PaO_2 88 mmHg, $PaCO_2$ 47 mmHg, and HCO_3 38 mEq/L. Pulses are strong and equal bilaterally, and the patient expectorates a small amount of white mucus into a tissue.	■ *Ineffective Breathing Pattern* related to exacerbation of asthma ■ *Impaired Gas Exchange* related to bronchoconstriction and mucus in airways ■ *Fatigue* related to ineffective sleep pattern ■ *Activity Intolerance* related to inadequate oxygenation (NANDA-I © 2014)	Together Nurse O'Hara and Ms. Mitchell agree on the following outcomes: ■ The patient's breathing will return to the green zone within 24 hours. ■ The patient's need for her rescue inhaler will decline within 3 days and return to baseline within 1 week. ■ The patient will maintain baseline respiratory rate and pattern sufficient to meet her ADLs within

IMPLEMENTATION

Ms. Mitchell's provider prescribes a higher-dose inhaled steroid to use 10–15 minutes after she uses her LABA. The provider also gives Ms. Mitchell a short, tapered course of prednisone. Ms. O'Hare initiates the following implementations:

■ Teaches Ms. Mitchell how to properly self-administer medications and about possible side effects associated with steroid use, including those that should be reported immediately
■ Explains the importance of taking the steroid as ordered and not stopping the medication suddenly
■ Provides strategies for managing fatigue, including a handout with written instructions

■ Teaches Ms.
hydration in a
■ Observes Ms
■ Reviews sign
and instructs
■ Schedules M
evaluation bu
or if she sees

Many exemplars contain **Nursing Care Plans**, and additional ones can be found in the Pearson eText in MyLab Nursing. The Nursing Care Plans follow the nursing process with sections on assessment, diagnosis, planning, implementation, and evaluation. They end with a series of Critical Thinking questions.

The **Multisystem Effects** features have been redesigned for the Third Edition. Each one highlights the effects that a disorder has on various systems of the body.

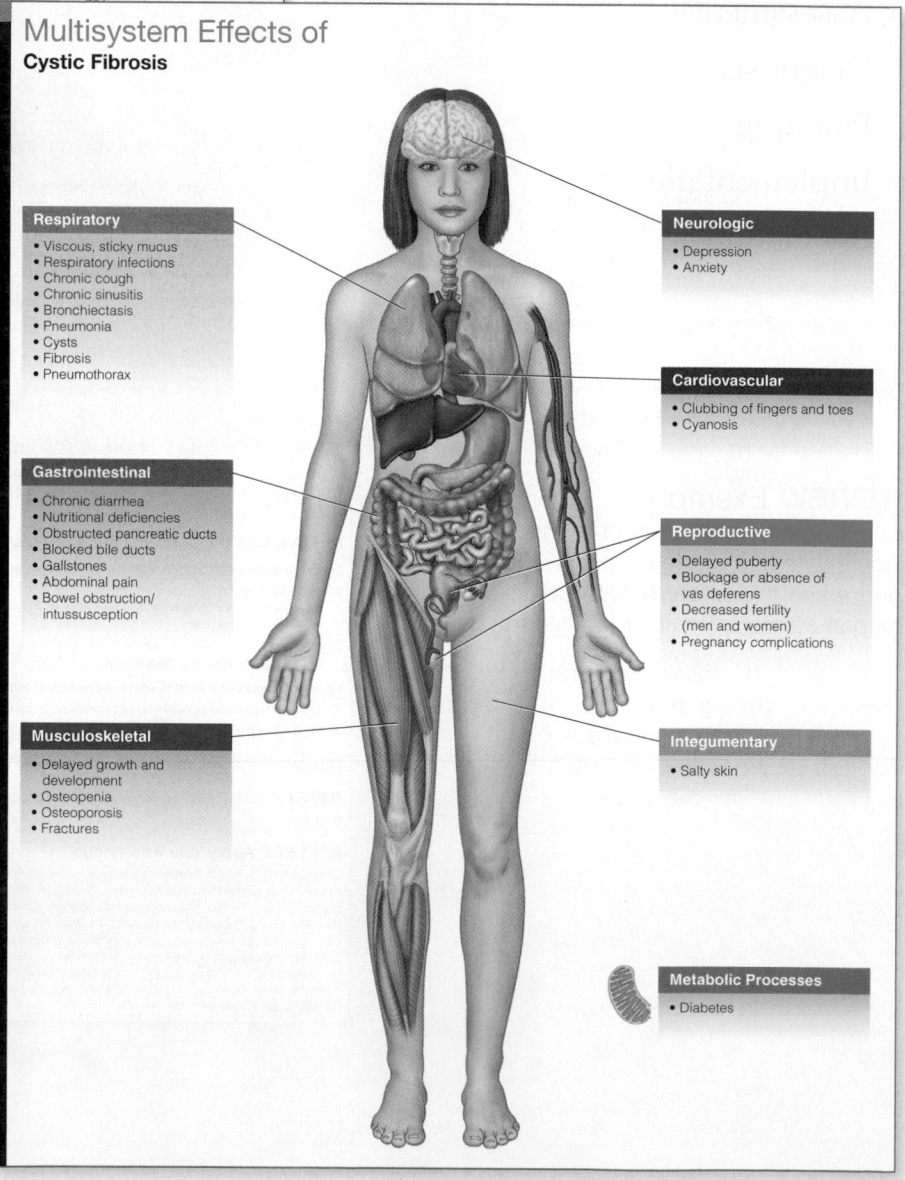

Multisystem Effects of
Cystic Fibrosis

Respiratory
- Viscous, sticky mucus
- Respiratory infections
- Chronic cough
- Chronic sinusitis
- Bronchiectasis
- Pneumonia
- Cysts
- Fibrosis
- Pneumothorax

Gastrointestinal
- Chronic diarrhea
- Nutritional deficiencies
- Obstructed pancreatic ducts
- Blocked bile ducts
- Gallstones
- Abdominal pain
- Bowel obstruction/intussusception

Musculoskeletal
- Delayed growth and development
- Osteopenia
- Osteoporosis
- Fractures

Neurologic
- Depression
- Anxiety

Cardiovascular
- Clubbing of fingers and toes
- Cyanosis

Reproductive
- Delayed puberty
- Blockage or absence of vas deferens
- Decreased fertility (men and women)
- Pregnancy complications

Integumentary
- Salty skin

Metabolic Processes
- Diabetes

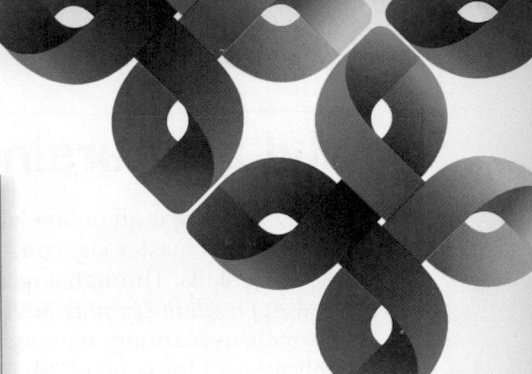

Focus on Integrative Health
Chronic Obstructive Pulmonary Disease

Complementary health approaches may be useful to help man-
[...] symptoms of COPD. Dietary measures, such as minimiz-
[...]ntake of dairy products and salt, may help reduce mucus
[...]uction and keep mucus more liquefied. Be sure to recom-
[...]d measures to replace the protein and calcium in dairy
[...]ucts to help maintain nutritional balance. Hot herbal teas
[...]e with peppermint may act as expectorants to help relieve
[...]t congestion.

[...]atients may be interested in trying complementary health
[...]oaches to assist them in quitting smoking. While additional
[...]es are needed to evaluate the effectiveness of comple-
[...]ary health approaches for use in quitting smoking, current
[...]rch suggests that acupuncture and hypnotherapy may be
[...]tive in promoting smoking cessation (Tahiri et al., 2012).
[...]wise, Hasan et al. (2014) found that hypnotherapy may be
[...]e effective than NRT for promotion of smoking cessation.

Focus on Diversity and Culture
Assessing for Cyanosis

When assessing for cyanosis, normal assessment findings vary
depending on the individual's normal skin tones. For example,
in a white or light-skinned individual, cyanosis due to hypoxemia most often manifests as a bluish discoloration of the lips,
oral mucosa, and nail beds. Among dark-skinned individuals,
cyanosis may be difficult to detect and may actually cause the
skin to appear darker. Typical manifestations of cyanosis in
dark-skinned individuals include pallor or an ash-gray discoloration of the skin surrounding the mouth. Conjunctivae appear
gray or blue-tinged among dark-skinned individuals. Among
patients whose normal skin tone is yellowish, cyanosis may
manifest as a gray–green skin discoloration (Sommers, 2011).

For the most part, care of patients from different cultures is covered in the basal text. **Focus on Diversity and Culture** features are used only for unique situations of which the nurse should be aware.

Focus on Integrative Health boxes highlight the use of complementary health approaches in addition to traditional nursing practice.

SAFETY ALERT Chronic cough and sputum are not normal occurrences. An individual experiencing chronic cough and sputum beyond 3–4 days should consult with a healthcare professional. Individuals with a smoking history as well as chronic cough and sputum production should have PFTs to determine lung function.

Each **Safety Alert** provides critical information the nurse needs to know to keep patients and staff safe.

≫ **Stay Current:** Visit the Safe to Sleep website at https://www.nichd.nih.gov/sts/Pages/default.aspxto learn more about SIDS prevention.

The **Stay Current** feature provides a weblink (which is a hot link in the eText) to a website that will keep students informed on the most recent updates.

The goal of the **Evidence-Based Practice** features is to show students the necessity of evidence driving practice. Each starts with a problem, delves into the research, presents implications for the nurse, and ends with critical thinking questions for the student.

Evidence-Based Practice
Compliance with Safe to Sleep Recommendations

Problem

Compared to previous recommendations for preventing SIDS, current recommendations are more complex. For example, the Safe to
Sleep guidelines address not only infant positioning but also maintaining a safe sleep environment and abstaining from co-sleeping
(bed sharing). The increased complexity of the recommendations
may lead to decreased parental compliance with current guidelines
for the prevention of SIDS (Goodstein, Bell, & Krugman, 2015).

Evidence

The Safe to Sleep recommendations include supine positioning during sleep, using a firm sleep surface, breastfeeding, room sharing
without co-sleeping, routine immunizations, and the use of a pacifier.
Items that should be avoided include soft bedding, toys, layered
clothing, and crib bumpers (USDHHS, 2015). Research suggests
that parental adherence to current recommendations for the prevention of SIDS is significantly increased when nurses model the behaviors that are reflective of all current guidelines for preventing SIDS and
obtain parental signatures on a document acknowledging receipt of
education related to current guidelines (Goodstein et al., 2015).

Implications

Nurses should demonstrate endorsement of all current recommendations for reducing SIDS-related deaths, including modeling and
implementing all recommendations as soon as the infant is clinically stable and up to discharge. Nurses working with parents of
newborns must provide additional patient teaching and follow-up,
as well as ensuring that parents understand the teaching. All parents should receive documented education on safe infant sleep
practices, including voluntary acknowledgement forms indicating
that education has been provided with regard to the specific current guidelines (Goodstein et al., 2015).

Critical Thinking Application

1. Identify barriers to educating parents and caregivers about
   current recommendations for preventing sleep-associated
   deaths.
2. Describe methods for evaluating parental understanding of
   the current guidelines for prevention of SIDS.

MyLab Nursing

MyLab Nursing is an online learning and practice environment that works with the text to help students master key concepts, prepare for the NCLEX-RN exam, and develop clinical reasoning skills. Through a new mobile experience, students can study *Nursing: A Concept-Based Approach to Learning* anytime, anywhere. New adaptive technology with remediation personalizes learning, moving students beyond memorization to true understanding and application of the content. MyLab Nursing contains the following features:

Dynamic Study Modules ... New adaptive learning modules with remediation that personalize the learning experience by allowing students to increase both their confidence and their performance while being assessed in real time.

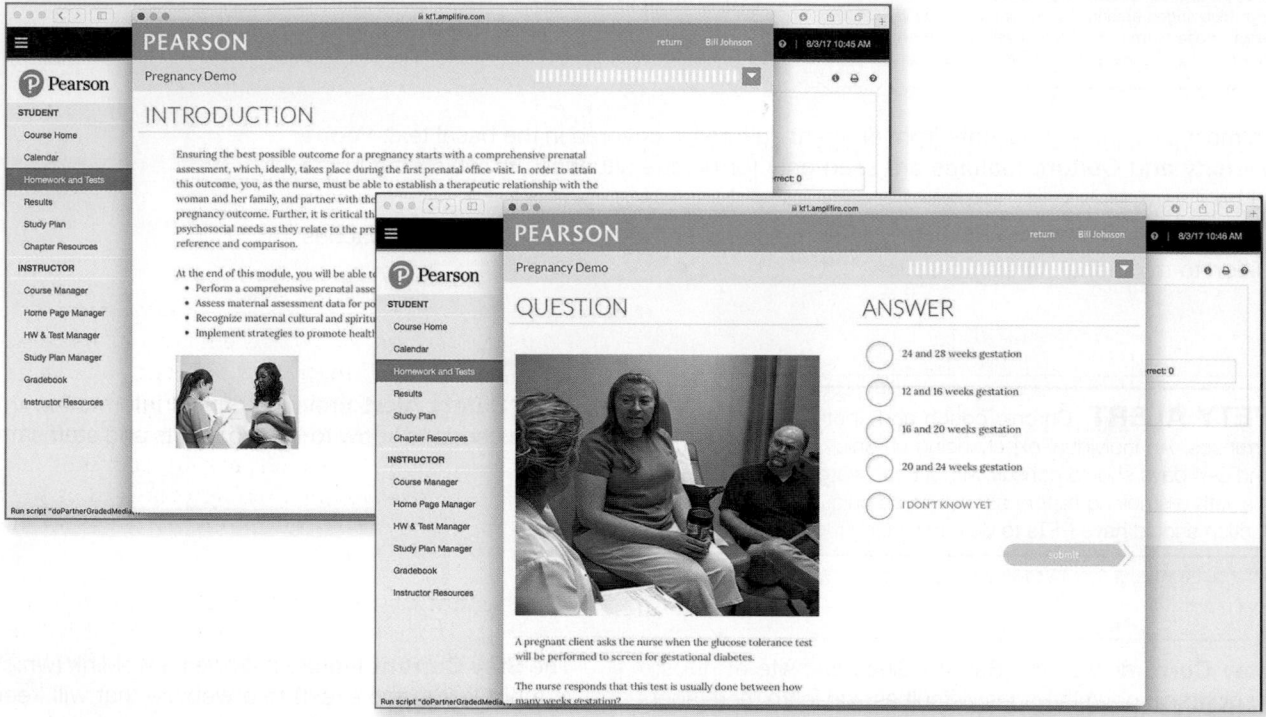

NCLEX-Style Questions ... Practice tests with more than 3000 NCLEX-style questions of various types build student confidence and prepare them for success on the NCLEX-RN exam. Questions are organized by Concept and Exemplar.

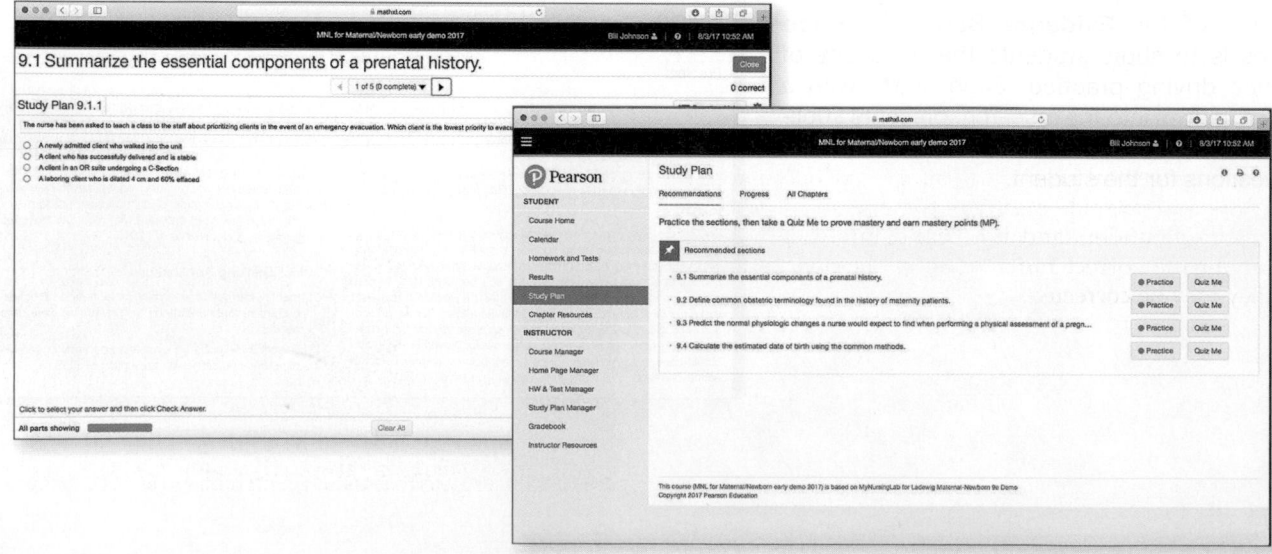

Decision Making Cases

... Clinical case studies that provide opportunities for students to practice analyzing information and making important decisions at key moments in patient care scenarios. These case studies are designed to help prepare students for clinical practice.

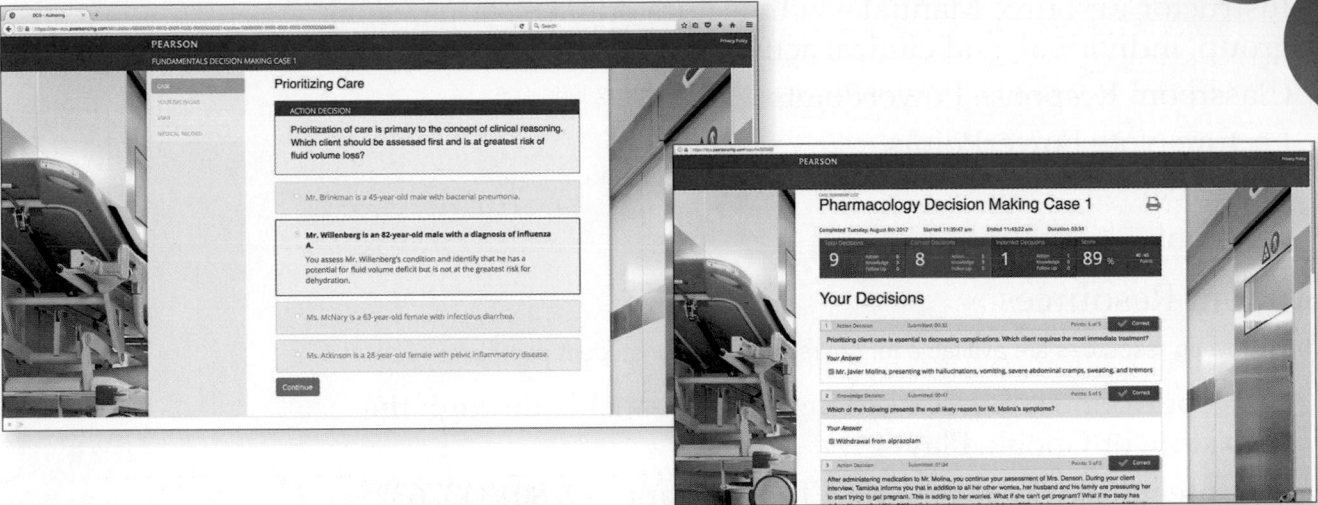

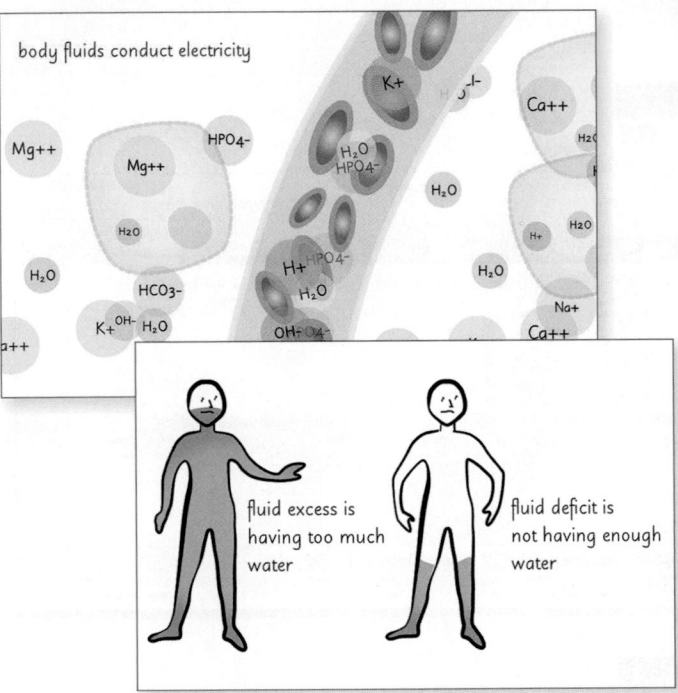

Pearson eText

... Enhances student learning both in and outside the classroom. Students can take notes, highlight, and bookmark important content, or engage with interactive and rich media to achieve greater conceptual understanding of the Concepts and their Exemplars. Interactive features include audio clips, pop-up definitions, figures, questions and answers, the nursing process, hotspots, and video animations. Some examples of video animations include:

- **Fluid and Electrolyte Animations** provide students with the necessary information about the balance and imbalance of fluids and electrolytes to think, reason, and make clinical judgments.

- **Congenital Heart Defect Animations** illustrate the many congenital heart defects that may occur in newborns and provide students the opportunity to see, hear, and understand how congenital heart defects impair the correct functioning of the heart and how they may be corrected.

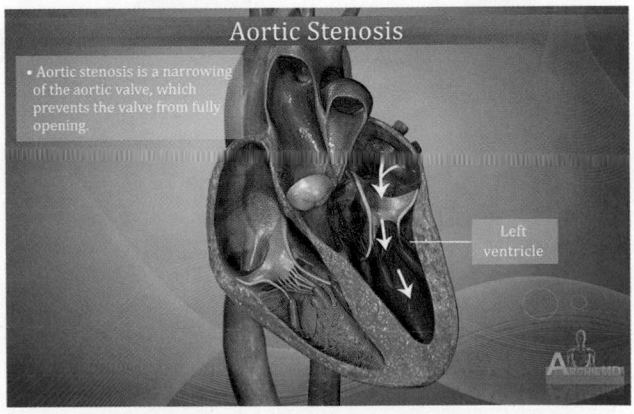

Resources

Instructor Resources

Instructor Resource Manual—with lecture outlines, large/small group, individual, and clinical activities

Classroom Response PowerPoints

Lecture Note PowerPoints

Image bank

Test bank

Student Resources

The following resources are available for course adoption or student purchase:

Concept Connections in Nursing app—available through the App store or Google Play

Comprehensive Review for NCLEX-RN app—9780134376325

RealEHRprep with iCare

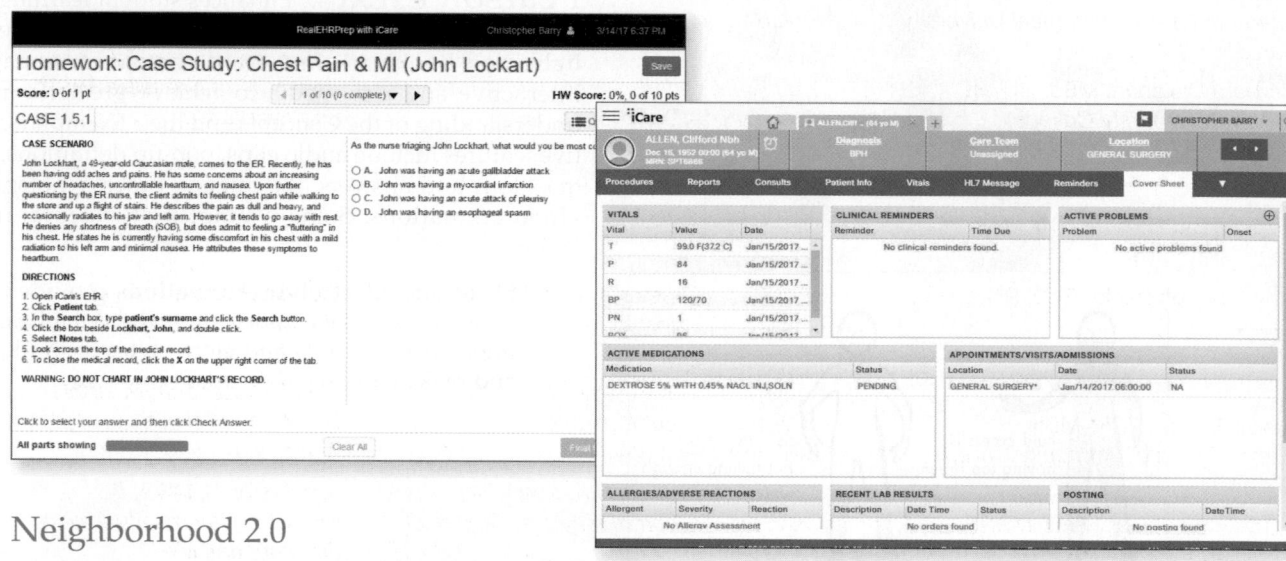

Neighborhood 2.0

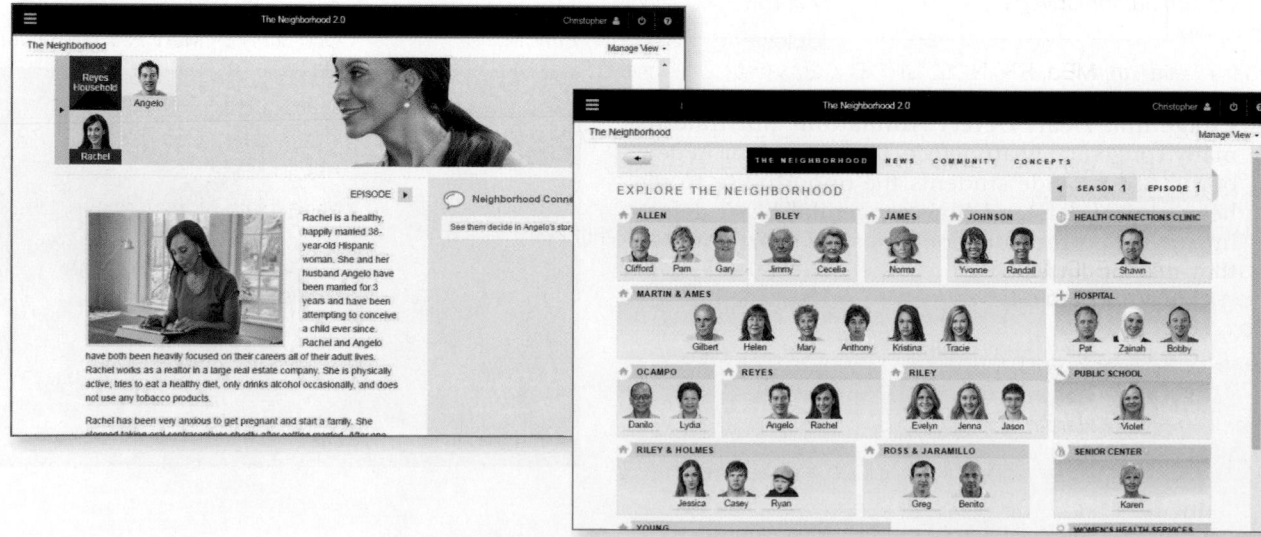

Acknowledgments

We would like to extend our heartfelt thanks to more than 80 instructors from schools of nursing across the country who have given their time generously during the past few years to help us create this concept-based learning package. The talented faculty on our Concepts Editorial Board and all of the Contributors and Reviewers helped us to develop this Third Edition through a variety of contributions and by answering myriad questions right up to the time of publication. *Nursing: A Concept-Based Approach to Learning*, Third Edition, has benefited immeasurably from their efforts, insights, suggestions, objections, encouragement, and inspiration, as well as from their vast experience as faculty and practicing nurses.

We would like to thank the editorial team, especially Julie Alexander, Publisher, for her continuous support throughout this process; Katrin Beacom, Director of Portfolio Management for championing this project; Erin Sullivan, the editorial assistant for helping to keep all the balls in the air; Bianca Sepulveda and Melissa Bashe for keeping us organized and putting together all of the components of the concepts program; and most of all, Laura Horowitz and Addy McCulloch, development editors, for their dedication and attention to detail that promoted an excellent outcome once again. Special thanks to the design team, led by Mary Siener, and Studio Montage for the thoughtful and integrated design of our concepts solution. Many thanks to Kelly Ricci and the Aptara team for producing this book with precision.

Concepts Editorial Board

Barbara Arnoldussen, MBA, BSN, RN, CPHQ
International Technological University
San Jose, CA

Barbara Callahan, MEd, RN, NCC, CHSE
Lenoir Community College
Kinston, NC

Linda K. Daley, PhD, RN, ANEF
The Ohio State University
Columbus, OH

Mark C. Hand, PhD, RN, MSN, CNE
East Carolina University
Greenville, NC

Pamela Phillips, PhD, RN
University of South Carolina Beaufort
Beaufort, SC

T. Kim Rodehorst, PhD, RN
University of Nebraska Medical Center
Scottsbluff, NE

Contributors

Michelle Aebersold, PhD, RN, CHSE, FAAN
University of Michigan
Ann Arbor, MI

Eleisa Bennett, RN, MSN
James Sprunt Community College
Kenansville, NC

Marlena Bushway, PhD, MSNEd, RN, CNE
New Mexico Junior College
Hobbs, NM

Barbara Callahan, MEd, RN, NCC, CHSE
Lenoir Community College
Kinston, NC

Linda Daley, PhD, RN
The Ohio State University
Columbus, OH

Christi Emerson, EdD, MSN, RN
University of Mary Hardin-Baylor
Belton, TX

Michele G. Hackney, EdD, MSN, RN, CNE
University of Mary Hardin-Baylor
Belton, TX

Elizabeth Johnston Taylor, PhD, RN
Loma Linda University
Loma Linda, CA

Amy Mitchell Kennedy, MSN, RN
Nursing Content Manager
Newport News, VA

Christine Kleckner, MA, MAN, RN
Minneapolis Community and Technical College
Minneapolis, MN

Juleann H. Miller, RN, PhD
St. Ambrose University
Davenport, IA

Jeanne Papa, MSN, MBE, ACNP
Neumann University
Aston, PA

Cynthia Parkman, PhD, RN
National University
San Diego, CA

Pamela Phillips, PhD, RN
University of South Carolina Beaufort
Beaufort, SC

T. Kim Rodehorst, PhD, RN
University of Nebraska Medical Center
Scottsbluff, NE

Judith Rolph, MSN, RN
MassBay Community College
Framingham, MA

Sharon Souter, RN, PhD, CNE
University of Mary Hardin-Baylor
Belton, TX

Patricia Vasquez, MSN, RN
Trinity Valley Community College
Kaufman, TX

Jacqueline M. Loversidge, PhD, RNC-AWHC, CNS
The Ohio State University
Columbus, OH

Reviewers

Folake Elizabeth Adelakun, RN, MSN, MBA-HC, DNP
Minneapolis Community and Technical College
Minneapolis, MN

Carol S. Amis, MSN, RN, CCRN
Minneapolis Community and Technical College
Minneapolis, MN

Barbara Arnoldussen, MBA, BSN, RN, CPHQ
International Technological University
San Jose, CA

Jacqueline Bencker, BSN, RN, CNOR
St. Mary Medical Center
Langhorne, PA

Eleisa Bennett, RN, MSN
James Sprunt Community College
Kenansville, NC

Shelley Layne Blackwood, EdS, MSN, RN-BC, PCCN
University of Mary Hardin-Baylor
Belton, TX

Karen Bledsoe, MSN, RN-C
University of Mary Hardin-Baylor
Belton, TX

Tracy Booth, MSEd, BSN, RN
University of Mary Hardin-Baylor
Belton, TX

Wendy Buchanan, RN, MSN-E
Southwestern Community College
Sylva, NC

Becky Bunn, MSN, RN
University of Mary Hardin-Baylor
Belton, TX

Regina Burgin, MSN, RN-BC
Sampson Community College
Clinton, NC

Marlena Bushway, PhD, MSNEd, RN, CNE
New Mexico Junior College
Hobbs, NM

Marcy Caplin, PhD, RN, CNE
Kent State University
Kent, OH

Kristine Carey, MSN, RN
Normandale Community College
Bloomington, MN

Diane Cohen, MSN, RN
MassBay Community College
Framingham, MA

Barbara E. Connell, RN, MSN
Southwestern Community College
Sylva, NC

Ann Crawford, RN, PhD, CNS, CEN, CPEN
University of Mary Hardin-Baylor
Belton, TX

Diane Daddario, MSN, ANP-C, ACNS-BC, RN, BC, CMSRN
Pennsylvania State University
University Park, PA

Linda Daley, PhD, RN
The Ohio State University
Columbus, OH

Carrie Dickson, MS, APRN, CNM, CNE
Normandale Community College
Bloomington, MN

Barbara Dixon, MSN, RN
University of Mary Hardin-Baylor
Belton, TX

Patricia Ann Durham-Taylor, RN, PhD
Truckee Meadows Community College
Reno, NV

Mary Ervi, MSN, RN, CNE
University of Mary Hardin-Baylor
Belton, TX

Vicki Evans, MSN, RN, CEN, CNE
University of Mary Hardin-Baylor
Belton, TX

Abimbola Farinde, PhD
Columbia Southern University
Orange Beach, AL

Pamela Fauskee, MN, RN, CNE
Anoka-Ramsey Community College
Cambridge, MN

James R. Fell, MSN, MBA, RN
The Breen School of Nursing, Ursuline University
Pepper Pike, OH

Judy Flowers, MSN, MS, RN
Catawba Valley Community College
Hickory, NC

Tobi Fuller, MSN, MS, RN
El Centro College
Dallas, TX

Frederick Gunzel
Independent Contractor
Farmingville, NY

Michele G. Hackney, EdD, MSN, RN, CNE
University of Mary Hardin-Baylor
Belton, TX

Mark C. Hand, PhD, RN, MSN, CNE
Durham Technical Community College
Durham, NC

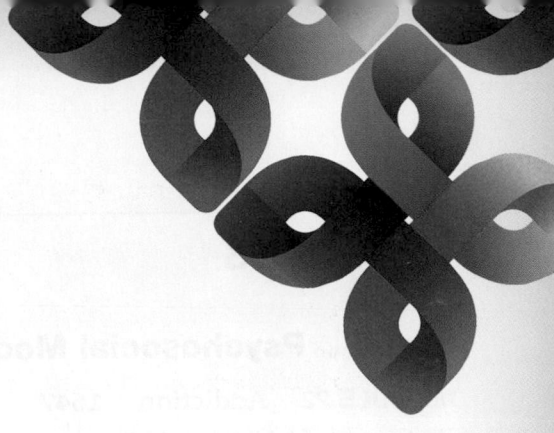

Lori Kelty, MSNEd, RN, CCRN, CEN, NE
Mercer County Community College
Windsor Township, NJ

Amy Mitchell Kennedy, MSN, RN
Nursing Content Manager
Newport News, VA

Christine Kleckner, MA, MAN, RN
Minneapolis Community and Technical
College
Minneapolis, MN

Dawna Martich, MSN, RN
Nursing Education Consultant
Pittsburgh, PA

Belle McGinty, MEd, RN, BSN
Brunswick Community College
Bolivia, NC

Kimi C. McMahan, RN, MSNEd
Southwestern Community College
Sylva, NC

Amy Mersiovsky, MSN, RN, BC
University of Mary Hardin-Baylor
Belton, TX

Juleann H. Miller, RN, PhD
St. Ambrose University
Davenport, IA

Michelle Natrop, RN, BAN, MSN
Normandale Community College
Bloomington, MN

Lynn Perkins, PhD, MSN, RN
Minneapolis Community and Technical
College
Minneapolis, MN

Margaret Prydun, PhD, RN, CNE
University of Mary Hardin-Baylor
Belton, TX

Judith Rolph, MSN, RN
MassBay Community College
Framingham, MA

John E. Scarbrough, PhD, PT,
RN, CNE
New Mexico State University
Las Cruces, NM

Cynthia K. Schweizer, MSN, RN
Brunswick Community College
Bolivia, NC

Amber J. Seidel, PhD
Pennsylvania State University
University Park, PA

Brenda L. Shostrom, RN, PhD
St. Ambrose University
Davenport, IA

Amy B. Sneed
Brunswick Community College
Bolivia, NC

Ami Stone, RN, MSN
University of Mary Hardin-Baylor
Belton, TX

Betsy Swinny, MSN, RN, CCRN
Baptist Health System
San Antonio, TX

Lori L. Thompson, APRN, MSN, NP-C
Vance–Granville Community College
Henderson, NC

Carolina Partners in Mental HealthCare
Wake Forest, NC

Patricia Vasquez, MSN, RN
Trinity Valley Community College
Kaufman, TX

Paulette Whitfield, PhD, RN, ANP-BC
University of Mary Hardin-Baylor
Belton, TX

Joanne Woods, BS, MSN
University of Mary Hardin-Baylor
Belton, TX

Contents

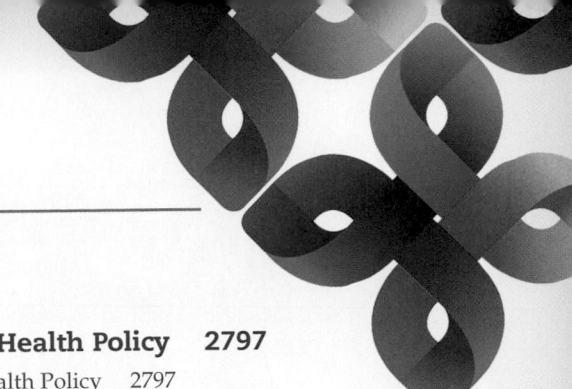

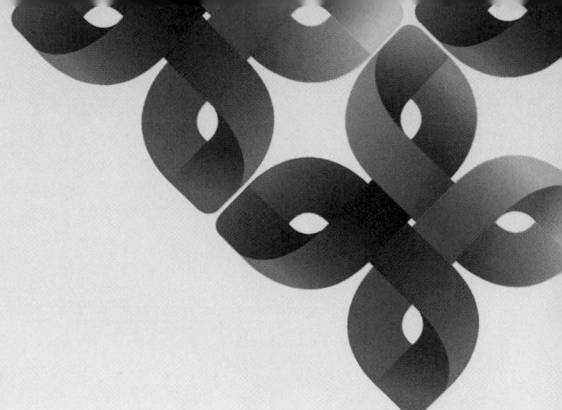

Part II
Psychosocial Modules

Part II consists of the psychosocial modules within the individual domain. Each module presents a concept that directly relates to sociologic or psychologic domains that impact patient health and well-being—such as cognition, family, and stress and coping—and selected alterations of that concept presented as exemplars. In the concept of cognition, for example, exemplars include Alzheimer disease, confusion, and schizophrenia. Each module addresses the impact of that concept and selected alterations on individuals across the lifespan, inclusive of cultural, gender, and developmental considerations.

Module 22
Addiction

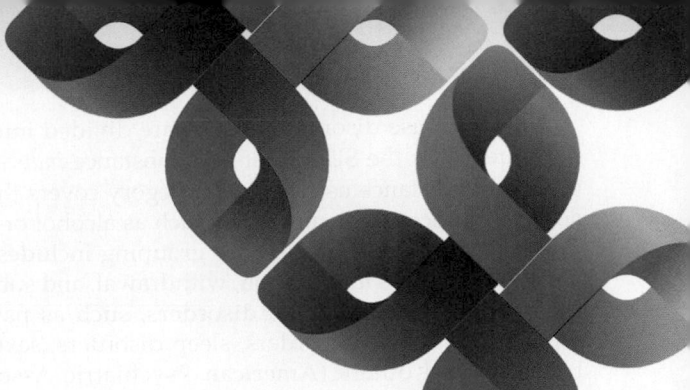

Module Outline and Learning Outcomes

The Concept of Addiction

Addiction

22.1 Summarize the processes involved in addiction.

Manifestations of Substance Use Disorders

22.2 Summarize manifestations of substance use disorders.

Concepts Related to Addiction

22.3 Outline the relationship between addiction and other concepts.

Health Promotion

22.4 Outline health promotion activities to reduce the risk for substance abuse and relapse.

Nursing Assessment

22.5 Differentiate common assessment procedures and tests used to examine individuals suspected of abusing a substance.

Independent Interventions

22.6 Analyze independent interventions nurses can implement for patients with substance use disorders.

Collaborative Therapies

22.7 Summarize collaborative therapies used by interprofessional teams for patients with substance use disorders.

Lifespan Considerations

22.8 Differentiate considerations related to the assessment and care of patients throughout the lifespan who abuse substances.

Addiction Exemplars

Exemplar 22.A Alcohol Abuse

22.A Analyze manifestations and treatment considerations for patients who abuse alcohol.

Exemplar 22.B Nicotine Use

22.B Analyze manifestations and treatment considerations for patients with an addiction to nicotine.

Exemplar 22.C Substance Abuse

22.C Analyze manifestations and treatment considerations for patients who abuse substances.

» The Concept of Addiction

Concept Key Terms

Abstinence, **1651**
Addiction, **1647**
Behavioral therapy, **1660**
Binge drinking, **1665**
Boundaries, **1652**
Brief strategic family therapy (BSFT), **1663**
Cognitive–behavioral therapy (CBT), **1660**
Codependence, **1651**

Contingency contracts, **1660**
Co-occurring disorders, **1651**
Delirium tremens (DTs), **1651**
Dependence, **1648**
Dialectical behavior therapy (DBT), **1661**
Enabling behavior, **1652**
Exercise addiction, **1654**

Extinction, **1660**
Family behavior therapy (FBT), **1663**
Functional family therapy (FFT), **1663**
Gambling disorder, **1653**
Group therapy, **1662**
Internet gaming disorder (IGD), **1654**
Intervention, **1660**
Milieu therapy, **1661**

Multidimensional family therapy (MDFT), **1663**
Multisystemic therapy (MST), **1663**
Online shopping addiction, **1654**
Polysubstance abuse, **1651**
Punishment, **1660**
Rational–emotive behavior therapy (REBT), **1661**

Recovery, **1658**
Reinforcement, **1660**
Sex addiction, **1654**
Sobriety, **1651**
Substance use disorder, **1647**
Teratogen, **1665**
Token economies, **1660**
Tolerance, **1648**

Addiction is defined as a psychologic or physical need for a substance (such as alcohol) or process (such as gambling) to the extent that the individual will risk negative consequences in an attempt to meet the need. Many individuals use substances recreationally to modify mood or behavior, and there are wide sociocultural variations in the acceptability of chemical use. Prescription medications include narcotics, sedatives, and stimulants and are dangerous when misused or abused. Illegal drugs include cocaine (including crack), heroin, hallucinogens, and inhalants. Marijuana/hashish use is illegal in many states. An individual may abuse any of these substances to the point of becoming addicted and unable to stop, despite dangerous, often life-threatening consequences. An individual who uses one or more substances to this extent may be diagnosed with a **substance use disorder**.

Substance use disorders (SUDs) are divided into one of two categories: the SUD itself and substance-*induced* disorders. The substance use disorder category covers the actual addictive process to a substance, such as alcohol or opiates. The substance-induced disorder grouping includes related conditions such as intoxication, withdrawal, and substance/medication–related mental disorders, such as psychosis, bipolar and related disorders, sleep disorders, sexual dysfunction, and others (American Psychiatric Association, 2013). Nursing interventions include providing acute care for patients with substance-induced disorders who are experiencing intoxication or withdrawal; educating patients and their family members about the disorder; and supporting recovery and abstinence in community-based programs.

The etiology of addiction is multifaceted. Childhood trauma, genetic variabilities, and other considerations are thought to play a role. Regardless of the reasons or etiology behind addiction, it can have grave consequences for both individuals and those who care for them.

The Surgeon General released a report in 2016 that stated:

> Historically, our society has treated addiction and misuse of alcohol and drugs as symptoms of moral weakness or as a willful rejection of societal norms, and these problems have been addressed primarily through the criminal justice system. Our health care system has not given the same level of attention to substance use disorders as it has to other health concerns that affect similar numbers of people. Substance use disorder treatment in the United States remains largely segregated from the rest of health care and serves only a fraction of those in need of treatment (Surgeon General, 2016, Executive Summary).

Nurses can play a role in prevention, education, and treatment of substance abuse and addiction.

Addiction

Addictive processes create cognitive, behavioral, and physiologic symptoms. The term *addiction* needs to be differentiated from dependence. **Dependence** is a physiologic need for a substance that the patient cannot control and that results in withdrawal symptoms if the drug or substance is stopped or withheld. Dependence on a substance also causes the user to develop a physiologic **tolerance** for the substance, requiring greater quantities of the substance to achieve the same pleasurable effects. In addition to physiologic symptoms, addiction also includes a psychologic need that causes affected individuals to seek the substance to which they are addicted—at any cost. Individuals with substance use disorders (often referred to as "addicts") may neglect their children, their work, or other responsibilities to meet their physiologic and psychologic needs.

Physiology and Psychology of Addiction

Various factors help explain why one person becomes addicted while another does not. The biopsychosocial model theorized by psychiatrist George L. Engel has been generally accepted as the most comprehensive theory for the process of addiction. Clinicians use his model as a foundation to link biological, genetic, psychologic, emotional, and sociocultural factors contributing to the development of addiction.

Biological Factors

E. Morton Jellinek (1946) first identified biological factors in his disease model of alcoholism. He hypothesized that addiction to alcohol had a biochemical basis and identified specific phases of the disease. Expanding on Jellinek's early work, researchers implicated low levels of dopamine and serotonin in the development of alcohol dependence (Czermak et al., 2004; Nellissery et al., 2003). More recent clinical studies have continued to confirm this finding (Kash, 2012).

Dopamine, dopamine receptor sites, and transporters, which recycle the neurotransmitter and cut off communication between neurons, are all intricately involved in the complex workings between the nervous system and substances of abuse (National Institute on Drug Abuse [NIDA], 2014a). Dopamine is a neurotransmitter present in regions of the brain that regulate movement, emotion, motivation, and feelings of pleasure. The limbic system, which links together a number of brain structures, contains the brain's reward circuit. The limbic system controls and regulates the ability to feel pleasure and mediates perception of other emotions, which helps to explain the mood-altering properties of many substances (NIDA, 2014a). When activated at normal levels, this system rewards natural human behaviors.

Overstimulating the reward system with drugs produces euphoric effects, which strongly reinforce the behavior of drug use (NIDA, 2014a). Most drugs that impact the biochemical mechanism of the brain affect one or more receptor sites (**Figure 22–1 »**). Most abused substances mimic or block the brain's most important neurotransmitters at these respective receptor sites. For example, heroin and other opiates mimic natural opiate-like neurotransmitters, such as endorphins. Cocaine and other stimulants block the reuptake of dopamine, serotonin, and norepinephrine, which causes the neurons to release abnormally large amounts of natural neurotransmitters or interferes with the normal reuptake of these neurotransmitters. These imbalances produce greatly amplified signals in the brain, ultimately permanently altering or disrupting neurons and neural pathways (NIDA, 2014a).

Whenever the reward circuit is activated, the brain encodes a memory, which encourages the individual to perform the same pleasurable act—or take the pleasurable substance—again and again. The reward experienced by the individual using the substance can be significant: For instance, cocaine can cause the release of 2 to 10 times the amount of dopamine released by eating or sexual intercourse (NIDA, 2014a). Neurobiological research into addiction postulates that addiction is the result of an increase in focus on a particular addictive behavior with a corresponding gradual loss of interest in other activities. The mesolimbic dopaminergic system is believed to play an important role in the search for rewarding stimuli, with a resulting increase in dopamine when the stimulus is received. Particular areas in the brain define something as pleasure. When these areas are stimulated as a result of addiction, the level of need for the substance or behavior is increased.

Other biological factors involved in addiction include other medical conditions and the individual's stage of development.

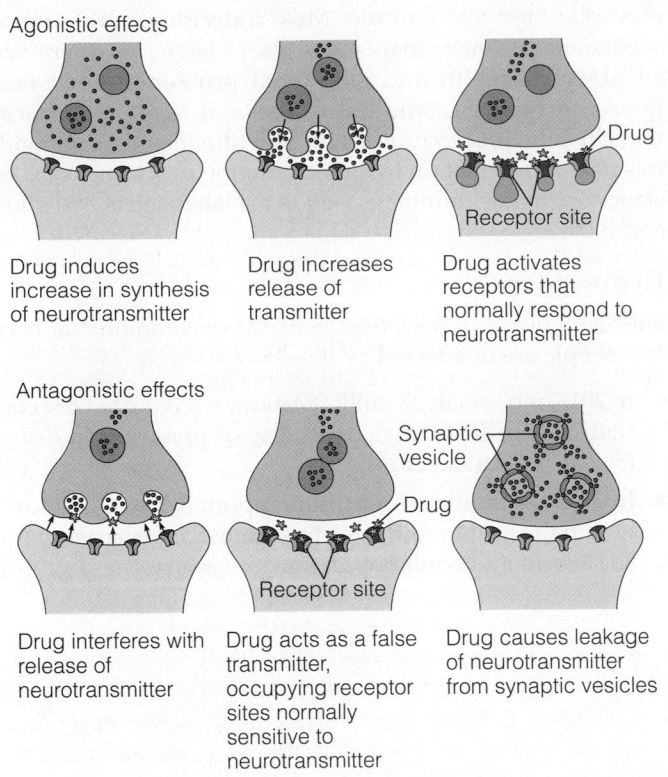

Agonistic effects

Drug induces increase in synthesis of neurotransmitter

Drug increases release of transmitter

Drug activates receptors that normally respond to neurotransmitter

Receptor site

Drug

Antagonistic effects

Synaptic vesicle

Drug

Receptor site

Drug interferes with release of neurotransmitter

Drug acts as a false transmitter, occupying receptor sites normally sensitive to neurotransmitter

Drug causes leakage of neurotransmitter from synaptic vesicles

Figure 22–1 》 Action of abused substances at brain receptor sites.

Mental disorders such as anxiety, depression, and schizophrenia may precede addiction; in other cases, drug abuse may trigger or exacerbate those mental disorders, particularly in people with specific vulnerabilities (NIDA, 2014a).

During adolescence, the prefrontal cortex—the part of the brain that helps individuals to assess situations, make sound decisions, and moderate emotions and impulses—is still developing. Thus, adolescents are at risk for making poor decisions about trying drugs or continuing to take them. Also, introducing drugs during this period of development may cause brain changes that have profound and long-lasting consequences (NIDA, 2014a). Abusing drugs during adolescence can interfere with meeting crucial social and developmental milestones and also compromise cognitive development. For example, heavy marijuana use in the teen years may cause a loss of several IQ points that are not regained even if users later quit in adulthood (NIDA, 2014e).

Genetic Factors

Genetic factors include an apparent hereditary factor that affects alcohol use and dependence. A link has been found between addiction and impulse control, although it is not fully understood. As stated earlier, addiction is strongly linked to the dopaminergic system of the brain's reward system. The speed with which someone becomes addicted depends on the substance, the frequency of use, the means of ingestion, the intensity of the high the person obtains, and the person's genetic and psychologic susceptibility. Adequate proof exists that addiction is, at least in part, genetically moderated. Researchers estimate that genetic factors account for between 40 and 60% of an individual's

vulnerability to addiction, a statistic that also accounts for the effects of environmental factors on the function and expression of a person's genes (NIDA, 2014a). Several genes have been identified that seem to influence the risk for alcohol dependence (Foroud & Phillips, 2012).

Psychologic Factors

No addictive personality type has been identified; however, several common factors seem to exist among alcoholics and drug users. Many individuals with substance use disorders experienced sexual or physical abuse in their childhood and, as a result, experience anxiety, low self-esteem, and difficulty expressing emotions. Research indicates a high correlation among substance use and childhood and adolescent trauma (NIDA, 2014a, 2014e). Therapist Peter Bernstein (2013) states "The vast majority of people with substance abuse problems have a traumatic past" (p. 16).

A link also exists between substance abuse and psychiatric disorders such as depression, bipolar disorder, anxiety, and antisocial and dependent personalities. The habit of using a substance becomes a form of self-medication to cope with day-to-day problems and develops into an addiction over time.

The pleasure model, proposed by Nils Bejerot, views addiction as an emotional fixation acquired through learning that is aimed at obtaining pleasure and avoiding discomfort. If the pleasure (euphoria) that results is sufficiently strong, it induces repetition and overcomes the person's natural drive, resulting in addiction. This model is the basis of zero tolerance for drugs as a prevention strategy.

Sociocultural Factors

Sociocultural factors are thought to play a strong role in the development of and tolerance for an addiction. Sociocultural factors often influence individuals' decisions as to when, what, and how they use substances. The way drugs are processed, the degree of acceptance or rejection of drug use, and an individual's financial resources influence what substance is used, how much is used, and what peer pressure the individual will face in his or her culture as the abuse becomes evident.

Family environment can increase a child's risk for developing addictive behaviors as an adolescent or adult. Parents or older family members who abuse alcohol or drugs or engage in criminal behavior can increase adolescents' risks of developing drug problems. Violence, physical and emotional abuse, and mental illness in the household also increase this risk (NIDA, 2014a, 2014e). Other factors include the availability of drugs within the neighborhood, community, and school and whether the adolescent's friends are using them (NIDA, 2014e). Academic failure or poor social skills can put a child at further risk for using or becoming addicted to drugs. Other factors predicting addiction are early use of substances and smoking a drug or injecting the substance into a vein, which increases its addictive potential. Smoked or injected drugs enter the brain within seconds and produce a powerful pleasure effect (NIDA, 2014a).

Sociocultural factors such as personality and religion/ spirituality appear to play a part in the risk profile for developing alcoholism in that interest in religion/spirituality practices have been correlated with lower alcohol use (Holt et al., 2015).

Research indicates that lesbian and bisexual women are at greater risk for alcohol and drug use disorders, whereas gay and bisexual men are at greater risk for illicit drug use. Affiliation with the gay culture and HIV status are correlated with increased substance abuse (Green & Feinstein, 2012).

Many factors place an individual at risk for substance use, abuse, and dependence. No single cause can explain why one individual develops a pattern of drug use and another person does not.

Manifestations of Substance Use Disorders

Specific behavioral and physiologic manifestations of substance use vary by substance. An overview of these manifestations and treatment options is provided in the Alterations and Therapies feature; further details can be found in the exemplars for this module. Most individuals who abuse substances for more than a few weeks begin to experience an array of health and emotional problems. They face increased risk for comorbid illness and family complications. It is helpful to nurses and practitioners working with this patient population to understand the prevalence of substance use in this country as well as the language of addiction and recovery.

Prevalence

Substance abuse in the United States is so common that very few people are unaffected by it.

- In 2015, more than 27 million Americans reported the current use of illicit drugs or misuse of prescription drugs (Surgeon General, 2016).
- In 2015, 66 million Americans reported binge drinking within the past month, which is almost one quarter of the adolescent and adult population (Surgeon General, 2016).

Alterations and Therapies
Addictions

ALTERATION	DESCRIPTION	TREATMENT
Nicotine addiction	Addiction to nicotine can result from smoking tobacco in the form of cigarettes, cigars, or pipes as well as from chewing tobacco.	■ Medications (e.g., bupropion [Zyban] and varenicline tartrate [Chantix]) ■ Nicotine replacement treatments (NRTs; e.g., nicotine gum/spray and the transdermal nicotine patch) ■ Behavior therapy ■ Support groups
Alcohol addiction	Chronic use of alcohol can lead to addiction, resulting in delirium tremens (DTs) if alcohol is not consumed.	■ Medications (e.g., disulfiram [Antabuse]) ■ Behavioral therapy ■ Support groups ■ 12-step program (e.g., Alcoholics Anonymous [AA]) ■ Detoxification ■ Milieu therapy ■ Family therapy
Substance addiction	Substance addiction may include abuse of heroin, cocaine, marijuana, crack, narcotics, barbiturates, inhalants, or any chemical substance that leads to addiction.	■ Behavior therapy ■ Support groups ■ Detoxification ■ Pharmacologic therapy, which may be required to minimize complications from withdrawal ■ Removal of peers providing substance ■ Milieu therapy ■ 12-step programs (e.g., Narcotics Anonymous [NA]) ■ Family therapy
Process addictions (sex, gambling, shopping, work)	Process addictions are those behaviors compulsively performed to reduce anxiety; they are considered by some to be a form of obsessive-compulsive disorder.	■ Psychotherapy ■ Behavior therapy ■ Milieu therapy ■ Support groups ■ 12-step programs (e.g., Gamblers Anonymous) ■ Family therapy

TABLE 22–1 Terminology Associated with Substance Abuse

Term	Definition
Abstinence	Voluntarily going without drugs or alcohol
Codependence	A cluster of maladaptive behaviors exhibited by significant others of a substance-abusing individual that serves to enable and protect the abuse at the expense of living a full and satisfying life
Co-occurring disorders	Concurrent diagnosis of a substance use disorder and a psychiatric disorder; one disorder can precede and cause the other, such as the theorized relationship between alcoholism and depression
Cross-tolerance	Tolerance to one drug conferring tolerance to another drug
Delirium tremens (DTs)	A medical emergency usually occurring 3–5 days following alcohol withdrawal and lasting 2–3 days; characterized by paranoia, disorientation, delusions, visual hallucinations, elevated vital signs, vomiting, diarrhea, and diaphoresis; also known as alcohol withdrawal delirium
Detoxification	The process of helping an addicted individual safely through withdrawal; commonly referred to as detox
Dual diagnosis	The coexistence of substance abuse/dependence and a psychiatric disorder in one individual (used interchangeably with dual disorder and co-occurring disorders)
Korsakoff psychosis	Secondary dementia caused by thiamine (B_1) deficiency that may be associated with chronic alcoholism; characterized by progressive cognitive deterioration, confabulation, peripheral neuropathy, and myopathy
Physical dependence	A state in which withdrawal syndrome will occur if drug use is discontinued
Polysubstance abuse	The simultaneous use of many substances
Psychologic dependence	An intensive, subjective need for a particular psychoactive drug
Sobriety	The state of habitually refraining from using alcohol or drugs
Tolerance	A state in which a particular dose elicits a smaller response than it formerly did; with increased tolerance, the individual needs higher and higher doses to obtain the desired response
Wernicke encephalopathy	Neurologic symptoms caused by biochemical lesions of the central nervous system after exhaustion of B-vitamin reserves, especially thiamine (vitamin B_1); symptoms often include ophthalmoplegia (abnormal eye movements), ataxia, and confusion
Withdrawal syndrome	A constellation of signs and symptoms that occurs in physically dependent individuals when they discontinue drug use

- Abuse of tobacco, alcohol, and illicit drugs is costly; in the United States, the costs related to crime, lost work productivity, and healthcare are estimated to be $249 billion annually for alcohol misuse and $193 billion annually for illicit drug use (Surgeon General, 2016).

- In 2014, 1.5 million people (0.6% of the population) age 12 or older were current users of cocaine; this figure included about 354,000 current users of crack (Center for Behavioral Health Statistics and Quality [CBHSQ], 2015).

- In 2014, an estimated 22.2 million Americans (8.4% of the population) age 12 or older were current users of marijuana. This represented an increase of 5.8% since 2007 (CBHSQ, 2015). The increase is likely due to the decriminalization and commercial sale of marijuana in several states.

- In 2014, about 435,000 people (0.2% of the population) age 12 or older were current heroin users (CBHSQ, 2015). Heroin has continued to grow as a drug of choice, and heroin-related overdose deaths increased fourfold between 2002 and 2013 (Centers for Disease Control and Prevention [CDC], 2015e).

These statistics only scratch the surface of the number of people dealing with addiction. These figures in combination with figures related to process addictions demonstrate the need for nurses to understand, recognize, and be able to screen patients for past and present addictions and behaviors.

The Language of Addiction and Recovery

The process of addiction and recovery has its own vocabulary. These terms are used by professionals from all aspects of healthcare who work with substance-abusing patients and their families. Many of these terms are appropriate regardless of the substance or process being abused. See **Table 22–1 》** for a list of some of these terms and their definitions.

Comorbidities

Substance abuse has a high rate of morbidity with both physical and mental illness (see the Concepts Related to Addiction feature). Imaging scans, chest x-rays, and blood tests show the damaging effects of drug abuse throughout the body. For example, tests show that tobacco smoke causes cancer of the mouth, throat, larynx, blood, lungs, stomach, pancreas, kidney, bladder, and cervix. Some drugs of abuse, such as inhalants, are toxic to nerve cells and may damage or destroy them either in the brain or in the peripheral nervous system.

Medical illnesses can be promoted or exacerbated by neglect of one's health and lack of preventive healthcare. Immunity is often compromised by malnutrition, poor hygiene, and risky behaviors related to addiction. Some infectious diseases, such as hepatitis A, B, and C, HIV and AIDS, and tuberculosis, are transmitted by substance abuse either directly or indirectly. Adverse central nervous system (CNS) effects are seen in manifestations of substance dependence, tolerance, craving, and withdrawal. Addiction behaviors affect the mental health and physical health of the addicted patient as well as the patient's family.

Individuals who abuse substances have a higher incidence of mental health disorders than the general population. Among the 20.7 million adults in the United States who experienced a substance use disorder in 2014, 40.7%—8.4 million adults—had a co-occurring mental illness (CBHSQ, 2015).

The depression that may be a part of the addiction process itself must be differentiated from a diagnosable mental illness. Because substance use disorder often co-occurs with other mental illnesses, patients presenting with one condition should be assessed for the other.

Individuals who abuse substances also commonly present with numerous social problems, ranging from dysfunctional family relationships to under- or unemployment or homelessness. Because of the scope of problems associated with chronic substance abuse and the staggering impact of untreated behavioral health conditions on individuals' lives and the cost of healthcare delivery, the Substance Abuse and Mental Health Services Administration (SAMHSA), the federal agency that spearheads the nation's behavioral health public health efforts, supports *integrative* care of co-occurring mental health and substance use disorders. Integration extends beyond health (including primary, specialty, emergency, and rehabilitative care) and behavioral health-care systems and also requires addressing patients' social needs, such as housing, employment, and transportation (SAMHSA, 2015a).

Effects of Addiction on Families

Substance abuse can have particularly devastating consequences for families, because it increases the family members' risk for social isolation and decreases their access to social supports that can be helpful to those experiencing addiction and their families. Typically, defensive coping mechanisms (particularly denial) arise as family members find themselves unable to cope with the addiction in a healthy way. Substance abuse can also interfere with normal family processes, from day-to-day activities related to parenting (such as not being able to drive for the carpool in the morning) to long-term changes such as role reversals, with older children taking on caregiving responsibilities.

Addiction within the family is often cloaked in secrecy and shame. An individual who is addicted is unable to control substance use (or, in the case of process addiction, excessive, compulsive behavior) and will use any means necessary to satisfy the overwhelming need for the substance. Family members, in an effort to protect the family and the addicted member from discovery, often close family ranks to the outside world.

Often, the term **boundaries** is used when talking about interpersonal relationships and addiction. Boundaries represent a type of relationship safety zone around a family and its members. Children and parents in healthy relationships have boundaries that are usually dictated by their role in the family. For example, the parent takes care of the children, the cohabiting adult couple has an intimate personal and physical relationship, and the child is a friend to peers and other children. Normally, boundaries around families are flexible, allowing members to interact with those outside of the family and with the community as needed and desired. Clear boundaries keep people safe within functional relationships. When addiction is present in a family, these boundaries often become rigid and inflexible. Such boundaries do not let information about the family needs or requests for needed assistance out and do not allow input or assistance from individuals or community agencies outside of the family.

Family members of addicts are often seen as enablers, inadvertently supporting the addict's behaviors. **Enabling behavior** is any action an individual takes that consciously or unconsciously facilitates substance dependence. Examples of enabling include family members making excuses to employers or teachers, or discontinuing their own social relationships with friends or neighbors in order to preserve the "healthy image" of the family in the community.

In families where addiction is present, communication is poor within and outside of the family system. Isolation results in an escalating cycle of addiction and dysfunction for the entire family. It is important for healthcare providers to recognize that shame and fear often lead to this isolation. A nonjudgmental approach to assessment and intervention, coupled with empathy and respect, is essential when working with those who are addicted to substances and their families. Substance abuse sometimes correlates with a history of abuse, economic instability, criminal behavior, and educational upheaval. Addiction is a family disease and should be viewed and treated within the context of the family. The longer the addiction continues, the more entrenched family members become in behaviors that further the addiction, such as denial and enabling. This codependency, in which the behaviors of the addict and those of the family revolve around the addiction and their shared behaviors in service of the addiction, harms the family. Children may carry these behaviors into adulthood, taking on specific characteristics beyond the family relationship. Characteristics of codependent individuals are described in **Box 22–1 》**. A number of support networks and groups, including Adult Children of Alcoholics and Al-Anon, exist to help family members learn about and recover from the effects of addiction.

Children growing up in a household with a parent who is addicted to drugs or alcohol face a number of challenges. Approximately 7.5 million children younger than the age of 18 (10.5% of all children) live with a parent who had an alcohol use disorder in the past year (CBHSQ, 2012). These

---

Box 22–1
Characteristics of Codependent Individuals

- Have low self-esteem.
- Have an exaggerated sense of responsibility for others' actions.
- Feel guilty when they assert themselves.
- Deny that they have a problem; think the problem is someone else or the situation.
- Tend to become hurt when their efforts aren't recognized.
- Do more than their share of work all of the time; have trouble saying "no" to anyone.
- Need approval and recognition.
- Fear being abandoned or alone.
- Have difficulty identifying their feelings despite experiencing painful emotions.
- Have difficulty adjusting to change.
- Struggle with intimacy and boundaries.
- Have poor communication skills.
- Have difficulty making decisions.
- Offer advice whether it has been asked for or not.
- Feel like a victim.
- Use manipulation, shame, or guilt to control others' behavior.

children are at a greater risk for depression, anxiety disorders, problems with cognitive and verbal skills, and parental abuse or neglect. Moreover, they are four times more likely than other children to develop alcohol problems themselves (CBHSQ, 2012). Similar issues exist with parents who abuse other substances or combine other substances with alcohol.

Parents often neglect their responsibilities for drugs, alcohol, or other behaviors, up to and including diverting household funds to pay for their addiction. Parents may disappear for hours or days at a time or may be emotionally and physically unavailable to their children even when at home. Compared with families in which substance abuse is not an issue, families with parents who abuse demonstrate poorer problem-solving abilities, both among the parents and within the family as a whole. These poor communication and problem-solving skills may be mechanisms through which lack of cohesion and increased conflict develop and escalate in affected families (National Association for Children of Alcoholics [NACOA], 2015). Children whose parents abuse substances are at risk for disruptive behavioral problems and are more likely to be sensation seeking, aggressive, and impulsive. Because of the secrecy and shame associated with substance abuse, many children of addicts are hesitant to talk about their own feelings, needs, and wants.

While some children growing up in families with addiction have obvious and apparent problems, others cope quite well. The level of dysfunction or resiliency of the nonabusing spouse is a key factor in the impact of the addiction on the children (NACOA, 2015). However, longitudinal research has confirmed the adverse lifelong psychosocial, behavioral, and developmental effects of growing up in a household headed by addicted parents.

Case Study >> Part 1

Paul is the 19-year-old son of Mark and Susan John. The Johns have been married for 20 years. Ms. John is a full-time stay-at-home mom. Paul's dad is a corporate attorney who has always been somewhat demanding of his wife and children. He drinks alcohol daily but has always been employed and has maintained a middle-class lifestyle for his family. Paul has two younger sisters: Mara, the younger of the two, has been treated for anorexia since the age of 12. His 15-year-old sister, Jess, is doing well in high school. Paul did well in high school, where he played varsity soccer and did fairly well academically.

Paul has just returned home from his first full year at college. His mother is concerned because he doesn't seem like his old self; he shows no interest in his old friends or in getting a summer job. On the other hand, he seems secretive and has left the house on many occasions claiming that he has new friends who "get it." He is very short tempered with his sisters, constantly irritable and discontented. He is very evasive when asked about his grades or any college activities. He has noticeable weight loss and appears unkempt. His father is intolerant of his behavior. His mother is concerned and has arranged to accompany him on a visit to his primary care provider. She is hoping to find out what his problem is so it can be treated before his father becomes angrier with him and his behavior. You are the nurse who is assessing Paul.

Clinical Reasoning Questions Level I

1. Describe the elements of the interview/assessment environment that you should consider before beginning Paul's patient assessment.

2. What questions would be appropriate in assessing Paul's physiologic, emotional, and psychologic status?

3. What elements of the family history might indicate a potential for substance use or abuse in Paul?

Clinical Reasoning Questions Level II

4. If substance abuse is suspected, how should you proceed to address any ego defense mechanisms displayed?

5. What diagnostic measures might be needed based on your assessment?

6. If depression is suspected, what further assessments would you perform?

Process Disorders

Although this chapter focuses on the care of patients with substance use disorders, it is important for nurses to also be able to recognize that individuals can become addicted to certain behaviors. Process disorders or addictions are groups of repetitive behaviors (e.g., gambling, shopping, internet gaming, exercise, sex) that activate biochemical reward systems similar to those activated by drugs of abuse. Process addictions produce behavioral symptoms comparable to those seen in substance use disorders (APA, 2013). One significant difference, however, is that the individual is not addicted to a substance, but to the behavior or the feeling brought about by the relevant action. In addition, the physical signs of drug addiction are absent in behavioral or process addiction (Alavi et al., 2012).

Gambling disorder is the only one of the repetitive processes with sufficient data to be included in the *Diagnostic and Statistical Manual of Mental Disorders* (5th ed.; DSM-5) as a diagnosable mental disorder (**Figure 22–2 >>**). The essential feature of gambling is the individual's willingness to risk something of value in the hope of obtaining something of greater value. The diagnostic criteria for gambling disorder highlight the similarities between a process addiction and a substance use disorder. To be diagnosed

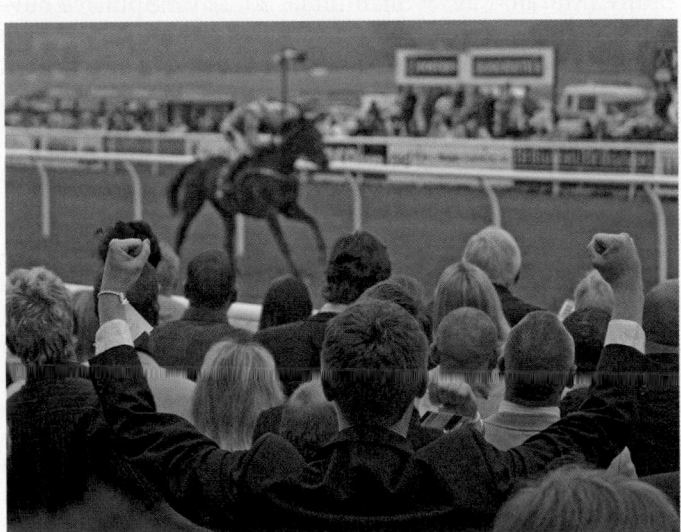

Source: Mikedabell/E+/Getty Images.

Figure 22–2 >> Gambling disorder, one of the process disorders, produces behavioral symptoms comparable to those seen in substance use disorders.

with gambling disorder, an individual must experience clinically significant impairment or distress related to the gambling; experience distress when trying to reduce or quit gambling; be preoccupied with gambling to the extent of jeopardizing income, employment, or significant relationships; and have a history of unsuccessful attempts to control or stop gambling (APA, 2013).

Other process addictions, which do not yet appear in the DSM-5 as diagnosable mental health disorders, also cause severe stress and strain to individuals and families. For example, in some individuals who initiate healthy levels of exercise, the practice later morphs into a full-blown **exercise addiction**. Research has suggested that an individual who is addicted to exercise will continue exercising regardless of physical injury, personal inconvenience, or disruption to other areas of life, including marital strain, interference with work, and lack of time for other activities (Landolfi, 2013). Individuals who become addicted to exercise are more likely than committed exercisers to exercise for intrinsic rewards and experience disturbing withdrawal sensations when unable to exercise. The characteristic personality traits in individuals with exercise addiction included high levels of excitement seeking and striving for achievement.

Excessive online shopping, often associated with overspending and aided by the internet, comprises compulsive and addictive forms of consumption and buying behavior. Review of the literature has shown that attributes associated with **online shopping addiction (OSA)** include low self-esteem, low self-regulation, negative emotional state, enjoyment, female gender, social anonymity, and cognitive overload (Rose & Dhandayudham, 2014). Increased accessibility, hyperstimulating marketing techniques, a loss of the protective delay between impulse and purchase, and over-valuing of the shopping process and objects purchased may all contribute to the potentially addictive nature of shopping (Hartston, 2012). Shopping addiction can adversely affect the individual's family, social, and occupational life. The addiction is associated with high rates of psychiatric comorbidity (Murali, Ray, & Shaffiullha, 2012). Compulsive buying has been linked with substance addiction, depression, and obsessive-compulsive disorder, as well as hoarding, but some research has found that excessive shopping is most closely related to addiction, that is, an increased sensitivity to reward (Lawrence, Ciorciari, & Kyrios, 2014).

Internet gaming disorder (IGD) is the persistent use of the internet to engage in games, often with other players, leading to clinically significant impairment or distress. Proposed criteria for diagnosis of IGD include preoccupation with gaming; withdrawal symptoms when gaming is taken away; tolerance (the need to spend increasing amounts of time in gaming or gaming-related activities); unsuccessful attempts to control use and participation; continued gaming despite distress or interference with other activities or interference with relationships; lying about time spent gaming; and using gaming to relieve a negative mood (APA, 2013).

There have been several proposed diagnostic labels for persistent, excessive sexual behaviors, often referred to as **sex addiction** or compulsive sexual behavior (CSB). Typical activities may include engaging in risky sexual practices with a number of partners; preoccupation with recurrent, intense, sexually arousing fantasies, sexual urges, or behaviors; visiting strip clubs; and engaging in phone sex (De Guzmán et al., 2016). These behaviors cannot be diagnosable as a paraphilia. CSB is estimated to affect up to 3 to 6% of the U.S. population (De Guzmán et al., 2016).

Clinicians have been researching how CSB can be escalated by the internet. Being online seems to facilitate and stimulate addictive tendencies in relation to sexual behavior, such as accessibility, affordability, anonymity, convenience, escape, and disinhibition. The internet has enabled behaviors that an individual would never imagine engaging in offline, such as cybersexual stalking, and has increased access to pornography (Cravens & Whiting, 2014; Griffiths, 2016). Moreover, personal communication devices such as cell phones make practices such as "sexting" (communicating sexually suggestive comments or photos) or engaging in cybersex chatrooms extremely convenient. Aside from the time consumed by a compulsion, hypersexual behavior, particularly time spent pursuing online sexual addictions, causes damage to interpersonal relationships and families. Many clinicians, even those trained in sexual disorders or addiction medicine, have difficulty detecting and diagnosing compulsive sexual behaviors and difficulty treating sexual compulsivity and cybersex addiction unless significant personal and social consequences have occurred that result in the individual seeking help.

Concepts Related to Addiction

Substance use disorder is not a self-contained disorder. Substance use can affect the physical, psychologic, and spiritual health of both the individual and the family. A few examples of systems and concepts that are related to substance abuse are outlined here.

Substance use impacts cognitive ability, including slowing reaction times, decreasing inhibitions, and impairing judgment and memory (SAMHSA, 2015b). Substance use also negatively impacts intellectual development in the children of abusing parents. Alcohol abuse is the primary factor contributing to the neurocognitive deficits and intellectual disabilities exhibited by children who have fetal alcohol spectrum disorders (FASD) because of in utero exposure to alcohol (Chokroborty-Hoque, Alberry, & Singh, 2014).

Gastrointestinal disorders (including the GI tract, liver, and pancreas) occur frequently with long-term substance use. For example, cocaine abuse can result in various gastrointestinal complications, including gastric ulcerations, retroperitoneal fibrosis, visceral infarction, intestinal ischemia, and gastrointestinal tract perforations (SAMHSA, 2015b). Long-term alcohol use often leads to cirrhosis of the liver, which impairs digestion of food and absorption of key nutrients.

Infectious diseases are common in individuals who abuse substances. Hepatitis C virus infection is the most common form of infectious hepatitis in patients with substance use disorders. At least 76% of patients who have used injectable drugs for less than 7 years are positive for hepatitis C, while 25% of patients who abuse alcohol and those who do not inject drugs also show serologic evidence of infection (SAMHSA, 2015b). Other infectious diseases associated with SUD are endocarditis, bacterial pneumonia, tuberculosis, skin infections resulting from administration of intravenous drugs (e.g., *Staphylococcus aureus* and *Streptococcus pyogenes*), and the sexually transmitted infections HIV/AIDS.

Individuals with SUD are prone to accidents of all kinds, with complications ranging from head trauma to falls with fractures. Chronic pain frequently is seen in patients as a result of trauma, poor health maintenance, or an inability to deal with pain without opioid drug use (SAMHSA, 2015b). Also, clinicians should also consider traumatic brain injury (TBI) when individuals with SUD present with neurologic impairment. People who abuse substances have a high risk of falls, motor vehicle accidents, gang violence, domestic violence, and so on, all of which may result in head injury (SAMHSA, 2015b).

Many individuals who experience overwhelming stress turn to substance use as a maladaptive coping mechanism. For example, researchers found that individuals of both genders who reported higher levels of stress tended to drink more. However, men turned to alcohol as a means for dealing with stress more often than women. For those who reported at least six stressful incidents, the percentage of men who engaged in binge drinking was about 1.5 times that of women, and alcohol abuse among men was 2.5 times higher than among women (National Institute on Alcohol Abuse and Alcoholism [NIAAA], 2012).

Veterans who have been in active combat are especially likely to turn to alcohol as a means of relieving stress. Post-traumatic stress disorder (PTSD) has been found in 14 to 22% of veterans returning from recent wars in Afghanistan and Iraq and has been linked to increased risk for alcohol abuse and dependence (NIAAA, 2012). Individuals who abuse substances and have experienced trauma have worse treatment outcomes for substance abuse than those without histories of trauma (SAMHSA, 2014a). Because traumatic experiences and their sequelae are closely tied to behavioral health problems, many clinicians have integrated trauma-informed care into addiction recovery programs (SAMHSA, 2014a). See the Evidence-Based Practice feature on trauma-informed care.

The Concepts Related to Addiction feature links some, but not all, of the concepts integral to addiction. They are presented in alphabetical order.

Concepts Related to
Addiction

CONCEPT	RELATIONSHIP TO ADDICTION	NURSING IMPLICATIONS
Cognition	↓ B_1 (thiamine) in the brain can cause changes in cognition, specifically confusion ↓ Memory, judgment, reaction times, cognitive ability	■ Assess for Wernicke encephalopathy, Korsakoff psychosis, and dementia. ■ Provide for patient safety. ■ Anticipate provision of thiamine therapy.
Family	↑ Substance use and abuse of family member → ↑ Family secrecy → ↑ Family isolation → ↓ Supportive resources available	■ Determine family understanding of substance abuse and addiction. ■ Communicate clearly, honestly, openly, and without judgment. ■ Anticipate involving the entire family in all aspects of the treatment process.
Infection	↑ Spread of infection through intravenous use of drugs, e.g., needle sharing ↑ Risk of sexually transmitted infections	■ Assess for hepatitis C, endocarditis, bacterial pneumonia, tuberculosis, skin infections resulting from administration of intravenous drugs. ■ Assess for sexually transmitted infections such as HIV/AIDS.
Nutrition	↓ Nutritional status → ↓ Body's ability to synthesize antibodies	■ Be alert to signs/symptoms of malnutrition and opportunistic infections. ■ Anticipate the need for a nutritional assessment, balanced diet, vitamin and mineral supplements. ■ Provide discharge planning that promotes patient's ability to meet nutritional needs.
Safety	↑ Risk-taking behaviors leads to ↑ risk for injury, violence, and HIV	■ Assess for risk behaviors, including driving under the influence, unprotected sex, or sharing needles. ■ Provide education related to safety. ■ Anticipate denial, family interference, or enabling.
Trauma	Substance abuse as coping mechanism → poorer outcomes Combat, TBI ↑ risk for PTSD → ↑ risk for substance abuse	■ Assess for patient and family safety. ■ Identify and refer to recovery programs that provide integrative, trauma-informed care. ■ Support family during recovery process.

Health Promotion

Prevention efforts related to substance abuse generally revolve around education. Federal initiatives include prevention efforts by SAMHSA and other federal organizations. Community and local initiatives, often sponsored as collaborations among law enforcement and local health and mental health professionals, may be developed to target needs in a specific community. At the individual level, nurses and other healthcare professionals assess patients' risk for substance abuse and provide education related to prevention, especially related to using healthy coping mechanisms and obtaining appropriate treatment for existing mental health disorders, such as depression.

Health promotion activities can be particularly important for patients who are in recovery from an addiction. Generally speaking, health promotion activities to help prevent patients from experiencing relapse include reviewing with patients the situations or feelings that triggered use in the past and helping patients recall and maintain healthy coping strategies that have been successful in helping them maintain sobriety. Nurses working with sober patients may need to help identify additional resources for patients during challenging times. For example, consider a mother with a history of substance use who gives birth to a premature newborn. Prior to discharge from the hospital, the nurse or case worker sets up early childhood intervention services. A nurse or early childhood intervention specialist will make weekly home visits to see how mother and baby are doing and provide supportive interventions that may include teaching feeding and parenting strategies. By reducing the stress level of the mother and promoting mother–child bonding, the mother will be at less risk for resuming addictive behaviors.

>> **Stay Current:** SAMHSA offers a registry of evidence-based prevention and treatment programs at http://nrepp.samhsa.gov.

Nursing Assessment

A trusting nurse–patient relationship, along with the nurse's ethical obligation to maintain confidentiality, may help the patient share information more freely. By including family members in the assessment process, nurses may uncover addictions or behaviors the patient is hiding. Nurses must help patients understand the importance of full disclosure of any addictions to protect them from potential treatment complications. All too often patients fail to admit addiction until permanent damage has already occurred. The nurse's responsibility is to recognize clues while complications are still preventable.

SAMHSA recommends that clinicians at all levels of treatment use SBIRT (screening, brief intervention, and referral to treatment) to identify patients with substance abuse issues (SAMHSA, 2015c). The goal is early intervention and treatment services for persons with substance use disorders, as well as those who are at risk of developing these disorders. *Screening* quickly assesses the severity of substance use and identifies the appropriate level of treatment. *Brief intervention* focuses on increasing insight and awareness regarding substance use and motivation toward

---

Box 22–2
Gender Differences Associated with Substance Use Disorder Treatment

During the past decade, SAMHSA has devoted research to discovering what features of substance treatment engage patients and promote recovery for different segments of the population. SAMHSA has issued treatment improvement protocols looking at gender differences between women and men seeking treatment for substance use issues.

For women, being responsible for the care of dependent children is one of the deterrents to treatment (SAMHSA, 2009). Women who do not have access to a treatment program that provides child care or who cannot arrange alternative child care may have to choose between caring for their children and entering treatment. Unfortunately, few programs allow mothers to bring their children or assist with services for children or child care (SAMHSA, 2009). Women who have children often fear that admitting a substance use problem will cause them to lose custody of their children. Clinicians need to be sensitive to this barrier, explore resources in the community, and help female patients deal with this issue.

For men, employment-related issues can strongly affect men's substance use/abuse, and men with substance use disorders are at greater risk for unemployment (SAMHSA, 2013). For men who are employed, their type of profession may affect the pattern and extent of their substance use. For example, research has shown a relationship between drinking and having positions that are typically male dominated. Men who work in production and craft jobs and jobs that require working with machinery or hazardous materials are more likely to use substances than those in positions that carry less risk (SAMHSA, 2013).

Men in particular have a fear of risking their employment to enter treatment. SAMHSA research has shown that men who needed substance abuse treatment were more than 16 times as likely as women who needed treatment to express concern that entering treatment would affect their jobs. Clinicians need to explore this fear with men and help them find treatment that will help safeguard existing employment.

---

behavioral change. *Referral to treatment* helps direct those who need more extensive treatment toward access to specialty care (SAMHSA, 2015c). In addition, SAMHSA has researched and recommended some gender-based treatment considerations (**Box 22–2 >>**).

Most clinicians use multidimensional assessment criteria developed by the American Society of Addiction Medicine (ASAM) when determining the most appropriate facility and level of care for initial placement, continued stay, and transfer/discharge of patients who abuse substances (ASAM, 2015). Assessment criteria include acute intoxication or withdrawal potential; biomedical conditions and complications; emotional, behavioral, or cognitive conditions and complications; readiness to change; relapse, continued use, or continued problem potential; and recovery/living environment (ASAM, 2015). The levels of care typically used in the United States range from ambulatory detoxification without extended onsite monitoring to medically managed intensive inpatient detoxification (SAMHSA, 2015b).

For individuals withdrawing from alcohol, sedative-hypnotics, or opioids, hospitalization (or some form of 24-hour medical care) is the preferred setting for detoxification, based on safety and symptom-relief concerns (SAMHSA, 2015b). Concurrent mental health issues, such as exacerbation of schizophrenia or bipolar disorder, may also require hospitalization for stabilization. Distressing physiologic symptoms also indicate the need for immediate hospitalization. These symptoms include, among others, a change in mental status, increasing anxiety and panic, hallucinations, seizures, temperature greater than 100.4°F (suggesting potential infection), significant increases and/or decreases in vital signs, abdominal pain, gastrointestinal bleeding, heightened deep tendon reflexes, and central nervous system irritability (SAMHSA, 2015b). Young individuals in good health, with no history of previous withdrawal reactions, may be able to manage withdrawal without medication. Nonmedical detoxification is a current trend because of cost effectiveness and inexpensive access to treatment for certain individuals seeking treatment (SAMHSA, 2015b).

SAFETY ALERT Clinicians need to assess for suicidality in individuals with substance use issues. Individuals with substance use disorders are about six times more likely to commit suicide than the general population (Ross, 2014). Roughly one in three individuals who commit suicide are under the influence of drugs, typically opiates such as oxycodone or heroin, or alcohol (Ross, 2014).

Observation and Patient Interview

Nurses who work with individuals with addiction issues often note observable manifestations at the first patient encounter. Familiar manifestations include unsteady gait and poor balance, lack of coordination, slurred speech, tremors, and unusual smells on the breath, body, or clothes. Other common manifestations include:

- Loss of interest in personal hygiene and grooming
- Watering or bloodshot eyes; large or small pupils
- Rhinorrhea (runny nose)
- Obvious weight loss or gain
- Inability to concentrate; hyperactivity, agitation, or giddiness
- Anger, frustration, or mood swings
- Appearing fearful, anxious, or paranoid with no reason
- Appearing lethargic or "spaced out."

These are only a few observable manifestations of substance use. Symptoms specific to certain substance addictions are described in more detail in following sections.

The nursing history plays an important role in determining potential addictive behavior. Patients may feel shame, contempt, or embarrassment about revealing their addiction. In addition, fear of legal reprisal may cause the patient to be reluctant to share information if the addiction is to an illegal substance.

Patients also may need to be assessed regarding the extent of crisis they are facing in their lives as the result of their substance use disorder, particularly if a crisis event or behavior motivates them to seek healthcare. The following list of questions provides a general crisis assessment that can be used in any problem-solving situation. It is of particular use for the patient whose crisis is the result of addiction behavior.

Individual Assessment

1. What is the most significant stress/problem occurring in your life right now?
2. Has this problem increased the frequency of substance use? (Quantify change in frequency or amount of substance used.)
3. Is your addiction behavior causing or contributing to the problem?
4. Who is the problem impacting? You? Your family? Your employer?
5. How long has this been a problem?
6. What does this problem mean to you?
7. What are the factors that cause this problem to continue?
8. Would the problem resolve if you stopped abusing the substance?
9. Have you had similar stresses/problems in the past?
10. What other stresses do you have in your life?
11. How are you managing your usual life roles (partner, parent, homemaker, worker, student, and so on)?
12. In what way has your life changed as a result of this problem?
13. Are you feeling as though you want to harm yourself or anyone else?
14. Describe how you have managed problems in the past.
15. What have you done to try to solve the problem so far? What happened when you tried this?
16. Describe possible resources (e.g., family, friends, employer, teacher; financial, spiritual).
17. Are you interested in abstaining from substance abuse? Are you considering a rehabilitation program?
18. What part of the overall problem is most important to deal with first?

Family Assessment

1. How do you perceive the current problem and the patient's addiction behavior?
2. In what way has the problem and the patient's addiction behavior affected your roles in the family?
3. How has your lifestyle changed since this problem began?
4. Describe communication within the family before and since this current problem began.
5. How does the family typically manage problems?
6. What has the family done to try to solve the problem so far?
7. What happened when you tried this?
8. How well do you believe the family is coping at this time?
9. Describe possible resources (e.g., extended family, friends; financial).
10. What are your expectations and hopes concerning this problem and the patient's addiction behavior?
11. Which part of the overall problem is most important to deal with first?
12. Can the problem be resolved without resolution of the addiction behavior?

Community Assessment

1. What are the living conditions of the neighborhood?
2. Are affordable child care services available?
3. Is there a community mental health center or rehabilitation center?
4. What support groups are available in the community?
5. Are there any possible funding resources?

Physical Examination

Physical assessment findings depend on the nature of the addiction and the substance being used. When performing a physical assessment, nurses must be alert for symptoms that are abnormal or not within expected boundaries and assess patient explanations for inconsistencies. Unless the patient comes to the provider under the influence or is referred by an employer, the physical examination may provide the first indications that an addiction is involved.

Diagnostic Tests

Diagnostic tests required for patients with addiction will be ordered based on the type of addiction they display. Specific diagnostic tests will be ordered for each type of addiction and may include serum drug levels; toxicology; chest x-rays for inhaled substances; organ biopsies related to damage caused by a substance; and urine, saliva, and serum testing for substance metabolites. Hair testing may be done to determine substance use within a period of 90 days.

Case Study >> Part 2

Paul is admitted to the emergency department (ED) at 2 a.m. on a Sunday morning in August as the result of a motor vehicle crash. His speech is slurred and his gate is ataxic. He is bleeding from a laceration on his left forehead, and he is complaining that his left arm is extremely painful and "falling off." A decision is made to admit Paul to the trauma unit. His father, as next of kin, is notified of the admission. His father states, "I knew this would happen. Let him rot." Paul becomes combative as you attempt to assess his state of consciousness and physical injuries.

Clinical Reasoning Questions Level I

1. You suspect substance use. What are your immediate concerns?
2. How will you promote Paul's cooperation with your assessment and eventual treatment?
3. What specific diagnostic tests will be appropriate related to both his suspected substance use and his physical injuries?

Clinical Reasoning Questions Level II

4. *Refer to the module on Legal Issues:* Are you able to begin assessment and treatment of Paul without consent from next of kin? What are the legal implications in this situation?
5. Paul's mother arrives in the ED. She is very upset and demanding to see him. Will you involve Paul's mother in his care? Why or why not?

Independent Interventions

Nurses may use a number of independent and collaborative caring interventions with patients who are addicted or who exhibit addiction behaviors. **Recovery** is generally defined as a state of voluntary sobriety in which the individual maintains personal health and functions normally within society without the use of the addictive substance or behavior. The goal of all interventions is to move the patient toward treatment and into recovery. Recovery is a lifelong process. Nurses must remember that no single intervention is sufficient to ensure permanent recovery, which requires substantial and continual work on the part of the individual.

Independent nursing interventions for patients with substance use disorders primarily focus around nursing care for any specific presenting symptoms, developing and maintaining the therapeutic nurse–patient relationship (including establishing and maintaining appropriate boundaries), and promoting healthy patient communication and coping skills. See the module on Stress and Coping for a discussion about defense mechanisms and nursing interventions to help patients develop healthy coping skills. As always, providing culturally competent care is critical to reducing barriers and improving outcomes (see the Focus on Diversity and Culture feature).

Promote Communication

Respect, empathy, and caring are essential components of caring for those with substance use disorders. Establishing a therapeutic nurse–patient relationship that places the patient at the center of all communication is essential for two reasons: (a) Many patients with substance use disorders have poor communication skills and rely on their addictive behaviors to avoid communicating with others, and (b) these patients are experienced at hiding their addictions and avoiding their addiction as the topic of discussion.

Because many individuals who abuse substances come from families with impaired communication, it is important that communication be simple, direct, and powerful (LaPierre, 2015). Many student and new clinicians will use euphemisms or talk too much when communicating with a substance

---

Focus on Diversity and Culture
Improving Cultural Competence Among Mental Health Clinicians

In 2014, the Substance Abuse and Mental Health Services Administration (SAMHSA) published a *Treatment Improvement Protocol: Improving Cultural Competence* to improve patient engagement in services, patient–provider therapeutic relationships, treatment retention, and outcomes. The protocol cites cultural competence as an essential ingredient in decreasing disparities in behavioral health. According to SAMHSA (2014b), culturally competent mental health and substance abuse clinicians:

- Frame issues in culturally relevant ways
- Allow for complexity of issues based on cultural context
- Make allowances for variations in the use of personal space
- Are respectful of culturally specific meanings of touch (e.g., hugging)
- Explore culturally based experiences of power and powerlessness
- Adjust communication styles to the patient's culture
- Interpret emotional expressions in light of the patient's culture.

abuser. Subtlety is counterproductive with many of these patients because they may not want to hear the message being conveyed and are often skilled in manipulating words and phrases as well as people (LaPierre, 2015). Recommended strategies for communicating with individuals who abuse substances include:

- Express concerns or pass along information without judgment. Correct any false ideas and fill in information gaps.

- Use "I" statements to describe concerns without singling out the substance-abusing individual.

- Remain calm without arguing or getting angry.

- Listen for contingency words such as "probably," "possibly," or "maybe" in conversations with individuals who abuse substances. These adverbs usually mean that the individual is not going to follow through on the topics being discussed.

- Hold patients accountable. If they agree to follow through on a task or plan, make a specific plan with them to encourage completion.

- Practice active listening skills. Notice when patients with substance use disorders are using defense mechanisms such as *deflecting* (turning the topic back on the speaker, changing the subject, or using humor to lighten the mood); *rationalizing* (explaining why a behavior or action that is clearly not acceptable is acceptable); *minimizing* (downplaying the extent of the addiction and its consequences); and *avoiding* (pretending not to hear or refusing to engage in discussion).

- Notice body language. Eye contact may indicate interest, while staring at the floor or other spots may indicate shame, exasperation, or refusal to engage. Other nonverbal indicators are muscle tension, indicating stress and fear; hand wringing, indicating anxiety and worry; and turning away, indicating termination of the conversation (British Columbia Schizophrenia Society, 2015; LaPierre, 2015).

Limit Setting and Boundary Violations

Limit setting refers to establishing parameters of desirable and acceptable patient behavior. Limit setting helps patients feel safe, advances therapeutic goals by eliminating nonproductive behaviors, promotes positive behavior change, and protects significant others and children of individuals who abuse substances from unacceptable behaviors (British Columbia Schizophrenia Society, 2015). Limit setting teaches the individual that there are choices, but there are also consequences for making poor decisions. The goal of setting limits is to teach patients how to consistently make good decisions. Unfortunately, setting limits can be challenging for both clinicians and family members, as substance users often respond with anger and resentment, with some even threatening to terminate the therapeutic or personal relationship. Clinicians and family members may feel defeated, angry, and frustrated when limits are breached (British Columbia Schizophrenia Society, 2015).

Often substance users have an unhealthy sense of personal boundaries and frequently cross them, by engaging in activities such as appropriating and selling or pawning a family member's property to pursue an addiction. Clinicians should encourage family members to set and enforce clear boundaries with defined consequences. Reluctance by family members to enforce personal boundaries is often related to poor communication and enmeshed, codependent behavior (Lander, Howsare, & Byrne, 2013; Mental Health America, 2015a).

Likewise, clinicians need to be aware of professional boundaries, which the patient can violate or exploit. Boundary crossing can involve inappropriate physical contact, giving and receiving gifts, contact outside of the normal therapy session, and use of provocative language, clothing, and proximity of the therapist and patient during sessions (Lander et al., 2013; Mental Health America, 2015b). The clinician also needs to guard against ambiguous relationships where multiple roles exist between a therapist and a patient, such as if the patient is also a student, friend, family member, employee, or business associate of the clinician.

Promote Adequate Nutrition

Patients who engage in any type of substance abuse are at risk for deficiencies in key nutrients. In the case of alcoholism, for example, thiamine deficiency can cause complications such as Wernicke syndrome. Nurses administer vitamins and dietary substances as ordered and monitor lab work (e.g., total albumin, complete blood count, urinalysis, electrolytes, and liver enzymes) and report significant changes to the provider. Nurses also collaborate with dietitians to determine the number of calories necessary for patients to maintain adequate nutrition and appropriate weight. In inpatient settings, nurses document intake, output, and calorie count and weigh patients daily if necessary. Nurses also teach patients with substance abuse about the importance of adequate nutrition and the physical effects of alcohol or substance abuse and related malnutrition on body systems. Nurses provide information about adequate nutrition using USDA recommendations.

Promote Participation in Treatment

Patients are more likely to participate in treatment when nurses and other clinicians are genuine, honest, and respectful of patients. Keep all promises and convey an attitude of acceptance. Do not accept the use of defense mechanisms such as rationalization or projection as the patient attempts to blame others or make excuses for his or her behavior. Encourage patients to examine how unhealthy coping mechanisms and maladaptive behaviors are impacting their lives and those they care about, and help them learn more healthy ways of coping and responding to stressful situations. Encourage patient participation in therapeutic group activities such as 12-step and support-group meetings with other people who are experiencing or have experienced similar problems. Patients often are more accepting of peer feedback than feedback from authority figures.

Collaborative Therapies

Treatment for addiction may be determined by level of severity and how the individual comes to seek treatment. Some patients are adjudicated to treatment by the judicial system. Patients with severe impairment of function may be involuntarily admitted or may be admitted for medical care associated with an injury. These are some of the many factors that influence individual patient plans of care.

Many clinicians routinely use the **5 A's** to help identify users and appropriate interventions based on the patient's willingness to quit (Agency for Healthcare Research and Quality [AHRQ], 2012). The steps are described below.

1. **Ask:** Identify and document substance use status for every patient at every visit.
2. **Advise:** In a clear, strong, and personalized manner, urge every substance user to quit.
3. **Assess:** Is the substance user willing to make a quit attempt at this time?
4. **Assist:** For the patient willing to make a quit attempt, use counseling and pharmacotherapy to help him or her quit. For those who need a higher level of care, for example, inpatient detoxification, make arrangements for admission.
5. **Arrange:** Schedule follow-up contact, in person or by telephone, preferably within the first week after the quit date (AHRQ, 2012).

In some cases, individuals seek care after being persuaded they need care through a process of confrontation called **intervention**. The goal of intervention is to prevent the addict from denying the problem and force him or her to face the negative aspects of behavior and enroll in treatment, typically in a residential treatment facility. In *family intervention,* the family enlists the help of a professional clinician to conduct the intervention with the participation of the family. The clinician and family meet with the individual together, with family members stating how the individual's addiction affects the family. Although the detoxification team can leverage the relationship the patient has with significant others, it is not recommended that clinicians use direct confrontation solely to force a person with a substance use disorder into treatment, because research has shown that treatment programs that rely on confrontational clinician techniques have yielded poor outcomes (SAMHSA, 2015b).

Frequently, individuals enter treatment because their inability to manage life skills and events results in a crisis. Often, these crises result in legal issues, such as impaired driving citations and vehicle crashes, child custody disputes, separation and divorce, and violent encounters. Other challenges such as job loss, financial difficulties, ruptured relationships, and distressing medical symptoms can also lead a patient with SUD to seek treatment. It is during crisis situations that patients with SUDs are most likely to be motivated to seek help. The inability to maintain emotional equilibrium is an important but short-lived feature of a crisis. Typically, the high level of anxiety created by a crisis forces the individual to return to the previous level of addiction; develop more constructive coping skills and seek help; or decompensate to a lower level of functioning.

While the process of detoxification, stabilization, and recovery frequently contains significant medical and pharmaceutical components, the motivation for long-term change often comes from psychosocial interventions. Psychosocial interventions for substance use disorders can be defined as interpersonal or informational activities, techniques, or strategies that target biological, behavioral, cognitive, emotional, interpersonal, social, or environmental factors with the aim of improving health functioning and well-being (Institute of Medicine [IOM], 2015).

The efficacy of psychosocial interventions, by themselves or combined with medication, has been well documented. Psychosocial interventions can address psychosocial problems that negatively impact adherence to medical treatments or can help the patient deal with the interpersonal and social challenges present during recovery. Not only are psychosocial interventions effective, but patients often prefer them to medications for SUD: 75% of patients, especially younger patients and women, preferred psychotherapy (McHugh et al., 2013). Psychosocial interventions also can be important to provide an alternative for those for whom medication is inadvisable (e.g., pregnant women, children, those with complex medical conditions); to enhance medication adherence; or to deal with the social and interpersonal issues that complicate recovery from mental health and substance use disorders (IOM, 2015). One such intervention is the incorporation of trauma-informed care into the overall treatment plan for individuals with alcohol or substance use disorders who have a history of trauma. See the Evidence-Based Practice feature for more information.

Behavior-Related Therapies

In **behavioral therapy**, patients learn techniques to modify or change their addictive behaviors. Classic *behavioral modification* therapy is based on the principle that all behavior has specific consequences. Thus, behavior can be changed by conditioning—a process of reinforcement, punishment, and extinction. Consequences that increase the likelihood of a particular behavior are referred to as **reinforcement**. *Positive reinforcement* provides a reward for the desired behavior, such as a token or treats for treatment compliance. *Negative reinforcement* removes a negative stimulus to increase the chances that the desired behavior will occur, such as when someone with a substance use disorder enters treatment and is able to separate from friends who are also abusing drugs.

Negative consequences that lead to a decrease in undesirable behavior are referred to as **punishment**. **Extinction** refers to the progressive weakening of an undesirable behavior through repeated nonreinforcement of the behavior. Most behavioral therapists believe that behavior changed through reinforcement is a more desirable clinical outcome than behavior changed through punishment. **Contingency contracts** may be an effective reinforcement process through which the patient is rewarded contingent upon meeting desired outcomes. Incentives found to be effective include both vouchers or cash equivalents (guaranteed payment) and "prize-based" approaches that feature the chance to earn a large prize (IOM, 2015). **Token economies** are formalized programs of contingency contracts common in behavior modification programs in which patients can accrue a number of token rewards to exchange for privileges or activities.

A more common approach is **cognitive–behavioral therapy (CBT),** which is used for a wide array of mental health and substance use disorders. It combines behavioral techniques with cognitive psychology—the scientific study of mental processes, such as perception, memory, reasoning, decision making, and problem solving (IOM, 2015). The goal is to replace maladaptive behavior and faulty cognitions

Evidence-Based Practice

Substance Use Disorders and Trauma-Informed Care

Problem

Trauma results from an event, series of events, or set of circumstances that an individual experiences as physically or emotionally harmful or threatening. Trauma can occur as a result of violence, abuse, neglect, loss, disaster, war and other negative events. Traumatic experiences affect all segments of society, regardless of age, gender, socioeconomic, status, race, ethnicity, geography, or sexual orientation. Trauma has lasting adverse effects on the individual's functioning and physical, social, emotional, or spiritual well-being and often causes the individual to seek alcohol or drugs to deal with psychic pain (SAMHSA, 2014b). People who abuse substances and have experienced trauma have worse treatment outcomes than those without histories of trauma.

Evidence

Many individuals with substance use disorders have experienced trauma as children or adults; conversely, substance abuse is known to predispose individuals to higher rates of traumas, such as dangerous situations and accidents, while under the influence and as a result of the lifestyle associated with substance abuse (SAMHSA, 2014a). During the past decade, which has featured natural disasters, overseas wars, and mass violence, clinicians have been focusing on how trauma, psychologic distress, quality of life, health, mental illness, and substance abuse are linked.

Research from two influential studies—the *Adverse Childhood Experiences Study* (CDC, 2013a) and the *Women, Co-occurring Disorders and Violence Study* (SAMHSA, 2007)—documented the relationships among exposure to traumatic events, impaired neurodevelopmental and immune systems responses, and subsequent health risk behaviors resulting in chronic physical or behavioral health disorders (SAMHSA, 2014a).

Implications

Patients with trauma histories were not responding to traditional therapies that focused solely on co-occurring mental health disorders and substance use. To address this treatment gap, trauma-informed therapies—known collectively as trauma-informed care (TIC)—have been created. Implementing trauma-informed services can improve screening and assessment, treatment planning, and placement while also decreasing the risk for retraumatization (SAMHSA, 2014a). TIC implementation may enhance patient–provider communication, thus decreasing risks associated with misunderstanding the patient's reactions and presenting problems or underestimating the need for appropriate referrals for evaluation or trauma-specific treatment (SAMHSA, 2014a).

The introduction of TIC has required re-education of mental health clinicians and increased sensitivity to patients' trauma histories. Personnel at public institutions and service systems such as schools and the court system are also being introduced to the concept of TIC and are being trained to identify patients with trauma histories and make appropriate referrals for mental health services.

Critical Thinking Application

1. Why were traditional therapies for substance use disorder unsuccessful with patients who abused alcohol and/or drugs and had trauma histories?

2. How does trauma relate to alcohol and substance use? Would it be better for patients with SUD to focus on trauma therapy or SUD therapy? Or should therapies be combined?

3. Which symptoms of trauma should school and court personnel be trained to recognize in children, adolescents, and adults?

4. Could mental health practices such as restraints and seclusion contribute to retraumatization? If yes, how?

---

with thoughts and self-statements that promote adaptive behavior. Variants of CBT include **rational–emotive behavior therapy (REBT)**, an active, solution-oriented therapy that focuses on resolving emotional, cognitive, and behavioral problems resulting from faulty evaluation of negative life events (Ellis, 2015), and **dialectical behavior therapy (DBT),** during which patients are taught how to regulate destructive emotions, practice mindfulness, and better tolerate distress (Linehan, 2015).

Behavior-oriented therapies are well suited to treating individuals with addictions because patients must alter familiar maladaptive coping mechanisms and find more successful methods of reducing anxiety. Because they spend a great deal of time with patients, nurses are in an ideal position to evaluate patient response to treatment and encourage developing patterns of positive behavioral change.

Milieu Therapy

A successful recovery environment supports behavior changes, teaches new coping measures, and helps the patient move from addiction to a sober life. This supportive environment is often referred to as **milieu therapy**. The milieu is a supportive environment in which clinicians and staff work with patients to provide safety and structure while assessing the patient's relationships and behavior (Menninger Clinic,

2015). Patients benefit because a consistent routine is maintained, which fosters predictability and trust. A milieu is considered therapeutic when the program's community provides a sense of civility, membership, belonging, care, and accountability (Menninger Clinic, 2015).

The structure of milieu therapy helps patients contain negative behavior and provides an opportunity to learn how to respond to challenging situations through staff and peer feedback and modeling constructive behavior. Other goals of milieu therapy include treating patients as responsible people, encouraging group and social interaction, emphasizing patients' rights to choose and participate in a variety of treatments, and accentuating informal relationships with healthcare professionals. Milieu therapy also supports clear communication and often features a tightly structured activity schedule with clear therapeutic goals. Patients are also taught how to use and access a support network. The overall goal behind all of these components is to support constructive, permanent behavioral change in the patient with SUD. The therapeutic milieu can be created in residential and inpatient programs as well as outpatient programs, such as group homes, community centers, or day programs.

Within the therapeutic milieu, the nurse plays a pivotal role by modeling and teaching desirable behaviors. Often, the nurse is the member of the patient's psychiatric team who spends the most time with, and around, the patient. The nurse's observations of, and interactions with, the patient provide information and opportunities critical to understanding the patient's addiction behavior and to helping the patient determine a successful path to recovery.

Group Therapy

Therapeutic groups provide support to individual members as they work through problems. During **group therapy**, which is facilitated by a professional group therapist, the group navigates psychologic, cognitive, behavioral, and spiritual dysfunctions. Irving Yalom is widely considered to be the father of modern group therapy. Through his work as a psychiatrist, Yalom defined many of the characteristics of successful groups, such as goal setting, group size, duration of therapy, and leader and member characteristics. Yalom recognized that the intensive group experience is a "powerful agent of change" (1974, p. 85), where members feel stimulated by the group, develop close bonds, and experience affective adjustments. Functional groups generate heightened emotional reflection, creating an atmosphere of group trust and support. Through interactions with others in the group, members practice valuable self-reflection (Yalom, 1974). Today, interactive group therapy is a mainstay in addiction recovery.

Groups can be held in the inpatient-unit or outpatient setting, community mental health centers, or other locations. Ballinger and Yalom (1995) identified mechanisms of change within a group and called them *curative factors* of group therapy. These factors provide a rationale for a variety of group interventions. **Table 22–2 》** describes the curative factors.

Nurses can function as group therapists in many different settings, leading groups to achieve desired outcomes. Certified advanced practice nurses can run interactive therapy groups and conduct psychotherapy with individuals, families, and groups. A single nurse may lead groups or share leadership responsibilities with a cotherapist. As the group leader, the nurse can unify the group members and help them relate to each other. Some important duties of the group leader include encouraging members to remain in the group, helping the group develop a sense of cohesiveness, and establishing a code of behavior and norms within the group (Ballinger & Yalom, 1995).

Adolescents can participate in group therapy and other peer support programs during and following treatment to help them achieve abstinence from substances (NIDA, 2014e). When led by trained clinicians following well-validated cognitive–behavioral therapy protocols, groups can provide positive social reinforcement through peer discussion. They can also help enforce incentives to avoid substance use and live a substance-free lifestyle. However, group treatment for adolescents carries a risk of unintended adverse effects: Group members may steer conversation toward talk that glorifies or extols substance use, thereby undermining recovery goals. Trained counselors need to be aware of that possibility and direct group activities and discussions in a more positive direction (NIDA, 2014e).

Support Groups

Because individuals with addictions typically have inadequate social networks, often restricted to fellow substance users, it is important for them to develop more functional support networks that can contribute to increased self-esteem and dignity, a sense of identity, and improved self-responsibility. Nurses frequently refer patients and their families to support groups that allow peers to share their thoughts and feelings and help one another examine issues and concerns. In support groups, members define their own needs, have equal power, and usually participate voluntarily. They may or may not be assisted by a mental health professional. For individuals with substance use issues, group recovery support generally consists of peer-based mentoring, education, and support services provided by individuals in recovery to individuals with substance use disorders or co-occurring substance use and mental disorders (Reif et al., 2014).

The support group SMART Recovery (Self-Management and Recovery Training) is based on the "scientifically

TABLE 22–2 Curative Factors of Group Therapy

Factor	Description
Instillation of hope	As patients observe other members further along in the therapeutic process, they begin to feel a sense of hope for themselves.
Universality	Through interaction with other group members, patients realize they are not alone in their problems or pain.
Imparting of information	Teaching and suggestions usually come from the group leader but may also be generated by the group members.
Altruism	Through the group process, patients recognize that they have something to give to the other group members.
Corrective recapitulation of the primary family group	Many patients have a history of dysfunctional family relationships. The therapy group is often like a family, and patients can learn more functional patterns of communication, interaction, and behavior.
Development of socializing techniques	Development of social skills takes place in groups. Group members give feedback about maladaptive social behavior. Patients learn more appropriate ways of socializing with others.
Imitative behavior	Patients often model their behavior after the leader or other group members. This trial process enables them to discover what behaviors work well for them as individuals.
Interpersonal learning	Through the group process, patients learn the positive benefits of good interpersonal relationships. Emotional healing takes place through this process.
Existential factors	The group provides opportunities for patients to explore the meaning of their life and their place in the world.
Catharsis	Patients learn how to express their own feelings in a goal-directed way, speak openly about what is bothering them, and express strong feelings about other members in a responsible way.
Group cohesiveness	Cohesiveness occurs when members feel a sense of belonging.

Source: Based on Yalom, I. D., & Leszcz, M. (2005). *The theory and practice of group psychotherapy* (5th ed.). New York, NY: Basic Books.

informed" use of psychologic treatments and legally prescribed psychiatric and addiction medication. The SMART program considers substance abuse and addiction to be complex maladaptive behaviors with possible physiologic factors and emphasizes teaching increasing self-reliance, rather than powerlessness (SMART Recovery, 2015). SMART features both face-to-face and online support. SMART's recovery program focuses on the following points: building and maintaining motivation; coping with urges; managing thoughts, feelings and behaviors; and living a balanced life (SMART Recovery, 2015).

Twelve-Step Programs

Twelve-step programs are support groups that offer a spiritual plan for recovery. These include Al-Anon, Narcotics Anonymous, Cocaine Anonymous, Adult Children of Alcoholics, Emotions Anonymous, Gamblers Anonymous, Overeaters Anonymous, and Sex Addicts Anonymous. Clinicians often employ 12-step facilitation therapy, an active engagement strategy designed to increase the likelihood that a substance user will join and participate in a 12-step group (NIDA, 2012b).

The 12-step program consists of prescribed beliefs, values, and behaviors. The sequential plan for recovery is stated in 12 steps. It begins with the individual admitting powerlessness over the substance and continues through steps that help individuals take responsibility for addictive behaviors and seek spiritual awakening in community with others. Step work is considered to be a lifelong process, usually facilitated by a peer sponsor. Twelve-step fellowship includes activities such as helping others, building relationships among members, and sharing joys and hardships. The only requirement for membership in 12-step programs is the sincere desire to change the target behavior.

>> **Stay Current:** The 12 Steps of Alcoholics Anonymous can be found at http://www.aa.org/assets/en_US/smf-121_en.pdf.

While many clinicians consider 12-step programs to be effective in treating individuals with substance use disorders (NIDA, 2012b), some researchers have found that 12-step groups may yield more modest outcomes (Reif et al., 2014). Studies do support findings that individuals who participate in 12-step programs have reduced relapse rates, increased treatment retention, improved relationships with treatment providers and social supports, and increased participant satisfaction with the overall treatment experience. However, research has uncovered concerns as to whether the benefits of 12-step peer recovery support can be distinguished from those of other concurrent recovery support activities (Reif et al., 2014).

Family Therapy

Family behavior therapy (FBT), which has demonstrated positive results in both adults and adolescents, addresses not only substance use problems but other co-occurring problems as well, including conduct disorders, mistreatment of children, depression, family conflict, and unemployment (NIDA, 2012b). In FBT, the patient and at least one significant other, such as a cohabiting partner or a parent (in the case of adolescents), try to apply the behavioral strategies taught in sessions and acquire new skills to improve the home environment.

In the treatment of adolescents, family involvement can be particularly important, since the adolescent will often be living with at least one parent and be subject to the parent's controls, rules, and/or supports (NIDA, 2012b, 2014e). Family-based approaches generally address a wide array of problems in addition to the substance problems, including family communication and conflict; co-occurring behavioral, mental health, and learning disorders; problems with school or work attendance; and peer networks. Research shows that family-based treatments are highly efficacious; some studies even suggest they are superior to other individual and group treatment approaches (NIDA, 2014e).

Family-based treatments can be adapted to various settings (e.g., mental health clinics, drug abuse treatment programs, social service settings, families' homes) and treatment modalities. **Brief strategic family therapy (BSFT)** is based on a family systems approach to treatment, in which one member's problem behaviors appear to stem from unhealthy family interactions. Over the course of 12 to 16 sessions, the BSFT counselor establishes a relationship with each family member, observes how the members behave with one another, and assists the family in changing negative interaction patterns (NIDA, 2014e). **Functional family therapy (FFT)** combines a family systems view of family functioning (e.g., unhealthy family interactions underlie an individual's problem behaviors) with behavioral techniques to improve communication, problem-solving, conflict resolution, and parenting skills. Principal treatment strategies include engaging families in the treatment process and enhancing their motivation for change, as well as modifying family members' behavior using CM techniques, communication and problem solving, behavioral contracts, and other methods (NIDA, 2014e).

Two other types of family therapy have been shown to be effective with adolescents and their families. Both are comprehensive, family-oriented, community-based therapies. **Multidimensional family therapy (MDFT)** has been shown to be effective even with more severe substance use disorders and can facilitate the reintegration of substance abusing juvenile detainees into the community (NIDA, 2014e). **Multisystemic therapy (MST)** has been shown to be effective even with adolescents whose substance abuse problems are severe and with those who engage in delinquent and/or violent behavior. The therapist may work with the family as a whole but will also conduct sessions with just the caregivers or the adolescent alone (NIDA, 2014e).

Pharmacologic Therapy

Pharmacologic therapies are available to treat and prevent symptoms of withdrawal and to treat overdose. Treating symptoms of withdrawal may involve reducing physiologic cravings for the drug of choice, but it may also involve reducing anxiety that serves as a stimulus for using a substance or to prevent dangerous symptoms associated with sudden withdrawal from powerful substances such as sedatives and hypnotics. A number of pharmacologic therapies are available. Many of these, however, have multiple drug interactions and should be used with caution. For example, disulfiram (Antabuse) should never be used during pregnancy and should be used with caution in patients taking phenytoin. See the Medications feature.

Medications

Used to Treat Addiction and Withdrawal Manifestations

CLASSIFICATION AND DRUG EXAMPLES	MECHANISMS OF ACTION	NURSING CONSIDERATIONS
Opioid Antagonists *Drug example:* Naloxone	Used to treat a narcotic overdose, these drugs block narcotic receptor sites and quickly reverse the effect of the narcotic if administered via IV therapy.	▪ Monitor patient condition, including respiratory rate, and anticipate the need for pain management as narcotic effects are reversed.
Benzodiazepines *Drug examples:* Chlordiazepoxide Diazepam Oxazepam Lorazepam	Diminishes anxiety; anticonvulsant qualities help provide safe withdrawal. May be ordered q4h or prn to manage effects from withdrawal; then dose is tapered to zero.	▪ Monitor for oversedation ▪ Caution patients not to mix with alcohol; can cause respiratory depression ▪ High potential for addiction; should be used for short term only ▪ Taper dosage; stopping abruptly may trigger seizures
Abstinence Medications *Drug examples:* Disulfiram Naltrexone Acamprosate Methadone	Diminishes cravings for alcohol and opioids; blocks cravings for heroin.	▪ Disulfiram can cause flushing of the face, headache, vomiting, and other unpleasant sensations if alcohol is consumed. ▪ Naltrexone will cause opioid withdrawal if given to an individual who has not detoxed. ▪ Methadone is addictive and can be abused. Monitor for cardiac arrhythmias. Overdose can cause respiratory depression, especially if mixed with alcohol.
Antiseizure Drugs *Drug examples:* Phenytoin Carbamazepine Valproic acid Phenobarbital Magnesium sulfate	Reduces and controls seizure activity resulting from withdrawal syndrome.	▪ Implement seizure precautions to maintain patient safety. If a seizure occurs, place a pillow under the patient's head and time the seizure, noting patient behavior during and after the event. ▪ Phenobarbital can cause a serious allergic reaction; monitor for hypersensitivity response. Phenobarbital is a teratogen and should not be taken by pregnant women. ▪ Magnesium sulfate can cause dizziness; flushing; irregular heartbeat; muscle paralysis or weakness. Patients should be assisted when standing or transferring.
Nicotine Replacement Therapy *Drug examples:* Nicotine patch Nicotine gum Nicotine lozenge Nicotine nasal spray Nicotine inhaler	Supplies the body with nicotine to support smoking cessation therapy.	▪ Patient support is an important element of smoking cessation, and patients benefit from behavior modification teaching in addition to pharmacotherapy.
Antidepressants *Drug examples:* Bupropion hydrochloride Fluoxetine Sertraline	Some antidepressants have been shown to reduce the craving for nicotine and support smoking cessation programs. Can also be administered to reduce depression occurring as the result of substance withdrawal.	▪ Monitor and assess for suicidal ideation. ▪ Assess for drug side effects, including drowsiness, insomnia, and blurred vision. ▪ Teach patient about self-administration of medications and symptoms to report. ▪ Teach patient not to mix drug with alcohol because of increased risk of seizures. ▪ Teach patient that antidepressants can take 3–4 weeks to become effective and not to discontinue abruptly; medication should be tapered off.

Medications *(continued)*

CLASSIFICATION AND DRUG EXAMPLES	MECHANISMS OF ACTION	NURSING CONSIDERATIONS
Nicotine Acetylcholine Receptor Agonists *Drug example:* Varenicline	Stimulates nicotine receptors more weakly than nicotine itself does, reducing cravings for and decreasing the pleasurable effects of tobacco.	▪ Assess for nicotine withdrawal symptoms such as depression, agitation, and exacerbation of preexisting mental health disorders. ▪ Suicide and suicidal ideation have been associated with use of varenicline. Assess patients for thoughts of suicide or changes in mood and affect.
Vitamins *Drug examples:* Thiamine (vitamin B$_1$) Folic acid Multivitamins	Prevents alcohol-related Wernicke encephalopathy. Corrects vitamin deficiency caused by heavy, long-term alcohol abuse.	▪ May not be absorbed properly in patients with impaired liver function. ▪ High-dose folic acid may increase risk of heart attack in some patients. ▪ Water-soluble vitamin overdoses can cause nausea and diarrhea.

SAFETY ALERT Drugs of abuse alter the brain's structure and function, resulting in changes that persist long after drug use has ceased. This may explain why individuals with substance use disorders are at risk for relapse even after long periods of abstinence and despite the potentially devastating consequences (NIDA, 2014a).

Lifespan Considerations

Addiction in Children and Adolescents

Research shows that many adolescents start to drink at very young ages. According to data from the 2012 *Monitoring the Future* study (Johnston et al., 2013), over half (54%) of 12th graders and more than one seventh (13%) of 8th graders report having been drunk at least once in their life. In 2012, 24% of 12th graders reported **binge drinking** (having five or more drinks in a row at least once in the prior 2 weeks). The survey also discovered that 1 in 15 (6.5%) high school seniors is a daily, or near-daily, marijuana user. As far as legal cigarettes, 1 in 6 (16%) 8th graders has tried smoking, and nearly 1 in 20 (5%) currently smoke. By 12th grade, more than a third (40%) have tried smoking, and nearly 1 in 6 (17%) is currently smoking.

The brain continues to develop well into the 20s, during which time it continues to establish important communication connections and further refines its function. Brain circuitry involving reward and memory and the prefrontal cortex, which governs emotional regulation and decision making, are still developing. This lengthy developmental period may help explain some of the risk-taking behavior that is characteristic of adolescence. Teenagers are highly motivated to pursue pleasure, but their judgment may be impaired, increasing the adolescent's risk for developing substance abuse. For some adolescents, thrill-seeking may include experimenting with alcohol and drugs. Developmental changes also offer a possible physiologic explanation for why teens act impulsively, often not recognizing that their risky behaviors have consequences.

Addiction in Pregnant Women

Among pregnant women age 15 to 44, 5.4% were current illicit drug users based on data averaged across 2012 and 2013, compared with 11.4% of women in this age group who were not pregnant (CBHSQ, 2015). Current illicit drug use was lower among pregnant women during the third trimester than during the first and second trimesters, with younger pregnant women age 15 to 17 reporting the highest use (CBHSQ, 2015). During 2011–2013, 10.2% of pregnant women reported using alcohol, and 3.2% had engaged in binge drinking in the past 30 days (Tan et al., 2015). By contrast, the prevalences of alcohol use and binge drinking among women who were not pregnant were 53.6% and 18.2%, respectively. Of significance, pregnant women who engaged in binge drinking reported a significantly higher frequency of binge drinking with a larger amount of alcohol consumed than women who were not pregnant (Tan et al., 2015).

Alcohol, nicotine, illicit drugs, and some prescription drugs are considered **teratogens**—agents that interrupt development or cause malformation in an embryo or fetus. Alcohol use during pregnancy can lead to fetal alcohol spectrum disorders (FASDs) and other adverse birth outcomes, while SUD can cause neonates to experience substance dependence and withdrawal symptoms, low birth weight, neurologic issues, developmental delays, and other issues (NIDA, 2015a; Tan et al., 2015). It is generally assumed that pregnant women who use alcohol or illicit drugs during pregnancy are continuing habits formed prior to their pregnancies. For this reason, health promotion related to substance use and abuse is important for all women seeking to become pregnant and at each healthcare interaction with the pregnant woman.

Addiction in Older Adults

Substance abuse in older adults is believed to be underestimated, underidentified, underdiagnosed, and undertreated. Until relatively recently, alcohol and prescription drug misuse, which affects a growing number of older adults, was not discussed in either the substance abuse or the geronto-logic literature. For example, alcohol use disorders affect 1 to 3% of older adults. But researchers believe that might still be an underestimate (Caputo et al., 2012).

Insufficient knowledge, limited research data, and hurried office visits are cited as causes for why healthcare providers often overlook substance abuse and misuse in this popula-tion. Diagnosis is often difficult because symptoms of sub-stance abuse in older individuals sometimes mimic symptoms of other medical and behavioral disorders com-mon among older adults, such as diabetes, dementia, and depression. In addition, many older adults do not seek treat-ment for substance abuse because they do not feel they need it (Hazelden Betty Ford Foundation, 2015).

Impaired Nurses

In 1982, the American Nurses Association (ANA) passed a resolution addressing alcohol and drug misuse and psycho-logic problems among nurses, with the intention of shifting the focus from punishment to rehabilitation. In 2002, the ANA adopted an updated resolution that called attention again to impaired nursing practice, stressing the need for peer assistance programs (Heise, 2003). The ANA currently joins with the International Nurses Society on Addictions to emphasize its commitment to the peer assistance programs offered by most—but not all—of the state boards of nursing. These programs offer comprehensive monitoring and sup-port services to reasonably ensure the safe rehabilitation and return of the nurse to her or his professional community (ANA, 2015).

Healthcare providers are as susceptible as anyone else to developing substance abuse. By the very nature of their roles, dentists, pharmacists, physicians, and nurses are in frequent contact with drugs and are at high risk for substance abuse

problems. As a rule, nurses experience many pressures in the workplace and have easy access to drugs. The American Nurses Association estimates that 10% of all nurses may be impaired or in recovery from alcohol or drug addiction; other researchers suggest that as many as 20% may have substance abuse issues (Starr, 2015). They also reported that the two best predictors of successful recovery from addiction are the length of treatment and the willingness of the nurse. Nurses who remained in treatment for at least a year are twice as likely to be drug free.

Substance abuse and dependence can lead to impaired professional practice; therefore, nurses must act responsibly when coworkers display signs of substance abuse. The American Nurses Association Code of Ethics for Nurses pro-vides a framework for patient safety. Four suggestions for implementing its philosophy are:

1. Do not ignore poor performance.
2. Do not lighten or change the nurse's patient assign-ment.
3. Do not accept excuses.
4. Do not allow yourself to be manipulated or fear con-fronting a nurse if patient safety is in jeopardy (Thomas & Siela, 2011).

If nurses are showing signs of a substance abuse problem, their colleagues can find information about impaired nurse programs through state boards of nursing. Warning signs of impaired nurses in the workplace are listed in **Table 22–3 》**.

The ANA (2015) has stated that nurses with substance abuse problems not only pose a potential threat to those for whom they care, but they also tend to neglect their own health and well-being. Nurses with addiction issues may be reluctant to report themselves because of shame, guilt, or fear of job loss. The ANA encourages nurses to self-report

TABLE 22–3 Warning Signs of Impaired Nurses in the Workplace

At-Risk Situations	Observable Warning Signs
Easy access to prescription drugs	Inaccurate narcotic counts or drugs frequently missing
	Patient complaints of ineffective pain control, denial of having received pain meds
	Excessive "wasting" of drugs
	Likelihood of volunteering to give medications to patients
	Frequent trips to the bathroom
Role strain	Frequent tardiness or absenteeism, especially before and after scheduled days off
	Haphazard, shoddy charting
	Judgment errors in patient care
	Unorganized, erratic behavior; unkempt appearance
Depression	Irritability, unable to focus or concentrate
	Abrupt mood swings
	Isolating self, taking long breaks
	Apathetic, depressed, lethargic
	Unexplained absences from assigned unit
Signs of alcohol or drug use	Smell of alcohol on breath
	Excessive use of perfumes, mouthwash, or mints
	Slurred speech, flushed face, reddened eyes, unsteady gait
	Long sleeves worn in hot weather to cover up arms
Signs of withdrawal	Tremors, restlessness, sweating
	Watery eyes, runny nose, stomachaches

and contact peer assistance programs offered by their state nursing organization or state board of nursing. Most state nurses' associations have peer assistance programs. Resources vary by state, but generally are accessible through each state association's website. Many state boards of nursing offer programs designed to guide nurses to sobriety, rather than instituting immediate disciplinary consequences. In addition, larger agencies may offer programs for employees, including employee assistance programs and support groups. Regardless, nurses who feel they are developing a substance abuse problem are ethically required to seek help in order to prevent mistakes in the workplace.

Case Study » Part 3

It is 36 hours post-ED admission, and Paul is being transferred from the trauma unit to a semiprivate room on a general medical-surgical unit. The scalp laceration is healing; there is no evidence of head injury. Paul's right humerus was fractured in the crash and a cast applied following a closed reduction. Laboratory studies revealed a blood alcohol level of 0.28 on admission. Paul now appears mildly anxious and has a mild visible tremor of his hands. He is being prepared for discharge tomorrow. Admission to a substance abuse treatment program is being considered.

Clinical Reasoning Questions Level I

1. List at least three nursing diagnoses that would apply to Paul.
2. What members of the interprofessional (IP) healthcare team should be involved in Paul's care and discharge planning? Delineate the role of each team member.
3. Consider the impact of Paul's addiction on him and on his entire family.
4. Can Paul be treated independently of his family?
5. Give some specific examples of how family involvement could be planned by members of the IP team.

Clinical Reasoning Questions Level II

6. Identify comprehensive, measurable long-term treatment goals for Paul and his family.
7. Discuss inpatient, outpatient, and community treatment options for Paul and his family. Consider the advantages and disadvantages of each.
8. Consider the impact of cognition (both Paul's and his family's) in Paul's long-term treatment plan.
9. What lifestyle changes may be necessary for Paul and his family?

REVIEW The Concept of Addiction

RELATE Link the Concepts

Linking the concept of addiction with the concept of family:

1. In a family with rigid boundaries—those in which rules and roles remain fixed under all circumstances—what approach(s) might be optimal for gaining trust in and building a therapeutic relationship?

2. Considering the many treatment options for those with addictions, design a comprehensive treatment plan to meet the needs of a family such as the one that we have been exploring through our case study, the John family.

Linking the concept of addiction with the concept of immunity:

3. Dietary support is an essential component of recovery. Describe the diagnostic assessment for deficiencies in the B-complex vitamins, particularly thiamin, folate, and B$_{12}$, and the fat-soluble vitamins, A, D, and E.

4. Why are individuals with addictions prone to opportunistic infection?

READY Go to Volume 3: Clinical Nursing Skills

- SKILL 1.1   Appearance and Mental Status: Assessing
- SKILLS 1.5–1.9 Vital Signs
- SKILL 1.22   Neurologic Status: Assessing
- SKILL 2.11   Medications: Preparing and Administering
- SKILL 2.28   Transdermal Patch Medication: Applying
- SKILL 4.5   Urine Specimen, Routine, 24-Hour: Obtaining
- SKILL 8.4   Capillary Blood Specimen for Glucose: Measuring
- SKILL 10.5   Nutrition: Assessing
- SKILL 15.3   Seizure Precautions: Implementing

REFER Go to Pearson MyLab Nursing and eText

- Additional review materials

REFLECT Apply Your Knowledge

George Brown is a 68-year-old man, in apparent good health with unremarkable lab work, who came to the ambulatory surgery center for elective gallbladder surgery. During the laparoscopic surgery, which started at 1 p.m., the surgeon noted some inflammation that made visualization of the gallbladder difficult. There was also more bleeding than expected. The surgeon converted the surgery into an open cholecystectomy, and the procedure was finished without any further issues.

After recovery in the perianesthesia unit, Mr. Brown is sent to the medical-surgical floor and arrives on the floor at 7:30 p.m. His wife joins him and remains at the bedside until 11 p.m. Aside from some occasional pain at the incision site, which is treated successfully with oral oxycodone/acetaminophen, Mr. Brown spends most of the night resting. On postoperative day 1, he is to ambulate. He receives two remaining doses of intravenous antibiotics because of the open surgery. If Mr. Brown progresses as anticipated, the surgeon expects to discharge him in the early evening.

When the day-shift nurse makes her initial morning assessment, Mr. Brown is restless but alert and oriented × 4. At 12 p.m., he is extremely restless, but knows he is in the hospital and reports some pain at the incision site. At 4 p.m., Mr. Brown is trying to get out of bed and leave the hospital; he knows who he is but thinks he is in the men's room at a local sports arena. By the time Ms. Brown arrives at 6:30 p.m., Mr. Brown is agitated and aggressive, trying to hit anyone approaching his bed. The attending physician is notified, and her adult nurse practitioner (ANP), who is rounding in the hospital, comes to Mr. Brown's room. After looking at recent vital signs of T 99.9°F, HR 110, and BP 165/98, the ANP orders a dose of intramuscular ziprasidone for agitation. After vigorously objecting to the shot, Mr. Brown eventually calms somewhat, but his eyes dart around the room and he hisses and startles occasionally, throwing his hands over his head. When asked, he reports seeing buzzards in the room. The ANP asks the night-shift nurse (who requests the CNA to stay with Mr. Brown while she left the room) and Ms. Brown to join her in a small family meeting room.

During the conference, the ANP states that she suspects Mr. Brown was going into alcohol withdrawal delirium. She asks

Ms. Brown about his social history. Ms. Brown reports that she and her husband moved to a nearby upscale retirement community 6 or 7 years ago. Mr. Brown had been suddenly retired from the investment firm he worked at in Chicago, when the company collapsed during the recession and was acquired by a competitor. Ms. Brown shares that they lost about a third of their retirement savings, but the move to a southern state stabilized their living expenses and they are now "comfortable." Mr. Brown had worked at his job for 35 years, was devoted to the company, and enjoyed his job. He was "devastated" when his job ended and was "anguished" when executives of his former company were vilified in the financial press for bad business decisions. Since his move, Mr. Brown has been a "little down," but he has thrown himself into charitable endeavors, serving on a number of boards and committees. Ms. Brown says that her husband is a "moderate" social drinker, who drinks four large vodka tonics every night and never appears to be drunk. She seems surprised that the ANP thinks her husband is withdrawing from alcohol.

1. Why do you think the ANP immediately suspected alcohol withdrawal? What were the clues that led her in that direction?

2. Do you think Mr. Brown has some unresolved psychosocial issues from his forced retirement? Are there any underlying mental health issues that may need treatment?

3. What will likely happen to Mr. Brown now? How will his hospital plan of care change? What orders are commonly on a detox protocol?

4. What will be Mr. Brown's discharge plan after he has been stabilized in the hospital? What will be Ms. Brown's role?

» Exemplar 22.A
Alcohol Abuse

Exemplar Learning Outcomes

22.A Analyze the manifestations and treatment considerations for patients who abuse alcohol.

- Describe the pathophysiology of alcohol abuse.
- Describe the etiology of alcohol abuse.
- Compare the risk factors and prevention of alcohol abuse.
- Identify the clinical manifestations of alcohol abuse.
- Identify the clinical manifestations of alcohol withdrawal.
- Summarize diagnostic tests and therapies used by interprofessional teams in the collaborative care of an individual with an alcohol use disorder.
- Differentiate the care of patients across the lifespan who abuse alcohol.
- Apply the nursing process to promote patient safety during withdrawal and detoxification.
- Apply the nursing process in providing culturally competent care to an individual with alcohol use disorder.

Exemplar Key Terms

Alcohol dependence, *1668*
Alcohol intoxication, *1671*
Alcohol poisoning, *1671*
Alcohol use disorder, *1668*
Alcohol withdrawal delirium, *1673*
Alcohol withdrawal syndrome, *1673*
Alcoholism, *1668*
Binge drinking, *1669*
Blackouts, *1673*
Confabulation, *1671*
Craving, *1670*

Overview

Alcohol includes liquor, beer, and wine. While much of society sees the use of nicotine and drugs as inappropriate, use of alcohol is still socially acceptable and often encouraged. Alcohol is frequently offered at weddings and other family events, beer is the favorite drink at sports venues across the country, and many grocery stores and restaurants now offer weekly or monthly wine tastings. Alcohol's availability may be the primary reason it is the most commonly used and abused substance in the United States. The most recent estimate of the economic costs of alcohol abuse in the United States is $235 billion (CDC, 2015c). These costs result from losses in workplace productivity, healthcare expenses for problems caused by excessive drinking, law enforcement and other criminal justice expenses related to excessive alcohol consumption, and motor vehicle crash costs from impaired driving (CDC, 2015c).

In 1992, the Joint Committee of the National Council on Alcoholism and Drug Dependence and the American Society of Addiction Medicine defined **alcoholism** as a "primary, chronic disease with genetic, psychosocial, and environmental factors influencing its development and manifestations" (Morse & Flavin, 1992). It is characterized by the behaviors discussed in the Concepts section of this module: inability to control the primary addictive behavior (drinking), fixation with the drug and continued use of it regardless of consequences, and impaired thought processes. The terms *alcoholism*, *alcohol abuse*, and *alcohol use* disorder are often used interchangeably. However, it should be noted that an individual can abuse alcohol to the extent that it impairs function and results in life-threatening symptoms without developing addiction behaviors or dependency. Alcoholism and **alcohol use disorder** more specifically refer to a chronic disease process with specific, identifiable manifestations and patterns. Clinicians following the guidelines of the American Society of Addiction Medicine may be more likely to use the term *alcoholism*, whereas those adhering to the DSM-5 may be more likely to use the term *alcohol use disorder*. Nurses working in all settings should be able to identify acute manifestations of both abuse and withdrawal, as well as patterns of dependence.

The pattern of **alcohol dependence** varies from person to person. Seven in 10 adults in the United States always drink

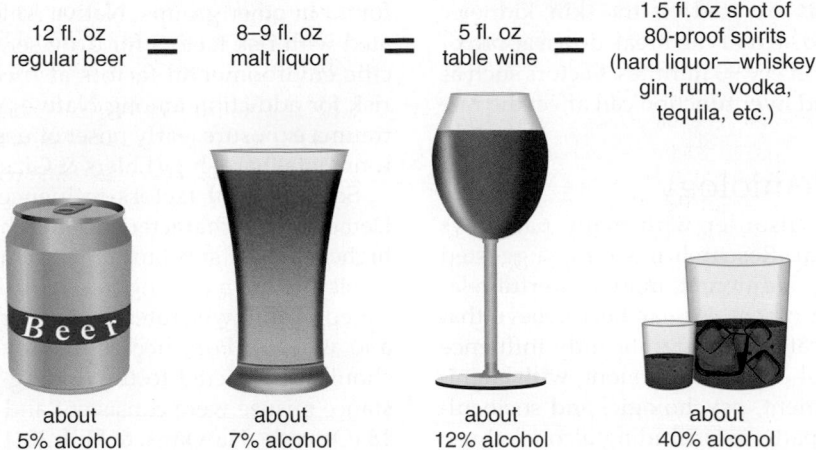

12 fl. oz
regular beer
=
8–9 fl. oz
malt liquor
=
5 fl. oz
table wine
=
1.5 fl. oz shot of
80-proof spirits
(hard liquor—whiskey,
gin, rum, vodka,
tequila, etc.)

about
5% alcohol

about
7% alcohol

about
12% alcohol

about
40% alcohol

Figure 22–3 》 One standard drink = ½ oz of ethyl alcohol.

at low-risk levels or do not drink at all (NIAAA, 2015a). Low-risk drinking is defined as no more than 4 drinks on any one day/no more than 14 drinks per week for men, and no more than 3 drinks on any one day/no more than 7 drinks per week for women (NIAAA, 2015a). The measurement of a standard drink is shown in **Figure 22–3 》**. Some people regularly drink large amounts of alcohol daily. Others restrict their use to heavy drinking on weekends or days off from work, often drinking copious amounts in a single session, a pattern of consumption known as **binge drinking**. Binge alcohol use is defined as drinking five or more drinks on the same occasion on at least 1 day in the past 30 days. Heavy alcohol use is defined as drinking five or more drinks on the same occasion on 5 or more days in the past 30 days (CBHSQ, 2014). Many individuals who engage in binge drinking begin doing so in college: College alcohol consumption has been linked with harmful consequences such as alcohol poisoning, drug overdoses, sexual assaults, and alcohol-impaired driving, which accounts for the majority of alcohol-related deaths among college students nationwide (NIAAA, 2015b).

Some people are able to abstain for long periods of time and then begin dysfunctional drinking patterns again. At times, individuals with alcohol dependence can drink with control; at other times, they cannot control their drinking behavior. As the course of alcoholism continues, addiction behaviors appear with increasing frequency. These may include starting the day off with a drink, sneaking drinks throughout the day, shifting from one alcoholic beverage to another, and hiding bottles at work and at home. An individual with alcoholism may find that drinking—or being sick from drinking—has often interfered with home or family duties, caused trouble at school or work, and created legal difficulties resulting from impaired driving (NIAAA, 2015a).

》 Stay Current: Visit the website of the National Institute on Alcohol Abuse and Alcoholism to see current research on alcohol dependence: http://www.niaaa.nih.gov/research.

Pathophysiology and Etiology

In 2014, a total of 139.7 million Americans age 12 or older reported current use of alcohol, 60.9 million reported binge alcohol use in the past month, and 16.3 million reported heavy alcohol use in the past month (CBHSQ, 2015). Long-term alcohol use contributes to more than 200 diseases and injury-related health conditions, including alcohol dependence, liver cirrhosis, cancers, and injuries. In 2012, 5.1% of the burden of disease and injury worldwide (139 million disability-adjusted life years) was attributable to alcohol consumption (NIAAA, 2015a).

Approximately 8.7 million people age 12 to 20 reported drinking alcohol, with some 5.3 million reporting binge drinking and 1.3 million reporting heavy alcohol use (CBHSQ, 2015). It is critical to understand the extent of alcohol use among those who are not of drinking age, because the negative consequences can be serious. In younger users, negative outcomes from alcohol use include interference with normal adolescent brain development, increased risk of developing an alcohol use disorder (AUD), sexual assaults, and injuries (NIAAA, 2015c). Among college-age alcohol users, negative consequences related to alcohol use include motor-vehicle crashes, assault by another student who has been drinking, alcohol-related sexual assault or date rape, and potential for developing an AUD (roughly 20% of college students do meet the criteria for an AUD). About 1 in 4 college students report academic consequences from drinking (NIAAA, 2015c).

Pathophysiology

Alcohol is a CNS depressant; as such, it acts on neurotransmitters in the brain, such as gamma-aminobutyric acid (GABA). GABA, the most prevalent inhibitory neurotransmitter in the brain, has a major role in decreasing neuronal excitability. Alcohol creates an additive effect with GABA, further inhibiting arousal and depressing the autonomic nervous system. Alcohol decreases glutamate activity, a major excitatory neurotransmitter. This may explain why cross-tolerance effects occur when alcohol and other CNS depressants are used in combination. When taken together, alcohol and other CNS depressants (e.g., benzodiazepines and barbiturates) can lead to respiratory depression and death.

Alcohol is absorbed in the mouth, stomach, and digestive tract. The liver metabolizes approximately 95% of the ingested alcohol; the rest is excreted via the skin, kidneys, and lungs. Generally, an individual can break down approximately 1 ounce of whiskey every 90 minutes. Factors such as body mass, food intake, and liver function can affect the rate of alcohol absorption.

Etiology and Epidemiology

Alcoholism is a complex disorder with many pathways leading to its development. Research has long suggested that certain people develop a different, more powerful relationship with alcohol than others. Researchers believe that genetic and other biological factors significantly influence the development of alcohol dependence, along with cognitive, behavioral, temperament, psychologic, and sociocultural factors. Alcohol use patterns, including alcohol abuse and alcohol dependence, are familial in nature, with genetics making up 50% of the risk for alcohol and drug dependence (NIAAA, 2015b). Similar styles of alcohol use and the presence of alcoholism are often found within the same family, running from parent to child and across multiple generations of biologically related individuals (NIAAA, 2015b).

Culturally, there are ethnic differences in alcohol use. In 2013, Whites were more likely than other racial/ethnic groups to report current use of alcohol (57.7%). The rates were 47.4% for persons reporting two or more races, 43.6% for Blacks, 43.0% for Hispanics, 38.4% for Native Hawaiians or other Pacific Islanders, 37.3% for American Indians or Alaska Natives, and 34.5% for Asians (CBHSQ, 2015). Researchers have examined biological differences among ethnic groups, including the effect of alcohol-metabolizing genes on drinking behaviors and the health effects of alcohol consumption in populations with health disparities, with no findings that have translated into treatment interventions (NIAAA, 2015c). Cultural factors such as poverty, geographic isolation, unemployment, difficulty in acculturation, social disadvantage, and alcohol availability also are significant factors that account for ethnic variability in alcohol abuse.

Mood and substance use disorders commonly co-occur with alcoholism (Pettinati, O'Brien, & Dundon, 2013). *Dual diagnosis* and *dual disorder* are older terms used to describe an individual who has both a diagnosis of substance abuse and a mental illness. For example, an individual with a depressive disorder may self-medicate with alcohol to treat the depression, or someone with alcoholism may become depressed. Research has found that medications for managing mood symptoms can be effective in individuals with substance abuse; however, these medications have not been found to impact the substance use disorder. One clinical study did find that combining one medication for depression with another for alcohol dependence reduced both the depression and the drinking simultaneously (Pettinati et al., 2013).

Risk Factors and Prevention

Native Americans experience alcoholism at higher rates than other populations. Genetics is a major contributing factor to Native American risk for alcohol abuse. Researchers found an overlap in the gene location for addiction and for the body mass index (BMI). This suggests that the combination could produce a "disorder of consumption." Native Americans also do not have the genes that alter alcohol-metabolizing enzymes, and they lack protective variants found in other groups. Native Americans' genes are associated with risk factors for drug sensitivity or tolerance. Specific environmental factors also contribute to an elevated risk for addiction among Native Americans. These include trauma exposure, early onset of use of substances, and environmental hardship (Ehlers & Gizer, 2013).

Sociocultural factors influence risk for alcohol abuse. Demographic characteristics that have been associated with higher rates of substance misuse include lower educational levels and not marrying by age 30. Becoming parents is associated with lower rates of substance misuse for both men and women. For successful prevention efforts, attention should be directed to the finding that the patterns of substance misuse were consistent and already observed by age 18 (Oesterle, Hawkins, & Hill, 2011). There is some evidence that stigma or discrimination may contribute to increased risk for alcohol abuse. Research has indicated that, when compared with the general population, LGBT (lesbian, gay, bisexual, and transgender) individuals are more likely to use alcohol and drugs, have higher rates of substance abuse, are less likely to abstain from use, and are more likely to continue heavy drinking into later life (SAMHSA, 2012a). Despite the fact that homosexuality is now considered a normal variation of human sexual and emotional expression, LGBT individuals experience discrimination and trauma at higher rates than other populations. Nurses should be careful to take a nonpathologic and nonprejudicial view of the LGBT community and, during assessment, sensitively explore for histories of trauma and alcohol and other substance abuse.

Another area that has received much research attention is that of the children of alcoholics (COAs). A study that contrasted the lifestyles of COAs with those who did not have that history found that COAs' families had higher unemployment rates. Even after controlling for their lower socioeconomic status, the COAs had significantly more mental health difficulties and a higher rate of substance use compared to the controls. Unhealthy lifestyle habits (e.g., lack of exercise, eating fast food, other poor food choices) were significantly more prevalent for COAs than for the controls. Female COAs reported more emotional and somatic symptoms than male COAs (Serec et al., 2012).

Clinical Manifestations of Alcohol Abuse

When used in moderation, certain types of alcohol can have positive physiologic effects by decreasing coronary artery disease and protecting against stroke. However, when consumed in excess, alcohol can lead to **craving** (a strong desire or urge to use alcohol), can severely diminish one's ability to function, and can ultimately lead to life-threatening conditions (APA, 2013).

Behavioral signs of alcohol abuse include (Mayo Clinic, 2015a):

- Being unable to limit the amount of alcohol consumed
- Trying to decrease the amount consumed with variable success
- Spending a lot of time drinking, getting alcohol, or recovering from alcohol use

- Feeling a strong craving or urge to drink alcohol
- Failing to fulfill major obligations at work, school, or home due to repeated alcohol use
- Continuing to drink alcohol even when it causes physical, social, or interpersonal problems
- Giving up or reducing social and work activities and hobbies
- Using alcohol in situations in which it is not safe, such as when driving or swimming

Some physiologic symptoms are developing a tolerance to alcohol so that the individual needs more alcohol to feel its effect or having a reduced effect from the same amount and experiencing withdrawal symptoms—such as nausea, sweating and shaking—when not consuming alcohol or drinking to avoid these symptoms (Mayo Clinic, 2015a).

Alcohol Intoxication and Overdose

Alcohol intoxication is the presence of clinically significant behavioral or psychologic changes due to alcohol use. Changes may include any combination of inappropriate sexual or aggressive behavior, mood lability, impaired judgment, and impaired social or occupational functioning (APA, 2013). Signs of alcohol intoxication include nausea, vomiting, lack of coordination, slurred speech, staggering, disorientation, irritability, short attention span, loud and frequent talking, poor judgment, lack of inhibition, and (for some) violent behavior. Alcohol intoxication may result in accidents or falls that cause contusions, sprains, fractures, and facial or head trauma. Evidence of mild intoxication can be seen after two drinks, with signs and symptoms of intoxication becoming more intense as the blood alcohol level (BAL or EtOH) increases (APA, 2013). High BALs may result in unconsciousness, coma, respiratory depression, and death.

Alcohol poisoning is a toxic condition that results from excessive consumption of large amounts of alcohol in a very short period of time. At BALs greater than 300 mg/dL, the symptoms of intoxication become greatly intensified. Signs and symptoms of alcohol poisoning include excessive sleepiness; amnesia; difficulty waking the patient; coma; serious decreases in pulse, temperature, blood pressure, and rate of breathing; urinary and bowel incontinence; and, eventually, death (APA, 2013). Advanced states of intoxication and alcohol poisoning are critical situations in the ED and necessitate careful triage and monitoring to prevent death or permanent disability.

BALs are highly predictive of CNS effects. At 0.10%, ataxia and dysarthria occur. From 0.20 to 0.25%, the person is unable to sit or stand upright without support. Between 0.3 and 0.4%, slipping into a coma is possible. Toxic levels in excess of 0.5% can cause death. Note that individuals with chronic alcoholism might have BALs in these ranges, but not have the same consequences, because of their developed tolerance to the effect of drinking (McNeece & DiNitto, 2012). In the United States, the legal level of intoxication is 0.08%.

Consequences of Chronic Use

Chronic use of alcohol can cause severe neurologic and psychiatric disorders. Severe damage to the liver occurs with chronic alcohol abuse, and that damage can progress from fatty liver to other liver diseases such as hepatitis and cirrhosis. Chronic alcoholism is the major cause of fatal cirrhosis. Chronic abuse of alcohol also can cause damaging effects to many other systems. These effects include myocardial disease, erosive gastritis, acute and chronic pancreatitis, sexual dysfunction, and an increased risk of breast cancer.

Malnutrition is another serious complication of chronic alcoholism. Thiamine (B$_1$) deficiency in particular can result in neurologic impairments, such as Wernicke-Korsakoff syndrome (WKS). WKS typically consists of two components, a short-lived and severe condition called Wernicke encephalopathy (WE), and a long-lasting and debilitating condition known as Korsakoff psychosis (Martin, Singleton, & Hiller-Sturmhöfel, 2015). WE is an acute life-threatening neurocognitive disorder with symptoms that include mental confusion, paralysis of the nerves that move the eyes, and impaired coordination (e.g., ataxia). Approximately 80 to 90% of individuals with WE develop Korsakoff psychosis, a chronic neuropsychiatric syndrome characterized by behavioral abnormalities and memory impairments. Patients with Korsakoff psychosis have difficulties remembering old information; they are also unable to acquire new information (Martin et al., 2015). They also frequently use **confabulation**, making up information to fill in memory blanks.

Another common consequence of thiamine deficiency and long-term alcohol consumption is cerebellar degeneration, caused by atrophy of certain regions of the cerebellum, the brain area involved in muscle coordination. Cerebellar degeneration is associated with difficulties in movement coordination and involuntary eye movements, such as nystagmus. Cerebellar degeneration is found both in alcoholics with WKS and in those without it (Martin et al., 2015).

Chronic consumption of alcohol not only produces tolerance, but it creates cross-tolerance to general anesthetics, barbiturates, benzodiazepines, and other CNS depressants. If alcohol is withdrawn abruptly, the brain becomes overly excited because previously inhibited receptors are no longer inhibited. This hyperexcitability manifests clinically as anxiety, tachycardia, hypertension, diaphoresis, nausea, vomiting, tremors, sleeplessness, and irritability. Severe manifestations of alcohol withdrawal include seizures, convulsions, and DTs. Complications of DTs include respiratory failure, aspiration pneumonitis, and cardiac arrhythmias.

Multisystem Effects

Alcohol is a chemical irritant that has a direct toxic effect on many organ systems. For example, toxic effects of alcohol on the liver may include alcoholic hepatitis, cirrhosis, cancer, hepatomegaly, and fatty liver. Alcohol dependence increases the individual's risk for pneumonia, bronchitis, and tuberculosis. In addition to the CNS effects already described, alcohol abuse can result in seizures, neuropathies, sleep disturbances, and alcoholic dementia. Alcohol abuse can also cause erectile problems, decreased testosterone, decreased sex drive, and menstrual irregularities.

Alcohol Abuse and Memory

Alcohol primarily interferes with the ability to form new long-term memories. Large amounts of alcohol, particularly

Clinical Manifestations and Therapies
Alcohol Abuse

ETIOLOGY	CLINICAL MANIFESTATIONS	CLINICAL THERAPIES
DTs as a result of sudden withdrawal of alcohol	■ Confusion ■ Disorientation ■ Agitation ■ Severe autonomic instability ■ Perceptual disturbances ■ Hallucinations (primarily visual but may be tactile) ■ Tremors of extremities ■ Anxiety, panic, and paranoia	■ Prescribe benzodiazepines. ■ Reduce stimuli, but keep well lit to minimize visual misinterpretations. ■ If present, treat with antiseizure medications.
Cirrhosis of the liver resulting from damage done by chronic alcoholism	■ Spider angiomata ■ Palmar erythema ■ Muehrcke nails, Terry nails, or clubbing ■ Hypertrophic osteoarthropathy ■ Dupuytren contracture ■ Gynecomastia ■ Hypogonadism ■ Hepatomegaly ■ Ascites ■ Splenomegaly ■ Jaundice ■ Asterixis ■ Weakness, fatigue, anorexia, weight loss	■ Explain that cirrhosis cannot be reversed, but abstaining from alcohol can delay or prevent further damage. ■ Emphasize abstaining from alcohol. ■ Stop any medications that are potentially damaging to the liver, such as acetaminophen. ■ Consider abdominocentesis to reduce ascites. ■ Monitor ammonia levels. ■ Prevent complications such as esophageal varices, hepatic encephalopathy, and hepatorenal syndrome. ■ Monitor for delayed coagulation times and apply pressure to punctures for 10 minutes.
Assaultive behaviors	■ Sexual assault in adolescents and young adults is commonly related to alcohol use. ■ Because of the release of inhibitions, control of emotions such as anger is reduced. ■ Access to weapons increases the risk of assaultive behavior becoming homicide. ■ Spousal or child abuse has strong link to alcohol ingestion.	■ Promote sobriety. ■ Encourage management classes. ■ Provide crisis intervention for family members who have been assaulted. ■ Provide follow-up counseling to reduce posttraumatic stress response.
Esophageal varices, which may result from portal hypertension due to cirrhosis	■ Hematemesis ranging from mild to severe ■ Heartburn ■ Black or tarry stools ■ Decreased urination secondary to hypotension ■ Light-headedness ■ Shock ■ Weight loss ■ Weakness, fatigue, jaundice ■ Pruritus of hands and feet ■ Edema of lower extremities ■ Mental confusion	■ Encourage abstinence from alcohol. ■ Perform emergency surgery to stop bleeding, involving removal of part of the esophagus or cauterization of varicosities. ■ Perform therapeutic endoscopy. ■ Monitor intake and output. ■ Take vital signs frequently during bleeding episodes to monitor for shock. ■ Administer fluids via IV therapy. ■ Administer beta-blockers if necessary to reduce incidence of bleeding.
Gastritis	■ Esophageal reflux ■ Decreased appetite ■ Recurrent diarrhea	■ Provide foods that will not exacerbate GI symptoms while meeting nutritional requirements. ■ Teach patient to remain upright for 3–4 hours following meals, eat small frequent meals, and avoid gas-producing foods. ■ Antidiarrheals, antacids, and H₂ blockers may be appropriate medications to reduce symptoms.
Wernicke encephalopathy	■ Ataxia ■ Abnormal eye movements ■ Mental confusion ■ Short-term memory loss	■ Provide for patient safety. ■ Place clocks and calendars to reduce mental confusion. ■ Assess cognition and document findings. ■ Administer IV or IM thiamine. ■ Avoid glucose administration until after thiamine administration. ■ Hydrate patient.

if consumed rapidly, can produce partial or complete **blackouts**, periods of memory loss for events that occurred while a person was drinking. Blackouts are much more common among social drinkers—including college drinkers—than was previously assumed, and blackouts have been found to encompass events ranging from conversations to sexual intercourse (White, 2015). Mechanisms underlying alcohol-induced memory impairments include disruption of activity in the hippocampus, a brain region that plays a central role in the formation of new memories (White, 2015). A more advanced CNS problem is Wernicke-Korsakoff syndrome, described previously.

Dementia occurs five times more often in older adults with alcoholism than in nondrinkers. On the plus side, prevention of drinking relapse in older adults with alcoholism is often better than that of younger patients. More than 20% of treated older alcohol-dependent individuals remain abstinent after 4 years (Caputo et al., 2012).

Alcohol Withdrawal

Mild alcohol withdrawal generally consists of anxiety, irritability, difficulty sleeping, and decreased appetite. The signs and symptoms of acute alcohol withdrawal generally start 6 to 24 hours after the individual takes the last drink. Alcohol withdrawal may begin when the patient still has significant blood alcohol concentrations. The signs and symptoms of acute alcohol withdrawal **(alcohol withdrawal syndrome)** may include the following: agitation; anorexia (lack of appetite), nausea, vomiting; tremor (shakiness), elevated heart rate, increased blood pressure; insomnia, intense dreaming, nightmares; poor concentration, impaired memory and judgment; increased sensitivity to sound, light, and tactile sensations; hallucinations (auditory, visual, or tactile); delusions, usually paranoid or persecutory; grand mal seizures, resulting in loss of consciousness, brief cessation of breathing, and muscle rigidity; hyperthermia; delirium with disorientation; and fluctuation in level of consciousness (SAMHSA, 2015b).

Alcohol withdrawal delirium, sometimes referred to as delirium tremens (DTs), usually occurs on days 2 and 3 but may appear as late as 14 days after the last drink consumed. The major goal of medical management is to avoid seizures and DTs, typically with aggressive use of higher doses of benzodiazepines coupled with antiseizure medications (SAMHSA, 2015b). DTs do not develop suddenly, but instead progress from earlier withdrawal symptoms. Properly administered medication and adherence to detoxification protocols will prevent DTs and limit possible overmedication (SAMHSA, 2015b). During acute withdrawal, the individual experiences confusion, disorientation, hallucinations, tachycardia, hypertension or hypotension, extreme tremors, agitation, diaphoresis, and fever. Death may result from cardiovascular collapse or hyperthermia. With intensive care and advanced pharmacology, the mortality rate related to alcohol withdrawal syndrome has dropped from 35% to 5% (Burns, 2013).

Collaboration

When caring for a patient who abuses alcohol, the nurse must work as a collaborative member of a team that may include physicians, psychologists, counselors, nutritionists, and assistive personnel who share the collaborative goal of helping the patient achieve sobriety. Many individuals seeking recovery work with a sponsor, a recovering alcoholic with several years of sobriety. Sponsors provide peer support and often attend AA or 12-step meetings with the individuals whom they sponsor.

Diagnostic Tests

The simplest method of detecting blood alcohol content is by using a Breathalyzer. BALs are the main biologic measures for assessment purposes. Knowledge of the symptoms associated with a range of BALs is helpful in ascertaining level of intoxication, level of tolerance, and whether the individual accurately reported recent drinking. At 0.10% (after 5–6 drinks in 1–2 hours), voluntary motor action becomes clumsy, resulting in ataxia and dysarthria. The degree of impairment varies with gender, weight, and food ingestion. Small women who drink alcohol on an empty stomach achieve intoxication more quickly than large men who have eaten a full meal. At 0.20 to 0.25% (after 10–12 drinks in 2–4 hours), function of the motor area in the brain is depressed, causing an inability to remain upright (McNeece & DiNitto, 2012). A level above 0.10% without associated behavioral symptoms indicates the presence of tolerance. High tolerance is a sign of physical dependence.

Assessing for withdrawal symptoms is important when the BAL is high. Medications given for treatment of withdrawal from alcohol are usually not started until the BAL is below a set norm (usually below 0.10%) unless withdrawal symptoms become severe. Measurement of BAL may be repeated several times, several hours apart, to determine the body's metabolism of alcohol and at what time it is safe to give the patient medication to minimize the withdrawal symptoms.

Biomarkers are lab tests that suggest heavy alcohol consumption by detecting the toxic effects that alcohol may have had on organ systems or body chemistry. Included in this class are the serum measures of gamma glutamyl transferase (GGT), aspartate amino transferase (AST), alanine amino transferase (ALT), and mean corpuscular volume (MCV) (SAMHSA, 2012b). The first three are serum enzymes produced by the liver. GGT elevation is often caused by liver enzyme induction by alcohol, liver damage, or many drugs, including prescription medications. Another indirect alcohol biomarker is carbohydrate-deficient transferrin (CDT); an elevation in CDT can indicate heavy alcohol consumption. Other biomarker laboratory tests include ethyl glucuronide (EtG) and ethyl sulfate (EtS), usually measured in urine. EtG and EtS are frequently used to monitor abstinence in clinical and justice system settings (SAMHSA, 2012b).

Treatment of Withdrawal

All CNS depressants, including alcohol, benzodiazepines, and barbiturates, have a potentially dangerous progression of withdrawal. Alcohol and the entire class of CNS depressants share the same withdrawal syndrome. Treatment of severe withdrawal during detoxification is mostly symptomatic through acetaminophen, vitamins, and medications to minimize discomfort.

In managing alcohol withdrawal, the goal is to minimize adverse outcomes such as patient discomfort, seizures, delirium tremens, and mortality and to avoid the adverse effects of withdrawal medications, such as excess sedation. Close monitoring is essential to ensure protection of the patient. Critical care monitoring may be indicated to manage alcohol withdrawal delirium, particularly when very high doses of benzodiazepines are needed or when significant concurrent medical conditions are present. Medications such as benzodiazepines are a first-line therapy, used to minimize the discomfort associated with alcohol withdrawal and to prevent serious adverse effects, particularly seizures (Manasco et al., 2012).

Clinicians may order one of several treatment approaches, including fixed-schedule dosing, symptom-triggered dosing, or a combination of the two. The Clinical Institute Withdrawal Assessment for Alcohol—Revised (CIWA-Ar) scale is currently recommended as the best scale for assessing the severity of symptoms of acute alcohol withdrawal (Manasco et al., 2012). Triage nurses can use that scale to determine the need for inpatient hospital admission, such as when the CIWA-Ar score is 10 points or higher. However, recent research indicates that the CIWA-Ar scale may underestimate the severity of alcohol withdrawal syndrome in certain ethnic groups, such as Native Americans (Rappaport et al., 2013).

SAFETY ALERT Close attention to vital signs and presence of withdrawal symptoms is essential when a patient is withdrawing from alcohol. Trending the vital signs and CIW-Ar scores over time can often show when an individual may be heading into *delirium tremens* (DTs). Preventive steps, such as aggressive use of prn medications and application of protocols, should be used to prevent DTs from occurring.

Two unique medications used to treat alcoholism are disulfiram (Antabuse) and naltrexone (ReVia, Depade). Disulfiram is a form of aversion therapy that prevents the breakdown of alcohol, causing physical illness (intense vomiting) if taken while drinking alcohol. All forms of alcohol, including over-the-counter cough and cold preparations, must be avoided. Naltrexone can help reduce the craving for alcohol by blocking the pathways to the brain that trigger a feeling of pleasure when alcohol and other narcotics are used. Because naltrexone blocks opiate receptors, patients should avoid taking any narcotics, such as codeine, morphine, or heroin, while on naltrexone. Patients also should discontinue all narcotics 7 to 10 days before starting on naltrexone; naltrexone taken while the individual is still on opioids will trigger withdrawal. It also is recommended that patients wear a medical alert bracelet stating that they are on naltrexone, in case of emergency medical treatment. Patients taking disulfiram or naltrexone must also participate in psychosocial treatments such as AA meetings, individual counseling, or group therapy because the desire to "take a break" from treatment can overcome the patient's motivation to continue taking the medication. AA meetings and therapy provide support and reinforce patients' efforts to continue treatment. Peer connections made through AA can be especially motivating.

Complementary Health Approaches

Alternative and complementary therapies are not usually employed as stand-alone methods for alcohol withdrawal. They are, however, generally used in a comprehensive, integrated substance abuse treatment system that promotes health and well-being, provides palliative symptom relief, and improves treatment retention (SAMHSA, 2015b). Acupuncture has been used to reduce the craving for a variety of substances, including alcohol, and appears to contribute to improved treatment retention rates. While electroencephalograph (EEG) biofeedback, also called *neurotherapy*, and herbal administration have been found to provide some benefit in the treatment of alcoholism, their use has not been supported by controlled studies (SAMHSA, 2015b). Many individuals addicted to alcohol also have found yoga to be helpful in the recovery process. Both neurotherapy and yoga may provide calming effects on the centers of the brain involved in anxiety and impulse control.

Lifespan Considerations

In recent years, alcohol researchers have focused their efforts on discovering the differences in how alcohol affects individuals at different ages, using subsequent findings to determine appropriate interventions and treatment protocols. Some of the characteristics of various ages and gender differences throughout the lifespan are detailed in this section.

Alcohol Abuse Among Adolescents

More youth in the United States drink alcohol than smoke tobacco or marijuana, making it the drug most used by American young people. The percentage of adolescents age 12 to 17 who were current alcohol users was 11.5% in 2014, which translated to 1 in 9 adolescents who were current alcohol users during that year. Nationally, 1 in 16 adolescents (1.5 million) engaged in binge drinking during the past month (CBHSQ, 2014).

Many adolescents start to drink at very young ages. In the United States, the average age at which young people age 12 to 17 begin to drink is 13 years old. Individuals who reported starting to drink before the age of 15 were four times more likely also to report meeting the criteria for alcohol dependence at some point in their lives (NIAAA, 2015d). The younger children and adolescents are when they start to drink, the more likely they will be to engage in risky behaviors. For example, frequent binge drinkers are more likely to use illicit substances, have sex with six or more partners, and earn poor grades in school (NIAAA, 2015d).

Physical, emotional, and lifestyle changes and developmental transitions, such as puberty and increasing independence, are strongly associated with the initiation of alcohol use and subsequent abuse of alcohol. These factors are discussed below.

- **Expectations.** Expectations influence drinking behaviors, including whether adolescents begin to drink and how much. An adolescent who expects drinking to be a pleasurable experience is more likely to drink than one who does not. Adolescents who drink the most also place the greatest emphasis on the positive effects of alcohol consumption (NIAAA, 2015d).

- *Sensitivity and tolerance to alcohol.* Differences between the adult brain and the brain of the maturing adolescent also may help to explain why many young drinkers are able to consume much larger amounts of alcohol than adults before experiencing the negative consequences of drinking, such as drowsiness, lack of coordination, and withdrawal/hangover effects. This unusual tolerance may help to explain the high rates of binge drinking among young adults. At the same time, adolescents appear to be particularly sensitive to the positive effects of drinking, such as feeling more at ease in social situations, and they may drink more than adults because of these positive social experiences (NIAAA, 2015d).

- *Personality characteristics and psychiatric comorbidity.* Children who begin to drink at a very early age (before age 12) often share similar personality characteristics, such as hyperactivity and aggression. These young people, as well as those who are depressive or anxious, may be at greatest risk for alcohol problems. Other behavior problems associated with alcohol use include rebelliousness, difficulty avoiding harmful situations, and acting out without regard for rules or the feelings of others (NIAAA, 2015d).

- *Environmental aspects.* Environmental factors, such as the influence of parents and peers, also play a role in alcohol use. For example, parents who drink more and who view drinking favorably may have children who drink more, and an adolescent girl with an older or adult boyfriend is more likely to use alcohol and other drugs and to engage in delinquent behaviors. The impact of the media is believed to be a significant influence. Greater exposure to alcohol advertising contributes to an increase in drinking among underage youth (NIAAA, 2015d).

Alcohol Abuse Among Women

Research has supported the concept that women are more vulnerable to the adverse consequences of alcohol abuse than men. No gender difference has been noted for age at onset of regular use, but women use alcohol for fewer years than men before entering treatment. The severity of drug and alcohol dependence has not been shown to differ by gender, but women have reported more severe psychiatric, medical, and employment complications than men (SAMHSA, 2009).

Compared with men, women experience greater cognitive impairment by alcohol and are more susceptible to alcohol-related organ damage. Women develop alcohol abuse and dependence in less time than do men, a phenomenon known as *telescoping*; women also develop damage at lower levels of consumption over a shorter period of time (SAMHSA, 2009). Women who drink the same amount as men will have higher blood alcohol concentrations because women have proportionately more body fat and a lower volume of body water to dilute the alcohol. In comparison with men, women have a lower first-pass metabolism of alcohol in the stomach and upper small intestine before it enters the bloodstream and reaches other body organs, including the liver (SAMHSA, 2009).

Women develop alcohol-induced liver disease over a shorter period of time and after consuming less alcohol, and

they are more likely than men to develop alcoholic hepatitis and to die from cirrhosis. Women who are dependent on alcohol or consume heavier amounts are more likely to die prematurely from cardiac-related conditions and have an increased risk of hypertension (SAMHSA, 2009). Numerous studies have documented associations and suggested causal relationships between alcohol consumption and breast cancer risk, especially among postmenopausal women who are moderate alcohol drinkers and who are using menopausal hormone therapy. Alcohol significantly increases the risks for many other cancers. Other negative side effects of alcohol abuse for women include osteoporosis, increased cognitive decline and brain atrophy, memory deficits, and an increased risk for Alzheimer disease (SAMHSA, 2009).

Alcohol Abuse Among Pregnant Women

Alcohol use can result in obstetric complications, miscarriage, or significant problems for the fetus. It is difficult to isolate the effects related solely to alcohol on fetal and infant development because women who abuse alcohol may be abusing other substances. Alcohol use is often accompanied by psychologic distress, victimization, and poverty. Moreover, these issues create additional demands and stressors for women, as well as guilt and shame about the use of alcohol and other substances during pregnancy (SAMHSA, 2009).

Above all other drugs, alcohol is the most common teratogen in pregnancy. Alcohol use is associated with an increased risk of spontaneous abortion, as well as increased rates of prematurity and *abruptio placentae* (premature separation of the placenta from the uterus). A study found that women who consumed five or more drinks per week were three times more likely to deliver a stillborn baby compared with those who had fewer than one drink per week (SAMHSA, 2009).

Alcohol contributes to a wide range of effects on exposed offspring, known as fetal alcohol spectrum disorders (FASDs). The most serious consequence is fetal alcohol syndrome (FAS), characterized by abnormal facial features, growth deficiencies, and central nervous system problems (see the module on Cognition for more information on FAS). Women who drink during breastfeeding pass alcohol on to the baby, which can create a variety of adverse outcomes.

Alcohol Abuse Among Older Adults

Some 41.7% of adults age 65 or older used alcohol in 2013, with 9.1% reporting binge drinking and 2.1% reporting heavy alcohol use (CBHSQ, 2014). Older adults who abuse alcohol have a greater risk for numerous physical problems and premature death. Public health clinicians have suggested that people over age 65 should have no more than 7 drinks a week and no more than 3 drinks on any one day (National Institute on Aging [NIA], 2012).

Chronic alcohol abuse is associated with irreversible tissue and organ damage. Alcohol interacts negatively with the natural aging process to increase risks for hypertension, certain cancers, liver damage and cirrhosis, immune system disorders, and brain damage (Caputo et al., 2012). Alcohol can worsen some health conditions such as osteoporosis, diabetes, hypertension, and ulcers. It can also cause changes in the heart and blood vessels, which can dull cardiac pain, leading to delayed diagnosis of impending heart attacks (NIA, 2012). Alcohol can cause older adults to be forgetful and confused, symptoms that could be mistaken for signs of Alzheimer disease, dementia, and depression (NIA, 2012).

Mixing prescription and over-the-counter medicines or herbal remedies with alcohol can be dangerous or even deadly for older adults, who routinely take medications for chronic health issues. Medications that cause problems when mixed with alcohol include aspirin, which increases the risk of stomach or intestinal bleeding; cold and allergy medicines containing antihistamines, which can cause drowsiness or sleepiness; and acetaminophen, which can cause liver damage (NIA, 2012). Cough syrups and laxatives that have a high alcohol content will create an additive effect with alcohol, causing the blood alcohol level to increase, and may cause intoxication. Alcohol combined with some sleeping pills, opioid pain pills, or anxiety/anti-depression medicine can cause respiratory difficulties leading to death (NIA, 2012).

Because depression and alcohol abuse are the most frequently found disorders in completed suicides, nurses should routinely screen older adults for concurrent substance abuse and mental disorders. Prevention of drinking relapse in older alcoholics can be more successful than in younger patients. One study found that more than 20% of treated older adults with alcohol dependency remained abstinent after 4 years (Caputo et al., 2012).

NURSING PROCESS

Nurses may interact with patients experiencing alcohol abuse or dependence in a variety of settings. The most common setting is an alcohol abuse treatment program where patients are hospitalized for an average of 10 to 15 days for detoxification and inpatient therapy. These patients may be voluntarily admitted or court ordered to undergo treatment after charges of driving under the influence or alcohol-related child abuse or neglect.

Patients with alcohol abuse or dependence have impaired senses and increased risk-taking behaviors, which can lead to injuries from falls and accidents requiring medical attention. Therefore, nurses will also encounter these patients in hospital EDs and medical-surgical units. Occupational nurses and community health nurses also interact with patients who abuse alcohol through employee assistance programs and community health departments. School nurses may encounter adolescents who abuse alcohol. Urgent care centers, pain clinics, and ambulatory care centers are other settings in which patients with alcohol abuse disorders frequently appear for minor health problems associated with chronic disorders related to alcohol abuse or dependence.

Assessment

A thorough history of the patient's past alcohol use is important to ascertain the possibility of tolerance, physical dependence, or withdrawal syndrome. The following questions are helpful in eliciting a pattern of substance use behavior:

- How many substances has the patient used simultaneously in the past?

- How often, how much, and when did the patient first use alcohol?
- Is there a history of blackouts, delirium, or seizures?
- Is there a history of withdrawal syndrome, overdoses, and complications from previous alcohol use?
- Has the patient ever been treated in an alcohol abuse clinic?
- Has the patient ever been arrested for DUI or charged with any criminal offense while using alcohol?
- Is there a family history of alcohol use?

The patient's medical history is another important area for assessment and should include the existence of any comorbid condition such as HIV, hepatitis, cirrhosis, Wernicke-Korsakoff syndrome, or a co-occurring mental illness. Information about prescribed and over-the-counter medications as well as any allergies or sensitivity to drugs is vital. Assess for history of abuse, family violence, or other trauma as well as history of suicide attempts. Ask if the patient is having any current thoughts of self-harm, suicide, or other violence.

Information about the patient's level of stress and other psychosocial concerns can help in assessing problems with alcohol use. Assess how the patient's alcohol use is affecting relationships at home and work; the patient's usual methods of coping with stress; and the patient's current support systems.

Several screening tools such as the Michigan Alcohol Screening Test (MAST) (Pokorny, Miller, & Kaplan, 1972) and the Brief Drug Abuse Screening Test (B-DAST) (Skinner, 1982) may help the nurse determine the degree of severity of alcohol abuse or dependence. The MAST Brief version is a 10-question self-administered questionnaire that takes 10 to 15 minutes to complete. An answer of yes to three or more questions indicates a potentially dangerous pattern of alcohol abuse. The CAGE questionnaire (Ewing, 1984) is useful when the patient may not recognize that he or she has an alcohol problem or is uncomfortable acknowledging it. This questionnaire is designed to be a self-report of drinking behavior, or it may be administered by a professional. One affirmative response raises concern and indicates the need for further discussion and follow-up. Two or more yes answers signify a problem with alcohol that may require treatment.

A nonthreatening question such as "How much alcohol do you drink?" is preferable to a more judgmental question, such as "You don't drink too much alcohol, do you?" Open-ended questions that elicit more than a simple yes or no answer help to determine the direction of future counseling. The professional should use therapeutic communication techniques to establish trust prior to the assessment process.

Nurses working in medical-surgical units, psychiatric units, and special alcohol abuse units routinely care for patients experiencing acute alcohol withdrawal. Several assessment tools are available to determine the severity of withdrawal symptoms and indicate the need for pharmacologic treatment to manage withdrawal symptoms. An example of a withdrawal assessment tool is the Clinical Institute Withdrawal Assessment for Alcohol—Revised (CIWA-Ar) scale discussed earlier (Sullivan et al., 1989) (**Figure 22–4 »**). This assessment is used widely in clinical and research settings for initial assessment and ongoing monitoring of alcohol withdrawal signs and symptoms.

Clinical Institute Withdrawal Assessment of Alcohol Scale, Revised (CIWA-Ar)

Patient:_____   Date: _____   Time: _____   (24 hour clock, midnight = 00:00)

Pulse or heart rate, taken for one minute:_____   Blood pressure:_____

NAUSEA AND VOMITING -- Ask "Do you feel sick to your stomach? Have you vomited?" Observation.
0 no nausea and no vomiting
1 mild nausea with no vomiting
2
3
4 intermittent nausea with dry heaves
5
6
7 constant nausea, frequent dry heaves and vomiting

TREMOR -- Arms extended and fingers spread apart. Observation.
0 no tremor
1 not visible, but can be felt fingertip to fingertip
2
3
4 moderate, with patient's arms extended
5
6
7 severe, even with arms not extended

PAROXYSMAL SWEATS -- Observation.
0 no sweat visible
1 barely perceptible sweating, palms moist
2
3
4 beads of sweat obvious on forehead
5
6
7 drenching sweats

ANXIETY -- Ask "Do you feel nervous?" Observation.
0 no anxiety, at ease
1 mild anxious
2
3
4 moderately anxious, or guarded, so anxiety is inferred
5
6
7 equivalent to acute panic states as seen in severe delirium or acute schizophrenic reactions

AGITATION -- Observation.
0 normal activity
1 somewhat more than normal activity
2
3
4 moderately fidgety and restless
5
6
7 paces back and forth during most of the interview, or constantly thrashes about

TACTILE DISTURBANCES -- Ask "Have you any itching, pins and needles sensations, any burning, any numbness, or do you feel bugs crawling on or under your skin?" Observation.
0 none
1 very mild itching, pins and needles, burning or numbness
2 mild itching, pins and needles, burning or numbness
3 moderate itching, pins and needles, burning or numbness
4 moderately severe hallucinations
5 severe hallucinations
6 extremely severe hallucinations
7 continuous hallucinations

AUDITORY DISTURBANCES -- Ask "Are you more aware of sounds around you? Are they harsh? Do they frighten you? Are you hearing anything that is disturbing to you? Are you hearing things you know are not there?" Observation.
0 not present
1 very mild harshness or ability to frighten
2 mild harshness or ability to frighten
3 moderate harshness or ability to frighten
4 moderately severe hallucinations
5 severe hallucinations
6 extremely severe hallucinations
7 continuous hallucinations

VISUAL DISTURBANCES -- Ask "Does the light appear to be too bright? Is its color different? Does it hurt your eyes? Are you seeing anything that is disturbing to you? Are you seeing things you know are not there?" Observation.
0 not present
1 very mild sensitivity
2 mild sensitivity
3 moderate sensitivity
4 moderately severe hallucinations
5 severe hallucinations
6 extremely severe hallucinations
7 continuous hallucinations

HEADACHE, FULLNESS IN HEAD -- Ask "Does your head feel different? Does it feel like there is a band around your head?" Do not rate for dizziness or lightheadedness. Otherwise, rate severity.
0 not present
1 very mild
2 mild
3 moderate
4 moderately severe
5 severe
6 very severe
7 extremely severe

ORIENTATION AND CLOUDING OF SENSORIUM -- Ask "What day is this? Where are you? Who am I?"
0 oriented and can do serial additions
1 cannot do serial additions or is uncertain about date
2 disoriented for date by no more than 2 calendar days
3 disoriented for date by more than 2 calendar days
4 disoriented for place/or person

Total CIWA-Ar Score _____
Rater's Initials _____
Maximum Possible Score 67

The CIWA-Ar is not copyrighted and may be reproduced freely. This assessment for monitoring withdrawal symptoms requires approximately 5 minutes to administer. The maximum score is 67 (see instrument). Patients scoring less than 10 do not usually need additional medication for withdrawal.

Source: From Sullivan, J.T., Sykora, K., Schneiderman, J., Naranjo, C.A., and Sellers, E.M. Assessment of alcohol withdrawal: The revised Clinical Institute Withdrawal Assessment for Alcohol scale (**CIWA-Ar**). *British Journal of Addiction* 84:1353–1357, 1989.

Figure 22–4 » Assessment tool for alcohol withdrawal.

The CIWA-Ar scale is a validated 10-item assessment tool that can be used to monitor and medicate patients going through alcohol withdrawal. The CIWA-Ar assesses for several alcohol withdrawal symptoms (e.g., high blood pressure, rapid pulse and respirations, tremors, insomnia, irritability, sweating, convulsions) and results in a score that is used to direct the administration of benzodiazepines or other drugs to relieve associated symptoms of withdrawal and to prevent seizures. A score of 8 points or fewer corresponds to mild withdrawal symptoms. Scores of 9 to 15 points indicate moderate withdrawal, whereas a score of 15 or greater denotes severe withdrawal and an increased risk of DTs and seizures.

SAFETY ALERT Alcohol withdrawal symptoms present within 8 hours after the last drink and usually peak within 24 to 72 hours. Patients with severe liver impairment and other physical complications may exhibit withdrawal symptoms for as long as a week after the last drink.

Diagnosis

Nursing diagnoses are individualized to specific patient needs. Primary diagnoses may include:

- *Injury, Risk for*
- *Violence, Risk for Other-Directed*
- *Denial, Ineffective*
- *Coping, Ineffective*
- *Imbalanced Nutrition: Less Than Body Requirements*
- *Knowledge, Deficient*
- *Liver Function, Risk for Impaired*
- *Family Processes, Dysfunctional*
- *Confusion, Acute*
- *Confusion, Chronic.*

(NANDA-I © 2014)

Planning

Goals for patient care depend on patient needs. The patient who denies a problem with alcohol will have far different needs than the patient experiencing withdrawal, participating in an alcohol abuse program, or facing serious complications from years of abuse. Possible goals may include the following:

- The patient will admit alcohol is controlling his or her life.
- The patient will agree to enter an alcohol treatment facility or outpatient program.
- The patient will experience no complications (or no further complications) as a result of alcohol abuse or alcohol withdrawal.
- The patient will achieve optimal nutritional status.
- The patient will remain sober.
- The patient will participate in support groups such as AA after discharge from treatment facility.

Implementation

During recent years, addiction specialists have sought to develop an efficient system of care that matches patients'

clinical needs with an appropriate care setting in the least confining and most cost-effective manner, a practice known as *least restrictive care* (SAMHSA, 2015c).

Unlike in the past, when patients in active withdrawal were always monitored in acute care settings, today's patients are more likely to withdraw from alcohol in community-based *social detoxification* programs with limited medical oversight (SAMHSA, 2015b). Sites of cares include residential rehabilitation programs, halfway houses, and partial hospitalization programs. Community and faith groups often operate social detoxification programs that may or may not have clear procedures for pursuing appropriate medical referral and emergency care. An advantage of these outpatient programs is that they provide structured environments while allowing the patient to maintain a viable presence in the community.

Another trend is *home detoxification*. ED and family physicians are now implementing outpatient alcohol detoxification guidelines with pharmacotherapy for individuals with mild to moderate alcohol withdrawal symptoms and no serious psychiatric or medical comorbidities (Muncie, Yasinian, & Oge, 2013). Many of these protocols advocate daily office visits or home visits. Because of the increasing array of treatment options, it is likely that nurses will perform more home or community visits or use telehealth to monitor patients withdrawing from alcohol in the future.

Withdrawal is often accompanied by poor physiologic and psychologic outcomes. As described earlier, withdrawal is a particularly high-risk event, when potentially dangerous withdrawal symptoms—confusion; seizures accompanied by rapid heartbeat, high blood pressure, and hyperthermia; delirium tremens; and coma leading to death—occur. Safety is a paramount concern. Equally important after detoxification are promoting physical recovery from alcohol addiction, enhancing coping skills, and providing referrals to services that prepare the patient for long-term abstinence from alcohol use. Among these necessary referrals are vocational counseling, self-help groups such as AA, and individual, group, and family therapy.

Patients who have histories of trauma may be ambivalent about treatment and feel "stuck," perceiving themselves as having fewer options (SAMHSA, 2014a). In addition, patients may avoid engaging in treatment because it is one step closer to addressing their trauma. These patients may exhibit challenging behaviors and need a longer course of treatment.

Caring interventions are based on the patient's need, diagnoses chosen, and goals set for care throughout the course of treatment. For all patients, nurses will work to promote healthy coping skills (see the module on Stress and Coping) to help patients reduce the need to use alcohol as a coping mechanism. In addition, patients who abuse alcohol require health promotion related to maintaining adequate nutrition, and in particular should take thiamine supplements as necessary to prevent complications from chronic alcoholism. Specific interventions to help patients begin the path to recovery from alcohol abuse follow.

Promote Patient Safety During Acute Withdrawal

- Observe the patient for withdrawal symptoms. Monitor vital signs frequently per protocol until the patient has stabilized. Provide adequate nutrition and hydration.

Take seizure precautions. These actions provide supportive physical care during detoxification.

- Assess blood alcohol level routinely and look for escalating signs of withdrawal, using an instrument such as the CIWA-Ar. Reliable information about withdrawal symptoms comes from BAL and vital signs; these measurements provide information about the need for prn medication to prevent DTs and other severe complications.

- Administer scheduled medications according to the detoxification protocol. Benzodiazepines help minimize the discomfort of withdrawal symptoms, anticonvulsants help prevent seizures, and vitamins and nutritional supplements support neurologic health.

- Assess the patient's level of orientation frequently. Orient and reassure the patient of safety in the presence of hallucinations, delusions, or illusions.

- Explain all interventions before approaching the patient. Use simple step-by-step instructions and face-to-face interaction. Minimize environmental distractions and talk softly to the patient. Excessive stimuli increase agitation.

- Provide positive reinforcement when thinking and behavior are appropriate or when the patient recognizes that delusions are not based in reality. Alcohol can interfere with the patient's perception of reality.

- Express reasonable doubt if the patient relays suspicious or paranoid beliefs. Reinforce accurate perception of people or situations. It is important to communicate that you do not share the false belief as reality.

- Do not argue with the patient who is experiencing delusions or hallucinations. Convey acceptance that the patient believes a situation to be true, but that you do not see or hear what is not there. Arguing with the patient or denying the belief serves no useful purpose because it does not eliminate the delusions.

- Talk to the patient about real events and real people. Respond to feelings and reassure the patient about being safe from harm. Discussions that focus on the delusions may aggravate the condition. Verbalization of feelings in a nonthreatening environment may help the patient develop insight.

Promote Safety in Outpatient and Home Settings

When an individual initiates outpatient or home care, obtain a drug history as well as urine and blood samples for laboratory analysis of substance content. Subjective history often is not accurate, and knowledge regarding substance use is important for accurate assessment and determining the appropriate care setting.

- Assess orientation and cognition. If the patient's level of cognitive functioning is not sufficient to implement the outpatient or home plan of care, contact a clinician who can evaluate the patient and assist in transfer to a higher level of care if needed.

- Have the patient (if able) or others in the home or community setting monitor vital signs frequently during the first day of detox using reliable home equipment, and several times per day subsequently. Teach the patient and

lay personnel about the signs and symptoms of severe withdrawal and make sure they understand when they should notify the clinician.

- Administer or teach the patient/others to administer scheduled medications according to the detoxification protocol. Monitor vital signs and symptoms such as increasing agitation and a change in level of consciousness to determine whether the patient should remain in outpatient or home care. Use vital signs to determine whether prn medications are indicated.

- Monitor for signs of alcohol intoxication. Some patients will start drinking again when withdrawal symptoms become too distressing.

- Suggest that the patient remain in a quiet room to decrease excessive stimuli. Monitor for excessive hyperactivity or agitation, which may indicate severe withdrawal symptoms, and suicidal ideation. These symptoms indicate that the patient may need emergency care.

- Determine specific risks to patient safety. Make sure that the patient is oriented to reality and the environment. Ensure that potentially harmful objects are stored outside the patient's immediate area, so that the patient cannot harm self or others if disoriented and confused.

Promote Healthy Self-Esteem

- Spend time with the patient and convey an attitude of acceptance. Encourage the patient to accept responsibility for his or her behaviors and feelings. An attitude of acceptance enhances self-worth.

- Encourage the patient to focus on strengths and accomplishments rather than weaknesses and failures. Minimize attention to negative ruminations.

- Encourage participation in therapeutic group activities. Offer recognition and positive feedback for actual achievements. Success and recognition increase self-esteem.

- Teach assertiveness techniques and effective communication techniques such as the use of "I feel" rather than "You make me feel" statements. Previous patterns of communication may have been aggressive and accusatory, causing barriers to interpersonal relationships.

Provide Patient Education

- Assess the patient's level of knowledge and readiness to learn the effects of alcohol on the body. Baseline assessment is required to develop appropriate teaching material.

- Develop a teaching plan that includes measurable objectives. Include significant others if possible. Lifestyle changes often affect all family members.

- Begin teaching with simple concepts and progress to more complex issues. Use interactive teaching strategies and written materials appropriate to the patient's educational level. Include information on the physiologic effects of alcohol, the propensity for physical and psychologic dependence, and risks to the fetus if the patient is pregnant. Active participation and handouts enhance retention of important concepts.

Patients are at highest risk for relapse within the first few months of stopping use of alcohol. An acronym that many therapists use to assist the patient in recognizing some behaviors that lead to relapse is **HALT**:

Hungry

Angry

Lonely

Tired.

Nurses should also emphasize the importance of a balanced diet, adequate sleep, healthy recreational activities, and a caring support system to prevent relapse.

Evaluation

The patient is evaluated on the ability to meet goals set during the planning stage of the nursing process. Potential expected outcomes include the following:

- The patient in the acute, community, or home setting undergoes withdrawal without physiologic complications.
- The patient controls anxiety to the extent the patient refrains from drinking when anxiety levels rise.
- The patient displays new coping mechanisms.
- The patient does not start using alcohol again.
- The patient does not experience any new physiologic or psychologic complications as a result of sobriety.
- The patient accepts responsibility for how his or her behavior impacts the family unit.

Over time, patients will maintain whatever coping supports they learned to continue abstinence and sobriety. Patients who do not address underlying psychologic issues will find sobriety challenging. Thus, the patient and clinician will need to evaluate progress at periodic intervals for an extended period of time.

New nurses may be surprised to see how often patients with an alcohol-use disorder return to drinking. An 8-year longitudinal study of 1162 people who entered treatment showed that extended abstinence does predict long-term recovery. This research showed that only about a third of people who are abstinent less than a year will remain abstinent, *while more than two thirds will relapse* (Dennis, Foss, & Scott, 2007). For those who achieve a year of sobriety, less than half will relapse. Patients who maintain 5 years of sobriety have a less than 15% chance of relapse.

When revaluating the plan of care, nurses should consider factors such as the patient's physiologic health, mental health, coping responses, legal involvement, vocational involvement, housing, peers, and social and spiritual support. Other factors hindering sobriety include the success of the transition from rehab to home, engagement with aftercare, motivation and ambivalence toward recovery, unrealistic expectations, and continued use of other substances. After considering all of these factors, the clinician should work with the patient to modify the plan of care to accommodate these new circumstances.

Nursing Care Plan
A Patient Experiencing Withdrawal from Alcohol

George Russell, age 58, fell at home and broke his arm. His wife took him to the emergency department where an open reduction and internal fixation of his right wrist was performed under general anesthesia in the operating room. He was admitted to the postoperative unit for observation following surgery because he required large amounts of anesthesia during the procedure.

Mr. Russell has a ruddy complexion and looks older than his stated age. He discloses that he was laid off from his factory job 2 years ago and has been working odd jobs until last week, when he was hired by a local assembly plant. His father was a recovering alcoholic, and his 30-year-old son has been treated for alcohol abuse in the past. Mr. Russell states that he knows alcoholism runs in the family, but he believes that he has his drinking under control. However, he cannot remember the events that led up to his fall and how he might have broken his arm.

ASSESSMENT	DIAGNOSES	PLANNING
During the nursing assessment, Mr. Russell is hesitant to provide information and refuses to make eye contact. Prior to his operation, a BAL was drawn because the ED nurse detected alcohol on his breath. His BAL was 0.40%, which is five times the legal limit for intoxication. His vital signs are within the upper limits of normal, but he is confused and disoriented with slurred speech and a slight tremor of the hands. He is 6 feet tall and weighs 140 pounds. His total albumin is 2.9 mg, and he has elevated liver enzymes. His wife states that he rarely eats the meals she prepares because he is usually drinking and has no appetite for food.	▪ *Ineffective Coping* related to possible hereditary factor and personal vulnerability ▪ *Risk for Injury* related to aggressive behavior, unsteady gait, and impaired motor responses ▪ *Ineffective Denial* related to inability to recognize maladaptive behaviors caused by substance use ▪ *Imbalanced Nutrition: Less Than Body Requirements* related to anorexia manifested by decreased weight and low serum protein levels (NANDA-I © 2014)	▪ The patient will express his true feelings associated with using alcohol as a method of coping with stressful situations. ▪ The patient will identify three adaptive coping mechanisms he can use as alternatives to alcohol in response to stress. ▪ The patient will verbalize the negative effects of alcohol and agree to seek professional help with his drinking. ▪ The patient will be free of injury as evidenced by steady gait and absence of subsequent falls. ▪ The patient will gain 1 pound (0.45 kilogram) per week without evidence of increased fluid retention. Serum albumin levels will return to normal range.

Nursing Care Plan (continued)

IMPLEMENTATION

- Establish a trusting relationship with the patient and spend time with him discussing his feelings, fears, and anxieties.

- Consult with a physician regarding a schedule for medications during detoxification, and observe the patient for signs of withdrawal syndrome.

- Explain the effects of alcohol abuse on the body, and emphasize that prognosis is closely associated with abstinence.

- Teach a relaxation technique that the patient believes is useful.

- Provide community resource information about self-help groups and, if the patient is receptive, a list of meeting times and phone numbers.

- Consult with a dietitian to determine the number of calories needed to provide adequate nutrition and a realistic weight. Document intake, output, and calorie count.

- Consult with a physician to begin vitamin B_1 (thiamine) and dietary supplements.

EVALUATION

Mr. Russell is discharged from the postoperative unit without complications. He successfully undergoes detoxification and contacts the employee assistance program at his new place of employment. He is on medical leave while his arm completely heals and now attends AA meetings 5 days a week. He reports that he enjoys taking long walks with his wife in the warm weather and that his appetite has returned. He has gained 10 pounds in the past 6 weeks and feels better physically than he has in many years.

CRITICAL THINKING

1. Explain why, during the initial nursing assessment, it would be important to ask questions about Mr. Russell's medication history and his use of other medications.

2. Mr. Russell asks you to explain the risks of taking disulfiram (Antabuse). What should you tell him?

3. Develop a care plan for Mr. Russell for the nursing diagnosis of *Imbalanced Nutrition: Less Than Body Requirements*. Why is this care plan necessary?

REVIEW Alcohol Abuse

RELATE Link the Concepts and Exemplars

Linking the exemplar of alcohol abuse with the concept of comfort:

1. Why might the patient who has detoxified from alcohol have trouble sleeping?

2. What nursing care might you provide to improve the patient's ability to sleep?

Linking the exemplar of alcohol abuse with the concept of infection:

3. What pathophysiology would increase the risk for infection in the patient who chronically abuses alcohol?

4. What nursing care would you provide this patient to reduce the risk of infection?

Linking the exemplar of alcohol abuse with the concept of legal issues:

5. The nurse, working in an ED, admits a patient accompanied by a police officer who requests that a serum BAL be drawn and tested for use in a court case related to the patient's driving while intoxicated. What are the patient's legal rights, and what legal obligations does the nurse have regarding this patient's rights of privacy?

Linking the exemplar of alcohol abuse with the concept of safety:

6. The nurse is caring for a patient who was brought to the ED with a BAL of 0.32%. The patient is somnolent, is speaking in incomplete sentences that are garbled and difficult to understand, and has a laceration on his forehead. He is admitted to the acute care facility for observation. How will you assess this patient's neurologic status to determine whether there is an alteration in level of consciousness reflecting a brain injury or alcohol intoxication?

READY Go to Volume 3: Clinical Nursing Skills

REFER Go to Pearson MyLab Nursing and eText

- Additional review materials

REFLECT Apply Your Knowledge

Candy Collins, a 46-year-old wife and mother of two, comes to her physician's office seeking help for alcohol abuse. She says her husband has threatened to leave her and take her children with him if she doesn't stop. The nurse determines that Mrs. Collins drinks at least five or six alcoholic beverages daily, usually starting after dinner, although sometimes she begins drinking after the children leave for school. The nurse learns that Mrs. Collins's behavior began 5 years ago, shortly after her youngest child began preschool. She denies having blackouts, although she reports occasionally waking in the morning with no memory of the night before.

1. What other data would you want to collect from Mrs. Collins related to her abuse of alcohol?

2. What treatment would you anticipate as appropriate for this patient?

3. What teaching would you provide both Mrs. Collins and her husband?

≫ Exemplar 22.B
Nicotine Use

Exemplar Learning Outcomes

22.B Analyze manifestations and treatment considerations for patients who use nicotine.

- Describe the pathophysiology of nicotine use.
- Describe the etiology of nicotine use.
- Compare the risk factors and prevention of nicotine use.
- Identify the clinical manifestations of nicotine use.
- Summarize diagnostic tests and therapies used by interprofessional teams in the collaborative care of an individual who uses nicotine.

- Differentiate care of patients who use nicotine across the lifespan.
- Apply the nursing process in providing culturally competent care to an individual who uses nicotine.

Exemplar Key Terms

Nicotine, *1682*
Nicotine replacement therapy (NRT), *1684*

Overview

Cigarette smoking is the single most preventable cause of disease and death in the United States. The CDC (2013d) estimates that 443,000 deaths each year are attributable to cigarette smoking. This estimate does not include patients exposed to secondhand smoke or patients who consume nicotine by using chewing tobacco.

Nicotine, a highly addictive chemical found in tobacco, is used worldwide and results in many complications (see the Focus on Diversity and Culture feature). Nicotine enters the body via the lungs (cigarettes, pipes, and cigars) and oral mucous membranes (chewing tobacco as well as smoking). Although smoking is legal, it has become increasingly socially unacceptable, as evidence of the danger of both smoking and breathing in others' secondhand smoke has been demonstrated. Burning of tobacco releases the active substances in the plant, making it available for absorption via the lungs into the bloodstream.

Commercial tobacco contains more than 4000 chemicals. Among these are nicotine (one of the most addictive substances known to humans); arsenic and hydrogen cyanide (poisons); acetone (a simple ketone that can irritate tissues and is a CNS depressant); and tar (which deposits on the lungs via cigarette smoke and reduces the elasticity of the alveoli, slowing air exchange). Cancer-causing agents in commercial tobacco include nitrosamines, cadmium, benzopyrene, polonium-210, nickel, urethane, and toluidine. As a result of the combination of chemicals entering the bloodstream, smoking has profound effects on virtually every organ system, ranging from hypertension due to vasoconstriction to suppression of the immune system.

A new public health concern is *vaping*, which uses battery-powered electronic cigarettes with an atomizer of liquid consisting of propylene glycol, glycerol, distilled water, flavorings (which may or may not be approved for food use), preservatives, and nicotine. The atomizer aerosolizes the liquid for inhalation (Farsalinos & Polosa, 2014). Consumers, known as *vapers*, may choose from several nicotine strengths, as well as non-nicotine liquids and flavorings. It remains to be proven whether e-cigarettes are actually safe or simply less harmful than tobacco, and debate rages about whether or how the devices should be regulated (Arnold, 2014). In many parts of the United States and the world, vaping is unregulated.

Of particular concern is the exploding popularity of e-cigarettes among teens and young adults (**Figure 22–5 ≫**). According to the CDC (2015b), e-cigarette use among middle and high school students tripled from 2013 to 2014, increasing from 4.5% in 2013 to 13.4% in 2014, rising from approximately 660,000 to 2 million students. Among middle school students, current e-cigarette use more than tripled from 1.1% in 2013 to 3.9% in 2014—an increase from approximately 120,000 to 450,000 students. In 2014, e-cigarette use surpassed current use of every other tobacco product overall, including conventional cigarettes. E-cigarettes were the most used tobacco product for non-Hispanic Whites, Hispanics, and non-Hispanic other race, while cigars were the most commonly used product among non-Hispanic Blacks (CDC, 2015b).

Pathophysiology and Epidemiology
Pathophysiology

In low doses, nicotine stimulates nicotinic receptors in the brain to release dopamine (a precursor to norepinephrine) and epinephrine, causing vasoconstriction. This increases the

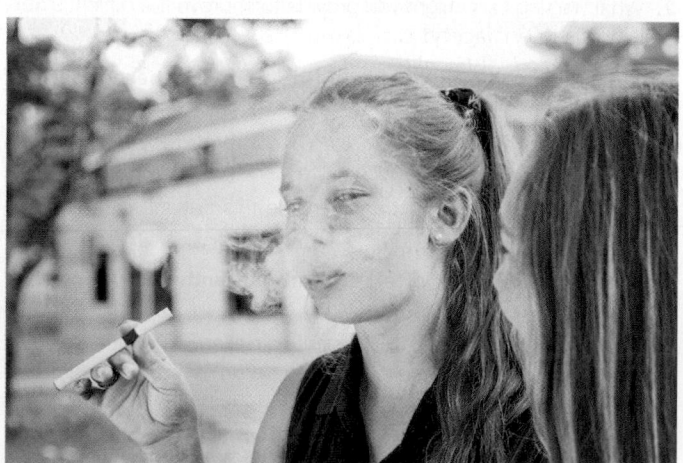

Source: Nicolas McComber/E+/Getty Images.

Figure 22–5 ≫ At least 2 million teens and young adults are using e-cigarettes. Researchers have yet to determine whether e-cigarettes are actually safe or are simply less harmful than tobacco.

Focus on Diversity and Culture
Nicotine Use: Still a Global Epidemic

In 2012, 21% of the global population age 15 and above smoked tobacco. Men smoked at five times the rate of women; the average rates were 36 and 7%, respectively (World Health Organization [WHO], 2015a). Smoking among men was highest in the WHO Western Pacific Region, with 48% of men smoking some form of tobacco. Smoking among women was highest (19%) in the WHO European Region

The rates at which adolescent girls age 13 to 15 use tobacco averaged around 8% globally. Among other regions, the highest prevalence among girls was seen in the WHO Region of the Americas, where almost 14% of young adolescent girls were already tobacco users. Boys age 13 to 15 in WHO South-East Asia Region and WHO Eastern Mediterranean Region used tobacco at higher rates than their counterparts in other regions, at over 20% in both regions (WHO, 2015a).

---

heart rate, blood pressure, and peripheral vascular resistance, increasing the heart's workload. Gastrointestinal effects include an increase in gastric acid secretion, an increase in the tone and motility of GI smooth muscle, nausea, and increased risk of vomiting.

In the CNS, nicotine occupies the receptors for acetylcholine in both dopamine and serotonin neural pathways. This causes the release of dopamine and norepinephrine. Initially, nicotine increases mental alertness and cognitive ability, but eventually it depresses those responses (Kneisl & Trigoboff, 2013).

Smokers can develop tolerance to nausea and dizziness, which may be experienced with initial use of nicotine, but not to the cardiovascular effects. Furthermore, because of the vasoconstriction, tissue oxygenation can be impaired in areas where vessels are already narrowed by atherosclerosis. Researchers have also found an association between ingredients in vaping liquids and lung disease. Diacetyl, a flavoring chemical linked to cases of severe respiratory disease, was found in more than 75% of flavored electronic cigarettes and refill liquids (Roeder, 2015). Inhaled diacetyl can cause the debilitating respiratory disease *bronchiolitis obliterans*, known as "popcorn lung" because it first appeared in workers who inhaled artificial butter flavor in microwave popcorn processing facilities.

Smokers often have more difficulty falling asleep than nonsmokers because nicotine acts as a stimulant. Smokers are usually easily aroused and often describe themselves as light sleepers. By refraining from smoking after the evening meal, the person usually sleeps better; moreover, many former smokers report that their sleeping patterns improve once they stop smoking.

Nicotine dependence results from chronic use. Research suggests that dopaminergic processes have a role in regulating the reinforcing effects of nicotine, making cessation difficult (Kneisl & Trigoboff, 2013). Withdrawal symptoms include craving, nervousness, restlessness, irritability, impatience, increased hostility, insomnia, impaired concentration, increased appetite, and weight gain. Gradual reduction in nicotine use seems to prolong suffering. Chronic health problems from smoking have been well established in the form of cancer, heart disease, emphysema, hypertension, and death.

Etiology and Epidemiology

Some of the most common factors that influence people to smoke are emotions, social pressure, alcohol use, lack of education, and age. Young people are more likely to use tobacco if they have access to smoking areas and tobacco products, especially to low-cost or free tobacco. They are also more likely to use tobacco if they have friends, brothers, or sisters who use tobacco; watch movies that have smoking in them; are not doing well in school or have friends who are not doing well in school; are not engaged in school or religious activities; and use other substances, such as alcohol or marijuana (CDC, 2012). People of lower socioeconomic status are more likely to smoke than those of higher socioeconomic status, partially because smoking is more socially acceptable in groups with fewer resources. Furthermore, these individuals are less successful in quitting smoking because they lack high-quality health education, lack support for quitting, and are exposed to smoking more often.

Approximately one in five U.S. adults smokes cigarettes, and smoking-related diseases claim more than 393,000 American lives each year (American Lung Association, 2013). Smoking is the most common form of recreational drug use, practiced by more than 1 billion people in the majority of human societies. According to a 2012 Surgeon General's report, *Preventing Tobacco Use Among Youth and Young Adults* (2012), more than 80% of adult smokers began smoking by 18 years of age, with 99% of them lighting up by age 26.

Risk Factors

As stated above, age, socioeconomic status and lack of engagement in activities are among the risk factors for smoking. Smoking itself is a risk factor for a number of diseases. It harms nearly every organ in the body and is a main cause of lung cancer and chronic obstructive pulmonary disease (COPD). Smoking is also a cause of coronary heart disease, stroke, and a host of other cancers and diseases (American Lung Association, 2013). Graves disease, infertility, early menopause, dysmenorrhea, impotence, osteoporosis, and degenerative disc disease have also been associated with smoking. Other less serious consequences include discolored teeth and fingernails, premature aging and wrinkling, bad breath, reduced sense of smell and taste, strong smell of smoke clinging to hair and clothing, and gum disease (Zhang & Wang, 2013). Smoking during pregnancy has been associated with preterm labor, spontaneous abortion, low-birth-weight infants, sudden infant death syndrome (SIDS), and learning disorders (Knopik et al., 2012).

Nonsmokers who are exposed to secondhand smoke at home or work increase their lung cancer risk by 20 to 30%. Concentrations of many cancer-causing and toxic chemicals are higher in secondhand smoke than in the smoke inhaled by smokers (CDC, 2013c). Secondhand smoke presents a number of dangers, particularly to children of smokers. According to the CDC (2013d), secondhand smoking increases children's risks for SIDS, otitis media, and asthma and other respiratory conditions. In addition, mothers who smoke and mothers who are exposed to secondhand smoke are more likely to have lower-birth-weight babies.

Prevention

Smoking and smokeless tobacco use are initiated and established primarily during adolescence. Adolescents and young adults are uniquely susceptible to social and environmental influences to use tobacco, and tobacco companies spend billions of dollars on cigarette and smokeless tobacco marketing. The Surgeon General's 2012 report provides evidence that coordinated, high-impact interventions, including mass media campaigns, price increases, and community-level changes protecting people from secondhand smoke, are effective in reducing the initiation and prevalence of smoking among youth.

National, state, and local program activities that have reduced and prevented youth tobacco use in the past have included combinations of the following: counteradvertising mass media campaigns (such as TV and radio commercials); comprehensive school-based tobacco-use prevention policies and programs; and higher costs of tobacco products through increased excise taxes.

Clinical Manifestations

Clinical manifestations of nicotine use are usually nonexistent in the early stages of use and are seen only when a complication such as COPD, cancer, or heart disease occurs. People who smoke for many years often have deep voices secondary to trauma to the vocal cords caused by the heat of the smoke and the chronic cough they often develop. See the exemplar on Lung Cancer in the module on Cellular

Regulation for manifestations of cancers associated with nicotine use; the exemplar on Chronic Obstructive Pulmonary Disease in the module on Oxygenation for the impact of smoking on lung function; and the exemplars on Coronary Artery Disease and Peripheral Vascular Disease in the module on Perfusion for information related to heart disease and peripheral vascular disease.

Collaboration

As with any addiction, the treatment process is a collaborative one. Individuals who are addicted to nicotine benefit from the support of family and friends, especially during times when they would usually be smoking or using tobacco. Although pharmacologic therapies are available over the counter, it is important for the patient to discuss treatment with healthcare providers to minimize symptoms of withdrawal and prevent interactions with prescribed medications. Some patients may seek complementary health approaches and support groups to help them quit smoking.

Nicotine Replacement Therapy

Nicotine replacement therapy (NRT) helps relieve some of the physiologic effects of withdrawal, including cravings, for patients trying to quit smoking or using tobacco. NRT transdermal patches and gums are available over the counter; nicotine inhalers and nasal sprays are available by prescription only. Use of these nicotine substitution products is not without complications. They do not treat underlying

Clinical Manifestations and Therapies
Nicotine Addiction

ETIOLOGY	CLINICAL MANIFESTATIONS	CLINICAL THERAPIES
Smoking: Cigarettes, cigars, pipes	*Early manifestations* ↑ Wrinkles in the skin, yellowing of fingers and fingernails due to impact on cellular radiation ↓ Sense of smell → Smell of smoke in hair, clothing ↑ Restlessness when cigarettes or smoking time curtailed *Late manifestations* ▪ Chronic cough ▪ COPD ▪ Increased mucus production ▪ Lung, stomach, bladder, oral, or laryngeal cancers	▪ Bronchodilators ▪ Expectorants ▪ Oxygen therapy ▪ Coughing and deep breathing ▪ Positioning ▪ Smoking cessation ▪ Nicotine replacement therapy ▪ Chemotherapy ▪ Radiation therapy ▪ Supportive care (group and individual support and/or therapy; motivational strategies) ▪ Pain management
Chewing tobacco	▪ Gum disease and gum recession ▪ Staining and wearing down of teeth ▪ Tooth decay, tooth loss ▪ ↑ Risk for cardiovascular disorders ▪ Oral cancers (gums, lips, tongue, floor and roof of mouth)	▪ Tobacco cessation programs ▪ Nicotine replacement therapy ▪ Daily dental hygiene and regular professional dental care ▪ Supportive care (group and individual support and/or therapy; motivational strategies) ▪ Cancer treatment as necessary ▪ Pain management as necessary

Patient Teaching
What Is Too Much Nicotine?

A potential issue with nicotine patches and gum in nicotine replacement therapy is that some of the transdermal patches and gum are designed for heavy smokers and may contain too large of a dose of nicotine. Depending on weight and customary nicotine usage, patients may experience unpleasant side effects from ingesting too much nicotine. Some of these signs include abdominal cramps, nausea, or vomiting; chest pain or difficulty breathing; rapid heart rate; panic attacks; dizziness; ringing in the ears; anxiety or agitation; headache; and muscle twitching.

Keep in mind that there is the possibility of nicotine poisoning with children who chew on patches or gum. This may present a medical emergency. Because of this risk, teach consumers to store NRT products out of the reach of children.

psychologic needs or address addictive behaviors associated with tobacco use. They also come with contraindications and warnings. Nurses should provide information about these contraindications and warnings to patients considering NRT. Nurses also should encourage patients to use nicotine therapy in combination with a smoking cessation program that will help them address the psychologic issues related to nicotine abuse.

Smoking Cessation Programs

Smoking cessation programs provide peer support, group therapy, and behavior therapy modifications that can help patients who smoke to quit smoking. The websites of the U.S. Surgeon General, the CDC, the American Heart Association, and the American Lung Association all provide information about smoking cessation programs and other means of quitting smoking.

》 Stay Current: The U.S. Department of Health and Human Services provides information and resources to help individuals quit smoking at the website http://betobaccofree.hhs.gov.

Complementary Health Approaches

A number of complementary therapies have been advocated as tools for quitting smoking, hypnotherapy and acupuncture among them. Generally speaking, any therapy that helps reduce patient anxiety levels, such as yoga and massage, will lower the likelihood that the patient will want to use nicotine to alleviate anxiety.

There is conflicting evidence about the success of hypnotherapy as a smoking cessation tool. As with any type of therapy, the qualifications and experience of the therapist have an effect on the success of the therapy. To increase the likelihood of success, nurses should encourage patients who are considering hypnotherapy also to participate in more traditional cessation programs.

Lifespan Considerations
Nicotine Addiction in Adolescents

In 2014, 1.7 million adolescents age 12 to 17 used tobacco products during the past month, and 1.2 million reported smoking cigarettes (CBHSQ, 2015). From 2002 to 2014, the percentage of adolescents who used tobacco in the past month declined roughly by half, from 15.2 to 7.0%. Similarly, the percentage of adolescents who were current cigarette smokers in 2014 was lower than the percentages in 2002 to 2013. In 2002, for example, about 1 in 8 adolescents were current cigarette smokers, while about 1 in 20 adolescents age 12 to 17 in 2014 were current cigarette smokers (CBHSQ, 2014). However, as mentioned previously, nicotine use reports have not yet included vaping use, which has exploded.

As seen with other substances, the teen years seem to be the gateway for nicotine use. Early research studies of the psychosocial risk factors for smoking indicated that stress, peer and family influences, ethnicity, and depression all served as risk factors for the development and maintenance of smoking in adolescents (Schepis & Rao, 2005). Protective factors include parental expectations and monitoring, religious activity, and sociopolitical factors such as tobacco-related marketing bans and higher cigarette taxes (CDC, 2012, 2013b). Neurobiological research has examined the concept of disinhibition as a risk factor for smoking in adolescents (Schepis & Rao, 2005).

Among young people, the short-term health consequences of smoking include respiratory and nonrespiratory effects, addiction to nicotine, and the associated risk of other drug use (World Health Organization [WHO], 2015b). Significantly, most young people who smoke regularly continue to smoke throughout adulthood. Smoking harms both performance and endurance in teen sports. Smoking reduces the rate of lung growth and reduces lung function: Teenage smokers experience shortness of breath almost three times more often than teens who do not smoke and produce phlegm more than twice as often as teens who do not smoke. Young adult smokers also show early vascular signs of heart disease and stroke and are at increased risk of lung cancer. The resting heart rates of young adult smokers are two to three beats per minute faster than those of nonsmokers. On average, someone who smokes a pack or more of cigarettes each day lives 7 years less than someone who never smoked (WHO, 2015b).

Smoking among adolescents is associated with increased risk for use of other substances. Teens who smoke are 3 times more likely than nonsmokers to use alcohol, 8 times more likely to use marijuana, and 22 times more likely to use cocaine. Smoking is associated with a host of other risky behaviors, such as fighting and engaging in unprotected sex (WHO, 2015b).

Nicotine Addiction in Pregnant Women

Generally speaking, pregnant women smoke at lower rates than women who are not pregnant, and this seems to hold true across all age groups. While there is some evidence of decline in smoking as pregnancy progresses, it is perhaps not enough: in 2012–2013, smoking rates of pregnant women age 15 to 44 were 19.9% in the first trimester, 13.4% in the second trimester, and 12.8% in the third trimester (CBHSQ, 2014).

There is a substantial body of literature documenting the dangers of maternal nicotine use for the fetus. First, there are the more than 4000 chemicals in cigarette smoke, more than

40 of which are known carcinogens. Nicotine crosses the placenta, and fetal concentrations of nicotine can be 15% higher than maternal concentrations (Knopik et al., 2012). Maternal cigarette smoking during pregnancy is associated with increased risk for spontaneous abortion, preterm delivery, respiratory disease, immune system difficulties such as asthma and allergies, and cancer later in life. Various studies link placental complications linked to prenatal exposure to cigarette smoke, including alterations to the development and function of the placenta. A body of research has suggested that prenatal tobacco exposure has been associated with serious neurodevelopmental and behavioral consequences in infants, children, and adolescents, including delayed psychomotor and mental development, increased physical aggression during early childhood, attention deficits, issues with learning and memory, increased impulsivity, and speech and language impairments (Knopik et al., 2012).

Nicotine Addiction in Older Adults

A 2012 survey of Medicare recipients found that 8.8% were current smokers; 44.7% and 46.5% of the sample, respectively, were former and never smokers (Choi & DiNitto, 2015). Current smokers had lower socioeconomic status, were more socially isolated, and had higher depressive symptoms than older adults who never smoked. Among the admitted smokers, 88.9% of them continued to smoke. The odds of successful smoking cessation increased if the individual received a new diagnosis of chronic illness (Choi & DiNitto, 2015). However, the odds decrease in those who are heavy smokers; these patients may require extended pharmacotherapy and counseling to be successful in smoking cessation.

Among people 50 and older, smokers are more likely to report health problems such as coughing, trouble breathing, and getting tired more easily than nonsmokers. Smoking often worsens existing medical conditions. Smoking increases the risk of many types of cancer, especially cancers along the respiratory and GI tracts (National Institutes of Health [NIH], 2015). Smoking has also been linked to diseases other than cancer in seniors, including pulmonary and cardiovascular diseases, diabetes complications, bone disease, bone density loss, cataracts, and stomach ulcers. Smokers are up to 10 times more likely to get cancer than a person who has never smoked (NIH, 2015).

NURSING PROCESS

Nurses may interact with patients addicted to nicotine in a variety of settings ranging from acute care to outpatient centers. Nurses often note the smell of smoke on a nicotine user and can implement a plan of care aimed at helping the patient make healthier lifestyle choices. Because of the high rate of smoking among patients with mental health disorders, psychiatric facilities are a common place to meet patients with nicotine addictions. It is not uncommon for patients to have addictions to multiple substances, and nurses should assess for other substance abuse problems. A nonjudgmental approach is important when caring for patients addicted to nicotine. Health promotion efforts are directed toward education about making healthy life choices and strategies to support the patient in abstaining from nicotine. Through

school programs, nurses can provide adolescents with ways to avoid peer pressure, thereby preventing nicotine use.

Assessment

When assessing patients who use nicotine, it is important to assess for amount and frequency of use, length of time nicotine has been used, and the presence of any symptoms indicating possible complications such as a chronic cough, shortness of breath, hypertension, chest pain, or unexpected symptoms. A comprehensive approach to the assessment of substance use is essential to ensure adequate and appropriate intervention. Three important areas to assess are a history of the patient's past substance use, medical and psychiatric history, and the presence of psychosocial concerns. Part of every assessment of individuals who abuse nicotine should be to determine their willingness and motivation to consider abstinence. Ask questions in a nonthreatening, matter-of-fact manner, phrased so as not to imply wrongdoing. Open-ended questions, such as the following, that elicit more than a simple yes or no answer help to determine the direction of future counseling:

- On average, how long have you used nicotine-containing products?

- On a typical day, how many cigarettes (cigars or pipes) do you smoke (or how much tobacco do you chew)?

- When did you last smoke or use tobacco?

- What kinds of problems has nicotine use caused for you and your family, friends, finances, and health? How much money do you think you spend on smoking or tobacco use?

- Tell me about any attempts you've made to quit using nicotine. How long did you quit? What made you return to nicotine use?

- How do you feel about the idea of being nicotine-free? Do you want help to quit now?

The patient's medical history is another important area for assessment and should include the existence of any concomitant physical or mental condition. Ask about prescribed and over-the-counter medications as well as any allergies or sensitivity to drugs. A brief overview of the patient's current mental status also is significant. Ask questions to assess patients for feelings of depression and thoughts of self-harm or harming others. Inquire about the use of nicotine by family members.

Information about the patient's level of stress and other psychosocial concerns can help in the assessment of substance use problems. Assess for the degree to which the patient's nicotine use is affecting relationships at home and work. Assess the patient's current coping mechanisms and support system.

Diagnosis

Every patient is unique, and the choice of the nursing diagnosis will depend on the type of complications the patient may be experiencing as a result of nicotine use. The needs of a patient being treated for lung cancer or heart disease after years of smoking will differ from the needs of the adolescent patient who may not yet be experiencing adverse effects from the newly begun habit. Possible nursing diagnoses include the following:

- *Injury, Risk for*
- *Denial, Ineffective*
- *Coping, Ineffective*
- *Airway Clearance, Ineffective*
- *Anxiety.*

(NANDA-I © 2014)

Planning

When designing the plan of care, the nurse must put the patient's needs, and no other expectations, at the forefront of the plan. If the patient has no motivation to make healthier life choices, the nurse must respect the choices the patient makes. Goals for patient care may include the following:

- The patient will verbalize the negative effects, both short term and cumulative, associated with smoking.
- The patient will voice strategies for support with quitting if/when the patient is ready to stop smoking.
- The patient will identify three activities that can aid in avoiding nicotine use.
- The patient will not experience complications as a result of nicotine use.

Implementation

The nurse's role regarding smoking is to (a) serve as a role model by not smoking, (b) provide educational information regarding the dangers of smoking, (c) help make smoking socially unacceptable (e.g., by posting no-smoking signs in patient lounges and offices), and (d) suggest resources such as hypnosis, lifestyle training, and behavior modification to patients who want to stop smoking. Nurses also can promote health related to tobacco by being aware of marketing efforts that target young adults. The tobacco industry has developed very effective campaigns to encourage smoking among young adults by advertising and sponsoring entertainment events.

Federal and state public policies have been some of the most effective tools at combating smoking. Some of these included making tobacco products less affordable; restricting tobacco marketing; banning smoking in public places, for example, workplaces, schools, day care centers, hospitals, restaurants, hotels, and parks; and requiring tobacco companies to label tobacco packages with information regarding health risks (CDC, 2012). Mass media campaigns against tobacco use, such as TV ads, have proven effective at helping prevent tobacco use by young people. Studies show that teens respond most to ads that trigger strong negative feelings, such as ads about the dangerous health effects of smoking and secondhand smoke and ads that expose the tobacco industry's marketing strategies that target young people (CDC, 2012). Even ads targeted for adult audiences help reduce tobacco use among young people. Finally, major league sports organizations have launched anti-tobacco media campaigns aimed at children and young adults. The focus of the campaigns has been athletes who use smokeless tobacco, implicated in oral, pancreatic, and esophageal cancers; mouth lesions; and tooth decay (Campaign for Tobacco-Free Kids, 2015). See the module on Oxygenation for additional interventions related to smoking cessation.

Evaluation

Patients are evaluated on the basis of the goals created during the planning stage. Expected outcomes may include the following:

- The patient describes feelings regarding nicotine use, abstinence, and methods of coping without the use of nicotine.
- The patient verbalizes negative effects on his or her own life and the lives of loved ones as a result of nicotine use.
- The patient is free of injury or complications resulting from nicotine use.
- The patient describes strategies that will be or can be useful when beginning a program to quit smoking.

Nurses should not be surprised when patients have difficulty quitting. The American Cancer Society (ACS) (2014) has noted that smoking cessation programs, like other programs that treat addictions, often have a fairly low success rate. The ACS has stated that only about 4 to 7% of people are able to successfully quit smoking on any given attempt without medications or other help. However, the success rate increases for patients who use adjunct therapies with nicotine replacement therapy. According to the ACS, studies in medical journals have reported that about 25% of smokers who use medications can stay smoke-free for more than 6 months. Clinicians should consider adding medications combined with counseling and other types of emotional support to boost success rates.

REVIEW Nicotine Use

RELATE Link the Concepts and Exemplars

Linking the exemplar of nicotine use with the concept of oxygenation:

1. Describe the pathophysiology of the respiratory system and the ability of the alveoli to oxygenate the tissues when a patient smokes.

2. While caring for a patient who is known to have smoked for more than 30 years, how would you amend your nursing plan of care as related to oxygenation?

Linking the exemplar of nicotine use with the concept of grief and loss:

3. The nurse is caring for a patient with terminal lung cancer and is talking with the family. The patient's daughter says, "If Dad wanted to stay around and be with us, he wouldn't have made the choice to smoke." How would you respond to this statement and help the family members deal with their anger over the patient's lifestyle choices?

4. Why might a patient with acute COPD who continues to smoke be denied a lung transplant? How can you help this patient

(and family) deal with the grief and loss they experience as a result of this decision?

READY Go to Volume 3: Clinical Nursing Skills

REFER Go to Pearson MyLab Nursing and eText

- Additional review materials
- Nursing Care Plan for a Patient with Nicotine Addiction

REFLECT Apply Your Knowledge

Mr. Wojikowski, a 50-year-old professional, has pneumonia and is currently being treated with antibiotics. He smokes two packs of cigarettes a day. Since this bout of pneumonia, he voices concern about his smoking and wonders if he should try to quit again. He states,

"I've tried everything and nothing works. The longest I last is about 1 month." He admits to being 30 pounds overweight and states that his wife and he have started walking 30 minutes every evening. His wife also has started making low-fat meals. He is concerned that if he quits smoking, he will gain more weight.

1. What information or knowledge is important for the nurse to remember when assisting a patient to advance to the next stage of change?

2. Each contact between a nurse and a patient is an opportunity for health promotion. Based on the knowledge or key concepts listed above, what question(s) would you ask Mr. Wojikowski?

3. In which state of change is Mr. Wojikowski relating to his cigarette smoking? What strategies could you, the nurse, consider?

» Exemplar 22.C
Substance Abuse

Exemplar Learning Outcomes

22.C Analyze manifestations and treatment considerations for patients who abuse substances.

- Describe the pathophysiology of substance abuse.
- Describe the etiology of substance abuse.
- Compare the risk factors and prevention of substance abuse.
- Identify clinical manifestations of substance abuse.
- Summarize diagnostic tests and therapies used by interprofessional teams in the collaborative care of an individual who abuses substances.
- Differentiate care of patients across the lifespan who abuse substances.
- Apply the nursing process in providing culturally competent care to an individual who abuses substances.

Exemplar Key Terms

Amphetamine, *1692*
Caffeine, *1690*
Cannabis sativa, *1691*
Central nervous system (CNS) depressants, *1691*
Craving, *1688*
Hallucinogens, *1692*
Impaired control, *1688*
Inhalants, *1693*
Kindling, *1689*
Neonatal abstinence syndrome (NAS), *1694*
Opiates, *1692*
Psychostimulants, *1691*
Risky use, *1688*
Social impairment, *1688*
Substance abuse, *1688*
Tolerance, *1689*
Withdrawal, *1689*

Overview

Substance abuse refers to the use of any chemical in a manner inconsistent with medical or culturally defined social norms despite physical, psychologic, or social adverse effects. A substance use disorder (SUD) is a cluster of cognitive, behavioral, and physiologic symptoms that indicate continued use of a substance despite significant negative consequences such as illness, functional impairment, or disruption of relationships (APA, 2013). Although all SUDs have common psychologic symptoms, researchers recently have been focusing on the underlying physiologic changes in brain circuitry that often persist even after detoxification, especially in individuals with severe disorders. It is believed that these permanent brain changes cause the behavioral effects characteristics of individuals with SUD, such as repeated relapses and intense substance craving (APA, 2013).

To be diagnosed with an SUD, an individual must exhibit a problematic pattern of substance use and a pathologic pattern of behaviors related to substance use. Patterns of symptoms recognized as part of the diagnostic criteria for SUD from the DSM-5 include symptoms related to impaired

control, social impairment, and risky use, as well as pharmacologic criteria (APA, 2013).

Symptoms of **impaired control** include taking a substance in larger amounts over a longer period of time; wanting to reduce use and reporting multiple unsuccessful attempts to cut down or quit; spending a lot of time obtaining, using, or recovering from the effects of the substance; and having daily activities that revolve around the substance. **Craving**, an intense desire for the substance, where it is difficult to think of anything else, also falls in the category of impaired control (APA, 2013). Craving often causes individuals to start using substances again.

Social impairment or dysfunction due to substance use may exhibit as failure to fulfill major roles at work, school, or home; continued substance use despite ongoing or recurrent social or interpersonal problems caused by the substance; and abandonment of or withdrawal from family, occupational, social, and/or recreational obligations and activities (APA, 2013).

Risky use is defined as repeated use of substances in situations in which it is physically hazardous and despite knowledge that the individual has a persistent physical or psychologic problem caused or worsened by substance use (APA, 2013). Pharmacologic criteria or symptoms include **tolerance**, needing a markedly larger dose of substance to achieve the desired effect of the substance. When attempting **withdrawal**, that is, abstinence from substances, the individual experiences uncomfortable withdrawal symptoms that often prompt resumed consumption of the substance (APA, 2013). Withdrawal occurs when an individual reduces or stops a drug that has been used heavily over a long period of time; it consists of a cluster of substance-specific behavioral symptoms with physiologic and cognitive components. Withdrawal causes clinically significant distress or impairment in social, occupational, or other important areas of function (APA, 2013). When an individual stops using a substance, uncomfortable, distressing, or even dangerous withdrawal symptoms can occur within hours. Depending on the amount of drugs consumed, withdrawal may put the patient in medical danger and may last up to several days.

The DSM-5 includes 10 separate classes of substances, ranging from alcohol, caffeine, and tobacco to cannabis, hallucinogens, opioids, sedatives, and stimulants (APA, 2013). For the purpose of this exemplar, the term *substance abuse* refers specifically to drugs, both legal and illegal, that lead to addiction and dependence. Because alcohol and nicotine are often abused, they are covered in separate exemplars in this concept. Three other commonly abused substances are cannabis (marijuana), opioids, and stimulants, which are discussed later in this exemplar.

Substance use disorders can range in severity from mild to severe, depending on the number of symptoms displayed by the individual. Substances can also induce disorders, such as psychosis experienced from taking hallucinogens. Substance use or abuse may co-occur with other mental health disorders, such as anxiety and depression. Approximately 20% of Americans with an anxiety or mood disorder such as depression also have an alcohol or other substance use disorder (Anxiety and Depression Association of America [ADAA], 2015). Substance use disorders by themselves are second only to mood disorders as the most frequent risk factors for suicidal behaviors (Office of the Surgeon General and National Action Alliance for Suicide Prevention, 2012).

Pathophysiology and Epidemiology

Pathophysiology

The pathophysiology of substance abuse was discussed earlier in the module. In summary, it is a complex, multifactorial process that involves a combination of biological, genetic, psychologic, and sociocultural factors. These factors and others may affect the process of recovery. For example, the craving that an individual has for a particular substance may be heightened by a phenomenon known as the kindling effect. **Kindling** refers to long-term changes in brain neurotransmission that occur after repeated detoxifications (Breese, Sinha, & Heilig, 2011). Recurrent detoxifications increase neuron sensitivity and are thought to intensify obsessive thoughts or cravings for a substance. Eventually, the brain responds spontaneously in a dysfunctional manner even when the substance is no longer being

used (Alterman, 2014). This phenomenon may explain why subsequent episodes of withdrawal from a substance tend to get progressively worse.

Etiology and Epidemiology

As stated earlier, the etiology of substance use is multifactorial, and it varies among individuals. Adolescents, for example, may begin to use if friends or peers are using, and then continue to use when they find that the drug activates the brain's reward center and results in a desired effect. In contrast, an adult who experiences a severe injury may initially take an opiate, such as OxyContin, for pain relief and find himself needing more of the drug to continue to cope with psychologic consequences of the injury well after the injury has physically healed. Regardless of the initial reasons for use, however, most individuals experience similar patterns of tolerance and dependency the longer they continue to use a substance. Individuals who use substances within the context of a drug culture may be more resistant to treatment and are at greater risk for relapse (see the Focus on Diversity and Culture feature).

As stated earlier, in 2015, more than 27 million Americans reported the current use of illicit drugs of misuse or prescription drugs (Surgeon General, 2016). The most commonly used illicit drug is marijuana. Approximately 22.5 million people age 22 or older used marijuana in 2014. An estimated 6.5 million people reported nonmedical use of psychotherapeutic drugs in the past month, including 4.3 million nonmedical users of prescription pain relievers. Thus, the number of current nonmedical users of pain relievers was second to marijuana among specific illicit drugs. Over half of first-time users (54.1%) were younger than age 18 when they first used, and more than half of new users were female. The 2013 average age of first use among those age 12 to 49 was 19.0 years. Of those using illicit drugs for the first time in 2013, 70.3% reported marijuana as their first drug (CBHSQ, 2014).

Substance use disorders in the United States cost over $700 billion a year, including the costs of treatment, related health problems, absenteeism, lost productivity, drug-related crime and incarceration, and education and prevention. This includes $224 billion for alcohol, and $193 billion for illicit drugs, and $295 billion for tobacco (NIDA, 2015b, 2015d). The relapse rates for drug addiction are 40–60%, comparable to relapse rates of other chronic illnesses, such as diabetes, hypertension, and asthma (NIDA, 2014a). Although cocaine, hallucinogens, inhalants, and heroin continue to be popular, marijuana use has experienced the greatest increase (CBHSQ, 2014).

In 2012, an estimated 2.1 million people in the United States experienced SUD related to prescription opioid pain relievers, and an estimated 467,000 were addicted to heroin (NIDA, 2014d). Use of prescription opioids (including OxyContin, hydrocodone, and morphine) is being increasingly examined, and individuals with chronic pain are being referred more often to pain specialists who frequently rely on nonopioid analgesics. Regulatory agencies and third-party payers have tightened control of prescriptions, and pharmaceutical manufacturers have introduced abuse-deterrent formulations of opioid medications. The result has been a transition to abuse of heroin, which is cheaper and in some communities easier to obtain than prescription opioids (NIDA, 2014d). Heroin abuse is dangerous because of the drug's addictiveness and its high risk for overdosing. With heroin, this danger is compounded by the lack of control over the purity of the injected drug and its possible contamination with other drugs. Heroin use has increased across the United States among men and women, most age groups, and all income levels. Some of the greatest increases occurred in demographic groups with historically low rates of heroin use: women, the privately insured, and people with higher incomes. As heroin use has increased, so have heroin-related overdose deaths. Between 2002 and 2013, the rate of heroin-related overdose deaths nearly quadrupled, and more than 8200 people died in 2013 (CDC, 2015e).

SAFETY ALERT Naloxone hydrochloride is a lifesaving medication that can stop or reverse the effects of an opioid or heroin overdose. Drug overdose deaths, driven largely by prescription drug overdoses, are now the leading cause of injury death in the United States—surpassing motor vehicle crashes. Naloxone (also known as Narcan) is available in nasal spray and injectable forms over the counter, can be used in adults or children, and is easily administered by anyone, even those without medical training (Food and Drug Administration, 2015). Family members and support persons of individuals with known addiction problems should acquire these rescue medications and prepare themselves to administer them in case of an overdose.

Focus on Diversity and Culture
Key Characteristics of a Drug Culture

Besides needing an understanding of current drug cultures—to help prevent infiltration of related behaviors and attitudes within the treatment environment—mental health clinicians also must help patients understand how such cultures support use and pose dynamic relapse risks (SAMHSA, 2014b). Drug cultures can change rapidly and vary across racial and ethnic groups, geographic areas, socioeconomic levels, and generations. Some of the questions used to obtain information about a particular drug culture center on the group's processes for establishing trust and credibility; socialization and values; obtaining status; gender roles and relationships; concepts of sanction, punishment, and conflict mediation; symbols, images, and dress; language and communication; and attitudes.

While there may be overlap among members, drug cultures differ based on substance used—even among people from similar ethnic and socioeconomic backgrounds (SAMHSA, 2014b). Drug cultures can differ according to geographic area as well as other social factors, such as socioeconomic status. For example, the drug culture of young, affluent people who use heroin can mirror the drug culture of street users, but it will also have notable differences. Finally, drug cultures change over time: Older people from New York who use heroin and who entered the drug culture in the 1950s or 1960s feel marginalized within the current drug scene, which they see as promoting a different set of values (SAMHSA, 2014b).

Risk Factors

Risk factors for drug abuse are multifactorial and can affect individuals of any age, gender, or economic status. Some factors that affect the likelihood and speed of developing an addiction include a family history of addiction; the presence of another mental disorder; the use of drugs as a coping mechanism to manage anxiety or depression; peer pressure; and lack of family involvement. Although men are more likely to experience problems with drugs than women, progression of addiction is faster among women than men (Mayo Clinic, 2015b).

Clinical Manifestations

Clinical manifestations, and their severity, depend on amount, frequency, and specific combination of substances used. Combining two CNS depressants, for example, will produce far more significant manifestations than using only one CNS depressant. Some symptoms can be alarming or even fatal. For example, long-term crack use can result in sensory hallucinations, and even the first use of cocaine can result in death for individuals with undiagnosed cardiac disorders. Clinical manifestations are linked to specific substances in the following sections.

Caffeine

Caffeine is a stimulant that increases the heart rate and acts as a diuretic. Although commonly consumed daily in soft drinks, coffee, tea, chocolate, and some pain relievers, an excessive amount of caffeine can cause negative physiologic effects, especially cardiac-related risks. Approximately 300 mg/day is safe for most healthy adults, but over 600 mg is considered excessive and is not recommended (Kneisl & Trigoboff, 2013). Individuals with a history of cardiac disease should be advised to cut down caffeine intake or eliminate it altogether. Caffeine, if consumed in large quantities, also can cause higher total cholesterol levels and insomnia.

Many individuals recognize the adverse effects of too much caffeine in their system and voluntarily cut down by drinking decaffeinated beverages. An individual who is addicted to caffeine and abruptly withdraws from it will most likely experience headaches and irritability. However, even with evidence of withdrawal symptoms, some clinicians do not consider caffeine as addicting, because it does not have a major action on the mesolimbic dopamine system (McNeece & DiNitto, 2012).

A rising number of adolescents are developing symptoms of caffeine dependence from consuming sizable quantities of caffeinated energy drinks. Energy drinks contain caffeine that ranges from 50 mg to 500 mg per can or bottle, compared with the average can of cola that has 35 mg (CDC, 2014). Researchers predict an increase in caffeine intoxication and problems with caffeine dependence and withdrawal, including sleep issues. Genetic factors may also play a role in these clinical manifestations.

According to the CDC (2014), young people who ingest energy drinks are more likely to participate in unhealthy behaviors, including alcohol use. Of particular concern are alcoholic beverages mixed with energy drinks, because the caffeine in these drinks can mask the depressant effects of alcohol. Individuals who consume alcohol mixed with energy drinks are three times more likely to binge drink and are twice as likely to report being taken advantage of sexually, to report taking advantage of someone else sexually, and to report riding with a driver who was under the influence of alcohol than drinkers who do not mix caffeine with alcohol (CDC, 2015a). Furthermore, researchers have found that recent traumatic brain injury (TBI) is more strongly related to consuming alcohol, energy drinks, and energy drinks and alcohol mixed. Consumption of these substances may be a coping mechanism to deal with the effects of TBI, or they may predispose adolescents to TBI, or both (Ilie et al., 2015).

Cannabis

Cannabis sativa is the source of marijuana. The greatest concentrations of psychoactive substances are in the flowering tops of the cannabis plant. Marijuana (also known as grass, weed, pot, dope, joint, and reefer) and hashish are the most common derivatives. The psychoactive component of marijuana is an oily chemical known as delta-9-tetrahydrocannabinol (THC). THC activates specific cannabinoid receptors in the brain and may act like opioids and cocaine in producing a pleasurable sensation.

The physiologic effects of cannabis are dose related and can cause an increase in heart rate and bronchodilation with short-term use. Chronic long-term use can lead to airway constriction and inflammation, and increased incidence of acute and chronic bronchitis (World Health Organization [WHO], 2013). Cannabis use also causes decreased spermatogenesis and testosterone levels in men and suppresses follicle-stimulating, luteinizing, and prolactin hormones in women, making breastfeeding impossible for new mothers. Birth defects also may be associated with cannabis use. Marijuana crosses the placental barrier and is spread to fetal tissues.

Euphoria and relaxation are the pleasurable effects most associated with marijuana use. Other subjective effects of marijuana include sedation and hallucinations. With increased use, marijuana can result in amotivational behaviors such as apathy, dullness, poor grooming, reduced interest in achievement, and disinterest. Memory impairment is common, because of the alteration of how information is processed in the hippocampus.

It is estimated that 9% of people who use marijuana will become dependent on it. The number increases to about 17% in those who start using at a young age (in their teens) and to 25 to 50% among daily users (NIDA, 2015c). Marijuana addiction is linked to a mild withdrawal syndrome, with frequent users reporting irritability, mood and sleep difficulties, decreased appetite, cravings, restlessness, and/or various forms of physical discomfort that peak within the first week after quitting and last up to 2 weeks.

A new health concern is the potency of cannabis, which has steadily increased over the past few decades. In the early 1990s, the average tetrahydrocannabinol (THC, a psychoactive substance) content in confiscated cannabis samples was roughly 3.7% for marijuana and 7.5% for *sinsemilla*, a higher-potency marijuana from specially tended female plants (NIDA, 2015c). In 2013, the THC content was 9.6% for marijuana and 16% for sinsemilla. Also, new methods of smoking or eating THC-rich hash oil extracted from the marijuana plant (a practice called "dabbing") may deliver very high levels of THC to the user. The average marijuana extract contains over 50% THC, with some samples exceeding 80% (NIDA, 2015c). These trends raise concerns that the consequences of marijuana use could be worse than in the past, particularly among new users or in young people, whose brains are still developing.

The 2013 *National Survey on Drug Use and Health* found that marijuana continues to be the most common illicit drug used (CBHSQ, 2014). In 2013, there were 19.8 million current users age 12 or older (7.5%), with as many as 11.7% of 8th graders reporting marijuana use in the past year. By 12th grade, 35.1% had used marijuana during the year prior to the survey and 21.2% were current users, with 5.8% saying they used marijuana daily or near daily (NIDA, 2015c).

Central Nervous System Depressants

Central nervous system (CNS) depressants, including barbiturates, benzodiazepines, paraldehyde, meprobamate, and chloral hydrate, also are subject to abuse. Cross-dependence exists among all CNS depressants, and cross-tolerance can develop to alcohol and general anesthetics. Chronic users of barbiturates require progressively higher doses to achieve subjective effects as tolerance develops, but they develop little tolerance to respiratory depression. The depressant effects related to barbiturates are dose dependent and range from mild sedation to sleep to coma to death. With larger doses over time and a combination of alcohol and barbiturates, the risk of death increases greatly.

The risk of accidental overdose and death resulting from barbiturates has resulted in decreased use, yet barbiturates are still clinically useful in treating seizure disorders and alcohol withdrawal. Benzodiazepines remain an option for short-term treatment of anxiety. Benzodiazepines alone are safer than barbiturates because an overdose of oral benzodiazepines rarely results in death. However, when taken together, CNS depressants (for example, alcohol and benzodiazepines) can result in death.

Psychostimulants

Psychostimulants such as cocaine and amphetamines have a high potential for abuse. Euphoria is the main subjective effect associated with cocaine and amphetamines, leading to addiction. Powdered cocaine has been "snorted" (inhaled through the nostrils) for thousands of years, but a more dangerous method is freebasing. Cocaine base (freebased cocaine, or "crack") is heat stable and is usually "cooked" in a baking soda solution and smoked (freebasing). Cocaine hydrochloride is diluted or cut before sale, and the pure form ("rocks") can be administered intranasally (snorted) or injected intravenously. "Skin popping" is a subcutaneous method that many substance abusers are using to administer drugs, perhaps leading to the formation of abscesses under the skin.

The duration of euphoria achieved by cocaine depends on the route of administration. Regardless, the pleasurable effects do not last long, and its highly addictive properties can easily lead to overdose. A mild overdose of cocaine produces agitation, dizziness, tremor, and blurred vision. A severe overdose produces anxiety, hyperpyrexia, convulsions, ventricular dysrhythmias, severe hypertension, and hemorrhagic stroke with possible angina or myocardial infarction.

Long-term intranasal use of cocaine can cause atrophy of the nasal mucosa, necrosis and perforation of the nasal septum, and lung damage. Crack cocaine injection requires serious attention because this drug use is associated with increased rates of high-risk behaviors (NIDA, 2013a).

Amphetamine is a powerful stimulant that poses a severe health risk to society because of its devastating physical and neurologic consequences, including amphetamine-induced mental disorders. Methamphetamine is a highly addictive form of amphetamine whose use is widespread because its manufacturing process can be carried out by individuals without special knowledge or expertise in chemistry. Methamphetamine is often taken in combination with other drugs such as cocaine and marijuana. Smoking or injection provides the greatest euphoria, although it may also be inhaled or ingested. Chronic use or abuse can result in paranoia, hallucinations, and compulsions. Some users experience delusions that insects are crawling over them, resulting in obsessive scratching. Psychosis characterized by violent behavior may also result (Partnership at Drugfree.org, 2013).

Amphetamines cause arousal and an elevation of mood with a sense of increased strength, mental capacity, and self-confidence and a decreased need for food and sleep. Tolerance to mood elevation, appetite suppression, and cardiovascular effects develops with amphetamines; however, dependence is more psychologic than physical.

Withdrawal from amphetamines produces dysphoria and craving with fatigue, prolonged sleep, excessive eating, and depression. Methamphetamine addiction can be successfully treated. Programs using a combination of individual and group therapy designed to promote behavioral changes as well as incentive-based programs have been cited as effective. Although there is currently no proven pharmacologic therapy, research in that area continues (NIDA, 2013b).

Opiates

Opiates such as morphine, meperidine, codeine, hydrocodone, oxymorphone, and oxycodone are narcotic analgesics. Some common brand names include Vicodin, Percocet, Oxy-Contin, and Opana. Narcotic analgesics are a type of pain reliever derived from natural or synthetic opiates. It is estimated that between 26.4 million and 36 million people abuse opioids worldwide, with an estimated 2.1 million people in the United States experiencing substance use disorders related to prescription opioid pain relievers in 2012 (NIDA, 2014d). The consequences of this abuse have been devastating. For

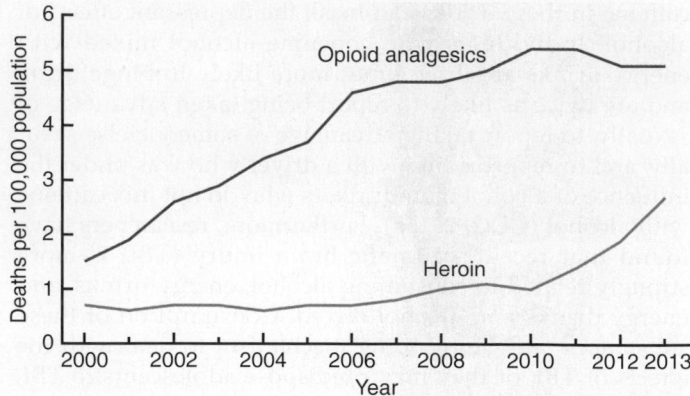

Source: From CDC. (2015). *Drug-poisoning deaths involving heroin: United States, 2000–2013.* Retrieved from http://www.cdc.gov/nchs/data/databriefs/db190.htm

Figure 22–6 》 While the age-adjusted rate for drug-poisoning deaths involving opioid analgesics has leveled in recent years, the rate for deaths involving heroin has almost tripled since 2010.

example, the number of unintentional overdose deaths from prescription pain relievers in the United States has more than quadrupled since 1999, although it is now leveling off (**Figure 22–6 》**). Further, drug abuse–related ED visits involving narcotic analgesics increased 153% in the nation from 2004 to 2011, with 420,040 ED visits in 2011 (Crane, 2015). Although the use of narcotic analgesics for acute pain management looks benign, long-term use has been associated with significant rates of abuse or addiction. Three problematic physiologic effects are hyperalgesia, hypogonadism, and sexual dysfunction (Manchikanti et al., 2010).

Heroin is an opiate that has been abused for many centuries and is usually administered intravenously. It induces a "rush" or "kick" that lasts less than a minute, followed by a sense of euphoria lasting several hours. Tolerance develops to the euphoria, respiratory depression, and nausea, but not to constipation and miosis. Physical dependence occurs with long-term use of opiates (**Figure 22–7 》**). Initial withdrawal symptoms such as drug craving, lacrimation (tear production), rhinorrhea, yawning, and diaphoresis usually take 10 days to run their course. The second phase of opiate withdrawal lasts for months, with insomnia, irritability, fatigue, and potential GI hyperactivity and premature ejaculation as problems.

Methadone is a synthetic opiate used to treat chronic pain and addiction to other opiates. Methadone does not hinder ability to function productively as other narcotics do, and it is a viable support for withdrawal (NIDA, 2014b).

Hallucinogens

Hallucinogens, also called *psychedelics,* include PCP, 3,4-MDMA, D-lysergic acid diethylamide (LSD), mescaline, dimethyltryptamine (DMT), and psilocin. Psychedelics bring on the same types of thoughts, perceptions, and feelings that occur in dreams. PCP (also called *angel dust*) was developed in the 1950s as an anesthetic similar to ketamine.

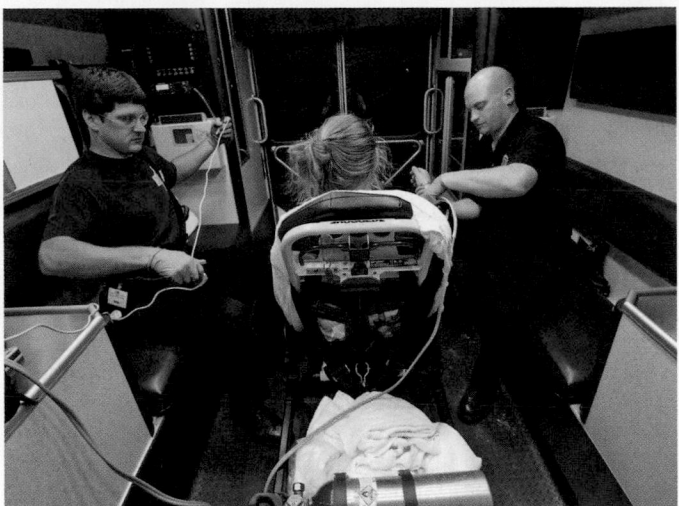

Source: Derek Davis/Portland Press Herald/Getty Images.

Figure 22–7 》 Paramedics monitor a 29-year-old woman after she was found unconscious from a heroin overdose. The woman thanked the paramedics, one of whom recognized her from an overdose about a month ago. "At least I still have my shoes this time" said the woman who told the paramedics that she normally uses ½ gram of heroin twice a day, but had cut her dose to ¼ gram that night because she had heard that it was stronger than usual.

Because of its severe side effects, its development for human use was discontinued. The most common route of administration is smoking tobacco, marijuana, or herbal cigarettes laced with PCP powder or the liquid form of PCP. In the clinical setting, patients experiencing PCP intoxication are often violent and difficult to control physically. A chemical restraint is frequently needed to protect other patients and staff from an agitated PCP user. Haloperidol (Haldol) has been evaluated as an effective medical intervention that does not cause harm to the patient (MacNeal et al., 2012).

MDMA, commonly known as Ecstasy, was very popular in the 1980s as a recreational "club drug" associated with dance clubs and "raves" and has reappeared in recent years as a date or rape drug. According to the 2013 *National Survey on Drug Use and Health* data, among people age 12 or older, 0.2%, some 609,000 people, used Ecstasy (CBHSQ, 2014). Ecstasy use from 2002 to 2014 has been fairly stable. Parties where other drugs such as marijuana and alcohol are present may lead to easier access or availability of Ecstasy, thereby increasing the chances for first-time Ecstasy use.

LSD affects serotonin receptors at multiple sites in the brain and spinal cord. LSD is usually taken orally but can be injected or smoked, as in tobacco- or marijuana-laced cigarettes. The individual's response to a trip, the experience of being high on LSD, cannot be predicted. Psychologic effects (e.g., seeing bursts of radiant colors and seeing objects that appear to breathe) and flashbacks are common. Serotonin imbalance is thought to affect impulse control and may be responsible for uninhibited sexual responses in women who

have been given the drug without their knowledge. Other hallucinogens are similar to LSD but have a different potency and course of action. Because physical dependence to hallucinogens does not appear to occur, withdrawal symptoms are not present.

Inhalants

Inhalants are categorized into three types: anesthetics, volatile nitrites, and organic solvents. Nitrous oxide (laughing gas) and ether are the most abused anesthetics. Amyl nitrite, butyl nitrite, and isobutyl nitrite are volatile nitrites used especially by homosexual men to induce venodilation and anal sphincter relaxation. Amyl nitrite is manufactured for medical use, but butyl and isobutyl nitrites are sold for recreational use. Other names for butyl and isobutyl nitrites are *climax*, *rush*, and *locker room*. Street names for amyl nitrite are *poppers* and *snappers*. Brain damage or sudden death can occur the 1st, 10th, or 100th time an individual uses an inhalant, resulting in "sudden sniffing death." This danger makes the use of inhalants more hazardous than some other substances. Inhalant use is highest among adolescents (NIDA, 2012a).

Another danger is the wide assortment of organic solvents that are available to and inhaled by young children. Organic solvents are ingested by three different methods: bagging, huffing, and sniffing. *Bagging* involves pouring the solvent in a plastic bag and inhaling the vapor. *Huffing* refers to pouring the solvent on a rag and inhaling. *Sniffing* refers to inhaling the solvent directly from the container. Common organic solvents are toluene, gasoline, lighter fluid, paint thinner, nail polish remover, benzene, acetone, chloroform, and model airplane glue. The effects from inhaling organic solvents are similar to those of alcohol. Prolonged use can lead to multiple toxicities. There are no antidotes for these inhalants; therefore, management of overdose is supportive.

Inhalant users have a compulsion to continue using inhalants, particularly if they have abused inhalants for prolonged periods. A mild withdrawal syndrome can occur with long-term inhalant abuse (NIDA, 2012a). Research suggests that inhalant users, on average, initiate use of cigarettes, alcohol, and almost all other drugs at younger ages and display a higher lifetime prevalence of substance use disorders, including abuse of prescription drugs, when compared with substance abusers without a history of inhalant use. Research has also discovered a link between eating disorders and inhalant use among both male and female students (NIDA, 2012a).

Collaboration

Effective treatment of substance abuse and dependence results from the efforts of an interprofessional team specializing in the treatment of psychiatric and substance use disorders. Therapies may include detoxification, aversion therapy to maintain abstinence, group and individual psychotherapy, psychotropic medications, cognitive–behavioral strategies, family counseling, and self-help groups. Patients who are abusing substances can be treated in either an inpatient or outpatient setting. A substance overdose is a life-threatening condition that requires emergency hospitalization to stabilize the patient medically before any of the interventions mentioned are implemented. Several diagnostic tests can provide valuable information about the patient's physical condition and set the course for treatment.

Diagnostic Tests

The body fluids most often tested for drug content are blood and urine, although saliva, perspiration, and hair may be tested. More invasive procedures such as serum drug levels are useful in the ED and other hospital settings to treat drug overdoses or complications. Urine drug screening (UDS), which is noninvasive, is the preferred method for detecting substances in the body. The length of time that drugs can be found in blood and urine varies from 24 hours to 30 days according to dosage and metabolic properties of the drug. THC, the psychoactive substance found in marijuana, is stored in fatty tissues (especially the brain and reproductive system) and can be detected in the body for up to 6 weeks (Kneisl & Trigoboff, 2013).

Pharmacologic Therapy

Common drugs used in the treatment of substance abuse and withdrawal are presented in the Medications feature in The Concept of Addiction.

Emergency Care for Overdose

Overdose of a patient on any substance is a serious medical emergency. Respiratory depression may require mechanical ventilation. The patient may become severely sedated and difficult to arouse. Every effort must be made to keep the patient awake; however, stupor and coma often result. A seizure is another serious complication that requires emergency treatment. If the overdose was intentional, the patient must be monitored constantly for further signs of suicidal ideation. An actively suicidal patient must never be left alone. Signs of overdose and withdrawal from major substances are summarized in **Table 22–4** >> along with recommended treatments.

Complementary Health Approaches

Auricular (ear) acupuncture has been used throughout the world as an adjunctive treatment during opioid detoxification for about 30 years. Although not subjected to rigorous controlled research, auricular acupuncture has been shown in smaller studies to benefit patients dependent on heroin. Patients with mild habits appeared to benefit more than those with severe withdrawal symptoms, which acupuncture did not alleviate. The 1997 National Institute of Health Consensus Statement on acupuncture stated that acupuncture treatment for addiction could be part of a comprehensive management program. The National Acupuncture Detoxification Association has developed protocols involving ear acupuncture in group settings that originated at Lincoln Hospital in the Bronx and are used by more than 400 drug treatment programs and 40% of drug courts (SAMHSA, 2015b).

Lifespan Considerations

At various stages of life, individuals become involved with substances for an assortment of reasons. Some of the salient lifespan factors associated with substance use disorder are discussed in the following section.

Substance Abuse in Adolescents

By the time they are seniors, 50% of high school students will have taken an illegal drug and more than 20% will have used a prescription drug for nonmedical reasons (NIDA, 2014e). Teens are particularly vulnerable to substance use disorders because of their developmental stage and because their brains are still developing and malleable until the mid-20s (NIDA, 2014e).

Adolescents use illicit substances for a variety of reasons, including the desire for new experiences, an attempt to deal with problems or perform better in school, and peer pressure. Many factors influence adolescent drug use, including the availability of drugs within the neighborhood, community, and school and whether the adolescent's friends are using drugs (NIDA, 2014e). Factors such as violence, physical or emotional abuse, mental illness, or drug use in the home increase the likelihood that an adolescent will use drugs. Adolescents who use drugs may have an inherited genetic vulnerability. Personality traits such as poor impulse control, a heightened need for excitement, and mental health conditions such as depression, anxiety, or ADHD make substance use more likely (NIDA, 2014e). Drug use at an early age is an important predictor of development of a substance use disorder later.

Substance Abuse in Pregnant Women

During pregnancy, the fetus is exposed to chemicals or substances that have the potential to harm the fetus. These teratogens can cause the fetus to experience alterations ranging from developmental delays to death. Substances commonly misused include cocaine, amphetamines, barbiturates, hallucinogens, club drugs, heroin, and other narcotics. Polysubstance use, which involves combining multiple substances with alcohol, tobacco, and illicit drugs, is common. Of pregnant women age 15 to 44, an estimated 5.4% annually are illicit drug users based on data averaged across 2012 and 2013 (CBHSQ, 2014). An overview of the potential effects of selected drugs is provided in **Table 22–5** >>.

Use of opiates during pregnancy can result in a drug withdrawal syndrome in newborns called **neonatal abstinence syndrome (NAS)**. NAS is occurring in epidemic numbers: There was a fivefold increase in the proportion of babies born with NAS from 2000 to 2012, when an estimated 21,732 infants were born with NAS—equivalent to one baby experiencing opiate withdrawal born every 25 minutes in the United States (NIDA, 2015a). Newborns with NAS are more likely than other babies to also have low birth weight and respiratory complications and require an average of 16.9 days in the hospital (compared to 2.1 days for other newborns), costing hospitals an estimated $1.5 billion. The majority of these charges (as high as 81%) are paid by state Medicaid programs, reflecting the tendency of opiate-abusing mothers to be from lower-income communities (NIDA, 2015a).

TABLE 22–4 Signs and Treatment of Overdose and Withdrawal

Drug	Overdose Signs	Overdose Treatment	Withdrawal Signs	Withdrawal Treatment
CNS Depressants				
Alcohol Barbiturates Benzodiazepines	Cardiovascular or respiratory depression or arrest (mostly with barbiturates) Coma Shock Convulsions Death	*If awake:* 1. Keep awake 2. Induce vomiting 3. Use activated charcoal to absorb drug 4. Vital signs (VS) q 15 minutes *Coma:* 1. Clear airway, intubate IV fluids 2. Perform gastric lavage 3. Take seizure precautions 4. Administer hemodialysis or peritoneal dialysis if ordered 5. Assess VS as ordered 6. Assess for shock and cardiac arrest.	Nausea and vomiting Tachycardia Diaphoresis Anxiety or agitation Tremors Marked insomnia Grand mal seizures Delirium (after 5–15 years of heavy use)	Carefully titrated detoxification with similar drug *Note:* Abrupt withdrawal can lead to death
Stimulants				
Cocaine/crack Amphetamines	Respiratory distress Ataxia Hyperpyrexia Convulsions Coma Stroke Myocardial infarction Death	Management for: 1. Hyperpyrexia 2. Convulsions 3. Respiratory distress 4. Cardiovascular shock 5. Acidic urine (ammonium chloride for amphetamine).	Fatigue Depression Agitation Apathy Anxiety Sleepiness Disorientation Lethargy Craving	Antidepressants (desipramine) Dopamine agonist Bromocriptine
Opiates				
Heroin Meperidine Morphine Methadone	Pupil dilation due to anoxia Respiratory depression arrest Coma Shock Convulsions Death	Narcotic antagonist (Narcan) quickly reverses CNS depression	Yawning, insomnia Irritability Rhinorrhea Panic Diaphoresis Cramps Nausea and vomiting Muscle aches Chills and fever Lacrimation Diarrhea	Methadone tapering Clonidine-naltrexone detoxification Buprenorphine substitution
Hallucinogens				
LSD	Psychosis Brain damage Death	1. Reduce environmental stimuli 2. Have one person "talk down patient"; reassure 3. Speak slowly and clearly 4. Administer diazepam or chloral hydrate for anxiety as ordered	No pattern of withdrawal	
PCP	Possible hypertensive crisis Respiratory arrest Hyperthermia Seizures	1. Acidify urine to help excrete drug (cranberry juice, ascorbic acid); in acute stage: ammonium chloride 2. Minimize stimuli 3. Do *not* attempt to talk down; speak slowly in low voice 4. Administer diazepam or Haldol as ordered	No pattern of withdrawal	
Inhalants				
Volatile solvents such as butane, paint thinner, airplane glue, and nail polish remover	Intoxication Agitation Drowsiness Disinhibition Staggering Light-headedness Death	Support affected systems	No pattern of withdrawal	
Nitrites	Enhanced sexual pleasure	Neurologic symptoms may respond to vitamin B_{12} and folate	No pattern of withdrawal	
Anesthetics such as nitrous oxide	Giggling, laughter Euphoria	Chronic users may experience polyneuropathy and myelopathy	No pattern of withdrawal	

TABLE 22–5 Potential Effects of Selected Drugs on Fetus/Newborn

Maternal Drug	Effect on Fetus/Newborn
Heroin	Withdrawal symptoms, convulsions, intrauterine growth restriction (IUGR), tremors, irritability, sneezing, vomiting, fever, diarrhea, and abnormal respiratory function
Methadone	Fetal distress, meconium aspiration; with abrupt termination of the drug, severe withdrawal symptoms, preterm labor, rapid labor, abruption
Phenobarbital	Withdrawal symptoms Fetal growth restriction
Phenothiazine derivatives	Withdrawal, extrapyramidal dysfunction, delayed respiratory onset, hyperbilirubinemia, hypotonia or hyperactivity, decreased platelet count
Diazepam (Valium)	Hypotonia, hypothermia, low Apgar score, respiratory depression, poor sucking reflex, cleft lip
Lithium	Congenital anomalies
Amphetamine sulfate (Benzedrine)	Generalized arthritis, learning disabilities, poor motor coordination, transposition of the great vessels, cleft palate
Dextroamphetamine sulfate (Dexedrine)	Congenital heart defects, biliary atresia, limb reduction defects
Cocaine	Cerebral infarctions, microcephaly, learning disabilities, poor state organization, decreased interactive behavior, CNS anomalies, cardiac anomalies, genitourinary anomalies, sudden infant death syndrome (SIDS)
Nicotine (half to one pack cigarettes/day)	Spontaneous abortion, placental abruption, small for gestational age (SGA), small head circumference, decreased length, SIDS, attention-deficit/hyperactivity disorder (ADHD) in school-age children
PCP ("angel dust")	Withdrawal symptoms Behavioral and developmental abnormalities
LSD	Chromosomal breakage
Marijuana	IUGR

Since the late 1980s, policymakers have debated the question of how society should deal with the problem of women's substance abuse during pregnancy. At the time of this writing, only one state, Tennessee, has specifically criminalized drug use during pregnancy; however, the state court systems have relied on existing criminal laws on the books to attack prenatal substance abuse (Guttmacher Institute, 2015). Several state supreme courts have upheld convictions ruling that a woman's substance abuse in pregnancy constitutes criminal child abuse. Meanwhile, other states have expanded civil child-welfare requirements to include prenatal substance abuse, so that prenatal drug exposure can provide grounds for terminating parental rights because of child abuse or neglect. To protect the fetus, some states have authorized civil commitment, such as forced admission to an inpatient treatment program, of pregnant women who use drugs and alcohol. Some states require healthcare professionals to report or test for prenatal drug exposure, which can be used as evidence in child-welfare proceedings. In order to receive federal child abuse prevention funds, states must require healthcare providers to notify child protective services when a provider who cares for an infant is affected by illegal substance abuse (Guttmacher Institute, 2015).

>> **Stay Current:** In 2014, the FDA published the Pregnancy and Lactation Labeling Rule, which requires that drug labels be formatted to assist healthcare providers in assessing risk versus benefit for pregnant women and nursing mothers who need to take medication. See samples of the new drug labels at http://www.fda.gov/Drugs/DevelopmentApprovalProcess/DevelopmentResources/Labeling/ucm093307.htm.

Substance Abuse in Older Adults

Substance abuse in older adults is likely to increase as the population ages: It is estimated that the number of adults 50 years and older with a substance use disorder will double from 2.8 million in 2006 to 5.7 million in 2020 (CBHSQ, 2014).

Individuals 65 years and older make up only 13% of the population, yet account for more than one third of total outpatient spending on prescription medications in the United States (NIDA, 2014c). Older patients are more likely to be prescribed long-term and multiple prescriptions, and some experience cognitive decline, which may lead to improper use of medications. Also, older adults on a fixed income may abuse another person's remaining medication to save money. The high rates of comorbid illnesses in older populations, age-related changes in drug metabolism, and the potential for drug interactions make these practices more dangerous than in younger populations.

The negative consequences of substance use are more critical in older adults. Substance abuse increases the risk of falls by affecting alertness, judgment, coordination, and reaction time. Substance abuse and dependence are less likely to be recognized in older adults because many of the symptoms of abuse (e.g., insomnia, depression, loss of memory, anxiety, musculoskeletal pain) may be confused with conditions commonly seen in older patients. This results in treating the symptoms of abuse rather than diagnosing and treating the abuse itself.

Older adults can have several potentially protective factors preventing illicit and nonmedical drug use: being married, never using alcohol or tobacco, and regularly attending religious services (SAMHSA, 2015b).

NURSING PROCESS

Nurses may interact with patients experiencing substance abuse or substance dependence in a variety of settings. The most common setting is an alcohol and drug abuse treatment program where patients are hospitalized for 20 to 30 days for detoxification and inpatient therapy. Patients in these settings may be admitted voluntarily or ordered by the court to undergo treatment. Patients with substance abuse or dependence have impaired senses and risk-taking behaviors that lead to injuries from falls and accidents requiring medical attention. Therefore, nurses frequently encounter them in emergency departments and medical-surgical units. Occupational nurses and community health nurses also interact with substance-abusing patients in outpatient or assertive community treatment programs, employee assistance programs, and community health departments. Urgent care centers, pain clinics, and ambulatory care centers are other settings in which patients with substance use disorders frequently appear for minor health problems associated with chronic disorders related to substance abuse or dependence.

Nursing care of the patient with substance abuse or dependence is challenging and requires a nonjudgmental atmosphere promoting trust and respect. Nurses should provide adults with information on healthy coping mechanisms and relaxation and stress reduction techniques to decrease the risks of substance abuse. Nurses have a responsibility to educate their patients about the physiologic effects of substances on the body. Nurses must encourage and support periods of abstinence while assisting patients to make major changes in lifestyles, habits, relationships, and coping methods.

Health promotion efforts are aimed at preventing drug use among children and adolescents and reducing the risks among adults. Adolescence is the most common phase for the first experience with drugs; therefore, teenagers are a vulnerable population, often succumbing to peer pressure. Healthy lifestyles, parental support, stress management, good nutrition, and information about ways to steer clear of peer pressure are important topics for the nurse to provide in school programs.

Assessment

Observation and Patient Interview

Many high-functioning substance abusers do not fit the stereotypical picture of someone who abuses drugs or alcohol. They are often members of the community, functioning in many responsible roles. They may not drink or use drugs every day. They may avoid the serious consequences that befall most individuals with addictions and their families. High-functioning individuals with SUDs can spend years, even decades, in denial. The high-functioning substance abuser's denial may be compounded by family and friends who fail to recognize or confront the problem.

A comprehensive approach to the assessment of all patients for substance use is essential to ensure adequate and appropriate intervention. Many patients who abuse substances struggle with communication and with trust, so it is essential that nurses use therapeutic communication techniques to establish trust prior to beginning the assessment process. Open-ended questions that elicit more than a simple yes or no answer are more effective in eliciting truthful information and may help determine the direction of future counseling. Examples of open-ended questions include:

- On average, how many days per week does the patient use substances?
- On a typical day when the patient uses, how much does he or she use?
- What is the greatest number of substances the patient has used at any one time during the past month?
- What specific substance(s) did the patient take before coming to the hospital or clinic?
- How long has the patient been using substances?
- How often and how much does the patient usually use?
- What problems has substance use caused for the patient and his/her family, friends, finances, and health?

History of Past Substance Use

A thorough history of the patient's past substance use is important in order to ascertain the possibility of tolerance, physical dependence, or withdrawal syndrome. The following questions are helpful in eliciting a pattern of substance use behavior:

- How many substances has the patient used simultaneously in the past?
- How often, how much, and when did the patient first use the substance(s)?
- Is there a history of blackouts, delirium, or seizures?
- Is there a history of withdrawal syndrome, overdoses, and complications from previous substance use?
- Has the patient ever been treated in a substance abuse clinic or program?
- Has the patient ever been arrested or charged with any criminal offense while using any substance?
- Is there a family history of substance abuse?

Medical and Psychiatric History

The patient's medical history is another important area for assessment and should include the existence of any concomitant physical or mental condition (e.g., HIV, hepatitis, cirrhosis, esophageal varices, pancreatitis, gastritis, Wernicke-Korsakoff syndrome, depression, schizophrenia, anxiety, or personality disorder). The nurse should ask about prescribed and over-the-counter medications as well as any allergies or sensitivity to drugs. A brief overview of the patient's current mental status is also significant, including any history of abuse, family violence, or other trauma; current feelings of anxiety, sadness, or depression; and history or presence of suicidal or homicidal ideation.

Psychosocial Issues

Information about the patient's level of stress and other psychosocial concerns can help in the assessment of substance use problems. Ask if the patient's substance use has affected relationships with others or the patient's ability to hold a job. Inquire about stress and coping mechanisms such as avenues of social support and activities.

Screening Tools

Screening tools such as the Brief Drug Abuse Screening Test (B-DAST or DAST) (Skinner, 1982) may help the nurse determine the degree of severity of substance abuse or dependence. Screening tools provide a nonjudgmental, brief, and easy method to ascertain patterns of substance abuse behaviors. The B-DAST is a yes/no self-administered 20-item questionnaire that is useful in identifying people who may be addicted to drugs other than alcohol. A positive response to one or more questions suggests significant drug abuse problems and warrants further evaluation. Because people do not always answer self-report tools truthfully, all patients who screen positive for drug addiction should be evaluated according to other diagnostic criteria.

Nurses working with patients who experience opiate withdrawal find two scales useful for assessing symptoms: First, the *Objective Opiate Withdrawal Scale (OOWS)* has the nurse rate 13 common, physically observable signs of opiate withdrawal as being either absent or present. Second, the *Subjective Opiate Withdrawal Scale (SOWS)* asks the patient to rate 16 symptoms on a scale of 0 (not at all) to 4 (extremely). In either case, the summed total score can be used to assess the intensity of opiate withdrawal and determine the extent of a patient's physical dependence on opioids. Higher scores mean a more intense withdrawal and more physical dependence (Handelsman et al., 1987). The two scales have also proven useful in clinical research studies in the 25 years since their creation. One example used the SOWS to measure withdrawal symptoms of patients with chronic low back pain taking extended-release hydromorphone (Jamison et al., 2013).

Diagnosis

Nursing diagnoses for patients with substance abuse problems are highly individualized depending on the substance abused, the length of time the patient has abused the chemical, and the sources of support available to the patient. Common diagnoses used in the care of these patients include the following:

- *Injury, Risk for*
- *Violence, Risk for Other- or Self-Directed*
- *Denial, Ineffective*
- *Coping, Ineffective*
- *Imbalanced Nutrition: Less Than Body Requirements*
- *Chronic or Situational Low Self-Esteem*
- *Knowledge, Deficient*
- *Family Processes, Dysfunctional*
- *Confusion, Acute or Chronic.*

(NANDA-I © 2014)

Planning

When planning care for a patient who is abusing substances, it is important to keep goals and expectations reasonable.

Substance abuse recovery takes many months and often requires several attempts before abstinence is obtained and maintained. As a result, setting both short- and long-term goals for the patient is often most effective.

Short-term goals may include the following:

- The patient will admit having a substance abuse problem and having lost control of her life as a result.
- The patient will seek help to stop using the substance.
- The patient will experience no complications as a result of drug withdrawal symptoms.
- The patient will enter a drug rehabilitation program to change the behavior.

Long-term goals may include the following:

- The patient will explore the impact of the substance addiction on family, job, and friends.
- The patient will describe and recognize her denial in avoiding the problems related to substance abuse.
- The patient will change her thinking and behavior as a result of understanding the negative consequences of substance abuse.
- The patient will regularly attend a support group to maintain sobriety from substance use.
- The patient will remain free of substance and maintain sobriety.

Implementation

Because patients with substance use disorders have difficulty communicating and maintaining relationships, it is important that the nurse convey an attitude of acceptance and promote healthy coping and appropriate behaviors. Teach and model assertive communication, as patients may have become dependent on unhealthy and less successful communication techniques. Set limits on manipulative behaviors and maintain consistency in responses. Encourage patients to focus on strengths and accomplishments rather than ruminating on weaknesses and failures. Minimize attention to any such ruminations. Help patients explore dealing with stressful situations rather than resorting to substance use, and teach healthy coping mechanisms such as physical exercise, deep breathing, meditation, and progressive muscle relaxation. Encourage participation in therapeutic group activities.

Other specific interventions for patients with substance abuse and addiction address patient safety related to abuse and withdrawal and adherence to treatment. The following interventions have implications for nursing care in both acute and home care settings.

Promote Safety

- Assess the patient's level of disorientation to determine specific risks to the safety of the patient, family members, and others.
- If the patient cannot withdraw from substances safely in the home or community setting, consider a higher level of care.

- Obtain a drug history as well as urine and blood samples for laboratory analysis of substance content. A patient may not admit to using drugs at all or may admit to using only one drug recreationally, when in truth, the patient is using one or more drugs regularly. Urine and blood samples provide accurate, objective information.

- Place the patient in a quiet, private room to decrease excessive stimuli and related agitation, but do not leave the patient alone if excessive hyperactivity or suicidal ideation is present.

- If the patient is disoriented, frequently orient the patient to reality and the environment, ensuring that potentially harmful objects are stored away from the patient. The patient may harm self or others if disoriented and confused.

- Monitor vital signs every 15 minutes until stable. If treatment is dependent on blood or urine levels of a specific drug, reevaluate as instructed by the treating physician.

Promote Patient Safety During Withdrawal

- Observe the patient for withdrawal symptoms. Monitor vital signs. Provide adequate nutrition and hydration. These actions provide supportive physical care during detoxification.

- Assess the patient's level of orientation frequently. Orient and reassure the patient of safety in the presence of hallucinations, delusions, or illusions.

- Explain all interventions before approaching the patient. Avoid loud noises and talk softly to the patient. Decrease external stimuli by dimming lights. Excessive stimuli increase agitation.

- Administer medications according to the detoxification schedule. Benzodiazepines may help minimize the discomfort of withdrawal symptoms.

- Provide positive reinforcement when thinking and behavior are appropriate or when the patient recognizes that delusions are not based in reality. Drugs and alcohol can interfere with the patient's perception of reality.

- Use simple step-by-step instructions and face-to-face interaction when communicating with the patient. The patient may be confused or disoriented.

- Express reasonable doubt if the patient relays suspicious or paranoid beliefs. Reinforce accurate perception of people or situations. It is important to communicate that you do not share the false beliefs as reality.

- Do not argue with the patient experiencing delusions or hallucinations. Convey acceptance that the patient believes a situation to be true, but that you do not see or hear what is not there. Arguing with the patient or denying the belief serves no useful purpose because it does not eliminate the delusions.

- Talk to the patient about real events and real people. Respond to feelings and reassure the patient that she is safe from harm. Discussions that focus on the delusions may aggravate the condition. Verbalization of feelings in a nonthreatening environment may help the patient develop insight.

Patient Teaching
Substance Abuse

Teach the patient and family the following:

- The negative effects of substance abuse, including physical and psychologic complications of substance abuse.
- The signs of relapse and the importance of aftercare programs and self-help groups to prevent relapse.
- Information about specific medications that help reduce cravings and maintain abstinence, including the potential side effects, possible drug interactions, and any special precautions to be taken (e.g., avoiding over-the-counter medications such as cough syrup that may contain alcohol).
- Ways to manage stress, including techniques such as progressive muscle relaxation, abdominal breathing techniques, imagery, meditation, and effective coping skills.

In addition, suggest resources such as the National Institute on Drug Abuse (NIDA; http://www.drugabuse.gov) for information on the science of addiction; AA, NA, and other self-help groups; employee assistance programs; individual, group, and family counseling; community rehabilitation programs; and the National Alliance for the Mentally Ill (NAMI).

Finally, for families of individuals with substance addiction issues, offer emotional support but do not enable the addiction; know your limits; and do not accept unacceptable behavior.

Provide Patient Education

- Assess the patient's level of knowledge and readiness to learn the effects of drugs and alcohol on the body. Baseline assessment is required to develop appropriate teaching material.

- Develop a teaching plan that includes measurable objectives. Include short-term goals so that the patient sees some level of success at an early stage. Include significant others if possible. Lifestyle changes often affect all family members.

- Begin with simple concepts and progress to more complex issues. Use interactive teaching strategies and written materials appropriate to the patient's educational level. Include information on physiologic effects of substances, the propensity for physical and psychologic dependence, and risks to the fetus if the patient is pregnant. Active participation and handouts enhance retention of important concepts.

Evaluation

The patient is evaluated based on the ability to meet goals designed during the planning phase of nursing care. Potential positive outcomes may include the following:

- The patient experiences no complications from withdrawing from substance.
- The patient admits a problem with substance abuse and seeks help.

- The patient enters a substance abuse program.
- The patient can describe choices made that contributed to substance abuse.
- The patient attends daily support group meetings after leaving the rehabilitation facility.
- The patient remains substance free for (insert time period—days, weeks, months—depending on progress and time sober).

While some sources have reported that as many as 90% of addicted individuals are unsuccessful in becoming substance free, the National Institute on Drug Abuse (NIDA, 2014a) estimated that the relapse rate of 40 to 60% for substance abuse is similar to that for other chronic illnesses, such as diabetes, hypertension, or asthma. NIDA has recommended that clinicians treat substance addiction like any other chronic illness for which relapse serves as a trigger for renewed intervention.

Nursing Care Plan
A Patient with Substance Abuse

Donna Smith is brought to the ED by her husband. She is agitated and can't stand still. Her husband tells the nurse that she has been getting high on crack cocaine on a regular basis. When she didn't come home last night, he called their cell phone company to activate her GPS and found her outside a motel on the highway. He took her home, where she began shouting, yelling, and throwing things and talking about the "men in the trees" who are after her. The nurse conducting the assessment determines that they have two children, ages 11 and 15, living at home.

ASSESSMENT

The nurse collects the following data during assessment:

Temperature 99.4°F axillary; pulse 114 bpm; respirations 20/min; BP 168/92 mmHg

Pupils constricted and equally responsive to light

Patient is muttering to herself in mostly unintelligible sentences, with phrases such as "men in trees," "gonna get me," and "don't worry" understood among gibberish words. Patient says she hears voices and points out things that are not there—apparently having both visual and auditory hallucinations.

Peripheral pulses are 3+ and bounding, sinus tachycardia is noted on ECG with frequent premature ventricular contractions, hyperreactive reflexes.

Patient is admitted to monitored unit (telemetry) for observation until cardiac and neurologic systems are stable.

DIAGNOSES

- *Injury, Risk for*
- *Family Processes, Interrupted*
- *Coping, Ineffective*
- *Confusion, Acute*
- *Violence, Risk for Other- or Self-Directed*

(NANDA-I © 2014)

PLANNING

Goals of care include the following:

- Experience no adverse cardiac event.
- Orient to time and place.
- ECG will return to normal sinus rhythm.
- Neurologic assessment will return to pre-substance use baseline.
- Agree to psychosocial intervention to assist in substance avoidance.

IMPLEMENTATION

- Monitor cardiorespiratory function.
- Assess orientation and maintain safety while hallucinating.
- Maintain low-stimulation environment until effects of drug subside.
- Maintain hydration to promote excretion of drug from system.
- Obtain complete history of substance use when patient's cognitive function returns.

- Administer sedatives and antiarrhythmics as required per orders.
- Refer Mr. Smith to a support program for spouses and children.
- Refer to substance abuse program to assist in abstinence once drugs have been cleared from system if patient is willing to participate.

EVALUATION

Evaluation of patient response may be based on the following expected outcomes:

- The patient experiences no cardiac event as the result of cocaine use.

- The patient's cognition returns to prior baseline.
- The patient admits to having a problem and agrees to seek treatment.

CRITICAL THINKING

1. While the patient is experiencing both auditory and visual hallucinations, how will the nurse respond if the patient insists there is something in the room that is not seen by the nurse?

2. What actions will the nurse implement to maintain the patient's safety?

3. After detoxification, the patient regains normal cognitive function and informs the nurse she is leaving the facility because she wants to "get high again." What is the nurse's legal obligation to this patient?

REVIEW Substance Abuse

RELATE Link the Concepts and Exemplars

Linking the exemplar of substance abuse with the concept of safety:

1. The nurse had surgery a few days ago and is taking a narcotic analgesic to control pain. Is it safe for the nurse to work assigned shifts while taking this medication? Why or why not?

2. You suspect that a coworker whom you admire for his experience and knowledge may be using an illegal drug. What is your best action to maintain patient safety? How would you handle this issue?

Linking the exemplar of substance abuse with the concept of trauma:

3. How does the abuse of substances affect the risk for violence committed by the patient?

4. When working in a substance abuse treatment facility, how can you, as the nurse, encourage spouses at risk for acts of domestic violence by your patients seek support for their own health?

READY Go to Volume 3: Clinical Nursing Skills

REFER Go to Pearson MyLab Nursing and eText

- Additional review materials

REFLECT Apply Your Knowledge

Casey Holmes is a physically fit 23-year-old man who had a troubled youth. His parents divorced when he was very young, and he bounced back and forth between parents—both of whom remarried. Growing up, he often saw his father hit his stepmother when angry. As an adolescent, Mr. Holmes became involved with a gang and was arrested a few times for petty crimes, such as shoplifting and vandalism. He never finished high school and moved out on his own at the age of 18. Since that time, he has held a number of odd jobs and has made an effort to stay out of trouble.

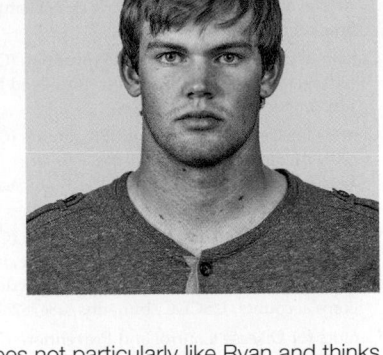

Mr. Holmes lives with his pregnant girlfriend Jessica Riley and her son Ryan. He does not particularly like Ryan and thinks Jessica spoils him. He is very proud of the fact that Jessica is pregnant with his baby. He is controlling of Jessica and does not want anybody else looking at her. On most days after work and into the evening, Mr. Holmes drinks beer and smokes dope with his buddies. He is irritated that Jessica does not party with him as much as she did when they first met. Mr. Holmes also uses other drugs when he can afford to buy them.

1. What are the priority nursing diagnoses for Mr. Holmes?

2. What are the implications of his substance abuse on the family?

3. Mr. Holmes accompanies Jessica to the clinic for one of her prenatal visits. The nurse is aware of Mr. Holmes's drug use, which Jessica admitted on a prior visit. What should the nurse say to Mr. Holmes during this visit regarding the impact of his behavior on Jessica and the baby?

References

Agency for Healthcare Research and Quality. (2012). Five major steps to intervention (the "5 A's"). Retrieved from http://www.ahrq.gov/professionals/clinicians-providers/guidelines-recommendations/tobacco/5steps.html

Alavi, S. S., Ferdosi, M., Jannatifard, F., Eslami, M., Alaghemandan, H., & Setare, M. (2012). Behavioral addiction versus substance addiction: Correspondence of psychiatric and psychological views. *International Journal of Preventive Medicine, 3*(4), 290–294.

Alterman, A. (2014). *Substance abuse and psychopathology.* New York, NY: Springer.

American Cancer Society. (2014). *A word about success rates for quitting smoking.* Retrieved from http://www.cancer.org/healthy/stayawayfromtobacco/guidetoquittingsmoking/guide-to-quitting-smoking-success-rates

American Lung Association. (2013). *Smoking.* Retrieved from http://www.lung.org/stop-smoking/about-smoking/health-effects/smoking.html

American Nurses Association. (2015). *Impaired nurse resource center.* Retrieved from http://www.nursingworld.org/MainMenuCategories/WorkplaceSafety/Healthy-Work-Environment/Work-Environment/ImpairedNurse

American Psychiatric Association. (2013). *Diagnostic and statistical manual of mental disorders* (5th ed.). Washington, DC: American Psychiatric Association.

American Society of Addiction Medicine. (2015). *What is the ASAM criteria?* Retrieved from http://www.asam.org/publications/the-asam-criteria/about/

Anxiety and Depression Association of America. (2015). *Substance use disorders.* Retrieved from http://www.adaa.org/understanding-anxiety/related-illnesses/substance-abuse

Arnold, C. (2014). Vaping and health: What do we know about e-cigarettes? *Environmental Health Perspectives, 122*(9), A245-A249. doi:10.1289/ehp.122-A244

Ballinger, B., & Yalom, I. D. (1995). *The theory and practice of group psychotherapy* (4th ed.). New York, NY: Basic Books.

Bernstein, P. M. (2013). *Trauma: Healing the hidden epidemic.* Petaluma, CA: Bernstein Institute for Integrative Psychotherapy and Trauma Treatment.

Breese, G. R., Sinha, R., & Heilig, M. (2011). Chronic alcohol neuroadaptation and stress contribute to susceptibility for alcohol craving and relapse. *Pharmacology and Therapeutics, 129*(2), 149–171. doi:10.1016/j.pharmthera.2010.09.007

British Columbia Schizophrenia Society. (2015). *Spouses handbook.* Retrieved from http://www.bcss.org/resources/topics-by-audience/family-friends/2004/05/spouses-handbook/#7

Burns, M. J. (2013). *Delirium tremens (DTs): Prognosis.* Retrieved from emedicine.medscape.com/article/166032

Campaign for Tobacco-Free Kids. (2015). *Knock tobacco out of the park.* Retrieved from http://tobaccofreebaseball.org/content/

Caputo, F., Vignoli, T., Leggio, L., Addolorato, G., Zoli, G., & Bernardi, M. (2012). Alcohol use disorders in the elderly: A brief overview from epidemiology to treatment options. *Experimental Gerontology, 47*(6), 411–416. doi:10.1016/j.exger.2012.03.019

Center for Behavioral Health Statistics and Quality (CBHSQ). (2012). *More than 7 million children live with a parent with alcohol problems.* Rockville, MD: Substance Abuse and Mental Health Services Administration.

Center for Behavioral Health Statistics and Quality (CBHSQ). (2014). *Substance use and mental health estimates from the 2013 National Survey on Drug Use and Health: Overview of findings.* (HHS Publication No. 14–4863). Rockville, MD: Substance Abuse and Mental Health Services Administration.

Center for Behavioral Health Statistics and Quality (CBHSQ). (2015). *Behavioral health trends in the United States: Results from the 2014 National Survey on Drug Use and Health.* (HHS Publication No. SMA 15-4927). Rockville, MD: Substance Abuse and Mental Health Services Administration.

Centers for Disease Control and Prevention (CDC). (2012). *A report of the Surgeon General: Preventing tobacco use among youth and young adults.* Atlanta, GA: Centers for Disease Control and Prevention.

Centers for Disease Control and Prevention (CDC). (2013a). *Adverse Childhood Experiences (ACE) Study.* Retrieved from http://www.cdc.gov/violenceprevention/acestudy/

Centers for Disease Control and Prevention (CDC). (2013b). *Celebrate moms who protect children's health.* Retrieved from http://www.cdc.gov/Features/SmokeFreeMoms

Centers for Disease Control and Prevention (CDC). (2013c). *Smoking and tobacco use.* Retrieved from http://www.cdc.gov/tobacco

Centers for Disease Control and Prevention (CDC). (2013d). *Smoking and tobacco use. Fast facts.* Retrieved from http://www.cdc.gov/tobacco/data_statistics/fact_sheets/fast_facts

Centers for Disease Control and Prevention (CDC). (2014). *CDC study: Youth perceptions about energy drinks.* Retrieved from http://content.govdelivery.com/accounts/USCDC/bulletins/a8e782

Centers for Disease Control and Prevention (CDC). (2015a). *Caffeine and alcohol.* Retrieved from http://www.cdc.gov/alcohol/fact-sheets/caffeine-and-alcohol.htm

Centers for Disease Control and Prevention (CDC). (2015b). *E-cigarette use triples among middle and high school students in just one year.* Retrieved from http://www.cdc.gov/media/releases/2015/p0416-e-cigarette-use.html

Centers for Disease Control and Prevention (CDC). (2015c). *Excessive alcohol use continues to be drain on American economy.* Retrieved from http://www.cdc.gov/media/releases/2015/p1015-excessive-alcohol.html

Centers for Disease Control and Prevention (CDC). (2015d). *Fact sheets: Underage drinking.* Retrieved from http://www.cdc.gov/alcohol/fact-sheets/underage-drinking.htm

Centers for Disease Control and Prevention (CDC). (2015e). *Today's heroin epidemic.* Retrieved from http://www.cdc.gov/vitalsigns/heroin/

Choi, N. G., & DiNitto, D. M. (2015). Role of new diagnosis, social isolation, and depression in older adults' smoking cessation. *The Gerontologist, 55*(5), 1–9. doi:10.1093/geront/gnu049

Chokroborty-Hoque, A., Alberry, B., & Singh, S. M. (2014). Exploring the complexity of intellectual disability in fetal alcohol spectrum disorders. *Frontiers in Pediatrics, 2*(90), 1–9. doi:10.3389/fped.2014.00090

Crane, E. H. (2015). Emergency department visits involving pain relievers. The CBHSQ report. *Center for Behavioral Health Statistics and Quality.* Retrieved from https://www.samhsa.gov/data/sites/default/files/report_2083/ShortReport-2083.html

Cravens, J. D., & Whiting, J. B. (2014). Clinical implications of internet infidelity: Where Facebook fits in. *American Journal of Family Therapy, 42*(4), 325–339. doi:10.1080/01926187.2013.874211

Czermak, C., Lehofer, M., Wagner, E. M., Prietl, B., Lemonis, L., Rohrhofer, A., … Liebmann, P. M. (2004). Reduced dopamine D$_4$ receptor mRNA expression in lymphocytes of long-term abstinent alcohol and heroin addicts. *Addiction, 99*(2), 251–257.

De Guzmán, I. N., Arnau, R. C., Green, B. A., Carnes, S., Carnes, P., & Jore, J. (2016). Empirical identification of psychological symptom subgroups of sex addicts: An application of latent profile analysis. *Sexual Addiction & Compulsivity, 23*(1), 34–55. doi:10.1080/10720162.2015.1095139

Dennis, M. L., Foss, M. A., & Scott, C. K. (2007). An eight-year perspective on the relationship between the duration of abstinence and other aspects of recovery. *Evaluation Review, 31*(6), 585–612. doi:10.1177/0193841X07307771

Ehlers, C. L., & Gizer, I. R. (2013). Evidence for a genetic component for substance dependence in Native Americans. *American Journal of Psychiatry, 170*(2), 154–164. doi:10.1176/appi.ajp.2012.12010113.

Ellis, A. (2015). *Rational emotive & cognitive-behavior therapy.* Retrieved from http://albertellis.org/rebt-cbt-therapy/

Ewing, J. A. (1984). Detecting alcoholism: The CAGE questionnaire. *Journal of the American Medical Association, 252*(14), 1905–1907.

Farsalinos, K. E., & Polosa, R. (2014). Safety evaluation and risk assessment of electronic cigarettes as tobacco cigarette substitutes: A systematic review. *Therapeutic Advances in Drug Safety, 5*(2), 67–86. doi:10.1177/2042098614524430

Food and Drug Administration. (2015). *FDA moves quickly to approve easy-to-use nasal spray to treat opioid overdose: Naloxone in nasal spray form provides important new alternative for family members, first responders.* Retrieved from http://www.fda.gov/NewsEvents/Newsroom/PressAnnouncements/ucm473505.htm

Foroud, T., & Phillips, T. J. (2012). *Assessing the genetic risk for alcohol use disorders.* Retrieved from National Institute on Alcohol Abuse and Alcoholism website: http://alcoholism.about.com/gi/dynamic/offsite.htm?site=http://www.niaaa.nih.gov

Green, K. E., & Feinstein, B. A. (2012). Substance use in lesbian, gay, and bisexual populations: An update on empirical research and implications for treatment. *Psychology of Addictive Behaviors, 26*(2), 265–278. doi:10.1037/a0025424

Griffiths, M. D. (2016). Compulsive sexual behaviour as a behavioural addiction: The impact of the internet and other issues. *Addiction.* doi:10.1111/add.13315

Guttmacher Institute. (2015). *Substance abuse during pregnancy. State Policies in Brief.* New York, NY: Guttmacher Institute.

Handelsman, L., Cochrane, K. J., Aronson, M. J., Ness, R., Rubinstein, K. J., & Kanof, P. D. (1987). Two new rating scales for opiate withdrawal. *American Journal of Drug and Alcohol Abuse, 13*(3), 293–308.

Hartston, H. (2012). The case for compulsive shopping as an addiction. *Journal of Psychoactive Drugs, 44*(1), 64-67. doi:10.1080/02791072.2012.660110

Hazelden Betty Ford Foundation. (2015). *Substance abuse among the elderly: A growing problem.* Retrieved from http://www.hazeldenbettyford.org/articles/substance-abuse-among-the-elderly-a-growing-problem

Heise, B. (2003). The historical context of addiction in the nursing profession: 1850–1982. *Journal of Addictions Nursing, 14*, 117–124.

Herdman, T. H. & Kamitsuru, S. (Eds.). *Nursing Diagnoses—Definitions and Classification 2015–2017.* Copyright © 2014, 1994–2014 NANDA International. Used by arrangement with John Wiley & Sons, Inc. Companion website: www.wiley.com/go/nursingdiagnoses

Holt, C. L., Roth, D. L., Huang, J., & Clark, E. (2015). Gender differences in the roles of religion and locus of control on alcohol use and smoking among African Americans. *Journal of Studies on Alcohol and Drugs, 76*(3), 482–492. doi:http://dx.doi.org/10.15288/jsad.2015.76.482

Ilie, G., Boak, A., Mann, R. E., Adlaf, E. M., Hamilton, H., Asbridge, M., … Cusimano, M. D. (2015). Energy drinks, alcohol, sports and traumatic brain injuries among adolescents. *PLoS One, 10*(9), e0135860. doi:10.1371/journal.pone.0135860

Institute of Medicine. (2015). *Psychosocial interventions for mental and substance use disorders: A framework for establishing evidence-based standards.* Washington, DC: National Academies Press.

Jamison, R. N., Edwards, R. R., Liu, X., Ross, E. L., Michna, E., Warnick, M., & Wasan, A. D. (2013). Relationship of negative affect and outcome of an opioid therapy trial among low back pain patients. *Pain Practices, 13*(3), 173–181. doi:10.1111/j.1533-2500.2012.00575.x

Jellinek, E. (1946). *Phases in the drinking history of alcoholics.* New Haven, CT: Hillhouse Press.

Johnston, L. D., O'Malley, P. M., Bachman, J. G., & Schulenberg, J. E. (2013). *Monitoring the future. National results on drug use: 2012 overview. Key findings on adolescent drug use.* Ann Arbor, MI: Ann Arbor Institute for Social Research, University of Michigan.

Kash, T. L. (2012). The role of biogenic amine signaling in the bed nucleus of the stria terminals in alcohol abuse. *Alcohol, 46*(4), 303–308. doi:10.1016/j.alcohol.2011.12.004

Kneisl, C. R., & Trigoboff, E. (2013). *Contemporary psychiatric–mental health nursing* (3rd ed.). Upper Saddle River, NJ: Pearson-Prentice Hall.

Knopik, V. S., Maccani, M. A., Francazio, S., & McGeary, J. E. (2012). The epigenetics of maternal cigarette smoking during pregnancy and effects on child development. *Development and Psychopathology, 24*(4), 1377–1390. doi:10.1017/S0954579412000776

Lander, L., Howsare, J., & Byrne, M. (2013). The impact of substance use disorders on families and children: From theory to practice. *Social Work in Health Care, 28*(0), 194–205. doi:10.1080/19371918.2013.759005

Landolfi, E. (2013). Exercise addiction. *Sports Medicine, 43*(2), 111–119. doi:10.1007/s40279-012-0013-x

LaPierre, J. (2015). *Communicating effectively with an active addict or alcoholic.* Retrieved from http://www.choosehelp.com/topics/living-with-an-addict/communicating-with-addict-alcoholic

Lawrence, L. M., Ciorciari, J., & Kyrios, M. (2014). Relationships that compulsive buying has with addiction, obsessive-compulsiveness, hoarding, and depression. *Comprehensive Psychiatry, 55*(5), 1137–1145. doi:http://dx.doi.org/10.1016/j.comppsych.2014.03.005

Linehan, M. M. (2015). *What is DBT?* Retrieved from http://behavioraltech.org/resources/whatisdbt.cfm

MacNeal, J. J., Cone, D. C., Sinha, V., & Tomassoni, A. J. (2012). Use of haloperidol in PCP-intoxicated individuals. *Clinical Toxicology, 50*(9), 851–853. doi:10.3109/15563650.2012.722222

Manasco, A., Chang, S., Larriviere, J., Hamm, L. L., & Glass, M. (2012). Alcohol withdrawal. *Southern Medical Journal, 105*(11), 607–612. doi:10.1097/SMJ.0b013e31826efb2d

Manchikanti, L., Fellows, B., Ailinani, H., & Pampati, V. (2010). Therapeutic use, abuse, and nonmedical use of opioids: A ten-year perspective. *Pain Physician, 13*(5), 401–435.

Martin, P. R., Singleton, C. K., & Hiller–Sturmhöfel, S. (2015). *The role of thiamine deficiency in alcoholic brain disease.* Retrieved from http://pubs.niaaa.nih.gov/publications/arh27-2/134-142.htm

Mayo Clinic. (2015a). *Alcohol use disorder.* Retrieved from http://www.mayoclinic.org/diseases-conditions/alcohol-use-disorder/basics/symptoms/con-20020866

Mayo Clinic. (2015b). *Drug addiction: Risk factors.* Retrieved from http://www.mayoclinic.org/diseases-conditions/drug-addiction/basics/risk-factors/con-20020970

McHugh, R. K., Whitton, S. W., Peckham, A. D., Welge, J. A., & Otto, M. W. (2013). Patient preference for psychological vs. pharmacological treatment of psychiatric disorders: A meta-analytic review. *Journal of Clinical Psychiatry, 74*(6), 595–602. doi:10.4088/JCP.12r07757

McNeece, C. A., & DiNitto, D. M. (2012). *Chemical dependency: A systems approach* (4th ed.). Upper Saddle River, NJ: Pearson.

Menninger Clinic. (2015). *Milieu therapy.* Retrieved from http://www.menningerclinic.com/patient-care/inpatient-treatment/professionals-in-crisis-program/milieu-therapy

Mental Health America. (2015a). *Co-dependency.* Retrieved from http://www.mentalhealthamerica.net/co-dependency

Mental Health America. (2015b). *Being an effective caregiver.* Retrieved from http://www.mentalhealthamerica.net/conditions/being-effective-caregiver

Morse, R. M., & Flavin, D. K. (1992). The definition of alcoholism. The Joint Committee of the National Council on Alcoholism and Drug Dependence and the American Society of Addiction Medicine to Study the Definition and Criteria for the Diagnosis of Alcoholism. *Journal of the American Medical Association, 268*(8), 1012–1014.

Muncie, H. L., Yasinian, Y., & Oge, L. (2013). Outpatient management of alcohol withdrawal syndrome. *American Family Physician, 88*(9), 590–595.

Murali, V., Ray, R., & Shaffiullha, M. (2012). Shopping addiction. *Advances in Psychiatric Treatment, 18*(4), 263–269. doi:10.1192/apt.bp.109.007880

National Association for Children of Alcoholics. (2015). *Children of alcoholics: Important facts.* Retrieved from http://www.nacoa.net/impfacts.htm

National Institute on Aging. (2012). *Alcohol use in older people.* Retrieved from https://d2cauhfh-6h4x0p.cloudfront.net/s3fs-public/alcohol_use_in_older_people_0.pdf

National Institute on Alcohol Abuse and Alcoholism (NIAAA). (2012). *The link between stress and alcohol.* (Alcohol Alert No. 85). Rockville, MD: National Institute on Alcohol Abuse and Alcoholism.

National Institute on Alcohol Abuse and Alcoholism (NIAAA). (2015a). *Rethinking drinking: Alcohol and your health* (NIH Publication No. 15-3770). Bethesda, MD: National Institute on Alcohol Abuse and Alcoholism.

National Institute on Alcohol Abuse and Alcoholism (NIAAA). (2015b). *Planning alcohol interventions using NIAAA's College AIM (Alcohol Intervention Matrix)* (NIH Publication No. 15-AA-8017). Bethesda, MD: National Institute on Alcohol Abuse and Alcoholism.

National Institute on Alcohol Abuse and Alcoholism (NIAAA). (2015c). *Alcohol facts and statistics.* Retrieved from http://www.niaaa.nih.gov/alcohol-health/overview-alcohol-consumption/alcohol-facts-and-statistics

National Institute on Alcohol Abuse and Alcoholism (NIAAA). (2015d). *Why do adolescents drink, what are the risks, and how can underage drinking be prevented?* Retrieved from http://pubs.niaaa.nih.gov/publications/AA67/AA67.htm

National Institute on Drug Abuse (NIDA). (2012a). *Inhalants* (NIH Publication No. 12-3818). Rockville, MD: National Institutes of Health.

National Institute on Drug Abuse (NIDA). (2012b). *Principles of drug addiction treatment: A research-based guide* (NIH Publication No. 12-4180). Rockville, MD: National Institutes of Health.

National Institute on Drug Abuse (NIDA). (2013a). *Drug facts: Cocaine.* Retrieved from http://www.drugabuse.gov/publications/drugfacts/cocaine

National Institute on Drug Abuse (NIDA). (2013b). *Methamphetamine* (NIH Publication No. 13-4210). Rockville, MD: National Institutes of Health.

National Institute on Drug Abuse (NIDA). (2014a). *Drugs, brains, and behavior: The science of addiction* (NIH Pub No. 14-5605). Rockville, MD: National Institutes of Health.

National Institute on Drug Abuse (NIDA). (2014b). *Heroin: What is heroin and how is it used?* (NIH Publication No. 15-0165). Rockville, MD: National Institutes of Health.

National Institute on Drug Abuse (NIDA). (2014c). *Prescription drug abuse: Older adults.* Retrieved from http://www.drugabuse.gov/publications/research-reports/prescription-drugs/trends-in-prescription-drug-abuse/older-adults

National Institute on Drug Abuse (NIDA). (2014d). *Prescription opioid and heroin abuse.* Retrieved from http://www.drugabuse.gov/about-nida/legislative-activities/testimony-to-congress/2015/prescription-opioid-heroin-abuse

National Institute on Drug Abuse (NIDA). (2014e). *Principles of adolescent substance use disorder treatment: A research-based guide* (NIH Publication Number 14-7953). Rockville, MD: National Institutes of Health.

National Institute on Drug Abuse (NIDA). (2015a). *Dramatic increases in maternal opioid use and neonatal abstinence syndrome.* Retrieved from http://www.drugabuse.gov/related-topics/trends-statistics/infographics/dramatic-increases-in-maternal-opioid-use-neonatal-abstinence-syndrome

National Institute on Drug Abuse (NIDA). (2015b). *Drug Facts: Nationwide trends.* Rockville, MD: National Institutes of Health.

National Institute on Drug Abuse (NIDA). (2015c). *Marijuana* (NIH Publication No. 15-3859). Rockville, MD: National Institutes of Health.

National Institute on Drug Abuse (NIDA). (2015d). *Trends and statistics.* Retrieved from http://www.drugabuse.gov/related-topics/trends-statistics

National Institutes of Health (NIH). (2015). *How smoking affects your health.* Retrieved from http://nihseniorhealth.gov/quittingsmoking/howsmokingaffectsyourhealth/01.html

Nellissery, M., Feinn, R. S., Covault, J., Gelernter, J., Anton, R. F., Pettinati, H., … Kranzler, H. R. (2003). Alleles of a functional serotonin transporter promoter polymorphism are associated with major depression in alcoholics. *Alcoholism: Clinical and Experimental Research, 27*(9), 1402–1408.

Oesterle, S., Hawkins, J. D., & Hill, K. G. (2011). Men's and women's pathways to adulthood and associated substance misuse. *Journal of Studies on Alcohol and Drugs, 72*(5), 763–773.

Office of the Surgeon General and National Action Alliance for Suicide Prevention. (2012). *2012 national strategy for suicide prevention: Goals and objectives for action.* Washington, DC: U.S. Department of Health and Human Services.

Partnership at Drugfree.org (2013). *Methamphetamine.* Retrieved from http://www.drugfree.org/drug-guide/methamphetamine

Pettinati, H. M., O'Brien, C. P., & Dundon, W. D. (2013). Current status of co-occurring mood and substance use disorders: A new therapeutic target. *American Journal of Psychiatry, 170*(1), 23–30. doi:10.1176/appi.ajp.2012.12010112

Pokorny, A. D., Miller, B. A., & Kaplan, H. B. (1972). The brief MAST: A shortened version of the Michigan Alcohol Screening Test. *American Journal of Psychiatry, 129*, 342–345.

Rappaport, D., Chuu, A., Hullett, C., Nematollahi, S., Teeple, M., Bhuyan, N., … Sanders, A. (2013). Assessment of alcohol withdrawal in Native American patients utilizing the Clinical Institute Withdrawal Assessment of Alcohol Revised Scale. *Journal of Addiction Medicine, 7*(3), 196–199.

Reif, S., Braude, L., Lyman, D. R., Dougherty, R. H., Daniels, A. S., Ghose, S. S., … Delphin-Rittmon, M. E. (2014). Peer recovery support for individuals with substance use disorders: Assessing the evidence. *Psychiatric Services, 65*(7), 853–861. doi:10.1176/appi.ps.201400047

Roeder, A. (2015). Chemical flavorings found in e-cigarettes linked to lung disease. *Harvard Gazette.* Retrieved from http://news.harvard.edu/gazette/story/2015/12/popcorn-lung-seen-in-e-cigarette-smokers/

Rose, S., & Dhandayudham, A. (2014). Towards an understanding of internet-based problem shopping behaviour: The concept of online shopping addiction and its proposed predictors. *Journal of Behavioral Addictions, 3*(2), 83–89. doi:10.1556/JBA.3.2014.003

Ross, C. C. (2014). Suicide: One of addiction's hidden risks. *Psychology Today.* Retrieved from https://www.psychologytoday.com/blog/real-healing/201402/suicide-one-addiction-s-hidden-risks

Schepis, T. S., & Rao, U. (2005). Epidemiology and etiology of adolescent smoking. *Current Opinions in Pediatrics, 17*(5), 607-612.

Serec, M., Svab, I., Kolšek, M., Svab, V., Moesgen, D., & Klein, M. (2012). Health-related lifestyle, physical and mental health in children of alcoholic parents. *Drug and Alcohol Review, 31*(7), 861–870. doi:10.1111/j.1465-3362.2012.00424.x

Skinner, H. A. (1982). *Drug abuse screening test (DAST)* (p. 363). Langford Lance, UK: Elsevier Science.

SMART Recovery. (2015). *SMART Recovery—Self management for addiction recovery.* Retrieved from http://www.smartrecovery.org

Starr, K. T. (2015). The sneaky prevalence of substance abuse in nursing. *Nursing, 45*(3), 16–17. Retrieved from http://journals.lww.com/nursing/Citation/2015/03000/The_sneaky_prevalence_of_substance_abuse_in.6.aspx

Substance Abuse and Mental Health Services Administration (SAMHSA). (2007). *The Women, Co-Occurring Disorders and Violence Study and Children's Subset Study: Program summary.* Rockville, MD: Author.

Substance Abuse and Mental Health Services Administration (SAMHSA). (2009). *Addressing the specific needs of women* (HHS Publication No. [SMA] 09-4426). Rockville, MD: Author.

Substance Abuse and Mental Health Services Administration (SAMHSA). (2012a). *A provider's introduction to substance abuse treatment for lesbian, gay, bisexual, and transgender individuals.* (HHS Publication No. [SMA] 12-4104). Rockville, MD: Author.

Substance Abuse and Mental Health Services Administration (SAMHSA). (2012b). *The role of biomarkers in the treatment of alcohol use disorders: 2012 revision* (HHS Publication No. [SMA] 12-4686). Rockville, MD: U.S. Department of Health and Human Services.

Substance Abuse and Mental Health Services Administration (SAMHSA). (2013). *Addressing the specific behavioral health needs of men* (HHS publication no. [SMA] 13-4736). Rockville, MD: Author.

Substance Abuse and Mental Health Services Administration (SAMHSA). (2014a). *Trauma-informed care in behavioral health services* (HHS Publication No. [SMA] 13-4801). Rockville, MD: Author.

Substance Abuse and Mental Health Services Administration (SAMHSA). (2014b). *Treatment improvement protocol: Improving cultural competence* (HHS Publication No. [SMA] 14-4849). Rockville, MD: Author.

Substance Abuse and Mental Health Services Administration (SAMHSA). (2015a). *Health care and health systems integration.* Retrieved from http://www.samhsa.gov/health-care-health-systems-integration

Substance Abuse and Mental Health Services Administration (SAMHSA). (2015b). *Detoxification and substance abuse treatment: A treatment improvement protocol* (HHS Publication No. [SMA] 15-4131). Rockville, MD: Author.

Substance Abuse and Mental Health Services Administration (SAMHSA). (2015c). *About screening, brief intervention, and referral to treatment (SBIRT).* Retrieved from http://www.samhsa.gov/sbirt/about

Sullivan, J. T., Sykora, K., Schneiderman, J., Naranjo, C. A., & Sellers, E. M. (1989). Assessment of alcohol withdrawal: The revised Clinical Institute Withdrawal Assessment for Alcohol Scale (CIWA-Ar). *British Journal of Addictions, 84,* 1353–1357.

Surgeon General. (2012). *Preventing tobacco use among youth and young adults: A report of the Surgeon General.* Retrieved from http://www.surgeon-general.gov/library/reports/preventing-youth-tobacco-use

Surgeon General. (2016). *Facing addiction in America: The Surgeon General's report on alcohol, drugs, and health.* Retrieved from https://addiction.surgeongeneral.gov

Tan, C. H., Denny, C. H., Cheal, N. E., Sniezek, J. E., & Kanny, D. (2015). *Alcohol use and binge drinking among women of childbearing age—United States, 2011–2013.* Atlanta, GA: Centers for Disease Control and Prevention.

Thomas, C. M., & Siela, D. (2011). The impaired nurse: Would you know what to do if you suspected substance abuse? *American Nurse Today, 6*(8). Retrieved from http://www.medscape.com/viewarticle/748598_7

White, A. M. (2015). *What happened? Alcohol, memory blackouts, and the brain.* Retrieved from http://pubs.niaaa.nih.gov/publications/arh27-2/186-196.htm

World Health Organization (WHO). (2013). *Management of substance abuse: Cannabis.* Retrieved from http://www.who.int/substance_abuse/facts/cannabis/en

World Health Organization (WHO). (2015a). *Prevalence of tobacco use.* Retrieved from http://www.who.int/gho/tobacco/use/en/

World Health Organization (WHO). (2015b). *Health effects of smoking among young people.* Retrieved from http://www.who.int/tobacco/research/youth/health_effects/en/

Yalom, I. D. (1974). Group therapy and alcoholism. *Annals of the New York Academy of Sciences, 233,* 85–103. doi:10.1111/j.1749-6632.1974.tb40286.x

Yalom, I. D., & Leszcz, M. (2005). *The theory and practice of group psychotherapy* (5th ed.). New York, NY: Basic Books.

Zhang, K., & Wang, X. (2013, May). Maternal smoking and increased risk of sudden infant death syndrome: A meta-analysis. *Legal Medicine (Tokyo, Japan), 15*(3), 115–321.

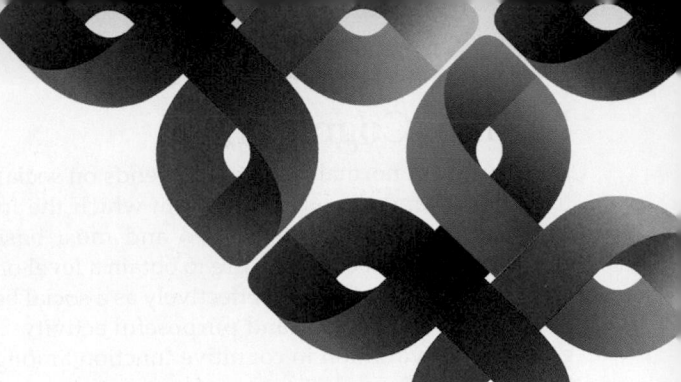

Module 23
Cognition

Module Outline and Learning Outcomes

The Concept of Cognition

Normal Cognition

23.1 Analyze the physiology of normal cognition.

Alterations to Cognition

23.2 Differentiate alterations in cognition.

Concepts Related to Cognition

23.3 Outline the relationship between cognition and other concepts.

Health Promotion

23.4 Explain measures to promote optimal cognition.

Nursing Assessment

23.5 Differentiate common assessment procedures and tests used to examine cognition.

Independent Interventions

23.6 Analyze independent interventions nurses can implement for patients with alterations in cognition.

Collaborative Therapies

23.7 Summarize collaborative therapies used by interprofessional teams for patients with alterations in cognition.

Lifespan Considerations

23.8 Differentiate considerations related to the assessment and care of patients with alterations in cognition throughout the lifespan.

Cognition Exemplars

Exemplar 23.A Alzheimer Disease

23.A Analyze Alzheimer disease as it relates to cognition.

Exemplar 23.B Delirium

23.B Analyze delirium as it relates to cognition.

Exemplar 23.C Schizophrenia

23.C Analyze schizophrenia as it relates to cognition.

» The Concept of Cognition

Concept Key Terms

Adaptive behavior, **1707**	Cognition, **1705**	Executive function, **1707**	Limbic system, **1707**	Praxis, **1707**
Agnosia, **1709**	Confabulation, **1709**	Fetal alcohol syndrome (FAS) , **1710**	Lobes, **1708**	Proprioceptive, **1706**
Alogia, **1709**	Confusion, **1708**		Long-term memory, **1707**	Psychosis, **1708**
Amnesia, **1709**	Delirium, **1714**	Fragile X syndrome, **1710**	Metacognition, **1705**	Sensory memory, **1706**
Anomia, **1709**	Delusions, **1708**	Hallucinations, **1708**	Neurons, **1707**	Short-term memory, **1706**
Aphasia, **1709**	Dementia, **1714**	Intellectual disability, **1710**	Neurotransmitters, **1707**	
Apraxia, **1709**	Down syndrome, **1710**		Orientation, **1706**	Social cognition, **1707**
Ataxia, **1709**	Dyspraxia, **1709**	Learning disabilities, **1710**	Physiologic tremor, **1709**	Tic, **1709**
Avolition, **1710**	Echolalia, **1709**			Tremor, **1709**
Carphologia, **1709**	Essential tremor, **1709**			Trisomy 21, **1711**

Cognition is the complex set of mental processes by which individuals acquire, store, retrieve, and use information. Cognition primarily involves activities that are controlled by the cerebral hemispheres, including perception, attention, memory, communication, decision making, and problem solving. The ability to think and reason is an essential component of human identity and function. **Metacognition** is a related term that refers to the human ability to think about thinking. A current understanding of cognition is drawn from the disciplines of cognitive psychology, neurology, computer science/artificial intelligence, philosophy, and anthropology.

Normal Cognition

A definition of normal cognition depends on social and cultural norms and the environment in which the individual operates. In general, the desired and most basic consequences of normal cognition are to obtain a level of survival and adaptation, to function effectively as a social being, and to engage in meaningful and purposeful activity. There is a great deal of variation in cognitive function among healthy individuals. Normal variations in cognition can be better understood by looking at some of the related components and categories associated with this concept. For an overview of cognitive development and related theories, see the module on Development.

Key Components and Categories

The key components that make up human cognition include perception, attention, and memory. Communication and social cognition, motor function, and planning, executive, and intellectual functions are broader categories of mental processing that are necessary for adaptive behavior.

Perception

Perception refers to an interpretation of stimuli or inputs that takes place in the brain. The process of perception depends on the sensory reception of internal and external data and is discussed in depth in the module on sensory perception. External stimuli or inputs include touch, taste, vision, hearing, and smell. Internal stimuli include **proprioceptive** sensations that contribute to motor function and spatial awareness. Perceptual variations are normal among individuals across the lifespan and can be influenced by factors such as genetics and culture. **Orientation** is a component of normal perception that includes four basic elements: person, place, time, and situation. *Orientation to person* is the ability to correctly identify one's own name. *Orientation to place* is the ability to identify one's location. *Orientation to time* is the ability to correctly identify the time of day, the date, and the season. *Orientation to situation* is the ability to describe the global circumstances surrounding a particular event.

Attention

Attention refers to the brain's ability to remain alert and aware while selectively prioritizing concentration on a stimulus (such as something that is seen or heard) or mental event (thinking and problem solving). The reticular activating system, thalamus, and frontal cortex are the structures that are primarily involved in arousal and attention. The neurotransmitters dopamine and norepinephrine both play a major role in regulating attention.

The human capacity to sustain attention and attend to multiple stimuli is limited. Variations in attention span are typical among healthy individuals and may be impacted by development, genetics, biological rhythms, culture, and other environmental factors (Rosenberg et al., 2015). Attention is significantly altered by the experience of illness or stress. An individual's level of awareness and attention span often signifies an underlying change or alteration in biophysical and psychosocial status. Individual safety depends on the ability to attend and focus.

Memory

Memory refers to the process by which individuals retain, store, and retrieve information gained from previous experiences. The ability to remember meaningful information provides the foundation for learning and adaptation from birth to death. Because memory represents the totality of human experience, alterations in memory have a significant impact on the holistic needs of the individual. Most models of memory classify subtypes according to their sequence and duration. These include sensory, short-term, and long-term memory (see **Figure 23–1 》**).

Sensory memory refers to the earliest stage of memory, in which visual input and auditory information are retained for less than a few seconds. Sensory information that receives attention from an individual passes into short-term memory.

Short-term memory refers to the active processing and manipulation of information in conscious awareness. Short-term memory only lasts several seconds, but it can be rehearsed or repeated and transferred into long-term memory. The total amount of information that can be managed in short-term memory is also finite. For example, most research has demonstrated that longer strings of information, such as a sequence of numbers exceeding 5 to 9 digits, cannot be retained (Freberg, 2016). One aspect of short-term memory

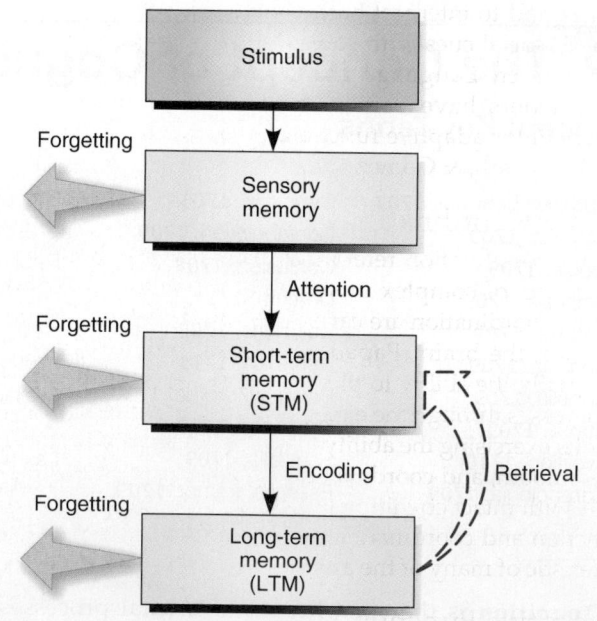

Figure 23–1 》 An information-processing model of memory. Many stimuli register in sensory memory. Those that are noticed are briefly stored in short-term memory, and those that are encoded are transferred to a more permanent facility. As shown, forgetting may be caused by failures of attention, encoding, or retrieval.

that deserves further explanation is *working memory*. Working memory is defined as the capacity to manipulate information stored in short-term memory. Examples include following a sequence of directions and performing mental mathematical calculations (D'Esposito & Postle, 2015; Ma, Husain, & Bays, 2014).

Long-term memory is used to describe the final sequence or destination of information that can be stored indefinitely. Long-term memory is further broken down into declarative and nondeclarative memories. *Declarative memories* are those that are explicit and can be consciously accessed; they are distinguished according to semantic and episodic types. *Semantic memory* consists of a collection of facts and verbal information. *Episodic memory* is composed of personal experiences. *Nondeclarative memories* are characterized by information that is outside of our conscious awareness. *Procedural memories* are a type of implicit memories that enable individuals to perform learned skills and tasks. Examples include such activities as walking, riding a bike, and driving a car (Zimmerman, 2014).

Communication and Social Cognition

The ability to receive, interpret, and express communication is an essential component of cognitive function (see the module on Communication). Memory plays a significant role in communication and speech.

Social cognition is the ability to process and apply social information accurately and effectively. It depends on the integrated function of the areas responsible for visual motor processing, language, and executive function. Scientists now believe that the neurohormone oxytocin plays an important role in social cognition (Lancaster et al., 2015). Individuals are normally able to apply an understanding of the needs of others and to interpret both verbal and nonverbal information or social cues with some degree of proficiency (American Speech Language and Hearing Association, 2016). Researchers have demonstrated that social cognition is essential for adaptive functioning across the lifespan (Bradford, Jentzsch, & Gomez, 2015).

Motor Coordination

Motor coordination refers to the planning, organizing, and execution of complex motor tasks. Cognitive function and motor coordination are carried out by shared neuronal pathways in the brain (Papadopoulos, Parrila, & Kirby, 2015). Normally the ability to plan and coordinate motor functions progresses through the expected stages of development, with adults exercising the ability to control movement in a deliberate, smooth, and coordinated fashion, called **praxis**. Individuals with intact cognition exhibit normal variations in motor function and coordination. Impaired motor function is characteristic of many of the alterations discussed in this module.

Executive Function

Executive function is an umbrella term that is used to describe the mental skills involved in planning and executing complex tasks. It incorporates coordination of the previously mentioned attributes of normal cognition, enabling individuals to selectively focus, control emotions, problem solve, and organize speech and motor activity. Examples include following multistep directions and prioritizing to manage time on a project.

Intellectual Function

Intelligence is a general term used to describe the mental capacity of the individual in relation to learning, reasoning, and problem solving. It is generally measured through the administration of one or more psychometric tests. The most commonly administered tests are the Stanford-Binet Intelligence Scales and Wechsler Intelligence Scales. Subtest scores for both are used to compare performance in areas such as general knowledge, quantitative and verbal reasoning, visual spatial processing, and working memory. The average of the scores is used to calculate an overall or full-scale intelligence quotient (IQ); however, subtest scores are also used to provide insight into individual strengths and weaknesses (Lerner & Johns, 2014).

Adaptive Behavior

Adaptive behavior refers to a set of practical skills people need to function in their everyday lives. Although the concept of adaptive behavior was originally intended to address the degree of limitations experienced by individuals with intellectual disabilities, the principles can be applied across the lifespan to patients experiencing alterations in cognitive function. The three categories of adaptive behavior are conceptual skills (use of language, reading, or telling time), social skills (ability to follow rules and interact appropriately with others) and practical skills (ability to engage in work and perform activities of daily living [ADLs]).

Physiology Review

Cognition largely depends on brain and nervous system functioning. The structural integrity of and complex physiologic processes that occur within the cerebral cortex are responsible for most aspects of the individual's ability to process sensory information. However, the **limbic system**, reticular activating system, and cerebellum also play a role in arousal, motivation, emotional regulation, and balance (see the module on Intracranial Regulation for more information).

The physiologic processes that occur in the brain have particular significance in the maintenance and regulation of cognitive processes. **Neurons** are the specialized cells of nervous system that have the capacity to carry messages through electrical and chemical signals. Microglia are the resident immune cells of the brain. They play an important role in regulating response to inflammation. **Neurotransmitters** are specialized chemicals that carry nerve impulses across the synaptic gaps between neurons. Research has demonstrated that abnormalities in cellular and neurotransmitter function are associated with many cognitive disorders. Various neurotransmitters are discussed in some detail in the modules on Mood and Affect and on Stress and Coping.

Normal Genetic Variations

Research demonstrates that genetic makeup accounts for up to 70% of the variations in cognition found in the general population. Different genes can be linked to particular components of cognitive function, such as attention in working memory in healthy adults (Störmer et al., 2012; Tucker-Drob, Briley, & Harden, 2013).

Alterations to Cognition

Although the etiology, presentation, and course of diseases impacting cognitive function vary, the key clinical manifestations of alterations in mental processing all relate to dysregulation of one or more of the key components or categories of normal cognition.

General Manifestations of Altered Cognitive Function

Alterations in perception, attention, memory, executive function, communication, social cognition, intellect, and adaptive behavior occur to varying degrees and are found in a number of conditions associated with this concept. The pathophysiology of these conditions is generally related to conditions causing abnormalities in the structure and function of the brain. An understanding of the general manifestations of cognitive dysfunction is essential for providing nursing care to individuals presenting with cognitive problems, regardless of the patient's specific medical diagnosis or condition.

Alterations in Perception

Altered perception and thinking are hallmarks of many of the conditions that impact cognition across the lifespan. Perceptual disturbances may be a function of structural and physiologic brain abnormalities in several areas of the cerebral cortex. They may be related to a primary cognitive disorder, such as dementia or schizophrenia, or to an underlying medical condition. Illogical thinking may be the result of frontal lobe dysfunction and dopamine imbalance. Distortions in perceptual processing are often the result of abnormalities in the **lobes** responsible for that aspect of sensory processing. Terms related to thinking and perception include the following:

- **Confusion** is a general term used to describe increased difficulty in thinking clearly, making judgments, and focusing attention.

- **Disorientation** is an element of confusion in which the individual is unable to correctly identify one or more of the following: person, place, time, and situation.

- **Psychosis** is a general term used to describe an abnormal mental state that alters an individual's thought processes and content in a manner that impacts the individual's perception of reality. Indicators of altered thought processes and content are most often observed through the patient's speech and behaviors. Common indicators of disorganized thinking are outlined in **Table 23–1 »**.

- **Delusions** are rigid, false beliefs—for example, believing that members of a healthcare team are actually government spies assigned to gather information that will be used to harm the patient or others. Common types of delusions include delusions of persecution, in which the individual believes that others are hostile or trying to harm him; delusions of reference, in which the individual falsely believes that public events or people are directly related to her; and delusions of grandeur, in which an individual has an inflated sense of self-worth and abilities.

- **Hallucinations** are sensory experiences that do not represent reality, such as hearing, seeing, feeling, or smelling things that are not actually present. Sometimes the type of hallucinations experienced by an individual provides clues to the underlying cause. Types of hallucinations include *auditory*, in which the individual hears voices or sounds that are not there; *visual*, in which the individual sees things that are not there or sees distortions of things that are there; or *tactile*, in which the individual feels things that are not present.

Alterations in Attention

Individuals with attention difficulties demonstrate deficits in the ability to focus, shift, and sustain attention consistently. Attention deficits are characteristic of many of the cognitive disorders discussed in this module and may also occur as a distinct disorder classified in the *Diagnostic and Statistical Manual of Mental Disorders* (DSM-5) as attention-deficit disorder (ADD) or attention-deficit/hyperactivity disorder (ADHD). More information on ADD and ADHD

TABLE 23–1 Indicators of Disordered Thinking

Indicator	Description
Loose associations	Pattern of speech in which a person's ideas slip off track onto another unrelated or obliquely related topic; also known as derailment.
Tangentiality	Occurs when a person digresses from the topic at hand and goes off on a tangent, starting an entirely new train of thought.
Incoherence/word salad/neologisms	Speaking in meaningless phrases with words that are seemingly randomly chosen, often made up, and not connected.
Illogicality	Refers to speech in which there is an absence of reason and rationality.
Circumstantiality	Occurs when the person goes into excessive detail about an event and has difficulty getting to the point of the conversation.
Pressured/distractible speech	Can be identified when the patient is speaking rapidly and there is an extreme sense of urgency or even frenzy as well as tangentiality. It is nearly impossible to interrupt the person.
Poverty of speech	The opposite of pressured speech; identified by the absence of spontaneous speech in an ordinary conversation. The person cannot engage in small talk and gives brief or empty responses.

Source: From Potter, M. L., & Moller, M. D. (2016). *Psychiatric–mental health nursing: From suffering to hope.* Reprinted and electronically reproduced by permission of Pearson Education, Inc., New York, NY.

can be found in the module on Development. Short-term difficulties with attention can also occur under conditions such as acute stress and anxiety and during periods of acute illness. Problems with attention can be related to any conditions that impact the structure and function of the brain. Such problems are manifested by alterations in one or more aspects of attention. For example, deficits in mental energy manifest in the ability to sustain effort required to complete certain tasks. Individuals with altered attention have difficulty determining what information is salient and connecting new information to what they already know. Issues in processing arise from the inability to control output—meaning that an individual may lack the ability to preview and inhibit an inappropriate or unsafe response or action.

Alterations in Memory

Individuals with cognitive alterations commonly have impairments in memory that may be an initial manifestation of a cognitive disorder with one or more memory functions impacted at any given time. Imbalances of acetylcholine, dopamine, gamma-aminobutyric acid (GABA), and glutamate have been implicated in memory problems (Khakpai, Nasehi, & Zarrindast, 2016; Marx & Gilon, 2014; Wu et al., 2014). Memory impairments may be temporary or chronic and may range from mild to severe. They may also be related to an underlying illness or trauma or be caused by a medical treatment or medication. **Amnesia** is a general term that is used to refer to the loss of recent or remote memory. Patients experiencing memory loss may unconsciously attempt to compensate for memory gaps by filling them in with fabricated events through a process known as **confabulation**.

Memory loss may manifest as problems related to short-term or long-term memory. Individuals with *short-term memory loss* may retain the ability to remember events that occurred 15 years ago but have difficulty recalling something that happened several minutes ago. Issues with working memory include difficulty following multistep directions, remembering the sequencing of numbers, or performing simple calculations. Individuals with *long-term memory problems* have difficulty recalling events and learning that occurred in the distant past. Examples include forgetting work skills that were learned 10 years ago or the inability to remember important life events, such as a wedding or the death of a loved one. Deficits in semantic memory can be manifested as **agnosia**, the inability to recognize objects through the use of one or more senses.

Alterations in Communication and Social Cognition

The ability to communicate with others is contingent on adequate perception, attention, and memory. In addition, any injury or insult to the areas of the brain responsible for the use of gestures and written and spoken words can impair communication and social cognition. Alterations in communication are common findings in many neurocognitive disorders. Common related terms include the following:

- **Aphasia** is the inability to use or understand language. Aphasia may be classified as expressive aphasia, receptive aphasia, or mixed (global) aphasia. Aphasia is discussed in greater depth in the module on Intracranial Regulation.

- **Anomia** is a type of aphasia where the individual is not able to recall the names of everyday objects and is often related to the progressive degeneration and loss of semantic memory that occurs with dementia.

- **Alogia** refers to a lack of (sometimes called impoverished) speech.

Frontal lobe and right brain dysfunction impact spatial awareness to the extent that affected individuals have difficulty gauging physical aspects of social communication, such as how close to stand to someone else. Impaired visual processing can result in the inability to accurately read and respond to nonverbal cues. Sometimes these individuals are mistakenly believed to be deliberately demonstrating rude or annoying behaviors. The deficits in communication and social function place patients at significant risk for health problems, social isolation, victimization, depression, and anxiety (Cacioppo & Cacioppo, 2014).

Alterations in Motor Coordination

The pathways used for cognitive processing and motor coordination and function are shared. Problems with the speed, fluency, and quality of movement are associated with many cognitive disorders and may be a side effect of medications that alter neurotransmitter function. **Dyspraxia** is a general term used to describe difficulty with the acquisition of motor learning and coordination through the process of growth and development. **Apraxia** refers to alterations in speech as a result of impaired motor function. **Ataxia** is a term used to describe problems with balance and coordination associated with neurologic dysfunction.

Involuntary movements include those that are not completely purposeful and occur without initiation by the patient, such as tics and tremors (Mansen & Gabiola, 2015). **Tics** are semi-involuntary movements that are sudden, repetitive, and non-rhythmic. They may involve muscle groups or vocalizations (motor or phonic). Suppression of a tic may be possible but results in discomfort or anxiety for the patient (Prastaro & Giratti, 2015). Sudden, brief, meaningless movements involving one muscle group are classified as simple tics. Examples of simple tics include eye blinking and head jerking (motor tics) and throat clearing and humming (phonic tics). Complex tics involve a cluster of movements that appear coordinated and more purposeful and thus may be more difficult to identify. Complex motor tics include pulling at clothing or touching people or objects; *echopraxia*, imitating the movements of others; *copropraxia*, performing obscene or forbidden gestures; and **carphologia**, lint-picking behavior that is often seen in dementia. Examples of complex phonic tics include **echolalia**, the meaningless repetition of phrases spoken by another (Mansen & Gabiola, 2015).

Tremors are unintentional rhythmic movements manifested in shaking of the affected part of the body. **Essential tremors** are those that are not associated with another condition and may be genetic in origin. **Physiologic tremors** occur normally as a result of physiologic exhaustion or emotional stress. Common tremors include *resting tremors*, a coarse, rhythmic tremor often observed in resting arms and hands that is characteristic of Parkinson disease and sometimes seen as a side effect of certain medications; and *dystonic tremors,* sustained involuntary muscle contractions causing twisting repetitive movements and painful or abnormal postures (Mansen & Gabiola, 2015).

Dyskinesia represents a general category of difficulty with or distortions of movement. It is may be associated with acquired disorders such as Parkinson disease or as side effect of some medications. Types of dyskinesias are:

- *Akathisia:* An internal feeling of restlessness that may lead to rocking, pacing, or other constant movement
- *Akinesia:* Diminished movement as a result of difficulty initiating movement
- *Bradykinesia:* Dyskinesia characterized by slow movement
- *Dystonia:* An acute episode of muscle contractions (may result from a neurodegenerative disease or a reaction to medication)
- *Rigidity:* Resistance to movement. *Cogwheel rigidity* refers to ratchet-like resistance when attempting to move the joints.

Alterations in Executive Function

Executive function is significantly affected by structural and physiologic abnormalities impacting the frontal cortex (Funahashi & Andreau, 2013; Hosenbocus & Chahal, 2012). Manifestations of impaired function include emotional dysregulation; poor judgment and decision making; reduced insight; forgetfulness; difficulty in planning, organizing, and concrete thinking; and personality changes. Difficulties can range from mild to severe. **Avolition** is decreased motivation, or the inability to initiate goal-directed activity, and may be in part related to deficits in executive dysfunction (Carpenter et al., 2016).

Alterations in Intellectual Function and Learning

Alterations in intellectual function and learning may be either developmental or acquired. The DSM-5 classifies both intellectual disabilities and specific learning disabilities that manifest in childhood as neurodevelopmental disorders (American Psychiatric Association [APA], 2013). Nurses should recognize that there are a broad range of issues impacting learning and intellectual function and that many individuals may demonstrate deficits in adaptive function without meeting the current diagnostic criteria (Gaddes, 2013). For more information on learning and associated problems, refer to the module on Development.

Learning disabilities are a group of disorders that impact an individual's ability to process information. The cause of learning disabilities is not entirely understood, but researchers believe that subtle variations in brain structure and function may be responsible. Both genetics and environmental factors probably contribute to these variations. In general, individuals with learning disabilities have average to above-average intelligence but demonstrate a gap between their actual and potential achievement. The impact of learning disabilities goes well beyond difficulty with basic academic skills. Most individuals with specific learning difficulties also experience one or more related problems with social cognition, executive function, memory, processing speed, attention, and motor coordination. As a result, they often face significant challenges with interpersonal relationships and other aspects of adaptive function (Learning Disabilities Association of America [LDA], 2016). Nurses are in a key position to assess for variations in development that may suggest an underlying learning issue.

Intellectual disabilities are characterized by significant limitations in intellectual functioning and adaptive behavior that begin prior to age 18. An IQ score of 70–75 or below is considered indicative of limited intellectual functioning. Intellectual disability can result from prenatal errors in central nervous system (CNS) development, external factors that damage the CNS, or pre- or postnatal changes in an individual's biological environment. Sometimes, these changes produce only mental limitations. Other times, intellectual disability is one of a constellation of symptoms linked to a particular cause (American Association of Intellectual and Developmental Disabilities, 2013).

Selected Alterations for Cognition

The exemplars included in this module represent only a fraction of the disorders that impair cognition. The classification of these disorders in the DSM-5 provides a context for understanding both similarities and differences in the exemplars and related conditions; however, the nursing care focuses primarily on supporting adaptive function and collaborating with healthcare professionals to provide holistic care that meets the unique needs of affected individuals regardless of medical diagnosis.

Selected Learning Disabilities

Although the DSM-5 has changed the classification of specific learning disabilities to include three specific categories limited to impairment in reading, impairment in written expression, and impairment in mathematics, many associated difficulties with cognitive function, such as communication processing disorders, have been reclassified under neurodevelopmental disorders (APA, 2013). **Table 23–2 》** identifies some of the most common learning issues nurses may encounter, using both common or umbrella terms and their associated DSM-5 classifications. Implications for nursing practice are included. For all patients with learning difficulties, support them and their families in seeking appropriate services and accommodations, and encourage activities that focus on strengths and build self-esteem.

Selected Intellectual Disabilities

Of the various conditions associated with intellectual disability, three deserve special mention because of the range of physical and cognitive alterations they involve. **Down syndrome**, **fragile X syndrome**, and **fetal alcohol syndrome (FAS)** are all caused by problems during prenatal development, although the first two conditions involve genetic errors while the third involves alcohol consumption during pregnancy. All three conditions are present at birth and affect an individual for the rest of his life. See **Table 23–3 》** for a summary of physical traits associated with these conditions.

Down Syndrome

Down syndrome occurs when an individual's cells contain a third full or partial copy of the 21st chromosome (National Down Syndrome Society, 2012). Usually, a full copy of the

Alterations and Therapies
Cognition

ALTERATION	DESCRIPTION	MANIFESTATIONS	INTERVENTIONS AND THERAPIES
Perceptual disturbances/ psychosis	Alterations in ability to interpret environmental stimuli, think clearly and logically, and maintain orientation to person, place, time, and situation	■ Hallucinations ■ Delusions ■ Disordered thinking ■ Disorientation/confusion	■ Identify and treat underlying cause ■ Reduce environmental stimulation ■ Reality orientation and validation therapy
Impaired attention	Difficulty sustaining or directing focus	■ Easily distracted ■ Avoids situations requiring sustained focus ■ Difficulty learning	■ Identify and treat underlying cause ■ Reduce distractions
Memory problems	Impairment in ability to recall information	■ Getting lost ■ Difficulty with word finding and recognition ■ Difficulty remembering recent events ■ Difficulty remembering remote events	■ Identify and treat underlying cause ■ Cognitive remediation ■ Provide compensatory strategies and memory aids
Problems with communication/ social cognition	Impairments in the ability to process social information and communicate with others	■ Difficulty adhering to social conventions ■ Receptive and expressive language problems	■ Refer for speech therapy ■ Provide accommodations and modifications ■ Provide social skills training
Problems with motor function/ control	Inability to carry out smooth, purposeful movement	■ Tic ■ Tremors ■ Dyskinesia	■ Identify and treat underlying cause ■ Provide environmental modifications ■ Refer for occupational therapy (OT) and physical therapy (PT)
Problems with executive function	Weaknesses in key mental skills required for adaptive function	■ Difficulty organizing ■ Difficulty planning ■ Poor impulse control ■ Problems with attention and memory	■ Provide compensatory strategies (lists, organizers) ■ Refer for OT ■ Support safety needs
Problems with intellectual function and learning	Problems with global intellectual function or acquisition of knowledge required for adaptive function	■ Low IQ ■ Problems with adaptive function ■ Academic problems ■ Social/emotional problems	■ Provide modifications and accommodations ■ Provide remediation ■ Focus on strengths

extra chromosome is present, a situation known as **trisomy 21**. In either case, the excess genetic material leads to intellectual disability and physical impairments that can range from mild to severe (**Figure 23-2 》**).

Individuals with Down syndrome are at increased risk of several problems not normally seen in childhood. Roughly 50% are born with congenital heart defects. Children with Down syndrome are also more likely to experience hearing loss, gastrointestinal blockages, celiac disease, vision problems, thyroid disease, skeletal abnormalities, orthodontic problems, leukemia, and eventual dementia. With appropriate support, affected individuals can lead healthy lives and sometimes live and work independently. Average life expectancy for individuals with Down syndrome is about 60 years, although some individuals live 10

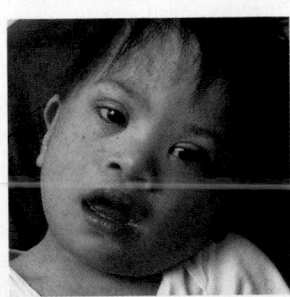

Source: George Dodson/Pearson Education, Inc.

Figure 23–2 》 A child with Down syndrome.

or even 20 years longer (Centers for Disease Control and Prevention, 2016; National Down Syndrome Society, 2012).

TABLE 23–2 Comparison of Common Learning Problems and Their Implications for Nurses

Common Terms and Associated DSM-5 Terms	Defining Characteristics	Nursing Implications
Common term ■ Auditory Processing Disorder (APD) and Language Processing Disorder (LPD) **DSM-5** ■ Communication Disorder: Language Disorder ■ Communication Disorder: Speech Sound Disorder	Individuals with APD and related language-based communication disorders have difficulty processing sounds and discriminating differences in where sounds come from. Problems learning verbally, focusing, remembering and applying auditory information and language.	■ Refer patients with communication deficits for evaluation. ■ Anticipate collaboration with speech pathologists and learning specialists. ■ Adapt teaching to show rather than tell. ■ Reduce auditory distractions. ■ Vary pitch and tone, space directives, and allow additional time for verbal processing.
Common term ■ Dyscalculia **DSM-5** ■ Specific Learning Disorder (in the area of mathematics)	Difficulty understanding numbers and learning math facts. Poor understanding of math symbols, difficulty with related tasks, such as telling time.	■ Refer patients with academic and occupational problems related to math for evaluation. ■ Recognize that patients may have difficulty calculating doses and taking medications on schedule. Encourage the use of devices (pill minders, single-dose dispensers) to promote safety.
Common term ■ Dysgraphia **DSM-5** ■ Specific Learning Disorder (in the area of written expression)	Disability impacting fine motor skills and the ability to write clearly and legibly. May have difficulty focusing or thinking while performing fine motor tasks.	■ Refer patients with academic/occupational problems related to written expression for evaluation. ■ Anticipate collaboration with occupational therapy. ■ Encourage the use of word processing devices, dictation software. ■ Recognize that patients may have difficulty performing fine motor skills necessary for self-care (e.g., dressing changes) and modify care to address.
Common term ■ Dyslexia **DSM-5** ■ Specific Learning Disorder (in the area of reading)	Difficulty with reading and language-based skills impacting reading fluency, decoding, and comprehension.	■ Refer patients with academic/ occupational problems related to reading for evaluation. ■ Anticipate collaboration with learning specialists. ■ Use nonverbal teaching strategies. ■ Recognize that the ability to follow written directions may be limited, supplement with visual aids, and record information if necessary.
Common term ■ Non-verbal Learning Disabilities (NVLD) **DSM-5** ■ Communication Disorder: Social/Pragmatic Communication Disorder ■ Motor Disorder: Developmental Coordination Disorder	Often a significant gap between high verbal skills and low perceptual skills (motor, visual-spatial skills, social skills). Typically impacts interpretation of nonverbal cues, such as body language. Difficulty understanding and adhering to social conventions. Difficulty integrating sensory information. Because of the devastating social implications of this disorder, individuals may present first with a mental health issue (e.g., depression, anxiety).	■ Screen for alterations in social development. ■ Consider learning issues when patients present with mental health issues. ■ Assess patient safety—may be at risk for bullying and abuse because of poor social skills and attempts to compensate with maladaptive behavior. ■ Anticipate collaboration with occupational therapy, speech pathology and psychologists, developmental pediatricians. ■ Use verbal strategies and avoid diagrams and images. ■ See strategies under associated problems: dyscalculia, dysgraphia, and visual perceptual motor deficit. ■ Teach social skills explicitly. ■ Assess for depression, anxiety, social isolation. ■ Recognize that the disorder may be poorly understood by family, teachers. and other healthcare professionals. Advocate for patient.
Common term ■ Visual Perceptual/Visual Motor Deficit **DSM-5** ■ Motor Disorder: Developmental Coordination Disorder	Difficulty performing tasks that require the integration of visual processing and application to motor tasks (e.g., copying, finding images in a field, keeping place, reading maps).	■ Address implications for self-care; provide lists for organizing items, navigating unfamiliar environments. ■ Anticipate collaboration with occupational therapy, physical therapy, speech pathology, and psychologists. ■ Recognize that patients may have difficulty adhering to treatments as a result of visual motor deficits. ■ Coordination disorders may discourage individuals from taking part in physical activity; encourage patients to find appropriate forms of exercise. ■ Preview before going to appointments in unfamiliar settings. ■ Use of devices such as pill organizers may promote safety. ■ Provide lists and step-by-step verbal instructions.
Common terms ■ Global Intellectual Delays ■ Previously called Mental Retardation **DSM-5** ■ Intellectual Disability: Intellectual Developmental Disorder	Impairment related to both IQ (below 70–75) and deficits in adaptive function/behavior.	■ Assess patient safety—may be at risk for bullying and abuse because of poor social skills and attempts to compensate with maladaptive behavior. ■ Anticipate collaboration with occupational therapy, speech pathology, psychologists, and developmental pediatricians ■ Address common comorbid health problems, including associated congenital defects (if present).

Sources: Data from American Psychiatric Association. (2013). *Diagnostic and statistical manual of mental disorders,* 5th ed. Washington, DC: Author; Learning Disabilities Association of America. (2016). Types of learning disabilities. Retrieved from http://ldaamerica.org/types-of-learning-disabilities; Mammarella, I. C., Ghisi, M. Bomba, M., Bottesi, G., Caviola, S. Broggi, F., & Nacinovich, R. (2016). Anxiety and depression in children with nonverbal learning disabilities, reading disabilities, or typical development. *Journal of Learning Disabilities, 49*(2), 130–139; Tuffrey-Wijne, I., Giatras, N., Goulding, L., Abraham, E., Fenwick, L., Edwards, C., & Hollins, S. (2013). Identifying the factors affecting the implementation of strategies to promote a safer environment for patients with learning disabilities in NHS hospitals: A mixed-methods study. *Health Services and Delivery Research,* No. 1.13. Retrieved from http://www.ncbi.nlm.nih.gov/books/NBK259489/

TABLE 23–3 Physical Traits Associated with Three Causes of Intellectual Disability

Down Syndrome See Figure 23–2	Fragile X Syndrome See Figure 23–3	Fetal Alcohol Syndrome See Figure 23–4
Broad hands with a single traverse palmar crease	Crossed eyes	Small eyes
Congenital cataracts	Enlarged testicles	Abnormal joints and bones
Decreased muscle tone	Epicanthic eye folds	CNS abnormalities
Epicanthic eye folds	Excessively flexible joints	Flattened nasal bridge
Flattened nose	High palate	Growth deficits
Hearing impairment	Increased likelihood of middle ear infections	Hearing impairment
Increased likelihood of diabetes, leukemia, and heart defects	Increased seizure risk	Lack of coordination
Protruding tongue	Large ears	Small nose that turns up at the tip
Short, stocky neck	Long head with protruding jaw	Small palpebral fissures
Small ears located low on the head	Scoliosis	Smooth philtrum
Small head		Thin vermillion border
Wide space between first two toes		

Fragile X Syndrome

Fragile X syndrome arises from a single recessive abnormality on the X chromosome. Specifically, a mutation in the *FMR-1* gene causes a small section of DNA to be repeated 200 or more times, rather than the normal 5–40 times. This change renders the gene unable to make its associated protein, and absence of the protein leads to errors in brain development and function (National Human Genome Research Institute, 2016).

A variety of signs and symptoms are associated with fragile X syndrome (**Figure 23-3 ≫**). The most notable is intellectual disability, typically accompanied by behavioral problems such as ADHD. Affected children may also exhibit autistic behaviors; speech problems; anxiety and mood problems; delays in learning to sit, walk, and talk; and enhanced sensitivity to environmental stimuli. Most individuals with fragile X syndrome are in generally good health and have a normal lifespan. Still, approximately 15% of affected males and 6–8% of females will experience seizures and require anticonvulsant medications (Consensus of the Fragile X Clinical & Research Consortium on Clinical Practices, 2012). Interestingly, boys usually experience the effects of fragile X syndrome to a much greater degree than girls. Because girls have two copies of the X chromosome, one X chromosome's *FMR-1* gene is able to produce enough protein to partially compensate for the amount normally produced by the other copy. Boys, however, have just one X chromosome, so no

compensatory mechanism is available (National Human Genome Research Institute, 2016).

Fetal Alcohol Syndrome

Unlike Down syndrome and fragile X syndrome, FAS is a completely preventable condition caused by maternal alcohol intake during pregnancy. (See the Patient Teaching feature.) FAS is the most severe of several fetal alcohol spectrum disorders (FASDs), all of which involve some degree of physical, intellectual, behavioral, and/or learning disability (**Figure 23-4 ≫**).

FAS and related disorders result from the presence of alcohol in a woman's bloodstream. Because alcohol crosses the placenta and the fetal liver cannot process it, the fetus has the same blood alcohol content as its mother, regardless of the type or amount of alcohol consumed (National Organization on Fetal Alcohol Syndrome, 2014a). Even small amounts of alcohol can dramatically disrupt prenatal development, causing facial, skeletal, and organ abnormalities, along with a variety of other problems. However, for a diagnosis of FAS (as opposed to another fetal alcohol spectrum disorder), a child must exhibit all of the following conditions:

- Growth deficits
- Characteristic facial abnormalities, including a smooth philtrum (ridge between the nose and upper lip), thin vermillion border (line between the lips and surrounding skin), and small palpebral fissures (separations between the upper and lower eyelids)

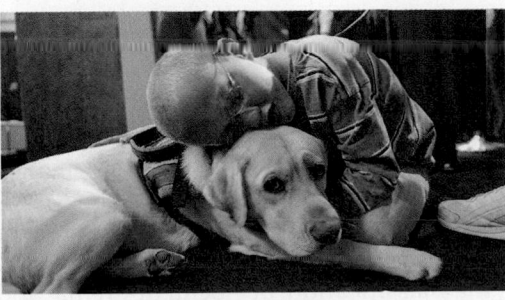

Source: ZUMA Press Inc/Alamy Stock Photo.

Figure 23–3 ≫ A child with fragile X syndrome.

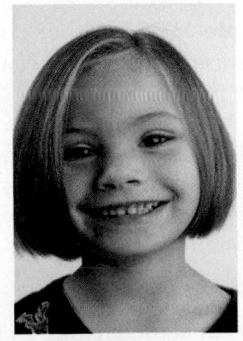

Source: Rick's Photography/Shutterstock.

Figure 23–4 ≫ A child with fetal alcohol syndrome.

Patient Teaching
Fetal Alcohol Syndrome

In the United States, about 1 in 10 women admit consuming at least one alcoholic drink during pregnancy, while about 2% report having five or more drinks at one time. These statistics indicate that all women need clear, timely messages about the damaging effects of alcohol on the fetus (Alshaarawy, Breslau, & Anthony, 2016).

Patient teaching must emphasize that the **only** way to prevent FAS is to abstain from all alcohol of all types for the entire duration of pregnancy. This message should be communicated to all female patients of childbearing age, including teenagers, so they understand how important it is to stop drinking immediately should they become pregnant. Nurses should also explain that the most dangerous time for fetal alcohol exposure may be early in pregnancy—often before a woman even knows she's expecting.

- Central nervous system abnormalities (structural, neurologic, and/or functional) (National Organization on Fetal Alcohol Syndrome, 2014b).

These nervous system abnormalities almost always result in some degree of mental impairment, such as intellectual disability, learning disability, communication problems, poor memory, or limited attention span. Although the many effects of FAS last a lifetime, early treatment can help lessen some symptoms and improve an affected individual's quality of life.

Other Preventable Causes of Intellectual Disability

- Maternal drug use, smoking, malnutrition, exposure to environmental toxins, and illness during pregnancy.

- Prematurity and low birth weight forecast disability more reliably than any other conditions. Difficulties at delivery, such as oxygen deprivation or birth injury, may also cause problems in intellectual functioning.

- Head injuries, near-drowning, and diseases such as whooping cough, chickenpox, measles, and *Haemophilus influenzae* type B (Hib) can damage the brain in childhood. Childhood exposure to lead, mercury, and other toxins can also cause irreparable damage to the nervous system.

- Malnutrition, childhood diseases, exposure to environmental health hazards, and a lack of intellectual stimulation early in life also are factors have been linked to intellectual disability.

In the United States and in other countries around the world, prevalence rates of intellectual disability have dropped thanks to public health measures that mandate newborn screening for phenylketonuria (PKU) and require vaccinations for Hib, measles, encephalitis, and rubella. Comprehensive prenatal care, including testing for diseases and administering folic acid to expectant mothers, also reduces the risk of intellectual disability.

Delirium

Delirium is usually an acute change in mental state that is characterized by confusion; inability to focus, shift, or sustain attention; disorientation; sleep-wake cycle disturbances; disorganized thinking; perceptual abnormalities; mood changes; and both psychomotor retardation and agitation. Delirium typically results from a medical condition, trauma, or chemical/substance exposure or withdrawal and is a common complication observed during stays in acute-care settings. Delirium is presented as an exemplar in this module.

Dementia

Dementia is a general term used to describe the loss of one or more cortical functions or cognitive attributes as a result of degeneration of the neurologic systems of the brain. The DSM-5 now uses the term *mild and major neurocognitive disorders* (NCDs) to replace the term *dementia*. Individuals with mild NCDs are those who demonstrate limited impairment and are able to maintain independent functioning with some modifications. They are often in the initial stages of disease progression. NCDs are classified as major when additional cortical functions are lost and the individual can no longer maintain independence (Blazer, 2013). Dementia can be caused or exacerbated by other conditions and variables, including metabolic problems, nutritional deficiencies, infections, poisoning, medications, and any conditions that compromise oxygenation and perfusion (National Institute for Neurological Disorders and Stroke, 2016). Subtypes of NCDs are classified by etiology and are discussed briefly below and in more detail in the exemplar on Alzheimer disease. The terms *major neurocognitive disorder* and *dementia* are both used in clinical practice and are used interchangeably in this module.

Alzheimer disease is the most common form of dementia, accounting for about 80% of all cases and affecting more than 5 million adults in the United States (Alzheimer's Association, 2014). Alzheimer-related NCD is included as an exemplar in this module. *Vascular* or *neurocognitive dementia* results from multiple small strokes or infarcts to the brain and is often manifested in a more abrupt change in cognitive function. Vascular dementia can occur alone or in combination with other forms of dementia and is thought to represent at least 10% of all cases of neurocognitive decline. Genetics and heritability appear to play a role in the development of most forms of dementia, although many impacted individuals have no family history. **Table 23–4 》** outlines other forms of dementia.

Nurses and other healthcare professionals need to recognize that a variety of conditions can mimic dementia, especially in older individuals. Depression and emotional problems may cause cognitive slowing and disorientation. It may be also difficult to distinguish symptoms of delirium from those of dementia. **Table 23–5 》** provides a comparison of the manifestations of delirium, dementia, and depression.

Schizophrenia Spectrum and Other Psychotic Disorders

As mentioned previously, psychotic disorders encompass a broad range of cognitive alterations that result in altered perceptions of reality and abnormal thinking in the absence of an underlying condition. Schizophrenia represents one type of psychotic disorder and is discussed in detail as an exemplar for cognition. The DSM-5 has been updated to change the classification of "Schizophrenia and Other Psychotic Disorders" to "Schizophrenia Spectrum and Other Psychotic Disorders," often collectively referred to as

TABLE 23–4 Selected Neurocognitive Disorders Resulting in Dementia

Disorder	Etiology	Clinical Manifestations	Onset/Course
Dementia due to HIV	Infection with HIV-1 produces a dementing illness called HIV-1-associated cognitive/motor complex.	Symptoms vary in early stages. Severe cognitive changes, particularly confusion, changes in behavior, and sometimes psychosis, are not uncommon in the later stages.	At first symptoms are subtle and may be overlooked. The severity of symptoms is associated with the extent of the brain pathology.
Dementia due to traumatic brain injury	Any type of head trauma.	Amnesia is the most common neuro-behavioral symptom following head trauma.	A degree of permanent disturbance may persist.
Dementia due to Parkinson disease	Parkinson disease is a neurologic condition resulting from the death of neurons, including those that produce dopamine, the chemical responsible for movement and coordination. It is characterized by tremor, rigidity, bradykinesia, and postural instability.	Dementia has been reported in approximately 20–60% of people with Parkinson disease and is characterized by cognitive and motor slowing, impaired memory, and impaired executive functioning.	Onset and course are slow and progressive.
Dementia due to Huntington disease	Huntington disease is an inherited, dominant gene, neurodegenerative disease. The first symptoms typically are choreic movements that involve facial contortions, twisting, turning, and tongue movements.	Cognitive symptoms include memory deficits, both recent and remote, as well as significant problems with frontal executive function, personality changes, and other signs of dementia.	The disease begins in the late 30s or early 40s and may last 10–20 years or more before death.
Lewy body dementia	This disorder is distinguished by the presence of Lewy bodies—eosinophilic inclusion bodies—seen in the cortex and brainstem.	Clinically, Lewy body disease is similar to Alzheimer disease; however, there is an earlier appearance of visual hallucinations and parkinsonian features.	Irreversible and progressive; tends to progress more rapidly than Alzheimer disease.

Sources: Based on Andreasen, N. C., & Black, D. W. (2006). *Introductory textbook of psychiatry* (4th ed.). Washington, DC: American Psychiatric Publishing; American Psychiatric Association. (2013). *Diagnostic and statistical manual of mental disorders* (5th ed.). Washington, DC: Author; Bourgeois, J. A., Seaman, J. S., & Servis, M. E. (2003). Delirium, dementia, and amnestic disorders. In R. E. Hales & S. C. Yudofsky (Eds.), *Textbook of clinical psychiatry* (4th ed.). Washington, DC: American Psychiatric Publishing; Sharon, I. (2010). *Huntington disease dementia*. Retrieved from http://emedicine.medscape.com/289706. Table first appeared in Potter, M. L., & Moller, M. D. (2016). *Psychiatric–mental health nursing: From suffering to hope.* Upper Saddle River, NJ: Pearson.

"SSDs" (APA, 2013). This change was partially intended to reflect a better understanding of the profound neurocognitive deficits associated with this disorder. Approximately 1–4% of the population experiences some type of psychotic disorder, and up to 1% of the worldwide population meets the criteria for schizophrenia (American Psychiatric Association, 2015). The DSM-5 identifies a number of psychotic disorders in addition to schizophrenia spectrum disorder. Because psychosis can result from an underlying medical condition or ingestion of one or more substances, diagnostic tests should be run to rule out any underlying illness or causative substance.

Risk Factors for Altered Cognitive Function

Although risk factors for impaired cognition vary according to the conditions described in this section, a few general principles apply. Most developmental and acquired cognitive disorders have a nonmodifiable familial/genetic component that predisposes individuals to the development of a specific disorder, such as dementia or schizophrenia. Other categories of risk factors include population-specific factors, lifestyle/behaviors, environmental exposures, and certain health conditions. Most cognitive disorders are believed to be multifactorial or the consequence of genetic factors and age, sex, lifestyle/behaviors, environmental exposures, or other health conditions.

Case Study >> Part 1

Victor Wallace is a 74-year-old man who was diagnosed with mild NCD due to Alzheimer disease 2 years ago. Mr. Wallace lives with his 50-year-old daughter, Anne Marie, who is his primary caregiver. His wife of 52 years died of pancreatic cancer 18 months ago.

TABLE 23–5 Comparison of Delirium, Dementia, and Depression

	Delirium	Dementia	Depression
Onset	Acute, sudden, rapid	Slow, progressive	Variable
Duration	Hours to days	Months to years	Episodic
Cognitive impairment	Memory, consciousness	Abstract thinking, memory	Memory and concentration
Mood	Rapid mood swings	Depression, apathy	Sadness, anxiety
Delusions/hallucinations	Both; often visual	May present in later stages	Delusions only
Outcome	Recovery possible	Poor	Recovery possible

Source: Potter, M. L., & Moller, M. D. (2016). *Psychiatric–mental health nursing: From suffering to hope.* Reprinted and electronically reproduced by permission of Pearson Education, Inc., New York, NY.

Mr. Wallace presents at his gerontologist's office at 9:30 on Thursday morning. Ms. Wallace requested the appointment because she is concerned about the changes she has seen in her father over the past month. As the nurse working with Mr. Wallace's gerontologist, you conduct an initial assessment and interview with Mr. Wallace and Ms. Wallace. Ms. Wallace reports that Mr. Wallace has exhibited increased confusion and anxiety at home and at the adult daycare center he attends each day while she is at work. In the past, Mr. Wallace had these problems only in unfamiliar settings. He is also experiencing a decline in language, increasingly using the wrong words to describe common objects and relying on scanning speech to find words. However, Ms. Wallace's main concern is her father's refusal to carry out the basic ADLs he is still capable of performing. When you ask Mr. Wallace about the ADLs, he says, "There's no point in trying because I won't be able to do them much longer."

As you observe Mr. Wallace, you note that he seems agitated. He is sitting on the edge of his chair, tapping his foot and rapping his hands on his knees. When you ask him basic questions, he has a hard time coming up with answers. When he can't find the words he wants, he just repeats the phrase, "That's how it is."

Mr. Wallace's vital signs and weight are normal, and his physical condition is good for a man his age. You administer the Cornell Scale for Depression in Dementia and his score is 17, indicating high probability of depression. The gerontologist maintains Mr. Wallace's current dose of 28 mg of memantine (Namenda) per day to slow the progression of his Alzheimer symptoms. She then adds sertraline (Zoloft), a selective serotonin reuptake inhibitor (SSRI), to treat his depression symptoms. Mr. Wallace is to start out taking 50 mg of sertraline per day, gradually working up to 150 mg per day over a 6-week period.

Clinical Reasoning Questions Level I

1. How do your observations of Mr. Wallace correlate with the changes Ms. Wallace reports?
2. What aspects of Mr. Wallace's presentation prompt you to test him for depression?
3. Why might Mr. Wallace's increased confusion in familiar settings be a concern for Ms. Wallace?

Clinical Reasoning Questions Level II

4. Why is it important to distinguish between Mr. Wallace's refusal to perform ADLs and an inability to do so?
5. Would speech therapy be an appropriate intervention for Mr. Wallace? Why or why not?
6. *Refer to the exemplar on Alzheimer disease in this module:* How would a change in Mr. Wallace's Alzheimer medication from an angiotensin-converting enzyme inhibitor, like memantine, to a cholinesterase inhibitor, like donepezil, affect the doctor's choice of SSRI for depression?

Concepts Related to Cognition

Cognitive function and other systems tend to be interdependent, so determining the extent to which other concepts or systems is involved can be difficult. For example, cerebral perfusion is necessary for normal cognitive functioning but depends on the adequate intake of oxygen and osmotic pressure needed to maintain adequate blood flow. Any condition that impairs cerebral perfusion will result in inflammation and metabolic changes that further impair cognition. Even subtle variations in perfusion can result in acute alterations in cognitive function, such as delirium, with older adults being more sensitive to these changes because of diminished functional reserves (Fogel & Greenberg, 2015). The possible causes of diminished cerebral tissue perfusion are many and range from cerebral edema to shock. Chronic cerebral hypoperfusion from decreased cardiac output and vascular changes have been implicated in Alzheimer disease and

other chronic and degenerative neurologic disorders (Alosco et al., 2013).

Cerebral perfusion and cognitive integrity depend on normal gas exchange. Decreased oxygenation leads to respiratory acidosis, in which levels of carbon dioxide increase and vasodilation of blood vessels occurs, resulting in increased intracranial pressure. Symptoms of acute oxygen deprivation include headaches, confusion, and irritability. Chronic and subtle mechanisms involved in decreased oxygen supply to the brain (as seen in chronic obstructive pulmonary disease [COPD] and anemia) can negatively impact the neurochemical signaling and synaptic plasticity necessary for normal cognitive development and function (Mukandala et al., 2016).

Fluid and electrolyte balance is also necessary to maintain adequate perfusion and to support cellular function in the brain. A change in mental status, memory, or attention is often an early sign of dehydration in older adults. Cerebral cells are the first to be impacted by the shift of fluids from the vascular to the intracellular space that occurs as a result of fluid volume excess. Early signs of cerebral edema include headache, nausea, and vomiting, with changes in mental status (McCance & Huether, 2014).

Brain function depends on complex metabolic processes required to meet the energy needs of neuronal cells and maintain the synthesis and function of neurochemicals in cognition. Any alteration in normal glucose supply or the excess or deficiency of other metabolic products can result in either acute or chronic cognitive dysfunction (González-Reyes et al., 2016). Both hypoglycemia and hyperglycemic ketoacidosis can result in confusion, hallucinations, and changes in consciousness. Infection, inflammation, and alterations in thermoregulation increase overall metabolic demands and can precipitate changes in cognitive function.

Inflammation appears to play a key role in altered cognitive function. Stress, infection, surgery, and cancer all result in an inflammatory response and the release of cytokines. Inflammation can occur in the brain and central nervous system as a direct result of trauma, cerebral infarction, or bacterial, viral, fungi, or prion infections. Peripheral inflammation (outside of the central nervous system) causes a cascade of physiologic events that alter glutamate, serotonin, dopamine, and acetylcholine systems considered central in cognition, with implications for an array of affective, cognitive, and behavioral responses (Benros et al., 2015). Initially, these changes are adaptive, enabling individuals to conserve energy necessary for healing. However, chronic or persistent inflammation can lead to irreversible neuronal changes.

Substances such as alcohol, illicit drugs, and some pharmaceuticals can impact cognitive function. Immediate consequences of alcohol intoxication include confusion, decreased attention, impaired judgment, loss of inhibition, disorientation, hallucinations, and memory loss. Chronic alcohol abuse can lead to hematologic changes that can limit oxygenation to the brain and lead to encephalopathy. Older adults are at a higher risk of permanent cognitive changes as a result of excessive alcohol consumption (Kim et al., 2012).

Permanent brain injury caused by trauma or acute oxygenation deprivation is a common source of cognitive pathophysiology. Cognitive disorders such as schizophrenia and learning disabilities are associated with both obvious and subtle anatomic differences in brain development and structure as well as developmental delays (Butterworth & Kovas, 2013; Ren et al., 2013).

Alterations in cognitive function have the potential to impact an individual's competency to make healthcare decisions and consent to certain treatments and procedures. Patients with mental health disorders, intellectual disabilities, and other cognitive conditions are often unable to advocate for themselves and are considered vulnerable populations. Establishing advance directives during mild stages of cognitive dysfunction or relapse is essential.

Individuals with a serious mental illness such as schizophrenia are at increased risk of involvement with the criminal justice system because of the behavioral manifestations of these disorders. Research demonstrates that individuals with psychotic disorders are overrepresented in the criminal justice system (Robertson et al., 2015).

The following feature links some, but not all, of the concepts related to cognition. They are presented in alphabetical order.

Concepts Related to Cognition

CONCEPT	RELATIONSHIP TO COGNITION	NURSING IMPLICATIONS
Addiction	Drugs and alcohol alter normal neuronal functioning, ↓ blood flow and/or waste removal → cognitive impairment.	■ Promote prevention of addiction behaviors, address risk factors. ■ Monitor vital signs. ■ Provide for patient safety. ■ Watch for symptoms of withdrawal and provide supportive care as necessary. ■ Pharmacotherapy, substance abuse counseling, patient education.
Development	Genetic factors, heredity, and environmental insults → cognitive dysfunction.	■ Refer for genetic counseling. ■ Screen for conditions that may impact cognitive development (e.g., metabolic disorders). ■ Assess for alterations in development. ■ Refer for evaluation. ■ Provide patient/family education and support; collaborate with special education services, psychologists, speech pathologists, occupational therapy, and others.
Inflammation	Inflammation → release of pro-inflammatory proteins that alter neurotransmitter function. Chronic and frequent inflammation → permanent cognitive decline.	■ Promote lifestyle behaviors that decrease inflammation (diet, exercise, prevention of infection, immunizations, injury prevention, use of helmets). ■ Assess for infection or injury that may be causing inflammation. ■ Implement measures to address inflammation/infection (antibiotics, anti-inflammatory agents).
Legal Issues	Recurring or chronic cognitive issues ↓ decision-making capacity and competency. Lack of appropriate services → involvement with the criminal justice system.	■ Provide safe environment. ■ Recognize that a history of incarceration alone does not predict violent behavior. ■ Advocate for community resources that can enable individuals with cognitive function to manage the symptoms of their disease and avoid encounters with the criminal justice system. ■ Monitor for signs of abuse, caregiver role strain. ■ Ask whether patient has established an advance directive or is interested in doing so. ■ Document the advance directives and all conversations about it in the patient's chart. ■ Advocate on the patient's behalf by ensuring that the advance directive is followed. ■ *Anticipate:* Patient, family community education, referral to counseling resources, case management services.
Oxygenation	Decreased O_2 reaching the brain → cognitive impairment, coma, and death.	■ Promote prevention of conditions that lead to impaired oxygenation; address modifiable risk factors. ■ Monitor vital signs, arterial blood gases (ABGs), airway clearance, and for signs of impaired perfusion. ■ Administer oxygen and carry out other interventions to support oxygenation.
Perfusion	Inadequate perfusion of brain tissue ↓ O_2 levels and → acute changes in cognitive function. Chronic impairments in perfusion and oxygenation ↑ risk for neurodegeneration.	■ Promote healthy lifestyle; address modifiable risk factors for alterations in perfusion. ■ Monitor vital signs, ABGs, and cardiac sounds. ■ Assess perfusion, including pulses, nail beds, and skin color. ■ *Anticipate:* Pharmacotherapy, intravenous (IV) fluids, stress/exercise tests, echocardiogram, possible cardiac catheterization and/or surgery.

Health Promotion

A health-promotion model for cognition views cognitive function on a continuum from optimal to impaired function, with the goal being to support independence and quality of life for all individuals at risk for or experiencing an alteration in cognitive function. The Centers for Disease Control has published the Healthy Brain Initiative (2013), which stresses the importance of proactive measures to address the public epidemic of cognitive disorders. Healthcare systems in the United States have largely emphasized the provision of services to individuals who require hospitalization or institutionalization. The focus is shifting toward allocating more resources to the prevention and early screening of cognitive disorders. When individuals are diagnosed with a cognitive disorder, the goal is to provide care that enables them to achieve their fullest potential, maintain their orientation to their families and communities, and live in environments that promote their inherent worth and self-efficacy.

Individuals with cognitive disorders are at greater risk for a variety of health problems as a result of both cognitive illnesses and their treatment. Research demonstrates that the health problems of individuals with cognitive problems are often ignored. Health promotion for individuals with cognitive disorders also incorporates the principle that no matter what the level of wellness, individuals have a right to care that addresses physiologic, psychosocial, and humanistic aspects of function.

Prevention

Prevention of cognitive disorders includes measures to reduce modifiable risk factors and enhance protective factors. *Universal prevention* of cognitive disorders targets the general population and includes interventions such as public health campaigns regarding the use of safety devices such as helmets and seatbelts. *Selective prevention* targets subgroups of the population whose risk of developing a cognitive disorder is higher than that of the general population based on an analysis of biological, psychologic, or socioeconomic factors. Examples include early intervention programs for children from disadvantaged backgrounds and counseling following exposure to trauma. *Indicated prevention* is aimed at individuals who have minimal but detectable manifestations of cognitive disorder. An example would be initiating treatment for an individual who demonstrates prodromal symptoms of schizophrenia or has biomarkers for a dementia.

Screening and Early Detection

The progression and or impact of many of the cognitive disorders described in this module can be positively impacted through early detection and intervention. A variety of screening tools are identified in the sections on assessment later in this module. Screening and detection of cognitive disorders occur in a number of settings, including but not limited to primary care settings, community health settings, and schools.

Nursing Assessment

A general assessment of cognitive status is an essential component of the nursing assessment of all patients. When a patient presents with the onset of any cognitive changes, the priority assessment focuses on addressing potentially life-threatening factors that may be contributing to the problem through physical assessment, history, and diagnostic procedures, such as laboratory values.

SAFETY ALERT Any changes in cognition require immediate attention. Cognitive disturbances put patients at increased risk of injury, so rapid institution of safety measures is critical. Also, prompt assessment of a patient's cognitive impairment may allow the healthcare team to more quickly identify and treat the underlying cause.

Cognitive assessment is performed both for the purposes of initial screening for the presence or absence of cognitive problems and for monitoring changes in cognition over time. An assessment of cognitive status should be performed during an initial provider or home care visit, following any changes in medical treatment and pharmacotherapy, during any transitions in care, and prior to obtaining consent for procedures. Certain individuals are at increased risk for cognitive problems and warrant more frequent assessment of cognitive status. For example, clinical guidelines published by Tullman, Fletcher, and Foreman (2012a) suggest that older adults who are hospitalized should be assessed for cognitive changes a minimum of every 8 hours and within 6 weeks of discharge from the hospital setting.

Observation and Patient Interview

Data gathering begins with the initial observation of the patient and focuses on appearance and behavioral manifestations that may be indicative of cognitive function. Appearance and dress can provide cues to the patient's mental state and ability to maintain self-care. The nurse may also make general observations related to social skills, motor function, activity level, ability to attend and focus on the assessment, and ability to provide logical and coherent responses to questions. The best source of information comes directly from the patient. However, when assessing pediatric patients or patients with moderate to severe cognitive impairment, a family member or caregiver may be asked to provide information.

During the patient interview, ask direct questions to elicit information related to biophysical and psychosocial history, development, family history, and environmental factors. Use judgment in direct questioning of individuals with established cognitive and perceptual problems, as some may not have the capacity to respond logically. In addition, cognitive problems such as perceptual problems and delusional thinking are likely to increase the patient's anxiety and may result in an escalation of inappropriate behaviors during the patient interview and examination.

Biophysical and Psychosocial History

The medical history includes gathering information about both the presenting problem and the presence or development of altered health patterns across the lifespan.

History of the Current Problem

Initial questions focus on the patient's perception of the problem and what brings the patient to the healthcare setting currently. Initial questions may proceed from broad questions about a typical day, including ADLs, self-care activities, and perceived level of health and wellness. When patients or family remembers report changes in cognitive function, ask non-threatening questions such as:

- Can you describe the changes?
- What do you think may be contributing to the changes?
- When did you begin experiencing these changes?
- Are these changes constant and, if not, how frequently do they occur?
- Have you previously sought medical advice or care related to these changes?

More focused questions include the following:

- Are you experiencing any changes in your ability to pay attention or remember things?
- Do you have difficulty planning and organizing things?
- Do you ever hear, see, or smell things that are not apparent to others?
- Have you been experiencing any problems that are making it difficult to learn or function in school (or work)?
- Have you been experiencing any problems expressing yourself or understanding others?
- Have you been diagnosed with any problems that might impact your thinking (e.g., learning disabilities, intellectual disabilities, Alzheimer or Parkinson disease, depression, mood disorders, anxiety, head injury, tumors, cerebral vascular problems, central nervous system infections)?

Depending on the patient's responses, seek additional detail about the impact on daily functioning, frequency and duration of symptoms, suspected causes or contributing factors, and how the patient has been treating or managing the symptoms. Be sure to obtain a list of all current medications with the dose, route, and frequency and to inquire about the use of any complementary health approaches.

History of Prior Biophysical and Psychosocial Alterations

Focused questions related to past medical history follow a structure similar to that under current medical history. Inquire about past health-related behaviors such as diet and exercise, access to routine care, and preventive health measures. Inquire about past use of alcohol and other substances, as these may have implications for care. Ask the patient about possible variables impacting prenatal health, childbirth and postnatal care, and childhood illnesses or exposures, and collect a psychosocial history to include evidence of overwhelming stressors, trauma, or violence.

Assess the patient's developmental history and developmental status, including evidence of achievement of expected milestones. This is especially important when performing an assessment of cognition in a child. Note any known factors that may impede normal growth and development, such as chronic illnesses and hospitalizations.

Ask if any family members had disorders such as dementia, schizophrenia, and/or developmental or learning problems. Because many patients may not have knowledge of the specific diagnoses in family members, use lay terms to ascertain whether any family members ever demonstrated unusual behavior, experienced confusion or memory loss, or required treatment or hospitalization for mental health issues.

Assess for environmental factors that may be contributing to the patient's cognitive status, including but not limited to social supports, ability to access healthcare and maintain a healthy diet and lifestyle, living situation and safety of the home environment, and any accommodations or services in place to support independent function. When assessing cognition in children, consider parenting techniques and capabilities, as well as access to activities and stimulation that promote cognitive development, such as age-appropriate activities and toys. Assess for any cultural factors that may impact cognition, including traditional health practices. Determine the possibility of any current or past exposures to toxic substances at home or at work.

Physical and Mental Status Examination

Once the interview is completed and the patient's history has been obtained, the nurse progresses to a physical assessment of the patient and a mental status examination. The physical examination incorporates an organized pattern of assessment to identify alterations that may be contributing to cognitive dysfunction. The mental status exam includes a series of procedures and tools used to detect alterations in perception and thinking.

Physical Examination

Because changes in cognitive function are often an early sign of decreased oxygenation, perfusion, or an alteration in another biophysical process, begin by obtaining a complete set of vital signs and assessing the patient's level of pain. Auscultation of the heart and lungs may reveal an underlying problem with gas exchange or perfusion. Murmurs in infants and young children may indicate congenital heart defects associated with other neurodevelopmental problems. An assessment of peripheral perfusion may indicate vascular problems that are compromising cerebral perfusion. An assessment of neurologic signs is an essential component of cognitive evaluation (detailed information can be found in the module on Intracranial Regulation). An evaluation of hearing, vision, touch, taste, and smell can help rule out perceptual problems related to impaired sensory function. Skin integrity can provide clues to the patient's nutritional status, fluid balance, and the possibility of injury or infection.

Physical development and height, weight, and fat distribution should be within normal limits for the patient's age. Observable physical alterations may be associated with many cognitive syndromes, including intellectual disabilities and schizophrenia (Cheng et al., 2014; Jones, Jones, & Del Campo, 2013; Moeschler et al., 2014; Tikka et al., 2013). Examples include small head circumference, wide or close-set eyes, prominent forehead, folds on the inner corners of the eyes (epicanthic skin folds), asymmetry or malformation of facial features and ears, tongue protrusion, palate and mouth abnormalities, flattened face or nose, limb abnormalities, small stature, poor muscle tone, some birthmarks, palmar folds, and altered posture.

An important component of the physical examination includes an assessment of motor function. Movements should be consistent with age and development. Any changes in gait or other evidence of movement disorders should be noted.

TABLE 23–6 Common Tools Used to Assess Cognition and Mental Status

Assessment Name	Description
Ages & Stages Questionnaires (ASQ),	Set of questionnaires tailored to detect alterations in development in young children.
American Academy of Pediatrics—Bright Futures	Kit for health promotion and prevention published by the American Academy of Pediatrics that includes schedules for screening and care and a variety of questionnaires used to detect health problems, including developmental alterations.
Confusion Assessment Method (CAM)	Interview-style exam that can be conducted in about 5 minutes, screens specifically for signs of delirium. Pediatric versions available for children 5 years and older (pCAM).
Cornell Assessment of Pediatric Delirium	Validated, rapid observational tool for screening children in intensive care for delirium.
Cornell Scale for Depression in Dementia	Nineteen-question tool that involves interviews with both patients and their caregivers, assesses for signs of depression in individuals known to have dementia.
Edinburgh Depression Scale	Validated 10-item questionnaire used to screen for the presence and severity of symptoms of postnatal depression.
Geriatric Depression Scale (GDS)	Brief questionnaire (15 or 30 items) that asks patients how they've felt over the past 7 days; assesses for depression in older adults.
Hamilton Rating Scale for Depression (HRSD)	Seventeen-question, 20-minute examination, assesses severity of depression in adult patients. The Weinberg Depression Scale for Children and Adolescents (WDSCA) and the Children's Depression Rating Scale (CDRS-R) are modeled on the HRSD and adapted for children over 5.
Mini–Mental State Examination (MMSE)	Thirty-question interview-style exam that assesses a patient's memory, language skills, attention level, and ability to engage in mental tasks, also known as the Folstein Mini–Mental State Examination. It may be modified for use in children after the age of 4.
Montreal Cognitive Assessment	One-page test that briefly assesses patient's ability in a variety of cognitive domains, including problem solving and sequencing (traits, similarities), attention (digit span, letter vigilance), memory (word list, orientation), visual-spatial construction and reasoning (cube, clock), and language (naming, repetition, word generation).
Nonverbal Learning Disabilities Scale (NVLD)	Deficits in the areas of motor skills, visual-spatial skills, and interpersonal skills.
Patient Health Questionnaire (PHQ)	Full-length 11-item tool that screens for depression and anxiety, somatic symptoms, and related disorders; abbreviated forms (PDQ-9 and PDQ-2) are used to more selectively screen for depression.
Positive and Negative Symptoms Scale (PANSS)	Registered nurses and other licensed healthcare providers can administer to detect positive, negative, and other manifestations of psychotic disorders and schizophrenia. May be useful in screening for perinatal psychosis.
Postpartum Depression Predictors Inventory (PDPI)	Validated short inventory that can be integrated into all phases of perinatal care to predict the risk of maternal depression.

Mental Status Examination

The mental status exam is a broad screening tool that is used to assess current cognitive functioning of the individual. Many specific tools exist to perform a mental status assessment, but most serve to capture data related to orientation, perception and thought content (including judgment and insight), attention and concentration, memory, speech/language/communication, mood and affect, and psychomotor activity. Other assessments may be used to rule out related conditions such as depression or other mood disorders or to gather information on developmental status or level of functional impairment. **Table 23–6 »** lists a variety of common assessment and screening tools that may be used by healthcare professionals to detect alterations in cognitive function. The Mental Status Assessment feature presents an example of an organized formal mental status examination with a description of normal and abnormal findings and the patient-centered considerations. Formal assessment often serves to validate findings gathered through observation.

Diagnostic Tests

Nurses collaborate with other disciplines to support diagnostic assessment of individuals for cognitive disorders. When individuals present with alterations in cognition, nurses can anticipate that a number of laboratory values

and diagnostic tests will be ordered to rule out an underlying medical condition. Priority diagnostic assessment focuses on life-threatening conditions that may manifest in cognitive alterations. Analysis of blood and cerebral spinal fluid can identify biomarkers associated with Alzheimer disease and schizophrenia, although this is not typically used for diagnosis. Relevant laboratory tests include the following:

- *Toxicology screens* to rule out alcohol or substances as a causative factor for changes in mental status
- *Drug levels* to rule out mental status changes related to toxic levels of therapeutic agents
- *Liver function tests (LFTs), complete blood count (CBC), thyroid function, B_1 (thiamine), sedimentation rate, urinalysis, HIV titer, and fluorescent treponemal antibody absorption (FTA-abs)* to rule out metabolic, inflammatory, and infectious conditions that may contribute to alterations in mental status
- *VeriPsych* blood test to identify biomarkers for schizophrenia
- *Cerebrospinal fluid (CSF)* and *blood markers* to identify biomarkers for Alzheimer disease
- *Genetic testing* to identify risk factors or underlying causes of a variety of cognitive disorders

Mental Status Assessment

ASSESSMENT/ METHOD	NORMAL FINDINGS	ABNORMAL FINDINGS	PATIENT-CENTERED CONSIDERATIONS
Step 1: Prepare the Patient			
Tell the patient you will be performing a series of tests. Describe what equipment you'll use. Explain that the exam should be comfortable, and ask the patient to inform you should difficulties arise. Provide an overview of the assessment activities and the order in which they will occur.	▪ Patient pays attention and asks questions as appropriate. ▪ Patient may be nervous, but this should not interfere with the assessment process.	▪ Patient displays high levels of confusion, anxiety, or agitation. ▪ Patient shows signs of delusions or hallucinations. ▪ Patient pays no attention to the information you provide. ▪ Patient is partially or fully uncommunicative.	▪ A number of assessment tools are available, with some tailored to specific conditions and/or populations. ▪ Direct questioning may not be appropriate for patients who are experiencing hallucinations, delusions, or extreme anxiety. ▪ Questions for children or individuals with intellectual disabilities should be modified.
Step 2: Position and Observe the Patient			
Take note of the patient's general appearance, including hygiene, posture, body language, and expression. Observe the patient's ability to follow your instructions.	▪ Patient follows directions. ▪ Patient's hygiene and overall appearance are acceptable. ▪ Patient's expressions and body language are appropriate to the situation.	▪ Poor hygiene and/or inappropriate expressions and body language might be reflective of depression, schizophrenia, dementia, or another cognitive disorder.	▪ In many cases, a patient's appearance and hygiene may be negatively affected by socioeconomic and cultural factors rather than mental status.
Step 3: Assess the Patient's Language Abilities			
Note the tone, rate, pronunciation and volume of the patient's speech throughout the course of the exam. Consider the patient's vocabulary and whether he seems to understand what you are saying.	▪ Patient's tone, rate, pronunciation, and volume are appropriate. ▪ Patient speaks easily and naturally, without searching for words. ▪ Patient understands what you are saying and indicates this through verbal and physical reactions. ▪ Social and language milestones have been met.	▪ Problems with language could be a result of anxiety, dementia, depression, or an expressive or receptive language disorder related to brain injury/illness.	▪ Consider whether the patient's hearing may be impaired, especially when working with older adults. ▪ Don't assume all patients are native English speakers. Some patients may simply be unable to communicate well in English. ▪ Consider the child's stage of development.
Step 4: Assess the Patient's Level of Orientation			
Check whether the patient knows the date and time. Ask if the patient knows where she is and why. Gauge the patient's level of consciousness.	▪ Patient knows the correct date and time, where she is, and why. ▪ Patient is fully conscious and alert.	▪ Reduced or varying consciousness may be due to hypoglycemia, stroke, seizure, delirium, or organic brain disease.	▪ Noticeable decreases in consciousness during the exam may necessitate immediate medical attention. ▪ Modify questions for children according to developmental level.
Step 5: Assess the Patient's Memory			
See whether the patient knows her name, birth date, and address. Ask the patient for a brief summary of places lived and jobs held. Attempt to verify all responses.	▪ Patient can recall basic personal information and provide an accurate biography appropriate to age and developmental level.	▪ Inability to recall events from one's past may be suggestive of dementia, especially Alzheimer disease.	▪ In Alzheimer disease, loss of short-term memory typically precedes loss of long-term memory. ▪ Alterations in memory in children may suggest a problem with learning or intellectual function.

(continued on next page)

Mental Status Assessment (continued)

ASSESSMENT/ METHOD	NORMAL FINDINGS	ABNORMAL FINDINGS	PATIENT-CENTERED CONSIDERATIONS
Step 6: Assess the Patient's Computational Ability			
Have the patient answer several arithmetic problems. Start with basic facts and work toward more complicated questions. The age and the developmental status of the patient should be considered.	▪ Patient can compute the correct values. Depending on age and cognitive stage, patient may be able to identify numeric symbols and count.	▪ Inability to perform simple calculations may be suggestive of brain disease or learning problems.	▪ Patient's responses may be negatively affected by language barriers, cognitive development, anxiety, and/or limited experience or education in mathematics.
Step 7: Assess the Patient's Emotions and Mood			
Note the patient's affect. Ask the patient how he feels and whether this is typical. If not, ask about events that may have prompted the change. Modify questions for children. Children may be asked to draw pictures of how they are feeling or to select from a visual scale.	▪ Patient's affect corresponds with the tone and content of his speech. ▪ Patient's emotions and mood are appropriate given past events and current situation and developmental status.	▪ Mismatch between the patient's affect and speech may reflect neurologic or psychologic problems. ▪ Absent, excessively subdued, or excessively animated expressions and responses may be indicative of psychologic disorders.	▪ Culture, temperament, and development impact emotional expression. Certain developmental stages are associated with increased lability.
Step 8: Assess the Patient's Perceptions and Thinking Abilities			
Note whether the patient's statements are complete, rational, and pertinent, and whether he/she seems aware of reality. Ask the patient to compare two different things or explain the meaning of a common phrase. Ask the patient if he sees, hears, smells, or feels things that are not apparent to others.	▪ Patient is aware of reality. ▪ Patient's statements are logical and complete. ▪ Patient correctly compares two objects and/or explains the meaning of a phrase. ▪ Patient denies hallucinations of any kind, or perceptual differences may be explained by level of cognitive development or sociocultural factors.	▪ Patients who are unaware of reality may be experiencing neurologic disturbances or a mental disorder. ▪ Illogical, incomplete statements suggest problems with concrete thought and may be indicative of a mental disorder. ▪ Absent or strange comparisons and explanations are frequent symptoms of psychologic disorders.	▪ Patient's responses may be negatively affected by language barriers, education level, and/or intellectual disability or level of cognitive development. ▪ Perceptual differences in young children may be related to magical thinking and animism. Children may have difficulty distinguishing between what is imagined and what is real.
Step 9: Assess the Patient's Decision-Making Ability			
Ask the patient about a personal situation that requires good judgment. Determine whether the patient's responses reflect consideration of viable options and logical decision making.	▪ Patient considers possible, probable, and appropriate options. ▪ Patient's thinking and decision-making capabilities are appropriate for age and stage of development.	▪ Patient considers impossible, improbable, or inappropriate options. ▪ Patient's decision reflects absent or inadequate consideration of available options.	▪ Consider whether the patient's options and decisions make sense—not whether they reflect the choice you would make. ▪ Decision-making capacity depends on the stage of cognitive development; refer to normal characteristics of thinking associated with each stage.

- *Metabolic screening*—Newborn screens for 26–40 metabolic disorders that can cause learning and intellectual disabilities
- *Diagnostic imaging* to detect conditions requiring emergency management, such as cerebral edema, cerebral vascular accidents, tumors, and traumatic injuries
- *MRIs and CT* to detect abnormalities that are suggestive of some neurocognitive, neurodevelopmental and psychotic disorders.

Psychometric tests include a variety of standardized tests that are usually administered by a psychologist or neuropsychologist to measure cognitive function in a variety of areas. Comprehensive neuropsychologic testing may include the use of a number of tests administered over a period of several days. Nurses, teachers, parents, and patients may be asked to complete one or more rating scales to contribute to an overall understanding of the presentation of the problem across a variety of domains.

Case Study » Part 2

In the winter after his visit to the gerontologist, Mr. Wallace begins experiencing increased agitation and wanders in the afternoons and evenings. One afternoon at the adult daycare center, Mr. Wallace slips out the door undetected. By the time the daycare providers realize he is gone, he has left the grounds and is wandering the neighborhood. The daycare providers call Ms. Wallace, his daughter, and 911, and a search for Mr. Wallace commences. Ms. Wallace and two police officers find Mr. Wallace 2 miles from the daycare center. He has no idea where he is or how he got there. He has taken a fall, and his face and hands are covered in scrapes.

The officers radio for an ambulance as Ms. Wallace attempts to talk to her father. Mr. Wallace panics because he does not recognize his daughter, and he pushes her to the ground. He then throws punches at the officers when they prevent him from running away. The paramedics arrive and restrain Mr. Wallace. Once he is restrained, Ms. Wallace is able to calm him down. He is then transported to the emergency department (ED), where you are the admitting nurse.

Mr. Wallace is calm on arrival to the hospital, and you are able to treat his injuries without incident. You attempt to speak with him, but he indicates he is tired and promptly falls asleep. You use this opportunity to interview Ms. Wallace. She states that aggression has become common during her father's increasingly frequent periods of confusion. Sometimes he doesn't recognize her; other times, he mistakes her for his sister. He is also increasingly unable to use basic objects—such as pencils, toothbrushes, and combs—and relies on Ms. Wallace for many basic ADLs. In addition, he occasionally experiences urinary and fecal incontinence. Ms. Wallace is shaken by the day's events and the situation in general, and she begins to cry.

When Mr. Wallace's gerontologist arrives in the ED, you inform her of these developments. She adds 7.5 mg of buspirone (BuSpar) two times daily (bid) to Mr. Wallace's treatment regimen to lessen his agitation and aggression. The doctor also tells Ms. Wallace that Mr. Wallace is starting to transition from moderate to severe Alzheimer disease, and she recommends that Ms. Wallace might consider looking for a nursing home that specializes in the care of individuals with this condition.

Clinical Reasoning Questions Level I
1. What are the priorities for Mr. Wallace's care to decrease his risk of wandering and injury during his remaining time at home?
2. What independent interventions can you perform to address the caregiver role strain felt by Ms. Wallace?
3. What additional information or education do you anticipate Ms. Wallace will need in light of the doctor's recommendation?

Clinical Reasoning Questions Level II
Referring to the exemplar on Alzheimer disease in this module:
4. Which of Mr. Wallace's symptoms indicate he is transitioning from moderate to severe AD?
5. What steps can Ms. Wallace take at home to lessen the incidence and severity of Mr. Wallace's sundowning episodes?
6. Why is it important for Ms. Wallace to find an institutional care situation for Mr. Wallace now rather than waiting until he reaches a more severe stage of AD?

Independent Interventions

Given an understanding of the importance of health promotion with respect to cognitive disorders, nurses should be prepared to carry out a variety of interventions across settings. Nursing interventions include teaching prevention, coordinating care and making appropriate referrals, implementing measures to promote individual/family safety and well-being, and advocating for the needs of individuals impacted by alterations in cognition.

Prevention and Coordination of Care

Nurses in community health and primary care settings play a critical role in addressing health-related behaviors and protective measures that can reduce the risk of developing cognitive disorders. Nurses accomplish this through teaching and providing anticipatory guidance. They also independently carry out routine assessments for cognitive problems using a variety of tools, and they refer patients for further diagnosis and treatment. Examples of independent interventions in this category include:

- Teaching about healthy diet, lifestyle, and the importance of preventive healthcare
- Ensuring that patients use protective headgear during sports and activities such as bike riding
- Stressing the importance of developmentally appropriate activities
- Administering routine developmental and cognitive screenings
- Making referrals to other members of the interprofessional team.

Promoting Safety and Well-Being

Nurses in all settings often plan care for individuals that promotes safety and adaptive functioning. For example, the home health nurse may work with individuals with schizophrenia or Alzheimer disease, monitoring adherence to treatment, providing emotional support to the patient and family, and assessing comorbid health conditions.

When patients do require hospitalization for acute changes in cognition, the priority is to identify and manage underlying conditions that may be contributing to the problem. Priority interventions address immediate safety. Secondary interventions include teaching patients and families about the illness and prescribed treatments, providing emotional support, and preparing for discharge to settings where they can receive the support necessary to achieve optimal functioning and prevent future hospitalization.

Even when patients are unable to return to their homes or families, nurses provide care that supports interpersonal functioning and the ability to engage in goal-directed activities. Examples of interventions across settings include:

- Evaluating risk of injury or suicide
- Implementing environmental modifications to support patient safety
- Educating patients and families about diseases, medications, and other therapeutic interventions
- Identifying patient and family strengths
- Encouraging the use of adaptive coping skills
- Supporting cultural and spiritual needs
- Providing ongoing emotional support to both patients and families
- Ensuring healthcare needs are met
- Monitoring the effectiveness of care.

Advocating for Patients

Because cognitive disorders have the potential to reduce decision-making capacity, nurses have a role in ensuring that patients are not abused or exploited and are able to partner in healthcare decisions to the greatest degree possible. This includes encouraging patients in remission or in the early stages of neurocognitive dysfunction to establish advance directives and providing teaching about legal protections that may apply to them (see the Patient Teaching feature). Other interventions related to advocacy include providing teaching related to legal rights and assisting caregivers and community members to understand cognitive disorders.

Collaborative Therapies

When working with individuals at risk for or experiencing alterations in cognitive function, nurses should anticipate collaborating with the patient, family, other members of the healthcare team, and potentially professionals from other

Patient Teaching
Legal Protections for Patients with Cognitive Dysfunction

Nurses should teach individuals with cognitive alterations and their families about several key laws that may affect them. For example:

- The Americans with Disabilities Act of 1990 ensures that individuals with disabilities have equal access to government services, employment, and public accommodations.
- The Education for All Handicapped Children Act of 1975 requires that children with any type of disability have access to free public education. An amendment to this act in 1986 provides federal funding to states that offer early intervention services.
- The Developmental Disabilities and Bill of Rights Act of 2000 provides federal funding to state, public, and nonprofit agencies that provide community-based training activities and education to individuals with developmental disabilities. The law also created the U.S. Administration on Developmental Disabilities to oversee these efforts.

disciplines, such as education and law. **Table 23–7** ⟩⟩ provides an overview of select members of the interprofessional team and their roles with respect to the collaboration and management of cognitive disorders. For a more extensive list, please refer to the module on Collaboration. Additional resources may be available through local chapters of organizations such as the LDA, the Alzheimer's Association, the American Psychiatric Association, the American Association of Intellectual and Developmental Disabilities, and the National Alliance on Mental Illness.

Pharmacologic Therapy

Nurses play a key role in medication administration, education, and adherence, and they must be familiar with the different classes of drugs prescribed to individuals with

TABLE 23–7 Selected Members of the Interprofessional Team for Management of Cognitive Disorders

Team Member	Role Description
Advocates (disability, patient care, special education advocates)	Individuals with varying levels of specialized training in advocacy for individuals with disabilities, mental illness, or related health concerns. Because levels of expertise and experience vary, patients should be encouraged to seek referrals from government agencies, reliable associations, and legal firms.
Developmental pediatricians	Board-certified pediatricians with specialized training and certification in the identification and management of developmental disorders that impact cognition and psychosocial function.
Occupational therapists	Master's prepared professionals that possess specialized education and training in determining and managing the impact of cognitive disorders on everyday functioning across the lifespan.
Neuropsychologists	Doctoral prepared clinical psychologists with specialized training in the area of central nervous system function and its relationship to human behavior. Qualified to perform comprehensive assessment and diagnosis of neurocognitive and neurodevelopmental function. Also collaborate with nurses and other professionals in the management of these disorders.
Special education professionals	Generally master's prepared educators with specialized training to work with students who have a wide range of learning, mental, emotional, and physical disabilities. Teach reading, writing, and math to students with mild and moderate disabilities through modified methods. Also, facilitate the acquisition of basic skills, such as literacy and communication techniques, to students with severe disabilities.
Speech language pathologists	Master's prepared professionals who have a primary role in the screening, assessment, diagnosis, and treatment of infants, children, adolescents, and adults with cognitive-communication disorders.
Psychiatric or psychosocial rehabilitation specialists	Assist patients with mental illness to function within the community. Levels of training vary, but most specialists have a master's degree in rehabilitation training. Additional certification as a Psychiatric Rehabilitation Practitioner can also be obtained through Psychiatric Rehabilitation Association (2016).

cognitive alterations. Drugs that are available for treating neurocognitive disorders are primarily aimed at slowing further brain changes. Medications used to treat psychosis, anxiety, and depression target the symptoms of the disorder. The Medications feature provides an overview of medications used to treat cognitive disorders and the implications for nursing practice.

SAFETY ALERT Nurses must assess patients with cognitive alterations to determine their ability to self-administer medication. Many patients will require caregiver administration of pharmaceuticals.

Missed doses may result in a return or exacerbation of symptoms and increase the patient's risk for injury. Long-acting formulations may enhance adherence. Assess for factors that affect adherence at each healthcare interaction.

Lifespan Considerations

Cognitive function is mediated by the interaction of genes and experience, both of which provide the foundation for cognitive changes that occur across the lifespan. Nurses use knowledge of these changes to modify assessment and interventions

Medications
Cognitive Disorders

CLASSIFICATION AND DRUG EXAMPLES	MECHANISMS OF ACTION	NURSING IMPLICATIONS
Acetylcholinesterase Inhibitors *Drug examples:* Donepezil (Aricept) Galantamine (Razadyne, Reminyl) Rivastigmine (Exelon) ***N*-Methyl-D-aspartate (NMDA) Receptor Antagonists** *Drug examples:* Memantine (Namenda) combination NMDA receptor antagonist and acetylcholinesterase inhibitors Memantine hydrochloride extended-release and donepezil hydrochloride (Namzaric)	Acetylcholinesterase inhibitors reduce acetylcholine breakdown, whereas NMDA receptor antagonists limit the effects of glutamate. Both drugs have a modest effect in slowing an individual's rate of cognitive decline in Alzheimer disease. **May also be used for:** ■ Vascular dementia ■ Parkinson-related dementia. Combination agent (Namzaric) used only after patients have been stabilized on memantine and donepezil	■ Explain the importance of taking medication as directed; teach about discontinuation and decline in function. ■ Provide patient education regarding dizziness, headache, gastrointestinal (GI) upset, and fatigue. ■ Promote adequate fluid intake. ■ Monitor patient's pulse rate. ■ Use with caution in patients with respiratory conditions (e.g., asthma, COPD). ■ Avoid the use of tricyclics and anticholinergic drugs because of their antagonistic effects.
Conventional Antipsychotics **Phenothiazines** *Drug examples:* Chlorpromazine (Thorazine) Fluphenazine Perphenazine Prochlorperazine (Compazine) Thioridazine Trifluoperazine **Nonphenothiazines** *Drug examples:* Haloperidol (Haldol) Loxapine (Loxitane) Pimozide (Orap) Thiothixene (Navene)	Both phenothiazines and nonphenothiazines block D_2 dopamine receptors in the brain, increasing synaptic levels of dopamine and leading to a decrease in symptoms of psychosis (including delusions and hallucinations). **May also be used for:** ■ Schizophrenia and other psychotic disorders ■ Tourette syndrome.	■ Monitor for anticholinergic symptoms, such as dry mouth, orthostatic hypotension, constipation, urinary retention, sedation, and sexual dysfunction. ■ Teach patient strategies to address anticholinergic effects (e.g., rising slowly, increasing fluid intake, and increasing fiber intake). ■ Monitor for extrapyramidal symptoms (EPS), such as acute dystonia, akathisia, parkinsonism, and tardive dyskinesia (TD). ■ Monitor for signs of hyperprolactemia (menstrual irregularities, decreased libido, gynecomastia, and osteoporosis). Adjunctive therapies, counseling, or changing to a different agent may improve some aspects of sexual dysfunction. ■ Monitor for autonomic instability associated with neuroleptic malignant syndrome. ■ Teach patients importance of adhering to medication regimen and not to abruptly discontinue medication. ■ Teach patients importance of wearing sunscreen.

(continued on next page)

Medications *(continued)*

CLASSIFICATION AND DRUG EXAMPLES	MECHANISMS OF ACTION	NURSING IMPLICATIONS
Atypical Antipsychotics *Drug examples:* Risperidone (Risperdal) Olanzapine (Zyprexa) Clozapine (Clozaril) Asenapine (Saphris) Paliperidone (Invega) Quetiapine (Seroquel) Ziprasidone (Geodon)	Block D_2 and serotonin receptors; treat both positive and negative symptoms of schizophrenia and psychotic disorders, exert mood-stabilizing effect. ***May also be used for:*** ■ Schizophrenia and other psychotic disorders ■ Bipolar disorder.	■ Monitor for adverse effects, such as alterations in glucose metabolism, hyperlipidemia, cardiovascular and cerebrovascular alterations and blood abnormalities. ■ Teach importance of healthy diet and exercise. ■ Monitor for EPS and neuroleptic malignant syndrome.
Third-generation Antipsychotics *Drug examples:* Aripiprazole (Abilify) Brexpiprazole (Rexulti)	Partial agonists of D_2 receptors, also block serotonin receptors.	■ Although generally well tolerated, patients should still be monitored for EPS, neuroleptic malignant syndrome (NMS), and medical effects associated with atypical antipsychotics. ■ Akathisia and restlessness may be more pronounced with this medication. ■ Teaching should address healthy diet and exercise, importance of adherence, and recognizing and reporting adverse effects.
Anxiolytics **Nonbenzodiazepines** *Drug examples:* Buspirone (BuSpar)	Probably inhibits serotonin reuptake and activates dopamine receptors in the brain, leading to a decrease in symptoms of anxiety.	■ Monitor for dependency, drowsiness, hypotension, tolerance, dizziness, and GI upset. ■ These agents may increase confusion. ■ Abrupt discontinuation may lead to rebound anxiety.
Selective Serotonin Reuptake Inhibitors (SSRIs) *Drug examples:* Sertraline (Zoloft), Fluoxetine (Prozac)	Inhibits reuptake of serotonin in the central nervous system, leading to a decrease in symptoms of depression and anxiety. ***May also be used for:*** ■ Depression ■ Anxiety ■ Obsessive-compulsive disorder ■ Posttraumatic stress disorder ■ Social anxiety disorder.	■ Monitor for suicide risk. ■ Monitor for serotonin syndrome. ■ Abrupt discontinuation may cause serotonin withdrawal. ■ Provide patient education regarding dizziness, insomnia, somnolence, GI upset, nausea or diarrhea, and avoiding over-the-counter (OTC) preparations that may increase risk of serotonin syndrome.
CNS Stimulants *Drug examples:* Methylphenidate (Ritalin) Amphetamine sulfate (Adderall)	It is believed that methylphenidate activates the brainstem arousal system and cortex. Also acts as a dopamine and norepinephrine reuptake inhibitor, resulting in a prolongation of dopamine receptor effects.	■ Monitor for insomnia, decreased appetite, increased heart rate, and hypertension or cardiac dysrhythmias. ■ Monitor patients with diabetes for decreased glycemic control. ■ Educate patients about the high potential for abuse.

Source: Based on Adams, M. P., Holland, L.N., & Urban, C. (2017). *Pharmacology for nurses: A pathophysiologic approach.* (5th ed.). Hoboken, NJ: Pearson Education.

with individuals who are at risk for or experiencing alterations in cognitive function. A major consideration is the impact of normal growth and development. **Figure 23–5** ≫ provides a timeline for normal brain development.

The best-known theory of cognitive development comes from the work of Swiss psychologist Jean Piaget (1896–1980). Piaget claimed that cognitive development is an orderly, sequential process in which children form adaptive cognitive structures—called *schemes*—in response to environmental stimuli. According to Piaget, as children learn more about the world by physically interacting with it, they actively revise their schemes to better fit with the reality they observe. Over time, as their brains mature and they are exposed to additional stimuli, children become capable of building more complex schemes—and as they do so, they move from one stage of development to the next. In fact, Piaget proposed that all children pass through four universal stages of cognitive development, as described in **Table 23–8** ≫: sensorimotor,

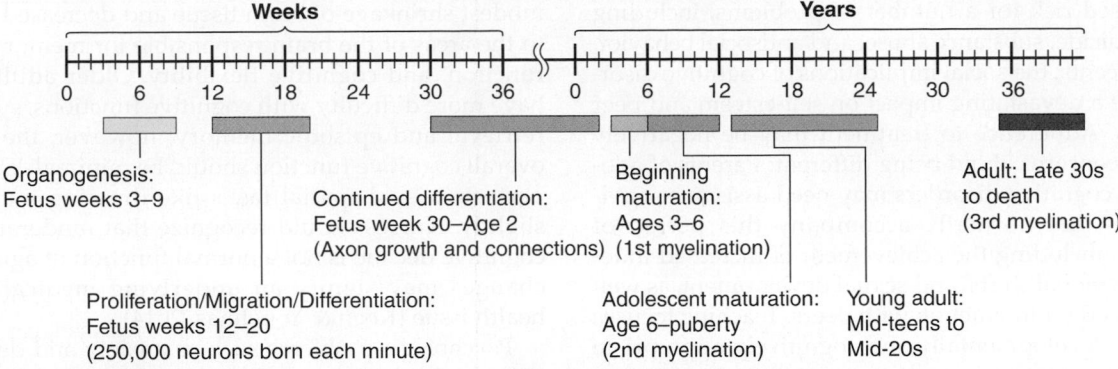

Source: Potter, M. L., & Moller, M. D. (2016). *Psychiatric–mental health nursing: From suffering to hope.* Reprinted and electronically reproduced by permission of Pearson Education, Inc., New York, NY.

Figure 23–5 ≫ Timeline of brain development.

preoperational, concrete operational, and formal operational (Piaget, 1966, 1972; Shaffer & Kipp, 2014).

Cognition from Conception to Adolescence

Simple neuronal connections that shape cognition first occur shortly after the period of conception. These simple connections are then followed by increasingly complex circuits. Any insults during the period of embryonic development, including exposure to toxic substances, maternal stress, nutritional deficits, and illness, can have a devastating impact on cognition (Harvard University Center on the Developing Child, 2016).

Rapid proliferation of neuronal connections occurs during the first few years of life and corresponds with the process through which children assimilate new information, revise cognitive constructs through a process called accommodation, and form new thinking structures or schemes to facilitate adaptation. One aspect of normal development is called *pruning*, a process by which unused connections are remodeled or eliminated in order to strengthen cognitive efficiency. Remodeling occurs during sensitive periods of time in brain development. During infancy and early childhood, for example, brains are primed for stimulation of visual pathways and language. If these pathways are not activated, the neuronal pathways required for them will be eliminated, impacting overall cognitive capabilities.

Both stress and illness predispose children to alterations in cognitive development and mental function. Nurses recognize that young children have some limitations in the functional reserves required to compensate for certain conditions, such as dehydration, fever, infection, and the effects of anesthesia. As a result, young children may be more likely to manifest cognitive changes such as confusion or hallucinations when any of these are present.

Cognition from Adolescence to Adulthood

Significant changes in brain structure continue to occur in adolescents, with another period of rapid generation of neuronal pathways and remodeling. Changes in activity in the limbic system are believed to account for increased sensation-seeking and need for arousal; at the same time, the underdeveloped prefrontal cortex is unable to mediate impulse control (Oettingen & Gollwitzer, 2015). Deficits in decision making can place adolescents at increased risk for head injuries. These deficits may also make adolescents more prone to use alcohol and other substances. Recent evidence, however, suggests that changes in dopamine systems shift adolescent orientation toward reward-seeking behavior, and that self-regulation may be enhanced through the provision of positive reinforcement (Steinberg, 2014).

Adolescents may experience a variety of alterations in cognition, including intellectual and learning disabilities. Alterations in neurocognitive function indicate early psychotic symptoms. Adolescents experiencing cognitive dysfunction

TABLE 23–8 Piaget's Stages of Cognitive Development

Stage and Age Range	Description	Developments
Sensorimotor Birth to 2 years	Infants use motor and sensory capabilities to explore the physical environment. Learning is largely trial and error.	Children develop a sense of "self" and "other" and come to understand object permanence. Behavioral schemes begin to produce images or mental schemes.
Preoperational 2–7 years	Young children use symbols (images and language) to explore their environment. Thought is egocentric, and children cannot adopt the perspectives of others.	Children participate in imaginative play and begin to recognize that others don't see the world the same way they do.
Concrete operational 7–11 years	Older children acquire cognitive operations, or mental activities that are an important part of rational thought. Logical reasoning is possible but limited to concrete (observable) problems.	Children are no longer fooled by appearances. They understand the basic properties of and relations among objects and events, and they are proficient at inferring motives.
Formal operational 11 years and beyond	Adolescents' cognitive operations are organized in a way that permits them to think about thinking. Thought is now systematic and abstract.	Logical thinking is no longer limited to the concrete or observable. Children engage in systematic, deductive reasoning and ponder hypothetical issues.

are at increased risk for a number of problems, including depression, suicide, substance abuse, and antisocial behavior.

For adolescents, the social implications of cognitive disorders can have a devastating impact on self-esteem and peer relationships. Adherence to treatment may be negatively impacted by concerns about being different. Parents of adolescents with cognitive disorders may need assistance navigating issues that normally accompany this period of development, including the achievement of increased independence, hormonal shifts, and sexual development, as well as a greater need for interaction with peers. Teaching focuses on providing developmentally and cognitively appropriate information on issues such as safety, sexuality, adaptive coping, and the management of the cognitive condition.

Cognition from Adulthood through Middle Age

Recent research suggests that brain maturation and, in particular, areas responsible for executive function are not fully mature until the mid- to late 20s (Friedman et al., 2016). Evidence also suggests that full maturation for men may not occur until the early 30s (Lim et al., 2015). Middle-aged adults demonstrate an enhanced ability to read other people's emotional state (Hartshorne & Germine, 2015). Vocabulary and other elements of accumulated facts and knowledge have been found to peak even later in life. Nurses can apply this information to dispel myths that surround the belief that cognitive decline is an inevitable aspect of aging, while focusing on cognitive strengths of patients across the lifespan.

Young adults with cognitive problems, such as intellectual disabilities or schizophrenia, often struggle to achieve the psychosocial tasks associated with this period of time. Nursing care should consider the patient's need to establish intimate relationships and pursue vocational goals. Teaching about family planning and sexually responsible behaviors should be incorporated into care.

Research is mixed related to the impact of pregnancy and childbirth on maternal cognition, with some studies indicating reduced function in the areas of processing speed, verbal recall, and attention (Henry & Sherwin, 2012; Logan et al., 2014). The hormonal shifts probably account for these changes and are largely adaptive, enabling the mother to be more in tune with the needs of the newborn. Fatigue and sleep deprivation may also contribute to cognitive alterations and may have a role in triggering other mental health issues.

Cognition in Older Adults

As the brain ages, typical changes account for subtle differences in cognitive processing. These may be caused by modest shrinkage of brain tissue and decreased blood flow to the areas of the brain responsible for memory, executive function, and cognitive flexibility. Older adults typically have more difficulty with cognitive functions, such as word retrieval and episodic memory; however, the impact on overall cognitive function should be minimal. The ability to perform visual-spatial tasks like drawing may diminish slightly. Nurses should recognize that moderate to severe cognitive decline is not a normal function of aging and that changes may signify an underlying medical or mental health issue (Koen & Yonelinas, 2014).

Psychologic problems such as anxiety and depression in older adults may also result in clinical manifestations that may be mistaken for dementia. Screening tools for depression and other mental health issues are used as part of a comprehensive assessment of cognition in older adults (see Table 23–7).

Case Study » Part 3

After his wandering episode, Mr. Wallace's condition rapidly declines. His communication skills are almost completely gone; he speaks infrequently and uses only two- or three-word sentences. He no longer recognizes Ms. Wallace, cannot perform ADLs, and is indifferent to food. His tendency toward wandering and aggression has disappeared. In fact, he rarely leaves his room. For his safety and to allow for provision of the care he needs, Mr. Wallace is admitted to an extended care facility that specializes in treating patients with Alzheimer disease.

You are the nurse assigned to care for Mr. Wallace. As part of his daily assessment, you obtain his vital signs, which include temperature 99.8°F oral, pulse 92 bpm, respirations 32/min, and blood pressure 108/74 mmHg. Auscultation of Mr. Wallace's lungs reveals faint bibasilar crackles. On reviewing his chart, you note that he has experienced a 5% weight loss since the previous month. You notify the attending physician about Mr. Wallace's vital signs, breath sounds, and weight loss. The physician orders a chest x-ray and CBC.

Clinical Reasoning Questions Level I

1. What is the significance of Mr. Wallace's vital signs and breath sounds?
2. What effect might Mr. Wallace's weight loss have on his cognitive condition?
3. What important pieces of information might be gleaned from tracking Mr. Wallace's food intake and weight?

Clinical Reasoning Questions Level II

4. What is the priority nursing diagnosis for Mr. Wallace at this time?
5. What independent interventions can you perform to optimize Mr. Wallace's respiratory status? What positive effects might these have on other aspects of his health?
6. *Refer to the exemplar on Alzheimer disease in this module:* Would Mr. Wallace's condition improve with the addition of a cholinesterase inhibitor to his treatment regimen? Why or why not?

REVIEW The Concept of Cognition

RELATE Link the Concepts

Linking the concept of cognition with the concept of perfusion:

1. Describe how alterations in perfusion can affect a patient's risk for specific types of dementia.
2. What measures might you implement when caring for a patient with impaired perfusion to limit the risk of dementia?

Linking the concept of cognition with the concept of development:

3. What considerations should a nurse apply when designing developmentally appropriate activities for an 8-year-old with Down syndrome?
4. What treatment measures used for patients with ADHD might also be useful for patients with fragile X syndrome? Why?

Linking the concept of cognition with the concept of family:

5. How might a family's normal processes and interactions be affected when one member is diagnosed with a cognitive disorder?

6. What actions can nurses take to support family members of patients with cognitive alterations?

READY Go to Volume 3: Companion Skills Manual

- SKILLS 1.5–1.9   Vital Signs
- SKILL 1.1   Appearance and Mental Status: Assessing
- SKILL 1.17   Heart and Central Vessels: Assessing
- SKILL 1.22   Neurologic Status: Assessing
- SKILL 1.24   Peripheral Vascular System: Assessing
- SKILL 1.27   Thorax and Lungs: Assessing
- SKILL 3.1   Pain in Newborn, Infant, Child, or Adult: Assessing
- SKILL 3.6   Sleep Promotion: Assisting
- SKILL 4.3   Urine Specimen, Clean-Catch, Closed Drainage System for Culture and Sensitivity: Obtaining
- SKILL 5.1   Intake and Output: Measuring
- SKILL 10.1   Body Mass Index (BMI): Assessing
- SKILL 11.8   Oxygen Delivery Systems: Using
- SKILL 15.1   Abuse: Newborn, Infant, Child, Older Adult, Assessing for
- SKILL 15.2   Fall Prevention: Assessing and Managing
- SKILL 15.4   Suicidal Patient: Caring for
- SKILL 15.5   Environmental Safety: Healthcare Facility, Community, Home

REFER Go to Pearson MyLab Nursing and eText

- Additional review material

REFLECT Apply Your Knowledge

Hannah Lister is a 6-year-old first-grade student who frequently presents to the school nurse's office with somatic complaints. Hannah's teacher is increasingly concerned that she is missing valuable class time. The nurse learns that Hannah has a history of learning and behavior problems and was recently diagnosed with nonverbal learning disability. The nurse and classroom teacher meet to discuss the issue with Hannah's parents. Hannah's mother is tearful as she talks about how anxious Hannah is. She states Hannah complains about having to go to school and complains that other students and teachers are "mean" to her. Hannah's mother says that her oldest child never had any of these problems, and she is at a loss as to how to help Hannah. Hannah's teacher believes that since Hannah is so articulate and has good reading skills, she is capable of doing much better in school. The teacher explains that she has worked with many children with learning disabilities who are not as bright as Hannah. She believes that Hannah should be held accountable for some of her rude and socially inappropriate behaviors and should receive consequences for missing class.

1. What might explain the teacher's misperceptions of Hannah's skills/capabilities?

2. What may make Hannah's learning problems different from those of students with language-based learning disabilities?

3. As the nurse, what kind of teaching could you provide to help teachers and parents understand some of the emotional and behavioral needs of children like Hannah?

4. When providing health teaching to Hannah, what kind of approach is most likely to be effective?

5. What types of independent and collaborative interventions may be appropriate to address Hannah's social and emotional needs?

≫ Exemplar 23.A
Alzheimer Disease

Exemplar Learning Objectives

23.A Analyze Alzheimer disease as it relates to cognition.

- Describe the pathophysiology of Alzheimer disease.
- Describe the etiology of Alzheimer disease.
- Compare the risk factors and prevention of Alzheimer disease.
- Identify the clinical manifestations of Alzheimer disease.
- Summarize diagnostic tests and therapies used by interprofessional teams in the collaborative care of an individual with Alzheimer disease.
- Differentiate care of patients with Alzheimer disease across the lifespan.
- Apply the nursing process in providing culturally competent care to an individual with Alzheimer disease.

Exemplar Key Terms

Alzheimer disease (AD), *1729*
Amyloid plaques, *1731*
Biomarkers, *1732*
Caregiver burden, *1730*
Early-onset familial AD (eFAD), *1730*
Neurofibrillary tangles, *1731*
Relocation syndrome (transfer trauma), *1737*
Sporadic AD, *1730*
Sundowning, *1732*

Overview

Alzheimer disease (AD) accounts for approximately 60–80% of all dementia cases in individuals age 65 and older. More than 5 million Americans suffer from AD, and this number is predicted to reach 7 million by 2025 and 14 million by 2050.

AD is currently the sixth leading cause of death in the United States (Alzheimer's Association, 2015).

Although AD usually manifests after age 65, some individuals experience symptoms as early as their 30s. Most individuals with AD survive between 4 and 8 years after diagnosis; those who are diagnosed at younger ages may live up to two decades. Patients typically spend more time in the moderate stage of AD than in any other stage. Eventually, they die from complications of the disease.

One important aspect of AD disease is **caregiver burden**. Caregiver burden refers to the psychologic, physical, and financial cost of caring for an individual with Alzheimer disease (Bevans & Sternberg, 2012). AD is associated with the higher levels of stress and caregiver burden than most other chronic illnesses. Nurses must consider both patient and caregiver needs when working with individuals with AD.

Pathophysiology and Etiology

Pathophysiology

There are two types of AD: familial and sporadic. **Early-onset familial AD (eFAD)** is an inherited disease. It is also called *early-onset AD* because it usually manifests before age 65. **Sporadic AD** shows no clear pattern of inheritance, although genetic factors may increase risk. Because it typically develops after age 65, sporadic AD is sometimes referred to as *late-onset AD*, and it is more common than its early-onset counterpart, accounting for 95% or more of all cases (Ridge, Ebbert, & Kauwe, 2013). Although the triggers may be different, eFAD and sporadic AD both involve the same set of pathophysiologic changes.

Individuals with AD show a pattern of degenerative changes related to neuronal death throughout the brain. The cells die in a characteristic order, beginning with neurons in the limbic system, including the hippocampus. Damage to this region results in emotional problems and loss of recent memory. From there, the destruction spreads up and out toward the cerebral surface (see **Figure 23–6 》**). Eventually, neuronal death in the cerebral lobes produces a range of symptoms, including loss of remote memory, as outlined in **Table 23–9 》**.

As AD progresses and more neurons die, two characteristic abnormalities develop in the brains of affected individuals. The first is thick protein clots called *neurofibrillary tangles*, and the second is insoluble deposits known as *amyloid plaques*. Researchers continue to investigate whether these abnormalities are a cause or a result of AD, as described in the section on etiology.

Etiology

Researchers are not sure why most cases of AD arise, although a variety of genetic and environmental factors appear to be involved. Moreover, the exact biochemical origins of AD remain unknown, even in patients who clearly have an inherited form of the disease. Researchers have therefore proposed several theories that seek to explain the disease process, including the cholinergic, amyloid, and tau hypotheses.

Cholinergic Hypothesis

The cholinergic hypothesis emerged in the early 1980s after nearly 20 years of investigation into the role of neurotransmitters. Researchers noted that lowered levels of acetylcholine (a cholinergic neurotransmitter) appeared to produce memory deficits. Autopsies also revealed that brains of indi-

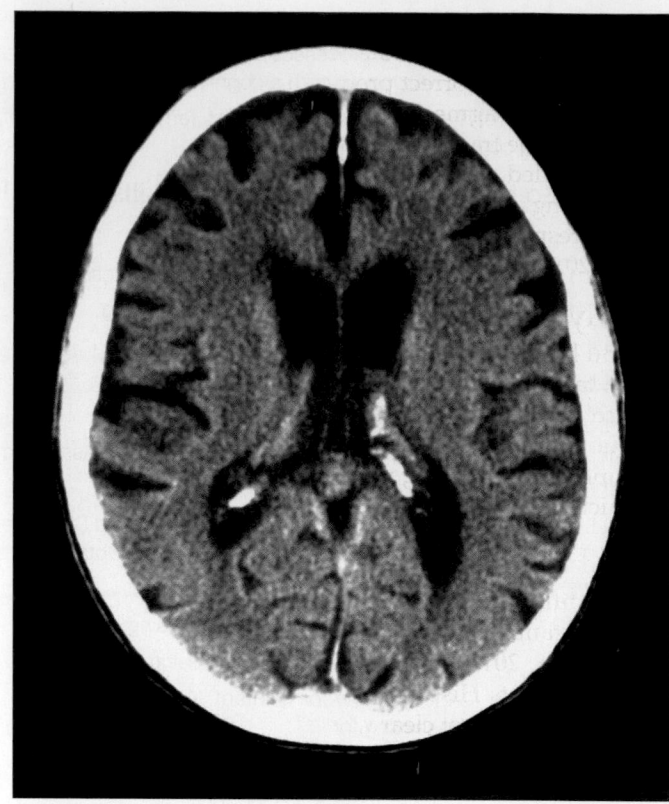

Source: Scott Camazine/Alamy Stock Photo.

Figure 23–6 》 CT scan of 84-year-old man with Alzheimer disease. Note atrophy of the brain.

viduals with AD had markers characteristic of decreased acetylcholine function. These findings suggested that AD was caused by below-normal production of acetylcholine in the brain and led to the development of acetylcholinesterase inhibitors. Because these agents have demonstrated only a modest effect on the disease, other theories have gained more attention (Rafii & Aisen, 2015).

Amyloid Hypothesis

Today, the amyloid and tau hypotheses are considered more likely explanations of the biochemistry of AD. The amyloid

TABLE 23–9 Cerebral Effects of AD

Region	Symptoms of Damage
Limbic system (including hippocampus)	Loss of memory (recent before remote); fluctuating emotions; depression; difficulty learning new information
Frontal lobe	Problems with intentional movement; difficulty planning; emotional lability; loss of walking, talking, and swallowing ability
Occipital lobe	Loss of reading comprehension; hallucinations
Parietal lobe	Difficulty recognizing places, people, and objects; hallucinations; seizures; unsteady movement; expressive aphasia; agraphia; agnosia
Temporal lobe	Impaired memory; difficulty learning new things; receptive aphasia

hypothesis states that AD arises when the brain cannot properly process a substance called *amyloid precursor protein (APP)*. Incorrect processing leads to the presence of short, sticky fragments of APP known as *beta-amyloid*. Eventually, the fragments clump together, forming insoluble deposits called **amyloid plaques**. These plaques damage the surrounding neurons, killing them and provoking an inflammatory response that may result in further brain damage (Khan, 2013).

Tau Hypothesis

The tau hypothesis focuses on a protein known as *tau*. Normally, tau holds together the microtubules responsible for intracellular transport within the axons of neurons. With AD, however, individuals have abnormal tau proteins that join and twist, forming **neurofibrillary tangles** instead of the microtubule network necessary for cellular survival.

Risk Factors

Nonmodifiable risk factors for Alzheimer disease include age, sex, family history, and genetic factors (Alzheimer's Association, 2016a, 2016b). Alzheimer disease disproportionately affects Hispanic and African American individuals, although it is not clear whether this relates to underlying biophysical characteristics or socioeconomic or cultural factors that increase modifiable risk factors. Individuals with a family history of AD are more likely to develop the disease, even in the absence of known genetic factors that predict or increase the risk of the disease. AD is almost 3 times more common in women than in men.

Although developing AD is not a normal or expected consequence of aging, the most prominent risk factor for Alzheimer disease is advancing age. Once an individual reaches the age of 65, the risk of developing the disease doubles every 5 years. After the age of 85, individuals have a 50% chance of developing the disease.

A summary of evidence recently conducted at the request of the Alzheimer's Association identifies a variety of modifiable risk factors associated with the disease that have been substantiated through valid and reliable research (Baumgart et al., 2015). For example, research has identified cardiovascular risk factors that include diabetes, mid-life obesity, mid-life hypertension, and hyperlipidemia. Evidence suggests that diabetes increases AD risk through both vascular and metabolic pathways (De Felice & Ferreira, 2014; Mushtaq, Khan, & Kamal, 2014, 2015). Mid-life obesity is correlated with vascular, metabolic, and inflammatory changes that appear to increase the risk of AD (Loef & Walach, 2013).

Lifestyle risk factors have been demonstrated to increase the risk of AD. There is a strong body of evidence linking cigarette smoking to cognitive decline and dementia. In addition, there is evidence to support the fact that individuals who lead a sedentary lifestyle are at increased risk for AD (Baumgart et al., 2015; Durazzo et al., 2014; Espeland et al., 2015).

Other risk factors appear to include lower level of formal education, a history of traumatic brain injury, depression, and disordered sleep. It is hypothesized that formal education provides a type of cognitive training that strengthens

neuronal cognitions and increases cognitive reserves (Sattler et al., 2012). Several strong and reliable studies have also linked the incidence of traumatic brain injury to AD, with individuals exposed to repeated trauma being at the greatest risk. It is believed that axonal injury, hypoxia, and inflammatory changes trigger neuronal degeneration associated with AD (Johnson, Stewart, & Smith, 2013; LoBue et al., 2015; Sivanandam & Thakur, 2012).

Depression is considered to be both a symptom of and risk factor for Alzheimer disease with overlapping neurobiological mechanisms responsible for both diseases (Wuwongse et al., 2013). There is research to suggest that the early management of depression with antidepressants may prevent cognitive decline associated with dementia (Chi et al., 2014). However, several new studies suggest that the use of antidepressants, especially SSRIs, may actually increase cortical changes associated with dementia and AD (Lebedev et al., 2014; Lee et al., 2016; Wang et al., 2016).

Another area of investigation has been the impact of sleep disorders on dementia and AD. Cohort and observational studies have linked sleep disorders to AD, with some research suggesting that the early use of continuous positive airway pressure (CPAP) in individuals with disorders such as apnea may reduce the incidence of decline (Osorio et al., 2015). Recent research also suggests that some of the agents used to treat insomnia, such as benzodiazepines and anticholinergic antihistamines, may actually accelerate cognitive deterioration (Defrancesco et al., 2015; Wurtman, 2015; Yaffe & Boustani, 2014).

Prevention

Evidence-based teaching for the general public with regard to increasing protective factors for AD includes reducing the incidence of cardiovascular disorders and other health problems by adopting a healthy lifestyle. For example, quitting smoking and using safety measures (e.g., safety belts) can reduce risk for developing Alzheimer disease, and even modest levels of exercise have been demonstrated to improve cognitive function (Baumgart et al., 2015; Intlekofer & Cotman, 2013). Other strategies include:

- ■ *Adopt a heart-healthy diet such as the Mediterranean diet.* Although many dietary studies are inconclusive, there is some evidence to suggest that antioxidant- and polyphenol-rich foods such as tea, cocoa, grapes, and colorful fruits and vegetables may interrupt formation of amyloid plaques and prevent AD (Feng et al., 2015; Pasinetti et al., 2015).

- ■ *Consume alcohol moderately.* Moderate alcohol consumption may be protective against AD. However, evidence is insufficient to suggest that individuals who do not already drink should start drinking (Baumgart et al., 2015).

- ■ *Stay socially active and connected with others.* Studies demonstrate that social engagement may improve cognitive function and have some protective effects against AD (Baumgart et al., 2015; Beckett, Ardern, & Rotondi, 2015; de Bruijn et al., 2015).

- ■ *Engage in activities that exercise cognitive function.* Evidence demonstrates that cognitive activities such as reading, completing puzzles, and learning new information or tasks build cognitive resilience and protect against cognitive decline (Beckett et al., 2015).

- **Utilize stress management techniques.** And seek appropriate treatment for depression and alterations in sleep.

Clinical Manifestations

The initial symptoms of AD emerge gradually and may be almost unnoticeable. The first manifestation is usually subtle memory loss that becomes increasingly apparent as time passes. Other early signs include difficulty finding words and performing familiar tasks; impaired judgment and abstract thinking; disorientation to time and place; and frequently misplacing things. These alterations go beyond the changes sometimes seen with normal aging, as described in the introduction to this module. Diurnal changes in cognitive function are typical, with patterns of diminished capacity in the evening (also known as **sundowning**). Changes in mood or personality are also common. Early in the course of AD, many individuals exhibit decreased initiative, odd behavior, and signs of depression. As the disease progresses, the continued deterioration in patients' cognition is accompanied by physical decline. At some point, affected individuals lose the ability to perform everyday tasks and must rely entirely on their caregivers.

AD is described in terms of three general stages: stage 1 (early), stage 2 (moderate), and stage 3 (severe). The Clinical Manifestations and Therapies feature outlines the clinical manifestations associated with each stage along with interventions. Individuals' rate of progression is affected by a variety of factors, including their overall health and the type of care they receive following diagnosis.

Collaboration

The care of patients with AD depends on collaboration among nurses, physicians, physical, occupational and speech therapists, psychologists, family members, volunteers, personal care assistants, social workers, and case managers. In the early to moderate stages of the disease, care is generally community based and involves outpatient visits to primary providers and a variety of services, including counseling, support groups, in-home care, daycare programs, and assisted living. When individuals are no longer able to be managed in the community setting, they may need to transition to a skilled nursing facility. In this section, diagnostic tests and therapies employed by members of the interprofessional team across settings are summarized.

Diagnostic Tests

There is no definitive way to diagnose AD other than performing a brain autopsy. Instead, practitioners rely on differential diagnosis, ruling out potential causes of a patient's symptoms until AD remains the most likely explanation. When individuals present with signs and symptoms of AD, the nurse can anticipate standard laboratory tests being ordered, including thyroid-stimulating hormone (TSH),

complete blood count (CBC), serum B_{12}, folate, complete metabolic panel, and testing for sexually transmitted infections. Screening tools and tests that aid in the diagnosis of AD are discussed in detail in the sections on assessment of and diagnosis of cognitive disorders.

Genetic testing may be conducted under certain clinical guidelines. Individuals with a parent with early-onset or eFAD have a 50/50 chance of inheriting the associated mutation. If genetic testing of offspring reveals the presence of the mutation, it confers an almost 100% probability of developing the disease. Individuals with a certain type of allele (ApOE4) are at a 12- to 15-fold increased *risk* of developing the disease and represent about 20% of all individuals impacted by the disease (Goldman et al., 2011; Loy et al., 2014). Other genetic factors are believed to be involved, and it is important to remember that lack of genetic findings does not mean that any individual will not develop the disease or that AD can be ruled out.

One emerging approach to diagnosis of AD that deserves mention is the analysis of biomarkers for the disease. **Biomarkers** are physiologic, chemical, or anatomic measures associated with certain conditions. Currently several biomarkers have been demonstrated to be associated with AD. These include morphologic or structural abnormalities detected through brain imaging techniques. Positron emission tomographic (PET) scan findings demonstrate hypometabolism and the presence of amyloid deposits in certain areas of the brain. In addition, an analysis of CSF may reveal the presence of certain proteins associated with neurodegeneration (Blennow & Zetterberg, 2013; Jack & Holtzman, 2013). Biomarkers for AD may be present even before the manifestations of the disease are present; therefore their identification in certain susceptible individuals may facilitate early intervention and planning.

Pharmacologic Therapy

There is currently no cure for AD. Two classes of medications are used to slow the progression of the disease. In addition, adjunctive agents may be prescribed to treat associated symptoms of depression, anxiety, or psychosis.

NMDA Receptor Antagonists and Combination Agents

Acetylcholinesterase (AChE) inhibitors have been standard treatment for over a decade. They work by reducing acetylcholine breakdown. Because individuals with Alzheimer disease are gradually losing neurons that communicate by using this substance, the presence of extra acetylcholine increases communication among the remaining neurons. This appears to temporarily stabilize symptoms related to language, memory, and reasoning for an average of 6 to 12 months.

Commonly prescribed acetylcholinesterase inhibitors include donepezil (Aricept), rivastigmine (Exelon), and galantamine (Razadyne). Rivastigmine and galantamine are approved for early to moderate stages of AD, while donepezil is approved for all stages. Although these drugs all act similarly, not all individuals respond to them in the same way. In fact, about half of individuals who take these drugs

Clinical Manifestations and Therapies
Alzheimer Disease

ETIOLOGY	CLINICAL MANIFESTATIONS	CLINICAL THERAPIES
Stage I Mild cognitive impairment	■ Reduced concentration and memory lapses noticeable by others ■ Difficulty learning new information ■ Problems functioning in work or social settings ■ Frequently losing or misplacing important objects ■ Difficulties with planning and organization ■ Forgetting familiar words or the locations of various objects	■ Patient/caregiver education and training ■ Environmental modifications to promote safety ■ Encourage planning for advanced stages of the disease while patients are still able to participate in decision making ■ Use of cuing devices such as to-do lists, calendars, written schedules, and verbal reminders ■ Cognitive Activity Kits ■ Deliberate establishment of and adherence to daily routines ■ Referral to community resources, support groups, and/or counseling services ■ Nonpharmacologic therapies such as healing touch, reality orientation, and reminiscence therapy ■ Counseling regarding possible retirement or withdrawal from the more challenging aspects of one's job
Stage II Moderate AD	■ Inability to carry out ADLs, such as preparing meals for oneself and choosing appropriate clothing ■ Loss of ability to live independently ■ Difficulty recalling one's address or phone number ■ Increased problems finding words and communicating clearly ■ Inability to recall information from recent memory ■ Increasing difficulty remembering details from remote memory ■ Disorientation to time and place ■ Increased tendency to become lost ■ Changes in ability to control bladder/ bowels ■ Changes in sleep patterns ■ Withdrawal from social situations and challenging mental activity ■ Increased moodiness, flat affect, or signs of depression and/or anxiety, paranoia	■ Behavioral interventions such as distraction, provision of meaningful activities ■ Continued use of cuing devices and established routines ■ Assistance with ADLs ■ Administration of anti-AD acetylcholinesterase inhibitors, including rivastigmine (Exelon), galantamine (Razadyne), and donepezil (Aricept); NDMA inhibitors may be added ■ Administration of SSRIs and/or anxiolytics to address mood-related symptoms ■ Occupational, physical, and speech therapy ■ Nonpharmacologic therapies such as healing touch, validation, and reminiscence therapy ■ Consultation with a dietitian or nutritionist ■ Respite care for family members and other caregivers ■ May require around-the-clock care or transition to a skilled nursing facility
Stage III Severe AD	■ Gradual inability to perform any ADLs, including bathing and toileting ■ Eventual urinary and fecal incontinence ■ Inability to identify family and caregivers ■ Extreme confusion and lack of awareness of one's surroundings ■ Gradual loss of remote memory and ability to speak ■ Inability to perform simple mental calculations ■ Dramatic personality changes, including extreme suspiciousness and fearfulness ■ Sundowning, delusions, compulsions, agitation, and violent outbursts ■ Gradual loss of ability to walk, sit unaided, and hold one's head up ■ Development of abnormal reflexes ■ Physical rigidity ■ Loss of swallowing ability	■ Assistance with all ADLs ■ Continuation of earlier behavioral and pharmacologic therapies ■ Addition of atypical antipsychotics, as appropriate ■ Round-the-clock care and/or admittance to a skilled nursing facility ■ Frequent repositioning ■ Liquid nutrition or feeding tubes as appropriate ■ Respite care for family members and other caregivers ■ End-of-life care

Source: Alzheimer's Association. (2016c). *Stages of Alzheimer's.* Retrieved from http://www.alz.org/alzheimers_disease_stages_of_alzheimers.asp; Budson, A. E., & Solomon, P. R. (2012). New diagnostic criteria for Alzheimer's disease and mild cognitive impairment for the practical neurologist. *Practical Neurology,* 12(2), 88–96; National Institutes of Health. (2015). *The changing brain in AD.* Retrieved from https://www.nia.nih.gov/alzheimers/publication/part-2-what-happensbrain-ad/changing-brain-ad see no delay in symptom progression. AChE inhibitors generally produce mild side effects such as decreased appetite, nausea, diarrhea, headaches, and dizziness. Adverse effects include GI bleeding and bradycardia. Teaching should include avoiding other medications that may increase the risk of GI bleeding and monitoring pulse rate. The patient's nutritional status and fluid balance should also be monitored. The dosage is slowly increased to minimize side effects. Patients and family members should be cautioned not to abruptly stop the medication, as this may cause a sudden worsening of symptoms. (Adams, Holland, & Urban, 2017).

NMDA Receptor Antagonists

NMDA receptor antagonists are believed to block the effects of glutamate, a neurotransmitter that is present with neuronal damage and appears to be involved in cognitive decline. NMDA receptor antagonists do not reverse existing damage, but they do slow the rate at which new damage occurs. Unlike acetylcholinesterase inhibitors, NMDA receptor antagonists generally are not prescribed until an individual is in the moderate to severe stages of AD.

Currently, memantine (Namenda) is the only NMDA receptor antagonist approved by the U.S. Food and Drug Administration (FDA). In 2014, a combination agent of memantine and donepezil (Namzaric) was approved for use in individuals with moderate to severe AD. Side effects of NMDA inhibitors are less common and usually milder than those associated with donepezil, rivastigmine, and galantamine. They include dizziness, constipation, confusion, headache, fatigue, and increased blood pressure. Patients and family members should be cautioned about performing activities requiring mental alertness or coordination until tolerance is established. The medication should be taken with food if stomach upset occurs (Adams et al., 2017; Alzheimer's Association, 2016d).

Other Medications Used to Treat AD Symptoms

Drug classes used to manage the symptoms of AD include antipsychotics (to treat delusions or hallucinations), anxiolytics (to treat anxiety), and SSRI antidepressants (to treat depression). Because there is some evidence that these agents may actually increase the risk of cognitive decline, patients and their families should be encouraged to discuss the risks versus benefits with their providers. For more details on these drugs, please refer to the Medications feature as well as the modules on Stress and Coping and Mood and Affect.

Nonpharmacologic Therapy

Nonpharmacologic interventions that have been demonstrated to be effective in treating AD include exercise, reality orientation therapy, validation therapy, and reminiscence therapy.

Reality Orientation

Reality orientation is a structured approach to orienting individuals to person, time, place, and situations at regular intervals and as needed through verbal communication and the use of visual cues (pictures, clocks, calendars, orientation boards). Reality orientation therapy is a collaborative intervention that is carried out by all members of the healthcare team. Reality orientation interventions have been demonstrated to improve cognitive function when used in combination with AChE inhibitors (Camargo, Justus, & Retzlaff, 2015). However, reorientation to certain situations or information may be upsetting in some cases and should be used judiciously.

Validation Therapy

Validation therapy involves searching for emotion or intended meaning in verbal expressions and behaviors. The basic premise is that seemingly purposeless behaviors and incoherent speech have significance to the patient and can be related to current needs (Feil, 2014). For example, if an individual is wandering and crying out for her mother, instead of reminding the patient that the mother is dead or unavailable, the nurse may say something like "You are looking for Mother. Is there something you need from her?" The goal is to elicit a response that identifies an unmet need, such as, "Yes, I need her to give me my dinner." The nurse can then address the wandering and associated anxiety by offering the patient something to eat or reassuring her that dinner will be available soon. Unlike reality orientation, validation therapy does not unnecessarily challenge the patient's perception of reality.

Reminiscence Therapy

Reminiscence therapy uses the process of purposely reflecting on past events. The nurse or other healthcare provider may encourage the patient to talk about events that occurred in the past, often by using scrapbooks, photo albums, music, or other items to facilitate the process. In addition to helping patients to retain long-term memory, reminiscence therapy may be comforting, provides a source of self-esteem, identity, and purpose, and can help to prevent isolation and withdrawal (Potter & Moller, 2016).

Complementary Health Approaches

The National Center for Complementary and Integrative Health (NCCIH) publishes findings derived from research about the safety and efficacy of alternative and complementary health practices for AD (see Focus on Integrative Health). Integrative therapies that have empirical evidence to support their efficacy in promoting comfort and relief from the symptoms of AD include art therapy, music therapy, healing touch, and reiki (Han et al., 2013; Livingston et al., 2014). Studies on the use of dietary supplements such as antioxidant vitamins, ginkgo biloba, resveratrol, omega-3 fatty acids, and medical food such as tramiprosate (Vivimind) and caprylic acid for the management of AD are inconclusive at best and associated with risks such as interaction with other drugs and toxicity. There is no convincing evidence to date that dietary supplements such as ginkgo, omega-3, vitamins B and E, ginseng, grape seed extract, or curcumin are beneficial in preventing or mitigating dementia or Alzheimer disease.

NURSING PROCESS

The application of the nursing process should be guided by clinical guidelines that are current and informed by the best available evidence. The primary goal of care is to provide a safe, supportive environment that meets patients' changing abilities and needs. The nurse must also take steps to support patients' family members as they cope with the emotional and physical demands of caring for a loved one with AD. Various tools and techniques for providing nursing care for patients and families with AD can be accessed from reliable sources such as The Hartford Institute for Geriatric Nursing, the Alzheimer's Association, and the Agency for Healthcare Research and Quality (AHRQ). Highlights of standards of current practice are provided in this section.

Assessment

Current clinical guidelines for the nursing assessment of individuals with AD include completion of a health history and assessment of physical status, cognitive function, functional status, behavioral presentation, and caregiver/environment (Fletcher, 2012). Serial assessments allow the nurse to monitor changes indicative of disease progression and the ability of the patient to manage safely in the current living environment.

Observation and Patient Interview

The nurse should start the assessment by observing the patient along with the caregivers. Patients with mild dementia may not present any signs or symptoms notable on appearance. At this stage, family members' reports of noticeable changes in memory or cognitive abilities in certain areas may be the first clue that there is a problem. As dementia progresses, patients exhibit signs of difficulty maintaining self-care, such as dressing inappropriately for the weather or an unkempt appearance; difficulty focusing on simple tasks or paying attention during the patient interview; and variable gait or changes in gait speed. The patient interview should address family history of AD and other dementias; medical history; current medications and use of any supplements; changes in cognition, communication, memory, and behavior; alterations in mood; sleep patterns; ability to perform ADLs; drug and alcohol use; and risk for or history of exposure to environmental toxins.

Cognitive Mental Status

For patients with AD, a thorough mental status examination is critical. Nurses can choose from a variety of assessment instruments, as described in the Assessment section. The MMSE is the test most commonly used to assess cognitive status.

Physical Examination

During the physical assessment, evaluate the patient's height, weight, vital signs, and overall physical condition. Throughout the exam, remain alert for possible signs of abuse, neglect, depression, malnutrition, elimination difficulties, and alterations in skin integrity, as AD increases the risk for all of these.

A number of other conditions can mimic the symptoms of dementia and AD. A useful mnemonic for remembering to assess for these conditions is **DEMENTIA:**

Drugs and alcohol

Eyes and ears

Metabolic and endocrine disorders

Emotional disorders

Neurologic disorders

Trauma or tumors

Infection

Arteriovascular disease

Functional Status

An assessment of functional status addresses any changes in ability to manage to day-to-day ADLs, such as eating or dressing, and instrumental activities of daily living (IADLs) such as cooking, managing housework, or taking care of finances. This can be addressed through direct questioning of patients or family members (e.g., "Over the past 7 days, have you noticed any changes in your family member's ability to complete getting dressed?"). Screening tools such as the Functional Activities Questionnaire (FAQ) may also be used (Cordell et al., 2013; Fletcher, 2012).

Behavioral Status

The behavioral assessment consists of direct observation of the patient and direct questioning of the patient and caregivers as well as the use of valid assessment tools. Assess for behavior changes associated with AD, including depression, anxiety, irritability, impulsivity, poor judgment, paranoia, delusions, and hallucinations. Inquire about events that precipitate any behavior changes so that potential triggers can be identified and eliminated. The Geriatric Depression Scale (GDS) may be used to detect changes in mood. The BEHAVE-AD is a 25-item assessment tool that nurses can use to elicit caregiver reports about a variety of behaviors. These are then scored to determine the magnitude of the disturbance in terms of patient and caregiver safety (Reisberg et al., 2014).

Caregiver/Living Environment

The final area of assessment addresses the needs of the caregiver and the adequacy of the living environment. Ask the caregiver(s) to share his perspective on the patient's ability to function in light of current support. It is also important to determine the impact that patient behaviors have on the caregiver and to gather data about the quality of the caregiving relationship. Two practical tools for assessing caregiver burden include the Zarit Burden Interview (ZBI) and the Caregiver Role Strain Index (CRI). Also assess current knowledge of effective caregiving interventions and the capacity to employ these interventions in the current living environment. Remember to assess for cultural values, beliefs, practices, and even barriers that may affect provision of care or the patient–family relationship (see Focus on Diversity and Culture: Addressing Cultural Factors That Increase Stigma and Caregiver Burden).

Diagnosis

Appropriate nursing diagnoses for patients with AD vary by stage of the disease and patient and family preferences and needs. Diagnoses should be prioritized to address physiologic

Focus on Diversity and Culture
Addressing Cultural Factors That Increase Stigma and Caregiver Burden

The stigma associated with having a family member with Alzheimer disease is influenced by a variety of cultural factors, and it has been demonstrated to increase caregiver burden by reinforcing negative emotional responses and limiting external sources of support (Parveen et al., 2015; Werner et al., 2012). Negative attitudes and beliefs about dementia and AD are common to many cultures. However, there are varying beliefs regarding the cause of the disease and appropriate management of care. Filial (family) values may reinforce the caregiver's sense that they have primary responsibility for caring for parents or other family members. Across various cultures, education and socioeconomic status are important mediators of the impact of stigma on caregivers. Nurses play a key role in assessing family/caregiver beliefs about AD. Family members may be asked open-ended questions such as "What do you or your family members believe caused this disease?" and "Who do you or your family members believe is responsible for caring for your parent/family member?" Once cultural barriers to care are identified, nurses can initiate teaching to address misperceptions and collaborate with other healthcare professionals to address barriers to care, such as lack of social support (Spector, 2017).

and safety needs first. The following list identifies some common nursing diagnoses:

- *Injury, Risk for*
- *Health Maintenance, Ineffective*
- *Self-care Deficit (specify)*
- *Imbalanced Nutrition: Less Than Body Requirements*
- *Memory: Impaired*
- *Communication: Verbal, Impaired*
- *Fear*
- *Caregiver Role Strain*
- *Swallowing, Impaired*
- *Physical Mobility, Impaired*
- *Wandering*
- *Compromised Human Dignity, Risk for*

(NANDA-I © 2014)

Planning

The planning portion of the nursing process involves identifying desired patient outcomes and formulating steps for achieving them. Appropriate goals and actions will vary depending on a patient's physical and mental status and current living situation, and they may include the following:

- Patient will remain free from injury.
- Patient will utilize lists, calendars, and other memory aids as needed.
- Patient will perform IADLs with caregiver assistance.
- Patient will exhibit reduced anxiety, agitation, and restlessness.
- Patient will take all medications as prescribed.

The nurse should also consider caregiver and family needs during the planning process. Some suggested outcomes are as follows:

- Caregiver will utilize respite care resources as necessary.
- Caregiver will learn effective strategies for coping with the stresses of supporting a loved one with AD.
- Caregiver will obtain the sleep and nutrition necessary to preserve personal health.

Implementation

Implementation of nursing interventions depends on patient and family needs and integrates an understanding of principles of health promotion in relation to the stages of the illness. The Progressively Lowered Stress Threshold (PLST) intervention model is supported by current clinical guidelines and is an approach that should guide nursing care during all stages of the illness (Fletcher, 2012). This model proposes that individuals with dementia and Alzheimer disease require a trajectory of environmental modifications in order to cope with progressive cognitive decline. An escalation in anxiety, depression, or behaviors such as wandering is likely to indicate inappropriate or inadequate environmental modifications.

With the advent of genetic testing and biomarker analysis, nurses increasingly provide care to patients who do not currently demonstrate signs of cognitive decline but who have a high likelihood of developing the disease. Changes in the diagnostic criteria for AD and other dementias now include recognition of mild forms of these disorders and provide opportunities for nurses and other healthcare providers to initiate early treatment to slow the progression of AD as well as increase opportunities for patient participation in advance planning.

Promote Safety and Physiologic Integrity

The safety and physiologic integrity of patients and family members, especially those providing care, is priority, even when significant changes in functional capacity have not yet occurred. The nurse should ensure that patients and families understand the role of health behaviors such as exercise and diet in slowing the progression of the disease. Emphasize the importance of adequate sleep, rest, nutrition, elimination, and pain control. Provide information on minimizing exposure to illness and the timely management of comorbid conditions that impact quality of life and may hasten the rate of cognitive decline.

Injury prevention requires a comprehensive approach that incorporates collaboration with other members of the healthcare team, including occupational and speech therapists. Principles of environmental safety are discussed in detail in the modules on Safety and Mobility and include but are not limited to identifying and removing hazards that increase the risk of falls, burns, drowning, skin breakdown, and ingestion or misuse of toxic substances. The risks and benefits of devices such as medic alert systems, patient tracking or alert systems, and locks should be discussed with patients and families. The use of physical and pharmacologic restraints should be avoided.

>> Stay Current: For more information on strategies that can be employed to avoid the use of restraints, see Avoiding Restraints in Patients with Dementia at the Hartford Institute for Geriatric Nursing at https://consultgeri.org/try-this/dementia/issue-d1.

Nurses should also address the patient's ability to continue occupational, recreational, and practical activities, such as driving, that may be negatively impacted by impaired cognition. Research shows that the rate of accidents in individuals in the first 2 years following an early diagnosis of AD is comparable to the general population but quickly increases thereafter (Alzheimer's Association, 2016e; Carter et al., 2015). Family members and caregivers should be alert to signs that driving is no longer safe, such as minor fender benders, getting lost, or ignoring stop signs or other traffic signals. Driver Rehabilitation specialists have expertise in evaluating driving abilities and making recommendations for terminating driving privileges.

>> **Stay Current:** For more information on assessment and intervention of driving in older adults with dementia and related disorders, visit http://seniordriving.aaa.com/evaluate-your-driving-ability/professional-assessment and http://www.alz.org/care/alzheimers-dementia-and-driving.asp

---

SAFETY ALERT The use of physical and pharmacologic restraints in individuals with AD and dementia significantly increases the risk of injury and death and is never considered therapeutic. Although safety is frequently cited as the rationale for using restraints, the risks of use clearly outweigh the benefits. The use of restraints and other measures to restrict movement can be avoided entirely through behavioral strategies such as distraction, consistent caregiving, provision of meaningful activities, and human monitoring.

Promote Adaptive Functioning and Coping

In the early stages of the disease, the nurse supports adaptive functioning by providing patient and family education and training, facilitating advanced planning, and supporting the emotional needs of both the family and the individual as they come to terms with the diagnosis.

>> **Stay Current:** For a nursing standard for addressing advance directives with patients, visit The Hartford Institute for Geriatric Nursing https://consultgeri.org/geriatric-topics/advance-directives.

Education centers on accessing health and financial resources, medication teaching, interventions to support optimal cognition and safety (e.g., cuing devices, calendars, lists, label, verbal reminders), and environmental modifications that may reduce stress. Communication strategies for individuals with AD include the following:

- Establish eye contact.
- Begin every interaction by introducing yourself and stating the patient's name.
- Talk in a calm reassuring tone.
- Use simple vocabulary and brief, straightforward sentences.
- Ask only one question at a time. Use questions that require yes or no answers, and provide sufficient response time.
- Repeat questions, explanations, and instructions as required.
- Be careful about challenging the patient's interpretation of reality, as this may lead to agitation and noncompliance.

As the disease progresses, the emphasis of nursing care focuses on addressing behavioral manifestations of the disease, including neuropsychiatric symptoms such as agitation, depression, and anxiety. Caregivers may need guidance in recognizing the unmet needs that behaviors such as wandering and restlessness represent. Prevention of fatigue, consistency in caregiving, using simple and direct communication, providing comforting and meaningful activities (art, music, reminiscence), scheduling quiet time, and reducing stimulation are effective behavioral strategies.

Nurses are often in a key position to counsel family members as they struggle with ambivalence and guilt related to the decision to transition the patient to a skilled nursing facility. It is important for the nurse to address cultural beliefs that may compound the difficulty associated with making such a decision. Nurses can guide caregivers to select services and placements that best meet the unique needs of the patient and the family and that optimize the family's ability to continue to participate in caregiving. Nurses should be cognizant of the phenomenon of **transfer trauma** or **relocation syndrome**—a worsening of symptoms associated with the stress of moving to a new environment. In addition to family participation in care, strategies to address the transition include retaining as many aspects of the home environment and previous routine as possible.

Provide End-of-Life Care

Nursing care for patients in the final stage of AD focuses on promoting quality of life and minimizing discomfort associated with physiologic decline and profound deficits in cognitive function. Principles of palliative care are discussed in detail in the modules on Comfort and on Grief and Loss and encompass a holistic approach to care. Palliative care with individuals with AD is challenged by the patient's inability to communicate needs. Family members and caregivers who have not resolved relationship issues during earlier stages of the illness may have more difficulty with treatment decisions and are at increased risk for complicated grieving.

Evaluation

Evaluation of patient outcomes is based on an understanding that patients may only be able to achieve a series of short-term outcomes based on the stage of disease progression. The focus is on ensuring that the patient and family achieve the optimal level of wellness for the particular stage of the disease. Evaluation also focuses on the caregivers' ability to manage the progression of the disease while meeting their own health and emotional needs. The following are examples of anticipated outcomes of care.

- The patient utilizes strategies to maintain independent functioning.
- The safety of the patient and others is maintained.
- The patient and/or family adheres to the prescribed treatment.
- Caregivers verbalize that self-care needs are met.

The unmet outcomes may indicate that the level of support being provided to the patient and family is no longer sufficient. In addition, it is possible that goals or certain interventions are no longer appropriate for the stage of the disease. In both cases the nurse would modify the plan of care.

Nursing Care Plan
A Patient with Alzheimer Disease

Sixty-one-year-old Loretta Gordon arrives at her general practitioner's office complaining of memory problems and depression that began about a month ago. Ms. Gordon is currently taking sertraline for her depression. She is afraid her medication is causing her current complaints, so she came to see the doctor.

ASSESSMENT

Gretchen Burchett, RN, obtains a patient history and conducts a physical examination of Ms. Gordon. Nurse Burchett notes that Ms. Gordon retired 2 years ago after 35 years as an elementary school music teacher. Shortly after retirement, Ms. Gordon began to experience depression and was prescribed sertraline; until recently, her symptoms were well controlled by the medication. Ms. Gordon receives a "comfortable pension" from the school and lives alone in a small house. She has never been married and has no children, but she maintains a close relationship with her brother, who is 15 years younger. Her primary social outlet is a group of women friends she's known since college, although she says she hasn't been attending their weekly get-togethers because she "has a hard time following the conversation." Ms. Gordon is an avid piano player but admits to recent frustration over her inability to follow sheet music.

Ms. Gordon is clean and well groomed, and her weight is healthy for someone her age and height. She struggles to find the right words when answering Nurse Burchett's questions. Nurse Burchett also notes a family history of AD and that Ms. Gordon sustained a serious head injury in a car accident 8 years ago. Ms. Gordon's vital signs include temperature 99.0°F oral; pulse 67 bpm; respirations 18/min; and blood pressure 116/72 mmHg.

Suspecting mild or early-stage AD, Nurse Burchett administers the MMSE. Ms. Gordon scores 23, indicating mild cognitive impairment. The physician orders blood tests to check for metabolic and endocrine problems and an MRI to assess for impaired blood flow and fluid accumulation in the brain. All of Ms. Gordon's test results are negative, and a diagnosis of probable mild or early-stage familial AD is made. The physician prescribes donepezil, 5 mg orally, increasing to 10 mg after 6 weeks. He also increases her sertraline from 150 mg orally to 175 mg and instructs her to return in 6 months.

DIAGNOSES

- *Risk for Injury* related to impaired cognitive function
- *Impaired Memory* related to diminished neurologic function
- *Chronic Confusion* related to deterioration of cognitive function
- *Impaired Verbal Communication* related to intellectual changes
- *Anxiety* related to awareness of physiologic and cognitive changes

(NANDA-I © 2014)

PLANNING

Goals for Ms. Gordon's care include:

- The patient will remain free from injury.
- The patient will verbalize an understanding of her disease and its stages.
- The patient will utilize lists, calendars, and other memory aids as needed.
- The patient will participate in speech and language therapy.
- The patient will exhibit decreased signs and symptoms of anxiety and depression.
- The patient will take all medications as prescribed.
- The patient will remain in the home environment as long as possible.

IMPLEMENTATION

- Teach about AD, and provide informational materials and recommendations for community resources.
- Collaborate with other members of the healthcare team to ensure advance planning and decision making, including advance directives, financial planning, and legal concerns related to guardianship and estate planning.
- Collaborate with the primary care provider and other members of the healthcare team about home visits to regularly assess the patient's functional capabilities and identify any safety concerns.
- Emphasize the use of calendars and electronic devices to record appointments and alert to important activities, such as medication administration.

- Instruct about the prescribed medications, potential side effects, and dietary changes that can minimize negative side effects.
- Refer to speech and occupational therapy.
- Teach about strategies to address behavioral changes and anxiety associated with AD, including decreasing environmental stress, regular sleep and meal schedules, redirection and distraction, minimizing unexpected changes, and counseling, relaxation, and music therapy for both patients and families.
- Promote therapeutic environments and activities that encourage physical, social, emotional, and cognitive well-being, including physical activity, diet, prevention and management of health problems, cognitive exercises, games, puzzles, and social engagement.

EVALUATION

Nurse Burchett refers Ms. Gordon to a speech therapist, and therapy sessions are scheduled for twice weekly. During therapy, Ms. Gordon engages in a series of exercises designed to slow her decline in communication skills. She has also mastered the electronic calendar and alarm on her cell phone, programming reminders for even basic daily functions. She enjoys an hour of music in the evenings, although she listens to recordings rather than playing her piano. After 6 months of pharmacologic treatment and speech therapy, Ms. Gordon's cognitive condition is stable and she once again scores 23 on her MMSE.

Ms. Gordon continues to display symptoms of depression, primarily stemming from the realization that there is no cure for her condition. She attends a local AD support group, which helps her verbalize and cope with her anxiety. With the help of her brother, who has invited Ms. Gordon to move into his home, she has created a long-term care plan.

Nursing Care Plan *(continued)*

CRITICAL THINKING

1. Ms. Gordon is fortunate that her brother is willing to be involved in her care. How would you adapt the care plan if Ms. Gordon had no family or her family was unwilling to be involved?

2. Ms. Gordon finds comfort in a support group for AD patients. Identify resources in your area that provide these kinds of services to AD patients and caregivers.

3. Develop a care plan for the nursing diagnosis of Self-Care Deficit related to cognitive decline and physical limitations.

REVIEW Alzheimer Disease

RELATE Link the Concepts and Exemplars

Linking the exemplar of Alzheimer disease with the concept of tissue integrity:

1. Why might patients with AD be at a heightened risk for impaired tissue integrity? What types of impairments would you most expect to see, and during which stages of AD would they most likely occur?

2. When caring for the patient with AD, what nursing interventions are appropriate when seeking to limit the risk of impaired tissue integrity?

Linking the exemplar of Alzheimer disease with the concept of spirituality:

3. How might a patient's spirituality be affected by a diagnosis of AD? How might a patient's diagnosis of AD affect her family and loved ones?

4. What nursing interventions might be appropriate for patients and families who are experiencing spiritual distress related to the cognitive and physical alterations associated with AD?

Linking the exemplar of Alzheimer disease with the concept of legal issues:

5. Why are issues of informed consent often problematic for individuals with AD?

6. What actions might nurses recommend to prevent such issues from arising?

READY Go to Volume 3: Clinical Nursing Skills

REFER Go to Pearson MyLab Nursing and eText

- Additional review material

REFLECT Apply Your Knowledge

Robert Moser, a 75-year-old man, is brought to the emergency department by State Trooper Kelly just before midnight. Law enforcement had received reports of a car driving erratically along the highway and pulled Mr. Moser over. Trooper Kelly tells you that when he stopped Mr. Moser, Mr. Moser was able to get out his wallet but unable to tell Trooper Kelly his name. Mr. Moser stated he was trying to find the hospital where his wife is located, but he could not name the hospital or say where it is. Trooper Kelly pulled up the list of contacts in Mr. Moser's cell phone. When Mr. Moser confirmed one of the contacts was his son, Trooper Kelly contacted the son and asked him to meet them at the hospital. The son, who informs Trooper Kelly that Mr. Moser recently was diagnosed with Alzheimer disease, lives out of town and will arrive in about an hour. Mr. Moser is polite and compliant, but he keeps asking "Is this a hospital?" over and over again. As you begin your assessment, Mr. Moser has difficulty finding the words he needs to respond.

1. What additional assessment information do you need?

2. Identify three other conditions that may produce symptoms that mimic dementia.

3. How will you go about the assessment given that Mr. Moser is unable to participate fully?

4. What are Mr. Moser's priorities for care *at this time*?

5. What stage of Alzheimer disease is Mr. Moser likely experiencing?

≫ Exemplar 23.B Delirium

Exemplar Learning Objectives

23.B Analyze delirium as it relates to cognition.

- Describe the pathophysiology of delirium.
- Describe the etiology of delirium.
- Compare the risk factors and prevention of delirium.
- Identify the clinical manifestations of delirium.
- Summarize diagnostic tests and therapies used by interprofessional teams in the collaborative care of an individual with a congenital heart defect.

- Differentiate care of patients with delirium across the lifespan.
- Apply the nursing process in providing culturally competent care to an individual with delirium.

Exemplar Key Terms

Confusion, *1740*
Confusion Assessment Method (CAM), *1743*
Delirium, *1740*
Sundowning, *1741*

Overview

Delirium is an abrupt, generally transient, and often fluctuating change in mental state and consciousness characterized by disorganized thinking, disorientation, perceptual disturbances, restlessness, agitation, and lability. **Confusion** is a closely related term, broadly used to describe increased difficulty in thinking clearly, making judgments, focusing attention, and maintaining orientation. The terms *acute confusion* and *delirium* have been used interchangeably; however, delirium is recognized as a distinct disorder and is classified by the DSM-5 according to the etiology.

The most important thing to remember about delirium is that it generally signals the presence of a reversible but potentially life-threatening condition. Delirium is associated with a number of adverse outcomes, including increased mortality, institutionalization, and dementia (Davis et al., 2013). The best patient outcomes are associated with the prevention of delirium; however, early detection and management may mitigate the consequences of the condition. It is believed that at least 1 of 10 hospitalized patients will experience delirium in the hospital setting, but the likelihood increases significantly according to age and variables such as diagnosis and treatment. Older adults experience delirium at rates up to 6 times that of the general hospital population. The incidence of delirium in long-term care settings is believed to be comparable, although the condition is often unrecognized. The incidence of delirium in community health settings is more elusive and possibly underestimated because of a lack of reliable measurement methods (Kalish, Gillham, & Unwin, 2014; Davis et al., 2013; Rooney et al., 2014).

Pathophysiology and Etiology

Pathophysiology

The exact pathophysiology of delirium is unknown. It is theorized that the conditions that lead to delirium increase cerebral oxidative stress and impair neurotransmitter action through a variety of structural, inflammatory, metabolic, and neurochemical pathways. For example, psychologic and physiologic stress both activate the sympathetic nervous system, impairing cholinergic transmission. The net result of these changes is diminished cerebral function and alterations in arousal mechanisms of the reticular activating system (RAS) and thalamus (Huang, 2013).

Etiology

A wide variety of conditions can result in delirium, including infections, metabolic imbalances, trauma, nutritional deficiencies, central nervous system disease, hypoxia, hypothermia, hyperthermia, circulatory problems, low blood glucose, toxin exposure, sleep deprivation, and drug and alcohol use and withdrawal (Rosen et al., 2015).

Iatrogenic (treatment-related) factors may also precipitate delirium and include the use of interventions such as medication, surgery and anesthesia, and electroconvulsive therapy (ECT). Hospitalized patients are much more likely to experience delirium because of the presence of predisposing illnesses, exposure to multiple medical interventions that may contribute to cognitive changes, and being in an environment that is unfamiliar, stimulating, and not conducive to maintaining normal diurnal rhythms. *Transfer trauma* or *relocation syndrome* is a major cause of stress in individuals of all ages and accounts, and a contributing factor to the high incidence of delirium in hospitalized patients. It should be noted that delirium occurs in 10–30% of the general hospital population, 15–50% of postoperative patients, and 70–80% of patients in the intensive care unit. Among hospitalized individuals over age 65, approximately 15–60% experience delirium, as do 20–90% of older patients with documented dementia (Fleet & Ernst, 2013; Solomon, Thilakan, & Jayakar, 2016).

Risk Factors

Although anyone can develop delirium, certain traits increase the likelihood of this condition. Age is a major risk factor. Older adults are at higher risk due to normal age-related cognitive decline. Age-related vision and hearing loss can contribute to delirium by impairing individuals' ability to accurately and effectively interpret their surroundings. Older patients are also more likely to experience many of the underlying physical causes of delirium, such as central nervous system and circulatory disease. Children are more prone to delirium than are adolescents and younger adults. Again, physiology is a primary factor, as children's bodies are less equipped to cope with insults such as fever, infection, and toxin exposure.

Other factors that can contribute to delirium include the presence of a chronic illness, onset of a new illness, or exacerbation of a current condition. The use of drugs, alcohol, or prescription medications such as hypnotics/sedatives, anxiolytics, antidepressants, anti-Parkinson drugs, anticonvulsants, or antispasmodics also increase the risk of delirium (Alagiakrishnan, 2015; Huang, 2013). Individuals with depression and other emotional disorders are at increased susceptibility as well, especially when faced with the added strain of illness, loss, or a change in environment such as hospitalization.

Prevention

Prevention focuses on reducing the incidence or presence of physiologic and psychosocial factors that lead to delirium, early detection of delirium, and a holistic approach to managing delirium in affected individuals. For individuals with predisposing conditions, proper medical management can reduce the likelihood of delirium. Standardized protocols should be implemented in healthcare settings to address the prevention, detection, and management of delirium (Tullman, Fletcher, & Foreman, 2012b).

Clinical Manifestations

Typical manifestations of delirium include reduced awareness, impaired thinking skills, and/or changes in activity level and behavior. See **Table 23–10 »** for an overview of common signs and symptoms from each of these categories. The intensity of manifestations varies, with some patients having only subtle symptoms and others experiencing acute loss of most or all cognitive function. Note that diagnostic markers of delirium may vary somewhat depending on the patient's cultural background (see Focus on Diversity and Culture: Delirium).

TABLE 23–10 Manifestations of Delirium

Category	Common Signs and Symptoms
Reduced awareness	■ Difficulty shifting attention from one topic to another ■ Limited or absent span of attention ■ High distractibility ■ Difficulty keeping track of what has been said ■ Inability to answer questions or engage in conversation ■ Little activity or response to the environment
Impaired thinking skills	■ Impaired memory (especially recent memory) ■ Disorganized thought ■ Disorientation to place, time, date, and/or person ■ Rambling, incoherent, illogical, or absent speech ■ Poor word-finding ability ■ Difficulty reading, writing, or understanding speech ■ Hallucinations and/or illusions
Changes in behavior	■ Agitation, irritability, restlessness, or combative behavior ■ Altered sleep patterns ■ Mood swings and extreme emotions ■ Fear, anxiety, and/or depression ■ Withdrawal

Sources: Data from Mayo Clinic. (2012). *Delirium.* Retrieved from http://www.mayoclinic.org/diseases-conditions/delirium/basics/definition/con-20033982; Tullman, D. F., Fletcher, K., & Foreman, M. D. (2012). Delirium: Prevention, early recognition, and treatment. In M. Boltz, E. Capezuti, T. T. Fulmer, D. Zwicker, & A. O'Meara (Eds.), *Evidence-based geriatric nursing protocols for best practice* (4th ed.). New York, NY: Springer; Osborn, K. S., Wraa, C. E., Watson, A., & Holleran, R. S. (2013). *Medical-surgical nursing: Preparation for practice* (2nd ed.). Upper Saddle River, NJ: Pearson.

Focus on Diversity and Culture
Delirium

Culture may also affect the diagnostic process. When working with patients from Hispanic, Asian, African American, and other cultural groups, the nurse must remember that these cultures may promote different conceptions of time, place, and person in comparison to Caucasian-American culture (Spector, 2017). Therefore, what the nurse might perceive as a lack of orientation to time might be perfectly normal, acceptable behavior to a patient and his family. Cultural beliefs may also impact the interpretation of manifestations such as hallucinations and incoherent speech. Patients and their families may view these experiences as spiritual or religious events rather than signs of illness (Spector, 2017). In such cases, the nurse must be careful not to discount or disparage the patient's cultural preferences and beliefs. Promotion of trust and acceptance is necessary for building an effective nurse–patient relationship.

Delirium is marked by vacillating symptoms. An individual may be largely unresponsive at one point in the day but hypervigilant just a few hours later, with a period of normal behavior in between. In addition, the individual's psychomotor activity may be hyperactive, hypoactive, or a mixture of both at various times throughout the day. Confusion that intensifies in the evening or at bedtime is referred to as **sundowning**. Sundowning is not a disorder in and of itself; rather, it is a feature of dementia that affects some individuals.

Clinical Manifestations and Therapies
Delirium

ETIOLOGY	CLINICAL MANIFESTATIONS	CLINICAL THERAPIES
Variable etiologies; may include the following: ■ Hospitalization or transfer to a new environment ■ Infection ■ Metabolic imbalance ■ Trauma ■ Nutritional deficiency ■ Central nervous system disease ■ Hypoxia ■ Hypothermia ■ Hyperthermia ■ Acute circulatory alteration ■ Hypoglycemia (decreased serum glucose) ■ Toxin exposure ■ Sleep deprivation ■ Drug and alcohol use or withdrawal	■ Reduced awareness, as evidenced by: ● Limited span of attention ● Difficulty focusing or logically shifting from one topic to another ● Inability to answer questions or engage in conversation ● Limited response to the environment ■ Impaired thinking skills, as evidenced by: ● Impaired memory ● Disorganized thought ● Disorientation to place, time, date, and/or person ● Impaired speaking, reading, and comprehension ability ■ Behavioral changes, such as: ● Hyperactivity, hypoactivity, or a combination thereof ● Hallucinations ● Agitation and/or restlessness ● Fear, anxiety, and/or depression ● Altered sleep patterns ● Mood swings ● Withdrawal ■ Acute onset and fluctuation of symptoms ■ Appearance of symptoms at specific times of day (e.g., sundowning)	■ Physical interventions aimed at correcting biological causes of delirium: ● Supplemental oxygen ● IV fluids and/or electrolytes ● Supplemental nutrition ■ Environmental interventions: ● Preventing under- or overstimulation ● Instituting safety measures ● Promoting consistency ■ Cognitive interventions: ● Orienting patient to place, time, date, and/or person ● Providing reassurance that delirium is temporary ■ Pharmacologic therapies aimed at the underlying cause of delirium (as appropriate) ■ Surgical treatment of the underlying cause of delirium (as appropriate)

Collaboration

Nurses must be familiar with a range of collaborative interventions related to delirium. These include diagnostic tests, medications, and nonpharmacologic therapies. Psychosocial considerations are directed toward both patients and their family members.

Diagnostic Tests

Medical professionals use any number of diagnostic procedures to determine the underlying source of a patient's delirium. The first steps usually include conducting a physical exam and obtaining a detailed medical history. Cognitive testing, such as the CAM test (described later in this exemplar), can also be useful for determining whether a patient is experiencing reversible confusion or another form of impairment.

Based on assessment data, the primary care provider will choose appropriate diagnostic procedures. Examples of tests that may be appropriate for identifying underlying causes of confusion include a detailed neurologic examination; drug and alcohol screening; laboratory tests for signs of infection and metabolic, nutritional, and other imbalances; and screening for depression and other psychiatric conditions.

Pharmacologic Therapy

No one drug or class of drugs is appropriate for all patients with delirium, but some medications may effectively treat the causative condition. For example, antipsychotics may be appropriate for patients with delirium related to an underlying psychotic disorder, and SSRIs and other antidepressants can help minimize delirium in some individuals with mood disorders. In other cases, discontinuation of medications may be the best course of action, especially for individuals who are experiencing drug-related delirium.

Nonpharmacologic Therapy and Integrative Care

Numerous nonpharmacologic interventions may benefit individuals with delirium, depending on their pathology. These interventions fall into three categories: physical, environmental, and cognitive.

- *Physical interventions* target anatomic or biological factors that may be contributing to delirium. Common physical interventions that promote enhanced cognition include oxygen administration, IV delivery of fluids and/or electrolytes, and provision of appropriate nutrition.
- *Environmental interventions* involve enhancing patients' level of comfort within their surroundings, as this helps minimize the likelihood of confusion. Often, these interventions focus on preventing under- or overstimulation, maintaining safety, and promoting consistency. (See the Nursing Process section.)
- *Cognitive interventions* involve orienting patients to person, place, and time, as well as providing reassurance that they are safe and that their delirium will be resolved. Validation therapy may also be an effective way of meeting patient needs (see exemplar on Alzheimer disease and the Nursing Process section below.)

There is some evidence to suggest that sensory interventions such as music therapy may assist in orienting patients experiencing delirium and/or reducing associated anxiety (Dzierba et al., 2015; American Geriatrics Society Expert Panel on Postoperative Delirium in Older Adults, 2015; Zhang et al., 2013). Given the complex nature of delirium and the ranges of patient variables impacting it, collaboration with a qualified music therapist is likely to result in the best outcomes. In addition, a recent meta-analysis of randomized controlled studies suggests that the use of exogenous melatonin may have a preventative effect on delirium (Chen et al., 2016).

SAFETY ALERT Older adults and individuals with dementia or other cognitive disorders and mental illnesses are at increased risk for a misdiagnosis related to the perception that changes in mental status are related to age or a psychiatric condition. In addition, it is easy to confuse diurnal changes in cognition (such as sundowning) with delirium caused by an underlying medical condition. Nurses should never assume that cognitive changes are related to age, mental health issues, or the time of day. A thorough assessment is essential to rule out underlying medical causes of any changes in mental status.

Lifespan Considerations

Although individuals of all ages are susceptible to delirium under certain conditions, risk factors and common etiologies of the condition are associated with different stages of the lifespan. Manifestations of delirium may also vary with different age groups.

Delirium in Children

Like older adults, children lack the functional reserves necessary to cope with both environmental and physiologic stressors and are at increased risk for delirium. In general, children with intellectual and developmental disabilities are at increased risk for delirium. The prevalence of delirium in hospitalized children ranges from 10 to 30% and is more common in younger and critically ill children or those emerging from anesthesia. Any febrile illness may cause symptoms of delirium, even in children being cared for at home. Manifestations of delirium may be confused with willful or oppositional behavior or be extremely frightening for parents. The Cornell Assessment of Pediatric Delirium can be used to detect delirium in children. Besides the prevention and management of the underlying medical condition, the presence of parents and family members has been found to reduce the incidence of delirium. Overall, the prognosis for children with delirium is better than that for older individuals (Schieveld et al., 2015).

Delirium in Adolescents

By adolescence, the ability to compensate for physiologic alterations that may precipitate delirium has improved; however, some of the common causes of delirium in adolescents are different. Adolescents may be at increased risk for head trauma as a result of participation in contact sports or a tendency toward impulsive, risk-taking behaviors. Drug and substance abuse and withdrawal are another common cause of delirium in this age group.

Delirium in Pregnant and Postpartum Women

Delirium during pregnancy or in the postpartum period is a serious sign and may indicate the presence of a life-threatening condition such as preeclampsia and HELLP syndrome, sepsis, hypo- or hyperglycemia, or fluid and electrolyte imbalance (possibly as a result of hyperemesis gravidarum). Delirium may also be associated with the stress of labor or the use of anesthetic agents. Symptoms of delirium may be difficult to distinguish from postpartum psychosis. Priority care focuses on the patient and determining the underlying cause. This includes monitoring fetal well-being as well as ensuring the safety of the newborn.

Delirium in Older Adults

In older patients, delirium may be confused with normal forgetfulness or dementia, especially when presenting in healthcare settings where staff are unfamiliar with the patient's history and prior cognitive status. Individuals with dementia are at increased risk of acute mental status changes associated with delirium, and therefore any change from baseline should be considered significant (Cole et al., 2015). Delirium is often the most prominent manifestation of conditions such as dehydration, respiratory tract infections, urinary tract infections, and urinary retention, and adverse drug events may occur in the absence of symptoms such as fever or discomfort. The possibility of intracranial events (stroke, bleeding) and acute pulmonary and myocardial events should also be considered. Prompt recognition and management of delirium is essential because the risk of long-term disability and death also increases exponentially in older adults (Ahmed, Leurent, & Sampson, 2014; Fick et al., 2013).

NURSING PROCESS

One of the nurse's primary duties in caring for a patient with delirium is to promote resolution of whatever condition is causing the patient's cognitive impairment. The nurse must also take steps to keep the patient safe, support cognitive functioning and comfort, and minimize the likelihood of further episodes of confusion. When assessing an individual's cognitive skills and orientation the nurse accounts for variables such as age and development, level of education, and culture.

Assessment

Nursing assessment for the patient with delirium typically involves three main elements: a health history, a physical examination, and a mental status examination.

Observation and Patient Interview

Observe the patient for behavioral manifestation of delirium, including extreme distractibility, disorganized thinking, rambling, irrelevant and incoherent speech, and purposeless motor activity. Fluctuations in psychomotor activity may also be observed with periods of restlessness and agitation to stupor, catatonia, and somnolence. Mood instability may be manifested by episodes of alternating distress or euphoria. The patient may also appear flushed and diaphoretic.

The history is critical to identifying potential causes of the patient's confusion and highlighting areas that require further assessment. Because the patient may not be able to provide a reliable history, a family member or caregiver may need to be interviewed. For the patient with delirium, basic components of the health history include the following:

- Age
- History of other disease processes
- Recent history of infection and/or fever
- Vision and/or hearing impairments
- Alcohol and drug use (including medications)
- Possible toxin exposure (e.g., in the workplace)
- Dietary patterns
- Untreated or undertreated pain
- History of depression or other mood disorders
- Recent life changes that may be contributing to cognitive and/or emotional upset

Physical Examination

During the physical examination, evaluate the patient's height, weight, vital signs, and overall condition. In addition to a focused assessment of perfusion, oxygenation, intracranial regulation, infection, and inflammation, assess for physical findings associated with any concerns brought up during the health history. For example, for a patient who reports that he is hard of hearing, attempt to determine the degree of impairment and explore the possibility that this impairment may be contributing to the patient's confusion.

To differentiate between delirium and dementia, the **Confusion Assessment Method (CAM)** may be used. The nurse should also screen the patient for depression, because this condition is often linked to confusion in older adults. For discussion of testing instruments designed for this purpose, refer to the Nursing Assessment section in this module.

>> **Stay Current:** A current version of the CAM can be accessed online at https://consultgeri.org/try-this/general-assessment/issue-13

Because delirium has a fluctuating course, ongoing assessment is important. The nurse should reassess patients with delirium frequently. Some patients may require one-on-one monitoring.

Diagnosis

Appropriate nursing diagnoses for patients with delirium vary, depending on the cause and severity of their condition. Still, some diagnoses are likely to apply to many, if not most, patients with acute confusion. These include:

- *Injury, Risk for*
- *Self-Care Deficit (Bathing, Dressing, Feeding, and/or Toileting)*
- *Disturbed Sleep Pattern*
- *Acute Confusion*
- *Verbal Communication, Impaired*
- *Social Interaction, Impaired*
- *Compromised Human Dignity, Risk for*

(NANDA-I © 2014)

Planning

The planning portion of the nursing process involves identifying desired outcomes and choosing evidence-based interventions that facilitate their achievement. Again, goals and interventions will vary depending on the cause and severity of a patient's delirium. Appropriate outcomes may include the following:

- Patient will remain free from injury.
- Patient will be oriented to time, place, date, and person.
- Patient will return to baseline cognitive status (i.e., status prior to onset of confusion).
- Patient will demonstrate the ability to communicate in a clear and logical manner.
- Patient will obtain adequate sleep and rest.
- Patient will exhibit reduced anxiety, agitation, and restlessness.
- Patient will be able to perform ADLs.

Implementation

Provide a Safe Environment for the Hospitalized Patient

Typically, nursing interventions for the patient with confusion revolve around providing of a safe, therapeutic environment that prevents further cognitive impairment and promotes resolution of the condition causing the patient's delirium. The following measures may be useful for most patients:

- Maintaining appropriate levels of noise and lighting in an attempt to prevent under- or overstimulation
- Preventing access to potential hazards (e.g., knives, guns, medications, lighters, and chemicals)
- Using behavioral interventions and monitoring systems to address wandering
- Promoting consistency by assigning the same caregivers and scheduling activities at the same time each day
- Providing an environment that supports normal sleep–wake cycles
- Ensuring access to assistive devices, including glasses and hearing aids
- Providing adequate pain management
- Keeping familiar items in the patient's environment without allowing the environment to become disorganized or cluttered
- Using calendars, clocks, and signs to help orient the patient to time, date, and place
- Encouraging loved ones to visit the patient

The nurse can also employ various communication strategies to limit confusion. The nurse should always wear a name tag and introduce himself during patient interactions. The nurse should then verbally orient the patient to date, time, and place. When talking with the patient, the nurse should speak clearly and allow time for response. All explanations of treatments or procedures should be brief and as easy to understand as possible. The nurse should reinforce reality by helping patients interpret confusing or unfamiliar stimuli. Any misconceptions of events or situations should be gently corrected. The nurse should also reassure patients that their delirium is temporary.

≫ Stay Current: The Hospital Elder Life Program (HELP) is a comprehensive, evidence-based patient-care program that provides optimal care for older persons in the hospital and has extensive resources for healthcare professionals on the prevention, identification and management of delirium in hospitalized patients. For more information visit: http://www.hospitalelderlifeprogram.org/for-clinicians/about-delirium/

SAFETY ALERT Challenging a patient who is delusional or misinterpreting reality has the potential to make a patient anxious and lead to agitation or aggressive behavior. Using validation techniques, the nurse can often determine the underlying need without unnecessarily upsetting the patient. Validating data are explained in detail in the module on Assessment.

Promote Safety in the Home

Teaching is especially important when patients have an ongoing health issue that predisposes them to delirium. For example, if patients are taking medications that increase their risk of cognitive changes, they and their loved ones should be informed of common symptoms of delirium and what to do when these symptoms arise. Similarly, patients with diabetes should be taught about signs of confusion related to abnormal blood glucose. In addition, family members and caregivers should be assisted with developing an action plan for assisting the patient during hyperglycemic or hypoglycemic episodes.

Evaluation

Ongoing evaluation is critical for all patients with delirium, as it allows nurses to monitor their condition and adjust the nursing plan of care as needed. Some examples of potential achieved outcomes include the following:

- Patient sustains no injuries.
- Patient is oriented to time, place, date, and person.
- Patient demonstrates an absence of manifestations of delirium.
- Patient communicates clearly and transitions logically between topics.
- Patient is able to perform ADLs.

Individuals with delirium may demonstrate permanent changes in neurocognitive function, especially when conditions such as dementia were already present. Family members and caregivers may be more aware of subtle differences indicating that the patient has not returned to her previous level of function. Even when cognitive status has improved, the nurse recognizes that individuals who have experienced delirium are at increased risk for future episodes. The resolution of delirium may allow the nurse to modify the plan of care and provide teaching that emphasizes the prevention, detection, and treatment of precipitating health issues.

REVIEW Delirium

RELATE Link the Concepts and Exemplars

Linking the exemplar of confusion with the concept of infection:

1. How might delirium increase the patient's risk for infection?

2. Why are patients with infection at a heightened risk for delirium? What types of infections do you think would most increase a patient's likelihood of delirium?

Linking the exemplar of confusion with the concept of stress and coping:

3. Why are patients more likely to experience delirium during periods of increased stress? What sorts of events are likely to be most stressful and thus result in confusion?

4. For the patient experiencing delirium, what nursing interventions could be implemented to help reduce stress and promote effective coping?

Linking the exemplar of delirium with the concept of safety:

5. How might caring for patients with delirium put a nurse's safety in jeopardy?

6. What interventions could a nurse implement to protect her own safety when caring for a patient with delirium? What legal or ethical issues are associated with these measures?

READY Go to Volume 3: Clinical Nursing Skills

REFER Go to Pearson MyLab Nursing and eText

- Additional review material

REFLECT Apply Your Knowledge

Clifford Allen is a 64-year-old man who has been married to his wife, Pam, for 40 years. Their only child, 24-year-old Gary, has Down syndrome and lives with them. Mr. Allen is a middle manager for a small manufacturing company where he has worked for the past 20 years.

Overall, Mr. Allen is in good health, although he has recently been undergoing conservative treatment for benign prostatic hyperplasia. He has a history of depression, including a brief episode during college for which he did not seek treatment. Mr. Allen had another episode shortly after his son was born, and at the encouragement of his wife, he sought treatment, which consisted of counseling and antidepressant medications. He quit taking the medications after 6 months and decided he would just learn to deal with depression on his own. Although he has had several mild episodes of depression since that

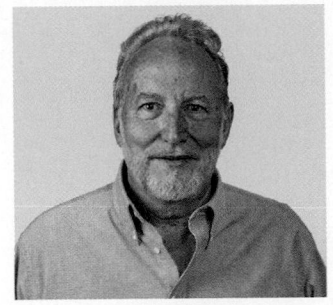 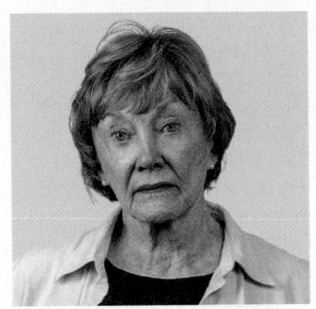

time, Mr. Allen has been unwilling to seek treatment because he fears the social stigma of being labeled medically depressed and is concerned that his employer will discover it through his use of his medical benefits. It is Mr. Allen's opinion that his employer would perceive depression as a sign of weakness. Overall, Mr. Allen has done well without the medications.

Mr. Allen has been thinking about retiring in the next few years. He and his wife have always planned to do some traveling, but mostly he looks forward to escaping his busy, stressful work environment. Mr. Allen and his son are involved in church activities; they also enjoy a walk each evening after supper. Mr. Allen belongs to a bowling league and is at the bowling alley a couple of evenings a week.

Mr. Allen is admitted to the acute care hospital for a transurethral resection of the prostate (TURP). He has been very anxious about the procedure because of the risk of impotence. The surgery goes smoothly, and he experiences no complications. In the immediate postoperative period, Mr. Allen has a three-way Foley catheter inserted, with continuous bladder irrigation. He experiences pain and occasional bladder spasms because of blood clots. The day after surgery, the nurse enters Mr. Allen's room, and he asks why the hospital bed was brought to his room and calls the nurse by his wife's name. He appears restless and agitated. The nurse assesses Mr. Allen and determines that he is experiencing delirium.

1. What factors may increase the risk of delirium in this patient?

2. What interventions would the nurse initiate for Mr. Allen?

3. What nursing diagnosis would be appropriate for Mr. Allen?

4. What assessment tools would the nurse use to assess Mr. Allen?

» Exemplar 23.C
Schizophrenia

Exemplar Learning Objectives

23.C Analyze schizophrenia as it relates to cognition.

- Describe the pathophysiology of schizophrenia.
- Describe the etiology of schizophrenia.
- Compare the risk factors and prevention of schizophrenia.
- Identify the clinical manifestations of schizophrenia.
- Summarize diagnostic tests and therapies used by interprofessional teams in the collaborative care of an individual with schizophrenia.

- Differentiate care of patients with schizophrenia across the lifespan.
- Apply the nursing process in providing culturally competent care to an individual with schizophrenia.

Exemplar Key Terms

Akathisia, *1753*
Alogia, *1749*
Anhedonia, *1749*
Assertive community treatment (ACT), *1754*

Overview

Schizophrenia is a profound neurobiological disorder that is characterized by psychotic symptoms, diminished capacity to relate to others, and behaviors that are appear odd or bizarre. Approximately 1% of persons living in the United States experience schizophrenia (National Institute of Mental Health, 2016). Although many people associate the disorder with perceptual alterations such as hallucinations, the most chronic and disabling aspects of the disease relate to functional deficits caused by alterations in communication, cognition, attention, memory, emotional regulation, initiative, and social interactions. (These manifestations are frequently classified as positive, negative, and cognitive symptoms and are discussed in more detail in the section on clinical manifestations.) Schizophrenia typically emerges during early adulthood, but it can also occur during childhood and adolescence or first manifest later in life. Schizophrenia is also associated with a 10- to 25-year reduction in life expectancy as a result of comorbid medical conditions and high rates of suicide (Laursen, Munk-Olsen, & Vestergaard, 2012). Historically, schizophrenia has been poorly understood, and the stigma associated with the disorder is perhaps one of the greatest challenges for individuals impacted by the disease (Gerlinger et al., 2013).

Even though schizophrenia is a single diagnosis, it is one of several disorders included in the DSM-5 within the category of "schizophrenia spectrum and other psychotic disorders" (APA, 2013). Manifestations of schizophrenia range in severity, and this disorder has symptoms and etiologies that overlap with other **psychotic disorders**.

Pathophysiology and Etiology
Pathophysiology

Currently the known pathologic mechanisms associated with schizophrenia include anatomic alterations, neurotransmitter abnormalities, and impairments in immune function. The relationship between these mechanisms is complex, and it is not always clear which alterations are a cause of or a consequence of the disease.

Structural Anatomic Alterations
Brain imaging studies of individuals with schizophrenia consistently reveal a pattern of structural abnormalities that include decreased volumes of gray matter in the prefrontal cortex, temporal lobes, hippocampus, and thalamus; enlarged ventricles and sulci; and decreased blood flow to the frontal lobe, thalamus, and temporal lobes (see **Table 23–11 》**). PET scan studies of individuals with schizophrenia reveal alterations in cerebral blood flow and glucose metabolism (Hayempour et al., 2013). Although brain abnormalities are present prior to the onset of symptoms, they are difficult to detect and become more pronounced with the first and subsequent episodes of psychotic symptoms.

Neurotransmitter Abnormalities

Abnormalities in neurotransmitter function contribute to the manifestations of schizophrenia. Alterations in the dopaminergic system have been implicated, in part because antipsychotic medications block the D_2 receptors norepinephrine and serotonin, and because GABA and acetylcholine neurotransmitter systems are also believed to be involved. Nicotinic acetylcholine receptors (nAChR) appear to be diminished in the hippocampus of individuals with schizophrenia, resulting in disturbances in inhibitory gateways. It has been proposed that nicotine stimulates these receptors, providing temporary relief of symptoms of schizophrenia (Mackowick et al., 2014). Research also implicates dysregulation in the NMDA subclass of glutamate receptors in the disease (Frankenburg, 2015; Hu et al., 2015; Moghaddam & Javitt, 2012). Glutamate is required for the degradation of dopamine and several other neurotransmitters that influence prefrontal information processing. Glutamate receptors also play an important role in migration of neurons during brain development. Individuals with schizophrenia have been shown to have abnormally low levels of glutamate in the CSF.

Immunologic and Inflammatory Pathways

Multiple studies support the involvement of inflammatory/immune pathways with an association with chronic oxidative stress (Okusaga, 2014). Microglia normally serve as a first line of defense against pathogenic invasion in the central nervous system. They are also involved in other essential brain functions, including the pruning and maintenance of synapses and the consumption of fragments of damaged cells. When activated, microglia produce inflammatory cytokines, resulting in a cascade of events that alter brain function. One consequence appears to be an interruption of

TABLE 23–11 Typical CNS Abnormalities Observed in Individuals with Schizophrenia

	Increased Size	Decreased Volume	Decreased Blood Flow	Decreased Blood Glucose	Decreased O$_2$ Use	Decreased Activity	Decreased Nicotinic Receptors
Ventricles	X						
Sulci	X						
Temporal lobes		X	X				
Hippocampus		X					X
Prefrontal cortex		X				X	
Thalamus		X					
Basal ganglia			X	X	X		
Frontal lobes			X	X	X		

metabolic processes responsible for NMDA receptor activity and dopamine regulation (Frankenburg, 2015; Martínez-Gras et al., 2012). It is known that individuals with schizophrenia have increased levels of cytokines, especially during periods of acute psychosis or relapse (Kirkpatrick & Miller, 2013). It is believed that additional insults such as illness and stress overwhelm an already compromised neuroimmune system, resulting in an exacerbation of cognitive dysfunction (Fineberg & Ellman, 2013; Horváth & Mirnics, 2014; van Venrooij et al., 2012).

Etiology

The exact causes of schizophrenia are not understood. The preponderance of evidence seems to suggest that some individuals have a polygenic predisposition and that a combination of factors, such as prenatal health issues and environmental factors, lead to manifestations of the disorder (Walder et al., 2014). Recent research also highlights an overlap in the genetic influences of schizophrenia and other neurodevelopmental disorders such as autism (De Lacy & King, 2013; Hommer & Swedo, 2015). The myelination of and reorganization of neuronal structures that typically occurs during adolescence seems to have an activating effect, possibly because the process depends on microglia that may have undergone pathologic changes earlier in development (Ahmed, Buckley, & Hanna, 2013; Catts et al., 2013; Fineberg & Ellman, 2013; Rapoport, Giedd, & Gogtay, 2012).

Previously, it was theorized that specific patterns of interaction in families played a key role in the development of schizophrenia. These **communication deviance** theories postulated that patterns of disorganized communication arose from repeated exposure to contradictory and conflicted messages. It is now believed that, in susceptible individuals, exposure to any overwhelming adversity stimulates a human stress of the hypothalamic–pituitary–adrenal (HPA) axis. This results in suppression of immune dysfunction and ultimately further decompensation of neuronal networks (Akdeniz, Tost, & Meyer-Lindenberg, 2014). It is important to remember that alterations in communication in family members of the individual with schizophrenia or any other psychiatric illness may be the result of the *bidirectional* nature of such conditions. That is, while family members may have a negative impact of the emotional health of the individual, the stress of coping with a family member

with a major mental illness can also lead to a breakdown in family interactions.

SAFETY ALERT Among individuals diagnosed with schizophrenia, an estimated 20 to 40% attempt suicide. Factors associated with this risk include (but are not limited to) greater awareness of the illness, younger age, recent loss, limited support, recent discharge, and treatment failure. Regardless of the treatment phase or the presence of additional risk factors, all individuals with schizophrenia should be closely monitored for suicide.

Risk Factors

Schizophrenia is a multifactorial disease influenced by a confluence of genetic, epigenetic, environmental, and developmental factors. One of the challenges of the disorder is that many of the associated risk factors lack the specificity or strength to guide preventative health measures.

Genetic Factors

Genetic factors significantly impact susceptibility and the risk for schizophrenia. Whereas members of the general population have a 1% risk of schizophrenia, individuals with an affected third-degree relative, such as a cousin, have a risk of 2%, and individuals with an affected second-degree relative (such as an aunt, uncle, half-sibling, or grandparent) have a risk of 2–6%. An individual who has a first-degree relative with schizophrenia (such as a parent or sibling) has a risk of schizophrenia of almost 50% (Light et al., 2014; Ripke et al., 2014). However, no single gene or set of genes has been implicated as a marker for the disorder, and approximately 60% of all individuals with schizophrenia have no known family history of the disease. The risk of schizophrenia increases incrementally with advancing paternal age as a result of cumulative mutations in sperm. Children born to fathers 60 years old and older have an almost twofold risk of developing the disorder (Ek et al., 2015; Frans, MacCabe, & Reichenberg, 2015; Hui et al., 2015; Jaffe et al., 2014; Smith, R., et al., 2013).

Epigenetic Factors

Most researchers now agree that external modifications to genes (**epigenetic** factors) must occur in order for schizophrenia to manifest. Many studies have focused on the impact of external events such as birth complications, in utero viral exposure, poor prenatal care, and marijuana use on gene expression in schizophrenia (Giovanoli et al., 2013; Kirkbride et al., 2012; Kundakovic, 2014; Sutterland et al., 2013). Recent research has implicated *Toxoplasma gondii* infection (toxoplasmosis) during pregnancy and early childhood in the development of the disease. *T. gondii* is spread via contact with cat feces, and it is recommended that pregnant women and children do not handle cat litter and that litter boxes be changed daily (Flegr, 2015; Torrey, Simmons, & Yolken, 2015).

Psychosocial Factors

Psychosocial factors such as early life adversity (including exposure to chronic and acute stressors such as poverty, violence, and trauma) have also been implicated in schizophrenia. Psychosocial risk factors are increased in instances where disparities in healthcare exist, such as with recent immigrant populations. Biochemical mechanisms involved in the stress response may have an epigenetic influence or exacerbate preexisting neuronal pathology (Kirkbride et al., 2012).

Developmental Factors

There is evidence to suggest that children and adolescents who display certain alterations in emotional, cognitive, language, and motor development are at an increased risk for developing schizophrenia. These findings may relate to manifestations of neurodevelopmental problems that precede the prodromal and active phases of the illness (Laurens et al., 2015). Stress that occurs during certain developmental periods such as early childhood or adolescence may confer a greater risk of developing the disorder.

Prevention

Primary prevention of schizophrenia includes comprehensive healthcare during pregnancy and childhood, and measures to reduce or eliminate adversity and environmental insults (e.g., poverty, abuse, trauma, injury, or exposure to environmental toxins). Secondary prevention of schizophrenia focuses on high-risk groups such as individuals who have a family history of the disorder or who demonstrate behaviors associated with progression to **psychosis**, acute periods of disordered thinking that affects the individual's perception of reality. Interventions include augmenting protective factors for the disease (e.g., teaching social skills or improving family interactions) and treating comorbid psychiatric conditions (Tandon et al., 2012). Research demonstrates that early screening and detection of cognitive, developmental, and behavioral alterations associated with schizophrenia and other mental illnesses may result in better outcomes for individuals, especially when nonpharmacologic interventions such as cognitive–behavioral therapy (CBT) are employed (Stafford et al., 2013; Tandon et al., 2012; Valmaggia et al., 2015). Some aspects of secondary prevention of schizophrenia present ethical challenges, such as the practice of initiating antipsychotic treatment when prodromal symptoms are apparent. The risks associated with labeling and treating individuals who may or may not go on to develop the disorder need to be considered (Appelbaum, 2015).

Tertiary prevention focuses on reducing the impact of the disease in individuals diagnosed with schizophrenia. A diagnosis of schizophrenia is devastating to both patients

and families. Holistic care aims to help patients to manage the disorder in the community, to provide support for family members and caregivers, and to prevent or manage comorbidities commonly associated with the disorder. Two critical components of health promotion for schizophrenia are an emphasis on **recovery** and **rehabilitation**. In the recovery phase, the symptoms of the disorder are present but under control. The emphasis for healthcare is on learning strategies to maintain health, such as adhering to treatment, reducing stress, and using effective coping strategies. The goal is the prevention of **relapse** (or a return to the acute phase of the illness). *Rehabilitation* refers to a level wellness in which symptoms of the condition are under control to the extent that the affected individual can engage in goal-directed activities (e.g., maintaining a job, carrying out self-care) (Potter & Moller, 2016).

Clinical Manifestations

The clinical manifestations of schizophrenia may be classified according to the stage of illness as well as the types of symptoms that are observed. Presenting symptoms may vary from person to person, with periods of exacerbation and remission. The trajectory of the illness must be recognized and understood in order to address the unique needs of individuals with the disorder. Many, but not all, individuals with schizophrenia experience sufficiently severe clinical manifestations that they have difficulty engaging in ADLs and functioning independently. These patients may benefit from in-home services, day treatment programs, group homes or residential care, or psychiatric rehabilitation through community services.

Symptom Types

The symptoms of schizophrenia are generally divided into positive, negative, and cognitive types, as depicted in **Figure 23–7 »**. There is some overlap in the classification of symptoms, and the presence of these manifestations does not necessarily indicate that an individual has schizophrenia. Affective symptoms are normally not included in these classifications but are common in schizophrenia and are also discussed in this section. The manifestation of symptoms varies according the phase of the illness.

Positive Symptoms

Positive symptoms are characterized by the psychotic features of the disorder that generally do not occur in healthy people and are outside of the range of normal experiences. Hallucinations, delusions, abnormal movements, and problems with speech or disordered thinking are all classified as positive symptoms.

Hallucinations are abnormal perceptual experiences that usually occur in the absence of external stimuli. Types of hallucinations are discussed in more detail in the Alterations section of this module. In individuals with schizophrenia, auditory hallucinations are generally most prevalent and often have threatening or accusatory content (Docherty et al., 2015).

Delusions are false beliefs that are based on faulty perceptions and inferences. The most common delusions seen in patients with schizophrenia are those of *reference*, which incorporate the belief that certain events occur for the benefit

✚ Positive Symptoms	━ Negative Symptoms	🧠 Cognitive Symptoms
Additions to normal experiences: • Delusions • Hallucinations • Abnormal movements • Formal thought disorder	Diminished affects and behaviors: • Flat or blunted affect • Thought blocking • Avolition • Poverty of speech • Social withdrawal	Cognitive issues may include: • Memory deficits • Attention deficits • Language difficulties • Loss of executive function

Source: Potter, M. L., & Moller, M. D. (2016). *Psychiatric–mental health nursing: From suffering to hope.* Reprinted and electronically reproduced by permission of Pearson Education, Inc., New York, NY.

Figure 23–7 》 The symptoms of schizophrenia have been categorized as positive, negative, and cognitive.

of the individual. Nihilistic delusions encompass beliefs that the individual is nonexistent or dead. Religious delusions involve the belief that the individual is a religious figure. Grandiose delusions involve beliefs that the individual has special power or significance. Persecutory delusions involve the belief that others wish to harm the individual. Delusions may take on bizarre or implausible features such as thought broadcasting (belief that others can hear thoughts), withdrawal (belief that others can remove thoughts), control (belief that others can control thoughts), and insertion (belief that others can insert thoughts into the person's mind).

Motor symptoms are common in individuals with schizophrenia and range from motor retardation or slowing to posturing and catatonic states. **Catatonia** is a state of unresponsiveness in an individual who is conscious. It may incorporate features such as *mutism* (lack of speech), *echopraxia* (repeating the movements of others), *echolalia* (repeating the words of others), *waxy flexibility* (maintaining whatever position the individual is placed in), and *automatic obedience* (automatic, robotic cooperation with requests). Catatonia can also manifest as an excited state that includes combativeness and impulsivity. Other motor symptoms may be the result of associated neurologic abnormalities and include oculomotor abnormalities, grimacing, and problems with motor sequencing and coordination (Damilou et al., 2016; Varambally, Venkatasubramanian, & Gangadhar, 2012).

Disorganized thinking is generally manifested in disruption of the form and organization of speech and is also referred to as a formal thought disorder (FTD). Individuals with an FTD lack appropriate, goal-directed thought processes and demonstrate a pattern of abnormal speech, including **loose associations**, tangentiality, incoherence, circumstantiality, and pressured speech. Table 23–1 provides definitions for these indicators of disorganized thinking.

Negative Symptoms

Negative symptoms refer to affects and behaviors that are diminished or absent in individuals with schizophrenia. These include having a flat or blunted affect, thought blocking (a sudden interruption in speech without explanation), **alogia** (poverty of thought and speech), **anhedonia** (inability to experience pleasure), **avolition** (lack of motivation or initiative), and social withdrawal. Negative symptoms tend to persist during all phases of the illness, are difficult to treat, and account for the some of the most disabling manifestations of the illness.

Cognitive Symptoms

Cognitive symptoms of schizophrenia include deficits in memory, attention, language, visual-spatial awareness, social and emotional perception, and intellectual and executive function. Memory deficits impact verbal processing, and individuals with schizophrenia may have difficulty with verbal fluency, pragmatics, and other aspects of spontaneous language. Visual memory deficits and impaired spatial processing also contribute to impaired social interactions. Individuals with schizophrenia often demonstrate poor facial recognition (facial agnosia) and may have difficulty with proxemics and nonverbal processing (e.g., modulating how close to stand to someone, interpreting nonverbal gestures). Individuals with schizophrenia demonstrate difficulty with attention and vigilance and may have difficulty concentrating on tasks that require a sustained focus. They are prone to sensory overload due to difficulty filtering out extraneous information. Studies have demonstrated an association between diminished global intellectual functioning and schizophrenia, with many affected individuals having difficulty with measures of both verbal and perceptual reasoning. Patients with schizophrenia frequently demonstrate **concrete thinking**, focusing on literal aspects of facts and details. They also typically exhibit limited insight due to deficits in theory of mind (Bora & Pantelis, 2013). Problems with executive functioning may manifest as difficulty with planning and organization, problem solving, and modulating impulses. Studies have shown that higher levels of cognitive impairment in individuals with schizophrenia are associated with poorer overall outcomes (Keefe & Harvey, 2012).

Affective Symptoms

In addition to positive, negative, and cognitive symptoms, patients with schizophrenia may also exhibit a number of affective symptoms, especially depression. Affective symptoms such as depression significantly increase the risk of suicide in patients with schizophrenia, especially in combination with other variables such as younger or older age, high IQ, higher levels of premorbid function, proximity to onset, male sex, and recent discharge from the hospital (Popovic et al., 2014).

Phases of the Illness

The classic course of schizophrenia consists of premorbid, prodromal, acute and residual phases. Research demonstrates that acute symptoms of the disorder appear to diminish as individuals grow older, with negative and cognitive symptoms becoming more pronounced and disabling. Some individuals may actually achieve complete remission of psychotic symptoms (Jeste & Maglione, 2013). Possible explanations for this include age-related dopaminergic activity changes.

Premorbid

Although 75% of patients with schizophrenia are diagnosed during adolescence or early adulthood, a number of alterations may be evident during childhood and the period immediately preceding the onset of the illness. *Premorbid* manifestations occurring in childhood include a number of nonspecific emotional, cognitive, and motor delays that have been identified in individuals who went on to develop schizophrenia (Stafford et al., 2013).

Prodromal Phase

The prodromal phase is a symptomatic period that signals a definite shift from premorbid functioning and continues until psychotic symptoms emerge. Manifestations include sleep disturbance, poor concentration, social withdrawal, perceptual abnormalities, and other attenuated or weakened symptoms of psychosis. A dramatic drop in functional or adaptive capabilities may occur with academic and vocational failure. The length of the prodromal period varies considerably, but for most individuals it lasts for 2 to 5 years (Fusar-Poli et al., 2014; Tandon et al., 2013).

Acute Phase

The acute phase of the illness is marked by the onset of florid psychotic/positive symptoms. It generally follows the prodromal period but in some instances appears suddenly. This period causes significant distress for the individual and is often the first time that help is sought. If the behavior represents a danger to the individual or others, short-term hospitalization may be required. The number of acute phases experienced by individuals is highly variable and depends, in part, on the ability to access high-quality treatment. In general, longer durations of untreated acute psychosis are associated with poorer long- and short-term patient outcomes (Chou et al., 2014).

Residual Phase

The **residual phase** of schizophrenia can be further broken down into the stabilization phase (6–18 months after the resolution of the acute phase) and the maintenance phase. The **stabilization phase** involves the immediate period of *recovery*, in which symptoms are under control but the individual is struggling to overcome exhaustion and cope with the impact of the illness. The **maintenance phase** corresponds with *rehabilitation* and a return to goal-directed activities and some level of functional status, such as holding down a job. It is important to remember that disabling cognitive and negative symptoms may persist during the residual phase. In addition, the patient may continue to demonstrate odd patterns of thinking and behavior. The level of dysfunction often increases with each subsequent episode of relapse. Patients often struggle with **side effects** of their medication and may lack the insight and or motivation required to adhere to treatment. Comprehensive treatment may reduce the risk of relapse, but it not always

possible to prevent it altogether. Careful monitoring of symptoms can often detect a shift toward the active state of the illness (Stahl et al., 2013).

Comorbid Disorders

Schizophrenia is associated with a number of psychiatric and medical comorbidities described in this section. The presence of these conditions adds to the overall burden of the illness and accounts for the significant reduction in lifespan for affected individuals. Contributing factors to comorbid illness include self-care deficits, sedentary lifestyles, social isolation, lack of access to quality healthcare, and poor dietary habits.

Individuals with schizophrenia are at increased risk for cardiovascular disease, diabetes, COPD, and many infectious diseases. Women with schizophrenia may have a higher incidence of medical problems and are more likely to experience more than one condition (Smith, D., et al., 2013). Approximately 80% of individuals with schizophrenia smoke cigarettes, possibly because of the short-term relief of symptoms associated with nicotine and its effect on nicotinic receptors (Brunzell & McIntosh, 2012). Some studies suggest that cardiovascular problems in patients with schizophrenia are frequently undertreated by healthcare providers (Crump et al., 2013; Smith, D., et al., 2013). Treatment with antipsychotic medications contributes to the overall risk of both cardiovascular disease and diabetes, as common effects include sedation, increased food intake, hyperlipidemia, and alterations in glucose regulation (Crump et al., 2013).

Comorbid substance abuse is found in almost 50% of all individuals with schizophrenia, a condition identified as **dual diagnosis**. Apart from caffeine and nicotine, the main substances of abuse used by individuals with schizophrenia are alcohol (20% over a lifetime), cannabis (lifetime prevalence 30%), and cocaine (lifetime prevalence 15–50%). As mentioned previously, the majority of individuals with schizophrenia smoke cigarettes and are far more likely to consume excess amounts of caffeine (>200 mg/day) than the general public (Thoma & Daum, 2013).

An estimated 25 to 60% of individuals with schizophrenia experience comorbid depression. Interestingly, multiple studies indicate that individuals with higher levels of premorbid function and greater awareness of the implications of their disorder are more likely to experience depression. Anxiety disorders also occur with greater frequency in schizophrenia, with approximately 10–15% of the population experiencing panic attacks and up to 20% having obsessive-compulsive disorder. Posttraumatic stress disorder may be seen in 12–19%. (Tsai & Rosenheck, 2013).

Collaboration

The management of schizophrenia is challenging for both patient and healthcare providers. A number of factors complicate treatment. These include characteristic clinical manifestations such as avolition and disordered thought processes and a fractured healthcare system. Although schizophrenia is a biological illness, many insurance policies continue to place restrictions on the types of services that can be accessed. State and federal funding for prevention and treatment of mental illness is not always a priority, as our society still retains many biases and misconceptions about mental illness.

Clinical Manifestations and Therapies

Schizophrenia

ETIOLOGY	CLINICAL MANIFESTATIONS	CLINICAL THERAPIES
Positive symptoms of psychosis	■ Hallucinations ■ Delusions ■ Thought disorders ■ Disorganized behavior ■ Movement disorders	■ Administration of conventional antipsychotics, atypical antipsychotics, and/or dopamine system stabilizers ■ CBT ■ Electroconvulsive therapy ■ Transcranial magnetic stimulation
Negative symptoms of psychosis	■ Anhedonia ■ Impaired memory ■ Flat affect ■ Avolition ■ Poverty of speech ■ Poor personal hygiene	■ Administration of atypical antipsychotics and/or dopamine system stabilizers ■ Psychiatric/psychosocial rehabilitation, including education about symptom management and signs of relapse and community service interventions such as assertive community treatment (ACT) ■ CBT; group, individual, and family therapy
Cognitive symptoms of schizophrenia	■ Concrete thinking ■ Impaired memory (problems with word finding and facial recognition) ■ Inattention and difficulty filtering out information ■ Poor planning, organization, and problem-solving skills	■ Cognitive remediation, CBT, social skills training ■ Modify the environment to reduce stimuli; break tasks down into small parts ■ Use lists and organizational aids ■ Psychosocial rehabilitation through community service models
Impaired social functioning	■ Withdrawal ■ Isolation ■ Difficulty maintaining relationships	■ Social skills training and guided practice in social situations ■ Psychosocial rehabilitation through community service models
Impaired occupational functioning	■ Unemployment, difficulty maintaining a job	■ Occupational therapy ■ Job training and placement

Another factor complicating the diagnosis and treatment of schizophrenia relates to cultural biases and influences. Providers often misinterpret cultural differences in behaviors and perceptions (see Focus on Diversity and Culture: Schizophrenia). In this section, collaborative care options are discussed, but nurses must recognize that vast improvements in our healthcare system, including cultural competency of providers, are needed to ensure that all patients have access to quality care.

Diagnostic Tests

Qualified mental health providers diagnose schizophrenia on the basis of findings obtained during a psychiatric evaluation of the patient. The evaluation generally includes a history and examination and may incorporate the use of screening tools and psychometric tests. Medical tests such as laboratory values and imaging studies are used to rule out other conditions. The patient must meet the criteria identified in the DSM-5, as exemplified by clinical manifestations described earlier. Diagnostic criteria specify that the individual must have experienced significant impairment of functioning for six or more months in one or more areas, such as home, work,

Focus on Diversity and Culture
Schizophrenia

Numerous studies have demonstrated that African and Latino Americans are up to three times more likely to be diagnosed with schizophrenia than are Caucasian Americans. Researchers have concluded that this phenomenon occurs even in the absence of a genetic predisposition to the disorder within these populations, leading the researchers to suggest that cultural biases play a significant role (Schwartz & Blankenship, 2014). Psychiatric diagnoses rely, in part, on clinician judgment about whether or not certain behaviors deviate from the norm. In many instances, providers do not account for cultural variances or the context in which the behaviors occur (Spector, 2017). It is possible that individuals from communities of color may be more reluctant to report affective symptoms that suggest other disorders. In addition, some perceptual experiences may be influenced by cultural beliefs. Nurses and other healthcare providers need to assess individual variables that may lead to misdiagnosis. Nursing care should not be dependent on diagnostic labels that may not consider patient-centered needs.

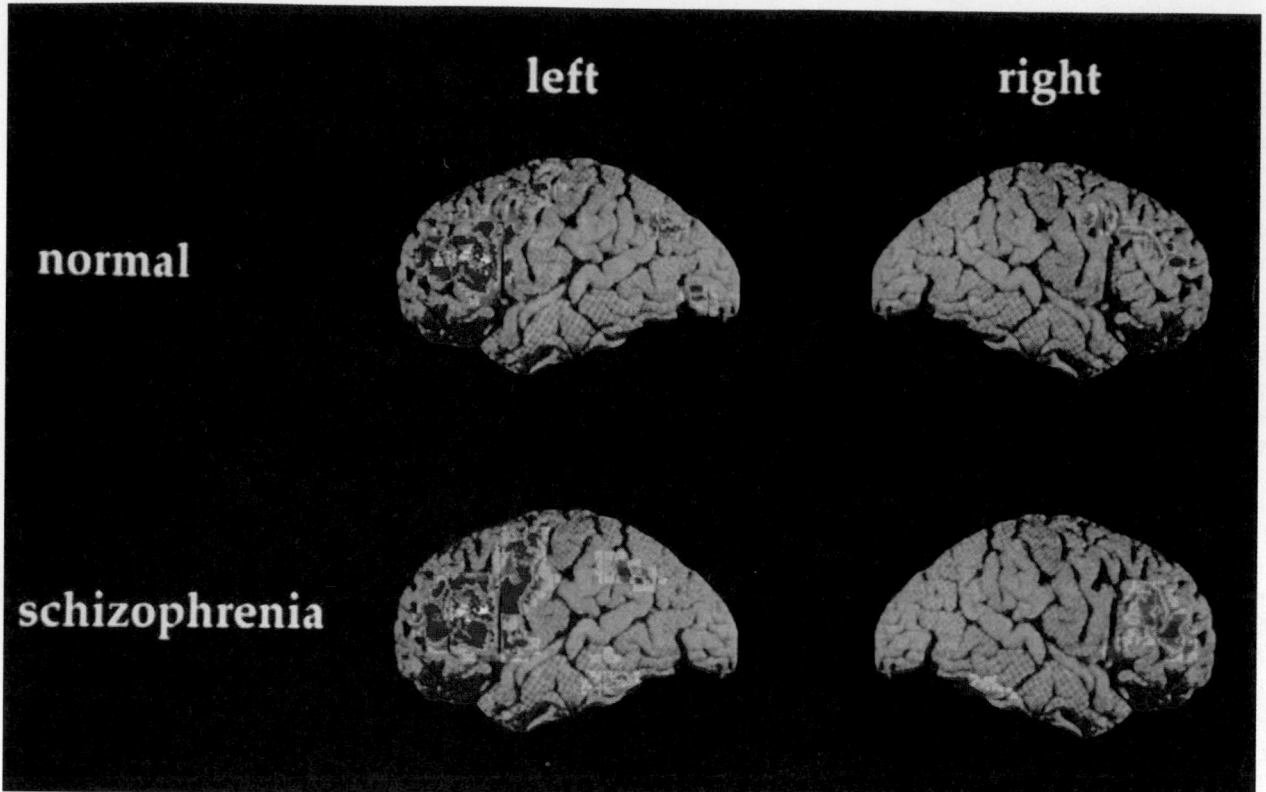

left right

normal

schizophrenia

Source: Wellcome Department of Cognitive Neurology/Science Source.

Figure 23–8 》 These PET scans show the difference between the brains of a normal patient and a patient with schizophrenia during a verbal fluency task—that is, the patients were asked to speak words. The red and yellow areas were activated when the subjects spoke the words. In the normal subject (top row), the brain shows much activity in the prefrontal and motor areas, and less activity in the parietal area on the left side. In the subject with schizophrenia (bottom row), there is also activity in the middle temporal gyrus (lower center of brain), which is not seen in the normal subject.

and self-care. Other mental disorders, such as bipolar disorder, and substance use also must be ruled out for a diagnosis of schizophrenia to be made (APA, 2013; Weickert et al., 2013).

Like other neurocognitive disorders discussed in this module, a number of biomarkers have been identified for schizophrenia, including the brain-imaging findings depicted in **Figure 23–8 》**. Presently biomarker analysis is used for research purposes, but in the future it may be used to confirm preclinical findings or to validate a diagnosis of schizophrenia.

Pharmacologic Therapy

The first line of intervention for schizophrenia is pharmacologic treatment with antipsychotic medications. The primary goal of pharmacotherapy is to decrease the positive symptoms of the disorder to a level that enables the individual to maintain social relationships and complete ADLs with minimal assistance. Antipsychotics do not cure schizophrenia, and complete remission is achieved in only about two thirds of patients taking these medications (Dold & Leucht, 2014). The relapse rate for individuals who discontinue the drugs is approximately 60–80% (Adams et al., 2017). Adherence to pharmacologic treatment is challenged by factors such as denial or poor insight into the illness, self-care deficits, and the incidence of common and serious adverse effects.

Antipsychotic medications include older, conventional agents called typical antipsychotics (first generation), atypical

antipsychotics (second generation), and dopamine system stabilizers (third generation) outlined in the Medications table in the section on Collaborative Therapies at the beginning of this module. Within each classification, different agents have properties that may make them more or less suitable for treating certain target symptoms. In addition, the profile of side effects and adverse effects may differ. When selecting an agent to treat psychotic symptoms clinicians, consider factors such as the severity of symptoms, prior degree of symptom response, adherence factors (e.g., dosing convenience, cost), side effect profile, and patient needs (Stahl et al., 2013). Long-acting injectable formulations may increase adherence. The efficacy of all classes of antipsychotics in treating the acute symptoms of the disease is about the same. An adequate treatment trial, with the full response to the medication being demonstrated, may take anywhere from 3 to 10 weeks and is necessary to evaluate efficacy, although symptoms such as hallucinations and delusions may diminish in days.

Typical or conventional antipsychotics consist of phenothiazine type (such as chlorpromazine) and nonphenothiazine (haloperidol). This is the "first generation" of drugs introduced to treat schizophrenia. The mechanism of action for both phenothiazine and nonphenothiazine antipsychotics is believed to be the blocking of postsynaptic D_2 receptors. Unfortunately, there are numerous adverse effects associated with typical antipsychotics that range from uncomfortable to disabling and life threatening. Anticholinergic effects occur, such as dry mouth, sedation, constipation, postural hypotension, and urinary retention. These effects are uncomfortable and place patients at increased risk of injury and infections. Sexual side effects such as ejaculation disorders and delay in achieving orgasm may be troubling for patients. Endocrine effects such as hyperprolactinemia can lead to osteoporosis, menstrual irregularities, decreased libido, gynecomastia, lactation, and erectile dysfunction.

Extrapyramidal symptoms (EPS) frequently occur with first-generation antipsychotics and include *acute dystonia*, *akathisia*, secondary *parkinsonism*, and *TD*. The most common EPS is **akathisia**, a feeling of uncomfortable restlessness that is often not recognized and managed appropriately. **Dystonia** often results in sudden and severe muscle spasms in the face, neck, and torso that can be frightening for patients and have the potential to lead to airway obstruction if not identified and reversed. Secondary parkinsonism is manifested by tremors, muscle rigidity, masked facies (lack of expression), stooped posture, and shuffling gait. **Tardive dyskinesia (TD)** is a potentially irreversible condition characterized by unusual facial movements, lip smacking, and wormlike movements of the tongue. **Neuroleptic malignant syndrome (NMS)** is a potentially fatal condition characterized by severe autonomic instability. Manifestations include high fever, confusion and changes in level of consciousness, muscle rigidity, and hyperthermia. Management of adverse effects such as anticholinergic symptoms and EPS often includes the use of anticholinergic medications such as benztropine (Cogentin). Antiparkinsonian/antimuscarinic drugs such as trihexyphenidyl (Artane) may be used to decrease stiffness and rigidity. Parenteral benztropine and diphenhydramine (Benadryl) can quickly reverse dystonia. Beta-adrenergic blockers and benzodiazepines may reduce the symptoms associated with akathisia. TD is usually managed with a reduction in dose or a switch to another agent. If NMS is suspected, antipsychotic agents are immediately discontinued and the patient is admitted to the intensive care unit (ICU) for supportive care.

Atypical antipsychotics (also called second-generation antipsychotics) are believed to also block D_2 receptors, although they have a weaker affinity that may account for the lower profile of certain side effects. In addition, atypical antipsychotics also block serotonin and alpha-adrenergic receptors. It is believed that these agents also treat some of the negative symptoms of the illness, although the clinical significance of this has recently come under question (Fusar-Poli et al., 2015). Examples include risperidone (Risperdal) and olanzapine (Zyprexa). One advantage of atypical antipsychotics seems to be a lower incidence of EPS and TD at therapeutic doses. However, adverse effects can still be quite severe, with an increased risk of medical problems such as metabolic syndrome, cardiovascular and cerebrovascular events, type 2 diabetes mellitus, blood dyscrasias, seizures, and sudden death. Anticholinergic effects, endocrine effects, TD, and NMS can also occur with these medications.

Dopamine-serotonin system stabilizers (DSSs—also called dopamine partial agonists or third-generation antipsychotics) have therapeutic benefits similar to those of atypical antipsychotics and an even lower profile of adverse effects. These agents are generally well tolerated, with very few anticholinergic side effects and a lower incidence of weight gain. They also seem to target affective symptoms and are often used to treat bipolar disorder and depression. Aripiprazole (Abilify) was the first drug approved from this class, and a new drug, brexpiprazole (Rexulti), was recently approved. Because of its similar therapeutic action, aripiprazole is included in the Medications feature with the atypical antipsychotics.

In addition to antipsychotics, individuals may be treated with adjunctive medications such as antianxiety agents, antidepressants, and mood stabilizers. These medications are discussed in the Collaborative Therapies section in the introduction to this module and in the modules on Stress and Coping and on Mood and Affect.

Nonpharmacologic Therapy

As mentioned previously, the recovery and rehabilitation model is the overarching approach to caring for individuals with schizophrenia outside of hospital and institutional settings. This model does not represent any single distinct pathway to care, but instead recognizes that each individual maintains their own life goals and should be provided with a variety of resources that will empower them to make informed decisions and build on their own strengths in order to regain control of their lives. Pharmacologic interventions alone are insufficient to address the complex needs of individuals with schizophrenia. Nurses providing care to patients with schizophrenia across all settings can anticipate interfacing with a variety of team members, including psychiatrists, social workers, occupational therapists, psychologists, psychiatric rehabilitation specialists, and mental health workers.

Family Intervention and Psychoeducation

Research demonstrates that the provision of family interventions, such as psychoeducation and counseling, can reduce the relapse rate for schizophrenia by up to 20% (Pitschel-Walz et al., 2015). Studies indicate that the best results are achieved when family interventions continue over several months and are combined with pharmacologic interventions and other treatment modalities. Some studies indicate that family psychoeducation in particular reduces the subjective burden of schizophrenia and leads to a more positive family atmosphere (Gühne et al., 2015).

Social Skills Training

Schizophrenia is characterized by deficits in social cognition that have a profound effect on the individual's ability to accurately read social cues and respond appropriately. Social skills training employs a systematic approach to teaching individuals with schizophrenia how to interact with others. One particularly effective approach is Social Cognition and Interaction Training (SCIT). SCIT is a group intervention delivered over a 6-month period. Participants work with trained therapists on three phases that consist of learning about emotions, figuring out situations, and practicing what was learned. Computerized exercises, videos, and other tools may be used to enhance learning. The overall effectiveness of such programs is still under investigation; however, early studies suggest that that the best results are achieved when SCIT is combined with cognitive remediation (Bowie et al., 2012; Gühne et al., 2015; Kurtz & Richardson, 2012; Roberts et al., 2014).

Cognitive–Behavioral Therapy

CBT is a psychosocial treatment that may be helpful in assisting patients with schizophrenia to cope with their symptoms by using distraction, positive self-talk, or behavioral processes such as exercising. In CBT, patients are encouraged to reframe symptoms of psychosis as attempts to cope. Problem-solving techniques are used to identify and make use of new coping strategies. Although earlier studies supported the efficacy of CBT for schizophrenia, a systematic review and meta-analysis conducted in 2014 indicates that CBT results in modest therapeutic effects (Jauhar et al., 2014). Some researchers argue that these findings are too restrictive, underestimating the benefits of more focused techniques and failing to consider benefits outside improvement in positive and negative symptoms (Mueser & Glynn, 2014; Thase, Kingdon, & Turkinton, 2014; Turner et al., 2014).

Cognitive Remediation

Cognitive remediation or rehabilitation includes strategies aimed to address cognitive deficits associated with schizophrenia. Techniques are similar to educational interventions employed in special education and focus on compensatory strategies as well as drill and practice techniques aimed at strengthening specific cognitive functions, such as working memory. Compensatory techniques include organizing and modifying the home environment to support adaptive function (labeling items, making lists, posting emergency numbers) and assisting patients to break down new skills into smaller steps that are then overlearned. Rehabilitation techniques include the use of computer programs that "exercise" certain cognitive functions through engaging games and activities. Because many models are used, the efficacy of these programs is difficult to measure; however, studies suggest that the most effective models address beliefs and motivation and incorporate opportunities for real-world practice (Bowie et al., 2012; Medalia & Saperstein, 2013).

Vocational Training

Vocational rehabilitation or training encompasses a variety of services aimed at increasing functional capacity and reducing unemployment for individuals with schizophrenia. Prevocational programs aim to increase employability by providing skills training. Supported employment programs assist patients to find and maintain employment. Vocational training may be incorporated into one of the community service models discussed in this section.

Community Service Models

A variety of community service models are available to address the needs of individuals with schizophrenia. Some of the most common models include crisis intervention teams, case management, and ACT.

Crisis intervention refers to short-term, intensive measures to address symptoms or behaviors that impact the safety and equilibrium of the patient and others. The portal of entry into crisis intervention may be the emergency department or through a mobile crisis intervention or outreach team. After an assessment is made, interventions such as medication adjustment, 24-hour monitoring, ECT, or a change in services are implemented in the least restrictive environment possible. For some patients, this may mean a short inpatient stay; for others, services may be provided in in the community in the patient's home, in a residential treatment center, or through a combination of partial day treatment and home care. *Mobile crisis outreach teams* consist of interprofessional team members who are deployed to the site of the crisis for assessment and intervention. They have special training that may be used to effectively de-escalate the situation and usually work in collaboration with law enforcement.

≫ **Stay Current:** For more information on mobile outreach teams and other crisis interventions services visit the National Alliance for the Mentally Ill (NAMI) "Getting Treatment During a Crisis" At https://www.nami.org/Learn-More/Treatment/Getting-Treatment-During-a-Crisis

Case management is a method of coordinating care by assigning each individual to a case manager or a qualified person who completes an assessment of patient needs, develops a plan, coordinates appropriate services, monitors the quality of care being provided, and maintains a collaborative relationship with the affected individual (see the module on Managing Care). Many variables impact the efficacy of this model, including availability of community resources, caseload, and clinician experience and training. These variables make it difficult to support or refute the overall effectiveness of these programs (Dadich, Fisher, & Muir, 2013).

Assertive community treatment (ACT) aims to meet many of the same goals as case management, but ACT is a service delivery model in which interprofessional team members share accountability for meeting patient needs in a collaborative and often intensive manner. Most individuals involved in ACT can expect to meet with more than one team member on a weekly basis. Services are available 24 hours a day and 7 days a week. ACT models follow a specific high-fidelity framework for meeting patient needs (such as medical care, housing, social support, and employment) by limiting team-member caseloads to no more than 10 individuals and by providing services directly rather than relying on referrals to agencies. The usefulness of ACT has been validated by research, which shows that ACT decreases patient hospitalization time and severity of symptoms while improving stability and quality of life (Bond & Drake, 2015; Schöttle et al., 2014).

≫ **Stay Current:** For more information on ACT programs and free evidence-based tool kits, visit the Substance Abuse and Mental Health Services Administration at http://store.samhsa.gov/product/Assertive-Community-Treatment-ACT-Evidence-Based-Practices-EBP-KIT/SMA08-4345

Individual, Family, and Group Therapy

The benefits of group, individual, and family therapies for other alterations in psychosocial function are discussed in the modules on Self, Stress and Coping, and Mood and Affect. Group interventions vary from self-help groups to those that have more focused on specific goals such as psychoeducation or social skills. The individual needs of the patient and family are used to determine which groups are most likely to provide the greatest benefits. Comprehensive care should include individual counseling for the patient with schizophrenia as well as counseling to address the unique burdens and challenges of the patient's family.

Electroconvulsive Therapy

Electroconvulsive therapy (ECT) is a procedure that delivers electronic impulses into the brain under general anesthesia. The goal of treatment is to induce seizure activity that, for the most part, is effective in treating affective disorders such as depression. ECT is not typically used to treat schizophrenia but appears to demonstrate some efficacy in treating certain symptoms of schizophrenia such as depression, paranoia, and catatonia (Zervas, Theleritis, & Soldatos, 2012). ECT is most effective when used in conjunction with medication. For more information on this procedure, refer to the module on Mood and Affect.

Repetitive Transcranial Magnetic Stimulation

Repetitive transcranial magnetic stimulation (rTMS) is a type of therapy that uses an electromagnet placed on the scalp to deliver pulses roughly equivalent to the strength of an MRI. The FDA approved rTMS for the treatment of depression in 2008. The efficacy of rTMS in treating auditory hallucinations and other symptoms of schizophrenia has been the subject of research for several years. A recent Cochrane review conducted by Dougall and colleagues (2015) concluded that, while some studies have suggested improvements in patients, there is currently insufficient robust evidence to conclude that rTMS is an effective standardized treatment for schizophrenia.

>> **Stay Current:** For more information on collaborative treatments used to treat schizophrenia, visit http://www.nami.org/Learn-More/Mental-Health-Conditions/Schizophrenia/Treatment

Complementary Health Approaches

Integrative and complementary treatments for schizophrenia include the use of nutritional interventions and supplements and the use of mind–body practices. There is no evidence to suggest that any of these treatments are effective alternatives to the collaborative interventions just discussed.

Research on nutritional interventions has focused on potential risks and benefits of supplementation with B vitamins, vitamin D, and omega-3 fatty acids. Currently the most positive and conclusive findings support the use of omega-3 fatty acids in the prodromal and residual phases of the disease (Arroll, Wilder & Neil, 2014; Chia et al., 2015). However, at least one randomized controlled study suggested that the use of omega fatty acids in the acute phase of the illness may actually exacerbate symptoms (Emsley et al., 2014). Safety and practical considerations should guide the use of nutritional interventions. The use of supplements should be discussed with providers so that an individual assessment of the risks versus potential benefits can be made.

Data regarding the effectiveness of mind–body interventions to manage the symptoms of schizophrenia is mixed. A systematic review conducted by Helgason and Sarris (2013) found mainly supportive evidence for music therapy, meditation, and other mindfulness techniques. Relaxation techniques, yoga, and mind–body groups had some supportive evidence. Evidence on the use of art therapy, drama, dance therapy, hypnosis, and biofeedback techniques was inconclusive at best.

Lifespan Considerations

As previously stated, the majority of individuals with schizophrenia experience an emergence of symptoms in early adulthood with a classic course preceded by prodromal symptoms and a lessening of positive symptoms with aging. The remainder of individuals with schizophrenia may be grouped into those with an early-onset schizophrenia (EOS) of the disorder (before the age of 18) or a pattern of later onset (after the age of 40), sometimes referred to as late-onset schizophrenia (LOS).

Early-Onset Schizophrenia

EOS generally refers to the emergence of symptoms of schizophrenia before 17 to 18 years of age. EOS accounts for approximately 4–5% of all individuals with schizophrenia. Onset prior to puberty is extremely rare, occurring in less than 0.04% of the population and is further classified as childhood-onset schizophrenia (COS). In general, childhood schizophrenia may be more difficult to diagnose. Hallucinations are less complex and may focus on childhood themes such as monsters and toys, making them difficult to distinguish from fantasy play. Symptoms such as disordered speech, motor deficits, cognitive deficits, and social withdrawal may overlap with manifestations of developmental disorders such as autism spectrum disorders (ASD) (Clemmenssen, Vernal, & Steinhausen, 2012).

Adolescents who experience EOS demonstrate symptoms similar to the adult variants of the disorder. Onset in adolescence seems to be at least slightly more prevalent in boys and is associated with an increased risk of suicide (Clemmenssen et al., 2012; Kelleher et al., 2012). The overall prognosis for both children and adolescents with EOS is poor and is associated with greater chronicity and higher levels of disability (Bartlett, 2014; Driver, Gogtay, & Rapoport, 2013). Management of EOS includes many of the same treatments and therapies that are used with adults with appropriate developmental modifications. Children are at increased risk of adverse effects from psychotropic medications, and many agents do not demonstrate the same efficacy as is observed in adults (Driver et al., 2013).

Late-Onset Schizophrenia

About 20–30% of all patients do not experience symptoms of schizophrenia until after age 40. The incidence of LOS seems to be greater in women, but other risk factors for the disease are comparable to those associated with an earlier onset. Typically, positive symptoms of the disease are more predominant, with paranoia, elaborate delusions, and hallucinations (Hanssen et al., 2015). Both cognitive and negative manifestations of the disease are higher than in the general population but lower than what is commonly observed in adult-onset schizophrenia. Patients with LOS often respond to lower doses of antipsychotic medication. These findings have led some scientists to suggest that late-onset schizophrenia may even represent a distinct disorder (Magliono, Thomas, & Josto, 2014).

When symptoms of schizophrenia do not emerge until after age 60, the condition is often referred to as very-late-onset schizophrenia (VLOS). VLOS can be distinguished from other variants by a lower genetic load and a higher level of premorbid function. The etiology of VLOS is believed to be neurodegenerative and organic factors. The incidence is higher in immigrant populations, suggesting that sociocultural factors also play a role (Nebhinani, Pareek, & Grover, 2014). Management may include lower-dose antipsychotics and psychosocial interventions.

NURSING PROCESS

The application of the nursing process depends on many factors, including the phase of the illness the patient is experiencing. Primarily, nursing goals for patients with schizophrenia include promoting symptom control and facilitating effective coping to help the patient achieve optimal mental, physical, and social functioning. Ideally, the patient will avoid further episodes of psychosis and be able to function successfully in the community to the greatest degree possible.

Assessment

Nursing assessment of a patient with schizophrenia typically involves three main elements: a patient interview, a physical examination, and a mental status examination.

Observation and Patient Interview

Nurses and others may notice the following in patients with schizophrenia: deteriorating personal appearance and neglect of personal hygiene; weight loss; unusual gestures; pacing; or incoherence characterized by making up words or speaking in sentences that make no sense (word salad). Many individuals with schizophrenia smoke, so a noticeable odor of smoke or tobacco may be present. A lack of insight is characteristic of schizophrenia, so patients may be unaware of these changes or actions.

The patient interview can reveal risk factors for schizophrenia, as well as help identify early signs of psychosis in patients who have not yet been diagnosed. For the patient with known or suspected schizophrenia, elements of the health history should include age; family history and paternal age; history of perinatal health problems or exposures, developmental delays, or exposure to trauma or adversity; history of behaviors such as substance abuse; history of positive, negative, cognitive, and affective manifestations; family coping; history of commonly comorbid mental illness (e.g., addiction, anxiety disorders, or mood disorders); and presence or emergence of major life stressors.

For the patient diagnosed with schizophrenia, ask about possible risk factors for exacerbations or signs of relapse, such as:

- Poor adherence to the prescribed treatment regimen (especially pharmacologic therapy)
- Possible development of resistance to antipsychotic medications
- Presence of mild to full-blown symptoms of psychosis
- Recent life events that may increase the likelihood of relapse

Physical Examination

Next, during the physical examination, evaluate the patient's overall physical condition. Throughout the physical exam, remain alert for possible signs of metabolic problems, cardiovascular problems, drug/alcohol abuse, and poor self-care, as schizophrenia increases the risk for all of these. Note any evidence of side effects from medications, such as movement problems, weight gain, or changes in vital signs.

Mental Status Examination

Finally, individuals with known or suspected schizophrenia should receive a thorough mental status examination. Nurses can choose from a variety of assessment instruments, as described in the Mental Assessment feature. Regardless of which tool is used, closely monitor for possible manifestations of schizophrenia throughout the mental status exam. Also keep in mind the patient's cultural and religious background, as this can affect an individual's description and interpretation of symptoms such as auditory and visual hallucinations.

Following the health history, physical exam, and mental status examination, several steps may be appropriate. For an individual suspected of having (but not yet diagnosed with) schizophrenia, referral to a psychologist or to a psychiatrist or other physician may be warranted. Laboratory testing and imaging studies may also be necessary to rule out other potential health problems. When working with a patient who has already been diagnosed with schizophrenia, note any significant changes in the patient's signs, symptoms, and behaviors since the last assessment. In addition, investigate the patient's living situation and adherence to the prescribed treatment regimen.

Diagnosis

Appropriate nursing diagnoses for patients with schizophrenia vary depending on symptoms and level of functioning. Still, some diagnoses are likely to apply to many, if not most, patients. Examples of these diagnoses include:

- *Suicide, Risk for*
- *Other-Directed Violence, Risk for*
- *Injury, Risk for*
- *Health Maintenance, Ineffective*
- *Self-Care Deficit (Bathing and/or Dressing)*
- *Verbal Communication, Impaired*
- *Social Interaction, Impaired*
- *Coping, Ineffective*
- *Noncompliance.*

(NANDA-I © 2014)

Planning

The planning portion of the nursing process involves identifying desired patient outcomes and formulating steps for achieving those outcomes. For patients with schizophrenia, appropriate nursing outcomes typically fall into one of three broad categories: symptom reduction, improved quality of life, and helping patients achieve life goals.

Outcomes Related to Symptom Reduction

- Patient will no longer experience hallucinations and delusions.
- Patient will experience a reduction in disordered thoughts.
- Patient will demonstrate appropriate affect.
- Patient will experience fewer negative symptoms of schizophrenia.
- Patient will take all medications as prescribed.

Outcomes Related to Quality of Life

- Patient will demonstrate appropriate self-care and personal hygiene.
- Patient will obtain adequate sleep.
- Patient will refrain from use of alcohol and/or illicit drugs.

- Patient will demonstrate improved coping skills.
- Patient will make a concerted effort to interact with others and avoid social isolation.

Outcomes Related to Achieving Life Goals
- Patient will cultivate appropriate occupational skills.
- Patient will find a job and maintain gainful employment.
- Patient will retain responsibility for personal finances.
- Patient will live independently in the community.

Implementation

Implementation involves evidence-based nursing interventions that facilitate the patient's achievement of identified goals of care. Although appropriate interventions will vary, the following principles apply to most patients diagnosed with schizophrenia.

Prevent Injury

The nurse's first priority of care should be to provide a safe environment for patients with schizophrenia and prevent them from engaging in violence toward self or others. When hallucinating or interpreting others' actions and statements from the standpoint of delusions, the patient may believe herself to be in danger, regardless of whether there is a factual basis for her fear. Under such circumstances, both the patient and perceived aggressors may be at risk for injury. Nursing interventions directed toward promoting safety and preventing injury may include administering antipsychotic medications as ordered, ensuring that the patient's surroundings are free of potentially harmful objects, minimizing environmental stimuli, and monitoring for suicidal behavior.

Provide Symptomatic Treatment

The nurse's second priority should be promoting control of the patient's current symptoms and minimizing the likelihood that additional symptoms will arise. Applicable nursing interventions may include orienting the patient to person and place; avoiding overwhelming or overstimulating the patient; remaining calm and consistent when speaking with the patient; and always informing the patient before touching him. When the patient appears to be experiencing hallucinations or delusions, the nurse should explain that she is not experiencing or thinking these things, yet she understands that they are real for the patient. Of course, the nurse must also ensure that patients understand and are able to follow all parts of their treatment regimen. Many times, patients will require referral to various community agencies that can assist patients with activities such as finding support groups, remembering to take their medications, and obtaining transportation to and from doctors' appointments and therapy sessions.

Educate Patients and Significant Others

Teaching and encouragement are another vital area of intervention for both patients with schizophrenia and their families. Inform patients and their loved ones about the symptoms and course of the disease, available therapeutic options and how they work, possible medication side effects, and potential signs of relapse. The nurse should also explore patients' and families' current communication and coping skills and encourage the development of new and potentially more effective strategies (see Patient Teaching: Communication Techniques for Families with a Member with Schizophrenia). Encourage patients to adopt healthier behaviors, such as discontinuing use of nicotine and alcohol, obtaining adequate sleep, and eating a balanced diet. Social skills training is often appropriate, as is encouraging patients to participate in activities that minimize their likelihood of social isolation and withdrawal. In addition, many individuals derive great benefit from training (or perhaps retraining) in how to perform various occupational skills and ADLs. To keep patients on the path toward fuller functioning and possibly even independent living, the nurse should be sure to provide frequent positive reinforcement for desired actions and behaviors.

Advocate for Patients

The nurse must take steps to advocate on behalf of patients with schizophrenia. For example, the nurse should ensure that all interventions and therapies are actually in a patient's best interests and not merely intended to ease the burden on the patient's family and caregivers. The nurse should also make sure patients understand their legal rights to the greatest degree possible. Because individuals with schizophrenia are often unable to understand or independently exercise these rights during periods of acute psychosis, they should be encouraged to develop advance directives and similar documents explaining their wishes for times when the disorder is not controlled.

Evaluation

Ongoing evaluation is critical for patients with schizophrenia, as it allows nurses to monitor their condition and adjust any patient-specific diagnoses, goals, and interventions as

---

Patient Teaching
Communication Techniques for Families with a Member with Schizophrenia

Families are often overwhelmed by the stress associated with having a member affected by schizophrenia. Without specific tools to cope, ineffective communication patterns can arise and have the potential to contribute to poor patient outcomes. Nurses can teach family members strategies to improve communication. For example, if a family is concerned about a patient's behavior, the nurse can guide them through the use of some of the following techniques:

- Using "I" language to express positive feelings (e.g., "I am happy when you decide to sit down for dinner with us")
- Engaging in active listening (e.g., asking questions and nodding in agreement when another person speaks)
- Making positive, specific requests for change that are linked to emotions (e.g., "I would really like it if you could play a game with us tonight")
- Expressing negative feelings with "I" rather than "you" language (e.g., saying "I'm worried that you may not be getting enough sleep" instead of "You never get enough sleep at night")

After teaching these skills, the nurse should have family members schedule a time for practice. It is also important for the nurse to emphasize that the more often family members use these skills, the more natural they will become.

necessary. Some general examples of potential achieved outcomes for patients with schizophrenia include the following:

- The patient adheres to the medication regimen.
- The patient demonstrates utilization of available community resources.
- The patient communicates clearly and transitions logically between topics.

- The patient reports an absence of hallucinations and/or delusions.
- The patient is able to perform ADLs.
- The patient refrains from use of nicotine, alcohol, and illicit drugs.
- The patient is able to work in a structured setting.

Nursing Care Plan
A Patient with Schizophrenia

Lauren Hildebrand, age 22, is brought to a private mental health center by her father, Peter, who is concerned about recent changes in her behavior. He reports that she is demonstrating increasing difficulty expressing her thoughts and that she often stops talking midsentence, as though she's forgotten what she was saying. He also states that Ms. Hildebrand dropped out of her graduate program in engineering 4 months ago because she suddenly was unable to maintain her grades. Mr. Hildebrand believes these problems are tied to cocaine use.

ASSESSMENT	DIAGNOSES	PLANNING
Angel Sanchez, the RN at the health center, obtains a patient history and physical examination of Ms. Hildebrand. Mr. Sanchez notes that Ms. Hildebrand was adopted as an infant and little is known about her birth mother beyond the fact that she was homeless at the time Ms. Hildebrand was born. Until 10 months ago, Ms. Hildebrand was an A student at the local university and was awarded a position as a graduate assistant in the engineering department. Shortly after beginning her assistantship, she began having problems expressing herself. At first, she simply seemed distracted, rapidly switching from one topic to another in conversation; this eventually segued into problems logically connecting thoughts and completing sentences. Within 6 months, Ms. Hildebrand was no longer able to maintain her grades and job responsibilities and was forced to drop out of the graduate program. Around this time, her friends became aware of her drug problem. Out of concern, they contacted her parents. Ms. Hildebrand's clothes are relatively new and fashionable, but they are rumpled and smell strongly of body odor. It appears that Ms. Hildebrand hasn't bathed or combed her hair in several days. Her affect is flat. Mr. Sanchez detects redness in and around Ms. Hildebrand's nostrils and notices that she frequently rubs her nose, both of which suggest insufflation of cocaine. Ms. Hildebrand admits that she uses cocaine but states that she hasn't used it in 3 days. She has difficulty answering Mr. Sanchez's other questions; her speech is garbled and relies heavily on rhyming words that do not make sense when strung together. Ms. Hildebrand is very thin, and the shape of her arm, hand, and clavicle bones stands out clearly under her skin. Her vital signs include T 100.1°F oral; P 95 bpm; R 22/min; and BP 131/88 mmHg. Based on his mental status assessment of Ms. Hildebrand, Mr. Sanchez suspects schizophrenia. The psychiatrist orders an MRI to rule out abnormalities such as brain tumors. Aside from slightly enlarged ventricles, Ms. Hildebrand's MRI does not reveal any unusual findings. After speaking with Ms. Hildebrand's father, the psychiatrist interviews Ms. Hildebrand, after which he diagnoses her with probable acute schizophrenia. Based on her mental state and substance abuse, the psychiatrist recommends Ms. Hildebrand complete a 28-day inpatient stay at the mental health center, where she will receive treatment for her psychiatric condition and substance abuse. He also prescribes olanzapine, 5 mg/day for 1 week, to be followed by 2.5 mg/day increases each week until Ms. Hildebrand exhibits improvement, not to exceed 20 mg/day.	- *Risk for Injury* related to disorganized thinking patterns and substance abuse - *Impaired Social Interaction* related to altered cognitive function - *Impaired Verbal Communication* related to perceptual and cognitive impairment - *Ineffective Health Maintenance* related to perceptual and cognitive impairment - *Self-Care Deficit* (*Bathing*) related to cognitive impairment and substance abuse - *Imbalanced Nutrition: Less Than Body Requirements* related to cognitive impairment and substance abuse (NANDA-I © 2014)	Goals for Ms. Hildebrand's care include: - The patient will remain free from injury. - The patient will demonstrate clear communication patterns. - The patient will verbalize logical thought processes. - The patient will exercise appropriate self-care and hygiene measures, including bathing or showering daily and completing oral hygiene care twice daily. - The patient will discontinue cocaine use. - The patient will gain 1 to 2 lb per week. - The patient will engage in appropriate rehabilitation and group therapy activities while hospitalized and after release.

Nursing Care Plan (continued)

IMPLEMENTATION

- Monitor the patient for indicators that suggest the potential for injury to self or others.
- Ensure the patient receives care that promotes physical and psychologic safety.
- Administer all medications as ordered.
- Monitor for signs and symptoms of cocaine withdrawal and address the need for substance abuse treatment.

- Assist the patient with establishing a pattern of self-care that includes adequate nutritional intake and hygiene.
- Teach patient and family members how to cope with schizophrenia and how to respond to signs of relapse.
- Encourage the patient to attend and engage in group therapy sessions.
- Ensure appropriate post-discharge services such as ACT.

EVALUATION

Mr. Sanchez works closely with Ms. Hildebrand during her stay at the mental health center. While at the center, Ms. Hildebrand receives education about her disorder, its causes and symptoms, and complications commonly associated with it. She also receives substance abuse counseling, CBT, and vocational counseling to prepare her to find a job after she is released. Her medication is gradually increased over the course of her stay until she reaches an effective dose of 12.5 mg/day. By the end of her inpatient stay, Ms. Hildebrand is able to demonstrate appropriate self-care skills related to hygiene, nutrition, and medication administration. She can also clearly and logically describe the symptoms of her condition and verbalize strategies for coping with them. She is scheduled to return to the center twice each week for group therapy and has an appointment to meet with an ACT provider.

CRITICAL THINKING

1. Based on the little we know of Ms. Hildebrand's birth mother, can we draw any conclusions about either Ms. Hildebrand's genetic predisposition to schizophrenia or environmental factors prior to her birth that may have predisposed her to this disorder? Why is it reasonable to draw these conclusions?
2. Research community services for individuals with schizophrenia in your geographical area. What types of services are offered, and which of these services would you recommend to Ms. Hildebrand if she were your patient? Why would you recommend them?
3. Develop a care plan for the nursing diagnosis Risk for Self-Directed Violence related to disruptions in cognitive processes.

REVIEW Schizophrenia

RELATE Link the Concepts and Exemplars

Linking the exemplar of schizophrenia with the concept of immunity:

1. Why might patients with schizophrenia be at a heightened risk of HIV infection and AIDS?
2. What measures might you implement when caring for a patient with schizophrenia to limit the risk of HIV exposure?

Linking the exemplar of schizophrenia with the concept of addiction:

3. Why are patients with schizophrenia more likely to abuse nicotine, alcohol, and illicit drugs? Be sure to explore physical, social, and psychologic factors in your response.
4. What special challenges might arise when addressing addiction behaviors in patients with schizophrenia (as opposed to other patients)? Why? How might the nurse attempt to overcome these challenges?

Linking the exemplar of schizophrenia with the concept of managing care:

5. Why are care coordination and case management especially important for patients with schizophrenia?
6. What sort of professionals might be involved in the overall plan of care for a patient with schizophrenia? How could the nurse promote better collaboration and communication among these providers?

READY Go to Volume 3: Clinical Nursing Skills

REFER Go to Pearson MyLab Nursing and eText

- Additional review material

REFLECT Apply Your Knowledge

Dwight Gibson, a 46-year-old man, is brought to the emergency department by his landlord, Ms. Alder. Ms. Alder is concerned about Mr. Gibson's current mental state. She reports that his behavior has always been eccentric for the 5 years she's known him. For example, he perpetually seems worried that someone is "out to get him" and has installed extra locks on his doors and windows.

Lately, however, Ms. Alder has felt that Mr. Gibson's behavior is progressing from merely unusual to severely disturbed. Ms. Alder explains that she lives in the apartment below Mr. Gibson's, and several times over the past month, she's heard him yelling. When Ms. Alder goes to check on him, he tells her he's arguing with the "voices," yet there's never anyone else in the apartment with him. Ms. Alder also mentions that Mr. Gibson seems to be letting garbage accumulate in his apartment, as it smells quite bad. Upon observation, Mr. Gibson's hair is dirty and his clothes are stained and torn. As the nurse conducting Mr. Gibson's initial assessment, you introduce yourself to him and ask how he is feeling. He replies that he is feeling fine. Next, you ask Mr. Gibson if you may check his blood pressure. He appears agitated and states, "They told you to do that, didn't they? They're trying to steal my spirit. They're afraid my spirit will tell me the truth. I will not let you do that."

1. What additional assessment information do you need?

2. How should you respond to Mr. Gibson's refusal to allow you to assess his blood pressure?

3. What are Mr. Gibson's priorities of care at this time?

4. Should Mr. Gibson be determined to be experiencing schizophrenia, what nursing diagnoses would be appropriate for inclusion in his plan of care?

References

Adams, M. P., Holland, L. N., & Urban, C. (2017). *Pharmacology for nurses: A pathophysiologic approach* (5th ed.). Hoboken, NJ: Pearson Education.

Ahmed, A. O., Buckley, P. F., & Hanna, M. (2013). Neuroimaging schizophrenia: A picture is worth a thousand words, but is it saying anything important? *Current Psychiatry Reports,* 15(3), 1–11.

Ahmed, S., Leurent, B., & Sampson, E. L. (2014). Risk factors for incident delirium among older people in acute hospital medical units: A systematic review and meta-analysis. *Age and Ageing,* afu022.

Akdeniz, C., Tost, H., & Meyer-Lindenberg, A. (2014). The neurobiology of social environmental risk for schizophrenia: An evolving research field. *Social Psychiatry and Psychiatric Epidemiology,* 49(4), 507–517.

Alagiakrishnan, K. (2015). *Delirium.* Retrieved from http://emedicine.medscape.com/article/288890-overview#a8

Alosco, M. L., Gunstad, J., Jerskey, B. A., Xu, X., Clark, U. S., Hassenstab, J., . . . Sweet, L. H. (2013). The adverse effects of reduced cerebral perfusion on cognition and brain structure in older adults with cardiovascular disease. *Brain and Behavior,* 3(6), 626–636.

Alshaarawy, O., Breslau, N., & Anthony, J. C. (2016). Monthly estimates of alcohol drinking during pregnancy: United States, 2002–2011. *Journal of Studies on Alcohol and Drugs,* 77(2), 272–276.

Alzheimer's Association. (2014). *What is Alzheimer's?* Retrieved from http://www.alz.org/alzheimers_disease_what_is_alzheimers.asp

Alzheimer's Association. (2015). *Facts and figures.* Retrieved from http://www.alz.org/facts/overview.asp

Alzheimer's Association. (2016a). *Prevention and risk of Alzheimer's and dementia.* Retrieved March 1, 2016 from http://www.alz.org/research/science/alzheimers_prevention_and_risk.asp

Alzheimer's Association. (2016b). *The search for causes and risk factors.* Retrieved from http://www.alz.org/research/science/alzheimers_disease_causes.asp

Alzheimer's Association. (2016c). *Stages of Alzheimer's.* Retrieved from http://www.alz.org/alzheimers_disease_stages_of_alzheimers.asp

Alzheimer's Association. (2016d). *Medications for memory loss.* Retrieved from http://www.alz.org/alzheimers_disease_standard_prescriptions.asp

Alzheimer's Association. (2016e). *Dementia and Driving Resource Center.* Retrieved from http://www.alz.org/care/alzheimers-dementia-and-driving.asp

American Association of Intellectual and Developmental Disabilities. (2013). *Definition of intellectual disability.* Retrieved from http://aaidd.org/intellectual-disability/definition#.VsNGSsfZrds

American Geriatrics Society Expert Panel on Postoperative Delirium in Older Adults. (2015). Postoperative delirium in older adults: Best Practice Statement from the American Geriatrics Society.

Journal of the American College of Surgeons, 220(2), 136–148.

American Psychiatric Association. (2013). *Diagnostic and statistical manual of mental disorders,* 5th ed. Washington, DC: Author.

American Psychiatric Association. (2015). *Schizophrenia spectrum and other psychotic disorders: DSM-5 selections.* Arlington, VA: American Psychiatric Publishing.

American Speech Language and Hearing Association. (2016). *Social language use (pragmatics).* Retrieved from http://www.asha.org/public/speech/development/Pragmatics/

Andreasen, N. C., & Black, D. W. (2006). *Introductory textbook of psychiatry* (4th ed.). Washington, DC: American Psychiatric Publishing.

Appelbaum, P. S. (2015). Ethical challenges in the primary prevention of schizophrenia. *Schizophrenia Bulletin,* 41(4), 773–775.

Arroll, M. A., Wilder, L., & Neil, J. (2014). Nutritional interventions for the adjunctive treatment of schizophrenia: A brief review. *Nutrition Journal,* 13(1), 1.

Bartlett, J. (2014). Childhood-onset schizophrenia: What do we really know? *Health Psychology and Behavioral Medicine,* 2(1), 735–747.

Baumgart, M., Snyder, H. M., Carrillo, M. C., Fazio, S., Kim, H., & Johns, H. (2015). Summary of the evidence on modifiable risk factors for cognitive decline and dementia: A population-based perspective. *Alzheimer's & Dementia,* 11(6), 718–726.

Beckett, M. W., Ardern, C. I., & Rotondi, M. A. (2015). A meta-analysis of prospective studies on the role of physical activity and the prevention of Alzheimer's disease in older adults. *BMC Geriatrics,* 15(1).

Benros, M. E., Sørensen, H. J., Nielsen, P. R., Nordentoft, M., Mortensen, P. B., & Petersen, L. (2015). The association between infections and general cognitive ability in young men—a nationwide study. *PLoS One,* 10(5), e0124005. doi:10.1371/journal.pone.0124005

Bevans, M., & Sternberg, E. M. (2012). Caregiving burden, stress, and health effects among family caregivers of adult cancer patients. *JAMA,* 307(4), 398–403.

Blazer, D. (2013). Neurocognitive disorders in DSM-5. *American Journal of Psychiatry Online.* doi/pdf/10.1176/appi.ajp.2013.13020179

Bond, G. R., & Drake, R. E. (2015). The critical ingredients of assertive community treatment. *World Psychiatry,* 14(2), 240–242.

Bora, E., & Pantelis, C. (2013). Theory of mind impairments in first-episode psychosis, individuals at ultra-high risk for psychosis and in first-degree relatives of schizophrenia: Systematic review and meta-analysis. *Schizophrenia Research,* 144(1), 31–36.

Bowie, C. R., McGurk, S. R., Mausbach, B., Patterson, T. L., & Harvey, P. D. (2012). Combined cognitive remediation and functional skills training for

schizophrenia: Effects on cognition, functional competence, and real-world behavior. *American Journal of Psychiatry,* 169(7), 710–718.

Bradford, E. E., Jentzsch, I., & Gomez, J. (2015). From self to social cognition: Theory of mind mechanisms and their relation to executive functioning. *Cognition,* 138, 21–34.

Blennow, K., & Zetterberg, H. (2013). The application of cerebrospinal fluid biomarkers in early diagnosis of Alzheimer disease. *Medical Clinics of North America,* 97(3), 369–376.

Brunzell, D. H., & McIntosh, J. M. (2012). Alpha7 nicotinic acetylcholine receptors modulate motivation to self-administer nicotine: implications for smoking and schizophrenia. *Neuropsychopharmacology,* 37(5), 1134–1143.

Budson, A. E., & Solomon, P. R. (2012). New diagnostic criteria for Alzheimer's disease and mild cognitive impairment for the practical neurologist. *Practical Neurology,* 12(2), 88–96.

Butterworth, B., & Kovas, Y. (2013). Understanding neurocognitive developmental disorders can improve education for all. *Science,* 340(6130), 300–305.

Cacioppo, J. T., & Cacioppo, S. (2014). Social relationships and health: The toxic effects of perceived social isolation. *Social and Personality Psychology Compass,* 8(2), 58–72.

Camargo, C., Justus, F., & Retzlaff, G. (2015). Effectiveness of reality orientation in the treatment of Alzheimer's disease (P6. 181). *Neurology,* 84(14 Supplement), P6–P181.

Carpenter, W. T., Frost, K. H., Whearty, K. M., & Strauss, G. P. (2016). Avolition, negative symptoms, and a clinical science journey and transition to the future. In M. Ling & W. D. Spaulding (Eds.), *The neuropsychopathology of schizophrenia* (pp. 133–158). New York, NY: Springer International.

Carter, K., Monaghan, S., O'Brien, J., Teodorczuk, A., Mosimann, U., & Taylor, J. P. (2015). Driving and dementia: A clinical decision pathway. *International Journal of Geriatric Psychiatry,* 30(2), 210–216.

Catts, V. S., Fung, S. J., Long., L. E., Joshi, D., Vercammen, A., Allen, K. M., . . . Shannon Weickert, C. S. (2013). Rethinking schizophrenia in the context of normal neurodevelopment. *Frontiers of Cellular Neuroscience* 7, 60.

Centers for Disease Control and Prevention. (2013). *The CDC Healthy Brain Initiative: Progress 2006-2011.* Atlanta, GA: Author.

Centers for Disease Control and Prevention. (2016). Facts about Down syndrome. Retrieved from https://www.cdc.gov/ncbddd/birthdefects/DownSyndrome.html

Chen, S., Shi, L., Liang, F., Xu, L., Desislava, D., Wu, Q., & Zhang, J. (2016). Exogenous melatonin for delirium prevention: A meta-analysis of randomized controlled trials. *Molecular Neurobiology,* 53(6), 4046–4053.

Cheng, H., Chang, C. C., Chang, Y. C., Lee, W. K., & Tzang, R. F. (2014). A pilot study: Association between minor physical anomalies in childhood and future mental problems. *Psychiatry Investigation*, 11(3), 228–231.

Chi, S., Yu, J. T., Tan, M. S., & Tan, L. (2014). Depression in Alzheimer's disease: Epidemiology, mechanisms, and management. *Journal of Alzheimer's Disease*, 42(3), 739–755.

Chia, S. C., Henry, J., Mok, Y. M., Honer, W. G., & Sim, K. (2015). Fatty acid and vitamin interventions in adults with schizophrenia: a systematic review of the current evidence. *Journal of Neural Transmission*, 122(12), 1721–1732.

Chou, P. H., Koike, S., Nishimura, Y., Kawasaki, S., Satomura, Y., Kinoshita, A., . . . Kasai, K. (2014). Distinct effects of duration of untreated psychosis on brain cortical activities in different treatment phases of schizophrenia: A multi-channel near-infrared spectroscopy study. *Progress in Neuro-Psychopharmacology and Biological Psychiatry*, 49, 63–69.

Clemmensen, L., Vernal, D. L., & Steinhausen, H. C. (2012). A systematic review of the long-term outcome of early onset schizophrenia. *BMC Psychiatry*, 12(1), 1.

Cole, M. G., Bailey, R., Bonnycastle, M., McCusker, J., Fung, S., Ciampi, A., . . . Bai, C. (2015). Partial and no recovery from delirium in older hospitalized adults: Frequency and baseline risk factors. *Journal of the American Geriatrics Society*, 63(11), 2340–2348.

Consensus of the Fragile X Clinical & Research Consortium on Clinical Practices. (2012). *Seizures in fragile X syndrome*. Retrieved from https://fragilex.org/wp-content/uploads/2012/08/Seizures-in-Fragile-X-Syndrome2012-Oct.pdf

Cordell, C. B., Borson, S., Boustani, M., Chodosh, J., Reuben, D., Verghese, J., . . . Medicare Detection of Cognitive Impairment Workgroup. (2013). Alzheimer's Association recommendations for operationalizing the detection of cognitive impairment during the Medicare Annual Wellness Visit in a primary care setting. *Alzheimers & Dementia*, 9(2), 141–145.

Crump, C., Winkleby, M. A., Sundquist, K., & Sundquist, J. (2013). Comorbidities and mortality in persons with schizophrenia: A Swedish national cohort study. *American Journal of Psychiatry*, 170(3), 324–333.

Dadich, A., Fisher, K. R., & Muir, K. (2013). How can non-clinical case management complement clinical support for people with chronic mental illness residing in the community? *Psychology, Health & Medicine*, 18(4), 482–489.

Damilou, A., Apostolakis, S., Thrapsanioti, E., Theleritis, C., & Smyrnis, N. (2016). Shared and distinct oculomotor function deficits in schizophrenia and obsessive compulsive disorder. *Psychophysiology*, 53(6), 796–805.

Davis, D. H., Kreisel, S. H., Terrera, G. M., Hall, A. J., Morandi, A., Boustani, M., . . . Brayne, C. (2013). The epidemiology of delirium: challenges and opportunities for population studies. *The American Journal of Geriatric Psychiatry*, 21(12), 1173–1189.

de Bruijn, R. F., Bos, M. J., Portegies, M. L., Hofman, A., Franco, O. H., Koudstaal, P. J., & Ikram, M. A. (2015). The potential for prevention of dementia across two decades: The prospective, population-based Rotterdam Study. *BMC Medicine*, 13(1), 1. doi:10.1186/s12916-015-0377-5

De Felice, F. G., & Ferreira, S. T. (2014). Inflammation, defective insulin signaling, and mitochondrial dysfunction as common molecular denominators connecting type 2 diabetes to Alzheimer disease. *Diabetes*, 63(7), 2262–2272.

Defrancesco, M., Marksteiner, J., Fleischhacker, W. W., & Blasko, I. (2015). Use of benzodiazepines in Alzheimer's disease: a systematic review of literature. *International Journal of Neuropsychopharmacology*, 18(10), pyv055.

De Lacy, N., & King, B. H. (2013). Revisiting the relationship between autism and schizophrenia: Toward an integrated neurobiology. *Annual Review of Clinical Psychology*, 9, 555–587.

D'Esposito, M., & Postle, B. R. (2015). The cognitive neuroscience of working memory. *Annual Review of Psychology*, 66, 115–142.

Docherty, N. M., Dinzeo, T. J., McCleery, A., Bell, E. K., Shakeel, M. K., & Moe, A. (2015). Internal versus external auditory hallucinations in schizophrenia: symptom and course correlates. *Cognitive Neuropsychiatry*, 20(3), 187–197.

Dold, M., & Leucht, S. (2014). Pharmacotherapy of treatment-resistant schizophrenia: a clinical perspective. *Evidence Based Mental Health*, 17(2), 33–37.

Dougall, N., Maayan, N., Soares-Weiser, K., McDermott, L. M., & McIntosh, A. (2015). Transcranial magnetic stimulation for schizophrenia. *Schizophrenia Bulletin*, 41(6), 1220–1222.

Driver, D. I., Gogtay, N., & Rapoport, J. L. (2013). Childhood onset schizophrenia and early onset schizophrenia spectrum disorders. *Child and Adolescent Psychiatric Clinics of North America*, 22(4), 539–555.

Durazzo, T. C., Mattsson, N., Weiner, M. W., & Alzheimer's Disease Neuroimaging Initiative. (2014). Smoking and increased Alzheimer's disease risk: A review of potential mechanisms. *Alzheimer's & Dementia*, 10(3), S122–S145.

Dzierba, A., Smithburger, P., Devlin, J., Swan, J., Kane-Gill, S., & Critical Care Pharmacotherapy Trials Network. (2015). 587: A national evaluation of ICU delirium identification, prevention and treatment practices. *Critical Care Medicine*, 43(12), 148.

Ek, M., Wicks, S., Svensson, A. C., Idring, S., & Dalman, C. (2015). Advancing paternal age and schizophrenia: the impact of delayed fatherhood. *Schizophrenia Bulletin*, 41(3), 708–714.

Emsley, R., Chiliza, B., Asmal, L., du Plessis, S., Phahladira, L., van Niekerk, E., . . . Harvey, B. H. (2014). A randomized, controlled trial of omega-3 fatty acids plus an antioxidant for relapse prevention after antipsychotic discontinuation in first-episode schizophrenia. *Schizophrenia Research*, 158(1), 230–235.

Espeland, M. A., Newman, A. B., Sink, K., Gill, T. M., King, A. C., Miller, M. E., . . . Reid, K. F. (2015). Associations between ankle-brachial index and cognitive function: Results from the Lifestyle Interventions and Independence for Elders Trial. *Journal of the American Medical Directors Association*, 16(8), 682–689.

Feil, N. (2014). Validation therapy with late-onset dementia populations. In G. M. M. Jones & B. L. L. Miensen (eds.), *Caregiving in dementia: Vol. 1: Research and Applications* (pp. 199–218). New York, NY: Routledge.

Feng, L., Chong, M. S., Lim, W. S., Lee, T. S., Kua, E. H., & Ng, T. P. (2015). Tea for Alzheimer prevention. *Journal of Prevention of Alzheimers Disease*, 2, 136–141.

Fick, D. M., Steis, M. R., Waller, J. L., & Inouye, S. K. (2013). Delirium superimposed on dementia is associated with prolonged length of stay and poor outcomes in hospitalized older adults. *Journal of Hospital Medicine*, 8(9), 500–505

Fineberg, A. M., & Ellman, L. M. (2013). Inflammatory cytokines and neurological and neurocognitive alterations in the course of schizophrenia. *Biological Psychiatry*, 73(10), 951–966.

Fleet, J., & Ernst, T. (2013) *Clinical Guideline: The prevention, recognition and management of delirium in adult patients*. Guys and St Thomas Foundation Trust, National Health Service, UK. Retrieved from https://www.gstt.nhs.uk/resources/our-services/acute-medicine-gi-surgery/elderly-care/delirium-adult-inpatients.pdf

Flegr, J. (2015). Schizophrenia and *Toxoplasma gondii*: An undervalued association? *Expert Review of Anti-infective Therapy*, 13(7), 817–820.

Fletcher, K. (2012). Dementia. In M. Boltz, E. Capezuti, T. T. Fulmer, D. Zwicker, & A. O'Meara (Eds.), *Evidence-based geriatric nursing protocols for best practice* (4th ed.). New York, NY: Springer. Retrieved from http://www.guideline.gov/content.aspx?id=4392

Fogel, B., & Greenberg, D. (2015). *Psychiatric care of the medical patient*. New York, NY: Oxford University Medical Press.

Frankenburg, F. (2015). *Schizophrenia: pathophysiology*. Retrieved from http://emedicine.medscape.com/article/288259-overview#a3

Frans, E., MacCabe, J. H., & Reichenberg, A. (2015). Advancing paternal age and psychiatric disorders. *World Psychiatry*, 14(1), 91–93.

Freberg, L. A. (2016). *Discovering behavioral neuroscience: An introduction to biological psychology* (3rd ed.). Boston, MA: Cengage Learning.

Friedman, N. P., Miyake, A., Altamirano, L. J., Corley, R. P., Young, S. E., Rhea, S. A., & Hewitt, J. K. (2016). Stability and change in executive function abilities from late adolescence to early adulthood: A longitudinal twin study. *Developmental Psychology*, 52(2), 326–340.

Funahashi, S., & Andreau, J. M. (2013). Prefrontal cortex and neural mechanisms of executive function. *Journal of Physiology—Paris*, 107(6), 471–482.

Fusar-Poli, P., Papanastasiou, E., Stahl, D., Rocchetti, M., Carpenter, W., Shergill, S., & McGuire, P. (2015). Treatments of negative symptoms in schizophrenia: meta-analysis of 168 randomized placebo-controlled trials. *Schizophrenia Bulletin*, 41(4), 892–899.

Fusar-Poli, P., Yung, A. R., McGorry, P., & Van Os, J. (2014). Lessons learned from the psychosis high-risk state: Towards a general staging model of prodromal intervention. *Psychological Medicine*, 44(01), 17–24.

Gaddes, W. H. (2013). *Learning disabilities and brain function: A neuropsychological approach*. New York, NY: Springer Science & Business Media.

Gerlinger, G., Hauser, M., Hert, M., Lacluyse, K., Wampers, M., & Correll, C. U. (2013). Personal stigma in schizophrenia spectrum disorders: A systematic review of prevalence rates, correlates, impact and interventions. *World Psychiatry*, 12(2), 155–164.

Giovanoli, S., Engler, H., Engler, A., Richetto, J., Voget, M., Willi, R., . . . Meyer, U. (2013). Stress in puberty unmasks latent neuropathological consequences of prenatal immune activation in mice. *Science*, 339(6123), 1095–1099.

Goldman, J. S., Hahn, S. E., Catania, J. W., Larusse-Eckert, S., Butson, M. B., Rumbaugh, M., . . . Bird, T. (2011). Genetic counseling and testing for Alzheimer disease: Joint practice guidelines of the American College of Medical Genetics and the National Society of Genetic Counselors. *Genetics in Medicine*, 13(6), 597–605.

González-Reyes, R. E., Aliev, G., Ávila-Rodrigues, M., & Barreto, G. E. (2016). Alterations in glucose metabolism on cognition: A possible link between diabetes and dementia. *Current Pharmaceutical Design*, 22(7), 812–818.

Gühne, U., Weinmann, S., Arnold, K., Becker, T., & Riedel-Heller, S. G. (2015). S3 guideline on psychosocial therapies in severe mental illness: evidence and recommendations. *European Archives of Psychiatry and Clinical Neuroscience, 265*(3), 173–188.

Han, J. H., Wilson, A., Vasilevskis, E. E., Shintani, A., Schnelle, J. F., Dittus, R. S., . . . Ely, E. W. (2013). Diagnosing delirium in older emergency department patients: Validity and reliability of the delirium triage screen and the brief confusion assessment method. *Annals of Emergency Medicine, 62*(5), 457–465.

Hanssen, M., van der Werf, M., Verkaaik, M., Arts, B., Myin-Germeys, I., van Os, J., . . . Outcome in Psychosis study group. (2015). Comparative study of clinical and neuropsychological characteristics between early-, late and very-late-onset schizophrenia-spectrum disorders. *American Journal of Geriatric Psychiatry, 23*(8), 852–862.

Hartshorne, J. K.,& Germine, L. T. (2015). When does cognitive functioning peak? The asynchronous rise and fall of different cognitive abilities across the life span. *Psychological Science, 26*(4), 433–443.

Harvard University Center on the Developing Child. (2016). *Brain architecture.* Retrieved from http://developingchild.harvard.edu/science/key-concepts/brain-architecture/

Hayempour, B. J., Cohen, S., Newberg, A., & Alavi, A. (2013). Neuromolecular imaging instrumentation demonstrating dysfunctional brain function in schizophrenic patients. *Journal of Alzheimer's Disease and Parkinsonism, 3,* 114. doi:10.4172/2161-0460.1000114

Helgason, C., & Sarris, J. (2013). Mind-body medicine for schizophrenia and psychotic disorders: a review of the evidence. *Clinical Schizophrenia & Related Psychoses, 7*(3), 138-148.

Henry, J., & Sherwin, B. (2012) Hormones and cognitive functioning during late pregnancy and postpartum: A longitudinal study. *Behavioral Neuroscience, 126*(1), 73–85. http://dx.doi.org/10.1037/a0025540

Herdman, T. H. & Kamitsuru, S. (Eds) *Nursing Diagnoses—Definitions and Classification 2015–2017.* Copyright © 2014, 1994–2014 NANDA International. Used by arrangement with John Wiley & Sons, Inc. Companion website: www.wiley.com/go/nursingdiagnoses

Hommer, R. E., & Swedo, S. E. (2015). Schizophrenia and autism—Related disorders. *Schizophrenia Bulletin,* sbu188.

Horváth, S., & Mirnics, K. (2014). Immune system disturbances in schizophrenia. *Biological Psychiatry, 75*(4), 316–323.

Hosenbocus, S., & Chahal, R. (2012). A review of executive function deficits and pharmacological management in children and adolescents. *Journal of the Canadian Academy of Child and Adolescent Psychiatry, 21*(3), 223–229.

Hu, W., MacDonald, M. L., Elswick, D. E., & Sweet, R. A. (2015). The glutamate hypothesis of schizophrenia: Evidence from human brain tissue studies. *Annals of the New York Academy of Sciences, 1338*(1), 38–57.

Huang, J. (2013). Delirium. In *Merck Manual Professional Version.* Retrieved from http://www.merckmanuals.com/professional/neurologic-disorders/delirium-and-dementia/delirium

Hui, C. L., Chiu, C. P., Li, Y. K., Law, C. W., Chang, W. C., Chan, S. K., . . . Chen, E. Y. (2015). The effect of paternal age on relapse in first-episode schizophrenia. *Canadian Journal of Psychiatry, 60*(8), 346–353.

Intlekofer, K. A., & Cotman, C. W. (2013). Exercise counteracts declining hippocampal function in aging and Alzheimer's disease. *Neurobiology of Disease, 57,* 47–55.

Jack, C. R., & Holtzman, D. M. (2013). Biomarker modeling of Alzheimer's disease. *Neuron, 80*(6), 1347–1358. doi:10.1016/j.neuron.2013.12.003

Jaffe, A. E., Eaton, W. W., Straub, R. E., Marenco, S., & Weinberger, D. R. (2014). Paternal age, de novo mutations and schizophrenia. *Molecular Psychiatry, 19*(3), 274.

Jauhar, S., McKenna, P. J., Radua, J., Fung, E., Salvador, R., & Laws, K. R. (2014). Cognitive-behavioural therapy for the symptoms of schizophrenia: Systematic review and meta-analysis with examination of potential bias. *British Journal of Psychiatry, 204*(1), 20–29.

Jeste, D. V., & Maglione, J. E. (2013). Treating older adults with schizophrenia: challenges and opportunities. *Schizophrenia Bulletin,* sbt043.

Johnson, V. E., Stewart, W., & Smith, D. H. (2013). Axonal pathology in traumatic brain injury. *Experimental Neurology.* doi:10.1016/j.expneurol.2012.01.013

Jones, K. L., Jones, M. C., & Del Campo, M. (2013). *Smith's recognizable patterns of human malformation.* St. Louis, MO: Elsevier Health Sciences.

Kalish, V. B., Gillham, J. E., & Unwin, B. K. (2014). Delirium in older persons: Evaluation and management. *American Family Physician, 90*(3), 150–158.

Keefe, R. S., & Harvey, P. D. (2012). Cognitive impairment in schizophrenia. In M. A. Geyer & G. Gross (Eds.), *Novel antischizophrenia treatments* (pp. 11–37). Berlin, Germany: Springer.

Kelleher, I., Lynch, F., Harley, M., Molloy, C., Roddy, S., Fitzpatrick, C., & Cannon, M. (2012). Psychotic symptoms in adolescence index risk for suicidal behavior: Findings from 2 population-based case-control clinical interview studies. *Archives of General Psychiatry, 69*(12), 1277–1283.

Khakpai, F., Nasehi, M., & Zarrindast, M. (2016). The role of NMDA receptors of the medial septum and dorsal hippocampus on memory acquisition. *Pharmacology Biochemistry and Behavior, 143,* 18–25.

Khan, A. (2013). *The amyloid hypothesis and potential treatments for Alzheimer's disease.* Retrieved from http://www.alzheimers.org.uk/site/scripts/documents_info.php?documentID=383&pageNumber=6

Kim, J. W., Lee, D. Y., Lee, B. C., Jung, M. H., Kim, H., Choi, Y. S., & Choi, I. G. (2012). Alcohol and cognition in the elderly: A review. *Psychiatry Investigation, 9*(1), 8–16.

Kirkbride, J. B., Susser, E., Kundakovic, M., Kresovich, J. K., Davey Smith, G., & Relton, C. L. (2012). Prenatal nutrition, epigenetics and schizophrenia risk: Can we test causal effects? *Epigenomics, 4*(3), 303–315.

Kirkpatrick, B., & Miller, B. J. (2013). Inflammation and schizophrenia. *Schizophrenia Bulletin, 39*(6), 1174–1179.

Koen, J. D., & Yonelinas, A. P. (2014). The effects of healthy aging, amnestic mild cognitive impairment, and Alzheimer's disease on recollection and familiarity: A meta-analytic review. *Neuropsychology Review, 24*(3), 332–354.

Kundakovic, M. (2014). Postnatal risk environments, epigenetics, and psychosis: Putting the pieces together. *Social Psychiatry and Psychiatric Epidemiology, 49*(10), 1535–1536.

Kurtz, M. M., & Richardson, C. L. (2012). Social cognitive training for schizophrenia: a meta-analytic investigation of controlled research. *Schizophrenia Bulletin, 38*(5), 1092–1104.

Lancaster, K., Carter, C. S., Pournajafi-Nazarloo, H., Karaoli, T., Lillard, T. S., Jack, A., . . . Connelly, J. J. (2015). Plasma oxytocin explains individual differences in neural substrates of social perception. *Frontiers in Human Neuroscience, 9,* 132. doi:10.3389/fnhum.2015.00132.

Laurens, K. R., Luo, L., Matheson, S. L., Carr, V. J., Raudino, A., Harris, F., & Green, M. J. (2015). Common or distinct pathways to psychosis? A systematic review of evidence from prospective studies for developmental risk factors and antecedents of the schizophrenia spectrum disorders and affective psychoses. *BMC Psychiatry, 15*(1), 205.

Laursen, T. M., Munk-Olsen, T., & Vestergaard, M. (2012). Life expectancy and cardiovascular mortality in persons with schizophrenia. *Current Opinion in Psychiatry, 25*(2), 83–88.

Learning Disabilities Association of America. (2016). *Types of learning disabilities.* Retrieved from http://ldaamerica.org/types-of-learning-disabilities

Lebedev, A. V., Beyer, M. K., Fritze, F., Westman, E., Ballard, C., & Aarsland, D. (2014). Cortical changes associated with depression and antidepressant use in Alzheimer and Lewy body dementia: An MRI surface-based morphometric study. *American Journal of Geriatric Psychiatry, 22*(1), 4–13.

Lee, C. W. S., Lin, C. L., Sung, F. C., Liang, J. A., & Kao, C. H. (2016). Antidepressant treatment and risk of dementia: A population-based, retrospective case-control study. *Journal of Clinical Psychiatry, 77*(1), 117–122.

Lerner J. & Johns, B. (2014). *Learning disabilities and related disabilities* (13th ed.). Boston, MA: Cengage Learning.

Light, G., Greenwood, T. A., Swerdlow, N. R., Calkins, M. E., Freedman, R., Green, M. F., . . . Olincy, A. (2014). Comparison of the heritability of schizophrenia and endophenotypes in the COGS-1 Family Study. *Schizophrenia Bulletin, 40*(6), 1404–1411.

Lim, S., Han, C. E., Uhlhaas, P. J., & Kaiser, M. (2015). Preferential detachment during human brain development: Age-and sex-specific structural connectivity in diffusion tensor imaging (DTI) data. *Cerebral Cortex, 25*(6), 1477–1489.

Livingston, G., Kelly, L., Lewis-Holmes, E., Baio, G., Morris, S., Patel, N., . . . Cooper, C. (2014). A systematic review of the clinical effectiveness and cost-effectiveness of sensory, psychological and behavioural interventions for managing agitation in older adults with dementia. *Health Technology and Assessment, 18*(39), 1–226, v–vi.

LoBue, C., Wilmoth, K., Cullum, C. M., Rossetti, H. C., Lacritz, L. H., Hynan, L. S., . . . Womack, K. B. (2015). Traumatic brain injury history is associated with earlier age of onset of frontotemporal dementia. *Journal of Neurology, Neurosurgery & Psychiatry.* doi:10.1136/jnnp-2015-311438

Loef, M., & Walach, H. (2013). Midlife obesity and dementia: Meta analysis and adjusted forecast of dementia prevalence in the United States and China. *Obesity, 21*(1), E1–E5.

Logan, D. M., Hill, K. R., Jones, R., Holt-Lunstad, J., & Larson, M. J. (2014). How do memory and attention change with pregnancy and childbirth? A controlled longitudinal examination of neuropsychological functioning in pregnant and postpartum women. *Journal of Clinical and Experimental Neuropsychology, 36*(5), 528–539.

Loy, C. T., Schofield, P. R., Turner, A. M., & Kwok, J. B. (2014). Genetics of dementia. *Lancet, 383*(9919), 828–840.

Ma, W. J., Husain, M., & Bays, P. M. (2014). Changing concepts of working memory. *Nature Neuroscience, 17*(3), 347–356.

Mackowick, K. M., Barr, M. S., Wing, V. C., Rabin, R. A., Ouellet-Plamondon, C., & George, T. P. (2014).

Neurocognitive endophenotypes in schizophrenia: modulation by nicotinic receptor systems. *Progress in Neuro-Psychopharmacology and Biological Psychiatry, 52*, 79–85.

Maglione, J. E., Thomas, S. E., & Jeste, D. V. (2014). Late-onset schizophrenia: do recent studies support categorizing LOS as a subtype of schizophrenia? *Current Opinion in Psychiatry, 27*(3), 173.

Mansen, T., & Gabiola, J. (2015). Patient focused assessment: The art and science of data gathering. Boston, MA: Pearson.

Martínez-Gras, I., García-Sánchez, F., Guaza, C., Rodríguez-Jiménez, R., Andrés-Esteban, E., Palomo, T., . . . Borrell, J. (2012). Altered immune function in unaffected first-degree biological relatives of schizophrenia patients. *Psychiatry Research, 200*(2), 1022–1025.

Marx, G., & Gilon, C. (2014). The molecular basis of memory. Part 3: Tagging with "emotive" neurotransmitters. *Frontiers in Aging Neuroscience, 6*, 58.

McCance, K. L, & Huether S. E (2014). Pathophysiology: The biologic basis for disease in adults and children. London, UK: Mosby.

Medalia, A., & Saperstein, A. M. (2013). Does cognitive remediation for schizophrenia improve functional outcomes? *Current Opinion in Psychiatry, 26*(2), 151–157.

Moeschler, J. B., Shevell, M., Saul, R. A., Chen, E., Freedenberg, D. L., Hamid, R., . . . Tarini, B. A. (2014). Comprehensive evaluation of the child with intellectual disability or global developmental delays. *Pediatrics, 134*(3), e903–e918.

Moghaddam, B., & Javitt, D. (2012). From revolution to evolution: The glutamate hypothesis of schizophrenia and its implication for treatment. *Neuropsychopharmacology, 37*(1), 4–15.

Mueser, K. T., & Glynn, S. M. (2014). Have the potential benefits of CBT for severe mental disorders been undersold? *World Psychiatry, 13*(3), 253–256.

Mukandala, G., Tynana, R., Lanigan, S., & O'Connor, J. J. (2016). The effects of hypoxia and inflammation on synaptic signaling in the CNS. *Brain Sciences, 6*(1), 6. http://doi.org/10.3390/brainsci6010006

Mushtaq, G., Khan, J. A., & Kamal, M. A. (2014). Biological mechanisms linking Alzheimer's disease and type-2 diabetes mellitus. *CNS & Neurological Disorders-Drug Targets (Formerly Current Drug Targets-CNS & Neurological Disorders), 13*(7), 1192–1201.

Mushtaq, G., Khan, J. A., & Kamal, M. A. (2015). Impaired glucose metabolism in Alzheimer's disease and diabetes. *Enzyme Engineering 4*, 124.

National Human Genome Research Institute. (2016). *Learning about fragile X syndrome.* Retrieved from https://www.genome.gov/19518828/

National Institute for Neurological Disorders and Stroke. (2016). *NINDS dementia information page.* Retrieved from http://www.ninds.nih.gov/disorders/dementias/dementia.htm

National Institute of Mental Health. (2016). *Schizophrenia.* Retrieved from http://www.nimh.nih.gov/health/statistics/prevalence/schizophrenia.shtml

National Down Syndrome Society. (2012). Down syndrome facts. Retrieved from http://www.ndss.org/Down-Syndrome/Down-Syndrome-Facts/

National Institutes of Health. (2015). The changing brain in AD. Retrieved from https://www.nia.nih.gov/alzheimers/publication/part-2-what-happens-brain-ad/changing-brain-ad

National Organization on Fetal Alcohol Syndrome. (2014a). *FASD: What everyone should know.* Retrieved from https://www.nofas.org/wp-content/uploads/2014/08/Fact-sheet-what-everyone-should-know_old_chart-new-chart1.pdf

National Organization on Fetal Alcohol Syndrome. (2014b). *FASD identification.* Retrieved from https://www.nofas.org/wp-content/uploads/2014/05/FASD-identification.pdf

Nebhinani, N., Pareek, V., & Grover, S. (2014). Late-life psychosis: An overview. *Journal of Geriatric Mental Health, 1*(2), 60.

Oettingen, G., & Gollwitzer, P. (2015). *Self-regulation in adolescence.* New York, NY: Cambridge University Press.

Okusaga, O. O. (2014). Accelerated aging in schizophrenia patients: The potential role of oxidative stress. *Aging and disease, 5*(4), 256-262.

Osorio, R. S., Gumb, T., Pirraglia, E., Varga, A. W., Lu, S. E., Lim, J., . . . Mosconi, L. (2015). Sleep-disordered breathing advances cognitive decline in the elderly. *Neurology, 84*(19), 1964–1971.

Papadopoulos, T., Parrila, R., & Kirby, J. (Eds.). (2015). *Cognition, intelligence, and achievement: A tribute to J. P. Das.* Salt Lake City, UT: Academic Press.

Parveen, S., Robins, J., Griffiths, A. W., & Oyebode, J. R. (2015). *Dementia detectives: Busting the myths.* Retrieved from https://www.researchgate.net/profile/Sahdia_Parveen/publication/279883193_Dementia_Detectives_Busting_the_myths/links/559d145008ae9dcf264f0786.pdf

Pasinetti, G. M., Wang, J., Ho, L., Zhao, W., & Dubner, L. (2015). Roles of resveratrol and other grape-derived polyphenols in Alzheimer's disease prevention and treatment. *Biochimica et Biophysica Acta (BBA)—Molecular Basis of Disease, 1852*(6), 1202–1208.

Piaget, J. (1966). *Origins of intelligence in children.* New York, NY: Norton.

Piaget, J. (1972). *The child's conception of the world.* Totowa, NJ: Littlefield, Adams.

Pitschel-Walz, G., Leucht, S., Bäuml, J., Kissling, W., & Engel, R. R. (2004). The effect of family interventions on relapse and rehospitalization in schizophrenia: a meta-analysis. *Focus, 2*(1), 78–94.

Popovic, D., Benabarre, A., Crespo, J. M., Goikolea, J. M., González Pinto, A., Gutiérrez Rojas, L., . . . Vieta, E. (2014). Risk factors for suicide in schizophrenia: Systematic review and clinical recommendations. *Acta Psychiatrica Scandinavica, 130*(6), 418–426.

Potter, M. L., & Moller, M. D. (2016). *Psychiatric–mental health nursing: From suffering to hope.* Upper Saddle River, NJ: Pearson.

Prastaro, M., & Girotti, F. (2015). Extrapyramidal diseases: Hyperkinetic movement disorders—tics and Tourette syndrome. In *Prognosis of Neurological Diseases* (pp. 381–383). Milan, Italy: Springer.

Psychiatric Rehabilitation Association. (2016). *Certification.* Retrieved from http://www.psychrehabassociation.org/cprp-certification/why-certification

Rafii, M. S., & Aisen, P. S. (2015). Advances in Alzheimer's disease drug development. *BMC Medicine, 13*(1), 62.

Rapoport, J. L., Giedd, J. N., & Gogtay, N. (2012). Neurodevelopmental model of schizophrenia: update 2012. *Molecular Psychiatry, 17*(12), 1228–1238.

Reisberg, B., Monteiro, I., Torossian, C., Auer, S., Shulman, M. B., Ghimire, S., . . . Xu, J. (2014). The BEHAVE-AD Assessment System: A perspective, a commentary on new findings, and a historical review. *Dementia and Geriatric Cognitive Disorders, 38*(1–2), 89–146. http://doi.org/10.1159/000357839

Ren, W., Lui, S., Deng, W., Li, F., Li, M., Huang, X., . . . Gong, Q. (2013). Anatomical and functional brain abnormalities in drug-naive first-episode schizophrenia. *American Journal of Psychiatry, 170*(11), 1308–1316.

Ridge, P. G., Ebbert, M. T., & Kauwe, J. S. (2013). Genetics of Alzheimer's disease. *BioMed Research International.* Retrieved from https://www.hindawi.com/journals/bmri/2013/254954/

Ripke, S., Neale, B. M., Corvin, A., Walters, J. T., Farh, K. H., Holmans, P. A., . . . Pers, T. H. (2014). Biological insights from 108 schizophrenia-associated genetic loci. *Nature, 511*(7510), 421.

Roberts, D. L., Combs, D. R., Willoughby, M., Mintz, J., Gibson, C., Rupp, B., & Penn, D. L. (2014). A randomized, controlled trial of Social Cognition and Interaction Training (SCIT) for outpatients with schizophrenia spectrum disorders. *British Journal of Clinical Psychology, 53*(3), 281–298.

Robertson, A. G., Swanson, J. W., Lin, H., Easter, M. M., Frisman, L. K., & Swartz, M. S. (2015). Influence of criminal justice involvement and psychiatric diagnoses on treatment costs among adults with serious mental illness. *Psychiatric Services, 66*(9), 907–909.

Rooney, S., Qadir, M., Adamis, D., & McCarthy, G. (2014). Diagnostic and treatment practices of delirium in a general hospital. *Aging Clinical and Experimental Research, 26*(6), 625–633.

Rosen, T., Connors, S., Clark, S., Halpern, A., Stern, M. E., DeWald, J., . . . Flomenbaum, N. (2015). Assessment and management of delirium in older adults in the emergency department: Literature review to inform development of a novel clinical protocol. *Advanced Emergency Nursing Journal, 37*(3), 183–196.

Rosenberg, M. D., Finn, E. S., Scheinost, D., Papademetris, X., Shen, X., Constable, R. T., & Chun, M. M. (2015). A neuromarker of sustained attention from whole-brain functional connectivity. *Nature Neuroscience, 19*(1), 165–171.

Sattler, C., Toro, P., Schönknecht, P., & Schröder, J. (2012). Cognitive activity, education and socioeconomic status as preventive factors for mild cognitive impairment and Alzheimer's disease. *Psychiatry Research, 196*(1), 90–95.

Schieveld, J. N. M., Ista, E., Knoester, H., & Molag, M. L. (2015). Pediatric delirium: A practical approach. In J. M. Rey (Ed.), *IACAPAP e-textbook of child and adolescent mental health.* Geneva, Switzerland: International Association for Child and Adolescent Psychiatry and Allied Professions.

Schöttle, D., Schimmelmann, B. G., Karow, A., Ruppelt, F., Sauerbier, A. L., Bussopulos, A., . . . Nika, E. (2014). Effectiveness of integrated care including therapeutic assertive community treatment in severe schizophrenia spectrum and bipolar I disorders: the 24-month follow-up ACCESS II study. *Journal of Clinical Psychiatry, 75*(12), 1–478.

Schwartz, R. C., & Blankenship, D. M. (2014). Racial disparities in psychotic disorder diagnosis: A review of empirical literature. *World Journal of Psychiatry, 4*(4), 133.

Shaffer, D. R., & Kipp, K. (2014). *Developmental psychology: Childhood and adolescence* (9th ed.). Belmont, CA: Wadsworth, Cengage Learning.

Sivanandam, T. M., & Thakur, M. K. (2012). Traumatic brain injury: a risk factor for Alzheimer's disease. *Neuroscience & Biobehavioral Reviews, 36*(5), 1376–1381.

Smith, D. J., Langan, J., McLean, G., Guthrie, B., & Mercer, S. W. (2013). Schizophrenia is associated with excess multiple physical-health comorbidities but low levels of recorded cardiovascular disease in primary care: cross-sectional study. *BMJ Open, 3*(4), e002808.

Smith, R., Reichenberg, A., Kember, R., Buxbaum, J., Schalkwyk, L., Fernandes, C., & Mill, J. (2013). Advanced paternal age is associated with altered DNA methylation at brain-expressed imprinted loci in inbred mice: Implications for neuropsychiatric disease [Letter to the editor]. *Molecular Psychiatry, 18*, 635–636.

Solomon, S., Thilakan, P., & Jayakar, J. (2016) Prevalence, phenomenology and etiology of delirium in medically ill patients. *International Journal of Research in Medical Sciences, 4*(3), 920–925. doi:10.18203/2320-6012.ijrms20160543

Spector, R. E. (2017). *Cultural diversity in health and illness* (9th ed.). Hoboken, NJ: Pearson Education.

Stafford, M. R., Jackson, H., Mayo-Wilson, E., Morrison, A. P., & Kendall, T. (2013). Early interventions to prevent psychosis: systematic review and meta-analysis. *BMJ, 346*, f185.

Stahl, S. M., Morrissette, D. A., Citrome, L., Saklad, S. R., Cummings, M. A., Meyer, J. M., . . . Warburton, K. D. (2013). "Meta-guidelines" for the management of patients with schizophrenia. *CNS Spectrums, 18*(3), 150–162.

Steinberg, L. (2014, January). *Adolescence* (13th ed.) [VitalSource Bookshelf Online]. Retrieved from https://bookshelf.vitalsource.com/#/books/0077798287/

Störmer, V., Passow, S., Biesenack, J., & Li, S. (2012). Dopaminergic and cholinergic modulations of visual-spatial attention and working memory: Insights from molecular genetic research and implications for adult cognitive development. *Developmental Psychology, 48*(3), 875–889.

Sutterland, A., Dieleman, J., Storosum, J., Voordouw, B., Kroon, J., Veldhuis, J., . . . Sturkenboom, M. (2013). Annual incidence rate of schizophrenia and schizophrenia spectrum disorders in a longitudinal population-based cohort study. *Social Psychiatry and Psychiatric Epidemiology, 48*(9), 1357–1365.

Tandon, N., Shah, J., Keshavan, M. S., & Tandon, R. (2012). Attenuated psychosis and the schizophrenia prodrome: Current status of risk identification and psychosis prevention. *Neuropsychiatry, 2*(4), 345–353.

Tandon, R., Gaebel, W., Barch, D. M., Bustillo, J., Gur, R. E., Heckers, S., . . . Carpenter, W. (2013). Definition and description of schizophrenia in the DSM-5. *Schizophrenia Research, 150*(1), 3–10.

Thase, M. E., Kingdon, D., & Turkington, D. (2014). The promise of cognitive behavior therapy for treatment of severe mental disorders: A review of recent developments. *World Psychiatry, 13*(3), 244–250.

Thoma, P., & Daum, I. (2013). Comorbid substance use disorder in schizophrenia: A selective overview of neurobiological and cognitive underpinnings. *Psychiatry and Clinical Neurosciences, 67*(6), 367–383.

Tikka, S. K., Nizamie, S. H., Das, B., Katshu, M. Z. U. H., & Goyal, N. (2013). Increased spontaneous gamma power and synchrony in schizophrenia patients having higher minor physical anomalies. *Psychiatry Research, 207*(3), 164–172.

Torrey, E. F., Simmons, W., & Yolken, R. H. (2015). Is childhood cat ownership a risk factor for schizophrenia later in life? *Schizophrenia Research, 165*(1), 1–2.

Tsai, J., & Rosenheck, R. A. (2013). Psychiatric comorbidity among adults with schizophrenia: A latent class analysis. *Psychiatry Research, 210*(1), 16–20. http://doi.org/10.1016/j.psychres.2013.05.013

Tucker-Drob, E. M., Briley, D. A., & Harden, K. P. (2013). Genetic and environmental influences on cognition across development and context. *Current Directions in Psychological Science, 22*(5), 349–355.

Tullman, D. F., Fletcher, K., & Foreman, M. D. (2012a). Delirium: Prevention, early recognition, and treatment. In M. Boltz, E. Capezuti, T. T. Fulmer, D. Zwicker, & A. O'Meara (Eds.), *Evidence-based geriatric nursing protocols for best practice* (4th ed.). New York, NY: Springer. Retrieved from https://consultgeri.org/geriatric-topics/delirium

Tullman, D. F., Fletcher, K., & Foreman, M. D. (2012b). Consult Geri RN: Nursing Standard of Practice Protocol: Delirium. Available at https://consultgeri.org/geriatric-topics/delirium

Turner, D. T., van der Gaag, M., Karyotaki, E., & Cuijpers, P. (2014). Psychological interventions for psychosis: A meta-analysis of comparative outcome studies. *American Journal of Psychiatry, 171*(5), 523–538.

Valmaggia, L. R., Byrne, M., Day, F., Broome, M. R., Johns, L., Howes, O., . . . McGuire, P. K. (2015). Duration of untreated psychosis and need for admission in patients who engage with mental health services in the prodromal phase. *British Journal of Psychiatry, 207*(2), 130–134.

van Venrooij, J. A., Fluitman, S. B., Lijmer, J. G., Kavelaars, A., Heijnen, C. J., Westenberg, H. G., . . . Gispen-de Wied, C. C. (2012). Impaired neuroendocrine and immune response to acute stress in medication-naive patients with a first episode of psychosis. *Schizophrenia Bulletin, 38*(2), 272–279.

Varambally, S., Venkatasubramanian, G., & Gangadhar, B. N. (2012). Neurological soft signs in schizophrenia—The past, the present and the future. *Indian Journal of Psychiatry, 54*(1), 73.

Walder, D. J., Faraone, S. V., Glatt, S. J., Tsuang, M. T., & Seidman, L. J. (2014). Genetic liability, prenatal health, stress and family environment: Risk factors in the Harvard Adolescent Family High Risk for Schizophrenia Study. *Schizophrenia Research, 157*(1), 142–148.

Wang, C., Gao, S., Hendrie, H. C., Kesterson, J., Campbell, N. L., Shekhar, A., & Callahan, C. M. (2016). Antidepressant use in the elderly is associated with an increased risk of dementia. *Alzheimer Disease and Associated Disorders.*

Weickert, C. S., Weickert, T. W., Pillai, A., & Buckley, P. F. (2013). Biomarkers in schizophrenia: a brief conceptual consideration. *Disease Markers, 35*(1), 3–9.

Werner, P., Mittelman, M. S., Goldstein, D., & Heinik, J. (2012). Family stigma and caregiver burden in Alzheimer's disease. *The Gerontologist, 52*(1), 89–97.

Wu, Z., Guo, Z., Gearing, M., & Chen, G. (2014). Tonic inhibition in dentate gyrus impairs long-term potentiation and memory in an Alzheimer's disease model. *Nature Communications, 5*, 4159.

Wurtman, R. J. (2015). How anticholinergic drugs might promote Alzheimer's disease: More amyloid-β and less phosphatidylcholine. *Journal of Alzheimer's Disease, 46*(4), 983–987.

Wuwongse, S., Cheng, S. S. Y., Wong, G. T. H., Hung, C. H. L., Zhang, N. Q., Ho, Y. S., . . . Chang, R. C. C. (2013). Effects of corticosterone and amyloid-beta on proteins essential for synaptic function: Implications for depression and Alzheimer's disease. *Biochimica et Biophysica Acta (BBA)—Molecular Basis of Disease, 1832*(12), 2245–2256.

Yaffe, K., & Boustani, M. (2014). Benzodiazepines and risk of Alzheimer's disease [Editorial]. *BMJ, 349*, g5312. doi:http://dx.doi.org/10.1136/bmj.g5312

Zervas, I. M., Theleritis, C., & Soldatos, C. R. (2012). Using ECT in schizophrenia: A review from a clinical perspective. *World Journal of Biological Psychiatry, 13*(2), 96–105.

Zhang, H., Lu, Y., Liu, M., Zou, Z., Wang, L., Xu, F. Y., & Shi, X. Y. (2013). Strategies for prevention of postoperative delirium: a systematic review and meta-analysis of randomized trials. *Critical Care, 17*(2), R47.

Zimmermann, B. (2014). *Procedural memory: Definition and examples.* Retrieved from http://www.livescience.com/43595-procedural-memory.html

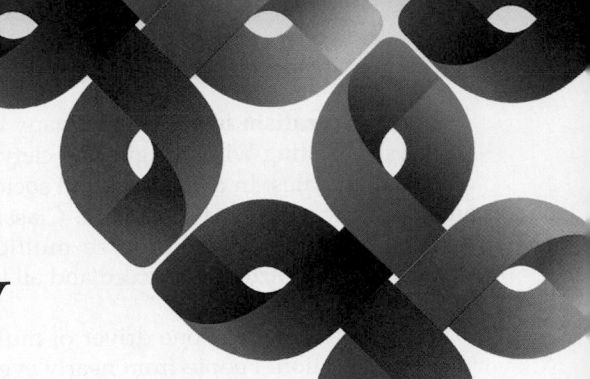

Module 24
Culture and Diversity

Module Outline and Learning Outcomes

The Concept of Culture and Diversity

Cultural Diversity

24.1 Describe the language used to describe cultural diversity.

Values and Beliefs

24.2 Analyze how values and beliefs are components of cultural diversity.

Disparities and Differences

24.3 Describe how cultural disparities and differences affect healthcare.

Concepts Related to Culture and Diversity

24.4 Outline the relationship between culture and diversity and other concepts.

Developing Cultural Competence

24.5 Analyze the need for developing cultural competence.

Nursing Process

24.6 Summarize the nursing process in the context of cultural competence.

>> The Concept of Culture and Diversity

Concept Key Terms

Acculturation, **1769**	Cultural	Enculturation, **1768**	Multiculturalism, **1766**	Social justice, **1769**
Ageism, **1772**	competence, **1776**	Ethnic groups, **1766**	Prejudice, **1778**	Stereotyping, **1769**
Alternative therapies, **1780**	Cultural groups, **1768**	Health	Race, **1770**	Subculture, **1765**
Assimilation, **1769**	Cultural humility, **1766**	disparity, **1773**	Racism, **1770**	Transgender, **1769**
Bias, **1770**	Cultural values, **1767**	Heterosexism, **1771**	Religion, **1774**	Vulnerable
Classism, **1770**	Culture, **1765**	Homophobia, **1771**	Sexism, **1770**	populations, **1773**
Complementary	Discrimination, **1765**	Intersex, **1769**	Sexual	Worldview, **1767**
therapies, **1780**	Diversity, **1765**	Minority, **1765**	orientation, **1771**	

Culture refers to the patterns of behavior and thinking that people living in social groups learn, develop, and share. The term **diversity** refers to the array of differences among individuals, groups, and communities. Today's nurses must be able to work with diverse populations of patients—patients of varying socioeconomic, cultural, and spiritual backgrounds and patients with varying values and belief systems. To be able to provide culturally aware nursing, nurses must examine their own cultural values and beliefs.

Cultural Diversity

Any discussion of culture and diversity must be informed by the terms and language that are part of that discussion. **Discrimination**, or the restriction of justice, rights, and privileges of individuals or minority groups, may occur when dominant groups reinforce their rules and regulations in a way that limits opportunities for others. A dominant group may be one that is dominant by reason of its numbers or as a result of having influence, power, money, and position to remain dominant while reinforcing rules and norms that benefit its own interests. The term **minority** usually refers to an individual or group of individuals who are outside the dominant group. Although demographics can vary from one area to another, in the United States, African Americans, Hispanics, and Native Americans are among those generally considered minority groups. **Subculture** is a term that refers to a group of people within a culture whose practices or beliefs are distinct or separate from the dominant or parent culture. Subculture is a term often defined more broadly and has been used to describe certain religious sects, ethnic groups, and even devotees of some genres of music or philosophy.

Multiculturalism is defined as many cultures and subcultures coexisting within a given society in which no one culture dominates. In a multicultural society, human differences are accepted and respected. Classrooms in an academic setting may be considered multicultural when all students are socialized to succeed and all learning styles are valued and understood.

In the United States, one driver of multiculturalism has been immigration. People from nearly every country in the world have come to the United States in search of a new way of life. Each year, approximately 1 million individuals obtain legal permanent resident status in the United States. The majority of those who immigrate are from Asian countries, primarily India (U.S. Department of Homeland Security, 2016).

Many individuals coming to America have sought freedom from an oppressive government. Others coming to our country have sought religious freedom, and still others freedom from poverty (**Figure 24–1 ≫**). In 2014, more than 1 million people came into the United States under legal status; of those, 96,066 claimed refugee status and 38,176 claimed asylum from political oppression (U.S. Department of Homeland Security, 2016). Many others come to the United States as refugees and claim family sponsorship. Nurses should take into consideration that some immigrants have fled such horrors as civil unrest, war, and oppression. Their psychologic scars may run deeper than the physical ones.

Each family or group of immigrants brings its own culture, adding to what has been described as the "melting pot" that is the United States. The image of a melting pot implies the assimilation of multiple ethnic groups and their cultural practices into a single national identity with national allegiance and values. However, as these groups become established in the American culture, part or all of their ethnic identity remains. Instead of a melting pot, the United States should be considered a salad bowl of different flavors or a mosaic of the unique qualities of the cultural groups, coming together to make one America.

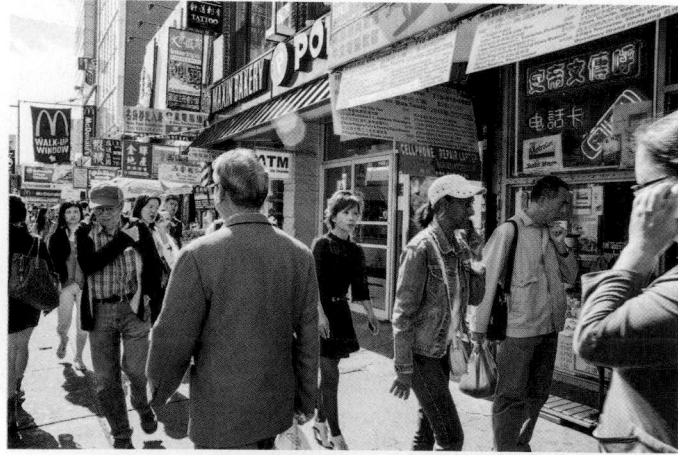

Source: sx70/iStock Editorial/Getty Images.

Figure 24–1 ≫ A crowded street in the Chinatown area of Flushing, Queens, New York. More than half a million Chinese-Americans live in New York City.

Members of each of these **ethnic groups** have common characteristics, including nationality, language, values, and customs, and they share a cultural heritage. Examples of ethnic groups are the large Cuban American population living in and around Miami, Florida; the Lakota Sioux, one of three major ethnic groups that make up the Great Sioux Nation; and the Hmong populations living in western North Carolina and in the Minneapolis-Saint Paul area in Minnesota.

In addition to different cultural and ethnic groups, individuals in the United States belong to one or more races. The U.S. Census Bureau (2013) identifies the following races:

- White
- Black or African American
- American Indian or Alaska Native
- Asian
- Native Hawaiian or Other Pacific Islander

Individuals of Hispanic, Latino, or Spanish origin may identify as members of any race.

Cultural, ethnic, racial, and other differences make nursing care both a privilege and a challenge. Nurses who are able to develop cultural competence and practice evidence-based care that is relevant to all of their patients will gain confidence in their abilities and greater personal benefit from their work with individual patients. A culturally competent practice begins with gaining a greater understanding of the differing values and beliefs of others (**Box 24–1 ≫**) and recognizing how these differing values and beliefs affect patients in all aspects of providing care.

Box 24–1
Nurses' Self-Awareness and Cultural Humility

Professional nurses must possess self-awareness. Self-awareness is critical to developing sensitivity to differences while supporting a sense of cultural humility rather than superiority over others. **Cultural humility** is the "ability to maintain an interpersonal stance that is other-oriented (or open to the other) in relation to aspects of cultural identity that are most important to the [person]" (Hook et al., 2013, p. 2)

As a nursing student, you may find your personal values to be in conflict with professional values. For example, you may find yourself uncomfortable with a certain ethnic group or religious faith. Yet a nurse, or any healthcare provider, cannot refuse to care for a person on the basis of cultural identity. Instead, your profession calls you to practice cultural humility, realizing that the person needs care, not judgment.

Following the June 2016 Orlando club shooting in which 49 people died and 53 others were wounded, one of the surgeons who was on duty the night of the shooting noted that he treated dozens of wounded people that night. He didn't know if any given patient was gay or straight, Hispanic or Black. He just knew that they needed care (Itkowitz, 2016). Similarly, military nurses have to care for wounded enemy combatants. Both nursing and military ethical codes require that enemy detainees are cared for without bias (Thompson et al., 2014). These examples illustrate the essence of cultural humility.

Values and Beliefs

Culture includes a society's values, beliefs, assumptions, principles, myths, legends, and norms. People living within a culture typically share many of the prevailing society's values and beliefs. People use these values and beliefs to help them define meaning, identify acceptable behaviors, choose emotional reactions, and determine appropriate actions in given situations. Values and belief systems are part of a culture, as are family relationships and roles. To understand patient behaviors in more depth, a nurse must identify which cultures are prevalent demographically in a given area, learn more about those cultures by reading or attending a class about them, and apply that knowledge and experience when providing patient care.

Values reflect an underlying system of beliefs. **Cultural values** describe preferred ways of behaving or thinking that are sustained over time and used to govern or guide a cultural group's actions and decisions. When people live together in a society, cultural values often determine the rules people live by each and every day. These rules may be variously stated, but they basically address similar values. Examples of some rules in Western culture (which usually refers to North America and parts of Europe) may include the following:

- Don't steal from others.
- Respect other people's property.
- Don't hurt others.
- Don't cheat on spouse or significant other.
- Share your food and clothing with those who are in need.
- Speak truthfully based on what you see.
- Respect your elders for their wisdom and experience.
- Respect God or a higher power.
- Respect nature and your environment.

Cultural characteristics include observable behaviors as well as the unseen values that influence those behaviors. Cultural practices have meanings that give the group its worldview and that reflects the social organization of the culture as a whole. The organization of a culture or society includes the following elements:

- **A physical element.** The geographic area in which a society is located
- **An infrastructure element.** The framework of the systems and processes that keep a society functioning
- **A behavioral element.** The way people in a society act and react to each other
- **A cultural element.** All the values, beliefs, assumptions, and norms that make up a code of conduct for acceptable behaviors within a society.

Each culture has its own worldview or understanding of the world. A **worldview** refers to how the people in a culture perceive ideas and attitudes about the world, other people, and life in general. A culture's worldview supports its overall *belief system*, which is developed to explain the mysteries of the universe and of life that each society tries to understand:

- What is the meaning of life?
- How do individuals know their purpose in life?
- What is reality?
- How much can be known about values and beliefs?
- Is there a God or power beyond me?
- How was the universe created?
- What happens after death?
- How do we care for the sick?

A cultural belief system influences an individual's decisions and actions in society regarding everything from preparing food and caring for the sick to rituals of death and burial. Scientific and medical advancements may or may not impact a culture's belief systems. Belief systems differ in every culture. The beliefs of a society are passed from generation to generation by word of mouth and by rituals, such as reading certain stories or books on holidays (**Figure 24–2 »**). In many cases, cultural practices are rooted in the individual's religious faith or practices (see the module on Spirituality). Children learn the belief system of their culture from parents and other family members who teach them any number of values and beliefs, including those about "right or wrong." Differing opinions may originate from religious beliefs or social conditions. People make decisions about "right or wrong," and as things change, people adapt and the culture evolves.

Belief systems are based on people's experiences and exposures to differences found in our world. As people's knowledge and understanding grow, their belief systems expand. Knowing why we believe what we believe builds self-awareness and understanding of differences in our own beliefs compared with the beliefs of others.

Culturally based beliefs and traditions can affect the course and outcome of disease and illness. Healthcare

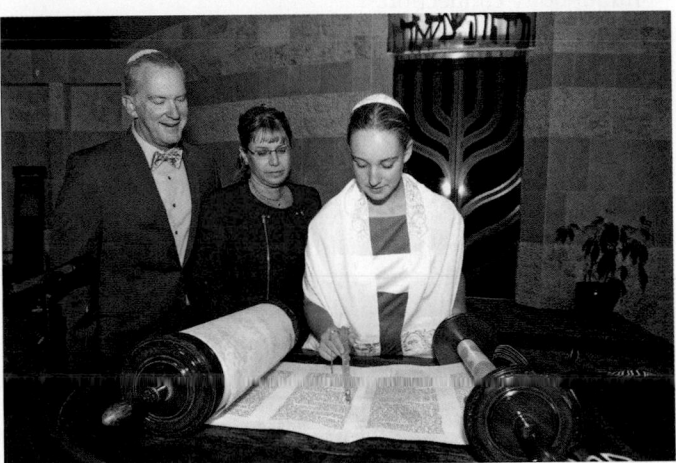

Source: 3bugsmom/iStock/Getty Images.

Figure 24–2 » Cultures try to understand and give meaning to life through spiritual beliefs, social values, and acceptable behaviors. In this picture, a 12-year-old girl is seen reading the Torah with her parents as she is acknowledged as a Bat Mitzvah, a Jewish adult.

TABLE 24–1 Examples of Differences in Core Beliefs

North American and Western Cultures	South American and Eastern Cultures
Health is viewed by many as the absence of disease.	Health is a state of harmony that encompasses the mind, body, and spirit.
Use of specialty practitioners (e.g., pediatricians, obstetricians)	Preference for respected healers from the culture of origin (e.g., herbalists, midwives, curanderos)
Recognition that food affects bio-physical processes, functions	Belief that food can restore imbalances
Independence, individualism, freedom are valued	Interdependence with family, community, and group acceptance are valued
Emphasis on use of modern (Western) healthcare practices to maintain or treat health issues	Emphasis on traditional methods of maintaining, protecting, and restoring health

Source: Based on Spector, R. E. (2017). *Cultural diversity in health and illness* (9th ed.). Hoboken, NJ: Pearson Education.

providers and patients bring their respective cultural backgrounds and expectations to each interaction. These differences can impact both the expectations and practices of the patient and the provision of services by nurses and other healthcare professionals. Some of these many differences are listed in **Table 24–1 》**.

Cultural differences can present barriers to necessary care. Some areas in which barriers can arise include the following (Spector, 2017):

- The importance, or lack of importance, of family members' involvement in managing illness and disease
- Lack of trust in the healthcare system and providers
- The belief that illnesses are not linked to scientific pathophysiology
- Refusal of modern healthcare providers to believe the mind–body connection
- Fear or denial of death or life after death
- Cultural assumptions about disease and illness that may influence the presentation of symptoms or the response to treatments.

Many cultures will not continue treatments and medications once they feel well (Carteret, n.d.). This is particularly true when discussing terminal illness and dying (Rollins & Huack, 2015). Although cultural beliefs and behaviors change over the years as a cultural group adapts to new ideas and conditions, some individuals may retain traditional behaviors and thinking and continue to follow the beliefs and practices as always. Tension can arise when different health belief systems conflict with each other. The result may be anxiety, anger, or fear. The healthcare provider may reduce a patient's discomfort and promote trust by showing a nonjudgmental attitude of respect. A nurse must also recognize the common defense mechanisms such as anger, avoidance, denial, intellectualization, or projection that may be used when an individual feels threatened (Berman & Snyder, 2012). See the module on Stress and Coping for information about defense mechanisms.

Professional nurses work with and care for people who have differing values and beliefs. It is important for nurses to understand how their own cultural beliefs and practices inform who they are as nurses, in part to strengthen their own value systems but also to ensure they are sufficiently self-aware to keep from projecting their own beliefs and values onto their patients.

Cultural Transmission

A society is a group of people who share a common culture, rules of behavior, and basic social organization. Culture is transmitted, or learned and shared, by people living together in a society. Cultural characteristics, such as customs, beliefs, values, language, and socialization patterns, are passed from generation to generation. **Cultural groups** can be categorized around racial, ethnic, religious, or socially common practice patterns. Race, however, does not equate with culture. Cultural groups often share common characteristics such as language, customs, beliefs, and values (Purnell, 2014; Spector, 2017). See **Box 24–2 》**.

Culture is transmitted from one generation to the next through language, material objects, rituals, customs, institutions, and art. Through the use of a common language, people learn how to live by the rules governing the society and how to earn money or trade goods or services to meet basic needs, such as food and shelter. Culture can influence everything the members of a society think and do.

Enculturation, or cultural transmission, is exemplified by a process children use to learn cultural characteristics from adults. These characteristics are often normalized, meaning that certain characteristics are used to define acceptable rules and procedures of behaviors. People biologically inherit physical traits and behavioral instincts, but they socially inherit cultural characteristics. An individual learns culture from other people in a society. Enculturation occurs in families until the children are ready to leave and establish their own values, beliefs, and practices through exposure to other cultural or societal practices through work, marriage, or higher education. However, enculturation may continue

Box 24–2
Cultural Characteristics

- History of origin
- Holiday customs
- Styles of dress
- General worldview
- Religious beliefs and practices
- Birth and death rituals and practices
- Food preferences and eating patterns
- Values
- Roles and patterns of relationships
- Leadership structure
- Health and illness beliefs and behaviors
- Social systems
- Concept of time
- Concept of personal space
- Gestures and facial expressions
- Concept of self
- Common language

among family members who live close to each other, celebrate religious holidays together, or otherwise work to maintain the culture within their family and limit their exposure to cultural differences. The great variety of cultural characteristics provides a broader perspective of cultural differences and respect.

People in a society have cultural characteristics that are embedded in art, music, food, religion, and traditions. Because culture is adaptive, these characteristics may be modified over the years as people use culture to adjust to changes in the world around them. Cultural behaviors are learned by:

- Observing others' actions
- Hearing instructions on what behaviors are right or wrong
- Imitating others doing a behavior
- Getting reinforcement (either positive or negative) for enacting a behavior
- Internalizing behaviors
- Spontaneously doing the behaviors without thinking about it

Different societies can come together and share or exchange cultures as well. People may evolve from one cultural group to another. **Assimilation** is the process of adapting to and integrating characteristics of the dominant culture as one's own. People typically benefit by exchanging ideas, natural resources, and goods. **Acculturation** is the process of not only adapting to another culture but also accepting the majority group's culture as one's own. Because culture is complex, members of a cultural group may engage in many behaviors and habits unconsciously, making them difficult to explain to others. Sometimes assimilation and acculturation are implicit and covert, whereas other times assimilation can be overt and coercive.

As individuals go through the process of acculturation, they may choose to discard some practices from their culture of origin in exchange for practices of the dominant culture. Therefore, nurses need to ask appropriate questions to assess individual cultural practices rather than make assumptions. For example, some patients of Chinese background may be practicing Buddhists who prefer traditional Chinese practices such as herbs and acupuncture; others may belong to a different faith and completely embrace Western medicine; while still others may blend practices in ways that make sense to them. Careful assessment of the individual patient is necessary to avoid making assumptions and stereotyping.

Diversity

Cultural differences are not the only hallmarks of diversity. Gender, race, class, sexual orientation, and age are just a few of the differences among individuals living in the United States. In many instances, these factors carry important implications for nursing. For example, African American women are at greater risk for heart disease than any other single population; older adults are at greater risk for injury due to falls; and children are at greater risk for accidental injury. Nurses must be prepared to work with each individual who walks in the door, regardless of that individual's personal background.

The concept of **social justice** recognizes that in society, not all groups are treated equally. Nursing has a long history and current mission to promote social justice by promoting a balance among groups in the sharing of resources, rights, and responsibilities (National League of Nursing, n.d.). Using a lens of social justice enables individuals and organizations to follow a code of ethics that promotes equitable distribution of resources and seeks equitable rights for all individuals, thus providing advocacy for people who lack access to resources. Culturally competent nurses should respect and advocate for human dignity. Stereotyping, prejudice, and discrimination can threaten the delivery of healthcare services and adversely affect patient outcomes. Nurses need to understand and recognize these attitudes in themselves and others in order to reduce their effects on the patients they serve. To overcome barriers to multiculturalism, nurses must have a deep understanding of vulnerable patients who are impacted by racism, sexism, classism, and heterosexism.

Gender

Traditionally gender has been dichotomized into two groups: men and women. However, it is now known that some people do not fit neatly into these categories of gender. **Intersex** is a general term used for a variety of conditions in which an individual is born with a reproductive or sexual anatomy that does not seem to fit the typical definitions of female or male (Intersex Society of North America [ISNA], n.d; Vanderbilt University, 2017). The term **transgender** refers to individuals who do not identify with the gender assigned to their body. *Genderqueer* or *gender nonconforming* are terms adapted by those who don't identify with either male or female; rather, they identify as both (Hein & Levitt, 2014). For example, an individual who identifies as transgender may have typical female anatomy but feel like a male and seek to become male by presenting as male and taking hormones or electing to have gender reassignment surgeries. A genderqueer person might have feelings of being both male and female.

Differences between men and women go beyond anatomy and physiology and cultural or social definitions. Compared to women, men typically are less verbal and more action oriented and have stronger skills in logic, mathematics, and coordination; women tend to be more skilled in languages, perceiving and responding to others' needs, and the arts. However, these are general tendencies and taking them at face value may lead to **stereotyping**. Stereotyping is an overgeneralization of group characteristics that reinforces societal biases and distorts individual characteristics (Grandbois & Sanders, 2012). Even within genders, individual diversity is expected; for example, some women may be highly coordinated, mathematically skilled, and uninterested in the arts. No conclusion about an individual can ever be drawn based on a simple term such as *woman* or *man*.

The genders also differ in access to and control over resources and decision-making power in the family and community. The extent of these differences is often cultural. Gender roles, often in interaction with socioeconomic circumstances, influence exposure to health risks, access to health information and services, health outcomes, and the social and economic consequences of ill health. This can be demonstrated by viewing the differences in mortality and morbidity between men and women of different cultures as well as their involvement in health prevention and health promotion programs. Therefore, nurses must recognize the root causes of gender inequities when designing a nursing plan of care. To obtain positive outcomes, health promotion and disease prevention and treatment need to address gender differences. For example, millions of women are injured as the result of spousal or significant other abuse, but the magnitude and health consequences of interpersonal violence against women have often been neglected in both research and policy.

Generally, there seems to be an assumption that interventions will be just as effective for men as for women. Many health promotion programs may be gender-blind and based on research that neither accounted for nor controlled for the gender of the study participants. Until the 1990s, many medications were tested only on White men, with no consideration that women or people of other ethnicities respond differently. Only in the mid-1990s did pharmaceutical companies begin to look at pharmacokinetic differences between males and females. Understanding the differences in responses between genders has led to research on how drugs affect women as well as those from different races and cultural backgrounds. As a result, scientists are finding that some drugs are more effective for women while others are more effective for men. In addition to the way in which men and women respond to health promotion, they also display different needs with regard to their response to the same diagnosis. For example, the traditional symptom of crushing chest pain as a primary indicator of myocardial infarction has been found to be primarily a male response. Women with myocardial infarction are more likely to experience extreme fatigue that extends to pain in the jaw, back, or shoulder if not treated early. Biological differences such as genetics, hormones, and metabolic influences combine to play a part in shaping different symptoms as well as morbidity and mortality rates (Casper et al., 2000; Schuiling & Likis, 2013).

By improving their understanding of how gender differences impact patient health, nurses can develop a plan of care that meets the specific and unique healthcare needs of each patient. It is important that nurses not allow their own gender bias or preconceived beliefs to affect their ability to assess and plan appropriate care for the individual patient. Health-promoting interventions aimed at inclusion in a safe and supportive environment promote a trusting nurse–patient relationship. Nurses should promote an environment in which patients can access essential services that address the differences between men and women in an equitable manner. When planning care, nurses who take into consideration the biological differences and social vulnerability of men and women are more likely to see positive outcomes for their patients.

Bias can be defined as favoring a group or individual over another. Gender bias results in **sexism** and occurs when male values, beliefs, or activities are preferred over female. Sexism may be overt or covert. Institutional bias related to gender results in sexist practices within an organization. Nurses need an awareness of cultural variations of gender, as they will be caring for diverse patient needs. What might

be considered sexism by one culture may not be in another. The wearing of a hijab, or head scarf, is an example. In some regions of the world, women are required by Islamic tradition to cover; however, in other areas of the world women have a choice to cover their heads. Some Muslim women find wearing the hijab empowering. Because their bodies are covered, they cannot be sexualized (Yusef, 2015). Because many women view wearing a hijab as an expression of faith, doing so should not necessarily be seen as a sign of sexism.

Another example of perceived sexism is that of the Hmong culture. In this culture, women typically do not make healthcare decisions, even regarding their own bodies. Typically, the woman's husband or father makes the decision, but sometimes, an elder man makes the healthcare decision for the woman. A woman could have an abscessed tooth, but the elder, not the patient, would determine if the tooth should be extracted because having males make medical decisions is preferred by many in this culture.

Race

The concept of race is complex. Historically, **race** has often been defined by physical attributes linked to continents of origin: Asia, Europe, Africa, and the Americas. Variations of skin color and hair texture have traditionally been used as markers of race. The dialogue about race and genetics is ongoing (Social Science Research Council, n.d.). However, the 2010 U.S. census data were collected by racial designation.

>> **Stay Current:** To learn more about the U.S. census racial categories, search the U.S. Census Bureau's website: https://www.census.gov/topics/population/race/about.html.

The oppression of a group of people based on perceived race is known as **racism**. Although racism is often perceived as overt acts of hostility, racism can also be insidious policies, procedures, traditions, and rules that benefit one group of people over another. For example, not providing translation services or not offering expensive diagnostic or treatment modalities based on race contributes to unequal treatment and injustice.

Class

Socioeconomic variations contribute to a society stratification based on money and access to resources. **Classism** is the oppression of groups of people based on their socioeconomic status. The lack of access to resources is apparent in some of the people at the lowest economic level such as the homeless, those living in poverty, or undocumented immigrants.

Homelessness

Among the most vulnerable patients are those who are homeless. Homeless patients present unique and complex challenges because they often live in dangerous, unsanitary conditions; have diets that are severely lacking in nutrients; and have very few resources for coping with illness. They must find shelter and food every day and cannot predict what the next day will bring. People who are homeless have difficulty obtaining, keeping, and storing medications. A high incidence of substance abuse and mental illness limits their ability to provide self-care. An important nursing intervention in addition to providing care to those who are homeless is to identify resources to help these patients.

>> **Stay Current:** The U.S. Department of Health and Human Services is the primary government agency for providing funds, research, and resources for the homeless. This website provides several resources and links on the subject of homelessness in the United States, including links to local and state agencies: http://www.hhs.gov/programs/social-services/homelessness/index.html.

Poverty

Although people who are homeless can be considered impoverished, many families with adequate shelter live in poverty. Children and those living in female-headed households are at greatest risk of living in poverty. Of those households living in poverty, 28.2% are headed by a woman, compared to 5.4% married couples and 14.9% male-headed households (U.S. Census Bureau, 2016).

- U.S. Census Bureau (2016) data indicate that the overall poverty rate is 13.5% with 43.1 million living in poverty. This is a decrease of 1.2% from the previous year, indicating that poverty rates have been improving over the past years.

- Median household income was $56,516 in 2015, which is a statistically significant 5.2% increase from 2014. This is the greatest change since 2007, the year of the last recession.

- The 2016 Census Bureau data also showed that 19.7% of children live in poverty, a decrease of 1.4%.

- Children of African American identity are more likely to live in poverty than their White counterparts. The poverty rates of Hispanic children continue to rise. Asian poverty statistics remain unchanged.

- The 2015 poverty rate for people age 65 and over was 8.8%, statistically unchanged for several years.

- More individuals are insured than in previous years, with only 9.1% reporting they are uninsured.

Undocumented Immigrants

Undocumented immigrants often do not seek healthcare until their condition becomes critical. This behavior results from a complex combination of factors. Many are uninsured, do not speak English, and have not yet learned the culture of their new homeland. Many believe that accessing healthcare will result in legal consequences, up to and including deportation. For some, the differences between the U.S. healthcare system and the medical practices and beliefs of their culture of origin create an additional barrier. These factors combine to create fear in the undocumented immigrant patient who needs medical attention (Ku & Jewers, 2013).

Special healthcare concerns related to this population include lack of preventive care, inadequate immunization status, and lack of past medical records. Because they enter the country without border screening, risks of diseases such as tuberculosis and HIV are much higher. Many feel more comfortable seeking help from traditional healers. Others receive their health information from television, the internet, community members, or family members, which can lead to misinformation and improper treatment.

States and regional politics vary across the country with regard to whether or not government or healthcare facilities are required to ask for proof of citizenship when providing care. Further, some states require reporting undocumented people, which also impedes those people's willingness to seek care. The nurse needs to be familiar with the laws within the state of nursing practice. When providing care to patients who may be or are known to be undocumented immigrants, the nurse has the ethical and moral imperative to deliver the same high-quality care delivered to any patient. Use of an interpreter or interpreter system will improve the quality of communication if the patient does not speak English or does not speak English well enough to understand the information presented. Thorough screening, nursing history, and assessment contribute to determining both current condition as well as risks, preventive care needs, and understanding of self-care upon discharge. Because access to healthcare for this population is unpredictable, nurses should maximize each opportunity to care for and teach self-care to these patients.

Sexual Orientation

Sexual orientation is a continuum ranging from those who have a strong preference for a partner of the same sex to those who strongly prefer someone of the opposite sex. *Homosexual* individuals prefer a partner of the same sex, with the term *lesbian* used to describe women who prefer to develop intimate relationships with other women. The term *gay* may refer to homosexual women or men, but is more commonly used to describe men who are homosexual. *Heterosexual* individuals prefer to develop an intimate relationship with a partner of the opposite sex. *Bisexual* individuals are physically attracted to both males and females. The most common biases related to sexual orientation are **homophobia** (fear, hatred, or mistrust of gays and lesbians often expressed in overt displays of discrimination) or **heterosexism** (view of heterosexuality as the only correct sexual orientation). In recent years, the American population has had a greater tolerance and acceptance of homosexuality. In a 2013 Pew Research Center survey, 55% of Americans were accepting of homosexuality. In the same survey, 92% of gays and lesbians reported feeling that society has become more accepting (Drake, 2013). Support for homosexuality and same-sex marriage in the United States remained at 55% following the Supreme Court's 2015 ruling that determined a constitutional right for homosexuals to marry (Fingerhut, 2016).

However, LGBTQ individuals (lesbian, gay, bisexual, transgender, and queer/questioning) continue to report discrimination and harassment, despite changing attitudes in society, even in the healthcare setting. A study showed that heterosexual nurses would much rather care for heterosexuals than gay men (Sabin, Riskind, & Nosek, 2015). Members of the LGBTQ community are also at greater risk for healthcare disparities and health issues. This is partially due to sexual practices, but also due to fear of discrimination and stigma. According to the Health Resources and Services Administration (n.d.), LGBTQ individuals are at higher risk for such health problems as obesity, mental health issues, substance abuse, and violence.

Transgender individuals face greater discrimination in healthcare than lesbians and gays. According to the National Transgender Discrimination Survey (Grant et al., 2011), 28% of transgender individuals delayed seeking healthcare for fear of discrimination, a far higher number than lesbians and gays report. The survey also found that 19% experienced refusal of care due to their gender status, and 28% experienced harassment in the healthcare setting (Grant et al., 2011). Sadly, transgender people are more likely to have mental health issues, including depression and anxiety, as well as abuse drugs and alcohol in order to cope with the difficulties involved in being transgender. The study found that 41% of those surveyed had attempted suicide; this is compared to 1.6% of the general public (Grant et al., 2011).

Social determinants affecting the health of LGBTQ individuals largely relate to oppression and discrimination. Examples include:

- Legal discrimination in access to health insurance, employment, housing, marriage, adoption, and retirement benefits

- Lack of laws protecting against bullying in schools

- Lack of social programs targeted to and/or appropriate for LGBTQ youth, adults, and older adults

- Shortage of healthcare providers who are knowledgeable about and culturally competent in providing LGBTQ healthcare.

Nurses must advocate for a physical environment that contributes to healthy LGBTQ individuals, including:

- Safe schools, neighborhoods, and housing

- Access to recreational facilities and activities

- Availability of safe meeting places

- Access to health services.

The Institute of Medicine (IOM) (2011) of the National Academies has published a book addressing LGBTQ health issues throughout the lifespan and found an ongoing need for healthcare professionals to improve culturally competent healthcare and to eliminate healthcare disparities. A follow-up report published in 2013 recognized even greater need for more research and promotion of health-seeking behaviors in the LBGTQ population (National Institutes of Health LGBT Research Coordinating Committee, 2013).

Disability Status

Many patients have physical or cognitive disabilities. During the past 30 years, various terms have been used to describe people with intellectual disabilities. Mental deficiency, mental retardation, mental handicap, developmental disability, and learning disability are examples. Patients with an intellectual disability and their families experience poorer healthcare compared with the general population. Living with an intellectual disability is often challenged by coexisting complex and chronic conditions and can lead to economic hardship and family conflict. Both intellectual and physical disability can impair the individual patient's ability to participate in health promotion and to provide self-care.

The American Association of People with Disabilities (2016) is the nation's largest cross-disability rights organization. It is an important advocacy, resource, and referral organization for individuals with disabilities and their families, friends, and advocates. Nurses working with patients with disabilities must develop trusting relationships so they can successfully assist patients with disabilities and their families and caregivers and enable them to find resources.

Age

Children and older adults are considered vulnerable populations. Both older adults and children often depend on others for nutrition, healthcare, transportation, and personal safety. Many older adults live on limited incomes. In 2014, there was a great disparity between men's and women's income for those over 65: the average income for a man was $31,169; for women it was $17,375 (Administration on Aging, 2015). More than 4.5 million (10%) older adults live in poverty, while 2.5 million (5.3%) live close to the poverty line (Administration on Aging, 2015). **Ageism** is defined as discrimination against older adults. U.S. culture places an emphasis on youth, beauty, and productivity, which minimizes respect and access to opportunities for older adults. The increasing use of the internet and technology as a primary means of sharing and retrieving information also has implications. More and more older adults are embracing technology and the internet, particularly in those with higher education and/or spouses (Vroman, Arthanat, & Lysack, 2015). However, those who have less education or do not have access to technology resources are left behind.

Disparities and Differences

In many ways the United States is a nation that celebrates culture and diversity. From Greek festivals to soul food to Tex-Mex, from gay pride parades to Chinese New Year, there is plenty of diverse heritage and society to celebrate. Unfortunately, these differences also give rise to disparities of opportunity, and these include disparities that relate to healthcare. In 2002, the Institute of Medicine released a report on disparities in the United States regarding the types and quality of health services that racial and ethnic groups receive. This historic report explored factors that may contribute to inequities in care and recommended policies and practices to eliminate these inequities. Fifteen years later, despite much progress, inequities still exist, and researchers are attempting to identify and prevent the causes of disparities (**Figure 24–3 »**). Nurses should be alert to practices in their work environment that impact the quality of care offered to individuals of any ethnic group. Healthcare practices should be accessible and culturally relevant, and patient preferences should be at the core of decision making. Nurses should work collaboratively to ensure quality care and provision of best-practice methods to all patients.

The recommendations for reducing these disparities in healthcare include increasing awareness of them among the public, healthcare providers, insurance companies, and policy makers. In addition, more diverse healthcare providers are needed in underserved communities, and more interpreters are needed in clinics and hospitals to improve the

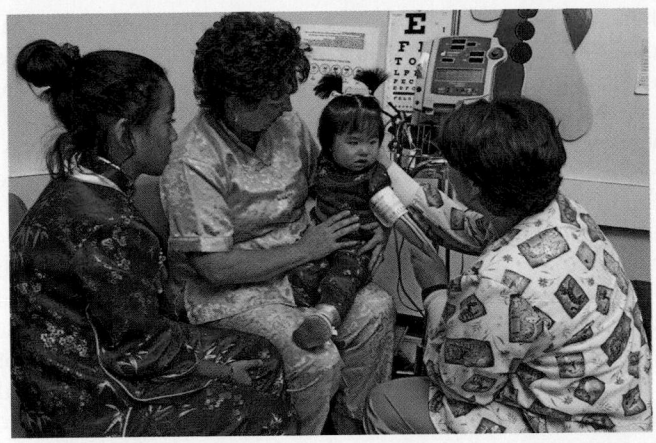

Figure 24–3 》》 Although much has been done to improve the quality of health services received by American cultural and ethnic minorities, these services are still in need of continued reform.

quality of care. The U.S. Department of Health and Human Services offers a free, online course to educate nurses and other healthcare workers on culturally competent care (https://www.thinkculturalhealth.hhs.gov/education/nurses) in order to help educate nurses and narrow the healthcare disparities gap and improve overall health in different populations.

》》 Stay Current: To read more on cultural competency, information on health equality, and other topics on minorities, explore http://minorityhealth.hhs.gov.

Vulnerable Populations

The concept of multiculturalism assumes that all cultural groups are equally valued and respected by others. Unfortunately, this is rarely the case. Historically, the United States has had norms, values, and even laws based on stratification of gender, race, and class divisions. The term **vulnerable population** refers to groups of people in our culture who are at greater risk for diseases and reduced lifespan due to lack resources and exposure to more risk factors. Poverty is a major culprit in vulnerable populations (World Health Organization, 2016). Persons in poverty are at risk for malnutrition, poor housing, violence, and limited or no access to healthcare. Other conditions associated with vulnerability include age, disability, health/disease state, education status, language spoken, and socioeconomic situation.

Oppression, or the systematic limitation of access to resources, may be covert or subtle and typically is linked to laws, education, or even healthcare norms and regional access to services and transportation. All vulnerable populations are less able than others to safeguard their needs and interests adequately. In conceptual terms, the most vulnerable are those households with the fewest choices and the greatest number of disabling factors.

Patients from vulnerable populations are more likely to develop health problems because they have the greatest number of risk factors and the fewest options for managing those risks. These individuals often have limited access to healthcare and are more dependent on others for helping

them meet their healthcare needs. Those from vulnerable populations are likely to be older, living in poverty, homeless, in abusive relationships, mentally ill, chronically ill, or children. It is not uncommon for vulnerable individuals to belong to more than one of these groups. They face multiple challenges, statistically poorer outcomes and shorter lifespans, and higher mortality and morbidity rates due to cumulative or combinations of risk factors. They may be from any culture, ethnicity, age, or gender, although they are more likely to be women than men. Nurses face many challenges when caring for individuals who are vulnerable. Their physical, social, and emotional needs are complex, and many have multiple chronic conditions that can complicate care still further. Assessing the patient from a vulnerable population requires the nurse to investigate all systems, determine stressors and coping mechanisms, and help the patient identify potential resources.

The welfare of vulnerable populations depends on the nation's willingness to provide the necessary programs to promote health and well-being. Other issues impacting the provision of healthcare to vulnerable populations include accessibility and transportation. Impoverished children living in very rural communities, for example, may not have access to fluoridated water and may be an hour from the nearest dentist who accepts Medicaid.

A primary focus of healthcare, as outlined by *Healthy People 2020*, is to reduce the disparity of access to healthcare among groups. *Healthy People 2020* defines a **health disparity** as "a particular type of health difference that is closely linked with social, economic, and/or environmental disadvantage. Health disparities adversely affect groups of people who have systematically experienced greater obstacles to health based on their racial or ethnic group; religion; socioeconomic status; gender; age; mental health; cognitive, sensory, or physical disability; sexual orientation or gender identity; geographic location; or other characteristics historically linked to discrimination or exclusion" (The Secretary's Advisory Committee on National Health Promotion and Disease Prevention Objectives for 2020, 2008, p. 28). Some examples of vulnerable group affiliations are highlighted in this module.

Social Differences

People learn the social behaviors practiced in their cultures and communities. These behaviors differ from culture to culture, from community to community. They may also be practiced by members of subcultures who decide to maintain traditional cultural practices, whereas others from the same culture living nearby may choose to adapt to the dominant culture (**Figure 24–4 》》**). The terms *subculture* and *minority* are sometimes used to label groups characterized by specific norms, beliefs, and values that coexist or even oppose those of the dominant culture. Some common social behavioral variations among people of different cultures involve communication, environmental control, hygiene, space, time, and social organization. These ethnic differences exist within smaller cultural groups within a larger society. Within the United States, social differences are evolving as individuals from different cultural groups relocate for college or work and interact with people from other cultures, and as the numbers of individuals of different cultural

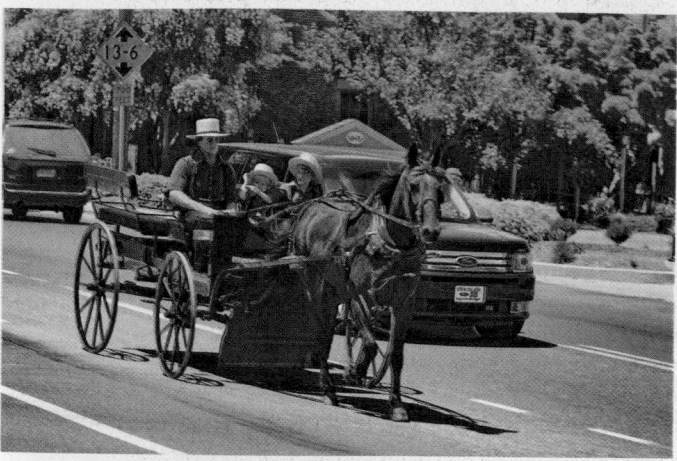

Source: gsheldon/iStock Editorial/Getty Images.

Figure 24–4 ❯❯ Subcultures can maintain heritage and identity through dress, foods eaten, and cultural festivities. This Amish family in Bird-in-Hand, Pennsylvania, wears traditional plain clothing and drives a horse-drawn buggy while sharing the road with the larger community of non-Amish Pennsylvanians who drive cars.

groups change over time. For instance, there has been a silent move of Native Americans from the reservations to the cities. This migration is partially due to violence on the reservations, poverty, and other socioeconomic factors (Williams, 2013). More Native Americans are living in cities than ever before, with roughly 70% living in metropolitan areas. With this, unfortunately, comes an increased poverty rate. Native Americans and Native Alaskans have the highest rate of poverty of all the races. In Minneapolis, Minnesota, the poverty rate for Native Americans is roughly 45%, compared to a national average for Native Americans of 27% (Macartney, Bishaw, & Fontenot, 2013; Williams, 2013). Yet, despite the higher poverty rates, Native leaders report that cities bring more opportunities than the reservations (Williams, 2013).

Communication

Cultural groups may speak a unique language or a variation of another language. The meaning of words can differ among various groups of people, and misunderstandings may result from lack of common communication. Languages vary in terms of references to time, gender, roles, or common concepts and definitions. Translation of concepts from one language to another may miss contextual embedded meanings and lead to misunderstandings. Misinterpretation of nonverbal communication also may lead to problems. Direct eye contact may show disrespect in some cultures and be a sign of interest and active listening in others. An example of a difference in nonverbal communication is when up-and-down head nodding does not reflect agreement, but instead is an attempt to acknowledge respect for authority.

Environmental Control

Relationship to the environment varies among cultures. Different health practices, values, and experiences with illness can be associated with an external or internal locus of control. Rotter (1966) theorized that individuals believe either

that they can control certain aspects of their lives (internal locus of control) or that outside sources control their lives (external locus of control). Those who believe in an internal locus of control over their health will be motivated to eat healthy, exercise, and make use of other wellness measures. For example, an American of European descent would more likely follow an internal locus of control based on the cultural belief of independence and care for self. Those who follow an internal locus of control tend to respond well to preventive medicine. Those with an external locus of control will feel that outside influences will care for their health. For example, some people who are Muslim believe the status of their health is Allah's will. Those who follow an external locus of control are less likely to be as engaged in preventive measures as they do not see themselves as being in control of their health.

Religious Variations

Many religions are practiced, including Protestant Christianity, Catholicism, Judaism, Hinduism, Islam, and Buddhism. **Religion** refers to a set of doctrines accepted by a group of people who gather together regularly to worship that offer a means to relate to God or a higher power, nature, and their spiritual being. Religion plays a greater role in some communities than in others. One town may sponsor a living nativity at Christmas, whereas the next may ban religious observances on government property altogether. See the module on Spirituality for more information.

Space

Culture defines an individual's perception of personal space. Comfort may result from honoring the boundaries of personal space, whereas anxiety can result when these boundaries are not followed. Practices regarding proximity to others, body movements, and touch differ among groups. Variations of intimate zones and social public distance occur among cultural groups, and a healthcare provider needs to be aware that what he perceives as normal or appropriate may be produce anxiety for others (Dayer-Berenson, 2011).

Time

The concepts of time, duration of time, and points in time vary among cultures. Past-oriented cultures, for example, value tradition. Individuals from cultures that closely follow tradition may not be receptive to new procedures or treatments. Present-oriented cultures focus on the here and now, and individuals from these cultures may not be receptive to preventive healthcare measures. Different cultures value time differently, and some may not emphasize being on time for appointments (Spector, 2017). Healthcare providers are very regulated by clock hours influencing wake, sleep, work, and mealtimes. Not all cultural groups are regulated by clock hours.

Biological Variations

People differ genetically and physiologically. These biological variations among individuals, families, and groups produce differences in susceptibility and response to various diseases among people of different cultures and all walks of life (**Figure 24–5 ❯❯**). The field of ethnopharmacology addresses variations in pharmacodynamics and

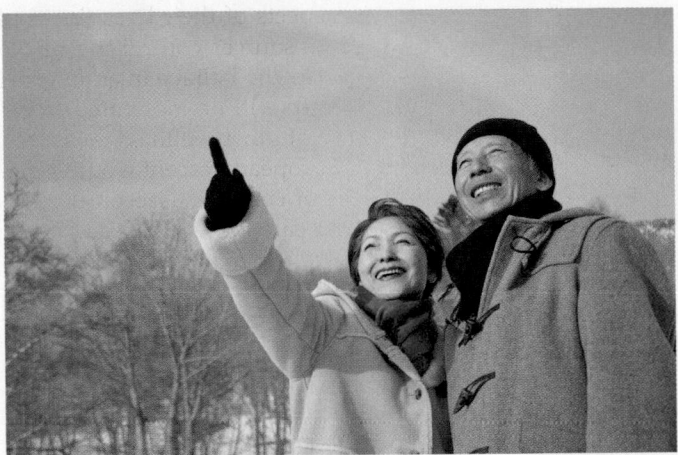

Source: TAGSTOCK1/iStock/Getty Images.

Figure 24–5 》 People from different cultures vary biologically. This couple of Japanese descent is likely to have higher blood glucose levels than people of other ethnic backgrounds.

pharmacokinetics among cultural groups. Nurses are responsible for monitoring patients' responses to the drugs they give and thus must be aware of these differences. In addition, some enzyme deficiencies occur more commonly in some cultural groups. For example, lactose deficiency (the inability to absorb milk by-products) or other malabsorption disorders are seen with increased incidence in Asian and African cultural groups.

Susceptibility to Disease

Certain ethnic groups or races may tend toward developing specific diseases. African Americans, for example, have a higher incidence of hypertension and sickle cell disease. Cystic fibrosis occurs almost exclusively in Caucasians. Native Americans have a higher incidence of diabetes (33%) than any other group (Spanakis & Golden, 2013). Sometimes, however, an individual's susceptibility to disease is not so obvious but may be discerned as a nurse takes a health history, including the health of any parents, grandparents, and siblings.

Skin Color

Historically, skin color has been associated with racial definitions. However, labeling of people based on their skin color should be avoided. Healthcare providers need to explore ethnic variations and not make assumptions based on skin color. As a nurse, when doing skin assessment, it is important to know that darker skin tones require closer inspection and enhanced lighting to observe changes (e.g., when assessing for changes in oxygenation). Skin color changes such as erythema and cyanosis are subtle, and palpation and lighting will need to be used for skin assessment. In addition, skin color does impact some prevalence statistics: African Americans and Native Americans have lower incidences of skin cancer due to higher levels of melanin.

Additional cultural and social differences are outlined in **Table 24–2 》**.

TABLE 24–2 Additional Cultural and Social Differences

Category	Implications
Hygiene	Cleanliness practices can vary among cultural groups. Whether or not body odor is disguised, ignored, or enhanced can vary by culture, as can hairstyles and grooming practices.
Nutrition	Food preferences can be an indicator of or cause of disease.
	Cooking techniques vary and may increase risk for disease in susceptible populations.
	Social patterns around eating and food choices also have implications for health promotion and direct nursing care.
Skeletal and growth and development differences	Skeletal variations occur across racial and cultural lines. For example, small-framed American women of European descent are at greater risk for osteoporosis. Pubertal developmental changes occur at different times.
Social organization	Across cultures and communities, the roles of older adults and the respect given them vary. Differences among who is the recognized head of household and gender roles also exist. Work and recreational patterns and norms vary. The role of adult children and caretaking expectations also vary among groups.

Clinical Example A

Susan Moore is a 16-year-old girl who comes to a local family practice clinic for a first-time appointment. She is complaining of painful, irregular, and heavy menstrual periods. Her mother comes with her to the clinic visit. Susan's assessment is notable for her lack of participation in regular medical care. Her parents homeschool Susan and her sisters, and her mother tells you that they hardly ever see a physician. Following a thorough nursing assessment and physical examination, the family nurse practitioner diagnoses Susan with endometriosis and recommends hormonal contraceptives. Susan's mother is adamant that Susan not take any medication, saying they believe in using only "natural" therapies and do not use prescription drugs. Susan begins to cry, complaining of how much pain she is in constantly, and she pleads with her mother to let her try the medication.

Critical Thinking Questions

1. What are the priorities for care for Susan based on the information presented here?
2. How can you show cultural sensitivity to Susan and her mother and promote evidence-based care?
3. Using therapeutic communication, what could you say or do to affect Susan's mother's decision regarding her daughter's treatment?

Concepts Related to Culture and Diversity

Differences among patients that are attributable to culture, ethnicity, race, gender, sexuality, and vulnerability impact the nursing care of patients in a variety of ways. Within the concept of communication, it is important to understand that patients use language differently, speak different languages, and recognize nonverbal cues differently. Therapeutic

Concepts Related to
Culture and Diversity

CONCEPT	RELATIONSHIP TO CULTURE AND DIVERSITY	NURSING IMPLICATIONS
Comfort	The verbalization of pain and preferred comfort measures may differ based on cultural expressions, gender norms, or other factors.	▪ Patients' reaction to pain may range from stoicism to hysterics. Nurses must assess and accept a variety of patient responses to pain and provide myriad interventions that include opioids, nonopioids, adjunct therapy, and complementary and alternative methods for reducing pain and increasing comfort.
Communication	Listening, clarification, reflection, and all therapeutic communication techniques are important when communicating with people different from you.	▪ Use therapeutic communication skills. ▪ Identify translation and interpreter resources in your organization. ▪ Use language that the patient understands.
Healthcare Systems	Availability of healthcare services for vulnerable populations may be low. Availability of resources varies by community.	▪ Unequal distribution of facilities and resources. ▪ Recognize cultural and group differences among healthcare providers. Seek to advocate for vulnerable populations. ▪ Refer patients in need of additional resources to social services and nonprofit service agencies.
Professional Behaviors	Recognize personal values and professional values.	▪ Self-awareness of cultural competence.
Sexuality	Sexual orientation, homophobia, heterosexism.	▪ Assist in advocating for LGBTQ healthcare needs and access. ▪ Recognize same-sex partners as family and patient support.
Spirituality	Recognize religious beliefs related to dietary regimen or times of fasting.	▪ Show respect for religious differences, leaders, and practice. ▪ Recognize that your personal spiritual and religious beliefs will not be universally shared with your patients. ▪ Be nonjudgmental of differences. ▪ Support patient religious practices.

communication, interpreters, shared languages, and awareness of nonverbal cues can help nurses communicate more effectively with patients from diverse backgrounds.

Within healthcare systems, the resources available to the different types of patients depend on a variety of factors, especially whether or not the patients have health insurance and access to resources such as transportation. Patients who live in poverty or who are homeless may need referrals to additional resources. Nurses must advocate for services, such as interpreters or mental health resources, for their patients who do not have the awareness or influence to ask on their own.

The professional behavior of nurses must be built on a moral and ethical code. Nursing as a discipline has a culture of its own. Nurses must understand collegial and regional differences to effectively work collaboratively with interprofessional teams. Self-awareness, emotional intelligence, and lifelong learning should be characteristics of a nurse's professional behavior.

Another concept related to culture and diversity is sexuality. Gender roles and the timing and type of sexual relationships vary among groups of people. Heterosexual and homosexual variations may also be culturally embedded.

Another concept related to culture and diversity is spirituality. Although spirituality may be defined more broadly

than religion, cultural variations exist around religious and church doctrines such as Hinduism, Judaism, Buddhists, Christianity, and Muslim practices. Religious practices commonly influence eating or fasting patterns, types of worship, and family roles and responsibilities. The Concepts Related to Culture and Diversity feature lists some, but not all, of the concepts integral to providing culturally aware nursing.

Developing Cultural Competence

Cultural competence is the ability to apply the knowledge and skills needed to provide high-quality, evidence-based care to patients of diverse backgrounds and beliefs to overcome barriers and access resources promoting health and wellness. Cultural competence has some basic characteristics:

1. Valuing diversity
2. Capacity for cultural self-assessment
3. Awareness of the different dynamics present when cultures interact
4. Knowledge about different cultures
5. Adaptability in providing nursing care that reflects an understanding of cultural diversity.

Cultural competence can be considered a process as well as an outcome, although no one person can be competent in dealing with all types of cultural variations. The American Association of Colleges of Nursing (2008) has identified five competencies considered essential for baccalaureate nursing graduates to provide culturally competent care in partnership with the interprofessional team:

- **Competency 1.** Apply knowledge of social and cultural factors that affect nursing and healthcare across multiple contexts.

- **Competency 2.** Use relevant data sources and best evidence in providing culturally competent care.

- **Competency 3.** Promote achievement of safe and quality outcomes of care for diverse populations.

- **Competency 4.** Advocate for social justice, including commitment to the health of vulnerable populations and the elimination of health disparities.

- **Competency 5.** Participate in continuous cultural competence development.

Because the concept of culture is very complex, scholars have identified models of cultural competence to facilitate the continuous process of cultural competence. The purpose of using a model is to help communicate and enhance the understanding of a complex concept. A theoretical model may provide a nurse or student with a deeper understanding of how concepts are related. Many models have been published. One of the oldest, yet still relevant, nursing theories regarding culture is Madeleine Leininger's (2002) Culture Care Diversity and Universality theory. Leininger developed this theory with a unique emphasis on cultural care and the nurse. See the module on Caring Interventions for more information regarding Leininger's Theory of Culture Care Diversity and Universality.

Another model is Rachel Spector's HeritageChain (2017), which outlines the variables that impact culturally competent care. These include the cultural heritage of the patient and the provider; the diversity of the area in which patient and provider live and work; the health panoramas of traditional cultural groups; and aspects of health and illness, such as traditional healing versus modern healthcare practices and family support and considerations (**Figure 24–6 》》**).

The nurse's journey toward cultural competency begins with self-awareness, with identifying areas in which the nurse can improve how she relates to and communicates with individuals with values and beliefs different from her own. See the Focus on Diversity and Culture feature for a values clarification checklist to help you begin to cultivate self-awareness.

The LEARN model (Association of American Medical Colleges, 2005; Berlin & Fowkes, 1983) can be used as a tool for developing cultural competency. Below is a modification

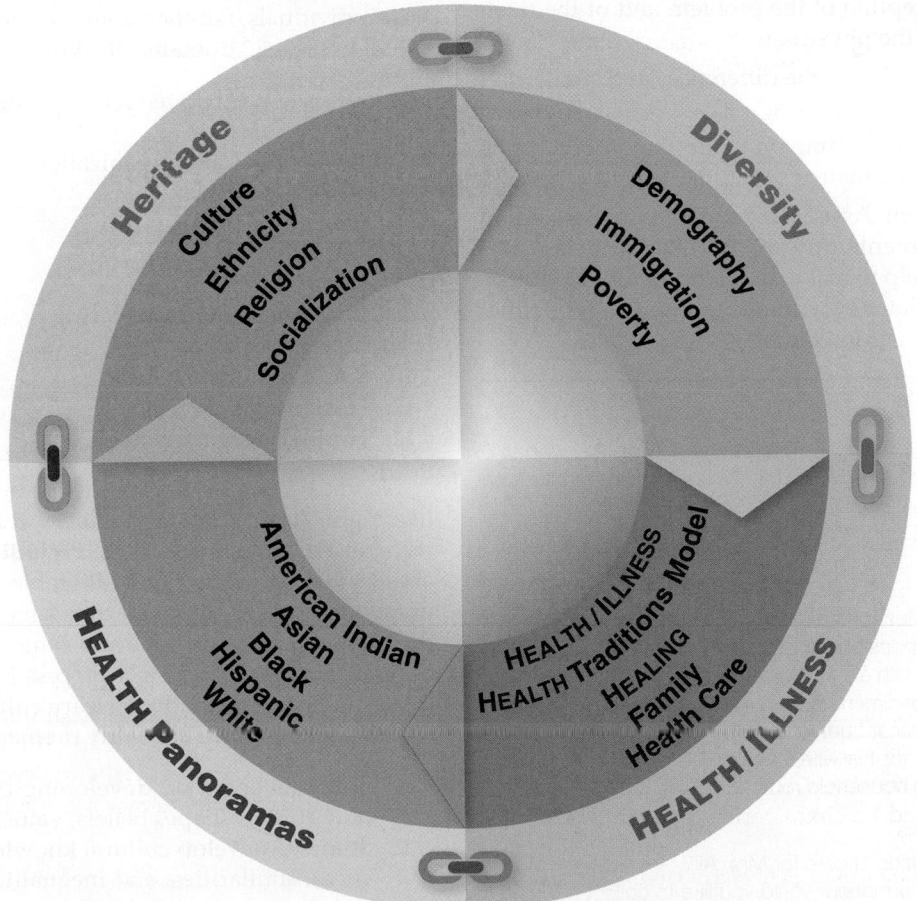

Figure 24–6 》》 The HeritageChain model of cultural competence developed by Rachel Spector (2017).

Focus on Diversity and Culture
How Culturally Competent Are You?

To help you identify areas where you can improve when providing nursing care to culturally different people, answer the following questions by checking "Yes" or "No":

____ Yes   ____ No   I accept values of others even when different from my own.

____ Yes   ____ No   I accept beliefs of others even when different from my own.

____ Yes   ____ No   I accept that the male and female roles may vary among different cultures.

____ Yes   ____ No   I accept that religious practices may influence how a patient responds to illness, health problems, and death.

____ Yes   ____ No   I accept that alternative medicine practices may influence a patient's response to illness and health problems.

____ Yes   ____ No   I accept cultural diversity in my patients.

____ Yes   ____ No   I attend educational programs to enhance my knowledge and skills in providing care to diverse cultural groups.

____ Yes   ____ No   I understand that patients who are unable to speak English may be very proficient in their own languages.

____ Yes   ____ No   I try to have written materials in the patient's language available when possible.

____ Yes   ____ No   I use interpreters when available to improve communication.

If you have more No responses than Yes responses, you may not be as culturally competent as you could be. The purpose of this self-assessment is to increase your awareness of areas where you can improve your cultural competence.

of the **LEARN** model that can help nurses include cultural behaviors in a patient's healthcare:

Listen to the patient's perception of the problem.

Explain your perception of the problem and of the treatments ordered by the physician.

Acknowledge and discuss the differences and similarities between these two perceptions.

Review the ordered treatments while remembering the patient's cultural parameters.

Negotiate agreement. Assist the patient in understanding the medical treatments ordered by the physician, and have the patient help to make decisions about those treatments as appropriate (e.g., choosing cultural foods that are permitted on an ordered diet).

Clinical Example B

Mr. and Mrs. Ali come to a local clinic because Mrs. Ali, who is 6 months pregnant, is not feeling well. Mr. Ali speaks English fluently, but his wife's proficiency in English is more limited. Both are dressed in American-style clothes. During the assessment, the registered nurse, Clea Smith, determines that the couple has a 9-month-old and a 2-year-old at home. Ms. Smith also learns that Mr. Ali is the head of the household, making most of the major decisions for the family, and that Mrs. Ali has sole responsibility for the family's care and daily living needs. Mrs. Ali presents with exhaustion and elevated blood pressure. After obtaining a urine specimen, the provider diagnoses toxemia and orders Mrs. Ali to be on strict bedrest and to return in 2 weeks. While Mr. Ali conveys concern for his wife's health, he is reluctant to have her treatment disrupt the household routine.

Critical Thinking Questions

1. What are the priorities of care for Mrs. Ali?
2. What additional information would you like to collect about this family?
3. Using the LEARN model, describe how the nurse working with this family could understand and address this situation and the physician's recommendations with both the husband and wife.

In addition to the LEARN model, nursing scholars have identified models that illuminate a variety of areas for nurses to explore to deepen their understanding of cultural competence.

Purnell's (2014) model of cultural competence identifies how individuals, families, communities, and the global society all possess 12 domains of culture:

1. Overview, inhabited localities, and topography
2. Communication
3. Family roles and organization
4. Workforce issues
5. Biocultural ecology
6. High-risk behaviors
7. Nutrition
8. Pregnancy and childbearing practices
9. Death rituals
10. Spirituality
11. Healthcare practices
12. Healthcare practitioners.

No one becomes culturally aware or culturally competent overnight. As healthcare providers, it is imperative that we recognize common prejudices. **Prejudices** are prejudgments about cultural groups or vulnerable populations that are unfavorable or false because they have been formed without the background knowledge and context on which to base an accurate opinion. There is a process by which nursing students (and other individuals) learn cultural confidence, with learning taking place in a fairly predictable sequence:

1. Students begin by developing cultural awareness of how culture shapes beliefs, values, and norms.
2. Students develop cultural knowledge about the differences, similarities, and inequalities in experience and practice among various societies.
3. Students develop cultural understanding of problems and issues facing societies and cultures when values, beliefs, and behaviors are compromised by another culture.

4. Students develop cultural sensitivity to the cultural beliefs, values, and behaviors of their patients. This reflects an awareness of their own cultural beliefs, values, and behaviors that may influence their nursing practice.

5. Students and nurses develop cultural competence and provide care that respects the cultural values, beliefs, and behaviors of their patients.

6. Nurses practice lifelong learning through ongoing education and exposure to cultural groups.

Standards of Competence

Maintaining cultural competence is an ongoing process. Nurses continually assess, modify, and evaluate the care provided to culturally diverse patients. In 2011, Douglas et al. addressed current standards for culturally competent nursing care. Their 12 standards are:

1. Social justice
2. Critical reflection
3. Knowledge of cultures
4. Culturally competent practice
5. Cultural competence in healthcare systems and organizations
6. Patient advocacy and empowerment
7. Multicultural workforce
8. Education and training in culturally competent care
9. Cross-cultural communication
10. Cross-cultural leadership
11. Policy development
12. Evidence-based practice and research.

Institutions such as hospitals also need to develop and implement cultural competence to address the cultural and language needs of an increasingly multicultural patient population. Purnell et al. (2011) developed a guide to assessing a culturally competent organization and suggested the following areas be addressed:

- **Administration and governance.** Some areas in which an organization may consider being culturally competent are congruence with a mission statement and implementation of policies and procedure. All administrators must walk the talk and promote organizational practices that promote cultural competence. Organizations should initiate a continuous monitoring process for assessment and evaluation of cultural and language needs. These practices may be hiring protocols, having an ethics or cultural committee to resolve conflicts, having a cafeteria with diverse food choices, and instituting effective communication policies. In addition, monies must be allocated to provide resources and training throughout the organization. Handouts and marketing plans should reflect diverse groups in their narrative, illustrations, and relevant terminology (Byrne et al., 2003).

- **Orientation and education.** The orientation or professional development for *all* employees should address concepts of cultural competency. An organization should have a philosophy of respect for all of its employees and have resources for multicultural and multilingual employees and community partners.

- **Language.** The United States is a country of many cultures, and healthcare professionals need to have a basic understanding of how language impacts healthcare delivery systems. Patients with limited proficiency in English often run into barriers when they try to enter the healthcare system. They may delay making an appointment because of difficulties communicating over the telephone, for example, and during this delay, the health problem may become more severe, requiring more expensive treatment. If the patient does make an appointment, there may be misunderstandings about the scheduled date, time, or location. Nurses need to know that translation services and interpreter access are federal mandates. Note, too, that translation services involve written communication, and interpreters refer to oral communication.

- **Staff competencies.** The last area for organizational cultural competency is providing opportunities for all staff to learn about a variety of cultural groups and become educated as culturally competent providers. Being competent is both an individual and organizational moral imperative for which the organization should provide resources and opportunities for education and multicultural experiences.

Using an Interpreter

Many patients do not speak English, and many who do speak some English are of limited proficiency. Any facility receiving federal funding from the U.S. Department of Health and Human Services is required to communicate effectively with patients or risk the loss of that funding. Having bilingual nurses available is one strategy to address the language barrier. Another strategy is providing access to language banks through electronic or telephone systems that nurses can dial for interpreter services. Unless a patient brings an interpreter with her, however, an interpreter may not have any previous knowledge of the patient. Nurses can ask a patient or family with limited English proficiency if the family works with any area service organizations that provide interpreters. These organizations attempt to provide competent interpreters who build relationships with families over time. However, the nurse should be aware that some cultures find it offensive to discuss medical issues with a member of the opposite gender or a younger person (Chang & Kelly, 2007). The nurse should collaborate with the patient and family regarding specifics for an interpreter.

Guidelines for using an interpreter include the following:

- When possible, use an interpreter to translate and provide meaning behind the words.

- To protect patient confidentiality and to guard against the possibility of the interpreter misunderstanding medical information, avoid using a family member as an interpreter.

- If possible, use an interpreter of the same gender as the patient.

- Address your questions to the patient, not the interpreter, but maintain eye contact with both the patient and the interpreter.

- Avoid using metaphors, medical jargon, similes, and idiomatic phrases.
- Observe the patient's nonverbal communication.
- Plan what to say, and avoid rephrasing or hesitating.
- Use short questions and comments. Ask one question at a time.
- Speak slowly and distinctly, but not loudly.
- Provide written materials in the patient's language as available.

>> **Stay Current:** Explore this website to learn about best practices for using interpreters in healthcare from the National Council on Interpreting in Health Care home page: http://www.ncihc.org.

Clinical Example C

Henry Lee is approximately 55 years old. Born in China, he has been living in the United States for the past 10 years, working as a professor at a local university. Following surgery for a broken arm, he refuses pain medication, explaining that his discomfort is bearable and he can survive without medication.

When you next check on him, you find him restless and uncomfortable. You have a standing order to administer medication as needed, and again offer to administer medication. Mr. Lee again refuses, saying that your other responsibilities are more important than his discomfort and he does not want to impose.

Critical Thinking Questions

1. What do you think is behind Mr. Lee's refusal to accept medication?
2. What can you do or say to change Mr. Lee's perception of the situation?
3. What additional information might influence your nursing care?

NURSING PROCESS

The nursing process is interwoven in providing culturally competent care. In each step, the nurse should be considerate of the patient's cultural background and practices. This holistic approach will help both the patient and the nurse create a therapeutic plan of care.

Assessment

The provision of culturally competent care begins with incorporating culture into the initial nursing assessment. Areas for assessment include the use of traditional healing practices such as herbal supplements or mind–body practices (e.g., cupping, acupuncture); cultural practices related to food preparation and preferences; religious or cultural practices at specific times of day or during the week; health beliefs; and preferences for care, such as whether or not women prefer to be examined by a female nurse.

When patients speak languages other than English or are not proficient in English, minimal assessment information from patients can be obtained with the following questions:

- What language do you speak? Do you speak any English?
- How long have you lived here?
- Describe the illness or problem that brings you here today.
- What do you think caused your problem?
- When did it start?
- Why do you think it started when it did?
- What does your sickness do to you?
- How severe is your sickness?
- What do you fear about your sickness?
- What helps make it better? Worse?
- What kind of treatment do you think you need?
- Are there any religious practices we need to know about?
- Who is your family?
- Who makes decisions most of the time?
- Who can you go to for help when you need it?

Assessment of cultural influences and practices is imperative because differences in cultural behaviors, beliefs, and values may result in barriers to patients achieving positive outcomes. Cultural misunderstandings or miscommunications also may result from different perceptions of health and of the illness diagnosed.

Nursing assessment of the patient's values and beliefs includes assessing for the use of complementary and alternative therapies. The term **complementary therapies** refers to any of a diverse array of practices, therapies, and supplements that are not considered part of conventional or traditional medicine and that are used *in addition to* conventional treatments. **Alternative therapies** is a term used to describe use of these diverse therapies *instead of* conventional therapies (see the Focus on Integrative Health feature). Assessing the patient for use of these therapies is important to determine patient preferences for care and if there are any therapies the patient is currently using that are contraindicated.

Diagnosis

Once the assessment is complete, nurses can begin to form diagnoses appropriate to the individual or family seeking care. Examples of NANDA International (NANDA-I) nursing diagnoses that may be appropriate for patients of different cultures include:

- *Powerlessness*
- *Spiritual Distress*
- *Religiosity, Risk for Impaired*
- *Fear*
- *Decisional Conflict*
- *Resilience, Risk for Impaired*
- *Anxiety*
- *Health Maintenance, Ineffective*
- *Coping, Ineffective*
- *Social Interaction, Impaired.*

(NANDA-I © 2014)

- Disturbed Thought Processes

Planning

Planning care in collaboration with the patient increases the likelihood that the patient will follow the care plan, particularly if the plan is culturally sensitive. At times it can be challenging to incorporate a patient's cultural preferences and practices into the care plan, especially in the hospital setting. For example, those patients whose origins are from India tend to have strong family ties. When a person becomes ill, several family members may come to the hospital and gather in the room, causing crowding. Typically, the mother will provide care for the patient. This can cause conflict, as many from India believe in self-medication and herbal medicines. The nurse, therefore, should collaborate with the patient and family to provide safe, effective care. Appropriate goals for patients will include the following:

- The patient will remain safe through the use of interpreters, educational materials written in the patient's primary language, and other cultural bridges of communication between the healthcare team and the patient.
- The patient will meet nutritional needs during hospitalization through meal accommodation, nutritional counseling, and incorporation of preferred foods in the meal plan.
- The patient will perform ADLs and increase mobility when appropriate.
- Both patient and family members will verbalize understanding of necessity of early mobility and independence with ADLs.

Implementation

Implementation should involve a care plan that incorporates the patient's cultural beliefs and practices.

Promote Safety

There is great potential for harm due to cultural and language issues. Patients who do not understand the language of the nurse may not adhere to safety instructions, including using a call light before getting out of bed. Family members may bring comfort foods from home that might interfere with fluid or diet restrictions. Some might want to complement the patient's care with traditional healing remedies that may interact with medications. The nurse must create an open channel of communication with family members and the patient in order to provide safe and culturally sensitive care. Additional assessment and patient teaching regarding safety procedures, medication side effects and interactions, and other areas of care may be necessary.

Provide Adequate Nutrition

In the hospital setting, ethnic foods are often not available. Many cultures see food as a way to provide healing and comfort. Some patients may not eat hospital food because it is foreign or taboo. For instance, those of Jewish heritage may not eat the food provided in a hospital if it is not prepared and served correctly in a kosher manner. Vietnamese patients may ignore Western food or diet recommendations if they follow traditional cultural practices regarding eating certain foods during illness. Regardless of the patient's background, carefully assess patient and family expectations and practices regarding foods and beverages and incorporate these into the plan of care when it is safe to do so.

Promote Physical Mobility

Many cultures believe that the sick must remain in bed with little physical activity until deemed well. The belief is that the sick person must gain strength. For example, some Filipinos believe that even showering is too strenuous for the patient and will bathe the family member in bed. The cultural belief of restricted activity may cause conflict with nurses who wish to promote activity to prevent skin integrity breakdown, clots, and other complications with immobility. The nurse can take this opportunity to educate as well as collaborate. The nurse should collaborate with the family to implement a plan that does include mobility, but also appreciates the cultural need for rest.

Evaluation

The evaluation of the nurse's plan of care will involve the underlying goals that include a culture component. Goals may include:

- The patient expresses that cultural needs were met.
- The patient is able to verbalize understanding of medical diagnosis and treatment plan.
- The patient is able to collaborate with the care team when using complementary therapies.
- The patient is able to meet nutritional needs.

Evaluating how successfully the patient is able to follow the treatment regimen while observing cultural practices and rituals is essential to determining patient outcomes but also provides a way for nurses to evaluate whether or not they provided culturally competent care that promoted improved patient outcomes.

Focus on Integrative Health
Overview of Complementary Health Approaches

The National Center for Complementary and Integrative Health (NCCIH) reports that approximately 33.2% of Americans use complementary and integrative health approaches (sometimes referred to as complementary and alternative medicine, or CAM) (Clarke et al., 2015). Types and examples of these approaches include:

- **Natural products.** Dietary supplements, including fish oil and herbal supplements such as turmeric
- **Mind and body practices.** Meditation, yoga, acupuncture, chiropractic medicine, massage therapy

≫ **Stay Current:** For more information on complementary and alternative therapies, go to the NCCIH website: https://nccih.nih.gov.

REVIEW The Concept of Culture and Diversity

RELATE Link the Concepts

Linking the concept of culture and diversity with the concept of development:

1. How might a pediatric patient's development be impacted if his or her mother is homeless?

2. How might an adolescent's development be impacted by the realization that he or she is homosexual?

You are a nurse working in a children's rehabilitation center. A 6-year-old girl who is recovering from a motor vehicle accident comes to your center for an extended stay. She speaks a little English. Her family has recently moved here from China, and her parents likewise have limited English. Although they are grateful for the help they are receiving, they are very stressed about their daughter's situation.

Linking the concept of culture and diversity with the concept of communication:

3. How might the nurse assess this family's values and beliefs in light of the family's inability to speak English?

4. How might involvement of an interpreter to facilitate communication impact the patient and her family's values and beliefs? How can you overcome this problem?

Linking the concept of culture and diversity with the concept of advocacy:

5. How can you advocate for this patient's values and beliefs while she is in the rehabilitation center?

6. The patient's family wishes to pray at the child's bedside using candles, which are not allowed because of the risk for fire related to oxygen use. How can you advocate for this family while maintaining safety?

REFER Go to Pearson MyLab Nursing and eText

- Additional review materials

REFLECT Apply Your Knowledge

Elam Avromovitch, a 76-year-old man, is visiting his son's family in the United States when he develops chest pain. A native of Israel and a follower of ultra-Orthodox Judaism, Mr. Avromovitch speaks Yiddish as his first language. Tests reveal he is having an acute myocardial infarction and needs intervention in a cardiac catheterization lab. The nurses on the cardiac floor are attempting to prepare him for the procedure while his son translates. The nurse attempts to call for a translator for the consent, but the son declines a translator, stating that he will serve instead. When attempting to undress Mr. Avromovitch for a required admission skin assessment before the procedure, the patient starts to "shoo" away the female nurses and tries to cover up. The son explains that women are not permitted to see him undressed, particularly women who are not of his faith.

1. Is the use of the son for interpretation valid for a legal consent for treatment?

2. How can the nurse respect Mr. Avromovitch's diversity requirements while maintaining facility policy and meeting the patient's healthcare needs?

3. What nursing diagnoses and interventions would be appropriate for Mr. Avromovitch's plan of care?

References

Administration on Aging. (2015). A profile of older Americans: 2015. U.S. Department of Health and Human Services. Retrieved from http://www.aoa.acl.gov/aging_statistics/profile/2015/docs/2015-Profile.pdf

American Association of Colleges of Nursing. (2008). *Cultural competency in baccalaureate nursing education.* Retrieved from http://www.aacn.nche.edu/leading-initiatives/education-resources/competency.pdf

American Association of People with Disabilities (AAPD). (2016). *Our focus.* Retrieved from http://www.aapd.com/our-focus/

Association of American Medical Colleges. (2005). *Cultural competence education.* Retrieved from https://www.aamc.org/download/54338/dataf

Berlin, E. A., & Fowkes, W. C. (1983). A teaching framework for cross-cultural health care. *Western Journal of Medicine, 139,* 934–938.

Berman, A., & Snyder, S. (2012). *Fundamentals of nursing: Concepts, process and practice.* Upper Saddle River, NJ: Pearson Education.

Byrne, M., Weddle, C., Davis, E., & McGinnis, P. (2003). The Byrne guide for inclusionary cultural content. *Journal of Nursing Education, 42*(6), 277–281.

Carteret, M. (n.d.). Cultural barriers to treatment and compliance. *Dimensions of culture: Cross cultural communications for healthcare professionals.* Retrieved from http://www.dimensionsofculture.com/2011/03/cultural-barriers-to-treatment-and-compliance/

Casper, M., Barnett, E., Halverson, J., Elmes, G., Braham, V., Majeed, Z., ... Stanley, S. (2000). *Women and heart disease: An atlas of racial and ethnic disparities in mortality* (2nd ed.). Morgantown, WV: Office for Social Environment and Health Research, West Virginia University.

Chang, M., & Kelly, A. E. (2007). Patient education: Addressing cultural diversity and health literacy issues. *Urological Nursing Journal, 27*(5), 411–417.

Clarke, T. C., Black, L. I., Stussman, B. J., Barnes, P. M., & Nahin, R. L. (2015). Trends in the use of complementary health approaches among adults: United States, 2002–2012. *National Health Statistics Report 79.* U.S. Department of Health and Human Services. Retrieved from http://www.cdc.gov/nchs/data/nhsr/nhsr079.pdf

Dayer-Berenson, L. (2011). *Cultural competencies for nurses: Impact on health and illness.* Sudbury, MA: Jones & Bartlett.

Douglas, M. K., Pierce, J. U., Rosenkoetter, M., Pacquiao, D., Callister, L. C., Hattar-Pollara, M., ... Purnell, L. (2011). Standards of practice for culturally competent nursing care: 2011 update. *Journal of Transcultural Nursing, 22*(4), 317–333. doi:10.1177/1043659611412965

Drake, B. (2013). How LGBT adults see society and how the public sees them. Pew Research Center. Retrieved from http://www.pewresearch.org/fact-tank/2013/06/25/how-lgbt-adults-see-society-and-how-the-public-sees-them/

Fingerhut, H. (2016). Support steady for same-sex marriage and acceptance of homosexuality. Pew Research Center. Retrieved from http://www.pewresearch.org/fact-tank/2016/05/12/support-steady-for-same-sex-marriage-and-acceptance-of-homosexuality/

Grandbois, D., & Sanders, G. (2012). Resilience and stereotyping: The experiences of Native American elders. *Journal of Transcultural Nursing, 23*(4), 389–396. doi:10.1177/1043659612451614

Grant, J. M., Mottet, L. M., Tanis, J., Harrison, J., Herman, J., & Keisling, M. (2011). *Injustice at every turn: A report of the national transgender discrimination survey.* Washington, DC: National Center for Transgender Equality and National Gay and Lesbian Task Force.

Health Resources and Services Administration (n.d.). *LGBT health.* Retrieved from http://www.hrsa.gov/lgbt/

Hein, L. C., & Levitt, N. (2014). Caring for ... transgender patients. *Nursing Made Incredibly Easy! 12*(6), 28–36. doi:10.1097/01.NME.0000454745.49841.76

Herdman, T. H. & Kamitsuru, S. (Eds.). *Nursing Diagnoses—Definitions and Classification 2015–2017.* Copyright © 2014, 1994–2014 NANDA International. Used by arrangement with John Wiley & Sons, Inc. Companion website: www.wiley.com/go/nursingdiagnoses

Hook, J. N., Davis, D. E., Owen, J., Worthington, E. L., Jr., & Utsey, S. O. (2013). Cultural humility: Measuring openness to culturally diverse clients. *Journal of Counseling Psychology, 60*(3), 353–366. doi:10.1037/a0032595

Itkowitz, C. (2016, June 21). An Orlando doctor's bloodied shoes — the story behind the viral story. *The Washington Post.* Retrieved from https://www.washingtonpost.com/news/inspired-life/wp/2016/06/21/im-carrying-them-on-me-all-the-time-the-orlando-doctor-whose-bloody-shoes-went-viral/

Institute of Medicine (IOM). (2002). *Unequal treatment: Confronting racial and ethnic disparities in health care.* Washington, DC: National Academy of Sciences.

Institute of Medicine (IOM). (2011). *The health of lesbian, gay, bisexual, and transgender people: Building a foundation for better understanding.* Washington, DC: National Academy of Sciences.

Intersex Society of North America (ISNA). (n.d.). *What is intersex?* Retrieved from http://www.isna.org/faq/what_is_intersex.

Ku, L.., & Jewers, M. (2013). *Healthcare for immigrant families: Current policies and issues.* Washington, DC: Migration Policy Institute. Retrieved from http://www.migrationpolicy.org/research/health-care-immigrant-families-current-policies-and-issues

Leininger, M. (2002). Culture care theory: A major contribution to advance transcultural nursing knowledge and practices. *Journal of Transcultural Nursing, 13,* 189–192. doi:10.1177/10459602013003005

Macartney, S. Bishaw, A., & Fontenot, K. (2013). Poverty rates for selected detailed race and Hispanic groups by state and place: 2007–2011. American Community Survey Briefs. *U.S. Census Bureau.* Retrieved from http://www.census.gov/prod/2013pubs/acsbr11-17.pdf

National Institutes of Health LGBT Research Coordinating Committee. (2013). Consideration of the Institute of Medicine (IOM) report on the health of lesbian, gay, bisexual, and transgender (LGBT) individuals. *National Institutes of Health.* Retrieved from https://report.nih.gov/UploadDocs/LGBT%20Health%20Report_FINAL_2013-01-03-508%20compliant.pdf

National League of Nursing. (n.d.). *Nursing is social justice advocacy.* Retrieved from http://www.nln.org/professional-development-programs/teaching-resources/toolkits/advocacy-teaching

Purnell, L., Davidhizar, R., Giger, J., Strickland, O., Fishman, D., & Allison, D. (2011). A guide to developing a culturally competent organization. *Journal of Transcultural Nursing, 22*(1), 7–14. doi:10.1177/1043659610387147

Purnell, L. D. (2014). *Guide to culturally competent health care* (3rd ed.). Philadelphia: FA Davis.

Rollins, L. K., & Huack, F. R. (2105). Delivering bad news in the context of culture: A patient-centered approach. *Journal of Communication, 22*(1), 21–26.

Rotter, J. B. (1966). Generalized expectancies for internal versus external control of reinforcement. *Psychological Monographs: General and Applied, 80*(1), 1–28. Retrieved from http://dx.doi.org/10.1037/h0092976

Sabin, J. A., Riskind, R. G., & Nosek, B. A. (2015). Health care providers' implicit and explicit attitudes toward lesbian women and gay men. *American Journal of Public Health, 105*(9), 1831–1841. doi:10.2105/AJPH.2015.302631

Schuiling, K. D., & Likis, F. E. (2013). *Women's gynecologic health* (2nd ed.). Sudbury, MA: Jones & Bartlett.

The Secretary's Advisory Committee on National Health Promotion and Disease Prevention Objectives for 2020. (2008). *Phase I report recommendations for the framework and format of Healthy People 2020.* Retrieved from https://www.healthypeople.gov/sites/default/files/PhaseI_0.pdf

Social Science Research Council. (n.d.). *Is race "real"?* Retrieved from http://raceandgenomics.ssrc.org

Spanakis, E. K., & Golden, S. H. (2013). Race/ethnic difference in diabetes and diabetic complications. *Current Diabetes Reports, 13*(6). Retrieved from http://doi.org/10.1007/s11892-013-0421-9

Spector, R. E. (2017). *Cultural diversity in health and illness* (9th ed.). Hoboken, NJ: Pearson Education.

Thompson, S., Duke, G., Haas, B., Vardaman, S., & Yarbrough, S. (2014). Military nurses caring for the enemy. *The International Journal for Human Caring,* 18(2): 61–70.

Vanderbilt University. (2017). Lesbian, Gay, Bisexual, Transgender, Queer, and Intersex Life: Definitions. Retrieved from https://www.vanderbilt.edu/lgbtqi/resources/definitions

U.S. Census Bureau. (2013). *Race: About.* Retrieved from http://www.census.gov/topics/population/race/about.html

U.S. Census Bureau. (2016, Sept. 13). *Income, poverty and health insurance coverage in the United States: 2015.* [Press Release CB16-158]. Retrieved from http://www.census.gov/newsroom/press-releases/2016/cb16-158.html

U.S. Department of Homeland Security. (2016). *Yearbook of immigration statistics: 2014.* Washington, D.C.: U.S. Department of Homeland Security, Office of Immigration Statistics. http://www.dhs.gov/xlibrary/assets/statistics/yearbook/2010/ois_yb_2010.pdf

Vanderbilt University. (2017). *Lesbian, gay, bisexual, transgender, queer, and intersex life: Definitions.* Retrieved from https://www.vanderbilt.edu/lgbtqi/resources/definitions

Vroman, K. G., Arthanat, S., & Lysack, C. (2015). "Who over 65 is online?" Older adults' dispositions toward information communication technology. *Computers in Human Behavior, 43,* 156–166. http://dx.doi.org/10.1016/j.chb.2014.10.018

Williams, T. (2013, April 13). Quietly, Indians reshape cities and reservations. *Star Tribune.* Retrieved from http://www.nytimes.com/2013/04/14/us/as-american-indians-move-to-cities-old-and-new-challenges-follow.html?_r=0

World Health Organization. (2016). *Vulnerable groups.* Retrieved from http://www.who.int/environmental_health_emergencies/vulnerable_groups/en/

Yusef, H. (2015, June 24). My hijab has nothing to do with oppression: It's a feminist statement. *The Guardian.* Retrieved from https://www.theguardian.com/commentisfree/video/2015/jun/24/hijab-not-oppression-feminist-statement-video

Module 25
Development

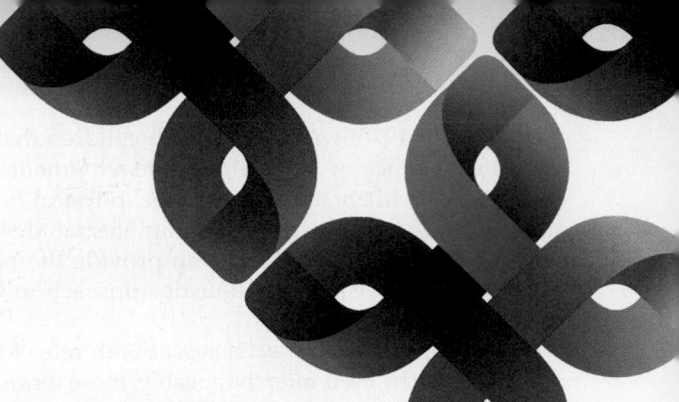

Module Outline and Learning Outcomes

The Concept of Development

Normal Development

25.1 Analyze the components and theories of normal development.

Growth and Development Through the Lifespan

25.2 Summarize the developmental milestones of individuals across the lifespan.

Alterations to Development

25.3 Differentiate alterations in development.

Concepts Related to Development

25.4 Outline the relationship between development and other concepts.

Health Promotion

25.5 Explain the promotion of healthy development.

Nursing Assessment

25.6 Differentiate common assessment procedures and tests used to examine development.

Independent Interventions

25.7 Analyze independent interventions nurses can implement for patients with alterations in development.

Collaborative Therapies

25.8 Summarize collaborative therapies used by interprofessional teams for patients with alterations in development.

Lifespan Considerations

25.9 Differentiate considerations related to the assessment and care of patients with alterations in development throughout the lifespan.

Development Exemplars

Exemplar 25.A Attention-Deficit/Hyperactivity Disorder

25.A Analyze ADHD as it relates to development.

Exemplar 25.B Autism Spectrum Disorder

25.B Analyze ASD as it relates to development.

Exemplar 25.C Cerebral Palsy

25.C Analyze CP as it relates to development.

Exemplar 25.D Failure to Thrive

25.D Analyze failure to thrive as it relates to development.

>> The Concept of Development

Concept Key Terms

Accommodation, **1790**	Conservation, **1798**	Ecologic theory, **1792**	Morality, **1792**	Puberty, **1802**
Adaptation, **1790**	Cooperative play, **1800**	Egocentrism, **1798**	Nature, **1792**	Receptive
Adaptation phase, **1792**	Development, **1786**	Expressive jargon, **1797**	Nurture, **1792**	speech, **1795**
Adjustment phase, **1792**	Developmental	Expressive	Object	Resilience, **1791**
Assimilation, **1790**	milestones, **1792**	speech, **1795**	permanence, **1798**	Risk factors, **1791**
Associative play, **1798**	Developmental	Growth, **1786**	Parallel play, **1796**	Self-efficacy, **1790**
Centration, **1798**	stage, **1786**	Magical thinking, **1798**	Personality, **1787**	Solitary play, **1793**
Cephalocaudal, **1786**	Developmental	Moral, **1792**	Protective	Temperament, **1790**
Cognitive development,	task, **1788**	Moral behavior, **1792**	factors, **1791**	Transductive
1789	Dramatic play, **1798**	Moral development, **1792**	Proximodistal, **1786**	reasoning, **1798**

Jean Piaget (1970) wrote: "It is with children that we have the best chance of studying the development of logical knowledge, mathematical knowledge, physical knowledge, and so forth" (p. 14). Understanding lifespan development and applying that knowledge can provide the nurse with valuable tools to provide a holistic approach to caring for patients of all ages.

The terms *growth* and *development* both refer to dynamic processes. Often used interchangeably, these terms have different meanings. **Growth** refers to physical change and increase in size. Indicators of growth include height, weight, bone size, and dentition. The pattern of physiologic growth is similar for all people. However, growth rates vary during different stages of growth and development. The growth rate is rapid during the prenatal, neonatal, infancy, and adolescent stages and slows during childhood. Physical growth is minimal during adulthood.

Development is an increase in the complexity of function and skill progression, the capacity and skill of an individual to adapt to the environment. Development is the behavioral aspect of growth (e.g., an individual develops the ability to walk, to talk, and to run).

Normal Development

Growth and development are independent, yet interrelated, processes. For example, an infant's muscles, bones, and nervous system must grow to a certain point before the infant is able to sit up or walk. Growth generally takes place during the first 20 years of life; development takes place throughout the lifespan. Principles of growth and development include:

- Growth and development are continuous, orderly, sequential processes influenced by maturational, environmental, and genetic factors.

- All humans follow the same pattern of growth and development.

- The sequence of each stage is predictable, although the time of onset, the length of the stage, and the effects of each stage vary with each individual.

- Each **developmental stage** (level of achievement) has its own characteristics. For example, Piaget suggested that in the sensorimotor stage (birth to 2 years) children learn to coordinate simple motor tasks.

- Growth and development occur in a **cephalocaudal** direction, that is, starting at the head and moving toward the trunk, legs, and feet (**Figure 25–1 》**). This pattern is particularly obvious at birth, when the head of the infant is disproportionately large.

- Growth and development occur in a **proximodistal** direction, that is, from the center of the body outward (see Figure 25–1). For example, infants can roll over before they can grasp an object with the thumb and second finger.

- Development proceeds from simple to complex, or from single acts to integrated acts. To accomplish the integrated act of drinking and swallowing from a cup, for example, the child must first learn a series of single acts: eye–hand coordination; grasping; hand–mouth coordination; controlled tipping of the cup; and then mouth, lip, and tongue movements to drink and swallow.

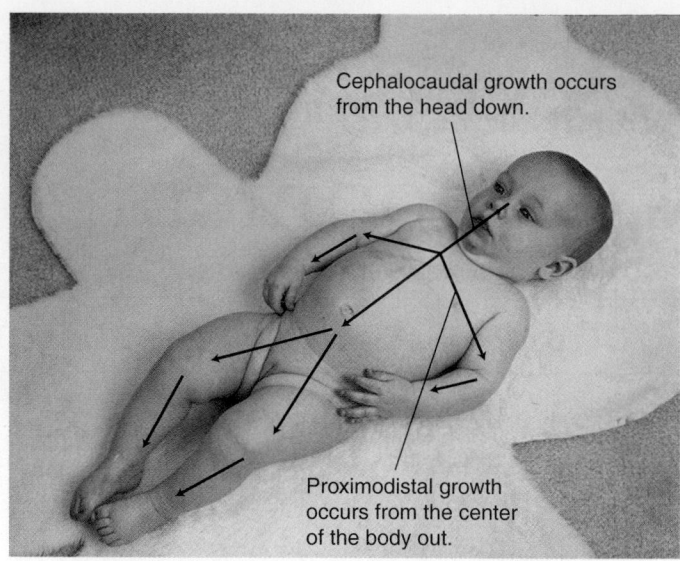

Cephalocaudal growth occurs from the head down.

Proximodistal growth occurs from the center of the body out.

Figure 25–1 》 In normal cephalocaudal growth, the child gains control of the head and neck before the trunk and limbs. In normal proximodistal growth, the child controls arm movements before hand movements. For example, the child reaches for objects before being able to grasp them. Children gain control of their hands before their fingers; that is, they can hold things with the entire hand before they can pick something up with just their fingers.

- Development becomes increasingly differentiated. Differentiated development begins with a generalized response and progresses to a specific skilled response. For example, an infant's initial response to a stimulus involves the total body, but a 5-year-old child can respond more specifically with laughter or fear.

- The pace of growth and development is uneven. It is known that growth is greater during infancy than during childhood. Asynchronous development is demonstrated by rapid growth of the head during infancy and the extremities at puberty.

- The rate of growth and development is highly individual; however, the sequence of growth and development is predictable. Stages of growth usually correspond to certain developmental changes (**Table 25–1 》》**).

Theories of Growth and Development

Theories help to explain one or more aspects of an individual's growth and development. Typically, theorists examine only one aspect of development, such as the cognitive, moral, or physical aspect. The area chosen for examination usually reflects the researcher's academic discipline and personal interest. The theorists may also limit the population that is studied to a particular part of the lifespan, such as infancy, childhood, or adulthood.

Although such theories can be useful, they have limitations. First, although a given theory may explain one aspect of the growth and development process, an individual does not develop in fragmented sections but rather as a whole human being. Thus, application of several theories may be

TABLE 25–1 Stages of Growth and Development

Stage	Age	Significant Characteristics	Nursing Implications
Neonatal	Birth–28 days	Behavior is largely reflexive and develops to more purposeful behavior.	Assist parents to identify and meet unmet needs.
Infancy	1 month–1 year	Physical growth is rapid.	Control the infant's environment so that physical and psychologic needs are met.
Toddlerhood	1–3 years	Motor development permits increased physical autonomy. Psychosocial skills increase.	Safety and risk-taking strategies must be balanced to permit growth.
Preschool	3–6 years	The preschooler's world is expanding. New experiences and the preschooler's social role are tried during play. Physical growth is slower.	Provide opportunities for play and social activity.
School age	6–12 years	This stage includes the preadolescent period (10–12 years). Peer group increasingly influences behavior. Physical growth is slower.	Allow time and energy for the school-age child to pursue hobbies and school activities. Recognize and support child's achievement.
Adolescence	12–18 years	Self-concept changes with biological development. Values are tested. Physical growth accelerates. Stress increases.	Assist adolescents to develop coping behaviors. Help adolescents develop strategies for resolving conflicts.
Young adulthood	18–40 years	A personal lifestyle develops. Individual establishes a relationship with a significant other and a commitment to something; many become parents. Physical growth slows and then stops (except for weight gain). Metabolism begins to slow down.	Accept adult's chosen lifestyle and assist with necessary adjustments relating to health. Recognize the individual's commitments. Support change as necessary for health.
Middle adulthood	40–65 years	Lifestyle changes because of other changes; for example, children leave home, occupational goals change. Physical changes may include weight gain, diminished vision and hearing, onset of wrinkles, hair loss in men. Risk for onset of chronic illness greatest during this time.	Assist patients to plan for anticipated changes in life, to recognize the risk factors related to health, and to focus on strengths rather than weaknesses.
Older adulthood			
Young-old	65–74 years	Adaptation to retirement and changing physical abilities is often necessary. Chronic illness may develop/continue.	Assist patients to keep mentally, physically, and socially active and to maintain peer group interactions.
Middle-old	75–84 years	Adaptation to decline in speed of movement, reaction time, and balance issues. Increasing dependence on others may be necessary.	Assist patients to cope with loss (e.g., hearing, sensory abilities, eyesight, death of loved one). Provide necessary safety measures.
Old-old	85 years and older	Increasing physical problems may develop. Many need help with self-care.	Assist patients with self-care as required, and with maintaining as much independence as possible.

necessary to gain insight about an individual's growth and development.

Another limitation of some theories is the suggestion that certain tasks are performed at a specific age. In most cases, the child or adult does accomplish the task at the time specified by the guidelines. In other cases, however, the nurse may find that an individual does not accomplish the task or meet the milestone at the exact time the theory suggests. Such individual differences are not easily defined or categorized by a single theory.

Growth and development are commonly thought of as having five major components: psychosocial, cognitive, moral, spiritual, and biophysical. Theorists have attempted to study and explain development through these lenses as well as others, including social learning, temperament and personality, and ecology. Researchers have advanced several theories about the various stages and aspects of growth and development, particularly with regard to infant and child development. A discussion of some of the major theories follows.

Psychosocial Theories

Psychosocial development refers to the development of personality. **Personality** can be considered an outward expression of the inner (intrapersonal) self; the enduring characteristic patterns of thinking, feeling, and behavior that make an individual unique. It encompasses an individual's temperament, feelings, character traits, independence, self-esteem, self-concept, behavior, ability to interact with others, and ability to adapt to life changes. Although personality is enduring over time, it may be influenced by or adapt to changes or differences in education, environments, and experiences.

Sigmund Freud (1856–1939) proposed many of the earliest theories regarding the development of personality. For nurses, the most relevant part of his work centers around the development of ego defense mechanisms, which are described in the module on Stress and Coping.

Erikson (1902–1994)

Erik H. Erikson (1963, 1968) proposed a theory of development that includes the entire lifespan, as he believed that people continue to develop throughout life. He described eight stages of development (**Table 25–2 >>**).

Erikson's theory proposes that life is a sequence of developmental stages or levels of achievement. Each stage signals a task that must be accomplished. The resolution of the task can be complete, partial, or unsuccessful. Erikson believed

TABLE 25–2 Erikson's Eight Stages of Development

Stage	Age	Primary Task	Outcomes of Successful Task Accomplishment	Outcomes of Failed Task Accomplishment
Infancy	Birth–18 months	Trust versus mistrust	Development of basic trust and sense of security	Lack of trust, sense of fear
Early childhood	18 months–3 years	Autonomy versus shame and doubt	Basic awareness of independence; sense of autonomy and self-control	Self-doubt, sense of helplessness, heightened dependence on caregivers
Late childhood	3–5 years	Initiative versus guilt	Emergence of basic sense of self-guidance and self-discipline	Impaired self-initiative, insecurity regarding leadership ability
School age	6–12 years	Industry versus inferiority	Confidence in ability to attain goals, initial formation of identity apart from nuclear family, successful peer group integration	Sense of incompetence, low self-esteem, difficulty integrating into peer groups
Adolescence	12–20 years	Identity versus role confusion	Formation of strong sense of identity as an individual and as a member of society, identification of personal and occupational goals	Role confusion, social alienation, potential substance abuse, potential development of antisocial personality disorder
Young adulthood	18–25 years	Intimacy versus isolation	Development of healthy romantic relationships without compromising personal identity	Avoidance of intimacy, fear of commitment, isolation
Adulthood	25–65 years	Generativity versus stagnation	Productivity and creativity, desire to care for and guide offspring (or, if childfree, to guide the next generation)	Self-preoccupation, primary attainment of pleasure through self-indulgence, stagnation
Maturity	65 years–death	Integrity versus despair	Sense of peace concerning life experiences, life choices framed within a meaningful context, development of wisdom	Life experiences framed by bitterness and/or regret; may progress to hopelessness and depression

Source: Based on Erikson, E. (1963). *Childhood and society.* New York, NY: W.W. Norton; Weber, J. R., & Kelley, J. H. (2010). *Health assessment in nursing* (4th ed.). Philadelphia, PA: Lippincott Williams & Wilkins; Watts, J., Cockcroft, K., & Duncan, N. (Eds.). (2010). *Developmental psychology* (2nd ed.). Cape Town, South Africa: UCT Press.

that the more successful an individual is at each developmental stage, the healthier the personality of the individual will be. Failure to complete any developmental stage interferes with the individual's ability to progress to the next level. These developmental stages can be viewed as a series of crises. Successful resolution of these crises supports healthy ego development. Failure to resolve the crises damages the ego.

Erikson's eight stages reflect both positive and negative aspects of the critical life periods. The resolution of the conflicts at each stage enables the individual to function effectively in society. Each phase has its own **developmental tasks** (skills or behavior patterns, such as walking or toileting independently, that are characteristic of that phase). At each stage, the individual must find a balance between, for example, trust and mistrust (stage 1) or integrity and despair (stage 8). See **Figures 25–2 》** and **25–3 》**.

According to Erikson, the environment is highly influential to development. Nurses can enhance a patient's development by being aware of the individual's developmental stage and assisting with the development of coping skills related to stressors experienced at that specific level. Nurses can strengthen a patient's positive resolution of a developmental task by providing the individual with appropriate opportunities and encouragement. For example, the nurse can encourage a 10-year-old child (industry versus inferiority) to be creative, to finish schoolwork, and to learn how to accomplish these tasks within the limitations imposed by health status. The nurse can encourage the older adult to maintain generativity (care for and connection with others) to avoid a sense of stagnation, or a feeling of disconnectedness that increases self-absorption and loneliness.

Erikson emphasized that people must change and adapt their behavior to maintain control over their lives. In his

view, no stage in personality development can be bypassed, and people can become fixated at one stage or regress to a previous stage under anxious or stressful conditions. For example, a middle-aged woman who has never satisfactorily resolved the identity versus role confusion task might

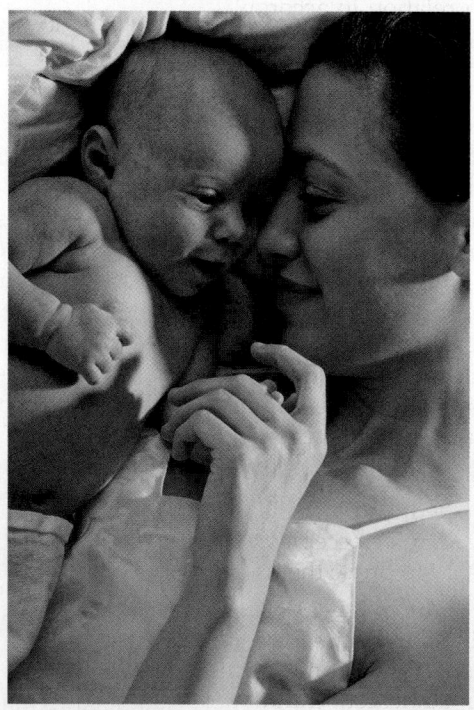

Source: Purestock/Getty Images.

Figure 25–2 》 This infant is clearly on his way to accomplishing a sense of basic trust in and security with his mother.

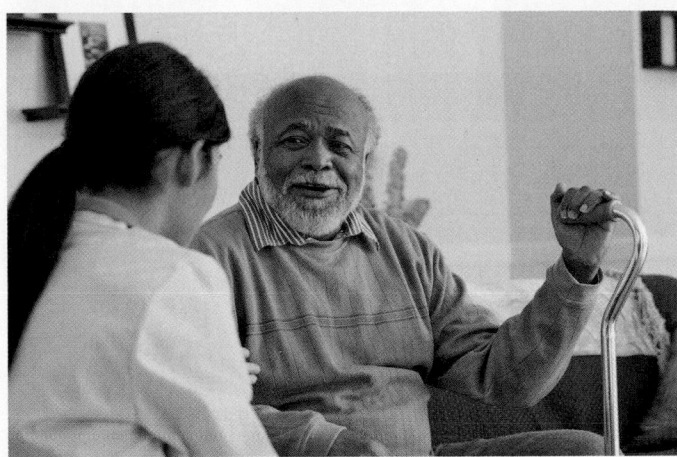

Source: Jupiter Images/Stockbyte/Getty Images.

Figure 25–3 》 Regular visits from a home health nurse can help older adults maintain their health and independence, contributing to the achievement of integrity versus despair.

regress to an earlier stage when stressed by an illness with which she cannot cope.

Gould (1935–)

Roger Gould is another theorist who has studied adult development. He believes that transformation is a central theme during adulthood: "Adults continue to change over the period of time considered to be adulthood and developmental phases may be found during the adult span of life" (Gould, 1972, p. 33). According to Gould, in his 20s the individual assumes new roles, in the 30s role confusion often occurs, in the 40s the individual becomes aware of time limitations in relation to accomplishing life's goals, and in the 50s the acceptance of each stage as a natural progression of life marks the path to adult maturity.

- *Stage 1 (ages 16–18).* Individuals consider themselves part of the family rather than individuals; they begin to want to separate from their parents.

- *Stage 2 (ages 18–22).* Although individuals have established autonomy, they feel it is in jeopardy; they feel they could be pulled back into their families.

- *Stage 3 (ages 22–28).* Individuals feel established as adults and autonomous from their families. They see themselves as well defined but still feel the need to prove themselves to their parents. They see this as the time for growing and building for the future.

- *Stage 4 (ages 28–34).* Marriage and careers are well established. Individuals question what life is all about and wish to be accepted as they are, no longer finding it necessary to prove themselves.

- *Stage 5 (ages 34–43).* This is a period of self-reflection. Individuals question long-held values as well as life itself. They see time as finite, with little time left to shape the lives of adolescent children.

- *Stage 6 (ages 43–50).* Personalities are seen as set. Time is accepted as finite. Individuals are interested in social activities with friends and spouse and desire both sympathy and affection from spouse.

- *Stage 7 (ages 50–60).* This is a period of transformation, with a realization of mortality and a concern for health. There is an increase in warmth and a decrease in negativism. The spouse is seen as a valuable companion (Gould, 1972, pp. 525–527).

Peck (1919–2002)

Theories and models about adult development are relatively recent compared with theories of infant and child development. Research into adult development has been stimulated by a number of factors, including increased longevity and healthier old age. In the past, development was viewed as complete by the time of physical maturity, and aging was considered a decline following maturity. The emphasis was on the negative rather than positive aspects of aging. However, Robert Peck (1968) believed that, although physical capabilities and functions decrease with old age, mental and social capacities tend to increase in the latter part of life.

Peck (1968) proposed three developmental tasks during old age, in contrast to Erikson's one (integrity versus despair):

1. *Ego differentiation versus work-role preoccupation.* An adult's identity and feelings of worth are highly dependent on that individual's work role. On retirement, people may experience feelings of worthlessness unless they derive their sense of identity from a sufficient number of roles that one such role can replace the work role or occupation as a source of self-esteem. For example, a man who likes to garden or golf can obtain ego rewards from those activities, replacing rewards formerly obtained from his occupation.

2. *Body transcendence versus body preoccupation.* This task calls for the individual to adjust to decreasing physical capacities and at the same time maintain feelings of well-being. Preoccupation with declining body functions reduces happiness and satisfaction with life.

3. *Ego transcendence versus ego preoccupation.* Ego transcendence is the acceptance without fear of one's death as inevitable. This acceptance includes being actively involved in one's own future beyond death. Ego preoccupation, by contrast, results in holding onto life and a preoccupation with self-gratification.

Cognitive Theory

Cognitive development refers to the manner in which people learn to think, reason, and use language. It involves a person's intelligence, perceptual ability, and ability to process information. Cognitive development represents a progression of mental abilities from illogical to logical thinking, from simple to complex problem solving, and from understanding concrete ideas to understanding abstract concepts. The most widely known cognitive theorist is Jean Piaget (1896–1980). His theory of cognitive development has contributed to other theories.

According to Piaget (1966), cognitive development is an orderly, sequential process in which a variety of new experiences (stimuli) must exist before intellectual abilities can develop. Piaget divides cognitive development into four major phases: the sensorimotor phase, the preoperational phase, the concrete operational phase, and the formal

TABLE 25-3 Piaget's Phases of Cognitive Development

Phases and Stages	Age	Significant Behavior
Sensorimotor phase	Birth–2 years	
Stage 1: Use of reflexes	Birth–1 month	Uses reflexes: sucking, rooting, grasping.
Stage 2: Primary circular reaction	1–4 months	Infant responds reflexively. Objects are extension of self.
Stage 3: Secondary circular reaction	4–8 months	Awareness of environment grows. Changes in the environment are actively made as infant recognizes cause and effect.
Stage 4: Coordination of secondary schemata	8–12 months	Intentional behavior occurs. Object permanence begins.
Stage 5: Tertiary circular reaction	12–18 months	Toddlers discover new goals and ways to attain goals. Rituals are important.
Stage 6: Mental combinations	18–24 months	Language gives toddlers a new tool to use.
Preoperational phase	2–7 years	Young children think by using words as symbols. Everything is significant and relates to "me." They explore the environment. Language development is rapid. Words are associated with objects.
		As children get older, egocentric thinking diminishes. They think of one idea at a time. Words express thoughts.
Concrete operational phase	7–11 years	Children solve concrete problems, begin to understand relationships such as size, understand right and left, and recognize various viewpoints.
Formal operational phase	11 years and up	Children use rational thinking. Reasoning is deductive and futuristic.

Source: Data from Piaget, J. (1966). *Origins of intelligence in children.* New York, NY: W.W. Norton. Copyright © 1966 International Universities Press, Inc.

operational phase. A detailed discussion of these phases, and how the nurse can incorporate his or her knowledge of them into nursing plans and interventions, can be found in the module on Cognition.

An individual develops through each of these phases; each phase has its own unique characteristics (**Table 25–3 »**). In each phase, the individual uses three primary abilities: assimilation, accommodation, and adaptation. **Assimilation** is the process through which humans encounter and react to new situations by using mechanisms they already possess. In this way, people acquire knowledge and skills as well as insights into the world around them. **Accommodation** is a process of change whereby cognitive processes mature sufficiently to allow the individual to solve problems that were unsolvable before. This adjustment is possible chiefly because new knowledge has been assimilated. **Adaptation**, or coping behavior, is the ability to handle the demands made by the environment.

Nurses can use Piaget's theory of cognitive development when developing teaching strategies. For example, a nurse can expect a toddler to be egocentric and literal; therefore, explanations to the toddler should focus on the needs of the toddler rather than on the needs of others. A 13-year-old can be expected to use rational thinking and to reason; therefore, when explaining the need for a medication, a nurse can outline the consequences of taking and not taking the medication, enabling the adolescent to make a rational decision. Nurses must remember, however, that the range of normal cognitive development is broad, despite the ages arbitrarily associated with each level. When teaching adults, nurses may become aware that some adults are more comfortable with concrete thought and are slower to acquire and apply new information than are other adults.

Behaviorism

Behaviorist theory states that learning takes place when an individual's reaction to a stimulus is either positively or negatively reinforced. The more rapid, consistent, and positive the reinforcement, the more likely a behavior is to be learned and retained.

B. F. Skinner (1904–1990) believed that organisms learn as they respond to or "operate on" their environment. His research led to the concept of *operant conditioning,* in which he maintained that rewarded or reinforced behavior will be repeated; behavior that is punished will be suppressed.

Social Learning Theory

Albert Bandura (1925–), a contemporary psychologist, believes that children learn attitudes, beliefs, customs, and values through their social contacts with adults and other children. Children imitate (or model) the behavior they see; if the behavior is positively reinforced, they tend to repeat it. However, Bandura also believes that people can consciously choose how to act, such as deciding to handle problems by talking rather than using violence. The external environment (the behavior of others) and the child's internal processes are both key elements in the behaviors the child manifests (Bandura, 1986, 1997a).

Bandura believes that an important determinant of behavior is **self-efficacy**, or the expectation that someone can produce a desired outcome. For example, if adolescents believe they can avoid use of drugs or alcohol, they are more likely to do so. A child who has confidence in his or her ability to exercise regularly or lose weight has a greater chance of success with these behavior changes. Parents who have confidence in their ability to care adequately for their infants are more likely to do so (Bandura, 1997b).

Temperament Theory

In contrast to personality, **temperament** refers to innate characteristics, such as nervousness or sensitivity, that do not change over time. Chess and Thomas (1995, 1996) recognize the innate qualities of personality that each individual brings to the events of daily life. They view the child as an individual who both influences and is influenced by the environment. However, Chess and Thomas focus on one specific aspect of development: the wide spectrum of behaviors possible in children and how they respond to daily events. Infants generally display clusters of responses, which Chess and Thomas have classified into three major personality types (**Box 25–1 »**). Although most children do not demonstrate all behaviors described for a particular type, they usually show a grouping indicative of one personality type (Chess & Thomas, 1995, 1996).

Longitudinal research has demonstrated that personality characteristics displayed during infancy are often consistent with those seen later in life. The ability to predict future characteristics is not possible, however, because of the complex and dynamic interaction of personality traits and environmental reactions.

Resiliency Theory

The concept of resilience first appeared in the literature in the early 1970s. Werner, Bierman, and French (1971) studied a cohort of children from Kauai, Hawaii, in efforts to understand why some children who grow up in poverty and other challenging situations did not follow in the footsteps of their parents, many of whom were alcoholics and/or had mental illness. The researchers felt those children grew up "resilient" to challenging situations (Werner et al., 1971). Resiliency theory examines the individual's characteristics as well as the interaction of those characteristics with the environment. **Resilience** is the ability to function with healthy responses, even when experiencing significant stress and adversity (Benard, 2014). In this model, the individual or family members experience a crisis that provides a source of stress, and the family interprets or deals with the crisis based on resources

---

Box 25–1
Patterns of Temperament—Chess and Thomas

- **"Easy" child.** The "easy" child is generally moderately active; shows regularity in patterns of eating, sleeping, and elimination; and is usually positive in mood and when subjected to new stimuli. The easy child adapts to new situations and is able to accept rules and work well with others. About 40% of children in the New York Longitudinal Study displayed this personality type.
- **"Difficult" child.** The "difficult" child displays irregular schedules for eating, sleeping, and elimination; adapts slowly to new situations and persons; and displays a predominantly negative mood. Intense reactions to the environment are common. The New York Longitudinal Study found that approximately 10% of children display this personality type.
- **"Slow-to-warm-up" child.** The "slow-to-warm-up" child has reactions of mild intensity and is slow to adapt to new situations. The child displays initial withdrawal followed by gradual, quiet, and slow interactions with the environment. About 15% of children in the New York Longitudinal Study displayed this personality type.

The remaining 35% of children studied showed some characteristics of each personality type.

Source: Data from Chess S., & Thomas, A. (1996). *Temperament: Theory and practice*, Philadelphia, PA: Brunner/Mazel.

---

available. Families and individuals have **protective factors** that provide strength and assistance in dealing with crises and **risk factors** that promote or contribute to their challenges (Cairns et al., 2014). Protective and risk factors can be identified in children, in their families, and in their communities. A

Evidence-Based Practice
Resiliency

Problem

Staff retention is an ever-present issue for intensive care units (ICUs). Nurses are faced with constant stress from many different sources, including but not limited to patient acuity, family dynamics, and ethical challenges. Those nurses who choose to work in critical care areas tend to have a higher incident of depression, anxiety, and posttraumatic stress disorder (PTSD).

Evidence

Mealer et al. (2014) conducted a small study of 27 nurses who worked in a variety of critical care settings. Prior to the study, the test subjects showed evidence of stress-related mental health conditions, including anxiety and depression. Of the 27 subjects, 11 scored positive for PTSD symptoms.

The group was divided into an intervention group (13 subjects) and control group (14 subjects). Those in the intervention group participated in a 2-day, multi-module resilience training that included writing therapy, mindfulness therapy, and self-care techniques. After 12 weeks, those who participated in the resilience training showed improvement in several mental health screening tools, including a significant decrease in depression, and reported greater skills in coping with the stresses of ICU nursing.

Implications

Providing resilience training, as well as prompting resilience and self-care techniques, is a worthy investment for nurse managers and healthcare facilities to make, as the outcomes of improved mental health and improved coping skills are likely to lower burnout and error rates and improve retention rates. Likewise, nurses, particularly those in critical care situations, should be aware that working in this specialty area calls for great resilience. Nurses can nurture their own personal resilience through different techniques, such as journaling and peer counseling. Nurses can apply this concept of resilience in several different ways.

Critical Thinking Application

1. You are working as the staff educator on an oncology unit. In what ways is this evidence-based resilience training applicable to your unit? Give a rationale for your answer.
2. You are working as a nurse manager of a 28-bed ICU. You want to incorporate resilience training for your staff. Should the training be part of the new hire orientation? Should the training be delayed until the new staff member is off probation and has been working on the unit for 6 or more months? Should resilience training be part of the yearly staff education? Give rationales for your answers.

typical crisis for a young child might be a transfer to a new child care provider. Protective factors for a child transferring to a new provider could involve past positive experiences with new people and an "easy" temperament. An additional protective factor might be the level of understanding the new child care provider has about the adaptation needs of young children to new experiences. Risk factors for a child experiencing this type of transition might include repeated moves to new care providers, limited close relationships with adults, and a "slow-to-warm-up" temperament.

Once confronted by a crisis, the child and family first experience the **adjustment phase**. This phase is characterized by disorganization and unsuccessful attempts at meeting the crisis. In the **adaptation phase**, the child and family meet the challenge and use resources to deal with the crisis (Walsh, 2011). Adaptation may lead to increasing resilience, as the child and family learn about new resources and inner strengths and develop the ability to deal more effectively with future crises.

Ecologic Theory

The relative importance in human development of heredity versus environment—or nature versus nurture—is controversial among theorists. **Nature** refers to the genetic or hereditary capability of an individual. **Nurture** refers to the effects of the environment on a person's performance. Contemporary developmental theories increasingly recognize the interaction of nature and nurture in determining the individual's development.

The ecologic theory of development was formulated by Urie Bronfenbrenner to explain the individual's unique relationship in all of life's settings, from close to remote (Bronfenbrenner, 1986, 2005; Bronfenbrenner et al., 1996). **Ecologic theory** emphasizes the presence of mutual interactions between the individual and these various settings. Neither nature nor nurture is considered more important. Bronfenbrenner believes each individual brings a unique set of genes—and specific attributes such as age, gender, health, and other characteristics—to his or her interactions with the environment. The individual then interacts in many settings at different levels or systems, such as family, school or work, and sports team or interest club. The systems the individual encounters affect both the individual and the other systems. For example, communication between the parent, the pediatrician's office, and the school may help ensure that a child has an asthma action plan in time for the school nurse to review it with the child's teachers and bus drivers.

Moral Theories

Moral development is a complex process that is not fully understood. It involves learning what a person should and should not do, but it is more than merely the imprinting of parents' rules and virtues or values on children. The term **moral** means "relating to right and wrong." The terms *morality*, *moral behavior*, and *moral development* need to be distinguished from each other. **Morality** refers to the requirements necessary for people to live together in society, **moral behavior** is the way an individual perceives and responds to those requirements, and **moral development** is the pattern of change in moral behavior with age. Refer to the exemplar on Morality in the module on Ethics for more information.

Kohlberg (1927–1987)

Lawrence Kohlberg's theory specifically addresses moral development in children and adults (Kohlberg, 1981, 1984). Kohlberg was not concerned with the morality of an individual's decision; rather, he focused on the reasons an individual makes a decision. According to Kohlberg, moral development progresses through three levels and six stages. Levels and stages are not always linked to a certain developmental stage, because some people progress to a higher level of moral development than others. It is worth noting that Kohlberg's theory of moral development has been criticized for a number of points, including emphasis on moral reasoning rather than moral action, failing to consider the role of the family in the development of the individual, sexual bias, and cultural insensitivity (Santrock, 2015). For example, after more than 10 years of research with female subjects, Carol Gilligan (1982) reported that women often consider the dilemmas Kohlberg used in research to be irrelevant.

Gilligan (1936–)

Gilligan proposed that moral development proceeds through three levels and two transitions, with each level representing a more complex understanding of the relationship of self and others and each transition resulting in a crucial reevaluation of the conflict between selfishness and responsibility (Campbell, 2010; Murray & Zentner, 2001, p. 251).

Gilligan (1982) proposes that because women often see morality in the integrity of relationships and caring, the moral problems they encounter are different from those of men. Men tend to consider what is right to be what is just, whereas for women what is right is taking responsibility for others as a self-chosen decision (p. 140). The ethic of justice, or fairness, is based on the idea of equality: Everyone should receive the same treatment. This is the development path usually followed by men and widely accepted by moral theorists. By contrast, the ethic of care is based on the premise of nonviolence: No one should be harmed. This is the path typically followed by women but given little attention in the literature of moral theory.

Spiritual Theories

The spiritual component of growth and development refers to individuals' understanding of their relationship with the universe and their perceptions about the direction and meaning of life. The most influential description of *spiritual development* was offered by Fowler (1981). Although Fowler used the term "faith development", he recognized faith as a universal human phenomenon that leads individuals to need and find meaning and an understanding of themselves in relation to their world. Refer to the module on Spirituality for more information on Fowler's description of spiritual development.

Growth and Development Through the Lifespan

Individuals constantly change and evolve throughout their lives. While some changes are subtle and highly individualized, others are apparent and represent **developmental milestones** common to all human beings at or near a specific phase of growth and development. The stages of sexual development are covered in the module on Sexuality.

Infants (Birth to 1 Year)

Immense changes occur during the child's first year of life. The child emerges totally dependent on others, his actions primarily reflexive in nature. By the end of his first year, the infant can walk and communicate. Never again in life is development so swift.

Physical Growth and Motor Development

The infant's birth weight usually doubles by about 5 months and triples by the end of the first year. Height increases by approximately 1 foot during this year. Teeth begin to erupt at about 6 months, and by the end of the first year, the infant has six to eight deciduous teeth. Physical growth is closely associated with type and quality of feeding. Likewise, culture and nutrition impact motor function. Angulo-Barroso et al. (2011) found that in cultures with diets high in iron, such as in Ghana, the infants reach motor milestones earlier than other infants of same age. On the other hand, in cultures with diets poor in iron, infants reach motor milestones (e.g., walking without assistance) at a later age.

Body organs and systems, although not fully mature at 1 year of age, function differently than they did at birth. Kidney and liver maturation helps the 1-year-old excrete drugs or other toxic substances more readily than in the first weeks of life. The changing body proportions mirror changes in developing internal organs (**Figure 25–4 》**). Maturation of the nervous system is demonstrated by increased control over body movements, enabling the infant to sit, stand, and walk. Sensory function also increases as the infant begins to discriminate visual images, sounds, and tastes (**Table 25–4 》**).

Cognitive Development

The brain continues to increase in complexity during the first year of life. Most of the growth involves maturation of cells, with only a small increase in cell number. This growth of the brain is accompanied by development of its functions, something easily understood when one compares the behavior of the newborn to that of the 1-year-old. The newborn's eyes widen in response to sound; the 1-year-old turns to the sound and recognizes its significance. The 2-month-old cries and coos; the 1-year-old says a few words and understands many more. The 6-week-old grasps a rattle for the first time; the 1-year-old reaches for toys and begins to feed herself.

The infant's behaviors provide clues about thought processes. Piaget's work outlines the infant's actions in a set of rapidly progressing changes in the first year of life. The infant receives stimulation through sight, sound, and feeling, which the maturing brain interprets. This input from the environment interacts with internal cognitive abilities to enhance cognitive functioning.

Psychosocial Development

The infant relies on interactions with primary care providers to meet needs and then begins to establish a sense of trust in other adults and in children. As trust develops, the infant becomes comfortable in interactions with a widening array of people.

Play

The play of infants begins in a reflexive manner. When infants move extremities or grasp objects, they experience the foundations of play. They gain pleasure from the feel and sound of these activities, and gradually perform them purposefully. For example, when a parent places a rattle in the hand of a 6-week-old infant, the infant grasps it reflexively. As the hands move randomly, the rattle makes an enjoyable sound. The infant learns to move the rattle to create the sound and then finally to grasp the toy at will to play with it.

The next phase of infant play focuses on manipulative behavior. The infant examines toys closely, looking at them, touching them, and placing them in his or her mouth. The infant learns a great deal about texture, qualities of objects, and all aspects of the surroundings. At the same time, interaction with others becomes an important part of play. The social nature of play is obvious as the infant plays with other children and adults. For example, when a parent walks by, the infant laughs and waves hands and feet wildly (**Figure 25–5 》**). The infant plays primarily alone with toys (**solitary play**) but enjoys the presence of adults or other children. Physical capabilities enable the infant to move toward and reach for objects of interest.

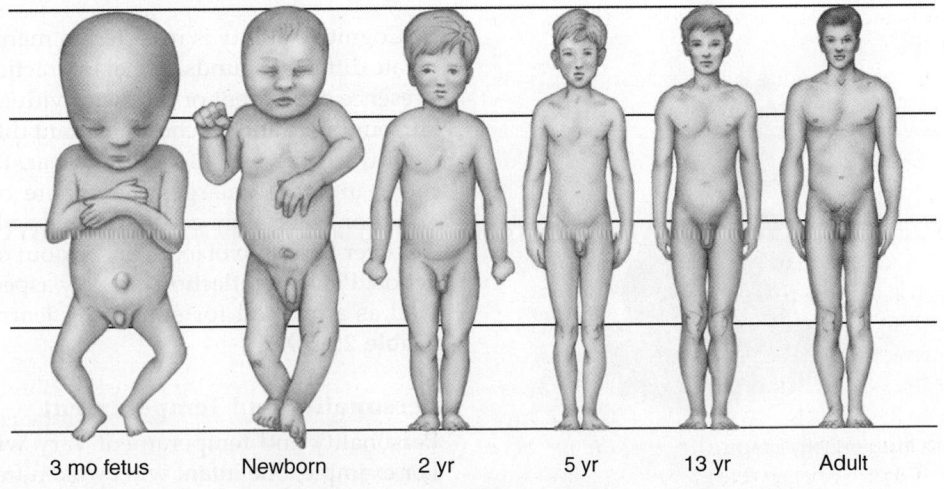

3 mo fetus   Newborn   2 yr   5 yr   13 yr   Adult

Figure 25–4 》 Body proportions at various ages.

TABLE 25-4 Growth and Development Milestones During Infancy

Age	Physical Growth	Fine Motor Ability	Gross Motor Ability	Sensory Ability
Birth–1 month	Gains 140–200 g (5–7 oz)/week. Grows 1.5 cm (1/2 in.) in first month. Head circumference increases 1.5 cm (1/2 in.)/month.	Forms hand into a fist. Draws arms and legs to body when crying.	Inborn reflexes such as startle and rooting are predominant activity. May lift head briefly if prone. Alerts to high-pitched voices. Comforts with touch.	Prefers to look at faces and black-and-white geometric designs. Follows objects in line of vision.
2–4 months	Gains 140–200 g (5–7 oz)/week. Grows 1.5 cm (1/2 in.)/month. Head circumference increases 1.5 cm (1/2 in.)/month. Posterior fontanel closes. Eats 120 mL/kg/24 hr (2 oz/lb/24 hr).	Holds rattle when placed in hand. Looks at and plays with own fingers. Brings hands to midline.	Moro reflex fading in strength. Can turn from side to back and then return. Head lag when pulled to sitting position decreases; sits with head held in midline with some bobbing. When prone, holds head and supports weight on forearms.	Follows objects 180 degrees. Turns head to look for voices and sounds.
4–6 months	Gains 140–200 g (5–7 oz)/week. Doubles birth weight in 5–6 months. Grows 1.5 cm (1/2 in.)/month. Head circumference increases 1.5 cm (1/2 in.)/month. Teeth may begin erupting by 6 months. Eats 100 mL/kg/24 hr (1 1/2 oz/lb/24 hr).	Grasps rattles and other objects at will; drops them to pick up another offered object. Mouths objects. Holds feet and pulls to mouth. Holds bottle. Grasps with whole hand (palmar grasp). Manipulates objects.	Holds head steady when sitting. Has no head lag when pulled to sitting. Turns from abdomen to back by 4 months and then back to abdomen by 6 months. When held standing, supports much of own weight.	Examines complex visual images. Watches the course of a falling object. Responds readily to sounds.
6–8 months	Gains 85–140 g (3–5 oz)/week. Grows 1 cm (3/8 in.)/month. Growth rate slower than first 6 months.	Bangs objects held in hands. Transfers objects from one hand to the other. Pincer grasp begins at times.	Most inborn reflexes extinguished. Sits alone steadily without support by 8 months. Likes to bounce on legs when held in standing position.	Recognizes own name and responds by looking and smiling. Enjoys playing with small and complex objects.
8–10 months	Gains 85–140 g (3–5 oz)/week. Grows 1 cm (3/8 in.)/month.	Picks up small objects. Uses pincer grasp well.	Crawls or pulls whole body along floor by arms. Creeps by using hands and knees to keep trunk off floor. Pulls self to standing and sitting by 10 months. Recovers balance when sitting.	Understands words such as "no" and "cracker." May say one word in addition to "mama" and "dada." Recognizes sound without difficulty.
10–12 months	Gains 85–140 g (3–5 oz)/week. Grows 1 cm (3/8 in.)/month. Head circumference equals chest circumference. Triples birth weight by 1 year.	May hold crayon or pencil and make mark on paper. Places objects into containers through holes.	Stands alone. Walks holding onto furniture. Sits down from standing.	Plays peek-a-boo and patty cake.

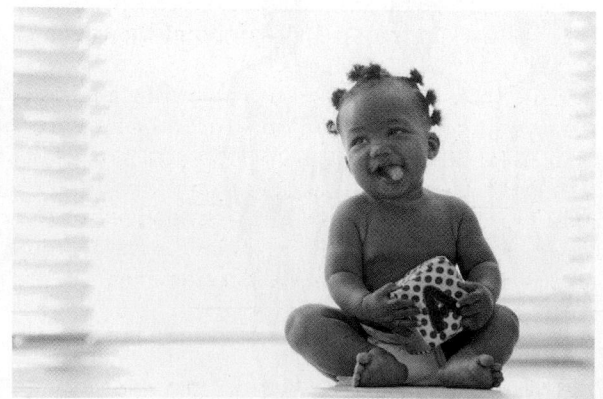

Source: Monkey Business Images/Getty Images.

Figure 25–5 ≫ This 9-month-old girl demonstrates physical, cognitive, and social capabilities while playing with blocks.

Cognitive ability is reflected in manipulation of blocks to create different sounds. Social interaction enhances play. The presence of a parent or other individual increases interest in surroundings and teaches the infant different ways to play.

Toward the end of the first year, the infant's ability to move in space enlarges the sphere of play. Once infants crawl or walk, they can get to new places, find new toys, discover forgotten objects, or seek out other people for interaction. Play is a reflection of every aspect of development, as well as a method for enhancing learning and maturation (**Table 25–5 ≫**).

Personality and Temperament

Personality and temperament vary widely among infants. For example, one infant will awaken frequently in the night, while another will sleep soundly for 8–10 hours. One infant may smile and react positively to interactions, while another

TABLE 25–5 Psychosocial Development During Infancy

Age	Play and Toys	Communication
Birth–3 months	■ Prefers visual stimuli of mobiles, black-and-white patterns, mirrors. ■ Responds to auditory stimuli such as music boxes, tape players, soft voices. ■ Responds to rocking and cuddling. ■ Moves legs and arms while adult sings and talks. ■ Likes varying stimuli—different rooms, sounds, visual images.	■ Coos. ■ Babbles. ■ Cries.
3–6 months	■ Prefers noise-making objects that are easily grasped, like rattles. ■ Enjoys stuffed animals and soft toys with contrasting colors.	■ Vocalizes during play and with familiar people. ■ Laughs. ■ Cries less. ■ Squeals and makes pleasure sounds. ■ Babbles multisyllabically (mamamamama).
6–9 months	■ Likes teething toys. ■ Increasingly desires social interaction with adults and other children. ■ Favors soft toys that can be manipulated and mouthed.	■ Increases vowel and consonant sounds. ■ Links syllables together. ■ Uses speechlike rhythm when vocalizing with others.
9–12 months	■ Enjoys large blocks, toys that pop apart and go back together, nesting cups and other objects. ■ Laughs at surprise toys like a jack-in-the-box. ■ Plays interactive games like peek-a-boo. ■ Uses push-and-pull toys.	■ Understands "no" and other simple commands. ■ Says "dada" and "mama" to identify parents. ■ Learns one or two other words. ■ Receptive speech surpasses expressive speech.

withdraws around unfamiliar people and frequently frowns and cries. Such differences in responses to the environment are believed to be inborn characteristics of temperament. Infants are born with a tendency to react in certain ways to noise and to interact differently with people. They may display varying degrees of regularity in activities of eating and sleeping, and manifest a capacity for concentrating on tasks for different amounts of time. Although an infant's temperament cannot be changed, parents can modify the environment to promote adaptation. Strategies include using only one or two consistent babysitters or caregivers, rather than engaging new or changing caregivers frequently, and feeding the infant in a quiet setting to encourage a focus on eating.

Focus on Diversity and Culture
Reaching Developmental Milestones

In some cultures, children are allowed to unfold and develop naturally at their own pace. Children wean and toilet train themselves with little interference or pressure from parents. The nurse should be sensitive to the childrearing practices of the family and support them in these culturally accepted practices.

For example, the developmental milestone for sleeping through the night is typically reached at age 4 to 5 months (Andrews & Boyle, 2016). However, in many cultures, including Native American, Alaskan Natives, and First Nations tribes, infants sleep with their mothers. Infants will wake and nurse typically every 4 hours through the night. The mothers are typically not disturbed by this on-demand feeding practice, so there is less motivation for the mother to have the child sleep through the night (Andrews & Boyle, 2016). Therefore, these infants do not reach the milestone of sleeping 8 hours a night until later in their development than infants who do not sleep with their mothers.

Communication

Communication skills are evident even at a few weeks of age. Infants communicate and engage in two-way interaction; they express comfort by soft sounds, cuddling, and eye contact. The infant displays discomfort by thrashing the extremities, arching the back, and crying vigorously. From these rudimentary skills, communication ability continues to develop until the infant speaks several words at the end of the first year of life (see Table 25–5). Nonverbal methods continue to be a primary method of communication between parent and child.

Nurses assess communication to identify possible abnormalities or developmental delays. Language ability may be assessed with a specialized language screening tool. Normal infants and toddlers understand (**receptive speech**) more words than they can speak (**expressive speech**). Abnormalities may be caused by a hearing deficit, developmental delay, or lack of verbal stimulation from caregivers. Further assessment may be required to pinpoint the cause of the abnormality.

Nursing interventions focus on providing a stimulating and comforting environment and encouraging parents to speak to infants and teach words. Hospital nurses should include the infant's known words when providing care, and provide nonverbal support by hugging and holding. Nurses planning interventions should consider the family's cultural patterns for communications and development.

Toddlers (1 to 3 Years)

Toddlerhood is sometimes called the first adolescence. The child from 1 to 3 years of age, who months before was merely an infant, is now displaying independence and negativism. Pride in newfound accomplishments emerges during this time.

TABLE 25–6 Growth and Development Milestones During Toddlerhood

Age	Physical Growth	Fine Motor Ability	Gross Motor Ability	Sensory Ability
1–2 years	■ Gains 227 g (8 oz) or more per month. ■ Grows 9–12 cm (3.5–5 in.) during this year. ■ Anterior fontanel closes.	■ By end of second year, builds a tower of four blocks. ■ Scribbles on paper. ■ Can undress self. ■ Throws a ball.	■ Runs. ■ Walks up and down stairs. ■ Likes push-and-pull toys.	Visual acuity 20/50
2–3 years	■ Gains 1.4–2.3 kg (3–5 lb)/year. ■ Grows 5–6.5 cm (2–2.5 in.)/year.	■ Draws a circle and other rudimentary forms. ■ Learns to pour. ■ Is learning to dress self.	■ Jumps. ■ Kicks ball. ■ Throws ball overhand.	

Physical Growth and Motor Development

The rate of growth slows during the second year of life. The child requires limited food intake during this time, a change that may cause concern to the parent. The nurse reassures parents with these concerns that this is a normal occurrence in their child's development. By age 2 years, the birth weight has usually quadrupled and the child is about one half of the adult height. Body proportions begin to change, with longer legs and a smaller head in proportion to body size than during infancy. The toddler has a pot-bellied appearance and stands with feet apart to provide a wide base of support. By approximately 33 months, eruption of the 20 deciduous teeth is complete.

Gross motor activity develops rapidly (**Table 25–6 »**) as the toddler progresses from walking to running, kicking, and riding a tricycle. As physical maturation occurs, the toddler develops the ability to control elimination patterns.

Cognitive Development

During the toddler years, the child moves from the sensorimotor to the preoperational stage of development. The early use of language awakens in the 1-year-old the ability to think about objects or people when they are absent. Object permanence is well developed.

At about 2 years of age, the increasing use of words as symbols enables the toddler to use preoperational thought. Rudimentary problem solving, creative thought, and an understanding of cause-and-effect relationships are now possible.

Psychosocial Development

The toddler is soundly rooted in a trusting relationship and feels more comfortable asserting autonomy and separating from primary care providers. It is important for toddlers to begin asserting their autonomy within the context of safe places and relationships that promote their interaction with both adults and other children.

Play

Patterns of play emerge and change between infancy and toddlerhood. The toddler's motor skills enable him to bang pegs into a pounding board with a hammer. The social nature of toddler play is also visible. Toddlers find the company of other children pleasurable, even though socially interactive play may not occur. Toddlers tend to play with similar objects side by side, occasionally trading toys and

words (**Figure 25–6 »**). This is called **parallel play**. Playing with other children assists toddlers to develop social skills. Toddlers engage in play activities they have seen at home, such as pounding with a hammer and talking on the phone. This imitative behavior helps them to learn new actions and skills.

Physical skills are manifested in play as toddlers push and pull objects, climb in and out and up and down, run, ride a Big Wheel, turn the pages of books, and scribble with a pen. Both gross motor and fine motor abilities are enhanced during this age period.

Cognitive understanding enables the toddler to manipulate objects and learn about their qualities. Stacking blocks and placing rings on a building tower teach spatial relationships and other lessons that provide a foundation for future learning. Various kinds of play objects should be provided for the toddler to meet play needs. These play needs can easily be met whether the child is hospitalized or at home (**Table 25–7 »**).

Personality and Temperament

The toddler retains most of the temperamental characteristics identified during infancy, but may demonstrate some changes. The normal developmental progression of toddlerhood plays a part in responses. For example, the infant who previously responded positively to stimuli, such as a new

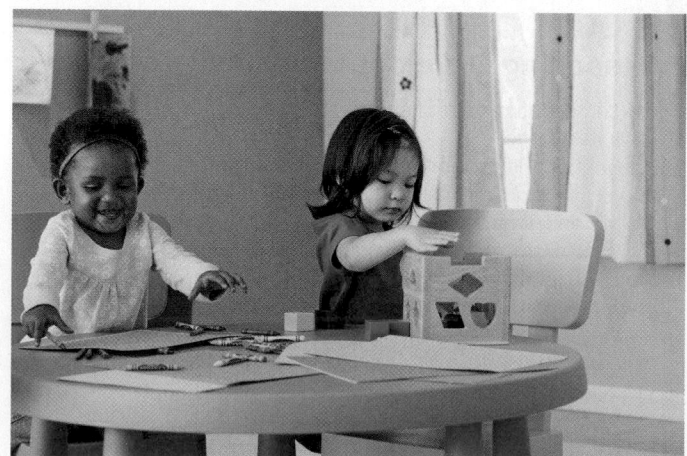

Source: Jupiter Images/Stockbyte/Getty Images.

Figure 25–6 » These toddlers display typical parallel play at daycare, playing next to but not with each other.

TABLE 25–7 Psychosocial Development During Toddlerhood

Age	Play and Toys	Communication
1–3 years	■ Refines fine motor skills by use of cloth books, large pencil and paper, wooden puzzles. ■ Facilitates imitative behavior by playing kitchen, grocery shopping, toy telephone. ■ Learns gross motor activities by riding Big Wheel tricycle, playing with a soft ball and bat, molding water and sand, tossing ball or beanbag. ■ Develops cognitive skills through exposure to educational television shows, music, stories, and books.	■ Increasingly enjoys talking. ■ Vocabulary grows exponentially, especially when spoken and read to. ■ Needs to release stress by pounding board, frequent gross motor activities, and occasional temper tantrums. ■ Likes contact with other children and learns interpersonal skills.

babysitter, may appear more negative in toddlerhood. The increasing independence characteristic of this age is shown by the toddler's use of the word *no*. The parent and child constantly adapt their responses to each other and learn anew how to communicate with each other.

Communication

Because the child's capacity for development of language skills is greatest during the toddler period, adults should communicate frequently with children in this age group. This communication is critical not only to the toddler's ability to communicate simple wants and needs, but also to cognitive and language development, which affects the toddler's future literacy. Toddlers also begin to learn the social interactions and nonverbal gestures that they observe.

At the beginning of toddlerhood, the child may use four to six words in addition to "mama" and "dada." Receptive speech (the ability to understand words) far outpaces expressive speech. By the end of toddlerhood, however, the 3-year-old has a vocabulary of almost 1000 words and uses short sentences. Toddler communication includes pointing, pulling an adult over to a room or object, and speaking in **expressive jargon** (using unintelligible words with normal speech intonations as if truly communicating in words). Other communication methods include crying, pounding or stamping feet, displaying a temper tantrum, or other means that illustrate dismay. These powerful communication methods can upset parents, who often need suggestions for handling them. Adults can best assist the toddler by verbalizing the feelings shown by the toddler, by saying things like "You must be very upset that you cannot have that candy. When you stop crying you can come out of your room." Verbalizing the child's feeling and then ignoring further negative behavior ensures that the parent is not unintentionally reinforcing the inappropriate behavior. While the toddler's search for autonomy and independence creates a need for such behavior, an upset toddler may respond well to holding, rocking, and stroking.

Parents and nurses can promote a toddler's communication by speaking frequently, naming objects, giving single-step directions, explaining procedures in simple terms, expressing feelings that the toddler seems to be displaying, and encouraging speech. The toddler is at an optimal age to learn two languages. For example, if the parents wish for their child to learn two languages, the toddler will benefit from a child care experience that will expose her to a second language in addition to the language her family speaks at home. Research continues to support the finding that those children who are bilingual have cognitive advantages over monolingual children (Ramírez & Kuhl, 2015).

The nurse who understands the communication skills of toddlers is able to assess expressive and receptive language and communicate effectively, thereby promoting positive healthcare experiences for these children. Parents often need suggestions for ways to communicate with the young child.

Preschool Children (3 to 6 Years)

The preschool years are a time of new initiative and independence. Most children are in a child care center or school for part of the day, and they learn a great deal from this social contact. Language skills are well developed, and the child is able to understand and speak clearly. Endless projects characterize the world of busy preschoolers. They may work with play dough to form animals, then cut out and paste paper, then draw and color.

Physical Growth and Motor Development

Preschoolers grow slowly and steadily, with most growth taking place in long bones of the arms and legs. The short, chubby toddler gradually gives way to a slender, long-legged preschooler (**Table 25–8** »).

Physical skills continue to develop. The preschooler runs with ease, holds a bat, and throws balls of various types. Writing ability increases, and the preschooler enjoys drawing and learning.

The preschool period is a good time to encourage good dental habits. Children can begin to brush their own teeth with parental supervision and help in reaching all tooth surfaces. Parents should floss children's teeth, give fluoride as prescribed if the water supply is not fluoridated, and schedule the first dental visit so the child can become accustomed to the routine of periodic dental care.

Cognitive Development

The preschooler exhibits characteristics of preoperational thought. Symbols or words are used to represent objects and people, enabling the young child to think about them. This is a milestone in intellectual development; however, the preschooler still has some limitations in thought (**Table 25–9** »). It is important to understand the preschooler's thought processes in order to plan appropriate teaching for healthcare and development of health habits.

TABLE 25–8 Growth and Development Milestones During the Preschool Years

Physical Growth	Fine Motor Ability		Gross Motor Ability	Sensory Ability
Gains 1.5–2.5 kg (3–5 lb)/year. Grows 4–6 cm (1 1/2–2 1/2 in.)/year.	Uses scissors. Draws circle, square, cross. Draws at least a six-part person. Enjoys art projects such as pasting, stringing beads, using clay. Learns to tie shoes at end of preschool years. Buttons clothes. Brushes teeth. Eats three meals, with snacks. Uses spoon, fork, and knife.		Throws a ball overhand. Climbs well. Rides tricycle.	Visual acuity continues to improve. Can focus on and learn letters and numbers.

Psychosocial Development

The preschooler is more independent in establishing relationships with others. The child interacts closely with children and adults and is able to plan and carry out activities.

Play

Play for the preschooler takes on a new dimension as he begins to interact with others. One child cuts out colored paper while his friend glues it on paper in a design. This new type of interaction is called **associative play**.

In addition to this social dimension, other aspects of play also differ. The preschooler enjoys large motor activities such as swinging, riding a tricycle, and throwing a ball (**Figure 25–7 ≫**). Preschoolers demonstrate increasing manual dexterity as they create more complex drawings and manipulations of blocks and modeling. Because fantasy life is so powerful at this age, the preschooler readily uses props to engage in **dramatic play** (the living out of the drama of human life).

The nurse can use playtime to assess the preschooler's developmental level, knowledge about healthcare, and emotions related to healthcare experiences. Observations about objects chosen for play, content of dramatic play, and pictures drawn can provide important assessment data. The nurse can also use play periods to teach the child about healthcare procedures and offer an outlet for expressing emotions (**Table 25–10 ≫**).

The use of media such as smartphones, tablets, and computers is becoming more of the preschooler's life than ever before. In a cross-sectional study of 350 children, Kabali et al. (2015) found that almost 96.6% of children ages 1–4 had used a mobile device, such as a smartphone, and that 75% had their own device. The nurse might find hospitalized children are easily soothed and distracted by portable media devices such as tablets (Radesky, Schumacher, & Zuckerman, 2015). However, the nurse should be aware that the research is very limited on what can be considered too much screen time. The American Academy of Pediatrics (AAP) recommends that parents and other caregivers discourage the use of screen time for children under 18 months unless it is for video chatting with a loved one. For older toddlers and preschoolers, the AAP recommends limiting screen time to

TABLE 25–9 Characteristics of Thought Identified by Piaget

Characteristic	Definition	Development Stage	Nursing Implications
Object permanence	Ability to understand that when something is out of sight it still exists	Sensorimotor period, especially in coordination of secondary schemes substage from 8 to 12 months	Before development of object permanence, babies will not look for toys or other objects out of sight; as the concept is developing they are concerned when a parent leaves, because they are not certain the parent will return.
Egocentrism	Ability to see things only from one's own point of view	Preoperational thought	Peers or others who have gone through an experience will not impress the preschooler; teaching should focus on what an experience will be like for the child himself.
Transductive reasoning	Connecting two events in a cause-and-effect relationship simply because they occur together in time	Preoperational thought	Ask the child what she thinks caused an occurrence; ask how the two events are connected; correct misconceptions to lessen child's guilt.
Centration	Focusing only on one particular aspect of a situation	Preoperational thought	Listen to the child's comments and deal with concerns in order to be able to present new concepts to the child.
Magical thinking	Believing that events occur because of one's thoughts or actions	Preoperational thought	Ask young children how they became ill, or what caused a parent's or sibling's illness. Correct misconceptions when the child blames self for causing problems by wishing someone ill or having bad behavior.
Conservation	Knowing that matter is not changed when its form is altered	Concrete operational thought	Before conservation of thought is reached, the child may think that gender can be changed when hair is cut, the leg under a cast is broken in separate pieces. Ask perceptions and clarify misconceptions.

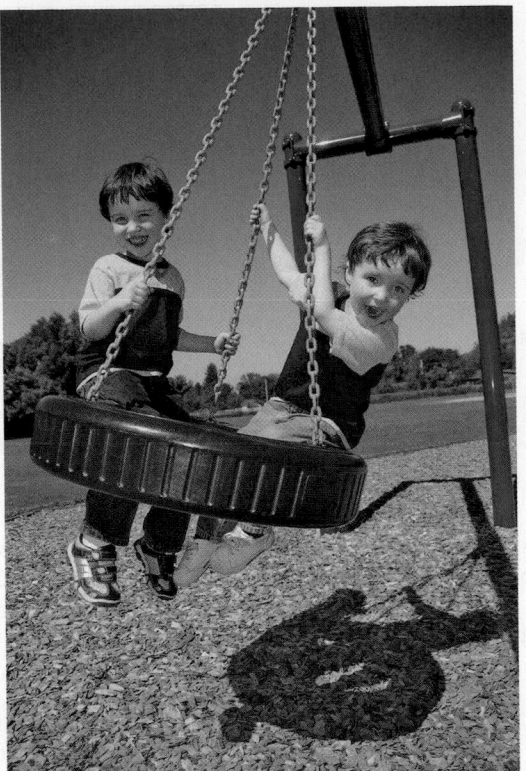

Source: Rossario/Shutterstock.

Figure 25–7 》 Preschoolers have well-developed large motor skills and enjoy activities such as swinging.

an hour a day and then only for educational programming or video chatting. Young children should not engage in screen time during meals and for at least an hour before bedtime (AAP, 2016).

As with television, it is crucial to ask how parents decide which technology and content is best for their children and how they monitor and set rules for use. Violence on mobile media should be avoided, and when encountered, parents and caregivers should help their children understand it. Providers can recommend age-appropriate, educational content and suggest the use of resources such as PBS Kids (www.pbskids.org), Sesame Workshop (www.sesameworkshop.org), or Common Sense Media (www.commonsensemedia.org) to guide media choices. Clinicians should strongly emphasize the benefits of parents and children using

interactive media together to enhance its educational value (Radesky et al., 2015, p. 2).

Personality and Temperament

Characteristics of personality observed in infancy tend to persist over time. The preschooler may need assistance as these characteristics are expressed in the new situations of preschool or nursery school. An excessively active child, for example, will need gentle, consistent handling to adjust to the structure of a classroom. Encourage parents to visit preschool programs to choose the one that would best foster growth in their child. Some preschoolers enjoy the structured learning of a program that focuses on cognitive skills, while others are happier and more open to learning in a small group that provides much time for free play. Nurses can help parents to identify their child's personality or temperament characteristics and to find the best environment for growth.

Communication

Language skills blossom during the preschool years. The vocabulary grows to over 2000 words, and children speak in complete sentences of several words and use all parts of speech. They practice these newfound language skills by endlessly talking and asking questions.

The sophisticated speech of preschoolers mirrors the development occurring in their minds and helps them to learn about the world around them. However, this speech can be quite deceptive. Although preschoolers use many words, their grasp of meaning is usually literal and may not match that of adults. These literal interpretations have important implications for healthcare providers. For example, the preschooler who is told she will be "put to sleep" for surgery may think of a pet recently euthanized; the child who is told that a dye will be injected for a diagnostic test may think he is going to die; mention of "a little stick" in the arm can cause images of tree branches rather than of a simple immunization.

Concrete visual aids such as pictures of a child undergoing the same procedure or a book to read together enhance teaching by meeting the child's developmental needs. Handling medical equipment such as intravenous bags and stethoscopes increases interest and helps the child to focus. Teaching may have to be done in several short sessions rather than one long session.

Some general approaches include the following:

- Allow time for the child to integrate explanations.
- Verbalize frequently to the child.

TABLE 25–10 Psychosocial Development During the Preschool Years

Age	Play and Toys	Communication
3–6 years	Associative play is facilitated by simple games, puzzles, nursery rhymes, songs. Dramatic play is fostered by dolls and doll clothes, play houses and hospitals, dress-up clothes, puppets. Stress is relieved by pens, paper, glue, scissors. Cognitive growth is fostered by educational television shows, music, stories and books.	Develops and uses all parts of speech, occasionally incorrectly. Communicates with a widening array of people. Play with other children is a favorite activity. Health professionals can: ■ Verbalize and explain procedures to children. ■ Use drawings and stories to explain care. ■ Use accurate names for bodily functions. ■ Allow the child to talk, ask questions, and make choices.

- Use drawings and stories to explain care.
- Use accurate names for bodily functions.
- Allow choices.

The preschooler's social growth and increased communication skills make these years the perfect time to introduce concepts related to problem solving and conflict resolution. Puzzles and manipulative toys help foster early problem-solving skills. Children in this age group can learn to calm themselves by learning how to take deep breaths and count to 3 or 5 when they are upset. Many preschool programs employ special curricula that help teachers and parents assist children in developing essential conflict resolution skills. Using language to resolve conflict is a protective factor that decreases the likelihood of children choosing inappropriate or violent behavior to try to get what they want or bring a distressing interaction to a close.

School-Age Children (6 to 12 Years)

School-age children demonstrate common characteristics of their age group. They are in a stage of industry in which it is important to the child to perform useful work. Meaningful activities take on great importance and are usually carried out in the company of peers. A sense of achievement in these activities is important to developing self-esteem and to preventing a sense of inferiority or poor self-worth.

Physical Growth and Motor Development

School age is the last period in which girls and boys are close in size and body proportions. As the long bones continue to grow, leg length increases (see Figure 25–4). Fat gives way to muscle, and the child appears leaner. Jaw proportions change as the first deciduous tooth is lost at 6 years and permanent teeth begin to erupt. Body organs and the immune system mature, resulting in fewer illnesses among school-age children. Medications are less likely to cause serious side effects, because they can be metabolized more easily. The urinary system can adjust to changes in fluid status. Physical skills are also refined as children begin to play sports, and fine motor skills are well developed through school activities.

Although it is commonly believed that the start of adolescence (age 12 years) heralds a growth spurt, the rapid increases in size commonly occur during school age. Girls may begin a growth spurt as early as 9 or 10 years of age and boys a year or so later (**Figure 25–8 》》**). Nutritional needs increase dramatically with this spurt.

The loss of the first deciduous teeth and the eruption of permanent teeth usually occur at about age 6 years, or at the beginning of the school-age period. Of the 32 permanent teeth, 22 to 26 erupt by age 12 years and the remaining molars follow during the teenage years. See the module on Health, Wellness, Illness, and Injury for a discussion of oral care for school-age children.

Cognitive Development

The child enters the stage of concrete operational thought at about age 7 years. This stage enables school-age children to consider alternative solutions and solve problems. However, school-age children continue to rely on concrete experiences and materials to form their thought content.

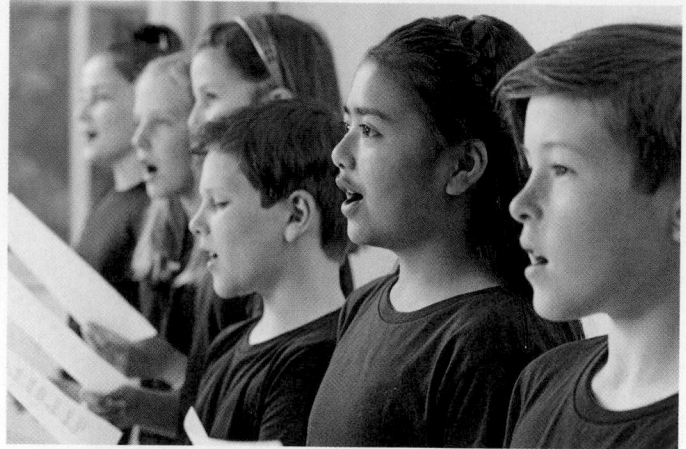

Source: Highwaystarz/iStock/Getty Images.

Figure 25–8 》》 Because girls have a growth spurt earlier than boys, girls often are taller than boys of the same age, as shown in this group of middle schoolers in a dress rehearsal for a choral performance.

During the school-age years, the child learns the concept of conservation (that matter is not changed when its form is altered). At earlier ages, a child believes that when water is poured from a short, wide glass into a tall, thin glass, there is more water in the taller glass. The school-age child recognizes that, although it may look like the taller glass holds more water, the quantity is the same. The concept of conservation is helpful when the nurse explains medical treatments. The school-age child understands that an incision will heal, that a cast will be removed, and that an arm will look the same as before once the intravenous infusion needle is removed. The child learns to read during this period and can concentrate for longer periods.

Psychosocial Development

The school-age child has many friends and cooperatively interacts with others to accomplish tasks. The child develops a sense of accomplishment from activities and relationships.

Play

Play for the school-age child is enhanced by increasing fine and gross motor skills. By 6 years of age, children have acquired the physical ability to hold the bat properly and may occasionally hit the ball. School-age children also understand that everyone has a role—the pitcher, the catcher, the batter, the outfielders. They cooperate with one another to form a team, are eager to learn the rules of the game, and want to ensure that these rules are followed exactly (**Table 25–11 》》**).

The characteristics of play exhibited by the school-age child include cooperation with others and the ability to play a part in order to contribute to a unified whole. This type of play is called **cooperative play**. The concrete nature of cognitive thought leads to a reliance on rules to provide structure and security. Children have an increasing desire to spend much of their playtime with friends, which demonstrates the social component of play. Play is an extremely important method of learning and living for the school-age child. Active physical play has decreased in recent years as

TABLE 25–11 Psychosocial Development During the School-Age Years

Age	Activities	Communication
6–12 years	Gross motor development is fostered by ball sports, skating, dance lessons, water and snow skiing/boarding, biking. A sense of industry is fostered by playing a musical instrument, gathering collections, starting hobbies, playing board and video games. Cognitive growth is facilitated by reading, crafts, word puzzles, schoolwork.	Use of language is mature. Is able to converse and discuss topics for increasing lengths of time. Spends many hours at school and with friends in sports or other activities. Health professionals can: ■ Assess child's knowledge before teaching. ■ Allow the child to select rewards following procedures. ■ Teach techniques such as counting or visualization to manage difficult situations. ■ Include both parent and child in healthcare decisions.

television viewing and playing of computer games have increased, leading to poor nutritional status and high rates of overweight among children.

When a child is hospitalized, the separation from playmates can lead to feelings of sadness and purposelessness. Normal, rewarding parts of play should be integrated into care. Friends should be encouraged to visit or call a hospitalized child. Discharge planning for the child who has had a cast or brace applied should address the activities in which the child can participate and those the child must avoid. Nurses should reinforce the importance of playing games with friends to both parents and children.

Personality and Temperament

Characteristics seen in earlier years tend to endure in the school years. The child classified as "difficult" at an earlier age may now have trouble in the classroom. Nurses may advise parents to provide a quiet setting for homework and to reward the child for concentration. For example, after completing homework, the child may be allowed to have "screen time" (play a video game, watch television, or play on the computer or tablet). Creative efforts and alternative methods of learning should be valued. Encourage parents to see their children as individuals who may not all learn in the same way. The "slow-to-warm-up" child may need encouragement to try new activities and to share experiences with others, whereas the "easy" child will readily adapt to new schools, people, and experiences.

Communication

During the school-age years, children should learn how to use language correctly, including correcting any lingering pronunciation or grammatical errors, and learning the pragmatic (social) uses of language. Vocabulary increases, and the child learns about parts of speech in school. Children also are becoming more technologically savvy with their communication. According to a 2013 study by the Pew Research Center, 78% of children 12 to 17 years of age have their own phone (Madden et al., 2013). The majority of "tweens" use their phones for texting rather than voice communications (Madden et al., 2013).

School-age children enjoy writing and, while in the hospital, can be encouraged to keep a journal of their experiences as a method of dealing with anxiety. The literal translation of words characteristic of preschoolers is uncommon among school-age children.

Some communication strategies helpful with the school-age child include:

- Provide concrete examples of pictures or materials to accompany verbal descriptions.
- Assess knowledge before planning the instruction.
- Allow child to select rewards following procedures.
- Teach techniques such as counting or visualization to manage difficult situations.
- Include child in discussions and history with parent.

Sexuality

Awareness of gender differences and sexuality becomes more pronounced during the school years. Although children become aware of sexual differences between genders during preschool years, they deal much more consciously with sexuality during the school-age years. As children mature physically, they need information about their bodily changes so that they can develop a healthy self-image and an understanding of the relationships between their bodies and sexuality. Children become interested in sexual issues and are often exposed to erroneous information on television shows, in magazines, from internet sources, or from friends and siblings. Schools and families need to use opportunities to teach school-age children factual information about sex and to foster healthy concepts of self and others. It is advisable to ask occasional questions about sexual issues to learn how much the child knows and to provide correct information when answers demonstrate confusion.

Both friends and the media are common sources of erroneous ideas. Appropriate and inappropriate touch should be discussed, with lists of trusted people who can be approached (teachers, clergy, school counselors, family members, neighbors) to discuss any episodes with which the child feels uncomfortable. Because even these trusted people can be implicated in inappropriate episodes, the nurse should encourage the child to go to more than one person, an important approach if the child is uncomfortable about a relationship with any individual.

Adolescents (12 to 18 Years)

Adolescence is a time of passage signaling the end of childhood and the beginning of adulthood. Although adolescents differ in behaviors and accomplishments, they are all in a period of identity formation. If a healthy identity and sense of self-worth are not developed during this period, role confusion and purposeless struggling will ensue. The adolescents in the healthcare setting will represent various degrees of identity formation, and each will offer unique challenges.

Physical Growth and Motor Development

The physical changes ending in **puberty**, or sexual maturity, begin near the end of the school-age period. The prepubescent period is marked by a growth spurt at an average age of 10 years for girls and 13 years for boys, although there is considerable variation among children. The increase in height and weight is generally remarkable and is completed in 2–3 years. The growth spurt in girls is accompanied by an increase in breast size and growth of pubic hair. Menstruation occurs last and signals achievement of puberty. In boys, the growth spurt is accompanied by growth in size of the penis and testes and by growth of pubic hair. Deepening of the voice and growth of facial hair occur later, at the time of puberty. For both boys and girls, some lack of coordination is common during growth spurts.

During adolescence children grow stronger and more muscular and establish characteristic male and female patterns of fat distribution. The apocrine and eccrine glands mature, leading to increased sweating and a distinct odor to perspiration. All body organs are now fully mature, enabling the adolescent to take adult doses of medications.

The adolescent must adapt to a rapidly changing body for several years. These physical changes and hormonal variations offer challenges to identity formation. See the Focus on Integrative Health.

Cognitive Development

Adolescence marks the beginning of Piaget's last stage of cognitive development, the stage of formal operational thought. The adolescent no longer depends on concrete experiences as the basis of thought but develops the ability to reason abstractly. The adolescent can understand concepts such as justice, truth, beauty, and power. The adolescent revels in this newfound ability and spends a great deal of time thinking, reading, and talking about abstract concepts.

Focus on Integrative Health
Weight Loss Supplements

Adolescents are major consumers of complementary and alternative medicine products, including dietary supplements and herbal therapies. The primary reason adolescents use herbal therapies is for weight loss. Unfortunately, many "holistic" products are unregulated and may be poisonous when not taken as directed or when taken in combination with other substances. These characteristics may escape the attention of the adolescent (Pomeranz et al., 2015). Dietary supplements, particularly those for weight loss and/or for energy, can cause cardiac symptoms, including chest pain, tachycardia, and heart palpitations (Geller et al., 2015). Adolescents are also less likely to report use of complementary medicines (National Center for Complementary and Integrative Health [NCCIH], 2016a). Therefore, the nurse should encourage both parents and adolescents to report any use of supplements, herbal remedies, or other complementary medicines.

Adolescents seek to establish their own identity and values. They may rebel against parental authority as they try out new activities and behaviors. Although this is normal for adolescents, it can create a number of difficulties at home and school as adolescents try to balance their need to express themselves against the expectations of parents, teachers, and other authority figures.

Psychosocial Development

The adolescent is mature in relationships with others. The key aspect that teens work on during relationships and activities is establishing a meaningful identity.

Activities

Activities represent a central focus for the adolescent. Maturity leads to new activities. Adolescents may drive, ride buses, or bike independently. They are less dependent on parents for transportation and spend more time with friends or doing activities. Activities include participation in sports and extracurricular school clubs, as well as "hanging out" and attending movies or concerts with friends. Activities also drive psychosocial development, as the peer group becomes the focus of activities, regardless of the teen's interests. Peers are important in establishing identity and providing meaning. Although same-sex interactions dominate, boy–girl relationships are more common than at earlier stages. Adolescents thus participate in and learn from social interactions fundamental to adult relationships. They also begin to develop abstract thought and analysis through conversations at home and at school.

Social media, texting, and other interactive technology has also become an integral part of the adolescent's social life and culture (Minges et al., 2015). Ninety-five percent of adolescents use the internet or other online media (Madden et al., 2013). Adolescents "hang out" not only in coffee shops and malls, but also in chat rooms, online games, and via group texts.

Personality and Temperament

Characteristics of temperament manifested during childhood usually remain stable in the teenage years. For instance, the adolescent who was a calm, scheduled infant and child often demonstrates initiative to regulate study times and other routines. Similarly, the adolescent who was an easily stimulated infant may now have a messy room, a harried schedule with assignments always completed late, and an interest in many activities. It is also common for an adolescent who was an easy child to become more difficult because of the psychologic changes of adolescence and the need to assert independence.

As during the child's earlier ages, the nurse's role may be to inform parents of different personality types and to help them support the teen's uniqueness while providing necessary structure and feedback. Nurses can help parents understand their teen's personality type and work with the adolescent to meet expectations of teachers and others in authority.

Communication

Adolescents understand and use all parts of speech. They commonly use colloquialisms and slang when speaking–or texting–with their peers.

The adolescent increasingly leaves the home base and establishes close ties with peers. These relationships become the basis for identity formation. A period of stress or crisis generally occurs before a strong identity can emerge. The adolescent may try out new roles by learning a new sport or other skills, experimenting with drugs or alcohol, wearing different styles of clothing, or trying other activities. It is important to provide positive role models and a variety of experiences to help the adolescent make wise choices.

The adolescent also has a need to leave the past, to be different, and to change from former patterns to establish a self-identity. Rules that are repeated constantly and dogmatically will probably be broken in the adolescent's quest for self-awareness. This poses difficulties when the adolescent has a health problem that requires ongoing care, such as diabetes or cardiac illness. Introducing the adolescent to other teens who manage the same problem appropriately usually is more successful in getting the adolescent to comply with a care plan than telling the adolescent what to do.

Teens need privacy during patient interviews or interventions. Even if a parent is present for part of a health history or examination, the adolescent should be given the opportunity to relay information to or ask questions of the healthcare provider alone. The adolescent should be given a choice of whether to have a parent present during an examination or while care is provided. Most information shared by an adolescent is confidential. Some states mandate disclosure of certain information to parents such as an adolescent's desire for an abortion. In these cases, the adolescent should be informed of what information will be disclosed to the parent.

In the hospital setting, nurses and care staff should allow adolescents the freedom of choice whenever possible, including preferences for evening or morning bathing, the type of clothes to wear while hospitalized, timing of treatments, and visitation guidelines. Use of contracts with adolescents may increase adherence with healthcare recommendations. Firmness, gentleness, choices, and respect must be balanced during care of adolescent patients.

Some specific communication strategies that help with the adolescent:

- Provide written and verbal explanations.
- Direct history and explanations to teen alone; then include parent.
- Allow for safe exploration of topics by suggesting that the teen is similar to other teens. ("Many teens with diabetes have questions about. . . . How about you?")
- Arrange meetings for discussions with other teens.

Sexuality

Sexuality is influenced by physical maturation and increased hormonal secretion, which are integral to the adolescent's development of physiologic sexual maturity. Psychosocially, this complex process involves growing interactions with members of the opposite sex, an interplay of the forces of society and family, and identity formation. The early adolescent progresses from attending dances and other social events with members of the opposite sex to the late adolescent who is mature sexually and may have regular sexual encounters.

Just as some adolescents are exploring their feelings for those of the opposite sex (heterosexual), others are finding that their attraction lies with those of the same gender (homosexual) or may begin to identify as bisexual (attracted to both genders). Most adolescents who feel supported and safe will have a positive adolescence (Centers for Disease Control and Prevention [CDC], 2014). Unfortunately, LGBTQ (lesbian, gay, bisexual, transgender, queer/questioning) youth have a great incidence of bullying, violence, and harassment (CDC, 2014). Partially because of negative interactions with peers and society, LGBTQ youth are more likely to abuse substances or report mental health problems such as anxiety and depression, and more likely to attempt suicide than their peers (CDC, 2014). Nurses are instrumental in helping LGBTQ youths by providing information for them and their parents, integrating LGBTQ content into sexual education curricula, and providing referrals for health and social care when needed. Nurses must examine their own beliefs and communication styles to provide culturally competent care. School nurses can play a particularly positive role in the safety and security of LGBTQ youths. School nurses can provide confidential healthcare and education to the LGBTQ student, collaborate with faculty and staff at a school, and provide support, education, and resources for parents and community members (National Association of School Nurses, 2016).

Trends indicate that adolescents are not as sexually active as in the past. According to the CDC (2016a), 41% of high school students have had sexual intercourse, a decrease from 47% in 2012 (CDC, 2012). Thirty percent of high school students reported having sex in the past 3 months (CDC, 2016a). Although fewer high school students are having sex, those who are sexually active are engaged in risky behaviors. For example, 43% reported not using a condom; 14% reported not using any form of birth control (CDC, 2016a). Many school districts now provide some teaching on STIs and HIV. Health histories include questions on sexual activity, STIs, and birth control use and understanding. Most hospitals routinely perform pregnancy screening on adolescent girls before elective procedures. More and more clinics are prophylactically screening teens for STIs with simple urine tests.

Adolescents will benefit from clear information about sexuality, an opportunity to develop relationships with adolescents in various settings, an open atmosphere at home and school where problems and issues can be discussed, and previous experience in problem solving and decision making. Alternatives and support for their decisions should be available.

In addition, the nurse who encounters a sexually active teenager should remember the nurse may be the very first healthcare provider with whom the teenager discusses his sexuality. The nurse who refrains from asserting her own personal beliefs and who emphasizes open communication and active listening will strengthen the teen's confidence in the healthcare system and increase the likelihood that the teen will seek help from a healthcare professional in the future.

Adults

The transition from adolescence to adulthood is complex. Unlike when individuals were infants and children with very clear milestones, adulthood does not have such defined markers. Yet, the adult continues to pass through stages or complete tasks that encompass the individual's physical, emotional, social, spiritual, and economic self.

Multisystem Effects of
Aging

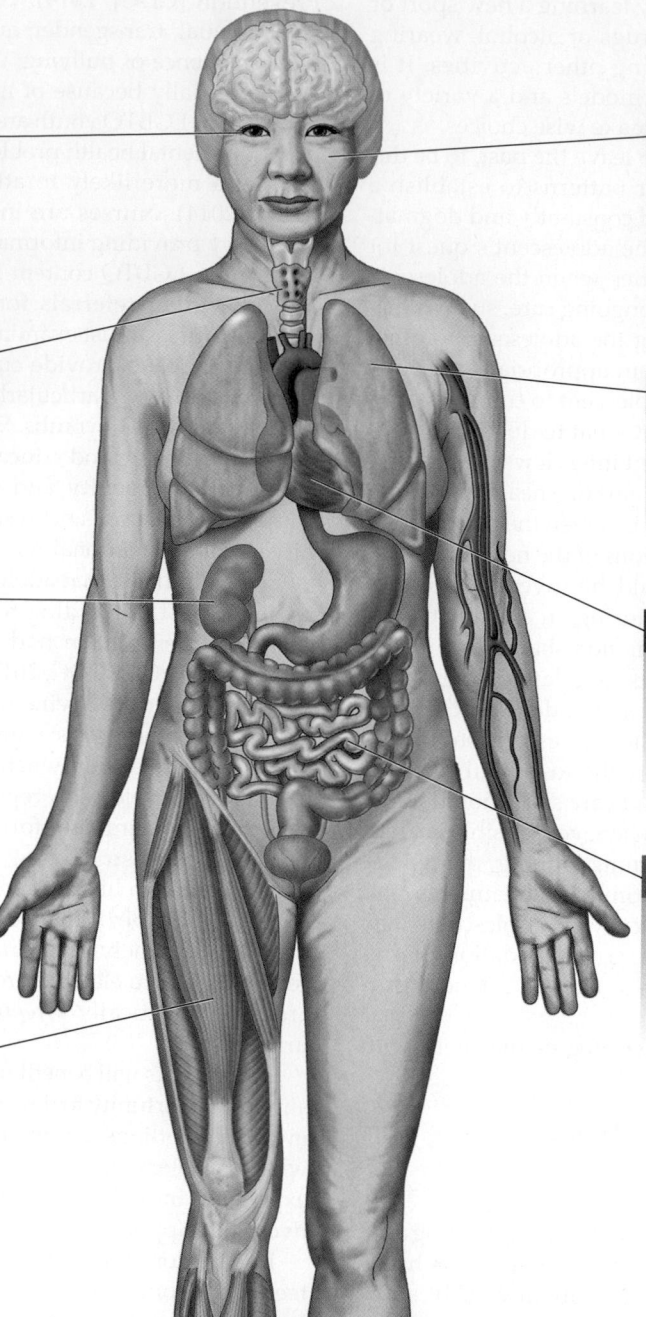

Sensory
- High frequency hearing loss
- Visual changes
- Sense of taste diminishes

Endocrine
- Gradual decrease in glucose tolerance

Urinary
- Kidneys become less efficient at removing waste from blood
- ↓ bladder capacity

Musculoskeletal
- ↓ muscle mass, especially in women
- Muscle mass decreases rapidly without exercise
- Thinning of intervertebral discs results in loss of height
- ↑ risk of osteoporosis (women)

Integumentary
- ↓ turgor, moisture, and subcutaneous fat
- Hairline recedes in men
- Loss of melanin in hair shaft causes graying

Respiratory
- Arteries stiffen and blood oxygenation levels decrease
- ↓ maximum breathing capacity

Cardiovascular
- Blood vessels lose elasticity
- ↑ systolic blood pressure
- Heart muscle thickens
- ↓ pumping rate

Gastrointestinal
- Large intestine gradually loses muscle tone
- Constipation
- ↓ gastric secretions

Young Adults

Many societies, such as those in the United States, consider adulthood to start at the age of 18 years. At this age, many adolescents begin to enjoy several adult privileges, such as voting and opening a bank account. At the age of 18, individuals can seek medical care without parental consent and can make medical decisions independently. With new laws regarding medical insurance in place, many young adults stay on their parents' insurance plans. The individual is still depending on the parents' insurance but is able to make medical decisions.

Economic status is no longer a sign of adulthood. In addition to staying on their parents' insurance plans, many young adults are staying with their parents into their mid-20s or later. Many are delaying marriage and childrearing until later in adulthood. The average age for first birth is 26.3, with a growing number of women having their first child between ages 30 and 35 (National Center for Health Statistics, 2016). Prominent life changes and stressors for young adults include going to (and paying for) college, choosing and establishing a career, and finding a significant other or spouse.

In terms of physical development, most individuals are still growing. In particular, men may not reach their full height until around age 20. Studies continue to show that the human brain is not fully mature until around the age of 25 (Arain et al., 2013). In the early to mid-20s, most individuals are at their peak physical condition. Causes of mortality and morbidity are mainly attributed to unintentional injury (i.e., motor vehicle crashes) and intentional trauma (homicide and suicide) (National Center for Health Statistics, 2015).

The health assessment of the young adult should include such vital signs as blood pressure, height, and weight (**Table 25–12 »**). Vision and hearing screenings should also be considered, particularly since many young people are of the "earbud generation." Assessment questions should address stressors, diet recall, activity level and exercise, family history, smoking history, and alcohol/substance use. Additional data necessary to appropriately assess young adults include sexual history and activity, menstrual concerns and patterns, and use of birth control, including condom use. As with the adolescent patient, the nurse should be open to questions and ready to educate the patient on sexual concerns. Health screenings should include STIs.

Middle Adults

The "middle" years of adulthood are typically considered to be between the ages of 40 and 65 years. Often called the "sandwich" generation, those who are in this stage of life often find themselves taking care of both their children (and sometimes, grandchildren) and their own aging parents. This creates a new set of stressors. In some cases, the individual must also cope with divorce or loss of a significant other.

In this stage of life, the body begins to experience changes related to aging (**Table 25–13 »**). Risk factors for heart disease, such as hypertension and elevated lipids, and related vascular problems start during this life period. Arthritis and back problems often arise during middle adulthood. Difficulty in mobility, most commonly due to spinal/back issues and arthritis, may cause disability in individuals in this age group (Courtney-Long et al., 2015).

The health assessment of the middle-aged adult should include vision and hearing screenings and vital signs, as well as height, weight, and BMI. Along with a complete physical assessment, these indicators can all be useful in

TABLE 25–12 Physical Status and Changes in the Young Adult Years

Assessment	Status During the 20s	Status During the 30s
Skin	Smooth, even temperature	Beginning of wrinkles
Hair	Slightly oily, shiny	Beginning of graying
	Beginning of balding	Balding
Vision	Snellen 20/20	Some loss of visual acuity and accommodation
Musculoskeletal	Strong, coordinated	Some loss of strength and muscle mass
Cardiovascular	Maximum cardiac output	Slight decline in cardiac output
	60–90 beats/min	60–90 beats/min
	Mean BP: 120/80	Mean BP: 120/80
Respiratory	Rate: 12–20	Rate: 12–20
	Full vital capacity	Decline in vital capacity

TABLE 25–13 Physical Changes in the Middle Adult Years

Assessment	Changes
Skin	■ Decreased turgor, moisture, and subcutaneous fat result in wrinkles.
	■ Fat is deposited in the abdominal and hip areas.
Hair	■ Loss of melanin in hair shaft causes graying.
	■ Hairline recedes in men.
Sensory	■ Visual acuity for near vision decreases (presbyopia) during the 40s.
	■ Auditory acuity for high-frequency sounds decreases (presbycusis); more common in men.
	■ Sense of taste diminishes.
Musculoskeletal	■ Skeletal muscle mass decreases by about age 60.
	■ Thinning of intervertebral discs results in loss of height (about 2.5 cm [1 in.]).
	■ Postmenopausal women may have loss of calcium and develop osteoporosis.
Cardiovascular	■ Blood vessels lose elasticity
	■ Systolic blood pressure may increase.
Respiratory	■ Loss of vital capacity (about 1 L from age 20 to 60) occurs.
Gastrointestinal	■ Large intestine gradually loses muscle tone; constipation may result.
	■ Gastric secretions are decreased.
Genitourinary	■ Hormonal changes occur: menopause, women (↓ estrogen); andropause, men (↓ testosterone).
Endocrine	■ Gradual decrease in glucose tolerance occurs.

establishing a baseline against which healthcare providers can compare changes over time. Assessment questions should address exercise and activity levels, diet and food choices, family history, alcohol/substance use, smoking history, and stressors. Sexual history and activity should be addressed in all individuals in this age group, even those who are married. Other health screenings that should be discussed with the adult patient include Pap smears, mammography, colonoscopy, fasting glucose, and lipid panels.

Older Adults

The World Health Organization (WHO) (2016) recognizes older adulthood as beginning at the age of 60. In the United States, the beginning of older adulthood is generally recognized as age 65, in part because at this age Americans qualify for Medicare benefits. The experiences of older adulthood vary considerably from one individual to the next. Some may retire at or before age 65, whereas others may work for many years afterward. Some older adults continue to be "sandwiched" with much older parents and younger generations of children and grandchildren.

Older adulthood is often thought of as a stage of loss and mourning. Many older adults experience loss of friends, relatives, and spouses. Some mourn physical loss, such as mobility due to arthritis or breasts due to cancer. Yet, many older adults continue to live healthy, active, happy lives. Older adults also continue to be sexually active well into their 80s and 90s. Because of advancements in preventive medicine and healthcare, many individuals are transitioning into older adulthood with few chronic conditions. However, as the body matures, chronic conditions can be complicated by the normal stages of aging. Risk for developing cardiovascular disease, cancer, type 2 diabetes (T2D), and neurocognitive disorders such as Alzheimer disease increases. Therefore, the nurse needs to be especially concerned about screening and further progression of a chronic disease.

As with all adults, the health assessment begins with vital signs. Height and weight are especially important, as it is during this stage in life that older adults start to experience degenerative changes in the spinal column, causing shrinking. Loss of muscle mass is common. Older adults are at greater risk for sensory losses, such as hearing or vision loss. Of course, a complete physical assessment of all systems should be included in the nurse's health assessment. Assessment questions should include exercise habits and tolerance, diet and appetite, ability to do activities of daily living, and tobacco/alcohol/substance use. According to the National Institutes of Health (n.d.), approximately 55% of older adults drink alcohol, which increases the older adult's risk for injury. Assessments of the older adult should include safety, functional status (e.g., self-care, mobility), and mental status to establish a baseline (see the module on Cognition). Normal age-related changes of aging are outlined in **Table 25–14))**.

Alterations to Development

Developmental disabilities are a cluster of conditions that occur as the result of impairment in motor function, speech and language development, behavioral patterns, or learning ability (CDC, 2015a). To recognize delays or deviations from normal patterns of development, the nurse must be knowledgeable about normal developmental milestones. Although this module focuses on impairments that affect pediatric development, it is important to remember that development continues throughout the lifespan and alterations may occur at any point. Any noted alteration should be investigated further. Management of developmental delays varies and may require use of an interprofessional team, depending on the nature of the alterations and the individual's needs. In addition, nurses assess each patient's individual developmental level and incorporate that into the plan of care. This is especially important when considering patient teaching and planning for the patient's care needs following discharge.

Alterations and Manifestations

Alterations in development may occur in a single area or multiple areas. Alterations may be referred to as a delay, a deficit, or a disorder. While developmental delays are primarily thought of as childhood disorders and improve or disappear with intervention and use and practice of skills, some (such as attention-deficit/hyperactivity disorder and autism spectrum disorder) will challenge the individual for the length of the lifespan. In addition, deficits in any area may occur in adulthood as the result of injury, stroke, or other trauma.

Communication

The term *communication disorder* refers to any delay or deficit in one of the following areas: speech, language, voice, or swallowing. Of these, speech and language disorders are the most prevalent (Black, Varhartian, & Hoffman, 2015). A child with a speech delay has difficulty making the sounds of language—that is, not being able to articulate specific sounds or speaking with a stutter. A child with a language delay may have difficulty accessing receptive language or may have difficulty expressing language. Language delays also encompass the acquisition of vocabulary. A child with a pragmatic language delay has difficulty using language in social contexts (American Speech-Language-Hearing Association, 2017).

Although hearing children may not necessarily benefit from learning sign language, research has shown that children with developmental delays and cognitive differences do benefit from learning sign language. Sign language has been particularly beneficial to those born with Down syndrome and autism as a nonverbal means of communication (Vandereet et al., 2011).

Motor Function

Motor delays are often more easily identified as a child fails to achieve certain milestones or experiences losses of previous gains. Motor delays may be seen in fine motor skills, gross motor skills, or both. Some 6% of children will experience developmental coordination disorder, which is usually identified when the child enters kindergarten. While some children will achieve all milestones, just at a later age, others, such as those with cerebral palsy, may never meet certain milestones (Noritz & Murphy, 2013). Tic disorders, such as Tourette syndrome, are characterized by rapid, recurrent movements or vocalizations and are considered a form of motor disorder. Tics are common in childhood but generally abate as the child matures (American Psychiatric Association [APA], 2013).

TABLE 25–14 Physical Changes in the Older Adult Years

Assessment	Changes
Skin	■ Decreased turgor and sebaceous gland activity result in dry, wrinkled skin. ■ Melanocytes cluster, causing "age spots" or "liver spots."
Hair and nails	■ Scalp, axillary, and pubic hair thins; nose and ear hair thickens. Women may develop facial hair. ■ Nails grow more slowly; may become thick and brittle.
Sensory	■ Visual field narrows, and depth perception is distorted. ■ Pupils are smaller, reducing night vision. ■ Lenses yellow and become opaque, resulting in distortion of green, blue, and violet tones and increased sensitivity to glare. ■ Production of tears decreases. ■ Sense of smell decreases. ■ Age-related hearing loss progresses, involving middle- and low-frequency sounds. ■ Threshold for pain and touch increases. ■ Alterations in proprioception (sense of physical position) may occur.
Musculoskeletal	■ Loss of overall mass, strength, and movement of muscles occurs; tremors may occur. ■ Loss of bone structure and deterioration of cartilage in joints result in increased risk of fractures and limitation of range of motion.
Cardiovascular	■ Systolic blood pressure rises. ■ Cardiac output decreases. ■ Peripheral resistance increases, and capillary walls thicken.
Respiratory	■ Loss of vital capacity continues as the lungs become less elastic and more rigid. ■ Anteroposterior chest diameter increases; kyphosis occurs. ■ Although blood carbon dioxide levels remain relatively constant, blood oxygen levels decrease by 10–15%.
Gastrointestinal	■ Production of saliva decreases, and declining number of taste buds reduces the number of accurate receptors for salt and sweet. ■ Gag reflex is decreased, and stomach motility and emptying are reduced. ■ Both large and small intestines undergo some atrophy, with decreased peristalsis. ■ The liver decreases in weight and storage capacity; incidence of gallstones increases; pancreatic enzymes decrease.
Genitourinary	■ Kidneys lose mass, and the glomerular filtration rate is reduced (by nearly 50% from young adulthood to old age). ■ Bladder capacity decreases, and the micturition reflex is delayed. Urinary retention is more common. ■ Women may have stress incontinence; men may have an enlarged prostate gland. ■ Reproductive changes in men include decreases in sperm count and testosterone; the testes becoming smaller; and an increase in the length of time to achieve an erection. ■ Reproductive changes in women include a decrease in estrogen levels, breast tissue, and vaginal lubrication; alkalinization of vaginal secretions; and atrophy of the vagina, uterus, ovaries, and urethra.
Endocrine	■ Pituitary gland loses weight and vascularity. ■ Thyroid gland becomes more fibrous, and plasma T_3 decreases. ■ Pancreas releases insulin more slowly; increased blood glucose levels are common. ■ Adrenal glands produce less cortisol.

For children having difficulty with fine motor skills, such as grasping and transferring objects, evaluation by an occupational therapist is recommended. Children who have difficulty meeting gross motor milestones will require evaluation by a physical therapist.

Cognition

A child experiencing a cognitive delay has difficulty with thinking and problem solving in relation to developmental milestones. For example, a 3-year-old who is unable to work with everyday objects (e.g., button, zipper), turn a door handle, or put together a three- or four-piece puzzle is showing evidence of not meeting developmental milestones for cognitive ability (CDC, 2016b). Preterm infants are at greater risk for cognitive delays than full-term infants (Lobo & Galloway, 2013). Cognitive delays are seen in children with a variety of disorders, including autism spectrum disorder, cerebral palsy, and Down syndrome. Children with intellectual disability will exhibit cognitive delays as well as difficulty with adaptive functioning. Children experiencing cognitive delays benefit from evaluation by an interprofessional team that includes a child psychologist, speech-language pathologist, occupational therapist, and physical therapist, as well as a nurse and the child's primary care provider.

Adaptive Functioning

Adaptive functioning encompasses life and social skills. Individuals who have difficulty adapting to different people and environments—at home, work, and school—face many challenges. Adaptive functioning and cognition are closely linked. For example, a small study of school-age children found that children who had difficulty controlling their inhibitions exhibited poorer adaptive functioning. Younger children in particular experienced greater teacher reports of inattention (Vuontela et al., 2013). While a number of studies have found a correlation between executive function and adaptive behavior in children with ADHD, researchers are also finding that poor executive functioning is associated with poor adaptive behavior in children with histories of heavy prenatal alcohol exposure (Ware et al., 2012). These children also benefit from evaluation by an interprofessional team.

Etiology

Certain alterations in development have a single manifestation; however, the alteration may stem from one of many different etiologies. For example, congenital anomalies, infantile glaucoma, and retinopathy of prematurity can all lead to visual impairment in neonates. In other cases, a single defect may manifest in an array of signs and symptoms. Fragile X syndrome (FXS) is a genetic disorder in which the absence of one protein impairs brain development and may yield multiple effects, including impairments related to language, learning, and social interaction (CDC, 2016c). Other developmental disabilities come about from exposure to fetal toxins, such as alcohol. Fetal alcohol spectrum disorders (FASDs) occur when pregnant mothers consume alcohol. Those born with FASDs have a host of challenges, including intellectual and neurologic, visual and hearing, as well as behavioral and mental health (CDC, 2015b). Infectious agents, such as viruses and bacteria, can cause fetal harm. Zika, a virus transmitted by certain breeds of mosquitoes, has been linked to miscarriage, impaired growth, microcephaly, neurologic deficits, eye damage, and hearing loss (CDC, 2016d).

Other developmental disabilities include attention-deficit/hyperactivity disorder (ADHD), intellectual disability (ID), Down syndrome (or trisomy 21), muscular dystrophy (MD), and Tourette syndrome. The exemplars in this module explore three developmental impairments commonly diagnosed initially in pediatric patients— ADHD, autism spectrum disorder (ASD), and cerebral palsy (CP)—and one seen in infants and older adults—failure to thrive (FTT).

>> **Stay Current:** For discussion of additional pediatric developmental disorders, visit the CDC's information center at http://www.cdc.gov/ncbddd/developmentaldisabilities/index.html.

Prevalence

Approximately 1 in 6 children in the United States is impaired by one or more developmental disabilities or by other forms of developmental delays (Boyle et al., 2011). Trends continue to show no significant change in disability rates other than in ASDs, which continue to rise (Van Naarden Braun et al., 2015). There are many different theories as to the cause of the rise in ASD diagnoses, including greater awareness of autism, better diagnostic tools, and change in the language used to poll parents (Zablotsky et al., 2015).

Other disabilities tracked by the CDC include ID, CP, vision impairment, and hearing loss. Currently, the CDC's Metropolitan Atlanta Developmental Disabilities Surveillance Program (MADDSP) is the hallmark tracking site for trends in childhood disabilities. Van Naarden Braun et al. (2015) found no significant change in the numbers of children with CP, at 3.5 per 1000 children. Approximately 13.6 per 1000 children have ID without ASD. Note that 28% of children who are identified as ID also have ASD. ASD is seen in 15.5 per 1000 children. In terms of ASD, boys are more

likely to have ASD, with approximately 1 in 40 boys compared with 1 in 182 girls (Van Naarden Braun et al., 2015).

Genetic Considerations and Nonmodifiable Risk Factors

In some cases, developmental delays are inevitable because of genetic abnormalities. Because chromosomes and genes carry messages that encode for certain characteristics, they also can carry diseases. Although some genetic mutations are incompatible with life and result in fetal death, live births can occur with others.

Chromosomal disorders may be caused by an array of factors, such as radiation exposure, parental age, exposure to infectious agents, or parental disease states; however, sometimes their causes cannot be determined. For example, there is increasing evidence linking genetics to ASD (Huquet, Ey, & Bourgeron, 2013). Some children inherit genes that lead to diseases such as cystic fibrosis; others may have a mutation that manifests in the disease. A family history of these diseases is usually present, but because genes sometimes mutate, an initial incidence of a genetic disorder may appear with no identifiable history.

Premature birth, multiple gestation, and low birth weight are also linked to an increased risk for several types of developmental disorders (CDC, 2015c). In all cases, early identification and referral to appropriate resources can help a patient to achieve the highest level of developmental functioning possible based on the abnormality.

Case Study » Part 1

Farah Mohamed, 24 years old, is a Somali refugee who immigrated to the United States at the age of 10. She is married and has a 2-year-old son, Amiir Yusef. She brings Amiir to the family practice clinic for his well-child visit. As his mother carries him from the lobby, you notice Amiir squirming the entire time. When you reach the examination room, Amiir screams in a high pitch and pulls away from his mother. During the assessment, you notice that Amiir is rocking back and forth on the floor as he sits with a toy vacuum, making R-noises. The mother remarks, "He loves vacuums. Sometimes, he screams and screams at the closet until I bring him the vacuum. I have to turn it on, and then he is happy. That toy vacuum is his favorite toy. He shows more love to the vacuum than he does to me."

When discussing Amiir's development, Ms. Mohamed tells you that he was born early, at 36 weeks, after she had been on bedrest for early cervical effacement. She shares that her pregnancy was difficult because she had hyperemesis gravidarum (intractable vomiting) through much of her pregnancy. She tells you that he was a quiet baby, and he did not like to be touched. She reports he still does not like to be held. She tells you, "I think he was angry I did not take better care of him when I was pregnant. He still is angry with me."

As your conversation and assessment progresses, you gather:

- Amiir was sitting by himself at 6 months.
- He did not crawl, but was able to pull himself up at 10 months.
- He walked independently at 13 months.
- He has difficulty holding a spoon and fork. Instead he likes to eat with his hands.
- His vocabulary is very limited.

Ms. Mohamed tells you she is worried about her son because he doesn't seem like other children. She shares, "My husband just graduated from college and is starting a new job. I am now going to college, and so I am not home much with Amiir. He spends most of his time with my mother. She does not speak English, and she puts Amiir in front of the television so that he will learn English. Is this why he doesn't really speak? Is it because he is confused about which language he should learn?"

Clinical Reasoning Questions Level I

1. Identify two or more developmental milestones that Amiir has met and two that he has not met. At what age should he have met the milestones that he has not met?
2. Using Erikson's theory of developmental stages, what is Amiir's current developmental task? What is Ms. Mohamed's developmental task?
3. Ms. Mohamed blames Amiir's vocabulary on the fact that he is growing up in a bilingual family. Could this indeed be the cause of Amiir's limited vocabulary? Why or why not?

Clinical Reasoning Questions Level II

4. Write two nursing diagnoses for this case study that could be used in the plan of care of Amiir and/or Ms. Mohamed.
5. Ms. Mohamed blames herself for Amiir's behavior. How would the nurse respond to her comments regarding blame for her difficult pregnancy?
6. After you complete your assessment, you are concerned that Amiir may have autism. What data collected during the assessment support or refute your suspicion? What additional data should be collected?

Concepts Related to Development

As stated earlier, most people with mild alterations in development, whether they occur in childhood or as the result of injury or trauma in adulthood, will be able to overcome them with appropriate interventions. For those with more significant delays or alterations, however, the implications for health, wellness, illness, injury, and functioning in all areas of life are great. The presence of a developmental disability increases the individual's risk for injury, abuse, and exploitation and increases difficulty with self-care, activities of daily living, and responding to and participating in treatment for acute or chronic illness.

Selected concepts integral to development are presented in the Concepts Related to Development feature. They are presented in alphabetical order.

Health Promotion

Health promotion to reduce risk for developmental disabilities in children focuses on maternal well-being. Preterm birth is the number one cause of long-term neurologic disabilities in children (CDC, 2015d). Several maternal factors have been linked with early deliveries, including age, race, socioeconomic status, health status, pregnancy abnormalities, and behavioral issues (CDC, 2015d). Behavioral factors include substance use, inadequate prenatal care, and psychologic influences (CDC, 2015d). Infants who are premature have immature body systems, requiring medical support in the newborn period.

Some developmental delays can be prevented by educating the pregnant patient in the care of her baby in utero. Education regarding proper prenatal care should start with the first prenatal visit. The nurse has the opportunity to begin the educational process of lifelong health promotion by starting with prenatal education. After birth, the focus shifts to helping parents raise a healthy child in a safe environment, giving that child the optimal ability to develop and thrive.

Prenatal Considerations

The mother's nutrition and general state of health play a part in pregnancy outcome. Even before the woman considers becoming pregnant, she should consider taking a prenatal vitamin with at least 400 mcg of folic acid for at least 1 month before conceiving to prevent such birth defects as anencephaly and spinal bifida (CDC, 2015e). The use of prenatal vitamins should continue throughout the pregnancy and postpartum stages to prevent anemia in the mother and baby, as well as other vitamin and mineral deficiencies.

Prescription medications, over-the-counter medications, and herbal supplements are not necessarily safe for the fetus. Differences in physiology related to gastric emptying, renal clearance, drug distribution, and other factors contribute to variations in pharmacokinetics during pregnancy. Drugs can cause teratogenesis (abnormal development of the fetus) or mutagenesis (permanent changes in the fetus's genetic material). Certain drugs can cause bleeding, stained teeth, impaired hearing, or other defects in the infant. In 2014, the U.S. Food and Drug Administration (FDA) published the Pregnancy and Lactation Labeling Rule, which requires that drug labels be formatted to assist healthcare providers in assessing risk versus benefit for pregnant women and nursing mothers who need to take medication (FDA, 2014).

>> Stay Current: See samples of the new drug labels at http://www.fda.gov/Drugs/DevelopmentApprovalProcess/DevelopmentResources/Labeling/ucm093307.htm.

Although some medications are safe during certain periods of the pregnancy, there is the potential for those same medications to be dangerous in other stages, depending on fetal development and approaching delivery. For example, ibuprofen, a nonsteroidal anti-inflammatory drug, has been found in a few studies to interfere with conception and cause miscarriages. In the later portion of the first trimester and second semester, there are no reported problems. However, after 30 weeks of pregnancy, the mother is advised not to take ibuprofen because of its potential to decrease of amniotic fluid and potential heart defects in the fetus (Organization of Teratology Information Specialists, 2014). To help healthcare providers and pharmacists provide evidence-based information regarding safe medication use by pregnant women and breastfeeding mothers, the CDC has paired with the Organization of Teratology Information Specialists (OTIS) to create a clearinghouse for information at www.mothertobaby.org

Some maternal illnesses are harmful to the developing fetus. Cytomegalovirus (CMV) infection is quite common in adults, children, and newborn babies. The CDC (2016d) estimates that 1 in 150 babies are born each year with this virus. Although many babies are infected via their mothers, few will have lasting effects. However, those who are infected, and affected, may be born with microcephaly, hearing loss, vision loss, intellectual disabilities, and major organ issues (CDC, 2016e). A fetus can also acquire chronic infections, such as AIDS and HIV infection or hepatitis B, from the mother.

Concepts Related to
Development

CONCEPT	RELATIONSHIP TO DEVELOPMENT	NURSING IMPLICATIONS
Assessment	Language, motor, cognitive, and adaptive functioning delays or deficits can make assessment a challenge.	■ Adapt the assessment to the individual's developmental level. ■ Include family and caregivers in the assessment as appropriate, but take care to promote autonomy on the part of the patient.
Family	Moderate to severe alterations in development may disrupt family processes as family members struggle to integrate the individual who is delayed or disabled into family activities and communication patterns. Families also must integrate therapies and interventions into their daily schedules.	■ Assess family functioning. ■ Assess family supports. ■ Provide referrals to area resources as needed.
Health, Wellness, Illness, and Injury	Individuals with developmental deficits or disorders benefit from appropriate nutrition, rest, and physical exercise. By reducing risk factors related to these areas, patients will be more likely to achieve better outcomes and integrate more successfully at home, work, and school. Illness can interfere with normal developmental processes. For example, toddlers who previously were toileting independently may regress during periods of hospitalization. In older adults, hospitalization can cause cognitive disturbances and impair functioning in other areas.	■ Assess sleep and rest patterns. ■ Assess meal patterns and dietary intake. ■ Assess level, amount, and type of exercise. ■ Encourage patients and families to participate in healthy behaviors related to sleep hygiene, eating habits, and exercise. ■ Provide referrals as needed for evaluation or support in these areas. ■ Assess functioning before hospitalization to establish baseline. ■ Communicate developmental level to providers who will be working with the patient. ■ Plan interventions and communications according to developmental level. ■ Assess for regression or deterioration at regular intervals. ■ Provide interventions necessary to promote return to functioning.
Safety	Deficits or delays may increase an individual's risk for injury or illness. For example, an individual with cognitive and adaptive functioning deficits may not recognize illness or injury requiring attention from a healthcare provider. Similarly, an individual with cognitive or adaptive functioning deficits may have difficulty following a treatment regimen without adequate supervision.	■ Assess personal, home, and environmental safety factors. ■ Link patients and families with resources that can promote skills that increase safety. ■ Simplify treatment instructions and regimen whenever possible.
Stress and Coping	Developmental delays or deficits can cause distress to the individual, caregivers/family, and those with whom the individual interacts at school and work.	■ Assess individual and family coping mechanisms. ■ Provide developmentally appropriate suggestions for improving coping skills.
Trauma	Individuals with developmental delays and disabilities are at increased risk for abuse from family members and strangers and at increased risk for sexual exploitation. Families and providers can be reluctant to discuss personal safety with these patients, putting them at even greater risk.	■ Assess patient and family understanding of the risks for abuse. ■ Provide patient and family education related to risks and personal safety practices.

Chronic maternal distress, anxiety, and/or depression can affect the fetus. A study by Bolten et al. (2011) showed that excess stress hormones such as cortisol pass through the placenta and can result in lower birth weight and size. Subsequent studies continue to show that maternal stress can affect the fetus and later child development. Maternal stress has even been linked to increased likelihood of childhood obesity (Liu et al., 2016).

The best outcomes for infants occur when mothers eat well; exercise regularly; seek early prenatal care; refrain from use of drugs, alcohol, tobacco, and excessive caffeine; and follow general principles of good health and infection prevention.

Environmental Factors

Adequate nutrition is an essential component of growth and development. For example, poorly nourished children are more likely to get infections than are well-nourished children. Infection, then, can cause further malnutrition as the individual may not want to eat or, because of such compensatory reactions such as diarrhea, may not be able to absorb nutrition. In addition, poorly nourished children may not attain their full height potential. Inadequate nutrition during pregnancy and the first few years of life may also impact brain development. See the module on Nutrition for more information.

Other environmental factors that can influence growth and development are the living conditions of the child (e.g., homelessness), socioeconomic status (e.g., poverty versus financial stability), climate, and community (e.g., providing developmental support versus exposing the child to hazards). Illness or injury can affect growth and development. Being hospitalized is stressful for a child and can affect the child's coping mechanisms. Prolonged or chronic illness may affect normal developmental processes, including psychosocial development. See the exemplar on Environmental Quality in the module on Advocacy for more information.

Screenings

Well-child visits are perhaps the most effective initial method of screening for developmental disorders. Through regularly assessing the child at set intervals, the healthcare provider is able to identify the child's degree of achievement of milestones related to growth and development. Developmental assessments are performed in the clinical setting, as well as in home, school, and community settings. In 2008, the National Early Childhood Technical Assistance Center (NECTAC) compiled a review of screening instruments that emphasized social and emotional development for young children ages birth through 5. The NECTAC listed 23 different instruments that may be selected and used by professionals, and another 15 instruments appropriate for use by caregivers or family members (Ringwalt, 2008). The Children's Health Fund of New York identified 50 different screening instruments for use with children ages birth to 72 months (Grant, Gracy, & Brito, 2010). Two of the more commonly used screening tools are the Ages and Stages Questionnaire (ASQ) and the Battelle Developmental Inventory Screening Test (BDIST). The ASQ is appropriate for children birth to 6 months and relies on the parent's report of the child's communication and motor skills, social skills, and problem solving ability. The BDIST is appropriate for children 12 to 60 months old and uses both parent report and direct observation of the child to assess skills in a variety of areas. Screening instruments used to screen for ASD and ADHD are outlined in those exemplars.

>> **Stay Current:** For more information on specific developmental screenings, visit the CDC's child development and screening information center at http://www.cdc.gov/ncbddd/childdevelopment/treematerials.html.

Anticipatory Guidance

Anticipatory guidance related to developmental and age-related risks for injury is discussed in the module on Safety.

Nursing Assessment

In nursing, developmental theories can be useful in guiding assessment, explaining behavior, and providing a direction for nursing interventions. An understanding of a child's intellectual ability helps a nurse to anticipate and explain certain reactions, responses, and needs. Nurses can then encourage patient behavior that is appropriate for that particular developmental stage.

In adult care, knowledge about the physical, cognitive, and psychologic aspects of the aging process is a fundamental aspect of administering sensitive nursing care. For example, nurses can use their familiarity with the theories of development to help patients understand and anticipate the psychosocial changes that take place after retirement or the physical limitations that come with aging.

Assessment of those with developmental differences requires that the nurse have not only a firm foundation in developmental theories and concepts, but also an understanding of the impact of those differences. For example, many cognitive tests require the individual to read or respond to pictures, actions that may not be possible for an individual with limited vision.

Pain is a subjective experience that is perceived differently across the lifespan. Healthcare providers often do not take into account Piaget's stages of cognitive development; yet, by doing so, the nurse can have a better understanding of the patient's perspective of pain and treat accordingly (Brain, 2000). For example, toddlers and young children in the preoperative phase are not able to connect illness with pain, and therefore will blame others for their pain. For example, a toddler will associate postoperative pain with the nurse who provides treatments.

Older adults see pain as a natural progression of aging. There is the misconception held by both patients and providers that pain is a normal of function of aging (Thielke, Sale, & Reid, 2012). Many elderly patients tend to downplay the extent of their pain for a variety of reasons, which leads to undertreatment of pain (Sale, Gignac, & Hawker, 2006). The nurse should be aware that when assessing for pain, the older adult might not rate his or her pain realistically.

Children with developmental delays or sensory deficits, such as those seen in ASD, often do not sense pain as others do. One child may giggle or laugh with shots, saying they "tickle," whereas another child will not tolerate the feel of mittens on the hands. Even though these children may not perceive pain as others might, they do experience pain. Unfortunately, many children with developmental delays and sensory deficits are not able to communicate their discomforts (Czarnecki et al., 2015). Allowing parents and caregivers to have an active role in pain management, such as in the case of surgery, is crucial in providing relief to these children, especially those who are nonverbal (Czarnecki et al., 2015).

Observation and Patient/Family Interview

Parents and caregivers of children are reliable resources of information about their child's behaviors and milestones (CDC, 2016b). The assessment should be conducted in a well-lit, quiet room with space for the family, patient, and nurse. Small spaces may make it difficult to observe the pediatric patient at play; dim rooms may make it difficult for the older patient to see.

The nurse should plan for plenty of time for the interview and should not rush the observation/interview process.

During the assessment interview, the nurse can observe the child for certain behaviors and physical traits. For example, the nurse would observe if an infant at the 6-month well-baby check can hold her head upright. With toddlers and older children, the nurse can provide age-appropriate toys, puzzles, and crayons, pencils, and paper. The nurse can observe for eye contact, overall appearance, interaction with family members and the nurse, and other visuals, such as body language, that can help the nurse gather the data to make an appropriate nursing plan.

The nursing interview is family-centered, culturally competent, and specific to the patient's age and developmental stage. Use open-ended questions and allow plenty of time for the patient and family members to answer questions and interject.

As necessary, provide an interpreter for patients whose primary language is not that of the nurse interviewer. Be aware of any cultural considerations during the interview and/or observation. In some cultures, the patient does not answer direct questions; rather, a spokesperson answers for the patient. In other cultures, the parents might find it disrespectful for the child to play while the nurse is doing the interview. The nurse can explain the importance of watching the child for certain developmental behaviors.

As with any nursing assessment, the interview should include complete health history. Interviews involving pediatric patients typically also include prenatal and birth history, including any complications. Biographical data and health history, including immunizations, current medications, and family history, should be included in this assessment, as well as a review of systems. See the module on Assessment for more information.

Nurses use information about developmental milestones to assess children, to identify those with delays, and to plan interventions that will foster development. Potential risks—such as prematurity, international adoption, and presence of health problems—necessitate a more frequent and in-depth assessment of observed milestones. Nurses compare the expected findings with assessment results, make referrals for further evaluation when appropriate, and use the results to plan nursing interventions.

Cultural Considerations

Culture influences development in numerous ways, including through traditional practices and genetic variations among some ethnic groups. The traditional customs of the many cultural groups represented in North America influence the development of children in these groups. Nutritional practices of various ethnic groups may influence the rate of growth for infants. In addition, development may be influenced by childrearing practices. In some cultures and families, children are carried next to the parent or caregiver rather than carried in a car seat or pushed in a stroller. It is important for nurses to take cultural practices into account when performing developmental screening; some tests may not be culturally sensitive and can inaccurately label a child as delayed when the pattern of development is simply different in the group, perhaps because of the family's childrearing practices. In other situations, the delay of a milestone might not be recognized because of culture. For

instance, a study showed that delays in ASD diagnosis in African American children were due to cultural practices and interpretations of behaviors (Burkett et al., 2015).

All cultural groups have rules regarding patterns of social interaction. Schedules of language acquisition are determined by the number of languages spoken and the amount of speech in the home. The particular social roles men and women assume in the culture affect school activities and ultimately career choices. Attitudes toward touching and other methods of encouraging developmental skills vary among cultures. Genetic traits common in certain ethnic or cultural groups may predispose children to being at the upper or lower ranges of growth and may influence other physical characteristics.

Physical Examination

The physical examination includes a review of systems as well as height, weight, and for children older than 2 years of age, a body mass index (BMI) assessment. In young children especially, any physical distress or change in weight/BMI or motor function may be an early indicator of nutritional or developmental issues. The feature on Development Assessment lists broad categories of areas to assess for individuals at various ages.

Diagnostic Tests

Laboratory diagnostic tests generally are not used to determine developmental status. Medical evaluations typically rule out organic reasons for developmental delays, such as lead poisoning, but from there, most developmental delays are diagnosed through other means. Observational tools, questionnaires, and screening tests are some of the tools that are most helpful in determining developmental status.

Case Study ›› Part 2

After you complete your assessment of Amiir Yusef, you share your findings with the nurse practitioner. The nurse practitioner also is concerned after her assessment. As you did, she found that Amiir would not make eye contact, showed affection toward an inanimate object, had limited vocabulary, skipped a milestone (crawling), and seems to not like tactile stimuli. She arranges for Amiir to have comprehensive testing by a child neuropsychologist.

As you are reviewing the discharge instructions with Ms. Mohamed, she begins to cry. She tells you, "I don't understand what this means. I have heard of this autism, but what is it? Is this from his vaccinations? I have heard in my community that I should not do vaccinations. What have I done? It is Allah's will."

Clinical Reasoning Questions Level I

1. Ms. Mohamed is visibly upset by the potential diagnosis of her son having autism. Reflect on therapeutic communication techniques to use when talking with Ms. Mohamed. What would you tell her to reassure her?

2. Ms. Mohamed, who is Muslim, made the comment, "It is Allah's will." What does that mean in terms of Ms. Mohamed's spiritual self?

Clinical Reasoning Questions Level II

3. *Refer to the exemplar on Autism.* How would you explain the definition of autism to Ms. Mohamed?

4. What are the causes of autism? How would you respond to Ms. Mohamed's question regarding vaccinations causing autism?

5. Ms. Mohamed requests information regarding diagnostic testing for autism. What information would you give Ms. Mohamed regarding how autism is diagnosed?

Development Assessment

GENERAL HEALTH	GROWTH AND DEVELOPMENT	PSYCHOSOCIAL HEALTH	NURSING CONSIDERATIONS
Newborns and Infants			
■ Feeding patterns and practices ■ Sleeping patterns and practices ■ Metabolic screening ■ Vision, hearing screenings ■ Immunizations ■ Tobacco/drug exposure ■ Risk for sudden infant death syndrome (SIDS) ■ Hand hygiene & infection prevention	■ Length, height, head circumference ■ Meets developmental milestones (Tables 25–4, 25–5)	■ Family attachment ■ Cultural practices ■ Self-soothing/self-regulation ■ Separation, stranger anxiety normal at this age	■ Be alert for significant changes from one well visit to the next–e.g., significant decrease or increase in percentile for length and weight requires evaluation ■ Lethargy or failure to meet milestones requires evaluation; may indicate poor nutritional intake.
Toddlers and Preschoolers			
■ Eating habits and meal patterns ■ Sleep and rest patterns ■ Immunizations ■ Oral health ■ Physical activity ■ Screen and TV time	■ Height and weight ■ Head circumference until 1 to 2 years old ■ Toilet training ■ Meets developmental milestones (Tables 25–6, 25–7, 25–8, 25–10)	■ Signs of independence vs. reliance ■ Parent and child interactions ■ Self-regulation ■ Beginning awareness of sex and gender ■ Self-regulation	■ <5th percentile weight or BMI or >85th percentile requires further evaluation ■ Provide anticipatory guidance related to changing risks for injury as child develops ■ Provide patient education regarding promoting healthy self-concept (e.g., praise, appreciation, limit-setting)
School-Age Children			
■ Eating habits and meal patterns ■ Sleep and rest patterns ■ Immunizations ■ Oral health ■ Physical activity ■ Screen and TV time, internet access and safety	■ Height, weight, BMI ■ Slow, steady growth normal until puberty ■ Assess risk and protective factors for obesity ■ Meets developmental milestones (Table 25–11)	■ Assess self-esteem, self-concept, including body image ■ Child should be exhibiting increasing independence, responsibility for self ■ Inquire about family relationships and stressors ■ Assess family supports and resources	■ Provide patient education regarding physical activity, making good food choices, and the need for parents to model healthy behaviors ■ Teaching for children at this age is most effective when children are actively engaged in learning. ■ Unusual complaints may require follow-up ■ Provide anticipatory guidance related to changing risks for injury as child develops
Adolescents			
■ Eating habits and meal patterns ■ Sleep and rest patterns ■ Immunizations ■ Oral health ■ Physical activity ■ Screen and TV time, internet access and safety ■ Extracurricular activities	■ Height, weight, BMI ■ Scoliosis screening ■ Sexual maturity rating (Tanner stages) ■ Breast/testicular exam ■ Sexually transmitted infection screenings, pelvic exam, Pap smear for those who are sexually active ■ Meets developmental milestones	■ Assess self-esteem, self-concept, including body image ■ Child should be exhibiting increasing independence, responsibility for self ■ Inquire about family relationships and stressors ■ Assess family supports and resources ■ Assess risks for injury related to extracurricular activities	■ Develop a partnership with the adolescent ■ Provide patient teaching relating to nutrition, physical activity, sleep hygiene ■ Provide anticipatory guidance related to changing risks for injury

(continued on next page)

Development Assessment *(continued)*

GENERAL HEALTH	GROWTH AND DEVELOPMENT	PSYCHOSOCIAL HEALTH	NURSING CONSIDERATIONS
Adults			
■ Eating habits and meal patterns ■ Sleep and rest patterns ■ Immunizations ■ Oral health ■ Physical activity ■ Risk and protective factors for health and mental health	■ Height, weight, BMI ■ Sexual activity/risks ■ Breast and pelvic or testicular exams ■ Use of tobacco, alcohol, drugs ■ Changes in health status are appropriate for age (Tables 25–12, 25–13)	■ Assess self-esteem, self-concept, including body image ■ Inquire about family relationships and stressors ■ Assess family supports and resources	■ Develop a therapeutic alliance with the patient ■ Provide anticipatory guidance and health teaching based on assessment and individual risk factors
Older Adults			
■ Eating habits and meal patterns ■ Sleep and rest patterns ■ Immunizations ■ Oral health ■ Physical activity ■ Risk and protective factors for health and mental health ■ Presence of chronic illness ■ Polypharmacy	■ Height, weight, BMI ■ Sexual activity/risks ■ Breast and pelvic or testicular exams ■ Use of tobacco, alcohol, drugs ■ Changes in health status are appropriate for age (Table 25–14)	■ Assess self-esteem, self-concept, including ability to engage in meaningful activity ■ Inquire about family relationships and stressors ■ Assess family supports and resources	■ Develop a therapeutic alliance ■ Assess for malnutrition, elder abuse ■ Assess ability to perform ADLs, access to resources

Independent Interventions

Often, patients with impaired development will demonstrate alterations in more than one area of function. For that reason, the treatment approach is varied.

As with all patient care, safety is the highest priority. All children with impaired mobility are at an exceptionally high risk for injury. For ambulatory children, the nurse should ensure that the child is assisted with activities as needed and that properly fitted orthotic devices are being effectively used. In addition, range-of-motion (ROM) exercises should be implemented in order to promote flexibility and reduce contracture formation. Families and caregivers should be instructed about injury prevention within the home, including keeping walkways free from loose rugs, electrical cords, or any other obstacles.

Patients affected by developmental impairment, as well as their caregivers and family members, face challenges that extend into the physical and psychosocial realm. For those individuals who require lifelong treatment of a severe condition, financial stress is a serious concern. The nurse caring for these individuals and their families should offer to facilitate connections with support groups and community resources, including agencies that offer assistance through financial aid or services.

As mentioned before, teaching patient safety will be based on the individual's needs, family situation, and home environment. General needs include the following:

■ **Health needs:** Provide demonstrations of interventions to be done at home (e.g., trach care or tube feedings) and ask for return demonstrations.

■ **Physical environment:** Provide safety instructions about smoke detectors, use of strobe lights as signals for the hearing impaired, and other safety devices. Provide patient and family education related to potential hazards in the home.

■ **Communication needs:** Develop a safety plan for emergencies that the parent and/or the patient and/or family can communicate and practice often with the patient. If the patient is nonverbal, collaborate with the family to create a visual or symbol safety plan for the patient.

● Instruct the family to contact the local emergency dispatch and have the house "flagged" that a patient with communication and/or other special needs lives at that number. Those with limited communication or cognitive delays can be taught to call 911 and know that help will arrive.

- Watch the patient demonstrate how to call 911. If possible, have the patient demonstrate how to call other important numbers.
- ***Cognitive needs:*** Encourage parents to let their child explore and experience his or her surroundings. Humans on all cognitive levels experience and learn via sensory input. Consult with school providers and other healthcare team members to find adaptive equipment that the child can use to participate in different activities safely.

Collaborative Therapies

Collaborative interventions for individuals with developmental delays and disabilities are highly individualized and yet are partially determined by the services available in the community. For individuals of all ages, the goal is to help the patient achieve the greatest level of independence in the least restrictive environment possible.

Early Intervention Services

In the United States, growth and development surveillance begins at birth. Nurses and other providers conduct routine and specific assessments following labor and delivery, prior to discharge, and in the neonatal intensive care unit. Early intervention services may begin that soon for children who are identified with a growth or development issue in the hospital. Early intervention services are designed to enhance both the health and development of infants and young children with or at risk for disabilities.

Developmental screenings continue at well-child visits and follow the recommendations of the AAP (2006). For children whose screenings suggest the need for further evaluation, the family is usually referred to the agency that oversees early intervention services in their community. Funding for early childhood intervention services is usually a combination of federal and state sources and is authorized under Part C of the Individuals with Disabilities in Education Act. Early intervention agencies employ nurses, pediatricians, child psychologists or other mental health professionals, speech-language pathologists (SLPs), occupational therapists (OTs), physical therapists (PTs), and other professionals as necessary to diagnose and meet the needs of children in their communities. Early childhood intervention agencies serve children ages 0 to 3. Together with the parent, the interprofessional team will develop an **individualized family service plan** (IFSP) that identifies the child and family's strengths and weaknesses and designs activities and goals to help the child meet developmental milestones. The family is included to ensure that parents receive appropriate education and to help them learn how to support their child's development.

Nurses working in early childhood intervention may assist with both physical and health screenings and assessments. In addition, they may provide direct follow-up services for children who are medically fragile or have a medical need with or without a co-occurring developmental issue. For example, a nurse from the local health department or the early childhood intervention agency may assist a child in daycare with parenteral feedings or administer growth hormone shots to a child who has been found to have a deficiency in growth hormone.

Early identification of children in need of these services is critical to ensure the best possible outcomes. In a systematic review of studies of occupational therapy services provided to young children, the reviewers noted that low-birth-weight infants who received early intervention services at home from birth to age 1 and then for an additional 2 years at child care centers had significantly higher cognitive function at age 3 (Frolek, Clark, & Schlaback, 2013). The reviewers also noted the importance of establishing partnerships between interprofessional early intervention team members and parents.

School-based Interventions

Once a child turns 3, responsibility for oversight of developmental delay interventions passes to the child's public school system. Public schools employ early childhood specialists, SLPs, OTs, PTs, and child mental health professionals to assist in diagnosis and planning for children with special needs. Children with special health needs may benefit from a 504 plan that the interprofessional team and parent develop. These plans may include accommodations (such as sitting at the front of the class) or ensure the provision of health-related interventions. For children who need educational support to address their developmental needs, the parent and the interprofessional team will develop an **individualized education plan** (IEP). As with early intervention services, most funding for IEP services is made possible by a combination of federal funding through the Individuals with Disabilities Act and state funds.

Illness, Injury, and Trauma

At any stage of life, the onset of acute or chronic illness, injury, or trauma can impair development or function. For all patients, nurses working in acute and long-term/rehabilitation settings conduct functional assessments and work to ensure that patients do not regress or lose ability to function. Adults who have lost or impaired functioning of a limb or body part require evaluation by an OT and/or PT. Adults who have lost any speech, language, or communication function due to stroke, injury, or other trauma should be evaluated by an SLP.

Lifespan Considerations

As stated earlier, many developmental delays may be overcome with timely and appropriate interventions. Some children, however, face long-term challenges and even disability. Individuals with developmental disability face greater risks for abuse and neglect, inappropriate treatment, and placement in more restrictive environments. At all ages and stages, the nurse acts as an advocate for the patient, seeking solutions that will help the patient live the fullest, best life in the least restrictive environment possible.

Adolescents and Younger Adults

The transition from childhood to adolescence and early adulthood is a challenging time for the individual and a stressful one for parents and family members. Just like their peers, teens with developmental differences typically seek greater independence from their parents, and parents and their growing children experience new stressors as the child matures toward adulthood (Rehm et al., 2012). Gaining independence is key for both parents and children alike. Some children with developmental impairments may have difficulty attaining independence and need greater support or encouragement than others.

Children "age out" of the system at 18 or on graduation from high school, and many of the supports once available to adolescents and their parents are no longer available. Challenges associated with this stage of development include transitioning to work or, for some, college; augmenting strained financial resources; and navigating disability program requirements and restrictions. Children with significant cognitive and/or adaptive impairments may leave home later in life; some may never leave home and will always require some level of supervision. Aging parents worry about how to plan for their adult child's safety after their deaths (Barron et al., 2016).

Risks for abuse and exploitation continue as the adolescent and young adult begins to take public transportation, go to work, or engage in new situations such as moving into a group home or various levels of assisted living situations. These housing alternatives can provide helpful, safe environments where adults with disabilities can thrive and gain independence.

Nurses working with adolescents and young adults with disabilities can provide support and encouragement to these patients and their families. Specific interventions may include assessing and providing information regarding personal and environmental safety; referring patients and families to peer support and vocational education programs; establishing case management services; and encouraging parents and families to make legal and financial arrangements for the patient (Rehm et al., 2012).

Pregnant Women

Evidence related to women with intellectual and developmental disabilities (IDD) during pregnancy appears to be limited. A study that compared the deliveries of 340 women with IDD and the general population found that pregnant women with IDD were more likely to be delivered by cesarean section and experience longer hospital stays. They experienced greater rates of adverse outcomes, and their babies were more likely to be low birth weight and premature (Parish et al., 2015). Specifically, mothers with FASD had higher mortality rate than non-FASD mothers (Li et al., 2011). Another study found that pregnant women with intellectual or developmental disability experienced greater social and health disparities during pregnancy (Brown et al., 2016). Despite the limited evidence, implications for nursing are clear: pregnant women with intellectual or developmental disability require careful interprofessional care during and following pregnancy. Nurses caring for these women must familiarize themselves with area resources in order to provide timely and helpful referrals.

Older Adults

One quarter of older adults with developmental disabilities live independently or with a spouse, with the majority living with a family member of some kind (Factor, Heller, & Janecki, 2012). Preexisting disability in the older adult increases the individual's risk for early symptom onset of chronic illness, inappropriate treatment, and placement in a more restrictive environment (Bishop & Lucchino, n.d.; Factor et al., 2012). For older adults with intellectual or developmental disabilities who present with symptoms of an emerging neurocognitive disorder, medical rule-outs are necessary to determine whether the adverse effects of a medication or environmental changes may be causing the alterations in cognition. Communication deficits can result in challenging behaviors in the older adult with a developmental disability. This, combined with the increased cost for care and often fragmented resources, creates an increased risk for patient frustration and caregiver burnout (Bishop & Lucchino, n.d.). Older adults with developmental disabilities also experience long wait lists for services (Factor et al., 2012). Nurses working with this population serve as advocates to help these patients navigate the services in their communities; assess patients' physical and mental health as well as adaptive and social functioning; and assess both patient and family needs.

Case Study » Part 3

Ms. Mohamed returns to the clinic for a follow-up appointment with her mother, Fartuun Eyl, and husband, Yuusef Yusef. Amiir has been diagnosed with autism by a pediatric neuropsychologist. During your initial interview, Mr. Yusef shares he does not trust the diagnosis of the neuropsychologist. He tells you, "This doctor, he did not know my son. How can he tell if my son has autism? I do not believe him."

While Mr. Yusef, is talking to you, his wife starts to cry. Amiir's grandmother starts speaking in Somali, and the family has a discussion in their primary language. During this time, Amiir is sitting on the ground, hugging his toy vacuum. The volume of the family discussing becomes louder. Amiir starts to scream in a high pitch. The family stops talking, and Ms. Mohamed attempts to comfort Amiir, but he pulls away. Mr. Yusef apologizes, telling you, "This is very hard for my wife and me. We love our son very much. We want only the best for him."

After meeting with the nurse practitioner regarding the results of the testing, the family meets with you for further education. Both Mr. Yusef and Ms. Mohamed express concern for Amiir's future. They tell you that in Somalia, children do not have autism, so the concept of autism is very new for them. The grandmother, who does not speak English, also asks questions through the daughter who interprets for her. The family is referred to a specialty center for different therapies.

Clinical Reasoning Questions Level I

1. *Refer to the exemplar on Autism and other resources.* Explain why Amiir began to scream when the family's discussion became louder. How can the family avoid such events in the future?
2. The family makes the statement that autism does not exist in Somalia. How does the nurse explain this discrepancy?
3. What resources are available in your own community to support children age 2 through 5 who are determined to be on the autism spectrum? Which of these might be appropriate for or helpful to Amiir and his family? Why?

Clinical Reasoning Questions Level II

4. *Refer to the module on Grief and Loss.* Is there a possibility that Amiir's caregivers are grieving his diagnosis? Why or why not? If the family is grieving, using a theory of grieving, categorize the family in a stage or phase of grieving. How can the nurse help the family cope with this diagnosis?
5. You notice that Ms. Mohamed and Mr. Yusef are translating for Ms. Eyl. She appears to have many questions. How should you respond to Ms. Eyl's language barrier?

REVIEW The Concept of Development

RELATE Link the Concepts

Linking the concept of development with the concept of infection:

1. Explain the impact of infection on prenatal development.

2. When caring for pregnant patients, how might the nurse promote infection prevention for both mother and fetus?

Linking the concept of development with the concept of family:

3. Explain the interrelationship between an individual's successful achievement of developmental milestones and the developmental health of the individual's family unit.

4. Describe specific aspects of family function that may be impacted when one family member is diagnosed with a developmental disorder.

Linking the concept of development with the concept of ethics:

5. You are caring for an 8-month-old infant who appears to be undernourished. Along the infant's arms and back, you note what appear to be bruises. The child's mother reports that she recently lost her job and can barely afford to pay her rent or other bills. As a nurse, what is the primary issue and what actions are required of you?

6. Identify potential ethical concerns that may arise as a result of using prenatal testing (e.g., amniocentesis and chorionic villus sampling) to diagnose developmental disorders in utero.

READY Go to Volume 3: Clinical Nursing Skills

- General assessment: SKILLS 1.1–1.4
- Vital signs: SKILLS 1.5–1.9
- Physical assessment: SKILLS 1.10–1.27
- SKILL 3.6   Sleep Promotion: Assisting
- SKILL 10.5   Nutrition: Assessing
- SKILL 15.5   Environmental Safety: Healthcare Facility, Community, Home

REFER Go to Pearson MyLab Nursing and eText

- Additional review materials

REFLECT Apply Your Knowledge

Abby is a 15-year-old girl who has recently graduated into the local high school. She has a diagnosis of Down syndrome and is considered moderate-to-high functioning. The school nurse is attending the girl's IEP meeting with the rest of the school team. When the mother of the girl is asked how about the transition from the small middle school to the larger high school, the mother relates, "I am worried about Abby. She has become so involved in so many things. She talks about new friends and wants to go to so many activities. She even has started dating! This boy has asked Abby to go to Homecoming, but I am nervous! Should I let her go?"

1. Why is the school nurse part of an IEP team?

2. How should the school nurse answer the mother's question?

3. What role can the school nurse have in Abby's development and safety? What education can the school nurse provide the mother? Provide Abby?

» Exemplar 25.A
Attention-Deficit/Hyperactivity Disorder

Exemplar Learning Outcomes

25.A Analyze ADHD as it relates to development.

- Describe the pathophysiology of ADHD.
- Describe the etiology of ADHD.
- Compare the risk factors and prevention of ADHD.
- Identify the clinical manifestations of ADHD.
- Summarize diagnostic tests and therapies used by interprofessional teams in the collaborative care of an individual with ADHD.
- Differentiate care of patients with ADHD across the lifespan.
- Apply the nursing process in providing culturally competent care to an individual with ADHD.

Exemplar Key Terms

Attention-deficit disorder (ADD), *1818*
Attention-deficit/hyperactivity disorder (ADHD), *1817*

Overview

At one time, **attention deficit/hyperactivity disorder (ADHD)** was considered a childhood condition, outgrown in adolescence and of little consequence for adults. Research indicates, however, that the disorder persists into adulthood in 30 to 70% of individuals. Classic characteristics exhibited by an individual with ADHD include difficulty completing tasks that require focused concentration, as well as hyperactivity, hyperkinesis (excessive movement), and impulsivity (APA, 2015; Roman-Urrestarazu et al., 2016). Hyperactivity and impulsivity may improve as the child nears adulthood, with inattentiveness appearing as the most persistent characteristic.

Studies have shown that while some adolescents may no longer meet diagnostic criteria or exhibit only mild symptoms, MRI scans continue to show brain abnormalities and deficits in memory function (Roman-Urrestarazu et al., 2016).

ADHD is often a missed diagnosis in the adolescent and adult. The adolescent's diagnosis is often complicated by other co-occurring behaviors and mental health diagnoses during this developmental stage (Children and Adults with Attention-Deficit/Hyperactivity Disorder [CHADD], 2016a). The adolescent may have difficulty due to the increasing cognitive demands of school and socialization. As a result, what is seen by parents, educators, and other adults as "just being a teen" or as defiant behavior might actually be ADHD. Among adults, ADHD is a known risk factor for antisocial behavior, substance abuse, involvement in serious accidents, academic underachievement, and low occupational success. In adults, inattention is more persistent than hyperactivity or impulsivity.

Roughly one third of adults with ADHD are not diagnosed until after 18 years of age. Approximately 41% of adults with ADHD go on to have a child with the disorder, suggesting a genetic component to the disease (American Academy of Child and Adolescent Psychiatry, 2016). Adult women in particular are misdiagnosed (CHADD, 2016b). Statistically, ADHD is equal between the genders and behaviors are very similar (Cortese et al., 2016), yet, females tend not to be diagnosed as readily as males throughout the lifespan. There are several rationales for this, especially the lack of hyperactivity exhibited in girls. Instead, many girls display inattentiveness and/or depression and stress (Rizzo, 2016; CHADD, 2016b).

The term **attention-deficit disorder (ADD)** is sometimes used to describe individuals who experience the inattentiveness and difficulty concentrating related to ADHD, but who are without the associated hyperactivity that accompanies ADHD. However, in the *Diagnostic and Statistical Manual of Mental Disorders* (DSM-5), the American Psychiatric Association officially recognizes only ADHD, the manifestations of which are described using specifiers (APA, 2013).

Pathophysiology and Etiology

Pathophysiology

The pathophysiology of ADHD is unclear, but some brain characteristics provide clues. Some children may have a deficit in the catecholamines dopamine and norepinephrine, which lowers the threshold for stimulus input. The disorder is marked by a delay in brain maturation in the areas of self-regulation. Increased input from stimuli and decreased self-regulation cause the hallmark inability to inhibit stimuli and motor activity. Some children exhibit additional problems such as aggressive behaviors, learning disabilities, and motor disorders.

Etiology

Although a variety of physical and neurologic disorders are associated with ADHD, children with identifiable causes represent a small proportion of this population. ADHD may result from several different mechanisms involving interaction of genetic, biological, and environmental risk factors. Examples of known associations include exposure to high levels of lead in childhood and prenatal exposure to alcohol or tobacco smoke. Studies have shown a strong association with preterm birth and that poor fetal growth is a contributing factor (Sucksdorff et al., 2015). Other prenatal factors associated with a higher incidence of ADHD include preterm labor, impaired placental functioning, and impaired oxygenation. Seizures and serious head injury are other potential associations.

Risk Factors

Genetic factors are implicated in the development of ADHD. Although ADHD occurs more commonly within families (25% have a first-degree relative with the disorder), a single

gene has not been located and a specific mechanism of genetic transmission is not known. It is believed that a genetic predisposition interacts with the child's environment, so that both factors contribute to the appearance of the condition. Family stress, poverty, and poor nutrition may be contributing factors in some cases.

Prevention

At this time, there is no known way to prevent the development of ADHD. Women should avoid smoking, drugs, and alcohol during pregnancy to help prevent behaviors that are similar to ADHD. Likewise, women should seek prenatal care to avoid preterm birth and monitor for low fetal growth. According to Sucksdorff et al. (2015), the risk for ADHD increased for each gestational week the infant is preterm.

Clinical Manifestations

Children with ADHD have problems related to decreased attention span, impulsiveness, and/or increased motor activity (**Figure 25–9 》**). Symptoms can range from mild to severe. The child has difficulty completing tasks, fidgets constantly, is frequently loud, and interrupts others. Sleep disturbances are common. Because of these behaviors, the child often has difficulty developing and maintaining social relationships and may be shunned or teased by other children. Furthermore, the child with ADHD is subjected to bullying not only in school, but also within the family by parents and siblings (Peasgood et al., 2016). Overall, those

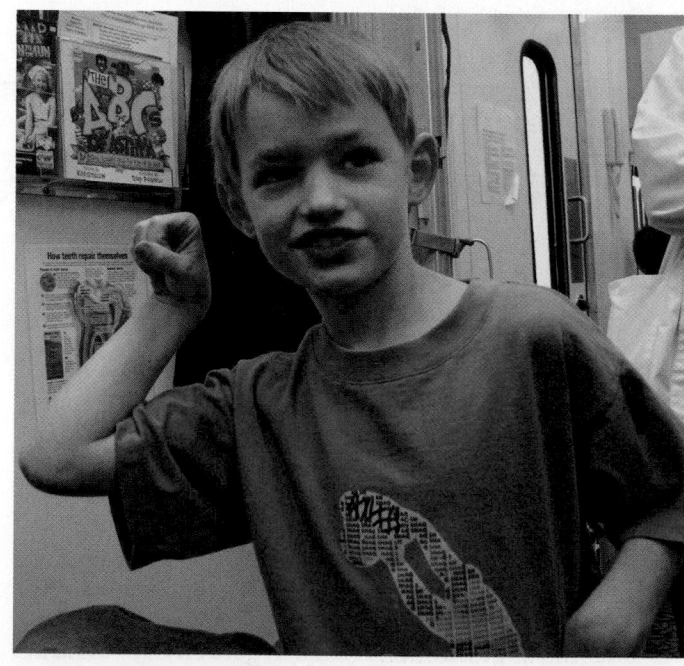

Source: George Dodson/Pearson Education, Inc.

Figure 25–9 》 This child with ADHD was challenged by a visit to a healthcare facility for dental care. He found it difficult to remain in the chair for the examination, and once it was over, he rapidly ran from one piece of equipment to another in the facility. He asked what things were for but did not wait for answers. His engaging personality emerged as he posed briefly for a picture. Such behaviors can be exhausting for parents to manage and may create safety hazards in the healthcare setting.

Clinical Manifestations and Therapies
ADHD

ETIOLOGY	CLINICAL MANIFESTATIONS	CLINICAL THERAPIES
ADHD may have a genetic basis; however, there is no clearly established cause for this disorder.	■ Symptoms of ADHD fall into three groups: Hyperactivity Impulsive behavior Lack of attention	■ Make environmental modifications. ■ Reduce environmental stimuli. ■ Encourage planned seating in classrooms, group settings. ■ Promote consistent limit setting. ■ Behavioral therapy: Reward appropriate behavior. Apply timely, appropriate consequences for inappropriate behavior. Teach strategies to improve focus, coping. ■ Medications: See Medications feature.

with ADHD report lower happiness and quality of life (Peasgood et al., 2016).

Typically, girls with ADHD show less aggression and impulsiveness than boys, but far more anxiety, mood swings, social withdrawal, rejection, and cognitive and language problems. Girls tend to be older at the time of diagnosis.

Collaboration

The successful diagnosis and treatment of the child or adult with ADHD requires a collaborative effort that may involve any combination of the following: parents, nurses, and physicians; teachers, school nurses, and school psychologists or other mental health specialists; and speech and language therapists.

Diagnostic Tests

Diagnosis begins with a careful history of the child, including family history, birth history, growth and developmental milestones, behaviors such as sleep and eating patterns, progression and patterns in school, social and environmental conditions, and reports from parents and teachers. A physical examination should be performed to rule out neurologic diseases and other health problems. The mental health specialist then tests the child and administers questionnaires to the parent and teacher. It is important to identify other conditions that may mimic ADHD or exist in conjunction with the disorders. These conditions may include depression, anxiety, learning disorder, conduct disorder, oppositional defiant disorder, or sleep disturbances (CHADD, 2016a).

Specific diagnostic criteria must be applied to all children with the potential diagnosis of ADHD (**Box 25–2 》》**). Behaviors at home and school or at daycare must be evaluated because abnormal patterns in two settings are needed for diagnosis. A variety of tests are available for the trained professional to use in establishing the diagnosis (**Table 25–15 》》**).

Based on the findings, desired outcomes are established for the child's performance and management of the disorder. Treatment is established to meet the desired behavioral

outcomes and includes a combination of approaches, such as environmental changes, behavior therapy, and pharmacotherapy. Pharmacotherapy is by far the most common approach across the lifespan with more than 70% of patients

Box 25–2
ADHD: A Closer Look

ADHD is marked by a persistent pattern of a cluster of symptoms that occur in multiple areas (e.g., home and school) of daily life and that fall within three categories: hyperactivity, impulsive behavior, and inattention. Symptoms must occur over a period of 6 months or more for a diagnosis of ADHD to be considered (APA, 2013; Mayo Clinic, 2017; National Institute of Mental Health [NIMH], 2016a).

Hyperactivity: Excessive movement characterizes the hyperactivity seen in ADHD. Examples include fidgeting, restlessness (especially in adolescents and adults), running or climbing at inappropriate times, inability to engage quietly in activities, and wearing others out with activity.

Impulsive behaviors: Examples of impulsive behaviors include interrupting others, intruding on others (e.g., taking another's toy), and having difficulty waiting turns. Impulsive talking or blurting out may also be observed. Impulsivity also may be characterized by poor decision making without regard to consequences.

Inattention: Inattention in the case of the individual with ADHD is not merely a lack of attention or a tendency to be easily distracted, although those certainly occur. The individual with ADHD may:

- Be unable to pay close attention; make careless mistakes
- Have difficulty focusing on those speaking to him or on activities
- Fail to follow directions or finish tasks
- Be disorganized
- Be reluctant to participate in activities that require effort
- Lose things or forget tasks

TABLE 25–15 Screening Tests for ADHD

Test	Source
Vanderbilt Parent and Teacher Scales	www.brightfutures.org/mentalhealth/pdf/professionals/bridges/adhd.pdf
Conners' Parent and Teacher Rating Scales—Revised—Long Form	http://www.mhs.com/product.aspx?gr=cli&id=overview&prod=conners3
Swanson, Nolan, and Pelham Questionnaire II Teacher and Parent Rating Scale (SNAP-IV)	www.ourgirlwednesday.com/downloads/snap-iv-instructions.pdf
Disruptive Behavior Disorder Scale	http://vinst.umdnj.edu/VAID/TestReport.asp?Code=DBRSF
ADHD Rating Scale	www.fmpe.org/en/documents/appendix/Appendix%201%20-%20ADHD%20Rating%20Scale.pdf
Revised Behavior Problem Checklist	http://vinst.umdnj.edu/VAID/TestReport.asp?Code=RBPC
Adult Self-Report Scale for ADHD	https://add.org/wp-content/uploads/2015/03/adhd-questionnaire-ASRS111.pdf

being prescribed a stimulant (Oehrlein et al., 2016). Treatment is expected to be long term.

Children are usually brought for evaluation when behaviors escalate to the point of interfering with the daily functioning of teachers or parents. When children have learning disabilities or anxiety disorders, the problem is commonly misdiagnosed as ADHD without further evaluation of the child's symptoms. ADHD can be diagnosed by a mental health professional or a medical provider. Careful management of ADHD in childhood may lead to better social functioning later in life, as well as better relationships with family and peers.

Pharmacologic Therapy

Children with moderate to severe ADHD are treated with pharmacotherapy (see the Medications feature). Stimulants are primarily prescribed; however, there are three nonstimulant medications approved by the FDA (2016) for children: Strattera (atomoxetine), Intuniv (guanfacine), and Kapvay (clonidine). Paradoxically, in patients with ADHD, psychostimulants help improve focus and attention, as opposed to yielding increased hyperactivity. Usually, a favorable response (a decrease in impulsive behaviors and an increase in the ability to sit still and attend to an activity for at least 15 minutes) is seen in the first 10 days of treatment and frequently with the first few doses. All psychostimulants are Schedule II drugs, which means that a monthly prescription must be obtained from a healthcare practitioner. Side effects include headaches, insomnia, tachycardia, and anorexia. A child's growth pattern should be carefully monitored while taking these medications. A "drug holiday," during which the child does not take the medication during weekends or over school breaks, can be considered and discussed with the prescribing provider.

SAFETY ALERT Many medications used to treat ADHD are central nervous system (CNS) stimulants. As such, they have a potential for abuse, especially among teens and young adults who take them as an appetite suppressant or in order to stay awake. In the adult population, the nurse should be aware of the increased risk of potentially fatal cardiovascular effects of stimulant medication (FDA, 2011).

Nonpharmacologic Therapy

Although medications are an important part of the treatment plan for the patient with ADHD, nonpharmacologic therapies are also integral components of care. Environmental modification and behavioral therapy can greatly improve outcomes for patients with ADHD and enhance their daily quality of life.

Environmental Modification

Children with ADHD often benefit from environmental changes. Decreasing stimulation by turning off the television, keeping the environment quiet, and maintaining an orderly and clutter-free desk or study area may help the child to stay focused on the task at hand. Another relatively simple change is appropriate classroom placement, preferably in a small class with a teacher who can provide close supervision and a structured daily routine. Consistent limits and expectations should be set for the child. Routines and signaled transitions help the child to feel organized. Children living in chaotic homes and communities may function better if the environment can be simplified. When aggressive behaviors occur, therapeutic approaches such as play and group therapy may be useful.

Behavioral Therapy

Behavioral therapy involves rewarding the child for desired behaviors and applying consequences for undesirable behaviors. Children may be rewarded by praise or earn points toward a movie or another desired outing for staying seated during meals or quietly listening in a classroom. Cues are established so that a child can subtly be reminded when impulsive or hyperactive behaviors are escalating. Behavioral therapy is most effective when all adults who are in close contact with the child, such as parents and teachers, are involved in and supportive of the program.

In a hallmark study conducted by NIMH, behavioral therapy in combination with medication has shown to be the best practice for treatment of ADHD (Molina et al., 2009). The AAP (2011) recommends that toddlers and small children should first be treated with behavioral therapy and later treated with medications if symptoms continue to be troublesome.

Complementary Health Approaches

According to the NCCIH (2016b), there is no scientific evidence supporting the use of complementary health approaches in the treatment of ADHD. Several areas of complementary medicine have been studied, including diet

Medications
ADHD

CLASSIFICATION AND DRUG EXAMPLES	MECHANISMS OF ACTION	NURSING CONSIDERATIONS
CNS Stimulants *Drug examples:* Amphetamine-dextroamphetamine (Adderall) Dexmethylphenidate (Focalin) Methylphenidate (Ritalin, Concerta) Dextroamphetamine (Dexedrine) Lisdexamfetamine (Vyvanse) Methamphetamine (Desoxyn)	The mechanisms of action for stimulants in the treatment of ADHD is poorly understood. It is thought to block the reuptake of dopamine and norepinephrine. *May also be used for:* Narcolepsy	▪ Teach patients and parents about side effects such as headaches, insomnia, and anorexia. ▪ Monitor patient's growth while on this medication. ▪ Ask about a "drug holiday" on weekends and school breaks. ▪ *Potential for abuse:* Some children will sell the drug at school.
Nonstimulants *Drug examples:* Atomoxetine (Strattera) Clonidine (Kapvay) Guanfacine (Intuniv)	The mechanism of action of nonstimulants in the treatment of ADHD is poorly understood. Atomoxetine is a selective norepinephrine reuptake inhibitor. Both clonidine and guanfacine are antihypertensives that are also used for ADHD. They are best used conjunctively with a stimulant.	▪ Has less abuse potential since nonstimulant. ▪ Teach parents to be alert for serious side effects, including psychosis and suicidal tendencies, particularly with atomoxetine. ▪ Monitor hepatic function while on atomoxetine. ▪ Monitor blood pressure while on clonidine or guanfacine. ▪ Use with caution in patients with heart disease.
Psychostimulant Skin Patch *Drug example:* Methylphenidate (Daytrana)	The mechanism of action for stimulants in the treatment of ADHD is poorly understood. It is thought to block the reuptake of dopamine and norepinephrine.	▪ Teach patients to alternate patch placement between left and right hips. ▪ Watch for skin irritations. ▪ Has been known to cause permanent leukoderma in some children. ▪ Teach patient to remove patch after 9 hours. ▪ Same side effect profile as oral medications.

Source: Data from Adams, M. P., Holland, L. N., & Urban, C. (2017). *Pharmacology for nurses: A pathophysiologic approach* (5th ed.). Hoboken, NJ: Pearson Education.

regimens, diet supplements, and neurofeedback (NCCIH, 2016b). Most of the popular supplements and special diets (such as the Feingold diet) have been disproved to alleviate the symptoms of ADHD.

Although it does not help reduce hyperactivity and other symptoms of ADHD, melatonin might help some patients who have difficulty with sleep. Mind/body therapies, such as yoga and massage likewise do not help with symptoms, but may help with sleep.

Lifespan Considerations

As stated in the Overview, although ADHD was once thought of as a childhood disorder, it is now being diagnosed in younger children and in adults. ADHD manifests in different ways across the lifespan. Nurses should be alert for the following signs of ADHD in patients of all ages.

ADHD in Toddlers and Preschoolers

Diagnosing ADHD in toddlers is difficult. Many of the normal behaviors of toddlers and preschoolers are similar to those seen in ADHD, such as trouble concentrating or taking turns. However, children as young as 3 years of age can be diagnosed with ADHD (NIMH, 2016a). Young children with ADHD tend to be more disruptive than those without. Some children are so disruptive they are expelled from preschool. Often, those children with ADHD tend to get special education placement. Young children with ADHD tend to have more injuries and take greater risks than their peers.

ADHD in School-Age Children and Adolescents

ADHD is typically diagnosed once the child reaches school age and the hyperactivity and impulsivity prevalent with this disorder manifest in the classroom setting. Children with ADHD often have academic difficulties regardless of their cognitive abilities. Creating peer relationships is an important part of development, but because of the behaviors of ADHD, children sometimes struggle with making and maintaining friends. Children with ADHD also are more prone to accidents and injuries due to risk-taking behaviors and lack of forethought.

As a child with ADHD progresses into adolescence, there is less hyperactivity but fidgeting and restless are still present. Impulsive behaviors and inattentiveness persist at this age and can continue into adulthood. Many of the behaviors of ADHD in adolescence could be considered antisocial, which in turn makes it difficult for the teen with ADHD to make and keep friends. School typically continues to be a challenge because of inability to focus and stay organized.

ADHD in Adults

The diagnosis of ADHD in the adult is often followed with a sense of relief. As children, these adults often exhibited mild symptoms, and therefore were not diagnosed. As they moved into adulthood, they continued to struggle with personal and social relationships, workplace responsibilities, and time management. Both young and older adults with ADHD exhibit antisocial behavior, have difficulties maintaining jobs, and participate in risky behaviors. The risky behaviors in particular are a concern for the nurse. Chemical dependency, assault, and trauma are commonly seen in adults with ADHD, particularly those who have gone undiagnosed and untreated. Compared to women without ADHD, adult women with ADHD are three times as likely to experience generalized anxiety, sexual abuse, suicidal thoughts, and chronic pain (Fuller-Thomson, Lewis, & Agbeyaka, 2016). Women with ADHD are twice as likely as their healthy counterparts to experience chemical dependency, poverty, and depression (Fuller-Thomson et al., 2016).

NURSING PROCESS

Especially when caring for pediatric patients, parents and caregivers are integral to each phase of the nursing process. In particular, because collection of assessment data depends largely on patient interviews, the nurse should establish effective communication patterns with the parents and caregivers.

Assessment

The nurse often encounters the family who is concerned about the child's behavior before a diagnosis has been made. Assessment of a patient with ADHD can sometimes be difficult, as ADHD is a complex neurodevelopmental disorder that is not always obvious. Moreover, the time a nurse spends with a patient is usually short, and the diagnosis of ADHD typically requires many interactions.

- **Observation and patient interview.** Because ADHD has two major presentations, inattentive or hyperactive/impulsive, the nurse should look for signs of either of these behaviors. Watch to see if the patient appears to be listening and/or paying attention to the nurse during discussions. Observe for sign of hyperactivity, such as fidgeting and inability to sit in one place. Listen for rapid, excessive speech patterns.

  Ask about family and birth history and have parents describe their child's behaviors. In the adult, the significant other or friends would be a good resource for behavior assessment. As appropriate, perform developmental screenings and look specifically for attention span and physical activity. Refer the family to their pediatric healthcare home for further assessment, then to a mental healthcare specialist

who is experienced in diagnosing ADHD. Adults can be diagnosed by either a mental health provider or a primary care provider, preferably someone with whom the patient has a long-term relationship.

The nurse may encounter the child with ADHD in the hospital when parents bring the child for treatment of an injury (e.g., fracture) or another problem. Explore in detail the parents' report of the child's attention span. Usually within a few minutes in an unstructured setting or waiting area, the child with ADHD becomes restless and searches for distraction. Gather information about the child's activity level and impulsiveness. Find out how the family manages at home and what treatments are being applied. For the hospitalized adult, data collection and assessment for ADHD are more complicated. Like the pediatric patient, the adult patient may become inattentive or restless and fidgety. Assess patient self-care and history of injuries consistent with ADHD behaviors.

- **Physical examination.** The physical exam of the patient with ADHD across the lifespan will not show any physical abnormalities unless the patient is being seen for injuries related to hyperactive and impulsive behaviors.

Diagnosis

Examples of nursing diagnoses that may be appropriate for both with a patient of any age who has ADHD include the following:

- *Injury, Risk for*
- *Imbalanced Nutrition: Less Than Body Requirements, Risk for*
- *Verbal Communication, Impaired*
- *Social Interaction, Impaired*
- *Self-Esteem, Chronic Low*
- *Caregiver Role Strain, Risk for.*

(NANDA-I © 2014)

Focus on Diversity and Culture
Differences in Ethnicity and ADHD Diagnosis

Past research into trends of ADHD and ethnicity and race had shown a greater percentage of White boys in middle to upper social economic classes being diagnosed with ADHD. However, current research indicates children of color of all socioeconomic status are underdiagnosed (Gómez-Benito et al., 2015; Siegel et al., 2016). Although the literature is inconclusive in regard to ethnic/racial trends of ADHD, it appears that ADHD is present in all ethnic and racial groups. Culture might play a significant factor in underdiagnosis. For example, in some cultures, energetic behaviors and fidgeting are not viewed as undesirable in children. As a result, parents might not seek out a diagnosis. Parenting style, which is influenced by culture, may also play a part in differential diagnosis. Practitioners of one culture might not appreciate the behaviors of a child of another culture. Other factors involved in diagnostic disparities may include financial means, lack of access to specialty providers, mistrust of providers from the dominant culture, and stigma.

Planning

Planning for the patient with ADHD may include the following goals:

- The pediatric patient will have a plan to facilitate learning and support appropriate behaviors at home and at school.
- The adult patient will have a plan in place to meet workplace expectations and responsibilities.
- The patient will remain safe from self-harm and/or physical injury.
- The patient will adhere to the treatment regimen.
- The patient and the patient's family will understand appropriate resources available in the community.

Implementation

Children with ADHD present a number of challenges to their parents and teachers. The nurse may need to provide patient teaching to both parents and teachers regarding medications and their side effects, the importance of decreasing stimuli and minimizing distractions, and the need for consistency and patience with behavior management plans. Some trial and error may be necessary before the child's treatment team (including parents and teachers) finds the combination of therapies that is most effective for the child.

Implementation of the nursing plan with the adult patient is even more of a challenge because much of the responsibility of follow-through is the patient's. Treatment adherence will be a high priority. The adult patient may not have the support system a child has and may benefit from case management to assist with medication adherence, support systems, and community resources.

Administer Pharmacologic Treatments

Stimulant and nonstimulant medications increase the patient's attention span and decrease distractibility. Interventions related to pharmacologic treatment include the following:

- Teach patient and parents or family members to be alert for the common side effects of these medications, including anorexia, insomnia, and tachycardia.
- Administer medication early in the day to help alleviate insomnia. Anorexia can be managed by giving medication at mealtimes.
- Perform careful periodic monitoring of weight, height, and blood pressure.
- Instruct families about the abuse potential of stimulant drugs; these drugs should be locked up and administered only as directed.

Minimize Environmental Distractions

Patients with ADHD benefit from fewer environmental distractions. For children:

- Keep potentially harmful equipment out of reach.
- Limit and monitor "screen" time.
- Provide a quiet, clutter-free area for study time.
- Use shades to darken the room during naps or at bedtime and minimize noise.

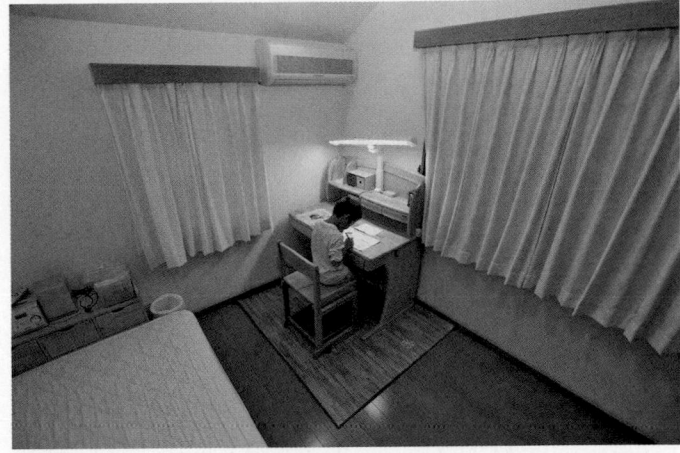

Source: MIXA next/Getty Images.

Figure 25–10 ❯❯ Managing the environment to provide quiet places with minimal distractions is often necessary for the child with ADHD. This boy reads and does homework in a room with no pictures, no music, and only his homework on his desk. He also is assisted by structure, such as a scheduled time for homework, with short breaks to walk around every 10 to 15 minutes.

- Teach parents to minimize distractions at home during periods when the child needs to concentrate (e.g., when doing schoolwork) (**Figure 25–10** ❯❯).
- When the child is hospitalized, minimizing environmental distractions may mean placement in a room with only one other child.

Adults may benefit from similar environmental modifications, including maintaining a quiet, clutter-free area for work and limiting screen time, especially when completing tasks and for an hour or more before bedtime.

Implement Behavioral Management Plans

Behavior modification programs can help reduce specific impulsive behaviors. An example is setting up a reward program for the child who has taken medication as ordered or completed a homework assignment. Depending on the child's age, the rewards may be daily as well as weekly or monthly. For example, one completed homework assignment might be rewarded with 30 minutes of basketball or a bike ride, and assignments completed for a week might be rewarded with participation in an activity of the child's choice on the weekend.

Provide Emotional Support

Family support is essential. Educate family members and patients about the importance of appropriate expectations and consequences of behaviors. Teach skills such as making lists of tasks to accomplish; following routines for eating, sleeping, recreation, and, for children, schoolwork; and minimizing stimuli in the environment when completing work.

When the child is hospitalized for another condition, the time may provide a brief respite from constant care by the parent. The activity, impulsivity, and general high energy of children with ADHD can fatigue parents. When the child is hospitalized, parents may want to spend a few hours each day at home or at a nearby residence for families. Ask them how they manage at home and offer ideas for respite care.

Patients who are diagnosed with ADHD as adults often need emotional support. While some are relieved to understand the cause of some of the hardships in their lives, others are dismayed by the diagnosis. Refer adult patients to mental health counselors as appropriate. Evidence-based practice has shown that cognitive-behavioral therapy combined with medications provides the best outcomes for adults with ADHD (Cherkasova et al., 2016).

Promote Self-Esteem

Patients with ADHD are easily frustrated, in part by their own behaviors and in part by the reactions of others. This frustration easily leads to loss of self-esteem. Nurses help patients with ADHD understand the disorder at a developmentally appropriate level, and also facilitate a trusting relationship with healthcare providers. Patients of all ages with ADHD who build healthy relationships with healthcare providers are more likely to seek help. Interventions to promote self-esteem may include:

- Emphasize the positive aspects of behavior and treat instances of negative behavior as learning opportunities.

- Encourage skills at which the patient excels and consider the use of support groups in school or in the community.

- Offer praise for successfully following tasks or meeting goals. For example, praise the adult patient whose spouse reports improved communication with children and other family members or the hospitalized child who helps carry toys around to other children.

Educate Families

Although families of all patients benefit from education about ADHD, parents of affected children need particular support to understand the diagnosis and to learn how to manage the child. Explain what the diagnosis is and what is known about attention-deficit disorders. Provide written materials, internet sites, and an opportunity to ask questions.

Emphasize the importance of a stable environment at home as well as at school. At home, the child may have difficulty staying on task. Parents need to consider the child's age and developmental appropriateness of tasks, give clear and simple instructions, and provide frequent reminders to ensure completion. Routines in the evening can promote good sleep patterns.

The nurse can serve as a liaison to teachers and school personnel or as the case manager for the child. See the Patient Teaching box for suggestions on how parents and teachers

---

Patient Teaching
Optimizing the Educational Experience for the Child with ADHD

Schools are now changing their perspective on children with ADHD. Prior to the DSM-5, ADHD was seen as a disruptive behavior disorder that highly impacted the school setting. Now that ADHD is seen as a neurodevelopmental disorder, schools are approaching the behaviors of ADHD students differently. The key to supporting the child with ADHD in school is a strong parent–teacher relationship. Parents can work with teachers to provide a school environment that fosters attention and learning. Some ideas that may be helpful include the following:

- Have the child sit near the front of the class, preferably away from doors or windows.

- Plan a reminder (for the child) that is apparent to the teacher and student but not to other children when the child needs to concentrate on attention. This might be an object placed on the student's desk or a light hand placed on the shoulder or arm.

- Go over assignments and tests with the child in person to explain areas that are understood and those that need attention. Give instructions verbally and in written form and repeat them more than once.

- Provide opportunities to take notes and make lists of assignments and mark off when accomplished. Have a planned

time to go through the child's backpack daily to find notices and to ensure that homework is completed and in a uniform location.

- Use computers, note-taking partners, or recording devices for making lists and taking notes.

- If the child has well-developed fine or gross motor skills, integrate motor movement into learning situations whenever possible. Allow the child to run occasional errands to provide additional opportunities for movement.

- Provide quiet places with minimal distraction for examinations. Offer additional time.

- Allow time for organizing clothing, desk, and other areas.

- Find the child's areas of excellence and allow for performance in these ways. Some children are talented in dance, others in art or extemporaneous speech.

- Never call the child names, make fun of behavior or performance, or call the child "hyperactive" in front of other children, teachers, or parents.

- Incorporate social and behavioral skills into the child's learning plan.

Sources: Based on Call-Schmidt, T., & Maharaj, G. (2004). Using nonpharmacological treatments in conjunction with stimulant medications for children with ADHD. *Journal of Pediatric Health Care, 18,* 255–259; National Alliance on Mental Illness (NAMI). (n.d.). ADHD and school: *Helping your child succeed in the classroom.* Retrieved from http://www.nami.org/Template.cfm?Section=ADHD&Template=/ContentManagement/ContentDisplay.cfm&ContentID=106379; Toplek, M. (2015). ADHD: Making a difference for children and youth in the schools. *Perspectives on Language and Literacy, 41*(1), 7–8.

can work together to optimize the child's educational experience. An IEP may be needed, with clear expected outcomes stated for the child's behaviors. IEPs or periods of instruction free from the distractions of the entire class may enable the child to improve school performance. Parents may have difficulty understanding the need for these approaches because the child often tests at above-average intelligence.

As the child grows older, provide explanations about the disorder and information about techniques that will assist in dealing with problems. Emphasize the importance of doing homework or other tasks requiring concentration in a quiet environment without background noise from a television or radio. Encourage children with ADHD to keep assignment notebooks and use checklists to help them accomplish specific tasks.

Evaluation

Expected outcomes of nursing care for the child with ADHD include the following:

- The parents and child demonstrate understanding of the disorder.

- The family accurately and safely manages medication administration.
- The child maintains a weight that is within normal limits.
- The child demonstrates an increase in attentiveness and a decrease in hyperactivity, impulsivity, and sleep disturbance.
- The child displays formation of a positive self-image.
- The child manifests formation of healthy social interactions with peers and family.
- The child achieves educational performance to maximum potential.

Expected outcomes for an adult with ADHD are very similar to that of a child and may also include:

- The patient remains safe and free from self-harm.
- The patient is adheres to the treatment regimen.
- The patient verbalizes responsibilities are being met, such as employment.

Nursing Care Plan
A Patient with ADHD

Melanie Taylor, age 8, visits her pediatrician's office for a routine checkup. Her mother, Mrs. Taylor, reports that Melanie is not doing well in school and that she is a difficult child to raise. Upon further questioning, Mrs. Taylor reports that her daughter is forgetful, has trouble focusing, and often does not respond to her name being called. She has to repeatedly ask her to perform her chores, get ready for bed, or do her homework. Melanie does not sleep well at night, and most nights she crawls into her parents' bed. One night Mrs. Taylor awoke to find Melanie watching TV at 2 a.m. in the family room. Melanie's teacher has suggested she be evaluated for possible ADHD.

ASSESSMENT	DIAGNOSES	PLANNING
The nurse interviews Melanie, who says she doesn't like school because "it's too hard" and the teacher "always tells me to sit still." Upon reviewing Melanie's medical history, the nurse finds the patient's growth and development have been normal to date. Mrs. Taylor's pregnancy and delivery were unremarkable. The physical examination is normal, although the nurse notes that Melanie often requires repetition of instructions such as "Touch your finger to your nose" before she complies. Both Melanie and her mother appear tired and yawn several times during the nurse's time with them. The provider speaks with Melanie and Mrs. Taylor, suggesting that the signs and symptoms are highly suspicious of ADHD, and provides a referral for the family to meet with a psychologist specializing in the care of patients with this disorder. The nurse provides Ms. Taylor with a Conners' Parent Rating Scale to complete and gives her a copy of the Teacher Rating Scale to give to Melanie's teacher for completion before seeing the counselor, who will evaluate the results.	■ *Self-Esteem, Situational Low, Risk for* ■ *Sleep Pattern, Disturbed* ■ *Caregiver Role Strain, Risk for* ■ *Fatigue* (NANDA-I © 2014)	■ The patient (Melanie) will sleep through the night, remaining in her own bed. ■ The patient will participate in a therapeutic regimen as recommended by the physician/healthcare provider. ■ The patient's parents and teachers will participate in the therapeutic regimen. ■ The patient will increase her ability to remain on task by 5-minute intervals over a period of 6–8 weeks, until she can remain on task for a minimum of 20 minutes at a time. ■ The patient will keep track of her belongings. ■ The patient will respond when spoken to the first time.

(continued on next page)

Nursing Care Plan (continued)

IMPLEMENTATION

- Explain diagnosis in terms Melanie can understand, and help Melanie understand that she is not "abnormal" but "unique" in how her brain works.
- Help Mrs. Taylor set rules related to sleep that will promote Melanie's sleep hygiene.
- Assist patient to understand how her potential diagnosis of ADHD impacts her thinking as well as how treatment can help her perform better in school.
- Determine if Melanie or Mrs. Taylor have questions related to ADHD.

- Suggest strategies for helping Melanie improve her concentration and memory.
- Teach positive behavioral skills through role play, role modeling, and discussion.
- Convey confidence in patient's and mother's ability to handle situation.
- Encourage increased responsibility for self, as appropriate.
- Encourage Melanie to accept new challenges.
- Monitor Melanie's statements of self-worth and frequency of self-negating verbalizations.

EVALUATION

Mrs. Taylor and Melanie return at the end of 3 months. Mrs. Taylor reports that Melanie is doing better at paying attention both at home and at school, and that she is able to maintain attention for 20 minutes "most of the time." Both of them are sleeping better. Melanie is able to answer the nurse's questions readily and describes things that she does to keep track of her belongings and try to stay on task. Melanie voices pride in her improvement at school.

CRITICAL THINKING

1. Mrs. Taylor asks the nurse, privately out of range of Melanie's hearing, if the diagnosis resulted from something she did as a parent or while pregnant. How would you respond?

2. Melanie tells the nurse, "I'm so stupid compared to the other kids in my class. I guess ADHD means I'm brain damaged." How would you respond?

3. Is it possible to adequately treat ADHD without the use of medications? Explain your answer.

REVIEW Attention-Deficit/Hyperactivity Disorder

RELATE Link the Concepts and Exemplars

Linking the exemplar of attention-deficit/hyperactivity disorder with the concept of family:

1. How can the nurse support the family of a child with ADHD?

2. What if the family is a single parent? A grandparent?

Linking the exemplar of attention-deficit/hyperactivity disorder with the concept of safety:

3. What interventions are important for the nurse to initiate to maintain the safety of a patient with ADHD?

4. When caring for an adolescent with ADHD, how would you teach automobile safety?

READY Go to Volume 3: Clinical Nursing Skills

REFER Go to Pearson MyLab Nursing and eText

- Additional review materials

REFLECT Apply Your Knowledge

Jason is an active, healthy 11-year-old boy. He is currently in fifth grade at the public elementary school near his home. He lives with his mother Evelyn and his 14-year-old sister Jenna. He has not had much contact with his father. Jason's home life has been somewhat stressful the past year or so because of ongoing fights between his mother and oldest sister Jessica; the conflict resulted in Jessica moving out of the house. Jason gets along well with his mother, but he has typical sibling conflicts with Jenna.

Jason has had problems in school for the past 3 years. Teachers report that he has difficulty staying on task and won't follow directions. Although he made some progress last year with his fourth-grade teacher, his grades have been consistently poor. His mother tries to help him with homework after school or in the evening; these sessions frequently turn into battlegrounds. It takes Jason hours to complete fairly simple assignments, resulting in a great deal of frustration for both Jason and his mother. The fact that he frequently comes home from school with headaches further aggravates the situation.

In addition to problems with academics, Jason has problems with social interactions. His teachers find him to be disruptive in the classroom. During the past year, he has often been sent to the principal's office for misbehaving. He has few friends and is a frequent target of teasing at school. Most of his time at home is spent playing video and computer games and watching TV.

1. What are the priorities of nursing care for Jason?

2. What outcomes would be appropriate for this patient?

3. What independent nursing interventions would you initiate for this patient?

» Exemplar 25.B
Autism Spectrum Disorder

Exemplar Learning Outcomes

25.B Analyze ASD as it relates to development.

- Describe the pathophysiology of ASD.
- Describe the etiology of ASD.
- Compare the risk factors and prevention of ASD.
- Identify the clinical manifestations of ASD.
- Summarize diagnostic tests and therapies used by interprofessional teams in the collaborative care of an individual with ASD.

- Differentiate care of patients with ASD across the lifespan.
- Apply the nursing process in providing culturally competent care to an individual with ASD.

Exemplar Key Terms

Autism spectrum disorder (ASD), *1827*
Echolalia, *1828*
Stereotypy, *1828*

Overview

The patient with **autism spectrum disorder (ASD)** characteristically demonstrates impaired communication and social interaction patterns, and the presence of repetitive, restrictive, and stereotyped behaviors. Manifestations of ASD range across a spectrum from mild to severe. Children and adults with ASD often experience impairments of language, cognition, and social skills that make them seem different from others. The prevalence of ASD is approximately 1 in 68 individuals in the United States. It is far more common in males (1 in 42) than females (1 in 189) (CDC, 2016f). A number of other conditions have a high co-occurrence with autism, including intellectual differences, mood or other mental health disorders, seizures, immune dysfunctions, and gastrointestinal issues (Autism Speaks, 2016). Managing ASD can be harrowing for both patients and family members. Nurses play an essential role in providing essential information and emotional support related to managing the diagnosis and promoting health and wellness for both the patient with autism and family members and caregivers.

» Stay Current: Keep abreast of statistics, research, and treatment at www.autismspeaks.org.

Pathophysiology and Etiology

Pathophysiology

The pathophysiology of autism is not well understood. What is known is that those with autism have defects in the genes and gene expression in the areas of cell-cycle expression. The construction of the brain is atypical in comparison to those without autism. MRIs and other imaging has shown there are abnormalities of neurons of the cerebral cortex. The frontal and temporal lobes are particularly susceptible to these abnormal neuron patches. The frontal lobe is responsible for social behaviors, motor function, problem solving, and other higher functions. The temporal lobe is responsible for language and sensory input. These neuron irregularities are thought to be responsible for the dysfunction and behaviors associated with autism. These abnormalities are created during fetal development. Because the infant brain continues to develop, with early intervention, the brain can develop neuron networking around the defective neuron

abnormalities and/or use pathways from nearby areas of the brain (Stoner et al., 2014).

Etiology

Although the etiology of ASD remains unknown, it is believed to be associated with a complex interplay between genetic, epigenetic, immunologic, and environmental factors. More than 800 ASD predisposition genes have been identified, and many of these implicate functional pathways related to synaptic organization and activity; chromatin remodeling; and Wnt signaling during development (Krumm et al., 2014; Yin & Schaaf, 2016).

Risk Factors

Without a specific etiology, determining risk for autism is difficult. However, research continues to point toward genetics and the influence of agents on genes. Children with genetic abnormalities such as tuberous sclerosis, fragile X syndrome, Down syndrome, congenital rubella syndrome, and neurofibromatosis have an increased occurrence of autism. Children who have family members with autism are more likely to be autistic. Boys have a higher rate of ASD than girls. Likewise, teratogens, such as valproic acid and thalidomide, have been linked to autism (CDC, 2016f).

Advanced maternal age has been associated with autism, but research is now finding that the ages of the both parents plays a factor. An extensive, global study found that mothers of age greater than 40 years and fathers of age greater than 50 years were more likely to have children with autism than those of other ages. Maternal age also played a factor in those children who were born to mothers younger than 20 years. The study also found that if there is a great age disparity between parents (greater than 10 years), there was a higher incidence of autism (Sandin et al., 2015).

Prevention

As with the prevention of any developmental condition, excellent prenatal care is essential to helping prevent autism. Prior to pregnancy, the woman should take folic acid and strive to be in good health. If the mother is on medication, including antiepileptics, she should discuss the benefits and risks of her medication and pregnancy. The woman should also discuss genetic counseling with her provider if there are family members with autism.

It is important to emphasize that multiple studies have found no link between immunizations and autism (Mayo Clinic, 2014; Stefano, Price, & Weintraub, 2013). Therefore, pregnant women should be vaccinated to prevent infection, a known cause of birth defects. During pregnancy, the mother should avoid alcohol, tobacco, infection, toxic substances, and other known causes of birth defects. While these measures might not necessarily prevent autism, they will help improve the chances of a healthy baby being born.

Clinical Manifestations

The essential features of autism typically become apparent by the time a child is 3 years of age. The core characteristics of autism are:

- Social deficits
- Language impairment
- Repetitive behaviors.

Social interactions are always complex and involve perceptions of the other individual as well as social behaviors. The patient with ASD does not learn the common characteristics of these social interchanges. As a result, the patient may be unable to converse normally, may fail to initiate conversations, and/or may fail to understand or observe nonverbal behavior.

Children with ASD manifest disturbances in the rate or sequence of development, with onset of abnormal functioning in at least one of the following areas prior to age 3: social interaction, language used in social interactions, and imaginative play.

In addition to difficulty relating to others or responding to social and emotional cues, **stereotypy**, or rigid and obsessive behavior, may be observed. Characteristically, these repetitive behaviors in affected children include head banging, twirling in circles, biting themselves, and flapping their hands or arms. The child's behavior may be self-stimulating or self-destructive. Responses to sensory stimuli are frequently abnormal and include an extreme aversion to touch, loud noises, and bright lights (**Figure 25–11 》**). Emotional lability (rapid, significant mood changes) is common.

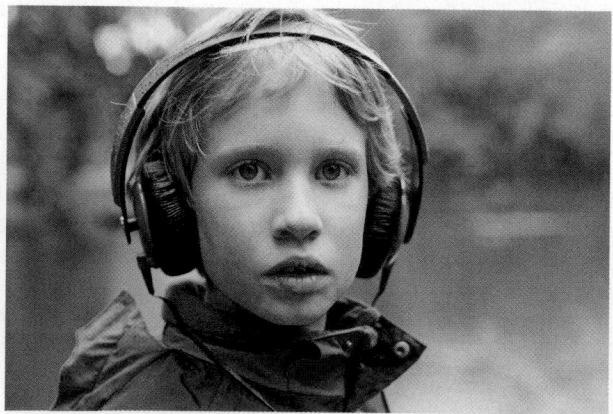

Source: Maria Dubova/iStock/Getty Images.

Figure 25–11 》 This child with autism chooses to wear headphones whenever he leaves the house because loud noises hurt his ears and frighten him. The headphones give him a sense of security, making it easier for him to go out and interact with others.

Communication difficulties or delays in speech and language are common and are often the first symptoms that lead to diagnosis. Absence of babbling and other communication by 1 year of age, absence of two-word phrases by 2 years, and deterioration of previous language skills are characteristic of autism. Language acquisition, including verbal and nonverbal communication patterns, such as eye contact, will vary based on the severity of the disorder. Some children and adults with ASD can participate fully in conversations, but may show characteristic behaviors such as marked lack of eye contact and lack of emotional reciprocity. They may or may not understand humor and other subtleties of language.

For children with ASD, speech patterns are likely to show certain abnormalities, such as the following:

- Using *you* in place of *I*
- Engaging in **echolalia** (a compulsive parroting of a word or phrase just spoken by another)
- Repeating questions rather than answering them
- Being fascinated with rhythmic, repetitive songs and verses.

Behaviors of children with ASDs show several differences from typically developing children's behaviors. Children with ASD may have a great difficulty dealing with new situations and typically show agitation and withdrawal when routines are changed. Children with ASD do not commonly explore objects, but have stereotyped behaviors. They may line up objects, play with the same objects over and over, and have certain rituals that must be performed. They often become upset if these normal routines are disrupted. Rituals may involve eating only certain types or colors of foods or eating in specific patterns.

Patients with ASD may manifest disturbances in the rate or sequence of development. Pediatric patients may be cognitively impaired, but they can demonstrate a wide range of intellectual ability and functioning. Cognitive impairment may be manifested early in life by slow developmental progression, particularly in social skills. Some children with ASD are of at least average intelligence, and some are highly gifted. Some children with ASD are impaired in particular areas of development, while others are above normal.

Most children with autism do not present with physical signs. Unfortunately, this can create problems for the higher functioning child, who might be perceived as "odd" or socially aloof. These individuals are often bullied and ostracized as a result. A minority of those with autism have macrocephaly, or brain overgrowth. Approximately 9.1% of individuals with autism will have a larger than normal head circumference. An analysis of several studies found the lower the level of functioning, the greater likelihood the autistic individual had macrocephaly (Sacco, Gabriele, & Persico, 2015).

The clinical manifestations and therapies for ASD are outlined in the following feature.

Collaboration

A number of agencies and resources are available to support the child with ASD. Many communities have an interprofessional committee or team that meets regularly to

Clinical Manifestations and Therapies

Autism Spectrum Disorder

ETIOLOGY	CLINICAL MANIFESTATIONS	CLINICAL THERAPIES
Level I	▪ Difficulty initiating social interactions ▪ Difficulty maintaining social interactions ▪ Inflexible behaviors affect functioning at home and/or school ▪ Problems with organization	▪ Visual cues and reminders ▪ Speech/language therapy ▪ Occupational therapy (gross and fine motor skills, ADLs) ▪ Behavioral therapy (e.g., applied behavior analysis [ABA]) or reinforcements
Level II	▪ Significant deficits in communication skills in all areas ▪ Reduced or unusual responses to social overtures from others ▪ Unable to initiate social interaction ▪ Difficulty coping with transitions or change ▪ Repetitive behaviors appear obvious to others and interfere with functioning in multiple situations ▪ Difficulty switching activities	▪ Visual cues and reminders ▪ Sign language ▪ Speech/language therapy ▪ Occupational therapy (gross and fine motor skills; ADLs) ▪ Behavioral therapy (ABA) or reinforcements
Level III	▪ Severe communication deficits ▪ Minimal response to social overtures ▪ Inflexible or restricted behaviors that severely impact functioning ▪ Marked distress on switching activities	▪ Visual cues and reminders ▪ Sign language ▪ Speech/language therapy ▪ Occupational therapy (gross and fine motor skills, ADLs) ▪ Behavioral therapy (ABA) or reinforcements

review services available in their area for children with special needs, including ASD. By law, public schools are charged with the responsibility of facilitating and providing services for children with ASD and other disabilities. For preschool-age children, services may be provided directly by the school system or in collaboration with a preschool developmental day center. Some private schools do accept and provide accommodations for children with autism, and some private schools are created exclusively for students with learning challenges. However, private schools are not required by law to provide accommodations for children with disabilities. Nurses frequently serve on interprofessional teams to ensure that medical and mental health needs of children with ASD are included in supportive plans. Team members may include parents, nurses, physicians, teachers, mental health professionals, occupational therapists, and physical therapists.

The overall prognosis for children with ASD to become functioning members of society is guarded. The extent to which adequate adjustment is achieved varies greatly. Successful adjustment is more likely for children with higher IQs, adequate speech, and access to specialized programs.

Diagnostic Tests

There is no laboratory test or imaging that can diagnose autism. Diagnosis is based on the presence of specific criteria, as described in the DSM-5. An early childhood intervention specialist, who may be a pediatrician or other licensed healthcare provider, may conduct an initial screening as well

as testing to rule out a medical cause of the child's behavior. Tests may include neuroimaging (CT scan or MRI), lead screening, DNA analysis, and electroencephalography.

Pharmacologic Therapy

It is important for the nurse to teach families and patients that there is no pill or medication that will "cure" autism. The FDA (2015) warns consumers of false advertising and cures for autism, including chelation therapy and mineral solutions. These "treatments" have been known to cause adverse effects, including nausea, vomiting, and electrolyte imbalances. One example is the Miracle Mineral Solution, which when mixed according to the directions, creates bleach that is then ingested by the unsuspecting consumer (FDA, 2015).

For some patients, medications are used to manage behaviors and associated symptoms. Medications used in the care of patients with ASD may include stimulants, selective serotonin reuptake inhibitors (SSRIs), and mood stabilizers. For example, fluoxetine, an SSRI, has been shown to help with repetitive behaviors; while risperidone, a second-generation antipsychotic, is used for ASD irritability (LeClerc & Easley, 2015).

SAFETY ALERT Children with autism might not respond to medications as other children do. Some negative behaviors might increase with medications. Other medications may cause severe depression and suicidal thoughts. Children with autism should be monitored closely when starting new medications.

Focus on Diversity and Culture
Disparities in Early Diagnosis

Current data show that in the United States, ASD is most common in non-Hispanic White children, followed by African American, Asian/Pacific Islander, Hispanic, and Native Indian/Native Alaskan (Christensen et al., 2016). However, autism may be more prevalent than is suspected in communities of color but underreported because of educational and cultural barriers. For example, Latina mothers are less likely to report their children not reaching milestones when seeking medical care for their children, making early detection of ASD or other developmental disorders difficult (Ratto, Reznick, & Turner-Brown, 2015). Diagnosis of children of color usually occurs at some point during the school-age years. As a consequence of the delayed diagnosis, these children tend to have more severe ASD. Several factors may be in play as to why parents of children with ASD do not seek diagnosis and treatment. Those factors include language barriers, lack of education regarding milestones and child behavior, social stigma of having a child with a disability, and challenges with healthcare, insurance, and/or financial resources (Christensen et al., 2016). As a result, more communities are creating centers focused on education, resources, and support for families of color with children with autism (Hewitt et al., 2013). Healthcare providers also play a part in late diagnosis of ASD in children of color. Again, language barriers play a key part. In addition, lack of cultural understanding on behalf of the provider may create a barrier and cause late diagnosis or misdiagnosis. Providers who educate themselves on cultural norms and barriers to care are more likely to be more effective in noting signs of autism. Screenings done with tools written in the language of the patient are less likely to lose meaning in translation. Educational material regarding developmental milestones and autism awareness at clinics and other community places should be printed in several languages. If possible, educational videos or multimedia education should also be available patients with low reading proficiency.

Nonpharmacologic Therapy

The infant brain is still developing and creating pathways and neurons. Research has shown a strong link between brain development and autism. As a result, early intervention to help facilitate healthy brain development is likely to decrease the severity of symptoms and behaviors in the young child with ASD. In addition, those children who receive intense therapies in early childhood have better long-term outcomes and maintain higher functionality (Estes et al., 2015).

Children are taught how to focus and apply learning. Treatment focuses on behavior management to reward appropriate behaviors, foster positive or adaptive coping skills, and facilitate effective communication. The goals of treatment are to reduce rigidity or stereotypy (repetitive, obsessive, machinelike movements) and other maladaptive behaviors.

Applied behavior analysis (ABA) is a commonly used treatment approach for autism. Based on the principles of B. F. Skinner's model that behaviors are reinforced with either positive or negative consequences, children with autism are taught behaviors with positive reinforcement or rewards. For example, a toddler who does not make eye contact may be taught to do so by being rewarded with a piece of cereal, or a 5-year-old might get a sticker on his shirt every time he completes a sentence.

ABA is very structured, intense, and lengthy, typically 6 to 8 hours a day for a minimum of 25 hours a week with a certified therapist. Parents are the continuation of the therapy when the therapist is not in the home. There are several types of ABA therapy, including Discrete Trial Training (DTT), Early Intensive Behavioral Intervention (EIBI), Pivotal Response Training (PRT), and Verbal Behavior Intervention (VBI) (CDC, 2015d).

Complementary Health Approaches

When faced with the diagnosis of autism in a child, many parents seek different therapies and treatments. It is estimated that approximately 30% of children with ASD have been treated with complementary and alternative therapies (Perrin et al., 2012), despite the fact that research continues to show that most complementary and alternative therapies are not effective in the treatment of autism (Brondino et al., 2015; CDC, 2015d; NCCIH, 2016c).

A popular option with parents of children with ASD is implementation of a gluten-free, casein-free (GFCF) diet. This has gained sufficient popularity that there are entire websites and programs devoted to this diet. Essentially, the GFCF diet eliminates the proteins gluten and casein from the patient's diet. Parents have reported improvement in behaviors in some children who follow this diet, and case studies have been documented (Elder et al., 2015). However, evidence to support this diet is lacking (Elder et al., 2015; CDC, 2015d). Nurses working with patients considering the GFCF diet should encourage them to consult with a nutritionist or registered dietitian who can help them make sure that they plan GFCF meals that will meet their child's nutritional needs.

Nurses can help parents evaluate studies on complementary care and encourage parents to initiate only one treatment at a time; the effectiveness of any one treatment cannot be measured properly if it is initiated in conjunction with other therapies. At each healthcare interaction, the nurse working with a patient with ASD should ask about therapies being used and discuss safeguards to avoid any undesired side effects.

Lifespan Considerations

Childhood ASD persists into adulthood. Children who receive timely intervention and whose parents and treatment teams collaborate to find the best treatment for them as individuals have the greatest chance of becoming successfully functioning adults. Even high-functioning adults with ASD continue to struggle with communication skills, especially understanding nonverbal communication and socialization. Adults with ASD are most successful when they seek employment opportunities and activities that play to their strengths.

Many communities provide job training and supervised work programs for adults with ASD. Many adults with less severe ASD are active community members, becoming fully employed and living independently. Others need more support and may choose to continue to live with their parents or to reside in a group living environment that provides additional support. A number of government programs exist to assist these individuals with financial support. Information on these programs is available from the Social Security Administration as well as local state and country social services. In addition, such nonprofit organizations as Easter Seals and Goodwill offer employment opportunities and resources. Finally, several internet resources, such as AutismSpeaks.org, are available for adults with autism to navigate different systems.

Few clinics exist that specifically treat adults with ASD, making it challenging for these adults to get the best level of care. Many adults with ASD who cannot function independently or whose families can no longer provide care for them end up being financially subsidized by the state. With the steady rise in the number of children diagnosed with this disorder comes a resulting increase in the number of adults with the disorder. The financial impact on state governments is significant and is likely to increase steadily for many years. This is all the more reason why children with ASD need to be identified early, so that they may have access to treatments and therapies that give them the best chance to become fully functioning adults.

As the person with autism matures, the likelihood of developing a mental health condition, such as anxiety or depression, also increases. The person with autism may not recognize the signs of mental illness; likewise, practitioners might not recognize signs of mental illness in the adult autistic patient (Moss et al., 2015). In turn, the individual with ASD may show decrease of functioning that is not related to autism, but rather, to undiagnosed mental illness. This adds to the burden of care.

Autism is a lifelong condition, but the greater concentration of research, resources, funding, and support is focused on children and young adults. Research on adults with ASD remains lacking, especially for the geriatric population. Diagnosis in the elderly population is rarely done. However, studies are showing that undiagnosed ASD may be hampering the quality of life in the elderly. Geurts, Stek, and Comijs (2016) found that in older adults, approximately 31% of patients with depression also show signs of autism. This study also concluded that like their younger counterparts, older adults with autism often develop mental illness.

NURSING PROCESS

Throughout application of the nursing process, the patient's parents or caregivers will be integral team members. Because much of the assessment data are collected by way of interview, the nurse should prioritize the establishment of effective, open communication patterns with the patient's primary caregivers and family members.

Assessment

The nurse may encounter the child with ASD when parents seek care for a suspected hearing impairment, speech difficulty, or developmental delay. Early and frequent developmental screening of all children can help in referral for thorough assessment and identification of cases.

- **Observation and patient/family interview.** Parents may report abnormal interaction such as lack of eye contact, disinterest in cuddling, minimal facial responsiveness, and failure to talk. Be alert to observations by the parents that the baby or young child does not look at them or provide other developmental or behavioral cues. Initial assessment focuses on language development, response

to others, and hearing acuity. Become familiar with the following "red flags" of the American Academy of Neurology and Child Neurology Society that require immediate evaluation (Pickles et al., 2009):

- No babbling or communication gestures by 12 months
- No single word by 16 months
- No spontaneous two words by 24 months
- Loss of language or social skills previously achieved.

Note both maternal and parental ages of the child at birth. Consider genetic history of autism or like behaviors in the patient's families. Ask about birth history, including possible neonatal exposure to medications such as antiepileptics, as well as exposure to toxins or alcohol. Carefully evaluate the child for history of developmental milestones and refer for abnormalities. Perform developmental screening that considers several areas of development, including motor activity, social skills, and language, or refer the family to a professional or community resource that provides such screenings. Recall that the child may have normal performance in one area such as motor skills, but delayed development in another area such as language skills. Likewise, language may be normal for age, but social interactions delayed. Include questions about adaptive skills such as toilet training and feeding patterns. Inquire about school performance, because some areas may be normal while others are delayed. Observe the child in play situations and evaluate the use of creative and exploratory play versus more repetitive patterns.

When a child with a diagnosis of ASD is hospitalized for a concurrent problem, obtain a history from the parents regarding the child's routines, rituals, and likes and dislikes, as well as ways to promote interaction and cooperation. Children with ASD may carry a special toy or object that they play with during times of stress. Ask parents about these objects and their use. Ask about the child's behaviors and observe them on admission. Obtain a history of acute and chronic illnesses and injuries. Ask about eating patterns and food restrictions. Inquire about complementary health approaches in a nonjudgmental and supportive manner.

For the adult patient with ASD, the nurse should remember that behaviors of other mental health conditions are similar and possibly overlap autism behaviors. These conditions include schizophrenia, ADHD, and obsessive-compulsive disorder (OCD) (NIMH, 2016b). Similar behaviors regarding ability to socialize, eye contact, sensory disorders, and repetitive behaviors will be present in the adult with ASD. Most adults who are diagnosed later in life will be considered higher functioning and very well may have careers and families. Many adults initiate the diagnosis with their provider. Some express relief after their diagnosis, as their behaviors have a etiology. Yet others may express sadness because there is no "cure" for ASD.

Just as with the evaluation of a child who potentially has autism, the nurse will question the adult patient regarding family history, neonatal exposures, birth history, and developmental history. Family members and others close to the patient are helpful in filling in any gaps the patient is unable to answer.

■ *Physical examination.* The physical exam for autism often will reveal no abnormalities because of the neurodevelopmental nature of this disorder. However, the nurse may face challenges in the physical assessment because of behavioral issues. Nurses will have to adapt the physical exam according to the patient's temperament, cognitive level, sensory perceptions, and developmental stage.

Patients with ASD who have sensory deficits or behaviors often do not like being touched. The patient might complain that a light touch hurts, yet giggle with immunizations. If asked to change into a gown, the patient may not like the material of the gown against the skin, becoming irritable or focused on the gown rather than the exam.

The patient may not sit still for the exam. The patient might also display flapping, rocking, or head-banging as a way to self-soothe during the exam. If the patient becomes irritable, the patient might have what is perceived as a temper tantrum, otherwise known as an "autistic meltdown" in some circles. The nurse will have to ensure the patient's safety during this time.

Many individuals with ASD do not like quick transitions. Just as with neurotypical children, the nurse should tell the patient before doing a certain assessment. For example, before assessing a patient's eyes with a penlight, the nurse should tell the patient first before shining a bright beam.

If the patient is nonverbal, the nurse should not assume the patient does not understand language. The nurse should continue to talk and explain things during the assessment. The nurse should also consider alternative communication tools in order to ask the patient questions. Some patients use such means as pictures, sign language, and technology (e.g., smartphone apps that convert pictures into spoken words) to communicate.

Encourage the patient or parents to bring something that brings comfort, such as a blanket or favorite object. Perform the exam in small, short steps, and consider giving the patient a reward, with each step (as typically done in ABA treatments). The nurse should never restrain a patient, particularly an older child or adult, to complete an exam. Examination of the adult patient will be very similar, but is likely to be less challenging than examining a child. However, many adults with ASD do have sensory perception issues, and others have difficulty with communication. The communication challenges maybe more along the lines of the social awkwardness of the exam. The patient might pull away from certain aspects of the physical exam. The nurse should advise the patient of each step of the exam, paying careful attention to transitions and actions.

Diagnosis

Nursing diagnoses must be tailored to fit the individual needs of the patient. Nursing diagnoses that may be appropriate for inclusion in the plan of care for the patient as well as the family include:

■ *Injury, Risk for*
■ *Development, Delayed*
■ *Knowledge Deficit*
■ *Verbal Communication, Impaired*

■ *Social Interaction, Impaired*
■ *Caregiver Role Strain*
■ *Family Coping, Compromised.*

(NANDA-I © 2014)

Planning

Nursing care of children with ASD focuses on preventing injury, stabilizing environmental stimuli, providing supportive care, enhancing communication, giving the parents anticipatory guidance, and providing emotional support. Appropriate outcomes for a child with ASD may include the following:

■ The child will remain free of injury.
■ The child will acquire communication strategies that enable communication with others.
■ The child will be able to perform self-care to maximum potential.
■ The child will demonstrate consistent developmental progress.
■ The child will participate in small group activities with family members or peers.
■ The child's symptoms will be managed successfully.

Nursing care of adults with a new diagnosis of ASD focuses on education and coping. Care of the adult with a current diagnosis of ASD focuses on assessing and promoting social interactions, continued education regarding diagnosis, and establishing and maintaining individual functions. Planning may include the following goals:

■ The patient will remain free from injury.
■ The patient will verbalize understanding of diagnosis.
■ The patient will demonstrate positive coping skills.
■ The patient will participate in social activities with peers, coworkers, and family members.
■ The patient will maintain independence to the full potential of the individual.

Implementation

Working with patients with ASD and their families requires patience, sensitivity, and understanding. Working with families, particularly with children and their parents, requires the nurse to remember that there is more than one patient involved in the treatment plan. While some parents may be aggressive about seeking information and resources, others may be too overwhelmed and exhausted from caring for their child to do this. For these parents, the nurse may be the most important, most accessible, and most caring resource available to them. Nurses must take the time to provide patient teaching and support and affirm parents' efforts to help their children.

Adults with ASD will want to have structure and a predictable course of action. Adults with ASD often are very punctual and time-conscious. Nurses should be aware that any delay in treatments may cause anxiety in the ASD adult. For example, if the nurse makes an appointment with the patient for 9:30 a.m., the nurse should strive to be on time. There is the possibility that some patients will become anxious at 9:32 a.m. Nurses will need to provide education for the adult patient, as well as any family members involved. Emotional support may be in order, particularly for the adult patient who will not benefit from ABA and other early interventions. Support services and groups also are not readily available for the adult patient. However, there are internet support groups through such websites as Autism Speaks and the National Autism Network. Case management services may help the adult with ASD navigate through the healthcare system.

Prevent Injury

Monitor children with ASD at all times, including bath time and bedtime. Close supervision ensures that the child does not obtain any harmful objects or engage in dangerous behaviors. For the child who engages in head banging or other harmful behaviors, bicycle helmets and hand mitts can be the least restrictive method for providing safety. They enable the child to participate in activities and engage in a social environment to the degree possible.

Provide Anticipatory Guidance

Many children with ASD will require lifelong supervision and support, especially if the disorder is accompanied by intellectual disability. Some children may grow up to lead independent lives, although they will have social limitations with impaired interpersonal relationships. Encourage parents to promote the child's development through behavior modification and specialized educational programs. The overall goal is to provide the child with the guidance, education, and support necessary for optimal functioning.

Address Environmental Issues

Patients with ASD interpret and respond to the environment differently than other individuals. Sounds that are not distressing to the average individual may be interpreted as loud, frightening, and overwhelming. They may respond to different sounds or environments by withdrawing, crying, or using ritualistic behaviors such as arm-flapping, which may or may not be self-injurious.

The patient needs to be oriented to new settings such as a hospital room and should be encouraged to bring familiar items from home. To avoid distressing the patient, minimize relocation of objects within the environment.

Provide Supportive Care

Developing a trusting relationship with the patient who has ASD is often difficult. Adjust communication techniques and teach to the patient's developmental level. Ask about the patient's usual home routines and maintain these routines as much as possible when the patient is out of the home.

Because self care abilities are often limited, the child or adult with ASD may need assistance to meet basic needs. When possible, schedule daily care and routine procedures at consistent times to maintain predictability. Identify rituals for naptime and bedtime and maintain them to promote rest and sleep. Integrate patterns that facilitate intake of nutritious foods at mealtimes.

For children, school programs and IEPs can help the child learn self-care skills. Parents are integral parts of the treatment team when the child's learning goals are established in early intervention or school programs. If the child is hospitalized, encourage parents to remain with the child and to participate in daily care planning.

All patients with ASD need emotional support. Children who are developing successfully may face new challenges with the onset of the emotional and hormonal changes of adolescence. As social circles develop in middle and high school, the adolescent with autism may become more painfully aware of being different from her peers. The nurse may see this when a parent brings in a child after a scuffle at school or for help with increasing self-destructive behaviors as the child struggles to deal with the many changes inherent in adolescence. The nurse can provide crucial information about the physical changes adolescents experience and help the parent modify the plan of care to include opportunities for building new skills the child needs to navigate this difficult time.

Enhance Communication

Because patients with autism have impaired communication skills, nursing care focuses on using and improving communication with the patient. When speaking, use short, direct sentences (Maher, 2012). If the patient responds well to visual cues, then pictures, computers, and other visual aids may form an important part of interaction. Some patients with limited verbal skills are able to learn and communicate through sign language, pictures, talking boxes, and smartphone apps.

Children with ASD benefit greatly from speech and language therapy. Encourage parents of these children to maintain close contact with speech therapists. Use of consistent communication techniques at home and at school provides further stability for the child and increases opportunities for successful communication.

Facilitate Community-based Care

Families need a great deal of support to cope with the challenges of caring for the child for adult family member with ASD. Many communities offer training programs for parents, in addition to support groups. Help parents identify resources for child care, such as special toddler programs and preschools. Provide resources for case management, respite care, and governmental services, including Social Security benefits to help with the added cost of ASD treatments.

Nurses working in these community training programs and support services can offer a variety of education for parents to cope with the stresses of having a child with ASD. Nurses can provide classes in stress-reduction techniques, stress management, self-care, and mind–body therapies.

The patient may need specialized transportation services or other social supports. The school-age child will need an IEP. The parent or primary caregiver often has difficulty obtaining respite care and may need assistance to find suitable resources. Siblings of children with autism may need help explaining the disorder to their friends or teachers. The nurse can be instrumental in assisting these siblings in understanding and explaining autism. Family support programs are available in some states to provide assistance to parents.

Local support groups for parents of autistic children are available in most areas. Families can also be referred local chapters of national autism programs. There are support groups for teens and adults with ASD as well. Many connect via social media networks and internet resources.

Social media is becoming a more popular way for those with ASD to socialize and plan get-togethers. While the research is in its early stages, those with ASD tend to be technologically savvy and use social media to find friends, which might be difficult in other social settings. Mazurek (2013) conducted a study to examine the use of social media networks by adults with ASD. Nearly 80% of those in the study used these networks to make social connections. Some of these connections led to face-to-face friendships. Social media may help the patient with ASD move past initial socialization awkwardness and help promote lasting friendships.

>> **Stay Current:** Patients of all ages with ASD and their families can find lots of support online and in their communities. Autism Speaks, https://www.autismspeaks.org; Autism Society of America, http://www.autism-society.org; and the National Autism Network, http://nationalautismnetwork.com/index.html are websites that are current on best practices for autism in several areas, including research, education, therapies, and other things related to autism.

Evaluation

At each healthcare interaction, the nurse discusses the child's progress with the parents, including any injuries that have occurred since the previous visit and the steps being taken to prevent recurrence. The nurse asks parents what type of environments the child is in during the day, paying particular attention to the frequency of transitions and changes in caregivers. For example, a child with ASD who attends school or an early intervention program at a preschool will do well having the same caregiver drop off the child in the morning and pick up the child at the end of the school day.

For children who are enrolled in early intervention programs or who have IEPs at school, the nurse should participate as part of the treatment team when possible. If this is not possible, the nurse should ask the parent how the child's treatment is progressing and continue to encourage open communication between the parents and the treatment team. For children who are taking medication to treat a comorbid disorder such as depression or ADHD, the nurse should, with parent permission, provide the necessary information to the treatment team so that the team is aware of potential side effects.

For adult patients with ASD, the nurse should inquire about coping strategies, workplace relationships, family relationships, anxieties, and social connections. Nurses may also ask about the usefulness of resources and support services. If the adult is taking medications, the nurse can evaluate for the desired effects and side effects of the medication.

REVIEW Autism Spectrum Disorder

RELATE Link the Concepts and Exemplars

Linking the exemplar of autism spectrum disorder with the concept of family:

1. How can the nurse support the family of a child with ASD?

2. How might other children in the family be impacted by a sibling with ASD?

Linking the exemplar of autism spectrum disorder with the concept of safety:

3. What interventions are important for the nurse to initiate to maintain the safety of a patient with autism?

4. What would be important at school?

READY Go to Volume 3: Clinical Nursing Skills

REFER Go to Pearson MyLab Nursing and eText

- Additional review materials

REFLECT Apply Your Knowledge

Chad, age 4, was recently diagnosed with autism spectrum disorder. Chad's mother keeps ruminating about her pregnancy, wondering what she did that "caused" Chad's illness. Chad recently became angry and reacted by banging his head against the wall. His parents told the nurse they do not believe that the doctor made the right diagnosis.

1. Based on the case study, what are the priorities of nursing care for Chad?

2. Based on the statement made by Chad's parents, what are his parents experiencing?

3. How might the nurse locate resources to help Chad's parents learn more about having a child with autism? What resources might the nurse find?

>> Exemplar 25.C Cerebral Palsy

Exemplar Learning Outcomes

25.C Analyze CP as it relates to development.

- Describe the pathophysiology of CP.
- Describe the etiology of CP.
- Compare the risk factors and prevention of CP.
- Identify the clinical manifestations of CP.
- Summarize diagnostic tests and therapies used by interprofessional teams in the collaborative care of an individual with CP.
- Differentiate care of patients with CP across the lifespan.
- Apply the nursing process in providing culturally competent care to an individual with CP.

Exemplar Key Term

Cerebral palsy (CP), *1835*

Overview

Cerebral palsy (CP) is a group of chronic conditions affecting body movement, coordination, and posture that results from a nonprogressive abnormality of the immature brain. CP often is the result of some type of insult to the developing brain of the fetus, neonate, or infant that occurs in the later stages of pregnancy, during birth, or within the first 2 years after birth. The impact of the disease can range from mild to profound mobility issues (**Figure 25–12 》**). CP may or may not include intellectual disability.

Cerebral palsy occurs in an estimated 1 per 323 births (Christensen et al., 2016). Four types of motor dysfunction are seen with CP—spastic, dyskinetic, ataxic, and mixed—and are related to the location of brain insult. Spastic CP, the most common type, affects approximately 80% of those diagnosed with CP (CDC, 2016g).

Pathophysiology and Etiology

Pathophysiology

Cerebral palsy involves abnormal development or damage to the immature brain that affects motor function and muscles (CDC, 2015e). There are two main categories: congenital and acquired. Congenital CP occurs during fetal development, birth, and the neonatal period. Acquired CP happens after the first 28 days of life. The specific insult leading to CP may not be identifiable if it occurs during the prenatal period. After

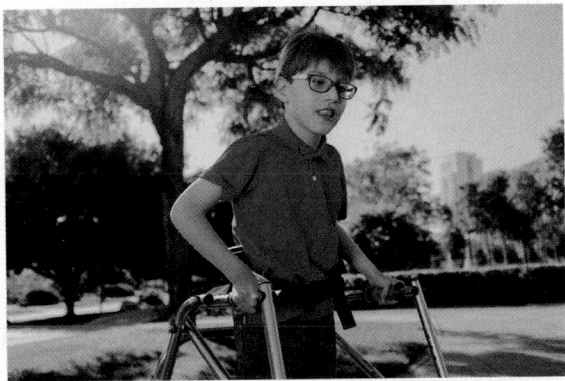

A

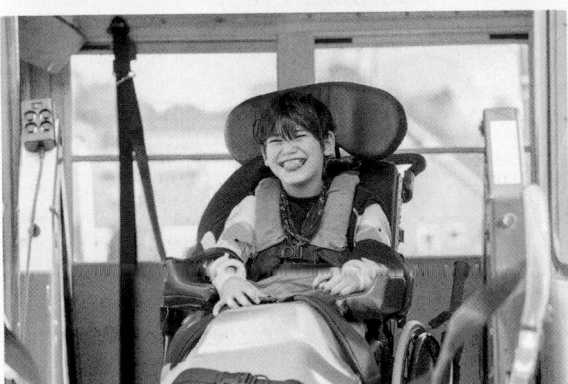

B

*Sources: **A,** Sweetmonster/iStock/Getty Images; **B,** Jaren Wicklund/iStock/Getty Images.*

Figure 25–12 》 Individuals with CP can have mild to profound mobility issues and may be able to walk unaided, need an assistive device **A,** or use a wheelchair **B.**

delivery, the cause of the damage (for example, encephalitis) is more likely to be identified. CP may result in decrease in muscle tone, muscle stretch reflexes, postural reactions, and primitive reflexes; it may also result in seizures, mental retardation, and/or hearing problems. The outcome depends on the area of the brain affected, the severity of the event, the duration of the insult, and the child's age at the time of the event.

Pathogenesis of CP is multifactorial and depends on the cause of the insult to the brain. Brain damage associated with cerebral palsy occurs in the motor areas of the brain, impairing the body's ability to control movement and adjust posture appropriately. CP is neither contagious nor inherited, and it is not progressive. It cannot be cured, but the associated symptoms can be managed.

CP often is identified when children fail to meet expected developmental milestones and diagnostic testing is ordered to pinpoint the reason for the delay. Symptoms and manifestations vary from person to person depending on the exact neurologic impact of the event.

Etiology

Approximately 85–90% of children with CP are diagnosed with congenital CP (CDC, 2015e). At one time, hypoxia was considered the primary culprit for congenital CP; however, research now indicates that it is only responsible for a small number of cases. Instead, pathogens, toxins, trauma, and genetic mutations that affect the development of the brain are now suspected causes of CP.

The pathology of the brain injury depends on the etiology. For instance, pathogens that directly attack the brain—such as *Streptococcus pneumoniae* (pneumococcus), which is responsible for the majority of meningitis in infants—cause cellular damage through the consumption of the brain's tissue and production of the by-product lactic acid. Trauma stretches and shears neural pathways and brain tissue. Neurotoxins, such as bilirubin, accumulate in the bloodstream and eventually injure the nerve cells in the brain.

The role of DNA in the development of CP is coming to greater light with the advancement of genetics. Genetic mutations have been found in individuals with CP in recent studies. In addition, males, who are considered vulnerable to genetic mutations because of the XY chromosome configuration, are more likely to have CP than females (MacLennan, Thompson, & Gecz, 2015).

Risk Factors

Risk factors for cerebral palsy include events and exposures that may cause damage to the developing brain. Risk factors do not necessarily mean, however, that the infant has or will develop cerebral palsy. For instance, children conceived via assisted reproductive technology (ART) have a greater incidence of cerebral palsy; however, many conceived via ART do not develop CP.

Risk factors associated with congenital CP occurring in utero include infections such as pelvic inflammatory disease (PID), rubella, chickenpox, CMV, and bacterial infections. Fevers in the mother prior to birth also may contribute to the development of CP. Cytokines, which are produced with fevers and certain infections, are thought to cause damage to neurons in the developing fetus's brain (CDC, 2015e). Blood type incompatibility between the fetus and mother may cause CP. If the mother is exposed to toxins, such as mercury, there is a greater chance of CP. Likewise, if the mother has such conditions as seizures, thyroid disease, or proteinuria, there is a slightly greater chance of CP (National Institute of Neurological Disorders and Stroke [NINDS], 2016).

Birth and the health of the neonate are significant factors that contribute to the risk of developing CP. Risk factors associated with delivery include breech delivery, tight and nuchal cords, shoulder dystocia, uterine rupture, placenta previa, and fetal stress and hypoxia (CDC, 2015e; NINDS, 2016; MacLennan et al., 2015).

Approximately 35% of CP cases occur in individuals with a history of preterm birth. Studies have found the earlier in gestational age the infant is born, the greater the likelihood the infant will have CP (MacLennan et al., 2015). Multiple fetuses are also at risk, partially due to the greater chance of preterm birth. Low birth weight, also associated with preterm birth and/or multiples, is also considered a risk factor. Neonates delivered with low Apgar scores have a greater risk of CP as well.

During the neonatal period, infants who have severe jaundice are at risk for developing CP due to hyperbilirubinemia. As mentioned previously, bilirubin is considered a neurotoxin and can damage the fragile neonatal brain on the cellular level. Because the neonatal immune system is immature, the infant is particularly susceptible to meningitis and encephalitis, two conditions also associated with CP.

Brain trauma is also a risk factor for CP. Neonates may experience trauma during birth from precipitous delivery, prolonged delivery, and other causes. After delivery, infants may experience trauma from shaken baby syndrome, being dropped, or improper placement in a car seat, as well as other means. The damage from these traumas puts the infant at risk for CP.

Prevention

The greatest risk for CP is preterm labor. Nurses should educate mothers-to-be on the prevention of preterm labor, including encouraging good prenatal care and visits with a provider. Nurses should also educate the pregnant patient on the signs and symptoms of preterm labor. Mothers with multiples in particular should have a close relationship with their providers to monitor the pregnancy. If the mother is placed on bedrest, the nurse should encourage the mother to comply with treatment in order to deliver a healthy baby.

Because maternal infection is associated with the development of CP, infection prevention, including maintaining good hand hygiene, is a primary goal. Keeping current with vaccinations is also a means by which a pregnant patient can reduce the risk for having a baby born with CP. After birth, parents should avoid exposure of their infant to the potential of infection, including using good hand hygiene when caring for the infant. Vaccinations are essential in preventing certain infections that may cause CP, including the *Haemophilus influenza* vaccination that helps prevent the most common form of bacterial meningitis.

Injury prevention, including properly securing infants during motor vehicle travel and taking measures to prevent falls, serves to protect the child from brain trauma. Nurses should also educate parents on stress reduction and prevention of shaken baby syndrome.

>> Stay Current: Shaken baby syndrome, also referred to as abusive head trauma or shaken infant syndrome, occurs when a parent or caregiver severely shakes a baby out of frustration. For more information, go to the National Center on Shaken Baby Syndrome, www. dontshake.org.

Clinical Manifestations

Cerebral palsy is characterized by abnormal muscle tone and lack of coordination, with spasticity found in the majority of cases. Children have a variety of symptoms depending on their age. See **Table 25–16 >>** for symptoms by type of central nervous system injury. Symptoms vary depending on the area of the brain involved and the degree of insult.

Children with CP usually are delayed in meeting developmental milestones. For example, at 6 months of age, they may have persistent back arching, show little spontaneous movement, and be unable to sit up. They frequently have other problems, including visual defects such as strabismus (abnormal alignment of the eyes or "crossed eyes"), nystagmus (involuntary rapid eye movement), or refractory errors; hearing loss; language delay; speech impediment; or seizures. Feeding may be difficult because of oral motor involvement. Intellectual impairment is seen in 30–50% of persons with CP. Intellectual challenges are more commonly seen in those with spastic quadriplegia; those with CP and a seizure disorder are most likely to have an intellectual disability.

Collaboration

Care of the patient with CP requires an interprofessional team of nurses, physical therapists, occupational therapists, physicians, speech therapists, dietitians, and social workers or case managers. Cerebral palsy is a lifelong condition that requires special consideration, particularly in the growing child who quickly outgrows assistive devices and must meet changing developmental needs.

TABLE 25–16 Clinical Characteristics of Cerebral Palsy

Clinical Characteristics	Definitions
Hypotonia	Floppiness, increased range of motion of joints, diminished reflex response
Hypertonia, rigidity, spasticity	Tense, tight muscles
	Uncoordinated, awkward, stiff movements; scissoring or crossing of the legs; exaggerated reflex reactions
Athetosis	Constant involuntary writhing motions that are more severe distally
Ataxia	Poor muscle control during voluntary movement, poor balance
Hemiplegia	Involvement of one side of the body, with the upper extremities being more dysfunctional than the lower extremities
Diplegia	Involvement of all extremities, but the lower extremities are more affected than the upper, usually spastic
Quadriplegia	Involvement of all extremities with the arms in flexion and legs in extension

Clinical Manifestations and Therapies
Cerebral Palsy

ETIOLOGY	CLINICAL MANIFESTATIONS	CLINICAL THERAPIES
Spastic	■ Persistent hypertonia, rigidity	■ Physical therapy ■ Muscle relaxants ■ Braces, splints, and orthotics
Cerebral cortex or pyramidal tract injury	■ Exaggerated deep tendon reflexes	■ In addition to therapies used for spastic CP, surgery may be required to loosen contractures or to repair curvature of the spine.
Most common form of CP, comprising 80% of cases (CDC, 2015e)	■ Persistent primitive reflexes ■ Leads to contractures and abnormal curvature of the spine	
Dyskinetic	■ Impairment of voluntary muscle control accompanied by appearance of involuntary movements (e.g., tics, chorea)	
Extrapyramidal, basal ganglia injury	■ Bizarre twisting movements ■ Tremors, difficulty with fine and purposeful motor movements ■ Exaggerated posturing ■ Rigid muscle tone when awake and normal or decreased muscle tone when asleep ■ Inconsistent muscle tone that may change hour to hour or day to day	
Ataxic cerebellar (extrapyramidal) injury	■ Abnormalities of voluntary movement involving balance and position of the trunk and limbs ■ Difficulty controlling hand and arm movements when reaching ■ Increased or decreased muscle tone ■ Hypotonia in infancy ■ Muscle instability and wide-based, unsteady gait	■ Canes, crutches, walkers, and other orthotics may be needed to promote mobility.
Mixed injuries to multiple areas	■ No dominant motor pattern ■ Unique compensatory movements and posture to maintain control over specific neuromotor deficits ■ Combination of characteristics from other types	

>> **Stay Current:** For more information on CP, visit the National Institutes of Health at www.nlm.nih.gov/medlineplus/cerebralpalsy.html.

Diagnostic Tests

Diagnosis is usually based on clinical findings. CP is difficult to diagnose in the early months of life, because it must be distinguished from other neurologic conditions and signs and may be subtle. Cerebral palsy is usually suspected between age 18 months to 2 years, and later confirmed around the age of 5 years (McIntyre, 2015; NINDS, 2016). However, earlier diagnosis is recommended, particularly in those children with high risk factors.

Suspicious findings include an infant who is small for his age or has a history of prematurity; low birth weight; low Apgar score (0–3 at 5 minutes); or the occurrence of an inflammatory, traumatic, or anoxic event (Ahlin et al., 2013). However, the majority of children who develop CP have normal Apgar scores at birth. Ultrasonography can be used to detect fetal and neonatal abnormalities of the brain, such as intraventricular hemorrhage. Neuromotor tests are used to evaluate the presence of normal movement patterns and absence of primitive reflexes and abnormal tone. Once CP is suspected, CT scans, MRI, and positron emission tomography may be performed.

Surgery

Surgical interventions may be required to improve function by balancing muscle power and stabilizing uncontrollable joints. The Achilles tendon may be lengthened to increase range of motion in the ankle, which allows the heel to touch the floor and thus improves ambulation. The hamstrings may be released to correct knee flexion contractures. Other procedures may be performed to improve hip adduction or correct the foot's natural position.

Selective dorsal rhizotomy (SDR) is a surgical procedure that disconnects afferent nerves in order to reduce spasticity. This is most commonly done in the spastic diplegia subtype of CP. Although this surgery helps reduce spastic muscles and has been shown to increase functionality, it can have troubling after-effects, including muscle weakness (Josenby et al., 2015).

Pharmacologic Therapy

Medications are given to control seizures, to control spasms (skeletal muscle relaxants, baclofen, and benzodiazepines), and to minimize gastrointestinal side effects (cimetidine or ranitidine). Baclofen is administered by intrathecal pump to decrease muscle tone and vasospasms when oral administration is ineffective or causes side effects (NINDS, 2016).

Botulinum toxin (BT-A) injections have been used in to decrease spasticity and are considered standard practice. BT-A helps relax the contracted muscle. Used in conjunction with a stretching program, those who undergo this treatment report good results. Several studies have also shown the effectiveness of this therapy, including the benefits of multiple injections (NINDS, 2016; Kahraman et al., 2016).

Nonpharmacologic Therapy

Clinical therapy focuses on helping the child develop to a maximum level of independence. Early intervention services are key and may include a combination of physical, occupational, and speech therapy, as well as special education to improve motor function and ability. Braces and splints, serial casting, and positioning devices (prone wedges, standers, and side-liers) are used to promote range of motion, skeletal alignment, stability, and control of involuntary movements. They are also used to prevent contractures. Physical therapy and occupational therapy promote optimal independent functioning. Interventions vary depending on the child's needs.

Lifespan Considerations

Many children with CP grow up to be independent, functioning adults with careers, families, and social support systems (**Figure 25–13 》**). Having CP does take a toll on the adult's body. Many adults with CP have chronic pain due to the contractions of the muscles, arthritis due to the wear and tear on the joints, and persistent fatigue due to the extended energy needed to work against the contracted muscles.

Because CP puts the body in a continual stress state, many adults experience premature aging. The majority of those with CP will have signs of premature aging, including atherosclerosis, osteoarthritis, and hypertension, by their early 40s (NINDS, 2016). As individuals with CP age, they are more prone to both urinary and bowel incontinence, which can hamper their quality of life. With all these factors affecting the patient with CP, depression is not uncommon. Comorbidities such as seizures and respiratory disorders often shorten the life of the person with CP.

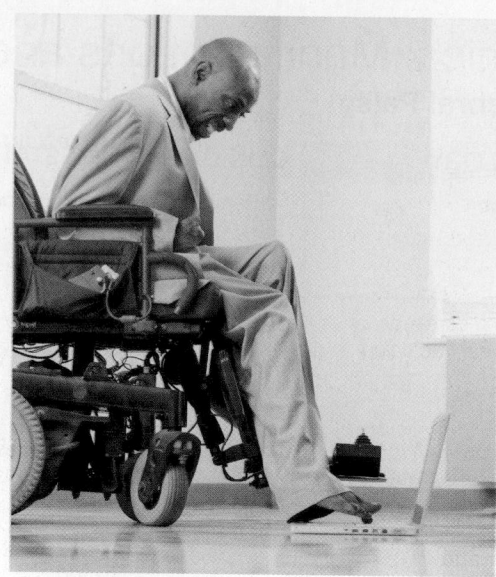

Source: Huntstock/Getty Images.

Figure 25–13 》 This man with CP uses a wheelchair and works on his laptop using his foot.

NURSING PROCESS

Nursing care focuses on early intervention, prevention of complications, and support of children and families to help them cope with the diagnosis of CP.

Assessment

Be alert for children whose histories indicate an increased risk for CP. It is not uncommon for children who are delayed in meeting developmental milestones or have neuromuscular abnormalities at 1 year of age to show gradual improvement in function. Studies have shown that assessment of general movements has a high predictive validity of CP among infants less than a year old (McIntyre, 2015).

Assess all children at each healthcare visit for developmental delays. Note any orthopedic, visual, auditory, or intellectual deficits. Assess for newborn reflexes, which may persist beyond the normal age in a child with CP. Identify infants who appear to have abnormal muscle tone or abnormal posture (child has an arched back, child becomes stiff when moving against gravity, child's neck or extremities have increased or decreased resistance to passive movement). A child with asymmetric or abnormal crawling using two or three extremities indicates a motor problem. Hand dominance before the preschool years is another sign of a motor problem. Record dietary intake as well as height and weight percentiles for children suspected to have or to be diagnosed with the condition.

Evaluate all infants who show symptoms of developmental delays, feeding difficulties caused by poor sucking, or abnormalities of muscle tone. Two simple screening assessments are helpful:

- Place a clean diaper on the 6- to 12-month-old infant's face. The infant without special needs will use two hands to remove it, but the infant with CP will use one hand or will not remove the cloth at all.

- Turn the infant's head to one side. A persistent asymmetric tonic neck reflex (beyond 6 months of age) indicates a pathologic condition. Suspect CP in any infant who has persistent primitive reflexes.

Diagnosis

Nursing diagnoses appropriate for inclusion in the care of the child with CP vary depending on the type of CP, the particular child's symptoms and age, and the family situation. Examples of nursing diagnoses relevant to caring for the patient with CP may include the following:

- *Injury, Risk for*
- *Mobility, Impaired*
- *Constipation, Risk for*
- *Tissue Integrity, Impaired*
- *Verbal Communication, Impaired*
- *Pain, Chronic*
- *Development, Delayed*
- *Caregiver Role Strain.*

(NANDA-I © 2014)

Planning

Because the condition can range from mild to severe and may involve numerous manifestations, care planning must be highly individualized on the basis of the specific needs of each individual. It may include the following goals:

- The patient will remain free from injury.
- The patient will demonstrate appropriate growth and development.
- The patient will maintain an appropriate diet to meet nutritional needs.
- The patient and family will monitor bony prominences to avoid altered skin integrity.

Implementation

Interventions need to be adapted to the particular child and family. Nursing care focuses on providing adequate nutrition, maintaining skin integrity, promoting physical mobility, promoting safety, promoting growth and development, teaching parents how to care for the child, and providing emotional support.

Prevent Injury

Patients with CP have varying degrees of mobility. The nurse should ensure that the patient receives the degree of assistance required for safe ambulation and that orthotic and assistive devices are properly used. Maintaining a safe environment includes eliminating all potential obstacles from walkways and providing adequate lighting. Assess caregivers and family members for awareness of safety precautions and provide teaching as needed.

Safety belts should be used for children in strollers and wheelchairs. An adaptive car safety seat may be needed to transport the child safely. A child with chronic seizures should wear a helmet to protect against further injury.

Promote Community-based Services

Children with CP need continuous support in the community. A case manager, such as the parent or a nurse, is often needed to coordinate care. Parents may need financial assistance to provide for the child's needs and to obtain appliances such as braces, wheelchairs, or adaptive utensils. As they grow, children need new adaptive devices, ongoing developmental assessment and care planning, and sometimes surgery. Although the brain lesion does not change, it manifests differently as the child grows. For example, once the child begins to walk, the extensor tone may cause tightening of the Achilles cord. Braces may decrease deformities, but surgery may be needed eventually. The nurse or healthcare provider is often the one to make referrals to early intervention programs to assist parents in meeting their child's needs. In addition, the nurse makes referrals, as appropriate, to support groups and organizations such as the United Cerebral Palsy Association and Shriners Hospitals.

An individualized transition plan developed during adolescence assists the family and adolescent with CP to develop plans for adult living. Vocational training options can be explored. The young adult (18–21 years) may be able to move into a group home or live independently if desired.

Provide Adequate Nutrition

Children with CP require high-calorie diets or supplements to the diet because of energy expenditure needed for movement and muscle contraction. Problems with swallowing, sucking, chewing, and movements in the mouth/jaw also cause nutritional challenges. Give the child soft foods in small amounts. Utensils with large, padded handles may be easier for the child to use. Oral hygiene can sometimes be an issue. Dental caries and gum disease are common in patients with CP because of difficulties with oral hygiene. This can also add to nutritional deficits if pain occurs with eating.

Maintain Skin Integrity

Take special care to protect the bony prominences from skin breakdown. Monitor the skin under splints and braces for redness. If the skin is red, the braces or splints should be removed and not replaced until the redness is gone.

Proper body alignment should be maintained at all times. Support the child with pillows, towels, and bolsters whether the child is in bed or in a chair. Support the head and body of a floppy infant. A child with spasticity may have scissored, extended legs, and a child with athetoid movements may be difficult to carry and transport.

Promote Physical Mobility

Range-of-motion exercises are essential to maintain joint flexibility and to prevent contractures. Consult with the child's physical therapist and help with recommended exercises. Teach parents to position the child to foster flexion rather than extension so that the child can more easily interact with the environment (for example, by bringing objects closer to the face). Consider the use of therapeutic massage and ROM exercise to help strengthen muscles and promote flexibility. A study showed that children who received scheduled therapeutic message and ROM exercises had less spasticity, stronger muscle strength, greater ROM, and higher function of ADLs (Yu et al., 2016).

As the child grows, adaptive and assistive technology may be needed to promote mobility and communication. Assistive technology is any item, equipment, or product customized for use to promote the functional capabilities and independence of an individual with disabilities. Examples include computers, adaptive utensils, and customized wheelchairs. Refer parents to the appropriate resources for help obtaining adaptive devices. Encourage parents to bring in the child's adaptive appliances (braces, positioning devices) for use during hospitalization.

Promote Growth and Development

Remember that many children with CP have physical disabilities but not necessarily intellectual disabilities. Use terminology appropriate for the child's developmental level. Help the child develop a positive self-image to ensure emotional health and social growth. Adaptive devices may be available to help the child with CP to communicate more independently. Children with a hearing impairment may need a referral to learn American Sign Language or other communication methods. Provide audio and visual activities for the child who is quadriplegic.

Provide Parent Education

Teach parents about the disorder and arrange sessions to teach them about all of the child's special needs. Teach administration, desired effects, and side effects of medications prescribed for seizures. Make sure parents are aware of the need for dental care for children, especially those taking anticonvulsants and other medications that can impact oral health.

Parents also may need suggestions for amending parenting strategies to promote the child's autonomy and abilities.

Provide Emotional Support

Parents require emotional support to help them cope with the diagnosis. Listen to the parents' concerns and encourage them to express their feelings and ask questions. Explain what they can expect from future treatment. Refer parents to individual and family counseling if appropriate. Work with other healthcare professionals to help families adjust to this chronic disease.

Evaluation

Patients are evaluated based on their ability to meet goals identified in the plan of care, which may include the following:

- Patient's growth is appropriate for age.
- Patient meets developmental milestones appropriate for age.
- Patient's nutritional status is adequate for age and energy needs.

Nursing Care Plan
A Patient with Cerebral Palsy

Justine McBride is a 2-year-old girl. Her mother was 41 when she delivered Justine, and Justine's father was 45. Justine is the seventh child in the family. Her mother works as a chemist in a local laboratory, and her father is an accountant for a large firm.

ASSESSMENT	DIAGNOSES	PLANNING
Justine's mother became concerned that Justine was not walking when she turned 14 months old; all of her other children were walking by 12 months of age. Diagnostic tests were performed, and Justine was diagnosed with spastic CP. Examination of Justine demonstrates scissoring of the legs when prone, stiff movements of arms and legs, hyperreflexia, and muscular rigidity.	■ *Mobility: Physical, Impaired* related to decreased muscle strength and control ■ *Imbalanced Nutrition: Less Than Body Requirements* related to difficulty in chewing and swallowing and high metabolic needs ■ *Health Management, Family, Ineffective,* related to excessive demands made on family with child's complex care needs (NANDA-I © 2014)	Goals for Justine's care include the following: ■ Justine will reach maximum physical mobility and all developmental milestones. ■ Justine will receive adequate visual sensory/perceptual input to maximize developmental outcome. ■ Justine will exhibit normal growth patterns for height, weight, and other physical parameters. ■ Justine's family will successfully support all of its members. ■ Justine will participate in activities to maximize development.

IMPLEMENTATION

Recreation Therapy: *Purposeful use of recreation to promote relaxation and enhancement of social skills.*

- Refer the family to an early intervention program. Encourage contact with other children through play groups or early intervention programs.
- Investigate recreational programs for children with disabilities and share information with the parents.

Family Mobilization: *Utilization of family strengths to influence Justine's health in a positive direction.*

- Allow chances for parents to verbalize the impact of CP on the family. Refer them to other parents and support groups.
- Explore community services for rehabilitation, respite care, child care, and other needs and refer family as appropriate.

Nursing Care Plan *(continued)*

- During home and office visits, review Justine's achievements and praise the family for care provided.
- Teach the family skills needed to manage Justine's care (e.g., medication administration, muscle stretching, physical rehabilitation, seizure management).
- Teach case management techniques.
- Assess needs of siblings; involve them in Justine's care as appropriate. Review with parents the needs of all children in the family.

Nutrition Management: *Assistance with or provision of a balanced dietary intake of foods and fluids.*

- Monitor height and weight and plot on a growth grid. Perform hydration status assessment.
- Teach the family techniques to promote caloric and nutrient intake.
- Position Justine upright for feedings.
- Place foods far back in the mouth to overcome tongue thrust.
- Use soft and blended foods.
- Allow extra time for chewing and swallowing.

- Obtain adaptive handles for utensils and encourage self-feeding skills.
- Apply manual jaw control technique if it helps the child to control jaw movement.
- Perform frequent respiratory assessment. Teach the family to avoid aspiration pneumonia.

Exercise Therapy, Joint Mobility: *Use of active and passive body movement to maintain or restore joint flexibility.*

- Perform development assessment and record age of achievement of milestones (e.g., reaching for objects, sitting).
- Plan activities to use gross and fine motor skills (e.g., holding a crayon or eating utensils, reaching for toys and rolling over).
- Allow time for the child to complete activities.
- Perform range-of-motion exercises every 4 hours for the child who is unable to move body parts. Position the child to promote tendon stretching (e.g., foot plantar flexion instead of dorsiflexion, legs extended instead of flexed at knees and hips).
- Arrange for and encourage parents to keep appointments with physical or rehabilitation therapist and other members of the collaborative team.

EVALUATION

The patient's progress in meeting the goals of care is based on the following expected outcomes:

- Justine reaches maximum physical mobility and all developmental milestones.
- Justine shows normal growth patterns for height, weight, and other physical parameters.

- Justine demonstrates appropriate growth and developmental progress. The family successfully supports all of its members.
- Justine engages in activities to maximize development.

CRITICAL THINKING

1. What support groups or professional organizations exist in your area that could help Justine's family cope with this diagnosis?
2. Why is involvement of the older siblings important?
3. How would you assess Justine's cognitive ability? Is cognition always impacted by CP?

REVIEW Cerebral Palsy

REVIEW Link the Concepts and Exemplars

Linking the exemplar of cerebral palsy with the concept of comfort:

1. How might you help to promote comfort in a child with CP who is required to wear braces and orthotics to bed at night?
2. If spasticity of muscles causes pain, what nonpharmacologic strategies might you recommend?

Linking the exemplar of cerebral palsy with the concept of cognition:

3. While caring for a child diagnosed with CP who also has mild cognitive impairment, how would you help the child become increasingly autonomous in performing range-of-motion exercises?
4. How might you encourage this child's parents to promote autonomy?

READY Go to Volume 3: Clinical Nursing Skills

REFER Go to Pearson MyLab Nursing and eText

- Additional review materials

REFLECT Apply Your Knowledge

Frangelica Gonzalez, 12 years old, was born with CP. She began working with physical therapists when she was less than 1 year old and has worn braces on her legs and used crutches to allow her greater mobility for as long as she can remember. Her mother and father have always told her she can overcome any challenge and do anything other children do if she tries hard enough. As a result of her parent's encouragement and support, Frangelica is a member of the school swim team, plays jazz piano, and has a large circle of friends. She has a younger brother who is 9 years old, an older brother who is 15 years old, and an identical twin sister who is healthy and does not have CP.

Lately her parents have noticed that Frangelica is moody, often seeming depressed, and her twin sister told their mother that Frangelica is "tired of being different." Frangelica has been waking in the morning offering various physical complaints as reasons why she can't go to school that day, ranging from a stomachache to a sore foot.

1. Why might Frangelica suddenly be feeling different and trying to find reasons not to go to school?

2. What strategies might you recommend to Frangelica's parents to help her cope with the developmental changes she is experiencing?

3. What strategies might you recommend to Frangelica to explore and cope with her feelings?

» Exemplar 25.D
Failure to Thrive

Exemplar Learning Outcomes

25.D Analyze failure to thrive as it relates to development.

- Describe the pathophysiology of failure to thrive.
- Describe the etiology of failure to thrive.
- Compare the risk factors and prevention of failure to thrive.
- Identify the clinical manifestations of failure to thrive.
- Summarize diagnostic tests and therapies used by interprofessional teams in the collaborative care of an individual with failure to thrive.

- Differentiate care of patients with failure to thrive across the lifespan.
- Apply the nursing process in providing culturally competent care to an individual with failure to thrive.

Exemplar Key Terms

Failure to thrive (FTT), *1842*
Geriatric failure to thrive (GFTT), *1842*

Overview

Failure to thrive (FTT) most commonly describes a syndrome in which an infant falls below the 5th percentile for weight and height on a standard growth chart or is falling in percentiles on a growth chart. The most common cause is malnutrition. Accurate statistics are not available because infants and children with FTT are typically undocumented (Sirotnak & Chiesa, 2016). This is because the majority of the parents of children with FTT do not or cannot seek proper and regular medical care. However, poverty rates are sometimes used, as many who live in poverty are food insecure.

Geriatric failure to thrive (GFTT) is a condition in which older patients experience a multidimensional decline in physical functioning that is characterized by weight loss of more than 5% of baseline body weight, decreased appetite, undernutrition and dehydration, depression, and cognitive and immune impairment. Similar to pediatric failure to thrive, GFTT can lead to death if left untreated.

Pathophysiology and Etiology

Pathophysiology

FTT and GFTT may stem from inadequate caloric intake, inadequate caloric absorption, or excessive caloric expenditure. In all cases, undernutrition results. Biological and psychosocial factors may also influence the development of FTT and GFTT.

GTT pathophysiology can be influenced by chronic diseases, including cancer, inflammatory diseases, chronic lung diseases, chronic renal insufficiency, and others. Medications, such as anticholinergic drugs, beta blockers, and SSRIs, can cause anorexia in the elderly patient.

Etiology

The cause of FTT can be organic, as in congenital AIDS, inborn errors of metabolism, neurologic disease, cleft palate, and esophageal reflux. However, most cases of FTT are nonorganic in origin. FTT resulting from nonorganic causes is called *feeding disorder of infancy or early childhood*.

Changes in body composition, imbalance between energy intake and demand, homeostatic dysregulation, and neurologic and psychologic changes are typical of GFTT. As the body ages, weight typically increases until late middle age and declines between ages 65 and 70. With this decline, lean body mass is lost. Fat mass, however, increases. The loss of lean body mass causes a decrease in the resting metabolic rate; in turn, older adults expend most of their energy performing activities of daily living (ADLs).

Certain age-related changes impact food intake and digestion. These include decreased sense of taste, decreased secretion of digestive enzymes, and decreased salivation. GI motility slows with aging, which also decreases metabolism. Dentition is also affected by aging, with older people at risk for losing teeth, having gum disease, and/or other painful mouth conditions. These changes make eating more difficult and less enjoyable; they also change older patients' sense of being full during meals. Ultimately, this leads older adults to consume fewer calories, which means they have less energy for performing ADLs.

At the same time that metabolic rate and energy consumption are changing, decreased efficiency of body systems makes it increasingly difficult for the body to maintain homeostasis. To compensate for these changes, homeostatic mechanisms require extra energy; this energy is not necessarily available in light of dietary changes. Neurologic and psychologic changes further compound these problems. Although many older adults experience good physical and cognitive health, some experience motor and cognitive decline, making it difficult to purchase food and prepare meals, and sometimes making it difficult to remember mealtimes and whether or not they've eaten.

Chronic diseases can also impact the older person's ability to maintain weight and nutritional status. Diabetes can cause malabsorption and end-organ damage. Parkinson disease can cause dysphagia and tremors that make it difficult to get food into the mouth. There are several other chronic diseases that can affect the body's ability to get and maintain nutrition.

Anorexia of aging, which can lead to GFTT, is a decrease in appetite and consequential decrease of nutrition intake (Landi et al., 2016). Vitamin and nutrient deficiencies are also common and decrease older patients' ability to recover from injury, illness, and infection. This impaired immunity makes older patients more susceptible to both chronic and acute illnesses; illness, in turn, makes patients more susceptible to GFTT.

Risk Factors

Infants who are deprived of mothering, especially those 3 to 15 months of age, will not learn to form significant relationships or to trust others. Touch, cuddling, and visual and auditory stimulation are all critical for the infant. Through these mechanisms, the baby comes to know self and the environment. Infants who fail to establish a loving, responsive relationship with a caregiver often fail to develop normally.

Infants and children whose parents or caregivers experience depression, substance abuse, mental retardation, or psychosis, or who have a history of abuse, are at risk for FTT. Their parents may be socially and emotionally isolated or may lack knowledge of infant nutritional and nurturing needs. A multifactorial and reciprocal interaction pattern may exist whereby the parent does not offer enough food or is not responsive to the infant's hunger cues and, as a result, the infant is irritable, not soothed, and does not give clear cues about hunger.

Children living in poverty are also at risk for FTT. When food is scarce, there is greater potential for undernutrition.

Risk factors for the older adult developing GFTT involve those conditions that lead to undernutrition. The presence of multiple chronic diseases, including diabetes, renal failure, cardiovascular disease, and neurologic disorders, increases risk for GFTT. There is a greater chance of anorexia that leads to malnutrition if the elderly patient is on more than four medications.

Sensory perception deficits can also lead to anorexia. Delirium can also cause the older adult not to have adequate nutrition. The geriatric patient who substitutes nutrition with alcohol or neglects to eat because of substance abuse is at risk for GFTT.

Mental health disorders put the older adult at risk for developing GFTT. Depression in particular is associated with GFTT. Residents in nursing homes, particularly veterans, show a greater risk of GFTT than those who live in the community (Ali, 2015).

Like children in poverty, adults who live in poor conditions and are food insecure are more likely to develop GFTT. Social isolation, widowhood, and abandonment by family/friends are also considered risk factors.

Prevention

Research suggests that educating caregivers regarding an infant's dietary and nutritional needs may help guard against development of FTT in children. Nurses can provide resources for family with food insecurity, including referrals to local food pantries, school meals, and state and federal food assistance. Likewise, home nursing visits have been shown to significantly impact caregivers' delivery of adequate nutrition to children within the home (Cole & Lanham, 2011). Parents should be encouraged to be part of the plan, rather than feeling ashamed, in order to have a successful outcome.

Prevention of GFTT is complicated. The nurse can review the patient's medications, being observant of those medications responsible for decreased appetite. Patients can be taught to eat high-calorie, nutritionally dense foods. Other nutritional strategies can also be discussed with the patient, including eating frequent, small meals.

Nurses can refer patients to social support groups to help decrease isolation. Various charity organizations can be used to help the senior have meals delivered to the home. Case management should be considered for those individuals with several chronic diseases, as well as for those in need of financial and/or transportation assistance to buy food.

Clinical Manifestations

The characteristics of FTT are persistent failure to eat adequately with no weight gain or with weight loss in a child under 6 years of age. While FTT may be caused by a physical disorder, in 80% of cases, no definitive underlying physical disorder is identified (Cole & Lanham, 2011). Infants with feeding disorders refuse food, may have erratic sleep patterns, are irritable and difficult to soothe, fall well under expected growth patterns, and are often developmentally delayed (**Figure 25–14 》》**).

Infants with inorganic FTT show delayed development without any physical cause. They are often malnourished and fail to gain weight and grow normally. Behavior may be apathetic and withdrawn, and the child may demonstrate poor eye contact and lack anticipated stranger danger.

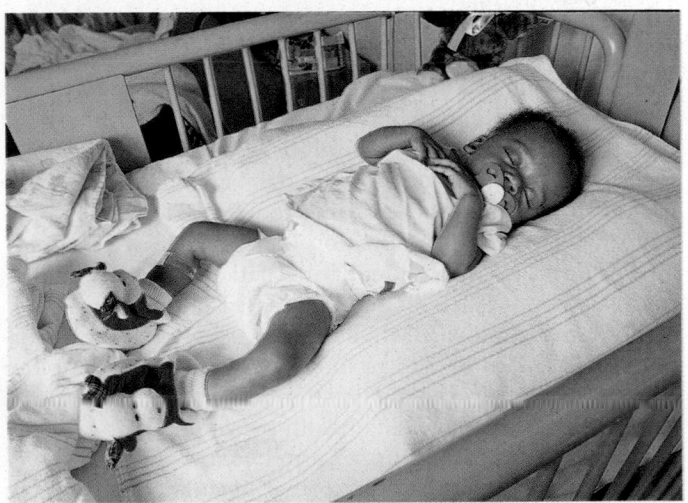

Figure 25–14 》》 Infants with failure to thrive may not look severely malnourished, but they fall well below the expected weight and height norms for their age and population. This infant, who appears to be about 4 months old, is actually 8 months old. He has been hospitalized for examination of his failure to thrive and treatment of an eating disorder.

Patients with GFTT typically present with unintended weight loss, lack of appetite and energy, and diminished physical activity and strength. Muscle tone is poor; limbs are cachectic, though fat deposits appear around the midsection. Skin is dry and scaly, and wounds heal slowly and poorly. Hair is thin and nails are weak, discolored, and misshapen. Patients may complain of bone or joint pain, and edema may be present. Blood tests reveal anemia, low serum albumin and prealbumin levels, and low serum cholesterol levels.

GFTT patients are sometimes described as being "wasted" or "frail." Wasting refers to gradual physical deterioration accompanied by a loss of strength and appetite. Frailty refers to cumulative physiologic decline that manifests itself in a wasted appearance, impaired physical abilities, decreased resistance to stressors, and diminished cognitive function. Resistance to stressors and cognitive functioning are important to consider when diagnosing GFTT because active older patients may consume fewer calories than required and experience weight loss, but be resilient to stress and have high cognitive functioning (White et al., 2012). In other words, weight loss alone is not indicative of GFTT.

Collaboration

A thorough history and physical examination are needed to rule out any chronic physical illness. The infant or child may be hospitalized so that healthcare providers can establish a routine for feeding and sleeping. The goals of treatment are to provide adequate caloric and nutritional intake, promote normal growth and development, and assist parents in developing feeding routines and responding to the infant's cues of physical and psychologic hunger.

>> **Stay Current:** For a description of a collaborative healthcare team addressing FTT, visit the website of the Kennedy Krieger Institute's Feeding Disorder Clinic at www.kennedykrieger.org/patient-care/patient-care-programs/outpatient-programs/feeding-disorders-clinic.

Diagnostic Tests

Diagnosis of FTT occurs primarily through assessment. In addition to clinical assessment, nutritional assessments are useful when evaluating patients for GFTT. Twenty-four hour recall is commonly used, though 7-day food diaries and food frequency questionnaires tend to be more accurate. The Malnutrition Universal Screening Tool (MUST), Mini Assessment (MNA), and Malnutrition Risk Scale (SCALES) may also be appropriate for identifying patients who are undernourished or at risk of being undernourished.

Body mass index (BMI) should be assessed; it is important, however, to recognize the limitations of BMI in older patients. Changes in height, posture, and muscle tone impact BMI's overall accuracy as a health measure. Tricipital skinfold measurement, mid-upper arm circumference, and biometric impedance analysis are other useful anthropometric assessments of lean mass and fat mass.

Psychosocial assessment is an important part of any GFTT assessment, especially if patients have risk factors for depression such as the loss of a spouse or a change in living arrangements. The Geriatric Depression Scale (GDS) is frequently used for such assessments; this online tool has both a short (15 question) and long (30 question) version. The Cornell Scale for Depression in Dementia may also be useful and is appropriate for patients with or without dementia.

>> **Stay Current:** See the Geriatric Depression Scale at http://www.medscape.com/viewarticle/447735.

Diagnostic laboratory tests also are appropriate when assessing for GFTT. Serum proteins—including albumin, transferrin, retinol-binding proteins, and thyroxine-binding prealbumin—are typically assessed. Decreases in any of these proteins can be indicative of GFTT. These values should be considered cautiously, however, because they also serve as markers for other problems commonly associated with aging, such as inflammation and infection. Serum cholesterol and vitamin levels are also assessed.

Surgery

Surgical management of the patient with FTT will vary based on the physiologic impairment. For example, possible surgical interventions may include cleft palate repair or alleviation of a bowel obstruction.

In some cases, medical conditions contributing to GFTT, such as esophageal strictures and bowel obstructions, may require surgical treatment. The type and appropriateness of such surgical interventions depend on the specific condition.

Pharmacologic Therapy

No medications are indicated for primary treatment of FTT. Rather, the approach to treatment includes identifying the cause, resolving any barriers to obtaining and absorbing adequate caloric intake, and providing nutritional supplementation to treat deficiencies.

Pharmacologic therapies for the treatment of GFTT typically involve vitamin regimens. Vitamins D, B_{12}, and folate are commonly prescribed supplements for GFTT patients. Vitamin D and folate deficiencies typically stem from altered dietary intake; B_{12} deficiencies, on the other hand, are most commonly caused by disease states.

In addition, if a GFTT patient is diagnosed with depression, pharmacologic therapy is likely to include tricyclic antidepressants, SSRIs, serotonin-norepinephrine reuptake inhibitors, or other second-generation antidepressants. In general, SSRIs are preferred because they have fewer adverse side effects in older patients. No matter the type of antidepressant prescribed, patients should be closely monitored for drug interactions (Wilson, Shannon & Shields, 2016).

Nonpharmacologic Therapy

Developmentally appropriate education for caregivers regarding nutrition and home care visits is believed to reduce the incidence of FTT among children. For patients who choose to breastfeed, the nurse should assess the patient's knowledge and efficacy and provide or facilitate the provision of additional teaching as needed.

Nonpharmacologic therapies tend to focus on improving oral intake of foods and fluids. Therapies may include providing smaller, more manageable portions to decrease patient anxiety about wasted food. Portions may be fortified with additional vitamins and nutrients, and they may be softer in texture for patients with dentition problems. Snacks should be offered, and patients should be allowed choice in menu selection whenever possible. Patients with alterations in mobility or illness should receive nursing assistance at mealtime.

For critically ill patients with GFTT, oral liquid, energy-dense, and high-quality protein supplements may be appropriate. For severely undernourished patients or those who cannot take food orally, enteral feeding is appropriate.

If underlying medical conditions contribute to GFTT, those must be treated with GFTT in mind. For example, restrictive therapeutic diets may cause weight loss; when GFTT is involved, the impacts of less restrictive diets on the two conditions should be assessed (Phillips, 2012).

NURSING PROCESS

Nursing care of the child with FTT is directed toward improving the child's nutritional intake with the end result of increasing the growth and health of the child. This may be accomplished through parent teaching; observation of child–parent interactions, especially during feeding times; and careful recording of height and weight on growth charts.

Nursing care of the older adult with GFTT involves both the acute care of the GFTT and the chronic care of any underlying disease processes. Assisting the patient to meet nutritional needs is a priority. This may include helping the patient make food choices that are nutritionally dense and easy to eat. Referral to a dietitian or nutritionist may be necessary. The nurse may also engage in therapeutic communication for the older adult who might be depressed, socially isolated, or coping with loss.

Assessment

Assessment of the child is essential for establishing the best intervention plan. Take accurate measurement of weight, height, BMI, and percentiles each time a child interacts with a healthcare provider to develop an important record of growth patterns over time. See the Focus on Diversity and Culture feature for more information on measuring growth. This helps to identify the child with an eating disorder. The child's activity level, developmental milestones, and interaction patterns also provide important information. When feeding the child, observe how the child indicates hunger or satiety, the ability of the child to be soothed, and general interaction patterns such as eye contact, touch, and cuddliness.

Ask parents about stressors in their lives that may prevent or interfere with appropriate interaction with the child. Questions about the pregnancy and delivery can elicit information about early disturbances in the child–parent relationship. Ask whether there are other children in the family and whether they have experienced feeding problems. It is important for the nurse to observe the child's and parents' behaviors when the parents feed the child; cues given by each individual and interactional modes such as rocking, singing, talking, and body postures are important.

For older adults, assess patients' opportunity for socializing during meals; intake tends to improve when others are present. In the home environment, assess the food preparation area to ensure that patients are physically capable of using necessary appliances and navigating the space. The

dining area should also be examined and any unneeded medical equipment removed. If patients in the home environment cannot prepare meals on their own, social services (e.g., "meals on wheels") should be considered (Phillips, 2012).

Diagnosis

Nursing diagnoses pertinent for the young child with FTT may include the following:

- *Imbalanced Nutrition: Less Than Body Requirements*
- *Development, Delayed*
- *Parenting, Risk for Impaired.*

Nursing diagnoses for the older adult with GFTT may include:

- *Fatigue.*
- *Imbalanced Nutrition: Less Than Body Requirements*
- *Self-Care Deficit.*

(NANDA-I © 2014)

Planning

The goals of nursing care for the child with FTT may include the following:

- Child will attain adequate growth and normal development.
- The parent–child relationship will improve.
- Parental understanding of the child's nutritional requirements will improve.
- Complications associated with poor nutrition will be prevented.

Goals for nursing care of older adults with GFTT may include:

- Patient will list five items that are nutritionally dense and include these items in a meal plan.
- Patient will have adequate mental health support and services.
- Patient will have stable sources of nutritious food and supplements as recommended by the healthcare provider.

Implementation

Nursing care centers on performing a thorough history and physical assessment, observing parent–child interactions during feeding times, and providing necessary teaching to enable parents to respond appropriately to their child's needs. Accurate weights, nutritional assessments, and developmental evaluation should be done to see if the child begins to grow more normally. Additional diagnostic tests may be given to rule out organic causes of the poor growth.

Once a diagnosis of nonorganic FTT is confirmed, parents become involved in feeding the child. Observations of feeding and continued careful physical assessments are needed. Teach parents to record carefully the child's intake at each meal or feeding. Teach parents how to understand and respond to the child's cues of hunger and satiety. Teach them to hold, rock, and touch the infant during feeding and to establish eye contact with infants and older children.

Upon discharge, refer parents to an early childhood intervention agency that can continue monitoring the home situation. Agency staff can observe feeding during a home visit and evaluate stresses and behavior patterns among family members. Frequent measurement of growth and development must be ensured so that the child is adequately nourished. Parents may need referral to community resources to help them manage stressful situations and to enhance their parenting skills.

For the older adult patient with GFTT, nursing care centers on weight gain and nutritional improvement. This will require the nurse to monitor input and output, paying mind to caloric intake and nutritional choices. Nurses should encourage nutritionally dense snacks and short, frequent meals. Addressing the underlying causes of the GFTT is also as important. For example, if the patient is prescribed several medications, the nurse can collaborate with a pharmacist and provider to evaluate the medication for anorexic side effects and consider alternatives. The nurse should consider case management for the patient. In nursing homes and transitional care units, the nurse should encourage the resident to participate in social activities, including eating with other residents.

Evaluation

The child's outcomes are largely evaluated based on the following:

- Growth and development of the child improve.
- The parent–child relationship improves.
- The parent voices a specific action plan to improve and maintain appropriate growth of child.
- The child experiences no long-term complications as a result of FTT.

Outcomes for older adults with GFTT may include:

- The patient achieves improved nutritional status.
- The patient has food security.
- The patient uses social support systems as necessary to promote health and functioning.

REVIEW Failure to Thrive

RELATE Link the Concepts and Exemplars

Linking the exemplar of failure to thrive with the concept of acid–base balance:

1. How might excessive protein metabolism as the result of inadequate sources of energy supply from dietary intake impact the patient's acid–base balance?

2. How might altered glucose metabolism as a result of inadequate caloric intake impact the patient's acid–base balance?

Linking the exemplar of failure to thrive with the concept of elimination:

3. How might inadequate caloric and nutrient intake impact elimination?

4. If caloric and nutrient intake is increased suddenly, how might the patient's elimination habits be impacted?

READY Go to Volume 3: Clinical Nursing Skills

REFER Go to Pearson MyLab Nursing and eText

- Additional review materials

REFLECT Apply Your Knowledge

Hilary is born 8 weeks prematurely at 32 weeks' gestation to a single adolescent mother. Hilary remains in the neonatal intensive care unit for 10 weeks until she is stable enough to be discharged. Her mother tries to visit at least once a week and is sometimes able to visit more often depending on whether someone can give her a ride to and from the hospital.

Hilary returns in 6 weeks following discharge and is found to have gained only 2 oz, increasing her weight from 2.32 kg (5 lb 2 oz) to 2.38 kg (5 lb 4 oz). The provider schedules a follow-up visit for 2 weeks later, and the nurse explains Hilary's nutritional requirements. When Hilary returns, she has lost 1 oz in weight.

1. Does Hilary qualify as having FTT? Explain your answer.

2. Do you suspect an organic or inorganic cause of her failure to gain weight?

3. Develop a nursing plan of care for Hilary.

REFLECT Apply Your Knowledge

Tom and Jenny Fordham, both in their 70s, have lived in the same home for more than 20 years. Mr. Fordham is a retired media professional; Mrs. Fordham a retired interior designer. In the past 3 years, both of them have experienced a decline in health. Mr. Fordham is now in the middle stages of Alzheimer disease. He is no longer able to drive and frequently needs to be reminded to do things like take a shower or take his medicine. Mrs. Fordham developed chronic obstructive pulmonary disease (COPD) several years ago. She now requires oxygen via cannula 24/7, and she uses her tiotropium bromide (Spiriva) and fluticasone (Flovent) inhalers daily as prescribed. She also takes calcium and vitamin D daily and ibandronate sodium (Boniva) once a month for osteoporosis. She continues to drive, although she finds it frustrating and does not like to go out often.

You are the nurse at Mrs. Fordham's primary care provider's office. When Mrs. Fordham comes for a routine checkup, you take her height and weight and find that she has lost 5 lb since she was in 3 months ago with acute bronchitis. She complains that Mr. Fordham is in the waiting room because she is too scared to leave him home alone. She relates that she has very little energy these days, and that taking care of him is "wearing me out."

1. What risk factors does Mr. Fordham have for GFTT? Mrs. Fordham?

2. What are your primary concerns about Mrs. Fordham at this time? Why?

3. What additional assessment data do you need to gather? Why?

References

Adams, M. P., Holland, L. N., & Urban, C. (2017). *Pharmacology for nurses: A pathophysiologic approach* (5th ed.). Hoboken, NJ: Pearson Education.

Ahlin, K., Himmelmann, K., Hagberg, G., Kacerovsky, M., Cobo, T., Wennerholm, U. B., & Jacobsson, B. (2013). Non-infectious risk factors for different types of cerebral palsy in term-born babies: A population-based, case–control study. *International Journal of Obstetrics & Gynaecology, 120*(6), 724–731.

Ali, N. (2015). Failure to thrive in elderly adults. *Medscape*. Retrieved from http://emedicine.medscape.com/article/2096163-overview#a5

American Academy of Child and Adolescent Psychiatry. (2016). *ADHD resource center*. Retrieved from https://www.aacap.org/aacap/families_and_youth/resource_centers/adhd_resource_center/Home.aspx.

American Academy of Pediatrics (AAP). (2006). Identifying infants and young children with developmental disorders in the medical home: An algorithm for developmental surveillance and screening. Council on Children with Disabilities Section on Developmental Behavioral Pediatrics, Bright Futures Steering Committee, Medical Home Initiatives for Children with Special Needs Project Advisory Committee. *Pediatrics, 118*(1). Retrieved from http://pediatrics.aappublications.org/content/118/1/405

American Academy of Pediatrics (AAP) Subcommittee on Attention-Deficit/Hyperactivity Disorder, Steering Committee on Quality Improvement and Management (2011). ADHD: Clinical practice guideline for the diagnosis, evaluation, and treatment of Attention-Deficit/Hyperactivity Disorder in children and adolescents. *Pediatrics, 128*(5), 1007–1022. doi:10.1542/peds.2011-2654

American Academy of Pediatrics (AAP). (2016). Media and young minds: A policy statement. Retrieved from http://pediatrics.aappublications.org/content/pediatrics/138/5/e20162591.full.pdf

American Psychiatric Association (APA). (2013). *Diagnostic and statistical manual of mental disorders* (5th ed.). Arlington, VA: Author.

American Psychiatric Association (APA). (2015). *What is ADHD?* Retrieved from https://www.psychiatry.org/patients-families/adhd/what-is-adhd

American Speech-Language-Hearing Association. (2017). *Social language use: Pragmatics*. Retrieved from http://www.asha.org/public/speech/development/Pragmatics/

Andrews, M. M., & Boyle, J. S. (2016). *Transcultural concepts in nursing care* (7th ed.). Philadelphia, PA: Wolters Kluwer.

Angulo-Barroso, R. M., Schapiro, L., Liang, W., Rodrigues, O., Shafir, T., Kaciroti, N., … Lozoff, B. (2011). Motor development in 9-month-old infants in relation to cultural differences and iron status. *Developmental Psychobiology, 53*(2), 196–210. Retrieved from http://doi.org/10.1002/dev20512

Arain, M., Hague, M., Johal, L., Mathur, P., Nel, W., Rais, A., … Sharma, S. (2013). Maturation of the adolescent brain. *Neuropsychiatric Disease and Treatment, 9*, 449–461.

Autism Speaks. (2016). *What are the symptoms of autism?* Retrieved from https://www.autismspeaks.org/what-autism/symptoms

Bandura, A. (1986). *Social foundations of thought and actions: A social cognitive theory*. Englewood Cliffs, NJ: Prentice Hall.

Bandura, A. (1997a). *Self-efficacy: The exercise of control*. New York, NY: W.H. Freeman.

Bandura, A. (1997b). *Self-efficacy in changing societies*. New York, NY: Cambridge University Press.

Barron, D. A., Coyle, D., Paliokosta, E., & Hassiotis, A. (2016). Transition for children with intellectual disabilities. University of Hertfordshire. Retrieved from http://www.intellectualdisability.info/life-stages/articles/transition-for-children-with-intellectual-disabilities

Benard, B. (2014). *The foundations of the resiliency framework*. Retrieved from http://www.resiliency.com/free-articles-resources/the-foundations-of-the-resiliency-framework/

Bishop, K. M., & Lucchino, R. (n.d.). Aging in individuals with a developmental disability. *Aging and Disabilities Resource Center Training for the Cross Network Collaboration of Florida*. Retrieved from http://elderaffairs.state.fl.us/doea/ARC/05c_Module_3_Aging_in_Individuals_with_a_Developmental_Disability.pdf

Black, L. I., Varhartian, A., & Hoffman, H. J. (2015). Communication disorders and use of intervention services among children aged 3–17 years: United States, 2012. *NCHS Data Brief No. 205*. Retrieved from https://www.cdc.gov/nchs/data/atabriefs/db205.pdf

Bolten, M. I., Wurmser, H., Buske-Kirschbaum, A., Papoušek, M., Pirke, K. M., & Hellhammer, D. (2011). Cortisol levels in pregnancy as a psychobiological predictor for birth weight. *Archives of Women's Mental Health, 14*(1), 33–41.

Boyle, C. A., Boulet, S., Schieve, L., Cohen, R. A., Blumberg, S. J., Yeargin-Allsopp, M., Visser, S., & Kogan, M. D. (2011). Trends in the prevalence of developmental disabilities in U.S. children, 1997–2008. *Pediatrics, 27*, 1034–1042.

Brain, C. (2000). *Advanced subsidiary psychology: Approaches and methods*. Cheltenham, U.K.: Nelson Thornes.

Brondino, N., Fusar-Poli, L., Rocchetti, M., Provenzani, U., Barale, F., & Politi, P. (2015). Complementary and alternative therapies for autism spectrum disorder. *Evidence-Based Complementary and Alternative Medicine, 2015*, 258589. Retrieved from http://doi.org/10.1155/2015/258589

Bronfenbrenner, U. (1986). Ecology of the family as a context for human development: Research perspectives. *Developmental Psychology, 22*, 723–742.

Bronfenbrenner, U. (Ed.). (2005). *Making human beings human: Bioecological perspectives on human development*. Thousand Oaks, CA: Sage.

Bronfenbrenner, U., McClelland, P. D., Ceci, S. J., Moen, P., & Wethington, E. (1996). *The state of Americans*. New York, NY: Free Press.

Brown, H. K., Lunsky, Y., Wilton, A. S., Cobigo, V., & Vigod, S. N. (2016). Pregnancy in women with intellectual and developmental disability. *Journal of Obstetrics and Gynecology Canada, 38*(1), 9–16.

Burkett, K., Morris, E., Manning-Courtney, P., Anthony, J., & Shambley-Ebron, D. (2015). African American families on autism diagnosis and treatment: The influence of culture. *Journal of Autism and Developmental Disorders, 45*(10), 3244–3254. doi:10.1007/s10803-015-2482-x

Cairns, K. E., Yap, M. B., Pilkington, D., & Jorm, A. F. (2014). Risk and protective factors for depression that adolescents can modify: A systematic review and meta-analysis of longitudinal studies. *Journal of Affective Disorders, 169C*, 61–75. doi:10.1016/j.jad.2014.08.006

Campbell, T. (2010). Ethics of care. In R. H. Corrigan & M. E. Farrell (Eds.), *Ethics: A university guide* (pp. 79–107). Gloucester, UK: Progressive Frontiers Press.

Centers for Disease Control and Prevention (CDC). (2012). Youth risk behavior surveillance—United States, 2011. *Morbidity and Mortality Weekly Report, 61*, SS-4.

Centers for Disease Control and Prevention (CDC). (2014). *LGBT youth*. Retrieved from http://www.cdc.gov/lgbthealth/youth.htm

Centers for Disease Control and Prevention (CDC). (2015a). *Facts about developmental disabilities*. Retrieved from http://www.cdc.gov/ncbddd/developmentaldisabilities/facts.html#ref

Centers for Disease Control and Prevention (CDC). (2015b). *Facts about FASDs*. Retrieved from http://www.cdc.gov/ncbddd/fasd/facts.html

Centers for Disease Control and Prevention (CDC). (2015c). *Premature birth*. Retrieved from http://www.cdc.gov/Features/Prematurebirth/

Centers for Disease Control and Prevention (CDC). (2015d). *Autism spectrum disorder: Treatments*. Retrieved from http://www.cdc.gov/ncbddd/autism/treatment.html#ref

Centers for Disease Control and Prevention (CDC). (2015e). *Folic acid*. Retrieved from https://www.cdc.gov/ncbddd/folicacid/faqs.html

Centers for Disease Control and Prevention (CDC). (2016a). *Sexual risk behaviors: HIV, STD, & teen pregnancy prevention*. Retrieved from http://www.cdc.gov/HealthyYouth/sexualbehaviors/

Centers for Disease Control and Prevention (CDC). (2016b). *Developmental milestones*. Retrieved from http://www.cdc.gov/ncbddd/actearly/milestones/index.html

Centers for Disease Control and Prevention (CDC). (2016c). *Facts about fragile X syndrome*. Retrieved from http://www.cdc.gov/ncbddd/fxs/facts.htm

Centers for Disease Control and Prevention (CDC). (2016d). *Zika virus*. Retrieved from http://www.cdc.gov/zika/index.html

Centers for Disease Control and Prevention (CDC). (2016e). *Babies born with CMV (congenital CMV infection)*. Retrieved from http://www.cdc.gov/cmv/congenital-infection.html

Centers for Disease Control and Prevention (CDC). (2016f). *Autism spectrum disorder (ASD)*. Retrieved from https://www.cdc.gov/ncbddd/autism/index.html

Centers for Disease Control and Prevention (CDC). (2016g). *Facts about cerebral palsy*. Retrieved from http://www.cdc.gov/ncbddd/cp/facts.html

Cherkasova, M. V., French, L. R., Syer, C. A., Cousins, L., Galina, H., Ahmadi-Kashani, Y., & Hechtman, L. (2016). Efficacy of cognitive behavioral therapy with and without medication for adults with ADHD: A randomized clinical trial. *Journal of Attention Disorders*. doi:10.1177/1087054716671197

Chess, S., & Thomas, A. (1995). *Temperament in clinical practice*. New York, NY: Guilford Press.

Chess, S., & Thomas, A. (1996). *Temperament: Theory and practice*. Philadelphia, PA: Brunner/Mazel.

Children and Adults with Attention-Deficit/Hyperactivity Disorder (CHADD). (2016a). *Diagnosing ADHD in adolescence*. Retrieved from http://www.chadd.org/Understanding-ADHD/For-Parents-Caregivers/Teens/Diagnosing-ADHD-in-Adolescence.aspx

Children and Adults with Attention-Deficit/Hyperactivity Disorder (CHADD). (2016b). *Women and girls.* Retrieved from http://www.chadd.org/Understanding-ADHD/For-Adults/Living-with-ADHD-A-Lifespan-Disorder/Women-and-Girls.aspx

Christensen, D. L., Baio, J., Braun, K. V., Van Naarden Braun, K., Bilder, D., Charles, J., ... Yeargin-Allsopp, M. (2016). Prevalence and characteristics of autism spectrum disorder among children aged 8 years—Autism and Developmental Disabilities Monitoring Network, 11 sites, United States, 2012. *Morbidity and Mortality Weekly Reports 65*(SS-3), 1–23. Retrieved from http://dx.doi.org/10.15585/mmwr.ss6503a1

Cole, S. Z., & Lanham, J. S. (2011). Failure to thrive: An update. *American Family Physician, 83*(7), 829–834.

Cortese, S., Faraone, S. V., Bernardi, S, Wang, S., & Blanco, C. (2016). Gender differences in adult attention-deficit/hyperactivity disorder: Results from the National Epidemiologic Survey on Alcohol and Related Conditions (NESARC). *Journal of Clinical Psychiatry, 77*(4):e421–e428. doi:10.4088/JCP.14m09630

Courtney-Long, E. A., Carroll, D. D., Zhang, Q. C., Stevens, A. C., Griffin-Blake, S., Armour, B. S., & Campbell, V. A. (2015, July 31). Prevalence of disability and disability type among adults—United States, 2013. *MMWR, Morbidity and Mortality Weekly Report.* Retrieved from https://www.cdc.gov/mmwr/preview/mmwrhtml/mm6429a2.htm

Czarnecki, M. L., Hainsworth, K. R., Jacobson, A. A., Simpson, P. M., & Weisman, S. J. (2015). Opioid administration for postoperative pain in children with developmental delay: Parent and nurse satisfaction. *Journal of Pediatric Surgical Nursing 4*(1), 15–27. doi:10.1097/JPS.0000000000000050

Elder, J. H., Kreider, C. M., Schaefer, N. M., & de Laosa, M. B. (2015). A review of gluten- and casein-free diets for treatment of autism: 2005–2015. *Nutrition and Dietary Supplements, 7,* 87–101.

Erikson, E. (1963). *Childhood and society.* New York, NY: W. W. Norton.

Erikson, E. (1968). *Identity: Youth and crisis.* New York, NY: W. W. Norton.

Estes, A., Munson, J., Rogers, S. J., Greenson, J., Winter, J., & Dawson, G. (2015). Long-term outcomes of early intervention in 6-year-old children with Autism Spectrum Disorder. *Journal of the American Academy of Child & Adolescent Psychiatry, 54*(7), 580–587. http://dx.doi.org/10.1016/j.jaac.2015.04.005

Factor, A., Heller, T., & Janicki, M. (2012). *Bridging the aging and developmental disabilities service networks: Challenges and best practices.* Chicago, IL: Institute on Disability and Human Development, University of Illinois at Chicago.

Food and Drug Administration. (2011). FDA drug safety communication: Safety review update of medications used to treat Attention-Deficit/Hyperactivity Disorder (ADHD) in adults. Retrieved from http://www.fda.gov/Drugs/DrugSafety/ucm279858.htm

Food & Drug Administration (FDA). (2014). *Pregnancy and lactation labeling (drugs) final rule.* Retrieved from http://www.fda.gov/Drugs/DevelopmentApprovalProcess/DevelopmentResources/Labeling/ucm093307.htm

Food and Drug Administration. (2015). *Beware of false or misleading claims for treating autism.* Retrieved from http://www.fda.gov/ForConsumers/ConsumerUpdates/ucm394757.htm

Food and Drug Administration. (2016). *Dealing with ADHD: What you need to know.* Retrieved from http://www.fda.gov/ForConsumers/ConsumerUpdates/ucm269188.htm

Fowler, J. W. (1981). *Stages of faith: The psychology of human development and the quest for meaning.* San Francisco, CA: Harper & Row.

Frolek Clark, G. J., & Schlaback, T. L. (2013). Systematic review of occupational therapy interventions to improve cognitive development in children ages birth–5 years. *American Journal of Occupational Therapy, 67*(4), 425–430.

Fuller-Thomson, E., Lewis, D. A., & Agbeyaka, S. K. (2016) Attention-deficit/hyperactivity disorder casts a long shadow: Findings from a population-based study of adult women with self-reported ADHD. *Child: Care, Health and Development, 42,* 918–927. doi:10.1111/cch.12380

Geller, A. I., Shehab, N., Weidle, N. J., Lovegrove, M. C., Wolpert, B. J., Timbo, B. B., ... Budnitz, D. S. (2015). Emergency department visits for adverse events related to dietary supplements. *New England Journal of Medicine, 373*(16), 1531–1540.

Geurts, H. M., Stek, M., & Comijs, H. (2016). Autism characteristics in older adults with depressive disorders. *American Journal of Geriatric Psychiatry, 24*(2), 161–169. doi:10.1016/j.jagp.2015.08.003

Gilligan, C. (1982). *In a different voice: Psychological theory and women's development.* Cambridge, MA: Harvard University Press.

Gómez-Benito, J., Van de Vijver, F. J. R., Balluerka, N., & Caterino, L. (2015). Cross-cultural and gender differences in ADHD among young adults. *Journal of Attention Disorders.* Advance online publication. doi:10.1177/1087054715611748

Gould, R. L. (1972). The phases of adult life: A study in developmental psychology. *American Journal of Psychiatry, 129,* 33–43. Published by American Psychiatric Association, © 1972.

Grant, R., Gracy, D., & Brito, A. (2010). Developmental and social-emotional screening instruments for use in pediatric primary care in infants and young children. *Children's Health Fund, New York, NY.* Retrieved from http://www.childrenshealthfund.org/sites/default/files/dev-and-mental-health-primary-care-screening-tools.pdf

Herdman, T. H. & Kamitsuru, S. (Eds.). *Nursing Diagnoses—Definitions and Classification 2015–2017.* Copyright © 2014, 1994–2014 NANDA International. Used by arrangement with John Wiley & Sons, Inc. Companion website: www.wiley.com/go/nursingdiagnoses

Hewitt, A., Gulaid, A., Hamre, K., Esler, A., Punyko, J., Reichle, J., & Reiff, M. (2013). *Minneapolis Somali autism spectrum disorder prevalence project: Community report 2013.* Minneapolis, MN: University of Minnesota, Institute on Community Integration, Research and Training Center on Community Living.

Huquet, G., Ey, E., & Bourgeron T. (2013). The genetic landscapes of autism spectrum disorders. *Annual Review of Genomics and Human Genetics, 14,* 191–213.

Josenby, A. L., Wagner, P., Jarnlo, G.-B., Westbom, L., & Nordmark, E. (2015), Functional performance in self-care and mobility after selective dorsal rhizotomy: A 10-year practice-based follow-up study. *Developmental Medicine and Child Neurology, 57*(3), 286–293. doi:10.1111/dmcn.12610

Kabali, H. K., Irigoyen, M. M., Nunez-Davis, R., Budacki, J. G., Mohanty, S. J., Leister, K. P., & Bonner, R. L. (2015). Exposure and use of mobile media devices by young children. *Pediatrics, 136*(6), 1–7. doi:10.1542/peds.2015-2151

Kahraman, A., Seyhan, K., Değer, Ü., Kutlutürk, S., & Mutlu, A. (2016). Should botulinum toxin A injections be repeated in children with cerebral palsy? A systematic review. *Developmental Medicine and Child Neurology, 58*(9), 910–917. doi:10.1111/dmcn.13135

Kohlberg, L. (1981). *Essays on moral development: Vol. 1. The philosophy of moral development.* San Francisco, CA: Harper & Row.

Kohlberg, L. (1984). *Essays on moral development: Vol. 2. The psychology of moral development.* San Francisco, CA: Harper & Row.

Krumm, N., O'Roak, B. J., Shendure, J., & Eichler, E. E. (2014). A de novo convergence of autism genetics and molecular neuroscience. *Trends in Neuroscience, 37*(2), 95–105.

Landi, F., Calvani, R., Tosato, M., Martone, A. M., Ortolani, E., Savera, G., ... Marzetti, E. (2016). Anorexia of aging: Risk factors, consequences, and potential treatments. *Nutrients, 8*(2), 69. doi:10.3390/nu8020069

LeClerc, S., & Easley, D. (2015). Pharmacological therapies for autism spectrum disorder: A review. *Pharmacy and Therapeutics, 40*(6), 389–397.

Li, Q., Fischer, W. W., Peng, C. Z., Williams, A. D., & Burd, L. (2011). Fetal alcohol spectrum disorders: A population based study of premature mortality rates in the mothers. *Maternal and Child Health Journal, 16*(6), 1332–1337. doi:10.1007/s10995-011-0844-3

Liu, T. G., Dancause, K. N., Elgbeili, G., Laplante, D. P., & King, S. (2016). Disaster-related prenatal maternal stress explains increasing amounts of variance in body composition through childhood and adolescence: Project Ice Storm. *Environmental Research, 150,* 1–7. http://dx.doi.org/10.1016/j.envres.2016.04.039

Lobo, M. A., & Galloway, J. C. (2013). Assessment and stability of early learning abilities in preterm and full-term infants across the first two years of life. *Research in Developmental Disability, 34*(5), 1721–1730.

MacLennan, A. H., Thompson, S. C., & Gecz, J. (2015). Cerebral palsy: Causes, pathways, and the role of genetic variants. *American Journal of Obstetrics and Gynecology, 213*(6), 779–788.

Madden, M., Lenhart, A., Duggan, M., Cortesi, S., & Gasser, U. (2013). *Teens and technology 2013.* Washington, DC: Pew Research Center. Retrieved from http://www.pewinternet.org/files/old-media/Files/Reports/2013/PIP_TeensandTechnology2013.pdf

Maher, E. M. (2012). Promoting social responsiveness within a developmental relationship-based approach with primary caregivers and young children with autism. *Neuropsychiatrie de l'Enfance et de l'Adolescence, 60*(5), S133–S134.

Mayo Clinic. (2014). *Autism spectrum disorder.* Retrieved from http://www.mayoclinic.org/diseases-conditions/autism-spectrum-disorder/basics/causes/con-20021148

Mayo Clinic. (2017). Attention-deficit/hyperactivity disorder (ADHD) in children. Retrieved from http://www.mayoclinic.org/diseases-conditions/adhd/symptoms-causes/dxc-20196181

Mazurek, M. O. (2013). Social media use among adults with autism spectrum disorders. *Computers in Human Behavior, 29*(4), 1709–1714.

McIntyre, S. (2015). How low can we go? Recognizing infants at high risk of cerebral palsy earlier. *Developmental Medicine and Child Neurology, 57*(10), 891.

Mealer, M., Conrad, D., Evans, J., Jooste, K., Solvnties, J., Rothbaum, B., & Moss, M. (2014). Feasibility and acceptability of a resilience training program for intensive care unit nurses. *American Journal of Critical Care, 23*(6), e97–e105. doi:10.4037/ajcc2014747

Minges, K. E., Salmon, J., Dunstan, D. W., Owen, N., Chao, A., & Whittemore, R. (2015). Reducing youth screen time: Qualitative metasynthesis of findings on barriers and facilitators. *Health Psychology, 34*(4), 381–397. http://doi.org/10.1037/hea0000172

Molina, B. S. G., Hinshaw, S. P., Swanson, J. M., Arnold, L. E., Vitiello, B., Jensen, P. S., ... MTA Cooperative Group. (2009). The MTA at 8 years: prospective follow-up of children treated for combined type ADHD in a multisite study. *Journal of the American Academy of Child and Adolescent Psychiatry, 48,* 484–500.

Moss, P., Howlin, P., Savage, S., Bolton, P., & Rutter, M. (2015). Self and informant reports of mental health difficulties among adults with autism findings from a long-term follow-up study. *Autism.* Retrieved from http://aut.sagepub.com/content/early/2015/05/22/1362361315585916.abstract

Murray, R. B., & Zentner, J. P. (2001). *Health promotion strategies through the life span* (7th ed.). Upper Saddle River, NJ: Prentice Hall.

National Alliance on Mental Illness (NAMI). (n.d.). *ADHD and school: Helping your child succeed in the classroom.* Retrieved from http://www.nami.org/Template.cfm?Section=ADHD&Template=/ContentManagement/ContentDisplay.cfm&ContentID=106379

National Association of School Nurses. (2016). *LGBTQ students: The role of the school nurse. Position statement.* Retrieved from https://www.nasn.org/PolicyAdvocacy/PositionPapersandReports/NASNPositionStatementsFullView/tabid/462/ArticleId/935/LGBTQ-Students-The-Role-of-the-School-Nurse-Revised-2016

National Center for Complementary and Integrative Health (NCCIH). (2016a). *Children and the use of complementary health approaches.* Retrieved from https://nccih.nih.gov/health/children

National Center for Complementary and Integrative Health (NCCIH). (2016b). *Attention-deficit hyperactivity disorder at a glance.* Retrieved from https://nccih.nih.gov/health/adhd/ataglance

National Center for Complementary and Integrative Health (NCCIH). (2016c). *Autism spectrum disorder and complementary health approaches.* Retrieved from https://nccih.nih.gov/health/providers/digest/autism-spectrum-disorder

National Center for Health Statistics. (2015). *Health, United States, 2015: With special feature on racial and ethnic health disparities* (Library of Congress Catalog No. 76–641496). Washington, DC: U.S. Government Printing Office.

National Center for Health Statistics. (2016). Mean age of mothers is on the rise: United States, 2000–2014. Retrieved from http://www.cdc.gov/nchs/products/databriefs/db232.htm

National Institutes of Health. (n.d.). *Alcohol use and older adults.* Retrieved from https://nihseniorhealth.gov/alcoholuse/alcoholandaging/01.html

National Institute of Mental Health (NIMH). (2016a). *Attention Deficit Hyperactivity Disorder.* Retrieved from https://www.nimh.nih.gov/health/topics/attention-deficit-hyperactivity-disorder-adhd/index.shtml

National Institute of Mental Health (NIMH). (2016b). *Autism spectrum disorder.* Retrieved from https://www.nimh.nih.gov/health/topics/autism-spectrum-disorders-asd/index.shtml?utm_source=rss_readersutm_medium=rssutm_campaign=rss_full

National Institute of Neurological Disorders and Stroke (NINDS). (2016). *Cerebral palsy: Hope through research.* Retrieved from http://www.ninds.nih.gov/disorders/cerebral_palsy/detail_cerebral_palsy.htm#3104_8

Noritz, G. H., & Murphy, N. A. (2013). Motor delays: Early identification and evaluation. *Pediatrics, 131*(6). Retrieved from: http://pediatrics.aappublications.org/content/131/6/e2016

Oehrlein, E. M., Burcu, M., Safer, D. J., & Zito, J. M. (2016). National trends in ADHD diagnosis and treatment: Comparison of youth and adult office-based visits. *Psychiatric Services, 67*(9), 964–969. http://dx.doi.org/10.1176/appi.ps.201500269

Organization of Teratology Information Specialists. (2014). *Fact sheet: Ibuprofen and pregnancy.* Retrieved from https://mothertobaby.org/fact-sheets/ibuprofen-pregnancy/pdf/

Parish, S. L., Mitra, M., Son, E., Bonardi, A., Swoboda, P. T., & Igdalsky, L. (2015). Pregnancy outcomes among U.S. women with intellectual disabilities. *American Journal of Intellectual and Developmental Disability, 120*(5), 433–443.

Peasgood, T., Bhardwaj, A., Biggs, K., Brazier, J. E., Coghill, D., Cooper, C. L., ... Sonuga-Barke, E. J. S. (2016). The impact of ADHD on the health and well-being of ADHD children and their siblings. *European Child & Adolescent Psychiatry 25*(11), 1217–1231. doi:10.1007/s00787-016-0841-6

Peck, R. (1968). Psychological developments in the second half of life. In B. L. Neugarten (Ed.), *Middle age and aging.* Chicago, IL: University of Chicago Press.

Perrin, J. M., Coury, D. L., Hyman, S. L., Cole, L., Reynolds, A. M., & Clemons, T. (2012). Complementary and alternative medicine use in a large pediatric autism sample. *Pediatrics, 130*(2):S77–S82. doi:10.1542/peds.2012-0900e

Phillips, R. M. (2012). Nutrition and depression in the community-based oldest-old. *Home Healthcare Nurse, 30*(8), 462–471.

Piaget, J. (1966). *Origins of intelligence in children.* New York, NY: W. W. Norton. Copyright © 1966 International Universities Press, Inc.

Piaget, J. (1970). *Genetic epistemology.* New York, NY: Norton & Co.

Pickles, A., Simonoff, E., Conti-Ramsden, G., Falcaro, M., Simkin, Z., Charman, T., ... Baird, G. (2009). Loss of language in early development of autism and specific language impairment. *Journal of Child Psychology and Psychiatry, 50*(7), 843–852. Published by Association for Child and Adolescent Mental Health, © 2009.

Pomeranz, J. L., Barbosa, G., Killian, C., & Austin, S. B. (2015). The dangerous mix of adolescents and dietary supplements for weight loss and muscle building: Legal strategies for state action. *Journal of Public Health Management & Practice, 21*(5), 496–503. doi:10.1097/PHH.0000000000000142

Radesky, J. S., Schumacher, J., & Zuckerman, B. (2015). Mobile and interactive media use by young children The good, the bad, and the unknown *Pediatrics, 135*(1), 1–3. doi:10.1542/peds.2014-2251

Ramírez, N. F., & Kuhl, P. K. (2016). *Bilingual language learning in children.* Seattle: University of Washington. Institute for Learning & Brain Sciences.

Ratto, A. B., Reznick, J. S., & Turner-Brown, L. (2015). Cultural effects on the diagnosis of autism spectrum disorder among Latinos. *Focus on Autism and Other Developmental Disabilities.* doi:10.1177/1088357615587501

Rehm, R. S., Fuentes-Afflick, E., Fisher, L. T., & Chesla, C. A. (2012). Parent and youth priorities during the transition to adulthood for youth with special health care needs and developmental disability. *Advances in Nursing Science, 35*(3), E57–E72. http://doi.org/10.1097/ANS.0b013e3182626180

Ringwalt, S. (2008). *Developmental screening and assessment instruments with an emphasis on social and emotional development for young children ages birth through five.* Chapel Hill: The University of North Carolina, FPG Child Development Institute, National Early Childhood Technical Assistance Center. Retrieved from http://www.nectac.org/~pdfs/pubs/screening.pdf

Rizzo, A. (2016). *Gender differences in ADHD diagnosis.* (Unpublished master's thesis). Rowan University. Paper 1409. Retrieved from http://rdw.rowan.edu/cgi/viewcontent.cgi?article=2410&context=etd

Roman-Urrestarazu, A., Lindholm, P., Moilanen, I., Kiviniemi, V., Miettunen, J., Jääskeläinen, E., ... Murray, G. K. (2016). Brain structural deficits and working memory fMRI dysfunction in young adults who were diagnosed with ADHD in adolescence. *European Child and Adolescent Psychiatry, 25*(5), 529–538. doi:10.1007/s00787-015-0755-8

Sacco, R., Gabriele, S., & Persico, A. M. (2015). Head circumference and brain size in autism spectrum disorder: A systematic review and meta-analysis. *Psychiatry Research: Neuroimaging, 234*(2), 239–251. http://dx.doi.org/10.1016/j.pscychresns.2015.08.016

Sale, J., Gignac, M., & Hawker, G. (2006). How "bad" does the pain have to be? A qualitative study examining adherence to pain medication in older adults with osteoarthritis. *Arthritis & Rheumatology, 55*(2), 272–278.

Sandin, S., Schendel, S., Magnusson, P. Hultman, C., Surén, P., Susser, E., ... Reichenberg, A. (2015). Autism risk associated with parental age and with increasing difference in age between the parents. *Molecular Psychiatry, 21,* 693–700. doi:10.1038/mp.2015.70

Santrock, J. (2015). *Life-span development* (15th ed.). Boston, MA: McGraw-Hill.

Siegel, C., Laska, E. M., Wanderling, J. A., Hernadez, J. C., & Levensen, R. B. (2016). Prevalence and diagnosis rates of childhood ADHD among racial-ethnic groups in a public mental health system. *Psychiatric Services, 67*(2), 199–205. Retrieved from http://dx.doi.org/10.1176/appi.ps.201400364

Sirotnak, A., & Chiesa, A. (2016). *Failure to thrive.* Retrieved from http://emedicine.medscape.com/article/915575-overview

Stefano, F., Price, C. S., & Weintraub, E. S. (2013). Increasing exposure to antibody-stimulating proteins and polysaccharides in vaccines is not associated with risk of autism. *Journal of Pediatrics, 163*(2), 561–567.

Stoner, R., Chow, M. L., Boyle, M. P., Sunkin, S. M., Mouton, P. R., Roy, S., ... Courchesne, E. (2014). Patches of disorganization in the neocortex of children with autism. *New England Journal of Medicine, 370,* 1209–1219. doi:10.1056/NEJMoa1307491

Sucksdorff, M., Lehtonen, L., Chudal, R., Suominen, A., Joelsson, P. Gissler, M., & Sourander, A. (2015). Preterm birth and poor fetal growth as risk factors of attention-deficit/hyperactivity disorder. *Pediatrics, 136*(3), e599–e608; doi:10.1542/peds.2015-1043

Thielke, S., Sale, J., & Reid, M. C. (2012). Aging: Are these 4 pain myths complicating care? *Journal of Family Practice, 61*(11), 666–670.

Toplek, M. (2015). ADHD: Making a difference for children and youth in the schools. *Perspectives on Language and Literacy, 41*(1), 7–8.

Van Naarden Braun, K., Christensen, D., Doernberg. N., Schieve, L., Rice, C., Wiggins, L., ... Yeargin-Allsopp, M. (2015). Trends in the prevalence of autism spectrum disorder, cerebral palsy, hearing loss, intellectual disability, and vision impairment, metropolitan Atlanta, 1991–2010. *PLoS One, 10*(4), e0124120. doi:10.1371/journal.pone.012412

Vandereet, J., Maes, B., Lembrechts, D., & Zink, I. (2011). Expressive vocabulary acquisition in children with intellectual disability: Speech or manual signs? *Journal of Intellectual and Developmental Disability, 36,* 91–104.

Vuontela, V., Carlson, S., Troberg, A. M., Fontell, T., Simola, P., Sarrinen, S., & Aronen, E. T. (2013). Working memory, attention, inhibition, and their relation to adaptive functioning and behavioral/emotional symptoms in school-aged children. *Child Psychiatry and Human Development, 44*(1), 105–122.

Walsh, F. (2011). Family resilience: A collaborative approach in response to stressful life challenges. In S. M. Southwick, B. T. Litz, D. Charney, & M. J. Friedman (Eds.), *Resilience and mental health: Challenges across the lifespan* (pp. 149–161). Cambridge, UK: Cambridge University Press.

Ware, A. L., Crocker, N., O'Brien, J. W., Deweese, B. N., Roeasch, S.C., Coles, C. D., ... Mattson, S. N. (2012). Executive function predicts adaptive behavior in children with histories of heavy prenatal alcohol exposure and attention-deficit/hyperactivity disorder. *Alcoholism Clinical and Experimental Research, 36*(3), 1431–1441.

Weber, J. R., & Kelley, J. H. (2010). *Health assessment in nursing* (4th ed.). Philadelphia, PA: Lippincott Williams & Wilkins.

Werner, E., Bierman, J., & French, F. (1971). *The children of Kauai: a longitudinal study from the prenatal period to age ten.* Honolulu: University of Hawaii Press.

White, J. V., Guenter, P., Jensen, G., Malone, A., & Schofield, M. (2012). Consensus statement of the Academy of Nutrition and Dietetics/American Society for Parenteral and Enteral Nutrition: Characteristics recommended for the identification and documentation of adult malnutrition (undernutrition). *Journal of the Academy of Nutrition and Dietetics 112*(5), 730–738. Retrieved from http://wvda.org/meeting2012/Malnutrition.pdf

Wilson, B., Shannon, M. & Shields, K. (2016). *Pearson nurse's drug guide.* New York, NY: Pearson Education.

World Health Organization (WHO). (2016). *Definition of an older or elderly person.* Retrieved from http://www.who.int/healthinfo/survey/ageingdefnolder/en/

Yin, J., & Schaaf, C. P. (2016). Autism genetics–an overview. *Prenatal Diagnosis.* Retrieved from http://dx.doi.org/10.1002/pd.4942

Yu, I., Seo, D., Kim, S., Im, J., Lee, J., & Bak, K. (2016). Effects of therapeutic massage program on range of motion, activities of daily living, strength in children with spastic cerebral palsy. *Journal of Korean Clinical Health Science, 4*(1), 542–549.

Zablotsky, B., Black, L. I., Maenner, M. J., Schieve, L. A., & Blumberg, S. J. (2015). *Estimated prevalence of autism and other developmental disabilities following questionnaire changes in the 2014 National Health Interview Survey.* National Health Statistic Report No. 87. Hyattsville, MD: National Center for Health Statistics.

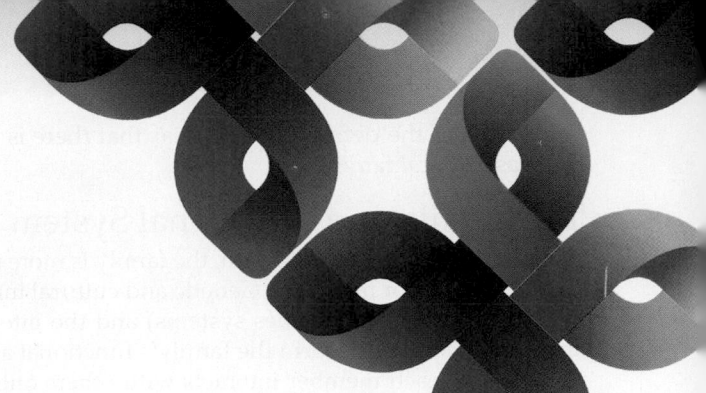

Module 26
Family

Module Outline and Learning Outcomes

The Concept of Family

Normal Presentation

26.1 Outline the makeup of the family structure.

Factors That Shape Family Development

26.2 Summarize the factors that shape family development.

Influence of Parenting on the Family System

26.3 Contrast how differences in parenting styles and strategies affect the family system.

Alterations in Family Function

26.4 Differentiate alterations in family.

Concepts Related to Family

26.5 Outline the relationship between family and other concepts.

Health Promotion

26.6 Explain family health promotion.

Nursing Assessment

26.7 Differentiate common assessment procedures and tests used to examine family.

Independent Interventions

26.8 Analyze independent interventions nurses can implement for patients with alterations in family.

Collaborative Practices

26.9 Summarize collaborative therapies used by interprofessional teams for patients with alterations in family.

Family Exemplar

Exemplar 26.A Family Response to Health Alterations

26.A Analyze family response to health alterations.

>> The Concept of Family

Concept Key Terms

Adolescent family, **1854**
Binuclear family, **1853**
Blended family, **1854**
Childfree family, **1854**
Discipline, **1859**
Ecomap, **1867**

Extended family, **1853**
Extended-kin network family, **1853**
Family, **1851**
Family-centered care, **1852**

Family cohesion, **1857**
Family communication, **1857**
Family coping mechanisms, **1857**
Family development, **1855**

Foster family, **1854**
Genogram, **1868**
Intergenerational family, **1854**
Joint custody, **1853**
Limit setting, **1858**

Nuclear family, **1853**
Punishment, **1859**
Resiliency, **1857**
Single-parent family, **1853**
Two-career family, **1853**

For most individuals, family serves as a primary developmental influence. Numerous family structures exist, from single-parent families to families headed by two mothers or two fathers. Regardless of structural variations, every family is subject to the challenges of life, including economic hardship, illness, and stress. This concept explores the role of the family in terms of development, childrearing, health promotion, and response to alterations in health status. In addition, the nurse's role in caring for the family unit is examined.

Normal Presentation

The Merriam-Webster dictionary gives no fewer than eight definitions of the word *family* (Merriam-Webster Dictionary,

2016). The basic unit of society, family can be defined as a group of people related to each other, by birth, by marriage, or by choice, who may or may not live together in the same household. The head of a family may be a single individual—for example, a grandfather or elder, or a single mother—or a couple who may or may not be married and who may or may not live under the same roof with all members of the family. The U.S. Census Bureau (2012) defines a **family** as two or more individuals who are joined together by marriage, birth, or adoption and are residing in the same household. More broadly, families are generally characterized by bonds of emotional closeness, sharing, and support. Beyond the Census Bureau's definition, there are legal, social, and psychologic definitions that also are commonly recognized.

Regardless of the definition, it is clear that there is no such thing as a *typical* family.

The Family as a Functional System

As with any unit or organization, the family is more than the sum of its parts or members. Genetic and cultural influences (including beliefs and values systems) and the interactions among its members inform the family's functional ability as well as how each member interacts with others outside the family. In other words, within a family, each individual is interconnected with and interdependent on the other members, both as individuals and as a group (Mellins et al., 2015). This is the heart of *family systems theory*. A *system* can be described as a set of parts or elements (or in the case of a family, individuals) that interact purposefully or orderly rather than randomly with each other (von Bertalanffy, 1981). Like any system, the family's purpose or goals are to maintain functioning—a steady state—and to adapt or respond successfully to change. Families that operate as *open systems* are able to exchange information (for example, by discussing and modeling acceptable behaviors) and resources (such as personal energy necessary to accomplish tasks) to meet problems and find solutions. Families that operate as *closed systems* often view change as a threat and have difficulty adapting to or overcoming change (Mellins et al., 2015; Kaakinen & Hanson, 2015).

Precisely because family members are so interconnected and interdependent, when nurses encounter any individual in need of care, they should approach the patient holistically, viewing the patient as part of a whole, as part of the family unit, and not simply as an individual. Consider the following examples:

- Parents caring for a toddler with a chronic illness. What hurdles might the child's parents face? What thoughts or feelings might they have? How might these impact care of other children? Their relationship as parents?

- A family whose oldest child has a serious mental illness, such as schizophrenia or bipolar disorder.

- A family whose main provider is in a motor vehicle crash and sustains significant head trauma.

- A woman who comes for a simple procedure (say, a mammogram or DEXA scan) at 3:30 and is still in the waiting room at 4:30 and must pick up her father from eldercare by 5:00 before picking up her teenager from soccer practice by 5:30.

Consider how even small issues can have a large impact and how the nurse and staff may view the issue differently from the patient, as in the last example provided. These and myriad other issues can impact functioning of the entire family system.

A family generally provides an environment for its members to learn group values, norms, and acceptable behaviors. Support and communication provide a way for families to maintain optimal health and functioning. In a healthy, functional family unit, roles include the following:

- Caring, nurturing, and educating children; teaching children how to get along in the world

- Maintaining the continuity of society by transmitting the family's knowledge, customs, traditions, values, and beliefs to children

- Receiving and giving love

- Preparing children to become productive members of society

- Meeting the needs of its members, including protection and economic support

- Serving as a buffer between family members and environmental and societal demands while advocating or addressing the interests and needs of the individual family members.

Individual family members take on certain social and gender roles and hold a designated status within the family based on the values and beliefs that bind the family together. These values and beliefs may evolve from the family's religious or cultural values and practices, social norms, education, and other influences to which parents were exposed during their childhood, adolescence, and early adult years. Parental roles, including childrearing practices and beliefs, are usually learned through a socialization process that occurs during childhood and adolescence.

Ideally, the family is a child's source of strength and support, the major constant in the child's life. Families are intimately involved in their children's physical and psychologic well-being, and they play a vital role in the health promotion and health maintenance of their children. Parents and children learn specific roles through a socialization process. By respecting the family's role, strengths, and experiences with the healthcare system, nurses have an opportunity to develop an effective partnership with the child and family as they make healthcare decisions that promote the child's health. This partnership between nurses and families is known as **family-centered care**. More recently, recognition of the advantages of involving patient and families across the lifespan directly in their care has resulted in patient- and family-centered care (PFCC). This concept identifies that the healthcare team needs to involve both the patient and the family in making mutually beneficial partnerships for the planning and implementation of healthcare in a variety of settings (Institute for Patient- and Family-Centered Care [IPFCC], 2015). Nursing care of the patient and family is core to nursing practice, and as such necessitates viewing this as a partnership in a comprehensive, holistic manner.

For many families, providing family-centered care also means providing culturally competent care. Families from different cultures are an integral part of North America's rich heritage. Each family has values and beliefs that are unique to its culture of origin and shape the family's structure, methods of interaction, healthcare practices, and coping mechanisms. These factors interact to influence the health of families. Families of a particular culture may cluster to form mutual support systems and to preserve their heritage; however, this practice may isolate them from the larger society (see **Figure 26–1 ≫**).

Diversity in Family Structures and Roles

Families consist of individuals (structure) and their responsibilities within the family (roles). Governmental data are grouped by types of *households*: married couples with children, married couples without children, other family households (single-parent families), men living alone, women living alone, lesbian and gay family households, and other

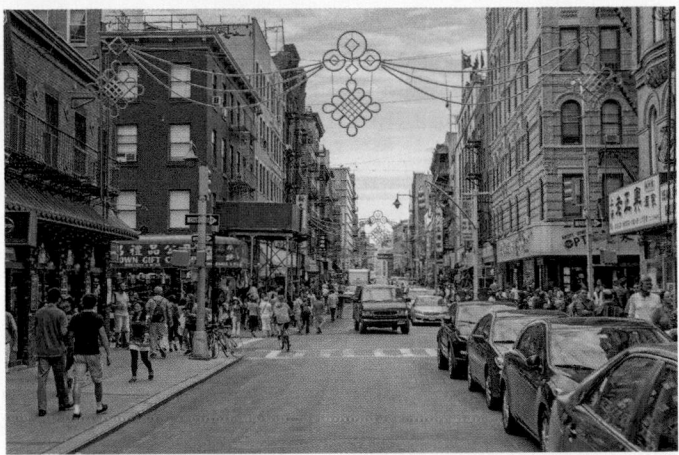

Source: Buffalo_Ghost/iStock/Getty Images.

Figure 26–1 》 An example of cultural clustering can be seen in New York's Chinatown in Manhattan.

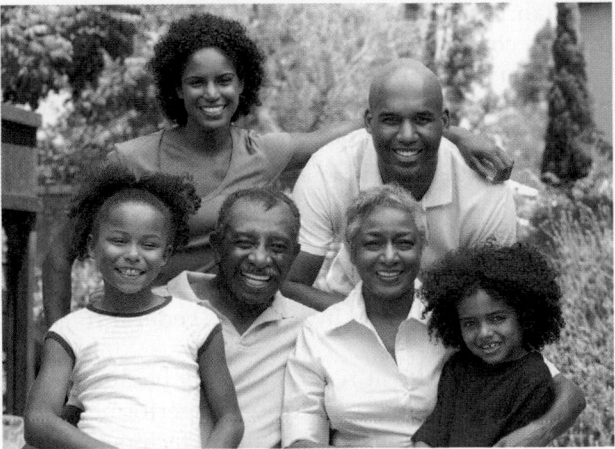

Source: © Monkey Business/Fotolia.

Figure 26–2 》 Three generations of a family enjoying a day in the park.

nonfamily households. Some families live in houses, some in apartments; some live in urban areas, some in rural towns, and some are homeless.

The family protects the physical health of its members by providing adequate nutrition and healthcare services. Family nutritional and lifestyle practices directly affect the developing health attitudes and lifestyle practices of the children. In most cases, the family's economic resources are secured by adult members.

When considering families from the standpoint of the tasks associated with functioning as a unit, many families are similar. However, family units in the United States are diverse in terms of structure and with regard to which family member assumes a given role.

Nuclear Family

A family structure of a mother and father and their offspring is known as the **nuclear family**. In 2014, 64% of children under the age of 18 lived in the same household with two married parents (Federal Interagency Forum on Child and Family Statistics, 2015).

When two biological parents divorce but continue to raise their children in partnership with one another, the family may be referred to as **binuclear**. Children in a binuclear family spend significant time with both parents, often going from one house to the other on a mutually agreed-upon schedule. In **joint custody**, both parents have equal legal rights and responsibility regardless of where the children live. The binuclear family model enables both parents to be involved in the children's upbringing and provides additional support and role models in the form of extended family members. Special nursing considerations in this family type involve ensuring that health promotion guidance and education for care of the child with an acute or chronic condition are communicated effectively to both biological parents.

Extended Family

The relatives of nuclear families, such as grandparents or aunts and uncles, compose the **extended family**. In some families, members of the extended family live with the family (see **Figure 26–2 》**). Although members of the extended family may live in different areas, they may be a source of emotional or financial support for the family. An extended family may share household and childrearing responsibilities with parents, siblings, or other relatives. In 2014, 1.6 million children in the United States lived with a grandparent (U.S. Census Bureau, 2015). Grandparents may raise children because the parents are unable to care for them. Grandparents endure emotional, physical, and financial stresses when taking on the childrearing role for one or more grandchildren.

One example of an extended family is the **extended-kin network family**. This is a specific form of an extended family in which two nuclear families of primary or unmarried kin live in proximity to each other. The family shares a social support network, chores, goods, and services. This type of family model is common in the Latino community. Multigenerational arrangements of this sort are more common in non-U.S. cultures and working-class families.

Two-Career Family

In **two-career families** (or dual-career families), both partners are employed by choice or by necessity. They may or may not have children. Two-career families have steadily increased since the 1960s because of increased career opportunities for women, a desire to increase the family's standard of living, and economic necessity. The U.S. Bureau of Labor Statistics (2012) reported that the percentage of married dual-career families rose to 58.5% in 2011. Two-career families have to address issues related to child care, household chores, and spending time together, with finding good-quality, affordable child care being one of the greatest stressors.

Single-Parent Family

In 2014, just over one-quarter of all children (28%) lived in a **single-parent family**, that is, a family with one parent only (Federal Interagency Forum on Child and Family Statistics, 2015). There are many reasons for single parenthood, including death of a spouse, separation, divorce, birth of a child to an unmarried woman (whether or not the pregnancy was planned), or adoption of a child by a single man or woman. The stresses of single parenthood are many: child care concerns, financial concerns, role overload and fatigue from managing daily tasks, and social isolation. Single-parent families may face difficulties because the sole parent may need assistance with childrearing issues, lack social and emotional support, or have financial issues. Single-parent families experience higher rates of poverty, which has important implications for the children. Poverty is highest among single-parent families headed by women, with 46% living in poverty. Only some 10% of children in married households live in poverty (Federal Interagency Forum, 2015).

Single mothers are at risk for poverty because of lack of child support, unequal pay for work performed, and the high costs of child care. Additional risk factors may include work skill deficiencies and cutbacks in social welfare programs, such as child-care subsidy programs. Nurses working with single parents assess their strengths and needs in providing care to the child, such as after-school and backup child care arrangements that enable the parent to fulfill work commitments. Nurses also determine if the family has access to all resources available to support growth and development, such as school breakfast and lunch programs that provide nutritional support.

Adolescent Family

The birth rate among teenagers peaked in 1991 and has decreased progressively since then to 34.2 births per 1000 women age 15–19 in 2010. This is the lowest birth rate for teenagers reported in more than 70 years (Martin, 2012). Rates are highest among Hispanic and Black females (Hamilton, Mathews, & Ventura, 2013). The parents in **adolescent families** are often developmentally, physically, emotionally, and financially ill prepared to undertake the responsibility of parenthood. Adolescent pregnancies frequently interrupt or stop formal education. Children born to adolescents are often at greater risk for health and social problems.

Foster Family

Children who can no longer live with their birth parents may require placement with a family that has agreed to include them temporarily. The legal agreement between the **foster family** and the court to care for the child includes the expectations of the foster parents and the financial compensation they will receive. A family (with or without its own children) may house more than one foster child at a time or different children over many years. Ideally, at some time the fostered child can either return to the birth parent(s) or be legally and permanently adopted by other parents.

Childfree Family

Childfree families are a growing trend. In some cases a family has no children by choice; in other cases, a family has no children because of issues related to infertility or other medical conditions that present risks to the woman or fetus should the woman become pregnant. According to the U.S. Census Bureau (2015), in 2014, more women in the United States (47.6% of those age 15 to 44) did not have children than at any other time since the government started tracking childbearing.

Blended Family

A **blended family** consists of two parents with biological children from previous relationships. The parents may be married or may cohabit. This family structure has become increasingly common in the United States because of high rates of divorce and remarriage. In 2014, of the 51.06 million children living with two parents in the United States, 8% (4.08 million) lived with a stepparent (U.S. Census Bureau, 2015).

Blended family models have both strengths and challenges. Blended families may have fewer financial issues than single parent homes and may offer a child a new support person and role model. Remarriage also provides a new opportunity for a successful relationship for the parents; however, the relationship between stepparents and stepchildren can be strained. Stresses can include discipline issues, adjustment problems, role ambiguity, strain with the other biological parent, and communication issues. When blended families with children form after the divorce or death of a parent, adjustment can be particularly challenged by the normal processes of grief and loss. An important nursing consideration is to direct families to resources that may help reduce the potential conflicts associated with different parenting styles, discipline, and manipulative behaviors of children that can develop within a blended family.

Intergenerational Family

In some cultures, and as people live longer, more than two generations may live together in an **intergenerational family**. Children may continue to live with their parents even after having their own children, or the grandparents may move in with their grown children's families after some years of living apart. In other situations, a generation is skipped or missing; that is, grandparents live with and care for their grandchildren, but the children's parents are not a part of this family. Many life events and choices can result in this type of family structure.

Cohabiting Family

Cohabiting (or communal) families consist of unrelated individuals or families who live under one roof. This may include never-married individuals as well as divorced or widowed persons. In 2014, 4% of children age 0 to 17 in the United States lived with two unmarried cohabiting parents. Others live with a single parent and a cohabiting partner (Federal Interagency Forum, 2015). Biological children may result from the relationship, or in some cases children of one parent are present and help form a blended cohabiting family.

An important nursing consideration for children who live in informal cohabiting families is that the nonbiological parent has no legal authority to seek emergency medical care for the child. However, in the case of a true emergency that could result in loss of life or diminished functioning, health professionals are obligated to provide care and obtain consent as soon as possible afterward. The nonbiological parent also may not have any knowledge of the child's medical history.

Gay and Lesbian Families

Gay and lesbian families can have all of the structures outlined previously (e.g., married, single parent, blended, intergenerational, cohabitation). They differ in that these families

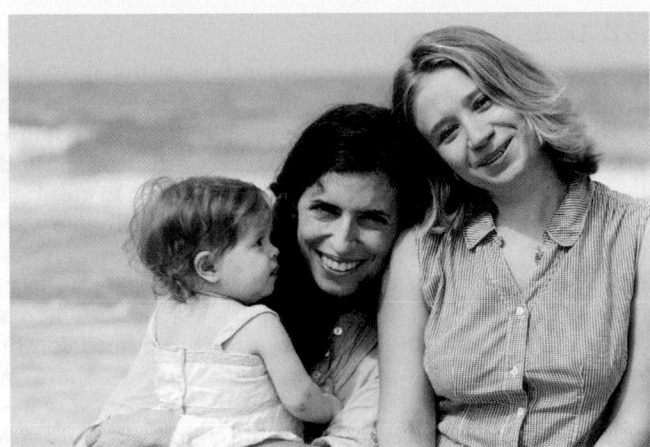

Source: © Dubova/Fotolia.

Figure 26–3 》》 A lesbian couple and their daughter.

have two or more people who share a same-sex orientation (see **Figure 26–3 》》**). Nearly 220,000 children in the United States live in a gay or lesbian household (Gates, 2013). Children in these families may be from a previous heterosexual union, or be born to or adopted by one or both member(s) of the same-sex couple. For example, a biological child may be born to one of the partners through artificial insemination or through a surrogate mother. Lesbian and gay couples function much like heterosexual couples, and children who are adopted or born into the family are highly valued. Although children raised in gay and lesbian families may face unique issues when interacting with peers and when revealing their parents' sexual orientation, they develop sex role orientations and behaviors similar to those of children in the general population.

These children have been found to have the same advantages and expectations for health, adjustment, and development as children born into heterosexual families. Lesbian and gay parents are believed to be as effective as heterosexual couples in providing a supportive and healthy environment for their children (American Academy of Pediatrics, 2013). In addition, Prickett, Martin-Storey, and Crosnoe (2015) reported that fathers of heterosexual marriages spent less time in child-focused activities than fathers of gay marriages. On average, same-sex parents spent 3.5 hours with their children, compared to 2.5 hours in households with a mother and a father.

SAFETY ALERT When obtaining consent to provide healthcare and medical treatments to children and adolescents, the healthcare provider should identify the biological or adoptive parent or confirm a caregiver's possession of legal documentation proving the right to make medical decisions on the child's behalf.

Children in these families typically have only one biological or adoptive legal parent even if they are legally married. In many states, the other partner is the coparent and has no legal parental status. Various states have now taken legislative action to ensure the security of children whose parents are gay or lesbian by guaranteeing access by the second parent to joint adoption rights. Coparent adoption provides for

either parent to give consent for healthcare and make other important decisions on behalf of the child. It also has implications for child custody and financial support in the event the parents separate or a death occurs, ensuring the child's right to a continuing relationship with and financial support from both parents. Nursing considerations for individuals in gay and lesbian families emphasize respect for the relationship between partners and recognition of the nurturing capacity in these families.

Legal issues for same-sex couples are significant and constantly changing. Many, but by no means all, companies and municipalities offer domestic partner benefits to employees. Domestic partner policies extend the same rights and privileges to the partner of a nonmarried employee of the same or opposite gender as would be offered to spouses. Health insurance is an example of a benefit that often is offered under domestic partner policies. California Family Code Section 297–297.5 defines *domestic partners* as "two adults who have chosen to share one another's lives in an intimate and committed relationship of mutual caring" (State of California Franchise Tax Board, 2013). Although numerous state and federal laws have been introduced in the United States to allow or prohibit same-sex marriages or civil unions, same-sex marriages have been legal nationwide since June 26, 2015. The nurse may find it challenging to keep current on how such legislation affects healthcare issues such as insurance coverage and the right to consent for healthcare.

》》 Stay Current: To view the up-to-date legislative policies on adoption by state, visit this website: www.childwelfare.gov/systemwide/laws_policies/state.

Single Adults Living Alone

Individuals who live by themselves represent a significant portion of today's society. According to the U.S. Census, in 2013, 27% of adults lived alone (U.S. Census Bureau, 2013). Singles include young self-supporting adults who have recently left their family of origin as well as older adults living alone. Young adults typically move in and out of living situations and may have membership in the family, nonfamily-household, and living-alone categories at different times. Older adults may find themselves single through divorce, separation, or the death of a spouse, but generally remain living alone for the remainder of their lives, especially women.

Stages of Family Development

Family development refers to the dynamics or changes that a family experiences over time, including changes in relationships, communication patterns, roles, and interactions. Although each family is unique, the members go through a set of fairly predictable changes. For example, Duvall (1977) developed an eight-stage family life cycle that describes the developmental process each family encounters. This model is based on the nuclear family (see **Table 26–1 》》**). The oldest child serves as a marker for the family's developmental stages except in the last two stages, when children are no longer present. Couples with more than one child may find themselves in overlapping stages, with developmental advances occurring simultaneously.

TABLE 26–1 Eight-Stage Family Life Cycle

Stage	Characteristics
Stage I	Beginning family, newly married couples*
Stage II	Childbearing family (oldest child is an infant through 30 months of age)
Stage III	Families with preschool children (oldest child is between 2.5 and 6 years of age)
Stage IV	Families with schoolchildren (oldest child is between 6 and 13 years of age)
Stage V	Families with teenagers (oldest child is between 13 and 20 years of age)
Stage VI	Families launching young adults (all children leave home)
Stage VII	Middle-aged parents (empty nest through retirement)
Stage VIII	Family in retirement and old age (retirement to death of both spouses)

*Keep in mind that this was the norm at the time the model was developed, but today families form through many different types of relationships.

Sources: Data from Duvall, E. M. (1977). *Marriage and family development* (5th ed.). Philadelphia, PA: Lippincott; Duvall, E. M., & Miller, B. C. (1985). *Marriage and family development* (6th ed.). New York, NY: Harper Row; Friedman, M. M., Bowden, V. R., & Jones, E. G. (2003). *Family nursing: Research, theory, and practice* (5th ed.). Upper Saddle River, NJ: Prentice Hall; Coehlo, D. P. (2015). Family child health nursing. In J. R. Kaakinen, D. P. Coehlo, R. Steele, A. Tabacco, & S. M. H. Hanson (Eds.), *Family health care nursing: Theory, practice, and research* (5th ed., pp. 387–432). Philadelphia, PA: F. A. Davis.

Other family development models have been developed to address the stages and developmental tasks facing the unattached young adult, the gay and lesbian family, those who divorce, and those who remarry.

Choosing to become a parent is a major life change for adults. Beginning when they first learn they are expecting a child (whether through pregnancy or adoption), parents experience stresses and challenges along with feelings of pride and excitement. Mothers and fathers adjust their lifestyles to give priority to parenting. Babies and very young children are dependent for total care 24 hours a day, and this often results in sleep deprivation, irritability, less personal time, and less time for the couple's relationship. In addition, the family with a new baby often experiences a change in financial status. Families progress in their development. Children grow up and, in many cases, initiate new generations of the family. Parents grow older, seeing their children leave the "nest" and progressing toward retirement. Factors that affect how families adjust to each stage include family communication patterns, resiliency, and parenting styles. These and other factors are outlined later in this module.

The family, like the individual, has developmental stages and tasks. Each new stage brings change, requiring adaptation; each stage also brings family-related risk factors for alterations in health and wellness. The nurse must consider the patient's needs both at specific developmental stages and within a family with specific developmental tasks.

Factors That Shape Family Development

Changes in the family structure, function, and processes can alter family development. These changes generally occur over time and may be planned or unplanned.

Cultural Practices

Family assessment requires consideration of the ages of all family members, as well as the cultural practices of the family. The age of the child or children will influence the family dynamic; for example, tasks associated with raising a toddler are vastly different from those pertinent to raising a teenager. Family activities and interaction will also vary depending on the age of the child. For example, when raising a toddler, a majority of the parents' focus may be on meeting the child's developmental and social needs, whereas a teenager will generally work to meet these needs on his own, and the parental roles incorporate guiding the teenager in making life choices.

Cultural practices may influence the child's diet, behavior, and even sleep patterns. Some cultural and religious traditions may involve vegetarianism (see **Figure 26–4))**), while others may involve periods of fasting. The manner in which a child is expected to behave in public and at home can be impacted by culture, as can the child's degree of respect for older adults. Culture can also affect the behavior of the entire family unit depending on matriarchal or patriarchal views. For example, in a matriarchal structure, the mother may be expected to take responsibility for making family healthcare decisions, to the near exclusion of the father and children. Although it is neither realistic nor necessary for the nurse to be an expert on each culture's beliefs, through open and

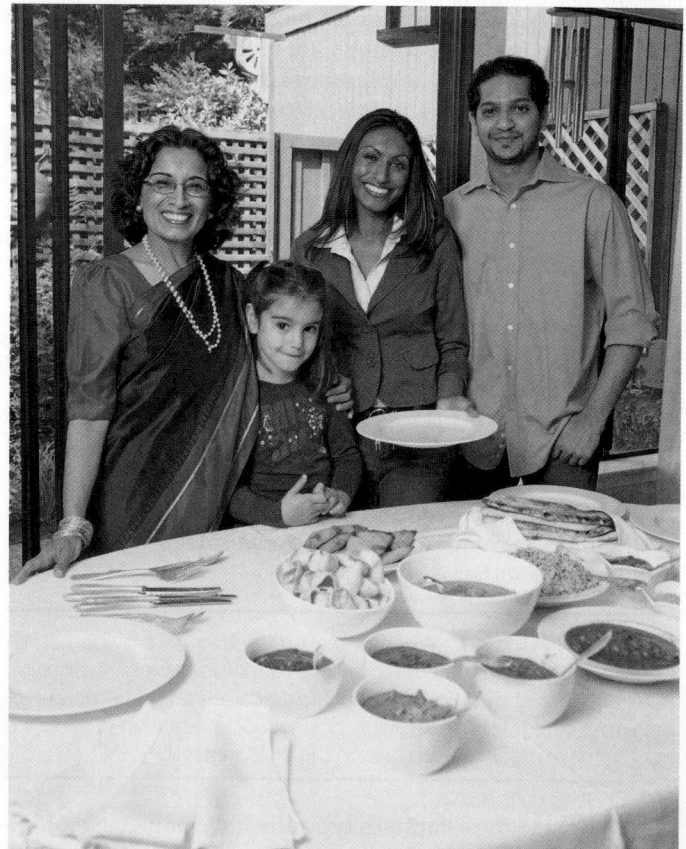

Source: Tanya Constantine/Blend Images/Getty Images.

Figure 26–4)) This extended family of Indian Americans are vegetarians In keeping with their Hindu religion's concept of nonviolence against all life forms.

nonjudgmental communication, the nurse can ascertain a great deal about the family's cultural influences.

Emotional Availability

Healthy coping among family members occurs when all members feel safe expressing their feelings—positive and negative—and the emotional environment of the family is one of respect, closeness, and predictability. Predictability refers to the inclusion of family routines on which family members can depend and in which they find comfort. Examples include a reasonably regular schedule of activities (e.g., reading before bed and a consistent bedtime). In a family with healthy coping, members are emotionally available to each other—that is, they have healthy emotional connections (Saunders, Kraus, Barone, & Biringen, 2015). Emotional availability is correlated to parenting ability (Yousafzai et al., 2015). Emotionally available parents are sensitive to their children's needs without being intrusive, provide structure for learning and exploration without exceeding the child's abilities, and are available but not interfering or hostile. These behaviors encourage child responsiveness, respect, and willingness to interact with parents and other family members (Biringen et al., 2014).

Family Communication Patterns

Family communication is a key factor in family development. Clear communication, problem solving, and sharing feelings associated with events within the family can help families achieve a high level of functioning and increase resilience (Walsh, 2016).

The effectiveness of family communication determines the family's ability to function as a cooperative, growth-producing unit. Messages are constantly being communicated among family members, both verbally and nonverbally. The information transmitted influences how members work together, fulfill their assigned roles in the family, incorporate family values, and develop skills to function in society. Intrafamily communication plays a significant role in the development of self-esteem, which is necessary for the growth of personality.

Family Cohesion

Family cohesion is defined as the emotional bonding between family members. Cohesion among family members can be visualized on a continuum from disengaged (very low cohesion and independence) to enmeshed (very high cohesion and dependence). A family unit may be very cohesive. In addition, there may be very cohesive or very disengaged dyadic or triadic relationships within the family. *Dyadic* refers to the dynamics in a relationship between two people; *triadic* to the dynamics among three people. For example, a dynamic triad may develop between one parent and two children when the other parent is called out of town for work and therefore absent on a regular basis.

Family Coping Mechanisms

Family coping mechanisms are the behaviors families use to deal with stress or changes imposed from either within or without the family. Coping mechanisms can be viewed as an active method of problem solving developed to meet life's challenges. The coping mechanisms families and family members develop reflect their individual resourcefulness. Families may use coping patterns rather consistently over time or may change their coping strategies when new demands are made on the family. The success of a family largely depends on how well it copes with the stresses it experiences.

Nurses working with families realize the importance of assessing coping mechanisms as a way of determining how families relate to stress. The resources available to the family also are important. Internal resources, such as knowledge, skills, effective communication patterns, and a sense of mutuality and purpose within the family, assist in the problem-solving process. In addition, external support systems promote coping and adaptation. These external systems may be extended family, friends, religious affiliations, healthcare professionals, or social service agencies. The development of social support systems is particularly valuable today because many families, because of stress, mobility, or poverty, are isolated from the resources that would traditionally have helped them cope with stress.

Family Size

The size of the family may influence the amount of attention parents are able to give individual children. In small families, parents often have more time to give attention to the children, encourage achievement, meet family expectations, and support involvement in community activities. In larger families, children may receive less personal attention from parents and turn to others in the family for needed support. Family finances may be more limited, which may help children learn about budgeting. Children may adopt a specialized family role to gain recognition, such as "the responsible one," "the clown," or "the black sheep." Children in larger families are encouraged to be cooperative to support family functioning.

Parent–Child Interaction

The qualities of family relationships and behaviors are important aspects of family strengths and functioning. Positive family relationships are characterized by parent–child warmth and supportiveness. Warm parent–child relationships can buffer children from stress and promote positive cognitive and social outcomes. Parents who are warm and place high demands on their children for appropriate behavior have children who tend to be content, self-reliant, self-controlled, and open to learning in school.

Mothers and fathers both contribute to the psychologic, emotional, and social health and development of their children. Both parents provide affection, nurturing, and comfort. They teach children life skills and healthy lifestyles. Both mothers and fathers promote the social competence, academic achievement, and problem-solving abilities of their children. More information on how parenting influences family development can be found later in this module.

Resiliency

Another factor important in shaping a family is the amount of **resiliency** the family has. Having resources and adaptive abilities increases the resilience of a family, thus helping them to overcome adversity, heal from adverse experiences, and progress beyond adversity to fulfillment (Walsh, 2016).

Life crises and developmental transitions can stimulate family growth and transformation. Resilient families make it through crises such as disability and death with a renewed sense of confidence and purpose. A qualitative study conducted by Ellis, Gergen, and Wohlgemuth (2016) found three factors that enhanced resilience in families who were dealing with long-term surgical stays: communication, expectations, and support. In addition, routine and consistent communication between all members of the healthcare team with all family members was one of the most prominent factors that enhanced resiliency. Allowing the family to support their family members through providing basic care or through identifying unique needs of their family member was seen as a supportive action to increase resilience.

Sibling Relationships

Siblings are a child's first peers, and siblings often have a lifelong relationship. Siblings, especially those of the same gender or who are close in age, tend to have a close relationship because they often share many common experiences through childhood and adolescence (see **Figure 26–5 》**).

Sibling rivalry between children exists at times in all families. Within the family, children learn to share, compete, and compromise with siblings. Some siblings take on roles such as protector, problem solver, friend, and supporter for dealing with issues in the family and in the environment. Some siblings learn to work well together to maintain privacy or to form a coalition for negotiating with the parents. An older sibling helps reinforce rules and roles in the family by prompting and inhibiting certain patterns of behavior in the younger siblings. However, one sibling may test the waters by breaking a previously implicit rule to determine what rule flexibility is allowed in the family.

Studies indicate that birth order may have an impact on intelligence, but it does not have an impact on personality. Using a within-family study design, Bleske-Rechek and Kelley (2013) identified that when evaluating five areas (openness, conscientiousness, extraversion, agreeableness, and neuroticism), parents did not see any difference in these traits

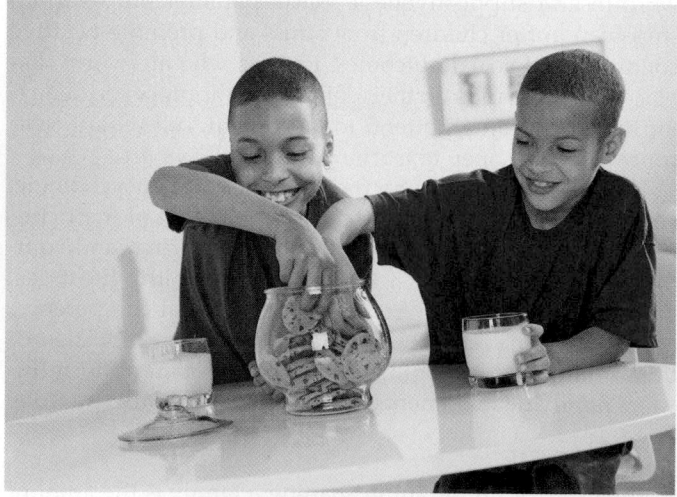

Source: Andersen Ross/Blend Images/Getty Images.

Figure 26–5 》 Same-gender siblings who are close in age tend to have close, lifelong relationships.

between their first- and last-born children as a function of their birth order. These authors conclude that the differences in personality may be due to genetic predispositions of the child and differences in environments that siblings do not necessarily share, such as peer groups. In a large study conducted on databases from Germany, Great Britain, and the United States (N = 20,186) using a within-family and between-family design, Rohrer, Egloff, and Schmukle (2015) found no differences in birth order in the following traits: extraversion, emotional stability, agreeableness, conscientiousness, and imagination. However, there was a small difference in self-reported intellect in this study.

Influence of Parenting on the Family System

Raising a family can be a difficult task. Every day, parents must balance change within the family, their role as parents, and the delicate nature of reward and stress when dealing with their children. Being flexible within the context of parenting is referred to as parenting flexibility (Moyer & Sandoz, 2014). Being able to deal with stressful issues without the need to control psychologic experiences can help the child to learn to cope and can provide the necessary structure for the parent–child relationship and the family unit to thrive.

Parenting Styles

Parents have responsibility for providing children stability through nurturance, safety, and structure in a family that undergoes frequent changes over time. The child needs to have physical and emotional space to grow and develop. Parents also provide their children with the values, beliefs, rituals, and behaviors learned and transmitted across family generations.

To be successful, parents should implement reasonable, consistent **limit setting** (established rules or guidelines for behavior) on children's autonomy while the children are still learning values and self-control. At the same time, parents need to foster their children's curiosity, initiative, and sense of competence. Parents use different styles to parent their children. Parental warmth and control are two major factors that are important in children's development. Parental warmth refers to the amount of affection and approval displayed. Parental control refers to how restrictive the parents are regarding rules. See **Table 26–2 》** for the characteristics associated with parental warmth and control.

Hughes (2013) identified four parenting styles. These include authoritarian, authoritative, permissive, and neglectful. Although families generally tend to use one style, they may vary their style for certain situations. Although helicopter parenting has not been identified as a specific and separate parenting style, research in this area is increasing. An overview of helicopter parenting can be found in **Box 26–1 》**.

Authoritarian Parents

Authoritarian parents tend to be punitive and adhere to rigid rules, or to be more dictatorial. This style sets firm limits, and those limits or rules are not negotiable or open to any discussion. Parents expect family beliefs and principles to be accepted without question. Children have no opportunity to

TABLE 26–2 Characteristics of Significant Parenting Attributes

Parenting Attribute	Parental Warmth	Parental Control
High level	■ Warm, nurturing ■ Expressing affection and smiling at children frequently ■ Limiting criticism, punishment ■ Expressing approval of child	■ Restrictive control of behavior ■ Surveying and enforcing compliance with rules ■ Encouraging children to fulfill their responsibilities ■ Sometimes limiting freedom of expression
Low level	■ Cool, hostile ■ Quick to criticize or punish ■ Ignoring children ■ Rarely expressing affection or approval ■ Sometimes rejecting children	■ Permissive, minimally controlling ■ Making fewer demands ■ Making fewer restrictions on behavior or expression of emotion ■ Permitting freedom in exploring environment

participate in the family decision-making process. Children with authoritarian parents do not develop the skills to examine why a certain behavior is desirable or how their actions might influence others.

Authoritative Parents

Authoritative parents use firm control to set limits, but they establish an atmosphere with open discussion or are more democratic than authoritarian parents. Limits for behavior are clear, consistent, and reasonable, but the children are encouraged to talk about why certain behaviors occurred and how the situations might be handled differently another time. Parents set and stick to established routines, so children have clear expectations of appropriate behavior. Authoritative parents provide explanations about inappropriate behaviors at a child's level of understanding. Children are allowed to express their opinions and objections, and some flexibility is permitted when appropriate. However, parents make it clear that they are the ultimate authority for

decisions. Children with authoritative parents develop a sense of social responsibility because they converse about their responsibilities and approaches.

Permissive Parents

Permissive parents show a great deal of warmth, but set few controls or restraints on the children's behavior. Parents are so intent on showing unconditional love that they fail to perform some important parenting functions. Children are allowed to regulate their own behavior. Discipline is inconsistent, and parents may threaten punishment but not follow through. Because the parents do not impose any controls on the children, the children end up controlling the parents.

Neglectful Parents

Neglectful parents do not display much interest in their children or in their roles as parents. They do not demonstrate affection or approval of their children, and they do not set limits or controls on them. This may occur because they do not care, or because their lives are so stressed that they have no time or energy left for the children.

Discipline and Limit Setting

Discipline is a method for teaching children the rules for how to behave in society and what is expected in different circumstances. **Punishment** is the action taken to enforce the rules when the child misbehaves. Parenting styles play an important role in the type of discipline and punishment parents use with children. When clear limits are set and consistently maintained, as with authoritative parenting, punishment may be needed less often. Limit setting and firm control of those limits are important discipline methods that allow children to learn to what extent they can safely and independently operate within the environment. Firm limits also help children feel secure; they are reassured by consistency and the sense of protection the limits are perceived to provide. Punishment helps children learn that misbehavior has consequences and may affect other individuals. This helps children develop a sense of responsibility for their behavior.

Alterations in Family Function

Any number of situations or factors can cause short- or long-term alterations in family function. Trauma, abuse, neglect, addiction, criminal activity, and military deployment are

---

Box 26–1
Helicopter Parenting

Overparenting, often referred to as helicopter parenting, refers to the overinvolvement of parents in their children's lives. A survey of 128 school counselors, teachers, and mental health professionals (Locke, Campbell, & Kavanagh, 2012) elicited a number of examples of overparenting behaviors, such as:

■ Low expectations and demands for children to develop independence, proceed along developmental milestones, or accept consequences for their actions
■ Constant monitoring, phoning, and intrusiveness in the child's life
■ A perception that their child is always right
■ Constant instruction regarding behavior, an intense focus on academics, and restriction of experiences with peers.

Although the effects of overparenting are still being studied and may vary from one child to the next, overparenting has been positively associated with increased parental anxiety. Among young adults and adults who experienced overparenting growing up, the overinvolvement of their parents was associated with an increase in ineffective coping skills, which in turn was associated with greater anxiety (Segrin et al., 2013).

Patient Teaching
Guidelines for Promoting Acceptable Behavior in Children

The nurse can assist parents in handling their child's misbehavior by helping them to:

- Set realistic expectations and directions for behavior based on the child's age and understanding; consistently enforce the expected directions and behaviors.

- Focus on promoting appropriate and desirable behaviors in the child.

- Model or suggest appropriate behavior.

- Review expected behavior for special situations, such as a family party, going to the movies, or other social event.

- Praise or reward the child using appropriate behaviors.

- Tell the child about his or her inappropriate behavior as soon as it begins, and offer guidelines for changing behavior or provide a distraction.

- When reprimanding the child, focus on the behavior rather than stating that the child is bad. Explain how the behavior is inappropriate and how it makes you, as the parent, and any other person involved feel. Avoid ridicule or accusation that can take the form of shame or criticism, because these actions can affect the child's self-esteem if repeated often enough. Stay calm.

- Remember that loud volume (yelling) is meant to warn of danger. Parents who discipline kindly have more success than those who discipline in anger or frustration.

- Be alert for situations when the child could misbehave, such as when tired or overexcited. Use a distraction to persuade or calm the child.

- Help children gain self-control with friendly reminders (e.g., count to 3, as soon as the clothes are on the doll, as soon as you finish the game) regarding the timing for transition to the next event of the day, such as bedtime, putting the toys away, or washing hands before dinner.

---

just a few of these situations. Resilient families may overcome such situations with time, patience, and understanding, and family and social support. Whenever a family experiences some kind of upheaval or alteration to family functioning, nurses assess for safety, coping mechanisms, and immediate and long-term needs, as well as providing support and making referrals as appropriate.

Abuse

Interpersonal (domestic) violence and child abuse and neglect have long-term implications for children and families. In addition to the risks of physical injury and even death, children who grow up with violence or neglect are at greater risk for delinquency, substance abuse, mental illness, and lower school achievement (Federal Interagency Forum, 2015). More information on the effects of abuse on children and families can be found in the module on Trauma.

Death of a Family Member

Death of an immediate family member can interrupt and even permanently alter family functioning and processes in a number of ways. The death of a parent brings both financial and practical concerns to the family as well as profound emotional loss. Loss of income and loss of another adult to assist with transportation to child care, school, doctor's appointments, and extracurricular activities combine to create new burdens for the remaining parent. In divorced families, death of a custodial parent can result in children relocating to new homes and schools. Death of a child has been identified as one of the most stressful events in an adult's life. For adults, death of a parent can result in an array of emotions and may also result in an adult child finding himself caring for the remaining parent, if the parent who died was a caregiver to the other parent.

Divorce

Nearly half of all children in the United States will experience the divorce of their parents (Anthony, DiPerna, & Amato, 2014). When the divorce is preceded by long periods of stress and tension between the parents, the family may experience some level of disruption or dysfunction well in advance of the actual divorce. Children may experience guilt in the form of feeling they did something that caused the divorce. If the divorce results in the children seeing significantly less of one parent, one or more of the children may experience feelings of abandonment. Young children especially may fear abandonment by the remaining parent. Divorce can bring disruption to daily schedules and even result in children changing schools or moving to another city or state. Children who lived in a stable household with both parents may find themselves moving in with grandparents or moving to another house or apartment. Disruptions associated with divorce can result in child adjustment, academic, or behavior problems (Arkes, 2015).

Effects of Stigma on Gay and Lesbian Families

In *Accelerating Acceptance 2016*, conducted by GLAAD, the authors report their findings of surveys conducted among non-LGBTQ Americans on their degree of acceptance of LGBTQ individuals. Between 27 and 32% of Americans reported they would feel either somewhat uncomfortable or very uncomfortable on learning a family member was LGBTQ. The stigma and discrimination that LGBTQ individuals in Americans feel is real, and it affects both LGBTQ individuals and their families.

Family Rejection of LGBTQ Youth

LGBTQ youth experience disparities in both physical and mental health compared to their heterosexual peers. This has significant implications for both the medical and the larger community, because some 3.2 million American youth age 8 to 18 identify as LGBTQ (Mallory et al., 2014). Factors cited as contributing to the increased risk of physical and mental illness among LGBTQ youth include rejection by families and peers and inadequate school and community supports (Mallory et al., 2014).

The significance of the role of the family in the health of the LGBTQ child or adolescent cannot be overstated. Compared with LGBTQ youth whose families were more accepting, youth who were rejected by their families were more than 8 times as likely to attempt suicide, almost 6 times as likely to report high levels of depression, more than 3 times as likely to report illegal drug use, and at much greater risk for acquiring HIV/AIDS and other sexually transmitted illnesses (Anonymous, n.d.).

Nurses working with families with an LGBTQ child or adolescent can support both the youth and the family by:

- Providing information on LGBTQ resources in the area
- Encouraging open, respectful communication among all family members
- Encouraging parents to allow their child access to LGBTQ friends and resources
- Helping the family understand that the young person is not to blame for any stigma the family experiences
- Encouraging the parents to talk with their child about her identity in an affirming manner
- Advocating in their communities for increased resources and support for LGBTQ children and adolescents.

LGBTQ Parents

Among the American media, there is an increased focus on LGBTQ parenting and on the specific question of whether children are worse off being raised by same-sex parents than by two heterosexual parents. A team of researchers reviewed the results of the 2011–2012 National Survey of Children's Health. They reviewed the responses of 95 female same-sex parent households with the responses of 95 different-sex parent households, with all households having children between 6 and 17 years old. No differences were observed in family relationships or child health outcomes, although the same-sex parents reported experiencing higher levels of parenting stress (Bos et al., 2016). As outlined earlier, parenting style and involvement, not the sexual attraction of the parents, seems to be the most important for child outcomes. However, children in gay and lesbian families may be at risk because of how they are treated by those in their communities. Nurses should be aware of support groups or other services to assist children in LGBTQ families who are misunderstood in their community.

Incarcerated Parents

The United States has 707 incarcerated people per 100,000 citizens and is the world leader in incarceration (American Psychological Association [APA], 2014). Children of incarcerated parents face many disadvantages that affect their emotional, physical, and mental health. Lee, Fang, and Luo (2013) identified that depression, anxiety, cholesterol, overall poor health, asthma, posttraumatic stress disorder (PTSD), migraines, and HIV were significantly associated with parental incarceration. Turney and Wildeman (2013) found that having an incarcerated father negatively impacted the relationship between the children and the

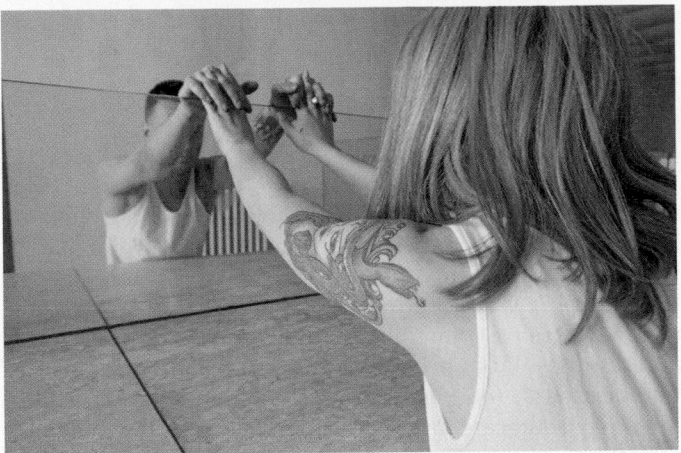

Source: C_FOR/ iStock/Getty Images.

Figure 26–6 ❯❯ Visiting day in prison is difficult for the incarcerated partner and the one left behind to care for the family.

father, as well as between the mother and the father. Separation and divorce are not uncommon when the father of the family is incarcerated and the mother is left to care for the children and take on the role responsibilities of the father (see **Figure 26–6 ❯❯**). In addition, all family members may be affected if the mother finds a new partner (Turney & Wildeman, 2013).

Military Deployment

Since the terrorist attack on September 11, 2001, many families have experienced having their loved ones deployed to Iraq, Afghanistan, and elsewhere. According to the Department of Defense, nearly 2 million children have at least one parent in the military (Department of Defense [DoD], 2012). Trautman, Alhusen, and Gross (2015) indicate that parental deployment is associated with increases in depressive symptoms, increased levels of parental stress, poorer general well-being, and greater use of mental health services (see **Figure 26–7 ❯❯**). Children have been shown to be at increased

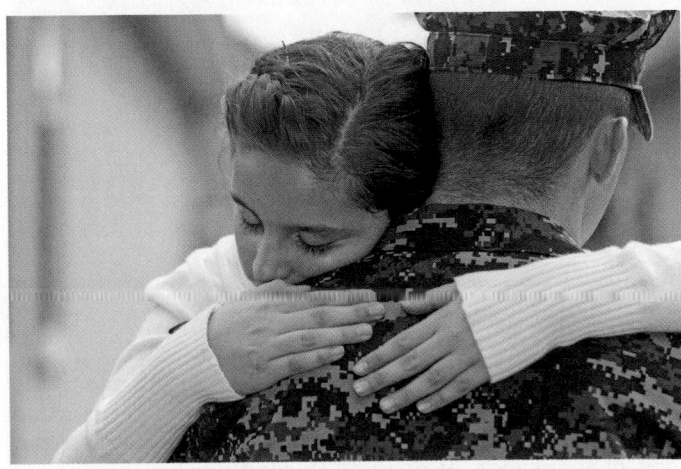

Source: Kali9/E+/Getty Images.

Figure 26–7 ❯❯ Parental military deployment puts children at increased risk for behavioral and emotional problems.

risk for behavioral and emotional problems and child maltreatment (Trautman et al., 2015).

Poverty

For 2013, the U.S. poverty threshold for a family of four with two children was $23,624. That same year, 20% of children lived below this threshold. Nearly half of these lived in families with extreme poverty. Extreme poverty is defined as below 50% of the poverty threshold (Federal Interagency Forum, 2015).

Poverty is associated with poor outcomes for children and families. First, it is linked with substandard housing, homelessness, food insecurity and malnutrition, lack of access to healthcare, unsafe neighborhoods, and inadequate school environments. Consider the issue of access to healthcare. Some may dismiss that as a nonissue because of the existence of Medicaid and Child Health Insurance Programs. But what of the child who lives in a rural area whose parent or parents does not have a car? That family's ability to access healthcare and other resources will be limited.

In children, poverty is associated with an array of short- and long-term consequences. The chronic stress of living in poverty leads to impaired concentration and memory. Poverty is also associated with lower academic achievement, increased dropout rates, increased risk for behavioral and emotional problems, and increased risk for physical illness (American Psychological Association [APA], 2016).

Trauma

When one or more family members experiences a traumatic event, it can upset the rhythms and relationships in the whole household and deplete individual and family coping mechanisms (see **Figure 26–8 >>**). Coping with

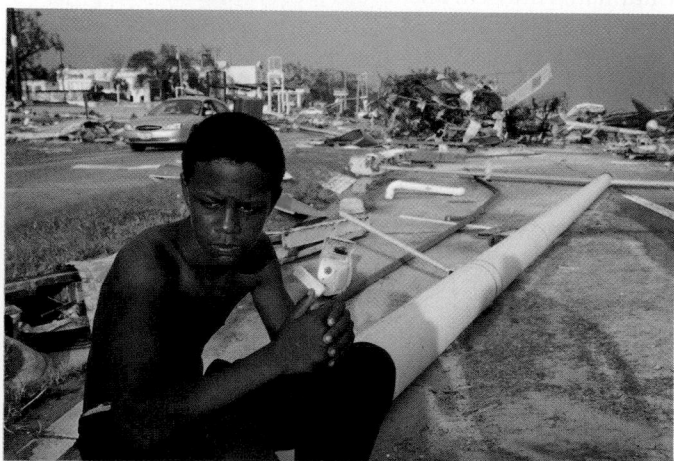

Source: Marvi Lacar/Getty Images News/Getty Images.

Figure 26–8 >> This 12-year-old boy sits at the site of his home in Biloxi, Mississippi, that was destroyed in Hurricane Katrina. In the year after Katrina struck, it is estimated that tens of thousands of children missed weeks, months, or even a full year of school. Many moved away from home never to return. Children from more fragile families are more likely to be traumatized and are more likely to recover slowly (Reckdahl, 2015).

trauma and its aftermath can leave little time and energy for the parents to initiate normal family activities or to provide comfort to children and other family members. Children who experience trauma are at risk for trauma-related problems and disorders that disrupt functioning (National Child Traumatic Stress Network, 2011; American Psychiatric Association, 2013).

Case Study >> Part 1

Maria Rodriguez, age 30, and her wife Daniella Marshall, age 32, were recently married and decided to start a family. Following donor insemination, Mrs. Rodriguez became pregnant. The couple arrives at the obstetrician's office for Mrs. Rodriguez's routine health exam. You are familiar with the couple and have provided care to them in the past. Today, you are assigned to care for Mrs. Rodriguez, who is now at 7 months' gestation. After talking to the couple for a few minutes, you notice that Mrs. Rodriguez is more reserved than usual and seems a bit depressed. When you ask how things are coming along with planning for the new arrival, both women are silent. Finally, Mrs. Marshall explains that they are struggling to cope with reactions from other participants of the birthing classes they have been attending, and it is making them both more stressed. Mrs. Rodriguez then tells you that she no longer wishes to attend the birthing classes, even though Mrs. Marshall wishes to complete the course.

Clinical Reasoning Questions Level I

1. What additional information would be useful in assessing the challenges faced by Mrs. Rodriguez and Mrs. Marshall?
2. Which characteristics of communication would best promote open discussion between you and this couple?
3. What are some societal challenges that same-sex couples face?

Clinical Reasoning Questions Level II

4. Describe two nursing diagnoses that may be applicable in the care of Mrs. Rodriguez and Mrs. Marshall.
5. What are some of the dangers of stress at this stage in Mrs. Rodriguez's pregnancy?
6. Explain some of the benefits of birthing classes in terms of both safe delivery of the child and family planning.

Concepts Related to Family

Any number of concepts can influence family dynamics. For example, when an individual suffers from addiction to illegal substances or alcohol, his addictive behaviors are likely to affect close family members in a number of ways. Life-threatening health conditions can result in anticipatory grieving, loss of financial security, and caregiver burden, increasing the stresses with which families cope on a daily basis. Alternatively, the birth of a child can result in the strengthening or weakening of bonds and relationships within the family. Family members may be drawn closer through shared interests in the welfare of the child. Conversely, the addition of a new family member can add financial and emotional stressors that strain familial relationships.

Culture and spirituality inform the lifestyles and decision-making process of many families. It is important to note, however, that even within a single family, individual members may engage in different beliefs and practices or

Alterations and Therapies
Family

ALTERATION	DESCRIPTION	MANIFESTATIONS	INTERVENTIONS AND THERAPIES
Abuse	Physical, emotional, or sexual abuse directed toward another individual	▪ Withdrawn emotions and a decrease in communication and/or socialization with family and friends ▪ Behavioral changes, such as anger, depression, acting out in school or at home, and changes in appetite or sleep patterns ▪ Bruises, broken bones, concussion, and other physical markers ▪ Fear of a specific person or situation (e.g., family events, arguments, school dances)	▪ Follow state laws and agency policies and procedures regarding the reporting of abuse and neglect. ▪ Treat physical injuries (e.g., broken bones, cuts, concussions) and emphasize the importance of follow-up care. ▪ Offer resources for emotional manifestations, for example, counseling or therapy. ▪ Provide proficient, nonjudgmental patient care.
Divorce	The separation of a couple from a marital bond with or without children	▪ Anxiety ▪ Depression ▪ Stress and resulting manifestations such as restlessness, weight loss, headaches, and sleeplessness ▪ Behavioral modifications in children (e.g., acting out in school, withdrawal, anger, confusion, nightmares)	▪ Provide information about counseling, therapy, and support groups. ▪ Advise about healthy coping mechanisms for stress—for example, exercise, new hobbies, and writing. ▪ Educate about the importance of health maintenance and nutrition even during times of high stress and anxiety.
Death of family member	The loss of a spouse, child, parent, or other family member	▪ Grief as evidenced by sadness, anger, denial, and pain associated with the loss ▪ Depression manifested in a lack of enjoyment of normal activities, intense feelings of sadness, and changes in appetite ▪ Sleeplessness ▪ Weight loss or weight gain ▪ Anxiety	▪ Provide information about therapy and support groups. ▪ Teach about healthy coping strategies. ▪ Assess for signs of complicated or traumatic grief. ▪ Facilitate referrals to grief counselors and other professional resources.
LGBTQ family member	Some 3.2 million children and youth identify as LGBTQ. Some 220,000 children live in households with same-sex parents.	▪ Shame, fear, anxiety, isolation associated with stigma and discrimination ▪ Homelessness ▪ Suicide	▪ Assess for safety and shelter, other supports. ▪ Honor preferences regarding names and titles. ▪ Promote family communication.
Incarceration	One or both parents are in jail for varying lengths of time	▪ Separation from one or both parents ▪ Possibility of repartnering of parent who is left to raise children ▪ Increase in physical and emotional concerns	▪ Facilitate communication with family counselor. ▪ Recognize changes in child's behavior indicating they are not coping with the situation. ▪ Provide nonjudgmental care and assistance.
Military deployment	Family with one or more members deployed from home (domestic or overseas deployment)	▪ Frequent separations and reunions ▪ Frequent family relocations ▪ Social considerations related to rank ▪ Lack of control over progress in employment, promotion	▪ Encourage and promote open family communication, use of alternative communication methods (e.g., video messaging, email). ▪ Assist family to identify previously helpful coping strategies. ▪ Encourage participation in social and community supports and activities. ▪ Assist family members in mutual goal setting.
Poverty	Individuals and families living near or below the federally designated poverty threshold.	▪ Overall poor health ▪ Increased stress ▪ Altered child development ▪ Increased risk for chronic illness	▪ Provide and encourage use of available resources. ▪ Identify support groups. ▪ Monitor child growth and development.

Concepts Related to
Family

CONCEPT	RELATIONSHIP TO FAMILY	NURSING IMPLICATIONS
Addiction	Substance and/or alcohol abuse can affect individual family members as well as the family unit as a whole. Potential stressors may be psychosocial, physiologic, financial, or spiritual in nature.	■ Be alert to the signs of addiction. ■ Propose interventions appropriate to addiction behavior. ■ Evaluate the individual's potential for being a danger to herself or others. ■ Recommend community resources to family members to help them process and cope with resultant complications.
Culture and Diversity	Cultural beliefs and practices may vary even among generations of the same family. They may impact decision-making processes, how patients and families view procedures, and day-to-day patient and family needs.	■ Explore meaning of culture and diversity as it impacts each family. ■ Identify resources available for families who are diverse or from a different culture.
Grief and Loss	Grief and loss may result in alterations in family dynamics, particularly if the deceased individual was in a position of family leadership or was the primary source of financial support. Grief reactions can also affect how family members relate to one another.	■ Be alert to the signs of intense grief reactions, such as lasting depression, anger, or denial. ■ Consider the nature of the loss and its possible ramifications. ■ Offer appropriate support and referral, such as therapy or grief counseling.
Reproduction	Addition of a family member may strengthen familial bonds through shared interests in the child's welfare or may instead strain relationships in terms of increased physical, emotional, and financial demands.	■ Teach about prenatal care and maternal health. ■ Encourage all family members to engage in educational activities. ■ Assess the involved individuals' responses to pregnancy and sensitively address potentially harmful issues, such as ineffective communication patterns. ■ Be alert to signs of postpartum depression. ■ Advise parents of potential jealousies and complications with toddlers and new infants.
Stress and Coping	Family stressors are many and may increase risks for physical and mental illness, caregiver burden, and successful family functioning.	■ Encourage open dialog among all family members. ■ Discuss what the issue means to family members. ■ Identify past coping mechanisms used by individual family members. ■ Help family members identify ways to find strength in the change. ■ Allow individuals to grieve. ■ Identify resources available.
Trauma	Trauma may be caused by physical abuse, or by emotional/verbal abuse or neglect. Trauma may also result from unintentional injuries. See the module on trauma for more information.	■ Identify and document physical findings associated with physical abuse/neglect. ■ Enlist the aid of counselors/clergy. ■ Provide support to all family members. ■ Encourage open communication.

experience different degrees of devotion to the culture, religion, or spiritual practices of the family. Generally speaking, the more recently a family has immigrated to this country, the more likely the family is to continue to practice traditional cultural and religious beliefs and practices (Spector, 2017). Culturally competent nursing practice is a critical part of nursing care for children and families. The Concepts Related to Family feature links some, but not all, of the concepts integral to family. They are presented in alphabetical order.

Health Promotion

Health and wellness promotion is an essential aspect of family health and focuses on increasing healthy behaviors and optimizing lifestyle choices. Educating patients and facilitating appropriate referrals (e.g., to nutritionists, educational programs, and community service providers) will not only improve the family's quality of life, but also reduce the risk of illness. Depending on the needs of the patient, nurses may collaborate with a variety of healthcare providers and professionals, including physicians, counselors, social workers, and mental health specialists.

Families may be most in need of health promotion and patient teaching during times of transition into new developmental or life stages. From teaching new parents the importance of skin-to-skin contact in the first hours after delivery to helping parents of teenagers identify signs of depression or addiction, nurses are uniquely placed to help parents parent their children successfully and to help families obtain optimal wellness and functioning. Settings in which nurses provide health promotion for patients and families include hospitals, physicians' offices and clinics, local health departments, and public schools.

Establishing a therapeutic relationship with the family is important in order to develop a rapport with the family that is characterized by empathy and trust. Having a trusting relationship also helps in development of mutually identified goals for the family's needs. The nurse provides information in a clear, timely, and sensitive manner. The nurse works with families by teaching them to identify solutions until they are able to problem solve independently. The family's ethnic and religious background needs to be considered in developing intervention recommendations.

When working with families, the nurse considers health and wellness not only from an individual perspective, but also in terms of the family unit. Family wellness promotion emphasizes addressing each individual family member's contribution to the health and well-being of the family and recognizing that if one member is affected, the entire family is affected. For example, any number of occupational or environmental problems could alter the individual's physical and emotional wellness. A physical ailment—such as a broken leg or lead poisoning—can be treated, but if occupational (e.g., physically demanding and personally unsatisfying hard labor) and environmental (e.g., house with lead-based paint in a dangerous neighborhood) aspects are not addressed, the health of the individual and the family remain at risk.

Family wellness and health promotion strategies involve empowering patients to make beneficial changes in their lives (Strout, 2012). Some common health promotion strategies include encouraging tobacco cessation, increased exercise, healthy eating habits, and use of stress reduction techniques. Each individual will have different needs and circumstances, requiring nurses to modify health promotion suggestions. For example, consider a stay-at-home mother of three who is seeking stress relief. For this patient, the nurse might suggest a community activity that promotes exercise (for stress relief) and a chance to connect with others in the community (for social wellness). Patients may decline to follow the nurse's suggestion; however, the nurse's role is to offer health- and wellness-promoting options without judgment and then allow the patient to decide.

Empowering patients requires nurses to help patients set goals for their own personal wellness and the wellness of their families. The choice of goals is dependent on the family's needs, both as individual members and as a unit. One family may set the goal of participating in a family game night once a week to promote emotional, social, and intellectual wellness, whereas another family could set the goal of going hiking or biking every 2 weeks as a family to promote physical and even spiritual wellness. Nurses can help families set goals by working to understand the needs and wants of the family (Strout, 2012).

Health promotion within the family unit can be challenging. In some cases, family members will respond positively to nursing suggestions and interventions; in other cases, patients may feel they are unable to change their lifestyle because of socioeconomic conditions, stress, or other factors. Individuals also may interpret health promotion as an attempt to control their behaviors. The nurse approaches families on a case-by-case basis, recognizing that each family unit will need different forms of care and different nursing approaches.

Risk and Protective Factors

Risk factors for family dysfunction may not always be evident. At times, the risk factors are masked by the absence of obvious problems. Stress, for example, can lead to many problems within a family, as the effects of unmanaged and unresolved stress can impact normal family functioning. Parental coping methods can also determine how children will learn to handle stress, because children often model the actions of their parents (APA, 2013). The response to stressors can be exacerbated by a real or perceived sense of powerlessness over circumstances, such as poverty, unemployment, or abuse. Other risk factors for family dysfunction include family separation, forced migration, and cultural and social isolation.

Protective factors for family health and function include stable living environments, healthy and consistent parenting and supervision, healthy family coping, social and community supports, and financial stability (e.g., adequate shelter, food and nutrition, and access to healthcare).

Recognition and awareness of risk and protective factors and knowledge of community supports can help the nurse identify and plan health and wellness promotion activities for families at risk of alterations in family coping, physical health, and mental health (see **Table 26–3 》》**).

Care in the Community

Nurses encounter families experiencing stress, trauma, poverty, acute health conditions, and chronic illnesses in all settings. Many times nurses are called on to assist families in finding resources to alleviate financial burdens or to help them access social supports. Although the names of local resource agencies may vary from one location to another, both public and private resources are available in most communities. Public resources include departments of social services, local health departments, departments of aging, and public schools. Private resources are often available through nonprofit organizations such as literacy centers, homeless and transition shelters, and nonprofits that serve the aging and the disabled. Nurses should be aware of the resources in their community that support the populations with which they work.

》》 Stay Current: The organization 2-1-1 is a free and confidential service that helps individuals find local resources: www.211.org

TABLE 26-3 Health and Wellness Promotion for the Family at Risk for Health Alterations

Developmental Stage and Associated Risk Factors	Potential Health Consequences	Health and Wellness Promotion Strategies
Individual, Couple, or Family with Infants and Preschoolers ■ Lack of knowledge about family planning, contraception, and sexual and marital roles ■ Inadequate prenatal care ■ Altered nutrition: inadequate nutrition, overweight, underweight ■ Smoking, alcohol/drug abuse ■ Lack of knowledge about child health and safety ■ Low socioeconomic status ■ First pregnancy before age 16 or after age 35	■ Premature pregnancy ■ Low-birth-weight infant ■ Birth defects ■ Injury to infant or child ■ Accidents	■ Promote preconception/prenatal care if applicable. ■ Obtain detailed history to uncover environmental issues and lifestyle practices that may impact health of individuals and family. ■ Provide education related to contraception and sexually transmitted infection (STI) prevention. ■ Facilitate nutritional assessment and counseling. ■ Offer referrals to appropriate resources for smoking cessation programs and alcohol/drug abuse counseling. ■ Educate about basic child health and safety protocols. ■ Identify resources for financial assistance and facilitate appropriate referrals. ■ Advocate for safe care of infants and their families.
Family with School-age Children ■ Unsafe home environment ■ Working parents with inappropriate or inadequate resources for child care ■ Low socioeconomic status ■ Child abuse or neglect ■ Multiple, closely spaced children ■ Repeated infections, accidents, and hospitalizations ■ Unrecognized and unattended health problems ■ Poor or inappropriate nutrition ■ Toxic substances in the home	■ Behavior problems ■ Speech and vision problems ■ Learning disabilities ■ Communicable diseases ■ Physical abuse ■ Developmental delay ■ Obesity, underweight	■ Educate about preventive healthcare measures. ■ Provide information about community assistance and healthcare programs. ■ Educate about contraception. ■ Provide information about adequate nutrition. ■ Provide education to children and families regarding risk of certain environmental hazards (i.e., risk of carbon monoxide [CO] poisoning and need for CO monitors in home).
Family with Adolescents and Young Adults ■ Family values of aggressiveness and competition ■ Lifestyle and behaviors that lead to chronic illness (substance abuse, inadequate diet) ■ Lack of problem-solving skills ■ Conflicts between parents and children	■ Violent death and injury ■ Alcohol/drug abuse ■ Unwanted pregnancy ■ Suicide ■ STIs ■ Domestic abuse	■ Promote healthy problem-solving skills. ■ Educate about healthy anger and emotion management techniques. ■ Provide information about healthcare resources. ■ Teach about contraception. ■ Facilitate learning about substance and alcohol abuse prevention.
Family with Middle-aged Adults ■ High-cholesterol diet ■ Obesity ■ Hypertension ■ Smoking, alcohol abuse ■ Physical inactivity ■ Personality patterns related to stress ■ Exposure to environment: sunlight, radiation, asbestos, or water or air pollution ■ Depression	■ Cardiovascular disease (coronary artery disease, cerebrovascular disease) ■ Cancer ■ Accidents ■ Suicide ■ Mental illness	■ Educate about nutrition and exercise and its relationship to cardiovascular disease, diabetes and certain forms of cancer. ■ Educate regarding changes in relationships, careers, and biologic changes that occur during this time. ■ Provide information about mental health counseling and facilitate referrals. ■ Suggest screening for hypertension, cardiac disease, osteoporosis, colon cancer, breast cancer. ■ Educate regarding occupational safety hazards and risk for exposure to potential carcinogens and risk of accidents (if applicable).
Family with Older Adults ■ Depression ■ Drug interactions ■ Chronic illness ■ Reduced income ■ Poor nutrition ■ Lack of exercise ■ Past environmental exposure to toxins and adverse lifestyle choices	■ Impaired vision and hearing ■ Hypertension ■ Acute illness ■ Chronic illness ■ Infectious diseases (influenza, pneumonia) ■ Injuries from burns and falls ■ Depression ■ Alcohol abuse ■ Adjusting to retirement, losses	■ Educate about nutrition and exercise. ■ Provide information about community-based programs for healthcare. ■ Facilitate mental health counseling. ■ Educate about illness prevention and health promotion (i.e., use of prescription medications with herbal remedies). ■ Encourage ways to stay involved and productive (i.e., volunteering, assisting with community projects). ■ Provide referrals regarding wills, advance directive, power of attorney.

Nursing Assessment

The purpose of family assessment is to determine the level of family functioning, clarify family interaction patterns, identify family strengths and weaknesses, and describe the health status of the family and its individual members. Also important are family living patterns, including communication, childrearing, coping strategies, and health practices. Family assessment gives an overview of the family process and helps the nurse identify areas that need further investigation. As the nurse becomes more acquainted with the family, the assessment continues in more targeted areas to further develop the nursing care plan.

Observation and Family Interview

To obtain an accurate and concise family assessment, the nurse needs to establish a trusting relationship with the parent(s) and the family. Data are best collected in a comfortable, private environment, free from interruptions. Typically this occurs in the family's home, but it may also occur in the clinic, hospital, or other similar setting.

Key to any good assessment and health history is observation of how family members interact with and respond to each other, what types of communication patterns they use, the amount of support they provide to one another, and the closeness/distance of each family member as they relate to one another. Interviewing family members individually or as a group, depending on the situation, provides additional valuable information about their knowledge regarding health promotion and illness prevention. The amount of cooperation, identification of norms within the family, and assessing for the potential for the family to engage in positive change are all other important aspects of observation and the interview (Rentfro, 2014). This information should be documented clearly on the electronic health record (EHR), whether the nurse is working with the family in the community or inpatient setting.

The family assessment provides important information about family structure and function, including which individuals are responsible for making healthcare decisions for specific family members. The following data may be useful in informing planning and care:

Family Structure

- Which adults spend the most time with the children? What is the nature of sibling relationships?
- Who has legal custody—that is, who is able to make healthcare decisions for the child?
- For older adults or those living with serious illness, has a family member been legally designated as having a healthcare power of attorney?

Family Roles/Functions/Resources

- Who provides for the child or family financially? Does the child/patient/family have health insurance?
- Who else helps the parent(s) care for the children? What other support systems does the family have in place?

Physical Health Status

- What is the health status of each member of the family? How do family members perceive their own health?

- What preventive practices does the family use (e.g., status of immunizations, oral hygiene practices, regularity of vision examinations)?
- To what extent do family members receive routine healthcare?

Mental Health Status

- What is the mental health status of each member of the family? How do family members perceive their own health?
- What protective factors are in place? What kind of family or community supports do family members access or participate in?
- What kind of coping mechanisms do individual members use? How does the family cope with stresses together?

Family Interactions and Values

- How do family members express feelings? Communicate with each other?
- What cultural and religious practices does the family observe? What relationship do these practices have to family health and well-being?
- What type of parenting style is preferred by the parent(s)? Do parents share caregiving responsibilities?
- What are the family's health values? How much emphasis is put on exercise, diet, and preventive healthcare? Are complementary health approaches included in their daily activities? Are they used to promote health and prevent illness?

Family Assessment Tools

In the context of wellness promotion, nursing assessment includes identifying and optimizing current positive behaviors and lifestyle choices, as well as recognizing the family's needs for disease prevention. In addition to patient interviews and observation of family processes, several tools are available for completing a multifaceted family assessment that takes into consideration a number of factors, including physiologic, psychosocial, spiritual, and environmental components. Presented are some of the more common tools that can be used by nurses to identify strengths and areas where families may need more support, education, or resources in order to strengthen the family unit.

Family Ecomap

How a family interacts within the community can provide useful information, especially when trying to determine how to support families who are having difficulty coping. **Ecomaps** are an assessment tool that can help nurses visualize how the family unit interacts with the external community environment, including schools, religious commitments, occupational duties, and recreational pursuits (see **Figure 26–9 》》**). The ecomap provides an opportunity to identify the organizational patterns of the family and the status of relationships within the family and community, as well as the community resources the family might access. As part of the assessment, the nurse observes intrafamily communication patterns closely, paying special attention to who does the talking for the family, which members are silent, how disagreements are handled, and how well the members listen to one another and encourage the participation of others. Nonverbal communication is important because it gives valuable clues about what people are feeling.

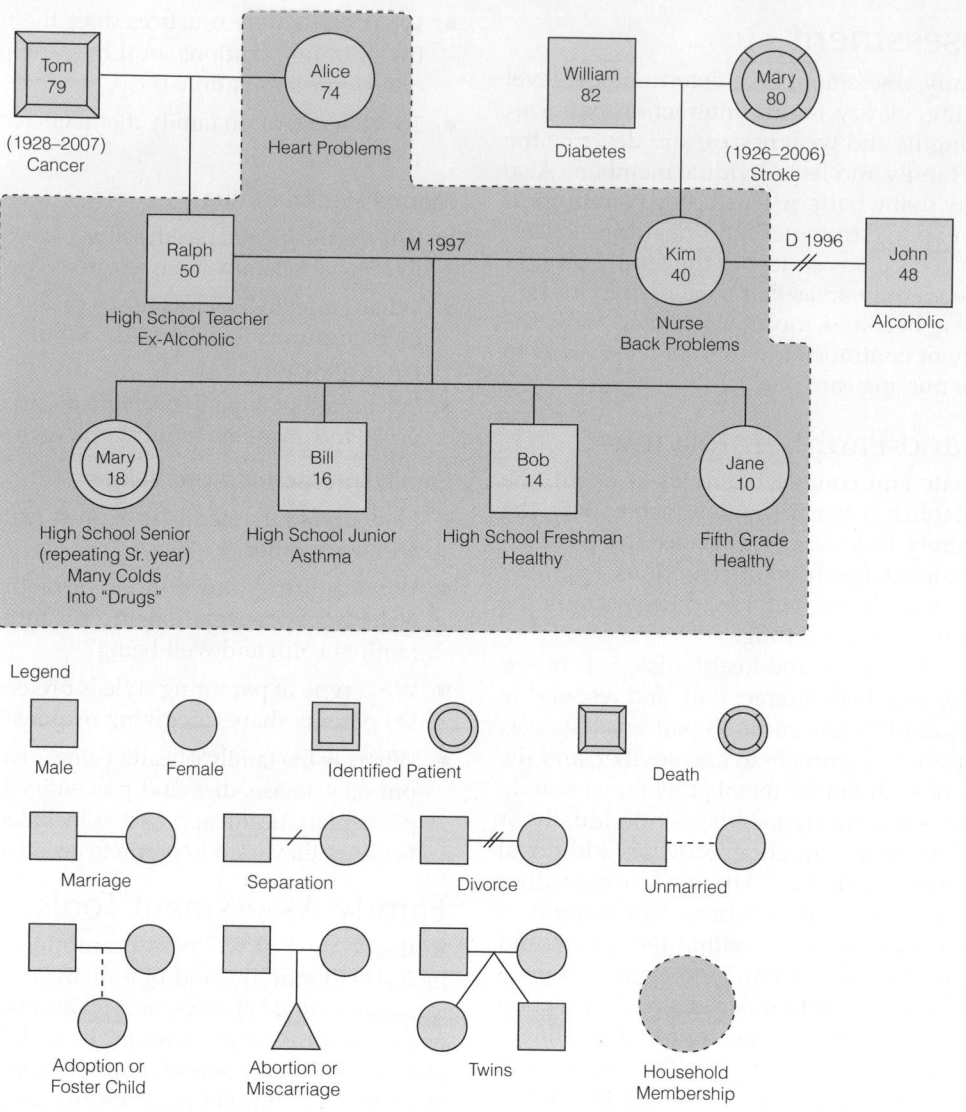

Figure 26–9 >> Example of a family genogram.

Family Genogram

Using a genogram assists the nurse to visualize familial relationships and patterns of chronic conditions occurring within the family unit. **Genograms** consist of visual representations of gender showing lines of birth descent through the generations (see **Figure 26–10 >>**).

Family APGAR

The Family APGAR is a quick, five-item questionnaire that may be used as an initial screening tool for family assessment. The five family concepts measured are family adaptability, partnership, growth, affection, and resolve (see **Table 26–4 >>**). This five-item questionnaire can be administered quickly to each family member over 10 years of age. Be concerned if the majority of responses fall in the "hardly ever" category or if responses vary a lot among family members. This may indicate a family that needs much more support to cope with the demands of daily life and may also provide insight into health maintenance and health promotion needs.

Home Observation for Measurement of the Environment

The HOME Inventory is an assessment tool developed to measure the quality and quantity of stimulation and support available in the home environment (Caldwell & Bradley, 1984). Four age-specific scales are available (birth to 3 years, 3 to 6 years, 6 to 10 years, and 10 to 15 years). Examples of subscales within each age-specific scale are parental responsiveness, acceptance of child, the physical environment, learning materials, variety in experience, and parental involvement. Data are collected during an informal, low-stress interview and observation over 45 to 90 minutes in the home setting. The child and his or her primary caregiver must be present and awake during the interview. Observation of the parent–child interaction is an essential part of the assessment. The intent is to allow family members to act normally. Assessment of the home environment will help to identify factors that promote the child's growth and development. Nursing interventions that could result from the HOME assessment include recommending items that can be

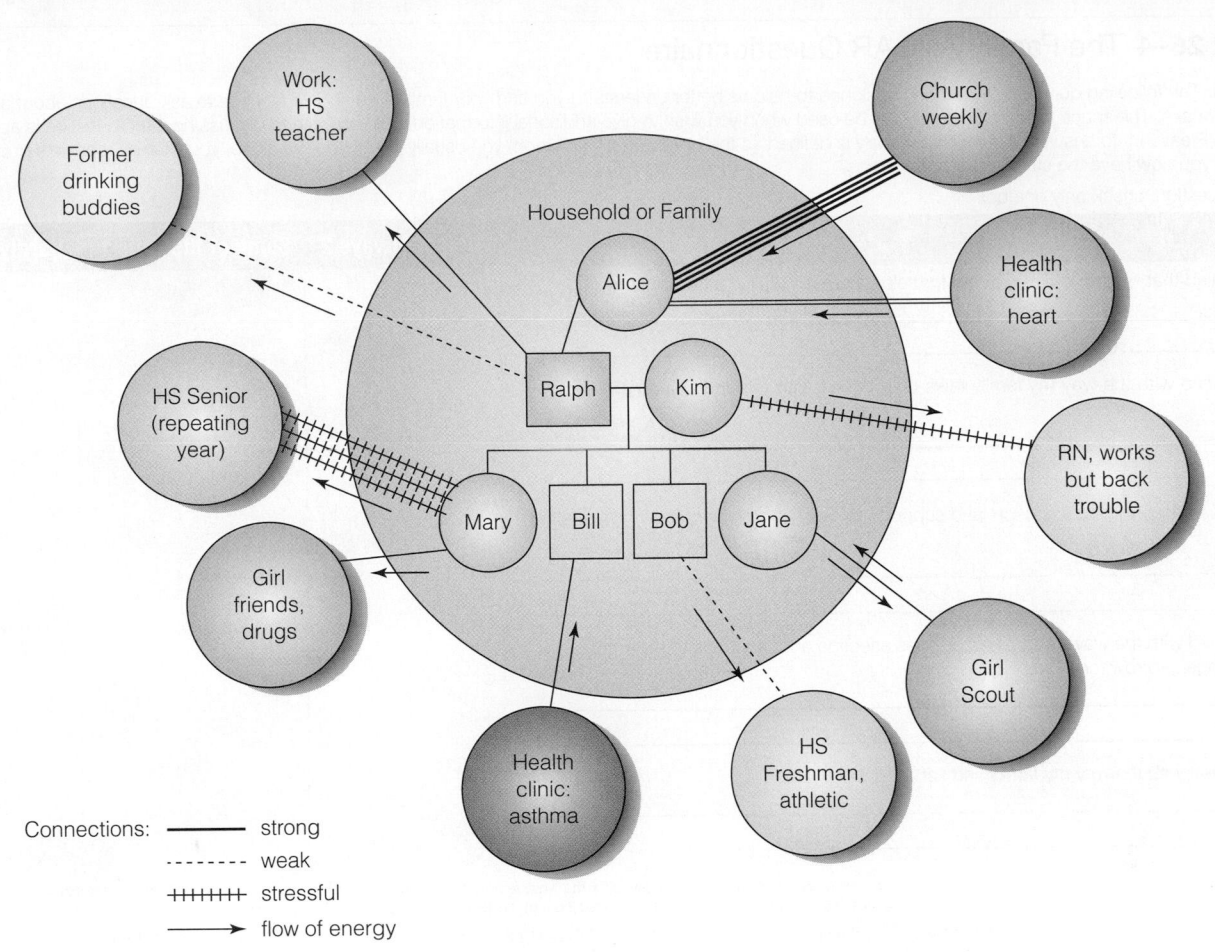

Connections:
——————— strong
-------- weak
++++++++ stressful
————▶ flow of energy

Figure 26–10 》 Example of a family ecomap. Many more components may be added to the map.

used in the home for toys and suggesting strategies for interacting with the child to promote learning.

The Friedman Family Assessment Tool

The Friedman Family Assessment Tool (FFAM), developed by Marilyn Friedman, was designed to assist nurses with family assessment. This tool provides a method for examining the whole family in the context of the larger community where the family resides. The interview collects information about a family's relationships, functioning, strengths, and problems.

》 Go to **Pearson MyLab Nursing and eText** to see a shortened version of the Friedman Family Assessment Tool.

Case Study 》 Part 2

After expressing concern for Mrs. Rodriguez and Mrs. Marshall, you begin to explore their birthing class experiences in greater detail. Mrs. Rodriguez explains that many of the other couples in the class are rude to her and her wife, and that the woman conducting the class is cold to them as well. The couple continues to tell you about similarly negative reactions they have experienced while searching for a birthing center. During the discussion, you notice that Mrs. Rodriguez becomes increasingly upset. When Mrs. Marshall asks for a few moments alone with Mrs. Rodriguez, you step out of the room. Upon your return, Mrs. Rodriguez apologizes for "losing control of my emotions." You assure her that she is welcome to express her emotions and that you are committed to providing her with the best possible

care, including recommending some potential alternatives to her current birthing classes. You continue your physical assessment of Mrs. Rodriguez. Her vital signs are T 98.8°F oral, P 86 bpm, R 24/min, and BP 168/90 mmHg. Mrs. Rodriguez denies any physical complaints or unusual changes in her condition. You leave the room to talk with the physician. The physician comes in to examine Mrs. Rodriguez and notes that everything appears to be fine but expresses concern about Mrs. Rodriguez's elevated blood pressure.

Clinical Reasoning Questions Level I
1. Presuming that Mrs. Rodriguez has no other health issues and no pregnancy-related complications, why might her blood pressure be elevated?
2. Identify three nursing actions described in this scenario that reflect respect and nonjudgmental care of this couple.

Clinical Reasoning Questions Level II
3. Describe two nursing interventions appropriate for inclusion in the care of this couple.
4. What steps might you take to assist Mrs. Rodriguez with identifying alternative providers of birthing classes?
5. What are some concerns associated with hypertension during the third trimester of pregnancy?

Independent Interventions

Families are shaped by multiple factors, including life experiences, current and past challenges, coping abilities, cultural

TABLE 26–4 The Family APGAR Questionnaire

Directions: The following questions have been designed to help us better understand you and your family. You should feel free to ask questions about any item in the questionnaire. The space for comments should be used when you wish to give additional information or if you wish to discuss how the question is applied to your family. Please try to answer all questions. Family is defined as the individual(s) with whom you usually live. If you live alone, your "family" consists of persons with whom you now have the strongest emotional ties.*

For each question, check only one box.

	Almost Always 2	Some of the Time 1	Hardly Ever 0
I am satisfied that I can turn to my family for help when something is troubling me. Comments: _____			
I am satisfied with the way my family talks over things with me and shares problems with me. Comments: _____			
I am satisfied that my family accepts and supports my wishes to take on new activities or directions. Comments: _____			
I am satisfied with the way my family expresses affection and responds to my emotions, such as anger, sorrow, and love. Comments: _____			
I am satisfied with the way my family and I share time together. Comments: _____			

*Note: Depending on which member of the family is being interviewed, the interviewer may substitute for the word *family* either *spouse, significant other, parents,* or *children*. Responses are scored 2, 1, 0 and totaled. The total score ranges from 0 to 10. The higher the score, the greater amount of satisfaction that family member has with family functioning.

Source: Adapted from Smilkstein, G. (1978). The family APGAR: A proposal for a family function test and its use by physicians. *Journal of Family Practice, 6,* 1231–1239. Reprinted with permission from Frontline Medical Communications, Inc.

diversity, individual personalities, and the age of the family members. Nurses can employ numerous interventions to assist families with navigating through challenges or difficult circumstances, as well as to promote the optimal use of each individual's strengths.

Explore Health Beliefs

Families have different and varying beliefs about health, illness, and ways and methods of treating illness. In some cases, these beliefs may be based in cultural or religious practices. As part of the assessment, the nurse asks open-ended questions in a nonjudgmental manner in an attempt to learn about the family's health beliefs, including the use of herbs and supplements and the use of home remedies. By exploring the family's health beliefs, nurses show respect for cultural and religious values and practice and can identify practices that may have a bearing on healthcare and family functioning. For example, consider the Muslim patient who has come in for assessment prior to scheduling a procedure. The nurse recognizes that the holy period of Ramadan is coming up and knows that observances for Ramadan include a month-long period of fasting from sunrise to sunset. One of the medications the patient will have to take during the postoperative period must be taken 4 times a day with food. Although the Muslim faith respects the need of those who are sick to abstain from fasting, the nurse consults with both the patient and the physician about whether or not the procedure may be scheduled after Ramadan.

Identify Resources

The nurse working with a family to develop a care plan identifies potential resources in the community that match the child's and the family's needs for support. The nurse will collaborate with the family to discuss those resources and to select the ones that are acceptable to the family, to increase the likelihood that the family will follow through with the plan. In some cases it may be necessary to collaborate with a multidisciplinary team, including social workers, to help the family obtain assistance to overcome, for example, transportation or financial problems or any others that interfere family functioning. The nurse may also assist the family in obtaining resources by such actions as role rehearsal, providing instructions and support when making an initial call, or connecting with another family support person who can help with resource linkage. The nurse will refer families with moderate or severe dysfunction to community resources for social support and counseling as appropriate.

Provide Patient and Family Education

Family members may have a lack of information or misinformation about health or disease. Because of the many advances in medicine and healthcare during the past few decades, patients may have outdated information about health, illness, treatment, and prevention. The addition of internet access has also caused a dramatic increase in the information available to families regarding health and illness (Hebda & Czar, 2014). The nurse is frequently in a position to give information or

Nursing Care Plan

A Single-Parent Family with Child Care Issues

ASSESSMENT	DIAGNOSES	PLANNING
Ms. Wilson, a newly divorced single mother, brings her 3-year-old son in for routine immunizations. After he has received his immunizations, while waiting the required 20 minutes before leaving, Ms. Wilson reveals that she recently lost her job because her company was bought by another. She says that she has found a new job, and that the salary is much higher, but the only available shift is from midnight to 7:00 a.m. She asks if there are any certified child-care providers who provide services during nighttime hours. She notes that her parents have offered to keep her son while she is at work, but she is worried about burdening her parents and being viewed as incapable of taking care of her child independently.	■ *Parenting, Readiness for Enhanced* ■ *Knowledge, Readiness for Enhanced* ■ *Decision Making, Readiness for Enhanced* (NANDA-I © 2014)	■ Ms. Wilson will be able to state the risks related to leaving a child home alone. ■ Ms. Wilson will learn of other resources available to help her care for her child in a safe environment. ■ Ms. Wilson will discuss available choices she has without risking her child's safety.

IMPLEMENTATION

- Explore patient's reluctance to accept her parents' offer to assist her.
- Assist with identifying additional sources of support, including support groups and classes geared toward meeting the needs of single parents.
- Reinforce and support the patient's concern for her child's well-being, including his physiologic and psychosocial wellness.
- Provide referrals to social services to help meet financial needs.
- Encourage and support patient's desire to be financially self-sufficient.
- Assess patient's knowledge of pediatric vaccination schedules and provide appropriate teaching, including in written form.

EVALUATION

Ms. Wilson agrees to explore the option of accepting her parents' offer to care for her child while she is at work. She also agrees to attend classes designed to educate and assist individuals with overcoming challenges that accompany single parenting.

CRITICAL THINKING

1. Is the nursing diagnosis of Readiness for Enhanced Parenting appropriate? Why or why not?
2. In what ways might Ms. Wilson's recent divorce have affected her family's level of wellness?
3. How might Ms. Wilson's fear of appearing dependent negatively impact her level of personal and family wellness?

---

correct misconceptions. This function is an important component of the nursing care plan. Referrals to other healthcare team members offer the nurse the ability to collaborate with others in providing the necessary care to families.

Collaborative Practices

The interconnectedness and interdependence that are inherent in each family underscore the importance of collaboration as part of family-centered nursing care. Armed with the information from the family assessment, the nurse advocates within the interprofessional care team on behalf of the family and helps family members learn how to advocate for themselves and each other. At all times, the nurse remembers that family members may perceive some needs, issues, and situations differently than the nurse or other members of the healthcare team. **Box 26–2** illustrates this aspect of family-centered care.

When working with families, nurses will often need to collaborate with other healthcare professionals. In some cases, collaboration may include working with experts who specialize in social work, psychology, or mental healthcare.

For families in need of counseling, financial assistance may be available. Generally, community-funded organizations offer free or discounted services. When making these recommendations, nurses should be aware of some stigmas surrounding therapy and counseling, and work to assure families of the potential benefits of these modes of care. For new or expectant parents, referral to parenting classes may be valuable. Families facing economic challenges should be made aware of community resources, including wellness clinics and food banks. Additional assistance and collaboration with the school nurse may also help those families whose children requires special care during the school day.

Family responsibilities for children do not necessarily end on the child's 18th birthday. This is particularly true for families with children with disability and families with children with *serious mental illness (SMI)*. Serious mental illnesses are those that create significant disability in an individual's ability to function and reach life goals. Many community and social supports for individuals with disability or mental illness end when the individual turns 18 or graduates from high school. Parents may find themselves at a loss to cope with an adult child who needs continued support and care. In particular,

Box 26–2
Family-Centered Collaborative Care

Kayla Harrison is a public health nurse who is part of the early childhood collaborative assessment and referral team in her community. The team also includes a child psychologist, a pediatrician, a speech and language therapist, and an early childhood specialist from the local public schools. The team is meeting with Coretta Simons, the grandmother and foster parent of Alex Simons, a 3-year-old who was referred for evaluation based on an obvious speech deficit and behavior problems reported by his preschool teacher. During the meeting, the team shares the results of Alex's evaluation and listens to Ms. Simon's concerns about her grandson. Ms. Simon is the foster parent for Alex and his two older siblings. She works 40 hours a week driving the van for the local eldercare center, taking older adults to and from the center for the day while their caregivers go to work. Ms. Simon reports that Alex is the youngest, and his behavioral problems are exhausting the entire family. Team members advise her that they would like for Alex to be enrolled in a part-day program offered by the school system. The program specializes in offering services for children based on an individual education plan. The team is also recommending that Alex see a child psychologist to begin to learn some coping skills and for Ms. Simon to participate in therapy as well. Ms. Simon shares she cannot take any more time off for work to attend to Alex's needs, in part because of the number of times she got calls at work from the preschool asking her to come to the center to help intervene with Alex's troublesome behaviors. She also says that she does not think a part-day program is best for Alex. That would mean he would have to be shuttled to and from his current preschool to the public school because she works all day. Ms. Simon does not see this as being appropriate for a 3-year-old.

Ms. Harrison, the nurse at the table, hears Ms. Simon's frustrations and recognizes quickly that Ms. Simon understands her needs, Alex's needs, and the needs of their family unit. The early childhood specialist, however, is pushing for Ms. Simon to make the therapy appointments happen, on the argument that this will help her learn to manage Alex's behaviors and help Alex learn some coping mechanisms as well. Ms. Harrison knows that the local preschool developmental day center has some grant funding to provide outreach mental health services to children in other preschool settings. Ms. Harrison suggests that the team begin Alex's treatment plan by starting with speech therapy and by signing Alex up for the outreach services so that a behavioral therapist can work with Alex at school. When possible, Ms. Simon can join in those sessions or observe and work with the therapist to find what works for Alex. Ms. Harrison suggests that the team try these options and meet again after a few weeks to see how the plan is working. Ms. Simon replies that this sounds feasible, that she would find it more helpful to meet with a therapist Ms. Harrison recommends at Alex's preschool instead of having to take him to and from appointments.

---

older adults who have been caring for adult children with disability or serious mental illness may experience increased distress as they plan for the care of their child beyond their own lives (Potter & Moller, 2016). Nurses may find themselves collaborating with these parents to help them find and access services for adult children. One advocacy organization, the Center for Parent Information and Resources, provides information for parents of individuals with disabilities.

>> **Stay Current:** The Center for Parent Information and Resources provides a list of organizations that offer resources or support for adults with disabilities. See http://www.parentcenterhub.org/repository/foradults/

Case Study >> Part 3

The physician requests that Mrs. Rodriguez remain at the office so that her blood pressure can be reassessed. While Mrs. Rodriguez is relaxing, you check with some of the staff and learn that a newly hired certified nurse midwife (CNM) offers a birthing class once per week. The CNM reports that two of her patients are a lesbian couple and that they are warmly welcomed by the other patients. You also consult with two of the physicians and compile a list of three birthing centers in the area that they prefer.

Upon return to Mrs. Rodriguez's room, you reassess her blood pressure, which is now 122/82 mmHg. You provide the couple with the information you have gathered about the birthing class and the three birthing centers. Both Mrs. Rodriguez and her wife express gratitude for your compassion and efforts to assist them. Mrs. Rodriquez is scheduled to return for a follow-up appointment in 2 weeks. She reports that she has a blood pressure monitor at home and tells you she'll check her blood pressure at least once daily. Mrs. Rodriguez agrees to contact the clinic if her blood pressure is elevated or if she has any unusual changes.

Clinical Reasoning Questions Level I
1. Do you think Mrs. Rodriguez and Mrs. Marshall are wellness oriented? Explain your answer.
2. What recommendations would you provide to help Mrs. Rodriguez keep her stress level down during her pregnancy?

Clinical Reasoning Questions Level II
3. What are some of the negative effects of stress on families?
4. According to the laws of your state, when the couple in this case study has their child, who will have parental rights?
5. If Mrs. Rodriguez's blood pressure had not decreased, what interventions could have been proposed?

REVIEW The Concept of Family

RELATE Link the Concepts

Linking the concept of family with the concept of culture:
1. Explain how culture influences the family unit. What are three values or beliefs that could impact how a family functions?
2. What impact does stereotyping have on family? Describe at least two negative effects stereotyping can have on the family unit.

3. How does the nurse incorporate the family's cultural beliefs into health promotion teaching?
4. How might the family's cultural beliefs impact their health behaviors?

Linking the concept of family with the concept of self:
5. What are two measures that could be implemented for a teenager you suspect is experiencing anorexia nervosa?

6. While you are providing care to a family of four (two parents, two children), the parents ask for advice on helping their daughter, who they believe has become bulimic. What suggestions do you provide the parents? Explain your answers.

Linking the concept of family with the concept of advocacy:

7. How can the nurse advocate for families from vulnerable populations in the community?

8. What responsibilities does the nurse have to advocate for families?

READY Go to Volume 3: Clinical Nursing Skills

- SKILL 1.1   Appearance and Mental Status: Assessing
- SKILL 3.6   Sleep Promotion: Assisting
- SKILL 10.5   Nutrition: Assessing
- SKILL 15.1   Abuse: Newborn, Infant, Child, Older Adult, Assessing for
- SKILL 15.5   Environmental Safety: Health Care Facility, Community, Home
- SKILL 15.6   Fire Safety: Health Care Facility, Community, Home

REFER Go to Pearson MyLab Nursing and eText

- Additional review materials
- Chart: Friedman Family Assessment Tool

REFLECT Apply Your Knowledge

The home health nurse has been visiting a 90-year-old woman and her younger sister who live together in a large farmhouse. The women have been active in caring for each other and their residence. During one of the home visits, they confide that the farm is too much for them, but they admit that they do not want to tell their families because they are afraid that they will be put into a nursing home.

1. What community resources are available to assist the sisters to live independently?

2. How should the family be involved in the decision making?

3. What signs can alert the nurse that the sisters are unable to care for themselves?

4. Should the nurse contact the family without the sisters' knowledge? Why or why not?

» Exemplar 26.A
Family Response to Health Alterations

Exemplar Learning Outcomes

26.A Analyze family response to health alterations.

- Describe the impact of illness on the family system.
- Identify the clinical manifestations of family response to health alterations.
- Outline aspects of collaboration necessary to the care of families experiencing health alterations.
- Apply the nursing process in providing culturally competent care to families with health alterations.

Exemplar Key Terms

Family burden, *1874*
Objective family burden, *1874*
Stigma, *1875*
Subjective family burden, *1874*

Overview

Although some patients are totally alone in the world, most have one or more people who are significant in their lives. These significant others may be related or bonded to the patient by birth, adoption, marriage, or friendship. Although not always meeting traditional definitions, people (or even pets) significant to the patient are the patient's family. The nurse includes the family as an integral component of care in all healthcare settings.

The Impact of Illness on the Family System

Illness of a family member is a crisis that affects the entire family system. The family is disrupted as members abandon their usual activities and focus their energy on restoring family equilibrium. Roles and responsibilities of the ill family member are delegated to other family members, or those functions remain undone for the duration of the illness. Family members experience anxiety about the sick individual and the resolution of the illness. This anxiety is compounded by additional responsibilities that leave less time or motivation to complete the normal tasks of daily living.

See **Box 26–3 »** for some factors that determine the impact of illness on the family unit.

The family's ability to deal with the stress of illness depends on the members' coping skills. Families with good communication skills are better able to discuss how they feel

---

Box 26–3
Factors Determining the Impact of Illness on the Family

- The nature of the illness, which can range from minor to life threatening
- The duration of the illness
- The residual effects of the illness, ranging from none to permanent disability
- The meaning of the illness to the family and its significance to family systems
- The financial impact of the illness, which is influenced by factors such as insurance and ability of the ill family member to return to work
- The effect of the illness on future family functioning (for instance, previous patterns may be restored or new patterns may be established).

about the illness and how it affects family functioning. They can plan for the future and are flexible in adapting these plans as the situation changes. An established social support network provides strength, encouragement, and services to the family during the illness. During health crises, families must realize that turning to others for support is a sign of strength rather than weakness. Nurses can be part of the support system for families, or they can identify other sources of support in the community.

During a crisis, families are often drawn together by a common purpose. In this time of closeness, family members have the opportunity to reaffirm personal and family values and their commitment to one another. Indeed, illness may provide a unique opportunity for family growth.

Nurses committed to family-centered care involve both the patient and the patient's family in the nursing process. Through their interaction with families, nurses can give support and information, although the patient needs to give permission regarding what information can be shared with family members. Nurses make sure that not only the patient but also each family member understands the disease, its management, and the effect of these two factors on family functioning.

The interconnected and interdependence of the family have considerable impact on patient care beyond the acute care setting. For example, changes in the dietary needs of one member may impact all family members. Nurses must assess the implications of treatment management on all members of the household, including siblings. Nurses must also be attuned to how family members are responding.

Nurses also support families as they try to find solutions, providing patient education about community resources and the Family Medical Leave Act (**Box 26–4 》》**).

Chronic Illness and the Family

Chronic illness has increased dramatically so much that nearly one half of the U.S. population experience a chronic condition, and more than one in four Americans have multiple chronic conditions (Murray & Lopez, 2013). The patient with a chronic illness may be hospitalized when experiencing an acute exacerbation, but the care of the patient is primarily and usually provided at home. Chronic illness in a family member is a major stressor that may cause changes in family structure and function, as well as in how family developmental tasks are performed.

Many different factors affect family responses to chronic illness; family responses in turn affect the patient's response to and perception of the illness. Factors influencing response to chronic illness include personal, social, and economic resources; the nature and course of the disease; and demands of the illness as perceived by family members. In a systematic review, Cousino and Hazen (2013) found that significantly greater parenting stress of caregivers of children with chronic illness was associated with greater caregiver responsibility for treatment management. Interestingly, duration and severity of illness were not found to be correlated with greater caregiver stress.

Patients with chronic illness, and their families, may be at risk for depression. Caregiver burden, loss of role function, and financial burden are just some of the factors that increase risk for depression in patients with chronic illness and their families. Nursing considerations for a patient with a chronic illness include being alert to symptoms of depression, both in the patient and in his or her close family members.

Serious Mental Illness and the Family

Caring for a family member with a mental illness can result in overwhelming emotional and economic stress on the family system, particularly if caregiver role strain becomes a contributing factor. Symptoms associated with SMI can significantly impair daily functioning, requiring a great deal of time and energy from family members who live with or care for the individual. Thus, it is common for the individual with SMI to become a large focus within the family dynamic, causing other members of the family to feel neglected or even ignored. In some situations this can cause a strain on the family unit as a whole (Mental Health America, 2013). In addition, a qualitative analysis by van der Sanden et al. (2015) found that family members of those who experienced mental illness were also stigmatized, increasing the stress felt by the family.

Family burden is the overall level of distress experienced as a result of the mental illness (Biegel & Schultz, 1999; Schene, 1990). **Objective burdens** are those that are measurable, such as disruption of family functioning and routines and financial costs of care. **Subjective burden** refers to the family or caregiver's perception of what is burdensome. Significantly higher family burden is associated with a number of variables. For example, the relapsing nature of schizophrenia has been associated with greater family burden than the more chronic, but perhaps more stable, symptoms of depression (Koujalgi & Patil, 2013). Acuity of patient symptoms is highly associated with caregiver burden, with sleep disturbances, lack of motivation, poor hygiene, acting out, and violent behaviors among a number of behaviors that increase family burden. Koutra et al. (2014) found that in families who have a member with psychosis, neither family cohesion nor flexibility was found to have significant direct

---

Box 26–4
Family and Medical Leave Act

Eligible parents of newborns and adopted children are entitled to 12 weeks of unpaid leave during any 12-month period, as initially authorized by the federal Family and Medical Leave Act of 1993. Vacation or sick leave may be used to pay for time away from work, depending on the employer's leave policies. This act also applies if a child, spouse, or parent of the employee develops a serious health condition. The employee is entitled to return to the previous position or an equivalent position with all the same pay, benefits, and other conditions. The act carries some additional conditions and requirements, including that employees are only eligible if they have worked for a covered employer for 1250 hours over the previous 12 months.

》》 Stay Current: More information on the Family and Medical Leave Act can be found at http://www.dol.gov/whd/fmla/employeeguide.htm

Source: Based on the Family and Medical Leave Act, Public Law 103-3, February 5, 1999. 5 U.S.C. 6381–6387; 5 CFR part 630, subpart L. Retrieved from http://www.opm.gov/pca/leave/HTMS/fmlafac2.asp.

effects on caregivers' psychologic distress; rather, this was mediated by family burden and caregivers' criticism.

The caregiving process itself can be stressful. Often community resources are not available, not satisfactory, or have long waiting lists. Insufficiency of these resources nationwide has resulted in high rates of homelessness, incarceration, and hospitalization of individuals with mental illness (Smith & Sederer, 2015). Some 40% of psychiatric patients have a history of criminal justice involvement related to decreased access to care, and rates of incarceration are high for individuals experiencing their first episode of mental illness, especially if it manifests as mania (Prince, Akincigil, & Bromet, 2007; Steadman et al., 2009). Families of the seriously mentally ill often find themselves negotiating the criminal justice system. Many times, the crimes are misdemeanors related to symptoms, such as disorderly conduct and intoxication.

Stigma describes patterns of negative attitudes that lead people to fear and discriminate against individuals with mental illness and their families. Because mental illness is so widely misunderstood, family members may isolate themselves from others who they feel are unsupportive or critical. Inability of some family members and friends to learn about and accept mental illness may lead to rejection. Further, discrimination resulting from stigma often extends to the family and caregivers (Pescosolido et al., 2013).

Feelings associated with subjective family burden include frustration, anxiety, hopelessness, and helplessness. Feels of depression and/or grief and loss may also be present. Chronic sorrow may take hold as family members experience the relapsing nature of the illness.

Families with healthy coping strategies are more likely to experience better outcomes and reduced caregiver burden. Healthy coping strategies when caring for a loved one with SMI include focusing on the positive response of the relationship, seeking social and community supports, reducing sources of conflict, and expressing affection. Moral support, practical support, and motivation to help the loved one improve in functional ability are essential to helping family members with SMI lower their symptom burdens and increase daily functioning (Aldersey, 2015). Families who act as stressors, increase or create conflict, display stigma and discrimination, or force treatment choices can impede the recovery of their loved one.

Pediatric Illness and the Family

Collaborating with families in providing healthcare is essential to promoting the best outcome when caring for children. Families have important knowledge to share about their child, their child's health condition, and how their child responds to various actions and events. They also need access to information that will make it possible for them to fully participate in planning and decision making.

Elements of family-centered care are outlined in **Table 26-5 »**.

Parents often need to assess their strengths in managing their ongoing family and caregiving responsibilities before planning how to add more caregiving responsibilities to their routine. Individuals who become family caregivers are at risk for considerable strain and stress, especially if they are unable to balance their own needs with those of the

---

Box 26–5
Guidelines for Effective Parent–Provider Collaboration

Parents have a role in developing an effective collaborative relationship with nurses and other health professionals. Parents often become experts in their child's health condition and learn to advocate for their child. They also must learn to communicate effectively with the health professionals caring for their child, and in the process develop a trusting relationship.

Tips for parents for improved communication are as follows:

- Keep a journal that includes your observations about your child's behavior, eating habits, illness, temperature, or anything else that might be helpful to the healthcare providers caring for your child.
- Keep a copy of your child's medical records, including test and procedure results.
- Write out questions or email healthcare providers, and do not hesitate to ask for clarification if you do not understand an answer provided.
- Be realistic about what you can expect from your child's nurses and doctors. They may not have all of the answers to your questions right away, but if you give them time, they will answer your questions. Try to let your healthcare providers know you appreciate their time and efforts on behalf of your child.

Communication tips for nurses include the following:

- Provide information and honestly discuss issues of concern to both the family and healthcare providers.
- Engage in creative problem solving and identify options for needed care that conform to the family's values and functioning.
- Demonstrate respect for the family's choices and methods for providing needed care.
- Continue to collaborate with the child and family and be willing to continue problem solving as new issues arise.

---

child. The nurse and parents should collaborate in developing the plan for the child's care, so as not to conflict with the family's cultural and ethnic illness-related behaviors, experiences, and beliefs. The child's opinions should also be integrated in the strategies for care. In almost all cases, the child leaves the healthcare setting and the family assumes responsibility for providing needed care in the home. The family caregivers must not feel alienated from a healthcare system they need for continuing assistance. See **Box 26–5 »** for guidelines for effective collaboration.

Family involvement is also valuable in the development of policies and guidelines for family-centered care in all types of healthcare settings. A family's experiences while receiving care may reveal valuable insights, perspectives, and realities that could lead to improved quality of care and satisfaction with care. Feedback could be provided on such issues as how comfortable they felt in the setting, their understanding of information provided to them, and the attitudes they sensed from health professionals. Parents who have been supported in developing leadership skills can be empowered to serve on advisory boards or councils representing the family and community perspectives (Warren, 2012).

TABLE 26–5 Elements of Family-Centered Care and Recommendations for Nursing Practice

Elements	Nursing Practice Recommendations
Family at the Center: ■ Incorporate into policy and practice the recognition that the family is the constant in a child's life, while the service systems and support personnel within those systems fluctuate, and that the illness or injury of a child affects all members of the family system.	■ Establish a therapeutic relationship with the family. ■ Perform a comprehensive family assessment in collaboration with the family, identifying both strengths and needs. ■ Use the family assessment when working with the family to plan, implement, and evaluate care, considering the impact of the child's illness or injury on the entire family, with special attention to the siblings. ■ Provide siblings with information about their sibling's illness/injury at an appropriate developmental level and answer questions honestly. ■ Promote sibling visitation in hospital settings and participation in home care activities. ■ Identify extended family members who should receive information and be included in the educational process.
Family–professional Collaboration: ■ Facilitate family–professional collaboration at all levels of hospital, home, and community care.	■ Develop provider–family relationships that are guided by the goals and expectations of both the family and the provider. ■ Ensure that parents are integral and critical collaborators in the decision-making process about their child's care. Involve children and adolescents in the decision-making process as appropriate for their cognitive and emotional development. ■ Ensure that parents have 24-hour access to their child, and facilitate their participation in the child's care. ■ Provide parents with the option to stay with their child during procedures and tests, and provide ways for parents to support the child during the procedure. ■ Provide comfort and hygiene facilities for families who spend long hours at the facility or travel great distances. ■ Promote the family's development of expertise in the special care of their child, fostering family independence and empowerment. ■ Incorporate parents and children into the quality assessment/improvement process. ■ Integrate family members into institutional and community advisory groups and involve them in policy development.
Family–professional Communication: ■ Exchange complete and unbiased information between families and professionals in a supportive manner at all times.	■ Provide information about the child's problem, prognosis, and needs in a manner that respects the child and family as individuals and promotes two-way dialogue. ■ Encourage the family to share information about the child and the illness/injury so that care planning and decisions are made in the most informed and collaborative manner.
Cultural Diversity of Families: ■ Incorporate into policy and practice the recognition and honoring of cultural diversity, strengths, and individuality within and across all families, including ethnic, racial, gender, spiritual, social, economic, educational, and geographic diversity.	■ Practice family-centered care in a culturally competent manner with respect and sensitivity for the wide range of families with diverse values and beliefs. ■ Seek to understand the family's beliefs and practices related to race, culture, gender, and ethnicity when developing relationships and collaborating in the child's healthcare. ■ Seek to understand and respect the family's religious/spiritual beliefs and practices and integrate these into the child's care, as the family desires. ■ Assist the family to address care issues related to socioeconomic status, insurance status, geography, and access to healthcare. ■ Integrate training programs on diversity, cultural understanding, and culturally competent care into staff development programs.
Coping Differences and Support: ■ Recognize and respect different methods of coping. Implement comprehensive policies and programs that provide families with the developmental, educational, emotional, spiritual, environmental, and financial support needed to meet their diverse needs.	■ Assess the strengths and weaknesses of the family's coping strategies and its resiliency factors and characteristics. Identify maladaptive coping mechanisms and help the family to augment its coping efforts. ■ Assess and support the family's needs and desires for support and assist the family in accessing and accepting assistance from support networks as needed or desired.
Family-centered Peer Support: ■ Encourage and facilitate family-to-family support and networking.	■ Educate parents about parent-to-parent and family support resources and help them to access such resources in the institution and community. ■ Provide access to psychoeducational groups that might be useful to parents, siblings, or ill/injured children.
Specialized Service and Support Systems: ■ Ensure that hospital, home, and community service and support systems for children needing specialized health and developmental care and their families are flexible, accessible, and comprehensive in responding to diverse family-identified needs.	■ Provide collaborative, flexible, accessible, comprehensive, and coordinated services to children and their families. ■ Provide comprehensive case management/care coordination for children and families with ongoing care needs. ■ Along with families, take an active role in advocating for the needs of ill and injured children.
Holistic Perspective of Family-centered Care: ■ Appreciate families as families and children as children, recognizing that they possess a wider range of strengths, concerns, emotions, and aspirations beyond their need for specialized health and developmental services and support.	■ Encourage attention to the normal developmental needs and developmental tasks of the entire family unit and individual family members. ■ Encourage and facilitate the development of individual and family identities beyond a focus on illness or injury. ■ Facilitate "normalization" as valued and desired by the family.

Source: Reprinted with permission from NAMI (2013). *NAMI Provider Education program.* Arlington, VA: National Alliance for the Mentally Ill. This is a 15-hour in-service training for direct case staff of mental health organizations. The course is taught by a trained team of family members, individuals living with mental illness, and a mental health professional who is also either a family member or living with a mental illness themselves. Copyright © 1999 by NAMI.

Some healthcare facilities are developing family resource centers to provide consumer information and support. In most cases, the resource center is a consumer-oriented health library with staffing, but peer support services may be coordinated through the center as well (Institute for Patient- and Family-Centered Care [IPFCC], 2016). Families can be supported in accessing useful information that helps them become informed decision makers about their child's care. Resources can often be provided in the preferred language and at an appropriate reading level.

When providing care to children, be aware that the family is central to all healthcare interventions with parents and child as the partners in care. It is important to consider how a healthcare setting's written policies, procedures, and literature for families refer to families and what attitudes these materials convey. Words like *policies*, *allowed*, and *not permitted* imply that hospital personnel have authority over families in matters concerning their children. Words like *guidelines*, *working together*, and *welcome* communicate an openness and appreciation for families in the care of their children.

Geriatric Illness and the Family

Adults who care for their own children and one or more of their own parents belong to a group that has come to be known as the "sandwich generation." This group of adults faces an incredible amount of stress trying to meet the diverse needs of young children and adolescents as well as aging parents. One of the chief sources of stress for these families is financial insecurity. A family with limited financial resources may face taking the aging parent into their own home or placing an aging parent who is no longer independent into a senior care facility that is below standard. If a family has very young children, taking an aging parent with dementia into the home can present either real or perceived hazards to the young children, increasing the stress level of the entire family. In addition, a member of the sandwich generation often faces additional stress addressing an older parent's needs while still trying to get children off to school and extracurricular activities and to maintain a full-time job. End-of-life issues can be a great source of stress and conflict for these families.

The needs of the family caring for an older adult who is ill will vary based on factors already detailed in this module.

In some cases, interventions needed are multiple and complex. But that should not stop nurses from helping family members identify needs that can be met in the short term with simple interventions. For example, caregivers may benefit from patient teaching regarding sleep hygiene to improve their own sleep or teaching about deep breathing and other relaxation techniques. Other nursing interventions may include referrals for respite care, hospice services, or counseling.

>> **Stay Current:** Older adults with neurologic disorders often experience sleep disruption. Research and advocacy organizations such as the Michael J. Fox Foundation for Parkinson's Research and the Alzheimer's Association offer resources to help both professionals and caregivers learn how to help their loved ones. See www.michaeljfox.org for resources for caregivers of individuals with Parkinson disease.

Risk Factors

The physical or mental illness of one family member places the entire family unit at risk for alterations in function. Among families, coping with illness may lead to family disputes, financial difficulties, and caregiver strain, as well as a number of other challenges. Financial challenges associated with illness are multifactorial; however, two common sources include medical bills and a member of the family leaving employment to help take care of another family member. Illness alone adds a considerable amount of stress to each family member's life—financial strains further compound the stress (Wadsworth & Rienks, 2012). High stress levels, especially among family caregivers, have been linked to health problems and an increased risk for premature mortality. Similarly, for the caregiver, impaired or inadequate coping function may lead to unhealthy choices, such as using tobacco and/or alcohol to manage stress levels (APA, 2013).

Prevention

Families who are made aware of the challenges associated with illness early in the process may benefit from having additional time to consider and plan for some of the upcoming circumstances. Talking about the illness as a family can be extremely beneficial, as can family counseling. Family support for one another is essential to get through this difficult time (Mental Health America, 2013). Nurses can help families by advising them of the challenges they will face and connecting them with the appropriate supportive resources, including counselors and sources of financial assistance as indicated.

Clinical Manifestations

Each family's reaction to a particular illness will vary based on their previous experiences, personal opinions, and cultural influences. Nurses must be alert to manifestations that signal the family is having difficulty coping with managing the illness and be able to respond appropriately to help family members improve their coping skills and access helpful resources (see the Clinical Manifestations and Therapies feature). Primary caregivers may benefit from education about techniques to relieve stress, participation in support groups, and respite care.

Clinical Manifestations and Therapies
Family Stressors

ETIOLOGY (PRIMARY STRESSOR)	CLINICAL MANIFESTATIONS	CLINICAL THERAPIES
Chronic illness in the family	■ Increased stress resulting in weight loss or gain, headaches, and anxiety ■ Lifestyle changes (e.g., job loss and financial difficulties) ■ Depression as evidenced by fatigue, lack of enjoyment, loss of interest in regular activities ■ Decreased participation in social activities; withdrawal ■ Unhealthy coping mechanisms (e.g., smoking, alcohol use, substance use)	■ Teach about healthy forms of stress management. ■ Provide resources for family counseling. ■ Educate about healthy eating habits to reduce risk for further illness and increase nutrition. ■ Discuss the benefits of exercise for stress relief and health.
Mental illness in the family	■ Confusion over changes occurring within the family unit ■ Stress related to helping the family member experiencing mental illness (possibly financial stress) ■ Anxiety ■ Depression ■ Feelings of loss related to changes in family member's behavior ■ Fear over the changes that are occurring ■ Changes in social activities, often resulting in decreased socialization	■ Educate about the benefits of counseling for the family to help with the changes that are occurring. ■ Advise about healthy stress management techniques. ■ Provide resources for support groups involving other families in similar circumstances. ■ Educate about the realities of the mental illness to dispel any misinformation and/or stigmas.
Illness of a child	■ Fear of death of the child ■ Anxiety, stress, depression in accordance with the child's illness and its effect on the parents and family ■ Decreased job performance, job loss, and financial difficulties resulting from taking the child to doctor appointments or spending time in the hospital ■ Confusion and anger resulting from a lack of control over the child's illness and health	■ Promote awareness of available counseling services. ■ Emphasize the importance of healthy eating habits and exercise. ■ Advise the primary caregivers to take time for themselves to avoid burnout. ■ Teach about healthy coping mechanisms and stress management. ■ Answer any questions the parents may have about their child's illness.
Caring for older parents	■ Criticism for not caring or not wanting to care for parent ■ Feeling censured because of reasons for caring for parent ■ Moral exclusion for not caring for parents	■ Suggest counseling for adult children of older adult as well as family members. ■ Provide resources such as respite care/day care for older adult and adult children.

Collaboration

Interventions vary based on the identified risks and actual or potential alterations in health. Nurses working with pediatric patients may collaborate with the school nurse, homebound teacher, guidance counselors, and other professionals. Collaboration with parents is key, because they often are the experts not only on their child but also on their child's illness, making them an extremely valuable member of the healthcare team. For older adults, nurses and other healthcare providers should continue to collaborate with the patient as long as the patient is able to participate in care.

However, the nurse and/or the healthcare team may increasingly collaborate with the older adult's primary caregiver in the event of progressive illness or deteriorating condition.

NURSING PROCESS

Nurses assess both the family and the patient when one family member is experiencing health problems. Families should be assessed for coping abilities, as well as possible complications that can arise from stress as a result of the family member's illness. Data from assessment of the patient and family will determine priorities for care.

Assessment

Assessment of the family facing challenges related to illness leads to the identification of family strengths and weaknesses. When indicated, the nurse also assesses the family's readiness and ability to provide continued care and supervision at home. Key components to consider when performing any family assessment and developing a patient's plan of care include the following:

- Cohesiveness and communication patterns within the family
- Family interactions that support self-care
- Number of friends and relatives available
- Family values and beliefs about health and illness
- Cultural and spiritual beliefs
- Developmental level of the patient and family.

Nursing assessment requires obtaining a complete family history, including genetic influences that may impact health. A family genogram (see Figure 26–9) may be helpful in collecting information, as detailed health histories should incorporate data regarding the patient's parents, siblings, grandparents, and even great-grandparents if information is available. If aunts, uncles, or cousins have had any health concerns, these should be noted as well. When assessing a family's history of mental illness, nurses should be aware that many individuals—especially from older generations—might not have volunteered knowledge about their mental illness. As a result, the patient may not know that a grandparent was diagnosed with a mental illness. Patients who were adopted and have no information about their birth parents will have no genetic health history to report, but information can be gathered about their health and environmental conditions during childhood, such as exposure to secondhand smoke, dietary patterns, or childhood illnesses.

Nurses are in a unique position to focus on care for an individual within the context of the family as partners. Being aware of issues that the family may face when one or more family members becomes ill can be helpful in guiding, teaching, and coordinating care for families. Being mindful of the impact of family function and structure in the particular family being cared for will provide a framework for identifying strengths of families as well as areas/resources needed by the family to recover and establish normal functioning patterns.

Diagnosis

Data gathered during a family assessment may lead to the following nursing diagnoses:

- *Family Processes, Interrupted*
- *Family Processes, Readiness for Enhanced*
- *Family Coping, Compromised*
- *Parenting, Impaired*
- *Parenting, Readiness for Enhanced*
- *Home Maintenance, Impaired*
- *Caregiver Role Strain.*

(NANDA-I © 2014)

Planning

Being sensitive to cultural differences is important in assessment and planning care. The nurse should determine who makes most of the decisions in the family, especially healthcare decisions, so he knows whom to obtain information from and whom to instruct. The extended family unit is found in many cultures, and different health beliefs and health practices may exist within the family. Building a trusting relationship with these families by talking with them about their beliefs and practices is the first step toward planning more effective care.

Nursing care includes assisting the family with planning realistic goals/outcomes and strategies that enhance family functioning, such as improving communication skills, identifying and using support systems, and developing and rehearsing parenting skills. Anticipatory guidance may assist well-functioning families in preparing for predictable developmental transitions that occur in the life of families.

To help families reintegrate the patient into the home following hospitalization or rehabilitation, nurses use data gathered during family assessment to identify family resources and deficits. By formulating mutually acceptable goals for reintegration, nurses help families cope with the realities of the illness and the changes it may have brought about. Such changes may include new roles and functions of family members or the need to provide continued medical care to the patient. Working together, nurses and families can create environments that restore or reorganize family functioning during illness and throughout the recovery process.

Implementation

Although teaching is a core nursing intervention, it is important to remember that standardized teaching plans may not be effective for patients with chronic illness and their families. These patients and their families should be encouraged to choose appropriate literature and to find self-help or support groups so they can interact with others who have the same illness.

For families who will be providing care in the home setting, extensive teaching may be required. When the plan of care includes medication administration and equipment use, family members and caregivers may feel overwhelmed by the technical aspects of the patient's care. As much as possible, teaching sessions should be organized and divided into segmented presentations to avoid overloading the family and caregivers with information. Teaching sessions may include demonstration of the family's ability to provide care to their family member. In addition, the nurses assists in identifying available resources that are socially and financially acceptable.

Evaluation

In evaluating the efficacy of the family nursing care plan, the nurse identifies the degree to which the family members have achieved the identified outcomes relevant to each nursing diagnosis. During evaluation, the nurse also examines all aspects of the nursing care plan to determine the effectiveness of nursing interventions, as well as to evaluate the continued relevance of original nursing diagnoses. Based on evaluation, the nursing care plan is modified to meet the family's current needs.

While the process of evaluation varies depending on the components of the family-specific nursing care plan, examples of criteria that may reflect successful achievement of identified outcomes include the following:

- Family members demonstrate the ability to identify realistic personal and family goals.

- Family members identify and demonstrate healthy coping strategies.
- Caregiver(s) demonstrate safe and effective implementation of care to their family member.
- Family members demonstrate support of the primary caregiver(s).

REVIEW Family Response to Health Alterations

RELATE Link the Concepts and Exemplars

Mrs. Ann Bell, an 82-year-old widow, was diagnosed with Alzheimer disease several years ago. She lives with her daughter and son-in-law and their two children, ages 16 and 10 years. Mrs. Bell has begun wandering, especially at night, and has started small fires when she attempts to cook and forgets about the pot on the stove. Mrs. Bell's daughter, Laura, accompanies her mother to her physician's appointment today and relates that the stress of caring for her mother, in addition to her other obligations to her husband and children, is becoming increasingly difficult.

Linking the exemplar of family response to health alterations with the concept of grief and loss:

1. How can the nurse help the family members to cope with the loss they feel related to Mrs. Bell's cognitive degeneration?

2. What strategies might help Mrs. Bell's grandchildren identify their feelings of grief and loss and work as a family to deal with these feelings?

Linking the exemplar of family response to health alterations with the concept of stress and coping:

3. What strategies can you suggest to help this family deal with the stress of Mrs. Bell's cognitive degeneration?

4. What referrals can you make to reduce Mrs. Bell's daughter's caregiver role strain?

REFER Go to Pearson MyLab Nursing and eText

- Additional review materials

REFLECT Apply Your Knowledge

Casey, a 16-year-old, is recuperating from injuries sustained in a motor vehicle crash in which he was the passenger. He was not wearing a seat belt and experienced a brain injury after striking the windshield. His cognitive and motor functions are impaired. After a 7-day acute care hospital stay, he was moved to an inpatient rehabilitation hospital, where he has been for the past 5 days. He is much more responsive to stimuli and to family members 12 days after his injury. Physical therapy is provided twice a day to promote range of motion and muscle tone and to prevent contractures. Plans are being made to discharge him home with outpatient rehabilitation care within the next 5 days. A case manager will be assigned to coordinate his healthcare services.

Casey lives with his mother, two half-brothers (10 and 6 years old), and stepfather. Both his mother and stepfather are employed full time and are trying to determine how to manage care for Casey once he returns home. Casey's father has not been actively involved in his life since his parents divorced 12 years ago. Casey's grandparents reside in the same town and may provide the family some support.

1. What family supports will Casey need as he continues his rehabilitation for the brain injury?

2. What family assessment information is needed to effectively plan nursing care for this adolescent and his family?

3. Identify two strengths and coping strategies that will help Casey's family members adapt to his disability.

Casey's family is coping with his initial survival of a serious brain injury and facing a long rehabilitation process. The family is just now recognizing that life as they have known it is changing. Casey is totally dependent for care, including bathing, toileting, feeding, and mobilizing. While he is expected to regain self-care abilities, the impact of the injury on his cognitive ability and future functioning is unknown.

Casey's extended family has provided support for the family during the past 12 days, but the level of support in the future weeks will decrease because of other family obligations. Casey's mother has already initiated a leave of absence from work so she can care for him when he returns home; however, this will mean the family has reduced income during that time period. Casey's younger brothers have been able to visit him, and they are very anxious because Casey cannot talk with them. They have been trying to avoid bothering their mother and father during this time, but they are wondering when life will be more normal and they can again participate in their usual afterschool activities.

4. What information about the family's strengths, needs, and resilience can be identified from the case study scenario?

5. What additional information would be helpful to know about family strengths and needs prior to developing a nursing care plan?

6. Based on your assessment of the family and challenges facing them, what is the priority nursing diagnosis for Casey and his family at this time? Why do you believe it is the priority?

7. Describe the use of family-centered care principles in planning Casey's nursing care in collaboration with the family.

8. What potential parenting issues could this family anticipate for Casey and his brothers?

References

Aldersey, H. M. (2015). Family influence in recovery from severe mental illness. *Community Mental Health Journal, 51*(4), 467–476. doi:10.1007/s10597-014-9783-y

American Academy of Pediatrics, Committee on the Psychosocial Aspects of Child and Family Health.

(2013). Promoting the well-being of children whose parents are gay or lesbian. *Pediatrics, 131*(4), 827–830.

American Psychiatric Association. (2013). *Diagnostic and statistical manual of mental disorders* (5th ed.). Washington, DC: Author.

American Psychological Association (APA). (2013). *Risks for family caregivers.* Retrieved from http://www.apa.org/pi/about/publications/caregivers/faq/risks.aspx

American Psychological Association (APA). (2014). The United States leads the world in incarceration.

A new report explores why—and offers recommendations for fixing the system. *Incarceration Nation (45)*9, 56. Retrieved from http://www.apa.org/monitor/2014/10/incarceration.aspx

American Psychological Association. (2016). *Effects of poverty, hunger, and homelessness on children and youth.* Retrieved from http://www.apa.org/pi/families/poverty.aspx

Anthony, C. J., DiPerna, J. C., & Amato, P. R. (2014). Divorce, approaches to learning, and children's academic achievement: A longitudinal analysis of mediated and moderated effects. *Journal of School Psychology, 52,* 249–261.

Arkes, J. (2015). The temporal effects of divorces and separations on children's academic achievement and problem behavior. *Journal of Divorce and Remarriage, 56,* 25–42.

Biegel, D. R., & Schultz, R. (1999). Caregiving and caregiver interventions in aging and mental illness. *Family Relationships, 48,* 345–355.

Biringen, Z., Derscheid, D., Vliegen, N., Closson, L., & Easterbrooks, A. E. (2014). Emotional availability (EA): Theoretical background, empirical research using the EA Scales, and clinical applications. *Developmental Review, 34,* 114–167. doi:10.1016/j.dr.2014.01.002

Bleske-Rechek, A., & Kelley, J. A. (2013). Birth order and personality: A within-family test using independent self-reports from both firstborn and laterborn siblings. *Personality and Individual Differences.* doi:http://dx.doi.org/10.1016/j.paid.2013.08.011

Bos, H. M. W., Knox, J. R., van Rijn-van Gelderen, L., & Gartrell, N. K. (2016). Same-sex and different-sex parent households and child health outcomes: Findings from the National Survey of Children's Health. *Journal of Developmental and Behavioral Pediatrics, 37*(3), 179–187.

Caldwell, B. M., & Bradley, R. H. (1984). The HOME Inventory and family demographics. *Developmental Psychology, 20*(2), 315–320.

Cousino, M. K., & Hazen, R. A. (2013). Parenting stress among caregivers of children with chronic illness: A Systematic Review. *Journal of Pediatric Psychology, 38*(8), 809-828.

Department of Defense (DoD). (2012). Demographics profile of the military community. Washington D. C.: Office of the Deputy Under Secretary of Defense. Retrieved from http://www.militaryonesource.mil/12038/MOS/Reports/2012_Demographics_Report.pdf.

Duvall, E. M. (1977). *Marriage and family development* (5th ed.). Philadelphia, PA: Lippincott.

Ellis, L., Gergen, J., & Wohlgemuth, L. (2016). Empowering the cheerers: Role of surgical intensive care nurses in enhancing family resilience. *American Journal of Critical Care, 25*(1), 39–45.

Federal Interagency Forum on Child and Family Statistics. (2015). *America's children: Key national indicators of well-being, 2015.* Retrieved from http://www.childstats.gov/pdf/ac2015/ac_15.pdf

Gates, G. J. (2013). *LGBT parenting in the United States: Executive summary.* Los Angeles, CA: The Williams Institute. Retrieved from http://williamsinstitute.law.ucla.edu/wp-content/uploads/LGBT-Parenting.pdf

Hamilton, B. E., Mathews, M. S., & Ventura, S. J. (2013). *Declines in state teen birth rates by race and Hispanic origin.* Retrieved from: http://www.cdc.gov/nchs/products/databriefs/db123.htm

Hebda, T. & Czar, P. (2014). *Handbook of informatics for nurses and health care professionals.* Upper Saddle River, NJ: Pearson.

Herdman, T. H. & Kamitsuru, S. (Eds.). *Nursing Diagnoses—Definitions and Classification 2015–2017.*

Copyright © 2014, 1994–2014 NANDA International. Used by arrangement with John Wiley & Sons, Inc. Companion website: www.wiley.com/go/nursingdiagnoses

Hughes, E. (2013). *Types of parenting styles and how to identify yours.* Retrieved from https://my.vanderbilt.edu/developmentalpsychologyblog/2013/12/types-of-parenting-styles-and-how-to-identify-yours

Institute for Patient- and Family-Centered Care (IPFCC). (2015). *Patient and family-centered care.* Retrieved from http://www.ipfcc.org/about/pfcc.html

Institute for Patient- and Family-Centered Care (IPFCC). (2016). *Patient and family resource centers.* Retrieved from: http://www.ipfcc.org/advance/topics/pafam-resource.html

Kaakinen, J. R. & Hanson, S. M. (2015). Family health care nursing: An introduction. In J. R. Kaakinen, D. P. Coehlo, R. Steele, A. Tabacco, & S. M. H, Hanson (Eds.), *Family health care nursing: Theory, practice and research* (5th ed., pp. 3–32). Philadelphia, PA: F. A. Davis.

Koujalgi, S. R., & Patil, S. R. (2013). Family burden in patients with schizophrenia and depressive disorder. *Indian Journal of Psychological Medicine, 35*(3), 251–255.

Koutra, S., Triliva, T., Roumeliotaki, Z., Stefanakis, M., Basta, C., Lionis, A., & Vgontzas, K. (2014). Family functioning in families of first-episode psychosis patients as compared to chronic mentally ill patients and healthy controls. *Psychiatry Research, 219*(3), 486–496.

Lee, R.D., Fang, X., & Luo, F. (2013). The impact of parental incarceration on physical and mental health of young adults. *Pediatrics, 131*(4), e1188–e1195.

Locke, J., Campbell, M. A., & Kavanagh, D. S. (2012). Can a parent do too much for their child? An examination by parenting professionals of the concept of overparenting. *Australian Journal of Guidance and Counselling, 22*(2), 249–265.

Mallory, C., Sears, B., Hasenbush, A., & Susman, A. (2014). *Ensuring access to mentoring programs for LGBTQ youth: A report of the Williams Institute.* Los Angeles, CA: UCLA School of Law.

Martin, M. E. (2012). Family structure and the intergenerational transmission of educational advantage. *Social Science Research, 41*(1), 33–47.

Mellins, R. B., Evans, D., Clark, N., Zimmerman, B., & Wiesemann, S. (2015). Developing and communicating a long-term treatment plan for asthma. *American Family Physician, 91,* 1–13.

Mental Health America. (2013). *Mental illness and the family: Recognizing warning signs and how to cope.* Retrieved from http://www.nmha.org/go/information/get-info/mi-and-the-family/recognizing-warning-signs-and-how-to-cope

Merriam-Webster Dictionary. (2016). *Family.* Retrieved from http://www.merriam-webster.com/dictionary/family

Moyer, D. N., & Sandoz, E. K. (2014). The role of psychological flexibility in the relationship between parent and adolescent distress. *Journal of Child and Family Studies, 24*(5), 1406–1418.

Murray, C. J. L., & Lopez, A. D. (2013). Measuring the global burden of disease. *New England Journal of Medicine, 369*(5), 448–457.

NAMI. (2013). *NAMI Provider Education program.* Arlington, VA: National Alliance for the Mentally Ill. This is a 15-hour in-service training for direct case staff of mental health organizations. The course is taught by a trained team of family members, indi-

viduals living with mental illness, and a mental health professional who is also either a family member or living with a mental illness themselves. Copyright © 1999 by NAMI.

National Child Traumatic Stress Network. (2011). *Trauma and families: Fact sheet for providers.* Retrieved from http://www.nctsn.org/sites/default/files/assets/pdfs/family_systems_factsheetproviders.pdf

Pescosolido, B., Medina, T., Martin J., & Long, J. (2013). The "backbone" of stigma: Identifying the global core of public prejudice associated with mental illness. *American Journal of Public Health, 103*(5), 853–860.

Potter, M. L., & Moller, M. D. (2016). *Psychiatric-mental health nursing: From suffering to hope.* New York, NY: Pearson Education, p. 698.

Prickett, K.C., Martin-Storey, A., & Crosnoe, R. (2015). A research note on time with children in different- and same-sex two-parent families. *Demography, 52*(3), 905–916. doi:10.1007/s13524-015-0385-2

Prince, J. D., Akincigil, A., & Bromet, E. (2007). Incarceration rates of persons with first-admission psychosis. *Psychiatric Services, 58*(9), 1173–1180.

Reckdahl, K. (2015, April 2). The lost children of Katrina. *The Atlantic.* Retrieved from http://www.theatlantic.com/education/archive/2015/04/the-lost-children-of-katrina/389345/

Rentfro, A. R. (2014). Health promotion and the family. In C. L. Edelman, E. C. Kudzma, & C. L. Mandle (Eds.), Health promotion throughout the life span (8th ed.). St. Louis, MO: Elsevier/Mosby.

Rohrer, J. M., Egloff, B., & Schmukle, S. C. (2015). Examining the effects of birth order on personality. *Proceedings of the National Academy of Sciences of the United States of America, 112*(46), 14224–14229. doi:10.1073/pnas.1506451112

Saunders, H., Kraus, A., Barone, L., & Biringen, Z. (2015). Emotional availability: Theory, research and intervention. *Frontiers in Psychology, 6,* 1089. doi:10.3389/fpsyg.2015.01069

Schene, A. H. (1990). Objective and subjective dimensions of family burden. Towards an integrative framework for research. *Social Psychiatry and Psychiatric Epidemiology, 25*(6), 289–297.

Segrin, C., Woszidlo, A., Givertz, M., & Montgomery, N. (2013). Parent and child traits associated with overparenting. *Journal of Social and Clinical Psychology, 32*(6). doi:10.1521/jscp.2013.32.6.569

Smith, T. E., & Sederer, L. I. (2015). A new kind of homelessness for individuals with serious mental illness? The need for a "mental health home." *Psychiatric Services, 60*(4), 528–533. doi:http://dx.doi.org/10.1176/ps.2009.60.4.528

Spector, R. E. (2017). *Cultural diversity in health and illness* (9th ed.). Hoboken, NJ: Pearson Education.

State of California Franchise Tax Board. (2013). *Domestic partners.* Retrieved from https://www.ftb.ca.gov/individuals/faq/dompart.shtml

Steadman, H., Osher, F., Robbins, P. C., Case, B., & Samuels, S. (2009). Prevalence of serious mental illness among jail inmates. *Psychiatric Services, 60*(2), 761–765.

Strout, K. (2012). Wellness promotion and the Institute of Medicine's future of nursing report: Are nurses ready? *Holistic Nursing Practice, 26*(3), 129–136.

Trautman, J., Alhusen, J., & Gross, D., (2015). Impact of deployment on military families with young children: A systematic review. *Nursing Outlook, 63*(6), 656–679. doi:http://dx.doi.org/10.1016/j.outlook.2015.06.002

Turney, K., & Wildeman, C. (2013). Redefining relationships: Explaining the countervailing consequences of parenteral incarceration for parenting. *American Sociological Review, 78*(6), 949–979. http://www.jstor.org/stable/43188367

U.S. Bureau of Labor Statistics. (2012). *Employment status of parents, 2011.* Retrieved from https://www.bls.gov/opub/ted/2012/ted_20120427.htm

U.S. Census Bureau. (2012). *America's family and living arrangements: 2012.* Retrieved from http://www.census.gov/hhes/families/data/cps2012.html

U.S. Census Bureau. (2013). *Families and living arrangements.* Retrieved from https://www.census.gov/hhes/families/data/cps2013H.html

U.S. Census Bureau. (2015). *Fertility: historical time series tables.* Retrieved from http://www.census.gov/hhes/fertility/data/cps/historical.html

van der Sanden, R. L. M., Bos, A. E. R., Stutterheim, S. E., Pryor, J. B., & Kok, G. (2015). Stigma by association among family members of people with a mental illness: A qualitative analysis. *Journal of Community & Applied Social Psychology, 25*(5), 400–417. doi:10.1002/casp.2221.

von Bertalanffy, L. (1981). *A systems view of man.* Boulder, CO: Westview Press.

Wadsworth, M. E., & Rienks, S. L. (2012). Stress as a mechanism of poverty's ill effects on children: Making a case for family strengthening interventions that counteract poverty-related stress. *American Psychological Association.* Retrieved from: http://www.apa.org/pi/families/resources/newsletter/2012/07/stress-mechanism.aspx

Walsh, F. (2016). *Strengthening family resilience.* New York, NY: Guilford Press.

Warren, N. (2012). Involving patient and family advisors in the patient and family-centered care model. *Medsurg Nursing, 21*(4), 233–239.

Yousafzai, A. K., Rasheed, M. A., Rizvi, A., Armstrong, R., & Bhutta, Z. A. (2015). Parenting skills and emotional availability: An RCT. *Pediatrics, 135*(5), 1. doi:10.1542/peds.2014-2335247-1257

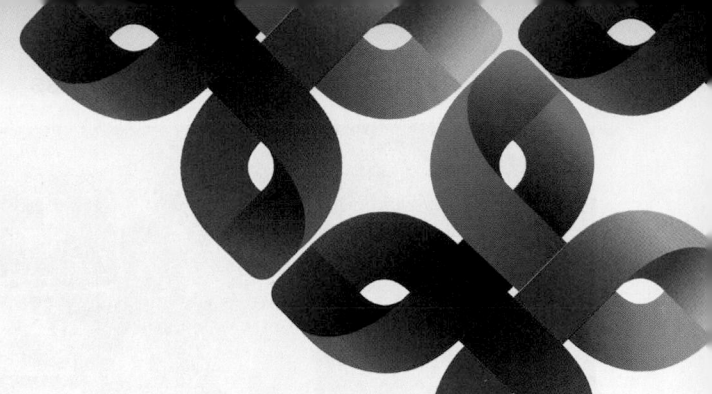

Module 27
Grief and Loss

Module Outline and Learning Outcomes

The Concept of Grief and Loss

The Process of Grieving

27.1 Analyze the process of grieving.

Factors That Affect the Grieving Process

27.2 Analyze factors that affect the grieving process.

Concepts Related to Grief and Loss

27.3 Outline the relationship between grief and loss and other concepts.

Nursing Assessment

27.4 Differentiate common assessment procedures used to examine patients or families who are grieving.

Independent Interventions

27.5 Analyze independent interventions nurses can implement for patients who are grieving.

Collaborative Therapies

27.6 Summarize collaborative therapies used by interprofessional teams for patients experiencing grief and loss.

Children's Grief Responses

27.7 Differentiate considerations related to the assessment and care of children who are dying or experiencing significant loss.

Perinatal Loss

27.8 Differentiate considerations related to the assessment and care of a family who experiences a perinatal loss.

Older Adults' Responses to Loss

27.9 Differentiate considerations related to the assessment and care of older adults experiencing a significant loss.

» The Concept of Grief and Loss

Concept Key Terms

Actual loss, **1884**	Childhood traumatic grief, **1897**	Disseminated intravascular coagulation (DIC), **1900**	Intrauterine fetal death (IUFD), **1899**	Perinatal loss, **1899**
Ageism, **1904**				Placental abruption, **1900**
Anticipatory grief, **1884**	Complicated grief, **1885**		Loss, **1883**	Rh disease, **1900**
Anticipatory loss, **1884**	Death anxiety, **1895**	Fetal demise, **1899**	Miscarriage, **1899**	Spontaneous abortion, **1899**
Bereavement, **1883**	Disenfranchised grief, **1884**	Grief, **1883**	Mourning, **1883**	
Blighted ovum, **1899**		Hospice, **1893**	Perceived loss, **1884**	Stillbirth, **1899**

Loss and grief are inherent in the human experience. Even so, reactions to loss and manifestations of grief vary widely. Each individual's methods of processing and coping with grief are influenced by numerous variables, including personality, age, culture, the nature of the loss, and the availability of a functional support system. **Loss** occurs when something or someone of value is rendered inaccessible or drastically changed. In addition to the loss of a loved one, numerous other sources of loss can also prompt grief reactions. Examples include the loss of a friend or relationship, loss of mobility, loss of independence, loss of a limb, and loss of hair from illness (**Figure 27–1 »**). By understanding the emotional and physical aspects associated with grief, nurses are better prepared to care for patients who have experienced loss, as well as to support these patients during the grieving process.

The Process of Grieving

Grief is the combination of various psychologic, biological, and behavioral responses to a loss. Psychologic responses may include anger, denial, and depression. Biological responses to grief include sleep disturbances, decreased appetite, and weight loss. Behavioral responses include personality changes and decreased socialization. Bereavement and mourning can also accompany grief. **Bereavement** is the response to having lost another through death. **Mourning** involves the processing and resolution of grief,

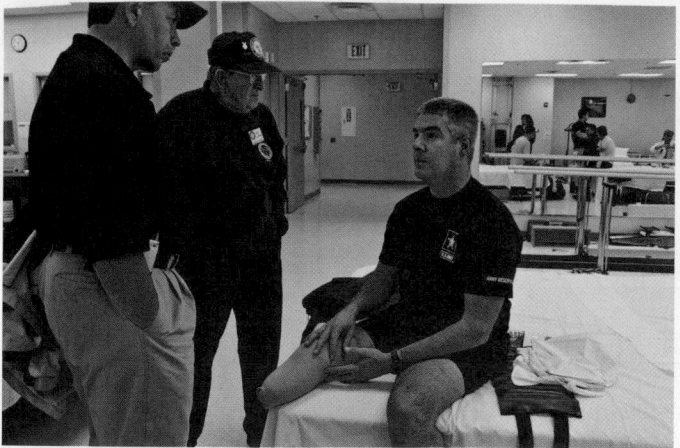

Source: David S. Holloway/Getty Images.

Figure 27–1 》 Loss of an aspect of self is common in those serving in the military, as loss of an appendage or a functional ability is one of the hazards of serving in combat.

generally through cultural and/or spiritual beliefs and practices. Grief can be triggered by any number of situations or occurrences, such as the loss of a loved one or acquaintance or being diagnosed with a terminal illness. Grief can also result from the end of a significant relationship with a partner or a close friend. In most cases, grief is a normal, healthy reaction to loss, as it helps the individual to process the situation. Grief should not be avoided, as avoidance often prolongs and intensifies the experience. For some individuals, the grieving process may also be prolonged by failure to mourn the loss according to an individual's cultural or spiritual practices.

The process of grieving is different for all who experience a loss. There is no correct way to grieve, nor is there a timetable for how long the grieving process should last. Manifestations associated with grief are highly individualized and depend on numerous factors such as the nature of the loss, the circumstances surrounding the loss, the developmental age and personality of the individual who is grieving, and the individual's history of grief and/or depression. Intense feelings of grief over the loss of a loved one are generally believed to lessen over a few months, and to resolve—or at least partly resolve—within 1–2 years (Walsh, 2012). This timetable does not apply in every case, and if the grief becomes complicated in any way—for example, when a loss is especially sudden or traumatic—resolution and acceptance take longer. Different types of grief should also be considered, as these often coincide with the type of loss experienced.

Types and Sources of Loss

Everyone experiences various types of loss over the course of a lifetime. The three main types of loss are **actual loss**, loss that is identified and recognized by others, such as the loss of a spouse; **anticipatory loss**, which occurs when an individual knows a loss is coming, such as the impending

death of a friend or family member from a fatal illness; and **perceived loss**, which is felt by an individual but cannot be verified as a loss from outside—for example, loss of control or loss of self-esteem.

The source of the loss may impact the range of an individual's emotional responses. For example, individuals who have lost a limb because of amputation lose an aspect of the self. They may experience disturbance of body image, depression, loss of independence, and frustration as they learn to live without use of the limb. Loss of an aspect of self can be very similar to loss of a loved one, in that the individual must learn to function despite the loss. Loss of independence itself is a serious loss, and it may occur with the loss of mobility due to injury or with debilitating illnesses such as dementia or multiple sclerosis.

Many individuals, families, and communities cope with grief and loss that is related to military conflicts. Examples include the loss and grief experienced by families who lost a loved one in the terror attacks of September 11, 2001, and loss and grief associated with military deployment. The deployment of military personnel carries a number of consequences that may result in grief responses. Long-term absence of a deployed parent creates additional responsibility for the parent remaining at home and a sense of loss for the entire family, as well as fear for the safety of the deployed family member. When both parents are deployed, children may be relocated away from their childhood home and support systems to live with other relatives. Personnel returning with traumatic physical and mental injuries may have difficulty rejoining the family unit. Finally, death of a family member overseas brings great loss to a family.

Types of Grief

Grief presents itself in many different forms, ranging from anticipatory grief to complicated grief. Similar to anticipatory loss, **anticipatory grief** is grief that is experienced before the event occurs. This can occur in anticipation of the death of a loved one, or in response to the diagnosis of an individual's own terminal illness. For example, a man's wife has a terminal illness and is expected to live only another 3 months. He may experience anticipatory grief in advance of his wife's death, grieving for her while she is still alive. Not all individuals experience anticipatory grief. Despite many debates on the subject, no conclusive studies have proven whether anticipatory grief actually lessens the grieving process after a loved one has died.

Disenfranchised grief occurs when individuals cannot acknowledge their loss to others, typically when the loss is not one that is socially recognized (sometimes referred to as an *ambiguous loss*). Disenfranchised grief may result from the loss of a partner in a socially unrecognized relationship, the loss of a child due to abortion, the loss of someone from suicide or a drug overdose, or even the loss of a pet. When a loss is considered socially unacceptable, the individual grieving the loss may experience not only intense grief but also feelings of isolation. Unable to participate in culturally appropriate expressions of mourning, the bereaved may find it very difficult to resolve their feelings and responses to the loss.

Individuals who are unable to process their grief to a point of resolution may experience **complicated grief**. Complicated grief is generally not diagnosed until 6 months after a loss. If at this time the grief has not diminished, has become debilitating, and makes daily activities difficult or impossible, the grief may be deemed complicated. Some have proposed renaming this type of grief *prolonged grief disorder (PGD)*. The two terms are sometimes used interchangeably (Robinaugh et al., 2012).

Theories of Grieving

Different theories have been proposed to explain the grieving process. Typically, these theories identify different stages of grief. Grief theorists include Elisabeth Kübler-Ross, George Engel, and Catherine Sanders.

Kübler-Ross and the Five Stages of Grief

One of the first grief theorists, Elisabeth Kübler-Ross (1969), proposed five stages of grief: denial, anger, bargaining, depression, and acceptance. A psychiatrist, Kübler-Ross based her theory on work she did with dying patients, so some criticism holds that these stages cannot, therefore, be ascribed to those mourning the loss of another. Other critics contend that the stages of grief do not always occur sequentially, as Kübler-Ross described them; stages can overlap or occur individually (Buglas, 2010, p. 45).

Denial, the first stage of grieving, may serve to soften the initial blow of the loss. A small amount of denial early in the grieving process is healthy, as it allows individuals who have undergone a loss to retreat into themselves so as to eventually accept the loss more fully. Nurses working with patients in denial should not force their patients to accept the loss; neither should they reinforce the denial. Denial generally occurs for only a short time, as most individuals eventually begin to accept the loss in their own way, so nurses should be understanding and supportive.

Anger is one of the most difficult stages for all those involved. During this stage, bereaved individuals direct their anger toward anyone who is around them, sometimes without even the slightest apology. Patients who are angry in their grief over a significant loss may direct their anger at staff, nurses, and doctors. This behavior should not be taken personally, as it usually has nothing to do with the actions of the nurse, doctor, or staff member.

The third stage is bargaining. Those who are in this phase of grieving try to make a bargain, generally with a higher power (such as God, Allah, or Mother Nature), or even with a doctor, for more time. Kübler-Ross found through interviews with patients that this stage sometimes results from the individual's guilt over something from the past. A nurse can help during this stage by listening sympathetically to the patient's expression of fears and guilt.

Depression follows the bargaining stage. Depression, a profound sense of deep and penetrating loss felt during the grieving period, is part of the normal work of loss. Nurses support patients during this phase by encouraging and allowing them to express their sadness and sometimes simply by sitting with them silently as they work through these emotions on their own.

After depression, the final stage of the grieving process is acceptance. During acceptance the patient is free from anger and depression; this is not a happy stage, but one almost lacking in emotions. Generally, during this time, a terminally ill patient's family needs more support and comfort than the patient, who often experiences a decreased desire for visits from family and loved ones. At this point, the dying individual has fully accepted the loss and gone through the various stages of grieving in order to arrive at acceptance.

Engel and Sanders

Other theories about the grieving process describe similar experiences with grief, but focus on the individual grieving for the loss of another as opposed to individuals grieving the loss of their own lives. George Engel's (1964) theory describes six stages of grief: shock, disbelief, awareness, restitution, idealization, and outcome. Shock and awareness are very similar to Kübler-Ross's stages of denial and anger, while restitution, idealization, and outcome deal primarily with the acceptance and understanding of the loss.

The work of Catherine Sanders (1998) focuses on the five distinct phases of grief: shock, awareness, conservation, healing, and renewal. The phases of shock and awareness resemble Kübler-Ross's stages of denial and anger, during which the patient is still working to come to terms with the loss. In the conservation/withdrawal phase, the individual begins to feel depressed and weakened from the loss, needing time to work through the emotions. Healing and renewal are the final stages, during which the emotions associated with grief begin to abate, and the individual is left with a feeling of acceptance.

Manifestations of Grief

Normal grief reactions are difficult to define, as all individuals grieve differently, but in general it is normal to experience sadness, anxiety, guilt, anger, confusion, sleep disturbances, and loss of appetite, among other reactions. The amount of time these emotions last varies. Typically, however, the intense feelings of grief begin to dissipate over the first 3–6 months following the loss, resurfacing on holidays, birthdays, and other important reminders of the loss. When grief becomes complicated, the intense emotions begin to impact the individual's ability to carry out daily activities. Similarly, these forms of grief may begin to affect the individual's health through loss of appetite, extreme depression, and sleeplessness. It is important for nurses to know the signs of different forms of grief reactions. Disenfranchised grief, described earlier, may result in a prolonged grief reaction, in part due to the individual's inability to mourn the loss in a socially acceptable way. Consider, for example, the case of a mother who gives up her child for adoption. Others do not know why she has made this decision, and individuals may assume that she did not want the child. Others are also likely to refrain from offering support or from asking questions, unsure how to treat the mother who is giving up her child. As a result, the birth mother may feel that society has told her she has no right to grieve the loss of this infant because she decided to give it up for adoption. Her grief may then become disenfranchised because she cannot acknowledge her loss to others. It is critical that nurses provide both physical care and psychosocial support to patients experiencing disenfranchised grief. When a mother has released her child for adoption, the nurse might mention the adoption, letting the patient know she is free to talk if she chooses. Often, the nurse's willingness to listen without offering advice helps the patient greatly by allowing her a safe, nonjudgmental place to grieve. The nurse could also offer the birth mother an opportunity to hold the infant and say good-bye, thus allowing a sense of closure (Aloi, 2009, p. 30).

For the individual experiencing complicated grief, the grieving process does not progress. Instead, an overwhelming sense of grief persists and sometimes worsens over a period of months. The individual may experience profound emotions associated with memories of the deceased, along with an inability to accept the reality of the loss. Auditory and visual hallucinations are not uncommon for those experiencing this form of prolonged grief. In addition to these symptoms, bereaved individuals may become distrustful or uncaring toward others, forcing themselves into a form of self-imposed isolation. Complicated grief arises in approximately 6–25% of the bereaved, who still feel intense, disruptive grief for a prolonged period of many months, or even years, while typically grief begins to lessen in intensity within 3–6 months. In the first 6 months after a loss, an individual is expected to experience some of the same symptoms seen in individuals with complicated grief, such as extreme distress and an inability to function normally in day-to-day activities. However, if after 6 months these symptoms have not lessened and individual functioning is significantly impaired or the individual is at an increased risk for suicide, then complicated grief may be diagnosed. The earliest this diagnosis can be made is 6 months; however, many still debate about how much time must elapse before this diagnosis can be made (Robinaugh et al., 2012).

Factors That Affect the Grieving Process

When considering the process of grieving, it is important to take into account the nature of the individual's loss as well as the support system. The nature of the loss and the individual's current health and financial status affect the amount and type of support needed. A loss that impacts daily functioning, such as the death of an income-earning spouse or of a primary caregiver, results in a variety of consequences. Individuals experiencing this type of loss typically require greater support than those who experience the loss of, say, a distant relative or casual acquaintance. Similarly, individuals who experience ambiguous losses—such as perinatal loss, the death of a pet, or the death of an ex-spouse—require a wholly different form of support. In general, individuals seek support from those who were close to the deceased or from those who have experienced similar losses. Researchers have found that among participants in a study of the importance of social support during bereavement, the majority of respondents said it was

helpful to talk to others who had undergone similar experiences, or who could truly understand the feelings of the individual grieving. In the same study, many participants reported that whether or not they took advantage of professional support such as therapy, they were comforted by knowing it was available to them if needed (Benkel, Wijk, & Molander, 2009, pp. 144–145).

Cumulative loss is defined as several losses within a short period, one after another after another. The individual who experiences cumulative loss may not recover from the initial loss before the next loss occurs. Each loss has the potential to compound the grief of previous loss to the point where the individual becomes paralyzed with grief (Thompson, 2012). An example of a cumulative loss would be an individual who experiences the death of a friend, then a short time later experiences the death of a spouse, and soon after is diagnosed with a serious illness. The individual may not be able to fully grieve the loss of the friend when having to then cope with the loss of the spouse. The grief then could be compounded with the diagnosis of a serious illness when the individual is faced with his or her own mortality.

Age

Children who experience loss at an early age are at greater risk of an intense grieving period, especially children who lose a parent or primary caregiver. This risk increases further when the remaining parent or caregiver fails to recognize the child's grief and assumes that the child is too young to be affected by the loss. If children do not receive support and explanation after a substantial loss, they may view the loss as a betrayal, giving rise to feelings of guilt and anger. This reaction may result in the development of trust issues later in life (Walsh, 2012, p. 33). Children's grief responses can also be more complicated if the individual lost was physically or mentally abusive, or both. In such cases, especially young children may find it difficult to process the loss because, while there is a considerable amount of sadness, there might also be some relief that the abuse is over. The guilt that comes with relief at the death of a loved one is difficult to handle at any age, but particularly for a young child, especially if the child is unable to express these feelings.

Adults' reactions to grief and loss can become abnormal if the loss cannot be, or is not, acknowledged by others, or if extreme grief responses do not lessen after a substantial amount of time. The complicated or disenfranchised grief responses in adults have more to do with personality, circumstance, support systems, and other factors. By middle adulthood, loss and grief begin to be expected and accepted as a normal occurrence. Although losses are certainly not easy, they typically are processed in a healthy manner. Older adults may be at greater risk for a complicated grief reaction because their support system may have become limited as a result of past losses, including the death of close family members and friends and even children and grandchildren (Walsh, 2012, p. 72). For example, an older adult who has already lost her husband may be more likely to experience complicated grief if her child dies, as she finds

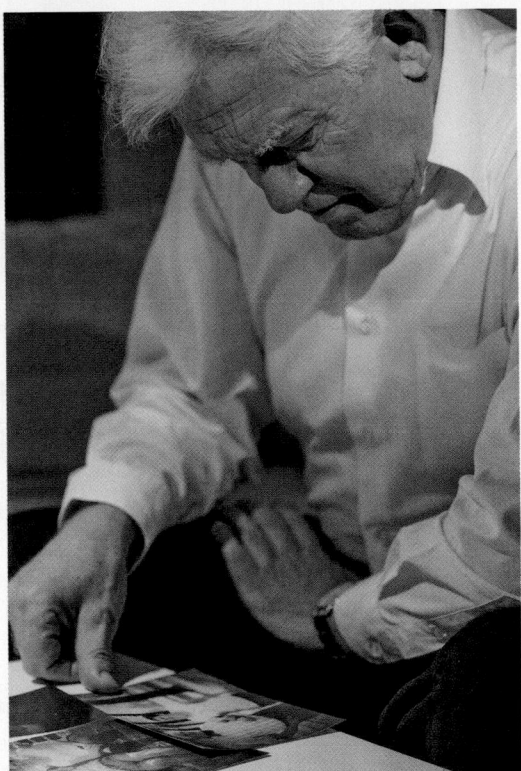

Source: KatarzynaBialasiewicz/iStock/Getty Images.

Figure 27–2 ❯❯ An elderly widower mourns the loss of his wife and needs to learn to cook for himself and clean the house, tasks his wife handled during their 60 years of marriage.

herself without her partner to help her mourn the loss of their child. As described earlier, these cumulative, substantial losses may result in complicated grieving. Having a past history of numerous losses may make the grieving process harder for older adults, as a new loss may serve as a reminder of past losses.

Symbolic losses are also more prevalent among older adults; for example, older adults are more at risk than other age groups of losing their independence, their memory, and their mobility, as well as other significant assets. Symbolic losses may occur as a consequence of the death of a spouse or caregiver. For example, a husband with limited mobility may rely on his wife for transportation, cooking, and assistance with daily living. If she dies, the husband faces a number of losses in addition to mourning her death (**Figure 27–2 ❯❯**).

Gender

Gender often is a factor in grief when society or culture influences how individuals perceive the grieving process. In some cultures, men cannot show sadness or tears, whereas women are expected to do so. In other cultures, only men can attend funerals, while women must stay at home and grieve privately (Purnell, 2014). Grief reactions in general, though, cannot truly be understood or analyzed based on the individual's gender alone. Factors such as age, personality, culture, family dynamics, and the nature of the loss must also be taken into account when assessing grief reactions.

Substance and Alcohol Abuse

Periods of grief and loss are very vulnerable times. Grief can have devastating effects that, if not acknowledged and dealt with, can result in various forms of self-medicating. Nurses encourage healthy coping mechanisms such as seeking counsel from support systems, seeking comfort from religious practices, going to support groups, and doing therapeutic writing. Unhealthy coping mechanisms can complicate grief, resulting in alcohol or drug use as a way to numb the pain of loss. The use of unhealthy coping mechanisms, including drugs or alcohol, can further prolong the grieving process. Because substance use only masks the pain and delays the work of grief, addiction may result quickly.

The signs of substance or alcohol abuse are not always easy to spot, especially in a patient who is going through a period of heightened grief. Some drugs used over a long period, or used in excess, can present in physical ways such as weight loss and a general physical deterioration. In situations where the nurse suspects alcohol or substance abuse, the nurse remains nonjudgmental and uses a therapeutic approach to ask how the patient has been handling the grief and adjusting to the loss. If patients admit to depending on alcohol or substances, the nurse can provide support and referral for the dependency and can also provide patient teaching related to healthy coping responses.

Resilience

Experiencing a loss, or many losses, can be a challenge for the individual to cope and recover. Resilience, in this case, is how quickly the individual can return to his or her normal state of being. Individual resilience depends on many factors. One impact on resilience is the cause of the loss. Those who experience loss unexpectedly or through trauma or violence may have more difficulty returning to normal than those who anticipate a loss due to illness (Boerner & Jopp, 2010). For example, a patient who must have an amputation because of a prolonged struggle with a non-healing wound will be more likely to cope than a patient who loses a limb in a car accident. Similarly, in the case of loss due to death, the relationship between the deceased and the bereaved can also be a factor in the individual's resilience in the situation.

The physical health of the individual at the time of loss can also affect resilience. A study found that bereaved spouses who were in good physical health were less likely to report somatic symptoms and/or depression after the loss of a spouse compared to those who were not in good health at the time of their spouse's death (Utz, Caserta, & Lund, 2012). Other factors that can influence an individual's resilience in the time of loss include mental and cognitive state, support systems, and spiritual strength.

Alterations and Therapies
Grief

ALTERATION	DESCRIPTION/DEFINITION	MANIFESTATIONS	INTERVENTIONS AND THERAPIES
Disenfranchised grief	The result of being unable to acknowledge a loss to others, generally because the grief is not socially recognized	<ul><li>Hiding grief from others as opposed to allowing support from friends and family</li><li>Not seeking support after a loss because of feelings of shame, guilt, or lack of recognition of the loss</li><li>Intensified emotions associated with grief as opposed to those found in a normal grief reaction</li><li>More pronounced feelings of anger and depression due to resentment over the unacknowledged loss</li></ul>	<ul><li>Refer the patient to support groups that acknowledge the loss and feelings of grief.</li><li>Recognize and support the patient's right to grieve the loss.</li><li>Facilitate the patient's spiritual and cultural needs.</li></ul>
Complicated grief	Prolonged or intensified grief causing an individual to be unable to proceed with the grieving process	<ul><li>Intense grieving for 6 months or more with little to no indication of grief resolution</li><li>Inability to proceed with daily activities after the loss</li><li>Visual and/or auditory hallucinations of the individual who has died</li><li>Growing distrust of friends and family members, making the individual seem cold or uncaring</li><li>Avoidance of places associated with memories of the deceased</li><li>Intense feelings of depression, at times accompanied by suicidal thoughts or tendencies</li></ul>	<ul><li>Psychotherapy</li><li>Monitoring for suicidal behaviors</li><li>Assessment for signs of alcohol and/or substance abuse</li><li>Appropriate referrals when signs of suicidal ideation and drug/alcohol abuse are present</li></ul>

Asking for Help

Depending on an individual's paradigm, as well as the views of society or an individual's culture, grief may carry a stigma. Neglecting to grieve or being unable to seek comfort and strength from support systems can lead to feelings of isolation. Nurses encourage patients to ask for help if they feel that the effects of loss are becoming overwhelming. Nurses also provide information about support systems and services available in the community. A strong support system can positively impact the grieving process.

Case Study >> Part 1

Josie Duncan is a 32-year-old woman whose 7-year-old daughter, Tasha, died 3 months ago after fighting leukemia. Mrs. Duncan took a week off from work after her daughter died and then returned to her job. She visits her primary care physician's office complaining of difficulty falling asleep over the past 2 weeks. After checking her vital signs, weight, and temperature, you notice that Mrs. Duncan has lost 15 pounds since her last visit 6 months ago. Her blood pressure and temperature are both normal. You observe that she looks exhausted and has deep circles under her eyes; the clothes she is wearing are at least a size too large. She also seems to be very distracted.

Clinical Reasoning Questions Level I

1. Why might Mrs. Duncan be having trouble sleeping?
2. What are some factors that influence an individual's grief response?
3. What additional questions would you want to ask Mrs. Duncan? Why?

Clinical Reasoning Questions Level II

4. Is Mrs. Duncan at risk for a complicated grief reaction? Explain your answer.
5. Do you think the doctor will prescribe medication for Mrs. Duncan's sleeplessness? What other interventions could be performed?

Concepts Related to Grief and Loss

Grief is an important consideration when working with end-of-life patients. Not only are these patients learning how to come to terms with the loss of their own lives, but also their families experience a variety of hardships during this time, from the financial burden of caring for the dying to anticipatory grieving. Nurses need to understand the grieving process in order to help end-of-life patients and their families work through grief. When working with grieving patients, it is equally important to obtain a full history in order to determine if those patients have a history of anxiety or depression, as these conditions can complicate or elongate the grieving process. Patients who have experienced a traumatic loss, such as a perinatal loss or a death due to violence, or who have witnessed a death are at risk for developing posttraumatic stress disorder (PTSD) and should be made aware of the signs. Similarly, patients who have a history of PTSD have a higher risk of developing a complicated grief reaction later in life. When grief becomes overwhelming, some individuals turn to alcohol or other substances to numb their emotions. Masking the impact of a loss only serves to prolong the grieving process.

The Concepts Related to Grief and Loss feature links some, but not all, of the concepts integral to grief and loss. They are presented in alphabetical order.

Concepts Related to
Grief and Loss

CONCEPT	RELATIONSHIP TO GRIEF AND LOSS	NURSING IMPLICATIONS
Addiction	Alcohol and substance abuse can mask the emotions associated with grief and cause a longer and sometimes more intensified grief reaction	▪ Look for signs of alcohol or substance use as an unhealthy coping mechanism for grief. ▪ Teach the patient about health coping mechanisms. ▪ Maintain a nonjudgmental attitude. ▪ Refer to a specialist.
Comfort	Palliative care can help further the grieving process for both patients and their families, providing both physical and psychologic comfort.	▪ Help dying patients to grieve for their own loss of life. ▪ Assist family members in understanding the signs of grief and acceptance of death. ▪ Provide referral to such assistance as hospice, support groups, and spiritual resources.
Culture and Diversity	Response to loss and the display of grief will be different from culture to culture. Culture also dictates how different family members, including males and females, are to respond to loss.	▪ Be aware that grief and loss response is culturally influenced. ▪ Ask the patient how his or her cultural needs can be met during the time of loss and grief.
Mood and Affect	Situational depression is common in those who experience loss. Those effects may include feelings of extreme sadness, guilt, worthlessness, and other such emotions. Physically the individual may complain of fatigue, lack of appetite, and sleep pattern disruption.	▪ Assess for suicidal ideation. ▪ Engage the patient in therapeutic communication. ▪ Provide resources for support groups. ▪ Refer the patient to a medical provider for evaluation and potential medications.
Nutrition	Those who are grieving often do not enjoy eating as they did previously. They are more likely to eat alone and eat less. Along with decreased caloric intake, bereaved people tend to have nutritional deficits as well.	▪ Assess the patient for signs of malnutrition. ▪ Monitor the patient's weight. ▪ Obtain a 24-hour food diary and make recommendations based on the findings. ▪ Provide and teach a nutrition plan based on the patient's needs. ▪ Suggest nutritionally dense, small meals to help promote weight stability and to meet nutritional needs.
Spirituality	Grief and loss can have either a positive or negative impact on the patient's spiritual foundation.	▪ Assess the patient's attitude and current state of spirituality. ▪ Refer the patient to a rabbi, priest, pastor, imam, or other spiritual counselor.
Stress and Coping	Existing anxiety disorders and PTSD can prolong or intensify the effects of grief.	▪ Assess patient's anxiety level and trauma history. ▪ Assess history of losses and level of current functioning. ▪ Encourage patients who are already in treatment to continue their treatment plan and to communicate their loss to their provider.

Nursing Assessment

Assessment related to grief and loss should include exploration of the patient's current grief, as well as interviewing the patient regarding any past significant losses. Obtaining a complete history of any medical conditions is also necessary. A mental health assessment and information about current coping abilities should also be obtained. A complete nursing assessment also includes identifying the patient's cultural and spiritual needs.

Observation and Patient Interview

Assessment of the patient who has experienced a loss includes assessing the many factors that contribute to an individual's grief reaction, such as the patient's age, coping mechanisms, support system, history of previous losses, history of depression, culture, and personality. When conducting an assessment, be attentive to the patient's needs and maintain a nonjudgmental attitude. If the patient has an extensive history of loss, ascertain how the patient dealt with those losses and whether the patient has achieved resolution or acceptance of them. A sensitive and thorough assessment promotes openness and creates an environment in which the patient can feel safe in discussing emotions. The following questions may be included in the patient interview.

Current Loss

- When did the loss occur?
- What was the nature of the loss?
- Are you having trouble carrying on with your normal activities?
- Have you experienced any trouble sleeping or eating?
- Have you talked to anyone about the loss (for example, a spouse, friends, family, or counselor)?
- Are you taking any medications and/or antidepressants?

History of Loss and Grief Reactions

- Have you experienced similar losses in the past?
- Did your grief manifest in ways similar to those for your grief for this loss?
- Are you experiencing any unresolved grief?

Lifestyle

- Do you have an active support system?
- Do you drink alcohol on a regular basis?
- What types of coping mechanisms have you employed to work through your grief?

Physical Examination

Physical examination of the grieving patient should include a complete physical assessment. Patients may have somatic complaints, such as abdominal pain or headaches, that will need focused assessments. Other focused assessments include looking for signs of self-harm, self-neglect, and nutritional status. Evaluate the patient's hair, skin, and nails for signs of malnutrition and wounds. Evaluate energy level, functional status, and mental status.

Assessing Family Functioning

Family bonds are often challenged when coping with loss. Some families are able to come together and grow stronger; other families become distant and detached. Assessment of the family unit is primarily an interview process. Questions to ask of family members include:

- What impact is the loss having on the family?
- What are the strengths of the family?
- What are the support systems of the family?
- What needs does the family have?
- How does the family perceive how they are coping?
- How are family members expressing their feelings?
- How is each family member's current health status?

>> *See the module on Family for more information regarding assessment of the family.*

Spiritual and Cultural Considerations

Accurate assessment of the grieving process requires awareness of an individual's cultural influences. While it would be unreasonable to expect nurses and other medical professionals to know the practices and beliefs of every culture, in many cases valuable information can be gleaned during a simple patient interview. Understanding the patient's culture may also give meaning to her or his reaction toward professionals who offer assistance, particularly as certain cultural or religious practices view seeking help as undesirable. The nurse should avoid the tendency to view individual behaviors and cultural practices through a personal, ethnocentric lens. By not understanding other cultures, the nurse is at risk of deeming the traditions and practices of others as odd because they do not fit into the nurse's own expectations and experiences. In most settings, patient populations offer a diversity of cultural backgrounds. Respect for the practices of others is essential to building trust, establishing a relationship, and, ultimately, providing effective patient care.

Awareness of the patient's cultural beliefs and values can prevent miscommunication and conflict. For example, some cultures see death as a beginning rather than an end and choose to celebrate the individual's life on earth and the movement to the next life. Misinterpretation of cultural belief may lead clinicians to try to promote coping mechanisms that may not have meaning to the individual patient. It is important to understand that patients view death and grief from their own perspective.

Mourning practices vary widely among cultures and religions. Some mourn openly and in public, while others mourn at home for a set period before moving back into society. In the Jewish faith, for example, followers practice the tradition of shivah, a 7-day mourning period during which the closest family members—such as parents, siblings, and spouse—stay together to mourn their loss and

Grief and Loss Assessment

ASSESSMENT/METHOD	NORMAL FINDINGS	ABNORMAL FINDINGS	LIFESPAN OR DEVELOPMENTAL CONSIDERATIONS
Loss Assessment			
Ask about previous losses. Discover the different types of losses, as well as their frequency.	Experiencing a number of losses is normal at almost any age. In the first few months after the loss, sadness, sleep disturbance, loneliness, and intermittent periods of decreased motivation or activity are to be expected.	■ Inability or unwillingness to process the loss ■ Denial of the loss for a prolonged time ■ Inability or unwillingness to discuss the loss ■ Accumulation of losses with little to no resolution ■ Grief that interferes with daily functioning and lasts 6 months or longer should trigger additional assessment.	■ Children are likely to process losses differently from adults; it should not be assumed that they do not understand loss because of their age. ■ Older adults are likely to develop numerous losses over their lifetime, and these can begin to have a cumulative effect.
Grief Assessment			
Assess patient's current and past grief reaction. Determine the nature of the loss causing the grief.	Grief is intense over the first 2–6 months after the loss and then begins to lessen. Resolution/acceptance generally occurs within 1–2 years after the loss.	■ *Complicated Grieving* ■ *Grief* related to traumatic loss ■ *Grief* related to disenfranchised loss ■ *Post-Trauma Syndrome*	■ Children and older adults are at a high risk for complicated grief. ■ Older adults are at high risk for depression. Loss of a spouse or caregiver may impact independence and requires additional assessment and referral.

receive visitors. Other cultures may emphasize the need to continue with normal activities, such as school or work, during the mourning period, in place of taking time away to mourn privately.

Similarly, cultural and religious practices are important to a patient who is dying. If a patient has specific spiritual or religious requests, such as seeing a priest or a rabbi or having ceremonial traditions performed by an elder of the religion, nurses and other staff should facilitate these requests whenever possible. Those who practice Catholicism, for example, believe the dying person should receive the Sacrament of the Sick (sometimes referred to as Last Rites) in order to receive God's grace before death. Some requests have greater impact on nursing and clinical staff than others. As part of Jewish practice, if the person dies on the Sabbath, the body cannot be removed from the place of death. This means the body cannot be removed from a hospital room until Sabbath is over. Some cultures and religions have ritualistic cleaning of the deceased by same-gender attendants. In those cases, opposite-gender nurses should not prepare a body for the morgue. Even more so, some faiths do not want those who are not of the faith to touch the deceased. When a Muslim person dies, the body is typically prepared for burial by Muslims of the same gender (Purnell, 2014), and nurses should limit the amount of contact with the deceased.

Case Study » Part 2

Mrs. Duncan tells you that she has been working a lot since her daughter died because she needs something to occupy her mind. For the last year of Tasha's life, Mrs. Duncan spent all of her free time taking Tasha to doctor appointments and treatments; now that Tasha is gone, Mrs. Duncan does not know what to do with her spare time. She reports that her appetite decreased before her daughter died, and she has not really had any desire to eat since then. Lately Mrs. Duncan has not wanted to see any of her friends because they act differently around her; they also have children, and Mrs. Duncan admits she does not want to be around children right now. She reports her sleeplessness started 2 weeks ago, shortly after the Christmas holiday. She and her husband tried to celebrate, but they felt it was not the same without their daughter. Mrs. Duncan admitted that she does not think her husband understands how upset she is over their loss.

Clinical Reasoning Questions Level I

1. Why was Mrs. Duncan's appetite poor before her daughter died?
2. What are two nursing diagnoses that apply to Mrs. Duncan?

Clinical Reasoning Questions Level II

3. Based on what you know about grief and loss, why do you think Mrs. Duncan began to experience sleep disturbances after Christmas?

4. How would you characterize Mrs. Duncan's support system? Is it strong, moderate, or weak? Explain your answer.

5. Do you think Mrs. Duncan is working through the grieving process, avoiding grief, or both? Justify your answer using data from the case study.

Independent Interventions

When an individual is grieving, it is sometimes hard to know what to say or do, and nurses may find themselves reluctant to pose questions that patients may see as an invasion of their privacy. It is important to know that there are many ways to offer a patient support and a forum to discuss any difficulties (**Figure 27–3 »**). Open-ended questions, such as asking how the patient has been doing since the loss or what challenges the patient is facing, may be effective for engaging the patient in discussion. Once the patient begins to speak, the nurse should use active listening techniques to show full engagement in the interaction. Body language also conveys the nurse's engagement in the conversation. A nurse's body language should be open and attentive, and when possible, both individuals should be positioned so they are at eye level with one another. (See the exemplar on Therapeutic Communication in the Communication module for a discussion of active listening techniques.)

Implementation of the patient's care depends on a number of factors, including the nature of the loss, the patient's health, the patient's use of coping mechanisms, and the patient's personality. Interventions helpful in working with adults and older adults who are grieving include:

- Teach the patient about the grieving process and its general progression.

- Discuss the benefits of different forms of therapy, as well as the differences between modes of therapy such as group therapy, psychotherapy, and one-on-one therapy.

- Inform the patient about the warning signs of intense depression and/or suicidal thoughts.

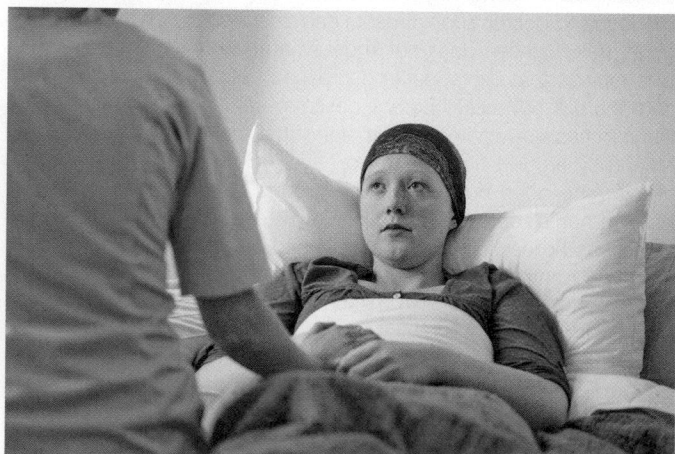

Source: KatarzynaBialasiewicz/iStock/Getty Images.

Figure 27–3 » Finding the time to talk with patients and actively listening to their concerns is an important component of nursing.

- Teach the patient about healthy coping mechanisms as opposed to unhealthy coping mechanisms.

- Provide a judgment-free area for the patient to discuss experiences and fears about grief.

- Encourage the patient to share emotions and fears with close family members or friends.

- Provide referral to resources that can assist the patient to maintain as much independence as possible.

Anticipatory Grief

With anticipatory grief, the individual begins to grieve before the actual loss occurs. For example, a family member may start the mourning process when given the news that another family member has a terminal condition. Sometimes, individuals complete the grieving process before the loss occurs and, as a result, become detached. As in the previous example, the family member of the individual who is diagnosed with the terminal illness may complete mourning for the individual before he or she has died. The family member may seem distant to the dying individual, causing isolation and loneliness for the terminally ill individual. The nurse can help both the family member and the dying individual with coping strategies for anticipatory grief. It is important for the nurse to educate those close to someone dying about the dying process. Likewise, the nurse can also promote healthy relationships between the dying and family members.

Helping the Patient to Cope with Death

The dying individual can be a hallmark example of someone experiencing anticipatory grief. Just as others will, the dying patient will experience stages of grief. The nurse can apply techniques and strategies for those experiencing the loss of their life just as others will be experiencing the loss of a loved one.

Preparing for one's own death is certainly a process that will be as unique as the individual. Some patients will embrace death as relief from their pain and find peace in death; others will be fearful of death and find despair. The nurse working with dying patients has a primary goal of providing comfort. This comfort is not exclusive to physical comfort: the nurse should help the patient cope in a holistic manner. Patients might feel a variety of things, including social distress, psychologic distress, and/or spiritual distress, along with physical distress (Hospice and Palliative Nurses Association, n.d.).

Some might find talking with a dying person awkward or uncomfortable. Acknowledging these feelings is important for the nurse to address. From there, the nurse should let the dying patient lead the conversation (Canadian Virtual Hospice, 2015). The nurse can offer support and provide care that the patient directs. If the patient expresses spiritual distress, the nurse can collaborate with a spiritual counselor; if the patient requests to relief from pain, the nurse can provide comfort measures. During these conversations with the dying patient, the nurse should always be honest regarding the patient's health status unless this is not culturally acceptable (some cultures do not believe in telling a person he or she is dying).

Coping with the Loss of a Patient

All nurses will encounter death of a patient at some point in their practice, although nurses in care settings such as oncology, hospice, the emergency department, and intensive care units will experience patient deaths with some frequency. Nurses are not immune to the effects of grief over the death of a patient. All nurses, but especially those who work with terminally ill patients, should assess their own needs to grieve and process a loss. If they do not, they could easily experience compassion fatigue, a type of burnout that occurs with emotional draining from caring for others, particularly dying, traumatized, and vulnerable patients (Boyle, 2011).

Nurses not accustomed to working with dying patients should also assess their own feelings regarding death. Peters et al. (2013) found that nurses who have strong anxiety regarding death tend to be more uncomfortable with caring for the dying patient. Nurses who are not comfortable with the topic of dying may not be prepared when confronted by a patient who is dying and in need of support. When this happens, nurses may cope by encouraging the patient or family member to talk about something else. While this may seem more conducive to the patient's happiness, it can be detrimental to the patient's overall well-being. Similarly, the nurse who is uncomfortable with the topic of death may try to avoid the topic by providing the patient with false hope, saying things such as "You are going to be fine; don't worry." This type of false reassurance is not beneficial to either the patient or the family (Berman & Snyder, 2016). Nurses need to honestly assess their own feelings about death and handle them properly so as not to impose these feelings on the patient. For example, a nurse who is obviously anxious about and fearful of death can make a patient more fearful of death.

When working with a patient who has a terminal illness, or a patient who has been fatally injured, it is easy for a nurse to form a bond with this individual. These bonds can result not only in normal feelings of grief, such as sorrow, but also in feelings of guilt, as nurses sometimes wonder if they could have done more to help their patients. In such cases, it is important that nurses acknowledge and process their feelings of guilt rather than ignore them. Similarly, nurses should seek support for any grief they may feel at the loss of a patient (**Figure 27–4 >>**). Resources for support may include coworkers, professional therapists or social workers, and grief counseling resources offered through employers. It is important that nurses make time to seek and find the support they need to process their own grief in a healthy manner. In acknowledging and processing their grief over a patient's death, nurses will be better able to help future patients and their families through the processes of death and grief.

Collaborative Therapies

Collaboration may include facilitating meetings between the hospital chaplain and the patient or the family, or requesting a referral to a social worker who can provide expert guidance about coping with loss or assist with linking patients with additional resources. Group therapy, bereavement

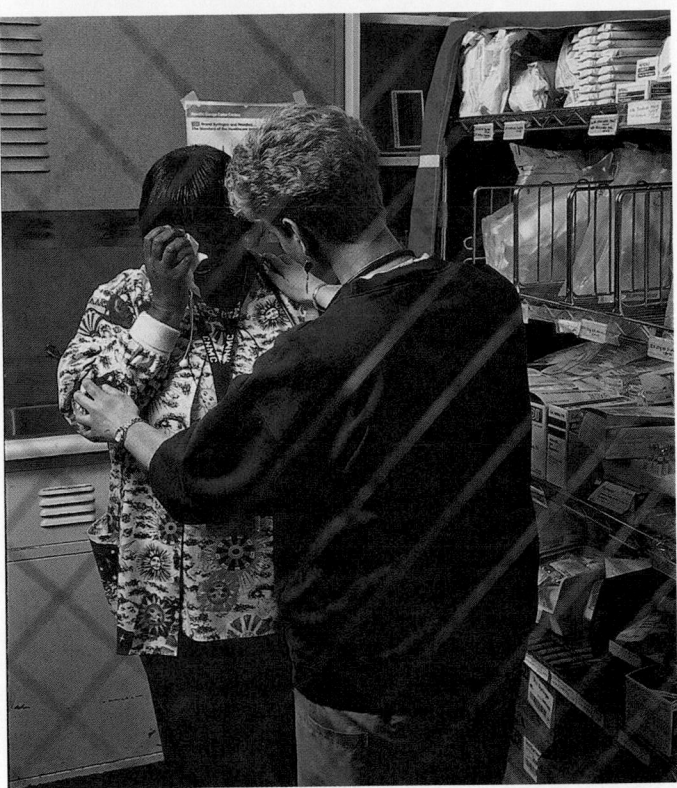

Figure 27–4 >> Nurses need to express their own grief in a supportive environment after a child's death. Sharing with colleagues the sadness and grief or futility of resuscitation efforts often helps nurses provide supportive care to the next family who needs it.

groups, and grief therapists can all be resources for patients who have experienced a loss. **Hospice** is an organization that provides end-of-life care for patients either in their homes or in a hospital setting. Area hospice programs also provide an array of other services, depending on the community resources available.

Treatment of complicated grief is often in the form of psychotherapy targeting specific symptoms related to the disorder. Physician Katherine Shear (Shear et al., 2005) developed Complicated Grief Treatment (CGT), a form of psychotherapy administered over 16 sessions in accordance with a published manual that describes this treatment. According to Shear, healing from a loss is composed of a loss-oriented process and a restoration-oriented process. During the first process, the individual accepts the loss; during the restoration process, the individual begins to move on to a life without the deceased (Robinaugh et al., 2012, p. 32). CGT has been shown to be helpful to patients on its own, but some have used it in combination with antidepressants. While recent studies have shown that antidepressants may be helpful to those with depression related to grief, they do not appear to be as effective for patients with complicated grief. However, combining the use of antidepressants with CGT has proved to be quite effective in helping patients to work through their grief.

Medications
Antidepressants

CLASSIFICATION AND DRUG EXAMPLES	MECHANISMS OF ACTION	NURSING CONSIDERATIONS
Antidepressants ■ Selective serotonin reuptake inhibitors (SSRIs) ■ Serotonin and norepinephrine reuptake inhibitors (SNRIs) ■ Tricyclic and tetracyclic antidepressants *Drug examples:* Escitalopram, fluoxetine, sertraline, duloxetine, doxepin	May be used to treat the symptoms of moderate or severe depression as the result of grief or loss. *May also be used for:* ■ Treatment of complicated grief in conjunction with psychotherapy	■ Monitor for signs of suicidal thoughts. ■ Teach patients about risks associated with specific antidepressants. ■ Monitor for signs of allergic reaction. ■ Monitor for signs of drug interactions.

Pharmacologic Therapy

If pharmacologic interventions are appropriate, antidepressant medications may be prescribed. Although impaired sleep patterns may be associated with grieving, medications to promote sleep usually are not indicated for these patients. In addition to the addictive potential of certain pharmacologic sleeping aids, these medications may be used to mask the patient's grief response, which can prolong the process. If these medications are prescribed, the patient should be carefully monitored for signs and symptoms that they are being used to blunt the emotional impact of grieving.

Nonpharmacologic Therapy

Finding support sources is one of the primary ways that the nurse can provide nonpharmacologic therapy for the person experiencing loss. Support can come in many forms, including support groups, family support, community support, faith community support, and individual counseling. The nurse can also provide support to the individual.

Complementary health approaches, including stress management techniques may be helpful. Those grieving might find comfort in gentle exercise, such as yoga and tai chi. Others might find massage and healing touch helpful. Aromatherapy might also be a useful tool to use for coping.

Case Study ≫ Part 3

Before the doctor talks with Mrs. Duncan, you discuss her complaints of sleeplessness and weight loss with him. You also inform him of Mrs. Duncan's difficulties since her daughter has died. After the doctor talks to Mrs. Duncan, he recommends that she consider talking with a grief counselor about the loss of her daughter. He also recommends that she try to eat more, and that she begin exercising at least three times a week—even if she only goes for a 10-minute walk. Mrs. Duncan and the doctor agree that she should try a combination of counseling, a healthy diet, and exercise before they consider the possibility of pharmacotherapy. Mrs. Duncan schedules a follow-up appointment for next month.

Clinical Reasoning Questions Level I

1. Why do you think the doctor recommended exercise?
2. What are some of the benefits of grief counseling?

Clinical Reasoning Questions Level II

3. Do you think Mrs. Duncan's grief reaction is normal after the loss of a child? Explain your answer.

4. Why did the doctor not prescribe pharmaceutical sleep aids immediately? What are some risk factors associated with taking controlled substances while grieving?
5. Do you think Mrs. Duncan has demonstrated healthy coping mechanisms for dealing with her grief?

Children's Grief Responses

Children and adults experience grief differently, and manifestations of grief vary across the lifespan (**Figure 27–5 ≫**). Children do not generally show or express their emotions regarding loss as openly as adults. Because young children may not express their grief in a way that is expected by an adult, they are sometimes believed to be too young to fully recognize the loss. However, this is not always the case. The child may be grieving in his or her own way and sometimes expresses this grief after the loss through art, imaginary games, playing, or behavioral changes. Behavioral changes, such as decreased socialization, irritability, and confusion, may occur more frequently in adolescents than in very young children (Walsh, 2012). Losses experienced by

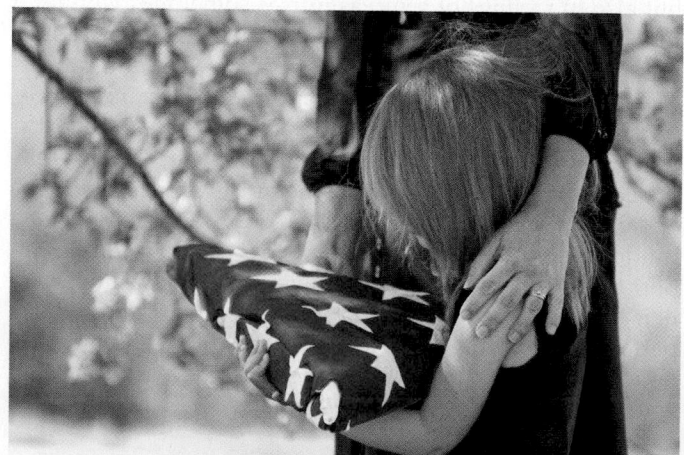

Source: Stephanie Frey/iStock/Getty Images.

Figure 27–5 ≫ Children who experience the death of a parent may be concerned about losing their other parent as well. Nurses can help by inviting children to talk about their grief and answering questions they may have.

children that may result in grieving include any of the following: loss of parent, grandparent, or sibling; loss of a pet; loss of a relationship with a parent due to divorce; loss of a childhood friend or mentor; and loss of support systems if the family relocates to another city or country.

Children's grief responses vary depending on a number of factors, most notably the child's developmental stage and the significance of the loss. When caring for a grieving child, it is important to remember that cognitive development greatly influences grief response. While young children have the capacity to understand loss to some degree, their grief is displayed in ways that differ from grief reactions seen in other age groups. Children also experience **death anxiety**, which manifests as feelings of fear and/or apprehension connected with death.

Developmental Stage

Children grieve differently at different stages of development. Quite a few similarities exist as well. Grief responses in children across the developmental stages are often behavioral: The child acts out emotionally or physically in one way or another.

Worden and Silverman (1996) proposed four tasks that help children adapt to loss:

1. Accept the loss and its permanence.
2. Experience the emotions associated with grief, such as anger, fear, sadness, guilt, and loneliness.
3. Adjust to daily life without the individual who has been lost.
4. Come to see the relationship with the deceased as one based on memories in place of continuing experience.

During the first task, the child must come to understand the loss. In the case of a death, the child must understand that the one who has been lost will not return. Many childhood movies, television shows, and books involve storylines in which an important character dies but is then magically brought back to life. Although a child may intellectually understand that this is not possible, the desire for the return of the individual who has been lost may be so great that it is easier for the child to believe that the individual will come back in some way. Although the child should not be forced to accept the death, nurses and other caregivers can explain and reinforce the reality that the beloved individual is not returning. During the second task, children experience emotions similarly to those of adults as they grieve loss. Nurses support children in this task by encouraging emotional expression and by helping parents to understand that these expressions are normal and appropriate. It also is helpful for adults to recognize that emotions can be triggered long after the loss by holidays, birthdays, or other special events. The third and fourth tasks of this model take time to process and accept (Howarth, 2011, pp. 23–24). Adults can help children in these tasks by listening, by helping children adjust to changes in routines, and by encouraging activities that promote new memories.

Age 2–4

Children age 2–4 cannot yet fully comprehend or express the ideas associated with loss. At this stage, they also see death as temporary or even reversible, believing that the individual or pet who has been lost will come home again. Reaction to grief at this age can also result in changes to sleeping and eating habits, as well as regression in the area of toilet training. Other habits also may change in reaction to loss; for example, the child may lose interest in normal activities or may crave more attention and affection. This type of behavior often manifests as the child becoming clingy or screaming when not being held. When dealing with loss at this age, it is best for caregivers to respond to the child's changes from grief by trying to maintain as normal a routine as possible. Similarly, providing extra reassurance and attention can also be helpful. It is easy to believe that children at such a young age do not understand the concept of loss or death, but they most certainly do notice and understand when change occurs. Therefore, it is important for parents to provide honest answers to questions about grief when they are asked.

Age 5–7

At this stage, children still view death as reversible. It is common during this age span for children to think of death as another place; according to this thinking, the loved one is still alive but has moved to a place the child cannot reach. Other common thought processes at this age revolve around feelings of guilt or blame. In the case of the death of a loved one, a child may fear having caused the death, especially as a result of negative thoughts about the individual or engaging in some type of misbehavior just before the death. Feelings of responsibility such as these are referred to as *magical thinking* and are quite normal in this stage of development. Children at this age may or may not verbalize these feelings, so parents or caregivers are advised to discuss the loss honestly and help the child realize the loss is not the child's fault. A child experiencing grief at this age may also act as though nothing has changed—this is a common reaction for children at this stage and is not by itself cause for alarm.

Grief responses for children age 5–7 may include changes in eating and sleeping patterns, as well as an increase in nightmares. It is also quite normal for the child to be concerned that other important individuals may die as well. Some children express these fears verbally, while others express them through artwork or even writing. Parents and caregivers can help children with reassurances about their safety and well-being, and also by inviting children to talk about their grief or ask any questions. It is best for adults to answer questions simply and honestly, providing the child with further explanations when needed.

Age 8–11

From around age 8 to age 11, children begin to understand that death means the individual is gone and will not be coming back. During this developmental stage, children become more curious about death and what happens after people (or pets) die. As in the previous developmental stage, children in this age group also tend to believe their thoughts or misbehaviors could be the cause of a loved one's death. It is common for a child to feel that the death of a loved one is a form of punishment for some misbehavior. Grief responses

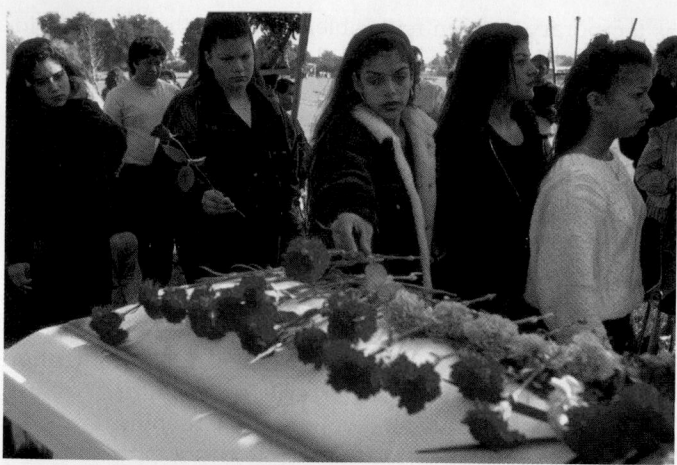

Source: A. Ramey/PhotoEdit Inc.

Figure 27–6 》》 Teenagers lay flowers on the casket of the victim of a drive-by shooting.

at this stage are typically behavioral and may involve becoming more aggressive, acting out in school, or misbehaving at home, or the child may respond by becoming more withdrawn and engaging in solitary activities.

Age 12–18

By the time children reach adolescence, they are more capable of understanding the abstract idea of death. During this time, children stop believing that their thoughts or behaviors can result in the death of others. Adolescent grief responses are very similar to those of most adults, and they may display a wide range of emotions, including depression, denial, and anger. It is very common for individuals in this age group to direct grief-related anger toward their parents. Adolescents should be encouraged, but not forced, to voice their feelings about the loss. Sometimes individuals in this age group feel more comfortable talking to peers or those outside the family (**Figure 27–6 》》**).

Significance of the Loss

The significance of a loss impacts the child's grief experience. For many children, their first encounter with loss is the death of a pet; regardless of the type of pet (fish or dog, cat or hamster), the loss carries meaning for the child. With the death of a pet, the child may react with an abbreviated grief response and, depending on age, ask a number of questions. For more significant losses, though, such as the death of a parent, grandparent, sibling, or friend, a child's grief response is likely to be much more developed.

Death of a Parent

Approximately 2.5 million children in the United States lose a parent before the age of 18 (Howarth, 2011, p. 21). In many ways the death of a parent, especially for a young child, is one of the most devastating losses the child will experience. The death of a parent is not only the loss of an important person; for many children the death results in the loss of an entire way of life. Children depend on their

parents or caregivers for almost everything, from their home, meals, and security to their sense of love and belonging. When a parent dies, children sense that all of those things are threatened. Children are very habit oriented, and a parent's death brings chaos and confusion to their daily routine. The death of one parent also puts numerous different stresses on the other parent, and the child may not receive as much attention or discipline as before. Depending on the developmental stage of the child, the death of one parent could also introduce profound fear that the other parent will die soon as well. This sense of impending loss can stimulate a great deal of anxiety for the child. How the surviving parent or guardian handles the adjustment period after the death has a large impact on how the child copes with the loss. Many children are said to adjust to a parent's death after about a year, but a large percentage still experience changes in behavior, such as social withdrawal and problems with schoolwork, well beyond the first year.

Death of a Grandparent

The death of a grandparent generally is one of the first significant losses children experience. How a child handles the death depends on the child's relationship with that grandparent. For example, if the child has met her grandfather only once because he lives in another state and does not visit often, the impact of the loss will be far less than if the grandparent has lived with and helped raise the child. In this case, the impact of the grandparent's death is similar to that of a parent dying. Children who realize the significance of the grandparent's relationship to their own parent may become concerned about the possibility of losing their parents.

Death of a Sibling

In many ways, the loss of a sibling can be as traumatic as losing a parent or primary caregiver. Siblings often spend much of their childhood together, and they share experiences and relationships with loved ones. For siblings who share a bedroom, the connection is intensified. At a minimum, the death of a sibling generates questions about mortality; related concerns may lead to fear and worry. If unaddressed, fear and worry may cause behavioral problems, developmental regression, and a heightened fear of anything the child believes may be harmful. Depending on the developmental stage of the child, feelings of guilt and confusion may also be associated with the death of a sibling. Children from ages 2 to 11 (and especially ages 2 to 7) often indulge in a certain amount of magical thinking, believing that their negative thoughts or wishes could be the cause of another's death. This type of thinking is particularly difficult in connection with siblings, as most siblings fight from time to time—so if a child's sister dies, he may believe that his mean thoughts toward her were the cause of her death.

Death of a Friend

Similar to the death of a sibling, the loss of a friend causes difficulties for children because it is the death of someone their own age. When a parent or grandparent dies, children often fear for the surviving adults; however, when another child dies, children fear for themselves and their friends. This fear can affect the child's sense of security in the world. If a child becomes friends with a schoolmate who is terminally ill, parents can work to prepare the child for the loss. If the death occurs suddenly, however, there is no time to prepare, and parents and caregivers should work to assure children of their safety.

Other Losses

Like adults, children experience losses other than death that can trigger a grief response. Parental divorce alone can be a significant loss, but it is further complicated if the divorce results in the child's separation from the noncustodial parent by a great distance. Similarly, deployment of a parent serving in the military or other parental absence creates a loss for the child and other family members. Moving can result in loss of school friends, teachers, and other support systems. Long-term or severe acute or chronic illness or injury may result in lifestyle modifications, loss of a limb or body part, or loss of independence. Children experiencing these losses need as much support as, and sometimes more support than, children who experience the death of a loved one.

Complications

Children can experience complications in the grief process as the result of circumstances surrounding the loss, or the significance of the loss. When children experience a significant or traumatic loss, they need a very strong support system to help them work through their feelings of grief, which are most likely difficult for them to understand. Children who do not receive the support they need are at an increased risk for developing a grief reaction that has been complicated in some way.

Children and adolescents who lose a parent are also at risk for premature death. A European study found that parental death, particularly those parents who die of traumatic or unexpected causes, was associated with early death of the child in young adulthood (Li et al., 2014). This may be attributed to genetic predisposition, impact on health caused by loss of a parent, and social well-being.

Complicated Grief Reactions

Loss of an abuser can lead to development of a complicated grief reaction. In such circumstances, feelings of grief are mixed with a sense of relief at knowing the abuse has ended. Regardless of age, coping with mixed emotions related to the death of an abuser presents serious challenges. For children, who lack the cognitive ability to fully understand death, the impact is even more complex. Furthermore, if the abuse has been hidden, the child's experience can be even more confusing. The child who is grappling with mixed emotions observes the others involved in mourning the loss. With no confidantes, the child has no one with whom to discuss the conflicted feelings. This need to hide emotions related to grief due to feelings of guilt or shame can result in a complicated grief reaction.

Childhood Traumatic Grief

Childhood traumatic grief is a grief reaction to the traumatic death of an individual who is important in a child's life or to witnessing a traumatic event (**Box 27-1** ≫). In addition, the child may find it traumatic to see a beloved individual's body after death. The child may associate thoughts of the beloved with the circumstances of the death and be unable to separate the beloved from the event (Finkelhor et al., 2013; Mannario & Cohen, 2011). This type of grief reaction results in both trauma and grief symptoms for the child. The child may begin to avoid activities that the child associates with the trauma. For example, if the child's mother died in an accident on the way to the grocery store, the child may associate riding in the car or going to the grocery store with death. Furthermore, the child may experience learning difficulties, behavioral issues, and mental health difficulties (Child Traumatic Stress Network, n.d.).

Not all children who witness trauma or violence, or lose a loved one to accidental death, develop traumatic grief. In fact, the majority of children recuperate from the loss with no lasting effects (Mannario & Cohen, 2011). However, those who do develop traumatic grief also often develop other mental health issues, including PTSD, depression, anxiety, and/or behavioral problems (Mannario & Cohen, 2011).

Clinical Manifestations

When children encounter death, they often do not grasp the idea entirely. As a result, their minds often work to protect them from the overwhelming feelings caused by grief. In some cases, children may not even react to loss outwardly. There is nothing wrong with this reaction: Their minds may act to protect them from experiencing emotions for which they have no point of reference. When children do react, though, their reactions often revolve around behavioral changes, which may include emotional and behavioral regression.

Behavioral Responses to Grief

Behavioral responses to grief vary depending on developmental age, temperament, and other factors already mentioned. Behavioral changes following loss may be immediate or may occur over an extended period of time. A child's behavior change often presents in one of two ways: withdrawal or acting out. Some children are more withdrawn at home but act out more frequently at school. The responses depend on the child. Some who withdraw will be quieter than usual and seem shy around others. Their primary method of play may be in activities they can do alone, such as drawing, reading, or simply engaging in solitary play. In rare cases, a school-age child may revert to total silence, refusing to speak to anyone. If this behavior goes on for an extended period, a doctor or therapist should be consulted.

Some children may respond to grief with anger and aggression. Anger typically is directed toward the individual who has passed away or at the loss itself but often is taken out on family, friends, or teachers. Other responses may involve trouble eating and sleeping or an overall feeling of anxiety. Adolescents who are grieving may turn to alcohol, tobacco, or drugs as a method of coping with the loss.

Watching a child's behavior change drastically after an individual has died can be terrifying for a parent or guardian. Nurses work to assure parents that the changes they are seeing in their children are a normal response to the loss and that each individual grieves differently. Nurses and other clinicians encourage parents to allow children to express their grief, either verbally or artistically, and provide parents with information about warning signs of unhealthy coping. For example, preoccupation with thoughts of death, engaging in dangerous activities, and drug or alcohol use are considered unhealthy coping mechanisms.

Cultural Considerations

How children handle their grief at the loss of a loved one is greatly influenced by the cultural or spiritual practices of the child's immediate family. For example, children may be raised to believe that someone who dies goes on to an afterlife. Other cultural traditions believe that an individual's soul is reincarnated in a new body after death. Some practices teach that no existence of any sort continues after death, and that death is simply the end of life (Spector, 2017). Nurses take the cultural and spiritual traditions of patients into consideration, especially when speaking to children about grief. For example, if a child's father has told her that the individual who has died will now be reincarnated in a new existence, and another individual who is not familiar with the family's culture tells the child that this individual is now in heaven, the child will most likely be very confused. The nurse who is unaware of a family's beliefs should avoid inadvertently imposing his own belief system on the child. Similarly, if the family has decided not to offer any explanation of an afterlife or lack thereof to the child, that is the parents' decision, and the nurse should not use spiritual beliefs to help the child work through her grief.

Collaboration

In most cases, childhood grief progresses naturally and in a healthy manner with the help of supportive family members and friends. Young children's minds are equipped to protect them from experiencing the full range of grief all at once and for prolonged periods. This is one of the many reasons children grieve differently from adults. When faced with a challenge that is beyond their emotional capacity, young children have defense mechanisms that allow them to compartmentalize the event. As a result, the child can focus on play or daily activities, as opposed to being overwhelmed.

Young children experience intense grief for short periods before their mind moves on to another focus (National Cancer Institute, 2013). In some cases, however, parents or guardians need to work with medical professionals to help their child process grief.

Pharmacologic Therapy

In most cases involving a child who is having difficulty working through grief, nonpharmacologic options such as therapy or group counseling are effective. Few pediatric patients will require pharmacologic intervention. Those who do need intervention for complicated grief typically have underlying mental health issues, such as anxiety (Melhem et al., 2007). Few studies have been done on the effectiveness of pharmacologic intervention for complicated grief in children and adolescents. Pharmacologic therapies can keep children from developing their own coping and healing mechanisms and may therefore cause problems later in life. In addition, many medications used as pharmacotherapy for extended grief responses must be tapered slowly. Parents or guardians should be informed of all the side effects of these medications so that they can make an informed decision. If cognitive–behavioral therapy and other nonpharmacologic interventions are given a significant trial and still prove ineffective, and if the child is at an increased risk for hurting himself or others, low doses of antidepressants and/or antianxiety medications may be suggested (Melhem et al., 2007). However, use of antidepressants may increase risk for suicidal ideation and behaviors in some children and adolescents, and this information should be provided to parents before they make a decision to begin antidepressant therapy (Potter & Moller, 2016). If the child is prescribed antidepressants, regular follow-up appointments should be scheduled for at least the first 12 weeks after beginning the medication. Antidepressants should also be used in combination with nonpharmacologic options to help the child work through grief and eventually move on to acceptance.

Nonpharmacologic Therapy

Individual sessions with a therapist or participation in a bereavement group can help children work through a difficult loss. Children's bereavement groups often include activities involving drawing, writing, or other forms of arts and crafts. During these activities, the child may be encouraged to draw expressions depicting how he feels about the loss. He may also be given the option of creating a scrapbook or a memory box about the individual who has died (Walsh, 2012, p. 113). Older children and adolescents may be encouraged to practice forms of writing therapy, which can involve keeping a journal about their feelings. Other activities in writing therapy include writing a letter to the deceased. In these writings, individuals are encouraged to be entirely honest without any fear of judgment from others or from themselves. The main idea behind this form of therapy is that writing about intense feelings of grief, pain, or trauma, will eventually cause the feelings to begin to subside. Many individuals are not comfortable talking about these emotions or thoughts and find it easier to express their emotions openly in writing. Therapeutic writing can also be suggested for terminally ill children as a way to express their fears and uncertainties.

Nursing Care

The nurse assesses the child's and the parents' history of previous losses, coping skills, psychosocial supports, and cultural and spiritual practices and preferences. In the case of a pediatric or adolescent child experiencing grief from a recent loss, the overall health and reactions of the child should be assessed. Some families have difficulty talking about death, and the nurse needs to assess the ability of family members to support the child's grief responses. Additional parent education and referral may be necessary to help parents support their child as she grieves the loss.

Nursing interventions for childhood grief include providing emotional support for both the patient and family as appropriate.

For a child who is dying, comfort measures are essential. Some comfort measures are:

- Provide pain medication as needed to keep the patient comfortable.
- Involve parents by suggesting measures to help the child, including massages, warm or cool blankets as needed, singing, and reading.
- Allow parents to stay with the child as much as possible.
- Offer resources for any spiritual or cultural traditions requested by the child or family.

Some emotional support measures are:

- Encourage the child and family to ask any questions they may have.
- Educate the parents about the signs of impending death.
- Provide information about the normal coping mechanisms generally displayed during the developmental stage of the child.
- Assist in helping the parents find meaning in the child's death; this has been shown to help facilitate acceptance.

For more information, see the exemplar on End-of-Life Care in the module on Comfort, particularly the section on End-of-Life Care for Children.

For a child who is grieving the loss of a loved one or friend, appropriate nursing interventions include the following:

- Encourage the child to honestly express any feelings about the loss.
- Assure the child that it is normal to feel angry, sad, and even confused when someone dies.
- Educate the child and parents about some healthy outlets for childhood grief, such as drawing, painting, or writing to the deceased.
- Provide the parents with information about explaining death in an honest and age-appropriate manner.

Perinatal Loss

Perinatal loss is the death of an infant or fetus at any time from the point of conception to 28 days after birth. Perinatal loss is a traumatic event for the infant's parents as well as other family members. In the past, some have proposed that perinatal loss results in less intense grief because the parents and family have not had time to form a close bond with the infant. This theory has since been proven incorrect. In fact, the grief associated with the loss of a child can be more intense than most other losses (Kersting & Wagner, 2012).

Causes of Perinatal Loss

Perinatal loss can be difficult for the mother both physically and emotionally. If the fetus is lost during the first 20 weeks of gestation, it is referred to as a **miscarriage** or a **spontaneous abortion**. This is a significant loss for the mother and should not be discounted for any reason. Loss of the infant after 20 weeks' gestation is known as **intrauterine fetal death (IUFD)** but is more commonly referred to as **fetal demise** or **stillbirth**. It is typical to assume that a stillbirth will produce a more difficult grief reaction for mothers. However, a study that looked at mothers experiencing miscarriages, stillbirths, and neonatal death found that the grief responses in the mothers were essentially the same (Kersting & Wagner, 2012). The grief response of fathers in perinatal loss has not been as well researched as that of mothers. What research has shown is that fathers do grieve like mothers, but with less intensity and for a shorter duration (Kersting & Wagner, 2012). In all cases, parents and other family members benefit from nursing care that provides a therapeutic presence and values parent and family statements and emotions (Potter & Moller, 2016).

The loss of a fetus while it is in the womb results from a variety of circumstances that can occur between conception and birth. These include biological conditions such as infection, an abnormality in the fetus, problems with the placenta, or accidents involving the umbilical cord. Environmental conditions also can contribute to, or cause, perinatal loss—for example, domestic abuse, motor vehicle crashes, or other accidents, such as a fall.

Miscarriage

One of the most common causes of miscarriage is **blighted ovum**, which occurs when the egg has been fertilized and both the membrane and placenta have formed, but the embryo has not formed. This condition sometimes results from chromosomal abnormalities in the fetus. Health conditions in the mother can also contribute to miscarriage—in particular, infections, hormonal problems, unmanaged diabetes, and thyroid disease. Other causes include drug and alcohol use, exposure to toxins, and smoking. Most miscarriages occur before the mother knows she is pregnant. Of pregnancies of which the mother is aware, approximately 15 to 20% will end in miscarriage, often around the 7th week of pregnancy (White, 2014).

Stillbirth

It may be impossible to know the reason for a stillbirth, even in the later stages of pregnancy. Some known factors that may contribute to and/or cause fetal demise include birth defects or chromosomal disorders, placental issues, infections, slow fetal growth, and umbilical cord problems.

Placental abruption occurs when the placenta detaches from the uterine wall before delivery. This condition does not always result in fetal demise, but the fetus's survival depends on the stage of development and prompt medical treatment. Umbilical cord abnormalities are relatively unusual, but if a knot in the cord occurs it could cause oxygen deprivation in the fetus. Another rare cause of fetal demise is **Rh disease**, where the mother is Rh negative and the child is Rh positive. If this condition arises, the mother's body sees the Rh-positive cells in the fetus as foreign and produces antibodies to fight off the Rh-positive cells. Rh disease results in the death of the fetus only in extreme cases.

Risk Factors and Prevention

Risk factors for perinatal loss include age, health conditions, and previous instances of perinatal loss. Increased age at the time of conception, particularly for women 40 or older, can increase the risk for complications during pregnancy. A woman's medical history also factors into the risk for complications. Generally having one past experience with a miscarriage or spontaneous abortion does not impact future pregnancies—depending on the cause—but past instances of multiple complications put a woman at higher risk. Similarly, contributing factors involving a weak cervix or other health conditions such as diabetes, obesity, or thyroid disease can lead to miscarriage or fetal demise (National Institutes of Health, 2013). The use of drugs, alcohol, tobacco, and/or caffeine increases the risk for pregnancy complications, as does exposure to harmful chemicals.

When fetal demise occurs and the mother does not go into labor naturally, labor is induced, or a cesarean section is performed. In cases of prolonged retention of the fetus, a condition known as **disseminated intravascular coagulation (DIC)** may occur. DIC is a disorder where the proteins controlling clotting of the blood become abnormally active, causing excessive clotting and then bleeding as available clotting factors are consumed. In addition to DIC, both infection and sepsis can set in if the dead fetus remains in the woman's womb for an extended period.

In the majority of cases it is not possible to prevent perinatal loss. As mentioned in the previous sections, many cases are circumstantial and/or biological and often cannot be detected until the miscarriage or fetal demise has occurred. The best prevention for parents is knowledge of factors that can compromise the mother's health. Women who are pregnant should avoid drugs, chemicals, tobacco, alcohol, and infectious diseases, as they may cause perinatal loss or other health complications for the fetus. Proper maternal care is also important, as some pregnancy complications can be caught early and treated before any harm is done to the fetus or mother.

Clinical Manifestations

The manifestations of perinatal loss involve both physical and emotional changes. The physical changes are either changes to the mother's body, including spotting, severe back pain, and cramping, or changes in fetal movement or heart rate. These manifestations indicate that something has occurred that could lead to fatal complications. After a peri-natal loss, the parents and family of the infant experience various, and often intense, forms of grief.

Changes in Fetal Activity

Some warning signs of pregnancy complications can be detected through fetal movement or fetal heartbeat. Mothers can generally first detect fetal movement between 18 and 20 weeks' gestation. From this point onward, fetal movement becomes more regular and predictable, with the mother detecting the greatest movement while sitting or lying down. A significant decrease in or stopping of fetal movement before labor may be a sign of complications, such as the fetus's receiving too little oxygen. Mothers should be observant of fetal movements, but not overly anxious. A fetus that does not move for an hour may be sleeping. Similarly, during the last trimester of pregnancy, the fetus may not move as much as in earlier weeks. When a significant decrease in fetal movement is detected, the clinician checks the fetal heart rate. If the heart rate is abnormal or cannot be detected, an ultrasound is done to check for complications. If complications are found and the fetus is still alive, early delivery or a cesarean section may be performed.

Grief

The loss of an infant during any stage of pregnancy can be an extremely traumatic event for both parents, and intense feelings of grief are to be expected. The intensity and duration of this grief depend on the individual, but it should not be assumed that this form of grief resolves quickly simply because the parents have not yet established a direct relationship with their baby. Studies have shown very little difference between the intensity of grief felt when a close family member dies and the grief felt after a perinatal death (Kersting & Wagner, 2012).

Grief in cases of perinatal loss may be intensified by the circumstances involving the loss. Many factors impact the parents' ability to resolve their emotions, including how the loss occurred, how the parents learned about the loss, and if the loss could have been prevented. Perinatal loss may also have a stigma attached to it, as some believe that it is unnecessary to mourn the loss of a child whom the parents have never come to know or raise. Beliefs such as these may hinder the parents' grieving process. These emotions can be further complicated for the mother if she feels guilt associated with the loss, and/or if postpartum depression becomes a factor.

Disenfranchised Grief

The loss of an infant before, or immediately following, birth may result in disenfranchised grief. Perinatal loss is often not a socially recognized loss, particularly if that loss occurred in the early stages of pregnancy. Early miscarriages are generally not discussed except between the parents and healthcare professionals; in such a case, the grief is unacknowledged socially. Losses that occur in the early stages of pregnancy can be more difficult to grieve, as no funeral services or other formal mourning traditions are practiced (Kersting & Wagner, 2012). The result may be that the parents feel they have no right to mourn or feel grief over the loss of their child. Disenfranchised or complicated grief can also occur if the pregnancy had to be terminated for health reasons. Many parents in this situation choose to tell friends and family that the loss of the child was due to miscarriage or fetal demise.

Postpartum Depression

Postpartum depression is a form of depression that occurs in the first few weeks after a child has been born. Many do not realize that postpartum depression can also occur in women who have sustained perinatal loss; in fact, two of the major risk factors for developing postpartum depression are experiencing complications during the pregnancy and sustaining a perinatal loss. The exact cause of postpartum depression is unknown, but the symptoms are similar to those of other forms of depression and may include anxiety, anger, difficulty concentrating, lack of enjoyment, feelings of inadequacy, sleeplessness or oversleeping, decreased or increase appetite, and suicidal thoughts (National Institute of Mental Health, n.d.). Experiencing these symptoms while trying to mourn the loss of a child can make both the grief and the depression worse. Women who are experiencing these emotions should be encouraged to discuss their thoughts and should be monitored closely for a worsening of symptoms.

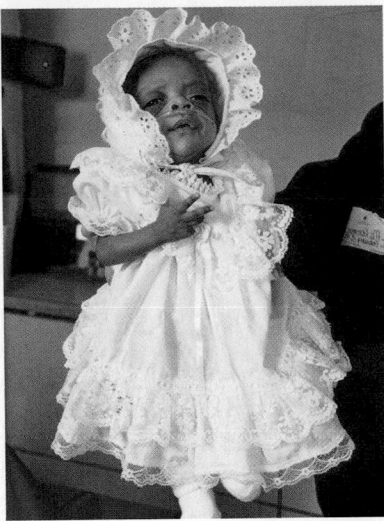

Figure 27–7 》 Religious rituals such as baptism and the blessing of an ill infant may provide great comfort to the family. When the infant is stable, a traditional baptism may be performed in the home or church with family and friends present. When the infant has a life-threatening illness, baptism may be performed in the hospital by a chaplain or health professional.

SAFETY ALERT Mothers who have lost a child and develop postpartum depression should be closely monitored for signs of serious depression and/or suicidal thoughts. Signs of depression include loss of interest in once-enjoyable activities, alterations in appetite, fatigue, and unexplainable crying spells. Suicidal thoughts may be evidenced by intense periods of depression accompanied by statements such as "everyone would be better off without me," or "I wish I was dead/had died instead." Some mothers will make very frank statements like, "That child needs her mother." Individuals contemplating suicide may also begin to give away items once valued, explaining that the items are not needed anymore.

Spiritual and Cultural Considerations

Parents who have lost a child may desire to speak with a religious or spiritual leader. Nurses can call for the hospital chaplain to meet with the parents or facilitate the presence of a spiritual leader of their choosing. If the infant is born alive but not expected to live long, the parents may want the child

to be baptized or to receive a form of blessing as soon as possible, depending on their beliefs (**Figure 27–7 》**). Nurses facilitate the family's participation in these rituals.

Religious or spiritual beliefs may affect how the parents mourn the loss of a child. Patients of the Catholic faith may worry if their child was stillborn and therefore unable to be baptized, and this may cause considerable anxiety. Some members of the Jewish faith observe the practice that parents and family members are not to mourn for a child who has been alive less than 30 days, and so parents of these babies are unable to hold any traditional services or burials (Dickstein, 1996; Tessler, 2014). Some traditions, such as Islam, believe the child is instantly admitted into heaven. Others, such as Buddhism and Hinduism, believe the child's soul will be reincarnated. Nurses should be respectful of patients' beliefs and offer to meet any needs that arise.

Focus on Diversity and Culture
Perinatal Loss

Perinatal death is considered to be death of the fetus at 20 weeks or greater. The neonatal period is considered as the first 28 days of life. Perinatal and neonatal deaths continue to remain steady in the United States, with an average of 5.96 fetal deaths per 1000 live births (MacDorman & Gregory, 2015). The United States ranks 26 out of 26 industrial nations in infant mortality (MacDorman et al., 2014). Fetal mortality is highest in mothers who are either in their teens or older than 35, in mothers who are unmarried, and in mothers carrying multiple fetuses (MacDorman & Gregory, 2015). In terms of race, non-Hispanic Blacks have the highest incidence of fetal death, with 10.53 per 1000 births, followed by American Indian or Alaska Natives with 6.22 per 1000 births. Mothers of Asian or Pacific Island race, and those of Cuban heritage, have the lowest, with 4.68 and 4.65 per 1000 births, respectively. Although the causative factors for the increase in perinatal deaths in non-Hispanic Blacks compared to other races have not been pinpointed, several possible causes include access to healthcare and prenatal care, maternal preconception, health, stress, income, infection, and cultural impact on pregnancy (MacDorman & Gregory, 2015).

Clinical Manifestations and Therapies
Perinatal Loss

ETIOLOGY	CLINICAL MANIFESTATIONS	CLINICAL THERAPIES
Miscarriage	▪ Spotting ▪ Cramping ▪ Lower back pain	▪ Antibiotics if an infection results
Placental abruption	▪ Back pain ▪ Uterine contractions ▪ Vaginal bleeding ▪ Abdominal pain	▪ IV fluids ▪ Blood transfusion ▪ Delivery of the fetus ▪ Antibiotics if infection occurs
Disseminated intravascular coagulation as a result of a retained fetus	▪ Bleeding ▪ Blood clots ▪ Drop in blood pressure	▪ Delivery of the fetus ▪ Treatment of clotting ▪ Plasma transfusions, if needed ▪ Antibiotics if sepsis occurs

Collaboration

After a perinatal loss, tests can be performed on both the mother and the fetus to determine the cause of the fetal demise. Some parents refuse this testing for personal or religious reasons, and that decision must be honored. Parents who have lost a child may also need additional support in the coming months: A large-scale epidemiologically based study found that women experiencing a stillbirth or early infant death (within the first 28 days of life) are 4 times as likely as live-birth mothers to exhibit symptoms of depression and 7 times as likely to exhibit symptoms of post-traumatic stress 9 months after the loss (Gold et al., 2016). Although many support groups and bereavement counselors can be recommended, this study suggests the need for follow-up after discharge, particularly for African American mothers, who were less likely to seek treatment for depressive or post-traumatic stress symptoms (Gold et al., 2016). Members of the interprofessional team caring for mothers experiencing perinatal loss should assess for resiliency factors, including support systems and access to follow-up care. Nurses should provide or ensure referrals for counseling and other resources are made before discharge.

Diagnostic Tests

A series of tests are available to determine the potential cause of fetal demise, but often it is impossible to determine the exact cause. After delivery, with the parents' consent, the fetus will undergo blood tests and placental tests, x-rays and MRIs, as well as chromosomal studies. These tests are done to determine a possible cause of the pregnancy complications and generally include an autopsy. Mothers also undergo a series of blood tests. These tests check to see if the mother has diabetes or thyroid disease, or if she has contracted any infectious disease that could have affected the fetus. A Betke-Kleihauer test may also be performed to check the mother's Rh antibodies to deter-

mine if Rh disease was a contributing factor. These tests can help the parents to know of possible similar problems with future pregnancies.

Pharmacologic Therapy

Depending on the circumstances surrounding the fetal demise, medications may be administered to treat the mother for any infections or complications. If a placental abruption has occurred, the mother may need IV fluids as well as a blood transfusion if the blood loss is substantial. In cases where the fetal demise goes untreated and the dead fetus is retained, disseminated intravascular coagulation may result, which requires treatment for the clotting, possible plasma transfusions, and treatment for sepsis, depending on how long the fetus has been retained. The mother may also need antibiotics if diagnostic tests indicate the presence of infection.

The mother is at risk for developing postpartum depression within the first 4 weeks after a perinatal loss. If this depression becomes overwhelming, especially in combination with the grief, two pharmacologic therapies may be recommended: antidepressants and hormone therapy. Antidepressants have been shown to be effective in the treatment of postpartum depression and can be used in combination with other forms of therapy and counseling. Hormone therapy, in the form of estrogen replacement, may help to dispel some of the symptoms of postpartum depression, but research on this treatment is sparse. Women should be made aware of the risks and benefits of all treatments so they may make an informed decision.

Nonpharmacologic Therapy

The grief resulting from perinatal loss can be intense and even overwhelming. Mothers may feel unnecessary guilt, believing that they, or their bodies, failed in some way and led to the infant's death. Intense grief and even feelings of guilt are entirely normal after the death of an infant and may last for a few weeks or possibly a few months. These emotions generally lessen on their own, but if they do not, or if the parents require further support, various forms of therapy can be helpful. Group therapy in cases of perinatal loss may be useful, or it may be more painful, depending on the patients. Some patients may find it therapeutic and reassuring to talk to other parents who have lost an infant, while others may see it as disorienting and painful to share others' experiences of such a traumatic event. In these cases, individual grief counseling is preferable.

Lifestyle changes may also assist mothers experiencing postpartum depression and grief. In place of isolation, mothers should seek out a strong support system after the loss; sharing their feelings about the loss as well as any trauma experienced has been proven to help prevent or alleviate any PTSD (Sutan et al., 2010). Physical activity and proper nutrition can also help to lessen the effects of depression.

Nursing Care

Perinatal loss can occur at any point in a pregnancy for a multitude of reasons. Mothers who are suspected of having sustained a perinatal loss should be evaluated immediately. A fetal heart monitor can be used to check the heart rate of the fetus. If a heartbeat cannot be found, an ultrasound should be done to determine if fetal demise has occurred. The safety of mother and fetus takes priority; if the assessment determines that the fetus is in distress, immediate action is necessary.

Following confirmation of fetal demise, the parents are informed. Institutional policies vary with regard to when parents are notified of fetal demise. In some cases, the parents are not informed until after the delivery. It is important to adhere to institutional policies and procedures.

The nurse begins assessing the parents' needs and resources as well as planning for needs that will arise during delivery. The nurse assesses the parents' spiritual needs by asking if they would like to speak to the hospital chaplain or if they would like the presence of another spiritual leader. Nurses also collaborate with social workers or grief counselors to provide further assistance to the parents after the birth.

Caring for Parents

When parents are admitted with a possible perinatal loss, they should be put in a private room as far away from the other mothers as possible. If it is determined that perinatal loss has occurred, the privacy provided is likely to benefit both parents. Once tests are performed and perinatal loss is confirmed, parents are informed of the test results and encouraged to ask any questions they may have. Nurses should allow parents time to process their grief before asking about the mother's birthing preferences. When the parents have indicated that they are ready to discuss the birthing process, the nurse should explain what will happen in the delivery of a stillborn infant; the parents should also be informed about the methods of inducing labor, if induction is to occur. The mother's birthing preferences determine how the birth takes place. Nurses consult her regarding how the room should be lit, who she would like in the birthing room with her, if she would like relaxing music playing, and what position she would prefer to give birth in. The moth-

er's comfort and understanding are an important priority for a nurse during the birthing process.

Before the child is born, the nurse should establish when and if the parents would like to see the infant. Parents should be gently encouraged to see the infant for their own sense of acceptance. If the parents wish to see the infant, the nurse should prepare them for how the child may look. For example, if the child is not fully developed, if the child is slightly blue or yellow from complications, or if the child is deformed in any way, the parents should be told before viewing the infant. It is important for nurses to respect parents' wishes if they would like time alone with the infant. The nurse also consults the parents to determine if they would like to take home keepsakes of the child, such as a picture, a lock of hair, or foot- or handprints.

After the birth has taken place and the parents have seen the infant, the nurse should again ask if they have any questions. The nurse assures both parents that any questions they may have are normal, even if the parents feel their questions are odd or morbid in some way. The nurse provides time and space for the parents to express their feelings, being careful to address feelings of guilt by explaining that most cases of perinatal loss cannot be prevented. Nurses provide information on discharge regarding the need to report any signs of infection, such as fever, chills, or dizziness. Nurses also make referrals for grief counseling and other sources of support the parents may require.

Caring for Siblings

If possible, the nurse should encourage parents to include siblings in the process of grieving for a stillborn baby. Siblings should be able to experience their newborn brother or sister, even if the infant is dead. Studies have shown that siblings who are able to experience the deceased brother or sister are able to mourn the death with less traumatic results (Avelin et al., 2012). In addition, having the older sibling create memories, such as taking pictures with or holding the deceased, also helped the older child cope with the loss. Children, however, should not be forced to hold, touch, or otherwise experience a deceased sibling. Rather, the parents and nurse should let the living sibling lead the encounter (Avelin et al., 2012).

Older Adults' Responses to Loss

Older adults' responses to grief and loss can be intricate because of inherent factors unique to this age demographic. Older adults are defined as anyone 65 years of age or older. At this point in life, the older adult has more than likely accumulated a number of losses, both symbolic and actual. This accumulation may compound any new grief felt by the individual: A new loss may bring up grief from one or more previous losses.

Sources of Loss

Grief and loss as experienced by older adults can be more complicated than at other ages. A single death may trigger multiple losses. For example, a woman in the early stages of Alzheimer disease may be able to live in her home while her husband is in good health. When he dies and she moves in with one of her children, her loss of independence may accelerate or she may experience relocation syndrome and a worsening of her dementia (see the exemplar on Alzheimer Disease in the module on Cognition for more information on relocation syndrome). Older adults also begin to lose friends and acquaintances in their age group, and as that happens they begin to anticipate their own death as well as the death of their partners (Walsh, 2012).

Losses associated with aging are varied and may include loss of independence, loss of mobility, loss of health, and loss of memory. Unfortunately, these create a misperception among some younger adults that aging brings frailty and deterioration of mental function. These misperceptions are considered a form of **ageism**, which involves forming stereotypes about older adults. Nurses must guard against such misperceptions. Many older adults live active, healthy, fulfilling lives.

Older adults are at greater risk of depression following significant real or symbolic losses. Depression in older adults is rarely the result of only one factor. Among the most common causes of depression in this population are the death of a loved one, loss of independence, illness, and isolation and loneliness. Untreated depression can worsen and is very serious. It can lead to the prolonging of other illnesses, and even to suicide. Unfortunately, death by suicide continues to be a factor in the aging population. Statistics show an increase of suicide in the geriatric population, 65 to 74 years of age, both men and women (Curtin, Warner, & Hedegaard, 2016). It should be noted there has been a slight decrease in suicides in those older than 75 years of age in the years 1999–2014 (Curtin et al., 2016). Grief is a powerful emotion, particularly when coupled with other losses. Older adults should be assessed for signs of serious depression and suicidal ideation, especially after the loss of a spouse or other loved one.

SAFETY ALERT Suicide in older adults is commonly the result of untreated depression. In the past, the chronic underdiagnosis of minor depression in older adults led to high suicide rates—particularly in men. Nurses in all settings should assess for signs of depression, even if it appears minor, and then assess for increased risk of suicide.

Clinical Manifestations

Manifestations of grief in older adults may be more profound than those observed in younger patients. Accumulating losses in combination with existing health conditions and medication side effects may contribute to a complicated grief reaction. As a result, grief in older adults that may present as a response to the loss of a single person, object, or freedom may actually be a reaction to numerous losses that have accumulated over time. How older adults handle loss depends on the circumstances of the loss, as well as the overall health of the individual—both physically and mentally.

Grief initially presents in older adults much as it presents in younger adults; anger, sadness, longing, disbelief, and depression may be present. The duration and intensity of these emotions vary from patient to patient. Older adults may seem to experience the emotional aspects of

grief more acutely than younger adults; for example, older adults may show pronounced and overwhelming feelings of anger or sadness in response to a death. It also is common for older adults—particularly those living alone—to respond to intense grief by neglecting their own needs. Eating habits, personal hygiene, and health maintenance may fluctuate during periods of bereavement. Nurses need to be particularly observant of these changes in regular nutrition, hygiene, and health, as they indicate that patients are not taking care of themselves and may need additional support.

Patient's History

In working with older adults who are experiencing grief, it is important to inquire about other recent losses, as well as any present health concerns such as dementia, Alzheimer disease, or a history of depression or suicide attempts. If a patient has recently experienced a number of losses, a common experience for older adults, the accumulation of these losses can be overwhelming. When assessing the span of loss in older adults, it is important to consider all losses. For example, the loss of mobility, the loss of independence, and even the loss of a beloved pet can all contribute to feelings of overwhelming grief.

For patients with dementia or Alzheimer disease, the death of a loved one is very complicated. The affected patient may have been told about the individual's death and been emotional, but may then have forgotten that this individual has died. Even in the early stages of Alzheimer disease, newly learned information is often forgotten quickly. A patient's loss of memory of a loved one's death can be hard on the nurse and/or the patient's caretaker, as the individual may ask to see the loved one who has died. Similarly, the patient may become very upset because the deceased has not come to visit. If the patient were to be reminded daily of the loss, then he would experience fresh grief for the individual who had died. With the progression of Alzheimer disease, the grieving process becomes virtually impossible as it constantly requires time to accept and process the loss.

Complicated Grief

Complicated grief in older adults manifests in feelings of unrelenting preoccupation and yearning resulting from the loss, experienced over an increased duration of time (at least 6 months or more). Memories, even those that are happy, elicit strong emotions, which may be coupled with an avoidance of familiar places or individuals who trigger thoughts of the deceased or regret for the loss. Patients may also manifest trust issues, suspecting once close friends and family members of judging their pain or not understanding their emotions. Because of these feelings of judgment or betrayal, the patients may appear distant and even uncaring. This may be especially true of older adults who have experienced a loss of independence or mobility. Nurses need to be observant of the progression of grief in older adults. If symptoms intensify or affect the patient's overall health, appropriate assessments and interventions need to be made. Signs of intense depression should also be monitored, as complicated grief and depression are often comorbid disorders (Robinaugh et al., 2012).

Spiritual and Cultural Considerations

Many older adults find deep meaning in their religious or spiritual beliefs and practices, possibly because they grew up during a time when religious practices were more widespread than they are today. Religious and spiritual practices can provide comfort for patients and their families. If the patient is in a nursing home, hospital, hospice, or an extended care facility and is working through grief, nurses should inquire if the patient would like to participate in any specific form of religious practice. Nurses should assist patients in meeting these needs when possible.

Sometimes, patients experience a disruption of their spiritual beliefs and/or values. This is known as spiritual distress. Rather than turning to religion in times of grief or loss, the patient may question or express anger toward the higher power or faith-base as to why the loss occurred. Nurses can encourage patients to regain a sense of spirituality. The nurse can guide the patient to address her spiritual distress, refer the patient to a spiritual leader or chaplain, and meet the patient's spiritual need requests when feasible. Those patients with a strong sense of spirituality have better coping mechanisms with serious illness, including less depression and better quality of life (Puchalski, 2012).

Collaboration

Older adults experiencing significant losses may require support in a variety of areas. Nurses must assess their need for support carefully. Patients might find it helpful to talk to others who have had similar losses, or they might want to speak individually with a professional therapist. Some patients may need referral to a social worker to learn more about means of financial support, including financial assistance with groceries or housing. Some patients may require pharmacologic therapy.

Pharmacologic Therapy

Two conditions involving grief may require pharmacologic therapies: depression and complicated grief. While many studies have been done regarding antidepressants in the elderly, studies regarding the use of antidepressants for treatment of complicated grief in the elderly are sparse (Shear, 2015). Treatment of depression begins with assessment to determine the underlying cause of the depression. Most of the time depression can be treated quite effectively through nonpharmacologic therapies, but if these prove ineffective, antidepressants may be used. Antidepressants should be used with caution in older adults, however, as various other medications have adverse reactions with some forms of antidepressants. Similarly, some conditions that are particularly prevalent in older adults—such as diabetes, dementia, and heart problems—can be made worse by antidepressants (Wiese, 2011; Wilson, Shannon, & Shields, 2017).

Treatment of complicated grief sometimes involves antidepressants, generally in the form of SSRIs. Some of the common SSRIs used are escitalopram, paroxetine, and nortriptyline. These are used in combination with Complicated Grief Treatment, as they have not proved effective when used alone to treat complicated grief (Robinaugh et al., 2012). Both escitalopram and nortriptyline are mildly contraindicated for use in older adults and are to be used with caution; similarly, paroxetine may cause negative side effects in patients with heart disease (Wilson et al., 2017). Older adults who are prescribed antidepressants for grief should be monitored closely for any side effects or complications.

Nonpharmacologic Therapy

Treatment of grief in older adults can be successful without medications. Group therapies can be quite effective, as they can be a means of support that the individual may be lacking, as well as a place where the patient can discuss any concerns in a judgment-free setting. This type of therapy can also be particularly helpful, as it introduces the patient to other individuals who have experienced the same loss and who may be having similar grief responses. For some patients, group therapy may not be a good option, but individual therapy may be helpful. Complicated grief is generally treated with a form of psychotherapy called Complicated Grief Treatment, a type of therapy in which the individual focuses on relationships and personal goals (Wetherell, 2012). Those who participate in Complicated Grief Treatment respond more quickly and have better outcomes than those using other therapies (Shear et al., 2005; Wetherell, 2012). Support groups have also proved effective in the treatment of complicated grief in older adults.

>> **Stay Current:** For more information on Complicated Grief Treatment, visit The Center for Complicated Grief at https://complicatedgrief.columbia.edu/

Focus on Diversity and Culture
Loss Among Older Adults

Nurses practice culturally sensitive care by assessing patients' cultural and spiritual beliefs and practices and incorporating them into the care plan appropriately. This aspect of nursing is particularly important in work with older adults experiencing loss. Culturally sensitive care requires assessing each individual patient's and family's beliefs and practices. Traditionally, however, certain cultures have had particular beliefs regarding the care of elders in the community (Purnell, 2014; Spector, 2017):

- Those who uphold traditional Asian cultural beliefs have a great respect for older adults and are expected to take care of their parents if they need assistance in later life.

- Muslims are instructed by the Qur'an to honor, respect, and care for their parents as they age. It might be considered dishonorable for an older Muslim adult to be placed in a retirement or nursing home if a child or grandchild is still available to see to the patient's care.

- In many Native American traditions, elders are considered the keepers of wisdom and knowledge. In some tribes, the care of the elderly is not just by immediate family, but also by extended family and community members.

American families of European descent are often scattered throughout the United States. Family members are sometimes faced with having to place an elderly relative in an assisted living or nursing home situation in order to provide care. Some American families bring the elderly family member into the home, but many times the elder is placed in a long-term care facility.

Nursing Care

Nursing care for older adults who are working through loss and grief requires a certain amount of sensitivity and understanding. Older adults may be reluctant to admit difficulty coping with grief, in part due to ageism and the stigma attached to conditions such as depression and dementia and mental health treatment. It is important for nurses to remember that, because of a patient's history with previous losses, a current loss that does not seem significant to the nurse may be very significant to the patient. Careful, holistic assessment is necessary for nurses to gain an accurate picture of the patient's care needs.

Nurses working with older adults who have experienced a loss and are subsequently grieving should complete a full assessment of the patient's history—both physical and mental health—as well as an assessment of the patient's coping mechanisms. Older adults, especially older adult men, are at a

particularly high risk for both depression and suicide, so the nurse should assess for signs of depression. The patient's support system should also be evaluated. Studies have found that the stronger the support of the patient, the quicker the return to normalcy. If the patient has been grieving for 6 months or more and the grief has not lessened, or has significantly increased, then the nurse should assess for signs of a complicated grief reaction. Collaboration with social workers can be quite helpful when working with patients who are grieving.

The nurse should provide the patient with assistance involving spiritual or cultural needs. If the patient would like to attend religious services or talk to a pastor, rabbi, or other spiritual leader, then the nurse should help to facilitate these needs. Similarly, the nurse should try to help the patient who mentions finding comfort in religious or spiritual texts, but not having access to them. Nursing interventions to assist older adults in coping with loss and grief are outlined in the Independent Interventions section earlier in the module.

Nursing Care Plan
Loss of a Parent by a Pediatric Patient

Justin Ferris, an 8 year-old boy, is brought in to his primary care provider's office by his father. Since Justin's mother died 8 months ago after a motor vehicle crash, Justin has been very withdrawn and quiet. In the last 2 weeks, he has stopped eating regularly, and his sleeping habits have been irregular.

ASSESSMENT

Mr. Ferris tells Justin's primary care nurse, an RN named Fatima Forez, that Johnny has been acting very strangely since his mother died. He has stopped playing with his regular friends or with anyone else. Justin has also been very quiet, only speaking to others if he is required to. The school has reported that Justin's grades have been declining. At first, Mr. Ferris thought Justin was experiencing normal grief reactions, but 2 weeks ago he stopped eating almost entirely, and he has been sleeping only a few hours a night.

Ms. Forez checks Justin's vitals and discovers that his blood pressure and temperature are both normal. When she checks Justin's weight, Ms. Forez notices that he has lost 7 pounds since his last visit 2 months ago. When Ms. Forez asks Justin why he has been having trouble eating and sleeping, he refuses to answer the question and looks down at the floor instead.

After discussing Justin's case with his primary care provider, Ms. Forez recommends that Justin start seeing a grief counselor once a week for help working through a probable complicated grief reaction.

DIAGNOSES

- *Complicated Grieving* related to psychosocial conflicts associated with coping with the loss of a parent
- *Imbalanced Nutrition: Less Than Body Requirements* related to loss of appetite secondary to grief and feelings of guilt
- *Disturbed Sleep Pattern* related to unexpressed emotions
- *Ineffective Coping* related to complicated grief reaction

(NANDA-I © 2014)

PLANNING

Goals for Justin's care include:
- The patient will keep weekly appointments with grief counselor.
- The patient will eat at least one full meal per day and eat whenever he feels hungry.
- The patient will regain a relatively normal sleep schedule.

IMPLEMENTATION

- Teach about complicated grief reactions.
- Emphasize the importance of eating to maintain and increase weight.
- Explain the benefits of grief counseling.

EVALUATION

Justin begins going to grief counseling every week. His therapist works with Justin to develop healthy coping mechanisms to work through his emotions and grief. Justin starts to get his appetite back, and his sleeping habits begin to improve. After 2 months of grief counseling, Justin goes to his follow-up appointment; his weight and disposition have returned to normal.

CRITICAL THINKING

1. If Justin had not improved after 2 months with a grief counselor, how would you change the nursing care plan?
2. What resources could the nurse provide to Justin's father other than individual grief counseling to help with Justin's needs?
3. What role could a school nurse play in Justin's recovery in collaboration with the primary care nurse?

REVIEW   The Concept of Grief and Loss

RELATE Link the Concepts

Linking the concept of grief and loss with the concept of violence:

1. You are caring for a 25-year-old woman who has sustained a perinatal loss as the result of domestic abuse. Describe at least four factors that put this patient at a high risk for a complicated grief reaction.

2. An 8-year-old boy has been physically abused by his father until 2 months ago, when the father died suddenly. What nursing interventions would be appropriate for this boy's grief? How could his history of abuse make the grief more difficult?

Linking children's response to loss with the concept of development:

3. While assessing a 4-year-old whose mother died 2 years ago, you find the child has some small delays in developmental milestones. Why might this have happened?

4. What interventions can you initiate to help this child meet future developmental milestones?

Linking older adult's response to loss with the concept of mobility:

5. What are your goals for the older adult patient who has lost the use of his or her legs?

6. Create a plan of care for an older adult patient who lives alone and is wheelchair bound.

READY Go to Volume 3: Clinical Nursing Skills

REFER Go to Pearson MyLab Nursing and eText

- Additional review materials

REFLECT Apply Your Knowledge

Carol Iverson, a 56-year-old woman, lives in a rural town with her husband, James. Their only child, James Iverson Jr., a Marine, was deployed in the Middle East where he was killed by an explosive device. While his remains were able to be returned to the family for burial, his casket was sealed. The community provided a hero's funeral with a great amount of support for Mr. and Mrs. Iverson and their extended family. However, within a few weeks, the town went back to its normal routine. Mrs. Iverson comes to the town's one health clinic 8 months later, complaining of lack of energy, little motivation, and poor appetite. She relates to the nurse that she hasn't had much closure with James Jr.'s death, even with the town's outpouring of grief. She reports that while her husband has been supportive, he too has gone back to his routine. She tells the nurse, "It seemed like everyone was there for me, and then the next minute, everyone was gone, just like James. I can't get over the last time I saw him, when he told me not to worry, and that he would be home soon. I believed him."

1. What would be a priority nursing diagnosis for Mrs. Iverson? What goals of care would be appropriate for her?

2. What factors play a role in Mrs. Iverson's grief response and possible development of complicated grief?

3. What would be the impact of resources for Mrs. Iverson living in a rural area versus an urban setting?

References

Aloi, J. A. (2009). Nursing the disenfranchised: Women who have relinquished an infant for adoption. *Journal of Psychiatric and Mental Health Nursing, 16,* 27–32.

Avelin, P., Erlandsson, K., Hildingsson, I., Bremborg, A. D., & Rådestad, I. (2012). Make the stillborn baby and the loss real for the siblings: Parents' advice on how the siblings of a stillborn baby can be supported. *The Journal of Perinatal Education, 21*(2), 90–98. Retrieved from http://doi.org/10.1891/1058-1243.21.2.90

Benkel, I., Wijk, H., & Molander, V. (2009). Family and friends provide most social support for the bereaved. *Palliative Medicine, 23,* 141–149.

Berman, A. J., Snyder, S. J., & Frandsen, G. (2016). *Kozier & Erb's fundamentals of nursing: Concepts, process, and practice* (10th ed.). Hoboken, NJ: Pearson Education.

Boerner, K., & Jopp, D. (2010). Resilience in response to loss. In J. W. Reich, A. J. Zautra, & J. S. Hall (Eds.), *Handbook of adult resilience* (pp. 126–145). New York, NY: Guilford Press.

Boyle, D. (2011). Countering compassion fatigue: A requisite nursing agenda. *The Online Journal of Issues in Nursing, 16*(1), Manuscript 2. doi:10.3912/OJIN.Vol16No01Man02

Buglas, E. (2010). Grief and bereavement theories. *Nursing Standard, 24*(41), 44–47.

Canadian Virtual Hospice. (2015). *Tips for talking with someone who is dying.* Retrieved from http://www.virtualhospice.ca/en_US/Main+Site+Navigation/Home/Topics/Topics/Communication/Tips+for+Talking+with+Someone+Who+is+Dying.aspx

Child Traumatic Stress Network. (n.d.). *Childhood traumatic grief for mental health professionals and providers.* Retrieved from http://www.nctsn.org/trauma-types/traumatic-grief/mental-health-professionals

Curtin, S. C., Warner, M., & Hedegaard, H. (2016). Increase in suicide in the United States, 1999–2014. NCHS data brief, no 241. Hyattsville, MD: National Center for Health Statistics.

Dickstein, S. (1996). Jewish ritual practice following a stillbirth. *The Committee on Jewish Law and Standards of the Rabbinical Assembly.* Retrieved from https://www.rabbinicalassembly.org/sites/default/files/public/halakhah/teshuvot/19912000/dickstein_stillbirth.pdf

Engel, G. L. (1964). Grief and grieving. *American Journal of Nursing, 64,* 93–98.

Finkelhor, D., Turner, H., Shattuck, A., & Hamby, S. (2015). Prevalence of childhood exposure to violence, crime, and abuse. *Journal of the American Medical Association. Pediatrics, 169*(8), 746–754. doi:10.1001/jamapediatrics.2015.0676

Gold, K. J., Leon, I., Boggs, M. E., & Sen, A. (2016). Depression and posttraumatic stress symptoms after perinatal loss in a population-based sample. *Journal of Women's Health, 25*(3), 263–269.

Herdman, T. H. & Kamitsuru, S. (Eds.). *Nursing Diagnoses—Definitions and Classification 2015–2017.* Copyright © 2014, 1994–2014 NANDA International. Used by arrangement with John Wiley & Sons, Inc. Companion website: www.wiley.com/go/nursingdiagnoses

Hospice and Palliative Nurses Association. (n.d.). *Home page.* Retrieved from http://hpna.advancing-expertcare.org

Howarth, R. A. (2011). Promoting the adjustment of parentally bereaved children. *Journal of Mental Health Counseling, 33*(1), 21–32.

Kersting, A., & Wagner, B. (2012). Complicated grief after perinatal loss. *Dialogues in Clinical Neuroscience, 14*(2), 187–194. Retrieved from http://www.ncbi.nlm.nih.gov/pmc/articles/PMC3384447/

Kübler-Ross, E. (1969). *On death and dying.* New York, NY: Macmillan.

Li, J., Vestergaard, M., Cnattingius, S., Gissler, M., Bech, B. H., Obel, C., & Olsen, J. (2014). Mortality after parental death in childhood: A nationwide cohort study from three Nordic countries. *PLoS Medicine, 11*(7), e1001679. Retrieved from http://dx.doi.org/10.1371/journal.pmed.1001679

MacDorman, M. F., & Gregory, E. C. W. (2015). Fetal and perinatal mortality: United States, 2013. *National Vital Statistics Report, 64*(8). Retrieved from http://www.cdc.gov/nchs/data/nvsr/nvsr64/nvsr64_08.pdf

MacDorman, M. F., Mathew, T. J., Mohangoo, A. D., & Zeitlin, J. (2014). International comparisons of infant mortality and relation factors: United States and Europe, 2010. *National Vital Statistics Reports, 63*(5). Retrieved from http://www.cdc.gov/nchs/data/nvsr/nvsr63/nvsr63_05.pdf

Mannario, A. P., & Cohen, J. A. (2011). Traumatic loss in children and adolescents. *Journal of Child and Adolescent Trauma, 4*(1), 22–33. Retrieved from http://dx.doi.org/10.1080/19361521.2011.545048

Melhem, N. M., Moritz, G., Walker, M., Shear, K., & Brent, D. (2007). Phenomenology and correlates of complicated grief in children and adolescents. *Child and Adolescent Psychiatry, 46*(4), 493–499. Retrieved from http://dx.doi.org/10.1097/chi.0b013e31803062a9

National Cancer Institute. (2013). *Children and grief.* Retrieved from http://www.cancer.gov/cancertopics/pdq/supportivecare/bereavement/Patient/page1/AllPages#6

National Institute of Mental Health. (n.d.). *Postpartum depression facts.* Retrieved from https://www.nimh.nih.gov/health/publications/postpartum-depression-facts/index.shtml

National Institutes of Health. (2013). *Pregnancy loss: Other FAQs.* Retrieved from https://www.nichd.nih.gov/health/topics/pregnancyloss/conditioninfo/Pages/faqs.aspx#health

Peters, L., Cant, R., Payne, S., O'Connor, M., McDermott, F., Hood, K., … Shimoinaba, K. (2013). How death anxiety impacts nurses' caring for patients at the end of life: A review of literature. *The Open Nursing Journal, 7*, 14–21. Retrieved from http://doi.org/10.2174/1874434601307010014

Potter, M. L., & Moller, M. D. (2016). *Psychiatric–mental health nursing care: From suffering to hope.* Upper Saddle River, NJ: Pearson Education.

Puchalski, C. M. (2012). Spirituality in the cancer trajectory. *Annals of Oncology, 23*(suppl 3), 49–55. doi:10.1093/annonc/mds088

Purnell, L. D. (2014). *A guide to culturally competent health care.* Philadelphia, PA: F.A. Davis.

Robinaugh, D. J., Marques, L., Bui, E., & Simon, N. M. (2012). Recognizing and treating complicated grief: Timing and severity of symptoms can help identify this distinct syndrome. *Current Psychiatry, 11*(8), 30–34.

Sanders, C. M. (1998). *Grief: The mourning after: Dealing with adult bereavement* (2nd ed.). New York, NY: Wiley.

Shear, K., Frank, E., Houck, P. R., & Reynolds, C. F. (2005). Treatment of complicated grief: A randomized controlled trial. *Journal of the American Medical Association, 293*(21), 2601–2608. Retrieved from http://jama.jamanetwork.com/article.aspx?articleid=200995

Shear, M. K. (2015). Complicated grief. *New England Journal of Medicine, 372,* 153–160. doi:10.1056/NEJMcp1315618

Spector, R. E. (2017). *Cultural diversity in health and illness* (9th ed.). Hoboken, NJ: Pearson Education.

Sutan, R., Amen, R. M., Ariffen, K. B., Teng, T. Z., Kamal, M. F., & Rusli, R. Z. (2010). Psychosocial impact of mothers with perinatal loss and its contributing factors: an insight. *Journal of Zhejiang University. Science. B, 11*(3), 209–217.

Tessler, I. (2014, October 8). New procedure allows parents to bury stillborn babies. Ynetnews.com. Retrieved from http://www.ynetnews.com/articles/0,7340,L-4557158,00.html

Thompson, N. (2012). *Grief and its challenges.* Hampshire, England: Palgrave Macmillan.

Utz, R. L., Caserta, M., & Lund, D. (2012). Grief, depressive symptoms, and physical health among recently bereaved spouses. *The Gerontologist, 52*(4), 460–471. doi:10.1093/geront/gnr110

Walsh, K. (2012). *Grief and loss: Theories and skills for the helping professions* (2nd ed.). Upper Saddle River, NJ: Pearson.

Wetherell, J. L. (2012). Complicated grief therapy as a new treatment approach. *Dialogues in Clinical Neuroscience, 14*(2), 159–166.

White, C. D. (2014). Miscarriage. *MedlinePlus.* Retrieved from https://medlineplus.gov/ency/article/001488.htm

Wiese, B. S. (2011). Geriatric depression: The use of antidepressants in the elderly. *BC Medical Journal, 53*(7), 341–347. Retrieved from http://www.bcmj.org/articles/geriatric-depression-use-antidepressants-elderly

Wilson, B. A., Shannon, M. T., & Shields, K. M. (2017). *Pearson nurse's drug guide 2017.* Upper Saddle River, NJ: Pearson.

Worden, J. W., & Silverman, P. R. (1996). Parental death and the adjustment of school-age children. *Omega: Journal of Death and Dying, 29*, 219–230.

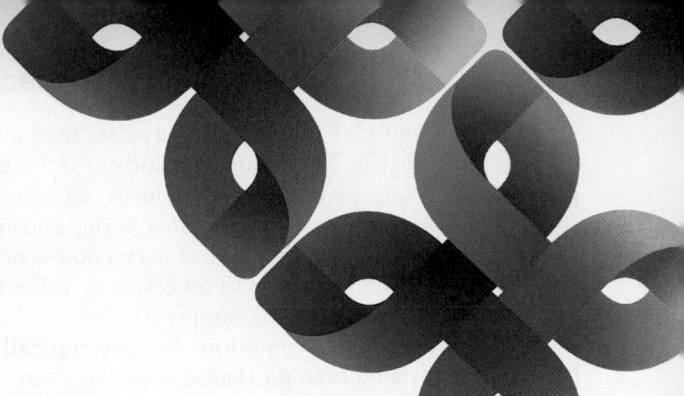

Module 28
Mood and Affect

Module Outline and Learning Outcomes

The Concept of Mood and Affect

Normal Mood and Affect

28.1 Summarize the characteristics of normal mood and affect.

Alterations to Mood and Affect

28.2 Differentiate alterations in mood and affect.

Concepts Related to Mood and Affect

28.3 Outline the relationship between mood and affect and other concepts.

Health Promotion

28.4 Explain the promotion of healthy mood and affect.

Nursing Assessment

28.5 Differentiate common assessment procedures and rating scales used to assess mood and affect.

Independent Interventions

28.6 Analyze independent interventions nurses can implement for patients with alterations in mood and affect.

Collaborative Therapies

28.7 Summarize collaborative therapies used by interprofessional teams for patients with alterations in mood and affect.

Lifespan Considerations

28.8 Differentiate considerations related to the assessment and care of patients with alterations in mood and affect throughout the lifespan.

Mood and Affect Exemplars

Exemplar 28.A Depression

28.A Analyze depressive disorders and relevant nursing care.

Exemplar 28.B Bipolar Disorders

28.B Analyze bipolar disorders and relevant nursing care.

Exemplar 28.C Postpartum Depression

28.C Analyze postpartum depression and relevant nursing care.

Exemplar 28.D Suicide

28.D Analyze the nurse's role in preventing and responding to patient suicide attempts.

» The Concept of Mood and Affect

Concept Key Terms

Adjustment disorder with depressed mood, **1914**	Bipolar disorder, **1914**	Euthymia, **1910**	Moods, **1910**	Postpartum psychosis, **1914**
Affect, **1910**	Circadian rhythms, **1915**	Hypomania, **1912**	Mood stabilizers, **1926**	Seasonal affective disorder (SAD), **1916**
Aggressive behavior, **1924**	Depressive disorder with peripartum onset, **1914**	Learned helplessness, **1916**	Passive behavior, **1924**	Serious mental illness, **1910**
Anhedonia, **1912**	Dysthymia, **1913**	Major depressive disorder (MDD), **1913**	Persistent depressive disorder, **1913**	Serotonin syndrome, **1926**
Anxious distress, **1912**	Electroconvulsive therapy (ECT), **1928**	Mania, **1910**	Postpartum blues, **1914**	Somatization, **1913**
Assertive behavior, **1924**	Emotions, **1909**	Mental health, **1910**	Postpartum depression, **1914**	Unipolar depression, **1913**
		Mental illness, **1910**		

Emotions, mood, and affect are critical elements of the human experience in that they shape and reflect our perceptions of and interactions with the world around us. Although often used interchangeably, each of these terms refers to unique psychosocial attributes (Ekkekakis, 2013).

Emotions are an individual's feeling responses to a wide variety of stimuli. An emotion is reactionary and linked to a specific event or object that can be identified by the person who is experiencing the emotion (Baumeister & Bushman, 2017). Emotions tend to be intense, focused, and relatively short lived. Examples include joy, surprise, fear, anger, and disgust (Liu, 2015). Frequently, an individual's emotions precipitate certain physiologic responses, such as smiling, frowning, clenching fists, pacing, sweating, and increased heart rate. Although an individual may choose not to verbally communicate emotions to others, it is difficult to prevent nonverbal expression of emotions.

Moods are similar to emotions but are typically longer lasting, less focused on a particular object or event, and less intense. A mood might have one trigger, multiple triggers, or no specific cause at all. Because **mood** is an enduring state of mind rather than a discrete reaction, it can shape a person's general expectations about the future (Liu, 2015). Unlike emotions, moods do not produce observable physiologic reactions. Therefore, only the individual is capable of describing mood; nurses and other clinicians must be careful not to assume they know a patient's mood based solely on their observations.

Affect refers to an individual's automatic reaction to an event or situation—the immediate, observable expression of mood. Like emotion, affect is evidenced by verbal and nonverbal responses; however, emotion involves a person's *conscious* reaction to an object or event, whereas affect involves a person's *unconscious* response to something as either good or bad. Affective reactions occur faster than emotional reactions, sometimes within a few microseconds. Individuals do not need to understand or even be familiar with something in order to have an affective response to it (Baumeister & Bushman, 2017).

Together, mood and affect play a large part in determining an individual's **mental health**, defined as a state of well-being in which an individual is able to work productively, cope with change and adversity, engage in meaningful relationships, and realize his or her own potential. Alterations in mood and affect can disrupt an individual's ability to accomplish one or more of these tasks. When these alterations are severe enough to have lasting detrimental effects on a person's life, they may rise to the level of mental illness. **Mental illness** can be defined as a condition that affects emotions, thinking, behavior, or any combination of the three. Mental illness is not typically confirmed until the individual experiences serious and lengthy impairment in the ability to function (American Psychiatric Association [APA], 2013).

This module explores the concept of mood and affect and provides exemplars that facilitate an understanding of impaired mood and affect. Both depression and bipolar disorder are classified as **serious mental illnesses** that increase the possibility the individual will experience serious dysfunction related to daily functioning and ability to achieve life goals (Potter & Moller, 2016). Information related to assessment of individuals with alterations in mood and affect, collaborative therapies, and nursing care is also provided.

Normal Mood and Affect

Defining or describing normal mood and affect can be challenging for a number of reasons. For one, standards of desired or acceptable attitudes and behavior vary widely among cultures as well as among individuals. Also, nearly

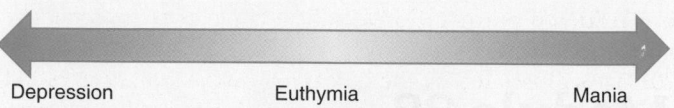

Depression   Euthymia   Mania

Figure 28–1 》 Range of mood states.

all individuals experience ongoing fluctuations in mood and affect in response to various biological, psychologic, sociologic, and cultural events and experiences (Potter & Moller, 2016).

In light of these complicating factors, mental health professionals typically describe mood and affect in terms of certain qualities rather than in terms of concrete categories of "normal" and "abnormal." Mood, as depicted in **Figure 28–1 》**, is said to exist on a continuum ranging from *depression* (an abnormally lowered mood characterized by sadness, emptiness, and irritability) to **mania** (an abnormally elevated mood that impairs functioning). Between these two extremes lies **euthymia**, or a stable range of mood that is neither elevated nor depressed. Although euthymic individuals experience occasional fluctuations in mood (for example, happiness at achieving a life goal or frustration associated with a temporary injury), these fluctuations are appropriate to the situation, are typical of the individual's usual pattern of response, and do not impair functional ability. Accordingly, an individual's mood is said to be "normal" if it falls somewhere in the central or euthymic portion of the continuum (Potter & Moller, 2016).

When evaluating a person's affect, healthcare professionals focus on several characteristics. *Appropriateness*, or *congruence*, refers to affect that matches the individual's emotional state and the immediate situation (Stuart, 2014). *Range* refers to the variety of feelings an individual conveys through affect. Most people exhibit a broad or full range of affect, meaning they are able to convey many different feelings using verbal and nonverbal responses. *Broad affect* is therefore considered normal. In contrast, individuals with *restricted affect* express only a limited range of feelings. For example, a patient who weeps when describing his wife's illness but shows no sign of happiness or excitement when discussing the birth of his child may have a restricted affect.

Intensity describes the degree of emotion displayed in a person's affect. Normal intensity means that the level of emotion expressed in an individual's affect is proportionate to the situation. In contrast, individuals with flat affect display no visible cues to their feelings whatsoever. Intensity may be described as:

- *Moderate.* The individual displays a level of emotion that is appropriate to the situation.
- *Overreactive.* The individual's level of emotion is disproportionate or extreme given the situation.
- *Blunted.* The individual displays a level of emotion that is dulled or muted given the situation.
- *Flat.* The individual's affect provides no visible cues to his emotions.

Stability refers to how often and how rapidly an individual's affect fluctuates. A stable affect, or one that remains consistent when there is no provocation in the environment, is considered normal. Conversely, a labile or rapidly changing affect is often suggestive of disease or disorder (Stuart, 2014). As illustrated by the preceding discussion, both mood and affect become dysfunctional when they are inappropriate to the situation, when they are out of proportion to the stimulus, and/or when they shift dramatically or rapidly out of proportion to external events.

Factors Contributing to Mood and Affect

Mood and affect are shaped by a number of internal and external factors, including neurologic function, personality, stress level, social interactions, day, time, gender, age, and illness status,. Each of these factors is briefly discussed below, and several are visited in greater depth later in the module in the section describing various theories of depression. Other factors that may influence mood and affect are identified in the Concepts Related to Mood and Affect section and within the specific exemplars.

Neurologic Function

Emotions, mood, and affect all originate deep within the brain, in an interconnected set of structures called the limbic system. Three structures of the limbic system—the hippocampus, the hypothalamus, and the amygdala—appear to be particularly important in the production and regulation of mood and affect. Under normal circumstances, limbic system activity is regulated by a nearby area of the brain called the medial prefrontal cortex (MPFC). If the MPFC fails to function properly, the limbic system may become overactive, and alterations in mood and affect may result. This is evidenced by brain imaging studies that show increased activity in the limbic systems of individuals with alterations in mood. Studies also reveal that these individuals tend to have decreased gray matter volume and lower metabolic activity in the MPFC, which helps explain why this structure is unable to properly control the limbic system (Field & Cartwright-Hatton, 2015; Grieve et al., 2013).

The exact cellular mechanisms of normal function within the MPFC and limbic system remain unclear. The prevailing theory is that alterations in neurotransmitter activity and/or neuronal receptivity to neurotransmitters contribute to the development of mood disorders such as depression and bipolar disorder (as described later in this module). Thus, normal neurotransmitter and neuronal function appears to be a key contributor to normal mood. Emerging research also suggests that proper glial cell function is necessary for normal mood and affect (Ongur et al., 2014).

Personality

Temperament and personality play a large role in shaping an individual's mood and affect. In general, high levels of neuroticism (emotional instability) and introversion and low levels of conscientiousness and agreeableness predispose individuals to negative affect, greater affect variability, and depressed mood. Conversely, low levels of neuroticism and high levels of extraversion, conscientiousness, and agreeableness are associated with greater likelihood of positive affect, lower affect variability, and elevated mood (Bowen et al., 2012; Hoerger, Chapman, & Duberstein, 2015; Komulainen et al., 2014).

Stress

Excessive stress and/or maladaptive coping responses are well-known contributors to alterations in mood and affect. When stress is chronic, it can lead to hormonal imbalances that disrupt normal brain function, especially in the hippocampus (Lucassen et al., 2016). Stress also appears to have a negative effect on the reward circuitry within the MPFC (Kumar et al., 2015). In addition, chronic stress increases a person's likelihood of inadequate sleep, poor dietary intake, and physical disease, which are themselves risk factors for altered mood and affect (as described later in this section).

Social Interactions

Social support and positive social interactions are clearly connected to stable, positive mood and affect: Multiple studies indicate that high-quality, positive social interactions themselves contribute to enhanced mood (Pemberton & Fuller Tyszkiewicz, 2016). Similarly, an individual's overall level of social support is often an important predictor of mood. Generally speaking, individuals who have greater levels of perceived support and larger, more diverse social networks tend to be at lower risk for depression and other alterations in mood and affect, which suggests that these factors offer a protective effect (Santini et al., 2015).

Day and Time

Both day of the week and time of day influence mood and affect. Most likely because of hormonal fluctuations associated with the body's circadian (24-hour) rhythms, people tend to experience lower mood in the morning. Most people's mood and affect then gradually become more positive throughout the day, reaching their peak in the afternoon hours before declining in the evening. This is true regardless of whether an individual is a so-called morning person or evening person. Interestingly, however, people with a preference for mornings tend to show better mood during all parts of the day than do people with a preference for evenings (Diaz-Morales, Escribano, & Jankowski, 2015; Jankowski, 2014).

Gender and Age

Research indicates that, as compared to men, women are more likely to physically express their emotions, are more comfortable discussing their feelings, and are more skilled at reading others' emotions (Fischer & LaFrance, 2015). Women are also more likely to experience negative emotions like guilt and shame (Else-Quest et al., 2012), and they tend to have stronger negative reactions to unpleasant stimuli (Gomez, von Gunten, & Danuser, 2013). In addition, research suggests that women tend to internalize and dwell on their emotions more than men (Chaplin & Aldao, 2013; Trives et al., 2016). In light of these factors, it is not surprising that women are more than 2 times as likely as men to experience mood disorders. However, the causes of these differences in emotional processing, mood, and affect remain an issue of debate, as described in the section on the gender bias theory of depression.

Age also tends to influence a person's mood and affect. As people grow into adulthood, the mood swings typical of early adolescence become less common (Maciejewski et al., 2015). Also, contrary to popular belief, older adults generally have more positive mood and affect than younger adults, perhaps because of their better use of various strategies of emotional regulation (English & Carstensten, 2014; Masumoto, Taishi, & Shiozaki, 2016; Stanley & Isaacowitz, 2011).

Illness Status

Given that overall health promotes normal mood and affect, it is not surprising that physical disease and injury are significant risk factors for alterations in mood and affect. In some cases, the nature of the disease or injury itself may account for the disruption. For example, conditions that affect the brain tissue or that cause alterations in hormone levels may be directly responsible for alterations in affect or unusually high or low mood. Research has also found a link between autoimmune diseases and mood disorders, which suggests that some alterations in mood may have an immunologic basis (Benros et al., 2013).

Individuals who have chronic conditions such as heart disease, diabetes, and cancer often face ongoing stress, physical limitations, alterations in self-concept, decreased quality of life, and/or concerns about mortality that contribute to negative mood. In fact, depression is one of the most common complications of chronic disease, and it can actually worsen the course of the disease if not promptly identified and addressed (DeJean et al., 2013; Gunn et al., 2012).

Alterations to Mood and Affect

An elevation or decrease in mood and affect may impair an individual's ability to cope with typical daily life stressors. Prolonged alterations may progress into a depressive or bipolar disorder and require professional intervention.

Individuals with depressive disorder exhibit depressed mood characterized by feelings of sadness or emptiness. Other core symptoms include **anhedonia** (a loss of interest or inability to experience pleasure with activities), fatigue and sleep disturbances, and somatic complaints. In children and adolescents, irritability is a common symptom of depression. In contrast, individuals with bipolar disorder typically experience a major depressive episode alternating with a period of mania or hypomania. **Mania** is an abnormal, persistent, expansive, elevated mood that lasts at least 1 week and that significantly impairs functioning, potentially requiring hospitalization. **Hypomania** is a similar impairment of mood that lasts at least four consecutive days; its symptoms, although significant, do not necessitate hospitalization (APA, 2013). Because of the degree to which mood disorders may impact daily functioning, they can affect individuals across a wide variety of systems and situations (see Concepts Related to Mood and Affect).

Anxious distress is associated with depressive and bipolar disorders with sufficient frequency that the *Diagnostic and Statistical Manual of Mental Disorders*, 5th ed. (DSM-5) (APA, 2013), includes it as a specifier clinicians may add to a diagnosis of depression or bipolar disorder. **Anxious distress** is a combination of symptoms associated with high anxiety, including restlessness, impaired concentration due to worry, fear of impending doom, and fear of losing control.

SAFETY ALERT Patients who experience anxious distress in combination with a depressive or bipolar disorder typically are harder to treat and at greater risk for suicide (APA, 2013).

The National Institute of Mental Health (NIMH) (n.d.a) reports that mood disorders affect nearly 10% of adults, with 45% of cases classified as severe. Mood disorders impact individuals of every race and age. Treatment is critical: Without it, patients are at increased risk for suicide. Mood disorders also carry economic costs. For example, depression is associated with lower rates of productivity, increased absenteeism, and increased rates of short-term disability (Greenberg et al., 2015). Patients with depressive and bipolar disorders are found in the community and in all clinical settings, and they frequently experience difficulties with their communication skills, family relationships, and ability or motivation to adhere to a treatment plan.

Pathophysiology of Altered Mood

As mentioned earlier, both the limbic system and the MPFC play a central role in normal mood and affect, so disruptions in either portion of the brain may result in altered mood. The cellular mechanisms that underlie these disruptions are an area of intense interest to researchers, although they are widely believed to involve alterations in neurotransmitter activity and/or neuronal receptivity to neurotransmitters.

Thus far, the so-called neurotransmitter hypothesis has largely focused on two monoamine neurotransmitters: serotonin and norepinephrine. Serotonin (5-HT) is involved in the regulation of aggression, mood, anxiety, impulsivity, appetite, sleep, and sex drive, whereas norepinephrine (NE) is involved in the regulation of attention, arousal, and behavior. Given that alterations in all of these areas are characteristic of mood disorders, dysregulation of both 5-HT and NE is thought to be a contributing factor to depression and bipolar disorder. This conclusion is supported by research showing decreased levels of both neurotransmitters in the brains of individuals with mood disorders (Patrick & Ames, 2015; Varcarolis, 2013).

More recently, scientists have also begun to investigate the potential contribution of other neurotransmitters, including dopamine (DA), acetylcholine (ACh), gamma-aminobutyric acid (GABA), and glutamate. DA is an essential component of the brain's reward circuitry, and ACh helps regulate the sleep–wake cycle. GABA reduces the ability of nerve cells to transmit information, whereas glutamate causes the opposite effect. Although all of these neurotransmitters—along with 5-HT and NE—appear to be involved in the pathophysiology of mood disorders, the exact nature of their roles remains unclear. Some studies suggest that abnormal levels of these substances contribute to depressive and bipolar disorders, while other studies suggest that altered neuronal receptivity to neurotransmitters may be to blame. Most likely, there are different combinations of problems with each of these neurotransmitter systems. It is also likely that the systems interact with one another in a variety of ways that scientists have yet to discover (Halter, 2014; Varcarolis, 2013; Werner & Covenas, 2015). As research continues to tease out the connections between these neurotransmitters and the cells on which they act, the underlying pathophysiology of mood disorders will no doubt become clearer.

Alterations and Manifestations

Alterations in mood and affect may be seen at any point across the lifespan. Brief periods of sadness, irritability, and excitement are common as individuals encounter hardship, challenge, and joy. At times, however, these periods extend beyond just a few days or weeks, depending on the nature of the stressor or situation and the individual's own ability to cope. In such instances, patients may demonstrate any number of manifestations of altered mood. Often, these manifestations exist independently of any diagnosable mental illness. Other times, they are part of a larger set of symptoms indicative of a mood disorder.

Common Manifestations of Altered Mood and Affect

As mentioned earlier, an individual's mood is considered altered if it is excessively elevated (manic) or excessively depressed. Similarly, affect is said to be altered if it is inappropriate (incongruent), narrowed, overreactive, blunted, and/or excessively labile. Beyond these basic indicators of abnormality, a number of other manifestations are common in individuals who are experiencing altered mood and affect.

Maladaptive Coping Responses

As previously described, high stress levels and maladaptive coping responses are well-known contributors to altered mood and affect, but they can also be manifestations of such alterations. Some of the most commonly observed maladaptive coping responses include avoidance (i.e., refusal to confront stressors), escape, rumination (i.e., persistent mental focus on stressful situations or symptoms and their implications), denial, helplessness, isolation, self-pity, self-blame, excessive dependency, and aggression. Note, however, that a wide range of other responses may also be considered maladaptive if they impair an individual's ability to function effectively when faced with life's demands (Michl et al., 2013; Skinner & Zimmer-Gembeck, 2016).

Altered Thought Processes

Altered thought processes can also be a manifestation of disrupted mood and affect. Decreased concentration, poor memory, impaired problem-solving ability, indecisiveness, and poor decision making are among the most common alterations. Less common but more drastic alterations in thought include paranoid thinking, hallucinations, and other forms of psychosis, all of which are associated with unstable mood (Marwaha et al., 2013).

Sleep Disturbances

Changes in sleep patterns are often observed in patients with altered mood and affect. In fact, sleep disturbances are a defining characteristic of nearly all mood disorders. People with manic or elevated mood tend to have difficulty sleeping, whereas individuals with low or depressed mood may experience either insomnia or excessive sleepiness. Even when patients with mood alterations are able to fall and remain asleep, they may not feel adequately rested or refreshed upon awakening (Potter & Moller, 2016).

Somatization

Somatization is the phenomenon in which individuals experience or express psychologic distress through physiologic responses. Although somatization may occur in the absence of mood disruptions, it is commonly associated with alterations in mood and affect. Examples of somatic symptoms frequently seen in individuals with mood alterations include fatigue, headache, heart distress, and dizziness.

Between 65 and 80% of individuals with depression report pain as a symptom. For some patients, pain may be an expression of their illness; for others, altered mood and affect may result from pain. Regardless of the exact circumstance, the complicated and likely bidirectional connection between mood and pain highlights the need to assess all patients with chronic pain for signs and symptoms of depression (de Heer et al., 2014; Potter & Moller, 2016).

Difficulties with Adaptive Functioning

Adaptive functioning refers to the ability to safely and independently participate in the demands of daily life—such as activities of daily living, maintaining home or living space, obtaining proper nutrition and medical care, managing finances, completing occupational tasks, planning for the future, and engaging in social interactions. Individuals with altered mood and affect commonly experience difficulties in one or more of these areas.

Disorders of Mood and Affect

When of sufficient duration and intensity, alterations in mood and affect may constitute a diagnosable disorder. Common mood disorders include depressive disorders, adjustment disorder with depressed mood, bipolar disorders, and postpartum mood disorders.

Depressive Disorders

Mental health practitioners recognize several types of depressive disorders, the most common of which is **major depressive disorder (MDD)**, also called **unipolar depression**. MDD is what most Americans think of when they hear the term "depression." MDD is diagnosed when the patient experiences either depressed mood or anhedonia most of the day, almost every day, during the same 2-week period. The depression or loss of interest must be accompanied by at least four of the following core symptoms:

- Sleep disturbances
- Significant weight change (5% or greater in either direction) or change in appetite
- Fatigue or loss of energy
- Feelings of worthlessness or guilt
- Change in activity level (either psychomotor agitation or retardation)
- Poor concentration
- Suicidal ideation or attempt.

MDD may involve just a single depressive episode, although most affected individuals experience multiple recurring episodes over the course of their lives (APA, 2013).

Persistent depressive disorder (dysthymia) is sometimes also referred to as depression, but the diagnostic criteria differ from those for MDD. Dysthymia may be diagnosed when a depressed mood is present for most of the day, more days than not, for at least 2 years. Symptoms of dysthymia are similar to but less severe than those of MDD (APA, 2013).

Adjustment Disorder with Depressed Mood

Individuals often experience dramatic life changes related to events such as death of a loved one, relocation, loss of autonomy, illness, and financial stress. One or more life changes or stressors may contribute to the development of **adjustment disorder with depressed mood**, also known as *situational depression*. Adjustment disorder with depressed mood is a maladaptive reaction to an identifiable psychosocial stressor (or stressors) that occurs within 3 months after the stressor occurs and persists for no longer than 6 months after termination of the stressor (APA, 2013). Symptoms of adjustment disorder with depressed mood are similar to those of the other depressive disorders but are less severe, although a higher level of anxiety may be present.

Bipolar Disorders

Bipolar-related disorders include bipolar I, bipolar II, cyclothymic disorder, and other related disorders. The medical diagnosis of **bipolar disorder** is given when an individual's mood alternates between the extremes of depression and mania or hypomania, interspersed with periods of normal mood. *Bipolar I disorder* is characterized by the occurrence of one or more manic episodes and one or more depressive episodes. *Bipolar II disorder* is characterized by one or more hypomanic episodes (less severe) and one or more depressive episodes.

Bipolar disorders may be further classified as follows (APA, 2013):

- *With mixed features.* The individual experiences symptoms of depression (e.g., depressed mood, anhedonia, and suicidal ideation or attempt) during episodes of mania or hypomania; or the individual experiences manic/hypomanic symptoms during the depressive episode.

- *With rapid cycling.* The individual experiences four or more mood episodes of illness (mania, hypomania, or depression) within a 12-month period, with at least 2 months between each episode OR with alternating episodes (e.g., a period of mania followed by a depressive episode). There is a higher risk of rapid cycling, cycle acceleration, and severity of mood episodes in women (Erol et al., 2015).

Postpartum Mood Disorders

Often, women can experience **postpartum blues** after childbirth, which includes symptoms such as mood swings, tearfulness, sleep disruptions, and increased anxiety. These symptoms usually occur within the first 2–3 days postpartum and may last up to a couple of weeks (Mayo Clinic, 2015a). When these symptoms are more severe and of longer duration, the woman may be diagnosed with **depressive disorder with peripartum onset**, often referred to as *peripartum* or **postpartum depression**.

Postpartum depression is defined as moderate to severe depression experienced during pregnancy and/or up to a year after giving birth. In up to 50% of cases, the depression begins during pregnancy. When postpartum depression arises after delivery, it usually starts within a few weeks after giving birth; however, sometimes the symptoms may present up to 12 months after birth (APA, 2013). Women who give birth to multiple children and/or to preterm children also are at higher risk for postpartum depression.

It is important to identify depression occurring during or following pregnancy as early as possible in order to try to prevent increasing duration and severity of symptoms. Symptoms of postpartum depression are outlined in the Alterations and Manifestations feature and the exemplar that appears later in this module. Symptoms may escalate to severe anxiety, panic attacks, and thoughts of suicide (suicidal ideation) or causing harm to the baby (Mayo Clinic, 2015a). Contributing factors include hormonal changes, family history of depression, feelings of being overwhelmed by parenting tasks, changes in family dynamics, and inadequate support.

Postpartum mood episodes accompanied by psychotic features occur in between 1 in 500 and 1 in 1000 deliveries. **Postpartum psychosis** is characterized by psychotic features associated with peripartum or (more commonly) postpartum depression. These episodes frequently involve command hallucinations or delusions. The command hallucinations may direct the mother to harm the infant, while the delusions may cause the mother to feel that the baby is possessed (APA, 2013).

Suicide

Suicide is itself a mood disorder and may be triggered by one or a series of event in individuals not previously diagnosed with a mood disorder. However, all major depressive episodes include the possibility of suicidal behavior. Suicide is the extreme of negative coping, leading to self-injurious behaviors causing death. The most reliable predictor of risk is a past history of suicidal threats or attempts. Other risk factors include gender (males are at higher risk), living alone, and persistent feelings of hopelessness (APA, 2013). It is critical that the nurse obtain a thorough history so that risk factors are identified and an appropriate plan of care may be developed. An individual who is actively suicidal requires inpatient hospitalization for safety and stabilization.

Theories of Depression

Depressive and bipolar disorders are currently thought to be caused by an interaction of individual genetic, biological, environmental, and psychosocial factors. Depressive disorders are considered spectrum disorders, occurring along a continuum of mild to severe. Most cases fall somewhere between these two extremes.

Both a patient's history (e.g., history of medical illness, trauma, and coping mechanisms) and current factors inform the clinical presentation of the patient's disorder, as well as how the individual copes with or responds to the disorder. For example, an individual may have a genetic predisposition to abnormalities in neurotransmission, but these abnormalities may occur only when certain psychologic mechanisms are present, or they may operate only when particular social interactions occur (Mullins et al., 2016). Furthermore, different forms of depression may have different risk factors. In some forms of depression, genetic predisposition may have a stronger role, whereas in other forms, stressors may have a greater role. Most likely, depression and other mood disorders represent a common final pathway of multiple underlying factors, with most affected individuals possessing more than one risk factor.

Alterations and Therapies
Mood and Affect

ALTERATION	DESCRIPTION	THERAPIES
Depression (including major depressive disorder and persistent depressive disorder)	Depressed mood that varies from mild to severe with severe phases lasting longer than 6 weeks. Symptoms include: ■ Feelings of sadness, hopelessness, powerlessness, apathy, or guilt ■ Changes in sleep and/or appetite ■ Anhedonia ■ Inability to concentrate ■ Psychomotor retardation or agitation	■ Antidepressant medications: SSRIs, SNRIs, bupropion, TCAs, MAOIs ■ Antidepressants may be combined with low-dose antipsychotic medication in resistant cases ■ Nonpharmacologic therapy: cognitive–behavioral therapy (CBT); electroconvulsive therapy (ECT); transcranial magnetic stimulation (TMS); vagus nerve stimulation (VNS)
Bipolar disorders	Extreme alterations in mood (mood swings) with intermittent periods of normal mood	■ Mood-stabilizing medication ■ Psychotherapy ■ Hospitalization or partial hospitalization during severe episodes
Depressive disorder with peripartum onset (postpartum depression)	Severe depression that appears during pregnancy or within the first year following the birth of a child. Symptoms include: ■ Sleep disturbances ■ Fatigue ■ Crying ■ Feelings of despair ■ Anxiety ■ Mood swings	Combination of antidepressants and psychosocial interventions is most effective.
Adjustment disorder with depressed mood (situational depression)	Hyperreaction to an identifiable, life-altering (but not life-threatening) stressor that occurs within 3 months after the onset of the stressor and persists for no more than 6 months after termination of the stressor; symptoms are similar to but less severe than those of major depressive disorder	Psychotherapy alone may be sufficient to relieve symptoms and return patient to premorbid level of functioning
Suicide	Self-injurious behaviors resulting in death	Inpatient hospitalization for safety and stabilization. Stabilization will include therapies for the diagnosed depressive disorders and any comorbid disorders, such as substance abuse

But precisely what factors (besides genetics) increase a person's likelihood of depression? Thus far, researchers have proposed several theories, each of which focuses on a different potential contributor and is described in the sections below. By remembering and applying elements from each of these theories, nurses can approach patients with depression from a more holistic perspective.

Biological Theories

Numerous studies demonstrate that depression has a biological basis. As explained earlier in the concept, specific alterations in structure, function, and neurotransmitter activity have been noted in the brains of individuals with depression. As described throughout the concept, depression also appears to be at least partially rooted in a person's genetics. Still, structural, functional, and genetic variations may not be the only biological contributors to depressive disorders. Other proposed contributors include disrupted biological rhythms, hormonal factors, and inflammation.

Biological Rhythms

Biological rhythms are regular fluctuations in the body's physiologic processes over a given period of time. When these fluctuations occur on a 24-hour cycle, they are known as **circadian rhythms**. Research suggests that for some individuals, internal desynchronization of the body's circadian rhythms may result in depression. The tendency toward internal desynchronization is probably inherited, but stresses, lifestyle, and normal aging also influence it. It is unclear, however, whether changes in circadian rhythms cause mood disturbances or whether changes in mood alter circadian rhythms (Baron & Reid, 2014; Bechtel, 2015). (See the module on Health, Wellness, Illness, and Injury for a more detailed discussion of circadian rhythms.)

Disruptions in the body's seasonal rhythms may also be problematic. For example, many people are at greater risk of depression during a specific time of year (typically, the winter months). This increased correlation between depressive symptoms and time of year is commonly referred to as **seasonal affective disorder (SAD)**, although the actual DSM-5 diagnosis is *major depressive disorder with seasonal pattern*. Common manifestations of SAD include decreased energy, increased periods of sleep, increased appetite, overeating, and weight gain (APA, 2013).

Hormonal Factors

Several lines of evidence support the theory that hormonal factors play a role in depression. One compelling finding is that individuals with depression tend to have increased levels of cortisol and corticotropin-releasing hormone. Both of these hormones are produced in the brain's hypothalamic–pituitary–adrenal (HPA) axis, which plays a major role in regulating mood and the body's response to stress. High levels of cortisol and corticotropin-releasing hormone are indicative of HPA hyperactivity, which (as described earlier) is commonly observed in individuals with mood disorders (Potter & Moller, 2016). Researchers aren't sure whether depression precipitates HPA hyperactivity and excess hormone production or whether HPA hyperactivity and excess hormone production precipitate depression. However, recent studies suggest that variations in the genes that code for corticotropin-releasing hormone may lead to increased susceptibility to major depression following negative life events (Liu et al., 2013; Waters et al., 2015).

The fact that women experience higher rates of depression than men indicates a connection between estrogen and depression. Decreased estrogen levels in particular seem to play a role, as evidenced by women's greater likelihood of depressive symptoms at certain points in the menstrual cycle, as well as at the onset of menopause. The exact nature of the estrogen–depression relationship remains unclear, however (Halter, 2014; Wharton et al., 2012).

Inflammation

Within the past decade, multiple research studies have noted that depressed individuals tend to have increased levels of inflammatory biomarkers called cytokines (Raison & Miller, 2012; Vogelzangs et al., 2014). Similar elevations have also been observed in individuals with bipolar disorder (Stertz, Magalhaes, & Kapczinski, 2012). These findings suggest that mood disorders have an inflammatory component, although scientists aren't yet sure of the precise connection between inflammation and depression. One factor complicating research in this area is the fact that elevated cytokine levels are not universal across all depressed individuals. Furthermore, many individuals who have elevated cytokine levels show no symptoms of depression. Together, these findings have led to the hypothesis that some (but not all) people with depression may have a genetic predisposition toward elevated cytokine production when faced with external stressors, as well as the hypothesis that other individuals may have genetic factors that protect them against the potentially mood-lowering effects of cytokines (Raison & Miller, 2012; Slavich & Irwin, 2014).

Interpersonal Theory

Interpersonal theory is rooted in the idea that all people have a basic inborn need for interpersonal relationships, because these attachments provide a sense of security and allow individuals to develop a healthy sense of self. When these relationships are threatened, individuals experience feelings of grief and anger. These emotions are a normal response to real or anticipated loss, but when they remain unrecognized or unresolved, depression may result (Verdeli & Weissman, 2014). Some interpersonal theorists believe that individuals who have been taught that it is inappropriate to experience and express anger learn to repress it. The result is that their anger is turned inward and against the self, triggering a depressive episode. Other theorists believe depression arises because of sadness and disappointment about failure to achieve desired goals, the loss of those goals, and/or a feeling of lack of control in life. Most interpersonal theorists also emphasize that there is a reciprocal relationship between depression and interpersonal problems. In other words, not only do threatened interpersonal attachments trigger depression, but depression itself can cause a person to interact with others in a way that promotes rejection, thus perpetuating the cycle and worsening the individual's depression (Hames, Hagan, & Joiner, 2013; Lipsitz & Markowitz, 2013).

Learning Theory

Learning theory states that individuals learn to be depressed in response to an external locus of control, in which they perceive themselves as having no ability to control the outcome of their life experiences. According to this theory, many individuals with depression have limited success in achieving gratification and little positive reinforcement for their attempts to cope with negative incidents. Over time, these repeated failures teach them that what they do has no effect on the final outcome of a situation. The more stressful their life events, the more these individuals' sense of helplessness is reinforced—a phenomenon referred to as **learned helplessness**. When these individuals reach the point of believing they have no control whatsoever, they no longer have the will or energy to cope with life, and a depressive state results (Halter, 2014; Potter & Moller, 2016).

Cognitive Theory

The cognitive theory of depression is based on the idea that internal thought processes influence the way individuals with mood disorders experience themselves and others. According to this theory, which comes largely from the work of Aaron Beck (1967), individuals with depression have skewed core views of themselves, of their environment, and of the future. Moreover, their characteristically negative way of thinking makes it impossible for these individuals to alter their behavior or even see the possibility for change at some point in the future. Consequently, people with depression have deeply held negative life views that tend to be based on cognitive distortions rather than reality (e.g., "I am a bad parent because I yelled at my child yesterday") (Potter & Moller, 2016).

Sociocultural Theory

Sociocultural theory emphasizes the role that social stressors play in the development of depression. These stressors take

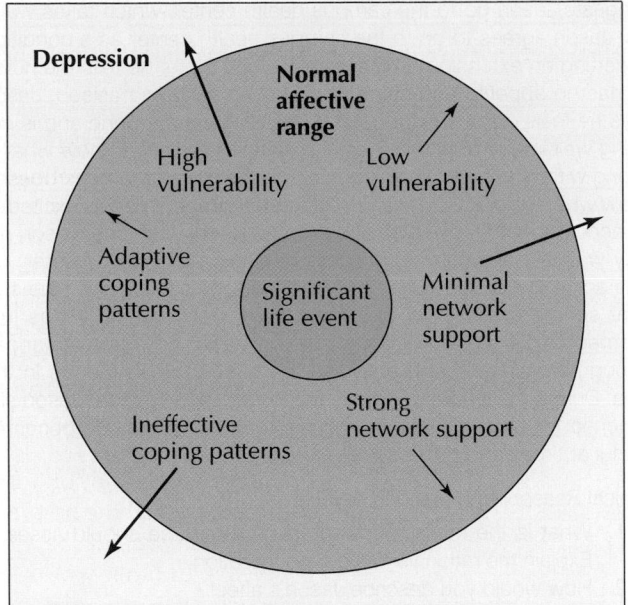

Figure 28–2 》 The relationship between life events and depression.

a variety of forms. Some are economic; common examples include poverty and job insecurity (Brown, 2012). Others involve a disruption in the family system, including divorce, children leaving home, or the death of a loved one. Some stressful life events involve a threat (e.g., illness, encounters with law enforcement), while others are emotionally exhausting (e.g., celebrating holidays, changing residences, or arguing with family and friends). Many individuals who experience stressful events do not become depressed. However, for those who are vulnerable to depression, stressors may play a significant role in the exacerbation and course of the disorder (Potter & Moller, 2016).

A number of factors influence the degree of stress that accompanies significant life events. **Figure 28–2 》** illustrates the relationship between life events and depression. The presence of a social support network can decrease the impact that an event may have on an individual. Individuals who have developed adaptive coping patterns such as problem solving, direct communication, and use of resources are more likely to maintain their normal mood. Those who feel out of control, are unable to problem solve, and ignore available resources are more apt to feel depressed. Thus, an individual's perception and interpretation of significant events may contribute to depression (Evans et al., 2015; Holden et al., 2012; Morris et al., 2015). Perception and interpretation of events may be informed by cultural or gender norms (see Focus on Diversity and Culture).

SAFETY ALERT Childhood sexual abuse (CSA) is a significant risk factor for depression during both childhood and adulthood, as well as for self-harming behaviors (e.g., cutting), posttraumatic stress disorder (PTSD), and suicide (Devries et al., 2014; National Center for PTSD, 2015). Therefore, depressed patients with a history of CSA should be assessed and closely monitored for self-harming and suicidal behaviors.

Focus on Diversity and Culture
Influence of Culture and Gender on Depressive Disorders

Throughout the world, women experience more depression than men. Certainly, there are cross-cultural similarities in the way women are socialized and in the inferior status they experience in many societies. Psychosocial stressors, including multiple work and family responsibilities, poverty, sexual and physical abuse, gender discrimination, unequal pay, lack of social supports, and traumatic life experience, may contribute to women's increased vulnerability to depression (Platt et al., 2015; World Health Organization, 2016a).

Gender socialization differences may also be a factor in the higher rate of depression in women. In many cultures, children are socialized to believe that girls are more influenced by emotions while boys are more influenced by reason. Similarly, girls are taught that it is acceptable to share their thoughts and feelings with others, while boys are encouraged to keep their emotions to themselves. Many societies also promote the idea that girls should be submissive and "nice" while boys should be tough and aggressive. Various disciplines—including psychology, sociology, nursing, and psychiatry—continue to study the effects that these differing messages have on children and adolescents, and how expectations related to gender roles impact men and women into adulthood. Many researchers have theorized that these messages create an environment in which women feel devalued, thus increasing their risk of depression. It is also likely that internalization of these societal messages has created a healthcare system in which both patients and practitioners are more likely to view depression as a "women's disorder," whether consciously or not. As a result, women are more likely to be diagnosed with depression even in the absence of severe symptoms, whereas men are less likely to be diagnosed and indeed less inclined to seek help for their symptoms in the first place (Swami, 2012; World Health Organization, 2016a).

Prevalence

According to the Centers for Disease Control and Prevention (CDC), 18.8 million American adults (9.5% of the adult population) will experience a depressive disorder. The CDC's National Center for Health Statistics (NCHS) reports that from 2009 to 2012, 7.6% of Americans age 12 and over reported moderate to severe depressive symptoms in the 2 weeks prior to the survey (CDC, 2014).

Major Depressive Disorder

Of the 7.6% of Americans age 12 and over who experience major depression adults age 40 to 59 experience the highest rates (9.8%), and adults age 60 and older experience the lowest rates (5.4%). Approximately 5.7% of adolescents experience major depressive disorder, and some 7.4% of young adults (those age 18 to 39) experience the disorder (CDC, 2014).

In every age group, females experience depression at higher rates than males. The highest rate of depression, 12.3%, is in women age 40–59. The lowest rates of depression are for males age 12–17 (4.0%) and age 60 and over (3.4%). According to the CDC (2014) and National Institute of Mental Health (NIMH) (2015), groups with the highest prevalence of depression include adults age 45 to 64; women; Native Americans,

Alaskan natives, and non-Hispanic Whites; and individuals living below the federal poverty level.

According to the CDC (2014), individuals living below the poverty line are more than twice as likely to experience depression than those who live above the poverty line. This difference may be in part due to poor access to healthcare, making those who live in poverty less likely to receive healthcare and obtain routine screenings. Without identification and treatment of medical issues, acute medical conditions may become chronic, and this can impact mental health. Other conditions associated with poverty can impact mental health, including difficulty maintaining a healthy lifestyle and accessing healthy food and exercise options.

Bipolar Disorders

Approximately 0.6% of people residing in the continental United States have been diagnosed with bipolar I disorder as defined by the DSM-5. The lifetime male-to-female ratio is approximately 1.1:1 (APA, 2013).

Postpartum Depression

According to the APA (2013), between 3 and 6% of women will experience the onset of a major depressive episode during pregnancy or within the months following pregnancy.

Suicide

According to the CDC (2015), suicide was the 10th leading cause of death in all age groups in 2015. In 2013, there were 41,149 suicides, or 113 suicides each day, or 1 suicide every 13 minutes. Furthermore, the CDC reports that males complete suicide 4 times more than females and represent 77.9% of all suicides. Suicide is the third leading cause of death in children age 10–14; second leading cause in persons age 15–34; fourth among persons age 35–44; fifth among 45–54; eighth among persons age 55–64; and seventh among those age 65 and older.

Genetic Considerations and Nonmodifiable Risk Factors

Increasingly, genetics and neurobiology have been found to play a role in the development of depressive and bipolar disorders. However, all individuals operate within the context of their environments. Genetics and neurobiology inform nursing care and treatment for individuals with mood disorders, but nurses and clinicians must not overlook other determinants when providing care.

According to the APA (2013), first-degree family members of an individual with major depressive disorder have a two- to fourfold increase in risk of being diagnosed with a similar disorder. Heritability is approximately 40%. For bipolar disorder, a family history of bipolar disorder is one of the most reliable indicators of increased risk. Individuals have a tenfold increase in risk of developing bipolar disorder if a relative has been diagnosed with bipolar disorder.

Case Study » Part 1

Jason is a 22-year-old college student. He has missed several classes and did not turn in a major paper. When contacted by his professor, Jason admits to feeling so depressed that he has not been able to concentrate on his course work and has not left his apartment for several days. His professor expresses concern and suggests Jason go to the campus health center, which takes walk-ins. Jason agrees to go to the campus health center as a condition of getting an extension on the paper. Once there, he tells the nurse he has no appetite and complains of difficulty falling asleep. Jason says he feels guilty for not getting his assignments done and is not doing well in any of his classes. He states he doesn't know what is wrong with him, he just can't seem to get motivated and he doesn't know why. He looked forward to going to college and was excited to be accepted and move away from home for the first time. Jason did very well last semester and in the beginning of this semester. He was active in several clubs and was thinking of running for the student senate and joining the track team, but recently things just seemed to fall apart. Although Jason has many acquaintances through his classes and activities, he has no close friends in the area. During the intake interview, the nurse observes that Jason sits hunched forward in his chair with his eyes downcast. He becomes tearful at times and never smiles.

Clinical Reasoning Questions Level I

1. What is the most important issue the nurse should assess? Explain the rationale for your prioritization.
2. How would you describe Jason's affect?
3. What are the physical health priorities for Jason at this time? If those physical needs are met by changes in lifestyle, for example, would Jason experience a sense of well-being?

Clinical Reasoning Questions Level II

4. What additional information would the healthcare providers need to determine the most likely cause of Jason's depressed mood? What is a good approach to obtaining relevant additional information?
5. What are the considerations in contacting Jason's family regarding his situation?
6. What sociocultural factors or stressors might be contributing to Jason's distress?

Concepts Related to Mood and Affect

Mood and affect are related to so many concepts and systems that a full discussion of these relationships is beyond the scope of this text. Selected examples of related concepts include addiction; cognition; health, wellness, illness, and injury; healthcare systems; stress and coping; and trauma.

The rate of comorbidity between mood disorders and substance use disorders is high. Results of the National Epidemiologic Survey on Alcohol and Related Conditions showed that 20.5% of those surveyed who were alcohol dependent also had an independent major depressive disorder. Respondents who reported alcohol dependence were 3.7 times more likely to have major depression than respondents who were not dependent on alcohol (Pettinati & Dundan, 2011). Similarly, bipolar disorders are associated with some of the highest rates of alcohol and substance abuse (Petrakis, Rosenheck, & Desai, 2011). Furthermore, suicide is the leading cause of death among individuals with substance abuse disorders (Substance Abuse and Mental Health Services Administration [SAMHSA], 2014).

As mentioned earlier in the module, disturbances in mood and affect frequently lead to alterations in an individual's normal thought processes. Individuals who are experiencing mania often have racing thoughts, whereas individuals who are experiencing depression are more likely to report that their thinking feels slow or cloudy. Other alterations in thought processes that may occur include decreased concentration and memory and impaired problem-solving and decision-making ability. Although far less common, hallucinations, delusions, and other forms of psychosis may also be manifestations of mood disorders (Marwaha et al., 2013; Potter & Moller, 2016).

Depressive and bipolar disorders impact functioning and overall wellness on a number of levels. Both categories of illness can manifest sleep disturbances. Numerous studies show a direct link between decreased amount and/or quality of sleep and negative mood and affect (Gobin et al., 2015; Minkel et al., 2012; Pemberton & Fuller Tyszkiewicz, 2016). On the other hand, regular physical activity appears to have a protective effect against depression and negative affect (Pemberton & Fuller Tyszkiewicz, 2016; Saneei et al., 2016). Individuals with moderate to severe alterations in mood and affect may neglect their physical health and personal hygiene and experience changes in eating patterns and weight gain or loss. Poor health outcomes can affect overall functioning.

Patients with mental illness may not have insurance to pay for health services; therefore, providing a list of free community resources (such as support groups) as well as scheduling appointments with community mental health centers may be necessary to assist the patient in securing increased access to care.

Individuals with depressive or bipolar disorder often have a history of trauma. By providing trauma-informed care to these patients, nurses can help protect them from retraumatization, assist them in understanding the manifestations of their illness in the context of their life experiences, and reframe their symptoms as a method of coping (Potter & Moller, 2016).

Similar to trauma, prolonged and overwhelming stress can result in depression or trigger a manic episode. Anxiety disorders often occur along with depression, and poorly managed anxiety can use up the coping reserves needed to prevent the onset of a depressive or manic episode.

The Concepts Related to Mood and Affect feature links some, but not all, of the concepts integral to mood and affect. They are presented in alphabetical order.

Health Promotion

There is no definitive way to prevent depression due to causative and contributing genetic and biological factors that cannot be modified. Some strategies can be useful, however, for modifying stressors and environmental factors that can contribute to depressive illnesses. For instance, research demonstrates that certain lifestyle choices can help protect individuals against the onset of mood disorders. Patients should be encouraged to reduce their intake of sugar, saturated fat, and refined foods and increase their consumption of fruits, vegetables, legumes, fish, and whole grains. Research also suggests that increased intake of certain nutrients—including omega-3 fatty acids, folic acid, vitamin D, selenium, and calcium—may play a protective role (Roca et al., 2016; Sanchez-Villegas & Martinez-Gonzales, 2013; Saneei et al., 2016; Whitaker et al., 2014; White, Horwath, & Conner, 2013). Similarly,

multiple studies emphasize the importance of adequate sleep and regular exercise in preventing mood alterations (Gobin et al., 2015; Minkel et al., 2012; Pemberton & Fuller Tyszkiewicz, 2016; Saneei et al., 2016). Additional research indicates that smoking cessation may decrease the risk of various mental disorders, including depression (Jacka, Mykleton, & Berk, 2012).

Additional primary prevention strategies focus on psychosocial factors rather than biological factors: Education about stress management, coping strategies, or positive parenting is a primary strategy that may be helpful to many individuals. Other strategies may need to be more community- or situation-specific: For example, veterans and people who live in communities where large-scale tragedy has occurred may benefit from measures that help them better cope with past traumatic events; and parents and children who are going through divorce or another stressful situation may benefit from facilitated discussion and use of coping strategies (Potter & Moller, 2016). Research also indicates that children of depressed parents are less likely to develop depression themselves after participating in family-based cognitive–behavioral interventions (Compas et al., 2015; de Angel et al., 2016).

Secondary and tertiary prevention strategies are similar to primary strategies that focus on psychosocial factors. Notable secondary approaches include regular screening (described in greater detail below); referring individuals with suspected mood disorders for accurate diagnosis and treatment; and counseling patients about their relative risks for developing mood disorders. Useful tertiary prevention measures include establishing collaborative care programs for patients with mood disorders; employing clinic- and home-based approaches to reducing depression among older adults and individuals with chronic health problems; and developing community-based programs that provide mental health services to homeless and impoverished individuals (Potter & Moller, 2016).

Screenings

The U.S. Preventive Services Task Force (USPSTF) recommends that all adults, including pregnant and postpartum women, be screened for depression by their primary care providers. Although the organization does not specify precisely when or how often screening should occur, it encourages nurses and clinicians to use a pragmatic approach that "might include screening all adults who have not been screened previously and using clinical judgment in consideration of risk factors, comorbid conditions, and life events to determine whether additional screening of high risk patients is warranted" (Siu & USPSTF, 2016a). A similar screening approach is recommended for adolescents between the ages of 12 and 18, but not for children age 11 and under (Siu & USPSTF, 2016b). According to the USPSTF (2016a, 2016b), research indicates that screening patients age 12 and up presents little to no risk of harm. Moreover, there is adequate evidence that early detection of depression followed by use of appropriate pharmacologic and/or psychotherapy decreases clinical morbidity and improves clinical outcomes.

Concepts Related to
Mood and Affect

CONCEPT	RELATIONSHIP TO MOOD AND AFFECT	NURSING IMPLICATIONS
Addiction	Addiction → depression Mood disorders → addiction Mood disorders + addiction = ↑ severity of both Mood disorders + addiction = ↑ suicidal behavior	▪ Assess for suicidal ideation. ▪ Assess for substance use. ▪ Provide concurrent treatment for mood disorders and substance abuse. ▪ Refer to community resources. ▪ Assess and educate family regarding codependency issues. ▪ Anticipate patient denial of substance use.
Cognition	Mood disorders → ↓ concentration, memory, problem solving, and decision making; ↑ risk of psychosis Depression → ↓ clarity and speed of thought processes Mania → ↑ flight of ideas and racing thoughts	▪ Conduct mental status examination. ▪ Provide patients who demonstrate slowed thinking adequate time to respond. ▪ Because patients may have trouble concentrating, simplify the communication process by offering limited choices. ▪ Do not challenge the patient's belief systems or values. ▪ Provide a safe environment and seek immediate medical intervention for patients with signs of psychosis.
Health, Wellness, Illness, and Injury	Depression = ↓ sleep/nutrition/ wellness → physical illness and functional status → ↑ depression	▪ Promote self-care, adequate rest and sleep, and exercise as appropriate. ▪ Assess for signs of physical illness and for somatic symptoms of depression (e.g., pain in the absence of injury). ▪ Promote routine health maintenance, screening, healthy lifestyle, and preventive care.
Healthcare Systems	↓ Access to healthcare → ↑ risk for depression and ↑ risk of suicide Depressive and/or manic symptoms ↑ individual use of healthcare systems Healthcare systems often ill-equipped to respond to comorbid psychiatric illness	▪ Conduct routine screenings for depression and suicidal ideation as recommended. ▪ Collaborate with interprofessional team to address psychologic needs of patients. ▪ Refer patient to a mental health professional for follow-up. ▪ Provide list of community services, including contact information. ▪ Make first appointment for the patient.
Stress and Coping	↑ Stress → depression or triggers mania Ineffective coping → depression and/or anxiety	▪ Assist patient in developing effective coping mechanisms. ▪ Assess for symptoms of anxiety. ▪ Assist patient in identifying triggers for anxiety symptoms. ▪ Teach stress reduction techniques.
Trauma	Experiencing violence → depression Exposure to trauma → depression and/or posttraumatic stress disorder	▪ Assess for suicide risk. ▪ Assess for history of violence. ▪ Assess for exposure to traumatic event. ▪ Provide safe environment. ▪ Educate regarding community resources.

A number of different instruments may be used when screening for depression and other mood disorders (**Table 28–1 »**). For example, the Patient Health Questionnaire (PHQ-9) is one of the most common instruments and can be used in a variety of settings to screen individuals to determine whether referral is necessary. The questionnaire is freely available in more than 30 languages (American Psychological Association, 2016a). Other screening tools that may be used in adult populations include the Hospital Anxiety and Depression Scales (for all adults), the Geriatric Depression Scale (for older adults), and the Edinburgh Postnatal Depression scale (for pregnant and postpartum patients) (Siu & USPSTF, 2016a). Providers may also choose from a number of screening instruments for children and adolescents, including the Patient Health Questionnaire for Adolescents (PHQ-A), the Mood and Feelings Questionnaire (MFQ), and the Children's

TABLE 28–1 Common Instruments Used to Screen for Depression and/or Bipolar Disorder

Screening Tools	Description
Children	
Children's Depression Inventory (CDI-2)	Short and long forms are available. The child or adolescent completes the self-report scale; parents and teachers complete separate forms.
Patient Health Questionnaire for Adolescents (PHQ-A)	41-question self-report scale assesses indicators of anxiety and depression.
Mood and Feelings Questionnaire (MFQ)	Short and long forms available; requires both child and parent(s) to complete a series of questions.
Center for Epidemiological Studies–Depression Scale for Children (CES-DC)	20-item self-report scale that screens for depression.
Mood Disorder Questionnaire (MDQ)	Brief self-report form used to screen adolescents for bipolar disorder.
Adults	
Patient Health Questionnaire (PHQ-9)	Commonly used, 10-question self-report scale used to screen adults for depression; may be used to monitor depression levels throughout treatment.
Beck Depression Inventory (BDI)	21-question self-report scale to screen adults for depression.
Center for Epidemiological Studies Depression Scale–Revised (CESD-R)	20-item self-report scale to screen adults for depression.
Older Adults	
Geriatric Depression Scale (GDS)	Individuals may complete the scale themselves or have a healthcare provider read it to them and score their answers. Long and short forms available.
Cornell Scale for Depression in Dementia (CSDD)	Clinicians use the CSDD to screen individuals with dementia for depression; clinicians use the scale with the caregiver and briefly interview the patient.
Postpartum Depression	
Edinburgh Postnatal Depression Scale (EPDS)	Self-report form that may be used in any setting to screen postpartum mother for depression.
Beck's Postpartum Depression Screening Scale (PDSS)	35-item response scale for use during routine care with all postpartum women to identify those who might be experiencing postpartum depression.

Depression Inventory (CDI-2) (Corona, McCarty, & Richardson, 2013). Regardless of which instrument is used, patients who score in the range indicative of depression or another mood disorder should be referred to a mental health professional for a thorough diagnostic evaluation.

>> **Stay Current:** Visit www.brightfutures.org/mentalhealth/pdf/professionals/bridges/ces_dc.pdf to see the CES-DC and http://cesd-r.com to see or take the CESD-R.

Care in the Community

Most people with mental illness are treated in the community. Deinstitutionalization has required more services to be available to the public at a lower level of care. Community services may include outpatient, intensive outpatient (part-day programs approximately 4 hours in duration), and partial-hospitalization (typically services are provided at the hospital daily or near daily for a full day and the patient goes home in the evenings). There are also a multitude of support groups and hotlines available for the public. Group homes (residences for individuals who are functional but chronically mentally ill) and half-way houses (usually a step-down from rehabilitation) are also part of community services.

Nursing Assessment

The first and most important aspect in conducting an assessment is to establish a therapeutic relationship based on mutual trust. The nurse should ask open-ended questions and allow adequate time for patient response. It is important that the nurse remain nonjudgmental and validate the patient's feelings. It may be necessary to reduce the patient's anxiety. The nurse should communicate with brief, clear statements, verify the patient's understanding, and clarify areas that may not be understood. Refer to the exemplar on Therapeutic Communication in the module on Communication for additional information.

The nurse conducting an assessment of the patient who reports feelings of sadness and irritability or exhibits symptoms of mania must remember that these disorders affect individuals in a variety of ways. More detail is provided below and in the exemplars that follow.

Observation and Patient Interview

Patients experiencing alterations in mood and affect may exhibit a variety of behavioral changes that will suggest the need for further assessment. For example, patients experiencing severe depressive or manic symptoms may exhibit poor hygiene. Other behavioral cues include incongruent verbal and nonverbal communication, irritability, exhaustion, lack of motivation, excitability, grandiosity, altered thought processes, pressured speech, and psychosis. Assess energy level, psychomotor symptoms such as agitation or retardation, and dietary and fluid intake.

During the patient interview, assess for previous diagnosis of mental illness, family history of mental illness, sleep quality, eating patterns, cognition, presence of chronic illness, and substance use.

Assess mood and affect, cognition and thought content, communication patterns, and pain and pain history. Obtain information about any mood fluctuations that may have occurred in the past. Assess the patient's perception of wellness and functioning. Is the patient's perception of health and mental health status congruent with the report of family members or caregivers? What is the patient's priority for care?

Assess coping patterns, home environment, and financial status as well as cultural beliefs and practices. These factors have important implications for treatment planning and patient adherence to treatment regimens.

Self-reporting scales are among the most common instruments used to screen for depression (see Table 28–1). These scales may be used as part of the assessment process but should not be used alone or out of context. Manifestations of altered mood may have their origins in other areas (such as physical illness or adverse effects of medications), and nurses must screen for the presence of these as well.

Cultural Considerations

Appropriate expressions of mood are largely culturally determined. For example, situations in which people are expected to experience sadness, anger, loneliness, frustration, joy, or happiness are defined by the culture. Culture also determines how people are to behave when experiencing a variety of feelings.

To effectively assess and care for patients with diverse backgrounds, it is important to learn and understand their societal norms related to thoughts, emotions, and behaviors. Furthermore, nurses must understand the impact of culture on both the expression of depression as well as the risks for depression. (See the Focus on Diversity and Culture feature.) Nurses should also remember that help-seeking behaviors can be culturally determined. For example, African Americans and Latinos often look to their family and faith communities for help before considering seeing a professional. There is a strong fear of hospitalization and involuntary commitment, both of which are more likely for African Americans and Latinos than for Caucasians. Both African Americans and Native Americans have reported greater distrust of the medical community and greater communication challenges (Spector, 2017). Members of communities of color continue to face greater financial hardship related to medical care. A report by the U.S. Census Bureau (2015) indicates that, in 2014, 11.8% of African Americans had no medical insurance at all, in contrast to 7.6% of the Caucasian population.

Although nurses need to take cultural factors into account during assessment (e.g., ensuring careful assessment that includes access to financial resources and attitudes toward the healthcare community), nurses must be careful not to stereotype patients during the assessment process. When nurses engage in stereotyping, they risk failing to assess for important indicators and are likely to increase barriers to trust and understanding when they should be building the therapeutic alliance and gaining patient trust.

Physical Examination

When conducting a physical examination of patients with diagnosed or suspected mood disorders, obtain a complete set of vital signs, including pain. Obtain a baseline weight and body mass index (BMI) to allow for the possibility of weight

Focus on Diversity and Culture
Depression in Recent Immigrants

Recent immigrants are at higher risk for depression as they cope with multiple stressors such as long-distance family relationships, unemployment or underemployment, discrimination, language problems, and a new environment. Immigrant children are at risk for depression as they are often expected to interpret the concerns of adult family members to outside authority figures such as physicians, nurses, teachers, and government officials (Guo et al., 2015; Smith, 2011).

monitoring if the treatment plan includes an antidepressant or mood stabilizer. Also be sure to assess sleep, nutrition, activity, and elimination patterns.

A thorough physical examination is necessary to rule out any medical or drug-related causes of presenting signs and symptoms and to identify any comorbid medical illnesses that require treatment. Some chronic medical conditions, especially those that cause pain and/or fatigue, increase the risk of depressive symptoms. Further, patients with depressive and bipolar disorders may be at greater risk of experiencing comorbid medical illness because their mental illness may impair functioning in the areas of self-care and nutrition.

Diagnostic Tests

Although no diagnostic laboratory or medical tests exist for mood disorders, a thorough workup is necessary to rule out any underlying medical conditions that could mimic or cause symptoms of mood disorders, as well as to detect comorbid medical illness that could contribute to symptoms and functional abnormalities. Diagnostic and laboratory tests may include hormone levels and thyroid function tests to rule out endocrine disorders, which can mimic depression or hypomania; electrolyte panels, urinalysis, and toxicology to rule out substance abuse; and liver function tests, because antidepressants are metabolized in the liver. Other tests may be ordered on the basis of the patient's individual symptoms and history (e.g., tests for specific nutritional deficiencies, presence of infection, or medication toxicity). A pregnancy test may be done in women of reproductive age because antidepressants may affect fetal development (Halverson et al., 2016; Tesar, 2010).

Case Study » Part 2

Following a clinical interview and administration of the Beck Depression Inventory, the healthcare provider at the campus health center diagnosed Jason with major depressive disorder and prescribed extended-release venlafaxine (Effexor XR). One month later, Jason comes to the health center for his follow-up appointment. The nurse notes that his behavior is nearly the opposite of what she observed at the initial visit. He describes his current mood as "fabulous." He states he is only sleeping about 2 hours a night but that "it's OK"—he feels great and is getting so much done in the extra hours of wakefulness. Jason also reports a heightened sexual desire and urges and attributes this to his decreased need for sleep. Jason tells the nurse that he completed his required paper and that it is so good, he is turning it into a book about the secret to the meaning of life, although he has not yet received a grade. He is running for student senate, tried out for the track team, and volunteered at the campus tutoring center. The increased participation in activities has resulted in making new friends with whom he goes drinking 2–3 nights a week. Jason is considering taking five accelerated courses during the summer.

During the interview, Jason's speech is loud, rapid, and pressured. He is restless, unable to sit still for more than 5 minutes. He offers to give the nurse his autograph because he is convinced his intended book will win a Pulitzer Prize. Jason denies side effects of the medication, and considers it a miracle drug because he feels better than he ever has in his entire life. When questioned about thoughts of suicide, he denies them stating, "A person as special as I am needs to be cloned, not killed!"

Clinical Reasoning Questions Level I

1. What else should the nurse assess?
2. How would you describe Jason's affect during this visit?
3. What are the priority health and safety considerations for Jason?

Clinical Reasoning Questions Level II

4. What could be responsible for Jason's remarkable change in mood, affect, and behavior?
5. What are the priority topics to address in Jason's healthcare teaching plan during this visit?
6. How would you rate Jason's risk for suicide? Given your assessment, what would be an effective care plan suggestion?

Independent Interventions

Nurses are in the singular position to provide a number of caring interventions for patients with depressive or bipolar disorders and their families. The most important of these are preventing patient suicide and promoting patient and family safety.

Although treatment of patients with depressive and bipolar disorders is best accomplished by an interprofessional team that includes nurses, mental health professionals, and primary providers, of those individuals who seek and receive treatment, many see only one provider. Nurses working in any setting should consider the following points of treatment management outlined in the APA (2015a) Practice Guidelines for the Treatment of Patients with Major Depressive Disorder. These points are valid for any patient with any alteration of mood and affect:

- Establish safety
- Promote treatment adherence
- Coordinate care
- Monitor responses to treatment
- Provide education to patients and families.

Prevent Suicide and Promote Safety

Patients experiencing alterations in mood are at increased risk for suicide. When the risk for self-directed violence is high, immediate intervention is necessary. The risk of suicide increases as patients in the severest stage of depression begin to improve; it is then that patients have sufficient energy and cognitive ability to plan and successfully implement a suicide plan. When a patient expresses suicidal ideation, confidentiality does *not* apply. It is the nurse's duty to report suicidal thoughts or actions to the treatment team, or take necessary steps to have the patient transported via ambulance or police to a community crisis screening center, hospital emergency department, or other appropriate facility according to state guidelines. See **Box 28–1** ⟫ for guidelines to help prevent inpatient suicide and promote safety.

Nurses should assist in the transition from hospital to home by helping patients identify situations or events that trigger feelings of altered moods and to learn to use coping methods they find helpful. Nurses also assist in the transition by helping patients develop a safety plan that includes these strategies as well as information on how to contact family members or their mental health professional if they are unable to return to stable mood without help from someone else.

Monitor Patient Response to Treatment

Nurses must closely monitor how patients with depressive or bipolar disorders respond to treatment. Close monitoring can help reveal whether patients are actually adhering to

Box 28–1
Preventing Inpatient Suicide and Promoting Safety

Check the policy and procedures of the individual inpatient treatment facility and implement those guidelines. For patients who express intent to kill themselves (with or without a plan) or who have made a suicide attempt within the past week, institute safety precautions and request a psychiatric consult as well (Columbia University Medical Center, n.d.).

- Evaluate the patient's level of suicide intent regularly and institute the appropriate level of staff supervision following unit protocol. Patients may deny suicidal ideation or underestimate their own risk (Knoll, 2012).
- Let suicidal patients know that the environment is safe for them. Remove sharp objects, razors, breakable glass items, mirrors, matches, and straps or belts and explain why these objects are being removed. Monitor the use of scissors, razors, and other potential weapons.
- Do not leave patients at risk for suicide alone. In acute care hospitals or residential settings, one-to-one observation must be instituted until a psychiatrist or qualified physician determines the patient is no longer at risk. Family members cannot substitute for staff in performing one-to-one observation. Some facilities use 15-minute checks, but these are not recommended for use with patients who are seriously suicidal or whose risk level is uncertain (Knoll, 2012).
- Be particularly alert during change of shifts and on holidays or other times when staffing is limited and during times of distraction, such as mealtimes and visiting hours.
- Examine items brought by visitors and monitor for safety. Many units have policies regarding what can and cannot be brought into the unit. Most prohibit food of any kind from outside of the facility.
- Facilitate the development of the therapeutic alliance and maintain a nonjudgmental attitude. Staff members' attitudes toward patients with mental illness can lead to breakdown of the therapeutic alliance and may indirectly increase patients' risk for attempting suicide (Knoll, 2012).
- Use a calm, reassuring approach and encourage patients to discuss all of their feelings. Patients need to know that all feelings are valid and that it benefits them to express their emotions appropriately.

their treatment regimen. If they are not, the nurse should investigate the reasons for nonadherence. When barriers to treatment are identified (e.g., financial constraints, trouble obtaining and/or taking medication, uncomfortable side effects), the nurse can work with the patient to develop strategies to overcome these barriers or possibly to seek another means of treatment. If the patient is adhering to the treatment plan but her condition is not improving, the nurse, patient, and other members of the healthcare team can collaborate to identify potential adjustments to the therapeutic regimen.

Monitoring the treatment response is also important for patients whose symptoms appear to be improving. In these cases, the nurse should consider whether the patient's recovery is occurring at an appropriate pace, whether any supplementary treatment approaches may be helpful, and/or whether any therapeutic measures are no longer necessary.

Support Family Functioning

The family members of an individual diagnosed with mental illness play an important role in treatment. The family member(s) also take responsibility for the patient's care, which can cause frustration and exhaustion, especially with repeated episodes. This care can lead to role strain as the family member(s) often have to care for children, work, and compensate for the mentally ill person's inability to perform usual tasks. It is important to involve the family member(s) as early in treatment as possible. They will be able to assist with maintaining the treatment plan while the nurse lends support when needed. Family, along with the affected individual, will need to have coping skills reinforced and will require education regarding the nature of the patient's illness and the treatment plan.

Teach Assertive Behavior

Nurses working with patients can model, encourage, and teach assertive behavior. Assertiveness is a learned behavior. Everyone has the potential to be assertive, but not everyone instinctively knows how. Children learn patterns of communicating from the adults around them. Individuals can unlearn poor communication patterns that do not work and learn new ones, which is the idea behind assertiveness training. The goal is to help individuals express themselves without fear of disapproval from others. Being assertive does not guarantee that others will agree, but it does provide an individual the satisfaction of offering a personal opinion without ignoring the opinions of others.

Aggressive behavior is directed toward getting what one wants without considering the feelings of others. Aggressive communicators want to get their own way at any cost and may use intimidation to do so. An example of aggressive behavior is insisting on going to a certain movie even though you know your companion does not enjoy that type of movie. The outcome of aggressive behavior is that although you may get what you want in the short run, others feel discredited and tend to avoid you.

Passive behavior consists of avoiding conflict at any cost, even at the expense of one's own happiness. An example of passive behavior is agreeing to go to a movie you do not want to see because your friend pressures you to go. Passive communicators hold their feelings in and allow anger to build up. Anger can explode suddenly or can be expressed

in passive–aggressive behavior. An example of passive–aggressive behavior is taking a long time to get ready to go out while your friend is waiting because you are angry at him for insisting on seeing a movie you do not want to see. The outcome is that the passive person gives up control and is left with resentment, which usually emerges in other ways that damage relationships.

Assertive behavior consists of expressing one's wishes and opinions, or taking care of oneself, but not at the expense of others. An example of assertive communication is saying, "I really don't care for violent movies. Let's look at the movie listings and see if there is something playing that we can both enjoy." The outcome of assertive behavior is self-confidence and self-esteem.

Maintain Professional Boundaries

Patients who are hopeless have a tendency to form dependent relationships. Nurses must work from the first contact with these patients to minimize the likelihood that maladaptive dependence occurs in the nurse–patient relationship. Strategies to minimize maladaptive dependence include the following:

- Emphasize the short-term nature of the relationship.
- Recognize that a patient who singles out one staff member exclusively and refuses to relate to others is developing dependence.
- Avoid giving patients the hope that the nurse–patient relationship can continue after therapy has ended.
- Refuse (kindly but firmly) requests for your address or telephone number.
- Remind patients that social contact will not be allowed.

If you find yourself wanting to continue relationships with certain patients, discuss these feelings with your instructor (if you are a student), your supervisor, or a respected professional peer (if you are a practicing nurse). It is essential that you separate your professional life from your social life.

Collaborative Therapies

Collaborative therapies for patients with mood disorders include pharmacotherapy, CBT and other psychotherapies, and complementary health approaches. Often, combining therapies leads to greater success. Nurses help patients determine what combination of therapies may be most helpful for them, encourage adherence to the treatment plan, and suggest alternatives if a sufficient trial of a treatment or therapy (typically at least 6 weeks) proves ineffective.

Pharmacologic Therapy for Depressive Disorders

Drugs used to treat depression by enhancing mood are categorized as antidepressants. Antidepressants are also sometimes prescribed to treat anxiety disorders. It is thought that antidepressants exert their effect through their action on certain neurotransmitters in the brain, including norepinephrine, dopamine, and serotonin. The two basic mechanisms of action are blocking the enzymatic breakdown of norepinephrine and slowing the reuptake of serotonin (see **Figure 28–3 》**). Nurses working with patients taking antidepressants must be

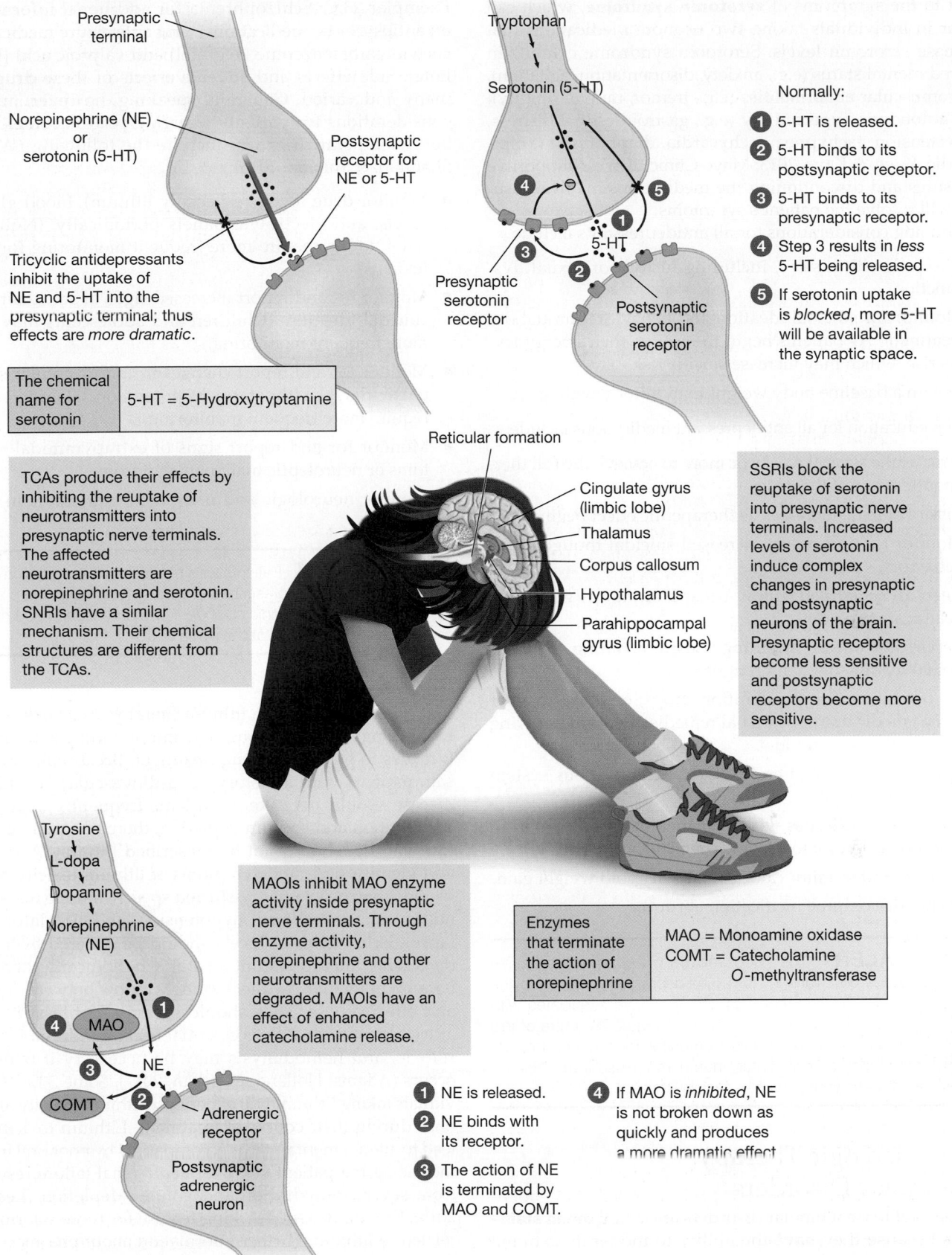

Presynaptic terminal

Norepinephrine (NE) or serotonin (5-HT)

Postsynaptic receptor for NE or 5-HT

Tricyclic antidepressants inhibit the uptake of NE and 5-HT into the presynaptic terminal; thus effects are *more dramatic*.

The chemical name for serotonin	5-HT = 5-Hydroxytryptamine

Tryptophan

Serotonin (5-HT)

Presynaptic serotonin receptor

Postsynaptic serotonin receptor

Normally:

1 5-HT is released.

2 5-HT binds to its postsynaptic receptor.

3 5-HT binds to its presynaptic receptor.

4 Step 3 results in *less* 5-HT being released.

5 If serotonin uptake is *blocked*, more 5-HT will be available in the synaptic space.

TCAs produce their effects by inhibiting the reuptake of neurotransmitters into presynaptic nerve terminals. The affected neurotransmitters are norepinephrine and serotonin. SNRIs have a similar mechanism. Their chemical structures are different from the TCAs.

Reticular formation

Cingulate gyrus (limbic lobe)

Thalamus

Corpus callosum

Hypothalamus

Parahippocampal gyrus (limbic lobe)

SSRIs block the reuptake of serotonin into presynaptic nerve terminals. Increased levels of serotonin induce complex changes in presynaptic and postsynaptic neurons of the brain. Presynaptic receptors become less sensitive and postsynaptic receptors become more sensitive.

Tyrosine

L-dopa

Dopamine

Norepinephrine (NE)

MAO

COMT

Adrenergic receptor

Postsynaptic adrenergic neuron

MAOIs inhibit MAO enzyme activity inside presynaptic nerve terminals. Through enzyme activity, norepinephrine and other neurotransmitters are degraded. MAOIs have an effect of enhanced catecholamine release.

Enzymes that terminate the action of norepinephrine	MAO = Monoamine oxidase COMT = Catecholamine O-methyltransferase

1 NE is released.

2 NE binds with its receptor.

3 The action of NE is terminated by MAO and COMT.

4 If MAO is *inhibited*, NE is not broken down as quickly and produces a more dramatic effect.

Figure 28–3 》 The mechanism of action of TCA, SSRI, and MAOI antidepression drugs.

alert to the symptoms of **serotonin syndrome**, which can occur in individuals taking two or more medications that increase serotonin levels. Serotonin syndrome exhibits in altered mental status (e.g., anxiety, disorientation, agitation); neuromuscular abnormalities (e.g., tremor, muscle rigidity); and autonomic hyperactivity (e.g., gastrointestinal distress, hypertension, tachypnea, tachycardia, diaphoresis) (Volpi-Abadie, Kaye, & Kaye, 2013; Mayo Clinic, 2017b). Supportive measures and discontinuing the medications involved usually will resolve the patient's symptoms.

Nursing considerations for all antidepressants include:

- Assess health history, including history of sexual dysfunction.
- Monitor for suicidal ideation and behaviors throughout treatment. As patients begin to recover, their energy levels rise, which may increase suicide risk.
- Obtain a baseline body weight to monitor weight gain.

Patient education for all antidepressant medications include:

- It may take several weeks or more to achieve the full therapeutic effect of the drug.
- Risk of suicide increases as therapeutic effect begins.
- Monitor for and report increased suicidal thoughts and behaviors.
- Keep all scheduled follow-up appointments with your healthcare provider.
- Report side effects, including nausea, vomiting, diarrhea, sexual dysfunction, and fatigue.
- Do not take other prescription drugs, over-the-counter (OTC) medications, or herbal remedies without notifying your healthcare provider.
- Avoid using alcohol and other central nervous system (CNS) depressants.
- Immediately discuss with your healthcare provider an intention or desire to become pregnant.
- Exercise and monitor caloric intake to avoid weight gain.
- Do not discontinue medication abruptly.

SAFETY ALERT The Food and Drug Administration (FDA) requires a "black box warning" for all antidepressants related to the increased risk for suicidal thoughts and behaviors associated with taking antidepressant medications. The nurse must be aware of this and educate patients and families to monitor for this and provide 24-hour emergency center contact numbers for use if this occurs. Patients age 24 and younger are especially at risk.

Pharmacologic Therapy for Bipolar Disorders

Drugs used to treat bipolar disorders are called **mood stabilizers** because they have the ability to moderate extreme shifts in emotions between mania and depression. Some anticonvulsive drugs are used for mood stabilization in patients with bipolar disorders. Medications commonly prescribed for the treatment of bipolar disorders include lithium carbonate (Eskalith); atypical antipsychotics, such as aripiprazole (Abilify) and olanzapine (Zyprexa) (see

Exemplar 23.C: Schizophrenia for additional information on antipsychotic medications); and antiseizure medications such as carbamazepine (Tegretol) and valproic acid (Depakote). Side effects and adverse effects of these drugs are many and varied. Generally speaking, however, nursing considerations for patients receiving pharmacologic therapy for bipolar disorders include the following (Wilson, Shannon, & Shields, 2016):

- Monitor drug levels (especially lithium), blood glucose levels, and electrolyte panels periodically. (Note that older adults require more frequent monitoring for drug toxicity.)
- Monitor for and report increased signs of suicidality and suicidal ideation. (Children and adolescents may need more frequent monitoring.)
- Monitor for and report changes in cardiovascular status, particularly orthostatic hypotension. (Older adults require more frequent monitoring.)
- Monitor for and report signs of extrapyramidal symptoms or neuroleptic malignant syndrome.
- Monitor neurologic and neuromuscular status in older adults.

SAFETY ALERT Patients with bipolar disorders who are in the depressive phase and prescribed only an antidepressant are at high risk for switching to a manic episode. For that reason, mood stabilizers are always prescribed at the same time.

Lithium Therapy

The role of the nurse in lithium therapy involves carefully monitoring a patient's condition and providing education as it relates to prescribed drug treatment. Because lithium is a salt, patients with a history of cardiovascular and kidney disease should not take it. Patients frequently experience dehydration and sodium depletion; therefore, patients on a low-salt diet should not be prescribed lithium. Assess for and identify signs and symptoms of lithium toxicity, which include diarrhea, lethargy, slurred speech, muscle weakness, ataxia, seizures, edema, hypotension, and circulatory collapse. Serum lithium levels should be ordered every 1–3 days when therapy is initiated and periodically thereafter because of the narrow therapeutic window between toxicity and effectiveness. They should be drawn at least 8 hours after the last dose. This is essential because lithium is nephrotoxic, and hemodialysis may be necessary if overdose occurs (Adams, Holland, & Urban, 2017). Some 30% of individuals taking lithium will experience lithium toxicity at least once during their course of treatment. Lithium toxicity can lead to altered mental status accompanied by poor oral intake, increasing the patient's risk for acute renal failure resulting from severe dehydration and volume depletion (Lederer, 2015). See the Patient Teaching feature for more information related to lithium. Further information about pharmacologic therapies for bipolar disorders is provided in Exemplar 28.B.

Nonpharmacologic Therapy

A nonpharmacologic approach to treatment for depression is commonly used in conjunction with pharmacologic therapy. Examples of nonpharmacologic therapies include

Medications

Antidepressants

CLASSIFICATION AND DRUG EXAMPLES	MECHANISM OF ACTION	NURSING CONSIDERATIONS
Selective Serotonin Reuptake Inhibitors (SSRIs) *Drug examples:* Citalopram, escitalopram, fluoxetine, paroxetine, sertraline, vilazodone	Slows the reuptake of serotonin into presynaptic nerve terminals. Increases the availability of serotonin in the synaptic cleft for post-synaptic receptors. ***May also be used for:*** ■ Anxiety disorders ■ Eating disorders	Take most SSRIs in the morning with food to avoid gastrointestinal upset and insomnia. If the patient complains of feeling sedated or tired, the SSRI may be taken in the evening. St. John's wort and *Ginkgo biloba* may cause serotonin syndrome when taken with SSRIs. Provide patient teaching related to suicidal ideation and serotonin syndrome.
Atypical Antidepressants (including SNRIs) *Drug examples:* Bupropion Duloxetine, venlafaxine, and mirtazapine are serotonin–norepinephrine reuptake inhibitors (SNRIs).	Bupropion works by inhibiting the uptake of dopamine, serotonin, and norepinephrine and elevating mood by increasing the levels of these neurotransmitters in the CNS. SNRIs inhibit the reabsorption of serotonin and norepinephrine and elevate mood by increasing the levels of serotonin, norepinephrine, and dopamine in the CNS. ***May also be used for:*** ■ Smoking cessation (bupropion "Zyban") ■ Anxiety disorders (duloxetine, venlafaxine) ■ Fibromyalgia, chronic musculoskeletal pain (duloxetine) ■ Neuropathic pain (duloxetine and off-label for bupropion and venlafaxine) ■ Attention-deficit disorder (venlafaxine, and off-label bupropion)	Take mirtazapine at bedtime because it usually causes excessive drowsiness, especially at lower doses. Should be used with caution in patients with seizure disorders because it lowers the seizure threshold. Monitor patients closely if a seizure disorder is present. Monitor for serotonin syndrome and neuroleptic malignant syndrome-like reactions. Increased risk of hepatotoxicity. Instruct patient on changing positions slowly secondary to potential for orthostatic hypotension. Should not be used as a single therapy for patients diagnosed with bipolar disorder, as it may worsen psychotic features or precipitate manic or hypomanic symptoms.
Tricyclic Antidepressants (TCAs) *Drug examples:* Amitriptyline, clomipramine, doxepin, imipramine, nortriptyline	Inhibits reuptake of both norepinephrine and serotonin into presynaptic nerve terminals ***May also be used for:*** ■ Anxiety ■ Neuropathy	TCAs may cause decreased sweating, along with anticholinergic side effects such as dry mouth, constipation, blurred vision, and increased heart rate. For patients over the age of 40, an electrocardiogram may be ordered prior to initiation of treatment to detect preexisting arrhythmias. TCAs are contraindicated in patients in the acute recovery phase of a myocardial infarction (MI), with heart block, or with a history of dysrhythmias because of the effects of TCAs on cardiac tissue. TCAs lower the seizure threshold, so patients with epilepsy should be closely monitored. Patients with urinary retention, narrow-angle glaucoma, or prostatic hypertrophy may not be good candidates for TCAs because of anticholinergic side effects.
Monoamine Oxidase Inhibitors (MAOIs) *Drug examples:* Selegiline, isocarboxazid, phenelzine, tranylcypromine	Inhibit monoamine oxidase, the enzyme that terminates the actions of neurotransmitters such as dopamine, norepinephrine, epinephrine, and serotonin.	Interacts with a large number of foods and other medications—sometimes with serious effects. Hypertensive crisis can occur when an MAOI is used concurrently with other antidepressants or sympathomimetic drugs. MAOIs also potentiate the hypoglycemic effects of insulin and oral antidiabetic drugs. A hypertensive crisis also can result from an interaction between MAOIs and foods containing tyramine, a form of the amino acid tyrosine. There must be at least a 14-day interval between the use of MAOIs and other drugs and food restrictions. Advise patient to wear a medic alert bracelet.

Source: Data from Adams, M. P., Holland, L. N., & Urban, C. (2017). *Pharmacology for nurses: A pathophysiologic approach.* (5th ed.). Hoboken, NJ: Pearson Education.

Patient Teaching

Lithium

The nurse should provide patients who take lithium with information related to their medication, including:

- Take medication as ordered because adherence is the key to successful treatment.
- Keep all scheduled laboratory visits to monitor lithium levels.
- Do not change diet or decrease fluid intake, because any changes in diet and fluid status can affect therapeutic drug levels.
- Avoid alcohol use.
- Do not take other prescription medications, OTC drugs, or herbal products without notifying your healthcare provider.
- Do not discontinue use except under the guidance of the healthcare provider.

---

psychotherapy, light therapy, support groups, and meditation. ECT may be used for treatment-resistant depression. Both medication and psychotherapy alone are effective in treating depression; however, the combination of both medication and psychotherapy is most effective. Therefore, psychotherapy is almost always recommended.

One of the most successful forms of psychotherapy is CBT. However, a number of different forms of psychotherapy can be considered. The best approach to psychotherapy is chosen based on the cause and symptoms of the depressive condition as well as the patient's needs and personality.

Cognitive–Behavioral Therapy

CBT focuses on skill training and problem solving to help patients reorient patterns of negative thinking and negative behaviors. The clinician or therapist works with patients to identify the most troubling problems in their lives and erroneous thought patterns or behaviors that may reinforce or exacerbate them. Therapists help patients problem solve by asking questions that help patients reflect and reconsider troubling situations. Examples of questions include: *What happens? What do you think when this happens? What do you do? Why do you think this happens to you? What would need to happen for you to feel differently? What might you do to change the situation?*

Cognitive–behavioral therapists use various techniques. One is *cognitive modification* of negative thought patterns. Every individual has automatic thought patterns, some of which are helpful and some of which are negative. An example is that of a teenage daughter who is 1 hour late for her curfew and has not called. The mother's automatic thought might be one of the following:

- "She must have been in an accident and can't call."
- "She cares so little for me that she can't call even though she knows how much I worry."
- "She is usually very responsible, so I am sure she will be home soon and will be able to tell me what happened."

Cognitive–behavioral therapists help patients identify these patterns of irrational thinking and find ways to replace them with more logical and fact-based patterns of thinking. For example, a mother experiencing depression may constantly choose to believe the worst in a number of given scenarios involving her children. In CBT, the therapist may help the mother view her children as they really are and begin to reorient her expectations. For example, the mother of a teen may change her thinking from "Something must have happened to Sarah!" to recognizing more likely scenarios: "Sarah is late for curfew, but she was at the football game with some friends. They probably went to get something to eat afterward and she's forgotten to call."

A technique promoted in CBT that may specifically help patients with depression is mindfulness training. Most people usually go through daily routines with little awareness or attention. *Mindfulness* is the art of conscious living by focusing one's full attention on the activity at hand. While it may be simple to practice mindfulness, it is not necessarily easy. Habitual unawareness is persistent, and mindfulness requires effort and discipline. Cognitive–behavioral therapists believe that the way for people to start changing their minds is not to force the change, but to watch it. Through the process of mindfulness, individuals can learn to identify destructive thought patterns, simply label them, and watch them pass by whenever they come to mind. As individuals learn how their brains "tell stories," they can begin to change their negative thought patterns.

Electroconvulsive Therapy

Electroconvulsive therapy (ECT) is a treatment procedure that passes an electric current through the brain to induce a seizure. It has been used clinically since the 1930s. It is usually given 2–3 times weekly for 3–4 weeks until a course of 6–12 treatments is completed. Research suggests that twice-weekly ECT is preferable, as it is roughly as effective as thrice-weekly administration but frequently requires fewer treatments and may be associated with longer-lasting therapeutic effects (Charlson et al., 2012). ECT is typically considered a second-line therapy for both treatment-resistant MDD and bipolar disorder, and it produces similar overall remission rates in patients with either condition (Dierckx et al., 2012). A systematic review of ECT (Allan & Ebmeier, 2011) cited the following findings from studies completed within the previous 10 years:

- ECT is effective in treating depression, with responses of over 80%.
- Response is even higher in patients who have depression with psychotic features.
- Response is relatively rapid (greater than 60% within 3 weeks).
- ECT is associated with improved mood, functional status, anxiety, and quality of life.
- Individuals of all ages, even older adults with cognitive impairment, tolerate and respond well to ECT.
- It does not cause a switch to mania when used to treat bipolar depression, and it may also be used in patients with bipolar disorder with mixed features.
- It is especially useful for patients with severe depression who are resistant to other treatments, those who are severely suicidal, and those with severe psychomotor retardation.

A review of ECT in pregnancy demonstrated its effectiveness in treating depression; however, it is linked with potential fetal and maternal complications such as premature labor, decreased fetal heart rate, and uterine contractions (Leiknes et al., 2015). Risks and benefits of ECT must be weighed carefully on an individual case basis before deciding to treat a pregnant woman with ECT.

ECT is administered while the patient is under anesthesia. A thorough medical examination is required prior to the procedure to clear the patient for anesthesia. Muscle relaxants are usually administered. The patient is ventilated during the procedure. Electroencephalogram (EEG) and electrocardiogram (ECG), oxygen saturation via pulse oximetry, and vital signs are monitored during the procedure, which only takes 5–10 minutes. Mild confusion following the procedure (a postictal state) is typical. Vital signs must be monitored frequently for several hours after the procedure. During a course of ECT, a transient short-term memory loss (anterograde amnesia) is expected. This is distressing to some patients, and they need to be reassured that memory is usually restored. In rare cases, however, retrograde amnesia occurs and may be permanent. There are the usual risks associated with anesthesia. It is essential that all the potential risks and benefits of ECT be explained to and understood by the patient. A written, informed consent form must be signed by the patient before the procedure. Patients have the right to refuse treatment at any time during the course of therapy.

Transcranial Magnetic Stimulation

Repetitive transcranial magnetic stimulation (rTMS) is an FDA-approved treatment for depression that involves the use of a magnetic field that passes through the skull, causing cells in the cerebral cortex to fire. The target area is the left prefrontal cortex, which is one part of the brain thought to be disrupted in depression. Targeting the opposite lobe, the right prefrontal cortex, has therapeutic effects in manic episodes. This therapy has a rapid onset of action of 1–2 weeks, which is faster than most psychotropic medications. Although rTMS produces fewer short-term adverse cognitive effects than ECT, numerous studies have found that its benefits are fewer and of shorter duration than those associated with ECT (Health Quality Ontario, 2016; Janicak & Dokucu, 2015; Minichino et al., 2012).

Complementary Health Approaches

In community surveys, depression, fatigue, insomnia, and anxiety are among the most commonly reported reasons for the use of alternative therapies. The following are some

---

Patient Teaching

Electroconvulsive Therapy (ECT)

Prior to ECT, the nurse will complete a medical history, a physical exam, and a mental health assessment. Tests that will be needed include blood work and an electrocardiogram (ECG). Upon arrival for the first ECT, the patient will need to be educated on what to expect, which will include the following:

- If part of your responsibility, educate patient about the procedure, potential side effects, and expected effects of ECT. Because ECT requires the administration of anesthesia, provide necessary information regarding anesthesia administration and recovery. Ensure that all necessary consent forms have been signed by the patient before continuing. Although informing patients and obtaining consent forms is legally a medical responsibility, in practice it is often shared by nurses.

- Inform the patient of the need to review his or her medical history and perform a short physical assessment.

- Ensure that the patient has had nothing by mouth for at least 4 hours before treatment.

- Just prior to treatment, request that the patient empty the bladder and remove contact lenses, jewelry, hairpins, and dentures.

- The nurse will initiate an IV, and electrodes will be placed on the patient's head.

During the ECT treatment, the patient should understand what will occur, including:

- Vital signs will be monitored and oxygenation will occur.

- General sedation will be given, oxygen will be administered via mask, and a mouth guard may be used to prevent breakage of teeth and biting of tongue.

- The anesthetic preparation usually consists of the following:
  a. Generally, an atropine like medication such as glycopyrrolate (Robinul) is given to decrease secretions and block cardiac vagal reflexes during the seizure.
  b. A short-acting anesthetic such as methohexital sodium (Brevital) is administered intravenously.
  c. Following induction, a skeletal muscle relaxant such as succinylcholine chloride (Anectine) is administered to prevent injuries during the seizure.
  d. The patient will be artificially ventilated until the muscle relaxant is fully metabolized, usually in 2–3 minutes. Oxygen is administered with a rubber bite block in place. If necessary, oxygen may be administered by positive pressure.

- An electric current is passed through the brain by means of unilateral or bilateral electrodes placed on the temples. This causes a generalized (or tonic–clonic) seizure that lasts for usually less than 60 seconds, the effects of which are masked by the muscle relaxant. Often the only observable signs of seizure are a fluttering of the eyelids and carpopedal spasms.

- The patient will have vital signs and brain activity monitored during the entire process.

Once the ECT is completed, the patient should understand that the following will occur:

- General anesthesia will begin to wear off.

- The nurse will monitor vital signs frequently.

- Upon awakening, the patient may experience some confusion and memory loss, which may be short term or permanent.

- Patients are recovered in the lateral recumbent position to facilitate drainage and to prevent aspiration. After they are fully recovered and have been reoriented by the nurse, they will be able to eat.

- After vital signs are stabilized, the patient is able to leave (if ECT is being performed on an outpatient basis).

- The patient should not drive for the remainder of the day and should also have someone with them for the day (Kellner et al., 2012; Mayo Clinic, 2017a).

complementary therapies used for mood disorders. Note that these types of therapies should be used as complementary, rather than alternative, therapies in patients experiencing significant disruption in functioning related to mood disorders. Patients taking pharmacologic therapy should be encouraged to consult their prescribing provider before trying herbs or dietary supplements.

Exercise

Research indicates that exercise can reduce anxiety and promote healthy behaviors and overall health (Bertisch et al., 2012; Herring, O'Connor, & Dishman, 2010). These benefits alone make exercise a key part of health promotion and patient teaching in patients with alterations in mood and affect. However, a Cochrane review of 39 studies with 2326 participants found no conclusive evidence that exercise improves symptoms of depression (Cooney et al., 2013), indicating that nurses should emphasize the overall health benefits of exercise rather than its use as a complementary or alternative therapy to patients with alterations in mood and affect. Still, exercise is recommended for people with mild to moderate depression, provided they are physically able to participate (Cooney et al., 2013; Josefsson, Lindwall, & Archer, 2014). Although some reviews indicate that no one form of exercise is best, others suggest that individuals with depressive symptoms should engage in moderate-intensity aerobic exercise three times a week for a minimum of 9 weeks. Exercise also appears to be most beneficial when used in combination with antidepressant medications (Danielsson et al., 2013; Stanton & Reaburn, 2013).

SAFETY ALERT St. John's wort is not a proven therapy for depression (National Center for Complementary and Integrative Health [NCCIH], 2016) and should not be used to postpone or replace conventional treatment. It should **not** be combined with prescription antidepressants. It also may interfere with the action of antiseizure medications. St. John's wort has been found to reduce the effectiveness of birth control pills and HIV medications, among others (NCCIH, 2016). If taken with SSRIs, TCAs, or some atypical antidepressants, serotonin syndrome may result.

Vitamin B

Low levels of the B vitamins have been linked to depression, as vitamin B plays a role in the development of serotonin and norepinephrine (Bottiglieri, 2013; Lewis et al., 2013). A systematic review found that short-term increase of folate or vitamin B_{12} is not helpful in the treatment of depression but may be helpful if taken for the long term (Almeida, Ford, & Flicker, 2015). There is inconsistent evidence that folic acid may improve the action of some antidepressants (Bedson et al., 2014; Coppen & Bailey, 2000).

Omega-3 Fatty Acids

A systemic review and meta-analysis of 13 randomized controlled trials that studied the role of omega-3 fatty acids as an adjuvant treatment for depression found no significant benefit when compared to placebo use, despite earlier reports of patients' experiences of mild to moderate improvements in mood (Bloch & Hannestad, 2012).

Acupuncture

Acupuncture is best known for pain relief but may be coupled with SSRI antidepressants for increased benefit. Clinical trials indicate that acupuncture, when used with SSRI antidepressants, enhances the therapeutic response, has an early onset of action, and is well tolerated compared to the use of SSRIs alone (Chan et al., 2015). Furthermore, patients who are treated with acupuncture coupled with SSRIs demonstrate a faster response time and decreased side effects (Liu et al., 2015). There is also some evidence that acupuncture may be beneficial in the treatment of depression in pregnant women when the acupuncture is targeted toward treatment of depression and not generalized (Sneizek & Siddiqui, 2013).

Case Study >> Part 3

Jason was admitted to the short-term acute care psychiatric unit of the local hospital. He was diagnosed with bipolar I disorder and started on aripiprazole (Abilify). Jason reports feeling as if he has to keep moving all the time, and he has mild dystonic symptoms involving muscle twitches in his hands. He is currently taking 20 mg of aripiprazole daily. He is attending individual and group therapy sessions. He is sleeping and eating more normally; his speech is no longer rapid and pressured. Jason no longer believes he has special talents. He says he now feels stupid about his previous behavior and ashamed that he ended up being hospitalized. He states, "I can't face anyone I know now that they know I am crazy. I don't want to live the rest of my life like this. What's the point?"

Clinical Reasoning Questions Level I

1. What symptoms should be reported to the physician and therapist?
2. Based on the information provided, what does the nurse need to assess immediately?
3. What is the probable cause of Jason's feelings of restlessness and muscle twitches? What additional treatments might be indicated to address them?

Clinical Reasoning Questions Level II

4. What do Jason's statements indicate and how should the nurse respond?
5. What is the priority nursing diagnosis for Jason at this time?
6. Why do you think Jason was not prescribed an antidepressant?

Lifespan Considerations
Mood and Affect in Children and Adolescents

Determinants of normal mood and affect in children and adolescents are generally the same as those for adults; however, a greater level of lability is common in younger patients and should not necessarily be considered suggestive of a mood disorder. Causes of "mood swings" among children and adolescents include anxiety about the physical changes they are experiencing; hormonal fluctuations associated with the onset of puberty; immaturity of the prefrontal cortex; and the pressures of adjusting to new roles and expectations (Balzer et al., 2015; Guyer, Silk, & Nelson, 2016; Larson, Csikszentmihalyi, & Graef, 2014). As adolescents progress toward adulthood, the mood swings typical of the teenage years become progressively less common (Maciejewski et al., 2015).

When a child's mood and affect fall outside the normal range for members of his age group, the possibility of a mood disorder should be considered. According to the NIMH (2013a), the 12-month prevalence of mood disorders among children age 8–15 is 3.7%. Girls are affected nearly twice as often as boys. Children experience depression, although onset typically occurs sometime between puberty and young adulthood; hence, depression rates rise during the later teenage years. In fact, according to the CDC (2014), 5.7% of adolescents age 12–17 experience depression. Bipolar disorder is rarely observed in this population, because onset nearly always occurs in late adolescence or when individuals are in their 20s (APA, 2013).

Initially, many parents choose to try psychotherapy alone to treat depressive disorders in their children and adolescents. However, if this proves unsuccessful, medication is indicated. Currently, fluoxetine (Prozac) is the only antidepressant that is FDA-approved for use in children. However, many healthcare providers prescribe other SSRIs for children with depression. For example, sertraline (Zoloft) is approved for use in treating obsessive-compulsive disorder in children but not depression. However, some providers may prescribe sertraline for children and adolescents with depression—an example of "off-label" use. Most prescribers will start children on a lower dose of antidepressant than is normally prescribed for adults and titrate up to a dose that is effective in symptom relief.

After a comprehensive review of published and unpublished controlled clinical trials of antidepressants in children and adolescents, the FDA issued a public warning in October 2004 regarding increased risk of suicidal thoughts or behavior in children and adolescents treated with SSRI antidepressant medications. However, several newer studies indicate that the benefits associated with taking antidepressants may be greater than the risk of suicide (Cooper et al., 2014; Gibbons et al., 2012; Isacsson & Rich, 2014).

SAFETY ALERT Note that the FDA does not recommend paroxetine (Paxil) to treat depression in children and adolescents (NIMH, 2013a). There are reports of increased suicidal thinking and behavior during initial treatment using paroxetine in children and adolescents. There is a "black box" warning secondary to these findings (FDA, 2014).

Mood and Affect in Pregnant Women

Manifestations and potential causes of depressive disorder with peripartum onset are detailed in the exemplar on Postpartum Depression. Generally speaking, new onset of depression during pregnancy appears to be related to anxiety about the fetus's health and the birth process, concern about relationship changes and adapting to the maternal role, and the many physical and hormonal changes of pregnancy. It is also important to note that many women who previously experienced depression either continue to experience symptoms or have a recurrence of symptoms during pregnancy (Fall, Goulet, & Vézina, 2013). When both women with existing mood disorders and women with new-onset

depression are considered, experts estimate that between 12 and 20% of women experience depression during the antepartum period. Many of these women remain undiagnosed or untreated, often because they feel ashamed to be depressed during a time in life when society expects them to be filled with joy and anticipation. Unfortunately, failure to seek treatment during pregnancy can have detrimental effects on both mother and child, including elevated likelihood of pregnancy complications, premature birth, high-risk maternal behavior, postpartum depression, intrauterine growth restriction, and developmental difficulties during childhood (Chan et al., 2014; Fall, Goulet, & Vézina, 2013; Syka, 2015).

Several treatment options are available for women who experience mood disorders during pregnancy. Many women opt for group therapy or psychotherapy, often because they are hesitant to pursue or continue pharmacologic treatment. A major reason for this hesitation is that, to date, no psychotropic drug has been assigned a Category A rating by the FDA. (A Category A rating indicates that there are no known fetal risks associated with a medication.) Research indicates, however, that many women and prescribers alike overestimate the risk associated with pharmacologic therapy during pregnancy. For example, SSRIs are among the most studied drugs in pregnant women, and substantial evidence exists that these drugs (with the exception of paroxetine [Paxil]) present low risk of major birth defects. Nonetheless, babies of mothers who took SSRIs during pregnancy do have a slightly elevated risk of persistent pulmonary hypertension in the newborn (PPHN) and neonatal withdrawal. TCAs are also considered low risk, although use of MAOI antidepressants is not recommended (Chan et al., 2014; Freeland & Shealy, 2014; Kalfoglou, 2016). For more information on the care and treatment of pregnant women with mood disorders, see the exemplars in this module.

Mood and Affect in Older Adults

Depression is not a normal part of aging; research suggests that older adults generally have more positive mood and affect than younger adults (English & Carstensen, 2014; Masumoto et al., 2016; Stanley & Isaacowitz, 2011). Thus, when older adults present with symptoms of depression, these symptoms need to be addressed. In many cases, these symptoms may be related to life changes, such as retirement; loss of aging friends, family, or spouse to death; downsizing or placement in assisted care; and loss of physical function. Major life-changing events can be precipitating factors to inability to cope leading to increased risk of depression (Potter & Moller, 2016). The presence of a chronic illness elevates the older adult's risk for depression.

When working with older patients, a thorough evaluation is necessary to rule out any underlying medical cause of mood alterations before medication is prescribed. As with most medications in older adults, the cardinal rule is to start with the lowest dose and increase slowly as tolerated and as needed to achieve therapeutic effect. Older adults may respond to a lower drug dose, but it is important to treat to remission. Also, because the majority of psychotropic medications are metabolized in the liver, caution must be taken in older adults with liver disease. For patients with depression, SSRIs are usually the drug of choice. Because psychotropic drugs lead to increased risk of orthostatic hypotension in older adults, patients should be educated to sit before standing and stand before walking to reduce their likelihood of falls. The patient and family should also be educated on fall-risk reduction strategies. In addition, a thorough medication history and periodic medication reconciliation should be conducted because of the risk of medication interactions and polypharmacy (Frank, 2014; Lindsey, 2009; Mulsant et al.,

2014). Most older adults with mood disorders respond well with antidepressants, psychotherapy, or a combination of the two (Potter & Moller, 2016).

SAFETY ALERT Atypical antipsychotics, often used to treat bipolar disorder, all have an FDA "black box" warning that they may increase mortality in older adults with dementia-related psychosis. Older adults taking these medications for bipolar disorder should be monitored carefully.

REVIEW The Concept of Mood and Affect

RELATE Link the Concepts

Linking the concept of mood and affect with the concept of development:

1. Explain how failure to master the developmental tasks of older adulthood could contribute to the development of depression (refer to developmental theories).

2. How can resiliency theory be applied to the development or prevention of depression?

Linking the concept of mood and affect with the concept of family:

3. How can the burden of having a family member with a severe mental illness such as bipolar disorder affect the family system?

4. How does the stage that the family is in affect family recovery from a mood disorder?

Linking the concept of mood and affect with the concept of self:

5. How would you assess self-esteem in a patient suspected of having a mood disorder?

6. What are some strategies that can be used to enhance the low self-esteem often experienced by patients with mood disorders?

READY Go to Volume 3: Clinical Nursing Skills

- SKILL 1.1   Appearance and Mental Status: Assessing
- SKILL 1.5–1.9   Vital Signs
- SKILL 1.22   Neurologic Status: Assessing
- SKILL 3.1   Pain in Newborn, Infant, Child, or Adult: Assessing
- SKILL 3.3   Pain Relief: Complementary Health Approaches
- SKILL 3.6   Sleep Promotion: Assisting
- SKILL 10.2   Diet, Therapeutic: Managing

- SKILL 10.5   Nutrition: Assessing
- SKILL 15.1   Abuse: Newborn, Infant, Child, Older Adult, Assessing for
- SKILL 15.4   Suicidal Patient: Caring for

REFER Go to Pearson MyLab Nursing and eText

- Additional review materials

REFLECT Apply Your Knowledge

Gerald Hanes is a 72-year-old widowed man who is brought in to his primary care provider's office by his daughter, who is worried about his unexplained weight loss. Gerald lives independently and is in good general health. Since Gerald's regular checkup 2 months ago, he has lost 20 pounds. He denies any concerns at this time. Gerald's daughter reports that he has not been attending church, which he used to do weekly. She further reports that ever since his wife died 3 months ago, he has not been maintaining his relationships with the family. She states that he still has most of the groceries left in the kitchen that she purchased for him 2 weeks ago. When asked if he is eating, Gerald states, "I'm just not hungry anymore." Gerald presents with a flat to sad affect and depressed mood. All laboratory test results are reported as negative or within normal limits.

Clinical Reasoning Questions Level I

1. What additional questions should the nurse ask Gerald during the assessment?

2. In further discussion with the daughter, she states that she knows that this is typical for the aging population. How should the nurse respond to this statement?

3. What are three appropriate nursing diagnoses for Gerald at this time?

» Exemplar 28.A
Depression

Exemplar Learning Outcomes

28.A Analyze depressive disorders and relevant nursing care.

- Describe the pathophysiology of depressive disorders.
- Describe the etiology of depressive disorders.
- Compare the risk factors and prevention of depressive disorders.
- Identify the clinical manifestations of depressive disorders.

- Summarize diagnostic tests and therapies used by interprofessional teams in the collaborative care of an individual with a depressive disorder.
- Differentiate care of patients with depressive disorders across the lifespan.
- Apply the nursing process in providing culturally competent care to an individual with a depressive disorder.

Exemplar Key Terms

Adjustment disorder with depressed mood, *1935*
Anhedonia, *1934*
Depression, *1933*
Dysthymia, *1935*
Hypersomnia, *1934*

Insomnia, *1934*
Major depressive disorder (MDD), *1934*
Major depressive episode, *1934*
Persistent depressive disorder, *1935*
Psychomotor retardation, *1935*
Seasonal affective disorder (SAD), *1935*
Situational depression, *1935*

Overview

Depression is a disorder characterized by a sad or despondent mood or loss of interest in usual activities. Many symptoms are associated with depression, including lack of energy; sleep disturbances; anxious distress; abnormal eating patterns; psychomotor retardation or agitation; and/or feelings of despair, guilt, and hopelessness. Depression is one of the most common mental health disorders and encompasses a variety of physical, emotional, cognitive, and social considerations. The Substance Abuse and Mental Health Services Administration (SAMHSA) (2015a) reports that just under 16 million American adults (approximately 6.6% of the population) will experience a major depressive episode in a given year. Treatment rate estimates for adults with depressive disorders are as low as 29% and as high as 41% (Olson, Blanco, & Marcus, 2016; SAMHSA, 2013).

The majority of patients who experience depression are found in mainstream everyday settings. Proper diagnosis and treatment require collaboration among healthcare providers. Because patients with depression are present in multiple settings and in all areas of practice, every nurse should be proficient in the assessment and nursing care of patients with this disorder.

Pathophysiology and Etiology

Pathophysiology

As described in the Concept section of this module, the exact pathophysiology of depression has yet to be determined. However, individuals with depression often have increased limbic system activity, along with decreased gray matter volume and lower metabolic activity in the MPFC (Field & Cartwright-Hatton, 2015; Grieve et al., 2013). Specific reasons for these findings remain unclear, although the working theory is that they involve alterations in neurotransmitter activity and/or neuronal receptivity to neurotransmitters. Several different neurotransmitters have been implicated in the pathophysiology of depression, including 5-HT, NE, DA, ACh, GABA, and glutamate (Halter, 2014; Patrick & Ames, 2015; Potter & Moller, 2016).

More recent studies have focused on a potential connection between depression and inflammation, based on the fact that many depressed individuals have increased levels of inflammatory biomarkers called cytokines (Raison & Miller, 2011; Vogelzangs et al., 2012). However, not all individuals with depression have elevated cytokine levels, and not all people with elevated cytokines have depression. Together, these findings have led to the hypothesis that some people with depression may have a genetic predisposition toward elevated cytokine production when faced with external stressors, as well as the hypothesis that other individuals may have genetic factors that protect them against the potentially mood-lowering effects of cytokines (Raison & Miller, 2011; Slavich & Irwin, 2014).

Hormonal factors also continue to be investigated as a possible cause of depression. Researchers have noted that individuals with depression tend to have increased levels of cortisol and corticotropin-releasing hormone, both of which are produced in the brain's HPA axis. High levels of cortisol and corticotropin-releasing hormone are indicative of HPA and limbic system hyperactivity, which (as described earlier) is commonly observed in individuals with depression (Potter & Moller, 2016). However, researchers aren't sure whether depression precipitates HPA hyperactivity and excess hormone production or whether HPA hyperactivity and excess hormone production precipitate depression.

Etiology

Depression has been linked to multiple possible causes. Genetics clearly plays some role, although the exact nature of this role remains unclear. Other potential causative mechanisms (many of which may have a genetic component) include hormonal imbalances, disruptions in biological rhythms, high stress levels, poor coping mechanisms, traumatic life events, unhealthy or insufficient interpersonal relationships, and internalization of unhealthy or unrealistic gender-based expectations. Refer to the "Theories of Depression" section in this module for more information on each of these possible contributors.

Risk Factors

Risk factors for depression include family history of depression or other mental illness, female gender, history of child abuse or trauma, unemployment, poverty, lower education, and lack of social supports (Andrews, 2016; Halverson, 2016). It should be noted that first-degree relatives of individuals with depression are three times as likely to develop depression than the general population (Halverson, 2016).

Prevention

As discussed at the beginning of this module, there is no definitive way to prevent depression, because of causative and contributing genetic and biological factors that cannot be modified. However, a number of approaches can be useful in controlling these factors. Individuals should be encouraged to eat a healthy diet, engage in regular exercise, avoid smoking, and obtain adequate sleep. Other primary prevention strategies include providing education about stress management and healthy emotional functioning; encouraging patients to participate in meaningful social relationships; providing targeted teaching and support to individuals who have experienced traumatic or otherwise life-altering events; and using family-based cognitive–behavioral interventions to reduce the likelihood of depression among children with depressed parents. Secondary prevention strategies include regular screening, counseling patients about their relative risks for depression, and referring individuals with suspected depression for accurate diagnosis and treatment. Finally, tertiary prevention focuses on provision of collaborative care and establishment of community-focused programs that target depressed and high-risk individuals. For a detailed discussion of all of these prevention approaches, refer to the Health Promotion section within this module.

Clinical Manifestations

Some of the clinical manifestations of depression seem fairly obvious: feelings of sadness and despair and sleep disturbances, for example. Others may not be as obvious, such as anger and physical complaints. Manifestations of depression also can differ according to culture, especially if mental illness is stigmatized within the culture. Mental illness is often displayed with somatic symptoms such as headaches, gastrointestinal discomfort, or sleep disturbances that may require assessment by a healthcare provider. Studies indicate that Chinese patients are more likely to report somatic symptoms when depressed than are Euro-Canadian patients (Dere et al., 2013). Depression is seen worldwide and is especially increased in post-conflict settings. For example, a study of post-conflict South Sudan reported rates of depression as high as 50% (Ameresekere & Henderson, 2012). It is important for nurses involved with patients with depression to know and recognize the symptoms.

Major Depressive Disorder

A **major depressive episode** is characterized by a change in several aspects of an individual's emotional state and functioning consistently over a period of 14 days or longer. The most important factor is the patient's mood, which the patient may not describe in terms of "depression." Instead, the patient may describe feelings of sadness, discouragement, or hopelessness. Some patients may report vague somatic (physical) complaints such as aches and pains; other patients may report increased anger, frustration, and irritability, with uncharacteristic outbursts over minor matters. It is not difficult to imagine that someone who looks and feels sad or empty is depressed. A diagnosis of depression is more likely to be missed when an individual simply seems anxious or irritable.

Major depressive disorder (MDD) may consist of a single episode or may exhibit as recurrent major depression at various points in life. Signs and symptoms of single-episode and recurrent major depression are found in **Box 28–2 »**. Onset of MDD generally occurs gradually, with symptoms progressing from anxiety and mild depression to a major depressive episode over a period of days, weeks, or months. The course of MDD is extremely variable, with some individuals experiencing remission for a period of months and others experiencing many years between episodes (APA, 2013). Individuals who experience MDD in the context of another disorder, such as substance abuse or borderline personality disorder, often experience symptoms that are more difficult to treat (APA, 2013). A diagnosis of MDD requires that the individual not have any previous episodes of mania or hypomania (which suggest a bipolar rather

Box 28–2
Symptoms of Major Depressive Disorder

- Significant distress or impairment of functioning
- Feelings of despair, hopelessness
- Sadness, crying
- Feelings of worthlessness, guilt
- Loss of self-esteem
- Loss of interest or pleasure in activities
- Substantial changes in weight or appetite over a short period of time
- Impairments in executive functioning (e.g., ability to plan, organize, solve problems, concentrate)
- Visible psychomotor agitation or retardation
- Aches and pains
- Excessive sleep loss or excessive sleeping
- Recurrent thoughts of death or suicide

Sources: American Psychiatric Association. (2013). *Diagnostic and statistical manual of mental disorders* (5th ed.). Washington, DC: Author; National Alliance on Mental Illness. (2017). *Depression.* Retrieved from http://www.nami.org/Learn-More/Mental-Health-Conditions/Depression; Snyder, H. R. (2013). Major depressive disorder is associated with broad impairments on neuropsychological measures of executive functioning: A meta-analysis and review. *Psychological Bulletin, 139*(1), 81–132.

than a depressive disorder) and be free of any medical disorder that might otherwise explain the symptoms the individual is experiencing (e.g., dementia) (APA, 2013).

SAFETY ALERT Healthcare providers often use language that is unfamiliar to patients and their families. To help patients and families understand the symptoms of a major depressive episode, nurses should discuss symptoms and characteristics using terms patients and families are more likely to understand. For example, rather than using the phrase "psychomotor retardation," nurses can inquire whether the patient is experiencing difficulty or slowness in speaking or in performing tasks.

Individuals with a history of a manic or hypomanic episodes are considered to have a bipolar disorder and are not classified under the categories of depressive disorders.

Individuals experiencing MDD often no longer enjoy activities that previously brought pleasure, such as hobbies, sports, and sex. This is a condition known as **anhedonia**. Changes in appetite, usually experienced as a reduction or loss of interest in food, are often seen, although increased appetite and cravings are also reported.

Sleep disturbances, particularly **insomnia** (inability to fall or stay asleep or, in some individuals, early morning awakening), are common in individuals with depression. Two types of insomnia are most often experienced by people having a major depressive episode. *Middle insomnia* refers to waking up during the night and having difficulty falling asleep again. *Terminal insomnia* refers to waking at the end of the night and being unable to return to sleep. Depressed patients also may report **hypersomnia**, in which the individual sleeps for prolonged periods at night as well as during the day but still wakes up tired or fatigued. These sleep disturbances are discussed at length in the module on Comfort.

Fatigue and decreased energy are characteristic symptoms of depression. Individuals with depression may report being tired upon awakening regardless of how long they have slept. Even the smallest task seems insurmountable, and routine activities require substantial effort and take longer to accomplish. Decreased energy may be manifested in **psychomotor retardation**, in which thinking and body movements are noticeably slowed and speech is slowed or absent. Psychomotor agitation also may occur, in which the individual cannot sit still; paces; wrings the hands; and picks at the fingernails, skin, clothing, bedclothes, or other objects.

Other common symptoms in individuals with moderate to severe depression include guilt or a sense of worthlessness, self-blame, impaired concentration and decision-making ability (even about trivial things), and suicidal ideation. Martin Seligman, PhD, was researching animal behaviors in 1967 and accidentally discovered what is now known as "learned helplessness." He found that learned helplessness occurs when an individual experiences unpredictable or uncontrollable events, which are usually traumatic, resulting in an internal perception of decreased ability to cope or change future situations (Overmier, 2013). Even if the individual may have the ability to avoid or control the adverse stimulus, the individual feels powerless and accepts the negative stimulus or situation. Learned helplessness is often a trigger for depression. The characteristics of a major depressive episode are illustrated in **Figure 28–4 ≫**.

Persistent Depressive Disorder

The term **persistent depressive disorder**, also known as **dysthymia** or *dysthymic disorder*, describes chronic depression for the majority of most days for at least 2 years (1 year for children and adolescents). Throughout those 2 years, no more than 2 months can be described as symptom-free. The symptoms of dysthymic disorder, while distressing, tend to be less severe than those of MDD, with fewer physiologic symptoms, but the degree of impact on individual functioning can be as great or greater than that of MDD. Individuals with persistent depressive disorder are at higher risk for developing other mental health disorders than those with MDD (APA, 2013).

Persistent depressive disorder often occurs in childhood, adolescence, or early adulthood and tends to be chronic. Whereas both girls and boys are equally affected as children, there are two to three times as many adult women as men

with dysthymic disorder. Factors that contribute to poorer long-term outcomes include the presence of a comorbid anxiety or conduct disorder, greater symptom severity, and greater impairment in functioning (APA, 2013).

Seasonal Affective Disorder

Seasonal affective disorder (SAD) is not an official DSM diagnosis, but rather a specifier of MDD "with seasonal pattern." Individuals with SAD typically experience symptoms, including sadness and low energy, during the winter months, when the days are shorter. Factors that increase a person's risk for SAD include female gender, age (with younger people being affected more often), and personal or family history of depression or bipolar disorder. Not surprisingly, the condition is also more common among people who live farther from the equator, where winters are longer (Melrose, 2015).

SAD arises due to biological fluctuations triggered by decreased exposure to natural light. People with SAD have elevated levels of SERT, a protein involved in serotonin transport in the brain. SERT binds with serotonin, so higher SERT levels lead to lower serotonin activity. SERT levels are naturally suppressed by exposure to sunlight, so when days grow shorter during the winter months, affected individuals' SERT levels rise, causing their serotonin activity to decline and their depressive symptoms to increase. Evidence also indicates that individuals with SAD overproduce melatonin. Melatonin is a hormone secreted by the pineal gland that causes sleepiness. Melatonin production increases in all people in response to darkness, but levels are particularly elevated in patients with SAD. Together, decreased serotonin and increased melatonin cause disruptions in affected individuals' circadian rhythms (Melrose, 2015).

Pharmacologic approaches to the treatment of SAD generally involve either bupropion (Wellbutrin) or SSRI antidepressants, with fluoxetine (Prozac) being the most common choice. Another common treatment approach is light therapy, also called phototherapy. With this approach, patients are exposed to a bright light that replicates natural outdoor lighting for 20–60 minutes each day. Light therapy is frequently the first-line treatment for SAD, as it generally has fewer adverse effects than drug therapy. However, recent research suggests that fluoxetine therapy is more cost-effective than light therapy and just as effective. Beyond pharmacologic and light therapy, counseling can also be useful in the treatment of SAD (Cheung et al., 2012; Melrose, 2015; Potter & Moller, 2016).

Adjustment Disorder with Depressed Mood

Adjustment disorder with depressed mood represents a change in mood and affect following a stressor, such as the end of a relationship, or multiple stressors; it may also be called **situational depression**. Symptoms generally begin 3 months after the event and typically last no more than 6 months. Adjustment disorder with depressed mood is differentiated from an appropriate change in mood following a sad or stressful event in that the distress experienced by the patient is out of proportion to the event and results in significant impairment in functioning (APA, 2013).

Mood depressed; Memory problems
Anxious; Apathetic; Appetite changes
"**J**ust no fun"
Occupational impairment
Restless; Ruminative

Doubts self; Difficulty making decisions
Empty feeling
Pessimistic; Persistent sadness; Psychomotor retardation
Reports vague pains
Energy gone
Suicidal thoughts and impulses
Sleep disturbances
Irritability; Inability to concentrate
Oppressive guilt
"**N**othing can help" (Hopelessness)

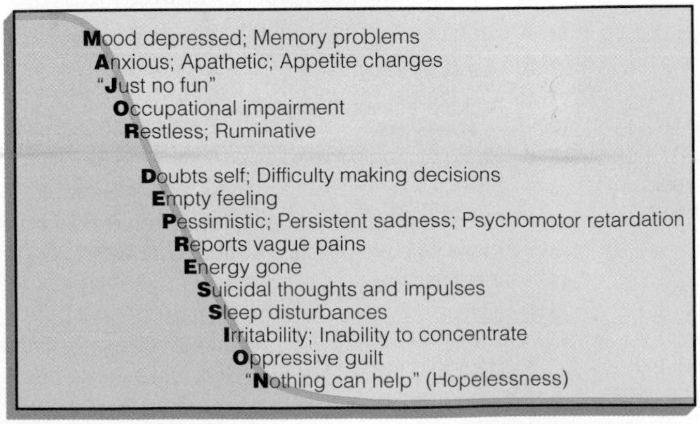

Figure 28–4 ≫ Characteristics of major depression.

Any life-altering event can create risk for the occurrence of adjustment disorder with depressed mood. This risk is further increased by a preexisting mental health issue, ineffective or unhealthy coping mechanisms, or lack of a support network. Patients with these preexisting conditions may find that adjustment disorder with depressed mood has exacerbated their condition. For example, in an attempt to diminish feelings of depression, a patient who has remained sober after a history of alcohol abuse may resume drinking as a coping mechanism following a stressful event.

Differentiating Depression from Grief

In some patients, depression and grief may present similarly on initial assessment. Nurses must distinguish whether a patient who exhibits sadness and anhedonia is depressed or grieving (**Table 28–2 》》**). Although this may appear to be easy, it can be difficult when working with new patients with whom the nurse has not yet developed a therapeutic relationship. Careful assessment includes determining if the feelings described by the patient were triggered by a loss or losses (such as the death of a family member).

Collaboration

As many as two thirds of those with depression may not receive appropriate treatment for their illness (Andrews, 2016). For those who do, many are treated in the community by a primary care provider or may go directly to a mental health provider for counseling but elect not to use prescription medications. In inpatient settings, nurses play an important role as a member of the interprofessional team that includes psychiatrists, social workers, occupational therapists, and other healthcare professionals. In outpatient settings, nurses may be the first healthcare provider to screen or assess an individual for depression. In any setting, nurses play an important role in providing patient education about therapies, in answering questions, and in encouraging patients to follow their treatment regimens.

Diagnostic Tests

Although there is no diagnostic test to determine depression, primary care clinicians typically perform a complete medical history and thorough physical exam to rule out the

Clinical Manifestations and Therapies
Depressive Disorders

ETIOLOGY	CLINICAL MANIFESTATIONS	CLINICAL THERAPIES
Major depressive disorder	Symptoms must last 14 days or longer and may include: ■ Feelings of sadness and hopelessness ■ Somatic complaints such as pain, stomachaches ■ Anxiety, anger, irritability ■ Loss of interest in pleasurable activities ■ Sleep disturbances	■ Pharmacologic therapies include: • Selective serotonin reuptake inhibitors (SSRIs). • Tricyclic antidepressants (TCAs). • Atypical antidepressants. • Electroconvulsive therapy (most often used for those who are resistant to treatment with medications). ■ CBT.
Adjustment disorder with depressed mood	Symptoms develop within 3 months in response to an identifiable stressor and may include: ■ Insomnia, hypersomnia ■ Crying ■ Avoiding pleasurable activities ■ Avoiding family and friends ■ Ignoring financial responsibilities ■ Performing poorly at work and school ■ Fighting, behaving recklessly	■ Improved sleep hygiene. ■ Short-term sedative. ■ CBT alone may be sufficient to help the individual return to normal. ■ Alternative therapies such as massage therapy may provide relief. ■ Antidepressant therapy. ■ CBT. ■ Family therapy. ■ Antidepressant therapy.
Persistent depressive disorder (dysthymic disorder)	Symptoms are not as severe as those of major depressive disorder, but last beyond 2 years with period of relief lasting less than 2 months.	■ Pharmacologic therapies are the same as for MDD. ■ Electroconvulsive therapy (most often used for those who are resistant to treatment with medications). ■ CBT.
Seasonal affective disorder	Depressive symptoms occur in relation to the seasons; usually during the winter months, when days are shorter.	■ Bupropion extended-release. ■ Light therapy. ■ CBT.

TABLE 28–2 Differences Between Depression and Grief

Trait	Depression	Grief
Trigger	Specific trigger not necessary, but may be present.	Trigger is usually loss or multiple losses.
Active/passive	Passive behavior tends to keep patient "stuck" in sadness.	Actively feel their emotional pain and emptiness.
Emotions	Generalized feeling of helplessness, hopelessness.	Experience a range of emotions that are usually intense.
Ability to laugh	Likely to be humorless and incapable of being happy or even temporarily cheered up; likely to resist support.	Sometimes will be able to laugh and enjoy humor; more likely to accept support.
Activities	Lacks interest in previously enjoyed activities.	Can be persuaded to participate in activities, especially as they begin to heal.
Self-esteem	Low self-esteem, low self-confidence; feels like a failure.	Self-esteem usually remains intact; does not feel like a failure unless it relates directly to the loss.
Feeling of failure	May dwell on past failures, catastrophize feelings.	Any self-blame or guilt relates directly to the loss; feelings resolve as they progress toward healing.

possibility of an underlying medical condition causing the patient's depressive symptoms. If no physical causes are found, the clinician can start the patient on the depression "treatment cascade": recognizing the clinical illness, initiating treatment, and evaluating the patient's response to treatment (Pence, O'Donnell, & Gaynes, 2012). Existing medical conditions, such as diabetes, may inform selection of medication therapy if determined appropriate.

Pharmacologic Therapy

Antidepressant medications are often prescribed for patients with depression. Because individuals experience different dysfunctions in neurotransmission, individuals respond differently to various antidepressants. A period of trial and error may be necessary to determine which medication is most effective for the patient. See the Collaborative Therapies section in the Concept section of this module for a more detailed discussion of these medications.

Psychotherapy

Psychotherapy often is used in combination with medications to treat major depression. Some of the psychosocial problems associated with depression (e.g., ability to relate to others, motivation, problem-solving ability) cannot be resolved with medications. Psychotherapy promotes effective coping skills and positive, helpful patterns of thinking and behavior. Patients with mild depression may benefit from therapy alone. CBT is the most effective type of psychotherapy for depression.

Other Therapies

As discussed earlier in this module, ECT and integrative therapies may be appropriate for the patient diagnosed with depression. Another therapy, magnetic seizure therapy (MST), is being studied for efficacy. This treatment uses a magnetic pulse to stimulate the brain to induce a seizure, similar to ECT, but early results show fewer side effects than ECT and reduced recovery time. MSTs are shorter in duration and are thought to cause less cognitive loss after treatment (Cretaz, Brunoni, & Lafer, 2015).

The nurse's role includes assessing for safety, assessing for potential contraindications, encouraging patient communication with all healthcare providers (e.g., primary care provider and mental health provider or therapist), and providing patient teaching related to types of therapies and the importance of adhering to the treatment plan.

Lifespan Considerations

Symptoms of depression can vary among age groups, although sadness and anhedonia are common at all ages. Treatment considerations also may vary.

Depressive Disorders in Children and Adolescents

Careful and thorough assessment of a child suspected of having depression is necessary to rule out physical illness that can be linked to depressive symptoms. Other tests, such as hearing and vision tests, may be indicated as well. It is essential to question parents, caregivers, or guardians regarding their observations of the child's behavior and recent changes or precipitating factors. Diagnostic evaluation must be performed by a child psychiatrist, psychiatric nurse practitioner, or other mental health professional experienced in the diagnosis and treatment of children and adolescents. A variety of scales and techniques are used; however, very little guidance is available relating to evaluation of children under 6 years of age. See the Concept section of this module for commonly used screening tools. Thorough assessment for both physical and mental health disorders is necessary because comorbidities (appearance with other disorders) are common. Examples of these include a history of bullying or substance abuse.

Depressive symptoms may vary with each age group. The following list indicates symptoms of depression with each age group through adolescence:

- Toddlers can show regressive behaviors in toileting and other activities.

- Preschoolers have fewer symbolic and other play activities and demonstrate self-destructive play themes. They may whine and show irritability, lack of interest, and lack of confidence.

- School-age children may show a decrease in academic performance, increased or decreased physical activity, somatic complaints, and loss of friends. The older school-age child may talk of running away or show signs of boredom and low self-esteem.

- The adolescent can have a wide array of symptoms (e.g., decreased social contact, poor school performance, lack of involvement in typical activities, poor self-care, difficulty with parents and teachers, or a focus on violence).

See the section Lifespan Considerations: Mood and Affect in Children and Adolescents for additional information on treatment for depression in children and adolescents.

Depressive Disorders in Pregnant Women

Depression can occur at any time during or after the course of a woman's pregnancy. See the exemplar on Postpartum Depression for a detailed outline of manifestations and treatment of women with peripartum depression.

Depressive Disorders in Older Adults

Depression is common among older adults, but it is important to note that it is not a normal part of aging. Manifestations of depression in older adults may include memory problems, social withdrawal, sleep disturbances, loss of appetite, and irritability. Some individuals may experience delusions or hallucinations. Depression in older adults can complicate treatment of other conditions because impairment of functioning due to depression may impair the individual's ability or motivation to participate in treatment. Other medical conditions can complicate treatment of depression if nurses and clinicians dismiss symptoms as related to another medical condition (or side effects of treatment) without doing a full assessment for depression.

Older adults are at risk for a depressive episode, especially when they experience two or more stressors in proximity. Development of a disabling illness (whether cognitive, physical, or otherwise), loss of a loved one, retirement, moving out of the home, or another stressful event may result in a depressive episode in the older adult (American Psychological Association, 2016b). Even those older adults who "see the glass as half full" are challenged by these types of stressors. The loss of driving privileges (due to physical or cognitive changes) is a huge loss to older adults, often putting a great deal of strain on family members who must accommodate the older adult who can no longer drive as well provide support as the individual learns to cope with this loss of independence.

Because of the increased risk older adults have for medical illness, careful assessment of the older adult is critical. Polypharmacy issues may make prescribing for older adults a challenge, and older adults taking psychotropic medications often require more frequent monitoring and laboratory tests (e.g., blood glucose levels). The Geriatric Depression Scale can be useful in screening older adults for depression and determining the need for further evaluation (Sheikh et al., 1991).

NURSING PROCESS

Priorities of nursing care focus on safety and meeting functional needs until the patient's condition improves. Risk of suicide must always be a consideration when caring for patients who are depressed. Patients with depression may not meet their daily hygiene, sleep, nutrition, or other needs. They are also at increased risk for accidental injury and

medical illness. The nurse can initiate strategies to help them until they are able to function autonomously.

Assessment

- **Observation and patient interview.** Assessment of patients with suspected depression begins with a thorough history and interview. Inquire about any past depressive, manic, or hypomanic episodes or behavior, as well as family history of mood disorders. Ask about and observe for the signs and symptoms discussed throughout the Concept section. Patients with depressive disorders may articulate any number of changes in mood and behavior: feelings of sadness, lack of interest in relationships and activities that previously brought pleasure, feelings of worthlessness or guilt, anxious distress, withdrawal, and/or social isolation. Patients may also articulate tearfulness and emotional outbursts.

  Cognitive alterations are another frequent feature of depression. Accordingly, be alert for signs or descriptions of problems such as impaired concentration, difficulty making decisions, poor memory, and impaired problem-solving ability. In severe cases, patients might also report or demonstrate paranoid thinking, delusions, and other forms of psychosis.

  The interview and history portion of the assessment is also a good time to observe for difficulties with adaptive functioning. Patients will often describe how long it takes them to complete activities that they formerly accomplished easily, such as preparing a simple meal. They may also neglect regular grooming and hygiene tasks, either skip meals or eat excessively, and/or respond inappropriately to social cues.

- **Physical examination.** The next step in assessment is to consider the patient's physical manifestations; in fact, somatic concerns are often the presenting complaint. Among the most common problems are fatigue, sleep disturbances or excessive sleep, and changes in appetite and/or weight. Patients with depression may complain of abdominal pains, headaches, and vague body aches. A problem with sexual functioning or lack of desire also may be a presenting complaint. Constipation is a common result of the general slowing of metabolism due to inactivity. Patients from some cultures are more likely to express symptoms of depression through complaints about body function and discomfort. See **Box 28–3 »** for information on how depression evidenced by somatic concerns can be detected in other settings. Possible medical problems that could be the cause of the patient's physical symptoms should always be investigated and ruled out before a diagnosis of depression is made.

Suicide Assessment

Assess all patients for suicide risk by using direct questioning. Ask whether the patient has thoughts of self-harm (*suicidal ideation*), how often these thoughts occur, and whether or not the person would act on these thoughts (intent). Inquire whether or not the patient has a plan regarding carrying out suicide (*plan/method*). If a plan exists, it is crucial to assess the lethality of the plan: degree of effort required, specificity of plan, accessibility of means to carry out the plan. Assess for

Box 28–3
Physical Complaints and Depression

Frequently, individuals will feel aches and pains more acutely when they are depressed. The natural reaction to pain is to seek help from a primary medical healthcare provider. There is a strong correlation between depression and pain, with either chronic pain causing depression or depression causing pain (Hall-Flavin, 2016). It is important for individuals who are experiencing depression to talk to their healthcare providers about other experiences and symptoms during their lifetime.

More than two thirds of patients diagnosed with depression express concerns with somatic symptoms and reports of pain (Bai et al., 2014; Bair et al., 2003). The implications of pain in patients with depression are serious: The presence of pain and other somatic symptoms may complicate recovery and remission (Karp et al., 2005; Kroenke et al., 2008). Traditionally, pain and somatic symptoms accompanying depression were attributed to a psychologic reaction. However, there is increasing evidence that neurobiology plays a role (Bai et al., 2014).

Many people—perhaps as many as two thirds of affected individuals—are unaware that they have depression (Andrews, 2016). They are more likely to assume that not enjoying their usual activities, experiencing changes in eating or sleeping habits, and feeling bad in one way or another are caused by a physical problem. Determining the real cause of distress will help to ensure effective responses to treatment.

history of prior suicide attempts or family history of suicide, as this signals increased risk. Note that asking about suicide will not "plant the idea" in the patient's mind. Rather, it is often a relief for the patient to be able to openly discuss these feelings and thoughts. See the Independent Interventions section and the exemplar on suicide for more information.

Assess for Comorbidities

Assess for the presence of medical illnesses. This is important not only to rule out the possibility of an underlying medical condition causing the patient's symptoms of depression, but also to identify illnesses that may trigger depression. These include autoimmune, oncologic, metabolic, and endocrine disorders. Chronic illnesses, such as asthma and diabetes, are associated with increased risk of depression. A diagnosis of a chronic or life-threatening illness may also trigger a depressive episode.

Alcohol, which is a CNS depressant, and certain legal and illegal drugs can cause or complicate depression. Through matter-of-fact questioning, obtain a complete list of all substances and medications the patient uses. A few prescription medications (such as beta-blockers and steroid medications) have depression as a side effect, and they should not be overlooked in the complete assessment (Halverson, 2016).

Diagnosis

A number of nursing diagnoses may be appropriate for patients with depression, including the following:

- *Self-Directed Violence, Risk for*
- *Situational Low Self-Esteem or Chronic Low Self-Esteem*
- *Hopelessness*
- *Social Isolation*
- *Health Maintenance, Ineffective*
- *Coping, Ineffective.*

(NANDA-I © 2014)

Planning

When planning care, the nurse's immediate priority should be to ensure that patients with depression remain free from injury and refrain from attempts to hurt themselves or others. Other high-priority goals include alleviating any vegetative symptoms, ensuring adequate nutritional intake, and promoting restful sleep. Then, together with the patient, the nurse should design a plan of care that may include any of the following objectives:

- The patient will engage in necessary daily self-care activities (e.g., eating three meals a day, wearing clean clothes, and bathing regularly).
- The patient will resume normal activity patterns, such as returning to work or school.
- The patient will seek and engage in meaningful social interactions.
- The patient will articulate taking steps to feeling better, such as adopting healthy lifestyle behaviors (e.g., exercise) or engaging in recreational activities or exercise *before* beginning to feel better.
- The patient will comply with all aspects of the treatment regimen, including pharmacologic and/or psychologic therapy.
- The patient will describe feelings of hope for the future.

Implementation

When implementing interventions designed to help patients with depression, keep two general principles in mind:

1. It is impossible to make patients with depression feel better by being cheerful. In fact, an overly cheerful attitude tends to make them feel even worse because it trivializes or minimizes the impact of their feelings. Try to adopt a more emotionally neutral attitude while maintaining confidence that they will feel better.
2. Recognize that working with patients with depression may eventually lower your own mood and make you feel "down" yourself. This is called *emotional contagion*. The nurse should be aware of personal feelings and, if necessary, ask to be assigned to a different type of patient for a time.

Interventions to address risk for suicide and self-harm are detailed in the exemplar on suicide. For patients with severe depression who manifest vegetative symptoms and altered thought processes, the nurse will facilitate pharmacologic and collaborative therapies as ordered; assess and facilitate orientation to person, place, time, and circumstance; promote adequate nutrition and rest; and take other actions to promote recovery such as reducing environmental stimuli and other potential triggers of anxiety.

Many patients with depression experience problems with self-esteem and social interaction as a result of their illness. Progression toward recovery requires that patients address these areas. Nursing interventions to promote self-esteem and social interaction follow.

Improve Self-Esteem

Although low self-esteem is a chronic problem, the nurse can take a number of actions to reduce negative thinking, thereby promoting improved self-esteem:

- Encourage patient participation in recreational activities. Simple conversation with a staff member or another patient helps interrupt the pattern of negative thoughts. Use care to identify activities that are not too complex for the patient's current level of functioning. Experiences of success, not more failures, are needed.

- Give positive, matter-of-fact reinforcement, such as "I notice that you combed your hair," rather than overly enthusiastic compliments or excessive praise such as "What a great hairstyle!" Appropriate recognition increases the likelihood that the patient will continue the positive behavior, while insincerity can be perceived as ridicule or infantilizing.

- Be accepting of patients' negative feelings, but set limits on the amount of time spent discussing accounts of past failures. Be alert for opportunities to interrupt negative conversational patterns with more neutral ones.

- Teach assertiveness techniques, such as the ability to say "no" to protect one's rights while respecting the rights of others. Patients with low self-esteem often allow others to take advantage of them. Practice these techniques with the patient, providing feedback on how it feels to be the recipient of assertive communication or an assertive action.

Instill Hope

It is equally important to help patients identify the aspects of their lives that are not within their control. Being able to accept what *cannot* be changed is just as essential as developing the ability to bring about positive change. This skill is particularly helpful in reorienting patients from feelings of hopelessness to a more hopeful aspect. Other interventions to help patients combat hopelessness include the following:

- Help patients identify their personal strengths. It may be useful to write these down. Recognize that it often takes time for patients to realize that they have any strengths. Recognizing strengths helps a patient design an activity or engagement plan that the patient is more likely to enjoy and find successful.

- Help patients weigh and choose alternatives. Taking responsibility even for small choices, such as when or where to eat, helps the patient regain self-esteem.

- Explore problem-solving models with the patient, including practicing problem solving. "When you found out the toaster was broken, you threw it against the wall. You said all that did was put a dent in the wall and make a mess for you to clean up. What might you do differently next time that might be more helpful?"

- Help patients to identify resources such as family, community, or friends who can provide support and encouragement in overcoming problems they identify.

Planning for discharge should begin with the first patient contact and is particularly important with hopeless, dependent patients. Help these patients and their families and significant others identify resources in the community they can use to build support systems. Support groups, therapy groups, and social groups can help patients separate from caregivers more readily when the time comes to end therapy.

Evaluation

Patient progress is evaluated based on the ability to meet the expected outcomes. These should be modified based on each patient's unique situation. Some examples of goal-based outcomes for patients with depression include:

- The patient does not express suicidal ideation or a desire to harm self or others.

- The patient is free from vegetative symptoms.

- The patient obtains adequate nutrition and sleep.

- The patient meets daily self-care needs.

- The patient resumes normal activity patterns.

- The patient participates in recreational activities and meaningful social interactions.

- The patient engages in specific steps intended to make him/her feel better.

- The patient adheres to all aspects of the treatment regimen.

Secondary interventions will need to be initiated if goals are not met with the current plan of care. Explore reasons that goals were not met, such as unresolved stressors, lack of adherence to the treatment regimen, or the possibility that a comorbid mental illness or an underlying medical condition has not been identified. If there are no identifiable causes of poor response to treatment, then secondary interventions will need to be implemented. These may include giving the patient additional time to allow the medication to take effect or to meet a goal or working with the treatment team to find a different medication or treatment approach.

Patient Teaching
Increasing Self-Esteem

Patients often believe that **when** they feel better, they will want to engage in activities. For patients who express this belief, implement patient teaching and explain that the patient must begin doing things **in order** to feel better. Being active promotes a more balanced feeling state. Encourage the patient to acknowledge that it takes self-discipline and energy to do something when he does not really feel like it. Other strategies that may help the patient increase self-esteem include helping the patient to set daily, weekly, and monthly goals that are easily achievable, which is likely to improve the patient's self-esteem as each goal is met. As self-esteem improves, the goals should become increasingly harder to meet but still achievable.

Nursing Care Plan
A Patient with Depression

ASSESSMENT

You are the hospice nurse assigned to Pam Allen, who is dying of cancer. During your assessment of her husband, Clifford Allen, he discloses the following:

- He was diagnosed with depression years ago but is not currently receiving treatment.
- Years ago his brother committed suicide.
- He feels helpless about Pam's situation. He says that he has been a terrible husband and father.
- He is not currently receiving any treatment for depression.
- He has two or three alcoholic drinks every night after Pam goes to bed.
- He is not sure how he is going to cope with caring for their son, Gary, who has Down syndrome, after Pam is gone.

DIAGNOSES

- *Powerlessness*
- *Grieving*
- *Situational Low Self-Esteem*
- *Caregiver Role Strain, Risk for*
- *Health Maintenance, Ineffective*
- *Anxiety*

(NANDA-I © 2014)

PLANNING

The next day the hospice nurse talks further with Mr. Allen. Together they create a plan of care that will help Mr. Allen:

- Investigate resources for helping him care for Gary.
- Develop a plan of exercise and recreation.
- Stop drinking.
- Begin treatment for depression as recommended by a mental health professional.

IMPLEMENTATION

- Provide teaching to Mr. Allen about the need to begin treatment for depression again in order to prevent deterioration in mood and affect.
- Refer Mr. Allen to a mental health professional for diagnosis and treatment.
- Encourage Mr. Allen to explore his feelings regarding his wife's terminal condition and what his life will be like after her death.
- Encourage Mr. Allen to talk with his wife about her wishes regarding her death and funeral care in order to take a more active role in meeting her needs.
- Educate Mr. Allen on the effects of alcohol as a central nervous system depressant.
- Educate Mr. Allen on how to implement effective coping skills and identify ineffective coping skills.

- Support Mr. Allen's need to grieve for his wife and help him recognize that sadness is a normal part of the process.
- Encourage Mr. Allen to see that maintaining his own health is an important contribution to both Pam's and Gary's care.
- Refer Mr. Allen to agencies serving patients with disabilities to determine what assistance may be available to help him care for Gary.
- Help Mr. Allen develop a plan of exercise and recreation.
- Support Mr. Allen's need to obtain assistance in caring for Pam and Gary to reduce caregiver role strain.
- Provide a list of community resources to Mr. Allen.

EVALUATION

- Mr. Allen demonstrates improvement by meeting the following expected outcomes:
- He begins seeing a mental health professional to treat depression.
- He is taking medications as prescribed.
- He has quit drinking alcohol.
- He finds a daycare program that specializes in treating adults with Down syndrome.

- He discusses his wife's terminal condition with her, her desires for end-of-life care, and her postmortem wishes.
- He learns that his medical insurance will pay for someone to come to the home to provide for Pam's care 4 hours a day and initiates these visits immediately.

CRITICAL THINKING

1. What expected outcome would you anticipate for Mr. Allen if he fails to obtain treatment for depression?

2. What community programs might you suggest to Mr. Allen to help him care for Gary and Pam?

3. What follow-up care can the hospice nurse provide Mr. Allen when making daily visits to Pam?

REVIEW Depression

RELATE Link the Concepts and Exemplars

Linking the exemplar of depressive disorders with the concept of addiction:

1. Why might dependence on alcohol promote depression?

2. What impact might dependence on nicotine have on mood and affect?

Linking the exemplar of depressive disorders with the concept of elimination:

3. What aspects of depression increase the risk for constipation?

4. How might alterations in elimination put an older patient at risk for depression?

READY Go to Volume 3: Clinical Nursing Skills

REFLECT Apply Your Knowledge

Melvin Thomas is a 14-year-old boy whose mother brings him to their family physician's office because this is the third day in a row that Melvin "hasn't felt well." Melvin has been getting in trouble at school for arguing with teachers, and he has missed a lot of school, complaining of stomachaches. Melvin's mother says that he rarely sees his dad but that her second husband tries to spend time with Melvin when he can. When they do spend time together, they go shooting at the gun range or play video games. Melvin's expression at the physician's office is sullen, and he keeps his arms crossed in front of him. He answers the nurse by giving one-syllable responses or by nodding or shaking his head.

1. What assessment findings would make you suspect Melvin is depressed?

2. What priority teaching would you want to provide Melvin's mother if the diagnosis of depression is confirmed?

3. What impact is depression having on Melvin's ability to meet developmental milestones?

≫ Exemplar 28.B
Bipolar Disorders

Exemplar Learning Outcomes

28.B Analyze bipolar disorders and relevant nursing care.

- Describe the pathophysiology of bipolar disorders.
- Describe the etiology of bipolar disorders.
- Compare the risk factors and prevention of bipolar disorders.
- Identify the clinical manifestations of bipolar disorders.
- Summarize diagnostic tests and therapies used by interprofessional teams in the collaborative care of an individual with bipolar disorder.

- Differentiate care of patients with bipolar disorder across the lifespan.
- Apply the nursing process in providing culturally competent care to an individual with bipolar disorder.

Exemplar Key Terms

Bipolar disorders, *1942*
Cyclothymic disorder, *1944*
Flight of ideas, *1943*
Hypomania, *1943*

Overview

The **bipolar disorders** are a group of mood disorders that are characterized by manic, hypomanic, and depressive episodes. Cyclothymic disorder, a related disorder, is characterized by alternating periods of hypomanic and depressive symptoms that are not significant enough to meet the criteria for hypomania or depression. Although less than 2% of the population is diagnosed with bipolar disorders, these types of disorders can have a tremendous impact on those closest to the person with the disorder (APA, 2013).

Pathophysiology and Etiology
Pathophysiology

No definitive cause or specific pathophysiology has been identified for bipolar spectrum disorders. Rather, they are thought to arise from a complex combination of genetic, physiologic, environmental, and psychosocial factors. Studies have not found significant evidence proving that bipolar disorder is localized to a specific area of the brain. However, studies in adults have found that the prefrontal cortex tends to be smaller with decreased functioning in those diagnosed with bipolar disorder (Phelps, 2014). Immunologic abnormalities, including unusual patterns of inflammation and glial cell activation, may contribute to the pathophysiology of mania and bipolar disorder (Stertz et al., 2012). Mitochondrial dysfunction and oxidative stress also may be involved in bipolar disorder (Andreazza et al., 2013; Morris & Berk, 2015). Children of parents with bipolar disorders have a 4–15% risk of having a bipolar disorder. Stressful life events (especially suicide of a family member); sleep cycle disruptions; family or caregivers with high expressed emotion; and an emotionally overinvolved, hostile, and critical communication pattern are factors associated with heritability. Bipolar disorders, schizophrenia, and major depressive disorders share biological susceptibility and inheritance patterns. Several genes and loci have been discovered that may be associated with bipolar disorders, including glycogen synthase kinase-3β (Price & Marzani-Nissen, 2012).

Bipolar I disorder consists of one or more manic or mixed episodes, and the course of illness is usually accompanied by major depressive episodes. *Bipolar II disorder* consists of one or more major depressive episodes accompanied by at least one hypomanic episode.

Etiology

Bipolar disorders tend to be recurrent and have the unusual tendency to increase in frequency as the individual ages. Many patients return to normal functioning during remission periods, but approximately 30% of those with bipolar disorder will exhibit functional impairment at work. Of patients with bipolar II disorder, at least 15% will continue to experience dysfunction between episodes, and up to 20% will not experience any recovery between alternating episodes of hypomania and depression (APA, 2013). Bipolar disorders typically appear between the ages of 15 and 30.

Risk Factors and Prevention

Risk factors include a family history of bipolar disorders, drug abuse, periods of very high stress, and a major life-altering event. Women and men are at equal risk of having bipolar disorders, although women are more likely to experience rapid cycling and depressive symptoms and are at greater risk for comorbid alcohol abuse than men (APA, 2013). There is no identifiable way to prevent bipolar disorders; however, seeking medical treatment immediately upon presentation of mental illness will assist in minimizing the effects and prevent symptoms from getting worse.

Clinical Manifestations

The manifestations experienced by the individual define the type of bipolar disorder. Nurses must recognize these manifestations, understand how patients respond during various stages, and provide patient and family teaching regarding symptoms and treatments.

Key Diagnostic Criteria

The DSM-5 diagnostic criteria for bipolar disorder include criteria for manic, hypomanic, and major depressive episodes. The criteria for major depressive episodes are the same as the criteria for diagnosing major depressive disorder (see Box 28–2). The DSM-5 characterizes manic episodes as (APA, 2013):

- Lasting most of the day, every day, for at least 1 week, or any duration if hospitalization is required
- Including some combination of symptoms and behaviors to the extent that the individual's changes in behavior are noticeable and impair social or occupational functioning. Examples of symptoms and behaviors characteristic of bipolar disorder include distractibility, racing thoughts (flight of ideas), psychomotor agitation, increase in goal-directed activity, pressured speech, disordered sleep patterns, and grandiosity.

As with MDD (and any other mental disorder), the symptoms cannot be attributed to a medical condition or the effects of a substance. At least one manic episode is necessary to diagnose bipolar I disorder. An individual experiencing hypomania does not experience impairment in functioning or require hospitalization. In the absence of mania, the individual with hypomania may be diagnosed with bipolar II disorder if other criteria are met (APA, 2013).

Mania and Hypomania

Mania is characterized by an abnormal and persistently elevated, expansive, or irritable mood and increased energy (or activity) present for most of the time, nearly every day, or a week or more and accompanied by specific symptoms as articulated in the DSM-5 and summarized above. **Flight of ideas** (rapidly changing, fragmented thoughts), pressured speech patterns, and increasing goal-directed activities are common during manic episodes. Psychotic symptoms such as delusions or hallucinations may be a feature of severe mania.

Hypomania is a less extreme form of mania that is not severe enough to markedly impair functioning or require hospitalization. Individuals experiencing hypomania feel wonderful, "on top of the world," and do not recognize changes in themselves. Those who know them well, however, are aware of the changes in mood and behavior. There are no psychotic features in hypomania.

The onset of manic episodes usually occurs in the early 20s but may begin at any age. It often follows a severe disappointment, embarrassment, or other psychic stressor. The mood of patients experiencing a manic episode is euphoric, or "high." Their behavior is excessive and out of bounds. During mania, individuals typically exhibit overly enthusiastic involvement in projects of an interpersonal, political, religious, or occupational nature. When someone or something gets in the way or appears to put a snag in their way, they become irritable. Moods alternate between euphoria and irritability. Increased sexual behaviors are common, including flirting, making sexual overtures, having inappropriate sexual relationships, and feeling compelled to seduce and be seduced. Women may dress in an uncharacteristically flashy or seductive manner and wear garish makeup. Grandiosity can reach delusional proportions. Patients with mania rarely believe they are sick, even when they are in financial or legal trouble, and may vehemently dispute the need for treatment. The characteristics of a manic episode are illustrated in **Figure 28–5 》**.

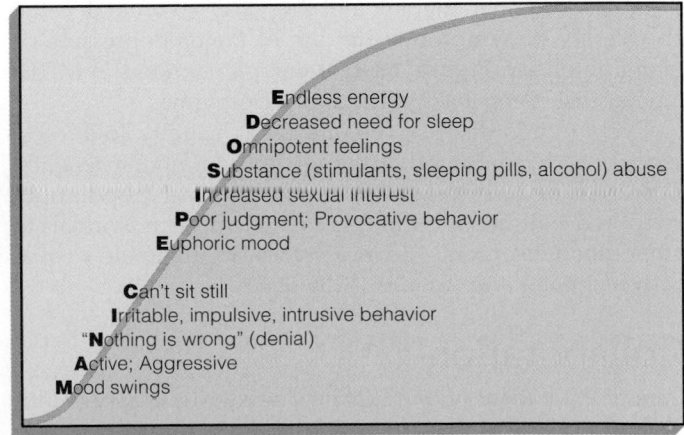

Endless energy
Decreased need for sleep
Omnipotent feelings
Substance (stimulants, sleeping pills, alcohol) abuse
Increased sexual interest
Poor judgment; Provocative behavior
Euphoric mood

Can't sit still
Irritable, impulsive, intrusive behavior
"**N**othing is wrong" (denial)
Active; Aggressive
Mood swings

Figure 28–5 》 Characteristics of a manic episode.

Depressive Episodes

A diagnosis of bipolar disorder does not always mean that manic or hypomanic behaviors will be manifested in the current episode of illness. Bipolar I and bipolar II disorder are characterized by periods of mania/hypomania alternating with major depressive episodes. Mood stabilizers are the drug of choice, so it is important when assessing patients who present with depression to determine if the patient has ever had a manic or hypomanic episode. Antidepressant medications should be used with care, at low doses, and only during the severe depressive episode to reduce the chance of switching to a manic state.

Many patients with bipolar disorders are not correctly diagnosed in a timely manner. This can mean that an individual loses years to an illness that could have been successfully managed if it had been correctly diagnosed and treated.

Mixed Features

The DSM-5 recognizes certain specifiers for bipolar and related disorders. These include a specifier *with mixed features*, which recognizes that depressive episodes may occur and be accompanied by symptoms of mania or hypomania, and manic or hypomanic episodes may occur and be accompanied by symptoms characteristic of depressive episodes (APA, 2013).

Rapid Cycling

Individuals with either bipolar I or bipolar II disorder may exhibit rapid cycling—four mood episodes occurring within a year with periods of partial or full remission of 2 months or more *or* with immediate alternate periods of mania/hypomania and depression. Individuals can experience episodes more than once a week and even more than once a day (NIMH, 2013b).

Cyclothymic Disorder

When patients have sustained at least 2 years of "chronic, fluctuating mood disturbance involving numerous periods of hypomanic symptoms and numerous periods of depressive symptoms," they are diagnosed with **cyclothymic disorder** (APA, 2013). They must be free of severe symptoms that qualify for the diagnosis of manic disorder or MDD. These individuals are often considered to be moody, unpredictable, or temperamental, and they may go on to develop an overlay of symptoms that are of major depressive or manic intensity. **Figure 28–6 >>** compares mood in MDD, bipolar disorders, dysthymia, and cyclothymia.

Cyclothymic disorder begins early, usually in adolescence or early adulthood. Although not common, with a lifetime risk of only 0.4–1.0% of the general population, cyclothymic disorder is thought to predispose individuals to other mood disorders. The incidence is approximately equal between males and females (APA, 2013).

Collaboration

Care of the patient with a bipolar disorder requires a multidisciplinary effort that includes the nurse, the patient, the primary care provider, a mental health specialist, a nurse case manager, and possibly a pharmacist as the team works to find a successful therapeutic regimen. The nurse should

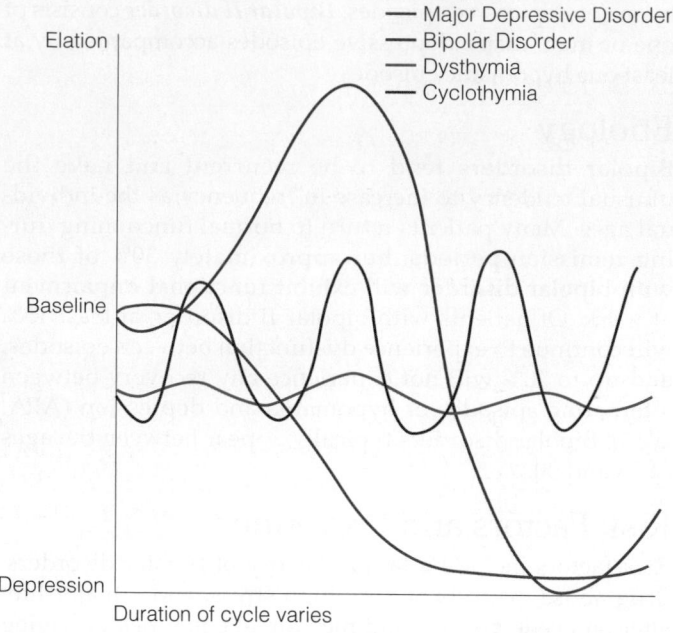

Figure 28–6 >> Comparison of affect (mood) in major depressive disorder, bipolar disorder, dysthymia, and cyclothymia.

take special care to encourage the patient to track feelings, behaviors, and side effects, especially during the first few weeks of trying a new medication.

Diagnostic Tests

There is no diagnostic test to determine bipolar and related disorders. Diagnosis is made on the basis of clinical manifestations and patient history. A physical examination, which may include drug testing, assists in ruling out the possibility of an underlying medical condition or substance abuse as the source of the patient's symptoms.

Pharmacologic Therapy

Hyperactive and agitated behavior usually responds fairly rapidly to antipsychotic mood stabilizers such as aripiprazole (Abilify), risperidone (Risperdal), and olanzapine (Zyprexa). The atypical antipsychotics, effective as mood-stabilizing medications, are often given in conjunction with anticonvulsive mood stabilizers. Because lithium takes 1–3 weeks before it is effective, atypical antipsychotics are used to help manage the symptoms of mania for individuals prescribed lithium until efficacy is achieved.

Nursing interventions include monitoring patients for adverse side effects of antipsychotic medications. These include extrapyramidal effects such as Parkinson-like symptoms (e.g., rigidity, tremor, or "pill rolling" movements of the fingers); dystonia, which is abnormal tonic contractions of the muscles (muscle spasms); and akathisia (subjective need to move, "jumping out of my skin"). Extrapyramidal symptoms should be reported and are usually treated by administration of an anticholinergic medication such as benztropine (Cogentin), diphenhydramine (Benadryl), or trihexyphenidyl (Artane). Acute dystonic reactions may be severe and require immediate medical intervention. These side effects can be distressing to the patient. The nurse must reassure the patient and explain what is occurring.

Clinical Manifestations and Therapies
Bipolar Disorders

ETIOLOGY	CLINICAL MANIFESTATIONS	CLINICAL THERAPIES
Mania/manic episode	Characterized by elevated, expansive, or irritable mood and increased activity or energy that significantly impairs social or occupational functioning and is accompanied by at least three of the following: ■ Increased self-esteem ■ Decreased need for sleep ■ Pressured speech ■ Flight of ideas ■ Distractibility ■ Increased involvement in goal-directed activities ■ Psychomotor agitation ■ Excessive involvement in pleasurable activities that carry a high risk of painful consequences	■ Assess for safety. ■ Administer mood stabilizers such as lithium. ■ Remove or limit environmental stimuli. ■ Set limits; teach limit setting. ■ Orient to self, place, and time.
Hypomania	■ Less extreme than mania; individuals describe themselves as feeling "wonderful" and do not recognize changes in their behavior, although friends and family can observe changes.	■ Assess for safety. ■ Administer mood stabilizers such as lithium. ■ Remove or limit environmental stimuli. ■ Set limits or teach limit setting.
Depressed episode	■ Symptoms of depression	■ Assess for safety. ■ Administer antidepressant with mood stabilizer.

SAFETY ALERT For patients with bipolar disorder, the orally disintegrating form of olanzapine may be prescribed to reduce instances of "med cheeking," where patients hide the tablet in their mouth or cheek until they can dispose of it. Valproic acid comes in liquid form, which can also assist with prevention of "med cheeking."

Several psychopharmacologic agents have proven effective in the long-term treatment of mania. One effective and widely used agent is lithium carbonate.

Lithium Carbonate

Lithium carbonate is an inorganic compound that has been used in the treatment and prevention of acute manic episodes since the 1960s.

Lithium alters neurotransmission in the CNS. It is thought to interfere with the ionic pump mechanism in brain cells, but its exact mode of action is unknown. Its use is not recommended during pregnancy and breastfeeding. Furthermore, it should not be used in patients with impaired renal function, congestive heart failure, sodium-restricted diets, or organic brain disease, as impaired CNS functioning secondary to these conditions places the patient at higher risk for lithium toxicity (Wilson et al., 2016). Administered orally, the onset of action ranges from 1 to 3 weeks. The dosage is gradually increased until the recommended therapeutic blood level of 0.8–1.2 mEq/L is achieved. Once the desired effect is achieved, the dosage is adjusted downward to the maintenance blood level of 0.6–1.2 mEq/L.

Patients who take lithium are at high risk for toxicity, because the difference between harmful and therapeutic lithium levels is quite small. Thus, patients' serum lithium levels should be determined prior to beginning drug therapy, then carefully monitored once therapy has begun. Note also that what is considered a therapeutic level for one patient might produce toxic effects in another patient. Accordingly, individual response to specific lithium doses must be carefully documented (Machado-Vieira et al., 2014). For example, individuals of Asian descent may respond to lower doses and blood levels of lithium, and therefore may experience toxicity at lower dosages than Caucasian patients (Quan et al., 2015). Monitor therapeutic effect as well as side effects.

Toxic symptoms begin appearing at blood levels above 1.5 mEq/L. Because there is such a narrow margin of safety, serum concentrations must be closely monitored until stabilized.

Antiseizure Medications

Medications used to treat seizures are often prescribed in combination with lithium or antipsychotic medications. Agents commonly used in the treatment of mania include valproic acid (Depakote, Depakene), lamotrigine (Lamictal), and carbamazepine (Tegretol). Side effects associated with antiseizure medications include drowsiness, fatigue, and weight gain. Typically, these side effects will decrease over time, but blood levels for some drugs must be regularly monitored to ensure that the patient is not experiencing toxicity. Pregnant women should not take these medications unless under the care of a healthcare provider. Caution patients not to discontinue these medications abruptly, but to consult with their prescribing provider regarding how to taper off gradually.

Atypical Antipsychotics

Aripiprazole (Abilify), olanzapine (Zyprexa), quetiapine (Seroquel), risperidone (Risperdal), asenapine (Saphris), and ziprasidone (Geodon) are among the atypical antipsychotics approved for bipolar mania and are becoming first-line treatments for bipolar mania. Olanzapine and aripiprazole come in an injectable form for use in acute agitation. These agents, especially the injectable forms, work quickly to calm the patient.

Lifespan Considerations

The rate of attempted suicide in those with bipolar disorders is high, as is co-occurrence with other disorders such as attention-deficit/hyperactivity disorder (ADHD), anxiety, and substance abuse, all of which complicate diagnosis (NIMH, 2013b).

Bipolar Disorders in Children

Children with bipolar disorders present with mood changes (such as being overly silly or joyful when that is unusual for the child) and behavioral changes (such as sleeping little but not feeling tired, and talking a lot and having racing thoughts) (American Academy of Child and Adolescent Psychiatry [AACAP], 2015). Some children may exhibit lengthy, violent temper tantrums. Older children may take on multiple tasks simultaneously and develop grandiose plans for their projects (APA, 2013). Children must be assessed based on their personal baseline, because children of the same age may be at different developmental stages. Taking into consideration the different developmental stages, it is difficult to define "normal" and "abnormal" behaviors.

Diagnosis of bipolar disorder may be made after other possibilities have been ruled out. Treatment of children with bipolar disorders may include medications to reduce severity of symptoms and psychotherapy to learn how to adapt to stressors and build relationships (AACAP, 2015). It is important that children be prescribed the fewest medications possible at the lowest effective doses.

Bipolar Disorders in Adolescents

The average age of onset of the first episode of mania, hypomania, or major depression is approximately 18 (APA, 2013), and the lifetime prevalence of bipolar disorders in adolescents is 0–3% (NIMH, 2013C). Treatment for adolescents will follow the same guidelines as are used for children. Because teenagers commonly show mood changes, including changes in sleeping and eating patterns, it is important not to mistake typical mood swings for bipolar disorder.

Bipolar Disorders in Pregnant Women

Studies suggest that women diagnosed with bipolar disorder are 5 to 10 times more likely to experience an episode during pregnancy. However, some women do experience their first episode while pregnant (NAMI, 2013). Stopping medications can worsen symptoms; therefore some healthcare providers will slowly taper the woman off medications, decrease the dose, or change the medication. If lithium is continued, serum lithium levels must be monitored frequently to prevent toxicity. The fetus should be assessed for potential heart defects, as risk for them increases with lithium use during the first trimester. In addition, lithium doses should be decreased at the onset of labor to avoid maternal toxicity at delivery. Women taking divalproex (Depakote) should be switched to another mood stabilizer before conception because of the higher-than-average risk for neural tube, cardiac, and craniofacial defects. Carbamazepine (Tegretol) is contraindicated in pregnancy (Freeland & Shealy, 2014).

Close monitoring is necessary for pregnant women with bipolar disorder throughout the pregnancy and during the postpartum period. Ultimately, the decision of whether to continue, begin, or adjust pharmacologic treatment for mood disorders is up to the patient herself. However, healthcare providers have a duty to educate pregnant women about the potential risks and benefits of both drug use and untreated mental illness (Kalfoglou, 2016).

Bipolar Disorders in Older Adults

Onset of bipolar disorder may occur at any time during life, including in the 60s or 70s. As with any patients, first episodes of manic symptoms presenting during midlife or late life indicate a need to perform medical testing to verify that there is not a medical or substance-related etiology. Treatment will be the same for older adults as for adults, although doses of medications may be lower. Older adults are also prone to experience more side effects and toxicity, requiring them to be monitored very closely. For example, lithium is contraindicated in older patients with kidney disease and should be used cautiously in patients with thyroid disease.

NURSING PROCESS

Because the nursing care of patients experiencing depressive symptoms is the same whether the diagnosis is a depressive disorder or a bipolar disorder, this section focuses on hypomania and mania, which constitute the other half of the bipolar continuum of behaviors. For all patients, assess personal history of cyclical patterns and triggers. Common triggers include changes in sleep patterns, negative life events (such a breaking up with a partner or losing a job), and use of alcohol or drugs. Early identification of triggers can assist with early identification of helpful interventions and improve patient outcomes (Koenders et al., 2014; Proudfoot et al., 2012).

Assessment

- ***Observation and patient interview.*** Assessment of patients with known or suspected bipolar disorder begins with a thorough history and interview. Inquire about any past manic or depressive episodes or behavior, as well as family history of mood disorders. Ask about and observe for the signs and symptoms discussed throughout the Concept section of this module, taking note of their severity, as they may range from mild (in hypomania) to extreme (in a frank manic episode). The nurse should also investigate the speed of onset for any symptoms, noting whether it is gradual or dramatic.

  Patients who are experiencing their first manic episode are most likely to be young people in their late teens or early 20s, although adolescents are sometimes affected. Affected individuals may demonstrate or articulate any number of changes in mood and behavior, including:

- Rapid changes in affect, such as going from elation in one moment to anger and irritability in the next.
- Inflated self-esteem, sometimes to the extent of having delusions of grandeur. Delusions of persecution also may be a feature.
- Ignorance or denial of fatigue, hunger, and even hygiene; being too involved in activity to focus on physiologic sensations.
- Rapid, loud, pressured speech.
- Unusual appearance (e.g., dressing inappropriately and using garish makeup or being disheveled and unkempt).
- A surprising sense of well-being. Individuals who are hypomanic and those early in manic episodes feel wonderful and do not understand why people are upset with their behavior.

Cognitive alterations are another frequent feature of mania. Be alert for changes in the patient's thought processes, evidenced by statements such as "I feel like my thoughts are racing." In addition to racing thoughts, other symptoms frequently common during manic episodes include an inability to concentrate and being easily distracted by the slightest stimulus in the environment. Some patients also experience hallucinations, delusions, and other forms of psychosis. Family members may report poor judgment and impulsivity, as evidenced by shopping sprees, drug use, or sexual activity that is out of character with the patient's usual behavior.

With bipolar I disorder, impairments in adaptive functioning are common. This includes difficulties in occupational function, which may result in being laid off from work, being placed on a leave of absence, or being fired because the behavior is disruptive in the workplace. Individuals who have mania cause interpersonal chaos by behaving manipulatively, testing limits, and playing one person against another. If their attempts at manipulation fail, they become irritable or hostile, and such behavior further alienates others.

- ***Physical examination.*** Assessment of the patient's physical manifestations is also critical. The hallmark of mania is constant motor activity. During a manic episode, patients may not stop to eat. Individuals in a manic state do not rest, have disordered sleep patterns, and may go for days without sleep. Bruises and other injuries sometimes result from the constant activity.

Patients who are in a manic state are not usually able to cooperate fully in the assessment process. In many cases, nurses find it necessary to rely on their own assessment skills and secondary sources, such as family members, to obtain essential assessment data. Family members often can provide detailed information about the onset and progression of symptoms, as well as information about any previous episodes.

Diagnosis

Several nursing diagnoses are common in the care of patients who have mania. These include the following:

- *Injury, Risk for*
- *Social Interaction, Impaired*
- *Impulse Control, Ineffective*

- *Impaired Mood Regulation*
- *Imbalanced Nutrition: Less than Body Requirements*
- *Self-Care Deficit, Bathing, Dressing, and Feeding*
- *Sleep Deprivation*
- *Suicide, Risk for*

(NANDA-I © 2014)

Although the nursing diagnosis *disturbed thought processes* is no longer recognized by NANDA International, some mental health agencies may continue to use it or a similar phrase to organize care for patients experiencing delusions or other disordered thought processes.

Planning

Outcomes for mood disorders include the expectation of a return to normal functioning. While these will vary by patient, appropriate outcomes for a patient with bipolar disorder include the following:

- The patient will remain free of injury.
- The patient will remain oriented.
- The patient will use appropriate behaviors in a variety of social settings.
- The patient will maintain self-care.
- The patient will no longer experience sleep disturbances.

Implementation

With patients who are manic, maintain a calm, relaxed, but firm and matter-of-fact demeanor, particularly when communicating limits. The nurse's behavior serves as a model and can be reassuring to out-of-control patients. As with all patients, building a trusting relationship is important.

Patients experiencing mania may unintentionally engage in behaviors that encroach on or violate boundaries or attempt to manipulate situations or individuals to their advantage. Nursing interventions, such as setting limits, promote patient security and often enable patients to curb their manipulative behavior or give it up entirely. Setting limits also assists in maintaining safety on the unit. Nurses should use self-reflection frequently to make sure they are maintaining their own boundaries of feelings and emotions.

Nurses design activities to facilitate the patient's ability to interact with others by identifying needed behavior changes and assigning tasks that will improve the patient's interactions with others. This may require mediating between the patient and others when the patient exhibits negative behavior. Nursing actions should encourage and demonstrate honesty and respect for others' rights.

Forming a therapeutic alliance with the patient, discovering her expectations, and providing opportunities for interpersonal interactions have been linked with positive long-term outcomes for people with bipolar disorders.

Promote Patient Safety

Taking steps to ensure the safety of patients and others in the environment is a priority.

- Provide the patient with community support by supplying names and phone numbers such as a local crisis hotline or the National Suicide Hotline (800-273-8255). Having access to support in the time of crisis may be a lifesaving intervention.

- Assist the patient in scheduling appointments with the mental health professional to ensure access has been established.

- Monitor activities. Scheduling a program of appropriate activity interspersed with rest periods helps provide an outlet for tension while protecting patients from exhaustion. Appropriate activities include walking, exercising, or dancing with the supervision of an activity therapist and supervised vacuuming or sweeping chores. Avoid highly competitive activities that bring out hostility and overtly aggressive behaviors.

- Set and enforce limits on unsafe or socially inappropriate behavior when patients are unable to control their impulses. Matter-of-fact intervention rather than angry scolding is the most effective approach. Patients may respond to verbal reminders or redirection to safer and more appropriate activities. Remember to reward appropriate behavior with positive reinforcement such as "I enjoyed our walk today because you were able to walk with me rather than running ahead."

- Provide a safe environment by reducing environmental stimuli. For hospitalized patients, this means providing a simply furnished private room that has had all unnecessary items removed. It should be in a quiet location to reduce noise stimulation. Low lighting also can be calming to the hyperactive patient.

- Monitor for safety hazards. Agitated patients are more apt to forget or disregard safety considerations such as safe use of smoking materials.

Promote Reality-based Thinking

The patient in a state of mania may demonstrate thinking that is out of touch with reality. It is important to give reality orientation to assist the patient into reality-based thinking.

- Present reality by spending time with patients. Identify yourself, the time and day, the location, and other orienting information as needed. Engage patients in reality-based, somewhat concrete activities (e.g., discussing a current event).

- Consistency is reassuring to patients with altered thought processes. Establish consistency by following a schedule to help patients understand what is expected of them. Consistency also is enhanced by assigning the same caregivers to work with the same patients whenever possible.

- It is not therapeutic to argue or try to reason with patients who are experiencing delusions or other altered thought processes. Arguing with a patient often serves to harden the belief system and can impair the development of trust. Instead, use statements such as "I find that hard to believe" or "That is extremely unusual" to instill reasonable doubt as a therapeutic intervention.

- When patients communicate perceptions of altered reality, reflect their statements back to them for validation. For example, asking "Are you saying that your husband is trying to poison you with monosodium glutamate?"

can help a patient understand how her perceptions sound to others. You will recognize that patients are becoming less delusional when they make statements such as "I know this sounds bizarre, but. . . ."

Promote Improved Self-Care

Self-care may become deficient during an exacerbation of symptoms of bipolar disorder. This includes activities of daily living such as nutrition, hygiene, rest, and elimination.

- Well-being is compromised when patients do not receive sufficient nourishment and fluids for extended periods of time, particularly during periods of hyperactivity. For the inpatient patient, work with a dietitian to ensure that high-calorie finger foods and nutritious liquids are available on the nursing unit until the patient is able to attend regular meals. For outpatient patients or those preparing for discharge, collaborate with the patient and dietitian to determine patient preferences and create a list of easily prepared foods that the patient finds palatable and can make or eat on the go.

- Assist hyperactive patients who are unwilling or unable to bathe, brush their teeth, shave, wash their hair, change clothes, or use the toilet. Autonomy is desirable, so allow patients to do as much for themselves as possible with verbal encouragement. Reinforce any attempts at self-care with recognition; for example, "I see you shaved today, Mr. Adams."

- During a manic phase, the patient may be awake for days at a time with minimal to no sleep. Sleep deprivation may occur, which impacts cognition and may lead to high blood pressure and cardiac disease. Decreasing stimulation in the milieu will help the patient rest, even if only for short periods of time. While the patient is awake, encourage him to perform tasks that require sitting down, even if only for a few minutes. For more information, see Enhancing Rest and Sleep in this section.

- Incontinence of urine or feces is occasionally seen in severely regressed patients during mania. This can be very disturbing to other patients and staff and insults the dignity of the patient who is experiencing incontinence. Nursing activities include establishing a schedule of frequent, regular toileting. Accompany the patient to the bathroom every hour or half hour until "accidents" no longer occur. A more common elimination problem is constipation. Hyperactive patients suppress the urge to defecate and may become severely constipated.

Set Limits

All staff members must agree on the established limits and enforce them consistently. Violations of limits must have established consequences, also agreed on by all staff members. Patients must know what behaviors are expected and what consequences will result if they exceed the limits. Inconsistent application of consequences will result in a failure to decrease manipulative behavior.

Nurses should expect patients to give charming explanations of why they exceeded this or that limit but should not be disarmed by these explanations. They are another form of manipulative behavior. Matter-of-fact limit enforcement and the consistent application of consequences are essential in promoting adaptive behaviors.

Enhance Rest and Sleep

Patients in the manic phase of bipolar disorder appear deceptively energetic when they may actually be nearing the point of exhaustion.

- Design nursing activities to facilitate regular sleep–wake cycles. Monitor patients closely for signs of fatigue and make provisions for rest periods. Promote nighttime sleeping by limiting extended daytime naps.

- Sleep may promote the rapid resolution of first episodes of mania. Prior to bedtime, decrease light and noise and encourage quiet activities and pre-sleep routines such as listening to soothing music. A warm bath and a snack may aid relaxation. Administer medications that do not suppress rapid-eye-movement (REM) sleep, such as zolpidem tartrate (Ambien), as prescribed.

- If patients experience extended nighttime wakefulness, avoid engaging them in long conversations or otherwise stimulating them or giving extra attention at night. Firmly encourage patients to stay in their darkened room with the expectation that they will fall asleep. If they will not stay in their room, assign a monotonous, repetitive task such as folding towels or sorting papers to encourage drowsiness.

- When patients are able to sleep, avoid waking them for nonessential care or activities. Allow for sleep cycles of at least 90 minutes.

Evaluation

Specific patient behaviors indicate that nursing interventions have been successful. Outcomes that indicate the patient has improved include:

- The patient remains free from injury.
- The patient is performing adequate self-care.
- The patient is able to sleep through the night.
- The patient is behaving appropriately in social settings.

Secondary interventions will need to be implemented if goals are not met. As with depression, the time frame may need to be extended. Combination pharmacologic therapy may need to be implemented by administering both antiseizure medications (mood stabilizers) and atypical antipsychotic medications. The initiation of clozapine (Clozaril) or ECT may be effective when first-line therapies are not successful. It is important for patients to understand that finding the medication regimen that is effective for them is a process and not to become frustrated when adjustments need to be made.

Nursing Care Plan
A Patient with Bipolar Disorder

Mr. Grey, a 52-year-old engineer, is brought to the emergency psychiatric clinic by two adult sons at 2 a.m. Their mother called them to come help with their father, who has not slept in 3 days. When they arrived at their parents' home, they found their father working on a large landscaping project in the backyard that involved stonework, a waterfall, a fish pond, and extensive plantings of trees, shrubs, and flowers.

ASSESSMENT	DIAGNOSES	PLANNING
According to the sons, Mr. Grey has had three prior episodes of manic behavior, beginning when he was in the army many years ago. He was stabilized on lithium carbonate for years but stopped taking it about a year ago because he felt so good. The current episode began about 1 week ago, after he was passed over for a promotion at work. He then took a leave of absence from his job to create what he called "the world's first home-based theme park." Any attempt by his wife to talk him out of the project has been met with anger and renewed resolve. Mr. Grey angrily tells the admitting nurse, "I don't know why these boys brought me here. I need to get back to work! I'm going to get millions for this franchise."	■ *Sleep Deprivation* ■ *Caregiver Role Strain* ■ *Interrupted Family Processes* ■ *Noncompliance* (NANDA-I © 2014) Other possible nursing diagnoses may include: ■ Disturbed thought processes ■ Nonadherence	Goals for care include: ■ The patient will comply with instructions for taking medications as ordered. ■ The patient will sleep through the night. ■ The patient will be oriented to time and place. ■ Family members will return to normal activities. ■ Family members will support medication administration.

IMPLEMENTATION

- With Mr. Grey and family members, develop a plan of activity that will help Mr. Grey disperse energy at appropriate times.

- Help family members set and enforce limits. For example, "From 8 p.m. until 6 a.m., Mr. Grey will remain indoors, engaged in sleep-promoting activities or sleeping."

- Refer Mr. Grey and his family to a therapist who can help them learn how to orient Mr. Grey to reality when his mind begins to stray.

- Help Mr. Grey and his wife learn how to promote sleep by decreasing environmental stimuli in the bedroom and engaging in good sleep hygiene.

(continued on next page)

Nursing Care Plan (continued)

EVALUATION

Expected outcomes to evaluate the patient's care include:

- The patient maintains therapeutic drug levels indicating compliance with medication regimen.
- The patient and family report that Mr. Grey obtains 6–8 hours of sleep per night.

- The patient demonstrates orientation to time and place.
- The family reports a return to normal daily routine.
- The patient regularly attends counseling sessions.

CRITICAL THINKING

1. What patient teaching can the nurse provide to reduce the risk of medication noncompliance once Mr. Grey feels well and is no longer symptomatic?
2. What teaching will the nurse provide the family to help them cope with the patient's diagnosis?

3. How can the nurse assist the patient to meet his nutritional needs during manic phases of the illness?

REVIEW Bipolar Disorders

RELATE Link the Concepts and Exemplars

Linking the exemplar of bipolar disorders with the concept of family:

1. How might bipolar disorder affect parenting styles?
2. How might different family processes affect a child's treatment for bipolar disorder?

Linking the exemplar of bipolar disorders with the concept of nutrition:

3. How might bipolar disorder affect a patient's nutritional status?

Linking the exemplar of bipolar disorders with the concept of health, wellness, and illness:

4. What consumer education resources are available to patients with bipolar disorders and their families to help them maintain their health during periods of relapse?

READY Go to Volume 3: Clinical Nursing Skills

REFER Go to Pearson MyLab Nursing and eText

- Additional review materials

REFLECT Apply Your Knowledge

Brittany Mathews, who is 21 years old and attending college, has been diagnosed with bipolar I disorder and is in the manic phase. Since admission 2 days ago, she has been averaging 2 hours of sleep a night. The rest of the night she spends pacing the hallways and talking to staff. She is in constant motion and brags about how much energy she has. Her clothing consists of startling bright miniskirts, low-cut sweaters, and high heels. Every few hours she changes clothes and reapplies her makeup to match.

1. What strategies might the nurse implement to maintain Ms. Mathews's safety at this time?
2. What risks to health does Ms. Mathews face during the manic phase of her illness, and how can the nurse reduce these risks?

» Exemplar 28.C
Postpartum Depression

Exemplar Learning Outcomes

28.C Analyze postpartum depression and relevant nursing care.

- Describe the processes of maternal role attainment and attachment.
- Identify the clinical manifestations of postpartum depression and psychosis.
- Summarize diagnostic tests and therapies used by interprofessional teams in the collaborative care of an individual with postpartum depression.
- Apply the nursing process in providing culturally competent care to an individual with postpartum depression.

Exemplar Key Terms

Major depressive disorder with peripartum onset, *1951*
Postpartum blues, *1951*
Postpartum depression, *1951*
Postpartum psychosis, *1953*
Puerperium, *1951*

Overview

The postpartum period is a time of readjustment and adaptation for the entire family, but especially for the mother. The woman experiences a variety of responses as she adjusts to a new family member, postpartum discomforts, changes in her body image, and the reality that she is no longer pregnant. Alterations in mood may occur at any time during pregnancy. Up to 50% of women identified with major depression during the postpartum period began experiencing depressive symptoms while pregnant. Therefore, clinical recommendations indicate that all pregnant women be assessed early in pregnancy for personal and family history of depressive disorders, bipolar disorders, peripartum or postpartum depression, and postpartum psychosis (see **Figure 28–7 》**) (ACOG, 2015).

The **puerperium** is that time immediately following childbirth when physiologic changes that occurred during pregnancy begin to return to normal. **Postpartum blues**, often referred to as "baby blues," are a common occurrence after childbirth and may affect up to 80% of women after giving birth. Symptoms include mood swings; feeling sad, anxious, or overwhelmed; crying spells (often for no reason); decreased appetite; and problems sleeping. These symptoms are not severe and do not require treatment. They usually resolve within a few days or a week (NIMH, n.d.b). **Postpartum depression**, a depressive disorder associated with pregnancy, is now recognized to begin *during* pregnancy approximately 50% of the time and is called **major depressive disorder with peripartum onset** in the DSM-5. Women who experience a depressive episode during pregnancy typically experience severe anxiety, and panic attacks are not uncommon. Mood and anxiety during pregnancy and postpartum blues are both associated with greater risk for postpartum depression (APA, 2013). This exemplar discusses the psychologic struggles that women face after giving birth and how nurses can support them during this critical time.

Postpartum Blues

As stated previously, the postpartum blues represent a transient period of depression that occurs in as many as 80% of women during the first few days following labor (NIMH, n.d.b). Postpartum blues may be manifested by mood swings, anger, weepiness, anorexia, difficulty sleeping, and a feeling of letdown. This mood change frequently occurs while the woman is still hospitalized, but it may occur at home. Changing hormone levels are a factor; psychologic adjustments, an unsupportive environment, and insecurity also have been identified as potential causes. In addition, fatigue, discomfort, and overstimulation may play a role. The postpartum blues usually resolve naturally within 10–14 days, but if symptoms persist or worsen, the woman may need evaluation for postpartum depression. If an assessment was not done previously, the nurse assesses the woman for predisposing factors during labor and the postpartum stay. Several depression scales are available for assessing postpartum depression. Depression screenings should be conducted on all women at least once during the perinatal period. Women with risk factors for perinatal depression should be monitored more closely (American College of Obstetricians and Gynecologists, 2015). For women whose screenings indicate possible depression, mental health treatment should be encouraged and provided (Yazici et al., 2015).

A key feature of postpartum blues is episodic tearfulness, often without an identifiable cause. Often when the woman is asked why she is crying, she responds that she does not know. Cunningham et al. (2010) speculate that several factors contribute to the blues:

- Emotional letdown that follows labor and childbirth
- Physical discomfort typical in the early postpartum period
- Fatigue
- Anxiety about caring for the newborn after discharge
- Depression during pregnancy or previous depression unrelated to pregnancy
- Severe PMS (premenstrual syndrome).

Validating the existence of this phenomenon, labeling it as a real but normal adjustment reaction, and providing reassurance can offer a measure of relief. Assistance with self-care and infant care, rest, good nutrition, information, and family support aids recovery. Encourage the mother's partner to watch for and report signs that the new mother is not returning to a normal mood but is instead slipping into a deeper depression.

The psychologic outcomes of the postpartum period are far more positive when the parents have access to a support network. Women and their partners may find that family relationships become increasingly important, but the increased family interaction itself can be a source of stress. New parents also may have increasing contact with other parents of small children but find that contact with coworkers declines. Of great concern are women and their partners who have no family or friends with whom to form a social network. Isolation at a time when the woman feels an increased need for support can result in tremendous stress and is often a contributing factor in situations of postpartum depression, child neglect, or abuse. New mother support groups are helpful for women who lack a social support system.

Postpartum doulas can be of great help during this critical time. Doulas are professionals trained to help the new

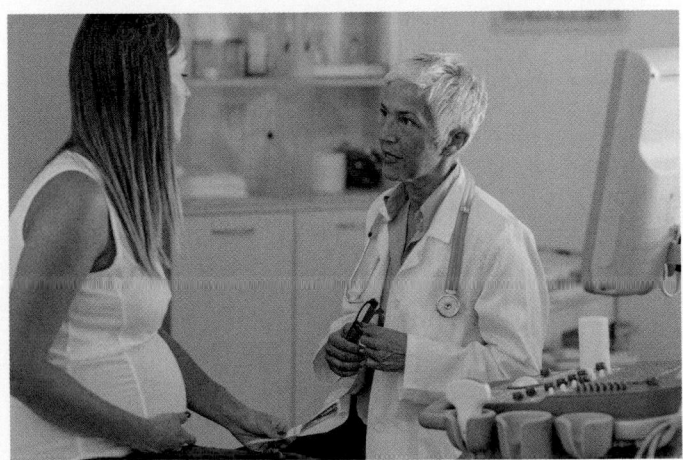

Source: Vgajic/E+/Getty Images.

Figure 28–7 》 All women should be assessed for depression during their pregnancies.

mother after the birth of the baby. As a "mother helper," a postpartum doula's services are tailored to help the new mother feel as rested as possible and be well nourished, and to place her household in good order so that she can focus her energy on her new baby.

Postpartum Mood Disorders

Postpartum Depression

Postpartum depression, or major depressive disorder with peripartum onset, is major depression that occurs during or in the first 4 weeks following birth. It has an overall prevalence rate of 3% to 6% in women during pregnancy or in the first 4 weeks following delivery (APA, 2013, p. 186). Postpartum depression may or may not be accompanied by psychotic symptoms.

Many of the symptoms of this major depression are indistinguishable from serious depression at other times in life: sadness, frequent crying, insomnia or excessive sleeping, appetite change, difficulty concentrating or making decisions, feelings of worthlessness, obsessive thoughts of inadequacy as an individual and parent, lack of interest in activities that are usually associated with pleasure (including sexual relations), and lack of concern about personal appearance. Persistent anxiety further contributes to the woman's feeling of being out of control. Irritability and hostility toward others, including the newborn, may be evident. Women participating in Beck's qualitative research on postpartum depression described a sense of living their daily life in a sort of fog, from which they believed they would never emerge. Once they improved, they often grieved over the time lost with their newborns while in this "fog." The duration of symptoms varies, but as many as half continue to be symptomatic at 6 months or longer.

Delayed treatment of major depression is associated with longer duration (Doucet et al., 2009).

Risk Factors and Prevention

Risk factors for postpartum depression include the following:

- History of depression, bipolar disorder, postpartum depression, or other mental illness
- Primiparity (first pregnancy)
- Ambivalence about maintaining the pregnancy
- Lack of social support
- Lack of a stable and supportive relationship with parents or partner
- The woman's lack of a supportive relationship with her parents, especially her father, as a child
- The woman's dissatisfaction with herself, including body image problems and eating disorders.

Women with postpartum depression are at risk for suicide, most prominently as they enter or exit the deeply depressed state. In a deep depression, the woman is unlikely to be able to plan and carry out suicide. For that reason, signs of improvement in depression should be celebrated with some caution. Whereas the woman with postpartum psychosis may attempt suicide because of illogical thought processes, the woman with major depression attempts suicide because her suffering is so great that dying seems a more favorable option than continuing to live in such pain. She also may attempt suicide to save her newborn from some perceived or real threat—including the possibility that she herself might harm the baby. The risk of suicide is greater in women who have attempted suicide previously, have a specific plan, and can access the means or weapon identified in the plan. The more specific the plan, the greater the probability of an attempt.

Patient Teaching
Primary Prevention Strategies for Postpartum Depression

Nurses can encourage pregnant women, new mothers, and parents to participate in a number of strategies to help prevent postpartum depression. Providing education to the woman's partner and primary support persons assists in the prevention or early identification of postpartum depression. Suggestions include the following:

- Celebrate childbirth but appreciate that it is a life-changing transition that can be stressful—at times it can seem overwhelming. Share your feelings with your partner and/or others.

- Consider keeping a journal in which you write down feelings. Not only is it emotionally cathartic, but it also provides a great memory book.

- Appreciate that you do not have to know everything to be a good parent—it is okay to seek advice during this transition.

- Connect to others who are parents—use them as a support and information network.

- Set a daily schedule and follow it even if you do not feel like it. Structuring activity helps counteract the inertia that comes with feeling sad or unsettled.

- Prioritize daily tasks. Decide what must be done and what can wait. Try to get one major thing done every day.

- Remember that you do not have to entertain or care for everyone who drops by. Doing something for someone else, however, often tends to make you feel better.

- If someone volunteers to lend a hand with tasks or baby care, accept the person's help. While your volunteer is in action, do something pleasurable or get some rest.

- Maintain outside interests. Plan some time every day—even if it is just 15 minutes—to do something exclusively for you that is pleasurable.

- Eat a healthy diet. Limit alcohol. Quit smoking. Get some exercise. (All of these can positively affect the immune system.)

- Get as much sleep as possible. Rest whenever you can, such as when the baby is napping. If you have other young children, bring them onto your bed to read or play quietly while you lie down.

- If things get overwhelming and you feel yourself slipping into depression, reach out to someone for help.

- Attend a postpartum support group if one is available. Also consider an international program such as Postpartum Support International, which provides an emergency contact phone number at 1-800-944-4PPD as well as a website at http://postpartum.net.

Focus on Diversity and Culture
Postpartum Depression

Postpartum depression is a universal phenomenon, not restricted to specific cultures. It is seen in both industrialized and nonindustrialized countries (O'Mahony & Donnelly, 2010).

The gender of an infant may influence the development of postpartum depression. In Sweden, births of boys were associated with recall of postpartum sadness in all ethnicities except those from the Middle East (Lagerberg & Magnusson, 2012). In Asia and some Middle Eastern countries, male offspring are highly preferred over female offspring (Grech, 2014; Purnell, 2014). Pakistani women who had already given birth to female children had an increased rate of depression when compared to those who had sons (Waqas et al., 2015).

An alarming cultural consideration in the United States is the disparity of healthcare for postpartum depression in low-income women. A study of more than 29,000 New Jersey Medicaid recipients found that Black and Latina women were significantly less likely than White women to initiate treatment for postpartum depression. Among those who did, Black and Latina women were less likely than White women to receive follow-up care, continue care, or refill antidepressant prescriptions (Kozhimannil et al., 2011).

Genetic Considerations

There is increasing support for the gene and environment interaction theory of depression and postpartum depression. Variants in genes that code enzymes affecting serotonin, dopamine, and noradrenalin (neurotransmitters affecting mood) were associated with development of depression in the peripartum period (Doornbos et al., 2009). Several studies implicated a serotonin-related transporter genotype in postpartum depression (Binder et al., 2010; Shapiro, Frasier, & Séguin, 2012). Other studies implicated monoamine oxidase–related genes in postpartum depression (Corwin et al., 2010). More research is needed to definitively identify the role of specific genes in postpartum depression.

Postpartum Psychosis

Postpartum psychosis (postpartum mood episodes with psychotic features) occurs in 1 in every 500 to 1000 deliveries (APA, 2013). The risk is increased in first deliveries, in women with prior postpartum depression, and in those with a history of depressive or bipolar disorder. Although relatively rare, postpartum psychosis gains considerable national attention when an incident of infanticide occurs.

Symptoms of postpartum psychosis include agitation, hyperactivity, insomnia, mood lability, confusion, irrationality, difficulty remembering or concentrating, poor judgment, delusions, and hallucinations that tend to be related to the infant. With appropriate treatment, most women experience improvement of symptoms within 2–3 months.

Postpartum psychosis is considered an emergency because of the risk of suicide and/or infanticide (Mayo Clinic, 2015a). The woman who is psychotic may experience delusions or hallucinations that support her perceptions that the infant should not be allowed to live. Illogical thinking or evidence of bonding difficulties may serve as cues to infanticide and suicide risk; however, this assessment is often challenging because of the lucidity seen in some psychotic patients.

Clinical Manifestations and Therapies
Postpartum Depression

ETIOLOGY	CLINICAL MANIFESTATIONS	CLINICAL THERAPIES
Postpartum blues	■ Mood swings ■ Feeling sad ■ Anxious or overwhelmed ■ Crying spells for no reason ■ Decreased appetite ■ Problems sleeping	■ Usually resolves without treatment within 3 to 14 days
Postpartum depression	■ Severe depression that occurs within the first year of giving birth, with increased incidence at about the fourth week postpartum, just before menses resumes, and upon weaning	■ Sertraline (Zoloft) or paroxetine (Paxil) ■ Support groups ■ Assistance with care of the newborn, taking care to promote self-confidence in mothering ■ Mental health counseling ■ Assistance with building self-esteem and self-confidence in mothering skills
Postpartum psychosis	■ Agitation ■ Hyperactivity ■ Insomnia ■ Mood lability ■ Confusion ■ Irrationality ■ Difficulty remembering or concentrating ■ Delusions and hallucinations that tend to be related to the infant	■ Lithium or antipsychotics ■ Should be supervised at all times when caring for infant or other children ■ Support groups ■ Short-term institutionalization may be required

SAFETY ALERT In all postpartum women, the presence of three symptoms of depression on 1 day or one symptom for 3 days may signal serious depression and requires immediate referral to a mental health professional.

Collaboration

It is not enough to simply refer women with a history of postpartum psychosis or depression or who are otherwise at high risk to a mental health professional for evaluation, counseling, and treatment between the second and sixth week postpartum. Clinical guidelines indicate these women require a detailed plan for psychiatric management during late pregnancy and during the early postpartum period. This plan should be shared (with consent) with the entire maternity team—e.g., obstetricians, nurses, and midwives. The plan should detail supports, contact information, and treatment considerations, including medications and breastfeeding.

Medication, individual or group psychotherapy, and practical assistance with child care and other demands of daily life are common treatment measures for both disorders; however, specific therapies may vary. Treatment of postpartum depression is not unlike treatment of any other significant depression: psychotherapy and antidepressant medications, usually SSRIs. The nurse's responsibilities as part of the healthcare team are discussed in detail in the Nursing Process section.

Diagnostic Tests

The routine use of a screening tool in a matter-of-fact approach significantly improves the diagnosis. The Edinburgh Postnatal Depression Scale (**Box 28–4 》**) and the Postpartum Depression Screening Scale (PDSS) are appropriate tools for use in assessing patients for postpartum depression. The PDSS is a 35-item scale that screens signs of postnatal depression such as cognitive impairment, sleeping and eating disturbances, emotional lability, guilt and shame, and thoughts of self-harm or suicide.

Pharmacologic Therapy

Treatment of postpartum psychosis is directed at the specific type of psychotic symptoms displayed and may include lithium, antipsychotics, or electroconvulsive therapy in combination with psychotherapy, removal of the infant, and social support. It is important for the nurse to realize that many of the drugs used in treating postpartum psychiatric conditions are contraindicated in breastfeeding women. However, systematic review concluded "(1) knowledge of pharmacokinetic characteristics are scarcely useful to assess safety and (2) the majority of antidepressants are

---

Box 28–4
Edinburgh Postnatal Depression Scale

In the past 7 days:

1. I have been able to laugh and see the funny side of things.
   As much as I always could
   Not quite so much now
   Definitely not so much now
   Not at all

2. I have looked forward with enjoyment of things.
   As much as I ever did
   Rather less than I used to
   Definitely less than I used to
   Hardly at all

*3. I have blamed myself unnecessarily when things went wrong.
   Yes, most of the time
   Yes, some of the time
   Not very often
   No, never

4. I have been anxious or worried for no good reason.
   No, not at all
   Hardly ever
   Yes, sometimes
   Yes, very often

*5. I have felt scared or panicky for no very good reason.
   Yes, quite a lot
   Yes, sometimes
   No, not much
   No, not at all

*6. Things have been getting on top of me.
   Yes, most of the time I haven't been able to cope at all
   Yes, sometimes I haven't been coping as well as usual
   No, I have been coping quite well
   No, I have been coping as well as ever

*7. I have been so unhappy that I have had difficulty sleeping.
   Yes, most of the time
   Yes, sometimes
   Not very often
   No, not at all

*8. I have felt sad or miserable.
   Yes, most of the time
   Yes, quite often
   Not very often
   No, not at all

*9. I have been so unhappy that I have been crying.
   Yes, most of the time
   Yes, quite often
   Only occasionally
   No, never

*10. The thought of harming myself has occurred to me.
   Yes, quite often
   Sometimes
   Hardly ever
   Never

Note: Response categories are scored 0, 1, 2, and 3 according to increased severity of the symptoms. Items marked with an asterisk are reverse-scored (3, 2, 1, 0). The total score is calculated by adding together the scores for each of the 10 items. A score above the threshold of 12 to 13 out of 30 indicates with 86% sensitivity that the woman is experiencing postpartum depression.

Source: From Cox, J. L., Holden, J. M., & Sagovsky, R. (1987). Detection of postnatal depression: Development of the 10-item Edinburgh Postnatal Depression Scale. *British Journal of Psychiatry, 150,* 782–786. Users may reproduce the scale without further permission provided they respect copyright by quoting the names of the authors, the title, and the source of the paper in all reproduced copies.

not usually contraindicated: (a) Selective serotonin reuptake inhibitors and nortriptyline have a better safety profile during lactation, (b) fluoxetine must be used carefully, (c) the tricyclic doxepin and the atypical nefazodone should be avoided, and (d) lithium, usually considered as contraindicated, has been recently rehabilitated" (Davanzo et al., 2011, p. 89). Recommendations are that a combination of antidepressants and psychosocial interventions be used regardless of whether or not the woman is breastfeeding. The woman and her partner should be reminded that antidepressants may take several weeks to have an effect. Providers may prefer to start antidepressants before the birth of the baby (usually at 36 weeks' gestation) so that a therapeutic blood level is achieved before the birth of the baby.

Support Groups

Support groups have proven to be successful adjuncts to pharmacologic treatment. In a support group of postpartum women and their partners, a couple may feel consolation that they are not alone in their experience. Moreover, the group provides a forum for exchanging information about postpartum depression, learning stress reduction measures, and experiencing renewed self-esteem and support. The most effective support groups provide for safe child care to facilitate attendance. If a support group is not available locally, the woman and her family may be encouraged to contact Depression After Delivery (DAD), now a national web-based support network that provides education and volunteers, or Postpartum Support International.

NURSING PROCESS

The priority of nursing care for the patient with postpartum depression is to maintain safety of both patient and family. Nurses may hesitate to assess patients for risk of harm to themselves or others for fear of introducing an idea that had not occurred to the patient. Not only is this not the case, but questioning the patient's thoughts of harming self or others can actually contribute to saving lives and should be a component of care for any patient experiencing depression.

Assessment

Because depression may occur during pregnancy, assessment of risk factors for depression and psychosis should be made early in the pregnancy and to encourage women who are at risk to seek professional mental health care (Yazici et al., 2015). In addition, pregnant women should be reassessed for manifestations of depression throughout the pregnancy and for up to 3 to 4 months following delivery. Questions designed to detect problems can be included as part of the routine prenatal history interview or questionnaire. Women with a personal or family history of psychiatric disease, particularly postpartum depression or psychosis, need prenatal instructions on the signs and symptoms of depression and may need additional emotional support. If one was not done previously, the nurse assesses the woman for predisposing factors during labor and the postpartum stay.

No matter what approach the nurse uses to assess for postpartum depression, enabling the woman to voice her feelings of maternal role transition and how she is adjusting in this vulnerable time is of inestimable value (Beck, 2008).

Listening to her story provides a critical emic (insider's) view of her circumstances as opposed to an etic (outsider's) view.

In providing daily care, the nurse observes the woman for objective signs of depression—anxiety, irritability, poor concentration, forgetfulness, sleep difficulties, appetite change, fatigue, and tearfulness—and listens for statements indicating feelings of failure and self-accusation. Severity and duration of symptoms should be noted. Report behavior and verbalizations that are bizarre or seem to indicate a potential for violence against herself or others, including the infant, as soon as possible for further evaluation.

The nurse needs to be aware that many normal physiologic changes of the puerperium are similar to symptoms of depression (lack of sexual interest, appetite change, fatigue). It is essential that observations be as specific and as objective as possible and that they be carefully documented. Beck and Indman (2005) found that anxiety was a prominent feature of illness for some women and suggested that women be assessed for their level of anxiety, particularly regarding infant care. Because of the strong association of interrupted sleep and postpartum depression and the finding that severe fatigue is an excellent predictor of postpartum depression (Corwin et al., 2005), assessing fatigue level at 2 weeks postpartum by telephone may be helpful in predicting depression risk early. Restorative sleep improves a woman's ability to cope and make decisions, thereby producing a sense of better self-control.

A central challenge for nursing is identifying women at risk of suicide. Asking the patient directly if she has thoughts of self-harm is best. If the patient responds "yes," she must be screened by a qualified mental health professional as soon as possible; she is not left alone until this has been accomplished. Family members also should be alert to signals that she may be intent on self-harm and advised that threats are to be taken seriously. Contact information for community mental health and crisis resources should be given to both the patient and family, along with the National Suicide Hotline toll-free number. Family members should be told to be especially vigilant for suicide when the woman seems to be feeling better.

Diagnosis

Possible nursing diagnoses that may apply to a woman with a postpartum psychiatric disorder include the following:

- *Coping, Ineffective*
- *Impaired Parenting, Risk for*
- *Risk for Violence: Self-Directed or Other-Directed.*

(NANDA-I © 2014)

Planning

Appropriate goals for the woman experiencing postpartum depression may include the following:

- The patient and family will remain free of injury.
- Family members and support persons will provide appropriate care for the newborn.
- The patient will articulate feelings and concerns.
- The patient will adhere to the plan of care.
- The patient will integrate the newborn into the family (with assistance as appropriate).

Implementation

Nurses working in antepartum settings (including the pediatrician's office) or teaching childbirth classes play indispensable roles in helping prospective parents appreciate the lifestyle changes and role demands associated with parenthood. Offering realistic information and anticipatory guidance and debunking myths about the perfect mother or perfect newborn may help prevent postpartum depression. Social support teaching guides are available for nurses to use in helping postpartum women explore their needs for postpartum support.

- Alert the mother, spouse, and other family members to the possibility of postpartum blues in the early days after birth and reassure them of the short-term nature of the condition.

- Describe symptoms of postpartum depression and encourage the mother to call her healthcare provider if symptoms become severe, if they fail to subside quickly, or if at any time she feels she is unable to function.

- Encourage the mother to plan how she will manage at home and provide concrete suggestions on how to cope in her adjustment to motherhood.

SAFETY ALERT Make an immediate referral for a mental health evaluation if the mother rejects the infant or makes a threat or an act of aggression against the infant. If any of these occurs, ensure that the infant is not left alone with the mother.

A diagnosis of postpartum depression or other psychiatric disorder poses major problems for the family. Depression interferes with the mother's ability to bond with the baby, which can cause the baby to have problems sleeping and eating and have future behavioral issues (NIMH, n.d.b). The father also often has a difficult time adjusting. The symptoms of these disorders are difficult to witness and may be harder to understand than physical problems such as hemorrhage and infection. The father may feel hurt by his partner's hostility; worry that she is becoming insane; or be baffled by her mood swings and lack of concern about herself, the newborn, or household responsibilities. He may be troubled by their lack of intimacy or deteriorating communication. Certainly, he has cause for concern about how the newborn and any other children are being affected. Very real practical matters—running the household; managing the children, including the totally dependent newborn; and caring for the mother—may be added to his usual routines and work responsibilities. It is not surprising that even in the most supportive families, relationships may suffer in response to these circumstances. It is often the father or another close family member who, in desperation, makes contact with the healthcare agency. This is especially difficult when the mother is reluctant to admit she is experiencing emotional difficulty or is too ill to recognize her own needs.

Information, emotional support, and assistance in providing or obtaining care for the infant may be needed. The nurse can assist family members by identifying community

---

Evidence-Based Practice
Prevention of, Identification of, and Interventions for Postpartum Depression

Problem

How can the risk of postpartum depression be identified early in a pregnancy? What is the most effective way to prevent postpartum depression? When it occurs, how can it be treated?

Evidence

Postpartum depression is a serious condition that occurs in 3 to 6% of women during pregnancy or in the first 4 weeks following delivery (APA, 2013). It often goes undetected, as symptoms may be hidden or misinterpreted. Untreated, the condition may have consequences for mothers, infants, and their families.

But what are the best methods for the prevention, detection, and/or treatment of postpartum depression? A Cochrane review examined this very question, and its results provide useful guidance for nurses and other healthcare professionals. In this review, Dennis and Dowswell (2013) analyzed 28 trials that collectively involved nearly 17,000 women. Some participants in these trials received standard pre- and postnatal care, while others received some sort of psychologic or psychosocial intervention. A variety of interventions were included in the review, including educational programs, CBT, interpersonal psychotherapy, nondirective counseling, and tangible in-person assistance. Some interventions were delivered in group settings, while others were delivered on an individual basis. Similarly, some occurred in the home while others occurred in the clinic, and some were delivered by professionals while others were delivered by laypeople.

In analyzing these interventions, the reviewers hoped to determine which programs and which delivery characteristics yielded the most beneficial outcomes. Their results were somewhat unexpected. In particular, there was no strong evidence indicating that pre- and post-birth classes, postpartum lay-based home visits,

early postpartum follow-up, continuity of care models, in-hospital debriefing, or CBT reduced participants' likelihood of postpartum depression. There was, however, evidence supporting the efficacy of professionally based home visits (e.g., from nurses or midwives), peer-based postpartum support via telephone, and interpersonal psychotherapy. These types of interventions were most successful when they included use of the Edinburgh Postnatal Depression Scale (EPDS) and when they specifically targeted at-risk women rather than the overall population of new mothers.

Implications

Nurses are in particularly good position to identify mothers at high risk for peripartum and postpartum depression. The EPDS should be an important part of these screening efforts. Once high-risk patients and/or patients who present with signs and symptoms of depression have been identified, they should be referred for additional support, ideally in the form of individually based interventions initiated postpartum. In-person interventions are most effective when delivered by a trained professional, whereas telephone interventions are effective when delivered by peers (Dennis & Dowswell, 2013). Some research also suggests that web-based, individualized, interactive interventions may yield beneficial results, but more research is needed before the usefulness of such programs can be confirmed (Haga et al., 2013).

Critical Thinking Application

1. Why do you think prepartum classes have little impact in preventing post-partum depression?

2. What advantages might peer-based postpartum support via telephone offer?

3. Why does postpartum care need to be individualized?

resources, making referrals to public health nursing services and social services, and providing a list of telephone numbers as well as emergency services that the mother may need. Postpartum follow-up is especially important, as are visits from a psychiatric home health nurse.

Evaluation

Expected outcomes of nursing care include the following:

- The patient's signs of depression are identified and she receives prompt intervention.
- The newborn is effectively cared for by the father or other support persons until the mother is able to provide care.

- The mother and newborn remain safe.
- The newborn is successfully integrated into the family unit.

Similar to major depressive disorder, postpartum depression may take time to resolve. The healthcare team will need to provide ongoing care for the mother, infant, and support persons, including integrating a mental health assessment into every postpartum follow-up appointment (O'Hara & McCabe, 2013). Regardless of the treatment provided, the safety of the infant, mother, and family must remain a priority for the healthcare team.

Nursing Care Plan
A Patient with Postpartum Depression

Salma al-Hussein, a 30-year-old woman who was born in Jordan but has lived in the United States for nearly 20 years, is brought to her primary care provider's office by her mother. Mrs. al-Hussein gave birth to her third child nearly 6 weeks ago. Her mother is worried because her daughter is showing almost no interest in the

baby and very little interest in her older children. Mrs. al-Hussein's mother and sister have been providing most of the care for the children. Mr. al-Hussein is a small business owner who works 10 to 12 hours per day, 6 days a week.

ASSESSMENT	DIAGNOSES	PLANNING
At first, Mrs. al-Hussein is slow to answer the nurse's questions and keeps her eyes on the floor during the assessment. Mrs. al-Hussein's mother says that her daughter is not normally like this, that she is usually full of life and outgoing and polite with others, even those she does not know well. With the encouragement of her mother, Mrs. al-Hussein becomes more cooperative. The nurse uses the Edinburgh Postnatal Depression Scale; Mrs. al-Hussein scores 14 out of 30.	■ *Parenting, Impaired* ■ *Powerlessness, Risk for* ■ *Impaired Social Interaction* ■ *Coping, Ineffective* (NANDA-I © 2014)	■ The patient will commit to safety. ■ The patient will express her feelings. ■ The patient will agree to participate in mental health counseling. ■ The family will continue to provide care for the children and support Mrs. al-Hussein as she begins the treatment process.

IMPLEMENTATION

- Refer to mental health professional.
- Attempt to persuade Mrs. al-Hussein to commit to safety for both herself and the children.
- Teach family to supervise mother's interaction with the infant and other children at all times to promote safety.
- Explain impact of postpartum depression to the family and help them cope with the impact on the family.
- Identify community resources for assisting with treatment.

- Encourage family to continue providing care for the infant and other children.
- Help Mrs. al-Hussein recognize the signs of depression and accept the diagnosis of postpartum depression.
- Explain to both Mrs. al-Hussein and her family members that postpartum depression is not uncommon and can be successfully treated, but risk for reoccurrence is high if she has additional children.

EVALUATION

Mrs. al-Hussein's care is evaluated based on the following expected outcomes:

- The patient begins treatment with a mental health counselor and is taking her medications as prescribed.

- Family members continue to provide supervision and care of the children until Mrs. al-Hussein's condition improves.
- The patient commits to safety for herself and her children.

CRITICAL THINKING

1. How would you persuade Mrs. al-Hussein to commit to safety for herself and her children?

2. What specific questions would you ask to determine if Mrs. al-Hussein is thinking about harming herself or her children?

3. If Mrs. al-Hussein admitted having fantasies of harming her children, how could you advocate for the family?

REVIEW Postpartum Depression

RELATE Link the Concepts and Exemplars

Linking the exemplar of postpartum depression with the concept of development:

1. How might a mother's postpartum depression impact the development of her 3-year-old daughter?

2. What is your priority developmental concern for the newborn when the mother has severe postpartum depression?

Linking the exemplar of postpartum depression with the concept of comfort:

3. What are your concerns for the mother who has postpartum depression regarding sleep and rest?

4. How will fatigue impact postpartum depression and the care of the newborn?

READY Go to Volume 3: Clinical Nursing Skills

REFER Go to Pearson MyLab Nursing and eText

■ Additional review materials

REFLECT Apply Your Knowledge

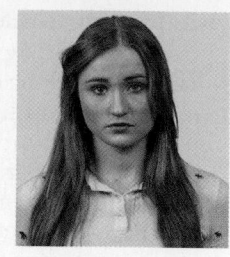

Jessica Riley is a single 17-year-old new mother of a 1-month-old infant son named Ryan whose father ended his relationship with Jessica when she was 4 months pregnant. Jessica's relationship with her mother has been strained for the past few years and worsened when she became pregnant. Because she was constantly fighting with her mother, Jessica moved to a small apartment when she was 6 months pregnant. Jessica's father left the family when Jessica was 7 years old. She recently completed her GED and is now trying to go to school part time for an associate's degree in cosmetology. She also works nearly full time as a waitress, but because she is supporting herself and her baby, she struggles financially.

1. What information in Jessica's history puts her at risk for postpartum depression?

2. How would you assess Jessica for potential postpartum depression?

3. What interventions can you implement to reduce Jessica's risk of postpartum depression?

» Exemplar 28.D
Suicide

Exemplar Learning Outcomes

28.D Analyze the nurse's role in preventing and responding to patient suicide attempts.

■ Describe the pathophysiology of suicide.

■ Describe the etiology of suicide.

■ Compare risk and protective factors for suicide.

■ Identify the clinical manifestations of suicidal ideation.

■ Summarize diagnostic tests and therapies used by interprofessional teams in the collaborative care of an individual at risk for suicide.

■ Differentiate care of patients at risk for suicide across the lifespan.

■ Apply the nursing process in providing culturally competent care to an individual at risk for suicide.

Exemplar Key Terms

Non-suicidal self-injury (NSSI), *1966*
Suicide, *1958*
Suicidal ideation, *1958*
Suicide attempt, *1958*

Overview

Suicide is the act of inflicting self-harm that results in death. When the act is not fatal, but the intent of the act was to cause death, it is referred to as a **suicide attempt**. Cases of an individual constantly considering, planning, or thinking about suicide are considered **suicidal ideation**. In the United States, suicide has become the 10th leading cause of death, even higher than homicide. In 2013, more than 41,000 individuals took their own lives, more than 1.3 million attempted suicide, and more than 9.3 million adults considered suicide (CDC, 2015).

Pathophysiology and Etiology

Depression is considered to play a role in many instances of suicide. Approximately half of those who take their own lives were confirmed as being depressed at the time of the incident (American Association of Suicidology [AAS], 2014). Further, an analysis of more than 46,000 responses to the Medical Expenditure Panel Surveys of U.S. Households in

2012 and 2013 found that only 28.7% of adults who screened positive for depression received treatment, and that uninsured adults, people of color, and men were less likely to receive treatment for depression than women and individuals with insurance (Olson et al., 2016). Lack of access to mental health care may result in underestimating the relationship between depression and suicide.

Influencing Factors

The majority of individuals who attempt or succeed at taking their own lives often cite a reason for wanting to die. However, suicide is generally influenced by a number of factors, not just one. By understanding the underlying causes of suicide, nurses can better recognize potential warning signs for suicidal behavior as well as identify individuals who are at greater risk.

Genetics and Neurobiology

Studies conducted over the past 15 to 20 years have indicated a familial aspect to suicidal tendencies in a number of cases. For example, an individual's risk for suicide is 5 times higher if a biological relative has committed suicide. Several neurobiological and genetic studies have proposed that genes and situational stressors work together to create the conditions for suicidal behavior. Parental suicide attempts appear to be among the most important factors contributing to suicidal tendencies, although there are inherent difficulties in teasing out how much of the increased risk is due to genetics and how much is due to dysfunctional family processes (Brent, Melhern, & Oquendo, 2015). Evidence also suggests that early traumatic experiences can lead to changes in gene expression (via epigenetic mechanisms) in the brain that render a person at increased risk for suicidal ideation (Rhodes et al., 2014).

The most commonly studied neurotransmitter thought to be connected with suicide is serotonin, which is also believed to play a central role in major depression. Suicidal individuals have been found to have decreased levels of serotonin, which can cause increased impulsivity and suicidal behavior (Larkin, 2016).

Interpersonal Factors

Individuals contemplating suicide can be influenced by a number of interpersonal factors, such as a history of being abused, a history of being raped, loneliness, a recent separation from a significant other, and grief from the passing of a friend or loved one. Any significant emotional disturbance can cause an individual to become depressed, and if the depression becomes unmanageable, that may lead to suicidal thoughts and behaviors. Loss and grief can be profound influencing factors for suicidal behavior, especially if loss is of significant importance. Individuals who have lost a partner—especially those without other close family ties—should be monitored closely for warning signs of dangerous behavior.

Situations that take away an aspect of an individual's control over life also may increase an individual's risk for suicide. Events such as unemployment and financial difficulties, the loss of a home, or another extremely stressful event can cause some individuals to despair of the possibility that life can improve or that they can feel something other than hopelessness. Feelings of hopelessness such as these are at the root of many cases of suicide. The individual may come to believe that the easiest, and only, way to handle the loss is to kill herself.

Comorbid Disorders

Approximately 90% of those who attempt or commit suicide have a comorbid disorder. Many of these disorders involve an element of depression, and it is estimated that approximately half of individuals who succeed at taking their own lives were experiencing depression at the time, or were in the recovery phase of depression (AAS, 2014). The most common comorbid disorders for suicide are bipolar disorder, borderline personality disorders, conduct disorders, schizophrenia, and drug and alcohol dependency. All of these disorders have aspects of impaired impulse control, depression, and altered consciousness, thus making them the primary disorders associated with suicide attempts and completion (Hooley et al., 2017).

Individuals with bipolar disorder are 15 to 20 times more likely to commit suicide than the general population. It is estimated that 25–50% of those with the disorder will attempt suicide at some point in their lives. Note that the risk for suicide among individuals with bipolar disorder decreases considerably with active treatment. The most commonly studied treatment associated with decreased suicide risk was administration of lithium (Lewitzka et al., 2015).

Numerous studies have shown that individuals with recurrent mood disorders have the highest risk of suicide. The general population has a 1.4% risk of committing suicide, whereas individuals with schizophrenia are shown to have a 10–13% risk. Those with alcohol dependency carry a 3–4% risk of suicide. Individuals with borderline personality disorder are often plagued with feelings of hopelessness and depression, making the prevalence of attempted and committed suicide quite high within that population. Similarly, conduct disorders and antisocial personality disorders are seen as predictors for suicidal behavior (Hooley et al., 2017).

Social Factors

Recessions, bullies, and/or dominant social beliefs can have an impact on individuals' mental health. Economic recessions can cause financial strain and job loss, which are both stressful events often cited as potential indicators of suicidal behavior. Economic recessions and high unemployment rates often lead to individuals defaulting on mortgages and losing their homes. Research indicates that there is a concealable stigma related to mortgage strain leading to feelings of shame and worthlessness. Concealing the mortgage strain due to the stigma leads to isolation, and isolation appeared to lead to the person's depression, anxiety, and emotional stress (Keene, Cowan, & Baker, 2015).

Bullying is another social factor that increases suicide risk. Bullies in schools or in the workplace are emotionally abusive toward their victims, harassing them to the point where the victims feel worthless or hopeless about life in general. Although many schools and community programs are working to eliminate bullying, it is still present across the country. Dominant social beliefs can also play a role. For example, bullying and discrimination have been linked to an increased risk for suicide among transgender and gender-nonconforming individuals (Haas, Rodgers, & Herman, 2014). Another study found that female refugees from areas sustaining genocide need preventive suicide measures (Levine et al., 2016). Additional groups that the Office of the Surgeon General (2012) reports at risk include individuals in the justice and child welfare settings; lesbian, gay, bisexual, and transgender (LGBT) populations; and members of the armed forces and veterans.

Etiology

A common theme that many suicide-attempt survivors report is that suicidal behavior comes from a feeling that death is the only option that will successfully solve the individual's current emotional strain (SAMHSA, 2015b). It is commonly said that suicide is a "cry for help," and while that may be true some of the time, suicide is a desire for a permanent solution to whatever catalyst has prompted the individual's behavior. Some who attempt suicide do so with the mindset that they would like to die, but if they do not, then at least others will realize how truly unhappy, or lonely, or desperate they feel. In cases such as these, a mild overdose of pharmaceuticals will often be used, or they will cause an injury that would be life threatening if no one found them in time.

Individuals who have only death in mind will generally use a gun, hang themselves, or jump from a tall building, because these methods are more likely to cause mortal injuries. Assessing lethality is important in determining patient suicide risk. Use of the scale for assessment of lethality of suicide attempt (SALSA) has proven to be useful in determining lethality. This scale has two components, with the first having four items indicating seriousness of attempt and consequences (for example, the method the individual has identified and the degree of medical intervention that will be needed if the patient uses this method). The second component is the global impression of lethality (Kar et al., 2014).

In cases where an individual has a comorbid disorder such as schizophrenia or bipolar disorder, the patient may report having been instructed by voices (e.g., command hallucinations) in their mind to commit suicide. If these voices have been present for the majority of the individual's life, the individual may find it difficult to ignore such commands. However, if some part of the individual's mind still has the desire to survive, he might employ less drastic means of suicide in an effort to both satisfy the voices and get help in stopping them if he is able to survive the suicide attempt.

Risk and Protective Factors

Risk factors for suicide in the United States include depression or other mental disorders; previous suicide attempt; a family history of abuse, violence, or suicide; substance abuse disorders; exposure to suicidal behavior; and firearms in the home. Other factors contributing to suicide risk include (APA, 2015b; Office of the Surgeon General, 2012; World Health Organization, 2016b):

- Social isolation; lack of support systems
- Recent unemployment
- Recent loss of a significant relationship
- Feelings of failure and hopelessness
- Access to lethal means (e.g., presence of a gun in the home)
- History of trauma or abuse
- Chronic physical illness, including chronic pain.

Other risk factors include gender and age. Men in the United States are more likely to die from suicide, whereas women are twice as likely to attempt suicide. Suicide is currently the seventh leading cause of death in males (Heron, 2016, p. 20). From the late 1980s to the early 2000s, older adults were at the highest risk for committing suicide of any age group. In 2014, the highest rate of suicide was among those age 85 and older, whereas the lowest rate of suicide was among those in the age group of 15–24 (American Foundation for Suicide Prevention, 2016).

Protective factors are "factors that make it less likely that individuals will develop a disorder. Protective factors may encompass biological, psychologic, or social factors in the individual, family, and environment" (Office of the Surgeon General, 2012). Examples of protective factors include the following:

- Strong family connections
- Community support
- Access to mental health providers
- Young children to care and provide for
- Strong ties to religions that denounce suicide.

Additional protective factors include caring for pets and use of healthy coping and decision-making skills (APA, 2015b; CDC, 2016a).

Clinical Manifestations

Although the clinical manifestations of suicidal ideation and behavior vary by age, culture, individual psychology, and life history, a few common factors underlie most suicidal behavior. Experts frequently cite impulsivity, aggression, pessimism, and an overall negative affect as personality traits associated with the condition. As stated earlier, negative events such as interpersonal crisis and financial catastrophe can play a role. The sense of a loss of meaning in life produces the painful, hopeless mental state conducive to suicide. Factors that predict suicidal behavior in the short term include major depression, psychic anxiety, delusions, and alcohol abuse. The fundamental clinical manifestation of suicidal ideation is the domination of the patient's consciousness by an unrelenting stream of painful thoughts. The suicidal person feels that death is the only possible solution to escape a mental life of unrelenting stress, anxiety, and depression (Hooley et al., 2017).

Behavior

Behavioral cues provide a window into the mind of an individual who may be contemplating suicide. Though not all people who commit suicide behave abnormally beforehand, many people provide clues that an attempt is imminent. An individual contemplating suicide may mention feeling helpless in the face of stress and may discuss life after death. He may also provide verbal cues such as "It won't matter for long" or "I can't take this much longer." Some behaviors may also demonstrate suicidal ideation, such as giving away personal possessions, withdrawing from relationships, and obtaining a means to end life such as purchasing a gun (Mayo Clinic, 2015b). It is important to note that some individuals may not demonstrate overt behaviors when suicidal. For example, data suggests that older adults may not report suicidal ideation (Cukrowicz et al., 2013).

The American Association of Suicidology (2016) developed a mnemonic device for the short-term indications of suicidal intent with the phrase **IS PATH WARM**. The letters in the phrase indicate the following terms:

Ideation	Purposelessness	Withdrawal
Substance abuse	Anxiety	Anger
	Trapped	Recklessness
	Hopelessness	Mood Changes

All of these terms are indicators of possible suicidal behavior, and concern for the patient's condition should increase if she exhibits more than one of these behaviors. An individual at immediate risk for suicide will often display the warnings signs of acute risk. These include talking of wanting to hurt herself; looking for access to firearms, pills, or other means of suicide; and talking or writing about death. If these symptoms are observed, the individual should not be left alone and a mental health professional should be contacted.

Cognition

Individuals who attempt suicide are more likely than their peers to experience distortions in cognition. Common distortions include (but are not limited to) unusually rigid thinking, dichotomous thinking, magnification, overgeneralization, externalization of self-worth, and "fortune telling," or predicting negative outcomes without considering the possibility of other, more positive outcomes (Jager-Hyman et al., 2014). After an unsuccessful suicide attempt, an easing of emotional stress typically takes place, especially if the attempt was expected to be lethal, and cognitive distortions often abate. Without appropriate treatment, however, this reduction in stress and distorted thinking is only temporary, and suicidal behavior frequently recurs. In fact, the year after an attempt, repetition of suicidal behavior occurs in 15–25% of cases, and there is an increased likelihood that the second or third attempt will be fatal. Long-term studies have shown that 7–10% of individuals who seriously attempt suicide will eventually kill themselves, a risk that is about 5 times greater than the average risk of 1.4% (Hooley et al., 2017).

Social Isolation

A common precipitant to suicidal behavior is social stress or isolation. An individual may become suicidal when he becomes alienated from family and friends, or even when he has difficulty adapting to the demands of new social roles. Loss of a loved one is a contributing factor related to suicide, as well as the loss of the ability to participate in once enjoyable activities. For older adults, the loss of autonomy, including a reliance on others to get around (e.g., loss of a drivers' license or loss of mobility) and feeling like they are a burden to others, contributes to the sense of social isolation and increases suicide risk (SAMHSA, 2015b).

Regardless of an individual's age, a stable social situation is essential to healthy mental functioning. The early 20th-century sociologist Emile Durkheim related the differences in suicide rates to differences in group cohesiveness and concluded that the best deterrent to suicide is a sense of involvement and identity with other people. Durkheim's thesis is confirmed by the prevalence of suicide among people living in disorganized families and people experiencing social isolation (Hooley et al., 2017). The link between suicide and weak group organization is also corroborated by the relationship between unemployment and suicidal ideation: Unemployed individuals are cut off from both their sense of purpose and their social network.

Cultural Considerations

Also within the United States, the various ethnic groups exhibit substantial differences in suicide rates. For example, American Indians and Alaska Natives have the highest rate of suicide, followed by non-Hispanic Whites. African Americans

Focus on Diversity and Culture
Suicide and LGBT Culture

Lesbian, gay, bisexual, and transgender (LGBT) individuals are at higher risk for suicide, in part, due to discrimination that they experience regularly from family, friends, colleagues, and society. Fear of non-acceptance may be a precipitant to depression and, if severe enough, has been known to lead to suicide.

- LGBT individuals are 2 times more likely to attempt suicide than heterosexual individuals.
- Gay and bisexual men are 4 times as likely to attempt suicide compared to heterosexual men.
- LGBT individuals are more likely to participate in suicide attempts and ideation compared to completed suicides.
- Increased risk for suicide in this population can be attributed to the presence of prejudice, stigmas, and discrimination.
- Adolescent LGBT individuals demonstrate a particularly high rate of suicide, attempted suicide, and suicidal ideation (CDC, 2017).

have the second lowest suicide rate, and the lowest rate is in the Hispanic population (NIMH, 2015). Suicide rates also vary significantly among national cultures. The United States currently has a suicide rate of about 13 per 100,000 (CDC, 2016b), whereas Greece, Spain, and the United Kingdom have rates of about 9 per 100,000. Hungary has a rate of about 40 per 100,000, the world's highest. Other European nations like Switzerland, Finland, Austria, Sweden, Denmark, and Germany have high rates due to a variety of cultural factors (Hooley et al., 2017).

Another cultural difference in the prevalence of suicide worldwide is gender disparity. Women are more likely to attempt suicide and men are more likely to complete suicide in the United States, but in India, Poland, and Finland, men are more likely to engage in nonfatal attempts. In China, India, and Papua New Guinea, women are more likely to complete suicide than men (Hooley et al., 2017).

Adherence to religious beliefs is considered to be a protective factor for suicide. Faiths such as Catholicism and Islam strongly forbid suicide, and rates of suicide in nations that follow these religions are accordingly low. Many societies have strong cultural taboos against suicide in addition to formal declarations. However, some nations provide cultural exceptions to the rule outlawing suicide. Japanese culture is one of the few societies in which suicide has been approved as a socially acceptable solution to certain problems of disgrace or social cohesion. The suicidal zeal for a political and religious cause has found a new form in the suicide bombings of Muslim extremists in the Middle East. Across cultures, suicide can be a violent expression of inner turmoil, or an act motivated by national or religious fervor (Hooley et al., 2017).

Collaboration

Suicide attempts and suicidal ideation, if caught early enough, can be addressed in a number of ways. The most common and effective method of treatment is to combine pharmaceutical interventions with talk or group therapy or counseling. For individuals who are also experiencing a

Clinical Manifestations and Therapies
Suicide

ETIOLOGY	CLINICAL MANIFESTATIONS	CLINICAL THERAPIES
Behavioral changes	■ Verbal cues indicating a desire to die or to "make it all stop" ■ Planning to commit suicide, including buying a gun, knife, or pills ■ Not participating in once-loved activities ■ Loss of interest in school or work ■ Participating in dangerous behavior such as drug use, driving too fast, or not taking safety precautions	■ Treat underlying condition ■ Behavioral therapy ■ Medication therapy ■ If a plan for suicide has been formed, make sure the person is not left alone ■ Educate about therapy options
Affect	■ Depression ■ Hopelessness ■ Loneliness ■ Anger ■ Anxiety	■ Treat underlying condition ■ Behavioral therapy ■ Medication therapy ■ Express a sincere desire to help the individual
Cognition	■ Rigid thinking ■ Fantasies about death or dying ■ Thought disorders ■ Preoccupation with death ■ "Fortune telling" and extreme negativity	■ Treat underlying condition ■ Behavioral therapy ■ Medication therapy
Social isolation	■ Life stressors ■ Poor support systems ■ Social pressure ■ Feeling as though there is no one to ask for help ■ Feeling alienated from society ■ End of a relationship ■ Death of a close friend, spouse, or family member	■ Behavioral therapy ■ Medication therapy ■ Group therapy to recognize that other individuals are experiencing similar issues
Biophysical changes	■ Sleep disturbances ■ Relapse or exacerbation of coexisting mental disorder ■ Potential physical evidence of self-harm (e.g., scars from cutting)	■ Address any immediate physical needs ■ Consider possible medical contributors to reoccurrence or exacerbation of mental disorder ■ Behavioral therapy ■ Medication therapy

comorbid disorder, the underlying disorder will need to be treated in addition to the suicidal behavior because the two conditions may exacerbate each other. Nurses will work with the patient, physicians, and therapists to create an effective plan of care.

Pharmacologic Therapy

Depending on the individual patient's manifestations and the presence of comorbid disorders, pharmacologic therapy may be appropriate for patients who are suicidal. The most likely choices of medications are antidepressants and mood stabilizers.

Antidepressants

The antidepressants most often used to treat depression (the underlying cause of the majority of suicide attempts) are fluoxetine (Prozac), citalopram (Celexa), sertraline (Zoloft), paroxetine (Paxil), and escitalopram (Lexapro). All five of these drugs are SSRIs and are used to balance and stabilize the neurotransmitters in the brain that affect mood and emotional responses. Although all of these medications are used to treat depression, they also have the potential side effect of causing suicidal tendencies. The use of antidepressants after a patient has attempted or seriously considered suicide should be combined with nonpharmacologic therapy.

Mood Stabilizers and Antipsychotics

Mood stabilizers commonly prescribed for bipolar disorder have the ability to moderate extreme shifts in emotions between mania and depression. Some antiseizure drugs are also used for mood stabilization in bipolar patients. For more on drugs for bipolar disorder, see the exemplar on Bipolar Disorders earlier in this module.

Antipsychotics (medications used in the treatment of schizophrenia) may be prescribed for patients who experience hallucinations and delusions or those with major depressive disorder with psychotic features. The treatment of these symptoms of the disease can help the suicidal patient immensely by eliminating one of the underlying causes of self-destructive thoughts. For more information about schizophrenia and antipsychotic medications, see the exemplar on Schizophrenia in the module on Cognition.

Nonpharmacologic Therapy

Therapeutic approaches to suicide prevention can be quite effective in many cases. The type of therapy employed will depend on both the patient and the therapist, but the three most common forms of therapy used for suicidal patients are group therapy, individualized therapy, and family therapy. All three of these forms can be combined to further help the patient work through her suicidal thoughts and behaviors. Family therapy will generally be used in tandem with either group or individualized therapy. The presence of the family can be very helpful in supporting the patient, especially because most individuals who are truly contemplating suicide will work to isolate themselves from friends and family before the event. Family therapy can also help the patient's family to understand what she is feeling and why she considered suicide, which can ultimately aid the family in taking an active role in supporting the patient's recovery.

Cognitive behavior psychotherapy for suicide prevention (CBT-SP) is sometimes used with adolescents who display serious suicidal ideation or have recently attempted suicide. CBT-SP works to help the individual develop skills to prevent suicidal behavior in the future. The therapy works with the adolescent patient to develop and employ healthy coping mechanisms and avoid all forms of self-harm (O'Connor et al., 2014).

Patients who are at risk for suicide or who have attempted suicide often benefit from therapeutic interventions addressing healthy coping mechanisms. Writing therapy can be employed to help the patient work through any suicidal thoughts or fantasies; similarly, a preoccupation with death and dying can be addressed through writing and keeping a journal. The journal will also serve to allow the patient to see the progress that has been made from the start of therapy until its completion, with the goal that the writing will change tone from potentially hopeless at the start to more positive and hopeful at the end.

Lifespan Considerations

In the United States in 2014, males were 3.6 times more likely to commit suicide than females. For adults, men between the ages of 25 and 44 committed suicide at a rate of 24.3 deaths per 100,000 individuals, and this increased to 29.7 deaths per 100,000 men between the ages of 45 and 64. Women between the ages of 25 and 44 committed suicide at a rate of 7.2 deaths per 100,000 individuals, and this increased to 9.8 deaths per 100,000 women between the ages of 45 and 64. Women between the ages of 45 and 64 had the highest suicide rate of any female age group (CDC, 2016b). Suicide rates for other age groups are provided in the following sections.

Firearms, suffocation, and poisoning are used for over 90% of all suicides. However, the preferred method of suicide

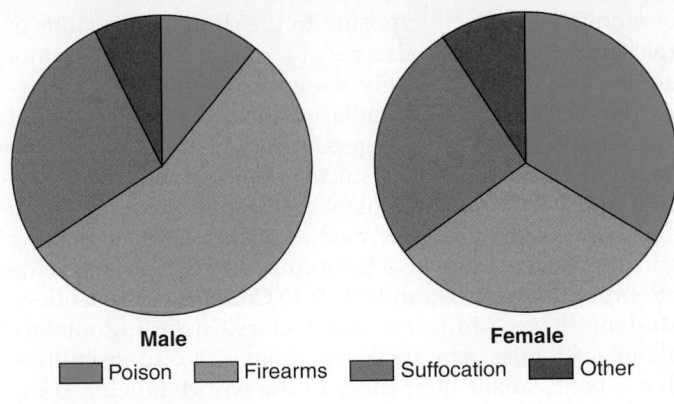

Male   **Female**

■ Poison   ■ Firearms   ■ Suffocation   ■ Other

Figure 28–8 ⟩⟩ Methods of suicide differ between men and women.

differs between males and females (see **Figure 28–8 ⟩⟩**). For the years in which the most recent data is available, 34.1% of females chose poisoning, 31.0% chose firearms, and 26.2% chose suffocation. In contrast, males predominantly used firearms (55.4%) compared to suffocation (26.8%) or poisoning (10.6%) (CDC, 2016b).

Suicide in Children

In 2014, boys between the ages of 10 and 14 committed suicide at a rate of 2.6 per 100,000 individuals, and girls in this age range committed suicide at a rate of 1.5 per 100,000 individuals. The increase from 0.5 (in 1999) to 1.5 (in 2014) suicides per 100,000 individuals represented the greatest increase in the suicide rate for females of any age group (CDC, 2016b). Children are at an increased risk for suicidal ideation if they have lost a parent, have been physically or sexually abused, have an unstable family, experience humiliation in school, or have lost a loved one. Psychopathology in childhood—including depression, antisocial behavior, ADHD, and impulsivity—is a strong predictor of childhood suicide. Suicide is the third leading cause of death in children age 10 to 14 (CDC, 2015). The most common means is hanging or strangulation. Statistics indicate that suicide is more common among Black children, especially Black males, than members of other ethnic and racial groups. Furthermore, more than a quarter of children who committed suicide discussed their intent to do so with someone else prior to their death. These findings highlight the importance of targeted prevention efforts, as well as not discounting the words of children who mention a desire to die (Sheftall et al., 2016).

Suicide in Adolescents and Young Adults

In 2014, males between the ages of 15 and 24 committed suicide at a rate of 18.2 per 100,000 individuals, and females in this age range committed suicide at a rate of 4.6 per 100,000 individuals (CDC, 2016b). Suicidal cognition in adolescents increases dramatically, most likely because of the collision of depression, anxiety, drug use, and conduct disorders in the teenage years. Adolescents and young adults may also attempt suicide because of a lack of meaningful relationships, sexual problems, and/or acute problems with parents or significant others. Exposure to the dramatic suicides of role-model celebrities also plays a role in the cognition of adolescents, who are highly susceptible to imitative behavior (Hooley et al., 2017). Similarly, suicide has an element of "contagion" among teenagers, meaning that adolescents are more likely to attempt suicide after learning of the suicide of a friend or acquaintance. In recent years, bullying and harassment via "new media" such as text messaging and the internet has also been linked to a rise in suicide attempts (Hawton, Saunders, & O'Connor, 2012). College students have additional risk factors, including anxiety about academics, new social situations and responsibilities, and anxiety about their place in the world. Suicide is the second leading cause of death among individuals age 15 to 34 (CDC, 2015).

Suicide in Pregnant Women

Suicide during pregnancy is not a common occurrence, despite the fact that pregnant women are at risk for depression with peripartum onset. The Centers for Disease Control and Prevention's Violent Death Reporting System indicates that there were approximately 43 women who committed suicide while pregnant between the years 2003 and 2007 (Georgia Health Sciences University, 2011). Relationship issues appeared to be contributing factors to more than half of these suicides. Older, White women were reported to be at greatest risk. Women are far more likely to attempt suicide in the postpartum period than during pregnancy, especially if they are experiencing postpartum depression or psychosis or if they have a history of mood disorders. In fact, suicide is believed to account for about 20% of deaths in women during the first year postpartum (Gentile, 2011).

Suicide in Older Adults

For older adults, men between the ages of 65 and 74 committed suicide at a rate of 26.6 deaths per 100,000 individuals, and this increased to 38.8 deaths per 100,000 men age 75 and older. Women between the ages of 65 and 74 committed suicide at a rate of 5.9 deaths per 100,000 individuals, and this decreased to 4.0 deaths per 100,000 women age 75 and older (CDC, 2016b). Men age 75 and older had the highest suicide rate of any other age group, and though older adults attempt suicide less often than individuals in other groups, they have a higher rate of completion because they use more lethal means. Further, many are not as resilient as younger adults. White men over the age of 65 make up 80% of those who commit suicide in late life (NIMH, 2015). One of the leading causes of suicide in the older population is depression, often undiagnosed, and the negative events that frequently come with long life: death of a loved one, illness, and isolation. Although most of the suicide attempts in this population are associated with mental illness, terminal illness increases the risk of depression and suicidal ideation or suicide. Terminal illness that causes pain and suffering is known to be a precursor to successful suicides. Suicide is the seventh leading cause of death in persons over the age of 65 (CDC, 2015). Interestingly, although older adults have higher suicide rates than younger populations, they are less likely to

mention suicidal ideation to their healthcare provider (Kiosses, Szanto, & Alexopoulos, 2014).

NURSING PROCESS

Appropriate, nonjudgmental nursing care of the patient who is suicidal is imperative. Nurses will work to ensure the patient's safety while helping empower the patient's need to refrain from self-harm. Every situation involving suicide is different, and nurses evaluate patients based on their individual cases and without any personal judgment or biases.

Assessment

Nurses working with patients who are considering suicide, or who have recently attempted suicide, should be direct but respectful when evaluating the patient and asking questions. It is a common misconception that talking about suicide directly can cause the patient to act in a suicidal manner. Individuals who are experiencing suicidal ideation respect direct acknowledgment of the situation as opposed to a restrained approach.

During assessment, obtain a full patient and family history, focusing in particular on any personal or family history of mood disorders. Inquire whether the patient has a history of suicide attempts or ideation, and if anyone in the patient's family has ever committed suicide.

Next, a thorough assessment to determine suicidality will need to occur. During this assessment, the nurse should evaluate the patient's mood and affect, behavior, cognition, and patterns of social interaction, looking specifically for the manifestations of suicidality described earlier. The nurse should also consider the various risk factors and protective factors outlined near the start of the exemplar. Questions to ask to assess suicidality may include (APA, 2016; Columbia University Medical Center, n.d.; Potter & Moller, 2016):

- Have you wished you were dead or that you could go to sleep and not wake up?
- Have you had any thoughts of killing yourself?
- Have you been thinking of how you might do this?
- Do you have any intent of acting on these thoughts?
- Have you started to work out the details of how you intend to carry out this plan?
- Do you have access to a means of suicide (e.g., gun, pills, vehicle)?
- Have you told anyone of your plan?
- Have you attempted to end your life in the past?
- What is happening in your life that makes you feel like you don't want to live?
- Has anyone in your family ever attempted or succeeded with suicide?

Once the presence of suicidality has been established, the nurse must assess the patient's level of intent and lethality. One frequently used tool in this area is the Columbia-Suicide Severity Rating Scale (C-SSRS), which has been administered to millions of individuals and has demonstrated success in reducing rates of patient suicide (The Joint Commission, 2016). The scale comes with a list of questions, many of which appear above, and recommendations for triage depending on the severity of the individual's suicidality. For example, a patient who has thought about killing himself or wished he was dead but does not express any intent to harm himself requires, at minimum, mental health referral at discharge. However, the patient who expresses intention to kill himself, with or without a plan, requires immediate safety monitoring and psychiatric consultation. For patients with a history of previous suicide attempt, interventions are determined by the amount of time that has lapsed since the previous attempt. These range from immediate monitoring for safety with a psychiatric consultation for the patient who attempted suicide within the last week to a referral to a mental health provider for the patient who attempted suicide more than a year ago (Columbia University Medical Center, n.d.). See Box 28–1 for an overview of safety precautions to reduce the risk of patient suicide in inpatient settings.

>> **Stay Current:** To download a copy of the C-SSRS and for more information, go to http://cssrs.columbia.edu

Another valuable tool for evaluating suicidality is the Suicide Assessment Five-Step Evaluation and Triage (SAFE-T). This assessment helps the nurse both determine the patient's risk level and select appropriate care interventions. The five steps involved in SAFE-T assessment are as follows:

1. Assess the patient's risk factors.
2. Assess the patient's protective factors.
3. Directly ask the patient about intent to commit suicide. This means the nurse should pose specific questions regarding the patient's thoughts, plans, behaviors, and intent.
4. Determine the patient's risk level and intervention. This determination should be based on the nurse's clinical judgment after completion of steps 1–3. Use of C-SSRS can also be helpful. Ultimately, the nurse should assign a risk level of low, moderate, or high.
5. Document the patient's risk level and treatment plan, along with the rationales for both.

Low-risk patients can be treated in an outpatient setting, while high-risk patients require immediate hospitalization and support. Following evaluation, individuals with a moderate level of risk can usually be treated in an outpatient setting or with partial hospitalization, but only if they can elaborate a plan for seeking immediate help should their desire to commit suicide increase. Note that the SAFE-T assessment should be conducted upon first contact with the patient and in subsequent contacts as appropriate, but particularly with any additional suicidal behaviors, increase in suicidal ideation, or pertinent clinical change. In addition, patients in inpatient settings should be assessed before increasing unit privileges and at discharge (SAMHSA, n.d.; Potter & Moller, 2016).

Diagnosis

The diagnoses for patients who demonstrate suicidal behavior or ideation or who have attempted suicide will change greatly depending on the assessment. Nurses recognize that each patient is an individual case. Some nursing diagnoses for patients are as follows:

- *Suicide, Risk for*
- *Self-Directed Violence, Risk for*
- *Vascular Trauma, Risk for*
- *Knowledge Deficit*
- *Hopelessness*
- *Powerlessness*
- *Self-Esteem: Situational Low or Chronic Low.*

(NANDA-I © 2014)

Planning

Involving the patient in the planning process can be beneficial depending on the individual's current emotional outlook. Empowering the patient to take control of the goals of his care can be a small step in working toward those goals. Some potential goals are:

- The patient will remain free from injury.
- The patient will ask for help when needed.
- The patient will discuss any extreme feelings of depression or hopelessness.
- The patient will participate in regularly scheduled meetings with his therapist.
- The patient will demonstrate healthy coping mechanisms.
- The patient will begin to demonstrate a desire to live.

Implementation

The majority of suicidal individuals are also depressed. Nurses will need to develop a therapeutic rapport with the patient, which will assist with adherence to the treatment plan. Prioritization of interventions is extremely critical, given the potentially lethal nature of the patient's condition. This means the nurse's first actions should focus on reducing the patient's risk for self-directed violence. After that, other interventions may be carried out as appropriate. These include encouraging patients to verbalize emotions and concerns; encouraging patients to attending individual, family, and group therapy sessions as scheduled; teaching effective coping skills; and teaching patients how to seek help when needed. Some agencies use no-harm contracts as an intervention (see **Box 28–5** >>).

Many patients at risk for suicide lack help-seeking behaviors, and feelings of hopelessness can skew perceptions and prevent patients from asking for help. Nurses can help patients identify sources for help and support and then provide opportunities for practice through role playing with the nurse, peers, or family members.

Promote Immediate Safety

- Ensure that patients who are actively experiencing suicidal ideation do not have access to any sharp objects, weapons, or modes that could be used to harm themselves.
- Ensure that the patient at high risk for suicide is never left alone. A nurse, healthcare professional, or other health-

Box 28–5
No-Harm Contracts and Safety Plans

Some agencies employ the use of no-harm contracts (sometimes referred to as behavioral contracts or individualized safety plans) to assist patients in identifying options other than self-harm when they experience feelings of suicide. Although there is a lack of evidence to support the use of no-harm contracts (APA, 2010), practice guidelines and competencies developed by The Joint Commission (2007), the American Psychiatric Nurses' Association (2015), and the U.S. Veterans' Administration (2013) include the development of individualized safety plans in collaboration with the patient. Individualized safety plans may help nurses and other clinicians to empower the patient, manage the suicidal crisis, strengthen the therapeutic alliance, provide an opportunity to educate the patient about warning signs and review coping strategies, and provide options for help and support (U.S. Veterans Administration, 2013; The Joint Commission, 2007). It is important for nurses and other providers to recognize that no-harm contracts and safety plans may be useful in these areas, but may not in and of themselves reduce a patient's risk for suicide. There is no guarantee that a patient who enters into a no-harm agreement will not attempt suicide. Further, no-harm contracts or safety plans should be used alongside, and not be substituted for, other essential nursing and clinical interventions.

1-800-799-4TTY (4889). Links to state websites can be found through the Suicide Prevention Resource Center (SPRC) at http://www.sprc.org.

SAFETY ALERT An individual who is contemplating suicide will generally not ask for help in obvious ways. However, the person's behavior will include clues associated with suicide, such as talking about wanting to die, giving away prized possessions, or saying that he will not be around much longer. These warning signs are the patient's way of asking for help, and nurses should be able to recognize them and respond effectively.

Assess and Monitor for Self-Injury Behaviors

Patients may present with **non-suicidal self-injury behaviors (NSSI)**. These are intentional self-inflicted acts of harm to body tissue without the intent of suicide. Self-mutilation and self-injury are used synonymously; however, currently, the preferred term is self-injury or NSSI (Kara et al., 2015). NSSI generally occurs during periods of painful moods, including guilt, sorrow, flashbacks, and depersonalization to physical pain. Additional reasons attributed to NSSI include self-punishment, attention seeking, imposing guilt, and adaptation to peers who also participate in NSSI (Kara et al., 2015). Patients demonstrating NSSI will need to be monitored closely and may be asked to sign a no-harm contract. Examples of NSSI include cutting, bruising, burning of the skin, trichotillomania, interfering with wound healing, and extreme nail biting (Emelianchik-Key, Byrd, & La Guardia, 2016).

Evaluation

The outcomes for patients demonstrating suicidal behavior can be varied. If the patient is responsive to treatment, then the outcome has a chance of being favorable. Some potential outcomes for the patient who is receiving treatment for suicidal ideation or attempted suicide include the following:

- The patient remains free from injury.
- The patient verbalizes emotions and concerns.
- The patient participates in all scheduled meetings with therapists and counselors.
- The patient demonstrates effective coping skills.
- The patient seeks help when needed.

If the patient remains actively suicidal, extreme caution must be taken, including the aforementioned steps to prevent self-directed violence.

Although many interventions can be employed when a patient demonstrates an unwillingness to live, none of these will prove successful if the individual does not have the desire to help himself. If a patient dies while in a nurse's care and there is an emotional or guilt response, then the nurse should find someone with whom to discuss her feelings in regard to this event. Other nurses, physicians, therapists, or counselors are good sources of support for nurses who have lost a patient.

care worker should be with the patient at all times until the risk for suicide decreases.

- Within the healthcare setting, instruct guests as to what objects they cannot have while visiting the patient, including knives, razor blades, and large quantities of pills.
- In homes, outpatient, or community settings, if a patient expresses that she is considering suicide, alert the appropriate people per agency protocols and applicable state laws: that can be the patient's family, the patient's primary healthcare provider, or a mental health service provider.

Increase Patient Knowledge

- Provide patient and family teaching about symptoms of depression, including feelings of helplessness, worthlessness, and lack of energy. Reassure patients that it takes time for feelings associated with depression to dissipate.
- Provide education to patients who have other comorbid disorders, especially bipolar disorder and schizophrenia.
- Provide medication education, including how the medication works; its intended purpose; how long it may take to experience the full, intended effect; and potential side effects.
- Education of family members and concerned individuals should include the telephone numbers of the National Suicide Prevention Lifeline: 1-800-273-TALK (8255),

Nursing Care Plan
A Patient Who Is Suicidal

Brandon Lewis, age 45, is admitted to the behavioral health unit after having threatened to attempt suicide. He was severely intoxi- cated at the time of his admission. Mr. Lewis is withdrawn and hes- itant to speak to anyone who approaches him.

ASSESSMENT

Danielle Serrano, an RN in the psychiatric department, enters Mr. Lewis's room to obtain a health history and suicide risk assess- ment. A nursing assistant is sitting in the room with Mr. Lewis. The hospital initiated suicide precautions when Mr. Lewis arrived, because his daughter reported that she had walked in on him try- ing to kill himself.

Mr. Lewis does not readily respond to the nurse's questions, so Ms. Serrano waits and begins talking to the patient about mun- dane topics such as the weather, a documentary she saw on tele- vision the evening before, and the lunch menu at the hospital for today. Eventually Ms. Serrano notices that Mr. Lewis seems to be more relaxed, so she asks him again if he would like to talk about what happened. When he does not reply, Ms. Serrano calmly explains that the patient's daughter told the nurse she found him with a large knife and a bottle of painkillers, and then called 911. Mr. Lewis asks if his daughter is still at the hospital, and the nurse responds that she will be back this evening.

The patient begins to explain that his wife left him 2 months ago, and then shortly after that he lost his job. Mr. Lewis has been drinking heavily for the past month. The night of his suicide attempt, he wanted all of the pain to stop, so he tried to kill himself. Mr. Lewis's daughter walked in and got the knife away from him, then called for help. The patient claims that he probably would not have tried to kill himself if he had not been intoxicated. Mr. Lewis has no previous history of suicide, depression, or any other comorbid disorders. Mr. Lewis denies any current thoughts of or intent to kill himself.

DIAGNOSIS

- *Suicide, Risk for*
- *Self-Directed Violence, Risk for*
- *Hopelessness*

(NANDA-I © 2014)

PLANNING

Identified outcomes for Mr. Lewis include:

- The patient will remain free from injury.
- The patient will discuss emo- tions and concerns.
- The patient will ask for help.
- The patient will demonstrate healthy coping mechanisms.
- The patient will participate in treatment for alcohol depen- dence.

IMPLEMENTATION

- Assist Mr. Lewis to decrease or eliminate self-abusive behaviors.
- Facilitate development of a positive outlook for the future.
- Provide for safety, stabilization, recovery, and maintenance until Mr. Lewis's depression improves.
- Administer antidepressants as ordered.
- Teach visitors about restricted items (razors, scissors, and so forth).
- Involve family, as patient allows, in discharge planning. Encour- age creation of a family safety plan.
- Educate patient and family about signs of increased suicidality, as well as available resources (e.g., suicide prevention hotlines, emergency psychiatric care).

- Initiate a multidisciplinary patient care conference to develop a plan of care.
- Refer to mental healthcare provider.
- Initiate suicide precautions (e.g., do not leave patient alone; make sure patient does not have access to potentially danger- ous objects).
- Encourage Mr. Lewis to verbalize feelings.
- Develop an individualized safety plan to help Mr. Lewis recognize and cope with triggers and warning signs using strategies other than self-harming.
- Limit access to windows.
- Consider strategies to decrease isolation.

EVALUATION

Mr. Lewis agrees that he needs help to abstain from alcohol and agrees to be admitted to an alcohol rehabilitation facility. He says he probably would never have tried to harm himself if he had not been drinking, but agrees counseling is required and talks with a psychologist.

CRITICAL THINKING

1. If you are the nurse caring for Mr. Lewis on the behavioral health unit, what actions will you take to keep the patient safe?

2. Will you notify Mr. Lewis's wife of his admission? Explain your answer.

3. What strategies would you promote to Mr. Lewis to reduce hopelessness and have hope for the future?

REVIEW Suicide

RELATE Link the Concepts and Exemplars

Linking the exemplar of suicide with the concept of health, wellness, illness and injury:

1. Explain the relationship between suicide and disrupted sleep pattern.

2. Explain the relationship between suicide and terminal illness.

Linking the exemplar of suicide with the concept of comfort:

3. Explain why the patient with chronic pain should be assessed for risk of suicide.

4. How will you assess the patient living with chronic pain for suicide risk?

READY Go to Volume 3: Clinical Nursing Skills

REFER Go to Pearson MyLab Nursing and eText

- Additional review materials

REFLECT Apply Your Knowledge

Jenny Vasquez, age 14, presents to the emergency department after having consumed a box of diphenhydramine (Benadryl) tablets. Her left wrist has also been cut horizontally; the amount of blood loss is unknown. Upon ED arrival, Jenny is lethargic. A security guard is present in the examination room. The physician begins to perform a physical assessment on Jenny.

Jenny's vital signs include temperature 96.2°F tympanic; pulse 118 bpm; and BP 152/96 mmHg. Respirations are 14 per minute, and Jenny does not appear to be in any acute respiratory distress. The ED physician quickly assesses Jenny's left wrist wound; there is no active bleeding and the wound is superficial with no deep tissue damage. A dressing is applied to the wound. Gastric lavage is performed immediately to remove the drugs from Jenny's stomach. Afterward, her wrist laceration is cleaned and sutured, and a sterile dressing is applied to the site.

Upon reassessment of Jenny, she speaks quietly and makes eye contact with the nurse. She explains that the teenagers at her school have been bullying her for the past year. Jenny is unsure about her sexual orientation, but was caught kissing another girl at the winter formal last year. Ever since then, she has been ostracized and teased constantly at school. The day of the suicide attempt, she arrived at her locker to find that someone had spray painted the words "queer," "freak," and "spic" in red paint. Seeing no other way to stop the abuse, Jenny tried to kill herself.

1. Based on the information provided about Jenny's situation, do you believe she is at especially high risk for attempting suicide again? Please explain your answer.

2. Do you believe that Jenny was actually trying to kill herself, or was this incident more of a "cry for help"? Justify your answer with evidence from the case study.

3. Identify three nursing diagnoses that are appropriate for inclusion in Jenny's plan of care.

References

Adams, M. P., Holland, L. N., & Urban, C. (2017). *Pharmacology for nurses: A pathophysiologic approach* (5th ed.). Hoboken, NJ: Pearson Education.

Allan, C. L., & Ebmeier, K. P. (2011). The use of ECT and MST in treating depression. *International Review of Psychiatry, 23*(5), 400–412.

Almeida, O. P., Ford, A. H., & Flicker, L. (2015). Systematic review and meta-analysis of randomized placebo-controlled trials of folate and vitamin B$_{12}$ for depression. *International Psychogenetics, 27*(5), 727–737.

Ameresekere, M., & Henderson, D. (2012). *Post-conflict mental health in South Sudan: Overview of common psychiatric disorders. Part 1: Depression and post-traumatic stress disorder.* Retrieved from http://www.southsudanmedicaljournal.com/archive/february-2012/post-conflict-mental-health-in-south-sudan-overview-of-common-psychiatric-disorders.-part-1-depression-and-post-traumatic-stress-disorder.html

American Academy of Child and Adolescent Psychiatry. (2015). *Bipolar disorder in children and teens.* Retrieved from: http://www.aacap.org/AACAP/Families_and_Youth/Facts_for_Families/FFF-Guide/Bipolar-Disorder-In-Children-And-Teens-038.aspx

American Association of Suicidology. (2014). *Depression and suicide risk.* Retrieved from http://www.suicidology.org/portals/14/docs/resources/factsheets/2011/depressionsuicide2014.pdf

American Association of Suicidology. (2016). *Warning signs.* Retrieved from http://www.suicidology.org/resources/warning-signs

American College of Obstetricians and Gynecologists (ACOG). (2015). *Committee Opinion No. 630: Screening for perinatal depression.* Retrieved from http://www.acog.org/Resources-And-Publications/Committee-Opinions/Committee-on-Obstetric-Practice/Screening-for-Perinatal-Depression

American Foundation for Suicide Prevention. (2016). *Suicide statistics.* Retrieved from http://afsp.org/about-suicide/suicide-statistics/

American Psychiatric Association (APA). (2010). *Practice guideline for the assessment and treatment of patients with suicidal behaviors.* Retrieved from http://psychiatryonline.org/pb/assets/raw/sitewide/practice_guidelines/guidelines/suicide.pdf

American Psychiatric Association (APA). (2013). *Diagnostic and statistical manual of mental disorders* (5th ed.). Washington, DC: Author.

American Psychiatric Association. (APA). (2015a). *Practice guidelines for the treatment of patients with major depressive disorder* (3rd ed.). Agency for Healthcare Research and Quality, National Guidelines Clearinghouse, NCG 008093. Retrieved from https://www.guideline.gov/summaries/summary/24158/practice-guideline-for-the-treatment-of-patients-with-major-depressive-disorder-third-edition

American Psychiatric Association (APA). (2015b). *Suicide prevention.* Retrieved from https://www.psychiatry.org/patients-families/suicide-prevention

American Psychiatric Association. (2016). *APA practice guidelines (2016) recommendations regarding assessment of suicide as part of the initial psychiatric assessment.* Retrieved from http://stopasuicide.org/assets/docs/APAPracticeGuidelines.pdf

American Psychiatric Nurses' Association. (2015). *Psychiatric mental health nurse essential competencies for assessment and management of individuals at risk for suicide.* Retrieved from https://www.apna.org/files/public/Resources/Suicide%20Competencies%20for%20Psychiatric-Mental%20Health%20Nurses(1).pdf

American Psychological Association. (2016a). *Mental and behavioral health and older Americans.* Retrieved from http://www.apa.org/about/gr/issues/aging/mental-health.aspx.

American Psychological Association. (2016b). *Patient Health Questionnaire (PHQ-9 & PHQ-2).* Retrieved from http://www.apa.org/pi/about/publications/caregivers/practice-settings/assessment/tools/patient-health.aspx

Andreazza, A. C., Wang, J. F., Salmasi, F., Shao, L., & Young, L. T. (2013). Specific subcellular changes in oxidative stress in prefrontal cortex from patients with bipolar disorder. *Journal of Neurochemistry, 127*, 552–561.

Andrews, L. B. (2016). Depression and suicide. *Medscape.* http://emedicine.medscape.com/article/805459-overview#a3

Bai, Y., Chiou, W., Su, T., Li, C., & Chen, M. (2014). Pro-inflammatory cytokine associated with somatic and pain symptoms in depression. *Journal of Affective Disorders, 155*, 28–34.

Bair, M. J., Robinson, R. L., Katon, W., & Kroenke, K. (2003). Depression and pain comorbidity: A literature review. *Archives of Internal Medicine, 163*(20), 2433–2445.

Balzer, B. W. R., Duke, S. A., Hawke, C. I., & Steinbeck, K. S. (2015). The effects of estradiol on mood and behavior in human female adolescents: A systematic review. *European Journal of Pediatrics, 174*(3), 289–298.

Baron, K. G., & Reid, K. J. (2014). Circadian misalignment and health. *International Review of Psychiatry, 26*(2), 139–154.

Baumeister, R. F., & Bushman, B. J. (2017). *Social psychology and human nature* (4th ed.). Boston, MA: Cengage.

Bechtel, W. (2015). Circadian rhythms and mood disorders: Are the phenomena and mechanisms causally related? *Frontiers in Psychiatry, 6*, 188.

Beck, A. (1967). *Depression: Clinical, experimental, and theoretical aspects.* New York, NY: Harper & Row.

Beck, C. T. (2008). *Postpartum mood and anxiety disorders: Case studies, research, and nursing care* (2nd ed.). Washington, DC: Association of Women's Health, Obstetric and Neonatal Nurses.

Beck, C. T., & Indman, P. (2005). The many faces of depression. *Journal of Obstetric, Gynecologic, and Neonatal Nursing, 34*(5), 569–576.

Bedson, E., Bell, D., Carr, D., Carter, B., Hughes, D., Jorgensen, A., . . . Williams, N. (2014, July). Folate Augmentation of Treatment—Evaluation for Depression (FolATED): randomised trial and economic evaluation. *NIHR Journals Library* (Health Technology Assessment, No. 18.48). Available at http://www.ncbi.nlm.nih.gov/books/NBK262306/;doi:10.3310/hta18480

Benros, M. E., Waltoft, B. L., Nordentoft, M., Ostergaard, S. D., Eaton, W. W., Krogh, J., & Mortensen, P. B. (2013). Autoimmune diseases and severe infections as risk factors for mood disorders: A nationwide study. *JAMA Psychiatry, 70*(8), 812–820.

Bertisch, S. M., Wells, R. E., Smith, M. T., & McCarthy, E. P. (2012). Use of relaxation techniques and complementary and alternative medicine by American adults with insomnia symptoms: Results from a national survey. *Journal of Clinical Sleep Medicine, 8*(6), 681–691. Retrieved from http://doi.org/10.5664/jcsm.2264

Binder, E. B., Jeffrey Newport, D., Zach, E. B., Smith, A. K., Deveau, T. C., Altshuler, L., . . . Cubells, J. F. (2010). A serotonin transporter gene polymorphism predicts peripartum depressive symptoms in an at-risk psychiatric cohort. *Journal of Psychiatric Research, 44*(10), 640–646.

Bloch, M.H., & Hannestad, J. (2012). Omega-3 fatty acids for the treatment of depression: systematic review and meta-analysis. *Molecular Psychiatry, 17*(12), 1272–1282. doi:10.1038/mp.2011.100

Bottiglieri, T. (2013). Folate, vitamin B$_{12}$, and *S*-adenosylmethionine. *Psychiatric Clinic North America, 36*, 1–13.

Bowen, R., Balbuena, L., Leuschen, C., & Baetz, M. (2012). Mood instability is the distinctive feature of neuroticism: Results from the British Health and Lifestyle Study (HALS). *Personality and Individual Differences, 53*(7), 896–900.

Brent, D. A., Melhem, N. M., & Oquendo, M. (2015). Familial pathways to early-onset suicide attempt: A 5.6-year prospective study. *JAMA Psychiatry, 72*(2), 160–168.

Brown, A. (2012). With poverty comes, depression, more than other illnesses. *Gallup.* Retrieved from http://www.gallup.com/poll/158417/poverty-comes-depression-illness.aspx

Centers for Disease Control and Prevention (CDC). (2014). *Depression in the U.S. household population.* Retrieved from http://www.cdc.gov/nchs/data/databriefs/db172.htm

Centers for Disease Control and Prevention (CDC). (2015). *Suicide facts at a glance.* Retrieved from http://www.cdc.gov/violenceprevention/pdf/suicide-datasheet-a.pdf

Centers for Disease Control and Prevention (CDC). (2016a). *Suicide: Risk and protective factors.* Retrieved from http://www.cdc.gov/violenceprevention/suicide/riskprotectivefactors.html

Centers for Disease Control and Prevention (CDC). (2016b). *Increase in suicide in the United States, 1999-2014.* Retrieved from http://www.cdc.gov/nchs/products/databriefs/db241.htm

Centers for Disease Control and Prevention (CDC). (2017). *Lesbian, gay, bisexual, and transgender health: LGBT youth.* Retrieved from http://www.cdc.gov/lgbthealth/youth.htm

Chan, J., Natekar, A., Einarson, A., & Koren, G. (2014). Risks of untreated depression in pregnancy. *Canadian Family Physician, 60*(3), 242–243.

Chan, Y. Y., Lo, W. Y., Yang, S. N., Chen, Y. H., & Lin, J. G. (2015). The benefit of combined acupuncture and antidepressant medication for depression: A systematic review and meta-analysis. *Journal of Affective Disorders, 176*, 106–117.

Chaplin, T. M., & Aldao, A. (2013). Gender differences in emotion expression in children: A meta-analytic review. *Psychological Bulletin, 139*(4), 735–765.

Charlson, F., Siskind, D., Doi, S. A. R., McCallum, E., Broome, A., & Lie, D. C. (2012). ECT efficacy and treatment course: A systematic review and meta-analysis of twice vs thrice weekly schedules. *Journal of Affective Disorders, 138*, 1–8.

Cheung, A., Dewa, C., Michalak, E. E., Browne, G., Levitt, A., Levitan, R. D., . . . Lam, R. W. (2012). Direct health care costs of treating seasonal affective disorder: A comparison of light therapy and fluoxetine. *Depression Research and Treatment, 2012*, 628434.

Columbia University Medical Center. (n.d.) Columbia-Suicide Severity Scale. Retrieved from http://cssrs.columbia.edu/

Compas, B. E., Forehand, R., Thigpen, J., Hardcastle, E., Garai, E., McKee, L., . . . Sterba, S. (2015). Efficacy and moderators of a family group cognitive-behavioral preventive intervention for children of depressed parents. *Journal of Consulting and Clinical Psychology, 83*(3), 541–553.

Cooney, G. M., Dwan, K., Greig, C. A., Lawlor, D. A., Rimer, J., Waugh, F. R., . . . Mead, G. E. (2013). Exercise for depression. *Cochrane Database of Systematic Reviews, 2013*(9), CD004366.

Cooper, W. O., Callahan, S. T., Shintani, A., Fuchs, D. C., Shelton, R. C., Dudley, J. A., . . . Ray, W. A. (2014). Antidepressants and suicide attempts in children. *Pediatrics, 133*(2), 204.

Coppen., A., & Bailey, J. (2000). Enhancement of the antidepressant action of fluoxetine by folic acid: A randomized, placebo-controlled trial. *Journal of Affective Disorders, 60*(2), 121–130.

Corona, M., McCarty, C. A., & Richardson, L. P. (2013). Screening adolescents for depression. *Contemporary Pediatrics, 30*(7), 24–30.

Corwin, E. J., Brownstead, J., Barton, N., Heckard, S., & Merin, K. (2005). The impact of fatigue on the development of postpartum depression. *Journal of Obstetric, Gynecologic, and Neonatal Nursing, 34*(5), 577–586.

Corwin, E., Kohen, R., Jarrett, M., & Stafford, B. (2010). The heritability of postpartum depression. *Biological Research for Nursing, 12*(1), 73–83.

Cretaz, E., Brunoni, A., & Lafer, B. (2015). *Magnetic seizure therapy for unipolar and bipolar depression: A systematic review.* Retrieved from http://www.hindawi.com/journals/np/2015/521398/

Cukrowicz, K., Jahn, D., Graham, R., Poindexter, E., & Williams, R. (2013). Suicide risk in older adults: Evaluating models of risk and predicting excess zeros in a primary care sample. *Journal of Abnormal Psychology, 122*(4), 1021–1030.

Cunningham, F. G., Leveno, K. J., Bloom, S. L., Hauth, J. C., Gilstrap, L. C., & Wenstrom, K. D. (2010). *Williams obstetrics* (23rd ed.). New York, NY: McGraw-Hill.

Danielsson, L., Noras, A., Waern, M., & Carlsson, J. (2013). Exercise in the treatment of major depression: A systematic review grading the quality of evidence. *Physiotherapy Theory and Practice, 29*(8), 573–585.

Davanzo, R., Copertino, M., De Cunto, A., Minen, F., & Amaddeo, A. (2011). Antidepressant medications and breastfeeding: A review of the literature. *Breastfeeding Medicine, 6*(2), 89–98.

de Angel, V., Prieto, F., Gladstone, T. R. G., Beardslee, W. R., & Irarrazaval, M. (2016). The feasibility and acceptability of a preventive intervention programme for children with depressed parents: Study protocol for a randomised controlled trial. *Trials, 17*, 237.

de Heer, E. W., Gerrits, M. M. J. G., Beekman, A. T. F., Dekker, J., van Marwijk, H. W. J., de Waal, M. W. M., . . . van der Feltz-Cornelis, C. M. (2014). The association of depression and anxiety with pain: A study from NESDA. *PLoS One, 9*(10), e106907.

DeJean, D., Giacomini, M., Vanstone, M., & Brundisini, F. (2013). Patient experiences of depression and anxiety with chronic disease: A systematic review and qualitative meta-synthesis. *Ontario Health Technology Assessment Series, 13*(16), 1–33.

Dennis, C. L., & Dowswell, T. (2013). Psychosocial and psychological interventions for preventing postpartum depression. *Cochrane Database of Systematic Reviews, 2013*(2), CD001134.

Dere, J., Sun, J., Zhao, Y., Persson, T., Zhu, X., Yao, S., . . . Ryder, A. (2013). Beyond "somatization" and "psychologization": Symptom level variation in depressed Han Chinese and Euro-Canadian outpatients. *Frontiers in Psychology, 4*, 377.

Devries, K., Mak, J., Child, J., Falder, G., Bacchus, L., Astbury, J., & Watts, C. (2014). Childhood sexual abuse and suicidal behavior: A meta-analysis. *Pediatrics, 133*(5), 1331–1344.

Diaz-Morales, J. F., Escribano, C., & Jankowski, K. S. (2015). Chronotype and time-of-day effects on mood during school day. *Chronobiology International, 32*(1), 37–42.

Dierckx, B., Heijnen, W. T., van den Broek, W. W., & Birkenhager, T. K. (2012). Efficacy of electroconvulsive therapy in bipolar versus unipolar major depression: A meta-analysis. *Bipolar Disorders, 14*(2), 146–150.

Doornbos, B., Dijck-Brouwer, D., Kema, I., Tanke, M., van Goor, S., Muskiet, F., & Korf, J. (2009). The development of peripartum depressive symptoms is associated with gene polymorphisms of MAOA, 5-HTT and COMT. *Progress in Neuro-Psychopharmacology & Biological Psychiatry, 33*(7), 1250–1254.

Doucet, S., Dennis, C. L., Letourneau, N., & Blackmore, E. R. (2009). Differentiation and clinical implications of postpartum depression and postpartum psychosis. *Journal of Obstetric, Gynecologic, and Neonatal Nursing, 38*(3), 269–279.

Ekkekakis, P. (2013). *The measurement of affect, mood, and emotion: A guide for health-behavioral research.* Cambridge, England: Cambridge University Press.

Else-Quest, N. M., Higgins, A., Allison, C., & Morton, L. C. (2012). Gender differences in self-conscious emotional experience: A meta-analysis. *Psychological Bulletin, 138*(5), 947–981.

Emelianchik-Key, K., Byrd, R., & La Guardia, A. (2016). Adolescent non-suicidal self-injury: Analysis of the youth risk behavior survey trends. *The Professional Counselor, 6*(1), 61–75.

English, T., & Carstensten, L. L. (2014). Emotional experience in the mornings and the evenings: Consideration of age differences in specific emotions by time of day. *Frontiers in Psychology, 5*, 185.

Erol, A., Winham, S. J., McElroy, S. L., Frye, M. A., Prieto, M. L., Cuellar-Barboza, A. B., . . . Bobo, W. V. (2015). Sex differences in the risk of rapid cycling and other indicators of adverse illness course in patients with bipolar I and II disorder. *Bipolar Disorders, 17*(6), 670–676.

Evans, L. D., Kouros, C., Frankel, S. A., McCauley, E., Diamond, G. S., Schloredt, K. A., & Garber, J. (2015). Longitudinal relations between stress and depressive symptoms in youth: Coping as a mediator. *Journal of Abnormal Child Psychology, 43*(2), 355–368.

Fall, A., Goulet, L., & Vézina, M. (2013). Comparative study of major depressive symptoms among pregnant women by employment status. *SpringerPlus, 2*(1), 201.

Field, M., & Cartwright-Hatton, S. (2015). *Essential abnormal and clinical psychology*. London, England: Sage.

Fischer, A., & LaFrance, M. (2015). What drives the smile and the tear: Why women are more emotionally expressive than men. *Emotion Review, 7*(1), 22–29.

Food and Drug Administration. (2014). *Antidepressant use in children, adolescents, and adults*. Retrieved from http://www.fda.gov/Drugs/DrugSafety/InformationbyDrugClass/UCM096273

Frank, C. (2014). Pharmacologic treatment of depression in the elderly. *Canadian Family Physician, 60*(2), 121–126.

Freeland, K. N., & Shealy, K. M. (2013). Toolbox: Psychotropic use in pregnancy and lactation. *Mental Health Clinician, 3*(2), 45–57.

Gentile, S. (2011). Suicidal mothers. *Injury and Violence, 3*(2), 90–97.

Georgia Health Sciences University. (2011, October 20). Homicide, suicide outpace traditional causes of death in pregnant, postpartum women. *Science-Daily*. Retrieved from www.sciencedaily.com/releases/2011/10/111020191854.htm

Gibbons, R. D., Brown, C. H., Hur, K., Davis, J., & Mann, J. J. (2012). Suicidal thoughts and behavior with antidepressant treatment: Reanalysis of the randomized placebo-controlled studies of fluoxetine and venlafaxine. *Archives of General Psychiatry, 69*(6), 580.

Gobin, C. M., Banks, J. B., Fins, A. I., & Tartar, J. L. (2015). Poor sleep quality is associated with a negative cognitive bias and decreased sustained attention. *Journal of Sleep Research, 24*(5), 535–542.

Gomez, P., von Gunten, A., & Danuser, B. (2013). Content-specific gender differences in emotion ratings from early to late adulthood. *Scandinavian Journal of Psychology, 54*(6), 451–458.

Grech, V. (2014). A global review of male offspring preference and gender bias in the caring of children. *Journal of the Malta College of Pharmacy Practice, 20*, 40–42.

Greenberg, P. E., Fournier, A-A., Sisitsky, T., Pike, C. T., & Kessler, R. C. (2015). The economic burden of adults with major depressive disorder in the United States (2005 and 2010). *Journal of Clinical Psychiatry, 76*(2), 155–162.

Grieve, S. M., Korgaonkar, M. S., Koslow, S. H., Gordon, E., & Williams, L. M. (2013). Widespread reductions in gray matter volume in depression. *NeuroImage: Clinical, 3*, 332–339.

Gunn, J. M., Ayton, D. R., Densley, K., Pallant, J. F., Chondros, P., Herrman, H. E., & Dowrick, C. F. (2012). The association between chronic illness, multimorbidity and depressive symptoms in an Australian primary care cohort. *Social Psychiatry and Psychiatric Epidemiology, 47*(2), 175–184.

Guo, J., Ren, X., Wang, X., Qu, Z., Zhou, Q., Ran, C., . . . & Hu, J. (2015). Depression among migrant and left-behind children in China in relation to the quality of parent-child and teacher-child relationships. *PLoS One, 10*(12), e0145606.

Guyer, A. E., Silk, J. S., & Nelson, E. E. (2016). The neurobiology of the emotional adolescent: From the inside out. *Neuroscience and Biobehavioral Reviews, S0149-7634*(16), 30160–30169.

Haas, A.P., Rodgers, P.L., & Herman, J.L. (2014). *Suicide attempts among transgender and gender nonconforming adults: Findings of the National Transgender Discrimination Survey*. Retrieved from http://williamsinstitute.law.ucla.edu/wp-content/uploads/AFSP-Williams-Suicide-Report-Final.pdf

Haga, S. M., Drozd, F., Brendryen, H., & Slinning, K. (2013). Mamma Mia: A feasibility study of a web-based intervention to reduce the risk of postpartum depression and enhance subjective well-being. *JMIR Research Protocols, 2*(2), e29.

Hall-Flavin, K. (2016). *Diseases and conditions: Depression (major depressive disorder)*. Retrieved from http://www.mayoclinic.org/diseases-conditions/depression/expert-answers/pain-and-depression/faq-20057823

Halter, M. J. (2014). *Varcarolis' foundations of psychiatric mental health nursing: A clinical approach* (7th ed.). St. Louis, MO: Elsevier Saunders.

Halverson, J. L. (2016). Depression. *Medscape*. Retrieved from http://emedicine.medscape.com/article/286759-overview#a4

Halverson, J. L., Bhalla, R., Andrews, L. B., Moraille-Bhalla, P., & Leonard, R. C. (2016). *Depression*. Retrieved from http://emedicine.medscape.com/article/286759-differential

Hames, J. L., Hagan, C. R., & Joiner, T. E. (2013). Interpersonal processes in depression. *Annual Review of Clinical Psychology, 9*, 355–377.

Hawton, K., Saunders, K. E., & O'Connor, R. C. (2012). Self-harm and suicide in adolescents. *The Lancet, 379*(9834), 2373–2382.

Health Quality Ontario. (2016). Repetitive transcranial magnetic stimulation for treatment-resistant depression: A systematic review and meta-analysis of randomized controlled trials. *Ontario Health Technology Assessment Series, 16*(5), 1–66.

Herdman, T. H. & Kamitsuru, S. (Eds.). *Nursing Diagnoses—Definitions and Classification 2015–2017.* Copyright © 2014, 1994–2014 NANDA International. Used by arrangement with John Wiley & Sons, Inc. Companion website: www.wiley.com/go/nursingdiagnoses

Heron, M. (2016). Deaths: Leading causes for 2013. *National Vital Statistics Reports, 65*(2). Retrieved from http://www.cdc.gov/nchs/data/nvsr/nvsr65/nvsr65_02.pdf

Herring, M. P., O'Connor, P. J., & Dishman, R. K. (2010). The effect of exercise training on anxiety symptoms among patients: a systematic review. *Arch Intern Med, 170*(4), 321–331.

Hoerger, M., Chapman, B., & Duberstein, P. (2015). Realistic affective forecasting: The role of personality. *Cognition and Emotion, 30*(7), 1304–1316.

Holden, K. B., Hall, S. P., Robinson, M., Triplett, S., Babalola, D., Plummer, V., . . . Bradford, L. D. (2012). Psychosocial and sociocultural correlates of depressive symptoms among diverse African American women. *Journal of the National Medical Association, 104*(11–12), 493–504.

Hooley, J. M., Butcher, J. N., Nock, M. K., & Mineka, S. M. (2017). *Abnormal psychology* (17th ed.). New York, NY: Pearson.

Isacsson, G., & Rich, C. L. (2014). Antidepressant drugs and the risk of suicide in children and adolescents. *Pediatric Drugs, 16*(2), 115–122.

Jacka, F. N., Mykletun, A., & Berk, M. (2012). Moving towards a population health approach to the primary prevention of common mental disorders. *BMC Medicine, 10*, 149.

Jager-Hyman, S., Cunningham, A., Wenzel, A., Mattei, S., Brown, G. K., & Beck, A. T. (2014). Cognitive distortions and suicide attempts. *Cognitive Therapy and Research, 38*(4), 369–374.

Janicak, P. G., & Dokucu, M. E. (2015). Transcranial magnetic stimulation for the treatment of major depression. *Neuropsychiatric Disease and Treatment, 11*, 1549–1560.

Jankowski, K. S. (2014). The role of temperament in the relationship between morningness–eveningness and mood. *Chronobiology International, 31*(1), 114–122.

Josefsson, T., Lindwall, M., & Archer, T. (2014). Physical exercise intervention in depressive disorders: Meta-analysis and systematic review. *Scandinavian Journal of Medicine and Science in Sports, 24*(2), 259–272.

Kalfoglou, A. L. (2016). Ethical and clinical dilemmas in using psychotropic medications during pregnancy. *AMA Journal of Ethics, 18*(6), 614–623.

Kar, N., Arun, M., Mohanty, M., & Bastia, B. (2014). Scale for assessment of lethality of suicide attempt. *Indian Journal of Psychiatry, 56*(4), 337–343.

Kara, K., Ozsoy, S., Teke, H., Congologlu, M., Turker, T., Renklidag, T., & Karapirli, M. (2015). Non-suicidal self-injurious behavior in forensic child and adolescent populations. *Neurosciences, 20*(1), 31–36.

Karp, J., Scott, J., Houck, P., Reynolds, C., Kupfer, D., & Frank, E. (2005). Pain predicts longer time to remission during treatment of recurrent depression. *Journal of Clinical Psychiatry, 66*(5), 591–597.

Keene, D., Cowan, S., & Baker, A. (2015). "When you're in a crisis like that, you don't want people to know": Mortgage strain, stigma, and mental health. *American Journal of Public Health, 105*(5), 1008–1012.

Kellner, C. H., Greenburg, R. M., Murrough, J. W., Bryson, E. O., Briggs, M. C., & Pasculli, R. M. (2012). ECT in treatment-resistant depression. *American Journal of Psychiatry, 169*(12), 1238–1244.

Kiosses, D. N., Szanto, K., & Alexopoulos, G. S. (2014). Suicide in older adults: The role of emotions and cognition. *Current Psychiatry Reports, 16*(11), 495.

Knoll, J. L. (2012). Inpatient suicide: identifying vulnerability in the hospital setting. *Psychiatric Times*, Retrieved from http://www.psychiatrictimes.com/suicide/inpatient-suicide-identifying-vulnerability-hospital-setting

Koenders, M. A., Giltay, E. J., Spijker, A. T., Hoencamp, E., Spinhoven, P., & Elzinga, B. M. (2014). Stressful life events in bipolar I and II disorder: Cause or consequence of mood symptoms? *Journal of Affective Disorders, 161*, 55–64.

Komulainen, E., Meskanen, K., Lipsanen, J., Lahti, J. M., Jylha, P., Melartin, T., . . . Ekelund, J. (2014). The effect of personality on daily life emotional processes. *PLoS One, 9*(10), e110907.

Kozhimannil, K. B., Trinacty, C. M., Busch, A. B., Huskamp, H. A., & Adams, A. S. (2011). Racial and ethnic disparities in postpartum depression care among low-income women. *Psychiatric Services, 62*(6), 619–625.

Kroenke, K., Shen, J., Oxman, T., William, J., & Dietrich, A. (2008). Impact of pain on the outcomes of depression treatment: Results from the RESPECT trial. *Pain, 134*(1–2), 209–215.

Kumar, P., Slavich, G. M., Berghorst, L. H., Treadway, M. T., Brooks, N. H., Dutra, S. J., . . . Pizzagalli, D. A. (2015). Perceived life stress exposure modulates reward-related medial prefrontal cortex responses to acute stress in depression. *Journal of Affective Disorders, 180,* 104–111.

Lagerberg, D., & Magnusson, M. (2012). Infant gender and postpartum sadness in the light of region of birth and some other factors: A contribution to the knowledge of postpartum depression. *Archives of Women's Mental Health, 15,* 121–130.

Larkin, M. (2016). Serotonin receptor binding potential tied to suicidal ideation and behavior. *Psych Congress Network.* Retrieved from http://www.psychcongress.com/article/serotonin-receptor-binding-potential-tied-suicidal-ideation-and-behavior

Larson, R., Csikszentmihalyi, M., & Graef, R. (2014). Mood variability and the psychosocial adjustment of adolescents. In M. Csikszentmihalyi (Ed.), *Applications of flow in human development and education.* Dordrecht, Germany: Springer.

Lederer, E. (2015). Lithium nephropathy. *Medscape.* Retrieved from http://emedicine.medscape.com/article/242772-overview#a5

Leiknes, K., Cooke, M., Jarosch-von Schweder, L., & Hoie, B. (2015). Electroconvulsive therapy during pregnancy: a systematic review of case studies. *Arch Womens Mental Health, 18*(1), 1–39.

Levine, S., Levav, I., Yoffe, R., Becher, Y., & Pugachova, I. (2016). Genocide exposure and subsequent suicide risk: A population based study. *PLoS One.* Retrieved from http://journals.plos.org/plosone/article?id=10.1371/journal.pone.0149524

Lewis, J. E., Tiozzo, E., Melillo, A. B., Leonard, S., Chen, L., Mendez, A., . . . Konefal, J. (2013). The effect of methylated vitamin B complex on depressive and anxiety symptoms and quality of life in adults with depression, *ISRN Psychiatry, 2013,* 621453.

Lewitzka, U., Severus, E., Bauer, R., Ritter, P., Muller-Oerlinghausen, & Bauer, M. (2015). The suicide prevention effect of lithium: More than 20 years of evidence—a narrative review. *International Journal of Bipolar Disorders, 3,* 15.

Lindsey, P. L. (2009). Psychotropic medication use among older adults: What all nurses need to know. *Journal of Gerontological Nursing, 35*(9), 28–38.

Lipsitz, J. D., & Markowitz, J. C. (2013). Mechanisms of change in interpersonal therapy (IPT). *Clinical Psychology Review, 33*(8), 1134–1147.

Liu, B. (2015). *Sentiment analysis: Mining opinions, sentiments, and emotions.* New York, NY: Cambridge University Press.

Liu, Y., Feng, H., Mo, Y., Gao, J., Mao, H., Song, M., . . . Liu, W. (2015). Effect of soothing-liver and nourishing-heart acupuncture on early selective serotonin reuptake inhibitor treatment onset for depressive disorder and related indicators of neuroimmunology: A randomized controlled clinical trial. *Journal of Traditional Chinese Medicine, 35*(5), 607–613.

Liu, Z., Liu, W., Yao, L., Yang, C., Xiao, L., Wan, Q., . . . Xiao, Z. (2013). Negative life events and corticotropin-releasing-hormone receptor 1 gene in recurrent major depressive disorder. *Scientific Reports, 3,* 1548.

Lucassen, P. J., Oomen, C. A., Schouten, M., Encinas, J. M., & Fitzsimons, C. P. (2016). Adult neurogenesis, chronic stress, and depression. In J. J. Canales (Ed.), *Adult neurogenesis in the hippocampus: Health, psychopathology, and brain disease.* London, England: Academic Press.

Machado-Vieira, R., Zanetti, M. V., De Sousa, R. T., Soeiro de Souza, M. G., Moreno, R. A., Busatto, G. F., & Gattaz, W. F. (2014). Lithium efficacy in bipolar depression with flexible dosing: A six-week, open-label, proof-of-concept study. *Experimental and Therapeutic Medicine, 8,* 1205–1208.

Maciejewski, D. F., van Lier, P. A. C., Branje, S. J. T., Meeus, W. H. J., & Koot, H. M. (2015). A 5-year longitudinal study on mood variability across adolescence using daily diaries. *Child Development 86*(6), 1908–1921.

Marwaha, S., Broome, M. R., Bebbington, P. E., Kuipers, E., & Freeman, D. (2013). Mood instability and psychosis: Analyses of British national survey data. *Schizophrenia Bulletin, 40*(2), 269–277.

Masumoto, K., Taishi, N., & Shiozaki, M. (2016). Age and gender differences in relationships among emotion regulation, mood, and mental health. *Gerontology and Geriatric Medicine, 2,* 2333721416637022.

Mayo Clinic. (2015a). *Postpartum depression.* Retrieved from http://www.mayoclinic.com/health/postpartum-depression/DS00546/DSECTION=symptoms

Mayo Clinic. (2015b). *Suicide and suicidal thoughts.* Retrieved from http://www.mayoclinic.org/disease4s-conditions/suicide/basics/symptoms/con-20033954

Mayo Clinic. (2017a). *Electroconvulsive therapy (ECT).* Retrieved from http://www.mayoclinic.org/tests-procedures/electroconvulsive-therapy/basics/definition/prc-20014161

Mayo Clinic. (2017b). *Serotonin syndrome: Symptoms.* Retrieved from http://www.mayoclinic.org/diseases-conditions/serotonin-syndrome/basics/symptoms/con-20028946

Melrose, S. (2015). Seasonal affective disorder: An overview of assessment and treatment approaches. *Depression Research and Treatment, 2015,* 178564.

Michl, L. C., McLaughlin, K. A., Shepherd, K., & Nolen-Hoeksema, S. (2013). Rumination as a mechanism linking stressful life events to symptoms of depression and anxiety: Longitudinal evidence in early adolescents and adults. *Journal of Abnormal Psychology, 122*(2), 339–352.

Minichino, A., Bersani, F. S., Capra, E., Pannese, R., Bonanno, C., Salviati, M., . . . Biondi, M. (2012). ECT, rTMS, and deep TMS in pharmacoresistant drug-free patients with unipolar depression: A comparative review. *Neuropsychiatric Disease and Treatment, 8,* 55–64.

Minkel, J. D., Banks, S., Htaik, O., Moreta, M. C., Jones, C. W., McGlinchey, E. L., . . . , Dinges, D. F. (2012). Sleep deprivation and stressors: Evidence for elevated negative affect in response to mild stressors when sleep deprived. *Emotion, 12*(5), 1015–1020.

Morris, G., & Berk, M. (2015). The many roads to mitochondrial dysfunction in neuroimmune and neuropsychiatric disorders. *BMC Medicine, 13,* 68.

Morris, M. C., Evans, L. D., Rao, U., & Garber, J. (2015). Executive function moderates the relation between coping and depressive symptoms. *Anxiety, Stress, and Coping, 28*(1), 31–49.

Mullins, N., Power, R. A., Fisher, H. L., Hanscombe, K. B., Euesden, J., Iniesta, R., . . . Lewis, C. M. (2016). Polygenic interactions with environmental adversity in the aetiology of major depressive disorder. *Psychological Medicine, 46,* 759–770.

Mulsant, B. H., Blumberger, D. M., Ismail, Z., Rabheru, K., & Rapoport, M. J. (2014). A systematic approach to the pharmacotherapy of geriatric major depression. *Clinics in Geriatric Medicine, 30*(3), 517–534.

National Alliance on Mental Illness (NAMI). (2013). *Pregnancy and bipolar disorder fact sheet.* Retrieved from http://www2.nami.org/factsheets/pregnancybipolar_factsheet.pdf

National Center for Complementary and Integrative Health. (2016). *St. John's wort and depression: In depth.* Retrieved from https://nccih.nih.gov/health/stjohnswort/sjw-and-depression.htm

National Center for PTSD. (2015). *Self-harm and trauma.* Retrieved from http://www.ptsd.va.gov/public/problems/self-harm.asp

National Institute of Mental Health (NIMH). (2013a). *Antidepressant medication for use in children and adolescents: Information for parents and caregivers.* Retrieved from http://www.nimh.nih.gov/health/topics/child-and-adolescent-mental-health/antidepressant-medications-for-children-and-adolescents-information-for-parents-and-caregivers.shtml

National Institute of Mental Health (NIMH). (2013b). *Bipolar disorder in children and teens: A parent's guide.* Retrieved from http://www.nimh.nih.gov/health/publications/bipolar-disorder-in-children-and-teens-a-parents-guide/index.shtml

National Institute of Mental Health (NIMH). (2013c). *Bipolar disorder among children.* Retrieved from http://www.nimh.nih.gov/statistics/1BIPOLAR_CHILD.shtml

National Institute of Mental Health (NIMH). (2015). *Suicide prevention.* Retrieved from http://www.nimh.nih.gov/health/topics/suicide-prevention/index.shtml

National Institute of Mental Health (NIMH). (n.d.a). *Any mood disorder in adults.* Retrieved from http://www.nimh.nih.gov/statistics/1ANYMOODDIS_ADULT.shtml

National Institute of Mental Health (NIMH). (n.d.b). *Postpartum depression facts.* Retrieved from http://www.nimh.nih.gov/health/publications/postpartum-depression-facts/index.shtml

O'Connor, S., Brausch, A., Anderson, A., & Jobes, D. (2014). Applying the Collaborative Assessment and Management of Suicidality (CAMS) to suicidal adolescents. *International Journal of Behavioral Consultation and Therapy, 9*(3), 53–58.

Office of the Surgeon General. (2012). *2012 national strategy of suicide prevention: Goals and objectives for action: A report of the U.S. Surgeon General and of the national action alliance for suicide prevention.* Retrieved from http://www.ncbi.nlm.nih.gov/pubmed/23136686

O'Hara, M. W., & McCabe, J. E. (2013). Postpartum depression: Current status and future directions. *Annual Review of Clinical Psychology, 9,* 279–407.

Olson, M., Blanco, C., & Marcus, S. C. (2016). Treatment of adult depression in the United States. *JAMA Internal Medicine.* doi:10.1001/jamainternmed.2016.5057

O'Mahony, J., & Donnelly, T. T. (2010). Immigrant and refugee women's post-partum depression help-seeking experiences and access to care: A review and analysis of the literature. *Journal of Psychiatric and Mental Health Nursing, 17,* 917–928.

Ongur, D., Bechtholt, A. J., Carlezon, W. A. Jr., & Cohen, B. M. (2014). Glial abnormalities in mood disorders. *Harvard Review of Psychiatry, 22*(6), 334–337.

Overmier, J. (2013). *Learned helplessness.* Retrieved from http://www.oxfordbibliographies.com/view/document/obo-9780199828340/obo-9780199828340-0112.xml

Patrick, R. P., & Ames, B. N. (2015). Vitamin D and the omega-3 fatty acids control serotonin synthesis and action, part 2: Relevance for ADHD, bipolar disorder, schizophrenia, and impulsive behavior. *FASEB Journal, 29*(6), 2207–2222.

Pemberton, R., & Fuller Tyszkiewicz, M. D. (2016). Factors contributing to depressive mood states in everyday life: A systematic review. *Journal of Affective Disorders, 200,* 103–110.

Pence, B. W., O'Donnell, J. K., & Gaynes, B. N. (2012). The depression treatment cascade in primary care: a public health perspective. *Current Psychiatry Rep, 14*(4), 328–338. doi:10.1007/s11920-012-0274-y

Petrakis, I., Rosenheck, R., & Desai, R. (2011). Substance use comorbidity among veterans with post-traumatic stress disorder and other psychiatric illness. *American Journal on Addictions, 20,* 185–189.

Pettinati, H., & Dundan, W. (2011). Comorbid depression and alcohol dependence: New approaches to dual therapy challenges and progress. *Psychiatric Times 28*(6), 1–8. Retrieved from http://www.nlm.nih.gov/medlineplus/ency/article/007215.htmetriev

Phelps, J. (2014). *Chapter 2: Brain differences in bipolar.* Retrieved from http://psycheducation.org/the-biologic-basis-of-bipolar-disorder/1035-2/

Platt, J., Prins, S., Bates, L., & Keyes, K. (2016). Unequal depression for equal work? How the wage gap explains gendered disparities in mood disorders. *Social Science and Medicine, 149,* 1–8.

Potter, M. L., & Moller, M. D. (2016). *Psychiatric-mental health nursing: From suffering to hope.* Hoboken, NJ: Pearson Education.

Price, A. L., & Marzani-Nissen, G. R. (2012). Bipolar disorder: A review. *American Family Physician, 85*(5), 483–493. Retrieved from http://www.aafp.org/afp/2012/0301/p483.html

Proudfoot, J., Whitton, A., Parker, G., Doran, J., Manicavasgar, V., & Delmas, K. (2012). Triggers of mania and depression in young adults with bipolar disorder. *Journal of Affective Disorders, 143*(1–3), 196–202.

Purnell, L. D. (2014). *Guide to culturally competent health care* (3rd ed.). Philadelphia, PA: F. A. Davis.

Quan, W., Wang, H., Jia, F., & Zhang, X.-H. (2015). Purpura associated with lithium intoxication. *Chinese Medical Journal, 128*(2), 284. Retrieved from http://doi.org/10.4103/0366-6999.149248

Raison, C. L., & Miller, A. H. (2011). Is depression an inflammatory disorder? *Current Psychiatry Reports, 13*(6), 467–475.

Rhodes, A. E., Boyle, M. H., Bridge, J. A., Sinyor, M., Links, P. S., Tommyr, L., . . . Szatmari, P. (2014). Antecedents and sex/gender differences in youth suicidal behavior. *World Journal of Psychiatry, 4*(4), 120–132.

Roca, M., Kohls, E., Gili, M., Watkins, E., Owens, M., Hegerl, U., . . . Penninx, B. W. (2016). Prevention of depression through nutritional strategies in high-risk persons: Rationale and design of the MooDFOOD prevention trial. *BMC Psychiatry, 16,* 192.

Sanchez-Villegas, A., & Martinez-Gonzales, M. A. (2013). Diet, a new target to prevent depression? *BMC Medicine, 11,* 3.

Saneei, P., Esmailzadeh, A., Keshteli, A. H., Reza Roohafza, H., Afshar, H., Feizi, A., & Adibi, P. (2016). Combined healthy lifestyle is inversely associated with psychological disorders among adults. *PLoS One, 11*(1), e00146888.

Santini, Z. I., Koyanagi, A., Tyrovolas, S., Mason, C., & Haro, J. M. (2015). The association between social relationships and depression: A systematic review. *Journal of Affective Disorders, 175,* 53–65.

Shapiro, G., Fraser, W., & Séguin, J. (2012). Emerging risk factors for postpartum depression: serotonin transporter genotype and omega-3 fatty acid status. *Canadian Journal of Psychiatry, 57*(11), 704–712.

Sheftall, A. H., Asti, L., Horowitz, L. M., Felts, A., Fontanella, C. A., Campo, J. V., & Bridge, J. A. (2016). Suicide in elementary school-aged children and early adolescents. *Pediatrics, 138*(4), e20160436.

Sheikh, J. I., Yesavage, J. A., Brooks, J. O., III, Friedman, L. F., Gratzinger, P., Hill, R. D., . . . Crook, T. (1991). Proposed factor structure of the Geriatric Depression Scale. *International Psychogeriatrics, 3,* 23–28.

Siu, A. L., & U.S. Preventive Services Task Force. (2016a). Screening for depression in adults: U.S. Preventive Services Task Force recommendation statement. *JAMA, 315*(4), 380–387.

Siu, A. L., & U.S. Preventive Services Task Force. (2016b). Screening for depression in children and adolescents: U.S. Preventive Services Task Force recommendation statement. *Annals of Internal Medicine, 164*(5), 360–366.

Skinner, E. A., & Zimmer-Gembeck, M. (2016). Coping. In H. S. Friedman (Ed.), *Encyclopedia of mental health* (2nd ed., pp. 350–357). Waltham, MA: Academic Press.

Slavich, G. M., & Irwin, M. R. (2014). From stress to inflammation and major depressive disorder: A social signal transduction theory of depression. *Psychological Bulletin, 140*(3), 774–815.

Smith, M. (2011). Immigration increases risk for depression. *Medpage Today.* Retrieved from http://www.medpagetoday.com/Psychiatry/Depression/25708

Sneizek, D. P., & Siddiqui, I. J. (2013). Acupuncture for treating anxiety and depression in women: A clinical systematic review. *Medical Acupuncture, 25*(3), 164–172.

Snyder, H. R. (2013). Major depressive disorder is associated with broad impairments on neuropsychological measures of executive functioning: A meta-analysis and review. *Psychological Bulletin, 139*(1), 81–132.

Spector, R. E. (2017). *Cultural diversity in health and illness* (9th ed.). Hoboken, NJ: Pearson Education.

Stanley, J. T., & Isaacowitz, D. M. (2011). Age-related differences in profiles of mood-change trajectories. *Developmental Psychology, 47*(2), 318–330.

Stanton, R., & Reaburn, P. (2013). Exercise and the treatment of depression: A review of the exercise program variables. *Journal of Science and Medicine in Sport, 17*(2), 177–182.

Stertz, L., Magalhaes, P. V. S., & Kapczinski, F. (2012). Is bipolar disorder an inflammatory condition? The relevance of microglial activation. *Current Opinion in Psychiatry, 26,* 19–26.

Stuart, G. W. (2014). *Principles and practice of psychiatric nursing* (10th ed.). St. Louis, MO: Elsevier Mosby.

Substance Abuse and Mental Health Services Administration. (SAMHSA). (2013). *Results from the 2012 National Survey on Drug Use and Health: Mental health findings.* NSDUH Series H-47, HHS Publication NO. (SMA) 13-4805. Rockville, MD: SAMHSA.

Substance Abuse and Mental Health Services Administration (SAMHSA). (2014). *Understanding the connection between suicide and substance abuse: What the research tells us.* Retrieved from http://www.samhsa.gov/capt/sites/default/files/resources/suicide-substance-abuse-research.pdf

Substance Abuse and Mental Health Services Administration (SAMHSA). (2015a). Behavioral health trends in the United States: Results from the 2014 national survey on drug use and health. Retrieved from http://www.samhsa.gov/data/sites/default/files/NSDUH-FRR1-2014/NSDUH-FRR1-2014.pdf

Substance Abuse and Mental Health Services Administration (SAMHSA). (2015b). *Promoting emotional health and preventing suicide.* Retrieved from http://store.samhsa.gov/shin/content/SMA15-4416/SMA15-4416.pdf

Substance Abuse and Mental Health Services Administration (SAMHSA). (n.d.). *Suicide assessment five-step evaluation and triage for mental health professionals.* Retrieved from http://www.integration.samhsa.gov/images/res/SAFE_T.pdf

Swami, V. (2012). Mental health literacy of depression: Gender differences and attitudinal antecedents in a representative British sample. *PLoS One, 7*(11), e49779.

Syka, A. (2015). Depression in pregnancy and ways of coping. *International Journal of Caring Sciences, 8*(1), 231–237.

Tesar, G. E. (2010). Recognition and treatment of depression. *Cleveland Clinic Center for Continuing Education.* Retrieved from http://www.clevelandclinicmeded.com/medicalpubs/diseasemanagement/psychiatry-psychology/recognition-treatment-of-depression/

The Joint Commission. (2007). *Screening for mental health: A resource guide for implementing the Joint Commission on Accreditation of Health Care Organizations' 2007 Patient Safety Goals on Suicide.* Retrieved from http://www.aha.org/content/00-10/JCAHOSafetyGoals2007.pdf

The Joint Commission. (2016). *Vital signs: The Columbia-Suicide Severity Rating Scale.* Retrieved from http://cssrs.columbia.edu/documents/jointcommission.pdf

Trives, J. J. R., Bravo, B. N., Postigo, J. M. L., Segura, L. R., & Watkins, E. (2016). Age and gender differences in emotion regulation strategies: Autobiographical memory, rumination, problem solving and distraction. *Spanish Journal of Psychology, 19,* e43.

U.S. Census Bureau. (2015). *Health insurance coverage in the United States: 2014.* Retrieved from https://www.census.gov/content/dam/Census/library/publications/2015/demo/p60-253.pdf.

U.S. Veterans Administration. (2013). *VA/DOD Clinical practice guideline for assessment and management of patients at risk for suicide.* Agency for Healthcare Research and Quality National Guidelines Clearinghouse, NGC 009978.

Varcarolis, E. M. (2013). *Essentials of psychiatric mental health nursing: A communication approach to evidence-based care* (2nd ed.). St. Louis, MO: Elsevier Saunders.

Verdeli, H., & Weissman, M. M. (2014). Interpersonal psychotherapy. In D. Wedding and R. J. Corsini (Eds.), *Current psychotherapies* (10th ed.). Belmont, CA: Brooks/Cole.

Vogelzangs, N., Beekman, A. T., van Reedt Dortland, A. K., Schoevers, R. A., Giltay, E. J., de Jonge, P., & Penninx, B. W. (2014). Inflammatory and metabolic dysregulation and the 2-year course of depressive disorders in antidepressant users. *Neuropsychopharmacology, 39*(7), 1624–1634. Retrieved from http://doi.org/10.1038/npp.2014.9

Volpi-Abadie, J., Kaye, A. M., & Kaye, A. D. (2013). Serotonin syndrome. *Ochsner Journal, 13*(4), 533–540.

Waqas, A., Raza, N., Lodhi, H. W., Muhammad, Z., Jamal, M., & Rehman, A. (2015). Psychosocial factors of antenatal anxiety and depression in Pakistan: Is social support a mediator? *PLoS One, 10*(1), e0116510. http://doi.org/10.1371/journal.pone.0116510

Waters, R. P., Rivalan, M., Bangasser, D. A., Deussing, J. M., Ising, M., Wood, S. K., . . . Summers, C. H. (2015). Evidence for the role of corticotropin-releasing factor in major depressive disorder. *Neuroscience and Biobehavioral Reviews, 58*, 63–78.

Werner, F. M., & Covenas, R. (2015). Treatment of bipolar disorder according to a neural network. *Journal of Cytology and Histology, 6*, 6.

Wharton, W., Gleason, C. E., Olson, S. R. M. S., Carlsson, C. M., & Asthana, S. (2012). Neurobiological underpinnings of the estrogen–mood relationship. *Current Psychiatry Reviews, 8*(3), 247–256.

Whitaker, K. M., Sharpe, P. A., Wilcox, S., & Hutto, B. E. (2014). Depressive symptoms are associated with dietary intake but not physical activity among overweight and obese women from disadvantaged neighborhoods. *Nutrition Research, 34*(4), 294–301.

White, B. A., Horwath, C. C., & Conner, T. S. (2013). Many apples a day keep the blues away: Daily experiences of negative and positive affect and food consumption in young adults. *British Journal of Health Psychology, 18*(4), 782–798.

Wilson, B., Shannon, M., & Shields, K. (Eds.). (2016). *Pearson nurse's drug guide*. New York, NY: Pearson Education.

World Health Organization. (2016a). *Gender and women's mental health*. Retrieved from http://www.who.int/mental_health/prevention/genderwomen/en/

World Health Organization. (2016b). *Suicide: Fact sheet*. Retrieved from http://www.who.int/mediacentre/factsheets/fs398/en/

Yazici, E., Kirkan, T., Aslan, P., Aydin, N., & Yazici, A. (2015). *Untreated depression in the first trimester of pregnancy leads to postpartum depression: high rates from a natural follow-up study*. Retrieved from http://www.ncbi.nlm.nih.gov/pmc/articles/PMC4344179/

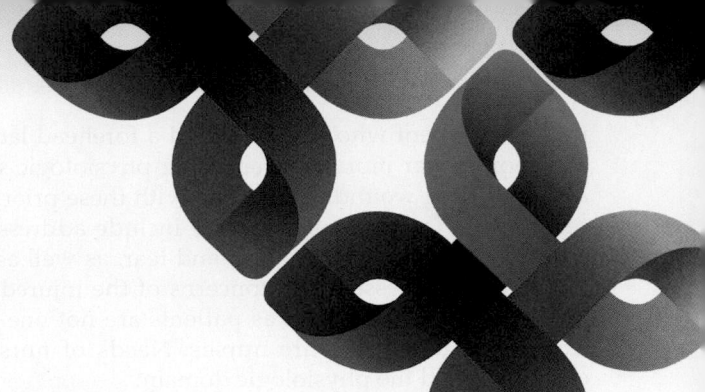

Module 29
Self

Module Outline and Learning Outcomes

The Concept of Self

Normal Presentation

29.1 Analyze the psychosocial processes related to self-concept.

Psychosocial Development Across the Lifespan

29.2 Differentiate considerations related to the development of self across the lifespan.

Alterations from Normal

29.3 Differentiate alterations in self-concept.

Concepts Related to Self

29.4 Outline the relationship between self-concept and other concepts.

Health Promotion

29.5 Explain the promotion of healthy self-concept.

Nursing Assessment

29.6 Differentiate common assessment procedures used to examine the individual's self-concept.

Independent Interventions

29.7 Analyze independent interventions nurses can implement for patients with alterations in self-concept.

Collaborative Therapies

29.8 Summarize collaborative therapies used by interprofessional teams for patients with alterations in self-concept.

Self Exemplars

Exemplar 29.A Feeding and Eating Disorders

29.A Analyze feeding and eating disorders and how they relate to self.

Exemplar 29.B Personality Disorders

29.B Analyze personality disorders and how they relate to self.

» The Concept of Self

Concept Key Terms

Anorexia nervosa (AN), **1980**	Global evaluative dimension of the self, **1978**	Personal identity, **1976**	Public self, **1976**	Role mastery, **1978**
Body image, **1976**		Personality disorder (PD), **1980**	Purging, **1981**	Role performance, **1977**
Bulimia nervosa (BN), **1980**	Global self-esteem, **1978**	Prader-Willi syndrome (PWS), **1980**	Real self, **1976**	Role strain, **1977**
Erik Erikson, **1978**	Ideal body image, **1977**		Role, **1977**	Self-awareness, **1978**
Feeding and eating disorders, **1980**	Ideal self, **1976**	Psychoanalytic theory, **1978**	Role ambiguity, **1977**	Self-concept, **1976**
	Introspection, **1978**		Role conflicts, **1977**	Self-esteem, **1978**
			Role development, **1977**	Specific self-esteem, **1978**

At the simplest level, caring for patients requires the nurse to be physically present in the care setting. Physical presence in the workplace requires adhering to a work schedule and honoring a commitment to an employer and to patients. However, the energy needed to maintain employment and to care for others requires that the nurse obtain adequate nutrition and rest. Likewise, the knowledge needed to apply the nursing process first requires education in the field of nursing.

On a deeper level, to assess and care for patients from a holistic perspective and to establish therapeutic relationships, the nurse must draw from psychosocial resources that include caring, empathy, and compassion, psychosocial resources whose attainment is far more personal than the attainment or use of time, energy, or knowledge. Nurses recognize that caring for others is not one dimensional in nature; that is, caring for a patient extends beyond the treatment of injury or illness. For example, treatment of a pediatric patient who has sustained a forehead laceration incorporates far more than ensuring physiologic stability and providing wound care. Along with these priority concerns, other facets of nursing care include addressing the wounded child's pain, anxiety, and fear, as well as recognizing and addressing the concerns of the injured child's family or loved ones. Just as patients are not one-dimensional beings, neither are nurses. Needs of nurses also extend beyond the physiologic domain.

To promote health and wellness in others, nurses must first recognize and understand their own thoughts, emotions, perceptions, abilities, and limitations. Recognition of one's own needs requires an understanding of the concept of self. *Self* can be described as the entirety of an individual's being, including body, sensations, emotions, and thoughts, as well as a conscious awareness of one's own being. Within the self are all personal traits, characteristics, beliefs, and behaviors. Accurate assessment of a patient's degree of psychosocial health requires that the nurse be capable of recognizing signs and symptoms of impairments and alterations. In addition, the nurse must be able to identify evidence-based interventions that are effective in the promotion of psychosocial well-being.

Both personally and professionally, wellness promotion requires the nurse to understand and apply principles related to the concept of self, which includes an individual's overall self-image and self-perception. This module explores the concept of self, as well as its various components.

Normal Presentation

Physiologic alterations often produce visible findings or manifestations that can be discerned through laboratory and diagnostic tests. The use of established parameters or guidelines can simplify the process of identifying abnormal findings.

In contrast, identification of abnormal psychosocial function requires a different approach. Rather than following objective algorithms and guidelines, normal parameters within the psychosocial realm often range along a continuum. Moreover, to identify what is normal or abnormal, the nurse must assess the degree to which the psychosocial concern is affecting the patient. *Normal* is more easily defined within the physiologic realm, whereas *healthy* is the term that more readily applies to the psychosocial realm.

Development of self is a dynamic process that is influenced by interpersonal interactions throughout an individual's lifetime. Numerous theorists, including famed psychologists Erik Erikson and Jean Piaget, proposed theories to describe the processes of human growth and development, including specific stages and tasks associated with each phase of life. From a broad standpoint, principles of growth and development apply to mastery of numerous tasks, as well as to achievement of milestones related to physiologic, cognitive, psychosocial, spiritual, and moral development. For many developmental tasks throughout the lifespan, successful task completion is rooted in interpersonal interaction.

Although this module offers an overview of the development of self, the primary focus includes exploring and describing the impact of self on patient health, as well as its importance to nursing care. (For in-depth discussion of theories related to psychosocial development, see the module on Development.)

Self-concept

Self-concept, which is integral to psychosocial development, is the personal perception of self that forms in response to interactions with others and the environment throughout the course of an individual's lifetime. Self-concept affects an individual mentally, physically, and spiritually. A negative self-concept can lead to struggles with adapting to change and building interpersonal relationships. In addition, a negative self-concept can increase an individual's susceptibility to physical and psychologic illnesses. Within the psychosocial domain, effective nursing care includes assessing patients' self-concept and assisting them with the development of a healthy, positive self-perception (Berman, Snyder, & Frandsen, 2016). Because each individual's self-concept impacts the nature and efficacy of her interpersonal interactions, including nurse–patient relationships, the nurse is responsible for exploring and optimizing her own self-concept. In nursing, components of self-concept are often considered to include personal identity, body image, role performance, self-esteem, and self-awareness, each of which will be discussed.

Personal Identity

Personal identity can be evaluated from the standpoint of three aspects of self: the ideal self, the real self, and the public self. The **ideal self** reflects qualities an individual believes he should possess, as well as those he aspires to develop. The **real self** represents the perceived true self (Ciccarelli & White, 2013). The real self may include observations about self or self-perceived qualities that the individual hides from others or does not readily share. For example, the real self may house perceptions such as "I am greedy" or "I am judgmental." The **public self** is formed on the basis of how the individual wishes to be perceived by others. For example, in the workplace, an individual's public self may lead to behaviors that inspire others to deem him as being friendly, competent, and team-oriented. While the ideal self reflects "who I should be and who I want to be," the real self represents "who I really am." The public self reflects "who I believe others think I am."

Characteristics that make up personal identity include objective descriptors, such as name, age, gender, marital status, and occupation. In addition, personal identity can include an individual's cultural background and ethnic origin. Values, beliefs, and self-expectations also shape personal identity. When an individual chooses values that he believes to be important and acts accordingly, his personal identity becomes stronger. This has a direct impact on nursing care, as congruence of the nurse's behavior with his own personal character and values impacts the extent to which patients and coworkers find him to be trustworthy (Riffkin, 2015).

Body Image

Body image is an individual's mental picture of her physical self. How an individual perceives the appearance and size of her body and emotional reaction to those perceptions are

TABLE 29–1 Elements of Body Image

Element	Description
Perceptual	Mental image of the body; includes perception of physical appearance and how one perceives his or her body when viewing it in a mirror.
Cognitive	Includes beliefs and attitudes about one's body, as well as the degree to which body image is valued and the individual's level of investment in physical appearance.
Behavioral	Encompasses behavioral manifestations that may reveal cues about an individual's feelings and perceptions about his or her body; for example, indicators may include wearing revealing clothing and engaging in activities that require physical exposure (e.g., wearing a swimsuit to the swimming pool).
Affective	Represents feelings about one's body, in terms of both appearance and function. May be negative (e.g., shame or embarrassment) or positive (e.g., pride or satisfaction).
Subjective satisfaction	Reflects an individual's degree of satisfaction with his or her body, both as a whole and in terms of individual parts or regions.

components of body image. However, the impact of an individual's body image extends far beyond these two components. Elements of body image include those within the perceptual, cognitive, behavioral, affective, and subjective satisfaction dimensions (see **Table 29–1 »**) (Ginis, Bassett-Gunter, & Conlin, 2012). Body image takes into account prosthetic devices, including hairpieces and artificial limbs, as well as assistive devices, such as wheelchairs, walkers, eyeglasses, and hearing aids (see **Figure 29–1 »**). The individual's perception of her need to use assistive devices is also part of body image.

Culture and society significantly impact body image, including the **ideal body image**, which is a mental representation of what an individual believes her body should look like. In particular, visual media—such as movies and magazine images—are viewed by some as promoting an unrealistic

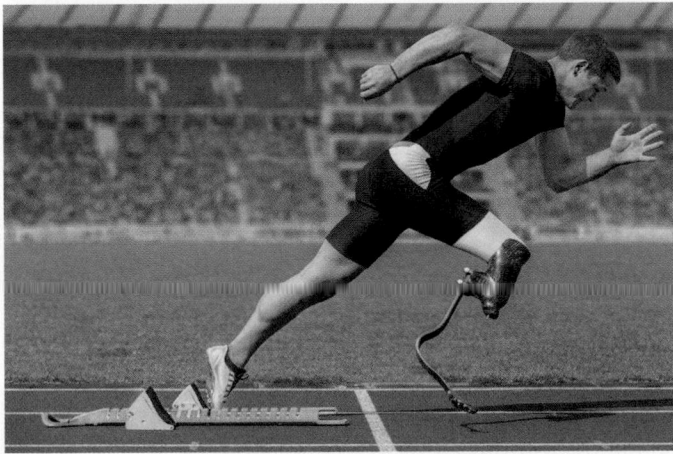

Source: Mezzotint_fotolia/Fotolia.

Figure 29–1 » Body image is the sum of a person's conscious and unconscious attitudes about his or her body. How do you think the runner pictured here views his body image?

ideal body image. For example, in the United States, the modeling and advertising industries often feature women who are extremely thin, which is an issue that has sparked cultural debate with regard to the effects of this practice on the development of ideal body image among young females. Typically, the more congruent an individual's perceived body image is with her ideal body image, the greater her level of satisfaction with body image will be.

Role Performance

A nursing student is also a son or daughter, perhaps a brother or sister, and may be a father or mother as well. Each of these positions or roles—student, offspring, sibling, and parent—is associated with certain behavioral expectations. A **role** encompasses a grouping of behavioral expectations associated with a specified societal or organizational position. Role expectations may be defined by numerous entities, including society, culture, religion, tribal leadership, an employer, or any organization of which the individual is a member. The demonstration of behaviors or actions associated with a given role is called **role performance**.

Teaching and modeling the behaviors needed to successfully assume a role are part of **role development**, which is essential for effective role performance. Role development also includes socialization of the individual who is preparing to assume a given role. For example, a graduate nurse who accepts a position in a medical–surgical hospital unit will most often complete an orientation program, which includes exposure of the newly employed nurse to basic aspects related to working in that clinical setting, such as institutional protocols and charting requirements. After orientation, the nurse usually will be assigned a preceptor who models expected nursing behaviors and assists the nurse with continued role development.

Ineffective role development can lead to **role ambiguity**, which occurs when an individual lacks clarity regarding the expectations, behaviors, or demands associated with fulfilling a given role. Individuals who feel incapable of fulfilling a role may experience **role strain**. In some cases, role strain may be the result of sexual stereotyping. For example, a female firefighter who is told or given the impression by male colleagues that she is physically incapable of handling the rigorous demands associated with a male-dominated occupation may experience role strain. Both role ambiguity and role strain can negatively impact self-concept.

When role-related expectations clash or are incongruent, **role conflicts** may occur. If needs for recognition, accomplishment, and independence are not met, the role conflict can produce embarrassment, increased stress, and decreased self-esteem (Berman et al., 2016). Conflicts may occur between one or more individuals (interpersonal) or within one individual (intrapersonal), as well as between groups and organizations. Forms of role conflict include the following:

- ***Interpersonal conflict.*** Occurs when individuals hold varying or conflicting expectations about tasks and behaviors associated with a specific role; for example, a husband and wife may have conflicting expectations about who is responsible for completing household chores and preparing meals.

- **Interrole conflict.** Occurs when roles create competing demands; for example, in the case of an individual who is balancing college courses with parenting, the demands associated with being a student may impinge on the demands of raising a child.

- **Person–role conflict.** Occurs when role expectations are in opposition to the values and beliefs of the one who fills the role; for example, despite the Western healthcare practice of promoting truth telling and autonomy, in some instances a family may ask that their family member not be informed that he has been diagnosed with a terminal illness (Coolen, 2012).

Role mastery occurs when an individual's behaviors within a role meet or exceed predetermined expectations. The inability to achieve role mastery can lead to stress, internal conflict, and impaired self-esteem (Berman et al., 2016).

Self-Esteem

Self-esteem, which is separate from self-concept, is an individual's opinion of himself. In essence, self-esteem describes the degree to which an individual approves of, values, or likes himself (Blascovich & Tomaka, 1991; Brown, 2014).

While self-concept reflects how an individual perceives himself, self-esteem, which is the evaluative component of self-concept (Berk, 2013), describes the individual's judgments and opinions about those perceived characteristics. Positive or high self-esteem is associated with greater levels of achievement, increased financial prosperity, and decreased incidence of depression (Orth & Robins, 2014).

Researchers have proposed two categories of self-esteem: global and specific. **Global self-esteem**, or the **global evaluative dimension of the self**, is the degree to which an individual likes herself overall, as a whole being. **Specific self-esteem**, however, reflects an individual's positive regard for certain aspects of herself (Brown, 2014; Gentile et al., 2009), such as physical appearance, athletic ability, parenting skills, or academic achievement.

Specific self-esteem influences global self-esteem (Berman et al., 2016). For example, if an individual who highly values athletic ability possesses exceptional athletic skills, that individual's athletic performance will impact his global self-esteem. However, if that same individual assigns little value to academic achievement, his global self-esteem will be minimally influenced by failing a college course.

In their landmark study, DeHart, Pelham, and Tennen (2006) identified early parent–child interactions as significantly influencing the development of self-esteem. Young adult children who reported exposure to greater levels of parental nurturing also reported higher self-esteem, while parental overprotectiveness was linked to lower self-esteem (DeHart et al., 2006). In addition, both behavioral and neural studies (using MRI scanning) have identified a link between an individual's perceived experience of rejection and the expression of a sense of low self-esteem (Kashdan et al., 2014; Leary, 2006). In studies of individuals between the ages of 14 and 30, high risk-taking behaviors, low sense of mastery, and poor health status effectively predicted lower levels of self-esteem. In older adults, self-esteem was higher among individuals who had completed more education (Orth & Robins, 2014).

Self-Awareness

For an individual to develop a reality-based perception of his real self requires **self-awareness**. Development of self-awareness begins in infancy, as infants learn to distinguish themselves from other individuals and objects in their environment. With the ability to differentiate his own voice and body from the voices and bodies of others, the infant's self-awareness increases (Berk, 2013). Developing self-awareness is an ongoing process that requires intense examination of one's personal perspectives, beliefs, and values. Moreover, self-awareness includes identifying relationships that connect actions to self. By establishing connections between past experiences and current actions or choices, the individual who is self-aware gains insight into the meaning of his behaviors. As opposed to viewing life experiences as being isolated events, many of which are perhaps inexplicable, development of self-awareness requires that actions and behaviors are viewed within the context of the individual's deep-seated values and beliefs (Demetriou & Kazi, 2013; Eckroth-Bucher, 2010). Essentially, the individual who is self-aware understands why he does what he does, and his behaviors and actions can be linked to his core beliefs and values.

The process of developing self-awareness requires **introspection**, which is personal exploration and evaluation of one's own thoughts, emotions, behaviors, and values. Introspection also incorporates both verbal and nonverbal feedback from others (Demetriou & Kazi, 2013; Eckroth-Bucher, 2010). While the process of introspection is intimate and personal in nature, the outcome of this process is greatly influenced by a number of external factors. In many ways, an individual's view of himself is significantly shaped by how others perceive him.

Development of Personality

Numerous behavioral theorists and scientists have proposed theories to describe the development of personality as a component of self. Among the most famous developmental theories are those originated by Sigmund Freud and Erik Erikson. Freud (1856–1939) is considered the founder of **psychoanalytic theory**, which provided the earliest framework for personality development and emphasized the presence of unconscious impulses and their influence on behaviors and the formation of self. Whereas Freud's theory is grounded in psychosexual elements and the human response to impulses, Erikson's theory incorporates social, cultural, and interpersonal components (Kneisl & Trigoboff, 2013).

The theory of psychosocial development originated by German-born psychologist and psychoanalyst **Erik Erikson** (1902–1994) is still widely taught today. Erikson (1950, 1963) developed the primary theory on psychosocial development in humans. His ideas were greatly influenced by Freud's theory regarding the structure and topography of personality (McLeod, 2013). Whereas Freud concentrated on internal conflicts, Erikson emphasized the role of culture and society and the conflicts that can influence personality. According to Erikson, the self develops as it successfully resolves crises that are distinctly social in nature. Three overriding themes in Erikson's theory are establishing trust in others, developing a sense of identity in society, and helping the next generation prepare for the future. Erikson extended Freudian theory by focusing on the adaptive and creative characteristics of the self and by expanding the notion of the stages of personality development to include the entire lifespan (McLeod, 2013). For more discussion of Erikson's developmental theory, see Table 25–2 in the module on Development.

Psychosocial Development Across the Lifespan

Early childhood experiences and brain circuitry development influence the child's developing central nervous system and have been linked to both risk and resiliency for psychopathology in adulthood (Potter & Moller, 2016). Environmental factors, such as toxins, early childhood maltreatment, diet, and stress can change gene activity and increase the risk for developing psychopathology later in life. Because approximately 75% of adult psychiatric disorders have their onset in childhood and adolescence, mental health promotion interventions that target these factors can change the course of development for children at risk for psychiatric disorders and alter the course of development along the psychologic, biological, sociologic, cultural, and spiritual domains (Potter & Moller, 2016). For example, interventions that promote healthy nutrition in pregnant women and in young children can reduce the risk for disorders or dysfunction in multiple areas of growth and development.

An important influence on psychosocial development is the occurrence of trauma at any life stage. The frequency and number of abusive and traumatic events, referred to as *complex trauma*, influence the severity of psychologic distress and can hinder development. Emotional experiences of trauma can be particularly overwhelming for children, especially if the home environment is the source of maltreatment (Potter & Moller, 2016). Interpersonal violence (IPV) is the primary source of trauma in adult women. Trauma can affect people of every race, ethnicity, age, sexual orientation, gender, psychosocial background, and geographic region (Substance Abuse and Mental Health Services Administration [SAMHSA], 2014).

Other key considerations at each developmental stage are discussed below.

Newborns and Infants (Birth to 1 Year)

During the first year of life, infants are uncertain about their environment and look to the primary caregiver for stability and consistency of care as they adjust to life outside the womb. If infants receive consistent, predictable, and reliable care, they will develop a sense of trust, which they will expect to occur in other relationships (McLeod, 2013). They will feel secure even in threatening situations and develop a sense of hope that other people will provide support.

Infants who do not feel secure will become fearful when dealing with new people and situations. They may mistrust others and lack confidence in the world around them or in their abilities to influence events. Lack of trust may result in anxiety, heightened insecurities, and a pervasive feeling of uneasiness (McLeod, 2013). Three influential theorists were Erikson (discussed below), who advanced strong views on the importance of trust for infants, and Bowlby (1969) and Ainsworth (1973), both of whom outlined how the quality of the early experience of attachment can affect relationships with others in later life (McLeod, 2013).

Toddlers (1 to 3 Years)

During this period, children are developing physically and becoming more mobile. Children will begin to assert their independence, develop skills, and engage in activities that promote growing independence and autonomy. Parents need to allow toddlers active exploration within an encouraging environment that is tolerant of failure, such as allowing children to don their own clothes without interference unless assistance is requested. The primary parental task at this stage is to foster independence while avoiding criticism of failures. By bolstering toddlers' self-esteem, parents will help children be supported in acquiring increased independence, thus becoming more confident and secure in their own ability to navigate in the world (McLeod, 2013).

Preschool Children (3 to 6 Years)

Around age 3 and continuing to age 5, children begin to assert themselves more frequently. They begin regularly interacting with other children and playing, which provides children with the opportunity to explore their interpersonal skills through initiating activities (McLeod, 2013). Children begin to plan activities, create games, and initiate activities with others, which help them begin to develop a sense of initiative and feel secure in their abilities to lead others and make decisions. However, if during this period children are overcontrolled or over-criticized, they may develop a sense of guilt and lack self-initiative (McLeod, 2013).

Children also begin to ask many questions to grow their knowledge base. If parents do not allow children to question and treat them as a nuisance, children may develop a sense of guilt that will influence interpersonal interactions and inhibit creativity. The parental balance at this point is to impose enough restriction on children that they begin to develop a conscience and self-control (McLeod, 2013).

School-Age Children (6 to 12 Years)

At age 6 to 12 years, the primary tasks of children are learning to read and write, to do math, and to perform activities on their own. Teachers begin to take an important role as they teach the specific skills (McLeod, 2013). At this stage, the child's peer group will gain greater significance and will become a major source of the child's self-esteem. The child now feels compelled to win approval by demonstrating specific competencies that are valued by society and begins to develop a sense of pride in acquired accomplishments (McLeod, 2013). Children age 5 to 9 exhibit increased control of emotions, form peer groups, and begin to understand how their actions affect others (Mental Health America [MHA], 2015).

Preteen adolescents of age 10 to 12 years commonly have emotional swings (feeling wonderful one minute, and sad or irritable the next). They begin to believe peer acceptance means being liked. They still rely on bonds with their parents but may not demonstrate closeness. They question rules and values, often saying things are "unfair." They may begin to focus more on their looks and dress (MHA, 2015). For preteens, it is important for parents and teachers to support their interests and their desire to acquire abilities and achieve goals. If this initiative is not encouraged or if it is restricted by parents or teacher, then the preteen begins to feel inferior, doubting his or her own abilities, and therefore may not reach full potential.

Adolescents (12 to 18 Years)

The major task of this life stage is to learn the roles required to become an adult. During this stage, the adolescent will reexamine personal identity, including sexual orientation and occupational roles (McLeod, 2013). Adolescents explore possibilities and begin to form their own identities based on the outcome of their explorations. Failure to establish a sense of identity within society can lead to role confusion, where the adolescent is uncertain regarding his or her place in society. In response to role confusion or identity crisis, an adolescent may begin to experiment with different lifestyles in such areas as work, education, drugs/alcohol, or political views (McLeod, 2013). Adolescents who are pressured into an identity have the potential to become unhappy and often rebel by establishing a negative identity.

Adolescents struggle with their sense of identity, worrying about being normal or "fitting in." They feel awkward about themselves and their body image and maintain high expectations for themselves. Although adolescents still rely on connectedness with their parents, they may complain that their parents interfere with their independence or behave rudely to their parents in front of others. Young teens begin testing rules and limits. As they develop more friendships with peers of both genders, they try to find a group of peers with whom they fit in and are accepted. Exposure to sex and drugs increases in adolescence. Moodiness is common, and young teens may return to childish behaviors when stressed. Intellectual efforts become more important (MHA, 2015).

Adults

In young adulthood (age 18 to 40 years), adults begin to share themselves more intimately with others, exploring relationships that lead toward longer term commitments with someone other than a family member. Successful completion of this stage can lead to comfortable relationships and a sense of commitment, safety, and care within a relationship (McLeod, 2013). Avoidance of intimacy and fear of commitment and relationships can lead to isolation, loneliness, and sometimes depression.

Researchers Erol and Orth (2011) studied levels of self-esteem in males and females between the ages of 14 and 30. Overall findings suggested that self-esteem increases during adolescence and, to a lesser degree, into young adulthood. Regardless of age, participants who were extraverted, emotionally stable, and conscientious reported higher self-esteem than did those participants who were deemed introverted, emotionally unstable, and less conscientious. In addition, among all ages studied, low risk-taking behaviors, high sense of mastery, and better health status reliably predicted higher levels of self-esteem.

During middle adulthood (age 40 to 65 years), adults establish careers, settle down within relationships, begin their own families, and develop a sense of being a part of the bigger picture. Adults give back to society through raising children, being productive at work, and becoming involved in community activities and organizations (McLeod, 2013). If adults fail to achieve these objectives, they become stagnant and feel unproductive.

As adults grow older (age 65+ years) and become senior citizens, they tend to slow down productivity and explore retirement options. If older adults see their lives as unproductive, feel guilty about the past, or perceive that they did not accomplish their life goals, they may become dissatisfied with life and develop despair, often leading to depression and hopelessness (McLeod, 2013).

In 2010, Orth, Trzesniewski, and Robins published findings of a study designed to evaluate the development of self-esteem between young adulthood and old age. Participants ranged in age from 25 to 104 years. Study findings included an apparent increase in self-esteem during young and middle adulthood, with self-esteem levels ultimately peaking around 60 years of age. After age 60, self-esteem declined. Higher self-esteem was reported by participants who had completed more education. Overall, results suggested that the declining self-esteem reported by older adults was primarily caused by changes in physical health and socioeconomic status (Orth et al., 2010).

Alterations from Normal

Alterations in self may stem from a variety of factors, including issues pertaining to the primary components of self-concept, self-esteem, and self-awareness. Within the component of self-concept, some researchers suggest that conflicts related to body image may lead to the development of feeding and eating disorders. Alterations in one or more components of self may manifest through the development of personality disorders.

Alterations and Manifestations

Feeding and Eating Disorders

Feeding and eating disorders are marked by chronic disturbances in eating or eating-related practices that result in impairment in food consumption or absorption to the extent that daily functioning is affected and physical and psychologic health are significantly impaired (American Psychiatric Association [APA], 2013). Feeding and eating disorders cause low self-esteem, self-hatred, fear, and hopelessness, and they put the individual at risk for a variety of physiologic problems. Affected individuals often also have other mental disorders such as anxiety disorders, substance abuse, or depression (National Institute of Mental Health [NIMH], 2014). Feeding and eating disorders can be fatal. Nurses should not underestimate the significance of these disorders.

The most common feeding and eating disorders include **anorexia nervosa, bulimia nervosa,** and binge-eating disorder, each of which is discussed in detail in the exemplar later in this module. The characteristic features of these three disorders are presented in **Table 29–2 ⟩⟩**. Other disorders that may impact body image include nocturnal sleep-related eating disorder and Prader-Willi syndrome. Additional disorders often clustered with the more prevalent feeding and eating disorders include pica, rumination disorder, and avoidant/restrictive food intake disorder.

TABLE 29–2 Characteristic Manifestations of Common Feeding and Eating Disorders

Eating Disorder	Characteristics
Anorexia Nervosa (AN)	■ Obsessive focus on weight and body size ■ Abnormally low body weight (usually 85% or less of the normal/expected weight) ■ Extreme fear of weight gain ■ May include **purging** behaviors (e.g., vomiting, diuretic use, laxative abuse) ■ Average age of onset 19 years
Bulimia Nervosa (BN)	■ Obsessive focus on weight and body size ■ Classified by presence or absence of purging behaviors ■ ***Purging type:*** includes episodes of binge eating followed by purging through self-induced vomiting or use of diuretics or laxatives ■ ***Nonpurging type:*** includes episodes of binge eating followed by fasting, intense and frequent exercise, or restrictive dieting ■ Average age of onset 20 years
Binge-Eating Disorder (BED)	■ Episodic compulsive consumption of excessive amounts of food within a 2-hour time period ■ Overeating typically conducted in private/secrecy ■ Not associated with purging behaviors ■ Average age at onset 25 years

Sources: Based on National Institute of Mental Health. (2014). *Eating disorders: About more than food.* Retrieved from https://www.nimh.nih.gov/health/publications/eating-disorders-new-trifold/index.shtml; Osborn, K. S., Wraa, C. E., Watson, A., & Holleran, R. S. (2013). *Medical–surgical nursing: Preparation for practice* (2nd ed.). Upper Saddle River, NJ: Pearson.

Nocturnal sleep-related eating disorder (NSRED) is characterized by an initial period of insomnia, followed by an episode of sleepwalking or semiconsciousness, during which time the affected individual consumes unusual foods or nonfood items. Primary manifestations associated with NSRED include obesity and difficulty losing weight. This sleep-related eating disorder is more common in women and typically starts when individuals are in their 20s. It often occurs in those who have restless leg syndrome and may be a related condition. NSRED may also be linked to other sleep disorders, such as obstructive sleep apnea, and has been associated with use of short-acting sleep medications, such as zolpidem (Mayo Clinic, 2014a). For these patients, interventions include referral to a nutritionist, evaluation of mood and stress, and screening for sleep-related disorders.

Pica refers to a continuing pattern of behavior in which the individual consumes nonnutritive, nonfood substances (e.g., chalk, paper, soap, dirt, metal, string, hair). Pica is more commonly reported in children, although it may appear in adults with intellectual disability or mental disorders. Pica may manifest in pregnancy related to cravings for nonfood substances (APA, 2013).

Rumination disorder describes the repeated regurgitation of food outside the presence of a medical condition (e.g., pyloric stenosis, gastroesophageal reflux). Onset may occur at any age, but if rumination begins in the first year of life, it may result in a medical emergency if it does not resolve spontaneously or if treatment is not initiated (APA, 2013).

Avoidant/restrictive food intake disorder is characterized as a disturbance in a eating patterns manifested by failure to meet nutritional needs. Significant weight loss, nutritional deficiency, and dependency on enteral feeding or nutritional supplements may be observed along with impairment of psychosocial functioning. This disorder is seen more commonly in children and may result in impaired family functioning because of the increased stress related to meals and around functions including meals (APA, 2013).

Prader-Willi syndrome (PWS) is a chromosomal disorder that usually manifests at about 2 years of age. The characteristic features include mental retardation, poor muscle tone, and an incessant desire to eat (Mayo Clinic, 2014b). Obesity occurs as a result of indiscriminate and excessive food consumption (Osborn et al., 2013). Because individuals with PWS have a constant sense of hunger and desire to eat, treatment includes ensuring good nutritional habits and providing the patient with the proper amount of food intake. Because of hormonal deficiencies, these patients exhibit impaired physical growth and hypogonadism (underdevelopment of the sex organs). Treatment for patients with PWS may include hormonal therapies, as well as mental health services to address comorbid conditions. Speech, physical, and occupational therapy may also be of benefit to these patients (Mayo Clinic, 2014c).

Personality Disorders

A **personality disorder (PD)** manifests as a pervasive pattern of behaviors, personal perceptions, and internal experiences that are significantly incongruent with an individual's cultural expectations. This persistent pattern of behaviors, perceptions, and experiences is relatively inflexible and causes distress or functional impairment (see **Figure 29–2 》**). Manifestations of the PD frequently lead to disruption of the individual's personal, social, and professional interactions. Typically, the onset of PDs is during adolescence or early adulthood (APA, 2013). At present, the American Psychiatric Association recognizes the following 10 forms of PD, each of which is discussed in the exemplar on Personality Disorders in this module (APA, 2013). Of these, borderline personality disorder (BPD) and antisocial personality disorder (ASPD) are the most challenging for patients, family members, and clinicians.

See the Alterations and Therapies feature for a summary of the manifestations and therapies for feeding and eating disorders and personality disorders.

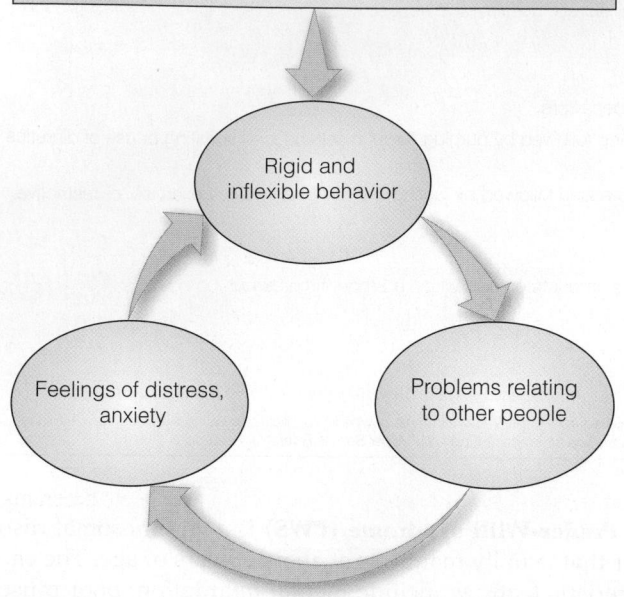

A person with a personality disorder has:

- Few strategies for relating to others
- Poor impulse control
- Different thought patterns and ways of perceiving
- Different range and intensity of affect from others in the culture.

Rigid and inflexible behavior

Feelings of distress, anxiety

Problems relating to other people

Figure 29–2 》 Vicious cycle of personality disorders.

Prevalence

Although feeding and eating disorders can impact individuals at any age, from the standpoint of patients who are officially diagnosed with an eating disorder, these conditions are reportedly more common among adolescents and young adults. In the United States, among adolescents between the ages of 13 and 17, an estimated 2.7% have an eating disorder. Bulimia nervosa is most prevalent among Hispanic adolescents, whereas anorexia nervosa is most prevalent among non-Hispanic White adolescents (Perez & Warren, 2013; Swanson et al., 2011). Bulimia nervosa (BN) is more common than is anorexia nervosa (AN) (APA, 2013). Lesbian, gay, and bisexual (LGB) identity has been associated with substantially elevated odds of purging and diet pill use in both male and female high school students, while bisexual females and males were also at elevated odds of obesity compared to same-gender heterosexuals (Austin et al., 2012).

Among individuals 18 years and older, an estimated 15% of all adults in the United States have at least one personality disorder (APA, 2013). Prevalence associated with specific PDs is discussed in the exemplar on Personality Disorders in this module.

Genetic Considerations and Nonmodifiable Risk Factors

Compared to boys, girls are more than twice as likely to develop an eating disorder (Swanson et al., 2011). Gender prevalence varies with regard to specific PDs.

Research suggests there is a genetic component in PDs, and selected PDs with paranoid and delusional features

may have a link with schizophrenia (APA, 2013). Certain personality characteristics can reflect the development of PDs, such as pervasive anxiety, fear, and aggression. Being a victim of childhood trauma or sexual abuse may promote the development of BPD. Adverse socioeconomic factors such as poverty and sociocultural factors such as migration can influence the development of a PD. A PD may be exacerbated following the loss of a significant support person, such as a spouse, or previously stabilizing social situations such as a job (APA, 2013).

Case Study 》 Part 1

Jocelyn LeMandre, a 28-year-old woman, is transported to the emergency department (ED) by a friend. Although Ms. LeMandre is alert, oriented, and denies any complaints, her friend reports that Ms. LeMandre "passed out during an aerobics class" and also notes Ms. LeMandre has been complaining of being light-headed for the past few weeks. Ms. LeMandre reports she is finishing her doctoral degree in chemistry and currently teaches university courses.

When questioned about her symptoms, Ms. LeMandre admits to "feeling a little light-headed" but also notes that she hasn't been drinking enough fluids lately. She reports that she exercises daily for 2 hours prior to teaching her first course and occasionally exercises for another hour before going to bed. When asked about her dietary habits, Ms. LeMandre quietly replies, "I eat almost anything I want to eat. I might as well—I'm still going to be fat," and then looks away. When asked, Ms. LeMandre reports her height and weight as 5'7" tall and 154 pounds. By observation, Ms. LeMandre's weight is relatively proportionate to her height. Upon assessment, Ms. LeMandre's vital signs, which are within normal limits, include temperature 97.8°F oral; pulse 89 bpm; respirations 20/min; and BP 92/52 mmHg.

Clinical Reasoning Questions Level I

1. Considering the report provided by Ms. LeMandre's friend and Ms. LeMandre's statements, what may be the cause of her light-headedness?
2. Based on Ms. LeMandre's educational background, occupation, and exercise regimen, what aspects of her personality are apparent?

Clinical Reasoning Questions Level II

3. At this time, what nursing diagnoses may be appropriate for inclusion in Ms. LeMandre's plan of care?
4. Based on the available information, what additional assessment data might you expect the primary healthcare provider to order for Ms. LeMandre?

Concepts Related to Self

An individual's self-concept and self-esteem may be affected by alterations in other systems. For example, someone who is challenged by alterations in mobility may experience difficulty with accomplishing simple tasks associated with daily living. Loss of independence and autonomy may negatively impact self-concept or self-esteem. Similarly, a positive self-concept and high self-esteem may help motivate the individual to move beyond the impairment and learn to adapt and function independently.

As discussed earlier, family plays a role in the development of healthy self-esteem. Overprotective parenting has been associated with lower self-esteem (McLeod, 2013). Authoritative parenting, interfamilial violence, and the loss of a close family member may also impact an individual's self-esteem.

Alterations and Therapies
Feeding and Eating Disorders and Personality Disorders

ALTERATION	DESCRIPTION	MANIFESTATIONS	INTERVENTIONS AND TREATMENTS
Feeding and eating disorders ■ Body image distortion	Impaired perception of body size and/or shape; e.g., a thin individual perceiving herself to be obese when she is excessively thin	■ Refusal to eat ■ Verbalized self-perception of obesity ■ Verbalized negative perception of body image	■ Cognitive–behavioral therapy (CBT) ■ Pharmacologic therapy for management of comorbid disorders or to treat acute symptoms of depression or anxiety
Feeding and eating disorders ■ Absence or loss of appetite	Extreme restriction or prohibition of oral intake through self-imposed starvation	■ Absence of appetite ■ Emaciation ■ Potential nutritional deficiencies, dehydration, and electrolyte imbalances ■ Potential death	■ CBT ■ In extreme cases, forced nutritional supplementation and hydration (e.g., through nasogastric feeding tube)
Feeding and eating disorders ■ Binge eating	Unrestrained consumption of excessive amounts of food within a 2-hour time period; eating continues even after sensing satiation	■ Weight exceeds recommended guidelines ■ If obesity is present, may have secondary physiologic alterations	■ CBT ■ Nutritional counseling and weight management programs
Feeding and eating disorders ■ Purging	Self-induced expulsion of food and/or products of digestion through use of forced vomiting, laxatives, enemas, and/or diuretics	■ Dental caries (cavities) and damage to tooth enamel due to caustic effects of stomach acid if frequent vomiting is occurring ■ Potential nutritional deficiencies, dehydration, and electrolyte imbalances; potassium and chloride levels due to frequent vomiting can lead to metabolic alkalosis ■ Relatively stable weight patterns ■ Relatively normal weight and body mass index (BMI)	■ CBT ■ Nutritional counseling, including encouragement to eat foods that provide replacement of electrolytes lost through vomiting (e.g., bananas, nuts, and dried cereals, and potatoes for potassium replacement)
Personality disorders ■ Absence or reduction of insight as to effects of behaviors ■ Externalized stress response ■ Failure to accept consequences of behaviors ■ May include egocentricity, grandiosity, or perfectionism	■ Pervasive pattern of behaviors, personal perceptions, and internal experiences that are significantly incongruent with an individual's cultural expectations ■ Behaviors, perceptions, and experiences are relatively inflexible and cause distress or functional impairment	■ Impaired function and disruption within personal, social, and professional realms ■ Impulsivity with disregard for consequences of actions ■ Outbursts of emotion, including anger and frustration ■ Attempts to control external environment, including other individuals ■ Potential self-directed violence ■ Potential suicidal ideations and suicide attempts ■ Potential other-directed violence ■ Potential psychosis	■ CBT ■ Dialectical behavioral therapy (DBT) ■ Schema-focused therapy (SFT) ■ Family-focused therapy ■ Expressive therapy ■ Pharmacologic treatment with antidepressants (e.g., selective serotonin reuptake inhibitors [SSRIs], such as fluoxetine) for management of obsessive-compulsive, aggressive, and self-destructive behaviors ■ Antipsychotics for cognitive-perceptual symptoms ■ Pharmacologic mood stabilizers for control of impulsive behavior and anger

Sources: Based on Potter, M. L., & Moller, M. D. (Eds.). (2014). *Psychiatric–mental health nursing: From suffering to hope.* Upper Saddle River, NJ: Pearson Education; Wilson, B. A., Shannon, M. T., & Shields, K. M. (2013). *Pearson nurse's drug guide.* Upper Saddle River, NJ: Pearson.

Decreased self-esteem has been associated with an increased risk for depression. Alterations in mood and affect influence an individual's level of resilience and coping abilities. Patients with personality disorders who have difficulty adhering to treatment regimens may experience negative consequences, including shame and stigmatization, as a result of their behaviors.

Nurses have an ethical responsibility to engage in self-care, as outlined by the American Nurses Association (ANA). In particular, Provision 5 of the ANA Code of Ethics for Nurses requires the nurse to provide the same level of self-care as that which he provides to others (Blum, 2014). Effectively caring for others requires first recognizing and adequately fulfilling one's own personal needs, including those within the physiologic, psychosocial, and spiritual realms.

The Concepts Related to Self feature links some, but not all, of the concepts related to Self. They are presented in alphabetical order.

Concepts Related to
Self

CONCEPT	RELATIONSHIP TO SELF	NURSING IMPLICATIONS
Advocacy	Being a member of a vulnerable and underserved population (e.g., the chronically mentally ill, the poor, LGBT populations, the homeless, certain ethnic groups) → ↓ access to healthcare services → poorer quality of life and ↓ health outcomes	■ Educate yourself on vulnerable and underserved populations in your region. ■ Join professional and community groups that try to address these issues. ■ As a nurse, advocate for outreach efforts to include these populations in healthcare services. ■ Advocate for increased funding and research to better serve these populations.
Development	Missed development stages → ↓ fulfillment of life roles and ↓ cognitive, physical, and psychosocial development → ↓ self-esteem	■ Screen patients for developmental delays and refer to appropriate healthcare community resources. ■ Develop appropriate accommodations for nonmodifiable disorders or presentations. ■ Educate the family on how to assist the family member with developmental delays and refer to appropriate community agencies for support.
Ethics	Nurses are required to administer self-care that is at the same level as that which they provide to others	■ Perform self-assessment and strive for self-awareness both personally and professionally. ■ Identify and meet personal needs in order to promote optimal physical, psychosocial, and spiritual self-wellness.
Family	↑ parental nurturing → ↑ self-esteem ↑ parental overprotectiveness → ↓ self-esteem	■ Interview the patient regarding his perception of his familial style of parenting. ■ Assess patient's level of self-esteem.
Mobility	Mobility → independence in daily living → ↑ self-esteem Impairment of mobility → increased dependence on others → may ↓ self-esteem and negatively impact self-concept High self-esteem and positive self-concept → greater resilience → increased likelihood for adaptation and achievement of optimal independence despite impairment	■ Assess self-concept and self-esteem in the patient with alterations in mobility. ■ Collaborate with other healthcare providers, including physical therapists and occupational therapists, to assist the patient with achieving maximum independence and autonomy. ■ Encourage the patient to focus on strengths and abilities, as opposed to limitations.
Mood and Affect	↓ self-esteem linked to ↑ risk for depression	■ Assess patients who exhibit low self-esteem for presence of signs and symptoms of depression. ■ In the clinical setting, report signs and symptoms of depression to the patient's primary care provider. ■ Facilitate referrals to mental health professionals for patients at risk for depression.
Stress and Coping	↑ stress → biogenic and psychosocial manifestations of stress → impaired physical and mental health	■ Assess patients for signs and symptoms of ineffective coping. ■ Refer patients for short-term pharmacologic interventions and CBT. ■ Refer patients to appropriate resources in the community.

Health Promotion

Promotion of healthy self-concept varies according to the individual. Early recognition of negative self-concept and poor self-esteem can assist nurses in identifying strategies that may promote healthy self-concept and self-esteem in individual patients. Because eating disorders and personality disorders have complex and multifactorial etiologies, there is no single way to prevent their development.

School-Based Interventions

With eating disorders, some experts recommend implementation of school-based interventions because schools play a vital role in promoting the intellectual, physical, social, and emotional development and well-being of children and adolescents (National Eating Disorders Collaboration [NEDC], 2014). Some of the suggested interventions include providing a body-image friendly environment and celebrating diversity; prohibiting appearance-related teasing, including cyber-bullying in school policy; ensuring no weighing, measuring, or anthropometric assessment of students in any context; providing an opportunity for all students to engage in regular physical activity in a noncompetitive, non–weight-loss focused, and safe environment; providing a balance of food options in the cafeteria; and displaying public material/posters including a wide diversity of body shapes, sizes, and ethnicities (NEDC, 2014).

Other school-based interventions include training all relevant teaching staff in the early identification and referral of students with serious body image concerns and suspected eating disorders. Training teachers, especially athletic coaches, on risk factors that are reinforced by social environments and to use body-friendly language in their interactions with students is also recommended (NEDC, 2014).

Promoting Healthy Self-Esteem

Although there is increasing research regarding the influence of genetics on the development of eating disorders and personality disorders, clinicians agree that a stable home environment, lack of exposure to trauma, and thoughtful parenting are protective factors. The promotion of healthy self-esteem throughout childhood and adolescence is also helpful in creating a stronger sense of self. Children with low self-esteem see temporary setbacks as permanent, intolerable conditions and maintain a sense of pessimism, which can increase their risk for experiencing stress, mental health problems, and difficulty with problem solving and meeting challenges (New, 2012). Children with healthy self-esteem tend to enjoy interacting with others and are comfortable in social settings. When challenges arise, they can work toward finding solutions and voice discontent without belittling themselves or others (New, 2012). These children are more likely to accept their strengths and weaknesses and are more optimistic.

Strategies nurses can offer to parents to promote healthy self-esteem in children include the following (New, 2012):

- Praise children not only for a job well done, but also for effort.
- When children lack certain skills, help them to use learning these skills as an opportunity to learn about themselves and appreciate what makes them unique.
- Be a role model by not being excessively harsh on yourself or pessimistic. Children mirror what they see.
- Identify and redirect inaccurate beliefs children have about themselves.
- Be spontaneous about giving affection, hugs, and praise. Give praise honestly without overdoing it. By praising children when they make good choices, you reinforce the good choices and encourage them to continue making good choices.
- Create a safe, loving home environment. Children exposed to parents who fight and argue repeatedly may feel they have no control over their environment and become helpless or depressed.
- Encourage children to participate in activities that require cooperation with others.

Screenings

Identification of manifestations associated with personality disorders and medical diagnosis of such is guided by the fifth edition of the American Psychiatric Association's *Diagnostic and Statistical Manual of Mental Disorders* (DSM-5) (APA, 2013). Screening for eating disorders may include administration of the SCOFF questionnaire (Morgan, Reid, & Lacey, 1999). The **SCOFF** questionnaire was developed in England and has been found to reliably identify core elements of early-stage anorexia nervosa and bulimia nervosa (Sim et al., 2010).

> **S:** Do you make yourself **S**ick because you feel uncomfortably full?
>
> **C:** Do you worry you have lost **C**ontrol over how much you eat?
>
> **O:** Have you recently lost more than **O**ne stone (14 pounds) in a 3-month period?
>
> **F:** Do you believe yourself to be **F**at when others say you are too thin?
>
> **F:** Would you say that **F**ood dominates your life?

One point for every "yes"; a score of 2 or higher indicates a likely case of anorexia nervosa or bulimia and the need for referral to a mental health specialist.

Nursing Assessment

Assessment of the patient with suspected impairments related to self requires giving priority consideration to establishing and maintaining a safe environment. Because certain PDs are associated with impulsive or aggressive behavior, the nurse should ensure that the patient, the nurse, or anyone else in the area is not at risk for physical injury throughout the patient's care. The second priority is establishing a therapeutic relationship, which requires the nurse to build trust and apply principles of therapeutic communication.

After establishing trust, the nursing assessment begins by tactfully interviewing the patient regarding components related to self-concept, self-esteem, and self-awareness. Although it is important to complete a thorough assessment, the nurse should avoid asking personal questions that are unlikely to substantially add to the assessment data. For examples of basic components of a psychosocial assessment, see **Table 29–3** 》.

TABLE 29–3 Sample Psychosocial Assessment Criteria

Dimension	Sample Assessment Criteria
Personal identity	Name
	Age
	Gender
	Marital status
	Occupation
	Cultural background, practices
	Ethnic origin
	Religious or spiritual affiliation, practices
	Self-perception: "How do you describe yourself?"
	Perceived image viewed by others: "How do others describe you?"
	Values: "In your life, what is most important to you?"
Physical history	Current physical illness
	History of physical illness
	Level of energy
	Disabilities
Communication skills and behaviors	Emotional tone
	Ability to follow conversation
	Verbal expression of emotion
	Verbal and nonverbal cues
Role performance	Current roles
	Presence of role conflicts, or recent changes (e.g., retirement, death of spouse)
	Level of congruence between current developmental life stage and role performance
	Past behaviors used in management of role conflict
Body image	*Perceptual:* "What do you think when you look at your body in a mirror?"
	Cognitive: "How important is physical appearance to you?"
	Behavioral: "Are you comfortable in clothing that exposes more of your body, such as a swimsuit?"
	Affective: "In one or two words, how do you feel about your body?"
	Subjective satisfaction: "Overall, how satisfied are you with your body? Which is your favorite body part or region? Which is your least favorite body part or region?"
Self-esteem	(Global) "How satisfied are you with yourself?"
	(Global) "Overall, do you feel you're the person you should be?"
	(Specific) "What do you like most about yourself?"
	(Specific) "What do you like least about yourself?"

Sources: Based on Berman, A., Snyder, S. J., & Frandsen, G. (2016). Pain management. In *Kozier and Erb's fundamentals of nursing: Concepts, process, and practice (10th ed.).* Hoboken, NJ: Pearson Education; Ginis, K. A. M., Bassett-Gunter, R. L., & Conlin, C. (2012). Body image and exercise. In E. O. Acevedo (Ed.), *The Oxford handbook of exercise psychology* (pp. 55–75). New York, NY: Oxford University Press; Kneisl, C. R., & Trigoboff, E. (2013). *Contemporary psychiatric–mental health nursing (3rd ed.).* Upper Saddle River, NJ: Pearson Education; Potter, M. L., & Moller, M. D. (Eds.). (2016). *Psychiatric–mental health nursing: From suffering to hope.* Upper Saddle River, NJ: Pearson Education.

Observation and Patient Interview

For many patients with alterations of self, observation may not yield visible clues. Exceptions do occur with patients who have eating disorders. For example, a patient with a restrictive eating disorder such as anorexia nervosa may appear skeletal, with downy hair (lanugo) on the face and limbs. Conversely, a patient who has bulimia or binge-eating disorder (BED) may present as overweight (BMI >25 to 30) or meet criteria for obesity (BMI >30) (Potter & Moller, 2016). When performing a patient history, the nurse may note that patients with anorexia display signs of reduced alertness and concentration and cognitive deficits as well as multiple physiologic characteristics, including poor sleep, sensitivity to the cold, and decreased energy (Potter & Moller, 2016). These signs and symptoms are discussed more fully in the exemplar on Feeding and Eating Disorders.

During the patient history, the nurse will assess the content of the patient's thinking patterns. In particular, patients with eating disorders exhibit distorted thinking regarding eating, calories, exercise, and body image. Patients with higher acuity will be unable to engage in normal activities and maintain productive relationships. A comprehensive nursing assessment also should determine the level of impairment and functioning within the family, relationships with peers, and performance in school or work (Potter & Moller, 2016). Any evidence of pica should be further investigated. In women, pica can lead to iron deficiency anemia. Ice pica may be indicative of an obsessive-compulsive or developmental disorder (Mesa, 2016).

It is less likely that a nurse will observe visible signs of a personality disorder upon initially meeting a patient. Because of the nature of PDs, clinicians are cautioned not to hurry a diagnosis. Although a single interview may confirm a prior assessment of a PD in a patient, clinicians are urged to assess the stability of personality traits over time across different situations (APA, 2013). Furthermore, assessment is complicated because patients often do not see personality characteristics reflecting psychopathology as problematic (APA, 2013).

Despite these considerations, some features of PDs may be apparent during an initial conversation. For example, patients with Cluster A traits, which include paranoid, schizoid, and schizotypal PDs, may appear odd or eccentric. Patients with Cluster B traits, which include antisocial, borderline, histrionic, and narcissistic PDs, may display dramatic, emotional, and erratic behaviors. Finally, patients with Cluster C traits, which include avoidant, dependent, and obsessive-disorder PDs, may appear as anxious or fearful (APA, 2013). During the assessment, careful attention to cultural considerations is necessary to prevent inadvertent mislabeling of behaviors (see the Focus on Diversity and Culture feature).

As part of the assessment, it may be necessary to interview family members or coworkers (with the patient's permission) to more fully assess the patient's perceptions of reality and behaviors as well as what manifestations or behaviors family members or coworkers find most challenging.

Physical Examination

When dealing with patients with eating disorders, the nurse should always remember that even though the etiologies of eating disorders are often psychologic, eating disorders have serious physiologic complications. For example, morbidity and mortality rates of anorexia are among the highest for all mental disorders (Potter & Moller, 2016). Thus, the assessment of patients with feeding and eating disorders requires thorough and ongoing medical monitoring. This includes frequently assessing vital signs, measuring height and weight, and repeating diagnostic tests such as complete blood count (CBC) and electrolytes and cardiac studies (e.g., electrocardiogram [ECG]).

A physical examination of a patient with a suspected PD is less likely to yield valuable clues, especially given that the treatments are primarily psychologic. If the patient has had a recent physical exam and any medical comorbidities are being managed by a healthcare provider, mental health clinicians will likely defer the physical exam. If a physical exam is conducted, it will include vital signs, assessment of the patient's appearance, and evidence of self-injurious behaviors (e.g., cutting), which are indicative of some Cluster B diagnoses.

Diagnostic Tests

In the diagnosis and treatment of patients with alterations in self, there are no specific laboratory diagnostics that can be used to conclusively confirm a diagnosis. For these patients, laboratory and diagnostic tests are initially used to rule out physiologic causes that might be the source of associated signs and symptoms.

For patients diagnosed with feeding and eating disorders, laboratory and diagnostic testing may be used to assess for additional impairments that have occurred as a result of the primary disorder. For example, in the care of a patient with anorexia nervosa who is severely dehydrated and malnourished, laboratory studies may include a CBC and electrolyte studies, as well as tests to assess kidney function, such as blood urea nitrogen (BUN) and creatinine, and liver function tests. Other diagnostic exams may include ECG, thyroid screening, arterial blood gas (ABG), and urinalysis.

Case Study » Part 2

After assessing Ms. LeMandre, the ED physician orders a CBC and serum electrolytes, as well as administration of intravenous fluids for treatment of acute dehydration. When you return to insert Ms. LeMandre's IV catheter, she asks if she can first use the restroom. You respond that she is welcome to use the restroom; however, because of her recent loss of consciousness and history of light-headedness, policy dictates that she must be transferred to the restroom by wheel-

chair. Ms. LeMandre replies, "That's ridiculous. I'm perfectly capable of walking to the restroom!" Against your wishes, Ms. LeMandre quickly rises from the ED gurney and proceeds to ambulate to the restroom with you following at her side. She staunchly refuses to allow you to assist her. As you wait outside the restroom door, you hear water running, followed by retching sounds. When you knock on the door and ask if she is okay, Ms. LeMandre replies, "I'm fine—I'll be out shortly."

Less than a minute later, Ms. LeMandre emerges with what appears to be a small amount of emesis on the front of her hospital gown. When you ask if she vomited, she replies, "I just ate too much before I worked out this morning. Sometimes, when I eat too much, I get an upset stomach."

Ms. LeMandre denies any further complaints and, at your insistence, she agrees to allow you to return her to her ED room via wheelchair. You insert her IV catheter without incident and begin infusion of 500 mL of lactated Ringer's solution, as ordered. Per Ms. LeMandre's request, you provide her with magazines to read while she awaits her lab draw and further assessment.

Clinical Reasoning Questions Level I

1. How does Ms. LeMandre's initial refusal to allow you to assist her to the restroom coincide with other aspects of her personality?
2. Does Ms. LeMandre's vomiting episode seem congruent with her explanation? How might Ms. LeMandre's vomiting contribute to her light-headedness?

Clinical Reasoning Questions Level II

3. Based on all available data, including nursing observations, what nursing diagnoses may be appropriate for inclusion in Ms. LeMandre's plan of care?
4. What actions should the nurse take next? What information should be reported to the primary care physician?

Independent Interventions

In the promotion of psychosocial wellness, nurses have the unique opportunity to build trusting relationships with patients and to create a safe environment in which the patient can openly discuss both positive and negative aspects of himself as a holistic being. Through assessment of a patient's psychosocial wellness, the nurse can assist patients with identifying areas of strength and weakness, which enhances the patient's level of self-awareness.

Establishing the Therapeutic Relationship

Establishment of trust and application of therapeutic communication techniques require the nurse to exercise authenticity. The principle of authenticity includes remaining committed to promoting the patient's health and well-being (Watson & Browning, 2012). In particular, for patients with alterations in self, trust and respect are keys to both assessment and treatment. When caring for these patients, building a therapeutic relationship can be especially challenging. Patients with PDs may already be impacted by the stigma and shame often associated with mental illness, and they may have limited social support systems. For patients with feeding and eating disorders, many of whom maintain their condition and behaviors in secrecy, speaking openly about their self-perceptions and eating patterns may be especially difficult. Recovery rates are poor and dropout rates are high among patients who receive inpatient treatment for feeding and eating disorders (Halmi, 2013).

Interventions for Patients with Eating Disorders

Interventions that focus on reducing stress and not specifically addressing the problematic eating behaviors may help initially to create a therapeutic nurse–patient relationship. At this stage, patient education about possible stressors that contribute to eating disorder behavior is also appropriate. While this approach does not directly confront the problem behavior, it does address the stressors that can lead to problem behaviors (Potter & Moller, 2016). Nursing interventions include decreasing exposure to environmental stress; decreasing anxiety by eliminating caffeine and other stimulants; helping patients increase social and familial connectedness through improving communication skills; and assessing and teaching coping strategies. As patients develop a therapeutic relationship and become more open to change, they can be referred to treatment using established methods such as CBT (Potter & Moller, 2016).

Patients with eating disorders often are paralyzed by low self-esteem. Nurses can promote self-worth and positive self-regard in these patients through a variety of interventions. When nurses provide positive reinforcement to patients who adhere to treatment and make efforts to meet goals, patients begin to view their efforts more optimistically (Potter & Moller, 2016). Helping patients set short-term, realistic goals helps patients to see and measure their treatment progress. Encouraging patients to reconnect with activities and experiences that they enjoy helps them begin to regain control over their own behaviors and begin to reexperience positive emotions (Potter & Moller, 2016).

Interventions for Patients with Personality Disorders

For patients with PDs, the priority interventions are directed to safety. Once safety is ensured, the nurse turns the focus toward building the therapeutic relationship, which, in turn, supports other nursing interventions in the areas of medication management, facilitating coping skills, strengthening reality orientation, maintaining professional boundaries, and milieu management (Potter & Moller, 2016). These interventions help patients begin to feel hopeful that they can progress in their treatment and improve their ability to function on a daily basis.

Regarding safety, the nurse will assess patients for suicidal ideation, history of suicide attempts, and desire and history of self-injurious behaviors (for detailed information, see the exemplar on Suicide in the module on Mood and Affect). If a patient does self-injure in some way, it is important for the nurse to remain objective and matter-of-fact. The nurse responds first with the necessary medical attention. Then, when the crisis is over, the nurse will process the event with the patient, looking for cues and feelings that may have contributed to or triggered the patient's desire to self-harm (Potter & Moller, 2016).

Self-awareness is an essential component of the therapeutic relationship when working with patients with PDs. Nurses must have a strong sense of identity, must be willing to set limits and reinforce boundaries, and should have supervision or collaborative relationships with colleagues with whom they can process their relationships with patients (Potter & Moller, 2016). Nurses working with these patients should frequently examine their patient relationships in order to maintain a consistent and therapeutic effect.

Nurses working with patients who have PDs should help reconnect patients with coping behaviors they have employed successfully in the past and teach patients new adaptive coping skills. For example, patients who act impulsively and aggressively may be taught to count until less angry, employ deep breathing exercises, and eventually to express anger verbally (Potter & Moller, 2016). Self-management, taking responsibility for one's own behavior and well-being, is another coping technique that can help bring a sense of order and empowerment to patients. Self-management behaviors promote social interaction and reduce disruptive behaviors and include adhering to the treatment plan and using appropriate social skills (Potter & Moller, 2016).

Collaborative Therapies

One problem among collaborative clinicians, especially when dealing with patients with personality disorders, is creating a therapeutic relationship that provides firm, consistent boundaries. Individuals diagnosed with PDs, especially BPD, often require limit setting to reinforce those boundaries (Potter & Moller, 2016). A consistent, firm approach reinforcing elements of the care plan and institutional policies is necessary. If reinforcement is inconsistent, a patient will often engage in splitting by playing one staff person against another (Potter & Moller, 2016). Therefore, nurses and other members of the treatment team need to consistently enforce interventions and boundaries and confront patients who are testing them. Specific interventions nurses and other members of the interprofessional team can take toward developing a therapeutic relationship include maintaining consistent staffing, following through on all agreements and promises, setting limits on inappropriate behavior, maintaining appropriate professional boundaries, and processing patient interactions with trusted colleagues (Potter & Moller, 2016).

Pharmacologic Therapy

Pharmacologic therapy normally is not the primary course of treatment for alterations in self, although it may be used to treat specific manifestations and/or comorbid conditions. For example, antipsychotic medications may be indicated in the care of patients with PDs who are experiencing delusions, hallucinations, or other manifestations associated with psychosis. Similarly, patients with feeding and eating disorders who experience comorbid anxiety or depression may also benefit from pharmacologic therapy.

Nonpharmacologic Therapy

For many patients with feeding and eating disorders or PDs, counseling and therapy are the mainstays of treatment. In particular, CBT, which emphasizes focusing on immediate problems and developing solutions through activities such as repatterning the patient's thinking or developing healthy coping behaviors to replace maladaptive ones, has been deemed useful in the treatment of the patients with feeding and eating disorders (NIMH, 2012). Other forms of therapy include DBT and SFT; these are discussed in the exemplar on Personality Disorders in this module.

Case Study » Part 3

You report Ms. LeMandre's vomiting episode to the ED physician. Shortly thereafter, Ms. LeMandre's CBC and serum electrolyte findings are available; all findings are within normal limits, although both her potassium level (3.7 mEq/L) and chloride level (99 mmol/L) are on the low end of the normal range. The physician diagnoses Ms. LeMandre with dehydration. However, in light of her laboratory results, rigorous exercise regimen, statements about her eating patterns, expressed body image, and vomiting episode, the physician is concerned that Ms. LeMandre's signs and symptoms may be manifestations of an eating disorder. He asks you to accompany him while he speaks with Ms. LeMandre. After speaking with her for several minutes about her dietary patterns and what she now describes as "occasionally getting sick when my stomach is too full," the physician asks Ms. LeMandre if he may ask her a few questions about her overall physical health and her views about food. Reluctantly, Ms. LeMandre agrees.

The physician proceeds to administer the SCOFF Questionnaire. Ms. LeMandre responds "yes" to two of the questions contained in the questionnaire: "Do you make yourself sick because you feel uncomfortably full?" and "Do you worry you have lost control over how much you eat?" Subsequently, the ED physician requests that Ms. LeMandre speak with the on-call psychiatrist.

Once again, Ms. LeMandre reluctantly agrees. Following the consultation, the psychiatrist diagnoses Ms. LeMandre with bulimia nervosa and schedules her for a follow-up appointment in 3 days for further evaluation and treatment.

Clinical Reasoning Questions Level I

1. What is the SCOFF Questionnaire? What criteria suggest the potential presence of anorexia nervosa or bulimia nervosa?
2. If Ms. LeMandre does have an eating disorder, why do you think her weight is within normal limits?
3. How does anorexia nervosa differ from bulimia nervosa?

Clinical Reasoning Questions Level II

4. Based on all available data, including nursing observations, what nursing diagnoses may be appropriate for inclusion in Ms. LeMandre's plan of care?
5. What is the most likely cause of Ms. LeMandre's near-hypokalemia (low serum potassium) and near-hypochloremia (low serum chloride)? In light of these deficiencies, what dietary recommendations might be appropriate for her?
6. What long-term risks are associated with feeding and eating disorders? How might Ms. LeMandre's personality traits affect her willingness to follow treatment protocols?

REVIEW The Concept of Self

RELATE Link the Concepts

Linking the concept of self with the concept of fluids and electrolytes:

1. Explain how alterations in self may affect fluid and electrolyte balance. Which personality disorders might lead the patient to be most vulnerable to alterations in fluid and electrolyte balance?
2. Describe at least three independent and collaborative nursing interventions that are appropriate for implementation in the plan of care for a patient with an alteration in fluid and electrolyte balance due to an eating disorder. Include discussion of diagnostic testing that may be useful for evaluating fluid and electrolyte balance in these patients.

Linking the concept of self with the concept of ethics:

3. Describe ethical considerations related to the nurse's self-care. How might a nurse's self-concept affect the ethical aspects of his behavior, both personally and professionally?
4. Describe ethical considerations that impact the care of a patient who is known or believed to be at risk for self-injury.
5. In the course of caring for a patient with an eating disorder who refuses to eat, what ethical considerations might the nurse face?

READY Go to Volume 3: Clinical Nursing Skills

- SKILL 1.1 Appearance and Mental Status: Assessing
- SKILLS 1.5–1.9 Vital Signs
- SKILL 1.22 Neurologic Status: Assessing
- SKILL 4.5 Urine Specimen, Routine, 24-Hour: Obtaining
- SKILL 8.4 Capillary Blood Specimen for Glucose: Measuring
- SKILL 10.5 Nutrition: Assessing
- SKILL 12.11 ECG, Strip: Interpreting
- SKILL 15.4 Suicidal Patient: Caring for

REFER Go to Pearson MyLab Nursing and eText

- Additional review materials

REFLECT Apply Your Knowledge

The family nurse practitioner (FNP) is seeing Caitlin Smith, a 26-year-old woman, who has come in for her annual checkup, primarily to renew her prescription for birth control pills. Caitlin is very well dressed and obviously overweight. She is 5'4" tall and weighs 188 pounds. The exam goes routinely until the FNP addresses Caitlin's weight, pointing out that her BMI of 32.3 makes her technically obese. Caitlin angrily explodes, saying loudly to the FNP, "When I want your opinion I will ask for it!" The FNP soothes Caitlin by saying she needs to discuss the weight because of the possible adverse health effects. Caitlin then starts crying. During additional questioning when Caitlin has calmed, the FNP finds out that Caitlin has a high-stress job in real estate management. She enjoys her job but feels that patients unfairly judge her because of her weight. Caitlin is vague about her dietary habits, but admits to being a stress eater and having a weakness for chocolate and sweets. "I can eat an entire chocolate cake at one sitting and not even be aware of it," she says. Sometimes after a stressful day, she goes home from work and eats snack foods continually until bedtime. She denies vomiting or overuse of laxatives. Caitlin also admits that her boyfriend recently broke up with her "because of my moods and anger. . . . I just think it is raging hormones." However, this is the fourth romantic relationship that has broken off abruptly since Caitlin graduated from college. Caitlin also worries about losing control or becoming angry at work.

1. Given Caitlin's statements and findings, she likely has which eating disorder?
2. The FNP will probably make which referrals for Caitlin's weight issue?
3. In a later visit, Caitlin discloses that she was sexually abused by an uncle during her preteen and early teen years. Caitlin's mother stopped the abuse when she found out about it, but it was never reported and Caitlin never received any counseling. Given her history of emotional lability, Caitlin may have or be at risk for developing which personality disorder?

» Exemplar 29.A
Feeding and Eating Disorders

Exemplar Learning Outcomes

29.A Analyze feeding and eating disorders and how they relate to self.

- Describe the pathophysiology of feeding and eating disorders.
- Describe the etiology of feeding and eating disorders.
- Compare the risk factors and prevention of feeding and eating disorders.
- Identify the clinical manifestations of feeding and eating disorders.
- Summarize diagnostic tests and therapies used by interprofessional teams in the collaborative care of an individual with feeding and eating disorders.
- Differentiate care of patients with feeding and eating disorders across the lifespan.

- Apply the nursing process in providing culturally competent care to an individual with a feeding and eating disorder.

Exemplar Key Terms

Anorexia nervosa (AN), *1993*
Binge eating, *1995*
Binge-eating disorder (BED), *1995*
Bulimia nervosa (BN), *1995*
Metabolism, *1990*
Nutrients, *1990*
Purging, *1993*

Overview

Food is essential to life. The body requires an adequate supply of **nutrients** to meet energy requirements such as thermoregulation, cellular regulation, and metabolism. Feeding and eating disorders are complex conditions that stem from myriad social, cultural, and psychologic causes and that culminate in the disruption of the body's nutrient supply. These disorders can cause either under- or overnutrition, both of which have negative physiologic effects. In the absence of a food source to use for energy, the body digests body fat and muscles. When it has excess food in proportion to energy use, weight gain and obesity result. Feeding and eating disorders produce biochemical and physiologic interruptions of the metabolism that endanger the whole body. **Metabolism** is the complex process by which the body breaks down and converts food and fluids into energy sources.

The three disorders discussed in this exemplar are anorexia nervosa, bulimia nervosa, and binge-eating disorder. Anorexia nervosa (AN) is a condition characterized by an extreme aversion to gaining weight, as well as physiologic and mental consequences associated with food restriction. Bulimia nervosa (BN) is characterized by a pernicious cycle of binging and purging. Binge-eating disorder (BED) is characterized by the consumption of large amounts of food and a feeling of loss of control during binges. These three conditions create biological, physiologic, and social imbalances that ravage an individual's health and self-concept. For individuals with feeding and eating disorders, the irregular supply of the nutrients necessary for physical health is compounded by psychologic states such as depression, isolation, and self-destructive tendencies.

» *See Chart 29–1: Clinical Manifestations and Therapies: Other Feeding and Eating Disorders at* **Pearson MyLab Nursing and eText.** *See the clinical manifestations and clinical therapies for pica, rumination, avoidant/restrictive food intake disorder (ARFID), and night eating syndrome (NES).*

Feeding and eating disorders are not defined by body weight and external appearance, but rather by the psychologic states that give rise to inadequate nutrition. There are many causes for feeding and eating disorders that are outcomes of biological, psychologic, and social processes. At present, researchers believe that an individual's family, social context, and culture provide triggers, but that hormones, brain chemicals, and genetics cause individuals to push themselves to starvation or obesity.

Pathophysiology

The biological aspects of eating disorders are complex and not fully understood. During active illness, there are known disturbances in neuroendocrine, neurochemistry, and neurotransmission circuitry and signal pathways (Monteleone & Maj, 2013). Investigators have found disturbances in serotonin and neuropeptide systems that modulate appetite, mood, cognitive function, impulse control, energy metabolism, and hormonal systems. As a result of their malnourished and emaciated state, individuals with AN have alterations of brain structure that are related to the course of the illness (Fonville et al., 2014), metabolism (Kaye, Bailer, & Klabunde, 2014), and neurochemistry. In contrast, those with BN have shown brain atrophy in imaging studies (Westmoreland, Krantz, & Mehler, 2016).

The genetic heritability of feeding and eating disorders is comparable to other biologically based mental illnesses. Twin studies in AN, BN, and BED estimate that 40 to 60% of the variance is accounted for by genetic factors (Fairweather-Schmidt & Wade, 2015; Trace et al., 2013). Furthermore, these studies revealed that puberty has a powerful impact in activating the genes of etiologic importance in feeding and eating disorders (Klump et al., 2012). Molecular genetic studies are beginning to identify chromosomal genes and regions that may contribute to the etiology of eating disorders. Areas on chromosomes 1, 4, and 10 may maintain risk genes for AN and BN (Trace et al., 2013). Additional risk for AN may be in the genes involved in the serotonin and opioid systems (Sestan-Pesa & Horvath, 2016).

The regulation of feeding behavior involves a complex integrative central and peripheral signaling network system of positive and negative feedback mechanisms that work to maintain energy homeostasis (Solon-Biet et al., 2014). Positive feedback signals are initiated by feeding behavior. In response, inhibitory or negative feedback signals, requiring greater potency, terminate an episode of eating (Halford & Harrold, 2012). In the case of binge eating, if there is a dysregulation in the relative potency of the negative feedback signaling mechanism, meal size and eating duration can be increased. Thus, binge eating may reflect a relative dysregulation in the negative feedback system. During meals, satiety-signaling neuropeptides—cholecystokinin (CCK) and glucagon-like peptide (GLP-1) from the gut (stomach and intestine)—generate sensory nerves impulses to the hindbrain. These satiation signals connect with neurons in the brain stem via synapses, where they influence meal size and duration (Potter & Moller, 2014).

Ghrelin, a gut peptide that increases appetite, acts on the vagus nerve and stimulates neurons in the hypothalamus. Short-acting satiation signals from the gut to the hindbrain also interact with the long-acting adiposity hormones, leptin and insulin, which are then released and circulate in the blood (Potter & Moller, 2016). These hormones gain access to the hypothalamus in response to the amount of fat stores and energy needs to maintain weight regulation, metabolism, and homeostasis. This higher-order integration evaluates inhibitory signals and metabolic state to determine energy storage needs for regulation, whereas the nucleus tractus solitarius in the caudal brainstem primarily controls the amount of food eaten. During food deprivation or restriction, the sensitivity of the short-acting satiation signals decreases. Therefore, it takes larger amounts of food to generate adequate signaling to terminate a meal (Halford & Harrold, 2012). These hormones can affect satiety by either increasing or decreasing the amount of food eaten.

Research has shown that in comparison to individuals without weight issues, those with feeding and eating disorders experience blunted or attenuated functioning in both the short- and long-acting signaling processes responsible for appetite and weight regulation. When individuals cease eating-disordered behaviors, these hormones may return to a normalized state. However, in some individuals these hormones may remain dysfunctional, indicating a trait-related phenomenon. Therefore, it remains to be determined whether these dysfunctions are a cause, consequence, or maintenance factor in eating disorders (Potter & Moller, 2016). When individuals who stop engaging in eating-disorder behaviors experience normalization of a hormone (such as CCK), this may indicate an adaptive response (Hannon-Engel, Filin, & Wolfe, 2012). It may be that a recalibration begins to effectively regulate and control the input of neuronal and hormonal signals to the hindbrain. As a result, homeostasis and the stability of the hormone system feedback loops are restored. The resulting responses are the absence of debilitating behaviors, such as binging or vomiting.

What is unclear is which adaptive mechanism(s) must be present and properly functioning for hormonal response to return to normal and for this behavior to remit. Understanding which biological adaptations must occur before remission and how these can be promoted and maintained is essential to the development of effective treatment strategies and relapse prevention, and it merits further investigation.

Etiology

Although many studies on the causes of feeding and eating disorders have been performed and published, there is no medical consensus on the etiology of these conditions. Biological and cognitive–behavioral theories are relevant to the development of these alterations. An understanding of these theories allows the nurse to take a holistic approach when caring for patients with feeding and eating disorders.

It seems clear that biology—including genetic and neurologic factors—plays a large part in the development of feeding and eating disorders. Research shows that relatives of patients with feeding and eating disorders are 5–10 times more likely to develop a disorder. Studies of twins have demonstrated that feeding and eating disorders occur for both twins at a rate of 40–60%, indicating that a genetic predisposition may play into the development of these conditions. Neurologic factors include neurotransmitter dysregulation. The neurotransmitter in question is 5-HT, or serotonin, which is synthesized partially of carbohydrates. A low level of 5-HT typically reduces an individual's satiety and increases the consumption of nutrients; a high level of the neurotransmitter increases satiety and decreases food intake. A current theory of binge eating holds that repeated binge episodes may result from a deficiency in serotonin, and that the tendency of individuals with bulimia to binge carbohydrate-rich foods is a manifestation of the body's attempt to replenish serotonin. However, 5-HT is not the only neurotransmitter involved in feeding and eating disorders. Norepinephrine and neuropeptide Y increase food consumption, while dopamine inhibits eating. In addition, endogenous opioids, such as endorphins, increase food intake and elevate mood. Individuals who are significantly underweight typically have significantly lower endorphin levels than individuals of normal weight. The fact that endorphin levels return to normal when weight returns to normal outlines the complex relationship between biology, nutrition, and psychology in feeding and eating disorders (Kneisl & Trigoboff, 2013).

Cognitive–behavioral theories view feeding and eating disorders as learned patterns of behavior based on irrational thought and beliefs. These theories look at the affected individual's cognition and behavior to stimuli, whether physiologic, psychologic, or social, and attempt to help the patient with the disorder by changing the maladaptive behavior and replacing it with a healthier response. An essential element of cognitive–behavioral theory is that the individual's thought patterns give rise to destructive behavioral patterns, and that irrational thoughts are at the heart of the network of problems that leads to feeding and eating disorders (Kneisl & Trigoboff, 2013; Potter & Moller, 2016).

Risk Factors

Because the origination of feeding and eating disorders is so complex, the risk factors for feeding and eating disorders are closely related to their etiologies. Biology, sociocultural factors, and family systems all contribute to the psychologic conditions that prime an individual for an eating disorder.

Increasingly, research is pointing to genetic factors as a major risk factor for feeding and eating disorders. Contemporary genetic research works with the behavioral, neurobiological, and temperamental variables that are core features of disorders. Behavioral conditions that may be related to genetics are perfectionism, orderliness, low tolerance for unfamiliar situations, low self-esteem, and high anxiety. The genetic underpinnings of these conditions can cause individuals to develop an eating disorder even when their culture does not commonly induce feeding and eating disorders (Kneisl & Trigoboff, 2013; Potter & Moller, 2016).

Sociocultural risk factors are elements of an individual's social and cultural context that exert the pressure that initiates an eating disorder. In the American culture, portrayals of men's and women's bodies in the media and a pervasive cultural understanding of a trim body as the "ideal" lead to the unrealistic expectation that everyone should have a low weight. In addition to glamorizing an unrealistically trim body shape, the cultural obsession with thinness leads to a bias against those who are overweight. These social factors diminish the self-esteem of those who believe they do not fit the "ideal" body shape and enhance self-worth for those who are deemed attractive. Girls and women are hardest hit by the cultural emphasis on thin bodies. Magazines targeted at adolescent girls present dieting as a sensible solution to the crises of adolescents and contain 90% more articles promoting weight control than magazines targeted at teenage boys. For many young women, self-esteem becomes centered on concerns about weight (Potter & Moller, 2016).

In recent years, the American ideal of male attractiveness has also shifted toward the unhealthy. Men and boys are confronted every day with images of male beauty that center on muscle-bound figures defined by their strength. The use of anabolic steroids is common among men with feeding and eating disorders, because in addition to seeking thinness they also seek improved muscle tone (National Association of Men With Eating Disorders, 2016). Because of the pressure that the media, social, and cultural expectations exert, feeding and eating disorders like anorexia and bulimia can be considered culture-reactive syndromes in the United States and the rest of the Western world. Negative body image, degraded self-worth, and body dissatisfaction create the stress that leads to feeding and eating disorders (Kneisl & Trigoboff, 2013; Potter & Moller, 2016).

Family systems theories do not necessarily hold that harmful family patterns cause feeding and eating disorders, but rather that the family enables maladaptive behaviors. Some individuals with feeding and eating disorders are survivors of childhood and adolescent abuse—including sexual abuse—much of which occurs in immediate and extended family systems. In addition to abuse, many families of patients with eating disorders have impaired conflict resolution skills. Another factor that enables the development of feeding and eating disorders is a family-wide emphasis on achievement and performance, with ambition for the family's success being one of the principal goals of the parents. Body shape frequently is related to success in these families, and an emphasis on fitness combined with a desire for control may become obsessive.

In addition to the family system impacting the development of an eating disorder, the appearance of a disorder can disrupt the fragile order of a family unit. After the diagnosis or appearance of a disorder such as anorexia, certain families become enmeshed: The boundaries between members become weak, interactions intensify, members become more dependent, and autonomy decreases. When these patterns occur, each family member becomes less stable and more involved with the other members' private concerns. The parents become overprotective, and food can take on extreme importance. A family's system of interpersonal relations influences the development of an eating disorder, and the presence of an eating disorder impacts the way a family conducts itself in a harmful cycle (Kneisl & Trigoboff, 2013; Potter & Moller, 2016).

Prevention

Prevention is a systematic attempt to change the circumstances that facilitate feeding and eating disorders. Prevention can involve reducing negative risk factors such as body dissatisfaction, depression, and basing self-esteem on appearance. Prevention also involves increasing protective factors

---

Patient Teaching
Sports and Eating Disorders: Warning Signs

Disordered eating behavior (DE) and eating disorders (EDs) frequently occur in children and adolescents participating in competitive sports. The reported prevalence of DE and EDs in athletic populations ranges from 18 to 45% in female athletes and up to 28% of all male athletes (Melin et al., 2014). The most common sports-related ED is **anorexia athletica**, a condition in which individuals seeking a lean body type engage in excessive exercise and calorie restriction. The condition may also be known as obligatory exercise or hypergymnasia because of excessive and compulsive exercise. Athletes experiencing sports anorexia overexercise to give themselves a sense of having control over their bodies.

Sports-related EDs have been associated with physical and mental health risks as well as impaired performance.

Warning signs of EDs associated with sports participation include the following findings (KidsHealth, 2016). The child or adolescent:

- Will not skip a workout, even if tired, sick, or injured.
- Seems anxious or guilty when missing even one workout.
- Is constantly preoccupied with weight and exercise routine.
- Does not like to sit still or relax because of worry that not enough calories are being expended.
- Has lost a significant amount of weight.
- Increases exercises after eating more.
- Skips seeing friends, gives up activities, and abandons responsibilities to make more time for exercise.
- Seems to base self-worth on the number of workouts completed and the effort put into training.
- Is never satisfied with own physical achievements.

Parents and coaches should be sensitive to encouraging restrictive eating behaviors to improve athletic performance and should practice using weight-neutral language when communicating with younger athletes. Parents and coaches should also be careful about putting too much pressure on young athletes, who have not yet developed effective coping mechanisms (KidsHealth, 2016).

such as basing self-esteem on factors other than appearance, and replacing unhealthy dieting with an appreciation for the body's natural functionality. A broad-based cultural emphasis on prevention is essential for the global reduction of the suffering associated with feeding and eating disorders (National Eating Disorders Association [NEDA], 2013).

Healthcare providers should target two types of audiences when implementing eating disorder prevention. Universal prevention, the first type, should be aimed at the general public, even at those individuals who show no signs of feeding and eating disorders. This type of prevention aims to promote healthy development and understanding of the many complex issues that cause these disorders, as a way of spreading the information that can cut them off before they begin. Targeted prevention, the second type of prevention, educates individuals who are beginning to show symptoms of feeding and eating disorders. These individuals may have high levels of body dissatisfaction. The goal of targeted prevention is to provide enough information to stop an eating disorder from developing (NEDA, 2013). Both universal and targeted programs have had success in preventing feeding and eating disorders, though targeted programs seem to be more effective.

Instruction and interventions interwoven and scaffolded by age throughout all years of K–12 education also seem to hold promise because teachers and coaches play an important role in promoting health and well-being within the school environment (see the Patient Teaching feature). Education about body image, disordered eating, and the risks of dieting and eating disorders are all important topics that should be addressed to help prevent an eating disorder from developing, ease the suffering of a young person in the early stages of an eating disorder, and reduce the stigma and misconceptions that surround eating disorders (NEDC, 2014). Proactive efforts to promote positive body image and healthy lifestyle choices should be integrated across the curriculum with the aim of helping to prevent eating disorders rather than simply responding reactively to existing issues (NEDC, 2014).

Clinical Manifestations

Clinical manifestations of the different feeding and eating disorders vary, but similarities include body image disturbance, anxiety, and ineffective coping skills. Commonly occurring feeding and eating disorders include anorexia nervosa, bulimia nervosa, and binge-eating disorder.

》 *An overview of clinical manifestations and therapies associated with less prevalent feeding and eating disorders can be found in Chart 29–1 at* **Pearson MyLab Nursing and eText.**

Anorexia Nervosa

Anorexia nervosa (AN) is a potentially deadly ED that compels individuals to lose more weight than is healthy for their age and height. Patients with anorexia have an intense fear of gaining weight, even when they show the symptoms of being dangerously underweight. Individuals with anorexia engage in dieting and exercising to the point of dangerous malnutrition to avoid gaining weight (PubMed Health, 2012a). Information related to the severity of anorexia nervosa and criteria for hospitalization are summarized in **Box 29–1** 》.

Box 29–1
Severity of Anorexia Nervosa and Criteria for Hospitalization

Clinical signs are important indicators of the severity of anorexia nervosa for two reasons: (1) Patients with anorexia nervosa often hide their symptoms and behaviors, and therefore may not always report reliably about the extent to which symptoms interfere with function or the duration of the symptoms; and (2) as the illness becomes more acute, the patient is at increased risk for physiologic dysfunction and even organ damage.

The DSM-5 identifies BMI (the weight in kilograms divided by the square of the height in meters) as an important clinical indicator of the severity of AN (APA, 2013):

Mild: BMI ≥ 17

Moderate: BMI 16–16.99

Severe: BMI 15–15.99

Extreme: BMI < 15

Providers with patients who have symptoms of anorexia nervosa with severe to extreme BMI deficits may determine a need for hospitalization based on the patient's BMI and other clinical signs, such as arrhythmia, systolic BP < 90 mmHg, and heart rate below 40 to 50 beats per minute (Harrington, Jimerson, Haxton, & Jimerson, 2015). Although specific clinical markers may vary by clinician or healthcare agency, the following indicators will likely necessitate admission (Harrington et al., 2015; Herpertz-Dhalman et al., 2015):

- Acute medical complication(s) requiring stabilization
- Refusal to eat
- Risk of self-harm or suicide
- Failure to respond to outpatient treatment

Anorexia nervosa typically begins during the teen years, and it is more commonly diagnosed in females. In particular, AN is more prevalent among White females with a history of high academic achievement. See the Evidence-Based Practice feature in the Collaboration section for a discussion of how those with feeding and eating disorders are affected by the internet. These women frequently have goal-oriented families or personalities, and they develop rigid "rules" that they use to control weight. These rituals can be simple, such as cutting food into tiny pieces, or elaborate, such as preparing lavish dinners for friends or family without consuming any food themselves. Criteria for diagnosis of AN include possessing an intense fear of weight gain, refusing to maintain a healthy weight, and perceiving a distorted body image. In previous years, amenorrhea (absence of menstruation for 3 or more months) was also a diagnostic criterion for AN; however, this is no longer the case. In order to maintain low body weight, individuals with anorexia severely limit food consumption and offset consumption with excessive exercise. Other behaviors include self-induced vomiting; refusing to eat in the presence of others; using diuretics, laxatives, and diet pills; and cutting food into small pieces as a way of pretending to eat (PubMed Health, 2012a).

Anorexia nervosa takes a toll on the entire body (see the Multisystem Effects feature). As an individual loses body weight and becomes malnourished, hair and nails become

Multisystem Effects of
Anorexia Nervosa

Endocrine
- Thyroid function slows
- Slow growth

Neurologic
- Damage to brain
- Impaired cognition

Urinary
- Kidney stones
- Kidney failure

Respiratory
- Breathing slows

Gastrointestinal
- Constipation
- Bloating

Cardiovascular
- Anemia
- Damage to heart
- Reduced heart rate
- Hypotension
- Dysrhythmias
- Heart failure

Musculoskeletal
- Osteoporosis
- Weak muscles
- Swollen joints
- Fractures

Reproductive
- Amenorrhea
- Difficulty getting pregnant
- Higher risk for miscarriage

Integumentary
- Brittle skin
- Dry, yellow, scaly skin
- Lanugo
- Brittle hair
- Loss of hair
- Brittle nails

Sensory
- Always feel cold
- Cold hands and feet

brittle, skin becomes dry and yellow, and a fine layer of hair called *lanugo* appears on previously hairless parts of the body. Individuals with anorexia may constantly feel cold, as the body loses its ability to retain heat. The starvation resulting from anorexia can cause damage to vital organs such as the brain, kidneys, and heart. Pulse rate and blood pressure drop, and irregular heart rhythms can cause heart failure. Loss of nutrients can lead to brittle bones and even changes in the brain, which in turn lead to impaired thinking. In the worst cases of anorexia, patients can starve themselves to death. The condition has the highest mortality rate of any mental illness, due to the complications of malnutrition and the high rate of suicide in the population (National Alliance on Mental Illness [NAMI], 2013a).

Bulimia Nervosa

Bulimia nervosa (BN) is a condition in which individuals binge on food or have episodes of overeating in which they feel a loss of control. After periods of binging, the individuals use methods such as vomiting or laxative abuse to prevent weight gain. Binging may also be followed by periods of extreme exercise. Many individuals who have bulimia also have anorexia nervosa. Individuals with bulimia are obsessed with their body appearance and engage in the destructive pattern of binging and purging to control weight (PubMed Health, 2012b). For diagnosis of bulimia nervosa, the individual must demonstrate binge eating in association with unhealthy compensatory behaviors (e.g., purging or excessive exercise) at least once per week over a 3-month period (APA, 2013).

Binge eating is the rapid consumption of an uncommonly large amount of food in a short amount of time, for example, over a 2-hour period (APA, 2013). Individuals who binge-eat feel out of control during the episode, and although eating binges may involve any kind of food, they usually consist of junk foods, fast foods, and high-calorie foods. Binging may be pleasant initially, but the individual who is binging quickly becomes distressed. A binge usually ends only when abdominal pain becomes powerful, when the individual is interrupted, or when the individual runs out of food. After the binge, the individual with bulimia feels guilt and engages in purging activities to rid the body of excess calories (NAMI, 2013b).

Purging behaviors are frequently dangerous and include a wide variety of activities that are meant to remove all food from the body, such as self-induced vomiting, enemas, or diuretics. Restrictive dieting and extreme exercising also are common. For many with bulimia, purging becomes a purification ritual and a means of regaining self-control in addition to a mechanism for emptying the body of nutrients (NAMI, 2013b).

Bulimia nervosa is frequently underdiagnosed because many of those who have the condition are either overweight or of normal weight. The typical age at onset is late adolescence or early adulthood. The disorder mainly affects females, although at least 1 in 10 individuals with the condition is male. BN is more common than anorexia, and it occurs in approximately 3% of the population. In addition, BN is often comorbid with other psychiatric disorders, such as mood disorders, anxiety disorders, substance abuse, and disorders of self-injurious behavior (NAMI, 2013b).

The principal indicator of BN is an incessant obsession with food and body weight. Other important indicators are physical signs of binging and purging. These include the trash produced by the large quantity of food required for binging, and the products—enemas and laxatives—used in purging. Individuals affected by BN may also experience menstrual irregularity and depressed mood, in addition to the unexplained stomach pain and sore throat that binging and purging produce. The signs of self-induced vomiting—unexplained damage to teeth, scarring on the backs of fingers, and swollen cheeks due to the damage to parotid glands—often indicate to doctors and dentists that there is a problem. Individuals who engage in chronic ingestion of syrup of ipecac (available over the counter and online) can experience toxicity, with the most serious adverse effects being lethal cardiac arrhythmias, low blood pressure, and heart failure.

Behaviors associated with BN can lead to severe physiologic damage, even if the individual's weight remains normal. Binging and purging cause unhealthy nutritional patterns, and self-induced vomiting can cause serious injury to the digestive tract. Tooth decay, esophageal and stomach injury, and acid reflux are all common in individuals with the condition.

Purging behaviors can lead to dehydration and changes in the body's electrolytes. Because stomach acid contains potassium and chloride, electrolyte disturbances associated with purging include low potassium (hypokalemia) and low chloride (hypochloremia). Frequent vomiting, diuretic use, or laxative abuse may cause hypokalemia; in each case, metabolic alkalosis may result (Potter & Moller, 2016). Bloating and slowed peristalsis (movement of gastric contents through the intestines) also may accompany BN. Complications stemming from electrolyte disturbances, severe dehydration, and undernutrition associated with BN may include cardiac arrhythmias, heart failure, and even death (NAMI, 2013b).

Binge-Eating Disorder

Persons with **binge-eating disorder (BED)** experience periods of rapid food consumption, episodes during which they are unable to stop eating. Individuals with the disorder may continue to eat until long after they are full, and they may experience embarrassment about their behavior. For some individuals with BED, binging can produce a sense a relief or fulfillment that gives way as the episode progresses into feelings of disgust, guilt, worthlessness, and depression (NAMI, 2013c).

There is no specific test that can diagnose someone with BED. Rather, a diagnosis is made by a mental health practitioner based on an assessment that includes a formal history and collateral information. Any patient diagnosed with the condition should have a full physical exam performed in order to screen for complications of the illness. These complications include obesity, high cholesterol, type 2 diabetes, and heart disease. In cases of

Clinical Manifestations and Therapies
Feeding and Eating Disorders

ETIOLOGY	CLINICAL MANIFESTATIONS	CLINICAL THERAPIES
Anorexia nervosa	■ Obsession over body shape and food ■ Extreme perfectionism ■ Rigidity, overcontrol, obsessive rituals ■ Significant weight loss ■ Body disturbances ■ Strenuous exercises ■ Reductions in heart rate, blood pressure, metabolic rate, and in production of estrogen or testosterone ■ Extreme sensitivity to cold ■ Feelings of depression	■ Antidepressants ■ Cognitive–behavioral therapy (CBT) ■ Group therapy ■ Family therapy
Bulimia nervosa	■ Cycle of binging and purging food ■ Body image disturbances ■ Abuse of laxatives, enemas, and diuretics ■ Extreme exercise to compensate for binging ■ Hoarding food ■ Secretive behaviors	■ Antidepressants ■ CBT ■ Family therapy
Binge-eating disorder	■ Binging once a week for at least 3 months ■ Absence of purging ■ Sense of loss of control ■ Allowing eating and weight to interfere with personal relationships ■ Sense of embarrassment, disgust after overeating	■ Antidepressants ■ CBT

extreme weight gain, complications can include arthritis, obstructive sleep apnea, and other weight-related conditions (NAMI, 2013c).

Collaboration

Feeding and eating disorders are diagnosed through a combination of laboratory tests to detect the effects of irregular nutrition and consultation with a medical professional. Once a disorder is diagnosed, reestablishment of adequate nutrition, cessation of binge–purge behaviors, and reduction of excessive exercise are the essential points of treating feeding and eating disorders. These goals are accomplished through a combination of pharmacologic and nonpharmacologic therapies, including psychotherapy. Treatment plans are tailored to individual needs but include counseling, medication, and, in extreme cases, hospitalization. Some patients require hospitalization to treat problems caused by severe malnutrition. An inpatient stay at a hospital can also be used to ensure that the patients are eating if they are severely underweight and to establish new eating patterns in a supportive environment (NIMH, 2012).

Diagnostic Tests

Laboratory tests can reveal the physiologic hallmarks of feeding and eating disorders. Screening for anorexia may include tests for albumin, total protein, electrolyte levels, CBC, and a bone density test to check for signs of osteoporosis. Other diagnostic exams include an electrocardiogram; kidney, thyroid, and liver function tests; and urinalysis. These exams determine whether there is a severe deficiency of any nutrients or any wasting of the body as a result of malnutrition (PubMed Health, 2012a).

Diagnostic tests for bulimia nervosa consider many more visible symptoms of disease than do the tests for anorexia because of the physical damage induced by purging. The dentist is often the first medical professional to identify signs of bulimia, including cavities and gum infections. The enamel of teeth may be worn or pitted because of exposure to the acid in vomit. Loss of stomach acid can lead to metabolic alkalosis. A physical exam may discover broken blood vessels in the eyes (from the stress of vomiting), a dry mouth, pouchlike cheeks, rashes and pimples, and cuts and calluses on the finger joints. Laboratory tests may show an electrolyte imbalance or dehydration from purging (PubMed Health, 2012b).

In order to diagnose a BED, a clinician typically conducts a physical exam, followed by blood and urine tests. A psychologic evaluation is necessary to complete the evaluation, including a discussion of the patient's eating habits. Following diagnosis, the other tests should be performed to check for the common health implications of

Evidence-Based Practice

Feeding and Eating Disorders and the Internet

Problem

For a patient coping with an ED, the internet can be perilous territory. Not only does the internet offer websites dedicated to encouraging and celebrating feeding and eating disorders, but some research suggests that sites provide erroneous diagnostic criteria that can be detrimental to patients and their families. Especially for adolescent patients who spend hours every day engaged with media, information on the internet can both prompt and exacerbate disordered eating behaviors.

Evidence

Approximately 92% of teens report daily internet use, with more than half (56%) of teens age 13 to 17 going online several times a day (Pew Research Center, 2015). Nearly three quarters of teens have or have access to a smartphone. African American teens are the most likely of any group of teens to have a smartphone, with 85% having access to one, compared with 71% of both White and Hispanic teens (Pew Research Center, 2015). African American and Hispanic youth report more frequent internet use than White teens. Among African American teens, 34% report going online almost constantly, as do 32% of Hispanic teens and 19% of White teens.

The overwhelming majority, 84%, of teens turn to the internet for health information (Center on Media and Human Development [CMHD], 2015). Teens report using online sources to learn more about puberty, drugs, sex, depression, and other issues. Nearly a third of teens (31%) visit medical websites for health information, with smaller numbers also relying on social media sites such as YouTube and Facebook. Forty-two percent of teens have researched fitness/exercise, followed by diet/nutrition (36%) and stress and anxiety (19%), with nearly one in three teens (32%) saying they have changed their behavior due to digital health information or tools (CMHD, 2015).

Digital media have become an important source of the social pressure, cultural expectations, and health misinformation that contribute to the development of feeding and eating disorders in adolescents. Many teens come across negative health information online, including drinking games (27%), getting tobacco or other nicotine products (25%), how to be anorexic or bulimic (17%), and how to get or make illegal drugs (14%) (CMHD, 2015).

With the prevalence of adolescent internet use, it is essential to consider that **more than 100** pro-eating-disorder websites not only encourage feeding and eating disorders, but also offer specific advice on anorexic and bulimic techniques, with pro-anorexia content composing almost 30% of the content on certain social media platforms (Rodgers et al., 2016). These pro–eating-disorder websites offer advice on binging, purging, and extreme forms of weight control, and they provide interactive resources such as message boards. Research indicates that the sites are alarmingly easy to access and understand (Rodgers et al., 2016). Pro–eating-disorder websites are readily accessible communities with dynamic, user-distributed content.

In addition to sites that provide information that explicitly promotes feeding and eating disorders, websites that purport to provide medical information can spread damaging information to individuals of all ages. Research shows that the quality of medical content related to the diagnosis and treatment of feeding and eating disorders is relatively low. Few sites fully describe the criteria for diagnosis, complications, and treatment options of any ED, and some provide a good deal of erroneous information. Some sites use inaccurate "diagnostic" terms—"bulimerexia," for example—as well as multiple "optimal" treatment options for each of the feeding and eating disorders. Inaccurate information is particularly dangerous for adolescents with disordered eating, and it may interfere with the family's decision to seek medical treatment (Smith et al., 2011).

Implications

The fact that almost all adolescents have easy access to the internet and its variety of viewpoints creates a new set of problems for parents and nurses. The web offers an interactive way for impressionable adolescents and young adults to engage with unhealthy cultural expectations of thinness. In addition, the myriad viewpoints expressed online include pathologic websites that support the damaging behaviors associated with anorexia and bulimia. Even sites that purport to present medical information and treatment options for EDs often contain flawed and medically inadequate information.

Critical Thinking Application

Consider a consultation with an adolescent female patient who has been exhibiting the behaviors associated with AN for the past 3 years. This patient has also been taking part in pro-anorexia message boards online for the past 2 years. She knows that anorexia is unhealthy but embraces the damage she deals her body by fasting and exercising, partly because she learned most of what she knows about the condition from websites full of incorrect "information." Identify a communication strategy that will enable you to correct her misconceptions about AN while attempting to communicate the grim reality of her disorder.

BED, including heart problems and gallbladder disease (Mayo Clinic, 2017).

Pharmacologic Therapy

There is currently no surgical treatment, aside from bariatric surgeries for extremely overweight patients, indicated as primary treatment for any of the feeding and eating disorders. Treating AN involves restoring the patient to a healthy weight, treating underlying psychologic issues, and eliminating behaviors that might lead to malnutrition and relapse. Research suggests that antidepressants, antipsychotics, or mood stabilizers may be modestly effective in treating patients with anorexia. Medications can treat some of the psychologic states that undergird the ED, but it is not yet clear whether medications are effective in preventing relapse. No medication has yet been shown to be effective in assisting weight gain.

The antidepressant fluoxetine (Prozac) is the only medication approved by the U.S. Food and Drug Administration for treating bulimia. This and other antidepressants may help individuals for whom depression and anxiety are at the root of bulimic behavior. Fluoxetine appears to lessen binging and purging behaviors, reduce the likelihood of relapse, and improve attitudes toward eating.

SAFETY ALERT Selective serotonin reuptake inhibitors (SSRIs), such as fluoxetine, which can be prescribed used to treat underlying depression in patients with EDs, carry an FDA-mandated black box warning regarding increased suicidality. The risk of suicide is especially increased in pediatric, adolescent, and young adult patients 18 to 24 years old. Parents should be made aware of this risk, know the symptoms of suicidal ideation, and know to contact the prescribing clinician immediately if symptoms present.

The pharmacologic options for treating BED are similar to the treatments for bulimia nervosa. Antidepressants, particularly fluoxetine, have been found to reduce binge-eating episodes and help ease depression (NIMH, 2012).

Nonpharmacologic Therapy

Although pharmacologic treatments may play a role in the treatment of feeding and eating disorders, therapies that do not make use of medication have proven to be more consistently effective. In the treatment of AN, individual, group, and family-based psychotherapy can address the psychologic reasons for the illness. A therapy called the *Maudsley approach* has been shown to be particularly effective in the treatment of adolescents with anorexia. In the Maudsley approach, the parents of the affected adolescent take responsibility for feeding the patient. Research shows that for patients with anorexia, a combined approach of medical attention and psychotherapy produces more complete recoveries than psychotherapy alone. There is no cure-all approach for AN, but evidence indicates that individualized treatment programs frequently achieve success and that specialized treatment may help reduce the risk of death.

The nonpharmacologic treatment of bulimia nervosa frequently involves a combination of options and depends on the needs of the individual patient. The most effective psychotherapy for patients with bulimia is CBT, which helps individuals focus on their present problems and how to solve them. CBT may be individualized or group-based, and it is effective in changing binge-and-purge behaviors and attitudes to eating. Systemic family therapy and family-based therapy are family-systems approaches that focus on family strengths and family narratives (Espie & Eisler, 2015). Family-based therapies are often used with adolescent anorexic patients, mobilizing the family as the primary resource in feeding and restoring health to an undernourished child.

Nonpharmacologic treatment options for BED are very similar to the options for bulimia nervosa. Psychotherapy, especially CBT that is individualized, has been shown to be effective in many cases with adolescent and adult patients (NIMH, 2012).

Treatment Settings

Day-patient programs are considered to be the first-line treatment approach when more a more structured program is needed for an anorexic patient. Day programs have advantages over inpatient programs in allowing continued engagement with the patient's educational, occupational, and social contexts. Day-patient settings are also more conducive to the active involvement of family members (including siblings) in treatment (Espie & Eisler, 2015).

Patients with high acuity must be treated with inpatient therapy. An inpatient stay provides a structured and contained environment in which patients have access to clinical support at all times. The close proximity of medical help reduces the chance of relapse while improving the chances of recovery. Inpatient programs are now frequently affiliated with daytime programs so that patients can move back and forth to the correct level of care. The majority of inpatient programs treat only patients with anorexia, bulimia, and BED so that the symptoms can be isolated and treated as effectively as possible (Academy for Eating Disorders, 2013). Inpatient settings also allow sufficient monitoring for *refeeding syndrome,* a dangerous and potentially fatal condition that can occur when patients who are severely malnourished begin eating again.

Criteria for admission include patients at immediate risk or for whom previous treatments have failed. Further indicators for hospital admission include less than 75% ideal body weight, ongoing weight loss despite intensive management, rapid or persistent decline in oral intake, and decline in weight despite maximally intensive outpatient intervention. Other considerations include physical parameters, such as hemodynamic instability, cardiovascular risk, and electrolyte abnormalities, as well as psychiatric assessment of such factors as risk of harm to self and others (Espie & Eisler, 2015).

Complementary Health Approaches

For individuals with feeding and eating disorders, a variety of complementary health approaches can help improve recovery outcomes. However, those with feeding and eating disorders sometimes use alternative medical techniques to achieve the unhealthy goals of disordered eating. For example, some individuals use herbal dietary substances as appetite suppressants or weight loss aids. Herbal supplements can be dangerous when they interact with other products, such as laxatives and diuretics, which are frequently used by those with feeding and eating disorders. Health professionals have not determined conclusively that any complementary or alternative therapies are helpful for individuals with anorexia, bulimia, or BED, but some research indicates that some therapies may help reduce anxiety. Acupuncture, massage, yoga, and meditation have been shown to improve mood and reduce the stress associated with feeding and eating disorders (Mayo Clinic, 2016).

Mindfulness-based approaches are growing in popularity as interventions for disordered eating and weight loss. Mindful meditation instructs the practitioner to become mindful of thoughts, feelings, and sensations and to observe them in a nonjudgmental way. Many alternative practitioners believe that mindfulness-based interventions, combined with other traditional weight loss strategies, have the potential to offer a long-term, holistic approach to wellness (Godsey, 2013). One meta-analysis found that mindfulness meditation effectively decreased binge eating and emotional eating in populations engaging in this behavior; however, evidence for its effect on weight loss was mixed (Katterman et al., 2014). Another study that implemented meditation training found that participants in the mindfulness intervention showed significantly greater decreases in food cravings, body image concern, emotional eating, and external eating than the control group (Alberts, Thewissen, & Raes, 2012).

Lifespan Considerations

Feeding and eating disorders are often thought of as conditions limited to adolescent and teen populations, but anorexia, bulimia, BED, and other feeding/eating disorders frequently affect other populations as well. BED differs from AN and BN in terms of age at onset, gender and racial distribution, psychiatric comorbidity, and association with obesity (Smink, Hocken, & Hoek, 2012). The *avoidant/restrictive food intake disorder* (ARFID) diagnosis addresses patients who struggle with impaired and distressing eating behaviors and symptoms and who lack the weight and body image–related concerns associated with AN and BN (Norris, Spettigue, & Katzman, 2016). Typically, patients with ARFID require the expertise of an interprofessional treatment team to provide the nutritional rehabilitation, medical management, and psychologic treatment characteristic of anorexia.

Some of the considerations related to EDs at various stages of the lifespan are discussed in the following section.

Feeding and Eating Disorders in Children

Of all the EDs, ARFID is the most significant diagnosis among this age group (Ornstein et al., 2013). Note that the diagnosis of ARFID is carefully distinguished from the "picky eating" often characteristic of infants and young children. Picky or fussy eating often includes limitations in the variety of foods eaten, unwillingness to try new foods (known as food "neophobia"), and aberrant eating behaviors, including rejection of foods of a particular texture, consistency, color, or smell (Norris et al., 2016). Prevalence rates for picky eating range from 14 to 50% in preschool children and from 7 to 27% in older children. The ARFID diagnosis eliminates picky eaters by identifying only those children with clinically significant restrictive eating problems that result in persistent failure to meet the child's nutritional and/or energy needs (APA, 2013).

Despite their high prevalence, associated morbidity and mortality, and available treatment options, EDs continue to be underdiagnosed by pediatric professionals (Campbell & Peebles, 2014). Higher rates of EDs are seen now in younger children, boys, and people of color; EDs are increasingly recognized in patients with previous histories of obesity. Furthermore, younger patients diagnosed with EDs are more likely to be boys, with a female-to-male ratio of 6:1, compared with a 10:1 ratio in adults (Campbell & Peebles, 2014).

Feeding and Eating Disorders in Adolescents and College-age Adults

According to the APA (2013), the 12-month prevalence of anorexia among young females is approximately 0.4%. For bulimia, the prior-year prevalence for young females was estimated to be 1–1.5%, with the highest prevalence occurring among young adults, because the disorder peaks in late adolescence and young adulthood (APA, 2013). The 12-month prevalence rate for binge eating among women was 1.6% (APA, 2013).

Young females at risk for developing anorexia often have co-occurring anxiety disorders or display obsessional traits in childhood (APA, 2013). Young women who develop bulimia often have temperamental traits such as weight concerns, low self-esteem, depressive symptoms, social anxiety disorder, and overanxious disorder of childhood. Risk factors for bulimia include thin body ideal; childhood sexual or physical abuse; and childhood obesity and early pubertal maturation. BED has the same psychopathology as AN and BN, but co-occurring disorders commonly associated with BED also include bipolar disorder, depressive disorders, anxiety disorders, and substance use disorders (APA, 2013). For all eating disorders, the severity of co-occurring psychiatric disorders will predict worse long-term outcomes.

Adolescence is a critical period of development and is a time of vulnerability during which EDs can develop. Research has indicated that a number of factors influence the development of an ED, such as perceived pressure to be thin, thin-ideal internalization, and body dissatisfaction (Rohde, Stice, & Marti, 2015). Dieting and negative affectivity also accelerate the development of an ED. Although these affective risk factors are present by early adolescence, EDs tend to emerge in late adolescence and early adulthood.

Feeding and Eating Disorders in Adults

Eating disorders, especially bulimia and binge eating behaviors, that are developed in adolescence and young adulthood often persist into adulthood. The risk factors and associated behaviors remain intact with one exception: Adults who have developed obesity from an eating disorder are now more likely than ever to undergo bariatric surgery as an intervention.

In one large study of 2266 individuals electing bariatric surgery, loss of control eating was reported by 43.4% and night eating syndrome by 17.7%; 15.7% satisfied criteria for BED and 2% for BN (Mitchell et al., 2015). Factors that independently increased the odds of BED were being a college graduate, eating more times per day, taking medication for psychiatric or emotional problems, and having symptoms of alcohol use disorder, lower self-esteem, and greater depressive symptoms. Before undergoing bariatric surgery, a substantial proportion of patients reported problematic eating behaviors. Several factors associated with BED were identified, most suggesting other mental health problems, including higher levels of depressive symptoms (Mitchell et al., 2015).

Whereas patients with obesity are having some success with bariatric surgery, adults with AN have notoriously poor outcomes, and treatment evidence is limited (Schmidt et al., 2015). There has been some limited clinical success with these patients with the Maudsley Model of Anorexia Nervosa Treatment for Adults (MANTRA), in which patients receive 20 to 30 weekly therapy sessions focusing on concerns specific to AN, including a need to avoid intense emotions; personality traits such as perfectionism; pro-anorexia beliefs (believing that the illness will help manage difficult emotions and the relationships that arouse them); and the response of families to the illness.

Feeding and Eating Disorders in Pregnant Women

Pregnancy and childbirth are major life events accompanied by profound biological, social, and psychologic changes. Research has indicated that disordered eating in pregnancy persists in a substantial proportion of women who have prepregnancy eating disorders. The presence of an eating disorder in this period may negatively affect the pregnancy (e.g., weight gain), delivery (e.g., cesarean delivery, preterm delivery), or offspring (e.g., birth weight) (Knoph et al., 2013).

Pregnancy may also influence the course of eating disorders. For the majority of women with AN and BN, pregnancy appears to lead to adaptive changes in eating behaviors, with the disorders often remitting during and after pregnancy. However, for some, pregnancy may lead to maladaptive changes in eating behavior. Research has found that pregnancy poses a risk for the onset of BED in vulnerable individuals, occurring in nearly 1 in every 20 women (Knoph et al., 2013; Watson et al., 2013). Obstetricians/gynecologists and clinicians need training to detect eating disorders and devise interventions to enhance pregnancy and neonatal outcomes.

Pica, the practice of eating nonfood items during pregnancy, has been documented in health literature for many years. One recent study of women of Mexican origin in the United States associated pica with iron deficiency, not anemia as customarily reported, and found the practice to be quite common, as over half the women reported ever engaging in pica (Roy et al., 2015). Yet another study associated increased pica in urban pregnant women with higher levels of lead in the blood (Thihalolipavan, Candalla, & Ehrlich, 2012). Finally, a large meta-analysis of pica found that the prevalence was higher in Africa compared with elsewhere in the world, increased as the prevalence of anemia increased, and decreased as educational attainment increased (Fawcett, Fawcett, & Mazmanian, 2016).

Feeding and Eating Disorders in Men

In the past, it has been believed that men have eating disorders less frequently than women. According to the APA (2013), anorexia and bulimia occur less frequently among males than females, with a 1:10 male-to-female ratio. However, some studies have contradicted this statistic, reporting up to 25% of ED patients being male (Campbell & Peebles, 2014). The APA (2013) has estimated that BED occurs in males at half the rate in females (0.8% and 1.6%, respectively). However, one ED study found that BED was more common among males than previously believed (Smink et al., 2012). Recent studies have attempted to better quantify prevalence in this population and to discover factors that distinguish male ED behaviors from that of females.

Research has found that men with EDs differ from women in their weight histories. Men frequently reported being mildly to moderately obese at some point in their lives before developing an eating disorder and were particularly susceptible if they were obese in childhood (Mitchell et al., 2012). In contrast, most women with EDs typically had a normal weight history. Compensatory behaviors, such as exercise, are also used more by men than women in order to avert the potential of developing medical complications that their fathers had developed (Mitchell et al., 2012). Most women use compensatory behaviors to achieve thinness. Compared with women, men with EDs are more often motivated to lose (or gain) weight to achieve optimal athletic performance and be eligible to compete in sports (Mitchell et al., 2012).

As is the case with women, many men with EDs have a history of sexual abuse. Research has demonstrated a strong correlation between sexual abuse and eating disorders, with an estimated 30% of eating-disordered patients having a history of sexual abuse (Mitchell et al., 2012). For men, sexual abuse has likely been underreported because of a disproportionate amount of shame and stigmatization that accompanies abuse for men versus women.

Factors predicting a male ED include childhood bullying; being gay or bisexual, which some studies have suggested may increase the likelihood of an ED by tenfold; depression and shame; excessive exercise coupled with increased diet success ("manorexia"); comorbid substance abuse, including the use of stimulants to lose weight; and media pressures resulting in male body dissatisfaction (Mitchell et al., 2012).

Feeding and Eating Disorders in Older Adults

The most common concern regarding older adults and disordered eating is the physiologic anorexia of aging. This process is characterized by a decrease in appetite and energy intake that occurs even in healthy people and is possibly caused by changes in the digestive tract, gastrointestinal hormone concentrations and activity, neurotransmitters, and cytokines (Soenen & Chapman, 2013). Unintentional weight loss in older people may be a result of protein-energy malnutrition, cachexia, the physiologic anorexia of aging, or any combination of these factors.

However, recent research has found that typical ED symptoms are also common in older adults. In a study of women age 50 and older, 62% of respondents said their weight or shape negatively impacts their life, and 64% think about their weight at least once a day (Gagne et al., 2012). Fully 13.3% of women age 50 and older exhibited ED symptoms. Binging and purging are both prevalent among women in their early 50s, but occur in women older than 75 as well. Research participants reported using unhealthy methods to lose weight and maintain thinness, including diet pills, excessive exercise, diuretics, laxatives, and vomiting. Feeding and eating disorders are detrimental to the health of individuals of all ages, but they can be particularly damaging to the bodies of older adults. The damaging effects of bulimia and anorexia exacerbate preexisting osteoporosis, cardiovascular problems, and gastroesophageal reflux disease (Gagne et al., 2012).

NURSING PROCESS

When assessing the patient with a known or suspected eating disorder, keep in mind that denial is often inherent to these conditions. Recognize that deceit and manipulation are characteristics of the disorder and not necessarily consciously chosen behaviors on the part of the patient.

Assessment

For the patient with an eating disorder, assessment combines a thorough review of both physiologic and psychosocial functioning as well as careful observations for the physiologic manifestations associated with feeding and eating disorders. When a patient presents with a significant weight gain or loss, do not automatically assume the patient has an eating disorder. Numerous physiologic conditions can lead to muscle wasting and weight loss, including cancer, hyperthyroidism, and impaired gastrointestinal function. Likewise, weight gain may occur due to a variety of causes, including endocrine disorders and medication side effects. Before the primary care provider establishes the diagnosis of an eating disorder, other causes for weight alteration must be ruled out (Kneisl & Trigoboff, 2013).

Focused assessment of the patient's nutritional status incorporates data obtained through the patient interview, physiologic assessment findings, and review of laboratory and diagnostic test results. Assessment of nutritional status includes height, weight, BMI, mid-arm circumference (MAC), and waist-to-hip ratio. It also includes assessment of the skin, the oral mucosa and tongue, the shape of the abdomen, and the nature and presence of bowel sounds. Assess the teeth and gums for any irregularities.

On physical assessment, patients with anorexia nervosa will appear emaciated. Their skin may be dry and covered by a fine layer of hair called *lanugo*, and they also may appear jaundiced (yellow-orange in color). As a result of malnourishment, hair and nails will appear to be brittle. Undernutrition may impair the function of any body system, including the brain, musculoskeletal system, kidneys, and heart. In particular, cardiovascular manifestations may include bradycardia, hypotension, and cardiac dysrhythmias (Potter & Moller, 2014). Because the potential effects of undernutrition are numerous, these patients require a complete physical assessment.

Assessment of patients with known or suspected bulimia nervosa usually includes completion of a physical exam by the primary healthcare provider, followed by psychologic evaluation and laboratory diagnostics. Patients with BN typically maintain a body weight that meets or exceeds normal weight limits. For these patients, focused assessment of the oral cavity can be very revealing. If purging behaviors include vomiting, patients' teeth may demonstrate pitting and enamel erosion, as well as an increased incidence of dental caries. Patients who purge by vomiting may also exhibit ruptured blood vessels in the eyes, as well as a hoarse voice due to throat irritation. Laboratory tests may reveal electrolyte imbalances or dehydration due to purging (PubMed Health, 2012b). In particular, patients with BN are susceptible to metabolic acidosis. If dehydrated, they may demonstrate a variety of manifestations, including hypotension, dry mouth, poor skin turgor, complaints of light-headedness or dizziness, general weakness, decreased urine production, and concentrated urine.

Diagnosis

Nursing diagnoses that may be appropriate for inclusion in the plan of care for the patient with an eating disorder may include the following:

- *Injury, Risk for,* related to orthostatic hypotension, fluid volume deficiency, and electrolyte imbalances
- *Fluid Volume, Deficient*
- *Imbalanced Nutrition: Less Than Body Requirements*
- *Cardiac Output, Decreased*

- *Mucous Membrane, Oral, Impaired*
- *Dentition, Impaired*
- *Body Image, Disturbed*
- *Coping, Ineffective*
- *Self-Esteem, Chronic Low*
- *Anxiety.*

(NANDA-I © 2014)

Planning

Primary long-term goals of care for the patient with an eating disorder include restoring nutritional status and fluid and electrolyte balance, maintenance of body weight within an acceptable range, and development of a healthy body image. Because these patients face significant psychosocial barriers, including body image distortion and rigid behavioral patterns, intensive psychologic care is often necessary for achieving long-term outcomes. Examples of short-term patient goals that may be applicable to the nursing plan of care for the patient with an ED include the following:

- The patient will remain free from injury.
- The patient will demonstrate manifestations of fluid volume balance, including adequate urine production, vital signs that range within normal limits, and absence of symptoms such as light-headedness or dizziness.
- The patient's laboratory testing will demonstrate electrolyte levels that are within normal limits.
- The patient will remain free of purging behaviors.
- The patient will actively participate in individual and/or group therapy.
- The patient will remain free of nonsuicidal self-injurious (NSSI) behaviors, such as cutting, and will report any suicidal ideation.

SAFETY ALERT Suicide attempts and repeated attempts are common among patients with eating disorders. For a number of years, anorexia nervosa has been consistently associated with high rates of suicide among adolescents and young adults. Findings also support that suicide risk appears elevated in bulimia nervosa and is perhaps even higher than individuals with anorexia. There seems to be an association with self-injurious behaviors, with a higher risk among individuals who binge and purge. Suicide risk should be routinely assessed with all patients with eating disorders (Kostro, Lerman, & Attia, 2014; Suokas et al., 2014).

Implementation

Care of the patient who is diagnosed with an eating disorder is highly complex. Priorities of care include protecting the patient from physiologic effects of the ED. However, the ultimate goal is identification and treatment of the cause of the alterations, which is the ED itself. For these patients, the primary intervention involves intensive therapy provided by a mental health professional who is specially trained in the treatment of patients with feeding and eating disorders. While recognizing the complexity of the origin and treatment of feeding and eating disorders, the nurse can promote wellness through preventing patient injury and encouraging healthy patient behaviors and thought patterns.

Prevent Injury

Patients with feeding and eating disorders are at constant or near-constant risk for injury due to undernutrition and its consequences. The effects of purging behaviors also keep the patient at risk for injury.

Behavioral contracts that outline prohibited actions and their consequences may prove effective in the care of patients who are at risk for injurious behaviors. However, especially early in the course of treatment, behavioral contracts may have adverse effects, particularly as asking patients to promise to control compulsive behaviors is unrealistic. For these patients, many of whom are already struggling with shame, the inability to adhere to the contract could serve to heighten the sense of shame and further diminish self-esteem. For patients in the clinical setting, constant monitoring and supervision may be necessary to ensure adequate nutritional intake and prevent purging behaviors.

Additional interventions include the following:

- Teach the patient to decrease exposure to environmental stress.
- Teach the patient to decrease anxiety by eliminating caffeine and other stimulants, such as energy drinks.
- Help to the patient increase social and familial connectedness through improving communication skills.
- Teach methods of self-soothing, such as watching TV, reading a book, listening to energizing music, calling a friend, or creating art.
- Encourage the patient to eliminate drugs or alcohol that can increase impulsivity (Potter & Moller, 2016).

In extreme cases, inpatient intake of nutrients and fluids may be medically ordered and administered to patients whose lives are at risk. For all patients, such issues raise ethical concerns and require the nurse to be aware of legal considerations related to forced care. Among experts in the field of feeding and eating disorders, the practice of forcing patient interventions to prevent injury (including death) is the subject of intense debate (Fox & Goss, 2012). If the patient is hospitalized for medical stabilization, the following interventions may be employed:

- Limit the patient's activity and energy expenditure, for example, no excessive exercise.
- Monitor vital signs, food and fluid intake/output, and electrolyte levels.
- Observe for signs of fluid overload, which may indicate refeeding syndrome.
- Monitor trips to the bathroom and look for food hoarding, for example, the patient has hidden food rather than eating it.
- Assess/monitor gastrointestinal and cardiac functioning, as necessary (Potter & Moller, 2016).

Promote a Therapeutic Relationship and Positive Self-Regard

Many patients with feeding and eating disorders have maintained secrecy with regard to their nutritional habits and purging behaviors. Treatment requires patients to be open about their behaviors, as well as to discuss sensitive topics and issues that may be psychologically painful. Transitioning from secrecy to openness is a major challenge that requires great courage on the part of the patient, as well as establishment of trust between the patient and the healthcare provider. With these patients, respect, consistency, and patience are keys to establishing trust, which is part of the foundation of a therapeutic relationship. Other interventions, which are equally appropriate in outpatient and inpatient settings, may include the following:

- Help the patient to identify triggers, such as troubling interpersonal relationships and turbulent internal emotional states, that promote disordered eating behaviors.
- Help the patient to reframe the feelings of purging behavior that contribute to a sense of empowerment, control, and relief from tension.
- Provide positive reinforcement when patients adhere to treatment and make efforts to meet goals.
- Help patients set short-term, realistic goals that they can easily achieve to foster opportunities for success and allow patients to see and measure their treatment progress.
- Encourage patients to reconnect with activities and experiences that they enjoy to help them begin to regain control over their own behaviors and begin to reexperience positive emotions (Potter & Moller, 2016).

Evaluation

Evaluation is a dynamic, ongoing feature of the nursing process that includes identifying the degree to which patients have achieved the goals and outcomes established in conjunction with each nursing diagnosis. While goals and outcomes for the patient with an eating disorder will vary based on patient individuality and the patient's nursing diagnoses, examples of potential outcomes relevant to the care of these patients may include the following:

- The patient remains free from injury.
- The patient's vital signs remain within normal limits.
- The patient's serum electrolytes remain within normal limits.
- The patient demonstrates production of non-concentrated urine.
- The patient denies light-headedness or dizziness.
- The patient does not demonstrate purging behaviors.
- The patient actively participates in individual and/or group therapy.

Many clinicians view recovery from eating disorders to be a cyclical rather than a linear process. Because eating disorders are complex with multifactorial influences, the care plan may need to be modified periodically if patients are not responding to planned interventions. Nurses and clinicians may need to reevaluate triggers and treatment regimens as well as help patients identify alternative methods of coping.

>> See Chart 29–2: Nursing Care Plan: A Patient with Anorexia Disorder at **Pearson MyLab Nursing and eText.**

REVIEW Feeding and Eating Disorders

RELATE Link the Concepts and Exemplars

Linking the exemplar on feeding and eating disorders with the concept of teaching and learning:

1. In the context of caring for a patient diagnosed with an eating disorder, describe the barriers the nurse faces with regard to teaching about nutrition.

2. The nurse is caring for a 17-year-old female patient who is diagnosed with anorexia nervosa. The patient's father states, "Once she starts eating regularly, she'll get better. She's just being stubborn." To effectively teach the father about the basis of AN, how should the nurse respond?

Linking the exemplar on feeding and eating disorders with the concept of acid–base balance:

3. How does purging by way of self-induced vomiting most often affect the individual's acid–base balance? How does purging through laxative abuse most often affect acid–base balance?

4. What potential cardiac complications may arise as a result of acid–base imbalances associated with feeding and eating disorders?

READY Go to Volume 3: Clinical Nursing Skills

REFER Go to Pearson MyLab Nursing and eText

- Additional review materials

- Chart 29–1: Clinical Manifestations and Therapies: Other Feeding and Eating Disorders
- Chart 29–2: Nursing Care Plan: A Patient with Anorexia Nervosa

REFLECT Apply Your Knowledge

Anisha Robinson is an 18-year-old college student who received a full scholarship for gymnastics. At 5′ 2″ and 101 pounds, Ms. Robinson is tiny, but she frequently complains about being overweight. When she is not practicing with the gymnastics team, she spends much of her time studying. Although her grades are outstanding, she worries that she will not be admitted into pharmacy school. Sometimes she is so anxious at night that she can't sleep. In order not to keep her roommate up, she'll go out and run 2–3 miles in the middle of the night. Her friends worry about her because they don't know how she can keep her strength up when she eats so little, despite the fact that she'll exercise for an hour or more after every meal. Her roommate becomes worried when they return from Thanksgiving break and she hears the gymnastics coach complaining that Ms. Robinson has gained 3 pounds over the holiday. Ms. Robinson tearfully resolves to eat less and work out more.

1. What are the priority nursing diagnoses for Ms. Robinson?

2. What nursing interventions may be appropriate for inclusion in Ms. Robinson's nursing plan of care?

3. What assessment findings may indicate that Ms. Robinson's health is deteriorating?

» Exemplar 29.B Personality Disorders

Exemplar Learning Outcomes

29.B Analyze personality disorders and how they relate to self.

- Describe the pathophysiology of personality disorders.
- Describe the etiology of personality disorders.
- Compare the risk factors and prevention of personality disorders.
- Identify the clinical manifestations of personality disorders.
- Summarize diagnostic tests and therapies used by interprofessional teams in the collaborative care of an individual with personality disorders.
- Differentiate care of patients with personality disorders across the lifespan.
- Apply the nursing process in providing culturally competent care to an individual with a personality disorder.

Exemplar Key Terms

Antisocial personality disorder (ASPD), *2000*
Avoidant personality disorder (APD), *2006*
Borderline personality disorder (BPD), *2006*
Dependent personality disorder (DPD), *2008*
Depersonalization, *2010*
Derealization, *2010*
Detachment, *2010*
Disinhibition, *2006*
Ego-syntonic, *2004*
Histrionic personality disorder (HPD), *2009*
Impulsiveness, *2004*
Manipulation, *2004*
Narcissism, *2004*
Narcissistic personality disorder (NPD), *2009*
Obsessive-compulsive personality disorder (OCPD), *2009*
Paranoid personality disorder (PPD), *2010*
Personality, *2003*
Personality disorder (PD), *2004*
Personality traits, *2003*
Psychoticism, *2010*
Schizoid personality disorder, *2010*
Schizotypal personality disorder, *2010*
Splitting, *2006*

Overview

The American Psychological Association (2013) defines **personality** as enduring characteristic patterns of thinking, feeling, and behavior that make an individual unique. These patterns begin to take shape in childhood and are set by early adulthood. Character and temperament constitute two important aspects of a person's personality. *Character* refers to moral and ethical value judgments, whereas *temperament* refers to innate characteristics, such as nervousness or sensitivity.

The elements that make up an individual's personality are called **personality traits**. They number in the hundreds, and examples include affability, impulsiveness, and honesty.

In the field of psychology, however, special emphasis has been placed on the five-factor model: neuroticism, extraversion, openness, agreeableness, and conscientiousness (Butcher, Mineka, & Hooley, 2013). Psychologists generally use these traits to describe an individual's personality, as they are considered to be universal; however, recent research raises questions as to their universality in non-Western, pre-industrialized societies (Gurven, von Rueden, & Massenkoff, 2013).

An individual's personality determines how that individual interacts with others. When established personality patterns result in repeated conflicts with others and impair the individual's ability to function in society, that individual is said to be experiencing a **personality disorder (PD)**. PDs affect all aspects of an individual's life and are marked by overly rigid and maladaptive behaviors that make it difficult for the individual to adapt to social demands and change. PDs are independent of mental disorders and substance abuse and are generally consistent over time and across varying situations.

Pathophysiology and Etiology

PDs typically manifest themselves during adolescence and continue throughout the lifespan, although in some cases symptoms diminish with age. Symptoms include interpersonal difficulties, identity problems that result in a weak sense of self, a lack of intimate relationships, and clumsy social skills that hinder cooperation. Individuals with PDs exhibit behaviors that may include **manipulation** (controlling and taking advantage of others); **narcissism** (believing oneself superior and worthy of special treatment); and **impulsiveness** (acting without regard to potential consequences) (Kneisl & Trigoboff, 2013).

Pathophysiology

The nature of these dysfunctions is not fully understood. The American Psychiatric Association has described a number of PDs, but because clinical definitions lack precision, there is often overlap. Consequently, individuals experiencing a PD are usually diagnosed with more than one. That said, all individuals with PDs demonstrate three common behaviors. First, they manage stress by attempting to change the environment rather than themselves; second, they fail to assume responsibility for the consequences of their actions; and third, they illustrate a lack of understanding as to how their behavior affects others. In effect, individuals with PDs are **ego-syntonic**, meaning that they behave according to the beliefs, desires, and values that concur with their disorder. In other words, they see themselves and their behavior as normal and view the problems that arise with others as external to themselves, often believing they are being victimized (Kneisl & Trigoboff, 2013).

PDs are also characterized by deficits in the areas of cognition, affect, interpersonal relationships, and impulse control; individuals with PDs manifest problems and difficulties in at least two of these areas of functioning (Kneisl & Trigoboff, 2013). In addition to this impairment, developing healthy coping strategies proves to be a challenge as individuals with PDs are typically inflexible. This lack of adaptability feeds into a continual negative cycle in which the same behaviors are consistently exhibited, sabotaging opportunities to gain new skills, and ultimately leading to social isolation.

Etiology

Much about PDs remains unknown, and studies on PDs are hampered by several factors. For example, the lack of diagnostic uniformity makes it difficult for researchers to define samples and replicate previous studies. Another problem is that most individuals experiencing PDs do not come to the attention of mental health professionals. Many individuals with PDs fail to recognize themselves as abnormal and see no need to seek out treatment (Potter & Moller, 2016). Consequently, mental health professionals often do not encounter individuals with PD unless behaviors are severe enough to warrant intervention by family members or the court system.

What is known is that the inflexible personality and behavioral patterns that characterize PDs appear to develop gradually, often with origins in childhood (Butcher et al., 2013). PDs do not appear to be the result of any one cause. Instead, they seem to be the result of an interaction between biological and environmental factors.

Genetics

There does appear to be a genetic causal relationship with certain PDs. According to the Mayo Clinic (2013a), a family history of schizotypal PD and/or schizophrenia increases the likelihood of an individual developing schizotypal PD. Other researchers have found clinical findings regarding genetics to be highly divergent, with some studies finding high heredity and others very low. One large-scale study that sought to remove interviewer bias, long thought to be a factor in variable results, showed that Cluster B personality disorders (e.g., antisocial borderline, narcissistic, and histrionic personality disorders) were strongly heritable, in the upper range of previous findings for mental disorders (Torgersen et al., 2012). In this study, familial environment scored very low in predicting risk of developing the disorders. A study on fraternal and identical twins with antisocial personality disorder (ASPD) found genetic factors to be a greater influence than environmental factors (Kendler, Aggen, & Patrick, 2012). The American Psychiatric Association (APA, 2013) reported on increasing evidence of the link among specific genes, obsessive-compulsive personality disorder (OCPD), and the personality traits of aggressiveness, anxiety, and fear.

Neurobiology

Research points to several neurobiological factors as contributors to the development of PDs. One comprehensive literature review on borderline personality disorder supported the following findings, which can be extrapolated to other PDs: The role of a genetic vulnerability in development of a PD is largely supported; gene–environment interactions had a high likelihood in the genesis of PDs; and plasticity genes (modifiable by environment and experiences) and vulnerability genes are likely both involved in the development of PDs (Amad et al., 2014). Another neuroimaging study found that trait anxiety may cause emotional interference and disrupt cognitive processing in individuals with borderline personality disorder (Holtmann et al., 2013).

Trauma History

Early life stress, including sexual abuse, physical abuse, emotional abuse, physical neglect, and emotional neglect, has been associated with the onset and severity of psychiatric disorders in adults. One meta-analysis showed that emotional abuse and physical neglect were demonstrated to be strongly associated with the development of personality disorders (Carr et al., 2013). Another study showed a strong correlation between childhood sexual abuse and the development of borderline PD (Bohus et al., 2013). Both studies showed that the link is stronger among females, although this may reflect more self-reporting of abuse among females than males. In summary, early life stress triggers aggravate, maintain, and increase the recurrence of PDs and other psychiatric diagnoses.

Exposure to interpersonal and accidental traumatic events and/or repeated episodes of trauma that result in posttraumatic stress disorder (PTSD) are also strongly linked to the development of PDs and other psychiatric diagnoses. The link between PTSD and development of borderline PD was significantly stronger than the link between PTSD and other psychiatric comorbidities (Amstadter et al., 2012). Although PTSD is a factor in the development of borderline PD, trauma also is strongly correlated with the development of avoidant, obsessive-compulsive, and dependent personality disorders (Friborg et al., 2013).

Intrapersonal Factors

Individuals with different PDs interact with others in a variety of ways. They may project their feelings onto those around them, demonstrate problems in developing genuine intimate relationships, lack a sense of guilt, or behave childishly, depending on their personality dysfunction (Kneisl & Trigoboff, 2013).

As discussed earlier in the concept, parent–child interactions can significantly affect a person's developing sense of self, and as a result, a child's perception of reality may become distorted if parents are insensitive to the child's needs. Individuals with a family background of criminality and parental separation, or a childhood marked by continually changing caregivers or care institutions, show a higher propensity for PDs. In one study, all PD dimensions were significantly related to various forms of family and school problems as well as child abuse (Hengartner et al., 2013). Poverty was uniquely associated with schizotypal PD; conflicts with parents with obsessive-compulsive PD; physical abuse with antisocial PD; and physical neglect with narcissistic PD. Sexual abuse was statistically significantly associated with schizotypal and borderline PD, but corresponding effect sizes were small (Hengartner et al., 2013).

The American Psychiatric Association (2013) also reported that individuals diagnosed with borderline PDs have a higher incidence of childhood sexual trauma. In addition, a longitudinal study of almost 800 mothers and their children showed that the incidence of borderline, narcissistic, obsessive-compulsive, and paranoid PDs increased threefold in children who were verbally abused by their mothers, independent of other factors such as sexual or physical abuse, the temperament of the child, and any coexisting psychiatric disorders (Johnson et al., 2001). Last, although mood and anxiety disorders are distinct from PDs, overlapping features among the three types of disorders exist, which makes the correlation between childhood verbal abuse by a parent and the later development of mood and anxiety disorders and PTSD noteworthy (Stevens et al., 2013).

Sociocultural Factors

The influence of social and cultural factors in personality disorders is not fully understood, yet it is known that they contribute to personal development. For example, when certain groups are discriminated against in a society, it is difficult for the members of that group to develop a healthy self-image. In traditional cultures, such as those found in Japan, there is societal pressure to conform and adhere to group norms. In the United States, on the other hand, emphasis is placed on the personal versus the communal, leading to the prevalence of a "me-first" mentality. Thus individuals from different parts of the world have a greater propensity for certain kinds of PDs according to their sociocultural backdrop.

There is evidence that histrionic disorders are less common in Asian cultures, where individuals tend to be more reserved, than in Hispanic cultures, where individuals tend to be more expressive. In the United States, African Americans and Caucasians are less prone to develop borderline PDs than Hispanics, but they differ with respect to schizotypal PD, with African Americans showing a greater propensity than Caucasians for developing such a disorder (Butcher et al., 2013).

Risk Factors

As discussed in the concept section of this module, both genetic and environmental factors are believed to influence the development of a PD. According to the Mayo Clinic (2013a), notable risk factors include genetics, such as having relatives diagnosed with a PD or another mental illness; family life, such as an unstable home life or parental loss via death or divorce; childhood abuse, such as verbal, physical, and sexual abuse or neglect; diagnosis of other disorders, such as childhood conduct disorder; and low socioeconomic status. That said, diagnosing PDs in children can prove to be challenging because the behavioral and thinking patterns that may indicate such a disorder could actually be the consequence of a developmental phase or the experimentation that often occurs during adolescence.

Prevention

PDs can be prevented if the developing patterns of behavior, feeling, and thought are identified before they become set. This generally requires intervention during childhood and early adolescence (Evans, 2012). Consequently, prevention programs have been created to address both developmental and environmental risk factors, and to break the cycle of repeating problematic patterns by providing interventions at school and in the home. Screening programs have been implemented in schools and primary care settings to help detect risk factors and identify patterns that indicate a PD may be forming (Evans, 2012).

In terms of interventions, there are several programs in the United States focused on imparting parenting skills to address aggressive and antisocial behaviors. The Nurse-Family Partnership Program is one of them. Under this program, registered nurses visit at-risk families with newborn children starting at the prenatal period and lasting through the child's second birthday. The nurses impart parenting skills and work with family members to change poor habits, such as smoking and unhealthy eating choices. Another is the Incredible Years Program, which uses video recordings of scenarios with parents to promote positive parent–child interactions. The program also includes a classroom management component for teachers and uses puppets to teach children social skills. A third program, New Beginnings, is designed to help children in the case of divorce by strengthening parenting skills; the program has reduced problem behaviors in children and improved parenting warmth and discipline. The parenting interventions included in these and other programs have demonstrated a positive correlation between sociable behavior and a child's self-esteem (Evans, 2012).

Barriers to these preventive measures include competing priorities, lack of infrastructure for implementation, lack of public education regarding mental health and the effectiveness of prevention, stigma, and a paucity of facilitating factors (Evans, 2012). Facilitators include leadership, flexible resources, linkage to healthcare reform or other legislation, coordination across agencies and governmental levels, and additional research.

Clinical Manifestations

The *Diagnostic and Statistical Manual*, Fifth Edition (DSM-5), specifies that individuals with PDs must exhibit dysfunctional behavior toward self and others, and they must also maintain persistent, rigid thoughts and beliefs that are incongruent with sociocultural norms (APA, 2013). Using a categorical approach, each of the 10 PDs is viewed as being a clinically distinct syndrome. However, the American Psychiatric Association also outlines criteria that are characteristic of PDs in general. These include that the individual exhibits a stable pattern of perceptions and behaviors that are out of line with cultural expectations and which occur in two or more areas: cognition, affect, impulse control, and personal relationships (APA, 2013). These patterns must not be consistent with any other psychiatric disorder or with any underlying medical illness or use or abuse of medications or substances.

The 10 personality disorders are categorized into three clusters: Cluster A includes those PDs that may be characterized by odd or eccentric behaviors; Cluster B includes the PDs characterized by dramatic, erratic, or emotional behaviors; and Cluster C includes those PDs typified by avoidant, dependent, or obsessive-compulsive behaviors (APA, 2013). The currently recognized PDs are presented in alphabetical order. For an overview of the primary PDs, see **Table 29–4 》**.

Antisocial Personality Disorder

One of the first named PDs was **antisocial personality disorder (ASPD)**, which is distinguished by the individual's propensity to manipulate or violate others' rights with a disregard for their feelings and/or the consequences (U.S. National Library of Medicine, 2012). Risk factors include having a caregiver who has antisocial PD or alcoholism and being a victim of child abuse. An estimated 3-4% of the U.S. population has ASPD, with approximately four times as many men having the disorder than women (Potter & Moller, 2016). Because of the lack of remorse and inclination for risk-taking behavior associated with ASPD, many individuals with this PD are found in prison and substance abuse treatment centers.

To confirm diagnosis of antisocial PD, an individual must illustrate dysfunction as illustrated by egocentric behaviors, including pleasure-seeking and unlawful behaviors. In addition, impairments must exist in interpersonal functioning either via a lack of empathy and remorse for wrongdoings or the inability to form and maintain intimate relationships, which often includes deceptive or coercive behaviors. Two trait domains are associated with antisocial PD: antagonism and **disinhibition**. In addition to the other general criteria for PDs, an individual with antisocial PD must be at least 18 years of age (APA, 2013). Often individuals younger than age 18 who demonstrate behaviors typical of antisocial PD have been diagnosed with a conduct disorder, such as oppositional defiant disorder, or attention-deficit/hyperactivity disorder (ADHD) (Potter & Moller, 2016).

Avoidant Personality Disorder

Avoidant personality disorder (APD) is characterized by extreme shyness and fear of rejection. Despite the desire to connect and bond with others, their insecurities and concern for other individuals' perception of them prevent individuals with this disorder from forming relationships of substance. Approximately 2.4% of individuals in the United States have APD (APA, 2013).

Low self-esteem, poor social skills, extreme sensitivity to criticism, and unrealistic expectations related to goal achievement and interacting in groups are characteristics of individuals with APD. They also typically experience a pronounced distrust of individuals' interest in relationship building. Detachment and negative affectivity are the two trait domains associated with APD, with negative affectivity being characterized by anxiety (APA, 2013).

Borderline Personality Disorder

In 1938, psychoanalyst Adolf Stern established the label of **borderline personality disorder (BPD)**, as he believed the symptoms of BPD sat on the dividing line or "border" between psychosis and neurosis. Currently, many mental healthcare professionals take exception with Stern's use of the term *borderline* because it can reinforce already existing negative perceptions of individuals with BPD (Kling, 2014).

Impulsivity, unstable emotions, and depression are key symptoms of BPD; self-harm is also common (see **Figure 29–3 》**), with suicide occurring in 8–10% of those with this disorder (NIMH, 2013a). **Splitting**, the inclination to perceive people or situations as one extreme or the other (e.g., all good or all bad), is also commonly found among individuals with BPD; this feature contributes to their frequent extreme shifts in mood (Oltmanns & Emery, 2012). Other core characteristics include identity disturbances; frantic attempts to prevent abandonment (real or perceived); impulsive behaviors; chronic feelings of emptiness; transient paranoia; and difficulty managing anger (APA, 2013).

TABLE 29–4 Personality Disorders and Associated Characteristics

Behavioral Traits	Affective Traits	Cognitive Traits	Social Traits
Antisocial Personality Disorder			
■ Impulsive; difficulty in delaying gratification ■ Dishonest ■ Irresponsible ■ Risk taking ■ Criminal behavior	■ Has no problems with self-expression yet remains detached in interactions ■ Lack of guilt and remorse for committing harmful acts ■ Callous ■ Easily agitated ■ Hostile ■ Failure to empathize	■ Egocentric ■ Grandiose ■ Despite lack of long-term planning, exhibits confidence in future success	■ Cannot form intimate relationships ■ Exploits others as form of interaction ■ Exhibits controlling and abusive behaviors ■ Aggressive
Avoidant Personality Disorder			
■ Intense discomfort in social situations ■ Avoids social contact unless feels will be fully accepted	■ Timid ■ Fearful of rejection ■ Intense worry and anxiety especially with regard to forming relationships	■ Hypersensitive to others' opinions of self ■ Acceptance of others' negative evaluations	■ Wants to have intimate relationships but an extreme fear of being embarrassed, judged, or rejected by others often prevents it ■ Possesses very few close relationships that are not familial
Borderline Personality Disorder			
■ Impulsive ■ Dangerous risk taking ■ Can self-mutilate and have suicidal tendencies ■ Unpredictable	■ Intense anxiety ■ Difficulty empathizing and feeling guilt ■ Psychotic episodes are common ■ Reactive moods ■ Difficulty in controlling anger ■ Consistently low mood; rarely experiences satisfaction or happiness	■ Unstable perception of self, ranging from grandiosity to self-loathing	■ Highly unstable relationships ■ Manipulative ■ Intense fear of abandonment ■ Mistrust ■ Behavior swings from all-encompassing interest in another individual to complete withdrawal
Dependent Personality Disorder			
■ Passive by nature ■ Seeks out others who are dominant and who will control the relationship	■ Strives to appear friendly and helpful ■ Will subordinate personal desires and needs and instead prioritize the desires and needs of others	■ Insecure with personal decision making ■ Pervasive sense of inferiority	■ Intense fear of rejection ■ Separation from the dominant other may produce extreme anxiety and depression
Histrionic Personality Disorder			
■ Flamboyant ■ Dramatic ■ Seeks to be the center of attention	■ Appears inconsiderate and incapable of empathy ■ Pervasive craving for excitement	■ Egocentric ■ Tends to prefer creative and artistic endeavors as opposed to academic achievement	■ May use sexual behaviors to manipulate others ■ May engage in high-risk sexual behaviors
Narcissistic Personality Disorder			
■ Very competitive in search of power, fame, and love ■ Arrogant ■ Manipulates others to achieve own ends	■ Difficulty in expressing emotions ■ Empathy is a challenge ■ Anxiety and fear in relation to failure	■ Grandiosity ■ Believes is better than others ■ Spends much time fantasizing about being powerful, famous, loved, and beautiful	■ Balanced reciprocal relationships are rare ■ Seeks out relationships as a way to boost own self-esteem
Obsessive-Compulsive Personality Disorder			
■ Perfectionist ■ Inflexible ■ Hardworking ■ High achiever ■ Compulsive; engages in repetitive or ritualistic checking	■ Difficulty in expressing emotions ■ Empathy is a challenge ■ Anxiety and fear in relation to failure	■ Extreme fear of making mistakes; may procrastinate or avoid tasks because of fear of failure	■ Tends to be controlling in relationships, which limits intimacy
Paranoid Personality Disorder			
■ Suspicious and mistrusting of others ■ Rigid, fixed worldview	■ Inflexible about beliefs, perceptions, and suspicions ■ Argumentative	■ Generally intelligent and highly capable of arguing in support of personal beliefs	■ Extreme jealousy may impair intimate relationships with significant others ■ Tends to believe every action by others is driven by malevolent intent or ulterior motive

(continued on next page)

TABLE 29–4 Personality Disorders and Associated Characteristics *(continued)*

Behavioral Traits	Affective Traits	Cognitive Traits	Social Traits
Schizoid Personality Disorder			
■ Loners; tend to prefer solitary activities ■ Uninterested in socialization	■ Generally appear apathetic ■ Flat (emotionless) affect	■ Generally indifferent to situations and circumstances ■ May appear to be cognitively impaired	■ Uninterested in intimate relationships ■ Prefers social isolation and avoids roles that require socialization
Schizotypal Personality Disorder			
■ Bizarre behaviors, appearance, and speech ■ Prefers solitary activities ■ Frequent lack of eye contact	■ Indifferent ■ Nonreactive or inappropriate in emotional situations	■ Extreme suspicion of others ■ Paranoid fears of persecution ■ Odd or distorted thoughts	■ Excessive anxiety in social situations ■ Fears intimate relationships ■ Alienation ■ Lacks the desire to form close relationships ■ Introverted

Sources: Based on Kneisl, C. R., & Trigoboff, E. (2013). *Contemporary psychiatric–mental health nursing (3rd ed.).* Upper Saddle River, NJ: Pearson Education; Mayo Clinic. (2016). *Personality disorders: Symptoms.* Retrieved from http://www.mayoclinic.org/diseases-conditions/personality-disorders/basics/symptoms/con-20030111; Potter, M. L., & Moller, M. D. (Eds.). (2016). *Psychiatric–mental health nursing: From suffering to hope.* Upper Saddle River, NJ: Pearson Education.

Gender plays a significant role in that 75% of diagnosed cases are in women (APA, 2013). Approximately 20% of psychiatric inpatients have BPD and 1.6% of the general population is affected; some estimates have ranged as high as 5.9% of the general population (APA, 2013). Risk factors include childhood abuse and abandonment and a strong genetic link: Individuals are five times more likely to be diagnosed with BPD if a first-degree relative also has the disorder. Antisocial personality disorder, mood disorders, and substance abuse disorders are also much more probable in families where individuals are affected with BPD (APA, 2013).

SAFETY ALERT Borderline personality disorder is often associated with self-mutilation, which can include cutting or carving into the skin (see Figure 29–3), burning, pulling out hair, and head banging, all known as nonsuicidal self-injury (NSSI). Nurses must be extremely cognizant of the signs of self-injury and demonstrate sensitivity when conducting an assessment. Patients often hide their injuries by wearing long sleeves or pants, even in warmer weather (Mayo Clinic, 2013b; NIMH, 2013b).

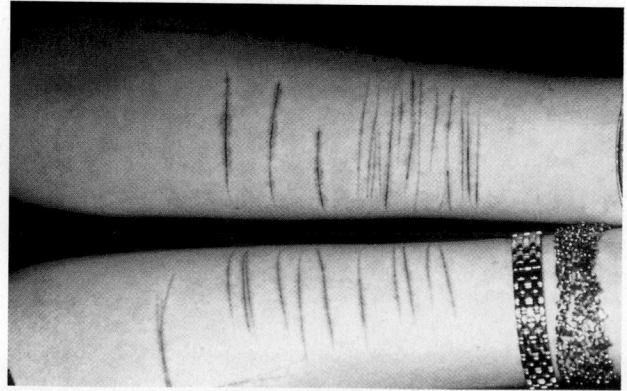

Source: Dr. P. Marazzi/Science Source.

Figure 29–3 》 Some individuals with borderline personality disorder engage in self-mutilating behavior, such as cutting.

Low self-esteem, intense self-criticism, and disassociation are associated with BPD. Interpersonal functioning is marked by the tendency to take offense easily or an intense fear of abandonment, which creates conflict-ridden and unstable relationships. The dysfunctional personality traits in BPD fall within the trait domains of negative affectivity (including emotional lability), disinhibition, and antagonism (APA, 2013). More information on borderline personality disorder can be found in **Box 29–2 》**.

Borderline personality disorder carries a great deal of stigma, even among mental health professionals. Kling (2014) found that a large portion of clinicians in the mental health field hold pejorative attitudes toward those with borderline personality disorder. Often, these attitudes become manifested through the use of stigmatizing language to describe patient behavior, such as "manipulative" and "attention seeking." In addition, Liebman and Burnette (2013) explored countertransference reactions to BPD in 560 clinicians via an online survey and found them to be markedly more negative than with any other disorder, which concurs with previous research.

Liebman and Burnette (2013) and McGrath and Dowling (2012) have recommended improved nurse training and education aimed at fostering a holistic view of BPD in order to better understand its causes and resulting behaviors. They cite CBT for nurses and BPD workshops as possible models. Kling (2014) voiced concerns on how stigmatizing language and attitudes affect the relationship between patient and clinician and how such language impacts recovery, and suggested self-governance measures that clinicians could use to improve patient interactions.

Dependent Personality Disorder

Central features of **dependent personality disorder (DPD)** include a pervasive need to be cared for, difficulty with decision making, separation anxiety, and impaired self-confidence. Individuals with DPD tend to seek out partners with dominant traits who will dictate decision making and choices (Potter & Moller, 2016). Individuals with DPD will

Box 29–2
Characteristics of Borderline Personality Disorder

Classified as a serious mental illness, borderline personality disorder impairs functioning in multiple areas because of the instability in mood, behavior, and self-image associated with the disorder. Characteristics of borderline PD include impulsive and often reckless behaviors, chronic feelings of emptiness, feelings of shame and guilt, and labile mood ranging from fear of abandonment to rage, as well as the increased risk for suicide or self-injurious behavior (SIB) (APA, 2013; Neacsiu et al., 2014). Symptoms must occur over time and not be attributed to another mental disorder or to substance use or medication side effects. In addition, individuals with borderline PD often have co-occurring mental illness. As a result, it is hardly surprising that a longitudinal study of 290 patients with borderline PD found significantly higher rates of participation in pharmacotherapy and more intensive treatment modalities (i.e., inpatient and day treatment programs associated with psychiatric hospitals) than patients with other personality disorders. The same study noted that treatment participation rates tend to decline within the first 8 years, with the notable exception of participation rates in pharmacotherapy (Zanarini et al., 2015).

Family members of patients with borderline PD need support and resources to learn how to help their loved one as well as to take care of themselves. The National Alliance on Mental Illness (2017) recommends several strategies for family members to follow:

- Find emotional support
- Take care of yourself—eat right, exercise, and avoid alcohol and drugs
- Encourage your loved one to continue treatment
- Learn and model techniques your loved one can use as coping strategies

Nurses can help family members by encouraging them to participate in their loved one's treatment plan, find local or online support groups, and maintain their own physical and mental health.

---

acquiesce to the wants and needs of others, often in an attempt to build or maintain a relationship. At times, these individuals will agree to perform undesirable tasks with the goal of receiving praise or acceptance from others (Kneisl & Trigoboff, 2013). Dependent personality disorder is found in between 0.49% and 0.6% of the general population and is diagnosed more frequently in women (APA, 2013). Chronic physical illness can predispose an individual to dependent personality disorder. Individuals with this disorder may experience mild impairment in occupational and social relationships in which independence is required (Potter & Moller, 2016)

Histrionic Personality Disorder

Characteristically, individuals with **histrionic personality disorder (HPD)** are self-centered (egocentric) and dramatic. In an attempt to garner attention, they may behave erratically, even going to extremes that appear "silly." Behind the attention-seeking behaviors is a strong sense of inadequacy and helplessness. In many cases, the individual with HPD's motivation for behaviors is rooted in a search for excitement and activity. For these patients, an apparent insincerity and inability to establish emotional commitment cause problems in the context of interpersonal relationships. The simultaneous need for love and reassurance experienced by the individual with HPD is counterbalanced by failure to demonstrate empathy and lack of consideration for significant others (Kneisl & Trigoboff, 2013). Their focus on themselves creates difficulty in establishing and maintaining relationships, and family members and caregivers may experience burnout (Potter & Moller, 2016).

Patients with HPD may demonstrate highly sexualized behaviors, appearing provocative and seductive. Seduction and sexuality serve as methods of manipulating others. For some patients with HPD, acting out may include impulsive sexual encounters and promiscuity, which lead to an increased risk for contracting and transmitting sexually transmitted infections (STIs). In addition, when needs for attention and affection are unfulfilled, the patient with HPD may act out through demonstration of suicidal behaviors (Kneisl & Trigoboff, 2013).

Narcissistic Personality Disorder

At the heart of **narcissistic personality disorder (NPD)** is a sense of grandiosity, an inability to empathize with others, and attention-seeking behaviors. Substance-abuse disorders (especially cocaine abuse), eating disorders (particularly anorexia nervosa), and depression, dysthymia, and social withdrawal are commonly found in conjunction with NPD (APA, 2013). More men than women are diagnosed, with 50–75% of the diagnoses being made in males. It is estimated that up to 6.2% of the general population experiences the disorder (APA, 2013).

Narcissistic personality disorder is characterized by extreme reliance on other individuals' perceptions and/or an inflated sense of self, or by approval seeking and either an extremely low or high set of personal standards. A failure to identify with others and their emotions or a hypersensitivity to others creates difficulty in developing meaningful relationships. NPD aligns with the trait domain of antagonism, specifically the trait facets of grandiosity and attention seeking (APA, 2013).

Obsessive-Compulsive Personality Disorder

Obsessive-compulsive personality disorder (OCPD) is characterized by significant impairments in social functioning and relationships and an all-consuming desire to achieve perfection in all tasks. It is important to note that OCPD is not the same as obsessive-compulsive disorder (OCD), which is covered in the module on Stress and Coping. Although they share similar traits, key differences exist. The International OCD Foundation (2012) specifies that individuals with OCPD do not see anything dysfunctional about their way of thinking or acting, whereas those with OCD recognize that their thoughts are disruptive and not normal, making them more likely to seek treatment. In addition, individuals with OCPD can demonstrate great productivity on the job, but their symptoms place strain on their interpersonal relationships; OCD generally causes disruptions in all areas. Men are twice as likely to experience OCPD as women, and approximately 2.1–7.9% of the general population is believed to have this disorder (APA, 2013).

Paranoid Personality Disorder

Individuals with **paranoid personality disorder (PPD)** tend to demonstrate an inability to trust others. Actions and intentions of others are perceived as having an underlying theme of malevolence. From the suspicious, mistrusting vantage point of the individual with PPD, others are viewed as being deceptive and disloyal. The pathologic jealousy sometimes associated with PPD can damage relationships with significant others. Tending toward being prejudicial and judgmental, individuals with PPD often maintain rigid, inflexible worldviews and will reject logic or proof that contradicts their beliefs. Hypervigilance combined with certainty that others' actions are prompted by hidden motives can lead to isolation for the patient with PPD (Kneisl & Trigoboff, 2013). Not surprisingly, the symptoms and behaviors associated with this disorder can result in family conflicts and occupational impairment (Potter & Moller, 2016). Prevalence rates for paranoid personality disorder are estimated at between 2.3% and 4.4% (APA, 2013). There is some evidence that there is increased prevalence of this disorder in first-degree relatives of individuals with schizophrenia and other psychotic disorders (APA, 2013).

Schizoid Personality Disorder

Central features of **schizoid personality disorder** include a seeming aloofness, a tendency to prefer solitary activities, absence of humor, and lack of interest in forming relationships, including those of a romantic nature. Generally disengaged and uninterested in social interaction, individuals with schizoid personality disorder may appear to be cognitively impaired and have difficulty working. Functional abilities and levels of adjustment vary among these patients; some are able to live independently and maintain marginal-to-adequate function within society, while others are institutionalized (Kneisl & Trigoboff, 2013).

Schizotypal Personality Disorder

Schizotypal personality disorder is distinguishable by extreme social anxiety and eccentric behavior. Commonly, **depersonalization** occurs, in which the individual feels apart from his body or an overall strangeness related to the physical self. Individuals with schizotypal personality disorder can also experience **derealization**, or feeling disconnected from their own body (Kneisl & Trigoboff, 2013). Schizotypal personality disorder and schizophrenia share similar criteria, but they are two different disorders, with schizophrenia being more severe. (For discussion of schizophrenia, see the module on Cognition.) For some individuals, symptoms of schizotypal personality disorder progress to a point where a diagnosis of schizophrenia is applied. Schizophrenia is commonly seen in families where another member is diagnosed with schizotypal personality disorder (Potter & Moller, 2016).

Individuals with schizotypal personality disorder experience difficulty in establishing boundaries between self and other individuals and frequently possess aims that are unrealistic or unclear. They frequently misunderstand other individuals' motives and actions, exhibit a lack of understanding of how their own behavior affects others, and experience challenges in establishing intimate relationships primarily because of anxiety and a lack of trust. The DSM-5 outlines three trait domains in schizotypal PD. The first is **psychoticism**, which is distinguished by eccentricity, cognitive and perceptual dysregulation, and unusual beliefs and experiences. The second trait domain is **detachment**, characterized by restricted affectivity and withdrawal, and the final trait domain is negative affectivity, which is defined by the trait facet of suspiciousness (APA, 2013).

>> **Stay Current:** In addition to the American Psychiatric Association's website, additional information about PDs can be found at www.MayoClinic.org and the National Institute for Mental Health at www.nimh.nih.gov.

Cultural Considerations

As environmental influences play a part in the development of personality, nurses and other healthcare professionals must take care not to deem a personality trait or behavior maladaptive or dysfunctional without first considering the influence of culture. For example: Individuals who are new to the United States may present as paranoid or overly suspicious of others when in fact their behavior could simply be a result of their unfamiliarity with American customs; some cultures condition girls and women to avoid social situations; and individuals from Latin cultures are generally much more expressive and exuberant than those from Britain. Cultural competence and being aware of one's own biases is crucial in providing quality care for patients. For additional examples, see the Focus on Diversity and Culture feature.

Collaboration

The treatment of PDs requires a collaborative effort that includes the patient, the interprofessional team responsible for the patient's care, and the patient's family. The team working with the patient may include a primary medical care provider; a psychiatrist or psychologist; a licensed mental health professional; an advanced practice nurse who specializes in psychiatric mental healthcare; the registered nurse; and other professionals. The registered nurse can fill several important functions, including providing education and follow-up related to the therapeutic regimen, and instilling hope in the patient and family that achieving a more normal level of functioning is possible.

Treating PDs is a considerable challenge and can generate frustration and try the patience of healthcare workers. All those involved, including nurses, must understand that an individual's personality developed over that individual's lifetime, reflecting learned experiences, and is therefore unlikely to change drastically. The aim instead should be realistic, short-term outcomes. Eventually, patients should be encouraged to seek long-term therapy, which is considered the most effective in the treatment of PDs. Long-term therapy demands time, dedication, and buy-in from the

Clinical Manifestations and Therapies
Personality Disorders

ETIOLOGY	CLINICAL MANIFESTATIONS	CLINICAL THERAPIES
Antisocial	▪ Impulsive ▪ Lack of remorse ▪ Failure to empathize ▪ Easily agitated, aggressive, and controlling	▪ Group therapy ▪ Anger management therapy ▪ Psychodynamic therapy ▪ Psychoeducation ▪ Pharmacologic therapy (antidepressants, mood stabilizers, antianxiety medications, antipsychotics)
Avoidant	▪ Extreme discomfort socially ▪ Hypersensitive ▪ Intense anxiety related to social contact ▪ Easily internalizes negative comments by others	▪ Social skills training ▪ Cognitive–behavioral therapy (CBT) ▪ Group therapy ▪ Pharmacologic therapy (antidepressants, antianxiety medications) ▪ Alternative therapy
Borderline	▪ Extreme risk-taking ▪ Impulsive ▪ Self-injury, suicidal ▪ Intense anxiety ▪ Consistently low mood ▪ Unstable relationships due to intense mistrust of others	▪ Schema-focused therapy (SFT) ▪ Dialectical behavior therapy (DBT) ▪ CBT ▪ Pharmacologic therapy (antidepressants, antianxiety medications, antipsychotics, mood stabilizers) ▪ Group therapy (e.g., STEPPS) ▪ Alternative therapy
Dependent	▪ Pervasive need to be under control by a dominant other ▪ Insecure about making decisions ▪ Chronic sense of inadequacy	▪ Psychotherapy ▪ Pharmacologic treatment of symptoms with antidepressants or anxiolytics; caution to monitor for dependence on medications
Histrionic	▪ Flamboyant, highly seductive in behavior and/or appearance ▪ May be sexually manipulative ▪ Demands to be center of attention ▪ Constantly seeks excitement and activity	▪ Psychotherapy may be effective ▪ Group therapy not recommended because of attention-seeking behaviors
Narcissistic	▪ Grandiosity ▪ Rage ▪ Depression, anxiety ▪ Manipulative ▪ Lack of empathy	▪ CBT ▪ Family-focused therapy (FFT) ▪ Pharmacologic therapy (antidepressants, antianxiety medications)
Obsessive-compulsive	▪ Inflexible, controlling ▪ Anxiety ▪ Difficulty with empathy ▪ Perfectionist	▪ CBT ▪ Pharmacologic therapy (SSRIs) ▪ Alternative therapy
Paranoid	▪ Unable to trust others ▪ Rigid, fixed worldview that often is conspiratorial in nature ▪ Believes others' actions are based on ulterior motives	▪ Psychotherapy ▪ If accepted by the patient, pharmacologic therapy may include antidepressants, anxiolytics, and antipsychotic medications
Schizoid	▪ Prefers solitude, uninterested in interpersonal relationships ▪ Generally unable to perceive or express strong emotions	▪ CBT ▪ Group therapy with others who are also learning interpersonal skills ▪ Pharmacologic treatment may include antidepressant and antipsychotic medications
Schizotypal	▪ Odd mannerisms and speech patterns ▪ Cold demeanor, inappropriate responses ▪ Lack of affect ▪ Distorted thoughts ▪ Intense anxiety in social situations ▪ Paranoid fears of persecution	▪ CBT ▪ FFT ▪ Pharmacologic therapy (antidepressants, antianxiety medications, antipsychotics) ▪ Alternative therapy

Focus on Diversity and Culture
Mental Health and Religious Beliefs

When caring for patients with personality disorders, nurses should be aware that some patients may interpret their condition in the context of deeply held religious and spiritual beliefs. More specifically, the symptoms of delusions and hallucinations may be viewed not as mental health issues, but rather as demonic possession or the work of evil spirits (Spector, 2017; Tajima-Pozo et al., 2011).

Complicating the issue is that many religious people from a variety of cultures may believe in otherworldly beings that can cause illness and misfortune. In the Muslim faith, for example, beliefs about jinn are held by some people with and without any signs of mental illness (Guthrie, Abraham, & Nawaz, 2016). Jinn are intelligent spirits of lower rank than the angels, able to appear in human and animal forms and capable of possessing humans, and can influence humans for good or evil.

In both the distant and recent past, the medical community viewed religious and spiritual influences as more likely to be harmful than helpful in patient care. As a consequence, individuals with personality disorders who maintained a strong spiritual or religious practice often chose not to enter the mental health system, either because of shame or fear of how their beliefs would be perceived, or because of their conviction that only religious and spiritual healing could help them (Pargament & Lomax, 2013). Today, the role of religion is viewed much differently. Partly because of a greater awareness of the need for cultural competence in mental healthcare, professional caregivers are more willing to integrate religious and spiritual elements into treatment (Pargament & Lomax, 2013). Many clinicians have realized that for some patients, religion instills hope, purpose, and meaning in their lives and also influences treatment compliance and outcomes (Grover, Davuluri, & Chakrabarti, 2014; Potter & Moller, 2016). Some therapists have begun to incorporate religious contexts and accommodations into CBT and other therapies with good results (Pargament & Lomax, 2013).

patient (Potter & Moller, 2016). Nurses should also be especially cognizant of establishing and maintaining firm, consistent boundaries with patients.

Diagnostic Tests

There is no one test mental health professionals use to diagnose PDs. Instead, PDs are typically diagnosed through an interview with the patient that covers issues such as symptoms, family history, and thoughts of violence, suicide, or self-injury. Although a single interview may be sufficient for an experienced clinician to make a diagnosis, it is more often necessary for the clinician to conduct more than one interview spaced over time to arrive at a definitive diagnosis (APA, 2013). A physical exam and laboratory tests (such as a toxicology screen) also help rule out other factors that could be the cause of abnormal behavior, such as drug and alcohol abuse (NIMH, 2013c; Mayo Clinic, 2013b).

Although mental health professionals refer to the specific diagnostic criteria for each PD found in the most recent version of the DSM, identifying the specific PD that a patient is experiencing can be complicated because of the frequent overlap of symptoms across disorders. The subjectivity of the patient's descriptions and the care provider's interpretation of those descriptions also pose a challenge (Mayo Clinic, 2013a). In this respect, there are a number of psychologic tests that can help mental health professionals arrive at a more definitive diagnosis, including personality inventories in a true/false or yes/no format, such as the Personality Diagnostic Questionnaire commonly used to identify NPD, and open-ended projective tests, such as the Thematic Apperception Test frequently used to identify personality traits (D'Agostino et al., 2012; Hopwood et al., 2012).

If the disorder becomes so pronounced that an individual is unable to provide self-care or is in imminent jeopardy of causing harm to self or others, especially with dangerous self-injurious behaviors or suicidal ideation, then the individual should be hospitalized. Different inpatient options exist, such as day hospitalization or residential treatment (Mayo Clinic, 2013b).

Pharmacologic Therapy

Individuals with PDs often are prescribed medications to control their symptoms. Obsessive-compulsive, aggressive, and self-destructive behaviors may be held in check with the use of SSRIs, such as fluoxetine (Prozac). Symptoms associated with avoidant and borderline disorders may be minimized with antidepressants, just as acute psychosis may be ameliorated with antipsychotic drugs. Medications, however, should be used to complement a comprehensive treatment plan that includes therapy (ideally long-term) that incorporates various approaches (Potter & Moller, 2016).

Psychotherapy

Long-term psychotherapy is the most highly recommended treatment for individuals with PDs. There are various different types of psychotherapy, some more suitable to certain types of PDs than others. Medical professionals usually draw from and combine elements of the different types of psychotherapy to meet a particular patient's needs (NIMH, 2013c). All of the therapies described here are generally available as both outpatient and inpatient services.

Cognitive–Behavioral Therapy

CBT combines cognitive aspects to change thoughts and beliefs with behavioral aspects to alter problematic action patterns. It focuses on skill training and problem solving. Typically, the therapist serves as a guide to assist the patient in recognizing harmful ways of thinking and erroneous beliefs and works with the individual to purge them by analyzing and reinterpreting both past and current experiences, thus helping the patient adopt positive behaviors and interactions with others.

If trauma has occurred, exposure therapy can be used. This is a behavioral therapy in which patients, guided by the therapist, repeatedly approach trauma-related thoughts, feelings, and situations that they have been avoiding because of the distress they cause. Repeated exposure to these thoughts, feelings, and situations helps reduce the power they have to cause distress (U.S. Department of Veterans Affairs, 2015). These therapies aim to reduce symptoms by offering patients the chance to develop concrete coping strategies in conjunction with the therapist. CBT can also help individuals with mood disorders recognize when their mood is about to shift, thus giving them the foresight to apply coping strategies to deal with these changes (APA, 2013; NIMH, 2013c).

Dialectical Behavioral Therapy

A combination of cognitive and behavior therapy, DBT originally was developed to treat individuals with suicidal thoughts. *Dialectical* refers to striking a balance between two extremes; the therapist displays understanding and validates the patient's behaviors and feelings while at the same time imposing limits and making the patient responsible for changing unhealthy patterns. It has proven effective in treating borderline personality disorder, showing lower dropout rates than other therapies and decreasing the frequency of suicide attempts. Through DBT, patients learn to accept things as they are and apply techniques to control strong emotions that might otherwise overwhelm them. Mindfulness is one such technique, where patients learn to become aware of and explore emotions without reacting to them. DBT also teaches patients emotional regulation and distress tolerance. This type of therapy usually relies on individual sessions to teach new skills and strategies, and then group sessions to apply them. Traditional and cognitive approaches are also used in conjunction with DBT to help patients foster better relationships with others (APA, 2013; NIMH, 2013c; Oltmanns & Emery, 2012).

Schema-Focused Therapy

Schema-focused therapy (SFT) combines aspects of CBT with other forms of psychotherapy to change a patient's self-perception. This is often applied to personality disorders, where the individual typically has a poor self-image. SFT aims to help patients view themselves differently so they can create new and more effective ways of interacting with their environment and others (NIMH, 2013c). Research has shown that SFT is an extremely effective treatment option for individuals with BPD, sometimes leading to recovery (Jacob & Arntz, 2013).

Group Therapy

Group therapy is also important to the treatment of certain PDs. For example, it can be helpful in strengthening empathic skills for individuals with ASPD in that it allows for feedback about the perceptions of the other group members (Potter & Moller, 2016). Another example of group therapy is the Systems Training for Emotional Predictability and Problem Solving (STEPPS), consisting of 20 two-hour sessions led by a social worker. According to the NIMH (2013c), the STEPPS program, when combined with other approaches, such as pharmacologic treatments and psychotherapy, has alleviated depression and improved the quality of life of individuals with borderline personality disorder.

Family-Focused Therapy

Family-focused therapy is often useful for the family members of patients with PD to participate in FFT so as to cope with the stress of living with a loved one with a personality disorder and avoid behaviors that might worsen the patient's condition. FFT educates family members about their loved one's disorder, giving them the necessary knowledge to improve interactions and play an active role in supporting the patient. For example, the patient's family can develop a course of action in case warning signs of a relapse appear. In addition, family therapy programs such as Family Connections address the needs and concerns of the patient's family members. DBT family therapy helps family members understand and support relatives with PD by teaching them skills and strategies and having them participate in the patient's treatment sessions (NIMH, 2013c).

Complementary Health Approaches

Although there is not a specific form of integrative therapy that is recommended for patients with PDs, complementary health approaches may provide some relief from certain symptoms, such as anxiety and depression. For instance, yoga, meditation, breathing exercises, and chamomile tea can help individuals with anxiety to relax, while vitamin B_{12} and omega-3 fatty acids can ease depression (National Center for Complementary and Integrative Health, 2016a). Studies indicate that omega-3 fatty acids may also serve to prevent psychosis from fully emerging in young individuals who show signs of developing such a disorder (National Center for Complementary and Integrative Health, 2016b).

Lifespan Considerations

Personality traits are enduring patterns of perceiving, relating to, and thinking about the environment that are exhibited in many social and personal contexts (APA, 2013). The essential diagnostic feature of a personality disorder is the enduring, inflexible pattern of inner experience and behavior and its effects on at least two of the following areas: cognition, affectivity, interpersonal functioning, or impulse control (APA, 2013). Characteristics of personality disorders at different ages during the lifespan are discussed below.

Personality Disorders in Childhood

Many times, traits of a PD that appear in childhood do not persist into adult life. However, a PD may be diagnosed in children or preadolescents in relatively unusual cases where the child's particular maladaptive personality traits appear to be pervasive, persistent, and unlikely to be limited to a specific development stage or another mental disorder (APA, 2013). For a PD to be diagnosed in childhood, the features must have been present for at least 1 year.

The exception is antisocial personality disorder, which cannot be diagnosed in someone under age 18. Often younger patients with similar behaviors are diagnosed with more age-appropriate disruptive, impulse-control, or conduct disorders prior to age 18 (APA, 2013). Research in this area has been focusing on the genetic, cognitive, emotional, biological, environmental, and personality characteristics of callous and unemotional traits displayed early in life by children with conduct disorders (Frick et al., 2014). Research has also been conducted to determine whether borderline personality-related characteristics observed in children are associated with increased risk for the development of borderline personality disorder. The research found that BPD related characteristics measured at age 12 years were highly heritable; were more common in children who had exhibited poor cognitive function, impulsivity, and more behavioral and emotional problems at age 5 years of age; and co-occurred with symptoms of conduct disorder, depression, anxiety, and psychosis (Belsky et al., 2012).

The avoidant behavior characteristics of Cluster C (avoidant and dependent personality disorders) often start in infancy or childhood, with display of shyness, isolation, and fear of strangers and new situations (APA, 2013). Although these behaviors are not uncommon in young children, they do tend to dissipate as most children age.

Personality Disorders in Adolescence and Early Adulthood

The features of a personality disorder become recognizable typically during adolescence or early adulthood. Cluster A disorders, such as paranoid, schizoid, and schizotypal PDs, may present in childhood and adolescence. These individuals will display characteristics such as solitariness, poor peer relationships, social anxiety, underachievement in school, hypersensitivity, peculiar thoughts and language, and idiosyncratic fantasies (APA, 2013).

Individuals diagnosed with Cluster B disorders, such as BPD, often overuse health- and mental-health–related resources. Individuals with BPD frequently display chronically unstable behaviors in early adulthood, with a serious lack of affective and impulse control. Impairment from the disorder and the risk for suicide are highest during the young-adult years (APA, 2013).

Individuals who will be later diagnosed with a Cluster C disorder (avoidant or dependent) will become increasingly shy during adolescence and early adulthood and avoid developing the social relationships characteristic of that developmental age (APA, 2013). However, clinicians caution against diagnosing children with dependent and avoidant disorders when the behaviors may actually be developmentally appropriate.

Personality Disorders in Pregnant Women

Little is known about the relationship of personality disorders and pregnancy. However, there has been some limited research on the relationship between hyperemesis gravidarum (HG), intractable nausea and vomiting during pregnancy, and psychiatric disorders, particularly anxiety and personality disorders. One study discovered that rates of major depression, generalized anxiety disorder, avoidant personality disorder, and obsessive-compulsive personality disorder were significantly higher in women with HG, with the onset of the disorder primarily occurring prior to pregnancy (Uguz et al., 2012).

Personality Disorders in Older Adults

Although by definition personality disorders have an onset no later than early adulthood, individuals with PDs may escape clinical attention until they are middle-aged or in later life. Often, loss of a significant support person or a stabilizing social situation, such as a job, exacerbates display of the disorder, and associated symptoms cause the individual to seek treatment (APA, 2013). A trained clinician should always evaluate personality changes in middle adulthood or later life to assess for medical conditions or previously undiagnosed substance use issues (APA, 2013).

Some types of personality disorders, such as antisocial and borderline PDs, become less evident or remit with age, particularly as an individual enters his or her 40s (APA, 2013). The risk of suicide also gradually wanes with age.

NURSING PROCESS

Just as the care of patients with personality disorders will be specific to each patient and the manifestations of the disorder, certain features of the nursing assessment will vary as well. Nurses working with patients with personality disorders should remember that some of the symptoms (e.g., labile affect and impairments in social skills) make it difficult to develop the nurse–patient relationship, especially when the patient denies the presence of symptoms or problems.

Assessment

Assessment data serves as the basis for application of the nursing process. However, assessment of the patient with a personality disorder may be complicated by a number of factors, including lack of insight or self-awareness; denial of the existence or manifestations of a disorder; inability to trust; and ineffective communication skills.

Within the realm of psychosocial assessment, the primary goals of assessment include identification of behaviors, beliefs, or thought patterns that disrupt the patient's social, professional, and personal life. When the patient lacks insight about the existence or effects of a PD, pertinent information may be gleaned from reports by family members or others who are closely associated with the patient. However, because maintenance of patient confidentiality is essential, the nurse must avoid overstepping the patient's personal and legal boundaries during data collection.

Data collection should include assessing work history; history of behavior problems, including violence directed at self or others; history of suicidal ideation; methods of resolving conflicts; alcohol and drug use; and nature of relationships with family members, coworkers, and friends. The nurse should ask questions that encourage the patient to describe aspects of self:

- When was the last time you were upset? What upset you? How did you handle it?
- How do others describe you?
- How would you describe yourself?
- What do you like about yourself? What would you like to change?
- How do you usually relate to others?

Assess for signs of self-directed violence, such as cutting (see Figure 29–3); assess for evidence of alcohol or drug use.

Diagnosis

Selection of nursing diagnoses depends on patient-specific needs and strengths, as well as on functional capability. For example, high-functioning patients who have insight into the nature and effects of their PD may be well suited for patient teaching, whereas patients who demonstrate significant functional impairment and lack of insight may not benefit from teaching. General examples of nursing diagnoses that may be appropriate for inclusion in the plan of care for the patient with a PD may include the following:

- *Injury, Risk for*
- *Self-Directed Violence, Risk for*
- *Other-Directed Violence, Risk for*
- *Self-Mutilation*
- *Coping, Ineffective*
- *Anxiety*
- *Social Isolation*
- *Social Interaction, Impaired*
- *Role Performance, Ineffective*
- *Disturbed Personal Identity*
- *Interrupted Family Processes.*

(NANDA-I © 2014)

Planning

Patient goals are measurable, patient-specific outcomes that allow for evaluation of the efficacy of nursing interventions. Goals of care should be realistic and tailored to the patient. Examples of patient goals that may be applicable to the nursing plan of care for the patient with a PD include the following:

- The patient will remain free from injury.
- The patient will refrain from violent behaviors.
- The patient will report a reduction in anxiety.
- The patient will verbalize emotions to staff.
- The patient will adhere to established rules and guidelines.
- The patient will actively participate in one-on-one and/or group therapy sessions.

Implementation

As with assessment and planning, implementation of the nursing plan of care will vary based on the manifestations and effects of the patient's PD. In general, nursing interventions for patients diagnosed with a PD will include preventing injury and maintaining physical safety of the patient, as well as protecting the safety of individuals with whom the patient interacts. In addition, promotion of comfort—both physical and psychosocial—is a priority of care. Psychosocial aspects of comfort promotion include building a therapeutic relationship with the patient and effectively managing conflicts. In a respectful, professional manner, the nurse establishes clear boundaries and limits for the patient. For patients who are amenable to socialization, the nurse identifies patient-specific interventions that will afford the patient the opportunity to learn and practice social skills.

Promote Safety

With all patients, priorities of care include injury prevention and safety promotion. For patients with PDs, some of whom are prone to self-destructive and impulsive behavior, the emphasis on injury prevention is heightened. Behavioral contracts that outline prohibited actions and the consequences of

those actions may be used to establish clear guidelines and expectations with regard to any form of behavior, including that related to injuring self or others. Basic precautions for patients in hospital settings include:

- Ensuring that the patient's environment is free from items that may be used to harm self or others
- Providing close supervision and monitoring
- Encouraging patients to seek assistance from members of the healthcare team when they need to process their feelings, including when they perceive that their stress levels are rising
- Encouraging patients to participate actively in therapy and groups.

In the community setting, clinicians also need to monitor patients for safety. Some considerations include the following points on medication safety and self-monitoring of mood and environment.

- Provide medication teaching regarding dosage and intervals, anticipated side effects, potential adverse reactions, and when to contact the healthcare provider for follow-up care.
- With adolescents and young adult patients, make sure that the patient and the family or support persons know that SSRIs carry an FDA black box warning regarding increased suicidality for that age group and are aware of the warning signs of increased suicidal ideation.
- Ensure that patients who engage in nonsuicidal self-injury (NSSI) know to contact their healthcare providers if they experience an increase in the occurrence or severity of these behaviors.
- Make sure that patients live in a safe environment where they will not be exposed to violence or financially or emotionally exploited. Patients who receive disability payments for their mental health disorders are often isolated and can be preyed on by coercive family or individuals in the community.

Promote the Therapeutic Relationship

The ineffective social skills and impaired perceptions that often accompany PDs can create unique challenges in the establishment of a therapeutic nurse–patient relationship. Moreover, for patients who struggle with trust issues, unplanned admission to a hospital or treatment center can exacerbate their anxiety and sense of mistrust. Consistency with patient care—including demonstration of respect for the patient at all times—is one of the first steps to building trust.

- Avoid stigmatizing the patient because of his illness. Individuals with PDs have a neurobiological imbalance in the brain, not a defective personality. Also, consider that many patients also have medical conditions and have experienced stress, trauma, severe childhood abuse, prolonged substance abuse, and exposure to toxins, and have genetically inherited traits.
- Balance flexibility with firmness. Patients may be unwilling to accept responsibility and unable to remember agreements, and they may be untrustworthy, difficult to understand, inconsistent with discipline, poor at keeping

appointments, and unpredictable emotionally. However, missed appointments, lying, and dangerous behaviors cannot be accepted. Precise oral and written communication is the best way to avoid misunderstandings.

- Focus on the strengths of the individual and his family system. Clinicians will have more success and reduce stress and stigmatization if they match interventions with patient strengths.

Establish Boundaries

Boundaries are limits that define what is acceptable to an individual in every facet of life, including the physical, mental, emotional, sexual, relational, spiritual, and professional realms. A breach of boundaries occurs when those limitations are ignored or exceeded. In many ways, definition of boundaries occurs during childhood, beginning in infancy, through experiencing interactions with others.

In the context of the nurse–patient relationship, establishing and maintaining healthy boundaries establishes a sense of safety and predictability for the patient. As the result of past experiences, including a history of abuse and a sense of shame that may accompany the stigmatization often associated with mental illness, the patient with a PD may have unhealthy, unclear, or nonexistent boundaries. The nurse can help the patient to understand and set healthy boundaries through interventions such as teaching, as well as through role playing with the patient. In helping the patient establish healthy boundaries, the nurse can use role play to simulate situations in which the patient is faced with potential boundary violations, assess the patient's coping skills, and teach the patient about healthy responses to attempted boundary violation (Potter & Moller, 2016).

Regardless of the patient's behaviors, the nurse is responsible for maintaining healthy professional boundaries. Provision 2 of the American Nurses Association's (ANA) Code of Ethics (2015) requires the nurse to establish and maintain boundaries, and to effectively set limits with patients. Establishing professional boundaries includes choosing which of the nurse's personal information is appropriate for sharing with the patient. Especially because of the intimate nature of the nurse–patient relationship, the patient also may ask personal questions—for example, whether or not the nurse is married or has children. Sharing some degree of background information in an appropriate, professional manner can strengthen the nurse–patient relationship; however, the oversharing of personal information is detrimental and nontherapeutic. Through sharing details of personal problems and struggles with the patient, the nurse can create an unnecessary—and unethical—burden for the patient, who is the one seeking care. Boundary violations occur when meeting the nurse's needs takes precedence over meeting the patient's needs. For further illustration of maintaining professional boundaries in nursing, see **Table 29–5 》》**.

》》 Stay Current: The National Council of State Boards of Nursing offers additional guidance and strategies regarding professional boundaries at https://www.ncsbn.org/professionalboundaries.htm

Evaluation

Evaluation is a dynamic, ongoing feature of the nursing process that includes identifying the degree to which patients have achieved the goals and outcomes established in relationship to each nursing diagnosis. While goals and outcomes for the patient with a PD will vary based on

TABLE 29–5 Maintaining Professional Boundaries in Nursing

Boundaries Maintained	Boundaries Breached
Keeping one's personal life private and focusing on the patient's needs	Sharing details of personal life, issues, and/or problems with a patient
Sharing limited details about basic background information when asked, such as marital status, number of children, educational background, and professional nursing background	Discussing the state of one's marriage (e.g., marital separation or currently in the process of divorce); sharing about one's children's behavioral problems or medical challenges; discussing personal, emotional, or legal problems or setbacks
Maintaining all patient-related information as confidential, and discussing only relevant aspects of the patient's condition and care with the necessary healthcare team members in the workplace	Revealing patient-related information to anyone who is not involved in planning or administering care to the patient
Limiting discussion of patients and their care to within the clinical setting	Discussing patients and their care in the hospital cafeteria, hallways, or other nonclinical areas; sharing any patient-related information through any format, including via social media
Interacting with the patient only during scheduled duty hours for professional intents and purposes	Visiting the patient during off-duty hours, in or away from the clinical setting; communicating with the patient by any means for purposes other than those directly related to the patient's plan of healthcare
Demonstrating respect for one's institution or organization, work policies, and other members of the healthcare team, and declining to discuss workplace-related conflicts or criticisms	Venting to the patient about issues or concerns regarding one's employer, work policies, or other members of the healthcare team
Facilitating referrals for patients with financial needs to appropriate organizations or assisting the patient in connecting with official agencies who can provide assistance	Giving patients personal items or financial assistance
Identification and referral to appropriate healthcare team members for resolution of the patient's personal conflicts	Choosing to side with a patient during conflict between patients and their spouses, family members, or significant others

Sources: Based on Potter, M. L. & Moller, M. D. (Eds.). (2016). *Psychiatric–mental health nursing: From suffering to hope.* Upper Saddle River, NJ; Remshardt, M. A. (2012). Do you know your professional boundaries? *Nursing Made Incredibly Easy, 10*(1), 5–6.

patient individuality and the nursing diagnoses included in the nursing plan of care, examples of achieved outcomes relevant to the evaluation of patient care may include the following:

- The patient remains free from injury.
- The patient does not demonstrate violent behaviors toward self or others.
- The patient verbalizes understanding of the concept of boundaries.
- The patient verbalizes understanding of the principles of respecting boundaries related to self and others.
- The patient actively participates in individual and/or group therapy.

Given that many of the personality disorders discussed in this section are resistive to treatment and the therapies are challenging and lengthy even for motivated patients, treatment failures do occur. In these cases, the clinician should reevaluate the plan of care. This includes conducting a strengths-based assessment of the patient and his or her supports: Has the patient's financial situation changed, necessitating more community services? Has a lifelong support died or disappeared from a patient's life, affecting his or her ability to cope? Are additional community services available that were not in place when the patient's last plan of care was constructed? Is the patient enthusiastic about the new plan of care, and is he or she capable of participating in the interventions proposed?

Nursing Care Plan
A Patient with Borderline Personality Disorder

Kathryn Harrison is a 20-year-old female patient transported to the emergency department (ED) by law enforcement. Officer Rick Natami, the attending police officer, reported that Ms. Harrison broke a window with her fist while arguing with her boyfriend. Subsequently, Ms. Harrison told her boyfriend she was going to kill herself. At that point, Ms. Harrison's boyfriend called 911. In addition to law enforcement, emergency medical personnel also responded to the call. Officer Natami reported that Ms. Harrison was combative at the scene and would not allow the paramedics to assess her injuries, nor would she permit them to transport her to the ED by ambulance. Her boyfriend had handed her a dish towel to wrap her hand, and while there is blood visible on the towel, the bleeding does not appear to be copious. As a result, because of her injuries and her threat to commit suicide, Officer Natami handcuffed and transported Ms. Harrison in his squad car for physical and psychiatric evaluation.

Upon arrival to the ED, Ms. Harrison is cursing at Officer Natami, as well as anyone with whom she makes eye contact, including her attending nurse. When the ED physician asks if he can assess Ms. Harrison's injuries, she replies, "Yeah, if you tell the cop to take these handcuffs off me and make him leave! You're cool, but he's a total jerk!" The ED physician tells Ms. Harrison he will ask the police officer to remove the handcuffs and stand outside the examination room, but only if she agrees to remain calm and noncombative. Ms. Harrison agrees, and the officer removes her handcuffs and steps outside the room. Because Ms. Harrison has previously been treated at the facility, her electronic medical record (EMR) is accessible. Based on her EMR, her past medical history includes borderline personality disorder and previous treatment for self-inflicted superficial leg lacerations. Before the ED physician evaluates Ms. Harrison's lacerations, he quietly asks the nurse to order a psychiatric consultation for the patient.

ASSESSMENT	DIAGNOSES	PLANNING
Following closure of her lacerations, Ms. Harrison agrees to allow the nurse to assess her vital signs and auscultate her heart and lungs. Vital signs include temperature 97.3°F oral, pulse 90 bpm, respirations 20/min, and BP 133/71 mmHg. Ms. Harrison's heart tones are normal; however, the nurse hears faint, bibasilar wheezes in her lungs. When the nurse asks if Ms. Harrison has had any recent respiratory problems, she replies, "I have no idea. I don't have health insurance and nobody cares anyway. I'm just a piece of garbage." Ms. Harrison begins to cry and states, "I don't know why I get so mad. I'm such an idiot! My boyfriend should dump me, just like everybody else does." The nurse verbally reassures Ms. Harrison that she is safe and will receive the best possible care. Ms. Harrison replies, "I'm sorry I called you names earlier—you're the nicest nurse I've ever met. The nurses on the psych floor are mean. They're only going to make me take a bunch of pills. I wish I could stay here, with you."	- *Injury, Risk for* - *Self-Directed Violence, Risk for* - *Other-Directed Violence, Risk for* - *Skin Integrity, Impaired* - *Self-Mutilation, Risk for* - *Coping, Ineffective* - *Suicide, Risk for* (NANDA-I © 2014)	- The patient will sustain no further physical injury. - The patient will not injure others. - The patient's wound will be closed and protected from further injury or contamination. - The patient will express her emotions to members of the healthcare team in a nondestructive manner. - The patient contracts for safety by agreeing to notify staff if she experiences any thoughts of nonsuicidal self-injury (NSSI) or suicide.

(continued on next page)

Nursing Care Plan (continued)

IMPLEMENTATION

- Maintain or delegate a team member to maintain constant observation of the patient to assess for and prevent injurious behavior.

- Outline behavioral guidelines for the patient, including the requirement that she cannot injure herself or attempt to injure others.

- Follow institutional guidelines for the application of physical restraints as needed.

- Seek to establish rapport with the patient through demonstrating respect and establishing therapeutic communication patterns.

- Enforce firm boundaries with the patient to prevent staff splitting.

- Encourage the patient to verbalize her emotions and use active listening techniques.

- Educate the patient about dressing changes and basic principles of wound care.

EVALUATION

Following evaluation by the on-call psychiatrist, Ms. Harrison was admitted to the psychiatric unit and hospitalized for 3 days. During her stay, she was argumentative with several of the staff nurses and patient care technicians, but she appeared to favor one of the nurses, Jim. When Jim was on duty, she first insisted that he be assigned to care for her but later refused to allow him to be her nurse, stating, "He's a jerk, just like my boyfriend." In meetings with the clinical psychologist, Ms. Harrison reported a history of physical abuse during childhood, including sexual abuse by an uncle, as well as several physically abusive dating relationships. When asked about abuse in her current relationship, Ms. Harrison denied any abuse and reported that her boyfriend was "the only person who ever cared" about her. The psychologist referred Ms. Harrison to a counselor who specialized in dialectical behavior therapy (DBT), but Ms. Harrison declined and stated, "I don't want to keep talking about stuff that happened when I was a kid. I just need to stop getting so mad at my boyfriend." She sustained no further injury during her hospitalization and was not physically abusive toward staff. Upon discharge, Ms. Harrison agreed to return to the ED in 7 days for suture removal.

CRITICAL THINKING

1. What other nursing interventions might be appropriate for inclusion in the plan of care for Ms. Harrison?

2. Describe two instances in which Ms. Harrison demonstrated splitting. How should the nurse address patients who demonstrate splitting behaviors?

3. Why did the psychologist recommend dialectical behavior therapy (DBT) for Ms. Harrison? How is DBT believed to be beneficial to patients diagnosed with BPD?

REVIEW Personality Disorders

RELATE Link the Concepts and Exemplars

Linking the exemplar on personality disorders with the concept of stress and coping:

1. In relationship to personality disorders (PDs), describe three behaviors that reflect impaired coping.

2. How does manipulation, which is a behavior associated with several PDs, affect the nurse's morale and stress level? Explain how the nurse can effectively cope with manipulation in the course of a therapeutic relationship.

Linking the exemplar on personality disorders with the concept of safety:

3. Which PDs are associated with a high risk for injury? How does impulsiveness increase the risk for injury?

4. A patient who is diagnosed with schizotypal personality disorder tells her nurse she hears voices that are ordering her to cut her wrists. How should the nurse respond? To protect the patient from injury, what actions should the nurse take?

READY Go to Volume 3: Clinical Nursing Skills

REFER Go to Pearson MyLab Nursing and eText

- Additional review materials

REFLECT Apply Your Knowledge

Steffan Richter, a 32-year-old man, recently was diagnosed with avoidant personality disorder. The psychiatrist who made the diagnosis recommended that Mr. Richter begin psychotherapy, but Mr. Richter declined after learning that group therapy may be indicated at some point during treatment. To Mr. Richter, psychotherapy would be almost unbearable, but talking about his issues in a group setting would be impossible.

Since graduating from college 10 years ago, Mr. Richter has worked as a mailroom clerk. Having earned a bachelor's degree in accounting, Mr. Richter is qualified to apply for other, higher-paying positions within the company. However, he chooses to maintain his current position, as his present job responsibilities greatly limit his need to interact with other individuals. Several years earlier, he was offered a supervisory position; however, he declined the offer. The promotion would have increased his salary significantly, but the job responsibilities included a great deal of interaction with the mailroom team and administrators.

During lunchtime, the mailroom shuts down operations so all employees can eat their meals together in the staff lounge. Because he finds the lunchtime social interaction in the staff lounge to be forced, unpleasant, and overwhelming, Mr. Richter remains in the quiet mailroom and reads a book during his break. Company policy restricts employees from eating in any areas other than the staff lounge, and employees are forbidden to leave the building during their work shift. Therefore, Mr. Richter never eats lunch during the week.

Because Mr. Richter is extremely shy and quiet, several of his coworkers refer to him as "the invisible man." He is also very underweight, and some of his coworkers tease him about his size. Although he finds his nickname and the teasing to be cruel and humiliating, Mr. Richter does not share his feelings; instead, he resolves to stay as far away as possible from the group. Several of his coworkers have invited him to join the group for social activities outside of work; however, he declines their invitations, as he knows his coworkers will only further demean and embarrass him. To avoid being humiliated or rejected, Mr. Richter does not build friendships at or away from his workplace.

1. How are the effects of avoidant personality disorder impacting Mr. Richter's occupational and professional advancement?

2. In what ways does avoidant personality disorder impact Mr. Richter socially, both in and out of his workplace?

3. How does avoidant personality disorder affect Mr. Richter's nutritional habits?

References

Academy for Eating Disorders. (2013). *Treatment.* Retrieved from http://www.aedweb.org/Treatment/1533.htm

Ainsworth, M. D. S. (1973). The development of infant-mother attachment. In B. Cardwell & H. Ricciuti (Eds.), *Review of child development research* (Vol. 3, pp. 1–94). Chicago, IL: University of Chicago Press.

Alberts, H. J. E. M., Thewissen, R., & Raes, L. (2012). Dealing with problematic eating behaviour: The effects of a mindfulness-based intervention on eating behaviour, food cravings, dichotomous thinking and body image concern. *Appetite, 58*(3), 847–851. doi:http://dx.doi.org/10.1016/j.appet.2012.01.009

Amad, A., Ramoz, N., Thomas, P., Jardri, R., & Gorwood, P. (2014). Genetics of borderline personality disorder: Systematic review and proposal of an integrative model. *Neuroscience & Biobehavioral Reviews, 40*, 6–19. doi:http://dx.doi.org/10.1016/j.neubiorev.2014.01.003

American Nurses Association. (2015). *Code of ethics for nurses with interpretive statements.* Silver Spring, MD: American Nurses Association.

American Psychiatric Association. (2013). *Diagnostic and statistical manual of mental disorders* (5th ed.). Arlington, VA: Author.

American Psychological Association. (2013). *Psychology topics: Personality.* Retrieved from http://www.apa.org/topics/personality/index.aspx

Amstadter, A. B., Aggen, S. H., Knudsen, G. P., Reichborn-Kjennerud, T., & Kendler, K. S. (2012). Potentially traumatic event exposure, posttraumatic stress disorder, and Axis I and II comorbidity in a population-based study of Norwegian young adults. *Social Psychiatry and Psychiatric Epidemiology, 48*(2), 215–223. doi:10.1007/s00127-012-0537-2

Austin, S. B., Nelson, L. A., Birkett, M. A., Calzo, J. P., & Everett, B. (2012). Eating disorder symptoms and obesity at the intersections of gender, ethnicity, and sexual orientation in US high school students. *American Journal of Public Health, 103*(2), e16–e22. doi:10.2105/ajph.2012.301150

Belsky, D. W., Caspi, A., Arseneault, L., Bleidorn, W., Fonagy, P., Goodman, M., & Moffitt, T. E. (2012). Etiological features of borderline personality related characteristics in a birth cohort of 12-year-old children. *Development and Psychopathology, 24*(01), 251–265. doi:doi:10.1017/S0954579411000812

Berk, L. E. (2013). *Exploring lifespan development* (3rd ed.). Boston, MA: Pearson.

Berman, A., Snyder, S. J., & Frandsen, G. (2016). Pain management. In *Kozier and Erb's fundamentals of nursing: Concepts, process, and practice* (10th ed.). Hoboken, NJ: Pearson Education.

Blascovich, J., & Tomaka, J. (1991). Measures of self-esteem. In J. P. Robinson, P. R. Shaver, & L. S.

Wrightsman (Eds.), *Measures of personality and social psychological attitudes* (Vol. 1, pp. 115–160). New York, NY: Academic Press.

Blum, C. A. (2014). Practicing self-care for nurses: A nursing program initiative. *OJIN: The Online Journal of Issues in Nursing, 19*(3). Retrieved from http://www.nursingworld.org/MainMenu Categories/ANAMarketplace/ANAPeriodicals/OJIN/TableofContents/Vol-19-2014/No3-Sept-2014/Practicing-Self-Care-for-Nurses.html

Bohus, M., Dyer, A. S., Priebe, K., Krüger, A., Kleindienst, N., Schmahl, C., & Steil, R. (2013). Dialectical Behaviour Therapy for post-traumatic stress disorder after childhood sexual abuse in patients with and without borderline personality disorder: A randomized controlled trial. *Psychotherapy and Psychosomatics, 82*(4), 221–233.

Bowlby, J. (1969). *Attachment and loss* (Vol. 1: Attachment). New York, NY: Basic Books.

Brown, J. D. (2014). Self-esteem and self-evaluation: Feeling is believing. In J. Suls (Ed.), *Psychological perspectives on the self: The self in social perspective* (Vol. 4, pp. 27–58). New York, NY: Psychology Press.

Butcher, J. N., Mineka, S., & Hooley, J. M. (2013). *Abnormal psychology* (15th ed.). Upper Saddle River, NJ: Pearson.

Campbell, K., & Peebles, R. (2014). Eating disorders in children and adolescents: State of the art review. *Pediatrics, 134*(3), 582–592. doi:10.1542/peds.2014-0194

Carr, C. P., Martins, C. M. S., Stingel, A. M., Lemgruber, V. B., & Juruena, M. F. (2013). The role of early life stress in adult psychiatric disorders: A systematic review according to childhood trauma subtypes. *Journal of Nervous and Mental Disease, 201*(12), 1007–1020. doi:10.1097/nmd.0000000000000049

Center on Media and Human Development (CMHD). (2015). *Teens turn to Internet to cope with health challenges.* Retrieved from http://www.northwestern.edu/newscenter/stories/2015/06/teens-turn-to-internet-to-cope-with-health-challenges.html

Ciccarelli, S. K., & White, J. N. (2013). *Psychology: An exploration* (3rd ed., Chap. 13). Upper Saddle River, NJ: Pearson.

Coolen, P. R. (2012). *Cultural relevance in end of life care.* Retrieved from http://ethnomed.org/clinical/end-of-life/cultural-relevance-in-end-of-life-care

D'Agostino, A., Manni, R., Limosani, I., Terzaghi, M., Cavallotti, S., & Scarone, S. (2012). Challenging the myth of REM sleep behavior disorder: No evidence of heightened aggressiveness in dreams. *Sleep Medicine, 13*(6), 714–719.

DeHart, T., Pelham, B. W., & Tennen, H. (2006). What lies beneath: Parenting style and implicit self-esteem. *Journal of Experimental Social Psychology, 42*(1), 1–17.

Demetriou, A., & Kazi, S. (2013). *Unity and modularity in the mind and self: Studies on the relationships between self-awareness, personality, and intellectual development from childhood to adolescence.* London, England: Routledge.

Eckroth-Bucher, M. (2010). Self-awareness: A review and analysis of a basic nursing concept. *Advances in Nursing Science, 33*(4), 297–309.

Erikson, E. (1950). *Childhood and society.* New York, NY: Norton.

Erikson, E. (1963). *Youth: Change and challenge.* New York, NY: Basic Books.

Erol, R. Y., & Orth, U. (2011). Self-esteem development from age 14 to 30 years: A longitudinal study. *Journal of Personality and Social Psychology, 101*(3), 607–619.

Espie, J., & Eisler, I. (2015). Focus on anorexia nervosa: Modern psychological treatment and guidelines for the adolescent patient. *Adolescent Health, Medicine and Therapeutics, 6*, 9–16. doi:10.2147/ahmt.s70300

Evans, M. E. (2012). Barriers and facilitators to implementation of the Institute of Medicine recommendations on preventing mental, emotional, and behavioral disorders among young people. *Journal of Child and Adolescent Psychiatric Nursing, 25*(2), 60–65. doi:10.1111/j.1744-6171.2012.00323.x

Fairweather-Schmidt, A. K., & Wade, T. D. (2015). Changes in genetic and environmental influences on disordered eating between early and late adolescence: A longitudinal twin study. *Psychological Medicine, 45*(15), 3249–3258. doi:http://dx.doi.org/10.1017/S0033291715001257

Fawcett, E. J., Fawcett, J. M., & Mazmanian, D. (2016). A meta-analysis of the worldwide prevalence of pica during pregnancy and the postpartum period. *International Journal of Gynecology and Obstetrics, 133*(3), 277–283. doi:10.1016/j.ijgo.2015.10.012

Fonville, L., Giampietro, V., Williams, S. C. R., Simmons, A., & Tchanturia, K. (2014). Alterations in brain structure in adults with anorexia nervosa and the impact of illness duration. *Psychological Medicine, 44*(9), 1965–1975. doi:http://dx.doi.org/10.1017/S0033291713002389

Fox, J. R. E., & Goss, K. (2012). *Eating and its disorders.* Sussex, England: Wiley.

Friborg, O., Martinussen, M., Kaiser, S., Øvergård, K. T., & Rosenvinge, J. H. (2013). Comorbidity of personality disorders in anxiety disorders: A meta-analysis of 30 years of research. *Journal of Affective Disorders, 145*(2), 143–155. doi:http://dx.doi.org/10.1016/j.jad.2012.07.004

Frick, P. J., Ray, J. V., Thornton, L. C., & Kahn, R. E. (2014). Can callous-unemotional traits enhance the understanding, diagnosis, and treatment of serious conduct problems in children and adolescents? A comprehensive review. *Psychological*

Bulletin, 140(1), 1–57. doi:http://psycnet.apa.org/doi/10.1037/a0033076

Gagne, D. A., Von Holle, A., Brownley, K. A., Runfola, C. D., Hofmeier, S., Branch, K. E., & Bulik, C. M. (2012). Eating disorder symptoms and weight and shape concerns in a large Web-based convenience sample of women ages 50 and above: Results of the gender and body image (GABI) study. International Journal of Eating Disorders, 45, 832–844.

Gentile, B., Grabe, S., Dolan-Pascoe, B., Twenge, J. M., Wells, B. E., & Maitino, A. (2009). Gender differences in domain-specific self-esteem: A meta-analysis. Review of General Psychology, 13(1), 34–45.

Ginis, K. A. M., Bassett-Gunter, R. L., & Conlin, C. (2012). Body image and exercise. In E. O. Acevedo (Ed.), The Oxford handbook of exercise psychology (pp. 55–75). New York, NY: Oxford University Press.

Godsey, J. (2013). The role of mindfulness based interventions in the treatment of obesity and eating disorders: An integrative review. Complementary Therapies in Medicine, 21(4), 430–439. doi:http://dx.doi.org/10.1016/j.ctim.2013.06.003

Grover, S., Davuluri, T., & Chakrabarti, S. (2014). Religion, spirituality, and schizophrenia: A review. Indian Journal of Psychological Medicine, 36(2), 119–124. doi:10.4103/0253-7176.130962

Gurven, M., von Rueden, C., & Massenkoff, M. (2013). How universal is the Big Five? Testing the five-factor model of personality variation among forager–farmers in the Bolivian Amazon. Journal of Personality and Social Psychology, 104(2), 354–370.

Guthrie, E., Abraham, S., & Nawaz, S. (2016). Process of determining the value of belief of jinn possession and whether or not they are a result of mental illness. BMJ Case Reports. Retrieved from https://www.ncbi.nlm.nih.gov/pubmed/26838303

Halford, J. C. G., & Harrold, J. A. (2012). Satiety-enhancing products for appetite control: Science and regulation of functional foods for weight management. Proceedings of the Nutrition Society, 71(2), 350–362. doi:http://dx.doi.org/10.1017/S0029665112000134

Halmi, K. A. (2013). Perplexities of treatment resistance in eating disorders. BMC Psychiatry, 13, 292. doi:10.1186/1471-244X-13-292

Hannon-Engel, S. L., Filin, E. E., & Wolfe, B. E. (2012). Role of altered CCK response in bulimia nervosa and following remission. Physiology & Behavior, 122, 56–61. doi:10.1016/j.physbeh.2013.08.014

Harrington, B. C., Jimerson, M., Haxton, C., & Jimerson, D. C. (2015). Initial evaluation, diagnosis, and treatment of anorexia nervosa and bulimia nervosa. American Family Physician, 91(1), 46–52.

Hengartner, M. P., Ajdacic-Gross, V., Rodgers, S., Müller, M., & Rössler, W. (2013). Childhood adversity in association with personality disorder dimensions: New findings in an old debate. European Psychiatry, 28(8), 476–482. doi:10.1016/j.eurpsy.2013.04.004

Herdman, T. H. & Kamitsuru, S. (Eds). Nursing Diagnoses—Definitions and Classification 2015–2017. Copyright © 2014, 1994–2014 NANDA International. Used by arrangement with John Wiley & Sons, Inc. Companion website: www.wiley.com/go/nursingdiagnoses.

Herpertz-Dahlman, B., von Elburg, A., Castro-Fornieles, J., & Schmidt., U. (2015). ESCAP Expert Paper: New developments in the diagnosis and treatment of adolescent anorexia nervosa—a European perspective. European Child & Adolescent Psychiatry, 24, 1153.

Holtmann, J., Herbort, M. C., Wüstenberg, T., Soch, J., Richter, S., Walter, H., . . . Schott, B. H. (2013). Trait

anxiety modulates fronto-limbic processing of emotional interference in borderline personality disorder. Frontiers in Human Neuroscience, 7(54). doi:10.3389

Hopwood, C. J., Donnellan, M. B., Ackerman, R. A., Thomas, K. M., Morey, L. C., & Skodol, A. E. (2012). The validity of the Personality Diagnostic Questionnaire–4 Narcissistic Personality Disorder Scale for assessing pathological grandiosity. Journal of Personality Assessment. doi:10.1080/00223891.2012.732637

International OCD Foundation. (2012). Obsessive-compulsive personality disorder (OCPD). Retrieved from http://www.ocfoundation.org/materials.aspx

Jacob, G. A., & Arntz, A. (2013). Schema therapy for personality disorders—A review. International Journal of Cognitive Therapy, 6(2), 171–185. doi:10.1521/ijct.2013.6.2.171

Johnson, J. G., Cohen, P., Smailes, E. M., Skodol, A. E., Brown, J., & Oldham, J. M. (2001). Childhood verbal abuse and risk for personality disorders during adolescence and early adulthood. Comprehensive Psychiatry, 42(1), 16–23.

Kashdan, T. B., DeWall, C. N., Masten, C. L., Pond, R. S., Powell, C., Combs, D., & Farmer, A. S. (2014). Who is most vulnerable to social rejection? The toxic combination of low self-esteem and lack of negative emotion differentiation on neural responses to rejection. PLoS One, 9(3), e90651. doi:10.1371/journal.pone.0090651

Katterman, S. N., Kleinman, B. M., Hood, M. M., Nackers, L. M., & Corsica, J. A. (2014). Mindfulness meditation as an intervention for binge eating, emotional eating, and weight loss: A systematic review. Eating Behaviors, 15(2), 197–204. doi:http://dx.doi.org/10.1016/j.eatbeh.2014.01.005

Kaye, W. H., Bailer, U. F., & Klabunde, M. (2014). Is anorexia nervosa an eating disorder? How neurobiology can help us understand the puzzling eating symptoms of anorexia nervosa. Retrieved from http://eatingdisorders.ucsd.edu/research/biocorrelates/PDFs/Kaye2010NeurobiologyofAN.pdf

Kendler, K. S., Aggen, S. H., & Patrick, C. J. (2012). A multivariate twin study of the DSM-IV criteria for antisocial personality disorder. Biological Psychiatry, 71(3), 247–253.

KidsHealth. (2016). Compulsive exercise. Retrieved from http://kidshealth.org/en/parents/compulsive-exercise.html#

Kling, R. (2014). Borderline personality disorder, language, and stigma. Ethical Human Psychology and Psychiatry, 16(2), 114–119. doi:10.1891/1559-4343.16.2.114

Klump, K. L., Culbert, K. M., Slane, J. D., Burt, S. A., Sisk, C. L., & Nigg, J. T. (2012). The effects of puberty on genetic risk for disordered eating: Evidence for a sex difference. Psychological Medicine, 42(3), 627–637. doi:10.1017/S0033291711001541

Kneisl, C. R., & Trigoboff, E. (2013). Contemporary psychiatric–mental health nursing (3rd ed.). Upper Saddle River, NJ: Pearson Education.

Knoph, C., Von Holle, A., Zerwas, S., Torgersen, L., Tambs, K., Stoltenberg, C., & Reichborn-Kjenne-rud, T. (2013). Course and predictors of maternal eating disorders in the postpartum period. International Journal of Eating Disorders, 46(4), 355–368. doi:10.1002/eat.22088

Kostro, K., Lerman, J. B., & Attia, E. (2014). The current status of suicide and self-injury in eating disorders: A narrative review. Journal of Eating Disorders, 2(1), 1–9. doi:10.1186/s40337-014-0019-x

Leary, M. (2006). Motivational and emotional aspects of the self. Annual Review of Psychology, 58, 317–344.

Liebman, R. E., & Burnette, M. (2013). It's not you, it's me: An examination of clinician- and patient-level influences on countertransference toward border-line personality disorder. American Journal of Orthopsychiatry, 83(1), 115–125. doi:10.1111.

Mayo Clinic. (2012). Binge eating disorder: Tests and diagnosis. Retrieved from http://www.mayoclinic.com/health/binge-eating-disorder/DS00608/DSECTION=tests-and-diagnosis

Mayo Clinic. (2013a). Personality disorders: Risk factors. Retrieved from http://www.mayoclinic.com/health/personality-disorders/DS00562/DSECTION=risk-factors

Mayo Clinic. (2013b). Self injury/cutting: Symptoms. Retrieved from http://www.mayoclinic.com/health/self-injury/DS00775/DSECTION=symptoms

Mayo Clinic. (2014a). Sleep-related eating disorder. Retrieved from http://www.mayoclinic.org/diseases-conditions/sleep-related-eating-disorder/basics/definition/con-20037290

Mayo Clinic. (2014b). Prader-Willi syndrome. Retrieved from http://www.mayoclinic.org/diseases-conditions/prader-willi-syndrome/basics/definition/con-20028982

Mayo Clinic. (2014c). Prader-Willi syndrome: Treatments and drugs. Retrieved from http://www.mayoclinic.org/diseases-conditions/prader-willi-syndrome/basics/treatment/con-20028982

Mayo Clinic. (2016). Eating disorders: Treatment. Retrieved from http://www.mayoclinic.org/diseases-conditions/eating-disorders/diagnosis-treatment/treatment/txc-20182967

McGrath, B., & Dowling, M. (2012). Exploring registered psychiatric nurses' responses towards service users with a diagnosis of borderline personality disorder. Nursing Research and Practice, 2012. Retrieved from http://www.hindawi.com/journals/nrp/2012/601918

McLeod, S. (2013). Erik Erikson. Retrieved from http://www.simplypsychology.org/Erik-Erikson.html

Melin, A., Torstveit, M. K., Burke, L. M., Marks, S., & Sundgot, J. (2014). Disordered eating and eating disorders in aquatic sports. International Journal of Sport Nutrition & Exercise Metabolism, 24, 250–259. doi:http://hdl.handle.net/11250/282104

Mental Health America (MHA). (2015). Healthy mental and emotional development. Retrieved from http://www.mentalhealthamerica.net/healthy-mental-and-emotional-development

Mesa, R. A. (2016). Is constantly craving and chewing ice a sign of anemia? Retrieved from http://www.mayo-clinic.org/diseases-conditions/iron-deficiency-anemia/expert-answers/chewing-ice/faq-20057982

Mitchell, J. E., King, W. C., Courcoulas, A., Dakin, G., Elder, K., Engel, S., & Wolfe, B. (2015). Eating behavior and eating disorders in adults before bariatric surgery. International Journal of Eating Disorders, 48(2), 215–222. doi:10.1002/eat.22275

Mitchell, K. S., Mazzeo, S. E., Schlesinger, M. R., Brewerton, T. D., & Smith, B. N. (2012). Comorbidity of partial and subthreshold PTSD among men and women with eating disorders in the National Comorbidity Survey—Replication study. International Journal of Eating Disorders, 45(3), 307–315. doi:10.1002/eat.20965

Monteleone, P., & Maj, M. (2013). Dysfunctions of leptin, ghrelin, BDNF and endocannabinoids in eating disorders: Beyond the homeostatic control of food intake. Psychoneuroendocrinology, 38(3), 312–330.

Morgan, J. F., Reid, F., & Lacey, J. H. (1999). The SCOFF questionnaire: Assessment of a new screening tool for eating disorders. BMJ, 319, 1467–1468.

National Alliance on Mental Illness. (2013a). Anorexia nervosa. Retrieved from http://www.nami.org/Template.cfm?Section=By_Illness&template=/

ContentManagement/ContentDisplay. cfm&ContentID=7409

National Alliance on Mental Illness. (2013b). *Bulimia nervosa*. Retrieved from http://www.nami.org/Content/ContentGroups/Helpline1/Bulimia.htm

National Alliance on Mental Illness. (2013c). *Binge eating disorder*. Retrieved from http://www.nami.org/Content/ContentGroups/Helpline1/Binge_Eating_Disorder.htm

National Alliance on Mental Illness. (2017). *Borderline personality disorder*. Retrieved from https://www.nami.org/Learn-More/Mental-Health-Conditions/Borderline-Personality-Disorder/Support

National Association of Men with Eating Disorders. (2016). *Anabolic steroid use among males with eating disorders*. Retrieved from http://namedinc.org/?page_id=36.

National Center for Complementary and Integrative Health. (2016a). *Stress and relaxation techniques: What the science says*. Retrieved from https://nccih.nih.gov/health/providers/digest/relaxation-science

National Center for Complementary and Integrative Health. (2016b). *Omega-3 supplements: In depth*. Retrieved from https://nccih.nih.gov/health/omega3/introduction.htm

National Eating Disorders Association. (2013). *Eating disorder prevention*. Retrieved from http://www.nationaleatingdisorders.org/eating-disorder-prevention

National Eating Disorders Collaboration. (2014). *Eating disorders in schools: Prevention, early identification and response*. Sydney, Australia: National Eating Disorders Collaboration.

National Institute of Mental Health (NIMH). (2012). *How are eating disorders treated?* Retrieved from http://www.nimh.nih.gov/health/publications/eating-disorders/how-are-eating-disorders-treated.shtml

National Institute of Mental Health (NIMH). (2013a). *Borderline personality disorder*. Retrieved from http://www.nimh.nih.gov/health/publications/borderline-personality-disorder/borderline_personality_disorder_508.pdf

National Institute of Mental Health (NIMH). (2013b). *Borderline personality disorder: What are the symptoms of borderline personality disorder?* Retrieved from http://www.nimh.nih.gov/health/publications/borderline-personality-disorder/what-are-the-symptoms-of-borderline-personality-disorder.shtml

National Institute of Mental Health (NIMH). (2013c). *Psychotherapies*. Retrieved from http://www.nimh.nih.gov/health/topics/psychotherapies/index.shtml

National Institute of Mental Health (NIMH). (2014). *Eating disorders: About more than food*. Retrieved from https://www.nimh.nih.gov/health/publications/eating-disorders-new-trifold/index.shtml

Neacsiu, A. D., Lungu, A., Hamed, M. S., Rizvi, S. L., & Linehan, M. M. (2014). Impact of dialectical behavior therapy versus community treatment by experts on emotional experience, expression, and acceptance in borderline personality disorder. *Behaviour Research and Therapy, 53*, 45–54.

New, M. (2012). *Developing your child's self-esteem*. Retrieved from http://kidshealth.org/parent/emotions/feelings/self_esteem.html#

Norris, M. L., Spettigue, W. J., & Katzman, D. K. (2016). Update on eating disorders: Current perspectives on avoidant/restrictive food intake disorder in children and youth. *Neuropsychiatric Disease and Treatment, 12*, 213–218. doi:10.2147/ndt.s82538

Oltmanns, T. F., & Emery, R. E. (2012). *Abnormal psychology*. Upper Saddle River, NJ: Pearson Education.

Ornstein, R. M., Rosen, D. S., Mammel, K. A., Callahan, S. T., Forman, S., Jay, M. S., . . . Walsh, B. T. (2013). Distribution of eating disorders in children and adolescents using the proposed DSM-5 criteria for feeding and eating disorders. *Journal of Adolescent Health, 53*(2), 303–305. doi:http://dx.doi.org/10.1016/j.jadohealth.2013.03.025

Orth, U., & Robins, R. W. (2014). The development of self-esteem. *Current Directions in Psychological Science, 23*(5), 381–387. doi:10.1177/0963721414547414

Orth, U., Trzesniewski, K. H., & Robins, R. W. (2010). Self-esteem development from young adulthood to old age: A cohort-sequential longitudinal study. *Journal of Personality and Social Psychology, 98*(4), 645–658.

Osborn, K. S., Wraa, C. E., Watson, A., & Holleran, R. S. (2013). *Medical-surgical nursing: Preparation for practice* (2nd ed.). Upper Saddle River, NJ: Pearson.

Paniagua, F. A., & Yamada, A. (Eds.). (2013). *Handbook of multicultural mental health: Assessment and treatment of diverse populations* (2nd ed.). San Diego, CA: Academic Press.

Pargament, K. I., & Lomax, J. W. (2013). Understanding and addressing religion among people with mental illness. *World Psychiatry, 12*(1), 26–32.

Perez, M., & Warren,. S. (2013). Assessing eating pathology in Hispanic Americans. In T. L. Benuto (Ed.), *Guide to psychological assessment with Hispanics* (pp. 201–214). Boston, MA: Springer US.

Pew Research Center. (2015). *Teens, social media & technology overview 2015*. Retrieved from http://www.pewinternet.org/2015/04/09/teens-social-media-technology-2015/

Potter, M. L., & Moller, M. D. (Eds.). (2016). *Psychiatric–mental health nursing: From suffering to hope*. Upper Saddle River, NJ: Pearson Education.

PubMed Health. (2012a). *Anorexia nervosa*. Retrieved from http://www.ncbi.nlm.nih.gov/pubmedhealth/PMH0001401/

PubMed Health. (2012b). *Bulimia*. Retrieved from http://www.ncbi.nlm.nih.gov/pubmedhealth/PMH0001381/

Riffkin, R. (2015). *Americans rate nurses highest on honesty, ethical standards*. Retrieved from http://www.gallup.com/poll/180260/americans-rate-nurses-highest-honesty-ethical-standards.aspx

Rodgers, R. F., Lowy, A. S., Halperin, D. M., & Franko, D. L. (2016). A meta-analysis examining the influence of pro-eating disorder websites on body image and eating pathology. *European Eating Disorders Review, 24*(1), 3–8. doi:10.1002/erv.2390

Rohde, P., Stice, E., & Marti, C. N. (2015). Development and predictive effects of eating disorder risk factors during adolescence: Implications for prevention efforts. *International Journal of Eating Disorders, 48*(2), 187–198. doi:10.1002/eat.22270

Roy, A., Fuentes-Afflick, E., Fernald, L., & Young, S. (2015). Pica is prevalent and strongly associated with iron deficiency, but not anemia, among Mexican-born pregnant women living in the United States. *FASEB Journal, 29*(1 Supplement).

Schmidt, U., Magill, N., Renwick, B., Keyes, A., Kenyon, M., Dejong, H., & Landau, S. (2015). The Maudsley Outpatient Study of Treatments for Anorexia Nervosa and Related Conditions (MOSAIC): Comparison of the Maudsley Model of Anorexia Nervosa Treatment for Adults (MANTRA) with specialist supportive clinical management (SSCM) in outpatients with broadly defined anorexia nervosa: A randomized controlled trial. *Journal of Consulting and Clinical Psychology, 83*(4), 796–807. doi:http://psycnet.apa.org/doi/10.1037/ccp0000019

Sestan-Pesa, M., & Horvath, T. L. (2016). Metabolism and mental illness. *Trends in Molecular Medicine, 22*(2), 174–183. doi:10.1016/j.molmed.2015.12.003

Sim, L. A., McAlpine, D. E., Grothe, K. B., Himes, S. M., Cockerill, R. G., & Clark, M. M. (2010). Identification and treatment of eating disorders in the primary care setting. *Mayo Clinic Proceedings, 85*(8), 746–751. http://doi.org/10.4065/mcp.2010.0070

Smink, F. R. E., Hoeken, D., & Hoek, H. W. (2012). Epidemiology of eating disorders: Incidence, prevalence and mortality rates. *Current Psychiatry Reports, 14*(4), 406–414. doi:10.1007/s11920-012-0282-y

Smith, A. T., Kelly-Weeder, S., Engel, J., McGowan, K. A., Anderson, B., & Wolfe, B. E. (2011). Quality of eating disorders Web sites: What adolescents and their families need to know. *Journal of Child and Adolescent Psychiatric Nursing, 24*, 33–37.

Soenen, S., & Chapman, I. M. (2013). Body weight, anorexia, and undernutrition in older people. *Journal of the American Medical Directors Association, 14*(9), 642–648. doi:http://dx.doi.org/10.1016/j.jamda.2013.02.004

Solon-Biet, S. M., McMahon, A. C., Ballard, J. W. O., Ruohonen, K., Wu, L. E., Cogger, V. C., & Simpson, S. J. (2014). The ratio of macronutrients, not caloric intake, dictates cardiometabolic health, aging, and longevity in ad libitum-fed mice. *Cell Metabolism, 19*(3), 418–430. doi:10.1016/j.cmet.2014.02.009

Spector, R. E. (2017). *Cultural diversity in health and illness* (9th ed.). Hoboken, NJ: Pearson Education.

Stevens, N. R., Gerhart, J., Goldsmith, R. E., Heath, N. M., Chesney, S. A., & Hobfoll, S. E. (2013). Emotion regulation difficulties, low social support, and interpersonal violence mediate the link between childhood abuse and posttraumatic stress symptoms. *Behavior Therapy, 44*(1), 152–161. doi:http://dx.doi.org/10.1016/j.beth.2012.09.003

Substance Abuse and Mental Health Services Administration. (2014). *Trauma-informed care in behavioral health services*. (HHS Publication No. [SMA] 13-4801). Rockville, MD: Substance Abuse and Mental Health Services Administration.

Suokas, J. T., Suvisaari, J. M., Grainger, M., Raevuori, A., Gissler, M., & Haukka, J. (2014). Suicide attempts and mortality in eating disorders: A follow-up study of eating disorder patients. *General Hospital Psychiatry, 36*(3), 355–357. doi:10.1016/j.genhosppsych.2014.01.002

Swanson, S. A., Crow, S. J., LeGrange, D., Swendsen, J., & Merikangas, K. R. (2011). Prevalence and correlates of eating disorders in adolescents: Results from the national comorbidity survey replication adolescent supplement. *Archives of General Psychiatry, 68*(7), 714–723.

Tajima-Pozo, K., Zambrano-Enriquez, D., de Anta, L., Moron, M. D., Carrasco, J. L., Lopez-Ibor, J. J., & Diaz-Marsá, M. (2011). Practicing exorcism in schizophrenia. *BMJ Case Reports*. doi:10.1136/bcr.10.2009.2350. Retrieved from http://www.ncbi.nlm.nih.gov/pmc/articles/PMC3062860/

Thihalolipavan, S., Candalla, B. M., & Ehrlich, J. (2012). Examining pica in NYC pregnant women with elevated blood lead levels. *Maternal and Child Health Journal, 17*(1), 49–55. doi:10.1007/s10995-012-0947-5

Torgersen, S., Myers, J., Reichborn-Kjennerud, T., Røysamb, E., Kubarych, T. S., & Kendler, K. S. (2012). The heritability of Cluster B personality disorders assessed both by personal interview and questionnaire. *Journal of Personality Disorders, 26*(6), 848–866. doi:10.1521/pedi.2012.26.6.848

Trace, S. E., Baker, J. H., Peñas-Lledó, E., & Bulik, C. M. (2013). The genetics of eating disorders. *Annual Review of Clinical Psychology, 9,* 589–620. doi:10.1146/annurev-clinpsy-050212-185546

Uguz, F., Gezginc, K., Kayhan, F., Cicek, E., & Kantarci, A. H. (2012). Is hyperemesis gravidarum associated with mood, anxiety and personality disorders: A case-control study. *General Hospital Psychiatry, 34*(4), 398–402. doi:10.1016/j.genhosppsych.2012.03.021

U.S. Department of Veterans Affairs. (2015). *Prolonged exposure therapy.* Retrieved from http://www.ptsd. va.gov/public/treatment/therapy-med/prolonged-exposure-therapy.asp

U.S. National Library of Medicine. (2012). *Diseases and conditions.* Retrieved from http://www.ncbi. nlm.nih.gov/pubmedhealth/s/diseases_and_conditions/a/

Watson, H. J., Von Holle, A., Hamer, R. M., Knoph Berg, C., Torgersen, L., Magnus, P., & Bulik, C. M. (2013). Remission, continuation and incidence of eating disorders during early pregnancy: A validation study in a population-based birth cohort. *Psychological Medicine, 43*(8), 1723-1–34. doi:10.1017/S0033291712002516

Watson, J., & Browning, R. (2012). Viewpoint: *Caring science meets heart science: A guide to authentic caring practice.* Retrieved from http://www.americannursetoday.com/viewpoint-caring-science-meets-heart-science-a-guide-to-authentic-caring-practice/

Westmoreland, P., Krantz, M. J., & Mehler, P. S. (2016). Medical complications of anorexia nervosa and bulimia. *American Journal of Medicine, 129*(1), 30–37. doi:http://dx.doi.org/10.1016/j.amjmed.2015.06.031

Zanarini, M. C., Frankenburg, F., Reich, D. B., Conkey, L. C., & Fitzmaurice, G. M. (2015). Treatment rates for patients with borderline personality disorder and other personality disorders: A 16-year study. *Psychiatry Online, 66*(1), 15–20. Retrieved from http://ps.psychiatryonline.org/doi/abs/10.1176/appi.ps.201400055

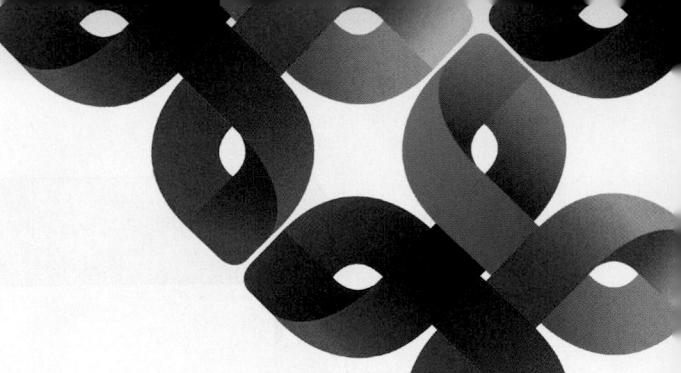

Module 30
Spirituality

Module Outline and Learning Outcomes

The Concept of Spirituality

Components of Spirituality

30.1 Analyze the components of spirituality.

Spirituality Throughout the Lifespan

30.2 Summarize the development of spirituality across the lifespan.

Concepts Related to Spirituality

30.3 Outline the relationship between spirituality and other concepts.

Health Promotion and Nursing Assessment

30.4 Explain the promotion of healthy spirituality and the techniques used to determine spiritual needs.

Spiritual Practices Affecting Nursing Care

30.5 Outline spiritual beliefs that can affect nursing care.

Independent Interventions and Collaborative Therapies

30.6 Summarize independent interventions and collaborative therapies used by healthcare teams for patients with spiritual needs.

Spirituality Exemplars

Exemplar 30.A Spiritual Distress

30.A Analyze spiritual distress as it relates to patient health.

Exemplar 30.B Religion

30.B Analyze religion as it relates to spirituality.

≫ The Concept of Spirituality

Concept Key Terms

Religion, **2024**	Spiritual distress, **2024**	Spirituality, **2023**
Spiritual development, **2025**	Spiritual well-being, **2024**	

Spirituality is a word derived from the Latin word *spirare*, which means "to blow" or "to breathe"; it has come to connote that which gives life or essence to being human. A definition of spirituality developed at an interprofessional, international consensus conference, recognized it as

a dynamic and intrinsic aspect of humanity through which persons seek ultimate meaning, purpose, and transcendence, and experience relationship to self, family, others, community, society, nature, and the significant or sacred. Spirituality is expressed through beliefs, values, traditions, and practices (Puchalski et al., 2014, p. 646).

Components of Spirituality

Because spirituality is a reflection of an inner experience that is expressed individually, it includes as many representations as there are human beings.

Spirituality, according to one classic source, can be described by measuring it, so to speak, on a "spirit titer" (Jourard, 1971). One's spirit titer is influenced by numerous factors, such as life experiences, coping skills, social supports, and individual belief systems. Individuals experience multiple changes and losses over their lifespan; if their spirit titer is low, they may become dispirited or depressed. If they have a high spirit titer, they will lean toward being inspired and becoming an inspiration to others in spite of hardships they experience (**Figure 30–1 ≫**). Nurses can aid healing when they assist patients in attaining and maintaining a high spirit titer.

Since 1989, more than 40 nurse scholars have conducted conceptual analyses of spirituality or closely related concepts to identify their constituent facets and characteristics. These analyses and definitions typically offered in the nursing literature consistently identify several core facets (e.g., Stephenson & Berry, 2014; Weathers, McArthur, & Coffey, 2016). Whether describing the spirituality of children or persons facing the end of life, these core facets include:

- Meaning (having purpose, making sense of life, having explanatory beliefs)
- Connecting (relating to others, nature, Ultimate Other, Higher Power, or God)
- Transcendence (appreciating a dimension that is beyond the self)

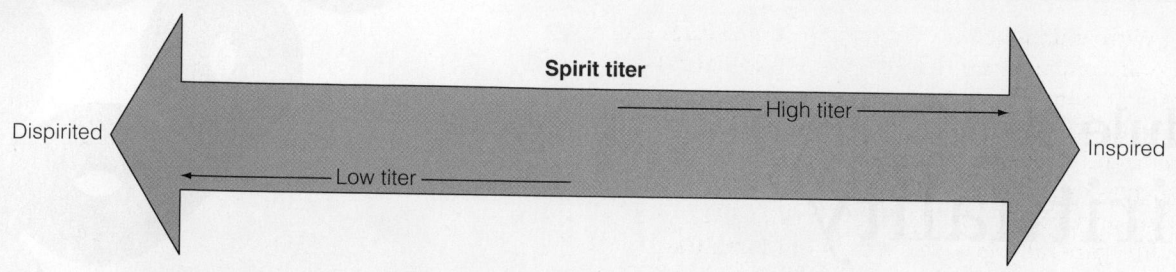

Figure 30–1 》 Each individual's spirit titer is influenced by their life experiences, coping skills, social support, and belief system.

Understanding how spirituality influences a patient's decision making and response to a health challenge, as well as how spirituality can be affected by illness, is crucial for nurses. Key components and expressions of spirituality include spiritual well-being, spiritual distress, spiritual needs, religion, and morality and ethics.

Spiritual Well-Being

Spiritual well-being, *wellness*, or *health* was defined by NANDA-I as a "pattern of experiencing and integrating meaning and purpose in life through connectedness with self, others, art, music, literature, nature, and/or a power greater than oneself that is sufficient for well-being and can be strengthened" (Carpenito-Moyet, 2013, p. 838). It is characterized by trusting relationships, inner strength, meaningfulness, and "motivation and commitment directed toward ultimate values of love, meaning, hope, beauty, and truth" (p. 838). According to one pioneer in the field, spiritual well-being is manifested by a feeling of being "generally alive, purposeful, and fulfilled" (Ellison, 1983, p. 332).

Spiritual Distress

Spiritual distress refers to a challenge to or feeling of dissatisfaction with one's spiritual well-being or with the belief system that provides strength, hope, and meaning to life. Some factors that may be associated with or contribute to an individual's spiritual distress include physiologic problems, treatment-related concerns, and situational concerns (e.g., death or illness of a significant other, inability to practice one's spiritual rituals, or feelings of embarrassment when practicing them) (Carpenito-Moyet, 2013).

Spiritual Needs

Just as every individual has a spiritual dimension, all patients have needs that reflect their spirituality. These needs are often accentuated by an illness or other health crisis. Patients who have well-defined spiritual beliefs may find that their beliefs are challenged by their health situation or may hold to their beliefs more firmly and appreciatively. Patients who have no defined beliefs may suddenly come face to face with challenging questions such as "Why me?" and others related to the meaning and purpose of life. Nurses need to be sensitive to indications of the patient's spiritual needs and respond appropriately. Examples of spiritual needs are listed in **Box 30–1 》**.

Religion

Although nurses may use the term *spirituality*, patients may equate it with religion. A **religion** is a system of beliefs that offer explanations and practices that allow one to cope with life's questions and challenges (Taylor, 2012). Thus, religions, whether institutionalized or not, provide means for gaining awareness of and expression of spirituality. Religious beliefs begin to answer questions about what is the nature of humankind and, how it came to be, what its purpose is, what is suffering, and what happens after death. Religious practices allow for the study and integration of these beliefs, and means and support for worshipping and

---

Box 30–1
Examples of Spiritual Needs

Needs Related to the Self

- Need for meaning and purpose
- Need to express creativity
- Need for hope
- Need to transcend life challenges
- Need for personal dignity
- Need for gratitude
- Need for vision
- Need to prepare for and accept death.

Needs Related to Others

- Need to forgive others
- Need to cope with loss of loved ones.

Needs Related to the Ultimate Other

- Need to be certain there is a God or Ultimate Power in the universe
- Need to believe that God is loving and personally present
- Need to worship.

Needs Among and Within Groups

- Need to contribute or improve one's community
- Need to be respected and valued
- Need to know what and when to give and take.

Source: From Taylor, E. J. (2002). *Spiritual care: Nursing theory, research, and practice.* Upper Saddle River, NJ: Prentice Hall. Reprinted by permission of Pearson Education, Inc., Upper Saddle River, New Jersey.

connecting with what is divine. Given this, it is natural that many religious practices are related to such life events as birth, transition from childhood to adulthood, marriage, illness, and death. Religious rules of conduct, typically influenced concurrently by culture, may also apply to matters of daily life such as dress, food, social interaction, childrearing, menstruation, and sexual relationships (Taylor, 2012).

Spirituality generally involves a belief in a relationship with some higher power, creative force, divine being, or infinite source of energy. For example, an individual may believe in God, Allah, the Great Spirit, or a Higher Power. Monotheism is the belief in the existence of one god, whereas polytheism is the belief in more than one god. An agnostic is an individual who doubts the existence of God or a supreme being or who believes that the existence of God has not been proved. An atheist is an individual who does not believe in any god.

Those who live in the United States of America are fairly religious. Surveys of U.S. Americans (The Association of Religion Data Archives, n.d.) revealed the following:

- 77% reported religion was an *important* part of their life

- 48% identified themselves as Protestant, 25% as Roman Catholic, 17% as "None," 8% as other (e.g., Buddhist, Muslim, Hindu), and 2% as Jewish (see **Figure 30–2 》**).

- 63% agreed that they had "no doubt that God exists," whereas 12% did so but with some doubt; 12% believed in "a Higher Power or cosmic force"

- 57% prayed at least once a day, 28% read sacred texts about weekly or more frequently, and 23% attended religious services at least once every week.

The frequency of religious practices does vary over the lifespan with an increase correlating directly with age. Indeed, various surveys suggest that older adults (especially those facing death), African Americans, and women tend to report more religiosity (e.g., Krause, 2011).

SAFETY ALERT Thinking about spirituality only as religion will cause an unethical stance toward nonreligious patients that is insensitive and domineering. Conversely, conceptualizing spirituality without religion will contribute to nursing care that is insensitive of patient religiosity and overlook this salient influence on religious patients' illness experiences (Pesut, 2016).

Morality and Ethics

Ethics guides the determination of what is "right" and "wrong" and deals with "oughts" and "shoulds" (Fowler, 2015). Morality refers to the rules a society has created for promoting ethical conduct, or right and virtuous behavior (see the module on Ethics). Considering that spirituality by definition recognizes individual needs for meaning and concern about supreme values, it certainly can be related to morality and ethics. Applying values and assigning meaning to things in life is inherent in ethical and moral decision making. The acts of valuing and finding meaning are acts involving and reflecting spirituality. When one asks ethical questions (e.g., "What is right in this situation? What ought I to do?"), one is also inevitably raising spiritual questions (e.g., "What is the source of truth for me?").

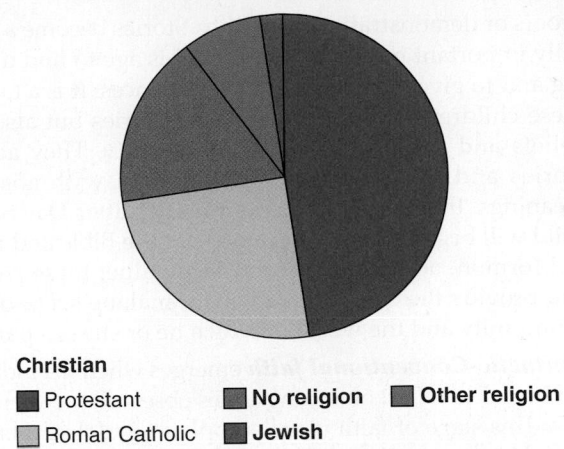

Christian
- ■ Protestant   ■ No religion   ■ Other religion
- ■ Roman Catholic   ■ Jewish

Source: Pew Research Center. (2016). If the U.S. had 100 people: Charting American's religious affiliations. Retrieved from http://www.pewresearch.org/fact-tank/2016/11/14/if-the-u-s-had-100-people-charting-americans-religious-affiliations/With the Figure: The Association of Religion Data Archives, n.d.

Figure 30–2 》 Religions of Americans (The Association of Religion Data Archives, n.d.).

Spirituality Throughout the Lifespan

Just as individuals develop physically, cognitively, and morally, they also develop spiritually. The most influential description of **spiritual development** was offered by Fowler (1981). Although Fowler used the term "faith" development, he recognized faith as a universal human phenomenon that leads individuals to need and find meaning and an understanding of themselves in relation to their world. Fowler arrived at these seven stages of faith development after analyzing in-depth interviews with more than 400 individuals who ranged in age from 3 to 84 years.

- **Undifferentiated faith** (infancy to 3 years): During this time, neonates and toddlers are acquiring the fundamental spiritual qualities of trust and mutuality, as well as courage, hope, and love. The transition to the next stage of faith begins when the child's language and thought start to converge, allowing for the use of symbolism. Sadly, these spiritual qualities can also be undermined, rather than developed, as may occur in situations of child abuse.

- **Intuitive-Projective faith** (3 to 7 years): This is the "fantasy-filled, imitative phase in which the child can be powerfully and permanently influenced by examples, moods, actions and stories of the visible faith" (Fowler, 1981, p. 133). During this stage, children relate intuitively to the ultimate conditions of existence through stories and images, the fusion of facts and feelings. Magical thinking and reality overlap during this stage. For a example, children at this age view Santa Claus as real and may view God as a big, smiling (or frowning) granddaddy in the sky (depending on the stories the important adults in the child's life tell).

- **Mythic-Literal faith** is found among school-age children (up to 12 years) but can linger even into adulthood. During this stage of faith, children are attempting to sort out what is fantasy from what is fact, by demanding proofs or demonstrations of reality. Stories become a critically important means for children this age to find meaning and to give organization to experiences. It is a task of these children to learn not only the stories but also the beliefs and practices of their community. They accept stories and beliefs literally rather than with abstract meanings. In this stage, for example, a Latter Day Saints child will begin learning the stories of the Bible and Book of Mormon, accepting them at face value; these stories will provide the child with a way of making sense of the community and the world of which he or she is a part.

- *Synthetic-Conventional faith* emerges when the individual begins to reflect on incongruities observed between stories. This stage of faith usually applies to adolescents and teens, but it can also characterize some adults. The synthetic-conventional stage accompanies the individual's experience of the world that is now beyond the family unit (e.g., school, media), and must provide a helpful understanding of this extended environment. While faith "must synthesize values and information; it must provide a basis for identity and outlook" (Fowler, 1981, p. 172). At this stage, individuals generally conform to the beliefs of those around them, because they have yet not reflected or studied these beliefs objectively. Thus, beliefs and values of teens are often held tacitly. For example, an adolescent or teen raised by observant Jews will likely continue to observe the Jewish practices of parents and accept parents' beliefs.

- *Individuative-Reflective faith* is typically observed among young adults, but may continue into later adulthood. This stage of faith is characterized by the development of a self-identity and worldview that is differentiated from those of others. The individual forms independent commitments, lifestyle, beliefs, and attitudes. The child who obediently attended Mom's Roman Catholic mass every Sunday will now examine independently what religious practices and beliefs to accept. Another characteristic of this stage of development is the demythologizing of symbols into conceptual meanings. To illustrate, the young adult who was taught as a child not to place anything on top of holy scriptures because of their sacredness, now understands that this is not religious edict, but rather an authority's attempt to teach respect for an object that informs the reader about what is sacred.

- *Conjunctive faith* usually is found among adults past midlife. At this stage, adults find new appreciation for their past, value their inner voices, and become aware of deep-seated myths, prejudices, and images that are indwelling because of their social background. An individual with conjunctive faith "strives to unify opposites in mind and experience" and allows "vulnerability to the strange truths of those who are 'other'" (Fowler, 1981, p. 198). For example, instead of trying to dissuade or avoid another with differing spiritual beliefs, a person in this stage of faith would embrace persons of other faith traditions, recognizing that in their faith may be new understanding. Also, an adult whose faith is conjunctive may practice prayer in a way that allows listening to the deeper self, instead of petitionary praying.

- *Universalizing* of faith is infrequently reached. Those in this stage of faith have a "sense of an ultimate environment [that] is inclusive of all being. They have become incarnators and actualizers of the spirit of an inclusive and fulfilled human community" (Fowler, 1981, p. 200). These persons work to unshackle social, political, economic, or ideologic burdens in society. They fully love life, yet simultaneously hold it loosely. Fowler identified Martin Luther King, Mahatma Gandhi, and Mother Teresa as examples of those having developed this level of faith.

From this descriptive theory, it is evident that the spirituality of children, adolescents, adults, and older adults will differ, although spiritual maturity can be stunted and change little for some. For example, the spirituality of adolescence may continue into adulthood, or the spirituality of mid-adulthood may not change as a person ages. Indeed, it is the crisis of illness, disability, or facing death that often causes individuals to revisit their spirituality and jumpstart continued development.

Another approach to theorizing how individuals develop spiritually is offered by psychologists influenced by theories about object relations and attachment (Hall et al., 2009; Harris et al., 2015). That is, it is proposed that how an individual has related to his mother or other significant caregivers during infancy and early childhood establishes a pattern for how he will relate to others, including a divinity or spiritual community, as an adult. Whereas there is evidence that individuals' ways of relating to God and others—with secure versus insecure attachment (e.g., avoiding or resisting)—corresponds with how they related to their parent figure(s), there is also evidence that compensatory attachments can also occur. For example, a person whose parent abused them as an infant can compensate by viewing God as the ideal parent.

Research by Hall and colleagues (2009, 2015) integrates these notions of correspondence and compensation. They proposed that explicit aspects of spirituality that can be chosen and controlled (e.g., religious beliefs and practices) can mediate implicit spirituality, which is based on the unconscious emotional information processing all persons have and which is influenced by early life experiences. For example, a patient who had an insecure attachment with a parent who was often absent, and coped with it by avoiding that parent, may experience the divine (e.g., God) as absent and avoid intimacy with God. Spiritual beliefs may, however, encourage the patient to use practices that allow this human–divine abyss to be approximated.

Spiritual Development of Children

Given the development of spirituality in children parallels their cognitive and psychosocial development, nursing care that supports spiritual well-being will consider what is age appropriate. Nurses can help ill or injured children to make sense of their health challenge by asking simple questions (e.g., "How are you like [name child's hero/heroine]?"), by actively listening, by offering opportunities to practice religious rituals the ways their parents do, and by providing materials for nonverbal expression (e.g., painting, play, music) (Petersen, 2014). For infants especially, it is imperative that nurses support parent–child bonding so that trust and a secure attachment can be encouraged. Secure attachment can be encouraged not only by allowing parents to be present with their child, but also by modeling or otherwise teaching parents about how to be fully and empathically present to their child.

Spiritual Development of Adolescents

Adolescents are, by nature, in the process of learning to differentiate themselves from their parents, form their own unique identity, and think independently and critically. Their spirituality will reflect this development. Adolescents are risk takers, seek to conform to others, and often make decisions that are focused in the present rather than on future possibilities or consequences (Magaldi-Dopman & Park-Taylor, 2013). Thus, adolescents may be inclined toward a spirituality or religiosity that "scratches these itches" (e.g., hyper-sensationalized worship experiences, cults, critically evaluating parental religiosity, choosing non-institutionalized expressions of spirituality). Yet evidence also indicates that adolescent religiosity generally corresponds with parental religiosity, especially if there is a warm, stable home environment and healthy parent–child relationship (Taylor et al., 2015). Nursing care for adolescents that supports spiritual well-being will recognize these characteristics. An example of a proven intervention for enhancing the spiritual well-being of adolescents with cancer is that of producing a music video. Working with a music therapist, adolescents can compose their lyrics, choose music, and select images or cast members and direct and produce their own videos (Robb et al., 2014).

Spiritual Development of Adults

Adulthood is a season of the lifespan when individuals typically form their own nuclear family and build a career and roles in their community. Meaning and connectedness are often related to these natural strivings. Thus, when the plan is ruined (e.g., by a significant loss or change such as divorce, chronic illness or disability, deadly accident, unemployment, or natural disaster), and the individual's sense of the world as safe and good is shattered, the person begins to reconstruct meaningfulness (Marris, 2016). Whereas some patients will "get stuck" asking existential questions and "Why me?", others will find illness to be a sacred journey and suffering to prompt spiritual transformation (Linders & Lancaster, 2013). As Fowler (1981) observed, some adults maintain the spirituality of their adolescence and young adulthood, while others grow spiritually.

Spiritual Development of Older Adults

There is evidence that spirituality increases among older adults, especially among women, starting as early as the late 50s (Krause, 2011; Wink & Dillon, 2003). Many older adults frequently use and highly value religious coping strategies such as prayer. Older adults may be especially concerned about living a purposeful life, about maintaining loving relationships to avoid social isolation, and about leaving a legacy and preparing for a peaceful death. Nursing care for older adults can support meaning-making activities. Some examples of meaning-making activities include conducting a life review or reminiscence therapy that allows the patient to weave together the strands of lived life; encouraging the patient to become dedicated to some social, political, religious, or artistic cause; and supporting the patient to leave a legacy or do an altruistic deed. As appropriate, nurses may also support older adults to reframe the "losses" of aging as "liberations." For example,

older adults possess great wisdom and are in a season of life that promotes spiritual growth.

Patients with dementia present special circumstances for spiritual caregiving. Nurses can help those with early stages of dementia to focus on the positives, the "haves" rather than the losses. Allowing older adults with dementia to tell their stories helps them to maintain some identity in the face of a disease that threatens the very sense of self. It also gives the nurse a window into the patient's world. Patients with dementia can also worship and express their hope and creativity through various art forms (e.g., movement, painting, music). These patients are often able to experience the compassion of others when they feel their caring touch or hear their soothing voice.

SAFETY ALERT Fowler (1981) observed that it is easy for individuals to have a disparaging view of those who are in a spiritual developmental phase from which they have just emerged. It is important for nurses to not view another as spiritually immature. Rather, it is helpful to remember that all persons are journeying as best they can through life (Brown, 2015).

Case Study ≫ Part 1

Tom Denton, a young adult male Jehovah's Witness, is brought into the emergency department (ED) with a gastrointestinal (GI) bleed. He is vomiting blood, hypotensive, pale, and diaphoretic, and his pulse is weak and thready. He is alert enough to hear Sharon Hynes, the ED physician, order a type and cross for four units of blood. Mr. Denton interrupts and states that he does not want the blood transfusion because of personal religious beliefs. Dr. Hynes orders volume-expanding agents to be used instead. Mr. Denton's wife Melissa arrives not long before he loses consciousness, and they discuss the use of the volume expanders versus blood transfusions. She agrees with his decision and tells him she loves him. He tells her he loves her also.

Clinical Reasoning Questions Level I

1. What are the primary concerns for Mr. and Mrs. Denton?
2. How are the staff and others likely to react to the couple's decision? Why?
3. How do the principles of autonomy affect this scenario?

Clinical Reasoning Questions Level II

4. Jehovah's Witnesses who receive a blood product against their will refer to that as "medical rape." In what ways might they experience rape trauma syndrome symptoms?
5. If Dr. Hynes had written a PRN order for blood "just in case Mr. or Mrs. Denton change their mind," what would be your role as a nurse advocate?
6. If Melissa had disagreed with Tom regarding this matter, how could an RN facilitate open and helpful communication between them?

Concepts Related to Spirituality

In today's busy healthcare environment, it can be easy for nurses and other healthcare providers to overlook a patient's spirituality. However, nurses understand that spiritual assessment can inform interventions that foster hope and incorporate a patient's spirituality as a resource for motivating patient change and improving patient outcomes (Neuman & Fawcett, 2002). As such, spirituality can be related to all aspects of a

Concepts Related to
Spirituality

CONCEPT	RELATIONSHIP TO SPIRITUALITY	NURSING IMPLICATIONS
Comfort	Spiritual/religious beliefs may dictate how to interpret and address pain and discomfort.	Assess how patients ascribe meaning to pain and suffering. Consider alternative therapies to manage discomfort if the patient wants to avoid opioids or other medications.
Culture and Diversity	Religion, an expression of spirituality, is integral to culture.	Be aware and sensitive to the diverse religious beliefs and practices of patients. If you don't know, assess (e.g., Please tell me about any religious beliefs or practices that should affect your healthcare).
Legal Issues	Western cultures, such as those in North America, have federal laws protecting personal religious liberties.	Clarify, advocate, and seek legal support if necessary, when a patient or colleague's religious liberties are threatened.
Nutrition	Spiritual/religious beliefs often prescribe a diet (e.g., vegetarianism, abstinence from alcohol). Some religious holidays are observed with fasting from all or certain specified foods.	Assess what diet the patient prefers.
Sexuality	Practices related to sexuality, such as family planning/birth control, may be influenced by spirituality.	When appropriate, assess the influence of spirituality on sexuality and associated practices. Provide care that is congruent with patients' spiritual/religious beliefs and practices.
Stress and Coping	People can use positive and negative religious coping strategies. Negative religious coping is associated with poor adjustment and outcomes.	Observe for expressions of negative religious coping (e.g., "God is punishing me" or "God/my church isn't there for me anymore"); make an appropriate referral (e.g., chaplain) if it is observed.

patient's health, mental health, and safety. For example, religious practices may include certain dietary restrictions or practices. These can affect prescribed diets, especially when the patient is a member of a family with limited funds for purchasing and organizing family meals. Spirituality may affect sexuality and reproduction if the patient adheres to sexual practices outlined by a religion. Spiritual practices and coping mechanisms can reduce stress and promote healthy coping, but there are some practices that may negatively impact a patient's ability to cope with stress.

The Concepts Related to Spirituality feature links some, but not all, of the concepts integral to spirituality. They are presented in alphabetical order.

Health Promotion and Nursing Assessment

Given that spirituality is an expression of the innate human yearning for meaningfulness, connection, and self-transcendence, it is no wonder that humans in their diversity have developed diverse ways for promoting their spiritual well-being or health. Whether individuals consider themselves as religious or spiritual, most prefer to have satisfactory responses to life's big questions, prefer to be at peace within and without, and want to be awed by something greater and more ultimate.

Until recently, spiritual practices tended to be religion and culture specific (Fowler et al., 2011). For example, Roman

Catholics primarily sought to promote their spiritual health by following the dictates of their church (e.g., regularly attending Mass, confession) and by praying in certain ways (e.g., with rosary, a string of beads that can be touched while saying a petitionary, memorized prayer). Likewise, Sikhs may have sought to become a baptized Khalsa (e.g., live a virtuous life dedicated to God, be prayerful, never cut any body hair, wear specific emblems). In fact, prior to modernization and the Enlightenment, most spiritual health promotion practices would have been religious.

In the world of internet, airplanes, and books, however, ideas are easily transmitted and spiritual practices are readily shared across cultures and continents. Concurrently, spirituality is no longer only within the domain of religion (Wuthnow, 1998). Today, many individuals have a "hyphenated" religiosity or a combination of self-selected spiritual practices that they find personally satisfying (Taylor, 2012). For example, an individual born and raised in a Seventh-day Adventist family may, as an adult, choose to worship weekly in an interfaith congregational church, read about and practice Buddhist meditation, and attend a monthly Baha'i fellowship meeting.

Although spiritual practices rooted in a religious tradition (at least originally) continue to be practiced in or out of a religion, many individuals also recognize secular (or nonreligious) approaches to spiritual health. Examples include spending time in nature, experiencing art and beauty, and gaining self-awareness through reflection and conversation.

Hodge (2015) and Taylor (2015) recommend a two-tiered approach to assessing patient spirituality. This approach typically involves the nurse first conducting an initial screening and a slightly more thorough spiritual history assessment. Next, an expert, typically the chaplain, will conduct a more in-depth interview, referred to as the spiritual assessment.

Screening

When a patient enters the healthcare system, a nurse can screen for the presence of any spiritual distress likely to interfere with healing. Fitchett and colleagues (King, Fitchett, & Berry, 2013) developed a screening protocol that is easily implemented. The protocol involves first asking the yes/no question, "Is spirituality or religion (S/R) important to you as you cope with illness?" If a patient responds with "yes," then the clinician can ask, "How much strength/comfort do you get now?" If spirituality or religiosity is important to the patient, but he is currently not receiving adequate strength or comfort from it, then the nurse can assume that spiritual distress is present and make a referral. If, however, the patient responds that S/R is unimportant, then the nurse can ask, "Has there ever been a time when S/R was important?" If the patient indicates that S/R has been important in the past, it is appropriate for the nurse to ask if the patient would like to visit with a chaplain. If S/R was never important or the patient receives adequate strength/comfort, then the nurse can infer there is no immediate spiritual crisis requiring support. When Fitchett's team studied the efficacy of this protocol, they found that the screening process was effective 92% of the time in correctly identifying patients with spiritual crisis.

Another approach to spiritual screening is to select a couple of general questions about the impact of spiritual or religious beliefs and practices on health and healthcare (e.g., "What spiritual beliefs or practices are important to you now while you live with illness?" and "How would you like your healthcare team to support you spiritually?"). Only patients who manifest some type of unhealthy spiritual need or who are at risk for spiritual distress need be subjected to a more thorough spiritual history or referred to a chaplain for an in-depth spiritual assessment.

SAFETY ALERT Because nurses are generalists in spiritual care (whereas chaplains, clergy, and others are spiritual care specialists), the role of the nurse in conducting spiritual assessment should be limited to that which is relevant to providing healthcare. It is inappropriate, unnecessary, and harmful to the patient–nurse relationship for a nurse to conduct a spiritual assessment because of personal curiosity or desire to proselytize.

Spiritual History and Observation

Data about a patient's spiritual beliefs are obtained from the patient's general history (religious preferences or orientation); through a nursing history; and by clinical observations of the patient's behavior, verbalizations, mood, and interactions with others. Nurses should never assume that a patient accepts all of the beliefs or follows all of the practices of the patient's stated religion.

When a more thorough assessment is needed (e.g., the patient is being admitted to the healthcare system and a more general assessment is appropriate, or the screening protocol reveals spiritual need), the nurse can assess further by conducting a spiritual history. Although the nurse will continually be assessing, the spiritual history is best taken at the end of the assessment process or following the psychosocial assessment, after the nurse has developed a relationship with the patient and/or the patient's support person. A nurse who has demonstrated sensitivity and personal warmth, earning some rapport, will be more successful during a spiritual assessment.

The most common spiritual history tool may be Puchalski's (2014) mnemonic **FICA**. This tool prompts the clinician to inquire about these four aspects of spirituality:

Faith or beliefs ("What spiritual beliefs are most important to you?")

Implications or influence ("How is your faith affecting the way you cope now?")

Community ("Is there a group of like-minded believers with whom you regularly meet?")

Address ("How would you like your healthcare team to support you spiritually?")

Many other questions, however, can be asked. For patients who are not religious, it will be important to select language that is not religious. Examples of questions to ask may include:

- What are your spiritual or religious beliefs or practices that would be important for your healthcare providers to know about?
- How is being sick or in the hospital challenging your spiritual or religious beliefs or practices?
- How is your faith helpful to you? In what ways is it important to you right now?
- What are your hopes and your sources of strength right now? What comforts you during hard times?
- In what ways can I boost your spirit?
- Would you like a visit from your spiritual counselor or the hospital chaplain?

Nurses can also observe for cues about patients' spiritual and religious preferences, strengths, concerns, or distress. These may be revealed by one or more of the following:

- **_Environment._** Does the patient have a Bible, Torah, Quran, other prayer book, devotional literature, religious medals, rosary, cross, Star of David, or religious get-well cards in the room? Does a church send altar flowers or Sunday bulletins? Is there a religious service that is televised or streamed over the internet that the patient would like to watch?
- **_Behavior._** Does the patient appear to pray before meals or at other times or read religious literature? Does the patient have nightmares and sleep disturbances or express anger at religious representatives or at a deity?
- **_Verbalization._** Does the patient mention God or a higher power, prayer, faith, a church, a synagogue, a temple, a spiritual or religious leader, or religious topics? Does the patient ask about a visit from the clergy? Does the patient express fear of death, concern with the meaning of life,

inner conflict about religious beliefs, concern about a relationship with a deity, questions about the meaning of existence or the meaning of suffering, or questions about the moral or ethical implications of therapy?

- **Affect and attitude.** Does the patient appear lonely, depressed, angry, anxious, agitated, apathetic, or preoccupied?
- **Interpersonal relationships.** Who visits? How does the patient respond to visitors? Does a minister or other spiritual mentor come? How does the patient relate to other patients and nursing personnel?

To provide holistic care, it is important for the nurse to understand the spiritual needs and beliefs of the patient. Understanding and support of a patient's spiritual beliefs and practices builds trust in the nurse–patient relationship, makes the patient feel more comfortable in strange environments, and individualizes the nursing plan of care to meet each individual's unique needs.

Case Study >> Part 2

Mr. Denton has slipped into a coma. Mrs. Denton is crying and begging her husband not to leave her. The staff members continue to treat the patient with the volume expanders, but there is no significant improvement. Dr. Hynes speaks to Mrs. Denton and asks whether she has changed her mind.

Clinical Reasoning Questions Level I

1. What would be an empathic and spiritually supportive comment an RN could offer to Mrs. Denton?
2. Who could be called to help Mrs. Denton during this time?
3. What resources are available to help Mrs. Denton?

Clinical Reasoning Questions Level II

4. How should the nurse assess the needs of Mr. and Mrs. Denton at this time?
5. Does Dr. Hynes have the right to ask Mrs. Denton this question? Why or why not?
6. What would be a healing environment for a patient in a coma?

Spiritual Practices Affecting Nursing Care

Patients frequently identify religious practices such as prayer as important strategies for coping with illness (Taylor, 2012). The most common practices affecting the nursing care of patients include practices associated with diet, healing, dress, birth, and death.

Beliefs Affecting Diet

Many religions have proscriptions regarding diet. There may be rules about which foods and beverages are allowed and which are prohibited. For example, Orthodox Jews are not to eat shellfish or pork, and Muslims are not to drink alcoholic beverages or eat pork. Members of the Church of Jesus Christ of Latter-Day Saints (Mormons), Seventh-day Adventists, and Hindus are not to drink coffee or alcoholic beverages. Older Catholics may choose not to eat meat on Fridays because it was prohibited in years past, and abstinence from meat is still required on some days during Lent. Many Buddhists and Hindus are generally vegetarian, not wanting to

take life to support life. Religious law may also dictate how food is prepared; for example, orthodox Jewish patients will request kosher food and Muslims will request halal. For these diets, food (especially meat) is to be obtained and prepared according to rules of the respective religious tradition.

Some solemn religious observances are marked by fasting, which is the abstinence from any or specified food for a specified period of time. Fasting in some religions may also require restricting beverages; others allow drinking of water or other sustaining beverages (e.g., fruit juice) on fast days. For example, Christians who are adherents of an Eastern Orthodox tradition observe numerous feast and holy days during the year. Each holy day has its rules regarding foods to eat; an oil-free and alcohol-free vegan diet will often meet these rules of fasting. During the month of Ramadan, devout Muslims eat no food and avoid beverages during daylight hours before breaking their fast after sunset. Members of Jewish synagogues fast on Yom Kippur, and devout Catholics may fast on the Lenten holy days of Ash Wednesday and Good Friday. Most religions lift the fasting requirements for seriously ill believers for whom fasting may be a detriment to health (e.g., patients with diabetes). Some religions may exempt nursing mothers or menstruating women from fasting requirements.

Healthcare providers should assess and incorporate patients' dietary and fasting beliefs prior to providing meals or prescribing diet plans.

Beliefs Related to Healing

Some patients attribute illness to a spiritual etiology. The most common attributions with spiritual or religious overtones may be those that construe benefit and punishment (Fowler et al., 2011). Examples of construed benefit include: "My illness is making me stronger inside," "This sickness is a wake-up call to get my life in order!" or "This health challenge is really making me draw closer to God and making me appreciate life more." Indeed, many religious traditions view illness and suffering as a test of faith and an opportunity for spiritual growth (Taylor, 2012).

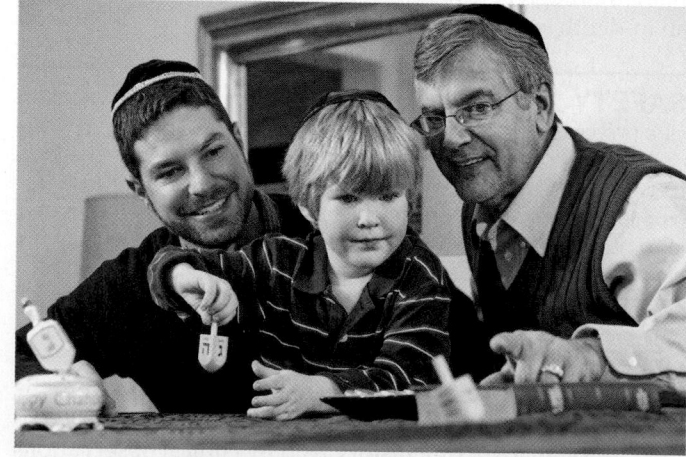

Source: GoldenKB/iStock/Getty Images.

Figure 30–3 >> Conservative and Orthodox Jewish men may wear a yarmulke at all times, even in the hospital. Reform Jews may wear yarmulkes only while praying and on religious occasions, such as this family celebrating Hanukkah.

Conversely, a health challenge can be thought of as a punishment, a reflection of a spiritual weakness, or as the result of an evil force. Illustrative patient statements could include: "If I hadn't been so wild and sinful as a youth (or so unfaithful as an adult), I wouldn't have this diagnosis now," or "Satan caused my sickness—and God allowed it." Although less than a quarter of patients likely make such negative attributions, they are detrimental to psychologic and spiritual well-being (Taylor, 2011). Patients who make such observations warrant further assessment and referral to a specialist. Indeed, clarifying that illness as punishment is not a belief congruent with the patient's religion (as is often the case) can bring enormous relief and spiritual healing.

Many religions offer healing rituals that symbolize the patient's choice to place their illness outcomes in the care of the divine (Taylor, 2011). Patients belonging to many Protestant denominations may request their local church minister and/or leaders to administer an "anointing." Similarly, Roman Catholics will appreciate a priest offering the Anointing of the Sick, as this is not just a ritual for the end of life. Healing rituals may involve reading scriptural passages offering hope and prayers for healing, usually with blessed oil being placed on the recipient's head. The family of a Hindu patient may visit the local temple and ask the priest for puja, a ritual involving a mantra said with the patient's name, lighting candles, burning incense, and offering fruit or flowers to an image of a deity. The family may be given a symbol (e.g., piece of sacred cloth) to give to the patient, who can wear it or place it above their bed. A more superstitious Jewish patient may tie a red string around the bedpost or place a psalm on the headboard. Orthodox and Roman Catholic patients, as well as many Protestants, will likely be eager to receive communion and confession from a priest or lay clergy. Patients who profess spirituality may adopt beliefs and rituals from a combination of sources, such as chanting, energy work, lighting candles, or burning sage. Despite the diversity of healing rituals and traditions patients may use, all reflect the human yearning for healing and blessing.

Beliefs Related to Dress

Many religions have laws or traditions that dictate dress. For example, Orthodox and Conservative Jewish men believe that it is important to have their heads covered at all times and therefore wear yarmulkes (**Figure 30–3 》**). Orthodox Jewish women cover their hair with a wig or scarf as a sign of respect to God (Orthodox-Jews.com, 2014). Mormons may wear temple undergarments in compliance with their religious dictates (Taylor, 2012). Some religions require women to dress in a conservative manner, which may include wearing sleeves and modestly cut tops, and skirts that cover the knees. Many Muslim women also cover most of their body in accordance with their particular ethnic or national background; conservative Muslim men and women ensure that the area between their navel and knees is always covered (Mujallad & Taylor, 2016). Hindu women accustomed to wearing saris prefer to cover all of the body except their arms and feet (**Figure 30–4 》**).

Women who wish to comply with religious dress codes may find wearing hospital gowns uneasy and uncomfortable.

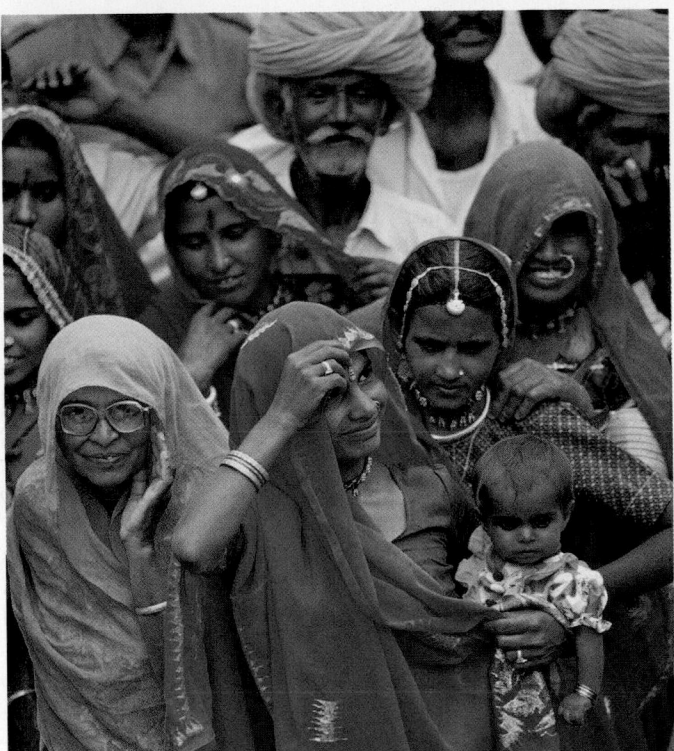

Figure 30–4 》 Many Hindu women cover all of their body except for their face, arms, and feet.

Patients may be especially disconcerted when undergoing diagnostic tests or treatments, such as mammography, that require body parts to be bared. Similarly, a Khalsid Sikh who has vowed to never cut body hair will be distraught if a nurse tries to do so in preparation for surgery or intravenous line insertion (Taylor, 2012).

Beliefs Related to Birth

Many religions have specific ritual ceremonies for a newborn that consecrate the infant to God (Taylor, 2012). For example, when a Muslim child is born, the father or other relative or cleric recites the Islamic call to prayer into the infant's ear. Hindus observe ceremonies for both the newborn and mother that involve symbolisms of purity and well wishes. A Jehovah's Witness will request that placental or umbilical cord blood be disposed of rather than extracted. Many Christians will christen or baptize their infant. Christian parents of seriously ill newborns may want baptism performed by the nurse or primary care provider if a chaplain or clergy person is not present. Religious dictates about circumcision vary. Whereas Hindus do not practice it, Muslims and Jews circumcise male infants. Christian traditions vary but generally leave the decision to parents (Taylor, 2012).

When nurses are aware of the religious needs of families and their infants, they can support families in fulfilling their religious obligations if necessary. This is especially important when the newborn infant is seriously ill or in danger of dying, because some individuals believe that if religious obligations are not fulfilled the infant will not be accepted into the community of the faithful after death.

Beliefs Related to Death

Spiritual and religious beliefs play a significant role in the believer's approach to death just as they do in other major life events (Taylor, 2012). Many believe that the individual who dies transcends this life for a better place or state of being. Some religions have special rituals surrounding dying and death that must be observed by the faithful. Observance of these rituals provides comfort to the dying individual and his or her loved ones. Some rituals are carried out while the individual is still alive and can include special prayers, singing or chants, and reading of sacred scriptures (e.g., Buddhists). Roman Catholic priests perform the sacrament of Anointing of the Sick (previously referred to as the Last Rites or Extreme Unction) when patients are very ill or near death. Muslims who are dying want their body or head turned toward Mecca and are encouraged to say the prayer recognizing their loyalty to Allah (God).

Bereavement rituals likewise vary across faith traditions (Taylor, 2012). For example, Jews have a tradition of burial within 24 hours following death, except on the Sabbath, and they sit Shiva (gather to pay respects). Tibetan Buddhists read the *Tibetan Book of the Dead* within 7 days of the death to release the soul of the deceased. Hindus cremate and Muslims bury the body within 24 hours ideally. Postmortem rituals and practices such as bathing and preparing the body for interment (e.g., especially for Jews and Muslims), saying specified prayers, and beliefs regarding methods for body disposal and what happens in an afterlife likewise vary by religion and culture. Religious symbols or objects should be treated with respect and kept with the body.

The nurse can help to support family members of the deceased by providing an environment conducive to the performance of their traditional death rituals. This will be possible if during the terminal illness, the patient and family are queried about observances or rituals surrounding the time of death.

Case Study » Part 3

Mr. Denton's minister arrives, and Mrs. Denton and the minister discuss the situation. They agree that the situation has been handled according to Mr. Denton's beliefs. Mr. Denton dies, and Mrs. Denton states, "He died as he believed; God's will has been done." Members of the ED staff are overheard saying things like "He was too young to die" and "If only they had allowed the blood transfusion."

Clinical Reasoning Questions Level I

1. What should the nurse do to help Mrs. Denton at this time?
2. How can an RN support community-based spiritual caregivers such as ministers?
3. What should the staff members do to help deal with their own feelings?

Clinical Reasoning Questions Level II

4. If the patient in the case study had been 10 years old and the parents had made the decision to treat with volume expanders only, with the same results, what would have been the staff's responsibility?
5. What ethical and legal issues would be involved in the decision-making process in this situation?
6. What end-of-life care would be appropriate before and after Mr. Denton's death?

Independent Interventions and Collaborative Therapies

When facilitating interventions or providing nursing therapeutics to nurture patient spiritual well-being, nurses should avoid unethically imposing personal spiritual beliefs on patients, whose circumstances inherently leave them vulnerable. Observing guidelines for ethical conduct in spiritual caregiving is essential. The following guidelines for nurses were offered by Winslow and Wehtje-Winslow (2007):

- First seek a basic understanding of patients' spiritual needs, resources, and preferences (i.e., assess).
- Follow the patient's expressed wishes regarding spiritual care.
- Do not prescribe or urge patients to adopt certain spiritual beliefs or practices, and do not pressure them to relinquish any of their beliefs or practices.
- Strive to understand personal spirituality and how it influences caregiving.
- Provide spiritual care in a way that is consonant with personal beliefs.

Although some patients are eager for nurses' overt offers of "spiritual care," others may be uncertain or opposed to such offers (Taylor, 2012). Patients often confuse religiosity with spirituality; this may contribute to their uncertainty about receiving spiritual care from nurses. Observing and using the patient's language for spirituality (e.g., "being at peace" or "faith") and exhibiting large measures of sensitivity and respect will help nurses to converse therapeutically with patients to provide spiritual care.

Before sharing personal beliefs or practices, a nurse must consider questions such as the following:

- For what purpose am I sharing my beliefs or practices? By doing so, am I meeting my needs or my patient's?
- Is my spiritual care reflecting a spiritual assessment?
- Am I preying on a vulnerable patient?
- Am I offering my beliefs or practices in a manner that allows my patient to comfortably refuse?
- Does my spiritual care hurt or contribute to a therapeutic relationship with the patient? (Taylor, 2012).

Prior to discussing ways nurses can support and nurture patient spirituality, it is also important to recognize how the spirituality of the nurse can impact the nurse–patient relationship (Taylor, 2012). How a nurse believes can affect the way that nurse provides care (Taylor, Gober, & Pfeiffer, 2014). For example, a nurse who believes God answers prayers for healing will likely be eager to pray for a patient (Minton, Isaacson, & Banik, 2016). The converse is also likely to be true. Therefore, it is important for the nurse to reflect on how his personal spirituality can ethically and effectively influence professional responsibilities. Also, the extent to which a nurse provides spiritual self-care may contribute to the extent with which that nurse is personally able to provide spiritual nurture (Taylor, 2012). See **Box 30–2 »** for suggestions for engaging in spiritual self-care.

Box 30–2
Spiritual Self-Care for Nurses

- Learn and practice mindfulness. That is, be tuned in mentally, emotionally, and physically to what you are experiencing in the present moment; do so without judgment about whether it is right or wrong. It will boost compassion for others and for yourself.
  - Classes, books, magazines, and internet sites offer much information about how to develop mindfulness.
  - Reflect on how mindful you are by taking the quiz at the Greater Good Science Center (http://greatergood.berkeley.edu/quizzes/take_quiz/4/).
- Recognize your own woundedness (e.g., fears, longings, obstructed goals). Know that it is this woundedness that allows you to be present to another's spiritual wounds. Although you do not need to have had the same experiences as your patients, you do need to be able to understand their emotions if you are to be compassionate—spiritually caring.
- Be as compassionate to yourself as you are to patients.
  - Helpful self-talk when you are hurting may include nonjudgmental, tender statements recognizing the pain as well as comforting comments (e.g., "This is hard; it is good to let myself admit this and feel it" and "My dear self, you are not alone; you are loved").

- Reflect on how kind you are to yourself by taking a 26-question Self-Compassion Scale available at http://self-compassion.org/test-how-self-compassionate-you-are/
- Experience self-compassion, the sacred source (a.k.a. God's love), when you are fully present to your woundedness. This may be felt as a softening of your "heart" when you are still.
- Remember there is a compassionate core in every person: "Call it the Buddha nature of love and compassion, the divinely bestowed image of God, the ever-present Beloved Lover, or simply the steady ember of our truest Self, a compassionate connection resides within every human heart—no matter how damaged or hardened that heart may become" (Rogers, 2015, p. 85).
- Notice the opening of your heart with compassion toward others when you realize that their woundedness essentially mirrors yours (e.g., you also have fears, longings, and obstructed goals).
- When you find yourself irritated or lacking compassion for a patient or colleague, appreciate that that person is functioning as a mirror and can teach you what needs compassion within yourself.

Engaging Community-based Spiritual Care Experts and Resources

If a patient is a member of a spiritual community, its leaders, members, and resources may provide support in various ways. For example, many religious traditions have systems in place for providing social support services to members in need (Taylor, 2012). These services may include respite care for caregivers, financial support, weekly visitations, or organizing meals and help with household duties.

Some religious traditions use lay leaders instead of trained clergy or may not have enough trained clergy to meet the needs of their congregants. Whether trained or untrained in pastoral counseling, a religious congregation or community will typically have someone whose role is to visit the sick (Taylor, 2012). Usually, it is the chaplain or family's prerogative to contact this religious leader.

Although not a prevalent resource, many large congregations (especially Christian) will have a faith community nurse (FCN) who is employed either by the congregation or by a local healthcare system. FCNs, or parish nurses, provide individual and community-oriented care for the congregation (e.g., home visits to the sick or elderly, health education or screening during church events) (Balint & George, 2015; Ziebarth, 2014). FCNs typically have received additional training in spiritual care. Their care is thought to help reduce hospital readmissions and lower healthcare costs (Yeaworth & Sailors, 2014; Ziebarth & Campbell, 2016).

Whether or not an FCN is present within a congregation, the faith community has often been found to be an excellent place for health promotion and disease screening, especially within African American Christian congregations. A number of health researchers have observed positive outcomes from health-related programs such as cancer or HIV screening, or lifestyle education for individuals with heart disease or diabetes (e.g., Brewer et al., 2016; Morris, 2015; Sattin et al., 2016). These typically integrate some aspect of the religion's beliefs into the program (e.g., reminding participants that their bodies are God's "temple").

Spiritual Therapies for Home or Hospital

There are several therapies that a nurse can recommend or facilitate that can promote spiritual well-being for a patient. Some of these are listed in **Table 30–1 》**.

SAFETY ALERT Nurses must recognize the limitations of their spiritual care abilities. Whereas some nurses may have knowledge and experience with a therapy, others may not. Nurses who do not have knowledge with a particular therapy may make tentative suggestions or call another nurse or expert to assist or follow up. Information from a trustworthy book or website may also be used.

Collaborating with Chaplains

Chaplains who are board certified are trained and credentialed in a religious tradition, as well as trained in counseling so that they can provide expert spiritual care regardless of a patient's spiritual or religious background. Chaplains provide assistance with religious rituals and support for patients and families with emotional, ethical, or spiritual concerns (Massey et al., 2015). Although a Swiss study of hospitalized patients found that the offer of a chaplain visit to a patient was half as likely to result in the acceptance of the offer if the offer was made by a nurse rather than a chaplain (Martinuz et al., 2013), nurses should still make such offers.

Research findings indicate that patients who are visited by a chaplain are more likely to be satisfied with the care

TABLE 30–1 Spiritual Therapies for Home or Hospital

Spiritual Therapy	Evidence/Rationale	Practice Suggestions
Altruism (Huber & MacDonald, 2012; Kahana et al., 2013; Marsh et al., 2015)	Oxytocin promotes altruism and altruism contributes to prosociality; it also is observed to predict life satisfaction and emotional and spiritual well-being.	■ Do a "random act of kindness" without expecting a reward, preferably one that involves some interaction with the recipient of the kindness ■ Savor the feeling of happiness the action provides (thereby creating a feedback loop) ■ Patients with limited abilities can phone or write to encourage others; smile at, listen empathically to, or pray for others; create inexpensive gifts to meet others' needs; and so forth
Awe (Piff et al., 2015; Van Cappelen & Saroglou, 2012)	Awe is "an emotional response to perceptually vast stimuli that transcend current frames of reference" (Piff et al.), and something that leaves one "feeling small." Awe is associated with greater prosociality, generosity, and ethical decision making. Awe may activate spiritual/religious feelings.	■ Provide virtual or real experiences in nature (e.g., video about galaxies, trip to local gorgeous place, sit under the night sky, National Geographic series) ■ Provide awe-inspiring music or other form of art, or stories that create a sense of awe (e.g., about a heroic act) ■ Remember that even gazing at the clouds out a hospital window or studying the dew on a blade of grass can stir awe ■ Recognize and cherish the feeling of awe for at least 15 seconds
Expressive artwork (Iliya, 2016; Robb et al., 2014; Yount, Rachlin, & Siegal, 2013)	Creating art is a means for self-expression and meaning making. It has been used in acute and community care settings with children, adolescents, individuals with mental health and disabilities, older adults, and individuals who have experienced trauma or displacement. Creative acts appear to lower cortisol (stress).	■ Expressive artwork can be completed individually or in a group setting ■ Depending on patient preferences, setting, and available resources, a type of art can be selected (e.g., digital media, drama, poetry, visual art) ■ An art, music, or play therapist, or recreation director may facilitate, or a nurse can simply provide materials and support ■ After the artwork is completed, it can be verbally discussed or performed—or kept private. If a patient wants to share, the nurse can ask the patient about what the artwork means or symbolizes for her ■ Reactions to the artwork are best if neutral and observational in nature
Dignity therapy (Chochinov et al., 2005; Fitchett et al., 2015)	Developed by psychiatrist Chochinov and evaluated in numerous settings and found to be effective for improving spiritual and emotional outcomes for patients at the end of life primarily. Encourages patients to tell their life story and construct meaning, and leave a legacy.	■ Listen deeply to patient's life stories, recognizing that they are attempts to make sense of one's life ■ Life stories can be recorded, transcribed, and compiled with photographs or other life mementos ■ Prompts can address what individuals view as important aspects or times in their lives, how they wish to be remembered, salient roles they have played in life, achievements, what they still want to say to others, what life lessons they wish to pass on ■ Whereas such extensive life storytelling is likely beyond the time resources of a nurse, a nurse can adapt the process or facilitate others (e.g., trained volunteers) to do this work
Gratitude (Emmons, 2013)	Affirming goodness and appreciating that this goodness comes from outside of yourself creates gratitude. It is associated with prosociality, emotional well-being, and other positive outcomes.	■ Intentionally look for opportunities to verbally express thanks to others (e.g., write a letter of gratitude) ■ Journal or make lists of graces for which one is thankful (e.g., journal five events at the end of each day that created meaning or gratitude) ■ Breathe deeply in a sense of grace and breathe out gratitude ■ Savor for 15 seconds the feeling accompanying acknowledgement of the grace and gratitude
Mindfulness, meditation (Boccia, Piccardi, & Guariglia, 2015; Buttle, 2015; Marchand, 2012)	Of Buddhist origin yet pervading Western societies, mindfulness meditation techniques have been adapted for Christian prayer and as a nonreligious lifestyle strategy for improving health and overall well-being. Numerous studies document various physical, psychologic, and spiritual benefits for those who practice mindfulness regularly.	Mindfulness techniques vary, but key elements include: ■ Focused attention on the present moment, the body's experience ■ Awareness, depth, and steadiness of breathing ■ Put judgmental and intrusive thoughts "on hold" ■ Mindfulness can be taught individually or in groups by a mindfulness expert; manualized training to nurses can prepare them to support patients to meditate
Writing a prayer or spiritual expression (Bennett & Elliott, 2013; Toussaint et al., 2014)	Writing about negative life events is known to improve emotional and physical well-being. Writing about negatives in the form of a prayer or as a spiritual expression may contribute to similar positive outcomes.	■ Encourage the patient to express feelings as well as facts; authenticity of expression may be an indicator of depth of the relationship with the divine ■ Writing can be put in a diary, laptop, or scratchpad; ensuring privacy for the written work is paramount ■ When writing a prayer (e.g., questions about suffering) to God, one can do so with the dominant hand; next, write with the nondominant hand any spontaneous thoughts that occur in response. These may be divinely inspired.

they receive at the hospital and be more likely to perceive that their emotional and spiritual needs were met (Marin et al., 2015; Sharma et al., 2016). Smith and colleagues (2013) explored how young persons with cancer who do not receive spiritual support from a chaplain were more likely to have worse quality of life, fatigue, and physical, emotional, social, and school/work function that those who did

receive spiritual services (N = 525, age 15–39). Although chaplains are increasingly generating evidence that their work produces positive outcomes, they often are not called until death is imminent (Choi, Curlin, & Cox, 2015). Nurses can be instrumental in making referrals to chaplains and collaborating with them to support patients' spiritual well-being at any stage of illness.

REVIEW The Concept of Spirituality

RELATE Link the Concepts

Linking the concept of spirituality with the concept of development:

1. How might a nurse address the spiritual needs of an 8-year-old child who has leukemia?

2. How might a nurse address the spiritual needs of a teenager with cystic fibrosis?

Linking the concept of spirituality with the concept of culture and diversity:

3. What could a nurse say to a Muslim patient who wants to fast during the day because it is the month of Ramadan, even though his physician has ordered a clear liquid diet?

4. How would you preoperatively prepare a Khalsid Sikh man for surgery requiring shaving of body hair when this man has vowed to never cut his hair?

REFER Go to Pearson MyLab Nursing and eText

- Additional review materials

REFLECT Apply Your Knowledge

Yasmeen is a 32-year-old woman who is 7 months pregnant. She presents to the emergency department complaining of moderate

vaginal bleeding and significant tenderness around her abdomen. She wears a long dress and scarf over her hair. While her husband, Khaled, is parking their car, Jonathan, her RN, quickly wheels her into a room and asks her to lie on a gurney. He pulls her gown up while simultaneously trying to protect her pelvic area from view by covering it with a blanket. He quickly works to expose her belly and apply a fetal monitor. Yasmeen appears very uncomfortable, but Jonathan assumes she is anxious because she could lose her baby. Just as the monitor begins to indicate signs of fetal distress, Khaled enters the room and insists that Jonathan leave immediately and get a female RN and MD for Yasmeen. He also quickly moves to cover Yasmeen's exposed belly and pull the falling scarf back over her hair.

1. The other female RNs in the ED are busy with a trauma patient, and time is of essence to care for Yasmeen and the fetus. What should Jonathan do?

2. Jonathan knows that the only ED physicians in house now are male. What should he say to Khaled?

3. If no female staff are available to help patient who refuses a male healthcare provider, what measures can be taken to promote modesty? How could you help a female patient who is disturbed by wearing a hospital gown that exposes her arms and legs?

4. If Yasmeen and Khaled's infant dies, what words or actions might comfort them?

≫ Exemplar 30.A
Spiritual Distress

Exemplar Learning Outcomes

30.A Analyze spiritual distress as it relates to patient health.

- Describe spiritual distress as the etiology.
- Apply the nursing process in providing culturally competent care to an individual with spiritual distress.

Exemplar Key Term

Presencing, *2036*

Overview

Spiritual beliefs and practices, whether religious or not, can be a strongly sustaining influence for critically or chronically ill patients and their families. As discussed earlier in this module, spiritual distress may be characterized by expressions of a deficit in meaning, purpose, hope, forgiveness, intimacy with the divine, and anger or a lack of interest about previously spiritually nurturing persons or

resources (Carpenito-Moyet, 2013). For example, "I'll never forgive myself/them!" "What good is it now to keep on living?" or "I'm never going to pray again, because what good did it do me?" No list of spiritual distress characteristics can be complete, however, considering the complexity and variability of individuals and their spiritual dimensions. By addressing spiritual distress (or the potential for spiritual distress), nurses are providing care that is truly healing and holistic.

Addressing Spiritual Distress

Spiritual distress may affect other areas of functioning and indicate other diagnoses. In these instances, spiritual distress may be the etiology. Examples of nursing diagnoses related to spiritual distress include the following:

- *Fear* related to apprehension about the soul's future after death and unpreparedness for death
- *Chronic* or *Situational Low Self-Esteem* related to failure to live within the precepts of one's faith
- *Disturbed Sleep Pattern* related to spiritual distress
- *Ineffective Coping* related to feelings of abandonment by God and loss of religious faith
- *Decisional Conflict* related to conflict between treatment plan and religious beliefs.

(NANDA-I © 2014)

NURSING PROCESS

Patients in spiritual distress require the nurse's thoughtful interventions to be performed in a timely manner. Although the nurse may not be able to provide the spiritual guidance patients require, the nurse can use sensitivity and therapeutic communication to help patients explore their feelings and work through their distress and help them talk with an individual who can provide the necessary spiritual guidance such as a religious leader, spiritual guide, or elder in their community.

Assessment

As part of the assessment of the patient, ask questions to determine the patient's spiritual beliefs and practices and how they affect or are affected by the patient's health condition. Asking open-ended questions such as "What was going on in your thoughts when you learned about the possible problems that can happen with your treatment?" serve to build the nurse–patient relationship as well as eliciting information the nurse will need to formulate the plan of care. Patient statements such as "Why is God doing this to me?" "I don't care anymore," and "I wish I were dead" indicate that the patient is in spiritual distress. A quality improvement project related screening for spiritual distress to patient satisfaction with and trust in their overall care for patients on an inpatient oncology unit (Blanchard, 2012). The findings concluded that nurses are interested in the spiritual well-being of their patients and assess for spiritual distress. When nurses were more likely to use referrals to chaplains after a brief spiritual screening protocol, patients reported improved patient outcomes and fewer harmful effects of spiritual distress.

Diagnosis

Carpenito-Moyet (2013) recognized three diagnoses related to spirituality: *Spiritual Distress*, *Readiness for Enhanced Spiritual Well-Being* (which recognizes that some individuals respond to adversity with an increased sensitivity to spirituality or spiritual maturation), and *Risk for Spiritual Distress* (which may be appropriate for a patient who currently shows no indication of this disruption of spirit yet may if a nurse fails to intervene).

Planning

In the planning phase, the nurse identifies interventions to help the patient achieve the overall goal of maintaining or restoring spiritual well-being so that the patient may realize spiritual strength, serenity, and satisfaction. Outcomes of care may include the following:

- The patient will fulfill religious obligations.
- The patient will find meaning in existence and the present situation.
- The patient will feel a sense of hope.
- The patient will have access to spiritual resources as needed.

Implementation

Spiritual care can include anything that supports spiritual well-being; it can be, for example, any of the following diverse actions:

- Recognize and validate the inner resources of an individual, such as coping methods, humor, motivation, self-determination, positive attitude, and optimism.
- Assist the patient to leave a legacy by storytelling and/or recording life stories for family and friends, and encouraging creative expression through art, music, and writing.
- Foster ways for patients to keep in touch with nature and maintain a sense of wonder.
- Facilitate a reunion with an estranged child.
- Provide a story about how someone in similar circumstances maintained hope and grew spiritually.
- Recognize that the seasons, the emergence of flowers in spring, the phases of the moon, and the migrations of birds provide examples of orderliness in the universe, even in the midst of chaos and loss.

Whereas there are spiritually nurturing activities and therapeutics that a nurse can introduce to a patient, what is likely most important is that the nurse is present to the patient in ways that communicate, "I hear you; I am with you; you are important; I will not judge you."

Provide Presence

Presencing refers to "just" being there or with a patient. Du Plessis (2016) observed that presencing can be the entering wedge for nurses wanting to provide spiritual care. That is, an inexperienced nurse who is uncomfortable with the intimate nature of spiritual care may be able to offer presencing. In a classic article about presencing, Pettigrew (1990) identified four distinguishing features: giving of self in the present moment, being available with all of the self, listening with full awareness of the privilege of doing so, and being there in a way that is meaningful to another individual.

To be fully present to a patient, a nurse must be purposefully attentive (Fahlberg & Roush, 2015). To be comfortable being fully present to another person, however, one must be comfortable being fully present to oneself (du Plessis, 2016). Strategies for increasing the ability to be present to a patient include:

- Slow down. Calm yourself.

- Make sure that in your "heart" you are willing to be present. Taking deep, slow breaths to center yourself. Nurses who listen attentively to patients yet fail to give of self (i.e., inwardly "make room") diminish their effectiveness.

- Sit down; keep your eye level at the same level as the patient's.

- Allow silence.

- Smile or exude positive energy while remaining respectful of the patient's emotional state (e.g., convey quiet, inner courage if the patient is experiencing sorrow or despair). Follow the patient's nonverbal cues.

- Focus. With whatever brief or long amount of time you have available, use it maximally by focusing completely on the patient. Be physically, emotionally, and mentally present.

- Empathize with the patient; actively and deeply listen (Fahlberg & Roush, 2015; Penque & Kearney, 2015; Taylor, 2007).

- Self-disclosure (e.g., telling the patient about how you overcame a similar situation) is never appropriate unless the patient requests it and it is shared with therapeutic intent rather than for self-serving reasons. (Ask, "Whose needs are being met here?")

Presencing is often the best and sometimes the only intervention to support a patient who suffers under circumstances that medical interventions cannot address. When a patient is helpless, powerless, and vulnerable, a nurse's presencing can be most beneficial. Rather than worrying about saying or doing "the right thing," nurses should focus on being fully present (Taylor, 2007).

Refer Patients for Spiritual Counseling

In some cases spiritual care is best referred to other members of the healthcare team. Referrals can be made for hospitalized patients and their families through the hospital chaplain's office if one is available. Nurses in home and community health settings can identify spiritual resources by checking directories of community service agencies, telephone directories, or religious directories that describe available spiritual counselors and the services provided through the religious community. Many religious counselors will provide assistance to members of their faith who are not members of their specific religious community. For example, a priest may attend a patient in the hospital or at home even though the individual is not a member of the priest's parish. The patient's permission is needed before seeking an outside counselor in order to protect the patient's right to confidentiality.

Referrals may be necessary when the nurse makes a diagnosis of spiritual distress. A nurse and religious counselor can work together to meet the patient's needs. One situation the nurse may encounter is patient refusal of necessary medical intervention because of religious tenets. In this case, the nurse encourages the patient, primary care provider, and spiritual adviser to discuss the conflict and consider alternative methods of therapy. The nurse's major roles are to provide information the patient needs to make an informed decision and to support and advocate for the patient's decision.

Evaluation

Using the measurable desired outcomes developed during the planning stage, the nurse collects data needed to judge whether patient goals and outcomes have been achieved. Appropriate outcomes for the patient who needs to maintain or be restored to spiritual health include the following:

- The patient identifies purposeful activities or ways of thinking.

- The patient articulates a sense of hopefulness about the future.

- The patient articulates how to access spiritual resources.

- The patient finds meaning and existence in the present situation.

Nursing Care Plan
A Patient with Spiritual Distress

ASSESSMENT	DIAGNOSES	PLANNING
Ms. Sally Horton is a 60-year-old hospitalized homemaker who is recovering from a right radical mastectomy. Her primary care provider told her yesterday that because of metastases of the cancer, her prognosis is poor. This morning her nurse finds her tearful, stating that she slept poorly and has no appetite. She asks the nurse, "Why has God done this to me? Perhaps it's because I have sinned in my life. I've not gone to church or spoken to a minister in several years. Is there a chapel in the hospital where I could go and pray? I'm terribly afraid of dying and what awaits me."	■ *Spiritual Distress* related to feelings of guilt and alienation from God as evidenced by questioning why "God has done this"; inquiries about praying in a chapel; insomnia; no appetite (NANDA-I © 2014)	■ The patient will interact with a spiritual leader from her faith. ■ The patient will read about spiritual practices that provide her comfort. ■ The patient will start a gratitude journal. ■ The patient will connect with others to share thoughts, feelings, and beliefs.

(continued on next page)

Nursing Care Plan (continued)

IMPLEMENTATION

- Create an accepting, nonjudgmental atmosphere.
- Assist her to express and reflect on her anger.
- Encourage the use of spiritual resources, if desired by the patient.

- Encourage verbalization of feelings, perceptions, and fears. Allow time for grieving.
- Referral to spiritual care expert of patient's choice to discuss self-forgiveness and perception that God may be punishing her.

EVALUATION

Ms. Horton has been visited on several occasions by her minister. She reads scripture each day and has found consolation in reading the book of Psalms. She states, "God is merciful and will help me bear my suffering."

CRITICAL THINKING

1. What spiritual resources might you recommend for this patient?
2. If Ms. Horton's husband believes that her disease is a result of sins committed throughout life, how could you help this patient?
3. If your religious beliefs would help this patient obtain spiritual well-being, what actions could you take to help this patient?

REVIEW Spiritual Distress

RELATE Link the Concepts and Exemplars

Linking the exemplar of spiritual distress with the concept of oxygenation:

1. Describe the risk for spiritual distress faced by the parents of a child who has just died from sudden infant death syndrome.

2. What caring interventions would you offer to the child's parents?

Linking the exemplar of spiritual distress with the concept of development:

3. What signals or words might indicate that an 8-year-old child from a Protestant Christian family is in spiritual distress? What caring interventions would be appropriate for a child this age?

4. How might a teenager communicate spiritual distress? What interventions would be appropriate for a teenager that would not be appropriate for a younger child?

REFER Go to Pearson MyLab Nursing and eText

- Additional review materials

REFLECT Apply Your Knowledge

Terry Mears is a 32-year-old man who received several pints of blood following an automobile crash 10 years ago. Five years ago he was diagnosed with AIDS, and he is now in the hospital with pneumonia and severe diarrhea. He is very ill and very discouraged. While you are caring for Mr. Mears, he comments, "I might as well die right now because I'm not going to get well. My folks were Methodist, but I guess I'm being punished because I'm not very religious."

1. Mr. Mears stated that he was "not very religious." Does that mean that he is not spiritual? Explain.

2. What data suggest that Mr. Mears may be experiencing spiritual distress?

3. How might illness affect one's spiritual beliefs? Religious beliefs?

4. How might a spiritual assessment be of benefit to both you and Mr. Mears?

≫ Exemplar 30.B
Religion

Exemplar Learning Outcomes

30.B Analyze religion as it relates to spirituality.

- List characteristics shared by all religions.
- Outline the components of religion.
- Compare the aspects of religion that affect medical care.

- Apply the nursing process in providing culturally competent care to a religious patient.

Exemplar Key Terms

Denomination, *2040*
Holy day, *2039*

Overview

Religion is an organized, communal approach to human spirituality. In its simplest terms, a religion provides its members with the constructs of beliefs, moral values, and spiritual practices that guide its members' expressions of their spirituality. Although religion is typically practiced in a community setting, such as a church, synagogue, or mosque, most religious individuals also practice their religion outside of this setting in various ways, and individuals who are separated from their religious community will often continue their observations of holy days and rituals in private.

Although there are many differences among religions, there are also many similarities. Characteristics common among all religions include:

- **Belief in god(s) or higher power.** Adherents of some religions, including Hinduism, Buddhism, and modern paganism, worship multiple gods.
- **Belief that the god or higher power has influence over humanity.**
- **Direct communication.** Members believe they communicate with the higher power, usually in the form of prayer that is expressive and receptive. Dreams, meditations, corporate worship, and rituals may also be means for human–divine communication and interaction.
- **Community.** Members typically worship collectively on a regular basis in a communal setting, such as a church, synagogue, gurdwara, temple, or mosque. Some religions use ritual rites of passage to admit new members (e.g., doctrinal or confirmation classes and baptism for most Christians).
- **Ethical or moral codes.** Probably the single best-known example of a religious moral code is the Ten Commandments.

Many societies have taboos or laws that prevent individuals or communities from expressing or practicing religion. Some countries have state religions (e.g., Islam in many Middle East countries, Eastern Orthodox traditions in Russia); these countries may or may not be welcoming to other religions. The U.S. Constitution mandates that religion be separate from government, yet how this doctrine of the separation of church and state is applied in society continues to be debated and interpreted.

Components of Religion

Religions also have similarities and differences about how to think about health, illness, suffering, and death. The very brief descriptions included later in this exemplar are mere snapshots intended to raise awareness of some important areas of health and healthcare that can be affected by an individual's religion. When appropriate, nurses should assess how patients' spiritual or religious beliefs and practices affect their approach to healthcare. These beliefs and practices often pertain to how patients relate to sacred time, scripture, symbols, and to the divine through prayer and other practices.

Holy Days

A **holy day** is a day set aside for special religious observance; all world religions observe certain holy days. For example, Christians (Catholics, Orthodox, and Protestants) observe Easter and Christmas, Jews observe Yom Kippur and Passover, Buddhists observe the birthday of the Buddha, Muslims observe the month-long holy period of Ramadan, and Hindus observe Mahashivratri, a celebration of Lord Shiva. Many religions require fasting, extended prayer, and reflection or ritual observances on sacred (or high holy) days. Believers who are seriously ill are often exempted from such requirements. Because many religions follow calendars other than the Gregorian calendar, a multifaith calendar can be used to identify the holy days of the various religious groups (Taylor, 2012).

The concept of the Sabbath is common to Christianity and Judaism, in response to the biblical commandment "Remember the Sabbath day to keep it holy." Most Christians view Sunday as "the Lord's day," whereas Jews and sabbatarian Christians (e.g., Seventh-day Adventists) observe their Sabbath on Saturday. Muslims (particularly men) traditionally gather on Friday at noon to worship and learn about their faith. Patients who are devout in their religious practices may want to avoid any special treatments or other intrusions on their day of rest and reflection.

Sacred Writings

Each religion has sacred and authoritative scriptures that provide guidance for its adherents' beliefs and behaviors. In addition, sacred writings frequently tell instructive stories of the religion's leaders, kings, and heroes. In most religions, these scriptures are thought to be the word of God or the Supreme Being as written down by prophets or other human representatives. Christians rely on the Bible, Jews on the Torah and Talmud, and Muslims on the Quran; Hindus have several holy texts, or Vedas; and Buddhists value the teachings of the Tripitakas. Scriptures generally set forth religious law in the form of admonitions and rules for living. This religious law may be interpreted in various ways by subgroups of a religion, and this may affect a patient's willingness to accept treatment suggestions.

Individuals often gain strength and hope from reading religious writings when they are ill or in crisis. Examples of scriptural stories that may give comfort to patients are Job's suffering, found in both the Jewish and Christian scriptures, and Jesus's healing of individuals who were physically or mentally ill, as outlined in the New Testament of the Bible.

Sacred Symbols

Sacred symbols include jewelry, medals, amulets, clothing, or body ornamentation (e.g., tattoos) that may be worn as a symbol of faith, for spiritual protection, or as a source of comfort and strength. Some individuals may wear religious medals at all times, and they may wish to wear them when they are undergoing diagnostic studies, medical treatment, or surgery. Individuals who are Roman Catholic may carry a rosary for prayer (see **Figure 30–5 》**); an individual who is Muslim may carry a mala, or string of prayer beads.

Individuals may have religious icons, altars, statues, totems, or other religious objects in their home, car, or place of work as a personal reminder of their faith or as part of a personal place of worship or meditation. Hospitalized patients or long-term care residents may wish to have their spiritual icons or objects with them as a source of comfort.

Prayer and Meditation

Prayer is "human communication with divine and spiritual entities" (Gill, 1987, p. 489). Some argue that because prayer requires a belief in a divine or spiritual entity, not all individuals pray, while others consider prayer a universal phenomenon that does not require such belief. Ulanov and Ulanov (1983), for example, proposed that everyone prays: "People pray whether or not they call it prayer. We pray

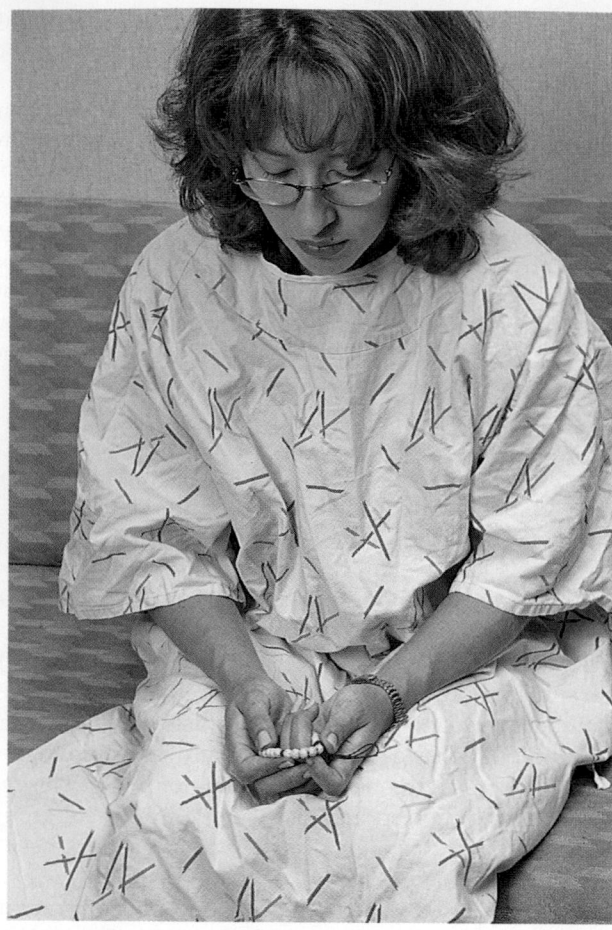

Figure 30–5 》 Patients may bring objects to the hospital to use in prayer or other religious rituals. Caregivers should respect such objects, because they usually have great significance for patients.

every time we ask for help, understanding, or strength, in or out of religion . . . who and what we are speak out of us. . . . To pray is to listen to and hear this self who is speaking" (p. 1). Prayer continues to be prevalent in American society. In a 2014 Pew Research Center survey, only 23% of those surveyed reported they seldom or never pray. The remaining respondents report praying daily (55%) or weekly or monthly (21%) (Pew Research Center, 2015).

Prayer experiences vary. Categories of prayer that still influence how researchers think about prayer have been identified by Poloma and Gallup (1991):

- **Ritual** (e.g., the Lord's Prayer, memorized prayers that can be repeated)

- **Petitionary** (e.g., "God, cure me!" or intercessory prayers when one is requesting something of the divine)

- **Colloquial** (i.e., conversational prayers)

- **Meditational** (e.g., moments of silence focused on nothing, a meaningful phrase, or a certain aspect of the divine).

Although meditational and colloquial prayer experiences have been found to be associated with spiritual well-being and good quality of life in healthy adults, ritual and petitionary prayer experiences may be most comforting and appropriate for those who are ill.

Some religions have prescribed prayers that are printed in a prayer book, such as the Anglican/Episcopal *Book of Common Prayer* or the Catholic missal. Some religious prayers are attributed to the source of faith; for example, the Lord's Prayer for Christians is attributed to Jesus, and the first sutra for Muslims is attributed to Mohammed.

Some religions require daily prayers or dictate specific times for prayer, meditation, or worship: the five daily prayers, or Salat, of the Muslims are performed while facing east toward Mecca at dawn, noon, midafternoon, sunset, and evening (see **Figure 30–6 》**). Other examples include the daily Kaddish of the Jews and the seven canonical prayers of the Roman Catholics. Individuals who are ill may want to continue or increase their prayer practices (Taylor, 2012). They may need uninterrupted quiet time during which they have their prayer books, rosaries, malas, or other icons available to them. Nurses can help patients by ensuring a quiet time for them to pray or meditate.

Aspects of Religion That Affect Medical Care

There are many categories (broad forms or types) of religions. Within each category are any number of **denominations**, subgroups with somewhat distinctive practices and beliefs. Even within a specific denomination, there may be further sects or denominations within the larger group. For example, there are Serbian, Greek, Russian, and other denominations of Eastern Orthodox Christians. There are Sunni, Shia, and Sufi Muslims as well as different types of Buddhists, Lutherans, Baptists, Jews, and so forth. Because of the great diversity of religious beliefs and practices even within one religious tradition or denomination, it is important to assess how patients interpret and apply their religion to their present health challenge (Taylor, 2012). Likewise, a patient who belonged to a particular religion as a child may have since modified her practices to suit her evolving beliefs.

The following sampling reviews some of the unique and salient religious beliefs and practices pertinent to healthcare. Although this information can help the nurse to be aware and supportive of each patient's religiosity, the nurse must always ask patients about their preferences.

Buddhism

Buddhism originated in Asia and spread throughout that continent, and many Asians are influenced by its teachings. Practicing Buddhists generally prefer Eastern medicine, believing that most illnesses can be cured through the mind and the use of herbs. This does not mean that Buddhists will refuse Western medicine. However, a Buddhist patient or patient of Asian origin may use traditional therapies in addition to those prescribed by a healthcare provider. Buddhists may be vegetarian, maintain an altar to Buddha, and practice a form of meditation.

Hinduism

Hinduism is a religion practiced by individuals from India and other parts of southern Asia. Typically, Hindus embrace Western medicine, but they will also employ alternative therapies from their culture such as yoga and various

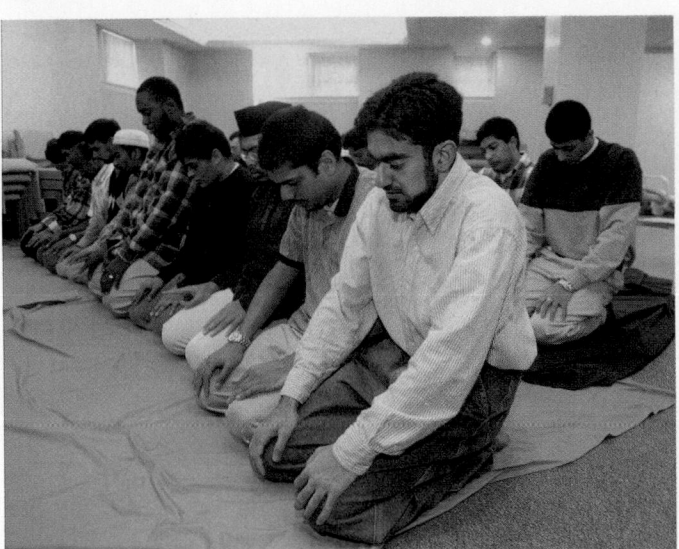

Source: John Gillis/AP Images.

Figure 30–6 >> Muslim students at Johns Hopkins University at their weekly prayer meeting.

Ayurvedic remedies. Hindus generally do not eat beef or much meat, and may prefer not to use medications that are derived from animals. Many will have food preferences and will want to achieve balance between foods thought to generate heat versus coolness within the body. Because Hindus greatly value cleanliness, nurses may need to offer support for specific cleansing rituals at the start of the day or before a meal. Hindus generally believe that they have more than one life, and as a result may choose not to participate in organ donation. As with many other religions, Hinduism has ceremonial rites that are practiced at the time of dying and immediately after death.

Islam

Islam is the second largest religion in the world, and those who practice Islam are called Muslims. Because many Muslims view events in their lives as a direct result of God's will, they may view illness or death as the will of God and therefore believe that healing can take place only through God's will. Cleanliness and modesty are of great importance in Islam. Respect modesty, avoid nakedness. Be scrupulous about keeping all but hands, face, and feet covered for the conservative Muslim woman. If possible, provide a nurse of the same gender to care for the patient. If not possible, allow a colleague or family member of the patient's gender to be present, leave a window or door ajar (if the patient is not exposed physically), and touch the patient only as necessary to conduct procedures (e.g., do not extend a handshake or caring touch). A male family member may request to remain present when a woman or girl is being examined or treated, as the role of protector is taken seriously. Practicing Muslims follow dietary practices that avoid overeating, alcohol, and pork and pork-based products. During the month of Ramadan, Muslims fast during daylight hours, although exceptions may be made for those who are weak or ill. Muslims are obligated to pray five times a day, so nurses working with Muslim patients should take these prayer times into consideration. These prayers occur at dawn, midday, late afternoon, after sunset, and late evening. Prior to prayer, ablutions (cleansing rituals) are performed; if the patient cannot use water, sand may be substituted. Prayers are made while facing the direction of Mecca, the Muslim holy city in Saudi Arabia.

Judaism

Typically, Jewish individuals participate actively in their medical care and seek treatment from modern Western doctors. Many Jews keep to a kosher diet to varying degrees (e.g., avoid pork and shellfish, do not mix dairy and meat). Sabbath observance varies (e.g., Orthodox Jews avoid traveling in vehicles, writing, turning on electric appliances and lights); some may refrain from healthcare activities, whereas others will want to not interrupt them. Traditionally Jews pray three times a day in a group; however, a nurse can pray with a Jew using "God" or "Lord" to address the divine. Because there are prescribed Jewish rituals for individuals who are near death and for the time of and after death, Jewish families will often request the presence of a rabbi, a Jewish spiritual leader, when they know a loved one is near death. Jewish burial customs require the dead to be buried as soon as possible, preferably within 24 hours.

Christianity

Although all Christians believe that Jesus was the Son of God and most accept a trinitarian God of Father, Son, and Holy Spirit, there are myriad Christian traditions. After Jesus was crucified, resurrected, and returned to His Father in heaven, the early Christian fellowship evolved into the western European branch of Roman Catholicism and the eastern branch of Orthodox Christianity, making those two denominations the earliest Christians. Then, in medieval times, a movement to reform the Roman Catholic church arose, leading to many subsequent Protestant denominations (e.g., Episcopalians, Methodists, Baptists, Lutherans, Presbyterians, and Anabaptists [e.g., Mennonites]) (see **Figure 30–7 >>**). In the 19th century in the United States, several churches emerged that are typically considered Protestant (e.g., Latter-Day Saints, Jehovah's Witnesses, Seventh-day Adventists, and Christian Scientists).

Like those of most world faiths, Christians in the United States (Catholics, Orthodox, and Protestants) believe their body is a "temple" of God and life is a grace. They generally embrace Western medicine, although they may differ in their views about birth control, abortion, same-sex marriage, and end-of-life care. A few of the unique religious practices not mentioned already in this module follow:

- Anabaptists denomination members may not have insurance coverage and rely on their religious community for support; however, they may refuse expensive healthcare, believing it is poor stewardship.

- Although most Christians will appreciate receiving the Eucharist or Holy Communion, Anglicans, Episcopalians, and Roman Catholics may be especially dutiful about receiving it. Communion is a ritual of ingesting bread and wine (or grape juice) led by clergy or lay leaders to commemorate the death of Jesus. The Lenten season (the 40 days from Ash Wednesday to Easter) may involve some degree of abstention from food.

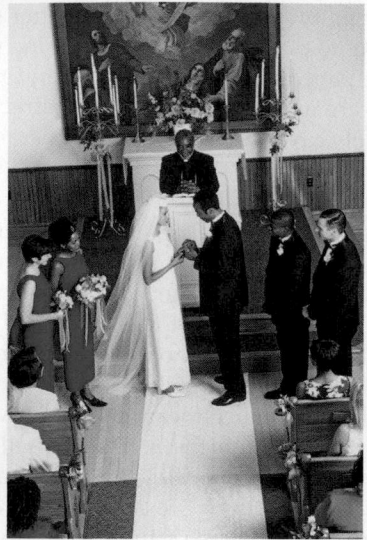 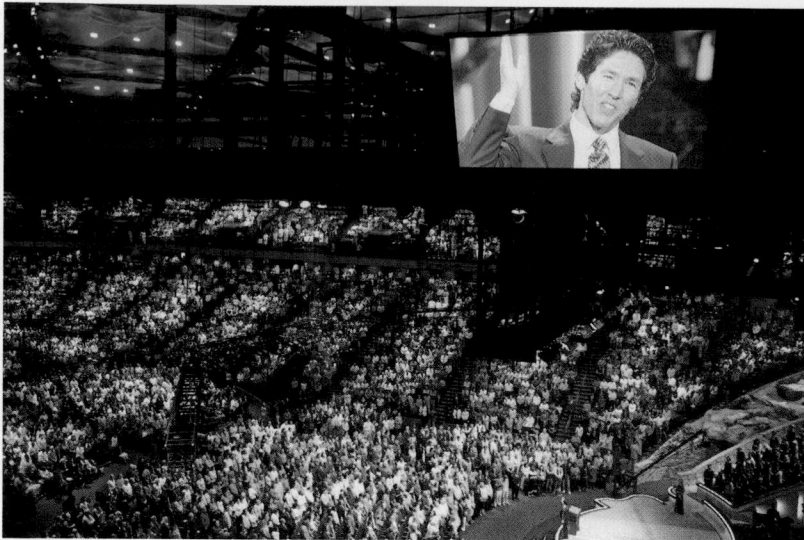

Source: ***A,*** Buccina Studios/Photodisc/Getty Images. ***B,*** Timothy Fadek/Corbis News/Getty Images.

Figure 30–7 》 There are more than 300,000 Protestant churches in the United States. Surveys show that 90% of them serve fewer than 350 people while the other 10% are megachurches with anywhere from 3000 to 30,000 worshippers each week. Half of all those who attend a Protestant church attend a megachurch (National Congregations Study, 2015).

- Christian Scientists typically oppose Western medical interventions, relying instead on lay and professional Christian Science practitioners. Faith and a positive attitude are paramount.

- Jehovah's Witnesses refuse most blood products. Alternative treatments such as blood conservation strategies, autologous techniques, hematopoietic agents, non-blood volume expanders, and so on can be discussed with the patient, who may want contact with the local Jehovah's Witness hospital liaison committee.

- Latter-Day Saints (LDS or Mormons) avoid alcohol, coffee, tea, and smoking. They may wear temple undergarments, which should be treated with respect.

- Seventh-Day Adventists likely will avoid unnecessary treatments on Sabbath, which begins at Friday sundown and ends at Saturday sundown. Adventists prefer restful, spirit-nurturing, family activities on Sabbaths. They are often vegetarian and abstain from caffeinated beverages, and do not smoke or drink alcohol.

- Roman Catholic doctrine posits that life begins at conception and should not be tampered with; therefore, abortion, euthanasia, and birth control are sinful. Confession of one's sins to a priest and accepting absolution from the priest is an important healing sacrament. Nurses working with a very sick or dying member of the Roman Catholic faith will want to make sure that the family has the opportunity to call for a priest to administer the sacrament of the Anointing of the Sick. Be aware that some patients may think that an offer of this sacrament means they are dying; in fact, it may be administered to anyone who is seriously ill or about to undergo a major operation.

- Orthodox Christians are urged to remain in contact with their local priest, rather than a hospital chaplain. Fasts from certain foods are often observed (i.e., most Wednesdays, Fridays, and Lent); these are relaxed for those who are ill, depending on their circumstances.

NURSING PROCESS

The nursing process can be applied to spiritual or religious care.

Assessment

As discussed in the Concept section of this module, assessment of the patient's spiritual or religious beliefs and practices occurs as part of the nursing history. The longer the patient's hospitalization or institutionalization, the more important this assessment becomes. In addition, any patient with an illness or injury that may result in a threat to life should be assessed for religious practices and spiritual needs. Depending on the patient's circumstances, nurses likely will need to inquire about religious practices related to:

- Diet (e.g., "What dietary preferences do you have? Are there specific foods or drinks you avoid, or certain diets for certain days that you try to keep?")

- Prayers, devotions, or worship desires (e.g., "What do you like to do to keep hopeful or find comfort?" or "How can we support you with any spiritual practices you like to do regularly? For example, do you like to pray, meditate, or read to be inspired or comforted?")

- Sacred objects (e.g., "Are there any personal items [sacred or religious objects or books or things] that we should make sure do not get lost here?")

- Prohibitions regarding medical procedures or treatments (if any).

Note the nonreligious language of the illustrative assessment questions.

Diagnosis

Any number of health challenges can threaten an individual's ability to practice his religion. NANDA International has three nursing diagnoses that reflect patient religious issues: *Impaired Religiosity, Risk for Impaired Religiosity,* and *Readiness for Enhanced Religiosity* (Carpenito-Moyet, 2013).

The religious patient and family may observe a number of religious practices at home, and these may be an essential part of each day in the life of the family. *Interrupted Family Processes* and *Readiness for Enhanced Family Coping* may also be appropriate diagnoses if these normal daily practices are disturbed by hospitalization. Because the individual's sense of self may be closely tied to his religious practices, *Risk for Compromised Human Dignity* and *Risk for Powerlessness* may also be appropriate diagnoses.

Impaired religiosity is the impaired ability to exercise reliance on religious beliefs and/or participate in rituals of a particular faith tradition. Illness or injury that disrupts religious practice can impair the patient's religiosity and result in emotional distress. An example of impaired religiosity might be the situation of the Roman Catholic patient who attends daily Mass but is on enforced bedrest or requires an extended hospitalization, or the Muslim patient who says evening prayers daily at the local mosque and is in the same situation.

In certain situations, a medical condition may require a decision that is in conflict with a patient's or family's religious practice. For example, a pregnant patient who believes that life begins at conception discovers at 20–22 weeks' gestation that she will not be able to carry the fetus to term and attempting to do so will most likely result in her death. How will she decide what to do? If she had been trying for years to get pregnant without success, how would that influence her decision? How would her decision be affected if she had two small children at home? In such a situation in which a medical condition presents a complication that is at odds with a patient's faith, the nursing diagnosis of *Risk for Impaired Religiosity* may be appropriate.

The relationship between the individual and her religion and religious practices is complex. Sometimes events that might threaten one individual's faith strengthen the faith of another. *Readiness for enhanced religiosity* is defined as the ability to increase reliance on religious beliefs and/or participate in rituals of a particular faith tradition.

Planning

When planning care, the nurse attempts to preserve the patient's and family's ability to observe their religious practices to every extent possible. This may include the following goals of care:

- The patient will be able to participate in religious observances as the patient desires.
- The patient will be able to participate in prayer at prescribed times without interruption.
- The patient will receive meals in keeping with religious dietary restrictions or requirements.
- The patient will have access to religious resources, including ministers, prayer partners, sacred texts, and sacred objects.

Implementation

Providing care related to the patient's religious needs must be done with great tact and sensitivity. The nurse's own religious beliefs may influence the approach to implementing care, but the nurse should never preach or proselytize his or her own beliefs and practices; rather, the nurse should focus on supporting the needs of the patient.

Support Religious Practices

Nurses need to consider specific religious practices that will affect nursing care, such as the patient's beliefs about birth, death, dress, diet, prayer, sacred symbols, sacred writings, and holy days. See **Box 30–3 »** for ways in which the nurse can help patients to continue their usual spiritual practices.

Assist Patients with Prayer

Prayer involves a sense of love and connection, as well as a reaching out. It offers a means for someone to talk to a greater power, a mechanism for expressing care, and a sense of serenity and connection with something greater. Evidence indicates that prayer boosts emotional and spiritual well-being (Jors & Bussing, 2015). From a national survey of Americans, Schafer (2013) found that when people knew that others were praying for them, they were more optimistic. Thus, this study suggests that telling patients that you are praying for them is a type of social support with positive impact.

Box 30–3
Supporting Religious Practices

- Create a trusting relationship with the patient so that any religious concerns or practices can be openly discussed and addressed.
- If unsure of the patient's religious needs, ask how nurses can assist in having these needs met. Avoid relying on personal assumptions when caring for patients.
- Do not discuss personal spiritual beliefs with a patient unless the patient requests it. Be sure to assess whether such self-disclosure contributes to a therapeutic nurse–patient relationship.
- Inform patients and family caregivers about spiritual support available at your institution (e.g., chapel or meditation room, chaplain services).
- Allow time and privacy for, and provide comfort measures prior to, private worship, prayer, meditation, reading, or other spiritual activities.
- Respect and ensure safety of the patient's religious articles (e.g., icons, amulets, clothing, jewelry).
- If desired by the patient, facilitate clergy or spiritual care specialist visitation. Collaborate with the chaplain (if available).
- Prepare the patient's environment for spiritual rituals or clergy visitations as needed (e.g., have a chair near the bedside for clergy, create private space).
- Make arrangements with the dietitian so that dietary needs can be met. If the institution cannot accommodate the patient's needs, ask the family to bring food. (Most religions have some recommendations about diet, such as espousing vegetarianism or rejecting alcohol.)
- Acquaint yourself with the religions, spiritual practices, and cultures of the area in which you are working.
- Facilitating/supporting a patient's religious practice does not require that you share the same beliefs or must participate in it yourself.
- Ask another nurse to assist if a particular religious practice makes you uncomfortable.
- All spiritual interventions must be done within agency guidelines.

Box 30–4
When a Patient Asks for Prayer

■ When a patient asks the nurse to pray, determine prayer preferences before starting (e.g., "How would you like to pray?"). Patients may prefer praying silently, while others may want the nurse to lead the prayer or to listen to the patient's prayer.

■ Assess how the patient approaches the addressee of prayer. For example, a Baptist may pray to Jesus, whereas a Jew would pray to God or Lord. Use terms such as "God" or "Sacred Source" until you know your patient's preference.

■ Before praying, assess what the patient would like you to pray (e.g., "For what would you like me to pray?"). The answer may provide greater insight into the patient's fears and concerns.

■ You may personalize the prayer by presenting your patient's name and personal concerns to the Divine.

■ If the prayer is colloquial, prayer can be used to summarize a conversation. This lets the patient know you have heard what was said. It may also help the patient to view circumstances more objectively.

■ Prayer may be the springboard to further discussion or catharsis. Stay with the patient after a prayer until there has been time for conversation.

■ Be mindful of one difference between magic and prayer. Magic invokes a greater power for personal gain. Prayer allows the greater power to do the greater good ("Thy will be done").

■ Praying with a patient may not involve verbalization. You may feel it will be more comfortable or appropriate if you remain quiet and fully present, praying silently.

■ Facilitate the patient's prayer practices. Schedule time when the patient will be undisturbed, palliate distressing symptoms that interfere with praying, help with articles that accompany prayers (e.g., rosaries, prayer garments, books of prayers), and so on.

■ In times of distress, a patient or loved one may not be able to construct a prayer spontaneously. You may want to model or teach a centering prayer that is very brief (e.g., "Lord, have mercy/healing"). Nurses can discuss with care recipients what prayer would benefit them most and encourage them to use it while alone. These prayers may be more beneficial when they are framed in a positive sense. To illustrate, "Jesus loves me" or "The Lord has mercy."

■ Encourage patients to think (privately or with you or a chaplain) about what prayer means to them. Offer questions such as these: What prompts you to pray? What do you expect from your praying? Are these expectations appropriate? How content are you with your prayer experiences? Is there a yearning for something more in your prayer experience?

Sources: Based on Taylor, E. J. (2012). *Religion: A clinical guide for nurses.* New York, NY: Springer; Hubbartt, B., Corey, D., & Kautz, D. D. (n.d.). *Nurse, please pray with me.* Retrieved from http://rnjournal.com/journal-of-nursing/nurse-please-pray-with-me; Taylor, E. J. (in press). Spiritual and religious support for persons living with cancer. In L. M. Gorman, & N. J. Bush (Eds.), *Psychosocial nursing care along the cancer continuum* (3rd ed.). Pittsburgh, PA: Oncology Nursing Society.

Illness can interfere with some patients' ability to pray (Taylor, 2012). Feelings such as anxiety, fear, guilt, grief, despair, and isolation can produce barriers to relationships in general and to the relationship the individual has with the Divine. In these instances, patients may ask the nurse to pray with them. Praying with patients should be done only when there is mutual agreement between the patients and those praying with them. Nurses who are unaccustomed to praying aloud or in public may find it helpful to have a formal prayer or a scriptural passage readily available. Because prayer can evoke deep feelings, the nurse may need to spend time with the patient following a prayer to enable the patient to express these feelings.

Patients may choose to participate in private prayer or may want group prayer with family, friends, or clergy. In these situations the nurse's major responsibility is to ensure a quiet environment and privacy. Nursing care may need to be adjusted to accommodate periods for prayer. Patients' preferences for prayer also reflect their personalities. That is, introverts may prefer being alone to pray, and their prayers will reflect their capacity for introspection. In contrast, extroverts' prayers may revolve around their relationships with others and be expressed in creative, verbal ways. Similarly, a prayer of a feeling-type patient may be emotion filled, whereas the prayer of a thinking-type patient may be based on ideas and logic. The nurse should support prayer according to the patient's preferences (see **Box 30–4 »**).

Evaluation

Expected outcomes of nursing care with regard to the patient's religious needs include the following:

■ The patient has been provided the opportunity to practice religious rituals, including prayers.

■ The nursing and dietary staff made appropriate considerations regarding dietary restrictions.

■ The patient successfully maintained connection with his or her religious practices and community of faith.

REVIEW Religion

RELATE Link the Concepts and Exemplars

Linking the exemplar of religion with the concept of stress and coping:

1. How might the patient's inability to perform customary religious rituals during times of illness result in anxiety?

2. How does helping the patient meet his or her religious needs, thus reducing anxiety, help the patient to recover more quickly?

Linking the exemplar of religion with the concept of development:

3. How might religious beliefs change as a patient ages?

4. In assisting the patient to meet his or her needs related to religion, how might the nurse's interventions differ based on the developmental stage of the patient?

REFER Go to Pearson MyLab Nursing and eText

■ Additional review materials

REFLECT Apply Your Knowledge

Olivia Rossi is an 80-year-old woman who attends Catholic Mass at her church every day. She enjoys shopping at the Italian market that is within walking distance of her home. A couple of years ago she was diagnosed with Parkinson disease. At first she did well, thanks to medication and therapy, but in the past few months her symptoms have become worse, and she is afraid to continue to live on her own. After going to visit several assisted living centers, she and her adult children chose one that is very nice, with a very well-qualified staff, but is a 15-minute drive from the nearest Catholic church. After a few weeks, the nurse working on Mrs. Rossi's floor notices that Mrs. Rossi has become depressed. The nurse approaches Mrs. Rossi and begins to talk with her about the changes she's experienced since moving to the center. Mrs. Rossi expresses her sadness at not being able to attend Mass and says that she misses her church community.

1. What are the priority nursing diagnoses for Mrs. Rossi?
2. What caring interventions could the nurse implement to help Mrs. Rossi?
3. What are the possible outcomes if Mrs. Rossi does not receive any nursing interventions?

References

Balint, K. A., & George, N. M. (2015). Faith community nursing scope of practice: Extending access to healthcare. *Journal of Christian Nursing, 32*(1), 34–40.

Bennett, P. R., & Elliott, M. (2013). God give me strength: Exploring prayer as self-disclosure. *Journal of Religion & Health, 52*(1), 128–142. doi:10.1007/s10943-011-9460-1

Blanchard, J. (2012). Screening for spiritual distress in the oncology inpatient: A quality improvement pilot project between nurses and chaplains. *Journal of Nursing Management, 20*(8), 1076–1084.

Boccia, M., Piccardi, L., & Guariglia, P. (2015). The meditative mind: A comprehensive meta-analysis of MRI studies. *Biomedical Research International, 419808*. doi:10.1155/2015/419808

Brewer, L. C., Balls-Berry, J. E., Dean, P., Lackore, K., Jenkins, S., & Hayes, S. N. (2016). Fostering African-American Improvement in Total Health (FAITH!): An application of the American Heart Association's Life's Simple 7 Among Midwestern African-Americans. *Journal of Racial and Ethnic Health Disparities, 4*(2), 269–281. doi:10.1007/s40615-016-0226-z

Brown, B. (2015). *Rising strong.* New York, NY: Penguin Random House.

Buttle, H. (2015). Measuring a journey without goal: Meditation, spirituality, and physiology. *Biomedical Research International, 891671*. doi:10.1155/2015/891671

Carpenito-Moyet, L. J. (2013). *Nursing diagnosis: Application to clinical practice* (15th ed.). Philadelphia, PA: Lippincott. Published by Lippincott Williams & Wilkins, © 2016.

Chochinov, H. M., Hack, T., Hassard, T., Kristjanson, L. J., McClement, S., & Harlos, M. (2005). Dignity therapy: A novel psychotherapeutic intervention for patients near the end of life. *Journal of Clinical Oncology, 23*(24), 5520–5525. doi:10.1200/jco.2005.08.391

Choi, P. J., Curlin, F. A., & Cox, C. E. (2015). "The patient is dying, please call the chaplain": The activities of chaplains in one medical center's intensive care units. *Journal of Pain & Symptom Management, 50*(4), 501–506. doi:10.1016/j.jpainsymman.2015.05.003

du Plessis, E. (2016). Presence: A step closer to spiritual care in nursing. *Holistic Nursing Practice, 30*(1), 47–53. doi:10.1097/hnp.0000000000000124

Ellison, C. W. (1983, April). Spiritual well-being: Conceptualization and measurement. *Journal of Psychology and Theology, 11*, 330–340.

Emmons, R. A. (2013). *Gratitude works! A 21-day program for creating emotional prosperity.* San Francisco, CA: Jossey-Bass.

Fahlberg, B., & Roush, T. (2016). Mindful presence: Being "with" in our nursing care. *Nursing, 46*(3), 14–15. doi:10.1097/01.nurse.0000480605.60511.09

Fitchett, G., Emanuel, L., Handzo, G., Boyken, L., & Wilkie, D. J. (2015). Care of the human spirit and the role of dignity therapy: A systematic review of dignity therapy research. *BMC Palliative Care, 14*, 8. doi:10.1186/s12904-015-0007-1

Fowler, J. W. (1981). *Stages of faith: The psychology of human development and the quest for meaning.* San Francisco, CA: Harper & Row.

Fowler, M., Kirkham-Reimer, S., Sawatzky, R., & Taylor, E. J. (2011). *Religion, religious ethics, and nursing.* New York, NY: Springer.

Fowler, M. D. M. (2015). *Guide to the code of ethics with interpretive statements.* Silver Spring, MD: American Nurses Association.

Gill, S. D. (1987). Prayer. In M. Eliade (Ed.), *The encyclopedia of religion* (pp. 489–492). New York, NY: Macmillan.

Hall, T. W., Edwards, E., & Wang, D. C. (2015). The spiritual development of emerging adults over the college years: A 4-year longitudinal investigation. *Psychology of Religion and Spirituality.* doi:10.1037/rel0000051

Hall, T. W., Fujikawa, A., Halcrow, S. R., Hill, P. C., & Delaney, H. D. (2009). Attachment to God and implicit spirituality: Clarifying correspondence and compensation models. *Journal of Psychology & Theology, 37*(4), 227–244.

Harris, J. I., Park, C. L., Currier, J. M., Usset, T. J., & Voecks, C. D. (2015). Moral injury and psychospiritual development: Considering the developmental context. *Spirituality in Clinical Practice, 2*(4), 256–266. doi:10.1037/scp0000045

Herdman, T. H. & Kamitsuru, S. (Eds.). *Nursing Diagnoses—Definitions and Classification 2015–2017.* Copyright © 2014, 1994–2014 NANDA International. Used by arrangement with John Wiley & Sons, Inc. Companion website: www.wiley.com/go/nursingdiagnoses

Hodge, D. R. (2015). Administering a two-stage spiritual assessment in healthcare settings: A necessary component of ethical and effective care. *Journal of Nursing Management, 23*(1), 27–38. doi:10.1111/jonm.12078

Hubbartt, B., Corey, D., & Kautz, D. D. (n.d.). *Nurse, please pray with me.* Retrieved from http://rnjournal.com/journal-of-nursing/nurse-please-pray-with-me

Huber, J. T., & MacDonald, D. A. (2012). An investigation of the relations between altruism, empathy, and spirituality. *Journal of Humanistic Psychology, 52*(2), 206–221. doi:10.1177/0022167811399442

Iliya, Y. A. (2016). Grief and the expressive arts: Practices for creating meaning. *Omega: Journal of Death & Dying, 72*(4), 362–365. doi:10.1177/0030222815598047

Jors, K., & Bussing, A. (2015). Personal prayer in patients dealing with chronic illness: A review of the research literature. *Evidence Based Complementary and Alternative Medicine, 2015, 927973.* doi:10.1155/2015/927973

Jourard, S. (1971). *The transparent self.* London, England: Van Nostrand.

Kahana, E., Bhatta, T., Lovegreen, L. D., Kahana, B., & Midlarsky, E. (2013). Altruism, helping, and volunteering: Pathways to well-being in late life. *Journal of Aging & Health, 25*(1), 159–187. doi:10.1177/0898264312469665

King, S. D., Fitchett, G., & Berry, D. L. (2013). Screening for religious/spiritual struggle in blood and marrow transplant patients. *Supportive Care in Cancer, 21*(4), 993–1001. doi:10.1007/s00520-012-1618-1

Krause, N. (2011). Assessing the prayer lives of older whites, older blacks and older Mexican Americans: A descriptive analysis. *International Journal for the Psychology of Religion, 22*(1), 60–78. doi:10.1080/10508619.2012.635060

Linders, E. H., & Lancaster, B. L. (2013). Sacred illness: Exploring transpersonal aspects in physical affliction and the role of the body in spiritual development. *Mental Health, Religion & Culture, 16*(10), 999–1008. doi:10.1080/13674676.2012.728578

Magaldi-Dopman, D., & Park-Taylor, J. (2013). Sacred adolescence: Practical suggestions for psychologists working with adolescents' religious and spiritual identity. *Spirituality in Clinical Practice, 1*(S), 40–52. doi:10.1037/2326-4500.1.S.40

Marchand, W. R. (2012). Mindfulness-based stress reduction, mindfulness-based cognitive therapy, and Zen meditation for depression, anxiety, pain, and psychological distress. *Journal of Psychiatric Practice, 18*(4), 233–252. doi:10.1097/01.pra.0000416014.53215.86

Marin, D. B., Sharma, V., Sosunov, E., Egorova, N., Goldstein, R., & Handzo, G. F. (2015). Relationship between chaplain visits and patient satisfaction. *Journal of Health Care Chaplaincy, 21*(1), 14–24. doi:10.1080/08854726.2014.981417

Marris, P. (2016). *Loss and change.* New York, NY: Routledge.

Marsh, N., Scheele, D., Gerhardt, H., Strang, S., Enax, L., Weber, B., . . . Hurlemann, R. (2015). The neuropeptide oxytocin induces a social altruism bias. *Journal of Neuroscience, 35*(47), 15696–15701. doi:10.1523/JNEUROSCI.3199-15.2015

Martinuz, M., Durst, A. V., Faouzi, M., Petremand, D., Reichel, V., Ortega, B., . . . Vollenweider, P. (2013). Do you want some spiritual support? Different rates of positive response to chaplains' versus nurses' offer. *Journal of Pastoral Care & Counseling, 67*(3–4), 3.

Massey, K., Barnes, M. J., Villines, D., Goldstein, J. D., Pierson, A. L., Scherer, C., . . . Summerfelt, W. T. (2015). What do I do? Developing a taxonomy of chaplaincy activities and interventions for spiritual care in intensive care unit palliative care. *BMC Palliative Care, 14,* 10. doi:10.1186/s12904-015-0008-0

Minton, M. E., Isaacson, M., & Banik, D. (2016). Prayer and the Registered Nurse (PRN): Nurses' reports of ease and dis-ease with patient-initiated prayer request. *Journal of Advanced Nursing, 72*(9), 2185–2195. doi:10.1111/jan.12990

Morris, G. S. (2015). Holistic health care for the medically uninsured: The Church Health Center of Memphis. *Ethnicity & Disease, 25*(4), 507–510. doi:10.18865/ed.25.4.507

Mujallad, A., & Taylor, E. J. (2016). Modesty among Muslim women: Implications for nursing care. *MEDSURG Nursing, 25*(3), 169–172.

National Congregations Study. (2015). *Religious congregations in 21st century America.* Retrieved from http://www.soc.duke.edu/natcong/

Neuman, B., & Fawcett, J. (2002). *The Neuman systems model* (4th ed.). Upper Saddle River, NJ: Prentice Hall.

Orthodox-Jews.com. (2014). *Culture: All about Orthodox Jewish women.* Retrieved from http://www.orthodox-jews.com/orthodox-jewish-women.html#axzz4Dg2s8PME

Poloma, M. M., & Gallup, G. H., Jr. (1991). *Varieties of prayer: A survey report.* Philadelphia, PA: Trinity Press International.

Penque, S., & Kearney, G. (2015). The effect of nursing presence on patient satisfaction. *Nursing Management, 46*(4), 38–44. doi:10.1097/01.numa.0000462367.98777.40

Pesut, B. (2016). There be dragons: Effects of unexplored religion on nurses' competence in spiritual care. *Nursing Inquiry, 23*(3), 191–199. doi:10.1111/nin.12135

Petersen, C. L. (2014). Spiritual care of the child with cancer at the end of life: A concept analysis. *Journal of Advanced Nursing, 70*(6), 1243–1253. doi:10.1111/jan.12257

Pettigrew, J. (1990). Intensive nursing care: The ministry of presence. *Critical Care Nursing Clinics of North America, 2,* 503–508.

Pew Research Center. (2015). *U.S. public becoming less religious.* Retrieved from http://www.pewforum.org/2015/11/03/chapter-2-religious-practices-and-experiences/#private-devotions

Piff, P. K., Dietze, P., Feinberg, M., Stancato, D. M., & Keltner, D. (2015). Awe, the small self, and prosocial behavior. *Journal of Personality and Social Psychology, 108*(6), 883–899. doi:10.1037/pspi0000018

Puchalski, C. M. (2014). The FICA spiritual history tool. *Journal of Palliative Medicine, 17*(1), 105–106. doi:10.1089/jpm.2013.9458

Puchalski, C. M., Vitillo, R., Hull, S. K., & Reller, N. (2014). Improving the spiritual dimension of whole person care: Reaching national and international consensus. *Journal of Palliative Medicine, 17*(6), 642–656. doi:10.1089/jpm.2014.9427. Published by Mary Ann Liebert, Inc., © 2014.

Robb, S. L., Burns, D. S., Stegenga, K. A., Haut, P. R., Monahan, P. O., Meza, J., . . . Haase, J. E. (2014). Randomized clinical trial of therapeutic music video intervention for resilience outcomes in adolescents/young adults undergoing hematopoietic stem cell transplant: A report from the children's oncology group. *Cancer, 120*(6), 909–917. doi:10.1002/cncr.28355

Rogers, F., Jr. (2015). *Practicing compassion.* Nashville, TN: Fresh Air Books.

Sattin, R. W., Williams, L. B., Dias, J., Garvin, J. T., Marion, L., Joshua, T. V., . . . Narayan, K. M. (2016). Community trial of a faith-based lifestyle intervention to prevent diabetes among African-Americans. *Journal of Community Health, 41*(1), 87–96. doi:10.1007/s10900-015-0071-8

Schafer, M. H. (2013). Close ties, intercessory prayer, and optimism among American adults: Locating God in the social support network. *Journal for the Scientific Study of Religion, 52*(1), 35–56. doi:10.1111/jssr.12010

Sharma, V., Marin, D. B., Sosunov, E., Ozbay, F., Goldstein, R., & Handzo, G. F. (2016). The differential effects of chaplain interventions on patient satisfaction. *Journal of Health Care Chaplaincy, 22*(3), 85–101. doi:10.1080/08854726.2015.1133203

Smith, A. W., Parsons, H. M., Kent, E. E., Bellizzi, K., Zebrack, B. J., Keel, G., . . . Keegan, T. H. (2013). Unmet support service needs and health-related quality of life among adolescents and young adults with cancer: The AYA HOPE Study. *Frontiers in Oncology, 3,* 75. doi:10.3389/fonc.2013.00075

Stephenson, P. S., & Berry, D. M. (2014). Describing spirituality at the end of life. *Western Journal of Nursing Research, 37*(9), 1229–1247. doi:10.1177/0193945914535509

Taylor, E. J. (2002). *Spiritual care: Nursing theory, research, and practice.* Upper Saddle River, NJ: Prentice Hall. Reprinted by permission of Pearson Education, Inc., Upper Saddle River, New Jersey.

Taylor, E. J. (2007). *What do I say? Talking with patients about spirituality.* Philadelphia, PA: Templeton.

Taylor, E. J. (2011). Religion and patient care. In M. Fowler, S. Kirkham-Reimer, R. Sawatzky, & E. J. Taylor (Eds.), *Religion, religious ethics, and nursing* (pp. 313–338). New York, NY: Springer.

Taylor, E. J. (2012). *Religion: A clinical guide for nurses.* New York, NY: Springer.

Taylor, E. J. (2015). Spiritual assessment. In B. R. Ferrell, N. Coyle, & J. A. Paice (Eds.), *Textbook of palliative nursing care* (4th ed., pp. 531–545). New York, NY: Oxford University Press.

Taylor, E. J., Gober, C., & Pfeiffer, J. B. (2014). Nurse religiosity and spiritual care. *Journal of Advanced Nursing. 70*(11), 2612–2621. doi:10.1111/jan.12446

Taylor, E. J., Petersen, C., Oyedele, O., & Haase, J. (2015). Spirituality and spiritual care of adolescents and young adults with cancer. *Seminars in Oncology Nursing, 31*(3), 227–241. doi:10.1016/j.soncn.2015.06.002

The Association of Religion Data Archives. (n.d.). *QuickStats.* Retrieved from http://thearda.com/quickstats/

Toussaint, L., Barry, M., Bornfriend, L., & Markman, M. (2014). Restore: The Journey Toward Self-Forgiveness: A randomized trial of patient education on self-forgiveness in cancer patients and caregivers. *Journal of Health Care Chaplaincy, 20*(2), 54–74. doi:10.1080/08854726.2014.902714

Ulanov, A., & Ulanov, B. (1983). *Primary speech: A psychology of prayer.* Atlanta, GA: John Knox Press.

Van Cappellen, P., & Saroglou, V. (2012). Awe activates religious and spiritual feelings and behavioral intentions. *Psychology of Religion and Spirituality, 4*(3), 223–236. doi:10.1037/a0025986

Weathers, E., McCarthy, G., & Coffey, A. (2016). Concept analysis of spirituality: An evolutionary approach. *Nursing Forum, 51*(2), 79–96. doi:10.1111/nuf.12128

Wink, P., & Dillon, M. (2003). Religious, spirituality, and psychosocial functioning in late adulthood: Findings from a longitudinal study. *Psychology and Aging, 18,* 916–924.

Winslow, G. R., & Wehtje-Winslow, B. J. (2007). Ethical boundaries of spiritual care. *Medical Journal of Australia, 186*(10 Suppl), S63–S66.

Wuthnow, R. (1998). *After Heaven: Spirituality in America since the 1950s.* Berkeley, CA: University of California Press.

Yeaworth, R. C., & Sailors, R. (2014). Faith community nursing: Real care, real cost savings. *Journal of Christian Nursing, 31*(3), 178–183.

Yount, G., Rachlin, K., & Siegel, J. (2013). Expressive arts therapy for hospitalized children: A pilot study measuring cortisol levels. *Pediatric Reports, 5*(2), 28–30. doi:10.4081/pr.2013.e7

Ziebarth, D. (2014). Evolutionary conceptual analysis: Faith community nursing. *Journal of Religion & Health, 53*(6), 1817–1835. doi:10.1007/s10943-014-9918-z

Ziebarth, D., & Campbell, K. P. (2016). A transitional care model using faith community nurses. *Journal of Christian Nursing, 33*(2), 112–118. doi:10.1097/cnj.0000000000000255

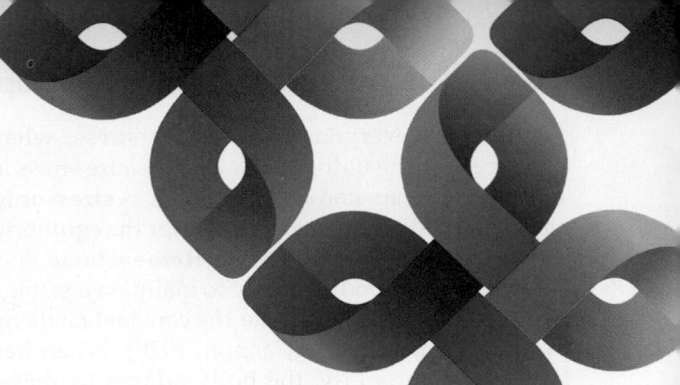

Module 31
Stress and Coping

Module Outline and Learning Outcomes

The Concept of Stress and Coping

Stress and Homeostasis

31.1 Contrast stress and homeostasis.

Stressors and the Coping Process

31.2 Explain types of stressors and the psychodynamics of coping.

Manifestations of Stress

31.3 Outline the manifestations and indicators of stress.

Concepts Related to Stress and Coping

31.4 Outline the relationship between stress and coping and other concepts.

Alterations from Normal Coping Responses

31.5 Differentiate alterations in coping.

Health Promotion

31.6 Explain the promotion of healthy coping and the prevention of stress-related illness.

Nursing Assessment

31.7 Differentiate among common assessment procedures and tests used to examine levels of stress and coping mechanisms.

Independent Interventions

31.8 Analyze independent interventions nurses can implement for patients with alterations in stress and coping.

Collaborative Therapies

31.9 Summarize collaborative therapies used by interprofessional teams for patients with stress-related illness and alterations in coping.

Lifespan Considerations

31.10 Differentiate considerations related to the care of patients with stress throughout the lifespan.

Stress and Coping Exemplars

Exemplar 31.A Anxiety Disorders

31.A Analyze anxiety disorders as they relate to stress and coping.

Exemplar 31.B Crisis

31.B Analyze crisis as it relates to stress and coping.

Exemplar 31.C Obsessive-Compulsive Disorder

31.C Analyze obsessive-compulsive disorder (OCD) as it relates to stress and coping.

>> The Concept of Stress and Coping

Concept Key Terms

Adaptation, 2051
Allostasis, 2048
Allostatic load, 2048
Anger, 2054
Anxiety, 2054
Approach coping, 2051
Avoidance coping, 2051
Biogenic stressors, 2049
Burnout, 2056
Cognitive appraisal, 2050
Cognitive structuring, 2054
Cognitive-behavioral therapy (CBT), 2063

Coping, 2048
Countershock phase, 2053
Depression, 2054
Diseases of adaptation, 2053
Distress, 2048
Ego defense mechanisms, 2056
Emotion-focused coping, 2051
Eustress, 2048
External environmental stressors, 2050

Fantasizing, 2056
Fear, 2054
General adaptation syndrome (GAS), 2052
Hassles, 2049
Hildegard Peplau, 2054
Homeostasis, 2048
Internal environment, 2050
Local adaptation syndrome (LAS), 2052
Maslow's hierarchy of needs, 2050

Meaning-focused coping, 2051
Nursing transactional model, 2053
Primary appraisal, 2050
Problem solving, 2054
Problem-focused coping, 2051
Psychosocial stressors, 2049
Reappraisal, 2051
Response-based stress model, 2052

Secondary appraisal, 2050
Self-control, 2056
Shock phase, 2052
Stage of exhaustion, 2053
Stage of resistance, 2053
Stimulus-based stress model, 2052
Stress, 2048
Stress mediators, 2048
Stress response, 2048
Stressor, 2048
Suppression, 2054

Although everyone experiences stress, what triggers stress in one individual may not cause stress in another. These triggers are known as stressors. A **stressor** is an external influence that threatens to disrupt the equilibrium necessary to maintain homeostasis. **Homeostasis** is classically described as the body's ability to maintain a stable, balanced internal environment despite the constant challenges posed by external influences (Cannon, 1929). When healthy and functioning properly, the body adapts to these external influences, or stressors, and promotes maintenance or restoration of homeostasis. Homeostasis is demonstrated by the body's ability to maintain fluid and electrolyte balance, oxygenation, and thermoregulation (the control of heat production and heat loss to maintain a steady body temperature). In particular, physiologic maintenance of the body's delicate acid–base balance provides a classic example of homeostasis in action (Cannon, 1932).

Stressors may be physical, mental, or emotional; they also may be positive or negative, depending on several variables, including the individual's perception of the experience. However, by definition, all stressors share one commonality: They have the capacity to cause stress.

Stress and Homeostasis

The term *stress* has appeared in the literature since approximately the 14th century, at which time it was applied in reference to hardship, adversity, or some form of affliction (Lumsden, 1981). However, the present-day understanding of the concept of stress was initially developed through the research and publications of Dr. Hans Selye (1907–1982). Selye was an endocrinologist and a pioneer in the study of stress and the stress response. Selye (1956) defined **stress** as the body's general, nonspecific response to the demands placed on it by a stressor. Selye further asserted that not all stress is bad; in some cases, stress can help an individual achieve desired goals or exceed self-imposed limitations (Cherry, 1978; Selye, 1956, 1976). Good stress, which Selye called **eustress**, is associated with accomplishment and victory. The opposite of eustress is **distress**, which is stress that is associated with inadequacy, insecurity, and loss (Cherry, 1978; Selye, 1956).

In further refining Cannon's conceptualization of homeostasis from a more holistic standpoint, Sterling and Eyer (1988) originated the term **allostasis**, which refers to the changes necessary to achieve the characteristic stability of homeostasis. During homeostasis, the body maintains vital functions such as heart and respiratory rates and oxygen and glucose levels within an ideal range. In contrast, current literature describes allostasis as the process the body uses to maintain a pathophysiologic deviation from the normal homeostatic operating level in the presence of stressors (Ramsay & Woods, 2014). This deviation from normal homeostasis allows the body to function as optimally as possible in the presence of major stressors. The process of allostasis includes the psychosocial and physiologic changes that occur in response to stress, many of which are triggered by activation of the sympathetic nervous system. In addition to other functions, the sympathetic nervous system triggers the body's "fight-or-flight" response, which is necessary for survival. Activation of the

sympathetic nervous system causes release of hormones such as epinephrine, which increases the heart rate and blood pressure to help deliver oxygen to tissues and organs. Epinephrine also causes bronchial dilation, which allows for increased oxygen uptake. This increase in oxygen uptake and delivery is intended to meet the increased metabolic demands associated with facing (fight) or escaping (flight) the stressor.

Formally referred to as the **stress response**, physiologic changes triggered by stress include activation of the neural, neuroendocrine, and endocrine systems as well as activation of target organs (Everly & Lating, 2013). The two primary stress mediators are glucocorticoids (e.g., cortisol) and catecholamines (e.g., epinephrine). These hormonal **stress mediators** are intended to promote adaptation (e.g., by triggering an increase in heart rate and blood pressure) when faced with physical danger.

Under ideal conditions, the stress response permits the body to compensate for the impact of stressors and ensure survival by either maintaining or regaining homeostasis. However, repeated activation of the stress response takes a toll on the individual. The physical cost of adaptation to physiologic or psychosocial stressors is referred to as the **allostatic load**. In addition to hormonal changes, the allostatic load also includes behavioral responses to stress. These can be favorable, as in participating in yoga or exercise, or unfavorable—for example, smoking or drinking alcohol. Chronic, prolonged overexposure to stress mediators, as well as inefficiency of the stress response and unhealthy behavioral responses to stress, can lead to illness (Robertson et al., 2015).

How an individual responds to stress varies and depends on both the individual and the stressor. **Coping** is a dynamic process through which an individual applies cognitive and behavioral measures to handle internal and external demands that the individual perceives as exceeding his available resources (Lazarus & Folkman, 1984). Individuals cope by integrating environmental and cognitive measures to mitigate or diminish the stress response (Everly & Lating, 2013). For example, a nursing student who is studying for final exams might cope with stress through environmental measures such as taking a walk or meeting a friend for coffee. Cognitively, the nursing student might alter her appraisal of the upcoming examination, choosing not to see it as an insurmountable barrier, but rather as a challenge for which she can prepare and that she can successfully master.

When an individual is unable to adapt to stress sufficiently to maintain homeostasis, functional impairment may occur. For example, a young child may become irritable and not be able to sit in the circle during morning carpet time at preschool, and may strike out at a classmate. An adult who fears the consequences of exposure to germs may compulsively wash his hands or clean the house, disrupting his ability to participate in normal activities. Individuals who experience impairment of functioning related to stress and coping may develop one of several stress or anxiety disorders. This module provides a discussion of stress and coping as well as a more detailed picture of specific related conditions, including anxiety disorders, phobias, and obsessive-compulsive disorder.

Stressors and the Coping Process

When patients in distress present to clinics, emergency departments, or mental health centers, nurses assist by assessing the source of the stress and the patient's response and by helping the patient cope with the stressor. To be able to respond appropriately, nurses must have a working knowledge of types of stressors; how human beings respond to or cope with stress; and theoretical models of stress and coping that provide insight into how nurses can support patients during types of stress.

Not everyone will agree as to what constitutes a stressor. For example, one individual may view bungee jumping as a terrifying, life-threatening event that should be avoided, but another individual views this activity to be an exhilarating form of stress release. Identification of a stressor depends on the individual's personal perception of the event or circumstance. However, certain stressors naturally evoke the physiologic stress response in all individuals, without regard to personal perception.

Types of Stressors

Stressors may be categorized using a variety of methods. From a broad standpoint, stressors often are categorized as being either biogenic or psychosocial (Everly & Lating, 2013).

Biogenic stressors directly trigger the stress response without any necessary cognitive process on the part of the individual; that is, the individual does not need to recognize the experience or circumstance as being stressful. Common examples of biogenic stressors include caffeine, amphetamines, and extreme temperatures (Everly & Lating, 2013). **Psychosocial stressors** may be either real or imagined. Rather than directly triggering the stress response, psychosocial stressors can facilitate its activation, depending on how the individual perceives the stressor (**cognitive appraisal**, discussed later in this module) (Everly & Lating, 2013). For example, an individual who has a fear of heights may respond to cleaning the gutters on her house differently than an individual who is not afraid of heights.

Just as the severity (or perceived severity) of a stressor impacts the magnitude of the stress response, so does the length of time to which the individual is exposed to the stressor. This is true regardless of whether the stressor is biogenic or psychosocial in nature—both can be equally powerful. In fact, anticipation of a stressor can produce the same physiologic response that occurs when faced with the stressor in reality (Matta, 2012). For example, anticipating or imagining a potential physical attack can evoke the release of the same stress hormones as those released during an actual physical fight.

From the standpoint of duration of exposure, stressors may be classified into four categories:

1. Acute and time limited
2. Sequential events following an initial stressor
3. Chronic intermittent
4. Chronic permanent.

See **Table 31–1 》** for examples of each classification.

To understand the reciprocal and dynamic relationship between the individual and the environment, it is necessary to consider sources of stress and types of stressors. The

TABLE 31–1 Classifications and Examples of Stressors

Classification of Stressors	Examples
1. Acute and time limited	Ankle sprain
	Nursing licensure exam
2. Sequential events following an initial stressor	Losing a job and subsequently filing for bankruptcy
3. Chronic intermittent	Strained relationship with in-laws
	Shared caregiving for an elderly parent
4. Chronic permanent	Paralysis
	Disability (e.g., blindness, deafness)

degree of a stressor's impact ranges from the benign (non-threatening) hassles of daily living to traumatic events within an individual, family, and society. Examples of traumatic events include rape, life-threatening illness or injury, and natural disasters such as hurricanes. **Box 31–1 》** lists some common stressors. Additional stressors related to lifespan and development are discussed in the section on Lifespan Considerations.

Daily Hassles

The individual day-to-day tensions that people face are commonly referred to in stress and coping research as **daily hassles**. Examples of daily hassles include making it through a work day or having to care for a small child after a poor night's sleep. Research indicates that hassles are more strongly correlated with somatic health and symptoms than more eventful stressors (DeLongis et al., 1982). A person's physical, emotional, and spiritual health affects whether or not the individual views a hassle as a minor inconvenience or a major strain. Alterations of health in any of these areas may overwhelm an individual's ability to cope with a specific stimulus or event, no matter how mild.

Box 31–1
Types of Stressors

Daily Hassles
- Roles of living
- Caring for children
- Pets
- Work responsibility
- Paying bills
- Traffic
- Neighbors

Internal Stressors
- Cognition (thoughts)
- Spirituality
- Emotions

Environmental Stressors
- Major cataclysmic changes affecting a large number of people (natural disasters, war, floods, hurricanes)
- Major changes affecting one or a few people (divorce, bereavement)

Internal Stressors

The **internal environment** includes the physical, spiritual, cognitive, emotional, and psychologic well-being of an individual and depends on the satisfaction of basic human needs. According to Lazarus and Folkman (1984), the drive to fulfill human needs internally sparks the stimulus to produce energy to seek gratification. When these internal needs are not met, individuals find it harder to cope with changes to their circumstances, including dealing with daily hassles, developmental stressors, or external stressors.

Dossey and Keegan (2016) address the spiritual dimension of the human condition as part of the individual's internal environment. The authors define *spirituality* as the essence of who we are and how we relate to the world. They incorporate elements of spirituality that include individual values, our place or fit in the world, and a sense of peace. Recent research has identified interconnectedness with the self, individuals, and the world around us as important components of spirituality. (See the module on Spirituality.)

Environmental Stressors

External environmental stressors include triggers outside of the individual that demand change or disrupt homeostasis. Positive stressors, such as graduation from college, generally produce eustress. Negative stressors, such as the inability to find employment, tend to cause distress. Stressors also may be simultaneously positive and negative, as with the combination of pending college graduation and imminent lack of employment. An event is a stressor if it creates a change in the individual or the individual's circumstances. **Table 31–2 》** outlines specific individual and environmental factors that affect an individual's response to a stressor.

The Coping Process

As stated earlier, **coping** is the process by which individuals can control or modify their responses to stressors. Successful coping allows individuals to maintain or return to homeostasis within a reasonable amount of time. Individuals who are unable to cope successfully may experience a range of symptoms requiring intervention from nurses and other healthcare professionals.

TABLE 31–2 Factors Affecting an Individual's Stress Response

Individual Factors	Environmental Factors
Genetic predisposition	Family support and connectedness
Past experience coping with stressors	Community support
Ability to meet own basic human needs	Financial resources
Cultural beliefs and customs	Community resources
Holistic health and well-being	Access to healthcare and education
Personal worldview and appraisal	Family appraisal
Coping mechanisms and history of coping successes	Social support

Cognitive Appraisal

Cognitive appraisal is a key factor in the patient's ability to cope with stressors. As the individual experiences exposure to a stressor, he appraises the stressor; that is, the individual mentally sorts, assesses, categorizes, evaluates, and frames the significance of an event or stressor with respect to his own well-being. The **primary appraisal** is the "first impression," occurring immediately on exposure to a stressor. Based on the transactional model, which is described in detail later in this module, there are three ways in which an individual categorizes a stimulus or demand: (1) irrelevant, (2) benign-positive, or (3) stressful. Irrelevant stressors are appraised as having no meaningful effect on the individual or his circumstance and are disregarded. Benign-positive stressors are demands for change that are perceived as preserving or enhancing well-being, such as taking a driver's education class. Stressors or stimuli categorized as stressful include those viewed as harmful, threatening, or disturbing, such as the death of a family member or a threat to life or safety.

During the **secondary appraisal**, the individual attempts to predict the impact, intensity, and duration of the coping behavior necessary to respond to the stressor. At this time, the individual selects a coping response.

In some cases, the intensity of an individual's stress response may appear to be incongruent with the stressor. For example, for some individuals, the loss of a family pet may be devastating and elicit an extreme stress response, whereas other individuals may demonstrate a response that is mild in intensity when faced with a similar loss. Likewise, some students may view earning a grade of "C" on an examination as being successful, because it is a passing grade; for others, earning anything less than an "A" is distressing. Keeping in mind that each individual is unique, **Maslow's hierarchy of needs** offers a model that is useful for understanding the significance of stressors within the context of human needs.

Maslow's Hierarchy of Needs

When Abraham Maslow introduced his hierarchy of needs in 1943, he proposed the existence of levels of human needs that could be organized into five categories: physiological, safety, love and belonging, self-esteem, and self-actualization (see **Figure 31–1 》**), listed in order of importance. Although Maslow later expanded his model to include self-transcendence as a sixth level of need (Koltko-Rivera, 2006; Maslow, 1968, 1987), the five-stage model is widely used to assist nurses and other professionals in identifying and prioritizing patient needs and interventions. According to Maslow, unmet lower-order needs will dominate the individual and prohibit higher-order needs from emerging. For example, for an individual who is experiencing extreme hunger or starvation, the quest for food becomes life's focus. As each category of needs is met, the individual's focus shifts to meeting higher-order needs: Once hunger is satiated, the need for safety and protection emerges and becomes the individual's primary goal. The satisfaction of both physiologic and safety needs allows for the emergence of needs related to love and belonging. This process continues as the individual is able to meet each stage of needs (Maslow, 1987).

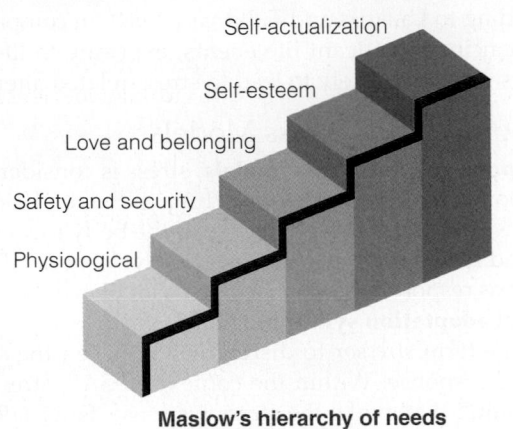

Self-actualization

Self-esteem

Love and belonging

Safety and security

Physiological

Maslow's hierarchy of needs

Figure 31–1 》 Maslow's hierarchy of needs.

It is important to note that individual traits and variations lead to flexibility with regard to the sequencing of Maslow's hierarchy of needs. As a result, the prioritization of needs may vary, depending on the individual (Maslow, 1987). As an example, for an individual who demonstrates an extremely powerful drive to achieve professional success, esteem needs (e.g., respect from others, empowerment, competence) may supersede needs related to love and belonging. Likewise, mental illness may lead to the exclusion of certain categories of needs (Maslow, 1987). For example, antisocial personality disorder is characterized by a lack of concern for the safety needs of self or others.

Effective Coping

Effective coping is a learned process, not an inherent personality trait. It includes all efforts mobilized by the individual to manage stressors. Coping involves constant change by the individual and includes spiritual, emotional, cognitive, and behavioral efforts to manage the demand. Lazarus and Folkman's (1984) transactional model describes coping as a means to manage or alter the problem causing the distress. The appraisal process allows the individual to inform the coping response by incorporating the person's own spiritual, cognitive, affective, and inherent vulnerability. In essence, every person responds to a stressor according to his or her unique worldview and condition.

Two forms of coping are (1) **problem-focused coping**, which is aimed at managing or altering the stressor, event, or circumstance; and (2) **emotion-focused coping**, which is directed at regulating the emotional response to the distress. Emotion-focused coping is used most when the stressor is perceived to be beyond the individual's control. In problem-focused coping, generally the perception is that the stressor can be changed (Lazarus & Folkman, 1984). Additional subcategories of coping include **avoidance coping** (using both behaviors and cognitive processes to avoid the stressor) and **approach coping** (confronting and trying to change the stressor by taking direct action). Finally, there is also **meaning-focused coping**, which involves re-evaluation to reduce the appraisal of a threat (Carver & Connor-Smith, 2010).

It is crucial for nurses to understand that any form of coping is an individual process influenced by the number of stressors; their source, type, intensity, and duration; and the individual's support, experience, and vulnerability. Nurses need to be aware of their own coping styles and maintain a nonjudgmental attitude about the coping mechanisms of individuals experiencing stressors. **Table 31–3 》** depicts various forms and examples of coping with stressors.

Healthcare professionals and researchers have clearly established the strong and complex relationship among stress, coping, and physical and psychologic illness (Cohen et al., 2012). Lazarus and Folkman (1984) note that it is the reaction to the demand, not the stimulus itself, that causes stress. The nursing transactional model allows the nurse to consider individual patient preferences, resources, culture, and environment in the assessment of the patient's abilities to respond to stress and to assist the patient in returning to homeostasis.

Reappraisal and Adaptation

Following attempts to cope with the stressor, the individual engages in a **reappraisal** process. During this time, the individual evaluates which coping mechanisms were successful and which were not. Ideally, the person begins another attempt to respond to the stressor and return to homeostasis. In terms of its effects on the body, stress is not viewed as "good" or "bad," but merely according to how much, what kinds, and under what conditions is it harmful or helpful (Lazarus & Folkman, 1984). **Adaptation** refers to the use of physiologic and psychologic processes to come to terms with the implications and outcomes of stressors (Biesecker

TABLE 31–3 Examples of Types of Coping

Types	Emotion-focused Coping (Defensive)	Problem-focused Coping	Avoidance	Approach	Meaning
Cognitive	Minimizing the event: "Oh, it's not that bad!"	Information gathering: "What are my odds of surviving?"	Denial of a situation or limiting information about stressful situations: "This is a bad dream!"	Confronting the situation	Identifying positive changes associated with stressful events; for example, personal illness that leads to increased family bonding
Behavioral	Performing physical activity to avoid thinking about a stressful situation	Adhering to a healthcare plan	Refusing to get a mammogram when a history of breast cancer runs in the family	Seeking means to exercise control	Attempting to fit into the environment: "I'll make the best of the situation."
Affective	Hoping for a miracle	Keeping feelings from interfering	Dealing with feelings later	Using feelings to motivate change	Seeking control of environment; regulating the emotional response to stress

et al., 2013). Adaptation and the development of health alterations are influenced by personal variables, with cognitive appraisal of the stressor, genetic predisposition to illness, and behavioral responses to stress being among the most significant factors (Herman, 2013).

Theoretical Models of Stress and Coping

Several theories and models exist to explain the phenomenon of stress. This section outlines stimulus-based and response-based stress models before presenting the transactional model in more detail.

Stimulus-based Stress Models

Stimulus-based stress models view "stress" as being synonymous with "stressor." These models define stress as being a life event that requires change or adaptation on the part of the individual who is experiencing the life event. Exposure to such life events leads to physiologic and psychologic "wear and tear" and can increase the individual's susceptibility to illness (Holmes & Rahe, 1967; Lyon, 2012). In their classic work, Holmes and Rahe (1967) proposed the Social Readjustment Rating Scale (SRRS), which quantified the impact of 43 significant life events—with none of the events classified as being either positive or negative—by assigning a numerical value to each individual experience. Examples of life events identified by Holmes and Rahe include death of a spouse or child, marriage, divorce, change of residence, and loss of a job. Variations of the SRRS questionnaire are still in use today. In 1997, a 77-item version of the SRRS was created (Miller & Rahe, 1997). In 2002, a shortened version was designed (Rahe & Tolles, 2002).

When considering the validity of the SRRS and similar scales, note that perception of a life event will vary among individuals, particularly with regard to cognitive appraisal of the event as being a stressor. Likewise, the impact of significant events must be considered from the standpoint of the individual's simultaneous exposure to routine stressors.

According to Lazarus and Folkman (1984), in comparison to experiencing significant life events, exposure to life's daily hassles was more likely to lead to stress-related alterations.

Response-based Stress Models

In **response-based stress models**, stress is considered to be a response to a stressor. According to Selye (1956, 1976), stress is "the nonspecific response of the body to any kind of demand made upon it" (1976, p. 1). Selye's model described the stress response as a three-stage chain of events called the **general adaptation syndrome (GAS)** or *stress response*. Selye used the term *stressor* to distinguish between the stimulus and the response. Within the context of GAS, stressors are any stimuli that evoke the stress response. Selye (1974) also proposed that not every instance of disruption of homeostasis qualifies as an occurrence of stress. For example, a close-flying insect that stimulates an individual to blink excessively may disturb the body's equilibrium, but this event does not necessarily trigger the GAS.

The stress response may be global (generalized) or local. A global response typically provokes physiologic changes that include hormone production and release and alterations in organs and structures. A local stress response, during which one organ or body system reacts to stress, may produce **local adaptation syndrome (LAS)**. For example, local inflammation in response to a scrape or minor laceration is an example of LAS. However, according to Selye (1976), both GAS and LAS produce a three-stage response: alarm reaction, resistance, and exhaustion (see **Figure 31–2 》》**).

Alarm Reaction

The body's initial response is the two-part alarm reaction, which begins with the **shock phase**. During the shock phase, as the body prepares for the cascade of physiologic reactions to the stressor, the sympathetic nervous system is suppressed and the individual may experience manifestations such as hypotension, decreased body temperature, and decreased muscle tone. During the second part of the alarm

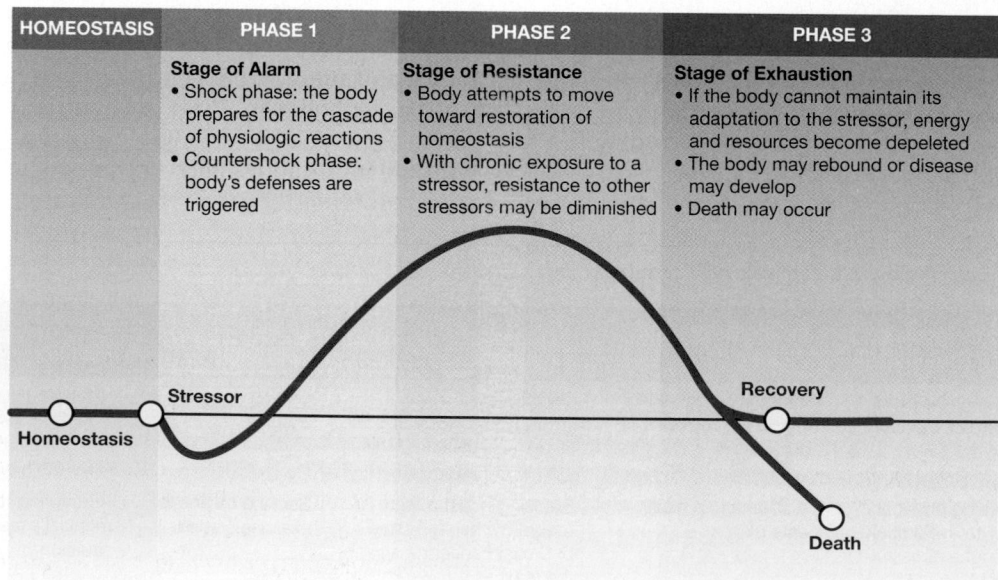

Figure 31–2 》》 The three stages of adaptation to stress: the alarm reaction, the stage of resistance, and the stage of exhaustion.

reaction, which is referred to as the **countershock phase**, sympathetic nervous system stimulation triggers the body's defenses, which in turn stimulates the hypothalamus. The hypothalamus releases corticotropin-releasing hormone (CRH), which stimulates the anterior pituitary gland to release adrenocorticotropic hormone (ACTH). This sympathetic stimulation, known as the HPA axis, results in secretion of catecholamines (epinephrine and norepinephrine) and glucocorticoids (cortisol) (see **Figure 31–3 »**). Significant body responses to epinephrine include increased myocardial activity, bronchial dilation, and increased fat mobilization. This adrenal hormonal activity prepares the individual for *fight or flight*. This primary response is short lived, lasting from 1 minute to 24 hours.

Stage of Resistance

During the second stage of the GAS, the **stage of resistance**, the body attempts to move toward restoration of homeostasis while continuing to respond to the stressor. With chronic exposure to a stressor, although the body may maintain resistance to the primary stressor, resistance to other stressors may be diminished. For example, an individual who is going through the divorce process may become emotionally and psychologically stable, giving an outward appearance of effectively coping with the emotional impact of the divorce. However, the prolonged physiologic stress response—which includes increased production of catecholamines (such as epinephrine and norepinephrine), glucose, and cortisol—may lead to increased susceptibility to physical illness, including peptic ulcers and hypertension. Selye (1946) called stress-related illnesses **diseases of adaptation**.

Stage of Exhaustion

During the third stage, the **stage of exhaustion**, if the body cannot maintain its adaptation to the stressor, the stressor will overwhelm the individual's ability to cope or mount a continued defense, resulting in the depletion of energy and resources. The body may rebound from the stressor after a period of rest, or disease may develop. Death also may ensue. The end of this stage depends largely on the adaptive energy resources of the individual, the severity of the stressor, and the external adaptive resources that are provided. An example of this can be seen in the patient who lives with chronic pain. The patient may be able to tolerate the pain during the day, but at night finds the pain far more stressful because energy resources are diminished to the point that the pain is intolerable.

Transactional Model

The transactional model of stress and coping emphasizes the individual's perception, or cognitive appraisal, of a given threat as being the most significant factor in the process. Proposed by Lazarus and Folkman (1984) in their landmark publication *Stress, Appraisal, and Coping,* this model incorporates variations among individuals in terms of the perception of stressors and the response to stress. Within the context of the Lazarus model, a perceived threat or stressor is an event or circumstance that has the ability to negatively impact well-being or that is appraised by the individual as exceeding the coping resources possessed by the individual. The primary danger posed by a stressor is that it threatens the individual's primary values and goals (Monat & Lazarus, 1991). According to Lazarus, the process of cognitive appraisal includes the following steps:

- *Primary appraisal:* evaluation of the transaction, which is the event or circumstance, in terms of its potential to harm, benefit, threaten, or challenge the individual
- *Secondary appraisal:* evaluation of the individual's available coping resources and potential options for responding to the event or circumstance
- *Coping:* application of available coping resources
- *Reappraisal:* ongoing evaluation and reinterpretation of the event or circumstance, as well as continued evaluation of the efficacy of the individual's coping strategies.

Culturally competent nursing care requires recognizing that cultural influences, as well as characteristics that are unique to the individual (including personality and temperament), impact both cognitive appraisal and coping styles.

The nursing transactional model is an adaptation of Lazarus and Folkman's work. The **nursing transactional model** is defined as the relationship between the nurse, the patient, and the environment in which they interact. This interaction or relationship is dynamic—with each transaction, the individual

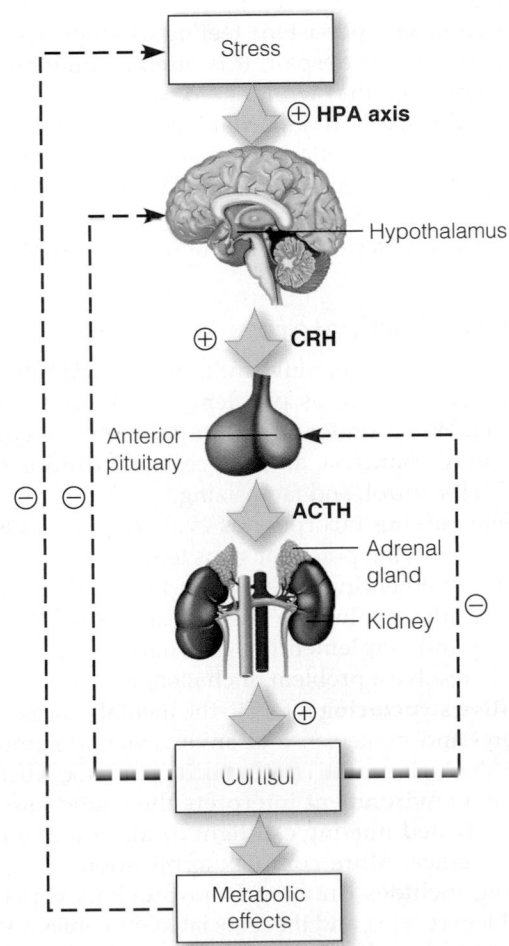

Figure 31–3 » Chronic stress results in overactivity of the hypothalamus-pituitary-adrenal (HPA) axis, which results in excessive release of cortisol, which results in more stress.

and the stressor engage to form a new transaction with a particular meaning. This model has numerous implications for the profession of nursing and care of the individual experiencing stress. The emphasis is on the relationship among stress, the patient, the nurse, and both the internal and external environment.

The nursing transactional model emphasizes communication and the development of an interpersonal relationship with the patient with the intent of decreasing the patient's anxiety and increasing or improving the patient's coping resources. This perspective and approach is largely based on the work of nursing theorist **Hildegard Peplau**, who is widely considered to be the mother of psychiatric nursing. In 1952, Peplau published her classic text, *Interpersonal Relations in Nursing*. As opposed to the task-oriented focus traditionally associated with nursing practice, Peplau viewed nursing as a therapeutic interpersonal process (Elder et al., 2013). As described in Peplau's theory, although the nurse begins as a stranger to the patient, during the course of the nurse–patient relationship, the nurse proceeds to assume several roles, including teacher, resource person, counselor, surrogate, and leader (Peplau, 1952).

Manifestations of Stress

Just as each individual is unique in terms of cognitive appraisal and coping methods, individuals also may vary in terms of the internal and external manifestations of stress. In addition to the physiologic domain, stress also may yield manifestations in various other domains, including psychologic and cognitive.

Physiologic Indicators

Physiologic manifestations of stress primarily result from stimulation of the sympathetic and neuroendocrine systems. As previously discussed, the individual's perception of the potential stressor triggers physiologic manifestations of stress. Prolonged exposure to perceived stressors and chronic activation of the stress response can lead to disease and may even be fatal. The relationship between this mind–body connection is illustrated in the Multisystem Effects of Stress feature.

Psychologic Indicators

Individual manifestations of stress within the psychologic domain may include fear, anxiety, anger, depression, and a variety of other responses.

Fear is a sense of apprehension triggered by a perceived threat to safety or well-being, including a painful stimulus or dangerous event. Fear may be aroused by memories of an actual past experience, exposure to a present threat, or anticipated exposure to an event or circumstance. Events that trigger fear may be real or perceived. For example, an individual who has never experienced a motor vehicle accident but who fears the possibility of one may fear driving a car. Even when the origin of fear is not based in reality or founded on an individual's actual experience, fear usually can be tied to a specific source.

Anxiety is characterized by apprehension, dread, mental uneasiness, and a sense of helplessness in response to an actual or perceived threat to the well-being of oneself or others. The degree of anxiety experienced by an individual may yield effects that range from minimal to debilitating. Unlike fear, an individual's anxiety may not have an apparent identifiable cause. Anxiety is discussed in greater detail in Exemplar 31.A.

Anger is a subjective sense of intense displeasure, irritation, or animosity. For those individuals who are taught that this emotion is unacceptable, development of anger may trigger a sense of guilt or shame. However, processing and expressing anger through constructive communication methods may lead to conflict resolution and personal growth. Constructive communication of anger requires clear identification of the source of the anger and a commitment to preventing escalation of anger during discussions.

Escalation of anger may lead to destructive emotions and behaviors, including hostility, aggression, or violence. Generally, hostility is characterized by open antagonism and may be expressed through both verbal and nonverbal means in combination with behaviors ranging from insensitive to destructive in nature. Aggression describes any behavior that is intended to harm another person, particularly when the other person is motivated to avoid the harm (Warburton & Anderson, 2015). The intended harm can be physical or emotional. Aggression associated with physical harm can lead to violence. Violence is the application of physical force with the intent to abuse or injure one or more individuals.

Depression is a persistent feeling of emptiness, hopelessness, sadness, or despair. It is often accompanied by a loss of interest (apathy) with regard to activities, including those related to daily living. Manifestations of depression include behavioral, emotional, and physical signs and symptoms. Chronic, recurrent, or extended periods of depression signal the need for evaluation and potential treatment (see the exemplar on Depression in the module on Mood and Affect).

Cognitive Indicators

In response to stress, cognitive indicators include changes in mental processes such as problem solving and cognitive structuring. When under stress, impairments in cognitive abilities may manifest as suppression, diminished or impaired self-control, and fantasizing.

Problem solving incorporates evaluating a challenging situation, identifying potential steps to resolve the situation, and then implementing those steps. In addition, problem solving includes evaluating the efficacy of solutions and identifying and implementing alternative approaches to adequately resolve a problem or challenge.

Cognitive structuring refers to the mental processes used to interpret and make sense of environmental stimuli. For example, through cognitive structuring, a nurse working in the hospital environment interprets the sound associated with an activated nursing call light to mean that a patient needs assistance. More complex application of cognitive structuring includes drawing from previous experiences with problem solving and the associated outcomes and then, through general application of those past experiences, forming a plan for resolving a present challenge.

Suppression, which is a defense mechanism, is the active, conscious process of denying unacceptable thoughts or emotions (Kneisl & Trigoboff, 2013). Suppression can be

Multisystem Effects of
Stress

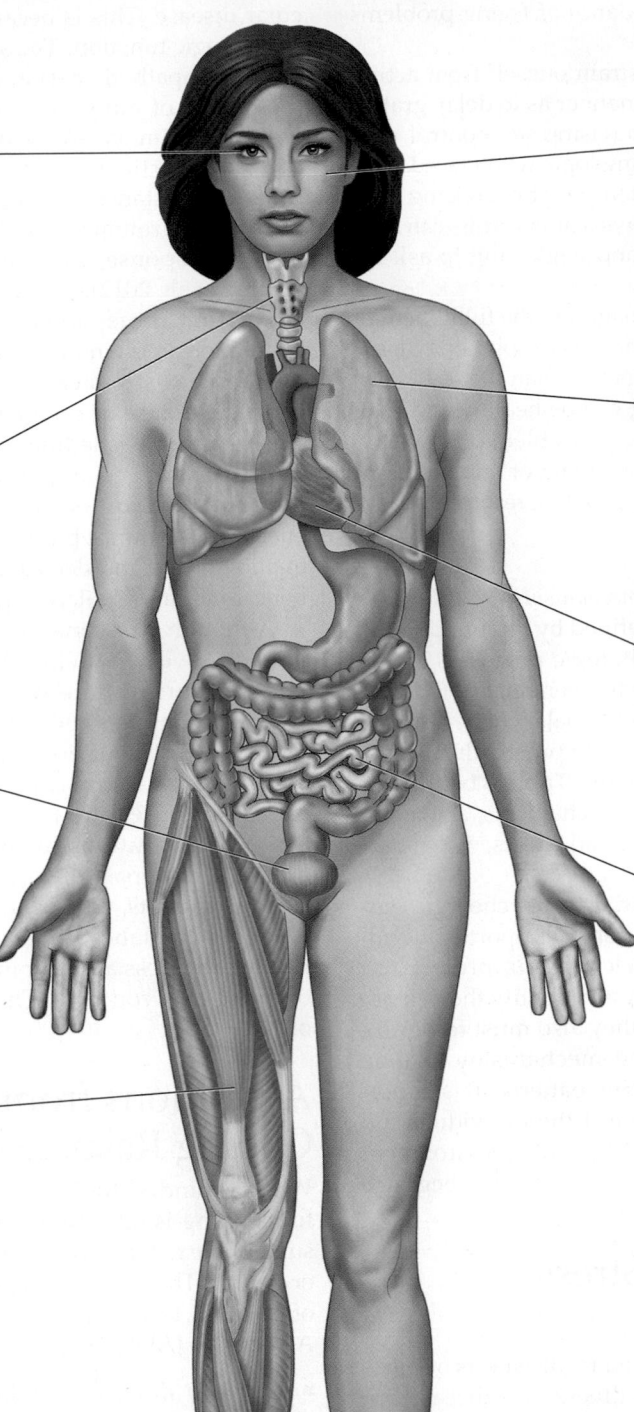

Sensory

- Pupillary dilation allows entrance of more light and enhanced visual perception
- Enhanced awareness and alertness in response to severe threats

Endocrine

- ↑ release of glucocorticoids and increased gluconeogenesis, which leads to increased serum glucose

Urinary

- ↑ sodium and water retention due to mineralocorticoid release, which leads to ↓ urine output and ↑ blood volume

Musculoskeletal

- ↑ muscular tension in preparation for fight or flight

Other Disorders

- Cancer
- Accident proneness
- Decreased immune response

Integumentary

- Diaphoresis to offset increased body temperature secondary to increased metabolism
- Skin pallor secondary to vasoconstrictive effects of norepinephrine

Respiratory

- ↑ respiratory rate and depth of respirations
- Dilation of bronchioles to facilitate increased oxygenation

Cardiovascular

- ↑ heart rate and cardiac output to promote transport of oxygen and nutrients throughout the body

Gastrointestinal

Inhibition of the parasympathetic nervous system leads to:

- ↓ peristalsis and possible constipation
- ↑ flatus
- ↓ salivation
- ↑ serotonin levels in the gut which leads to feelings of nausea

healthy; for example, an individual may suppress anger related to a disagreement with his significant other in order to effectively perform his work-related duties and demonstrate a positive attitude toward his coworkers. However, suppression may also lead to avoidance of facing problems or challenges.

Self-control is the ability to restrain oneself from acting on impulse or to behave in such a manner as to delay gratification. In an extreme example, exercising self-control may prevent fear or panic from overriding logic when faced with a stressful situation. However, attempts at exercising self-control—or a desire to appear to have self-control—can lead to ignoring or denying emotions and neglecting to ask for needed assistance.

Fantasizing, or *daydreaming*, is imagining the fulfillment of desires or wishes or mentally picturing the resolution of a situation in a manner that is more favorable than the resolution that occurred in reality. Fantasizing can be healthy and may even lead to identifying solutions to problems. However, excessive use of fantasy as a form of coping or in an attempt to avoid facing challenges can delay problem resolution.

Ego Defense Mechanisms

Frequently referred to as *defense mechanisms*, **ego defense mechanisms** were proposed and defined by Sigmund Freud (1946) as being unconscious psychologic processes developed for the purpose of defending the personality (or self). Individuals use defense mechanisms to balance the tensions that emerge during times of stress and to protect themselves from anxiety and its adverse effects. See **Table 31–4 》** for a description of the primary defense mechanisms, as well as examples of their functional purpose and effects, which may be positive or negative.

Defense mechanisms are essential to psychologic survival. Just as the fight-or-flight response supports individual physical survival, defense mechanisms protect our psychologic state. Nurses must not only identify the defense mechanisms used by patients, but they also must recognize how they themselves use defense mechanisms to gain insight into their own defensive coping patterns. It is important to remember that defenses protect the individual and the ego. Providing a safe and nonjudgmental environment helps patients let go of protective defenses and begin to cope with reality.

Concepts Related to Stress and Coping

Stress and coping are integrally linked to all aspects of nursing care. Patients who experience illness and disease are exposed to increased physical and emotional stress compared to their healthy counterparts, and this stress may extend to their caregivers (American Psychological Association, 2012). Individuals who have been exposed to personal loss or trauma are also susceptible to increased stress. Even on the joyful occasion of a new baby, new parents and siblings experience stress related to disrupted sleep patterns, exhaustion, caregiving demands, and decreased attention to self. This stress is heightened even more for the family if the infant has health problems, especially if it is a chronic illness that will affect the child for years (Cousino & Hazen, 2013).

Individuals exposed to high levels of stress due to personal health problems, caregiving responsibilities, or daily life struggles are more susceptible to emotional and physical health problems such as depression, obesity, and cardiovascular disease. This is because stress is intricately linked to physiologic function. The stress response triggers activation of the sympathetic nervous system, which in turn prompts the release of numerous neurotransmitters and hormones, with the primary stress mediators being catecholamines and glucocorticoids. The development of glucocorticoid receptor resistance associated with chronic stress may produce an environment that fails to downregulate the inflammatory response, thus leading to disease susceptibility (Cohen et al., 2012).

Nursing professionals are not exempt from the stress related to caregiving duties. Left unmanaged, what initially manifests as stress can translate into something far more serious. Because of occupation-specific demands, including irregular work schedules and increased workloads due to staffing shortages, nurses are at particularly high risk for **burnout**. In addition to adverse emotional and physical effects on the nurse, burnout is also associated with reduced quality of care and decreased patient satisfaction with nursing care (Stimpfel, Sloane, & Aiken, 2012).

Although stress may not be a primary diagnosis for all patients, every patient who seeks medical attention and requires nursing care will benefit from knowledge about coping techniques related to their unique situation. Individuals who experience chronic stress are more likely to engage in unhealthy coping behaviors. In contrast, nurses can support healthy coping behaviors by implementing caring interventions, using therapeutic communication, and providing patient teaching. In addition, they can advocate for patients, caregivers, and other nursing professionals when collaborative care is needed. The Concepts Related to Stress and Coping feature lists some, but not all, of the related concepts. They are presented in alphabetical order.

Alterations from Normal Coping Responses

When an individual experiences stress so disabling that functioning is adversely affected, the individual is highly susceptible to the development of a disorder of anxiety, stress, or trauma. The DSM-5 recognizes three different classifications of disorders related to stress and coping (American Psychiatric Association [APA], 2013):

- *Anxiety disorders,* which include separation anxiety disorder, selective mutism, specific phobia, social anxiety disorder (social phobia), panic disorder, agoraphobia, generalized anxiety disorder, substance/medication-induced anxiety disorder, anxiety disorder due to another medical condition, other specified anxiety disorder, and unspecified anxiety disorder. Anxiety disorders and phobias are discussed in detail in Exemplar 31.A.

- *Obsessive-compulsive and related disorders,* which include obsessive-compulsive disorder, body dysmorphic disorder, hoarding disorder, trichotillomania (hair-pulling disorder), excoriation (skin-picking disorder),

TABLE 31–4 Ego Defense Mechanisms

Defense Mechanism	Example(s)	Use/Purpose
Compensation: covering up weaknesses by emphasizing a more desirable trait or by overachievement in a more comfortable area	A high school student too small to play football becomes the star long-distance runner for the track team.	Allows an individual to overcome weakness and achieve success
Denial: attempting to screen or ignore unacceptable realities by refusing to acknowledge them	A woman, though told her father has metastatic cancer, continues to plan a family reunion 18 months in advance.	Temporarily isolates an individual from the full impact of a traumatic situation
Displacement: transferring or discharging emotional reactions from one object or person to another object or person	A husband and wife are fighting, and the husband becomes so angry he hits a door instead of his wife. A student gets a C on a paper she worked hard on and goes home and yells at her family.	Allows for feelings to be expressed through or to less dangerous objects or people
Identification: attempting to manage anxiety by imitating the behavior of someone feared or respected	A student nurse imitates the nurturing behavior she observes one of her instructors using with patients.	Helps an individual avoid self-devaluation
Intellectualization: evading the emotional response that normally would accompany an uncomfortable or painful incident by using rational explanations that remove from the incident any personal significance and feelings	The pain over a parent's sudden death is reduced by saying, "He wouldn't have wanted to live disabled."	Protects an individual from pain and traumatic events
Introjection: a form of identification that allows for the acceptance of others' norms and values into oneself, even when contrary to one's previous assumptions	A 7-year-old tells his little sister, "Don't talk to strangers." He has introjected this value from the instructions of parents and teachers.	Helps an individual avoid social retaliation and punishment; particularly important for the child's development of superego
Minimization: not acknowledging the significance of one's behavior	An individual says, "Don't believe everything my wife tells you. I wasn't so drunk I couldn't drive."	Allows an individual to decrease responsibility for his or her own behavior
Projection: blaming others or the environment for unacceptable desires, thoughts, shortcomings, and mistakes	A mother is told her child must repeat a grade in school, and she blames this on the teacher's poor instruction. A husband forgets to pay a bill and blames his wife for not giving it to him earlier.	Allows an individual to deny the existence of shortcomings and mistakes; protects self-image
Rationalization: justifying certain behaviors by faulty logic and ascription of motives that are socially acceptable but did not in fact inspire the behavior	A mother spanks her toddler too hard and says it was all right because he couldn't feel it through the diapers anyway.	Helps an individual cope with the inability to meet goals or certain standards
Reaction formation: a mechanism that causes people to act exactly opposite to the way they feel	An executive resents his bosses for calling in a consulting firm to make recommendations for change in his department, but verbalizes complete support of the idea and is exceedingly polite and cooperative.	Aids in reinforcing repression by allowing feelings to be acted out in a more acceptable way
Regression: resorting to an earlier, more comfortable level of functioning that is characteristically less demanding and responsible	An adult throws a temper tantrum when he does not get his own way. A critically ill patient allows the nurse to bathe and feed him.	Allows an individual to return to a point in development when nurturing and dependency were needed and accepted with comfort
Repression: an unconscious mechanism by which threatening thoughts, feelings, and desires are kept from becoming conscious; the repressed material is denied entry into consciousness	A teenager, seeing his best friend killed in a car crash, becomes amnesic about the circumstances surrounding the accident.	Protects an individual from a traumatic experience until he or she has the resources to cope
Sublimation: displacing energy associated with more primitive sexual or aggressive drives into socially acceptable activities	An individual with excessive, primitive sexual drives invests psychic energy into a well-defined religious value system.	Protects an individual from behaving in irrational, impulsive ways
Substitution: replacing a highly valued, unacceptable, or unavailable object with a less valuable, acceptable, or available object	A woman wants to marry a man exactly like her dead father and settles for someone who looks a little bit like him.	Helps an individual achieve goals and minimizes frustration and disappointment
Undoing: performing an action or using words designed to cancel some disapproved thoughts, impulses, or acts in which the person relieves guilt by making reparation	A father spanks his child and the next evening brings home a present for him. A teacher writes an examination that is far too difficult, then constructs a grading curve that makes it easy to earn a high grade.	Allows an individual to appease guilty feelings and atone for mistakes

substance/medication-induced obsessive-compulsive and related disorder, obsessive-compulsive and related disorder due to another medical condition, other specified and obsessive-compulsive and related disorder, and unspecified obsessive-compulsive and related disorder. Obsessive-compulsive disorder (OCD) is discussed in detail in Exemplar 31.C.

- **Trauma- and stressor-related disorders,** which include reactive attachment disorder, disinhibited social engagement disorder, posttraumatic stress disorder, acute stress disorder, adjustment disorders, and other specified trauma- and stressor-related disorder. Posttraumatic stress disorder is discussed in an exemplar in the module on Trauma.

Concepts Related to
Stress and Coping

CONCEPT	RELATIONSHIP TO STRESS AND COPING	NURSING IMPLICATIONS
Addiction	High chronic stress → unhealthy coping behaviors → ↑ alcohol, nicotine, or substance abuse	■ Assess all patients and caregivers for signs of addiction. ■ Educate patients and caregivers about the harmful effects of substance use and addictive behaviors. ■ Refer patients and caregivers to counseling or support groups as needed.
Collaboration	Multiple health issues → ↑ stress for the patient → ↑ need for collaboration between healthcare providers Conflict between family members or between patients and healthcare providers → ↑ stress for all parties involved → ↑ need for collaboration with a neutral third party	■ Assess stress levels and coping habits of patients with multiple health issues. ■ Identify collaborators who may be able to provide information or patient teaching that will help reduce the patient's stress level and increase the use of healthy coping techniques. For example, a patient with high stress levels related to obesity, diabetes mellitus, and cardiovascular disease may benefit from collaboration with a nutritionist. ■ Assess families for signs of family conflict that may be increasing the stress level for patients and caregivers. ■ Refer patients and families struggling with family conflict to family therapists or mediators.
Mood and Affect	Depression → ↑ stress → ↑ depression ↑ depression → ↑ risk for suicide	■ Assess the coping techniques of patients with mood and affective disorders and their caregivers. ■ Use therapeutic communication to encourage patients to engage in positive coping and adhere to their recommended treatment regimen. ■ Refer patients and caregivers to counseling or support groups as needed.
Perfusion	Stress response → release of catecholamines epinephrine and norepinephrine → ↑ blood pressure and ↑ heart rate	■ Assess patients for hypertension and tachycardia. ■ Be aware that prolonged exposure to stress can lead to long-term hypertension and secondary complications, including cardiovascular disease, cerebrovascular accident (CVA, or stroke), and renal damage. ■ Educate patients about stress management techniques, including regular physical exercise. ■ Facilitate referrals to counselors as ordered.
Reproduction	Changing hormone levels associated with pregnancy and childbirth → ↑ feelings of being overwhelmed → ↓ ability to cope Responsibilities associated with caring for a newborn → ↑ stress	■ Assess pregnant women for self-care activities and emotional health. ■ Assess mothers with newborns for self-care activities, sleep patterns, and emotional health. ■ Assess mothers with newborns for postpartum depression. ■ Assess mothers and fathers with premature newborns for signs of stress and inadequate coping techniques. ■ Provide patient teaching on newborn care techniques, breastfeeding, infant sleeping patterns, and other topics that may be contributing to stress in new parents.
Self	Stress → ↑ incidence of feeding and eating disorders	■ Assess individuals with stress for abnormal weight gain or loss. ■ Assess patients' eating habits, including whether stress makes them eat more or less than normal. ■ Provide patient teaching about healthy eating habits to individuals who use unhealthy eating habits to cope with stress. ■ Refer patients and caregivers to counseling or support groups as needed.
Teaching and Learning	Patient teaching about coping techniques → ↓ stress → ↑ healthy coping behaviors → ↑ overall health Mentoring less experienced healthcare providers → ↓ stress → ↑ job performance → ↑ patient satisfaction and health	■ Teach patients and family members struggling with high levels of stress about healthy coping techniques, including relaxation techniques and therapeutic communication. ■ Provide mentoring and encouragement to other healthcare providers to reduce stress. ■ Teach coping techniques to other healthcare providers, which can reduce on-the-job stress, prevent burnout, and increase job performance.

Alterations and Therapies
Stress and Coping

ALTERATION	DESCRIPTION	MANIFESTATIONS	INTERVENTIONS AND THERAPIES
Generalized anxiety disorder	Excessive worry about everyday problems for at least 6 months, with anxiety that is more intense than the situation warrants	■ Anticipation of disaster and preoccupation with health issues, money, familial problems, or challenges at work ■ Difficulty relaxing, tendency to startle easily, trouble concentrating and falling asleep ■ Various somatic complaints, which may include fatigue, headache, muscle tension and aches, digestive issues, irritability, shortness of breath or dyspnea, and hot flashes	■ Psychotherapy, including cognitive–behavioral therapy (CBT) ■ Pharmacotherapy, which may include antidepressants (e.g., selective serotonin reuptake inhibitors [SSRIs]), anxiolytic medications (e.g., benzodiazepines), beta-blockers, and antipsychotic medications ■ Relaxation techniques, such as massage and guided imagery ■ Mental health counseling
Phobias	An intense, persistent, irrational fear or dread of an object, situation, or activity that elicits panic and automatic avoidance of or compelling urge to stay away	■ Fear and anxiety in response to exposure (or, in some cases, imagined exposure) to the phobia-related object, situation, or activity	■ Pharmacotherapy, which may include short-term use of benzodiazepines, or administration of SSRIs or tricyclic antidepressants ■ CBT ■ Desensitization and implosion therapy for specific phobias ■ Dietary changes, including alcohol and caffeine restrictions
Panic disorder	A sudden attack of terror that can produce a sense of unreality, impending doom, or a fear of losing control	■ Somatic manifestations may include pounding heart, rapid heart rate (tachycardia), rapid respirations (tachypnea), weakness, sweatiness, light-headedness, or dizziness	■ Reduced environmental stimuli or placement in a quiet, nonstimulating environment ■ CBT ■ Pharmacotherapy, which may include antidepressants (e.g., SSRIs or tricyclic antidepressants), anxiolytic medications (e.g., benzodiazepines), beta-blockers, and antipsychotic medications ■ Relaxation techniques, such as massage and guided imagery ■ Mental health counseling
Obsessive-compulsive disorder (OCD)	Characterized by obsessive thoughts and compulsive repetitive behaviors formed in response to the obsessive thoughts to lower the level of anxiety experienced	■ Signs and symptoms vary depending on the theme of the specific obsessions and compulsions (see Exemplar 31.C). For example, OCD that features a theme of excessive cleanliness may include a fixation on the need to clean oneself and/or the environment (and fear of contamination), along with repetitive behaviors related to cleaning.	■ CBT ■ Antidepressants

Prevalence

According to the Anxiety and Depression Association of America (ADAA, 2014), anxiety disorders are the most common mental health disorders in the United States. The prevalence of anxiety disorders is approximately 18%, impacting 40 million individuals (ADAA, 2014). Generalized anxiety disorder (GAD) affects 6.8 million adults in the United States, and twice as many women as men. The disorder can develop at any time in the life cycle, although individuals in early adulthood are at greatest risk for developing it (ADAA, 2015a). Additional U.S. prevalence rates for disorders that are discussed in this module's exemplars include the following (ADAA, 2014):

■ Obsessive-compulsive disorder (OCD) affects approximately 2.2 million individuals or an estimated 1.0% of the population.

■ Phobias affect an estimated 19 million individuals, which is approximately 8.7% of the population.

Genetic Considerations and Risk Factors

Gender is a significant risk factor associated with anxiety and stress-related disorders. Overall, women are about twice as likely as men to develop an anxiety disorder. This may be because women are more sensitive to low levels of the stress hormone corticotropin-releasing factor (CRF) (ADAA, n.d.a). However, women are not more susceptible to every type of anxiety disorder. For example, OCD and social anxiety disorder are equally common in men and women (ADAA, 2014).

Both genetic factors and life experiences contribute to anxiety disorders. Anxiety disorders tend to run in families, a trend related partially to genetics and partially to environment. Up to 50% of patients with panic disorder and 40% of people with GAD have close relatives with the disorder, and individuals with close relatives who have OCD are 9 times more likely to develop OCD themselves (University of Maryland Medical Center [UMMC], 2013). In addition, many children develop fears and anxiety that are similar to those of their parents. For some patients, exposure to trauma or a significant event may trigger an anxiety disorder in individuals who are genetically susceptible (Cleveland Clinic, 2014).

Other factors that influence the development of anxiety disorders include personality-related characteristics; for example, shy children are at an increased risk (Mayo Clinic, 2014a). Traumatic events, including a history of spousal or childhood abuse and being bullied, also increase the risk of impairment. Social factors, especially limited or absent socialization and living in a threatening environment, increase an individual's susceptibility to developing an anxiety disorder. Even hypersensitivity of the amygdala—which is the brain's "fear center"—is believed to be a potential factor that may increase the likelihood for development of an anxiety-related disorder (UMMC, 2013).

Case Study » Part 1

Kevin DeLarno is a 23-year-old student who is completing his second year of graduate school in the study of anatomy and physiology. He presents to the university student health services center with complaints of frequent headaches, including a current headache that he describes as "a throbbing in the front of my head." He rates his pain as 7 on a scale of 0 to 10, with 10 being the worst imaginable pain. During his patient interview, he denies any past medical history or any additional complaints, including trauma, visual disturbances, dizziness, weakness, or neurologic changes. According to Mr. DeLarno, his headaches are "interfering with my study schedule. I have exams every week and I can't concentrate on studying. If I don't get these headaches under control, I'm going to end up failing at least one class this semester." He reports that he drinks "about a pot of coffee a day" and occasionally smokes a cigar when he is socializing with his friends.

Upon arrival, Mr. DeLarno's vital signs include temperature 97.9°F oral; pulse 92 bpm; respirations 18/min; and BP 153/82 mmHg. Auscultation of his heart and lungs reveals no abnormal findings. Mr. DeLarno insists he is "fine, except for these stupid headaches. I'm sure it's just stress. I need something to help me get them under control so I can get my work done." During his assessment interview, the nurse asks if Mr. DeLarno has made any recent changes to his daily routine or health habits. He replies, "There aren't any recent changes, but soon, there will be. I'm getting married in 3 months and my fiancé and I will be moving off campus. We're in the process of buying a house."

Mr. DeLarno further states that he is "excited about getting married," but feels the wedding planning has gotten out of hand, as he and his fiancé have already exceeded their wedding budget. When asked what activities he engages in for enjoyment and recreation, he replies, "I don't have time for anything except classes and studying. I used to work out and play racquetball three times a week, but I don't have the time for that right now."

Clinical Reasoning Questions Level I

1. Based on Mr. DeLarno's statements, what are his current potential sources of stress?
2. In addition to his complaints of recurrent headaches, which assessment data might reflect manifestations of the stress response?
3. Describe the effects of coffee and nicotine intake, including how these effects are similar to those evoked by the stress response.

Clinical Reasoning Questions Level II

4. Do positive stressors and negative stressors differ in terms of physiologic effects? Explain your answer.
5. Presuming Mr. DeLarno's headaches are stress related, what nursing diagnoses would be appropriate for inclusion in his nursing plan of care?
6. What nursing interventions could be implemented to promote stress reduction for Mr. DeLarno?

Health Promotion

Health promotion for individuals experiencing anxiety focuses on decreasing exacerbation of symptoms and identifying healthy coping behaviors that the patient is motivated to use. It is important to note that patients who are experiencing severe or panic levels of anxiety will not be able to retain new information and will require different interventions. For those who are able to focus on new information, topics for patient teaching can be found in the Patient Teaching feature.

Family wellness promotion is also essential to enhancing physiologic and psychosocial outcomes for patients of all ages (see the module on Family). The link between the development of mental illness and childhood abuse and neglect serves to emphasize this point. Research suggests that childhood abuse is associated with an increased risk for physical and psychologic disorders, including depression and anxiety. These increased risks remain in effect decades after the abuse occurs (Herringa et al., 2013). Even when overt abuse and neglect are not factors, family dynamics and parenting styles can pose serious threats to a child's psychosocial well-being. For example, frequent changes in caregivers may predispose a child to the development of separation anxiety disorder or reactive attachment disorder (APA, 2013; Mayo Clinic, 2014b).

Nursing Assessment

Just as individuals evaluate (appraise) and prioritize stressors, the nurse assesses and prioritizes health concerns. During the assessment, the nurse will help patients identify stressors that trigger unhealthy coping responses as well as the potential effects of those responses.

Many patients with anxiety will present complaining of physical symptoms. In the case study example, Mr. DeLarno's presenting complaint is a headache, which he then attributes to "just stress." Some patients, however, will be unable to

Patient Teaching
Wellness Promotion for Patients with Stress-Related Disorders

Nurses should provide patient teaching to patients with stress-related disorders to promote wellness and healthy coping techniques. Topics for teaching may include:

- *Physical exercise:* Educate the patient about the benefits of physical exercise (see the module on Health, Wellness, Illness, and Injury). Physiologic benefits of regular physical exercises include improved cardiac and pulmonary function, enhanced muscle tone and joint mobility, and weight control. Psychologic benefits include tension relief, stress reduction, enhanced sense of well-being, and promotion of relaxation following activity.

- *Sleep/rest patterns:* Promote a healthy balance between sleep/rest and activity and teach relaxation techniques to promote relaxation and sleep. Adequate sleep and rest are essential to survival, allow for physical healing and restoration, and enhance cognitive function. Sleep also helps remove free radicals, which are believed to be associated with illness and disease. Promote good sleep hygiene (see the Patient Teaching feature on Sleep Hygiene in the module on Comfort). Consider providing patient teaching about breathing exercises, imagery, muscle relaxation, movement techniques, and biofeedback.

- *Nutrition:* Provide education related to balanced nutrition and facilitate referrals to dietary professionals and nutritionists. Teach patients that inadequate nutrition reduces physical resistance to illness and increases susceptibility to disease and illness (see the module on Nutrition). Teach patients that the excessive intake of caffeine and use of nicotine may interfere with sleep/rest patterns.

- *Time management:* Teach patients how to balance fulfilling personal responsibilities (e.g., work, family, school) with time for rest, socialization, and extracurricular activities. Teach patients that effective time management is associated with an increased sense of control and decreased sense of stress.

- *Boundary setting:* Teach patients how to identify potential stressors and how to implement personal boundaries. Setting up personal boundaries can aid the patient in determining the appropriateness of requests/demands made by others and can allow the individual to identify which requests/demands can be fulfilled while still maintaining wellness.

---

articulate anxiety, because of a lack of either awareness or understanding of the source of their symptoms or because of a reluctance to disclose what they consider very personal information. Through developing the therapeutic nurse–patient relationship, the nurse may be able to encourage reluctant patients to disclose necessary information or come to an awareness of how stress and anxiety are impacting their health.

During the nursing assessment, the nurse acknowledges and affirms the patient's concerns. **Box 31–2** >> describes application of the nursing transactional model with regard to specific communication strategies that may be appropriate for use during assessment of the patient with anxiety.

Observation and Patient Interview

The patient interview should include collection of data related to the patient's current and past illnesses, specific physical complaints, general health history, patient-perceived stressors or stressful incidents, manifestations of stress, and past and present coping strategies. In addition to an assessment interview, the nurse may use a simple checklist while talking with and observing the patient to note indications of stress (see **Box 31–3** >> for a sample checklist). The first step in mediating the effect of a stressor is conscious awareness of the manifestations of stress. Review the symptom checklist to increase your awareness of and assess your own stress reactions and behaviors.

SAFETY ALERT Legal requirements to maintain patient confidentiality do not apply in the event of a patient's threat to harm self or others. If a patient indicates during the patient interview or any time during the assessment that he or she intends to injure self or others, the nurse has the responsibility to report this information to the proper authorities.

Box 31–2
Application of the Nursing Transactional Model to Assessment of the Patient with Anxiety

In the nursing transactional model, the nurse is part of the anxious patient's environment and can influence changes in the patient with both verbal and nonverbal cues. From the very first interaction with the patient, the nurse's demeanor conveys a great deal of information to the patient about how the patient can expect to be treated. Initial nursing actions that inspire patient confidence and that may help calm anxious patients include the following:

- Focus on the person: Make eye contact as appropriate and minimize distractions.
- Take a nonthreatening stance.
- Validate the patient's feelings: "I know you are very uncomfortable; we will do everything we can to help you feel better."

- Determine and address the patient's immediate concerns: "What can I do right away to help you?"
- Remember to address the patient by name. Some patients find terms of endearment such as "Honey" or "Sweetie" impersonal or demeaning. Using the patient's first name may be seen as patronizing if the patient is expected to use the nurse's last name. On the other hand, some patients respond positively to the informality of first-name use. Ask patients how they would prefer to be addressed, and never use the first name of anyone over age 18 without permission.

Box 31–3
Stress Assessment Checklist

Behavioral	Cognitive	Emotional	Physical
Always doing too much	Ambivalence	Agitation/anger	Constipation
Argumentativeness	Difficulty concentrating or listening	Anxiety and feeling pressured	Diaphoresis
Grinds teeth during sleep	Fear of the unknown	Crying	Diarrhea
Increase in compulsive behaviors (eating, drinking, nail biting, sexual activity, smoking)	Forgetfulness	Defensiveness	Difficulty falling asleep
Looks at watch or clock often	Lack of creativity	Easily annoyed	Dry mouth
Loud voice	Lack of initiative	Fear	Fatigue
Pacing	Lack of a sense of humor	Feeling overwhelmed	Gastrointestinal upsets or butterflies
Talks too fast	Memory lapses/loss	Feeling powerless	Headaches
Vigilance	Short attention span	Hostility	Increase in blood sugar levels
Withdrawal	Trouble thinking	Irritability	Increase in respiration rate
Work on multiple projects simultaneously	Wanting to run away	Isolation	Insomnia
	Worrying	Jumpiness and nervousness	Muscular stiffness and tension
		Sadness	Pallor
		Suspiciousness	Racing or pounding heart
			Restlessness
			Shakiness
			Sweaty palms
			Urinary frequency

Screening tests are available for use in the identification of many anxiety and stress-related disorders, including GAD, OCD, and specific phobias.

>> **Stay Current:** To view a sample of these screening tools, visit the Anxiety and Depression Association of America's online library at www.adaa.org/living-with-anxiety/ask-and-learn/screenings.

Physical Examination

Physical assessment of the patient should include observation and testing of the body systems for physical manifestations of stress. Gastrointestinal signs and symptoms of stress may include constipation, diarrhea, dry mouth, and nausea. Integumentary signs may include diaphoresis and pallor. Neurologic symptoms may include insomnia, fatigue, headaches, and restlessness. Cardiovascular and respiratory signs may include tachycardia and hyperpnea. Endocrine and urinary signs may include hyperglycemia and urinary frequency. Motor symptoms may include sluggish or stiff movements and muscle tension. Stress and anxiety may also manifest in behavioral habits that can be observed, such as cutting, fingernail biting, or evidence of crying. Remember that physical manifestations of distress may not be apparent when cognitive coping is effective.

Diagnostic Tests

For identification of disorders of anxiety and stress-related disorders, diagnostic criteria are collected primarily through patient interviews and reports of subjective symptoms. Medical testing may be conducted to rule out a medical etiology such

Focus on Diversity and Culture
Assessing Patients from Different Cultures

When working with patients from different cultures, nurses must take care not to inadvertently attribute a normal, healthy cultural response as inappropriate or maladaptive. Cultural expressions of distress vary. For example, some Chinese immigrants are less likely to discuss stress but will complain of somatic illnesses as a result (Lee, Suchday, & Wylie-Rosett, 2012). Therefore, a thorough assessment of stressors, the individual patient's perception of the stressors and cultural background, and the patient's efforts to seek help or reduce distress will help distinguish each patient's individual stress responses.

The Cultural Formulation Interview (CFI) outlined in the DSM-5 may be used to assist healthcare providers in interviewing patients as part of a comprehensive mental health assessment. The CFI is a series of 16 questions designed to assess patients in four areas (APA, 2013):

- Cultural definition of the problem

- Cultural perceptions of cause and support

- Cultural factors affecting coping and past help-seeking behaviors

- Cultural factors affecting current help-seeking behaviors.

as cardiovascular dysfunction or an adverse response to a medication. Patients with disorders related to stress and coping, particularly children, may present with somatic (physical) complaints and may not initially articulate any anxiety or trauma. Although patients may present to primary care providers with complaints that appear to be related to exposure to stress or due to impaired coping mechanisms, diagnosis of associated psychiatric disorders requires evaluation by a trained mental health professional, such as a psychiatrist or advanced practice psychiatric nurse.

Case Study >> Part 2

Mr. DeLarno is awaiting evaluation by the university healthcare clinic's nurse practitioner. He agrees to dimming of his room lights while he waits. After resting quietly for 10 minutes, he falls asleep. When the nurse awakens Mr. DeLarno to reassess him, he states, "I'm surprised I fell asleep. Usually, I can't fall asleep no matter how hard I try to relax. I'm only sleeping a couple of hours each night." He reports his headache "feels quite a bit better, but I know it's going to come back with a vengeance as soon as I start studying again." He rates his pain as 3 on a scale of 0 to 10, with 10 being the worst imaginable pain. His blood pressure has decreased to 128/72 mmHg and his pulse is now 78 bpm.

Upon arriving to assess Mr. DeLarno, the nurse practitioner introduces herself and asks the patient to describe his current complaints, as well as any similar problems he has experienced in the past. Mr. DeLarno states, "My headache is better, but I need something to help me control it when I'm studying. I think alprazolam would help—I have a friend who takes that when he gets stressed." The nurse practitioner responds by noting that she would like to further assess Mr. DeLarno, as well as ask him a few questions before making any treatment recommendations. Mr. DeLarno replies, "The nurse I saw earlier already listened to my heart and lungs, and she already asked me a bunch of questions. Headaches are my only problem—I don't need any additional workup. I can't stay here all day. Are you able to help me or not?"

Clinical Reasoning Questions Level I

1. Explain the most likely reasons for Mr. DeLarno's decreased headache and decrease in blood pressure and heart rate.
2. What is the significance of Mr. DeLarno's reported sleep habits?

Clinical Reasoning Questions Level II

3. In the event that Mr. DeLarno's complaints are related to anxiety, is a prescription for alprazolam a preferable first approach to treatment? Why or why not?
4. How should the nurse practitioner respond to Mr. DeLarno's seeming frustration with the need for additional assessment?

Independent Interventions

Nursing care of patients with alterations in stress and coping includes independent interventions such as using therapeutic communication, encouraging the patient to maintain or achieve optimal health, and assisting the patient with identifying strategies that will help him meet his goals.

Additional independent nursing interventions include implementing cognitive–behavioral interventions, such as teaching nonpharmacologic relaxation techniques, as well as encouraging patient and family participation in support groups. Validating the patient's feelings is essential to building self-esteem and fostering healthy coping. Reinforcing positive coping efforts, offering hope and reassurance to the

patient about her ability to cope, and helping her identify successes in life can provide a sense of personal power and hope. Spiritual distress occurs when an individual loses hope of ever resolving the problem or coping more adaptively. The chronic nature of anxiety disorders can be devastating and can erode an individual's sense of power and self-worth.

In the care of patients diagnosed with mental illness, one of the nurse's most crucial roles is patient advocacy. Covert discrimination against individuals with mental illness still exists today in society and the healthcare system. According to the U.S. Department of Housing and Urban Development (HUD, 2014), in 2013–2014, an estimated 20% of homeless individuals were experiencing mental illness. Even when provided with housing, these individuals were unlikely to remain off the streets unless they received access to continued healthcare treatment and services. Every individual and nurse who cares enough about the plight of individuals living with mental illnesses has the ability to impact public policy. Organizations such as the National Alliance on Mental Illness (NAMI) provide a platform for individuals to work collaboratively.

>> **Stay Current:** To learn more about advocating for individuals with mental illnesses, visit NAMI's website, www.nami.org. NAMI is the nation's largest organization for individuals experiencing mental illness and their families. NAMI has affiliates in every state and in about 1000 communities across the country.

Collaborative Therapies

Collaborative interventions for patients experiencing moderate to severe difficulty coping with stressors include administration of prescribed pharmacologic therapies and facilitation of counseling, psychotherapy, and other therapies as ordered. In addition to being well informed about various interventions and treatment options, such as psychotherapy, nurses should be able to recognize and manage their own responses to stress.

Psychotherapy

Psychotherapy is a preferred method of treating anxiety and other psychiatric disorders. Psychotherapy involves talking with a mental health professional, such as a psychiatrist, mental health nurse, advanced practice psychiatric nurse, psychologist, social worker, or counselor, to explore the nature and symptom management of the disorder (National Institute of Mental Health [NIMH], 2015). The severity of symptoms may warrant hospitalization in a safe therapeutic milieu, or social setting, for the individual. Such an intervention provides needed protection from environmental stressors and the additional support of group therapy. The impact of overwhelming and disabling anxiety can create vulnerability to depression, suicidal thoughts, or self-harm.

Cognitive–Behavioral Therapy

Cognitive–behavioral therapy (CBT) combines cognitive techniques and behavior modification to change detrimental beliefs and thought patterns. The goals of CBT include enhancing problem-solving and coping skills. Usually, the therapist guides the patient in identifying detrimental or distorted thought patterns and assists her with restructuring these thoughts and beliefs. Through analysis and reinterpretation of past and current experiences, the patient is able to learn and apply new skills that promote healthy behaviors and positive interpersonal interactions (APA, 2013; NIMH, 2013a).

Exposure-based CBT combines the techniques used in CBT with exposure of the patient to a controlled version of the situation that triggers the anxiety. By inducing mild anxiety under the supervision of a mental health expert, exposure-based CBT can help an individual with panic disorder learn that his panic attacks are not heart attacks, for example (NIMH, 2015). Additional cognitive–behavioral techniques are listed in **Box 31–4 》**.

Box 31–4
Additional Cognitive–Behavioral Therapeutic Techniques

The following techniques are also commonly used as a part of CBT:

- *A comprehensive assessment interview* is the first step in developing a contract with the goal of behavioral change. The purpose of the interview is to develop a complete picture of the patient's stress responses (e.g., negative thought patterns, feelings of worry or fear, or maladaptive behaviors such as repeated hand washing), so that strategies for changing these responses may be targeted. The interview process identifies problematic behavior and divides it into four areas:
  - The behavioral area, which asks what the patient is doing
  - The cognitive component, which asks what the patient is thinking
  - The affective component, which asks what the patient is feeling
  - The physiologic component, which probes the physical reality of the situation.
- *Thought stopping* is a technique that is used to help the patient change her thinking processes. Many individuals who experience anxiety have difficulty with repetitive, maladaptive thinking, and thought stopping is used to halt destructive thoughts before they get out of control. In this technique, the patient learns to stop destructive thoughts by visualizing a specific image, sensation, or circumstance. The thought-stopping agent can be the image of a traffic stop sign, the sound of the word *stop*, the tactile sensation of leaning against a closed door, or the visualization of pushing one's negative thoughts out the back door. Successful thought stopping should be implemented whenever maladaptive thoughts occur, so that over time, the patient learns to stop such thoughts reflexively.
- *A behavioral contract* outlines the behavioral changes that the patient and the mental health professional agree should take place. When negotiating a behavioral contract, a mental health provider engages the patient and family as colleagues, avoids jargon, and ensures that the patient and family are comfortable with the contract. Possible problems with behavioral contracts include a lack of understanding, a lack of commitment, a lack of adequate follow-up, and the lack of a defined plan of care. Continuing assessment, regular evaluation, and troubleshooting meetings can determine whether adjustments to the contract are necessary. Contracts can be adjusted in many ways, from changes in the prioritization of objectives to the appropriate revision of goals.

Source: Based on Kneisl, C. R., & Trigoboff, E. (2013). *Contemporary psychiatric–mental health nursing* (3rd ed.). Upper Saddle River, NJ: Pearson Education.

Pharmacologic Therapy

The therapeutic goal of psychopharmacology is to manage symptoms and alleviate distress. Generally speaking, pharmacologic therapies are most successful when used in combination with psychotherapy. Many patients require medication for only short periods of time. Some patients, however, may require longer courses of medication. Many patients with anxiety disorders can lead normal, fulfilling lives if they receive proper treatment (NIMH, 2015).

Medications used in the treatment of anxiety disorders include benzodiazepines. These medications may be used for short-term treatment during an acute phase of an anxiety disorder. Patients experiencing anxiety secondary to short-term medical therapies, such as mechanical ventilation, also may find benzodiazepines helpful. Benzodiazepines are generally not recommended for use beyond a few weeks because of their addictive properties. In addition, some research suggests that long-term use of benzodiazepines may cause permanent cognitive dysfunction, including in the areas of information processing and verbal learning (Stewart, 2005). Despite current guidelines that recommend the use of benzodiazepines primarily during the acute phase of treatment for anxiety, in reality these medications sometimes are prescribed for long-term use (Olfson, King, & Schoenbaum, 2015). Patients should consult with their prescribing provider about the potential side effects of long-term benzodiazepine use.

For long-term management of certain anxiety disorders, prescribers may consider an antidepressant. SSRIs are helpful in the treatment of phobias, symptoms of OCD, and panic symptoms. Fluoxetine (Prozac), paroxetine (Paxil), and sertraline (Zoloft) are examples of SSRIs that may be used in the treatment of patients with disorders of anxiety and stress. Tricyclic antidepressants, such as imipramine (Tofranil) or amitriptyline (Elavil), may also be used. These are contraindicated in patients with a history of heart dysfunction or heart attack (Adams, Holland, & Urban, 2017).

Monoamine oxidase inhibitors (MAOIs) such as phenelzine (Nardil), atypical antidepressants such as serotonin–norepinephrine reuptake inhibitors (SNRIs), and antipsychotic agents may also be prescribed for the treatment of these disorders. Beta-blockers may be used to block the effects of sympathetic nervous system stimulation and reduce manifestations of anxiety. See the Medications feature.

Herbal supplements, including valerian, kava, and passion flower, are used by some individuals in the treatment of anxiety. However, these medications have not been conclusively proven to be effective and may cause various side effects (Mayo Clinic, 2012a). The nurse should caution the patient to consult with his primary healthcare provider before adding herbal supplements to his medication regimen.

SAFETY ALERT The antihistamine diphenhydramine (Benadryl) is not suitable for use in the long-term treatment of anxiety-related disorders. Although diphenhydramine does produce sedation, research suggests that this drug's sedative effects are not effective for achieving anxiolysis (reduction of anxiety) (Baas et al., 2009). Moreover, cessation of diphenhydramine after long-term use can cause withdrawal symptoms. Patients with anxiety-related signs and symptoms should seek professional evaluation and guidance.

Medications

Anxiety- and Obsessive-Compulsive-Related Disorders

CLASSIFICATION AND DRUG EXAMPLES	MECHANISMS OF ACTION/ INDICATIONS FOR USE	NURSING CONSIDERATIONS
Antidepressants *Drug examples:* - SSRIs, such as citalopram (Celexa), escitalopram (Lexapro), fluoxetine (Prozac), paroxetine (Paxil), and sertraline (Zoloft) - Tricyclic antidepressants, such as imipramine (Tofranil)	SSRIs inhibit reuptake of the neurotransmitter serotonin in the brain, resulting in circulation of increased levels of serotonin. Although primarily used for treatment of depression, certain SSRIs are also effective in the treatment of patients with anxiety, OCD, and panic disorder. Tricyclic antidepressants block presynaptic neuronal reuptake of serotonin and norepinephrine, resulting in increased circulating levels of these neurotransmitters. Tricyclic antidepressants may be used in the treatment of patients with panic disorders.	- Monitor for development of suicidal ideation or worsening of symptoms. - Assess for adverse effects, including dizziness or drowsiness. - Counsel patients to avoid alcohol in combination with SSRIs or tricyclic antidepressants. - Periodically obtain complete blood count (CBC) with differential, serum electrolyte panel, and liver and kidney function studies. - Do not start SSRIs within 14 days of discontinuing MAOI drugs. - Women who are pregnant or breastfeeding should not take SSRIs or TCAs.
Atypical Antipsychotics *Drug examples:* Olanzapine (Zyprexa) Risperidone (Risperdal)	Interfere with action of serotonin and dopamine in the brain; as a result, for some patients, they promote reduction of compulsive behaviors and decreased agitation. In conjunction with other therapies, may be used in the treatment of patients with OCD or panic disorders.	- Monitor for neuroleptic malignant syndrome and tardive dyskinesia, and immediately report signs and symptoms of these conditions. - Assess for side effects, including drowsiness, excess sedation, somnolence, or increased agitation. - Monitor CBC, kidney and liver function studies, serum electrolytes, and serum glucose level. - Use of atypical antipsychotics is associated with weight gain and obesity, so monitor weight over time.
Nonbenzodiazepines *Drug examples:* Buspirone (Buspar) Zolpidem (Ambien)	Some act as a dopamine agonist in the brain and also inhibit serotonin reuptake (leading to increased circulating serotonin), producing antianxiety effect. Others are specific to the gamma-aminobutyric acid (GABA) receptor to produce relaxation and anxiolytic effects. Used to treat GAD.	- Assess for side effects, including nausea, headaches, and dizziness. - Use with caution in individuals with impaired liver or kidney function. - Advise patient this medication requires daily administration for several weeks to produce antianxiety effect.
Benzodiazepines *Drug examples:* Alprazolam (Xanax) Clonazepam (Klonopin) Diazepam (Valium) Lorazepam (Ativan) Temazepam (Restoril)	Potentiate the effect of the naturally occurring inhibitory neurotransmitter GABA, leading to promotion of relaxation and a decrease in the subjective experience of anxiety.	- Not recommended for long-term use because of habit-forming properties. - Monitor patient for excess sedation and dizziness. - Use cautiously in patients with impaired hepatic function and monitor liver function studies for these patients. - Counsel patient to avoid alcohol in combination medications in this classification.
Beta-Blockers *Drug example:* Propranolol (Inderal)	Selectively block cardiac and bronchial beta receptors, compete with epinephrine and norepinephrine, and reduce effects of sympathetic nervous system stimulation, such as increased heart rate, increased cardiac contractility, and increased blood pressure. Unlabeled uses include management of anxiety states and prevention of acute panic states (such as those related to public speaking).	- Assess blood pressure and heart rate prior to administration. Withhold medication if systolic blood pressure <90 mmHg or apical pulse rate <60 bpm, or if blood pressure and apical pulse rate do not meet parameters defined by the prescribing provider. - Monitor for adverse effects, including bradycardia, confusion, fatigue, and drowsiness. - Beta blockers may cause hypoglycemia or hyperglycemia and mask the symptoms of hypoglycemia in patients with diabetes, so any patient with diabetes who is using beta-blockers should be monitored carefully.

Source: Based on Adams, M. P., Holland, L.N., & Urban, C. (2017). *Pharmacology for nurses: A pathophysiologic approach.* (5th ed.). Hoboken, NJ: Pearson Education.

Case Study >> Part 3

Following Mr. DeLarno's assertion that he cannot "stay here all day" and his prompting for rapid treatment, the nurse practitioner replies, "I can imagine that your headaches are interfering with every aspect of your life, Mr. DeLarno. In particular, it must be miserable to try to study while you have a pounding headache, much less to take an exam. I want to help you find the best solution, which means I'll need some more information from you." She further explains to Mr. DeLarno that additional assessment is needed to accurately identify the cause of his headaches, as well as to choose the appropriate treatment approach. Initially, Mr. DeLarno is disappointed about not receiving a prescription for alprazolam, which he again suggests will fully resolve his headaches. However, after talking with the nurse practitioner, he agrees with the plan for further assessment.

The nurse practitioner performs a focused neurologic assessment, including assessing Mr. DeLarno's pupillary response to light and his extremity strength. She also interviews him as to the presence of any alterations in sensory perception, including numbness, tingling, or other unusual sensations. With the exception of his headache and sleep disturbances, which Mr. DeLarno reports began about 8 months earlier, his assessment findings reveal no abnormalities.

Based on assessment findings, the nurse practitioner suspects Mr. DeLarno may have developed generalized anxiety disorder (GAD). For further evaluation and treatment, she refers him to a mental health specialist affiliated with the university clinic. She further instructs Mr. DeLarno to avoid caffeine and nicotine and to contact the clinic if his headaches worsen or if he experiences any alterations in sensory perception. In addition, she offers to refer Mr. DeLarno to a local massage therapist who offers one free massage to students referred by the university student health services center. The patient agrees to follow up with the student wellness center and pleasantly accepts the referral for massage, stating, "I'm calling the massage therapist as soon as I walk out of here."

Clinical Reasoning Questions Level I

1. Which of the nurse practitioner's statements represent validation of the patient's complaints? Explain how validation can serve to diffuse a tense verbal interaction with a patient.

2. How could the staff nurse support and facilitate the interventions prescribed by the nurse practitioner?

Clinical Reasoning Questions Level II

3. Identify three nursing diagnoses that are appropriate for inclusion in Mr. DeLarno's nursing plan of care.

4. What additional recommendations could be offered by the staff nurse to promote healthy sleep/rest patterns for this patient?

Lifespan Considerations

Each stage of the lifespan comes with its own developmental stressors (see **Box 31–5** >>). The individual's response to those stressors and the coping mechanisms used to deal with each stressor will differ on the basis of the developmental stage, personality, and environment.

Stress and Coping in Children and Adolescents

Stressors in children and adolescents can be divided into normative and nonnormative stressors. Normative stressors that are common to all children include separation from parents or caregivers, starting school, and making new friends. Normative stressors may also be stressors that many but not all children face, such as being overweight, parents fighting, and getting bad grades (Rice, 2012). Normative stressors for children may also include situations that would not be considered stressful for an adult, including not having enough to do and not spending enough time with parents (Lewis, Siegel, & Lewis, 1984).

Normative stressors change as the child ages. For example, the transition from childhood to adolescence involves stressors such as navigating relationships with peers and completing performance-related tasks, such as academic assignments that require public speaking. Researchers who

Box 31–5
Developmental Stressors Across the Lifespan

Infants and Toddlers
- Separation from primary caregiver
- Cold stress, heat exposure
- Premature birth
- Maternal consumption of substances, toxins
- Feeding issues
- Impaired maternal bonding or attachment

Children
- Starting school
- Playing with peers/making friends
- Separation from parents/caregivers
- Conflict with parents/siblings

Adolescents
- Puberty
- Performance (sports, academics, arts)
- Independence (driving, job, social life)
- Relationships (peers, friends, dating, teachers, parents)
- Peer pressure
- Spiritual development

Adults
- Dating/marriage
- Birth or death of children
- Career
- Purchasing a house
- Health changes
- Divorce or death of spouse

Pregnant Women
- Hormone changes
- Body changes
- Childbirth
- Financial fears
- Fear of having an unhealthy baby or miscarriage

Older Adult
- Aging
- Retirement
- Loss of independence
- Terminal illness or multiple chronic illnesses
- Loneliness and isolation
- Death of peers or spouse

studied the impact of adolescent challenges in relationship to the stress response have determined that peer rejection stimulates an increase in systolic blood pressure and in the production of saliva α-amylase (sAA), which is an enzyme that is reflective of sympathetic nervous system activation. In addition, stressors related to performance-based challenges are associated with increased cortisol production and increased diastolic blood pressure (Stroud et al., 2009).

In contrast, nonnormative stressors are those that very few children and adolescents face but that produce higher stress levels. Nonnormative stressors may include serious illness of the child or a close family member, death of a parent, child abuse, natural disasters, or homelessness (Rice, 2012). Nonnormative stress can become "toxic" if the child or adolescent does not receive the adult support he needs. Toxic stress can influence a child's health into adulthood, increasing the risk for developing chronic diseases such as cardiovascular disease, cancer, asthma, and depression (Johnson, Riley, Granger, & Riis, 2013). Prevention of toxic stress often requires intervention at the levels of family, society, and government rather than at the biological level (Johnson et al., 2013).

In the early stages of development, some degree of anxiety is normal, particularly when children are separated from their parents or caregivers. Stranger anxiety is most pronounced during the first 2 years of life. Many young children have not yet developed normal coping processes, so they frequently cry or throw a temper tantrum when faced with stressful situations. However, as a result of normal cognitive development, usually around the toddler stage, children become better able to distinguish between dangerous and nondangerous situations, and fears begin to abate. Along with this developing sense of discernment, toddlers also begin to learn how to cope with fear (Berk, 2012).

As children learn to cope with stressors, they face new stressors such as starting school, making new friends, and feeling pressured to get good grades. Later in childhood, especially during adolescence, stressors often include changes related to puberty, performance, and conflict with parents. If the child does not learn how to cope with these stressors or does not receive appropriate support from a parent or other caregiver (see the Focus on Diversity and Culture feature), anxiety disorders may develop. A child or adolescent whose anxiety or fear persists beyond the expected age of resolution or endures for 6 months or longer may have developed an anxiety disorder and will benefit from referral to a mental health specialist (APA, 2013).

When working with children and adolescents, the challenge for the nurse is to differentiate between true anxiety disorders and normal developmental stressors and fears. Therefore, it is vital to assess not only the presence of emotional and behavioral cues related to stress but also the duration, severity, and timing of symptoms. Psychosocial assessment of the pediatric patient should be age and developmentally specific (see the module on Development) and should take into consideration that children may exhibit manifestations of disorders in ways that vary significantly from those demonstrated by adult patients. Signs of stress or anxiety in children may include irritability, withdrawal from pleasurable activities, clinging to a parent, frequent complaining about feeling ill, new or recurring fears, crying,

Focus on Diversity and Culture
Latchkey Children

Latchkey children are children and adolescents who spend hours at home alone each day between when they get home from school and when a parent or other adult arrives home from work. Latchkey children often come from families with two working parents or from single-parent families in which the parent works long hours at one or more jobs to support the family. In most cases, families with latchkey children cannot afford afterschool care and do not have adequate family or community support to provide the needed child care. Often older latchkey children become responsible for caring for younger children, sometimes even including providing meals and snacks for themselves and their siblings. Latchkey children who are unsupervised for more than 2 hours per day are at high risk of developing physical and social problems and anxiety. They are more likely to become involved in substance abuse and petty crimes when adult supervision is lacking, and they are more prone to aggressive behaviors and somatic complaints. The likelihood of developing negative coping strategies is higher for latchkey children who are experiencing a mental illness or who are genetically or environmentally susceptible to developing a mental illness.

Sources: Data from Potts, N. L., & Mandleco, B. L. (2012). *Pediatric nursing: Caring for children and their families* (3rd ed.). Clifton Park, NY: Cengage Learning; Ruiz-Casares, M., Rousseau, C., Currie, J. L., & Heymann, J. (2012). "I hold on to my teddy bear really tight": Children's experiences when they are home alone. *American Journal of Orthopsychiatry, 82*(1), 97–103; Na, K-S., Lee, S. I., Hong, H. J., Oh, M-J., Bahn, G. H., Ha, K., . . . Kyung, Y-M. (2014). The influence of unsupervised time on elementary school children at high risk for inattention and problem behaviors. *Child Abuse & Neglect, 38*(6), 1120–1127.

sleeping or eating too much or too little, bedwetting, and declining grades at school (American Psychological Association, n.d.a). Signs of stress or anxiety in adolescents may include excessive tiredness, anger and defiance, refusing to participate in favorite activities, becoming involved in substance abuse or criminal activities, sudden drops in grades at school, and social withdrawal.

When assessing children, nurses need to be aware of the language children use to express their stress or anxiety because children often use terms different from those used by adults. Children may not understand the concept of stress, so they may use terms such as "worry," "confused," or "mad" to describe their feelings. They may also convey stressful feelings by expressing negative thoughts about themselves or their environment (American Psychological Association, n.d.a). In addition, nurses should be aware that children and adults have different views of what types of circumstances are stressful to children. Children often find constant, minor stressors to be more stressful than one-time, large stressors. In addition, the anticipation of a major stressor may be more stressful to children than the actual experience of the stressor (Lewis et al., 1984). Nurses should also assess how the child's parents cope with stress, because children often mimic what they see.

When performing a nursing assessment on adolescents, the assessment should include interviewing both the patient and the guardian individually with the approval of the guardian. Adolescents may feel more comfortable discussing stressful situations when their parents are not present. The nurse should encourage adolescents to be truthful about stressors they are exposed to, including peer pressure to participate in sexual activities, criminal activities, and substance abuse. Because adolescents may feel more comfortable discussing these issues with a healthcare provider of the same gender, the nurse should always ask the patient and the guardian whether a provider of the same gender is preferred.

Several tools are available for nurses to assess the stress levels of children and adolescents. The most widely used diagnostic tool is the Anxiety Disorders Interview Schedule for children and parents (ADIS-C/P). However, the ADIS-C/P follows DSM-IV criteria rather than DSM-5. Another common assessment tool is the Screen for Child Anxiety Related Emotional Disorders-71 (SCARED-71), which may be used to identify anxiety disorders in individuals age 8 to 18 years (Bodden, Bogels, & Muris, 2009). Other tools include the Revised Children's Anxiety and Depression Scale (RCADS) and the Spence Children's Anxiety Scale (SCAS) (Creswell, Waite, & Cooper, 2014). In addition, the Children's Sources of Stress Scale (Ryan-Wenger, Sharrer, & Campbell, 2005) identifies sources of stress that relate to school-age children, and the Feel Bad Scale (FBS) is a 20-item list containing 17 normative stressors and 3 nonnormative stressors (Lewis et al., 1984). These scales were developed by determining what types of situations are most stressful to children rather than using an adult's opinion of what they think causes stress in children. Therefore, they are more applicable to assessing childhood stressors.

If a child or adolescent is experiencing elevated levels of stress, the nurse can teach coping strategies to both the child and the parents. Strategies that may be beneficial for children to practice include talking about their problems with a parent or other trusted adult; practicing relaxation exercises such as listening to calm music, taking deep breaths, or practicing a hobby or favorite activity; participating in physical activity; setting realistic expectations; and asking for help to manage stress. Strategies that may be beneficial for parents to practice to help their child cope with stress include providing a safe and secure home environment, being selective about television programming that young children watch (to decrease their exposure to violence and potential fears), spending time with their child, listening to their child and encouraging the child to talk about fears or worries, building the child's sense of self-worth, and keeping the child informed during potentially stressful changes (Kaneshiro, 2014).

In addition to teaching coping strategies, the nurse, along with the physician, may recommend CBT as a treatment method for childhood and adolescent anxiety. Treatment of children and adolescents with CBT is often based on Kendall's "Coping Cat," a method that involves psycho-education, modification of negative thoughts, exposure to feared stimuli, and training in coping skills (Creswell et al., 2014).

When discussing treatment methods for children and adolescents with alterations in stress and coping, treatment should focus on teaching multiple coping strategies rather than on pharmacologic intervention. Many antianxiety and antidepressant medications are not approved for children and adolescents, and some medications increase the risk of depression and suicide (NIMH, n.d.a). Therefore, medications are used only in severe cases of anxiety in children and adolescents. If the patient is prescribed an anxiolytic medication or antidepressant, the nurse should teach the patient and guardian about the risks associated with medication use.

Stress and Coping in Older Adults

Stressors for older adults are often related to changes associated with aging: loss of mobility, loss of independence, retirement, loss of peers or a spouse, or being diagnosed with a terminal illness or multiple chronic illnesses. Older adults who experience a loss of mobility or who have lost friends or a spouse to death may also feel a sense of isolation or loneliness, which can cause additional stress. Even the advancement of everyday technology can be a stressor for older adults who don't understand how to use computers or cell phones.

Signs and symptoms of stress in older adults include alterations in sleep patterns, eating habits, and self-care; headaches or other pains; tachycardia; gastrointestinal problems; negative feelings or attitudes; mood swings; social isolation; frequent crying; poor judgment; and lack of concentration. Older adults are more likely to report physical discomforts before they will report mental or cognitive problems. However, the diagnosis of anxiety-related disorders can be complicated by preexisting physical illness or cognitive changes in this population. For example, changes in self-care habits may be in response to stress, or they may be in response to cognitive changes that decrease the patient's ability to remember how to use basic grooming tools. Fear of stigmatization is also a significant consideration. Because many older adults were raised during a time when mental illness carried a heavy stigma, they may be especially resistant to reporting any symptoms of mental disorders (ADAA, n.d.b). Alterations due to anxiety and stress may also be difficult to identify in older adults because older adults often have better emotional control and coping strategies than younger adults (Miller, 2012).

When faced with stressors, older adults tend to use more passive emotion-focused coping strategies, including denial or acceptance. Older adults often choose carefully the events or situations that they worry about because they are attempting to conserve energy for the most important situations. Thus, they may tend to avoid some problems or withdraw from normal activities rather than face the situation that causes anxiety (Miller, 2012). For example, an older adult who has anxiety related to incontinence will often avoid leaving the house in order to prevent potential embarrassment related to their incontinence. This can lead to isolation and depression.

Older adults who maintain their social circles and remain physically active have better mental and physical health than those who isolate themselves (Miller, 2012). Social coping strategies tend to have a greater effect in reducing stress and anxiety than individual or personal coping strategies (McDougle, Konrath, Walk, & Handy, 2015). Nurses can promote wellness in older adults by encouraging them to remain socially and physically active and pursue activities that bring them joy and fulfillment. Older adults will benefit from spending time with family and friends or by participating in religious practices or volunteering. This support system can help older adults maintain their mental health and feel a sense of well-being rather than a sense of anxiety or stress.

Depending on the individual and the level of stress, some older adults may also be candidates for CBT or medication. However, medications should be used carefully because of potential drug interactions that may occur in older adults who are taking multiple other medications.

REVIEW The Concept of Stress and Coping

RELATE Link the Concepts

Linking the concept of stress and coping with the concept of communication:

1. Describe the application of therapeutic communication in the nursing care of patients with disorders related to stress and coping.

2. Particularly during the care of patients with disorders related to stress and coping, why is giving advice contraindicated? What specific communication strategies are recommended for these patients?

Linking the concept of stress and coping with the concept of ethics:

3. What is patient confidentiality, and how does this principle pertain to patients who seek treatment for alterations related to stress and coping? Under what circumstances is the requirement to maintain patient confidentiality not applicable?

4. While in the hospital cafeteria, a nurse overhears a nursing colleague discussing a patient's recent hospital admission for treatment related to an unusual phobia. Although the nursing colleague does not specify the patient's name, she includes a detailed discussion of the patient's complaints. How should this situation be addressed?

READY Go to Volume 3: Clinical Nursing Skills

- SKILL 1.1   Appearance and Mental Status: Assessing
- SKILL 1.5   Blood Pressure: Newborn, Infant, Child, Adult, Obtaining
- SKILL 1.6   Pulse, Apical and Peripheral: Obtaining
- SKILL 1.8   Respirations: Newborn, Infant, Child, Adult, Obtaining
- SKILL 1.25   Skin: Assessing
- SKILL 2.11   Medications: Preparing and Administering
- SKILL 3.1   Pain in Newborn, Infant, Child, or Adult: Assessing
- SKILL 3.3   Pain Relief: Complementary Health Approaches
- SKILL 3.6   Sleep Promotion: Assisting
- SKILL 15.1   Abuse: Newborn, Infant, Child, Older Adult, Assessing for
- SKILL 15.5   Environmental Safety: Healthcare Facility, Community, Home

REFER Go to Pearson MyLab Nursing and eText

- Additional review materials

REFLECT Apply Your Knowledge

Martina Carrillo is a sixth grader at Longview Middle School. Over the past month, she has been to see the school nurse several times with complaints of a stomachache. She has not complained about any other physical symptoms, and her stomachache has not led to vomiting. However, the school nurse notes that her heart rate and respiratory rate have increased slightly over the month. Based on school records and talking with Martina, the school nurse knows that Martina is the oldest of four children in an immigrant family. Her father is still in Mexico, and her mother works a shift from 3 p.m. to 11 p.m. at a local factory. Martina is on the free lunch program at school. In spite of speaking both English and Spanish fluently, Martina's grades have been declining over the past 3 months. When asked about this, Martina states that she often doesn't understand her homework and doesn't have time to spend on it because she is caring for her younger siblings in the evenings after school.

1. What potential stressors might Martina be facing each day in addition to those listed in the case study that the nurse might need to ask Martina about?

2. What physiologic processes might be leading to Martina's complaint of a stomachache?

3. What coping strategies may be advantageous for the school nurse to teach Martina?

4. How can the school nurse be an advocate for Martina during this time?

» Exemplar 31.A Anxiety Disorders

Exemplar Learning Outcomes

31.A Analyze anxiety disorders as they relate to stress and coping.

- Describe the pathophysiology of anxiety disorders.
- Describe the etiology of anxiety disorders.
- Compare the risk factors for and prevention of anxiety disorders.
- Identify the clinical manifestations of anxiety disorders.
- Summarize diagnostic tests and therapies used by interprofessional teams in the collaborative care of individuals with anxiety disorders.
- Differentiate considerations for care of patients with anxiety disorders across the lifespan.
- Apply the nursing process in providing culturally competent care to an individual with an anxiety disorder.

Exemplar Key Terms

Anxiety, *2070*
External locus of control, *2074*
Free-floating anxiety, *2070*
Generalized anxiety disorder (GAD), *2072*
Internal locus of control, *2074*
Panic disorder, *2073*
Phobia, *2073*
Vulnerability, *2070*

Overview

Anxiety is a response arising in anticipation of a perceived or actual threat to oneself or significant relationships. Anxiety is characterized by feelings of mental uneasiness, apprehension, dread, foreboding, and feelings of helplessness. Generally, anxiety helps people cope; it is a reaction to a stressor and is part of daily living. Anxious energy is a productive force for most people, and the experience of anxiety is influenced by an individual's genetic makeup as well as emotional, developmental, physical, cognitive, sociocultural, and spiritual factors.

Anxiety disorders may occur when normal feelings of anxiety get out of control and begin to impair individual functioning. Anxiety disorders are mental illnesses characterized by feelings of distress or fear during everyday situations. Fear is typically a heightened physical and emotional response to imminent danger, real or perceived (APA, 2013). Left untreated, anxiety disorders can damage personal relationships and the ability to work. Anxiety disorders impair daily activity and can lead to low self-esteem, drug abuse, and social isolation. Anxiety disorders are the most common mental illnesses in the United States, typically afflicting around 20% of the population. Effective treatments exist for anxiety disorders, but many people do not seek treatment because they do not realize how severe their symptoms are or because family, friends, and even physicians have difficulty recognizing the symptoms (NAMI, 2012).

The ability to differentiate healthy and expected stress responses from those that are harmful is an essential psychosocial competency for all nurses. Every individual experiences anxiety at times. The individual's anxiety is no longer healthy when the anxiety level reaches the point at which it prevents the individual from returning to homeostasis through healthy coping and adaptation.

Pathophysiology and Etiology

Pathophysiology

Research suggests that people are more likely to experience anxiety disorders if their parents have anxiety disorders. However, it is not clear whether biological or environmental factors play a greater role in the development of these conditions. Research suggests that traumatic brain injury may increase an individual's susceptibility for development of an anxiety disorder. In any case, scientists have found that certain areas of the brain, including the amygdala, function differently in people with anxiety disorders (NAMI, 2012).

The appearance of an anxiety disorder in an individual of any age requires attention by both healthcare professionals and caregivers. Family and friends may be the first to notice anxiety symptoms. Healthcare professionals recognize that many medical problems—including hormonal and neurologic conditions—may cause symptoms of anxiety. The primary symptom of anxiety disorders is what psychiatrists sometimes refer to as **free-floating anxiety**. This is characterized by excessive worry that is hard to control and whose focus may shift from moment to moment. Free-floating anxiety is anxiety that is not connected to a specific stimulus (Kneisl & Trigoboff, 2013). Examples of anxiety disorders are listed in the Concept section earlier in this module. This exemplar discusses three of them: generalized anxiety disorder, panic disorder, and phobias.

Etiology

Across the range of anxiety disorders, there are some important similarities in the basic causes of the anxiety response. Biological causes seem to play a significant role in the development of anxiety disorders. Abnormal function of structures in the limbic system and certain parts of the cortex appear to be involved. The neurotransmitters most closely involved with the anxiety response are GABA, norepinephrine, and serotonin. Genetic contributions play a role as well, with at least part of the genetic vulnerability being nonspecific, or common across the disorders. Psychosocial and behavioral factors include the classical conditioning of fear and a perception of lack of control over one's environment, an attitude that begins in childhood (Butcher, Mineka, & Hooley, 2013).

Vulnerability refers to the individual's susceptibility to react to a specific stressor. Individual vulnerability stems from biological and environmental sources, both of which have been the subjects of etiologic research. (See Focus on Diversity and Culture: Anxiety Disorders in Immigrant Populations.) Current explanations of the origin of anxiety disorders include neurobiological, neurochemical, psychosocial, behavioral, genetic, and humanistic theories.

Neurobiological Theories

Several areas of the brain orchestrate the experience of anxiety and the expression of the symptoms (see **Figure 31–4** »). The amygdala is known as the "emotional brain" and is the focus of much research related to feelings of anxiety, fear, and anger, which are elicited in this area. The hippocampus stores memory related to fear. The locus coeruleus stimulates arousal and contains almost half of all the neurons that use norepinephrine as a neurotransmitter. Stimulating an animal's locus coeruleus produces anxious behaviors. Heart rate and respirations are regulated by the brainstem, and the hypothalamus activates the entire response. The frontal cortex assists with appraisal of a threat and is the center of cognitive processes. The thalamus integrates all sensory stimuli, and the basal ganglia are responsible for the tremors associated with anxiety (Dubuc, 2013). Individual differences in the structure of the brain or injury to the brain will also alter the anxiety response.

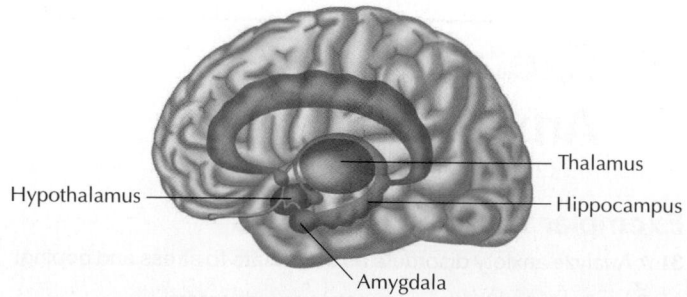

Source: From Mansen, Thomas. Patient Focused Assessment: The Art and Science of Clinical Data Gathering. Copyright © 2015 by Pearson Education.

Figure 31–4 » The limbic system. Just above the inner core, yet surrounded by the cerebral cortex, the limbic system plays a role in motivation, emotion, and memory. The system is composed of many structures, including the thalamus, amygdala, hippocampus, and hypothalamus.

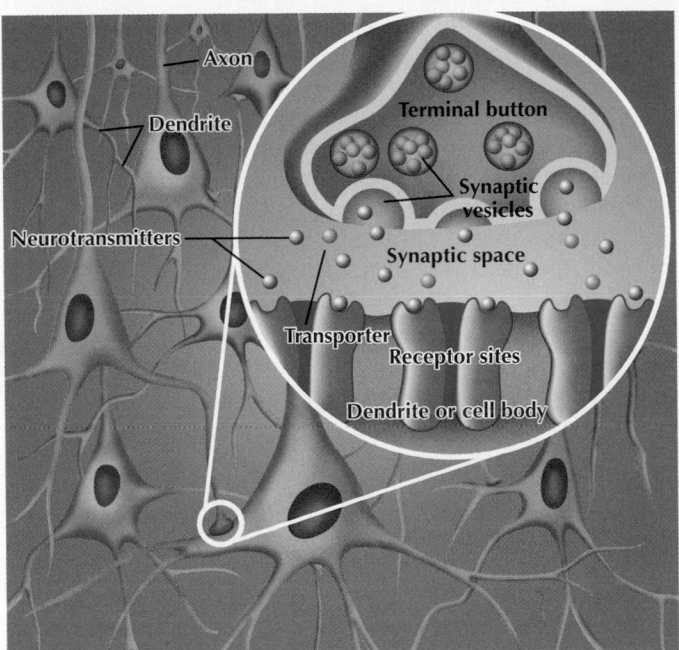

Figure 31–5 》 Neurotransmission: How neurons communicate.

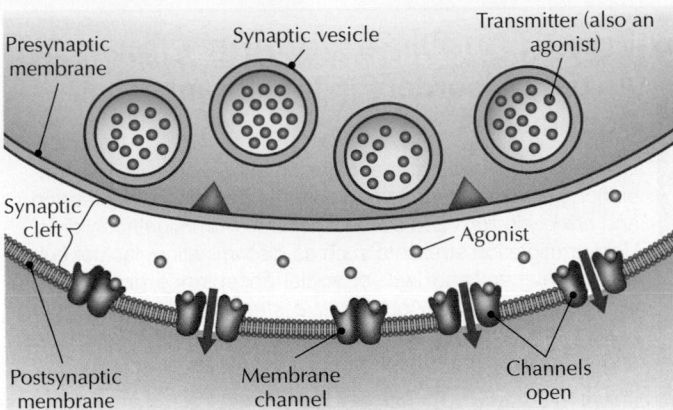

A, Strong agonist activates receptors without transmission.

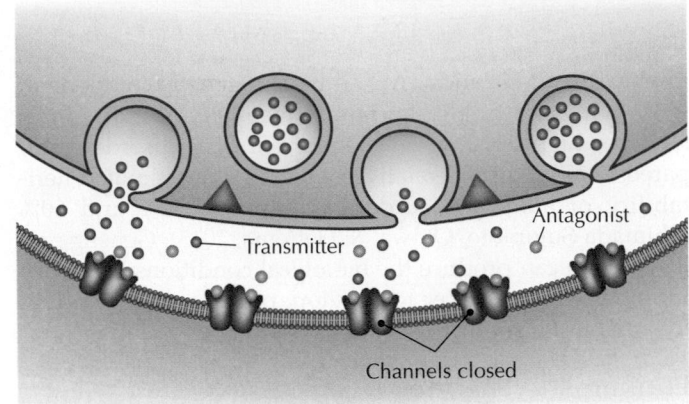

B, Antagonist blocks receptors. Agonist cannot act.

Figure 31–6 》 Ligands: Agonists and antagonists. Agonists and antagonists bind to the same binding site as transmitters. **A,** An agonist has potency, so it activates the cell biologically, while **B,** antagonists bind and have no potency. An antagonist produces its effect by blocking the binding site, preventing a transmitter from binding and producing its biological effect.

Neurochemical Theories

Communication within the brain occurs between neurons through the transmission of electrical stimuli (see **Figures 31–5 》** and **31–6 》**). To transmit a signal, a neuron releases chemicals called neurotransmitters. These chemicals deliver messages by binding to the receptors on the surface of another neuron, causing the neuron to fire and transmit the electrical impulse. Once the message is delivered, the neurotransmitter is taken back to a vesicle in the presynaptic cell (NIMH, 2013b). Any disruption in these transporters, binding sites, or cell structure can cause an alteration in cell functioning, leading to misfiring.

Structural anatomic differences, dysregulation of neurotransmitters, sensitivity of neuronal receptor sites, and the balance of neurotransmitters in the synaptic cleft all have an effect on the anxiety reaction. The brain's benzodiazepine receptor system enhances the activity of GABA, an inhibitory neurotransmitter that "shuts down" or slows excitability in the cell. It is present in the locus coeruleus, where norepinephrine is produced. Norepinephrine is an excitatory neurotransmitter that signals arousal and hyperarousal. Researchers believe that an imbalance in the regulation of these two neurotransmitters produces anxiety disorders: When GABA is decreased and norepinephrine is increased, anxiety results (Kneisl & Trigoboff, 2013). Serotonin is also implicated in the pathology of anxiety. It is thought to produce a feeling of well-being and is believed to be correlated with a decrease in anxiety (Butcher et al., 2013).

Psychosocial Theories

Psychoanalytic theory views anxiety as a sign of internal conflict resulting from the threatened emergence of repressed emotions into consciousness. According to the theory, an individual fears expressing forbidden emotions and so becomes anxious. Neo-Freudian analytical views of anxiety believe that it can be traced back to birth trauma, whereas interpersonal theorists stress the importance of the transmission of the mother's anxiety to the child (Kneisl & Trigoboff, 2013). Psychosocial theorists actively debate the origin of anxiety, but these debates typically have little to do with clinical practice.

Behavioral Theories

Behaviorists believe that faulty thinking and behavior are learned dysfunctional responses to stressors. They believe individuals can unlearn unhealthy behaviors by engaging in behavior modification, a treatment approach that teaches patients new ways to behave in response to stress. Behavior modification therapies use conditioning techniques—positive and negative reinforcements—in order to produce systematic desensitization, a process in which the patient builds up tolerance to anxiety through gradual exposure to a series of anxiety-provoking stimuli.

Genetic Theories

As stated earlier, research suggests that genetic predisposition may play a part in the development of anxiety disorders. According to twin and family studies, panic disorder, phobic disorders, and GAD all have a genetic component, with twins and first-order family members of individuals having a higher risk of developing the same disorder compared to more distant relatives. Overall, the estimated heritability of anxiety disorders is between 30% and 60% (Shimada-Sugimoto, Otowa, & Hettema, 2015). Genetic predisposition can produce the biological conditions necessary for an anxiety disorder to develop, priming an individual for anxious behavior.

Humanistic Theories

A humanistic, holistic explanation of anxiety disorders argues that biological, psychologic, behavioral, and genetic causes do not exist in isolation—they interact with one another to produce the complex of symptoms we call anxiety disorders. The humanistic perspective has generated a nuanced approach to patient care that integrates psychotherapeutic interventions, steps to develop social support systems, techniques to reduce external stress, and psychopharmacologic therapy.

Risk Factors

Risk factors for anxiety disorders include the dysregulation of neurotransmitters such as serotonin, norepinephrine, GABA, and a neuropeptide known as cholecystokinin. Other risk factors include the following:

- Childhood adversity, including witnessing traumatic events
- Family history of anxiety disorders
- Social factors, such as lack of social connection
- Serious or chronic illness
- Traumatic events
- Personality factors such as shyness and worrying
- Multiple stressors, such as chronic illness concurrent with loss of employment (UMMC, 2013).

Prevention

Prevention of anxiety disorders depends on an individual's ability to recognize her own growing anxiety. Individuals at risk for anxiety disorders should seek medical help early,

because these conditions become harder to treat as they progress. Keeping track of patterns of worrying can also help stop anxiety before it grows out of control. Mental health professionals advise that individuals at risk for anxiety disorders keep journals to catalog stressors and sources of relief and to manage priorities. Finally, individuals with multiple risk factors should avoid unhealthy substance use, including the abuse of alcohol, illegal drugs, and even nicotine and caffeine. These drugs can stimulate anxiety, and for people who are addicted, quitting can worsen anxiety (Mayo Clinic, 2012b).

Clinical Manifestations

Anxiety disorders are clustered around a range of physiologic, psychologic, behavioral, and cognitive manifestations. Although each of the disorders is distinct (GAD is completely distinct from acute stress disorder, and so on), the symptoms of all the disorders cluster around excessive, irrational fear and dread (NIMH, 2015). Worry is a major component of each of the anxiety disorders. Individuals in anxiety states experience the emotion both as a subjective condition and as a range of physical symptoms resulting from muscular tension and autonomic nervous system activity. Chronic anxiety can lead to physical manifestations and disabilities, including constipation, diarrhea, epigastric distress, and heartburn, as well as musculoskeletal aches and pains. Anxiety can develop suddenly or gradually, and it may be expressed as relatively mild physiologic symptoms or as an incapacitating episode of acute anxiety (Kneisl & Trigoboff, 2013). See **Table 31–5 》** for an overview of three types of anxiety disorders; each is discussed in more detail in the following sections.

Generalized Anxiety Disorder

Individuals with **generalized anxiety disorder (GAD)** go through their days filled with intense tension and worry, even if no external stressors are present. They anticipate disaster and are preoccupied with health issues, money, familial problems, or challenges at work. GAD may be diagnosed when excessive worrying is out of proportion to stressors (perceived or actual), interferes with daily functioning, and occurs for a period of at least 6 months (APA, 2013). Individuals with GAD cannot rid themselves of their anxious state, although they can usually recognize that their anxiety is more intense than the situation requires. They have difficulty relaxing, startle easily, and have trouble concentrating and falling asleep (see **Figure 31–7 》》**). Somatic symptoms of GAD include fatigue, headache, muscle tension and aches, digestive issues, irritability, feeling out of breath, and hot flashes. Sleep disturbances are common. Adults with mild or well-controlled GAD can function in social situations and hold down jobs, but those with severe, poorly controlled GAD have great difficulty carrying out daily tasks. GAD affects 6.8 million adults in the United States, and twice as many women as men. The disorder can develop at any time in the life cycle, although people are at the highest risk for the condition in early adulthood, between childhood and middle age (NIMH, n.d.b).

GAD can manifest in children with all the same symptoms as in adults. Children with GAD feel significantly distressed and, as with adults, the principal sign of GAD is

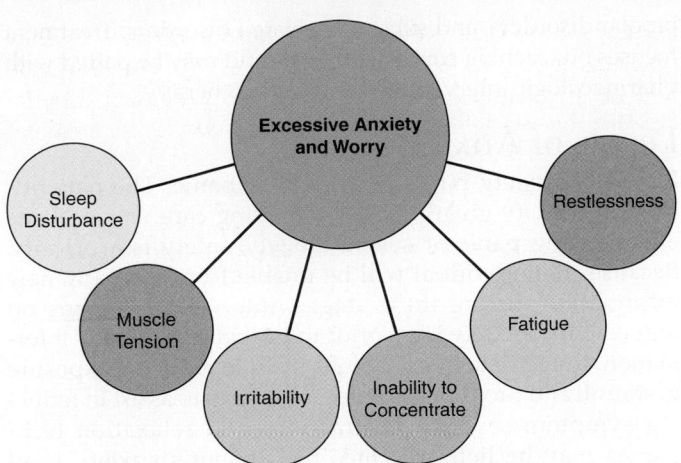

Source: From Potter, M. L., & Moller, M. D. (2016). Psychiatric–mental health nursing: From suffering to hope. (1st ed.). Upper Saddle River, NJ: Pearson.

Figure 31–7 ›› Key symptoms of generalized anxiety disorder.

intense worry over a long period of time. GAD is common among children and adolescents and is treated mostly with psychotherapy, the goal of which is to build up healthy and constructive responses to anxiety (Boston Children's Hospital, 2012).

Panic Disorder

Panic disorder is characterized by sudden attacks of terror, sometimes accompanied by a pounding heart, sweating, fainting, or dizziness. In a panic attack, an individual will feel flushed or chilled, his hands will tingle or become numb, and he may experience nausea, chest pain, and a sense of breathlessness, in addition to a sense of unreality, a fear of impending death, and a terror of losing control. A

fear of one's own unexplained symptoms is itself a symptom of panic disorder. Individuals in the grip of a panic attack sometimes believe they are dying or losing their minds; between episodes, they may worry intensely about the next panic attack (APA, 2013; NIMH, n.d.c). Attacks can occur at any time of day and even during sleep. An attack usually lasts only around 10 minutes, but some symptoms may last much longer. The disorder affects around 6 million people in the United States and is twice as common in women as men (NIMH, n.d.c).

People who have full-fledged panic disorder can become incapacitated by their condition and should seek treatment before they start to avoid situations where attacks have occurred. In severe cases, people who have panic attacks avoid normal activities. One third of people who have panic disorder become housebound and are able to confront a feared situation only when accompanied by a loved one or trusted friend. If the patient seeks treatment early, however, and the illness is correctly diagnosed, the disorder can usually be cleared up, because panic disorder is one of the most treatable anxiety disorders (NIMH, n.d.c).

SAFETY ALERT Panic attacks and heart attacks have many common symptoms, making it difficult to discern one from the other. Any patient experiencing sudden, severe chest pain should be treated according to your organization's heart attack protocols.

Phobias

Individuals with **phobias** experience intense, persistent fear or anxiety associated with a particular object or situation, called a stressor, and tend to avoid that stressor at all costs. Contact with the stressor produces severe panic. Stressors can be anything; needles and syringes, airplanes, spiders, dogs, closed areas, performing, and social activities are a

TABLE 31–5 Summary of Criteria for Anxiety Disorders

The following are summaries of the criteria for the anxiety disorders discussed in this exemplar. Refer to the DSM-5 for the complete diagnostic criteria.

Disorder	Summary
Generalized anxiety disorder	▪ Characterized by intense tension and worry, even in the absence of external stressors.
	▪ May demonstrate anticipation of disaster and/or preoccupation with health issues, money, familial problems, or work-related challenges.
	▪ Affected individuals usually recognize that their anxiety is disproportionate to the circumstances.
	▪ Manifestations include difficulty relaxing, pronounced startling, trouble concentrating, and difficulty falling asleep.
	▪ Somatic symptoms include fatigue, headache, muscle tension and aches, digestive issues, irritability, feeling out of breath, and hot flashes.
	▪ Diagnostic criteria include excessive anxiety about everyday problems for at least 6 months.
Panic disorder	▪ Recurrent unexpected panic attacks, when at least one of the attacks has been followed by 1 month of persistent concern about having more attacks, worry about the implications of the attack, or a significant change in behavior related to the attacks.
	▪ The attacks are not due to the physiologic effects of a substance.
	▪ The attacks are not better accounted for by another mental disorder.

Phobias
  Specific phobia
  Agoraphobia
  Social anxiety disorder
	▪ Intense, persistent, irrational fear of an object or situation that compels the individual to avoid the stressor that elicits the fear.

	▪ Exposure to the stressor produces an anxiety response that may take the form of a panic attack.
	▪ Anxiety about the stressor is out of proportion to the actual threat of danger posed by the object or situation, after accounting for cultural contextual factors.
	▪ Symptoms must last at least 6 months for patients regardless of age.

Sources: Based on BehaveNet. (2013). *Panic disorder without agoraphobia.* Retrieved from http://behavenet.com/panic-disorder-without-agoraphobia; National Institute of Mental Health (NIMH). (2015). *Anxiety disorders.* Retrieved from http://www.nimh.nih.gov/health/topics/anxiety-disorders/index.shtml; BehaveNet. (2015). *Phobia.* Retrieved from http://behavenet.com/phobia; and American Psychiatric Association (APA). (2013). *Diagnostic and statistical manual of mental disorders* (5th ed.). Arlington, VA: Author.

few examples. Phobias adversely impact quality of social, occupational, and academic function and also interfere with activities of daily living (APA, 2013). An estimated 8.7% of the U.S. population is affected by a specific phobia, and women are twice as likely to develop a specific phobia as men (ADAA, 2014).

Individuals with phobias and other forms of anxiety may exhibit an external locus of control. Lazarus and Folkman (1984) describe *locus of control* as the extent to which an individual believes he has control over the events in his life. Individuals with an **internal locus of control** believe their actions, choices, and behaviors impact life events. Those with an **external locus of control** believe that powers outside of themselves, such as luck or fate, determine life events.

There are three primary categories of phobias: specific phobia, agoraphobia, and social anxiety disorder (formerly known as social phobia). Specific phobia is intense or extreme fear with regard to a particular object or situation such as spiders, snakes, flying, or heights. *Agoraphobia* is characterized by anxiety associated with two or more of the following situations: being in enclosed spaces, being in open spaces, using public transportation, being in a crowd or standing in a line of people, or being alone outside the home environment (APA, 2013). Social anxiety disorder is characterized by pervasive, extreme fear of one or more social situations that may lead to scrutiny by others.

Phobias are frequently comorbid with other psychiatric alterations, including depressive disorders, anxiety disorders, bipolar disorders, and substance-related disorders. Treatment focuses on teaching coping strategies and may be paired with pharmacologic interventions and psychotherapy.

Levels of Anxiety

Levels of anxiety range from mild to panic. The patient's level of anxiety greatly impacts nursing care. For patients experiencing panic or severe anxiety, safety is a priority. Because the individual will be unable to take in any new information during these stages, interventions focus on reducing the anxiety level prior to providing any new information. Immediate interventions include reducing exposure to stimuli and providing comfort measures to assist in reducing symptom severity. Distractions and relaxation techniques may be helpful. Once the patient's anxiety level decreases, additional interventions to reduce anxiety, such as beginning a course of medication and starting psychotherapy, may be introduced. Patients who experience mild anxiety may benefit from nonpharmacologic interventions, such as yoga, deep breathing, and journaling.

Collaboration

With the exception of panic disorder, the treatment of anxiety disorders occurs more frequently in the home and community than in the hospital. Considering the level of distress that accompanies anxiety disorders, it is not difficult to understand the vulnerability of individuals with anxiety to

Evidence-Based Practice
Anxiety Disorders and Oxidative Stress
Problem

Psychologic stress has been associated with oxidative stress (OS), which is a loss of balance in the body's oxidation–reduction reactions. In OS, production of reactive oxygen species (ROS) and reactive nitrogen species (RNS) outpaces production of counteracting antioxidants. The result is cellular and molecular damage. Because of its high level of oxygen consumption and its lipid-rich nature, the brain is especially susceptible to OS. Research suggests a connection between OS and anxiety and depression, though the nature of this connection remains unclear (Salim, 2014).

Evidence

OS produces an inflammatory response; when this response occurs in the brain, it is known as neuroinflammation. Research indicates that chronic stress leads to chronic neuroinflammation, which damages neurons. This damage is associated with anxiety behaviors and depression (Xu, Wang, Klabnik, & O'Donnell, 2014).

Studies in mice further suggest that OS progressively increases with repeated exposure to stress, and that chronic stress alters expression of the genes that regulate antioxidant systems (Seo et al., 2012). The hippocampus and frontal cortex of the brain appear to be most affected by the negative effects of OS, but it is unclear whether OS is a side effect or cause of psychologic distress (Xu et al., 2014). Although the causal relationship between the two has yet to be determined, the link between them is well established, with much research focusing on the importance of excess ROS in anxiety (Salim, 2014).

Implications

Antidepressants are often prescribed for anxiety because of their primary effects on norepinephrine and serotonin. Research now suggests that the secondary antioxidant effects of these medications may also be beneficial to patients with anxiety. Few trials have been conducted with human subjects, but animal studies in this area are promising (Xu et al., 2014).

There is also a lack of research into the safety of antioxidants in amounts greater than those found in food (Xu et al., 2014). For patients with anxiety, the principal source of antioxidants remains diet. Vitamin C, vitamin E, carotenoids, selenium, and manganese all have antioxidant properties, as do flavonoids and phenols. Plant-based foods are the best dietary sources of these antioxidants and include fruits, vegetables, whole grains, nuts, and legumes (Harvard School of Public Health, n.d.). In addition, the nutrients found in these foods may benefit health for reasons other than their antioxidant properties.

Critical Thinking Application

1. Consider the relationship of OS and anxiety. How do you think this relates to an individual's environment and upbringing?
2. Do you think OS is triggered by an individual's lifestyle, or might a state of OS impact the way an individual handles stressors in his or her environment?
3. Is the OS theory of anxiety relevant to clinical practice? With this theory in mind, would you recommend dietary or lifestyle changes to patients with anxiety?

Clinical Manifestations and Therapies
Anxiety Disorders

LEVEL OF SEVERITY OF ANXIETY	CLINICAL MANIFESTATIONS	CLINICAL THERAPIES
Mild	■ Increase in sensory perception and arousal ■ Increase in alertness ■ Sleeplessness ■ Increase in motivation ■ Restlessness and irritability	■ Mild anxiety typically is resolved by an individual's coping mechanisms. Mild anxiety may be helpful to the patient to accentuate focus and concentration. ■ Patients who are distressed by mild anxiety may benefit from Improved sleep hygiene Relaxation techniques Behavior therapy Massage Aromatherapy.
Moderate	■ Narrowing of perceptual field and attention span (a process called "selective inattention") ■ Reduction in alertness and awareness of surroundings ■ Feeling of discomfort and irritability with others ■ Self-absorption ■ Increased restlessness ■ Increase in respirations, heart rate, and muscle tension ■ Increase in perspiration ■ Rapid speech, louder tone, and higher pitch	■ Cognitive and behavior therapy to identify triggers and learn improved coping techniques. ■ Relaxation techniques. ■ Integrative therapies such as yoga, acupuncture, massage. ■ Low-dose antianxiety medications if symptoms do not improve with other therapies or if the medications exacerbate chronic conditions.
Severe	■ Perceptual field greatly reduced ■ Difficulty following directions ■ Feelings of dread, horror ■ Need to relieve anxiety ■ Headache ■ Dizziness ■ Nausea, trembling, insomnia ■ Palpitations, tachycardia, hyperventilating, diarrhea	■ Cognitive and behavior therapy to learn to identify triggers and to learn better coping techniques. ■ Antianxiety medications (may include benzodiazepines). ■ Relaxation techniques. ■ Integrative therapies such as yoga, acupuncture, massage. ■ Hospitalization may be required initially to manage severe anxiety until improved coping mechanisms are developed.
Panic	■ Inability to focus ■ Perception distorted ■ Terror ■ Feelings of doom ■ Bizarre behavior ■ Dilated pupils ■ Trembling, sleeplessness, palpitations, pallor, diaphoresis, muscular incoordination ■ Immobility or hyperactivity, incoherence	Immediate, structured intervention required. ■ Immediate therapies include the following: Placing patient in a quiet, less stimulating environment Use of repetitive or physical task to diffuse energy Administration of antianxiety medications. ■ Long-term therapies include the following: Psychotherapy (cognitive, behavioral, or CBT) Pharmacologic therapy Relaxation techniques Improved sleep hygiene Integrative health therapies such as massage, acupuncture, yoga, hydrotherapy Nutrition consultation Mental health counseling.

substance abuse and/or depression. This combination is a threat to treatment success and positive outcomes for the individual. Because the individual is part of a family and a larger community, nurses need to support positive outcomes for individuals by involving both the individual and his or her family in the treatment process. Such treatment is multimodal and involves the assessment of age, education, health and health practices, spirituality, and culturally specific needs (NIMH, 2013a).

Diagnostic Tests

Evaluation of an individual with symptoms of an anxiety disorder includes a complete medical history and physical exam. Currently no laboratory tests are available to diagnose any of the anxiety disorders, but various diagnostic tests may be used to rule out physical illness as the cause of the symptoms. If no physical illness is found, the patient may be referred to a mental health professional trained to diagnose and treat mental illnesses. Mental health providers use specially designed interview and assessment tools to evaluate an individual for an anxiety disorder. The mental health professional bases the diagnosis on the patient's subjective report of the duration and intensity of symptoms, including any interference with daily functioning. The diagnosis is typically made according to the criteria in the DSM-5.

Pharmacologic Therapy

Medication does not cure anxiety disorders, but it can control or diminish the severity of the associated signs and symptoms while the patient enters psychotherapy. Medication may be prescribed by a psychiatrist, advanced practice psychiatric/mental health nurse, or primary care provider (e.g., physician, nurse practitioner). The medications usually used for anxiety disorders are antidepressants, antianxiety drugs, and beta-blockers, although antipsychotics are sometimes used. See the Medications feature in this module's Concept section for more information.

Antidepressants were developed to treat depression, but they are also effective for anxiety disorders. Although they begin to alter brain chemistry after the first dose, their full effect requires a few weeks because a series of neurobiological changes must take place before antidepressants achieve efficacy. SSRIs alter the levels of the neurotransmitter serotonin in the brain and are commonly prescribed for anxiety disorders. SSRIs are generally started at low doses and then increased as their effectiveness becomes apparent. SSRIs have fewer side effects than previous generations of antidepressants, but they sometimes generate nausea, agitation, and occasionally sexual dysfunction. Related to the SSRIs, SNRIs inhibit the reabsorption of serotonin and norepinephrine to elevate mood. Examples of SNRIs include venlafaxine and duloxetine.

The most commonly used antianxiety drugs are benzodiazepines. When used for a short time, these drugs have few side effects other than drowsiness. However, higher and higher doses may be necessary over a long period of time, so benzodiazepines are typically not prescribed for long-term use. Because they take only hours to reach efficacy, they often are prescribed for patients experiencing severe or panic levels of anxiety. Patients with panic disorder can typically take benzodiazepines for up to a year without harm. Examples of benzodiazepines used in the treatment of anxiety include alprazolam (Xanax), diazepam (Valium), lorazepam (Ativan), and chlordiazepoxide (Librium) (Adams et al., 2017).

Some patients experience withdrawal symptoms if they stop taking benzodiazepines abruptly, and anxiety can return immediately after cessation. Their potential for tolerance and withdrawal have led some physicians to avoid prescriptions for benzodiazepines. Buspirone (Buspar), an azapirone, is a newer antianxiety medication used to treat GAD. It has the benefit of no risk of dependence. Possible side effects include nausea, headaches, and dizziness. Unlike benzodiazepines, buspirone must be taken consistently for at least 2 weeks to achieve an antianxiety effect.

SAFETY ALERT Benzodiazepines can be habit forming and should be used cautiously in individuals with a history of drug or alcohol addiction. Abruptly discontinuing use of benzodiazepines can result in withdrawal, and patients discontinuing benzodiazepines should slowly taper down following their doctor's instructions. In addition, benzodiazepine use in older adults is linked to an increased incidence of dementia, so they should be used with caution in older adults (de Gage et al., 2012)

MAOIs may be used to treat anxiety. MAOIs inhibit the action of monoamine oxidase (MAO), which is responsible for terminating the action of neurotransmitters such as serotonin, norepinephrine, and dopamine. Because of their high side effect profile (e.g., insomnia, hypertensive crisis, sexual dysfunction, respiratory and circulatory collapse, and serotonin syndrome), MAOIs are often the last line of treatment for patients who do not respond to other treatments. MAOIs also have several drug–drug interactions and food–drug interactions that make their use more complicated in patients with multiple diseases.

Beta-blockers, such as propranolol (which is used to treat heart conditions), can prevent the physical abnormalities (such as blushing and hyperventilation) that accompany certain anxiety disorders, particularly social anxiety disorder. When a feared situation can be predicted (such as speaking before a large group or flying in an airplane), the physician may prescribe a beta-blocker to manage the physical symptoms of anxiety (NIMH, n.d.d).

At times, antipsychotic medications—drugs typically reserved for conditions such as bipolar disorder and schizophrenia—are used to treat anxiety disorders. Typical antipsychotics, the first drugs of this type, include haloperidol, chlorpromazine, and loxapine. These drugs have been shown to produce a significant reduction in neurotic anxiety. Atypical antipsychotics, a later generation of antipsychotics, provide potential benefits for patients with GAD. Extended-release quetiapine has been shown to prevent relapse anxiety in patients with GAD, but more studies need to be performed to examine the risks and benefits of using antipsychotic medications for anxiety disorders (Jewell, 2015).

Nonpharmacologic Therapy

Nonpharmacologic therapy is very effective in the treatment of anxiety disorders. Integrative health practices can be used in conjunction with pharmacotherapy to bring relief to patients with anxiety disorders, but the most effective non-pharmacologic therapy is psychotherapy, including CBT. Psychotherapy involves talking with a mental health professional, (e.g., psychiatrist, psychologist, advanced practice psychiatric nurse, social worker, counselor) to uncover what triggers the anxiety disorder and to determine how to work through its symptoms. The most effective treatment strategy for most people with anxiety disorders is a combination of CBT and medication (NIMH, 2015).

Cognitive–behavioral Therapy

CBT is a useful nonpharmacologic intervention for treating anxiety disorders. The cognitive aspect of this treatment helps the patient recognize and change the thought patterns that support his fears, and the behavioral aspect helps the patient change the way he reacts to anxiety-provoking situations. This intervention has been proven to reduce the symptoms of all types of anxiety disorders. For additional discussion of CBT, refer to the Concept section of this module.

Integrative Health

Although conventional medical therapies have been consistently shown to ease the symptoms of anxiety disorders, integrative therapies also have been shown to ease the symptoms of anxiety. These therapies include herbal preparations, massage and touch, and yoga and meditation.

Herbal Preparations

Overall, herbal preparations show little promise as potential therapies for the symptoms of anxiety. However, a few different plant species seem to have moderate effects on anxiety disorders. Scientific studies provide evidence that kava, a member of the pepper family, may be beneficial for anxiety management, but the U.S. Food and Drug Administration (FDA) has warned that kava supplements have been linked to a risk of severe liver damage. In addition, kava has been associated with cases of dystonia, drowsiness, and scaly, yellowed skin. It is also suspected to interact with drugs used to treat Parkinson disease.

Lavender is commonly used for aromatherapy, in which the essential oil from the flowers is inhaled. Dried lavender flowers can be used to make teas or liquid extracts that can be taken orally. Small studies on lavender show mixed results, and topical use of diluted lavender and the use of the oil for aromatherapy is considered safe for adults. However, the undiluted oil irritates skin, is poisonous by mouth, and may cause drowsiness (National Center for Complementary and Integrative Health [NCCIH], 2012).

Chamomile is a traditional remedy in widespread use, and a recent study has found that the plant has modest benefits for some people with mild to moderate GAD. Chamomile is generally well tolerated. However, there are reports of allergic reactions in people who have eaten chamomile products, especially individuals who are allergic to plants in the daisy family, including ragweed, chrysanthemums, marigolds, and daisies (UMMC, 2015).

Massage and Therapeutic Touch

Scientific research on massage and touch therapy is limited, but evidence suggests that massage may benefit some patients. A single session of massage therapy can reduce state anxiety (a reaction to a particular situation), blood pressure, and heart rate, and multiple sessions can reduce "trait anxiety" (an individual's predisposition to anxiety), depression, and pain. It is not currently known how massage therapy has these effects on the body. *Gate control theory*, for instance, suggests that massage may provide stimulation to block pain signals sent to the brain. Other theories suggest that massage may stimulate the release of chemicals such as serotonin or endorphins or cause mechanical changes in the body.

Relaxation Techniques, Yoga, and Meditation

In addition to being a state of mind, relaxation physically changes the way the body functions, relieving stress in the process. When the body relaxes, breathing slows, blood pressure and oxygen consumption decrease, and well-being increases. Being able to produce the relaxation response by using relaxation techniques may counteract the long-term stress that can lead to anxiety disorders. Relaxation techniques often combine breathing and focused attention to calm the mind and body, and usually only require brief instruction from a practitioner before they can be done without assistance. Common relaxation techniques include autogenic training, biofeedback, deep breathing, guided imagery, progressive relation, and self-hypnosis.

Yoga, a tradition linked to Indian spiritual practice, can also be used to produce a relaxation response. Yoga is currently widely used as an integrative health practice and for exercise purposes. Many people who practice yoga do so to maintain well-being, improve fitness, and relieve stress, in addition to addressing specific health conditions such as back pain, arthritis, and anxiety (NCCIH, 2013).

Evidence also suggests that religious or secular meditation can be used to combat the effects of anxiety. Several studies have found that transcendental meditation (TM) helped participants decrease psychologic distress and increase coping ability. In one particular study, TM was shown effective for reducing stress, burnout, and depression in teachers and support staff working with students who have behavioral problems (Elder, Nidich, Moriarty, & Nidich, 2014).

Lifespan Considerations

Anxiety is common in every age group, but stressors, coping mechanisms, and treatment options are different depending on the patient's developmental level. For children, adolescents, pregnant women, and older adults, specific knowledge of their unique situations is required in order to provide appropriate care.

Anxiety in Children

Symptoms of anxiety disorders in childhood are more prevalent in girls and children from low socioeconomic backgrounds. All children from disadvantaged socioeconomic backgrounds are more vulnerable to emotional illness than their more advantaged peers. Familial predisposition is also a contributing vulnerability factor. Studies suggest that, in general, 3–5% of children and adolescents have an anxiety disorder of some kind. Similar to adults, children with anxiety disorders run the risk of

TABLE 31–6 Symptoms of Anxiety in Children and Adolescents

Symptoms common to both children and adolescents	■ Excessive worrying ■ Headaches and body aches ■ Stomachaches ■ Muscle tension
Symptoms common in children	■ Frequently missing school or social activities ■ Tiredness/exhaustion/fatigue ■ Declining grades at school ■ Trouble sleeping/nightmares ■ Restlessness ■ Trouble concentrating ■ Irritability ■ Extreme homesickness when away from family ■ Shyness ■ Frequent crying
Symptoms common in adolescents	■ Withdrawal from social activities ■ Inner restlessness ■ Continual nervousness ■ Perform poorly in school ■ Dependency ■ Easily startle, sweat, blotch, or flush ■ Engage in substance abuse ■ Impulsive sexual behavior ■ May also have depression or an eating disorder ■ Interferes with their ability to function ■ Suicidal ideations ■ Changes in eating habits and sleeping patterns ■ Self-injury/cutting ■ Trembling ■ Frequent need to urinate

developing other anxiety disorders, depression, and substance abuse (UMMC, 2013). Common signs and symptoms of anxiety in children are listed in **Table 31–6 ⟫**.

One of the most common anxiety disorders in children is separation anxiety disorder (SAD). Children with SAD fear being lost from their family or fear something bad happening to a loved one. They may have inappropriate or excessive worry about being apart from people to whom they are most attached, may refuse to sleep alone or have repeated nightmares with a theme of separation, may worry excessively about family members, and may refuse to go to school. Other symptoms may include a reluctance to be alone, frequent physical complaints, muscle aches, excessive worry, and an excessive "clinginess" even when at home. Symptoms of fear must be powerful enough to interfere with everyday life and must last for at least 4 weeks to be considered SAD.

Symptoms of SAD are more severe than those of normal separation anxiety, which is a developmental phase that most children experience between the ages of 18 months and 3 years. SAD is also distinct from stranger anxiety, which is normal for children between 7 and 11 years old. In children, SAD occurs equally in boys and girls, and the first indications of the condition often occur between the ages of 7 and 9. Approximately 4% of younger children have SAD, and the

estimate for adolescents is slightly lower (Children's Hospital of Pittsburgh, 2013). In some cases, separation anxiety can persist or recur in adulthood as adult separation anxiety (ASAD), though ASAD may have its first onset in adulthood (Milrod et al., 2014). Some phobias also develop during childhood. Social anxiety disorder, for example, typically develops between the ages of 11 and 15 and almost never after the age of 25. Situational phobias, on the other hand, generally develop by the mid-20s. Unlike adults with phobic disorders, children are not always able to understand that the fear created by a phobic stressor is irrational.

Anxiety in children is often treated with CBT, medication, or a combination of both. SSRIs are the medications of choice for children with anxiety. Tricyclic antidepressants and benzodiazepines are less commonly used to treat children. Other forms of therapy, including acceptance and commitment therapy (ACT) and dialectical behavioral therapy (DBT), may also be used in children in place of CBT (ADAA, n.d.c). However, the most effective treatment is a combination of SSRIs with CBT. Children may also benefit from family therapy and parent education (Cleveland Clinic, 2013).

Anxiety in Adolescents

An estimated 8% of adolescents between ages 13 and 18 have an anxiety disorder, with symptoms often manifesting in childhood. Only 18% of adolescents with a diagnosed anxiety disorder receive professional mental healthcare (NIMH, n.d.e). The difficulty in distinguishing anxiety from the normal developmental challenges of adolescence contributes to this low rate of treatment. Girls are more than twice as likely as boys to be diagnosed with anxiety during adolescence (Steingard, 2014).

Issues of social acceptance and independence are common stressors for adolescents, as is dissatisfaction with physical changes to the body during the teen years. Adolescents with anxiety disorders may appear shy or withdrawn in social situations and may refuse to engage in new experiences. They may also avoid activities that they previously enjoyed. Extremes of emotion may occur, with responses being either overly emotional or overly restrained. In an attempt to lessen feelings of anxiety, individuals may engage in dangerous or uncharacteristic behaviors. Anxiety tends to be comorbid with other mental health problems, and adolescents believed to have an anxiety disorder should be assessed for depression, developmental conditions, and language problems (Creswell et al., 2014). Treatment of anxiety in adolescents is similar to treatment of anxiety in children.

SAFETY ALERT Studies have indicated that adolescents, as well as some children, have an increased risk of developing suicidal ideations when taking SSRIs (Gibbons et al., 2015), so medical professionals should discuss the risks and rewards of pharmacologic therapy with adolescents and their parents before prescribing SSRIs.

Anxiety in Pregnant Women

Psychologic stress is common during pregnancy, with mild anxiety presenting frequently both before and after giving birth. Reliable data about the prevalence of prenatal anxiety do not exist; however, one study estimates that as many as 18% of pregnant women and 20% of new mothers develop severe anxiety (George et al., 2013). Maternal anxiety leads to negative physical outcomes for mother and child and inhibits parental bonding.

Common stressors during pregnancy include concerns about resources, employment, and personal responsibilities, as well as fears related to the birth process and pregnancy complications. In addition, individuals at the greatest risk for anxiety during pregnancy tend to be insecure in personal relationships, have a history of infertility, and lack psychosocial resources (Schetter & Tanner, 2012). Common symptoms of anxiety such as fatigue and sleep disturbance are not reliable predictors of anxiety in pregnancy because they are commonly experienced during pregnancy; other symptoms such as panic attacks and muscle tension may be indicative of maternal anxiety.

Pregnant women must be very careful about treating anxiety with medication. Studies indicate that birth defects occur two to three times more frequently in babies born to women who took certain SSRIs during early pregnancy, specifically fluoxetine and paroxetine. However, other SSRIs, including sertraline, do not carry these same effects (Reefhuis et al., 2015). In addition, use of SSRIs in the third trimester is associated with an increased risk of pulmonary hypertension and other problems in the newborn (ADAA, 2015b). However, abruptly stopping SSRI use could be harmful for both mother and baby, so women with mild anxiety who are considering getting pregnant should taper off anxiety medications several months before attempting to become pregnant. Untreated anxiety in a pregnant woman is also hazardous, potentially leading to low birth weight, premature birth, and difficulty adapting to life outside the womb for the infant and to pregnancy termination, postpartum depression, impaired attachment to the baby, substance abuse, and other complications for the mother. Therefore, nonpharmacologic approaches such as CBT and relaxation techniques are a high priority for treatment of anxiety in pregnant women. In addition, women with severe anxiety may decide to continue their medication after discussing all options with their healthcare provider, because even though the risk of birth defects is higher for women who take SSRIs and other antianxiety medications, the risk is still very low (less than 1%).

Anxiety in Older Adults

Older adults with cognitive impairments or one or more chronic physical impairments are at increased risk for developing anxiety. Significant emotional loss, such as the death of a spouse, also increases the older adult's risk for anxiety. In older adults, manifestations of anxiety may overlap with medical illness, resulting in older adults presenting first to their primary care provider. Although the prevalence rates of anxiety disorders in older adults are lower than in the general population, this may be due to misdiagnosis rather than to an actual lower rate of anxiety in older adults. Risk factors for anxiety disorders in older adults include lower education levels, presence of multiple chronic illnesses, and being unmarried (D'Arrigo, 2013).

Older adults have differences in drug absorption, action, metabolism, and excretion compared with younger adults. They also are more likely to experience side effects associated with antianxiety medications, especially if they take medications for physical illnesses that may have drug–drug interactions with medications prescribed for anxiety. Pharmacologic treatment should begin with low doses in this population and be titrated to higher doses based on effectiveness and occurrence of side effects. In addition, benzodiazepines should be avoided in the older population because of harmful side effects such as a decrease in cognition. Similar to other age groups, older adults may find that CBT is effective for treating their anxiety.

NURSING PROCESS

Nursing interventions are focused on reducing the severity of the symptoms of anxiety. Specific interventions include establishing a rapport, communicating therapeutically, supporting and enhancing coping skills, assessing and identifying maladaptive coping, fostering mental health, maintaining a therapeutic milieu, minimizing the deleterious effects of anxiety, and promoting the health of the individual. The generalist nurse provides case management, home healthcare, psychoeducation, and medication administration.

Assessment

- **Observation and patient interview.** Assessment of patients with anxiety includes interviewing the patient with regard to current and previous illnesses, medication (and supplement) regimen, and past and present stressors. In addition, the nurse should tactfully interview the patient about current and previous methods of coping, including the use of alcohol and drugs, particularly because certain coping methods may actually compound the individual's sense of anxiety and may predispose the patient to developing an illness or other health alteration.

In particular, the nursing assessment for individuals experiencing mild anxiety should focus on appraisal. To gain understanding about the individual, the nurse acquires information about how the person appraises and prioritizes stressors. To facilitate the adaptive coping process, the nurse critically evaluates thoughts that may be increasing the person's anxiety. In addition, the nurse should do the following when appraising the patient's anxiety or fear:

- Observe for physical symptoms associated with anxiety. Muscle tension or twitching, trembling, body aches and soreness, cold or clammy hands, dry mouth, and sweating are common in individuals with anxiety disorders. Nausea, diarrhea, and urinary frequency may also occur (UMMC, 2013).
- Review the medical history for conditions that commonly occur with anxiety. Depression, bipolar disorder, substance abuse, and eating disorders often occur in addition to anxiety disorders (UMMC, 2013).
- Consider family history of anxiety disorders or depression. Individuals with blood relations diagnosed with anxiety or depression are more likely to have these conditions (UMMC, 2013).
- Assess the patient's emotional and psychologic well-being. Levels of life satisfaction and happiness are often lower in individuals with excessive anxiety (Centers

for Disease Control and Prevention [CDC], 2013). Self-acceptance, openness to new experiences, hopefulness, and sense of purpose are impacted by anxiety. The number and positive or negative nature of personal relationships should also be considered (CDC, 2013).

- Gauge the patient's social well-being. Anxiety may affect an individual's sense of social acceptance and usefulness to society, as well as his or her beliefs about society as a whole (CDC, 2013).
- Consider socioeconomic pressures the patient is facing. Pressures such as unemployment or financial loss pose risks to individual mental health and create anxiety (World Health Organization [WHO], 2014).
- Assess the patient's home and work conditions. Stressful or violent home life, high-pressure work conditions, and rapid change in either the home or workplace contribute to anxiety (WHO, 2014).

- ***Physical examination.*** Physical assessment should include a general assessment, as well as a focused assessment of any body systems that are relevant to the patient's current complaints.

Diagnosis

Selection of nursing diagnoses should be patient-specific and depends on numerous factors, including the degree to which anxiety is impacting the patient's daily life and social interaction. Examples of nursing diagnoses that may be appropriate for inclusion in the plan of care for the patient with an anxiety or a phobic disorder may include the following:

- *Anxiety*
- *Fear*
- *Knowledge, Deficient*
- *Coping, Ineffective*
- *Social Interaction, Impaired*
- *Sleep Pattern, Disturbed*
- *Health Management, Ineffective.*

(NANDA-I © 2014)

Planning

The nursing plan of care, designed in collaboration with the patient, may include the following goals:

- The patient will report a decrease in level of anxiety and frequency of anxiety episodes.
- The patient will report a decrease in the frequency and severity of phobic episodes.
- The patient will articulate successful coping mechanisms.
- The patient will report increasing use of successful coping mechanisms.
- The patient will verbalize healthy ways of responding to fear.
- The patient will demonstrate effective implementation of relaxation techniques.
- The patient will participate in psychotherapy or group counseling activities as outlined by the primary care provider.

Implementation

Interventions appropriate for patients with anxiety symptoms vary depending primarily on the severity of the individual's symptoms. Patients with severe anxiety or panic require immediate intervention and close supervision. The safety of the individual is at risk because of the narrowing of perception and inability to process information and think rationally. Patients with mild or moderate anxiety can benefit from several nursing interventions, including helping them identify triggers for their anxiety, providing patient teaching, and promoting effective coping and healthy behaviors (see **Figure 31–8 》**). Patients with severe anxiety or panic will also benefit from these interventions when their anxiety has subsided to a manageable level.

Interventions for Mild Anxiety

Patients experiencing mild anxiety are often able to learn information and acquire new behaviors easily. The nurse is able to provide valuable information to these patients, teaching them ways to manage stress and modify thinking processes and behaviors. The nurse should review the following when teaching the patient about anxiety disorders:

- How to recognize triggers and symptoms of anxiety. Early recognition of triggers can help patients respond with healthy coping strategies before anxiety levels rise.
- How to identify anxiety levels. Mild levels of anxiety can sometimes improve motivation and learning, whereas moderate and severe anxiety impact concentration and perception. Differentiating among the various levels helps patients determine if they are having a useful, appropriate anxiety response or an inappropriate anxiety response with potentially negative effects.
- Self-management and diversion techniques for coping with anxiety. Stepping back from a situation in order to reassess it and learning to accept that some things cannot be controlled are important self-management skills. Exercising, engaging in hobbies, and spending time with friends or family are often effective diversions. Both types of techniques help the patient refocus the mind away from stressors to lessen anxiety (Mayo Clinic, 2014b).

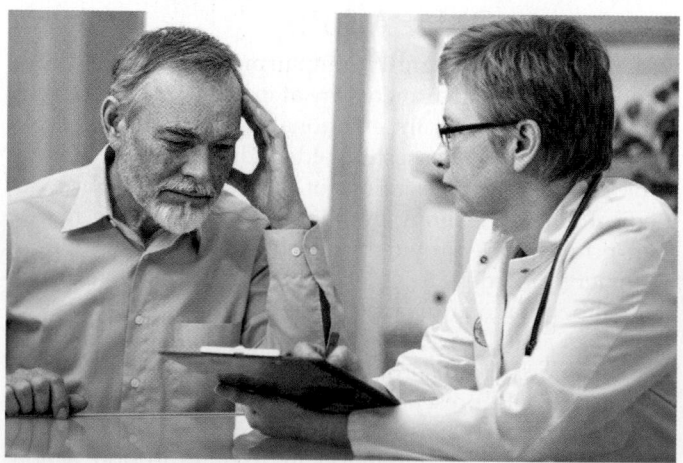

Source: Alexander Raths/Shutterstock.

Figure 31–8 》 Nurses can help patients cope with anxiety through a number of interventions.

- Introducing the concept of positive self-talk for coping with anxiety. Positive self-talk helps patients replace anxious thoughts with more rational and realistic ones. Self-talk typically involves the patient repeating a set of statements to herself in an effort to curtail anxiety. The first statement is generally a firm but gentle admonition designed to stop anxious thoughts. This may be followed by one or more positive coping statements.

- Encouraging the use of muscle relaxation and mental visualization to refocus attention away from anxiety. Meditation, deep breathing, and yoga are popular relaxation techniques that patients can do in their own homes (UMMC, 2013).

- The importance of taking medications as prescribed. The majority of medications used to treat anxiety disorders influence activity of neurotransmitters and typically take up to several weeks to achieve efficacy. Skipping a dose on days when anxiety levels are low will negatively impact a medication's overall effectiveness. It may also increase the patient's risk for relapse of anxiety symptoms. Medication should only be discontinued as instructed by a healthcare provider.

- The importance of attending therapy sessions as prescribed. The goal of psychotherapy and CBT is the reduction of anxiety symptoms. Throughout the therapy process, symptoms improve as initial successes are built upon. Failure to participate in therapy sessions hinders the building process (Mayo Clinic, 2014b).

- Information about community resources for everyday and emergency situations. Everyday resources include support groups, message boards, and local and national organizations dedicated to anxiety disorders. Emergency resources include crisis hotlines, emergency departments, and trusted mental health professionals familiar with the patient's disorder.

For additional information, see the Patient Teaching feature.

Interventions for Moderate Anxiety

Patients with moderate anxiety need appropriate intervention to prevent escalation of symptoms. Interventions may include:

- Encourage participation in diversional activities, such as exercise, to reduce stress. For example, walking briskly, running, or working out large muscle groups assists the individual to manage her own physical responses to anxiety.

- Help the patient identify current stressors. When the patient knows and can identify the situations that cause anxiety, he can develop a systematic approach to addressing or eliminating the stressor. Eliminating the stressor rather than simply avoiding it reduces the anxiety associated with it in the long term.

- Help the patient identify what coping strategies have been successful in the past. When the patient knows and can identify strategies he has used successfully in the past, he may be able to return to earlier patterns that are helpful in reducing his anxiety.

- Encourage the patient to adhere to the treatment regimen and discuss the addition of integrative therapies with the primary care provider. Patients can become discouraged while waiting for pharmacologic interventions to take full effect or while learning new strategies for coping in psychotherapy. Adding one or more integrative therapies as adjuvant treatment may help relieve symptoms of anxiety until medications or psychotherapy begin to take effect.

Interventions for Severe Anxiety

Patients with severe anxiety benefit from clear, direct communication and simple questions rather than questions or instructions that require the patient to process more than one thing at a time. Some interventions for moderate anxiety, such as identifying triggers and determining helpful strategies that have worked in the past, are also appropriate when working with patients with severe anxiety. As always, the nurse should administer medications as ordered and encourage patients to adhere to the therapeutic regimen (e.g., therapy, exercise, use of previously identified integrative therapies such as yoga). Some patients may require inpatient hospitalization until they are able to reduce their anxiety level and develop new strategies for coping.

Interventions for Panic

Patients who are at a panic level of anxiety require active supervision and clear, direct communication. Remain with the patient to ensure his own and others' safety. Patients at this stage may require assistance from the nurse to meet basic needs, such as nutrition and fluids, pain relief, elimination, or rest.

- Maintain a calm demeanor. Speak slowly using a low-pitched voice. High-pitched voices can increase anxiety, and the nurse's calm presence may help reduce patient anxiety and fear.

- Reduce environmental stimuli. A calm environment promotes calmness in the patient.

- Reinforce reality when thought processes are altered because of fear. Help the patient focus on what is real.

- Set limits as necessary to ensure safety. Use simple statements and speak in an authoritative voice.

- Allow pacing or harmless repetitive physical tasks, as these can help diffuse negative energy.

- Administer medications as ordered.

Patient Teaching
Techniques to Reduce Anxiety

Essential teaching for the individual experiencing an anxiety disorder or phobia includes deep breathing and progressive relaxation techniques to lower anxiety responses. Avoidance of stimulants, caffeine, and nicotine is essential. Instructing the patient on the use of cognitive techniques can be helpful in lowering the individual's response to the threat. Strategies such as thought blocking, self-talk, and conversation with a support person all assist the individual to manage and empower more adaptive coping skills. Physical exercise that makes use of large muscle groups, such as walking, running, weight lifting, hiking, and various sport activities, can dissipate pent-up energy. Exercising also releases natural chemicals such as endorphins, improving mood and natural pain relief.

Evaluation

Evaluation of the patient experiencing anxiety is based on the symptoms with which she presented and her strengths and weaknesses. Suggested expected outcomes may include:

- The patient's anxiety has diminished as reflected by vital signs returning to baseline and patient's report of a decreased level of anxiety.

- The patient demonstrates new or improved coping measures to reduce anxiety.

- The patient self-moderates the anxiety response when stressors occur.

- The patient engages in healthy behaviors related to sleep, exercise, and nutrition.

- The patient demonstrates a desire to overcome anxiety and a willingness to follow the treatment regimen.

If the patient is still experiencing anxiety during the evaluation phase, the nurse should provide secondary interventions. In all cases of unresolved anxiety, the nurse should provide patient teaching related to additional nonpharmacologic coping techniques that the patient may use. For example, if the patient was taught only relaxation exercises, the nurse may advocate for CBT or teach deep breathing exercises. If the patient has tried CBT with little success, the nurse may advocate with the physician to prescribe an antianxiety medication. Using multiple coping strategies in addition to nonpharmacologic and pharmacologic therapies may be needed to successfully reduce anxiety over the long term in patients with anxiety disorders.

Nursing Care Plan

A Patient with Agoraphobia

Mrs. Randolph is 43 years old, married, and the mother of four daughters in their late teens and early twenties. She is referred to the psychiatric outpatient clinic from the local emergency department following an acute panic attack with symptoms of racing heartbeat, sweating, feeling faint, and the belief that she was dying.

ASSESSMENT	DIAGNOSES	PLANNING
She could not identify any events, thoughts, or feelings that precipitated the incident; it seemed to occur "out of the blue." She felt unable to cope with the severity of the symptoms of the attack: "I tried to talk myself out of it; to tell myself it would go away, but it only got worse." Mrs. Randolph reports she has had similar attacks lasting from 2 minutes to 2 hours in the past with no physical cause found by her family physician. Her daily routine has become restricted, and she will not leave the house without a family member. She is not comfortable alone in her home and can't sleep if any family member is still out. She is ashamed and angry about her growing disability and often tries to cover up her fears to friends and family. Recent life events include a hysterectomy 4 weeks ago and loss of employment resulting from hospitalization; the second anniversary of her father's sudden death is upcoming. She has no other history of mental health issues. She saw a therapist for her panic disorder when the attacks first started, "about the time I left home to marry," but did not follow up because she felt ashamed ("I've always been a strong and effective person!"), because the episodes were not so severe then, and because she found relief from the panic attacks after she had children. Her mother rarely left the house, never participating in social events unless they were in the home. She described her relationship with her husband as emotionally warm and supportive. She dreads seeing her daughters move from home. Assessment findings: - Is an attractive, carefully groomed woman who looks her stated age. - Appears somewhat tense. - Answers questions cooperatively, but at times with some hesitation, as if expecting criticism or judgment from the interviewer. - Oriented to time, place, and person. - Memory intact, good recall, no difficulty with calculations. - Affect appears normal, with occasional evidence of anger in the form of irritability or sarcasm. Mood is within normal limits. - Speech normal in flow and volume, pressured at times when she corrects an impression. - Posture rigid at times, but she relaxes as she becomes more comfortable with the interview.	- *Role Performance, Ineffective* related to fear and anxiety level - *Coping, Ineffective* related to overwhelming fears (NANDA-I © 2014) - Disturbed thought processes related to high level of anxiety	Goals of care include: - The patient will describe specific changes in role function. - The patient will demonstrate appropriate decision making. - The patient will demonstrate effective coping as evidenced by employing behaviors to reduce stress and reporting fewer negative feelings.

Nursing Care Plan (continued)

IMPLEMENTATION

- Maintain a calm manner.
- Stay with the patient.
- Use short, simple sentences.
- Direct patient's attention to a repetitive or physical task.
- Administer pharmacologic agents as ordered.

- Encourage patient to identify previous coping skills.
- Help patient identify coping resources (including social supports).
- Teach patient relaxation techniques.
- Encourage patient to verbalize feelings.

EVALUATION

Expected outcomes to evaluate the patient's response to care include:

- The patient demonstrates role performance as evidenced by the ability to meet role expectations, knowledge of role transition periods, and reported strategies for role changes.

- The patient demonstrates ability to choose between two or more alternatives.
- The patient uses actions to manage stressors that tax personal resources.

CRITICAL THINKING

1. What factors may be contributing to Mrs. Randolph's agoraphobia?

2. What interview questions would you like to ask Mrs. Randolph's family?

3. What strategies would you recommend to help Mrs. Randolph overcome her fear of leaving her house alone?

REVIEW Anxiety Disorders

RELATE Link the Concepts and Exemplars

Linking the exemplar of anxiety disorders with the concept of perfusion:

1. What impact does anxiety have on perfusion?

2. What medications normally prescribed for anxiety would be contraindicated for an individual with a history of heart disease?

Linking the exemplar of anxiety disorders with the concept of acid–base balance:

3. How might anxiety impact acid–base balance?

4. What nursing interventions might the nurse recommend for the patient with anxiety that is altering acid–base balance?

READY Go to Volume 3: Clinical Nursing Skills

REFER Go to Pearson MyLab Nursing and eText

- Additional review materials

REFLECT Apply Your Knowledge

Heather O'Malley is a 34-year-old woman who is newly separated from her husband. She has been a stay-at-home mother of children ages 7, 5, and 4, along with a 3-month-old infant. Her days are very busy caring for her young children, and she wonders how she will manage on her own, especially because she will need to find a job in order to provide for the financial needs of the household now that her husband has moved out. Although he is paying court-ordered child support, it is not enough to meet the living expenses of Ms. O'Malley and all four children. Her attempts to work with a lawyer to get additional money in the form of alimony are on hold because she does not have money to pay the lawyer.

Ms. O'Malley worked as a nurse before quitting when the oldest child was born. She looks into taking a refresher course so she can return to nursing and learns that several hospitals provide the course free of charge if she agrees to work for them after successful completion. She applies to one of these hospitals and is called for an interview. Ms. O'Malley wakes up early on the morning of the interview, feeds the older children and sends them to school, then takes the youngest child to the house of a neighbor who has agreed to babysit. She returns home to dress for her interview, thinking about how she will find good child care if she takes a full-time job and trying to figure out what salary she will need to meet her financial obligations if they are to stay in their home. As she is starting the car, Ms. O'Malley suddenly finds she can't catch her breath, feels light-headed and dizzy, and has acute chest pressure. She sits in the car concentrating on her breathing until the feeling subsides and then returns to the house to cancel her interview. She reschedules twice, and each time the same physical symptoms begin before she can get to the interview. When she calls to reschedule a third time the hospital declines to set up another interview.

1. What stressors are impacting Ms. O'Malley at this time?

2. If Ms. O'Malley came to the clinic and you were admitting her to the office, what assessment questions would you ask to explore her methods of coping?

3. Describe three nursing diagnoses that may be appropriate for inclusion in Ms. O'Malley's nursing plan of care.

4. For each nursing diagnosis, list at least two relevant nursing interventions.

Exemplar 31.B
Crisis

Exemplar Learning Outcomes

31.B Analyze crisis as it relates to stress and coping.

- Describe the characteristics of crisis.
- Describe factors that affect individual response to crisis.
- Identify the clinical manifestations of a crisis response.
- Summarize diagnostic tests and therapies used by interprofessional teams in the collaborative care of an individual in crisis.
- Differentiate considerations for care of patients in crisis across the lifespan.
- Apply the nursing process in providing culturally competent care to an individual in crisis.

Exemplar Key Terms

Anticipatory guidance, *2094*
Crisis, *2084*
Crisis counseling, *2088*
Crisis intervention, *2088*
Crisis intervention centers, *2089*
Maturational crisis, *2085*
Resilience, *2085*
Scaling, *2091*
Situational crisis, *2084*

Overview

By necessity, life and the human condition include the experience of crisis. A **crisis** occurs when an event or circumstance overwhelms an individual's inherent ability to resolve, manage, or process the event. A crisis refers to any acute incident that can evolve from a situation or event and that overwhelms an individual's normal coping process. Such a situation or event may involve a developmental, biological, psychosocial, environmental, or spiritual stressor. Crises occur when the typical or normal methods an individual uses to cope with stressful situations no longer reduce the anxiety or resolve the situation. This failure produces an acute state of emotional and psychologic turmoil. Adaptation and successful resolution of a crisis may involve a number of adjustments and may result in a change in the individual's coping process. A crisis also affords the individual an opportunity to grow and change as a result of successful adaptation to the crisis.

Crisis as an Individual Event

Characteristics of Crisis

A crisis is, by definition, an acute situation and is precipitated by an event that creates disequilibrium. Crises occur in the lives of all individuals. The experience of crisis is an individual event. What is a crisis for one person may not constitute a crisis for someone else. The characteristics of a crisis are:

- Something all individuals will experience as a part of living
- Presence of a specific stimulus or event
- Defined individually
- Acute event that will resolve (usually 4–6 weeks)
- Affords the opportunity for growth or deterioration

All crises provide opportunities for growth or deterioration (Townsend, 2014). Typically, an individual resolves a crisis in one of three ways: (1) adapt to the crisis and return to the previous level of functioning, (2) use the opportunity to improve as an individual and cope with life more effectively, or (3) deteriorate to a lower level of functioning. The first possible resolution preserves the individual's status quo, the second changes it for the better, and the third changes it for the worse.

The contributions of Caplan (1964) to the prevention of mental illness have long provided the groundwork on which to build what is known today as *crisis theory*. Individuals interact constantly with the environment; internally, they struggle to meet Maslow's hierarchy of needs (see Figure 31–1). These needs—physical, psychologic, social, and spiritual—manifest differently as an individual progresses through the lifespan. The individual's ability to fulfill needs, maintain homeostasis, regulate affect, mobilize resources, and maintain reality testing affects the individual's capability for adaptation. The individual's perception of the crisis, resources, support, and ego strength all influence his or her capacity to return to prior levels of functioning after crisis.

Types of crises include both situational and maturational crises. A **situational crisis** involves an unexpected stressor or circumstance that occurs in the course of daily living (see **Figure 31–9**). Acute stressors may arise from the external

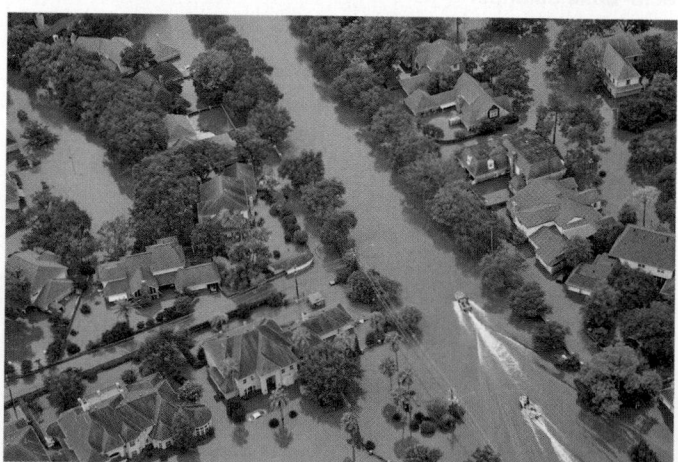

Source: DIIMSA Researcher/Shutterstock.

Figure 31–9 In August and September of 2017, hurricane Harvey hit the Houston area of Texas (shown here) and hurricane Irma hit lower Florida, and the winds, rain, and storm surges damaged and/or flooded hundreds of thousands of homes, creating crises for many families.

environment, such as tornadoes or earthquakes; the internal environment, such as critical illness or disfigurement; and interpersonal sources, such as the death of a loved one or a lost relationship. **Maturational crisis** occurs normally as individuals progress through the life cycle. Everyone experiences predictable stages of human growth and development as outlined by Erikson (1968) (see Table 25.2 in the module on Development). During each stage, the individual is subject to unique stressors. A failure at any one stage compromises the next stage of development.

Holistically, achievement of growth and development milestones requires a tremendous amount of energy. Unexpected life events may alter the person's ability to adapt successfully to either a maturational or a situational crisis. This increases an individual's vulnerability, often requiring supportive interventions from healthcare providers.

Resilience

The American Psychological Association defines **resilience** as "the process of adapting well in the face of adversity, trauma, tragedy, threats or significant sources of stress" (American Psychological Association, n.d.b). Although resilience may be thought of variously as a trait, a process, or an outcome, it involves numerous biological, psychologic, social, and cultural factors and determinants (Southwick et al., 2014). As a process, resilience is the way in which individuals adapt successfully to crisis events to develop positive outcomes (Reyes et al., 2015). Resilience exists on a continuum, manifesting in varying degrees at different times depending on the event and the individual (Southwick et al., 2014). Resilience is dynamic in nature. That is, an individual may demonstrate varying degrees of resilience when exposed to the same or similar stressors throughout the lifespan. Individuals may also be more or less resilient in different domains of life—better able to adapt to stress in their professional life than in their personal life, for example (Southwick et al., 2014).

Individual resilience is strongly influenced by the person's optimistic sense of perceived self-efficacy (see **Figure 31–10 >>**). Psychologist Dr. Albert Bandura posited that an individual must have a strong feeling of personal efficacy to successfully persevere in the face of adversity (Bandura, 1994). Optimism refers to a sense of confidence and hope with regard to positive or favorable resolution of a situation or set of circumstances. Perceived self-efficacy refers to an individual's beliefs concerning his or her capability to influence and exercise control over the events that shape his or her life (Bandura, 1994).

Bandura, whose contributions to the field of psychology include his famous *social learning theory*, conducted in-depth research in the area of self-efficacy. According to Bandura (1994), an individual's perception of self efficacy is shaped by the following influences:

- **Mastery experiences:** Personal experiences with conquering obstacles through tenacious efforts and perseverance; a pattern of easy achievement of success may lead an individual to expect victory and to be discouraged by failure.
- **Vicarious experiences:** When observing the success or failure of someone similar to himself performing a task, an individual will tend to believe that he will perform similarly given the same task.

- **Social persuasion:** The extent to which an individual is verbally persuaded by others to believe he or she is capable of achieving success and to accomplish given tasks.
- **Somatic and emotional states:** Incorporates self-judgments regarding an individual's stress response and physical abilities, as well as mood state. Individuals may be self-critical of their stress response or sense of tension when faced with stressors; in turn, these same individuals may perceive their physical response to stress as rendering them susceptible to failure. In comparison to a negative mood, a positive mood is associated with greater perceived self-efficacy (Bandura, 1994).

Resilience, along with factors such as cognitive appraisal and coping style (as discussed in the Concept section of this module), affects both the physical and psychologic manifestations of an individual's response to crisis.

Clinical Manifestations

Individuals in crisis need immediate assistance and support. The Clinical Manifestations and Therapies feature outlines the common clinical symptoms and manifestations of individuals in crisis.

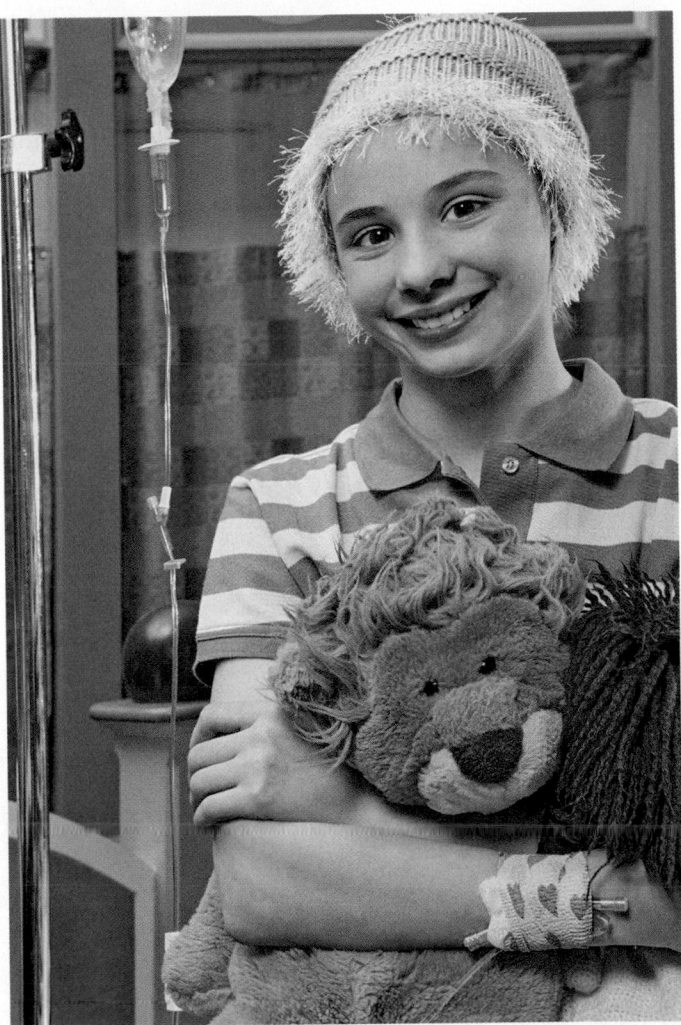

Source: XiXinXing/iStock/Getty Images

Figure 31–10 >> Resilience is the ability to adapt successfully in the face of adversity.

Clinical Manifestations and Therapies
Crisis

ETIOLOGY	CLINICAL MANIFESTATIONS	CLINICAL THERAPIES
▪ Physical trauma (including rape, assault, and exposure to violence)	▪ Difficulty problem solving	▪ Counseling
▪ Emotional trauma (including psychologic and verbal abuse)	▪ Disorganized thought processes with difficulty processing information	▪ Crisis intervention
▪ Exposure to violence, including in the school or workplace settings	▪ Disorientation	▪ Inpatient hospitalization and intensive counseling
▪ Illness- and health-related alterations	▪ Vulnerability	▪ Couple, family, and/or group therapy
▪ Significant loss (including death of a loved one or significant other)	▪ Increased tension and helplessness	▪ Pharmacologic treatment for specific stress-related manifestations, if indicated (e.g., short-term administration of benzodiazepines for treatment of anxiety) or as indicated based on patient-specific needs (e.g., prophylactic antibiotics)
▪ Exposure to natural and environmental disasters	▪ Fearfulness and sense of being overwhelmed	
▪ Exposure to acts of terrorism	▪ Intense emotional reactions	
▪ Financial stressors	▪ Increased sensory input and bombardment	
▪ Legal stressors (including divorce, child custody disputes, and identity theft)	▪ Hypervigilance	
	▪ Intense physical reactions depicted in the fight-or-flight response	
	▪ By definition, event usually is time limited and resolves within 6 weeks	

The goal in crisis is to stabilize the reactions of the individual, thereby initiating the process of adaptation by reducing the disruption created by the crisis. To facilitate adaptive coping, it is essential that nurses encourage patients to express their feelings and listen attentively and supportively. The nurse is an active participant in the intervention process. The generalist nurse serves as communicator, facilitator, and resource expert for the patient.

Collaboration

Caring for patients during times of crisis may include facilitating counseling referrals, connecting patients and families with community agencies, and implementing crisis interventions. For some patients, an extended or severe response to crisis may warrant pharmacologic intervention.

Diagnostic Tests

The patient interview and physical assessment provide the most valuable data for use in planning patient care. In addition, tools are available for use in evaluating the impact of a crisis event. For example, the Horowitz Impact of Event Scale (IES), which originally was developed in 1979 and revised in 1997, allows for measurement of an individual's stress response following traumatic or impactful life experiences (Horowitz, Wilner, & Alverez, 1979; Weiss & Marmer, 1997). Some researchers found the IES-R to be especially useful in helping to identify signs and symptoms associated with posttraumatic stress disorder (PTSD).

>> **Stay Current:** To view the IES-R, visit http://consultgerirn.org/uploads/File/trythis/try_this_19.pdf

Focus on Diversity and Culture
Expression of Emotion

Cultural factors may influence how an individual expresses emotions. In certain cultures, expressions of pain, sorrow, or fear are viewed as signs of weakness. The nurse should be aware of the patient's cultural background and, while maintaining respect for the patient's privacy, gently offer the patient the opportunity to express himself.

Emotional expression tends to be congruent with what the culture values. Individuals in a culture that values independence and individuality will be more likely to express emotions such as irritation and anger in a time of crisis (De Leersnyder, Boiger, & Mesquita, 2013). In contrast, individuals from cultures that value relationships will be more likely to express emotions such as guilt or shame (De Leersnyder et al., 2013). Therefore, individuals from relationship-focused cultures may be at greater risk for suicide if they feel that the poor choices of others are their fault, such as a mother taking responsibility for the poor choices of her children (Galanti, 2015).

Nurses need to be aware of cultural differences in values and how these may affect the expression of emotions during a time of crisis. Some individuals may openly express their feelings, whereas others may interpret their emotions in terms of physical symptoms (Galanti, 2015) or fail to show an emotional response at all. In some cases, lack of an emotional response or failure to engage with a healthcare provider may be a result of previous negative experiences with the healthcare system (Spector, 2017). Taking the time to understand each patient's emotions through the patient's cultural viewpoint can help provide a supportive and calming environment for the patient.

Pharmacologic Therapy

Pharmacologic therapies may be prescribed to address immediate medical needs, which vary widely depending on the nature of the crisis. Immediate needs that may require pharmacologic treatment include:

- Pain following injury (e.g., associated with a motor vehicle crash)
- Threat of infection following injury or exposure to a bacterial infection (e.g., prophylactic treatment for tuberculosis following a lengthy stay in a hurricane shelter)
- Sleep disturbance
- Anxiety or depression

For additional discussion about medications used in the treatment of patients with manifestations such as anxiety and depression, see the Medications feature in the Concept section of this module.

Nonpharmacologic Therapy

Nursing care of patients in crisis includes:

- Establishing a therapeutic relationship
- Ensuring patient safety from the first moment of contact
- Mobilizing support through the significant other, family, relatives, friends, church support groups, healthcare institutions, and organizations such as the American Red Cross
- Collaborating with mental health professionals

Directive suggestion may be helpful, such as gently advising the mother of a critically sick child to go home and sleep while assuring her that she will be called immediately if her child's condition changes. Offering time, attention, and direction is most critical during a crisis. An arrangement for a follow-up care appointment suggests concern for the individual's well-being. The opportunities to offer care in crisis are endless and may involve only a moment of time.

Therapeutic Communication

Communicating with individuals in crisis requires frequent, brief, simple, and often directive communication. Biologically, the brain of the individual in crisis is in the process of being bombarded with electrochemical reactions. Concentration and the ability to remember and retain information can be impaired. The nurse must continually reassess what the individual has heard or interpreted. In applying the transactional model, it is important to remember primary appraisal. What does the individual believe is happening? How can the nurse add resources and information to the reappraisal process to facilitate adaptive coping? Continual observation of patterns of communication within the family and/or group is essential. Because of the hyperarousal that occurs during the crisis, the nurse must monitor and assess nonverbal communication, tone, inflection, and mannerisms while communicating. See **Box 31–6 >>** for guidelines concerning how to conduct effective therapeutic communication with patients. For more information, see the exemplar on Therapeutic Communication in the module on Communication.

Box 31–6
Guidelines for Therapeutic Communication in Crisis

- Incorporate verbal and nonverbal communication.
- Maintain eye contact, nod when appropriate, and avoid distractions to signal genuine concern for the patient.
- Maintain congruence between the verbal and nonverbal messages communicated by the nurse (Kourkouta & Papathanasiou, 2014).
- Paraphrase and repeat the patient's statements to validate the nurse's understanding of the patient and seek clarification; for example: "I hear you saying that you feel like everything's a mess." "Tell me what that means to you."
- Avoid making statements or comments that invalidate or judge the patient's experience instead of listening to and trying to understand it. Examples include statements such as "That doesn't sound important" or "I doubt it happened like that."
- Although encouraging the expression of emotions is important, when appropriate, silence is also an effective communication tool. In addition to demonstrating respect for the patient's privacy and willingness to share, periods of silence also allow the patient to reflect on her thoughts and emotions in order to more effectively express them.

In times of crisis, the nurse may be the one responsible for communicating bad news regarding injury or death of loved ones. As in all care settings, the nurse uses therapeutic communication strategies to impart this information and to provide support to family or friends as they process the information (see **Box 31–7 >>**).

Box 31–7
Communicating Painful Information

One of the uncomfortable roles of the nurse is to communicate painful information to individuals. This task can be unnerving. A few simple guidelines convey a professional attitude of concern and care for those receiving dire news:

1. Greet the individuals with warmth, a kind smile, and an introduction.
2. Inform them that you are there and will assist during this difficult time.
3. Provide privacy, go to a place to sit down to discuss the information, and offer tissues and drinks.
4. Inquire about what they know, answer questions, and provide support.
5. Apprise them of the current circumstances in terms that they can understand.
6. Respond to their feelings and offer support.
7. Ask what they need from you and what has helped them in the past to cope with difficult situations.
8. Incorporate cultural and religious practices of the individuals in crisis to provide comfort.
9. Inform them you will facilitate communication and provide direction about the best means of accessing information.
10. Focus on the immediate reaction and needs of the individuals in crisis.
11. Write down specific contact numbers and instructions.
12. Check back with them as needed to see how they are doing and update them with any new information.

Crisis Counseling

Crisis counseling is focused on brief solutions, focused interventions, and supportive care. During the course of a crisis, nurses should consider each individual's physical vulnerability and degree of emotional stability, with special emphasis on determining the patient's risk for self-harm or potential for harming others. While prioritizing the safety of the patient and others, the nurse should assess the patient's perception of and response to the crisis while also ensuring that the patient's basic needs are met. The alarm reaction, anxiety, and fear may prevent the person from resting, sleeping, or eating. In hospital and other clinical settings, important members of the healthcare team during a crisis may include the hospital chaplain or family minister, a grief counselor, a social worker, a child and family therapist, and a teacher. However, crisis counseling is often performed in a community context. For example, the Federal Emergency Management Agency's Crisis Counseling Program (2015) emphasizes that crisis counseling should be:

- *Outreach oriented,* delivering counseling services in the communities affected instead of waiting for survivors to seek out the services themselves

- *Conducted in nontraditional settings,* contacting survivors in their homes and communities, outside of clinical or office settings

- *Designed to strengthen existing community support systems,* supplementing and supporting existing community response systems

See **Box 31–8 »** for an overview of the components of crisis counseling.

Crisis Intervention

A **crisis intervention** is an emergent approach to care that is intended to assist patients with recognizing a crisis situation and identifying and implementing an immediate, short-term solution. For the patient, the ultimate goal of crisis intervention is restoration to a level of functioning that is at or above the level of the precrisis state. This approach often incorporates the patient's family members and loved ones as well as those individuals who are significant to the patient in terms of providing social support. Depending on the circumstances, a crisis intervention also may include professionals from a variety of specialties, such as school guidance counselors, law enforcement or probation officers, rescue workers, and clergy members. Successful completion of a crisis intervention depends on the patient's needs; for example, some crisis interventions may culminate in the patient's receiving outpatient counseling or guidance, while others may require immediate hospital admission or transfer to a facility that provides treatment for patients with substance abuse disorders. Crisis interventions may happen in a community setting outside of a hospital context if that is what an individual patient's particular needs dictate. For example, the Minnesota Department of Human Services (DHS) lists potential mobile crisis intervention services as (Minnesota DHS, 2013):

- Coping with immediate stressors to lessen suffering

- Identifying and using available resources as well as the strengths of the individual receiving the intervention

- Avoiding unnecessary hospitalization and the loss of the ability to live independently

---

Box 31–8
ABCs of Crisis Counseling

Achieve Rapport

In the first stage of crisis counseling, the nurse or therapist works to achieve rapport with the patient by using therapeutic communication. Helping patients clarify feelings and perceptions of the event first will assist them in venting initial emotions, lower their anxiety levels, and create an environment that will support building of the therapeutic relationship and development of a plan of care. Additional goals at this stage include assessing immediate needs and ensuring the patient's immediate physical and emotional safety.

Boil Down the Problem (Identify, Validate, and Intervene)

At this stage, the nurse or therapist helps the patient identify the problem, providing validation and intervention. Communication with the patient at this stage focuses on identifying the problem, assessing how the patient is thinking and feeling about the problem, and evaluating the patient's functional ability since the crisis event. Goals at this stage include helping patients identify their most pressing problems, encouraging patients to talk about the present, and assessing and addressing ongoing safety concerns, such as risk for suicide, abuse, and substance abuse.

In some situations, patients may not have a previous experience and coping mechanisms that they can articulate. Giving patients small choices, such as asking what they would like to drink or if they would like to make a phone call, can help build their confidence.

Assessment and intervention will vary greatly depending on the patient and the crisis. The safety assessment of a patient with asthma following a natural disaster will be very different from the safety assessment of a patient who is being abused by her partner.

Cope with the Problem (Resolution and Referral)

At this stage, the nurse or therapist determines what is necessary to help the patient cope with the problem. Using Maslow's hierarchy of needs to focus on the patient's basic needs of shelter, food, water, and physiologic safety is a good framework to use when prioritizing care for patients in crisis. For patients who are victims of violence, physiologic and emotional safety needs will be very closely related. Consider both short- and long-term needs for resolution and referral. Goals at this stage include determining what the patient wants to happen and what will help the patient to meet his or her needs and to support the patient's need for validation and hope for the future.

Sources: Jones, W. L. (1968). The A-B-C method of crisis management. *Mental Hygiene, 52*(1), 87–89; Kanel, K. (2015). *A guide to crisis intervention* (5th ed.). Stamford, CT: Cengage Learning; Mental Health Academy. (n.d.) *Crisis counseling: The ABC model.* Retrieved from https://www.mentalhealthacademy.com.au/video_details.php?catid=15&vid=68.

- Developing action plans
- Returning the individual to a precrisis level of functioning

Crisis intervention centers provide telephone consultation for patients in crisis. Some organizations also offer consultation by way of email and online chatting. In most cases, call-in crisis intervention centers, also known as crisis hotlines, are staffed by trained volunteers who follow protocols to assist the patient and who have professional consultation available to them, such as mental health counselors and psychologists. These 24-hour services allow callers to remain anonymous. For individuals who use crisis hotline services, primary goals include preventing the caller from inflicting harm directed at herself or others, giving the individual an opportunity to share her emotions and conflicts, and encouraging follow-up care with a local mental health professional if needed.

A step-by-step intervention is outlined in **Box 31-9 »**. A crisis connection provides a lifeline for the patient in crisis and allows the nurse to determine immediate needs.

Temporary Relocation

Patients in crisis—in particular, those who are homeless and those who are subject to abuse—may require assistance with meeting one of the most basic needs: finding shelter. Nurses should be aware of community organizations and representatives who can assist patients with finding emergency living arrangements.

Lifespan Considerations

The response to trauma varies throughout the lifespan. For all age groups, nurses should carefully assess the particular cultural, social, and family factors that may influence how each patient speaks about their feelings and needs. Nurses may also identify and recommend community resources and organizations that can assist patients in crisis in their area.

Children and Adolescents in Crisis

Children and adolescents are highly susceptible to crisis. Because of their developmental level and lack of experience dealing with crises, they are less able to cope with extreme circumstances than are adults. This is especially true for children with disabilities. Types of crises to which children and adolescents may be exposed include bullying, divorce or separation of parents, child abuse, school shootings, death of a parent or sibling, failed attempts at suicide, friends committing suicide, unexpected pregnancy, and trauma from accidents, natural disasters, sports, and other events.

Box 31-9
Crisis Connection

1. Make contact and connect with the individual.
2. Assess immediate safety needs.
3. Determine thought processes.
4. Scan for physical distress.
5. Listen intently, supporting emotional reactions.
6. Explore perceptions of the crisis.
7. Identify coping strengths.
8. Develop a support plan and a follow-up plan.

Focus on Integrative Health
Prayer

As discussed in the Concept section of this module, the mind–body connection has been established through research. Elicitation of the stress response by way of cognitive appraisal of a stressor is a classic example of this connection. Building on this relationship, a holistic approach to nursing care acknowledges a connection between not only the mind and body, but also the spirit.

In the United States, a study of findings from the adult Alternative Medicine supplement of the National Health Interview Survey (NHIS) in 2002 and 2007 focusing on the use of prayer as an integrative treatment for depression revealed that general prayer among those surveyed increased from 40.2 to 45.7% between those years. Compared to those who were neither depressed nor prayed, women, unmarried individuals, individuals with a high school education, and individuals age 50–64 were more likely to use prayer while depressed. The study suggested that it is essential for healthcare providers to be aware of their patients' use of prayer as a means of coping with depression as well as with other healthcare concerns (Wachholtz & Sambamthoori, 2013). Concerning the effects of prayer on healing and wellness, research is hindered by obvious limitations, including that psychosocial wellness is largely subjective and, as such, is difficult to measure quantitatively. Moreover, the inclusion of treatments that are in addition to prayer, such as pharmacologic interventions, complicates the study of the effects of prayer alone. What is clear is that prayer is a widely used approach in the quest for healing. For nurses, the implications of this finding include assessing and respecting the spiritual beliefs of each individual patient, including those who are atheists.

Children and adolescents will respond to and cope with crisis events differently depending on their age, developmental maturity, support resources, life experiences, and association with the event. Nurses should work closely with parents to assess and care for children and adolescents after a crisis, because parents know their children best and can report changes in behavior that may signal a poor coping response to the crisis that requires additional intervention.

All children and adolescents dealing with crisis should receive emotional support from parents and healthcare professionals. Nurses can provide support by reassuring the child that he is safe; encouraging the child to express her feelings; telling the child that it is appropriate to feel emotions such as sadness, anger, grief, or fear; and keeping the child informed about what is happening in the crisis situation. Nurses should encourage parents to spend extra time with their child, talk to the child about the event at a developmentally appropriate level, monitor the child for changes in behavior, limit their child's television viewing about the event, and help the child maintain a normal routine. Nurses should teach parents that behavior changes often associated with crisis events that may signal a poor coping response include clinginess, nightmares, bedwetting, irritability, a decrease in normal play activity, changes in eating patterns, reporting headaches or stomachaches, aggression, and behavior problems at school. Adolescents should be monitored carefully for signs of depression and risk for suicide.

If a child or adolescent continues to respond to the crisis event with abnormal behavior and poor coping beyond a reasonable time for the severity of the event, the nurse should advocate for the child and family to receive additional counseling from a child or family mental health professional. The nurse may also encourage the child and family to find creative ways to respond to the crisis. For example, the death of a sibling or friend may be commemorated by planting a tree in their honor or making a donation to their favorite charity.

Pregnant Women in Crisis

In addition to crises that other adults face, pregnant women may face crises related to miscarriage, having a child with a disability or other chronic illness, and preterm birth. Some pregnant women may experience a crisis if they are pregnant as the result of a rape, and teen mothers may experience crisis related to rejection by family and friends and the fear of raising the child while still in school. Other women may experience a crisis if they decide to have an abortion or give up the baby for adoption. These crises may take on an even greater magnitude if the pregnant woman does not receive support from the child's father.

Nurses can provide a safe and calming environment in which the pregnant woman can express her fears and other emotions. Nurses should validate the pregnant woman's emotions and correct any misconceptions the woman might have. Nurses should provide pregnant women with information specific to their situation. For example, if a pregnant woman has been told she will have a child with Down syndrome, the nurse can provide the woman with literature about what to expect when caring for a child with Down syndrome. Nursing interventions that increase knowledge about the crisis situation will increase the woman's ability to cope with the stressor.

For women who are pregnant as a result of rape, the nurse can encourage the woman to work with the police and court personnel and provide support and a listening ear as the woman expresses her distress over the situation. If the pregnant woman is a teenager, the nurse can ensure that the teen's parents will provide a stable environment for the teen and baby or work with the teen and social system to find a stable home for the new family.

If a pregnant woman must deal with a crisis unrelated to her pregnancy, she may be more open to receiving nursing care and more likely to implement suggestions for maintaining her emotional and physical health (Littleton-Gibbs & Engebretson, 2013). However, pregnant women experience many hormonal changes during pregnancy that can affect their moods and their ability to deal with crisis situations. For example, they may be more susceptible to depression and anxiety disorders. In addition, behavioral and physical changes, especially changes that affect the pregnant woman's health, can affect the development of the baby. For example, high blood pressure from high levels of stress increases the potential for preterm labor or a low-birth-weight infant (National Institutes of Health, 2012). Coping with a crisis situation by drinking alcohol or smoking can lead to fetal alcohol

spectrum disorders or problems with placental attachment (American Congress of Obstetricians and Gynecologists [ACOG] 2013). Therefore, pregnant women in crisis should be monitored carefully, and the nurse should provide support for the mother and baby throughout the pregnancy and after birth.

Older Adults in Crisis

Older adults are often more susceptible to injury during crisis events that involve natural disasters, home fires, motor vehicle accidents, wandering from home, and other traumatic events. Older adults also have higher incidence of chronic disorders such as diabetes and heart disease, so they are more susceptible to changes in health related to lack of access to medications and nutrition. Older adults may be more susceptible to confusion and disorientation.

The nurse caring for an older adult during a crisis should begin by orienting the older adult to person, time, and place, and asking what the patient remembers about the crisis event. If the older adult is properly oriented, the nurse should provide any emergency care needed and begin a full physical, mental, and emotional assessment. In particular, the nurse should determine the older adult's health history and gain access to any medications the older adult might need during the time they are in the nurse's care. The nurse should encourage the older adult's family and friends to provide support during and after the crisis, as isolation and loneliness can lead to further deterioration of the patient's physical and mental health.

NURSING PROCESS

Initially, the primary focus of crisis intervention is to ensure safety. Once safety is established, the ideal goals include helping the patient acknowledge and manage the crisis and assisting the patient to identify and access resources needed to achieve resolution.

Assessment

The nurse systematically assesses the patient in crisis, beginning with making contact and connecting with the patient. Assess and identify patient safety issues such as:

- Safe and adequate shelter
- Access to food and healthcare
- Feelings of hopelessness or threat to self or others
- Risk for harm or violence (to/from self or others).

To ensure the patient's safety, emergent admission to a hospital or treatment center may be necessary. Ideally, assessment also includes interviewing the patient's family or significant others.

Individual Assessment

During the assessment process, the nurse must determine the patient's thought processes, orientation, and ability to process information. Assessment of the patient's physical condition includes any physical complaints and determining if the patient is able to fulfill basic needs such as eating, resting, sleeping, and self-care. Because of the intensity of the fight-or-flight reaction, vulnerable individuals may be at risk for physical illness during a crisis.

Psychosocial assessment includes assessing the patient's perception of the precipitating event, impact of the crisis, and his ability to cope with the crisis. The nurse should also interview the patient regarding his current and past coping methods, as well as his support system. Particularly for disaster survivors, the issue of survivor's guilt should be explored. For these patients, guilt may stem from the act of surviving while knowing others have died. Survivors may also harbor guilt as a result of the actions they took to survive.

Scaling assessment questions involve asking the patient to rate the severity of symptoms or problems. This allows the nurse to determine the perceptions of the patient. For example, the nurse may ask, "Mr. Smith, on a scale of 0 to 10, with 10 being absolutely intolerable, how would you score your distress right now?" Assessment information is prioritized on the basis of input from the individual.

It is important to remember that the expression of feelings about and interpretations of an event are culturally influenced and must be considered within the context of the individual's life. Sociocultural factors greatly impact an individual's interpretation of a crisis or traumatic event, as well as her response to the event. For example, among members of some cultures, persistent anxiety is considered to be a sign of weakness, as opposed to being a potential sign of a stress-related disorder. This belief is particularly prevalent among some women in the Pacific Islander and Asian cultures; as a result, these women may not reach out for help until they enter a crisis stage (Nydegger, 2012).

Cultural competence extends beyond the identification of a patient's cultural and ethnic background; it encompasses being aware of a patient's health practices and beliefs and demonstrating respect for the patient's preferences. However, the nurse also has a responsibility to identify health practices that may be detrimental to the patient's well-being. Identification and evaluation of the patient's culturally based health practices requires sensitive, nonjudgmental exploration of the topic. For example, the patient interview may include items such as "I want to try to understand how this experience may be affecting you. Please tell me more about how you feel," and "How would you expect your family or close friends to react to a similar experience?"

Family Assessment

House fires, motor vehicle crashes, serious illness or injury or death of an immediate family member, and natural disasters are just a few of the crises that families can experience. Emotional crises such as divorce, bankruptcy, and abuse also affect families. Each individual family member's response to a crisis will impact family functioning. Family communication patterns may promote or hinder family members' response to crises. Nurses working with families in crisis situations will benefit from assessing how family members have coped in previous crises as well as assessing immediate individual and family needs. If the crisis results in serious injury or illness to one or more family members, nurses can assist by offering a variety of interventions, including:

- Obtaining and providing information regarding the health status of the loved one

- Facilitating communication between the family and the healthcare team
- Ensuring access to and promoting communication with the loved one
- Providing privacy and emotional support (Ball, Bindler, Cowan, 2017, p. 449).

Community Assessment

Nurses may be among the first civilians called on to offer assistance in the wake of a disaster. For the community faced with crisis, assessment begins with triage and treatment of patients in need. Next follows assessment of living conditions and availability of basic resources, such as food, water, and shelter. Identification of the community's mental health and support resources, as well as the availability of financial and organizational resources (such as disaster assistance organizations), is also essential.

Diagnosis

Selection of nursing diagnoses depends on the patient's crisis response and associated manifestations. Examples of nursing diagnoses that may be appropriate for inclusion in the nursing plan of care for a patient in a state of crisis may include the following:

- *Injury, Risk for*
- *Anxiety*
- *Self-Neglect*
- *Coping, Ineffective*
- *Confusion, Acute.*

  (NANDA-I © 2014)

Planning

Planning involves the selection of realistic goals and identified outcomes that promote resolution of the selected nursing diagnoses. Examples of patient goals and outcomes that may be relevant to the nursing care of a patient in crisis may include the following:

- The patient will remain free from injury.
- The patient will identify and use necessary resources and social support.
- The patient will report a reduction in perceived anxiety.
- The patient will actively participate in counseling and group therapy activities as outlined by the primary care provider.
- The patient will express understanding of coping techniques that can be used during times of crisis.
- The patient will respond appropriately to questions and conversation and show no signs of confusion.

Implementation

Implementation involves assisting patients with meeting needs identified in the assessment phase. Establishment of trust and application of therapeutic communication techniques serve as the foundation for building a relationship with the patient in crisis. The nurse should avoid minimizing the patient's feelings or offering false reassurances of hope.

Reduce Risk for Injury

Patients may be at greater risk of injury during a crisis because they are overwhelmed and unable to properly cope with or respond to changes in their environment. Depending on the type of crisis, patients may be at risk for injury directly due to the crisis, or they may be at risk for injury inflicted by self or others. For example, a woman who has been beaten by her husband may be at risk for further injury from her husband either at the hospital or when she returns home. Similarly, that same woman may be at risk for self-inflicted injury if she decides to attempt suicide. To reduce the risk for injury:

- Identify risk factors for injury in the patient's home environment that the patient can control and remove. Depending on the patient's situation, this may include fixing stairs, installing lights, removing hazardous materials, and removing weapons, among other interventions. Discuss potential risk factors with patients to make them aware of ways to reduce their risk for injury.

- Monitor the patient's community for ongoing threats and changes that could produce new risk factors. Especially in a crisis situation affecting the community at large when the crisis and the response to it are ongoing, the situation on the ground could change rapidly.

- Isolate patients from any potential sources of injury. If the potential injury is from another person, isolate the patient from the threatening individual. If the potential injury is from self, remove any potential weapons from the patient's immediate surroundings. If the potential source of injury is the environment, remove the patient from the environment and place the patient in a safe location.

- If the patient is in a hospital environment and the patient is a source of risk for injury to self, a patient companion may be assigned to the patient, the patient may be moved to a location where he can be easily observed by nursing staff, or restraints may be used as a last resort. Use of restraints should always be consistent with the level of risk and the patient's need to be kept from harm.

SAFETY ALERT Nurses need to be constantly aware of the potential dangers and risk of injury involved in responding to patients in crisis. These threats may come from the environment, particularly if the crisis is a natural disaster or community crisis; or threats may come from other people involved in the crisis, and even from the patients themselves. Also, nurses must be careful to ensure that in responding to crises they are aware of the possibility of becoming overwhelmed psychologically, emotionally, or physically themselves, to the point where they are no longer able to monitor effectively for risks to their safety.

Decrease Anxiety

Anxiety may accompany the patient's feeling of being overwhelmed by the crisis and unable to properly cope and make recovery from the crisis difficult. Almost all patients who are dealing with a crisis will experience anxiety at some point, although when they experience anxiety, the magnitude of anxiety that they experience and how they cope with it will differ with each individual. To learn more about nursing interventions associated with anxiety, see Exemplar 31.A.

Promote Self-Care

A crisis creates a strong potential for patients to fall into habits of self-neglect, with overwhelmed individuals falling out of established routines of self-care. Patients may ignore self-care activities such as bathing and other hygiene rituals, neglect home responsibilities such as caring for family or paying bills, or neglect work responsibilities that could result in loss of a job and further crisis. To promote patient self-care and reduce the risk for self-neglect:

- Encourage family members to assist the patient in meeting self-care needs. Monitor for signs of self-neglect such as unwashed hair or clothing the patient has worn for several days or that is mismatched, inadequate, or inappropriate.

- Encourage family and friends to help with home responsibilities such as providing child care or making sure bills are paid to prevent further crisis for the patient.

- Ensure the patient is eating and hydrating enough at home and has support from family or friends in ensuring proper routines of hydration and nutrition. If needed, recommend community nutrition resources such as Meals on Wheels.

- Help patients reduce stress associated with returning to work during a time of crisis. Help patients research family leave, vacation, and other work resources that may allow them to be away from work for an extended period of time without losing their jobs.

- In a hospital setting, encourage patients to follow routines of self-care that are within their control. Also ensure that they are taking in appropriate nutrition and hydration.

Promote Effective Coping

Depending on the type of crisis, the patient or the patient's family members and friends may display ineffective coping. Ineffective coping is often evidenced by blank emotions, shock, a lack of appetite, self-neglect, ineffective communication, ineffectual learning, excessive crying, or hysteria. The nurse can promote effective coping by:

- Providing information about community resources that may help the patient return to independence after a crisis. This may include resources for housing, furniture and clothing, transportation, food, jobs, physical therapy, counseling, and support groups (see Patient Teaching feature). Resources needed will vary depending on the patient's situation.

- Presenting a calm and collected demeanor to the patient and family at all times. Seeing others display calmness can help calm individuals who are anxious or upset.

- Removing the patient or the patient's family from visual reminders of the crisis situation. For example, the patient should be taken to a hotel or hospital after their house has burned down rather than being allowed to stay at the site. Similarly, nurses may discourage parents from viewing procedures that are required to care for a child who has been in a severe motor vehicle accident, especially if the child is unconscious and will not benefit from the presence of the parent. Placing the patient or the patient's family in a quiet environment and minimizing external stimuli will help them achieve a sense of calmness.

- Encouraging the patient or the patient's family members to drink water and eat small snacks to sustain nutrition and hydration.

- Encouraging the patient or the patient's family members to participate in self-care activities such as sleeping and bathing. The nurse may need to encourage family members of hospitalized patients to go home to get some sleep or a change of clothing.

- Contacting next of kin for the patient to reduce isolation and provide a support system for the patient.

- Providing patients or their family members with small, simple tasks that they can perform. Completing simple tasks may help them feel like they are helping or achieving some control over the situation.

- Keeping patients informed about their medical status or the medical status of their loved one using therapeutic communication techniques. See Boxes 31–6 and 31–7. Consider also providing written information about the patient's situation or status so that patients or family members with ineffective learning can review the information when they are more emotionally stable. Offer to answer any questions and be available to talk with the family as needed.

Decrease Acute Confusion

Patients who have had a head injury or a major shock associated with a crisis may display acute confusion. This confusion may pertain to disorientation about location, events, time and date, or even personal identity. The nurse can decrease a patient's confusion by:

- Providing orienting information, such as a reminder about the events that caused the crisis or a reminder of the individual's location and the time and date.

- Providing written instructions related to treatments and care.

- Helping patients remember who they are (if their identity is known by the nurse). This may include showing patients their own ID card, such as a driver's license, or allowing them to see family and friends.

- Repeating information as needed in a calm and soothing manner until the patient begins to feel oriented to the situation and less confused.

Evaluation

Expected outcomes that may be appropriate for the patient experiencing a crisis include:

- The patient has identified and removed risk factors for injury from the environment.

- The patient reports using community resources and sources of social support such as family and friends.

- The patient reports feeling less anxiety associated with the crisis.

- The patient maintains proper hygiene, nutrition, hydration, and other self-care tasks, as evidenced by lack of

Patient Teaching
Benefits of Support Groups

Nurses should be ready to provide patients with information and recommendations regarding support groups that may be helpful in general or helpful specifically for people coping with their particular crisis. Potential benefits of support groups include:

- Participation in regular, judgment-free contact with people whose needs are similar to the patient's

- Empowerment and a feeling of being in control

- Improved coping skills and better adjustment increases the chance of moving forward from the crisis

- Freedom to speak openly and honestly

- A support network and sounding board for emotional responses to crisis

- A reduction in feelings of distress, depression, anxiety, or fatigue caused by putting problems in perspective

- An increase in feelings of self-worth and self-esteem, improved assertiveness, and improved personal relationships

- A reduction in feelings of isolation caused by realizing that others are struggling with the same problems, leading to increased social reconnection

- Development of a better understanding of the patient's situation, including providing a space for the patient to break down misconceptions and reduce harmful self-talk

- Practical advice and information about treatment options, including integrative treatments

- Diversity within the group gives new perspectives on how to approach the problem

- Comparison of notes regarding resource and physician options.

Source: Data from Mayo Clinic. (2015a). *Support groups: make connections, get help.* Retrieved from http://www.mayoclinic.org/healthy-lifestyle/stress-management/in-depth/support-groups/art-20044655; American Psychological Association. (n.d.c). *Psychotherapy: Understanding group therapy.* Retrieved from http://www.apa.org/helpcenter/group-therapy.aspx; Graham, L., Powell, R., & Karam, A. (n.d.). *The power of social connection.* Retrieved from http://www.nsvrc.org/sites/default/files/the-power-of-social-connection.pdf.

fatigue, maintenance of appropriate weight, and clean clothes and body.

- The patient displays effective coping techniques that are appropriate to the situation and expresses a regained sense of control over the crisis.

- The patient is independently oriented to self, time, place, and can describe the precipitating event.

The nurse may have to evaluate the patient in crisis multiple times before the situation is resolved and the patient appears to be in good health again. Each time, the nurse should reevaluate the patient for safety, adequate self-care, anxiety levels, coping techniques, and social support. Any areas that still require improvement to stabilize the patient should be prioritized to promote the patient's physical and mental health. Once the patient is stabilized, additional nursing interventions for milder symptoms or needs can be implemented.

Nursing Care Plan
A Patient in Crisis

ASSESSMENT

Deborah Smith is a 30-year-old woman who comes to the emergency department following a fall down the stairs outside her apartment. She breaks down in tears during the assessment. Not only is her ankle painful and swollen, but the father of her two small children has recently been arrested for nearly killing his girlfriend. She has no idea when he will be able to pay child support again, and she is afraid she will not be able to return to work at her job as a waitress if her ankle is sprained. The physical assessment reveals the following:

- Vital signs include temperature 99.0°F oral; pulse 96 bpm; respirations 18/min; and BP 136/86 mmHg.
- Hands are trembling, patient is tearful and crying
- Circular scars noted on both forearms the size of pencil erasers
- Left ankle is edematous and painful to touch, unable to perform range of motion in ankle
- Abrasions on the palm of the right hand, left elbow, and both knees.

DIAGNOSES

- *Pain, Acute*
- *Anxiety*
- *Caregiver Role Strain, Risk for*
- *Impaired Resilience, Risk for.*

(NANDA-I © 2014)

PLANNING

- Identify community resources that can provide assistance until Ms. Smith can return to work.
- Identify Ms. Smith's strengths in terms of available resources and family support.
- Manage pain to allow Ms. Smith to maintain comfort.
- Teach patient crutch walking and self-care for injured ankle.

IMPLEMENTATION

- Encourage Ms. Smith to express her feelings.
- Ask Ms. Smith whom she can look to for help. Are the children's grandparents supportive? Does she have a supportive spiritual community? Does her workplace have a sick leave policy? Are there resources within the community that can provide support and assistance?
- Provide referral to the hospital's department of social services to determine potential community resources.

- Encourage Ms. Smith to identify her strengths that can help her resolve her current crisis.
- Establish a follow-up plan for Ms. Smith's physical as well as psychosocial needs.
- Provide teaching on care of ankle injury, symptoms to report to provider immediately, crutch walking, and wound care.

EVALUATION

Social services assisted Ms. Smith in obtaining unemployment insurance during her medical leave of absence and provided **anticipatory guidance** to help her retain her job until she was able to return. Ms. Smith developed a stronger relationship with her church community, whose members assisted in picking up the children from school, delivered meals, and helped to perform tasks such as laundry that Ms. Smith could not perform with limited mobility.

CRITICAL THINKING

1. If you were the nurse caring for Ms. Smith and lived in the same community, would it be appropriate for you to offer to provide home care for her and the children when you had time available? Why or why not?

2. Is it appropriate for you, as the nurse caring for Ms. Smith, to solve problems for her? Explain your answer.

3. What functions can social service provide to help patients in crisis like Ms. Smith?

REVIEW Crisis

RELATE Link the Concepts and Exemplars

Linking the exemplar of crisis with the concept of addiction:

1. When a crisis results from addiction behavior, what is the nurse's priority intervention? Explain your answer.

2. When a patient's spouse is demonstrating addiction behavior that has caused the patient's crisis, what community referrals might you consider suggesting to help the patient?

Linking the exemplar of crisis with the concept of culture and diversity:

3. Why might one series of events trigger a crisis for one patient but not another?

4. How do coping strategies differ during times of crisis for patients from vulnerable populations versus those who are less vulnerable? How would your nursing interventions differ for each patient?

READY Go to Volume 3: Clinical Nursing Skills

REFER Go to Pearson MyLab Nursing and eText

- Additional review materials

REFLECT Apply Your Knowledge

Carol Holland is a 51-year-old mother of three. She is a nurse educator and works full time at a community college. Her son Paul recently moved back to live with her to attend college full time. Along with Paul,

Mrs. Holland lives with her husband Tom and their other son Mike. Her oldest and only daughter Angela lives in an apartment nearby. The Hollands receive a call in the wee hours of the morning. One of Mike's friends tells them that Mike has been in a terrible accident, and they need to come to the hospital immediately. Arriving at the trauma unit at 3:00 a.m., the Hollands and their son Paul enter the satellite unit. Mike is intubated and requires mechanical ventilation. Mrs. Holland scans Mike's body for signs of independent life, but he is motionless. His face is so swollen that he is nearly unrecognizable to her. What appears to be a blue cable cord holds together a laceration that encompasses most of his head. His left arm is swollen three times its size, and is blue and seeping from lacerations. As Paul collapses in a nearby chair and

begins weeping, the nurse quietly gathers vital information from Mrs. Holland. She directs Mike's family to the lounge where they will wait during a procedure to insert a ventricular shunt. The neurosurgeon is unsure Mike will survive the night.

1. What type of crisis is this family experiencing?
2. Given the information presented thus far, which nursing diagnoses might be applicable?
3. What are some possible psychosocial interventions for the patient and the family?
4. What basic needs might this family have throughout the night?

≫ Exemplar 31.C
Obsessive-Compulsive Disorder

Exemplar Learning Outcomes

31.C Analyze obsessive-compulsive disorder (OCD) as it relates to stress and coping.

- Describe the pathophysiology of OCD.
- Describe the etiology of OCD.
- Compare the risk factors for and prevention of OCD.
- Identify the clinical manifestations of OCD.
- Summarize diagnostic tests and therapies used by interprofessional teams in the collaborative care of an individual with OCD.

- Differentiate considerations for care of patients with OCD across the lifespan.
- Apply the nursing process in providing culturally competent care to an individual with OCD.

Exemplar Key Terms

Compulsion, *2095*
Obsession, *2095*
Obsessive-compulsive disorder (OCD), *2095*

Overview

Obsessive-compulsive disorder (OCD) is a disabling disorder characterized by obsessive thoughts and compulsive, repetitive behaviors that dominate an individual's life (see **Figure 31–11 ≫**). An **obsession** is a recurrent, unwanted, and often distressing thought or image that leads to feelings of fear and anxiety. A **compulsion** is a repetitive behavior or mental activity (such as counting) used in an attempt to mitigate the obsessive thoughts and reduce feelings of anxiety (APA, 2013). To be diagnosed with OCD, the individual must experience distress and lose time (more than 1 hour a day) due to the consuming rituals and repetitive behaviors associated with the disorder (APA, 2013).

Pathophysiology and Etiology

Pathophysiology

A malfunction in the cortico-striato-thalamo-cortical (CSTC) circuit in the brain is the possible cause for OCD (see **Figure 31–12 ≫**); the neurotransmitters serotonin, dopamine, and glutamate are all involved in OCD (Bokor & Anderson, 2014). A specific gene has not yet been isolated, but research has identified many candidate genes and found that some regions of the genome might include disease genes (Privitera et al., 2015). The neurobiology of OCD involves several areas of the brain: the orbitofrontal cortex, anterior cingulate gyrus, and basal ganglia (Bokor & Anderson, 2014). Neuroimages of individuals with OCD indicate abnormalities in the basal ganglia and the orbitofrontal cortex. Imaging data, genomic studies, and animal models of aberrant grooming behavior have contributed to the idea that the glutamatergic system plays a role in OCD. These findings are compatible

with circuit-based theories of OCD and have driven interest in testing the efficacy of pharmacologic treatments for OCD that modulate glutamate function (Goodman et al., 2014). Over the past decade, studies of OCD's pathogenesis have produced mounting evidence that increased immune system activation plays an important role (Rao et al., 2015).

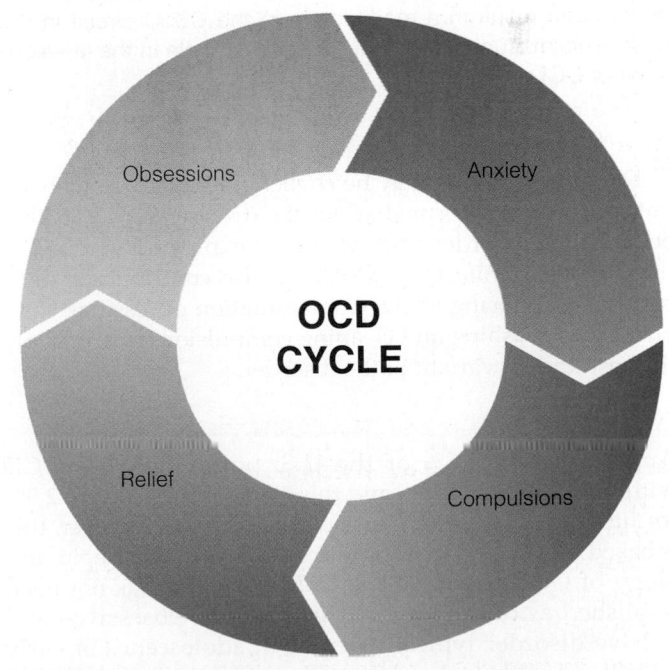

Figure 31–11 ≫ Individual resilience is influenced by the person's own confidence in, and hope for, a positive resolution to stressful circumstances.

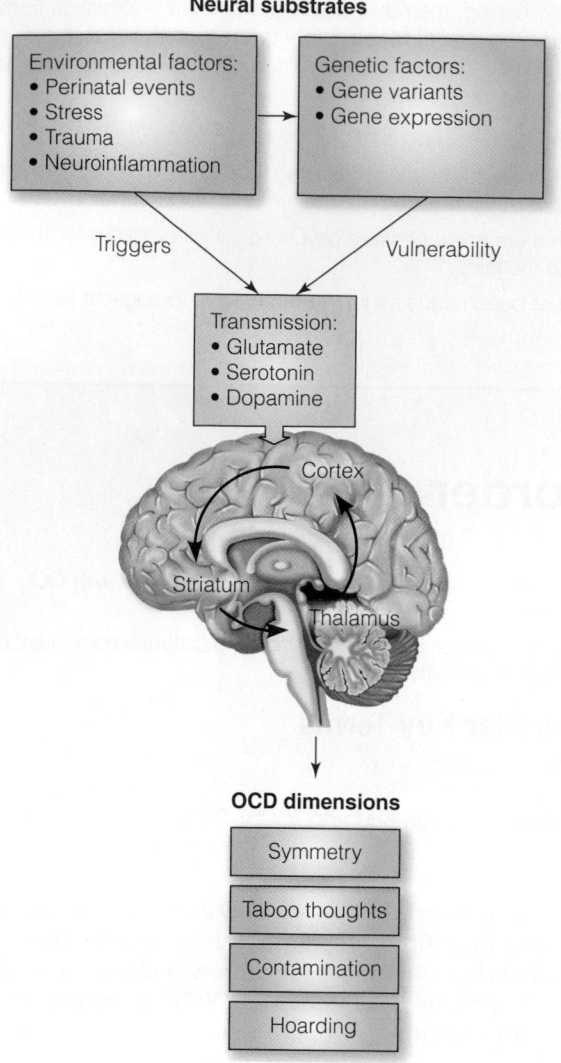

Figure 31–12 » A combination of environmental and genetic factors can result in a malfunction in the CSTC circuit in the brain. This malfunction is thought to play a role in the development of OCD.

Diagnosis of OCD may be challenging for those who are untrained or uninformed about the disease. Variances that occur in the disorder, and which are explained in detail in the Clinical Manifestations section, also contribute to difficulty in diagnosing OCD. Contamination obsessions combined with washing and cleaning compulsions are probably the best-known variant of the disorder.

Etiology

Approximately 1.2% of the U.S. population has OCD within a 12-month span, and this number increases to 2.3% for lifetime prevalence (Ruscio et al., 2010). However, this is based on DSM-IV criteria; a true analysis of the epidemiology of OCD based on the DSM-5 criteria has not been published as of the time of this writing. Obsessive-compulsive disorder typically begins in adolescence or early adulthood, although some cases do begin in childhood. OCD affects men and women equally, but men develop the disorder earlier. Among males, approximately 25% of

those with OCD demonstrate onset before 10 years of age (APA, 2013). Without treatment, the rate of remission is estimated to be low. However, for individuals who experience childhood onset of OCD, approximately 40% may experience remission by the time they reach early adulthood (APA, 2013).

Risk Factors

Risk factors for OCD include having a first-degree relative with the disorder. A history of childhood sexual or physical abuse also increases the risk, as does exposure to other stressful or traumatic events during childhood (APA, 2013).

Clinical Manifestations

Obsessive-compulsive disorder is not to be confused with *obsessive-compulsive personality disorder*. The clinical manifestations of the personality disorder involve more of a preoccupation with perfection and are characterized by inflexibility.

The most frequently reported obsessions in OCD are repeated thoughts about contamination from shaking hands; repeated doubts with fear of having hurt someone or leaving a door unlocked; and a need to have things in a certain order. Common themes of the associated intrusive, repetitive thoughts include those which are considered by the individual to be forbidden or taboo; for example, religious or sexual obsessions and fears related to self-harm or injury of others (APA, 2013). Aggressive impulses are often of a sexual nature or obscene. The obsessions are not rational or real-life problems. The patient with OCD is, at some point, aware that the obsessions are not real (APA, 2013).

Compulsions are also part of OCD. Commonly reported repetitive behaviors include hand washing, ordering, checking, and counting. Note that hoarding, a behavior associated with OCD in DSM-IV, is recognized in DSM-5 as a distinct and separate disorder, hoarding disorder, within the category of Obsessive-Compulsive and Related Disorders (APA, 2013). For additional examples of commonly occurring obsessions and their related compulsions, see the Clinical Manifestations and Therapies feature. Compulsive behavior does not produce a sense of pleasure for the patient with OCD. Rather, the individual feels driven to perform the compulsion to reduce the anxiety produced by the obsession.

Collaboration

Diagnosis of OCD is made by a licensed clinical mental health professional. Care often occurs in the community and may include the nurse in collaboration with the patient's mental health provider, primary care provider, and school counselor or social worker. Because the impact of OCD can range from mild to disabling, the patient's needs will vary. The most common therapy for OCD is pharmacotherapy, followed by psychotherapies. Guidelines for treatment of OCD are summarized in **Box 31–10 »**.

Diagnostic Tests

No definitive laboratory findings have been identified for diagnosing OCD.

Clinical Manifestations and Therapies
Obsessive-Compulsive Disorder

ETIOLOGY (OBSESSIONS)	CLINICAL MANIFESTATIONS (COMPULSIONS)	CLINICAL THERAPIES
Aggressive, sexual, and religious obsessions with checking compulsions	■ Checks doors, locks, appliances, written work ■ Confesses frequently (to anything) ■ Needs to ask others repeatedly for assurance	■ Pharmacologic therapies include SSRIs: 　fluoxetine (Prozac) 　sertraline (Zoloft) 　fluvoxamine (Luvox) 　paroxetine (Paxil) ■ Antipsychotic medications such as risperidone (Risperdal) may be helpful for those who do not respond to SSRIs. ■ Cognitive behavior therapy may include desensitization therapy, in which the person is carefully exposed over a period of time to an object that promotes fear. For example, the therapist and patient may, at an appropriate time, agree that the patient will touch the doorknob. ■ Other therapies such as deep brain stimulation may be helpful to those who are treatment resistant.
Symmetry obsessions with ordering, arranging, and repeating compulsions	■ Needs to have objects in fixed and symmetrical positions ■ Repeats movements, such as going in and out of doorways, getting in and out of chairs, touching objects ■ Counts or spells silently or aloud	
Contamination obsessions with washing and cleaning compulsions	■ Repeatedly washes hands, showers, bathes, brushes teeth ■ Cleans personal space frequently	

Focus on Diversity and Culture
Lack of Diversity in Research

Evaluation of clinical studies on OCD shows that the majority of studies focus on White populations. Black and Hispanic populations are underrepresented in many clinical studies, even though prevalence rates and many manifestations of OCD of those populations are similar to those experienced by White populations (Wetterneck et al., 2012; Williams, Elstein et al., 2012). Limited studies on cultural differences between White and other cultural or ethnic groups indicate that Blacks and Hispanics are less likely to receive treatment for OCD based on the negative stigma associated with mental health conditions and socioeconomic barriers (Wetterneck et al., 2012; Williams, Domanico et al., 2012). However, Black patients report contamination symptoms more frequently than White patients and are twice as likely to report excessive concerns about animals (Williams, Elstein et al., 2012). In addition, religious differences often have a role in the development of OCD: Individuals who adhere to religions that practice rituals, such as Jewish, Catholic, and Islamic faiths, are more likely to develop OCD with repeated and excessive practice of religious rituals such that they interfere with everyday obligations (Himle, Taylor, & Chatters, 2012; Grant, 2014).

Pharmacologic Therapy

For the patient with OCD, SSRIs are often prescribed as part of the treatment regimen. Clomipramine, which is a tricyclic antidepressant (TCA), also may be administered (Mayo Clinic, 2015b). While SSRIs tend to have fewer side effects than TCAs, all medications carry risks and potential adverse effects. The nurse's role includes educating the patient about the safe administration of medications, as well as the potential side effects.

Nonpharmacologic Therapy

Psychotherapy is an integral component of treatment for the patient with OCD. In addition to focusing on the patient, therapy and counseling sessions may include the patient's family members or significant others. In particular, a kind of CBT called ERP has proven to be most effective for patients with OCD. Using ERP, the affected individual is gradually exposed to the object of his or her obsession or fear and is taught healthy methods of coping with the associated anxiety (Mayo Clinic, 2013). Other CBT therapies, especially those that involve restructuring thought patterns and behavior, have been found effective for these patients. For a discussion of CBT, refer to the Concept section of this module.

Box 31–10
Guidelines for the Treatment of Individuals with OCD

- **Psychiatric management.** OCD is usually a chronic illness. Treatment is necessary when the symptoms interfere with functioning or cause significant distress. Therapeutic management consists of a variety of therapeutic interventions throughout the course of the illness.
- **Psychiatric assessment.** The psychiatrist or psychiatric nurse practitioner will usually consider a medical evaluation and assessment of common comorbid conditions, such as depression, bipolar symptoms, other anxiety disorders, tics, impulse-control disorders, anorexia nervosa, bulimia nervosa, alcohol use, attention-deficit/hyperactivity disorder, and a history of panic attacks.

- **Pharmacotherapy.** Successful medication treatment should be continued for 1–2 years before gradually tapering and while observing for symptom exacerbation. Clomipramine, fluoxetine, fluvoxamine, paroxetine, and sertraline are approved by the FDA for treatment of OCD. The SSRIs have fewer side effects than clomipramine and are recommended for the first medication trial.
- **Psychotherapy.** CBT that relies primarily on behavioral techniques such as exposure and response prevention (ERP) is recommended because it has the best evidentiary support. Family therapy may reduce interfamily tensions due to the individual's OCD symptoms.

Source: American Psychiatric Association. (2007). *Practice guideline for the treatment of patients with obsessive compulsive disorder (p. 570).* Arlington, VA: Author. (Guidelines reaffirmed in 2012); Greenberg, W. M. (2015). *Obsessive-compulsive disorder treatment & management.* Retrieved from http://emedicine.medscape.com/article/1934139-treatment#showall; Mayo Clinic. (2013). *Obsessive-compulsive disorder (OCD).* Retrieved from http://www.mayoclinic.org/diseases-conditions/ocd/basics/definition/con-20027827.

Lifespan Considerations

OCD most commonly begins in children, adolescents, and young adults. Understanding the differences in younger and older populations of individuals with OCD is essential to the proper care of these individuals.

OCD in Children and Adolescents

The mean age of onset of OCD symptoms in children is around age 7.5, but it is often not recognized or diagnosed until much later. Diagnosis of OCD generally peaks in prepubescent children and then again in early adulthood. An estimated 1 to 2% of school-aged children have OCD (Geller & March, 2012). In children and adolescents, boys appear to develop symptoms of OCD earlier than girls, but the ratio of boys to girls with OCD evens out as children age and go through puberty.

Symptoms of OCD in children are often hidden or ill defined, causing them to be missed by parents and clinicians. Younger children in particular are not able to articulate their fears, which often relate to fear of a major disaster such as the loss of a parent (Geller & March, 2012). Obsessions and compulsions are often similar to those experienced by adults, but they may change over time, with the same individual experiencing different obsessions or compulsions as they age. Compulsions are often related to sensory stimuli, including the perception of both physical (tactile, musculoskeletal) and mental (tactile, auditory, visual) sensations (Geller & March, 2012). Children and adolescents are also more likely than adults to experience rage attacks in relation to their OCD, a phenomenon that is enhanced if their family accommodates or reinforces their OCD behaviors (Storch et al., 2012).

Studies conducted by the U.S. Surgeon General, as well as other researchers, suggest that the development of OCD in some children may be linked to streptococcal infection (Swedo, Leckman, & Rose, 2012). Initially referred to by the acronym PANDAS, which stands for pediatric autoimmune neuropsychiatric disorders associated with streptococcal infections, researchers have proposed revision of this condition to pediatric acute-onset neuropsychiatric syndrome (PANS). Its hallmark is a sudden and abrupt exacerbation of OCD symptoms after a strep infection. The cause of this form of OCD appears to be antibodies mistakenly attacking a region of the brain. Another major risk factor for the development of OCD in children is association with a first-order relative (parent or sibling) who also has OCD (Geller & March, 2012).

Many children with OCD will spontaneously resolve their symptoms as they age. However, a younger age of onset, increased duration of OCD, inpatient treatment, and some subsets of symptoms tend to persist (Geller & March, 2012). When possible, CBT and ERP therapy should be used as a first-line treatment for OCD in children. For more severe cases, such as children with declining grades and stronger compulsions in a school setting, medication may be needed. SSRIs appear effective in alleviating symptoms of OCD in children. Several randomized, controlled trials revealed SSRIs to be effective in treating children and adolescents with OCD (Geller & March, 2012).

OCD in Older Adults

Older adults are more likely to report their physical complaints and avoid discussing their mental complaints (ADAA, n.d.d). As a result, it is commonly thought that symptoms of anxiety and related disorders decrease with age. However, OCD and subclinical obsessive-compulsive symptoms (OCS) are common in older adults, especially those with depression and decreased mental and social functioning (Klenfeldt et al., 2014). Subclinical obsessive and compulsive symptoms appear to be much more frequent than clinical OCD in older adults, and the patients often find these symptoms very distressing (Pulular, Levy, & Stewart, 2013).

Because older adults are less likely to discuss their mental symptoms, a general assessment of older adults should include assessment for changes in mental status, including obsessive and compulsive symptoms. Older adults with one or more mental or anxiety disorders should be given a thorough psychiatric assessment, because OCD is often comorbid with other mental disorders. This comorbidity may interfere with responsiveness to treatment and increase the time it takes for medications to be effective in older adults.

NURSING PROCESS

The primary nursing goals for the patient with OCD are to ensure patient safety and to alleviate anxiety and distress. Care must be taken not to prevent the performance of rituals that the patient uses to reduce anxiety but rather to promote new behavioral patterns and coping mechanisms to make the rituals unnecessary while maintaining the safety of the patient.

Assessment

- ***Observation and patient interview.*** The nursing assessment interviews of patients with OCD share many similarities to those used with patients who have anxiety disorders. Suggested interview questions include:

Current and Past Medical History

- Does anyone in your family experience an anxiety disorder?
- Have you experienced intrusive or unwanted thoughts? Please describe the nature of the unwanted thoughts.
- Do you find yourself performing repetitive actions and behaviors to alleviate your anxiety? Please describe.
- Describe how these compulsions have interfered with your life.
- How old were you when you first experienced these obsessive-compulsive thoughts and behaviors? Age at diagnosis?
- Approximately how much time out of your day is spent dealing with these obsessions and compulsions?
- On a scale of 0–10, please rate your current level of distress (0 = no distress, 10 = intolerable anxiety).
- What have you tried in the past to alleviate the anxiety? What do you think was successful?
- Describe any repetitive or ritualistic behaviors.
- Do you use counting when feeling anxious?
- Have you experienced depression? Have you considered suicide? If yes, please rate on a scale from 0 to 10 how likely you are to act on these thoughts or impulses (0 = not at all, 10 = I will kill myself).
- Do you drink or use illicit drugs to manage your anxiety? If so, please list name, frequency, and amount.

Activities of Daily Living

- Is your health at risk as a result of the obsessions and compulsions?
- Describe a typical day (sleep, eating, activities, employment).
- How has this disorder affected your relationships?
- How has this disorder affected your spirituality?
- How has this disorder affected your emotional well-being and mental health?
- ***Physical examination.*** A thorough examination may determine physical problems resulting from manifestations of OCD. For example, excessive hand washing or the use of irritating cleansing agents may result in loss of tissue integrity.

Diagnosis

Appropriate nursing diagnoses for OCD may vary depending on the nature of the obsessive thoughts and compulsive behaviors and the severity of the illness. In addition to *Anxiety*, possible nursing diagnoses for OCD patients include the following:

- *Fear*
- *Coping, Ineffective*
- *Role Performance, Ineffective*
- *Impaired Tissue Integrity, Risk for*
- *Social Interaction, Impaired.*

(NANDA-I © 2014)

Planning

Planning in collaboration with the patient should be prioritized according to what the patient identifies as most important and may include the following goals:

- The patient will identify triggers for obsessive-compulsive behaviors.
- The patient will experience reduced anxiety without performing associated compulsive behaviors.
- The patient will incorporate coping techniques to decrease the need to perform compulsive behaviors.
- The patient will decrease time spent performing compulsive behaviors so that they no longer interfere with everyday role performance.
- The patient will participate in appropriate social activities previously avoided because of obsessive or compulsive tendencies.

Implementation

A supportive and nonjudgmental demeanor is essential when working with patients with OCD. Often the individual is aware that the compulsive behaviors are unreasonable and feels embarrassed. Compulsive behaviors serve as coping mechanisms to lower the level of anxiety or defensively "undo" the obsessive thoughts. Interrupting an individual during a ritual or compulsive behavior creates more anxiety and frequently leads to the individual redoing or repeating the behavior to reduce anxiety. If a patient with OCD is admitted to the hospital, the hospital staff may need to collaborate with the patient to accommodate the rituals until the patient experiences relief from anxiety. Administration of medications to lower anxiety and reevaluation of the patient's response to the medication are the responsibility of the nurse in collaboration with the healthcare provider and the patient.

Alleviate Fear

Patients with OCD often perform ritualistic behaviors to help alleviate fears associated with contamination or causing harm to others. These fears are often based on distortions of reality that the patient believes. Most of the time, the patient is aware that the compulsions are unnecessary. The patient's mental health professional will help the patient work to alter beliefs and correct perceptions. However, the nurse can implement several nursing interventions to help reduce a patient's fears:

- Provide a calm presence for the patient that will encourage the patient to verbalize fears. Validate the patient's feelings without encouraging the patient's belief in a distorted reality.

- Provide facts related to the patient's fears that are based in reality. For example, a patient who is afraid of contamination may benefit from knowledge about the immune system and the benefit of limited exposure to germs.

- For patients who are hospitalized for treatment of their OCD or for any other reason, take steps to reduce environmental stimulation. Remove or hide items associated with any triggers associated with the patient's obsession or compulsion. Teach patients to remove triggers from their home or work environment as much as possible.

Promote Effective Coping

When patients with OCD experience fears or obsessions, they are unable to use normal coping strategies to prevent the practice of compulsive behaviors. Instead, they perform compulsive behaviors as a coping mechanism. This often disrupts the performance of normal roles and may cause them to feel embarrassed or isolated from society. Nurses can teach patients effective coping behaviors, as described in the Patient Teaching feature.

Promote Effective Role Performance

The ritualistic behaviors and shame associated with OCD often interfere with the ability of the patient to perform normal roles, including family, home, and work responsibilities. OCD behaviors may also interfere with the patient's ability to perform self-care activities. The nurse can help patients adequately perform their roles by:

- Encouraging patients to have healthy conversations with their family members about the disorder.

- Listening to the patient describe how the ritualistic behaviors are disrupting his or her ability to perform normal roles. This includes having the patient describe normal roles that the patient is not performing because of the disorder. This may help the patient discover why he or she feels compelled to perform compulsive behaviors and to discuss ways in which the patient can begin to perform normal roles again in the future.

- Promoting self-awareness for the patient to understand his reaction to environmental triggers. Understanding his own thought processes and the reasons behind those thoughts can promote changes in thought patterns necessary to decrease disruptive behaviors and increase performance of normal roles.

- Encouraging the patient to participate in individual or family behavioral therapy or counseling. In addition to medication, therapy or counseling is one of the most effective ways to help patients with OCD regain control over their life and behaviors. The nurse can provide references to therapists or counselors who specialize in the treatment of OCD.

SAFETY ALERT   Patients who perform excessive washing rituals are at a high risk for impaired tissue integrity, especially on the hands. Excessive handwashing with soaps and antibacterial gels can dry the skin and leave it susceptible to cracking and bleeding. Teach the patient about consequences of excessive hand washing and techniques to help maintain skin integrity, including the regular use of lotions.

Promote Social Interaction

Patients with OCD who spend hours each day performing ritualistic behaviors may find that they are no longer able to participate in social activities. Performing rituals or checking behaviors often delays the patient's arrival at an event or prevents the patient from leaving home altogether. Friends may avoid spending time with the patient because of the patient's odd behaviors and time wasting. As patients progress through treatment, nurses can promote social interaction of the patient by teaching time management techniques so patients can plan to arrive at social events on time and encouraging patients to be open with their friends about the disorder and to enlist their support during social interactions. The nurse may also encourage the patient to invite close friends and family to a counseling session so they can be a part of the healing process.

Evaluation

Patients with OCD have a low rate of successful response to treatment; about 50% improve with treatment, but only 10% recover completely (Harvard Health Publications, 2009). Therefore, the nurse will need to continually evaluate the patient and develop new nursing diagnoses and interventions. Successful response to nursing care may be evaluated by using the following expected outcomes:

- The patient verbalizes a reduction in anxiety associated with the compulsive need to perform ritualistic behaviors.

- The patient demonstrates an understanding of appropriate coping behaviors and verbalizes successful use of healthy coping behaviors to reduce the need to perform compulsive behaviors.

- The patient demonstrates an ability to effectively perform expected roles, including family, home, and work roles.

- The patient verbalizes increased social interaction and a decrease in missed events due to the performance of ritualistic behaviors.

Patient Teaching

Adaptive Coping

Establishing a therapeutic relationship provides the nurse with an opportunity to promote healthy adaptive coping. Patient teaching about the nature of obsessive thinking is critical to lowering the patient's feelings of shame and anxiety. The nurse can help the patient realize that fears arise from the disease, not from any real threat. Nurses can help patients reframe how they think about their disease and help them reframe thought processes in order to reduce ritual performance, such as helping the patient meditate instead of performing a ritual and then recognizing that nothing bad happened as a result of the absence of the ritual. The nurse has an essential role in helping the patient with OCD understand that he or she can decrease anxiety and gain control over the disease through pharmacologic and behavior therapies.

The nurse should understand that complete healing from OCD will likely take many years for most patients. During this time, the nurse should continually reevaluate the patient and suggest changes in treatment modalities depending on the success or failure of previous treatment plans. The nurse may need to teach additional coping strategies or advocate for the patient to receive different medication or to add CBT or family counseling to the treatment plan. Importantly, the nurse should encourage the patient to continue treatment, not give up, and not accept the disorder as normal or inevitable.

REVIEW Obsessive-Compulsive Disorder

RELATE Link the Concepts and Exemplars

Linking the exemplar of obsessive-compulsive disorder with the concept of mood and affect:

1. How might mood be impacted in the patient who is unable to control his ritualistic compulsive disorders?

2. Is assessment for suicidal ideation important when admitting a new patient with OCD? Why or why not?

Linking the exemplar of obsessive-compulsive disorder with the concept of advocacy:

3. If a patient's rituals involve an act that places her in danger, what actions can the nurse take to advocate for the patient while not causing increased anxiety that can result from not being able to perform the ritual?

4. While working on a medical unit in a local hospital, you admit an adult patient for surgery. While collecting the admission assessment, you note what you suspect is ritualistic compulsive behavior. How can you best advocate for this patient?

READY Go to Volume 3: Clinical Nursing Skills

REFER Go to Pearson MyLab Nursing and eText

- Additional review materials

REFLECT Apply Your Knowledge

Karleen Lassiter, a married, 40-year-old mother of three children, is admitted to a hospital psychiatric unit with complaints of anxiety, inability to relax, and intrusive thoughts that she states are "horrific." When asked to describe her thoughts, she states, "I'm afraid I'm going to hell as punishment for what goes through my mind sometimes. It's really dark stuff." In conjunction with her intrusive thoughts, Ms. Lassiter recites the same prayer up to 50 times daily. Ms. Lassiter is trained as a respiratory therapist, but she has not practiced in the clinical setting for the past 5 years. In part, she reports that her departure from her position as a respiratory therapist was related to her need to complete her prayer rituals. Ms. Lassiter explains that her employment was terminated due to her being late for work on several occasions, because "I needed to finish praying before I could leave for work." She is aware that her behavior is irrational and that it is negatively impacting her life; however, she is unable to control or cease the behavior.

Ms. Lassiter's medical history includes panic attacks between the ages of 18 and 21, during college enrollment. She denies suicidal ideation; however, she states, "I don't think I can handle living like this. My husband and kids think I'm crazy, and they're right."

1. Based on the available assessment data, identify Ms. Lassiter's apparent obsessions and compulsions.

2. Describe appropriate communication strategies for encouraging Ms. Lassiter to further describe her intrusive thoughts.

3. Based on the patient's statements, identify the priority nursing diagnosis for Ms. Lassiter.

References

Adams, M. P., Holland, L. N., & Urban, C. (2017). *Pharmacology for nurses: A pathophysiologic approach* (5th ed.). Hoboken, NJ: Pearson Education.

American Congress of Obstetricians and Gynecologists (ACOG). (2013). *Tobacco, alcohol, drugs, and pregnancy*. Retrieved from http://www.acog.org/Patients/FAQs/Tobacco-Alcohol-Drugs-and-Pregnancy

American Psychiatric Association (APA). (2007). (Guidelines reaffirmed in 2012) *Practice guideline for the treatment of patients with obsessive compulsive disorder* (p. 570). Arlington, VA: Author.

American Psychiatric Association (APA). (2013). *Diagnostic and statistical manual of mental disorders* (5th ed.). Arlington, VA: Author.

American Psychological Association. (2012). *Stress in America: Our health at risk*. Washington, DC: Author.

American Psychological Association. (n.d.a). *Identifying signs of stress in your children and teens*. Retrieved from http://www.apa.org/helpcenter/stress-children.aspx

American Psychological Association. (n.d.b). *The road to resilience*. Retrieved from http://www.apa.org/helpcenter/road-resilience.aspx

American Psychological Association. (n.d.c). *Psychotherapy: Understanding group therapy*. Retrieved from http://www.apa.org/helpcenter/group-therapy.aspx

Anxiety and Depression Association of America (ADAA). (2014). *Facts & statistics*. Retrieved from http://www.adaa.org/about-adaa/press-room/facts-statistics

Anxiety and Depression Association of America (ADAA). (2015a). *Generalized anxiety disorder (GAD)*. Retrieved from http://www.adaa.org/generalized-anxiety-disorder-gad

Anxiety and Depression Association of America (ADAA). (2015b). *Pregnancy and medication*. Retrieved from http://www.adaa.org/living-with-anxiety/women/pregnancy-and-medication

Anxiety and Depression Association of America (ADAA). (n.d.a). *Women: Facts*. Retrieved from http://www.adaa.org/living-with-anxiety/women/facts

Anxiety and Depression Association of America (ADAA). (n.d.b). *Living and thriving with anxiety or depression means conquering your symptoms: Older adults—Symptoms*. Retrieved from http://www.adaa.org/living-with-anxiety/older-adults/symptoms

Anxiety and Depression Association of America (ADAA). (n.d.c). *Treatment*. Retrieved from http://www.adaa.org/living-with-anxiety/children/treatment

Anxiety and Depression Association of America (ADAA). (n.d.d). *Older adults*. Retrieved from http://www.adaa.org/living-with-anxiety/older-adults

Baas, J. M. P., Mol, N., Kenemans, J. L., Prinssen, E. P., Niklson, I., Xia-Chen, C., . . . van Gerven J. (2009). Validating a human model for anxiety using startle potentiated by cue and context: The effects of alprazolam, pregabalin, and diphenhydramine. *Psychopharmacology (Berlin), 205*(1), 73–84.

Ball, J. W., Bindler, R. C., Cowen, K., & Shaw, M. (2017). *Principles of pediatric nursing: Caring for children,* (7th ed.). Hoboken, NJ: Pearson Education.

Bandura, A. (1994). Self-efficacy. In V. S. Ramachandran (Ed.), *Encyclopedia of human behavior* (Vol. 4, pp. 71–81). New York, NY: Academic Press.

BehaveNet. (2015). *Phobia.* Retrieved from http://behavenet.com/phobia

Biesecker, B. B., Erby, L. H., Woolford, S., Adcock, J. Y., Cohen, J. S., Lamb, A., . . . Reeve, B. B. (2013). Development and validation of the Psychological Adaptation Scale (PAS): Use in six studies of adaptation to a health condition or risk. *Patient Education & Counseling, 93*(2), 248–254.

Berk, L. (2012). *Child development* (9th ed.). Upper Saddle River, NJ: Prentice Hall.

Bodden, D. H., Bogels, S. M., & Muris, P. (2009). The diagnostic utility of the Screen for Child Anxiety Related Emotional Disorders-71 (SCARED-71). *Behavior Research and Therapy, 47*(5), 418–425.

Bokor, G., & Anderson, P. D. (2014). Obsessive-compulsive disorder. *Journal of Pharmacy Practice, 27*(2), 116–130.

Boston Children's Hospital. (2012). *Generalized anxiety disorder (GAD).* Retrieved from http://www.childrenshospital.org/az/Site948/mainpageS948P0.html

Butcher, J. N., Mineka, S., & Hooley, J. M. (2013). *Abnormal psychology* (15th ed.). Upper Saddle River, NJ: Pearson.

Cannon, W. B. (1929). Organization for physiological homeostasis. *Physiological Reviews, 9*(3), 399–431.

Cannon, W. B. (1932). *The wisdom of the body.* New York, NY: W. W. Norton.

Caplan, G. (1964). *Principles of preventive psychiatry.* New York, NY: Basic Books.

Carver, C. S., & Connor-Smith, J. (2010). Personality and coping. *Annual Review of Psychology, 61*, 679–704.

Centers for Disease Control and Prevention (CDC). (2013). *Mental health basics.* Retrieved from http://www.cdc.gov/mentalhealth/basics.htm

Cherry, L. (1978). On the real benefits of eustress: An interview with Hans Selye. *Psychology Today, 11*(10), 60–70.

Children's Hospital of Pittsburgh. (2013). *Separation anxiety disorder.* Retrieved from http://www.chp.edu/CHP/P02582

Cleveland Clinic. (2013). *Treating anxiety disorders in children and adolescents.* Retrieved from https://my.clevelandclinic.org/childrens-hospital/health-info/ages-stages/childhood/hic_Treating-Anxiety_Disorders_in_Children_and_Adolescents

Cleveland Clinic. (2014). *Anxiety disorders.* Retrieved from http://my.clevelandclinic.org/services/neurological_institute/center-for-behavorial-health/disease-conditions/hic-anxiety-disorders

Cohen, S., Janicki-Deverts, D., Doyle, W. J., Miller, G. E., Frank, E., Rabin, B. S., & Turner, R. B. (2012). Chronic stress, glucocorticoid receptor resistance, inflammation, and disease risk. *Proceedings of the National Academy of Sciences, 109*(16), 5995–5999.

Cousino, M. K., & Hazen, R. A. (2013). Parenting stress among caregivers of children with chronic illness: A systematic review. *Journal of Pediatric Psychology, 38*(8), 809–828.

Creswell, C., Waite, P., & Cooper, P. (2014). Assessment and management of anxiety disorders in children and adolescents. *Archives of Disease in Childhood, 99*(7), 674–678.

D'Arrigo, T. (2013). *Finesse required to treat anxiety in the elderly.* Retrieved from http://www.acpinternist.org/archives/2013/01/elderly.htm

De Gage, S. B., Begaud, B., Bazin, F., Verdoux, H., Dartigues, J-F., Peres, K., . . . Pariente, A. (2012). Benzodiazepine use and risk of dementia: Prospective population based study. *BMJ, 345*, e6231.

De Leersnyder, J., Boiger, M., & Mesquita, B. (2013). Cultural regulation of emotion: Individual, relational, and structural sources. *Frontiers in Psychology, 4*, 55.

DeLongis, A., Coyne, J. C., Dakof, G., Folkman, S., & Lazarus, R. (1982). Relationship of daily hassles, uplifts, and major life events to health status. *Health Psychology, 1*(2), 119–136.

Dossey, B. M., & Keegan, L. (2016). *Holistic nursing: A handbook for practice* (7th ed.). Burlington, MA: Jones & Bartlett.

Dubuc, B. (2013). *Brain abnormalities associated with anxiety disorders.* Retrieved from http://thebrain.mcgill.ca/flash/i/i_08/i_08_cr/i_08_cr_anx/i_08_cr_anx.html

Elder, C., Nidich, S., Moriarty, F., & Nidich, R. (2014). Effect of transcendental meditation on employee stress, depression, and burnout: A randomized controlled study. *The Permanente Journal, 18*(1), 19–23. Retrieved from http://www.ncbi.nlm.nih.gov/pmc/articles/PMC3951026/

Elder, R., Evans, K., Nizette, D., & Trenoweth, S. (2013). *Psychiatric and mental health nursing* (3rd ed.). Sydney, Australia: Elsevier.

Erikson, E. H. (1968). *Identity: Youth and crisis.* New York, NY: Norton.

Everly, G. S., & Lating, J. M. (2013). *A clinical guide to the treatment of the human stress response* (3rd ed.). New York, NY: Springer.

Federal Emergency Management Agency. (2015). *Crisis counseling assistance & training program.* Retrieved from https://www.fema.gov/recovery-directorate/crisis-counseling-assistance-training-program

Freud, S. (1946). *The ego and mechanisms of defense.* New York, NY: International Universities Press.

Galanti, G-A. (2015). *Caring for patients from different cultures* (5th ed.). Philadelphia, PA: University of Pennsylvania Press.

Geller, D. A., & March, J. (2012). Practice parameter for the assessment and treatment of children and adolescents with obsessive-compulsive disorder. *Journal of the American Academy of Child & Adolescent Psychiatry, 51*(1), 98–113.

George, A., Luz, R., De Tychey, C., Thilly, N., & Spitz, E. (2013). Anxiety symptoms and coping strategies in the perinatal period. *BMC Pregnancy and Childbirth, 13*(233). Retrieved from http://www.medscape.com/viewarticle/819791_2

Gibbons, R. D., Perraillon, M. C., Hur, K., Conti, R. M., Valuck, R. J., & Brent, D. A. (2015). Antidepressant treatment and suicide attempts and self-inflicted injury in children and adolescents. *Pharmacoepidemiology and Drug Safety, 24*(2), 208–214.

Goodman, W. K., Grice, D. E., Lanidus, K. A., & Coffey, B. J. (2014). Obsessive-compulsive disorder. *Psychiatric Clinics of North America, 37*(3), 257–267.

Grant, J. E. (2014). Obsessive-compulsive disorder. *New England Journal of Medicine, 371*, 646–653.

Greenberg, W. M. (2015). *Obsessive-compulsive disorder treatment & management.* Retrieved from http://emedicine.medscape.com/article/1934139-treatment#showall

Harvard Health Publications. (2009). *Treating obsessive-compulsive disorder.* Retrieved from http://www.health.harvard.edu/mind-and-mood/treating-obsessive-compulsive-disorder

Harvard School of Public Health. (n.d.). *Antioxidants: Beyond the hype.* Retrieved from http://www.hsph.harvard.edu/nutritionsource/antioxidants/.

Herdman, T. H. & Kamitsuru, S. (Eds.). *Nursing Diagnoses—Definitions and Classification 2015–2017.* Copyright © 2014, 1994–2014 NANDA International. Used by arrangement with John Wiley & Sons, Inc. Companion website: www.wiley.com/go/nursingdiagnoses

Herman, J. P. (2013). Neural control of chronic stress adaptation. *Frontiers in Behavioral Neuroscience, 7*, 61.

Herringa, R. J., Birn, R. M., Ruttle, P. L., Burghy, C. A., Stodola, D. E., Davidson, R. J., & Essex, M. J. (2013). Childhood maltreatment is associated with altered fear circuitry and increased internalizing symptoms by late adolescence. *Proceedings of the National Academy of Sciences, 110*(47), 19119–19124.

Himle, J. A., Taylor, R. J., & Chatters, L. M. (2012). Religious involvement and obsessive compulsive disorder among African Americans and Black Caribbeans. *Journal of Anxiety Disorders, 26*(4), 502–510.

Holmes, T. H., & Rahe, R. H. (1967). The social readjustment rating scale. *Journal of Psychosomatic Research, 11*, 213–218.

Horowitz, M. J., Wilner, M., & Alverez, W. (1979). Impact of events scale: A measure of subjective stress. *Psychosomatic Medicine, 41*(3), 209–218.

Jewell, S. (2015). *Antipsychotics for anxiety.* Livestrong.com. Retrieved from http://www.livestrong.com/article/183286-antipsychotics-for-anxiety

Johnson, S. B., Riley, A. W., Granger, D. A., & Riis, J. (2013). The science of early life toxic stress for pediatric practice and advocacy. *Pediatrics, 131*(2), 319–327.

Kaneshiro, N. K. (2014). *Stress in childhood.* Retrieved from https://www.nlm.nih.gov/medlineplus/ency/article/002059.htm

Kneisl, C. R., & Trigoboff, E. (2013). *Contemporary psychiatric–mental health nursing* (3rd ed.). Upper Saddle River, NJ: Pearson Education.

Koltko-Rivera, M. E. (2006). Rediscovering the later version of Maslow's hierarchy of needs: Self-transcendence and opportunities for theory, research, and unification. *Review of General Psychology, 10*(4), 302–317.

Kourkouta, L., & Papathanasiou, I. V. (2014). Communication in nursing practice. *Materiasociomedica, 26*(1), 65–67.

Lazarus, R. S., & Folkman, S. (1984). *Stress, appraisal, and coping.* New York, NY: Springer.

Lee, C., Suchday, S., & Wylie-Rosett, J. (2012). Perceived social support, coping styles, and Chinese immigrants' cardiovascular responses to stress. *International Journal of Behavioral Medicine, 19*(2), 174–185. doi.org/10.1007/s12529-011-9156-7

Leon, A. (2014). Immigration and stress: The relationship between parents' acculturative stress and young children's anxiety symptoms. *Student Pulse, 6*(3). Retrieved from http://www.studentpulse.com/a?id=861

Lewis, C. E., Siegel, J. M., & Lewis, M. A. (1984). Feeling bad: Exploring sources of distress among pre-adolescent children. *American Journal of Public Health, 74*(2), 117–122.

Littleton-Gibbs, L. Y., & Engebretson, J. C. (2013). *Maternity nursing care* (2nd ed.). Clifton Park, NY: Cengage Learning.

Lumsden, D. P. (1981). Is the concept of "stress" of any use, anymore? In *Contributions to primary prevention in mental health: Working papers.* Toronto, ON: Toronto National Office of the Canadian Mental Health Association.

Lyon, B. L. (2012). Stress, coping, and health: A conceptual overview. In V. H. Rice (Ed.), *Handbook of stress, coping, and health: Implications for nursing research, theory, and practice* (2nd ed., pp. 1–20). Thousand Oaks, CA: Sage.

Maslow, A. (1943). A theory of human motivation. *Psychological Review, 50*(4), 370–396.

Maslow, A. H. (1968). *Toward a psychology of being* (2nd ed.). New York, NY: Van Nostrand Reinhold.

Maslow, A. H. (1987). *Motivation and personality* (3rd ed.). New York, NY: Harper & Row.

Matta, C. (2012). *The stress response: How dialectical behavior therapy can free you from needless anxiety, worry, anger & other symptoms of stress.* Oakland, CA: New Harbinger Publications.

Mayo Clinic. (2012a). *Anxiety.* Retrieved from http://www.mayoclinic.com/health/anxiety/DS01187/DSECTION=alternative-medicine

Mayo Clinic. (2012b). *Anxiety: Prevention.* Retrieved from http://www.mayoclinic.com/health/anxiety/DS01187/DSECTION=prevention

Mayo Clinic. (2013). *Obsessive-compulsive disorder (OCD).* Retrieved from http://www.mayoclinic.org/diseases-conditions/ocd/basics/definition/con-20027827

Mayo Clinic. (2014a). *Social anxiety disorder (social phobia).* Retrieved from http://www.mayoclinic.org/diseases-conditions/social-anxiety-disorder/basics/definition/con-20032524

Mayo Clinic. (2014b). *Diseases and conditions: Anxiety.* Retrieved from http://www.mayoclinic.org/diseases-conditions/anxiety/basics/symptoms/con-20026282

Mayo Clinic. (2015a). Support groups: Make connections, get help. Retrieved from http://www.mayoclinic.org/healthy-lifestyle/stress-management/in-depth/support-groups/art-20044655

Mayo Clinic. (2015b). *Clomipramine.* Retrieved from http://www.mayoclinic.org/drugs-supplements/clomipramine-oral-route/description/drg-20072005

McDougle, L., Konrath, S., Walk, M., & Handy, F. (2015). Religious and secular coping strategies and mortality risk among older adults. *Social Indicators Research.* doi:10.1007/s11205-014-0852-y.

Mental Health Academy. (n.d.) *Crisis counseling: The ABC model.* Retrieved from https://www.mentalhealthacademy.com.au/video_details.php?catid=15&vid=68

Miller, C. A. (2012). Nursing for wellness in older adults (6th ed.). Philadelphia, PA: Lippincott Williams & Wilkins.

Miller, M. A., & Rahe, R. H. (1997). Life changes scaling for the 1990s. *Journal of Psychosomatic Research, 43,* 279–292.

Milrod, B., Markowitz, J., Gerber, A., Cyranowski, J., Altemus, M., Shapiro, T., . . . Glatt, C. (2014). Childhood separation anxiety and the pathogenesis and treatment of adult anxiety. *American Journal of Psychiatry, 171*(1), 34–43. Retrieved from http://ajp.psychiatryonline.org/doi/full/10.1176/appi.ajp.2013.13060781

Minnesota Department of Human Services. (2013). *General MHCP non-enrollable mental health provider requirements.* Retrieved from http://www.dhs.state.mn.us/main/idcplg?IdcService=GET_DYNAMIC_CONVERSION&RevisionSelectionMethod=LatestReleased&dDocName=dhs16_136715

Monat, A., & Lazarus, R. S. (1991). *Stress and coping* (3rd ed.). New York, NY: Columbia University Press.

Na, K-S., Lee, S. I., Hong, H. J., Oh, M-J., Bahn, G. H., Ha, K., . . . Kyung, Y-M. (2014). The influence of unsupervised time on elementary school children at high risk for inattention and problem behaviors. *Child Abuse & Neglect, 38*(6), 1120–1127.

National Alliance on Mental Illness (NAMI). (2012). *Mental illnesses: Anxiety disorders.* Retrieved from http://www.nami.org/Template.cfm?Section=By_Illness&Template=/ContentManagement/ContentDisplay.cfm&ContentID=142543

National Center for Complementary and Integrative Health (NCCIH). (2012). *Lavender.* Retrieved from https://nccih.nih.gov/health/lavender/ataglance.htm

National Center for Complementary and Integrative Health (NCCIH). (2013). *Yoga for health.* Retrieved from https://nccih.nih.gov/health/yoga/introduction.htm

National Institutes of Health. (2012). *Will stress during pregnancy affect my baby?* Retrieved from https://www.nichd.nih.gov/health/topics/preconceptioncare/conditioninfo/pages/stress.aspx

National Institute of Mental Health (NIMH). (2013a). *Psychotherapies.* Retrieved from http://www.nimh.nih.gov/health/topics/psychotherapies/index.shtml.

National Institute of Mental Health (NIMH). (2013b). *Brain basics.* Retrieved from http://www.nimh.nih.gov/health/educational-resources/brain-basics/brain-basics.shtml

National Institute of Mental Health (NIMH). (2015). *Anxiety disorders.* Retrieved from http://www.nimh.nih.gov/health/topics/anxiety-disorders/index.shtml

National Institute of Mental Health (NIMH). (n.d.a) *Antidepressant medications for children and adolescents: Information for parents and caregivers.* Retrieved from http://www.nimh.nih.gov/health/topics/child-and-adolescent-mental-health/antidepressant-medications-for-children-and-adolescents-information-for-parents-and-caregivers.shtml

National Institute of Mental Health (NIMH). (n.d.b) *Generalized anxiety disorder (GAD).* Retrieved from http://www.nimh.nih.gov/health/topics/generalized-anxiety-disorder-gad/index.shtml

National Institute of Mental Health (NIMH). (n.d.c). *Panic disorder.* Retrieved from http://www.nimh.nih.gov/health/topics/panic-disorder/index.shtml

National Institute of Mental Health (NIMH). (n.d.d). *Social phobia (social anxiety disorder).* Retrieved from http://www.nimh.nih.gov/health/topics/social-phobia-social-anxiety-disorder/index.shtml

National Institute of Mental Health (NIMH). (n.d.e) *Anxiety disorders in children and adolescents (fact sheet).* Retrieved from http://www.nimh.nih.gov/health/publications/anxiety-disorders-in-children-and-adolescents/index.shtml

Nydegger, R. (2012). *Dealing with anxiety and related disorders: Understanding, coping, and prevention.* Santa Barbara, CA: ABC-CLIO.

Olfson, M., King, M., & Schoenbaum, M. (2015). Benzodiazepine use in the United States. *JAMA Psychiatry, 72*(2), 136–142.

Peplau, H. (1952). *Interpersonal relations in nursing.* New York, NY: Putnam.

Privitera, A. P., Distefano, R., Wefer, H. A., Ferro, A., Pulvirenti, A., & Giugno, R. (2015). OCDB: A database collecting genes, miRNAs and drugs for obsessive-compulsive disorder. *Database (Oxford).* doi:10.1093/database/bav069

Pulular, A., Levy, R., & Stewart, R. (2013). Obsessive and compulsive symptoms in a national sample of older people: Prevalence, comorbidity, and associations with cognitive function. *American Journal of Geriatric Psychiatry, 21*(3), 263–271.

Rahe, R., & Tolles, R. (2002). The brief stress and coping inventory: A useful stress management instrument. *International Journal of Stress Management, 9*(2), 61–70.

Ramsay, D. S., & Woods, S. C. (2014). Clarifying the roles of homeostasis and allostasis in physiological regulation. *Psychological Review, 121*(2), 225–247.

Rao, N. P., Venkatasubramanian, G., Ravi, V., Kalmady, S., Cherian, A., & Yc, J. R. (2015). Plasma cytokine abnormalities in drug-naïve, comorbidity-free obsessive-compulsive disorder. *Psychiatry Research, 229*(3), 949–952. doi:10.1016/j.psychres.2015.07.009

Reefhuis, J., Devine, O., Friedman, J. M., Louik, C., & Honein, M. A. (2015). Specific SSRIs and birth defects: Bayesian analysis to interpret new data in the context of previous reports. *BMJ, 350,* h3190.

Reyes, A. T., Andrusyszyn, M. A., Iwasiw, C. Forchuk, C., & Babenko-Mould, Y. (2015). Nursing students' understanding and enactment of resilience: A grounded theory study. *Journal of Advanced Nursing, 71*(11), 2633–2633. doi:10.1111/jan.12730

Rice, V. H. (2012). *Handbook of stress, coping, and health* (2nd ed.). Thousand Oaks, CA: Sage.

Robertson, T., Benzeval, M, Whitley, E., & Popham, F. (2015). The role of material, psychosocial and behavioral factors in mediating the association between socioeconomic position and allostatic load (measured by cardiovascular, metabolic and inflammatory markers). *Brain, Behavior, and Immunity, 45,* 41–49.

Ruscio, A. M., Stein, D. J., Chiu, W. T., & Kessler, R. C. (2010). The epidemiology of obsessive-compulsive disorder in the National Comorbidity Survey Replication. *Molecular Psychiatry, 15*(1), 53–63.

Ryan-Wenger, N. A., Sharrer, V. W., & Campbell, K. K. (2005). Changes in children's stressors over the past 30 years. *Pediatric Nursing, 31*(4), 282–288.

Salim, S. (2014). Oxidative stress and psychological disorders. *Current Neuropharmacology, 12*(2), 140–147. Retrieved from http://www.ncbi.nlm.nih.gov/pmc/articles/PMC3964745/

Schetter, C. D., & Tanner, L. (2012). Anxiety, depression and stress in pregnancy: Implications for mothers, children, research, and practice. *Current Opinion in Psychiatry, 25*(2), 141–148.

Selye, H. (1946). The general adaptation syndrome and the diseases of adaptation. *Journal of Clinical Endocrinology, 6*(1), 117–231.

Selye, H. (1956). *The stress of life.* New York, NY. McGraw-Hill.

Selye, H. (1974). *Stress without distress.* Philadelphia, PA: J. B. Lippincott.

Selye, H. (1976). *The stress of life* (revised ed.). New York, NY: McGraw-Hill. Published by American Psychiatric Association, © 2013.

Seo, J., Park, J., Choi, J., Kim, T., Shin, J., Lee, J., & Han, P. (2012). NADPH oxidase mediates depressive behavior induced by chronic stress in mice. *Journal of Neuroscience, 32*(28), 9690–9699.

Shimada-Sugimoto, M., Otowa, T., & Hettema, J. M. (2015). Genetics of anxiety disorders: Genetic epidemiological and molecular studies in humans. *Psychiatry and Clinical Neurosciences, 69*(7), 388–401.

Southwick, S. M., Bonanno, G. A., Masten, A. S., Panter-Brick, C., & Yehuda, R. (2014). Resilience definitions, theory, and challenges: Interdisciplinary perspectives. *European Journal of Psychotraumatology, 5,* 25338.

Spector, R. E. (2017). *Cultural diversity in health and illness* (9th ed., pp. 231–232, 166–167). Hoboken, NJ: Pearson Education.

Steingard, R. (2014). *Mood disorders and teenage girls.* Retrieved from http://www.childmind.org/en/posts/articles/mood-disorders-teenage-girls-anxiety-depression

Sterling, P., & Eyer, J. (1988). Allostasis: A new paradigm to explain arousal pathology. In S. Fisher & J. Reason (Eds.), *Handbook of life stress, cognition and health* (pp. 629–649). New York, NY: Wiley.

Stewart, S. A. (2005). The effects of benzodiazepines on cognition. *Journal of Clinical Psychiatry, 66*(Suppl. 2), 9–13.

Stimpfel, A. W., Sloane, D. M., & Aiken, L. H. (2012). The longer the shifts for hospital nurses, the higher the levels of burnout and patient dissatisfaction. *Health Affairs, 31*(11), 2501–2509.

Storch, E. A., Jones, A. M., Lack, C. W., Ale, C. M., Sulkowski, M. L., Lewin, A. B., . . . Murphy, T. K. (2012). Rage attacks in pediatric obsessive-compulsive disorder: Phenomenology and clinical correlates. *Journal of the American Academy of Child & Adolescent Psychiatry, 51*(6), 582–592.

Stroud, L. R., Foster, E., Papandonatos, G. D., Handwerger, K., Granger, D. A., Kivlighan, K. T., & Niaura, R. (2009). Stress response and the adolescent transition: Performance versus peer rejection stressors. *Development and Psychopathology, 21*(1), 47–68.

Swedo, S., Leckman, J. F., & Rose, N. R. (2012). From research subgroup to clinical syndrome: Modifying the PANDAS criteria to describe PANS (pediatric acute-onset neuropsychiatric syndrome). *Pediatrics & Therapeutics, 2*(2), 1–8.

Townsend, M. (2014). *Psychiatric mental health nursing: Concepts of care in evidence based practice* (7th ed.). Philadelphia, PA: F. A. Davis.

University of Maryland Medical Center (UMMC). (2013). *Anxiety disorders*. Retrieved from http://umm.edu/health/medical/reports/articles/anxiety-disorders

University of Maryland Medical Center (UMMC). (2015). *German chamomile*. Retrieved from https://umm.edu/health/medical/altmed/herb/german-chamomile

U.S. Department of Housing and Urban Development (HUD). (2014). *HUD's 2014 continuum of care homeless assistance programs: Homeless populations and subpopulations*. Washington, DC: Author.

Wachholtz, A. B., & Sambamthoori, U. (2013). National trends in prayer use as a coping mechanism for depression: Changes from 2002 to 2007. *Journal of Religion and Health, 52*(4), 1356–1368.

Warburton, W. A., & Anderson, C. A. (2015). Aggression, social psychology of. In J. D. Wright (Ed.), *International encyclopedia of the social & behavioral sciences* (2nd ed., Vol. 1, pp. 373–380). Amsterdam. The Netherlands: Elsevier.

Weiss, D. S., & Marmer, C. R. (1997). The impact of event scale—Revised. In J. P. Wilson & T. M. Keane (Eds.), *Assessing psychological trauma and PTSD: A handbook for practitioners* (pp. 399–411). New York, NY: Guilford Press.

Wetterneck, C. T., Little, T. E., Rinehart, K. L., Cervantes, M. E., Hyde, E., & Williams, M. (2012). Latinos with obsessive-compulsive disorder: Mental healthcare utilization and inclusion in clinical trials. *Journal of Obsessive-Compulsive and Related Disorders, 1*(2), 85–97.

Williams, M. T., Domanico, J., Marques, L., Leblanc, N. J., & Turkheimer, E. (2012). Barriers to treatment among African Americans with obsessive-compulsive disorder. *Journal of Anxiety Disorders, 26*(4), 555–563.

Williams, M. T., Elstein, J., Buckner, E., Abelson, J. M., & Himle, J. A. (2012). Symptom dimensions in two samples of African Americans with obsessive-compulsive disorder. *Journal of Obsessive-Compulsive and Related Disorders, 1*(3), 145–152.

World Health Organization (WHO). (2014). *Mental health: Strengthening our response*. Retrieved from http://www.who.int/mediacentre/factsheets/fs220/en/

Xu, Y., Wang, C., Klabnik, J, & O'Donnell, M. (2014). Novel therapeutic targets in depression and anxiety: Antioxidants as a candidate treatment. *Current Neuropharmacology, 12*(2), 109–119.

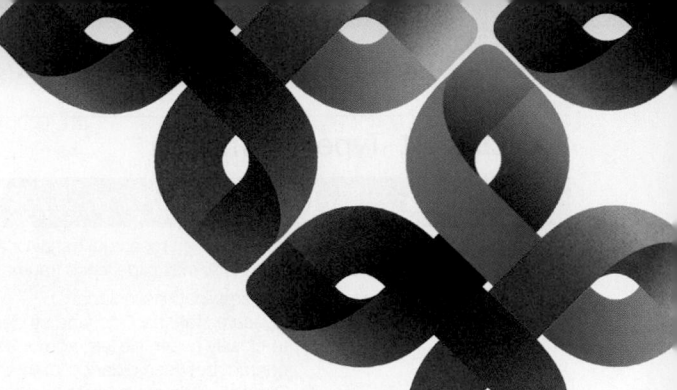

Module 32
Trauma

Module Outline and Learning Outcomes

The Concept of Trauma

Interpersonal Violence

32.1 Analyze interpersonal violence as a component of trauma.

Community and Systemic Violence

32.2 Analyze community and systemic violence as components of trauma.

Unintentional Trauma

32.3 Analyze unintentional trauma.

Concepts Related to Trauma

32.4 Outline the relationship between trauma and other concepts.

Health Promotion

32.5 Summarize health promotion as it relates to trauma.

Nursing Assessment

32.6 Differentiate common assessment procedures and tests used to examine trauma.

Independent Interventions

32.7 Analyze independent interventions nurses can implement for patients who have experienced trauma.

Collaborative Therapies

32.8 Summarize collaborative therapies used by interprofessional teams for patients who have experienced trauma.

Trauma Exemplars

Exemplar 32.A Abuse

32.A Analyze abuse as it relates to trauma.

Exemplar 32.B Multisystem Trauma

32.B Analyze multisystem trauma as it relates to trauma.

Exemplar 32.C Posttraumatic Stress Disorder

32.C Analyze PTSD as it relates to trauma.

Exemplar 32.D Rape and Rape-Trauma Syndrome

32.D Analyze rape and rape-trauma syndrome as they relate to trauma.

 ## The Concept of Trauma

Concept Key Terms

According to the Substance Abuse and Mental Health Services Administration (SAMHSA) (2015), **trauma** "results from an event, series of events, or set of circumstances that is experienced by an individual as physically or emotionally harmful or life threatening and that has lasting adverse effects on the individual's functioning and mental, physical, social, emotional, or spiritual well-being." The term *trauma* has been associated with the word *accident*. Accident means that the injury occurred without intent. In contrast, trauma professionals generally define trauma as either intentional or unintentional. Intentional and unintentional trauma encompass a variety of physical and emotional injuries resulting from motor vehicle crashes, pedestrian injuries, gunshot wounds, falls, violence toward others, or self-inflicted violence (see **Table 32–1 》**).

Trauma can be either acute or chronic. Acute trauma occurs when a person experiences a traumatic event that occurs only once. Examples include being a victim or witness to a violent act; natural disasters such as hurricanes, tornadoes, earthquakes, and fires; a motor vehicle crash; or the loss of a loved one. Repeated exposure to traumatic events, such as war, abuse, neglect, or an accumulation of traumatic events throughout the lifetime, may result in chronic trauma.

TABLE 32-1 Types of Trauma

Type of Trauma	Description
Bullying	Aggressive (often repeated) behavior among school-age children related to a perceived imbalance of power. Both children, the bullied and the bully, may experience trauma leading to mental illness, substance abuse, and suicide. Nursing implications include: ■ Educate staff, parents, and students on how to identify signs of bullying and what actions to take if it is identified; on the need to closely supervise large groups of children such as at recess; and on the need to maintain age-appropriate groups, limiting the contact between older children and younger children. ■ Report bullying to parents and proper authorities per established facility protocol and state guidelines.
Emotional abuse or psychologic maltreatment	Verbal or emotional abuse or excessive demands and expectations in which the individuals may experience behavioral, emotional, affective, and other mental disturbances.
Forced displacement	Forced displacement of individuals or communities from their homes due to conflict, violence, persecution, or human rights violations. Forced displacement is long term or permanent, and many individuals become immigrants or refugees. Nursing implications include: ■ Work with authorities per established facility protocol and state/federal guidelines (World Bank, 2015).
Historical trauma	Cumulative emotional and psychologic injuries as a result of traumatic experiences spanning across generations in a community. This is often associated with racial or ethnic groups that have sustained major losses and attacks on or discrimination against their culture or well-being.
Military trauma	Results from the effects of deployment and trauma-related stress on military personnel and their families. Returning service personnel may experience mental illness and substance abuse issues. Nursing implications include: ■ Assess for safety. ■ Assess individual and family mental health needs. ■ Make referrals as necessary.
Natural or manmade disasters	Trauma resulting from a major accident or disaster such as tornadoes, hurricanes, mudslides, earthquakes, floods, wildfires, and drought. There are also human causes of this type of trauma, such as mass shootings, chemical spills, and terrorist attacks. Nursing implications include: ■ Work with authorities for identification of survivors as well as assisting patients in locating family members per established facility protocols. ■ Provide for immediate safety and psychologic needs.
Neglect	Failing to provide basic human needs such as food, clothing, or shelter as well as medical treatments and medication. Exposing someone to dangerous environments, abandonment, or forcing the individual out of the home are also forms of neglect. Neglect is the most common form of abuse reported to child welfare authorities; however, neglect can also occur with caregivers not meeting the needs of adults even though they have the means to do so.
Physical abuse or assault	Causing or attempting to cause physical pain or injury to another by physical means such as hitting, punching, burning, kicking, or striking with an object.
School violence	Violence that occurs in a school setting, which includes school shootings, bullying, violence, and suicide.
Serious accident, illness, or medical procedure	Unintentional injury or accident, illness, or medical procedures such as surgery that result in extreme pain; may be life threatening.
Sexual abuse or assault	The U.S. Department of Justice's (DOJ's) Office on Violence Against Women defines sexual assault as "any type of sexual contact or behavior that occurs without the explicit consent of the recipient to include forced sexual intercourse, forcible sodomy, child molestation, incest, fondling, and attempted rape" (DOJ, 2016). The U.S. Government defines human trafficking as a two-part statement: "Sex trafficking in which a commercial sex act is induced by force, fraud, or coercion, or in which the person induced to perform such act has not attained 18 years of age; *and* the recruitment, harboring, transportation, provision, or obtaining of a person for labor or services, through the use of force, fraud, or coercion for the purpose of subjection to involuntary servitude, peonage, debt bondage, or slavery" (National Institute of Justice, 2012).
System-induced trauma and retraumatization	Systems in place to assist and protect the public may cause trauma. For example, the Child Welfare Department abruptly removing children from their home, causing separation of siblings and time in foster care, may traumatize children. Another example would be the use of seclusion or mechanical restraints on a previously traumatized individual, which may cause traumatic memories to surface or potentiate a relapse of an existing mental illness.
Traumatic grief of separation	Death, abrupt and/or unexpected or accidental death, premature death, or homicide of a family member, caretaker, or friend; unexplained indefinite separation from a parent, caretaker, family member, or friend due to circumstances beyond control. Nursing implications include: ■ Provide support services for both the patient and the family to include support related to grief and potential survivor's guilt (a survivor may experience guilt associated with having survived a situation when another or others have died).
Victim of or witness to domestic or family violence	According to DOJ's Office on Violence Against Women (DOJ, 2014), domestic violence is defined as: "a pattern of abusive behavior in any relationship that is used by one partner to gain or maintain power and control over another intimate partner. Domestic violence can be physical, sexual, emotional, economic, or psychologic actions or threats of actions that influence another person. This includes any behaviors that intimidate, manipulate, humiliate, isolate, frighten, terrorize, coerce, threaten, blame, hurt, injure, or wound someone."
Victim of or witness to extreme personal violence	Witnessing or experiencing extreme violence, including homicide, suicide, or any other violent acts. Nursing implications include: ■ Provide support services for both the patient and the family, including support related to grief and potential survivor's guilt.
War, terrorism, or political violence	Exposure to war, terrorism, or politically motivated acts of violence such as bombings, shootings, and looting.

Sources: Based on Substance Abuse and Mental Health Services Administration (SAMHSA). (2016). *Types of trauma and violence.* Retrieved from http://www.samhsa.gov/trauma-violence/types; National Child Traumatic Stress Network (NCTSN). (n.d.a). *Types of traumatic stress.* Retrieved from http://www.nctsn.org/trauma-types; Center for Early Childhood Mental Health Consultation. (n.d.). *Types of traumatic experiences.* Retrieved from http://www.ecmhc.org/tutorials/trauma/mod1_3.html.

Nurses are an integral part of medical care for all trauma victims. The nurse must know the fundamental care of all types of trauma victims. There is no way to provide an all-inclusive list of nursing implications, as each situation and each individual will present differently, and the nursing care plan will need to be adapted to each patient. However, there is one common nursing implication for all trauma cases that is critical: Assess and monitor for safety. The nurse will also ensure that every patient who experiences trauma is provided with a supportive, safe environment during care while remaining culturally sensitive to the patient's needs.

For patients experiencing physical trauma, interventions will include the following: Assess the patient, identify injuries sustained; prioritize care of each injury; assess and monitor pain level; assess and monitor mental status; and document clearly and precisely, including all specifics about wounds, as the documentation may be used for legal purposes at a later date.

Interventions appropriate for patients experiencing emotional trauma include the following: Assess and monitor mental status; prioritize mental health needs; validate expressed feelings; and provide community support services information, including a crisis hotline number.

Nursing implications for all criminally related situations (e.g., abuse, neglect, sexual assault) include reporting to proper authorities per established facility protocol and state guidelines; verifying the patient has a safety plan established; ensuring the patient has a safe environment to go to following discharge; and, as stated earlier, documenting wounds and injuries clearly and precisely, as the documentation will likely be used in a legal manner.

Interpersonal Violence

Interpersonal violence is violence that occurs within relationships between family members (also called *family violence*), intimate partners (*intimate partner violence*), and acquaintances or strangers (*community violence*) that does not aim to further the goals of a formal group or cause. Violence of this nature may include physical or sexual assault, abusive relationships, stalking, or homicide (World Health Organization [WHO], 2013a).

A violent crime can involve one of four offenses: murder, rape, robbery, or aggravated assault. Of the most recent data available, aggravated assaults constituted 62.4% of these crimes, robbery represented 29.4%, rape accounted for 6.9%, and murder made up the final 1.2% (Federal Bureau of Investigation [FBI], 2012a). However, violence also represents all instances of abuse, including sexual abuse, child abuse, elder abuse, intimate partner abuse, physical abuse, and emotional abuse.

Violence may result in minor or major trauma. **Minor trauma** involves minor injury to a single part or system of the body. A fracture of the clavicle, a small second-degree burn, and a laceration requiring sutures are examples of minor trauma. **Major trauma** involves serious single-system injury (such as the amputation of a leg) or multiple-system injuries (simultaneous injuries such as a punctured lung, traumatic brain injury, and crushed bones in the arms and legs; also called **multisystem trauma**). Multisystem trauma is often the result of a motor vehicle crash.

Violence may also result in blunt or penetrating trauma. **Blunt trauma** occurs when there is no communication between the damaged tissues and the outside environment. For example, a baseball batter being hit by a pitch may cause damage to the underlying vascular tissue, muscles, and bones. Blunt trauma is frequently caused by motor vehicle crashes, falls, assaults, and sports activities. **Penetrating trauma** occurs when a foreign object enters the body, causing damage to body structures. Examples of penetrating trauma are gunshot or stab wounds and impalement.

Both the attacker and the victim in an incident of interpersonal violence feel aggression during the encounter. Baron and Richardson (1994) offer the following definition of aggression: "any form of behavior directed toward the goal of harming or injuring another living being who is motivated to avoid such treatment." Frequently, a display of aggression is associated with feelings of anger or stress and an overall high emotional response. However, aggression involved in interpersonal violence can also be **instrumental aggression**, which is aggression executed in the absence of emotional arousal. Instrumental aggression frequently takes place in individuals with antisocial disorders. A chronic physiologic activation in response to stress can be one of the causes of the development of an aggressive personality. Stress can also lead to depression characterized by anxiety, anger, and aggressive outbursts, especially if early life experiences such as maltreatment or neglect are involved (Buchanan et al., 2012).

Particularly in families or among intimate partners, violence may occur with a patterned frequency, generally referred to as the **cycle of violence**. The cycle of violence consists of three phases. In the first phase, tension builds between individuals in a relationship as communication fails or expectations are not met. An abusive or threatening incident occurs in the second phase. During this phase, the victim feels traumatized and the aggressor blames the victim for the incident. The third phase of the cycle is known as the honeymoon period, a time during which the aggressor may show love and affection and may also promise to change. During this phase, the victim may feel responsible for the abuse, consider reconciliation, and recant or minimize the incident. However, if the relationship or attitudes are not repaired, communication often fails again, starting the cycle over.

Sometimes, the phrase *cycle of violence* (or cycle of abuse) refers to violence that occurs across multiple generations within a family. In this context, children witness or are subjected to patterned family violence committed by their parents. Physical or emotional damage incurred by children during these experiences increases the likelihood of subjecting their own children to maltreatment (Child Welfare Information Gateway, n.d.).

Although violence in the United States may not be on the rise (see Focus on Diversity and Culture), it is certainly a cause for concern that impacts both the law enforcement community and the healthcare community. Victims of violent acts may seek treatment at emergency departments, urgent care centers, or physician's offices. For injuries that are psychologic in nature, individuals may seek treatment from counselors, therapists, or other mental health specialists.

Abuse and Neglect

Both victims and perpetrators of abuse are seen across all age, race, and socioeconomic groups. Therefore, nurses must continually assess for signs of abuse while caring for patients, especially those from vulnerable populations such as children, older adults, and the disabled.

Federal law defines child abuse as "Any recent act or failure to act on the part of a parent or caretaker which results in death, serious physical or emotional harm, sexual abuse or exploitation" of a child or "An act or failure to act which presents an imminent risk of serious harm" to a child (U.S. Department of Health and Human Services [USDHHS], 2010). Child abuse involves any intentional mistreatment of a child under the age of 18 by someone in a custodial role. It is the state's responsibility to define definitions of child abuse and neglect. Most states recognize four types of child abuse: physical abuse, neglect, sexual abuse, and emotional abuse.

Elder abuse represents the abuse and neglect of individuals 65 years of age and older. The perpetrator is typically the individual's trusted caregiver. Failure of the intended caregiver to provide care or protect an older adult from harm also constitutes maltreatment. Types of elder abuse include physical abuse, sexual abuse, emotional or psychologic abuse, neglect, abandonment, and financial or material exploitation (National Center on Elder Abuse, n.d.a).

Another group of individuals vulnerable to abuse and neglect include those with developmental disabilities. Children with disabilities are 1.68 times more likely to experience abuse or neglect than children without disabilities (Child Welfare Information Gateway, 2012). Furthermore, the U.S. Department of Justice (2015) reports that adults with disabilities, with the exception of those 65 years of age and older, are victim to abuse and neglect at more than double the rate of those without disabilities. Individuals age 65 years and older with developmental delays showed no significant statistical difference from those without disabilities.

Physical Abuse

Healthcare providers must be able to identify manifestations of all forms of abuse. One indicator noted with all age groups is withdrawal from friends, other family members, and activities. Other common, less overt, symptoms of abuse include behavioral changes, depression, and even suicide attempts. Children and teenagers may miss school and scheduled activities. They also may attempt to run away from home. More recognizable symptoms of physical abuse include unexplained injuries, bruising, or fractures. Incongruence between the explanation of the injury and the injury itself is a red flag that may indicate abuse.

Neglect

Assessing for neglect is just as important as assessing for other types of abuse. Symptoms of neglect may present differently based on the age group and population. For example, a child who lives in an area with cold winters may be wearing a coat that is not warm enough or may not have warm clothing at all. Poor hygiene, lack of medical or dental care, poor growth and development of a child, or weight loss of a dependent or older adult are indicative of neglect. Behavioral issues, such as inability to focus or pay attention, stealing food, and apathy, may also be observed.

Sexual Abuse

Sexual abuse differs from sexual assault. With sexual abuse, an individual who has perceived power over the victim (e.g., parent, teacher, coach, family friend, or relative) takes advantage of the trust established, luring the victim into sexual activity. The victim of sexual abuse is usually compliant and may even be protective of the perpetrator. In contrast, sexual assault is forced, and the possible violent, nonconsensual sexual act may result in serious emotional and physical injury to the victim. Overt symptoms of sexual abuse may include knowledge about sexually related topics that are inappropriate for the child's age, minors who present with pregnancy or sexually transmitted diseases, appearing to be experiencing pain upon sitting or walking, and blood in underwear. When a child sexually abuses another child, it may indicate that the abuser has also been a victim of sexual abuse (Mayo Clinic, 2015). Because overt symptoms of sexual abuse are not always present, the nurse must also observe for passive manifestations common with sexual abuse, including depression, anxiety, fear, shame, guilt, nightmares, eating disorders, self-neglect, withdrawal, and mistrust of adults. Sexual promiscuity and substance abuse are also common behaviors for victims of sexual abuse.

Emotional Abuse

Symptoms of emotional abuse may not be easy to identify, as the manifestations are emotional in nature without identifiable injuries. Social withdrawal, apathy, and diminished self-confidence and self-esteem may be noted. Children may not want to go to school or may avoid certain situations. The child may also have an intense desire to obtain attention and affection. Psychosomatic issues, such as complaints of not feeling well, unexplained headaches, and stomachaches, may also be reported. A pattern of these behaviors warrants assessment. Victims of domestic violence should also be assessed for the presence of emotional abuse.

Complex Trauma

Complex traumas are interpersonal traumas that generally begin in childhood. These traumas occur repeatedly and are cumulative. Generally, complex trauma occurs from direct harm, such as severe abuse, neglect, abandonment, and exploitation (Firestone, 2012). Effects of complex trauma include children having difficulty forming attachments and relationships. They may have difficulty later in life maintaining romantic relationships and friendships, and they may have problems with authority figures. Becoming over-reactive or over-responsive to a normal daily stressor may become prevalent. Children may exhibit somatic complaints, whereas adults may turn to risky behaviors such as substance abuse. Children who have sustained complex trauma may also have difficulty controlling their emotions and may have limited ability to express emotions. Dissociation is another reaction when faced with a traumatic situation. For instance, if a child with a history of past sexual abuse is exposed to another episode of sexual abuse, the child may undergo dissociation as a form of self-preservation. During dissociation, the child becomes mentally separated from the event. Children who experience complex trauma often demonstrate inability to reason or make decisions, and they frequently have learning disabilities (NCTSN, n.d.b).

In 2005, the media brought national attention to the true story of "The Girl in the Window," Danielle, a 6-year-old girl who was reported to law enforcement as a possible child neglect case. She had experienced a lifetime of complex trauma. When she was found, she was so severely neglected that she couldn't speak; was covered in feces, bug bites, and sores; had matted, lice-infested hair; had a swollen diaper on; was emaciated at only 46 pounds; and could only drink from a bottle. After tests were performed, she had no physical ailments and there was no organic cause for her severe delays. She will be developmentally delayed for life due to the degree of neglect she experienced. She continues to have tantrums, rarely speaks, is food aggressive, and has difficulty with forming relationships or socializing, especially with women. This is an extreme case demonstrating lifelong effects of complex trauma sustained during the developmental years.

Physical Assault

Assault is defined by the Bureau of Justice Statistics (BJS, 2016a) as "An unlawful physical attack or threat of attack. Assaults may be classified as aggravated or simple. Rape, attempted rape, and sexual assaults are excluded from this category, as well as robbery and attempted robbery. The severity of assaults ranges from minor threats to nearly fatal incidents." A **simple assault** is generally considered a physical attack by an individual against another in which a weapon is not used and the attack does not result in serious physical injury. In contrast, **aggravated assault** is "An attack or attempted attack with a weapon, regardless of whether an injury occurred, and an attack without a weapon when serious injury results" (BJS, 2016a).

Sexual Assault and Rape

Sexual assault is any type of sexual contact without the consent of the victim, such as fondling and molestation. Rape is nonconsensual penetration orally, vaginally, or anally. The victim may experience physical and emotional trauma related to the acts of sexual assault or rape. Rape-Trauma Syndrome is a psychologic response that elicits negative emotional and physical responses that can last months after the rape or assault. In the United States, an estimated 32.3% of multiracial women were raped during their lifetime, followed closely by American Indian/Alaska Native women at 27.5%. Non-Hispanic Black women (21.2%) and non-Hispanic White women (20.5%) in the United States had nearly the same report of lifetime prevalence of rape. Hispanic women in the United States had the lowest reported lifetime prevalence of rape at 13.6% (Centers for Disease Control and Prevention [CDC], 2014a).

Human sex trafficking is a major domestic and international concern. Sex trafficking has come to the attention of authorities, human rights advocates, policymakers, and the public only in recent years. The Department of Justice's Bureau of Justice Assistance (n.d.) reports that human trafficking is one of the most profitable organized crimes and is growing rapidly. The FBI (n.d.a) reports that over the past decade, they have arrested more than 2000 sex traffickers. The National Human Trafficking Resource Center (2016) reports that in the first quarter of 2016, there were 1654 human trafficking cases reported in the United States, with California reporting the highest occurrence with 305 cases.

Homicide

Homicide occurs when the unlawful acts of a perpetrator result in the death of a victim. In addition to caring for the victims of assault and attempted homicide, nurses may also be responsible for caring for the perpetrators. Nurses provide the same high quality of care for all patients regardless of the events that have led them to seek medical treatment.

SAFETY ALERT In situations where patients have the potential to become violent toward the healthcare professionals working to treat their injuries, nurses should take appropriate precautions. In the clinical setting, security personnel or police officers should be present when needed.

Prevalence

In the United States, trauma-related events are a widespread problem that affects people of all ages. More than 3 million suspected child maltreatment cases are reported to state and local agencies each year, with almost 700,000 cases of confirmed maltreatment (CDC, 2014b). In addition, almost 800,000 youth are hospitalized annually because of violence (CDC, 2016a). Data about maltreatment of older adults is harder to assess, largely because it is extremely underreported and often occurs at the hands of the person's intended caregiver. A study conducted in 2011 reported that 7.6–10% of older adults had experienced abuse in the year prior to the study (National Center on Elder Abuse, n.d.b).

Emergency departments handle 42 million trauma-related visits each year in the United States. Each year, roughly 2 million people are admitted to hospitals because of trauma. Violence accounts for about 10% of all traumatic brain injuries, including shaken baby syndrome, gunshot wounds, intimate partner violence (IPV; also called domestic violence), and child maltreatment (National Trauma Institute, 2012).

Genetic Considerations and Risk Factors

To better understand the causes and risk factors of the occurrence of trauma, specifically related to violence, researchers have conducted studies about the influence that genetic predisposition, age, and gender have on people who commit violent acts. Each of these lenses explores the scope of violent behavior.

Genetic Predispositions Toward Violence

Researchers continue to study whether a genetic predisposition toward violent behavior exists. They have found that although genetics may increase the risk that an individual will become violent, environment is often a cofactor in its manifestation. For example, prior abuse and exposure to violence increase an individual's risk of becoming violent (CDC, 2016b).

Genetic disorders that relate to social and mental health are often discussed in conjunction with studies that look at the genetic predisposition toward violence. Included in this discussion are bipolar disorder, paranoid schizophrenia, impulse control disorder, and depression. Mental illness alone is not a predictor of future violent behavior. However, studies have shown that individuals diagnosed with a mental illness that goes untreated can manifest violent behaviors (Treatment Advocacy Center, 2015).

Age

According to the CDC (2014a), many victims of sexual violence and IPV were first victimized at a young age, with 78.7% of rapes occurring before the age of 25 years. A number of behaviors displayed in youth are considered risk factors for becoming a violent perpetrator. These include a history of being a victim of violence, low IQ, substance use or abuse, history of early aggressive behaviors, deficits in social cognitive or information-processing abilities, and exposure to violence and conflict in the family (CDC, 2016b).

Gender

Gender has a strong influence on violence, according to statistics. Although individuals of any gender may become victims of violence, women are victims of IPV and sexual violence more frequently than men are. In recent studies, women accounted for four of every five victims of IPV. Although still prevalent in the United States, IPV has declined by over 60% for males and females in recent years. Severe physical violence at the hands of an intimate partner affected 24.3% of female intimate partner victims versus 13.8% of male victims (CDC, 2013a).

When it comes to IPV, several factors contribute to male aggression. Factors that relate to the family include having a criminal father figure, coming from a disrupted family, and having poor parental relationships. Individual risk predictors include impulsive behaviors and aggressiveness. Research has shown that these factors, when present in early childhood, can predict IPV in men. In addition, men who engaged in IPV often had struggles with employment, alcoholism, and drugs (CDC, 2015a).

SAFETY ALERT Nurses will encounter violent patients at times; therefore, it is important to monitor for and identify warning signs that a patient that may be escalating so that nurses and other staff can act to de-escalate the patient's behaviors. Some indications that a patient may become aggressive include pacing, loud voice, reddened face, clenched fists, and rigid posture.

Case Study ›› Part 1

A gunshot victim is en route to the emergency department (ED) by ambulance. You will be the patient's admitting nurse. At present, you have minimal information about the patient. The paramedics report that the bleeding is controlled and the patient is alert with temperature 97.0°F oral; pulse 92 bpm; respirations 22/min; and BP 105/75 mmHg. It is currently unclear how much blood loss the patient has sustained. The ambulance ETA (estimated time of arrival) is 5 minutes.

Clinical Reasoning Questions Level I

1. How would severe blood loss affect the patient's blood pressure?
2. What are the primary nursing considerations for this patient?

Clinical Reasoning Questions Level II

3. Consider your perceptions of this patient, knowing only that this individual is a gunshot victim. What is your initial response?
4. How would your perceptions change if the patient is a victim of IPV? A criminal assailant? Someone who was injured while protecting another individual from harm? Explain your perceptions for each category.
5. Describe the symptoms of severe blood loss and shock. Describe the nursing interventions for a patient who presents with severe blood loss.

Community and Systemic Violence

Although violence often occurs between two individuals, violence can also occur at a community level and within specific organizations such as the workplace or school. Community and systemic violence often involves multiple victims with varying degrees of trauma. This can put a strain on emergency department resources and healthcare workers because of the rapid influx of a large number of patients, some of whom will likely have life-threatening injuries.

Community Violence

The NCTSN (n.d.a) defines *community violence* as "predatory violence (such as robbery) and violence that comes from personal conflicts between people who are not family members. It may include brutal acts such as shootings, rapes, stabbings, and beatings. Children may experience trauma as victims, witnesses, or perpetrators."

Hate crimes and gang-related violence also fall into the category of community violence. Hate crimes are crimes against a person or property with the underlying motivation of bias against a race, religion, disability, sexual orientation, ethnicity, gender, or gender identity (FBI, n.d.b). Of the 5922 single-bias hate crimes reported in 2013, 48.5% were racially motivated, 20.8% were due to sexual orientation, 17.4% were religiously motivated, 11.1% were associated with ethnicity, 1.4% were disability related, and 0.3% were against a gender (FBI, 2014). Gang violence includes approximately 33,000 street gangs, motorcycle gangs, and prison gangs, encompassing approximately 1.4 million criminally active members. These gangs operate by using violence for control of their community to increase their illegal money-making activities (FBI, n.d.c).

Focus on Diversity and Culture
Extremists and Hate Groups

Some cultures are more prone to assault and homicide than others due to circumstances and adherent belief systems. Religious and/or political extremists such as the Islamic State of Iraq and Syria (ISIS) and hate groups such as the Ku Klux Klan and Aryan Brotherhood are similarly known for their propensity for violent acts toward others. These groups often assault or even murder other individuals based on their religion, race, or sexual orientation. Religious and political extremists who seek to injure or kill others as an act of homage to their belief system or as an act of revenge against a political decision pose a threat to all who encounter them. The level of violence within these particular groups has increased during the past decade (Meadows, 2013). Nurses need to be aware that they may need to provide care to a member of an extremist or hate group who may react violently toward healthcare members from diverse backgrounds (Meadows, 2013).

Workplace Violence

Workplace violence is a widespread issue that has more recently come to the attention of authorities, health professionals, media, and the public, mostly due to mass fatality occurrences; however, most incidents do not result in mass fatalities or even a single homicide. The Bureau of Justice's (2011) Statistics Special Report indicated that 1.7 million workplace violence episodes occurred each year from 1993 to 1999. Aggravated assaults accounted for the majority of these reported incidents.

The National Safety Council (2014) reported that 15.1 of every 10,000 full-time healthcare and social assistance workers required time off from work for workplace violence–related injuries in 2012. This report further stated that contributing factors for violent episodes included long wait times, patients with psychiatric problems, patients under the influence of drugs or alcohol, and patients with a history of violent behaviors. States are now passing legislation to protect their healthcare workers; for example, Idaho passed a bill making it a felony to assault a healthcare worker, with a penalty of up to 3 years in prison.

Horizontal violence is also an issue in the workplace. The Crisis Prevention Institute (CPI) (2016) defines *horizontal violence*, also known as lateral violence, as "hostile or aggressive behavior by an individual or group toward other group members. It is usually nonviolent, but can cause psychological or emotional damage to employees." Behaviors may include sabotage, criticism, and harassment. Horizontal violence often results in nurse bullying, which has become so prevalent that The Joint Commission developed standards that went into effect in 2009 to address this issue (CPI, 2016). Novice nurses and seasoned nurses can both fall prey to nurse bullying.

Young nurses with less than 3 years of professional experience are more likely to receive negative criticism of their

Evidence-Based Practice
Nurses Assaulted in the Workplace
Problem

Emergency department and psychiatric unit nurses experience high levels of assault at the hands of patients. This problem has not been decreasing in recent years, with some wondering if the problem is actually increasing. Physical assaults on nurses by patients are overwhelmingly underreported.

Evidence

The National Advisory Council on Nurse Education and Practice (2007) has reported that "health care workers are more likely to be attacked than prison guards and police officers." A risk for assault from a patient is present for all nurses, but emergency department and psychiatric unit nurses carry the highest levels of risk. One study concluded that 76% of nurses surveyed experienced a form of violence within the past 12 months (Speroni et al., 2014). The types of violence reported included physical violence, verbal abuse, and verbal threats by both patients and visitors.

Implications

High incidences of assault in the workplace lead to low job satisfaction, low retention rates, difficult recruitment, and detrimental effects on patient care. According to a study performed by Roldan and colleagues (2013), physical violence encountered in the work environment is linked to anxiety, feelings of low personal accomplishment, and burnout.

Critical Thinking Application

Identify ways in which instances of violence in emergency departments and psychiatric units could be decreased. Consider how patient care is affected by violent behavior. Describe some collaborative efforts that could be taken within the hospital setting to decrease cases of assault.

work, are more isolated from institutional activities, and face more challenges in proving themselves (Ovayolu, Ovayolu, & Karadag, 2014). Effective functioning of the team requires that all nurses, both novice and experienced, respect each other, treat each other fairly, remain empathetic, and maintain focus as to why they are working as a nurse—to assist in achieving positive patient outcomes.

School Violence

The BJS (2016a) annual report on "Indicators of School Crime and Safety" presents 23 indicators of crime and safety from a number of sources, including the perspectives of students, teachers, and administrators in the school systems. The topics addressed are specific to the school environment and include victimization, injuries sustained by teachers, bullying and cyber-bullying, fights, availability of weapons, use of substances by students, and students' perceptions of safety and crime. This report indicates that in 2014, children between the ages of 12 and 18 years were victims of 486,400 nonfatal violent crimes. According to the CDC (2014c), only 1–2% of all homicides of school-age children happen on the grounds of schools or on the way to or from a school-sponsored event; therefore, most students will never experience lethal violence at school. These findings minimize the importance of school-related violence prevention.

Bullying

Bullying occurs when the perpetrator perceives the victim as being weaker or more vulnerable than they are. Bullying can be overt, such as the perpetrator being physically aggressive toward the victim, taunting, calling the victim names, and teasing. However, more passive bullying methods are also prevalent, such as intentionally leaving the victim out of a group or activity, spreading malicious rumors, and encouraging other students to shun or alienate the victim.

According to the CDC (2014d), children who report both being bullied and participating in bullying are at high, long-term risk for suicide. Children involved in bullying in any way are at increased risk for an array of negative outcomes, including mental illness, poor school performance, and involvement in interpersonal or sexual violence. Children who are the frequent victims of bullies have an increased risk of suicidal behaviors as well as increased negative physical and emotional outcomes.

Although there is no way to validate that bullying directly causes suicide, there are enough data to support the potential correlation. As one example, Jessica Logan, an 18-year old senior in an Ohio high school, sent a nude picture to her boyfriend in a text message. After they broke up, the ex-boyfriend shared the picture with other people, which is when the bullying, taunting, and cyber-bullying began. After attending a funeral of a boy who committed suicide, Jessica went home and hanged herself. Greater attention to cases such as Jessica's are leading to the development of preventive measures. For instance, Ohio passed the "Jessica Logan Act" in November 2012, which mandates that the State Board of Education establish and implement guidelines for defining and establishing policies related to cyber-bullying. Before this, school administrators had no ability to hold students accountable for bullying behaviors that occurred using technology (e.g., internet, texting, and social media). Continued efforts need to be made to address bullying behaviors, minimize the opportunities for bullying to occur, and increase accountability for bullying behaviors.

Mass Shooter Incidents

The FBI (2013b) states that mass shooting incidents involve an "active shooter," and has defined active shooter as "an individual actively engaged in killing or attempting to kill people in a confined and populated area." The FBI further reports that approximately 160 active shooter incidents occurred between 2000 and 2013. During the first 7 years of this period, there was an average of 6.4 shootings per year. This percentage drastically increased to 16.4 active shooter incidents in the next 7 years. These same incidents either killed or injured 1043 victims, a total that does not include the shooters. Mass shootings are defined as killing three or more people, and 40% of the active shooter incidents were deemed mass shootings. Of the total shooters in these active shooter incidents, 40% committed suicide. Of the 160 active shooter incidents, an alarming 24% occurred in the educational environment (preschool through institutions of higher learning). The most deadly

mass shooting in the United States occurred June 12, 2016, in an Orlando, Florida, nightclub, where the active shooter killed 50 people, with an additional 53 people injured (Alvarez & Pérez-Peña, 2016). The second and third most deadly mass shootings were both in educational environments, with 32 killed at Virginia Tech in 2007 and 27 killed at Sandy Hook Elementary School in 2012.

Systemic Violence

Systemic violence occurs when there is a deliberate attempt to cause social injustice or inequality that could result in injury or death. Several examples of systemic violence include racism, sexism, slavery, and genocide. Systemic violence resulting in injury, death, or violation of human rights that is committed in the United States is federally prosecuted.

Unintentional Trauma

Unintentional trauma is caused by unintentional action and is not associated with medical conditions. Trauma-related and stressor-related disorders may also be associated with a major accident, a medical incident that is sudden and catastrophic (e.g., waking during surgery or anaphylactic reaction), or continuous stressors such as a persistent, painful illness (American Psychiatric Association [APA], 2013). Physical and emotional trauma may coincide with each other; therefore, it is important for nurses to understand the impact of physical trauma on patients, including how the physical trauma may precipitate emotional trauma.

Major Illness or Injury

Serious accidents, injuries, persistent painful medical conditions, and sudden, catastrophic medical conditions have a major physical and emotional impact on patients. Multisystem trauma occurs when injury involves multiple body systems, such as to the cardiac, respiratory, integumentary, or musculoskeletal systems (frequently associated with motor vehicle crashes), and may be attributed to trauma and stressor-related disorders (see Exemplar 32.B on Multisystem Trauma). Trauma-related and stressor-related disorders associated with an injury or medical event include posttraumatic stress disorder and acute stress disorder. Major illnesses, especially those associated with pain, may be a precursor to an adjustment disorder, which is also classified as a trauma and stressor-related disorder (APA, 2013).

Natural Disasters

Natural disasters, such as earthquakes, floods, tornadoes, and hurricanes, affect thousands of people every year. All natural disasters have the ability to cause severe emotional and physical trauma, major destruction, and death. Survivors of natural disasters will exhibit a mild to moderate stress response during and immediately after the emergency due to recognizing the grave danger associated with the disaster. Generally, survivors show resiliency after disasters, and the stress responses do not become chronic or debilitating; however, some people may be more affected by the disaster and will require medical intervention. The likelihood of developing PTSD is multifactorial, including the amount and extent of exposure and the nature of the individual (U.S. Department of Veterans Affairs [VA], 2016a).

Alterations and Therapies

Trauma

ALTERATION	DESCRIPTION	MANIFESTATIONS	INTERVENTIONS AND THERAPIES
Physical injury	■ Physical injuries include minor and major intentional and unintentional injuries and medical (sudden and catastrophic or terminal/life threatening) injuries.	■ Lacerations and contusions ■ Sprains, strains, dislocations, and fractures ■ Amputations ■ Puncture wounds ■ Internal injuries or bleeding (laceration of spleen) ■ Shock ■ Hypovolemia ■ Head trauma ■ Loss of senses ■ Respiratory impairment ■ Exposure (chemical, radiation)	■ Assess patient, identifying injuries sustained ■ Prioritize care of each injury ■ Assess and monitor pain level ■ Assess and monitor mental status
Emotional injury	Emotional stress that evolves after exposure to a traumatic or overwhelming event in which an individual's physical and mental health are endangered. Although most people show resiliency after a traumatic event, some may have symptoms that evolve into exaggerated stress responses.	Immediately following event: ■ Feeling numb or dazed ■ Confusion or disorientation ■ Disbelief and despair ■ Anxiety, nervousness, and fear of the event reoccurring ■ Unresolved emotional responses that evolve into acute stress disorder or PTSD ■ May include flashbacks, nightmares, and recurrent, intrusive memories of the adverse event(s); hypervigilance or the appearance of "being on edge"; avoidance of stimuli associated with the traumatic event ■ May include intense physiologic reactions when exposed to cues that are similar to or representative of some part of the traumatic experience ■ Manifestations may include some form of dissociation; for example, viewing oneself from the perspective of another individual or being unable to recall certain events related to the traumatic event (APA, 2013)	■ Support groups ■ Community support ■ Individual therapy ■ Cognitive–behavioral therapy (CBT) ■ Exposure-based CBT (application of principles of CBT combined with reexposure to the stressful event, including use of imagination, verbal discussion, or written exercises) (National Institute of Mental Health [NIMH], 2016) ■ Eye movement desensitization and reprocessing (EMDR) ■ Pharmacologic treatments, which may include antipsychotic agents, antidepressants (e.g., selective serotonin reuptake inhibitors [SSRIs]), and anxiolytics (e.g., benzodiazepines) (Mayo Clinic, 2014a) ■ Relaxation techniques, such as massage and guided imagery ■ Mental health counseling
Loss of community	■ Displaced from home due to any cause that was not by choice (e.g., natural disaster, war, forced immigration, and IPV) ■ Loss of ability to communicate secondary to destruction of means of communication or congestion of telephone service ■ Destruction of roadways ■ Destruction of stores or markets resulting in a loss of availability of required supplies, food, water, and medicines	■ Feelings of helplessness and complete loss of control ■ Anger ■ Confusion, disorientation ■ Anxiety, nervousness ■ Feeling vulnerable, lack of shelter or safety ■ Basic needs not being met (food, water, shelter, hygiene)	■ Ensure safety and shelter ■ Provide method of communication when available ■ Provide food, water, and medications as available ■ Offer support ■ Refer to community services (Red Cross or other organizations providing aid) ■ Assist with disaster registries to help reunite separated loved ones

(continued on next page)

Alterations and Therapies (continued)

ALTERATION	DESCRIPTION	MANIFESTATIONS	INTERVENTIONS AND THERAPIES
Complicated grief	■ Grief is a natural response to loss of a loved one. Generally, as time passes, the symptoms of grief diminish or resolve so that the survivor can accept and move forward ■ For some people, the feelings of grief are so severe and debilitating that they do not improve with time (Mayo Clinic, 2014b) ■ A risk factor associated with grief includes being the survivor of disaster. They may know that their loved one has died or their loved one may be missing and presumed dead ■ A sudden loss of life due to unexpected illness or accident may be traumatic ■ Suicide survivors also experience trauma-related grief.	■ Intense sorrow ■ Focus is on the death of the loved one ■ Numbness or detachment ■ Bitterness, agitation, and irritability ■ Lack of trust in others ■ Anhedonia and inability to think of positive experiences with the loved one	■ Psychotherapy (similar to what is used for PTSD) ■ CBT ■ Pharmacologic treatments, which may include antidepressants

Concepts Related to Trauma

Trauma is related to various nursing practices, among them the concepts of communication, sexuality, and stress and coping. Communication is vital in all areas of nursing, especially when violence is a contributing factor. Patients who have been exposed to a traumatic situation are likely to be experiencing pain (both physical and emotional) and significant amounts of stress. Nurses need to employ therapeutic communication to help patients work through the stress and fear and ultimately accept that the situation they experienced cannot be reversed. If the patient has experienced any form of sexual trauma, the patient could also be experiencing fear regarding sexually transmitted infections as well as the possibility of unwanted pregnancy.

In addition, the concepts of comfort, development, grief, and ethics are associated with trauma. Comfort measures will need to be employed to address the physical discomfort and emotional trauma. If tragedy strikes a child, development could be altered. Traumatic events may cause such strong responses that they may impair normal emotional development. Grief is a normal response to death; however, experiencing the death of a loved one caused by a traumatic event is a risk factor associated with complicated grief. Ethical principles will guide practice related to trauma victims. Treatment requires informed consent; however, trauma victims are often unable to give consent, so the healthcare provider will need to obtain alternate consent, such as from a parent, caregiver, spouse, or designated healthcare advocate. Some, but not all, of the concepts related to trauma are outlined in the Concepts Related to Trauma feature. They are presented in alphabetical order.

Health Promotion

Trauma often results from a combination of predisposing, precipitating, and protective factors in several areas. **Predisposing factors** are those that increase an individual's risk of being a victim of a traumatic experience or causing a traumatic experience for others (i.e., perpetrating violence). Predisposing factors may be categorized as vulnerability factors or risk factors. In the context of violence, **vulnerability factors** increase an individual's risk of being a victim; **risk factors** increase the potential that someone will become a perpetrator. **Precipitating factors** are factors that give rise to a specific incident. **Protective factors**, on the other hand, decrease the risk of perpetration and victimization. For example, connectedness to school has been found to be a protective factor for youth violence (CDC, 2016b). Areas to be addressed in examining factors contributing to societal violence include biophysical, psychologic, physical, environmental, sociocultural, behavioral, and healthcare system considerations.

Many factors influence an individual's response to traumatic events, in terms of both vulnerability factors and risk factors. Influencing factors do not cause destructive behavior, nor do they wholly determine that an individual will become a victim; rather, factors such as these can define trends and warning signs. For example, an individual may have a childhood history of being abused, reacting with anger, and experiencing academic failures from a young age. All of these elements are predisposing factors to violent behavior, but they are not determining factors (Office of Mental Health, 2012).

Concepts Related to
Trauma

CONCEPT	RELATIONSHIP TO TRAUMA	NURSING IMPLICATIONS
Comfort	Physical needs will need to be met so that psychologic needs may be addressed. Pain will need to be assessed and controlled. There may be a need for providing basic needs such as food, shelter, and the ability to meet basic hygiene needs.	▪ Assess and monitor pain; administer analgesics as prescribed. ▪ Employ comfort measures to decrease stress, such as warm blankets, relaxation techniques, and reassurance of safety. ▪ Provide supplies and opportunity to tend to basic hygiene.
Communication	Clear and therapeutic communication with patients after a violent or traumatic experience can help alleviate stress and facilitate acceptance.	▪ Use therapeutic communication to facilitate healing and acceptance. ▪ Encourage the patient to ask questions. ▪ Explain any procedures or tests suggested to the patient. ▪ Use appropriate nonverbal communication (body language) to encourage open communication.
Development	The neurobiological impact of a traumatic event is contingent on the developmental stage of a child having experienced a traumatic event, or a series of traumatic events.	▪ Use therapeutic communication to promote trust and feelings of safety; use age-appropriate terminology. ▪ Provide reassurance. ▪ Encourage child to ask questions. ▪ Explain any procedures or tests suggested to the patient. ▪ Maintain therapeutic environment with decreased stimulation to assist in feelings of safety.
Ethics	Traumatic situations require principles of ethical nursing care so that effective treatment may be obtained by the victims; this promotes the most positive outcomes possible.	Promote principles of ethical nursing care: ▪ Autonomy—allow patients to make decisions for themselves; informed consent. ▪ Beneficence—compassionate care such as administering analgesics to control physical pain. ▪ Nonmaleficence—Follow institutional guidelines and established best practice while administering care. ▪ Fidelity—Demonstrate truthfulness, loyalty, fairness, and advocacy for the patient. ▪ Justice—Equal and fair treatment; prioritizing victims' injuries accurately. ▪ Paternalism—Providing information based on patient's best interest. (American Nurses Association, n.d.)
Grief and Loss	Trauma-related incidents, especially related to disasters and sudden unexpected death of a loved one, are risk factors associated with complicated grief.	▪ Assess for safety. ▪ Use therapeutic communication. ▪ Promote trust. ▪ Validate patient feelings. ▪ Assess spiritual needs. ▪ Assist with disaster registries to find missing loved ones.
Sexuality	Sexual trauma is a form of violence that can cause both psychologic and physical trauma. Sexual trauma can also result in diseases, infections, and unwanted pregnancy.	▪ For victims of sexual assault, assessment may include use of a sexual assault evidence collection kit (also known as a rape kit), if permitted by the patient. ▪ Educate about options regarding the possibility of unwanted pregnancy (e.g., emergency contraception). ▪ Educate about tests for sexually transmitted infections and diseases. ▪ Facilitate referrals to resources such as support groups, therapy, and counseling.
Stress and Coping	All forms of trauma can cause stress, potentially leading to exacerbation of the injury and increased emotional strain.	▪ Communicate with the patient regarding needs and wants, especially those in relation to stress relief (e.g., the presence of a family member or friend). ▪ Answer questions regarding treatment and injuries calmly and honestly.

Predisposing Factors

Predisposing factors for trauma include environmental, psychologic, cultural, and behavioral variables. Geographical and environmental factors can deeply affect other aspects of an individual's life. Living in an impoverished community, especially one with a strong presence of gangs and drugs, puts an individual at increased risk for witnessing, experiencing, or even committing acts of violence (CDC, 2016b; Office of Mental Health, 2012). These environmental situations can also become cyclical, with multiple generations feeling trapped in the same community with the same high levels of violence. Over time, the stress and constant danger become traumatic, often feeding into more violence within the community, as well as within individual families.

Families themselves can be a predisposing factor to violence, especially if there is a history of abuse and neglect within the family or if family members are involved in drug or alcohol abuse. Other influencing variables are individual or behavioral in nature, such as a preoccupation with danger or violence, a history of abusing or torturing animals, or a history of bullying (either as the bully or as the bullied). Psychologic factors should also be considered, including aggressive tendencies, uncontrolled anger, extreme emotional distress, emotional instability, and depression (CDC, 2016b; Office of Mental Health, 2012).

When a disaster occurs, stress reactions are typically the same reactions seen with any trauma. Predisposing factors may have an impact on a victim, making their stress reaction more intense and long-lasting. The amount of exposure that a victim experiences has a direct impact on future mental health disorders. For example, directly experiencing the threat of severe injury or death increases the risk for needing professional mental healthcare (VA, 2016b). Females are more likely than males to have extreme reactions, and extreme reactions are more prevalent in people age 40–60 years, which is attributed to having more responsibility related to family and jobs. Examples of factors that predict the worst outcomes include severe injury or death of a loved one, separation from family (especially children), extreme loss of property, and forced displacement (VA, 2016b).

Protective Factors

In opposition to predisposing factors to violence and trauma, protective factors reduce the risk of becoming a perpetrator or experiencing debilitating responses to traumatic situations. Many of these protective factors apply to adolescents. According to the CDC (2016b), some variables that decrease the risk associated with violence include:

- Determination and success in school
- Healthy and positive social relationships
- Parents who show interest in their child's experiences
- Involvement in the community
- Participation in family activities
- Participation in cultural or religious practices
- Strong emotional support from friends and family.

There are protective factors associated with victims of disastrous events as well. Over time, most people will recover and move forward with their lives without having severe, chronic mental health issues. Factors that can increase resiliency include a strong, well-developed support system; effective coping skills and the positive belief that one can survive; and hope, including optimism, spiritual belief, and practical resources (VA, 2016b).

Promoting Safety

Anyone can become a perpetrator or victim of violence or abuse, and anyone can develop chronic mental health issues following traumatic situations. Knowing the warning signs of violent behavior can help promote safety. Warning signs of potentially violent behavior include uncontrolled anger, threatening language, and aggression. Similarly, recognizing the indicators of violence can help individuals avoid potentially dangerous situations by implementing protective measures. Protective measures include not walking or running alone in deserted areas, asking for help when being abused, and reporting violent behaviors or abusive situations.

Promoting a healthy community involves changing the roots of negative behavior in individual homes, in schools, and within the community. Community programs should focus on education regarding abuse, bullying, and neighborhood violence. Middle and high schools should include a curriculum about dating violence, bullying, and overall safety. Youth centers devoted to healthy recreational and educational activities can help prevent youth violence. According to the National Crime Prevention Council (2016), the incidence of personal violence has decreased over the past three decades; they attribute this decrease to vigilance and use of precautions.

Nurses can help promote safety by educating patients about high-risk situations, such as spouses who have been abusive in the past and the dangers of date rape and violence. Assessing the signs of abuse and offering interventions can also help establish safety. Nurses working in schools or other community settings can help dispel myths about aggression and abuse, assuring patients that it is never acceptable for someone to control or injure them. Assessing for inadequate coping mechanisms, signs of inadequate anger management, or inappropriate behavior can help identify risk factors and implement behavior therapy before someone is victimized.

Traumatic situations can occur at any time and to anyone; however, some traumatic situations can be prepared for because they are predictable. For example, earthquakes are more likely to occur on the West Coast, tropical storms and hurricanes are more likely on the coasts, and tornadoes are more common in the Midwest. People living in susceptible regions should be educated on how to prepare for potential disaster situations. Being prepared with supplies, communication plans, and family meeting places are protective measures to decrease long-lasting effects. Nurses must remain current with new, evidence-based practice initiatives to help promote safety for individuals, patients, facilities, and the community during and after traumatic events.

Modifiable Risk Factors

Abuse can be stopped, but many victims feel powerless against their abusers. By recognizing the signs of distress and injury that accompany abuse, nurses can assist victims in making their environment safer. Promoting safe behaviors and preparedness and identifying risk factors may decrease traumatic mental illnesses and trauma-related injuries and death.

Abuse Prevention

Nurses in all areas of practice need to take a proactive role in prevention, identification, and treatment of violence-related trauma. Early screening of vulnerable individuals and efforts to promote a change in attitudes and beliefs about family violence are essential. If they are to assist victims effectively, nurses must be aware of their own feelings about family violence. Nurses who are unclear about their own feelings about family violence may deny its existence, blame the victim in crisis, or minimize the effects of the violence. Nurses may be providing medical care to perpetrators and must perform self-reflection regarding their personal biases, allowing the nurse to maintain a nonjudgmental and unbiased attitude while providing medical care.

Nurses can be instrumental as advocates for developing policies and programs and providing in-service training and education to healthcare professionals and the public. Comprehensive violence prevention programs require a variety of disciplines and organizations working together, such as healthcare agencies, criminal justice agencies, and social service agencies.

Trauma Prevention

Areas of health promotion and trauma prevention interventions for individuals and communities include the following:

- **Motor vehicle safety:** Use seat belts and helmets as appropriate, have properly functioning air bags, avoid driving under the influence of alcohol or drugs, refrain from reckless driving, test for visual or cognitive deficits in older adults, avoid cell phone use while driving, avoid driving while fatigued, reduce distraction of young drivers by limiting the number of passengers
- **Relationships:** Teach communities how to recognize IPV, child abuse, elder abuse, abuse of developmentally delayed persons, or neglect
- **Communities:** Promote gun control, reduce participation in gangs, improve the condition of streets, promote neighborhood safety, review child abuse and fatalities for trends.

One example of a community trauma prevention strategy or intervention is the multidisciplinary child abuse or child fatality prevention team. Communities may develop teams such as these to review child abuse or child fatality cases to determine whether recommendations need to be made at the state level. Examples of recommendations include requirements for car seat or bicycle helmet use. Team members frequently include community health nurses, school nurses, preschool directors and school principals, members of law enforcement, and representatives of the district attorney's office.

Trauma-Informed Care

SAMHSA (2014) uses a trauma-informed approach that includes six key principles when addressing the needs of trauma victims. These principles are generalized for different settings, events, and areas:

1. Safety
2. Trustworthiness and Transparency
3. Peer Support
4. Collaboration and Mutuality
5. Empowerment, Voice and Choice
6. Cultural, Historical, and Gender Issues.

Trauma-specific interventions should meet the needs of the survivor, including treating the individual with respect and providing information, connectivity, and hope regarding recovery. Nurses should also understand the interrelation between trauma and substance abuse and mental health issues. Last, nurses need to work with the survivor, family and friends, and human service agencies to empower the survivor.

Nursing Assessment

Assessment of a trauma victim will depend on the nature and extent of the injuries. Because both acute trauma and chronic trauma can lead to long-standing mental health issues such as depression, anxiety, and posttraumatic stress disorder, the nurse not only must address the physical injuries identified, but also should perform a mental health assessment. During the assessment phase, it is imperative for nurses to consider the patient's cultural and spiritual practices, because these can have bearing on further treatment, interventions, and outcomes.

To begin the physical assessment, the priority when assessing any patient always begins with the **ABCs**:

Airway

Breathing

Circulation

For patients with severe physical injuries, the nurse may need to implement primary CAB (compressions, airway, breathing) protocols within the Basic Life Support guidelines and the ABC protocols within the Advanced Cardiac Life Support guidelines. Only when these priority needs have been met will the nurse go on to conduct a more complete assessment. Abuse and trauma assessments are the most common assessments for violence-related trauma. Nurses consider patients on a case-by-case basis; injuries from trauma manifest differently depending on the patient's overall disposition, experience, age, and history. Stereotypical mindsets regarding abuse victims have no place in nursing; all patients who present with signs of abuse should be assessed for abuse.

Abuse Assessment

Often the nurse is the first person to discover that the patient has been abused. Some victims may not disclose the abuse, may deny it despite obvious symptoms, or may minimize its impact. However, it is the nurse's responsibility to be alert for symptoms of abuse in all patients without allowing personal bias to influence assessments. During the assessment interview, the nurse must ensure privacy and safety from the perpetrator. The patient may be unwilling to admit to the reality of family violence until a trusting nurse–patient relationship evolves. The nurse should assure the patient of a genuine desire to help the entire family system. The nurse should approach this topic with a professional and calm demeanor, as if it were any other health risk. The nurse can also offer the option of answering questions about incidents of abuse with "sometimes" instead of "yes" or "no." This may encourage the patient to make a first step to acknowledge the abuse.

Victims of violence-related trauma or abuse require healthcare for a variety of conditions. Common physical complaints include chronic pelvic pain, headache, irritable bowel syndrome, arthritis, pelvic inflammatory disease, and neurologic damage. Psychiatric illness (e.g., alcoholism) may be the result of sexual or physical abuse. Depression is also common. The assessment interview should include a detailed nursing history and a description of current symptoms.

Victims of physical abuse may sustain a variety of injuries. During a head-to-toe assessment, the nurse may observe for indications of abuse, such as the following:

- **Head:** bald patches on the scalp where hair has been pulled out; evidence of trauma from blows to the head, such as hematoma, facial bruises, facial fractures, bruised or swollen eyes, hemorrhages into the eyes; petechiae around the eyes from attempted strangulation
- **Skin:** swelling or tenderness, bruises, burns, or scars of past injuries on the skin, genitals, and rectal areas (these injuries could also be in various stages of healing)
- **Musculoskeletal system:** fractures or evidence of previous fractures, particularly of the face, arms/legs, and ribs; dislocated joints, especially in the shoulder when the victim is grabbed or pulled by the arm
- **Abdomen:** bruises, wounds, or intra-abdominal injuries, especially if the person is pregnant
- **Neurologic system:** hyperactive reflexes due to neurologic damage; paresthesias, numbness, or pain from old injuries.

If the nursing assessment reveals possible IPV, a team assessment needs to take place. The victim's medical condition and emotional state must be assessed. The severity and potential fatality of the situation must be considered as well as the legal ramifications and the needs of dependent children. The nurse must follow state regulations and institutional policies related to mandatory reporting.

Trauma Assessment

Violence or disaster-related events result in traumatic injury that may involve multiple systems. Because of the serious consequences of trauma, it is important to identify the patient's injuries and institute appropriate interventions immediately. When caring for the trauma victim, the nurse must always prioritize assessments with the **ABCDEs** as the highest priority concerns (American College of Surgeons Committee on Trauma [ACSCOT], 2017):

Airway maintenance with cervical spine protection

Breathing and ventilation

Circulation with hemorrhage control

Disability and neurologic assessment

Exposure and environmental control

Only after assessing the ABCDEs can the nurse go on to perform a detailed assessment of other systems or a focused assessment of the involved area of trauma.

Trauma usually occurs suddenly, leaving the patient and family with little time to prepare for its consequences. Nurses provide a vital link in both the physical and psychosocial care of an injured patient and family. In caring for the patient who has experienced trauma, nurses must consider not only the initial physical injury but also its

long-term consequences, including rehabilitation and (in cases of accidents, abuse, or assault) prevention. Trauma may alter the patient's previous way of life, potentially affecting independence, mobility, cognitive thinking, and appearance. Therefore, the nurse should assess the patient in each of these areas.

Death is a common result of serious traumatic injury and may be immediate, early, or late. Immediate death happens at the scene from such injuries as a torn thoracic aorta or decapitation. Early death occurs within several hours of the injury from, for example, shock or delay in recognizing injuries. Late death generally occurs one or more days after the injury and may result from multiple organ failure, sepsis, head trauma, or blood loss.

Trauma may result in death or cause injury serious enough to alter both the patient's and the family's lives. The suddenness and seriousness of the event are precipitating factors in the development of a psychologic crisis. Nurses working with the patient who has experienced trauma should assess the family for a variety of needs, including immediate social and spiritual support. For patients who will require long-term rehabilitation, nurses may provide family members with referrals for counseling or financial support services. Assessment of patients' religious preferences regarding treatment and rehabilitation is critical (see the Focus on Diversity and Culture feature).

Nurses may call on the hospital chaplain, foreign language interpreter, dietitian, social worker, victim's advocate, or other professional to assist a patient who is the victim of violence or trauma and/or the patient's family. Law enforcement officers are also integral to cases of trauma, but they are not a required healthcare provider; therefore, their investigation should occur once the patient is stable (unless questioning is critical for safety purposes). Although these officials are trained for investigations, officers may, on occasion, become an obstacle to providing effective care to a victim. They may also overstimulate the victim, causing emotional decompensation. The nurse will need to advocate for the victim and intervene following hospital protocol.

Focus on Diversity and Culture
Religious Practice Considerations for Violence-Related Trauma

Cultural and spiritual considerations in treatments for violence-related trauma are numerous and will vary based on the incident (e.g., abuse vs. extensive trauma). For example, Christian Scientists believe that healing is a matter of faith and find that they can live happy and healthy lives without drugs and traditional medical interventions (Christian Science, 2016). Jehovah's Witnesses believe it is in defiance of their religious scripture to accept blood transfusions, even as a lifesaving procedure (Jehovah's Witnesses, 2016). If a patient participates in a religion that prohibits blood transfusions or any life saving procedure, nurses and physicians should explain the dangers and potential outcomes of not accepting the procedure, as well as educate the patient and family on alternative options, but ultimately the care team must honor the patient's decision (Chand, Subramanya, & Rao, 2014).

Numerous factors help healthcare providers determine the seriousness of a patient's injuries and the potential for survival when violence results in serious trauma. Scoring systems such as the Champion Revised Trauma Score system can be helpful. A rapid but comprehensive trauma assessment, completed on the scene, includes the following:

- *Airway and breathing assessments* to determine if the airway is patent, maintainable, or nonmaintainable and if ventilations are impeded in any way, such as by rib fractures or a pneumothorax
- *Circulation assessment* to palpate peripheral and central pulses; to assess capillary refill, skin color, and temperature; and to identify any external sources of bleeding
- *Level of consciousness* and *pupillary function assessments*
- *Assessment for any obvious injuries.*

The Glasgow Coma Scale is another scoring system that is used to quantify the level of consciousness following traumatic brain injury (TBI). For more information on the Glasgow Coma Scale, see the module on Intracranial Regulation.

Diagnostic Tests

The diagnostic tests ordered once the patient reaches the hospital depend on the type of injury the patient has sustained. Tests that may be ordered for victims of trauma include the following:

- *Blood type and crossmatch* involves typing the patient's blood for ABO antigens and Rh factor, screening the blood for antibodies, and crossmatching the patient's serum and donor red blood cells.
- *Blood alcohol level* measures the amount of alcohol in a patient's blood. Alcohol alters the patient's level of consciousness and response to pain.
- *Urine drug screen* may also be ordered. Like alcohol, drugs such as cocaine alter the patient's level of consciousness and overall response to the primary survey.
- *Pregnancy test* for any woman of childbearing age rules out the potential for pregnancy and fetal injury.
- *Focused assessment by sonography in trauma (FAST)* exam evaluates the presence of blood in body cavities. Primary focus is on the peritoneum. It is also helpful in identification of blood in the pleura and pericardium.
- *Diagnostic peritoneal lavage* determines the presence of blood in the peritoneal cavity, which may indicate abdominal injury. This test is generally done in the emergency department, but has been used less frequently since the inception of the FAST exam.
- *Computerized tomography (CT) scans* can reveal injuries to the brain, skull, spine, spinal cord, chest, and abdomen.
- *Magnetic resonance imaging (MRI) scans* can reveal injuries to the brain and spinal cord.
- *X-rays* can reveal bone fractures.

Case Study » Part 2

The ambulance arrives at the ED and paramedics emerge with the patient, Mark Alvarez, a 32-year-old police officer. Officer Alvarez was shot during a routine traffic stop, sustaining a bullet wound to his right shoulder. Upon arrival, the patient is awake and alert. His clear speech suggests a patent airway. His respirations are regular and nonlabored. His skin is pink, warm, and dry. You obtain another set of vital signs, which include temperature 97.2°F oral; pulse 90 bpm; respirations 20/min; and BP 100/72 mmHg. Following a thorough medical assessment by the ED physician, Officer Alvarez is declared stable. He will require surgical intervention to explore and treat his shoulder injury. The ED physician orders laboratory diagnostics, including complete blood count (CBC), serum electrolytes, and type and crossmatch for possible administration of blood products.

Following assessment and evaluation by the trauma surgeon, Officer Alvarez is scheduled for immediate surgical exploration of his right shoulder.

You remain with Officer Alvarez while he is waiting to be taken to surgery. The patient seems slightly anxious. When you ask if he has any questions about his surgery, Officer Alvarez responds by asking if his wife has arrived yet. You report that she has not. Officer Alvarez seems disappointed to hear this; he asks you to make sure she is told he is going to surgery and you assure him she will be informed as soon as she arrives. A nurse from the operating room arrives to transport Officer Alvarez to surgery.

Clinical Reasoning Questions Level I

1. Explain two possible reasons for Officer Alvarez's decrease in blood pressure.
2. Why do you think Officer Alvarez seems more concerned about his wife's absence than his impending surgery?
3. How would the case have changed if Officer Alvarez's airway had not been patent?

Clinical Reasoning Questions Level II

4. Would Officer Alvarez's injury have been worse had he been shot in the left shoulder? Explain your answer.
5. Describe three long-term interventions for Officer Alvarez's care after surgery.
6. Describe two possible complications that could arise during the patient's surgery.

Independent Interventions

Caring for patients who have experienced traumatic events may evoke strong emotional responses from the nurse. However challenging the situation, the nurse must maintain focus on the patient to provide effective, high-quality care. Interventions for all types of trauma-related care will be both independent and collaborative, but the nurse may have first contact with the patient, during which time several independent interventions can be employed.

Interventions for Victims of Abuse

In cases of abuse, the nurse may be the first professional to have contact with the patient, so it is essential for the nurse to (a) assess safety by determining the immediacy of danger, (b) convey that the patient is not to blame and has the right to be safe, (c) explore options for help, and (d) provide information regarding available services. The nurse must avoid a judgmental attitude and support the individual's choice about whether to leave the unsafe situation or return to the abusive relationship. Because severely battered women are at risk for homicide, the nurse needs to inform the patient about associated risk factors and determine the immediacy of danger.

Nurses must familiarize themselves with agency protocols and resources available for victims of IPV. Most municipalities have crisis help lines and hotlines to assist victims of abuse. The nurse should also keep a record of telephone numbers for transition houses and rape crisis centers, alcohol and drug abuse information, support groups, religious organizations, and legal services. In addition, several national organizations offer toll-free contacts, such as the National Organization for Victim Assistance, the National Coalition Against Domestic Violence (in the United States), and the National Clearinghouse on Family Violence (in Canada).

The priority nursing consideration regarding the child who is abused is to ensure safety. Once the child's safety is ensured, developing a trusting relationship will allow the child to discuss his or her feelings and describe the abusive event(s). The child should not be required to repeat the story for multiple reports, because each retelling carries the possibility of creating trauma for the child. All hospitals and agencies working with children who are abused have standard protocols that provide a supportive environment and ensure that adequate information needed by law enforcement is obtained without further victimization of children through a repetitive or unfriendly process.

The nurse working with a child who is a victim of abuse needs to convey belief in the child's story; the nurse also must assure the child that he or she has done nothing wrong. The nurse should avoid making negative comments about the abuser and must follow established protocols for mandatory reporting, documentation, and use of available support services (e.g., the police department, social service agencies, and child welfare agency).

Short-term interventions for older adults the nurse suspects of being abused include developing a positive relationship with both the victim and the abuser, exploring ways for the older adult to maximize independence, and exploring the need for additional home care services or alternative living arrangements.

Interventions for Victims of Trauma

Victims of trauma often present in the emergency department with life-threatening injuries, including hypovolemia due to blood loss, organ damage, and multisystem complications. The patient will often be in both physical and psychologic shock. Medical care for the patient in shock focuses on treating the underlying cause, increasing arterial oxygenation, and improving tissue perfusion. Depending on the cause and type of shock, interventions include emergency care measures, oxygen therapy, fluid replacement, and medication administration.

The nurse's role in trauma care begins with **triage**, the process of determining which patient most urgently needs medical intervention. Triage is based on the ABCDEs of trauma care. The nurse begins the triage process by performing a rapid general assessment, including vital signs, level of consciousness, and a head-to-toe review looking for obvious physical alterations (ACSCOT, 2017).

When caring for a patient who has experienced trauma, maintaining a patent airway and monitoring breathing and circulation are ongoing responsibilities. If the patient has experienced blood loss, is in shock, or is in unstable condition, the initiation of an IV line is often a high priority because it allows for administration of medications, fluid, and blood products. Changes in the patient's condition are often marked by subtle alterations, so the nurse's primary role is in performing ongoing assessments in order to correct problems before they become more acute.

Collaborative Therapies

Care of the trauma patient depends on a team approach. Providing trauma care with a team focus helps each team member know his or her role. Prompt delegation of tasks and responsibilities improves the patient's chances for survival and decreases the morbidity that may result from traumatic injuries. For more information on delegation, refer to the exemplar on Delegation in the module on Managing Care.

The initial focus of care for the patient with a traumatic injury is physiologic stabilization. During this time, physical injuries are identified and treated. From the psychosocial standpoint, the best treatment for families experiencing trauma or violence generally involves an interprofessional approach with nurses, physicians, social workers, spiritual leaders, law enforcement, protective services personnel, community resource organizations, and, often, lawyers. Most families are more open to accepting help during a time of crisis than at other times. Patients being treated for violence-related trauma will most likely be willing to develop new behavior patterns for a short time following a traumatic event. If families are not helped during that time, they will likely return to previous behavior patterns, including violence.

Nurses should know the laws associated with reporting abuse. In the United States and Canada, nurses are required to report any suspected child abuse. The courts and child protective agencies make decisions in the child's interest. They may allow a child to remain in the home but under court supervision; they may remove the child from the home; or, in instances of very severe abuse or repeated abuse despite intervention, they may terminate parental rights. Adult victims of IPV generally will make the decision whether they want to report the violent episode(s) to law enforcement. It is important that the nurse educate the victim on all options and resources available so that an informed decision can be made.

The nurse plays a critical role on a multidisciplinary team working with families involved in traumatic injuries. The nurse is often the healthcare worker who spends the most time with patients and forms a trusting nurse–patient relationship. As a result, the patient may feel most comfortable when talking with the nurse and be more likely to relate details of the traumatic event. The nurse's role may include teaching, support, or role modeling behavior. For example, if a child is transferred to foster care, the nurse may provide patient teaching to the foster family to provide for the child's healthcare needs.

Adults and older adults experiencing abuse or a traumatic event need similar collaborative interventions, including physicians, social workers, counselors, spiritual leaders, law enforcement, and lawyers. Nurses facilitate referrals and honestly answer any questions asked by the patient.

Medications

Trauma

CLASSIFICATION AND DRUG EXAMPLES	MECHANISMS OF ACTION	NURSING CONSIDERATIONS
Inotropic drugs **Drug examples:** Dopamine (Intropin) Dobutamine (Dobutrex) Isoproterenol (Isuprel)	Inotropic drugs (drugs that increase myocardial contractility) may be given to increase cardiac output and improve tissue perfusion.	■ Administer only after fluid volume restoration. ■ Monitor for signs of extravasation, and stop infusion immediately if it occurs. ■ Watch for any side effects such as pain, irregular heartbeat, or rise in diastolic pressure.
Vasopressors **Drug examples:** Dopamine Epinephrine Norepinephrine Phenylephrine	Vasopressors may be administered in conjunction with fluid replacement to treat neurogenic, septic, or anaphylactic shock.	■ Monitor cardiovascular response to medications, including heart rate and rhythm and blood pressure. ■ Use cautiously in children, volume-depleted patients (e.g., severely dehydrated or those who have sustained significant blood loss), and older adults. ■ Watch for signs of confusion and headache, which could be signs of water intoxication.
Opioid Analgesics **Drug example:** Morphine	Opioids are used to treat pain. However, the effects of the pain medications may alter patient responses to injury and mask potential injuries. For this reason, patient assessment generally is performed prior to administration of opioids or other medications that may produce sedative effects.	■ Monitor for respiratory depression and administer reversal agent (naloxone) if needed. ■ Use cautiously in patients with head trauma.

Source: Based on Adams, M. P., Holland, L. N., & Urban, C. (2017). *Pharmacology for nurses: A pathophysiologic approach* (5th ed.). Hoboken, NJ: Pearson Education.

Surgery

Surgical intervention may be required to treat injuries related to trauma. Some injuries require emergency surgery to stop bleeding or repair organ damage. Nurses will work to keep patients stable while preparing them for surgery, diagnostic testing, or other treatments to repair their injuries. Whereas some injuries sustained from trauma will require basic surgical interventions, other injuries will require more complex surgery.

Pharmacologic Therapy

Pharmacologic treatment for trauma patients may include administering analgesics for pain; however, because analgesics may cause sedation, physical and neurologic assessments are usually conducted prior to administering these medications. Depending on the severity of the patient's injury, inotropic agents and vasopressors also may be indicated (see the Medications feature).

Nonpharmacologic Therapy

A common issue with physical trauma is pain control. A patient who does not have effective pain management may require longer hospitalization, experience additional complications, and have poor outcomes. Along with pharmacologic pain management, the nurse will also need to employ nonpharmacologic pain management techniques.

For more information on nonpharmacologic pain control, see the module on Comfort.

Complementary Health Approaches

Complementary health approaches may be added to the traditional treatment to assist in symptom management. Patients with a long treatment trajectory (for example, extensive physical therapy and rehabilitation) may benefit from complementary strategies such as stress reduction techniques or acupuncture to help alleviate pain. Patients who face long-term disability will benefit from referrals to organizations that provide education and support in obtaining assistive devices, including service animals. The nurse will need to educate the patient to inform all healthcare providers if using complementary health approaches, especially herbal remedies or supplements, because of the possibility that such approaches may be contraindicated with prescription medications.

Case Study ›› Part 3

One month following his right shoulder injury and surgery, Officer Alvarez presents to the clinic for his post-op visit. His surgery was successful; the bullet was excised, and damage to the surrounding tissues was minimal. Officer Alvarez has been attending physical therapy sessions, which he describes as "sort of helpful, but my shoulder swells a little bit after my therapy appointments." He reports that he is gaining range of motion in his right shoulder. On a scale of 0 to 10 (with 10 being extreme pain), Officer Alvarez rates his pain as 2.

When asked about his anticipated return to work, Officer Alvarez becomes very quiet. After a pause, he tells you he is expected to return to work in 3 days. He explains that he will be on light duty, which entails working in an administrative role inside the police department until he has fully recovered. You notice that Officer Alvarez seems uncomfortable discussing his return to work, so you tactfully explore the topic. You begin by asking how he feels about returning to work. Officer Alvarez reports that he feels fine physically; however, he has been having nightmares about the shooting. When you ask if he has discussed his nightmares or the actual shooting with anyone, he replies, "It's not something I really want to talk about. I have an appointment with the department shrink tomorrow, though. They're making me see her before I can go back to work." When you ask if he would like to speak with a counselor outside his department, Officer Alvarez replies, "I really don't

want to talk about anything with anybody. I just want my shoulder to heal up."

Clinical Reasoning Questions Level I

1. What nursing interventions could you suggest to Officer Alvarez to promote comfort in his shoulder following therapy sessions?

2. What concerns might Officer Alvarez have with regard to his return to work, both in the psychosocial and physical realms?

Clinical Reasoning Questions Level II

3. Is Officer Alvarez at risk for developing posttraumatic stress disorder? Explain your answer.

4. In light of Officer Alvarez's statements, should the nurse proceed with exploring psychosocial considerations related to his injury? Why or why not?

REVIEW The Concept of Trauma

RELATE Link the Concepts

Linking the concept of trauma with the concept of cognition:

1. Describe how untreated schizophrenia could lead to instances of violence and/or violent behavior.

2. How would you assess and diagnose abuse in a patient with advanced Alzheimer disease? What signs and symptoms would you look for in particular?

Linking the concept of trauma with the concept of mood and affect:

3. What assessment questions would you want to ask the patient who was admitted after sustaining injuries from domestic violence whose mood appears sad with a tearful affect?

4. Could a woman experiencing postpartum depression be at increased risk for abusing her children or spouse? Explain your answer.

Linking the concept of trauma with the concept of clinical decision making:

5. You are working in the emergency department when several ambulances arrive simultaneously because of a nearby apartment fire. When triaging the patients, you find that there are patients with fractures, second- and third-degree burns, and respiratory distress. Another patient is unconscious. Which of the patients require priority care? Explain your answer.

6. A patient has been admitted to the emergency department following a motor vehicle crash. The patient has an open fracture of the femur, deep facial lacerations, and broken ribs coupled with a pneumothorax. What priority nursing interventions would you implement first? Explain your answer.

READY Go to Volume 3: Clinical Nursing Skills

- SKILL 1.1   Appearance and Mental Status: Assessing
- SKILL 1.5–1.9   Vital Signs
- SKILL 1.19   Musculoskeletal System: Assessing
- SKILL 1.22   Neurologic Status: Assessing
- SKILL 1.25   Skin: Assessing
- SKILL 1.27   Thorax and Lungs: Assessing
- SKILL 3.1   Pain in Newborn, Infant, Child, or Adult: Assessing

- SKILL 7.1   Glasgow Coma Scale: Using
- SKILL 9.16   Cast, Initial: Caring for
- SKILL 15.1   Abuse: Newborn, Infant, Child, Older Adult, Assessing for
- SKILL 15.4   Suicidal Patient: Caring for
- SKILL 15.5   Environmental Safety: Healthcare Facility, Community, Home

REFER Go to Pearson MyLab Nursing and eText

- Additional review materials

REFLECT Apply Your Knowledge

A family of four was vacationing on the West Coast when a major earthquake occurred. The destruction where their hotel was located was severe, and many buildings were damaged, including their hotel. The parents and 13-year-old daughter were unharmed; however, the 9-year-old son, James, sustained severe physical trauma with obvious open fractures and profuse bleeding from the head. James was unconscious when the rescue team found him. The disaster response team triaged James and immediately transported him, via ambulance, to Los Angeles, the nearest city that remained operational, for medical care. Upon arrival, James' respirations were 26 per minute, blood pressure was 68/40 mmHg, and pulse was 140 bpm. James has regained consciousness and is being sent for x-rays and a CT scan of the brain. Test results show fractures of the left femur and tibia, the left humerus, radius and ulna, and a skull fracture. The CT scan reports a contusion of the brain with no other anomalies. James will need to have surgery to correct placement of the open, complete fractures. After surgery, he will need to remain in the hospital for additional tests, stabilization, and monitoring. The parents and sister have arrived and are displaced. The entire family is traumatized (crying, confused, and in a state of disbelief) and the nurse noted that the mother was clenching her prayer beads.

1. What three priority nursing diagnoses would you select for James?

2. Whom should the nurse contact regarding arrangements that can be made for the family so that they can remain close to James during his stay in the hospital? What might these arrangements include?

3. What other healthcare professionals and ancillary staff members should the nurse involve in the care of James and his family?

>> Exemplar 32.A
Abuse

Exemplar Learning Outcomes

32.A Analyze abuse as it relates to trauma.

- Describe the pathophysiology of abuse.
- Describe the etiology of abuse.
- Compare the risk factors and prevention of abuse.
- Outline the types of abuse perpetrated throughout the lifespan.
- Identify the clinical manifestations of abuse.
- Summarize diagnostic tests and therapies used by interprofessional teams in the collaborative care of an individual who has been abused.
- Apply the nursing process in providing culturally competent care to an individual who has been abused.

Exemplar Key Terms

Bullying, *2126*
Child abuse, *2126*
Cyber-bullying, *2127*
Elder abuse, *2128*
Intimate partner violence (IPV), *2127*
Neglect, *2124*
Physical abuse, *2124*
Psychologic abuse, *2124*
Sexual abuse, *2124*
Youth violence, *2127*

Overview

Abuse can happen to individuals of any age and from any demographic or sociocultural background. Abuse does not only happen to those with supposedly *weak* personalities; individuals with strong or dominant personalities can fall victim to abuse as well. Predisposing risk factors to become an abuser exist for all forms of abuse; however, even if all identified factors are present, the person may not become an abuser. Abuse is a growing concern in the United States, with many cases going unreported because of fear of or threats from the abuser.

Pathophysiology and Etiology

Abuse is often related to control (see **Figure 32–1** >>). When one individual attempts to control another individual, a form of abuse must occur. The four types of abuse that most

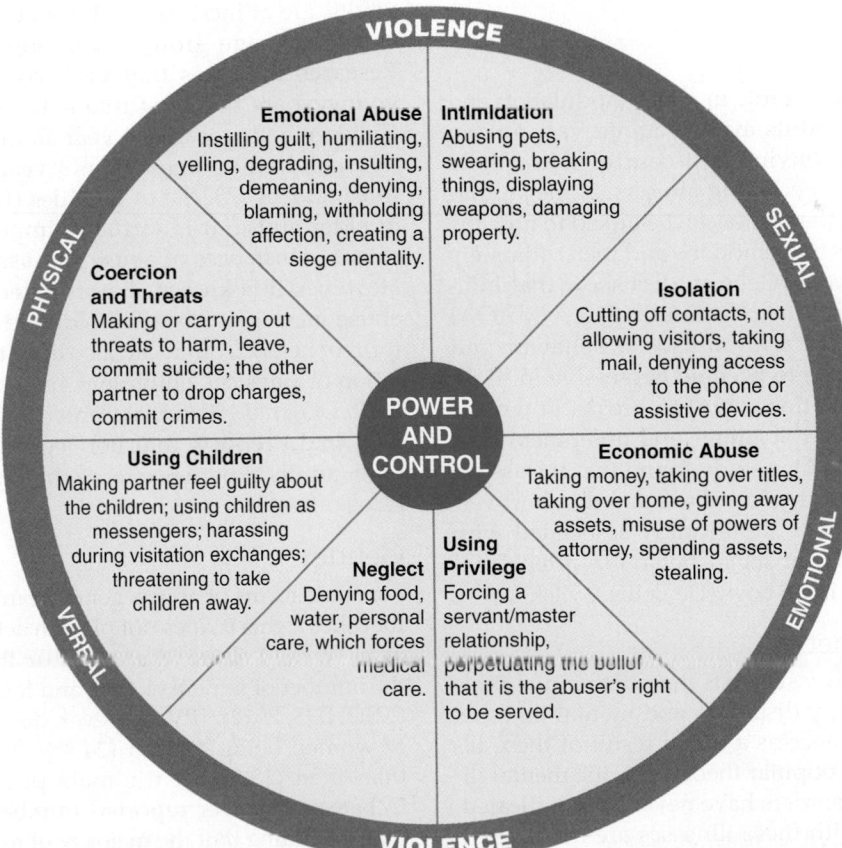

Source: Potter, M. L., & Moller, M. D. (2016). *Psychiatric-mental health nursing: From suffering to hope.* Hoboken, NJ: Pearson Education. Reprinted and Electronically reproduced by permission of Pearson Education, Inc., New York, NY.

Figure 32–1 >> The power and control wheel illustrates the strategies one partner may use to intimidate, control, and harm another.

states identify are **physical abuse**, **psychologic abuse**, **sexual abuse**, and **neglect** (see Table 32–1 for definitions). All of these can work to break down an individual's self-confidence and self-worth. Some common elements of abuse are humiliation, intimidation, and physical injury (Benedictis, Jaffe, & Segal, 2012). Each type of abuse has unique characteristics and requires individual approaches to diagnosis and management (Medscape, 2015). Abuse sometimes start as emotional abuse—such as telling the victim he is not smart enough, or that no one will ever love him—but over time, emotional abuse can escalate to physical abuse or even sexual abuse. Physical abuse is generally accompanied by psychologic abuse. In cases of sexual abuse, especially childhood sexual abuse, victims will often be exposed to forms of psychologic abuse whereby the perpetrator will use the child's need for love and approval against him in order to force the child to submit (American Psychological Association, 2013). Ultimately, cases of abuse involve both the use of control and manipulation.

Etiology

Many theories exist concerning the motivation for violent behavior and abuse within families. Some of those theories propose that individuals are genetically predisposed to violence, whereas other theories discuss the influences of society and family structure. No definite causes of family violence have ever been agreed on, but neurobiology, psychopathology theory, and social learning theory lead into one another to help highlight some contributing factors to abusive behavior.

Neurobiology

Genetics is believed to play a role in anger modulation and emotion control. Anger and its manifestations vary among individuals, with some having self-control and others expressing their anger by becoming abusers. Some studies have therefore suggested that genes can be linked to how the brain processes situations and emotions and then ultimately produces a reaction of anger. Gene studies show that individuals with low levels of the monoamine oxidize A (MAOA) genotype (often associated with antisocial behavior and aggression) are more prone to become aggressive in high-anxiety or emotional situations. MAOA breaks down the biogenic amines serotonin, dopamine, and norepinephrine, which influences behavior. One study found that the association between neglect and physical abuse and the short version of the MAOA gene was significantly associated with mental health problems, antisocial behavior, attentional problems, and hyperactivity in boys (De Bellis & Zisk, 2014).

Psychopathology Theory

The psychopathology theory suggests that some individuals who experience personality disorders and mental illnesses participate in family violence as a direct result of these illnesses. Although this is a popular theory, specific mental illnesses and personality disorders have never been indicated, and many individuals with these illnesses are not violent. Some personality disorders and emotional illnesses when left untreated can result in violent tendencies (e.g., bipolar disorder, schizophrenia, paranoid personality disorder) (Treatment Advocacy Center, 2015); however, as with risk factors, having an untreated mental illness does not always result in abuse or violence.

Social Learning Theory

Social learning theory explains that individuals learn violent tendencies through association with others and a reinforcement of the abusive behavior. Children are especially susceptible to this form of learning, because they model the behaviors of those around them. Children often model the behaviors of parents, siblings, other adults, or actions they see on television. Therefore, children have a high likelihood of adopting abusive tendencies perpetrated by their parents or siblings, thus furthering a cycle of abuse within the family. Relationship factors, including a family environment characterized by physical violence and a childhood history of abuse or neglect, are risk factors for perpetration (CDC, 2016c).

Risk Factors

Risk factors associated with perpetration of abuse include individual (e.g., parents' history of child maltreatment), family (e.g., family disorganization, dissolution, and violence), and community. Risk factors associated with victimization include very young children, older adults, and individuals with special needs (CDC, 2016c).

Age

Some age groups, particularly younger children and older adults, are at increased risk for abuse because abusers consider these age groups to be more helpless than others. Research indicates that very young children (age 4 and younger) are the most frequent victims of child fatalities. Children younger than 1 year accounted for 46.5% of fatalities; children younger than 3 years accounted for almost three fourths (73.9%) of fatalities (USDHHS, 2013). In cases of elder abuse, it is virtually impossible to know the full extent of instances of abuse because many are not reported. However, it is known that as older adults age, the risk for abuse increases. Abuse in older adults is commonly in the form of neglect, but it can also be in terms of financial exploitation or physical, emotional, or sexual abuse (Anetzberger, 2012; DOJ, n.d.; National Center on Elder Abuse, n.d.b). The DOJ (n.d.) reports that between 30% and 40% of abused older adults experience more than one form of abuse by the same offender.

Gender

For some forms of abuse, gender can be a risk factor, whereas for other forms it does not play an active role. For example, in cases of child abuse, there is virtually no difference between the number of female victims and the number of male victims (USDHHS, 2012). IPV, however, does show a higher instance of women being abused (24.3% of the female population) than men (13.8% of the male population) (CDC, 2013a). Debates exist over reported numbers of IPV victims, with many claiming that the majority of male victims do not report being abused by their spouse. Trends in elder abuse, though, show a clear delineation of women being abused more often than men (National Center on Elder Abuse, n.d.b).

Testosterone has been correlated with higher aggression levels in humans, which helps explain why many offenders are young men with muscular physiques. These individuals typically have high levels of testosterone and low levels of serotonin, the neurotransmitter commonly associated with satisfaction.

Physiologic Development

Physiologic illnesses and disabilities may present one of the highest risk factors for all forms of abuse. Individuals with disabilities are more likely to be seen as easy targets for abuse, with perpetrators assuming that the victim will not, or cannot, report the crime. Some common reported disabilities associated with cases of abuse include intellectual disabilities, physical and learning disabilities, visual or hearing impairments, dementia, and Alzheimer disease (National Center on Elder Abuse, n.d.b; USDHHS, 2012). Approximately 11% of all child abuse victims had a physical or emotional disability of some kind. A study of women with disabilities found that 67% had been subjected to physical abuse and 53% had been sexually abused at some point in their lives. A similar study was conducted in men with disabilities and found that 55% had been physically abused at some time in their lives. It has also been discovered that IPV among individuals with disabilities is increasingly prevalent and even disproportionate (National Center on Elder Abuse, n.d.b).

Cultural Factors

An individual's culture can also be a risk factor for abuse, with some cultures condoning acts that Western culture considers to be abusive. For example, some Asian cultures use shame as a method of teaching children respect or for controlling individuals within the family unit. Shame in these instances could be considered a form of psychologic abuse, as the individual being shamed may be continually verbally confronted with his supposed shortcomings and mistakes. Parents from Asian cultures frequently practice the honor and shame practice even when they migrate to the United States, and this practice is passed down from generation to generation. This practice leaves some children needing mental health treatment for low self-esteem, depression, and anxiety; however, because of a perception that mental illness may tarnish the family reputation, many children go untreated (Louie, 2014). Physical abuse can also be a matter of cultural significance, with some cultures employing and condoning punishments of a physical nature toward their children or spouses.

Within cultures that are strictly patriarchal (or matriarchal), IPV may be more prevalent. In these situations, one member of the relationship has more power than the other, creating tension that could lead to physical or psychologic violence. In other cultures, the husband or male partner is strictly in control of the relationship and all members of the family, thus giving him the right to use punishments that he considers necessary. Stress is not a reason for violence. Abuse and violence are an explanation of the "privileges of men's experiences over women's" (Asian Pacific Institute on Gender-Based Violence [APIBGBV], n.d.).

In rare but increasingly prevalent instances, some cultures may practice ritualistic forms of abuse. Many of these cultures acknowledge a belief and worship of Satan or another devil-like deity. Within the practices of these cultures, children (or new inductees) are continuously terrorized and tortured as a mode of control. Physical, emotional, sexual, and spiritual abuse are all parts of ritualistic abuse. Examples of ritualistic physical abuse include beatings, torture, confinement, and forced ingestion. Methods of emotional abuse include manipulating, lying to, and blaming the victim. Sexual abuse may include forcing sex on children or nonconsenting adults, as well as forcing others to commit sex acts against children or nonconsenting adults. Spiritual abuse may present as reversal of good and evil and infringement on freedom of thought (Ritual Abuse, Ritual Crime and Healing, 2016). If a nurse suspects a patient is being abused, regardless of the source of the abuse, the nurse must follow state and agency reporting policies.

Socioeconomic Factors

Some researchers consider poverty to be the largest risk factor and predictor of child abuse and neglect. The stress and feelings of inevitability that come with poverty can lead to frustration, anger, and potentially physical and emotional abuse. Living in poverty or an economically depressed area contributes significantly to the probability of an individual engaging in or becoming the victim of an assault. However, individuals from high socioeconomic backgrounds can also become the victims and perpetrators of abuse.

Substance Abuse

Substance or alcohol abuse is not necessarily a predictor of abusive behavior, but the excessive use of any mind-altering substance can make abusive situations much worse. Alcohol can contribute to the aggressive behavior that leads to violent behaviors by reducing inhibitions and modifying the functioning of neurotransmitters, including a decrease in serotonin function (Ciccarelli & White, 2013). For example, if an individual is already being extremely emotionally abusive, the use of illegal substances or alcohol could push the perpetrator to physical or sexual abuse, or the emotional abuse could become intensified. Alcohol and other substances do not create an abusive situation; other factors also need to be considered, such as the personality of the individual using the substances. However, substance and/or alcohol abuse is one of the leading risk factors for perpetrators of all forms of abuse.

SAFETY ALERT A patient who is under the influence of an illegal substance and/or alcohol is highly unpredictable, which increases the risk for violent behavior. The nurse will need to monitor the patient at all times and assess for signs of escalating behavior. If there is potential for violence, it is important that the healthcare team and security be made aware for safety purposes.

Firearms in the Home

It is controversial and virtually impossible to assign statistics for an increased risk for mortality in cases of abuse when a gun is present in the house, because these statistics depend on too many reported variables such as the type of firearm, the storage of the firearm, and the location of the incident. However, according to the FBI (n.d.d), the following 2014 statistics were reported regarding intimate partner homicide, firearm violence, and related factors:

- 35.5% of female victims (for whom the murderer was known) were killed by a husband or boyfriend.
- 40.4% of all murder victims (for whom the circumstance was known) were killed during arguments—including romantic arguments.
- 68.5% of weapons used during all murders were handguns.

Prevention

The prevention of abuse must come from various levels, including individual, community, society, relationship, and parenting. In addition, the many factors that contribute to abusive relationships need to be addressed in order to stop abuse. Often, abuse is part of a familial or personal cycle that has been going on for years, and until the abuser acknowledges or realizes the cycle, it is likely to continue. Nurses can help prevent abuse by observing for the signs and symptoms of abuse and then working to address the situation. When children are involved, nurses must report the abuse per facility protocol and state regulations; but in cases of IPV, it is ultimately the individual's choice to seek help in stopping the situation. In cases in which the patient does desire help to stop a violent and abusive situation, nurses can work to facilitate referrals to shelters, other healthcare providers, law enforcement, and lawyers. For patients who want to leave an abusive home or relationship, nurses can provide patient teaching regarding the development of a safety plan (see the Patient Teaching feature).

SAFETY ALERT Sudden unemployment or other forms of financial stress can greatly increase an individual's stress and thus create a large risk factor for participating in abusive behavior toward another individual.

Patient Teaching
Developing a Safety Plan

Developing a safety plan will help an individual who lives in an abusive environment to plan an escape. Elements of a safety plan may include:

1. Practice how to get out safely. Know the easiest escape route from the current location (exiting through doors, windows, fire escapes).
2. Keep purse or wallet and keys easily accessible at all times.
3. Have a contact person(s) and number(s) available who can be notified to call police.
4. Teach children to call police or 911.
5. Have a code word to indicate a violent situation so that friends, family, or children know to call police.
6. Move to a low-risk area in the event of an argument (rooms with access to outside door and not in bathroom, kitchen, or room with weapons).
7. Use judgment. If the situation is serious, give the partner what is being demanded to calm them down.

Source: Based on Domestic Violence Resource Center. (2014). *Safety planning.* Retrieved from http://www.dvrc-or.org/safety-planning/; National Center on Domestic and Sexual Violence. (n.d.). *Domestic violence personalized safety plan.* Retrieved from http://mnadv.org/_mnadvWeb/wp-content/uploads/2011/07/DV_Safety_Plan.pdf; Rape, Abuse, and Incest National Network. (2016). *Safety planning.* Retrieved from https://rainn.org/articles/safety-planning.

Abuse Throughout the Lifespan

Categorizing abuse is often done in terms of the age of the victim or the form of abuse being perpetrated. Infant abuse, child abuse, bullying, youth violence, IPV, sexual abuse, and elder abuse are the main categories discussed in this section. Each type of mistreatment presents differently within the life of the victim and has a common perpetrator; for example, child abuse is commonly committed by parents or caregivers. The physical and emotional manifestations of these types of abuse are presented in detail later in the exemplar.

Infant Abuse

Infants are prone to abuse because they are completely dependent and vulnerable. Their needs sometimes outweigh the patience of a parent, especially if the pregnancy was unwanted or if the parent is young, has poor coping skills, or has a poor support system. Infants under 12 months of age had the highest prevalence of victimization in 2013 (USDHHS, 2013). Abusive head trauma (AHT), which includes shaken baby syndrome, is the leading cause of child abuse deaths in children under 5 years of age. Babies less than a year old are at greatest risk for AHT, which is likely because the most common trigger is inconsolable crying (CDC, 2016d). AHT often happens when the caregiver or parent becomes angry or frustrated, and then shakes the child or hits or slams child's head into something in order to stop the crying. Nearly all victims of AHT experience long-term physical consequences, and approximately 25% of all victims die from their injuries (CDC, 2016d).

Child Abuse

According to the Child Abuse Prevention and Treatment Act (CAPTA), **child abuse** and neglect are defined as "any recent act or failure to act on the part of a parent or caretaker which results in death, serious physical or emotional harm, sexual abuse or exploitation" of a child or "an act or failure to act which presents an imminent risk of serious harm" to a child (USDHHS, 2010). In 2013, approximately 3.5 million children (age newborn to 17) were reported to be victims of child abuse in the United States, with one fifth of reports being substantiated. Of the reports made, 61.6% were made by professionals (USDHHS, 2013). However, many cases of child abuse still go unnoticed and unreported.

Children of all races and ethnicities may be victims of child abuse. Child abuse is often defined as having three forms: neglect, physical abuse, or sexual abuse. In 2013, neglect accounted for the highest percentage of child mistreatment cases in the United States at 79.5%. Approximately 83% of the perpetrators were between the ages of 18 and 44 years, and 53.9% of perpetrators were women (USDHHS, 2013).

Bullying

School-age children frequently find themselves the victims of bullying. The CDC (2016e) defines **bullying** as "any unwanted aggressive behavior(s) by another youth or group of youths, who are not siblings or current dating partners, involving an observed or perceived power imbalance that is repeated multiple times or is highly likely to be repeated." Bullying may result in physical injuries and emotional distress, and it may disturb academic progress. Bullying can occur in the presence of the victim as well as through the use of technology such as text messages, email, cell phone applications, chat rooms, and social media, which are all forms of **cyber-bullying**. Although electronic media are helpful in allowing youth to communicate with family and friends easily and regularly, youth can also use this technology to threaten, embarrass, and harass their peers. Technology has also made it possible for the bully to be anonymous, making it difficult for parents or authorities to confront this behavior. Bullying has been addressed by most states' boards of education by making bullying a punishable offense by school authorities; however, cyber-bullying has been challenging for school officials to address because the act often does not occur on school grounds. Regulations are beginning to catch up with technology with some states, such as Ohio's "Jessica Logan Act" (see Community and Systemic Violence—Bullying earlier in this module) putting mandates in place that require the state board of education to establish and implement policies related to cyber-bullying. Recent research suggests that youth who are victims of electronic aggression are more likely to experience victimization in person, including sexual harassment, psychologic or emotional abuse by a caregiver, witnessing an assault with a weapon, and rape (CDC, 2016f).

Although there is not a direct link between being a bully or being bullied and suicidal behavior, there is a correlation between the two. One study indicates that 22% of bullies, 29% of victims of bullying, and 38% of bully victims reported suicidal thinking or a suicide attempt (Borowsky, Taliaferro, & McMorris, 2013).

SAFETY ALERT Screenings of all youth at school and healthcare settings should include questions related to bullying, as the bully, the bullied, or both, for identification of these risk factors so that intervention can occur.

Youth Violence

Youth violence occurs in minors and may continue into young adulthood. Youth violence may include being a victim of violence, a violent offender, or a witness to violence. According to the CDC (2015b), in 2012, more than 599,000 youth, age 10–24 years, received medical treatment for injuries related to assault. Violence has a negative effect on communities, increases healthcare costs, decreases property values, and disrupts social services (CDC, 2015b). Violence perpetrated by youths is one of the most visible forms of violence in society. In the United States and around the world, violence by youths flourishes in gangs, schools, and public areas.

As with assault and homicide committed by individuals in any age demographic, the problem of youth violence cannot be viewed as isolated from other problem behaviors. Violent adolescents and young adults exhibit a range of problems, from truancy and dropping out of school to substance abuse, compulsive lying, reckless driving, and contraction of sexually transmitted diseases. The recklessness and instability of adolescence is partially responsible for high levels of youth violence, but there are close links between youth violence and experience in childhood. Witnessing violence in the family, being abused, and prolonged exposure to a community culture

of violence can all condition children and adolescents to view violence as an acceptable means of solving problems (WHO, 2013b). Adolescents and young adults are most likely to commit and be victimized by assault and homicide, but other groups are at risk as well.

Intimate Partner Violence

Intimate partner violence (IPV) is the act of inflicting sexual, emotional, or physical harm on a current or previous partner or spouse. IPV can occur in any couple, including same-sex couples, adolescent couples, and older adult couples. The four main forms include physical violence such as punching, kicking, or biting; sexual violence that includes forced sexual acts or physically violent sexual contact; threats of both physical and/or sexual violence; and emotional abuse such as humiliating the victim or controlling the victim by diminishing self-esteem. Stalking can also be a form of IPV and is defined by the CDC (2016g) as "a pattern of repeated, unwanted attention and contact that causes fear or concern for one's own safety or the safety of someone else (e.g., family member or friend)." Some examples of stalking include the stalker sending the target continuous unwanted gifts and the stalker watching from a distance or showing up at a place where the target does not want them to be. The stalker may also instill fear by threatening to harm the target's friends, family, or pet or damage property or by sneaking into the targeted individual's home.

Although IPV is commonly believed to be committed primarily by men, research does not support this perception. Approximately 27.3% of women and 11.5% of men in the United States have been victims of IPV. Furthermore, 22.3% of women and 14% of men age 18 and older reported being a victim of severe physical violence by an intimate partner (CDC, 2015c).

When assessing an individual for IPV, nurses must remain nonjudgmental regardless of gender, sexual orientation, culture, or the socioeconomic status of the patient. IPV can result in long-lasting physical and emotional complications, and if the individual feels helpless or as though she will not be believed, then the violence is likely to continue. Most cases of IPV begin as mild emotional or physical abuse, but they eventually escalate to more severe violence and can even end in death. Nurses can help prevent this form of violence by being observant for the manifestations of IPV (discussed later in this section) and helping to empower the victim.

≫ Stay Current: Jacquelyn C. Campbell, PhD, RN, FAAN, and Nancy Glass, PhD, MPH, RN, FAAN, have created an instrument that helps determine the level of risk an abused woman has of being killed by her intimate partner. Visit their website at http://dangerassessment.org to learn more about it.

Sexual Abuse

Sexual abuse is defined by the DOJ as "any type of sexual contact or behavior that occurs without the explicit consent of the recipient to include forced sexual intercourse, forcible sodomy, child molestation, incest, fondling, and attempted rape" (DOJ, 2016). Sexual assault falls under the category of "Sexual Violence," which includes the following types: "Completed or attempted forced penetration of a victim;

completed or attempted alcohol/drug-facilitated penetration of a victim; completed or attempted forced acts in which a victim is made to penetrate a perpetrator or someone else; completed or attempted alcohol/drug-facilitated acts in which a victim is made to penetrate a perpetrator or someone else; non-physically forced penetration, which occurs after a person is pressured verbally or through intimidation or misuse of authority to consent or acquiesce; unwanted sexual contact; and non-contact unwanted sexual experiences" (CDC, 2016h). All individuals can be at risk for sexual violence regardless of gender, age, education, IQ, or socioeconomic status. Sexual abuse is often perpetrated by an individual the victim knows, such as an acquaintance, family member, teacher, authority figure, parent, sibling, or spouse. The majority of offenders involved in child sexual abuse are family members or are known to the child in some manner (American Psychological Association, 2013).

Elder Abuse

Elder abuse is the intentional physical, emotional, or sexual mistreatment or neglect of an individual 65 years of age or older. Although other forms of abuse have been declining over recent years, elder abuse has been on the rise. It is believed that this upward trend is due to increased reporting of elder abuse as the problem receives more attention. Even so, recent studies estimate that only one in every 14 cases of elder abuse is actually reported. The reasons behind decreased reporting are numerous but are believed to be the result of an unwillingness to report family members—who are the primary perpetrators of elder abuse. Other reasons for low reporting involve the physical or mental inability to report the abuse, as well as a fear of retaliation from the abuser (National Center on Elder Abuse, n.d.b). The older adult may also fear that they will not have a place to live if they report the abuser. The abuser may have even threatened to place the patient in a residential nursing facility if they report the abuse. The nurse will need to assure the patient that they will be protected and that safety is a priority.

The abuse of older adults—whether it is physical, emotional, or sexual—results in numerous consequences, including decreased health, inability to heal from broken bones, and an increased risk for mortality. Studies have also shown that elder abuse that results in hospitalization for the victim often leads to the individual being discharged to a nursing home or long-term care facility as opposed to returning home (Anetzberger, 2012). Nursing homes and other facilities are also not immune to mistreatment. The National Institute of Justice (2015) reports that the most common form of abuse sustained by older adults in residential care facilities was verbal and psychologic abuse by staff, although they found these incidents to be relatively uncommon. Nurses need to be vigilant in assessing for cases of maltreatment in older adults.

Clinical Manifestations

The signs of abuse can vary based on the population being abused as well as the type of abuse. IPV, for example, will often manifest with signs of intense fear and control, such as the victim not having access to cash and losing all contact with friends and family. The signs of physical and emotional abuse will also vary among populations, with children

reacting to psychologic abuse differently than adults. In cases of sexual abuse, however, the signs are primarily consistent across age demographics. Nurses should be vigilant in assessing for signs of abuse in all patients.

Manifestations of Physical Abuse

Infants have the highest prevalence of fatality due to physical abuse, which is likely related to the infant's small body and occurrences of AHT. "Shaken baby syndrome" occurs in as little as 5 seconds of violent shaking. This action causes the infant's brain to bounce back and forth against the skull, leading to bruising, swelling, pressure, and bleeding in the brain, all of which may lead to permanent brain damage. Shaking an infant may also lead to other injuries such as damage to the neck, spine, and eyes (U.S. National Library of Medicine, 2016). Gentle bouncing, playing, swinging, and bouncing associated with jogging while holding the infant do not cause AHT. If an infant falls or is accidentally dropped, it will cause a different type of brain trauma than that associated with shaken baby syndrome.

Many of the manifestations of physical abuse of a child are apparent, such as broken or fractured bones in different stages of healing, AHT, excessive bruising, and burns or scars in specific shapes (**Figure 32–2 》》**). More of these physical indicators are outlined in the Clinical Manifestations and Therapies table. Signs of long-term traumatic physical abuse can be evidenced by poor language, cognitive, and emotional development, primarily caused by the stress of abuse as an infant or young child. Advanced visual and motor impairment—such as blindness and spinal cord injuries—can also be indicators of physical abuse at a young age. A child who is being abused may also present with

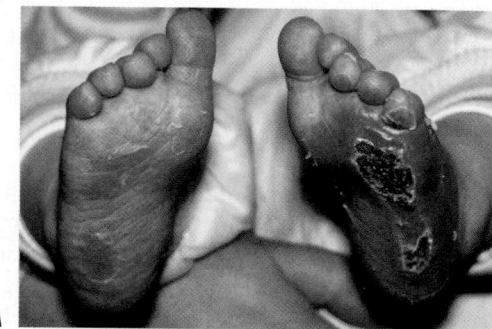

A

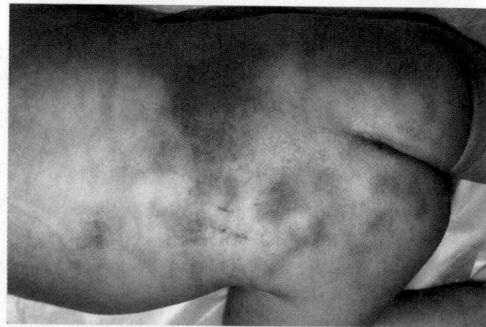

B

Source: **A,** Biophoto Associates/Science Source. **B,** SPL/Science Source.

Figure 32–2 》》 Examples of child abuse. **A,** This child's feet were burned when the parent held the feet against a heater. **B,** Battered child showing bruises and lacerations.

behavioral changes. Some common changes include trouble sleeping, changes in eating habits, wetting the bed, avoiding specific situations or individuals (e.g., family gatherings, a once-trusted friend or relative), and participation in high-risk behavior (drugs, alcohol, dangerous sports) (CDC, 2016i; Meadows, 2013).

Youth violence can also result in physical harm to a child. According to a survey by the CDC (2016a), in the 30 days preceding the survey, 7% of high school students reported not attending school on one or more days because of not feeling safe. Youth violence is a nationwide issue that causes injury and death to youth victims. This violence also causes issues within the community, such as decreased property values. There are potential warning signs of violent behavior that cannot be modified, such as being a victim of bullying, being young at the onset of the first violent episode, witnessing violence at home, or having a major mental illness (American Psychological Association, 2016). Additional factors that may precipitate violence include substance abuse, gang involvement, and feelings of rejection and disrespect. The American Psychological Association also reports that new or active signs associated with youth violence include increased drug or alcohol use, frequent physical altercations, declining school performance, and carrying a weapon (2016).

IPV presents with physical manifestations similar to those of other forms of violence, such as bruises, broken bones, knife wounds, head injuries, and headaches. Individuals experiencing this form of abuse may begin using alcohol and other substances to cope with the abuse. Depression, suicide attempts, fear, and avoidance of social situations are common. Victims of IPV are often cut off from any form of support by their abuser; they are generally not encouraged to have relationships with family members or friends, and their freedoms are limited. Interestingly, victims of IPV and their children are at increased risk for being victims of violence, including homicide, when they are leaving the perpetrator.

Manifestations of physical abuse in older adults include bruises, contusions, or broken bones; however, these symptoms can also be explained away by a simple fall. Therefore, all major injuries in older adults need to be investigated for the possibility of physical abuse.

Manifestations of Psychologic Abuse

Bullying can include either physical or psychologic abuse or both. It is not always obvious that a child is a victim of bullying. A child may fear telling parents or authorities about the attacks because of fear of retaliation from the bully. Most symptoms of bullying are passive and could be overlooked. A child may experience an acute change in behavior and may decline participating in activities they previously found enjoyable (if the bully is present at these functions). Also, the child may begin to dislike school, have increased absenteeism, or experience a decrease in academic performance. Other manifestations include low self-esteem, loneliness, anxiety, depression, and suicidal ideations. There may also be somatic complaints such as frequent headaches and stomachaches (CDC, 2016j).

IPV abusers will seek to control victims' finances and decision-making abilities in order to prevent them from leaving the relationship. Some perpetrators will even work to get their partner (or themselves) pregnant and then threaten to keep the child if the victim leaves. Individuals involved in IPV are likely to be intimidated by their abuser and reluctant to seek or accept help. Controlling abusers will likely accompany the victim to the hospital or treatment center for treatment of their injuries to ensure that the patient does not ask for help, and, depending on the type of abuse, to demonstrate repentance for the injuries (Benedictis et al., 2012). In situations such as these, it may be very difficult or even impossible for the nurse to talk to the patient alone. Nurses could try to schedule a follow-up appointment or express a willingness to help the patient at a later date if the patient wishes to come back alone.

In addition to assessing for typical signs of abuse, psychologic, or emotional, abuse should be assessed. General symptoms may include acute changes of behavior or frequent arguments between the caregiver and patient. The nurse may witness threatening, controlling, or belittling behaviors of the caregiver toward the patient. Another manifestation is the patient exhibiting dementia-like symptoms such as rocking, sucking, or mumbling to self (HelpGuide. org, 2016).

Manifestations of Sexual Abuse

Victims of sexual abuse may be withdrawn or combative, acting out in various situations. Emotions such as guilt, anxiety, depression, suicidal thoughts, and fear are quite common. In children who have experienced sexual abuse, one of the most pronounced indicators is an early sexual knowledge or early interest in sexual acts. Other children may regress instead, demonstrating behavioral difficulties, bedwetting, and insomnia. Physical manifestations of sexual abuse at any age include injuries to genitals or anus, swollen genitals, bladder or kidney infections, sexually transmitted infections or diseases, unintended pregnancies, and pelvic inflammatory disease (National Sex Offender Public Website [NSOPW], n.d.).

In addition, there are warning signs that may be suggestive of a perpetrator of sexual abuse. Some examples of these behaviors include ignoring social, emotional, or physical boundaries; oversharing adult issues with a child; being overly interested in the sexuality of a teen; frequently walking in on children/teens in the bathroom; and exposing a child to adult sexual interaction with lack of regard (NSOPW, n.d.). If the nurse observes any of these behaviors in an older teen or adult, the nurse should assess the situation further.

Manifestations of Neglect

Some signs of neglect of an infant may include uncared-for diaper rash, dirty diapers, poor hygiene, poor eye contact or detachment, failure to thrive, and skin sores, rashes, and flea bites (National Society for the Prevention of Cruelty to Children [NSPCC], 2016). Healthcare providers need to be mindful when assessing infants, as some of these conditions may develop unrelated to neglect; therefore, if neglect is suspected, a further, more in-depth assessment must occur.

Children may display signs of neglect in various ways. Neglect may include anything from leaving a child home alone to more critical situations such as malnutrition. Poor hygiene, dirty clothing, clothing that is too small or inappropriate for weather conditions, and appearing hungry or presenting with no money for lunch at school are all signs of neglect. Health and developmental problems may present as untreated medical or dental issues, not reaching developmental milestones, and poor language development. Living conditions may indicate neglect of a child as well, such as living in an unsanitary environment that has animal feces or urine that is not cleaned up, infestations of bugs leaving bites on the child, or even having to care for other family members at a young age (NSPCC, 2016).

Neglect in an adult relationship may also occur. Generally, emotional neglect is difficult to determine, as the symptoms may not be present or overt and usually consists of omissions (failing to meet the needs of the partner). An example of emotional neglect may involve one partner spending more time at work or with others than the other partner. Another example is a partner consistently not providing the emotional support that the other needs (Cohen, 2013).

Neglect is the most common form of abuse of the older adult (Ayalon, 2015). Similar to that in children, neglect of an older adult comprises physical needs not being met or care being intentionally withheld. Neglect in older adults may be difficult to identify and is underreported because many victims are unable to report due to physical, cognitive, or mental deficits. Because family members frequently are caregivers, the victim may also be reluctant to tell because they don't want them to get into trouble. Manifestations of neglect of older adults may include unexplained weight loss, dehydration, poor hygiene, unsanitary conditions, untreated medical issues, decubiti, unsafe living conditions (no electricity, heat, or running water), or desertion of the older adult (HelpGuide.org, 2016).

SAFETY ALERT Older adults often go unheard when complaints of abuse occur; claims are often dismissed because the listener thinks the older adult is confused or disoriented. As a nurse, you must explore and report any complaint related to any form of abuse. It is not the job of the nurse to determine whether abuse is occurring, but rather to advocate for the patient by obtaining as much information as possible and reporting the potential abuse per institution protocol and state regulations.

Cultural Considerations

Cultural considerations in cases of abuse are twofold, with some acts or traditions presenting as signs of abuse (such as cupping or coin rubbing), and other cultures partaking in acts that Western culture considers abusive (hitting one's wife for disobedience or hitting children with objects as a form of punishment). In cases of suspected abuse due to marks on the patient's body, nurses must take cultural healing practices into consideration. The practices of cupping and coin rubbing—generally practiced by many Asian cultures, as well as individuals who participate in holistic healing—can both create marks on the body that could be misinterpreted as signs of abuse (**Figure 32–3 >>**) (Ward et al., 2013). Cupping is the act of placing a glass cup on the skin and then using heat to create suction; often this is performed to promote blood flow and overall healing. The

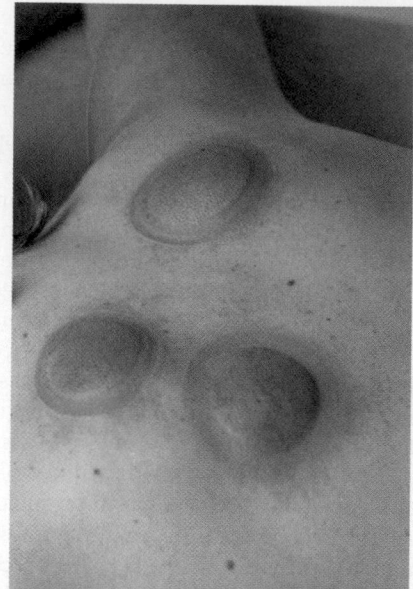

A

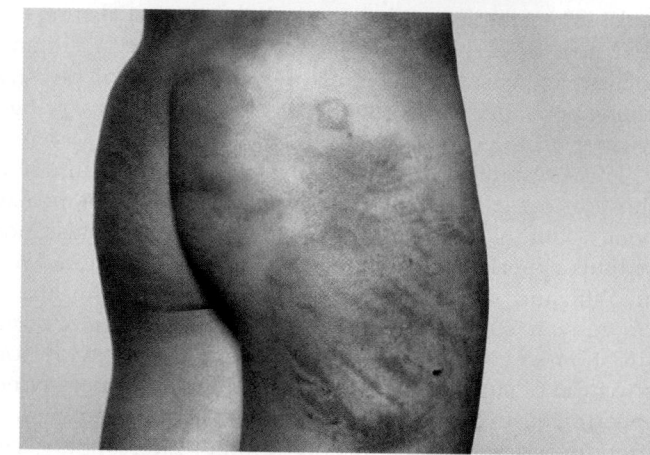

B

Source: Used with permission of the American Academy of Pediatrics, "Visual Diagnosis of Child Abuse Slide Kit." Copyright © AAP/Kempe. *A,* Norbert Reismann/doc-stock/Alamy Stock Photo *B,* Biophoto Associates/Science Source.

Figure 32–3 >> It is important to differentiate cultural practices such as *A,* cupping, and *B,* coining, from signs of child abuse.

result of the procedure can be circular red welts or even dark bruising, which are often found along the individual's back. Coin rubbing is used to treat a multitude of ailments from headaches and fevers to minor illnesses, but it also leaves marks on the skin. In this treatment, warm oil is rubbed on the skin and then a coin is rubbed in a diagonal line until long marks appear. If these marks are seen without knowledge of their origin, they may look almost like marks from a whip. Neither of these treatments are abusive in nature but are instead a form of healing.

Some cultural conceptions of punishment can be considered child abuse. Physical punishment of a child varies among cultures from spanking or hitting their hand, to burning the child, to even hitting the child with a cord to leave cuts (see the Focus on Diversity and Culture feature). Many of these practices may not seem acceptable from a Western perspective, but in some areas of Trinidad and

Focus on Diversity and Culture
Cultural Interpretations of Abuse

■ Some Latin American cultures discipline children by having them kneel on uncooked rice for a short period of time. Practices similar to this are common in many cultures and are not considered to be harmful (Pennsylvania Family Support Alliance, 2016).

■ Elder abuse is a growing problem around the world, and it is overlooked and ignored in numerous cultures (WHO, 2013c).

■ Certain interpretations of holy scripture and teachings by different religions allow for women to be hit by their husbands. Women of those belief systems may be reluctant to report their abuse based on religious grounds.

■ Many victims of IPV from other countries who live in the United States do not report abuse because of a fear of deportation for themselves or their families.

■ Some individuals do not report IPV because it would dishonor or shame their families. Individuals who reported this custom were originally from South Asia, Bangladesh, China, Japan, Jordan, Latin America, and Vietnam (Montalvo-Liendo, 2009).

Nigeria, hitting a child with a cord is a common form of punishment. Similarly, in many cultures—particularly Chinese and Vietnamese—it is acceptable to discipline a child with the use of sticks. Burning a child, particularly with a shaped object, could be a tradition of punishment passed down within an individual family, whereby the mother was burned as a child so she deems it acceptable to do the same to her child. In cases of suspected culturally influenced abuse, nurses recognize that parents may not see the injuries to their child as inappropriate or even abusive but rather as an unfortunate result of the child's behavior. It is not a nurse's place to judge; however, nurses are mandated reporters of child abuse and should follow the state regulations and facility protocol on reporting, even if it is a cultural form of discipline.

Collaboration

Usually, the best way to treat abusive families is to use an interprofessional approach involving nurses, physicians, social workers, protective services personnel, law enforcement, and, often, lawyers. Most families are more open to accepting help and may be willing to develop new behavior patterns for a short time following a crisis, but changing behaviors over time requires more work and support. It is common for family members to return to previous, unhealthy behavior patterns, including those that condone or promote abuse.

The nurse plays an important role in the interprofessional team providing treatment to the child who is the victim of abuse. The nurse should ensure that the team creates a safe environment in which the child feels supported at home, at school, and in the therapeutic environment. Children of abuse are often deprived of control, so it is important to shift control back to the child while helping the child feel empowered. Building trust is also imperative, because it will help the nurse develop a rapport with the young patient. Building trust with a child should never involve lying or making false promises; for example, do not promise that the child's parent(s) will not *get in trouble*—that is for Child Protective Services and the courts to decide. Nurses are also "mandatory reporters," so if a child discloses information about abuse, the nurse must report the situation; therefore, it would also be a false promise to say, or imply, that information will be kept between the nurse and the child. For more information, see the exemplar on Mandatory Reporting in the module on Legal Issues.

As part of the interprofessional team, the nurse should plan interventions that will encourage affective release in a supportive environment. Play therapy helps these children explore traumatic themes, fears, and distorted beliefs. It is a nonthreatening way to process thoughts and feelings associated with abuse. Art therapy provides an opportunity to express feelings for which the children have no words. Therapeutic stories can be used to present the traumatic issues of abuse, link victims' feelings to their behaviors, and describe new coping methods. Journal writing can help older children cope with intrusive thoughts and feelings. They often choose to bring their journal into therapy sessions.

Diagnostic Tests

Diagnostic tests cannot prove that an individual is being abused, but some tests, such as x-rays, MRIs, and CT scans, can show indicators of possible abuse. In most cases, tests are used to diagnose the full extent of the damage in order to properly treat the patient. In cases of physical abuse, an ultrasound or a CT scan of the abdomen can check for abdominal or organ injuries, CT scans of the head will show hemorrhage or skull fractures, and an MRI of the spine will show any spinal injuries. For sexual abuse, swabs for DNA are needed to provide the abuser's identity, and urine samples will show bladder or kidney infections. Tests for sexually transmitted infection should be conducted. Pregnancy tests should be administered to females of childbearing age who are victims of sexual abuse. The range of testing to be conducted will depend on the type of abuse, injuries, and consent of the victim.

Pharmacologic Therapy

Because injuries associated with abuse vary greatly depending on the situation and type of abuse, pharmacologic therapies also vary. Physical injuries such as broken bones and dislocations will require pain medication, sedatives, and anti-inflammatories while setting the injury and for resultant pain. Stabbings, gunshot wounds, or other penetrating injuries will require medications to prevent or heal infections as well as fluids to correct fluid volume deficit. Tetanus boosters or vaccines will be needed for most deep penetrating wounds. In cases of physical and emotional abuse, the patient may experience posttraumatic stress disorder (PTSD), which could require medication in addition to therapy interventions (see Exemplar 32.C on PTSD).

Nonpharmacologic Therapy

The physical effects of abuse will often heal long before the emotional effects have even begun to fade; therefore,

Clinical Manifestations and Therapies
Abuse

ETIOLOGY	CLINICAL MANIFESTATIONS	CLINICAL THERAPIES
Infant abuse	▪ Untreated diaper rash; lengthy time spent in soiled diapers; poor hygiene ▪ Poor eye contact; detachment ▪ Frequent ear infections (from bottle propping) ▪ Failure to thrive ▪ Sores; rashes; flea bites ▪ Fractures (multiple or in various stages of healing, inconsistent with explanations of injury); bruises; welts ▪ AHT; shaken baby syndrome	▪ Treat physical injuries. ▪ Give antibiotics for any infections as prescribed. ▪ Reporting of the abuse is mandatory. ▪ Ensure the safety and security of the child.
Child abuse and youth violence	▪ Bruises or welts in unusual places or in several stages of healing; distinctive shapes ▪ Wary of physical contact with adults ▪ Behavioral extremes of withdrawal or aggression ▪ Burns (especially cigarette burns; immersion burns of hands, feet, or buttocks; rope burns; or distinctively shaped burns) ▪ Apprehensive when other children cry ▪ Fractures (multiple or in various stages of healing, inconsistent with explanations of injury) ▪ Joint swelling or limited mobility ▪ Long-bone deformities ▪ Lacerations and abrasions to the mouth, lip, gums, eye, genitalia ▪ Human bite marks ▪ Signs of AHT ▪ Deformed or displaced nasal septum ▪ Bleeding or fluid drainage from the ears or ruptured eardrums ▪ Broken, loose, or missing teeth ▪ Difficulty in respirations, tenderness or crepitus over ribs ▪ Abdominal pain or tenderness ▪ Recurrent urinary tract infection ▪ Emotional and/or behavioral problems ▪ Increased absenteeism from school ▪ Severe injuries such as penetrating wounds or gunshot wounds	▪ Treat physical injuries. ▪ Give antibiotics for any infections as prescribed. ▪ Therapy may be behavioral, cognitive, group, or play therapy depending on developmental stage. ▪ Reporting of the abuse is mandatory. ▪ Ensure the safety and security of the child.
Bullying	▪ Acute change in behavior ▪ Decreased participation in previously enjoyed activities ▪ Disliking school; increased absenteeism; decrease in academic performance ▪ Low self-esteem; loneliness; anxiety ▪ Depression; thoughts or plans for suicide ▪ Frequent somatic complaints	▪ Allow child to express feelings; give validation of concerns. ▪ Notify proper authorities (teacher, school administrators) so that adequate supervision may occur. ▪ Therapy for depression; may be behavioral, cognitive, group, or play therapy depending on developmental stage. ▪ Ensure the safety and security of the child.
Sexual Abuse	▪ Torn, stained, or bloody underwear ▪ Pain or itching in genital areas ▪ Bruises or bleeding from external genitalia, vagina, rectum ▪ Poor peer relationships ▪ Withdrawal ▪ Sexually transmitted disease ▪ Unwilling to participate in physical activities ▪ Swollen or red cervix, vulva, or perineum ▪ Wears long sleeves and several layers of clothing even in hot weather ▪ Semen around the mouth or genitalia or on clothing ▪ Pregnancy ▪ Delinquency or running away ▪ Inappropriate sexual behavior or mannerisms ▪ Regressive behaviors	▪ Treat physical injuries. ▪ Test for sexually transmitted diseases and infections. ▪ Administer pregnancy test. ▪ Take DNA swabs for identification of the perpetrator. ▪ Treat for depression and/or suicidal behavior. ▪ Therapy may be behavioral, cognitive, group, or play, depending on developmental stage. ▪ Educate on rights and ability to report to authorities. ▪ Consider behavioral therapy for perpetrators.

Clinical Manifestations and Therapies *(continued)*

ETIOLOGY	CLINICAL MANIFESTATIONS	CLINICAL THERAPIES
Intimate partner violence (IPV)	■ Chronic fatigue ■ Casual response to serious pain ■ Vague complaints, aches, and injury or excessively emotional response to a relatively minor injury ■ Frequent injuries ■ Recurrent sexually transmitted diseases ■ Frequent ambulatory or emergency department visits ■ Muscle tension ■ Nightmares ■ Facial lacerations ■ Depression ■ Injuries to chest, breasts, back, abdomen, or genitalia ■ Anorexia or other eating disorder ■ Bilateral injuries of arms or legs ■ Anxiety ■ Symmetric injuries ■ Drug or alcohol abuse ■ Obvious patterns of belt buckles, bite marks, fist or hand marks ■ Suicide attempts ■ Poor self-esteem ■ Burns of hands, feet, buttocks, or with distinctive patterns ■ Headaches ■ Gastrointestinal or stress ulcers	■ Treat physical injuries and physiologic conditions. ■ Treat psychologic effects such as depression with medication or therapy. ■ Suggest substance abuse counseling for perpetrator and victim, as needed. ■ Provide referrals for community services, support groups, and shelters.
Elder abuse	■ Constant hunger or malnutrition ■ Listlessness ■ Poor hygiene ■ Social isolation ■ Inappropriate dress for the weather ■ Chronic fatigue ■ Unattended medical needs ■ Poor skin integrity or decubiti ■ Contractures ■ Urine burns/excoriation ■ Dehydration ■ Fecal impaction ■ Bruises and welts ■ Withdrawal ■ Burns ■ Confusion ■ Fractures ■ Fear or suspicion of caretaker, family members, healthcare providers ■ Sprains or dislocations ■ Lacerations or abrasions ■ Evidence of oversedation ■ Failure to meet financial obligations	■ Treat physical injuries. ■ Treat dehydration and malnutrition with increased fluids and food intake. ■ Treat psychologic effects such as depression with medication or therapy. ■ Arrange for respite services. ■ Consider adult day care. ■ Reporting of the abuse is mandatory. ■ Ensure the safety and security of the older adult. ■ Refer perpetrators to treatment or therapy. ■ Arrange transfer of legal authority.

nonpharmacologic therapies used with victims of abuse are numerous and important for the patient. Therapy, counseling, and support groups are the most commonly prescribed forms of treatment in cases of abuse. The type of therapy will depend on the personality, needs, and desires of the patient.

Domestic Violence Shelters

Domestic violence shelters offer a broad array of services for patients of all ages, including immediate shelter for victims and their children and referrals to agencies that provide group therapy for parents and children, advocacy, and parent training. Some shelters may be gender specific, but most offer shelter regardless of gender. Many shelters offer lists of attorneys and other professionals who offer services with sliding-scale fees. Many programs offer outreach services, including education and training on workplace violence and elder abuse. Nurses working in all settings should have contact information available for community domestic violence shelters.

NURSING PROCESS

Care of an individual who has been abused will vary depending on the type of abuse and the age of the individual. A patient's reaction to the abuse will also affect care, especially if fear, shame, and/or self-blaming are present. Nurses treat individuals on a patient-by-patient basis, assessing the need of a specific individual rather than the needs of a supposedly *typical* abuse victim.

Assessment

The nurse's assessment in cases of abuse will be in order of the severity of the injuries. Life-threatening injuries will be assessed first, and other injuries will be assessed after the patient's safety is ensured. A complete medical history will be performed to determine if the patient has a history of injuries that could be the result of abuse. Nurses need to consider the patient's emotional state; victims of abuse could be scared of their abuser or of being blamed for the abuse. Similarly, some patients may be more nervous around staff of the same gender as the abuser; if possible, make adjustments to the staff directly caring for that patient. Some hospitals now assess victims of violence on locked units to minimize exposure of victims and hospital staff to perpetrators.

Diagnosis

Nursing diagnoses are dependent on the patient's current physical and psychosocial status. Patients who have experienced abuse could have a range of diagnoses, depending on the mode of abuse. Diagnoses relevant to actual or suspected victims of child abuse, elder abuse, or interpersonal violence may include, but are not limited to, the following:

- *Pain, Acute*
- *Powerlessness*
- *Post-Trauma Syndrome*
- *Sexual Dysfunction*
- *Social Isolation.*

(NANDA-I © 2014)

Planning

Goals for a patient who has experienced abuse will change according to the nursing diagnoses and the individual. The age of the patient will also affect how an individual reacts to having been injured as the result of abuse. Examples of goals for the patient who has experienced abuse are as follows:

- The patient will be safe and free from harm.
- The patient will report mild to no pain.
- The patient will ask for help in safely resolving the abusive situation.
- The patient will honestly convey feelings of fear, helplessness, anger, or depression.
- The patient will report any suicidal ideation.
- The patient will acknowledge that she is not responsible for the abuse.
- The patient will practice healthy coping mechanisms.

Implementation

The nurse's ability to implement care measures will depend on the patient's willingness to accept help in leaving or reconciling the abusive situation. In most states, some forms of abuse, such as child abuse and elder abuse, must be reported to the proper authorities. However, reporting other forms of abuse—including IPV and certain instances of sexual abuse—is often left to the discretion of the victim.

Promote Safety

In cases of abuse, the patient's safety is the primary concern. Because of mandatory reporting laws, nurses must report all suspected cases of child abuse. In some states, it is also legally mandated for nurses to report the abuse or neglect of an older adult. Cases of IPV are often left to the victim to report, but some areas have laws concerning mandatory reporting of IPV. The use of specific weapons and the nature of the injuries are often factors for mandatory reporting of IPV in states with those laws. Nurses must be aware of regulations within the state where they are practicing and abide by those laws. When abuse is suspected, the nurse should follow institutional policies and guidelines for reporting. In the clinical setting, the nurse usually is required to notify a supervisor to begin the reporting process.

When mandatory reporting is not indicated, it is imperative for nurses to provide the patient with information about resources for seeking help. Adults who have experienced a form of abuse can be gently encouraged to seek assistance in promoting their own safety. If the patient chooses not to seek assistance, then information should be provided in case assistance is ever needed. Resources can be in the form of the patient's friends and family members or community liaisons who can work to help the individual find a secure living environment. Other resources can be offered, such as police, lawyers, and agencies that can provide ongoing assistance for the victim. Nurses encourage the patient to accept help in seeking an abuse-free living situation, but the decision ultimately lies with the patient. Some individuals will not be ready to seek help, and while the nurse may disagree with this decision, he must refrain from judgment and be respectful of the patient's decision. All nurses can do in these situations is offer assistance and resources; this lets the victim know that help is available if it is needed in the future.

Establish a Therapeutic Relationship

Establishing appropriate modes of interaction with a patient who has been abused is vital. A large factor in establishing a therapeutic relationship is establishing trust. Many cases of physical abuse involve psychologic abuse, which often belittles an individual's sense of self-worth and self-love, sometimes to the point that they feel it is impossible for them to do anything correctly. A healthcare worker who appears to be angry or disappointed in a patient for not choosing to seek assistance in leaving an abusive situation will shatter all forms of trust that had been established with that patient. Nurses need to work to establish a trusting relationship with adults who have been abused, assuring them that they are in a judgment-free and safe setting.

When nurses suspect child abuse, age-specific considerations must be employed. The child needs to feel safe and secure, particularly from the potential abuser. All early conclusions about the situation should be dismissed, because it is unwise to assume knowledge of a situation until all the details are presented. Child abuse is a very serious situation and should never be taken lightly; however, nurses should be aware that cases of false reporting do exist. The majority of these cases are not malicious on the part of the child but are rather the result of a misunderstanding or a leading question on the part of the healthcare professional. All forms of leading questions should be avoided when talking to children about abuse. It is appropriate to ask a child how she hit her head; it is inappropriate to ask a child if her mother slammed her head into a kitchen counter. Children in high-stress situations will sometimes work to tell an adult what they think that adult wants to hear. With this in mind, nurses should ask open-ended questions with no indication of the answer they expect to receive. It is imperative for nurses to follow organizational protocols with regard to suspected child abuse interviews.

Facilitate Communication

Accepting help after having experienced abuse for weeks, months, or years is sometimes exceptionally difficult for victims. Elements of fear of their abuser, lack of social support, decreased financial resources, and a sense of hopelessness all contribute to an apparent disinclination to accept assistance. Nurses need to understand these fears to better assist patients in this difficult situation. Many resources can be offered to help combat these individual reservations. For example, the patient can be put in contact with local law enforcement agencies to file an order of protection against the abuser to ensure some degree of safety from retaliation. Connections can also be fostered with social workers, counselors, and community liaisons to find safe housing and assist with social and financial support. Nurses reassure patients that options and resources are available to help them move away from the abusive situation being experienced.

Promote Empowerment

Helping patients achieve a sense of control within the situation is one of the first steps in helping them accept assistance. All forms of abuse include an element of control on the part of the perpetrator and generally result in taking control away from the victim. In working to help patients regain that sense of control, nurses can help empower them to leave the situation. Support groups and individual therapy are recommended to help the patient talk about the abuse and potentially connect with others who have experienced similar situations. Education should occur to ensure that the patient is aware of community services, support groups, and law enforcement numbers. Ensuring that a safety plan is developed will also aid in empowering the patient (see Patient Teaching: Developing a Safety Plan). Interventions vary depending on the individual's age and circumstances, so referrals are made on a case-by-case basis.

Evaluation

All forms and cases of abuse are different depending on the age of the victim and the circumstances of the abuse; therefore, the outcomes in these cases will vary. It is important to set realistic goals for patients. Some desired outcomes include the following:

- The patient remains free from injury or harm.
- The patient has a safety plan in place.
- The patient seeks assistance when needed.
- The patient demonstrates knowledge of the resources available to individuals in abusive situations.
- The patient verbalizes awareness that she is not responsible for or deserving of abuse.
- The patient openly communicates her fears with regard to the abusive situation.

Individuals with severe injuries related to abuse may need additional evaluation and follow-up, including potential surgical interventions. The nurse should treat these patients like other patients undergoing surgery, including prepping the patient for surgery and providing aseptic care of the surgical wound. In addition, nurses may need to continue to suggest counseling or group therapy or other types of emotional support to individuals who seem reluctant to get help for emotional trauma. When a nurse sees a patient repeatedly because of injuries from abuse, the nurse should continue to advocate for patient safety and encourage the patient to seek help. The patient may not be receptive to help after a first or second instance of abuse, but the patient may be more likely to want help if the abuse has happened repeatedly. Continued evaluation and support of the patient sustaining abuse is necessary to promote the most positive outcome possible.

REVIEW Abuse

RELATE Link the Concepts and Exemplars

Linking the exemplar of abuse with the concept of development:

1. What protective factors would indicate a child probably has not experienced abuse? At age 3? At age 15?
2. What factors would put a child at risk for abuse?

Linking the exemplar of abuse with the concept of mood and affect:

3. What mood and affect would you anticipate a victim of abuse might display?

4. What nursing assessment regarding mood and affect would be a priority when admitting a patient who was abused by a family member?

READY Go to Volume 3: Clinical Nursing Skills

REFER Go to Pearson MyLab Nursing and eText

- Additional review materials

REFLECT Apply Your Knowledge

Lucy Barnes, a 30-year-old woman who is 25 weeks pregnant, comes to the emergency department of Parkfield Community Hospital. She says she fell and hit her head at home and is having head-aches. During the assessment, the nurse notices multiple bruises in various stages of healing over her body and asks Lucy how she got them. Lucy says that she is just clumsy and falls a lot. While the nurse is assessing Lucy, another nurse enters the room to tell Lucy that her boyfriend is there to take her back home. At that point, Lucy becomes frightened and tells the nurse that her boyfriend has hit her many times before and had knocked her down today. She says he has threatened to kill her if she tells anyone, and she does not want to leave with him.

1. Identify questions that the nurse could use in continuing her assessment and in documenting the discussion with Lucy.
2. What other people should be involved in Lucy's care in the emergency department?
3. Who should make the decision about where Lucy should go?

Exemplar 32.B
Multisystem Trauma

Exemplar Learning Outcomes

32.B Analyze multisystem trauma as it relates to trauma.

- Describe the etiology of multisystem trauma.
- Compare the risk factors and prevention of multisystem trauma.
- Identify the clinical manifestations of multisystem trauma.
- Summarize diagnostic tests and therapies used by interprofessional teams in the collaborative care of an individual with multisystem trauma.

- Differentiate care of patients with multisystem trauma across the lifespan.
- Apply the nursing process in providing culturally competent care to an individual with multisystem trauma.

Exemplar Key Terms

Motor vehicle crash (MVC), *2136*
Multisystem trauma, *2136*
Traumatic brain injury (TBI), *2139*
Whiplash, *2139*

Overview

Multisystem trauma refers to injuries affecting multiple body systems such as the neurologic, respiratory, and circulatory systems. There are many causes of multisystem trauma, such as abuse, motor vehicle crashes, poisonings, drownings, falls, natural disasters, human-caused disasters, homicide, and suicide. Nearly 80% of pediatric multisystem trauma victims include head trauma. The CDC (2015d) further reports unintentional injuries as the leading cause of death in the United States for people age 1–44 years. According to the CDC (2016k), unintentional poisonings are the leading cause of injury-related deaths, followed by **motor vehicle crashes (MVCs)**.

Etiology

Poisonings are the leading cause of injury death in the United States, with 47,055 people losing their lives to drug poisoning in 2014 (CDC, 2016l) (see **Figure 32–4 >>**). Prescription and illicit drugs cause the majority of these poisonings. MVCs are a major concern because of the significance of injuries sustained. The leading causes of death related to MVCs include teenage drivers, distracted driving, and alcohol- or drug-impaired driving (CDC, 2015e, 2016m). Note that the leading causes of death in the United States also indicate the prevalence of nonfatal injuries related to the same cause. In addition, all causes of fatal injuries are also causes of multisystem trauma.

Risk Factors

Although there is no way to fully cover all risk factors associated with multisystem trauma, some of the major causes of injury and death are discussed in this section.

The CDC (2016l) indicates that 1.6 times more males died from poisonings than females, with the highest death rate

being between the ages of 45 and 54 years. Opioid analgesics accounted for 40% of all drug-related poisonings.

While some MVCs are influenced by forces of nature, such as a deer or other forms of wildlife running across the road or a sudden ice or rain storm, the primary cause of accidents is human error. Some of the main risk factors for motor vehicle incidents include age, speeding, distraction, aggressive driving, and impaired driving.

Both young and older drivers are at particular risk for motor vehicle crashes. Beginning drivers age 16–19 are still gaining experience with a variety of driving conditions and situations (**Figure 32–5 >>**). They are also more likely to take risks while driving. Individuals in this age group are three

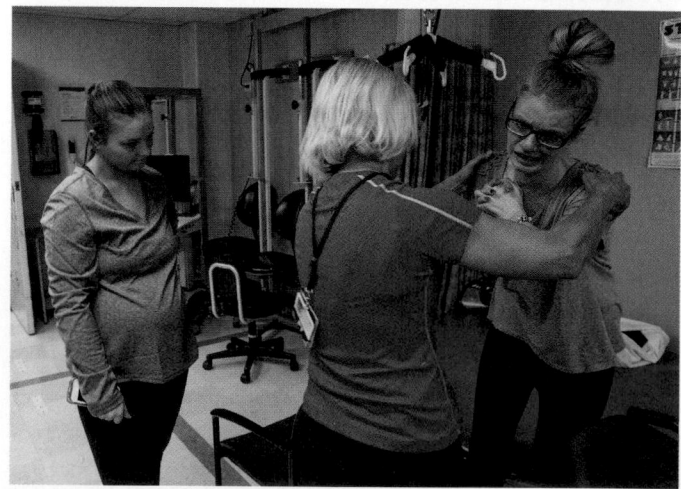

Source: Nikki Kahn/The Washington Post/Getty Images.

Figure 32–4 >> A physical therapist works with a 19-year-old as she learns to walk after experiencing a heroin overdose 2 years earlier.

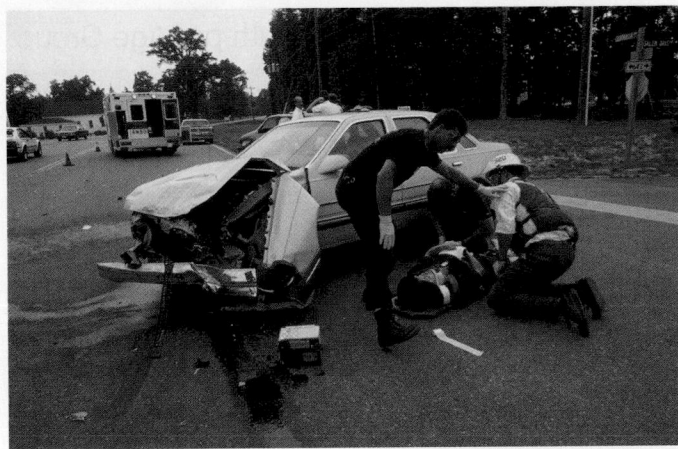

Source: Tim Wright/Corbis Historical/Getty Images.

Figure 32–5 》 Beginning drivers take more risks and are three times more likely to be involved in a crash.

times more likely to be involved in a crash than drivers age 20 and older (CDC, 2015e). Older adult drivers (age 65 and older) are at risk for MVCs because of preexisting health conditions that can flare up while driving (such as heart or respiratory problems) and decreases in sensory perception (reduced eyesight and hearing).

Unsafe driving practices are a risk within every age group. Speeding and impaired driving in particular contribute to the majority of MVCs. When a motor vehicle is moving too quickly, it is impossible to stop effectively if there is a sudden incident on the road—such as a car stopping suddenly, an animal walking across the road, or a pedestrian unexpectedly crossing the street. Impaired driving limits the individual's ability to react quickly, potentially leading to an accident due to delayed response time. Other driving traits that represent a risk for MVCs are driver distraction and aggressive driving. Distraction can result from using a phone, dropping a beverage or food item while driving, or even having talking or crying children in the car. Aggressive driving leads to tailgating and other dangerous driving habits that increase the risk for accidents.

Refer to the following sections in this module for additional information related to risk factors for multisystem trauma related to these etiologies: Interpersonal Violence, Community and Systemic Violence, and Accidental/Incidental Trauma.

Prevention

Knowledge of the causes and at-risk groups directs prevention efforts. Trauma-related injuries and deaths are preventable. Injury is the greatest health hazard for most age groups; therefore, injury prevention must be integrated into every health contact with all patients.

Poisonings can be prevented by following the prescription and by not taking too much or not taking it too frequently. Make sure that all medications are kept in a protected area and, if children are in the home, that childproof lids are used. Turn on the light when taking medications and keep medication in the original container. Medications for children, teenagers, and older adults should be monitored to ensure that no errors occur during administration. Substance abuse may also lead to poisoning;

therefore, it is important to encourage the abuser to obtain substance abuse treatment and not enable the abuse by providing the drug or money for the drug.

Many teens learn to drive and have a license by 16 years of age. They often transport friends, get distracted by social interactions in the car, have little experience with actions to take if a car slides or has mechanical problems, may drink and drive, and are often tired when driving. Several states have instituted graduated driver licensing to help decrease some risks. Graduated driver licensing is an approach used to decrease MVCs among novice teen drivers. Common approaches are to increase the period required for a learner's permit, decrease driving after dark, and limit passengers in the car. Another method that has been suggested to improve safety records is to involve parents in practice driving times. Driving should always be presented as a privilege and a responsibility. Serious consequences such as losing the ability to drive for a time after any infraction can be suggested to parents. Because of the great risk of injury and death from MVCs, ask at each health visit if the teen drives or rides with other teens, what rules parents have established about driving, and whether the teen ever drinks and drives or rides with someone who does. Reinforce the need to wear a safety belt at all times and to never drink and drive. Many injuries can be prevented by using protective gear and following safety guidelines.

Prevention efforts among older adults can be in the form of regular eye and hearing examinations as well as considerations of side effects of any medications being taken. Various injury prevention efforts for all ages are listed in **Table 32–2 》**.

SAFETY ALERT Older adults are frequently on multiple medications that may cause vertigo, drowsiness, or orthostatic hypotension. The patient should be educated on the side effects of the medications and be advised of the dangers of driving while taking the medication.

Patient Teaching
Pool Safety for Children

Parents of children who have easy access to a swimming pool or body of water should be educated on water safety:

1. Never leave children unattended around water. Provide constant, undistracted supervision.
2. Ensure that all children know how to swim (enroll in swim lessons).
3. Have inexperienced swimmers wear Coast Guard–approved life jackets.
4. Prevent unsupervised access to pools (install locks, alarms, monitoring system and fencing).
5. Learn first aid and CPR.
6. Educate children to not play around drains or suction devices.
7. If a child is missing, check the water first.

Sources: Based on American Red Cross. (2016). *Water safety.* Retrieved from http://www.redcross.org/get-help/preparefor-emergencies/types-of-emergencies/watersafety; National Safety Council. (2016). *Drowning: It can happen in an instant.* Retrieved from http://www.nsc.org/learn/safety knowledge/Pages/news-and-resources-water-safety.aspx; National Water Safety Month. (2016). *Water safety tips from our friends at the International Swimming Hall of Fame (ISHOF).* Retrieved from http://www.nationalwatersafety-month.org/water-safety-tips

TABLE 32–2 Strategies for Preventing Injuries Based on Top Three Causes of Death per Age Group

At-Risk Group or Behavior and Top Three Causes of Death	Injury Prevention Strategy
Newborns/infants: *0–12 months:* Unintentional suffocation Homicide (unspecified) Homicide (other specified)	■ Never place a newborn or infant face down on soft surfaces. ■ Do not use soft bedding, pillows, or crib bumpers, and ensure the mattress is the correct size and not covered in plastic and that no plastic bags are accessible. ■ Broken balloons are a choke hazard, so it is important to make sure that infants are unable to reach a balloon or any broken pieces. ■ Choose an infant-only car seat or a convertible seat suitable for an infant. Always have infant ride in a rear-facing car seat. Never place a rear-facing car safety seat in the front seat with an active passenger air bag. ■ Ensure that parents and caregivers have necessary resources to properly care for an infant. Make sure that they have adequate assistance in caring for the child to prevent exhaustion, frustrations, and resentment. ■ If a parent has a mental illness, make sure that the mental illness is effectively treated and the parent is stable, especially while taking care of infants and young children. ■ Report any suspected abuse of a newborn or infant to the proper authorities.
Toddlers and preschoolers: *1–4 years:* Unintentional drowning MVC Homicide (unspecified)	■ Monitor toddlers at all times, especially during bath time or around any water. Toddlers can drown in as little as 1 inch of water. ■ If there is a swimming pool accessible, it is important to have a protective gate around the pool and to have pool alarms indicating unexpected motion in the water. If the toddler or preschooler's home is near a body of water such as a pond or a lake, a protective barrier (such as a fence) should be installed. The toddler/preschooler should be attended at all times while outside. See the Patient Teaching feature for more information on pool safety. ■ Enroll toddlers and preschoolers in swimming lessons. They will be taught safety around water as well as basic life-saving techniques such as floating. ■ Insist on safety seat use for all trips. Use an approved safety seat only. Know the laws in your state. Some states now require children up to age 2 to be in rear-facing car seats (Pennsylvania Department of Transportation, 2016). Toddlers and preschoolers are not large enough to use car seat belts. ■ Report any suspected abuse of toddlers or preschoolers to the proper authorities.
School-age: *5–9 years:* MVC Unintentional drowning Unintentional fire/burn *10–14 years:* MVC Suicide (suffocation) Suicide (firearm)	■ Verify that the school-age child is belted in properly before starting car. Forward-facing car seats and booster seats are used in the backseat. These child restraint systems must be used until the child is 57 inches tall (or 8–12 years of age) and can safely use regular car safety belts. The backseat is preferred for all children and should be the only location used for children 12 years and younger. ■ Always use both lap and shoulder belts. Make sure the lap belt fits low and tight across the lap/upper thigh area and the shoulder belt is snug across the chest and shoulder to avoid abdominal injuries. ■ Use locking mechanisms on hot tubs. Install fencing or a barrier to prevent children from gaining access to a pool or body of water. ■ Do not allow children to dive into pools less than 9 feet deep, and teach them to not play around drains. ■ Always supervise children, even if a lifeguard is present. At large bodies of water (e.g., ocean or lake) make sure that the child wears an approved flotation device. ■ Fire detectors should be working in all homes regardless of age group. The detector should be tested monthly. ■ Have a developed fire escape plan and test it routinely. Have an identified meeting place outside the home. Teach children to stay low when smoke is present. ■ Maintain the home's water heater at 120 degrees to prevent scalding. ■ Use the back burner on the stove, keeping pan handles facing back so that children cannot reach. Monitor stove and oven at all times while in use. ■ Educate children that steam can also cause burns. Microwaves easily cause food to heat quickly and let off steam; therefore, a child needs to understand microwave safety as well as being careful with microwave-prepared foods.
Adolescents and young adults: *15–24 years:* MVC Homicide (firearm) Unintentional poisoning	■ Promote school-based education programs. ■ Enforce rules about safe driving, including use of seat belts for every trip. ■ Discourage drug and alcohol use. ■ The best way to protect adolescents from gun violence is to remove all guns from the home. If there are guns in the home, they should be stored in a securely locked container, with the ammunition stored in a separate locked container. ■ Monitor for warning signs of suicide such as behavioral changes, low self-esteem, and hopelessness. Obtain professional assistance if warning signs are present. ■ Parents should maintain involvement with their teens and provide a safe, stable home. Maintain a supportive yet non-intrusive relationship. ■ Teens should be encouraged to be involved in extracurricular activities.
Adults: *25–34 years:* Unintentional poisoning MVC Homicide (firearm) *35–64 years:* Unintentional poisoning MVC Suicide (firearm)	■ Take prescription medications as directed. ■ If substance abuse is present, encourage treatment. ■ Use seat belts for every trip. Drive following all laws such as speed limit, stopping at all stops signs/lights, and so forth. ■ Do not drive under the influence of prescription medication, illicit drugs, or alcohol. Maintain focus and do not use cell phone while driving to eliminate being a distracted driver. ■ Monitor for warning signs of depression (see the module on Mood and Affect). Intervention should immediately occur if suicidal ideation is present. ■ Monitor for warning signs of aggression (see the Concept section of this module).

TABLE 32–2 Strategies for Preventing Injuries Based on Top Three Causes of Death per Age Group *(continued)*

At-Risk Group or Behavior and Top Three Causes of Death	Injury Prevention Strategy
Older adults: **65+ years:** Unintentional fall MVC Suicide (firearm)	■ Encourage regular vision exams, driving ability screenings, and community programs. ■ Evaluate potential effects of medications for both driving purposes and determining fall risk potential. ■ Encourage exercise to maintain strength and endurance while ambulating. ■ Eliminate trip hazards such as rugs and items placed in walkways or on stairwells, and keep walkways illuminated at night. ■ Monitor for warning signs of depression (see the module on Mood and Affect). Intervention should immediately occur if suicidal ideation is present.

Clinical Manifestations

MVCs, violence, abuse, and disaster-related events often result in a combination of physical and emotional injuries. Physical injuries can range from mild (minor scrapes and contusions) to severe (broken bones, head injuries, and even fatal injuries). When emotional injuries are present, they are often in the form of acute trauma syndrome (especially if other victims were severely or fatally injured) or a fear of exposure to the same event. Nurses will see a wide range of injuries as the result of trauma-related events.

Common Injuries

Injuries are very common as the result of trauma, with some of the more prevalent injuries being whiplash, **traumatic brain injury (TBI)**, spinal cord injuries, facial injuries, internal organ damage, and fractures. **Whiplash** results when a sudden impact to a motor vehicle causes an individual's head and neck to be forcibly contorted, resulting in injury to the spine. Spinal injuries are common in trauma and can result in partial or complete paralysis. Facial injuries and *traumatic brain injuries* (brain trauma that occurs after a sudden blow to the head) often occur in trauma-related events due to the individual's head hitting the dashboard, steering wheel, or air bag; blunt trauma from a violent assault; or objects falling on the victim's head.

Although wearing a seat belt can save a life, seat belts also can cause injuries during a crash. Common injuries from a seat belt are fractured ribs, fractured collarbone, internal injuries, and organ damage, as well as the potential for a punctured lung secondary to broken ribs.

Collaboration

Collaborative care of the patient who has sustained multisystem traumatic injury depends on a team approach (**Figure 32–6 》**). The team includes health personnel on site and the nurses, physicians, and surgeons at the hospital. Providing trauma care with a team focus helps each team member know his or her role. Prompt delegation of tasks and responsibilities improves the patient's chances for survival and decreases the morbidity that may result from traumatic injuries.

》 Stay Current: Many organizations such as the Society of Trauma Nurses and the American College of Surgeons offer courses in trauma care for nurses. For more information, visit the Advanced Trauma Care for Nurses page at http://www.traumanurses.org/atcn and the Advanced Trauma Life Support page at www.facs.org/trauma/atls/about.html.

Community awareness and health promotion efforts require collaboration as well. Healthcare institutions along with local fire departments, law enforcement, and health departments will often combine to offer awareness campaigns regarding issues related to motor vehicle crashes, violence prevention, and disaster readiness. Communities have disaster readiness plans and train healthcare professionals and volunteers on emergency readiness and response.

Diagnostic Tests

Because trauma-related injuries vary widely, so do the diagnostic tests used to assess the severity of those injuries. Common diagnostic procedures include MRIs, CT scans, x-rays, and ultrasounds. These procedures can help determine the severity of head, neck, and back injuries and to identify internal bleeding, broken bones, or torn muscles. An EEG can be used to diagnose changes in brain activity.

Surgery

The life-threatening nature of traumatic incidents will often lead to a patient needing surgery to repair damage and/or stop internal bleeding. If internal organ damage is indicated—due either to organ rupture or to a foreign object puncturing the abdominal cavity—emergency surgery will be needed to

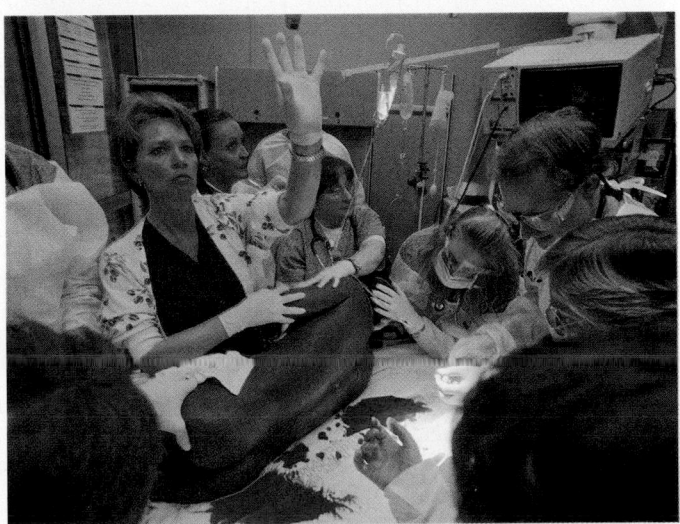

Source: Robert Tirey/Alamy Stock Photo.

Figure 32–6 》 A nurse in the emergency department asks for a wipe to clean off blood from the victim of a stabbing.

Clinical Manifestations and Therapies
Multisystem Trauma

ETIOLOGY	CLINICAL MANIFESTATIONS	CLINICAL THERAPIES
Mild head injury	▪ Headache ▪ Sensitivity to light, blurred vision ▪ Nausea, dizziness, balance problems ▪ Changes in memory	▪ CT, MRI, and/or electroencephalogram (EEG) to determine the extent of the injury. ▪ Application of ice. ▪ Stitches for open wounds. ▪ Elevation of head of bed to 30 degrees.
Traumatic brain injury (TBI)	▪ Loss of consciousness ▪ Headache; repeated nausea and vomiting ▪ Dilation of one or both pupils ▪ Confusion ▪ Seizures and coma ▪ Possible death	▪ Same clinical therapies as for mild head injury. ▪ Pharmacologic therapies such as diuretics and anticonvulsant medications. ▪ Surgery to remove hematomas, repair skull fractures, or remove skull fragments from the brain, and cutting out a section of skull to allow for swelling of brain, which diminishes the pressure on the brain. ▪ Physical and/or speech therapy depending on the severity of the injury.
Whiplash	▪ Neck stiffness and pain ▪ Dizziness, blurred vision, headaches, ringing in the ears ▪ Concentration and memory problems	▪ Prescription pain relievers such as hydrocodone or oxycodone. ▪ Muscle relaxants to relieve muscle spasms. ▪ Lidocaine injections into the affected muscle to relieve pain and muscle spasms. ▪ Ice and heat therapy. ▪ Physical therapy. ▪ Immobilization collar to promote proper healing.
Spinal cord injury, either incomplete or complete	▪ Loss of sensation and movement below affected area ▪ Pain if nerve damage is present ▪ Breathing difficulty ▪ Loss of bladder and bowel control ▪ Numbness and tingling in extremities	▪ Immobilization of the spine with a neck collar. ▪ Sedation to prevent further damage to the spine, if necessary. ▪ Methylprednisolone (Medrol) to decrease inflammation and nerve damage. ▪ Surgery if possible. ▪ Physical therapy and rehabilitation. ▪ Pain medications.

repair the damage or stabilize the patient until a transplantation can be performed.

Injuries involving severe head or spinal trauma may require surgery depending on the circumstances. Head injuries will not always need surgery; however, if an intracranial hemorrhage (ICH) is present and the bleeding does not stop on its own, surgery may be the only solution. Intracranial pressure (ICP) will be monitored when a head injury is present, and if the pressure rises to dangerous levels, surgery will be performed to release some of the pressure. Spinal injuries are often irreversible once they have occurred, but in most cases surgery will be needed to remove bone fragments and stabilize the spine.

Pharmacologic Therapy

The majority of injuries sustained will be painful to patients and will require pain management. Less severe injuries involving sprains, minor cuts, and mild concussions do not require strong pain medicines but rather a form of ibuprofen. Deep cuts requiring sutures usually will be treated with lidocaine as a numbing agent. In cases of more severe injuries, particularly those that require surgery, stronger pain medications—most often opioids—are administered. Sedation may be necessary if the patient's reaction to the injuries or the pain puts her in danger of further injury. Nurses will follow proper sedation protocols, ensuring that the patient is not oversedated.

Nonpharmacologic Therapy

Physical therapy and rehabilitation are often required for severe injuries, including broken bones (especially compound fractures), spinal injuries, and some traumatic brain injuries. If the patient falls into a coma or is put into a drug-induced coma, physical therapy and rehabilitation will be needed if muscle tone decreased significantly while the patient was unconscious. Patients with impairments in neurologic, motor, speech, and/or language functioning may require speech therapy. Patients with TBI or another injury that impairs self-care and other abilities may work with an occupational therapist to relearn some of those activities.

Individuals will be provided with a referral and resources for therapy and counseling to help with emotional trauma resulting from the accident.

Complementary Health Approaches

Complementary health approaches are normally not recommended for anything other than mild injuries, although some pain reduction strategies, such as mindfulness meditation, may be used in conjunction with pharmacologic therapy with provider approval. For patients requiring rehabilitation, therapists may use integrative therapy that is tailored to the patient's specific needs. Thorough assessment of patient preferences regarding the use of complementary health approaches is necessary at each stage of assessment and treatment for patients with multisystem trauma.

Lifespan Considerations

Infants and Toddlers with Multisystem Trauma

Traffic accidents are the leading cause for multisystem trauma in infants and toddlers (**Figure 32–7 》**). Infants and children are more susceptible to multisystem trauma than adults because of their small body size and, with infants, open cranial sutures and fontanels; however, they recover better than adults, especially from head trauma (Children's Health, 2016). The open fontanels allow for increased intracranial mass or brain swelling, which may mask symptoms of injury until a rapid decompensation occurs; therefore, bulging fontanels indicate a severe injury and should be treated as such. The nurse needs to be alert for signs of child abuse. Injuries such as fractured ribs, multicolored bruises, evidence of previous, healed injuries,

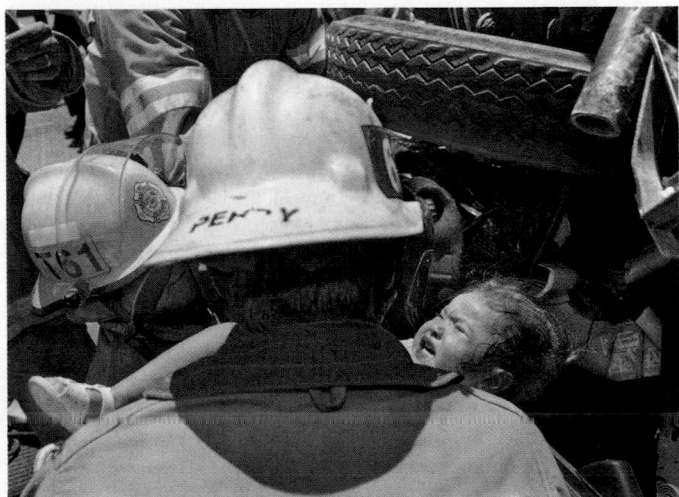

Source: Kari Rene Hall/Los Angeles Times/Getty Images.

Figure 32–7 》 Motor vehicle crashes are the leading cause of multisystem trauma in infants and toddlers. This 2-year-old girl was trapped under a tractor-trailer and had to be extricated using the Jaws of Life. She was in a car seat strapped in the backseat of her mother's car, and she sustained moderate injuries.

fractures of long bones in children younger than 3 years, and retinal hemorrhages may indicate maltreatment and warrant an intensive investigation.

Children and Adolescents with Multisystem Trauma

Assessment priorities for a child are the same as for an adult; however, there may be even more serious effects of trauma in the pediatric patient because of the anatomical and physical characteristics of the younger patient (ACSCOT, 2017). Children are still growing, which means that after a traumatic injury, their body must not only heal from the injury, but also continue to develop.

Children are more likely to experience seizures after head trauma. These seizures usually resolve, but they require diagnostic testing with a CT scan. Injuries to the pancreas, small bowel perforations, and bladder ruptures are more common in children. These injuries are generally from blunt impact such as from bicycle handlebars and seat belts from a motor vehicle crash.

When a child has a fractured bone, the bone will heal, but the bone's growth plate may be affected, causing that affected bone to quit growing. Children are at high risk for tension pneumothorax secondary to mobility of the mediastinal structures. If a pneumothorax is identified, treatment is the same as for adults. The nurse also needs to be alert for signs of maltreatment.

Pregnant Women with Multisystem Trauma

There are two patients when a pregnant woman sustains multisystem trauma—the mother and the fetus; however, treatment priorities are the same for a pregnant woman as for a nonpregnant woman (ACSCOT, 2017). The best treatment for the fetus is resuscitation of the mother. The mother should be assessed, followed by an assessment of the fetus, and then the secondary assessment of the mother.

An increase in blood volume occurs in the pregnant woman. In cases of severe blood loss, the fetus may be in distress and the placenta deprived of oxygen before symptoms (tachycardia, hypotension, and other signs of hypovolemia) occur in the mother. The mother's condition and vital signs may appear stable initially with hypovolemia. It is also important to keep uterine compression of the vena cava from occurring. This can be completed by manually displacing the uterus to the left side, which relieves pressure on the inferior vena cava.

The main cause of fetal demise is maternal shock or death. Abdominal examination is also a priority. In 30% of trauma cases, placenta abruption occurs, which is the second leading cause of fetal death. Fetal heart rate should be monitored closely. A normal fetal heart rate is 120–160 beats/min. It is important to note that abruption of the placenta or other fetal demise does not always cause vaginal bleeding.

Older Adults with Multisystem Trauma

Older adults are less likely to be injured than younger adults; however, they are more likely to have a fatal outcome (ACSCOT, 2017). Falls are the most common cause of multisystem trauma resulting in death (CDC, 2016k). Older adults may be wearing dentures, which could interfere with maintaining airway. Broken dentures should be removed while leaving well-fitted dentures in place. Monitoring the respiratory system closely is critical secondary to the decreased respiratory reserve due to the aging process. A blood pressure reading that is within normal limits may be misleading. Blood pressure generally increases with age; therefore, a systolic reading of 120 mmHg may actually be indicative of hypovolemia. Another consideration regarding the older adult includes obtaining a medication history, as the patient may be on multiple medications. The nurse should always be alert to the increased risk of abuse for this vulnerable population.

NURSING PROCESS

Nursing care of the patient who has been injured begins with a primary assessment and the initiation of collaborative interventions for any life-threatening injuries. Nursing care is directed toward the patient's specific responses to trauma.

Assessment

For the patient who has sustained a traumatic injury, primary consideration should be given to the airway: Assess if the airway is patent, maintainable, or nonmaintainable. Assess for manifestations of airway obstruction: stridor, tachypnea, bradypnea, cough, cyanosis, dyspnea, decreased or absent breath sounds, changes in oxygen levels, and changes in level of consciousness. Assessing the airway and initiating interventions are the first steps in managing the patient with multiple injuries. Cervical and spinal immobilization should be maintained to reduce risk of spinal cord injury. Cervical and spinal immobilization should be discontinued only by physician's order after determining that the patient has not sustained a spinal injury. Although not always needed, this determination may require evaluation of the patient's spine using CT scanning.

Diagnosis

The trauma patient has many complex and interrelated actual or potential alterations in health. The nursing care in this section focuses on patient and family problems with respirations, infection, immobility, spirituality, and stress. Potential nursing diagnoses, which are numerous, may include the following:

- *Airway Clearance, Ineffective*
- *Breathing Pattern, Ineffective*
- *Tissue Perfusion, Risk for Decreased Cardiac*
- *Tissue Perfusion, Risk for Ineffective Peripheral*
- *Fluid Volume, Risk for Deficient*
- *Infection, Risk for*
- *Mobility: Physical, Impaired*
- *Spiritual Distress*
- *Post-Trauma Syndrome.*

(NANDA-I © 2014)

Planning

Goals are based on individualized patient needs and the type and amount of trauma sustained. Goals may include the following:

- The patient's airway will remain patent.
- The patient will demonstrate regular, non-labored respirations and oxygen saturation levels of 95% or greater.
- The patient's blood pressure will be maintained within normal limits.
- The patient will not develop cardiac dysrhythmias.
- The patient will remain free of signs or symptoms of infection.
- The patient will remain free of sensory deficits.
- The patient will retain or regain mobility.

Implementation

As with any traumatic injury, nursing interventions begin with the ABCDEs. Only after ensuring an intact airway, appropriate breathing, and adequate circulation are other issues addressed.

Maintain Airway Patency and Ventilation

The patient with multiple injuries is at great risk for developing airway obstruction and apnea. Facial injuries, loose teeth, blood, and vomitus increase the risk for aspiration and obstruction. Neurologic injuries and cerebral edema alter the patient's respiratory drive and ability to keep the airway clear.

- For patients who do not require tracheal intubation and controlled or assisted ventilation, administer supplemental oxygen per hospital protocols by way of face mask or nasal cannula.
- Monitor oxygen saturation by applying a pulse oximeter. Adjust oxygen flow to maintain oxygen saturation from 95 to 100%. Decreased oxygen saturation readings despite a patent airway may indicate inadequate ventilation or ineffective oxygen exchange.

SAFETY ALERT Pulse oximetry in patients who have been exposed to carbon monoxide (i.e., house fires) is unreliable because it cannot differentiate carboxyhemoglobin from oxyhemoglobin.

- Monitor level of consciousness. An early sign of an ineffective airway is change in the patient's behavior. If the patient becomes restless, anxious, combative, or unresponsive, the effectiveness of the airway needs to be evaluated immediately and appropriate interventions initiated.

Assess for Neurologic Deficits and Expose Obscured Areas

For a trauma assessment, neurologic status and exposure are also assessed.

- Neurologic assessment includes identifying altered level of consciousness, abnormal pupillary response to light, impaired or diminished mobility, and decreased or absent sensation.

- Exposure requires removal of the patient's clothing to allow for identification of injuries that may be obscured. Expose the patient only as needed for assessment and treatment.

- Full assessment requires that the patient be rolled to one side for inspection of the back and posterior of the body. When rolling the patient to one side, the trauma team will use a technique known as "logrolling," which allows for maintenance of neutral alignment of the spine.

- To prevent hypothermia, warm blankets may be used to cover the patient, and the room temperature may be increased during periods for which exposure is required.

Promote Fluid Volume Balance

Both blood loss and the shifting of fluid from the intravascular space can lead to hypovolemia, which, if left untreated, may progress to cardiovascular shock. Therefore, the plan of care for patients who sustain significant traumatic injuries includes:

- Insertion of a large-bore IV catheter (at minimum, 18-gauge or larger in diameter) for administration of fluids, medications, and blood products.

- Administration of IV fluid and blood products as per the physician's orders.

- Insertion of a Foley catheter for continued assessment of urine production, which is an indirect reflection of the patient's kidney function and fluid volume status.

Prevent Infection

Traumatic injuries are considered dirty wounds. Projectiles enter the body through dirty surfaces and clothing, carrying dirt and debris into the wound. Open fractures provide a portal for the entry of bacteria and dirt. Even with surgical intervention, the wounds often remain contaminated. Risk factors for wound infection include contamination, inadequate wound care, and the condition of the wound at the time of closure. Aseptic techniques used in applying and changing dressings reduce the entry of organisms:

- Use careful hand hygiene practices. Hand hygiene remains the single most important factor in preventing the spread of infection.

- Use strict standard precautions and aseptic technique when caring for wounds. Standard precautions are essential to protect the patient and the nurse from infection. In addition, perform the following:
  a. Monitor wounds for odor, redness, heat, swelling, and copious or purulent drainage.
  b. Monitor hidden wounds, such as those under casts, by asking the patient whether the pain has increased and observing for increased drainage and heat over the area of the wound.
  c. Ensure that cross-contamination between wounds does not occur. Collect drainage in ostomy bags if it is copious.

- Take and record vital signs, including temperature, every 2–4 hours. Abnormal vital signs, particularly an elevated body temperature, indicate the presence of an infection.

- Provide adequate fluids and nutrition. Adequate fluids, calories, and protein are essential to wound healing.

- Assess for manifestations of gas gangrene: fever, pain, and swelling in traumatized tissues and drainage with a foul odor. Gas gangrene is usually caused by the organism *Clostridium perfringens*. This bacterium is found in the soil and can be introduced into the body during a traumatic injury. The organism grows in the tissues, causing necrosis; hydrogen and carbon dioxide are released, with resultant swelling of tissues. If the infection continues, tissues are progressively destroyed, and sepsis and death may result.

- Assess status of tetanus immunization and administer tetanus toxoid or human toxin-antitoxin as prescribed.

- Use strict aseptic technique when inserting catheters, suctioning, administering parenteral medications, or performing any other invasive procedure. Using aseptic technique during invasive procedures reduces the chances of infection.

Promote Mobility

The patient with trauma injuries is often unable to change positions independently and is at risk for complications of the integumentary, cardiovascular, gastrointestinal, respiratory, musculoskeletal, and renal systems. Patients at greatest risk are those who have multiple injuries, spinal cord injuries, peripheral nerve injuries, or traumatic amputations. Collaborate with the physical therapist and occupational therapist (if available) to determine the most effective types and schedule of exercises and assistive devices:

- If active bleeding or edema is not present, provide active or passive exercises to affected and unaffected extremities at least once every 8 hours. Exercise improves muscle tone, maintains joint mobility, improves circulation, and prevents contractures.

- Help the patient turn, cough, and breathe deeply, and use the incentive spirometer at least every 2 hours. Changing positions, coughing, deep breathing, and incentive spirometry reduce the risk of integumentary and respiratory complications.

- If the patient is unable to be moved and positioned, consider a specialty bed, such as the kinetic continuous rotation bed. The kinetic continuous rotation bed allows continuous turning of the patient; the motion decreases pulmonary complications, venous stasis, postural hypotension, urinary stasis, muscle wasting, development of decubiti, and bone demineralization.

- Monitor the lower extremities each day for manifestations of deep venous thrombosis: heat, swelling, and pain. Measure and record the circumference of the thigh and calf each day. If anti-embolic stockings or intermittent compression stockings are used, remove them for 1 hour during each shift and assess the skin. Venous stasis results when surrounding muscles are unable to contract and help move the blood through the veins. Thrombus (clot) formation in deep veins is a major risk for pulmonary embolism.

Offer Spiritual Comfort Measures

Trauma generally strikes without warning and carries potentially devastating consequences, including death or severe alterations in the lives of the victim and family. The traumatic death of a loved one may be the most difficult event a family will ever experience. The decision to cease life support systems or to donate organs challenges the family's belief systems and psychologic stability. Nursing care of the family (or patient) experiencing spiritual distress includes:

- Give the family information about the option to donate the patient's organs. The decision to donate organs needs to be based on information about the patient's condition, prognosis, and criteria by which brain death is determined. It is important to convey to family members that organ donation is only an option and that the choice is up to them.

- Encourage the family members to ask questions and express their feelings about the traumatic event and/or organ donation. Allowing families to express their feelings may help prevent long-term consequences such as guilt.

- Refer the family for follow-up care. Long-term follow-up is important for the family facing the sudden death of a loved one. Grieving is not an overnight process, and providing the family with resources that may be used in the future may prevent future crises and dysfunction.

- Provide the family of the dying or deceased patient a place and time to pray or observe faith rituals together. Provide the family the opportunity to call for the family minister or spiritual leader. Praying or observing faith rituals helps the family begin a healthy process of grieving.

- Be present for the family. By providing presence, the nurse provides a level of support and assures the family that they and their loved one are valued and respected. More information about providing spiritual support can be found in the module on Spirituality.

Promote Psychosocial Well-Being

Acute stress disorder is an immediate, intense, sustained emotional response to a disastrous event. It is characterized by emotions that range from anger to fear and by flashbacks or psychic numbing. The patient may be calm or may express feelings of anger, disbelief, terror, and shock, which may last from 3 days up to 1 month. Some individuals who witness or experience a traumatic event may develop PTSD, characterized by flashbacks and nightmares of the traumatic event (see the exemplar that follows). The patient may use ineffective coping mechanisms, such as alcohol or drugs, and withdraw from relationships. Appropriate interventions may include the following:

- Assess emotional responses while providing physical care. Observe for crying, sleep problems, suspiciousness, and fear during the initial phase of treatment. If the patient is unconscious, encourage family members and friends to express their feelings. These assessments provide valuable information about the patient's ability to cope with the trauma.

- Be available if the patient wishes to talk about the trauma, and encourage expression of feelings. The patient may initially deny negative feelings; this denial is a coping mechanism in the initial phase of recovery.

- Teach relaxation techniques, such as deep breathing, progressive muscle relaxation, or imagery. These techniques are often useful in coping when thoughts of the trauma recur.

- Refer the patient and family members for counseling, psychotherapy, or support groups as appropriate. Continued therapy may be necessary to assist the patient and family to resolve the acute and long-term effects of trauma.

Facilitate Community-Based Care

Address the following topics to prepare the patient and family for home care:

- The type of home environment to which the patient will be returning, including any changes that will be required to let the patient function in that environment

- Medications, dressings, wound care, equipment, and supplies

- Special diet, if needed

- Rehabilitation plan and its effect on the patient's family

- Follow-up appointments with the provider or at the trauma clinic

- Emotional changes that the patient may undergo as a result of the trauma

- Helpful resources include home healthcare, community support groups, and the National Institute of Neurological Disorders and Stroke.

Evaluation

The reaction and future care of each patient will vary based on the type and severity of injuries. In some cases, the patient will be discharged the same day as the injury, whereas other patients will need treatment for a longer period. Some desired outcomes for patients include the following:

- The patient's airway remains free of obstruction.

- The patient's respiratory rate remains within normal limits.

- The patient's oxygen saturation is maintained at 95% or greater.

- The patient develops no cardiac dysrhythmias.

- The patient's blood pressure is maintained within normal limits.

- The patient remains free of signs or symptoms of infection.

- The patient develops no neurovascular deficits.

- The patient retains mobility.

- The patient verbally expresses emotions and concerns.

If outcomes are not met, another evaluation will need to occur to determine what is preventing the patient from meeting established goals. For example, if the patient is not able to bear weight in the set amount of time, there may be an unidentified injury or complications related to a post-surgical procedure. Another example would be that the patient's vital signs do not stabilize after surgery. An assessment will need to occur to determine the cause of the decompensation, which may be an unidentified internal hemorrhage.

Nursing Care Plan
A Patient with Multiple Injuries

Jane Souza is a 25-year-old married woman with two children who provides day care for preschool children in her home. As she is driving the interstate at 65 miles per hour, a car crosses the median and strikes her vehicle head-on. Ms. Souza, who is not wearing a seat belt, is thrown forward against the steering wheel. The front of her car is pushed up against her by the car that struck her, entrapping her lower extremities. After extensive efforts to extricate her from the car, Ms. Souza is transported to the local trauma center. She is still conscious, is receiving high-flow oxygen by mask, and has one intravenous line in place. Her vital signs are a palpable systolic blood pressure of 80 mmHg, a pulse rate of 120 bpm, and a respiratory rate of 36/min. On arrival, she states that she is having difficulty breathing.

ASSESSMENT

- *Airway:* Maintainable with high-flow oxygen in place.
- *Breathing:* Respiratory rate of 36/min, multiple bruising and abrasions on right side of her chest, decreased breath sounds on the right side.
- *Circulation:* No palpable radial pulses; palpable brachial pulses. Monitor shows sinus tachycardia. No active external bleeding noted. Skin color pale, cool to the touch, and diaphoretic.
- *Neurologic:* Moved her fingers when asked; complains of difficulty breathing; denies that she is hurt. Pupils 4 mm, equal, and react to light. Has a broken right arm and an open fracture of the left ankle; because of these injuries, extremity movement is limited.

Because of Ms. Souza's respiratory distress, she is intubated and ventilated with 100% oxygen. Another intravenous line is inserted and O-negative blood administered.

DIAGNOSES

- *Ineffective Breathing Pattern* related to multiple bruises and abrasions on the right side of the chest, and respiratory difficulty
- *Deficient Fluid Volume* related to acute internal blood loss (presumed because no active bleeding can be found)
- *Risk for Injury* related to trauma resuscitation

(NANDA-I © 2014)

PLANNING

Patient goals include:

- The patient will maintain adequate oxygenation.
- The patient will maintain adequate circulating blood volume.

IMPLEMENTATION

- Monitor airway and assist in any needed airway management.
- Explain all procedures.
- Monitor the effects of fluid and blood administration, including any changes in blood pressure and pulse.
- Prepare for transfer to the operating room for emergency surgery.
- Keep family informed about her condition.

EVALUATION

Ms. Souza is transferred to the operating room, where it is determined that she has a ruptured spleen and a serious pelvic fracture.

Ms. Souza's treatment continues in the operating room.

CRITICAL THINKING

1. Is the nursing diagnosis of Deficient Fluid Volume appropriate for Ms. Souza? Why or why not?
2. The assessment of a patient who has experienced trauma is ABCDE. What is the rationale for this sequence?
3. Following surgery, Ms. Souza is moved to the surgical intensive care unit. She is very anxious and restless. What assessments would you make to identify the cause of her restlessness?
4. Infection is a common complication for the trauma patient. Describe five risks for infection that are present from the time of injury to the time of hospital discharge.

REVIEW Multisystem Trauma

RELATE Link the Concepts and Exemplars

Linking the exemplar of multisystem trauma with the concept of intracranial regulation:

1. What is the priority of care when your patient who experienced a head injury in a car crash has a blood pressure of 90/60 mmHg and a heart rate of 51 bpm?
2. What nursing interventions would be appropriate for inclusion in the plan of care for the patient who has a head injury from a car crash to prevent the rise of intracranial pressure?

Linking the exemplar of multisystem trauma with the concept of perfusion:

3. Describe potential threats to a patient's perfusion as a result of a motor vehicle crash. How would perfusion be impacted if the patient's mobility was altered because of traction or other immobilizing treatments?
4. How can you promote mobility for a patient involved in a motor vehicle crash who has a casted left leg and right arm? How would this plan change if the patient were an older adult with diminished mobility prior to the trauma?

READY Go to Volume 3: Clinical Nursing Skills

REFER Go to Pearson MyLab Nursing and eText

- Additional review materials

REFLECT Apply Your Knowledge

Lilia Hoffman, age 25, was the driver of a vehicle that was struck by another vehicle at an intersection. The driver of the car that hit her ran a red light. Ms. Hoffman was extracted from her car using the Jaws of Life and was moaning when initially removed but did not respond to verbal commands. Her pupils were pinpoint and reactive to light. The paramedics at the scene provided initial emergent care. Her vital signs included temperature 96.2°F oral; pulse 110 bpm; respirations 12/min; and BP 90/50 mmHg. She had bleeding from facial and scalp lacerations as well as suspected rib fractures. Her lung sounds were clear and equal bilaterally, and her oxygen saturation was 97%. Ms. Hoffman's airway was determined to be patent and oxygen was administered via face mask at 10 liters per minute.

The air bag in Ms. Hoffman's car deployed. It was unknown whether she sustained a head or neck injury. One of the paramedics immediately administered manual stabilization of Ms. Hoffman's cervical spine until a cervical collar (c-collar) was applied. In addition to c-spine immobilization, Ms. Hoffman was placed on a long spinal board to prepare for transport to the local emergency department. Circulatory status was assessed and an 18-gauge intravenous catheter was inserted in her left forearm, followed by intravenous administration of 0.9% normal saline at a rate of 150 mL/hr.

In the emergency department, Ms. Hoffman's vital signs were temperature 98°F oral; pulse 118 bpm; respirations 14/min; and BP 98/50 mmHg. An IV bolus of 250 mL of normal saline was administered and a Foley catheter inserted. Her airway remained patent and oxygen was continued.

1. What are three priority nursing diagnoses for Ms. Hoffman?
2. What laboratory and diagnostic tests should the nurse anticipate being ordered?
3. Under what circumstances can Ms. Hoffman's spinal precautions (cervical collar and longboard spinal immobilization) be discontinued?

 # Exemplar 32.C
Posttraumatic Stress Disorder

Exemplar Learning Outcomes

32.C Analyze PTSD as it relates to trauma.

- Describe the pathophysiology of PTSD.
- Describe the etiology of PTSD.
- Compare the risk factors and prevention of PTSD.
- Identify the clinical manifestations of PTSD.
- Summarize therapies used by interprofessional teams in the collaborative care of an individual with PTSD.

- Differentiate care of patients with PTSD across the lifespan.
- Apply the nursing process in providing culturally competent care to an individual with PTSD.

Exemplar Key Terms

Acute stress disorder, *2147*
Depersonalization, *2148*
Eye movement desensitization and reprocessing (EMDR), *2149*
Flashbacks, *2147*
Posttraumatic stress disorder (PTSD), *2146*

Overview

Each individual responds to traumatic events differently based on their own personal history, coping mechanisms, and the exact circumstances surrounding the nature of the traumatic event. For an individual to be diagnosed with a trauma or stressor-related disorder (e.g., acute stress disorder or PTSD), the individual must meet specific criteria for diagnosis, of which the first is exposure to a traumatic or stressful event. There is a close relationship between trauma-related disorders and anxiety, obsessive-compulsive, and dissociative disorders. Depending on the individual, emotional symptoms of trauma or stressor-related disorders can vary greatly from fear and anxiety to agitation and dysphoria. **Posttraumatic stress disorder (PTSD)** is commonly associated with military personnel, specifically those returning from war; however, PTSD can affect any individual from any background across the lifespan.

The APA (2013) characterizes PTSD as a disorder in which an individual who is exposed to a traumatic event develops intrusive symptoms, such as recurrent nightmares; patterns of persistent efforts to avoid stimuli associated with

or reminiscent of the traumatic event; negative changes in cognition or mood; and marked changes in reactivity or arousal, such as hypervigilance or impaired concentration. For an individual to be diagnosed, these symptoms must occur for more than 1 month beyond the precipitating event.

Along with PTSD, this class of disorders also includes (APA, 2013):

- Reactive attachment disorder, which is a rare disorder in young children that is often associated with neglect; manifests as an apparent aversion to engaging in interaction with adults.

- Disinhibited social engagement disorder, which is most commonly diagnosed in young children and is associated with neglect. Manifestations include an abnormal propensity for the child to interact with unfamiliar adults.

- Acute stress disorder, which is similar to PTSD, but the symptoms only last from 3 days to 1 month following exposure to one or more traumatic events such as war, experiencing assault, being kidnapped, or natural or human-caused disasters.

- Adjustment disorders, which are characterized according to the patient's manifestations (e.g., depressed mood, anxiety, disturbance of conduct), begin approximately 3 months after a stressor, and resolve within 6 months.

Pathophysiology and Etiology

Pathophysiology

In the United States, recent events have brought discussion of PTSD to the forefront. For example, some of those who experienced, witnessed, or attended to survivors of the World Trade Center attacks on September 11, 2001, have spoken publicly about their personal experiences with PTSD. Recent wars and conflicts, particularly in the Middle East, have resulted in a significant rise in PTSD in military and civilian personnel (**Figure 32–8 》**). Natural disasters, such as hurricanes and fires, also provide sources of trauma, as do the increasing incidences of mass shootings such as the 2012 shootings in a theater in Aurora, Colorado, and an elementary school in Newtown, Connecticut; and more recently, a night club shooting in Orlando, Florida, in 2016.

Traumatic events that may trigger PTSD include violent personal assaults, natural or human-caused disasters, motor vehicle crashes, military combat, being taken hostage or being tortured, imprisonment, dismemberment, incest, and child abuse. PTSD also can stem from sexual assault or being subjected to sexual experiences during childhood (APA, 2013). Even threats of violence or injury may prompt the development of PTSD. However, intentional infliction of harm or violence, such as torture or rape, is associated with a higher incidence of this disorder (APA, 2013).

PTSD may manifest through numerous signs and symptoms, including fear-based reexperiencing of the event; alterations in emotional and behavioral states; dysphoric mood and negative cognitive states; and alterations in arousal and reactivity (APA, 2013). Some patients will experience manifestations that predominantly reflect one

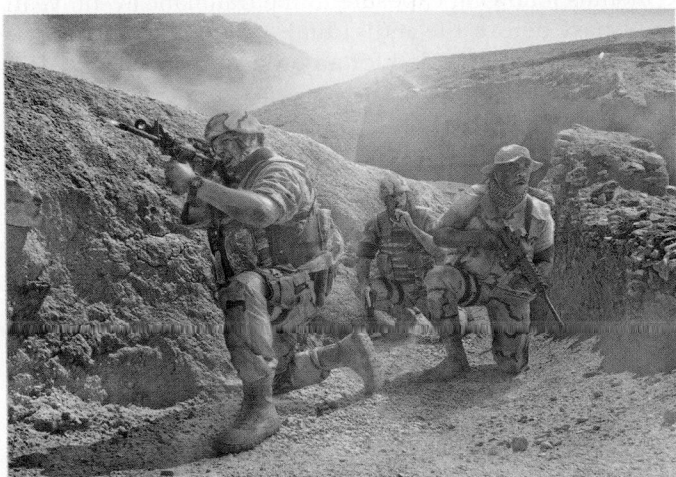

Source: Blend Images/Alamy Stock Photo.

Figure 32–8 》 Many military personnel in or returning from the wars in Iraq and Afghanistan experience PTSD.

Box 32–1
Overview of Acute Stress Disorder

Although there are similarities between **acute stress disorder** and PTSD, the two disorders are separate and distinct from one another. The individual with acute stress disorder experiences symptoms for 3 days to 1 month immediately after exposure to a traumatic event. In contrast, patients with PTSD experience symptoms for more than 1 month, with the onset of symptoms usually occurring 3 months or more after exposure to the trauma (APA, 2013).

Acute stress disorder stems from an individual experiencing, learning of, or witnessing an extremely stressful event that involves the threat of death, actual or threatened serious injury, or actual physical or sexual violation. The individual is said to be experiencing acute stress disorder if he experiences nine (or more) symptoms from any of five categories—intrusion (intrusive distressing memories), negative mood, dissociation (an altered sense or reality or dissociative amnesia), avoidance, and arousal (such as sleep disturbances, irritability, or poor concentration)—that begin or get worse after the traumatic event (APA, 2013).

category of alterations, whereas others will experience a combination of manifestations (APA, 2013).

When reexperiencing the traumatic event, the individual with PTSD may experience **flashbacks**, the recurrence of images, sounds, smells, or feelings from the traumatic event. Flashbacks are often triggered by daily events, such as a car backfiring on the street or the smell of a perpetrator's cologne. In the affected individual's mind, flashbacks may be so lifelike that they appear to be happening in reality. Frequently, the individual experiences recurrent nightmares or intrusive memories related to the traumatic event.

Some individuals who experience trauma may experience acute stress during the immediate aftermath of the trauma. An acute stress or anxiety response sufficient to impair functioning may result in acute stress disorder, discussed in **Box 32–1 》**. Acute stress disorder shares several factors with PTSD, but is of a much shorter duration.

Etiology

Exposure to an overwhelming stressor can occur at any age. Childhood trauma, abuse, and molestation can create enduring effects and clinical symptoms that last into adulthood. Additional factors that contribute to the development of PTSD are an individual history of a psychiatric disorder or a lack of emotional support or resources during the trauma. Among adults in the United States, the prevalence of PTSD is about 3.5% (NIMH, n.d.), with women being more susceptible to its development (APA, 2013). Incidence among veterans is particularly high: One report documents that, of military personnel who had been deployed in overseas combat presenting for treatment at VA healthcare centers, 21% were treated for PTSD. Incidence increases when TBI is present: 75% of combat personnel who experienced TBI had a concurrent diagnosis of PTSD (Congressional Budget Office, 2012).

Focus on Diversity and Culture
Refugee Trauma

In 2013, a total of 69,909 refugees were admitted into the United States (Homeland Security, Office of Immigration Statistics, 2014). Refugee trauma is a form of PTSD that is specific to the traumatic events experienced by individuals during war or persecution that may have lifelong effects. Child refugees may exhibit symptoms such as nightmares, anxiety, psychosomatic symptoms, hopelessness, and disrupted sleep patterns (NCTSN, n.d.c). Adult refugees frequently experience negative manifestations of PTSD and depression (Harvard Program in Refugee Trauma, n.d.). The refugees will also need to be assessed for physical trauma secondary to possible torture and other forms of violence endured (see **Figure 32–9 》》**).

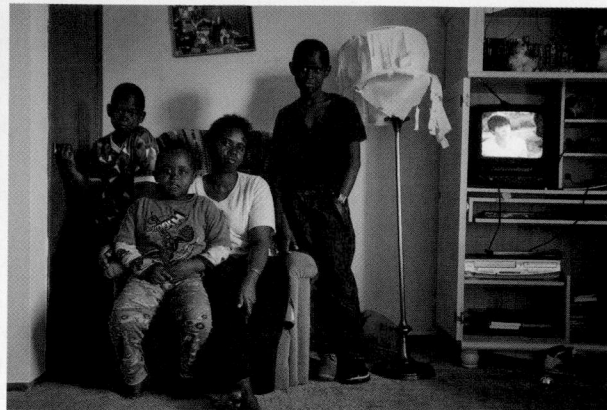

Source: Christophe Calais/Corbis Historical/Getty Images.

Figure 32–9 》 This family, originally from the Democratic Republic of Congo, was living in a refugee camp in Burundi called Gatumba in 2004. One night, armed factions attacked the refugee camp, killed 166 people, and injured another 116. The oldest boy in this family had a leg amputated. Since that night, 525 Gatumba survivors have been relocated to North America. This family lives in Boise, Idaho, where the mother works as a chambermaid.

Risk Factors

Individuals of any age and any cultural group may develop PTSD. In the United States, the incidence of this disorder is higher among military veterans, law enforcement officers, firefighters, and emergency medical personnel (APA, 2013). Risk factors for PTSD include the following:

- The severity of the event itself, including whether or not the individual was harmed or watched others be harmed or killed

- Little or no social or psychologic support following the trauma

- Additional stressors immediately following the event, such as loss of a spouse or family member or loss of employment

- Presence of preexisting mental illness.

Prevention

The most effective way to prevent the development of PTSD is for the individual to use their support system after exposure to a traumatic event. This may mean reaching out to family and friends or seeking professional help. Obtaining help and support as soon as possible after exposure is integral in preventing normal stress reactions from developing into acute stress disorder or longer term PTSD. Obtaining support will aid the individual in using positive, effective coping skills and prevent her from succumbing to ineffective coping skills such as self-medicating with drugs and alcohol (Mayo Clinic, 2014c).

Clinical Manifestations

Patients who experience flashbacks may lose touch with reality and may cognitively return to the traumatic incident as if it is happening again. Some may experience **depersonalization**, an emotional numbing and a loss of their sense of reality, feelings, and sense of self in relation to others. Patients who experience depersonalization may have difficulty in interpersonal relationships and with trusting or being affectionate. Things they formerly enjoyed may not provide pleasure for them anymore. Individuals may express uncharacteristic irritability, aggression, and violence.

Hyperarousal and hypervigilance are associated with PTSD, rendering the affected individual in a near-constant state of "high alert." The individual may experience sleep disturbances and become restless. He may also feel a strong sense of agitation and have poor concentration. Dissociation, in which the individual blocks emotions related to the traumatic event, or dissociative amnesia, in which certain elements of the traumatic event are blocked altogether, may occur. The emotional numbness that can occur leads to impairment in establishing and maintaining social relationships. As with other anxiety disorders, depression may accompany PTSD. Likewise, individuals with PTSD may abuse alcohol or other substances to alleviate their symptoms.

Although manifestations of PTSD usually emerge within 3 months following exposure to the traumatic event, years may pass before the individual's signs and symptoms meet the criteria needed for an official diagnosis of PTSD (APA, 2013).

Collaboration

Caring for the patient with PTSD requires the skillful ability to assess and facilitate the care of patients, families, and communities. As a patient advocate, the nurse must effectively connect individuals with the resources they need to recover successfully from trauma. These resources may include financial resources, such as social services; medical resources, such as free clinics and mental health providers who treat uninsured patients on a sliding-scale basis; and agencies that provide food and shelter. If support from a spiritual leader is requested, it should be provided.

Because of the all-encompassing impact of trauma on an individual's life, a holistic approach to treatment may be most effective, combining pharmacologic and alternative therapies, such as relaxation techniques, CBT, eye movement

Clinical Manifestations and Therapies
Acute and Posttraumatic Stress Disorders

ETIOLOGY	CLINICAL MANIFESTATIONS	CLINICAL THERAPIES
Acute Stress Disorder Anxiety disorder that evolves from exposure to actual trauma or threat of physical harm. Recovery varies from 3 days to 1 month.	■ Intrusive distressing memories ■ Negative mood ■ Dissociation ■ Avoidance ■ Arousal problems	■ Ensure the safety of the patient and provide basic needs. ■ Promote support by family and friends. ■ Provide patient teaching related to coping mechanisms. ■ Provide emotional support. ■ Administer medications as prescribed to decrease arousal. ■ Holistic approach to treatment includes CBT.
PTSD Anxiety disorder that evolves from exposure to actual trauma or threat of physical harm. Recovery varies from 1 month to several years. Comorbidity may include depression, substance abuse, or other anxiety disorders.	■ Persistent frightening thoughts and memories or flashbacks of the event: images, sounds, smells, or feelings ■ Emotional numbing ■ Sleep disorders ■ Hypervigilance and exaggerated startle response ■ Reexperiencing the event ■ Trouble with affection ■ Irritability, aggressiveness, or violence ■ Avoidance of trauma-related situations or general social contacts ■ Drug and alcohol abuse ■ Depression ■ Suicidal thoughts or violence	■ Holistic approach to treatment includes CBT. ■ Eye movement desensitization and reprocessing. ■ Supportive therapy. ■ Group therapy. ■ Pharmacologic therapy, including benzodiazepines, SSRIs, and antipsychotic agents. ■ Prazosin, which is an antihypertensive medication that also inhibits the brain's response to norepinephrine, may be prescribed for treatment and prevention of nightmares (Mayo Clinic, 2014a).

desensitization and response therapy (discussed below), and support from a multiagency team of providers.

Pharmacologic Therapy

Depending on the severity and nature of a patient's PTSD manifestations, SSRIs are often used in conjunction with psychotherapy as a treatment. The only two SSRIs approved by the U.S. Food and Drug Administration (FDA) for the treatment of PTSD are sertraline (Zoloft) and paroxetine (Paxil). Prazosin, which is an antihypertensive medication, is effective in the reduction of nightmares associated with PTSD (Mayo Clinic, 2014a).

SAFETY ALERT SSRI medications may produce undesirable side effects; therefore, it is important to educate the patient that most side effects will diminish after the first few weeks. If the patient does not understand this, the risk of nonadherence to the medication regimen increases, leaving the patient untreated and susceptible to decompensation of illness.

Nonpharmacologic Therapy

Eye movement desensitization and reprocessing (EMDR) is a form of psychotherapy that contains elements of several types of therapy, including CBT and body-centered therapy. It is so named because one of the elements involves dual attention stimulus using eye movements, taps, or tones. *Dual attention stimulus* allows the patient to reprocess or reappraise the trauma by focusing internally on the traumatic event or another stressor while simultaneously focusing on a different external stimulus (EMDR Institute, n.d.).

Exposure therapy assists the patient by gradually exposing them to elements of the traumatic event, which enables them to face their fears. This form of treatment uses writing, pictures, and possibly visiting the place where the traumatic event occurred (NIMH, 2016). This form of therapy allows the patient to develop effective coping skills in a safe, controlled environment. The use of virtual reality also assists the patient in revisiting the site where the traumatic event occurred without having to go back to the real site (Mayo Clinic, 2014a).

Preliminary research indicates that acupuncture may be effective in treating patients with PTSD. Patients may need to participate in acupuncture on a regular basis for a period of 3 months or more (National Center for Complementary and Integrative Health [NCCIH], 2014). Nurses working with patients who are interested in trying acupuncture as a treatment for PTSD should encourage the patients to add

Focus on Integrative Health
PTSD

The U.S. Department of Veterans Affairs and Department of Defense identify psychopharmacology, stress inoculation, exposure, and/or CBT as the front-line, best standard approach to PTSD (International Society for Traumatic Stress Studies, 2016). Complementary integrative health (CIH) approaches, such as yoga and meditation, can also be taught to the patient. Stress inoculation is a form of psychotherapy in which the therapist educates the patient on the stress that they may endure, including the negative outcomes. This enables the patient to have an effective plan to address the negative obstacles he may encounter (Mills, Reiss, & Dombeck, n.d.). Prolonged exposure therapy (PE) is a type of exposure therapy that has four components to assist the patient in working through the feelings associated with the traumatic event. The first component is educating the patient on PTSD, including responses and symptoms. Breathing retraining is another component that teaches the patient how to control breathing while experiencing the stressful feelings. Real-world training is another part of PE that helps by having the patient practice situations that they may have been avoiding (e.g., a veteran who may fear driving because of hitting a roadside bomb while at war). Last, talking through the trauma assists the patient in not being fearful of his memories (VA, 2015).

acupuncture as an adjunctive therapy and not to abandon CBT and more traditional therapies.

Lifespan Considerations
PTSD in Children

Manifestations of PTSD in young children vary significantly from those demonstrated by adult patients. For example, children with PTSD who are under the age of 6 years may reexperience the trauma through play in such a way as to overtly or indirectly recreate the traumatic event. Some children may reexperience trauma by drawing pictures that symbolize the trauma. Children with PTSD may also behave recklessly or aggressively, or they may withdraw from interacting with others. Because of their undeveloped ability to express thoughts or identify emotions, expressions of PTSD in very young children often occur through changes in mood (APA, 2013).

Additional symptoms that may be seen in children under the age of 6 years may include nocturnal enuresis after the child has already been toilet trained, forgetting how to talk or not talking at all, acting out the traumatic event during activities with other children, and being exceptionally needy or clingy.

PTSD in Adolescents

Older children and adolescents have manifestations similar to those that the adult experiences; however, they may also demonstrate disruptive, disrespectful, or destructive behaviors (NIMH, 2016). Adolescents may engage in traumatic reenactment where the traumatic event(s) have been injected into their daily life. Impulsive and aggressive behaviors are more typical of this age group as well (VA, 2016c). Furthermore, there is an increased risk of suicide, substance abuse, poor social support, poor concentration, academic problems, and poor physical health with adolescents diagnosed with PTSD (Nooner et al., 2012).

PTSD in Older Adults

PTSD in older adults is not limited to veterans, although it is often associated with the experiences of a soldier. According to the VA, 70–90% of adults age 65 and older have experienced at least one traumatic event during their lifetime (VA, 2016d). Older veterans may report more somatic complaints, fewer typical PTSD general symptoms, and less depression, hostility, and guilt than younger veterans (VA, 2016d).

A complete mental status exam, including cognitive screening, is recommended when assessing the older adult. Assessment of the history of trauma and symptomatology should be performed routinely, as these patients may minimize the significance of this history or not report it at all, as it likely occurred a long time ago. Note that older patients may report somatic symptoms as opposed to emotional symptoms. The older adult who may be experiencing PTSD symptoms should be assessed using a valid PTSD measuring tool and be assessed for suicidal thoughts and behaviors, because they are at increased risk of suicide compared with middle-aged adults (VA, 2016e).

NURSING PROCESS

Patients with PTSD experiencing hyperarousal and vigilance may exhibit unpredictable, aggressive, or bizarre behavior. The nursing priorities for these patients are ensuring the safety of the patient and others while quickly lowering patient anxiety levels. The patient with PTSD exhibiting extreme anxiety needs immediate pharmacologic intervention, a quiet and calm environment, and reassurance that he or she is safe. Once anxiety levels are reduced, the healthcare team can help the patient learn a new process of appraisal and coping mechanisms.

Because of the complexity of trauma, families may also experience PTSD and require the nurse's assistance and support. Evaluation of the impact on the family must also be included in the assessment, evaluation, and decision-making process. Families play a key role in the support of the individual. In the case of national disasters, entire communities may be involved in the trauma.

Assessment

Assessing a patient for PTSD will involve both physical and psychologic approaches. Identify risk and protective factors and assess immediate and long-term safety concerns. Multiple tools are available for use in screening for PTSD; some have been developed for use with children. Specific interview questions to ascertain the diagnosis of PTSD are aimed at the following clinical manifestations: reexperiencing or flashbacks, hyperarousal and vigilance, an exaggerated startle response, and sleep disturbances. For example, an interview question might be: "Have you experienced painful images or memories of combat or other trauma which you couldn't get out of your mind, even though you may have wanted to? Have these been recurrent?" (VA, 2016e). Identification of PTSD in children is improved when they are questioned directly about their experiences. Assessment of younger children involves questioning the child and/or the parents about significant changes in behavior and sleeping patterns. For children and vulnerable patients who are believed to be victims of abuse, the nurse should follow organizational protocols for reporting these situations. Questions may include:

- How would you describe your mood?
- When do you feel most content? When do you feel least content?
- What are your favorite activities?
- What activities help you relax?
- How often do you socialize or participate in activities with others?
- Describe your sleep habits. Do you sleep soundly through the night? Do you feel rested when you awaken?
- Do you have friends or other individuals with whom you can be open and honest about your thoughts and emotions?
- How important is being able to share your thoughts and feelings?
- Are you currently working? If so, what type of work are you engaged in?

Because of the traumatization experienced by these patients, as well as the subsequent potential for emotional and physical isolation, establishment of trust can be especially challenging. For example, many military personnel and veterans are resistant to openly sharing their thoughts and emotions even with their colleagues and fellow veterans. During the assessment and throughout the care of all patients with PTSD, the nurse should be aware that direct questioning of the patient with regard to traumatic experiences may inhibit establishment of a trusting relationship and can even provoke frustration and anger in the patient. The nursing assessment should include interview questions that allow for patient assessment without pressuring the patient to reveal information he is not ready or able to share. Through the inclusion of open-ended questions, the nurse affords the patient the opportunity to express himself to the degree with which he is comfortable while demonstrating respect for the patient's personal boundaries.

SAFETY ALERT Safety is always a priority. The nurse must remember that a patient diagnosed with PTSD may demonstrate agitation, aggressiveness, and even violence. The nurse will need to educate the family on the need for a safety plan in the event that the patient becomes violent.

Diagnosis

Evaluating assessment data for an individual with PTSD can be challenging. For some patients with PTSD, manifestations of the disorder can be compounded by substance abuse, depression, and insomnia. Appropriate diagnoses for the patient with PTSD may include any of the following:

- *Violence: Self-Directed, Risk for*
- *Violence: Other Directed, Risk for*
- *Post-Trauma Syndrome*
- *Anxiety*
- *Fear*
- *Coping, Ineffective*
- *Coping: Family, Compromised*
- *Sleep Pattern, Disturbed.*

(NANDA-I © 2014)

The nurse must explore the specific assessment questions directed at PTSD in order not to overlook the possibility of this diagnosis. It is important for the healthcare provider to involve the individual in the decision-making process and to facilitate the individual's preferences.

Planning

Planning includes identification of measurable, realistic patient goals that are relevant to the selected nursing diagnoses. Examples of patient goals that may be relevant to the care of the patient with PTSD include the following:

- The patient will remain free from injury or harm.
- The patient will report a decreased perception of anxiety.
- The patient will report a reduction or cessation of nightmares.
- The patient will discuss emotions related to traumatic experiences with at least one trusted mental health specialist or counseling professional.
- The patient will verbalize awareness of nonpharmacologic stress reduction techniques.

Implementation

The presence of PTSD is not an inevitable outcome of a traumatic event. Some individuals may require only limited interventions. Clinically significant indicators are the severity of the event itself and the severity of the individual's initial response. For patients who develop this disorder, in addition to the interventions described previously, it is important to recognize the profound impact PTSD exerts on components related to multiple aspects of daily life, including an impact on the social, interpersonal, and occupational domains. These patients may benefit from being connected with organizations and community resources that can facilitate long-term assistance and that can offer sensitive guidance to the process for building trusting relationships with others. The nurse should also reinforce understanding of effective coping strategies and encourage their use, which may assist in decreasing anxiety (see the module on Stress and Coping).

Patient Teaching
Typical Human Responses to Traumatic Events

Patients with PTSD should be given ample information about the typical human responses to traumatic events. Education about the process helps patients normalize the experience and gain information for reappraisal. Information and resources can lead to adaptive coping; conversely, a lack of resources may induce maladaptive coping. It is the nurse's responsibility to provide information about the treatments available and support resources for PTSD to help the individual and family make informed choices.

SAFETY ALERT Compassion fatigue (CF) often occurs in healthcare providers who perform caregiving work on a regular basis. Relating to people who are helpless, suffering, or traumatized can precipitate CF. Symptoms of CF include excessive blaming, isolation from others, receiving an unusual amount of complaints, self-medicating with drugs or alcohol, poor concentration, and apathy (Compassion Fatigue Awareness Project, 2013). Once CF is identi-fied, the nurse has already made the first step in overcoming the issue. Actions such as taking care of oneself, expressing needs, and clarifying boundaries will assist in eliminating these negative emotions.

Evaluation

The nurse evaluates the patient's response to treatment using these suggested expected outcomes:

- The patient uses self-calming techniques.
- The patient experiences fewer cognitive distortions and fewer repetitive thoughts (ruminations) or obsessions.
- The patient decreases time spent ruminating over worries, verbalizing more accurate predictions of future events.

If patient outcomes are not met, additional measures should be taken, including evaluation of medication efficacy and adherence to treatment regimen. The patient may need to journal daily events in order to identify triggers, allowing effective coping skills to be incorporated. The patient may need to be encouraged to avoid triggers while learning coping strategies.

Nursing Care Plan
A Patient with Posttraumatic Stress Disorder

Sarah Green is a 44-year-old nurse whose 14-year-old son was killed in a motor vehicle crash (MVC) just over 6 months ago. At the time of the MVC, Ms. Green was driving her son to soccer practice when another vehicle crossed the interstate median and struck her vehicle. Her son died at the scene, and Ms. Green sustained serious injuries. Ms. Green also has a 17-year-old daughter and a 19-year-old son.

ASSESSMENT	DIAGNOSES	PLANNING
At present, Ms. Green attends a support group for grieving parents, which she finds to be therapeutic. However, she has been having flashbacks about the night of the accident and can barely control herself when she knows one of her children is driving or riding in a car. Usually, when one of the children asks to borrow the car she just says "no" to avoid having to worry about them. Ms. Green knows she needs to see someone. She talks to a friend who is also a coworker, who recommends that she talk with an occupational health counselor at work. Ms. Green does not want anyone at work to know she is having trouble, but she agrees to see a mental health nurse that her friend recommends. At her initial appointment, Ms. Green freely shares her experiences with the flashbacks, which happen two or three times a week, usually at night. She says that when she knows her children are going anywhere, she can feel her heart racing, her breathing speeding up, and her palms getting sweaty. She tells the mental health nurse that she gets through these episodes by lying down and saying the Lord's Prayer out loud.	The mental health nurse develops the following nursing diagnoses: - *Post-Trauma Syndrome* - *Anxiety* - *Fear* (NANDA-I © 2014)	Goals for Ms. Green's care include the following: - The patient will use deep breathing to control escalating anxiety. - The patient will express fears clearly. - The patient will describe the symptoms associated with the various levels of anxiety. - The patient will demonstrate breathing exercises to reduce anxiety.

Nursing Care Plan *(continued)*

IMPLEMENTATION

- Teach Ms. Green how to monitor her physiologic level of arousal.
- Teach use of abdominal breathing at first sign of anxiety.
- Help patient to express fears that interfere with her life.
- Encourage patient to search for, confront, and relieve the source of the original anxiety.
- Teach distraction techniques that can control moderate levels of anxiety.

- Teach the use of positive imagery.
- Teach calming techniques such as muscle relaxation.
- Teach positive affirmations such as "I am calm and happy" or "I am very relaxed."
- Identify safe physical outlets for negative feelings, such as exercise.

EVALUATION

- The patient expresses feelings appropriately.
- The patient spends less time thinking about the accident and instead turns thoughts to more positive memories.

- The patient allows her adolescent children to borrow the car, setting reasonable limits to reduce her anxiety.

CRITICAL THINKING

1. What impact does Ms. Green's PTSD have on her children's development?

2. How would you teach Ms. Green relaxation techniques?

REVIEW Posttraumatic Stress Disorder

RELATE Link the Concepts and Exemplars

Linking the exemplar of posttraumatic stress disorder with the concept of development:

Explore the incidence of childhood abuse, molestation, and incest in the Unites States.

1. What impact does childhood abuse, molestation, and incest have on the growth and development of a child?

2. Childhood abuse, molestation, and incest can negatively affect the physical, emotional, spiritual, and cognitive processes of individuals. What alterations in health are associated with abuse later in life?

Linking the exemplar of posttraumatic stress disorder with the concept of mood and affect:

3. What questions should be asked of a patient who is experiencing manifestations of PTSD and expresses hopelessness?

4. What nursing interventions should be employed if the patient with PTSD is expressing suicidal ideation?

READY Go to Volume 3: Clinical Nursing Skills

REFER Go to Pearson MyLab Nursing and eText

- Additional review materials

REFLECT Apply Your Knowledge

Melinda Burns lives in Manhattan. She is engaged to be married to a man she says she loves very much, and although this should be the happiest time of her life, she is feeling very anxious and stressed.

She was 12 years old on September 11, 2001, when terrorists attacked the United States. She was in school when the planes hit the World Trade Center. They had to evacuate the school after the collapse of the buildings because the ash was so thick it made breathing difficult. Her father picked her up, and they went to a hotel room in New Jersey because their apartment was also covered in ash. They weren't allowed to go home until several weeks later. Ms. Burns' grandmother stayed with her in the hotel room while her father tried to find her mother, who worked on the 92nd floor of the North Tower. Her dad never found her mother, and she never came home. Ms. Burns says the worst part is that her mother's body was never identified from the wreckage, so she feels like she has no closure or confirmation that her mother is really dead. One of the New York firemen came to their home almost a year later to return a necklace that was found, and the engraving helped them identify it as her mom's. Ms. Burns treasures the necklace even though it is badly damaged and burned.

Ms. Burns is seeking care because she is having trouble functioning and difficulty performing ADLs. She reports severe anxiety whenever she hears a siren, she has been waking from nightmares related to the World Trade Center several times a week, and she can't bring herself to watch any television programs or movies about the terrorist attack because they always make her cry. She has turned down a number of jobs because she can't bring herself to work on the upper levels of tall buildings. She says lately she has been having trouble concentrating, even when planning her wedding, because she can't seem to think about anything other than the World Trade Center and what her mother's final minutes must have been like.

1. What nursing diagnoses are appropriate for Ms. Burns?

2. What collaborative actions can the healthcare team take to help Ms. Burns?

3. What independent nursing interventions would you initiate if Ms. Burns was your patient?

» Exemplar 32.D
Rape and Rape-Trauma Syndrome

Exemplar Learning Outcomes

32.D Analyze rape and rape-trauma syndrome as they relate to trauma.

- Describe the pathophysiology of rape and rape-trauma syndrome.
- Describe the etiology of rape and rape-trauma syndrome.
- Compare the risk factors and prevention of rape and rape-trauma syndrome.
- Identify the clinical manifestations of rape and rape-trauma syndrome.
- Summarize diagnostic tests and therapies used by interprofessional teams in the collaborative care of an individual who has been raped.

- Differentiate care of patients across the lifespan who have been raped.
- Apply the nursing process in providing culturally competent care to an individual who has been raped.

Exemplar Key Terms

Acquaintance rape, 2155
Marital rape, 2155
Rape, 2154
Rape-trauma syndrome (RTS), 2154

Overview

Rape is one form of sexual violence. According to the FBI (2012c), **rape** is "penetration, no matter how slight, of the vagina or anus with any body part or object, or oral penetration by a sex organ of another person, without the consent of the victim." Because rape occurs at the hands of another and involves loss of control, individuals who are raped are often referred to as "victims" by law enforcement, as seen in the definition provided by the FBI. However, healthcare and mental health professionals working with individuals who have been raped commonly use the term "survivor" for empowerment purposes.

Each individual who is raped will have a unique reaction to the incident. Variations in reactions can be due to the individual's past history, personality, the circumstances of the event, whether infection or pregnancy occurs, and many other factors. For decades, clinicians working with rape survivors have recognized **rape-trauma syndrome (RTS)**, a series of psychologic sequelae that many individuals experience following rape in addition to physiologic sequelae. Although symptoms and reactions vary widely, most survivors of rape experience great emotional and physical impact. Many initially exhibit shock and disbelief, followed by fear, humiliation, shame, self-blame, and distrust in others (CDC, 2016n). Emotional detachment, sleep disturbances, flashbacks, and mental replay of the rape are common. Physical symptoms may include gastrointestinal disorders, chronic pain, sexually transmitted infections, cervical cancer, and genital injury. Another major health issue is that more than 32,000 pregnancies per year result from rape (CDC, 2016n). Some survivors of rape may go on to experience emotional symptoms so severe that they impact functioning to the extent that the survivor may develop PTSD (APA, 2013).

Pathophysiology and Etiology

Rape can occur under a number of circumstances and can include physically violent elements (such as being threatened with a weapon or tortured) as well as psychologic elements (such as survivors being told the rape was their own fault, being called berating names, or being threatened with harm to their loved ones if they report the rape to authorities). Regardless of the circumstances of the rape, survivors will need to heal emotionally and physically. After being raped, survivors may feel as though they have little to no control over what happens to them and as though they have lost a part of themselves. Elements of fear, guilt, and anxiety will also often be present (CDC, 2016n).

Influencing Factors

Those who commit rape will often know their victim, who is often a spouse, an ex-spouse, an acquaintance, a friend, or a relative. A majority of individuals who have experienced rape knew their attacker, with only 13.8% of women and 15.1% of men reporting a stranger as their attacker (CDC, 2012). Some factors influencing those who commit rape are environmental or social in nature, while others pertain to the individual's psychologic well-being. It is imperative to remember that both men and women can commit rape and be raped.

Intrapersonal and Interpersonal Factors

Multiple types of rapists exist, including those who know the victim and those who are strangers. To become a rapist, an individual needs to overcome the moral and ethical dilemma of taking away another individual's right to say no. Often this decision comes about through the use of drugs or alcohol; through powerful emotions such as anger, revenge, or a sense of entitlement; or through the use of self-delusion, convincing themselves that their victim actually wants to go through with the act despite protests. Depending on the rapist's own justifications, the act will either be physically violent with a result of profuse injuries to the victim, or emotionally violent with the perpetrator using verbal coercion and only enough physical force to complete the rape.

No one form of rape is easier than another; however, different types of rapists cause varied reactions in their targets.

For example, if the rapist was someone the individual knows on a personal level (e.g., a friend, relative, or spouse), the survivor is likely to have serious trust issues as a result of the experience. Individuals who had a prior romantic relationship with the rapist are also prone to developing low self-esteem and higher levels of guilt, believing that their supposed poor character judgment led to the event (DeAngelis, 2013).

Sociocultural Factors

For an individual to commit rape, a precipitating force needs to be present. This force could be emotional or substance based, or it could even be biological or environmental. Biological factors would include psychologic disorders that cause impaired decision making or deficient impulse control. Environmental factors that could influence an individual's decision to commit rape include growing up in a setting where physical, emotional, or sexual violence was common and perhaps even accepted. Similarly, being raised in a culture where women or men are seen as possessions rather than individuals could cause individuals to believe they have the right to take what they would like from others despite objections from the victim. Areas that have high crime rates and a seemingly increased tolerance for violence are also more prone to having a higher percentage of rape cases (CDC, 2016o).

Etiology

Approximately 79,770 girls and women were forcibly raped in 2013 in the United States (FBI, 2013c); overall, the incidents of rape have been decreasing steadily during the past 20 years. A national survey of adults has shown that approximately 1 in 5 women and 1 in 71 men have reported being raped at some point in their lives. Of female victims, 42.2% were first raped before age 18, and 37.4% were first raped between ages 18 and 24. Of male victims, 27.8% reported being raped before the age of 11 (CDC, 2012).

Marital rape occurs when one spouse forces the other to have sex against his or her will. Marital rape is considered a crime in all 50 states and can occur with both physical and emotional abuse. **Acquaintance rape** is a rather broad term used to describe a rape committed by an acquaintance or other familiar individual. The largest percentage of acquaintance rape cases occurs on college campuses, with many of them including factors such as the consumption of alcohol and illegal substances (by the perpetrator, the victim, or both) (Meadows, 2013).

Acquaintance rape can involve the use of "date rape" drugs or "club drugs." The three most common date rape drugs are gamma-hydroxybutyric acid (GHB), flunitrazepam (Rohypnol—slang "roofie"), and ketamine hydrochloride (ketamine). These three drugs are odorless and tasteless and thus can be easily added to a victim's drink without detection. After consuming the drugs, the victim will feel mildly euphoric and sedated and will often experience memory loss (Meadows, 2013). It is important to remember that even if the victim drank alcohol or consumed drugs willingly, he or she is *not* at fault for being assaulted.

Focus on Diversity and Culture
Rape of Vulnerable Populations

The homeless population, an identified vulnerable population, has an increased prevalence of sexual violence compared to women nationally. One study indicates that 13% of homeless women admitted to being raped in the past year, with half of those same women stating that they were raped at least twice (The White House Council on Women and Girls, 2014). This same report also indicates that homeless women are at increased risk of human sex trafficking as well.

The disabled population is also at higher risk for sexual violence. The White House Council on Women and Girls (2014) reports that women who have a disability are three times more likely to experience sexual violence than those without a disability.

The intense trauma associated with rape can lead to physical injuries as well as intense emotional injuries such as RTS. Individuals who have had a traumatic experience may display signs of shock and denial shortly after the experience.

Risk Factors

Individuals can be at a higher risk for rape if they are under the influence of drugs and/or alcohol, but these factors do not cause rape to occur. Similarly, being young could be considered a risk factor for rape, but only because a large percentage of survivors report having been raped before they were 18 years old.

The risk factors for committing a rape are also difficult to determine. Even if an individual has all of the risk factors, it does not necessarily mean that individual will become a rapist. Protective factors may lessen the risk of becoming a sexually violent perpetrator and may occur at the individual, relationship, community, or societal level. Risk and protective factors for sexual violence perpetration are listed in **Table 32–3 》**.

Prevention

The majority of preventive programs involving rape focus on stopping the perpetrator from committing the act. Programs such as these are often aimed at those who have committed sexual assault in the past, and they try to help the individual accept responsibility for the crime. Preventive measures for victims include knowledge and awareness about situations that could foster those looking to commit rape, such as crowded bars, parties, raves, and fraternity or sorority parties on college campuses. Paying attention to surroundings and traveling in pairs or groups can also deter an individual looking to rape a single unsuspecting victim. Self-defense classes and training aid in fighting off an individual attempting to commit sexual assault, which could give the victim a better chance of escaping (CDC, 2013b). For tips on avoiding date rape drugs, see the Patient Teaching feature.

TABLE 32–3 Risk and Protective Factors for Perpetration of Sexual Violence

Risk Factors for Perpetration			
Individual	**Relationship**	**Community**	**Societal**
■ Alcohol and drug use ■ Delinquency ■ Empathic deficits ■ General aggressiveness and acceptance of violence ■ Early sexual initiation ■ Coercive sexual fantasies ■ Preference for impersonal sex and sexual risk taking ■ Exposure to sexually explicit media ■ Hostility toward women ■ Adherence to traditional gender role norms ■ Hyper-masculinity ■ Suicidal behavior ■ Prior sexual victimization or perpetration	■ Family environment characterized by physical violence and conflict ■ Childhood history of physical, sexual, or emotional abuse ■ Emotionally unsupportive family environment ■ Poor parent–child relationships, particularly with fathers ■ Association with sexually aggressive, hypermasculine, and delinquent peers ■ Involvement in a violent or abusive intimate relationship	■ Poverty ■ Lack of employment opportunities ■ Lack of institutional support from police and judicial system ■ General tolerance of sexual violence within the community ■ Weak community sanctions against sexual violence perpetrators	■ Societal norms that support sexual violence ■ Societal norms that support male superiority and sexual entitlement ■ Societal norms that maintain women's inferiority and sexual submissiveness ■ Weak laws and policies related to sexual violence and gender equity ■ High levels of crime and other forms of violence
Protective Factors for Perpetration			
■ Parental use of reasoning to resolve family conflict ■ Emotional health and connectedness ■ Academic achievement ■ Empathy and concern for how one's actions affect others			

Source: Data from Centers for Disease Control and Prevention (CDC). (2016o). *Sexual violence: Risk and protective factors.* Retrieved from http://www.cdc.gov/violenceprevention/sexualviolence/riskprotectivefactors.html.

Clinical Manifestations

The clinical manifestations of rape vary depending on the genders of the assailant and the victim, the physical violence involved in the rape, and the type of rape. Common manifestations include oral, vaginal, or anal injuries and/or physical injuries with the presence of semen not belonging to the victim. Individuals who have been raped will also demonstrate psychologic symptoms such as shock, denial, and confusion directly following the event.

Physical Injuries

Common physical injuries in rape victims include swelling, redness, and lacerations around the vagina or anus; injuries to the throat from forced oral sex or restraint; bruises; broken bones; and knife and gunshot wounds. Defensive and restraint injuries will present as wounds to the hands, arms, feet, and legs, often in the form of bruises, lacerations, and/or fractured bones. If the victim was restrained (often with rope, handcuffs, or plastic zip ties), additional injuries will

Patient Teaching
Date Rape Drugs

Date rape drugs are being used to make a person vulnerable to being raped. The nurse should teach the patient methods of prevention and what to do if they suspect they have been drugged:

1. Always keep your drink with you; never leave it unattended.
2. Do not accept premade or open drinks from someone you don't know.
3. Watch your drink being made by the bartender.
4. Inspect drinks (Rohypnol now releases a blue dye when mixed in light-colored drinks; however, it is important to know that other drugs, including generic versions of Rohypnol, may not be detectable) (National Institute on Drug Abuse [NIDA] for Teens, 2015).
5. Do not leave a location if you are alone or with someone that you do not know or explicitly trust.

Symptoms of being drugged include:

1. Becoming sleepy or confused; feeling more drunk than warranted by the amount of alcohol consumed.
2. Feelings of weakness or loss of coordination.
3. Nausea, vomiting, headaches (National Crime Prevention Council, n.d.).

If you feel that you have been drugged, get help immediately. Seek out a friend, security, or even the bartender. Do not leave with the person you suspect may have drugged you, and seek medical attention immediately (Crime Prevention Tips, 2013).

be found around the wrists, ankles, and possibly the neck. Internal injuries and bleeding could be present if the patient was beaten before or after the rape, or raped with an object such as a bottle.

Long-term physical complications often present as pelvic pain, back pain, frequent headaches, gastrointestinal disorders, and potential pregnancy complications in women. Some of these long-term symptoms—such as headaches, gastrointestinal upset, and even back pain—can be caused by a mix of intense stress and injuries from the rape (CDC, 2016n). Other long-term effects could be the result of sexually transmitted diseases or infections, such as herpes or HIV.

Immediate Response

Initial responses to rape generally include feelings of shock, denial, and disbelief. Other early responses involve fear, anger, guilt, embarrassment, helplessness, loss of control, confusion, anxiety, and nervousness (CDC, 2016n; Meadows, 2013). The survivor will likely be hesitant to trust others, especially those of the same gender as the attacker. Nurses understand this fear and work to reassure patients of their safety. If a woman has been raped by a male attacker, it may be necessary to have primarily female healthcare professionals working with her. If a male staff member is needed, a female nurse should accompany him to provide reassurance to the patient.

An individual's first response after a rape is often to shower in an attempt to wash away the incident as well as what is left of the attacker's physical presence (such as the individual's body odor and fluids). If consulted, nurses advise patients not to shower before being examined because this will remove potential evidence that could be collected and used to identify the attacker. Nurses should recognize that this request is difficult for the patient and provide reassurance that a shower will be provided as soon as the examination is complete.

Some patients will present themselves as though nothing has happened while acting unfazed by the situation. Nurses realize that this reaction is often an effect of shock and denial. Patients who react in this manner should be treated as sensitively as other patients who outwardly display their emotions. All procedures, tests, and examinations should be explained to the patient in detail, and the patient should be asked to give consent before any test or examination is performed. Nurses should work to empower the patient's decision-making process. The staff involved in the care of a rape victim needs training on giving physical and emotional support to rape victims.

Long term Response

After the initial shock of the incident subsides, patients will begin to accept that the rape has occurred. In the weeks following the incident, a variety of emotional responses will be present, and these responses will differ depending on the personality of the patient. Common responses include anger, flashbacks of the incident, avoidance of previously enjoyed activities, avoidance of the setting where the rape occurred, insomnia, eating disturbances, sexual dysfunction, and depression (Meadows, 2013). Some individuals will cut all emotional ties to friends and family members, whereas others will seek the comfort of familiarity and respond very negatively to being alone. The emotional distress of the incident can trigger the use of unhealthy coping mechanisms such as using drugs and alcohol or participating in high-risk sexual behavior. Pregnancy is also a concern for those who have been raped; more than 32,000 pregnancies occur each year as the result of forced sexual encounters (CDC, 2016n). How the patient responds to the pregnancy depends on the emotional trauma associated with the incident as well as the personality of the individual. Emotional difficulties will likely coincide with the progression of the pregnancy.

Depression and suicidal thoughts or actions are common after rape. Nurses should be mindful of the warning signs of suicide (see the module on Mood and Affect) and employ appropriate interventions. All individuals who have experienced rape should be provided with resources for therapy, support groups, and counseling. Whether patients choose to use these resources is their decision, but the nurse is responsible to provide patients with the means to seek help.

SAFETY ALERT Rape survivors are at a high risk for developing an eating disorder, including anorexia, bulimia, or a crossover between the two. Eating disorders do not always develop out of an individual's desire to lose weight; often they come from an emotional disturbance. One of the main components of both anorexia and bulimia is control over what the individual is consuming and over the nutrients that stay in the body or are forcefully discarded. In a rape situation, anger and stress can lead to eating disorders (CDC, 2016p).

Cultural Considerations

The cultural considerations in rape often involve the culture's dominant definition of rape and what that act entails. Not all members of a culture will have the same beliefs about one particular topic. Cultures that demonstrate male superiority and devalue the thoughts and rights of women will likely not consider the forcible rape of a woman or girl a matter of great importance. Conversely, feminist cultures will view the rape of a woman or girl as an injustice (Kalra & Buhgra, 2013).

Marital rape is not acknowledged in many cultures around the world. If two individuals are married, then any sexual contact is considered legal and warranted. Individuals from these cultures would be hesitant to seek help if they were raped by their spouse; it could even be considered dishonorable to the victim's family to imply that a crime was committed. Marital rapes often go unreported; however, 9% of all rapes reported are perpetrated by a husband or ex-husband (Health Research Funding, 2014).

Individuals in the sex industry (e.g., prostitutes or exotic dancers) can also be raped. Regardless of whether an individual's job includes having sexual relations with others, if someone states an unwillingness to continue and the other person does not stop, then the act becomes rape. Nurses do not judge patients who say they have been raped; they provide quality care to all individuals.

Clinical Manifestations and Therapies
Rape-Trauma Syndrome

ETIOLOGY	CLINICAL MANIFESTATIONS	CLINICAL THERAPIES
Acute phase of RTS	Expressive styles vary: ▪ Open expression of feelings—confusion, fear, crying, sobbing, pacing, hostility, inappropriate laughter ▪ Controlled style—numbness, shock, disbelief, withdrawal ▪ Compound reaction—reactivated symptoms of previous conditions, for example, psychotic behavior, depression, suicidal behavior, substance abuse ▪ Somatic reactions—tension headache, fatigue, increased startle reaction, nausea, gagging ▪ Outward appearance of adjustment with an attempt to restore equilibrium ▪ Life activities are renewed, but superficially and mechanically ▪ Periods of anxiety, fear, nightmares, depression, guilt, shame, vulnerability, helplessness, isolation, sexual dysfunctions	▪ Counseling ▪ Therapy ▪ Follow-up care for emotional and physical trauma ▪ Medication
Reorganization phase of RTS	▪ Anger at the assailant, at society, and at the judicial system ▪ The need to talk to resolve feelings ▪ The survivor seeks family and professional support	▪ Therapy ▪ Support groups
PTSD (if unable to recover)	▪ Anxiety ▪ Flashbacks ▪ Depression ▪ Nightmares ▪ Withdrawal	▪ CBT ▪ Support groups ▪ Antidepressants

SAFETY ALERT Rape survivors may experience long-term effects that include depression and suicidal ideations. The nurse should provide referrals for support groups and other community services, including crisis hotline numbers, which may assist the patient in coping effectively with the traumatic event.

Collaboration

An interprofessional team caring for patients who have been raped includes law enforcement personnel immediately after the rape and nurses, physicians, and mental health professionals for ongoing treatment. Sexual Assault Nurse Examiners (SANE) often participate in the assessment process. Many communities have victims' advocates who are available to guide rape victims through the process of prosecuting their attacker. These are sometimes volunteers trained by local health departments and district attorneys' offices. Some law enforcement agencies or district attorneys' offices employ trained staff to serve as victim's advocates. It is important that the nurse validate that all policies and procedures are followed with precision and that meticulous documentation is completed, as the information may be presented in legal proceedings.

>> **Stay Current:** Visit the website of the International Association of Forensic Nurses (IAFN) at www.iafn.org to learn more about becoming a Sexual Assault Nursing Examiner.

Diagnostic Tests

Although not diagnostic in nature, a rape kit will likely be completed for the purpose of convicting the rapist, if caught. As a result, chain-of-custody laws must be followed, and these vary within jurisdictions. The rape kit may take several hours to complete, and the healthcare provider cannot leave the rape kit at any time during the process. The rape kit has a special number assigned to it and contains 16 separate steps in collecting evidence. Each evidence envelope or bag has the same rape kit number. The victim will be given the number to this rape kit, but it will only be processed if the victim makes a report to the police. Specimens will include the following:

- Vaginal, oral, and anal swabs for DNA material (it is important that the victim be asked whether they have had any consensual sexual relations in the last 5 days so that the consensual partner and perpetrator can be differentiated) (Forensics for Survivors, 2015)

- Scrapings from under the patient's fingernails for skin samples if the patient scratched the rapist

- Combing of pubic hair for rapist's DNA

- Clothing worn by the victim (if the individual is brought directly to the ED following the rape).

In addition to the specimens collected for legal purposes, the victim is tested for sexually transmitted infections and potential pregnancy. Baseline testing is performed at the time of the initial examination, and follow-up HIV testing is done at 3, 6, and 12 months. Pregnancy testing related to the rape cannot be accurately performed until the woman has missed her first menstrual period; however, emergency contraception is available to prevent pregnancy

Pharmacologic Therapy

Women who have been raped can be offered emergency contraception in order to prevent unwanted pregnancy. The contraceptive is more likely to be successful if taken within 3 days of the attack. Some individuals will be opposed to using contraception; the nurse will explain the patient's options and then be respectful of whatever decision the patient makes.

Numerous sexually transmitted diseases and infections can be contracted during a rape—regardless of whether the attacker used a condom or not. The most common and treatable infections are listed below, along with their prescribed pharmacologic treatment:

- Syphilis, treated with penicillin (CDC, 2015f)
- Chlamydia, treated with a dose of azithromycin or a week of doxycycline (CDC, 2015g)
- Gonorrhea, treated with a combination of ceftriaxone and azithromycin (CDC, 2015h)
- Trichomoniasis, treated with metronidazole or tinidazole (CDC, 2015i).

Nonpharmacologic Therapy

Support groups, therapy, and counseling are recommended to patients who have experienced a forced sexual encounter or are experiencing RTS. Some patients will be more receptive to support groups where others who have had similar experiences come together to discuss the aftermath of the event and how they are working to heal from the experience. Other patients will prefer a more private setting and choose to work individually with a therapist to process their own personal experiences. While attending therapy, patients will develop healthy coping mechanisms to process their emotions and will work to release feelings of self-blame.

Lifespan Considerations

Treatment will predominantly be the same for victims of rape, regardless of gender or age; however, there may be slight variances in care. For instance, a young child, a postmenopausal woman, or a male victim will need physical treatment and emotional support, but they will not need emergency contraception. Younger and older individuals who are living with a caregiver may need help creating a post-discharge safety plan, especially if the perpetrator was the caregiver. The approach in explaining the rape kit, treatment, and follow-up will vary; age-appropriate terminology will need to be used.

NURSING PROCESS

Nursing care for a patient who has been raped depends on a number of factors, including the physical violence inflicted during the incident, the patient's emotional state, and the patient's willingness to allow an examination. Nurses know that this is an extremely difficult situation for the patient, so they must be both patient and understanding.

Assessment

When conducting a nursing assessment for a patient who has been raped, nurses first need to ensure the patient's safety. If knife or gunshot wounds, organ damage, and/or severe head trauma are present, those injuries need to be assessed and treated first before any minor physical injuries or psychologic injuries are assessed. Injuries to the vagina, anus, and throat are likely to be present and should be assessed. The patient may be in shock or outwardly emotionally distraught. Nurses should be aware that patients' reactions to rape vary greatly in accordance with the situation and the developmental age and personality of the patient.

Once the physical safety of the patient is ensured, nurses work to comfort and empower the patient by explaining the patient's choices for examination and providing information about resources. Individuals who have been raped do not have to allow the nurse to complete a rape kit, nor do they have to talk to a counselor; however, nurses should encourage both of these. If the patient agrees to an examination and the collection of evidence, nurses will explain every step of the process and ask permission during the examination itself. Although the patient may be willing to allow evidence collection and DNA swabbing, she may not want any pictures taken of the injuries. Nurses need to remain supportive of the patient's decisions. Disease, infection, and pregnancy testing and treatment should be discussed with the patient, and interventions should be planned accordingly.

The nurse assesses the patient's emotional needs, asking if the person would like a parent, friend, or rape advocate present during the examination. Police involvement is also offered if the patient chooses to file a statement about the incident.

Diagnosis

The patient's diagnosis is contingent on the injuries and emotional state of the individual. Some potential nursing diagnoses include:

- *Infection, Risk for*
- *Rape-Trauma Syndrome*
- *Fear*
- *Pain, Acute*
- *Powerlessness*
- *Coping, Ineffective*
- *Self-Esteem, Situational Low*

(NANDA-I © 2014)

Planning

It is critical for the patient who is the victim of rape to have control over the planning process. The patient's input regarding short-term and long-term goals is essential to prevent revictimization and to help the patient regain control over self and environment. Appropriate short-term goals include:

- The patient will receive treatment for physical injuries sustained during the rape.
- The patient will participate in follow-up care for physical injuries.
- The patient will follow a safety plan following release from medical care.

It may be more than the patient can manage to think beyond the first few days following the rape. The nurse can provide follow-up care to determine when the patient is ready to engage in further planning. This follow-up care also allows the nurse to reassess how the patient is meeting short-term goals. Appropriate long-term goals may include the following:

- The patient will gain control over remembering—experiencing decreased flashbacks and nightmares.
- The patient will work toward affect tolerance—ability to name feelings, feel them, and endure them without overwhelming arousal or numbing.
- The patient will gain mastery over symptoms—anxiety, fear, depression, and sexual problems will decrease or become more tolerable.
- The patient will reconnect—increasing his or her ability to trust and attach to others.
- The patient will discover or attach some kind of meaning to the event, finding empowerment.

Implementation

Patients who are victims of rape will require extensive nursing care. First, nurses must provide comfort for the patient, including providing privacy and ensuring the patient's safety. The nurse will also help facilitate evidence collection and help treat physical trauma. The nurse also can also help empower the patient to recover emotionally and psychologically from the event.

Provide Comfort

Upon admission, individuals who have been raped are placed in a private room. Access to the patient is restricted to only necessary personnel, and a family member or friend can be present to provide emotional support at the patient's request. Patients are assured of their safety and privacy, and nurses do not judge or make assumptions about the individual who has been raped or their decisions involving treatment and evaluation. Patients should be given emotional support, and pain medication can be administered as needed once appropriate assessments are completed.

Facilitate Evidence Collection

Nurses determine if the patient has taken a shower or changed clothing. The nurse works with the patient to relay the details of the incident, including whether a condom was used and the type(s) of rape. If the patient chooses to have evidence collected, nurses explain every step of the process as it is being performed. Individuals are informed that they can ask to stop at any point in the process. Typically, a Sexual Assault Nurse Examiner (SANE) nurse will be involved with the forensic process of evidence collection. DNA swabs and hair and skin samples are taken in an effort to identify the attacker.

Treat Physical Injuries

All physical injuries, including broken bones, lacerations, bruises, and other wounds, are treated in order of severity. Tests for sexually transmitted diseases and infections are performed, and patients are informed about appropriate treatments. Emergency contraception for cases of potential pregnancy is explained to the patient and offered. The need for continued HIV testing at regular intervals during the next year is discussed, and the patient is informed about potential outcomes.

Empower the Patient

Nurses provide referrals to social workers, counselors, support groups, and law enforcement. If patients choose not to use these referrals, that is their decision, but nurses explain their options for seeking help, which will begin the process of empowerment. The nurse should educate the patient on the importance of and assist in developing a safety plan *prior* to discharge from the hospital (see Patient Teaching: Developing a Safety Plan in Exemplar 32.A on Abuse).

Evaluation

Patients are encouraged to ask any questions they may have, either about the examination process or about future testing and resources. Nurses explore all options with the patient as appropriate. Some potential outcomes are as follows:

- The patient expresses emotions regarding the rape.
- The patient is empowered to take control of the situation.
- The patient discusses any fears or questions about the examination.
- The patient employs healthy coping mechanisms.
- The patient asks for, and accepts, help when needed.
- The patient acknowledges that the rape was not his or her fault.

If outcomes are not met, the nurse should reassess the patient to determine if the patient needs additional time to meet the outcomes or if the outcomes were unrealistic. Working with survivors of rape requires compassion and understanding, because each person will cope differently. The patient is likely to be traumatized, which may interfere with their ability to understand or retain information. The nurse should demonstrate patience and review information as necessary.

Nursing Care Plan
A Patient Who Has Been Raped

Renee Meyers, age 23, comes into the emergency department after having been raped by her ex-boyfriend. She explains that the incident happened 4 hours ago, but she was hesitant to ask for help because she feels some responsibility for the attack.

ASSESSMENT

Camilla Wright, an RN in the ED, escorts Ms. Meyers to a private examination room. Ms. Meyers is resistant to talking about the events, repeating multiple times that she feels that the attack was her own fault and that she cannot believe this could have happened. Nurse Wright is patient and tells the patient to take her time in relaying the events as they occurred. The nurse also reassures the patient that she is perfectly safe in the hospital and that no action will be taken without her permission.

After approximately 30 minutes, Ms. Meyers begins to discuss the details of the rape, reporting that her ex-boyfriend forced her to have sexual intercourse with him. When Ms. Meyers tried to resist, her attacker struck her repeatedly in the face with his fists. Nurse Wright notices slight discoloration near the patient's right eye, and the left side of her face is moderately swollen. The patient is visibly shaking, and she is fighting back tears. Ms. Meyers explains that the attacker did not use a condom and says she is very worried about becoming pregnant.

Nurse Wright does not interrupt while Ms. Meyers is relaying the events; when she is finished, she asks if the patient has showered since the incident. Ms. Meyers reports that she has not showered. Nurse Wright then explains the process of collecting evidence and testing for sexually transmitted infections, and asks Ms. Meyers if she is willing to consent to the examination and completion of a rape kit. At first, Ms. Meyers is hesitant, but Nurse Wright does not try to pressure her into consent; instead, she asks the patient if she would like some time alone to think it over.

Ms. Meyers takes some time alone and then informs Nurse Wright that she would like to have evidence collected. The patient also requests to be tested for sexually transmitted infections.

DIAGNOSES

- *Risk for Infection* related to STIs
- *Rape-Trauma Syndrome*
- *Fear* related to possible pregnancy
- *Acute Pain* related to physical trauma
- *Powerlessness*
- *Ineffective Coping.*

(NANDA-I © 2014)

PLANNING

Goals for Ms. Meyers' care include:

- The patient will be tested and treated for any potential infections.
- The patient will make an informed decision with regard to emergency contraceptive treatment.
- The patient will report physical pain as absent or tolerable, as evidenced by patient rating of pain as 3 or less on a scale of 0–10.
- The patient will make an informed decision with regard to reporting the sexual assault to law enforcement officials.
- The patient will make an informed decision with regard to evidence collection for potential future prosecution of the perpetrator.
- The patient will openly express emotions and concerns to trusted confidantes.
- The patient will seek follow-up counseling and psychosocial care.
- The patient will develop a safety plan prior to discharge.

IMPLEMENTATION

- Refer to rape advocacy program.
- Administer prescribed analgesics as needed for pain control.
- Administer medications as needed or desired to prevent sexually transmitted infections and pregnancy if patient agrees.
- Support and educate about the physical examination and specimen collection process.
- Assist in collection of specimens following chain of custody using a rape evidence kit.
- Inform of HIV testing.
- Educate about legal procedures available to patient.
- Educate on importance of and assist with completion of safety plan.

EVALUATION

Ms. Meyers consented to collection of specimens and physical examination, which will aid in conviction of the rapist. She verbalizes pain as a 3 on a scale of 0–10 (with 0 being absence of pain and 10 being severe pain). Ms. Meyers agreed to speak with the rape victim advocate and was given community support phone numbers and addresses. She has verbalized understanding of the need for future HIV and pregnancy testing and has completed a safety plan. She has called her best friend, Beth Adams, to drive her home when discharged.

CRITICAL THINKING

1. How should the nurse respond to Ms. Meyers if she refused to have specimens collected or a physical examination at this time?

2. Explain how the nurse should describe emergency contraceptives and their actions.

3. How might this patient's emotional state change over the next 24–48 hours?

REVIEW Rape and Rape-Trauma Syndrome

RELATE Link the Concepts and Exemplars

Linking the exemplar of rape and rape-trauma syndrome with the concept of stress and coping:

1. What teaching would you provide a patient with rape-trauma syndrome about managing anxiety?

2. Describe the differences in communication strategy to assess for rape in a 12-year-old child versus a 30-year-old woman.

Linking the exemplar of rape and rape-trauma syndrome with the concept of self:

3. How will you plan to assist the victim of rape to regain her self-esteem?

4. When collecting specimens for use by law enforcement during the investigation of potential rape, what nursing interventions can be implemented to help the patient maintain a positive self-concept?

READY Go to Volume 3: Clinical Nursing Skills

REFER Go to Pearson MyLab Nursing and eText

- Additional review materials

REFLECT Apply Your Knowledge

Damien Harris, a 31-year-old man, transports himself to the ED after having been raped near a local bar. Mr. Harris has numerous bruises to his back, face, and ribs; he also has a shallow cut along his neck. He tells the nurse that a man approached him while he was outside a local bar having a cigarette; the man claimed to be having car trouble. Mr. Harris offered to help the stranger with his car, but once they were away from the bar, the man began attacking him. The attacker put a knife to Mr. Harris's throat and threatened to kill him if he resisted. After the rape, the attacker struck Mr. Harris on the head and left him unconscious. Both his wallet and cell phone were taken by the attacker. Mr. Harris explains that his ribs hurt when he breathes and his head has begun throbbing since he regained consciousness. He has requested the use of a phone to call a friend.

1. What are the three primary nursing interventions for this patient?

2. What resources can be offered to Mr. Harris?

3. Would the nursing care plan be any different if the patient in this scenario were a woman? Explain your answer.

References

Alvarez, L., & Pérez-Peña, R. (2016). Orlando gunman attacks gay nightclub, leaving 50 dead. *The New York Times*, June 12, 2016. Retrieved from https://www.nytimes.com/2016/06/13/us/orlando-nightclub-shooting.html

American College of Surgeons Committee on Trauma. (2017). *Advanced trauma life support* (10th ed.). Chicago, IL: American College of Surgeons.

American Nurses Association. (n.d.). *Short definitions of ethical principles and theories: Familiar words, what do they mean?* Retrieved from http://www.nursing-world.org/MainMenuCategories/EthicsStan-dards/Resources/Ethics-Definitions.pdf.

American Psychiatric Association (APA). (2013). *Diagnostic and statistical manual of mental disorders* (5th ed.). Arlington, VA: Author.

American Psychological Association. (2013). *Understanding child sexual abuse: Education, prevention, and recovery.* Retrieved from http://www.apa.org/pubs/info/brochures/sex-abuse.aspx#

American Psychological Association. (2016). *Warning signs of youth violence.* Retrieved from http://www.apa.org/helpcenter/warning-signs.aspx

Anetzberger, G. J. (2012). An update on the nature and scope of elder abuse. *Journal of the American Society on Aging, 36*(3), 12–20.

Asian Pacific Institute on Gender-Based Violence (APIGBV). (n.d.). *Domestic violence.* Retrieved from http://www.api-gbv.org/violence/domestic-violence.php

Ayalon, L. (2015). Reports of elder neglect by older adults, their family caregivers, and their home care workers: A test of measurement invariance. *Journal of Gerontology, 70*(3), 432–442.

Baron, R. A., & Richardson, D. R. (1994). *Human aggression* (2nd ed.). New York, NY: Plenum.

Benedictis, T. D., Jaffe, J., & Segal, J. (2012). Domestic violence and abuse: Types, signs, symptoms, causes, and effects. *American Academy of Experts in Traumatic Stress.* Retrieved from http://www.aaets.org/article144.htm

Borowski, I., Taliaferro, L., & McMorris, B. (2013). Suicidal thinking and behavior among youth involved in verbal and social bullying: Risk and protective factors. *Journal of Adolescent Health, 53*(1), S4–S12.

Buchanan, T. W., Bagley, S. L., Standfield, R. B., & Preston, S. D. (2012). The emphatic, physiological resonance of stress. *Social Neuroscience, 7*(2), 191–201. doi:10.1080/17470919.2011.588723

Bureau of Justice. (2011). *Workplace violence: 1993–2009.* Retrieved from http://www.bjs.gov/index.cfm?ty=pbdetail&iid=2377

Bureau of Justice Assistance. (n.d.). *Anti-human trafficking task force initiative.* Retrieved from https://www.bja.gov/ProgramDetails.aspx?Program_ID=51

Bureau of Justice Statistics. (2015). *Violent crime rate remained unchanged while property crime rate declined in 2014.* Retrieved from http://www.bjs.gov/content/pub/press/cv14pr.cfm

Bureau of Justice Statistics. (2016a). *Indicators of school crime and safety: 2015.* Retrieved from http://www.bjs.gov/index.cfm?ty=pbdetail&iid=5599

Bureau of Justice Statistics. (2016b). *Violent crime.* Retrieved from http://www.bjs.gov/index.cfm?ty=tp&tid=31

Centers for Disease Control and Prevention (CDC). (2012). *Sexual violence.* Retrieved from https://www.cdc.gov/violenceprevention/pdf/sv-datasheet-a.pdf

Centers for Disease Control and Prevention (CDC). (2013a). *The National Intimate Partner and Sexual Violence Survey.* Retrieved from http://www.cdc.gov/violenceprevention/nisvs

Centers for Disease Control and Prevention (CDC). (2013b). *Sexual violence: Prevention strategies.* Retrieved from http://www.cdc.gov/violenceprevention/sexualviolence/prevention.html

Centers for Disease Control and Prevention (CDC). (2014a). *Prevalence and characteristics of sexual violence, stalking, and intimate partner violence victimization—National Intimate Partner and Sexual Violence Survey, United States, 2011.* Retrieved from http://www.cdc.gov/mmwr/preview/mmwrhtml/ss6308a1.htm

Centers for Disease Control and Prevention (CDC). (2014b). *Child maltreatment: Facts at a glance.* Retrieved from http://www.cdc.gov/violenceprevention/pdf/childmaltreatment-facts-at-a-glance.pdf

Centers for Disease Control and Prevention (CDC). (2014c). *School violence: Data and statistics.* Retrieved from http://www.cdc.gov/violenceprevention/youthviolence/schoolviolence/data_stats.html

Centers for Disease Control and Prevention (CDC). (2014d). *The relationship between bullying and suicide: What we know and what it means for schools.* Retrieved from http://www.cdc.gov/violenceprevention/pdf/bullying-suicide-translation-final-a.pdf

Centers for Disease Control and Prevention (CDC). (2015a). *Intimate partner violence: Risk and protective factors.* Retrieved from http://www.cdc.gov/violenceprevention/intimatepartnerviolence/riskprotectivefactors.html

Centers for Disease Control and Prevention (CDC). (2015b). *Understanding youth violence.* Retrieved from http://www.cdc.gov/violenceprevention/pdf/yv-factsheet-a.pdf

Centers for Disease Control and Prevention (CDC). (2015c). *Intimate partner violence: Consequences.* Retrieved from http://www.cdc.gov/violenceprevention/intimatepartnerviolence/consequences.html

Centers for Disease Control and Prevention (CDC). (2015d). *Health, United States, 2015: With special feature on racial and ethnic disparities.* Retrieved from http://www.cdc.gov/nchs/data/hus/hus15.pdf#019

Centers for Disease Control and Prevention (CDC). (2015e). *Teen drivers: Get the facts.* Retrieved from http://www.cdc.gov/motorvehiclesafety/teen_drivers/teendrivers_factsheet.html

Centers for Disease Control and Prevention (CDC). (2015f). *2015 sexually transmitted diseases treatment guidelines: Syphilis treatment and care.* Retrieved from http://www.cdc.gov/std/syphilis/treatment.htm

Centers for Disease Control and Prevention (CDC). (2015g). *2015 sexually transmitted diseases treatment guidelines: Chlamydial infections.* Retrieved from http://www.cdc.gov/std/tg2015/chlamydia.htm

Centers for Disease Control and Prevention (CDC). (2015h). *2015 sexually transmitted diseases treatment guidelines: Gonococcal infections in adolescents and adults.* Retrieved from http://www.cdc.gov/std/tg2015/gonorrhea.htm

Centers for Disease Control and Prevention (CDC). (2015i). *2015 sexually transmitted diseases treatment guidelines: Trichomoniasis.* Retrieved from http://www.cdc.gov/std/tg2015/trichomoniasis.htm

Centers for Disease Control and Prevention (CDC). (2016a). *Youth violence: Consequences.* Retrieved from http://www.cdc.gov/violenceprevention/youthviolence/consequences.html

Centers for Disease Control and Prevention (CDC). (2016b). *Youth violence: Risk and protective factors.* Retrieved from http://www.cdc.gov/violenceprevention/youthviolence/riskprotectivefactors.html

Centers for Disease Control and Prevention (CDC). (2016c). *Child abuse and neglect: Risk and protective factors.* Retrieved from http://www.cdc.gov/violenceprevention/childmaltreatment/riskprotectivefactors.html

Centers for Disease Control and Prevention (CDC). (2016d). *Preventing abusive head trauma in children.* Retrieved from http://www.cdc.gov/violenceprevention/childmaltreatment/abusivehead-trauma.html

Centers for Disease Control and Prevention (CDC). (2016e). *Featured topic: Bullying research.* Retrieved from http://www.cdc.gov/violenceprevention/youthviolence/bullyingresearch/

Centers for Disease Control and Prevention (CDC). (2016f). *Electronic aggression.* Retrieved from http://www.cdc.gov/violenceprevention/youthviolence/electronicaggression/index.html

Centers for Disease Control and Prevention (CDC). (2016g). *Intimate partner violence: Definitions.* Retrieved from http://www.cdc.gov/violenceprevention/intimatepartnerviolence/definitions.html

Centers for Disease Control and Prevention (CDC). (2016h). *Sexual violence: Definitions.* Retrieved from http://www.cdc.gov/violenceprevention/sexualviolence/definitions.html

Centers for Disease Control and Prevention (CDC). (2016i). *Child abuse and neglect: Consequences.* Retrieved from http://www.cdc.gov/violenceprevention/childmaltreatment/consequences.html

Centers for Disease Control and Prevention (CDC). (2016j). *Bullying.* Retrieved from http://www.cdc.gov/ncbddd/disabilityandsafety/bullying.html

Centers for Disease Control and Prevention (CDC). (2016k). *10 leading causes of injury deaths by age groups highlighting unintentional injury deaths, United States—2014.* Retrieved from http://www.cdc.gov/injury/images/lc-charts/leading_causes_of_injury_deaths_unintentional_injury_2014_1040w740h.gif

Centers for Disease Control and Prevention (CDC). (2016l). *NCHS data on drug-poisoning deaths.* Retrieved from http://www.cdc.gov/nchs/data/factsheets/factsheet_drug_poisoning.htm

Centers for Disease Control and Prevention (CDC). (2016m). *Distracted driving.* Retrieved from http://www.cdc.gov/motorvehiclesafety/distracted_driving/

Centers for Disease Control and Prevention (CDC). (2016n). *Sexual violence: Consequences.* Retrieved from http://www.cdc.gov/violenceprevention/sexualviolence/consequences.html

Centers for Disease Control and Prevention (CDC). (2016o). *Sexual violence: Risk and protective factors.* Retrieved from http://www.cdc.gov/violenceprevention/sexualviolence/riskprotectivefactors.html

Centers for Disease Control and Prevention (CDC). (2016p). *Sexual violence.* Retrieved from http://www.cdc.gov/features/sexualviolence/

Chand, M., Subramanya, H., & Rao, G. (2014). *Management of patients who refuse blood transfusion.* Retrieved from http://www.ncbi.nlm.nih.gov/pmc/articles/PMC4260316/

Child Welfare Information Gateway. (2012). *The risk and prevention of maltreatment of children with disabilities.* Retrieved from https://www.childwelfare.gov/pubPDFs/focus.pdf

Child Welfare Information Gateway. (n.d.). *Cycle of abuse.* Retrieved from https://www.childwelfare.gov/topics/can/impact/long-term-consequences-of-child-abuse-and-neglect/abuse/

Children's Health. (2016). *Multisystem trauma.* Retrieved from https://www.childrens.com/for-healthcare-professionals/departments-institutes-programs/critical-care-picu/multi-system-trauma

Christian Science. (2016). *How can I be healed?* Retrieved from http://www.christianscience.com/what-is-christian-science/how-can-i-be-healed

Ciccarelli, S. K., & White, J. N. (2013). *Psychology: An exploration* (2nd ed.). Upper Saddle River, NJ: Pearson Education.

Cohen, E. (2013). *What is emotional neglect? How to tell if your partner is emotionally neglectful.* Retrieved from https://www.psychologytoday.com/blog/what-would-aristotle-do/201311/what-is-emotional-neglect

Compassion Fatigue Awareness Project. (2013). *Recognizing compassion fatigue.* Retrieved from http://www.compassionfatigue.org/pages/symptoms.html

Congressional Budget Office. (2012). *The Veteran's Health Administration's treatment of PTSD and traumatic brain injury among recent combat veterans.* Retrieved from https://www.cbo.gov/sites/default/files/cbofiles/attachments/02-09-PTSD.pdf

Crime Prevention Tips. (2013). *Date rape drugs.* Retrieved from http://www.crimepreventiontips.org/college-campus-safety/date-rape-drugs.html

Crisis Prevention Institute (CPI). (2016). *Horizontal violence in hospitals.* Retrieved from http://www.crisisprevention.com/Resources/Knowledge-Base/Horizontal-Violence-in-Hospitals. Published by Sage Publications (U.S.), © 2007.

DeAngelis, T. (2013). *Rape takes global toll on women's lives, study finds.* Retrieved from http://www.apa.org/monitor/2013/01/rape.aspx

De Bellis, M., & Zisk, A. (2014). *The biological effects of childhood trauma.* Retrieved from http://www.ncbi.nlm.nih.gov/pmc/articles/PMC3968319/

EMDR Institute. (n.d.). *Dual attention stimuli.* Retrieved from http://www.emdr.com/?s=dual+stimulation

Federal Bureau of Investigation (FBI). (2012a). *Violent crime.* Retrieved from http://www.fbi.gov/about-us/cjis/ucr/crime-in-the-u.s/2011/crime-in-the-u.s.-2011/violent-crime/violent-crime

Federal Bureau of Investigation (FBI). (2012b). *Annual crime in the U.S. report released.* Retrieved from http://www.fbi.gov/news/stories/2012/october/annual-crime-in-the-u.s.-report-released

Federal Bureau of Investigation (FBI). (2012c). *UCR program changes definition of rape.* Retrieved from http://www.fbi.gov/about-us/cjis/cjis-link/march-2012/ucr-program-changes-definition-of-rape

Federal Bureau of Investigation (FBI). (2013a). *Crime in the United States 2013: By state.* Retrieved from https://www.fbi.gov/about-us/cjis/ucr/crime-in-the-u.s/2013/crime-in-the-u.s.-2013/tables/5tabledatadecpdf/table_5_crime_in_the_united_states_by_state_2013.xls

Federal Bureau of Investigation (FBI). (2013b). *A study of active shooter incidents in the United States between 2000 and 2013.* Retrieved from https://www.fbi.gov/about-us/office-of-partner-engagement/active-shooter-incidents/a-study-of-active-shooter-incidents-in-the-u.s.-2000-2013

Federal Bureau of Investigation (FBI). (2013c). *Crime in the United States 2013: Rape.* Retrieved from https://www.fbi.gov/about-us/cjis/ucr/crime-in-the-u.s/2013/crime-in-the-u.s.-2013/violent-crime/rape

Federal Bureau of Investigation (FBI). (2014). *Latest hate crime statistics report released.* Retrieved from https://www.fbi.gov/news/stories/2014/december/latest-hate-crime-statistics-report-released

Federal Bureau of Investigation (FBI). (n.d.a). *Human trafficking.* Retrieved from https://www.fbi.gov/about-us/investigate/civilrights/human_trafficking

Federal Bureau of Investigation (FBI). (n.d.b). *Hate crimes—overview.* Retrieved from https://www.fbi.gov/about-us/investigate/civilrights/hate_crimes/overview

Federal Bureau of Investigation (FBI). (n.d.c). *Gangs.* Retrieved from https://www.fbi.gov/about-us/investigate/vc_majorthefts/gangs

Federal Bureau of Investigation (FBI). (n.d.d). *2014 crime in the United States.* Retrieved from https://www.fbi.gov/about-us/cjis/ucr/crime-in-the-u.s/2014/crime-in-the-u.s.-2014/offenses-known-to-law-enforcement/expanded-homicide

Firestone, L. (2012). *Recognizing complex trauma.* Retrieved from https://www.psychologytoday.com/blog/compassion-matters/201207/recognizing-complex-trauma

Forensics for Survivors. (2015). *The rape exam.* Retrieved from http://www.surviverape.org/forensics/sexual-assault-forensics/rape-exam

Harvard Program in Refugee Trauma. (n.d.). *Treatment plan.* Retrieved from http://hprt-cambridge.org/clinical/treatment-plan/

Health Research Funding. (2014). *21 amazing spousal rape statistics.* Retrieved from http://health-researchfunding.org/21-spousal-rape-statistics/

HelpGuide.org. (2016). *Elder abuse and neglect.* Retrieved from http://www.helpguide.org/articles/abuse/elder-abuse-and-neglect.htm

Herdman, T. H. & Kamitsuru, S. (Eds). *Nursing Diagnoses—Definitions and Classification 2015–2017.* Copyright © 2014, 1994–2014 NANDA International. Used by arrangement with John Wiley & Sons, Inc. Companion website: www.wiley.com/go/nursingdiagnoses

Homeland Security: Office of Immigration Statistics. (2014). *Refugees and asylees: 2013.* Retrieved from https://www.dhs.gov/sites/default/files/publications/ois_rfa_fr_2013.pdf

International Society for Traumatic Stress Studies. (2016). *Military matters: Complementary integrative health in the movement towards transforming patient centered care in the VA.* Retrieved from http://www.istss.org/education-research/traumatic-stresspoints/2016-june/military-matters-complementary-integrative-health.aspx

Jehovah's Witness. (2016). *Why don't Jehovah's Witness accept blood transfusions?* Retrieved from https://www.jw.org/en/jehovahs-witnesses/faq/jehovahs-witnesses-why-no-blood-transfusions/

Kalra, G., & Buhgra, D. (2013). Sexual violence against women: Understanding cross-cultural intersections. *Indian Journal of Psychiatry, 55*(3), 244–249.

Louie, S. (2014). *Asian honor and suicide: The difference between the East and the West.* Retrieved by https://www.psychologytoday.com/blog/minority-report/201406/asian-honor-and-suicide

Mayo Clinic. (2014a). *Post-traumatic stress disorder: Treatments and drugs.* Retrieved from http://www.mayoclinic.org/diseases-conditions/post-traumatic-stress-disorder/basics/treatment/con-20022540.

Mayo Clinic. (2014b). *Complicated grief: Definition.* Retrieved from http://www.mayoclinic.org/diseases-conditions/complicated-grief/basics/definition/con-20032765.

Mayo Clinic. (2014c). *Post-traumatic stress disorder: Prevention.* Retrieved from http://www.mayoclinic.org/diseases-conditions/post-traumatic-stress-disorder/basics/prevention/con-20022540.

Mayo Clinic. (2015). *Child abuse: Symptoms.* Retrieved from http://www.mayoclinic.org/diseases-conditions/child-abuse/basics/symptoms/con-20033789.

Meadows, R. J. (2013). *Understanding violence and victimization* (6th ed.). Boston, MA: Pearson Education.

Medscape. (2015). *Child abuse.* Retrieved from http://emedicine.medscape.com/article/800657-overview#a5

Mills, H., Reiss, N., & Dombeck, M. (n.d.). *Stress reduction and management: Stress inoculation therapy.* Retrieved from http://www.gulfbend.org/poc/view_doc.php?type=doc&id=15683&cn=117

Montalvo-Liendo, N. (2009). Cross-cultural factors in disclosure of intimate partner violence: An integrated review. *Journal of Advanced Nursing, 65*(1), 20–34. doi:10.1111/j.1365-2648.2008.04850.x

National Advisory Council on Nurse Education and Practice. (2007). *Violence against nurses: An assessment of causes and impacts of violence in nursing education and practice.* Retrieved from http://www.hrsa.gov/advisorycommittees/bhpradvisory/nacnep/Reports/fifthreport.pdf

National Center for Complementary and Integrative Health (NCCIH). (2014). *Acupuncture may help symptoms of post-traumatic stress disorder.* Retrieved from https://nccih.nih.gov/research/results/spotlight/092107.htm

National Center on Elder Abuse. (n.d.a) *Types of Abuse.* Retrieved from http://www.ncea.aoa.gov/FAQ/Type_Abuse/index.aspx

National Center on Elder Abuse. (n.d.b). *Statistics/data.* Retrieved from http://www.ncea.aoa.gov/Library/Data/index.aspx

National Child Traumatic Stress Network (NCTSN). (n.d.a). *Types of traumatic stress.* Retrieved from http://www.nctsn.org/trauma-types

National Child Traumatic Stress Network (NCTSN). (n.d.b). *Effects of complex trauma.* Retrieved from http://www.nctsn.org/trauma-types/complex-trauma/effects-of-complex-trauma

National Child Traumatic Stress Network (NCTSN). (n.d.c). *Refugees and trauma.* Retrieved from http://nctsn.org/trauma-types/refugee-trauma/learn-about-refugee-trauma

National Crime Prevention Council. (2016). *Violent crime and personal safety.* Retrieved from https://www.ncpc.org/topics/violent-crime-and-personal-safety

National Crime Prevention Council. (n.d.). *If date rape happens to you.* Retrieved from https://www.sjpd.org/BFO/Community/Crimeprev/crimeprevention%20forms/date_rape.pdf

National Human Trafficking Resource Center. (2016). *Hotline statistics.* Retrieved https://traffickingresourcecenter.org/states

National Institute of Justice. (2012). *Human trafficking.* Retrieved from http://www.nij.gov/topics/crime/human-trafficking/pages/welcome.aspx

National Institute of Justice. (2015). *Extent of elder abuse victimization.* Retrieved from http://www.nij.gov/topics/crime/elder-abuse/pages/extent.aspx

National Institute on Drug Abuse (NIDA) for Teens. (2015). *What are date rape drugs and how do you avoid them?* Retrieved from https://teens.drugabuse.gov/blog/post/what-are-date-rape-drugs-and-how-do-you-avoid-them

National Institute of Mental Health (NIMH). (2016). *Post-traumatic stress disorder.* Retrieved from http://www.nimh.nih.gov/health/topics/post-traumatic-stress-disorder-ptsd/index.shtml

National Institute of Mental Health (NIMH). (n.d.). *Post-traumatic stress disorder among adults.* http://www.nimh.nih.gov/health/statistics/prevalence/post-traumatic-stress-disorder-among-adults.shtml

National Safety Council. (2014). *Workplace violence in healthcare.* Retrieved from http://www.safetyandhealthmagazine.com/articles/11172-workplace-violence-in-health-care-nurses

National Sex Offender Public Website (NSOPW). (n.d.). *Recognizing sexual abuse.* Retrieved from https://www.nsopw.gov/en/education/recognizingsexualabuse?AspxAutoDetectCookieSupport=1

National Society for the Prevention of Cruelty to Children (NSPCC). (2016). *Neglect: Signs, symptoms and effects.* Retrieved from https://www.nspcc.org.uk/preventing-abuse/child-abuse-and-neglect/neglect/signs-symptoms-effects-neglect/

National Trauma Institute. (2012). *Trauma statistics.* Retrieved from http://www.nationaltraumainstitute.org/home/trauma_statistics.html

Nooner, K., Linares, L., Batinjane, J., Kramer, R., Silva, R., & Cloitre, M. (2012). Factors related to post-traumatic stress disorder in adolescents. *Trauma, Violence, & Abuse, 13*(3), 153–166.

Office of Mental Health. (2012). *Violence prevention: Risk factors.* Retrieved from http://www.omh.ny.gov/omhweb/sv/risk.htm

Ovayolu, O., Ovayolu, N., & Karadag, G. (2014). Workplace bullying in nursing. *Workplace Health and Safety, 62*(9) 370–374.

Pennsylvania Department of Transportation. (2016). *Child passenger safety.* Retrieved from http://www.penndot.gov/TravelInPA/Safety/TrafficSafetyAndDriverTopics/Pages/Child-Passenger-Safety.aspx

Pennsylvania Family Support Alliance. (2016). *Discipline, parenting styles and abuse.* Retrieved from http://www.pa-fsa.org/Parents-Caregivers/Preventing-Child-Abuse-Neglect/Discipline-Parenting-Styles-and-Abuse

Potter, M. L., & Moller, M. D. (2016). *Psychiatric-mental health nursing: From suffering to hope.* Hoboken, NJ: Pearson Education. Reprinted and Electronically reproduced by permission of Pearson Education, Inc., New York, NY.

Ritual Abuse, Ritual Crime and Healing. (2016). *Ritual abuse.* Retrieved from http://ra-info.org/faqs/

Roldan, G., Salazar, I., Garrido, L., & Ramos, J. (2013). Violence at work and its relationship with burnout, depression and anxiety in healthcare professionals of the emergency services. *Health, 5*(2), 193–199.

Speroni, K., Fitch, T., Dawson, E., Dugan, L., & Atherton, M. (2014). Incidence and cost of nurse workplace violence perpetrated by hospital patients or patient visitors. *Journal of Emergency Nursing, 40*(3), 218–228.

Substance Abuse and Mental Health Services Administration (SAMHSA). (2014). *SAMHSA's concept of trauma and guidance for a trauma-informed approach.* Retrieved from http://store.samhsa.gov/shin/content/SMA14-4884/SMA14-4884.pdf. Published by Substance Abuse and Mental Health Services Administration, © 2014.

Substance Abuse and Mental Health Services Administration (SAMHSA). (2015). *About NCTIC.* Retrieved from http://www.samhsa.gov/nctic/about.

Treatment Advocacy Center. (2015). *Consequences of non-treatment.* Retrieved from http://www.treatmentadvocacycenter.org/resources/consequences-of-lack-of-treatment/violence/1384

U.S. Department of Health and Human Services (USDHHS). (2010). *Definitions of child abuse and neglect in federal law.* Retrieved from https://www.childwelfare.gov/can/defining/federal.cfm

U.S. Department of Health and Human Services (USDHHS). (2012). *Child maltreatment 2011.* Retrieved from http://www.acf.hhs.gov/sites/default/files/cb/cm11.pdf.

U.S. Department of Justice. (2014). *Office on violence against women.* Retrieved from https://www.justice.gov/ovw/areas-focus.

U.S. Department of Justice. (2015). *Crime against persons with disabilities, 2009–2013, statistical tables.* Retrieved from http://www.bjs.gov/content/pub/pdf/capd0913st.pdf.

U.S. Department of Justice. (2016). *Sexual assault.* Retrieved from https://www.justice.gov/ovw/sexual-assault.

U.S. Department of Justice. (n.d.). *Financial exploitation FAQs.* Retrieved from https://www.justice.gov/elderjustice/financial/faq.html#what-is-the-definition-of-elder-financial-exploitation.

U.S. Department of Veterans Affairs (VA). (2015). *Prolonged exposure therapy.* Retrieved from http://www.ptsd.va.gov/public/treatment/therapy-med/prolonged-exposure-therapy.asp.

U.S. Department of Veterans Affairs (VA). (2016a). *Effects of traumatic stress after mass violence, terror, or disaster.* Retrieved from http://www.ptsd.va.gov/professional/trauma/disaster-terrorism/stress-mv-t-dhtml.asp

U.S. Department of Veterans Affairs (VA). (2016b). *Effects of disasters: Risks and resiliency factors.* Retrieved from http://www.ptsd.va.gov/public/types/disasters/effects_of_disasters_risk_and_resilience_factors.asp

U.S. Department of Veterans Affairs (VA). (2016c). *PTSD in children and adolescents.* Retrieved from http://www.ptsd.va.gov/professional/treatment/children/ptsd_in_children_and_adolescents_overview_for_professionals.asp

U.S. Department of Veterans Affairs (VA). (2016d). *Posttraumatic stress symptoms of older adults: A review.* Retrieved from http://www.ptsd.va.gov/professional/treatment/older/ptsd_symptoms_older_adults.asp

U.S. Department of Veterans Affairs. (2016e). *PTSD assessment and treatment in older adults.* Retrieved from http://www.ptsd.va.gov/professional/treatment/older/assessment_tx_older_adults.asp

U.S. National Library of Medicine. (2016). *Shaken baby syndrome*. Retrieved from https://www.nlm.nih.gov/medlineplus/ency/article/007578.htm

Ward, M., Ornstein, A., Niec, A., Murray, C., & Canadian Paediatric Society, Child and Youth Maltreatment Section. (2013). The medical assessment of bruising in suspected child maltreatment cases: A clinical perspective. *Paediatric and Child Health, 18*(8), 433–437.

White House Council on Women and Girls. (2014). *Rape and sexual assault: A renewed call to action*. Retrieved from https://www.whitehouse.gov/sites/default/files/docs/sexual_assault_report_1-21-14.pdf

World Bank. (2015). *Forced displacement: A growing world crisis FAQs*. Retrieved from http://www.worldbank.org/en/topic/fragilityconflictviolence/brief/forced-displacement-a-growing-global-crisis-faqs

World Health Organization (WHO). (2013a). *Definition and typology of violence*. Retrieved from http://www.who.int/violenceprevention/approach/definition/en

World Health Organization (WHO). (2013b). *World report on violence and health*. Retrieved from http://www.who.int/violence_injury_prevention/violence/world_report/en/index.html

World Health Organization (WHO). (2013c). *Elder abuse*. Retrieved from http://www.who.int/ageing/projects/elder_abuse/en

Part III
Reproduction Module

Part III consists of the module on reproduction, which falls within the individual domain. This module presents the concept of reproduction, with exemplars designed to take the nursing student through the stages of pregnancy to caring for the newborn and the baby who is born prematurely. This module addresses care for newborn, mother, and family, including biophysical and psychosocial needs.

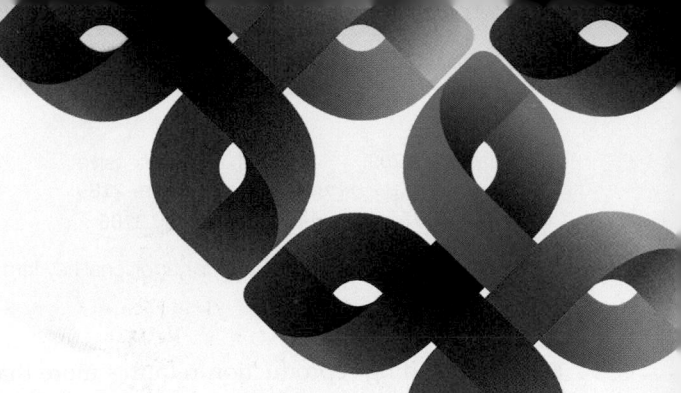

Module 33
Reproduction

Module Outline and Learning Outcomes

The Concept of Reproduction

Normal Presentation of the Female Reproductive System

33.1 Analyze the physiology of the reproductive system.

Conception and Embryonic Development

33.2 Explain the processes of conception and embryonic development.

Embryonic and Fetal Development

33.3 Explain the processes of embryonic and fetal development.

Physical and Psychologic Changes of Pregnancy

33.4 Analyze the physical and psychologic changes of pregnancy.

Concepts Related to Reproduction

33.5 Outline the relationship between reproduction and other concepts.

Health Promotion

33.6 Explain the promotion of healthy reproduction.

Nursing Assessment

33.7 Differentiate among common assessment procedures and tests used to examine reproduction.

Independent Interventions

33.8 Analyze independent interventions nurses can implement for patients with alterations in reproduction.

Collaborative Therapies

33.9 Summarize collaborative therapies used by inter-professional teams for patients with alterations in reproduction.

Lifespan Considerations

33.10 Differentiate considerations related to the care of patients with alterations in reproduction throughout the lifespan.

Reproduction Exemplars

Exemplar 33.A Antepartum Care

33.A Summarize antepartum care of the pregnant woman.

Exemplar 33.B Intrapartum Care

33.B Summarize intrapartum care of the pregnant woman.

Exemplar 33.C Postpartum Care

33.C Summarize postpartum care of the mother.

Exemplar 33.D Newborn Care

33.D Summarize care of newborns.

Exemplar 33.E Prematurity

33.E Summarize care of premature newborns.

>> The Concept of Reproduction

Concept Key Terms

Acrosomal reaction, **2179**	Chloasma, **2190**	Embryonic membranes, **2180**	Gametogenesis, **2178**	Obstetric conjugate, **2172**
Amnion, **2181**	Chorion, **2180**	Estimated date of birth (EDB), **2185**	Goodell sign, **2188**	Oogenesis, **2178**
Amniotic fluid, **2181**	Conjugate vera, **2172**		Graafian follicle, **2176**	Ovulation, **2173**
Aortocaval compression, **2189**	Corpus luteum, **2176**	False pelvis, **2171**	Hegar sign, **2190**	Pelvic inlet, **2172**
Ballottement, **2194**	Cotyledons, **2183**	Female reproductive cycle, **2173**	McDonald sign, **2193**	Pelvic outlet, **2172**
Blastocyst, **2179**	Diagonal conjugate, **2172**		Meiosis, **2177**	Physiologic anemia of pregnancy, **2189**
Braxton Hicks contractions, **2183**	Diastasis recti, **2191**	Fertilization, **2178**	Melasma gravidarum, **2190**	Placenta, **2182**
Capacitation, **2179**	Ductus arteriosus, **2185**	Fetus, **2187**	Mitosis, **2177**	Postconception age, **2186**
Chadwick sign, **2188**	Ductus venosus, **2185**	Foramen ovale, **2185**	Morning sickness, **2193**	Prenatal education, **2221**
	Embryo, **2186**	Gametes, **2170**	Morula, **2179**	Quickening, **2193**
			Nägele rule, **2209**	

(continued on next page)

Understanding reproduction requires more than understanding sexual intercourse or the process by which the female and male sex cells unite. The nurse also must be familiar with the structures and functions that make childbearing possible and the phenomena that initiate it. The primary functions of both female and male reproductive systems are to produce sex cells and transport them to locations where their union can occur. The sex cells, called **gametes**, are produced by specialized organs called *gonads*. A series of ducts and glands in both the male and female reproductive systems contribute to the production and transport of the gametes.

Normal Presentation of the Female Reproductive System

The female reproductive system is described in detail in the module on Sexuality. Two key components of the female reproductive system are discussed here in relation to their importance to conception and childbearing: the bony pelvis and the female reproductive cycle.

Bony Pelvis

The female bony pelvis has two unique functions:

- To support and protect the pelvic contents
- To form the relatively fixed axis of the birth passage.

The structure of the pelvis must be clearly understood because it is an essential component of the childbirth process.

Bony Structure

The pelvis is composed of four bones: two innominate bones, the sacrum, and the coccyx. The pelvis resembles a bowl or basin; its sides are the innominate bones, and its back is the sacrum and coccyx. Lined with fibrocartilage and held tightly together by ligaments, the four bones join at the symphysis pubis, the two sacroiliac joints, and the sacrococcygeal joints (**Figure 33–1 》**).

The innominate bones, also known as the hip bones, are made up of three separate bones: the ilium, ischium, and pubis. These bones fuse to form a circular cavity, the acetabulum, which articulates with the femur.

The ilium is the broad, upper prominence of the hip. The iliac crest is the margin of the ilium. The ischial spines, the foremost projections nearest the groin, are the site of attachment for ligaments and muscles.

The ischium, the strongest bone, is under the ilium and below the acetabulum. The L-shaped ischium ends in a marked protuberance, the ischial tuberosity, on which the weight of a seated body rests. The ischial spines arise near the junction of the ilium and ischium and jut into the pelvic cavity. The shortest diameter of the pelvic cavity is between the ischial spines. The ischial spines serve as reference points

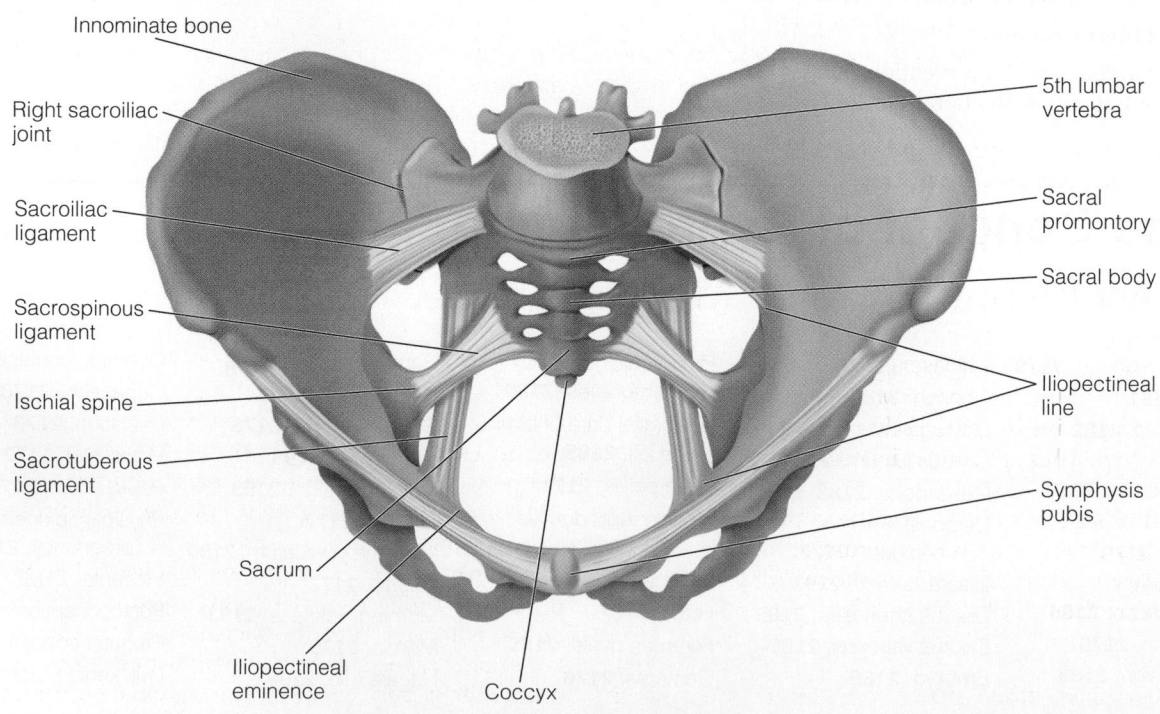

Figure 33–1 》 Pelvic bones with supporting ligaments.

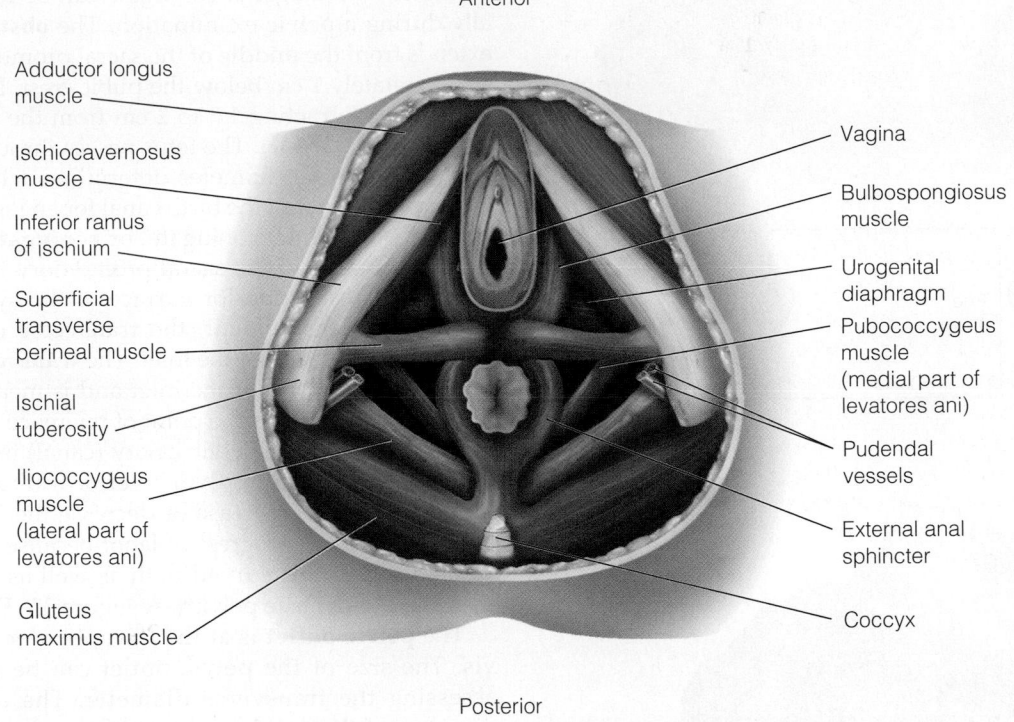

Anterior

Adductor longus muscle

Ischiocavernosus muscle

Inferior ramus of ischium

Superficial transverse perineal muscle

Ischial tuberosity

Iliococcygeus muscle (lateral part of levatores ani)

Gluteus maximus muscle

Vagina

Bulbospongiosus muscle

Urogenital diaphragm

Pubococcygeus muscle (medial part of levatores ani)

Pudendal vessels

External anal sphincter

Coccyx

Posterior

Figure 33–2 >> Muscles of the pelvic floor. (The puborectalis, pubovaginalis, and coccygeal muscles cannot be seen from this view.)

during labor to evaluate the descent of the fetal head into the birth canal.

The pubis forms the slightly bowed front portion of the innominate bone. Extending medially from the acetabulum to the midpoint of the bony pelvis, each pubis meets the other to form a joint called the *symphysis pubis*. The triangular space below this junction is known as the *pubic arch*. The fetal head passes under this arch during birth. The symphysis pubis is formed by heavy fibrocartilage and the superior and inferior pubic ligaments. The mobility of the inferior ligament increases during a woman's first pregnancy and increases further in subsequent pregnancies.

The sacroiliac joints also have a degree of mobility that increases near the end of pregnancy as the result of an upward gliding movement. The pelvic outlet may be increased by 1.5–2 cm in the squatting and sitting positions. This relaxation of the joints is induced by *relaxin*, which is a pregnancy hormone.

The sacrum is a wedge-shaped bone formed by the fusion of five vertebrae. On the anterior upper portion of the sacrum is a projection into the pelvic cavity known as the *sacral promontory*. This projection is a guide in determining pelvic measurements.

The small triangular bone last on the vertebral column is the coccyx. It articulates with the sacrum at the sacrococcygeal joint. The coccyx usually moves backward during labor to provide more room for the fetus.

Pelvic Floor

The muscular pelvic floor of the bony pelvis is designed to overcome the force of gravity exerted on the pelvic organs. It acts as a supporting structure to the irregularly shaped pelvic outlet, providing stability and support for surrounding structures.

Deep fascia, the levator ani, and coccygeal muscles form the part of the pelvic floor known as the pelvic diaphragm. The components of the pelvic diaphragm function as a whole, yet they are able to move over one another. This physiology provides an exceptional capacity for dilation during birth and return to prepregnancy condition following birth. Above the pelvic diaphragm is the pelvic cavity; below and behind it is the perineum. The sacrum is located posteriorly.

The levator ani muscle makes up the major portion of the pelvic diaphragm and consists of four muscles: the iliococcygeus, pubococcygeus, puborectalis, and pubovaginalis. The iliococcygeal muscle, a thin muscular sheet underlying the sacrospinous ligament, helps the levator ani support the pelvic organs. Muscles of the pelvic floor are shown in **Figure 33–2** >>.

Pelvic Division

The pelvic cavity is divided into the false pelvis and the true pelvis. The **false pelvis** (**Figure 33–3A** >>), the portion above the pelvic brim, or linea terminalis, supports the weight of the enlarged pregnant uterus and directs the presenting fetal part into the true pelvis below.

The **true pelvis** is the portion that lies below the linea terminalis (pelvic brim). The bony circumference of the true pelvis is made up of the sacrum, coccyx, and innominate bones and represents the bony limits of the birth canal. The relationship between the true pelvic cavity and the fetal head is of paramount importance: The size and shape of the true pelvis must be adequate for normal fetal passage during

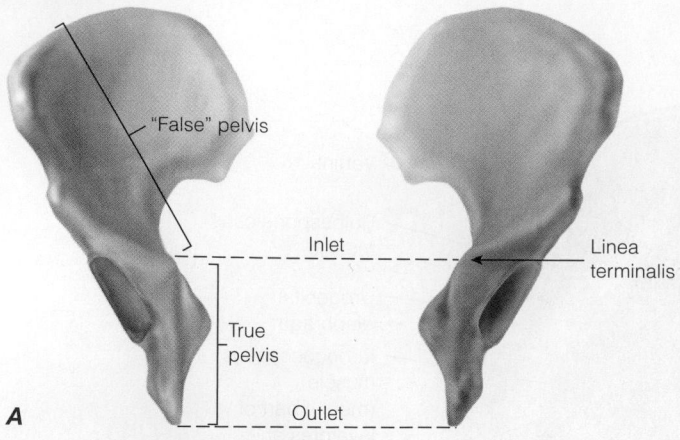

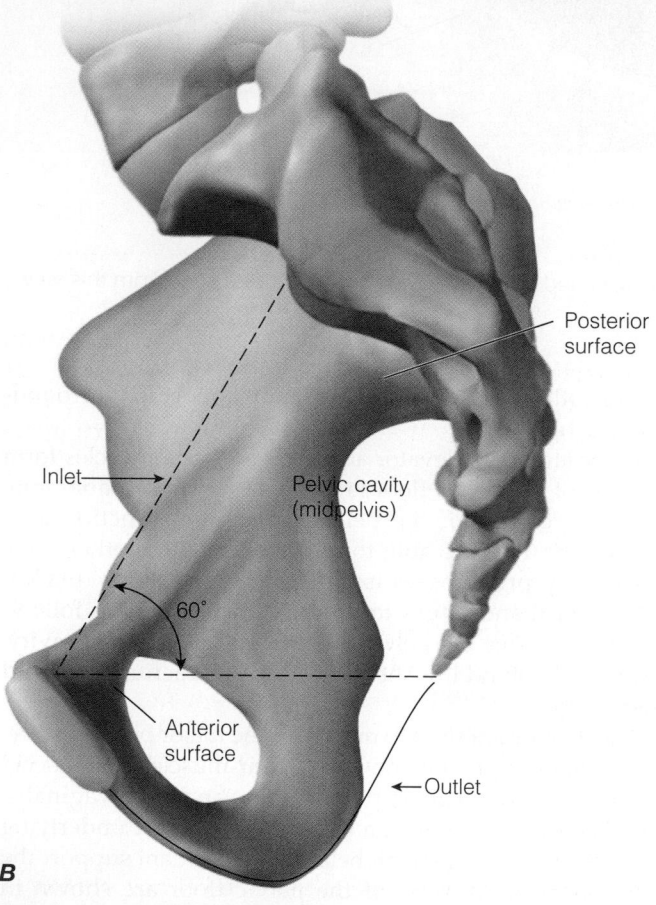

Figure 33–3 ⟩⟩ Female pelvis. **A,** False pelvis is a shallow cavity above the inlet; true pelvis is the deeper portion of the cavity below the inlet. **B,** True pelvis consists of inlet, cavity (midpelvis), and outlet.

labor and at birth. The true pelvis consists of three parts: the inlet, the pelvic cavity, and the outlet (Figure 33–3B). Each part has distinct measurements that aid in evaluating the adequacy of the pelvis for childbirth.

The **pelvic inlet** is the upper border of the true pelvis and is typically rounded. Its size and shape are determined by assessing three anteroposterior diameters. The **diagonal conjugate** extends from the subpubic angle to the middle of the sacral promontory and is typically 12.5 to 13 cm in

diameter. The diagonal conjugate can be measured manually during a pelvic examination. The **obstetric conjugate** extends from the middle of the sacral promontory to an area approximately 1 cm below the pubic crest. Its length is estimated by subtracting 1.5 to 2 cm from the diagonal conjugate (**Figure 33–4 ⟩⟩**). The fetus passes through the obstetric conjugate, whose diameter determines whether the fetus can move down into the birth canal for engagement to occur. The true (anatomic) conjugate, or **conjugate vera**, extends from the middle of the sacral promontory to the middle of the pubic crest (superior surface of the symphysis). One additional measurement, the transverse diameter, helps determine the shape of the inlet. The **transverse diameter** is the largest diameter of the inlet and is measured by using the linea terminalis as the point of reference.

The midpelvis or pelvic cavity (canal) is a curved canal with a longer posterior than anterior wall. A change in the lumbar curve can increase or decrease the tilt of the pelvis and influence the progress of labor because the fetus has to adjust itself to this curved path as well as to the different diameters of the true pelvis (see Figure 33–3B).

The **pelvic outlet** is at the lower border of the true pelvis. The size of the pelvic outlet can be determined by assessing the transverse diameter. The anteroposterior diameter of the pelvic outlet increases during birth as the presenting part of the fetus pushes the coccyx posteriorly at the mobile sacrococcygeal joint. Decreased mobility, a large fetal head, and/or a forceful birth can cause the coccyx to break. As the fetus' head emerges, the long diameter of the head (occipital frontal) parallels the long diameter of the outlet (anteroposterior).

The transverse diameter (bi-ischial or intertuberous) extends from the inner surface of one ischial tuberosity to the other. It is the shortest diameter of the pelvic outlet and is even shorter in a woman who has a narrowed pubic arch. The pubic arch is of great importance because the fetus must pass under it during birth. If it is narrow, the baby's head may be pushed backward toward the coccyx, making extension of the head difficult. This situation, known as outlet dystocia, may require the use of forceps or a cesarean birth. The shoulders of a large baby also may become wedged under the pubic arch, making birth more difficult.

Pelvic Types

The Caldwell–Moloy classification of pelves is still sometimes used to differentiate bony pelvic types (Caldwell & Moloy, 1933). The four basic types are gynecoid, android, anthropoid, and platypelloid (**Figure 33–5 ⟩⟩**). However, variations in the female pelvis are so great that classic types are not usual. Each type has a characteristic shape, and each shape has implications for labor and birth. The types are described here, along with their implications for labor and birth.

Gynecoid Pelvis

The most common female pelvis is the gynecoid type. All of the inlet diameters are at least adequate for a vaginal birth. The gynecoid pelvic outlet has a wide and round pubic arch; the inferior pubic rami are short and concave. The anteroposterior diameter is long; the transverse diameter, adequate. The overall capacity of the outlet is adequate

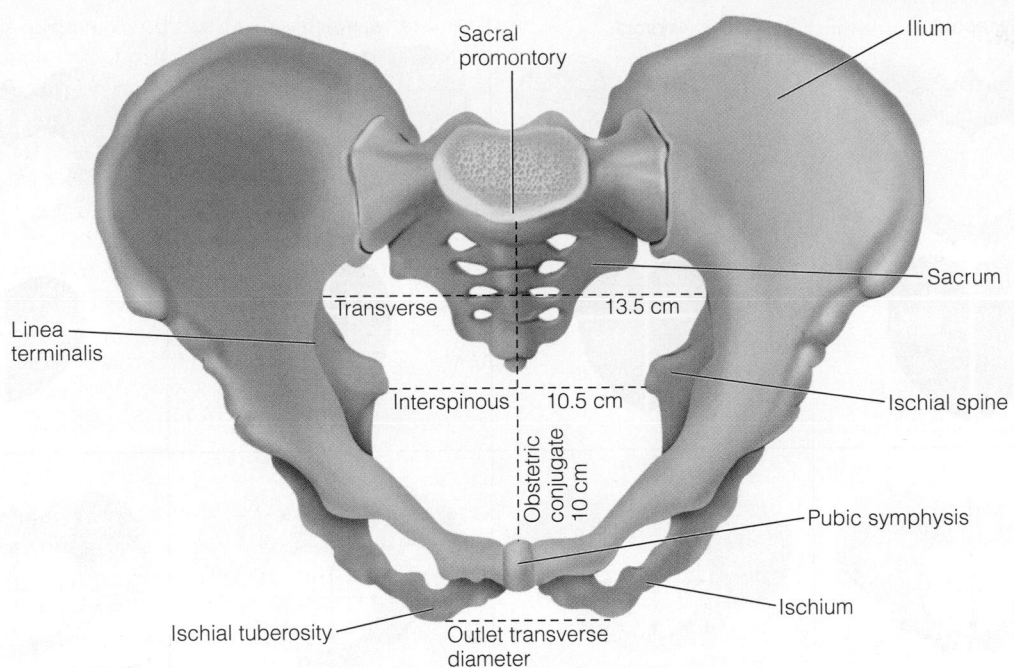

Figure 33–4 》》 Pelvic planes: coronal section and diameters of the bony pelvis.

for a vaginal birth. Approximately 50% of female pelves are classified as gynecoid (Caldwell & Moloy, 1933).

Android Pelvis

The normal male pelvis is the android type; this type is occasionally seen in females. The inlet is heart shaped. The anteroposterior and transverse diameters are adequate for a vaginal birth, but the posterior sagittal diameter is too short, and the anterior sagittal diameter is long. The android outlet has a narrow, sharp, and deep pubic arch; the inferior pubic rami are straight and long. The anteroposterior diameter is short, and the transverse diameter is narrow. The capacity of the outlet is reduced. Approximately 20% of female pelves are classified as android (Caldwell & Moloy, 1933). The structure of an android pelvis is not favorable for a vaginal birth. Cesarean birth may be required.

Anthropoid Pelvis

The inlet of an anthropoid pelvis is oval, with a long anteroposterior diameter and an adequate but rather short transverse diameter. The midpelvic diameters are at least adequate, making its capacity adequate for a vaginal birth. The anthropoid outlet has a normal or moderately narrow pubic arch; the interior pubic rami are long and narrow. The outlet capacity is adequate. Approximately 25% of female pelves are classified as anthropoid (Caldwell & Moloy, 1933).

Platypelloid Pelvis

The platypelloid type refers to the flat female pelvis. The inlet is a distinctly transverse oval with a short anteroposterior and extremely short transverse diameter. The transverse diameter is wide, but the anteroposterior diameter is short. The outlet capacity may be inadequate for a vaginal birth. The platypelloid bones are similar to those of a gynecoid pelvis. Only 5% of female pelves are classified as platypelloid (Caldwell & Moloy, 1933).

Female Reproductive Cycle

The **female reproductive cycle** is composed of the ovarian cycle, during which **ovulation**, the release of a mature egg from an ovary, occurs, and the uterine cycle, during which menstruation occurs. These two cycles take place simultaneously (**Figure 33–6 》》**).

Effects of Female Hormones

After menarche, a female undergoes a cyclic pattern of ovulation and menstruation, which is disrupted only by pregnancy, for a period of 30–40 years. This cycle is an orderly process under neurohormonal control. Each month multiple oocytes mature, with typically one, and sometimes more than one, rupturing from the ovary and entering the fallopian tube. The ovary, vagina, uterus, and fallopian tubes are major target organs for female hormones.

Estrogen

The ovaries produce mature gametes and secrete hormones (estrogens, progesterone, and testosterone). Estrogens cause the uterus to increase in size and weight because of increased glycogen, amino acids, electrolytes, and water. Blood supply is expanded as well. Under the influence of estrogens, myometrial contractility increases in both the uterus and fallopian tubes. Uterine sensitivity to oxytocin also increases. Estrogens inhibit follicle-stimulating hormone (FSH) production and stimulate luteinizing hormone (LH) production.

Estrogens have effects on many hormones and other carrier proteins. For example, they contribute to the increased amount of protein bound iodine in pregnant women and in women who use oral contraceptives containing estrogen. Estrogens decrease the excitability of the hypothalamus, which may cause an increase in sexual desire.

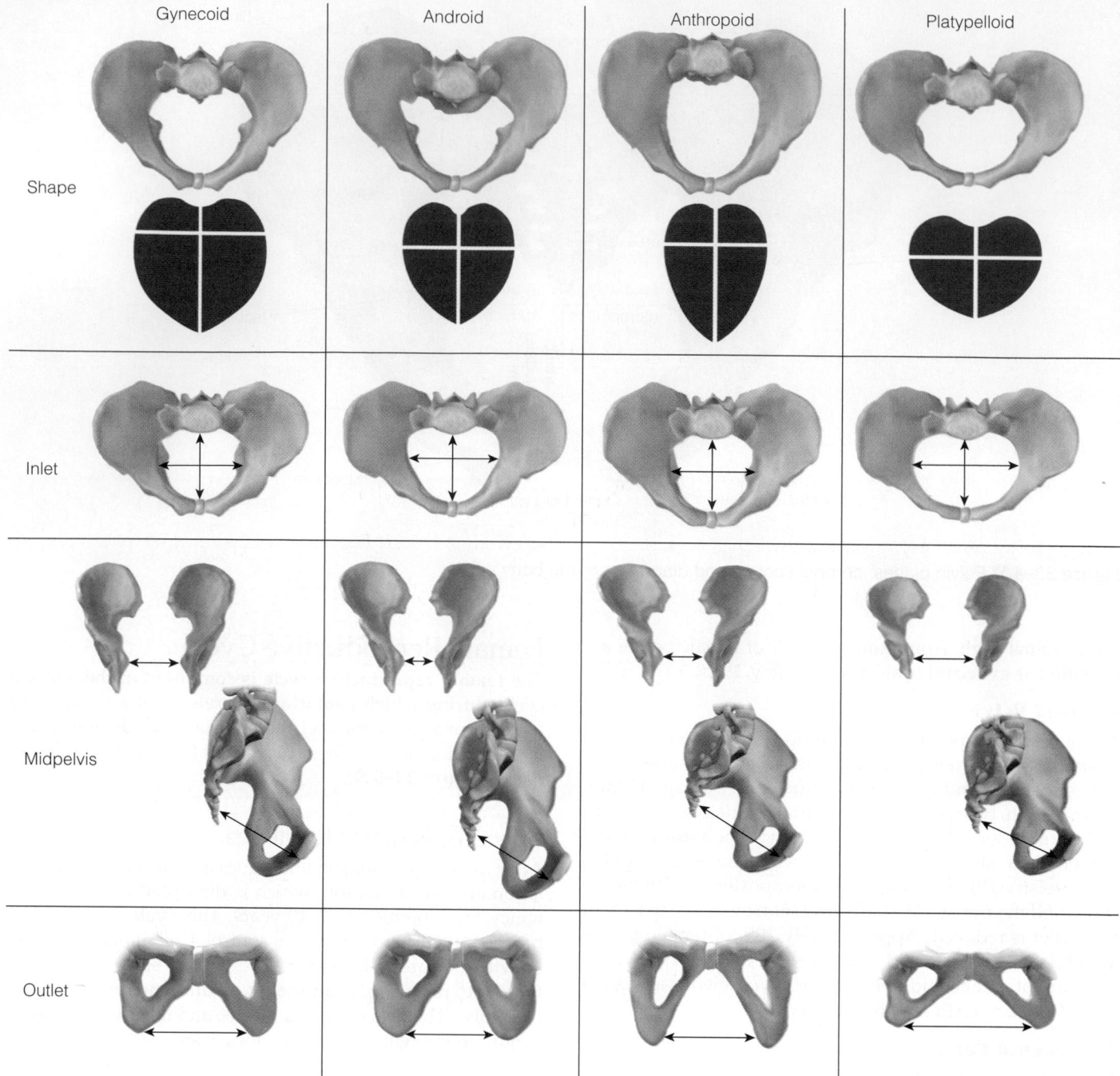

Figure 33–5 » Comparison of Caldwell–Moloy pelvic types.

Progesterone

Progesterone is secreted by the corpus luteum and is found in greatest amounts during the secretory (luteal or progestational) phase of the menstrual cycle. Progesterone is often called the *hormone of pregnancy* because its effects on the uterus allow pregnancy to be maintained. Under the influence of progesterone, the vaginal epithelium proliferates, the cervix secretes thick, viscous mucus, and contractility of the uterus is suppressed. Breast glandular tissue increases in size and complexity. Progesterone also prepares the breasts for lactation and may contribute to constipation in pregnancy due to relaxation of smooth muscle, which results in decreased peristalsis.

Prostaglandins

Prostaglandins (PGs), which are oxygenated fatty acids, are produced by the cells of the endometrium. They are classified as hormones. Prostaglandins have varied action in the body. The two primary types of PGs are groups E and F. Generally, PGE relaxes smooth muscles and is a potent vasodilator; PGF is a potent vasoconstrictor and increases the contractility of muscles and arteries. Although the primary actions of PGE and PGF seem antagonistic, their basic regulatory functions in cells are achieved through an intricate pattern of reciprocal events.

Prostaglandin production increases during follicular maturation, is dependent on gonadotropins, and seems to be

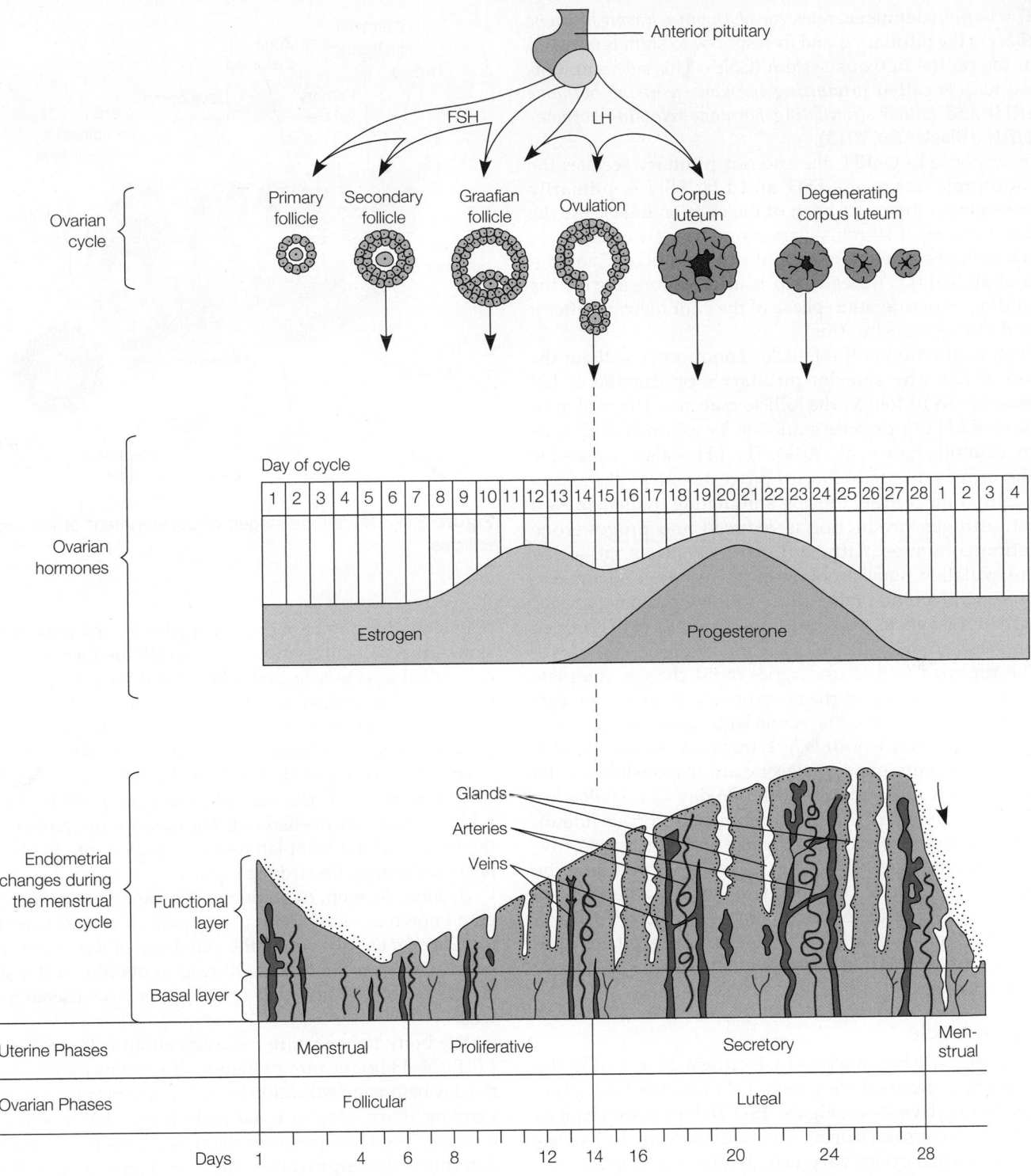

Figure 33-6 » Female reproductive cycle: interrelationships of hormones with the three phases of the uterine cycle and the two phases of the ovarian cycle in an ideal 28-day cycle.

critical to follicular rupture (Cunningham et al., 2014). Extrusion of the ovum, resulting from follicular swelling and increased contractility of the smooth muscle in the theca externa layer of the mature follicle, is thought to be caused in part by $PGF_{2\alpha}$. Significant amounts of PGs are found in and around the follicle at the time of ovulation.

Neurohumoral Basis of the Female Reproductive Cycle

The female reproductive cycle is controlled by complex interactions between the nervous and endocrine systems and their target tissues. These interactions involve the hypothalamus, anterior pituitary, and ovaries.

The hypothalamus secretes *gonadotropin-releasing hormone (GnRH)* to the pituitary gland in response to signals received from the central nervous system (CNS). This releasing hormone also is called *luteinizing hormone-releasing hormone (LHRH)* and *follicle-stimulating hormone-releasing hormone (FSHRH)* (Blackburn, 2013).

In response to GnRH, the anterior pituitary secretes the gonadotropic hormones FSH and LH. FSH is primarily responsible for the maturation of the ovarian follicle. As the follicle matures, it secretes increasing amounts of estrogen, which enhances the development of the follicle (Cunningham et al., 2014). This estrogen is also responsible for the rebuilding or proliferation phase of the endometrium after it is shed during menstruation.

Final maturation of the follicle cannot occur without the action of LH. The anterior pituitary's production of LH increases 6- to 10-fold as the follicle matures. The peak production of LH can precede ovulation by as much as 12 to 24 hours (Cunningham et al., 2014). The LH is also responsible for the increase in production of progesterone by the granulosa cells of the follicle, thereby stimulating ovulation. As a result, estrogen production is reduced and progesterone secretion continues. Although estrogen levels fall a day before ovulation, small amounts of progesterone continue to be present. Ovulation takes place following the very rapid growth of the follicle, as the sustained high level of estrogen diminishes and progesterone secretion begins.

The ruptured follicle undergoes rapid change, complete luteinization occurs, and the mass of cells becomes the **corpus luteum**. The lutein cells secrete large amounts of progesterone with smaller amounts of estrogen. Concurrently, the excessive amounts of progesterone are responsible for the secretory phase of the uterine cycle. On day 7 or 8 following ovulation, if pregnancy does not occur, the corpus luteum begins to involute, or decrease in size and functional activity. It loses its secretory function, severely diminishing the production of progesterone and estrogen. The anterior pituitary responds with increasingly large amounts of FSH, and LH production begins a few days later. As a result, new follicles become responsive to subsequent ovarian cycles and begin maturing.

Ovarian Cycle

The ovarian cycle has two phases. During a 28-day cycle, the *follicular phase* occurs during days 1–14 and the *luteal phase* occurs during days 15–28. **Figure 33–7 ≫** depicts the changes the follicle undergoes during the ovarian cycle. In women whose menstrual cycles vary, usually only the length of the follicular phase varies because the luteal phase is of fixed length. During the follicular phase, the immature follicle matures as a result of FSH. Within the follicle, the oocyte grows.

A mature **graafian follicle** appears about the 14th day under dual control of FSH and LH. It is a large structure, measuring about 5 to 10 mm, which produces increasing amounts of estrogen. In the mature graafian follicle, the cells surrounding the fluid-filled antral cavity are called granulosa cells. The mass of granulosa cells surrounding the oocyte and follicular fluid is called the cumulus oophorus. In the fully mature graafian follicle, the zona pellucida, a thick elastic capsule, develops around the oocyte. Just before

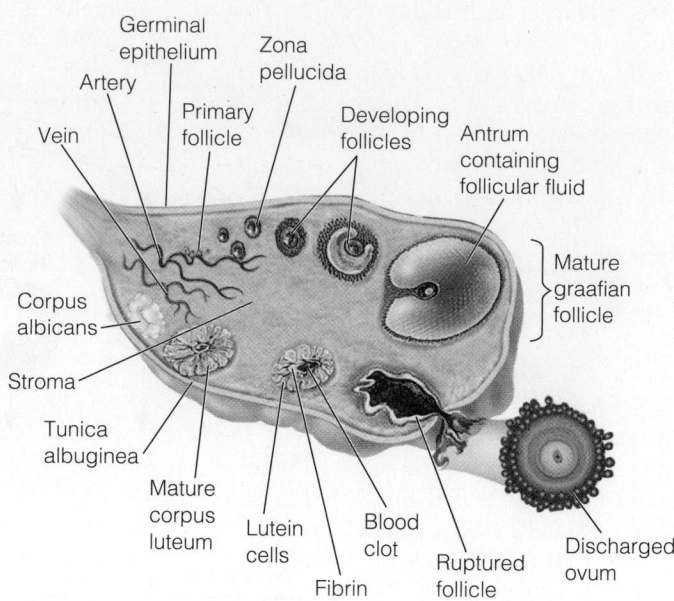

Figure 33–7 ≫ Various stages of development of the ovarian follicles.

ovulation, the mature oocyte completes its first meiotic division. As a result of this division, two cells are formed: a small cell, called a *polar body,* and a larger cell, called a secondary oocyte. The secondary oocyte matures into the ovum.

As the graafian follicle matures and enlarges, it comes close to the surface of the ovary. The ovary surface forms a blister-like protrusion 10–15 mm in diameter, and the follicle walls become thin. The secondary oocyte, polar body, and follicular fluid are pushed out. The ovum is discharged near the fimbria of the fallopian tube and pulled into the tube to begin its journey toward the uterus.

In some women, ovulation is accompanied by midcycle pain known as *mittelschmerz.* This pain may be caused by a local peritoneal reaction to the expulsion of the ovum. Vaginal discharge may increase during ovulation, and a small amount of blood (midcycle spotting) may be discharged as well.

The body temperature increases about 0.3°–0.6°C (0.5°–1.0°F) 24–48 hours after ovulation. It remains elevated until the day before menstruation begins. There may be an accompanying sharp drop in basal body temperature before the increase. These temperature changes are useful clinically to determine the approximate time ovulation occurs (Blackburn, 2013).

Generally, the ovum takes several minutes to travel through the ruptured follicle to the fallopian tube opening. The contractions of the tube's smooth muscle and its ciliary action propel the ovum through the tube. The ovum remains in the ampulla, where, if it is fertilized, cleavage can begin. The ovum is thought to be fertile for only 6–24 hours. It reaches the uterus 72–96 hours after its release from the ovary.

• The luteal phase begins when the ovum leaves its follicle. Under the influence of LH, the corpus luteum develops from the ruptured follicle. Within 2 or 3 days, the corpus luteum becomes yellowish and spherical and increases in vascularity.

If the ovum is fertilized and implants in the endometrium, the fertilized egg begins to secrete *human chorionic gonadotropin (hCG)*, which is needed to maintain the corpus luteum. If fertilization does not occur, within about a week after ovulation, the corpus luteum begins to degenerate, eventually becoming a connective tissue scar called the corpus albicans. With degeneration comes a decrease in estrogen and progesterone. This triggers the hypothalamus to release *gonadotropin-releasing hormone (GnRH)*, which stimulates the synthesis and secretion of LH and FSH. This process initiates a new ovulatory cycle.

Menstrual Cycle

Menstruation is cyclic uterine bleeding in response to cyclic hormonal changes. Menstruation occurs when the ovum is not fertilized and begins about 14 days after ovulation in an ideal 28-day cycle. The menstrual discharge, also referred to as the menses or menstrual flow, is composed of blood mixed with fluid, cervical and vaginal secretions, bacteria, mucus, leukocytes, and other cellular debris. The menstrual discharge is dark red and has a distinctive odor.

Menstrual parameters vary greatly among individuals. Generally, menstruation occurs every 29 days, but the cycle varies from 21 to 35 days. Some women have longer cycles, which can skew standard calculations of the estimated date of birth (EDB). Emotional and physical factors such as illness, excessive fatigue, stress or anxiety, and vigorous exercise programs can alter the cycle interval. Certain environmental factors such as temperature and altitude also may affect the cycle. The duration of menses is from 2 to 8 days, with the blood loss averaging 25–60 mL and the loss of iron averaging 0.5–1 mg daily.

The uterine (menstrual) cycle has three phases: menstrual, proliferative, and secretory. Menstruation occurs during the *menstrual phase*. Some endometrial areas are shed, although others remain. Some of the remaining tips of the endometrial glands begin to regenerate. The endometrium is in a resting state following menstruation. Estrogen levels are low, and the endometrium is 1–2 mm deep. During this part of the cycle, the cervical mucus is scanty, viscous, and opaque.

The *proliferative phase* begins when the endometrial glands enlarge, becoming twisted and longer in response to increasing amounts of estrogen. The blood vessels become prominent and dilated, and the endometrium increases in thickness six- to eightfold. This gradual process reaches its peak just before ovulation. The cervical mucus becomes thin, clear, watery, and more alkaline, making the mucosa more favorable to spermatozoa. As ovulation nears, the cervical mucus shows increased elasticity, called *spinnbarkeit*. At ovulation, the mucus will stretch more than 5 cm. The pH of the cervical mucus increases from below 7.0 to 7.5 at the time of ovulation. On microscopic examination, the mucus shows a characteristic ferning pattern (**Figure 33–8 》》**). This fern pattern is useful in assessing ovulation time.

The *secretory phase* follows ovulation. The endometrium, under estrogenic influence, undergoes slight cellular growth. Progesterone, however, causes such marked swelling and growth that the epithelium is warped into folds. The amount of tissue glycogen increases. The glandular epithelial cells begin to fill with cellular debris, become twisted, and dilate. The glands secrete small quantities of endometrial fluid in preparation for

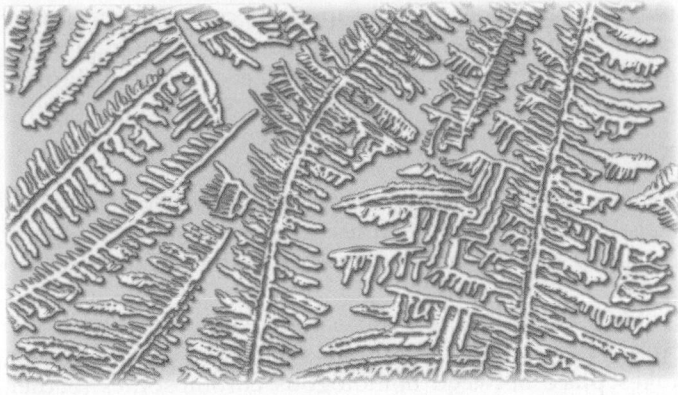

Figure 33–8 》》 Ferning pattern.

a fertilized ovum. The vascularity of the entire uterus increases greatly, providing a nourishing bed for implantation. If implantation occurs, the endometrium, under the influence of progesterone, continues to develop and becomes even.

If fertilization does not occur, the *menstrual phase* begins. The corpus luteum begins to degenerate, and as a result, both estrogen and progesterone levels fall. Areas of necrosis appear under the epithelial lining. Extensive vascular changes also occur. Small blood vessels rupture, and the spiral arteries constrict and retract, causing a deficiency of blood in the endometrium, which becomes pale. This phase is characterized by the escape of blood into the stromal cells of the uterus. The menstrual flow begins, thus beginning the menstrual cycle again. After menstruation, the basal layer remains so that the tips of the glands can regenerate the new functional endometrial layer. (For more about the female reproductive cycle, see the module on Sexuality.)

Conception and Embryonic Development

Each human begins life as a single cell called a fertilized ovum, or zygote. This single cell reproduces itself and, in turn, each resulting cell reproduces itself in a continuing process. The new cells are similar to the cells from which they came. Cells are reproduced by mitosis or meiosis, two different but related processes.

Mitosis results in the production of diploid body (somatic) cells, which are exact copies of the original cell. Mitosis makes growth and development possible, and in mature individuals, it is the process by which the body's cells continue to divide and replace themselves. **Meiosis** is a process of cell division leading to the development of the eggs and sperm needed to produce a new organism. Unlike cells produced during mitosis, the cells produced during meiosis contain only half the genetic material or number of chromosomes (the haploid number).

Mitosis

During mitosis, the cell undergoes several changes, ending in cell division. As the last phase of cell division nears completion, a furrow develops in the cell cytoplasm, which divides it into two daughter cells, each with its own nucleus. Daughter cells have the same diploid number of chromosomes

(46) and same genetic makeup as the cell from which they came. After a cell with 46 chromosomes goes through mitosis, the result is two identical cells, each with 46 chromosomes.

Meiosis

Meiosis is a special type of cell division by which diploid cells in the testes and ovaries give rise to gametes (sperm and ova) with the haploid number of chromosomes, which is 23.

Meiosis consists of two successive cell divisions. In the first division, the chromosomes replicate. Next, a pairing takes place between homologous chromosomes (Sadler, 2015). Instead of separating immediately, as in mitosis, the chromosomes become closely intertwined. At each point of contact, a physical exchange of genetic material takes place between the chromatids (the arms of the chromosomes). New combinations are provided by the newly formed chromosomes; these combinations account for the wide variation of traits in people (e.g., hair and eye color). The chromosome pairs then separate, and the members of the pair move to opposite sides of the cell. In contrast, during mitosis, the chromatids of each chromosome separate and move to opposite poles. The cell divides, forming two daughter cells, each with 23 double-structured chromosomes; thus each contains the same amount of deoxyribonucleic acid (DNA) as a normal somatic cell. In the second division, the chromatids of each chromosome separate and move to opposite poles of each of the daughter cells. Cell division occurs, resulting in the formation of four cells, each containing 23 single chromosomes, identified as the haploid number of chromosomes. These daughter cells contain only half the DNA of a normal somatic cell (Sadler, 2015).

Mutations may occur during the second meiotic division if two of the chromatids do not move apart rapidly enough when the cell divides. The still-paired chromatids are carried into one of the daughter cells and eventually form an extra chromosome. This condition, autosomal nondisjunction (chromosomal mutation), is harmful to the offspring that may result should fertilization occur. Another type of chromosomal mutation can occur if chromosomes break during meiosis. If the broken segment is lost, the result is a shorter chromosome—a situation known as deletion. If the broken segment becomes attached to another chromosome, a harmful mutation called a translocation results.

Gametogenesis

Meiosis occurs during **gametogenesis**, the process by which germ cells, or gametes (*ovum* and *sperm*), are produced. These cells contain only half the genetic material of a typical body cell. The gametes must have a haploid number (23) of chromosomes so that when the female gamete (egg or ovum) and the male gamete (sperm or spermatozoon) unite to form the **zygote** (fertilized ovum), the normal human diploid number of chromosomes (46) is reestablished.

Oogenesis

Oogenesis is the process that produces the female gamete, called an ovum (egg). The ovaries begin to develop early in the fetal life of the female. All of the ova that the female will produce in her lifetime are present at birth. The ovary gives rise to oogonial cells, which develop into oocytes. Meiosis begins in all oocytes before the female fetus is born, but stops before the first division is complete and remains in this arrested phase until puberty. During puberty, the mature primary oocyte proceeds (by oogenesis) through the first meiotic division in the graafian follicle of the ovary.

The first meiotic division produces two cells of unequal size with different amounts of cytoplasm but with the same number of chromosomes. These two cells are the secondary oocyte and the first polar body. Both the secondary oocyte and the first polar body contain 22 double-structured autosomal chromosomes and one double-structured sex chromosome (X).

At ovulation, a second meiotic division begins immediately and proceeds as the oocyte moves down the fallopian tube. Division is again not equal, and the secondary oocyte moves into the metaphase stage of cell division, where its meiotic division is arrested until and unless the oocyte is fertilized.

When the secondary oocyte completes the second meiotic division after fertilization, the result is a mature ovum with the haploid number of chromosomes and virtually all of the cytoplasm. In addition, the second polar body (also haploid) forms at this time. The first polar body now has also divided, producing two additional polar bodies. Thus, at the completion of meiosis, four haploid cells have been produced: the three polar bodies, which eventually disintegrate, and one ovum (Sadler, 2015).

Spermatogenesis

During puberty, the germinal epithelium in the seminiferous tubules of the testes begins the process of **spermatogenesis**, which produces the male gamete (sperm). The diploid spermatogonium replicates before it enters the first meiotic division, during which it is called the primary spermatocyte. During this first meiotic division, the spermatogonium replicates and forms two haploid cells called secondary spermatocytes, each of which contains 22 double-structured autosomal chromosomes and either a double-structured X sex chromosome or a double-structured Y sex chromosome. During the second meiotic division, they divide to form four spermatids, each with the haploid number of chromosomes. The spermatids undergo a series of changes during which they lose most of their cytoplasm and become sperm (spermatozoa). The nucleus becomes compacted into the head of the sperm, which is covered by a cap called an acrosome that is, in turn, covered by a plasma membrane. A long tail is produced from one of the centrioles.

Fertilization

Fertilization is the process by which a sperm fuses with an ovum to form a new diploid cell, or zygote. The zygote begins life as a single cell with a complete set of genetic material, 23 chromosomes from the mother's ovum and 23 chromosomes from the father's sperm for a total of 46 chromosomes. The following events lead to fertilization.

Preparation for Fertilization

The mature ovum and spermatozoon have only a brief time to unite. Ova are considered fertile for about 12–24 hours after ovulation. Sperm can survive in the female reproductive tract for 48–72 hours, but they are believed to be healthy and highly fertile for only the first 24 hours.

The ovum's cell membrane is surrounded by two layers of tissue. The layer closest to the cell membrane is called the *zona pellucida*. It is a clear, noncellular layer whose thickness influences the fertilization rate. Surrounding the zona pellucida is a ring of elongated cells, called the *corona radiata* because they radiate from the ovum like the gaseous corona around the sun. These cells are held together by hyaluronic acid. The ovum has no inherent power of movement. During ovulation, high estrogen levels increase peristalsis in the fallopian tubes, which helps move the ovum through the tube toward the uterus. The high estrogen levels also cause a thinning of the cervical mucus, facilitating movement of the sperm through the cervix, into the uterus, and up the fallopian tube.

The process of fertilization takes place in the ampulla (outer third) of the fallopian tube. In a single ejaculation, the male deposits approximately 200–500 million spermatozoa into the vagina, of which only approximately one thousand sperm actually reach the ampulla (Sadler, 2015). Fructose in the semen, secreted by the seminal vesicles, is the energy source for the sperm. The spermatozoa propel themselves up the female tract by the flagellar movement of their tails. Transit time from the cervix into the fallopian tube can be as short as 5 minutes but usually takes an average of 2–7 hours after ejaculation (Sadler, 2015). Prostaglandins in the semen may increase uterine smooth muscle contractions, which help transport the sperm. The fallopian tubes have a dual ciliary action that facilitates movement of the ovum toward the uterus and movement of the sperm from the uterus toward the ovary.

The sperm must undergo two processes before fertilization can occur: capacitation and the acrosomal reaction. **Capacitation** is the removal of the plasma membrane overlying the spermatozoa's acrosomal area and the loss of seminal plasma proteins. If the glycoprotein coat is not removed, the sperm will not be able to fertilize the ovum (Sadler, 2015). Capacitation occurs in the female reproductive tract (aided by uterine enzymes) and is thought to take about 7 hours. Sperm that undergo capacitation take on three characteristics: (1) the ability to undergo the acrosomal reaction, (2) the ability to bind to the zona pellucida, and (3) the acquisition of hypermotility.

The **acrosomal reaction** follows capacitation, whereby the acrosomes of the sperm surrounding the ovum release their enzymes (hyaluronidase, a protease called acrosin, and trypsinlike substances) and thus break down the hyaluronic acid in the ovum's corona radiata (Sadler, 2015). Approximately a thousand acrosomes must rupture before enough hyaluronic acid is cleared for a single sperm to penetrate the ovum's zona pellucida successfully.

At the moment of penetration by a fertilizing sperm, the zona pellucida undergoes a reaction that prevents additional sperm from entering a single ovum. This is known as the block to polyspermy. This cellular change is mediated by release of materials from the cortical granules, organelles found just below the ovum's surface, and is called the *cortical reaction*.

The Moment of Fertilization

After the sperm enters the ovum, a chemical signal prompts the secondary oocyte to complete the second meiotic division, forming the nucleus of the ovum and ejecting the second polar body. Then the nuclei of the ovum and sperm swell and approach each other. The true moment of fertilization occurs as the nuclei unite. Their individual nuclear membranes disappear, and their chromosomes pair up to produce the diploid zygote. Because each nucleus contains a haploid number of chromosomes (23), this union restores the diploid number (46). The zygote contains a new combination of genetic material that results in an individual different from either parent and from anyone else.

The sex of the zygote is determined at the moment of fertilization. The two chromosomes (the sex chromosomes) of the 23rd pair—either XX or XY—determine the sex of an individual. The X chromosome is larger and bears more genes than the Y chromosome. Females have two X chromosomes, and males have an X and a Y chromosome. Whereas the mature ovum produced by oogenesis can have only one type of sex chromosome—an X—spermatogenesis produces two sperm with an X chromosome and two sperm with a Y chromosome. When each gamete contributes an X chromosome, the resulting zygote is female. When the ovum contributes an X and the sperm contributes a Y chromosome, the resulting zygote is male. Certain traits are termed *sex-linked* because they are controlled by the genes on the X sex chromosome. Two examples of sex-linked traits are color blindness and hemophilia.

Preembryonic Development

The first 14 days of development, starting the day the ovum is fertilized (conception), make up the preembryonic stage, or the stage of the ovum. Development after fertilization can be divided into two phases: cellular multiplication and cellular differentiation. These phases are characterized by rapid cellular multiplication and differentiation and establishment of the primary germ layers and embryonic membranes. Synchronized development of the endometrium and the embryo is a prerequisite for implantation to succeed (Moore, Persaud, & Torchia, 2016). These phases and the process of implantation (nidation), which occurs between them, are discussed next.

Cellular Multiplication

Cellular multiplication begins as the zygote moves through the fallopian tube toward the cavity of the uterus. This transport takes 3 days or more and is accomplished mainly by a weak fluid current in the fallopian tube resulting from the beating action of the ciliated epithelia that line the tube.

The zygote now enters a period of rapid mitotic divisions called cleavage, during which it divides into 2 cells, 4 cells, 8 cells, and so on. These cells, called blastomeres, are so small that the developing cell mass is only slightly larger than the original zygote. The blastomeres are held together by the zona pellucida, which is under the corona radiata. The blastomeres eventually form a solid ball of 12–32 cells called the **morula**.

As the morula enters the uterus, two things happen: The intracellular fluid in the morula increases, and a central cavity forms within the cell mass. Inside this cavity is an inner solid mass of cells called the **blastocyst**. The outer layer of cells that surrounds the cavity and replaces the zona pellucida is the **trophoblast**. Eventually, the trophoblast develops

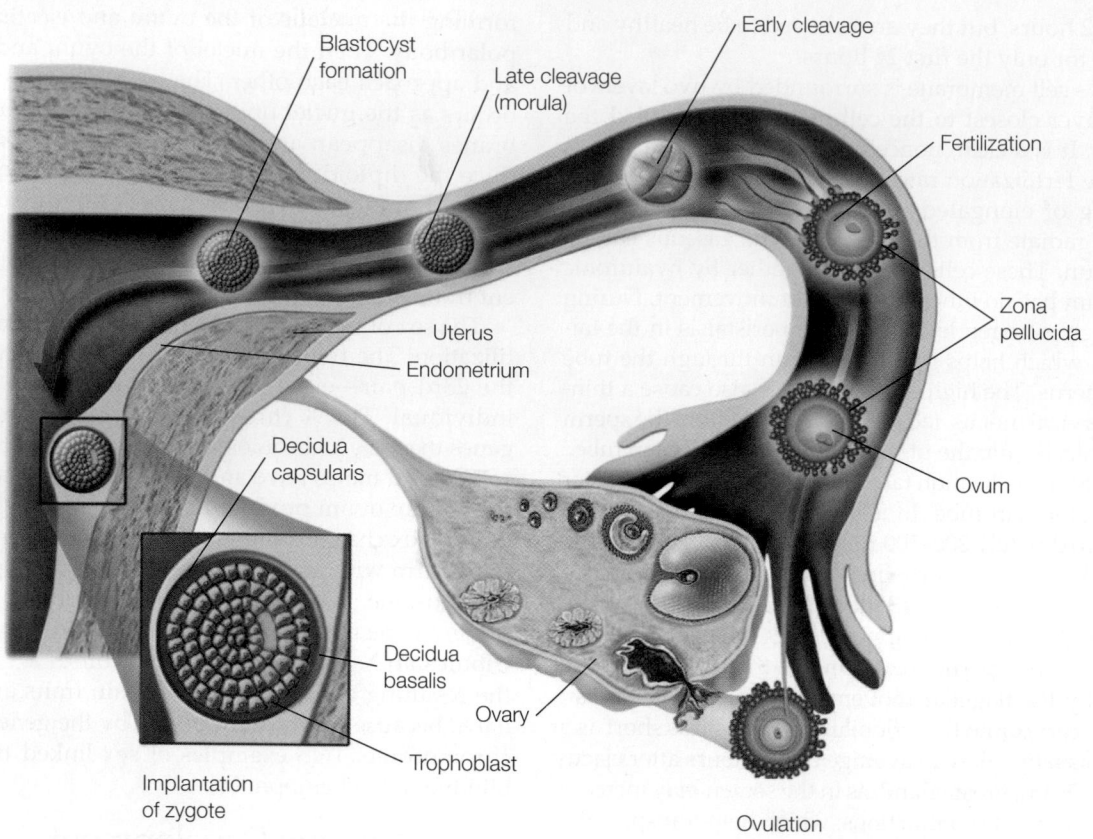

Figure 33–9 》 During ovulation, the ovum leaves the ovary and enters the fallopian tube. Fertilization generally occurs in the outer third of the fallopian tube. The figure depicts subsequent changes in the fertilized ovum from conception to implantation.

into one of the two embryonic membranes, the *chorion*. The blastocyst develops into a double layer of cells called the embryonic disc, from which the *embryo* and the *amnion* (embryonic membrane) develop. The journey of the fertilized ovum to its destination in the uterus is illustrated in **Figure 33–9 》**.

Early pregnancy factor (EPF), an immunosuppressant protein, is secreted by the trophoblastic cells. This factor appears in the maternal serum within 24–48 hours after fertilization and forms the basis of a pregnancy test during the first 10 days of development (Caudle, 2014; Moore et al., 2016).

Implantation (Nidation)

While floating in the uterine cavity, the blastocyst is nourished by the uterine glands, which secrete a mixture of lipids, mucopolysaccharides, and glycogen. The trophoblast attaches to the surface of the endometrium for further nourishment. The most frequent site of attachment is the upper part of the posterior uterine wall. Between 7 and 10 days after fertilization, the zona pellucida disappears and the blastocyst implants itself by burrowing into the uterine lining and penetrating down toward the maternal capillaries until it is completely covered (Moore et al., 2016). The lining of the uterus thickens below the implanted blastocyst, and the cells of the trophoblast grow down into the thickened lining, forming processes that are called *chorionic villi*.

Under the influence of progesterone, the endometrium increases in thickness and vascularity in preparation for implantation and nutrition of the ovum. After implantation,

the endometrium is called the decidua. The portion of the decidua that covers the blastocyst is called the decidua capsularis, the portion directly under the implanted blastocyst is the decidua basalis, and the portion that lines the rest of the uterine cavity is the decidua vera (parietalis). The maternal part of the placenta develops from the decidua basalis, which contains large numbers of blood vessels (magnified inset in Figure 33–9) (London et al., 2017). The chorionic villi (discussed shortly) in contact with the decidua basalis will form the fetal portion of the placenta.

Cellular Differentiation

Primary Germ Layers

About the 10th to 14th day after conception, the homogeneous mass of blastocyst cells differentiates into the primary germ layers. These three layers—the ectoderm, mesoderm, and endoderm—are formed at the same time as the embryonic membranes. All tissues, organs, and organ systems will develop from these primary germ cell layers.

Embryonic Membranes

The **embryonic membranes** begin to form at the time of implantation (**Figure 33–10 》**). These membranes protect and support the embryo as it grows and develops inside the uterus. The first and outermost membrane to form is the **chorion**. This thick membrane develops from the trophoblast and has many fingerlike projections called chorionic villi on its surface. These chorionic villi can be used for early genetic testing of the embryo at 10–11 weeks' gestation by

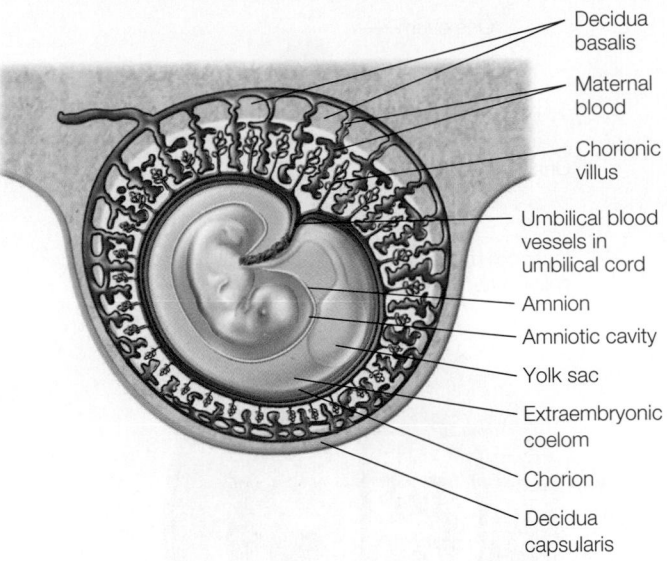

Decidua basalis
Maternal blood
Chorionic villus
Umbilical blood vessels in umbilical cord
Amnion
Amniotic cavity
Yolk sac
Extraembryonic coelom
Chorion
Decidua capsularis

Figure 33–10 》 Early development of primary embryonic membranes. At 4½ weeks, the decidua capsularis (placental portion enclosing the embryo on the uterine surface) and decidua basalis (placental portion encompassing the elaborate chorionic villi and maternal endometrium) are well formed. The chorionic villi lie in blood-filled intervillous spaces within the endometrium. The amnion and yolk sac are well developed.

chorionic villus sampling (CVS). As the pregnancy progresses, the chorionic villi begin to degenerate, except for those just under the embryo, which grow and branch into depressions in the uterine wall, forming the fetal portion of the placenta. By the fourth month of pregnancy, the surface of the chorion is smooth except at the place of attachment to the uterine wall.

The second membrane to form, the amnion, originates from the ectoderm, a primary germ layer, during the early stages of embryonic development. The **amnion** is a thin protective membrane that contains amniotic fluid. The space between the membrane and the embryo is the amniotic cavity. This cavity surrounds the embryo and yolk sac, except where the developing embryo (germ-layer disc) attaches to the trophoblast via the umbilical cord. As the embryo grows, the amnion expands until it comes in contact with the chorion. These two slightly adherent membranes form the fluid-filled amniotic sac, which protects the floating embryo.

Amniotic Fluid

The primary functions of **amniotic fluid** are to:

- Act as a cushion to protect the fetus against mechanical injury during pregnancy and labor.
- Help control the embryo's temperature (the embryo relies on the mother to release heat).
- Permit symmetrical external growth and development of the embryo.
- Prevent adherence of the embryo–fetus to the amnion (decreases chance of amniotic band syndrome) to allow freedom of movement so that the embryo–fetus can change position (flexion and extension), thus aiding in musculoskeletal development.

- Allow the umbilical cord to be relatively free of compression.
- Act as an extension of fetal extracellular space (hydropic fetuses have increased amniotic fluid).
- Permit fetal swallowing and excretion, thus serving as a waste repository.

Amniotic fluid is slightly alkaline and contains albumin, urea, uric acid, creatinine, lecithin, sphingomyelin, bilirubin, fat, fructose, leukocytes, proteins, epithelial cells, enzymes, and fine hair called lanugo. The amount of amniotic fluid at 10 weeks is about 30 mL, and it increases to 210 mL at 16 weeks (Cunningham et al., 2014). After 28 weeks, the volume ranges from 700 to 1000 mL. As the pregnancy continues, the fetus influences the volume of amniotic fluid by swallowing the fluid and excreting lung fluid and urine into the amniotic fluid (London et al., 2017). The fetus swallows up to 262 mL/kg/day. Between 29 and 30 weeks, the amniotic fluid volume changes very little. After 39 weeks the amniotic fluid begins to dramatically decrease. Abnormal variations are *oligohydramnios* (too little amniotic fluid) and *polyhydramnios* (too much amniotic fluid or an amniotic fluid index greater than the 97.5 percentile for the corresponding gestational age). Polyhydramnios is also called *hydramnios*.

Yolk Sac

In humans, the yolk sac is small, and it functions only in early embryonic life. It develops as a second cavity in the blastocyst on about day 8 or 9 after conception. It forms primitive red blood cells (RBCs) during the first 6 weeks of development, until the embryo's liver takes over the process. As the embryo develops, the yolk sac is incorporated into the umbilical cord, where it can be seen as a degenerated structure after birth.

Umbilical Cord

As the placenta develops, the **umbilical cord** is being formed from the mesoderm and is covered by the amnion. The body stalk, which attaches the embryo to the yolk sac, contains blood vessels that extend into the chorionic villi. The body stalk fuses with the embryonic portion of the placenta to provide a circulatory pathway from the chorionic villi to the embryo. As the body stalk elongates to become the umbilical cord, the vessels in the cord decrease to one large vein and two smaller arteries. About 1% of umbilical cords have only two vessels: an artery and a vein. This condition may be associated with congenital malformations primarily of the renal, gastrointestinal, and cardiovascular systems. A specialized connective tissue known as **Wharton jelly** surrounds the blood vessels in the umbilical cord. This tissue, in addition to the high blood volume pulsating through the vessels, prevents compression of the umbilical cord in utero. The umbilical cord has no sensory or motor innervation, so cutting the cord after birth is not painful. At term (37–42 weeks' gestation), the average cord is 2 cm (0.8 in.) across and about 55 cm (22 in.) long. The cord can attach itself to the placenta at various sites. Central insertion into the placenta is considered normal.

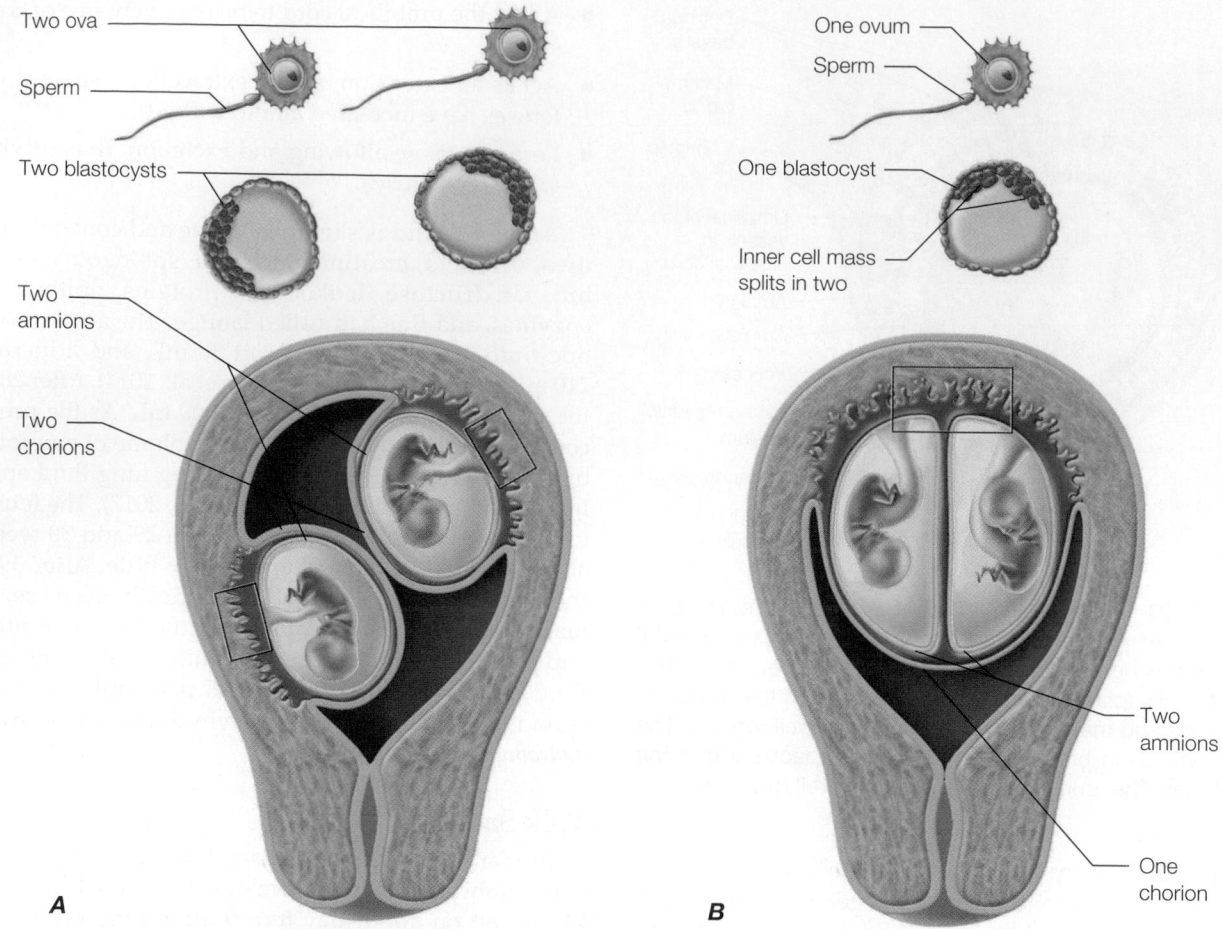

Figure 33–11 » ***A,*** Dizygotic (fraternal) twins. (Note separate placentas.) ***B,*** Monozygotic (identical) twins.

Umbilical cords appear twisted or spiraled, which is most likely caused by fetal movement. A true knot in the umbilical cord rarely occurs; if it does, the cord is longer than usual. More common are so-called false knots, caused by the folding of cord vessels. A *nuchal cord* is said to exist when the umbilical cord encircles the fetal neck.

Twins

Twins normally occur in approximately 1 in 80 pregnancies, and triplets occur in 1 in 8000 pregnancies. The current rate of twinning is attributed to delayed childbearing and the use of artificial reproductive treatments (London et al., 2017). Twins may be fraternal or identical (**Figure 33–11 »**).

» *Go to **Pearson MyLab Nursing and eText** for a MiniModule on twins.*

Development and Functions of the Placenta

The **placenta** is the means of metabolic and nutrient exchange between the embryonic and maternal circulations. Placental development and circulation do not begin until the third week of embryonic development. The placenta develops at the site where the embryo attaches to the uterine wall. Expansion of the placenta continues until about 20 weeks, when it covers approximately one half of the internal surface of the uterus. After 20 weeks' gestation, the placenta becomes thicker but not wider. At 40 weeks' gestation, the placenta is about 15–20 cm (5.9–7.9 in.) in diameter and 2.5–3 cm (1–1.2 in.) in thickness. At that time, it weighs about 400–600 g (14–21 oz).

The placenta has two parts: the maternal and fetal portions. The maternal portion consists of the decidua basalis and its circulation. Its surface is red and fleshlike. The fetal portion consists of the chorionic villi and their circulation. The fetal surface of the placenta is covered by the amnion, which gives it a shiny gray appearance (**Figures 33–12 »** and **33–13 »**).

Development of the placenta begins with the chorionic villi. The trophoblastic cells of the chorionic villi form spaces in the tissue of the decidua basalis. These spaces fill with maternal blood, and the chorionic villi grow into them. As the chorionic villi differentiate, two trophoblastic layers appear: an outer layer, called the syncytium (consisting of syncytiotrophoblasts), and an inner layer, known as the cytotrophoblast. The cytotrophoblast thins out and disappears around the fifth month, leaving only a single layer of syncytium covering the chorionic villi. The syncytium is in direct contact with the maternal blood in the intervillous spaces. It is the functional layer of the placenta, and it secretes the placental hormones of pregnancy.

A third inner layer of connective mesoderm develops in the chorionic villi, forming anchoring villi. These anchoring

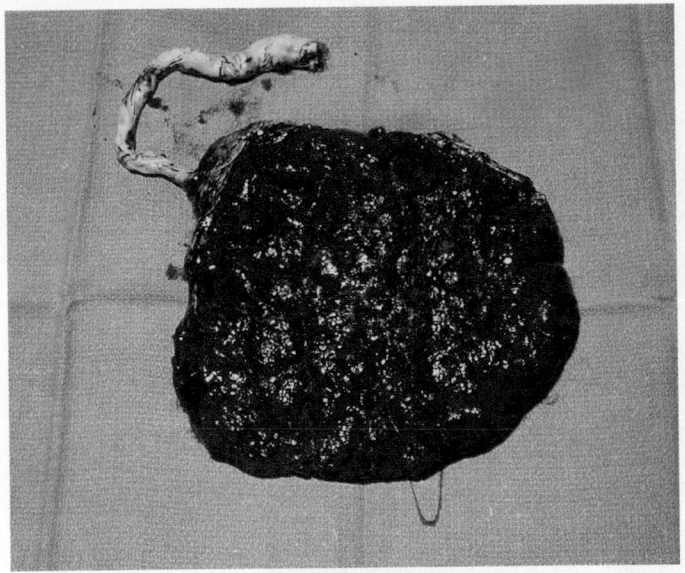

Source: Courtesy of Marcia London.

Figure 33–12 》 Maternal side of placenta.

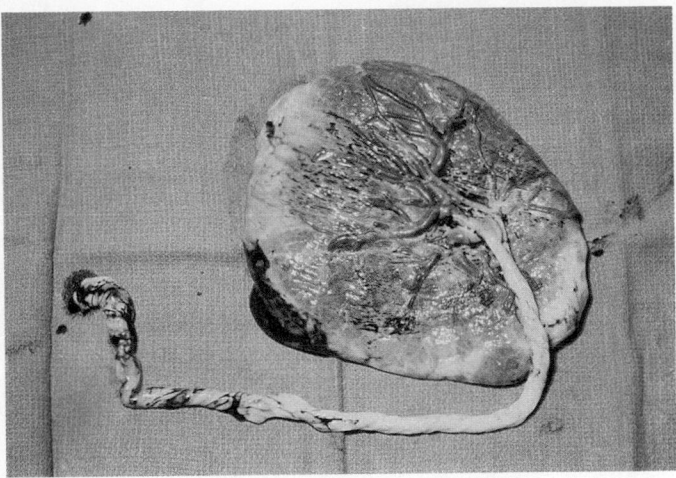

Source: Courtesy of Marcia London.

Figure 33–13 》 Fetal side of placenta.

villi eventually form the septa (partitions) of the placenta. The septa divide the mature placenta into 15–20 segments called **cotyledons** (subdivisions of the placenta made up of anchoring villi and decidual tissue). In each cotyledon, the branching villi form a highly complex vascular system that allows compartmentalization of the uteroplacental circulation. The exchange of gases and nutrients takes place across these vascular systems.

Placental Circulation

After implantation of the blastocyst, the cells distinguish themselves into fetal cells and trophoblastic cells. The proliferating trophoblast successfully invades the decidua basalis of the endometrium, first opening the uterine capillaries and later opening the larger uterine vessels. The chorionic villi are an outgrowth of the blastocystic tissue. As these villi continue to grow and divide, the fetal vessels begin to form. The intervillous spaces in the decidua basalis develop as the endometrial spiral arteries are opened.

By the end of the fourth week, the placenta has begun to function as a means of metabolic exchange between embryo and mother. The completion of the maternal–placental–fetal circulation occurs about 17 days after conception, when the embryonic heart begins functioning (Moore et al., 2016). By 14 weeks, the placenta is a discrete organ. It has grown in thickness as a result of growth in the length and size of the chorionic villi and accompanying expansion of the intervillous space.

In the fully developed placenta's umbilical cord, fetal blood flows through the two umbilical arteries to the capillaries of the villi, becomes oxygen enriched, and then flows back through the umbilical vein into the fetus (**Figure 33–14 》**). Late in pregnancy a soft blowing sound (funic souffle) can be heard over the area of the umbilical cord. The sound is synchronous with the fetal heartbeat and fetal blood flow through the umbilical arteries.

Maternal blood, rich in oxygen and nutrients, moves from the arcuate artery to the radial artery to the uterine spiral arteries and then spurts into the intervillous spaces. These spurts are produced by the maternal blood pressure. The spurt of blood is directed toward the chorionic plate, and as the blood loses pressure, it becomes lateral (spreads out). Fresh blood enters continuously and exerts pressure on the contents of the intervillous spaces, pushing blood toward the exits in the basal plate. The blood then drains through the uterine and other pelvic veins. A uterine souffle, timed precisely with the mother's pulse, also is heard just above the mother's symphysis pubis during the last months of pregnancy. This souffle is caused by the augmented blood flow entering the dilated uterine arteries.

Braxton Hicks contractions are intermittent painless uterine contractions that may occur every 10–20 minutes; they occur more frequently near the end of pregnancy. These contractions are believed to facilitate placental circulation by enhancing the movement of blood from the center of the cotyledon through the intervillous space. Placental blood flow is enhanced when the woman is lying on her left side because venous return from the lower extremities is not compromised (Blackburn, 2013).

Placental Functions

Placental exchange functions occur only in those fetal vessels that are in intimate contact with the covering syncytial membrane. The syncytium villi have brush borders containing many microvilli, which greatly increase the exchange rate between maternal and fetal circulation (Blackburn, 2013; Sadler, 2015).

The placental functions, many of which begin soon after implantation, include fetal respiration, nutrition, and excretion. To carry out these functions, the placenta is involved in metabolic and transfer activities. In addition, it has

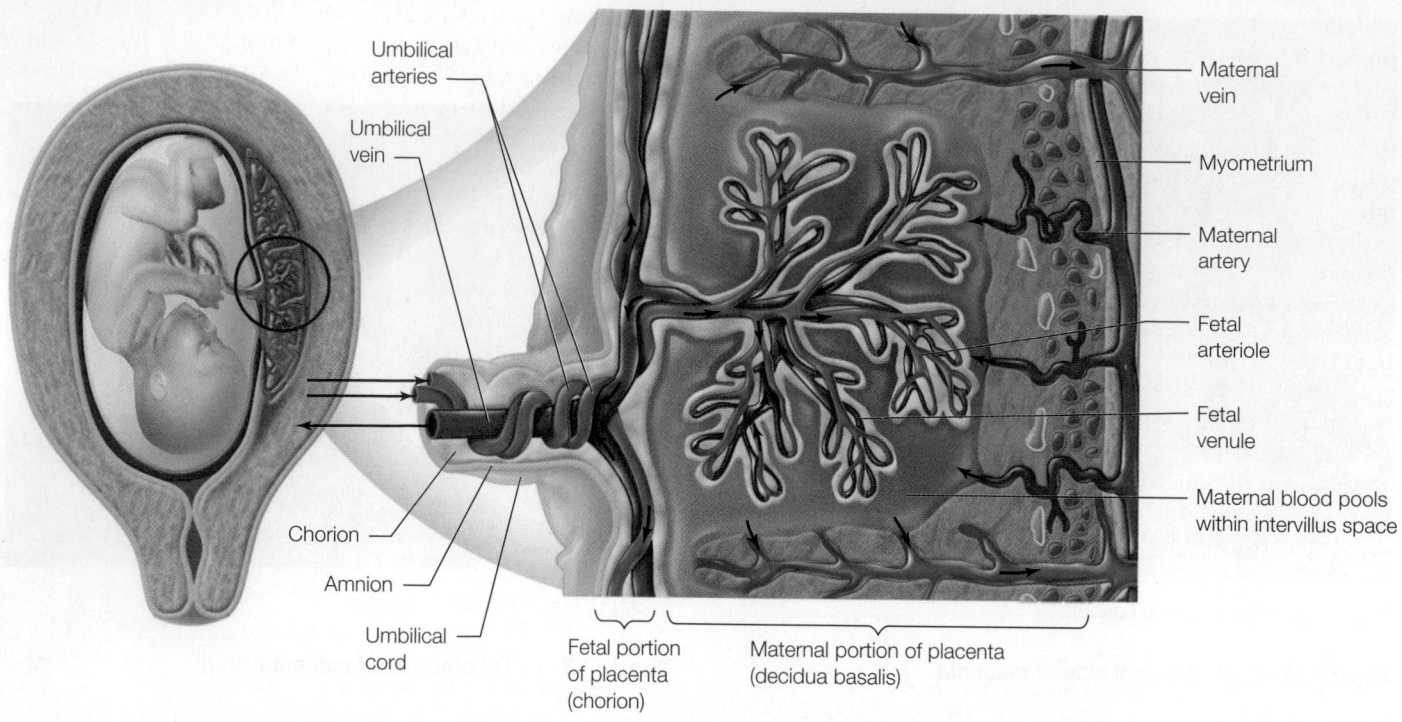

Umbilical arteries

Umbilical vein

Maternal vein

Myometrium

Maternal artery

Fetal arteriole

Fetal venule

Maternal blood pools within intervillus space

Chorion

Amnion

Umbilical cord

Fetal portion of placenta (chorion)

Maternal portion of placenta (decidua basalis)

Figure 33–14 》 Vascular arrangement of the placenta. *Arrows* indicate the direction of blood flow. Maternal blood flows through the uterine arteries to the intervillous spaces of the placenta and returns through the uterine veins to maternal circulation. Fetal blood flows through the umbilical arteries into the villous capillaries of the placenta and returns through the umbilical vein to the fetal circulation.

endocrine functions and special immunologic properties. (See the discussion later in this section.)

Metabolic Activities

The placenta continuously produces glycogen, cholesterol, and fatty acids for fetal use and hormone production. The placenta also produces numerous enzymes, such as sulfatase, which enhances excretion of fetal estrogen precursors, and insulinase, which increases the barrier to insulin. These enzymes are required for fetoplacental transfer. The placenta breaks down certain substances such as epinephrine and histamine (Blackburn, 2013). In addition, it stores glycogen and iron.

Transport Function

The placental membranes actively control the transfer of a wide range of substances by a variety of transport mechanisms.

■ *Simple diffusion* moves substances from an area of higher concentration to an area of lower concentration. Substances that move across the placenta by simple diffusion include water, oxygen, carbon dioxide, electrolytes (sodium and chloride), anesthetic gases, and drugs. Insulin and steroid hormones originating from the adrenals, as well as thyroid hormones, also cross the placenta. However, this happens at a very slow rate. The rate of oxygen transfer across the placental membrane is greater than that allowed by simple diffusion, indicating that oxygen also is transferred by some type of facilitated diffusion transport. Unfortunately, many substances of

abuse, such as cocaine and heroin, cross the placenta via simple diffusion.

■ *Facilitated transport* involves a carrier system to move molecules from an area of greater concentration to an area of lower concentration. Molecules such as glucose, galactose, and some oxygen are transported by this method. Ordinarily, the glucose level in the fetal blood is approximately 20–30% lower than the glucose level in the maternal blood because the fetus is metabolizing glucose rapidly. This, in turn, causes rapid transport of additional glucose from the maternal blood to the fetal blood.

■ *Active transport* can work against a concentration gradient and allows molecules to move from areas of lower concentration to areas of higher concentration. Amino acids, calcium, iron, iodine, water-soluble vitamins, and glucose are transferred across the placenta this way. The measured amino acid content of fetal blood is greater than that of maternal blood, and calcium and inorganic phosphate occur in greater concentration in fetal blood than in maternal blood (Blackburn, 2013).

In addition, fetal RBCs can pass into the maternal circulation through breaks in the capillaries and placental membrane, particularly during labor and birth. Certain cells (e.g., maternal leukocytes) and microorganisms such as viruses (e.g., HIV, which causes AIDS), and the bacterium *Treponema pallidum* (which causes syphilis), can cross the placental membrane under their own power (Moore et al., 2016). Some bacteria and protozoa infect the placenta by causing lesions and then entering the fetal blood system.

Reduction of the placental surface area, as with abruptio placentae (partial or complete premature separation of the placenta), lessens the area that is functional for exchange. Placental diffusion distance also affects exchange. In conditions such as diabetes and placental infection, edema of the villi increases the diffusion distance, thus increasing the distance the substance must be transferred.

Blood flow alteration changes the transfer rate of substances. Decreased blood flow in the intervillous space is seen in labor and with certain maternal diseases such as hypertension. Mild fetal hypoxia increases the umbilical blood flow, but severe hypoxia results in decreased blood flow.

As the maternal blood picks up fetal waste products and carbon dioxide, it drains back into the maternal circulation through the veins in the basal plate. Fetal blood is hypoxic in comparison to maternal blood; therefore, it attracts oxygen from the mother's blood. Affinity for oxygen increases as the fetal blood gives up its carbon dioxide, which also decreases its acidity.

Endocrine Functions

The placenta produces hormones that are vital to the survival of the fetus. These include hCG; human placental lactogen (hPL); and two steroid hormones, estrogen and progesterone.

The hormone hCG is similar to LH and prevents the normal involution of the corpus luteum at the end of the menstrual cycle. If the corpus luteum stops functioning before the 11th week of pregnancy, spontaneous abortion occurs. The hCG also causes the corpus luteum to secrete increased amounts of estrogen and progesterone.

After the 11th week, the placenta produces enough progesterone and estrogen to maintain pregnancy. In the male fetus, hCG also exerts an interstitial cell-stimulating effect on the testes, resulting in the production of testosterone. This small secretion of testosterone during embryonic development is the factor that causes male sex organs to grow. The hormone hCG may play a role in the trophoblast's immunologic capabilities (ability to exempt the placenta and embryo from rejection by the mother's system). This hormone is used as a basis for pregnancy tests. (Placental hormones are discussed further in the Endocrine System section.)

Development of the Fetal Circulatory System

The circulatory system of the fetus has several unique features that, by maintaining the blood flow to the placenta, provide the fetus with oxygen and nutrients while removing carbon dioxide and other waste products.

Most of the blood supply bypasses the fetal lungs because they do not carry out respiratory gas exchange. The placenta assumes the function of the fetal lungs by supplying oxygen and allowing the fetus to excrete carbon dioxide into the maternal bloodstream. **Figure 33–15 》** shows the fetal circulatory system. The blood from the placenta flows through the umbilical vein, which enters the abdominal wall of the fetus at the site that, after birth, is the umbilicus (belly button). As umbilical venous blood approaches the liver, a small portion of the blood enters the liver sinusoids, mixes with blood from the portal circulation, and then enters the inferior

vena cava via hepatic veins. Most of the umbilical vein's blood flows through the **ductus venosus** directly into the inferior vena cava, bypassing the liver. This blood then enters the right atrium, passes through the **foramen ovale** into the left atrium, and pours into the left ventricle, which pumps blood into the aorta. Some blood returning from the head and upper extremities by way of the superior vena cava is emptied into the right atrium and passes through the tricuspid valve into the right ventricle. This blood is pumped into the pulmonary artery, and a small amount passes to the lungs for nourishment only. The larger portion of blood passes from the pulmonary artery through the **ductus arteriosus** into the descending aorta, bypassing the lungs. Finally, blood returns to the placenta through the two umbilical arteries, and the process is repeated.

The fetus obtains oxygen via diffusion from the maternal circulation because of the gradient difference of 50 mmHg PO_2 in maternal blood in the placenta to 30 mmHg PO_2 in the fetus. At term, the fetus receives oxygen from the mother's circulation at a rate of 20–30 mL/min (Sadler, 2015). Fetal hemoglobin facilitates obtaining oxygen from the maternal circulation because it carries as much as 20–30% more oxygen than adult hemoglobin.

Fetal circulation delivers the highest available oxygen concentration to the head, neck, brain, and heart (coronary circulation) and a lesser amount of oxygenated blood to the abdominal organs and the lower body. This circulatory pattern leads to cephalocaudal (head-to-tail) development in the fetus.

Fetal Heart

The heart of the fetus, like that of the adult, is controlled by its own pacemaker. The sinoatrial (SA) node sets the rate and is supplied by the vagus nerve. Bridging the atrium and the ventricle is the atrioventricular (AV) node, also supplied by the vagus nerve. Baseline changes in the fetal heartbeat have been shown to be under the influence of this nerve. When the fetus is stressed, the sympathetic nervous system causes the release of norepinephrine, which increases the fetal heart rate. To counteract the increase in blood pressure, baroreceptors, which respond to the increase in pressure, are present in the vessel walls at the junction of the internal and external carotid arteries. When stimulated, these receptors, under the influence of the vagus and glossopharyngeal nerves, cause the heart rate to slow. Chemoreceptors in the fetal peripheral and central nervous systems respond to decreased oxygen tensions and to increased carbon dioxide tensions, leading to fetal tachycardia and an increase in blood pressure. The CNS also has control over heart rate. Increased activity of the fetus in a wakeful period is exhibited in an *increase* in the variability of the fetal heart baseline. Sleep patterns involve a *decrease* in the baseline variability. In cases of severe hypoxia, the release of epinephrine and norepinephrine will cause an increase in the fetal heart rate.

Embryonic and Fetal Development

Pregnancy is calculated to last an average of 10 lunar months: 40 weeks, or 280 days. This period of 280 days is calculated from the onset of the last normal menstrual period to the time of birth. **Estimated date of birth (EDB)**, the date

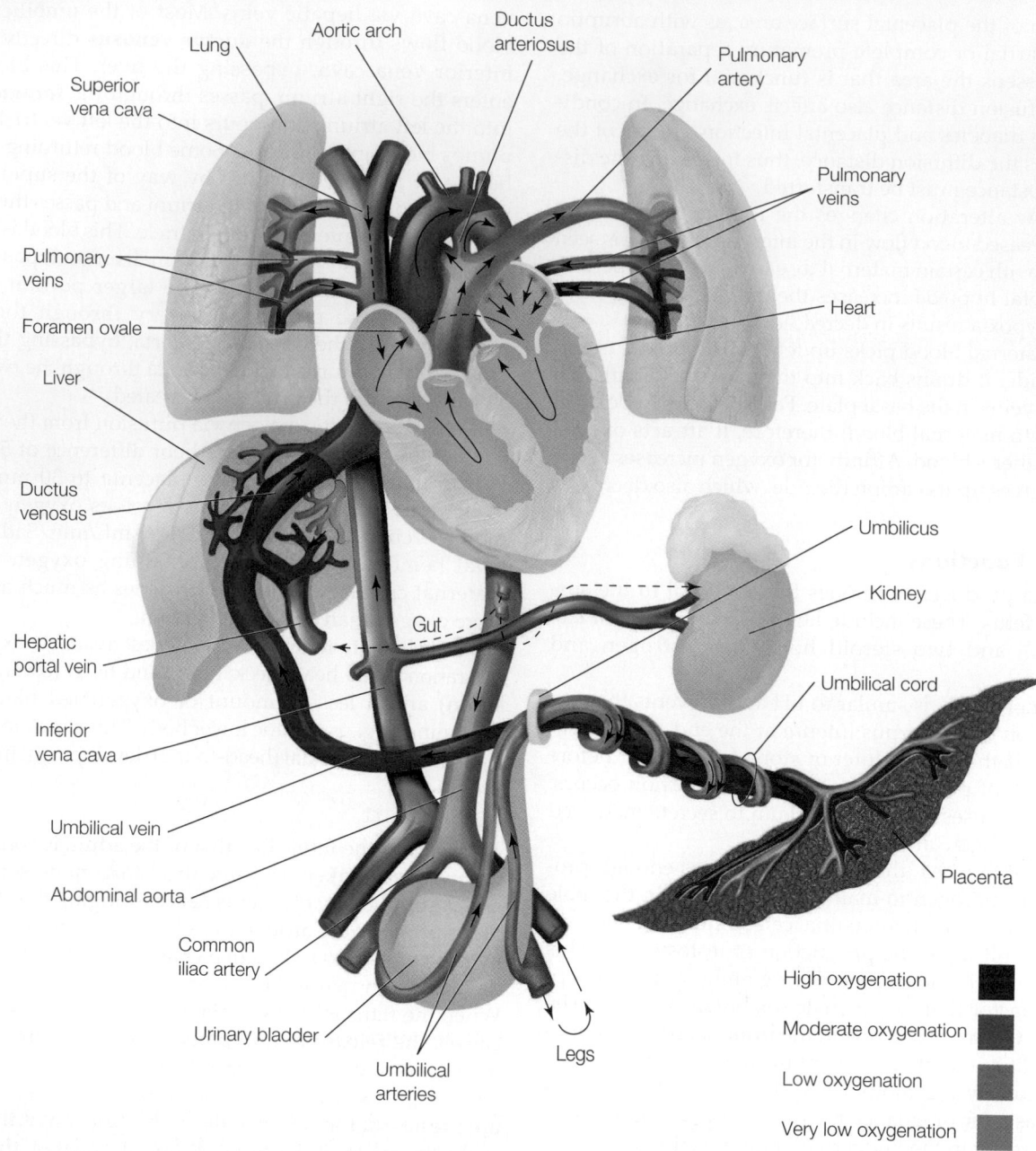

Lung
Aortic arch
Ductus arteriosus
Pulmonary artery
Superior vena cava
Pulmonary veins
Pulmonary veins
Foramen ovale
Heart
Liver
Ductus venosus
Umbilicus
Kidney
Gut
Hepatic portal vein
Umbilical cord
Inferior vena cava
Umbilical vein
Placenta
Abdominal aorta
Common iliac artery
Urinary bladder
Legs
Umbilical arteries

High oxygenation
Moderate oxygenation
Low oxygenation
Very low oxygenation

Figure 33–15 ≫ Fetal circulation. Blood leaves the placenta and enters the fetus through the umbilical vein. After circulating through the fetus, the blood returns to the placenta through the umbilical arteries. The ductus venosus, the foramen ovale, and the ductus arteriosus allow the blood to bypass the fetal liver and lungs.

around which childbirth will occur, and sometimes referred to as the estimated date of delivery (EDD), usually is calculated by this method. Most fetuses are born within 10–14 days of the calculated date of birth. The fertilization age (or **postconception age**) of the fetus is calculated to be about 2 weeks less, or 266 days (38 weeks), or 9.5 calendar months. The latter measurement is more accurate because it measures time from the fertilization of the ovum, or conception.

≫ Go to **Pearson MyLab Nursing and eText** for Chart 1: Organ Development in the Embryo and Fetus.

In review, human development follows three stages. The preembryonic stage, as discussed earlier in this module,

consists of the first 14 days of development after the ovum is fertilized. The embryonic stage covers the period from day 15 until approximately the end of the eighth week, and the fetal stage extends from the end of the eighth week until birth (**Figure 33–16 ≫**).

Embryonic Stage

The stage of the **embryo** starts on day 15 (the beginning of the third week after conception) and continues until approximately the eighth week, or until the embryo reaches a crown–rump length (CRL) of 3 cm (1.2 in.). This length is usually reached about 56 days after fertilization (the end of the eighth gestational week). During the embryonic stage,

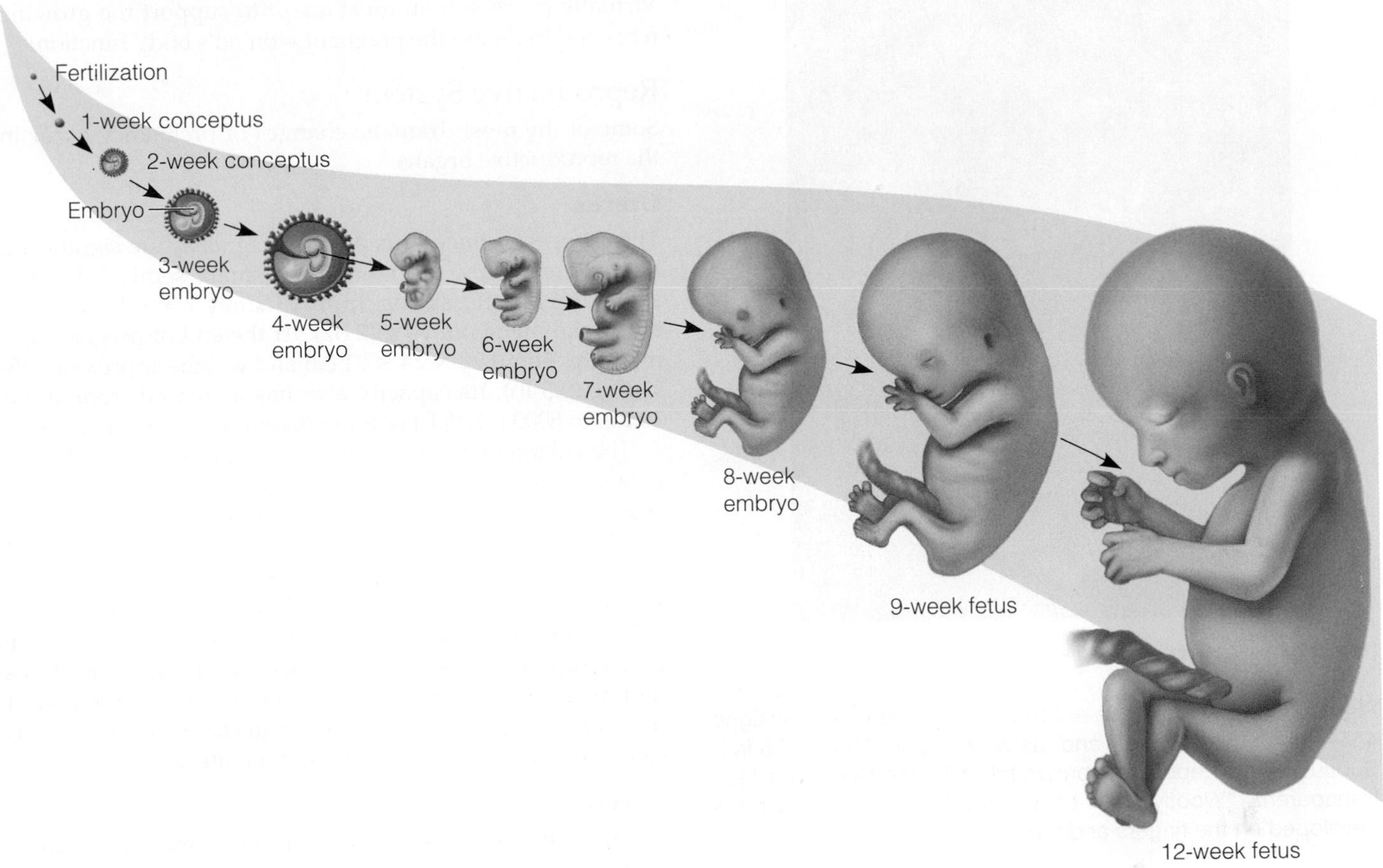

Fertilization

1-week conceptus

2-week conceptus

Embryo

3-week embryo

4-week embryo

5-week embryo

6-week embryo

7-week embryo

8-week embryo

9-week fetus

12-week fetus

Figure 33–16 ≫ The actual size of a human conceptus from fertilization to the early fetal stage. The embryonic stage begins in the third week after fertilization; the fetal stage begins in the ninth week.

tissues differentiate into essential organs and the main external features develop. The embryo is most vulnerable to *teratogens* during this period (**Figure 33–17 ≫**).

Fetal Stage

By the end of the eighth week, the embryo is sufficiently developed to be called a **fetus**. Every organ system and external structure that will be found in the full-term newborn is present. The remainder of gestation is devoted to refining structures and perfecting function. **Figure 33–18 ≫** shows the fetus at 20 weeks' gestation.

Full Term

The fetus is considered full term at 37 completed weeks and up to 40 weeks. The crown–heel length (CHL) varies from 48 to 52 cm (19 to 21 in.), with males usually longer than females. Males also usually weigh more than females. The weight at term is about 3000–3600 g (6 lb 10 oz–7 lb 15 oz) and varies in different ethnic groups. Skin color also varies and has a smooth, polished look. The only lanugo left is on the upper arms and shoulders. The hair on the head is no longer woolly, but is coarse and about 2.5 cm (1 in.) long. Vernix caseosa is present, with heavier deposits remaining in the creases and folds of the skin. The body and extremities are plump, with good skin turgor, and the fingernails extend beyond the fingertips. The chest is prominent but still a little smaller than the head, and mammary glands protrude in

both sexes. In males, the testes are in the scrotum or are palpable in the inguinal canals.

As the fetus enlarges, amniotic fluid diminishes to about 500 mL or less and the fetal body mass fills the uterine cavity.

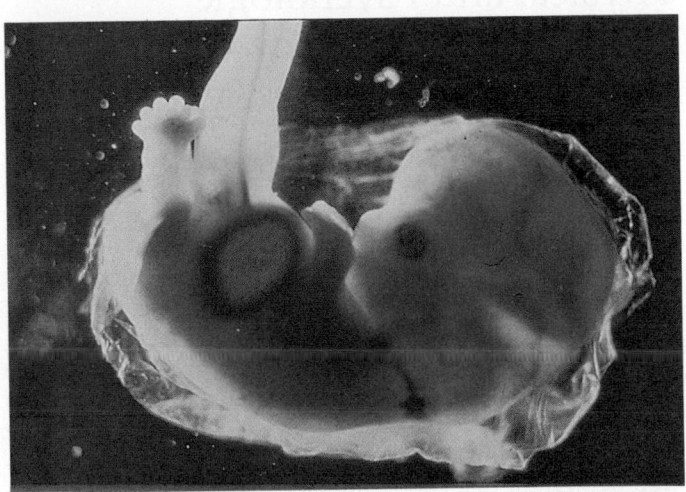

Source: Petit Format/Science Source.

Figure 33–17 ≫ The embryo at 7 weeks. The head is rounded and nearly erect. The eyes have shifted forward and closer together, and the eyelids begin to form.

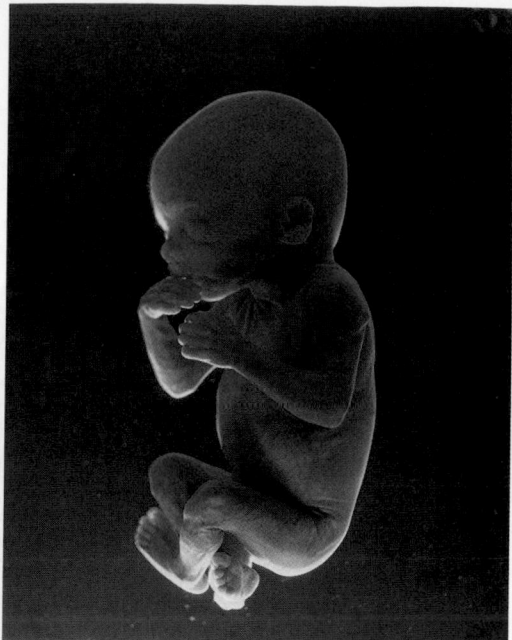

Source: James Stevenson/Science Source.

Figure 33–18 》 The fetus at 20 weeks. The fetus now weighs 435–465 g (15.2–16.3 oz) and measures about 19 cm (7.5 in.). Subcutaneous deposits of brown fat make the skin a little less transparent. "Woolly" hair covers the head, and nails have developed on the fingers and toes.

The fetus assumes what is called its *position of comfort*, or *lie*. The head is generally pointed downward, following the shape of the uterus (and possibly because the head is heavier than the feet). The extremities, and often the head, are well flexed. After 5 months, patterns in feeding, sleeping, and activity become established; so at term, the fetus has its own body rhythms and individual style of response.

Physical and Psychologic Changes of Pregnancy

The growth of the developing fetus and the physical and psychologic changes that occur in the pregnant mother continue to inspire feelings of awe and amazement, not to mention curiosity. First, it is nothing short of a miracle that the union of two microscopic entities—an ovum and a sperm—can produce a living being. Second, the woman's body must undergo extraordinary physical changes to maintain a pregnancy.

Pregnancy is divided into three trimesters, each approximately a 3-month period. Each trimester brings predictable changes for both mother and fetus. This section describes these physical and psychologic changes. It also presents the various cultural factors that can affect a pregnant woman's well-being.

Anatomy and Physiology of Pregnancy

The changes that occur in the pregnant woman's body may result from hormonal influences, the growth of the fetus, and the mother's physiologic adaptation to the pregnancy.

Virtually every system must adapt to support the growing fetus and maintain the pregnant woman's body functions.

Reproductive System

Some of the most dramatic changes of pregnancy occur in the reproductive organs.

Uterus

The changes in the uterus during pregnancy are significant. Before pregnancy, the uterus is a small, semisolid, pear-shaped organ measuring approximately 7.5 × 5 × 2.5 cm and weighing about 60 g (2 oz). At the end of pregnancy, it measures about 28 × 24 × 21 cm and weighs approximately 1100 g (2.5 lb); its capacity also has increased from about 10 mL to 5000 mL (5 L) or more (Cunningham et al., 2014).

The enlargement of the uterus is primarily caused by the enlargement (hypertrophy) of the preexisting myometrial cells as a result of the stimulating influence of estrogen and the distention caused by the growing fetus. Only a limited increase in cell number (hyperplasia) occurs. The fibrous tissue between the muscle bands increases markedly, which adds to the strength and elasticity of the muscle wall. The enlarging uterus, developing placenta, and growing fetus require additional blood flow to the uterus. By the end of pregnancy, one sixth of the total maternal blood volume is contained in the vascular system of the uterus.

Cervix

Estrogen stimulates the glandular tissue of the cervix, which increases in cell number and becomes hyperactive. The endocervical glands secrete a thick, sticky mucus that accumulates and forms a mucous plug, which seals the endocervical canal and prevents the ascent of microorganisms into the uterus. This plug is expelled when cervical dilation begins. The hyperactivity of the glandular tissue also increases the normal physiologic mucorrhea, at times resulting in profuse discharge. Increased cervical vascularity also causes both the softening of the cervix (**Goodell sign**) and its blue-purple discoloration (**Chadwick sign**).

Ovaries

The ovaries stop producing ova during pregnancy. During early pregnancy, hCG maintains the corpus luteum, which persists and produces hormones until weeks 6–8 of pregnancy. The corpus luteum secretes progesterone to maintain the endometrium until the placenta produces enough progesterone to maintain the pregnancy. The corpus luteum then begins to disintegrate slowly.

Vagina

Estrogen causes a thickening of the vaginal mucosa, a loosening of the connective tissue, and an increase in vaginal secretions. These secretions are thick, white, and acidic (pH 3.5–6.0). The acid pH helps prevent bacterial infection but favors the growth of yeast organisms. Thus, the pregnant woman is more susceptible to *Candida* infection than usual.

The supportive connective tissue of the vagina loosens throughout pregnancy. By the end of pregnancy, the vagina and perineal body are sufficiently relaxed to permit passage of the baby. Because blood flow to the vagina is increased, the vagina may show the same blue-purple color (Chadwick sign) as the cervix.

Breasts

Estrogen and progesterone cause many changes in the breasts. They enlarge and become more nodular as the milk producing glands increase in size and number in preparation for lactation. Superficial veins become more prominent, the nipples become more erectile, and the areolas darken. Montgomery's follicles (sebaceous glands) enlarge, and **striae** (reddish stretch marks that slowly turn silver after childbirth) may develop.

Colostrum, an antibody-rich yellow secretion, may leak or be expressed from the breasts during the last trimester. Colostrum gradually converts to mature milk during the first few days after childbirth.

Respiratory System

Many respiratory changes occur to meet the increased oxygen requirements of a pregnant woman. The volume of air breathed each minute increases 30–40%. In addition, progesterone decreases airway resistance, permitting a 15–20% increase in oxygen consumption as well as increases in carbon dioxide production and in the respiratory functional reserve.

As the uterus enlarges, it presses upward and elevates the diaphragm. The subcostal angle increases, so that the rib cage flares. The anteroposterior diameter increases, and the chest circumference expands by as much as 6 cm; as a result, there is no significant loss of intrathoracic volume. Breathing changes from abdominal to thoracic as pregnancy progresses, and descent of the diaphragm on inspiration becomes less possible. Some hyperventilation and difficulty in breathing may occur.

Nasal stuffiness and epistaxis (nosebleeds) also may occur because of estrogen-induced edema and vascular congestion of the nasal mucosa.

Cardiovascular System

During pregnancy, blood flow increases to organ systems with an increased workload. Thus, blood flow increases to the uterus, placenta, and breasts, whereas hepatic and cerebral flow remains unchanged. Cardiac output begins to increase early in pregnancy and peaks at 25–30 weeks' gestation at 30–50% above prepregnancy levels. It generally remains elevated in the third trimester.

The pulse may increase by as many as 10–15 beats/min at term. The blood pressure decreases slightly, reaching its lowest point during the second trimester. It gradually increases to near prepregnancy levels by the end of the third trimester.

The enlarging uterus puts pressure on pelvic and femoral vessels, interfering with returning blood flow and causing stasis of blood in the lower extremities. This condition may lead to dependent edema and varicosity of the veins in the legs, vulva, and rectum (hemorrhoids) in late pregnancy. This increased blood volume in the lower legs also may make the pregnant woman prone to postural hypotension.

When the pregnant woman lies supine, the enlarging uterus may press on the vena cava. This reduces blood flow to the right atrium; lowers blood pressure; and causes dizziness, pallor, and clamminess. Research indicates that the enlarging uterus also may press on the aorta and its collateral

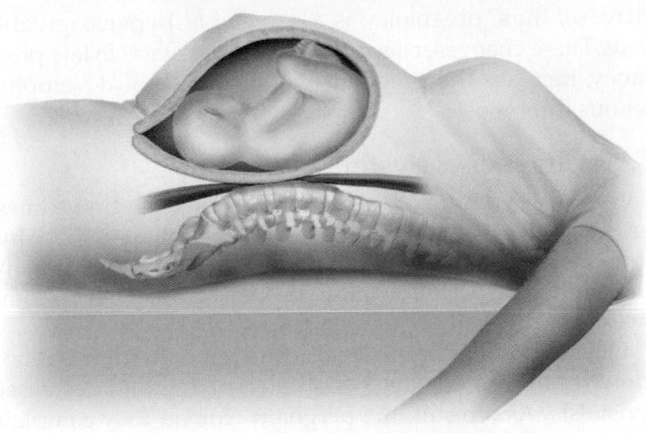

Figure 33–19 》 Vena caval syndrome. The gravid uterus compresses the vena cava when the woman is supine. This reduces the blood flow returning to the heart and may cause maternal hypotension.

circulation (Cunningham et al., 2014). This condition is called **supine hypotensive syndrome**. It also may be referred to as **vena caval syndrome** or **aortocaval compression (Figure 33–19 》)**. It can be corrected by having the woman lie on her side, preferably on her left. Blood volume progressively increases beginning in the first trimester, increases rapidly until about 30–34 weeks' gestation, and then plateaus until birth at about 40–50% above nonpregnancy levels. This increase occurs because of increases in both erythrocytes and plasma (Cao & O'Brien, 2013).

The total erythrocyte (RBC) volume increases by about 25%. This increase in erythrocytes is necessary to transport the additional oxygen required during pregnancy. However, the increase in plasma volume during pregnancy averages about 50%. Because the plasma volume increase (50%) is greater than the erythrocyte increase (25%), the hematocrit, which measures the concentration of RBCs in the plasma, decreases slightly (Cao & O'Brien, 2013). This decrease is referred to as the **physiologic anemia of pregnancy** (pseudoanemia).

Iron is necessary for hemoglobin formation, and hemoglobin is the oxygen-carrying component of erythrocytes. Thus, the increase in erythrocyte levels results in the pregnant woman's increased need for iron. Even though the gastrointestinal absorption of iron is moderately increased during pregnancy, it is usually necessary to add supplemental iron to the diet to meet the expanded RBC and fetal needs. Women who are diagnosed with anemia prior to pregnancy may require more iron supplementation.

Leukocyte production increases slightly to an average of 8500 mm³, with a range of 5600–12,200 mm³. During labor and the early postpartum period, these levels may reach 25,000/mm³ or higher (Gordon, 2012). Although the cause of leukocytosis is not known, this increase is a normal finding (Cunningham et al., 2014).

Both the fibrin and plasma fibrinogen levels increase during pregnancy. Although the blood-clotting time of a pregnant woman does not differ significantly from that of a nonpregnant woman, clotting factors VII, VIII, IX, and X increase; thus, pregnancy is a somewhat hypercoagulable state. These changes, coupled with venous stasis in late pregnancy, increase the pregnant woman's risk of developing venous thrombosis.

Gastrointestinal System

Nausea and vomiting are common during the first trimester because of elevated hCG levels and changed carbohydrate metabolism. Gum tissue may soften and bleed easily. The secretion of saliva may increase and even become excessive (ptyalism).

Elevated progesterone levels cause smooth muscle relaxation, resulting in delayed gastric emptying and decreased peristalsis. As a result, the pregnant woman may complain of bloating and constipation. These symptoms are aggravated as the enlarging uterus displaces the stomach upward and the intestines are moved laterally and posteriorly. The cardiac sphincter also relaxes, and heartburn (pyrosis) may occur because of reflux of acidic secretions into the lower esophagus. Hemorrhoids frequently develop in late pregnancy from constipation and from pressure on vessels below the level of the uterus.

Only minor liver changes occur with pregnancy. Plasma albumin concentrations and serum cholinesterase activity decrease with normal pregnancy, as with certain liver diseases.

The emptying time of the gallbladder is prolonged during pregnancy as a result of smooth muscle relaxation from progesterone. This, coupled with the elevated levels of cholesterol in the bile, can predispose the woman to gallstone formation.

Urinary Tract

During the first trimester, the enlarging uterus is still a pelvic organ and presses against the bladder, producing urinary frequency. This symptom decreases during the second trimester, when the uterus becomes an abdominal organ and pressure against the bladder lessens. Frequency reappears during the third trimester, when the presenting part descends into the pelvis and again presses on the bladder, reducing bladder capacity, contributing to hyperemia, and irritating the bladder.

The ureters (especially the right ureter) elongate and dilate above the pelvic brim. The glomerular filtration rate (GFR) rises by as much as 50% beginning in the second trimester and remains elevated until birth. To compensate for this increase, renal tubular reabsorption also increases. However, glycosuria sometimes is seen during pregnancy because of the kidneys' inability to reabsorb all of the glucose filtered by the glomeruli. Glycosuria may be normal or may indicate *gestational diabetes mellitus (GDM)* (diabetes mellitus with onset or first recognition during pregnancy), so it always warrants further testing.

Skin and Hair

Changes in skin pigmentation commonly occur during pregnancy. Increased estrogen, progesterone, and α-melanocyte-stimulating hormone levels are thought to stimulate these changes. Pigmentation of the skin increases primarily in areas that are already hyperpigmented: the areola, the nipples, the vulva, the perianal area, and the linea alba. The linea alba refers to the midline of the abdomen from the pubic area to the umbilicus and above. During

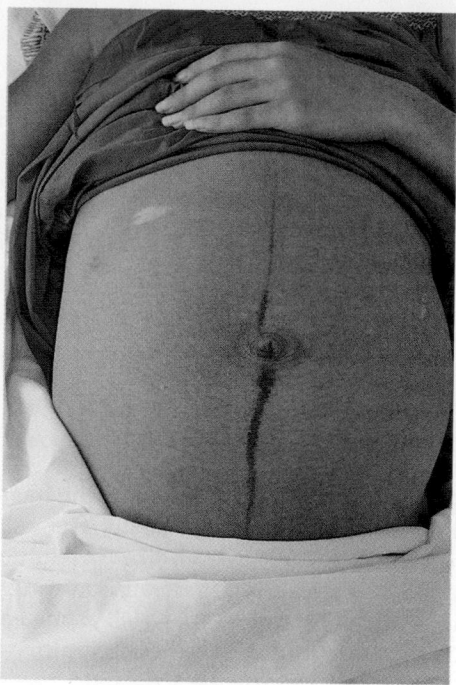

Figure 33–20 ⟩⟩ Linea nigra.

pregnancy, this area darkens and is referred to as the *linea nigra* (**Figure 33–20 ⟩⟩**). Facial **chloasma**, or **melasma gravidarum** (also known as the "mask of pregnancy"), a darkening of the skin over the cheeks, nose, and forehead, may develop. Chloasma or melasma is more prominent in dark-haired women and is aggravated by exposure to the sun. The condition fades or becomes less prominent soon after childbirth, when the hormonal influence of pregnancy subsides.

The sweat and sebaceous glands are often hyperactive during pregnancy. Some women may notice heavy perspiration, night sweats, and the development of acne even if they have never experienced these symptoms before.

Striae may appear on the abdomen, thighs, buttocks, and breasts. They result from reduced connective tissue strength because of elevated adrenal steroid levels.

Vascular spider nevi—small, bright red elevations of the skin radiating from a central body—may develop on the chest, neck, face, arms, and legs. They may be caused by increased subcutaneous blood flow in response to elevated estrogen levels.

The rate of hair growth may decrease during pregnancy; the number of hair follicles in the resting or dormant phase also decreases. After birth, the number of hair follicles in the resting phase increases sharply and the woman may notice increased hair shedding for 1–4 months. However, practically all hair is replaced within 6–12 months (Cunningham et al., 2014).

Musculoskeletal System

No demonstrable changes occur in the teeth of pregnant women. The dental caries that sometimes accompany pregnancy are probably caused by inadequate oral hygiene and dental care, especially if the woman has problems with bleeding gums or nausea and vomiting.

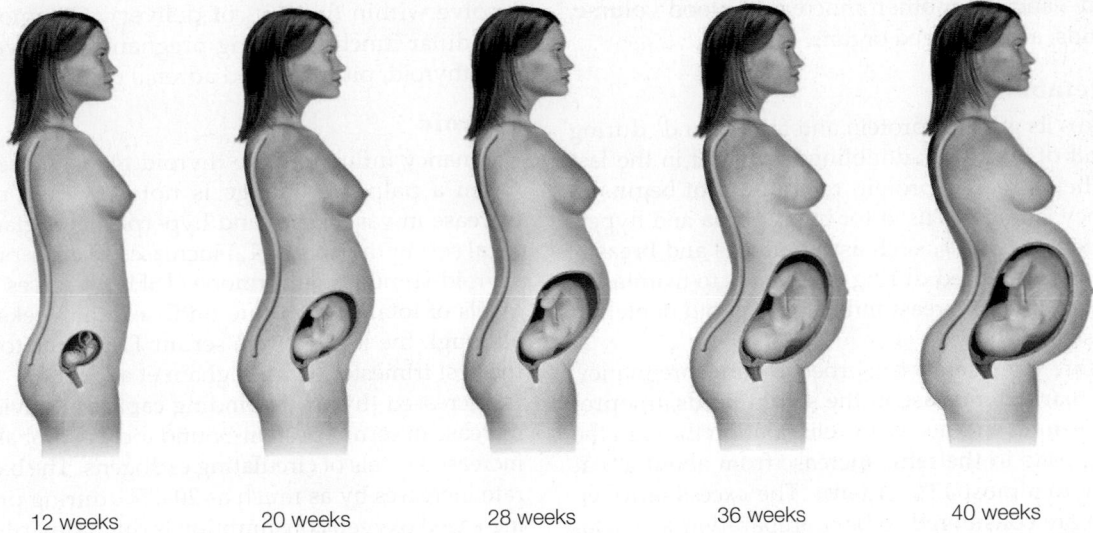

| 12 weeks | 20 weeks | 28 weeks | 36 weeks | 40 weeks |

Figure 33–21 》 Postural changes during pregnancy. Note the increasing lordosis of the lumbosacral spine and the increasing curvature of the thoracic area.

The joints of the pelvis relax somewhat because of hormonal influences. The result is often a waddling gait. As the pregnant woman's center of gravity gradually changes, the lumbodorsal spinal curve becomes accentuated and her posture changes (**Figure 33–21 》**). This posture change compensates for the increased weight of the uterus anteriorly and frequently results in low backache.

Pressure of the enlarging uterus on the abdominal muscles may cause the rectus abdominis muscle to separate, producing **diastasis recti**. If the separation is severe and muscle tone is not regained postpartum, subsequent pregnancies will not have adequate support and the woman's abdomen may appear pendulous.

Eyes

Two changes generally occur in the eyes during pregnancy. First, intraocular pressure decreases, probably as a result of increased vitreous outflow. Second, a slight thickening of the cornea occurs, which is generally attributed to fluid retention (Gordon, 2012). Although these changes are not readily perceived, some pregnant women experience difficulty wearing previously comfortable contact lenses. The change in the corneas generally disappears by 6 weeks postpartum (Davidson, London, & Ladewig, 2017).

Central Nervous System

Pregnant women frequently describe decreased attention, concentration, and memory during and shortly after pregnancy, but few studies have explored this phenomenon. One study did compare a group of pregnant women and a control group, finding a decline in memory among the pregnant women that could not be attributed to depression, anxiety, sleep deprivation, or other physical changes of pregnancy. This memory loss disappeared soon after childbirth. Another study found that sleep problems are common in pregnancy. These include difficulty going to sleep, frequent awakenings, fewer hours of night sleep, and reduced sleep efficiency (Cunningham et al., 2014).

Metabolism

Most metabolic functions accelerate during pregnancy to support the additional demands of the growing fetus and its support system. The expectant mother must meet her own tissue replacement needs, those of the fetus, and tissue changes preparatory for labor and lactation. No other event in life induces such profound metabolic changes.

Weight Gain

Growth of the uterus and its contents, growth of the breasts, and increases in intravascular fluids account for most of the weight gain in pregnancy. In addition, extra water, fat, and protein are stored; these are called *maternal reserves*.

Adequate nutrition and weight gain are important during pregnancy. The recommended total weight gain during pregnancy for a woman of normal weight before pregnancy is 11.5–16 kg (25–35 lb); for women who were overweight before becoming pregnant, the recommended gain is 6.8–11.5 kg (15–25 lb). Obese women are advised to limit weight gain to 5–9 kg (11–20 lb). Underweight women are advised to gain 12.7–18.1 kg (28–40 lb) (American College of Obstetricians and Gynecologists [ACOG], 2013a). Weight may decrease slightly during the first trimester because of nausea, vomiting, and food intolerances of early pregnancy. The lost weight is soon regained, and for normal women, the ACOG (2013a) recommends a gain of 0.5–2 kg (1.1–4.4 lb) during the first trimester, followed by an average gain of about 0.45 kg (1 lb) per week during the last two trimesters.

Water Metabolism

Increased water retention is a basic chemical alteration of pregnancy. Several interrelated factors cause this phenomenon. The increased level of steroid sex hormones affects sodium and fluid retention. The lowered serum protein also influences the fluid balance, as do the increased intracapillary pressure and permeability. The extra water is needed for the products of conception—the fetus, placenta, and amniotic fluid—and the mother's increased blood volume, interstitial fluids, and enlarged organs.

Nutrient Metabolism

The fetus makes its greatest protein and fat demands during the second half of gestation, doubling in weight in the last 6–8 weeks. The increased protein retention that begins in early pregnancy is initially used for hyperplasia and hypertrophy of maternal tissues, such as the uterus and breasts. Protein must also be stored during pregnancy to maintain a constant level within the breast milk and to avoid depletion of maternal tissues.

Fats are more completely absorbed during pregnancy, resulting in a marked increase in the serum lipids, lipoproteins, and cholesterol and decreased elimination through the bowel. Fat deposits in the fetus increase from about 2% at midpregnancy to almost 12% at term. The excess nitrogen and lipidemia are considered to be a preparation for lactation. In addition, the woman's body switches from glucose metabolism to lipid metabolism once glucose from food intake has been used up. This leads to an increased tendency to develop ketosis between meals and overnight. The demand for carbohydrate increases, especially during the last two trimesters. Intermittent glycosuria is not uncommon during pregnancy. When it is not accompanied by a rise in blood sugar levels, glycosuria is secondary to the increased glomerular filtration rate. Fasting blood sugar levels tend to fall slightly, returning to more normal levels by the sixth postpartum month. The oral glucose tolerance test shows no change with pregnancy.

The possibility of diabetes during pregnancy must not be overlooked. Plasma levels of insulin increase during pregnancy (probably because of hormonal changes that cause increased tissue resistance) and rapid destruction of insulin takes place within the placenta. The woman's insulin production must increase during the second trimester, and any marginal pancreatic function quickly becomes apparent. The woman with diabetes often experiences increased exogenous insulin demands during pregnancy.

The demand for iron during pregnancy is accelerated, and the pregnant woman needs to guard against anemia. Iron is necessary for the increase in erythrocytes, hemoglobin, and blood volume, as well as for the increased tissue demands of both woman and fetus. Iron transfer takes place at the placenta in only one direction: toward the fetus. It has been demonstrated that approximately five sixths of the iron stored in the fetal liver is assimilated during the last trimester of pregnancy. This stored iron in the fetal liver compensates in the first 4 months of neonatal life for the normal inadequate amounts of iron available in breast milk and non-iron-fortified formulas.

The progressive absorption and retention of calcium during pregnancy have been noted. The maternal plasma concentration of bound calcium decreases as the levels of bindable plasma proteins fall. Approximately 30 g of calcium is retained in maternal bone for fetal deposition late in pregnancy.

Endocrine System

Hormonal changes of pregnancy affect endocrine function in various ways. Alterations are typically temporary and resolve within 6 weeks of delivery. Common changes in glandular function during pregnancy involve the thyroid, parathyroid, pituitary, and adrenal glands.

Thyroid

Pregnancy influences the thyroid gland's size and activity. Often a palpable change is noted, which represents an increase in vascularity and hyperplasia of glandular tissue. Total serum thyroxine (T_4) increases in early pregnancy, and thyroid-stimulating hormone (TSH) decreases. The elevated levels of total T_4 continue until several weeks postpartum, although the level of free serum T_4 returns to normal after the first trimester (Cunningham et al., 2014).

Increased thyroxine-binding capacity is evidenced by an increase in serum protein-bound iodine, probably due to the increased levels of circulating estrogens. The basal metabolic rate increases by as much as 20–25% during pregnancy. The increased oxygen consumption is due primarily to fetal metabolic activity.

Parathyroid

The concentration of the parathyroid hormone and the size of the parathyroid glands increase, paralleling the fetal calcium requirements. Parathyroid hormone concentration reaches its highest level of approximately twofold between 15 and 35 weeks of gestation, returning to a normal or even subnormal level before childbirth.

Pituitary

Pregnancy is made possible by the hypothalamic stimulation of the anterior pituitary gland. The anterior pituitary produces *FSH*, which stimulates follicle growth in the ovary, and *LH*, which affects ovulation. Stimulation of the pituitary also prolongs the ovary's corpus luteal phase, which maintains the secretory endometrium in preparation for pregnancy. *Prolactin*, another anterior pituitary hormone, is responsible for initial lactation.

The posterior pituitary secretes *vasopressin* (antidiuretic hormone) and *oxytocin*. Vasopressin causes vasoconstriction, which results in increased blood pressure; it also helps regulate water balance. Oxytocin promotes uterine contractility and stimulates ejection of milk from the breasts (the let-down reflex) in the postpartum period.

Adrenals

Little structural change occurs in the adrenal glands during a normal pregnancy. Estrogen-induced increases in the levels of circulating cortisol result primarily from lowered renal excretion. The circulating cortisol levels regulate carbohydrate and protein metabolism. A normal level resumes 1–6 weeks postpartum.

The adrenals secrete increased levels of aldosterone by the early part of the second trimester. The levels of secretion are even more elevated in the woman on a sodium-restricted diet. This increase in aldosterone in a normal pregnancy may be the body's protective response to the increased sodium excretion associated with progesterone (Cunningham et al., 2014).

Pancreas

The islets of Langerhans are stressed to meet the increased demand for insulin during pregnancy, and a latent deficiency may become apparent during pregnancy, producing symptoms of gestational diabetes.

Hormones in Pregnancy

Several hormones are required to maintain pregnancy. Most of these are produced initially by the corpus luteum; the placenta then assumes production.

- **Human chorionic gonadotropin:** The trophoblast secretes hCG in early pregnancy. This hormone stimulates progesterone and estrogen production by the corpus luteum to maintain the pregnancy until the placenta is developed sufficiently to assume that function.

- **Human placental lactogen:** Also called human chorionic somatomammotropin (hCS), hPL is produced by the syncytiotrophoblast. This hormone is an antagonist of insulin; it increases the amount of circulating free fatty acids for maternal metabolic needs and decreases maternal metabolism of glucose to favor fetal growth.

- **Estrogen:** Secreted originally by the corpus luteum, estrogen is produced primarily by the placenta as early as the seventh week of pregnancy. Estrogen stimulates uterine development to provide a suitable environment for the fetus. It also helps to develop the ductal system of the breasts in preparation for lactation.

- **Progesterone:** Progesterone, also produced initially by the corpus luteum and then by the placenta, plays the greatest role in maintaining pregnancy. It maintains the endometrium and also inhibits spontaneous uterine contractility, thus preventing early spontaneous abortion due to uterine activity. In addition, progesterone helps develop the ductal system of the breasts in preparation for lactation.

- **Relaxin:** Relaxin is detectable in the serum of a pregnant woman by the time of the first missed menstrual period. Relaxin inhibits uterine activity, diminishes the strength of uterine contractions, aids in the softening of the cervix, and has the long-term effect of remodeling collagen. Its primary source is the corpus luteum, but small amounts are believed to be produced by the placenta and uterine decidua throughout pregnancy.

Prostaglandins in Pregnancy

Prostaglandins (PGs) are lipid substances that can arise from most body tissues but occur in high concentrations in the female reproductive tract and are present in the decidua during pregnancy. Although their exact functions during pregnancy are still unknown, it has been proposed that PGs are responsible for maintaining reduced placental vascular resistance. Decreased PG levels may contribute to hypertension and preeclampsia. Prostaglandins are also believed to play a role in the complex biochemistry that initiates labor, although their specific functions are still being defined.

Signs of Pregnancy

Many of the changes women experience during pregnancy are used to diagnose the pregnancy itself. They are called the subjective, or presumptive, changes; the objective, or probable, changes; and the diagnostic, or positive, changes of pregnancy.

Subjective (Presumptive) Changes

The subjective changes of pregnancy are the symptoms the woman experiences and reports. Because they can be caused by other conditions, they cannot be considered proof of pregnancy.

>> Go to **Pearson MyLab Nursing and eText** for Chart 2: Differential Diagnosis of Pregnancy—Subjective Changes.

Amenorrhea, or the absence of menses, is the earliest symptom of pregnancy. The missing of more than one menstrual period, especially in a woman whose cycle is ordinarily regular, is an especially useful diagnostic clue. Excessive fatigue may be noted within a few weeks after the first missed menstrual period and may persist throughout the first trimester. Urinary frequency is experienced during the first trimester as the enlarging uterus presses on the bladder. This improves during the second trimester when the enlarging uterus escapes the pelvis, and then recurs in the third trimester when the growing fetus presses on the bladder.

Nausea and vomiting in pregnancy (NVP) occur frequently during the first trimester and may be the result of elevated hCG levels and changed carbohydrate metabolism. Because these symptoms often occur in the early part of the day, they are commonly referred to as **morning sickness**. In reality, the symptoms may occur at any time and can range from a mere distaste for food to severe vomiting.

Changes in the breasts are frequently noted in early pregnancy. These changes include tenderness and tingling sensations, increased pigmentation of the areola and nipple, and changes in the Montgomery glands. The veins in the breasts also become more visible and form a bluish pattern beneath the skin.

Quickening, or the mother's perception of fetal movement, occurs about 18–20 weeks after the last menstrual period (LMP) in a woman pregnant for the first time, but may occur as early as 16 weeks in a woman who has been pregnant before. Quickening is a fluttering sensation in the abdomen that gradually increases in intensity and frequency.

Objective (Probable) Changes

An examiner can perceive the objective changes that occur in pregnancy. Because these changes also have other causes, they do not confirm pregnancy.

>> Go to **Pearson MyLab Nursing and eText** for Chart 3: Differential Diagnosis of Pregnancy—Objective Changes.

The only physical changes detectable during the first 3 months of pregnancy are caused by increased vascular congestion. These changes are noted on pelvic examination. As noted earlier, there is a softening of the cervix called the Goodell sign. The Chadwick sign is a bluish, purple, or deep red discoloration of the mucous membranes of the cervix, vagina, and vulva. (Some sources consider this a presumptive sign.) The **Hegar sign** is a softening of the isthmus of the uterus, the area between the cervix and the body of the uterus. The **McDonald sign** is an ease in flexing the body of the uterus against the cervix.

General enlargement and softening of the body of the uterus can be noted after the eighth week of pregnancy. The fundus of the uterus is palpable just above the symphysis

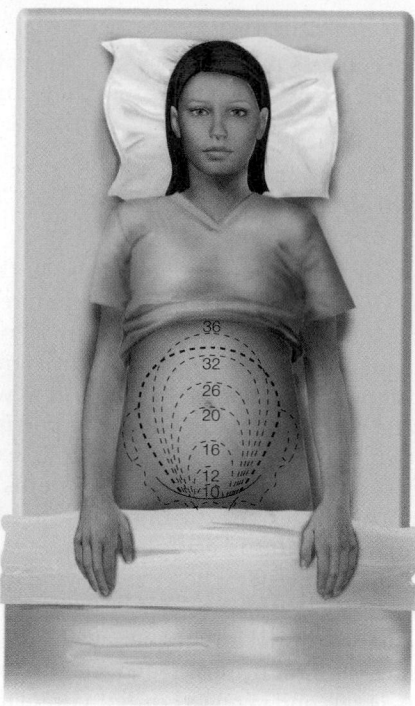

Figure 33–22 》》 Approximate height of the fundus at various weeks of pregnancy.

pubis at about 10–12 weeks' gestation and at the level of the umbilicus at 20–22 weeks' gestation (**Figure 33–22 》》**).

Enlargement of the abdomen during the childbearing years is usually regarded as evidence of pregnancy, especially if it is continuous and accompanied by amenorrhea. Braxton Hicks contractions are palpable with abdominal palpation after week 28. As the woman approaches the end of pregnancy, these contractions may become uncomfortable.

Uterine souffle may be heard when the examiner auscultates the abdomen over the uterus. It is a soft blowing sound that occurs at the same rate as the maternal pulse. The funic souffle occurs at the same rate as the fetal heart rate (FHR).

The fetal outline may be identified by palpation in many pregnant women after 24 weeks' gestation. **Ballottement** is the passive fetal movement elicited when the examiner inserts two gloved fingers into the vagina and pushes against the cervix. This action pushes the fetal body up, and as it falls back, the examiner feels a rebound.

Pregnancy tests are based on analysis of maternal blood or urine for the detection of hCG, the hormone secreted by the trophoblast. These tests are not considered positive signs of pregnancy because the similarity of hCG and the pituitary-secreted LH occasionally results in cross-reactions. In addition, certain conditions other than pregnancy can cause elevated levels of hCG.

Clinical Pregnancy Tests

The most commonly used assay for pregnancy diagnosis is measuring the beta subunit of hCG in either urine or serum. Currently four main hCG tests are used: (1) *radioimmunoassay*, (2) immunoradiometric assay, (3) enzyme-linked immunosorbent assay (ELISA), and (4) fluoroimmunoassay. hCG is detectable in more than 97% of patients (Greene et al.,

2013). False-negative or false-positive results can also occur. In pregnancy, levels normally peak at 10–12 weeks' gestation, and this initial rise is important in monitoring high-risk pregnancies where viability has not been documented. Failure to observe the expected rise may suggest an ectopic pregnancy or spontaneous abortion. An abnormally high level or accelerated rise can also prompt investigation into possible disorders such as molar pregnancy, multiple gestations, or chromosomal abnormalities. There is a rapid decline in the hCG levels until 22 weeks' gestation when another gradual rise occurs (Cunningham et al., 2014).

Diagnostic (Positive) Changes

The positive signs of pregnancy are completely objective, cannot be confused with a pathologic state, and offer conclusive proof of pregnancy.

The fetal heartbeat can be detected with a fetoscope by approximately weeks 17–20 of pregnancy. With an electronic Doppler device, the fetal heartbeat can be detected as early as weeks 10–12. The fetal heart rate is between 110 and 160 beats/min and must be counted and compared with the maternal pulse for differentiation. Auscultation of the abdomen may reveal sounds other than that of the fetal heart. The maternal pulse, emanating from the abdominal aorta, may be unusually loud, or a uterine souffle may be heard.

Fetal movement is actively palpable by a trained examiner after about 20 weeks' gestation. The movements vary from a faint flutter in the early months to more vigorous movements late in pregnancy.

Visualization of the fetus by ultrasound confirms a pregnancy. The gestational sac can be observed by 4–5 weeks' gestation (2–3 weeks after conception). Fetal parts and fetal heart movement can be seen as early as 8 weeks. A transvaginal ultrasound has been used to detect a gestational sac as early as 10 days after implantation (Cunningham et al., 2014).

Psychologic Response of the Expectant Family to Pregnancy

Pregnancy is a turning point in a family's life, accompanied by stress and anxiety, whether the pregnancy is desired or not. Especially when this is their first child, the expectant parents may be unaware of the physical, emotional, and cognitive changes of pregnancy and may anticipate no problems from such a normal event. Thus, they may be confused and distressed by new feelings and behaviors that are essentially normal.

For beginning families, pregnancy is the transition period from childlessness to parenthood. If the expectant woman is married or has a stable partner, she is no longer only a mate, but also must assume the role of mother. Her partner, whether male or female, will become a parent, too. The anticipation of parenthood brings significant role changes for them. Career goals and mobility may be affected, and the couple's relationship takes on a different meaning to them and within the larger family and community. If the pregnancy results in the birth of a child, the couple enters a new, irreversible stage of their life together. With each subsequent pregnancy, routines and family dynamics are again altered, requiring readjustment and realignment.

In most pregnancies, finances are an important consideration. Pregnant women with or without stable partners recognize the financial impact of a child and may be concerned about financial issues. Decisions about financial matters need to be made at this time. Will both parents work outside the home during the pregnancy or after the child is born? If so, who will provide child care? Couples also may need to decide about the division of domestic tasks. Any differences of opinion must be discussed openly and resolved so that the family can meet the needs of its members.

If the pregnant woman has no stable partner, she must deal with the role changes, fears, and adjustments of pregnancy, as well as financial uncertainty, alone or seek support from family or friends. She also faces the reality of planning for the future as a single parent. Even if the pregnant woman plans to relinquish her baby, she still must deal with the adjustments of pregnancy. This can be especially difficult without a good support system.

Developmental Tasks of the Expectant Couple

Pregnancy can be viewed as a developmental stage with its own distinct developmental tasks. For a couple, it can be a time of support or conflict depending on the amount of adjustment each is willing to make to maintain the family's equilibrium.

During a first pregnancy, the couple plans together for the child's arrival, collecting information on how to be parents. At the same time, each member of the couple continues to participate in some separate activities with friends or family members. The availability of social support is an important factor in psychosocial well-being during pregnancy. The social network is often a major source of advice for the pregnant woman; however, both sound and unsound information may be conveyed.

During pregnancy, the expectant parents face significant changes and must deal with major psychosocial adjustments. Other family members, especially other children of the woman or couple and the grandparents-to-be, also must adjust to the pregnancy.

>> Go to **Pearson MyLab Nursing and eText** to see Chart 4: Parental Reactions to Pregnancy.

For some individuals or couples, pregnancy is more than a developmental stage; it is a crisis. Crisis can be defined as "a disturbance or conflict in which the individual cannot maintain a state of equilibrium." Pregnancy can be considered a *maturational crisis*, because it is a common event in the normal growth and development of the family. During such a crisis, the individual or family is in disequilibrium. Egos weaken, usual defense mechanisms are not effective, unresolved issues from the past reappear, and relationships shift. This period of disequilibrium and disorganization is marked by unsuccessful attempts to solve the perceived problems. If the crisis is not resolved, it will result in maladaptive behaviors in one or more family members and possible disintegration of the family. Families that are able to resolve a maturational crisis will return successfully to normal functioning and can even strengthen the bonds in the family relationship.

The Mother

Pregnancy is a condition that alters body image and necessitates a reordering of social relationships and changes in the roles of family members. The way each woman meets the stresses of pregnancy is influenced by her emotional makeup, her sociologic and cultural background, and her acceptance or rejection of the pregnancy. However, many women manifest similar psychologic and emotional responses during pregnancy, including ambivalence, acceptance, introversion, mood swings, and changes in body image.

A woman's attitude toward her pregnancy can be a significant factor in its outcome. Even if the pregnancy is planned, there is an element of surprise at first. Many women commonly experience feelings of ambivalence during early pregnancy. This ambivalence may be related to feelings that the timing is somehow wrong; worries about the need to modify existing relationships or career plans; fears about assuming a new role; unresolved emotional conflicts with the woman's own mother; and fears about pregnancy, labor, and birth. These feelings may be more pronounced if the pregnancy is unplanned or unwanted. Indirect expressions of ambivalence include complaints about considerable physical discomfort, prolonged or frequent depression, significant dissatisfaction with changing body shape, excessive mood swings, and difficulty in accepting the life changes resulting from the pregnancy.

Many pregnancies are unintended, but not all unintended pregnancies are unwanted. A pregnancy can be unintended and wanted at the same time. However, an unintended pregnancy can be a risk factor for depression. Higher levels of depression are also found in women who report more negative responses to pregnancy, who believe the pregnancy has greater consequences, and who experience more symptoms, especially in the third trimester (Jessop, Craig, & Ayers, 2014).

Conflicts about adapting to pregnancy are no more pronounced for older pregnant women (age 35 and over) than for younger ones. Moreover, older pregnant women tend to be less concerned about the normal physical changes of pregnancy and are confident about handling issues that arise during pregnancy and parenting. This difference may result because older pregnant women have more experience with problem solving. However, older pregnant women may have fewer pregnant peers and thus may have fewer people with whom to share concerns and expectations.

Pregnancy produces marked changes in a woman's body within a relatively short period of time. Pregnant women experience changes in body image because of physical alterations and may feel a loss of control over their bodies during pregnancy and later during childbirth. These perceptions are related to a certain extent to personality factors, social network responses, and attitudes toward pregnancy. Although changes in body image are normal, they can be very stressful for the woman. Explanation and discussion of the changes may help both the woman and her partner deal with the stress associated with this aspect of pregnancy.

Fantasies about the unborn child are common among pregnant women. The themes of the fantasies (baby's appearance, gender, traits, impact on parents, and so on) vary by trimester and differ among women who are pregnant for the first time and women who already have children.

First Trimester

During the first trimester, feelings of disbelief and ambivalence are common. The woman's baby does not seem real, and she focuses on herself and her pregnancy. She may experience one or more of the early symptoms of pregnancy, such as breast tenderness or morning sickness, which are unsettling and at times unpleasant.

At this time, the expectant mother also begins to exhibit some characteristic behavioral changes. She may become increasingly introspective and passive. She may be emotionally labile, with characteristic mood swings from joy to despair. She may fantasize about a miscarriage and feel guilty because of these fantasies. She may worry that these thoughts will harm the baby in some way. Nursing responsibilities at this time include helping the mother to identify coping strategies and providing options and counseling for women experiencing a pregnancy that is both unintended and unwanted.

Second Trimester

During the second trimester, quickening occurs around 20 weeks. This perception of fetal movement helps the woman think of her baby as a separate individual, and she generally becomes excited about the pregnancy even if she had not been looking forward to the pregnancy earlier. The woman becomes increasingly introspective as she evaluates her life, her plans, and her child's future. This introspection helps the woman prepare for her new mothering role. Emotional lability, which may be unsettling to her partner, persists. In some instances, the partner may react by withdrawing. This withdrawal is especially distressing to the woman because she needs increased love and affection. Once the couple understands that these behaviors are characteristic of pregnancy, it is easier for the couple to deal with them effectively, although to some extent they may be sources of stress throughout pregnancy. As pregnancy becomes more noticeable, the woman's body image changes. She may feel great pride, embarrassment, or concern. Generally, women feel best during the second trimester, which is a relatively tranquil time.

Third Trimester

In the third trimester, the woman feels both pride about her pregnancy and anxiety about labor and birth. Physical discomforts increase, and the woman is eager for the pregnancy to end. She experiences increased fatigue, her body movements are more awkward, and her interest in sexual activity may decrease. During this time, the woman tends to be concerned about the health and safety of her unborn child and may worry that she will not cope well during childbirth. Toward the end of this period, the woman often experiences a surge of energy as she prepares for childbirth. Many women report bursts of energy, during which they vigorously clean and organize the home ("nesting").

Psychologic Tasks of the Mother

Rubin (1984) identified four major tasks that the pregnant woman undertakes to maintain her intactness and that of her family and at the same time to incorporate her new child into the family system. These tasks form the foundation for a mutually gratifying relationship with her baby:

1. ***Ensuring safe passage through pregnancy, labor, and birth.*** The pregnant woman feels concern for her unborn child and for herself. She looks for competent prenatal care to provide a sense of control. She may seek information from literature, observe other pregnant women and new mothers, and discuss with others. She also attempts to ensure safe passage by engaging in self-care activities related to diet, exercise, alcohol consumption, and the like. In the third trimester, she becomes more aware of external threats in the environment—a toy on the stairs, the awkwardness of an escalator—that pose a threat to her well-being. She may worry if her partner is late or if she is home alone. Sleep becomes more difficult, and she longs for birth even though it, too, is frightening.

2. ***Seeking acceptance of this child by others.*** The birth of a child alters a woman's primary support group (her family) and her secondary affiliate groups. The woman slowly and subtly alters her network to meet the needs of her pregnancy. In this adjustment, the woman's partner is the most important figure. The partner's support and acceptance help form a maternal identity. If there are other children in the home, the mother also works to ensure their acceptance of the coming child. Acceptance of the anticipated change is sometimes stressful, and the woman may work to maintain special time with her partner or older children. The woman without a partner looks to others, such as a family member or friend, for this support.

3. ***Seeking commitment and acceptance of herself as mother to the newborn (binding in).*** During the first trimester, the child remains a rather abstract concept. With quickening, however, the child begins to become a real individual, and the mother begins to develop bonds of attachment. The mother experiences the movement of the child within her in an intimate, exclusive way, and out of this experience, bonds of love form. This binding-in process, characterized by its strong emotional component, motivates the pregnant woman to become competent in her role and provides satisfaction for her in the role of mother. This possessive love increases her maternal commitment to protect her fetus now and her child after he or she is born.

4. ***Learning to give of oneself on behalf of one's child.*** Childbirth involves many acts of giving. A man "gives" a child to a woman; she in turn "gives" a child to her partner. Life is given to a baby; a sibling is given to older children of the family. The woman begins to develop a capacity for self-denial and learns to delay immediate personal gratification to meet the needs of another. Baby showers and gifts are acts of giving that increase the mother's self-esteem and help her recognize the separateness and needs of the coming baby.

Accomplishment of these tasks helps the expectant woman develop her self-concept as a mother. The expectant woman who was well nurtured by her own mother may view her mother as a role model and emulate her; the woman who views her mother as a poor mother may worry that she will make similar mistakes. A woman's self-concept as a mother expands with experience and continues to grow through subsequent childbearing and childrearing.

The Father

Until fairly recently, the expectant father or partner was often viewed as a "bystander" or observer of the pregnancy. He was necessary for conception, for bill paying, and for providing male guidance as his child matured. This view has changed, and the father is now expected to be a nurturing, caring, involved parent as well as a provider. In response to societal pressures, the influence of the feminist movement, and the economic pressures that have resulted in more women being employed outside the home, shared parenting and shared breadwinning have become more common. Many men have actively sought to be more involved in the experience of childbirth and parenting.

Expectant fathers experience many of the same feelings and conflicts experienced by expectant mothers when the pregnancy has been confirmed. Initially, expectant fathers may feel pride in their virility, which pregnancy confirms, but also have ambivalent feelings. The extent of ambivalence depends on many factors, including the father's relationship with his partner, his previous experience with pregnancy, his age, his economic stability, and whether the pregnancy was planned. The expectant father must first deal with the reality of the pregnancy and then struggle to gain recognition as a parent from his partner, family, friends, coworkers, society—and from his baby as well. The expectant mother can help her partner be a participant and not merely a helpmate to her if she has a definite sense of the experience as *their* pregnancy and *their* baby and not *her* pregnancy and *her* baby.

Men whose partners are pregnant following a previous pregnancy loss may experience a variety of emotions attributable to the loss. These emotions might include an increased sense of risk, feelings of increased concern about the outcome of the current pregnancy, the recognition that something could go wrong again, and the sense that increased vigilance is essential. These fathers may call home more often to check on the mother's condition and the baby and may also feel an increased need to be involved more actively in the current pregnancy.

In general, the expectant father faces psychologic stress as he makes the transition from nonparent to parent or from parent of one to parent of two or more. Sources of stress include financial issues, unexpected events during pregnancy, concern that the baby will not be healthy and normal, worry about the pain the partner will experience in childbirth, and his role during labor and birth. Other sources of stress for expectant fathers include concern over the changing relationship with their partners, diminished sexual responsiveness in their partners or in themselves, changes in relationships with their families or male friends, and their ability to parent.

The role of the father is crucial both prenatally and postnatally. Healthcare providers need to encourage and welcome the father's involvement during the pregnancy. It is important to educate fathers about the role they can play in promoting healthy child development and how they can best support the mother during pregnancy to enhance healthy outcomes (Alio et al., 2013).

The expectant father must establish a fatherhood role just as the expectant mother develops a motherhood role. The mother experiences biologic changes of pregnancy that aid in the transition to motherhood. Fathers may feel left out because they are unable to experience what their partner is experiencing. The fathers who are most successful at developing a fatherhood role generally like children, are excited about the prospect of fatherhood, are eager to nurture a child, have confidence in their ability to be a parent, and share the experiences of pregnancy and childbirth with their partners. Fathers may have a lack of understanding of their role if they came from dysfunctional families, if they lacked positive role models, or if there was a general lack of education available to them (Alio et al., 2013).

First Trimester

After the initial excitement of announcing the pregnancy to friends and relatives and receiving their congratulations, an expectant father may begin to feel left out of the pregnancy. He is also often confused by his partner's mood changes and perhaps bewildered by his responses to her changing body. He may resent the attention given to the woman and the changes in their relationship as she experiences fatigue and a decreased interest in sex.

During this time, his child is a "potential baby." Fathers often picture interacting with a child of age 5 or 6 rather than a newborn. Even the pregnancy itself may seem unreal until the woman shows more physical signs.

Second Trimester

The father's role in the pregnancy is still vague in the second trimester, but his involvement can be increased by his watching and feeling fetal movement. It is helpful if the father, as well as the mother, has the opportunity to hear the fetal heartbeat. That requires a visit to the healthcare provider's office. Involvement of fathers in antepartum care is increasing and may even be an expectation of their partner. For many men, seeing the fetus on ultrasound is an important experience in accepting the reality of the pregnancy.

Like expectant mothers, expectant fathers need to confront and resolve some of their own conflicts about the fathering they received. A father needs to sort out those behaviors in his own fathering that he wants to imitate and those he wishes to avoid.

The anxiety experienced by the father-to-be is lessened if both parents agree on the support role the man is to assume during pregnancy and on his projected paternal role. For example, if both see his role as that of breadwinner, the man's stress is low. However, if the man views his role as that of breadwinner and the woman expects him to be actively involved in preparations and child care, his stress increases. An open and honest discussion about the expectations each parent has about their roles will help the father-to-be in his transition to fatherhood (London et al., 2017).

The woman's appearance begins to alter at this time, and men react differently to the physical change. For some it decreases sexual interest; for others it may have the opposite effect. Both partners experience a multitude of emotions, and it continues to be important for them to communicate and accept each other's feelings and concerns. In situations in which the expectant mother's demands dominate the relationship, the expectant father's resentment may increase to the point that he is spending more time at work, involved in a hobby, or with his friends. The behavior is even more likely if the expectant father did not want the pregnancy or if the relationship was not a good one before the pregnancy.

Third Trimester

If the couple have communicated their concerns and feelings to one another and grown in their relationship, the third trimester is a special and rewarding time. A more clearly defined role evolves at this time for the expectant father, and it becomes more obvious how the couple can prepare together for the coming event. They may become involved in childbirth education classes and make concrete preparations for the arrival of the baby, such as shopping for a crib, car seat, and other equipment. If the expectant father has developed a detached attitude about the pregnancy before this time, however, it is unlikely that he will become a willing participant even though his role becomes more obvious.

Concerns and fears may recur. Many men are afraid of hurting the unborn baby during intercourse. The father may also begin to have anxiety and fantasies about what could happen to his partner and the unborn baby during labor and birth and feels a great sense of responsibility. The questions asked earlier in pregnancy emerge again. What kind of parents will he and his partner be? Will he really be able to help his partner in labor? Can they afford to have a baby?

The nurse needs to be prepared to meet the needs of lesbian or gay families as well. While all 50 states in the United States now recognize same-sex marriage, these couples may still face unique challenges in completing their developmental tasks.

Siblings

The introduction of a new baby into the family often leads to sibling rivalry, which results from children's fear of change in the security of their relationships with their parents. Some of the behaviors demonstrating feelings of sibling rivalry may even be directed toward the mother during the pregnancy as she experiences more fatigue and less patience with her toddler, for example. Parents who recognize the situation early in pregnancy and make constructive responses can help minimize the problems of sibling rivalry.

Preparation of the young child for a new sibling should begin several weeks before the anticipated birth and is best designed according to the age and experience of the child. The mother may let the child feel the fetus moving in her uterus, explaining that this is "a special place where babies grow." The child can help the parents put the baby clothes in drawers or prepare the baby's room. Because they do not have a clear concept of time, young children should not be told too early about the pregnancy.

Consistency is important in dealing with young children. They need reassurance that certain people, special things, and familiar places will continue to exist after the new baby

arrives. The crib is an important though transient object in a child's life. If it is to be given to the new baby, the parents should thoughtfully help the child adjust to this change. Any move from crib to bed or from one room to another should precede the baby's birth by several weeks or more. If the new baby is to share a room with one or more siblings, the parents must discuss this with them.

Some parents advocate cosleeping or bed sharing (one or both parents sleeping with their baby or young child), and so the crib is less of an issue. Cosleeping (newborn/infant sleeping in the same bed with the mother), which is common in many non-Western cultures, is on the increase in the United States. Opinion varies sharply about the advantages and risks of the practice. In 2005 the American Academy of Pediatrics (AAP) issued a policy statement recommending against cosleeping because of the increased risk of sudden infant death syndrome (SIDS) (Blair, 2015). The AAP and forensic researchers recommend that the safest place for the baby to sleep is in the parents' room with the baby in a crib in proximity to the parents for the first 6 months of life (Blair, 2015).

If the sibling is ready for toilet training, it is most effectively done several months before or after the baby's arrival. Parents should know that the older, toilet-trained child may regress to wetting or soiling because he or she sees the new baby getting attention for such behavior. The older, weaned child may want to drink from the breast or bottle again after the new baby comes. If the new mother anticipates these behaviors, they will be less frustrating during her early postpartum days.

During the pregnancy, older children should be introduced to a new baby for short periods to get an idea of what a new baby is like. This introduction dispels fantasies that the new arrival will be big enough to be a playmate. Pregnant women may also find it helpful to bring their children to a prenatal visit after they have been told about the expected baby. The children are encouraged to become involved in prenatal care and to ask any questions they may have. They are also given the opportunity to hear the fetal heartbeat, either with a stethoscope or with the Doppler device. This helps make the baby more real to them.

If siblings are school-age children, the pregnancy should be viewed as a family affair. Teaching about the pregnancy should be based on the child's level of understanding and interest. Overeager parents may go into longer and more in-depth responses than the child is able to understand. Some children are more curious than others. Books at their level of understanding can be made available in the home. Involvement in family discussions, attendance at sibling preparation classes, encouragement to feel fetal movement, and an opportunity to listen to the fetal heart supplement the learning process and help make the school-age child feel part of the pregnancy. Sibling preparation classes assist in the transition process for both parents and children. After attending the classes, children often exhibit an increased ability to express their feelings and less anxiety.

Older children or adolescents may appear to have a sophisticated knowledge base, but it may be intermingled with many misconceptions. Thus, parents should make opportunities to discuss their concerns and should involve the children in preparation for the new baby.

Even after the birth, siblings need to feel that they are part of a family event. Changes in hospital regulations allowing siblings to be present at the birth or to visit their mother and the new baby facilitate this process. Participation in special programs for siblings may help in this process. On arrival at home, siblings can share in "showing off" the new baby.

Sibling preparation for the arrival of a new baby is essential, but other factors are equally important. These include the amount of parental attention focused on the new arrival, the amount of parental attention given the older child after the birth of the new arrival, and parental skill in dealing effectively with regressive or aggressive behavior.

Grandparents

The first relatives told about a pregnancy are usually the grandparents. Often the expectant grandparents become increasingly supportive of the couple even if conflicts existed previously. But even sensitive grandparents may have difficulty knowing how deeply to become involved in the childrearing process.

Because grandparenting can occur over a wide expanse of years, people's response to this role varies considerably. Younger grandparents leading active lives may not demonstrate as much interest as the young couple would like. In other cases, expectant grandparents may freely give advice and gifts, sometimes to excess. For grandparents, conflict may be related to the expectant couple's need to feel in control of their lives, or it may stem from events signaling changing roles in the grandparents' lives (e.g., retirement, financial concerns, menopause, or death of a friend). Some parents of expectant couples may already be grandparents with a developed style of grandparenting. This influences their response to the pregnancy.

Because childbearing and childrearing practices have changed, family cohesiveness is promoted by effective communication and frank discussion between young couples and interested grandparents about the changes and the reasons for those changes. Clarifying the role of the grandparents ensures a comfortable situation for all.

Classes for grandparents may provide information about changes in birth and parenting practices. These classes help familiarize grandparents with new parents' needs and may offer suggestions for ways in which the grandparents can support the childbearing couple.

Cultural Values and Pregnancy

A universal tendency exists to create ceremonial rituals or rites around important life events. Thus, rituals are often tied to pregnancy, childbirth, marriage, and death. The rituals and customs of a group are a reflection of the group's values. Therefore, the identification of cultural values is useful in predicting reactions to pregnancy. An understanding of male and female roles, family lifestyles, religious values, or the meaning of children in a culture may explain reactions of joy or shame.

Generalization about cultural characteristics or values is difficult because not every individual in a culture may display these characteristics. Just as variations are seen

---

Focus on Diversity and Culture
Providing Culturally Competent Care

Nurses who are interacting with expectant families from a different culture or ethnic group can provide more effective, culturally competent nursing care by

- Critically examining their own cultural beliefs
- Identifying personal biases, attitudes, stereotypes, and prejudices
- Making a conscious commitment to respect and study the values and beliefs of others
- Using sensitive, current language when describing others' cultures
- Learning the rituals, customs, and practices of the major cultural and ethnic groups with whom they have contact
- Including cultural assessment and assessment of the family's expectations of the healthcare system as a routine part of prenatal nursing care
- Incorporating the family's cultural and spiritual practices into prenatal care as much as possible
- Fostering an attitude of respect for and cooperation with alternative healers and caregivers when possible
- Providing for the services of an interpreter when language barriers exist
- Learning the language (or at least several key phrases) of at least one of the cultural groups with whom they interact
- Recognizing that ultimately it is the woman's right to make her own healthcare choices
- Evaluating whether the woman's healthcare beliefs have any potential negative consequences for her health.

---

between cultures, they are also seen within cultures. For example, because of their exposure to the American culture, a third-generation Chinese American family might have different values and beliefs from those of a Chinese family that has recently immigrated to America. For this reason, the nurse needs to supplement a general knowledge of cultural values and practices with a complete assessment of the individual's values and practices. Focus on Diversity and Culture: Providing Culturally Competent Care summarizes the key actions a nurse can take to become more culturally aware.

Cultural assessment is an important aspect of prenatal care. Increasingly, healthcare professionals know that they must address cultural needs during a prenatal assessment to provide culturally competent healthcare during pregnancy. The nurse needs to identify the prospective parents' main beliefs, values, and behaviors related to pregnancy and childbearing. This includes information about ethnic background, degree of affiliation with the ethnic group, patterns of decision making, religious preference, language, communication style, and common etiquette practices. The nurse also can explore the woman's (or family's) expectations of the healthcare system. Once this information has been gathered, the nurse can plan and provide care that is appropriate and responsive to a family's needs.

Case Study » Part 1

Emma Halleck is a 22-year-old woman who presented at the antepartum clinic on June 15. She suspects that she is pregnant: A home pregnancy test was positive. Her last menstrual period began on April 10. She reports having urinary frequency, breast tenderness, fatigue, and occasional nausea and vomiting. She has begun to have some light-headedness and dizziness when she first gets up after sitting or sleeping.

Mrs. Halleck tells you she is married and states that this is her second pregnancy. She miscarried at 10 weeks approximately 6 months ago. She denies any history of drug or alcohol use, sexually transmitted infections (STIs), multiple partners, family violence, medical–surgical disorders, or mental illness. Mrs. Halleck is excited about the pregnancy, and she reports that her husband is, too. She does express concern over her ability to carry the pregnancy to term, although she feels relieved that she is beyond the time of her first pregnancy loss. This pregnancy was a planned pregnancy. Mrs. Halleck is a college graduate, employed as a teacher, and has group health insurance through the local public school system.

Exam

Weight 122 lb (prepregnant weight usually between 115 and 120 lb)

Height 5′4″

BP 110/60 mmHg, P 82 beats/min, R 16/min

Hgb 12, Hct 33%, WBC 5000

UA, blood glucose, and protein all negative

Rubella titer—immune

HIV, STIs—negative

Hepatitis antibody—negative

Immunoassay pregnancy test—positive

Mother: O Rh negative; father: O Rh positive.

On pelvic exam, the physician determines that Mrs. Halleck's uterus is enlarged and at the top of the symphysis pubis. The lower uterine segment is soft; the cervix is soft and bluish in color. There is an increase in vaginal and cervical secretions. The physician determines that Mrs. Halleck's pelvis is adequate for a normal vaginal birth. Vaginal ultrasound confirms pregnancy with fetal heart tones at 120 beats per minute.

Clinical Reasoning Questions Level I

1. Why is Mrs. Halleck experiencing urinary frequency?
2. Why is Mrs. Halleck having breast tenderness at this time?
3. Are light-headedness and dizziness normal? Why or why not? What nursing intervention should be taught to all pregnant women to avoid these symptoms?

Clinical Reasoning Questions Level II

4. Are the uterine changes assessed on examination considered normal? Why or why not?
5. How does the body maintain pregnancy during the first 12 weeks?
6. Which developmental stage of pregnancy is Mrs. Halleck in? How did you determine this?
7. How would you assess whether fetal attachment is occurring?

Concepts Related to Reproduction

Pregnancy is directly related to reproduction, but affects all body systems and many concepts. Changes and alterations may involve multiple aspects of health. A holistic model of nursing care assists the nurse to engage in patient-centered care focusing on the physical, psychosocial, and spiritual needs of the patient. The Concepts Related to Reproduction feature outlines some, but not all, of the concepts that are integral to pregnancy. They are presented in alphabetical order.

Sexuality is a key concept in reproductive health, as intercourse is the means by which conception occurs. Anatomic and hormonal changes of pregnancy may alter sexual activity between partners, affecting intimacy and relationships. An additional concern is the potential for unprotected sex before or during pregnancy. Unprotected sex may lead to STIs, which could result in infertility, fetal loss, or complications for mother and fetus. Sexuality is considered as families plan the timing of pregnancies and consider future pregnancies.

Expected physiologic changes in pregnancy often result in discomfort. Anatomic adjustments occur over time as the fetus grows and maternal tissues and structures adapt to physical and hormonal changes. Chronic pain caused by existing diagnoses may increase as pregnancy progresses. During labor, contractions, cervical dilation, and vaginal distention cause pain that may be managed using nonpharmacologic and pharmacologic interventions. The source of postpartum pain varies depending on the length of labor and pushing, types of delivery, and potential perineal trauma. Cramping and discomfort that may accompany breastfeeding are also possible.

Antepartum monitoring includes methods to assess perfusion of mother and fetus. Because poor tissue perfusion decreases the amount of oxygen that reaches the tissues, it is important to maintain normal hemoglobin and hematocrit levels to promote the production and function of red blood cells. In addition, screening allows for early identification of conditions that may impair perfusion, including congenital anomalies, abnormalities of the placenta, and nutritional deficits. Hypertensive disorders of pregnancy may decrease perfusion, resulting in poor fetal growth or neurologic risks for the mother. Conditions that threaten the viability of mother or fetus may require preterm delivery.

Prenatal nutrition is crucial for adequate growth and development of fetal tissues. Nutritional assessment occurs throughout pregnancy via laboratory values and monitoring of weight gain. Nutritional deficits may occur in vulnerable populations or for those diagnosed with hyperemesis or other gastrointestinal disorders. Adequate nutrition is also required for the production of nutrient-dense breast milk and continues to be a critical component of continued growth and development of the newborn.

Hormonal influences may alter carbohydrate metabolism during pregnancy, leading to the development of gestational diabetes mellitus (GDM). Increased maternal glucose levels may cause the fetus to become large for gestational age (LGA), leading to potential complications for mother and fetus during and after delivery. Patients with an existing diagnosis of diabetes mellitus (DM) may develop vascular changes that impair fetal perfusion, resulting in a newborn that is small for gestational age (SGA). Glucose tolerance tests occur during pregnancy to screen for and diagnose GDM. (GDM is discussed in detail in Exemplar 33.A.)

Oxygenation is essential for normal tissue growth and function. Alterations in oxygenation may cause fetal acidosis, which could result in impaired function of the newborn or fetal loss (see the module on Acid–Base Balance). Existing

Concepts Related to
Reproduction

CONCEPT	RELATIONSHIP TO REPRODUCTION	NURSING IMPLICATIONS
Comfort	Pregnancy discomforts Labor pain Postpartum pain.	■ Pregnancy: provide comfort measures for common discomforts. ■ Labor: provide comfort measures for labor (relaxation, hot/cold, positioning, ambulating, birthing balls, hydrotherapy), medications for pain relief, including IVP and epidurals. ■ Postpartum: Provide instruction on Kegel exercises, sitz baths.
Metabolism	Diabetes, gestational diabetes ↑ risks to both mother and baby.	■ Assess for signs/symptoms of hypoglycemia and hyperglycemia. ■ Encourage 30 minutes of exercise after each meal. ■ Conduct fetal kick counts twice daily beginning at 28 weeks. ■ Teach blood glucose monitoring. ■ Refer to dietitian. ■ Encourage frequent prenatal visits. ■ Encourage verbalization of feelings related to diabetes diagnosis.

Nutrition	Prenatal nutrition is critical for a healthy fetus.
	Breastfeeding.
		■ Educate patient on need to increase calories and fluid intake and on safe food consumption during pregnancy.
		■ Provide health promotion strategies to enhance fetal/neonatal health:
		  ● Easily digested foods
		  ● Decreased allergies, risk for illness
		  ● Promotion of self-regulation of feedings.

Oxygenation	Untreated or undertreated respiratory disease ↑ risk of inadequate oxygenation to fetus.	■ Educate patient regarding need to adhere to therapeutic regimen for respiratory conditions such as asthma. ■ Refer patients who need specialized care who do not already have a provider (e.g., pulmonologist). ■ Assess respiratory status, patient signs/symptoms at each healthcare interaction.
Perfusion	↓ tissue perfusion creates oxygen deficit to organs.	■ Assess perfusion, including pulses, nail beds, color, body position for comfort, orientation. ■ Be alert for tachycardia, then hypotension, cool clammy skin, altered level of consciousness (LOC). ■ Administer oxygen. ■ Replace IV fluids. ■ Weigh pads. ■ Administer pharmacotherapy to contract uterus.
Sexuality	Unprotected intercourse ↑ likelihood of pregnancy, ↑ risk for sexually transmitted infections. Anatomic and hormonal changes.	■ Educate patient regarding safe sex practices. ■ Assess risk factors. ■ Provide additional education related to risk factors. ■ Educate couple about normal alterations affecting intimacy.
Stress and Coping	Emotional and relational changes occur with growth of the family. Responsibilities expand with incorporation of a new child. Expected physical changes may impact self-esteem. Pregnancy, delivery, and recovery may not meet expectations. (i.e., birth experience and idealized child).	■ Encourage expression of concerns. ■ Assess patient's and family's past coping strategies. ■ Reinforce adaptive coping. ■ Reinforce realistic expectations.
Teaching and Learning	Patient/couples education enhances pregnancy outcomes.	■ Educate patient/couple about labor and comfort measures. ■ Inform patient about expected physiologic and psychologic changes associated with pregnancy. ■ Provide information about purpose and significance of findings.

maternal diagnoses such as asthma may cause poor maternal oxygenation, which, in turn, disrupts placental gas exchange for the fetus. Assessment of fetal oxygenation occurs via monitoring of the fetal heart rate, and takes place in the clinic, antepartum testing unit, or the labor and delivery unit. Adequate maternal nutrition, avoidance of the supine position, and treatment of respiratory conditions help to maintain oxygenation of the mother and fetus.

The addition of a child to the family unit requires role transitions for each family member. Impaired coping may disrupt normal family processes and relationships as members adjust to pregnancy, prepare for delivery, and incorporate the new child into the family. Ineffective coping skills may result in alterations in family dynamics and relationships as members compare the reality of the birth experience with expectations. Negative responses to expected physical changes of pregnancy may also have an impact on body image, which could result in unhealthy behaviors involving nutrition and physical activity.

Effective teaching and learning are key factors that may improve patient outcomes. Pregnant women, especially those who are pregnant for the first time, require a great deal of education and support from healthcare providers. Patient understanding of the need for antepartal testing and regular clinic visits improves compliance and leads to better patient outcomes. Anticipation of expected changes of pregnancy may enhance the pregnancy experience, especially if both the mother and father understand the physiology of pregnancy and normal changes that may occur. The labor process may be enriched if couples attend childbirth classes in preparation for the delivery.

Health Promotion

The nurse can help promote maternal and fetal well-being by providing expectant couples with accurate, complete information about health behaviors and issues that can affect pregnancy and childbirth. Health behaviors, such as breast care, rest, sexual activity, and exercise, help protect both the fetus and the mother and decrease the discomfort of the mother during both pregnancy and labor. Issues that can affect pregnancy range from clothing to employment to travel. The nurse working with pregnant women needs to be able to provide patient teaching in all of these areas.

Breast Care

Whether the pregnant woman plans to formula-feed or breastfeed her baby, support of the breasts is important to promote comfort and prevent back strain, particularly if the breasts become large and pendulous. The sensitivity of the breasts in pregnancy is frequently relieved by good support.

Wearing a well-fitting, supportive brassiere that has the following qualities is essential:

- The straps are wide and do not stretch (elastic straps soon lose their tautness with the weight of the breasts and frequent washing).
- The cup holds all breast tissue comfortably.
- Tucks or other devices allow the brassiere to expand, thus accommodating the enlarging chest circumference.

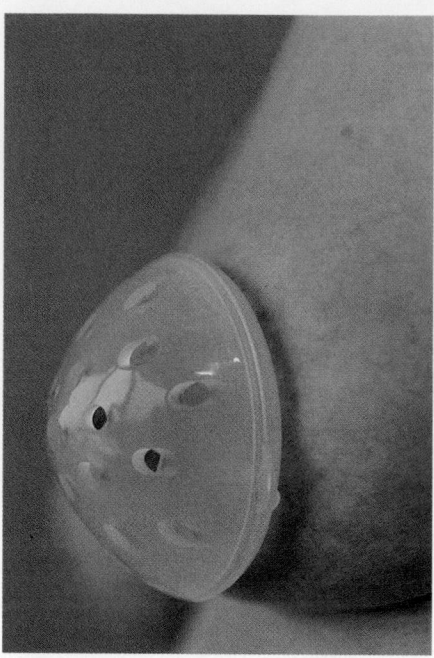

Figure 33–23 ❯❯ This breast shell is designed to increase the protractility of inverted nipples. Worn the last 3–4 weeks of pregnancy, it exerts gentle pulling pressure at the edge of the areola, gradually forcing the nipple through the center of the shield. It may be used after birth if necessary.

- The brassiere supports the nipple line approximately midway between the elbow and shoulder but is not pulled up in the back by the weight of the breasts.

Cleanliness of the breasts also is important, especially if they begin leaking colostrum, which may occur during the last trimester (or earlier in women pregnant with multiples). If colostrum crusts on the nipples, it can be removed with warm water. The woman planning to breastfeed is advised not to use soap on her nipples because of its drying effect.

Some women have flat or inverted nipples. True nipple inversion, which is rare, is usually diagnosed during the initial prenatal assessment. Breast shells designed to correct inverted nipples are effective for some women, but others gain no benefit from them (**Figure 33–23 ❯❯**).

Activity and Rest

Exercise during pregnancy helps maintain maternal fitness and muscle tone, leads to improved self-image, promotes regular bowel function, increases energy, improves sleep, relieves tension, helps control weight gain, and is associated with improved postpartum recovery. Normal participation in exercise can continue throughout an uncomplicated pregnancy and, in fact, is encouraged.

The woman can check with her certified nurse-midwife (CNM) or obstetrician about taking part in strenuous sports, such as skiing and horseback riding. In general, the skilled sportswoman is not discouraged from participating in these activities if her pregnancy is uncomplicated. However, pregnancy is not the appropriate time to learn a new sport.

Certain conditions contraindicate exercise. These conditions include rupture of the membranes, preeclampsia–eclampsia,

Patient Teaching
Pregnant Women and Exercise

The following guidelines are helpful in counseling pregnant women about exercise:

- Even mild to moderate exercise is beneficial during pregnancy. Regular exercise—at least 30 minutes of moderate exercise daily or most days—is preferred (Kimberly, Neibyl, & Johnson, 2012).

- After the first trimester, women should avoid exercising in the supine position. In most pregnant women, the supine position is associated with decreased cardiac output. Because uterine blood flow is reduced during exercise as blood is shunted from the visceral organs to the muscles, the remaining cardiac output is further decreased. Similarly, women should avoid standing motionless for prolonged periods (Katz, 2012).

- Because decreased oxygen is available for aerobic exercise during pregnancy, women should modify the intensity of their exercise based on their symptoms, should stop when they become fatigued, and should avoid exercising to the point of exhaustion. Non-weight-bearing exercises, such as swimming and cycling, are recommended because they decrease the risk of injury and provide fitness with comfort.

- As pregnancy progresses and the center of gravity changes, especially in the third trimester, women should avoid exercises in which the loss of balance could pose a risk to mother or fetus. Similarly, women should avoid any type of exercise that might result in even mild abdominal trauma.

- A normal pregnancy requires an additional 300 kcal/day of nutritional intake. Women who exercise regularly during pregnancy should be careful to ensure that they consume an adequate diet.

- To augment heat dissipation, especially during the first trimester, pregnant women should wear clothing that is comfortable and loose while exercising, ensure adequate hydration, and avoid prolonged overheating. For the same reason, pregnant women are advised to avoid hot tubs and saunas. If a pregnant woman is unable to talk or feels unable to breathe, the exercise effort is too high.

- As a result of the cardiovascular changes of pregnancy, heart rate is not an accurate indicator in pregnant women for the intensity of exercise. If a pregnant woman is unable to maintain a conversation while exercising, then her exercise effort is too high (Field, 2012).

Focus on Integrative Health
Yoga During Pregnancy

Yoga may build strength and alleviate stress and physiologic discomforts in pregnancy. Pregnant women should attend only yoga classes designed for pregnancy unless they are familiar with potentially harmful yoga positions and can avoid them when attending regular yoga classes. The following advice is important for women who practice yoga during pregnancy (Field, 2012):

- During pregnancy, some yoga poses or positions are contraindicated. Pregnant women should avoid poses that put pressure on the uterus as well as any extreme stretching positions.

- Because of the changed center of gravity that occurs as pregnancy progresses, pregnant women need to be especially careful to maintain balance when stretching.

- Pregnant women should avoid stomach-lying for any poses. After 20 weeks of gestation, they should lie on their side rather than on their back for floor positions.

- In the last trimester, pregnant women may experience vena caval syndrome resulting in reduced blood flow back to the heart as the growing fetus puts pressure on the major vessels when lying flat on their backs.

- Pregnant women should immediately stop any pose that is uncomfortable.

- Warning signs that indicate the need to contact the healthcare provider immediately include dizziness, extreme shortness of breath, sudden swelling, contractions, leaking of fluid, and vaginal bleeding.

shortened cervix on transvaginal ultrasound or cerclage placement, persistent vaginal bleeding in the second and third trimesters, risk factors for preterm labor or a history of preterm labor in a prior or current pregnancy, placenta previa after 23 weeks of gestation, and chronic medical conditions that might be negatively impacted by vigorous exercise, such as significant heart disease (American Academy of Pediatrics & American College of Obstetricians and Gynecologists [AAP & ACOG], 2012). See Patient Teaching: Pregnant Women and Exercise.

The nurse may suggest that the woman wear a supportive bra and appropriate shoes when exercising. The nurse should advise the woman to warm up and stretch to help prepare the joints for activity and, after exercising, to cool down with a period of mild activity to help restore circulation and avoid pooling of blood. A moderate, rhythmic exercise routine involving large muscle groups, such as swimming, cycling, or brisk walking, is best. Jogging or running is acceptable for women already conditioned to these activities as long as they avoid exercising at maximum effort and overheating. See Focus on Integrative Health: Yoga During Pregnancy.

During exercise, warning signs include pain of any kind, difficulty walking, dizziness, headache, muscle weakness, dyspnea before exertion, uterine contractions, vaginal bleeding, or fluid loss from the vagina (AAP & ACOG, 2012). The woman should stop exercising if these symptoms occur and modify her exercise program. If the symptoms persist, the woman should contact her healthcare provider.

Adequate rest in pregnancy is important for both physical and emotional health. Women need more sleep throughout pregnancy, particularly in the first and last trimesters when they tire easily. Without adequate rest, pregnant women have less resilience. Finding time to rest during the day may be difficult for women who work outside the home or have small children. The nurse can help the expectant mother examine her daily schedule to develop a realistic plan for short periods of rest and relaxation.

Sleeping becomes more difficult during the last trimester because of the enlarged abdomen, increased frequency of urination, and greater activity of the fetus. Finding a comfortable position becomes difficult for the pregnant woman.

Progressive relaxation techniques similar to those taught in childbirth classes can help prepare the woman for sleep.

Sexual Activity

As a result of the physiologic, anatomic, and emotional changes of pregnancy, couples usually have many questions and concerns about sexual activity during pregnancy. Often, these questions are about possible injury to the baby or the woman during intercourse and about changes in the desire each partner feels.

In the past, couples often were warned to avoid sexual intercourse during the last 6–8 weeks of pregnancy in order to prevent complications, such as infection or premature rupture of the membranes. However, these fears seem to be unfounded. In a healthy pregnancy, there is no medical reason to limit sexual activity. Intercourse is contraindicated for medical reasons, such as rupture of membranes, placenta previa, threatened spontaneous abortion, or the risk of preterm labor (Cunningham et al., 2014).

The expectant mother may experience changes in sexual desire and response. Often, these changes are related to the various discomforts that occur throughout pregnancy. For instance, during the first trimester, fatigue or nausea and vomiting may decrease desire, and breast tenderness may make the woman less responsive to fondling of her breasts. During the second trimester, many of the discomforts have lessened, and with the vascular congestion of the pelvis, the woman may experience greater sexual satisfaction than she experienced before pregnancy.

During the third trimester, interest in coitus may again decrease as the woman becomes more uncomfortable and fatigued. In addition, shortness of breath, painful pelvic ligaments, urinary frequency, leg cramps, and decreased mobility may lessen sexual desire and activity. If they are not already doing so, the heterosexual couple should consider coital positions other than male superior, such as side by side, female superior, and vaginal rear entry.

Sexual activity does not have to include intercourse. Many of the nurturing and sexual needs of the pregnant woman can be satisfied by cuddling, kissing, and being held. The warm, sensual feelings that accompany these activities can be an end in themselves. Her partner, however, may choose to masturbate.

The sexual desires of partners of pregnant women are also affected by many factors in pregnancy. These factors include the previous relationship with the partner, acceptance of the pregnancy, attitudes toward the partner's change of appearance, and concern about hurting the expectant mother or baby. Some find it difficult to view their partners as sexually appealing while they are adjusting to the concept of their partners as mothers. Others find their partners' pregnancies arousing and experience feelings of increased happiness, intimacy, and closeness.

The expectant couple should be aware of their changing sexual desires, the normality of these changes, and the importance of communicating these changes to each other so that they can make nurturing adaptations. The nurse has an important role in helping the expectant couple adapt. The couple should feel free to express concerns about sexual activity, and the nurse should be able to respond and give anticipatory guidance in a comfortable manner. See Patient Teaching: Sexual Activity During Pregnancy.

Dental Care

Proper dental hygiene is important in pregnancy because ensuring a healthy oral environment is essential to overall health. Periodontal disease is a contributing factor to preterm labor (ACOG, 2013b). In spite of such discomforts as nausea and vomiting, gum hypertrophy and tenderness, possible ptyalism (excessive, often bitter salivation), and heartburn, pregnant women need to maintain regular oral hygiene by brushing at least twice a day and flossing daily.

The nurse should encourage the pregnant woman to have a dental checkup early in her pregnancy. Dentistry should proceed as needed in pregnancy. Local anesthesia is fine, but epinephrine should not be used. The woman should inform her dentist of her pregnancy so that she is not exposed to teratogenic substances. See the exemplar on Oral Health in the module on Health, Wellness, Illness, and Injury.

Other Health Promotion Measures

A number of health promotion measures not directly related to pregnancy are necessary to ensure the health of the mother and fetus. Some of these measures relate to immunizations, clothing, bathing, maternal employment, and travel.

Immunizations

All women of childbearing age need to be aware of the risks of receiving certain immunizations if pregnancy is possible. The influenza and Tdap vaccines are recommended for pregnant women (Centers for Disease Control and Prevention [CDC], 2014a). Immunizations with attenuated live viruses, such as rubella vaccine, should not be given in pregnancy because of the teratogenic effect of the live viruses on the developing embryo. The most current recommendations on vaccines related to pregnancy should be obtained from the CDC website (www.cdc.gov).

Clothing

Traditionally, maternity clothes have been constructed with fuller lines to allow for the increase in abdominal size during pregnancy. However, maternity wear has changed in recent years and now also includes clothes that are more fitted, with little attempt to hide the pregnant abdomen. Maternity clothing can be expensive, and it is worn for a relatively short time. Women can economize by sharing clothes with friends, sewing their own garments, or buying used maternity clothes.

High-heeled shoes tend to aggravate back discomfort by increasing the curvature of the lower back. They are best avoided if the woman experiences backache or has problems with balance. Shoes should fit properly and feel comfortable.

Bathing

Because perspiration and mucoid vaginal discharge increase during pregnancy, hygiene is important. Practices related to cleansing the body are often influenced by cultural norms; thus, a pregnant woman may choose to cleanse only some portions of her body daily or may elect to take daily showers or tub baths. Caution is needed during tub baths because balance becomes a problem in late pregnancy. Rubber mats

Patient Teaching

Sexual Activity During Pregnancy

Discussion about various sexual activities requires that the nurse be comfortable with his or her sexuality and also be tactful. A discussion of sexuality and sexual activity should stress the importance of open communication so that the couple feels comfortable expressing feelings, preferences, and concerns. The nurse can assist the couple regarding sexual activity during pregnancy with the following patient teaching:

- Begin by explaining that the pregnant woman may experience changes in desire during the course of pregnancy. During the first trimester, discomforts such as nausea, fatigue, and breast tenderness may make intercourse less desirable for many pregnant women. Universal statements that give permission, such as "Many couples experience changes in sexual desire during pregnancy. What kind of changes have you experienced?" are often effective in starting discussion. Depending on the woman's (or couple's) level of knowledge and sophistication, part or all of this discussion may be necessary.

- In the second trimester, as symptoms decrease, desire may increase. In the third trimester, discomfort and fatigue may lead to decreased desire in the pregnant woman. If the partner is present, approach the partner in the same nonjudgmental way discussed previously. If not, ask the pregnant woman if she has noticed any changes in her partner or if her partner has expressed any concerns.

- Explain that partners of pregnant women may notice changes in their level of desire, too. Among other things, this change may be related to feelings about their partner's changing appearance, their belief about the acceptability of sexual activity with a pregnant woman, or concern about hurting the woman or fetus. Some partners find the changes of pregnancy erotic; others must adjust to the notion of their partners as mothers. Deal with any specific questions about the physical and psychologic changes that the couple may have.

- Explain that the woman may notice that orgasms are much more intense during the last weeks of pregnancy and may be followed by cramping. Because of the pressure of the enlarging uterus on the vena cava, the pregnant woman should not lie flat on her back for intercourse after about the fourth month. If the couple prefers that position, a pillow should be placed under the pregnant woman's right hip to displace the uterus. Alternative positions such as side by side, female superior, or vaginal rear entry may become necessary as her uterus enlarges.

- Stress that sexual activities both partners enjoy are generally acceptable. It is not advisable, however, for couples who favor anal sex to go from anal penetration to vaginal penetration because of the risk of introducing *Escherichia coli* into the vagina. The couple may be content with these approaches to meeting their sexual needs, or they may require assurance that such approaches are indeed "normal."

- Suggest that alternative methods of expressing intimacy and affection, such as cuddling, holding and stroking each other, and kissing, may help maintain the couple's feelings of warmth and closeness. If the partner feels desire for further sexual release, the pregnant woman may help her partner masturbate to climax, or the partner may prefer to masturbate in private.

- Advise the pregnant woman who is interested in masturbation as a form of gratification that the orgasmic contractions may be especially intense during later pregnancy.

- Stress that sexual intercourse is contraindicated once the membranes have ruptured or if bleeding is present. Pregnant women with a history of preterm labor may be advised to avoid intercourse, because the oxytocin that is released with orgasm stimulates uterine contractions and may trigger preterm labor. Because oxytocin is also released with nipple stimulation, fondling the breasts may be contraindicated in those cases as well.

- Some couples are skilled at expressing their feelings about sexual activity. Others find it difficult and can benefit from specific suggestions. The nurse should provide opportunities for discussion throughout the talk. An explanation of the contraindications accompanied by their rationale provides specific guidelines that most couples find helpful. Specific handouts on sexual activity are helpful for couples and may address topics that were not discussed.

and hand grips are important safety devices. Vasodilation caused by warm water may make the woman feel faint when she attempts to get out of the tub, so she may require assistance, especially during the last trimester. During the first trimester, pregnant women should avoid hyperthermia associated with the use of a hot tub or Jacuzzi, because it may increase the risk for miscarriage or neural tube defects (Snijder et al., 2012).

Employment

Pregnant women who have no complications can usually continue to work until they go into labor (AAP & ACOG, 2012). Although pregnant women who are employed in jobs that require prolonged standing (>5 hours) do have a higher incidence of preterm birth, prolonged standing has no effect on fetal growth (Snijder et al., 2012).

Fetotoxic hazards are always a concern to the expectant couple. The pregnant woman (or the woman contemplating pregnancy) who works in industry should contact her company physician or nurse about possible hazards in her work environment and do her own reading and research on environmental hazards as well. Similarly, a male partner can seek information about hazards in his workplace that might affect his sperm.

Travel

If medical or pregnancy complications are not present, there are no restrictions on travel. Pregnant women are advised to avoid travel if they have a history of bleeding or preeclampsia or if multiple births are anticipated. Availability of medical care at the destination is an important factor for the near-term woman who travels. It may be helpful to travel with a copy of the woman's medical record.

Travel by automobile can be especially fatiguing, aggravating many of the discomforts of pregnancy. The pregnant woman needs frequent opportunities to get out of the car and walk. (A good pattern is to stop every 2 hours and walk around for approximately 10 minutes.) She should wear both lap and shoulder belts; the lap belt should fit snugly and be positioned under the abdomen and across the upper thighs. The shoulder strap should rest comfortably between the woman's breasts. Seat belts play an important role in preventing fetal and maternal morbidity and mortality with subsequent fetal death (Cunningham et al., 2014). Fetal death in car crashes is related to placental separation (abruptio placentae) as a result of uterine trauma. Use of the shoulder belt decreases the risk of traumatic flexion of the woman's body, thereby decreasing the risk of placental separation.

As pregnancy progresses, long-distance trips are best taken by plane or train. Currently, flying is considered to be safe up to 36 weeks of gestation in the absence of any complications (AAP & ACOG, 2012). Before flying, the woman should check with her airline to see if they have any travel restrictions. Prolonged air travel may lead to edema in the lower extremities and the development of venous thrombolytic events. To minimize complications, the traveler should consider wearing support stockings, maintain oral hydration, periodically move the lower extremities, change positions frequently, and move about the cabin at least every 2 hours when conditions are favorable (AAP & ACOG, 2012).

SAFETY ALERT Although the Zika virus was discovered in the 1940s, the recently identified adverse effects on fetal development resulted in research involving transmission and pregnancy risks. Researchers determined that the virus is transmitted directly from mother to fetus through the placenta, resulting in neural damage.

Transmission of the Zika virus occurs via mosquito bites and through sexual contact. Only one in five people with Zika infection will exhibit symptoms. Once infected, individuals are protected from future infection.

Symptoms of Zika infection include mild fever, maculopapular rash, headache, arthralgia (joint pain), and myalgia (muscle pain).

Prevention of infection includes:

Wearing long-sleeved shirts and pants

Using mosquito bed nets or window screens

Applying topical products containing DEET

Eliminating standing water, which is where mosquitoes breed

Avoiding traveling to areas where the virus is actively circulating.

Source: Hamel, M. S., & Hughes, B. L. (2016). Zika infection in pregnancy. *Contemporary OB/GYN, 61*(8), 16–42.

Complementary Health Approaches

Many pregnant women elect to use complementary health approaches, such as homeopathy, herbal medicine, acupressure and acupuncture, biofeedback, therapeutic touch, massage, and chiropractic, as part of a holistic approach to their healthcare regimens. The nurse should inquire about the use of complementary health approaches as part of a routine nursing assessment. The nurse working with pregnant women and childbearing families should develop a general understanding of the more commonly used therapies in order to be able to answer basic questions and provide resources as needed.

Pregnant women should understand that herbs are considered to be dietary supplements and are not regulated through the U.S. Food and Drug Administration (FDA), as prescription or over-the-counter (OTC) drugs are. Because of limited scientific evaluation of potential harmful effects on the fetus, herbal supplements should be avoided, particularly in the first trimester (Romm, 2011).

›› Stay Current: Additional information about herbs, homeopathic remedies, and other alternative options may be accessed at the website of the National Center for Complementary and Integrative Health, http://nccam.nih.gov.

Teratogenic Substances

Substances that adversely affect the normal growth and development of the fetus are called **teratogens**. The nurse who is caring for the pregnant woman, or for the woman who is trying to become pregnant, should teach her about teratogenic substances, including alcohol, and emphasize the need for the woman to discuss the use of any and all medications, including psychotropic drugs, with her obstetrician. Obstetricians and nurse-midwives are the most informed about the potential effects of medications on the fetus. The nurse should also instruct the patient with a chronic condition, such as asthma or diabetes, to inform her treating physician if she is (or is trying to become) pregnant. The pregnant woman with a chronic condition should be encouraged to use a single pharmacy and to inform the pharmacy staff that she is pregnant. Discussing potential hazards in the work and home environments, such as pesticides and exposure to x-rays in the first trimester, is important for preventing teratogenic effects on the fetus.

For a more thorough discussion of the risks of substance abuse during pregnancy, see the exemplar on Substance Abuse in the module on Addiction. An overview of the risks associated with tobacco use is provided here.

Tobacco

In the United States, smoking tobacco during pregnancy is one of the most significant, modifiable causes of poor pregnancy outcomes. Smoking during pregnancy has a strong association with low-birth-weight neonates. In addition, mothers who smoke have an increased risk of preterm birth, premature rupture of the membranes, fetal demise, placentae previa, abruptio placentae, premature rupture of membranes, and preterm birth (Cunningham et al., 2014). Pregnant women who smoke tobacco and participate in other unhealthy behaviors, such as alcohol use, further increase their risk for low-birth-weight newborns (Barron, 2014). Research also links maternal tobacco smoking, both during and after pregnancy, with an increased risk of SIDS. Maternal smoking exposes young children to other risks of secondhand smoke, including middle ear infections, acute and chronic respiratory tract illnesses, and behavioral and learning disabilities (Al-Sayed & Ibrahim, 2014).

Nursing Assessment

The nurse caring for a woman who is pregnant establishes an environment of comfort and open communication with each antepartum visit. The nurse conveys interest in the woman as an individual and discusses the woman's concerns and desires. Typically, the registered nurse may complete many areas of prenatal assessment. Advanced practice nurses such as CNMs and certified women's health nurse practitioners have the education and skill to perform full and complete antepartum assessments. This section focuses on the initial prenatal assessment.

Box 33–1
Definition of Terms

The following terms are used in recording the history of prenatal patients:

Abortion: Spontaneous loss or termination of pregnancy that occurs before the end of 20 weeks' gestation or the birth of a fetus–newborn who weighs less than 500 g (Cunningham et al., 2014)

Antepartum: Time between conception and the onset of labor; often used to describe the period during which a woman is pregnant; used interchangeably with *prenatal*

Gestation: The number of weeks since the first day of the last menstrual period

Gravida*: The number of pregnancies in the woman's lifetime, regardless of duration, including current pregnancy

Intrapartum: Time from the onset of true labor until the birth of the baby and placenta

Multigravida: A woman who is in her second or any subsequent pregnancy

Multipara: A woman who has had two or more births at more than 20 weeks' gestation

Nulligravida: A woman who has never been pregnant

Nullipara: A woman who has had no births at more than 20 weeks' gestation

Para*: Birth after 20 weeks' gestation regardless of whether the baby is born alive or dead

Postpartum: Time from birth until the woman's body returns to an essentially prepregnant condition

Postterm labor: Labor that occurs after 42 weeks' gestation

Prenatal: Time between conception and the onset of labor; antepartum

Preterm or premature labor: Labor that occurs after 20 weeks' gestation but before completion of 37 weeks' gestation

Primigravida: A woman who is pregnant for the first time

Primipara: A woman who has had one birth at more than 20 weeks' gestation, regardless of whether the baby was born alive or dead

Stillbirth: A baby born dead after at least 20 weeks' gestation

Term: A word that was formerly used to identify the normal duration of pregnancy. The stand-alone use of this word is now discouraged because it represents such a wide range of time and related risks (Spong, 2013). ACOG (2013c) recommends that the following definitions be used:

- Late preterm: births that occur before 34 0/7 through 36 6/7 weeks' gestation
- Early term: births that occur between 37 weeks 0 days and 38 weeks 6 days
- Full term: births that occur between 39 weeks 0 days and 40 weeks 6 days

*The terms *gravida* and *para* are used in relation to pregnancies, not the number of fetuses. Thus, twins, triplets, and so on, count as one pregnancy and one birth.

Patient Interview

The course of a pregnancy depends on a number of factors, including the woman's prepregnancy health, the presence of disease states, the woman's emotional status, and her past healthcare. A thorough history is useful in determining the status of a woman's prepregnancy health. Terms useful for recording the history of prenatal patients are listed in **Box 33–1 »**.

Patient Profile

The history is essentially a screening tool that identifies factors that may place the mother or fetus at risk during the pregnancy. The following information is obtained for each pregnant woman at the first prenatal assessment:

1. ***Current Pregnancy***
   - First day of last normal menstrual period (Is she sure or unsure of the date? Do her cycles normally occur every 28 days, or do her cycles tend to be longer?)
   - Presence of cramping, bleeding, or spotting since LMP
   - Woman's opinion about the time when conception occurred and when baby is due
   - Woman's attitude toward pregnancy (Is this pregnancy planned? Wanted?)
   - Results of pregnancy tests, if completed
   - Any discomforts since LMP (e.g., nausea, vomiting, urinary frequency, fatigue, or breast tenderness)

2. ***Past Pregnancies***
   - Number of pregnancies
   - Number of abortions, spontaneous or therapeutic
   - Number of living children
   - History of previous pregnancies, length of pregnancy, length of labor and birth, type of birth (vaginal, forceps- or vacuum-assisted, or cesarean), type of anesthesia used (if any), woman's perception of the experience, and complications (antepartum, intrapartum, and postpartum)
   - Neonatal status of previous children: Apgar scores (see Exemplar 33.D, Newborn Care, for a discussion of Apgar scoring), birth weights, general development, complications, and feeding patterns (breast milk or formula)
   - Loss of a child (miscarriage, elective or medically indicated abortion, stillbirth, neonatal death, relinquishment, or death after the neonatal period) (What was the experience like for her? What coping skills helped? How did her partner, if involved, respond?)
   - If Rh negative, was Rh immune globulin received during pregnancy and/or after birth/miscarriage/abortion to prevent sensitization?
   - Prenatal education classes and resources (books)

3. ***Gynecologic History***
   - Date of last Pap smear; any history of abnormal Pap smear; any follow-up therapy completed

- Previous infections: vaginal, cervical, tubal, sexually transmitted (see the exemplar on Sexually Transmitted Infections in the module on Sexuality)
- Previous surgery (uterine/ovarian)
- Age at menarche
- Regularity, frequency, and duration of menstrual flow
- History of dysmenorrhea
- Sexual history
- Contraceptive history (If birth control pills were used, did pregnancy occur immediately following cessation of pills? If not, how long after?)
- Any issues related to infertility or fertility treatments

4. **Current Medical History**
   - Weight
   - Blood type and Rh factor if known
   - General health, including nutrition (dietary practices such as vegetarianism) and regular exercise program (type, frequency, and duration)
   - Any medications currently being taken (including nonprescription, homeopathic, or herbal medications) or taken since the onset of pregnancy
   - Previous or present use of alcohol, tobacco, or caffeine (Ask specifically about the amount of alcohol, cigarettes, and caffeine [specify coffee, tea, cola, and chocolate] consumed each day)
   - Illicit drug use or abuse (Ask about specific drugs such as cocaine, crack, methamphetamines, and marijuana)
   - Drug allergies and other allergies (Ask about latex allergies or sensitivities)
   - Potential teratogenic insults to this pregnancy, such as viral infections, medications, x-ray examinations, surgery, or cats in the home (possible source of toxoplasmosis)
   - Presence of disease conditions such as diabetes, hypertension, cardiovascular disease, renal problems, or thyroid disorder
   - Record of immunizations
   - Presence of any abnormal symptoms

5. **Past Medical History**
   - Childhood diseases
   - Past treatment for any disease condition
   - Surgical procedures
   - Presence of bleeding disorders or tendencies
   - Accidents requiring hospitalizations
   - Blood transfusions

6. **Family Medical History**
   - Presence of diabetes, cardiovascular disease, cancer, hypertension, hematologic disorders, tuberculosis, or preeclampsia–eclampsia
   - Occurrence of multiple births
   - History of congenital diseases or deformities
   - History of mental illness
   - Causes of death of deceased parents or siblings
   - Occurrence of cesarean births and cause if known

7. **Religious, Spiritual, and Cultural History**
   - Does the woman want to specify a religious preference on her chart? Does she have any spiritual beliefs or practices that might influence her healthcare or that of her child, such as prohibition against receiving blood products, dietary considerations, or circumcision rites?
   - What practices are important to maintaining her spiritual well-being?
   - Might practices in her culture or that of her partner influence her care or that of her child?

8. **Occupational History**
   - Occupation
   - Physical demands (Does she stand all day, or are there opportunities to sit and elevate her legs? Any heavy lifting?)
   - Exposure to chemicals or other harmful substances
   - Opportunity for regular meals and breaks for nutritious snacks
   - Provision for maternity or family leave

9. **Partner's History**
   - Presence of genetic conditions or diseases in him or in his family history, if partner is the father
   - Age
   - Significant health problems
   - Previous or current alcohol intake, drug use, or tobacco use
   - Blood type and Rh factor, if partner is the father
   - Occupation
   - Educational level; methods by which the partner learns best
   - Attitude toward the pregnancy

10. **Personal information about the mother (social history)**
    - Age
    - Educational level; methods by which she learns best
    - Race or ethnic group (to identify need for prenatal genetic screening and racially or ethnically related risk factors)
    - Housing; stability of living conditions
    - Economic level
    - Acceptance of pregnancy, whether intended or unintended
    - Any history of emotional or physical deprivation or abuse of herself or children or any abuse in her current relationship (Ask specifically whether she has been hit, slapped, kicked, or hurt within the past year or since she has become pregnant. Ask whether she is afraid of her partner or anyone else. If yes, of whom is she afraid? *Note:* Ask these questions when the woman is alone)
    - History of emotional problems
    - Support systems
    - Personal preferences about the birth (expectations of both the woman and her partner, presence of others, and so on)
    - Plans for care of child following birth
    - Feeding preference for the baby (breast milk or formula?)

Obtaining Data

In many instances, a questionnaire is used to obtain information. The woman should complete the questionnaire in a quiet place with a minimum of distractions. The nurse can obtain further information in an interview, which allows the pregnant woman to clarify her responses to questions and gives the nurse and the woman the opportunity to develop rapport.

The expectant father or partner can be encouraged to attend the prenatal examinations; the individual is often able to contribute to the history. The nurse should encourage partners to use the opportunity to ask questions or express concerns that are important to them.

Prenatal High-Risk Screening

Risk factors are any findings that suggest that the pregnancy may have a negative outcome, for either the woman or her unborn child. Screening for risk factors is an important part of the prenatal assessment. Many risk factors can be identified during the initial assessment; others may be detected during subsequent prenatal visits. It is important to identify high-risk pregnancies early so that appropriate interventions can be started promptly. Not all risk factors threaten a pregnancy equally; thus, many agencies use a scoring sheet to determine the degree of risk. Information must be updated throughout the pregnancy as necessary. A pregnancy may begin as low risk and change to high risk because of complications.

Obstetric History

The nurse interviews the patient regarding previous pregnancies, which affect the woman's plan of care. A woman who has experienced previous miscarriages or complications of pregnancy may require increased monitoring and a greater level of support than a woman who has already had one or more successful pregnancies without complication.

The terms *gravida* and *para* are used in relation to pregnancies, not to the number of fetuses. Thus, twins, triplets, and other multiples count as one pregnancy and one birth. Miscarriages and fetal losses before viability at 24 weeks of gestation are called fetal demise. Those before 20 weeks are called abortions.

The following examples illustrate how these terms are applied in clinical situations:

1. Jean Sanchez has one child born at 38 weeks of gestation and is pregnant for the second time. At her initial prenatal visit, the nurse indicates her obstetric history as "gravida 2 para 1 ab 0." Jean Sanchez's present pregnancy terminates at 16 weeks of gestation. She is now "gravida 2 para 1 ab 1."
2. Tracy Hopkins is pregnant for the fourth time. At home, she has a child who was born at term. Her second pregnancy ended at 10 weeks of gestation. She then gave birth to twins at 35 weeks of gestation. One of the twins died soon after birth. At her antepartum assessment, the nurse records her obstetric history as "gravida 4 para 2 ab 1."

To avoid confusion, it is best for practicing nurses to clarify the recording system used at their facilities.

A useful acronym for remembering the detailed system is **G TPAL**:

G: number of pregnancies (**G**ravida)

T: number of **T**erm babies born—that is, the number of babies born after 37 weeks of gestation

P: number of **P**reterm babies born—that is, the number of babies born after 20 weeks but before the completion of 37 weeks of gestation

A: number of pregnancies ending in either spontaneous or therapeutic **A**bortion

L: number of currently **L**iving children

Using this approach, the nurse would have initially described Jean Sanchez (see the first example) as "gravida 2 para 1001." Following Jean's spontaneous abortion, she would be "gravida 2 para 1011." Tracy Hopkins would be described as "gravida 4 para 1212." **Figure 33–24 》》** illustrates this method.

SAFETY ALERT In general, it is best to avoid an initial discussion of a woman's obstetric history in front of her partner. It is possible that the woman had a previous pregnancy she has not mentioned to her partner, and revealing this information could violate her right to privacy.

Determining Due Date

Families generally want to know the "due date," or the date around which childbirth will occur. Historically, the due date has been called the estimated date of confinement (EDC). However, the concept of *confinement* is rather negative, and many caregivers avoid it by referring to the due date as the estimated date of delivery. Even then, childbirth educators often stress that babies are not "delivered" like a package; they are born. In keeping with a view that emphasizes the normalcy of the process, this text refers to the due date as the estimated date of birth (EDB).

To calculate the EDB, it is helpful to know the date of the woman's last menstrual period. However, some women have episodes of irregular bleeding or fail to keep track of menstrual cycles. Thus, other techniques also help determine how far along a woman is in her pregnancy—that is, at how many weeks of gestation she is. These techniques include evaluating uterine size, determining when quickening occurs, and auscultating FHR with a Doppler device or ultrasound and, later, with a fetoscope.

The most common method of determining the EDB is to use the **Nägele rule**. To use this method, one begins with the

Name	Gravida	Term	Preterm	Abortions	Living Children
Jean Sanchez	2	1	0	1	1
Tracy Hopkins	4	1	2	1	2

Figure 33–24 》》 The **G TPAL** approach provides detailed information about a woman's pregnancy history.

first day of the last menstrual period (LMP), subtracts 3 months, and adds 7 days. For example:

First day of LMP	November 21
Subtract 3 months	−3 months
	August 21
Add 7 days	+7 days
EDB	August 28

It is simpler to change the months to numeric terms:

November 21 becomes	11–21
Subtract 3 months	−3
	8–21
Add 7 days	+7
EDB	8–28

A gestation calculator or wheel permits the caregiver to calculate the EDB even more quickly (**Figure 33–25 》**).

If a woman with a history of menses every 28 days remembers her last menstrual period and was not taking oral contraceptives before becoming pregnant, the Nägele rule may be a fairly accurate determiner of the EDB. However, ovulation usually occurs 14 days before the onset of the next menses, not 14 days after the previous menses. Consequently, if the woman's cycle is irregular or is more than 28 days long, the time of ovulation may be delayed. If she has been using oral contraceptives, ovulation may be delayed for several weeks following her last menses. Then, too, a postpartum woman who is breastfeeding may resume ovulating but be amenorrheic for a time, making calculation impossible. Thus, the Nägele rule, although helpful, is not foolproof.

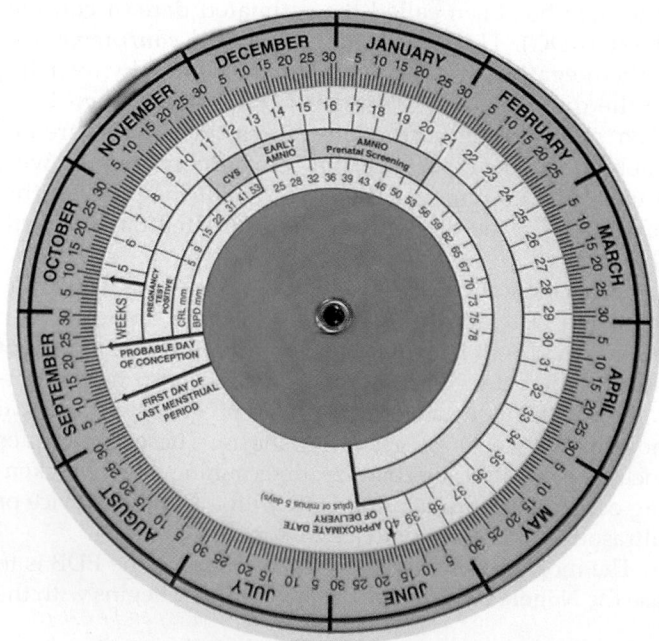

Source: George Dodson/Pearson Education, Inc.

Figure 33–25 》 The EDB wheel can be used to calculate the due date. To use it, place the arrow labeled "1st day of last period" on the date of the woman's last menstrual period (LMP). Then read the EDB at the arrow labeled "40." In this case, the LMP is September 8 and the EDB is June 16.

It is important to determine the EDB as accurately as possible, as the gestational age at which many prenatal screenings are done is extremely important. The most common reason for false-positive results on aneuploidy and neural tube defect screening is inaccurate calculation of gestational age (Messerlian, Farina, & Palomaki, 2016). It is also essential for evaluating fetal growth and deciding on the timing of intervention for postterm pregnancies. The most accurate estimation of gestational age is a 7–10 week crown–rump length (CRL) measurement consistent with LMP dating. If there is a discrepancy of more than 3 days between early ultrasound and LMP, the pregnancy is dated by the ultrasound (MacKenzie, Stephenson, & Funai, 2016).

Physical Examination

The physical examination begins with assessment of vital signs; then the woman's body is examined. The pelvic examination is performed last. Before the examination, the woman should provide a clean urine specimen. When her bladder is empty, the woman is more comfortable during the pelvic examination and the examiner can palpate the pelvic organs more easily. After the woman has emptied her bladder, the nurse asks her to disrobe and gives her a gown and sheet or some other protective covering.

Increasing numbers of nurses (e.g., CNMs and other nurses in advanced practice) are prepared to perform complete physical examinations. The nurse who does not yet possess advanced assessment skills can assess the woman's vital signs, explain the procedures to allay apprehension, position her for examination, and assist the examiner as necessary. Each nurse is responsible for operating at the expected standard for his or her skill and knowledge base.

Thoroughness and a systematic procedure are the most important considerations when performing the physical portion of a prenatal examination. To promote completeness, the Prenatal Assessment feature is organized in three columns that address the areas to be assessed and the normal findings, the variations or alterations that may be observed and their possible causes, and nursing responses to the data. The nurse should be aware that certain organs and systems are assessed concurrently with others during the physical portion of the examination.

Uterine Assessment

Physical Examination

When a woman is examined in the first 10–12 weeks of pregnancy and her uterine size is compatible with her menstrual history, uterine size may be the single most important clinical method for dating her pregnancy. In many cases, however, women do not seek prenatal care until well into their second trimester, when it becomes more difficult to evaluate specific uterine size. In women with obesity, it is difficult to determine uterine size early in a pregnancy because the uterus is more difficult to palpate.

Fundal Height

Fundal height may be used as an indicator of uterine size, although this method is less accurate late in pregnancy. A centimeter tape measure is used to measure the distance abdominally from the top of the symphysis pubis to the top of the

Prenatal Assessment

PHYSICAL ASSESSMENT/ NORMAL FINDINGS	ALTERATIONS AND POSSIBLE CAUSES*	NURSING RESPONSES TO DATA†
Vital Signs		
Blood pressure (BP): less than or equal to 140/90 mmHg	High BP (essential hypertension; renal disease; gestational hypertension, apprehension or anxiety associated with pregnancy diagnosis, exam, or other crises; preeclampsia if initial assessment not done until after 20 weeks' gestation)	BP greater than 140/90 mmHg requires immediate consideration; establish woman's BP; refer to healthcare provider if necessary. Assess woman's knowledge about high BP; counsel on self-care and medical management.
Pulse: 60–100 beats/min; rate may increase 10 beats/min during pregnancy	Increased pulse rate (excitement or anxiety, cardiac disorders)	Count for 1 full minute; note irregularities.
Respirations: 12–20 breaths/min (or pulse rate divided by 4); pregnancy may induce a degree of hyperventilation; thoracic breathing predominant	Marked tachypnea or abnormal patterns	Assess for respiratory disease.
Temperature: 36.0°–38.5°C (96.8°–101.3°F)	Elevated temperature (infection)	Assess for infection process of disease state, or ruptured membranes, if temperature is elevated; refer to healthcare provider.
Body Mass Index (BMI)		
Between 18.5 and 24.9 based on prepregnant weight or weight on presentation to care if prepregnant weight is unknown	Less than 18.5 or greater than 30	Evaluate need for nutritional counseling; obtain information on eating habits, cooking practices, food regularly eaten, income limitations, need for food supplements, pica and other abnormal food habits. Note initial weight to establish baseline for weight gain throughout pregnancy.
Skin		
Color: consistent with racial background; pink nail beds	Pallor (anemia); bronze, yellow (hepatic disease; other causes of jaundice) Bluish, reddish, mottled; dusky appearance or pallor of palms and nail beds in dark-skinned women (anemia)	The following tests should be performed: complete blood count (CBC), bilirubin level, urinalysis, and blood urea nitrogen (BUN). If abnormal, refer to healthcare provider.
Condition: absence of edema (slight edema of lower extremities is normal during pregnancy)	Edema (possible preeclampsia); rashes, dermatitis (allergic response)	Counsel on relief measures for slight edema. Initiate preeclampsia assessment; refer to healthcare provider.
Lesions: absence of lesions	Ulceration (varicose veins, decreased circulation)	Further assess circulatory status; refer to healthcare provider if lesion is severe.
Spider nevi common in pregnancy	Petechiae, multiple bruises, ecchymosis (hemorrhagic disorders; abuse) Change in size or color (carcinoma)	Evaluate for bleeding or clotting disorder. Provide opportunities to discuss abuse if suspected. Refer to healthcare provider.
Pigmentation: pigmentation changes of pregnancy include linea nigra, striae gravidarum, melasma		Assure woman that these are normal manifestations of pregnancy and explain the physiologic basis for the changes.
Café-au-lait spots	Six or more (Albright syndrome or neurofibromatosis)	Consult with healthcare provider.
	*Possible causes of alterations are identified in parentheses.	†This column provides guidelines for further assessment and initial nursing intervention.

(continued on next page)

Prenatal Assessment *(continued)*

PHYSICAL ASSESSMENT/ NORMAL FINDINGS	ALTERATIONS AND POSSIBLE CAUSES*	NURSING RESPONSES TO DATA†
Nose		
Character of mucosa: redder than oral mucosa; in pregnancy, nasal mucosa is edematous in response to increased estrogen, resulting in nasal stuffiness (rhinitis of pregnancy) and nosebleeds (epistaxis)	Olfactory loss (first cranial nerve deficit)	Counsel woman about possible relief measures for nasal stuffiness and nosebleeds; refer to healthcare provider for olfactory loss.
Mouth		
May note hypertrophy of gingival tissue because of estrogen	Edema, inflammation (infection); pale in color (anemia)	Assess hematocrit for anemia; counsel regarding dental hygiene habits. Refer to healthcare provider or dentist if necessary. Routine dental care is appropriate during pregnancy (no epinephrine, no nitrous anesthesia). Dental x-rays can be done during the second trimester if needed.
Neck		
Nodes: small, mobile, nontender nodes	Tender, hard, fixed, or prominent nodes (infection, carcinoma)	Examine for local infection; refer to healthcare provider.
Thyroid: small, smooth, lateral lobes palpable on either side of trachea; slight hyperplasia by third month of pregnancy	Enlargement or nodule tenderness (hyperthyroidism)	Listen over thyroid for bruits, which may indicate hyperthyroidism. Question woman about dietary habits (iodine intake). Ascertain history of thyroid problems; refer to healthcare provider.
Chest and Lungs		
Chest: symmetric, elliptic, smaller AP than transverse diameter	Increased AP diameter, funnel chest, pigeon chest (emphysema, asthma, chronic obstructive pulmonary disease [COPD])	Evaluate for emphysema, asthma, COPD.
Ribs: slope downward from nipple line	More horizontal (COPD) angular bumps (rachitic rosary) (vitamin C deficiency)	Evaluate for COPD. Evaluate for fractures. Consult healthcare provider. Consult nutritionist.
Inspection and palpation: no retraction or bulging of intercostal spaces (ICS) during inspiration or expiration; symmetric expansion	ICS retractions with inspirations, bulging with expiration; unequal expansion (respiratory disease)	Do thorough initial assessment. Refer to healthcare provider.
Tactile fremitus	Tachypnea, hyperpnea, Cheyne-Stokes respirations (respiratory disease)	Refer to healthcare provider.
Percussion: bilateral symmetry in tone	Flatness of percussion, which may be affected by chest wall thickness	Evaluate for pleural effusions, consolidations, or tumor.
Low-pitched resonance of moderate intensity	High diaphragm (atelectasis or paralysis), pleural effusion	Refer to healthcare provider.
Auscultation: upper lobes: bronchovesicular sounds above sternum and scapulas; equal expiratory and inspiratory phases	Abnormal if heard over any other area of chest	Refer to healthcare provider.
Remainder of chest: vesicular breath sounds heard; inspiratory phase longer (3:1)	Rales, rhonchi, wheezes; pleural friction rub; absence of breath sounds; bronchophony, egophony, whispered pectoriloquy	Refer to healthcare provider.
	*Possible causes of alterations are identified in parentheses.	†This column provides guidelines for further assessment and initial nursing intervention.

Prenatal Assessment *(continued)*

PHYSICAL ASSESSMENT/ NORMAL FINDINGS	ALTERATIONS AND POSSIBLE CAUSES*	NURSING RESPONSES TO DATA†
Breasts		
Supple: symmetric in size and contour; darker pigmentation of nipple and areola; may have supernumerary nipples. Axillary nodes unpalpable or pellet-sized	"Pigskin" or orange-peel appearance, nipple retractions, swelling, hardness (carcinoma); redness, heat, tenderness, cracked or fissured nipple (infection) Tenderness, enlargement, hard node (carcinoma); may be visible bump (infection)	Encourage monthly self-examination; instruct woman how to examine her breasts. Refer to healthcare provider if evidence of inflammation.
Pregnancy changes: 1. Size increase noted primarily in first 20 weeks. 2. Become nodular. 3. Tingling sensation may be felt during first and third trimester; woman may report feeling of heaviness. 4. Pigmentation of nipples and areolae darkens. 5. Superficial veins dilate and become more prominent. 6. Striae seen in multiparas. 7. Tubercles of Montgomery enlarge. 8. Colostrum may be present after 12th week. 9. Secondary areola appears at 20 weeks, characterized by series of washed-out spots surrounding primary areola. 10. Breasts less firm, old striae may be present in multiparas.		Discuss normalcy of changes and their meaning. Teach and/or institute appropriate relief measures. Encourage use of supportive, well-fitting brassiere.
Heart		
Normal rate, rhythm, and heart sounds	Enlargement, thrills, thrusts, gross irregularity or skipped beats, gallop rhythm or extra sounds (cardiac disease)	Complete an initial assessment. Explain normal pregnancy-induced changes. Refer to healthcare provider if indicated.
Pregnancy changes: 1. Palpitations may occur due to sympathetic nervous system disturbance 2. Short systolic murmurs that increase in held expiration are normal due to increased volume		
Abdomen		
Normal appearance, skin texture, and hair distribution; liver nonpalpable; abdomen nontender	Muscle guarding (anxiety, acute tenderness); tenderness, mass (ectopic pregnancy, inflammation, carcinoma)	Assure woman of normalcy of diastasis. Provide initial information about appropriate prenatal and postpartum exercises. Evaluate woman's anxiety level. Refer to healthcare provider if indicated.
	*Possible causes of alterations are identified in parentheses.	†This column provides guidelines for further assessment and initial nursing intervention.

(continued on next page)

Prenatal Assessment (continued)

PHYSICAL ASSESSMENT/ NORMAL FINDINGS	ALTERATIONS AND POSSIBLE CAUSES*	NURSING RESPONSES TO DATA[†]
Pregnancy changes: 1. Purple striae may be present (or silver striae on a multipara) as well as linea nigra. 2. Diastasis of the rectus muscles late in pregnancy. 3. Size: flat or rotund abdomen; progressive enlargement of uterus due to pregnancy. 10–12 weeks: fundus slightly above symphysis pubis. 16 weeks: fundus halfway between symphysis and umbilicus. 20–22 weeks: fundus at umbilicus. 28 weeks: fundus three finger breadths above umbilicus. 36 weeks: fundus just below ensiform cartilage.	Size of uterus inconsistent with length of gestation (IUGR, multiple pregnancy, fetal demise, hydatidiform mole, polyhydramnios, inaccurate dating)	Reassess menstrual history regarding pregnancy dating. Use ultrasound to establish diagnosis.
4. Fetal heart rate: 110–160 beats/min may be heard with Doppler at 10–12 weeks' gestation; may be heard with fetoscope at 17–20 weeks.	Failure to hear fetal heartbeat with Doppler (fetal demise, hydatidiform mole)	Refer to healthcare provider. Administer pregnancy tests. Use ultrasound to establish diagnosis.
5. Fetal movement palpable by a trained examiner after 18th week. 6. Ballottement: during fourth to fifth month, fetus rises and then rebounds to original position when uterus is tapped sharply.	Failure to feel fetal movements after 20 weeks' gestation (fetal demise, hydatidiform mole) No ballottement (oligohydramnios)	Refer to healthcare provider for evaluation of fetal status. Refer to healthcare provider for evaluation of fetal status.

Extremities

Skin warm, pulses palpable, full range of motion; may be some edema of hands and ankles in late pregnancy; varicose veins may become more pronounced; palmar erythema may be present	Unpalpable or diminished pulses (arterial insufficiency); marked edema (preeclampsia)	Evaluate for other symptoms of heart disease; initiate follow-up if woman mentions that her rings feel tight. Discuss prevention and self-treatment measures for varicose veins; refer to healthcare provider if indicated.

Spine

Normal spinal curves: concave cervical, convex thoracic, concave lumbar	Abnormal spinal curves; flatness, kyphosis, lordosis	Refer to healthcare provider for assessment of cephalopelvic disproportion.
In pregnancy, lumbar spinal curve may be accentuated	Backache	May have implications for administration of spinal anesthetics.
Shoulders and iliac crests should be even	Uneven shoulders and iliac crests (scoliosis)	Refer very young women to healthcare provider; discuss back-stretching exercise with older women.

Reflexes

Normal and symmetric	Hyperactivity, clonus (preeclampsia)	Evaluate for other symptoms of preeclampsia.

Pelvic Area

External female genitals: normally formed with female hair distribution; in multiparas, labia majora loose and pigmented; urinary and vaginal orifices visible and appropriately located	Lesions, hematomas, varicosities, inflammation of the Bartholin glands; clitoral hypertrophy	Explain pelvic examination procedure. Encourage woman to minimize her discomfort by relaxing her hips. Provide privacy.
	*Possible causes of alterations are identified in parentheses.	[†]This column provides guidelines for further assessment and initial nursing intervention.

Prenatal Assessment *(continued)*

PHYSICAL ASSESSMENT/ NORMAL FINDINGS	ALTERATIONS AND POSSIBLE CAUSES*	NURSING RESPONSES TO DATA†
Vagina: pink or dark pink, vaginal discharge odorless, nonirritating; in multiparas, vaginal folds smooth and flattened; may have episiotomy scar	Abnormal discharge associated with vaginal infections	Obtain vaginal smear. Provide understandable verbal and written instructions about treatment for woman and partner if indicated.
Cervix: pink color; os closed except in multiparas, in whom os admits fingertip	Eversion, reddish erosion, nabothian or retention cysts, cervical polyp; granular area that bleeds (carcinoma of cervix); lesions (herpes, human papilloma virus [HPV]); presence of string or plastic tip from cervix (intrauterine device [IUD] in uterus)	Provide woman with a hand mirror and identify genital structures for her; encourage her to view her cervix if she wishes. Refer to healthcare provider if indicated. Advise woman of potential serious risks of leaving an IUD in place during pregnancy; refer to healthcare provider for removal.
Pregnancy changes: *1–4 weeks' gestation:* enlargement in AP diameter *4–6 weeks' gestation:* softening of cervix (Goodell sign); softening of isthmus of uterus (Hegar sign); cervix takes on bluish coloring (Chadwick sign) *8–12 weeks' gestation:* vagina and cervix appear bluish violet in color (Chadwick sign)	Absence of Goodell sign (inflammatory conditions, carcinoma)	Refer to healthcare provider.
Uterus: pear-shaped, mobile; smooth surface	Fixed (pelvic inflammatory disease [PID]); nodular surface (fibromas)	Refer to healthcare provider.
Ovaries: small, walnut-shaped, nontender (ovaries and fallopian tubes are located in adnexal areas)	Pain on movement of cervix (PID); enlarged or nodular ovaries (cyst, tumor, tubal pregnancy, corpus luteum of pregnancy)	Evaluate adnexal areas; refer to healthcare provider.

Pelvic Measurements

Internal measurements: 1. Diagonal conjugate is at least 11.5 cm. 2. Obstetric conjugate is estimated by subtracting 1.5–2.0 cm from diagonal conjugate. 3. Inclination of sacrum. 4. Motility of coccyx; external intertubular diameter is greater than 8 cm.	Measurement below normal Disproportion of pubic arch Abnormal curvature of sacrum Fixed or malposition of coccyx	May be considered as a factor in protraction or arrest of labor.

Anus and Rectum

No lumps, rashes, excoriation, tenderness; cervix may be felt through rectal wall	Hemorrhoids, rectal prolapse; nodular lesion (carcinoma)	Counsel about appropriate prevention and relief measures; refer to healthcare provider for further evaluation.

Laboratory Evaluation

Hemoglobin: 12–16 g/dL; women residing in areas of high altitude may have higher levels of hemoglobin	Less than 11 g/dL (anemia)	*Note.* Wear nonlatex gloves when drawing blood. Hemoglobin less than 12 g/dL requires nutritional counseling; less than 11 g/dL requires iron supplementation.
	*Possible causes of alterations are identified in parentheses.	†This column provides guidelines for further assessment and initial nursing intervention.

(continued on next page)

Prenatal Assessment *(continued)*

PHYSICAL ASSESSMENT/ NORMAL FINDINGS	ALTERATIONS AND POSSIBLE CAUSES*	NURSING RESPONSES TO DATA†
ABO and Rh typing: normal distribution of blood types	Rh negative	If Rh negative, check for presence of anti-Rh antibodies. Discuss the need for measurement of antibody titers during pregnancy, management during the intrapartum period, and possible need for Rh immune globulin. Determine the father's Rh status if possible.
CBC: Hematocrit: 38–47% physiologic anemia (pseudoanemia) may occur	Marked anemia or blood dyscrasias	Perform CBC and Schilling differential cell count. Consider iron studies and hemoglobin electrophoresis
RBCs: 4.2–5.4 million/microliter		
White blood cells (WBCs): 5000–12,000/microliter	Presence of infection; may be elevated in pregnancy and with labor	Evaluate for other signs of infection.
Differential Neutrophils: 40–60% Bands: up to 5% Eosinophils: 1–3% Basophils: up to 1% Lymphocytes: 20–40% Monocytes: 4–8%		
Syphilis tests: serologic tests for syphilis (STS), complement fixation test, Venereal Disease Research Laboratory (VDRL) test—nonreactive	Positive reaction STS—tests may have 25–45% incidence of biologic false-positive results; false results may occur in individuals who have acute viral or bacterial infections, hypersensitivity reactions, recent vaccinations, collagen disease, malaria, or tuberculosis	Positive results may be confirmed with the fluorescent treponemal antibody-absorption (FTA-ABS) test; all tests for syphilis give positive results in the secondary stage of the disease; antibiotic tests may cause negative test results.
First trimester integrated screen	Abnormal fetal nasal bone and/or nuchal fold on ultrasound combined with abnormal lab values as the quad screen.	Offered to all pregnant women at the gestational age appropriate for each test. If abnormal, further testing such as ultrasound or amniocentesis is offered.
Noninvasive prenatal testing (NIPT)/cell-free fetal DNA (cffDNA)	Detection of abnormal fetal alleles in maternal serum	Refer to healthcare provider
Quad screen (Evaluates four factors—maternal serum alpha-fetoprotein [MSAFP], unconjugated estriol [UE], human chorionic gonadotropin [hCG], and inhibin-A: normal levels)	Elevated MSAFP (neural tube defect, underestimated gestational age, multiple gestation). Lower than normal MSAFP (Down syndrome, trisomy 18). Higher than normal hCG and inhibin-A (Down syndrome). Lower than normal UE (Down syndrome)	Refer to healthcare provider for possible amniocentesis.
Indirect Coombs Test: done on all pregnant women at the initial prenatal visit and repeated at 28 weeks for Rh negative women	Red blood cell (RBC) antibodies present (either Rhesus or non-Rhesus)	A number of RBC antigens may cause isoimmunization and fetal and newborn hemolytic disease. The most common of these is the D antigen, which may occur when an Rh-negative mother carries an Rh-positive fetus. This may be prevented through prenatal administration of Rh immune globulin (RhoGAM).
	*Possible causes of alterations are identified in parentheses.	†This column provides guidelines for further assessment and initial nursing intervention.

Prenatal Assessment *(continued)*

PHYSICAL ASSESSMENT/ NORMAL FINDINGS	ALTERATIONS AND POSSIBLE CAUSES*	NURSING RESPONSES TO DATA†
Screening for Group B Streptococcus (GBS): Rectal and vaginal swabs obtained at 35–37 weeks' gestation for all pregnant women	Positive culture (maternal colonization)	Antibiotics administered during labor for infection prophylaxis in the neonate.
Glucose Tolerance Test: 50-g 1-hour glucose screen (done between 24 and 28 weeks' gestation)	Plasma glucose level greater than 130–140 mg/dL is considered abnormal, depending on provider preference. Be aware of your institution's guidelines.	Refer for a diagnostic 3-hour glucose tolerance test.
Urinalysis: normal color; specific gravity; pH 4.6–8.0	Abnormal color (porphyria, hemoglobinuria, bilirubinemia); alkaline urine (metabolic alkalemia, *Proteus* infection, old specimen)	Repeat urinalysis; refer to healthcare provider.
Urinalysis: negative for protein, RBCs, WBCs, casts	Positive findings (contaminated specimen, kidney disease)	Repeat urinalysis; refer to healthcare provider.
Urinalysis: glucose: negative (a small degree of glycosuria may occur in pregnancy)	Glycosuria (physiologic secondary to increased glomerular filtration of pregnancy for glucose, diabetes mellitus)	Assess blood glucose level; test urine for ketones.
Rubella titer: hemagglutination-inhibition (HAI) test—1:10 or above indicates woman is immune	HAI titer less than 1:10	Immunization will be given postpartum or within 6 weeks after childbirth. Instruct woman whose titers are less than 1:10 to avoid children who have rubella.
Hepatitis B screen for hepatitis B surface antigen (HbsAg): negative	Positive	If negative, consider referral for hepatitis B vaccine postpartum. If positive, refer to physician. Babies born to women who test positive are given hepatitis B immune globulin soon after birth, followed by first dose of hepatitis B vaccine.
HIV screen: offered to all women; encouraged for those at risk; negative	Positive	Refer to healthcare provider.
Illicit drug screen: offered to all women; negative	Positive	Refer to healthcare provider.
Hemoglobin screen for patients of African, Mediterranean, or south Asian descent: negative	Positive; test results would include a description of cells	Refer to healthcare provider.
Pap smear: negative	Test results that show atypical cells	Refer to healthcare provider. Discuss with the woman the meaning of the findings and the importance of follow-up.
Gonorrhea culture: negative	Positive	Refer for treatment.
	*Possible causes of alterations are identified in parentheses.	†This column provides guidelines for further assessment and initial nursing intervention.

(continued on next page)

Prenatal Assessment (continued)

CULTURAL ASSESSMENT§	VARIATIONS TO CONSIDER	NURSING RESPONSE TO DATA§§
Determine the woman's fluency in written and oral English	Woman may be fluent in language other than English	Work with a knowledgeable translator to provide information and answer questions.
Ask the woman how she prefers to be addressed	Some women prefer informality; others prefer to use titles	Address the woman according to her preference. Maintain formality in introducing oneself if that seems preferred.
Determine customs and practices regarding prenatal care:	Practices are influenced by individual preference, cultural expectations, or religious beliefs	Honor a woman's practices and provide for specific preferences unless they are contraindicated for safety reasons.
■ Ask the woman if there are certain practices she expects to follow when she is pregnant	Some women believe they should perform certain acts related to sleep, activity, or clothing	Have information printed in the language of different cultural groups that live in the area.
■ Ask the woman if there are any activities she cannot do while she is pregnant	Some women have restrictions or taboos they follow related to work, activity, sexual, environmental, or emotional factors	Provide alternate activities if needed.
■ Ask the woman whether there are certain foods she is expected to eat or avoid while she is pregnant. Determine whether she has lactose intolerance	Foods are an important cultural factor. Some women may have certain foods they must eat or avoid; many women have lactose intolerance and have difficulty consuming sufficient calcium	Respect the woman's food preferences, help her plan an adequate prenatal diet within the framework of her preferences, and refer to a dietitian if necessary.
■ Ask the woman whether the gender of her caregiver is of concern	Some women are comfortable only with a female caregiver	Arrange for a female caregiver if it is the woman's preference.
■ Ask the woman about the degree of involvement in her pregnancy that she expects or wants from her support person, mother, and other significant people	A woman may not want her partner involved in the pregnancy. The role may fall to the woman's mother or a female relative or friend	Respect the woman's preferences about her partner's involvement; avoid imposing personal values or expectations.
■ Ask the woman about her sources of support and counseling during pregnancy	Some women seek advice from a family member or traditional healer	Respect and honor the woman's sources of support.
Psychologic Status		
Excitement and/or apprehension, ambivalence	Marked anxiety (fear of pregnancy diagnosis, fear of medical facility)	Establish lines of communication. Active listening is useful. Establish trusting relationship. Encourage woman to take active part in her care.
	Apathy; display of anger with pregnancy diagnosis	Establish communication and begin counseling. Use active listening techniques.
Educational Needs		
May have questions about pregnancy or may need time to adjust to reality of pregnancy		Establish educational, supporting environment that can be expanded throughout pregnancy.
Support System		
Can identify at least two or three individuals with whom she is emotionally intimate (partner, parent, sibling, friend)	Isolated (no telephone, unlisted number); cannot name a neighbor or friend whom she can call on in an emergency; does not perceive parents as part of her support system	Institute support system through community groups. Help woman to develop trusting relationship with healthcare professionals.
§These are only a few suggestions. We do not mean to imply that this is a comprehensive cultural assessment; rather, it is a tool to encourage cultural competence.		§§This column provides guidelines for further assessment and initial nursing intervention.

Prenatal Assessment *(continued)*

CULTURAL ASSESSMENT[§]	VARIATIONS TO CONSIDER	NURSING RESPONSE TO DATA[§§]
Family Functioning		
Emotionally supportive Adequate communication Mutually satisfying Cohesiveness in times of trouble	Long-term problems or specific problems related to this pregnancy, potential stressors within the family, pessimistic attitudes, unilateral decision making, unrealistic expectations of this pregnancy or child	Help identify the problems and stressors, encourage communication, and discuss role changes and adaptations.
Economic Status		
Source of income is stable and sufficient to meet basic needs of daily living and medical needs	Limited prenatal care; poor physical health; limited use of healthcare system; unstable economic status	Discuss available resources for health maintenance and the birth. Institute appropriate referral for meeting expanding family's needs (e.g., food stamps).
Stability of Living Conditions		
Adequate, stable housing for expanding family's needs	Crowded living conditions; questionable supportive environment for newborn	Refer to appropriate community agency. Work with family on self-help ways to improve situation.
[§]These are only a few suggestions. We do not mean to imply that this is a comprehensive cultural assessment; rather, it is a tool to encourage cultural competence.		[§§]This column provides guidelines for further assessment and initial nursing intervention.

uterine fundus (the McDonald method) (**Figure 33–26 »**). Fundal height in centimeters correlates well with weeks of gestation after 20 weeks. The normal variation is gestational weeks plus or minus 2 cm. Thus, at 26 weeks' gestation, fundal height is 24–28 cm depending on fetal position and maternal body habitus. The woman should have voided within 30 minutes of the exam and should lie in the same position each time. In the third trimester, variations in fetal weight decrease the accuracy of fundal height measurements. A lag in progression of measurements of fundal height from month to month and from week to week may signal a fetus that is small for gestational age (SGA). A sudden increase in fundal height may indicate twins or hydramnios.

Small for gestational age is defined as a fetal weight estimated by ultrasound or a baby's actual birth weight that is less than the 10th percentile for gestational age. When no cause for this can be identified and the fetus or newborn shows no evidence of compromise, it may be concluded that it is constitutionally small. When a fetus is SGA in the setting of some pathology, this is called *intrauterine growth restriction (IUGR)*. Causes include congenital anomalies, exposure to teratogens, maternal smoking and substance abuse, malnutrition, abnormal formation of the placenta, and decreased placental perfusion (King et al., 2013).

Leopold Maneuvers

Leopold maneuvers are a system of palpating the uterus externally, starting at the fundus and moving downward, to assess the baby's position and orientation. In the first maneuver, the examiner grips the fundus with both hands and identifies the fetal parts in the fundus. The second maneuver consists of palpating the sides of the uterus to locate the fetal back and legs. The third maneuver consists of grasping the lower portion of the uterus to identify the fetal part that is lowest in the pelvis, called the presenting part. It should be the head in the third trimester. The fourth maneuver consists of identifying the position of the fetal brow or occiput to determine the degree of flexion or extension of the head (Gabbe et al., 2012).

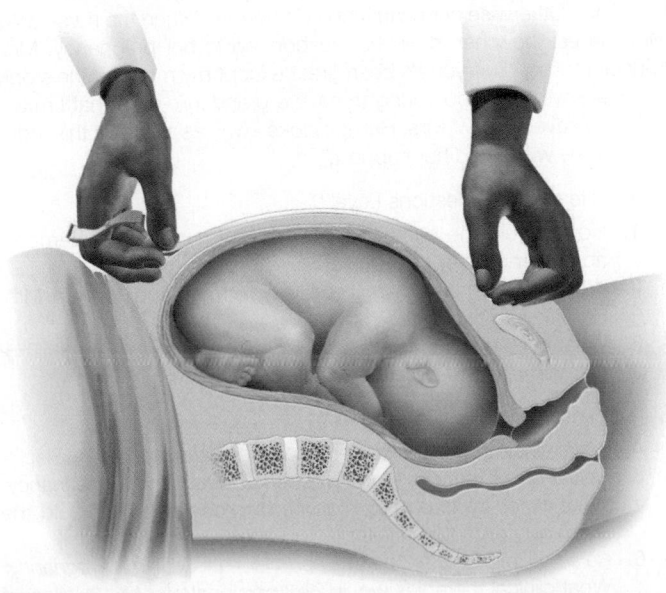

Figure 33–26 » A cross-sectional view of fetal position when the McDonald method is used to assess the fundal height.

Assessment of Fetal Development

Fetal assessment occurs at various points in gestation to determine fetal development and well-being. Methods include subjective and objective findings, such as fetal movement, fetal heartbeat, and ultrasound. Healthcare providers compare findings to gestational age and expected developmental milestones. Providers use findings to develop a plan of care to promote positive pregnancy outcomes.

Quickening

The first perception of fetal movement by the mother is termed quickening. Quickening may indicate that the fetus is nearing 20 weeks' gestation. However, quickening may be experienced between 16 and 22 weeks' gestation, so this method is not completely accurate.

Fetal Heartbeat

An ultrasonic Doppler device (**Figure 33–27 》**) is the primary tool for assessing fetal heartbeat. It can detect fetal heartbeat, on average, at 8–12 weeks' gestation. If such a device is not available, a fetoscope may be used, although in current practice it is seldom necessary. The fetal heartbeat can be detected by fetoscope as early as week 16 and usually by 19 or 20 weeks' gestation.

Ultrasound

In the first trimester, ultrasound scanning can detect a gestational sac as early as 5–6 weeks after the LMP, fetal heart activity by 6–7 weeks, and fetal breathing movement by 10–11 weeks of pregnancy. Crown-to-rump measurements can be made to assess fetal age until the fetal head can be visualized clearly. Biparietal diameter (BPD) can then be used. The BPD measures the diameter across the fetus's skull from one parietal bone to the other. BPD measurements can be made by approximately 12–13 weeks and are most accurate between 20 and 30 weeks, when rapid growth in the BPD occurs. Measurements and visualization of structures in the fetal body are used to determine appropriate growth, development, and function.

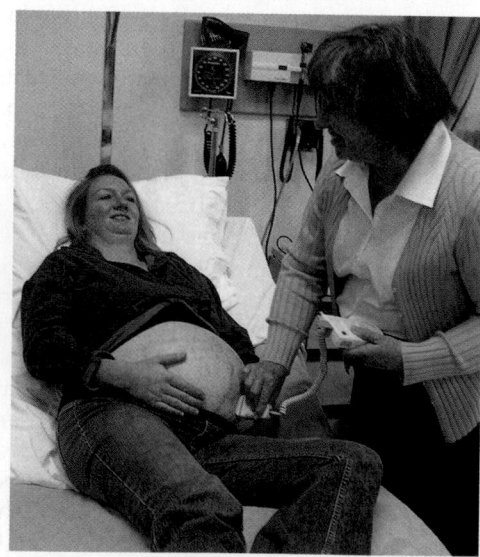

Figure 33–27 》 Listening to the fetal heartbeat with a Doppler device.

Assessment of Pelvic Adequacy (Clinical Pelvimetry)

The pelvis can be assessed vaginally by a process called *clinical pelvimetry*. It is performed by physicians or by advanced practice nurses such as CNMs or nurse practitioners. Some caregivers assess the pelvis as part of the initial physical examination. Others wait until later in the pregnancy, when hormonal effects are greatest and it is possible to make some determination of fetal size. However, pelvic adequacy can be reliably determined only by a trial of labor. Both radiographic and physical assessments of pelvic adequacy are poor predictors of the course of labor and birth.

Prenatal Tests

A number of tests may be used to detect hCG during pregnancy. In addition, a number of diagnostic and screening tests allow healthcare professionals (and the pregnant woman) to monitor the safety of both mother and child. These tests are summarized in **Table 33–1 》**; some of them are discussed in greater detail in Exemplar 33.A.

Nursing care for the woman who is undergoing prenatal testing focuses on outcomes to ensure that she understands the reasons for the test, understands the test results, and has support during the test. In addition, other objectives include completing the tests without complication and ensuring that the safety of the mother and her unborn child has been maintained.

Case Study 》 Part 2

When Mrs. Halleck returns to the clinic at 32 weeks' gestation, she says, "I feel like I need to pee all the time." Mrs. Halleck also states that she doesn't feel like exercising as much as she used to. She used to go to the gym three or four times a week, but now she only goes on the weekend, saying "I just don't feel like it. I keep getting these dull headaches, and all I seem to be able to do is sit on the sofa and eat and go to the bathroom." On examination, Mrs. Halleck has gained 12 pounds since her last appointment and her current weight is 150 lb. Her vital signs are T_O 98.6°F, BP 139/90 mmHg, P 84 beats/min, R 21/min. Otherwise her examination is normal. When the nurse asks Mrs. Halleck how her family has responded to her pregnancy, Mrs. Halleck replies, "Everyone's been great except my mother. She's only 45. She says she's too young to have a grandchild, and that I'm too young to have a baby." Mrs. Halleck looks away as she says this, adding, "I really wish I had her support."

Clinical Reasoning Questions Level I

1. How should the nurse respond to Mrs. Halleck's statements about her mother?
2. What interventions can the nurse recommend to help Mrs. Halleck with her nausea?
3. What interventions can the nurse recommend to Mrs. Halleck in response to her complaint about urinary frequency?

Clinical Reasoning Questions Level II

4. Which findings should concern the nurse caring for Mrs. Halleck?
5. *Referring to Exemplar 16.H, Hypertensive Disorders in Pregnancy:* What other signs and symptoms of preeclampsia should the nurse assess in Mrs. Halleck?
6. *Referring to Exemplar 16.H, Hypertensive Disorders in Pregnancy:* What clinical therapies would be appropriate for Mrs. Halleck if the nurse observes edema in her extremities in addition to her high blood pressure?

TABLE 33–1 Summary of Selected Antenatal Surveillance and Screening

Goal	Test	Timing
To confirm intrauterine pregnancy and viability	Ultrasound: gestational sac volume	5 or 6 weeks after LMP by transvaginal ultrasound
To determine gestational age	Ultrasound: crown/rump length	6–10 weeks' gestation
	Ultrasound: BPD and fetal body measurement rations	Greater than or equal to 14 weeks
To evaluate fetal growth	Ultrasound: BPD	
	Ultrasound: fetal body measurement ratios	Greater than or equal to 14 weeks
	Ultrasound: estimated fetal weight	About 23–42 weeks' gestation
To detect congenital anomalies and problems	Nuchal translucency testing	11–13 weeks' gestation
	Ultrasound	Greater than or equal to 18 weeks
	Chorionic villus sampling	10–12 weeks' gestation
	Amniocentesis	After 15 weeks' gestation
	First trimester integrated screen	10–13 weeks' gestation
	Cell-free fetal DNA (cffDNA)	From 9 weeks onward
To determine placental location	Ultrasound	18–20 weeks initially. Repeated at 28–32 weeks for re-evaluation if needed
To assess fetal status	Biophysical profile	Approximately 23 weeks to birth
	Maternal assessment of fetal activity	Approximately 28 weeks to birth
	Nonstress test	Approximately 28 weeks to birth
To diagnose cardiac problems	Fetal echocardiography	Second and third trimesters
To assess fetal lung maturity with amniocentesis or vaginal pool sampled amniotic fluid	L/S ratio	32–39 weeks
	Phosphatidylglycerol	32–39 weeks
	Phosphatidylcholine	32–39 weeks
	Lamellar body counts	32–39 weeks
To determine fetal presentation	Ultrasound	At term or on admission for labor and birth

Independent Interventions

Caring interventions for the pregnant woman are focused on teaching the patient appropriate self-care techniques, especially with regard to protecting the fetus and relieving discomfort. Many of these interventions are discussed in Exemplars 33.A and 33.B on antepartum and intrapartum care, respectively. Those that are covered here are related to fetal safety and to some of the most common discomforts experienced by the pregnant woman.

It is important to recognize that pregnancy is usually a normal process that ends with the delivery of a healthy newborn. The nurse's role in these cases is health promotion and patient teaching. However, alterations can result in injury to either the fetus or the woman or both. The nurse assesses patients at each encounter in order to rapidly intervene, to minimize complications, and promote expected outcomes. Holistic, culturally appropriate care is important to make the experience as positive as possible for the woman and her family.

Prenatal Education

Prenatal education programs provide important opportunities to share information about pregnancy and childbirth and to enhance the parents' decision-making skills. The content of each class is generally directed by the overall goals of the program. For example, in classes that aim to provide preconceptional information, preparations for becoming pregnant and optimizing the woman's health status are the major topics. Other classes may be directed toward childbirth choices available today, preparation of the mother and her partner for pregnancy and birth, preparation for a vaginal birth after a previous cesarean (VBAC) birth, and preparation for the birth by specific people such as grandparents or siblings. The nurse who knows the types of prenatal programs available in the community can direct expectant parents to programs that meet their special needs and learning goals.

From the expectant parents' point of view, class content is best presented in chronology with the pregnancy. It is important to begin the classes by finding out what each parent wants to learn and including a discussion of related choices. Classes that provide an environment supportive of practicing newly learned techniques and the freedom to ask questions and receive explanations are beneficial in helping class participants obtain these goals (Davidson et al., 2017).

Relief of the Common Discomforts of Pregnancy

The common discomforts of pregnancy result from physiologic and anatomic changes and are fairly specific to each of the three trimesters. See Table 33–2 in Exemplar 33.A for a summary of the common discomforts of pregnancy, their possible causes, and the self-care measures that might relieve discomfort. Health professionals often refer to these discomforts as minor, but they are not minor to the pregnant woman. They can make her quite uncomfortable and, if they are unexpected, anxious.

Nausea and Vomiting

Nausea and vomiting are early, very common symptoms occurring in up to 80% of pregnant women (Fantasia, 2014). These symptoms appear sometime after the first missed menstrual period and usually cease by the fourth missed menstrual period. Some women develop an aversion to specific foods, many experience nausea on arising in the morning, and others experience nausea throughout the day or in the evening.

The exact cause of nausea and vomiting in pregnancy (NVP) is unknown, but it is thought to be multifactorial. An elevated hCG level is believed to be a major factor, but changes in carbohydrate metabolism, fatigue, and emotional factors also may play a role. Research suggests that pregnant women should start taking a multivitamin before reaching 6 weeks' gestation to reduce the effects of NVP (ACOG, 2015a).

In addition to the self-care measures identified in Table 33–2, certain complementary therapies may be useful. For example, many women find that acupressure applied to pressure points in the wrists is helpful. Ginger also may relieve NVP (see Focus on Integrative Health: Ginger for Morning Sickness). Pyridoxine (vitamin B$_6$) or vitamin B$_6$ plus doxylamine (Unisom), an OTC antihistamine, is considered a first-line treatment. This is now available by prescription as a combined tablet under the brand name Diclegis. Antihistamine H$_1$-receptor blockers, phenothiazines, and antinausea medications such as promethazine (Phenergan), metoclopramide (Reglan), and ondansetron (Zofran) are considered safe and effective for treating refractory cases. In severe cases, methylprednisolone, a steroid, may be used, but as a last resort because it poses a potential risk to the fetus (ACOG, 2015a).

Focus on Integrative Health
Ginger for Morning Sickness

Women who experience NVP often try alternative approaches to relieve their symptoms because they are reluctant to take medication for fear of harming their fetus. Ginger has long been used as a traditional remedy for treating nausea and vomiting associated with early pregnancy (Tiran, 2012). It has few side effects when taken in small doses (National Center for Complementary and Integrative Health [NCCIH], 2012). Ginger is available in a variety of forms, including the fresh root, capsules, tea, candy, cookies, crystals, inhaled powdered ginger, and sugared ginger.

The nurse should advise a woman to contact her healthcare provider if she vomits more than once a day or shows signs of dehydration such as dry mouth and concentrated urine. In such cases, the healthcare provider might order an antiemetic such as promethazine (Phenergan).

Urinary Frequency

Urinary frequency, a common discomfort of pregnancy, occurs early in pregnancy and again during the third trimester because of pressure of the enlarging uterus on the bladder. Although frequency is considered normal during the first and third trimesters, the woman is advised to report to her healthcare provider signs of bladder infection such as pain, burning with voiding, or blood in the urine. Fluid intake should never be decreased to prevent frequency. The woman needs to maintain an adequate fluid intake—at least 2000 mL (eight to ten 8-oz glasses) per day. The nurse should also encourage her to empty her bladder frequently (about every 2 hours while awake).

Backache

Nearly 70% of women experience backache during pregnancy (King et al., 2013). Backache is due primarily to exaggeration of the lumbosacral curve that occurs as the uterus enlarges and becomes heavier. Maintaining good posture and using proper body mechanics throughout pregnancy can help prevent backache. The pregnant woman is advised to avoid bending over at the waist to pick up objects and should bend from the knees instead. She should place her feet 12–18 inches apart to maintain body balance. If the woman uses work surfaces that require her to bend, the nurse can advise her to adjust the height of the surfaces.

Collaborative Therapies

According to the American Association of Colleges of Nursing (AACN, 2016), "Collaboration emanates from an understanding and appreciation of the roles and contributions that each discipline brings to the care delivery experience." A diversity of disciplines, as well as treatment team members, enhances care by broadening available expertise and innovative ideas.

Members of the interprofessional team collaborate to coordinate high-quality, safe, and evidence-based care. Team members may include perinatologists, neonatologists, certified nurse-midwives, women's health practitioners, obstetricians, pediatricians, dietitians, social workers, mental healthcare providers, pharmacists, endocrinologists, cardiologists, lactation consultants, and registered nurses.

Pharmacologic Therapy

A number of pharmacologic therapies may be safely used to protect the health and safety of the mother and fetus. A pregnant woman who lives with chronic illness or disease needs to discuss the treatment of her illness during her pregnancy with both her obstetrician and her treating physician. The nurse's responsibility is to elicit information about any preexisting illness when obtaining the patient's health history. Particular consideration should be given to women with existing respiratory or cardiac disease, diabetes mellitus, or HIV. Pregnant women living with a chronic disease require additional teaching regarding management of their disease during pregnancy. Collaboration among all of the healthcare professionals working with these patients is essential to promoting patient self-care and fetal well-being.

Medications

The use of medications during pregnancy, including prescriptions, OTC drugs, and herbal remedies, is of great concern because maternal drug exposure is associated with birth defects. Many pregnant women need medication for therapeutic purposes, such as the treatment of infections, allergies, or other pathologic processes. In these situations, the problem can be complex. Known teratogenic agents are not prescribed and usually can be replaced with medications that are considered safe. Even when a woman is highly motivated to avoid taking any medications, she may have taken potentially teratogenic medications before her pregnancy was confirmed, especially if she has an irregular menstrual cycle.

The greatest potential for gross abnormalities in the fetus occurs during the first trimester of pregnancy, when fetal organs are first developing. Many factors influence teratogenic effects, including the specific type of teratogen and the dose, the stage of embryonic development, and the genetic sensitivity of the mother and fetus. For example, the commonly prescribed acne medication isotretinoin (Accutane) is associated with a high incidence of spontaneous abortion and congenital malformations if taken early in pregnancy.

To provide information for caregivers and patients, the FDA has developed a labeling system for medications administered during pregnancy. Medications were previously listed under a five-category system (Categories A, B, C, D, and X) to assist patients and caregivers to make informed decisions about the safety of medication to treat conditions during pregnancy. In 2014, the FDA amended its regulations governing the labeling to prescription drugs and biologic products for women who are pregnant or lactating. These regulations became effective in June 2015. According to the new requirements, three categories have been specified (U.S. Food and Drug Administration [FDA], 2014):

- ***Pregnancy.*** If the drug is absorbed systemically, labeling must include a risk summary of adverse developmental outcomes that includes data from all relevant sources, including human, animal, and/or pharmacologic information. The labeling must also contain relevant information to help healthcare providers counsel women about the use of the drug during pregnancy. In addition, if there is a pregnancy exposure registry for the drug, the labeling should include a specific statement to that effect followed by contact information needed to obtain information about the registry or to enroll.

- ***Lactation.*** For drugs that are absorbed systemically, labeling must include a summary of the risks of using a drug when the woman is lactating. To the extent that information is available, the summary should include relevant information about the drug's presence in human milk, the effects of the drug on milk production, and the effects of the drug on the breastfed child.

- ***Females and Males of Reproductive Potential.*** This section must include information when human or animal data suggests drug-associated effects on fertility. It should also specify when contraception or pregnancy testing is required or recommended, such as before, during, or after the drug therapy.

Although the first trimester is the critical period for teratogenesis, some medications are known to have a teratogenic effect when taken in the second and third trimesters. For example, tetracycline taken in late pregnancy is commonly associated with staining of teeth in children and has been shown to depress skeletal growth, especially in premature babies. Sulfonamides taken in the last few weeks of pregnancy are known to compete with bilirubin attachment of protein-binding sites, increasing the risk of jaundice in the newborn (Niebyl & Simpson, 2012).

Pregnant women need to avoid all medications—prescribed, homeopathic, or OTC—if possible. If no alternative exists, it is wisest to select a well-known medication rather than a newer drug whose potential teratogenic effects may not be known. When possible, the oral form of a drug should be used, and it should be prescribed in the lowest possible therapeutic dose for the shortest time possible. The advantage of using a particular medication must outweigh the risk. Any medication with possible teratogenic effects is best avoided.

Nonpharmacologic Therapy and Complementary Health Approaches

Nonpharmacologic therapies are considered safe and effective for use during pregnancy for women with depression, chronic headaches, sleep disturbances, back pain, and nausea and vomiting of pregnancy. Examples include relaxation therapy, physical therapy, massage therapy, cognitive–behavioral therapy, and hydrotherapy. Many women use complementary and alternative medicine (CAM), such as homeopathy, herbal therapy, acupressure, acupuncture, biofeedback, therapeutic touch, massage, and chiropractic, as part of a holistic approach to their healthcare regimen. Nurses are in a unique position to bridge the gap between conventional therapies and CAM therapies. As patient advocates, nurses are able to provide patients with information needed to make informed decisions about their health and healthcare. Using a nonjudgmental approach, the nurse should inquire about the use of CAM as part of a routine antepartum assessment. It is important that nurses working with pregnant women and their families develop a general understanding of the more commonly used therapies to be able to answer questions and provide resources as needed.

It is important for the pregnant woman to understand that herbs are considered to be dietary supplements and are not regulated as prescription or OTC drugs by the FDA. In general, it is best to advise pregnant women not to ingest any herbs, except ginger, during the first trimester of pregnancy. The website of the National Center for Complementary and Integrative Health is a reliable source for information about herbs, homeopathic remedies, and other alternative options.

Lifespan Considerations

Although pregnancy is a normal process for many women, it can carry increased risk for adolescents and women over age 35. These special populations require additional considerations throughout the childbearing process. Considerations may include additional testing, monitoring, and the assessment of psychosocial needs.

Adolescent Pregnancy

Over the past decade, U.S. adolescent birth rates have steadily decreased; however, the rate is substantially higher than in other Western industrialized countries (CDC, 2016). As recently as 2014, a total of 249,078 babies were born to females age 15–19 years, for a birth rate of 24.2 per 1000 women in this age group (CDC, 2016).

Adolescent pregnancy is a health and social issue with no single cause or cure. For the adolescent, pregnancy comes at a time when her physical development and the developmental tasks of adolescence are incomplete. She may not be prepared physically, psychologically, or economically for parenthood. Thus both she and her child are at high risk for a number of adverse outcomes. Compared with women of similar socioeconomic status who postpone childbearing, teen mothers are less likely to finish high school, less likely to go to college, more likely to be single, less likely to receive child support, and more likely to require public assistance. Babies of adolescent mothers are at an increased risk for preterm birth, low birth weight, and newborn/infant mortality. In addition, children of teen mothers tend to score lower on assessments of knowledge, language development, and cognition. They are also more likely to grow up without a father. In addition, children of adolescent mothers are at an increased risk for abuse and neglect (Born, 2012).

Pregnancy Over Age 35

An increasing number of women are choosing to have their first baby after age 35. Many factors contribute to this trend, including the following:

- The availability of effective birth control methods
- The expanded roles and career options available to women
- The increased number of women obtaining advanced education, pursuing careers, and delaying parenthood until they are established professionally
- The increased incidence of later marriage and second marriage
- The high cost of living, which causes some young couples to delay childbearing until they are more secure financially
- The increased availability of specialized fertilization procedures, which offers opportunities for women who had previously been considered infertile.

There are advantages to having a first baby after the age of 35. Single women or couples who delay childbearing until they are older tend to be well educated and financially secure. Usually their decision to have a baby was deliberately and thoughtfully made. Because of their life experiences, they are also more aware of the realities of having a child than younger women, and they recognize what it means to have a baby at their age. This delay in family allows for women to pursue advanced educational degrees and prepare financially for the impact children will have on their lives. Some women are ready to make a change in their lives, desiring to stay home with a new baby. Those who plan to continue working outside the home are typically able to afford good child care.

Special Concerns of the Expectant Couple Over Age 35

No matter what their age, most expectant couples have concerns regarding the well-being of the fetus and their ability to parent. The older couple has additional concerns related to their age, especially if they are over 40. Some couples are concerned about whether they will have enough energy to care for a new baby. Of greater concern is their ability to deal with the needs of the older child as they themselves age.

The financial concerns of an older couple are usually different from those of a younger couple. The older couple is generally more financially secure than the younger couple. However, when their "baby" is ready for college, the older couple may be near retirement and might not have the means to provide for their child.

While considering their financial future and future retirement, the older couple may be forced to face their own mortality. Certainly this is not uncommon in midlife, but instead of confronting this issue at 40–45 years of age or later, the older expectant couple may confront the issue several years earlier as they consider what will happen as their child grows.

The older couple facing pregnancy following a late or second marriage or after therapy for infertility may find themselves somewhat isolated socially. They may feel "different" because they are often the only couple in their peer group expecting their first baby. In fact, many of their peers are likely to be parents of adolescents or young adults and may be grandparents as well.

The response of older couples who already have children to learning that the woman is pregnant may vary greatly depending on whether the pregnancy was planned or unexpected. Other factors influencing their response include the attitudes of the couple's children, family, and friends to the pregnancy; the impact on their lifestyle; and the financial implications of having another child. Sometimes couples who had previously been married to other mates will choose to have a child together. The concept of blended family applies to situations in which "her" children, "his" children, and "their" children come together as a new family group.

The woman who has delayed pregnancy may be concerned about the limited amount of time that she has to bear children. When pregnancy does not occur as quickly as she hoped, the older woman may become increasingly anxious as time slips away on her "biological clock." When an older woman becomes pregnant but experiences a spontaneous abortion, her grief for the loss of her unborn child is exacerbated by her anxiety about her ability to conceive again in the time remaining to her.

Healthcare professionals may treat the older expectant couple differently than they would a younger couple. Older women may be offered more medical procedures, such as amniocentesis and ultrasound, than younger women. An older woman may be prevented from using a birthing room or birthing center even if she is healthy, because her age is considered to put her at risk.

Medical risks for the pregnant woman over age 35 are discussed in Exemplar 33.A, Antepartum Care.

Case Study » Part 3

Mrs. Halleck is at the clinic for a weekly follow-up appointment. She reports that she has been taking her blood pressure at home, and her readings during the past 2 weeks have been consistently around 130/85 mmHg. On examination, her weight is 151 lb, T_O 98.5°F, BP 131/84 mmHg, P 85 beats/min, R 20/min. Mrs. Halleck reports that is very stressed about her blood pressure. She has already lost a baby and she is afraid she may lose this one. In addition, as a relatively young teacher, she does not have a lot of sick time built up and if she cannot return to work, she doesn't know how she and her husband will be able to pay their bills. "My parents won't help," she says, "My mother is still more worried about her image than she is about me." Mrs. Halleck begins to cry and states, "I cry all the time now. I can't sleep. My husband says he doesn't know what to do

with me. I knew we should've waited before we tried to have another baby!"

Clinical Thinking Questions Level I

1. What is the priority for care for Mrs. Halleck at this time?
2. Based on the history of her pregnancy and the findings at this visit, what screenings do you anticipate the healthcare provider will order for Mrs. Halleck?
3. What do you think the nurse's responsibility to Mr. Halleck is at this time?

Clinical Thinking Questions Level II

4. What independent nursing interventions can the nurse implement to assist Mrs. Halleck at this time?
5. *Referring to Exemplar 28.C, Postpartum Depression:* What risk factors does Mrs. Halleck have for postpartum depression?
6. *Referring to Exemplar 28.C, Postpartum Depression:* What could the nurse do to assess Mrs. Halleck for possible depression with peripartum onset? The Edinburgh Postnatal Depression Scale and the Postpartum Depression Predictors Inventory may provide additional information to aid the nurse and the healthcare provider in determining if Mrs. Halleck needs further intervention at this time.

REVIEW The Concept of Reproduction

RELATE Link the Concepts

Linking the concept of reproduction with the concept of family:

1. Identify specific examples that demonstrate how the childbearing family is meeting developmental tasks of pregnancy.
2. Discuss family adaptation to pregnancy.
3. Describe the impact of family stressors on pregnancy.

Linking the concept of reproduction with the concept of nutrition:

4. Develop health promotion strategies to promote optimal nutrition during pregnancy, postpartum, and throughout the first year of life.
5. Analyze the impact of nutritional deficits on birth outcomes.
6. Identify motivational strategies to improve nutritional status throughout the childbearing period.

Linking the concept of reproduction with the concept of perfusion:

7. Analyze fetal assessments to determine placental perfusion and fetal well-being.
8. Discuss the impact of poor perfusion on maternal–fetal outcomes.
9. Prioritize nursing care according to severity of postpartum hemorrhage.

READY Go to Volume 3: Clinical Nursing Skills

- SKILL 14.1   Amniocentesis: Assisting
- SKILL 14.2   Antepartum, Maternal and Fetal: Assessing
- SKILL 14.3   Antepartum Pelvic Examination: Assisting
- SKILL 14.4   Deep Tendon Reflexes and Clonus: Assessing
- SKILL 14.5   Fetal Well-Being, Nonstress Test and Biophysical Profile: Assessing
- SKILL 14.6   Rh Immune Globulin: Administering
- SKILL 14.7   Amniotomy (Artificial Rupture of Membranes): Assisting

- SKILL 14.8   Epidural: Assisting and Caring for Patient
- SKILL 14.9   Fetal External Electronic: Monitoring
- SKILL 14.10 Fetal Heart Rate: Auscultating
- SKILL 14.11 Fetal Internal Scalp Electrode Placement: Monitoring
- SKILL 14.12 Induction of Labor with Oxytocin and Other Agents: Assisting and Caring for Patient
- SKILL 14.13 Intrapartum, Maternal and Fetal: Assessing
- SKILL 14.14 Intrapartum Pelvic Examination: Assisting
- SKILL 14.15 Prolapsed Cord: Caring for Patient
- SKILL 14.16 Breastfeeding: Assisting
- SKILL 14.17 Lochia: Evaluating
- SKILL 14.18 Postpartum, Maternal: Assessing
- SKILL 14.19 Postpartum, Perineum: Assessing
- SKILL 14.20 Uterine Fundus, After Vaginal or Caesarean Birth: Assessing
- SKILL 14.21 Apgar Score: Assessing
- SKILL 14.22 Circumcision: Caring for
- SKILL 14.23 Newborn: Assessing
- SKILL 14.24 Newborn, Initial Bathing
- SKILL 14.25 Newborn Thermoregulation: Assisting
- SKILL 14.26 Phototherapy, Newborn, Infant: Providing
- SKILL 14.27 Umbilical Cord Clamp: Caring for

REFER Go to Pearson MyLab Nursing and eText

- Additional review materials
- MiniModule: Twins
- Chart 1: Organ Development in the Embryo and Fetus
- Chart 2: Differential Diagnosis of Pregnancy—Subjective Changes

- Chart 3: Differential Diagnosis of Pregnancy—Objective Changes
- Chart 4: Parental Reactions to Pregnancy

REFLECT Apply Your Knowledge

Mrs. Patterson, 41, is a G1P0 with a history of infertility. She currently works as an account manager for a pharmaceutical company and has been promoted to International Sales Director. She typically works long hours and must travel on occasion. She and her husband, 43, married for 15 years, are anticipating the arrival of their first child, but have expressed some concerns. Mrs. Patterson's height is 167.6 cm (5 ft, 6 in.); weight, 64.9 kg (143 lb); fundal height, 26 cm; ultrasound results show an intrauterine pregnancy at 25 weeks' gestation. No fetal abnormalities were noted. She has no existing medical diagnoses. Mrs. Patterson voices concerns about balancing motherhood with her career. She states that her husband is supportive, but recognizes that a new child may alter their routine and lifestyle. Mrs. Patterson also states that she is worried that her busy schedule may compromise the pregnancy.

1. What are the priority concerns for Mrs. Patterson?
2. Given the current findings, what interventions would be most therapeutic?
3. What resources might be appropriate for this patient?
4. What independent nursing interventions can the nurse implement to assist Mrs. Patterson at this time?

≫ Exemplar 33.A
Antepartum Care

Exemplar Learning Outcomes

33.A Summarize antepartum care of the pregnant woman.

- Summarize relief of the common discomforts of pregnancy.
- Describe commonly occurring alterations related to pregnancy.
- Summarize maternal and fetal risk factors related to pregnancy.
- Compare diagnostic tests used to assess fetal well-being.
- Describe factors that influence maternal nutrition and weight gain.
- Differentiate considerations related to the assessment and care of pregnant adolescents and women over 35.
- Illustrate the nursing process in providing culturally competent care to the pregnant woman and her family.

Exemplar Key Terms

Amniocentesis, 2244
Contraction stress test (CST), 2243
Dietary Reference Intakes (DRIs), 2246
Fetal movement record, 2238
Folic acid, 2228
Gestational diabetes mellitus (GDM), 2230
Kegel exercises, 2266
Lactase deficiency, 2252
Lacto-ovovegetarians, 2250
Lactose intolerance, 2252
Lactovegetarians, 2250
Lecithin/sphingomyelin (L/S) ratio, 2245
Nonstress test (NST), 2241
Pelvic tilt, 2265
Penta screen, 2246
Pica, 2250
Quadruple screen, 2245
Surfactant, 2244
Ultrasound, 2239
Vegans, 2250

Overview

From the moment a woman finds out she is pregnant, she faces a future marked by dramatic changes. Her appearance will alter. Her relationships will change. Even her psychologic state will be affected. She will need to make adjustments in her daily life to cope with these changes. So, too, will her family. The roles and responsibilities of family members, for example, may alter as the woman's ability to perform certain activities changes. The family also must adapt psychologically to the expected arrival of a new member.

The expectant woman and her family will probably have many questions about the pregnancy and its impact on all of them, especially if this is a first pregnancy. Their daily activities and healthcare practices may affect the well-being of the unborn child. Addressing self-care and discomforts related to pregnancy, performing ongoing assessment to ensure fetal and maternal health and safety, and preparing for childbirth are the nursing priorities for the woman experiencing a normal pregnancy.

Relief of the Common Discomforts of Pregnancy

The common discomforts of pregnancy result from physiologic and anatomic changes and are fairly specific to each of the three trimesters (**Table 33–2 ≫**). Health professionals often refer to these discomforts as minor, but they are not minor to the pregnant woman. In fact, they can make her quite uncomfortable and, if they are unexpected, anxious.

At each prenatal visit, focus patient teaching on changes or possible discomforts the pregnant woman might encounter during the coming month and the next trimester. If the pregnancy is progressing normally, spend a few minutes describing her baby at that particular stage of development. In regard to culture and diversity, discuss potential self-care techniques to promote safe practices and encourage incorporation of traditions supportive of patient needs. See Focus on Diversity and Culture: Self-Care Techniques During Pregnancy.

TABLE 33–2 Self-care Measures for Common Discomforts of Pregnancy

Discomfort	Influencing Factors	Self-Care Measures
First Trimester		
Nausea and vomiting	Increased levels of hCG Changes in carbohydrate metabolism Emotional factors Fatigue	Avoid odors or causative factors. Eat dry crackers or toast before arising in morning. Have small but frequent meals. Avoid greasy or highly seasoned foods. Take dry meals with fluids between meals. Drink carbonated beverages.
Urinary frequency	Pressure of uterus on bladder in both first and third trimesters	Void when urge is felt. Increase fluid intake during the day. Decrease fluid intake *only* in the evening to decrease nocturia.
Fatigue	Specific causative factors unknown May be aggravated by nocturia due to urinary frequency	Plan time for a nap or rest period daily. Go to bed early. Seek family support and assistance with responsibilities so that more time is available to rest.
Breast tenderness	Increased levels of estrogen and progesterone	Wear well-fitting, supportive bra.
Increased vaginal discharge	Hyperplasia of vaginal mucosa and increased production of mucus by the endocervical glands due to the increase in estrogen levels	Promote cleanliness by daily bathing. Avoid douching, nylon underpants, and pantyhose; cotton underpants are more absorbent.
Nasal stuffiness and nosebleed (epistaxis)	Elevated estrogen levels	May be unresponsive, but cool-air vaporizer may help; avoid use of nasal sprays and decongestants.
Ptyalism (excessive, often bitter salivation)	Specific causative factors unknown	Use astringent mouthwashes, chew gum, or suck hard candy. Carry tissues or a small towel to spit into when necessary.
Second and Third Trimesters		
Heartburn (pyrosis)	Increased production of progesterone, decreasing gastrointestinal motility and increasing relaxation of cardiac sphincter, displacement of stomach by enlarging uterus, thus regurgitation of acidic gastric contents into the esophagus	Eat small and more frequent meals. Use low-sodium antacids if approved by healthcare provider. Avoid overeating, fatty and fried foods, lying down after eating, and sodium bicarbonate.
Ankle edema	Prolonged standing or sitting Increased levels of sodium due to hormonal influences Circulatory congestion of lower extremities Increased capillary permeability Varicose veins	Practice frequent dorsiflexion of feet when prolonged sitting or standing is necessary. Elevate legs when sitting or resting. Avoid tight garters or restrictive bands around legs.
Varicose veins	Venous congestion in the lower veins that increases with pregnancy Hereditary factors (weakening of walls of veins, faulty valves) Increased age and weight gain	Elevate legs frequently. Wear supportive hose. Avoid crossing legs at the knees, standing for long periods, garters, and hosiery with constrictive bands.
Hemorrhoids	Constipation (see following discussion) Increased pressure from gravid uterus on hemorrhoidal veins	Avoid constipation. Apply ice packs, topical ointments, anesthetic agents, warm soaks, or sitz baths; gently reinsert hemorrhoid into rectum as necessary.
Constipation	Increased levels of progesterone, which cause general bowel sluggishness Pressure of enlarging uterus on intestine Iron supplements Diet, lack of exercise, and decreased fluids	Increase fluid intake, fiber in the diet, and exercise. Develop regular bowel habits. Use stool softeners as recommended by healthcare provider.
Backache	Increased curvature of the lumbosacral vertebrae as the uterus enlarges Increased levels of hormones, which cause softening of cartilage in body joints Fatigue Poor body mechanics	Use proper body mechanics. Practice the pelvic-tilt exercise. Avoid uncomfortable working heights, high-heeled shoes, lifting of heavy loads, and fatigue.
Leg cramps	Imbalance of calcium/phosphorus ratio Increased pressure of uterus on nerves Fatigue Poor circulation to lower extremities Pointing the toes	Practice dorsiflexion of feet to stretch affected muscle. Evaluate diet. Apply heat to affected muscles. Arise slowly from resting position.

(continued on next page)

TABLE 33–2 Self-care Measures for Common Discomforts of Pregnancy *(continued)*

Discomfort	Influencing Factors	Self-Care Measures
Faintness	Postural hypotension Sudden change of position causing venous pooling in dependent veins Standing for long periods in warm area Anemia	Avoid prolonged standing in warm or stuffy environments. Evaluate hematocrit and hemoglobin.
Dyspnea	Decreased vital capacity from pressure of enlarging uterus on the diaphragm	Use proper posture when sitting and standing. Sleep propped up with pillows for relief if problem occurs at night.
Flatulence	Decreased gastrointestinal motility leading to delayed emptying time Pressure of growing uterus on large intestine Air swallowing	Avoid gas-forming foods. Chew food thoroughly. Get regular daily exercise. Maintain normal bowel habits.
Carpal tunnel syndrome	Compression of median nerve in carpal tunnel of wrist Aggravated by repetitive hand movements	Avoid aggravating hand movements. Use splint as prescribed. Elevate affected arm.

Source: Davidson, M., London, M., & Ladewig, P. (2017). *Olds' maternal–newborn nursing & women's health across the lifespan* (10th ed.), Key Points: Health Promotion Education: Self-Care Measures for Common Discomforts of Pregnancy, pp. 289–290. Hoboken, NJ: Pearson.

Alterations of Pregnancy

Even though pregnancy is a normal process, for some women it may become a life-threatening event because of potential or existing complications. These complications can result from factors such as age, parity, blood type, socioeconomic status, psychologic health, or preexisting chronic illnesses. Alterations or complications may involve pregestational factors related to a variety of concepts, such as metabolism, perfusion, oxygenation, immunity, nutrition, and coping. Some alterations arise during pregnancy and potentially result in additional complications related to an increased risk for preterm delivery or perinatal loss. Effective prenatal care is directed toward identifying factors that increase a pregnant woman's risk and developing supportive therapies that promote optimal health of the mother and her fetus.

Anemia During Pregnancy

Anemia indicates inadequate levels of hemoglobin (Hb) in the blood. Anemia is defined as hemoglobin less than 12 g/dL in nonpregnant women and less than 11 g/dL in pregnant women (ACOG, 2015b). Ethnicity, altitude, smoking, nutrition, and medications can affect the normal limits of hemoglobin. The lower limit of normal tends to be higher for women who smoke and those who live at higher altitudes because their bodies require a greater quantity of red blood cells to maintain their tissue oxygen levels. The common anemias of pregnancy are due either to insufficient hemoglobin production related to nutritional deficiency in iron or folic acid during pregnancy, or to hemoglobin destruction in inherited disorders, specifically sickle cell disease and thalassemia.

Iron Deficiency Anemia

Iron deficiency anemia is the most common medical complication of pregnancy. Low iron stores in the body may result in diminished red blood cell production (Short & Domagalski, 2014). This is primarily a consequence of expansion of plasma volume without normal expansion of maternal

hemoglobin mass (ACOG, 2015b). The greatest need for increased iron intake occurs in the second half of pregnancy. When the iron needs of pregnancy are not met, maternal hemoglobin falls below 11 g/dL. Serum ferritin levels, indicating iron stores, are below 12 mg/L.

The woman with iron deficiency anemia may be asymptomatic, but she is more susceptible to perinatal infection and has an increased chance preeclampsia and bleeding. There is evidence of increased risk of low birth weight, prematurity, stillbirth, and neonatal death in babies of women with severe iron deficiency (maternal Hb less than 6 g/dL). The newborn is not iron deficient at birth because of active transport of iron across the placenta, even when maternal iron stores are low. However, these babies do have lower iron stores and are at increased risk for developing iron deficiency during the newborn period and infancy (Abu-Ouf & Jan, 2015).

The first goal of healthcare is to prevent iron deficiency anemia. To prevent anemia, the AAP and ACOG (2012) recommend that pregnant women supplement their diet with at least 30 mg of iron daily. This amount is contained in most prenatal vitamins. In addition, the woman should be encouraged to eat an iron-rich diet. If anemia is diagnosed, the dosage should be increased to 60–120 mg/day of iron. If the woman remains anemic after 1 month of therapy, further evaluation is indicated.

Folic Acid Deficiency Anemia

Folate deficiency is the most common cause of megaloblastic anemia during pregnancy. **Folic acid** is needed for deoxyribonucleic acid (DNA) and ribonucleic acid (RNA) synthesis and cell duplication. In its absence, immature red blood cells fail to divide, become enlarged (megaloblastic), and are fewer in number. Even more significantly, an inadequate intake of folic acid has been associated with neural tube defects (NTDs) (spina bifida, anencephaly, myelomeningocele) in the fetus or newborn. With the tremendous cell multiplication that occurs

Focus on Diversity and Culture
Self-care Techniques During Pregnancy*

Belief or Practice	Nursing Considerations
Home Remedies	
■ Pregnant women of Native American background may use herbal remedies. An example is the dandelion, which contains a milky juice in its stem believed to increase breast milk flow in mothers who choose to breastfeed (Spector, 2017). ■ Patients of Chinese descent may drink ginseng tea for faintness after childbirth or as a sedative when mixed with bamboo leaves. ■ Some individuals of African heritage may use self-medication for pregnancy discomforts—for example, laxatives to prevent or treat constipation (Purnell, 2014).	Find out what medications and home remedies your patient is using, and counsel her regarding their overall effects. It is common for individuals to avoid telling healthcare workers about home remedies, because the patient may feel the use of such remedies will be judged unfavorably. Phrase your questions in a sensitive, accepting way.
Nutrition	
■ Some women of Italian background may believe it is necessary to satisfy desires for certain foods in order to prevent congenital anomalies. Also, they may believe they must eat food that they smell, or else the fetus will move "inside," which will result in a miscarriage. ■ Some pregnant women of African descent may continue the tradition of eating clay, dirt, or starch, which they believe will benefit the mother and fetus (Carmoney, 2014).	Discuss the woman's beliefs and practices in regard to nutrition during pregnancy. Obtain a diet history from the patient. Discuss the importance of a well-balanced diet during pregnancy, with consideration of the woman's cultural beliefs and practices. In some cases, you might want to suggest remedies that may be more effective— for example, eating high-fiber foods to reduce constipation. If the home remedy is not harmful, there is no reason to ask a patient to discontinue this practice.
Alternative Healthcare Providers	
■ Some pregnant women of Mexican background may choose to seek out the care of a *partera* (midwife) for prenatal and intrapartum care. A *partera* speaks their language, shares a similar culture, and can care for pregnant women at home or in a birthing center instead of a hospital. ■ Some individuals in Hispanic-American communities may use a *curandero* (folk healer). A *curandero* frequently uses herbs, massage, and religious artifacts for treatment (Spector, 2017).	Discuss the variety of choices for healthcare providers available to the pregnant woman. Contrast the benefits and risks of different settings for prenatal care and birth. Provide reassurance that the goal of healthcare during pregnancy and birth is a healthy outcome for mother and baby, with respect for the specific cultural beliefs and practices of the mother.
Exercise	
■ Some pregnant women of Italian descent may fear changing their body position in certain ways because they believe this may cause the fetus to develop abnormally. Some individuals of European, African, and Mexican descent believe that reaching over the head during pregnancy can harm the baby.	Ask the woman whether she is afraid of any activities because of the pregnancy. Assure her that reaching over her head will not harm the baby, and evaluate other activities for their effect on the pregnancy.
Spirituality	
■ Native Americans are aware of the mind–soul connection and may try to follow certain practices to have a healthy pregnancy and birth. These practices could include a focus on peace and positive thoughts as well as certain types of prayers and ceremonies. A traditional healer may assist them (Ogburn et al., 2012). ■ Some individuals of European background may tend to pay more attention to spirituality in their life to alleviate fears and ensure a safe birth.	Encourage the use of support systems and spiritual aids that provide comfort for the pregnant woman.

*Note: This information is meant only to provide examples of the behaviors that may be found within certain cultures. Not all members of a culture practice the behaviors described.

in pregnancy, an adequate amount of folic acid is crucial. However, increased urinary excretion of folic acid and fetal uptake can rapidly result in folic acid deficiency.

Diagnosis of folic acid deficiency anemia may be difficult, and it is usually not detected until late in pregnancy or the early puerperium. This is because serum folate levels normally fall as pregnancy progresses. Even though folate levels are lower with deficiency, they will fluctuate with diet. Measurement of erythrocyte folate status is more reliable but indicates the folate status of several weeks previously. Women with true folic acid deficiency anemia often present with nausea, vomiting, and anorexia. Hemoglobin levels as low as 3–5 g/dL may be found. Typically the blood smear reveals that the newly formed erythrocytes are macrocytic.

Folic acid deficiency during pregnancy is prevented by a daily supplement of 0.4 mg of folate. Treatment of deficiency consists of 1-mg folic acid supplements. Because iron deficiency anemia almost always coexists with folic acid deficiency, the woman also needs iron supplements. The Food and Drug Administration (FDA) requires the addition of folic acid for all foods labeled "enriched." Even with this addition, the U.S. Public Health Service recommends that all women of childbearing age (15–45 years) consume 0.4 mg of folic acid daily. This recommendation is important because half of all U.S. pregnancies are unplanned and NTDs occur very early in pregnancy (3–4 weeks after conception), before most women realize they are pregnant (AAP & ACOG, 2012). Nurses can play a crucial role in helping young women become aware of this important recommendation.

Sickle Cell Disease

Sickle cell disease (SCD) is an autosomal recessive disorder in which the normal adult hemoglobin, hemoglobin A (HbA), is abnormally formed. This abnormal hemoglobin is called hemoglobin S (HbS). Approximately 1 in 12 African Americans has sickle cell trait and 1 in every 300 African American newborns has some form of sickle cell disease (ACOG, 2015b). Diagnosis is confirmed by hemoglobin electrophoresis or a test to induce sickling in a blood sample. Prenatal diagnosis and newborn screening for sickle cell disease are important components of perinatal care (ACOG, 2015b).

Women with sickle cell trait have a good prognosis for pregnancy if they have adequate nutrition and prenatal care. Maternal mortality due to sickle cell disease is rare. Women with sickle cell disease may have experienced severe complications by the time they reach childbearing age (James, 2014). Complications include anemia requiring blood transfusion, infections, and emergency cesarean births. Acute chest syndrome, congestive heart failure, or acute renal failure may also occur. Prematurity and intrauterine growth restriction (IUGR) are also associated with sickle cell disease. Fetal death is believed to be due to sickling attacks in the placenta.

Because the woman with sickle cell disease maintains her hemoglobin levels by intense erythropoiesis, additional folic acid supplements (4 mg/day) are required. Maternal infection should be treated promptly because dehydration and fever can trigger sickling and crisis. Vaso-occlusive crisis is best treated by a perinatal team in a medical center. Proper management requires close observation and evaluation of all symptoms. Women with sickle cell disease are at higher risk of developing *sickle cell crisis*, which may increase rates of maternal morbidity and mortality (Alayed et al., 2014).

Diabetes During Pregnancy

Carbohydrate metabolism is affected early in pregnancy by a rise in serum levels of estrogen, progesterone, and other hormones. These hormones stimulate maternal insulin production and increase tissue response to insulin; therefore, anabolism (building up) of glycogen stores in the liver and other tissues occurs.

In the second half of pregnancy, the woman demonstrates prolonged hyperglycemia and hyperinsulinemia (increased secretion of insulin) following a meal. Although the mother is producing more insulin, placental secretion of hPL and prolactin (from the decidua), as well as elevated levels of

cortisol (an adrenal hormone) and glycogen, causes increased maternal peripheral resistance to insulin. This resistance helps ensure that a sustained supply of glucose is available for the fetus. This glucose is transported across the placenta to the fetus, which uses it as a major source of fuel. Maternal amino acids are also actively transported by the placenta from the mother to her fetus. The fetus uses these amino acids for protein synthesis and as a source of energy. In addition to ensuring that glucose is available to the fetus, the increased maternal resistance to insulin means that the pregnant woman has a lower peripheral uptake of glucose to meet her own needs. This results in a catabolic (destructive) state during fasting periods (e.g., during the night and after meal absorption). Because increasing amounts of circulating maternal glucose are being diverted to the fetus, maternal fat is metabolized (lipolysis) during fasting periods much more readily than in a nonpregnant individual. This process is called *accelerated starvation*. Ketones may be present in the urine as a result of lipolysis.

The delicate system of checks and balances that exists between glucose production and glucose use is stressed by the growing fetus, who derives energy from glucose taken from the mother, and by maternal resistance to the insulin her body produces. This stress is referred to as the *diabetogenic effect of pregnancy*. Thus any preexisting disruption in carbohydrate metabolism is augmented by pregnancy, and any diabetic potential may precipitate gestational diabetes mellitus.

Gestational Diabetes Mellitus

Gestational diabetes mellitus (GDM) is defined as a carbohydrate intolerance of variable severity with onset or first recognition during pregnancy. It results from (1) an unidentified preexisting disease or (2) the unmasking of a compensated metabolic abnormality by the added stress of pregnancy, or (3) it is a direct consequence of the altered maternal metabolism stemming from changing hormonal levels. Diagnosis of GDM is important because even mild diabetes increases the risk of perinatal morbidity and mortality. Many women with GDM progress over time to overt type 2 diabetes mellitus (T2D).

Influence of Preexisting and Gestational Diabetes During Pregnancy

Pregnancy can affect diabetes significantly. First, the physiologic changes of pregnancy can drastically alter insulin requirements. Second, pregnancy may accelerate the progress of vascular disease secondary to diabetes.

The disease may be more difficult to control during pregnancy because insulin requirements are changeable. Insulin needs frequently decrease early in the first trimester. Levels of hPL, an insulin antagonist, are low; energy demands of the embryo/fetus are minimal; and the woman may be consuming less food because of nausea and vomiting. Nausea and vomiting may also cause dietary fluctuations, which can increase the risk of hypoglycemia or insulin shock. Insulin requirements usually begin to rise late in the first trimester as glucose use and glycogen storage by the woman and fetus increase. As a result of placental maturation and production of hPL and other hormones, insulin requirements may double or quadruple by the end of pregnancy.

Because her energy needs increase during labor, the woman with diabetes may require more insulin at that time to balance intravenous glucose. After delivery of the placenta, insulin requirements usually decrease abruptly with loss of hPL in the maternal circulation.

Other factors contribute to the difficulty in controlling the disease. As pregnancy progresses, the renal threshold for glucose decreases. There is an increased risk of ketoacidosis, which may occur at lower serum glucose levels in the pregnant woman with diabetes than in the nonpregnant woman with diabetes. The vascular disease that accompanies diabetes may progress during pregnancy. Hypertension may occur. Nephropathy may result from renal blood vessel impairment, and retinopathy may develop (from occlusion of the microscopic blood vessels of the eye).

Influence of Preexisting Diabetes and Gestational Diabetes on Pregnancy Outcome

The pregnancy of a woman who has diabetes carries a higher risk of complications than a normal pregnancy, especially perinatal mortality and congenital anomalies. The risk has been reduced by the recent recognition of the importance of tight metabolic control (fasting, premeal, and bedtime blood glucose levels of 60–95 mg/dL; peak postprandial blood glucose levels of 100–129 mg/dL; and glycohemoglobin less than 6%). New techniques for monitoring blood glucose, delivering insulin, and monitoring the fetus have also reduced perinatal mortality (ACOG, 2013d).

Maternal Risks

Maternal health problems in diabetic pregnancy have been greatly reduced by the team approach to preconception planning and early prenatal care and by the increased emphasis on maintaining tight control of blood glucose levels. The prognosis for the pregnant woman with gestational, type 1, or type 2 diabetes that has not resulted in significant vascular damage is positive. However, diabetic pregnancy still carries higher risks for complications than normal pregnancy.

Hydramnios, or an increase in the volume of amniotic fluid, occurs in 10–20% of pregnant women with diabetes. It is thought to be a result of excessive fetal urination because of fetal hyperglycemia (ACOG, 2013d). *Preeclampsia–eclampsia* occurs more often in diabetic pregnancies, especially when diabetes-related vascular changes already exist.

Hyperglycemia due to insufficient amounts of insulin can lead to *ketoacidosis* as a result of the increase in ketone bodies (which are acidic) in the blood released when fatty acids are metabolized. Ketoacidosis usually develops slowly, but it may develop more rapidly in the pregnant woman because of the hyperketonemia associated with accelerated starvation in the fasting state. The tendency for higher postprandial glucose levels because of decreased gastric motility and the contrainsulin effects of hPL also predispose the woman to ketoacidosis. If the ketoacidosis is not treated, it can lead to coma and death of both mother and fetus.

Another risk to the pregnant woman with diabetes is a difficult labor (*dystocia*), caused by fetopelvic disproportion if fetal macrosomia (>4000 g) exists. The pregnant woman with diabetes is also at increased risk for recurrent monilial vaginitis (yeast infection) and urinary tract infections because of increased glycosuria, which contributes to a favorable environment for bacterial growth. If untreated, asymptomatic bacteriuria can lead to pyelonephritis, a serious kidney infection.

Several studies have demonstrated that pregnancy worsens *retinopathy* in women with diabetes. Most investigators agree that during a diabetic pregnancy, good control of blood glucose levels and the use of laser photocoagulation (a treatment used to prevent retinal hemorrhage when the retina shows changes in the blood vessels) when indicated minimize the risk of the negative effects of pregnancy. Hence, women with preexisting diabetes should be referred to an ophthalmologist for evaluation during pregnancy.

Fetal–Neonatal Risks

Many of the problems of the newborn result directly from high maternal plasma glucose levels. The incidence of *congenital anomalies* in diabetic pregnancies is 6–12% and is the major cause of death for babies of mothers with diabetes. Research suggests that this increased incidence of congenital anomalies is related to multiple factors, including high glucose levels in early pregnancy (ACOG, 2013d). The anomalies often involve the heart, central nervous system (CNS), and skeletal system. Septal defects, coarctation of the aorta, and transposition of the great vessels are the most common heart lesions seen. CNS anomalies include hydrocephalus, meningomyelocele, and anencephaly. One anomaly, *sacral agenesis*, appears only in babies of mothers with diabetes. In sacral agenesis, the sacrum and lumbar spine fail to develop and the lower extremities develop incompletely. To reduce the incidence of congenital anomalies, preconception counseling and strict diabetes control before conception and in the early weeks of pregnancy are indicated.

Approximately 18% of newborns of mothers with diabetes are large for gestational age (LGA) as a result of high levels of fetal insulin production stimulated by the high levels of glucose crossing the placenta from the mother. Sustained fetal hyperinsulinism and hyperglycemia ultimately lead to *macrosomia* and deposition of fat. If born vaginally, the macrosomic newborn is at increased risk for birth trauma such as fractured clavicle or brachial plexus injuries due to shoulder dystocia. Shoulder dystocia occurs when, following birth of the head, the anterior shoulder of the macrosomic fetus does not emerge either spontaneously or with gentle traction (ACOG, 2013d). Macrosomia can be significantly reduced by tight maternal blood glucose control.

After birth, the umbilical cord is severed and, thus, the generous maternal blood glucose supply is eliminated. However, continued islet cell hyperactivity leads to excessive insulin levels and depleted blood glucose (hypoglycemia) within 2–4 hours after birth in the neonate. Babies of mothers with diabetes with vascular involvement (see the module on Metabolism) may demonstrate IUGR. This occurs because vascular changes in the mother decrease the efficiency of placental perfusion, and the fetus is not as well sustained in utero. *Respiratory distress syndrome* appears to result from inhibition, by high levels of fetal insulin, of some fetal enzymes necessary for surfactant production. Polycythemia in the newborn is due primarily to the diminished ability of glycosylated hemoglobin in the mother's blood to release oxygen. *Hyperbilirubinemia* is a result of the inability of immature liver enzymes to metabolize the increased bilirubin resulting from the polycythemia. Hypocalcemia, characterized by signs of irritability or even tetany, may occur. The cause of these low calcium levels in newborns of mothers with diabetes is not known.

Clinical Therapy

Gestational diabetes is more common than preexisting diabetes. It is estimated to occur in from 6 to 7% of pregnancies, depending on the population studied (ACOG, 2013d). Therefore, screening for its detection is a standard part of prenatal care. If diabetes is suspected, further testing is undertaken for diagnosis.

All pregnant women should have their risk of diabetes assessed at the first prenatal visit (see Exemplar 12.A, Type 1 Diabetes Mellitus, in the module on Metabolism). Women at high risk (prior history of GDM or birth of an LGA baby, marked obesity, diagnosis of polycystic ovarian syndrome, presence of glycosuria, or a strong family history of type 2 diabetes mellitus [T2D]) should be screened for diabetes as soon as possible. In early pregnancy, the screening criteria for nonpregnant individuals is used: Hb A1C equal to or greater than 6.5% would be considered diagnostic as would a fasting plasma glucose level equal to or greater than 126 mg/dL (American Diabetes Association [ADA], 2014).

If there is no preexisting diabetes, screening for GDM is done using one of two approaches performed at 24 to 28 weeks' gestation (ADA, 2014). In the two-step approach, the first step is to give the woman a non-fasting, 50-g, 1-hour oral glucose tolerance test (OGTT). The oral glucose load can be given at any time of the day with no requirement for fasting. One hour later, plasma glucose is measured. If plasma glucose levels are elevated (equal to or greater than 140 mg/dL, depending on the laboratory used), a 100-g, 3-hour glucose test is done. In the second step, a 100-g, 3-hour OGTT is administered. The woman eats an unrestricted diet, consuming at least 150 g of carbohydrates per day for at least 3 days before her scheduled test. She then ingests a 100-g oral glucose solution in the morning after an overnight fast. Plasma glucose is measured fasting and at 1, 2, and 3 hours. A diagnosis of GDM occurs if two or more of the following values are met or exceeded:

Fasting	95 mg/dL
1 hour	180 mg/dL
2 hours	155 mg/dL
3 hours	140 mg/dL

In the one-step approach, the woman ingests a 75-g oral glucose solution in the morning after an overnight fast. Plasma glucose levels are determined fasting and at 1 and 2 hours. A diagnosis of GDM occurs if any one of the following values are equaled or exceeded:

Fasting	92 mg/dL
1 hour	180 mg/dL
2 hours	153 mg/dL

Laboratory Assessment of Long-term Glucose Control

Glycosylated hemoglobin (hemoglobin A1C) is a laboratory test that loosely reflects glucose control over the previous 4–8 weeks. It measures the percentage of glycohemoglobin in the blood. Glycohemoglobin is the hemoglobin to which a glucose molecule is attached. The test is not reliable for screening for gestational diabetes and is not recommended at this time.

In women with known pregestational diabetes, however, abnormal hemoglobin A1C values correlate directly with the frequency of spontaneous abortion and fetal congenital anomalies. Consequently, women with preexisting diabetes who plan to become pregnant should work to achieve hemoglobin A1C levels at target levels (less than 6%) without significant hypoglycemia (ADA, 2014). Once the woman is pregnant, her hemoglobin A1C levels should be tested at the initial prenatal visit and every 2–3 months if target levels have been achieved (ADA, 2014).

Diet therapy and regular exercise form the cornerstone of intervention for GDM. Insulin therapy is indicated when dietary management is unable to achieve a 1-hour postprandial blood glucose value of less than 130–140 mg/dL, a 2-hour postprandial level of less than 120 mg/dL, or a fasting glucose of less than 95 mg/dL. In most instances, the overt diabetic manifestation disappears postpartum, though subtle manifestations of impaired insulin secretory capacity may remain.

Oral hypoglycemics are used during pregnancy when needed, with Glyburide being the most common.

Evaluation of Fetal Status

Information about the well-being, maturation, and size of the fetus is important for planning the course of the pregnancy and the timing of birth. Because pregnancies complicated by preexisting diabetes are at increased risk of neural tube defects, a quadruple screen, which includes testing for maternal serum α-*fetoprotein (AFP)*, is offered at weeks 16–20 of gestation. Daily maternal evaluation of *fetal activity*, begun at about 28 weeks, is effective and simple to do. The woman is taught a particular method for counting fetal movements.

Nonstress testing (NST) may be started at about 28 weeks. If evidence of IUGR, preeclampsia, oligohydramnios, or poorly controlled blood glucose exists, testing may begin as early as 23 weeks and may be done more often. NSTs are increased to twice weekly at 32 weeks' gestation. If the NST is nonreactive, a fetal biophysical profile is performed. If the woman requires hospitalization (for example, to control glycemia or for complications), NSTs may be done daily.

Ultrasound at 18 weeks confirms gestational age and diagnoses multiple pregnancy or congenital anomalies. It is repeated at 28 weeks to monitor fetal growth for IUGR or macrosomia. Some physicians order *fetal biophysical profiles* (ultrasound evaluation of fetal well-being in which fetal breathing movements, fetal activity, reactivity, muscle tone, and amniotic fluid volume are assessed) as part of an ongoing evaluation of fetal status.

Alterations and Therapies

Pregnancy

ALTERATION	DESCRIPTION	THERAPY
Pregestational Factors		
Prenatal substance abuse	Use of tobacco, alcohol, or illegal substances, including cocaine, methamphetamines, narcotics, or abuse of prescription medications. Such use can be profoundly harmful to the fetus.	■ Nursing care is focused on motivating the patient to abstain from substance use and on supporting the patient through the withdrawal-and-recovery period. ■ For more information, see Exemplar 22.C, Substance Abuse, in the module on Addiction.
Diabetes mellitus	An endocrine disorder of carbohydrate metabolism resulting from inadequate production or use of insulin. The patient may be diagnosed with diabetes before becoming pregnant or develop gestational diabetes during pregnancy.	■ Patient teaching is important to promote self-care focused on stable glucose levels using a balance of diet, exercise, medications, and frequent monitoring. ■ For more information, see Exemplar 12.A, Type 1 Diabetes Mellitus, in the module on Metabolism.
Anemia	Inadequate levels of hemoglobin in the blood, defined as levels of <11 g/dL during pregnancy (ACOG, 2015b) caused by either insufficient hemoglobin production related to nutritional deficiency in iron or folic acid or to hemoglobin destruction in inherited disorders, such as sickle cell disease.	■ Monitor patients for symptoms of anemia (fatigue, pallor, shortness of breath, and alterations in level of consciousness). ■ Promote good nutrition in order to meet the body's metabolic needs. For more information, see Exemplar 2.B, Anemia, in the module on Cellular Regulation.
HIV/AIDS	Viral infection caused by the human immunodeficiency virus (HIV); called AIDS (acquired immunodeficiency syndrome) when symptoms of the disease appear.	■ Reassure the pregnant woman that risk of transmission to the fetus can be reduced by use of antiretroviral medication, that pregnancy is not believed to accelerate progression of the disease, and that most medications used to treat HIV can be safely taken during pregnancy. ■ Cesarean birth and abstaining from breastfeeding are recommended to reduce the risk of transmission to the baby. ■ For more information, see Exemplar 8.A, HIV and AIDS, in the module on Immunity.
Heart disease	Pregnancy increases cardiac output, heart rate, and blood volume, which the normal heart can adapt to but which may put stress on the heart of a patient with decreased cardiac reserve. Women in Class I or II usually experience a normal pregnancy; those in Class III or IV are at risk for more severe complications.	■ Assess the stress of pregnancy on functional capacity of the heart during all antepartum visits. This includes monitoring vital signs and comparing them with prepregnancy levels, activity level, and factors that increase strain on the heart, such as anemia, infection, anxiety, lack of a support system, and lifestyle demands (career, home life, and other children to care for). ■ For more information, see the module on Perfusion.
Asthma	An obstructive lung condition that can improve symptoms in some pregnant women and worsen symptoms in others. Asthma has also been linked with higher rates of hyperemesis gravidarum, preeclampsia, uterine hemorrhage, and perinatal mortality.	■ Promote oxygenation to prevent hypoxia in both the mother and the fetus. ■ Teach the woman how to recognize signs of preterm labor, because the rate of premature birth is higher in patients with asthma. ■ The goal of therapy is to prevent maternal exacerbations, because even a mild exacerbation can cause severe hypoxia-related complications in the fetus. If an exacerbation occurs, inhaled albuterol may be recommended by the healthcare provider. ■ For more information, see Exemplar 15.B, Asthma, in the module on Oxygenation.

(continued on next page)

Alterations and Therapies (continued)

ALTERATION	DESCRIPTION	THERAPY
Epilepsy	Chronic disorder characterized by seizures. Many women have uneventful pregnancies with excellent outcomes. Those with more frequent seizures before pregnancy may have exacerbations during pregnancy. Encourage patients to consult with their neurologists before and during pregnancy.	■ Teach the patient to continue taking recommended antiseizure medication as well as supplementing with folic acid and vitamin K throughout the pregnancy to improve fetal outcome. ■ For more information, see Exemplar 11.B, Seizure Disorders, in the module on Intracranial Regulation.
Hyperthyroidism	Enlarged, overactive thyroid gland. This can increase the risk for preeclampsia and postpartum hemorrhage in the mother and for abortion, intrauterine death, and stillbirth in the fetus if not well controlled. Even low doses of antithyroid drug in the mother may produce a mild fetal/neonatal hypothyroidism; higher dose may produce a goiter or mental deficiencies. Fetal loss is not increased in women who are euthyroid.	■ Nursing care is focused on early identification and treatment. ■ For more information, see Exemplar 12.F, Thyroid Disease, in the module on Metabolism.
Hypothyroidism	Characterized by inadequate thyroid secretions (decreased thyroxine [T_4]:thyroxine-binding globulin [TBG] ratio), elevated thyroid-stimulating hormone (TSH), lowered basal metabolic rate, and enlarged thyroid gland (goiter). Long-term replacement therapy usually continues during pregnancy at the same dosage as before. If the mother is untreated, the rate of fetal loss is 50%, with a high risk for congenital goiter or true cretinism. Therefore, newborns are screened for T_4 level. Mild TSH elevations present little risk because TSH does not cross the placenta.	■ Nursing care is focused on early identification and treatment to prevent potential complications. ■ Teach the patient the importance of taking a thyroid hormone supplement regularly to maintain stable levels. ■ For more information, see Exemplar 12.F, Thyroid Disease, in the module on Metabolism.
Multiple sclerosis	Neurologic disorder that destroys the myelin sheath of nerve fibers and affects primarily young women. Pregnancy is associated with remission and slightly increased relapse rates postpartum. Uterine contraction strength is not diminished, but labor may be almost painless because of diminished sensation.	■ Nursing care is focused on promoting rest and nutrition. ■ For more information, see Exemplar 13.D, Multiple Sclerosis, in the module on Mobility.
Rheumatoid arthritis	Chronic inflammatory disease believed to have a genetic component. Remission of symptoms is common during the antepartum period, with relapse in the postpartum period. Heavy salicylate use may prolong gestation and lengthen labor. Salicylates may have possible teratogenic effects.	■ Monitor for anemia secondary to blood loss from salicylate therapy. ■ Encourage rest to relieve weight-bearing joints, but the patient needs to continue range-of-motion exercises. ■ The patient in remission may be advised to stop medications during pregnancy. ■ For more information, see Exemplar 8.C, Rheumatoid Arthritis, in the module on Immunity.
Systemic lupus erythematosus (SLE)	Autoimmune collagen disease characterized by exacerbations and remissions. Women who conceive when the disease is in remission appear to have little risk for adverse outcomes. Those with active disease have less favorable outcomes, although pregnancy does not appear to alter the long-term prognosis (Nili et al., 2013). Increased incidence of spontaneous abortion, stillbirth, prematurity, and intrauterine growth restriction (IUGR). Babies born to women with SLE may have characteristic skin rash, which usually disappears by 12 months. Neonates are at increased risk for complete congenital heart block, a condition that can be diagnosed prenatally (Nili et al., 2013). When diagnosed, the mother is given corticosteroids that cross the placenta and decrease fetal heart inflammation (Davidson et al., 2017).	■ Nursing care is focused on providing emotional support throughout the pregnancy and monitoring fetal well-being. Women with SLE have often experienced prenatal loss and may be very fearful about the outcome of pregnancy. ■ For more information, see Exemplar 8.D, Systemic Lupus Erythematosus, in the module on Immunity.

Alterations and Therapies (continued)

ALTERATION	DESCRIPTION	THERAPY
Tuberculosis (TB)	An infection caused by *Mycobacterium tuberculosis*, which often affects the lungs. There has been a significant increase in diagnosis of TB, often associated with HIV infection, living in homeless shelters, and illicit drug use (Cunningham et al., 2014). Eighty percent of new cases are found in developing countries, primarily in Africa and Asia. In the United States, the majority of cases occur in foreign-born people (CDC, 2013). The relapse rate does not increase if TB is inactive because of prior treatment. Isoniazid crosses the placenta, but most studies show no teratogenic effects. Rifampin also crosses the placenta, and the possibility of harmful effects is still being studied.	■ When isoniazid is used during pregnancy, the woman should take supplemental pyridoxine (vitamin B_6). ■ Extra rest and limited contact with others are required until the disease becomes inactive. ■ If maternal TB is inactive, the mother may breastfeed and care for her baby. If TB is active, the newborn should not have direct contact with the mother until she is noninfectious. ■ For more information, see Exemplar 9.G, Tuberculosis, in the module on Infection.
Gestational Onset		
Vaginal bleeding	Primarily the result of abortion (miscarriage) during the first and second trimesters. Bleeding can also result from complications, such as ectopic pregnancy or gestational trophoblastic disease. In the second half of pregnancy, bleeding is often caused by placenta previa and abruptio placentae.	■ Monitor blood pressure and pulse frequently. ■ Observe the woman for behaviors indicative of shock, such as pallor, clammy skin, perspiration, dyspnea, or restlessness. ■ Count and weigh pads to assess amount of bleeding over a given time period; save any tissue or clots expelled. ■ If at 12 weeks' gestation or beyond, assess fetal heart tones with a Doppler. ■ Prepare the woman for intravenous (IV) therapy. There may be standing orders to begin IV therapy on patients who are bleeding. ■ Prepare equipment for examination. ■ For more information, see Exemplar 16.L, Shock, in the module on Perfusion; and Exemplar 19.D, Menstrual Dysfunction, in the module on Sexuality.
Spontaneous abortion (miscarriage)	Many pregnancies end in the first trimester by spontaneous abortion, often without the woman's awareness that she was even pregnant. Most miscarriages result from chromosomal abnormalities. Other causes include teratogens, faulty implantation because of an abnormal reproductive tract, weakened cervix, placental abnormalities, chronic maternal diseases, endocrine imbalances, and maternal infections.	■ Miscarriage during the first trimester can rarely be reversed, so nursing care is focused on providing emotional support and preventing complications. ■ Discourage use of hot tubs, because hyperthermia increases risk.
Ectopic pregnancy	Implantation of the fertilized ovum in a site other than the endometrial lining of the uterus. Ectopic pregnancy has many associated risk factors, including tubal damage caused by pelvic inflammatory disease, previous tubal surgery, congenital anomalies of the tube, endometriosis, previous ectopic pregnancy, presence of an intrauterine device, and in utero exposure to diethylstilbestrol.	■ Nursing care is focused on early identification, providing emotional support, and preventing complications secondary to blood loss. ■ Pain management is an important nursing intervention. ■ Assess human chorionic gonadotropin (hCG) levels (often lower with ectopic pregnancy and do not increase normally). ■ Prepare the patient for surgery. ■ Provide postoperative reassurance that pregnancy is still possible with one remaining fallopian tube.
Gestational trophoblastic disease (GTD)	Pathologic proliferation of trophoblastic cells (the trophoblast is the outermost layer of embryonic cells). This includes hydatidiform mole, invasive mole (chorioadenoma destruens), and choriocarcinoma.	■ Teach the woman about the need for regular screening for choriocarcinoma. ■ Assess all pregnant women for symptoms of GTD, including vaginal bleeding that is brown with greater uterine enlargement than expected for gestational age. ■ Follow quantitative hCG levels (discussed in greater detail in the Concept section of the module on Sexuality).

(continued on next page)

Alterations and Therapies (continued)

ALTERATION	DESCRIPTION	THERAPY
Hyperemesis gravidarum	Excessive vomiting during pregnancy that progress to a point at which the woman not only vomits everything she swallows but also retches between meals. Increased hCG levels may play a role.	■ Assess hydration. ■ Administer IV fluids. ■ Assess nutritional status. ■ Total parenteral nutrition may be administered to prevent malnutrition. ■ Keep patient away from food odors that may increase nausea and vomiting. ■ Maintain oral hygiene. ■ For more information on treating dehydration, see Exemplar 9.A, Fluid and Electrolyte Imbalance, in the module on Fluids and Electrolytes.
Hypertensive disorders	Preeclampsia, eclampsia, chronic hypertension, and gestational hypertension.	■ Nursing care focuses on prevention and early detection. ■ For more information, see Exemplar 16.H, Hypertensive Disorders in Pregnancy, in the module on Perfusion.
Alloimmunization	Destruction of fetal hemoglobin. When the mother is Rh negative and the fetus is Rh positive, alloimmunization may occur in second and successive pregnancies if maternal-fetal blood mixture occurs, whether the pregnancy was carried to term or not. Alloimmunization causes fetal anemia, resulting in marked fetal edema (hydrops fetalis). Congestive heart failure may result. Marked jaundice leading to neurologic damage is also a risk.	■ Administer Rh immunoglobulin at 28 weeks of gestation if the pregnancy continues, or immediately following a spontaneous miscarriage if the mother is Rh negative and the father is Rh positive, or within 72 hours after delivery if the mother is Rh negative and the baby is Rh positive. ■ Assess lab results for positive Coombs test, indicating sensitization, in which case Rh immunoglobulin is not administered.
ABO incompatibility	When a woman who has type O blood becomes pregnant with a type A, B, or AB fetus, causing interaction of antibodies present in maternal serum and the antigen sites on the fetal red blood cells. ABO incompatibility does not normally cause the severity of hemolysis seen with Rh incompatibility.	■ Assess blood type during prenatal care, and document so that the newborn can be followed after birth for potential hyperbilirubinemia if ABO incompatibility is likely.
Herpes simplex virus	Viral infection causing painful lesions in the genital area; may also occur on the cervix. This infection can profoundly affect the fetus. Primary infection has been associated with spontaneous abortion, low birth weight, and preterm birth. Transmission to the fetus usually occurs with membrane rupture and rarely via transplacental infection. If the fetus is infected, symptoms may include fever or hypothermia, jaundice, seizures, and poor feeding.	■ Prepare the mother for the need for cesarean birth if active lesions are present when she goes into labor.
Group B streptococcal (GBS) infection	Bacterial infection is found in the lower gastrointestinal or urogenital tracts of 10–40% of pregnant women (AAP & ACOG, 2012). Women may transmit GBS infection to their fetus in utero or during childbirth. GBS is one of the major causes of early-onset neonatal infection. Newborns become infected by vertical transmission from the mother during birth or by horizontal transmission from colonized nursing personnel or colonized babies. GBS causes severe, invasive disease in newborns.	■ Nursing care is focused on detection and early intervention during pregnancy in order to resolve the infection before delivery and, if not resolved prior, through prescribed IV antibiotics during labor.

Alterations and Therapies (continued)

ALTERATION	DESCRIPTION	THERAPY
Urinary tract infections	Dysuria, urgency, frequency; low-grade fever and hematuria. If not treated, infection may ascend and lead to acute pyelonephritis, which is associated with increased risk of premature birth and IUGR.	▪ Nursing care is focused on teaching the woman the signs to report in order to allow quick intervention and to prevent potential complications. ▪ Oral sulfonamides taken in the last few weeks of pregnancy may lead to neonatal hyperbilirubinemia and kernicterus.
Vulvovaginal candidiasis	Fungal infection manifested by thick, white, curdy discharge as well as by severe itching, dysuria, and dyspareunia. If the infection is present at birth and the fetus is born vaginally, the fetus may contract thrush.	▪ Nursing care is focused on teaching the woman the signs and symptoms of infection, preventive measures, and rapid recognition so that treatment can be initiated quickly.
Syphilis	Sexually transmitted infection manifested by chancre lasting 3–6 weeks, then often asymptomatic until Stage III. Syphilis can be passed transplacentally to the fetus. If untreated, one of the following can occur: second trimester abortion, stillborn baby at term, congenitally infected baby, or uninfected live newborn. (For more information, see Exemplar 19.E, Sexually Transmitted Infections, in the module on Sexuality.)	▪ Screening for infections should be part of prenatal care in order to treat and eliminate the infection before delivery.

Assessment of Fetal Well-being

A number of tests are used to obtain accurate and helpful data about the developing fetus. At times, just one test is done; in other circumstances, a combination of testing is necessary. Some of these assessment techniques pose risks to the fetus and, possibly, to the pregnant woman; the risk to both should be considered before deciding to perform the test. The healthcare provider must be certain that the advantages outweigh the potential risks and added expense. In addition, the diagnostic accuracy and applicability of these tests may vary. Although some tests are for *screening* purposes, meaning that they indicate the fetus may be at risk for a certain disorder or anomaly, others are *diagnostic*, meaning that they can diagnose the abnormality. Not all high-risk pregnancies require the same tests.

Before administration of any screening or diagnostic test, the nurse should use the following guide to ensure that the patient knows the reason for performing the procedure:

1. Assess whether the woman knows the reason why the screening or diagnostic test is being recommended:
   - "Has your physician or nurse-midwife told you why this test is necessary?"
   - "Sometimes tests are done for many different reasons. Can you tell me why you are having this test?"
   - "What is your understanding about what the test will show?"

2. Provide an opportunity for questions:
   - "Do you have any questions about the test?"
   - "Is there anything that is not clear to you?"

3. Explain* the test procedure, paying particular attention to any preparation the woman needs before the test:
   - "The test that has been ordered for you is designed to _____." (*Add specific information about the particular test. Give the explanation in simple language.*)

4. Validate the woman's understanding of the preparation:
   - "Tell me what you will have to do to get ready for this test."

5. Give permission for the woman to continue to ask questions if needed:
   - "I'll be with you during the test. If you have any questions at any time, please don't hesitate to ask."

Selected conditions that indicate a pregnancy is at risk include the following:

- Maternal age less than 16 or more than 35 years
- Chronic maternal hypertension, preeclampsia, diabetes mellitus, or heart disease
- Presence of Rh isoimmunization (immune response to foreign antigen Rh-positive cells)
- Maternal history of fetal demise (stillbirth)
- Suspected IUGR
- Pregnancy prolonged past 42 weeks of gestation
- Multiple gestation
- Prior preterm birth
- Previous pregnancy losses before 20 weeks' gestation or diagnosed cervical insufficiency.

---

*For any procedure that requires consent, the healthcare provider should explain the procedure, not the nurse.

Maternal Assessment of Fetal Activity

Clinicians now generally agree that vigorous fetal activity provides reassurance of fetal well-being and that a marked decrease in activity or cessation of movement may indicate possible fetal compromise (or even death), requiring immediate follow-up (Blackburn, 2013). Maternal assessment is typically used to monitor fetal well-being beginning at approximately 28 weeks of gestation. It provides a low-technology, inexpensive means to evaluate fetal well-being. A reduction of fetal movement has been associated with fetal hypoxia, fetal growth restriction, and fetal death (Malm et al., 2014).

Although there is no standard definition of how many movements should occur within a specified time, if there are fewer than 10 movements in a 12-hour period, or fewer than three in a 1-hour period, or if the amount of movement is significantly less than normal, the woman should immediately notify her healthcare provider. A maternal perception of decreased movement occurring during a 24-hour period should cause concern and warrant antepartum fetal testing.

Fetuses spend approximately 25% of their time making gross body movements. Fetal movements are directly related to the fetus's sleep–wake cycle and vary from the maternal sleep–wake cycle (Blackburn, 2013; O'Neill & Thorp, 2012). Fetuses may react to maternal hypoglycemia by decreasing their activity level. In women with a multiple gestation, daily fetal movements are significantly higher. After 38 weeks, fetuses spend 75% of their time in a quiet-sleep or active-sleep state. Other factors affecting fetal movement include sound, cigarette smoking, and drugs.

A variety of methods for tracking fetal activity have been developed. These methods focus on having the pregnant woman keep a fetal movement record, such as the Cardiff Count-to-Ten method (**Figure 33–28 ≫**) or the Daily Fetal Movement Record (DFMR). A **fetal movement record** is a

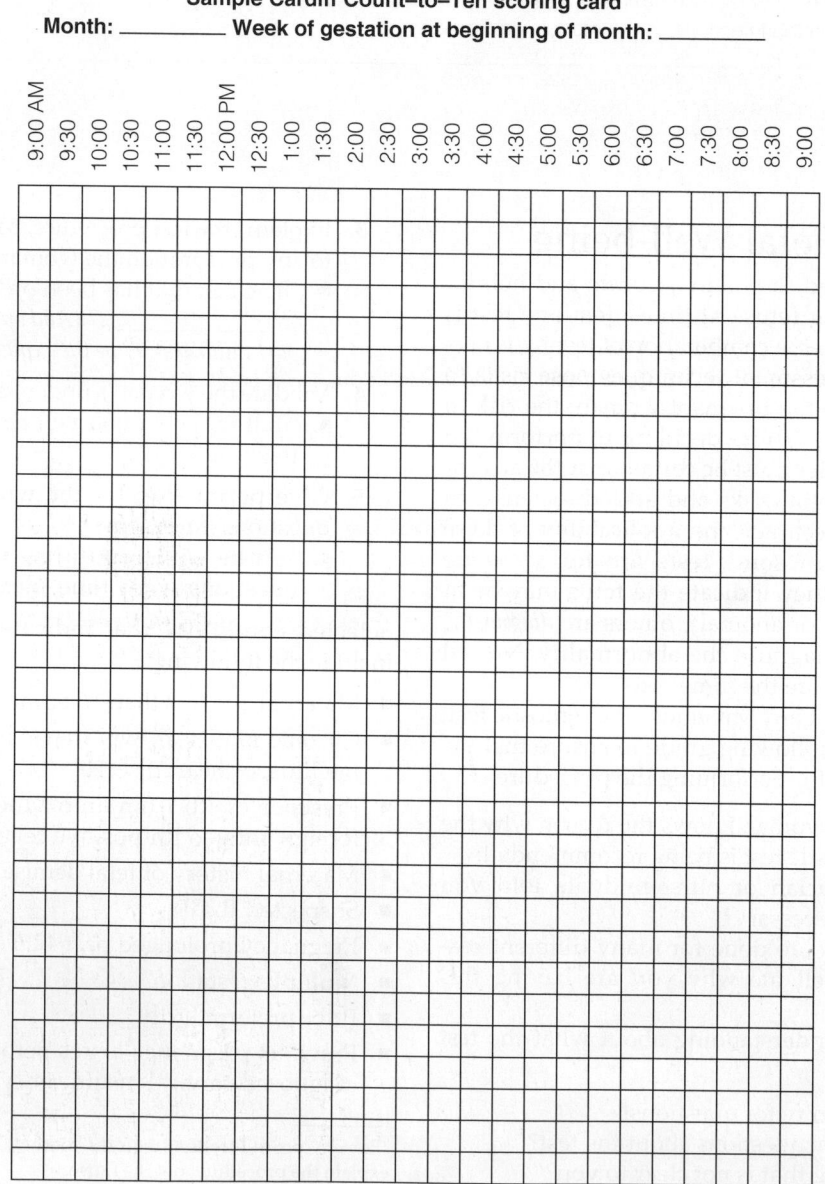

Figure 33–28 ≫ An adaptation of the Cardiff Count-to-Ten scoring card for assessment of fetal movement.

Patient Teaching
Maternal Assessment of Fetal Activity

- Explain that fetal movements are first felt around 18 weeks of gestation. This is called *quickening*. From that time, the fetal movements get stronger and easier to detect. A slowing or stopping of fetal movement may be an indication that the fetus needs some attention and evaluation. The mother's perception of decreased fetal movement is sufficient in most cases. Formal tracking of fetal movement does not lead to improved outcomes in low-risk pregnancies but may have value in high-risk situations.

- Describe the procedures, and demonstrate how to assess fetal movement. Sit beside the woman and show her how to place her hand on the fundus to feel fetal movement. Advise the woman to keep a daily record of fetal movements beginning at about 28 weeks of gestation.

- Explain the procedure for the Cardiff Count-to-Ten method:
  a. Beginning at the same time each day, have the woman place an X on the Cardiff card (Figure 33–28) for each fetal movement she perceives during normal everyday activity until she has recorded 10 of them.
  b. Movement varies considerably, but the woman should feel fetal movement at least 10 times in 12 hours, and many women will feel 10 fetal movements in much less time, possibly 2 hours or less.

- Explain the procedure for the Daily Fetal Movement Record (DFMR) method:

  a. The woman should begin counting at about the same time each day, after taking food.
  b. She should lie quietly in a side-lying position.
  c. The woman should feel at least three fetal movements within 1 hour.

- Instruct the woman to contact her care provider in the following situations:
  a. Using the Cardiff method: If there are fewer than 10 movements in 12 hours.
  b. Using the DFMR method: If there are fewer than three movements in 1 hour.
  c. Both methods: If overall the fetus's movements are slowing, and it takes much longer each day to note the minimum number of movements in the specified time period, and if there are no movements in the morning.
  d. If there are fewer than three movements in 8 hours.

- Whichever method she is using, encourage the woman to complete her fetal movement record daily and to bring it with her during each prenatal visit. Assure her that the record will be discussed at each prenatal visit and that questions may be addressed at that time if desired.

- Provide the woman with a name and phone number in case she has further questions.

---

noninvasive technique that enables the pregnant woman to monitor and record movements easily and without expense. See Patient Teaching: Maternal Assessment of Fetal Activity.

The expectant mother's perception of fetal movements and her commitment to completing a fetal movement record may vary. When a woman understands the purpose of the assessment, how to complete the form, whom to call with questions, and what to report—and has the opportunity for follow-up during each visit—she generally views completing the fetal movement record as an important activity. The nurse should be available to answer questions and clarify areas of concern.

Ultrasound

Valuable information about the fetus may be obtained from **ultrasound** testing, in which intermittent ultrasonic waves (high-frequency sound waves) are transmitted by an alternating current to a transducer, which is applied to the woman's abdomen. The ultrasonic waves are deflected by tissues within the patient's abdomen, showing structures of varying densities (**Figures 33–29 ≫** and **33–30 ≫**).

Diagnostic ultrasound has several advantages. It is noninvasive, painless, and nonradiating to both the woman and the fetus. Serial studies (several ultrasound tests done over a span of time) may be done for assessment and comparison.

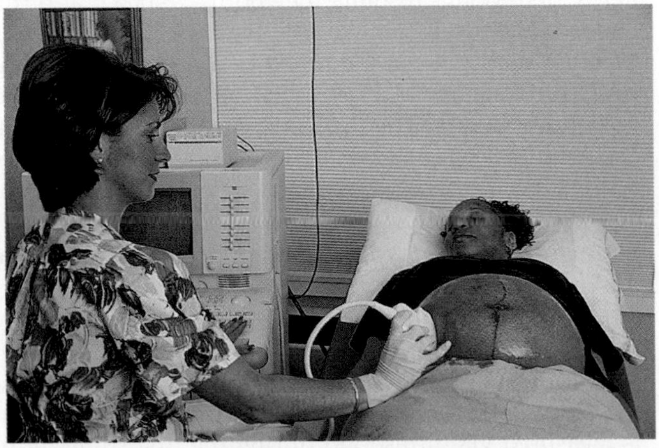

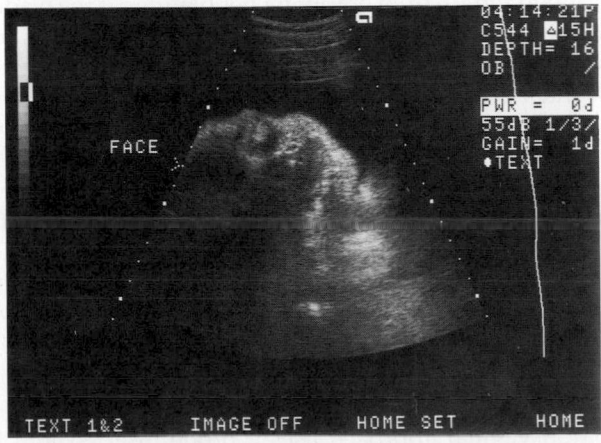

Figure 33–29 ≫ Ultrasound scanning permits visualization of the fetus in utero.

Figure 33–30 ≫ Ultrasound of fetal face.

Soft-tissue masses (e.g., tumors) can be differentiated, the fetus can be visualized, fetal growth can be followed (especially in the presence of multiple gestation), cervical length and impending cervical insufficiency can be detected, and a number of other potential problems can be averted. In addition, the results are immediately available to the ultrasonographer and physician.

The use of four-dimensional ultrasound may eventually be able to generate future research regarding fetal well-being. Four-dimensional ultrasound combines the components of three-dimensional ultrasound with a fourth dimension, time, because it monitors live action. The technology produces images of photo-like quality, allowing healthcare providers to better visualize fetal structures and producing better guidance during invasive intrauterine procedures, such as amniocentesis and chorionic villus sampling. However, advanced 3D/4D techniques can increase the incidence of artifacts, or distortions, which could increase the need for additional scanning and increase parental anxiety (Malhotra et al., 2014).

Although ultrasound is believed to serve as a useful tool in monitoring the fetus throughout pregnancy, it does have limitations. Ultrasound is limited by maternal body habitus, fetal positioning, and technician or physician skill. Another limitation is that ultrasound cannot guarantee that a fetus does not have certain disorders or defects. Even though certain fetal problems can be diagnosed via the technology, sometimes abnormalities go unrecognized. A "normal" ultrasound is reassuring for the parents and the healthcare team, but it is important for parents to realize that a normal sonogram is not 100% reliable.

The two most common methods of ultrasound scanning are transabdominal and transvaginal.

Transabdominal Ultrasound

In the transabdominal approach, a transducer is moved across the patient's abdomen. The woman is often scanned with a full bladder, because when the bladder is full, the examiner can assess other structures, especially the vagina and cervix, in relation to the bladder. The ability to see the lower portion of the uterus and cervix is particularly important when vaginal bleeding is noted and placenta previa is the suspected cause. The patient is directed to drink 1–1.5 quarts of water approximately 2 hours before the examination and to refrain from emptying her bladder. If the bladder is not sufficiently filled, she is asked to drink three to four 8-oz glasses of water and is rescanned 30–45 minutes later.

A water-based transmission gel is generously spread over the woman's abdomen, and the sonographer slowly moves a transducer over the abdomen to obtain a picture of the uterine contents and surrounding structures. Ultrasound testing takes 20–30 minutes. The patient may feel discomfort caused by pressure applied over a full bladder. In addition, if the woman lies on her back during the test, she may develop shortness of breath. This may be relieved by elevating her upper body during the test.

Transvaginal Ultrasound

The transvaginal approach uses a probe inserted into the vagina. Once inserted, the transvaginal probe is close to the structures being imaged; therefore, it produces a clearer, more defined image. The improved images obtained by transvaginal ultrasound have enabled sonographers to identify struc-

tures and fetal characteristics earlier in pregnancy. Internal visualization can also be used as a predictor for preterm birth in high-risk patients (Cunningham et al., 2014). Use of the ultrasound technique to detect shortened cervical length or funneling (a cone-shaped indentation in the cervical os) is helpful in predicting preterm labor, especially in patients who have a history of preterm birth (Cunningham et al., 2014).

After the procedure is fully explained to the woman, she is prepared in the same manner as for a pelvic examination: in the lithotomy position, with appropriate drapes to provide privacy, and a female attendant in the room. It is important that her buttocks be at the end of the table so that, once inserted, the probe can be moved in various directions. A small, lightweight vaginal transducer is covered with a specially fitted sterile sheath, a condom, or one finger of a glove. Ultrasound gel is then applied to both the inside and outside of the covering, making insertion into the vagina easier and providing a medium for enhancing the ultrasound image. The transvaginal procedure can be accomplished with an empty bladder, and most women do not feel discomfort during the exam. The probe is smaller than a speculum, so insertion is usually completed with ease. The woman may feel the movement of the probe during the exam as various structures are imaged. Some patients may want to insert the probe themselves to enhance their comfort, whereas others would feel embarrassed even to be asked. The CNM, physician, or ultrasonographer offers the choice based on personal rapport with the patient.

Ultrasound testing can be of benefit in the following ways:

- ***Early identification of pregnancy.*** Pregnancy may be detected as early as the fifth or sixth week after the last menstrual period by assessing the gestational sac and the presence of a fetal heart rate (FHR) after 6 weeks of gestation.

- ***Observation of fetal heartbeat and fetal breathing movements.*** Fetal breathing movements have been observed as early as 11 weeks of gestation.

- ***Identification of more than one embryo or fetus.***

- ***Comparison of the biparietal diameter of the fetal head, head circumference, abdominal circumference, and femur length to assess growth patterns.*** These measurements help determine the gestational age of the fetus and identify IUGR.

- ***Clinical estimations of birth weight.*** This assessment helps identify macrosomia (newborns > 4000 g at birth) and low-birth-weight newborns (babies < 2500 g at birth). Macrosomia has been identified as a predictor of birth-related trauma and is a risk factor for both maternal and fetal morbidity (Jazayeri, 2012). It is used only as a guideline in clinical decision making. Antenatal estimates of fetal weight are poor predictors of both actual fetal weight and outcomes in labor and birth.

- ***Detection of fetal anomalies such as anencephaly and hydrocephalus.***

- ***Examination of nuchal translucency in the first trimester to assess for Down syndrome and other fetal structural anomalies*** (Sahota et al., 2012). Nuchal translucency describes an area in the back of the fetal neck that is measured via ultrasound during the first trimester of pregnancy. Nuchal translucency testing (NTT), also known as nuchal testing or nuchal fold testing, is performed at 11–13 weeks of gestation to screen for trisomies 13, 18, and 21 (Miguelez et al., 2012).

- *Examination of fetal cardiac structures (echocardiography).*
- *Length of fetal nasal bone.* The length of the fetal nasal bone during the NTT is used to indicate a risk factor for Down syndrome. Fetuses with a nonvisualized or shortened nasal bone are more likely to have trisomy 21 than are those with a normal-length nasal bone (Sonek et al., 2012).
- *Identification of amniotic fluid index (AFI).* Ultrasound can provide a rough measurement of the amount of amniotic fluid, which is an indicator of fetal well-being. The maternal abdomen is divided into quadrants using the umbilicus as the center point. The vertical diameter of the largest amniotic fluid pocket in each quadrant is measured. All measurements are totaled to obtain the AFI in centimeters. Women with an AFI of more than 24 cm are considered to have polyhydramnios (an excessive amount of amniotic fluid in the amniotic sac), and women with an AFI of less than 5 cm at term are considered to have oligohydramnios (not enough amniotic fluid). An AFI of between 5 and 24 cm is considered to be normal. After 39 weeks of gestation, the amniotic fluid volume begins to decline (Magann & Ross, 2014). Both polyhydramnios and oligohydramnios are associated with increased risk to the fetus, including nonreassuring fetal status, IUGR, meconium-stained amniotic fluid, and an increase in admissions to the neonatal intensive care unit.
- *Location of the placenta.* The placenta is located before amniocentesis to avoid puncturing it during the procedure. Ultrasound is valuable in identifying and evaluating placenta previa (Cunningham et al., 2014).
- *Placental grading.* As the fetus matures, the placenta calcifies. These changes can be detected by ultrasound and graded according to the degree of calcification. Placental grading can be used to identify internal placental vasculature, in which abnormalities can be associated with preeclampsia and chronic hypertension.
- *Detection of fetal death.* Inability to visualize the fetal heart beating and the separation of the bones in the fetal head are signs of fetal death.
- *Determination of fetal position and presentation.*
- *Accompanying procedures.* Ultrasound guidance is used in a variety of intrauterine procedures, including amniocentesis and chorionic villus sampling.

Nonstress Test

The **nonstress test (NST)**, a widely used method of evaluating fetal status, may be used alone or as part of a more comprehensive diagnostic assessment called a biophysical profile. The NST is based on the knowledge that when the fetus has adequate oxygenation and an intact CNS, accelerations of the FHR occur with fetal movement. An NST requires an external electronic fetal monitor to observe and record these FHR accelerations. A nonreactive NST is fairly consistent in identifying at-risk fetuses (Cunningham et al., 2014).

The advantages of the NST include the following:

- It is quick to perform, permits easy interpretation, and is inexpensive.

- It can be done in an office or clinic setting.
- It is a noninvasive procedure.
- There are no known side effects.

The disadvantages of the NST include the following:

- It is sometimes difficult to obtain a suitable tracing.
- The woman has to remain relatively still for at least 20 minutes.

Procedure for NST

The test can be done with the patient in a reclining chair or in bed with the patient in a left-tilted semi-Fowler or side-lying position. Research has shown that certain maternal positions can help produce more favorable results. Patients in left-tilted semi-Fowler, sitting, and left lateral positions are more likely to have a reactive tracing. Patients should not be placed in a supine position, because it decreases cardiac output and uterine perfusion, maternal back pain, and maternal shortness of breath (Cunningham et al., 2014). An electronic fetal monitor is used to obtain a tracing of the FHR and fetal movement. The nurse places the monitor under the woman's clothing. Privacy should be provided. The examiner puts two elastic belts on the patient's abdomen. One belt holds a device that detects uterine or fetal movement; the other belt holds a device that detects the FHR. As the NST is done, each fetal movement is documented so that associated or simultaneous FHR changes can be evaluated.

Interpretation of NST Results

An NST is indicated after 32 weeks at any time fetal well-being needs to be established. It may be used between 26 and 32 weeks with modified criteria for interpretation. The results of the NST are interpreted as follows:

- *Reactive test.* A reactive NST shows at least two accelerations of FHR with fetal movements of 15 beats/min, lasting 15 seconds or more, over 20 minutes (**Figure 33–31 》**). This is the desired result.
- *Nonreactive test.* In a nonreactive test, the reactive criteria are not met. For example, the accelerations do not meet the requirements of 15 beats/min or do not last 15 seconds (**Figure 33–32 》**).
- *Unsatisfactory test.* An NST is unsatisfactory if the data cannot be interpreted or there was inadequate fetal activity.

It is important that anyone who performs the NST understand the significance of any decelerations of the FHR during testing. If decelerations are noted, the healthcare provider should be notified for further evaluation of fetal status.

Fetal Acoustic and Vibroacoustic Stimulation Tests

Acoustic (sound) and vibroacoustic (vibration and sound) stimulation of the fetus can be used as an adjunct to the NST. A handheld, battery-operated device is applied to the woman's abdomen over the area of the fetal head. This device generates a low-frequency vibration and a buzzing sound. These are intended to induce movement and associated accelerations of

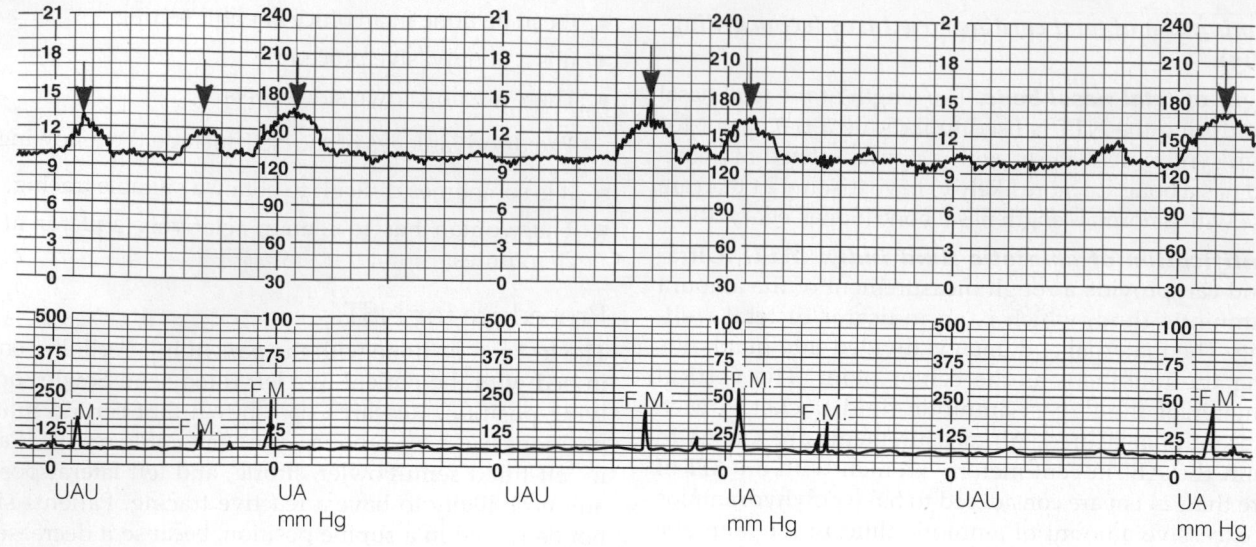

Figure 33–31 》 Example of a reactive nonstress test: accelerations of 15 beats/min lasting 15 seconds with each fetal movement (FM). Top of strip shows fetal heart rate (FHR); bottom of strip shows uterine activity tracing. Note that FHR increases (above the baseline) at least 15 beats and remains at that rate for at least 15 seconds before returning to the former baseline.

the FHR in fetuses with a nonreactive NST and in fetuses with decreased variability of the FHR during labor. The sound stimulus persists for 1 second; if no accelerations occur, it is then repeated at 1-minute intervals up to two times and then progresses to 2 seconds waiting 1 minute if no accelerations occur after the stimulus. Whether the fetus responds more to the vibration or to the sound is not known. Two FHR accelerations of 15 beats/min, lasting 15 seconds, in a 20-minute period indicate a reactive test (Cunningham et al., 2014).

Advantages of the fetal acoustic stimulation test and the vibroacoustic stimulation test include the following:

- Both are noninvasive techniques and are easy to perform.
- Results are rapidly available.
- Time for the NST is shortened.

Biophysical Profile

Use of the biophysical profile is indicated when there is risk of placental insufficiency or fetal compromise. The biophysical profile is a comprehensive assessment of five biophysical variables over a 30-minute period:

1. Fetal breathing movement
2. Fetal movements of body or limbs
3. Fetal tone (extension and flexion of extremities)
4. Amniotic fluid volume (visualized as pockets of fluid around the fetus)
5. FHR accelerations with activity (reactive NST).

The first four variables are assessed by ultrasound scanning; FHR reactivity is assessed with the NST. By combining

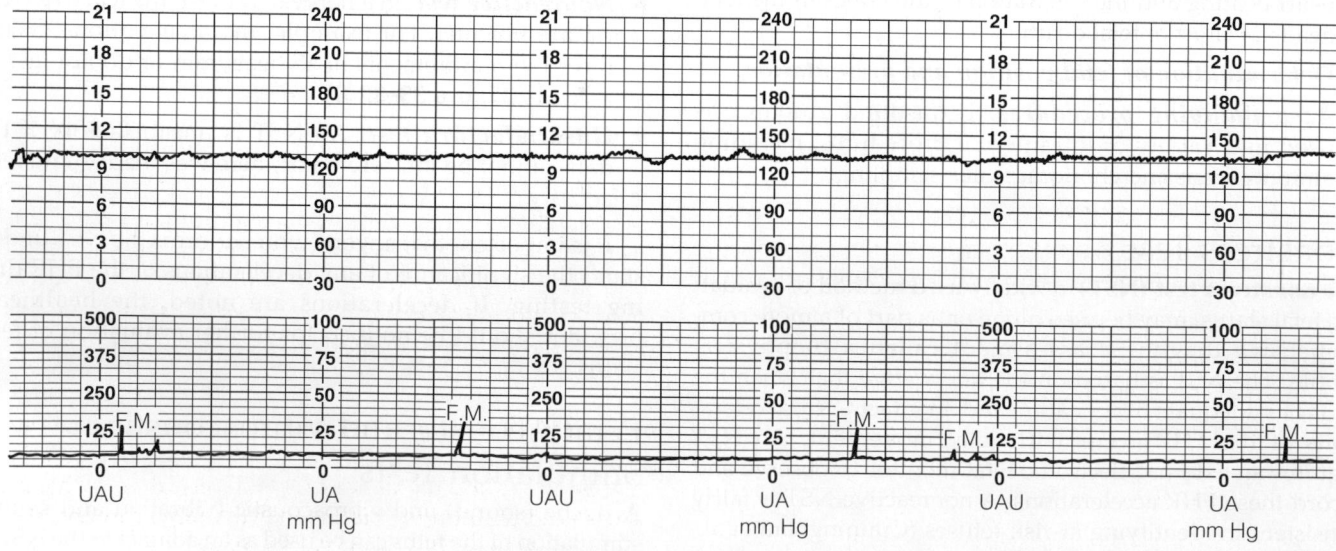

Figure 33–32 》 Example of a nonreactive nonstress test. There are no accelerations of the fetal heart rate (FHR) with fetal movement (FM). Baseline FHR is 130 beats/min. The tracing of uterine activity is on the bottom of the strip.

TABLE 33–3 Criteria for Biophysical Profile Scoring

Component	Normal (Score = 2)	Abnormal (Score = 0)
Fetal breathing movements	≥1 episode of rhythmic breathing lasting ≥30 seconds within 30 minutes	≤30 seconds of breathing in 30 minutes
Gross body movements	≥3 discrete body or limb movements in 30 minutes (episodes of active continuous movement considered as single movement)	≤2 movements in 30 minutes
Fetal tone	≥1 episode of extension of a fetal extremity with return to flexion or opening or closing of hand	No movements or extension/flexion
Amniotic fluid volume	Single vertical pocket >2 cm AFI >5 cm	Largest single vertical pocket ≤2 cm AFI <5 cm
Nonstress test	≥2 accelerations of ≥15 beats/min for ≥15 seconds in 20–40 minutes	0 or 1 acceleration in 20–40 minutes

these five assessments, the biophysical profile helps to identify the compromised fetus or to confirm the healthy fetus and also provides an assessment of placental functioning.

Specific criteria for normal and abnormal assessments are presented in **Table 33–3 》**. A score of 2 is assigned to each normal finding, and a score of 0 to each abnormal one, for a maximum score of 10. Scores of 8 and 10 are considered to be normal. Such scores have the least chance of being associated with a compromised fetus unless oligohydramnios is noted, in which case delivery of the fetus may be indicated (Thompson, Kuller, & Rhee, 2012).

Use of the biophysical profile may be indicated in the following conditions when there is risk of placental insufficiency or fetal compromise:

- IUGR
- Maternal diabetes mellitus
- Maternal heart disease
- Maternal chronic hypertension
- Maternal preeclampsia or eclampsia
- Maternal sickle cell disease
- Suspected fetal postmaturity (>42 weeks of gestation)
- History of previous stillbirths
- Rh sensitization
- Abnormal estriol excretion
- Hyperthyroidism
- Renal disease
- Nonreactive NST.

Contraction Stress Test

The **contraction stress test (CST)** is a means of evaluating the respiratory function (oxygen and carbon dioxide exchange) of the placenta. It enables the healthcare team to identify the fetus at risk for intrauterine asphyxia by observing the response of the FHR to the stress of uterine contractions (spontaneous or induced). During contractions, intrauterine pressure increases, and blood flow to the intervillous space of the placenta is momentarily reduced, thereby decreasing oxygen transport to the fetus. A healthy fetus usually tolerates this reduction well and maintains moderate variability. If the placental reserve is insufficient, however, then fetal hypoxia, depression of the myocardium, and a decrease in variability to minimal or absent may occur, indicating an altered state in fetal oxygen reserve.

In many areas, the CST has given way to the biophysical profile. It is still used, however, in areas where the availability of other technology is reduced (e.g., during night shifts) or limited (e.g., at small community hospitals or birthing centers). It may also be used as an adjunct to other forms of fetal assessment.

The CST is contraindicated in the patient with third-trimester bleeding from placenta previa, marginal abruptio placentae or unexplained vaginal bleeding, previous cesarean section with classic incision (vertical incision in the fundus of the uterus), premature rupture of the membranes, cervical insufficiency, cerclage in place (gathering stitch around cervix), anomalies of the maternal reproductive organs, history of preterm labor (if being done before term), or multiple gestation.

The critical component of the CST is the presence of uterine contractions. These contractions may occur spontaneously, which is unusual before the onset of labor, or they may be induced (stimulated) with oxytocin (Pitocin) administered intravenously (also known as an oxytocin challenge test). A natural method of obtaining oxytocin is through the use of breast stimulation (either via nipple self-stimulation or application of an electric breast pump); the posterior pituitary produces oxytocin in response to stimulation of the breasts or nipples.

An electronic fetal monitor is used to provide continuous data about the FHR and uterine contractions. After a 15-minute baseline recording of uterine activity and FHR, the tracing is evaluated for evidence of spontaneous contractions. If three spontaneous contractions of good quality and lasting 40–60 seconds occur in a 10-minute window, the results are evaluated, and the test is concluded. If no contractions occur, or if the contractions that do occur are insufficient for interpretation, then intravenous administration of oxytocin, breast self-stimulation, or application of an electric breast pump is done to produce contractions of good quality. The CST should be conducted only in a setting where tocolytic medications are available if a tachysystole pattern occurs or if labor is stimulated from the test.

The CST is classified as follows:

- **Negative.** A negative CST shows three contractions of good quality lasting 40 seconds or longer in a 10-minute period without evidence of late decelerations. This is the desired result and implies that the fetus can handle the hypoxic stress of uterine contractions.

- **Positive.** A positive CST shows repetitive, persistent, late decelerations, in which the fetal heart rate decreases after

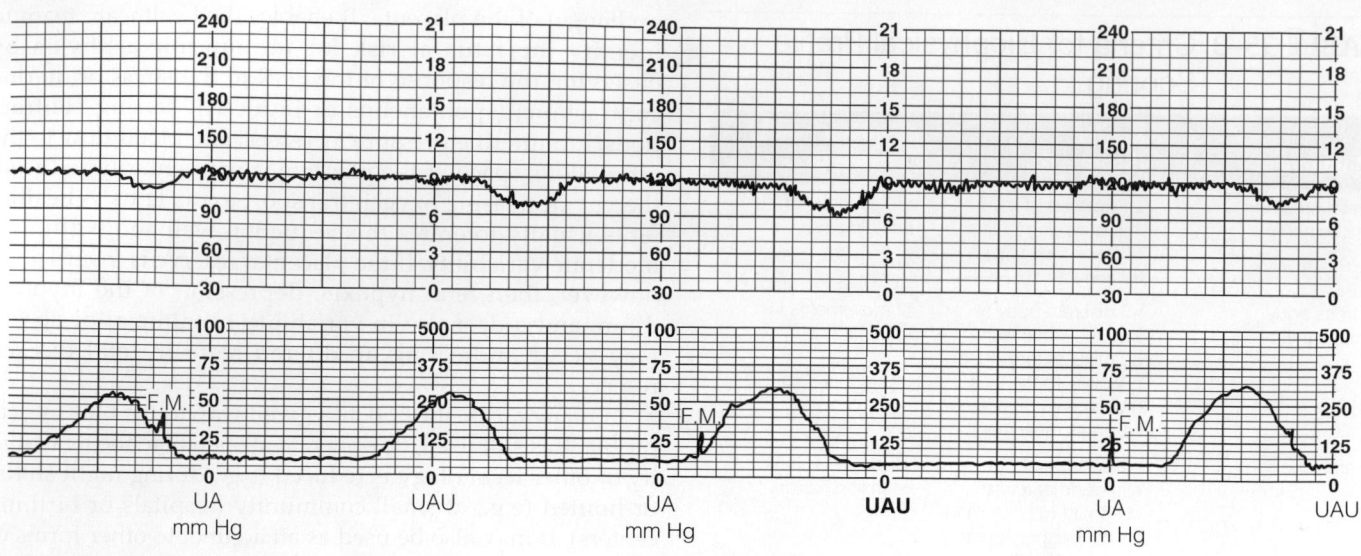

Figure 33–33 》》 Example of a positive contraction stress test. Repetitive late decelerations occur with each contraction. Note that there are no accelerations of fetal heart rate (FHR) with three fetal movements (FM). The baseline FHR is 120 beats/min. Uterine contractions (bottom half of strip) occurred four times in 12 minutes.

the onset of a contraction and recovers after the completion of a contraction, with more than 50% of the contractions (**Figure 33–33 》》**). This is not a desired result. The hypoxic stress of the uterine contraction causes a slowing of the FHR. The pattern will not improve, and will most likely get worse with additional contractions.

- *Equivocal.* An equivocal–suspicious test has non-persistent late decelerations associated with tachysystole (contraction frequency of every 2 minutes or duration lasting longer than 90 seconds). When this test result occurs, more information is needed (Davidson et al., 2017).

- *Unsatisfactory.* In an unsatisfactory CST, the quality of the tracing is too poor to accurately interpret FHR with contractions or the frequency of three contractions lasting 40–60 seconds occurring in a 10-minute window of time cannot be obtained for the end point of the test.

A negative CST implies that the placenta is functioning normally, fetal oxygenation is adequate, and the fetus will probably be able to withstand the stress of labor. If labor does not occur in the ensuing week, further testing is done.

A positive CST with a nonreactive NST presents evidence that the fetus will not likely withstand the stress of labor. A positive CST may be able to identify a compromised fetus earlier than a nonreactive NST because of the stimulated interruption of intervillous blood flow (Blackburn, 2013). Although a negative CST is reliable in predicting fetal status, a positive result needs to be verified, such as with a biophysical profile.

Amniotic Fluid Analysis

Amniocentesis is a procedure used to obtain amniotic fluid for genetic testing to determine fetal abnormalities or fetal lung maturity in the third trimester of pregnancy. During an amniocentesis, the physician scans the uterus using ultrasound to identify the fetal and placental positions and to identify adequate pockets of amniotic fluid. The skin is then cleaned with a Betadine solution. The use of a local anesthesia at the needle insertion site is optional. A 22-gauge needle is then inserted into the uterine cavity to withdraw amniotic fluid (**Figure 33–34 》》**). After 15–20 mL of fluid has been removed, the needle is withdrawn, and the site is assessed for streaming (movement of fluid), which is an indication of bleeding. The FHR and maternal vital signs are then assessed. Rh immune globulin is given to all Rh-negative women. The analysis of amniotic fluid provides valuable information about fetal status. Amniocentesis is a fairly simple procedure, although complications do occur on rare occasions (<1% of cases).

A number of studies can be performed on amniotic fluid. These tests can provide information about genetic disorders, fetal health, and fetal lung maturity. Concentrations of certain substances in amniotic fluid provide information about the health status of the fetus. An amniocentesis is 99% accurate in diagnosing genetic abnormalities. Because gestational age, birth weight, and the rate of development of organ systems do not necessarily correspond, amniotic fluid may also be analyzed to determine the maturity of the fetal lungs. Determination of fetal lung maturity is important when making clinical decisions regarding the timing of birth for women who may have complications, such as preeclampsia or diabetes.

Lecithin/Sphingomyelin Ratio

The alveoli of the lungs are lined with a substance called **surfactant**, which is composed of phospholipids. Surfactant lowers the surface tension of the alveoli when the newborn exhales. When a neonate with mature pulmonary function takes its first breath, a tremendously high pressure is needed to open the lungs. By lowering the alveolar surface tension, surfactant stabilizes the alveoli, and a certain amount of air always remains in the alveoli during expiration. Thus, when the neonate exhales, the lungs do not collapse. A baby born before synthesis of surfactant is complete, however, is unable

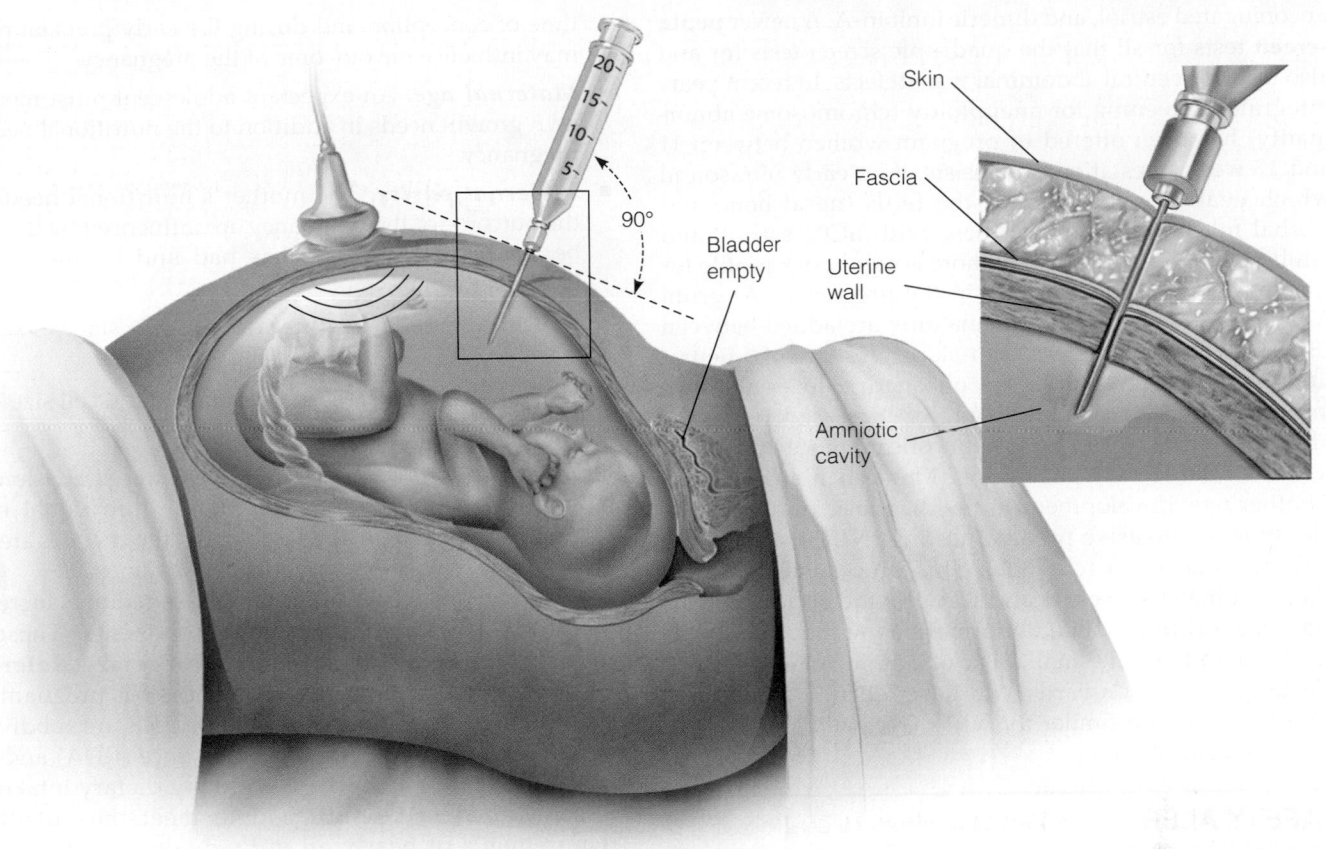

Figure 33–34 》 Amniocentesis. The woman is scanned by ultrasound to determine the placenta site and to locate a pocket of amniotic fluid. The needle is then inserted into the uterine cavity to withdraw amniotic fluid.

to maintain lung stability. Each breath requires the same effort as the first. This results in underinflation of the lungs and the development of respiratory distress syndrome.

Fetal lung maturity can be ascertained by determining the **lecithin/sphingomyelin (L/S) ratio**. Lecithin and sphingomyelin are two components of surfactant. Early in pregnancy, the sphingomyelin concentration in amniotic fluid is greater than the concentration of lecithin, and so the L/S ratio is low (i.e., lecithin levels are low, and sphingomyelin levels are high). At approximately 32 weeks of gestation, sphingomyelin levels begin to fall, and the amount of lecithin begins to increase. By 35 weeks of gestation, an L/S ratio of 4:1 is usually achieved in the normal fetus. An L/S ratio of 2:1 indicates that the risk of respiratory distress syndrome is very low. Under certain conditions of stress, such as a physiologic problem in the mother, placenta, and/or fetus (e.g., hypertension or placental insufficiency), the fetal lungs mature more rapidly (Angelini & Lafontaine, 2012).

Phosphatidylglycerol

Phosphatidylglycerol (PG) is another phospholipid in surfactant. PG is not present in the fetal lung fluid early in gestation. It appears when fetal lung maturity has been attained, at approximately 34 weeks of gestation. Because the presence of PG is associated with fetal lung maturity, when it is present, the risk of respiratory distress syndrome is low. Determination of PG is also useful in blood-contaminated specimens. Because PG is not present in blood or vaginal fluids, its presence is reliable in predicting fetal lung maturity.

Chorionic Villus Sampling

Chorionic villus sampling (CVS) involves obtaining a small sample of chorionic villi from the developing placenta.

The advantages of this procedure are early diagnosis and a short waiting time for results. Whereas amniocentesis is not done until at least 14 weeks of gestation, CVS is typically performed between 10 and 12 weeks of gestation. Previous studies that evaluated the use of CVS at 9 weeks of gestation found a possible association between limb-reduction birth defects and early CVS. Based on these findings, most practitioners do not recommend early CVS before 10 weeks of gestation (Cunningham et al., 2014). Risks of CVS include failure to obtain tissue, rupture of membranes, leakage of amniotic fluid, bleeding, intrauterine infection, maternal tissue contamination of the specimen, and Rh isoimmunization.

Because CVS testing is performed so early in the pregnancy, it cannot detect neural tube defects. Patients who desire screening for neural tube defects would need a quadruple screening or the AFP component of first trimester integrated screening at 15–20 weeks of gestation.

The **quadruple screen** is a widely used test to screen for Down syndrome (trisomy 21), trisomy 18, and neural tube defects. The serum test assesses for appropriate levels of alpha-fetoprotein, human chorionic gonadotropin, unconjugated estriol, and dimeric inhibin-A. A newer **penta screen** tests for all that the quadruple screen tests for and also tests for ventral abdominal wall defects. In recent years integrated screening for aneuploidy (chromosome abnormality) has been offered to pregnant women between 11 and 13 weeks' gestation. It consists of an early ultrasound which evaluates markers on the fetus (nasal bone and nuchal fold) and combines these with hCG, estriol, and inhibin A values to generate a more accurate risk profile for trisomy 13, 18, and 21 earlier in the pregnancy. A serum AFP and ultrasound for fetal anatomy are added between 18 and 20 weeks to determine risk or presence of a neural tube defect. Abnormal values on quadruple, penta, and integrated screens are indicators of increased risk only. They must be followed by a diagnostic amniocentesis from which a fetal karyotype is done (Messerlian et al., 2016). Another new development in the diagnosis of fetal aneuploidy is noninvasive prenatal testing (NIPT), also called cell free fetal DNA (cffDNA). This process detects fetal alleles in maternal serum and can provide accurate information on chromosomal abnormalities without the invasiveness and, albeit small, risk of amniocentesis from 9 weeks gestation onward (Wolfberg, 2016). Aneuploidy detection rates are similar for NIPT, CVS, and amniocentesis (King et al., 2013).

SAFETY ALERT When explaining options for genetic testing to expectant parents, inform them that even if a CVS shows no chromosomal abnormality, it cannot screen for neural tube defects. Patients who have a normal CVS and an abnormal quadruple screen test are to be offered amniocentesis. Patients with risk factors for neural tube defects may want to consider amniocentesis instead of CVS because amniocentesis screens for both types of disorders.

The nurse assists the physician during the amniocentesis or CVS and supports the woman undergoing the procedure. Although the physician has explained the procedure in advance so that the patient can give informed consent, the woman is likely to be apprehensive, both about the procedure itself and about the information it may reveal. She may become anxious during the procedure and need additional emotional support. The nurse can provide support by further clarifying the physician's instructions or explanations, by relieving the patient's physical discomfort when possible, and by responding verbally and physically to the woman's need for reassurance.

Factors Affecting Maternal Nutrition

A woman's nutritional status before and during pregnancy can significantly influence her health and that of her fetus. In most prenatal clinics and offices, nurses offer nutritional counseling directly or work closely with a nutritionist to provide nutritional assessment and teaching.

The following factors influence the pregnant woman's ability to achieve good prenatal nutrition:

- *General nutritional status before pregnancy.* Nutritional deficits, such as folic acid deficiency, present at the

time of conception and during the early prenatal period may influence the outcome of the pregnancy.

- *Maternal age.* An expectant adolescent must meet her own growth needs in addition to the nutritional needs of pregnancy.
- *Maternal parity.* The mother's nutritional needs and the outcome of the pregnancy are influenced by the number of pregnancies she has had and by the interval between them.

Fetal growth occurs in three overlapping stages:

1. Growth by increase in cell number
2. Growth by increases in cell number and cell size
3. Growth by increase in cell size alone.

Nutritional problems that interfere with cell division may have permanent consequences. If the nutritional insult occurs when cells are mainly enlarging, the changes are usually reversible when normal nutrition resumes.

Growth of fetal and maternal tissues requires increased quantities of essential dietary components. These are listed in the federal government's **Dietary Reference Intakes (DRIs)** as specific allowances for pregnant and lactating women (**Table 33–4 》**). The DRIs are subdivided into the recommended dietary allowance (RDA) and adequate intake (AI). An RDA is the daily dietary intake that is considered to be sufficient to meet the nutritional requirements of nearly all individuals in a specific life stage and gender group. An AI is the value cited for a nutrient when the data are not sufficient to calculate an estimated average requirement. Most of the recommended nutrients can be obtained by eating a well-balanced diet each day. **Table 33–5 》** is a sample daily food plan for pregnancy and lactation.

It is important to consider the many factors that affect a woman's nutrition. What environmental risks should the woman consider? What are her age, lifestyle, and culture? What food beliefs and habits does she have? What an individual eats is determined by availability, economics, and symbolism. These factors and others influence the expectant mother's acceptance of the nurse's intervention. For more information, see the module on Nutrition.

Socioeconomic Influences

Socioeconomic level may be a determinant of nutritional status. Families living at the poverty level cannot afford the same foods that higher-income families can. Thus, pregnant women with low incomes are frequently at risk for poor nutrition. Because access to healthy proteins and fresh fruits and vegetables is critical for pregnant women and very young children, federal, state, and local programs exist to provide at-risk women and their children with nutritional support. The largest program assisting low-income families and individuals is the Supplemental Nutrition Assistance Program (SNAP). This program works with state agencies, communities, educators, and faith-based organizations to provide nutrition assistance to those who qualify for benefits (U.S. Department of Agriculture, 2016). The largest program available for women and children is the Special Supplemental Nutrition

TABLE 33–4 Dietary Reference Intakes (DRIs) for Nonpregnant, Pregnant, and Lactating Females, Vitamins and Elements

	Age	Vitamin A (mcg/day)	Vitamin C (mg/day)	Vitamin D (mcg/day)	Vitamin E* (mg/day)
Females	9–13 yr	600	45	15	11
	14–18 yr	700	65	15	15
	19–70 yr	700	75	15	15
	>70 yr	700	75	20	15
Pregnancy	14–18 yr	750	80	15	15
	19–50 yr	770	85	15	15
Lactation	14–18 yr	1200	115	15	19
	19–50 yr	1300	120	15	19

	Age	Vitamin K (mcg/day)	Thiamine (mg/day)	Riboflavin (mg/day)	Niacin (mg/day)
Females	9–13 yr	60*	0.9	0.9	12
	14–18 yr	75*	1.0	1.0	14
	19–70 yr	90*	1.1	1.1	14
Pregnancy	14–18 yr	75*	1.4	1.4	18
	19–50 yr	90*	1.4	1.4	18
Lactation	14–18 yr	75*	1.4	1.6	17
	19–50 yr	90*	1.4	1.6	17

	Age	Vitamin B_6 (mg/day)	Folate[†] (mcg/day)	Vitamin B_{12} (mcg/day)	Calcium (mg/day)
Females	9–13 yr	1.0	300	1.8	1300*
	14–18 yr	1.2	400	2.4	1300*
	19–50 yr	1.3	400	2.4	1000*
	51– ≥70 yr	1.5	400	2.4	1200*
Pregnancy	14–18 yr	1.9	600	2.6	1300*
	19–50 yr	1.9	600	2.6	1000*
Lactation	14–18 yr	2.0	500	2.8	1300*
	19–50 yr	2.0	500	2.8	1000*

	Age	Iodine (mcg/day)	Iron (mg/day)	Magnesium (mg/day)	Phosphorus (mg/day)
Females	9–13 yr	120	8	240	1250
	14–18 yr	150	15	360	1250
	19–30 yr	150	18	310	700
	31–50 yr	150	18	320	700
	51– ≥70 yr	150	8	320	700
Pregnancy	≤18 yr	220	27	400	1250
	19–30 yr	220	27	350	700
	31–50 yr	220	27	360	700
Lactation	≤18 yr	290	10	360	1250
	19–30 yr	290	9	310	700
	31–50 yr	290	9	320	700

(continued on next page)

TABLE 33–4 Dietary Reference Intakes (DRIs) for Nonpregnant, Pregnant, and Lactating Females, Vitamins and Elements (continued)

	Age	Selenium (mcg/day)	Zinc (mg/day)
Females	9–13 yr	40	8
	14–18 yr	55	9
	19–30 yr	55	8
	31–70 yr	55	8
	>70 yr	55	12
Pregnancy	<18–30 yr	60	11
	31–50 yr	60	13
Lactation	≤18 – 50 yr	70	12

*Values are adequate intakes rather than recommended dietary allowances (RDAs). All other values on the chart are RDAs.

†In view of evidence linking folate intake with neural tube defects in the fetus, it is recommended that all women capable of becoming pregnant consume 400 mcg from supplements or fortified foods in addition to intake of food folate from a varied diet.

Source: Based on Institute of Medicine (IOM). (2010). *Dietary reference intakes (DRIs): Recommended dietary allowances and adequate intakes, vitamins and elements*. Washington, DC: Food and Nutrition Board, Institute of Medicine, National Academies.

Program for Women, Infants and Children (WIC) program, a federal program administered at the state level. WIC provides food vouchers and nutrition education to low-income and at-risk pregnant and postpartum women and for at-risk newborns/infants and children up to 5 years old.

》Stay Current: More information about the WIC program can be found at the program's website, www.fns.usda.gov/wic.

Cultural, Ethnic, and Religious Influences

Cultural, ethnic, and religious backgrounds determine an individual's experiences with food and influence that individual's food preferences and habits (**Figure 33–35 》**). Individuals of different nationalities are accustomed to eating different foods because of the kinds of foodstuffs available in their countries of origin. The way food is prepared varies depending on the customs and traditions of the ethnic and cultural group. In addition, the laws of certain religions sanction particular foods, prohibit others, and direct the preparation and serving of meals. For an example, see the accompanying Focus on Diversity and Culture feature.

In each culture, certain foods have symbolic significance. Generally these symbolic foods are related to major life experiences such as birth and death. Although generalizations have been made about the food practices of ethnic and religious groups, there are many variations. The extent to which individuals continue to consume traditional ethnic foods and follow food-related ethnic customs

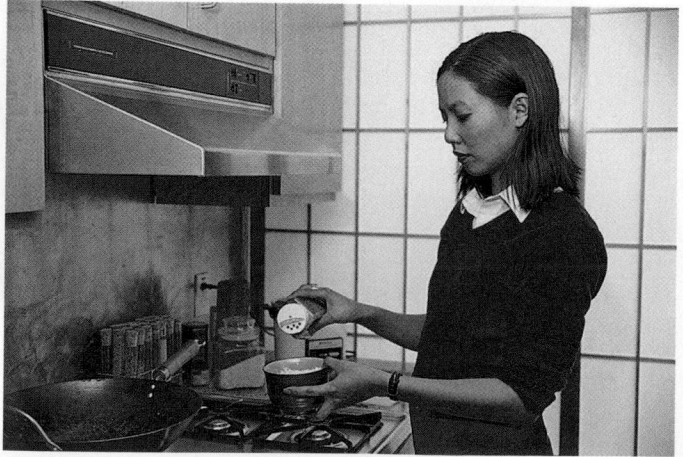

Figure 33–35 》 Cultural factors affect food preferences and habits.

Focus on Diversity and Culture
The Kosher Diet

The kosher diet followed by many Jewish individuals forbids the eating of pork products and shellfish. Certain cuts of meat from sheep and cattle are allowed, as are fish with fins and scales. In addition, many Jews believe that meat and dairy products should not be mixed and eaten at the same meal. Findings from a study of Jewish women in southern Israel indicate that iron deficiency anemia is the most prevalent type of anemia among Jewish women (Treister-Goltzman, Peleg, & Biderman, 2015). Those who follow a kosher diet acknowledge the need for increased protein, vitamins, and other nutrients during pregnancy. The Jewish community encourages intake of healthy sources of nutrients in alignment with the practices defined in kosher dietary guidelines. Acceptable food choices include protein from fish, eggs, and some meat and poultry, as well as legumes combined with whole grains. Additional recommendations include the consumption of at least one serving of leafy green vegetables and one serving of orange vegetables each day.

TABLE 33–5 Daily Food Plan for Pregnancy and Lactation

Food Group	Nutrients Provided	Food Source	Recommended Daily Amount During Pregnancy	Recommended Daily Amount During Lactation
Dairy products	Protein; riboflavin; vitamins A, D, and others; calcium; phosphorus; zinc; magnesium	Milk—whole, 2%, skim, dry, buttermilk	Four 8-oz cups (five for teenagers) used plain or with flavoring, in shakes, soups, puddings, custards, cocoa	Four 8-oz cups (five for teenagers); equivalent amount of cheese, yogurt, and so forth
		Cheeses—hard, semisoft, cottage	Calcium in 1 cup of milk equivalent to 1 1/2 cups of cottage cheese; 1 1/2 oz of hard or semisoft cheese; 1 cup of yogurt; 1 1/2 cups of ice cream (high in fat and sugar)	
		Yogurt—plain, low-fat		
		Soybean milk		
Meat and meat alternatives	Protein; iron; thiamine, niacin, and other vitamins; minerals	Beef, pork, veal, lamb, poultry, animal organ meats, fish, eggs; legumes; nuts, seeds, peanut butter, grains in proper vegetarian combination (vitamin B_{12} supplement needed)	Three servings (one serving = 2 oz), combination in amounts necessary for same nutrient equivalent (varies greatly)	Two servings
Grain products, whole grain or enriched	B vitamins; iron; whole grain also has zinc, magnesium, and other trace elements; provides fiber	Breads and bread products such as cornbread, muffins, waffles, hotcakes, biscuits, dumplings, cereals, pastas, and rice	6–11 servings daily: one serving = one slice bread, 3/4 cup or 1 oz of dry cereal; 1/2 cup of rice or pasta	Same as for pregnancy
Fruits and fruit juices	Vitamins A and C; minerals; raw fruits for roughage	Citrus fruits and juices, melons, berries, all other fruits and juices	Two to four servings (one serving for vitamin C): one serving = one medium fruit, 1/2–1 cup of fruit; 4 oz of orange or grapefruit juice	Same as for pregnancy
Vegetables and vegetable juices	Vitamins A and C; minerals; provides roughage	Leafy green vegetables; deep yellow or orange vegetables such as carrots, sweet potatoes, squash, tomatoes; green vegetables, such as peas, green beans, and broccoli; other vegetables, such as beets, cabbage, potatoes, corn, and lima beans	Three to five servings (one serving of dark green or deep yellow vegetable for vitamin A): one serving = 1/2 – 1 cup of vegetables; two tomatoes; one medium potato	Same as for pregnancy
Fats	Vitamins A and D; linoleic acid	Butter, cream cheese, fortified table spreads; cream, whipped cream, whipped toppings; avocado, mayonnaise, oil, nuts	As desired in moderation (high in calories): one serving = 1 tbsp butter or enriched margarine	Same as for pregnancy
Sugar and sweets		Sugar, brown sugar, honey, molasses, agave syrup	Occasionally, if desired	Same as for pregnancy
Desserts		Nutritious desserts such as fruits, puddings, custards, fruit whips, and crisps; other rich, sweet desserts and pastries	Occasionally, if desired	Same as for pregnancy
Beverages	Fluid	Coffee, decaffeinated beverages, tea, bouillon, carbonated drinks	As desired, in moderation	Same as for pregnancy
Miscellaneous		Iodized salt, herbs, spices, condiments	As desired	Same as for pregnancy

Note: The pregnant woman should eat regularly, three meals a day, with nutritious snacks of fruit, cheese, milk, or other foods between meals if desired. (More frequent but smaller meals are also recommended.) Between four and six 8-oz glasses of water, and a total of between eight and ten 8-oz cups of total fluid intake, should be consumed daily. Water is an essential nutrient.

is affected by the extent of their exposure to other cultures and by the availability, quality, and cost of traditional foods.

When working with pregnant women from any ethnic background, the nurse should understand the impact of the woman's cultural and spiritual beliefs on her eating habits and identify any beliefs she may have about food and pregnancy. Talking with the woman can help the nurse determine the level of influence that traditional food customs exert. The nurse can then provide dietary advice that is meaningful to the woman and her family.

Psychosocial Influences

The nurse should be aware of the various psychosocial factors that influence a woman's food choices. The sharing of food has long been a symbol of friendliness, warmth, and social acceptance in many cultures. Some foods and food practices are associated with status. Some foods are prepared "just for company"; others are served only on special occasions or holidays.

Knowledge about the basic components of a balanced diet is essential. Often, educational level is related to economic status, but even individuals with very limited incomes can prepare well-balanced meals if their knowledge of nutrition is adequate.

The expectant woman's attitudes and feelings about her pregnancy influence her nutritional status. For example, foods may be used as a substitute for expressing emotions, such as anger or frustration, or as a way of expressing feelings of joy. The woman who is depressed or does not wish to be pregnant may manifest these feelings through loss of appetite or overindulgence in certain foods.

Eating Disorders

Two serious eating disorders, anorexia nervosa and bulimia nervosa, develop most commonly in adolescent girls and young women. These conditions are described fully in Exemplar 29.A, Feeding and Eating Disorders, in the module on Self.

Women with eating disorders who become pregnant are at risk for a variety of complications. The consequences of the restricting, bingeing, and purging behaviors characteristic of eating disorders can result in a lack of nutrients being available for the fetus. These patients are at increased risk for miscarriage, hyperemesis gravidarum, preeclampsia, and birth complications, whereas their babies have an increased incidence of preterm birth, low birth weight, low Apgar scores (see Exemplar 33.D, Newborn Care, for a discussion of Apgar scores), and intrauterine death (Micali et al., 2012).

Pregnancy can be an especially difficult time for the woman with an eating disorder, even if she has long desired a child. The consumption of additional food and the expectations that she will gain additional weight can result in feelings of fear, anxiety, depression, and guilt. Women with eating disorders also have high rates of postpartum depression (Micali et al., 2012).

When a pregnant woman has an eating disorder, education and individualized meal plans can help the patient increase her dietary intake while maintaining a sense of control. A multidisciplinary approach to treatment, involving medical, nursing, psychiatric, and dietetic practitioners, is indicated. Pregnant women with eating disorders need to be closely monitored and supported throughout their pregnancies.

Pica

Pica is the craving for and persistent eating of nonnutritive substances not ordinarily considered to be edible or nutritionally valuable, such as soil, clay, and soap. Pica appears to occur worldwide but is underreported because women are often embarrassed to discuss it. In the United States, pica is more common among women who are economically disadvantaged, are of African American descent, live in rural areas, practiced pica before pregnancy, belong to a culture that encourages pica as important for fertility, and have family members who also practice pica (Ellis & Schnoes, 2012).

Iron deficiency anemia is the most common concern in pica. The connection of ice pica to iron deficiency is well known, but it is unclear if ingestion of large amounts of ice is a sign of iron deficiency or a contributing factor. However, the pica often resolves with iron supplementation (King et al., 2013). The ingestion of laundry starch or certain types of clay may contribute to iron deficiency because they interfere with iron absorption. The ingestion of large quantities of clay could fill the intestine and cause fecal impaction, and the ingestion of starch may be associated with excessive weight gain. Lead poisoning, one of the most serious complications that can result from *geophagia* (eating soil or clay), may affect both the mother and her fetus. Geophagia may produce soil-borne parasitic infections, such as toxoplasmosis and toxocariasis. Gastrointestinal (GI) tract complications resulting from pica can be mechanical bowel problems, constipation, ulcerations, perforations, and intestinal obstructions. It also can result in impaired cognitive functioning, kidney damage, and encephalopathy. Consequently, blood lead levels should be determined in cases of diagnosed or suspected geophagia.

The nurse should be aware of pica and its implications for the woman and fetus. Assessment for pica is an important part of a nutritional history. However, a patient may be embarrassed about her cravings or reluctant to discuss them for fear of criticism. Using a nonjudgmental approach, the nurse can provide the woman with information that is useful in decreasing or eliminating this practice.

Vegetarianism

Vegetarianism is the dietary choice of many individuals for religious, health, or ethical reasons. There are several types of vegetarians. **Lacto-ovovegetarians** include milk, dairy products, and eggs in their diets. **Lactovegetarians** include dairy products but no eggs in their diets. **Vegans** will not eat any food from animal sources.

The expectant woman who is vegetarian must eat the proper combination of foods to obtain adequate nutrients. If her diet allows, the woman can obtain ample and complete proteins from dairy products and eggs. Plant protein quality can be improved if it is consumed with these animal proteins.

If the woman follows a vegan diet, careful planning is necessary to obtain complete proteins and sufficient calories. An adequate, pure vegan diet contains protein from unrefined grains (brown rice, whole wheat), legumes (beans, split peas, lentils), nuts in large quantities, and a variety of cooked and fresh vegetables and fruits. Adequate dietary protein can be obtained by consuming a varied diet with complementary amino acids, which together provide complete proteins. Complete proteins can be obtained by eating different types of plant-based proteins, such as beans and rice, peanut butter on whole-grain bread, and whole-grain cereal with soy milk, either in the same meal or over a day. Seeds may provide adequate protein in the vegetarian diet if the quantity is large enough. Obtaining sufficient calories to ensure adequate weight gain can be difficult, however, because vegan diets tend to be high in fiber and therefore filling. **Figure 33–36 ❯❯** depicts a vegetarian food pyramid with suggestions for daily servings.

Both lacto-ovovegetarians and vegans should eat four servings of vitamin B_{12}–fortified foods (meat substitutes, tofu, cereals, soy milk, and nutritional yeast) daily. A daily supplement of vitamin B_{12} is also recommended during pregnancy and while breastfeeding (London et al., 2017).

The best sources of iron and zinc are animal products; consequently, vegan diets may also be low in these minerals. In addition, a high fiber intake may reduce mineral (calcium,

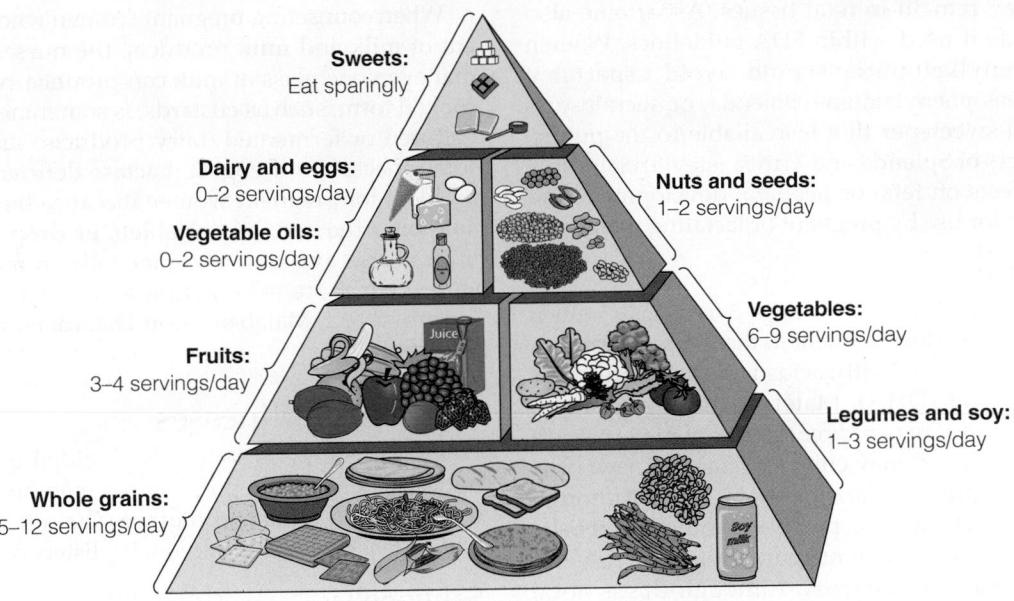

Figure 33–36 » The vegetarian food pyramid.

iron, and zinc) bioavailability. Thus, pregnant women who are vegetarians should be advised to have approximately 1200–1500 mg/day of calcium, which is higher than the recommended levels for patients who are omnivores. Vitamin D supplements may be indicated for women who do not have adequate exposure to sunlight (Baggerly et al., 2015).

To achieve optimal nutrition, the nurse should emphasize the use of foods that are nutrient dense and that provide a balanced diet. A vegetarian food group guide appears in **Table 33–6 »**.

Special Dietary Considerations

The pregnant woman must carefully consider choices regarding foods and food additives. These include maintaining adequate levels of folic acid, use of artificial sweeteners, mercury levels in fish, and lactose intolerance.

Folic Acid

Folic acid, or folate, is required for normal growth, reproduction, and lactation and prevents the macrocytic, megaloblastic anemia of pregnancy. Megaloblastic anemia caused by folate deficiency is rarely found in the United States, but it does occur.

Even more significantly, an inadequate intake of folic acid has been associated with fetal neural tube defects (spina bifida, meningomyelocele). Although these defects are considered to be multifactorial, research indicates that 50–70% of spina bifida and anencephaly cases could be prevented by adequate intake of folic acid (ACOG, 2014; CDC, 2015a). Experts recommend that all women of childbearing age (15–45 years) consume 400 mcg of folic acid daily because half of all U.S. pregnancies are unplanned and neural tube defects occur very early in pregnancy (3–4 weeks after conception), before most women realize they are pregnant (CDC, 2015a). The best food sources of folate are fresh green leafy vegetables, liver, peanuts, and whole-grain breads and cereals. Folic acid can be made inactive by oxidation, ultraviolet light, and heating. It can easily be lost during improper storage and cooking. To prevent unnecessary loss, foods should be stored covered to protect them from light, cooked with only a small amount of water, and not overcooked.

Use of Artificial Sweeteners

Sweeteners classified as *Generally Recognized as Safe (GRAS)* by the FDA are acceptable for use during pregnancy. As with other foods, moderation should be exercised when using artificial sweeteners, such as saccharin, which can cross the

TABLE 33–6 Vegetarian Food Groups

Food Group	Mixed Diet	Lacto-Ovovegetarian	Lactovegetarian	Vegan
Grain	Bread, cereal, rice, pasta	Bread, cereal, rice, pasta	Bread, cereal, rice, pasta	Bread, cereal, rice, pasta
Fruit	Fruit, fruit juices	Fruit, fruit juices	Fruit, fruit juices	Fruit, fruit juices
Vegetable	Vegetables, vegetable juices	Vegetables, vegetable juices	Vegetables, vegetable juices	Vegetables, vegetable juices
Dairy and dairy alternatives	Milk, yogurt, cheese	Milk, yogurt, cheese	Milk, yogurt, cheese	Fortified soy milk, rice milk, almond milk
Meat and meat alternatives	Meat, fish, poultry, eggs, legumes, tofu, nuts, nut butters	Eggs, legumes, tofu, nuts, nut butters	Legumes, tofu, nuts, nut butters	Legumes, tofu, nuts, nut butters

placenta and may remain in fetal tissues. Aspartame also appears to be safe if used within FDA guidelines. Women affected by phenylketonuria should avoid aspartame because it contains phenylalanine. Splenda, or sucralose, is another artificial sweetener that is available to the public. The manufacturers of Splenda and Truvia (stevia) claim that they have no effects on fetal or neonatal development and are therefore safe for use by pregnant or lactating women.

Mercury in Fish

Seafood is an important source of omega-3 fatty acids, which are essential for neural development in the fetus. Of particular interest are the omega-3 fatty acids and their derivative, docosahexaenoic acid (DHA). Maternal dietary intake of DHA during pregnancy may reduce the risk of preterm birth and low birth weight and may enhance fetal and newborn/infant brain development (Carlson et al., 2013). Although the omega-3 in fish is beneficial, pregnant women need to be aware that fish can also contain mercury. Nearly all fish and shellfish contain traces of mercury. Although this is not a concern for most individuals, some fish and shellfish contain higher levels of mercury than others, and mercury can pose a threat to the developing nervous system of a fetus or young child. Mercury exposure also can have a negative effect on cognitive functioning, resulting in deficiencies in language, attention, motor function, memory, and visual–spatial abilities (Solan & Lindow, 2014). Consequently, pregnant women need information about the importance of seafood in their diet, but also need to know that they should consume seafood that is low in mercury. The U.S. government has issued the following guidelines for women who are pregnant or may become pregnant, breastfeeding mothers, and young children (Agency for Toxic Substance and Disease Registry [ATSDR], 2013):

- Do not eat swordfish, shark, tilefish, or king mackerel, because these fish contain high levels of mercury.

- Eat up to 12 oz/week (two average meals) of a variety of shellfish and fish that are lower in mercury. Commonly eaten fish that are lower in mercury include canned light tuna, shrimp, salmon, catfish, and pollack. Albacore (white) tuna has more mercury than canned light tuna; therefore, only 6 oz/week of albacore tuna is recommended.

- Check local advisories about the mercury content of fish caught by family and friends. If no information is available, limit fish caught in local areas to 6 oz/week, and avoid consuming additional fish that week.

Lactase Deficiency (Lactose Intolerance)

Some individuals have difficulty digesting milk and milk products. This condition, known as **lactase deficiency** or **lactose intolerance**, results from an inadequate amount of the enzyme lactase, which breaks down the milk sugar lactose into smaller, digestible substances.

Lactase deficiency is found in many adults of African, Mexican, Native American, Ashkenazi Jewish, and Asian descent and, indeed, in many other adults worldwide. Individuals who are not affected are mainly of northern European heritage. Symptoms include abdominal distention, discomfort, nausea, vomiting, loose stools, and cramps.

When counseling pregnant women who might be intolerant of milk and milk products, the nurse should be aware that even one glass of milk can produce symptoms. Milk in cooked form, such as custards, is sometimes tolerated, as are cultured or fermented dairy products, such as buttermilk, some cheeses, and yogurt. Lactase deficiency need not be a problem for pregnant women, because the enzyme is available over the counter in tablets or drops. Lactase-treated milk is also available commercially in most large grocery stores. For more information about lactase deficiency, see Exemplar 4.C, Malabsorption Disorders, in the module on Digestion.

Foodborne Illnesses

Foodborne illnesses should be avoided by any individual, but especially by the pregnant woman because they pose a threat to both fetus and mother. The nurse should provide patient teaching about salmonella, listeriosis, and hepatitis E.

Salmonella

Because of the risk for *Salmonella* contamination in raw eggs, advise pregnant women to avoid eating or tasting foods that may contain raw or lightly cooked eggs. These foods include cake batter; homemade eggnog; sauces made with raw eggs, such as Caesar salad dressing; and homemade ice cream (FDA, 2013).

Listeriosis

Listeria monocytogenes is another bacterium that poses a threat to an expectant mother and her fetus. *Listeria* is especially challenging because the organism can be found in refrigerated, ready-to-eat foods, such as unpasteurized milk and dairy products, meat, poultry, and seafood. To prevent listeriosis, advise pregnant women to do the following (FDA, 2013):

- Maintain the refrigerator at a temperature of 4°C (40°F) or below and the freezer at −18°C (0°F).

- Refrigerate or freeze prepared foods, leftovers, and perishables within 2 hours after eating or preparation.

- Do not eat hot dogs, deli meats, or luncheon meats unless they are reheated until steaming hot.

- Avoid soft cheeses, such as feta, brie, Camembert, blue-veined cheeses, queso fresco, or queso blanco (a soft cheese often used in Hispanic cooking) unless the label clearly states that they are made with pasteurized milk.

- Do not eat refrigerated pâtés or meat spreads or foods that contain raw (unpasteurized) milk. Do not drink unpasteurized milk.

- Avoid eating refrigerated smoked seafood, such as salmon, trout, cod, tuna, or mackerel, unless it is in a cooked dish, such as a casserole. Canned or shelf-stable pates, meat spreads, and smoked seafood are considered safe.

Hepatitis E

Hepatitis E is a viral infection found most often in developing countries. This disease is spread through the feces of infected people or animals and is transmitted most often through unclean drinking water, but it can also be contracted by eating contaminated food. Hepatitis E is often more severe in pregnant women, especially during the third trimester, and may lead to maternal death (Gurley et al., 2012).

To prevent hepatitis E, pregnant women should wash their hands thoroughly after using the bathroom, changing diapers, or handling raw foods. When traveling to areas where the quality of the water is uncertain, they should avoid eating raw foods, unpeeled fruit, and uncooked fish. They should also avoid drinking tap water or using ice made with tap water. Rather, they should use bottled or boiled water for drinking, tooth brushing, and formula preparation (Gurley et al., 2012).

Maternal Weight Gain

Maternal weight gain is an important factor in fetal growth and neonatal birth weight. The optimal weight gain depends on the woman's weight for height (body mass index [BMI]) and her prepregnant nutritional state. An adequate weight gain indicates an adequate caloric intake. It does not, however, ensure that the woman has a sufficient nutrient intake. The pregnant woman must maintain the nutritional quality of her diet as her weight gain progresses.

The Institute of Medicine (2009) recommends weight gains in terms of optimal ranges based on prepregnant BMI, and ACOG (2013e) supports these recommendations. The IOM recommendations are shown in **Table 33–7 》**.

The pattern of weight gain is important. The ideal pattern for a normal-weight woman consists of a gain of 0.9–1.8 kg (2.0–4.0 lb) during the first trimester, followed by a gain of approximately 0.3–0.5 kg (0.8–1 lb) per week during the second and third trimesters. The rate of weight gain in the second and third trimesters needs to be slightly higher for underweight women, and slightly lower (0.5–0.7 lb/week) for overweight women and 0.4–0.6 lb/week for women with obesity (ACOG, 2013e; IOM, 2009). A normal-weight woman who is expecting twins is advised to gain approximately 0.7 kg (1.5 lb) per week during the second and third trimesters of her pregnancy. Inadequate maternal weight gain has been associated with preterm birth and its associated problems for the newborn (ACOG, 2013e; IOM, 2009).

Obesity is becoming a major health problem in many developed countries, and more and more women are entering pregnancy already overweight or obese. Pregnant women who are obese are at an increased risk for medical and pregnancy-related complications, such as spontaneous abortion, gestational diabetes, preeclampsia, labor induc-

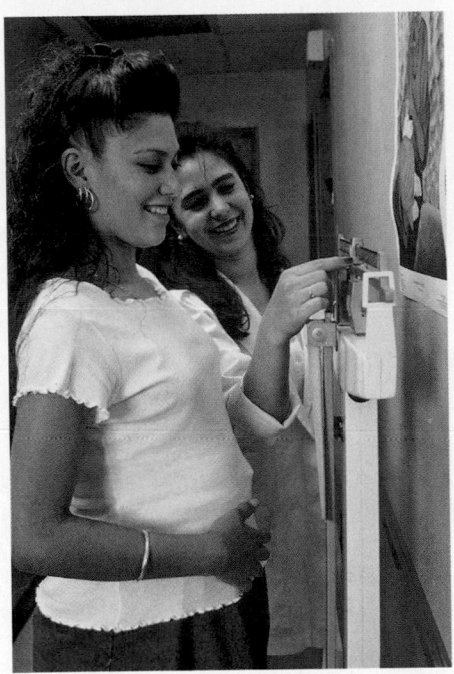

Figure 33–37 》 It is important to monitor a pregnant woman's weight over time.

tion, and cesarean birth. They also have a higher incidence of fetal anomalies. They should be considered to be at high risk and counseled accordingly (ACOG, 2013e).

Maternal obesity also has implications for children. The children of mothers who are overweight and obese are predisposed to developing obesity and its related health concerns. In fact, the child of an overweight mother is three times more likely to be overweight by the age of 7 than is a child of a normal-weight mother (Ballogh, 2015).

Because of the association between maternal weight gain and pregnancy outcome, most healthcare providers pay close attention to weight gain during pregnancy (**Figure 33–37 》**). Weight gain charts can be useful in monitoring the rate and pattern of weight gain over time.

Excessive weight gain during pregnancy also has long-term implications because weight gain during pregnancy is by far the most important predictor of the amount of weight that a woman will retain following childbirth (ACOG, 2013e). Counseling the pregnant woman to eat a variety of

TABLE 33–7 Institute of Medicine Weight Gain Recommendations for Pregnancy

Prepregnancy Weight Category	Body Mass Index*	Recommended Range of Total Weight (lb)	Recommended Rates of Weight Gain[†] in the Second and Third Trimesters (lb) (Mean Range [lb/wk])
Underweight	<18.5	28–40	1 (1–1.3)
Normal weight	18.5–24.9	25–35	1 (0.8–1)
Overweight	25–29.9	15–25	0.6 (0.5–0.7)
Obese (includes all classes)	30+	11–20	0.5 (0.4–0.6)

*Body mass index is calculated as weight in kilograms divided by height in meters squared, or as weight in pounds multiplied by 703 divided by square of height in inches.

[†]Calculations assume a 1.1- to 4.4-lb weight gain in the first trimester.

Source: Based on Institute of Medicine. (2009). *Weight gain during pregnancy: Reexamining the guidelines.* Washington, DC: National Academies Press. ©2009 National Academy of Sciences. Retrieved from http://www.nationalacademies.org/hmd/~/media/Files/Report%20Files/2009/Weight-Gain-During-Pregnancy-Reexamining-the-Guidelines/Report%20Brief%20-%20Weight%20Gain%20During%20Pregnancy.pdf

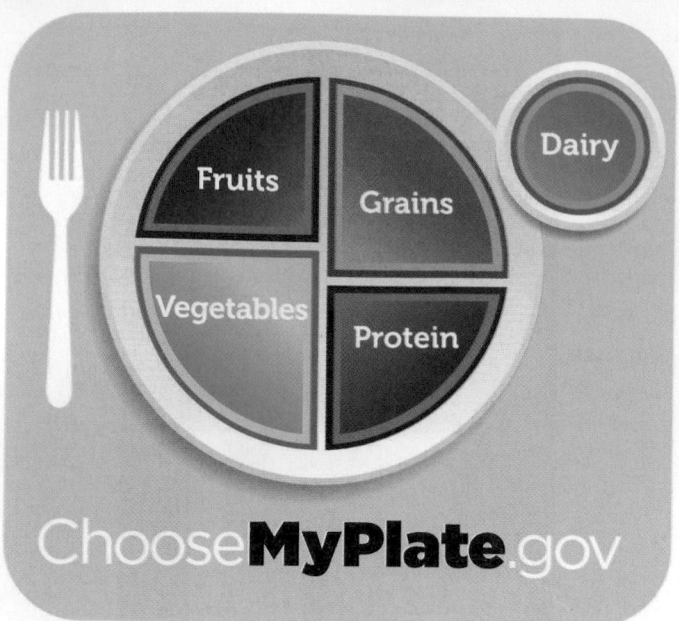

Source: U.S. Department of Agriculture; U.S. Department of Health and Human Services.

Figure 33–38 ❯❯ ChooseMyPlate identifies the basic food groups and provides guidance about healthful eating. Grains, vegetables, and fruits are emphasized, with slightly less emphasis on dairy and protein. MyPlate is designed to remind Americans to eat healthfully.

nutrients from each of the food groups places less emphasis on the amount of her weight gain and more on the quality of her intake. It may also be helpful to encourage the woman to begin a simple exercise program such as walking.

The federal government's newly designed food choice program, ChooseMyPlate, offers users a colorful plan that emphasizes variety, proportionality, moderation, and physical activity. It is also designed to help guide individuals to make healthier choices (**Figure 33–38 ❯❯**).

❯❯ Stay Current: Go to www.choosemyplate.gov/pregnancy-breast-feeding.html to see the USDA's nutrition recommendations for pregnant women and to https://www.choosemyplate.gov/MyPlate-Daily-Checklist to see how women can get a personalized "MyPlate Daily Checklist" using ChooseMyPlate's SuperTracker.

SAFETY ALERT Weight varies with time of day, amount of clothing, inaccurate scale adjustment, or weighing error. Do not overemphasize a single weight; rather, pay attention to the overall pattern of weight gain.

Lifespan Considerations

The adolescent and the woman over age 35 have specific physiologic, psychologic, and care concerns during their pregnancies. Some of those considerations are discussed in this section.

Considerations for Adolescent Pregnancy

Nutritional care of the pregnant adolescent is of particular concern to healthcare professionals. Many adolescents are nutritionally at risk because of a variety of complex and interrelated emotional, social, and economic factors. Important nutrition-related factors to assess in pregnant adolescents include low prepregnant weight, low weight gain during pregnancy, young age at menarche, smoking, excessive prepregnant weight, anemia, unhealthy lifestyle (drug or alcohol use), chronic disease, and history of an eating disorder.

Estimates regarding the nutritional needs of adolescents are generally determined by using the DRIs for nonpregnant teenagers (age 11–14 or 15–18) and adding nutrient amounts recommended for all pregnant women (see Table 33–4). If the pregnant adolescent is physiologically mature (> 4 years since menarche), her nutritional needs approach those reported for pregnant adults. However, adolescents who become pregnant less than 4 years after menarche are at risk because of their physiologic and anatomic immaturity. These adolescents are more likely than older adolescents to still be growing, which can affect the fetus's development. Thus, young adolescents (age 14 and younger) need to gain more weight than older adolescents (age 18 and older) to produce babies of equal size.

In determining the optimal weight gain for the pregnant adolescent, the nurse adds the recommended weight gain for an adult pregnancy to that expected during the postmenarchal year in which the pregnancy occurs. If the teenager is underweight, additional weight gain is recommended to bring her to a normal weight for her height.

Specific Nutrient Concerns

Caloric needs of pregnant adolescents vary widely. Major factors in determining caloric needs include the physical activity level of the individual and whether her growth is complete. Figures as high as 50 kcal/kg have been suggested for young, pregnant adolescents who are very active physically. A satisfactory weight gain usually confirms an adequate caloric intake.

An inadequate iron intake is a major concern with the adolescent diet. Iron needs are high for the pregnant teen because of the requirement for iron by the enlarging maternal muscle mass and blood volume. Iron supplements—providing between 30 and 60 mg of elemental iron—are definitely indicated.

Calcium is another nutrient that demands special attention from pregnant adolescents. Inadequate intake of calcium is frequently a problem in this age group. Adequate calcium intake is necessary to support the normal growth and development of the fetus and the growth and maintenance of calcium stores in the adolescent. An extra serving of dairy products or other calcium-rich foods is usually suggested for teenagers. Calcium supplementation is indicated for teens who do not consume dairy products or other significant calcium sources in sufficient quantities.

Because folic acid plays a role in cell reproduction, it is also an important nutrient for pregnant teens. As previously indicated, a supplement is usually recommended for all pregnant women, regardless of age.

Other nutrients and vitamins must be considered when evaluating the overall nutritional quality of the teenager's diet. Nutrients that have been found to be deficient in this age group include zinc and vitamins A, D, and B_6. Inclusion of a wide variety of foods—especially fresh and lightly processed foods—is helpful in obtaining adequate amounts of trace minerals, fiber, and vitamins.

Dietary Patterns

Healthy adolescents often have irregular eating patterns. Many skip breakfast, and most tend to be frequent snackers. Teens rarely follow the traditional three-meals-a-day pattern. Their day-to-day intake often varies drastically, and many eat food combinations that may seem bizarre to adults. Despite these practices, adolescents usually achieve a better nutritional balance than most adults would expect.

In assessing the diet of the pregnant adolescent, the nurse should consider the eating pattern over time, not simply a single day's intake. Once the pattern is identified, the nurse can direct counseling toward correcting deficiencies.

Counseling Issues

Counseling about nutrition and healthy eating practices is an important element of care for pregnant teenagers that nurses can provide effectively in a community setting. This counseling may be individualized, involve other teens, or provide a combination of both approaches. If an adolescent's family member does most of the meal preparation, it may be useful to include that individual in the discussion if the adolescent agrees. Involving the expectant father in counseling may also be beneficial. Clinics and schools often offer classes and focused activities designed to address this topic.

The pregnant teenager's understanding of nutrition will influence not only her well-being but also that of her child. However, teens tend to live in the present, and counseling that stresses long-term changes may be less effective than more concrete approaches. In many cases, group classes are effective, especially those that include other teens. In a group atmosphere, adolescents often work together to plan adequate meals, including foods that are special favorites.

Risks to the Adolescent Mother

There may be physiologic, psychologic, and sociologic risks for the pregnant adolescent.

Physiologic Risks

Adolescents older than 15 years who receive early, thorough prenatal care are at no greater risk during pregnancy than women older than age 20. Unfortunately, adolescents often begin prenatal care later in pregnancy than other age groups. Thus, risks for pregnant adolescents include preterm births, low-birth-weight newborns, cephalopelvic disproportion, iron deficiency anemia, and preeclampsia and its sequelae. In the adolescent age group, prenatal care is the critical factor that most influences pregnancy outcome.

Teenagers age 15 to 19 have a high incidence of STIs, including herpes virus, syphilis, and gonorrhea (U.S. Preventive Services Task Force, 2014). The incidence of chlamydial infection is also increased in this age group. The presence of such infections during a pregnancy greatly increases the risk to the fetus. Other problems seen in adolescents are cigarette smoking and drug use. By the time pregnancy is confirmed, the fetus may already have been harmed by these substances.

Psychologic Risks

The major psychologic risk to the pregnant adolescent is the interruption of her developmental tasks. Adding the tasks of pregnancy to her own developmental tasks creates a huge amount of psychologic work, the completion of which will affect the adolescent's and her newborn's futures. **Table 33–8** >> suggests typical behaviors of the adolescent when she becomes aware of her pregnancy. In reviewing

TABLE 33–8 Initial Reaction to Awareness of Pregnancy

Age	Adolescent Behavior	Nursing Implications
Early adolescent (14 years and younger)	Fears rejection by family and peers. Enters healthcare system with an adult, most likely mother (parents still seen as locus of control). Value system closely reflects that of parents, so teen turns to parents for decisions or approval of decisions. Pregnancy probably not a result of intimate relationship. Is self-conscious about normal adolescent changes in body. Self-consciousness and low self-esteem likely to increase with rapid breast enlargement and abdominal enlargement of pregnancy.	Be nonjudgmental in approach to care. Focus on needs and concerns of adolescent, but if parent accompanies daughter, include parent in plan of care. Encourage both to express concerns and feelings regarding pregnancy and options: abortion, maintaining pregnancy, adoption. Be realistic and concrete in discussing implications of each option. During physical exam of adolescent, respect increased sense of modesty. Explain in simple and concrete terms physical changes that are produced by pregnancy versus puberty. Explain each step of physical exam in simple and concrete terms.
Middle adolescent (15–17 years)	Fears rejection by peers and parents. Unsure of whom to confide in. May seek confirmation of pregnancy on own with increased awareness of options and services, such as over-the-counter pregnancy kits and Planned Parenthood. If in an ongoing, caring relationship with partner (peer), may choose him as confidant. Economic dependence on parents may determine if and when parents are told. Future educational plans and perception of parental support or lack of support are significant factors in decision regarding termination or maintenance of the pregnancy. Possible conflict between parental and own developing value system.	Be nonjudgmental in approach to care. Reassure the adolescent that confidentiality will be maintained. Help adolescent identify significant individuals in whom she can confide to help make a decision about the pregnancy. Be aware of state laws regarding requirement of parental notification if abortion intended. Also be aware of state laws regarding requirements for marriage: usually, minimum age for both parties is 18; 16- and 17-year-olds are, in most states, allowed to marry only with consent of parents. Encourage adolescent to be realistic about parental response to pregnancy.
Late adolescent (18–19 years)	Most likely to confirm pregnancy on own and at an earlier date due to increased acceptance and awareness of consequences of behavior. Likely to use pregnancy kit for confirmation. Relationship with father of baby, future educational plans, and personal value system are among significant determinants of decision about pregnancy.	Be nonjudgmental in approach to care. Reassure the adolescent that confidentiality will be maintained. Encourage adolescent to identify significant individuals in whom she can confide. Refer to counseling as appropriate. Encourage adolescent to be realistic about parental response to pregnancy.

Source: London et al. (2017). *Maternal & Child Nursing Care* (5th ed.). Hoboken, NJ: Pearson Education.

these behaviors, the nurse should realize that other factors may influence individual responses.

Sociologic Risks

Being forced into adult roles before completing adolescent developmental tasks causes a series of events that may result in prolonged dependence on parents, lack of stable relationships with the opposite sex, and lack of economic and social stability. Many teenage mothers drop out of school during their pregnancy, and then are less likely to complete their schooling. Similarly, they are less likely to go to college. In fact, fewer than 2% of teenagers who give birth before age 18 attain a college degree by age 30 (Alan Guttmacher Institute [AGI], 2016). In addition, teenage mothers are more likely to have big families and more likely to be single. Lack of education in turn reduces the quality of jobs available and leads to more tenuous employment and increased poverty (Herrman & Nandakumar, 2012).

Some pregnant adolescents choose to marry the father of the baby, who may also be a teenager. Unfortunately, most teenage marriages end in divorce. This fact should not be surprising, because pregnancy and marriage interrupt the adolescents' childhood and basic education. Lack of maturity in dealing with an intimate relationship also contributes to marital breakdown.

Dating violence is often an issue for teens. When surveyed, 10.3% of adolescents report some level of physical dating violence, and 10.4% experience some form of sexual dating violence ranging from touching and kidding to forced intercourse (Kann et al., 2014). The violence increases in pregnant teens. However, research suggests that this number is significantly lower than the actual number because teens are far less likely to report domestic violence than are adults.

The increased incidence of maternal complications, preterm birth, and low-birth-weight babies among teen mothers also affects society because many of these mothers are dependent on government programs. In the United States, the results of teenage childbearing costs tax payers $9.4 billion annually (Ventura, Hamilton, & Mathews, 2014). Much of this cost comes from Medicaid, state health department, maternal care clinics, federal monies for Aid to Families with Dependent Children, the Supplemental Nutritional Assistance Program (SNAP), and direct payments to healthcare providers. The need for increased financial support for good prenatal care and nutritional programs remains critical.

Early, middle, and late adolescents respond differently to the developmental tasks of pregnancy, reflecting their age and maturity. In addition to her maturational level, the amount of nurturing the pregnant adolescent receives is a critical factor in the way she handles pregnancy and motherhood.

The early-adolescent girl (younger than 15 years) tends to think in a more concrete manner and usually has only a minimal ability to anticipate consequences of her behavior and see herself in the future. In addition, some degree of discomfort with normal body changes and body image may exist. The middle-adolescent girl (15 to 17 years) is prone to experimentation (i.e., drugs, alcohol, and sex), seeks independence, and frequently turns to her peer group for support, information, and advice. Pregnancy at this age can force

parental dependency and interfere with attempts at independence. Middle adolescents are capable of abstract thinking but may struggle with anticipating the long-term implications of their behavior. Finally, the late adolescent (17 to 19 years) is developing individuality and can picture herself in control. More sophisticated abstract thinking and an ability to anticipate consequences contributes to the development of problem-solving and decision-making skills (Borca et al., 2015).

>> Go to **Pearson MyLab Nursing and eText** to see Chart 5: The Early Adolescent's Response to the Developmental Tasks of Pregnancy.

Considerations for the Pregnant Woman Over Age 35

In the United States and Canada the risk of death in childbirth has declined dramatically for women of all ages since 1950 because of advances in maternal health and obstetric practice. There are, however, medical risks for the pregnant woman over age 35 that must be considered.

Medical Risks

The risk of maternal death is significantly higher for women over age 35 and is even higher for women age 40 and older. These women are more likely to have chronic medical conditions that can complicate a pregnancy. Preexisting medical conditions such as hypertension or diabetes probably play a more significant role than age in maternal well-being and the outcome of pregnancy. In addition, the rate of miscarriage, still birth, preterm birth, low birth weight, and perinatal morbidity and mortality is higher in pregnant women over age 35 (Carolan, 2013). Nevertheless, while the risk of pregnancy complications is higher in women over age 35 who have a chronic condition such as hypertension or diabetes or who are in poor general health, the risks are much lower than previously believed for physically fit women without preexisting medical problems (Cunningham et al., 2014).

The incidence of low-birth-weight newborns, very preterm births, and perinatal death is higher among women age 35 and older (Kenny et al., 2013). Women over age 35 who become pregnant also have an increased risk for gestational diabetes mellitus, hypertension, placenta previa, difficult labor, and newborn complications (March of Dimes [MOD], 2016).

The cesarean birth rate is also increased in women over age 35. This practice may be related to pregnancy complications as well as to increased concern by the woman and physician about the pregnancy outcome (MOD, 2016).

The risk of conceiving a child with Down syndrome increases with maternal age, especially when the mother is over age 35. ACOG (2016a) recommends that all pregnant women, regardless of age, be offered screening for Down syndrome. Research has focused on the use of quadruple screening to detect Down syndrome and trisomy 18. First-trimester ultrasound assessment of the thickness of fetal nuchal folds (nuchal translucency, or NT) combined with serum screens of free beta-hCG and pregnancy-associated plasma protein A (PAPP-A) is increasing the detection of Down syndrome, trisomy 18, and trisomy 13. If the screening results are not in the normal range, follow-up testing using ultrasound and amniocentesis is often indicated (ACOG, 2016a).

Amniocentesis or noninvasive prenatal testing through cell free fetal DNA (cffDNA) are routinely offered to all women over age 35 to permit the early detection of several chromosomal abnormalities, including Down syndrome. Routine genetic testing has not been offered to couples when the only risk is advanced paternal age, because there is insufficient evidence to determine a specific paternal age at which to start genetic testing. Advanced paternal age is associated with adverse fetal and neonatal outcomes, including an increased risk for autism spectrum disorder (Kovac et al., 2013).

Additional Concerns of the Pregnant Woman Over Age 35

The increased medical risks that the pregnant woman over age 35 faces, combined with social, familial, and other healthcare concerns, place many of these patients and their families at risk for impaired family processes. In particular, women who are mothers of older children and who provide some level of care for their own older parents may find themselves at their wits' ends trying to find a way to juggle their many responsibilities. The arrival of a new baby in a blended family may cause jealousy among older siblings or strain relationships with in-laws or former partners. The nurse should engage in active listening with these women and their partners, help them prioritize their concerns, and provide referrals to supportive resources as appropriate.

Often, because of their established routines, couples expecting their first child require assistance in understanding how to integrate a newborn into their daily routines. Secondary to increased risk to both the fetus and the pregnant woman, the family is often anxious, and this anxiety can create stress in the household. Encourage the couple to express their fears and concerns and provide support and reassurance. Anxiety may be particularly high when they are waiting for diagnostic test results. Couples may report that they are fighting more than usual. The nurse should help these patients recognize that the role anxiety plays in disrupting their relationships is often an important step to improving the relationship.

If the couple has other children, especially if the siblings are in the teen or preteen age, they may find their older children are embarrassed by the pregnancy. Older siblings may also fear being asked to contribute to the newborn's care. It is important for the couple to take time to understand their older children's concerns and make it clear to the siblings that the newborn will be the responsibility of the parents, not the responsibility of the older children. Siblings should be welcomed to participate in newborn care but should not be placed in the position of taking on a majority of the responsibility. The nurse can provide a supportive role in this process by encouraging open family communication and trust.

NURSING PROCESS

A written care plan or clinical pathway that incorporates the prenatal record, nursing diagnoses, and patient goals is essential to ensure continuity of care. Prenatal care, especially for women with low-risk pregnancies, is community based, typically in a clinic or a private office. The healthcare community recognizes the value of providing a primary care nurse in these settings to coordinate holistic care for each childbearing family. The nurse in a clinic or health maintenance organization may be the only source of continuity for the woman, who may see a different healthcare provider at each visit.

Assessment

The nurse can complete many areas of prenatal assessment. Advanced practice nurses, such as CNMs and certified women's health nurse practitioners, have the education and skill to perform full and complete antepartum assessments. Areas of assessment may include the following:

- The woman's physical status
- The woman's understanding of pregnancy and the changes that accompany it
- The woman or family's attitudes about the pregnancy and expectations of the impact a baby will have on their lives
- Any health teaching needs
- The degree of support the woman has available to her
- The woman's knowledge of newborn/infant care.

While gathering data, the nurse also has an opportunity to discuss important aspects of nutrition within the context of the family's needs and lifestyle. In addition, the nurse seeks information about psychologic, cultural, and socioeconomic factors that may influence food intake.

At subsequent prenatal visits, the nurse continues to gather data about the course of the pregnancy to date and the woman's responses to it. The nurse also asks about the adjustment of the support person and of other children, if any, in the family. As the pregnancy progresses, the nurse inquires about the preparations the family has made for the new baby. The nurse asks specifically whether the woman has experienced any discomfort, especially the kinds of discomfort that are often seen at specific times during a pregnancy. The nurse also inquires about physical changes that relate directly to the pregnancy, such as fetal movement, and asks about the danger signs of pregnancy (**Table 33–9 ⟫**).

SAFETY ALERT Pregnancy is a high-risk period for intimate partner violence (IPV). It is important for the nurse to assess the woman with suspicious or unexplained injuries for this possibility.

Other pertinent information includes any exposure to contagious illnesses, medical treatment and therapy prescribed for medical problems since the last visit, and any prescription or OTC medications or herbal supplements that were not prescribed as part of the woman's prenatal care.

During the antepartum period, it is essential for the nurse to begin assessing the readiness of the woman and her partner (if possible) to assume their responsibilities as parents successfully. **Box 33–2 ⟫** identifies areas for assessment of parenting ability.

TABLE 33–9 Danger Signs in Pregnancy

Danger Sign	Possible Cause
Sudden gush of fluid from vagina	Premature rupture of membranes
Vaginal bleeding	Abruptio placentae, placenta previa, lesions of cervix or vagina, "bloody show"
Abdominal pain	Premature labor, abruptio placentae
Temperature above 38.3°C (101°F) and chills	Infection
Dizziness, blurred vision, double vision, spots before eyes	Hypertension, preeclampsia
Persistent vomiting	Hyperemesis gravidarum
Severe headache	Hypertension, preeclampsia
Edema of hands, face, legs, and feet	Preeclampsia
Reflex irritability, convulsions	Preeclampsia, eclampsia
Epigastric pain	Preeclampsia, ischemia in major abdominal vessel
Oliguria	Renal impairment, decreased fluid intake, preeclampsia
Dysuria	Urinary tract infection
Absence of fetal movement	Maternal medication, obesity, fetal death

Box 33–2
Prenatal Assessment of Parenting Ability

Perception of Complexities of Mothering

A. Desires baby for itself.

Positive:

1. The pregnancy is a planned or desired extension of a stable home life.

Negative:

1. Wants baby to meet own needs, such as someone to love her, someone to get her out of unhappy home, a way to repair faltering relationship.
2. The pregnancy is unwanted.
    - Was the pregnancy planned or a surprise?
    - How do you feel about being a mother?
    - Have you considered terminating the pregnancy or placing the baby for adoption?

B. Expresses consideration of the impact of mothering role on other roles (relationship, career, school).

Positive:

1. Realistic expectations of how baby will affect job, career, school, and personal goals.
2. Interested in learning about child care.

Negative:

1. Lacks insight regarding the physical, emotional, and social demands of parenting.
2. Uninterested in learning about the needs of a baby.

C. Makes lifestyle changes for the baby's benefit.

Positive:

1. Gives up routines not good for baby (quits smoking, adjusts eating habits).
    - What do you think it will be like to take care of a baby?
    - How do you think your life will be different after you have your baby?
    - How do you feel this baby will affect your job, career, school, and personal goals?

- How will the baby affect your relationship with your significant other?
- What can you do to help yourself and the baby be as healthy as possible?
- What can you do to prepare for being a mother?

2. Initiates positive, proactive routines (childbirth classes, prenatal exercise classes, stress reduction).

Negative:

- Rationalizes or denies behavior that places the baby at risk.
- Expresses inability for or lack of interest in proactive behavior.

Attachment

A. Strong feelings regarding gender of baby.

Positive:

1. Verbalizes love and acceptance of either gender.

Negative:

1. Believes baby will be like negative aspects of self and partner.
2. Verbalizes belief that she will be unable to parent a child of a particular gender.
3. Considers a particular gender as conferring more or less status on the family.
    - Why do you prefer a certain gender?
    - How will you feel and what will you do differently if your baby is a boy/girl?

B. Interested in data regarding fetus (e.g., growth and development, heart tones).

Positive:

1. Verbalizes positive thoughts about the baby.
2. Asks questions about the baby's development and status.

Negative:

1. Shows no interest in fetal growth and development, quickening, and fetal heart tones.
2. Expresses negative feelings about fetus.

Box 33–2 *(continued)*

3. Rejects counseling regarding nutrition, rest, hygiene.
   - Encourage interest in the fetus. Point out normal development.
   - Explore the mother's reasons for negative feelings and/or rejection of counseling.

C. Fantasizes about baby.

Positive:

1. Prepares for the addition of a baby to her household.
2. Speaks of the baby as her child and her other children's brother and sister.
3. Talks to the baby in utero.
4. Makes positive speculations about the baby's appearance and disposition.

Negative:

1. Bonding conditional depending on gender, age of baby, and/or labor and birth experience.
2. Woman considers only own needs when making plans for baby.
3. Exhibits no attachment behaviors.
4. Failure to prepare.
   - What did you think or feel when you first felt the baby move?
   - Have you started preparing for the baby?
   - What do you think your baby will look like?
   - How would you like your new baby to look?
   - Does this baby have a name?

Acceptance of Child by Significant Others

A. Acknowledges acceptance by significant others of the new responsibility.

Positive:

1. Acknowledges unconditional acceptance of pregnancy and baby by significant others.
2. Partner accepts new responsibility for child.
3. Shares experience of pregnancy with significant others.

Negative:

1. Significant others not supportively involved with pregnancy.
2. Conditional acceptance of pregnancy by significant others depending on gender, ethnicity, age of baby.
3. Decision making does not take in needs of fetus (e.g., food money spent on new car).
4. Partner and family with no/little responsibility for needs of pregnancy, woman/fetus.
   - How does your partner feel about this pregnancy?
   - How do your parents feel?
   - What do your friends think?

- Does your partner have a preference regarding the baby's gender? If so, why?
- How does your partner feel about being a parent?
- What do you think your partner will be like as a parent?
- What do you think your partner will do to help you with child care?
- Have you and your partner talked about how the baby might change your lives?
- Who have you told about your pregnancy?
- Do you have family or friends who can help you take care of a new baby?

B. Concrete demonstration of acceptance of pregnancy/baby by significant others (e.g., baby shower, significant other involved in prenatal education).

Positive:

1. Baby shower.
2. Significant other attends prenatal class with woman.
3. Commitment from the mother's community to help take care of the new baby (watch older children when she is in labor and immediately postpartum, meal planning, housework).
   - If partner attends clinic with woman, note partner's degree of interest (e.g., listens to heart tones).
   - Significant other plans to be with woman during labor and birth.
   - Partner is contributing financially.

Ensures Physical Well-Being

A. Concerns about having normal pregnancy, labor and birth, and baby.

Positive:

1. Preparing for labor and birth, attends prenatal classes, interested in labor and birth.
2. Aware of danger signs during pregnancy.
3. Seeks and uses appropriate healthcare (e.g., time of initial visit, keeps appointments, follows through on recommendations).

Negative:

1. Denies signs and symptoms that might suggest complications of pregnancy.
2. Verbalizes extreme fear of labor and birth—refuses to talk about labor and birth.
3. Misses appointments, fails to follow instructions, refuses to attend prenatal classes.
   - Encourage expression of fears so they can be addressed.
   - Ask about reasons for missed appointments in order to assist with obtaining services (medical transportation, social working, home health nurse).

Note: When "Negative" is not listed in a section, the reader may assume that negative is the absence of positive responses.

Source: Modified and used with permission of the Minneapolis Health Department, Minneapolis, MN.

The accompanying Subsequent Prenatal Assessment feature provides a systematic approach to the regular physical examinations the pregnant woman should undergo for optimal antepartum care and also provides a model for evaluating both the pregnant woman and the expectant partner, if the partner is involved in the pregnancy.

SAFETY ALERT When assessing blood pressure, have the pregnant woman sit up with her arm resting on a table so that her arm is at the level of her heart. Expect a decrease in her blood pressure from baseline during the second trimester because of normal physiologic changes. If this decrease does not occur, evaluate further for signs of preeclampsia.

Subsequent Prenatal Assessment

PHYSICAL ASSESSMENT/ NORMAL FINDINGS	ALTERATIONS AND POSSIBLE CAUSES*	NURSING RESPONSES TO DATA†
Vital Signs		
Temperature: 36.2°–37.6°C (97°–99.6°F)	Elevated temperature (infection)	Evaluate for signs of infection. Refer to healthcare provider.
Pulse: 60–100 beats/min Rate may increase 10 beats/min during pregnancy	Increased pulse rate (anxiety, cardiac disorders)	Note irregularities. Assess for anxiety and stress.
Respiration: 12–20 breaths/min	Marked tachypnea or abnormal patterns (respiratory disease)	Refer to healthcare provider.
Blood pressure: less than 140/90 mmHg (falls in second trimester)	Greater than 140/90 mmHg	Assess for headache, edema, proteinuria, and hyperreflexia. Refer to healthcare provider. Schedule appointments more frequently.
Weight Gain		
First trimester: 1.6–2.3 kg (3.5–5 lb)	Inadequate weight gain (poor nutrition, nausea, small for gestational age)	Discuss appropriate weight gain.
Second trimester: 5.5–6.8 kg (12–15 lb)	Excessive weight gain (excessive caloric intake, edema, preeclampsia)	Provide nutritional counseling. Assess for presence of edema or anemia.
Third trimester: 5.5–6.8 kg (12–15 lb)		
Edema		
Small amount of dependent edema, especially in last weeks of pregnancy	Edema in hands, face, legs, and feet (preeclampsia)	Identify any correlation between edema and activities, blood pressure, or proteinuria. Refer to healthcare provider if indicated.
Uterine Size		
See the Initial Prenatal Assessment feature in the Concept section for normal changes during pregnancy	Unusually rapid growth (multiple gestation, hydatidiform mole, hydramnios, miscalculation of estimated date of birth)	Evaluate fetal status. Determine height of fundus. Use diagnostic ultrasound.
Fetal Heartbeat		
110–160 beats/min Funic souffle	Absence of fetal heartbeat after 20 weeks of gestation (maternal obesity, fetal demise)	Evaluate fetal status.
Laboratory Evaluation		
Hemoglobin: 12–16 g/dL Pseudoanemia of pregnancy	Less than 11 g/dL (anemia)	Provide nutritional counseling. Hemoglobin check is repeated at 28–36 weeks of gestation. Consider a hemoglobin screen for women of Mediterranean, African, or South Asian descent.
Quad marker screen: blood test performed at 15–22 weeks of gestation. Evaluates four factors—maternal serum alpha-fetoprotein (MSAFP), unconjugated estriol (UE), human chorionic gonadotropin (hCG), and inhibin-A: normal levels	Elevated MSAFP (neural tube defect, underestimated gestational age, multiple gestation); lower-than-normal MSAFP (Down syndrome, trisomy 18); higher-than-normal hCG and inhibin-A (Down syndrome); lower-than-normal UE (Down syndrome)	Recommended for all pregnant women; especially indicated for women with any of the following risk factors: age 35 or over, family history of birth defects, previous child with a birth defect, insulin-dependent diabetes before pregnancy (Medline Plus, 2012). If quad screen abnormal, further testing such as ultrasound or amniocentesis may be indicated.
	*Possible causes of alterations are identified in parentheses.	†This column provides guidelines for further assessment and initial nursing intervention.

Subsequent Prenatal Assessment *(continued)*

PHYSICAL ASSESSMENT/ NORMAL FINDINGS	ALTERATIONS AND POSSIBLE CAUSES*	NURSING RESPONSES TO DATA†
First trimester integrated screen	Provides the same information as the quad screen in a more accurate and timely fashion as information on trisomy 13, 18 and 21 is available between 11 and 13 weeks' gestation and laboratory tests are combined with ultrasound of the fetal nasal bone and nuchal fold	
NIPT/cell free fetal DNA (cffDNA)	Allows analysis of fetal alleles in maternal serum. Provides information on chromosomal anomalies	
Repeat indirect Coombs test done on Rh-negative women: negative (done at 28 weeks of gestation)	Rh antibodies present (maternal sensitization has occurred)	If Rh negative and unsensitized, Rh immune globulin is given. If Rh antibodies are present, Rh immune globulin is not given; fetus is monitored closely for isoimmune hemolytic disease.
50-g, 1-hour glucose screen (done between 24 and 28 weeks of gestation)	Plasma glucose level greater than 140 mg/dL (GDM) *Note:* Some facilities use a level of greater than 130 mg/dL, which identifies 90% of women with GDM	Discuss implications of gestational diabetes mellitus (GDM). Refer for a diagnostic 100-g oral glucose tolerance test.
Urinalysis: See the Initial Prenatal Assessment feature in the Concept section for normal findings	See the Initial Prenatal Assessment feature in the Concept section for deviations	Repeat urinalysis at 7 months of gestation. Repeat dipstick test at each visit.
Protein: negative	Proteinuria, albuminuria (contamination by vaginal discharge, urinary tract infection, preeclampsia)	Obtain dipstick urine sample. Refer to healthcare provider if deviations are present.
Glucose: negative *Note:* Glycosuria may be present because of physiologic alterations in glomerular filtration rate and renal threshold.	Persistent glycosuria (diabetes mellitus)	Refer to healthcare provider.
Screening for Group B streptococcus: rectal and vaginal swabs obtained at 35–37 weeks of gestation for all pregnant women	Positive culture (maternal colonization)	Explain fetal/neonatal risks and the need for antibiotic prophylaxis in labor. Refer to healthcare provider for therapy.
	*Possible causes of alterations are identified in parentheses.	†This column provides guidelines for further assessment and initial nursing intervention.

CULTURAL ASSESSMENT§	VARIATIONS TO CONSIDER	NURSING RESPONSES TO DATA†
Determine the mother's (and family's) attitudes about the gender of the unborn child	Some women have no preference about the gender of the child; others do. In many cultures, boys are especially valued as firstborn children	Provide opportunities to discuss preferences and expectations; avoid a judgmental attitude to the response.
Ask about the woman's expectations of childbirth. Will she want someone with her for the birth? Whom does she choose? What is the role of her partner?	Some women want their partner present for labor and birth; others prefer a female relative or friend Some women expect to be separated from their partner once cervical dilation has occurred	Provide information on birth options, but accept the woman's decision about who will attend.
§These are only a few suggestions. We do not mean to imply that this is a comprehensive cultural assessment; rather, it is a tool to encourage cultural competence.		†This column provides guidelines for further assessment and initial nursing intervention.

(continued on next page)

Subsequent Prenatal Assessment (continued)

CULTURAL ASSESSMENT§	VARIATIONS TO CONSIDER	NURSING RESPONSES TO DATA†
Ask about preparations for the baby; determine what is customary for the woman	Some women may have a fully prepared nursery; others may not have a separate room for the baby	Explore reasons for not preparing for the baby. Support the mother's preferences, and provide information about possible sources of assistance if the decision is related to a lack of resources.

Expectant Mother

Psychologic status	Increased stress and anxiety	Encourage woman to take an active part in her care.
First trimester: Incorporates idea of pregnancy; may feel ambivalent, especially if she must give up desired role; usually looks for signs of verification of pregnancy, such as increase in abdominal size or fetal movement	Inability to establish communication; inability to accept pregnancy; inappropriate response or actions; denial of pregnancy; inability to cope	Establish lines of communication. Establish a trusting relationship. Counsel as necessary. Refer to appropriate professional as needed.
Second trimester: Baby becomes more real to woman as abdominal size increases and she feels movement; she begins to turn inward, becoming more introspective		
Third trimester: Begins to think of the baby as a separate being; may feel restless, and may feel that the time of labor will never come; remains self-centered and concentrates on preparing place for baby		
Educational needs: Self-care measures and knowledge about the following: Health promotion Breast care Hygiene Rest Exercise Nutrition Relief measures for common discomforts of pregnancy Danger signs in pregnancy (see Table 33–9)	Inadequate information	Provide information and counseling.
Sexual activity: Woman knows how pregnancy affects sexual activity	Lack of information about effects of pregnancy and/or alternative positions during sexual intercourse	Provide counseling.
Preparation for parenting: appropriate preparation	Lack of preparation (denial, failure to adjust to baby, unwanted child)	Counsel. If lack of preparation is caused by inadequacy of information, provide information.
Preparation for childbirth: Patient is aware of the following: 1. Prepared childbirth techniques 2. Normal processes and changes during childbirth 3. Problems that may occur as a result of drug and alcohol use and of smoking	Continued abuse of drugs and alcohol; denial of possible effect on self and baby	If couple chooses a particular technique, refer to childbirth classes. Encourage prenatal class attendance. Educate woman during visits based on current physical status. Provide reading list for more specific information. Refer for thorough evaluation of substance abuse.
Woman has met other physician or nurse-midwife who may be attending her birth in the absence of primary caregiver	Introduction of new individual at birth may increase stress and anxiety for woman and partner.	Introduce woman to all members of group practice.
§These are only a few suggestions. We do not mean to imply that this is a comprehensive cultural assessment; rather, it is a tool to encourage cultural competence.		†This column provides guidelines for further assessment and initial nursing intervention.

Subsequent Prenatal Assessment *(continued)*

CULTURAL ASSESSMENT§	VARIATIONS TO CONSIDER	NURSING RESPONSES TO DATA†
Impending labor: Patient knows signs of impending labor: 1. Uterine contractions that increase in frequency, duration, and intensity 2. Bloody show 3. Expulsion of mucous plug 4. Rupture of membranes	Lack of information	Provide appropriate teaching, stressing importance of seeking appropriate medical assistance.
Expectant Partner		
Psychologic status		
First trimester: May express excitement over confirmation of pregnancy; male partner may be pleased with evidence of his virility; concerns move toward providing for financial needs; energetic, may identify with some discomforts of pregnancy, and may even exhibit symptoms	Increasing stress and anxiety; inability to establish communication; inability to accept pregnancy diagnosis; withdrawal of support; abandonment of the mother	Encourage expectant partner to come to prenatal visits. Establish line of communication. Establish trusting relationship.
Second trimester: May feel more confident and be less concerned with financial matters; may have concerns about expectant mother's changing size and shape, her increasing introspection		Counsel. Let expectant partner know that it is normal to experience these feelings.
Third trimester: May have feelings of rivalry with fetus, especially during sexual activity; may make changes in physical appearance and exhibit more interest in self; may become more energetic; fantasizes about child, but usually imagines older child; fears mutilation and death of woman and child		Include expectant partner in pregnancy activities as the partner desires. Provide education, information, and support. Increasing numbers of expectant partners are demonstrating desire to be involved in many or all aspects of prenatal care, education, and preparation.
§These are only a few suggestions. We do not mean to imply that this is a comprehensive cultural assessment; rather, it is a tool to encourage cultural competence.		†This column provides guidelines for further assessment and initial nursing intervention.

The woman's individual needs and the assessment of her risks should determine the frequency of subsequent visits. Generally, the recommended frequency of antepartum visits is as follows:

- Every 4 weeks for the first 28 weeks of gestation
- Every 2 weeks until 36 weeks of gestation
- After week 36, every week until childbirth.

During the subsequent antepartum assessments, most women demonstrate ongoing psychologic adjustment to pregnancy. However, some women may exhibit signs of possible psychologic problems, such as the following:

- Increasing anxiety
- Inability to establish communication
- Inappropriate responses or actions
- Denial of pregnancy
- Inability to cope with stress

- Intense preoccupation with the gender of the baby
- Failure to acknowledge quickening
- Failure to plan and prepare for the baby (e.g., living arrangements, clothing, and feeding methods)
- Indications of substance abuse.

If the woman's behavior indicates possible psychologic problems, the nurse can provide ongoing support and counseling and also refer the woman to appropriate professionals.

Diagnoses

Nursing diagnoses, of course, vary from pregnancy to pregnancy but may include the following:

- *Deficient Knowledge* related to self-care
- *Deficient Fluid Volume* secondary to vomiting/hyperemesis gravidarum
- *Decisional Conflict* related to unexpected pregnancy

- *Anxiety* related to change in role, deficient knowledge, reaction of family members, and so forth
- *Imbalanced Nutrition: Less Than Body Requirements,* related to nausea and vomiting
- *Risk for Overweight* related to excessive caloric intake
- *Readiness for Enhanced Parenting*
- *Readiness for Enhanced Family Processes.*

(NANDA-I © 2014)

Planning

Together, the nurse and patient will establish the plan of care. Sometimes, priorities of care are based on the most immediate needs or concerns expressed by the woman. For example, during the first trimester, when she is experiencing nausea or is concerned about sexual intimacy with her partner, the woman likely will not want to hear about labor and birth. At other times, priorities may develop from findings during a prenatal examination. For example, a woman who is showing signs of preeclampsia may feel physically well and find it hard to accept the nurse's emphasis on the need for frequent rest periods.

Potential goals of nursing care during pregnancy may include the following:

- The woman will increase her daily intake of calcium to the DRI level.
- The woman will articulate the danger signs during pregnancy and when to call the physician's office or seek emergency care.
- The woman will have the opportunity to express concerns and ask questions.
- The woman will articulate methods of self-care.
- The woman with a chronic condition will consult with her obstetrician and her treating physician during the pregnancy.

Implementation

When providing patient care, the nurse should be sensitive to religious or spiritual, cultural, and socioeconomic factors that may influence a family's response to pregnancy as well as to the woman's expectations of the healthcare system. The nurse can avoid stereotyping patients simply by asking each woman about her expectations for the antepartum period. Although many women's responses may reflect what are thought to be traditional norms, other women may have decidedly different views or expectations that represent a blending of beliefs or cultures.

Promote Knowledge Related to Self-care

The nurse may see a pregnant woman only once every 4–6 weeks during the first several months of her pregnancy, during which time it is important to establish an environment of comfort and open communication with each antepartum visit. The nurse conveys interest in the woman as an individual and discusses her concerns and desires. The nurse can be extremely effective in working with the expectant family by answering questions; providing comprehensive information about pregnancy, prenatal healthcare activities,

and community resources; and supporting the healthcare activities of the woman and her family.

Communities often have a wealth of services and educational opportunities available for pregnant women and their families, and the knowledgeable nurse can help expectant families to assess and access these services. A community-based approach supports the family's assumption of equal responsibility with healthcare providers in working toward their common goal of a positive birth experience.

Home care can be of benefit to any pregnant woman, but it is especially effective in removing barriers for women who have difficulty accessing healthcare. These barriers may include lack of locally available healthcare facilities, problems with transportation to the facility, or schedule conflicts with available appointment times because of employment hours or family responsibilities. A prenatal home care visit or phone contact can also be useful for women who anticipate a short inpatient stay after childbirth. At the prenatal contact, the nurse explains the perinatal program and answers any questions the woman or her family have. Currently, home care is most often used for women with prenatal complications that can be managed without hospitalization if effective nursing assessment and care are provided in the home.

Throughout the prenatal period, the nurse shares information with the family, both verbally and through written materials. This information is designed to help the family carry out self-care and wellness measures as needed and report changes that may indicate a health problem. The nurse also provides anticipatory guidance to help the family plan for changes that will occur after childbirth. The expectant woman and her partner and/or other family members are encouraged to identify and discuss issues that could be sources of postpartum stress. Issues to be addressed before the birth may include sharing of baby and household chores, help during the first few days after childbirth, options for babysitting to allow the mother (and couple) some free time, the mother's return to work after the baby's birth, and sibling rivalry. Families resolve these issues in different ways, but the postpartum adjustment period tends to be easier for those who agree on the issues beforehand than for those who do not confront and resolve these issues.

Childbirth education classes are important in promoting adaptation to the event of childbirth for expectant couples. Classes for pregnant adolescents and expectant parents over age 35 are now available in many communities.

Important topics for patient teaching include the following:

- Self-care to promote positive outcomes (e.g., nutrition, activity, avoiding OTC medications, and delegating care of the litter box to other family members)
- Strategies to minimize the discomforts of pregnancy
- Childbirth preparation classes
- Danger signs to report to the provider
- Signs and symptoms of labor.

Exercises to Prepare for Childbirth

Certain exercises help strengthen muscle tone in preparation for birth and promote more rapid restoration of muscle tone after birth. Some physical changes of pregnancy can be minimized by faithfully practicing prescribed body-conditioning exercises. Many body-conditioning exercises for pregnancy are taught; a few of the more common ones are discussed here.

Handouts are a valuable tool for providing information, as are pictures. When combined, they are especially useful. The nurse can develop a handout that describes the correct way to perform prenatal exercises, and include drawings or photos. For exercises that may be new to a woman, such as the pelvic tilt, the nurse can provide a handout for later reference, but also demonstrate the exercise and have the woman do a return demonstration.

PELVIC TILT The **pelvic tilt**, or pelvic rocking, is an exercise that helps prevent or reduce back strain as it strengthens abdominal muscles. To do the pelvic tilt in early pregnancy, the woman lies on her back and puts her feet flat on the floor. This flexes the knees and helps prevent strain or discomfort. The woman decreases the curvature in her back by pressing her spine toward the floor. With her back pressed to the floor, the woman then tightens her abdominal muscles as she tightens and tucks in her buttocks. In the second and third trimesters of pregnancy, the woman can also perform the pelvic tilt while on her hands and knees (**Figure 33–39 》**), sitting in a chair, or standing with her back against a wall. The body

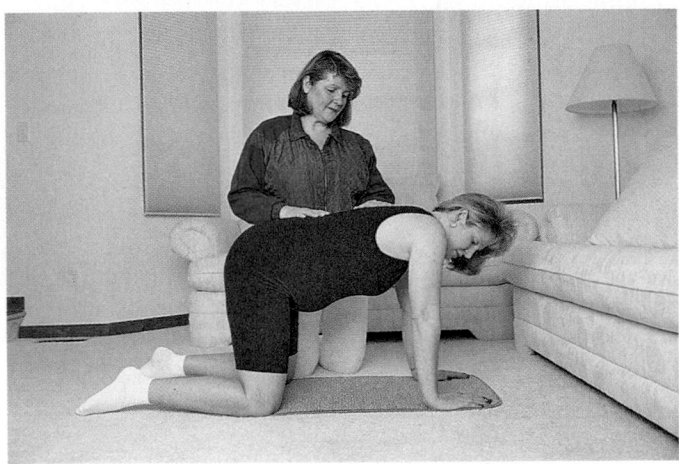

A

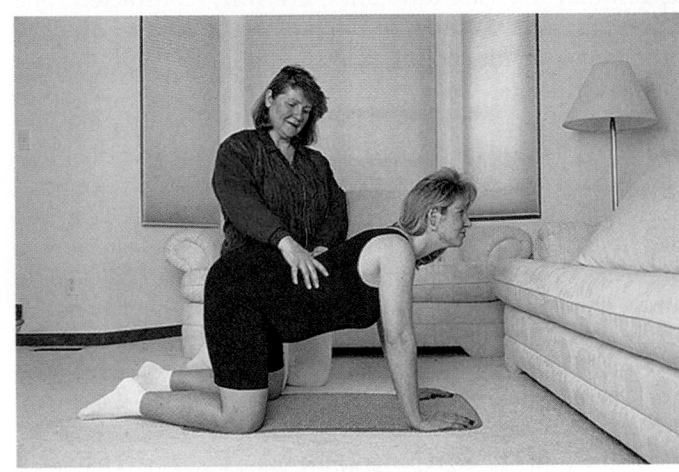

B

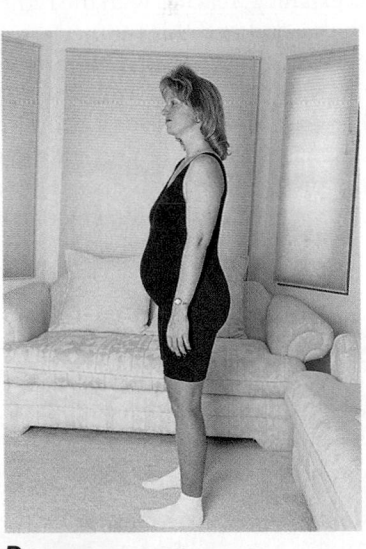

C

D

Figure 33–39 》 A, Starting position when the pelvic tilt is done on hands and knees. The back is flat and parallel to the floor, the hands are below the head, and the knees are directly below the buttocks. **B,** A prenatal yoga instructor offers pointers for proper positioning for the first part of the tilt: head up, neck long and separated from the shoulders, buttocks up, and pelvis thrust back, allowing the back to drop and release on an inhaled breath. **C,** The instructor helps the woman assume the correct position for the next part of the tilt. It is done on a long exhalation, allowing the pregnant woman to arch her back, drop her head loosely, push away from her hands, and draw in the muscles of her abdomen to strengthen them. Note that in this position, the pelvis and buttocks are tucked under, and the buttock muscles are tightened. **D,** Proper posture. The knees are slightly bent but not locked, and the pelvis and buttocks are tucked under, thereby lengthening the spine and helping support the weighty abdomen. With her chin tucked in, this woman's neck, shoulders, hips, knees, and feet are all in a straight line perpendicular to the floor. Her feet are parallel. This is also the starting position for doing the pelvic tilt while standing.

alignment that results when the pelvic tilt is done correctly should be maintained as much as possible throughout the day.

SAFETY ALERT Doing the pelvic tilt on hands and knees may aggravate back strain. Teach women with a history of minor back problems to do the pelvic tilt only in the standing position.

ABDOMINAL EXERCISES A basic exercise to increase abdominal muscle tone is tightening abdominal muscles with each breath. This exercise can be done in any position, but it is best learned during early pregnancy. The woman lies supine with knees flexed and feet flat on the floor. The woman expands her abdomen and slowly takes a deep breath. Exhaling slowly, she gradually pulls in her abdominal muscles until they are fully contracted. She relaxes for a few seconds and then repeats the exercise. The pregnant woman should avoid the supine position after the first trimester.

Partial sit-ups strengthen abdominal muscle tone and can be done if there is no preexisting diastasis recti. In early pregnancy, partial sit-ups must be done with the knees flexed and the feet flat on the floor to avoid strain on the lower back. The woman stretches her arms toward her knees as she slowly pulls her head and shoulders off the floor to a comfortable level (if she has poor abdominal muscle tone, she may not be able to pull up very far). She then slowly returns to the starting position, takes a deep breath, and repeats the exercise while exhaling. To strengthen the oblique abdominal muscles, the woman repeats the process but stretches the left arm to the side of her right knee, returns to the floor, takes a deep breath, and then, while exhaling, reaches with the right arm to the left knee. During the second and third trimesters, these exercises can be done on a large exercise ball. They can be done approximately five times in a sequence, and the sequence can be repeated at other times during the day as desired. It is important to do the exercises slowly to prevent muscle strain and overtiring. If the pregnant woman does have diastasis recti, isometric abdominal exercises should be done instead.

PERINEAL EXERCISES Perineal muscle tightening, also called **Kegel exercises**, strengthens the pubococcygeus muscle and increases its elasticity (**Figure 33–40 》**). The woman can feel the specific muscle group to be exercised by stopping urination midstream. Doing Kegel exercises while urinating is discouraged because this practice has been associated with urinary stasis and urinary tract infection.

Childbirth educators sometimes use the following technique to teach Kegel exercises: Tell the woman to think of her perineal muscles as an elevator. When she relaxes, the elevator is on the first floor. To do the exercises, she contracts, bringing the elevator to the second, third, and fourth floors. She keeps the elevator on the fourth floor for a few seconds and then gradually relaxes the area. If the exercise is properly done, the woman does not contract the muscles of the buttocks and thighs.

Kegel exercises can be done at almost any time. Some women use ordinary events—for instance, stopping at a red light—as a cue to remember to do the exercise. Others do Kegel exercises while waiting in a checkout line, talking on the telephone, or watching television.

INNER THIGH STRETCH The nurse can advise the pregnant woman to assume a seated position with the knees bent and the bottoms of the feet together. This "tailor sit" stretches the muscles of the inner thighs in preparation for labor and birth.

Evaluate Readiness for Enhanced Family Processes

The problems and concerns of the pregnant woman, the relief of her discomforts, and the maintenance of her physical, psychologic, and spiritual health receive much attention during the antepartum period. However, her well-being is intertwined with the well-being of those to whom she is closest. Thus, the nurse also addresses the needs of the woman's family to help maintain the integrity of the family unit.

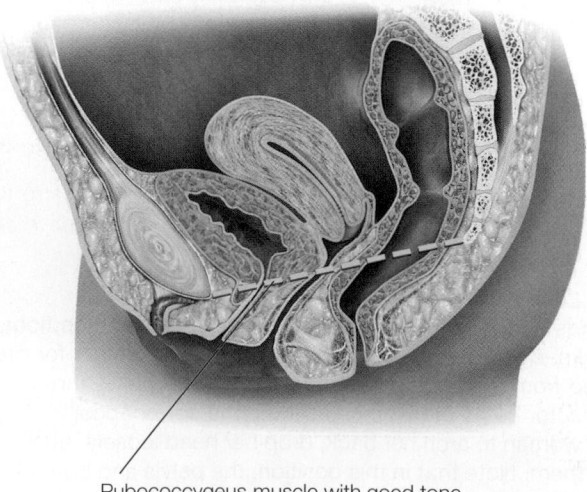

Pubococcygeus muscle with good tone

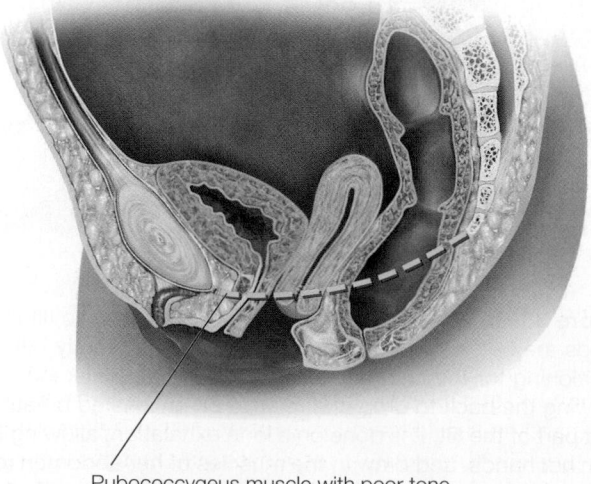

Pubococcygeus muscle with poor tone

Figure 33–40 》 Kegel exercises. The woman tightens the pubococcygeus muscle to improve support to the pelvic organs.

Periodic prenatal examinations offer the nurse an opportunity to assess the woman's psychologic needs and emotional status. If the woman's partner attends the antepartum visits, the nurse can also identify the partner's needs and concerns. The interchange between the nurse and the woman or her partner will be facilitated if it takes place in a friendly, trusting environment. The woman should have sufficient time to ask questions and air concerns. If the nurse provides the time and demonstrates genuine interest, the woman will be more at ease bringing up questions that she may believe are silly or has been afraid to verbalize. The nurse who has an accurate understanding of all the changes of pregnancy is most able to answer questions and provide information.

CARE OF THE PARTNER While the pregnant woman's partner is present in most cases, the partner's presence cannot be assumed. It is important to assess the woman's support system to determine which significant individuals in her life will play a major role during her childbearing experience.

Anticipatory guidance of the expectant woman's partner, if the partner is involved in the pregnancy, is a necessary part of any plan of care. The partner may need information about the anatomic, physiologic, and emotional changes that occur during and after pregnancy, the couple's sexuality and sexual response, and the reactions that the partner is experiencing. The partner may wish to express feelings about breastfeeding versus formula feeding, the gender of the child, the partner's own ability to parent, and other topics.

If it is culturally acceptable to the couple and personally acceptable to the partner, the nurse may refer the couple to expectant parents' classes. These classes provide valuable information about pregnancy and childbirth using a variety of teaching strategies, such as discussion, films, demonstrations with educational models, and written handouts. Some classes even give the partner the opportunity to get a "feel" for pregnancy by wearing a pregnancy simulator. Such classes also offer the couple an opportunity to gain support from other couples.

The nurse assesses the partner's intended degree of participation during labor and birth and knowledge of what to expect. If the couple prefers that the partner's participation be minimal or restricted, the nurse must support the decision. With this type of consideration and collaboration, the partner is less apt to develop feelings of alienation, helplessness, and guilt during the pregnancy. As the couple's relationship is strengthened and the partner's self-esteem increases, the partner is better able to provide physical and emotional support to the woman during labor and birth.

CARE OF SIBLINGS AND OTHER FAMILY MEMBERS The responses of siblings and other family members to the pregnancy are discussed in detail in the Concept section of this module. Briefly, these responses may include feelings of insecurity and even hostility. Thus, in the plan for prenatal care, the nurse incorporates a discussion about the negative feelings some children develop when anticipating the arrival of a sibling. Parents may be distressed to see an older child regress to "babyish" behavior or become aggressive toward the newborn. Parents who are unprepared for the older child's feelings of insecurity, anger, jealousy, and rejection may respond inappropriately in their confusion and surprise. The nurse emphasizes that open communication between parents and children (or acting out feelings with a doll if the child is too young to verbalize) helps children master their feelings. Children may feel less neglected and more secure if they know that their parents are willing to help with their anger and aggressiveness.

It is important not to make assumptions about a woman's beliefs, because cultural norms vary greatly both within a culture and from generation to generation. The nurse should observe the woman carefully and take the time to ask questions. Patients will benefit greatly from the nurse's increased awareness of their cultural beliefs and practices.

Identify Concerns and Promote Strengths

The nurse needs to discuss risks, identify concerns, and promote strengths. It is helpful in promoting a sense of well-being for the nurse to treat the pregnancy as normal unless specific health risks are identified. As the pregnancy continues, the nurse identifies and discusses concerns the woman may have related to her age or to specific health problems.

The common discomforts of pregnancy, such as nausea and vomiting, urinary frequency, fatigue, breast tenderness, heartburn, ankle edema, and other problems, can contribute to an unpleasant pregnancy for the woman. At each prenatal visit, the nurse can focus teaching on ways to cope with the potential discomforts the woman may experience.

The nurse can support couples who decide to have amniocentesis by providing information and answering questions about the procedure and by providing comfort and emotional support during the amniocentesis. If the results indicate that the fetus has Down syndrome or another genetic abnormality, the nurse can ensure that the couple has complete information about the condition, its range of possible manifestations, and its developmental implications.

Evaluation

Anticipated outcomes of nursing care include the following:

- The woman and her partner are knowledgeable about the pregnancy and express confidence in their ability to make appropriate healthcare choices.

- The expectant woman and her partner and their children, if any, are able to cope with the pregnancy and its implications for the future.

- The woman receives effective healthcare throughout her pregnancy as well as during birth and the postpartum period.

- The woman and her partner develop skills in child care and parenting.

Nursing Care Plan
The Pregnant Patient

Martina de Herrara and her husband arrived in the United States from Puerto Rico 6 months ago. This is her first prenatal visit since her pregnancy was confirmed 2 days earlier. Mrs. de Herrara's first child is 3 years old and was born in Puerto Rico. Their families live in Puerto Rico, but Mrs. de Herrara's mother has come to visit and help her get settled in their new home. Mrs. de Herrara's husband speaks some English but is unable to attend the prenatal visit, so she has brought her mother to the prenatal clinic. Mrs. de Herrara's native language is Spanish. Both women speak very little English and seem uncomfortable as they wait for the provider. The nurse needs to complete a health history, collect some laboratory specimens, and get Mrs. de Herrara scheduled for her next appointment.

ASSESSMENT	DIAGNOSIS	PLANNING
Subjective: Shaking head side to side, no eye contact, anxious Objective: BP 128/82 mmHg, pulse 84 beats/min, respirations 16/min, height 5′4″, weight 140 lb, urine negative for protein and glucose	■ *Deficient Knowledge* about prenatal care related to barriers in communication and sociocultural factors. (NANDA-I © 2014)	■ The woman will demonstrate understanding of health information received during prenatal visits.

IMPLEMENTATION

- Schedule an interpreter during prenatal visits.
- Refer to posters with pictures to explain routine care and procedures during the prenatal exam.
- Use teaching models to demonstrate procedures.
- Provide brochures about prenatal care in the patient's native language.
- Refer the woman to prenatal classes taught in her native language.
- Involve other members of the healthcare team to assist with prenatal care.

EVALUATION

- The woman responds appropriately to the nurse by using an interpreter.
- The woman demonstrates understanding by pointing to pictures and phrases on posters.
- The woman uses hand gestures to demonstrate understanding.

CRITICAL THINKING

1. Because of the loss of easily understandable tone and correlation with body language in this situation as the patient speaks, how can the nurse assess the woman's anxiety after providing patient teaching?
2. Using an interpreter, how can the nurse determine the woman's understanding of patient teaching?
3. What questions would you ask to assess the patient's cultural beliefs and needs related to her culture?

REVIEW Antepartum Care

RELATE Link the Concepts and Exemplars

Linking the exemplar of antepartum care with the concept of fluids and electrolytes:

1. What recommendations would you make to reduce the risk of dehydration for the pregnant woman who reports vomiting one or two times per day?

2. What electrolyte levels would you want to monitor in the pregnant woman with frequent morning sickness and vomiting?

Linking the exemplar of antepartum care with the concept of stress and coping:

3. You are caring for a woman with four children who had a tubal ligation after delivery of her last baby. During this visit, the woman finds she is pregnant. How can you help her to cope with the discovery and reduce anxiety enough to allow decision making?

4. You are caring for a woman who has been receiving infertility treatments for the past 2 years without success and has just learned she is pregnant. The woman is very anxious about fetal well-being and the possibility of miscarriage. Design a plan of care to promote anxiety reduction.

READY Go to Volume 3: Clinical Nursing Skills

REFER Go to Pearson MyLab Nursing and eText

- Additional review materials
- Chart 5: The Early Adolescent's Response to the Developmental Tasks of Pregnancy

REFLECT Apply Your Knowledge

Jessica Riley is a single, 18-year-old mother with a 1-year-old son, Ryan. Jessica has had no contact with Ryan's father since before

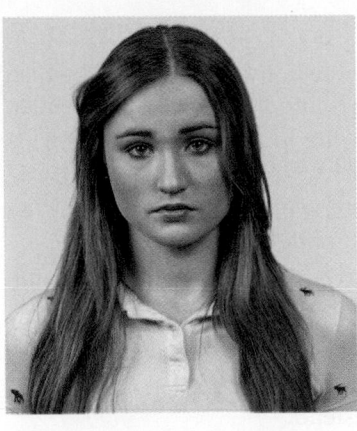

Ryan was born. Jessica and Ryan live in a small, one-bedroom apartment with Jessica's boyfriend, Casey. Jessica is now 6 months pregnant with Casey's child. Although Jessica works full time at a restaurant, she has struggled financially. She is glad Casey contributes to paying the bills and is not sure how she could financially make it without him. Her mother, Evelyn, helps by watching Ryan in the evenings. In addition, Jessica has government assistance in the form of WIC coupons and Medicaid. Ryan attends a government-assisted day care program.

Jessica goes to her 24-week prenatal visit. She continues to see the same midwife and likes her a lot because she makes Jessica feel comfortable. Jessica's history indicates she does not exercise and eats mostly fast foods. Jessica smoked about half a pack of cigarettes a day and drank alcohol socially when she partied.

Jessica tells the nurse who admits her that she tried to stop smoking but hasn't been able to. When asked about alcohol intake, Jessica tells the nurse she is no longer drinking. She shares with the nurse that Casey was giving her a hard time about not drinking, so she has been pretending to drink to keep him happy. While taking Jessica's blood pressure, the nurse notes bruises in the form of fingerprints on her upper arms. While helping Jessica prepare for the examination, the nurse also notes a bruise on her abdomen. When she asks Jessica how it happened, Jessica blushes, stutters, then looks down and mumbles, "I must have bumped into something."

1. Would you assess Jessica further to determine if she has been abused? If so, what specific questions would you ask?

2. What risk factors have you identified related to Jessica's fetus? What nursing strategies can you implement to reduce these risks?

3. What patient teaching would you provide at this prenatal visit?

» Exemplar 33.B
Intrapartum Care

Exemplar Learning Outcomes

33.B Summarize intrapartum care of the pregnant woman.

- Summarize factors important to labor and birth.
- Describe the physiology of labor.
- Outline the stages of labor and birth.
- Summarize the maternal and fetal response to labor.
- Describe maternal and fetal alterations during the intrapartum period.
- Differentiate considerations related to the assessment and care pregnant adolescents and women over 35.
- Illustrate the nursing process in providing culturally competent care to the pregnant woman and her family.

Exemplar Key Terms

Accelerations, *2311*
Artificial rupture of membranes, *2278*
Asynclitism, *2272*
Baseline fetal heart rate, *2309*
Baseline FHR variability, *2309*
Bloody show, *2278*
Braxton Hicks contractions, *2278*
Cardinal movements, *2281*
Cervical ripening, *2286*
Cesarean birth, *2290*
Crowning, *2281*
Decelerations, *2311*
Doula, *2322*
Duration, *2275*
Early deceleration, *2286*
Effacement, *2276*

Electronic fetal monitoring, *2306*
Engagement, *2272*
Episiotomy, *2289*
Family-centered care, *2270*
Fetal attitude, *2271*
Fetal bradycardia, *2309*
Fetal lie, *2271*
Fetal position, *2273*
Fetal presentation, *2271*
Fetal tachycardia, *2309*
Fontanels, *2271*
Forceps-assisted birth, *2288*
Frequency, *2273*
Hyperventilation, *2322*
Intensity, *2275*
Intrauterine pressure catheter, *2305*
Labor induction, *2288*
Late deceleration, *2313*
Leopold maneuvers, *2306*
Lightening, *2277*
Malpresentations, *2271*
Molding, *2271*
Premature rupture of membranes (PROM), *2278*
Presenting part, *2271*
Preterm premature rupture of membranes (PPROM), *2278*
Spontaneous rupture of membranes (SROM), *2278*
Station, *2273*
Sutures, *2271*
Synclitism, *2272*
Vacuum extraction, *2289*
Vaginal birth after cesarean (VBAC), *2294*
Variable decelerations, *2313*

Overview

In the final weeks of pregnancy, both mother and baby begin to prepare for birth. The fetus develops and grows in readiness for life outside of the womb. At the same time, the expectant woman undergoes various physiologic and psychologic changes that prepare her for childbirth. During her prenatal visits, the mother is instructed to call her healthcare provider if any of the following occur:

- Rupture of membranes
- Regular, frequent uterine contractions (nulliparas, 5 minutes apart for 1 hour; multiparas, 6–8 minutes apart for 1 hour)
- Any vaginal bleeding
- Decreased fetal movement.

Increasingly, pregnant women and their families are seeking out family-centered care. **Family-centered care** is a model of care based on the philosophy that the physical, sociocultural, spiritual, and economic needs are combined and considered collectively when planning care for the childbearing family (Katz, 2012). To reflect the consumer demand for family-centered care, most birthing centers now have *birthing rooms*, single rooms where the woman and her partner or other family members will stay for the labor, birth, recovery, and possibly the postpartum period. These rooms may also be called labor, delivery, recovery, and postpartum (LDRP) rooms or single-room maternity care.

The atmosphere of a birthing room is more relaxed than that of a traditional hospital room, and families seem to feel more comfortable in birthing rooms. Another benefit is that the woman does not have to be transferred from one area to another for the actual birth. A birthing room setting not only helps the laboring woman create her own space to labor in, it also enhances the family's comfort and involvement. Birthing rooms usually have beds that can be adapted for birth by removing a small section near the foot. The decor is designed to produce a homelike atmosphere in which families can feel both safe and at ease.

This exemplar discusses in detail the normal progression of labor and culturally appropriate, family-centered care for the laboring mother, fetus, and close family members. A brief discussion of alterations that may occur in the intrapartum period is also provided.

Factors Important to Labor and Birth

The progress of labor is critically dependent on the complementary relationship among the following five factors:

1. Birth passage
2. Fetus
3. Relationship between birth passage and fetus
4. Physiologic forces of labor
5. Psychologic considerations.

Abnormalities affecting any one of these factors can alter the outcome of labor and jeopardize both the expectant woman and her baby.

Birth Passage

The true pelvis, which forms the bony canal through which the fetus must pass, is divided into three sections: the inlet, the pelvic cavity (midpelvis), and the outlet. Factors specific to the birth passage are the following:

- Size of the maternal pelvis, including diameters of the pelvic inlet, midpelvis, and outlet
- Type of maternal pelvis (gynecoid, android, anthropoid, platypelloid, or a combination)
- Ability of the cervix to dilate and efface
- Ability of the vaginal canal and external opening of the vagina (the introitus) to distend.

Fetus

Several aspects of the fetal body and position are critical to the outcome of labor. These include the fetal head, fetal attitude, fetal lie, and fetal presentation. Primary among these are the size and orientation of the fetal head.

Fetal Head

The head is the least compressible and largest part of the fetus. The size of the fetal head is a significant factor in the passage of the fetus during delivery. Once the fetal head has been born, the birth of the rest of the body is rarely delayed. The fetal skull (cranium) has three major parts:

1. Face
2. Base of the skull
3. Vault of the cranium (roof).

The bones of the face and cranial base are well fused and essentially fixed. The base of the cranium is composed of the two temporal bones, each with a sphenoid and ethmoid bone. The bones composing the vault are the two frontal bones, the two parietal bones, and the occipital bone (**Figure 33–41 》**). These bones are not fused, allowing this

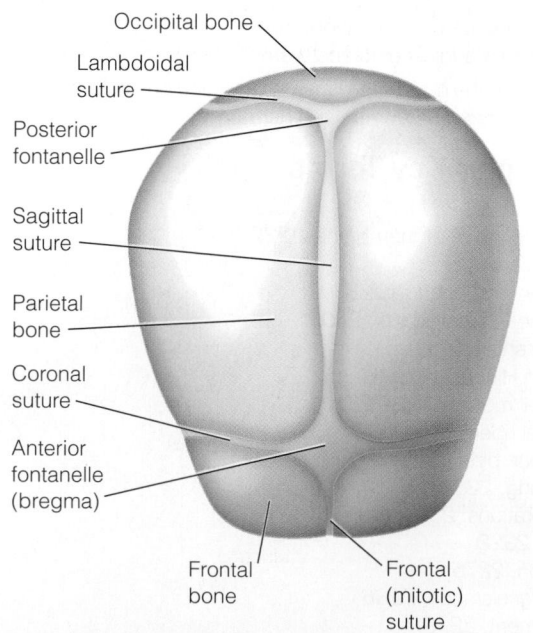

Occipital bone
Lambdoidal suture
Posterior fontanelle
Sagittal suture
Parietal bone
Coronal suture
Anterior fontanelle (bregma)
Frontal bone
Frontal (mitotic) suture

Figure 33–41 》 Superior view of the fetal skull.

portion of the head to adjust in shape as the presenting part passes through the narrow portions of the pelvis. The cranial bones overlap under pressure of the powers of labor and the resistance of the pelvis. This overlapping is called **molding**.

The **sutures** of the fetal skull are membranous spaces between the cranial bones. The intersections of these sutures are called **fontanels**. Cranial sutures allow molding of the fetal head during birth and help the clinician to identify the position of the fetal head during vaginal examination. The important sutures of the cranial vault are as follows (see Figure 33–41):

- *Frontal (mitotic) suture.* Located between the two frontal bones, this becomes the anterior continuation of the sagittal suture.
- *Sagittal suture.* Located between the parietal bones, this divides the skull into left and right halves; it runs anteroposteriorly, connecting the two fontanels.
- *Coronal suture.* Located between the frontal and parietal bones, this extends transversely left and right from the anterior fontanel.
- *Lambdoidal suture.* Located between the two parietal bones and the occipital bone, this extends transversely left and right from the posterior fontanel.

The anterior and posterior fontanels (along with the sutures) are clinically useful in identifying the position of the fetal head in the pelvis and in assessing the neurologic and hydration status of the newborn after birth. The anterior fontanel is diamond shaped and measures approximately 2 by 3 cm. It permits growth of the brain by remaining unossified for as long as 18 months. The posterior fontanel is much smaller and closes within 8–12 weeks after birth. It is shaped like a small triangle and marks the meeting point of the sagittal suture and the lambdoidal suture.

Following are several important landmarks of the fetal skull (**Figure 33–42 ≫**):

- *Mentum.* This is the fetal chin.
- *Sinciput.* This anterior area is known as the brow.

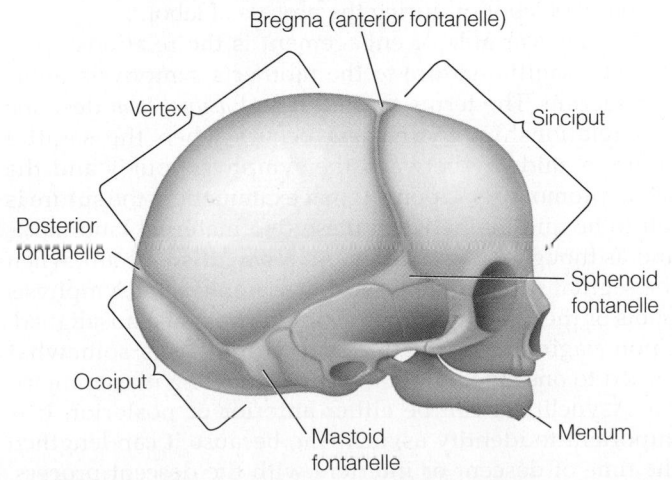

Figure 33–42 ≫ Lateral view of the fetal skull identifying the landmarks that have significance during birth.

- *Bregma.* This is a large diamond-shaped anterior fontanel.
- *Vertex.* This is the area between the anterior and posterior fontanels.
- *Posterior fontanel.* This is the intersection between posterior cranial sutures.
- *Occiput.* This is the area of the fetal skull occupied by the occipital bone, beneath the posterior fontanel.

The diameters of the fetal skull vary considerably within its normal limits. Some diameters shorten and others lengthen as the head is molded during labor. Fetal head diameters are measured between the various landmarks on the skull. For example, the suboccipitobregmatic diameter is the distance from the undersurface of the occiput to the center of the bregma, or anterior fontanel.

Fetal Attitude

Fetal attitude refers to the relation of the fetal parts to one another, including flexion or extension of the fetal body and extremities. The normal attitude of the fetus is one of moderate flexion of the head, flexion of the arms onto the chest, and flexion of the legs onto the abdomen.

Fetal Lie

Fetal lie refers to the relationship of the cephalocaudal (spinal column) axis of the fetus to the cephalocaudal axis of the woman. The fetus may assume either a longitudinal (vertical) lie or a transverse horizontal lie. A longitudinal lie occurs when the cephalocaudal axis of the fetus is parallel to the woman's spine. A transverse lie occurs when the cephalocaudal axis of the fetus is at a right angle to the woman's spine.

Fetal Presentation

Fetal presentation is determined by fetal lie and by the body part of the fetus that enters the pelvic passage first. This portion of the fetus is referred to as the **presenting part**. Fetal presentation may be cephalic, breech, or shoulder. The most common presentation is cephalic. When this presentation occurs, labor and birth are likely to proceed normally. Breech and shoulder presentations are called **malpresentations** because they are associated with difficulties during labor. With a malpresentation, labor does not proceed as expected.

The fetal head presents itself to the passage in approximately 97% of term births. The cephalic presentation can be further classified according to the degree of flexion or extension of the fetal head (attitude) as follows:

- *Vertex presentation.* The fetal head is completely flexed onto the chest, and the smallest diameter of the fetal head (suboccipitobregmatic) presents to the maternal pelvis (**Figure 33–43A ≫**). The occiput is the presenting part. Vertex is the most common type of presentation.
- *Military presentation.* The fetal head is neither flexed nor extended. The occipitofrontal diameter presents to the maternal pelvis (Figure 33–43B). The top of the head is the presenting part.
- *Brow presentation.* The fetal head is partially extended. The occipitomental diameter, the largest anteroposterior

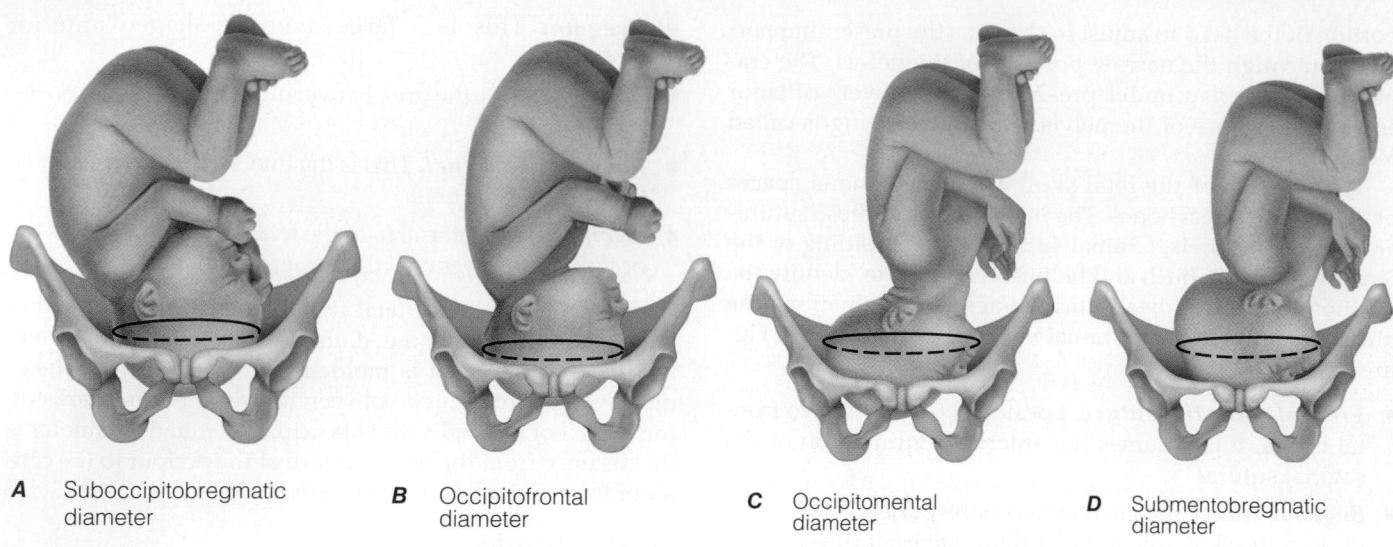

| **A** Suboccipitobregmatic diameter | **B** Occipitofrontal diameter | **C** Occipitomental diameter | **D** Submentobregmatic diameter |

Figure 33–43 ≫ Cephalic presentation. **A,** Vertex presentation. Complete flexion of the head allows the suboccipitobregmatic diameter to present to the pelvis. **B,** Military (median vertex) presentation with no flexion or extension. The occipitofrontal diameter presents to the pelvis. **C,** Brow presentation. The fetal head is in partial (halfway) extension. The occipitomental diameter, which is the largest diameter of the fetal head, presents to the pelvis. **D,** Face presentation. The fetal head is in complete extension, and the submentobregmatic diameter presents to the pelvis.

diameter, is presented to the maternal pelvis (Figure 33–43C). The sinciput is the presenting part (refer to Figure 33–42).

- **Face presentation.** The fetal head is hyperextended (complete extension). The submentobregmatic diameter presents to the maternal pelvis (Figure 33–43D). The face is the presenting part.

Breech presentations occur in 3% of all births (Cunningham et al., 2014). In all variations of the breech presentation, the sacrum is the landmark to be noted. These presentations are classified according to the attitude of the fetus's hips and knees:

- **Complete breech.** The fetal knees and hips are both flexed, the thighs are on the abdomen, and the calves are on the posterior aspect of the thighs. The buttocks and feet of the fetus present to the maternal pelvis.

- **Frank breech.** The fetal hips are flexed, and the knees are extended. The buttocks of the fetus present to the maternal pelvis.

- **Footling breech.** The fetal hips and legs are extended, and the feet of the fetus present to the maternal pelvis. In a single footling breech, one foot presents; in a double footling breech, both feet present.

A shoulder presentation is also called a transverse lie. Most frequently, the shoulder is the presenting part, and the acromion process of the scapula is the landmark to be noted. However, the fetal arm, back, abdomen, or side may present in a transverse lie. The incidence of shoulder presentation is 0.1% of all births (Gabbe et al., 2012).

Relationship Between the Birth Passage and the Fetus

When assessing the relationship of the maternal pelvis and the presenting part of the fetal body, the nurse considers the engagement of the fetal presenting part, the station or location of the fetal presenting part in the maternal pelvis in relation to the ischial spine, and the fetal position or relationship of the presenting part to one of the four quadrants of the maternal pelvis.

Engagement

Engagement of the presenting part occurs when the largest diameter of the presenting part reaches or passes through the pelvic inlet. Whereas engagement confirms the adequacy of the pelvic inlet, it does not indicate whether the midpelvis and outlet are also adequate.

Engagement can be determined by vaginal examinations and Leopold maneuvers. In primigravidas, engagement occurs approximately 2 weeks before term. Multiparas, however, may experience engagement several weeks before the onset of labor or during the process of labor.

Another variable of engagement is the relationship of the fetal sagittal suture to the mother's symphysis pubis and sacrum. The terms *synclitism* and *asynclitism* describe this relationship. **Synclitism** occurs when the sagittal suture is midway between the symphysis pubis and the sacral promontory. Upon vaginal examination, the suture is felt to be midline between these two maternal landmarks and as though it is in alignment. **Asynclitism** occurs when the sagittal suture is directed toward either the symphysis pubis or the sacral promontory and is felt to be misaligned. Upon vaginal examination, the suture feels somewhat turned to one side within the pelvis, making it asymmetrical. Asynclitism can be either anterior or posterior. It is important to identify asynclitism, because it can lengthen the time of descent or interfere with the descent process. Sometimes, this can lead to inability of the fetal head to fit through the birth canal and can result in the need for a cesarean birth.

Station

Station refers to the relationship of the presenting part to an imaginary line drawn between the ischial spines of the maternal pelvis. In a normal pelvis, the ischial spines mark the narrowest diameter through which the fetus must pass. As a landmark, the ischial spines have been designated as zero (0) station (**Figure 33–44 》**). If the presenting part is higher than the ischial spines, a negative number is assigned, noting the number of centimeters above zero station. Engagement is represented when the fetal head reaches zero station. Positive numbers indicate that the presenting part has passed the ischial spines. Station –5 is at the pelvic inlet, and station +5 is at the outlet.

During labor, the presenting part should move progressively from the negative stations to the midpelvis at zero station and into the positive stations. If the presenting part can be seen at the woman's perineum, birth is imminent. Failure of the presenting part to descend in the presence of strong contractions may be caused by disproportion between the maternal pelvis and the fetal presenting part, malpresentation, asynclitism, or multiple fetuses. Station is assessed by vaginal examination.

Fetal Position

Fetal position refers to the relationship between a designated landmark on the presenting fetal part and the front, sides, or back of the maternal pelvis. The chosen landmarks differ according to presentation as follows:

- The landmark for vertex presentations is the occiput.
- The landmark for face presentations is the mentum.

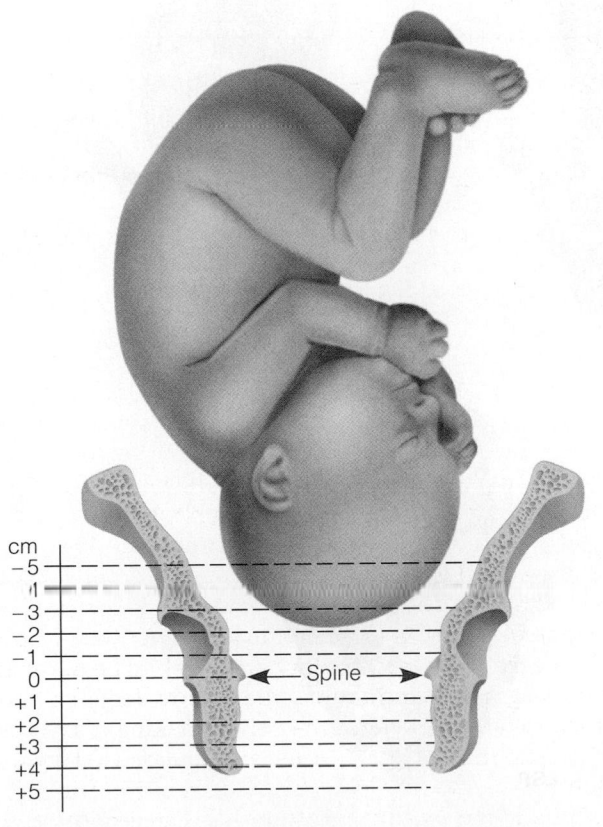

cm
-5
-4
-3
-2
-1
0 ←— Spine —→
+1
+2
+3
+4
+5

Figure 33–44 》 Measuring the station of the fetal head while it is descending. In this view, the station is –2/–3.

- The landmark for breech presentations is the sacrum.
- The landmark for shoulder presentations is the acromion process on the scapula.

To determine position, the nurse notes which quadrant of the maternal pelvis the appropriate landmark is directed toward: left anterior, right anterior, left posterior, or right posterior. If the landmark is directed toward the side of the pelvis, fetal position is designated as transverse rather than anterior or posterior. In documentation, the following abbreviations are used:

- Right (R) or left (L) side of the maternal pelvis
- The landmark of the fetal presenting part: occiput (O), mentum (M), sacrum (S), or acromion process (A)
- Anterior (A), posterior (P), or transverse (T), depending on whether the landmark is in the front, back, or side of the pelvis.

These abbreviations help the healthcare team communicate the fetal position. For example, when the fetal occiput is directed toward the back and to the left of the birth passage, the abbreviation used is LOP (left-occiput-posterior). In the setting of a transverse lie, the fetal spine may be either superior or inferior. This is simply described as *back up* or *back down*, respectively (Strauss, 2015).

Assessment techniques to determine fetal position include inspection and palpation of the maternal abdomen and vaginal examination. The most common fetal presentation is occiput anterior. When this presentation occurs, labor and birth are likely to proceed normally. Presentations other than occiput anterior are more frequently associated with problems during labor; therefore, they are called malpresentations. Presentations and malpresentations are illustrated in **Figure 33–45 》**.

Physiologic Forces of Labor

Primary and secondary forces work together to achieve birth of the fetus, fetal membranes, and placenta. The primary force is uterine muscular contractions, which cause the changes of the first stage of labor: complete effacement and dilation of the cervix. The secondary force is the use of abdominal muscles to push during the second stage of labor, which also is known as bearing down.

Contractions

In labor, uterine contractions are rhythmic but intermittent. Between contractions, there is a period of relaxation. This allows the uterine muscles to rest and provides respite for the laboring woman. It also restores uteroplacental circulation, which is important to fetal oxygenation and adequate circulation in the uterine blood vessels.

Each contraction has three phases:

1. *Increment:* the building up of the contraction (the longest phase)
2. *Acme:* the peak of the contraction
3. *Decrement:* the letting up of the contraction.

When describing uterine contractions during labor, healthcare providers use the terms *frequency, duration,* and *intensity* (**Figure 33–46 》**). **Frequency** refers to the time between the beginning of one contraction and the beginning

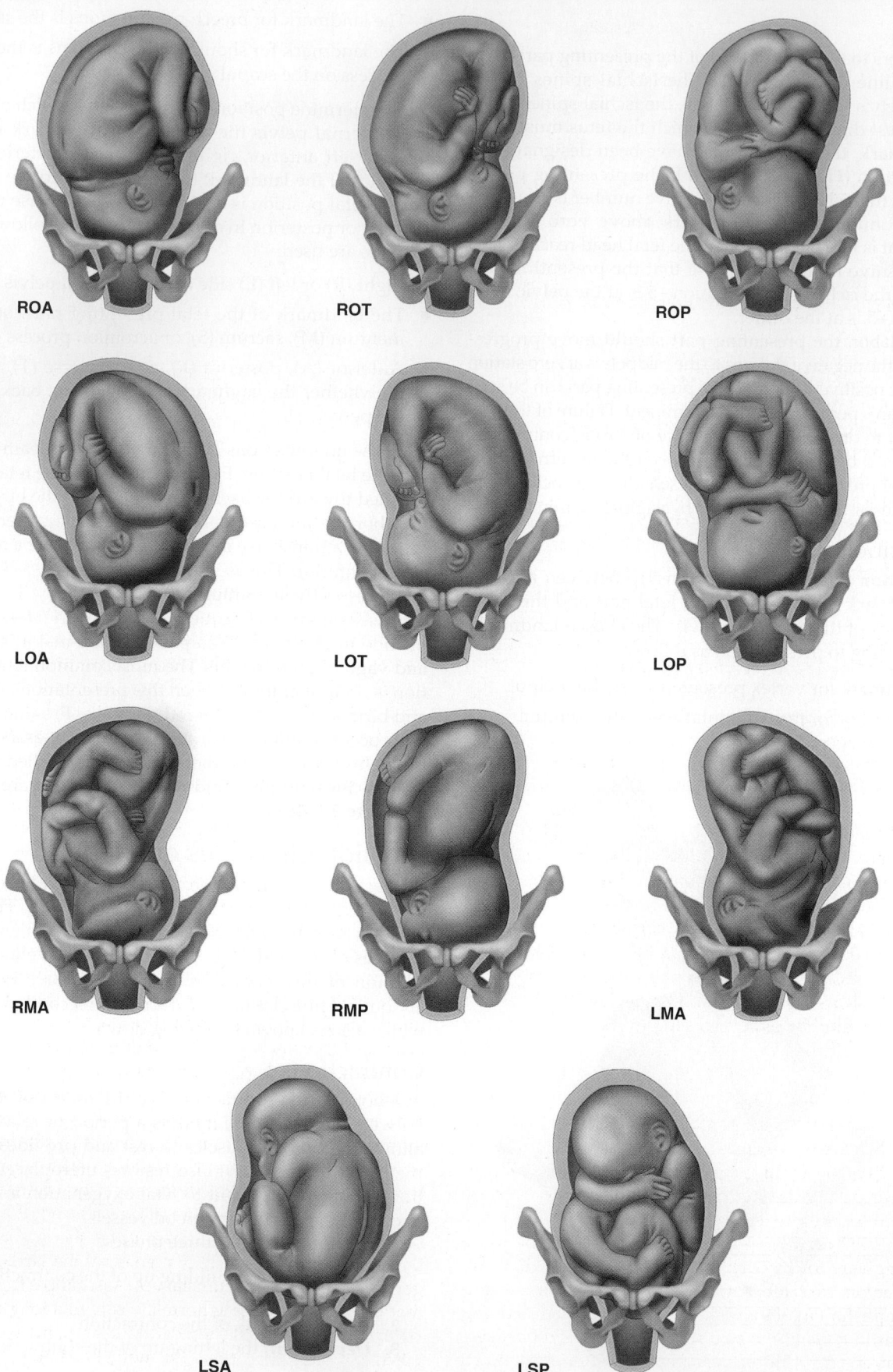

Figure 33–45 》 Presentations and malpresentations. *Key:* FIRST LETTER: R = right, L = left. SECOND LETTER: O = occiput, M = mentum, S = sacrum, A = acromion process. THIRD LETTER: A = anterior, P = posterior, T = transverse.

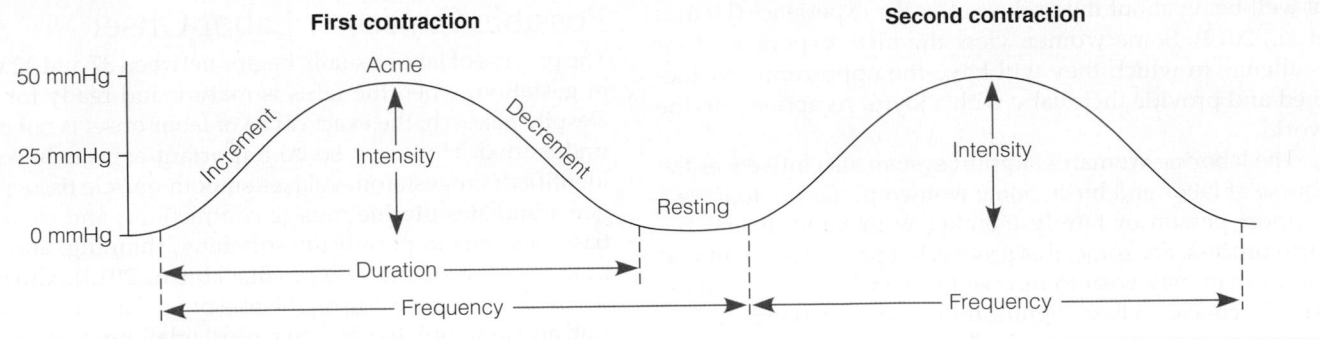

Figure 33–46 » Characteristics of uterine contractions.

of the next contraction. **Duration** is measured from the beginning of a contraction to the completion of that same contraction. **Intensity** refers to the strength of the contraction during acme. In most instances, intensity can be estimated by an experienced examiner palpating the uterine fundus during a contraction, but it may be measured directly with an intrauterine catheter. When intensity is measured with an intrauterine catheter, the normal resting pressure in the uterus (between contractions) averages 10–12 mmHg. During acme, the intensity ranges from 25 to 40 mmHg in early labor, 50 to 70 mmHg in active labor, 80 to 100 mmHg during transition, and more than 100 mmHg while the woman is pushing in the second stage (Blackburn, 2013).

At the beginning of labor, the contractions are usually mild. As labor progresses, the duration, intensity, and frequency of the contractions increase. Because the contractions are involuntary, the laboring woman cannot control their duration, frequency, or intensity.

Bearing Down

After the cervix is completely dilated and the fetus has descended enough to stimulate a maternal urge to push, the maternal abdominal muscles contract as the woman pushes (Goer & Romano, 2012). This pushing action (also called *bearing down*) aids in expulsion of the fetus and placenta. If the cervix is not completely dilated, however, bearing down can cause cervical edema, which retards dilation, and may cause tearing and bruising of the cervix and maternal exhaustion.

Psychosocial Considerations

The final critical factor is the parents' psychosocial readiness, including their fears, anxieties, birth fantasies, excitement level, feelings of joy and anticipation, and level of social support. These psychosocial factors affect both parents. Both are making a transition into a new role, and both have expectations of themselves during the labor and birth experience and as caregivers for their child and their new family. Psychosocial factors that affect labor and birth include the couple's accomplishment of the tasks of pregnancy, usual coping mechanisms in response to stressful life events, support system, preparation for childbirth, and cultural influences. Even pregnant women and partners who attend childbirth preparation classes and have a solid support system can be concerned about what labor will be like. Many couples, even in the intense happiness and excitement of the event, may be concerned about whether they will be able to perform the way they expect, whether the pain will be more than the mother expects or can cope with, and whether the partner can provide helpful support. Although birth is usually a happy and joyful event, it is also a time of physical and emotional stress. Whether that stress is positive or negative, it can affect a couple's responses to the labor itself.

A woman approaching her first labor faces a totally new experience, and the woman who has given birth before knows that this labor might be very different from her previous experience. Most women wonder whether they will live up to their expectations for themselves, whether they will experience a physical injury (e.g., lacerations, episiotomy, or cesarean incision), and whether significant others will be supportive. Many women are excited and happy that labor has begun; however, they may have concerns about the labor process itself.

Expectant women mentally prepare for labor through meaningful action and imaginary rehearsal. The actions frequently consist of "nesting behavior" (housecleaning, decorating the nursery) and a "psyching up" for the labor, which varies depending on the woman's self-confidence, self-esteem, and previous experiences with stress. Specific actions to prepare for labor may focus on becoming better informed and prepared. In addition, just as a woman tries on the maternal role during pregnancy, fantasizing about labor seems to help her understand and become better prepared for it. Fantasies about the excitement of the baby's birth and the sharing of the experience involve the woman in constructive preparation. Many pregnant women have dreams about their baby, labor, birth, and parenting. Some women may fear the pain of contractions, whereas others may welcome the opportunity to feel the birth process. Some women view the pain as threatening and associate it with a loss of control over their bodies and emotions. Others see the pain as a rite of passage into motherhood and a necessary means to an end. It is helpful for the woman to realize that she is safe and that labor pain is not the same sign of danger as pain in other circumstances. Assurances from the nurse that labor is progressing normally can go a long way toward reducing anxiety (and thereby reducing pain) and providing positive reinforcement that the mother is doing a good job.

Empowerment and having control over one's body play a key role in determining whether the woman views her labor and birth positively. Women who viewed their birth experiences as being positive were also more likely to have a sense of well-being about themselves after the experience (Haines et al., 2013). Some women view the birth experience as a challenge in which they will have the opportunity to succeed and provide their baby with a joyful reception into the world.

The laboring woman's support system also influences the course of labor and birth. Some women prefer not to have a support person or family member with them during the birth process. For some, this process is a private moment that the woman may wish to reserve for herself. However, most women choose to have significant individuals (family members, partner, or friend) with them during labor and birth. This social support tends to have a positive effect. For some families, the birth event is a celebration in which they may want as many significant others present as possible. Some women may want to create a joyful, festive atmosphere that includes the grandparents, friends, and other children. A labor partner's presence at the bedside provides a means to enhance communication and to demonstrate feelings of love. Communication needs may include talking and the use of affectionate and reassuring words from the partner. Affection may also take the form of holding hands, hugging, touching, or gentle reassurance for the laboring woman.

How the woman views the birth experience in hindsight may affect her mothering behaviors. It appears that any activities by the expectant woman or by healthcare providers that enhance the birth experience benefit the mother–baby connection. Studies have shown that when some women are disappointed with their birth experience, they may have some initial difficulties and be at higher risk for postpartum mood disorders (Gurber et al., 2012). The partner's experience of the birth and opportunities for bonding may have important implications for parenting as well. Psychosocial factors associated with a positive birth experience are summarized in **Box 33–3 》》**.

Physiology of Labor

In addition to considering the five critical factors affecting the progress of labor and birth, it is essential to explore the physiology of the normal birth experience.

Box 33–3
Factors Associated with a Positive Birth Experience

- Motivation for the pregnancy
- Attendance at childbirth education classes
- A sense of competence or mastery
- Self-confidence and self-esteem
- Feelings of empowerment
- Positive relationship with mate
- Maintaining control during labor
- Support from partner or other individual during labor
- Not being left alone in labor
- Trust in the medical/nursing staff
- Having personal control of breathing patterns, comfort measures
- Choosing a healthcare provider who has a compatible philosophy of care
- Receiving clear information regarding procedures

Possible Causes of Labor Onset

The process of labor usually begins between 37 and 42 weeks of gestation, when the fetus is mature and ready for birth. Despite research, the exact cause of labor onset is not clearly understood. However, some important aspects have been identified: Progesterone relaxes smooth muscle tissue; estrogen stimulates uterine muscle contractions; and connective tissue loosens to permit the softening, thinning, and eventual opening of the cervix (Blackburn, 2013). Currently, researchers are focusing on the role of fetal membranes (chorion and amnion), the decidua, prostaglandin, corticotropin-releasing hormone, and progesterone withdrawal in relation to labor onset (Blackburn, 2013).

Myometrial Activity

In true labor, with each contraction the muscles of the upper uterine segment shorten and exert a longitudinal traction on the cervix, causing effacement. **Effacement** is thinning of the cervix as it is drawn upward into the uterine side walls. The cervix changes progressively from a long, thick structure to a structure that is tissue-paper thin (**Figure 33–47 》》**). In primigravidas, effacement usually precedes dilation.

Contractions are stimulated by the hormone oxytocin. Oxytocin is a potent uterine stimulant and is frequently used as an agent to induce or augment labor in term fetuses or when delivery is necessitated. Uterine sensitivity to oxytocin is increased during pregnancy (Blackburn, 2013). Oxytocin is produced in the hypothalamus and secreted into the bloodstream, but it is also produced in uterine tissues during late gestation, with concentrations increasing at the onset of labor. Oxytocin receptors are most likely formed in the gestational tissues, which when stimulated produce myometrial activity (Cunningham et al., 2014).

The uterus shortens with each contraction, which in turn pulls the lower uterine segment upward. This shortening causes flexion of the fetal body, thrusting the presenting part down toward the lower uterine segment and the cervix. The pressure exerted by the fetus is called the fetal axis pressure. As the uterus shortens, the longitudinal muscle fibers elongate, and the lower uterine segment becomes more distensible and removes resistance on the presenting part as the uterus is pulled upward. This action and the hydrostatic pressure of the fetal membranes cause cervical dilation. The cervical os and cervical canal widen from less than 1 cm to approximately 10 cm, allowing birth of the fetus. When the cervix is completely dilated and retracted into the lower uterine segment, it can no longer be palpated. At the same time, the round ligament pulls the fundus forward, aligning the fetus with the bony pelvis.

Note that the metric system is used for measurement in labor and delivery. Dilation of the cervix is measured in centimeters, for example.

Changes in the Pelvic Floor

Direct pressure from the fetal head pushes the rectum and vagina downward and forward with each contraction along the curve of the pelvic floor. As the fetal head descends to the pelvic floor, the pressure of the presenting part causes the perineal structure, which was once approximately 5 cm

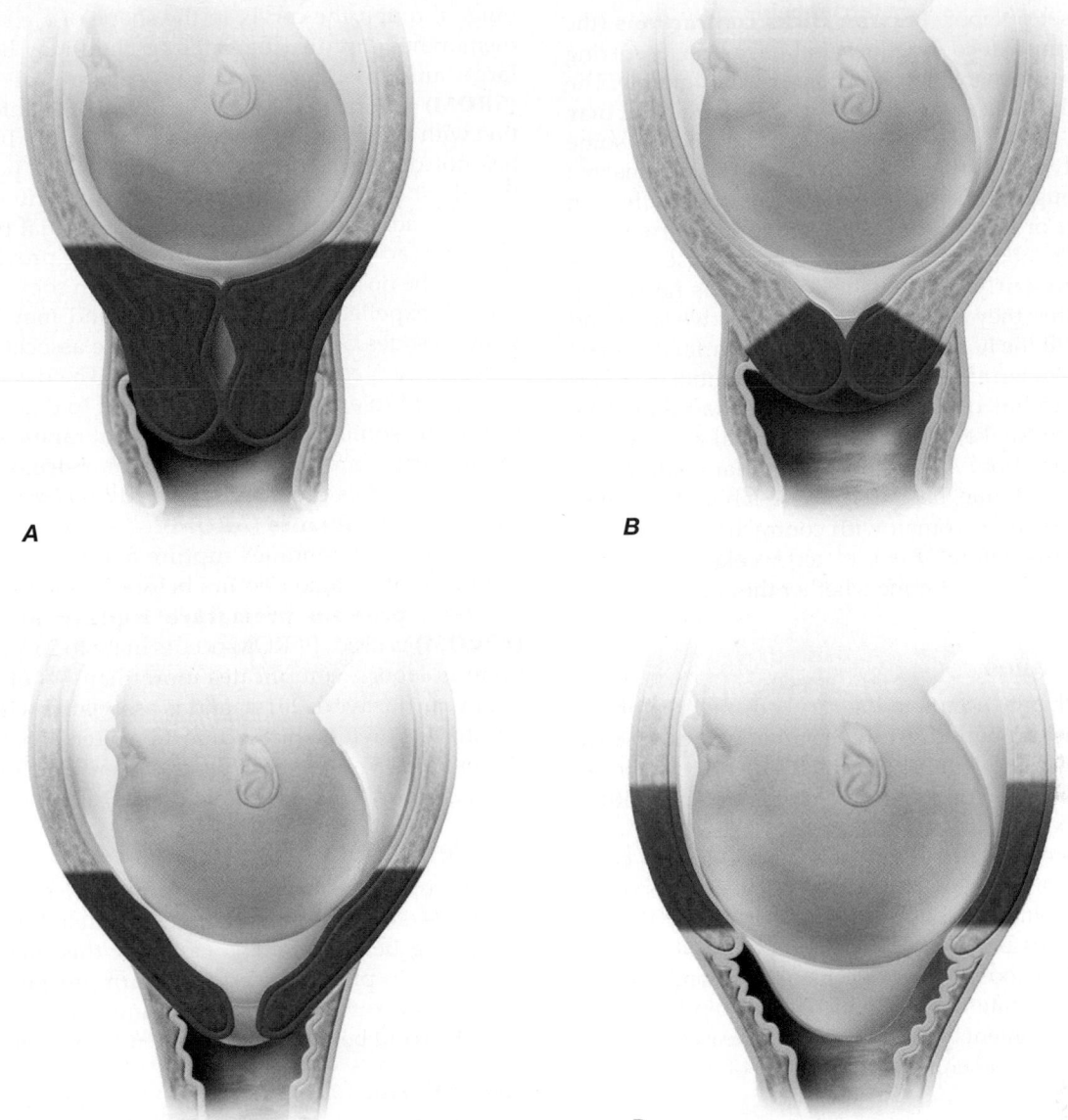

Figure 33–47 》 Effacement of the cervix in the primigravida. **A,** Beginning of labor. There is no cervical effacement or dilation. The fetal head is cushioned by amniotic fluid. **B,** Beginning cervical effacement. As the cervix begins to efface, more amniotic fluid collects below the fetal head. **C,** Cervix is about one-half (50%) effaced and slightly dilated. The increasing amount of amniotic fluid below the fetal head exerts hydrostatic pressure on the cervix. **D,** Complete effacement and dilation.

in thickness, to change to a structure less than 1 cm thick. A normal physiologic anesthesia is produced as a result of the decreased blood supply to the area. The anus everts, exposing the interior rectal wall as the fetal head descends forward (Blackburn, 2013).

Premonitory Signs of Labor

Most primigravidas and many multiparas experience the following signs and symptoms of impending labor: lightening, Braxton Hicks contractions, cervical changes, bloody show, rupture of membranes, and a sudden burst of energy.

Lightening

Lightening describes the effects that occur when the fetus begins to settle into the pelvic inlet (engagement). With fetal

descent, the uterus moves downward, and the fundus no longer presses on the diaphragm, so breathing is eased. However, with increased downward pressure of the presenting part, the woman may notice the following:

- Leg cramps or pains caused by pressure on the nerves that course through the obturator foramen in the pelvis
- Increased pelvic pressure
- Increased urinary frequency
- Increased venous stasis, leading to edema in the lower extremities
- Increased vaginal secretions resulting from congestion of the vaginal mucous membranes.

Braxton Hicks Contractions

Before the onset of labor, **Braxton Hicks contractions** (the irregular, intermittent contractions that have been occurring throughout the pregnancy) may become uncomfortable. The pain seems to be focused in the abdomen and groin but may feel like the "drawing" sensations experienced by some women with dysmenorrhea. Braxton Hicks contractions that are strong enough to disturb the mother without affecting cervical change or fetal descent are sometimes referred to as "false" labor. Prelabor contractions may be exhausting. If the contractions are fairly regular, the woman has no way of knowing whether they are the beginning of active labor and she may come to the hospital or birthing center for a vaginal examination to determine whether cervical dilation is occurring. These prelabor contractions may be exacerbated by inadequate fluid intake, a full bladder, sexual activity, or a urinary tract infection. An episode of regular contractions may resolve or continue, becoming active labor. It is important to remember that women with contractions that occur on a regular basis before 37 completed weeks of gestation should be assessed to determine whether they are experiencing preterm labor.

Cervical Changes

Considerable change occurs in the cervix during the prenatal and intrapartum period. At the beginning of pregnancy, the cervix is rigid and firm, and it must soften so that it can stretch and dilate to allow passage of the fetus. This softening of the cervix is called ripening.

As term approaches, the action of enzymes, such as collagenase and elastase, breaks down the collagen fibers of the cervix. As the collagen fibers change, their ability to bind together decreases because of increasing amounts of hyaluronic acid, which loosely binds collagen fibrils, and decreasing amounts of dermatan sulfate, which tightly binds collagen fibrils. The water content of the cervix also increases. All these changes result in a weakening and softening of the cervix.

Bloody Show

During pregnancy, cervical secretions accumulate in the cervical canal to form a barrier called a mucous plug. With softening and effacement of the cervix, the mucous plug is often expelled, resulting in a small amount of blood loss from the exposed cervical capillaries. The resulting pink-tinged secretions are called **bloody show**. Bloody show is considered to be a sign that labor will begin within 24–48 hours. Vaginal examination that includes manipulation of the cervix may also result in a blood-tinged discharge, which is sometimes confused with bloody show.

Rupture of Membranes (ROM)

In approximately 12% of women, the amniotic membranes rupture before the onset of labor. After membranes rupture, 90% of women will experience spontaneous labor within 24 hours (Jazayeri, 2014). Membrane rupture prior to the onset of labor is referred to as **premature rupture of membranes (PROM)**. Many clinicians recommend induction of labor in the setting of term PROM to avoid intra-amniotic infection. There is, however, no quality evidence to support this practice, and patients should be given the option of awaiting spontaneous labor (Goer & Romano, 2012).

At the beginning of labor, the amniotic membranes may bulge through the cervix in the shape of a cone. When the membranes rupture, the amniotic fluid may be expelled in large amounts. **Spontaneous rupture of membranes (SROM)** generally occurs at the height of an intense contraction with a gush of the fluid out of the vagina. If engagement has not occurred, the danger exists that a portion of the umbilical cord may be expelled with the fluid (prolapsed cord). In addition, because of these potential problems, the woman is advised to notify her healthcare provider and proceed to the hospital or birthing center. In some instances the fluid is expelled in small amounts and may be confused with episodes of urinary incontinence associated with urinary urgency, coughing, or sneezing. The discharge should be checked to ascertain its source and to determine further action. In some instances, the membranes are ruptured by the healthcare provider, using an instrument called an amniohook. This procedure is called *amniotomy* or **artificial rupture of membranes (AROM)**.

When the membranes rupture and leakage of amniotic fluid from the vagina occurs before 37 weeks of gestation, the term **preterm premature rupture of membranes (PPROM)** is used. PPROM occurs in up to 25% of all cases of preterm labors, complicates more than 3% of pregnancies each year (Jazayeri, 2014), and is associated with more than one third of preterm births. Infection often precedes PPROM. When PPROM is suspected, strict sterile technique should be used in any vaginal examination.

Sudden Burst of Energy

Some women report a sudden burst of energy approximately 24–48 hours before labor. This often finds expression in nesting behaviors. The cause of this energy spurt is unknown. In prenatal teaching, warn prospective mothers not to overexert themselves during this energy burst in order to avoid being overtired when labor begins.

Other Signs

Additional premonitory signs include the following:

- Weight loss of 1–3 lb resulting from fluid loss and electrolyte shifts produced by changes in estrogen and progesterone levels.

- Diarrhea, indigestion, or nausea and vomiting just before onset of labor. The cause of these signs is unknown.

Differences Between True and False Labor

The contractions of true labor produce progressive dilation and effacement of the cervix. They occur regularly and increase in frequency, duration, and intensity. The discomfort of true labor contractions usually starts in the back and radiates around to the abdomen. The pain is not relieved by ambulation; in fact, walking may intensify the pain.

The contractions of false labor do not produce progressive cervical effacement and dilation. Classically, they are irregular and do not increase in frequency, duration, and intensity. The contractions may be perceived as a hardening or "balling up" without discomfort, or discomfort may occur mainly in the lower abdomen and groin. The discomfort may be

TABLE 33–10 Comparison of True and False Labor

True Labor	False Labor
Contractions are at regular intervals.	Contractions are irregular.
Intervals between contractions gradually shorten.	Usually no change.
Contractions increase in duration and intensity.	Usually no change.
Discomfort begins in back and radiates around to abdomen.	Discomfort is usually in abdomen.
Intensity usually increases with change in activity.	Change of activity has no effect on contractions.
Cervical dilation and effacement are progressive.	No change.
Contractions do not decrease with rest or warm tub bath.	Rest and warm tub lessen contractions.

relieved by ambulation, changing positions, drinking a large amount of water, or taking a warm shower or tub bath.

The pregnant woman will find it helpful to know the characteristics of true labor contractions as well as the premonitory signs of ensuing labor. At times, however, the only way to differentiate accurately between true and false labor is to assess dilation. The woman must feel free to come in for accurate assessment of labor and should be counseled not to feel foolish if the labor is false. The nurse must reassure the woman that false labor is common and that it often cannot be distinguished from true labor except by vaginal examination. **Table 33–10 >>** provides a comparison of true and false labor.

Stages of Labor and Birth

To assist healthcare providers, common terms have been developed as benchmarks to subdivide the labor process into phases and stages of labor. It is important to note, however, that these represent theoretical separations in the process. A laboring woman will not usually experience distinct differences from one stage to another.

The first stage begins with the onset of true labor and ends when the cervix is completely dilated at 10 cm and the mother has the urge to push. The second stage begins with urge to push in the setting of complete dilation and ends with the birth of the newborn. The third stage begins with the birth of the newborn and ends with the delivery of the placenta.

Some clinicians identify a fourth stage. During this stage, which lasts 1–4 hours after delivery of the placenta, the uterus effectively contracts to control bleeding at the placental site (Cunningham et al., 2014).

First Stage

The first stage of labor is divided into the latent, active, and transition phases. Each phase of labor is characterized by physical and psychologic changes and is summarized in **Table 33–11 >>**.

Latent Phase

The latent (or prodromal) phase starts with the beginning of regular contractions, which are usually mild. The woman feels able to cope with the discomfort. She may be relieved that labor has finally started and that the end of pregnancy has come. Although she may be anxious, she is able to recognize and express those feelings of anxiety. The woman is often smiling and eager to talk about herself and answer questions. Excitement is high, and her partner or other support person is often equally elated.

TABLE 33–11 Characteristics of Labor

	First Stage			Second Stage
	Latent Phase	**Active Phase**	**Transition Phase**	
Labor				
Nullipara	<20 hr in most cases	1.1–3.8 hr	1–3.2 hr	≤3 hr, may be longer than 3 hours with epidural anesthesia
Multipara	<14 hr in most cases	0.9–3.2 hr	0.6–2 hr	<1 hr, may be as much as 2 hours with epidural
Cervical dilation	0–6 cm	6–8 cm	8–10 cm	
Contractions				
Note: Contractions patterns may vary considerably. Patterns that do not fit the parameters outlined here are only classified as pathologic in the setting of protraction or arrest of labor.				
Frequency	Every 10–30 min	Every 2–5 min	Every 1.5–2.0 min	Every 1.5–2.0 min
Duration	30–40 sec	40–60 sec	60–90 sec	60–90 sec
Intensity	Begin as mild and progress to moderate; 25–40 mmHg by intrauterine pressure catheter (IUPC)	Begin as moderate and progress to strong; 50–70 mmHg by IUPC	Strong by palpation; 70–90 mmHg by IUPC	Strong by palpation; 70–100 mmHg by IUPC

Uterine contractions become established during the latent phase and increase in frequency, duration, and intensity. They may start as mild contractions lasting 30 seconds with a frequency of 10–30 minutes and progress to moderate ones lasting 30–40 seconds with a frequency of 5–7 minutes. As the cervix begins to dilate, it also effaces, although little or no fetal descent is evident. For a woman in her first labor (nullipara), the latent phase of the first stage of labor averages 8.6 hours but does not typically exceed 20 hours. The latent phase in multiparas averages 5.3 hours and does not typically exceed 14 hours. Such specific descriptions of the latent/prodromal phase are guidelines and the actual experiences of women prior to the active phase vary widely. Timing and duration of contractions and time elapsed before the onset of the active phase do not, in themselves, require intervention or influence management. Maternal exhaustion may call for therapeutic rest or in-hospital hydration (King et al., 2013).

Active Phase

When the woman enters the early active phase, her anxiety and her sense of the need for energy and focus tend to increase as she senses the intensification of contractions and pain. She may begin to fear a loss of control or may feel the need to "really work and focus" on the contractions. Women will use a variety of coping mechanisms. Some women exhibit a sense of purpose and the need for regrouping, whereas others may feel a decreased ability to cope or a sense of helplessness. Women who have support persons and family available often experience greater satisfaction and have less anxiety compared to women without support.

During this phase, the cervix dilates from approximately 6 to 8 cm (1.6 to 2.8 in.). Fetal descent is progressive and the rate of cervical dilation most often increases. During the active phase, contractions become more frequent and longer in duration, and they increase in intensity. By the end of the active phase, contractions may have a frequency of 2–5 minutes, a duration of 40–60 seconds, and strong intensity.

Transition Phase

The transition phase is the last part of the first stage of labor. When the woman enters the transition phase, she may demonstrate an acute awareness of the need for her energy and attention to be completely focused on the task at hand. She may experience significant anxiety or feel out of control. She becomes acutely aware of the increasing force and intensity of the contractions. Irritability and feelings of self-doubt may occur. She may become restless, frequently changing position in an attempt to get comfortable. The nurse should recognize these behaviors as normal and communicate such to the laboring woman and her support person.

By the time the woman enters the transition phase, she is inner directed and often tired. She may not want to be left alone; at the same time, the support person may be feeling the need for a break. The nurse should reassure the woman that she will not be left alone. It is crucial that the nurse be available as relief support at this time and keep the patient informed about where her labor support people are if they leave the room. Some women have the intuition that the end of labor is occurring and know that birth is near; an instinct to have support people remain often occurs.

During the transition phase, contractions have a frequency of approximately every 1.5–2 minutes, a duration of 60–90 seconds, and strong intensity. The transition phase does not usually last longer than 3 hours for nulliparas or longer than 1 hour for multiparas (King et al., 2013). The total duration of the first stage may be increased by approximately 1 hour if epidural anesthesia is used.

As dilation approaches 10 cm, there may be increased rectal pressure and an uncontrollable desire to bear down, an increased amount of bloody show, and rupture of membranes (if it has not already occurred). With the peak of a contraction, the woman may experience a sensation of intense pressure. If laboring without anesthesia, she may fear that she will be "torn open" or "split apart." She may also fear that the sensations indicate that something is wrong. The nurse should inform the patient that what she is feeling is normal in this stage of labor. Even with assurance, however, the woman may increasingly doubt her ability to cope with labor and may become apprehensive, irritable, and withdrawn. She may be terrified of being left alone, though she might not want anyone to talk to or touch her. However, with the next contraction, she may ask for verbal and physical support.

Other characteristics of this phase may include the following:

- Increasing bloody show
- Hyperventilation
- Generalized discomfort, including low backache, shaking and cramping in legs, and increased sensitivity to touch
- Increased need for partner's and/or nurse's presence and support
- Restlessness
- Increased apprehension and irritability
- An inner focusing on her contractions
- A sense of bewilderment, frustration, and anger at the contractions
- Requests for medication
- Hiccupping, belching, nausea, or vomiting
- Beads of perspiration on the upper lip or brow
- Increasing rectal pressure and feeling the urge to bear down.

The woman in this phase is anxious to "get it over with." She may be amnesic and sleep between her now-frequent contractions. Her support persons may start to feel fatigue and may feel helpless, and they may want more participation from the nurse as their efforts to alleviate the woman's discomfort seem less effective.

Second Stage

The second stage of labor begins with complete cervical dilation and ends with birth of the baby. For primigravidas, the second stage should be completed within 3–4 hours after the cervix becomes fully dilated; for multiparas, the second stage is often less than 15 minutes long. Contractions continue with a frequency of about every 1.5–2 minutes, a duration of 60–90 seconds, and strong intensity (Cheng, 2014). Descent of the fetal presenting part continues until it reaches the perineal floor.

As the fetal head descends, the woman usually has the urge to push because of pressure from the fetal head on the sacral and obturator nerves. As she pushes, intra-abdominal pressure is exerted from contraction of the maternal abdominal muscles. As the fetal head continues its descent, the perineum begins to bulge, flatten, and move anteriorly. Most women feel acute, increasingly severe pain and a burning sensation as the perineum distends. The amount of bloody show may increase. The labia begin to part with each contraction, and between contractions, the fetal head appears to recede. With succeeding contractions and maternal pushing effort, the fetal head descends farther. **Crowning** occurs when the head no longer recedes and remains visible at the vaginal introitus between contractions; this means that birth is imminent.

The woman may feel some relief that the transition phase of the first stage is over, the birth is near, and she can push. Some women feel a sense of purpose now that they can be actively involved. The woman may be focused and should be encouraged to center all her energy into pushing. The nurse should encourage resting between contractions as well. The support person can offer ice chips, fan the woman, who is often overheated and fatigued, offer verbal encouragement, and provide support to the legs.

For women without childbirth preparation, this stage can become frightening. The nurse should encourage the woman to work with her contractions and not fight them. A support person who has never seen a labor may also become disconcerted during this time. The nurse can assist the support person in performing activities and offering encouragement that assists the woman during the birth process. The woman may feel she has lost her ability to cope and may become embarrassed, or she may demonstrate extreme irritability toward the staff or her supporters as she attempts to regain control over her body. Some women feel a great sense of purpose and are unrelenting in their efforts to work with each and every contraction, and some women will be very forceful with and directive of staff and support persons. Although not as common, some women may not experience an overwhelming urge to push and will require guidance and encouragement by the nurse to effectively push during contractions. All of these reactions and emotions are normal and should be supported as the woman works toward the birth.

Positional Changes of the Fetus

For the fetus to pass through the birth canal, the fetal head and body must adjust to the passage by certain positional changes. These changes, called **cardinal movements** or mechanisms of labor, are described here in the order in which they occur (**Figure 33–48 》**):

- **Descent.** This occurs because of four forces: (1) pressure of the amniotic fluid, (2) direct pressure of the uterine fundus on the breech, (3) contraction of the abdominal muscles, and (4) extension and straightening of the fetal body. The head enters the inlet in the occiput transverse or oblique position because the pelvic inlet is widest from side to side. The sagittal suture is equidistant from the maternal symphysis pubis and the sacral promontory.

- **Flexion.** This occurs as the fetal head descends and meets resistance from the soft tissues of the pelvis, the muscles

of the pelvic floor, and the cervix. As a result of the resistance, the fetal chin flexes downward onto the chest.

- **Internal rotation.** The fetal head must rotate to fit the diameter of the pelvic cavity, which is widest in the anteroposterior diameter. As the occiput of the fetal head meets resistance from the levator ani muscles and their fascia, the occiput rotates—usually from left to right—and the sagittal suture aligns in the anteroposterior pelvic diameter.

- **Extension.** The resistance of the pelvic floor and the mechanical movement of the vulva opening anteriorly and forward assist with extension of the fetal head as it passes under the symphysis pubis. With this positional change, the occiput, and then the brow and face, emerge from the vagina.

- **Restitution.** The shoulders of the fetus enter the pelvis inlet obliquely and remain oblique when the head rotates to the anteroposterior diameter through internal rotation. Because of this rotation, the neck becomes twisted. Once the head is born and is free of pelvic resistance, the neck untwists, turning the head to one side (restitution), and aligns with the position of the back in the birth canal.

- **External rotation.** As the shoulders rotate to the anteroposterior position in the pelvis, the head turns farther to one side (external rotation).

- **Expulsion.** After the external rotation, and through the pushing efforts of the laboring woman, the anterior shoulder meets the undersurface of the symphysis pubis and slips under it. As lateral flexion of the shoulder and head occurs, the anterior shoulder is born before the posterior shoulder. The body follows quickly.

Spontaneous Birth (Vertex Presentation)

As the fetal head distends the vulva with each contraction, the perineum becomes extremely thin, and the anus stretches and protrudes. With time, the head extends under the symphysis pubis and is born. When the anterior shoulder meets the underside of the symphysis pubis, a gentle push by the mother aids in the birth of the shoulders. The body then follows. See a birth sequence in **Figure 33–49 》**.

Third Stage

The third stage of labor is defined as the period of time from the birth of the baby until the completed delivery of the placenta, and should be completed within 30 minutes of the birth of the baby. Intervention is required if separation of the placenta from the uterine wall has not occurred after 30 minutes (see *Retained placenta* in the Alterations and Therapies feature).

Placental Separation

After the baby is born, the uterus contracts firmly, diminishing its capacity and the surface area of placental attachment. The placenta begins to separate because of this decrease in surface area. As this separation occurs, bleeding results in formation of a hematoma between the placental tissue and the remaining decidua. This hematoma accelerates the separation process. The membranes are the last to separate. They are peeled off the uterine wall as the placenta descends into the vagina.

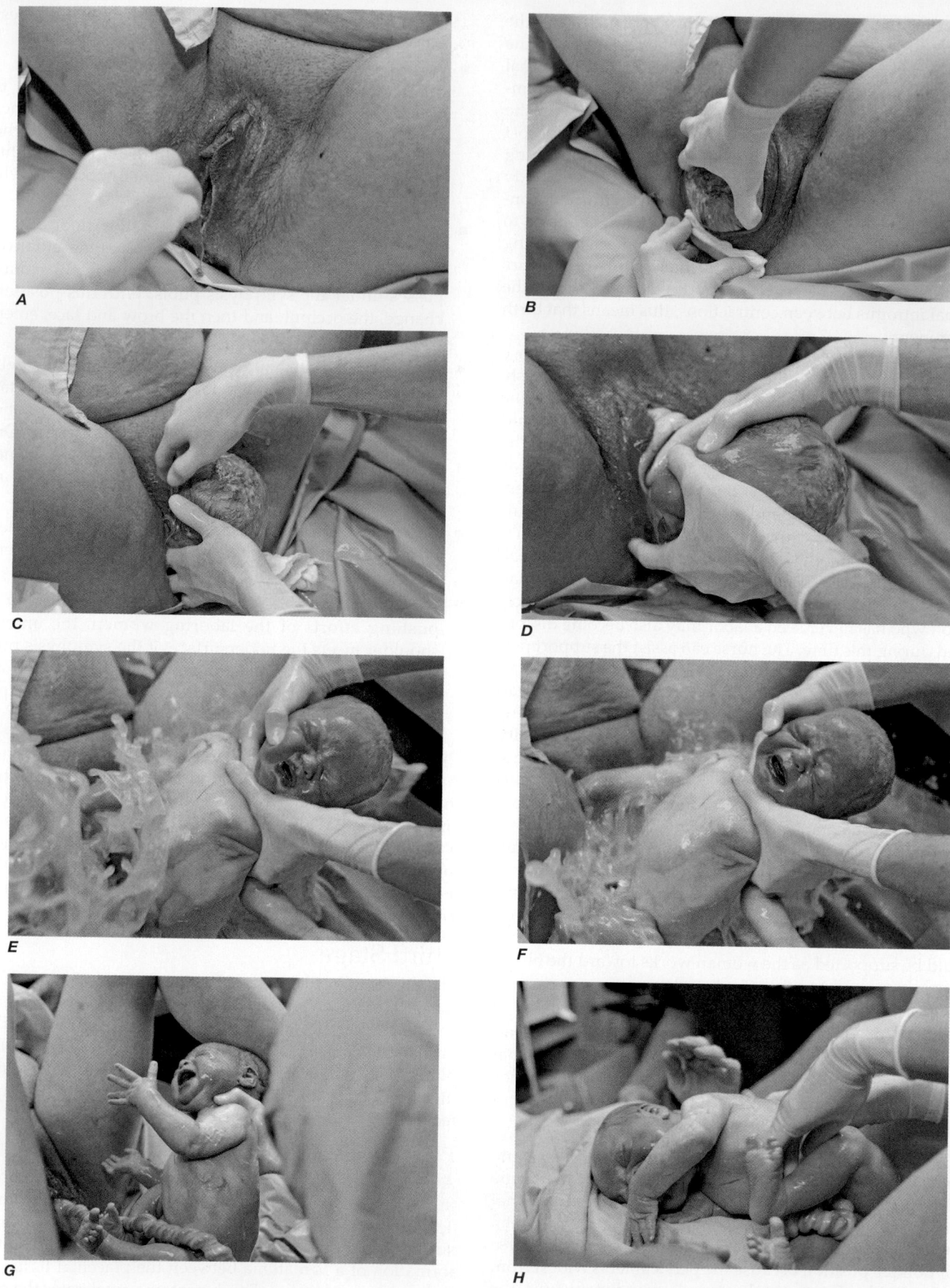

Source: Michele Davidson.

Figure 33–48 》 A birth sequence.

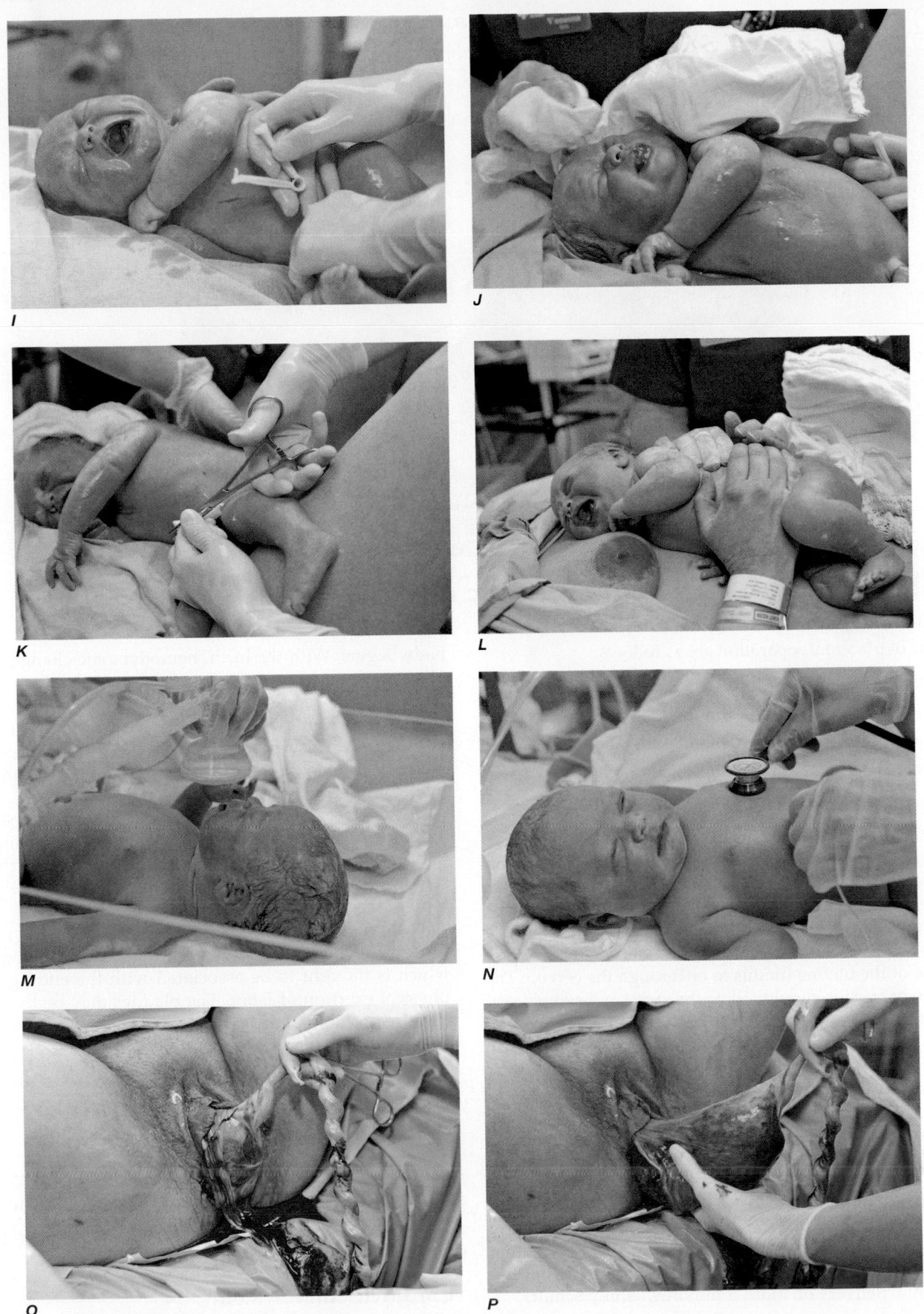

Figure 33–48 ›› A birth sequence. *(continued)*

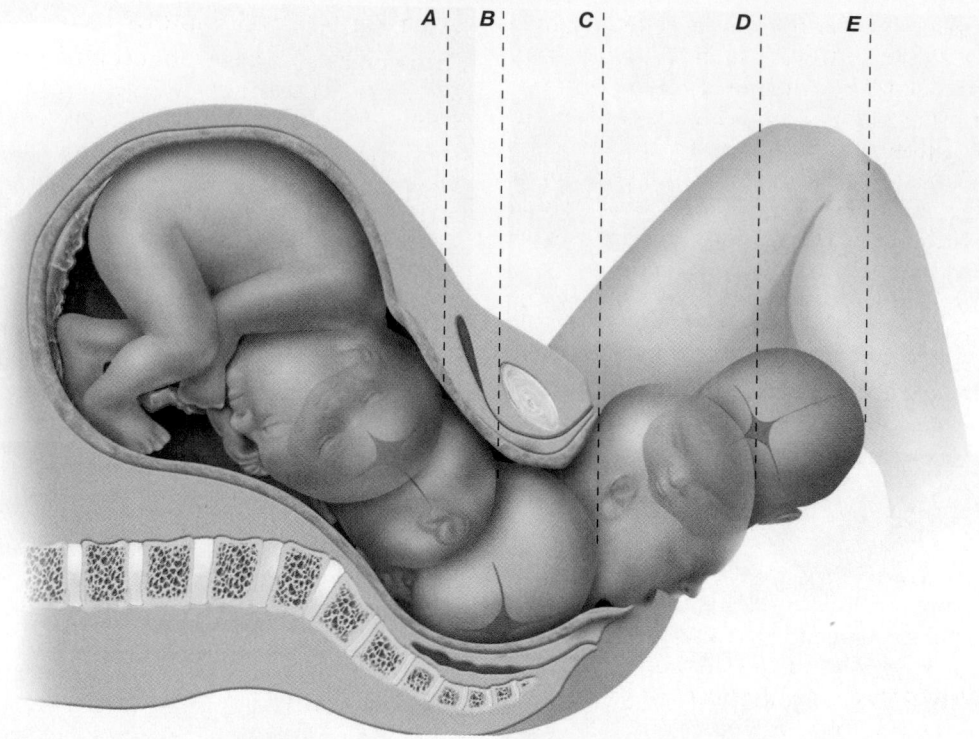

Figure 33–49 》 Mechanisms of labor. **A,** Descent. **B,** Flexion. **C,** Internal rotation. **D,** Extension. **E,** External rotation.

Signs of placental separation are as follows:

- A globular uterus
- A rise of the fundus in the abdomen
- A sudden gush or trickle of blood
- Further protrusion of the umbilical cord out of the vagina.

Placental Delivery

When the signs of placental separation appear, the woman may bear down to aid in placental expulsion. If this fails and the healthcare provider has ascertained that the fundus is firm, gentle traction may be applied to the cord while counterpressure is exerted on the lower uterine segment with the provider's opposite hand to guard against uterine inversion (a prolapse of the uterine fundus to or through the cervix). The direction of traction should follow the sacral and symphyseal curves, and care should be taken to avoid allowing the placenta to fall into the collection pan in an uncontrolled fashion. This may snap off adherent membranes, leaving them in the uterus to cause infection and/or abnormal bleeding.

If the placenta separates from the outer margins inward, it will roll up and present sideways, with the maternal surface delivering first. This is known as the Duncan mechanism of placental delivery and, because the placental surface is rough, is commonly called "dirty Duncan" (see Figure 33–12). If the placenta separates from the inside to the outer margins, it is delivered with the fetal (shiny) side presenting (see Figure 33–13). This is known as the Schultz mechanism of placental delivery or, more commonly, "shiny Schultz."

Fourth Stage

The fourth stage of labor is the time, from 1 to 4 hours after birth, during which physiologic readjustment of the mother's body begins. With the birth, hemodynamic changes occur. Normal blood loss may be as much as 500 mL. With this blood loss and removal of the weight of the pregnant uterus from the surrounding vessels, blood is redistributed into venous beds. This results in a moderate drop in both systolic and diastolic blood pressure, increased pulse pressure, and moderate tachycardia (Cunningham et al., 2014).

The uterus remains contracted in the midline of the abdomen. The fundus is usually midway between the symphysis pubis and umbilicus. Its contracted state constricts the vessels at the site of placental implantation. Immediately after birth of the placenta, the cervix remains open.

Nausea and vomiting usually cease. The woman may be thirsty and hungry. She may experience a shaking chill, which is thought to be associated with the ending of the physical exertion of labor. The bladder may be hypotonic because of trauma during the second stage and/or administration of anesthetics that decrease sensations. Hypotonic bladder can lead to urinary retention.

Maternal and Fetal Response to Labor

Maternal Systemic Response to Labor

The labor and birth process affects nearly all maternal physiologic systems.

Cardiovascular System

The mother's cardiovascular system is stressed both by the uterine contractions and by the pain, anxiety, and apprehension she experiences. During pregnancy, circulating blood volume increases by 50%. The increase in cardiac output peaks between the second and third trimester, although during labor there is a significant increase in cardiac output. With each contraction, 300–500 mL of blood volume is forced back into the maternal circulation, which results in an increase in cardiac output of as much as 10–15% over the typical third-trimester levels (Blackburn, 2013). Further increases in cardiac output occur as the laboring woman experiences pain with uterine contractions and her anxiety and apprehension increase.

Maternal position also affects cardiac output. In the supine position, cardiac output decreases, heart rate increases, and stroke volume decreases. When the mother turns to a lateral (side-lying) position, cardiac output increases. Women with preexisting heart disease have higher rates of arrhythmias in labor (Blackburn, 2013).

Blood Pressure

As a result of increased cardiac output, blood pressure (both systolic and diastolic) rises during uterine contractions. In the first stage of labor, systolic pressure may increase by 35 mmHg and diastolic pressure may increase by approximately 25 mmHg during a contraction. There may be further increases in the second stage during pushing (Blackburn, 2013). The nurse should ensure that blood pressure measurements are not obtained during uterine contractions because they can result in inaccurate readings.

Respiratory System

Oxygen demand and consumption increase at the onset of labor because of the presence of uterine contractions. As anxiety and pain from contractions increase, hyperventilation frequently occurs. With hyperventilation, the arterial partial pressure of carbon dioxide ($PaCO_2$) falls, and respiratory alkalosis results (Powrie, Greene, & Camann, 2012).

By the end of the first stage of labor, most women develop a mild metabolic acidosis that is compensated for by respiratory alkalosis (see the module on Acid–Base Balance). As the woman pushes in the second stage of labor, her $PaCO_2$ levels may rise along with her blood lactate levels (because of muscular activity), leading to mild respiratory acidosis. By the time the baby is born (end of the second stage), the metabolic acidosis is uncompensated for by respiratory alkalosis (Blackburn, 2013).

The changes in acid–base status that occur in labor quickly reverse in the fourth stage because of changes in the woman's respiratory rate. Acid–base levels return to pregnancy levels by 24 hours after birth and to nonpregnant levels by a few weeks after birth (Blackburn, 2013; Powrie et al., 2012).

Renal System

During labor, increases are seen in the maternal renin level, plasma renin activity, and angiotensinogen level. These elevations are thought to be important in the control of uteroplacental blood flow during birth and the early postpartum period (Blackburn, 2013).

Structurally, the base of the bladder is pushed forward and upward when engagement occurs. The pressure from the presenting part may impair blood and lymph drainage from the base of the bladder, leading to edema (Cunningham et al., 2014).

Gastrointestinal System

During labor, gastric motility and absorption of solid food are reduced. Gastric emptying time is prolonged, and gastric volume (amount of contents that remain in the stomach) remains increased, regardless of the time the last meal was taken (Blackburn, 2013). Some narcotics also delay gastric emptying time and add to the risk of aspiration if general anesthesia is used.

Immune System and Other Blood Values

The white blood cell (WBC) count increases to 25,000–30,000 cells/mm^3 during labor and the early postpartum period. The change in WBCs is mostly because of increased neutrophils resulting from a physiologic response to stress. The increased WBC count makes it difficult to identify the presence of an infection.

Maternal blood glucose levels decrease during labor because glucose is used as an energy source during uterine contractions. The decreased blood glucose levels lead to a decrease in insulin requirements (Blackburn, 2013).

Pain

Pain during labor comes from a complexity of physical causes. Each mother experiences and copes with pain differently. Past experiences coping with pain will likely influence how the woman copes with pain during the labor process. Multiple factors affect a patient's reaction to labor pain.

Causes of Pain During Labor

The pain associated with the first stage of labor is unique in that it accompanies a normal physiologic process. Even though perception of the pain of childbirth varies among women, a physiologic basis exists for discomfort during labor. Pain during the first stage of labor arises from dilation of the cervix, which is the primary source of pain; stretching of the lower uterine segment; pressure on adjacent structures; and hypoxia of the uterine muscle cells during contraction (Blackburn, 2013). The areas of pain include the lower abdominal wall and the areas over the lower lumbar region and the upper sacrum.

During the second stage of labor, pain is caused by hypoxia of the contracting uterine muscle cells, distention of the vagina and perineum, and pressure on adjacent structures. Pain during the third stage of labor results from uterine contractions and cervical dilation as the placenta is expelled. This stage of labor is short, and afterward, anesthesia is needed primarily for episiotomy repair.

Factors Affecting Response to Pain

Many factors affect the individual's perception of and response to pain. For example, childbirth preparation classes may reduce the need for analgesia during labor. Preparing for labor and birth through reading, talking with others, or attending a childbirth preparation class frequently has positive effects for the laboring woman and her partner. The woman who knows what to expect and what techniques she may use to increase comfort tends to be less anxious during the labor. A tour of the birthing center and an opportunity to see and feel the environment also help reduce anxiety (especially with the first child), because during admission many new things are happening and they seem to occur all at once.

In addition, individuals tend to respond to painful stimuli in the way that is acceptable in their culture. In some cultures, it is natural for members to communicate pain, no matter how mild, whereas in other cultures, members stoically accept pain, either out of fear or because it is expected. Nurses need to be aware of cultural norms and demonstrate culturally competent care to women and their families in the intrapartum setting to facilitate satisfying birth experiences.

Response to pain may also be influenced by fatigue and sleep deprivation. The fatigued patient has less energy and ability to use such strategies as distraction or imagination to deal with pain. As a result, she may lose her ability to cope with labor and choose analgesics or other medications to relieve the discomfort.

A woman's previous experience with pain and anxiety also affects her ability to manage current and future pain. Women who have had experience with pain seem to be more sensitive to painful stimuli compared to those who have not. Unfamiliar surroundings and events may increase anxiety, as may separation from family and loved ones. Anticipation of discomfort and questions about whether the mother can cope with the contractions may increase anxiety as well.

Both attention and distraction influence the perception of pain. When the sensation of pain is the focus of attention, the perceived intensity is greater. A sensory stimulus, such as a back rub, can provide distraction and help refocus the woman's attention on the stimulus rather than the pain. Randomized controlled trials have shown that the continuous presence of a support person improves the woman's coping ability and perception of her experience. Furthermore, consistent provision of social support and comfort measures shortens the duration of labor, decreases use of analgesia and anesthesia, and reduces the rate of operative delivery (King et al., 2013).

Fetal Response to Labor

When the fetus is healthy, the mechanical and hemodynamic changes of normal labor have no adverse effects. However, certain physiologic responses, including heart rate, acid–base, hemodynamic changes, and fetal sensation experiences do occur.

Heart Rate

Fetal heart rate decelerations (periodic decreases in FHR from the normal baseline) can occur with intracranial pressures of 40–55 mmHg as the head pushes against the cervix. The currently accepted explanation of this **early deceleration** is hypoxic depression of the central nervous system, which is under vagal control. The absence of these head-compression decelerations in some fetuses during labor is explained by the existence of a threshold that is reached more gradually in the presence of intact membranes and lack of maternal resistance. These early decelerations are harmless in a normal fetus.

Acid–Base Status

Blood flow is decreased to the fetus at the peak of each contraction, leading to a slow decrease in pH status. During the second stage of labor, as uterine contractions become longer and stronger and the woman often holds her breath to push, the fetal pH decreases more rapidly. Although women are encouraged to maintain slow, evenly paced breathing, holding of the breath often occurs. As the base deficit increases, fetal oxygen saturation drops by approximately 10% (Blackburn, 2013).

Hemodynamic Changes

The adequate exchange of nutrients and gases in the fetal capillaries and intervillous spaces depends, in part, on the fetal blood pressure. Fetal blood pressure is a protective mechanism for the normal fetus in the anoxic periods caused by the contracting uterus during labor. The fetal and placental reserves are usually enough to ensure that the fetus comes through these anoxic periods unharmed (Blackburn, 2013).

Fetal Sensation

Beginning at approximately 37 or 38 weeks of gestation (full term), the fetus is able to experience sensations of light, sound, and touch. The full-term fetus is able to hear music and the maternal voice. Even in utero, the fetus is sensitive to light and will move away from a bright light source. In addition, the full-term fetus is aware of pressure sensations during labor, such as the touch of the healthcare provider during a vaginal exam or the pressure on the head as a contraction occurs. Although the fetus may not be able to process this input, it is important to note that as the woman labors, the fetus also experiences the labor.

Alterations During Intrapartum Care

Most births occur without the need for operative obstetric intervention. In some instances, however, procedures are necessary to maintain the safety of the woman and the fetus. The most common of these procedures are labor induction, episiotomy, cesarean birth, and vaginal birth after cesarean (VBAC).

Generally, women are aware of the possible need for an obstetric procedure during their labor and birth. However, some women expect to have a normal, physiologic experience and feel disappointed, angry, or even guilty when an unanticipated procedure becomes necessary. This conflict between expectation and the need for intervention presents a challenge to maternity nurses. To support patient-centered care, the nurse provides information regarding any procedure to help the woman and her partner or other support person understand what is proposed, the anticipated benefits and possible risks, and any alternatives.

Cervical Ripening

Induction of labor may be necessary or beneficial in certain clinical situations. When the cervix is unfavorable (usually defined as a Bishop score less than 6; see **Table 33–12** »), the use of cervical ripening agents increases the likelihood of a successful induction of labor. Misoprostol (Cytotec) and formulations of prostaglandin E_2 (PGE$_2$) gel for **cervical ripening** (softening and effacing of the cervix) are drugs that may be used for the pregnant woman at or near term when there is a medical or obstetric indication for induction of labor. Mechanical methods designed to ripen the cervix include the use of balloon catheters to encourage mechanical dilation.

TABLE 33–12 Bishop Scoring System

Score	Dilation (cm)	Position of Cervix	Effacement (%)	Station (from −3 to +3)	Cervical Consistency
0	Closed	Posterior	0–30	−3	Firm
1	1–2	Midposition	40–50	−2	Medium
2	3–4	Anterior	60–70	−1, 0	Soft
3	5–6	—	80	+1, +2	—

Source: Data from Bishop, E. H. (1964). Pelvic scoring for elective inductions. *Obstetrics & Gynecology, 24,* 266.

Use of Misoprostol

Misoprostol (Cytotec) is a synthetic PGE_1 analogue that can be used to soften and ripen the cervix and to induce labor. It is available as a tablet that is inserted into the vagina, or it can be taken orally or sublingually. The use of Cytotec for cervical ripening has fluctuated. Cytotec was widely used in the 1990s for cervical ripening and induction of labor until several reports showed an increase in the rates of uterine rupture. However, there is now a large body of research that supports its safety and efficacy when used appropriately (Phend, 2013). Cytotec is approved by the FDA for prevention of peptic ulcer disease and has had special labeling for indication of cervical ripening and induction of labor since 2002 (Phend, 2013).

Research has shown that the use of Cytotec for ripening the cervix and inducing labor is more effective than the use of oxytocin or prostaglandin agents and is less costly. Women who receive Cytotec to induce labor typically deliver within 24 hours of administration. The use of Cytotec is also associated with lower cesarean birthrates. When compared with women who have been induced using prostaglandin agents or oxytocin, the adverse outcomes do not differ among the three methods (ACOG, 2013f). Most adverse maternal and fetal outcomes associated with misoprostol have been associated with the use of doses larger than the recommended 25 mcg. Intravaginal misoprostol has been found to be as efficacious as or superior to dinoprostone gel (Cunningham et al., 2014). Guidelines for misoprostol induction include the following (ACOG, 2013f):

- The initial dosage should be 25 mcg.
- Recurrent administration should not exceed dosing intervals of more than 3–6 hours.
- Oxytocin should not be administered less than 4 hours after the last Cytotec dose.
- Cytotec should be administered only where the uterine activity and FHR can be monitored continuously for an initial observation period.

Contraindications for Cytotec include the following:

- Nonreassuring FHR tracing
- Frequent uterine contractions of moderate intensity.

Use of Prostaglandin Agents

The two most commonly used types of prostaglandin gel are Prepidil and Cervidil. Prepidil gel contains 0.5 mg dinoprostone (a form of prostaglandin E_2 for intracervical application) and is placed intracervically. Cervidil is packaged in an intravaginal insert that resembles a 2-cm-square piece of cardboard. It is placed in the posterior vagina and is left in place to provide a slow release of 10 mg dinoprostone at a rate of 0.3 mg/hr over 12 hours.

The advantage of Cervidil is that it can be removed easily if an adverse reaction occurs. Both preparations have been demonstrated to cause cervical ripening, shorter labor, and lower requirements for oxytocin during labor induction (ACOG, 2013f). Vaginal birth is achieved within 24 hours for most women. The incidence of cesarean birth is reduced when prostaglandin agents are used before labor induction.

Risks of prostaglandin administration include uterine tachysystole (more than five contractions in 10 minutes), nonreassuring fetal status, higher incidence of postpartum hemorrhage, and uterine rupture that can occur even in the absence of a previous uterine incision (Creasy et al., 2014). Women with a previous uterine incision should not receive prostaglandin agents, because the risk of uterine rupture is greatly increased (ACOG, 2013f). Prostaglandin should be used with caution in women with compromised cardiovascular, hepatic, or renal function and in women with asthma or glaucoma (Creasy et al., 2014).

Use of Mechanical Methods

Balloon catheters are the safest and most common mechanical method of cervical ripening, though laminaria may still be used in some institutions. Advantages of mechanical agents for cervical ripening are similar efficacy when compared to hormonal agents, less cost, lower incidence of systemic side effects, and lower incidence of uterine tachysystole (Davidson, 2013).

Balloon catheters have been used for cervical ripening for many years to promote mechanical dilation. A Foley catheter with a 25- to 80-mL balloon is passed through the undilated cervix and then inflated. The weighted balloon applies pressure on the internal os of the cervix and acts to ripen the cervix. This technique can be used alone or in conjunction with pharmacologic or additional mechanical methods. Advantages of the balloon catheter include higher vaginal birth rates and lower rates of hypersystolic labor when combined with PGE_2 gel (Goldberg, 2015). One study examined cervical ripening after Foley catheter insertion and found that the mean change in the Bishop score was 3.56 after placement of a Foley bulb catheter. The average time from

Foley bulb expulsion until birth was 8 hours and 27 minutes, which indicates that Foley bulb induction is a safe and effective means to induce cervical ripening (Posner, Black, & Jones, 2013). A systematic review of the evidence of mechanical methods of cervical ripening and induction found that in women with an unfavorable cervix, Foley catheter placement prior to induction with oxytocin significantly reduced the duration of labor and reduced the risk of a cesarean section (Posner et al., 2013).

Nursing Care During Cervical Ripening

Physicians, CNMs, and labor and delivery nurses who have had special education and training may administer agents for cervical ripening. Maternal vital signs are assessed for a baseline, and an electronic fetal monitor is applied for at least 20 minutes to obtain an external tracing of uterine activity, FHR pattern, and a reactive nonstress test (NST). If a nonreactive test is obtained, consultation with the healthcare provider is required. After the gel, intravaginal insert, or tablet has been inserted, the woman is instructed to remain lying down with a rolled blanket or hip wedge under her right hip to tip the uterus slightly to the left for the first 30–60 minutes to maintain the cervical ripening agent in place. Gel may leak from the endocervix. The nurse monitors the woman for uterine tachysystole and FHR abnormalities (changes in baseline rate, variability [fluctuations in the FHR], and presence of decelerations) for 30 minutes to 2 hours if a prostaglandin gel agent is used (ACOG, 2013f). If tachysystole occurs, the woman is positioned on her left side and oxygen is administered if fetal stress is noted. The administration of a tocolytic agent (such as a subcutaneous injection of 0.25 mg terbutaline) should be considered if the uterine tachysystole pattern continues. The gel may be removed if severe nausea, vomiting, or tachysystole develops (Wilson, Shannon, & Shields, 2017). Treatment with antiemetics, antipyretics, and antidiarrheal agents usually is not indicated. Women who receive Cervidil or Cytotec tend to remain in the acute care setting so the contraction pattern and fetal status can be monitored continuously for an initial observation period (ACOG, 2013f).

Women undergoing induction via balloon catheters do not need continuous fetal monitoring. The nurse can perform intermittent monitoring along with the maternal vital signs. The nurse should also assess the location of the catheter to ensure that the catheter has not become displaced. This can be achieved by marking the catheter tubing at the introitus and noting whether movement has occurred. Vaginal examinations should not be performed.

Labor Induction

The ACOG defines **labor induction** as the stimulation of uterine contractions before the spontaneous onset of labor, with or without ruptured fetal membranes, for the purpose of accomplishing birth. Induction may be indicated in the presence of the following (Cunningham et al., 2014):

- Diabetes mellitus
- Renal disease
- Preeclampsia–eclampsia
- Chronic pulmonary disease

- Premature rupture of membranes
- Chorioamnionitis
- Postterm gestation greater than 42 weeks
- Mild abruptio placentae without evidence of nonreassuring fetal status
- Intrauterine fetal demise
- Intrauterine fetal growth restriction
- Isoimmunization
- Oligohydramnios
- Nonreassuring fetal status
- Nonreassuring antepartum testing.

Relative indications include chronic hypertension, systemic lupus erythematosus, gestational diabetes, coagulation disorders, cholestasis of pregnancy, polyhydramnios, fetal anomalies requiring specialized neonatal care, logistical factors (risk of rapid birth, distance from hospital), psychologic factors, advanced cervical dilation, previous stillbirth, and postterm gestation greater than 41 weeks (Cunningham et al., 2014).

All contraindications to spontaneous labor and vaginal birth are contraindications to the induction of labor. Maternal contraindications include, but are not limited to, the following (Cunningham et al., 2014):

- Patient refusal
- Placenta previa or vasa previa
- Transverse fetal lie
- Previous classic uterine incision (or any vertical incision in the upper portion of the uterus)
- Active genital herpes infection
- Umbilical cord prolapse
- Absolute cephalopelvic disproportion.

Before induction is attempted, appropriate assessment must indicate that both the woman and the fetus are ready for the onset of labor. This includes evaluation of fetal maturity and cervical readiness. The gestational age of the fetus is best evaluated by accurate maternal menstrual dating and early ultrasound exams. Amniotic fluid studies provide valuable information regarding fetal lung maturity.

Forceps-assisted Birth

Forceps are designed to assist the birth of a fetus by providing traction or by providing the means to rotate the fetal head to an occipitoanterior position. In medical literature and practice, **forceps-assisted birth** is also known as *instrumental delivery*, *operative delivery*, or *operative vaginal delivery*. There are many different types of forceps, each with special functions. The type of forceps used is determined by the physician assisting with the birth and the clinical situation.

Indications for Use of Forceps

Indications for the use of forceps include the presence of any condition that threatens the mother or fetus and that can be relieved by birth. Conditions that put the woman at risk include heart disease, acute pulmonary edema or pulmonary compromise, certain neurologic conditions, intrapartum infection, prolonged second stage, or exhaustion. Fetal conditions include premature placental separation, prolapsed umbilical cord, and nonreassuring fetal status. Forceps may be used when the fetal station is very low to shorten the second stage of labor and spare the woman's pushing effort (when exhaustion or heart disease is present) or when regional anesthesia or paralysis has affected the woman's motor innervation, and she cannot push effectively (Cunningham et al., 2014).

Risk factors for a forceps- or vacuum-assisted birth (discussion to follow) are as follows (Cunningham et al., 2014):

- Nulliparity
- Maternal age (35 and over)
- Maternal height of less than 150 cm (4 ft 11 in.)
- Pregnancy weight gain of more than 15 kg (33 lb)
- Postdate gestation (41 weeks or more)
- Epidural anesthesia
- Fetal presentation other than occipitoanterior
- Presence of dystocia (labor dysfunction)
- Presence of a midline episiotomy
- Abnormal FHR tracing.

Neonatal and Maternal Risks

Some newborns may develop a small area of ecchymosis or edema, or both, along the sides of the face as a result of forceps application. Cephalohematoma (and subsequent hyperbilirubinemia) may occur as well as transient facial paralysis. Other reported complications include low Apgar scores, retinal hemorrhage, corneal abrasions, ocular trauma, other trauma (Erb palsy, fractured clavicle), elevated neonatal bilirubin levels, and prolonged hospital stay (Cunningham et al., 2014).

Maternal risks may include trauma such as lacerations of the birth canal, periurethral lacerations, and extensions of a median episiotomy into the anus, resulting in increased bleeding, bruising, hematomas, and pelvic floor injuries. Women who give birth with the assistance of forceps are more likely to have a third- or fourth-degree laceration and report more perineal pain and sexual problems in the postpartum period (Cunningham et al., 2014). In addition, an increase in postpartum infections, cervical lacerations, and prolonged hospital stays has been reported (Cunningham et al., 2014). Women who give birth with the assistance of forceps may also experience urinary and rectal incontinence, anal sphincter injury, and postpartum metritis (Cunningham et al., 2014).

Vacuum Extraction

Vacuum extraction is an obstetric procedure used by physicians and CNMs to assist the birth of a fetus by applying suction to the fetal head. The vacuum extractor accounts for 68% of all operative vaginal births. Its use has increased by 41% since 1990 and continues to rise (Cunningham et al., 2014). The vacuum extractor is composed of a soft suction cup attached to a suction bottle (pump) by tubing. The suction cup, which comes in various sizes, is placed against the occiput of the fetal head, avoiding the fontanels. Care must be taken to ensure that no cervical or vaginal tissue is trapped under the cup. The pump is used to create negative pressure (suction) of approximately 50–60 mmHg in a stepwise sequence or rapid application. An artificial caput ("chignon") is formed as the fetal scalp is pulled into the cup.

The longer the duration of suction, the more likely the newborn is to have a scalp injury. Although there are no data on the duration of use, ACOG advises a 30-minute time limit (Simpson & Creehan, 2013). Although there are no specifications on the number of attempts, failure to descend with multiple attempts is an indicator that a cesarean birth may be needed. In addition, if more than three "pop-offs" occur (the suction cup pops off the fetal head), the procedure should be discontinued. The most common indication for the use of the vacuum extractor is a prolonged second stage of labor or nonreassuring FHR pattern. Vacuum extraction is also used to relieve the woman of pushing effort, or when analgesia or fatigue interferes with her ability to push effectively, or in cases of nonreassuring fetal status when prompt birth is indicated. The vacuum extractor is preferred to forceps in cases of suspected cephalopelvic disproportion (CPD), when successful passage of the fetal head requires all potential space inside the vaginal canal. True CPD is an absolute contraindication to vacuum extraction. Other contraindications include nonvertex presentations, maternal or suspected fetal coagulation defects, known or suspected hydrocephalus, and fetal scalp trauma (Cunningham et al., 2014). Relative contraindications include suspected fetal macrosomia, high fetal station, face or breech presentation, gestation less than 34 weeks, incompletely dilated cervix, and previous fetal scalp blood sampling (Cunningham et al., 2014).

Neonatal complications include scalp lacerations, bruising, subgaleal hematomas, cephalohematomas, intracranial hemorrhages, subconjunctival hemorrhages, neonatal jaundice, fractured clavicle, Erb palsy, damage to the sixth and seventh cranial nerves, retinal hemorrhage, and fetal death. In addition, shoulder dystocia occurs more often (Cunningham et al., 2014). There appear to be more neonatal complications and injuries with use of a metal suction cup device than with soft cup devices. In the presence of a preterm gestation, risk of periventricular-intraventricular hemorrhage (PV-IVH) has been a concern, and some studies provide conflicting recommendations. Maternal complications include perineal trauma, edema, third- and fourth-degree lacerations, postpartum pain, and infection (Simpson & Creehan, 2013). Women who give birth with the aid of a vacuum extractor report more sexual difficulties in the postpartum period. Maternal genital tract and anal sphincter injuries occur less frequently with the vacuum extractor than with forceps.

Episiotomy

An **episiotomy** is a surgical incision of the perineal body to enlarge the outlet. The episiotomy has long been thought to minimize the risk of lacerations of the perineum and overstretching of perineal tissues. However, episiotomy may actually increase the risk of fourth-degree perineal lacerations (Blackburn, 2013). Research suggests, first, that rather than protecting the perineum from lacerations, the presence of an episiotomy makes it more likely that the woman will have anal sphincter tears and, second, that perineal lacerations heal more quickly than deep perineal tears (Blackburn, 2013). In clinical practice, research has shown that the incidence of major perineal trauma (extension to or through the anal sphincter) is more likely to happen if a midline episiotomy is done (Gurol-Urganci et al., 2013). Women with previous episiotomies that resulted in a third- or fourth-degree extension were more likely to have a repeat occurrence when episiotomy was used initially compared to women who had a spontaneous laceration without the use of episiotomy (Yogev et al., 2014). Additional complications associated with episiotomy are blood loss, infection, pain, and perineal discomfort that may continue for days or weeks past birth, including painful intercourse (Lyndon et al., 2012). Episiotomy is indicated for protection against injury to the anterior external genitalia, expediting delivery in the setting of non-reassuring fetal status, or enlarging the space in which to apply forceps or disimpact the fetal anterior shoulder. The ACOG discourages the use of episiotomy when it is not indicated. Rates have fallen from over 60% in 1979 to 12% in 2012 (Robinson, 2015).

Overall factors that place a woman at increased risk for episiotomy are primigravid status, large or macrosomic fetus, occipitoposterior position, use of forceps or vacuum extractor, and shoulder dystocia. Other factors that may be mitigated by nurses, physicians, and CNMs include the following:

- Use of lithotomy and other recumbent positions (causes excessive and uneven stretching of the perineum)

- Encouraging or requiring sustained breath holding during second-stage pushing (causes excessive and rapid perineal stretching, can adversely affect blood flow in mother and fetus, and requires woman to be responsive to caregiver directions rather than to her own urges to push spontaneously)

- Arbitrary time limit placed by the physician or CNM on the length of the second stage.

Preventive Measures

General tips to help reduce the incidence of lacerations and episiotomies include the following:

- Perineal massage during pregnancy for nulliparous women

- Natural pushing during labor and avoiding the lithotomy position or pulling back on legs, which tightens the perineum

- Side-lying position for pushing, which helps slow birth and diminish tears

- Warm or hot compresses on the perineum and firm counterpressure

- Encouraging a gradual expulsion of the baby at the time of birth by encouraging the mother to "push, take a breath, push, take a breath," thereby easing the baby out slowly

- Avoiding immediate pushing after epidural placement.

Episiotomy Procedure

The two types of episiotomy are midline and mediolateral, with midline being the most common in current use. Just before birth, when approximately 3–4 cm (1.2–1.6 in.) of the fetal head is visible during a contraction, the episiotomy is performed by using sharp scissors with rounded points (Cunningham et al., 2014). The midline incision begins at the bottom center of the perineal body and extends straight down the midline to the fibers of the rectal sphincter. The mediolateral incision begins in the midline of the posterior fourchette and extends at a 45° angle downward to the right or left.

The episiotomy is usually performed with regional or local anesthesia but may be done without anesthesia in emergency situations. It is generally proposed that as crowning occurs, the distention of the tissues causes numbing. Repair of the episiotomy and any lacerations is completed either during the period between birth of the baby and expulsion of the placenta or after expulsion of the placenta. Adequate anesthesia must be given for the repair.

Cesarean Birth

Cesarean birth (the birth of the baby through an abdominal and uterine incision) is one of the oldest known surgical procedures. Until the 20th century, cesarean procedures were used primarily to save the fetus of a dying woman. As the maternal and perinatal morbidity and mortality rates associated with cesarean birth steadily decreased throughout the 20th century, the proportion of cesarean births increased. Beginning in the early 1970s the cesarean birth rate rose steadily for almost two decades. In 1989, however, in an effort to control healthcare costs, the number of cesarean births began to decline, but from 2010–2012, the rate of cesarean births performed in the United States reached an all-time high of 32.8% (Martin et al., 2015). Since then, the rate has dropped to 32.2% in 2014 (CDC, 2015b).

Cesarean birth rates differ dramatically in other parts of the world. Worldwide, women living in urban areas are four times more likely to have a cesarean compared to women living in rural areas. Countries with low cesarean birth rates (less than 17%) include the Netherlands, Finland, and Norway. The highest rates were found in Italy, Portugal, and the United States, with rates greater than 30%. Overall, the incidence of cesarean birth has continued to increase worldwide (World Health Organization [WHO], 2015).

The increasing rate of cesarean births in the United States is linked to a rise in repeat cesarean births fueled by concerns about the risk of uterine rupture with a vaginal birth after a previous cesarean birth. There is also an increase in requests from women for cesarean births so that they can avoid the pain of labor and vaginal birth. Statements in some medical literature that vaginal births could result in pelvic floor damage during the birth process have led some women to consider cesarean births (King et al., 2013). There is an emerging trend as well to "schedule" birth by cesarean section to meet specific needs of the parents, such as coordinating work projects, arranging for babysitting of older children, or allowing relatives who must travel from other geographic locations to be present for the birth itself.

Cesarean birth on request is associated with a reduction in maternal hemorrhage risk; however, it is also associated with increases in neonatal respiratory problems, longer hospitalizations, and increased complications in subsequent pregnancies, including placenta implantation problems and uterine rupture (ACOG, 2013g). Cesarean birth without medical indications should not be recommended for women desiring several children, for women less than 39 weeks of gestation, or when pregnancy dating is unknown or may be inaccurate. It should also not be motivated by the potential lack of anesthesia availability in an institution (ACOG, 2013g).

Many other factors have contributed to the rise in the cesarean birth rate and need to be considered in any discussion about decreasing the rate. These factors include an increased use of epidural anesthesia, maternal age over 35, failed labor inductions, decline in vaginal breech deliveries, decreases in operative vaginal deliveries, increased repeat cesarean rates, reduced vaginal birth after cesarean birth rates, increased physician scheduling of cesarean births for personal convenience, political pressure from malpractice insurance carriers who attempt to dictate practice standards, and fear of litigation (ACOG, 2013g).

Indications

Commonly accepted indications for cesarean birth include complete placenta previa, breech presentation, transverse lie, placental abruption accompanied by nonreassuring fetal status, active genital herpes, umbilical cord prolapse, arrest of descent and/or arrest of dilation, nonreassuring fetal status, previous classic incision on the uterus (either previous cesarean birth or myomectomy), more than one previous cesarean birth, benign and malignant tumors that obstruct the birth canal, and cervical cerclage.

Certain maternal medical conditions are contraindications to a vaginal birth and warrant a cesarean birth (Society for Maternal-Fetal Medicine, 2012). These medical conditions include the following:

- Cardiac disorders
- Severe maternal respiratory disease
- Central nervous system disorders that increase intracranial pressure
- Mechanical vaginal obstruction, such as an ovarian mass or lower uterine segment fibroids
- HIV infection in the mother
- Severe mental illness that results in an altered state of consciousness.

Other indications that are now commonly associated with cesarean birth, although in some circumstances may allow the child to be delivered vaginally, include breech presentation, previous cesarean birth, major congenital anomalies, and severe Rh isoimmunization.

Maternal Mortality and Morbidity

Cesarean births have a higher maternal mortality rate than vaginal births. In the United States, women undergoing a cesarean birth have a twofold risk of most complications associated with delivery compared with women who give birth vaginally (Cunningham et al., 2014; Stranges, Wier, & Elixhauser, 2012). In England, emergency cesarean birth is associated with a ninefold risk of death when compared with vaginal delivery, and elective cesarean births have a threefold risk (Cunningham et al., 2014). Perinatal morbidity is also considerably higher in women who have had a cesarean.

Common postoperative complications include infection, reactions to anesthesia agents, blood clots, and bleeding. Women who have had a cesarean birth are twice as likely to be rehospitalized within 60 days of birth when compared with women who have had a vaginal birth. Other sources of maternal morbidity that are directly associated with cesarean birth include ureteral injury, bladder laceration, and wound infection (Cunningham et al., 2014).

Skin Incisions

The skin incision for a cesarean birth is either transverse (Pfannenstiel) or vertical, and it is not indicative of the type of incision made into the uterus. Time factors, patient preference, previous vertical skin incision, or physician preference determines the type of skin incision.

The transverse incision is made across the lowest and narrowest part of the abdomen. Because the incision is made just below the pubic hairline, it is almost invisible after healing. The limitation of this type of skin incision is that it does not allow extension of the incision if needed. Because it usually requires more time to make and repair, this incision is used when time is not of the essence (e.g., with arrest of descent and/or arrest of dilation and stable fetal and maternal status).

The vertical incision is made between the navel and the symphysis pubis. This type of incision is quicker and, therefore, is preferred in cases of nonreassuring fetal status when rapid birth is indicated, with preterm or macrosomic babies, or when the woman is significantly obese (Cunningham et al., 2014; Posner et al., 2013).

Uterine Incisions

The two major locations of uterine incisions are in the lower uterine segment and in the upper segment of the uterine corpus. The type of uterine incision depends on the need for the cesarean. The choice of incision affects the woman's opportunity for a subsequent vaginal birth and her risks of a ruptured uterine scar with a subsequent pregnancy.

The lower uterine segment incision most commonly used is a transverse incision. The lower uterine segment transverse incision is preferred for the following reasons (Cunningham et al., 2014):

- The lower segment is the thinnest portion of the uterus and involves less blood loss.
- It requires only moderate dissection of the bladder from the underlying myometrium.
- It is easier to repair, although repair takes longer.
- The site is less likely to rupture during subsequent pregnancies.
- There is a decreased chance for adherence of bowel or omentum to the incision line.

Disadvantages of this type of segment incision include the following:

- It takes longer to make a transverse incision.
- It is limited in size because of the presence of major vessels on either side of the uterus.
- It has a greater tendency to extend laterally into the uterine vessels.

- The incision may stretch and become a thin window, but it usually does not create problems clinically until subsequent labor ensues.

The lower uterine segment vertical incision is preferred for multiple gestation, abnormal presentation, placenta previa, nonreassuring fetal status, and preterm and macrosomic fetuses. Disadvantages of this type of incision include the following:

- The incision may extend downward into the cervix.
- More extensive dissection of the bladder is needed to keep the incision in the lower uterine segment; hemostasis and closure are more difficult.
- The vertical incision carries a higher risk of rupture with subsequent labor. Consequently, once a vertical incision is performed, future births need to be via cesarean.

One other incision, the classic incision, was the method of choice for many years but is used infrequently today. This vertical incision was made into the upper uterine segment. It resulted in greater blood loss and was more difficult to repair. Most important, it carried an increased risk of uterine rupture with subsequent pregnancy, labor, and birth, because the upper uterine segment is the most contractile portion of the uterus.

Analgesia and Anesthesia

There is no perfect anesthesia for cesarean birth. Each has its advantages, disadvantages, possible risks, and side effects. Goals for the administration of analgesia and anesthesia include safety, comfort, and emotional satisfaction for the patient.

Preparation for Cesarean Birth

Because one of every four births is a cesarean, preparation for this possibility should be an integral part of all prenatal education. The nurse should encourage pregnant women and their partners to discuss the possibility of a cesarean birth, and their specific needs and desires under those circumstances, with their healthcare provider. Their preferences may include the following:

- Participating in the choice of anesthetic
- Partner or significant other being present during the procedures and/or birth
- Partner or significant other being present in the recovery or postpartum room
- Video recording and/or taking pictures of the birth
- Delayed instillation of eye drops to promote eye contact between parent and newborn in the first hours after birth
- Physical contact or holding the newborn while in the operating and/or recovery room (by the partner if the mother cannot hold the baby)
- Breastfeeding in the recovery area within the first hour of birth.

Information that couples need about cesarean birth includes the following:

- What preparatory procedures to expect
- Description or viewing of the birthing room

- Types of anesthesia for birth and analgesia available postpartum
- Sensations that may be experienced
- Roles of significant others
- Interaction with newborn
- Immediate recovery phase
- Postpartum phase.

Preparing the woman and her family for cesarean birth involves more than the procedures of establishing an intravenous line, instilling a urinary indwelling catheter, and performing an abdominal prep. Good communication skills are essential in preparing the woman and her support person. The use of therapeutic touch and direct eye contact (if culturally acceptable and possible) assists the woman in maintaining a sense of control and lessens her anxiety.

If the cesarean birth is scheduled and not an emergency procedure, the nurse has ample time for preoperative teaching and to provide an opportunity for the woman and her support person to express their concerns, ask questions, and develop a relationship with the nurse.

In preparation for surgery, the woman is given nothing by mouth. To reduce the likelihood of serious pulmonary damage if gastric contents are aspirated, antacids may be administered within 30 minutes of surgery. If epidural anesthesia is used, the nurse may assist with the procedure, monitor the woman's blood pressure and response, and continue electronic fetal monitoring. An abdominal and perineal prep is done, and an indwelling catheter is inserted to prevent bladder distention. An intravenous line is started with a large-bore needle to permit rapid administration of blood if that becomes necessary. Preoperative medication may be ordered. The pediatrician should be notified and preparation made to receive the new baby. The nurse ensures that the neonatal radiant warmer is working and that resuscitation equipment is available.

The nurse assists in positioning the woman on the operating table. Fetal heart rate is assessed before surgery and during preparation because fetal hypoxia can result from the mother lying in the supine position. The operating room table is adjusted so that it slants slightly to one side, or a hip wedge (folded blanket or towels) is placed under the right hip to tip the uterus slightly and reduce compression of blood vessels. The uterus should be displaced 15 degrees from the midline. This helps relieve the pressure of the heavy uterus on the vena cava and lessens the incidence of vena cava compression and maternal supine hypotension. The suction should be in working order, and the urine collection bag should be positioned under the operating table to obtain proper drainage. Auscultation or electronic fetal monitoring of the fetal heart rate is continued until immediately before the procedure. If the fetus was monitored internally, a last-minute check is done to ensure that the fetal scalp electrode has been removed.

The nurse continues to provide reassurance and to describe the various procedures being performed (along with their rationales) to ease anxiety and give the woman a sense of control.

Women undergoing elective cesarean birth can be given information about the postoperative experience before their birth experience. Important components of patient education that can be emphasized before birth include dealing with postoperative discomfort, splinting the incision to decrease pain, frequent deep breathing and coughing, and the importance of early ambulation. Patients who receive this information before the birth are more apt to remember it when the information is reviewed in the early postpartum period.

Preparation for Repeat Cesarean Birth

When the parents are anticipating a repeat cesarean birth, they have a general understanding of what will occur, which can help them make informed choices about their birth experience. Those who have had previous negative experiences need an opportunity to describe what they felt. Encourage the parents to identify what they would like to be different and to list options that would make the experience more positive. Those who have already had positive experiences need reassurance that their needs and desires will be met in a similar manner. Provide all families the opportunity to discuss any fears or anxieties. For women who previously labored and then had an unexpected cesarean birth, the experience may be perceived as negative. Emphasize the positive aspects of a repeat cesarean birth. These include participation in selecting the birth date, lack of fatigue related to labor, ability to prepare and make arrangements for other children, and the ability for other family members or friends to be present at the hospital during or immediately after birth if desired by the couple.

Preparation for Emergency Cesarean Birth

When the need for a cesarean birth emerges suddenly, the period preceding surgery must be used to its greatest advantage. It is imperative that the nurse use the most effective communication skills in supporting the parents. The nurse describes what they may anticipate during the next few hours and gives the woman information about (and the rationale for) any procedure before it begins. It is essential for the nurse to explain what is going to happen, why it is being done, and what sensations the woman may experience. This allows the woman to be informed and to consent to the procedure, which gives her a sense of control and reduces her feelings of helplessness.

Supporting the Partner

Every effort should be made to include the partner in the birth experience. When attending a cesarean birth, the partner wears protective coverings similar to those worn by others in the operating suite. A stool can be placed beside the woman's head so that the partner can sit nearby to provide physical touch, visual contact, and verbal reassurance.

To promote the participation of the partner who chooses not to be in the operating suite, the nurse can do the following:

- Allow the partner to be nearby, where the partner can hear the newborn's first cry.
- Encourage the partner to carry or accompany the newborn to the nursery for the initial assessment.
- Involve the partner in postpartum care in the recovery room.

In some emergency circumstances, a support person may not be permitted in the operating room. Some facilities have policies that prohibit a support person from being in the operating room if the woman requires general anesthesia or if an emergency birth is being performed. In these situations, the support person should receive a thorough explanation of what is happening and why, be advised when the staff will return to provide information, know the expected length of time for the procedure, and be reassured that the mother is receiving the care she and the baby need. Because this exclusion is stressful for family members, the staff needs to provide information as soon as possible after providing emergency care to the mother.

Immediate Postnatal Recovery Period

After birth, the nurse assesses the Apgar score (Apgar scoring is described fully in Exemplar 33.D, Newborn Care) and completes the same initial assessment and identification procedures used for vaginal births.

Identification bands must be placed on the newborn and the mother (as well as on the support person, if present) before removing the baby from the operating room. The nurse should make every effort to assist the parents in bonding with their baby. If the mother is awake, one of her arms can be freed to enable her to touch and stroke the baby. The newborn may be placed on the mother's chest or held in an *en face* (face-to-face) position. If physical contact is not possible, the nurse should provide a running narrative so that the mother knows what is happening with her baby. The nurse assists the anesthesiologist or nurse anesthetist with raising the mother's head so that she can see her baby immediately after birth. The parents can be encouraged to talk to the baby, and the partner can hold the baby until the family is taken to the recovery room.

The nurse caring for the postpartum woman assesses the mother's vital signs every 5 minutes until they are stable, then every 15 minutes for an hour, and then every 30 minutes until the woman is discharged to the postpartum unit. The nurse remains with the woman until she is stable.

The nurse evaluates the dressing and perineal pad every 15 minutes for at least an hour. Gently palpate the fundus to determine whether it is remaining firm; palpation may be performed by placing a hand to support the incision. Intravenous oxytocin is usually administered to promote the contractility of the uterine musculature. If the mother has been under general anesthesia, she should be positioned on her side to facilitate drainage of secretions, turned, and assisted with coughing and deep breathing every 2 hours for at least 24 hours. If she has received a spinal or epidural anesthetic, the level of anesthesia is checked every 15 minutes for the first 2 hours and then hourly until full sensation has returned. It is important for the nurse to monitor intake and output and to observe the urine for a bloody tinge, which could mean surgical trauma to the bladder. The healthcare provider prescribes medication to relieve the mother's pain and nausea, and that medication is administered as needed.

Bonding can be promoted by encouraging mother and baby skin-to-skin contact for the first hour uninterrupted and performing all assessments and procedures on the newborn at the mother's bedside if both are stable.

Vaginal Birth After Cesarean

In the late 1980s there was an increasing trend to have a *trial of labor after cesarean (TOLAC)* and **vaginal birth after cesarean (VBAC)** in cases of nonrecurring indications for a cesarean (for example, twins, umbilical cord prolapse, placenta previa, nonreassuring fetal status). This trend was influenced by consumer demand and studies that support VBAC as a viable and safe alternative. VBAC rates peaked in the late 1990s and then the practice came under renewed scrutiny, causing rates to decline into the 2000s. This prompted the National Institutes of Health to review the matter and issue a statement on the safety of TOLAC. Consensus among providers is that all women who meet eligibility criteria should be offered TOLAC (King et al., 2013). The average VBAC success rate is 60–80% (ACOG, 2015c). The ACOG guidelines (2015c) state that the following aspects should be met when identifying candidates for a trial of labor:

- No contraindications for vaginal birth
- A woman with one or two previous cesarean births and a low transverse uterine incision
- A clinically adequate pelvis based on clinical pelvimetry or prior vaginal birth
- A woman with one previous cesarean birth with an undocumented uterine scar unless there is a high suspicion there was a classic incision performed previously
- Absence of other uterine scars or history of previous uterine rupture
- A physician who is able to do a cesarean needs to be available throughout active labor
- In-house anesthesia personnel are available for an emergency cesarean birth if warranted.

The absolute risks of VBAC are small. The incidence of uterine rupture is 0.9% of all TOLACs (ACOG, 2015c). Risks associated with VBAC are listed in **Box 33–4 »**.

The nursing care of a woman undergoing VBAC varies according to institutional protocols. Generally, if the woman is at low risk (has had one previous cesarean with a lower uterine segment incision), her blood count, type, and screen are obtained on admission; a heparin lock is inserted for intravenous access if needed; continuous electronic fetal monitoring (EFM) is used; and clear fluids may be taken. If the woman is at higher risk, NPO status should be maintained, and, in addition to the care listed, an intrauterine catheter may be inserted to monitor intrauterine pressures during labor.

Supportive and comfort measures are very important. The woman may be excited about this opportunity to experience labor and vaginal birth but apprehensive if she does not know what to expect from labor. The nurse provides information and encouragement for the laboring woman and her partner.

Intrapartum Risk Factors

A number of other alterations may occur during the intrapartum period. These include precipitous birth, abruptio placentae, placenta previa, premature rupture of membranes, preterm and postterm labor, hypertonic labor, hypotonic labor patterns, fetal malpresentation, fetal macrosomia, nonreassuring fetal status, prolapsed umbilical cord, anaphylactoid syndrome of pregnancy (amniotic fluid embolism), cephalopelvic disproportion, retained placenta, lacerations, placenta accreta, shoulder dystocia, and perinatal loss. These alterations are described in the Alterations and Therapies feature. Perinatal loss is discussed in the module on Grief and Loss.

>> Go to **Pearson MyLab Nursing and eText** for Chart 6, *Intrapartum High-Risk Factors.*

Lifespan Considerations

Lifespan considerations during labor and delivery primarily relate to a woman's age. Young women of adolescent years and women over the age of 35 pose some unique considerations for the nurse.

The Adolescent During Labor and Delivery

As with all women, each adolescent in labor is different. The nurse must assess what each teen brings to the experience as follows:

- Has the young woman received prenatal care?
- What are her attitudes and feelings about the pregnancy?
- Who will attend the birth, and what is each individual's relationship to the woman?
- What preparation has she had for the experience?
- What are her expectations and fears regarding labor and birth?
- How has her culture influenced her?
- What are her usual coping mechanisms?
- What are her plans for the newborn?

Any adolescent who has not had prenatal care requires close observation during labor. Fetal well-being is established by fetal monitoring. Adolescent women are at risk for pregnancy and labor complications and must be assessed carefully. The nurse must be especially alert for any physiologic complications of labor. The young woman's prenatal record is carefully reviewed for risks, and the adolescent is screened for preeclampsia, cephalopelvic disproportion, anemia, cigarette smoking, alcohol and drugs ingested during pregnancy, sexually transmitted infections (see the exemplar on Sexually Transmitted Infections in the module on Sexuality), and size–date discrepancies.

Box 33–4
Risks Associated with Vaginal Birth After Cesarean

- Uterine rupture
- Scar dehiscence
- Hysterectomy
- Uterine infection
- Neonatal death
- Intrauterine fetal demise
- Stillbirth
- Transfusion
- Hypoxic ischemic encephalopathy

Alterations and Therapies
Intrapartum

ALTERATION	DESCRIPTION	THERAPIES
Precipitous birth	Rapid progression of labor, with birth occurring within 3 hours or less.	■ The nurse's primary responsibility is to provide a physically and psychologically safe experience for the woman and her baby. ■ If birth is imminent, do not leave the mother alone, even for a minute. ■ Provide reassurance, and send auxiliary personnel to retrieve the emergency birth pack.
Abruptio placentae	Premature separation of a normally implanted placenta from the uterine wall; may be a catastrophic event depending on the severity of the resulting hemorrhage, which may be vaginal or may be unseen because it collects in the uterus or abdomen.	■ Monitor uterine resting tone, which is frequently increased with abruptio placentae. ■ Monitor abdominal girth measurements to determine internal blood collection. ■ Monitor vital signs, hemoglobin and hematocrit, and urine output.
Placenta previa	Implantation of the placenta in the lower uterine segment rather than the upper portion, resulting in placental separation with dilation of the cervix.	■ Teach all pregnant women the importance of reporting any bright-red vaginal bleeding, often scant at first. ■ Avoid vaginal examination if placenta previa is suspected. ■ Assess blood loss, pain, vital signs, fetal well-being, and uterine contractility. ■ Provide emotional support for the mother and family.
Premature rupture of membranes	Spontaneous rupture of the membranes before the onset of labor. Preterm PROM (PPROM) is the rupture of membranes occurring before 37 weeks of gestation associated with infection, previous history of PPROM, hydramnios, multiple pregnancy, urinary tract infection, amniocentesis, placenta previa, abruptio placentae, trauma, cervical insufficiency, bleeding during pregnancy, and maternal genital tract anomalies.	■ Assess for duration of rupture, appearance of amniotic fluid, and fetal well-being. ■ Monitor woman for signs of infection, including WBC count and vital signs. ■ Assess for potential cord compression if witnessed rupture. ■ Educate the woman and her partner regarding implications of PROM and all treatments.
Preterm labor	Labor that occurs between 20 and 36 completed weeks of pregnancy. Patients are admitted if at high risk for delivery in the setting of advanced cervical dilation, history of preterm delivery, or positive fetal fibronectin (fFN), a protein in the membranes found in vaginal secretions before 20 weeks and after 37 weeks. Detection of fFN on a vaginal swab between 24 and 34 weeks gestation increases suspicion of preterm labor (King et al., 2013); if at low risk for imminent delivery, patients are sent home on pelvic rest and normal activity.	■ Administer IV magnesium sulfate for 12 hours maximum for fetal neuroprotection, and IM betamethasone. ■ Monitor blood pressure every 10–15 minutes, serum magnesium levels, reflexes, respiratory rate, urinary output, and level of sedation, and be prepared to administer calcium if toxicity is suspected. ■ Provide emotional support to the woman, who may be fearful for fetal well-being. ■ Teach woman to recognize onset of labor, to perform home uterine activity monitoring, to evaluate contraction activity, and symptoms to report.
Postterm labor	A pregnancy that exceeds 42 weeks, occurring most frequently in primigravidas, women with history of postterm pregnancies, or fetal anencephaly.	■ Conduct ongoing assessment of fetal well-being. ■ Assess fluid for meconium following rupture of membranes. ■ Provide patient education. ■ Provide emotional support, encouragement, and recognition of the woman's anxiety.
Hypertonic labor	Ineffective uterine contractions of poor quality occurring in the latent phase of labor with increased resting tone of the myometrium and frequent contractions.	■ Provide comfort and support to the laboring woman and her partner. ■ Provide supportive measures such as change of position, quiet environment, back rubs, or guided imagery. ■ Consider therapeutic rest.

(continued on next page)

Alterations and Therapies (continued)

ALTERATION	DESCRIPTION	THERAPIES
Hypotonic labor patterns	Usually developing in the active phase of labor, characterized by fewer than two to three contractions in a 10-minute period of low intensity causing minimal discomfort; often the result of overstretching of the uterus, bowel or bladder distention, arrest of descent, or fetal malposition.	■ Assess contractions, maternal vital signs, and FHR, watching for signs of infection or dehydration. ■ Promote maternal–fetal well-being. ■ Monitor for maternal exhaustion. ■ Assess for meconium if rupture of membranes. ■ Consider augmentation of labor.
Fetal malpresentation	Any presentation that is not right-occiput-anterior (ROA), occiput-anterior (OA), or left-occiput-anterior (LOA), which may prolong labor or require a cesarean section.	■ Assist with position change to promote fetal repositioning. ■ Promote rest if labor is prolonged. ■ Provide patient education. ■ Prepare for surgery if cesarean section is required.
Fetal macrosomia	A newborn weight of > 4000 g at birth, often associated with excessive maternal weight gain, maternal obesity, uncontrolled maternal diabetes, grand multiparity, prolonged gestation, or those with a previous baby with macrosomia >4000 g (Cunningham et al., 2014).	■ Identify women at risk, and assess FHR for nonreassuring fetal status. ■ Assess for labor dysfunction or lack of fetal descent. ■ Provide support, encouragement, and education. ■ Monitor for hemorrhage postpartum. ■ Assess newborn after delivery for cephalohematoma.
Nonreassuring fetal status	When the oxygen supply is insufficient to meet the physiologic needs of the fetus, a nonreassuring fetal status may result, which may be transient or chronic. Demonstrated by change in FHR, decreased fetal movement, meconium-stained amniotic fluid, or ominous FHR patterns.	■ Review prenatal history, and note any risk factors. ■ Assess fetal heart rate, and note characteristics of amniotic fluid with rupture. ■ Promote maternal positioning to maximize ureteroplacental fetal blood flow.
Prolapsed umbilical cord	The umbilical cord precedes the fetal presenting part, placing pressure on the cord and reducing or stopping blood flow to and from the fetus. Of greatest risk when rupture of membranes occurs before engagement of fetal presenting part.	■ Assess FHR, and observe for prolapse for a full minute when membranes rupture. If loop of cord is discovered, a gloved hand elevates the fetal presenting part to relieve pressure until the cesarean delivery can be accomplished. ■ Administer oxygen by face mask to increase fetal oxygenation. ■ If the presenting part is well applied to the cervix, then ambulation should be encouraged. If the presenting part is not well applied to the cervix, the woman is at an increased risk of cord prolapse and ambulation should be discouraged; however, the woman can sit with the head of the bed elevated or in a rocking chair to facilitate gravity.
Anaphylactoid syndrome of pregnancy (amniotic fluid embolism)	In the presence of a small tear in the amnion or chorion high in the uterus, an area of separation in the placenta, or cervical tear, a small amount of amniotic fluid may leak into the chorionic plate and enter the maternal circulatory system as an amniotic fluid embolism. The more debris in the amniotic fluid (e.g., meconium), the greater the maternal danger.	■ Administer oxygen under positive pressure, and summon emergency assistance. ■ Establish intravenous access quickly. ■ Perform cardiopulmonary resuscitation if respiratory and cardiac arrest occur. ■ Call anesthesiologist immediately. ■ Provide support to the woman's partner and family members.
Cephalopelvic disproportion (CPD)	Occurs when the fetal head is too large to pass through any part of the birth passage, which can result in prolonged labor, uterine rupture, necrosis of maternal soft tissues, cord prolapse, excessive molding of the fetal head, or damage to the fetal skull and central nervous system.	■ Assess adequacy of maternal pelvis for a vaginal birth, size of the fetus, and its presentation and position. ■ Suspect CPD when labor is prolonged, cervical dilation and effacement are slow, and engagement of the presenting part is delayed. ■ Provide support to the couple, and keep them informed of what is happening and about the procedures being performed. ■ Assess cervical dilation and fetal descent more frequently. ■ Monitor contractions and fetal well-being continuously. ■ Position to optimize pelvic diameters.

Alterations and Therapies (continued)

ALTERATION	DESCRIPTION	THERAPIES
Retained placenta	Retention of the placenta beyond 30 minutes after birth, resulting in bleeding that may lead to shock.	▪ Assess for excessive bleeding and uterine contraction after delivery. ▪ Monitor maternal vital signs.
Lacerations	Tearing of the cervix or vagina, indicated by bright-red vaginal bleeding in the presence of a well-contracted uterus. The highest risk is in young ...liparous women and during operative vaginal delivery (forceps or vacuum assisted).	▪ Monitor for bright-red blood during labor. ▪ Promote perineal massage prenatally. ▪ If lacerations occur, manage pain and apply ice to the area after delivery to reduce edema. ▪ Teach the mother to rinse the perineum after every elimination and use sitz baths to reduce discomfort.
Placenta accreta	The chorionic villi attach directly to the myometrium of the uterus in placenta accreta. Two other types of placental adherence are *placenta increta*, in which the myometrium is invaded, and *placenta percreta*, in which the myometrium is penetrated. The adherence itself may be total, partial, or focal, depending on the amount of placental involvement.	▪ Assess for bleeding. ▪ Monitor vital signs. ▪ Prepare woman for surgical intervention and possible hysterectomy.
Shoulder dystocia	Impaction of the fetal anterior shoulder behind the maternal pubic bone after the birth of the head. Risk factors include macrosomia, history of shoulder dystocia, and rapid labor. However, most shoulder dystocias are not predictable. Pressure from the maternal bone on the fetal brachial plexus can result in paralysis of the arm. Failure to resolve the problem may lead to fetal hypoxia, encephalopathy, and death.	▪ The healthcare provider will perform maneuvers to free the shoulder. ▪ Call for assistance from the unit and nursery staff. ▪ Maintain an orderly atmosphere and clear communication. ▪ Emphasize the importance of and helping the mother to cooperate with maneuvers and avoid pushing. ▪ Monitor fetal status. ▪ Monitor time from birth of the head to fetal expulsion. ▪ Reposition the mother to maximize pelvic diameters. ▪ Apply suprapubic pressure on provider request to assist in dislodging the shoulder.
Perinatal loss	Death of a fetus or newborn from the time of conception through the end of the newborn period 28 days after delivery.	▪ Discussed in detail in the module on Grief and Loss.

The support role of the nurse depends on the young woman's support system during labor. The adolescent may not be accompanied by someone who will stay with her during childbirth, or she may have her mother, the father of the baby, or a close friend as her labor partner. Regardless of whether the teen has a support person, the nurse needs to establish a trusting relationship with her. In this way, the nurse can help the teen understand what is happening to her. Establishing a nurturing rapport is essential. Some nurses may view adolescent pregnancy as a negative event; however, it is important to treat the young woman with respect. The adolescent who is given positive reinforcement will leave the experience with increased self-esteem despite the emotional problems that may accompany her situation.

If a support person accompanies the adolescent, that individual also needs the nurse's encouragement and support. The nurse must explain changes in the young woman's behavior, substantiate her wishes, and describe ways the support person can be of help. The nursing staff needs to reinforce the adolescent's feelings that she is wanted and important.

The adolescent who has taken childbirth education classes is generally better prepared for labor compared to the adolescent who has not. However, the nurse must keep in mind that the younger the adolescent, the less she may be able to participate actively in the process, even if she has taken prenatal classes.

The very young adolescent (ages 14 and younger) has fewer coping mechanisms and less experience to draw on than her older counterparts. Because her cognitive development is incomplete, the younger adolescent may have fewer problem-solving capabilities. Her ego integrity may be more threatened by the experience of labor, and she may be more vulnerable to stress and discomfort. She may be more childlike and dependent than older teens. As a result, the very young adolescent needs someone to rely on at all times during labor. The nurse must be sure that instructions and explanations are simple and concrete. During the transition phase, the adolescent may become withdrawn and unable to express her need to be nurtured. Touch, soothing encouragement, and measures to provide comfort help her maintain control and meet her needs for dependence. During the second stage of labor, the young adolescent may feel as if she is losing control and may reach out to those around her. By remaining calm and giving directions, the nurse helps her cope with feelings of helplessness.

The middle adolescent (ages 15–17 years) often attempts to remain calm and unflinching during labor. The experienced nurse realizes that a caring attitude will still help the young woman. Many older adolescents believe that they "know it all," but they may be no more prepared for childbirth than their younger counterparts. The nurse's reinforcement and nonjudgmental manner will help them save face. If the adolescent has not taken childbirth preparation classes, she may require preparation and explanations.

The older teenager (ages 18–19 years) responds to the stresses of labor in a manner similar to that of the adult woman.

Adolescents, regardless of their age, need ongoing education throughout labor and in the early postpartum period. Provide clear explanations. Encourage these patients in particular to ask questions and seek information.

Even if the adolescent is planning to relinquish her newborn, she should be given the option of seeing and holding the baby. She may be reluctant to do this at first, but the grieving process is facilitated if the mother sees the baby. However, seeing or holding the newborn should be the young woman's choice.

Adolescents need individualized care for the issues that they face in the postpartum period. They may experience additional psychosocial issues unique to their age group and their developmental level. Adolescents are also at an increased risk for unintended subsequent pregnancies and abortions. Proper discharge teaching includes contraceptive options (Gavin et al., 2013).

Labor and Delivery Over Age 35

Generally, women over age 35 respond to the stresses of labor similarly to their younger counterparts.

In the United States and Canada, the risk of death during labor and delivery has declined dramatically during the past 30 years for women of all ages. However, the risk of maternal death is higher for women over age 35 and even higher for women age 40 and older. These women are more likely to have a chronic medical condition that can complicate pregnancy. Preexisting medical conditions such as hypertension or diabetes probably play a more significant role than age in maternal well-being and the outcome of pregnancy. In addition, the rates of miscarriage, stillbirth, preterm birth, low birth weight, and perinatal morbidity and mortality are higher in pregnant women over age 35 (Carolan, 2013). Nevertheless, while the risk of pregnancy complications is higher in women over age 35 who have a chronic condition such as hypertension or diabetes or who are in poor general health, the risks are much lower than previously believed for physically fit women without preexisting medical problems (Cunningham et al., 2014).

NURSING PROCESS

Maternal–newborn nursing has kept pace with the changing philosophy of childbirth. Nurses who choose positions in a birthing area are presented with opportunities to interact with patients in a wide variety of situations, ranging from a family that wants maximum interaction to one that wants to be left alone as much as possible. In addition, despite the increasing focus on family-centered care, the nurse must always be ready to meet the needs and concerns of the woman who is laboring alone. In every case, nurses strive to provide high-quality, individualized care.

The physiologic and psychologic events that occur during labor call for continual and rapid adaptations by the mother and fetus. Frequent and accurate assessments are crucial to the progress of these adaptations. In current nursing practice, the traditional assessment techniques of observation, palpation, and auscultation are augmented by the judicious use of technology, such as ultrasound and electronic monitoring. These tools may provide more detailed information for assessment; however, it is important for the nurse to remember that the technology only provides data. It is the nurse who truly monitors the mother and her baby.

Maternal Assessment

Assessment of the mother begins with a patient history and screening for intrapartum risk factors. The nurse obtains a brief oral history when the woman is admitted to the birthing area. Typically, the nurse assesses the maternal and fetal vital signs immediately (**Table 33–13 »**). If the vital signs are within normal limits, the interview continues. If a problem is identified, nursing care is then prioritized.

TABLE 33–13 Nursing Assessments in the First Stage

Phase	Mother	Fetus
Latent	Blood pressure and respirations each hour if in normal range. Temperature every 4 hours unless over 37.5°C (99.6°F) or membranes ruptured, then every 2 hours. Uterine contractions every 30 minutes.	FHR every 60 minutes for low-risk women and every 30 minutes for high-risk women if normal characteristics are present (average variability, baseline in the 110–160 beats/min range, without late or variable decelerations) or assess the heart rate every 30 minutes if the provider orders intermittent auscultation in a low-risk setting. Note fetal activity. If electronic fetal monitor is in place, assess for reactive nonstress test.
Active	Blood pressure, pulse, and respirations every hour if in normal range. Uterine contractions palpated every 15–30 minutes.	FHR every 30 minutes for low-risk women and every 15 minutes for high-risk women if normal characteristics are present.
Transition	Blood pressure, pulse, and respirations every hour. Contractions palpated every 15–30 minutes.	FHR every 15–30 minutes if normal characteristics are present.

It is common for the healthcare provider to send the prenatal records to the labor and birthing unit before the woman's due date. Review this information to ensure that changes have not occurred since the information was documented. During the initial interview, the nurse is building a trusting relationship. It is often helpful if the nurse sits down and appears unrushed, makes direct eye contact (if culturally appropriate), and begins the interview with a statement such as "I am going to be asking you some very personal and specific questions so that we can provide the best care for both you and your baby." This conveys a nonjudgmental approach, shows respect, and makes the expectant mother feel more at ease. Each agency has its own admission forms, but they usually include the following information:

- Woman's name and age
- Religious preference and spiritual practices
- Last menstrual period and estimated date of birth
- Attending physician or CNM
- Personal data: blood type; Rh factor; results of serology testing; prepregnant and present weight; allergies to medications, foods, or other substances; prescribed and OTC medications taken during the pregnancy; and history of drug and alcohol use and smoking during the pregnancy
- History of previous illness, such as tuberculosis, heart disease, diabetes, convulsive disorders, and thyroid disorders; asthma; sickle cell, Tay-Sachs, and other inherited disorders; or pregnancy-related complications (e.g., preterm labor, gestational diabetes, preeclampsia, or low platelets)
- Problems in the prenatal period, such as elevated blood pressure, bleeding problems, recurrent urinary tract infections, other infections, abnormal laboratory findings (e.g., abnormal glucose screen indicating gestational diabetes or low hemoglobin or hematocrit indicating anemia), or sexually transmitted infections
- Pregnancy data: gravida, para, abortions, and neonatal deaths
- Method chosen for newborn/infant feeding
- Type of childbirth education or newborn/infant care classes
- Previous newborn/infant care experience
- Woman's preferences regarding labor and birth, such as no episiotomy, no analgesics or anesthetics, or the presence or absence of the partner or others at the birth
- Pediatrician, family practice physician, or nurse practitioner
- Additional data: history of special tests, such as nonstress test, biophysical profile, or ultrasound; history of any preterm labor; onset of labor; amniotic fluid membrane status; and brief description of any previous labor and birth
- Onset of labor, status of amniotic membranes (intact, ruptured, time of rupture, color, and odor).

Because of the prevalence of domestic violence in our society (see the exemplar on Abuse, in the module on Trauma), the nurse needs to consider the possibility that the pregnant woman may have experienced abuse at some point in her life. Many victims of domestic violence, sexual assault, or childhood abuse may be anxious about the labor process or may experience anxiety during labor. Therefore, it is essential to review the woman's prenatal record and any other available records for information that may indicate abuse or a history of victimization by violence.

Intrapartum High-risk Screening

Screening for intrapartum high-risk factors is an integral part of assessing the woman in labor. As the history is obtained, the nurse notes the presence of any potential risk factors that may be considered high-risk conditions. For example, the woman who reports a physical symptom such as intermittent bleeding needs further assessment to rule out abruptio placentae or placenta previa before the admission process continues. It is important to determine the difference between vaginal bleeding and bloody show. In addition to identifying the presence of a high-risk condition, the nurse must recognize the implications of the condition for the laboring woman and her fetus. For example, if there is an abnormal fetal position, the nurse understands that the labor may be prolonged and that prolapse of the umbilical cord is more likely, thereby increasing the possibility of a cesarean birth.

Although physical conditions are frequently listed as the major factors that increase risk during the intrapartum period, socioeconomic and cultural variables, such as poverty, nutrition, the amount of prenatal care, living conditions, cultural beliefs regarding pregnancy, and communication patterns, may also precipitate a high-risk situation. Mental illness is a risk factor as well, because it can result in episodic prenatal care or the need to take psychotropic medications during the pregnancy (Davidson, 2013). In addition, research indicates that women who experience posttraumatic stress disorder (PTSD) may be at increased risk for some pregnancy complications (Onoye et al., 2013). (See the exemplar on Posttraumatic Stress Disorder, in the module on Trauma.) Other risk factors include smoking, drug use, and consumption of alcohol during pregnancy. The nurse can quickly review the prenatal record for number of prenatal visits; weight gain during pregnancy; progression of fundal height; assistance, such as Medicaid and WIC participation; exposure to environmental agents; and history of traumatic life events, including abuse.

A partial list of intrapartum risk factors appears in **Box 33–5 》**. Keep these factors in mind during the assessment.

Box 33–5
Selected Intrapartum Risk Factors

- Intermittent bleeding
- Abnormal fetal presentation
- Poverty
- Poor nutrition
- Lack of prenatal care
- Mental illness
- PTSD
- Smoking
- Drug use
- Alcohol use

Intrapartum Physical and Psychosociocultural Assessment

A physical examination is part of the admission procedure and part of the ongoing care of the patient. Although the intrapartum physical assessment is not as complete and thorough as the initial prenatal physical examination (see the Concepts section of this module), it does involve assessment of some body systems and the actual labor process.

The physical assessment portion includes assessments performed immediately on admission as well as ongoing assessments. Nurses conduct ongoing assessments in all clinical situations. For example, when the woman is changing into her gown, the nurse can assess the skin for bruises, needle marks, burns, or other abnormalities. The nurse can also determine whether the woman appears to be undernourished or overnourished. When labor is progressing rapidly, however, the nurse may not have time for a complete assessment. In that case, the critical physical assessments include maternal vital signs, labor status, fetal status, and laboratory findings.

Assessment of psychosocial history is a critical component of intrapartum nursing assessment. An estimated one third of all pregnant women are exposed to some type of psychotropic medication during their pregnancies. In addition, an estimated 10% of pregnant women meet the criteria for major depressive disorder during pregnancy and another 18% have depressive symptoms while pregnant (Dalfen, 2014). Perinatal depression is a common complication of pregnancy with potentially devastating consequences if it goes unrecognized and untreated (ACOG, 2015d). Any mental illness can play a role in how the woman copes with the labor and birth experience and should be assessed by the admitting nurse. Women with identified disorders will need ongoing assessment during the labor and birth.

The nurse can begin gathering data about sociocultural factors as the woman enters the birthing area. The nurse observes the communication pattern between the woman and her support person and their responses to admission questions and initial teaching. If the woman and her support person do not speak English and translators are not available among the birthing unit staff, the course of labor and the nurse's ability to interact and provide support and education are affected. The couple must receive information in their primary language to make informed decisions (see Nursing Care Plan in Exemplar 33.A). Communication may also be affected by cultural practices, such as beliefs about when to speak, who should ask questions, or whether it is acceptable to let others know about discomfort. People from certain cultures may want to experience birth naturally and may decline pain medications. In some cultures, the partner is not expected to be present in the birthing area. Nurses need to be culturally competent so that this is not interpreted as lack of interest in the birth, the mother, or the baby (Spector, 2017).

Individualized nursing care can best be planned and implemented when nurses know and honor the values and beliefs of the laboring woman (Spector, 2017). To avoid stereotyping patients, the nurse always asks the woman and her family about individual beliefs and preferences. Nurses who feel uncertain about what to ask or to consider need to explore the varying cultural values and beliefs of the people residing in their community. Although some communities have a prominent culture that may follow certain rituals, the nurse should still ask each patient about her own individual beliefs and preferences.

The final section of the assessment guide addresses ideas, knowledge, fantasies, and fears about childbearing. The nurse should ask the patient whether she has any special needs. However, because some women may not know what needs may arise, ongoing assessment is imperative. It is important for the nurse to pay specific attention to body language, eye contact, and other nonverbal cues that may indicate the woman is experiencing anxiety or other feelings. By assessing the patient's cultural and psychosocial status, the nurse can better meet the woman's needs for information and support. The nurse can then assist the woman and her partner; in the absence of a partner, the nurse may become the support person.

The Intrapartum Assessment feature provides a framework the nurse can use when examining the laboring woman.

Assessment of Contractions

Once contractions begin, the nurse must assess the nature of the contractions and any accompanying pain. When palpating a woman's uterus during a contraction, compare the consistency to your nose, chin, and forehead to determine the intensity. Many experienced nurses note that the feel during mild contractions is similar in consistency to the tip of the nose, moderate contractions feel more like the chin, and with strong contractions, the uterus feels firm, much like the forehead.

It is also important to assess the laboring woman's perception of pain. How does she describe the pain? What is her affect? Is this contraction more uncomfortable than the last one? Is the nurse's palpation of intensity congruent with the woman's perception? (For instance, the nurse might evaluate a contraction as mild in intensity, whereas the laboring woman evaluates it as very strong.) A nurse's assessment is not complete unless the laboring woman's affect and response to the contractions are also noted and charted.

Electronic monitoring of uterine contractions provides continuous data. Electronic monitoring is routinely used in many birth settings for high-risk patients and those having oxytocin-induced labor. Electronic monitoring may be done externally, with a device that is placed against the maternal abdomen, or internally, with an intrauterine pressure catheter.

EXTERNAL ELECTRONIC MONITORING OF CONTRACTIONS When monitoring contractions by external means, the portion of the monitoring equipment called a tocodynamometer, or "toco," is positioned against the fundus of the uterus and held in place with an elastic belt. The toco contains a flexible disk that responds to pressure. When the uterus contracts, the fundus tightens and the change in pressure against the toco is amplified and transmitted to the electronic fetal monitor. The monitor displays the uterine contraction as a pattern on graph paper.

External monitoring offers several advantages, including a continuous recording of the frequency and duration of uterine contractions, and it is noninvasive. However, it does

Intrapartum Assessment: First Stage of Labor

PHYSICAL ASSESSMENT/ NORMAL FINDINGS	ALTERATIONS AND POSSIBLE CAUSES*	NURSING RESPONSES TO DATA†
Vital Signs		
Blood pressure (BP): less than 140 systolic and 90 and greater than 90/50 diastolic	High blood pressure (essential hypertension, preeclampsia, renal disease, apprehension, anxiety, or pain) Low blood pressure (supine hypotension) Hemorrhage/hypovolemia Shock Drugs Side effect of epidural anesthesia	Evaluate history of preexisting disorders, and check for presence of other signs of preeclampsia. Do not assess during contractions; implement measures to decrease anxiety and reassess. Provide quiet environment. Have O_2 available. Notify anesthesiologist.
Pulse: 60–100 beats/min (normal, nonpregnant) Additional 10–20 beats/min during pregnancy	Increased pulse rate (excitement or anxiety, cardiac disorders, early shock, drug use)	Evaluate cause, reassess to see if rate continues; report to healthcare provider.
Respirations: 16–24 breaths/min (or pulse rate divided by 4)	Marked tachypnea (respiratory disease), hyperventilation in transition phase Decreased respirations (narcotics)	Assess between contractions; if marked tachypnea continues, assess for signs of respiratory disease or respiratory distress.
	Hyperventilation (anxiety/pain)	Encourage slow breaths if woman is hyperventilating.
Pulse oximetry 95% or greater	Pulse oximetry less than 90%: hypoxia, hypotension, hemorrhage	Administer O_2; notify healthcare provider.
Temperature: 36.2°–37.6°C (97°–99.6°F)	Elevated temperature (infection, dehydration, prolonged rupture of membranes, epidural regional block)	Assess for other signs of infection or dehydration.
Weight		
25–35 lb greater than prepregnant weight	Weight gain greater than 35 lb (fluid retention, obesity, large baby, diabetes mellitus, preeclampsia) Weight gain less than 15 lb (small for gestational age, substance abuse, psychosocial problems)	Assess for signs of edema. Evaluate dietary patterns from prenatal record.
Lungs		
Normal breath sounds, clear and equal	Rales, rhonchi, friction rub (infection), pulmonary edema, asthma	Reassess; refer to healthcare provider.
Fundus		
At 40 weeks of gestation, located just below the xiphoid process	Uterine size not compatible with estimated date of birth (small for gestational age, large for gestational age, hydramnios, multiple pregnancy, placental/fetal anomalies, malpresentation)	Reevaluate history regarding pregnancy dating. Refer to healthcare provider for additional assessment.
Edema		
Slight amount of dependent edema	Pitting edema of face, hands, legs, abdomen, sacral area (preeclampsia)	Check deep tendon reflexes for hyperactivity; check for clonus; refer to healthcare provider.
Hydration		
Normal skin turgor, elastic	Poor skin turgor (dehydration)	Assess skin turgor; refer to healthcare provider for deviations. Provide fluids per healthcare provider orders.
	*Possible causes of alterations are identified in parentheses.	†This column provides guidelines for further assessment and initial nursing intervention.

(continued on next page)

Intrapartum Assessment: First Stage of Labor (continued)

PHYSICAL ASSESSMENT/ NORMAL FINDINGS	ALTERATIONS AND POSSIBLE CAUSES*	NURSING RESPONSES TO DATA†
Perineum		
Tissues smooth, pink color	Varicose veins of vulva, herpes lesions/genital warts	Note on patient record need for follow-up in postpartum period; reassess after birth, refer to healthcare provider.
Clear mucus; may be blood tinged with earthy or human odor	Profuse, purulent, foul-smelling drainage	Suspected gonorrhea or chorioamnionitis; report to healthcare provider; initiate care to newborn's eyes; notify neonatal nursing staff and pediatrician.
Presence of small amount of bloody show that gradually increases with further cervical dilation	Hemorrhage	Assess BP and pulse, pallor, diaphoresis, report any marked changes. Standard precautions.
Labor Status		
Uterine contractions: regular pattern	Failure to establish a regular pattern, prolonged latent phase Hypertonicity Hypotonicity Dehydration	Evaluate whether woman is in true labor. Ambulate if in early labor. Evaluate patient status and contractile pattern. Obtain a 20-minute electronic fetal monitoring strip. Notify healthcare provider. Provide hydration.
Cervical dilation: progressive cervical dilation from size of fingertip to 10 cm (3.9 in.)	Rigidity of cervix (frequent cervical infections, scar tissue, failure of presenting part to descend)	Evaluate contractions, fetal engagement, position, and cervical dilation. Inform patient of progress.
Cervical effacement: progressive thinning of cervix	Failure to efface (rigidity of cervix, failure of presenting part to engage); cervical edema (pushing effort by woman before cervix is fully dilated and effaced, trapped cervix)	Evaluate contractions, fetal engagement, and position. Notify healthcare provider if cervix is becoming edematous; work with woman to prevent pushing until cervix is completely dilated. Keep vaginal exams to a minimum.
Fetal descent: progressive descent of fetal presenting part from station −5 to + 4	Arrest of descent (abnormal fetal position or presentation, macrosomic fetus, inadequate pelvic measurements)	Evaluate fetal position, presentation, and size.
Membranes: may rupture before or during labor	Rupture of membranes more than 12–24 hours before onset of labor	Assess for ruptured membranes using Nitrazine test tape before doing vaginal exam. Follow standard precautions. Keep vaginal exams to a minimum to prevent infection. When membranes rupture in the birth setting, immediately assess FHR to detect changes associated with prolapse of umbilical cord (FHR slows).
Findings on Nitrazine test tape: Membranes probably intact: Yellow pH 5.0 Olive pH 5.5 Olive green pH 6.0	False-positive results may be obtained if large amount of bloody show is present, previous vaginal examination has been done using lubricant, or tape is touched by nurse's fingers	Assess fluid for consistency, amount, odor; assess FHR frequently. Assess fluid at regular intervals for presence of meconium staining. Follow standard precautions while assessing amniotic fluid.
Membranes probably ruptured: Blue-green pH 6.5 Blue-gray pH 7.0 Deep blue pH 7.5		Teach woman that amniotic fluid is continually produced (to allay fear of "dry birth"). Teach woman that she may feel amniotic fluid trickle or gush with contractions. Change pads often.
	*Possible causes of alterations are identified in parentheses.	†This column provides guidelines for further assessment and initial nursing intervention.

Intrapartum Assessment: First Stage of Labor (continued)

PHYSICAL ASSESSMENT/ NORMAL FINDINGS	ALTERATIONS AND POSSIBLE CAUSES*	NURSING RESPONSES TO DATA†
Amniotic fluid clear, with earthy or human odor, no foul-smelling odor	Greenish amniotic fluid (fetal stress) Bloody fluid (vasa previa, abruptio placentae) Strong or foul odor (amnionitis)	Assess FHR; do vaginal exam to evaluate for prolapsed cord; apply fetal monitor for continuous data; report to healthcare provider. Take woman's temperature and report to healthcare provider.

Fetal Status

FHR: 110–160 beats/min	Less than 110 or greater than 160 beats/min (nonreassuring fetal status); abnormal patterns on fetal monitor: decreased variability, late decelerations, variable decelerations, absence of accelerations with fetal movement	Initiate interventions based on particular FHR pattern.
Presentation: cephalic, 97%; breech, 3%	Face, brow, breech, or shoulder presentation	Report to healthcare provider; after presentation is confirmed as face, brow, breech, or shoulder, woman may be prepared for cesarean birth.
Position: left-occiput-anterior (LOA) most common	Persistent occipital-posterior (OP) position; transverse arrest	Carefully monitor maternal and fetal status. Reposition mother in side-lying or on hands and knees position to promote rotation of fetal head.
Activity: fetal movement	Hyperactivity (may precede fetal hypoxia) Complete lack of movement (nonreassuring fetal status or fetal demise)	Carefully evaluate FHR; apply fetal monitor. Carefully evaluate FHR; apply fetal monitor. Report to healthcare provider.
	*Possible causes of alterations are identified in parentheses.	†This column provides guidelines for further assessment and initial nursing intervention.

CULTURAL ASSESSMENT§	VARIATIONS TO CONSIDER	NURSING RESPONSES TO DATA§§
Cultural influences determine customs and practices regarding intrapartum care.	Individual preferences may vary.	
Ask the following questions: ■ Who would you like to remain with you during your labor and birth?	She may prefer only her partner or other support person to remain or may also want family and/or friends.	Provide support for her wishes by encouraging desired people to stay. Provide information to others (with the woman's permission) who are not in the room.
■ What would you like to wear during labor?	She may be more comfortable in her own clothes.	Offer supportive materials, such as disposable pads, if needed to protect her clothing. Avoid subtle signals to the woman that she should not have chosen to remain in her own clothes. Have other clothing available if the woman desires. If her clothing becomes contaminated, it will be simple to place it in a plastic bag.
■ What activity would you like during labor?	She may want to ambulate most of the time, stand in the shower, sit in the Jacuzzi, sit on a chair/stool/birthing ball, remain on the bed, and so forth.	Support the woman's wishes; provide encouragement and complete assessments in a manner so her activity and positional wishes are disturbed as little as possible.
■ What position would you like for the birth?	She may feel more comfortable in lithotomy position with stirrups and her upper body elevated, side-lying or sitting in a birthing bed, standing, or squatting, or on hands and knees.	Collect any supplies and equipment needed to support her in her chosen birthing position. Provide information to the support person regarding any changes that may be needed based on the chosen position.
§These are only a few suggestions. We do not mean to imply that this is a comprehensive cultural assessment; rather, it is a tool to encourage cultural competence.		§§This column provides guidelines for further assessment and initial nursing intervention.

(continued on next page)

Intrapartum Assessment: First Stage of Labor (continued)

CULTURAL ASSESSMENT§	VARIATIONS TO CONSIDER	NURSING RESPONSES TO DATA§§
■ Is there anything special you would like?	She may want the room darkened or to have curtains and windows open, music playing, her support person to cut the umbilical cord, to save a portion of the umbilical cord, to save the placenta, to videotape the birth, or other particular preferences.	Support requests, and communicate requests to any other nursing or medical personnel (so requests can continue to be supported and not questioned). If another nurse or physician does not honor the request, act as advocate for the woman by continuing to support her unless her desire is truly unsafe.
Ask the woman if she would like fluids, and ask what temperature she prefers.	She may prefer clear fluids other than water (tea, clear juice). She may prefer iced, room temperature, or warmed fluids.	Provide fluids as desired.
Observe the woman's response when privacy is difficult to maintain and her body is exposed.	Some women do not seem to mind being exposed during an exam or procedure; others feel acute discomfort.	Maintain privacy and respect the woman's sense of privacy. If the woman is unable to provide specific information, the nurse may draw from general information regarding cultural variation: Southeast Asian women may not want any family member in the room during exam or procedures. The woman's partner may not be involved with coaching activities during labor or birth. Muslim women may need to remain covered during the labor and birth and avoid exposure of any body part. The husband may need to be in the room but remain behind a curtain or screen so he does not view his wife at this time.
If the woman is to breastfeed, ask if she would like to feed her baby immediately after birth.	She may want to feed her baby right away or may want to wait a little while.	
§These are only a few suggestions. We do not mean to imply that this is a comprehensive cultural assessment; rather, it is a tool to encourage cultural competence.		§§This column provides guidelines for further assessment and initial nursing intervention.

PSYCHOSOCIAL ASSESSMENT	VARIATIONS TO CONSIDER	NURSING RESPONSES TO DATA††
Preparation for Childbirth		
Does the woman have some information regarding process of normal labor and birth?	Some women do not have any information regarding childbirth.	Add to present information base.
Does the woman have breathing and/or relaxation techniques to use during labor?	Some women do not have any method of relaxation or breathing to use, and some do not desire them.	Support breathing and relaxation techniques that the patient is using; provide information if needed.
Have the woman and support person done extensive preparation for childbirth?	Some women have strong opinions regarding labor and birth preparation.	Support the woman's wishes to participate in her birth experience; support the woman's birth plan.
Response to Labor		
Latent phase: relaxed, excited, anxious for labor to be well established	May feel unable to cope with contractions because of fear, anxiety, or lack of information.	Provide support and encouragement, establish trusting relationship.
Active phase: becomes more intense, begins to tire	May remain quiet and without any sign of discomfort or anxiety, may insist that she is unable to continue with the birthing process.	Provide support and coaching if needed.
		††This column provides guidelines for further assessment and initial nursing intervention.

Intrapartum Assessment: First Stage of Labor (continued)

PSYCHOSOCIAL ASSESSMENT	VARIATIONS TO CONSIDER	NURSING RESPONSES TO DATA[††]
Transitional phase: feels tired, may feel unable to cope, needs frequent coaching to maintain breathing patterns		
Coping mechanisms: ability to cope with labor through use of support system, breathing, relaxation techniques, and comfort measures, including frequent position changes in labor, immersion in warm water, and massage	May feel marked anxiety and apprehension, may not have coping mechanisms that can be brought into this experience, or may be unable to use them at this time. Survivors of sexual abuse may demonstrate fear of intravenous lines or needles, may recoil when touched, may insist on a female caregiver, may be very sensitive to body fluids and cleanliness, and may be unable to labor lying down.	Support coping mechanisms if they are working for the woman; provide information and support if she exhibits anxiety or needs alternative to present coping methods. Encourage participation of partner or other individual if a supportive relationship seems apparent. Establish rapport and a trusting relationship. Provide information that is true and offer your presence.
Anxiety		
Some anxiety and apprehension is within normal limits.	May show anxiety through rapid breathing, nervous tremors, frowning, grimacing, clenching of teeth, thrashing movements, crying, increased pulse and blood pressure	Provide support, encouragement, and information. Teach relaxation techniques. Support controlled breathing efforts. May need to provide a paper bag to breathe into if woman says her lips are tingling. Note FHR.
Sounds During Labor		
	Some women are very quiet; others moan or make a variety of noises.	Provide a supportive environment. Encourage woman to do what feels right for her.
Support System		
Physical intimacy between mother and partner (or mother and support person/doula); caretaking activities, such as soothing conversation and touching	Some women would prefer no contact; others may show clinging behaviors.	Encourage caretaking activities that appear to comfort the woman; encourage support for the woman; if support is limited, the nurse may take a more active role.
Support person stays in proximity	Limited interaction may come from a desire for quiet.	Encourage support person to stay close (if this seems appropriate).
Relationship between mother and partner or support person: involved interaction	The support person may seem to be detached and maintain little support, attention, or conversation.	Support interactions; if interaction is limited, the nurse may provide more information and support. Ensure that the support person has short breaks, especially before transition.
		[††]This column provides guidelines for further assessment and initial nursing intervention.

not accurately record the intensity of the uterine contraction, and it is difficult to obtain an accurate fetal heart rate in some women, such as those who are very obese, those who have hydramnios, or those with a very active fetus. In addition, the woman may be bothered by the belt if it requires frequent readjustment when she changes position. Electronic monitoring allows the nurse to continually monitor the fetus if concerns arise based on the fetal heart rate. It also enables the nurse and physician or CNM to observe the pattern of the FHR over a period of time by examining the electronic fetal monitoring strip.

INTERNAL ELECTRONIC MONITORING OF CONTRACTIONS Internal intrauterine monitoring provides the same data as external monitoring, as well as accurate measurement of uterine contraction intensity (the strength of the contraction and the actual pressure within the uterus). After membranes have ruptured, the physician or CNM (or the nurse in some facilities) inserts the **intrauterine pressure catheter** into the uterine cavity and connects it by a cable to the electronic fetal monitor. It is important to first assess the fetal position and to review a past ultrasound to determine the location of the placenta, because the internal monitor should be placed away from the placenta. If an ultrasound has not been previously obtained, the healthcare provider may wish to obtain one on the unit or have the sonographer perform such an exam.

The pressure within the uterus in the resting state and during each contraction is measured by a small micropressure device located in the tip of the catheter. Internal electronic monitoring is used when it is imperative to have accurate intrauterine pressure readings to evaluate the stress on the uterus or to determine the adequacy of contractions. The advantage of the intrauterine pressure monitor is that it can directly measure the intensity of the contraction. It can be used when the external monitor may not be accurately assessing the contraction strength, such as in cases of maternal obesity. It can also be used when oxytocin is being administered to ensure that uterine contractions are adequate.

During internal electronic monitoring, the nurse should also evaluate the woman's labor status by palpating the intensity and resting tone of the uterine fundus during contractions. Technology is a useful tool if used as an adjunct to good assessment skills, but it is not a replacement for those skills.

Cervical Assessment

Cervical dilation and effacement are evaluated directly by vaginal examination. The vaginal examination can provide information about the adequacy of the maternal pelvis, membrane status, characteristics of amniotic fluid, and fetal position and station.

Fetal Assessment

A complete intrapartum fetal assessment requires determination of the fetal position and presentation as well as evaluation of the fetal status.

Assessment of Fetal Position

Fetal position is determined in the following ways:

- Inspection of the woman's abdomen
- Palpation of the woman's abdomen
- Vaginal examination to determine the presenting part
- Ultrasound
- Auscultation of fetal heart rate.

INSPECTION Observe the woman's abdomen for size and shape. Assess the lie of the fetus by noting whether the uterus projects up and down (longitudinal lie) or left to right (transverse lie).

PALPATION: LEOPOLD MANEUVERS **Leopold maneuvers** are a systematic way to evaluate the maternal abdomen. Frequent practice increases the examiner's skill in determining fetal position by palpation. (See the Concepts section for information on how to perform Leopold maneuvers.) Leopold maneuvers may be difficult to perform on women who are obese or those who have excessive amniotic fluid (hydramnios). Before performing Leopold maneuvers, the nurse should have the woman empty her bladder and then lie on her back with her feet on the bed and her knees bent.

VAGINAL EXAMINATION AND ULTRASOUND Other assessment techniques to determine fetal position and presentation include vaginal examination and the use of ultrasound to visualize the fetus. During the vaginal examination, the examiner can palpate the presenting part if the cervix is dilated. Information about the position of the fetus and the degree of flexion of its head (in cephalic presentations) can also be obtained. Visualization by ultrasound is used when the fetal position cannot be determined by abdominal palpation.

AUSCULTATION OF FETAL HEART RATE The handheld Doppler ultrasound is used to auscultate the FHR between, during, and immediately after uterine contractions. A fetoscope may also be used. Instead of listening haphazardly over the woman's abdomen for the FHR, the nurse may choose to perform Leopold maneuvers first. Leopold maneuvers not only indicate the probable location of the FHR but also help determine the presence of multiple fetuses, fetal lie, and fetal presentation.

The FHR is heard most clearly at the fetal back (**Figure 33–50 ≫**). In a cephalic presentation, the FHR is best heard in the lower quadrants of the maternal abdomen. In a breech presentation, it is heard at or above the level of the maternal umbilicus. In a transverse lie, the FHR may be heard best just above or just below the umbilicus. As the presenting part descends and rotates through the pelvic structure during labor, the location of the FHR tends to descend and move toward the midline.

After the FHR is located, it is usually counted for 30 seconds, starting at the acme or immediately after a contraction, and multiplied by 2 in order to obtain the number of beats per minute. It is also appropriate to listen for a full minute, particularly after a change in status such as rupture of membranes (Freeman et al., 2012). If the FHR is irregular or has changed markedly from the last assessment, or if an audible deceleration is heard, the nurse listens for a full minute, through and immediately after a contraction. In these situations, continuous electronic fetal monitoring is warranted (Menihan & Kopel, 2014). It is important to note that intermittent auscultation has been found to be as effective as the electronic method for fetal surveillance.

Electronic Monitoring of Fetal Heart Rate

Electronic fetal monitoring produces a continuous tracing of the FHR, which allows many characteristics of the FHR to be visually assessed. A growing number of physicians and nurses, however, are beginning to question the widespread use of this technology. Although fetuses who are monitored continuously have a reduction in seizures, there is no reduction in cerebral palsy, newborn/infant mortality, or adverse neonatal outcomes. Women who receive continuous fetal monitoring are more likely to undergo a cesarean birth or an instrument-assisted birth (Resnik, 2013).

INDICATIONS FOR ELECTRONIC MONITORING If one or more of the following factors are present, the FHR and contractions are monitored electronically:

- Previous history of a stillbirth at 38 or more weeks of gestation

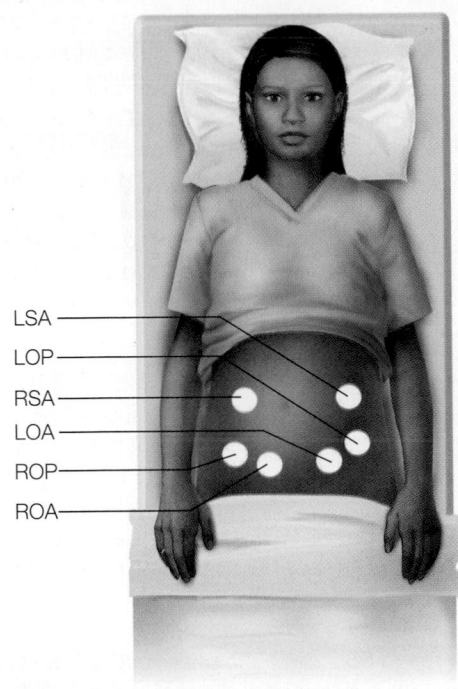

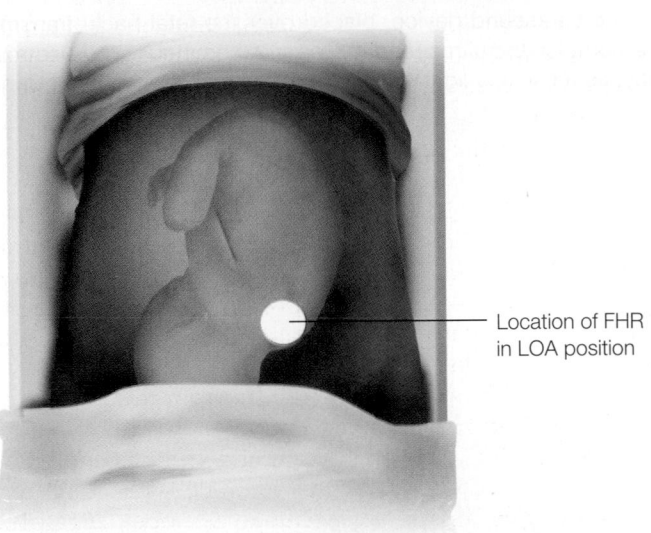

Figure 33–50 》 Location of fetal heart rate in relation to the more commonly seen fetal positions. The FHR is heard more clearly over the fetal back.

- Presence of a complication of pregnancy (e.g., preeclampsia, placenta previa, abruptio placentae, multiple gestation, and prolonged or premature rupture of membranes)
- Induction of labor (labor that is begun as a result of some type of intervention [e.g., an intravenous infusion of oxytocin])
- Preterm labor
- Decreased fetal movement
- Nonreassuring fetal status
- Meconium staining of amniotic fluid (meconium has been released into the amniotic fluid by the fetus, which may indicate a problem)
- Trial of labor following a previous cesarean birth (Menihan & Kopel, 2014)

- Maternal fever
- Placental problems.

METHODS OF ELECTRONIC MONITORING External monitoring of the fetus is usually accomplished by ultrasound. A transducer, which emits continuous sound waves, is placed on the maternal abdomen. When placed correctly, the sound waves bounce off the fetal heart and are picked up by the electronic monitor. The actual moment-by-moment FHR is displayed graphically on a screen (**Figure 33–51 》**). In some instances, the monitor may track the maternal heart rate instead of the FHR. However, the nurse can avoid this error by comparing the maternal pulse to the FHR.

Recent advances in technology have led to the development of new ambulatory methods of external monitoring. Using a telemetry system, a small, battery-operated transducer transmits signals to a receiver connected to the monitor. This system, which is held in place with a shoulder strap, allows the patient to ambulate, helping her to feel more comfortable and less confined during labor. Many of the newer models can also be worn in the tub and can be completely submerged in water, making a more natural birthing experience possible even for women who require continuous monitoring for medical indications. In contrast, the system depicted in Figure 33–51 requires the laboring woman to remain close to the electrical power source for the monitor.

Internal monitoring requires an internal spiral electrode. Women who require internal monitoring are typically confined to bed and cannot ambulate. To place the fetal scalp electrode (FSE) on the fetal occiput, the amniotic membranes must be ruptured, the cervix must be dilated at least 2 cm (0.08 in.), the presenting part must be down against the cervix, and the presenting part must be known (i.e., the nurse must be able to detect the actual part of the fetus that is down against the cervix). If all these factors are present, the labor and birth nurse (if specialty training has been completed), physician, or CNM inserts a sterile internal spiral electrode into the vagina and places it against the fetal head. The spiral electrode is rotated clockwise until it is attached to the scalp. It is essential that the electrode not be placed over the eye or a fontanel, so the fetal position must be determined before a scalp electrode is applied. Wires that extend from the spiral electrode are attached to a leg plate (placed on the woman's thigh) and then attached to the electronic fetal monitor. This method of monitoring the FHR provides more accurate continuous data than external monitoring because the signal is clearer and movement of the fetus or the woman does not interrupt it (**Figure 33–52 》**).

Internal monitoring has both risks and benefits. It provides a more accurate fetal tracing and is more effective in monitoring the fetal status. In rare cases, the scalp electrode can be placed on the fetal fontanel or, if the fetus is in a face presentation, on an eye, thus causing fetal injury. Women with certain medical conditions, such as HIV infection, should not be monitored with internal monitoring, because it can increase the risk of viral transmission.

The FHR tracing at the top of **Figure 33–53 》** was obtained by internal monitoring with a spiral electrode; the uterine contraction tracing at the bottom of the figure was obtained by external monitoring with a toco. Note that the

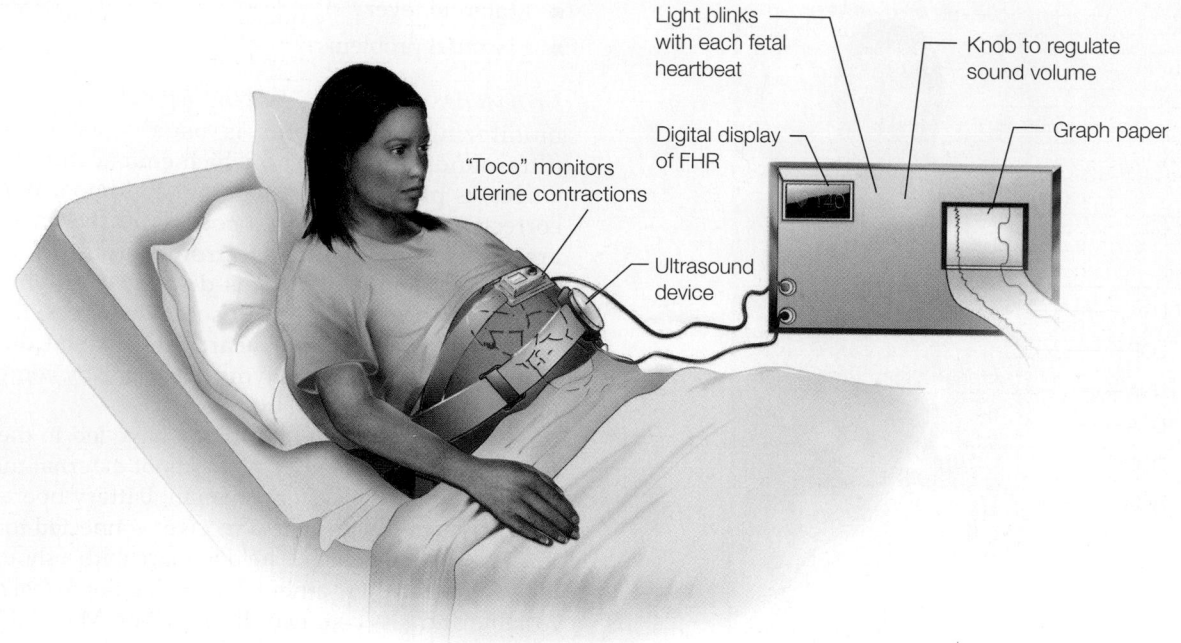

Light blinks with each fetal heartbeat

Knob to regulate sound volume

Digital display of FHR

Graph paper

"Toco" monitors uterine contractions

Ultrasound device

Figure 33–51 》 Electronic fetal monitoring by external technique. The ultrasound device, placed over the fetal back, transmits information on the fetal heart rate. Information from both the tocodynamometer and ultrasound device is transmitted to the electronic fetal monitor. The FHR is indicated in four ways: on the digital display, as a blinking light, by sound, and on special monitor paper. The uterine contractions are displayed on the graph paper.

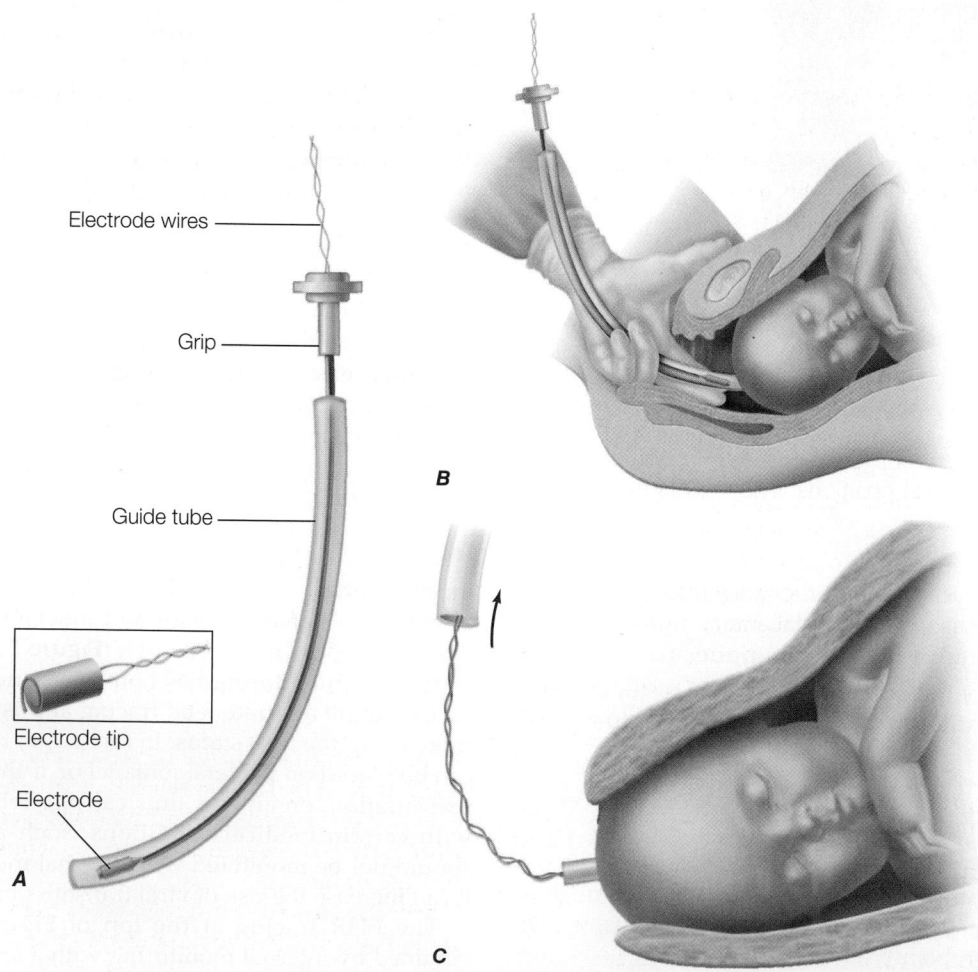

Electrode wires

Grip

Guide tube

Electrode tip

Electrode

A

B

C

Figure 33–52 》 Technique for internal, direct fetal monitoring. *A,* Spiral electrode. *B,* Attaching the spiral electrode to the scalp. *C,* Attached spiral electrode with the guide tube removed.

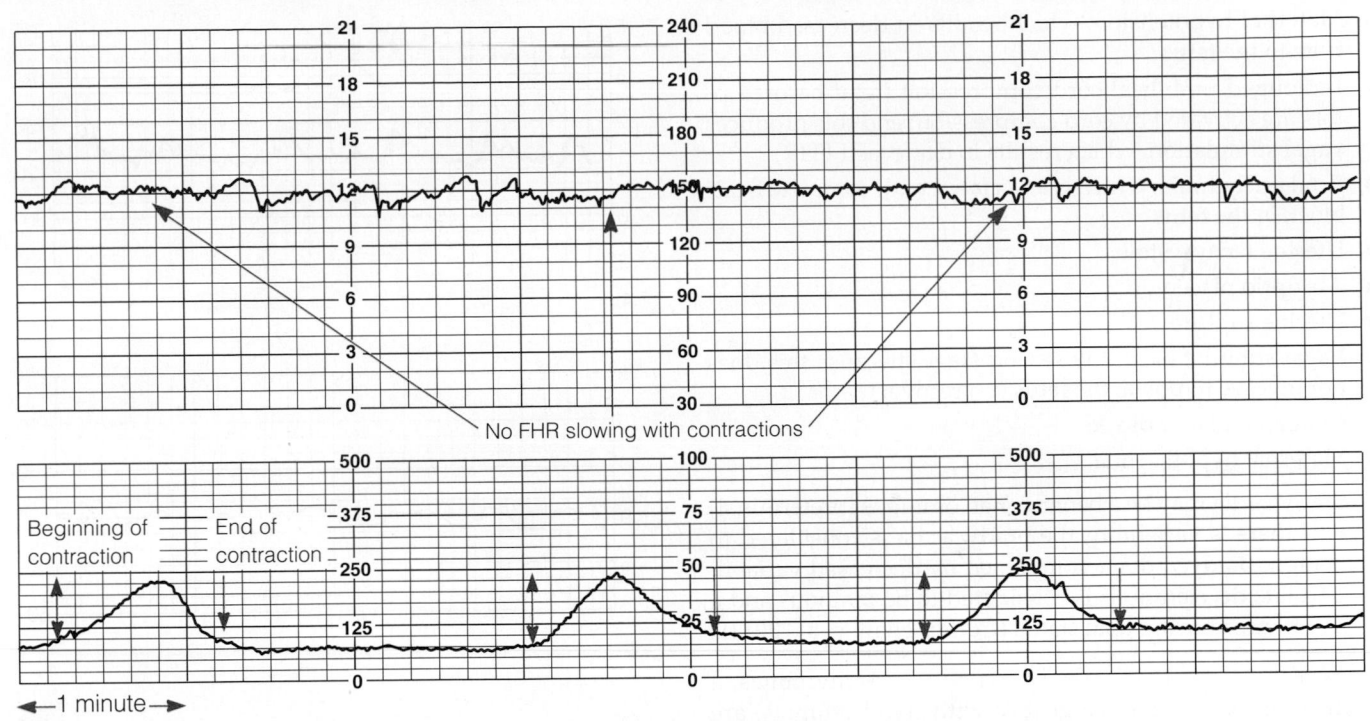

Figure 33–53 ≫ Normal fetal heart rate range is from 110 to 160 beats/min. The FHR tracing in the upper portion of the graph indicates an FHR range of 140–155 beats/min. The bottom portion depicts uterine contractions. Each dark vertical line marks 1 minute, and each small rectangle represents 10 seconds. The contraction frequency is about every 2.5 minutes, and the duration of the contractions is 50–60 seconds.

FHR is variable (the tracing moves up and down instead of in a straight line). In Figure 33–53, each dark vertical line represents 1 minute; therefore, contractions are occurring about every 2.5–3 minutes. The FHR is evaluated by assessing an electronic monitor tracing for baseline rate, baseline variability, and periodic changes.

BASELINE FETAL HEART RATE The **baseline fetal heart rate** refers to the average FHR rounded to increments of 5 beats/min observed during a 10-minute period of monitoring. This excludes periodic or episodic changes, periods of marked variability, and segments of the baseline that differ by more than 25 beats/min. The duration should be at least 2 minutes (Menihan & Kopel, 2014). Normal FHR (baseline rate) ranges from 110 to 160 beats/min. There are two abnormal variations of the baseline rate—those above 160 beats/min (tachycardia) and those below 110 beats/min (bradycardia). Another change affecting the baseline is called **baseline FHR variability**, which is fluctuation in the FHR baseline of 2 cycles per minute or greater, with irregular amplitude and inconstant frequency (Cunningham et al., 2014).

A *wandering baseline* fluctuates between 120 and 160 beats/min in an unsteady wandering pattern and can be associated with neurologic impairment of the fetus or a preterminal event (Cunningham et al., 2014). Possible causes for this pattern include congenital defects or metabolic acidosis. Immediate interventions are needed in order to enhance fetal oxygenation. Birth should be anticipated (Hamilton & Warrick, 2013).

Fetal tachycardia is a sustained rate of 161 beats/min or above. Marked tachycardia is 180 beats/min or above.

Causes of tachycardia include the following (Cunningham et al., 2014):

- Early fetal hypoxia, which leads to stimulation of the sympathetic system as the fetus compensates for reduced blood flow
- Maternal fever, which accelerates the metabolism of the fetus
- Maternal dehydration
- Beta-sympathomimetic drugs, such as ritodrine, terbutaline, atropine, and isoxsuprine, which have a cardiac stimulant effect
- Chorioamnionitis (fetal tachycardia may be the first sign of developing intrauterine infection)
- Maternal hyperthyroidism (thyroid-stimulating hormones may cross the placenta and stimulate FHR)
- Fetal anemia (the heart rate is increased as a compensatory mechanism to improve tissue perfusion)
- Tachydysrhythmias (fetal dysrhythmias occur in less than 1% of all pregnancies).

Tachycardia is considered to be an ominous sign if it is accompanied by late decelerations, severe variable decelerations, or decreased variability. If tachycardia is associated with maternal fever, treatment may consist of antipyretics and/or antibiotics.

Fetal bradycardia is a rate of less than 110 beats/min during a 10-minute period or longer. Causes of fetal bradycardia include the following (Cunningham et al., 2014):

- Late (profound) fetal hypoxia (depression of myocardial activity)

- Maternal hypotension, which results in decreased blood flow to the fetus
- Prolonged umbilical cord compression (fetal baroreceptors are activated by cord compression, and this produces vagal stimulation, which results in decreased FHR)
- Fetal arrhythmia, which is associated with complete heart block in the fetus
- Uterine tachysystole
- Abruptio placentae
- Uterine rupture
- Vagal stimulation in the second stage (because this does not involve hypoxia, the fetus can recover)
- Congenital heart block
- Maternal hypothermia.

Bradycardia may be a benign or an ominous (preterminal) sign. If there is variability, the bradycardia is considered to be benign. Bradycardia accompanied by decreased variability and late decelerations is considered to be ominous and a sign of nonreassuring fetal status (Cunningham et al., 2014).

ARRHYTHMIAS AND DYSRHYTHMIAS Arrhythmias, a term often used interchangeably with dysrhythmias, are disturbances in the FHR pattern that are not associated with abnormal electrical impulse formation or conduction in the fetal cardiac tissue but are related to a structural abnormality or congenital heart disease. The majority of fetal arrhythmias are irregular rhythms (Anderson & Stone, 2013). Fetal arrhythmias may be detected when listening to the FHR on a fetal monitor. It is important to rule out artifacts or electrical interference, which may occur. Most true arrhythmias are accompanied by baseline bradycardia, baseline tachycardia, or an abrupt baseline spiking. Whereas 90% of dysrhythmias are benign, 10% can be life threatening and require the consultation of a neonatal or pediatric cardiology expert (Miller, Miller, & Tucker, 2013).

VARIABILITY Baseline variability is a measure of the interplay (the push–pull effect) between the sympathetic and parasympathetic nervous systems. Baseline variability is fluctuations in the FHR of two cycles per minute or greater. **Figure 33–54 »** depicts the different ranges of variability. The amplitudes of the peaks and troughs in beats per minute are defined as follows (Papadakis, McPhee, & Rabow, 2014):

- *Absent:* amplitude undetectable
- *Minimal:* amplitude detectable but less than 5 beats/min
- *Moderate:* amplitude 6–25 beats/min
- *Marked:* amplitude greater than 25 beats/min.

Reduced variability is the best single predictor for determining fetal compromise (Cunningham et al., 2014). Fetal acidosis and subsequent hypoxia are highest in fetuses that have absent or minimal variability.

Causes of decreased variability include the following (Cunningham et al., 2014):

- Hypoxia and acidosis (decreased blood flow to the fetus)
- Administration of drugs such as meperidine hydrochloride (Demerol), diazepam (Valium), or hydroxyzine (Vistaril) that depress the fetal central nervous system

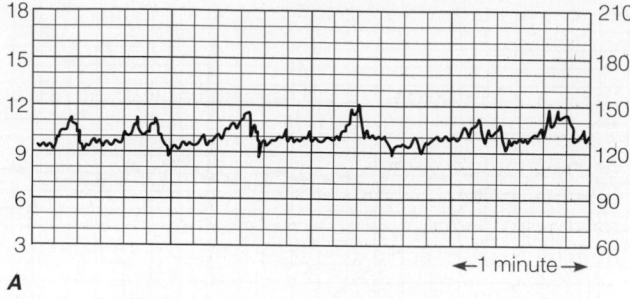

A

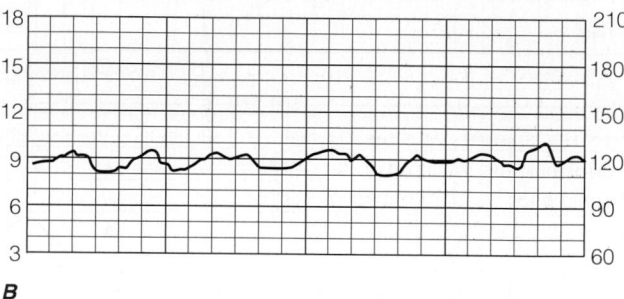

B

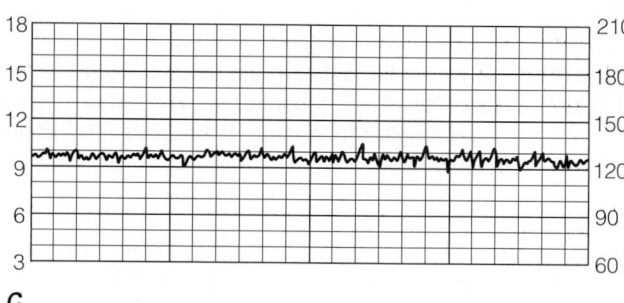

C

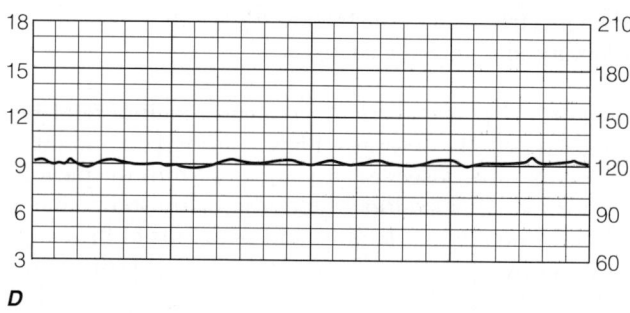

D

Figure 33–54 » Variability. *A,* Marked variability. *B,* Moderate variability. *C,* Minimal variability. *D,* Absent variability.

- Fetal sleep cycle (during fetal sleep, variability is decreased; fetal sleep cycles usually last for 20–40 minutes each hour)
- Fetus of less than 32 weeks of gestation (fetal neurologic control of heart rate is immature)
- Fetal dysrhythmias
- Fetal anomalies affecting the heart, central nervous system, or autonomic nervous system
- Previous neurologic insult
- Tachycardia.

Causes of marked variability include the following (King et al., 2013):

- Early mild hypoxia (variability increases as a result of compensatory mechanism)
- Fetal stimulation or activity (stimulation of autonomic nervous system because of abdominal palpation, maternal vaginal examination, application of spiral electrode on fetal head, or acoustic stimulation)
- Fetal breathing movements
- Advancing gestational age (greater than 30 weeks of gestation).

Absent variability that does not appear to be associated with a fetal sleep cycle or the administration of drugs is a warning sign of nonreassuring fetal status. It is especially ominous if absent or minimal variability is accompanied by late decelerations (explained shortly). If decreased variability is noted on monitoring, consider application of a spiral electrode to obtain more accurate information.

ACCELERATIONS **Accelerations** are transient increases in the FHR normally caused by fetal movement. When the fetus moves, its heart rate increases, just as the heart rates of adults increase during exercise. Often, accelerations accompany uterine contractions, usually because the fetus moves in response to the pressure of the contractions. Accelerations of this type are thought to be a sign of fetal well-being and adequate oxygen reserve. The accelerations with fetal movement are the basis for nonstress tests.

DECELERATIONS **Decelerations** are periodic decreases in FHR from the normal baseline. They are categorized as early, late, and variable according to the time of their occurrence in the contraction cycle and their waveform (**Figure 33–55 »**). Nursing interventions for decelerations are outlined in **Table 33–14 »**.

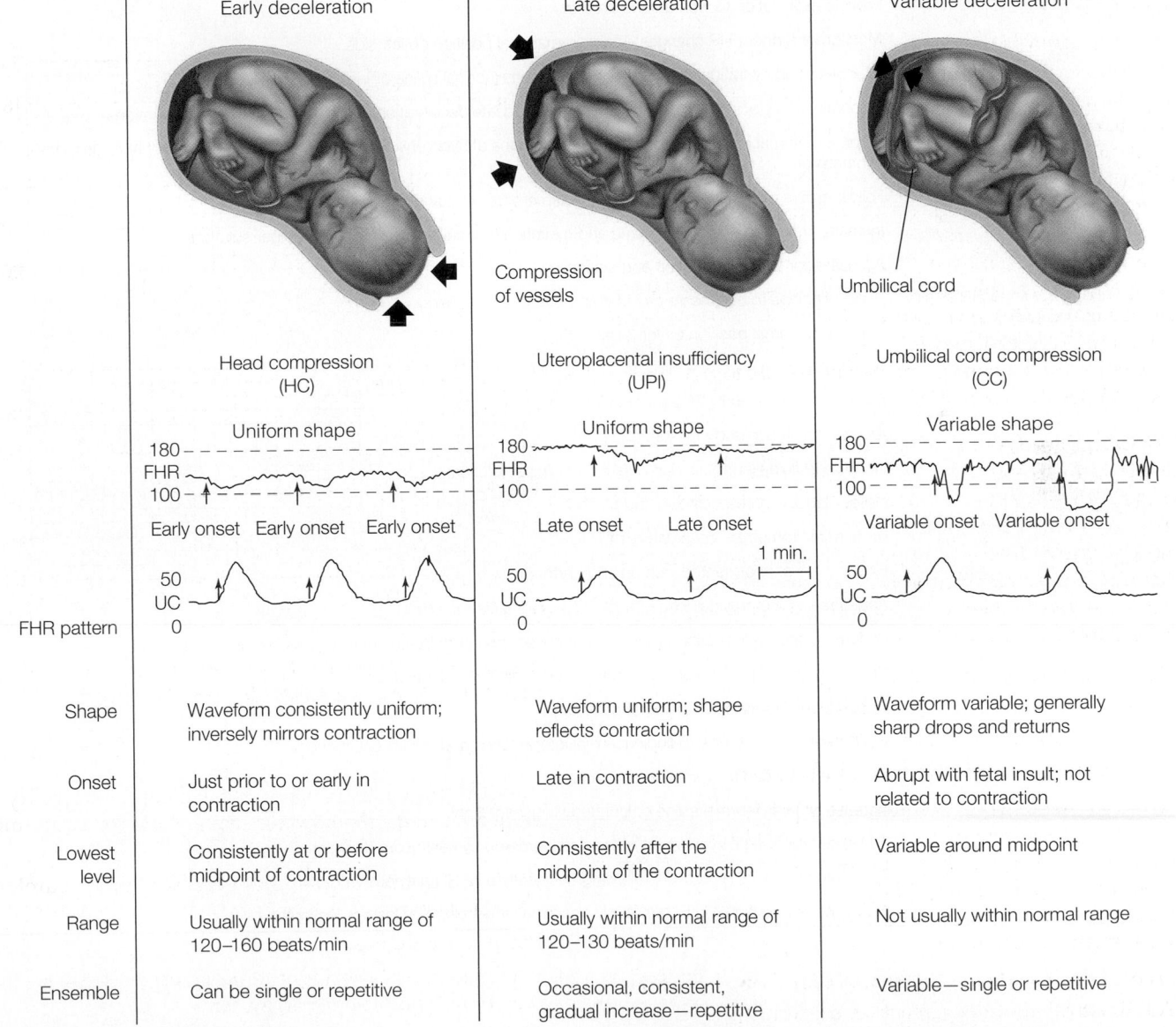

	Early deceleration	Late deceleration	Variable deceleration
	Head compression (HC)	Uteroplacental insufficiency (UPI)	Umbilical cord compression (CC)
Shape	Waveform consistently uniform; inversely mirrors contraction	Waveform uniform; shape reflects contraction	Waveform variable; generally sharp drops and returns
Onset	Just prior to or early in contraction	Late in contraction	Abrupt with fetal insult; not related to contraction
Lowest level	Consistently at or before midpoint of contraction	Consistently after the midpoint of the contraction	Variable around midpoint
Range	Usually within normal range of 120–160 beats/min	Usually within normal range of 120–130 beats/min	Not usually within normal range
Ensemble	Can be single or repetitive	Occasional, consistent, gradual increase—repetitive	Variable—single or repetitive

Figure 33–55 » Types and characteristics of early, late, and variable decelerations.

TABLE 33–14 Guidelines for Management of Variable, Late, and Prolonged Deceleration Patterns

Pattern	Nursing Interventions
Variable decelerations (Cause: umbilical cord compression)	Report findings to healthcare provider and document in chart.
	Provide explanation to woman and partner.
Isolated or occasional, moderate	Change maternal position to one in which FHR pattern is most improved.
	Perform vaginal examination to assess for prolapsed cord or change in labor progress.
	Monitor FHR continuously to assess current status and for further changes in FHR pattern.
Variable decelerations, severe and uncorrectable (Cause: umbilical cord compression)	Administer oxygen by face mask at 7–10 L/min.
	Report findings to healthcare provider and document in chart.
	Provide explanation to woman and partner.
	Prepare for probable cesarean birth. Follow interventions previously listed.
	Prepare for vaginal birth unless baseline variability is decreasing or FHR is progressively rising, in which case cesarean, forceps, or vacuum birth is indicated.
	Maintain good hydration with intravenous (IV) fluids (normal saline or lactated Ringer solution).
Late decelerations (Cause: uteroplacental insufficiency)	Administer oxygen by face mask at 7–10 L/min.
	Report findings to healthcare provider and document in chart.
	Provide explanation to woman and partner.
	Monitor for further FHR changes. Maintain maternal position on left side.
	Maintain good hydration with intravenous (IV) fluids (normal saline or lactated Ringer solution).
	Discontinue oxytocin if it is being administered and late decelerations persist despite other interventions.
	Monitor maternal blood pressure and pulse for signs of hypotension; possibly increase flow rate of IV fluids to treat hypotension.
	Follow orders of healthcare provider for treatment for hypotension if present.
	Increase IV fluids to maintain volume and hydration (normal saline or lactated Ringer solution).
	Assess labor progress (dilation and station).
Late decelerations with tachycardia or decreasing variability (Cause: uteroplacental insufficiency)	Report findings to healthcare provider and document in chart.
	Maintain maternal position on left side.
	Administer oxygen by face mask at 7–10 L/min.
	Discontinue oxytocin if it is being administered.
	Assess maternal blood pressure and pulse.
	Increase IV fluids (normal saline or lactated Ringer solution).
	Assess labor progress (dilation and station).
	Prepare for immediate cesarean birth.
	Explain plan of treatment to woman and partner.
	Assist healthcare provider with fetal blood sampling (if ordered).
Prolonged decelerations (Cause: multiple issues that result in prolonged impaired perfusion)	Perform vaginal examination to rule out prolapsed cord or to determine progress in labor status.
	Change maternal position as needed to try to alleviate decelerations.
	Discontinue oxytocin if it is being administered.
	Notify healthcare provider of findings/initial interventions and document in chart.
	Provide explanation to woman and partner.
	Increase IV fluids (normal saline or lactated Ringer solution).
	Administer tocolytic if hypertonus noted and if ordered by healthcare provider.
	Anticipate normal FHR recovery following deceleration if FHR previously normal.
	Anticipate intervention if FHR previously abnormal or deceleration lasts > 3 minutes.

When the fetal head is compressed, cerebral blood flow is decreased, which leads to central vagal stimulation and results in early deceleration. The onset of early deceleration is associated with the onset of the uterine contraction. This type of deceleration is of uniform shape, is usually considered to be benign, and does not require intervention.

SAFETY ALERT The presence of repetitive early decelerations may be a sign of advanced dilation or the beginning of the second stage of labor (King et al., 2013). If the monitoring strip shows recurring early decelerations, ask the laboring woman whether she is experiencing any pressure. Pressure that occurs only with the contractions typically indicates advanced dilation. Intense pressure that does not change or ease up when the contractions cease may indicate the beginning of the second stage. A vaginal examination may be performed to establish the amount of dilation.

Late deceleration is caused by uteroplacental insufficiency resulting from decreased blood flow and oxygen transfer to the fetus through the intervillous spaces during uterine contractions. The most common causes of late decelerations are maternal hypotension resulting from the administration of epidural anesthesia and uterine tachysystole associated with oxytocin infusion (Groll, 2012). The onset of the deceleration occurs after the onset of a uterine contraction and is of a uniform shape that tends to reflect associated uterine contractions. The late deceleration pattern is considered to be a nonreassuring sign and requires continuous assessment. If late decelerations continue and birth is not imminent, a cesarean birth may be indicated.

Variable decelerations occur if the umbilical cord becomes compressed, reducing blood flow between the placenta and fetus. The resulting increase in peripheral resistance in the fetal circulation causes fetal hypertension. Fetal hypertension stimulates the baroreceptors in the aortic arch and carotid sinuses, slowing the FHR. The onset of variable decelerations differs in timing with the onset of the contraction, and the decelerations are variable in shape. This pattern requires further assessment.

A sinusoidal pattern appears similar to a waveform. The characteristics of this pattern include absence of variability and the presence of a smooth, wavelike shape. The pattern resembles a perfect letter "S" lying on its side. These patterns can be pseudosinusoidal (benign) or true sinusoidal. The true pattern is associated with Rh alloimmunization, fetal anemia, severe fetal hypoxia, umbilical cord occlusion, twin-to-twin transfusion, or a chronic fetal bleed. Pseudosinusoidal patterns are usually temporary and commonly occur with the administration of medications such as meperidine (Demerol) or butorphanol tartrate (Stadol) (Groll, 2012).

Decelerations are also classified based on the rate in which the FHR leaves the baseline FHR:

- **Abrupt decelerations** occur in less than 30 seconds (King et al., 2013)
- **Variable decelerations** descend abruptly.
- **Gradual decelerations** require 30 seconds or more to descend. Both early and late decelerations descend gradually (King et al., 2013).

- **Episodic decelerations** occur independently of the uterine contractions and are frequently the result of external stimulations, such as vaginal exams.
- **Periodic decelerations** refer to decelerations that occur with the contractions and are considered to be repetitive if they occur with 50% of the contractions (King et al., 2013).
- **Prolonged decelerations** are those that leave the baseline for more than 2 minutes but less than 10 minutes.

EVALUATION OF FETAL HEART RATE TRACINGS Evaluation of the electronic monitor tracing begins by looking at the uterine contraction pattern. To evaluate the contraction pattern, the nurse does the following:

1. Determine the uterine resting tone.
2. Assess the contractions: What is the frequency? What is the duration? What is the intensity?

The next step is to evaluate the FHR tracing as follows:

1. Determine the baseline: Is the baseline within the normal range? Is there evidence of tachycardia? Is there evidence of bradycardia?
2. Determine FHR variability: Is variability absent? Minimal? Moderate? Marked?
3. Determine whether a sinusoidal pattern is present.
4. Determine whether there are periodic changes: Are accelerations present? Do they meet the criteria for a reactive nonstress test? Are decelerations present? Are they uniform in shape? If so, determine whether they are early or late decelerations. Are they nonuniform in shape? If so, determine whether they are variable decelerations.

After evaluating the FHR tracing for the factors just listed, the nurse may further classify the tracing as reassuring (normal) or nonreassuring (worrisome). Reassuring patterns contain normal parameters and do not require additional treatment or intervention. Characteristics of reassuring FHR patterns include the following:

- Baseline rate is 110–160 beats/min.
- Variability is moderate.
- Periodic patterns consist of accelerations with fetal movement, and early decelerations may be present.

Nonreassuring patterns may indicate that the fetus is becoming stressed and intervention is needed. Characteristics of nonreassuring patterns include the following:

- Severe variable decelerations (FHR drops below 70 beats/min for longer than 30–45 seconds and is accompanied by rising baseline or decreasing variability or slow return to baseline.)
- Late decelerations of any magnitude
- Absence of variability
- Prolonged deceleration (a deceleration that lasts 60–90 seconds or more)
- Severe (marked) bradycardia (FHR baseline of 70 beats/min or less).

Nonreassuring patterns may require continuous monitoring and more involved treatment and intervention (see Table 33–14).

Box 33–6
The Three-Tier Fetal Heart Rate Interpretation System

Category I

Category I FHR tracings include *all* of the following:

- Baseline rate: 110–160 beats/min
- Baseline FHR variability: moderate
- Late or variable decelerations: absent
- Early decelerations: present or absent
- Accelerations: present or absent.

Category II

Category II FHR tracings include all FHR tracings not categorized as Category I or Category III. Category II tracings may represent an appreciable fraction of those encountered in clinical care. Examples of Category II FHR tracings include any of the following:

- Baseline rate
  - Bradycardia not accompanied by absent baseline variability
  - Tachycardia
- Baseline FHR variability
  - Minimal baseline variability
  - Absent baseline variability not accompanied by recurrent decelerations
  - Marked baseline variability

- Accelerations
  - Absence of induced accelerations after fetal stimulation
- Periodic or episodic decelerations
  - Recurrent variable decelerations accompanied by minimal or moderate baseline variability
  - Prolonged deceleration of 2 minutes or more but less than 10 minutes
  - Recurrent late decelerations with moderate baseline variability
  - Variable decelerations with other characteristics, such as slow return to baseline, "overshoots," or "shoulders."

Category III

Category III FHR tracings include:

- Absent baseline FHR variability and any of the following:
  - Recurrent late decelerations
  - Recurrent variable decelerations
  - Bradycardia
- Sinusoidal pattern.

Source: Data from American College of Obstetricians & Gynecologists (ACOG) (2009, reaffirmed 2013). *Intrapartum fetal heart rate monitoring: Nomenclature, interpretation, and general management principles.* (ACOG Practice Bulletin No. 106.) Washington, DC: ACOG.

After evaluating the FHR tracing for the factors listed, the nurse may categorize the tracing according to the Three-Tier Fetal Heart Rate Interpretation System shown in **Box 33–6** ≫. The three-tier system for the categorization of FHR patterns is recommended by ACOG, Association of Women's Health, Obstetric, and Neonatal Nurses (AWHONN), and the National Institute of Child Health and Human Development (Callahan & Caughley, 2013). Categorization of the FHR tracing evaluates the fetus at that point in time; tracing patterns can and will change. An FHR tracing may move back and forth between categories depending on the clinical situation and management strategies employed.

- ***Category I FHR tracings are normal.*** They are strongly predictive of normal fetal acid–base status at the time of observation. The FHR tracings may be followed in a routine manner, and no specific action is required.

- ***Category II FHR tracings are indeterminate.*** They are not predictive of abnormal fetal acid–base status, yet we do not have adequate evidence at present to classify these as Category I or Category III. Category II tracings require evaluation and continued surveillance and reevaluation, taking into account all of the associated clinical circumstances.

- ***Category III FHR tracings are abnormal.*** They are predictive of abnormal fetal acid–base status at the time of observation. They require prompt evaluation. Depending on the clinical situation, efforts to expeditiously resolve the abnormal FHR pattern may include, but are not limited to, provision of maternal oxygen, change in maternal position, discontinuation of labor stimulation, and treatment of maternal hypotension.

It is important to provide information to the laboring woman regarding the FHR pattern and the interventions that will help her fetus. Sharing information with the laboring woman reassures her that a potential or actual problem has been identified and that she is an active participant in the interventions. Occasionally, a problem arises that requires immediate intervention. In that case, the nurse can say something like "It is important for you to turn on your side right now because the baby is having a little difficulty. I'll explain what is happening in just a few moments." This type of response lets the woman know that although an action needs to be accomplished rapidly, information will soon be provided. In the haste to act quickly, the nurse must not forget that it is the woman's body and her baby.

Labor and birth nurses must be skilled and competent in evaluating electronic FHR patterns and responding appropriately (see Table 33–14). Competence can be maintained through frequent in-services, formal courses, and continuing education programs.

RESPONSES TO ELECTRONIC MONITORING Responses to electronic fetal monitoring can be varied and complex. Many women have little knowledge of monitoring unless they have attended a prenatal class that dealt with this subject. Some women react to electronic monitoring positively, viewing it as a reassurance that "the baby is okay." They may also feel the monitor helps identify problems that develop in labor. Other women may have ambivalent or even negative feelings about the monitor. They may think the monitor is interfering with a natural process, and they do not want the intrusion. They may resent the time and attention that the monitor requires—time that could otherwise be spent providing nursing care. Some women may find that the equipment, wires, and sounds increase their anxiety. The discomfort of lying in one position and fear of injury to the baby are other objections.

Diagnosis

In the first stage of labor, appropriate nursing diagnoses may include the following:

■ *Fear* related to discomfort of labor and unknown labor outcome

■ *Anxiety* related to discomfort of labor and unknown labor outcome

■ *Pain, Acute,* related to uterine contractions, cervical dilation, and fetal descent

■ *Childbearing Process, Readiness for Enhanced,* related to the normal labor process and comfort measures.

(NANDA-I © 2014)

In the second and third stages of labor, appropriate nursing diagnoses may include the following:

■ *Pain, Acute,* related to uterine contractions, the birth process, and/or perineal trauma from birth

■ *Childbearing Process, Readiness for Enhanced,* related to pushing methods to assist in the birth

■ *Anxiety* related to the outcome of the birth process.

(NANDA-I © 2014)

In the fourth stage of labor, possible nursing diagnoses include the following:

■ *Pain, Acute,* related to perineal trauma

■ *Childbearing Process, Readiness for Enhanced,* related to the involution process and self-care needs

■ *Family Processes, Readiness for Enhanced,* related to incorporation of the newborn into the family.

(NANDA-I © 2014)

Planning

When a plan of care is devised for the intrapartum period, the nurse can develop a general plan that encompasses the total process, from the beginning of labor through the fourth stage, or a plan can be developed for each stage of labor and birth. It is imperative that the nurse assess the couple's understanding of the labor process and provide brief explanations as labor progresses in accordance with the couple's learning needs. The overriding goal is to provide a safe environment for the mother and fetus. Additional goals for care may include:

■ Support the mother and family by offering reassurance and information as needed throughout the labor and birth experience

■ Promote maternal coping behaviors

■ Provide comfort measures to promote pain relief as needed

■ Acknowledge and support the mother's desires and choices throughout labor, whenever possible

■ Create an environment that is sensitive and supportive of the biophysical, psychosocial, spiritual, and cultural needs of the mother and her family.

Labor can be both an exciting and anxiety-producing time for the mother and her family. Feelings of ambivalence are relatively common as the laboring mother and her partner or support person experience a variety of assessments, care activities, and technologies. Orienting the mother and her family to what to expect can promote feelings of well-being during the labor and birth process (see Patient Teaching: What to Expect During Labor).

Patient Teaching

What to Expect During Labor

■ Provide information on the basic assessment and care activities. Allow time for questions and discussion as the progress of labor permits. Describe aspects of the admission process, including the following:

● Taking an abbreviated history

● Physical assessment (maternal vital signs [VS], FHR, contraction status, status of membranes)

● Assessment of uterine contractions (frequency, duration, intensity)

● Orientation to surroundings

● Introductions to other support staff

● Determination of woman's and any support person's expectations of the nurse.

■ Present aspects of ongoing physical care, such as when to expect assessment of maternal VS, FHR, and contractions.

■ If the electronic fetal monitor is used, describe how it works and the information it provides. Demonstrate the fetal monitor. Orient the woman to the sights and sounds of the monitor. Explain what "normal" data will look like and what characteristics are being watched for.

■ Note that assessments will increase as the labor progresses, especially during the transition phase (usually the time the woman would like to be left alone), to help keep the mother and baby safe by noting deviations from the normal course.

■ Describe the vaginal examination and the information it elicits. Use a cervical dilation chart to illustrate the amount of dilation.

■ Review comfort techniques that may be used in labor, and ascertain what the woman thinks will promote comfort. Focus on open discussion.

■ Review the childbirth preparation the woman has learned so that you will be able to support her in their use. Ask the woman to demonstrate the techniques she has learned.

■ Review comfort and support measures, such as positioning, back rub, touch, distraction techniques, and ambulation.

■ If the woman is in early labor, offer her a tour of the birthing area, and explain equipment and routines. Include the woman's partner.

Implementation

The woman in labor and her partner or support person tend to be concerned about arriving at the birth center in time for the birth. Sometimes, the labor is advanced and birth is imminent, but usually the woman is in early labor at admission. If time permits and the family is not familiar with what will occur during labor, the nurse can provide necessary information (see the Patient Teaching feature).

Integrate Cultural Beliefs

Knowledge of values, customs, and practices of various cultures is as important during labor as it is in the prenatal period. Without this knowledge, a nurse is less likely to understand a family's behavior and may attempt to impose his or her personal values and beliefs on the woman and her family. As cultural sensitivity and competence increase, so does the likelihood of providing satisfying, high-quality care (Spector, 2017). In providing culturally appropriate care, it is important to familiarize yourself with cultural beliefs from various cultures, but also important to avoid making generalizations based on a patient's perceived ethnicity, culture, or identity (Ingraham, Wingo, Foster, & Roberts, 2017). The nurse must always remain aware that an individual example of a birthing practice will never be pertinent to all women in a given group.

MODESTY Modesty is an important consideration for most women regardless of culture. Many women from a variety of backgrounds find it uncomfortable to be physically examined, so respecting the need for privacy with draping, asking the woman if she would like family members to leave the room, or making other accommodations as needed should be done whenever possible. Some women may be uncomfortable when men are present; others may be uncomfortable with exposure regardless of the gender of the healthcare providers. It is prudent to assume that embarrassment will occur with exposure and take measures to provide privacy rather than to assume that it will not matter to the woman if she is exposed.

When a woman identifies a cultural or religious preference, it is important to ask questions to gain a specific understanding of what that means to her and how she sees it impacting her care needs. For example, according to the Orthodox Jewish law of *Tznuit*, women should maintain modesty in order to preserve dignity. For some women, this may be accomplished by providing a long sleeve gown that covers her elbows and knees, whereas other Orthodox Jewish women may voice no preferences. It is important that the nurse balances knowledge of cultural and religious beliefs with verbal or behavioral cues that support a woman's preferences. For example, offering to pull the curtain while a woman changes into her patient gown shows understanding that some women prefer not to change in front of their husbands. For those who do not adhere to this belief, it provides an opportunity for the woman to verbally decline, thus providing cues on her own belief and preferences (Neis, 2017).

EXPRESSION AND MEANING OF PAIN The manner in which a woman chooses to deal with the discomfort of labor varies widely. Some women seem to turn inward and remain very quiet or cease conversation completely. Others may be very vocal, with behaviors such as counting out loud, moaning, crying, or shouting. They may also turn from side to side or change positions frequently, often appearing restless. While some cultural influences impact the labor process, women react to labor based on a variety of factors, with culture being only a single variable; therefore, generalizations should not be used to anticipate a woman's responses.

For example, while silence may be culturally more common in some Chinese societies, it does not mean that all Chinese women will desire to labor quietly.

Different cultures also have differing beliefs about the meaning and value of labor pain. Some Latina women view pain during labor as a symbol of love toward the baby—the more intense the pain, the more intense the love. As in all cultures, beliefs that were strongly held by one generation may change over time. In the past, many Native American women viewed labor pain as natural and many used meditation, self-control, or indigenous plants or herbs, such as black cohosh, throughout their labor to aid them during birth (Spector, 2017). While some Native women may still adhere to these practices, others may no longer adhere to these beliefs and may want more modern approaches used to control pain. Labor and delivery nurses can provide culturally competent care by becoming acquainted with the beliefs and practices of the various subcultures while assessing each woman for her own unique preferences within a cultural context. In the birthing situation, the truly effective nurse supports the family's cultural practices as long as it is safe to do so.

It is important to explore each patient's desires for her labor and to inquire how she would like to manage her pain. This is important because adverse birth events increase the risk for postpartum mood disorders and can even create trauma, which can cause psychological issues that persist for future pregnancies (DeGroot & Vik, 2017).

Provide Nursing Care on Admission

The manner in which the maternity nurse greets the laboring woman and her partner influences the course of the woman's hospital stay. The arrival at the healthcare setting and the sometimes impersonal and technical aspects of admission can produce profound stress, fear, and anxiety. If women and their families are greeted in a brusque, harried manner, they are less likely to look to the nurse for support. A calm, pleasant manner indicates to the woman that she is important. It helps to instill in the couple a sense of confidence in the staff's ability to provide quality care during this critical time.

Following the initial greeting, the nurse escorts the woman and support person to the birthing room and provides a quick yet thorough orientation to the facility, including the location of the restrooms, public phones, and nurse-call or emergency-call system. These simple steps can go a long way toward helping the couple feel more at ease. The nurse also explains the monitoring equipment or other unfamiliar technology. Every effort needs to be made to demystify the environment for the laboring woman and her support person. Some women prefer that their partner remain with them during the admission process, although others prefer to have the partner wait outside.

As the nurse helps the woman undress and get into a hospital gown, he or she can start to develop rapport and begin

Focus on Diversity and Culture
Childbirth Customs

Various cultures have different customs and beliefs surrounding childbearing and childbirth. Generalizations regarding cultural perspectives are discussed with examples designed to provide students with ways to integrate cultural customs into specific individualized labor and birth options for women.

Some Hmong women from Laos may prefer to stay active during labor and to squat during the second stage of labor. It is not unusual for the partner to be present and actively involved in providing comfort. Some laboring women may prefer only "hot" foods and warm water to drink (Spector, 2017). For some Hmong women, the family may request that the mother be given a soft-boiled egg to restore her energy as soon as birth occurs. The nurse may ask the woman about her own cultural beliefs and obtain specific requests for labor positioning, ambulation in labor, who she would like to provide labor support, preferred birth positions, temperature of oral fluids preferred, and advise her that a regular diet with her own food preferences can begin immediately following a vaginal birth.

Some Vietnamese women may show a strong sense of self-control throughout labor. They may prefer to walk during labor and to give birth in a squatting position. Like many people from other Asian cultures, some may view labor as a "hot condition" and prefer cold beverages; however, during the postpartum period, which is viewed as a "cold" condition, they may prefer warm liquids (Kim, 2017). In some cultures, newborn praise can be perceived negatively, sometimes being referred to as is the "evil eye" which is associated with jealousy (Lloreda-Garcia, 2017).

Some Latina women desire to have their partners present during labor and birth to show their love and to speak using affectionate words. Many Latina women also typically want their mothers present during the birth process (Attanasio, Hardeman, Kozhimannil, & Kjerulff, 2017). Again, knowledge of traditional cultural norms can help the nurse effectively coordinate care for the woman and her family. Cultural norms should guide, not dictate, the assessment process.

Some Muslim women may have their husband present, whereas others may desire a female friend or relative with them during childbirth. Because modesty is of great concern for many Muslim women, care must be taken to cover the woman as much as possible (Spector, 2017). Some women may want to put their *khimar* (head covering) on before a male enters the room. For some Muslim families, it may be important for a female nurse, physician, or CNM to perform examinations when possible. For women who express a preference for female care providers, it is important to discuss the possibility that a female provider may not always be present and that if a male is required, every effort to provide privacy and advanced notice will be given (Davidson, Ladewig, London, 2017). For some Muslim patients, traditions such as calling praise to Allah (*adhan*) into the newborn's right ear may be requested (Spector, 2017).

Different religious practices are observed throughout the world. Some Orthodox Jewish women observe the law of *niddah*, which begins with the onset of regular uterine contractions or the appearance of bloody show or membrane rupture. Once this occurs, the *niddah* law mandates a physical separation of husband and wife (Neis, 2017). The nurse should inquire about specific observations so the best support and encouragement for the mother can be provided. If couples describe the preference for limited physical contact, the nurse will need to assist the woman and serve as the primary caretaker. Sometimes, the laboring woman's mother or another female friend or relative may be present (Neis, 2017). During this time period, the father may read prayers, choose not to observe the birth, and wait to reenter the room until after the woman has completed the third stage of labor and has been assisted in resuming a comfortable position in bed.

---

the assessment process. The experienced labor and birth nurse can obtain essential information about the woman and her pregnancy, initiate any immediate interventions needed, and establish individualized priorities and preferences within a few minutes after admission. Forming realistic objectives for laboring women is a major challenge for nurses, because each woman has different coping mechanisms and support systems.

Laboring women often face a number of unfamiliar procedures that may seem routine for healthcare providers. It is important to remember that all patients have the right to accept or reject care measures. The patient's informed consent is needed before any procedure that involves touching her body. The admission process, therefore, includes signing an informed consent for treatment and providing information regarding advance directives. Typically, an identification bracelet and an allergy band are attached to the expectant woman's wrist.

Laboring families have specific expectations of the labor and birth experience, of themselves, of the nurse, and of the physician or CNM. Sometimes, families have unrealistic expectations, which can increase anxiety, create stress, and end in disappointment if expectations are not met. The nurse should encourage all families to discuss their preferences and special requests. Some families may present to the birthing center with a birth plan. Reviewing the plan provides the nurse with the opportunity to explore the family's wishes. If requests cannot be met, explain the reasons thoroughly. All members of the healthcare team need to be informed of the family's requests.

Some families want the nurse present at all times, whereas others desire privacy and want to spend time alone. Couples may want a great deal of support if they have not attended childbirth education classes or if they are anxious. Others may want to enjoy the experience as a couple, with as few outside interruptions as possible. In this case, the nurse informs the couple of the nurse's availability and of the need to make intermittent assessments.

If indicated, the nurse assists the woman into bed. A side-lying or semi-Fowler position rather than a supine position is most comfortable and prevents supine hypotensive syndrome (vena caval syndrome). After obtaining the essential information from the patient and her records, the nurse begins the intrapartum assessment. Once the assessment is complete, the nurse can make effective nursing decisions about intrapartum care, including the following:

- Should ambulation, bedrest, or a combination of the two be encouraged?
- Is more frequent or continuous electronic fetal monitoring needed?
- What preferences does the woman have for her labor and birth?
- Is a support person available?
- What special needs do this woman and her partner have?

The nurse auscultates the FHR. The nurse assesses the woman's blood pressure, pulse, respirations, oral temperature, and level of pain or discomfort. The nurse also assesses contraction frequency, duration, and intensity (possibly while gathering other data). Before the vaginal examination, the nurse informs the woman about the procedure and its purpose and obtains her consent; afterward, the nurse conveys the findings.

If signs of advanced labor are observed, a vaginal examination must be done immediately upon admission. If the woman shows signs of excessive bleeding or reports episodes of painless bleeding in the last trimester, refrain from performing a vaginal examination and notify the healthcare provider immediately.

Results of the FHR assessment, uterine contraction evaluation, and vaginal examination help determine whether the rest of the admission process can proceed at a leisurely pace or whether additional interventions are required. For example, an FHR of less than 110 beats/min on auscultation indicates that a fetal monitor should be applied immediately to obtain additional data and that continuous fetal monitoring should be performed. The patient's vital signs can be assessed once the monitor is in place.

SAFETY ALERT If the fetal monitor is no longer recording the fetal heart tracing, check for adequate gel under the transducer and reposition it before assuming there is a problem with the fetus. Maternal and fetal movement are the most common causes of an inability to trace the FHR.

The admission process includes collecting a clean, voided, midstream urine specimen. The woman with intact membranes may collect her specimen in the bathroom. Decisions regarding activity level are generally based on physical findings, clinician orders, the patient's desires, agency policy, and safety concerns.

The nurse may test the woman's urine for the presence of protein, ketones, and glucose by using a dipstick before sending the sample to the laboratory. This procedure is especially important if edema or elevated blood pressure is noted on admission. Proteinuria of +1 or more may be a sign of impending preeclampsia. Glycosuria is frequently found in pregnant women because of the increased glomerular filtration rate in the proximal tubules and the inability of these tubules to increase reabsorption of glucose. It may also be associated with gestational diabetes, however, and should not be discounted. While the woman is collecting the urine specimen, the nurse can gather the equipment for any preparation procedures ordered by the healthcare provider.

Laboratory tests are done during early admission. Hemoglobin and hematocrit values help determine the oxygen-carrying capacity of the circulatory system and the woman's ability to withstand blood loss at birth. Elevation of the hematocrit may indicate hemoconcentration of blood, which occurs with edema or dehydration. A low hemoglobin value, in the absence of other evidence of bleeding, suggests anemia. Blood may be typed and cross-matched if the woman is in a high-risk category. Platelets are evaluated as well, because low platelets can lead to bleeding problems. Low platelets are also a contraindication

for epidural anesthesia. In addition, a type and screen is performed in case an obstetric emergency arises and the woman needs to get blood products. Additional serologic testing may be performed as indicated. Offer HIV testing to all women who have not been previously screened (AIDS. gov, 2015).

Depending on how rapidly labor is progressing, the nurse notifies the healthcare provider before or after completing the admission procedures. The report includes the following information:

- Parity
- Cervical dilation and effacement
- Station
- Presenting part
- Status of the membranes
- Contraction pattern
- FHR
- Vital signs that are not in the normal range
- Any significant prenatal history
- Woman's birth preferences
- Woman's reaction to labor
- Woman's preferences for pain relief.

The nurse also enters an admission note into the computer or the charting system. The admission note should include the reason for admission, the date and time of the woman's arrival and notification of the healthcare provider, the condition of the woman and her baby, and labor and membrane status.

Provide Nursing Care During the First Stage of Labor

The nurse needs to evaluate physical parameters of the woman and her fetus. Maternal temperature is monitored every 2–4 hours unless the temperature is over 37.5°C (99.6°F), in which case it is taken every hour. When the amniotic membranes have ruptured, maternal temperature is assessed every 1–2 hours, depending on the policy of the institution. Blood pressure, pulse, respirations, and response to pain are monitored as indicated or according to unit policy. If the woman's blood pressure is greater than or equal to 140/90 mmHg or her pulse is more than 100 beats/min, the nurse must notify the healthcare provider and reevaluate the blood pressure and pulse more frequently. Monitor the woman's pain level continually, because increased pain can elevate the blood pressure and pulse, especially during contractions.

The nurse palpates uterine contractions for frequency, intensity, and duration every 30 minutes. The nurse also auscultates the FHR every 30 minutes in active labor for low-risk women and every 15 minutes for high-risk women as long as the FHR remains between 110 and 160 beats/min and is reassuring (Miller et al., 2012). Auscultate the FHR throughout one contraction and for approximately 15 seconds after the contraction to ensure there are no decelerations. If the FHR baseline is not in the range of 110–160 beats/min or if decelerations are heard, continuous electronic monitoring is recommended (see Table 33–14).

» Visit *Pearson MyLab Nursing and eText* for Chart 7: Psychologic Characteristics and Nursing Support During the First and Second Stages of Labor.

LATENT PHASE The nurse offers food and fluids as desired unless complications exist that may necessitate general anesthesia. Avoiding both liquids and solids during labor, which was once standard practice, is no longer necessary, because evidence-based practice research and new guidelines indicate that clear fluids can be consumed throughout labor and up to 2 hours before an elective cesarean birth. Recent findings suggest that consumption of clear fluids about 1 hour before cesarean section did not increase the risk of regurgitation or aspiration (Ghorashi et al., 2014). In a low-risk setting, it is not necessary to restrict intake in any way.

ACTIVE PHASE During the active phase, the contractions have a frequency of 2–5 minutes, a duration of 40–60 seconds, and a moderate to strong intensity. As the contractions become more frequent and intense, a woman who has been ambulatory may choose to sit in a chair or lie down. Contractions need to be palpated every 30 minutes.

Vaginal exams may be performed to assess cervical dilation and effacement as well as fetal station and position. Vaginal examinations should be limited, however, because they introduce bacteria, which can lead to maternal infection. During the active phase, the cervix dilates from 6 to 8 cm, and vaginal discharge and bloody show increase; thus, the nurse needs to change the perineal pads more frequently.

The FHR is auscultated and evaluated every 30 minutes for low-risk women and every 15 minutes for high-risk women (Malhotra et al., 2014). Maternal blood pressure, pulse, and respirations are monitored during the FHR assessment or more frequently if indicated. The mother's level of pain and coping mechanisms are assessed continuously.

The woman is encouraged to void because a full bladder can interfere with fetal descent. If she is unable to void, catheterization or insertion of an indwelling Foley catheter may be necessary.

If the amniotic membranes have not ruptured previously, they may do so during this phase. When the membranes rupture, the nurse notes the amount, color, odor, and consistency of the amniotic fluid and the time of rupture and immediately auscultates the FHR. The fluid should be clear, with no odor. Nonreassuring fetal status may lead to intestinal and anal sphincter relaxation. This may result in the release of meconium into the amniotic fluid, which turns the fluid greenish brown. When the nurse notes meconium-stained fluid, an electronic monitor is applied to assess the FHR continuously. Current management of membrane rupture without labor varies. Providers may opt to deliver the fetus within 24–48 hours, or allow the pregnancy to continue while administering antibiotics to the mother, or allow the pregnancy to continue with no intervention other than monitoring unless the mother develops signs of infection. In this case, the Group B streptococcus status is evaluated, and intrapartum antibiotics are administered as indicated. Labor induction may be initiated on a case-by-case basis (ACOG, 2016b).

SAFETY ALERT The highest-priority assessment following rupture of membranes is to check the fetal heart rate. As amniotic fluid is evacuated, the umbilical cord may become trapped between the fetal head and the maternal pelvis. The pressure on the umbilical cord slows or completely stops all blood flow to the fetus, which will be evidenced by a drop in FHR and ultimate fetal demise if not properly managed.

An additional potential issue during this phase is prolapse of the umbilical cord, which may occur when membranes rupture and the fetal presenting part is not well applied to the cervix. The concern is that the amniotic fluid coming through the cervix will propel the umbilical cord through the cervix (prolapsed cord). The FHR is auscultated because a drop in FHR might indicate an undetected prolapsed cord. Immediate intervention is necessary to remove pressure on a prolapsed umbilical cord.

» Visit *Pearson MyLab Nursing and eText* for Chart 8: Deviations from Normal Labor Process Requiring Immediate Intervention.

TRANSITION PHASE During transition, the contraction frequency may be every 1.5–2 minutes, duration is 60–90 seconds, and intensity is strong. Cervical dilation increases from 8 to 10 cm, effacement is complete (100%), and a heavy amount of bloody show is usually present. Contractions are palpated at least every 30 minutes. Sterile vaginal examinations may be done more frequently because this stage of labor usually is accompanied by rapid change. The FHR is auscultated every 30 minutes for low-risk women and every 15 minutes for high-risk women; maternal blood pressure, pulse, and respirations are monitored when the FHR is assessed or according to unit policy. Note that women may receive more frequent assessments based on individualized needs. The woman's pain level is monitored continuously.

Comfort measures become very important in this phase of labor, but continual assessment is required to ensure appropriate intervention. Women may also shake uncontrollably, feel nausea, or vomit during this stage. The woman may rapidly change from wanting a back rub and other hands-on care to wanting to be left completely alone. The support person and the nurse need to follow the woman's cues and change interventions as needed. Because the woman is breathing more rapidly, the nurse can increase the woman's comfort by offering small spoons of ice chips to moisten her mouth or applying an emollient to dry lips. The nurse can encourage the woman to rest between contractions. If analgesics have been administered, a quiet environment enhances the quality of rest between contractions.

Some women have difficulty coping during this time and need help with their breathing. Either the support person or the nurse can breathe along with the woman during each contraction to help her maintain her pattern. A gentle reminder to "slow down your breathing" can help to prevent hyperventilation. It is helpful to encourage the woman and to assure her that she is doing a good job. The woman will begin to feel increased rectal pressure as the fetal presenting part moves down the birth canal. The nurse encourages the woman to refrain from pushing until the cervix is completely dilated. To help the woman avoid involuntary pushing during contractions, the nurse can encourage pant–blow breathing, suggesting that the woman "pant like a puppy" or "blow in short breaths as if you were blowing out a candle." This measure helps prevent cervical edema.

The end of the transition phase and the beginning of the second stage may be indicated by a change in the woman's voice or the sounds that she is making. As the fetus moves down and the woman feels increased pressure and a bearing-down sensation, her voice tends to deepen. If she moans during a contraction, it takes on a more guttural quality. Experienced nurses recognize this sound as a sign of changes in the woman.

PROMOTION OF COMFORT　The nurse identifies factors that may contribute to discomfort for the laboring woman. These factors include uncomfortable positions or infrequent position changes, diaphoresis, continual leaking of amniotic fluid, a full bladder, a dry mouth, anxiety, and fear. The nurse and patient together plan interventions to minimize the effects of these factors.

Women in labor have many types of responses to pain. As the intensity of the contractions increases with the progress of labor, the woman becomes less aware of the environment and may have difficulty hearing and understanding verbal instructions. Some women may become irritable during this time. The pattern of coping with labor contractions varies from the use of highly structured breathing techniques to turning inward. As stated previously, the woman's responses to pain may have a cultural basis. Low moaning that begins deep in the throat, rocking or swaying, counting, facial grimacing, and using loud vocalizations are all effective means of dealing with the discomfort of labor and birth. Some women feel that making sounds helps them cope and do the work of labor, whereas others make loud sounds only as they lose their perception of control.

The most frequent physiologic manifestations of pain are increased pulse and respiratory rates, dilated pupils, increased blood pressure, and muscle tension. During labor, these reactions are transitory because the pain is intermittent. Increased muscle tension is most significant because it may impede the labor process. Women in labor frequently tighten skeletal muscles voluntarily during a contraction and remain motionless. This method of dealing with the contractions may actually increase her discomfort, but the woman may believe it is the only acceptable way to cope with the pain.

A woman generally wants touching, massage, and other forms of physical contact during the first part of labor, but when she moves into the transition phase, she may pull away. Alternatively, the woman may beseech her partner or the nurse to hold her hand or rub her back, or she may even reach out and grasp the support person. Some women are uncomfortable with being touched at all, regardless of the phase of labor; others do not welcome touch from a nonfamily member. It is important to validate the unique strengths and coping techniques of the individual and to meet each family on their own terms, always keeping in mind that this is their experience. Cultural influences can also affect how a woman will react to support and touch in labor. The nurse

takes cues from the woman and makes adjustments in her care to meet the patient's specific needs.

- ***General comfort.*** General comfort measures are of great importance during labor. By relieving minor discomforts, the nurse helps the woman optimize her coping abilities to deal with pain. The woman is encouraged to ambulate as long as there are no contraindications, such as vaginal bleeding or rupture of membranes before the fetus is engaged in the pelvis. Ambulation can increase comfort and aid in fetal descent. Even if the woman prefers not to walk around, upright positions, such as sitting in a rocker or leaning against a wall or bed, can enhance comfort. If the woman stays in bed, the nurse can encourage her to assume positions that she finds comfortable.

If the woman is more comfortable on her back, the nurse should elevate the head of the bed to relieve the pressure of the uterus on the vena cava. Pillows may be placed under each arm and under the knees to provide support. Because a pregnant woman is at increased risk for thrombophlebitis, it is important to avoid excessive pressure behind the knee and calf. The nurse needs to assess pressure points often. Frequent changes of position contribute to comfort and relaxation. The hands-and-knees posture may be used to relieve persistent back pain during labor.

Wearing socks or slippers may alleviate cold feet, and adjusting the room's thermostat can offset excessive warmth. Attention to such details allows the woman to focus on the more important issues of giving birth. The woman may be offered a warmed or cooled facial cloth, which is placed on her forehead or across or behind her neck. Providing a toothbrush and toothpaste for oral care can also increase comfort.

Diaphoresis and the constant leaking of amniotic fluid can dampen the woman's gown and bed linen. Offering fresh, smooth, dry bed linen promotes comfort. To avoid having to change the bottom sheet following rupture of the membranes, the nurse may replace absorbent underpads at frequent intervals (following standard precautions). To promote comfort and prevent infection, keep the perineal area as clean and dry as possible. A full bladder adds to discomfort during a contraction and may prolong labor by interfering with the descent of the fetus. The bladder should be kept as empty as possible. Even if the woman is voiding, urine may be retained because of the pressure from the fetal presenting part. The nurse can detect a full bladder by palpating directly over the symphysis pubis. Encourage the woman to empty her bladder every 1–2 hours. Some of the regional procedures for analgesia and anesthesia during labor contribute to the inability to void, and catheterization may be necessary.

The support person and any family members in attendance also need to be encouraged to maintain their own comfort. Because their attention is directed toward the laboring woman, they may forget their own needs. The nurse may have to encourage them to take breaks, to maintain food and fluid intake, and to rest. Many support persons and family members are reluctant to leave the woman unattended while they meet their own personal needs. Offer to stay with the woman during their absence. This provides reassurance to the support person or family member that the woman will be well cared for in his or her absence.

■ *Handling anxiety.* The anxiety experienced by women beginning labor is related to a combination of factors inherent to the process. A moderate amount of anxiety about pain enhances the woman's ability to deal with it. However, an excessive degree of anxiety decreases her ability to cope with the pain. Women in the latent phase of labor who are experiencing increased levels of anxiety about their ability to cope and their own personal safety are much more likely to describe their pain as unbearable. Women at risk for greater anxiety during labor include those who are young, poor, and lacking in social support. Women with preexisting mental illness, such as depression and anxiety, are at a greater risk for developing posttraumatic stress disorder related to their labor and birth experience (Modarres et al., 2012). Women with mental illness issues may need additional support to assist them with identifying effective coping mechanisms during the labor and birth process.

Ways to decrease anxiety not related to pain are to give information, which eases fear of the unknown; to establish rapport with the couple, which helps them preserve their personal integrity; and to express confidence in the couple's ability to work with the labor process. In addition to being a good listener, the nurse must demonstrate genuine concern for the laboring woman. Remaining with the woman as much as possible conveys a caring attitude and dispels fears of abandonment. Praise for breathing, relaxation, and pushing efforts not only encourages repetition of the behavior but also decreases anxiety about the ability to cope with labor.

■ *Patient teaching.* Providing truthful information about the nature of the discomfort that will occur during labor is important. Stressing the intermittent nature and maximum duration of the contractions can be helpful. The woman can cope with pain better when she knows that a period of relief will follow. Describing the type of discomfort and specific sensations that will occur as labor progresses helps the woman recognize these sensations as normal and expected when she does experience them.

Advise the woman that although the strength and intensity of contractions are different for each woman, they may feel like a tightening sensation or a menstrual cramp initially. Over time, as the labor progresses, the contractions become more intense and more uncomfortable, with the uterus tightening and becoming very hard and with the pain radiating from the back around to the front. For some women, the pain takes their breath away, or they may feel anxiety and fear. As the contractions become more painful, they also occur closer together. The sensation of having to push occurs as the head progresses into the pelvis and feels like the woman has to have a bowel movement. Once the contraction goes away, this intense feeling of having to have a bowel movement usually lets up somewhat.

Descriptions of sensations are best accompanied by information on specific comfort measures. As previously noted, some women experience the urge to push during the transition phase, when the cervix is not fully dilated and effaced. This sensation can be controlled by pant–blow breathing (it is difficult to pant or blow and bear down at the same time); the nurse should provide instructions about this technique before it is required.

Thorough orientation and explanation of surroundings, procedures, and equipment being used also decrease anxiety, thereby reducing pain. Attachment to an electronic monitor may produce fear because the woman may associate equipment of this type with people who are critically ill. It may also limit the woman's ability to move about and comfort herself with position changes and ambulation. If continuous electronic fetal monitoring is needed, the nurse can explain the beeps, clicks, and other strange noises and give a simplified explanation of the monitor strip. The nurse emphasizes that use of the fetal monitor provides a way to assess the well-being of the fetus during the course of labor. If available, a less intrusive telemetry monitor may be applied so that the woman has more freedom to move about. In addition, the nurse can show the woman and her partner or support person how the monitor can help them identify the beginnings of contractions. The nurse should encourage the woman to begin her breathing technique at the onset of each contraction; this may help lessen her perception of pain.

Labor and childbirth may be a critical time for the woman with a history of childhood physical, emotional, and/or sexual abuse or rape. To develop a competent plan of care, all laboring women should be evaluated on admission for a history of childhood abuse or rape. Depending on their cultural background, women may need specific examples of abuse to determine whether they have had these types of experiences, because some behaviors that are considered to be abusive in our society may be thought of as normal patterns of behavior in other cultures. Women may or may not be able to address this issue with the nurse because sharing such personal information is difficult and may stir up painful memories. It is therefore especially important for the nurse to be alert for nonverbal cues, such as excessive unexplained anxiety, unrelenting pain, and/or intense fear during vaginal exams, and to be prepared to offer additional teaching to help offset the woman's anxiety.

■ *Supportive relaxation techniques.* Tense muscles increase resistance to the descent of the fetus and contribute to maternal fatigue. This fatigue increases pain perception and decreases the woman's ability to cope with the pain. Comfort measures, massage, techniques for decreasing anxiety, and patient teaching can contribute to relaxation. Adequate sleep and rest are also important. The laboring woman needs to be encouraged to use the period between contractions for rest and relaxation. A prolonged prodromal phase of labor (also known as false labor or Braxton Hicks contractions) may interfere with sleep. An aura of excitement naturally accompanies the onset of labor, making it difficult for the woman to sleep even though the contractions are mild and infrequent. The nurse may have to act as an advocate for the woman to limit the number of visitors, interruptions, and phone calls.

Distraction is another method of increasing relaxation and coping with discomfort. During early labor, conversation or activities such as watching television, light reading, or playing cards or other games can serve as distractions. One technique that is effective for relieving moderate pain is to have the woman concentrate on a pleasant experience she has had in the past. Other techniques include the use of a specific visual or mental focal point (e.g., a picture of a loved one), breathing techniques, counting or humming, or visualization.

Touch is another type of distraction. Although some women regard touching as an invasion of privacy or a threat to their independence, many want to touch and be touched during a painful experience. To determine whether the woman desires touch, the nurse can place a hand on the side of the bed within the woman's reach. The woman who needs touch will reach out for contact, and the nurse can follow through with this behavioral cue.

Back pain associated with labor may be relieved by firm pressure on the lower back or sacral area. To apply firm pressure, the nurse can place his or her hand or a rolled, warmed towel or blanket in the small of the woman's back or can instruct the woman's support person to do so.

In some instances, analgesics or regional anesthetic blocks may be used to enhance comfort and relaxation during labor. The nurse may also enhance the woman's relaxation by providing encouragement and support for her controlled breathing techniques.

- **Breathing techniques.** Breathing techniques may help the laboring woman. Used correctly, they raise the woman's pain threshold, permit relaxation, enhance her ability to cope with contractions, provide a sense of control, and allow the uterus to function more efficiently.

Various types of breathing techniques can be used in labor. Many women learn patterned-paced breathing during prenatal education classes. This type of controlled breathing often has three levels. The woman tends to begin with the first level and then proceed to the next when she feels the need. Regardless of the level of breathing used, a cleansing breath (involving only the chest) begins and ends each pattern. The cleansing breath consists of inhaling slowly through the nose until a sense of fullness in the lungs occurs, and then exhaling slowly through pursed lips. The first pattern may also be called slow, deep breathing or slow-paced breathing. During the breathing movements, only the chest moves. The woman inhales slowly through her nose, moves her chest up and out during the inhalation, and exhales through pursed lips. The breathing rate is 6–9 breaths per minute.

The second pattern may be called shallow or modified-paced breathing. The woman begins with a cleansing breath. At the end of the cleansing breath, she pushes out a short breath. She then inhales and exhales through the mouth at a rate of about four breaths every 5 seconds. This pattern can be altered into a more rapid rate that does not exceed 2–2.5 breaths every second.

The third pattern, introduced earlier, is called pant–blow or patterned-paced breathing. It is similar to modified-paced breathing except that the breathing is punctuated every few breaths by a forceful exhalation through pursed lips. A pattern of four breaths may be used to begin. All breaths are kept equal and rhythmic. As the contraction becomes more intense, the woman may adjust the pattern as needed to 3:1, 2:1, and finally 1:1.

Abdominal breathing is another technique that can be effective in labor. In abdominal breathing, the woman moves the abdominal wall outward as she inhales and inward as she exhales. This method tends to lift the abdominal wall off the contracting uterus and thus helps to provide pain relief. The breathing is deep and rhythmic and typically relaxing. As transition approaches, the woman using abdominal breathing may feel the urge to breathe more rapidly. The pant–blow pattern discussed earlier can be suggested to slow the breathing and help the woman avoid the urge to bear down.

- **Hyperventilation. Hyperventilation** is the result of an imbalance of oxygen and carbon dioxide (i.e., too much carbon dioxide is exhaled, and too much oxygen remains in the body). Hyperventilation may occur when a woman breathes very rapidly over a prolonged period. The signs and symptoms of hyperventilation are tingling or numbness in the tip of the nose, lips, fingers, or toes; dizziness; spots before the eyes; or spasms of the hands or feet (carpopedal spasms). If hyperventilation occurs, the nurse encourages the woman to slow her breathing rate and take shallow breaths. With instruction and encouragement, many women are able to change their breathing to correct the problem. Encouraging the woman to relax and counting out loud for her so that she can pace her breathing during contractions are also helpful actions. If the signs and symptoms continue or become more severe, the woman is treated for hyperventilation as appropriate. The nurse remains with the woman to reassure her, because hyperventilation can increase anxiety levels.

ROLE OF THE DOULA   Throughout the first stage of labor, the nurse assesses and supports the interaction between the woman and her partner. In the absence of a partner, or when the partner desires a less active role, it is becoming more common for women to employ a paid caregiver who has experience in caring for laboring women. This caregiver, often called a **doula**, has typically received special training and may even be certified. The doula's role is to enhance the laboring woman's comfort and decrease her anxiety. A doula can be a valuable advocate for the laboring woman and her family as well as an asset to the labor nurse. For example, the doula might support the woman by helping identify the beginning of each contraction and encouraging her as she breathes through it. A constant presence offering continued encouragement and support with each contraction throughout labor has immeasurable benefits.

Provide Nursing Care During the Second Stage of Labor

The second stage is reached when the cervix is completely dilated (10 cm [3.9 in.]). The uterine contractions continue as in the transition phase. Maternal pulse, blood pressure, and FHR are assessed every 5 minutes; some protocols recommend assessment after each contraction (Anderson & Stone, 2013). Once the second stage is reached, the nurse remains with the woman continually and generally does not leave the room. Nursing care during the second stage focuses on providing care, promoting comfort, and assisting during the birth.

As the woman pushes during the second stage, she may make a variety of sounds. A low-pitched, grunting sound ("uhhh") usually indicates that the woman is working with the pushing. The nurse who feels comfortable with maternal sounds and stays sensitive to changes in the sounds may be able to detect if the woman is losing her ability to cope. For instance, if the woman feels afraid of the sensations produced by her pushing effort, her sound may change to a high-pitched cry or whimper.

It is not uncommon for the woman to be afraid to push. In these situations, the woman may talk or cry out during the contraction instead of actively pushing. During this time, the nurse provides support, reassurance, and clear directions for the woman to follow. Often, it is helpful to direct the woman to concentrate on a single voice, listen for suggestions, and let her body do the work. Many women find this type of interaction comforting because it allows them to focus on one individual.

When teaching the effective technique for pushing, instruct the woman to bear down and push into her bottom as if she is having a bowel movement. Watch the woman's perineum and rectum while she is pushing, and give verbal praise and encouragement when change in the perineum or rectum is seen, indicating she is successfully pushing.

During the second stage, the woman may feel intense rectal pressure. The instinctive response is to resist and to tighten muscles rather than bear down (push). A sensation of "splitting apart" or burning also occurs in the latter part of the second stage when the woman is pushing. The woman who expects these sensations and who understands that bearing down contributes to progress at this stage is more likely to do so.

When the urge to bear down becomes uncontrollable and pushing begins, the nurse can help by encouraging the woman and by supporting her efforts. Most women push spontaneously and effectively in response to messages from their body. This more natural approach, which lets the mother wait to bear down until she feels an urge to push, may shorten the pushing phase, thereby reducing the incidence of physiologic stress in the mother and acidosis in the newborn. This technique also decreases the incidence of instrument births and damage to maternal perineal tissue (Ara et al., 2015). In some settings, however, sustained, forceful pushing may be useful. In that case, when the contraction begins, the nurse tells the woman to take a cleansing breath or two, then to take a third large breath and hold it while pushing down with her abdominal muscles (called the Valsalva maneuver).

A nullipara is usually prepared for birth when perineal bulging is noted. A multipara usually progresses much more. As the birth approaches, the woman's partner or support person also prepares.

The nurse monitors the woman's blood pressure and the FHR between contractions, and the nurse assesses the contractions at least every 5 minutes until the birth. The nurse continually assesses the woman's level of pain or her ability to cope with the discomfort of labor. The nurse continues to assist the woman in her pushing efforts to keep both the woman and the support person informed of procedures and progress and to support them both throughout the birth.

PROMOTION OF COMFORT Most of the comfort measures that were used during the first stage remain appropriate during the second stage. Applying cool cloths to the face and forehead may help to cool the woman involved in the intense physical exertion of pushing. The woman may feel hot and want to remove some of her clothing or bed linens. Care still needs to be taken to provide privacy even though covers are removed. The nurse encourages the woman to rest and relax all muscles during the periods between contractions. The nurse and support person can assist the woman into a pushing position with each contraction to further conserve energy. Between contractions, the woman should be assisted into a comfortable position. Sips of fluids or ice chips may be used to provide moisture and relieve dryness of the mouth. Positive reinforcement and encouragement should be continually provided.

For some women, but especially those with epidural anesthesia, the urge to push may not occur spontaneously. The question then becomes whether to encourage passive descent of the fetus versus active pushing (see Evidence-Based Practice: Passive Descent Versus Active Pushing in Women with Epidural Anesthesia).

ASSISTING DURING BIRTH In addition to assisting the woman and her partner, the nurse assists the healthcare provider in preparing for the birth. The provider dons a sterile gown and gloves and may place sterile drapes over the woman's abdomen and legs. An episiotomy may be performed just before the actual birth.

Shortly before the birth, the birthing room or delivery room is prepared with the equipment and materials that may be needed. These materials typically come in a prepackaged kit and contain the instruments and disposable drapes, gowns, and containers that will be used during the birth. The nurse ensures that all supplies and a pair of sterile gloves are placed on the instrument table. This table can be prepared before the birth and covered with a sterile drape. If the birth is to occur in a birthing room, family members do not need to change into other clothing; if the birth is to occur in a delivery room or surgery suite, they don a disposable scrub suit or scrubs provided by the facility. Thorough hand hygiene is required of the nurses and physician or CNM. Nurses who will be in direct contact with the mother at the time of birth need to wear protective clothing, such as an apron or gown with a splash apron, disposable gloves, and eye covering. The physician or CNM also needs to wear a plastic apron or a gown with a splash apron, eye covering, and sterile gloves.

SAFETY ALERT Some physicians and CNMs routinely use other equipment or supplies during the birth. Examples of such equipment include mineral oil, warm water, and clean washcloths for perineal massage. Gathering these supplies early can save time and enable the nurse to stay with the woman during pushing.

If for any reason the laboring woman is to give birth in a location other than the birthing room (e.g., in the case of a

Evidence-Based Practice

Passive Descent Versus Active Pushing in Women with Epidural Anesthesia

Problem

Which method of pushing—passive descent or active pushing as soon as full cervical dilation is achieved—provides the most benefit for mothers with epidural anesthesia?

Epidural analgesia is a common method of pain management during active labor, but one of its side effects is a decrease in a woman's lower body sensations. This may inhibit the natural urge to push upon full cervical dilation. Women have traditionally been directed to push immediately once cervical dilation reaches 10 cm, whether they felt the urge to push or not. The chief concern leading to this practice was that an extended second stage of labor was deleterious for both mother and baby, leading to acidosis, maternal exhaustion, and neonatal morbidity.

The natural second stage of labor includes a period of time in which the fetus descends, which the literature refers to as "passive descent." Passive descent allows the woman to delay pushing until she feels the urge to push or until the head is visible.

Evidence

Evidence to support the delay of bearing down for women without the urge to push has existed for decades. Immediate pushing does not reduce the incidence of acidosis or shorten the second stage of labor. Indeed, prolonged active pushing has been shown to increase the incidence of fetal and maternal acidosis, increase the

risk of having an instrument-assisted birth, and decrease the chance a woman would have a spontaneous vaginal birth. Immediate pushing often lengthens the second stage of labor as compared to allowing the fetus to descend via the primary power of uterine contractions (Osborne & Hanson, 2014).

Furthermore, passive descent has additional benefits in that it allows for further fetal descent and rotation, better situating the fetus in the woman's pelvis. It also causes further release of oxytocin that augments the progress of labor.

Implications

These findings suggest that the duration of active pushing should be limited, not the duration of the second stage of labor.

Critical Thinking Application

1. How can the nurse help the mother recognize the urge to push at an effective time when epidural analgesia is in place?

2. How does a rest period during pushing influence perinatal outcomes?

3. What risk factors are associated with active pushing during the second stage of labor?

4. What are the evidence-based nursing interventions related to the second stage of labor?

---

forceps-assisted birth where a quick transition to cesarean delivery may be necessary), she is moved on her bed or a cart shortly before birth. It is important that the woman move from one bed to another between contractions. During the contraction, the woman feels increased discomfort and may be involved in pushing efforts. Perineal bulging may be occurring, which adds to the discomfort and difficulty in moving. Take care to preserve her privacy during the transfer, and provide safety by raising the side rails. The bed itself should be placed in a locked position. The labor bed or transfer cart must be carefully braced against the delivery table to ensure the woman's safety during the transfer.

Even though the operating room setting is different from that of a birthing room, the family can still be together during the birth. It is important for nurses to provide encouragement for family members to participate, because the delivery room environment may be unfamiliar and seem intimidating. The family member may hesitate to continue providing support because of fear of interfering or being in the way. The nurse provides clear, simple directions that help the support person participate throughout the birth process. The nurse can ensure the support person is sitting as close as possible to the woman. The nurse can also encourage hand holding and touching or stroking of the woman's face.

■ ***Maternal birthing positions.*** The upright posture for birth was considered to be normal in most societies until modern times. Women variously selected squatting, kneeling, standing, and sitting positions for birth. During the mid-20th century, the recumbent position (lithotomy

position) became common in North American hospitals because of the convenience it offered when applying new technology. In recent years, however, consumers and healthcare professionals have begun searching for alternative positions, refocusing on the comfort of the laboring woman rather than on the convenience of the physician or CNM.

❯❯ See **Pearson MyLab Nursing and eText** for Chart 9: Comparison of Birthing Positions.

Evidence-based practice research has shown that the squatting position results in fewer instrumental deliveries, fewer episiotomy extensions, and fewer perineal tears compared to the lithotomy position (Ara et al., 2015). An upright position, which has been found to be the most effective birthing position, is possible even for women who have epidural anesthesia.

The woman may be positioned for birth on a bed with use of leg supports in a squatting position, or perhaps on her hands and knees. If a birthing bed is used, the back is elevated 30–60 degrees to help the woman bear down. Stirrups, if needed and used, are padded to alleviate pressure. If the nurse is assisting the woman to place her legs in the stirrups, both the woman's legs should be lifted simultaneously to avoid strain on the abdominal, back, and perineal muscles. Stirrups are sometimes needed if the woman is unable to control her legs following epidural anesthesia, if forceps or a vacuum extractor is being used, or if a difficult birth is anticipated. The nurse should adjust the stirrups to fit the woman's legs. The feet are supported in the stirrup holders. The height and angle of the stirrups are adjusted so there is no pressure on the back of the knees or the calves, which might cause discomfort and postpartum vascular problems. Some practitioners may opt to leave the bed assembled and, instead, lower the foot of the bed into a lower position. Many times, women are more comfortable in this position. When stirrups are not used for the birth, the woman's legs may be placed in stirrups after the birth if a repair of the perineum is needed.

- **Cleansing the perineum.** After the mother has been positioned for the birth, her vulvar and perineal area are cleansed to increase her comfort, to remove the bloody discharge that is present before the actual birth, and to prevent infection. Perineal cleansing methods range from use of warm, soapy water to aseptic technique depending on the agency protocol or on physician or CNM orders. Once the cleansing has been completed, the woman returns to the desired birthing position.

- **Supporting the couple.** Both the woman's partner or support person and the nurse who has been with the woman during the labor continue to provide support during contractions. They encourage the woman to push with each contraction, and as the fetal head emerges, ask her to take shallow breaths or to pant to prevent pushing. The physician or CNM may instruct the woman to "push and breathe, push and breathe" in an effort to ease the fetal head out to prevent perineal trauma and tearing. While supporting the head, the physician or CNM assesses whether the umbilical cord is around the fetal neck and removes it if it is, then suctions the mouth and nose with a bulb syringe if there are any obvious obstructions to spontaneous breathing. The mouth is suctioned first to prevent reflex inhalation of mucus when the sensitive nares are touched with the bulb syringe tip. The woman is encouraged to push again as the rest of the newborn's body is born.

Provide Nursing Care During the Third Stage of Labor

Nursing care during the third stage of labor focuses on initial care of the newborn, enhancing attachment, assisting with delivery of the placenta, and providing care for the mother. Newborn care is discussed in Exemplar 33.D; this section discusses maternal care.

DELIVERY OF THE PLACENTA   After birth, the healthcare provider prepares for the delivery of the placenta. The following signs suggest placental separation:

- The uterus rises upward in the abdomen.
- As the placenta moves downward, the umbilical cord lengthens.
- A sudden trickle or spurt of blood appears.
- The shape of the uterus changes from a disk to a globe.

While waiting for these signs, the nurse palpates the uterus to check for bogginess (soft or mushy feeling) and fullness caused by uterine relaxation and subsequent bleeding into the uterine cavity. After the placenta has separated, the woman may be asked to bear down to aid delivery of the placenta.

Oxytocics are frequently given at the time of the delivery of the placenta so that the uterus will contract and bleeding will be minimized. Oxytocin (Pitocin), 20 units, may be added to an intravenous infusion, or 10 units may be given intramuscularly. In the presence of hemorrhage caused by uterine atony, some healthcare providers may order up to 40 units of oxytocin in a liter of intravenous fluid; methylergonovine maleate (Methergine), 0.2 mg, administered intramuscularly; or carboprost tromethamine (Hemabate), 250 mcg/mL, administered intramuscularly. Cytotec has been commonly used when other pharmacologic interventions have failed. Cytotec is administered rectally in dosages of 800–1000 mcg (Hofmeyr, Gülmezoglu, & Pileggi, 2013). In addition to administering the ordered medications, the nurse assesses and records maternal blood pressure before and after administration of oxytocics and assesses the amount of bleeding.

After delivery of the placenta, the healthcare provider inspects the placenta and membranes to make sure they are intact and that all cotyledons are present. If there is a defect or a part missing from the placenta, a manual uterine examination or uterine exploration is done. The nurse notes on the birth record the time of delivery of the placenta.

Cord Blood Analysis at Birth

When significant abnormal FHR patterns have been noted, meconium-stained amniotic fluid is present, or the newborn is depressed at birth, umbilical cord blood may be analyzed immediately following the birth to determine whether acidosis is present. ACOG (2012a) recommends performing cord blood analyses when the Apgar score is below 7 at 5 minutes of age (normal Apgar score is 7–10) (see Exemplar 33.D for an in-depth discussion of the Apgar scoring system).

The cord is clamped before the neonate takes the first breath. Using a Kelly clamp, the healthcare provider clamps a 20- to 25-cm (8- to 10-in.) portion of the umbilical cord. A small amount of blood (1.0 mL is required for a full panel) is aspirated with a syringe from one of the umbilical arteries or from an artery and a vein. If the cord blood will not be analyzed immediately, a heparinized syringe should be used. Normal fetal blood pH is above 7.25 (ACOG, 2012b). Lower levels indicate acidosis and hypoxia. Many healthcare providers order cord blood analysis to minimize medicolegal exposure.

Provide Nursing Care During the Fourth Stage of Labor

The healthcare provider inspects the vagina, cervix, and perineum for lacerations and makes any necessary repairs. The episiotomy or laceration may be repaired now if it was not done previously.

The nurse assesses the uterus for firmness by palpating the fundus. The normal position is at the midline and below the umbilicus. A displaced fundus may be caused by a full bladder or by blood collected in the uterus. The clots or blood accumulation in the uterus may be expelled by grasping the uterus transabdominally with one hand anteriorly and posteriorly and then squeezing. The nurse continues to palpate the uterine fundus at frequent intervals for at least 4 hours to ensure that it remains firmly contracted (**Figure 33–56 》**), but it is not massaged unless it is soft (boggy). If the uterine fundus becomes soft (uterine atony) or

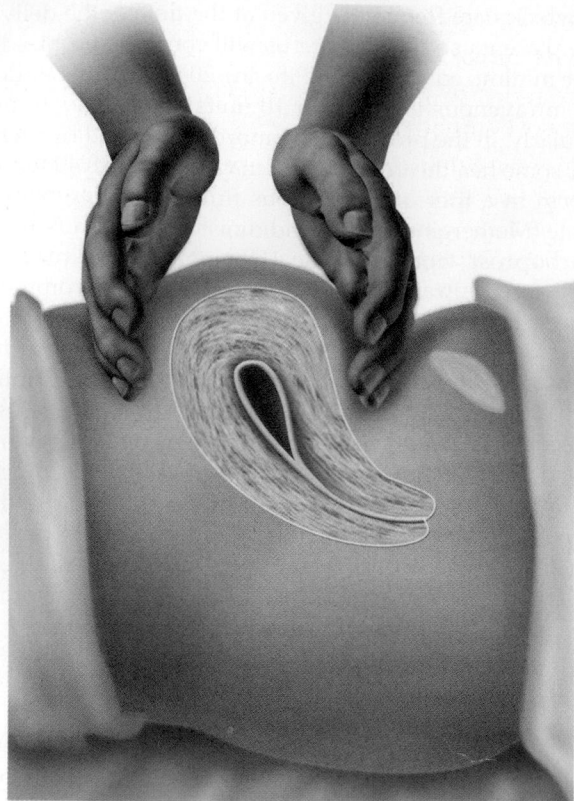

Figure 33–56 » Suggested method of palpating the fundus of the uterus during the fourth stage. The left hand is placed just above the symphysis pubis, and gentle downward pressure is exerted. The right hand is cupped around the uterine fundus.

appears to rise in the abdomen, the nurse massages it until firm; then, the nurse exerts firm pressure on the fundus in an attempt to express retained clots. During all aspects of fundal massage, the nurse uses one hand to provide support for the lower portion of the uterus and prevent damage to the round ligaments and uterine eversion. The uterus is very tender at this time; all palpation and massage should be performed as gently as possible.

The nurse washes the woman's perineum with gauze squares and warmed solution and then dries the area well with a towel before placing the sanitary pad. Many times, an ice pack is also placed against the perineum to promote comfort and decrease swelling. If stirrups have been used, the woman's legs are removed from the stirrups at the same time to avoid muscle strain. The woman is encouraged to move her legs gently up and down in a bicycle motion. The woman remains in the same bed or is transferred to a recovery room bed, and the nurse helps her don a clean gown. Soiled linens are removed, and the woman is typically offered something to drink.

During the recovery period (1–4 hours) the nurse monitors the woman closely. The perineum is inspected for edema and hematoma formation, and frequent checking of vital signs for deviations from normal is required. The maternal blood pressure is monitored at 5- to 15-minute intervals to detect any changes. Blood pressure should return to the prelabor level because an increased volume of blood is returning to the maternal circulation from the uteroplacental shunt. Pulse rate

should be slightly lower than it was during labor. Baroreceptors cause a vagal response, which slows the pulse. A rise in blood pressure may be a response to oxytocic drugs or may be caused by preeclampsia. Blood loss may be reflected by a lowered blood pressure and a rising pulse rate (**Table 33–15** »).

The nurse also monitors the woman's temperature. Frequently, women have tremors or uncontrollable shaking in the immediate postpartum period that may be caused by a difference in internal and external body temperatures (higher temperature inside the body than outside). Another theory is that the woman is reacting to the fetal cells that have entered the maternal circulation at the placental site. The nurse may place a heated blanket next to the woman's skin to alleviate the problem; this can be replaced as often as the mother desires.

The nurse assesses the mother's pain level. If the woman is experiencing any type of discomfort, pain medications can be administered as ordered. The nurse also assists with comfort measures, such as position changes, frequent ice pack changes, and administration of topical medications that are often ordered to reduce perineal edema and discomfort.

The nurse inspects the bloody vaginal discharge for amount and charts it as minimal, moderate, or heavy and as with or without clots. This discharge (lochia rubra) should be bright red. A soaked perineal pad contains approximately 100 mL of blood. If the perineal pad becomes soaked in a 15-minute period or if blood pools under the buttocks, continuous observation is necessary. When the fundus is firm, a continuous trickle of blood may signal laceration of the vagina or cervix or an unligated vessel in the episiotomy.

If the fundus rises and displaces to the right, the nurse must be concerned about two factors:

1. As the uterus rises, the uterine contractions become less effective and increased bleeding may occur.
2. The most common cause of uterine displacement is bladder distention.

The nurse palpates the bladder to determine whether it is distended. The bladder fills rapidly with the extra fluid

TABLE 33–15 Maternal Adaptations Following Birth

Characteristic	Normal Finding
Blood pressure	Returns to prelabor level
Pulse	Slightly lower than in labor
Uterine fundus	In the midline at the umbilicus, or 1–2 fingerbreadths below the umbilicus
Lochia	Red (rubra), small to moderate amount (from spotting on pads to 1/4–1/2 of pad covered in 15 minutes); does not exceed saturation of one pad in first hour
Bladder	Nonpalpable
Perineum	Without hematomas or open lacerations. Mild to moderate bruising and/or edema is common.
Appetite/Thirst	Variations possible. Increased hunger is typical due to the high level of energy expenditure during the labor and birth process. Increased thirst is due to loss of fluids (blood, sweat, urine) and fluid shifts associated with birth process.
Emotional state	Wide variation, including excited, exhilarated, smiling, crying, fatigued, verbal, quiet, pensive, and sleepy

volume returned from the uteroplacental circulation (and with any fluid received intravenously during labor and birth). The postpartum woman may not realize that her bladder is full, because trauma to the bladder and urethra during childbirth and the use of regional anesthesia decrease bladder tone and the urge to void.

All measures should be taken to enable the mother to void. The nurse may place a warm towel across the lower abdomen or pour warm water over the perineum to relax the urinary sphincter and facilitate voiding. The woman may also try running warm water over her hand. If the woman is unable to void, catheterization is necessary.

SAFETY ALERT In the immediate postbirth recovery period, report the following conditions to the healthcare provider:

- Hypotension
- Tachycardia
- Uterine atony
- Excessive bleeding
- Hematoma.

The woman and her partner or support person may be tired, hungry, and thirsty. Some agencies serve them a meal. Most women are very hungry after birth. The tired mother will probably drift off into a welcome sleep. The partner can also be encouraged to rest, because the supporting role is physically and mentally tiring. If the mother is not in a birthing room, she is usually transferred from the birthing unit to the postpartum or mother–baby area after 1 hour or more, depending on agency policy and whether the following criteria are met:

- Stable vital signs
- Stable bleeding

- Undistended bladder
- Firm fundus
- Sensations fully recovered from any anesthetic agent received during birth.

For some women, the childbirth experience has been extremely painful, filled with hours of feeling powerless or out of control. In this circumstance, the woman is at higher risk for developing posttraumatic stress disorder (Harris & Ayers, 2012).

Evaluation

Evaluation provides an opportunity to determine the effectiveness of nursing care. As a result of comprehensive nursing care during the intrapartum period, the following outcomes may be anticipated:

- The mother's physical and psychologic well-being has been maintained and supported.
- The baby's physical and psychologic well-being has been protected and supported.
- The mother and her family members have had input into the birth process and have participated as much as they desired.
- The mother and her baby have had a safe birth.

An additional purpose of care evaluation is to determine if further care is needed based on maternal or neonatal outcomes. If the outcomes are not being met, the nurse may choose to continue or revise the plan of care for optimal outcome attainment. For example, if the mother's or newborn's physical well-being is compromised, transferring them to a more intensive care setting such as an ICU or NICU may be warranted. Likewise, if the mother's psychologic well-being is compromised, a psychologic consult may be needed and safety measures initiated.

Nursing Care Plan
A Patient Requiring Induction of Labor

Lakshmi Pandey is being admitted to labor and childbirth this morning for an induction. She is accompanied by her husband, Nitya. Mrs. Pandey is a primigravida at 42 weeks of gestation. She has been experiencing Braxton Hicks contractions during the past week, but a contraction pattern has not been established. Mrs. Pandey's membranes are intact, and her vital signs are within normal limits. Her cervix is soft and pliable, 80% effaced, and 3 cm dilated. Fetal station is –1. The nurse places an external fetal monitor to obtain a baseline fetal heart rate pattern and evaluate uterine activity.

ASSESSMENT	DIAGNOSES	PLANNING
Subjective: Braxton Hicks contractions, restlessness, backache, apprehension. Pain level reported as 5 out of 10. Objective: Cervix is 3 cm dilated, 80% effaced; –1 station; amniotic membranes are intact. BP 120/84 mmHg, temperature 37.1°C (98.8°F), pulse 94 beats/min, respirations 14/min, FHR 144 with average variability.	■ *Risk for Injury* related to tachysystole of uterus caused by induction of labor ■ *Anxiety* related to discomfort of labor and unknown labor outcome (NANDA-I © 2014)	■ The patient will progress through the stages of labor without difficulty or complications. ■ The patient will have contractions every 2–3 minutes, with duration of 40–60 seconds, and moderate intensity. ■ The patient's labor will progress with cervical dilation, effacement, and fetal descent. ■ The patient's resting tone will return to baseline between contractions. ■ The patient's vital signs will remain within normal limits.

(continued on next page)

Nursing Care Plan (continued)

IMPLEMENTATION

- Obtain a baseline for maternal blood pressure, pulse, respirations, temperature, and pain level.
- Confirm medical, surgical, obstetric, and prenatal history; confirm any allergies with patient.
- Place patient on external fetal monitor for 20 minutes to obtain a baseline for FHR, variability, and periodic changes (accelerations or decelerations).
- Insert intravenous line, and begin primary infusion with 1000 mL of electrolyte solution.
- Piggyback oxytocin solution into primary intravenous tubing, via pump, in the port closest to the intravenous insertion site.
- Monitor infusion pump and connections.
- Monitor and evaluate maternal blood pressure and pulse before each increase in the oxytocin infusion rate.

- Evaluate urine output.
- Evaluate and document FHR before each increase in the oxytocin infusion rate.
- Evaluate and document contraction pattern before each increase of the oxytocin infusion rate.
- Increase the oxytocin infusion dosage until adequate contractions are achieved or the maximum dose per agency protocol is reached.
- Evaluate contraction frequency, duration, and intensity before increasing the infusion rate. Discontinue the oxytocin infusion and infuse primary solution if signs of tachysystole of the uterus are detected.
- Initiate treatment measures to reverse the effects of the oxytocin infusion if fetal tachycardia or bradycardia occurs.

EVALUATION

- Contractions increased in frequency, duration, and intensity.
- Increase in cervical dilation, effacement, and intensity was achieved.

- Uterus remained soft between contractions.

CRITICAL THINKING

1. Mrs. Pandey has been receiving an oxytocin infusion for the past 4 hours and is currently receiving 6 milliunits/min. Your assessment of Mrs. Pandey's contractions includes frequency every 3 minutes, lasting 60 seconds, with moderate intensity. FHR ranges from 140 to 155 beats/min with average variability. Her cervix is now 6 cm (2.4 in.) dilated, 100% effaced, anterior, and the station is 0. Will you continue to monitor at the same infusion rate, increase the rate, or decrease the rate?

2. While monitoring a woman with an oxytocin infusion, you assess that the woman's contractions are now every 2 minutes and that the FHR has dropped to 100 beats/min with a decrease in variability. Several late decelerations are also assessed. What is your initial nursing action?

REVIEW Intrapartum Care

RELATE Link the Concepts and Exemplars

Linking the exemplar of intrapartum care with the concept of comfort:

You are caring for a mother in the transition stage of labor when she begins crying and says, "It hurts so much. I don't know if I can take this anymore." As you were admitting her, when contractions were less frequent and intense, the woman told you it was very important to her that she deliver the baby without taking any pain medication and that she would feel like a failure if she gave in and took a narcotic.

1. Will you offer her a narcotic analgesic to reduce her discomfort? Explain your answer.

2. What nonpharmacologic strategies can you implement to help her manage her pain?

Linking the exemplar of intrapartum care with the concept of culture and diversity:

3. When admitting a patient to the labor unit, what cultural assessment will you perform?

4. The woman tells you a cultural belief in her family is that a candle must be burning when the baby is born, because they believe the

baby will move toward the light, thereby making labor easier and the baby will be born faster. How will you respond to this request?

READY Go to Volume 3: Clinical Nursing Skills

REFER Go to Pearson MyLab Nursing and eText

- Additional review materials
- Chart 6: Intrapartum High-Risk Factors
- Chart 7: Psychologic Characteristics and Nursing Support During the First and Second Stages of Labor
- Chart 8: Deviations from Normal Labor Process Requiring Immediate Intervention
- Chart 9: Comparison of Birthing Positions

REFLECT Apply Your Knowledge

It's a busy night, and you admit two patients, one right after the other. The first patient is a 24-year-old single woman in labor with her first pregnancy. Her contractions are 8 minutes apart, she is dilated 2 cm (0.8 in.), and is at the +3 station. She tells you the pain is almost more than she can stand during contractions and asks how soon the physician can start the epidural. The second patient is 28 years old and in labor with her fourth child. Her contractions are also 8 minutes apart, and she is dilated to 2 cm (0.8 in.) and at the +2 station. She is laughing and joking with her partner between contractions and asks if it would be okay if they play cards while they wait for labor to progress.

1. What factors may be influencing the different responses of these women to the pain of labor?
2. How would your nursing care differ for these women?
3. Which woman do you anticipate is likely to deliver first? Explain your answer.

» Exemplar 33.C Postpartum Care

Exemplar Learning Outcomes

33.C Summarize postpartum care of the mother.

- Summarize physical adaptations of the body systems postpartum.
- Describe the psychologic adaptations of the mother postpartum.
- Outline the nutrition requirements for new mothers.
- Summarize alterations in the postpartum period.
- Differentiate considerations related to the assessment and care of pregnant adolescents and women over 35.
- Illustrate the nursing process in providing culturally competent care to the new mother and her family.

Exemplar Key Terms

Afterpains, *2330*
Colostrum, *2332*

Overview

During the **puerperium**, or postpartum period, the woman readjusts, both physically and psychologically, from pregnancy and birth. The period begins immediately after birth and continues for approximately 6 weeks, or until the body has returned to a near prepregnant state.

Physical Adaptations

The physiologic changes of pregnancy are numerous and take place over several months. Likewise, after delivery, the woman's body goes through many changes as it begins to return to a nonpregnant state.

Reproductive System

Specific changes to the woman's reproductive system include involution of the uterus, discharge of lochia, cervical, vaginal, and perineal changes, the return of ovulation and menstruation, abdominal changes, and lactogenesis and breast changes. In addition, changes to the gastrointestinal, urinary, cardiovascular, neurologic, and immunologic systems occur.

Involution

The term **involution** describes the rapid reduction in size of the uterus and the return of the uterus to a nonpregnant state. Following separation of the placenta, the decidua of the uterus is irregular, jagged, and varied in thickness. The spongy layer of the decidua is cast off as lochia (uterine discharge of the debris remaining after birth), and the basal layer of the decidua remains in the uterus to become differentiated into two layers. This occurs within the first 48–72 hours after birth. The outermost layer becomes necrotic and is sloughed off in the lochia. The layer closest to the myometrium contains the fundi of the uterine endometrial glands. These glands lay the foundation for the new endometrium. Except at the placenta site, this process is completed in approximately 3 weeks. Healing at the placenta site occurs gradually over 6 weeks, at which point the site is completely healed (Cunningham et al., 2014). Bleeding from the larger uterine vessels of the placenta site is controlled by compression of the contracted uterine muscle fibers. The clotted blood is gradually absorbed by the body. Some of these uterine vessels are eventually obliterated and replaced by new vessels with smaller lumens.

The placenta site heals by a process of exfoliation and growth of endometrial tissue. This occurs with upward endometrial growth in the decidua basalis under the placenta site, with simultaneous growth of endometrial tissue from the margins of the site. The infarcted superficial tissue then becomes necrotic and is sloughed off (Blackburn, 2013). Exfoliation is a very important aspect of involution; if healing of the placenta site leaves a fibrous scar, the area available for future implantation is limited, as is the number of possible pregnancies.

With the dramatic decrease in the levels of circulating estrogen and progesterone following placental separation, the uterine cells atrophy, and the hyperplasia of pregnancy begins to reverse. Proteolytic enzymes are released, and macrophages migrate to the uterus to promote autolysis (self-digestion), which breaks down and absorbs protein material in the uterine wall. Factors that enhance involution include an uncomplicated labor and birth, complete expulsion of the placenta and membranes, breastfeeding, manual removal of the placenta during a cesarean birth, and early ambulation.

>> Go to **Pearson MyLab Nursing and eText** for Chart 10: Factors That Slow Uterine Involution.

The **fundus** (top portion of the uterus) is situated in the midline and is palpable below the umbilicus (**Figure 33–57 >>**). Following expulsion of the placenta, the uterus contracts to the size of a large grapefruit. The uterine blood vessels are firmly compressed by the myometrium. Blood and clots that remain within the uterus and changes in support of the uterus by the ligaments cause the fundus of the uterus to rise to the level of the umbilicus within 6–12 hours after birth.

A fundus that is above the umbilicus and is boggy (feels soft and spongy rather than firm and well contracted) is associated with excessive uterine bleeding. As blood collects and forms clots within the uterus, the fundus rises, interrupting firm contractions of the uterus and exacerbates **uterine atony** (relaxation of uterine muscle tone).

When the fundus is higher than expected on palpation and is not in the midline (usually deviated to the right), distention of the bladder should be suspected; the bladder should be emptied immediately and the uterus reassessed. If the woman is unable to void, in-and-out catheterization of the bladder may be required. In the immediate postpartum period, many women may not be aware of a full bladder. Because the uterine ligaments are still stretched, a full bladder can move the uterus. By the end of the puerperium, these ligaments regain their nonpregnant length and tension.

After birth, the top of the fundus remains at the level of the umbilicus for about half a day. On the first day postpartum, the top of the fundus is located about 1 cm (0.4 in.) below the umbilicus. The top of the fundus descends approximately one fingerbreadth (width of the index, second, or third finger), or 1 cm (0.4 in.), per day until it descends into the pelvis on about the 10th day.

If the mother is breastfeeding, the release of endogenous oxytocin from the posterior pituitary in response to suckling hastens involution of the uterus. Barring complications, such as infection or retained placental fragments, the uterus approaches its prepregnant size and location by 5–6 weeks. In women who had an oversized uterus during the pregnancy (because of hydramnios, birth of a large-for-gestational-age baby, or multiple gestation), the time frame for an immediate uterine involution process is lengthened. If intrauterine infection is present, foul-smelling lochia or vaginal discharge results. The infection irritates the uterine muscle, causing the fundus to descend much more slowly. When infection is suspected, other clinical signs, such as fever and tachycardia, and fundal tenderness must be assessed. Any slowing of descent is called **subinvolution**.

Afterpains (cramplike pains caused by intermittent contractions of the uterus that occur after childbirth) are often more severe in multiparas than in primiparas. These afterpains may cause the mother severe discomfort for 2–3 days after birth. The administration of uterotonic agents (intravenous infusion with oxytocin or oral administration of methylergonovine maleate) stimulates uterine contraction and increases the discomfort of the afterpains. A warm water bottle placed against the lower abdomen may reduce this discomfort. In addition, the breastfeeding mother may find it helpful to take a mild analgesic agent approximately 1 hour before feeding her baby. The nurse can assure the mother who is breastfeeding that the prescribed analgesics are not harmful to the newborn and help improve the quality of the breastfeeding experience. If afterpains are interfering with the mother's rest, she may find it helpful to take an analgesic at bedtime.

Lochia

The uterus rids itself of the debris remaining after birth through a discharge called **lochia**, which is classified according to its appearance and contents. These classifications are lochia rubra, lochia serosa, and lochia alba.

Lochia rubra is dark red. It occurs for the first 2–3 days and contains epithelial cells, erythrocytes, leukocytes, shreds of decidua, and occasionally fetal meconium, lanugo, and vernix. Clotting is often the result of blood pooling in the upper portion of the vagina. A few small clots (no larger than a nickel) are common, particularly in the first few days after birth. However, lochia should not contain large (plumsize) clots; if it does, the cause should be investigated without delay.

Lochia serosa is a pinkish color. It follows from approximately day 3 until day 10. Lochia serosa is composed of

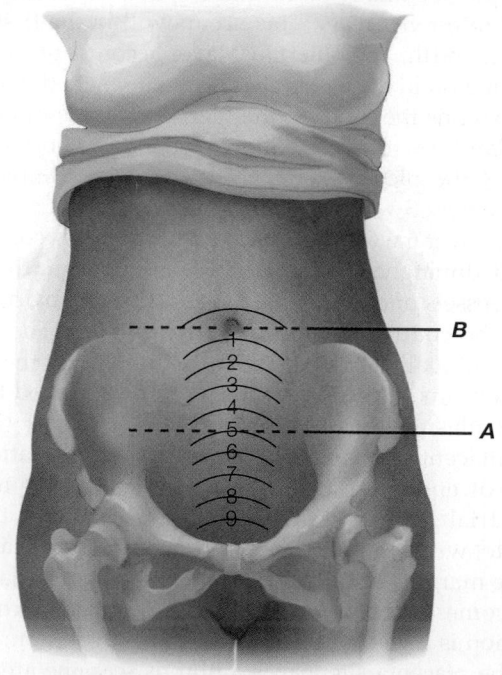

Figure 33–57 >> Involution of the uterus. **A,** Immediately after delivery of the placenta, the top of the fundus is in the midline and approximately halfway between the symphysis pubis and the umbilicus. Approximately 6–12 hours after birth, the fundus is at the level of the umbilicus. **B,** The height of the fundus then decreases about one fingerbreadth (~1 cm) each day.

serous exudate, shreds of degenerating decidua, erythrocytes, leukocytes, cervical mucus, and numerous microorganisms (Blackburn, 2013).

The red blood cell component decreases gradually, and a creamy or yellowish discharge persists for an additional week or two. This final discharge, termed **lochia alba** (from the Latin word for *white*), is composed primarily of leukocytes, decidual cells, epithelial cells, fat, cervical mucus, cholesterol crystals, and bacteria. Variation in the duration of lochia discharge is not uncommon; however, the trend should be toward a lighter amount of flow and a lighter color of discharge. When the lochia flow stops, the cervix is considered to be closed, and chances of infection ascending from the vagina to the uterus decrease.

Like menstrual discharge, lochia flow has a musty, stale odor that is not offensive. Microorganisms are always present in the vaginal lochia and contaminate the uterus with vaginal bacteria by the second day following birth. It is thought that infection does not develop because the organisms involved are relatively nonvirulent. Any foul smell to the lochia or used peripad suggests infection and the need for prompt additional assessment, such as white blood cell count and differential and assessment for uterine tenderness and fever.

The total average volume of lochia is approximately 225 mL, and the daily volume gradually decreases (Blackburn, 2013). Discharge is greater in the morning because of pooling in the vagina and uterus while the mother lies sleeping. The amount of lochia may also be increased by exertion or breastfeeding. Multiparous women usually have more lochia than first-time mothers. Women who undergo a cesarean birth typically have less lochia than women who give birth vaginally (Blackburn, 2013).

Evaluation of lochia is necessary not only to determine whether hemorrhage is present but also to assess uterine involution. The type, amount, and consistency of lochia determine the stage of healing of the placenta site; a progressive change from bright red at birth to dark red, then to pink, and then to white or clear discharge should be observed. Persistent discharge of lochia rubra or a return to lochia rubra may indicate subinvolution or late postpartum hemorrhage.

The nurse should exercise caution in evaluating bleeding immediately after birth. The continuous seepage of blood is more consistent with cervical or vaginal lacerations and may be effectively diagnosed when the bleeding is evaluated in conjunction with uterine consistency. Lacerations should be suspected if the uterus is firm and of expected size and if no clots can be expressed.

Cervical Changes

Following birth, the cervix is flabby, formless, and may appear bruised. The lateral aspects of the external os are sometimes lacerated during the birth process (Cunningham et al., 2014). The external os is markedly irregular and closes slowly. It admits two fingers for a few days following birth, but by the end of the first week, it admits only a fingertip.

The first childbearing permanently changes the shape of the external os. The characteristic dimple-like os of the nullipara changes to the transverse slit (fish-mouth) os of the multipara. After significant cervical laceration or several lacerations, the cervix may appear lopsided. Because of the slight change in the size of the cervix, changes in maternal weight, muscle tone, and pelvic architecture, a diaphragm or cervical cap will need to be refitted if the woman uses one of these methods of contraception.

Vaginal Changes

The vagina appears edematous and may be bruised following birth. The apparent bruising is caused by pelvic congestion and trauma and quickly disappears. Small, superficial lacerations may be evident, and the rugae are obliterated. The hymen, torn and jagged, heals irregularly, leaving small tags called carunculae myrtiformes.

The size of the vagina decreases, and rugae return within 3–4 weeks (Blackburn, 2013; James, 2014). This facilitates the gradual return to smaller, although not nulliparous, dimensions. By 6 weeks, the vagina of a woman who is not breastfeeding usually appears normal. The lactating woman is in a hypoestrogenic state because of ovarian suppression, and her vaginal mucosa may be pale and without rugae. The effects of the lowered estrogen level may lead to dyspareunia (painful intercourse), which may be reduced by the addition of a water-soluble personal lubricant.

Tone and contractility of the vaginal orifice may be improved by perineal tightening exercises, such as Kegel exercises (discussed in Exemplar 33.A). The woman may begin these soon after birth. The labia majora and labia minora are more flaccid in the woman who has borne a child than in the nullipara.

Perineal Changes

During the early postpartum period, the soft tissue in and around the perineum may appear edematous, with some bruising. If an episiotomy or a laceration is present, the edges should be approximated. Initial healing of the episiotomy or laceration occurs in 2–3 weeks after the birth, although complete healing may take up to 4–6 months (Blackburn, 2013). Perineal discomfort may be present during this time.

Ovulation and Menstruation

The return of ovulation and menstruation varies for each postpartum woman. Menstruation generally returns as soon as 7 weeks in 70% and by 12 weeks in all nonlactating mothers or as late as 3 years in 70% of breastfeeding mothers (Pessel & Tsai, 2013). The return of ovulation is directly associated with a rise in the serum progesterone level.

The return of ovulation and menstruation in breastfeeding mothers is usually prolonged. It is associated with the length of time the woman breastfeeds and whether formula supplements are used. If a mother breastfeeds for less than 1 month, the return of menstruation and ovulation is similar to that in the woman who is not breastfeeding. Women who exclusively breastfeed usually experience a delay in menstruation of at least 3 months. Suckling by the baby typically results in alterations in the gonadotropin-releasing hormone production, which is thought to be the cause of amenorrhea (Blackburn, 2013). Although exclusive breastfeeding helps to reduce the risk of pregnancy for the first 6 months after birth, it should be relied on only temporarily and if it meets the criteria for the lactational amenorrhea method. Furthermore, because ovulation precedes menstruation and because women often supplement breastfeeding with bottles and pacifiers, breastfeeding is not considered to be a reliable means of contraception.

Abdomen

The uterine ligaments (notably the round and broad ligaments) are stretched and require the length of the puerperium to recover. Although the stretched abdominal wall appears loose and flabby, it responds to exercise within 2–3 months. However, the abdomen may fail to regain good tone and will remain flabby in the grand multipara, in the woman whose abdomen is overdistended, or in the woman with poor muscle tone before pregnancy. **Diastasis recti abdominis** (a separation of the abdominal muscle) may occur with pregnancy, especially in women with poor abdominal muscle tone. If diastasis occurs, part of the abdominal wall has no muscular support and is formed only by skin, subcutaneous fat, fascia, and peritoneum. This may be especially pronounced in women who have undergone a cesarean section, during which the rectus abdominis muscles are manually separated to access the uterine muscle. Improvement depends on the physical condition of the mother, the total number of pregnancies, pregnancy spacing, and the type and amount of physical exercise. Diastasis may result in a pendulous abdomen and increased maternal backache. Fortunately, diastasis responds well to exercise, and abdominal muscle tone can improve significantly.

The striae (stretch marks), which occur as a result of stretching and rupture of the elastic fibers of the skin, take on different colors based on the mother's skin color. The striae of light-skinned mothers are red to purple at the time of birth, then gradually fade to silver or white. The striae of mothers with darker skin, in contrast, are darker than the surrounding skin and remain darker. Striae gradually fade after a time, but they do remain visible.

Breasts and Lactogenesis

During pregnancy, increased levels of estrogen stimulate breast duct proliferation and development, and elevated progesterone levels promote the development of lobules and alveoli in preparation for lactation. Prolactin levels rise from approximately 10 mcg/mL before pregnancy to 200 mcg/mL at term. However, lactation is suppressed during pregnancy by elevated progesterone levels secreted by the placenta. Once the placenta is expelled at birth, progesterone levels fall, and the inhibition is removed, triggering milk production. This occurs whether the mother has breast stimulation or not. If breast stimulation is not occurring by the third or fourth day, however, prolactin levels begin to drop. By 2 weeks postpartum, if there is no stimulation, prolactin levels will be back to prepregnancy levels, and milk production will cease (Walker, 2016).

Initially, lactation is under endocrine control. The hormone prolactin is released from the anterior pituitary in response to breast stimulation from suckling or the use of a breast pump. Prolactin stimulates the milk-secreting cells in the alveoli to produce milk, then rapidly drops back to baseline. If more than approximately 3 hours elapse between stimulation, prolactin levels begin to drop below baseline. To reverse the overall decline in prolactin level, the mother can be encouraged to stimulate her breasts more frequently (e.g., every 1.5–2.0 hours). Mothers should be strongly encouraged to stimulate their breasts frequently if their babies are not effective feeders or if they are separated from their babies. Prolactin receptors are established during the first 2 weeks postpartum in response to frequency of breast stimulation (Human Milk Banking Association of North America, 2011). Inadequate development of prolactin receptors during this time is likely to negatively impact the mother's long-term milk volume.

Colostrum is the initial milk that begins to be secreted during midpregnancy and that is immediately available to the baby at birth. It provides the newborn with all the nutrition required until the mother's milk becomes more abundant in a few days. No routine supplementation of other fluids is necessary unless there is a medical indication. Colostrum is a thick, creamy, yellowish fluid with concentrated amounts of protein, fat-soluble vitamins, and minerals; it has lower amounts of fat and lactose compared with mature milk. It also contains antioxidants and high levels of lactoferrin and secretory IgA. It promotes the establishment of *Lactobacillus bifidus* flora in the digestive tract, which helps protect the baby from disease and illness. Colostrum also has a laxative effect on the newborn, which helps the baby pass meconium stools, which in turn helps decrease hyperbilirubinemia (Ladewig, London, & Davidson, 2017).

The milk that flows from the breast at the start of a feeding or pumping session is called *foremilk*. The foremilk is watery milk that is high in protein and low in fat (1–2%). This milk has trickled down from the alveoli between feedings to fill the lactiferous ducts, and it is low in fat because the fat globules made in the alveoli stick to each other and to the walls of the alveoli and do not trickle down. In addition to prolactin release, stretching of the nipple and compression of the areola signal the hypothalamus to trigger the posterior pituitary gland to release oxytocin. Oxytocin acts to cause the myoepithelial cells surrounding the alveoli in the breast tissue to contract, ejecting milk (including the fat globules present) into the ducts. This process is called the milk-ejection reflex but is better known in lay terms as the "let-down" reflex (response). The average initial let-down response occurs about 2 minutes after a baby begins to suckle, and between 4 and 10 let-down responses will occur during a feeding session. The milk that flows during "let-down" is called *hindmilk*. Hindmilk is rich in fat (which can exceed 10%) and, therefore, is high in calories. In a sample of expressed breast milk, the average total fat concentration is approximately 4% and the total caloric content is approximately 20 calories/oz.

By 6 months of breastfeeding, prolactin levels are only 5–10 mcg/mL, yet milk production continues. A whey protein called feedback inhibitor of lactation (FIL) has been identified as influencing milk production through a negative feedback loop. FIL is present in breast milk and functions to decrease milk production. The more milk that remains in the breast for a longer period of time, the more milk production is decreased. On the other hand, the more often the breasts are emptied, the lower the level of FIL and the faster milk is produced. This mechanism of regulating milk at the local level is called autocrine control. This process is key to understanding how a mother maintains or loses her milk supply (Riordan, 2016). A number of factors can delay or impair lactogenesis. Maternal factors include the following (Janke, 2014):

- Cesarean birth
- Postpartum hemorrhage
- Type 1 diabetes
- Untreated hypothyroidism
- Obesity
- Polycystic ovary syndrome
- Retained placenta fragments
- Vitamin B_6 deficiency
- History of previous breast surgery
- Insufficient glandular breast tissue
- Significant stress.

Other factors that can interfere with breastfeeding include smoking, use of alcohol, and use of some prescription and OTC medications (e.g., antihistamines and combined birth control pills).

Stages of Human Milk

During the establishment of lactation, there are three stages of human milk:

1. Colostrum
2. Transitional milk
3. Mature milk.

After 30–72 hours of colostrum production, maternal milk production normally becomes noticeably more abundant. The milk "coming in" is called **transitional milk** and has qualities intermediate between those of colostrum and mature milk. It is still light yellow in color but is more copious than colostrum and contains more fat, lactose, water-soluble vitamins, and calories. By day 5, most mothers are producing approximately 500 mL/day.

Mature milk is white or slightly blue-tinged in color. It is present by 2 weeks postpartum and continues thereafter until lactation ceases. Mature milk contains approximately 13% solids (carbohydrates, proteins, and fats) and 87% water. Mature human milk's appearance, similar to that of skim cow's milk, may cause mothers to question whether their milk is "rich enough." The nurse should reassure the mother that this is the normal appearance of mature human milk and that mature milk provides the baby with all the necessary nutrients. Although gradual changes in composition do occur continuously over periods of weeks to accommodate the needs of the growing newborn, the composition of mature milk in general is fairly consistent with the exception of the fat content as noted previously. Milk production continues to increase slowly during the first month. By 6 months postpartum, a mother produces approximately 800 mL/day (Blackburn, 2013).

Gastrointestinal System

Following birth, the mother may be hungry and may enjoy a light meal. Frequently, she is quite thirsty and will drink large amounts of fluid. Drinking fluids helps replace those lost during labor, in the urine, and through perspiration.

The bowels tend to be sluggish following birth because of the lingering effects of progesterone, decreased abdominal muscle tone, and bowel evacuation associated with the labor and birth process. Women who have had an episiotomy or who have lacerations or hemorrhoids may tend to delay elimination because they fear increasing their pain or believe their stitches will be torn if they bear down. However, refusing or delaying the bowel movement may cause increased constipation and more pain when bowel elimination finally occurs.

There is no evidence in favor of restricting oral intake following a cesarean birth. While institutional policies may vary, evidence suggests that advancing the diet as desired restores the gastrointestinal system to a normal state more quickly than withholding solids and does not lead to an increased rate of complications (King et al., 2013). The woman may experience some initial discomfort from flatulence. This can be relieved by early ambulation and use of antiflatulence medications. Chamomile or peppermint tea may also be helpful in reducing discomfort from flatulence. It may take a few days for the bowel to regain its tone, especially if general anesthesia was used. The woman who has had a cesarean or a difficult birth may benefit from stool softeners.

Urinary System

The postpartum woman has increased bladder capacity, swelling and bruising of the tissue around the urethra, decreased sensitivity to fluid pressure, and decreased sensation of bladder filling. Consequently, she is at risk for overdistention, incomplete bladder emptying, and buildup of residual urine. Women who have had neuraxial anesthesia, such as an epidural or spinal, have inhibited neural functioning of the bladder and are more susceptible to bladder distention, difficulty voiding, and bladder infections. In addition, use of oxytocin to facilitate uterine contractions following expulsion of the placenta has an antidiuretic effect. Following cessation of the oxytocin, the woman will experience rapid bladder filling.

Urinary output increases during the early postpartum period (first 12–24 hours) because of postpartum diuresis. The kidneys must eliminate an estimated 2000–3000 mL of extracellular fluid with the normal pregnancy, which causes rapid filling of the bladder (Blackburn, 2013). Adequate bladder elimination is an immediate concern. Women with preeclampsia, chronic hypertension, and diabetes experience greater fluid retention than do other women, and postpartum diuresis is increased accordingly.

If urinary stasis exists, chances for urinary tract infection increase because of bacteriuria and the presence of dilated ureters and renal pelves, which persist for approximately 6 weeks after birth. A full bladder may also increase the tendency of the uterus to relax by displacing the uterus and interfering with its contractility, leading to hemorrhage. In the absence of infection, the dilated ureters and renal pelves return to prepregnant size by the end of the sixth week.

Vital Signs

With the possible exception of the first 24 hours after birth, the woman should be afebrile during the postpartum period. Epidural anesthesia for labor, which can interfere with heat dissipation, has a direct effect on maternal temperature but rarely results in overt fever (Shatken, Greenough, & McPherson, 2012). A maternal temperature of up to 38°C (100.4°F) may occur after childbirth as a result of the exertion and dehydration of labor. An increase in temperature to between 37.8°C and 39°C (100° and 102.2°F) may also occur during the first 24 hours after the mother's milk comes in (Cunningham et al., 2014). However, in women not meeting these criteria, infection must be considered in the presence of an increased temperature.

Immediately following childbirth, many women experience a transient rise in both systolic and diastolic blood pressures, which spontaneously return to the prepregnancy baseline during the next few days (James, 2014). A decrease may indicate physiologic readjustment to decreased intrapelvic pressure, or it may be related to uterine hemorrhage. Orthostatic hypotension, as indicated by feelings of faintness or dizziness immediately after standing up, can develop in the first 48 hours as a result of abdominal engorgement that may occur after birth. A low or decreasing blood pressure may reflect hypovolemia secondary to hemorrhage, but it is a late sign (see discussion of hypovolemia in the module on Fluids and Electrolytes). Blood pressure elevations may result from excessive use of oxytocin or vasopressor medications. Because preeclampsia can persist into or occur first in the postpartum period, routine evaluation of blood pressure is needed. If a woman complains of headache, hypertension must be ruled out before analgesics are administered.

Puerperal bradycardia with rates of 50–70 beats/min commonly occurs during the first 6–10 days of the postpartum period. This may be related to decreased cardiac effort, decreased blood volume following placental separation and contraction of the uterus, and increased stroke volume. A pulse rate of greater than 100 beats/min may indicate hypovolemia, infection, fear, or pain and requires further assessment.

Frequently, the mother experiences intense tremors that resemble shivering from a chill immediately after birth. This shivering has been explained as a

- result of the sudden release of pressure on the pelvic nerves after birth,

- response to a fetus-to-mother transfusion that occurred during placental separation,

- reaction to maternal adrenaline production during labor and birth, or

- reaction to epidural anesthesia.

If not followed by fever, this chill is of no clinical concern, but it is uncomfortable for the woman. The nurse can increase the woman's comfort by covering her with a warmed blanket and reassuring her that the shivering is a common, self-limiting situation. If the woman allows herself to go with the shaking, the shivering will last only a short time. Some women may find a warm beverage to be helpful. Later in the puerperium, chill and fever indicate infection and require further evaluation.

Blood Values

Blood values should return to the prepregnant state by the end of the postpartum period. Pregnancy-associated activation of coagulation factors may continue for variable amounts of time after birth. This condition, in conjunction with trauma, immobility, sepsis, obesity, African American ethnicity, diabetes, smoking, and advanced maternal age, predisposes the woman to development of thromboembolism (King et al., 2013). The incidence of thromboembolism is reduced by early ambulation.

Nonpathologic leukocytosis often occurs during labor and in the immediate postpartum period, with white blood cell counts of 25,000–30,000 cells/mm^3 (Cunningham et al., 2014). These values typically return to normal levels by the end of the first postpartum week. Leukocytosis combined with the normal increase in erythrocyte sedimentation rate may obscure the diagnosis of acute infection at this time (James, 2014).

Hemoglobin and hematocrit levels may be difficult to interpret during the first 2 days after birth because of the changing blood volume. The loss of blood in the first 24 hours accounts for half the red blood cell volume gained during the course of the pregnancy. Blood loss averages 200–500 mL with a vaginal birth and nearly 1000 mL with a cesarean birth (Pessel & Tsai, 2013). Lochia constitutes less than 25% of this blood loss (James, 2014). As extracellular fluid is excreted, hemoconcentration occurs, with a concomitant rise in hematocrit. A drop in values indicates an abnormal blood loss. The following is a convenient rule to remember: A two to three percentage point drop in hematocrit equals a blood loss of 500 mL (James, 2014). After 3–4 days, mobilization of interstitial fluid leads to a slight increase in plasma volume. This hemodilution leads to a decrease in hemoglobin, hematocrit, and plasma protein by the end of the first postpartum week. Decreases in plasma volume reach nonpregnant levels by 4–6 weeks postpartum (Blackburn, 2013).

Platelet levels typically fall as a result of placental separation. They then begin to increase by the third to fourth day postpartum, gradually returning to normal by the sixth week postpartum. Fibrinolytic activity typically returns to normal during the hours following birth. The hemostatic system as a whole reaches its normal prepregnant status by 3–4 weeks postpartum; however, the diameter of deep veins can take up to 6 weeks to return to prepregnant levels (Blackburn, 2013). This explains the prolonged risk of thromboembolism in the first 6 weeks following birth.

Cardiovascular Changes

The mother's cardiovascular system undergoes dramatic changes during the birth that can result in cardiovascular instability because of an increase in cardiac output. The cardiac output typically stabilizes and returns to pregnancy levels within an hour following birth. Maternal hypervolemia acts to protect the mother from excessive blood loss. Cardiac output declines by 30% in the first 2 weeks and reaches normal levels by 6–12 weeks (Blackburn, 2013).

Diuresis in the first 2–5 days after birth assists in decreasing the extracellular fluid and results in a weight loss of 3 kg (6.6 lb) (James, 2014). Failure to have diuresis in the immediate postpartum period can lead to pulmonary edema and subsequent cardiac problems. This is seen more commonly in women with a history of preeclampsia or preexisting cardiac problems (Blackburn, 2013; James, 2014).

Neurologic and Immunologic Changes

Neurologic problems and disorders can predispose women to higher rates of morbidity and mortality during pregnancy and the postpartum period. Headaches are the most common neurologic symptoms encountered by postpartum women. Headaches may result from fluid shifts in the first week after birth, leakage of cerebrospinal fluid into the extradural space during spinal anesthesia, gestational hypertension, or stress (James, 2014). Migraine headaches may persist during pregnancy and postpartum (Hoshiyama et al., 2012). It is more likely that a woman will have a seizure during labor or in the first 24 hours after birth than during pregnancy (Sibai, 2012). Women with epilepsy also have more feeding difficulties, irritability, and lethargy.

Psychologic Adaptations

The postpartum period is a time of readjustment and adaptation for the entire childbearing family but especially for the mother. The woman experiences a variety of responses as she adjusts to a new family member, postpartum discomforts, changes in her body image, and the reality that she is no longer pregnant.

The first day or two after birth, the mother may seem passive about the event and may seem more concerned with her own needs. Food and sleep are priority needs, and she begins to process the event. By the second or third day, the new mother is ready to resume control of her mothering and of her body and life in general. At this stage, however, she may experience anxiety and require assurance that she is doing well as a mother. Difficulties with feedings may be a particular source of anxiety.

Maternal Role Attainment

Maternal role attainment (MRA) is the process by which a woman learns mothering behaviors and becomes comfortable with her identity as a mother. Formation of a maternal identity occurs with each child a woman bears. As the mother grows to know this child and forms a relationship, the mother's maternal identity gradually and systematically evolves, and she "binds in" to the newborn (Rubin, 1984).

Maternal role attainment often occurs in four stages (Mercer, 1995):

1. **The anticipatory stage** occurs during pregnancy. The woman looks to role models, especially her own mother, for examples of how to mother.
2. **The formal stage** begins when the child is born. The woman is still influenced by the guidance of others and tries to act as she believes others expect her to act.
3. **The informal stage** begins when the mother starts making her own choices about mothering. The woman begins to develop her own style of mothering and finds ways of functioning that work well for her.
4. **The personal stage** is the final stage of maternal role attainment. When the woman reaches this stage, she is comfortable with the notion of herself as "mother."

In most cases, MRA occurs within 3–10 months after birth. Social support, the woman's age and personality traits, the marital relationship, the presence of underlying anxiety or depression, the woman's previous child care experiences, the temperament of her infant, and the family's socioeconomic status all influence the woman's success in attaining the maternal role.

The postpartum woman faces a number of challenges as she adjusts to her new role (Mercer, 1995):

- For many women, finding time for themselves is one of the greatest challenges of motherhood. It is often difficult for the new mother to find time to read a book, talk to her partner, or even eat a meal without interruption.
- Women also report feelings of incompetence because they have not mastered all aspects of the mothering role. Many times mothers find themselves unsure of what to do in a given situation.
- The next greatest challenge involves fatigue resulting from sleep deprivation. The demands of nighttime care are tremendously draining, especially when the woman has other children.
- Another challenge for the new mother involves the feeling of responsibility that having a child brings. A woman experiences a sense of lost freedom, an awareness that she will never again be quite as carefree as she was before becoming a mother.
- Finding time for older children following the birth of a new baby also presents challenges. Many women feel guilty because the new baby takes up so much of their time. Sibling rivalry or ill feelings about the baby from other children can put additional stress on the mother.
- Mothers sometimes cite the infant's behavior as a challenge, especially when the child is about 8 months old. The baby develops stranger anxiety, begins crawling and getting into things, and may be fussy from teething. In addition, the baby's tendency to put things in the mouth requires constant vigilance by the parent.

In 2004, Mercer proposed replacing the term *maternal role attainment (MRA)* with the term *becoming a mother (BAM)*. She stated that BAM "more accurately encompasses the dynamic transformation and evolution of a woman's persona than does MRA, and the term MRA should be discontinued."

A mother's first interaction with her newborn is influenced by many factors, including her involvement with her family of origin, her relationships, the stability of her home environment, the communication patterns she has developed, and the degree of nurturing she received as a child. These factors shaped the person she has become. The following personal characteristics are also important:

- *Level of trust.* What level of trust has this mother developed in response to her life experiences? What is her philosophy of childrearing? Will she be able to treat her baby as a unique individual with changing needs that should be met as much as possible?
- *Level of self-esteem.* How much does she value herself as a woman and a mother? Is she generally able to cope with the adjustments of life?
- *Capacity for enjoying herself.* Is the mother able to find pleasure in everyday activities and human relationships?
- *Adequacy of knowledge about childbearing and childrearing.* What beliefs about the course of pregnancy, the

capabilities of newborns, previous experiences with infants or children, and the nature of her emotions may influence her behavior at first contact with her newborn and later?

- **Prevailing mood or usual feeling tone.** Is the woman predominantly content, angry, depressed, or anxious? Is she sensitive to her own feelings and those of others? Will she be able to accept her own needs and to obtain support in meeting them?

- **Reactions to the present pregnancy.** Was the pregnancy planned? Did it go smoothly? Were there ongoing life events that enhanced her pregnancy or depleted her reserves of energy? How have other life roles changed because of her pregnancy and motherhood?

By the time of birth, each mother has developed some kind of emotional orientation to the baby based on these factors.

Initially after birth during the *taking-in* period, the woman tends to be passive and somewhat dependent. She follows suggestions, hesitates to make decisions, and is still rather preoccupied with her needs (Rubin, 1984). She may have a great need to talk about her perceptions of her labor and birth. This helps her work through the process, sort out the reality from her fantasized experience, and clarify anything that she did not understand. Food and sleep are major needs.

By the second or third day after birth, the new mother is often ready to resume control of her body, her mothering, and her life in general. Rubin (1984) labeled this the *taking-hold* period. If she is breastfeeding, she may worry about her technique or the quality of her milk. If her baby spits up after a feeding, she may view it as a personal failure. She may also feel demoralized by the fact that the nurse or an older family member handles her baby proficiently while she feels unsure and tentative. She requires assurance that she is doing well as a mother. Today's mothers seem to be more independent and adjust more rapidly, exhibiting behaviors of "taking-in" and "taking-hold" in shorter periods of time than those previously identified.

Development of Family Attachment

Nurses caring for families in the postpartum stage need to be aware of the long-term adjustments and stresses that the family faces as its members adjust to new and different roles. Nurses can help by providing anticipatory guidance about the realities of being a parent and by giving the postpartum family parenting literature for reference at home. Ongoing parenting groups give parents an opportunity to discuss problems and become comfortable in new roles.

Father–Newborn Interactions

In Western cultures, commitment to family-centered maternity care has fostered interest in understanding the feelings and experiences of the new father. Evidence suggests that the father has a strong attraction to his newborn and that the feelings he experiences are similar to the mother's feelings of attachment. The father's characteristic sense of absorption, preoccupation, and interests in the newborn demonstrated during early contact is termed *engrossment*. Engrossment occurs after birth when the father and the newborn bond. Engrossment is not only the effect of the father caring for the baby, such as holding and comforting, but the emotional effect that the baby has on the father (Sears & Sears, 2016). Differences in involvement still exist among fathers in Western culture and may be influenced by factors other than culture (e.g., previous experience with paternal role or exposure to male/father role models).

Siblings and Others

Babies are capable of maintaining a number of strong attachments without loss of quality. These attachments may include siblings, grandparents, aunts, and uncles. The social setting and personality of the individual seem to be significant factors in the development of multiple attachments. Birth centers are especially geared toward the family's inclusion in the birth process. In the hospital setting, the advent of open visiting hours and rooming-in permits siblings and others to participate in the attachment process.

Initial Maternal Attachment Behavior

After labor and birth, a new mother demonstrates a fairly regular pattern of maternal behaviors as she continues to familiarize herself with her newborn. In a progression of touching activities, the mother proceeds from fingertip exploration of the newborn's extremities toward palmar contact with larger body areas and finally to enfolding the newborn with the whole hand and arm. The time she takes to accomplish these steps varies from minutes to days. The mother increases the proportion of time spent in the *en face* position—she arranges herself or the newborn so that she has direct face-to-face and eye-to-eye contact (**Figure 33–58 》**). There is an intense interest in having the newborn's eyes open. When the newborn's eyes are open, the mother characteristically greets and talks to the baby in high-pitched tones.

In most instances, the mother relies heavily on her senses of sight, touch, and hearing in getting to know what her baby is really like. She also tends to respond verbally to any sounds emitted by the newborn, such as cries, coughs, sneezes, and grunts. The sense of smell may be involved as well.

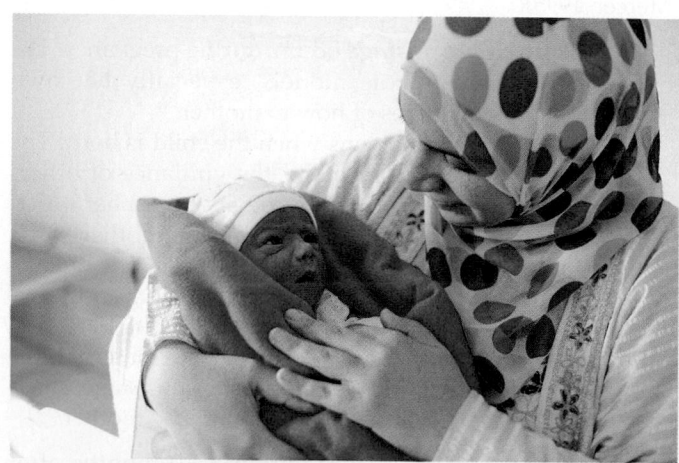

Source: ZouZou/Shutterstock.

Figure 33–58 》 A mother *en face* with her newborn.

The nurse plays a key role in assessing and assisting the mother–newborn bond. As discussed in detail in Exemplar 33.D, the nurse facilitates a number of activities that help strengthen maternal attachment, including feeding, bathing, and recognizing the baby's specific cues related to sleep and activity. Ongoing assessment of the mother's psychologic adaptation is critical because it allows the nurse to evaluate what patient teaching needs to be provided. Nursing interventions that foster the process of becoming a mother include the following categories:

- Instructing for newborn/infant caregiving
- Building awareness of and responsiveness to newborn/infant interactive capabilities
- Promoting maternal–newborn attachment
- Preparing the woman for the maternal social role preparation
- Encouraging interactive therapeutic nurse–patient relationships

Maternal/social role preparation and interactive therapeutic nurse–patient relationships may have a greater impact on the progress of becoming a mother than formal teaching. A detailed discussion of psychologic assessment of the postpartum mother is included in the Nursing Process section of this exemplar.

Postpartum Weight and Nutrition

An initial weight loss of approximately 4.5–5.4 kg (10–12 lb) occurs as a result of birth of the baby and expulsion of the placenta and amniotic fluid. Diuresis accounts for the loss of an additional 2.3 kg (5 lb) during the early puerperium. By the sixth to eighth week after birth, many women have returned to approximately their prepregnant weight if they had gained the average 11.4–13.6 kg (25–30 lb) during pregnancy. For others, a return to prepregnant weight may take longer. Women often express concern about the slow pace of their postpartum weight loss. Multiparas tend to be more positive than primiparas, probably because a multipara's previous experience has prepared her for the fact that the body does not immediately return to a prepregnant state.

Nutritional needs change following childbirth. Nutrient requirements vary depending on whether the mother decides to breastfeed. An assessment of postpartum nutritional status is necessary before giving nutritional guidance. Postpartum nutritional status is determined primarily by assessing the new mother's weight, hemoglobin and hematocrit levels, clinical signs, and dietary history.

Postpartum Nutritional Status

The amount of weight gained during pregnancy is a major determinant of weight loss after childbirth. Generally, women who gain excessive weight during pregnancy are more likely to sustain a weight gain 1 year following childbirth, putting them at increased risk of long-term overweight or obesity. The mother's weight should be considered in terms of ideal weight, prepregnancy weight, and weight gain during pregnancy. Women who desire information about weight reduction can be referred to a dietitian or nutritionist for individual counseling or to community-based educational programs. Educational programs need to address a variety of issues, such as the significance of the quality of food eaten rather than its quantity; the importance of regular physical activity in improving health, building lean muscle mass, and increasing metabolism; and the value of meal planning to ensure that healthy foods are readily available and to avoid pitfalls such as opting for fast foods, which are often high in fat.

Hemoglobin and erythrocyte levels should return to normal within 2–6 weeks after childbirth. Hematocrit levels gradually rise because of hemoconcentration as extracellular fluid is excreted. Iron supplements are generally continued for 2–3 months following childbirth to replenish stores depleted by pregnancy.

The nurse assesses clinical symptoms the new mother may be experiencing. Constipation is a common problem following birth. The nurse can encourage the woman to maintain a high fluid intake to keep the stool soft. Dietary sources of fiber, such as whole grains, fruits, and vegetables, are also helpful in preventing constipation.

The nurse obtains specific information on dietary intake and eating habits directly from the woman. Visiting the mother during mealtimes provides an opportunity for unobtrusive nutritional assessment. Which foods has the woman selected? Is her diet nutritionally sound? A comment focusing on a positive aspect of her meal selection may initiate a discussion of nutrition.

The nurse needs to inform the dietitian if a woman's cultural or religious beliefs require specific foods so that appropriate meals can be prepared for her. The nurse may also refer women with unusual eating habits or numerous questions about good nutrition. In addition, the nurse provides literature on nutrition so that the woman will have a source of appropriate information at home.

During the childbearing years, the risk for obesity becomes especially problematic for women. Consequently, it is critical to use the postpartum period to change behaviors and help promote effective weight management in women.

Nutritional Care of Formula-feeding Mothers

After birth, the formula-feeding mother's dietary requirements return to prepregnancy levels. If the mother has a good understanding of nutritional principles, it is sufficient to advise her to reduce her daily caloric intake by approximately 300 kcal and to return to prepregnancy levels for other nutrients.

If the mother has a limited understanding of nutrition, now is the time to teach her the basic principles and importance of a well-balanced diet. Her eating habits and dietary practices will eventually be reflected in the diet of her child.

If the mother has gained excessive weight during pregnancy (or perhaps was overweight before pregnancy) and wishes to lose weight, the nurse should refer her to a dietitian or a nutritionist. A weight-reduction diet can be designed to meet nutritional needs and food preferences. Weight loss goals of 0.45–0.9 kg (1–2 lb) per week are usually suggested.

In addition to meeting her own nutritional needs, the new mother is usually interested in learning how to provide for her baby's nutritional needs. A discussion of newborn/infant feeding that includes topics such as selecting newborn/infant formulas, formula preparation, and vitamin and mineral supplementation is appropriate and generally well received.

Nutritional Care of Breastfeeding Mothers

The nutritional needs of the mother are increased during breastfeeding. In Exemplar 33.A, Table 33–4 lists the Dietary Reference Intakes during breastfeeding for specific nutrients, and Table 33–5 provides a sample daily food plan for lactating women. It is especially important for the breastfeeding mother to consume sufficient calories because inadequate caloric intake can reduce milk volume. However, milk quality generally remains unaffected. The breastfeeding mother should increase her calories by approximately 200 kcal over her pregnancy requirement or 500 kcal over her prepregnancy requirement. This results in a total of approximately 2500–2700 kcal/day for most women.

Because protein is an important ingredient in breast milk, an adequate intake while breastfeeding is essential. An intake of 65 g/day during the first 6 months of breastfeeding, and of 62 g/day during the second 6 months, is recommended. As in pregnancy, it is important for the mother to consume adequate nonprotein calories to prevent the use of protein as an energy source.

Calcium is an important ingredient in milk production, and requirements during lactation remain the same as those during pregnancy—that is, an increase of 1000 mg/day. If the intake of calcium from food sources is not adequate, calcium supplements are recommended.

Liquids are especially important during lactation, because inadequate fluid intake may decrease milk volume. Fluid recommendations while breastfeeding are eight to ten 8-oz glasses daily, including water, juice, milk, and soups.

In addition to counseling nursing mothers on how to meet their increased nutrient needs during breastfeeding, it is important to discuss a few issues related to newborn/infant feeding. For example, many breastfeeding mothers are concerned about how specific foods they eat may affect their babies. Generally, the nursing mother need not avoid any foods except those to which she might be allergic. Occasionally, however, some nursing mothers find that certain foods may cause the baby to be colicky or to develop a skin rash. Onions, turnips, cabbage, chocolate, spices, and seasonings are common offenders. The best advice to give the nursing mother is to avoid those foods that she suspects cause distress in her baby. For the most part, however, she should be able to eat any nourishing food she wants without fear that her baby will be affected.

Alterations in the Postpartum Period

Two common postpartum alterations are hemorrhage and endometritis. **Early (primary) postpartum hemorrhage** occurs in the first 24 hours after childbirth and is the more common of the two types of postpartum hemorrhage. **Late (secondary) postpartum hemorrhage** occurs from 24 hours to 6 weeks after birth. Postpartum hemorrhage (PPH) continues to be a cause of significant maternal mortality and morbidity, although there has been a decrease in the Western world over recent years.

The traditional definition of PPH has been a blood loss of greater than 500 mL following childbirth. That definition is currently being questioned, however, because careful quantification indicates that the average blood loss in a vaginal birth is actually greater than 500 mL, and the average blood loss after a cesarean childbirth exceeds 1000 mL (Harvey & Dildy, 2013). Clinically, PPH can be defined as a drop in maternal hematocrit levels of 10% or more from predelivery baseline or excessive bleeding that causes hemodynamic instability or the need for a blood transfusion (Sosa, 2014). Some common causes of PPH include overdistention of the uterus, abruptio placentae, placenta previa, precipitous labor, prolonged labor, retained placental tissue, and birth trauma.

Uterine atony (relaxation of the uterus) is the leading cause of early PPH. If external or internal uterine massage is not effective in controlling excessive bleeding, uterine stimulants such as oxytocin, misoprostol, ergotamine, and prostaglandin analog and will be administered (Thorp & Laughton, 2014).

>> Go to **Pearson MyLab Nursing and eText** for Chart 11: Uterine Stimulants Used to Prevent and Manage Uterine Atony.

Postpartum endometritis (metritis), an inflammation of the endometrium portion of the uterine lining occurring anytime up to 6 weeks postpartum, may occur in 30–35% of those who give birth by cesarean after an extended period of labor and ruptured membranes (Duff, 2014). Postpartum infection from vaginal delivery primarily affects the placental implantation site, the decidua, and adjacent myometrium. Bacteria that colonize the cervix and vagina gain access to the amniotic fluid during labor and postpartum and begin to invade devitalized tissue (the lower uterine segment, lacerations, and incisions). The same pathogenesis, polymicrobial proliferation and tissue invasion, is associated with cesarean delivery, but surgical trauma, additional devitalization of tissue, blood and serum accumulation, and foreign bodies (suture, staples) provide additional favorable anaerobic bacterial conditions.

Assessment findings consistent with endometritis are foul-smelling lochia, sawtooth fever (usually between 38.3°C [101.0°F] and 40°C [104°F]), uterine tenderness on palpation, lower abdominal pain, tachycardia that parallels the temperature increase, and chills (James, 2014).

Alterations in health during the antepartum and intrapartum period may cause increased risk during the postpartum period. **Table 33–16 >>** lists risks associated with various conditions.

Lifespan Considerations

Although the nurse considers all new mothers' physical and psychosocial needs, the adolescent mother and the mother over the age of 35 may require specific care and guidance.

Nursing Care of the Postpartum Adolescent

The adolescent mother may have special postpartum needs, depending on her level of maturity and her support system. The nurse needs to assess maternal–newborn interaction, roles of support people, plans for discharge, knowledge of childrearing, and plans for follow-up care. It is imperative

TABLE 33–16 Postpartum High-Risk Factors

Risk Factor	Condition
Preeclampsia	↑ Blood pressure
	↑ Central nervous system irritability
	↑ Need for bedrest → ↑ risk thrombophlebitis
	↑ Risk of seizures
Diabetes	Need for insulin regulation
	Episodes of hypoglycemia or hyperglycemia
	↓ Healing
Cardiac disease	↑ Maternal exhaustion
Cesarean birth	↑ Recovery time
	↑ Pain from incision
	↑ Risk of infection
	↑ Length of hospitalization
Overdistention of uterus (multiple gestation, hydramnios)	↑ Risk of hemorrhage
	↑ Risk of thrombophlebitis
	↑ Risk of anemia
	↑ Risk of breastfeeding problems (cesarean section risk)
	↑ Stretching of abdominal muscles
	↑ Incidence and severity of afterpains
Abruptio placentae, placenta previa	Hemorrhage → anemia
	↑ Uterine contractility after birth → ↑ infection risk
Precipitous labor (<3 hours)	↑ Risk of lacerations to birth canal → hemorrhage
Prolonged labor (>24 hours)	Exhaustion
	↑ Risk of hemorrhage
	Nutritional and fluid depletion
	↑ Bladder atony and/or trauma
	Endometritis
	Uterine inversion
Trauma due to difficult birth	Exhaustion
	↑ Risk of perineal lacerations
	↑ Risk of hematomas
	↑ Risk of hemorrhage → anemia
Extended period of time in stirrups at birth	↑ Risk of thrombophlebitis
	↑ Risk of muscle, tendon, ligament, and nerve injury
Retained placenta	↑ Risk of hemorrhage
	↑ Risk of infection
Uterine atony	↑ Risk of hemorrhage

that a community health service contact the adolescent shortly after discharge.

Contraception counseling is an important part of teaching the adolescent mother. The incidence of repeat pregnancies during adolescence is high. The younger the adolescent, the more likely she is to become pregnant again, and the more likely the mother is to experience complicated pregnancy and birth (Sedgh et al., 2015; Torvie et al., 2015). Nurses should be aware of the state laws that govern their jurisdiction in order to determine if providing contraception without parental consent is allowed. In states where adolescents can obtain birth control without parental consent, it is often more comfortable for the adolescent to address these issues without others being present. Adolescents also may encounter obstacles when attempting to obtain contraceptives

themselves. These may include embarrassment about discussing the topic; concerns about confidentiality, such as not wanting their parents to know or having to give permission; and lack of knowledge regarding available methods. Nurses can play a key role in overcoming these obstacles by providing teaching and referrals that address these barriers. See the exemplar on Family Planning in the module on Sexuality.

The nurse has many opportunities for teaching the adolescent about her newborn in the postpartum unit. Because the nurse is a role model, the manner in which the nurse handles a newborn greatly influences the young mother. If the father is present, he should be included in as much of the teaching as possible. If the grandparents are going to take an active role in caring for the baby, they should also be included in teaching if this is desired by the new mother.

As with older parents, a newborn examination done at the bedside gives adolescents information about their baby's health and shows possible positions for handling the baby. The nurse can also use this time to provide information about newborn and infant behavior. Parents who have some idea of what to expect from their baby are less frustrated with the baby's behavior.

The adolescent mother appreciates positive feedback about her newborn and her developing maternal responses. Praise and encouragement will increase her confidence and self-esteem. Young mothers with low self-esteem, family conflict, and few social supports are more likely to encounter postpartum depression (Cherry & Dillon, 2014). Careful assessment of these factors should be made during the postpartum period so that appropriate referrals can be provided before discharge.

Group classes for adolescent mothers should include information about newborn/infant care skills, such as taking the baby's temperature, clearing the nose and mouth, monitoring growth and development, feeding the baby, providing well-baby care, and identifying danger signals in the ill newborn. These classes can also address unique needs of teen mothers, such as peer relationships, added responsibilities, and goal setting.

Ideally, teenage mothers should visit adolescent clinics for assessments of themselves and their children for several years after birth. In this way, the adolescent's enrollment in classes on parenting, need for vocational guidance, and school attendance can be supported and followed closely. Classes in the school system for young mothers are an excellent way of helping adolescents finish school and learn how to parent at the same time. Some public high schools have on-site child care centers to assist adolescent mothers and to provide an opportunity for them to learn important child development principles and child-care tasks.

Nursing Care of the Postpartum Mother Over Age 35

The mother over age 35 may have special postpartum needs based on her birth experience, personal expectation, and lifestyle choices. Women may delay childbearing for a variety of reasons such as relationship choices, educational opportunities, career options, and financial considerations. In addition, physiologic conditions may impair normal reproductive processes. Because of their greater life experiences, older parents may also be more aware of the realities of having a child and what it means to have a baby at their age (Ladewig et al., 2017).

Although women over 35 experience the same involution process as younger mothers, they may have life experiences and education that better prepare them for parenthood. Despite the potential advantage of more life experiences, older couples must be made aware that the addition of a newborn will alter established routines and practices. In addition to routine postpartum follow-up, some women over 35 with pre-existing conditions or complications may need additional follow-up with healthcare providers other than their obstetrician.

NURSING PROCESS

During the first several postpartum weeks, the woman must accomplish the following physical and developmental tasks:

- Restore physical condition.
- Develop competence in caring for and meeting the needs of her baby.
- Establish a relationship with her new child.
- Adapt to altered lifestyles and family structure resulting from the addition of a new member.

Assessment

Postpartum Physical Examination

Comprehensive care is based on a thorough assessment that identifies individual needs or potential problems. The nurse should remember the following principles in preparing for and completing the assessment of the postpartum woman:

- Use universal precautions, including wearing gloves during this exam.
- Select a time that will provide the most accurate data. Palpating the fundus when the woman has a full bladder, for example, may give false information about the progress of involution. Ask the woman to void before assessment.
- Explain the purpose of regular assessment.
- Ensure that the woman is relaxed before starting. Perform the procedures as gently as possible to avoid unnecessary discomfort.
- Record and report the results as clearly as possible.
- Take appropriate precautions to prevent exposure to body fluids.

While performing the physical assessment, the nurse should also be teaching the woman. The assessment provides an excellent time to provide information about the body's postpartum physical and anatomic changes as well as the danger signs to report. Because the time that new mothers spend in the postpartum unit is limited, nurses need to use every available opportunity for patient education about self-care. To assist nurses in recognizing these opportunities, examples of patient teaching during the assessment are provided throughout the following discussion. See Postpartum Assessment: First 24 Hours After Birth.

Psychologic Assessment

Adequate assessment of the mother's psychologic adjustment is an integral part of postpartum evaluation. This assessment focuses on the mother's general attitude, feelings of competence, available support systems, and caregiving skills. It also evaluates her fatigue level, sense of satisfaction, and ability to accomplish her developmental tasks.

PSYCHOLOGIC ASSESSMENT RISK FACTORS Some new mothers have little or no experience with newborns and may feel totally overwhelmed. They may show these feelings by asking questions and reading all available material or by becoming passive and quiet, because they simply cannot deal with their feelings of inadequacy. Unless a nurse questions the woman about her plans and previous experience in a supportive, nonjudgmental way, the nurse might conclude that the woman is uninterested, withdrawn, or depressed. Clues indicating adjustment difficulties include the following:

- Excessive continued fatigue
- Marked depression
- Excessive preoccupation with physical status or discomfort
- Evidence of low self-esteem
- Lack of support systems
- Marital problems
- Inability to care for or nurture the newborn
- Current family crises, such as illness or unemployment.

These characteristics frequently indicate a potential for maladaptive parenting, which may lead to child abuse or neglect (physical, emotional, or intellectual) and cannot be ignored. Referrals to public health nurses or other available community resources may provide greatly needed assistance and alleviate potentially dangerous situations.

ASSESSMENT OF EARLY ATTACHMENT A nurse in any postpartum setting can periodically observe and note progress toward attachment. Research shows that fathers experience attachment feelings similar to those experienced by mothers, and the assessment should include both parents when possible. This section, however, focuses primarily on the mother's attachment process.

The following questions can be addressed in the course of nurse–patient interaction:

- Is the mother demonstrating attachment behaviors toward her newborn? To what extent does she seek face-to-face contact and eye contact? Has she progressed from fingertip touch, to palmar contact, to enfolding the baby close to her own body? Is attachment increasing or decreasing? If the mother does not exhibit increasing attachment, why not? Do the reasons lie primarily within her, the baby, or the environment?
- Is the mother inclined to nurture her baby by feeding every 2–3 hours?
- Is she progressing in her interactions with her newborn?
- Does the mother act consistently? If not, is the source of unpredictability within her or her baby?
- Does she seek information and evaluate it objectively? Does she develop solutions based on adequate knowledge of valid data? Does she evaluate the effectiveness of her maternal care and adjust appropriately?
- Is the mother sensitive to the newborn's needs as they arise? How quickly does she interpret her baby's behavior and react to cues? Does she seem happy and satisfied with the baby's responses to her efforts? Is she pleased

Postpartum Assessment: First 24 Hours After Birth

PHYSICAL ASSESSMENT/ NORMAL FINDINGS	ALTERATIONS AND POSSIBLE CAUSES*	NURSING RESPONSES TO DATA†
Vital Signs		
Blood pressure (BP): should remain consistent with baseline BP during pregnancy	High BP (preeclampsia, essential hypertension, renal disease, anxiety); drop in BP (may be normal; uterine hemorrhage)	Evaluate history of preexisting disorders and check for other signs of preeclampsia (edema, proteinuria). Assess for other signs of hemorrhage (↑ pulse, cool clammy skin).
Pulse: 60–100 beats/min	Tachycardia (difficult labor and birth, hemorrhage)	Evaluate for other signs of hemorrhage (↓ BP; cool, clammy skin).
Respirations: 12–20 breaths/min	Marked tachypnea (respiratory disease)	Assess for other signs of respiratory disease.
Temperature: 36.6°–38.0°C (98°–100.4°F)	After first 24 hours, temperature of 38.0°C (100.4°F) or higher suggests infection	Assess for other signs of infection; notify healthcare provider.
Breasts		
General appearance: smooth, even pigmentation; changes of pregnancy still apparent; one may appear larger	Reddened area (mastitis)	Assess further for signs of infection.
Palpation: depending on postpartum day, may be soft, filling, full, or engorged	Palpable mass (caked breast, mastitis); engorgement (venous stasis); tenderness, heat, edema (engorgement, caked breast, mastitis)	Assess for other signs of infection: If blocked duct, consider heat, massage, and position change for breastfeeding. Assess for further signs. Report mastitis to healthcare provider.
Nipples: supple, pigmented, intact; become erect when stimulated	Fissures, cracks, soreness (problems with breastfeeding); not erectile with stimulation (inverted nipples)	Reassess technique; recommend appropriate interventions.
Lungs		
Sounds: clear to bases bilaterally	Diminished (fluid overload, asthma, pulmonary embolus, pulmonary edema)	Assess for other signs of respiratory distress.
Abdomen		
Musculature: abdomen may be soft, have a "doughy" texture; rectus muscle intact	Separation in musculature (diastasis recti abdominis)	Evaluate size of diastasis; teach appropriate exercises for decreasing the separation.
Fundus: firm, midline; following expected process of involution	Boggy (full bladder, uterine bleeding, retained products of conception)	Massage until firm. Assess bladder, and have woman void if needed. Attempt to express clots when firm. If bogginess remains or recurs, report to healthcare provider.
May be tender when palpated	Constant tenderness (infection)	Assess for evidence of endometritis.
Cesarean section incision dressing: dry and intact	Moderate to large amount of blood or serosanguineous drainage on dressing	Assess for hemorrhage. Reinforce dressing and notify healthcare provider.
Lochia		
Scant to moderate amount, earthy odor; no clots	Large amount, clots (hemorrhage) Foul-smelling lochia (infection)	Assess for firmness and express additional clots. Begin peripad count. Assess for other signs of infection; report to healthcare provider.
Normal progression: first 1–3 days: rubra	Failure to progress normally or return to rubra from serosa (subinvolution)	Report to healthcare provider.
Following rubra: days 3–10: serosa (alba seldom seen in hospital)		
	*Possible causes of alterations are identified in parentheses.	†This column provides guidelines for further assessment and initial nursing actions.

(continued on next page)

Postpartum Assessment: First 24 Hours After Birth (continued)

PHYSICAL ASSESSMENT/ NORMAL FINDINGS	ALTERATIONS AND POSSIBLE CAUSES*	NURSING RESPONSES TO DATA†
Perineum		
Slight edema and bruising in intact perineum	Marked fullness, bruising, increasing pain (vulvar hematoma)	Assess size. Apply ice glove or ice pack. Report to healthcare provider.
Episiotomy: no redness, edema, ecchymosis, or discharge; edges well approximated	Redness, edema, ecchymosis, discharge, or gaping stitches (infection)	Encourage sitz baths; review perineal care and appropriate wiping techniques.
Hemorrhoids: none present (if present, should be small and nontender)	Full, tender, inflamed hemorrhoids	Encourage sitz baths, side-lying position, Tucks pads, anesthetic ointments, manual replacement of hemorrhoids, stool softeners, and increased fluid intake.
Costovertebral Angle (CVA) Tenderness		
None	Present (kidney infection)	Assess for other symptoms of urinary tract infection (UTI); obtain clean-catch urine. Report to healthcare provider.
Lower Extremities		
No pain with palpation; negative calf pain on ambulation	Positive findings (thrombophlebitis)	Report to healthcare provider.
Elimination		
Urinary output: voiding in sufficient quantities at least every 4–6 hours; bladder not palpable	Inability to void (urinary retention); symptoms of urgency, frequency, dysuria (UTI)	Employ nursing interventions to promote voiding; if not successful, obtain order for catheterization.
		Report symptoms of UTI to healthcare provider.
Bowel elimination: should have normal bowel movement by second or third day after birth	Inability to pass feces (constipation caused by fear of pain from episiotomy, hemorrhoids, perineal trauma)	Encourage fluids, ambulation, roughage in diet, and sitz baths to promote healing of perineum; obtain order for stool softener.
	*Possible causes of alterations are identified in parentheses.	†This column provides guidelines for further assessment and initial nursing actions.
CULTURAL ASSESSMENT§	**VARIATIONS TO CONSIDER**	**NURSING RESPONSES TO DATA§§**
Determine customs and practices regarding postpartum care. Ask the mother whether she would like fluids, and ask what temperature she prefers.	Individual preference may include room-temperature or warmed fluids rather than iced drinks.	Provide for specific request if possible. If woman is unable to provide specific information, the nurse may draw from general information regarding cultural variation.
Ask the mother what foods she would like.	Special foods or fluids to hasten healing after childbirth.	Mexican women may want food and fluids that restore hot–cold balance to the body. Women of European background may ask for iced fluids.
Ask the mother whether she would prefer to be alone during breastfeeding.	Some women may be hesitant to have someone with them when their breast is exposed.	Provide privacy as desired by the mother.
§These are only a few suggestions. We do not mean to imply this is a comprehensive cultural assessment; rather, it is a tool to encourage cultural competence.		§§This column provides guidelines for further assessment and initial nursing intervention.

Postpartum Assessment: First 24 Hours After Birth (continued)

PSYCHOSOCIAL ASSESSMENT/NORMAL FINDINGS	VARIATIONS TO CONSIDER*	NURSING RESPONSES TO DATA†
Psychologic Adaptation		
During first 24 hours: passive; preoccupied with own needs; may talk about her labor and birth experience; may be talkative, elated, or very quiet (the taking-in phase)	Very quiet and passive; sleeps frequently (fatigue from long labor; feelings of disappointment about some aspect of the experience; may be following cultural expectation)	Provide opportunities for adequate rest, nutritious meals and snacks that are consistent with what the woman desires to eat and drink, and opportunities to discuss birth experience in nonjudgmental atmosphere if the woman desires to do so.
Usually by 12 hours: beginning to assume responsibility; some women eager to learn; easily feels overwhelmed (the taking-hold phase)	Excessive weepiness, mood swings, pronounced irritability (postpartum blues, feelings of inadequacy, culturally proscribed behavior)	Explain postpartum blues; provide supportive atmosphere. Determine support available for mother. Consider referral for evidence of profound depression.
Attachment		
En face position, holds baby close, cuddles and soothes, calls by name, identifies characteristics of family members in newborn, may be awkward in providing care. Initially may express disappointment over gender or appearance of baby but within 1–2 days demonstrates attachment behaviors.	Continued expressions of disappointment with gender, appearance of baby; refusal to care for baby; derogatory comments; lack of bonding behaviors (difficulty in attachment, following expectations of cultural/ethnic group)	Provide reinforcement and support for newborn caregiving behaviors; maintain nonjudgmental approach and gather more information if caregiving behaviors are not evident.
Patient Education		
Has basic understanding of self-care activities and newborn care needs; can identify signs of complications that should be reported.	Unable to demonstrate basic self-care and newborn care activities (deficient knowledge; postpartum blues; following prescribed cultural behavior; may be cared for by grandmother or other family member)	Identify predominant learning style. Determine whether woman understands English, and provide interpreter if needed. Provide reinforcement of information through conversation and written material (remember that some women and their families may not be able to understand written materials because of language difficulties or inability to read). Provide information regarding newborn/infant care skills that are culturally consistent. Give woman an opportunity to express her feelings. Consider social service home referral for women who have no family or other support, are unable to take in information about self-care and baby care, and demonstrate no caregiving activities.
	*Possible causes of alterations are identified in parentheses.	†This column provides guidelines for further assessment and initial nursing actions.

with feeding behaviors? How much of this ability and willingness to respond is related to the baby's nature and how much to her own?

- Does the woman state that she is pleased with her baby's appearance and gender? Is she reporting experiencing pleasure during interactions with her newborn? What interferes with the enjoyment? Does she speak to the baby frequently and affectionately? Does she call him or her by name? Does she point out family traits or characteristics she sees in the newborn?

- Are there any cultural factors that might modify the mother's response? For instance, is it customary for the

grandmother to assume most of the child care responsibilities while the mother recovers from childbirth?

When these questions have been addressed and the facts assembled, the nurse's intuition and knowledge should combine to answer three more questions:

1. Is there a problem in attachment?
2. If so, what is the problem?
3. What is its source?

The nurse can then devise a creative approach to the problem as it presents itself in the context of a unique, developing mother–newborn relationship.

Diagnosis

Typical diagnoses related to the mother's needs may include any of the following:

- *Urinary Elimination, Impaired*
- *Breastfeeding, Ineffective*
- *Constipation*
- *Pain, Acute*
- *Sleep Pattern, Disturbed*

(NANDA-I © 2014)

The postpartum family's needs, which should be identified during assessment, are also frequently used for developing nursing diagnoses. Examples of these diagnoses include the following:

- *Deficient Knowledge* related to information about newborn/infant care
- *Anxiety* related to role transition
- *Family Processes, Readiness for Enhanced*

(NANDA-I © 2014)

Planning

Goals for care may include:

- The mother will demonstrate bonding with newborn as evidenced by using the *en face* position.
- The mother will meet the baby's needs as they arise.
- The mother will demonstrate adequate self-care to meet her needs as they arise.
- The mother will seek assistance as needed to care for self and newborn.
- The mother's physical condition returns to a nonpregnant state.
- The mother will gain competence in caregiving and confidence in herself as a parent.

Implementation

Care of the mother during the postpartum period requires a great deal of patient teaching in order to prepare her for discharge.

Provide Patient Teaching

An important component of postpartum nursing care is patient teaching, which must be individualized to the learning capability and readiness of the parents. Meeting the educational needs of the new mother and her family can be challenging. Each woman's educational needs will depend on her age, background, educational level, experience, and expectations. However, because the mother spends only a brief period of time in the postpartum area, it can be difficult for the nurse to identify and address individual instructional needs. Effective education provides the childbearing family with sufficient knowledge to meet many of its own health needs and to seek assistance if necessary. The nurse should have the mother exercise her choices when possible and support those choices, with the help of cultural awareness and a sound knowledge base (see Focus on Diversity and Culture: Postpartum Care).

The nurse first assesses the learning needs of the new mother through observation, sensitivity to nonverbal cues,

Focus on Diversity and Culture
Postpartum Care

In many cultures, women and their families may embrace practices involving rest, seclusion, and dietary restraint, designed to assist the woman and her baby during the period of postpartum vulnerability. Chou (2017) notes a systematic review of over 50 studies concluded that globally, most cultures identify a specified postpartum period, ranging 7 and 42 days, in which these practices are common threads. In some cultures, there is also a period of seclusion which coincides with the period of lochial flow or postpartum bleeding. It should be noted that there are multifaceted variables that formulate a woman's personal beliefs and while cultural traditions will vary, the period of physiological recovery appears to coincide with the need for physical recovery in most cultures (Chou, 2017).

and tactfully phrased questions. For example, "What plans have you made for handling things when you get home?" may elicit a response of several words and provide the opportunity for some information sharing and guidance. Some agencies also use checklists of common concerns for new mothers. The woman can check the concerns that are of interest to her.

Teaching during the postpartum period is a continuous process in which the nurse takes opportunities during interactions with the new parents to identify learning opportunities and offer teaching interventions. The nurse can also plan and implement teaching in a logical, nonthreatening way based on knowledge of and respect for the family's cultural values and beliefs. Unless the nurse believes a culturally related activity would be harmful, it can be supported and encouraged.

Nurses need to consider the mother's physical and psychosocial needs when conducting postpartum teaching. Initially, the woman may be exhausted from the birth experience, and her concentration may be impaired. Later, the new mother may be preoccupied with visitors and phone calls. Information should be delivered a little at a time and repeated to make sure that the parents understand what the nurse has discussed with them. Repetition is a valuable tool in the postpartum environment. In addition, many women are discharged during the first 48 hours after birth, making postpartum education difficult.

When the nurse is performing teaching sessions, the schedule of the woman's partner must also be considered. If the partner returns to work during the immediate postpartum period, teaching sessions in the late afternoon or early evening may be more convenient. In some cultures, such as the Hispanic culture, female relatives often assist the new mother and baby, so it is important to include any care providers in the teaching session.

Postpartum units use a variety of instructional methods, including handouts, formal classes, videos, and individual interaction. Printed materials are helpful for new mothers to consult if questions arise at home. Some facilities offer a hotline service that new mothers can call with questions or concerns. As the cultural diversity in the United States continues to grow, the need for culturally competent information is imperative. Along with culturally diverse material, teaching aids should be presented in the woman's native language when possible. Written materials should be available, and translators or language lines should be used. Many patients are now accustomed to using the internet and may prefer to visit support groups and access educational materials online. As technology expands, the nurse must remain current with the changing technology and the resources it creates. Evaluation of learning may also take several forms, such as return demonstrations, question-and-answer sessions, and even formal evaluation tools. Follow-up phone calls after discharge provide additional evaluative information and continue the helping process for the family.

Teaching content should include information on role changes and psychologic adjustments as well as skills. Risk factors and signs of postpartum depression should be reviewed with every woman. Information is also essential for women with specialized educational needs, such as mothers who have had a cesarean birth, parents of twins, parents of a newborn with congenital anomalies, parents with other young children, parents with a child who will require long-term hospitalization, and so on. More and more women with disabilities are now having children, and they may require additional support and education. Anticipatory guidance can help prepare parents for the many changes they will experience with a new family member.

Following discharge, various services are available in most communities to meet the needs of the postpartum family. These services range from educational, such as classes on nutrition, exercise, newborn/infant care, and parenting, to specific healthcare programs, such as well-baby checks, immunization clinics, family-planning services, new-mother support groups, and more. Some are offered by private caregivers, whereas others are the domain of city, county, state, or federal agencies. In all cases, the goal is to help ensure that all family members have the opportunity to meet healthcare needs, regardless of their resources.

Home healthcare is an important form of community-based nursing care offered to postpartum families. Home care visits and phone contacts help ensure that new parents have the necessary skills and resources to care for their baby.

Promote Comfort and Well-Being

The nurse can promote and restore maternal physical well-being by monitoring uterine status, vital signs, cardiovascular status, elimination patterns, nutritional needs, sleep and rest, and learning needs. Some women also require medication to relieve pain, treat anemia, provide immunity to rubella, and prevent development of antibodies in the nonsensitized Rh-negative woman. To promote immunization status, the CDC (2014a) recommends that postpartum patients receive TdaP, and, depending on the time of year, the flu vaccine as indicated. Most postpartum women need nursing interventions to promote their comfort and relieve stress.

>> Go to **Pearson MyLab Nursing and eText** for Chart 12: Essential Information for Common Postpartum Drugs.

It is important to ask the woman if she believes any special measures will be particularly effective and to offer her choices when possible. It is also important to remember that in some cultures or religions, such as Orthodox Judaism, women are prohibited from certain activities during the Sabbath, such as turning on electric lights and signing consent forms, and may need assistance with opening the wrappers of sanitary pads, tearing toilet paper, and using the call button to summon the nurse. The nurse and patient should discuss this prior to the start of the Sabbath.

Focus on Integrative Health
Lysine

Lysine, an essential amino acid, has been identified as a supplement that decreases the incidence of pain following an episiotomy. Lysine is available as a supplement. The recommended adult dosage is 12 mg/kg per day. It is also present in dietary sources, including meat, cheese, fish, eggs, soybeans, and nuts.

Many nursing interventions are available for the relief of perineal discomfort. Before selecting a method, the nurse needs to assess the perineum to determine the degree of edema and other problems. Application of ice to an episiotomy can promote comfort. The warmth of the water in the sitz bath provides comfort, decreases pain, and promotes circulation to the tissues, which promotes healing and reduces the incidence of infection. Gel pads, ice packs, and cool sitz baths have been found to be effective in reducing perineal edema and reducing the response of nerve endings that cause perineal discomfort (Brincat et al., 2015).

Complementary health approaches such as the use of lysine may be helpful in decreasing discomfort associated with an episiotomy (see Focus on Integrative Health: Lysine). In addition, patient teaching is imperative to promote healing of the perineum following delivery (see Patient Teaching: Perineal Care).

Some mothers experience hemorrhoidal pain after giving birth. Relief measures include the use of sitz baths, topical anesthetic ointments, rectal suppositories, or witch hazel pads applied directly to the anal area. The woman may be taught to digitally replace external hemorrhoids back into

Patient Teaching
Perineal Care

Many women do not consider the episiotomy to be a surgical incision. Discussion helps them understand the importance of good wound care.

- Describe the process of wound healing. Discuss the risk of contamination of the episiotomy or laceration repair by bacteria from the anal area.
- Explain techniques that are used to keep the episiotomy clean and promote healing, such as
  a. sitz bath, or
  b. use of a peribottle following each voiding or defecation. Wash with soap and water at least once every 24 hours. Change peripads at least four times per day.
- Demonstrate correct use of the peribottle or sitz bath if necessary.
- Describe comfort measures:
  a. Ice pack, glove, or tea pad immediately following birth
  b. Sitz bath
  c. Judicious use of analgesics or topical anesthetics
  d. Tightening buttocks before sitting
- Identify signs of suture line infection. Advise the woman to contact her caregiver if infection develops.
- Encourage discussion, and provide printed handouts. Some of this content may also be covered during a small postpartum class.

Patient Teaching
Common Postpartum Concerns

Several postpartum occurrences cause special concern for mothers. The nurse will frequently be asked about the following events:

Source of Concern	Explanation
Gush of blood that sometimes occurs when she first arises	Result of normal pooling of blood in the vagina when the woman lies down to rest or sleep. Gravity causes blood to flow out when she stands.
Passing clots	Blood pools at the top of the vagina and forms clots that are passed upon rising or sitting on the toilet.
Night sweats	Normal physiologic occurrence that results as the body attempts to eliminate excess fluids that were present during pregnancy. May be aggravated by a plastic mattress pad.
Afterpains	More common in multiparas. Caused by contractions and relaxation of uterus. Increased by oxytocin and breastfeeding. Relieved with mild analgesics and time.
"Large stomach" after birth and failure to lose all weight gained during pregnancy	The baby, amniotic fluid, and placenta account for only a portion of the weight gained during pregnancy. The remainder takes approximately 6 weeks to lose. Abdomen also appears large because of decreased muscle tone. Postpartum exercises will help.

her rectum. Hand washing to prevent contamination to the vagina is essential. The woman may also find it helpful to maintain a side-lying position when possible and to avoid prolonged sitting. The mother is encouraged to maintain an adequate fluid intake, and stool softeners are administered to ensure greater comfort with bowel movements. Mothers should be advised to avoid straining with bowel movements, because this can increase the severity and discomfort associated with hemorrhoids. The hemorrhoids usually disappear a few weeks after birth if the woman did not have them before her pregnancy.

To reduce afterpains, the nurse can suggest that the woman lie prone, with a small pillow under her lower abdomen, and explain that the discomfort may feel intensified for approximately 5 minutes but then diminishes greatly, if not completely. The prone position applies pressure to the uterus and, therefore, stimulates contractions. When the uterus maintains a constant contraction, the afterpains cease. Additional nursing interventions include a sitz bath (for warmth), positioning, ambulation, or administration of an analgesic agent. For breastfeeding mothers, an analgesic administered 30 minutes to an hour before nursing helps promote comfort and enhances maternal–newborn interaction.

Discomfort may be caused by immobility. The woman who has been in stirrups or has pulled back on her legs for an extended period of time may experience muscular aches from such extreme positioning. It is not unusual for women to experience joint pains and muscular pain in both arms and legs, depending on the effort exerted during the second stage of labor. Early ambulation is encouraged to help reduce the incidence of complications, such as constipation and thrombophlebitis. It also helps promote a feeling of general wellbeing. The nurse provides information about ambulation and the importance of monitoring any signs of dizziness or weakness. Despite best efforts by the nurse to teach the mother about postpartum care and anticipated changes following delivery, certain occurrences may cause concern for mothers (see Patient Teaching: Common Postpartum Concerns).

Enhance Attachment

The first few hours—and even minutes—after birth are an important period for the attachment of mother and newborn.

If contact can occur during the first hour after birth, the newborn will be in a quiet state and able to interact with parents by looking at them. Newborns also turn their heads in response to a voice. If possible and desired by the mother, the nurse may place the newborn on the woman's chest so that she can directly see her baby (**Figure 33–59 »**). This early interaction, particularly skin-to-skin contact between mother and baby, promotes attachment, early breastfeeding, and family interaction.

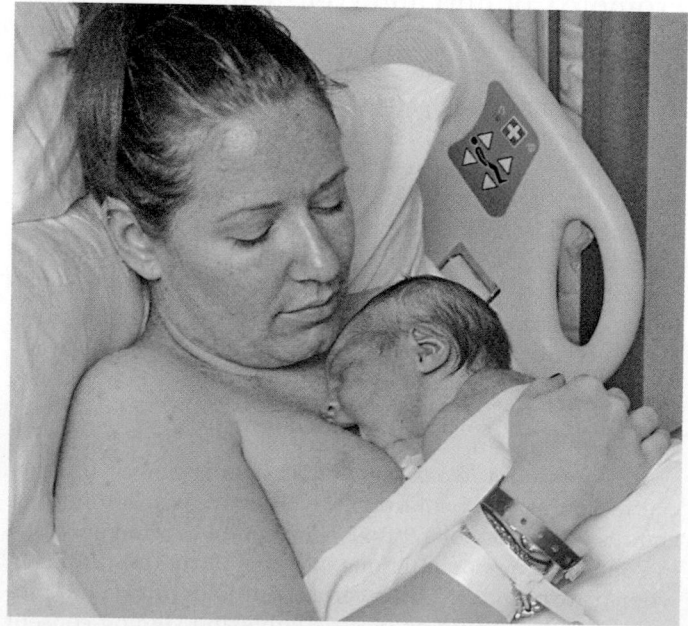

Source: Courtesy of Brigitte Hall, RNC, MSN, IBCLC.

Figure 33–59 » Mother and newborn skin-to-skin.

The first parent–newborn contact may be brief (a few minutes), and it may be followed by a more extended contact after the mother completes other uncomfortable procedures (expulsion of the placenta and suturing of the episiotomy or laceration). When the newborn is returned to the mother, the nurse can assist her to begin breastfeeding if the woman so desires. The baby may seek out the mother's breast, and early contact between mother and newborn can greatly affect breastfeeding success. Even if the newborn does not actively nurse, he or she can lick, taste, and smell the mother's skin. This activity by the newborn stimulates the maternal release of prolactin, which promotes the onset of lactation. These early interactions are associated with greater breastfeeding success.

Darkening the birthing room by turning out most of the lights causes newborns to open their eyes and gaze around. This in turn enhances eye-to-eye contact with the parents. (*Note:* If the healthcare provider needs a light source, the spotlight can be left on.) Treatment of the newborn's eyes with antibiotic eye ointment may also be delayed up to an hour after birth (AAP, 2016a). Many parents who establish eye contact with the newborn are content to quietly gaze at their baby. Others may show more active involvement by touching or inspecting the newborn. Some mothers talk to their babies in a high-pitched voice, which seems to be soothing to newborns. Some couples verbally express amazement and pride when they see they have produced a beautiful, healthy baby. Their verbalization enhances feelings of accomplishment and ecstasy.

Encourage both parents to do whatever they feel most comfortable doing. Some parents prefer only limited contact with the newborn immediately after birth and, instead, desire private time together in a quiet environment. In spite of the current zeal for providing immediate attachment opportunities, nursing personnel need to be aware of parents' wishes. The desire to delay interaction with the newborn does not necessarily imply a decreased ability of the parents to bond with their newborn.

Discuss Suppression of Lactation

For the woman who chooses not to breastfeed, lactation may be suppressed by mechanical inhibition. Although signs of engorgement do not usually appear until the second or third day postpartum, engorgement is best prevented by beginning mechanical methods of lactation suppression as soon as possible after birth. Ideally, this involves having the woman begin wearing a supportive, well-fitting bra within 6 hours after birth. Some women may prefer a tight-fitting sports bra. The woman should wear the bra continuously until lactation is suppressed (usually 5–7 days) and remove it only to shower. The bra provides support and eases the discomfort that can occur with tension on the breasts because of fullness. Ice packs should be applied over the axillary area of each breast for 20 minutes four times daily. This practice should begin soon after birth. In addition, ice is useful in relieving discomfort if engorgement occurs.

The nurse should advise the mother to avoid any stimulation of her breasts by her baby, herself, breast pumps, or her sexual partner until the sensation of fullness has passed. Such stimulation increases milk production and delays the suppression process. Heat is avoided for the same reason; therefore, the mother is encouraged to let shower water flow over her back rather than her breasts.

Some mothers may inquire about suppression medications used in the past for nonnursing mothers. The nurse should inform these patients that because of concerns related to side effects, such medications are no longer used. Mechanical, rather than pharmacologic, methods are now employed.

Relieve Emotional Stress

The birth of a child, with the changes in role and the increased responsibilities it produces, is a time of emotional stress for the new mother. During the early postpartum period, the mother may be emotionally labile; mood swings and tearfulness are common. Initially the mother may repeatedly discuss her experiences of labor and birth. This allows the mother to integrate her experiences. If she believes that she did not cope well with labor, she may have feelings of inadequacy and may benefit from reassurance that she did well. Some women feel that they did not have any perception of time during the labor and birth and want to know how long it really lasted, or they may not remember the entire experience. In this case, it is helpful for the nurse to talk with the woman and provide the information that she is missing and desires.

During this time, the new mother must also adjust to the loss of her fantasized child and accept the child she actually has. This task may be more difficult if the child is not of the desired gender or if the baby has birth defects. Women who gave birth prematurely may experience guilt or have feelings of inadequacy. Immediately after the birth (the taking-in period), the mother is focused on bodily concerns and may not be fully ready to learn about personal and newborn care. Following the initial dependent period, the mother becomes very concerned about her ability to be a successful parent (the taking-hold period). During this time, the mother requires reassurance that she is effective. She also tends to be receptive to teaching and demonstration designed to assist her in mothering successfully.

The depression, weepiness, and "let-down feeling" that characterize the postpartum blues are often a surprise for the new mother. She requires reassurance that these feelings are normal, an explanation of why they occur, and a supportive environment that permits her to cry without feeling guilty. The Edinburgh Postnatal Depression Scale (EPDS) (see Box 28–4 in the exemplar on Postpartum Depression in the module on Mood and Affect) is a widely used, validated screening tool that provides the nurse with clear information differentiating normal postpartum adjustment from postpartum depression. It consists of a 10-item questionnaire in which each patient response is given a score from 0 to 3. A total score greater than 12 is strongly associated with depression and indicates a need for intervention (Roy-Burne, 2016). See the exemplar on Postpartum Depression in the module on Mood and Affect for an in-depth discussion of postpartum depression.

Promote Rest

Energy is needed to make the psychologic adjustments to a new baby and to assume new roles, so it is helpful for the new mother to know that fatigue may persist for several weeks or even months. Although most new mothers feel tired, if they have perceived the pregnancy and birth as a natural process, they tend to view themselves as healthy and well. Mothers who have other children may feel overwhelmed trying to meet the needs of the larger family.

Physical fatigue can affect other adjustments and functions of the new mother as well. For example, fatigue can reduce milk flow, thereby increasing problems with establishing breastfeeding. Persistent fatigue is especially common when mothers attempt to perform activities while the baby is napping instead of resting themselves. The nurse teaches women that failure to get adequate rest can lead to chronic fatigue and should be avoided. Fatigue can be a symptom of postpartum depression and should be discussed with the healthcare provider if symptoms continue or are accompanied by other signs of depression. Severe ongoing fatigue can also be a symptom of a thyroid disorder and should be evaluated by a healthcare provider (Gabbe et al., 2012).

Most mothers view the postpartum period as a time for recuperation. In many non-Western cultures, the 40 days following the birth are a time of recovery, when female relatives or friends assist the new mother in her daily activities (Zerwekh & Garneau, 2014). In Mexico, during the first 7 days, non–household members are not permitted to visit or enter the home. Mothers receive help with housework and eat special foods. It is recommended that they not be exposed to wind, and bathing is prohibited.

Specific groups of mothers at a higher risk for postpartum fatigue include the following:

- Mothers of multiples
- Mothers with babies who are still hospitalized and who engage in multiple trips to the hospital to visit their babies
- Mothers of newborns with birth defects or special needs
- Mothers who lack social and familial support
- Mothers who return to work before the advised 6-week time period
- Mothers who have been on extended bedrest during the pregnancy.

Discuss Sexual Activity and Contraception

Typically, postpartum couples resume sexual intercourse once the episiotomy is healed and the lochial flow has stopped (Leeman & Rogers, 2012). Because this usually occurs by the end of the third week, before the 6-week follow-up, it is important that the woman and her partner have

Evidence-Based Practice
Optimizing Adherence to the Postpartum Plan of Care

Problem

In the weeks following birth, the plan for postpartum care may become fragmented among healthcare providers due to inconsistent communication between the inpatient and outpatient settings. As a result, as many as 40% of women do not attend a postpartum visit (ACOG, 2016c).

Evidence

The postpartum visit provides the opportunity for the patient and the healthcare provider to discuss both physical and psychosocial concerns, to establish a plan for contraception, and to determine which healthcare provider will assume primary care. In addition, a full physical examination is conducted, including a gynecologic exam, Pap smear, breast exam, and evaluation of general health after delivery (Haran et al., 2014). Women diagnosed with gestational diabetes, hypertensive disorders of pregnancy, or preterm birth should be counseled about these disorders and the associated risks for future pregnancies. The postpartum visit provides an opportunity for women to ask questions about their labor experience, the childbirth process, and any complications that may have occurred (ACOG, 2016c).

Implications

The American College of Obstetricians and Gynecologists (ACOG, 2016c) make the following recommendations regarding optimizing postpartum care:

- Provide anticipatory guidance during antenatal visits to initiate the postpartum plan of care
- Establish a single healthcare provider to assume responsibility for coordinating the woman's postpartum care, including contact information and written instructions
- Discuss pregnancy complications with respect to risks for future pregnancies and recommendations to optimize maternal health

- Emphasize the need for early postpartum follow-up for women with hypertensive disorders and other complications of pregnancy
- Explain the need for a comprehensive postpartum visit within the first 6 weeks after birth, including a full assessment of physical, social, and psychologic well-being
- Establish a system to ensure that women who desire long-acting reversible contraception, or any other form of contraception, receive it during the postpartum visit
- Recommend anticipatory guidance at the postpartum visit that includes newborn/infant feeding, expressing breast milk if returning to work or school, postpartum weight retention, sexuality, physical activity, and nutrition
- Determine who will assume primary responsibility for the woman's ongoing care (Ob-Gyn or other healthcare provider)

Critical Thinking Application

1. Do you have any biases that may hinder your ability to provide adequate anticipatory guidance for optimization of postpartum care? Think about a variety of situations that may present opportunities for bias, including caring for patients of different cultures and spiritual backgrounds, patients from different age groups, patients from different sexual orientations and marital status, and patients experiencing dysfunctional family dynamics.

2. How will you act as an advocate for a woman who chooses to either breastfeed or bottle feed her baby?

3. How would you approach postpartum teaching about contraceptives for a 17-year-old single mother and a 27-year-old married mother with two children?

4. What are some strategies to improve adherence to the postpartum plan of care? Consider the nurse–patient relationship and how it relates to communication, patient teaching, and collaboration.

information about what to expect. The nurse may inform the couple that because the vaginal vault is "dry" (lacking estrogen), some form of water-soluble lubrication, such as K-Y jelly or Astroglide, may be necessary during intercourse. The woman-superior and side-lying coital positions may be preferable, because they allow the woman to control the depth of penile penetration. Couples should be counseled that intercourse may be uncomfortable for the woman for some time and that patience is imperative.

Breastfeeding couples should be cautioned that during orgasm, milk may spurt from the nipples because of the release of oxytocin. Some couples find this spurt to be pleasurable or amusing, but others choose to have the woman wear a bra during sexual activity. Nursing the baby before lovemaking reduces the chance of milk release.

Other factors may inhibit satisfactory sexual experiences. For example, the baby's crying may be a distraction, the woman's changed body may seem unattractive to her or her partner, maternal sleep deprivation may reduce the woman's desire, or the woman's physiologic response to sexual stimulation may be altered because of hormonal changes. By 3 months postpartum, many couples return to prepregnant levels of sexual interest and activity; however, this is highly variable. It is not abnormal for women, especially when breastfeeding, to experience decreased libido for several months. Decreased libido can be associated with hormonal changes, fatigue, stress, and lack of time because of family and work demands.

With anticipatory guidance during the prenatal and postpartum periods, the couple can be forewarned of potential temporary problems. Anticipatory guidance is enhanced if the couple can discuss their feelings and reactions as they experience them.

》 Go to **Pearson MyLab Nursing and eText** for Chart 13: Resuming Sexual Activity After Childbirth.

Information on contraception should be provided as part of discharge teaching if it is permissible within the healthcare agency. The nurse can also be an important resource for the woman and her partner during postpartum follow-up. Couples typically choose to use contraception to control the number of children they will have or to determine the spacing of future children. Some religious-based hospital facilities prohibit nurses and other healthcare providers from discussing contraception. If the nurse is discussing birth control, it is important to emphasize that in choosing a specific method, consistency of use is essential. The nurse needs to identify the advantages, disadvantages, risks, and contraindications of the various methods to help the couple, or the single mother, make an informed choice about the most practical and compatible method. Breastfeeding women are commonly concerned that a contraceptive method will interfere with their ability to breastfeed. Breastfeeding women should be given available options and choose the method that best fits their lifestyle, financial situation, and personal preference.

Promote Well-being After Cesarean Birth

The mother who has a cesarean birth usually does extremely well postoperatively. Most women are ambulating by the day after the surgery. By the second postpartum day, the woman usually can shower, which seems to provide a mental as well as physical lift. Most women are discharged by the third day after birth.

The chances of pulmonary infection, however, are increased after a cesarean birth because of immobility after the use of narcotics and sedatives and because of the altered immune response in postoperative patients. Therefore, nurses should encourage the woman to cough and deep breathe every 2–4 hours while awake until she is ambulating frequently.

Nurses should also encourage leg exercises every 2 hours until the woman is ambulating. These exercises increase circulation, help prevent thrombophlebitis, and aid intestinal motility by tightening abdominal muscles.

Many of the complications that historically occurred after a cesarean birth were related to postpartum care practices in which mothers were encouraged to stay in bed for prolonged periods of time. Early ambulation, eating a low-roughage diet shortly after birth, and breastfeeding or newborn feeding soon after birth all enhance the recovery of the mother and decrease complications in the postoperative period. Even though a cesarean birth is an operative procedure, most women giving birth are relatively healthy and, therefore, are less likely to experience postoperative complications when compared with other surgical patients.

The nurse monitors and manages the woman's pain experience during the postpartum period. Sources of pain include incisional pain, gas pain, referred shoulder pain, periodic uterine contractions (afterbirth pains), discomfort related to breastfeeding, and pain from voiding, defecation, or constipation. Nursing interventions are oriented toward preventing or alleviating pain or helping the woman cope with pain and include the following:

- Administer analgesics as needed, especially during the first 24–72 hours after childbirth. Use of analgesics relieves the woman's pain and enables her to be more mobile and active. Some facilities administer ibuprofen on a continuous basis in the early postpartum period to decrease swelling, reduce pain, and lower the need for, or frequency of, narcotic agents.

- Promote comfort through proper positioning, frequent changes of position, massage, back rubs, oral care, and reduction of noxious stimuli, such as noise and unpleasant odors.

- Encourage visits by significant others, including the newborn and older children. These visits distract the woman from the painful sensations and help reduce her fear and anxiety.

- Encourage the use of breathing, relaxation, guided imagery, and distraction (e.g., stimulation of cutaneous tissue) techniques taught in childbirth preparation class.

Epidural analgesia administered just after the cesarean birth is an effective method of pain relief for most women in the first 24 hours following birth. Other methods of pain relief that may be ordered by the physician include patient-controlled analgesia and a continuous peripheral nerve block. A continuous epidural infusion is administered via an electric pump through an epidural catheter that is left in place following birth. The device has a button the woman can depress if additional pain relief is needed. Nursing assessments are hourly for women with a continuous epidural infusion in place and include vital signs, level of pain, amount of drug received, and amount of self-administration. The tubing is inspected to ensure that connections are maintained, because movement by the woman in bed could disrupt the line. The epidural site should also be assessed to ensure that the catheter has not been displaced.

Although the use of general anesthesia continues to decline, women who receive general anesthesia warrant additional assessments in the immediate postpartum period. Vital signs should be monitored continually until the woman has regained consciousness. Cardiopulmonary equipment should be in close range, with cardiac monitoring available as needed. The pulse oximeter should be used to determine the woman's oxygen status.

If a general anesthetic was used, abdominal distention may produce marked discomfort for the woman during the first few postpartum days. Measures to prevent or minimize abdominal distention include leg exercises, abdominal tightening, ambulation, avoiding carbonated or very hot or cold beverages, and avoiding the use of straws. Medical intervention for gas pain includes using rectal suppositories and enemas to stimulate passage of flatus and stool and encouraging the woman to lie on her left side. Lying on the left side allows the gas to pass from the descending colon to the sigmoid colon so that it can be expelled more readily.

Many physicians also order a nonsteroidal anti-inflammatory drug (NSAID) in addition to the previously mentioned agents once the woman is tolerating oral fluids well. NSAIDs assist with decreasing inflammation and do not have the negative side effects associated with many narcotics, such as sedation and constipation. NSAIDs are often given in combination with narcotic agents during the immediate postpartum period and often result in a decreased intake of narcotic agents.

Sometimes, women who have a cesarean birth have other discomforts that can be relieved with pharmacologic interventions. The nurse assesses the woman for other symptoms, such as nausea, itching (typically related to the morphine used in the epidural), and headache. If the woman is experiencing nausea, an antiemetic can be administered. Itching can also be relieved with pharmacologic interventions. NSAIDs are effective in managing headaches and other body aches.

The nurse can minimize discomfort and promote satisfaction as the mother assumes the activities of her new role. Instruction and assistance in assuming comfortable positions when holding or breastfeeding the baby will do much to increase the mother's sense of competence and comfort. The nurse should teach the woman to splint her incision when she ambulates to decrease pulling on the incision and the discomfort created by contraction of the abdominal muscles.

Other measures are aimed at needs that are unique to the woman who has had an operative birth. These measures include the following:

- Assess for the return of bowel sounds in all four quadrants every 4 hours, and assess the consistency of the abdomen. Women with a firm, distended abdomen may have difficulty passing flatus or stool.
- Assess the intravenous site, flow rate, and patency of the intravenous tubing.
- Monitor the condition of surgical dressings or the incision site using the REEDA scale (redness, edema, ecchymosis, discharge, and approximation of the suture line) along with skin temperature at and around the incision line.

Provide Care for the Woman Who Places Newborn for Adoption

Women who choose to place their babies for adoption are more likely to be single, Caucasian, never married adolescents than Hispanic or African American women of any age. The majority of women who relinquish their children have higher education and income levels, higher future educational or career goals, and mothers and fathers who favor adoption. Still others may feel that they are not emotionally ready for the responsibilities of parenthood, or their partner may strongly disapprove of the pregnancy. These and many other reasons may prompt the woman to relinquish her baby. The number of women who give their babies up voluntarily, however, is shrinking because of an increase in the acceptability of single motherhood and teenage parenting (Martin et al., 2015). Less than 1% of all births in the United States result in an adoption (Center for American Progress, 2015).

Increasingly, babies are being placed in foster care because of the mother's illicit drug use, past history of abusing children, or incarceration. The number of babies placed for adoption because of these circumstances is unknown, but several factors must be met, including clear evidence that the parent is unfit and that severing the parental rights is in the best interest of the child (Child Welfare Information Gateway, 2013a). Many of these babies may be placed with relatives or in long-term foster care.

In the 1990s, a number of babies were abandoned and left to die because the mothers did not want them and did not want others to know of their pregnancies. Starting in 1997, Infant Safe Haven Acts were passed that provided a means for a mother to place her baby up for adoption anonymously. The legislation was enacted to protect newborns from death caused by abandonment. Today, all 50 states plus the District of Columbia and Puerto Rico have legislation in place to ensure that relinquished babies are left with safe providers who can care for them and provide medical services. The relinquishing mother is protected from prosecution for neglect or abandonment under the law (Child Welfare Information Gateway, 2013b).

The mother who places her baby for adoption usually experiences intense ambivalence. Several factors contribute to this. First, there are social pressures against giving up one's child. In addition, the woman has usually made considerable adjustments in her lifestyle to carry and give birth to this child, and she may be unaware of the growing bond between her and her child. Her attachment feelings may peak upon seeing her baby. At the same time, she may not have told friends and relatives about the pregnancy and, therefore, may lack a support system to help her work through her feelings and support her decision making. After childbirth, the mother needs to complete a grieving process to work through her loss and its accompanying grief, loneliness, guilt, and other feelings. Mothers who relinquish their newborns and have open adoptions experience less grief than those who have closed adoptions (Castle, 2012). When the relinquishing mother is admitted to the birthing unit, the nurse should be informed about the mother's decision to relinquish the baby. The nurse needs to respect any special requests for the birth and encourage the woman to express her emotions. After the birth, the mother should be allowed access to the baby; she is the one who will decide whether she wants to see the newborn. Seeing the newborn often aids in the grieving process and provides an opportunity for the birth mother to say good-bye. When the mother sees her baby, she may feel strong attachment and love. The nurse needs to assure the woman that these feelings do not mean that her decision to relinquish the child is wrong; relinquishment is often a painful act of love.

Postpartum nursing care also includes arranging ongoing care for the relinquishing mother. Some mothers may request an early discharge or a transfer to another medical unit. When possible, the nurse supports these requests.

Evaluation

Anticipated outcomes of comprehensive nursing care of the postpartum family include the following:

- The mother is reasonably comfortable and has learned pain relief measures.

- The mother is rested and understands how to add more activity during the next few days and weeks.

- The mother's physiologic and psychologic well-being have been supported.

- The mother verbalizes her understanding of self-care measures.

- The new parents demonstrate how to care for their baby.

- The new parents have had opportunities to form attachment with their baby.

- The new parents have information and access to community resources. This includes adoptive and relinquishing parents.

An additional purpose of care evaluation is to determine if further care is needed based on the postpartum family's outcomes. If the outcomes are not being met, the nurse may choose to continue or revise the plan of care for optimal outcome attainment (see Nursing Care Plan: A Postpartum Patient).

Nursing Care Plan
A Postpartum Patient

Cathy McGhee delivered Callie, a healthy girl, 4 days ago. At the time of birth, Ms. McGhee was able to put the newborn to breast within the first hour. Callie was very alert at birth, latching on without difficulty. Ms. McGhee was able to breastfeed successfully during the remainder of her hospital stay. Today, Ms. McGhee has returned to the clinic complaining of pain and swelling in both breasts and a low-grade fever. She has also had trouble getting Callie to latch on.

ASSESSMENT	DIAGNOSIS	PLANNING
Subjective: Breast pain and tenderness, anxiety Objective: Temperature 38°C (100.4°F). Breast tissue is firm, warm, and skin is shiny and taut. Swelling in axillary area and flattened nipples.	■ *Acute Pain* related to increased breast fullness secondary to increased blood supply to breast tissue causing swelling of tissue around milk ducts (NANDA-I © 2014)	■ The patient will remain free of breast fullness and pain. ■ The patient will experience decreased swelling of breast tissue. ■ The patient will exhibit no signs of breast tenderness or firmness.

IMPLEMENTATION

- Instruct woman to breastfeed frequently.
- Instruct woman to breastfeed at least 10–15 minutes on each breast per feeding.
- Assist woman to pre-express milk onto nipple or baby's lips.
- Initiate pumping or manually express milk at the beginning of the feeding.

- Instruct woman to pump, hand express, or massage to empty breast when feedings are missed.
- Administer analgesics before breastfeeding.
- Apply warm and/or cold compresses before breastfeeding.
- Apply fresh cabbage leaves to the breast between feedings.

EVALUATION

- No evidence of swelling found in breast tissue.
- Pain has decreased.

- Breast tissue is soft and without tenderness.

CRITICAL THINKING

1. The nurse preparing Ms. McGhee for discharge notices that Callie was breastfed 3 hours ago but for only 3–4 minutes on each breast. Ms. McGhee states that the baby is very sleepy and has slept most of the day. She says she will wait to breastfeed again until she is home and more comfortable, because her breasts hurt and are swollen. The nurse assesses the woman's breasts, which are firm and tender, with some swelling under the arm. What should the nurse instruct the patient to do before discharge? What can Ms. McGhee do to minimize the breast fullness and discomfort?

2. A postpartum nurse is teaching a breastfeeding class to new mothers. During the class, one woman states she had a problem with engorgement after the birth of her first child and wants to know what she can do differently this time in order to avoid the problem again. What strategies can the nurse suggest to help prevent engorgement?

REVIEW Postpartum Care

RELATE Link the Concepts and Exemplars

Linking the exemplar of postpartum care with the concept of family:

1. What challenges would you anticipate for the new family following the delivery of twins or triplets?

2. How might you assess a family's ability to incorporate a newborn into the family unit?

Linking the exemplar of postpartum care with the concept of stress and coping:

3. What stressors must the mother of a newborn cope with after discharge?

4. How do these stressors impact the risk for child abuse? What nursing implementations and strategies can the nurse offer the new family to reduce this risk?

READY Go to Volume 3: Clinical Nursing Skills

READY Go to Pearson MyLab Nursing and eText

- Additional review materials
- Chart 10: Factors That Slow Uterine Involution
- Chart 11: Uterine Stimulants Used to Prevent and Manage Uterine Atony
- Chart 12: Essential Information for Common Postpartum Drugs
- Chart 13: Resuming Sexual Activity After Childbirth

REFLECT Apply Your Knowledge

Jessica Riley is a single, 18-year-old mother with a 1-year-old son, Ryan. Jessica has had no contact with Ryan's father since before Ryan was born. Jessica and Ryan live in a small, one-bedroom apartment with Jessica's boyfriend, Casey. She is currently pregnant with Casey's baby.

Jessica took the evening off from work because she was feeling very tired. She fixes dinner for Casey before he has to go to work. While she is fixing dinner, Ryan begins crying in the other room, and Jessica interrupts making dinner to attend to his needs.

When they all finally sit down to eat, Casey throws his plate against the wall and screams at her for making a "lousy dinner." He then proceeds to yank her out of her chair, hit her in the back, and knock her to the floor. She gets up crying, and he hits her in the abdomen and says, "You care more about these damn brats than me and what I want." She falls to the floor, and he kicks her in the abdomen. Jessica screams in

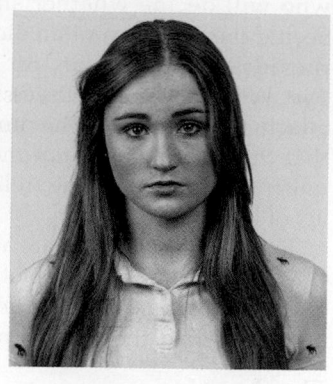

pain. She somehow gets off the floor and makes it into the bedroom. The neighbor in the next apartment hears the commotion and calls the police.

When the police arrive, they find Jessica on the bed doubled over and crying, Ryan in his crib crying, and Casey watching TV while smoking a joint. The police note that Jessica is pregnant and call for an ambulance. They ask her whether she was hit, and she tells them no. The police tell Jessica they are taking Casey in for drug possession and further questioning. Jessica calls her mother and asks her to come get Ryan and then meet her at the hospital.

When the paramedics arrive, they start an intravenous line, place Jessica on oxygen, and transport her to the hospital. At the hospital, the OB triage nurse sends her directly to the labor and delivery unit. Jessica delivers a healthy baby girl later in the evening. Because Jessica sustained a small abruption to the placenta, the midwife and physician suspect trauma from abuse.

In the immediate postpartum period, the midwife talks with Jessica privately. Jessica is told that she had a small abruption and that the placenta had an infarct. The midwife tells Jessica that in these situations, trauma is suspected. The midwife also shares with Jessica that sometimes women in abusive relationships get hit or kicked in the abdomen. Jessica cries and admits to the midwife that this is what happened, but she insists that Casey didn't mean to do it and is sure he will never do it again. She tells the midwife she will not press charges.

Social work is called for referral before Jessica goes home. The nurse midwife tells Jessica that a social work referral is required because of the risk of intimate partner violence and drug charges against Casey. Jessica worries about this, fearing that Casey will be angry. The social worker makes a visit the day after Jessica and the baby are discharged; Jessica is relieved that Casey is not home. Jessica tells the social worker everything is fine and that there are really no problems.

1. As the nurse caring for Jessica, what nursing diagnosis would be appropriate for the plan of care?

2. What risks to parental attachment do you anticipate for Jessica and her new daughter?

3. Create a teaching plan for Jessica before discharge.

» Exemplar 33.D
Newborn Care

Exemplar Learning Outcomes

33.D Summarize care of newborns.

- Summarize the adaptations of the newborn to extrauterine life.
- Outline alterations found in newborns.
- Summarize collaborative therapies used by interprofessional teams for newborns with alterations.
- Illustrate the nursing process in providing culturally competent care to the newborn.

Exemplar Key Terms

Acrocyanosis, 2356
Active acquired immunity, 2364
Apgar score, 2374
Barlow maneuver, 2391
Brazelton Neonatal Behavioral Assessment Scale, 2393
Caput succedaneum, 2386
Cephalohematoma, 2385
Chemical conjunctivitis, 2386

Overview

The newborn (neonatal) period is the time from birth through the 28th day of life. During this period, the newborn adjusts from intrauterine to extrauterine life. The transition from fetus to newborn is the most complex physiologic adaptation that occurs in the human experience and involves virtually every organ system of the body (Hillman, Kallapur, & Jobe, 2012). The nurse needs to be knowledgeable about a newborn's normal physiologic and behavioral adaptations and be able to recognize alterations.

Adaptations to Extrauterine Life

The first 6 hours of life, in which the newborn's body systems adapt to extrauterine life, is called the period of **neonatal transition**. The respiratory and cardiac systems undergo the most dramatic changes within the first minutes after birth.

Respiratory Adaptations

To begin life as a separate being, the newborn must immediately establish respiratory gas exchange in conjunction with marked circulatory changes. These radical and rapid changes are crucial to the maintenance of extrauterine life.

Initiation of Respiration

To maintain life, the lungs must function immediately after birth. Two changes are necessary for this to happen:

1. Pulmonary ventilation must be established through lung expansion.
2. A marked increase in the pulmonary circulation must occur.

The first breath of life—the gasp in response to mechanical and reabsorptive, chemical, thermal, and sensory changes associated with birth—initiates the serial opening of the alveoli. So begins the transition of the newborn from a fluid-filled environment to an air-breathing, independent, extrauterine life. **Figure 33–60 》** summarizes the initiation of respiration.

During the latter half of gestation, the fetal lungs continuously produce fluid. This fluid expands the lungs almost completely, filling the air spaces. Production and maintenance of a normal volume of fetal lung fluid are essential for normal lung growth (Fraser, 2014). Through intermittent fetal breathing movements, the fetus practices respiration, develops the chest wall muscles and the diaphragm, and regulates lung fluid volume. Some of the lung fluid moves up into the trachea and into the amniotic fluid; it is then swallowed by the fetus.

During delivery, the fetal chest is compressed, increasing intrathoracic pressure and squeezing a small amount of the fluid out of the lungs. After the birth of the newborn's trunk, the chest wall recoils. This chest recoil creates a negative intrathoracic pressure, which is thought to produce a small, passive inspiration of air that replaces the fluid in the large airways that is squeezed out.

After this first inspiration, the newborn exhales, with crying, against a partially closed glottis, creating positive intrathoracic pressure. The high positive intrathoracic pressure distributes the inspired air throughout the alveoli and begins to establish functional residual capacity (FRC), which is the air left in the lungs at the end of a normal expiration. The higher intrathoracic pressure also increases absorption of fluid via the capillaries and lymphatic system. The negative intrathoracic pressure created when the diaphragm moves down with inspiration causes lung fluid to flow from the alveoli across the alveolar membranes into the pulmonary interstitial tissue.

At birth, the alveolar epithelium is temporarily more permeable. This permeability, combined with decreased cellular resistance at the onset of breathing, may facilitate passive liquid absorption. With each succeeding breath, the lungs continue to expand, stretching the alveolar walls and increasing the alveolar volume.

Protein molecules are too large to pass through capillary walls. The presence of more protein molecules in the pulmonary capillaries than in the interstitial tissue creates oncotic pressure. This pressure draws the interstitial fluid into the capillaries and lymphatic tissue to balance the concentration of protein. Lung expansion helps the remaining lung fluid move into the interstitial tissue. As pulmonary vascular resistance decreases, pulmonary blood flow increases, and more interstitial fluid is absorbed into the bloodstream. In the healthy term newborn, lung fluid moves rapidly into the

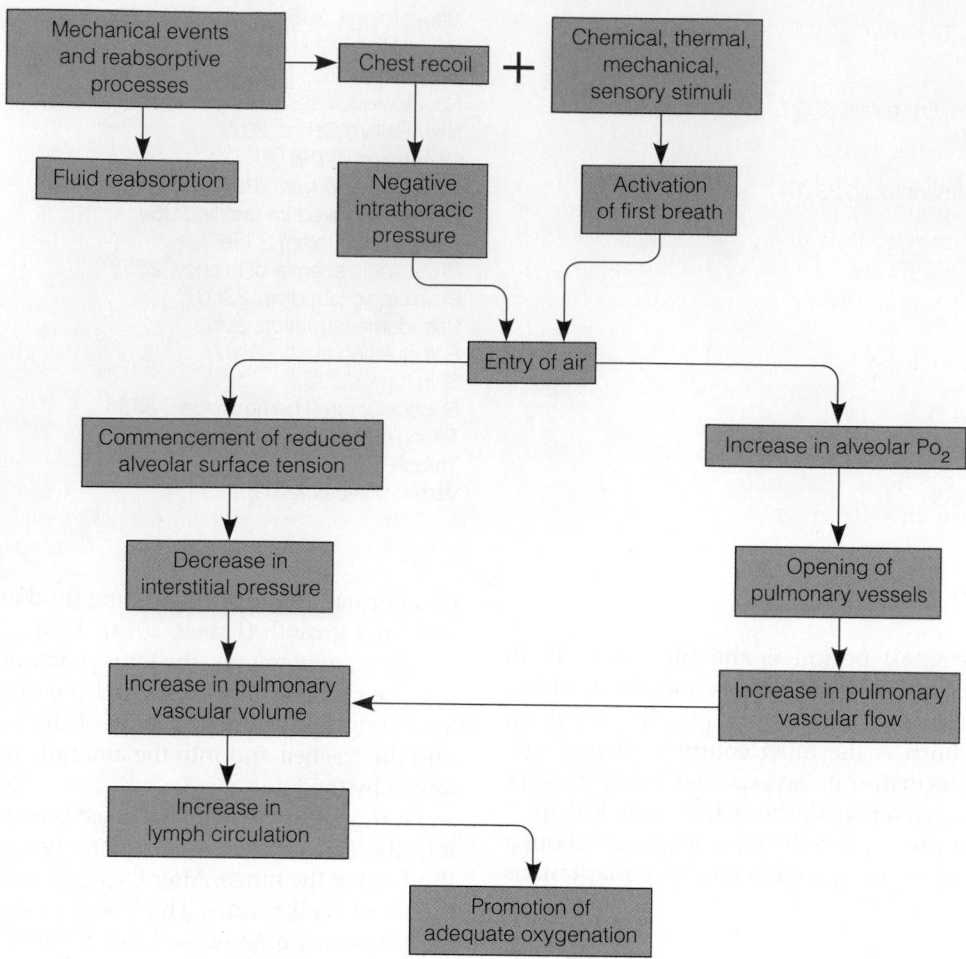

Figure 33–60 ⟫ Initiation of respiration in the newborn.

interstitial tissue, but it may take several hours to move into the lymph and blood vessels. By 30 minutes of age most newborns have a normal FRC with uniform lung expansion. Surfactant is essential for a normal FRC (Rosenberg, 2013).

Although the initial chest recoil assists in clearing the airways of accumulated fluid and permits further inspiration, most healthcare providers believe mucus and fluid should be suctioned from the newborn's mouth, nose, and throat. These providers use a bulb syringe to suction the mouth and nose as soon as the newborn's head and shoulders are delivered and again as the newborn adapts to extrauterine life and stabilizes.

Newborns may have problems clearing the fluid in the lungs and beginning respiration for a variety of reasons:

- The lymphatic system may be underdeveloped, thus decreasing the rate at which the fluid is absorbed from the lungs.

- Complications may occur before or during labor and birth that interfere with adequate lung expansion; thus, the decrease in pulmonary vascular resistance fails to occur, resulting in decreased pulmonary blood flow. These complications include the following:

  a. Inadequate compression of the chest wall in very small newborns (small for gestational age or very low birth weight) because of immature muscular development

  b. The absence of chest wall compression in a neonate born by cesarean birth, although this compression can be externally applied by skilled healthcare providers as they deliver the newborn from the uterus

  c. Respiratory depression because of maternal analgesia or anesthesia agents

  d. Aspiration of amniotic fluid, meconium, or blood.

Several chemical factors contribute to the onset of breathing. One of the most important is asphyxia of the fetus and newborn. The first breath is an inspiratory gasp, the result of central nervous system (CNS) reaction to sudden pressure, temperature change, and other external stimuli. This first breath is triggered by the slight elevation in partial pressure of carbon dioxide and decrease in pH and partial pressure of oxygen (PO_2), which are the natural result of a vaginal labor and birth. These changes, which are present in all newborns to some degree, stimulate the aortic and carotid chemoreceptors, initiating impulses that trigger the medulla's respiratory center. Although this brief period of asphyxia is a significant stimulator, prolonged asphyxia is abnormal and depresses respiration. Early cord clamping before the initiation of respirations may result in reflex bradycardia and the need for resuscitative efforts (Gruneberg & Crozier, 2015). As a result, it is appropriate for newborns to vigorously cry and be active before the cord is clamped or the placenta separates.

A significant decrease in environmental temperature after birth, from 37°C to between 21° and 23.9°C (98.6°F to 70°–75°F), results in sudden chilling of the moist newborn (Blackburn, 2013). The cold stimulates skin nerve endings, and the newborn responds with rhythmic respirations. Normal temperature changes that occur at birth are within acceptable physiologic limits. Excessive cooling may result in profound respiratory depression and evidence of cold stress.

Upon birth the newborn experiences light, new sounds, and the full effects of gravity for the first time. As the fetus moves from the womb's familiar, comfortable, and quiet environment to one of sensory abundance, a number of physical and sensory influences help respiration begin. These stimuli include the following:

- The actual experience of birth, with its numerous tactile, auditory, and visual stimuli
- Joint movement, which results in enhanced proprioceptor stimulation to the respiratory center to sustain respirations
- Thorough drying of the newborn and placing the baby on the mother's chest and abdomen for skin-to-skin contact provides ample stimulation in a comforting way and also decreases heat loss.

Factors Opposing Initiation of Respiration

Three major factors may inhibit the initiation of respiratory activity:

- The contracting force between alveoli (alveolar surface tension)
- Viscosity of lung fluid within the respiratory tract, which is influenced by surfactant levels
- The ease with which the lungs are able to fill with air (lung compliance).

Alveolar surface tension is the contracting force between the moist surfaces of the alveoli. This tension, which is necessary for healthy respiratory function, would nevertheless cause the small airways and alveoli to collapse between each inspiration were it not for the presence of surfactant. By reducing the attracting force between alveoli, surfactant prevents the alveoli from completely collapsing with each expiration and thus promotes lung expansion. Similarly, surfactant promotes lung compliance (the ability of the lung to fill with air easily). When surfactant decreases, compliance also decreases. Decreased compliance, combined with the small radii of the newborn's airway, results in an increase in the pressure needed to expand the alveoli with air.

The first breath usually establishes a functional residual capacity that is 30–40% of the fully expanded lung volume. This functional residual capacity allows alveolar sacs to remain partially expanded on expiration, decreasing the need for continuous high pressures for each of the following breaths. Subsequent breaths require only 6–8 cm H_2O of pressure to open alveoli during inspiration. Therefore, the first breath of life is usually the most difficult.

Cardiopulmonary Physiology

As air enters the lungs, PO_2 rises in the alveoli, which stimulates the relaxation of the pulmonary arteries and triggers a decrease in pulmonary vascular resistance. As pulmonary vascular resistance decreases, the vascular flow in the lung increases rapidly and achieves 100% normal flow at 24 hours of life. This delivery of greater blood volume to the lungs contributes to the conversion from fetal circulation to newborn circulation.

After pulmonary circulation is established, blood is distributed throughout the lungs, although the alveoli may or may not be fully open. For adequate oxygenation to occur, the heart must deliver sufficient blood to functional, open alveoli. Shunting of blood is common in the early newborn period. Bidirectional blood flow, or right-to-left shunting through the ductus arteriosus, may divert a significant amount of blood away from the lungs, depending on the pressure changes of respiration, crying, and the cardiac cycle. This shunting in the newborn period is also responsible for the unstable transitional period in cardiopulmonary function.

Oxygen Transport

The transportation of oxygen to the peripheral tissues depends on the type of hemoglobin in the red blood cells (RBCs). In the fetus and newborn, a variety of hemoglobins exist, the most significant being fetal hemoglobin (HbF) and adult hemoglobin (HbA). Approximately 70–90% of the hemoglobin in the fetus and newborn is of the fetal variety. The greatest difference between HbF and HbA relates to the transport of oxygen.

Because HbF has a greater affinity for oxygen than does HbA, the oxygen saturation in the newborn's blood is greater than that in the adult's, but the amount of oxygen available to the tissues is less. This situation is beneficial prenatally because the fetus must maintain adequate oxygen uptake in the presence of very low oxygen tension (umbilical venous PO_2 cannot exceed uterine venous PO_2). However, this high concentration of oxygen in the blood makes hypoxia in the newborn particularly difficult to recognize. Clinical manifestations of cyanosis (bluish discoloration of skin and mucous membranes) do not appear until low blood levels of oxygen are present. In addition, alkalosis (increased pH) and hypothermia can result in less oxygen being available to the body tissues, whereas acidosis, hypercarbia, and hyperthermia can result in less oxygen being bound to hemoglobin and more oxygen being released to the body tissues. (See the module on Acid–Base Balance.)

Maintaining Respiratory Function

The lung's ability to maintain oxygenation and ventilation (the exchange of oxygen and carbon dioxide) is influenced by such factors as lung compliance and airway resistance. Lung compliance is influenced by the elastic recoil of the lung tissue and anatomic differences in the newborn. The newborn has a relatively large heart and mediastinal structures that reduce available lung space. Also, the newborn chest is equipped with weak intercostal muscles and a rigid rib cage, with horizontal ribs and a high diaphragm, which restrict the space available for lung expansion. The large abdomen further encroaches on the high diaphragm to decrease lung space. Another factor that limits ventilation is airway resistance, which depends on the radii, length, and number of airways. Airway resistance is increased in the newborn compared with that in adults.

Characteristics of Newborn Respiration

Initial respirations may be largely diaphragmatic, shallow, and irregular in depth and rhythm. The abdomen's movements are synchronous with the chest movements. When the breathing pattern is characterized by pauses lasting 5–15 seconds, **periodic breathing** is occurring. Periodic breathing is rarely associated with differences in skin color or heart rate changes, and it has no prognostic significance. Tactile or other sensory stimulation increases the inspired oxygen and converts periodic breathing patterns to normal breathing patterns during neonatal transition. With deep sleep, the pattern is reasonably regular. Periodic breathing occurs with rapid-eye-movement (REM) sleep, and grossly irregular breathing is evident with motor activity, sucking, and crying. Cessation of breathing lasting more than 20 seconds is defined as apnea and is abnormal in term newborns. Apnea may or may not be associated with changes in skin color or bradycardia (drop below 100 beats/min). Apnea always needs to be further evaluated.

Newborns tend to be obligatory nose breathers: The nasal route is the primary route of air entry because of the high position of the epiglottis and the position of the soft palate (Blackburn, 2013). Although many term newborns can breathe orally, nasal obstructions can cause respiratory distress. Therefore, it is important to keep the nose and throat clear.

Immediately after birth, and for approximately the next 2 hours, respiratory rates of 60–70 breaths/minute are normal.

Some cyanosis and **acrocyanosis** (bluish discoloration of hands and feet) are normal for several hours; thereafter, the newborn's color improves steadily. If respirations drop below 30 or exceed 60 breaths/min when the neonate is at rest, or if retractions, cyanosis, or nasal flaring and expiratory grunting occur, the healthcare provider should be notified. Any increased use of the intercostal muscles (retractions) may indicate respiratory distress, which should be reported immediately.

Cardiovascular Adaptations

During fetal life, blood with higher oxygen content is diverted to the heart and brain. Blood in the descending aorta is less oxygenated and supplies the kidney and intestinal tract before it is returned to the placenta. Limited amounts of blood, pumped from the right ventricle toward the lungs, enter the pulmonary vessels. In the fetus, increased pulmonary resistance forces most of this blood through the ductus arteriosus into the descending aorta.

>> Go to **Pearson MyLab Nursing and eText** to see Chart 14: Fetal and Neonatal Circulation.

Marked changes occur in the cardiovascular system at birth. Expansion of the lungs with the first breath decreases pulmonary vascular resistance and increases pulmonary blood flow. Pressure in the left atrium increases as blood returns from the pulmonary veins. Pressure in the right atrium drops, and systematic vascular resistance increases as umbilical venous blood flow is halted when the cord is clamped. These physiologic mechanisms mark the transition from fetal to neonatal circulation and show the interplay of cardiovascular and respiratory systems (**Figure 33–61** >>).

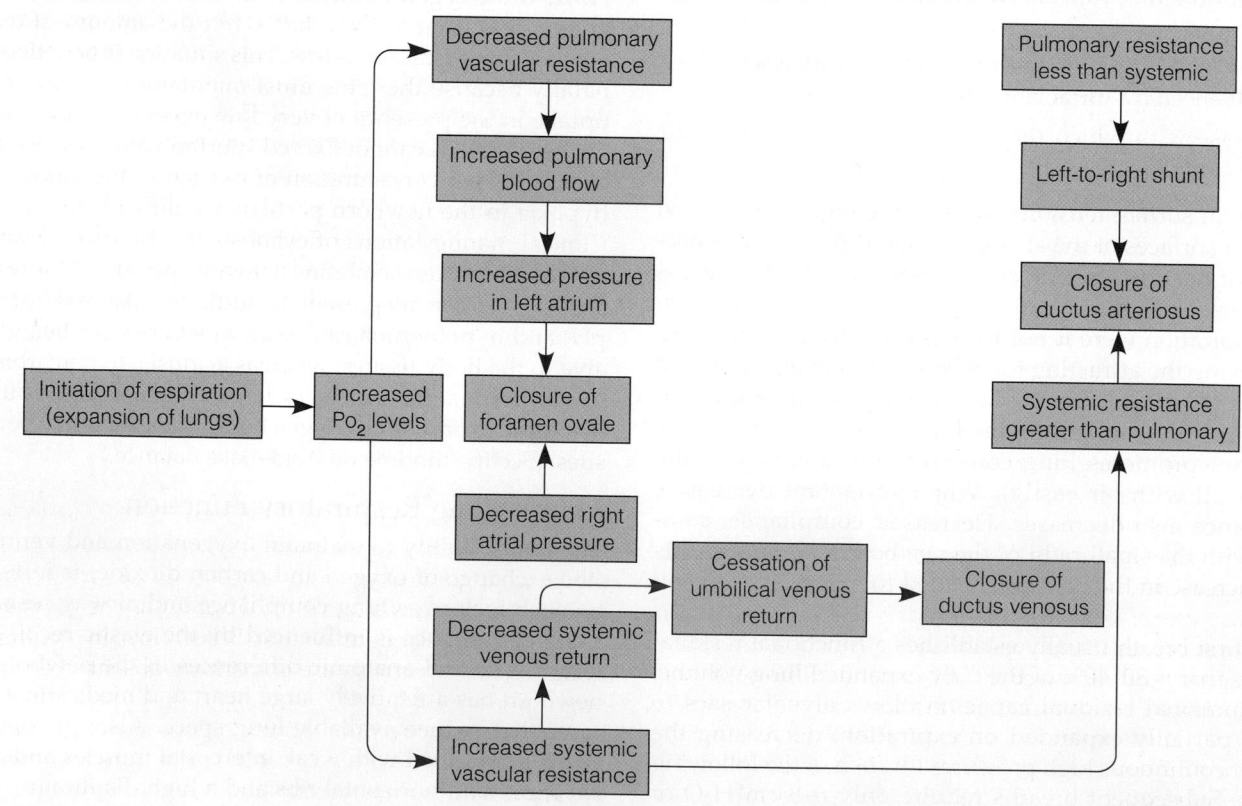

Figure 33–61 >> Transitional circulation: conversion from fetal to neonatal circulation.

Five major areas of change occur in cardiopulmonary adaptation:

1. ***Increased aortic pressure and decreased venous pressure.*** Clamping of the umbilical cord eliminates the placental vascular bed and reduces the intravascular space. Consequently, aortic (systemic) blood pressure increases. At the same time, blood return via the inferior vena cava decreases, resulting in a decreased right atrial pressure and a small decrease in pressure within the venous circulation.

2. ***Increased systemic pressure and decreased pulmonary artery pressure.*** With loss of the low-resistance placenta, systemic resistance pressure increases, resulting in greater systemic pressure. At the same time, lung expansion increases pulmonary blood flow, and the increased blood PO_2 associated with initiation of respirations dilates pulmonary blood vessels. The combination of vasodilation and increased pulmonary blood flow decreases pulmonary artery resistance. As the pulmonary vascular beds open, the systemic vascular pressure increases, enhancing perfusion of the other body systems.

3. ***Closure of the foramen ovale.*** Closure of the foramen ovale is a function of changing atrial pressures. In utero, pressure is greater in the right atrium, and the foramen ovale is open after birth. Decreased pulmonary resistance and increased pulmonary blood flow increase the pulmonary venous return into the left atrium, thereby increasing left atrial pressure slightly. The decreased pulmonary vascular resistance and the decreased umbilical venous return to the right atrium also decrease right atrial pressure. The pressure gradients across the atria are now reversed, with the left atrial pressure now greater, and the foramen ovale is functionally closed 1–2 hours after birth. However, a slight right-to-left shunting may occur in the early newborn period. Any increase in pulmonary resistance or right atrial pressure, such as occurs with crying, acidosis, or cold stress, may cause the foramen ovale to reopen, resulting in a temporary right-to-left shunt. Anatomic closure occurs within 30 months (Blackburn, 2013).

4. ***Closure of the ductus arteriosus.*** Initial elevation of the systemic vascular pressure above the pulmonary vascular pressure increases pulmonary blood flow by reversing the flow through the ductus arteriosus. Blood now flows from the aorta into the pulmonary artery. Furthermore, although the presence of oxygen causes the pulmonary arterioles to dilate, an increase in blood PO_2 triggers the opposite response in the ductus arteriosus—that is, it constricts.

   In utero, the placenta provides prostaglandin E_2, which causes ductus vasodilation. With the loss of the placenta and increased pulmonary blood flow, prostaglandin E_2 levels drop, leaving the active constriction by PO_2 unopposed. If the lungs fail to expand or if PO_2 levels drop, the ductus remains patent. Functional closure starts within 18 hours after birth, and fibrosis of the ductus occurs within 2–3 weeks after birth (Blackburn, 2013; Fraser, 2014).

5. ***Closure of the ductus venosus.*** Although the mechanism initiating closure of the ductus venosus is not known, it appears to be related to mechanical pressure changes after severing of the cord, redistribution of blood, and cardiac output. Closure of the bypass forces perfusion of the liver. Fibrosis of the ductus venosus occurs within 2 months.

Assessment of the newborn's heart rate, blood pressure, heart sounds, and cardiac workload provides data for evaluating cardiac function. The newborn's blood pressure tends to be highest immediately after birth and then descends to its lowest level at about 3 hours of age. By days 4–6, the blood pressure rises and then plateaus at a level approximately the same as the initial level. Blood pressure is sensitive to the changes in blood volume that occur in the transition to newborn circulation. Peripheral perfusion pressure is a particularly sensitive indicator of the newborn's ability to compensate for alterations in blood volume before changes in blood pressure. Capillary refill should be less than 3 seconds when the skin is blanched.

Blood pressure values during the first 12 hours of life vary with the birth weight and gestational age. The average mean blood pressure is 31–61 mmHg in the full-term, resting newborn over 3 kg (6.6 lb) during the first 12 hours of life (Gomella, 2013). Crying may cause an elevation of in both the systolic and diastolic blood pressure; thus, accuracy is more likely in the quiet newborn. Currently two-point pulse oximetry (right hand and either foot) is recommended to screen for congenital heart disease. An SpO_2 of <95% needs to be referred to a cardiology clinic (Bradshaw et al., 2012; Goetz & Hokanson, 2011).

Shortly after the first cry and the start of changes in cardiopulmonary circulation, the newborn heart rate can accelerate to 180 beats/min. The average resting heart rate in the first week of life is 110 to 160 beats/min in a healthy full-term newborn but may vary significantly during deep sleep or active awake states. In full-term newborns, the heart rate may drop to a low of 80 to 100 beats/min during deep sleep (Van Woudenberg, Wills, & Rubarth, 2012).

Murmurs are produced by turbulent blood flow. Murmurs may be heard when blood flows across an abnormal valve or across a stenosed valve, when an atrial or ventricular septal defect is present, or when the flow across a normal valve is increased.

In newborns, 90% of all murmurs are transient and not associated with anomalies. These murmurs usually involve incomplete closure of the ductus arteriosus or foramen ovale. Soft murmurs may be heard as the pulmonary branch arteries increase their blood flow from 7% to 50% of the combined ventricular output during transition, causing a physiologic peripheral pulmonary stenosis. Clicks may normally be heard at the lower left sternal border as the great vessels dilate to accommodate systolic blood flow in the first few hours of life. Murmurs are sometimes absent even in seriously malformed hearts.

Before birth, the right ventricle does approximately two thirds of the cardiac work, resulting in increased size and thickness of the right ventricle at birth. In the first 2 hours after birth, when the ductus arteriosus remains mostly patent, about one third of the left ventricular output is returned to the pulmonary circulation. As a result, the left ventricle has a significantly greater increase in volume load than the right ventricle after birth, and it needs to progressively increase in both size and thickness. This may explain why right-sided heart defects are better tolerated than left-sided ones and why left-sided heart defects rapidly become symptomatic after birth.

Hematopoietic Adaptations

In the first days of life, hematocrit may rise 1–2 g/dL above fetal levels as a result of placental transfusion, low oral fluid intake, and diminished extracellular fluid volume. By 1 week after birth, peripheral hemoglobin is comparable to fetal blood counts. The hemoglobin level declines progressively over the first 2 months of life (Blackburn, 2013). This initial decline in hemoglobin creates a phenomenon known as **physiologic anemia of infancy**. A factor that influences the degree of physiologic anemia is the nutritional status of the newborn. Supplies of vitamin E, folic acid, and iron may be inadequate given the amount of growth in the later part of the first year of life. Hemoglobin values fall, mainly from a decrease in red cell mass rather than from the dilutional effect of increasing plasma volume. The facts that red cell survival is lower in newborns than in adults and that red cell production is less also contribute to this anemia. Neonatal RBCs have a lifespan of 60–70 days, approximately one-half to two-thirds the lifespan of adult RBCs (Bagwell, 2014). The normal RBC count in a term newborn is in the range of 5.1–5.3 million per milliliter during the first 24–48 hours of life (Bagwell, 2014).

Leukocytosis is a normal finding, because the stress of birth stimulates increased production of neutrophils during the first few days of life. Neutrophils then decrease to 35% of the total leukocyte count by 2 weeks of age. Lymphocytes play a role in antibody formation and eventually become the predominant type of leukocyte, and the total WBC count falls.

Blood volume is approximately 85 mL/kg for a term neonate (Diab & Luchtman-Jones, 2015). For example, a 3.6-kg (8-lb) newborn has a blood volume of 306 mL. Blood volume varies based on the amount of placental transfusion received during the delivery of the placenta as well as other factors, including the following:

- Delayed cord clamping and the normal shift of plasma to the extravascular spaces
- Gestational age
- Prenatal and/or perinatal hemorrhage
- Site of the blood sample.

SAFETY ALERT Laboratory results may vary between capillary collection and venous collection. Greater variances can be expected if capillary collection was difficult or good blood flow was not obtained and the heel was squeezed excessively, which increases the risk of cellular damage within the specimen, increased serum levels, and micro blood clots.

Temperature Regulation

Newborns are homeothermic: They attempt to stabilize their internal (core) body temperatures within a narrow range in spite of significant temperature variations in their environment.

Thermoregulation in the newborn is closely related to the rate of metabolism and oxygen consumption. Within a specific environmental temperature range, called the **neutral thermal environment (NTE)**, the rates of oxygen consumption and metabolism are minimal, and internal body temperature is maintained because of thermal balance (Blackburn, 2013). Thus, the normal newborn requires higher environmental temperatures to maintain a thermoneutral environment.

Several newborn characteristics affect the establishment of thermal stability:

- The newborn has a thinner epidermis and less subcutaneous fat than an adult.
- Blood vessels in the newborn are closer to the skin than the blood vessels of an adult. Therefore, the circulating blood is influenced by changes in environmental temperature and, in turn, influences the hypothalamic temperature-regulating center.
- The flexed posture of the term newborn decreases the surface area exposed to the environment, thereby reducing heat loss.
- Shivering, a form of muscular activity that generates body heat, is common in the cold adult, but is rarely seen in the newborn.

Size and age may also affect the establishment of an NTE. For example, the small-for-gestational-age newborn has less adipose tissue and is hypoflexed and, therefore, requires higher environmental temperatures to achieve an NTE. Larger, well-insulated newborns may be able to cope with lower environmental temperatures. If the environmental temperature falls below the lower limits of the NTE, the newborn responds with increased oxygen consumption and metabolism, which results in greater heat production. As a result, prolonged exposure to the cold may result in depleted glycogen stores and acidosis. Oxygen consumption also increases if the environmental temperature is above the NTE.

A newborn is at a distinct disadvantage in maintaining a normal temperature. With a large body surface in relation to mass and a limited amount of insulating subcutaneous fat, the term newborn loses heat at about four times the rate of an adult. The newborn's poor thermal stability is primarily because of excessive heat loss rather than impaired heat production. Because of the risk of hypothermia and possible cold stress, minimizing heat loss in the newborn after birth is essential (see Evidence-Based Practice: Thermoregulation and Heat Loss Prevention in Newborns). This topic is covered in more detail in the module on Thermoregulation.

Hepatic Adaptations

In the newborn, the liver is frequently palpable 2–3 cm (0.8–1.2 in.) below the right costal margin. It is relatively large and occupies approximately 40% of the abdominal cavity. The newborn liver plays a significant role in iron storage, carbohydrate metabolism, conjugation of bilirubin, and coagulation. Additional essential functions of the liver include the production of bile, regulation of plasma proteins and glucose, and the biotransformation of drugs and toxins. The neonate has less than 20% of the hepatocytes that are

Evidence-Based Practice
Thermoregulation and Heat Loss Prevention in Newborns

Problem

What is the best way to support thermoregulation in the newborn immediately after birth?

Evidence

Newborns have several risk factors for hypothermia after birth: a large surface-to-mass ratio, minimal subcutaneous tissue, and wet skin. The challenge of thermoregulation is increased if the newborn is low birth weight, preterm, or sick. Cold stress can lead to harmful side effects or even death. Several systematic reviews of research on newborn thermoregulation have been published by professional groups interested in neonatal health: AWHONN, the American College of Nurse Midwives, and the American College of Pediatricians (Lunze & Hamer, 2012; Moore et al., 2012; Turnbull & Petty, 2013). These reviews have focused on healthy newborns as well as on newborns at risk. Multiple systematic reviews of multisite, randomized trials provide the strongest level of evidence for nursing practice.

Skin-to-skin contact of the newborn with its mother after birth is recommended as the mainstay of thermoregulation for most healthy newborns. When placed skin to skin, the baby gets heat directly from its mother via conduction. Skin-to-skin care is associated with both short- and long-term benefits, and it has been shown to be an effective method of thermoregulation for babies as small as 1200 g. For smaller babies, or babies who are too ill to be placed on their mother's skin, resuscitation and other treatments may allow evaporative heat loss. Prewarming the delivery suite to 80°F and placing the newborn in a plastic bag up to the neck during physiologic stabilization prevents heat loss in high-risk babies. Heated mattresses are also effective in preventing hypothermia.

While plastic barriers have been shown to avoid hypothermia in high-risk newborns, no studies have demonstrated that these interventions reduce the long-term risk of death, brain injury, mean duration of oxygen therapy, or hospitalization. Some barrier methods (e.g., occlusive dressings) result in hyperthermia. Continuous monitoring of the newborn's body temperature should accompany any of the heat loss barrier methods.

Implications

Family-centered birth care provides the best environment for the newborn, including support of thermoregulation. You can avoid hypothermia in healthy newborns by drying the baby with a towel, placing the bare newborn in direct contact with the mother's bare skin, and placing a blanket over them both. Babies who are too small or too sick for skin-to-skin contact should be dried, placed on a heated mattress, and wrapped in plastic wrap up to the neck. A small cut can be made in the plastic for access to the umbilicus. In the case of plastic barriers, continuous monitoring of the baby's temperature is necessary to avoid overheating. Temperature can be continuously monitored using a temperature probe on the newborn's skin connected to a monitoring device.

Critical Thinking Application

1. Discuss the evidence related to thermoregulation with skin-to-skin contact immediately after birth.
2. Identify nursing interventions that promote thermoregulation in the newborn.
3. Describe complications of cold stress in each physiologic system in the newborn.

---

present in the adult liver, and liver growth continues after birth until it reaches its mature size.

Iron Storage

As RBCs are destroyed after birth, the iron is stored in the liver until needed for new RBC production. Newborn iron stores are determined by total body hemoglobin content and length of gestation. The term newborn has approximately 270 mg of iron at birth, and approximately 140–170 mg of this amount is in the hemoglobin. If the mother's iron intake has been adequate, enough iron will be stored to last until the baby is about 5 months of age. After about 6 months of age, the infant requires foods containing iron or iron supplements to prevent anemia.

Carbohydrate Metabolism

At term, the newborn's cord blood glucose level is 15 mg/dL lower than the maternal blood glucose level (Rosenberg, 2013). Newborn carbohydrate reserves are relatively low. One third of this reserve is in the form of liver glycogen. Newborn glycogen stores are twice those of the adult. The newborn enters an energy crunch at the time of birth, with the removal of the maternal glucose supply and the increased energy expenditure associated with the birth process and extrauterine life. The newborn consumes fuel sources at a faster rate because of the work of breathing, loss of heat when exposed to cold, activity, and activation of muscle

tone. Glucose is the main source of energy in the first 4–6 hours after birth. During the first 2 hours of life, the serum blood glucose level declines, then rises, and finally reaches a steady state by 3 hours after birth (Rosenberg, 2013).

The nurse may assess the newborn's glucose level on admission if risk factors are present or per agency protocol. As stores of liver and muscle glycogen and blood glucose decrease, the newborn compensates by changing from a predominantly carbohydrate metabolism to fat metabolism. This allows the newborn to derive energy from fat and protein as well as from carbohydrates. The amount and availability of each of these "fuel substrates" depend on the ability of immature metabolic pathways, which lack specific enzymes or hormones, to function in the first few days of life.

Conjugation of Bilirubin

Conjugation of bilirubin is the conversion of yellow lipid-soluble pigment into water-soluble pigment. Unconjugated (indirect) bilirubin is a breakdown product derived from hemoglobin released primarily from destroyed RBCs. Unconjugated bilirubin is not in an excretable form and is a potential toxin. Total serum bilirubin is the sum of conjugated (direct) and unconjugated (indirect) bilirubin.

Fetal unconjugated bilirubin crosses the placenta to be excreted, so the fetus does not need to conjugate bilirubin. Total bilirubin at birth is usually less than 3 mg/dL unless an abnormal hemolytic process has been present in utero.

After birth, the newborn's liver must begin to conjugate bilirubin. This produces a normal rise in serum bilirubin levels in the first few days of life.

The bilirubin formed after RBCs are destroyed is transported in the blood bound to albumin. The bilirubin is transferred into the hepatocytes and bound to intracellular proteins. These proteins determine the amount of bilirubin held in a liver cell for processing and, consequently, the amount of bilirubin uptake into the liver. Direct bilirubin is excreted into the tiny bile ducts, then into the common duct and duodenum. The conjugated (direct) bilirubin then progresses down the intestines, where bacteria transform it into urobilinogen (urine bilirubin) and stercobilinogen. Stercobilinogen is not reabsorbed; rather, it is excreted as a yellow-brown pigment in the stools.

Even after the bilirubin has been conjugated and bound, it can be changed back to unconjugated bilirubin via the enterohepatic circulation. In the intestines, beta-glucuronidase enzyme acts to split off (deconjugate) the bilirubin from glucuronic acid if it has not first been acted on by gut bacteria to produce urobilinogen. The free bilirubin is then reabsorbed through the intestinal wall and brought back to the liver via portal vein circulation. This recycling of the bilirubin and decreased ability to clear bilirubin from the system are prevalent in babies with very high beta-D-glucuronidase activity levels, those who are exclusively breastfed, and those with delayed bacterial colonization of the gut (e.g., because of the use of antibiotics). Very high beta-D-glucuronidase activity levels further increase the newborn's susceptibility to jaundice (yellow pigmentation of body tissues due to high bilirubin levels).

The newborn liver has relatively less glucuronyl transferase activity in the first few weeks of life than an adult liver. This reduction in hepatic activity, along with a relatively large bilirubin load, decreases the liver's ability to conjugate bilirubin and increases susceptibility to jaundice.

Coagulation

The liver plays an important part in blood coagulation during fetal life, and it continues this function following birth. Coagulation factors II, VII, IX, and X (synthesized in the liver) are activated under the influence of vitamin K and, therefore, are considered to be vitamin K dependent. The absence of normal flora needed to synthesize vitamin K in the newborn gut results in low levels of vitamin K, which in turn results in a transient blood coagulation alteration between the second and fifth day of life. From a low point at approximately 2–3 days after birth, these coagulation factors rise slowly, but they do not approach adult levels until 9 months of age or later (Bagwell, 2014). Other coagulation factors with low umbilical cord blood levels are factors XI, XII, and XIII. Fibrinogen and factors V and VII are near adult levels. Although newborn bleeding problems are rare, an injection of vitamin K (AquaMEPHYTON) is given prophylactically on the day of birth to combat potential clinical bleeding problems.

Platelet counts at birth are in the same range as for older children, but newborns may manifest mild transient difficulty in platelet aggregation functioning. This platelet problem is accentuated by phototherapy. Prenatal maternal therapy with phenytoin sodium (Dilantin) or phenobarbital also causes abnormal clotting studies and newborn bleeding in the first

24 hours after birth. Neonates born to mothers receiving warfarin (Coumadin) compounds may bleed because these agents cross the placenta and accentuate existing vitamin K–dependent factor deficiencies; therefore, most pregnant women in need of anticoagulant therapy receive heparin, which does not cross the placental barrier (Yarrington, Valente, & Economy, 2015). Transient neonatal thrombocytopenia may occur in newborns born to mothers with severe hypertension or HELLP (*h*emolysis, *e*levated *l*iver enzymes, and *l*ow *p*latelet count) syndrome and in newborns born to mothers who have idiopathic isoimmune thrombocytopenic purpura.

Physiologic Jaundice

Physiologic jaundice (nonpathologic unconjugated hyperbilirubinemia) is caused by accelerated destruction of fetal RBCs, impaired conjugation of bilirubin, and increased bilirubin reabsorption from the intestinal tract. This condition does not have a pathologic basis but is a normal biological response of the newborn.

Muchowski (2014) describes six factors—several of which can also be related to pathologic events—whose interaction may give rise to physiologic jaundice:

1. *Increased amounts of bilirubin delivered to the liver.* The increased blood volume because of delayed cord clamping combined with faster RBC destruction in the newborn leads to an increased bilirubin level in the blood. A proportionately larger amount of nonerythrocyte bilirubin forms in the newborn. Therefore, newborns have two to three times greater production or breakdown of bilirubin than adults. The use of forceps or vacuum extraction, which sometimes causes facial bruising or cephalohematoma (entrapped hemorrhage), can increase the amount of bilirubin to be handled by the liver.

2. *Defective hepatic uptake of bilirubin from the plasma.* If the newborn does not ingest adequate calories, the formation of hepatic binding proteins diminishes, resulting in higher bilirubin levels.

3. *Defective conjugation of bilirubin.* Decreased uridine-diphosphoglucuronosyl activity, as in hypothyroidism or inadequate caloric intake, causes the intracellular binding proteins to remain saturated and results in greater unconjugated bilirubin levels in the blood. The fatty acids in breast milk are thought to compete with bilirubin for albumin-binding sites and, therefore, to impede bilirubin processing.

4. *Defective excretion of bilirubin.* A congenital infection may cause impaired excretion of conjugated bilirubin. Delay in introduction of bacterial flora and decreased intestinal motility can also delay excretion and increase enterohepatic circulation of bilirubin.

5. *Inadequate hepatic circulation.* Decreased oxygen supplies to the liver associated with neonatal hypoxia or congenital heart disease lead to a rise in the bilirubin level.

6. *Increased reabsorption of bilirubin from the intestine.* Reduced bowel motility, intestinal obstruction, or delayed passage of meconium (the first stool) increases the circulation of bilirubin in the enterohepatic pathway, thereby resulting in higher bilirubin values.

Approximately 40% of full-term newborns exhibit physiologic jaundice on about the second or third day after birth, and it may last as long as 5 days (Zaja et al., 2014). This condition does not have a pathologic basis, but rather is a normal biologic response of the newborn. The characteristic yellow color results from increased levels of unconjugated (indirect) bilirubin, which are a normal product of RBC breakdown and reflect the body's temporary inability to eliminate bilirubin. Bruising, feeding patterns, and gastrointestinal activity can influence serum bilirubin levels (Ladewig et al., 2017). Serum levels of bilirubin reach approximately 4–6 mg/dL before the yellow coloration of the skin and sclera appear. The signs of physiologic jaundice appear after the first 24 hours postnatally. This time frame differentiates physiologic jaundice from pathologic jaundice, which is clinically seen at birth or within the first 24 hours of postnatal life. Generally, physiologic jaundice is more prevalent than pathologic jaundice. Hypothermia, hypoglycemia, maternal use of medications such as sulfa drugs and salicylates, and prematurity contribute to the development of physiologic jaundice (Ladewig et al., 2017). A major risk factor for developing severe hyperbilirubinemia in term neonates is a total serum or transcutaneous level in the high-risk zone on a bilirubin nomogram. The nomogram created by Bhutani, Johnson, and Sivieri (1999) and approved by the American Academy of Pediatrics (2004) is frequently used, as are bilirubin calculation tools available via the internet.

≫ **Stay Current:** Visit www.bilitool.org to see a bilirubin calculation tool based on the nomogram by Bhutani et al. (1999).

There is no consistent definition of neonatal hyperbilirubinemia; what is considered to be in that range varies with population characteristics and age (Blackburn, 2013). Peak bilirubin levels are reached between days 3 and 5 in the full-term newborn. These values are established for European and American White newborns. Chinese, Japanese, Korean, and Native American newborns have considerably higher bilirubin levels that are not as apparent and that persist for longer periods with no apparent ill effects (Blackburn, 2013).

The nursery or postpartum room environment, including lighting, may hinder early detection of the degree and type of jaundice. Pink walls and artificial lights mask the beginning of jaundice in newborns. Daylight assists the observer in early recognition by eliminating distortions caused by artificial light.

If jaundice is suspected, the nurse can quickly assess the newborn's coloring by pressing the skin, generally on the forehead or nose, with a finger. As blanching occurs, the nurse can observe the icterus (yellow coloring).

Several newborn care procedures will decrease the probability of high bilirubin levels:

■ Maintain the newborn's skin temperature at 36.5°C (97.8°F) or above, because cold stress results in acidosis. Acidosis in turn decreases available serum albumin-binding sites, weakens albumin-binding powers, and causes elevated unconjugated bilirubin levels.

■ Monitor stool for amount and characteristics. Bilirubin is eliminated in the feces; inadequate stooling may result in reabsorption and recycling of bilirubin. Encourage early breastfeeding, because the laxative effect of colostrum increases the excretion of meconium and transitional stool.

■ Encourage early feedings to promote intestinal elimination and bacterial colonization and provide the caloric intake necessary for formation of hepatic binding proteins.

If jaundice becomes apparent, nursing care is directed toward keeping the newborn well hydrated and promoting intestinal elimination.

Physiologic jaundice may be very upsetting to parents; they require emotional support and a thorough explanation of the condition. If the baby is placed under phototherapy, a few additional days of hospitalization may be required; this may also be disturbing to parents. The nurse can encourage parents to provide for the emotional needs of their newborn by continuing to feed, hold, and caress the baby. If the mother is discharged, the parents are encouraged to return for feedings and to telephone or visit when possible. In many instances, the mother, especially if she is breastfeeding, may elect to remain hospitalized with her newborn; the nurse should support this decision. If insurance limitations make this unrealistic, it may be possible to find an empty room for the discharged mother and her family to use while visiting the newborn. As an alternative to continued hospitalization, the newborn may be treated with home phototherapy.

Breastfeeding and Breast Milk Jaundice

Breastfeeding is implicated in prolonged jaundice in some newborns. *Breastfeeding jaundice* occurs during the first days of life in breastfed newborns. It appears to be related to inadequate fluid intake with some element of dehydration and not with any abnormality in milk composition (Hardy, D'Agata, & McGrath, 2016). Prevention of early breastfeeding jaundice includes encouraging frequent (every 2–3 hours) breastfeeding, avoiding supplementation if the newborn is not dehydrated, and accessing maternal lactation counseling. Breastfeeding jaundice is self-limiting; it peaks around day 3 as enteral intake increases, then resolves.

In *breast milk jaundice*, the bilirubin level begins to rise after the first week of life, when physiologic jaundice is waning after the mother's milk has come in. The level peaks at 5–10 mg/dL at 2–3 weeks of age and then declines over the first several months of life (Hardy et al., 2016).

In contrast to breastfeeding jaundice, breast milk jaundice is related to milk composition. Some women's breast milk contains several times the normal concentration of certain free fatty acids. These free fatty acids may compete with bilirubin for binding sites on albumin and inhibit the conjugation of bilirubin or increase lipase activity, which disrupts the RBC membrane. Increased lipase activity enhances absorption of bile across the gastrointestinal tract membrane, thereby increasing the enterohepatic circulation of bilirubin. Newborns with breastfeeding jaundice appear well, and at present, development of kernicterus (toxic levels of bilirubin in the brain) has not been documented. Temporary cessation of breastfeeding may be advised if bilirubin reaches presumed toxic levels of approximately 20 mg/dL or if the interruption is necessary to establish the cause of the hyperbilirubinemia. Most providers believe that breastfeeding may be resumed once other causes of jaundice have been ruled out and as long as serum bilirubin levels remain below 20 mg/dL. In cases of breast milk jaundice, the newborn's serum bilirubin levels begin to fall dramatically within 24–36 hours after breastfeeding is discontinued. With resumption of breastfeeding, the bilirubin concentration may have a slight rise of 2–3 mg/dL, with a subsequent decline. Breastfeeding mothers need encouragement and support in their desire to breastfeed their babies, assistance and instruction regarding pumping and expressing milk during the interrupted nursing period, and reassurance that they are capable of feeding and nurturing their babies (Lauwers & Swisher, 2016). To diminish misunderstandings by mothers from a variety of cultural backgrounds, careful explanations about newborn jaundice are warranted (see Focus on Diversity and Culture: Interpreting Illness Through Cultural Beliefs).

Gastrointestinal Adaptations

The term newborn has sufficient intestinal and pancreatic enzymes to digest most simple carbohydrates, proteins, and fats. The carbohydrates requiring digestion in the newborn are usually disaccharides (lactose, maltose, and sucrose), which are split into monosaccharides (galactose, fructose, and glucose) by the enzymes of the intestinal mucosa. Lactose is the primary carbohydrate in the breastfeeding newborn and generally is easily digested and well absorbed. The only enzyme lacking in the newborn is pancreatic amylase, which remains relatively deficient during the first few months of life. Newborns have trouble digesting starches (changing more complex carbohydrates into maltose), so they should not be fed solid foods until at least 4 to 6 months of age (AAP, 2016b; Mayo Clinic, 2016).

Although proteins require more digestion than carbohydrates, they are well digested and absorbed from the newborn intestine. The newborn digests and absorbs fats less efficiently because of the minimal activity of the pancreatic enzyme lipase. The newborn excretes approximately 10–20% of the dietary fat intake, compared with 10% for the adult. The newborn absorbs the fat in breast milk more completely than the fat in cow's milk because breast milk consists of more medium-chain triglycerides and contains lipase.

Focus on Diversity and Culture
Interpreting Illness Through Cultural Beliefs

Cultural beliefs lead mothers to interpret illness within their cultural framework, especially when instructions are not given clearly or are not understood by the mother (Lauderdale, 2012; Andrews & Boyle, 2016). For example, different cultures have different beliefs and practices about activity during pregnancy. These may influence when to have the baby shower, what position the mother sleeps in, and even what foods the mother eats during pregnancy. Careful assessment of the mother's cultural beliefs and practices can minimize misunderstandings as well as negative or unrealistic maternal reactions.

By birth, the newborn has experienced swallowing, gastric emptying, and intestinal propulsion. In utero, fetal swallowing is accompanied by gastric emptying and peristalsis of the fetal intestinal tract. By the end of gestation, peristalsis becomes much more active in preparation for extrauterine life. Fetal peristalsis is also stimulated by anoxia, causing the expulsion of meconium into the amniotic fluid by more mature fetuses.

Air enters the stomach immediately after birth. The small intestine is filled with air within 2–12 hours, and the large bowel is filled within 24 hours. The salivary glands are immature at birth, and the newborn produces little saliva until about 3 months of age. The newborn's stomach has a capacity of approximately 50–60 mL. It empties intermittently, starting within a few minutes of the beginning of a feeding and ending 2–4 hours after a feeding. Bowel sounds are present within the first 30–60 minutes of birth; the newborn can successfully feed during this time. The newborn's gastric pH becomes less acidic about a week after birth and remains less acidic than that of adults for the next 2–3 months.

The cardiac sphincter is immature, as is neural control of the stomach. Therefore, some regurgitation may be noted in the newborn period. Regurgitation of the first few feedings during the first day or two of life can usually be lessened by avoiding overfeeding and by burping the newborn well both during and after the feeding.

When no other signs and symptoms are evident, vomiting is limited and ceases within the first few days of life. Continuous vomiting or regurgitation should be observed closely. If the newborn has swallowed bloody or purulent amniotic fluid, lavage of the stomach may be indicated in the term newborn to relieve the problem. Bilious vomiting is abnormal and must be evaluated thoroughly; it may represent a condition that warrants prompt surgical intervention.

Adequate digestion and absorption are essential for newborn growth and development. If optimal nutritional support is available, postnatal growth should parallel intrauterine growth; that is, after 30 weeks of gestation, the fetus gains 30 g per day and adds 1.2 cm (0.5 in.) to body length daily. To gain weight at the intrauterine rate, the term newborn requires 120 calories/kg per day. After birth, caloric intake is often insufficient for weight gain until the newborn is 5–10 days old. During this time, the term newborn may experience a weight loss of 5–10%. Because insensible water loss and a shift of intracellular water to extracellular space account for the 5–10% weight loss, failure to lose weight when caloric intake is inadequate may indicate fluid retention.

Term newborns usually pass **meconium** (their first stool) within 8–24 hours of life and almost always within 48 hours. Meconium is formed in utero from the amniotic fluid and its constituents, intestinal secretions, and shed mucosal cells. It is recognized by its thick, tarry-black or dark green appearance (**Figure 33–62A ⟫**). Transitional (thin brown to green) stools consisting of part meconium and part fecal material are passed for the next day or two (Figure 33–62B), and then the stools become entirely fecal (Figure 33–62C). Generally, the stools of a breastfed newborn are pale yellow (but may be pasty green); they are more liquid and more frequent

(A) Day 1 and Day 2

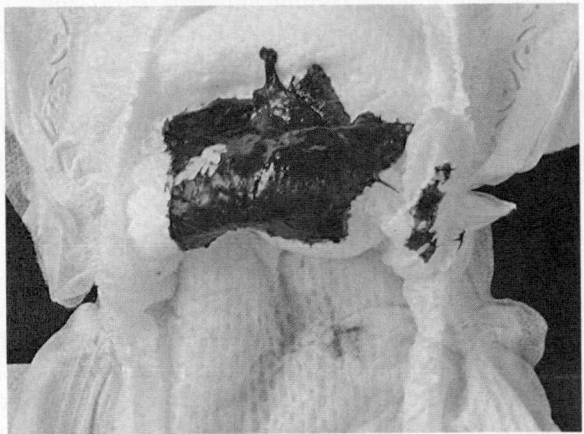

(B) Day 3 and Day 4

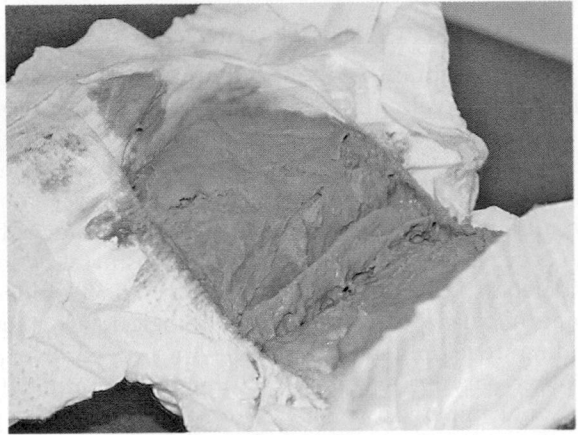

(C) Day 5

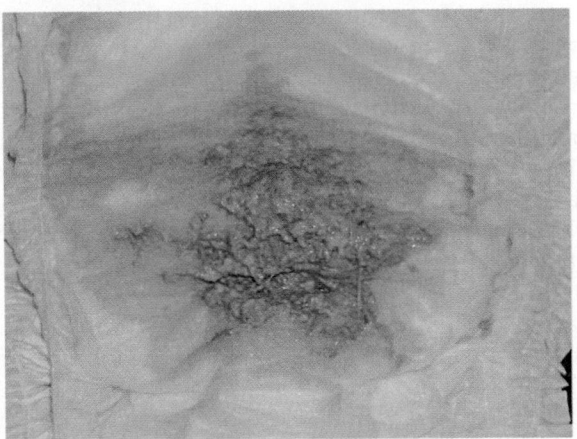

Source: Courtesy of Brigitte Hall, RNC, MSN, IBCLC.

Figure 33–62 ≫ Examples of newborn stools. **A,** Meconium. **B,** Transitional stools. **C,** Fecal stools.

than those of formula-fed newborns, whose stools are paler. Frequency of bowel movement varies but ranges from one every 2–3 days to as many as 10 daily. Mothers should be counseled that the newborn is not constipated as long as the bowel movement remains soft.

Urinary Tract Adaptations

Certain physiologic features of the newborn's kidneys influence the newborn's ability to handle body fluids and excrete urine:

- The term newborn's kidneys have a full complement of functioning nephrons by 34–36 weeks of gestation.

- The glomerular filtration rate of the newborn's kidney is low in comparison with the adult rate. Because of this physiologic decrease in kidney glomerular filtration, the newborn's kidney is unable to dispose of water rapidly when necessary.

- The juxtamedullary portion of the nephron has limited capacity to reabsorb HCO_3^+ and H^+ and to concentrate urine (reabsorb water back into the blood). The limitation of tubular reabsorption can lead to inappropriate loss of substances present in the glomerular filtrate, such as amino acids, bicarbonate, glucose, and sodium.

Full-term newborns are less able than adults to concentrate urine because their tubules are short and narrow. The limited tubular reabsorption of water and limited excretion of solutes (principally sodium, potassium, chloride, bicarbonate, urea, and phosphate) in growing newborns also reduce their ability to concentrate urine. Although feeding practices may affect the osmolarity of the urine, they have limited effect on the concentration of the urine. The ability to concentrate urine fully is attained by 3 months of age.

The newborn's difficulty concentrating urine makes the effect of excessive insensible water loss or restricted fluid intake unpredictable. The newborn kidney is also limited in its dilutional capabilities. Concentrating and dilutional limitations of renal function are important considerations in monitoring fluid therapy to prevent dehydration or overhydration.

Many newborns void immediately after birth; this voiding frequently goes unnoticed. A newborn who has not voided by 48 hours should be assessed for adequacy of fluid intake, bladder distention, restlessness, and symptoms of pain. The appropriate clinical personnel should be notified if indicated (Gabbe et al., 2012).

The initial bladder volume is 6–44 mL of urine. Unless edema is present, normal urinary output is often limited, and voidings are scanty until fluid intake increases. (The fluid of edema is eliminated by the kidneys, so newborns with edema have a much higher urinary output.) During the first 2 days after birth, the newborn voids 2–6 times daily, with a urine output of 15 mL/kg per day. The newborn subsequently voids 5–25 times every 24 hours, with a volume of 25 mL/kg per day.

Following the first voiding, the newborn's urine frequently appears cloudy (because of mucus content) and has a high specific gravity, which decreases as fluid intake increases. Occasionally, pink stains ("brick dust spots") appear on the diaper. These are caused by urates and are innocuous. Blood or whitish discharge may occasionally be observed on the diapers of female newborns; this **pseudomenstruation** is related to the withdrawal of maternal hormones. Males who are circumcised may have bloody spotting following the procedure. In the absence of apparent causes for bleeding, the healthcare provider should be notified. During the early neonatal period, normal urine is straw colored and almost odorless, although odor does occur when certain drugs are given, metabolic disorders exist, or infection is present. **Box 33–7** ≫ contains urinalysis values for the normal newborn.

Immunologic Adaptations

The newborn's immune system is not fully activated until sometime after birth. Limitations in the newborn's inflammatory response result in failure to recognize, localize, and destroy invasive bacteria. As a result, the signs and symptoms of infection are often subtle and nonspecific in the newborn. The newborn also has a poor hypothalamic response to pyrogens; therefore, fever is not a reliable indicator of infection. In the neonatal period, hypothermia is a more reliable sign of infection.

Of the three major types of immunoglobulins that are primarily involved in immunity—IgG, IgA, and IgM—only IgG crosses the placenta. When the pregnant woman forms antibodies in response to illness or immunization, this process is called **active acquired immunity**. When IgG antibodies are transferred from the pregnant woman to the fetus in utero, **passive acquired immunity** results because the fetus does not produce the antibodies itself. IgG antibodies are very active against bacterial toxins.

Because the maternal IgG is transferred primarily during the third trimester, preterm newborns (especially those born before 34 weeks of gestation) may be more susceptible to infection than term newborns. In general, newborns have immunity to tetanus, diphtheria, smallpox, measles, mumps, poliomyelitis, and a variety of other bacterial and viral diseases. The period of resistance varies: Immunity against common viral infections, such as measles, may last 4–8 months; immunity to certain bacteria may disappear within 4–8 weeks.

The normal newborn can produce a protective immune response to vaccines, such as hepatitis B immunoglobulin vaccine, when given as early as a few hours after birth. It is customary to begin the majority of routine immunizations at 2 months of age so that the infant can develop active acquired immunity.

The IgM antibodies are produced in response to blood group antigens, gram-negative enteric organisms, and some viruses in the expectant mother. Because IgM does not normally cross the placenta, most or all of it is produced by the fetus beginning at 10–15 weeks of gestation. Elevated levels of IgM at birth may indicate placental leaks or, more commonly, antigenic stimulation in utero. Consequently, elevations of IgM suggest that the newborn was exposed to an intrauterine infection, such as syphilis or TORCH syndrome (*to*xoplasmosis, *r*ubella, *c*ytomegalovirus, *h*erpesvirus hominis type 2 infection). The lack of available maternal IgM in the newborn also accounts for the susceptibility to gram-negative enteric organisms, such as *Escherichia coli*.

The functions of IgA immunoglobulins are not fully understood. IgA appears to provide protection mainly on secreting surfaces, such as the respiratory tract, gastrointestinal tract, and eyes. Serum IgA does not cross the placenta and is not normally produced by the fetus in utero. Unlike the other immunoglobulins, IgA is not affected by gastric action. Colostrum (the forerunner of breast milk) is very high in the secretory form of IgA. Consequently, it may be of significance in providing some passive immunity to the neonate of a breastfeeding mother. Newborns begin to produce secretory IgA in their intestinal mucosa approximately 4 weeks after birth.

Neurologic and Sensory–Perceptual Function

The newborn's brain is about one quarter the size of an adult's, and myelination of nerve fibers is incomplete. Unlike the cardiovascular and respiratory systems, which undergo tremendous changes at birth, the nervous system is minimally influenced by the actual birth process.

Because many biochemical and histologic changes have yet to occur in the newborn's brain, the postnatal period is considered to be a time of risk with regard to development of the brain and nervous system. For neurologic development—including development of intellect—to proceed, the brain and other nervous system structures must mature in an orderly, unhampered fashion.

Intrauterine Experience

Newborns respond to and interact with the environment in a predictable pattern of behavior that is somewhat shaped by their intrauterine experience. This intrauterine experience is affected by intrinsic factors, such as maternal nutrition, and by external factors, such as the mother's physical environment. Depending on the newborn's intrauterine experience and individual temperament, neonatal behavioral responses to different stresses vary. Some newborns react quietly to stimulation, others become overreactive and tense, and still others exhibit a combination of the two.

Factors such as exposure to intense auditory stimuli in utero may eventually manifest in the behavior of the newborn. For example, the fetal heart rate initially increases when the pregnant woman is exposed to auditory stimuli, but repetition of the stimuli leads to decreased fetal heart rate. Thus, the newborn who was exposed to intense noise during fetal life is significantly less reactive to loud sounds after birth.

Characteristics of Newborn Neurologic Function

Normal newborns are usually in a position of partially flexed extremities, with the legs near the abdomen. When awake, the newborn may exhibit purposeless, uncoordinated bilateral movements of the extremities. The organization and quality of the newborn's motor activity are influenced by a number of factors, including the following (Nugent, 2013):

- Intrauterine growth restriction
- Prenatal stress
- Environmental chemicals
- Obstetric medications
- Acute fetal distress
- Gestational and pregestational diabetes
- Intrauterine drug exposure
- Prematurity and low birth weight.

Eye movements are observable during the first few days of life. An alert newborn is able to fixate on faces and geometric objects or patterns, such as black-and-white stripes. A bright light shining in the newborn's eyes elicits the blinking reflex.

The cry of the newborn should be lusty and vigorous. High-pitched cries, weak cries, and no cries are causes for concern.

The newborn's body growth progresses in a cephalocaudal (head-to-toe), proximal–distal fashion. The newborn is somewhat hypertonic—that is, there is resistance to extending the elbow and knee joints. Muscle tone should be symmetric. Diminished muscle tone and flaccidity may indicate neurologic dysfunction.

Specific symmetric deep tendon reflexes can be elicited in the newborn. The knee-jerk reflex is brisk; a normal ankle clonus may involve three to four beats. Plantar flexion is present. Other reflexes, including the Moro, grasping, Babinski, rooting, and sucking reflexes, are characteristic of neurologic integrity. **Table 33–17** >> provides a summary of stimulus, and response, for the common newborn reflexes.

Performance of complex behavioral patterns reflects the newborn's neurologic maturation and integration. Newborns who can bring a hand to their mouth may be demonstrating motor coordination as well as a self-quieting technique, thus increasing the complexity of the behavioral response. Newborns also possess complex, organized, defensive motor patterns, as exhibited by the ability to remove an obstruction, such as a cloth across the face.

Periods of Reactivity

The behavior of the newborn can be divided into three categories, the sleep state, the transitional state, and the alert state (McGrath & Vittner, 2015). These postnatal behavioral states are similar to those that have been identified during pregnancy. Subcategories are identified under each major category.

Sleep States

The sleep states are as follows:

- **Deep or quiet sleep.** Deep sleep is characterized by closed eyes with no eye movements; regular, even breathing; and jerky motions or startles at regular intervals. Behavioral responses to external stimuli are likely to be delayed. Startles are rapidly suppressed, and changes in state are not likely to occur. Heart rate may range from 100 to 120 beats/min.
- **Active or light sleep (rapid eye movement [REM] sleep).** The baby has irregular respirations; eyes closed, with REM; irregular sucking motions; minimal activity; and irregular but smooth movement of the extremities. Environmental and internal stimuli may initiate a startle reaction and a change of state.

Newborn sleep cycles have been recognized and defined according to duration. The length of the sleep cycle depends on the age of the newborn. At term, REM active sleep and quiet sleep occur in intervals of 50–60 minutes (Gardner, Goldson, & Hernandez, 2016). Approximately 45–50% of the newborn's total sleep is active sleep, 35–45% is quiet sleep, and 10% is transitional between these two periods. Growth hormone secretion depends on regular sleep patterns. Any disturbance of the sleep–wake cycle can result in irregular spikes of growth hormone. REM sleep stimulates the highest peaks of growth hormone and the growth of the neural system. Over a period of time, the newborn's sleep–wake patterns become diurnal (the newborn sleeps at night and stays awake during the day).

Alert States

In the first 30–60 minutes after birth, many newborns display a quiet alert state. After a sleep phase that lasts from a few minutes to between 2 and 4 hours, a second alert state occurs. This second alert period lasts 4 to 6 hours in the normal newborn. The nurse should use these alert states to encourage bonding and breastfeeding.

The newborn's periods of alertness tend to be shorter during the first 2 days after birth; this allows the baby to recover from the birth process. Subsequent alert states are of choice or of necessity. Increasing choice of wakefulness by the newborn indicates a maturing capacity to achieve and maintain consciousness. Heat, cold, and hunger are but a few of the stimuli that can cause wakefulness by necessity. Once the disturbing stimuli have been removed, the baby tends to fall back asleep.

The following are subcategories of the alert state (McGrath & Vittner, 2015):

- **Drowsy.** The behaviors common to the drowsy state are open or closed eyes; fluttering eyelids; semidozing appearance; and slow, regular movements of the extremities. Mild startles may be noted from time to time. Although the reaction to a sensory stimulus is delayed, a change of state often results.
- **Quiet alert.** In the quiet-alert state, the newborn is alert and follows and fixates on attractive objects, faces, or auditory stimuli. Motor activity is minimal, and the response to external stimuli is delayed.
- **Active alert.** In the active-alert state, the newborn's eyes are open, and motor activity is quite intense, with thrusting movements of the extremities. Environmental stimuli increase startles or motor activity, but individual reactions are difficult to distinguish because of the generally high activity level (**Figure 33–63** >>).
- **Crying.** Intense crying is accompanied by jerky motor movements. Crying serves several purposes for the newborn. It may be a distraction from disturbing stimuli, such as hunger and pain. Fussiness often allows the newborn to discharge energy and reorganize behavior. Most important, crying elicits an appropriate response of help from the parents.

TABLE 33–17 Common Reflexes of the Newborn

Reflex	Stimulus and Response	Visual
Rooting	Elicited when the side of the newborn's mouth or cheek is touched. In response, the newborn turns toward that side and opens the lips to suck (if not fed recently).	
Sucking	Elicited when an object is placed in the newborn's mouth or anything touches the lips. Newborns suck even while sleeping; this is called *nonnutritive sucking*, and it can have a quieting effect on the baby. Disappears by 12 months.	
Moro	Elicited when the newborn is startled by a loud noise or lifted slightly above the crib and then suddenly lowered. In response, the newborn straightens arms and hands outward while the knees flex. Slowly the arms return to the chest, as in an embrace. The fingers spread, forming a C, and the newborn may cry. This reflex may persist until about 6 months of age.	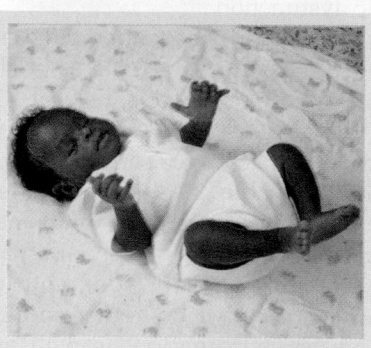
Tonic neck (fencer position)	Elicited when the newborn is supine and the head is turned to one side. In response, the extremities on the same side straighten, whereas on the opposite side they flex. This reflex may not be seen during the early newborn period, but once it appears it persists until about the third month.	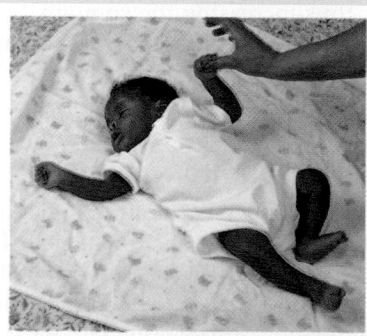
Stepping	When held upright with one foot touching a flat surface, the newborn puts one foot in front of the other and "walks" (*stepping reflex*). This reflex is more pronounced at birth and is lost in 4–8 weeks.	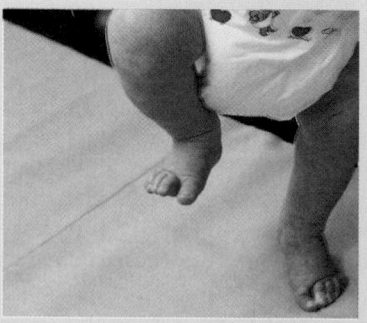

TABLE 33–17 Common Reflexes of the Newborn *(continued)*

Reflex	Stimulus and Response	Visual
Palmar grasping	Elicited by stimulating the newborn's palm with a finger or an object; the newborn grasps and holds the object or finger firmly enough to be lifted momentarily from the crib.	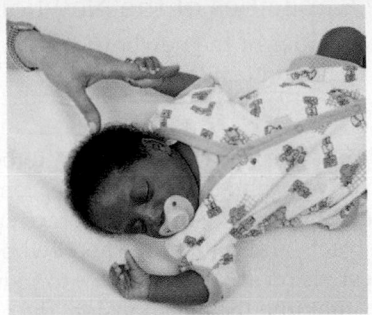
Babinski	Fanning and hyperextension of all toes and dorsiflexion of the big toe occurs when the lateral aspect of the sole is stroked from the heel upward across the ball of the foot. In children older than 24 months, an abnormal response is extension or fanning of the toes; this Babinski response indicates upper motor neuron abnormalities.	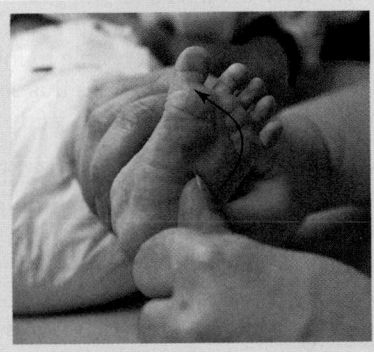
Blinking	Flash of light causes eyelids to close.	
Pupillary	Flash of light causes pupils to constrict.	
Startle	Loud noise evokes flexion in arms with fists clenched.	
Abdominal	Tactile stimulation causes abdominal muscles to contract.	
Withdrawal	Slight pinprick to sole of foot causes leg to flex.	
Plantar (toe-grasping) reflex	Pressure applied against the ball of the foot elicits plantar flexion of the toes. Disappears by 12 months.	
Trunk incurvation (Galant reflex)	Stroking the spine of the prone newborn causes the pelvis to turn to the stimulated side.	

Sources: American Academy of Pediatrics. (2013). Newborn reflexes. Retrieved from http://www.healthychildren.org/English/ages-stages/baby/pages/Newborn-Reflexes.aspx; Ladewig, P. A. W., London, M. L., & Davidson, M. R. (2017). Table 24–2 in *Contemporary Maternal-Newborn Nursing Care*, 9th ed. Hoboken, NJ: Pearson; MedlinePlus. (2011). Infant reflexes. Retrieved from http://www.nlm.nih.gov/medlineplus/ency/article/003292.htm.

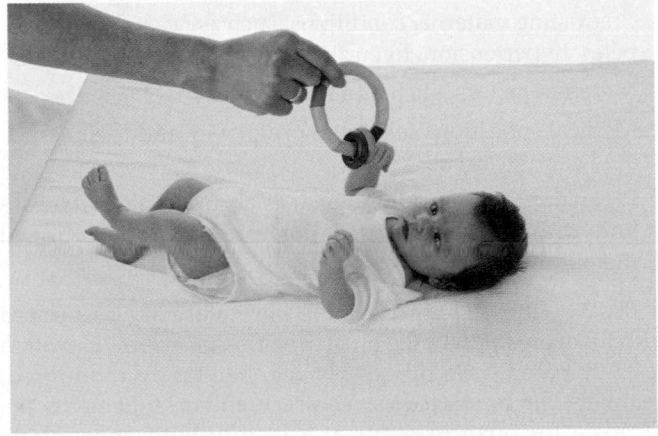

Source: Jules Selmes/Pearson Education, Inc.

Figure 33–63 ›> Newborn in active alert state turning his head to follow an object.

Behavioral Capacities of the Newborn

Newborns have several behavioral capacities that assist them in adapting to extrauterine life. For example, **self-quieting ability** is the ability of newborns to use their own resources to quiet and comfort themselves. Their repertoire includes hand-to-mouth movements, sucking on a fist or tongue, and attending to external stimuli. Neurologically impaired newborns are unable to use self-quieting activities and require more frequent comforting from caregivers when stimulated. For example, drug-positive newborns often exhibit abnormal sleep and feeding patterns and irritability.

Habituation is the newborn's ability to process and respond to complex stimulation. For example, when a bright light is flashed into the newborn's eyes, the initial response is blinking, constriction of the pupil, and perhaps a slight startle reaction. However, with repeated stimulation the newborn's response repertoire gradually diminishes and disappears. The capacity to ignore repetitious, disturbing stimuli is a newborn defense mechanism that is readily apparent in the noisy, well-lit nursery.

Sensory Capacities of the Newborn

Sensory capacities of the newborn include visual, auditory, olfactory, taste, and tactile capacities.

Visual Capacity

Orientation is the newborn's ability to be alert to, follow, and fixate on appealing and attractive, complex visual stimuli. The newborn prefers the human face and eyes and high-contrast objects and patterns. The newborn is nearsighted and has best vision at a distance of 8 to 15 inches. As the face or object comes into the line of vision, the newborn responds with bright, wide eyes as well as still limbs and a fixed stare. This intense visual involvement may last several minutes. During this time, the newborn is able to follow the stimulus from side to side. The newborn uses this sensory capacity to become familiar with family, friends, and surroundings.

Auditory Capacity

The newborn responds to auditory stimulation with a definite, organized behavioral repertoire. The stimulus used to assess auditory response should be selected to match the state of the newborn. A rattle is appropriate for light sleep, a voice for an awake state, and a clap for deep sleep. As the newborn hears the sound, the cardiac rate rises; a minimal startle reflex may be observed. If the sound is appealing, the newborn will become alert and search for the site of the auditory stimulus. Lack of auditory development is associated with an increased risk of sudden infant death syndrome. The CDC (2015c) currently recommends that newborns be screened for hearing loss no later than 1 month of age.

Olfactory Capacity

Newborns not only select their mother by smell, they apparently also can select other individuals by smell (Lehtonen, 2015). Newborns are able to distinguish their mothers' breast pads from those of other mothers as early as 1 week after birth.

Taste and Sucking

The newborn responds differently to varying tastes. Sugar, for example, increases sucking. Newborns fed with a rubber nipple versus the breast also show sucking pattern variations. When breastfeeding, the newborn sucks in bursts, with frequent regular pauses. The bottle-fed newborn, however, tends to suck at a regular rate, with infrequent pauses.

When awake and hungry, the newborn displays rapid searching motions in response to the rooting reflex. Once feeding begins, the newborn establishes a sucking pattern according to the method of feeding. Finger sucking is seen in utero as well as after birth. The newborn frequently uses nonnutritive sucking as a self-quieting activity, which assists in the development of self-regulation. For bottle-fed babies, there is no reason to discourage nonnutritive sucking with a pacifier. Pacifiers should be offered to breastfed babies only after breastfeeding is well established. If the pacifier is offered too soon, a phenomenon called "nipple confusion" may occur, in which the breastfed baby has difficulty learning to suck from the breast and will nurse less.

Tactile Capacity

The newborn is very sensitive to being touched, cuddled, and held. Often, a mother's first response to an upset or crying newborn is touching or holding. Swaddling, placing a hand on the abdomen, or holding the arms to prevent a startle reflex are other methods of soothing the newborn. The quieted newborn is then able to attend to and interact with the environment. Touch is also used to rouse a drowsy newborn, making him or her more alert for feeding.

Alterations of the Newborn Period

Neonatology is the field of medicine providing care for sick and premature neonates. Many levels of nursery care have evolved in response to increasing knowledge about at-risk newborns: special care, intensive care, and convalescent or transitional care. Along with the newborn's parents, the nurse is an important caregiver in all these settings. As a member of the multidisciplinary healthcare team, the nurse is a technically competent professional who contributes the high-touch, human care necessary in the high-tech perinatal environment.

Various factors influence the outcome of at-risk neonates, including the following:

- Birth weight
- Gestational age
- Type and length of illness
- Environmental factors
- Maternal factors
- Maternal–newborn separation.

An at-risk newborn is one susceptible to illness (morbidity) or even death (mortality) because of dysmaturity, immaturity, physical disorders, or complications during or after birth. In most cases, the neonate is the product of a pregnancy involving one or more predictable risk factors, including the following:

- Low socioeconomic level of the mother
- Limited access to healthcare or no prenatal care
- Exposure to environmental dangers, such as toxic chemicals and illicit drugs
- Preexisting maternal conditions, such as heart disease, diabetes, hypertension, hyperthyroidism, and renal disease
- Maternal factors, such as age and parity
- Medical conditions related to pregnancy and their associated complications
- Pregnancy complications, such as abruptio placentae, oligohydramnios, preterm labor, premature rupture of membranes, and preeclampsia.

Because these factors and the perinatal risks associated with them are known, the birth of at-risk newborns can often be anticipated. The pregnancy can be closely monitored, treatment can be started as necessary, and arrangements can be made for birth to occur at a facility with appropriate resources to care for both mother and baby.

Whether or not prenatal assessment indicates that the fetus is at risk, the course of labor and birth, as well as the newborn's ability to withstand the stress of labor, cannot be predicted. Thus, the nurse's use of electronic fetal heart monitoring or fetal heart auscultation by Doppler plays a significant role in detecting stress or distress in the fetus. Immediately after birth, the Apgar score may help identify the at-risk newborn, but it is not the only indicator of possible long-term outcome.

The newborn classification and neonatal mortality risk chart is another useful tool for identifying newborns at risk. Before this classification tool was developed, birth weight of less than 2500 g was the sole criterion for determining prematurity. Healthcare providers then recognized that a newborn could weigh more than 2500 g and still be premature. Conversely, a newborn weighing less than 2500 g might be functionally at term or beyond. As a result, birth weight and gestational age together are now the criteria used to assess neonatal maturity, morbidity, and mortality risk.

According to the newborn classification and neonatal mortality risk chart, gestation (postmenstrual age) is divided as follows:

- **Preterm:** less than 37 (completed) weeks
- **Term:** 37–41 6/7 (completed) weeks
- **Postterm:** greater than 42 weeks.

Late preterm is an emerging classification that refers to subgroups of newborns between 34 and 37 weeks of gestation. As shown in **Figure 33–64 》**, large-for-gestational-age newborns are those who plot above the 90th percentile curve

on an intrauterine growth chart. Appropriate-for-gestational-age newborns are those who plot between the 10th percentile and 90th percentile growth curves. Small-for-gestational-age newborns are those that plot below the 10th percentile growth curve. A newborn is assigned to a category depending on birth weight, length, occipitofrontal head circumference, and gestational age. For example, a newborn classified as Pr SGA is preterm and small for gestational age. The term newborn whose weight is appropriate for gestational age is classified F AGA. It is important to note that intrauterine growth charts are influenced by altitude and by the ethnicity of the newborn population used to create the chart. Also, the assigned newborn classification may vary according to the intrauterine growth curve chart used; therefore, the chart used should correlate with the characteristics of the patient population.

Neonatal mortality risk is a baby's chance of death within the newborn period—that is, within the first 28 days of life. As indicated in **Figure 33–65 》**, the neonatal mortality risk decreases as both gestational age and birth weight increase. Neonates who are preterm and small for gestational age have the highest mortality risk. The previously high mortality rates for large-for-gestational-age newborns have decreased at most perinatal centers because of both improved management of diabetes in pregnancy and increased recognition of potential complications of these newborns.

Neonatal morbidity can be anticipated based on birth weight and gestational age. In Figure 33–65, the newborn's birth weight is located on the vertical axis, and the gestational age in weeks is found along the horizontal axis. The area where the two meet on the graph identifies common problems. This tool assists in determining the needs of particular newborns for special observation and care. For example, a newborn of 2000 g at 40 weeks of gestation should be carefully assessed for evidence of distress, hypoglycemia, congenital anomalies, congenital infection, and polycythemia.

Exemplar 33.E discusses care of the premature newborn. Common alterations seen in the newborn are described in Alterations and Therapies: Newborn Care.

》 Go to **Pearson MyLab Nursing and eText** to see Chart 15: Potential Birth Injuries and Chart 16: Congenital Anomalies: Identification and Care in the Newborn Period.

Collaboration

The healthcare team, composed of members from various disciplines, works together to care for the newborn. The team commonly includes a pediatrician or neonatal specialist, a nurse, a lactation consultant, and an audiology specialist. The nurse's role is described in detail in the Nursing Process section that follows. Needs of the newborn differ dramatically in the 4-hour period following birth versus later time periods. Assessment and interventions involve all body systems as the neonate transitions from intrauterine to extrauterine life. As a result, care is divided into initial care, subsequent care, and preparation for discharge. Complications in the newborn may require referral to additional specialists.

NURSING PROCESS

As with any patient, the plan of care for the newborn is based on thorough and ongoing assessment. Thermoregulation and respiratory and cardiac function are the nurse's

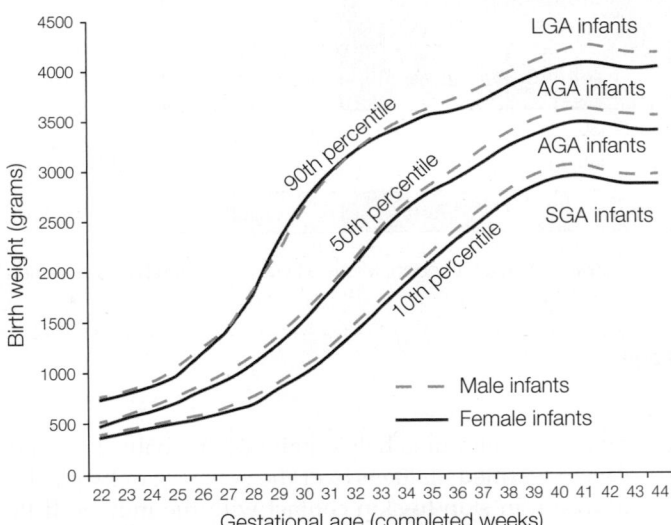

Source: From Oken, E., Kleinman, K. P., Rich-Edwards, J., & Gillman, M. W. (2003). A nearly continuous measure of birth weight for gestational age using a United States national reference. *BMC Pediatrics, 3*, 6. Retrieved from http://www.biomedcentral.com/1471-2431/3/6© 2003 Oken et al.; licensee BioMed Central Ltd. This is an Open Access article: verbatim copying and redistribution of this article are permitted in all media for any purpose, provided this notice is preserved along with the article's original URL.

Figure 33–64 》 Classification of newborns by birth weight and gestational age. Select reference percentiles for birth weight at each gestational age from 22 to 44 completed weeks for male and female singleton newborns: 10th, 50th, and 90th percentiles. Data from 3,423,215 male and 3,267,502 female newborns in the 1999–2000 U.S. Natality datasets.

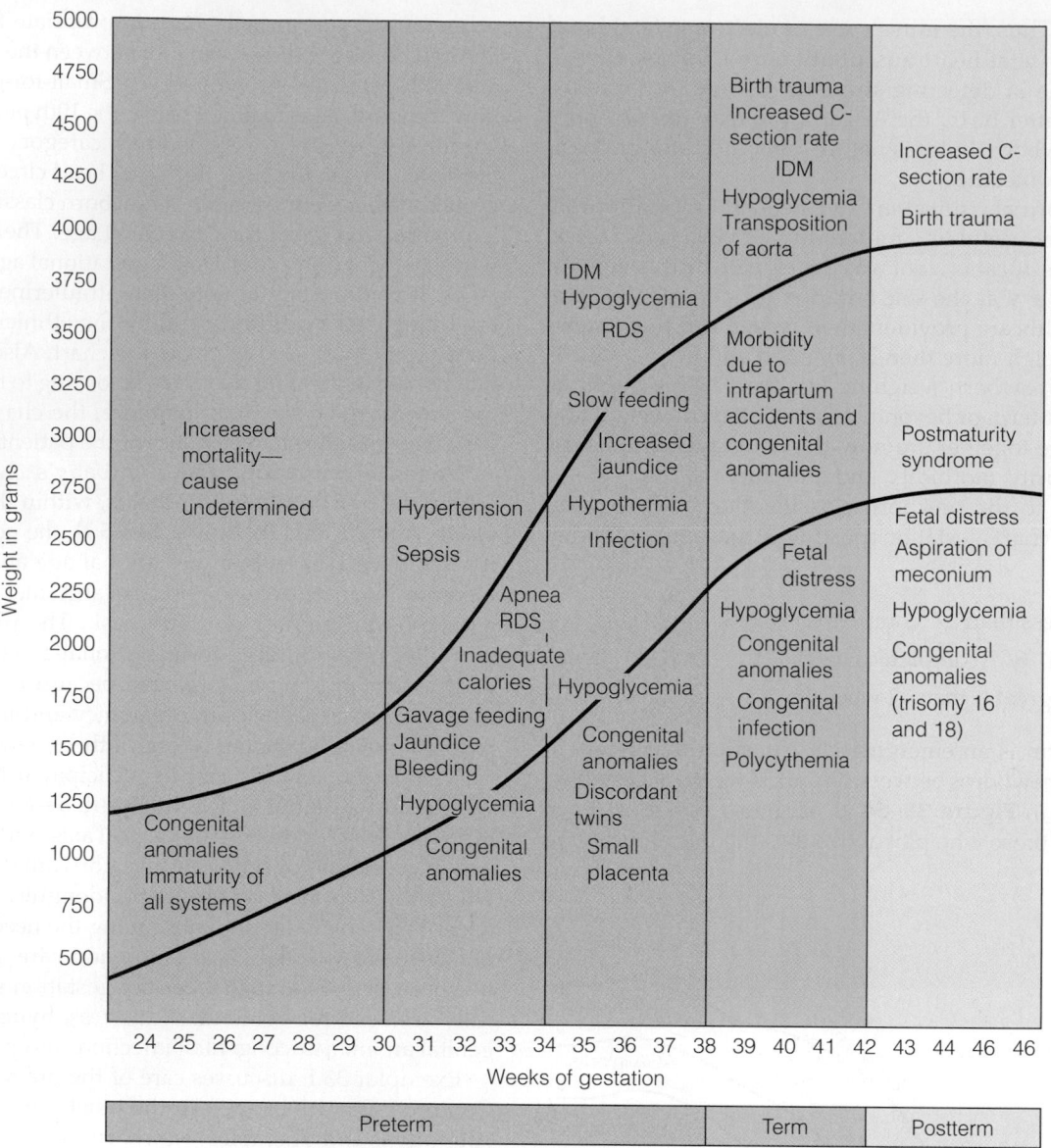

Source: From *Contemporary Maternal-Newborn Nursing* 7th edition, by Patricia W Ladewig; Marcia L London; Michele Davidson. Published by Pearson Education © 2009.

Figure 33–65 》 Neonatal morbidity by birth weight and gestational age.

primary concerns. These and other interventions are discussed in this section.

Initial Care of the Newborn

Immediately after birth, the provider places the newborn on the mother's abdomen or under the radiant heat unit. Placing the newborn on the maternal abdomen promotes attachment and bonding and gives the mother the opportunity to immediately interact with her baby. Placing the baby on the mother's chest also promotes early breastfeeding opportunities. Even though the baby may not breastfeed immediately, placement on the mother's chest enables the baby to smell, touch, and lick the mother's nipples. The newborn is maintained in a modified Trendelenburg position, which aids drainage of mucus from the nasopharynx and trachea by gravity. The newborn is dried immediately, and wet blankets

are removed. The nurse helps maintain the baby's warmth by placing warmed blankets over the newborn or by placing the newborn in skin-to-skin contact with the mother. If the newborn is under a radiant-heated unit, he or she is dried, placed on a dry blanket, and left uncovered under the radiant heat. Because radiant heat warms the outer surface of objects, a newborn wrapped in blankets will receive no benefit from radiant heat.

The newborn's nose and mouth are suctioned with a bulb syringe as needed. Most immediate care of the newborn can be accomplished while the newborn is in the parent's arms or under the radiant-heated unit. Many women request that their babies be left on their abdomens or chests while initial care is given. Unless a medical complication exists, the nurse should complete assessments in this position to promote parental attachment.

Alterations and Therapies
Newborn Care

ALTERATION	DESCRIPTION	THERAPIES
Growth		
Small for gestational age (SGA)	Less than the 10th percentile for birth weight; the newborn may be preterm, term, or postterm; often seen in women who smoke, have high blood pressure, or any condition that reduces blood flow to the fetus. Increased risk of perinatal asphyxia, perinatal mortality, polycythemia, and hypoglycemia.	■ Care is aimed at promoting growth. ■ Requires ongoing screening for potential complications related to SGA, including polycythemia, cold stress, asphyxia, hypothermia, and hyperbilirubinemia. ■ Assess parents and family members because SGA may be an expected finding if short stature runs in the family.
Very small for gestational age (VSGA)	Less than the third percentile for birth weight; the newborn may be preterm, term, or postterm.	■ Promote weight gain. ■ Monitor blood sugar levels for hypoglycemia. ■ Promote smoking cessation or substance abstinence if that is a factor in the newborn's VSGA status.
Large for gestational age (LGA)	Newborn's weight is at or above the 90th percentile; often associated with maternal diabetes, genetic predisposition, multiparous women, erythroblastosis fetalis, Beckwith-Wiedemann syndrome, or transposition of the great vessels.	■ Accurate estimation of gestational age is important to determining LGA status. ■ Carefully assess for potential birth trauma, including effects of cephalopelvic disproportion and macrosomia, fractured clavicle or humerus, or damage to the brachial plexus nerves as a result of shoulder dystocia. ■ Monitor for hypoglycemia, polycythemia, and hyperbilirubinemia.
Intrauterine growth restriction (IUGR)	Pregnancy circumstances of advanced gestation and limited fetal growth most commonly associated with lack of prenatal care, age extremes in the mother, low socioeconomic status, hypertension, multiple-gestation pregnancy, grand multiparity, and primiparity. Environmental factors such as excessive exercise, exposure to toxins, high altitudes, and maternal drug use have also been implicated.	■ Early identification is important to early intervention. ■ If IUGR is unexplained, an in utero infection must be ruled out. ■ Monitor newborn for hypoglycemia. ■ Provide patient teaching to promote growth after discharge and participation in neonatal stimulation programs to promote neurologic function.
Conditions Present at Birth		
Newborn of a mother with diabetes	Babies born to mothers with diabetes are often LGA, macrosomic, ruddy in color, and have excessive adipose tissue, decreased total body water, edema, cardiomegaly, and often trouble regulating blood sugar levels initially because of higher-than-normal insulin production in utero to cope with the mother's elevated blood sugar levels.	■ Assess blood sugar levels frequently. ■ Monitor for signs of hypoglycemia, including tremors, cyanosis, apnea, temperature instability, poor feeding, and hypotonia. ■ Seizures may occur in severe cases. ■ Assess lab results for hypocalcemia, hyperbilirubinemia, and polycythemia. ■ Initial assessment should observe for birth trauma due to large size.
Postterm newborn	Newborn born after 42 weeks of gestation; most often seen in those of Australian, Greek, and Italian heritage. Most are normal size but large because they continued to grow in utero and face higher risk for morbidity, with a 2–3 times higher mortality rate. Potential complications include hypoglycemia, meconium aspiration, polycythemia, congenital anomalies, seizures, and cold stress.	■ Many postterm neonates will adapt well to extrauterine life. ■ Monitor serum blood sugar. ■ Assess respiratory status, especially in the presence of possible meconium aspiration. ■ Maintain neutral thermal environment until newborn demonstrates temperature stability.

(continued on next page)

Alterations and Therapies (continued)

ALTERATION	DESCRIPTION	THERAPIES
Newborns with prenatal substance abuse exposure	Substance exposure may include tobacco, marijuana, prescription medications, narcotics, or any number of illegal substances.	■ Babies are at risk for IUGR, meconium aspiration, reduced birth weight, vomiting, seizures, or irritability depending on the substances the fetus was exposed to. ■ Sedate newborns to decrease irritability and tremors. ■ Provide IV fluid therapy for hydration. ■ Possibly advise against breastfeeding. ■ Care of newborns and infants with prenatal substance abuse is discussed in detail in the module on Addiction.
Newborns born to mothers with HIV/AIDS	HIV can be transmitted through the fetal circulation, but the mother who begins antiretroviral medications early in her pregnancy can reduce the risk to the newborn.	■ Advise mother that taking most HIV medications during pregnancy is safe. ■ Neonates may be given prophylactic antiretroviral therapy to decrease risk of active infection. ■ Advise against breastfeeding. ■ This concept is discussed in detail in the exemplar on HIV and AIDS, in the module on Immunity.
Congenital heart defects	Any number of abnormalities can impact the heart during fetal development, increasing the challenge for newborn adaptation to extrauterine life.	■ One third of neonates born with congenital heart defects develop life-threatening symptoms in the first few days of life. ■ Therapies range from palliative care to surgery. ■ This topic is discussed in more detail in the exemplar on Congenital Heart Defects in the module on Perfusion.
Phenylketonuria (PKU)	Amino acid disorders, in which phenylalanine found in dietary protein cannot be converted to tyrosine, result in accumulation of phenylalanine in the blood, which, in turn, results in damage to brain tissue that leads to progressive mental retardation.	■ Collect routine screening blood sample before discharge (24–48 hours after first enteral feeding). ■ Instruct parents that a second screening may be required if initial collection occurs before the initiation of enteral feedings. This follow-up screening often occurs between 7 and 14 days of life.
Maple syrup urine disease	Rapidly progressing and often fatal disease, when untreated, caused by enzymatic defect in the metabolism of the branched-chain amino acids leucine, isoleucine, and alloisoleucine.	■ Diagnosed by routine newborn screening and confirmed by plasma amino acid assay. ■ Instruct parents on importance of obtaining second screening exam, as noted for PKU.
Galactosemia	An inborn error of carbohydrate metabolism in which the body is unable to use the sugars galactose and lactose. Enzyme pathways in liver cells normally convert galactose and lactose to glucose. In galactosemia, one step in that conversion pathway is absent because of the lack of either the enzyme galactose 1-phosphate uridyl transferase or the enzyme galactokinase. High levels of unusable galactose circulate in the blood, resulting in cataracts, brain damage, and liver damage.	■ Instruct parents on importance of routine newborn screening for inborn errors of metabolism.
Homocystinuria	Disorder caused by a deficiency of the enzyme cystathionine beta-synthase, which causes an elevated excretion of homocysteine and methionine.	■ Screening is included in the Recommended Uniform Screening Panel (RUSP) and is considered an amino acid disorder (U.S. Department of Health and Human Services, 2015). ■ No symptoms are usually seen in the newborn period.
Birth-Related Stressors		
Asphyxia	Asphyxia can occur for a number of reasons, including, but not limited to, abruptio placentae, prolapsed cord, maternal hypoxia or death, difficult or prolonged labor, meconium in the amniotic fluid, intrapartum bleeding, maternal infection, prematurity, multiple births, or narcotic use during labor.	■ Promote oxygenation, airway clearance, and breathing to reduce newborn hypoxia, which often includes resuscitation. ■ Monitor blood gas status. ■ Support parents and family. ■ Provide cardiorespiratory monitoring. ■ Newborn is usually taken to the neonatal intensive care unit.

Alterations and Therapies (continued)

ALTERATION	DESCRIPTION	THERAPIES
Respiratory distress	May result from inadequate production of surfactant, prematurity, excessive airway secretions, narcotic administration to the mother during labor, meconium aspiration, or congenital anomalies, among other factors. Parenchymal damage results in hyaline membrane disease compounded by mechanical ventilation if required.	▪ Continuous monitoring is conducted with a cardiorespiratory monitor. ▪ Continuous oxygen saturation monitoring is provided. ▪ Determine arterial blood gas levels frequently until stable. ▪ May require assistance with respiration in the form of mechanical ventilation, continuous positive airway pressure (CPAP), bilevel positive airway pressure (BiPAP), and/or oxygen administration. ▪ Parents and family members require emotional support because it can be very frightening to see a small baby who is so sick and who requires mechanical ventilation.
Transient tachypnea of the newborn	Of particular risk to the LGA and late-preterm neonate because of inadequate clearing of the airways; the newborn will display increased work of breathing 1–6 hours after birth, with rapid respirations, grunting, nasal flaring, and/or mild respiratory and metabolic acidosis. Improvement is usually seen after 24–48 hours.	▪ Monitor newborn's respiratory adaptation to extrauterine life, and report any signs of distress immediately to primary healthcare provider. ▪ Administration of oxygen should be in conjunction with oxygen saturation monitoring to prevent complications related to oxygen toxicity. ▪ Promote parental attachment because a newborn requiring oxygen may not be able to feed or spend as much time with parents until breathing improves.
Meconium aspiration syndrome (MAS)	Meconium is passed in utero secondary to stress and/or hypoxia. This fluid may be aspirated into the tracheobronchial tree in utero or during the first few breaths taken by the newborn. Meconium causes chemical irritation and also forms small balls that become lodged in terminal airways, allowing some air to enter the alveoli but not allowing air to escape. As alveoli continue to expand, they eventually rupture. Complete respiratory collapse may be seen in severe cases.	▪ Avoid positive end-expiratory pressure, which forces more air into the lungs and increases chance that alveoli might rupture. ▪ Mechanical ventilation may be inadequate, and oscillating ventilators that administer 300–400 breaths/minute in small waves of air may be required. ▪ Continuous cardiorespiratory and oxygen saturation monitoring is indicated. ▪ Reduce oxygen demands by keeping the baby quiet; sedation may be required. ▪ Hypoxic newborns should not be fed because oxygen is shunted from the gut; total parenteral nutrition may be administered to meet nutritional demands.
Cold stress	Results from inadequate temperature regulation; can progress to respiratory distress.	▪ Thermoregulation is discussed in the Nursing Process section that follows and in detail in the module on Thermoregulation.
Hypoglycemia	Abnormally low blood sugar (40 mg/dL) can result from a number of conditions, including a mother with diabetes, prematurity, or cold stress.	▪ If possible, feed the baby to raise blood sugar levels. ▪ If unable to feed, 10% dextrose in water ($D_{10}W$) may be administered intravenously. ▪ Observe for signs of hypoglycemia, including jitteriness, crying, or in severe cases, seizures.
Polycythemia	Abnormally high hemoglobin levels; can result from placental transfusion caused by delayed cord clamping or cord stripping, fetal asphyxia, or twin-to-twin blood transfusion in utero.	▪ Encourage fluids. ▪ Monitor cardiorespiratory status for tachycardia or congestive heart failure, respiratory distress. ▪ Assess jaundice caused by increased red blood cell breakdown. ▪ May require patience with feeding because of feeding intolerance, poor feeding, and vomiting.

TABLE 33–18 The Apgar Scoring System

Sign	Score 0	Score 1	Score 2
Heart rate	Absent	Slow—below 100 beats/min	Above 100 beats/min
Respiratory effort	Absent	Slow—irregular	Good crying
Muscle tone	Flaccid	Some flexion of extremities	Active motion
Reflex irritability	None	Grimace	Vigorous cry
Color	Pale blue	Body pink, blue extremities	Completely pink

Source: Data from Apgar, V. (1966, August). The newborn (Apgar) scoring system, reflections and advice. *Pediatric Clinics of North America, 13,* 645.

Apgar Scoring System

The Apgar scoring system (**Table 33–18 »**) is used to evaluate the physical condition of the newborn at birth. The newborn is rated 1 minute after birth and again at 5 minutes and receives a total score (**Apgar score**) ranging from 0 to 10 based on the following assessments:

- **Heart rate** is auscultated or palpated at the junction of the umbilical cord and skin. This is the most important assessment. A newborn heart rate of less than 100 beats/min indicates the need for immediate resuscitation.

- **Respiratory effort** is the second most important Apgar assessment. Complete absence of respirations is termed apnea. A vigorous cry indicates adequate respirations.

- **Muscle tone** is determined by evaluating the degree of flexion and resistance to straightening of the extremities. A normal newborn's elbows and hips are flexed, with the knees positioned up toward the abdomen.

- **Reflex irritability** is evaluated by stroking the baby's back along the spine or by flicking the soles of the feet. A cry merits a full score of 2. A grimace is given 1 point, and no response is scored as 0.

- **Skin color** is inspected for cyanosis and pallor. Generally, newborns have blue extremities with a pink body, which merits a score of 1. This condition is termed acrocyanosis and is present in 85% of normal newborns at 1 minute after birth. A completely pink newborn scores a 2, and a totally cyanotic, pale neonate scores a 0. Newborns with darker skin pigmentation will not be pink in color. Their skin color is assessed for pallor and acrocyanosis, and a score is selected on the basis of the assessment.

A score of 7–10 indicates a newborn in good condition who requires only nasopharyngeal suctioning and, perhaps, some oxygen near the face (called "blow-by" oxygen). If the Apgar score is less than 7 at 5 minutes, the scoring should be repeated every 5 minutes up to 20 minutes (AAP & ACOG, 2012), and resuscitative measures may need to be instituted. Apgar scores of less than 3 at 5 minutes may correlate with neonatal mortality (Assuncao et al., 2012).

Clamping the Cord

If the healthcare provider has not placed some type of cord clamp on the newborn's umbilical cord, the nurse must do so. Before applying the cord clamp, the nurse examines the cut end of the cord for the presence of two arteries and one vein. The umbilical vein is the largest vessel; the arteries are seen as smaller vessels. The number of vessels is recorded on the birth and newborn records. The cord is clamped approximately 1.3–2.5 cm (0.5–1 in.) from the abdomen to allow room between the abdomen and clamp as the cord dries. Abdominal skin must not be clamped, because this will cause necrosis of the tissue. The most common type of cord clamp is the plastic Hollister cord clamp (**Figure 33–66 »**). The Hollister clamp is removed in the newborn nursery approximately 24 hours after the cord has dried.

Evidence-based practice suggests that delayed clamping may yield more benefits than immediate cord clamping (ACOG, 2012a). Delaying cord clamping for at least 30–60 seconds produces increased blood volume, reduced need from blood transfusions, decreased incidence of intracranial hemorrhage, and a lower frequency of iron deficiency anemia (ACOG, 2012a). One concern with delayed clamping is

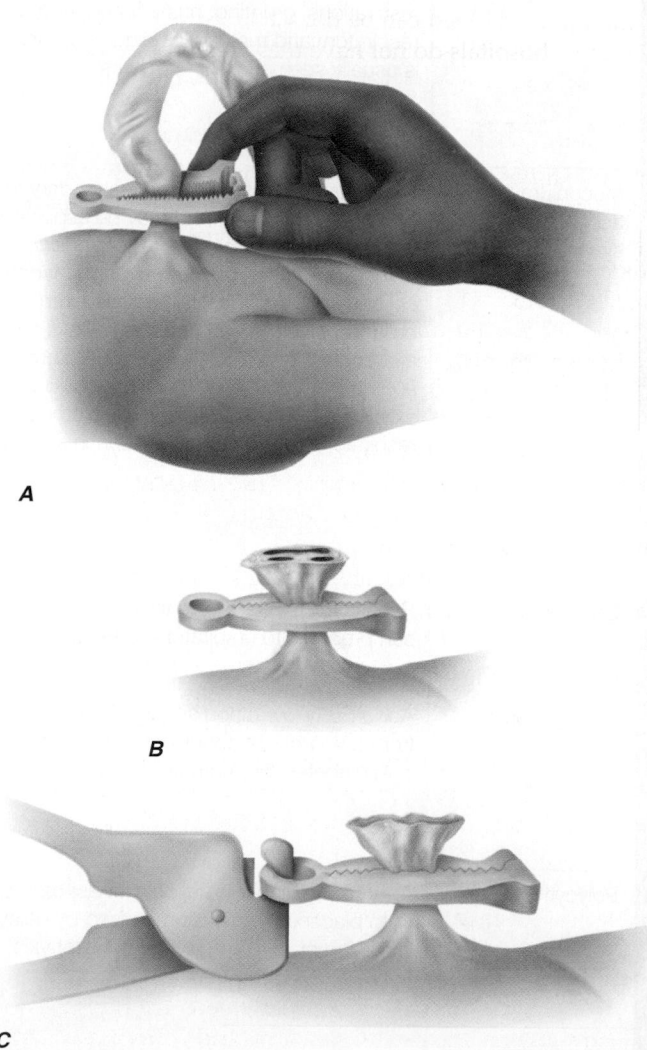

A

B

C

Figure 33–66 » Hollister cord clamp. *A,* Clamp is positioned 1/2–1 in. from the abdomen and then secured. *B,* Cut cord. The one vein and two arteries can be seen. *C,* Plastic device for removing the clamp after the cord has dried. After the cord is cut, the nurse grasps the Hollister clamp on either side of the cut area and gently separates it.

polycythemia, which is benign. Other concerns include delayed resuscitation of the newborn and interfering with cord blood banking collection (ACOG, 2012a).

Banking Cord Blood

A growing number of parents are arranging for cord blood banking. Parents obtain a special container from the Cord Blood Registry, which they bring with them for the birth. Immediately after the newborn's umbilical cord is clamped and cut, the healthcare provider withdraws blood from the remaining umbilical cord by inserting a large-gauge needle into the umbilical vein. The needle allows the blood to be collected into the container. The nurse labels the specimen immediately and follows the directions required for storage and pickup. The collected cord blood can then be used to treat childhood cancers, rare genetic disorders, and cerebral palsy. There are both public and private cord blood banks. At private banks, the cord blood is stored for possible later use by the donor. Alternatively, cord blood may be donated to public banks for use by anyone in need, much like blood donations. Although cord blood can be donated at some hospital facilities, most hospitals do not have these services available. The main drawback of cord blood banking remains the cost.

Newborn Identification and Security

Identification bands typically come in a set of four, all preprinted with identical numbers. The nurse places two bands on the newborn—one on the wrist and one on the ankle. The newborn bands must fit snugly to prevent their loss. The nurse then gives the mother and partner each a band. The band number is documented in the maternal and newborn medical records. The bands allow access to the newborn care areas; they must not be removed until the newborn is discharged. In most facilities, as a security measure, only individuals with a band are given unlimited access to the newborn. Some facilities also include an umbilical clamp with a preprinted number identical to the number printed on the bands.

Although some institutions rely on an umbilical band system to ensure the safety of newborns, others attach an alarm to the ankle band (**Figure 33–67 》**). The alarm is triggered if the device is tampered with or if the newborn is removed from the perimeters of the security field.

Additional hospital security measures are now commonplace in maternity settings. This includes mandating that all staff wear appropriate identification at all times. Parents are instructed that individuals without appropriate identification should not be allowed to remove their baby under any circumstances. The nurse also advises the parents to place their baby on the side of the bed away from the window and to have the baby returned to the nursery whenever the mother naps or showers and no other family member is present.

Although hospital newborn abductions are rare, they are catastrophic for the family, hospital, and community. Many abductors pose as medical personnel to gain access to the mother and baby. Women should be advised to ask all hospital personnel for proper identification. If the mother or family feels unsure of the individual, they should immediately use the call bell to alert the nurse and ask for other verification. If a woman is reluctant to allow a student nurse to transport her baby, the staff nurse should be asked to assist the student.

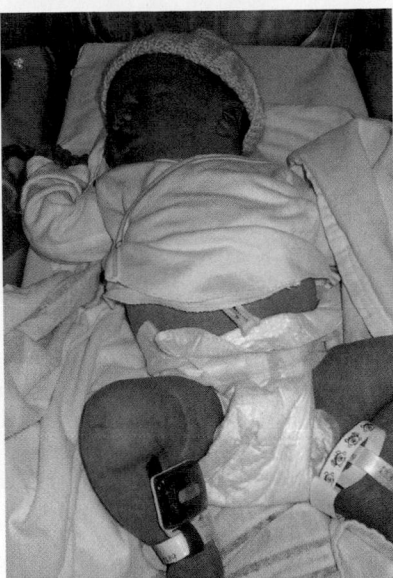

Source: Anne Garcia.

Figure 33–67 》 Newborn with security device in place on one ankle.

Assessment

Unlike the adult, the newborn communicates needs primarily by behavior. Because nurses are the most consistent professional observers of the newborn, they can translate this behavior into information about the newborn's condition and respond with appropriate nursing interventions.

Assessment of the newborn is a continuous process designed to evaluate development and adjustments to extrauterine life. In the birth setting, the Apgar scoring procedure and careful observation form the basis of assessment and are correlated with information such as the following:

- Maternal prenatal care history
- Birthing history
- Maternal analgesia and anesthesia
- Complications of labor or birth
- Treatment instituted immediately after birth, in conjunction with determination of clinical gestational age
- Consideration of the classification of newborns by weight and gestational age and by neonatal mortality risk
- Physical examination of the newborn.

During the first 1–4 hours after birth, the nurse incorporates data from these sources with the assessment findings to formulate a plan for nursing intervention.

The various newborn assessments and the data obtained from them are valuable only to the degree to which they are shared with the parents. The parents must be included in the assessment process from the moment of their child's birth. The Apgar score and its meaning should be explained immediately to the family. As soon as possible, the parents should take part in the physical and behavioral assessments as well.

The nurse encourages the parents to identify the unique behavioral characteristics of their newborn and to learn nurturing activities. Attachment is promoted when parents have an opportunity to explore their newborn in private and identify individual physical and behavioral characteristics themselves. It is essential that the nurse provide supportive responses to parents' questions and observations throughout the assessment process. The newborn physical examination is the beginning of newborn health surveillance and health education for the newborn's family that will continue beyond discharge.

Timing of Newborn Assessments

During the first 24 hours of life, the newborn makes the critical transition from intrauterine to extrauterine life. The risk of mortality and morbidity is statistically high during this period. Assessment of the newborn is essential to ensure that the transition proceeds successfully.

There are three major time frames for assessments of newborns while they are in the birth facility:

1. The first assessment is done in the birthing area immediately after birth to determine the need for resuscitation or other interventions. The stable newborn can stay with the family after birth in order to initiate early attachment. The newborn with complications is usually taken to the nursery for further evaluation and intervention.
2. A second assessment is done by the nursery nurse as part of routine admission procedures. During this assessment, the nurse carries out a brief physical examination to estimate gestational age and evaluate the newborn's adaptation to extrauterine life. No later than 2 hours after birth, the admitting nursery nurse should evaluate the newborn's status and any problems that place the newborn at risk (AAP & ACOG, 2012).
3. Before discharge, a CNM, physician, or nurse practitioner will carry out a behavioral assessment and a complete physical examination to detect any emerging or potential problems. A general assessment is also done at this time.

Initial Physical Assessment

The nurse performs an abbreviated but systematic physical assessment in the birthing area to detect any abnormalities (**Table 33–19** ≫). First, the nurse notes the size of the newborn as well as the contour and size of the head in relationship to the rest of the body. The newborn's posture and movements indicate tone and neurologic functioning.

TABLE 33–19 Initial Newborn Evaluation

Assess	Normal Findings
Respirations	30–60 breaths/min, irregular
	No retractions, no grunting
Apical pulse	110–160 beats/min, somewhat irregular
Temperature	Skin temp above 36.5°C (97.8°F)
Skin color	Body pink with bluish extremities
Umbilical cord	Two arteries and one vein
Gestational age	Should be 37–42 weeks to remain with parents for an extended time
Sole creases	Sole creases that involve the heel

The nurse inspects the skin for discoloration, presence of vernix caseosa and lanugo, and evidence of trauma and desquamation (peeling of skin). **Vernix caseosa** is a white, cheesy substance found normally on newborns. It is absorbed within 24 hours after birth. Vernix is abundant on preterm babies and absent on postterm newborns. **Lanugo** (fine hair) is seen on preterm newborns, especially on the shoulders, foreheads, backs, and cheeks. Desquamation of the skin is seen in postterm newborns.

In general, expect a scant amount of vernix on upper back, axilla, and groin; lanugo only on upper back; ears with incurving of upper two thirds of pinnae and thin cartilage that springs back from folding; male genitals—testes palpated in upper or lower scrotum; female genitals—labia majora larger, clitoris nearly covered.

In the following situations, the newborn may require stabilization by the nursing staff or the NICU team and may need to be temporarily removed from the birth area.

- Apgar score of less than 8 at 1 minute and less than 9 at 5 minutes or baby requires resuscitation measures
- Respirations below 30 or above 60 breaths/min, with retractions and/or grunting
- Apical pulse below 110 or above 160 beats/min, with marked irregularities
- Skin temperature below 36.5°C (97.8°F)
- Skin color pale blue or circumoral pallor
- Baby less than 37 weeks or more than 42 weeks of gestation
- SGA or LGA newborns
- Congenital anomalies involving open areas in the skin (meningomyelocele).

The nurse observes the nares for flaring and, as the newborn cries, inspects the palate for cleft palate. The nurse looks for mucus in the nose and mouth and removes it with a bulb syringe as needed. The nurse inspects the chest for respiratory rate and the presence of retractions. If retractions are present, the nurse assesses the newborn for grunting or stridor. A normal respiratory rate is 30–60 breaths/min. It is important to note that during the first few hours of life the newborn's respiratory rate may be as high as 80 breaths/min. The nurse auscultates the lungs bilaterally for breath sounds. Absence of breath sounds on one side could indicate a pneumothorax. Because a small amount of fluid may remain in the lungs, rales may be heard immediately after birth; this fluid will be absorbed. Rhonchi indicate aspiration of oral secretions. If there is excessive mucus or respiratory distress, the nurse suctions the newborn with a mucous trap or wall suction. The nurse notes and records elimination of urine or meconium on the newborn record.

Establishing Gestational Age

The nurse must establish the newborn's gestational age in the first 4 hours after birth so that careful attention can be given to age-related problems. Once learned, the procedure can be done in a few minutes. Clinical **gestational age assessment tools** have two components:

1. External physical characteristics
2. Neurologic or neuromuscular development.

Physical characteristics generally include sole creases, amount of breast tissue, amount of lanugo, cartilaginous development of the ear, and testicular descent and scrotal rugae or labial development. These objective clinical criteria are not influenced by labor and birth and do not change significantly within the first 12 hours after birth.

Neurologic examination facilitates assessment of functional or physiologic maturation in addition to physical development. However, the newborn's nervous system is unstable during the first 24 hours of life. Therefore, neurologic evaluation findings based on reflexes or assessments that are dependent on the higher brain centers may not be reliable. If the neurologic findings drastically deviate from the gestational age derived by evaluation of external characteristics, a second assessment is done in 24 hours.

The neurologic assessment components (excluding reflexes) can aid in assessing the gestational age of newborns of less than 34 weeks of gestation. Between 26 and 34 weeks, neurologic changes are significant, whereas significant physical changes are less evident. One significant neuromuscular change is that muscle tone progresses from extensor tone to flexor tone in the extremities because the neurologic system matures in a caudocephalad (tail-to-head) progression.

SAFETY ALERT It is essential for the nurse to wear gloves when assessing the newborn in the early hours after birth and before the first bath until amniotic fluid, as well as vaginal and bloody secretions, on the skin are removed.

Ballard et al. (1991) developed the estimation of gestational age by maturity rating, a simplified version of the well-researched **Dubowitz tool**. The Ballard tool omits some of the neuromuscular tone assessments, such as head lag, ventral suspension (difficult to assess in very ill newborns or those on respirators), and leg recoil. In the Ballard tool, each physical and neuromuscular finding is given a value, and the total score is matched to a gestational age. The maximum score on the Ballard tool is 50, which corresponds to a gestational age of 44 weeks.

Postnatal gestational age assessment tools can overestimate preterm gestational age and underestimate postterm gestational age. The tools have been shown to lose accuracy when newborns of less than 28 weeks or more than 43 weeks of gestation are assessed. Ballard et al. (1991), in the **New Ballard Score**, added criteria for more accurate assessment of the gestational age of newborns between 20 and 28 weeks of gestation and less than 1500 g. They suggest that the assessments should be made within 12 hours of birth to optimize accuracy, especially in newborns with a gestational age of less than 26 weeks. Also, the Ballard assessment may be overstimulating to neonates of less than 27 weeks of gestation. Some maternal conditions, such as preeclampsia, diabetes, and maternal analgesia and anesthesia, may affect certain gestational assessment components and warrant further evaluation. Maternal diabetes, although it appears to accelerate fetal physical growth, seems to retard maturation. Maternal hypertension states, which retard fetal physical growth, seem to speed maturation.

Newborns of women with preeclampsia have a poor correlation with the criteria involving active muscle tone and edema. Maternal analgesia and anesthesia may cause respiratory depression in the baby. Babies with respiratory distress syndrome tend to be flaccid and edematous and to assume a "frog-like" posture. These characteristics affect the scoring of the neuromuscular components of the assessment tool used.

ASSESSING PHYSICAL MATURITY CHARACTERISTICS The nurse first evaluates observable characteristics without disturbing the baby. Selected physical maturity characteristics common to the Dubowitz and Ballard gestational assessment tools are presented in **Figure 33–68 ≫** in the order in which they might be most effectively evaluated.

Other physical characteristics assessed by some gestational age scoring tools include the following:

- **Vernix** covers the preterm newborn. The postterm newborn has no vernix. After noting vernix distribution, the birthing area nurse (wearing gloves) dries the newborn to prevent evaporative heat loss, thus disturbing the vernix and potentially altering this gestational age criterion.

- **Hair** of the preterm newborn has the consistency of matted wool or fur and lies in bunches rather than in the silky, single strands of the term newborn's hair.

- **Skull firmness** increases as the fetus matures. In a term newborn, the bones are hard, and the sutures are not easily displaced. The nurse should not attempt to displace the sutures forcibly.

- **Nails** appear and cover the nail bed at about 20 weeks of gestation. Nails extending beyond the fingertips may indicate a postterm newborn.

ASSESSING NEUROMUSCULAR MATURITY CHARACTERISTICS The CNS of the fetus matures at a fairly constant rate. Tests have been designed to evaluate neurologic status as manifested by development of neuromuscular tone. As noted earlier, neuromuscular tone in the fetus develops in a caudocephalad direction, from the lower to the upper extremities.

The neuromuscular evaluation of the newborn requires more manipulation and disturbances than the physical evaluation. The neuromuscular evaluation is best performed when the newborn has stabilized. Selected neuromuscular maturity characteristics common to the Dubowitz and Ballard gestational assessment tools are presented in **Figure 33–69 ≫**.

Other neuromuscular characteristics assessed by some gestational age scoring tools include the following:

- **Head lag** (neck flexor) is measured by pulling the newborn to a sitting position and noting the degree of head lag. Total lag is common in newborns up to 34 weeks of gestation, whereas postterm newborns (>42 weeks) hold their heads in front of their body lines. Full-term newborns can support their heads momentarily.

- **Ventral suspension** (horizontal position) is evaluated by holding the newborn prone on the nurse's hand. The position of the head and back and the degree of flexion in the arms and legs are noted. Some flexion of arms and legs indicates 36–38 weeks of gestation; fully flexed extremities, with the head and back even, are characteristic of a term newborn.

Physical Characteristics of Gestational Age

Skin

Assess for thickness, transparency, and texture.

The preterm newborn's skin appears thin and transparent, and has visible blood vessels.

As the newborn approaches term, the skin is thicker and appears opaque because of increased subcutaneous tissue.

Disappearance of the protective vernix caseosa promotes skin desquamation; this is commonly seen in postmature neonates and those showing signs of placental insufficiency.

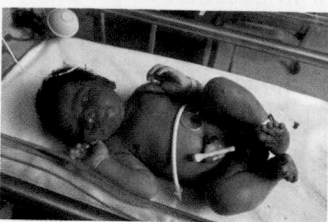

A. Preterm skin

Source: ©Tom McCarthy/PhotoEdit.

B. Term skin

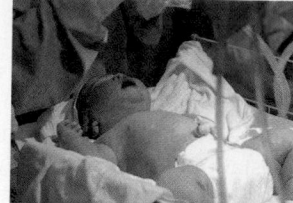

Source: Glenn Kraushar/Alamy Stock Photo.

C. Postterm skin

Lanugo

Assess for the quantity of lanugo, the fine soft hair covering the fetus during intrauterine development.

This hair begins to appear at approximately 19–20 weeks' gestation and is most prominent at 27–28 weeks' gestation.

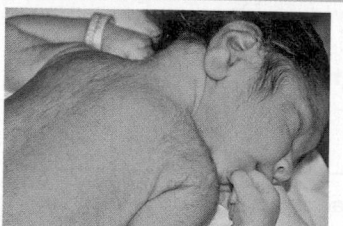

It is mostly shed by 37 weeks' gestation. It first begins to thin over the lower back and then disappears last from the shoulders.

Source: Vanessa Howell, RN, MSN.

D. Lanugo

Plantar surfaces

Assess the number of sole creases over the bottom of the foot. They are reliable indicators of gestational age in the first 12 hours of life.

Plantar creases vary with ethnicity; in newborns of African descent, sole creases may be less developed at term.

A few creases appear on the anterior portion of the foot and the heel is smooth at approximately 34 weeks' gestation *(Ballard score 2)*.

By 36 weeks' gestation, a deeper network of creases cover the anterior two thirds of the foot and the heel is smooth *(Ballard score 3)*.

At term, deep creases cover the entire foot, including the heel *(Ballard score 4)*.

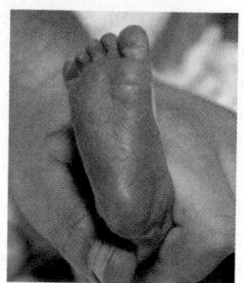

E. Plantar surface, 34 weeks gestation

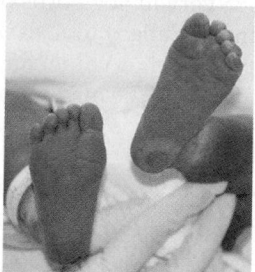

F. Plantar surface, 36 weeks gestation

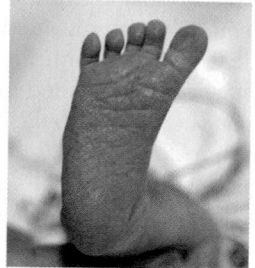

G. Plantar surface, term

Breast

Assess the chest for visibility of the nipple and areola. Then assess the size of the breast bud when grasped between the thumb and forefinger. The extremely preterm neonate has no visible nipple and areola. The nipple and areola become more defined and raised by 34 weeks' gestation. A small breast bud appears by 36 weeks' gestation.

The nurse should not grasp the nipple firmly, because skin and subcutaneous tissue will prevent accurate estimation of size. The nurse must do this procedure gently to avoid causing trauma to the breast tissue.

At 38 weeks' gestation, the breast bud is 4 mm *(Ballard score 3)*.

At term, it grows to 5–10 mm *(Ballard score 4)*.

As gestation progresses, the breast tissue mass and areola enlarge. However, a large breast tissue mass can occur as a result of specific conditions other than advanced gestational age or the effects of maternal hormones on the baby. In the LGA neonate, the accelerated development of breast tissue in a mother with diabetes is a reflection of subcutaneous fat deposits. SGA term or postterm newborns may have used subcutaneous fat, which would have been deposited as breast tissue, to survive in utero; as a result, their lack of breast tissue may indicate a gestational age of 34–35 weeks even though other factors indicate a term or postterm newborn.

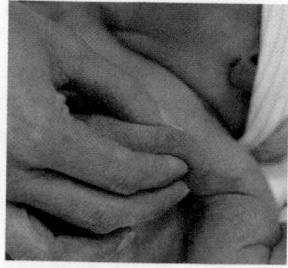

H. Breast bud, 38 weeks' gestation

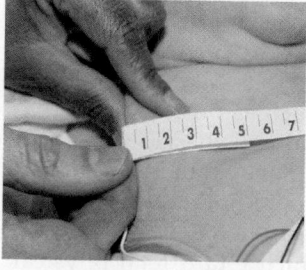

I. Breast bud, term

Figure 33–68 ›› Physical characteristics of gestational age.

Eyes and ears

Assess the eye opening. In extremely preterm neonates, the eyelids are examined with gentle flexion to determine the amount of fusion. Eye opening begins at 22 weeks, and the lids are completely unfused by 28 weeks' gestation.

Assess the formation of the ear cartilage and curving of the pinna. At earlier gestational ages the lack of cartilage allows the ear to fold easily and retain the fold. As gestational age increases, the resistance of the ear to folding increases and recoil is seen. In extremely preterm neonates the pinnae are flat. Incurving proceeds from the top down toward the lobes with advancing gestational age.

The ear of the newborn at approximately 36 weeks gestation shows incurving of the upper two thirds of the pinna *(Ballard score 2)*.

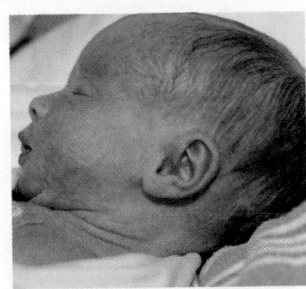

J. Ear at 36 weeks gestation

Newborn at term shows well-defined incurving of the entire pinna *(Ballard score 3)*.

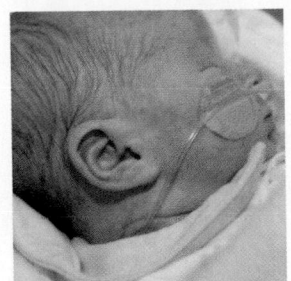

K. Ear at term

The pinna is folded toward the face and released. If the auricle stays in the position in which it is pressed or returns slowly to its original position, it usually means the gestational age is less than 38 weeks.

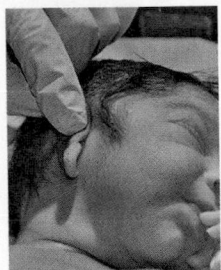

Source: Vanessa Howell, RN, MSN.

L. Assessing the pinna

Male genitals

Assess for size of the scrotal sac, presence of rugae (wrinkles and ridges in the scrotum), and descent of the testes.

Before 36 weeks of gestation, the scrotum has few rugae, and the testes are palpable in the inguinal canal not within the scrotum *(Ballard score 2)*.

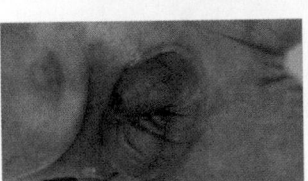

M. Male genitals, preterm

By 36–38 weeks, the testes are in the upper scrotum, and rugae have developed over the anterior portion of the scrotum. By term, the testes are fully descended in the lower scrotum, which is pendulous and covered with rugae *(Ballard score 3)*.

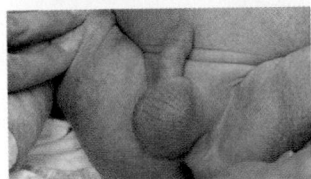

N. Male genitals, term

Female genitals

Assess labial development. Genital appearance depends in part on subcutaneous fat deposition and, therefore, relates to fetal nutritional status. The clitoris varies in size and, occasionally, is so swollen that it is difficult to identify the sex of the newborn. This swelling may be caused by adrenogenital syndrome, which causes the adrenals to secrete excessive amounts of androgen and other hormones.

At 32 weeks of gestation, the clitoris is prominent and the labia minora are flat *(Ballard score 1)*.

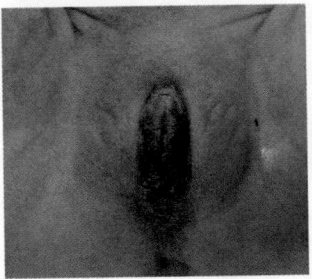

O. Female genitals, 32 weeks gestation

By 36 weeks' gestation, the labia majora are larger and the clitoris is nearly covered *(Ballard score 2)*.

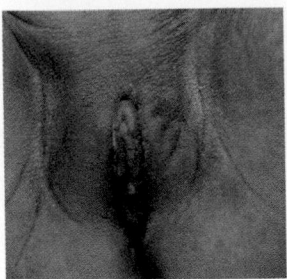

P. Female genitals, 36 weeks' gestation

At term, the labia majora are well developed and cover both the clitoris and labia minora *(Ballard score 3)*.

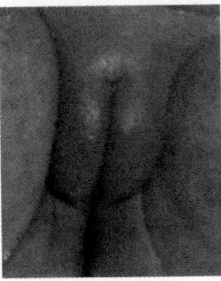

Source: Christine Anderson.

Q. Female genitals, term

Figure 33–68 》 Physical characteristics of gestational age. *(continued)*

Neuromuscular Characteristics of Gestational Age

Resting posture

Assess the posture that the supine newborn assumes at rest. The extremely preterm neonate will lie with arms and legs extended or in any position placed.

At approximately 31 weeks' gestation, the newborn has slightly more flexion in the arms and legs (*Ballard score 1 or 2*).

At approximately 35 weeks' gestation, the newborn exhibits stronger flexion of the arms, hips, and thighs (*Ballard score 3*).

At term, the newborn exhibits hypertonic flexion of all extremities with arms flexed to the chest, hands fisted, and legs flexed toward the abdomen (*Ballard score 4*).

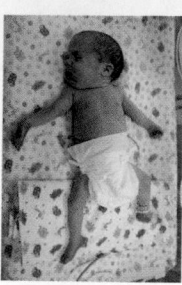

A. Resting posture, 31 weeks' gestation

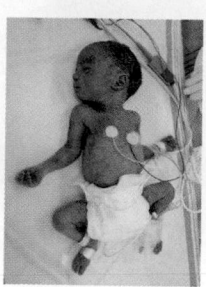

B. Resting posture, 35 weeks' gestation

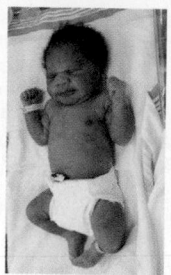

C. Resting posture, term

Square window sign

Assess the angle of the wrist when the palm is flexed toward the forearm until resistance is felt. The angle formed at the wrist is measured. The extremely preterm neonate has no flexor tone and cannot achieve a 90-degree angle. The preterm neonate has poor flexion and is unable to flex the arm at the elbow more than 90 degrees.

At 28–32 weeks' gestation, the angle is 90 degrees (*Ballard score 0*).

At 38–40 weeks' gestation, the angle is 30- to 40-degrees (*Ballard score 2 to 3*).

A 0- to 15-degree angle occurs in newborns from 40–42 weeks' gestation (*Ballard score 4*).

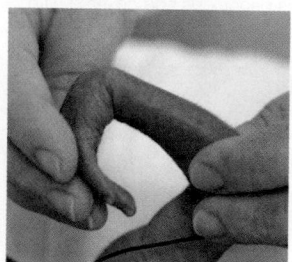

D. Square window sign, 28–32 weeks' gestation

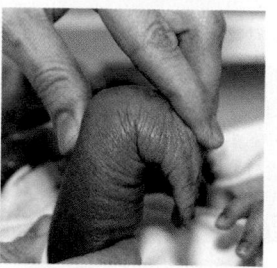

E. Square window sign, 38–40 weeks' gestation

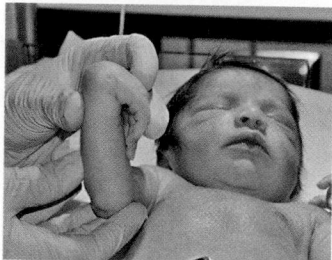

Source: Vanessa Howell, RN, MSN.

F. Square window sign, 40–42 weeks' gestation

Recoil of extremities

Very preterm neonates do not resist extension. They respond with weak and delayed flexion in a small arc. Term newborns resist extension and briskly return their arms to the flexed position.

Arm recoil may be slower in healthy but fatigued newborns after birth; therefore, arm recoil is best elicited after the first hour postbirth, when the baby has had time to recover from the stress of the birth. The deep sleep state also decreases the arm recoil response. Assessment of arm recoil should be bilateral to rule out brachial palsy.

Assess the amount of arm flexion by flexing both arms at the elbows for 5 seconds. Then extend the arms at the elbows

Release the arms to see the amount of recoil

Because flexion first develops in the lower extremities, recoil generally is first tested in the legs. Place the newborn supine on a flat surface. With a hand on the newborn's knees, place the baby's legs in flexion and extend them parallel to each other and flat on the surface. The response to this maneuver is recoil of the newborn's legs. According to gestational age, they may not move or may return slowly or quickly to the flexed position. Preterm neonates have less muscle tone than term neonates, so preterm neonates have less recoil.

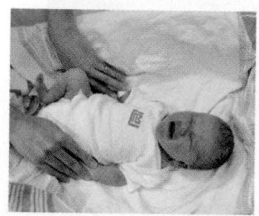

G. Extend arms at elbows

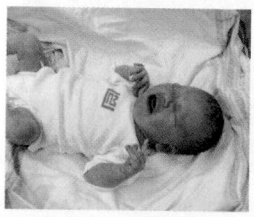

H. Release arms to see recoil

Figure 33–69 》 Neuromuscular characteristics of gestational age.

Popliteal angle

Assess the angle of the knee in the supine newborn. The angle formed is then measured.

Holding the pelvis flat, flex and hold the thigh to the abdomen while extending the leg at the knee until resistance is met

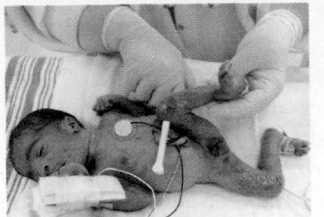

I. Popliteal angle

The newborn with more advanced gestational age has greater flexion. Results vary from no resistance in the very immature newborn to an 80-degree angle in the term newborn.

Scarf sign

Assess the newborn's resistance to pulling the arm across the chest toward the opposite shoulder. The newborn's elbow moves closer to the opposite shoulder with decreasing gestational age.

Until approximately 30 weeks' gestation, the elbow moves past the midline with no resistance *(Ballard score 1)*.

At 36–40 weeks' gestation, the elbow is at midline *(Ballard score 2)*.

The term newborn's elbow will not cross the midline of the chest *(Ballard score 4)*.

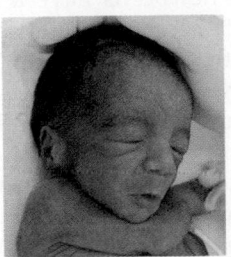

J. Scarf sign, 30 weeks' gestation

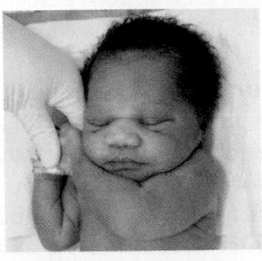

K. Scarf sign, 36–40 weeks' gestation

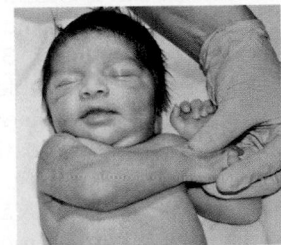

Source: Vanessa Howell, RN, MSN.

L. Scarf sign, term

Heel-to-ear extension

Assess by placing the newborn in a supine position and then gently drawing the foot toward the ear on the same side until resistance is felt. Allow the knee to bend during the test and hold the buttocks down to keep from rolling the baby. Both the proximity of foot to ear and the degree of knee extension are assessed.

A preterm, immature newborn's leg will remain straight, and the foot will go to the ear or beyond *(Ballard score 0)*.

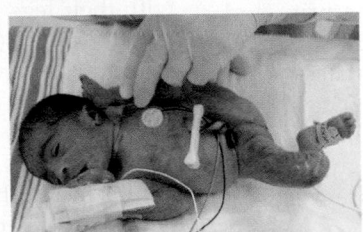

M. Heel-to-ear extension

With advancing gestational age, the newborn demonstrates increasing resistance to this maneuver. Maneuvers involving the lower extremities of newborns who had frank breech presentation should be delayed to allow for resolution of leg positioning.

Ankle dorsiflexion

Assess by flexing the ankle on the shin. Use a thumb to push on the sole of the newborn's foot while the fingers support the back of the leg. Then, measure the angle formed by the foot and the interior leg.

A 45-degree angle indicates 32 to 36 weeks' gestation *(Ballard score 1)*.

A 20-degree angle indicates 36–40 weeks' gestation (Ballard score 2 to 3). A 15- to 0-degree angle is common at 40 weeks or more of gestation *(Ballard score 4)*.

Ankle dorsiflexion findings can be influenced by intrauterine position and congenital deformities.

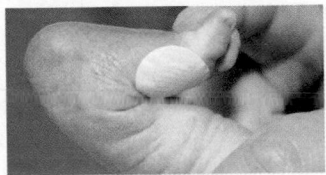

N. Ankle dorsiflexion, 32–36 weeks' gestation.

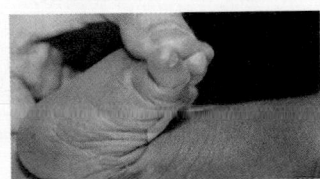

O. Ankle dorsiflexion, 40 or more weeks' gestation.

Figure 33–69 ≫ Neuromuscular characteristics of gestational age. *(continued)*

■ *Major reflexes,* such as sucking, rooting, grasping, Moro, tonic neck, Babinski, and others, are evaluated during the newborn exam (see Table 33–17).

ADDITIONAL METHODS FOR ESTIMATING GESTATIONAL AGE A supplementary method for estimating gestational age (done by the physician or nurse practitioner) is to view the vascular network of the cornea with an ophthalmoscope. The nurse may need to delay administration of prophylactic eye ointment in preterm neonates until after this vascular eye exam has been done. The amount of vascularity present over the surface of the lens assists in identifying neonates with a gestational age of 27–34 weeks (Rosenberg, 2013).

When the gestational age determination and birth weight are considered together, the newborn can be identified as one whose growth is classified as SGA (below 10th percentile), AGA (between 10th and 90th percentile), or LGA (above 90th percentile) (see Figure 33–64).

This determination enables the nurse to anticipate possible physiologic problems and is used in conjunction with a complete physical examination to establish an appropriate plan of care for the individual newborn. For example, newborns who are SGA or LGA are at risk for hypoglycemia and therefore often require frequent glucose monitoring and early feedings started soon after birth.

The nurse also plots the gestational age against the newborn's length, head circumference, and weight on an appropriate growth chart to determine if these measurements fall within the average range—the 10th to 90th percentile for the corresponding gestational age. These correlations further document the level of maturity and appropriate category for the newborn. The comparison of the newborn's weight–length ratio further facilitates identification of SGA newborns as having symmetric or asymmetric growth restriction. Measuring weight and height often aggravates newborns and may alter their vital signs. For better accuracy, take the newborn's vital signs before weighing and measuring the neonate.

Subsequent Physical Assessment

Once the initial assessment process is complete and gestational age has been established, the nurse carries out a thorough, systematic assessment of the newborn. Completing the physical assessment in the presence of the parents provides an opportunity to acquaint them with their unique newborn. The examination is performed in a systematic, head-to-toe manner, and all findings are recorded. When assessing the physical and neurologic status of the newborn, the nurse should first consider general appearance and then proceed to specific areas.

GENERAL APPEARANCE The newborn's head is disproportionately large for its body. The neck looks short because the chin rests on the chest. Newborns have a prominent abdomen, sloping shoulders, narrow hips, and rounded chests. The center of the baby's body is the umbilicus rather than the symphysis pubis, as in the adult. The body appears long and the extremities short.

Newborns tend to stay in a flexed position similar to the one maintained in utero and will offer resistance to straightening of the extremities. This flexed position contributes to the short appearance of the extremities. The hands are tightly clenched. After a breech birth, the feet are usually dorsiflexed, and it may take several weeks for the newborn to assume the typical newborn posture.

WEIGHT AND MEASUREMENT The normal, full-term newborn has an average birth weight of 3405 g (7 lb, 8 oz). Other factors that influence weight are age and size of the parents, health of the mother (smoking and malnutrition decrease birth weight), and the interval between pregnancies (short intervals, such as every year, result in lower birth weight). After the first week, and for the first 6 months, the baby's weight increases about 198 g (7 oz) weekly.

Approximately 70–75% of the newborn's body weight is water. During the initial newborn period (the first 3–4 days), term newborns have a physiologic weight loss of about 5–10% because of fluid shifts. For the term newborn, weight loss that is greater than 10% indicates the need for clinical appraisal. Large babies also tend to lose more weight because of greater fluid loss in proportion to birth weight. Factors contributing to weight loss include insufficient fluid intake resulting from delayed breastfeeding or a slow adjustment to the formula, increased volume of meconium excreted, and urination. Weight loss may be marked in the presence of temperature elevation (because of associated dehydration) or consistent chilling (because of nonshivering thermogenesis).

The length of the average newborn is difficult to measure because the legs are flexed and tensed. To measure length, the nurse should place newborns flat on their backs with their legs extended as much as possible. The average length is 50 cm (20 in.), and the range is 46–56 cm (18–22 in.). The newborn will grow approximately 2.5 cm (1 in.) a month for the next 6 months. This is the period of most rapid growth.

At birth, the newborn's head is one third the size of an adult's head. The circumference (biparietal diameter) of the newborn's head is 32–37 cm (12.5–14.5 in.). For accurate measurement, the nurse places the tape over the most prominent part of the occiput and brings it just above the eyebrows. The circumference of the newborn's head is approximately 2 cm (0.8 in.) greater than the circumference of the newborn's chest at birth and will remain in this proportion for the next few months. It is best to take another head circumference measurement on the second day if the newborn experienced significant head molding or developed a caput from the birth process.

The average circumference of the chest is 32 cm (12.5 in.) and ranges from 30 to 35 cm (12 to 14 in.). Chest measurements are taken with the tape measure placed at the lower edge of the scapulas and brought around anteriorly, directly over the nipple line. The abdominal circumference, or girth, may also be measured at this time by placing the tape around the newborn's abdomen at the level of the umbilicus, with the bottom edge of the tape at the top edge of the umbilicus.

TEMPERATURE Initial assessment of the newborn's temperature is critical; if no heat conservation measures are started, skin temperature decreases markedly within

10 minutes after exposure to room air. The newborn's temperature should stabilize within 8–12 hours.

Temperature is monitored when the newborn is admitted to the nursery and at least every 30 minutes until the newborn's status has remained stable for 2 hours. Thereafter, the nurse should assess temperature at least once every 8 hours, or according to institutional policy (AAP & ACOG, 2012). For neonates who have been exposed to Group B hemolytic streptococcus, more frequent temperature monitoring may be required.

Temperature can be assessed by the axillary skin method, a continuous skin probe, the rectal route, or a tympanic thermometer. Axillary temperatures are the preferred method and are considered to be a close estimation of the rectal temperature. Axillary temperature ranges from 36.5° to 37.0°C (97.7° to 98.6°F). Skin temperature is measured most accurately by means of a continuous skin probe, but this method generally is used only with small or sick newborns placed under radiant warmers or in isolettes. Normal skin temperature is 36°–36.5°C (96.8°–97.7°F). Rectal temperature is assumed to be the closest approximation to core temperature, but the accuracy of this method depends on the depth to which the thermometer is inserted. The rectal temperature is often measured during the initial newborn assessment to determine patency. This method is not recommended for routine use because of the risk of irritation to the rectal mucosa and increased chances of perforation (Blackburn, 2013). Normal rectal temperature is 36.6°–37.2°C (97.8°–99°F).

Temperature instability (a deviation of more than 1°C [2°F] from one reading to the next) or a subnormal temperature may indicate an infection. In contrast to an elevated temperature in older children, an increased temperature in a newborn may indicate a reaction to too many coverings, too hot a room, or dehydration. Dehydration, which tends to increase body temperature, occurs in newborns whose feedings have been delayed for any reason. Newborns may respond to overheating (temperature of >37.5°C [99.5°F]) by increased restlessness and, eventually, by perspiration after 35–40 minutes of exposure (Blackburn, 2013). The perspiration appears initially on the head and face and then on the chest.

SKIN CHARACTERISTICS Although the newborn's skin color varies with genetic background, all healthy newborns have a pink tinge to their skin. The ruddy hue results from increased RBC concentrations in the blood vessels and limited subcutaneous fat deposits.

Skin pigmentation is slight in the newborn period, so color changes may be seen even in darker-skinned babies. Caucasian newborns have a pinkish-red skin tone a few hours after birth, and African American newborns have pinkish-red to reddish-brown skin color. Hispanic and Asian newborns may have an olive skin tone (Vargo, 2014). Skin pigmentation deepens over time; therefore, variations in skin color indicating illness are more difficult to evaluate in African American and Asian newborns (Vargo, 2014). A newborn who is cyanotic at rest and pink only with crying may have choanal atresia (congenital blockage of the passageway between the nose and pharynx). If crying increases the cyanosis, heart or lung problems should be suspected. Very pale newborns may be anemic or have hypovolemia (low blood pressure) (see discussion of hypovolemia in the module on Fluids and Electrolytes) and should be evaluated for these problems.

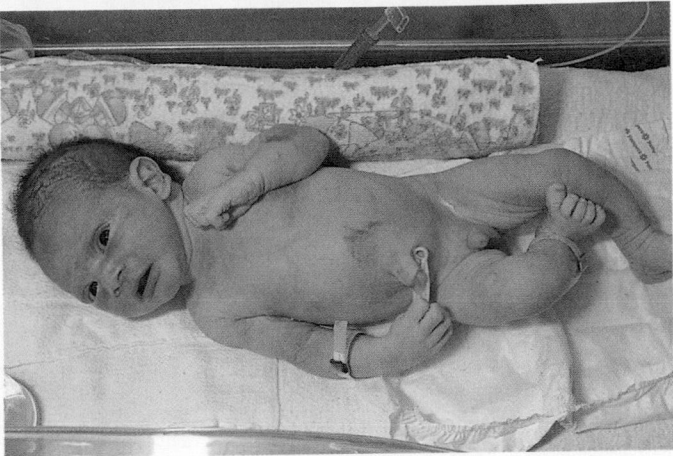

Source: George Dodson/Pearson Education, Inc.

Figure 33–70 》 Newborn with acrocyanosis.

Acrocyanosis may be present in the first 24–48 hours after birth (**Figure 33–70 》》**). This condition, bluish discoloration of the hands and feet, is caused by poor peripheral circulation, which results in vasomotor instability and capillary stasis, especially when the baby is exposed to cold. Blue hands and nails are a poor indicator of decreased oxygenation in a newborn. If the central circulation is adequate, the blood supply should return quickly (2–3 seconds) to the extremity after the skin is blanched with a finger. The nurse should assess the face and mucous membranes for pinkness that reflects adequate oxygenation.

Mottling (lacy pattern of dilated blood vessels under the skin) occurs as a result of general circulation fluctuations. It may last several hours to several weeks, or it may come and go periodically. Mottling may be related to chilling or prolonged apnea, sepsis, or hypothyroidism.

Harlequin sign (clown) color change is occasionally noted: A deep red color develops over one side of the newborn's body while the other side remains pale, so the skin resembles a clown's suit. This color change results from a vasomotor disturbance in which blood vessels on one side dilate while the blood vessels on the other side constrict. It usually lasts from 1 to 20 minutes. Affected newborns may have single or multiple episodes, but they are transient and clinically insignificant. The nurse should document each occurrence.

Jaundice is yellow pigmentation of body tissues caused by the presence of bile pigments. It is first detectable on the face (where skin overlies cartilage) and the mucous membranes of the mouth, and it has a head-to-toe progression (Vargo, 2014). Jaundice regresses in the opposite direction (from toe to head). It is evaluated by blanching the tip of the nose, the forehead, the sternum, or the gum line. This procedure must be carried out in appropriate lighting. If jaundice is present, the area will appear yellowish immediately after blanching. Another area to assess for jaundice is the sclera. Evaluation and determination of the cause of jaundice must be initiated immediately to prevent possibly serious sequelae. The jaundice may be related to breastfeeding (extremely rare), hematomas, immature liver function, or bruises from forceps, or it may be caused by blood incompatibility, oxytocin (Pitocin) augmentation or

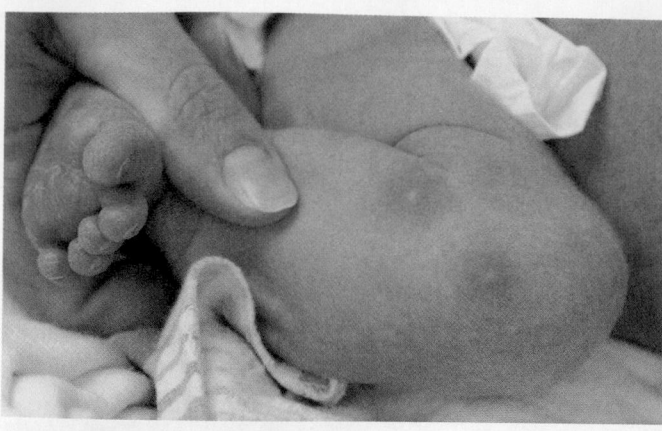

Source: George Dodson/Pearson Education, Inc.

Figure 33–71 》 Erythema toxicum on leg.

induction, or a severe hemolytic process. Any jaundice noted before a newborn is 24 hours of age should be reported to the physician or neonatal nurse practitioner.

Erythema toxicum is an eruption of lesions in the area surrounding a hair follicle that are firm, vary in size from 1 to 3 mm, and consist of a white or pale yellow papule or pustule with an erythematous base. It is often called "newborn rash" or "flea bite" dermatitis. The rash may appear suddenly, usually over the trunk and diaper area, and is frequently widespread (**Figure 33–71 》**). The lesions do not appear on the palms of the hands or the soles of the feet. The peak incidence is at 24–48 hours of life. The condition rarely presents at birth or after 5 days of life. The cause is unknown, and no treatment is necessary. Some healthcare providers believe it may be caused by irritation from clothing. The lesions disappear in a few hours or days. If a maculopapular rash appears, a smear of the aspirated papule will show numerous eosinophils on staining; no bacteria will be cultured.

Milia (exposed sebaceous glands) appear as raised white spots on the face, especially across the nose (**Figure 33–72 》**). No treatment is necessary, because they will clear spontaneously within the first month. Newborns of African heritage

have a similar condition called transient neonatal pustular melanosis (Silverman, 2012).

Skin turgor (the elasticity of the skin) is assessed to determine hydration status, the need to initiate early feedings, and the presence of any infectious processes. The usual place to assess skin turgor is over the abdomen, forearm, or thigh. Skin should be elastic and return rapidly to its original shape.

Forceps marks may be present after a difficult forceps birth. The newborn may have reddened areas over the cheeks and jaws. It is important to reassure the parents that these marks will disappear, usually within 1 or 2 days. Transient facial paralysis resulting from the forceps pressure is a rare complication. Vacuum extractor suction marks on the vertex of the scalp are often seen when vacuum extractors are used to assist with the birth; these marks are benign and do not indicate underlying brain lesions.

BIRTHMARKS Birthmarks are frequently a cause of concern and guilt for parents. The mother may be especially anxious, fearing that she is to blame ("Is my baby 'marked' because of something I did?"). Birthmarks should be identified and explained to the parents. By providing appropriate information about the cause and course of birthmarks, the nurse can relieve the fears and anxieties of the family. The nurse should note any bruises, abrasions, or birthmarks seen on admission to the nursery.

Telangiectatic nevi (stork bites) appear as pale pink or red spots and are frequently found on the eyelids, nose, lower occipital bone, and nape of the neck. These lesions are common in newborns with light complexions and are more noticeable during periods of crying. These areas have no clinical significance and usually fade by the second birthday.

Mongolian spots are macular areas of bluish-black or gray-blue pigmentation on the dorsal area and the buttocks (**Figure 33–73 》**). They are common in newborns of Asian, Hispanic, and African descent and in any newborn with darker skin. They gradually fade during the first or second year of life. They may be mistaken for bruises and should be documented in the newborn's chart.

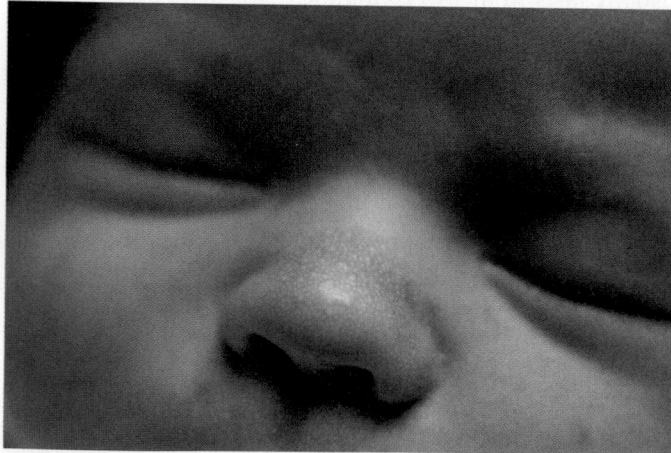

Source: Jack Sullivan/Alamy Stock Photo.

Figure 33–72 》 Facial milia.

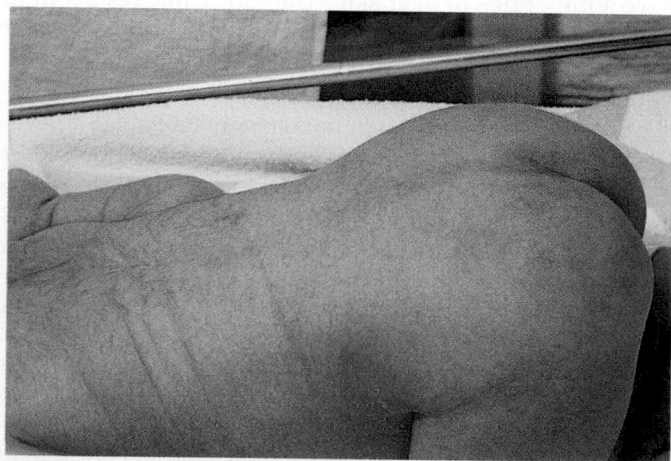

Source: George Dodson/Pearson Education, Inc.

Figure 33–73 》 Mongolian spots.

Nevus flammeus (port-wine stain) is a capillary angioma directly below the epidermis. It is a nonelevated, sharply demarcated, red-to-purple area of dense capillaries. In newborns of African descent, it may appear as a purple-black stain. The size and shape vary, but it commonly appears on the face. It does not grow in size, does not fade with time, and as a rule, does not blanch. The birthmark may be concealed by using an opaque cosmetic cream. **Nevus vasculosus (strawberry mark)** is a capillary hemangioma. It consists of newly formed and enlarged capillaries in the dermal and subdermal layers. It is a raised, clearly delineated, dark red, rough-surfaced birthmark commonly found in the head region. Such marks usually grow (often rapidly) starting in the second or third week of life, and they may not reach their full size until about 6 months (Witt, 2015). They begin to shrink and start to resolve spontaneously several weeks to months after they reach peak growth. A pale purple or gray spot on the surface of the hemangioma signals the start of resolution. The best cosmetic effect is achieved when the lesions are allowed to resolve spontaneously.

HEAD The newborn's head is large (approximately one fourth of the body size), with soft, pliable skull bones. For most term neonates, the occipitofrontal circumference is 32–37 cm (12.6–14.6 in.).

The head may appear asymmetric in the newborn of a vertex birth. This asymmetry, called **molding**, is caused by overriding of the cranial bones during labor and birth. The degree of molding varies with the amount and length of pressure exerted on the head. Within a few days after birth, the overriding usually diminishes, and the suture lines become palpable. Because head measurements are affected by molding, a second measurement is indicated a few days after birth.

The heads of breech-born newborns and of those delivered by elective cesarean are characteristically round and well shaped because no pressure was exerted on them during birth. Any extreme differences in head size may indicate microcephaly (abnormally small head) or hydrocephalus (an abnormal buildup of fluid in the brain). Variations in the shape, size, or appearance of the head measurements may be caused by craniosynostosis (premature closure of the cranial sutures), which will need to be corrected through surgery to allow brain growth, and plagiocephaly (asymmetry caused by pressure on the fetal head during gestation) (Johnson, 2015).

Two fontanels ("soft spots") may be palpated on the newborn's head. Fontanels, which are openings at the juncture of the cranial bones, can be measured with the fingers. Accurate measurement necessitates that the examiner's finger be measured in centimeters. The assessment should be carried out with the newborn in a sitting position and not crying. The diamond-shaped anterior fontanel is approximately 3–4 cm (1.2–1.6 in.) long by 2–3 cm (0.8–1.2 in.) wide. It is located at the juncture of the frontal and parietal bones. The posterior fontanel, smaller and triangular, is formed by the parietal bones and the occipital bone and is 0.5 by 1 cm. Because of molding, the fontanels are smaller immediately after birth than they are several days later. The anterior fontanel closes within 18 months, whereas the posterior fontanel closes within 8–12 weeks.

The fontanels are a useful indicator of the newborn's condition. The anterior fontanel may swell when the newborn cries or passes a stool or may pulsate with the heartbeat, which is normal. A bulging fontanel usually signifies increased intracranial pressure, and a depressed fontanel indicates dehydration (Vargo, 2014).

The sutures between the cranial bones should be palpated for the amount of overlapping. In newborns whose growth has been restricted, the sutures may be wider than normal, and the fontanels may also be larger because of impaired growth of the cranial bones. In addition to inspecting the newborn's head for degree of molding and size, the nurse should evaluate it for soft-tissue edema and bruising.

Cephalohematoma is a collection of blood resulting from ruptured blood vessels between the surface of a cranial bone (usually parietal) and the periosteal membrane (**Figure 33–74 》**). The scalp in these areas feels loose and slightly edematous. These areas emerge as defined hematomas between the first and second days. Although external

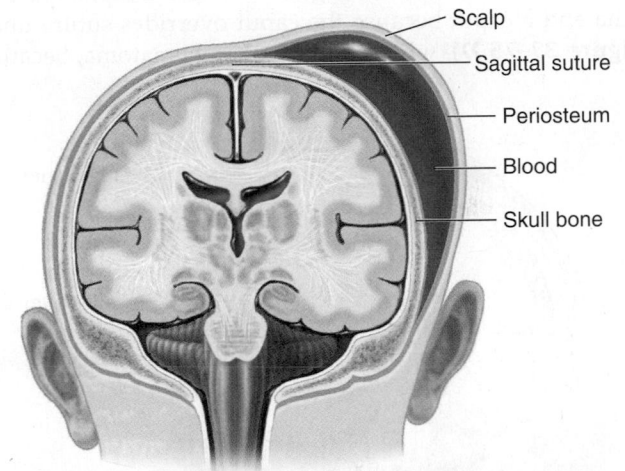

Scalp
Sagittal suture
Periosteum
Blood
Skull bone

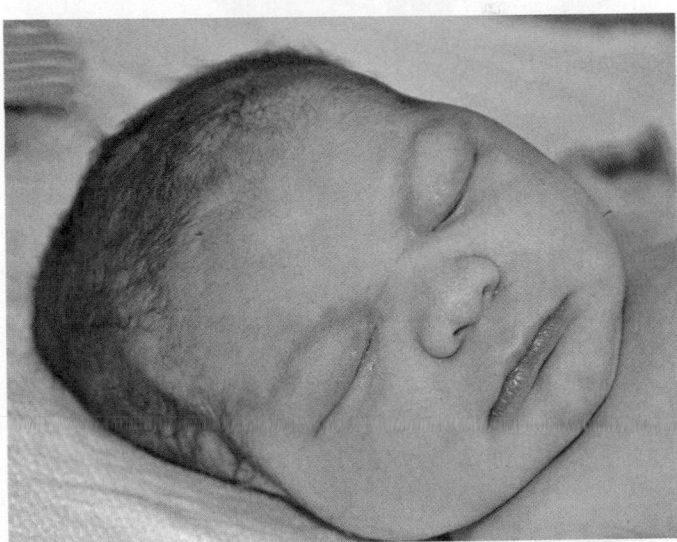

Source: Courtesy of Jo Engle, RN, MSN, NNP-BC, and Vanessa Howell RN, MSN.

Figure 33–74 》 Cephalohematoma is a collection of blood between the surface of a cranial bone and the periosteal membrane. This is a cephalohematoma over the left parietal bone.

pressure may cause the mass to fluctuate, it does not increase in size when the newborn cries. Cephalohematomas may be unilateral or bilateral and do not cross suture lines. They are relatively common in vertex births and may disappear within 2 weeks to 3 months. They may be associated with physiologic jaundice because extra RBCs are being destroyed within the cephalohematoma. A large cephalohematoma can lead to anemia and hypotension.

Caput succedaneum is a localized, easily identifiable, soft area of the scalp, generally resulting from a long and difficult labor or vacuum extraction. The sustained pressure of the presenting part against the cervix results in compression of local blood vessels, and venous return is slowed. This results in an increase of tissue fluids, edematous swelling, and occasional bleeding under the periosteum. The caput may vary from a small area to a severely elongated head. The fluid in the caput is reabsorbed within 12 hours to a few days after birth. Caputs resulting from vacuum extractors are sharply outlined, circular areas up to 2 cm (0.8 in.) thick. They disappear more slowly than naturally occurring edema. It is possible to distinguish between a cephalohematoma and a caput because the caput overrides suture lines (**Figure 33–75 »**), whereas the cephalohematoma, because

of its location, never crosses a suture line. Also, caput succedaneum is present at birth, whereas cephalohematoma generally is not.

» Go to **Pearson MyLab Nursing and eText** to see Chart 17: Comparison of Cephalohematoma and Caput Succedaneum.

FACE The newborn's face is well designed to help the newborn suckle. Sucking (fat) pads are located in the cheeks, and a labial tubercle (sucking callus) is frequently found in the center of the upper lip. The chin is recessed, and the nose is flattened. The lips are sensitive to touch, and the sucking reflex is easily initiated.

Symmetry of the eyes, nose, and ears is evaluated. Symmetry of facial movement should be assessed to determine the presence of facial palsy.

Facial paralysis appears when the newborn cries: The affected side is immobile, and the palpebral (eyelid) fissure widens. Paralysis may result from forceps-assisted birth or pressure on the facial nerve caused by the maternal pelvis during birth. Facial paralysis usually disappears within a few days to 3 weeks, although in some cases it may be permanent.

EYES The eyes of the newborn range from a blue- or slate-gray color to a dark brown color. Scleral color tends to be bluish white in all newborns because of its relative thinness. A blue sclera is associated with osteogenesis imperfecta. The infant's eye color is usually established at approximately 3 months, although it may change any time up to 1 year.

The eyes should be checked for size, equality of pupil size, reaction of pupils to light, blink reflex to light, and edema and inflammation of the eyelids. The eyelids are usually edematous during the first few days of life because of the pressure associated with birth.

Erythromycin is frequently used prophylactically to reduce risk from bacteria to which the neonate may have been exposed during the birth process. Erythromycin is preferred over the once-popular silver nitrate because erythromycin does not usually cause chemical irritation of the eye. The instillation of silver nitrate drops in the newborn's eyes may cause edema, and **chemical conjunctivitis** (irritation of the conjunctiva by chemicals used to treat the eyes, resulting in a purulent greenish yellow discharge exudate) may appear a few hours after instillation but disappears in 1–2 days. Tetracycline is still used in some institutions (AAP & ACOG, 2012).

If infectious conjunctivitis exists, the newborn has the same purulent discharge exudate as in chemical conjunctivitis, but it is caused by gonococcus, *Chlamydia*, staphylococci, or a variety of gram-negative bacteria. It requires treatment with ophthalmic antibiotics. Onset is usually after the second day. Edema of the orbits or eyelids may persist for several days until the newborn's kidneys can eliminate the fluid.

Small **subconjunctival hemorrhages** appear in approximately 10% of newborns and are commonly found on the sclera. These hemorrhages are caused by the changes in vascular tension or ocular pressure during birth. They will remain for a few weeks and are of no pathologic significance.

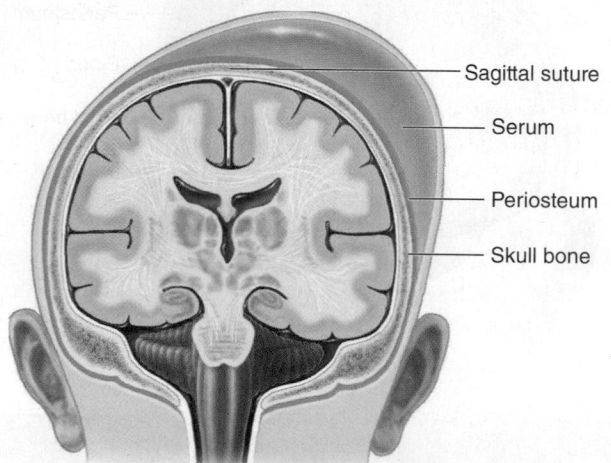

Sagittal suture

Serum

Periosteum

Skull bone

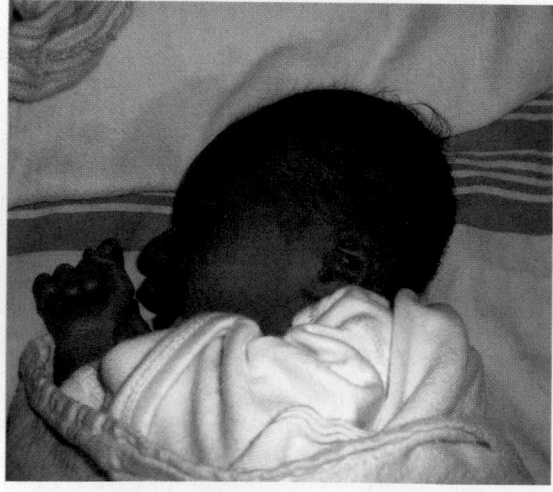

Source: Michele Davidson.

Figure 33–75 » Caput succedaneum is a collection of fluid (serum) under the scalp.

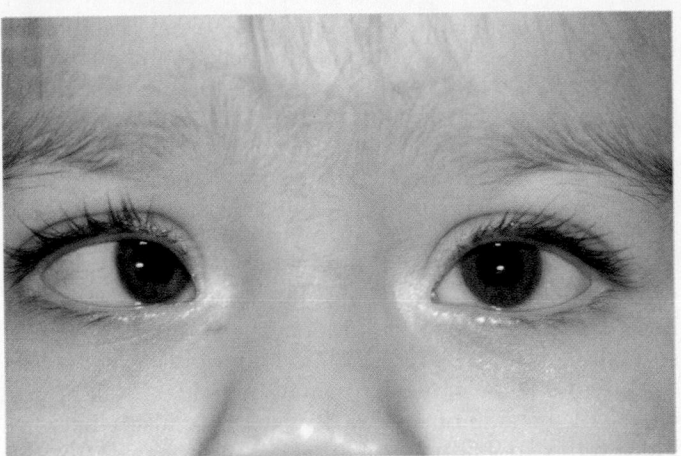

Figure 33–76 》 Transient strabismus may be present in the newborn because of poor neuromuscular control.

Parents need reassurance that the newborn is not bleeding from within the eye and that vision will not be impaired.

The newborn may demonstrate transient strabismus caused by poor neuromuscular control of eye muscles (**Figure 33–76** 》). It gradually dissipates in 3–4 months. The "doll's-eye" phenomenon is also present for approximately 10 days after birth. As the newborn's head position is changed to the left and then to the right, the eyes move to the opposite direction. "Doll's eye" results from underdeveloped integration of head–eye coordination.

The nurse should observe the newborn's pupils for opacities or whiteness and for the absence of a normal red retinal reflex. Red retinal reflex is a red-orange flash of color observed when an ophthalmoscope light reflects off the retina. In a newborn with dark skin color, the retina may appear paler or more grayish. Absence of red reflex occurs with cataracts. Congenital cataracts should be suspected in newborns of mothers with a history of rubella, cytomegalic inclusion disease, or syphilis. Brushfield spots (black or white spots on the periphery of the iris) can be associated with Down syndrome (Vargo, 2014).

The cry of the newborn is commonly tearless because the lacrimal structures are immature at birth and are not usually fully functional until the second month of life. However, some babies produce tears during the newborn period.

Although poor oculomotor coordination and absence of accommodation limit visual abilities, newborns have peripheral vision, can fixate on objects near (20.3–38.1 cm [8–15 in.]) and in front of their face for short periods, can accommodate to large objects (7.6 cm [3 in.] tall × 7.6 cm [3 in.] wide), and can seek out high-contrast geometric shapes. Newborns can perceive faces, shapes, and colors, and they begin to show visual preferences early. Newborns generally blink in response to bright lights, to a tap on the bridge of the nose (glabellar reflex), or to a light touch on the eyelids. Pupillary light reflex is also present. Examination of the eye is best accomplished by rocking the newborn from an upright position to the horizontal a few times or by other methods, such as dimming overhead lights, which elicit an opened-eye response.

NOSE The newborn's nose is small and narrow. Babies are characteristically nose breathers for the first few months of life and generally remove obstructions by sneezing. Nasal patency is ensured if the newborn breathes easily with the mouth closed. If respiratory difficulty occurs, the nurse checks for choanal atresia (congenital blockage of the passageway between nose and pharynx). This can be done by observing the newborn feeding or by gently occluding each of the nares (Cavaliere & Sansoucie, 2014).

The newborn has the ability to smell after the nasal passages have been cleared of amniotic fluid and mucus. Newborns demonstrate this ability by the search for milk. Newborns turn their heads toward a milk source, whether bottle or breast. Newborns react to strong odors, such as alcohol, by turning their heads away or blinking.

MOUTH The lips of the newborn should be pink. A touch on the lips should produce sucking motions. Saliva is normally scant. The taste buds develop before birth, and the newborn can easily discriminate between sweet and bitter flavors.

The easiest way to examine the mouth completely is to stimulate the baby to cry by gently depressing the tongue, thereby causing the newborn to open the mouth fully. It is extremely important to examine the entire mouth to check for a cleft palate, which can be present even in the absence of a cleft lip. The examiner moves a gloved index finger along the hard and soft palate to feel for any openings. If the facility still provides gloves with powder, the glove powder should always be removed before examining the newborn's mouth.

Occasionally, an examination of the gums will reveal precocious teeth over the area where the lower central incisors will erupt. If they appear loose, they should be removed by the provider to prevent aspiration. Gray-white lesions (inclusion cysts) on the gums may be confused with teeth. On the hard palate and gum margins, **Epstein pearls** (small, glistening, white specks [keratin-containing cysts] that feel hard to the touch) are often present. They usually disappear in a few weeks and are of no significance. **Thrush** may appear as white patches that look like milk curds adhering to the mucous membranes, and bleeding may occur when patches are removed. Thrush is caused by *Candida albicans*, often acquired from an infected vaginal tract during birth, antibiotic use, or poor hand washing when the mother handles her newborn. Thrush is treated with an oral preparation of nystatin (Mycostatin).

A newborn who has ankyloglossia (tongue tied) has a ridge of frenulum tissue attached to the underside of the tongue at varying lengths from its base, causing a heart shape at the tip of the tongue. "Clipping the tongue," or cutting the ridge of tissue, is recommended only in severe cases. This ridge generally does not affect speech or eating, and cutting creates an entry for infection.

Transient nerve paralysis resulting from birth trauma may be manifested by asymmetric mouth movements when the newborn cries or by difficulty with sucking and feeding.

EARS The ears of the newborn are soft and pliable and should recoil readily when folded and released. In the

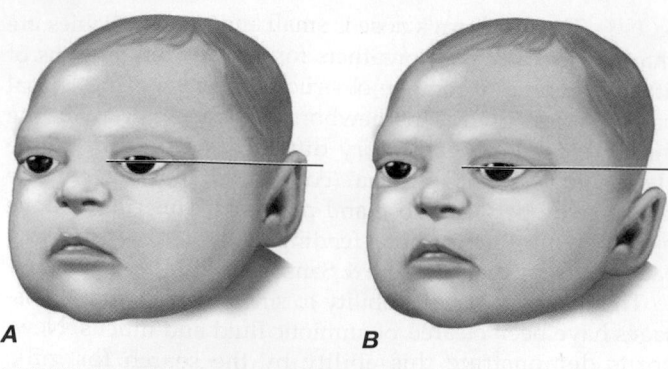

A **B**

Figure 33–77 》》 The position of the external ear may be assessed by drawing a line across the inner and outer canthus of the eye to the insertion of the ear. **A,** Normal position. **B,** True low-set position.

normal newborn, the top of the ear (pinna) should be parallel to the outer and inner canthus of the eye. The ears should be inspected for shape, size, firmness of cartilage, and position. Low-set ears (**Figure 33–77 》》**) are characteristic of many syndromes. Although most often associated with Down syndrome, low-set ears may indicate other chromosomal abnormalities, intellectual disability, and internal organ abnormalities, especially bilateral renal agenesis. Preauricular skin tags may be present just in front of the ear. Visualization of the tympanic membrane typically is not done soon after birth because blood and vernix block the ear canal.

The first cry helps initiate hearing improvement as mucus from the middle ear is absorbed, the eustachian tube becomes aerated, and the tympanic membrane becomes visible. Newborns, especially when awake, should startle or respond to loud noise. Although this is not a completely accurate test, absence of this response requires further evaluation. This is one of the reasons why the AAP has endorsed universal newborn hearing screening before discharge from the birthing unit as the standard of care (AAP & ACOG, 2012; Johnson, 2015). If the birth occurs in the home or an alternative birthing center, referral for screening should be made within 1 month of birth. The current goal is to screen all babies by 1 month of age, confirm hearing loss with audiologic examination by 3 months of age, and treat with comprehensive early intervention services before 6 months of age (AAP & ACOG, 2012). Families need to be educated about appropriate interpretation of screening test results and the suitable steps for follow-up.

The newborn can discriminate the individual characteristics of the human voice and is especially sensitive to sound levels within the normal conversational range. The newborn in a noisy nursery may habituate to the sounds and not stir unless the sound is sudden or much louder than usual.

NECK A short neck, creased with skinfolds, is characteristic of the normal newborn. Because muscle tone is not well developed, the neck cannot support the full weight of the head, which rotates freely. The head lags considerably when the newborn is pulled from a supine to a sitting position, but the prone newborn is able to raise the head slightly. The neck is palpated for masses and the presence of lymph nodes and is also inspected for webbing. Adequacy of range of motion and neck muscle function is determined by fully extending the head in all directions. Injury to the sternocleidomastoid muscle (congenital torticollis) must be considered in the presence of neck rigidity.

The nurse evaluates the clavicles for evidence of fractures, which occasionally occur during difficult births or in newborns with broad shoulders. The normal clavicle is straight. If it is fractured, a lump and a grating sensation (crepitus) during movements may be palpated along the course of the side of the break. The nurse also elicits the Moro reflex to evaluate bilateral equal movement of the arms. If the clavicle is fractured, the response will be demonstrated only on the unaffected side.

CHEST The thorax is cylindrical and symmetric at birth, and the ribs are flexible. The general appearance of the chest should be assessed. A protrusion at the lower end of the sternum, called the xiphoid cartilage, is frequently seen. It is under the skin and will become less apparent after several weeks as adipose tissue accumulates.

Engorged breasts occur frequently in both male and female newborns. This condition, which occurs by the third day, is a result of maternal hormonal influences and may last up to 2 weeks (**Figure 33–78 》》**). A whitish secretion from the nipples may also be noted. The newborn's breast should not be massaged or squeezed, because this may cause a breast abscess. Extra, or supernumerary, nipples are occasionally noted below and medial to the true nipples. These harmless pink or (in dark-skinned newborns) brown spots vary in size and do not contain glandular tissue. Accessory nipples can be differentiated from a pigmented nevus (mole) by placing the fingertips alongside the accessory nipple and pulling the adjacent tissue laterally. The accessory nipple will appear dimpled. At puberty, the accessory nipple may darken.

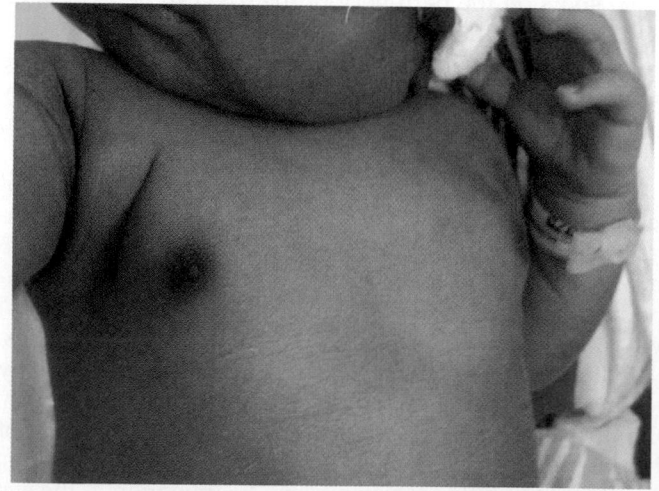

Source: Michele Davidson.

Figure 33–78 》》 Breast hypertrophy.

CRY The newborn's cry should be strong, lusty, and of medium pitch. A high-pitched, shrill cry is abnormal and may indicate neurologic disorders or hypoglycemia. Periods of crying usually vary in length after consoling measures are used. Babies' cries are an important method of communication; alerting caregivers to changes in a baby's condition and needs.

RESPIRATIONS Normal respiration for a term newborn is 30–60 breaths/minute and is predominantly diaphragmatic, with associated rising and falling of the abdomen during inspiration and expiration. The nurse notes any signs of respiratory distress, nasal flaring, intercostal or xiphoid retraction, expiratory grunt or sigh, seesaw respirations, or tachypnea (>60 breaths/minute). Hyperextension (chest appears high) or hypoextension (chest appears low) of the anteroposterior diameter of the chest should also be noted. The nurse auscultates both the anterior and posterior chest. Some breath sounds are heard best when the newborn is crying, but localizing and identifying breath sounds are difficult in the newborn. Upper airway noises and bowel sounds can be heard over the chest wall, making auscultation difficult. Because sounds may be transmitted from the unaffected lung to the affected lung, the absence of breath sounds may not be diagnosed. Air entry may be noisy in the first couple of hours until lung fluid resolves, especially after cesarean births. Brief periods of apnea (periodic breathing) occur, but no color or heart rate changes occur in healthy, term newborns. Sepsis should be suspected in term newborns experiencing apneic episodes.

HEART The nurse examines the heart for rate and rhythm, position of the apical impulse, and heart sound intensity. The pulse rate is variable and is influenced by physical activity, crying, state of wakefulness, and body temperature. The nurse auscultates the entire chest region (precordium) below the left axilla, and below the scapula. Auscultation for a full minute, preferably when the newborn is asleep, allows the nurse to obtain apical pulse rates.

A shift of heart tones in the mediastinal area to either side may indicate pneumothorax, dextrocardia (heart placement on the right side of the chest), or a diaphragmatic hernia. The nurse should auscultate heart sounds using both the bell and the diaphragm of the stethoscope. A slur or slushing sound (usually after the first sound) may indicate a murmur. Although 90% of all murmurs are transient and are considered to be normal, the nurse should document and report them. Many murmurs are secondary to closing of a patent ductus arteriosus or a patent foramen ovale, which should close 1–2 days after birth. A low-pitched, musical murmur just to the right of the apex of the heart is fairly common. Occasionally, significant murmurs are heard, such as the murmur of a patent ductus arteriosus, aortic or pulmonary stenosis, or small ventricular septal defect. Congenital cardiac defects are discussed in the module on Perfusion.

The nurse evaluates peripheral pulses (brachial, femoral, and pedal) to detect any lags or unusual characteristics.

Brachial pulses are palpated bilaterally for equality and compared with the femoral pulses. Femoral pulses are palpated by applying gentle pressure with the middle finger over the femoral canal (**Figure 33–79 ⟩⟩**). Decreased or absent femoral pulses may indicate coarctation of the aorta or hypovolemia and require additional evaluation. A wide difference in blood pressure between the upper and lower extremities also indicates coarctation of the aorta.

The measurement of blood pressure is best accomplished by using a noninvasive blood pressure device. If a blood pressure cuff is used, the newborn's extremities must be immobilized during the assessment, and the cuff should cover two thirds of the upper arm or upper leg. Movement, crying, and inappropriate cuff size can give inaccurate measurements of the blood pressure.

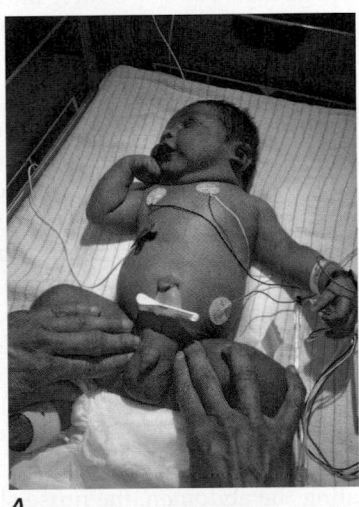

A

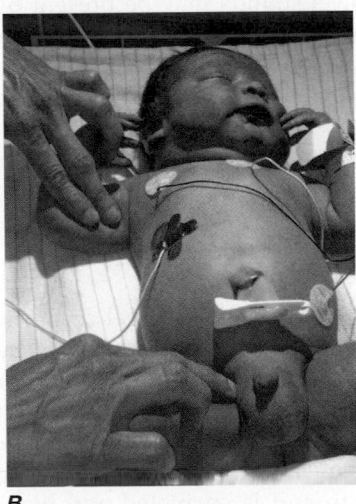

B

Source: Carol Harrigan, RNC, MSN, NNP.

Figure 33–79 ⟩⟩ *A,* Bilaterally palpate the femoral arteries for rate and intensity of the pulses. Press fingertip gently at the groin as shown. ***B,*** Compare the femoral pulses to the brachial pulses by palpating the pulses simultaneously for comparison of rate and intensity.

If possible, obtain blood pressure measurements during the quiet sleep or sleep state. Place the cuff on the neonate's arm or leg, and give the neonate time to quiet. Obtain an average of two to three measurements when making clinical decisions. Follow mean blood pressure to monitor changes, because the mean blood pressure is less likely to be erroneous. Noninvasive blood pressure may overestimate blood pressure in very-low-birth-weight neonates.

It is essential to measure blood pressure routinely for newborns who are in distress, premature, or suspected of having a cardiac anomaly (Vargo, 2014). Neonates who have birth asphyxia and are on ventilators have significantly lower systolic and diastolic blood pressures compared with healthy neonates. If a cardiac anomaly is suspected, blood pressure is measured in all four extremities. At birth, systolic values usually range from 70 to 50 mmHg and diastolic values from 45 to 30 mmHg. By the 10th day of life, blood pressure rises to 90/50 mmHg.

ABDOMEN   The nurse can learn a great deal about the newborn's abdomen without disturbing the neonate. The abdomen should be cylindrical, protrude slightly, and move with respiration. A certain amount of laxness of the abdominal muscles is normal. A scaphoid (hollow-shaped) appearance suggests the absence of abdominal contents (often seen in diaphragmatic hernias). No cyanosis should be present, and few, if any, blood vessels should be apparent to the eye. There should be no gross distention or bulging. The more distended the abdomen, the tighter the skin becomes, with engorged vessels appearing. Distention is the first sign of many gastrointestinal abnormalities.

Before palpating the abdomen, the nurse should auscultate for the presence or absence of bowel sounds in all four quadrants. Bowel sounds may be present by 1 hour after birth. Palpation can cause a transient decrease in the intensity of bowel sounds.

The nurse palpates the abdomen systematically, assessing each of the four abdominal quadrants and moving in a clockwise direction until all four quadrants have been palpated for softness, tenderness, and the presence of masses. The nurse should place one hand under the newborn's back for support during palpation.

UMBILICAL CORD   The umbilical cord initially appears white and gelatinous, with the two umbilical arteries and one umbilical vein readily apparent. Because a single umbilical artery is frequently associated with congenital anomalies, the nurse should count the vessels during the newborn assessment. The cord begins drying within 1 or 2 hours of birth and is shriveled and blackened by the second or third day. Within 7–10 days, it sloughs off, although a granulating area may remain for a few days longer.

Cord bleeding is abnormal and may result because the cord was inadvertently pulled or the cord clamp was loosened. Foul-smelling drainage is also abnormal and is generally caused by infection, which requires immediate treatment to prevent septicemia. If the newborn has a patent urachus (abnormal connection between the umbilicus and bladder),

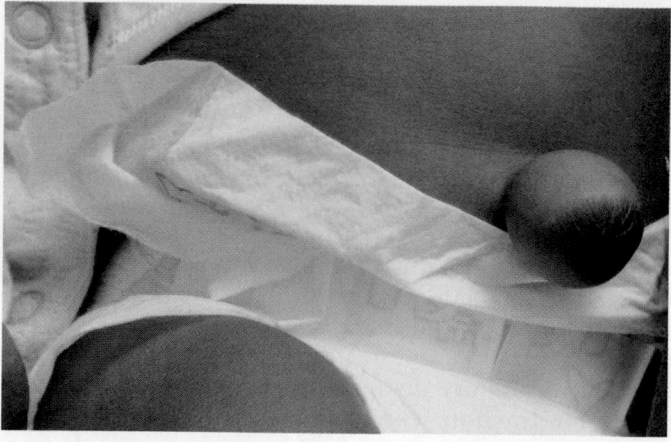

Source: George Dodson/Pearson Education, Inc.

Figure 33–80 》 Umbilical hernia.

moistness or draining urine may be apparent at the base of the cord. Another umbilical cord anomaly that can occur is umbilical cord hernia and associated patent omphalomesenteric duct (**Figure 33–80 》**). Umbilical hernias are more common in newborns of African American descent than in Caucasian babies (Goodwin, 2015).

GENITALS   For female neonates, the nurse examines the labia majora, labia minora, and clitoris and notes whether the size of each is appropriate for gestational age. A vaginal tag or hymenal tag is often evident and will usually disappear in a few weeks. During the first week of life, the female newborn may have a vaginal discharge composed of thick, whitish mucus. This discharge, which can become tinged with blood, is called pseudomenstruation and is caused by the withdrawal of maternal hormones. Smegma (a white, cheeselike substance) is often present between the labia. Removing it may traumatize tender tissue.

For male neonates, the nurse inspects the penis to determine whether the urinary orifice is positioned correctly. Possible alterations include *hypospadias*, which occurs when the urinary meatus is located on the ventral surface of the penis, and *epispadias*, in which the meatus is located on the dorsal surface of the glans. Hypospadias occurs most commonly among individuals of Western European descent. *Phimosis* is a condition in which the opening of the foreskin (prepuce) is small and the foreskin cannot be pulled back over the glans at all. This condition may interfere with urination, so the adequacy of the urinary stream should be evaluated.

The nurse then inspects the scrotum for size and symmetry. Scrotal color variations are especially prominent in African American, Indian, and Hispanic newborns (Vargo, 2014). Palpation allows the nurse to verify the presence of both testes and to rule out cryptorchidism (failure of testes to descend). The nurse palpates the testes separately between the thumb and forefinger, with the thumb and forefinger of the other hand placed together over the inguinal canal. Scrotal edema and discoloration are common in breech births. *Hydrocele* (a collection of fluid surrounding the testes in the scrotum) is common in newborns and should be identified. It usually resolves without intervention.

The nurse should report the presence of a discolored or dusky scrotum and solid testis, because this may indicate testicular torsion.

ANUS It is essential to inspect the anal area to verify that it is patent and has no fissure. Imperforate anus and rectal atresia may be ruled out by observation and through an initial rectal temperature. Digital examination, if necessary, is done by a physician or nurse practitioner. The nurse also notes the passage of the first meconium stool. Atresia of the gastrointestinal tract or meconium ileus with resultant obstruction must be considered if the newborn does not pass meconium in the first 24 hours of life.

EXTREMITIES The nurse assesses the newborn's extremities for gross deformities, extra digits or webbing, clubfoot, and range of motion. Normal newborn extremities appear short, are generally flexible, and move symmetrically. Abnormalities should be noted so that the plan of care may be created.

Nails extend beyond the fingertips in term newborns. The nurse should count fingers and toes. Polydactyly is the presence of extra digits on either the hands or the feet. Syndactyly refers to fusion (webbing) of fingers or toes. The hands are inspected for normal palmar creases; a single palmar crease, called a simian line (**Figure 33–81 》**), is frequently present in children with Down syndrome.

Brachial palsy, paralysis of portions of the arm, results from trauma to the brachial plexus during a difficult birth. It occurs commonly when strong traction is exerted on the head of the newborn in an attempt to deliver a shoulder lodged behind the symphysis pubis in the presence of shoulder dystocia. Brachial palsy may also occur during a breech birth if an arm becomes trapped over the head and traction is exerted.

The portion of the arm affected is determined by the nerves damaged. **Erb-Duchenne paralysis (Erb palsy)** involves damage to the upper arm (fifth and sixth cervical nerves) and is the most common type. Injury to the eighth cervical and first thoracic nerve roots and the lower portion of the plexus produces the relatively rare lower arm injury. The whole-arm type results from damage to the entire plexus.

With Erb-Duchenne paralysis, the newborn's arm lies limply at the side. The elbow is held in extension, with the forearm pronated. The newborn is unable to elevate the arm. Lower arm injury causes paralysis of the hand and wrist; complete paralysis of the limb occurs with the whole-arm type.

The nurse carefully instructs the parents in the correct method of performing passive range-of-motion (ROM) exercises (to prevent muscle contractures and restore function) and arranges supervised practice sessions for the parents and referral to physical therapy follow-up within 2 weeks of discharge. In more severe cases, splinting of the arm is indicated until the edema decreases. The arm is held in a position of abduction and external rotation, with the elbow flexed 90 degrees; this is often called the "Statue of Liberty" position. The "Statue of Liberty" splint is commonly used, although similar results are obtained by attaching a strip of muslin to the head of the crib and tying the other end around the wrist, thereby holding the arm up.

Prognosis is related to the degree of nerve damage resulting from trauma and hemorrhage within the nerve sheath. With minimal trauma, complete recovery occurs within a few months. Moderate trauma may result in partial paralysis. With severe trauma, recovery is unlikely, and muscle wasting may develop.

The legs of the newborn should be of equal length, with symmetric skinfolds. However, they may assume a "fetal posture" secondary to position in utero, and it may take several days for the legs to relax into a normal position. To evaluate for hip dislocation or hip instability, the Ortolani and Barlow maneuvers are performed. The nurse (or, more commonly, the physician or nurse practitioner) performs the **Ortolani maneuver** to rule out the possibility of developmental dysplastic hip, also called congenital hip dysplasia (hip dislocatability). With the newborn relaxed, quiet, and on a firm surface, with hips and knees flexed at a 90-degree angle, the experienced nurse grasps the neonate's thigh with the middle finger over the greater trochanter and then lifts the thigh to bring the femoral head from its posterior position toward the acetabulum. With gentle abduction of the thigh, the femoral head is returned to the acetabulum. Simultaneously, the examiner feels a sense of reduction or a "clunk" as the femoral head returns. This reduction is palpable and may be heard. With the **Barlow maneuver**, the healthcare provider grasps and adducts the neonate's thigh and then applies gentle downward pressure. Dislocation is felt as the femoral head slips out of the acetabulum. The femoral head is then returned to the acetabulum using the Ortolani maneuver, confirming the diagnosis of an unstable or dislocatable hip (**Figure 33–82 》**).

The feet are then examined for evidence of a talipes deformity (clubfoot). Intrauterine position frequently causes the feet to appear to turn inward (**Figure 33–83 》**); this is termed a "positional" clubfoot. If the feet can easily be returned to the midline by manipulation, no treatment is indicated, and the nurse teaches ROM exercises to the family. Further evaluation is indicated when the foot will not turn

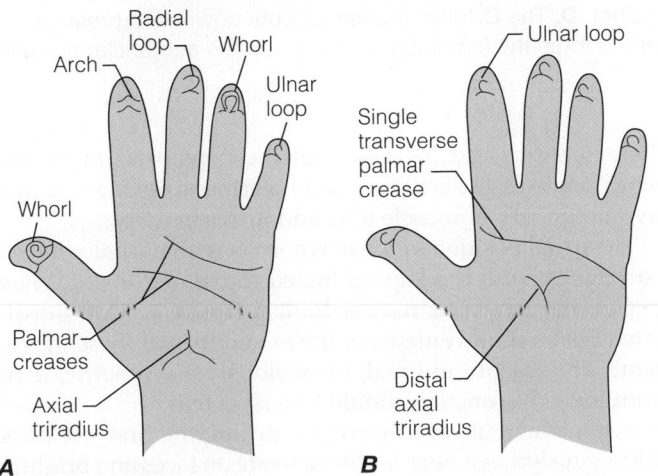

Figure 33–81 》 Dermatoglyphic patterns of the hands in **A**, a normal individual, and **B**, a child with Down syndrome. Note the single transverse palmar crease, distally placed axial triradius, and increased number of ulnar loops.

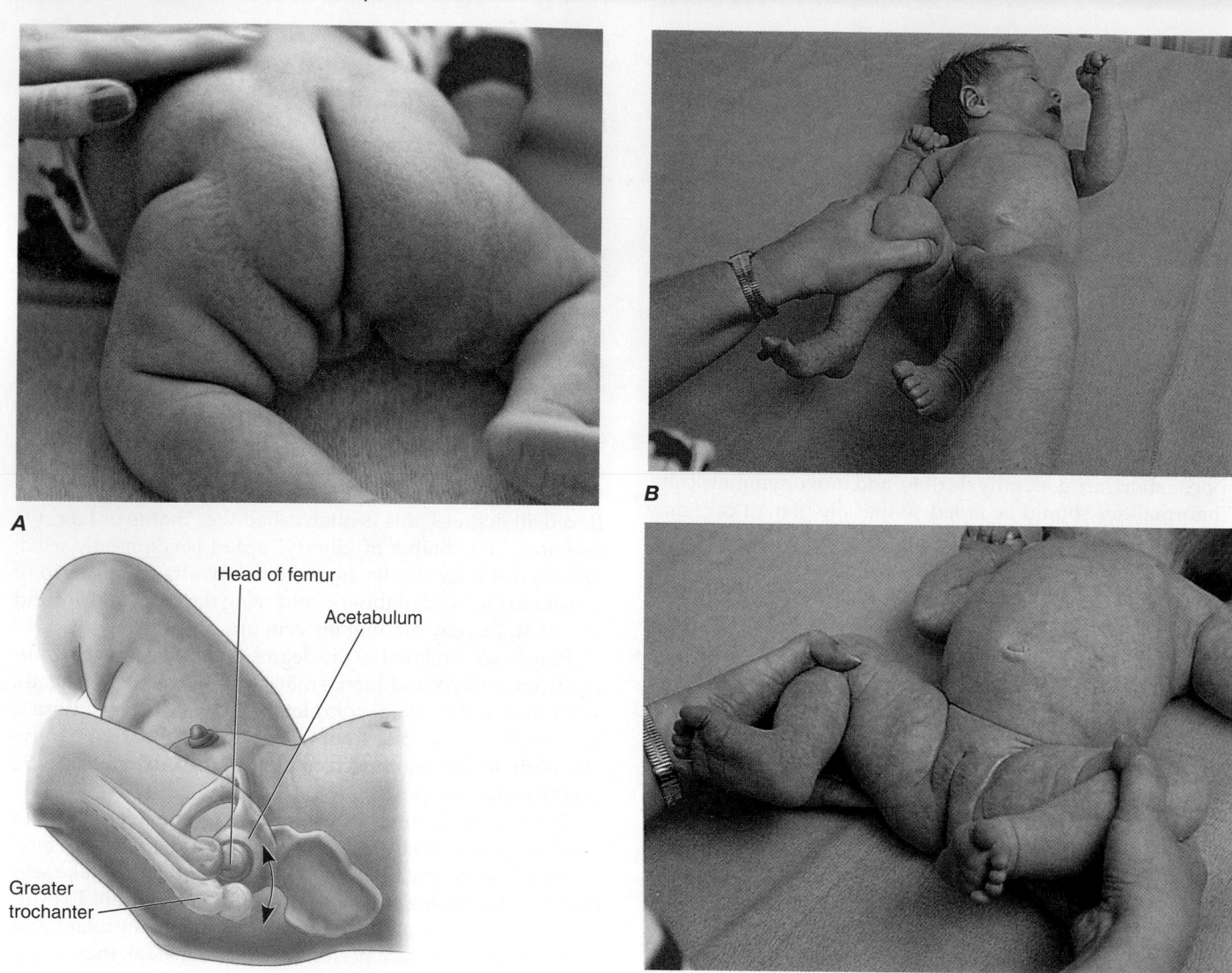

Source: (**A, B,** and **D**) George Dodson/Pearson Education, Inc.

Figure 33–82 ≫ A, The asymmetry of gluteal and thigh fat folds seen in a baby with left developmental dysplasia of the hip. **B,** The Barlow (dislocation) maneuver. The baby's thigh is grasped and adducted (placed together) with gentle downward pressure. **C,** Dislocation is palpable as the femoral head slips out of the acetabulum. **D,** The Ortolani maneuver puts downward pressure on the hip and then inward rotation. If the hip is dislocated, this maneuver will force the femoral head back into the acetabular rim with a noticeable "clunk."

to a midline position or align readily. This is considered the most severe type of "true clubfoot," or talipes equinovarus.

BACK   With the newborn prone, the nurse examines the back. The spine should appear straight and flat, because the lumbar and sacral curves do not develop until the newborn begins to sit. The base of the spine is examined for a dermal sinus. A nevus pilosus ("hairy mole") is occasionally found at the base of the spine. This is significant because it is frequently associated with spina bifida. A pilonidal dimple should be examined to ascertain that there is no connection to the spinal canal.

Assessing Neurologic Status

The nurse should begin the neurologic examination with a period of observation, noting the general physical characteristics and behaviors of the newborn. Important behaviors to assess are the state of alertness, resting posture, cry, and quality of muscle tone and motor activity.

The usual position of the newborn is with partially flexed extremities, with the legs abducted to the abdomen. When awake, the newborn may exhibit purposeless, uncoordinated bilateral movements of the extremities. If these movements are absent, minimal, or obviously asymmetric, then neurologic dysfunction should be suspected.

Eye movements are observable during the first few days of life. An alert newborn is able to fixate on faces and brightly colored objects. Shining a bright light in the newborn's eyes elicits the blinking response.

The nurse evaluates muscle tone by moving various parts of the body while the head of the newborn is in a neutral position. The newborn is somewhat hypertonic; that is, there

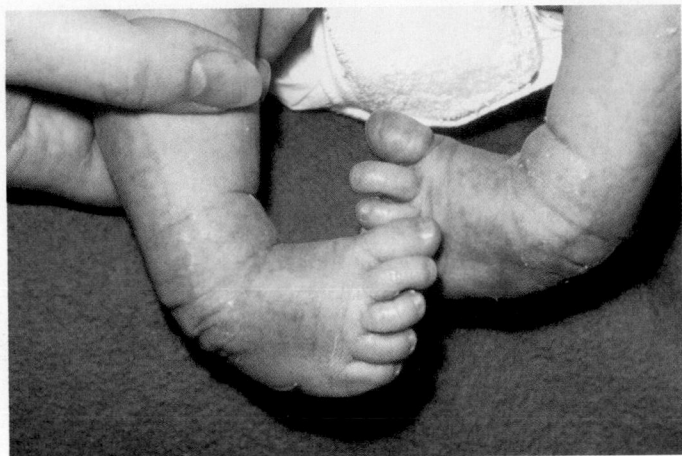

A

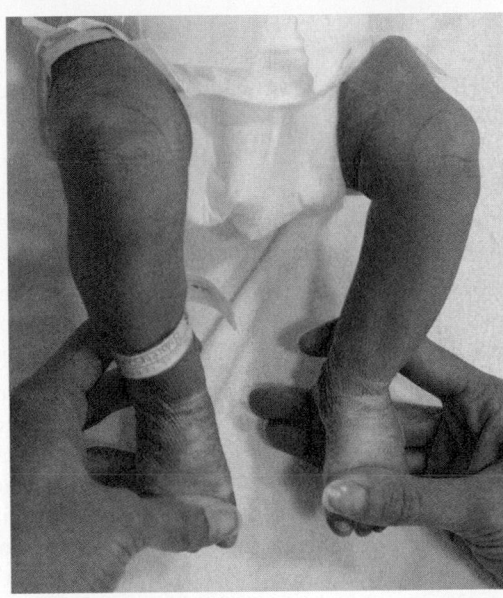

B

Source: A, Jim Stevenson/Science Source. *B,* George Dodson/Pearson Education, Inc.

Figure 33–83 》 A, Unilateral talipes equinovarus (clubfoot). **B,** To determine the presence of clubfoot, the nurse moves the foot to the midline. Resistance indicates true clubfoot.

should be resistance to extending the elbow and knee joints. Muscle tone should be symmetric. Diminished muscle tone and flaccidity require further evaluation.

Tremors or jitteriness (tremor-like movements) in the term newborn must be evaluated to differentiate the tremors from convulsions. Tremors may also be related to hypoglycemia, hypocalcemia, or substance withdrawal. Environmental stimuli may initiate tremors. Jitteriness may be distinguished from tonic–clonic seizure activity because it usually can be stopped by the baby's sucking on the extremity or by the nurse holding or flexing the involved extremity. A fine jumping of the muscle is likely to be a CNS disorder and requires further evaluation. Newborn seizures may consist of no more than chewing or swallowing movements, deviations of the eyes, rigidity, or flaccidity because of CNS immaturity. In contrast to tremors, seizures are not usually initiated by stimuli, and they cannot be stopped by holding.

Specific deep tendon reflexes can be elicited in the newborn but have limited value unless they are obviously asymmetric. The knee jerk is typically brisk; a normal ankle clonus may involve three or four beats. Plantar flexion is present.

The newborn's immature CNS is characterized by a variety of reflexes. Because the newborn's movements are uncoordinated, methods of communication are limited, and control of bodily functions is restricted, the reflexes serve a variety of purposes. Some are protective (blink, gag, and sneeze), some aid in feeding (rooting and sucking) and may not be very active if the newborn has eaten recently, and some stimulate human interaction (grasping). See Table 33–17 for commonly found reflexes in the normal newborn.

The nurse assesses CNS integration as follows:

1. The nurse inserts a gloved finger into the newborn's mouth to elicit a sucking reflex.
2. As soon as the newborn is sucking vigorously, the nurse assesses hearing and vision responses by noting changes in sucking in the presence of a light, a rattle, and a voice.
3. The newborn should respond to such stimuli with a brief cessation of sucking, followed by continuous sucking with repeated stimulation.

This CNS integration exam demonstrates auditory and visual integrity as well as the ability to conduct complex behavioral interactions.

As healthcare providers carry out the newborn physical and neurologic assessment, they are always on the alert to recognize possible alterations and possible injuries related to the birth process that require further investigation and intervention.

Assessing Newborn Behavior

The **Brazelton Neonatal Behavioral Assessment Scale** provides valuable guidelines for assessing the newborn's state changes, temperament, and individual behavioral patterns (Brazelton, 1984). It provides a way for the nurse, in conjunction with the parents (primary caregivers), to identify and understand the individual newborn's states and capabilities. Families learn which responses, interventions, or activities best meet the special needs of their newborn, and this understanding fosters positive attachment experiences.

The Brazelton assessment tool identifies the newborn's repertoire of behavioral responses to the environment and also documents the newborn's neurologic adequacy and capabilities. The examination usually takes 20–30 minutes and involves approximately 30 tests. Some items are scored according to the newborn's response to specific stimuli. Others, such as consolability and alertness, are scored as a result of continuous behavioral observations throughout the assessment. (For a complete discussion of all test items and maneuvers, see Brazelton & Nugent, 1995.)

Because the first few days after birth are a period of behavioral disorganization, the complete assessment should be done on the third day after birth. The nurse should make every effort to elicit the best response. This may be accomplished by repeating tests at different times or by testing during situations that facilitate the best possible response, such as when the parents are holding, cuddling, rocking, and/or singing to their baby.

Assessment of the newborn should be carried out initially in a quiet, dimly lighted room, if possible. The nurse should first determine the newborn's state of consciousness, because scoring and introduction of the test items are correlated with the sleep or waking state (discussed previously). The newborn's state depends on physiologic variables, such as the amount of time from the last feeding, positioning, environmental temperature, and health status; the presence of such external stimuli as noises and bright lights; and the sleep–wake cycle of the neonate. An important characteristic of the newborn period is the pattern of states, as well as the transitions from one state to another. The pattern of states is a predictor of the newborn's receptivity and ability to respond to stimuli in a cognitive manner. Babies learn best in a quiet, alert state and in an environment that is supportive and protective and that provides appropriate stimuli.

The nurse should observe the newborn's sleep–wake patterns, including the rapidity with which the newborn moves from one state to another, the newborn's ability to be consoled, and the newborn's ability to diminish the impact of disturbing stimuli. The following questions may provide the nurse with a framework for assessment:

- Does the newborn's response style and ability to adapt to stimuli indicate a need for parental interventions that will alert the newborn to the environment so that he or she can grow socially and cognitively?

- Are parental interventions necessary to lessen the outside stimuli, as in the case of the baby who responds to sensory input with intensity?

- Can the baby control the amount of sensory input that he or she must deal with?

The behaviors, and the sleep–wake states in which they are assessed, are categorized as follows:

- *Habituation.* The nurse assesses the newborn's ability to diminish or shut down innate responses to specific repeated stimuli, such as a rattle, bell, light, or pinprick to the heel.

- *Orientation to inanimate and animate visual and auditory assessment stimuli.* The nurse observes how often and where the newborn attends to auditory and visual stimuli. Orientation to the environment is determined by an ability to respond to clues given by others and by a natural ability to fix on and follow a visual object both horizontally and vertically. This capacity and the parental appreciation of it are important for positive communication between newborn and parents; the parents' visual (*en face*) and auditory (soft, continuous voice) presence stimulates their newborn to orient to them. Inability or a lack of response may indicate visual or auditory problems. It is important for parents to know that their newborn can turn to voices soon after birth or by 3 days of age and can become alert at different times with a varying degree of intensity in response to sounds.

- *Motor activity.* Several components are evaluated. Motor tone of the newborn is assessed in the most characteristic state of responsiveness. This summary assessment includes overall use of tone as the newborn responds to being

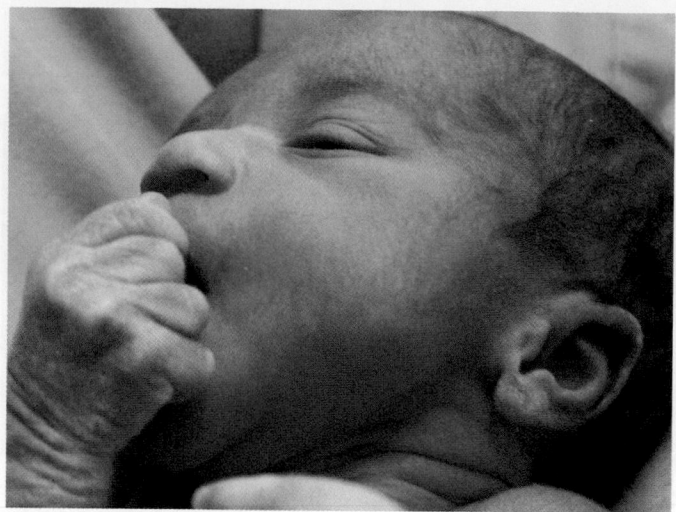

Source: George Dodson/Pearson Education, Inc.

Figure 33–84 》 The newborn can bring hand to mouth as a self-soothing activity.

handled—whether during spontaneous activity, prone placement, or horizontal holding—and overall assessment of body tone as the newborn reacts to all stimuli.

- *Variations.* Frequency of alert states, state changes, color changes (throughout all states as examination progresses), activity, and peaks of excitement are assessed.

- *Self-quieting activity.* This assessment is based on how often, how quickly, and how effectively newborns can use their resources to quiet and console themselves when upset or distressed. Considered in this assessment are such self-consolatory activities as putting a hand to mouth, sucking on a fist or the tongue, and attuning to an object or sound (**Figure 33–84 》**). The newborn's need for outside consolation must also be considered (e.g., seeing a face; being rocked, held, or dressed; using a pacifier; and being swaddled).

- *Cuddliness or social behaviors.* This area encompasses the newborn's need for, and response to, being held. These behaviors influence the couple's self-esteem and feelings of acceptance or rejection. Cuddling also appears to be an indicator of personality. Cuddlers appear to enjoy, accept, and seek physical contact; are easier to placate; sleep more; and form earlier and more intense attachments. Noncuddlers are active, restless, have accelerated motor development, and are intolerant of physical restraint. Smiling, even as a grimace reflex, greatly influences parent–newborn feedback. Parents identify this response as positive.

Once assessment has been completed, the nurse reviews the data and analyzes it to determine the newborn's specific needs.

Diagnosis

Nursing diagnoses of the newborn during the transition period are based on an analysis of the assessment findings. Physiologic alterations of the newborn form the basis of many nursing diagnoses, as does the family members' incorporation of them in caring for the new baby. Nursing diagnoses that may apply to newborns include the following:

- *Ineffective Airway Clearance* related to presence of mucus and retained lung fluid
- *Ineffective Thermoregulation* related to evaporative, radiant, conductive, convective heat losses, immature hypothalamic response
- *Acute Pain* related to heelsticks for glucose or hematocrit tests or a vitamin K injection.

(NANDA-I © 2014)

Examples of nursing diagnoses that may apply during daily care of the newborn include the following:

- *Ineffective Breathing Pattern* related to periodic breathing
- *Imbalanced Nutrition: Less Than Body Requirements* related to limited nutritional and fluid intake and increased caloric expenditure
- *Impaired Urinary Elimination* related to meatal edema secondary to circumcision
- *Risk for Infection* related to umbilical cord healing, circumcision site, immature immune system, or potential birth trauma (forceps or vacuum extraction birth)
- *Readiness for Enhanced Breastfeeding* related to lack of information about breastfeeding
- *Readiness for Enhanced Parenting* related to lack of information about basic baby care, male circumcision, and formula feeding
- *Interrupted Family Processes* related to integration of newborn into family or demands of newborn care and feeding
- *Risk for Injury* related to reabsorption of bilirubin and decreased defecation.

Nursing diagnoses that may apply to the newborn's family include the following:

- *Readiness for Enhanced Parenting* related to appropriate behavioral expectations for the newborn
- *Readiness for Enhanced Family Processes* related to integration of newborn into family unit or demands of newborn care and feeding

(NANDA-I © 2014).

Planning

The broad goals of nursing care during this period are the following:

- The newborn will be healthy and well.
- The family unit will function well.

The nurse meets the first goal by providing comprehensive care to the newborn in the mother–baby unit. The nurse meets the second goal by teaching family members how to care for their new baby and by supporting their efforts so that they feel confident and competent. The nurse must be knowledgeable about family adjustments that need to be made as well as about the healthcare needs of the newborn. It is important for the family to return home with the positive

feeling that they have the support, information, and skills to care for their newborn. Equally important is the need for each member of the family to begin a unique relationship with the newborn. The cultural and social expectations of individual families and communities affect the way in which normal newborn care is carried out.

Implementation

At the moment of birth, numerous physiologic adaptations begin to take place in the newborn's body. Because of these dramatic changes, newborns require close observation to determine how smoothly they are making the transition to extrauterine life. Newborns also require specific care that enhances their chances of making this transition successfully. Immediately after birth, the baby is formally admitted to the healthcare facility by the nurse.

The nurse reviews the mother's prenatal record for information concerning possible risk factors for the newborn. These include infectious diseases screening results, drug or alcohol use, alterations to normal pregnancy and delivery, prolonged rupture of membranes, instrument or vacuum delivery, use of narcotic analgesia, presence of meconium, psychosocial concerns such as depression or anxiety, and any other maternal data that may impact the newborn's ability to successfully transition to the extrauterine environment.

Care of the newborn is based on an analysis of assessment findings and the goals of the plan of care. This section covers some of the more common or essential interventions, both in the initial period immediately following birth and in the transition period that continues until the newborn and family are discharged.

Initial Care of the Newborn

The nurse responsible for the newborn first checks and confirms the newborn's identification with the mother's identification and then obtains and records all significant information.

MAINTENANCE OF A CLEAR AIRWAY For the neonate with any initial respiratory distress or excessive oral secretions, the nurse should position the newborn on the back (or the side if secretions are copious) and suction the airway using a bulb syringe. When possible, this procedure should be delayed for 10–15 minutes after birth to reduce the potential for severe vasovagal reflex apnea. Excessive secretions should be reported to the primary healthcare provider because they may indicate tracheoesophageal fistula.

MEASUREMENT OF VITAL SIGNS In the absence of any newborn distress, the nurse continues to admit the newborn by measuring vital signs. The vital signs for a healthy term newborn should be monitored at least every 30 minutes until the newborn's condition has remained stable for 2 hours (AAP & ACOG, 2012). The newborn's respirations may be irregular yet still be considered normal. Periodic breathing, lasting only 5–15 seconds with no color or heart rate changes, is considered to be normal. The normal pulse range is 110–160 beats/min (a pulse anywhere from 100 to 205 beats/min may be considered normal), and the normal respiratory range is 30–60 breaths/min (during the first several hours after birth it is not uncommon for the newborn to have a respiratory rate as high as 80 breaths/min).

PROMOTION OF THERMOREGULATION An NTE is best achieved by performing the newborn assessment and interventions with the newborn unclothed and under a radiant warmer. The radiant warmer's thermostat is controlled by the thermal skin sensor taped to the newborn's abdomen, upper thigh, or arm. The sensor indicates when the newborn's temperature exceeds or falls below the acceptable temperature range. The nurse should be aware that leaning over the newborn may block the radiant heat waves from reaching the neonate. In addition to placing the baby under a radiant warmer, it is common practice in some institutions to cover the newborn's head with a cap to prevent further evaporative heat loss (Blackburn, 2013).

When the newborn's temperature is normal and vital signs are stable (2–4 hours after birth), the baby may be given a sponge bath. However, this admission bath may be postponed for some hours if the newborn's condition dictates or if the parents wish to give the first bath. In light of early discharge practices (12–48 hours), healthy term newborns can be bathed safely immediately after the admission assessment is completed. The baby is bathed while still under the radiant warmer. The newborn may be bathed in the parents' room and by the parents. Bathing the newborn offers an excellent opportunity for the nurse to teach and welcome parents' involvement in the care of their baby.

The nurse rechecks the baby's temperature after the bath and, if it is stable, dresses and places the newborn in an open crib at room temperature. If the baby's axillary temperature is below 36.5°C (97.7°F), the nurse returns the baby to the radiant warmer. The rewarming process should be gradual to prevent hyperthermia. Once the newborn is rewarmed, the nurse implements measures to prevent further neonatal heat loss, such as keeping the newborn dry, swaddled in one or two blankets with a hat on, and away from cool surfaces or instruments. Newborns are often "double-wrapped" in two or more blankets for temperature maintenance.

VITAMIN K DEFICIENCY A prophylactic injection of phytonadione (vitamin K) is recommended to prevent hemorrhage, which can occur because of low prothrombin levels in the first few days of life. The potential for hemorrhage is considered to result from the absence of intestinal bacterial flora, which influences the production of vitamin K in the newborn. Newborns should receive a single parenteral dose of 0.5–1 mg of phytonadione within 1 hour of birth; this dose may be delayed until after the first breastfeeding in the childbirth/birthing area (AAP & ACOG, 2012; Marcewicz, 2014). Current recommendations underscore the need for treatment in babies who are exclusively breastfed (Blackburn, 2013).

The phytonadione injection is given intramuscularly in the middle third of the vastus lateralis muscle, located in the lateral aspect of the thigh (**Figure 33–85 >>**). Before injecting, the nurse must thoroughly clean the newborn's

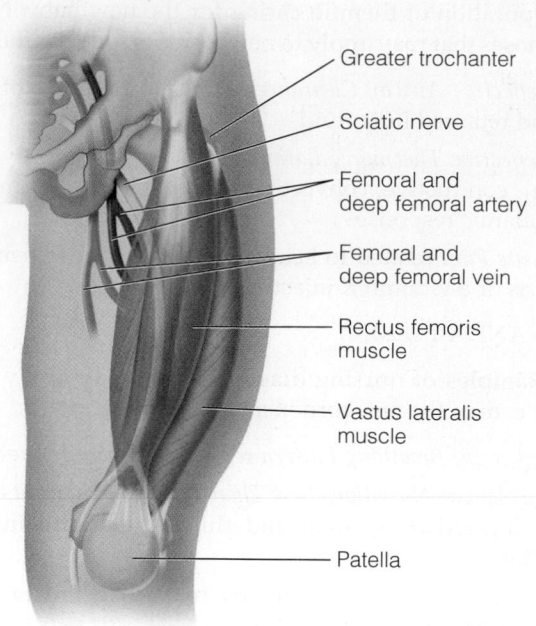

Greater trochanter
Sciatic nerve
Femoral and deep femoral artery
Femoral and deep femoral vein
Rectus femoris muscle
Vastus lateralis muscle
Patella

Figure 33–85 >> Injection sites. The middle third of the vastus lateralis muscle is the preferred site for intramuscular injection in the newborn.

skin site for the injection with a small alcohol swab. The nurse uses a 27-gauge, 1/2 in. to 5/8 in. needle for the injection (**Figure 33–86 >>**). An alternative site is the rectus femoris muscle in the anterior aspect of the thigh. However, this site is near the sciatic nerve and femoral artery, so injections here should be done with caution.

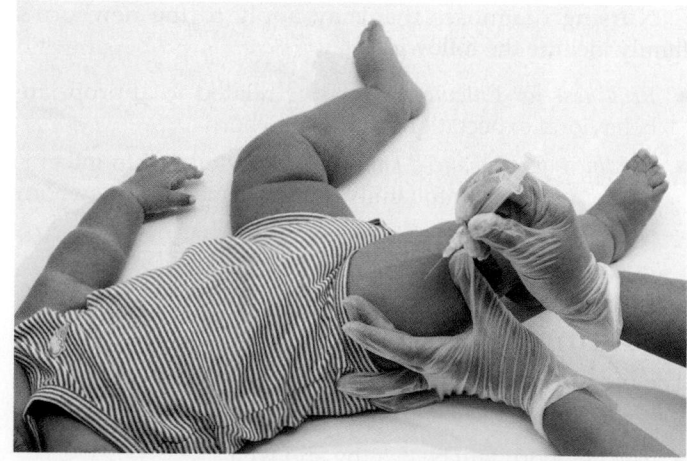

Source: Marlon Lopez/MMG1 Design/Shutterstock.

Figure 33–86 >> Procedure for vitamin K injection. Cleanse the area thoroughly with an alcohol swab and allow the skin to dry. Hold the tissue of the upper outer thigh (vastus lateralis muscle) taut, and quickly insert a 27-gauge, 1/2 in. to 5/8 in. needle at a 90-degree angle to the thigh. Aspirate, then slowly inject the solution to distribute the medication evenly and minimize the baby's discomfort. Remove the needle and gently massage the site with an alcohol swab.

PREVENTION OF EYE INFECTION The nurse is responsible for giving the legally required prophylactic eye treatment for *Neisseria gonorrhoeae*, which may have infected the newborn of an infected mother during the birth process. A variety of topical agents appear to be equally effective. Ophthalmic ointments that are used include 0.5% erythromycin (Ilotycin Ophthalmic), 1% tetracycline, or per agency protocol (AAP & ACOG, 2012). All of these ointments are also effective against chlamydia, which has a higher incidence rate than gonorrhea.

Successful eye prophylaxis requires that the medication be instilled into the lower conjunctival sac of each eye (**Figure 33–87 ≫**). The nurse massages the eyelid gently to distribute the ointment. Instillation may be delayed up to 1 hour after birth to allow eye contact during parent–newborn bonding.

Eye prophylaxis medications can cause chemical conjunctivitis, which gives the newborn some discomfort and may interfere with the newborn's ability to focus on the parents' faces. The resulting edema, inflammation, and discharge may cause concern if the parents have not been informed that the side effects will clear in 24–48 hours and that this prophylactic eye treatment is necessary for the newborn's well-being.

EARLY ASSESSMENT OF NEONATAL DISTRESS During the first 24 hours of life, the nurse is constantly alert for signs of distress. If the newborn is with the parents during this period, the nurse must take extra care to teach them how to maintain their newborn's temperature, recognize the hallmarks of newborn distress, and respond immediately to signs of respiratory problems. The parents learn to observe the newborn for changes in color or activity, grunting or "sighing" sounds with breathing, rapid breathing with chest retractions, or facial grimacing. Their interventions include nasal and oral suctioning with a bulb syringe, positioning, and vigorous fingertip stroking of the newborn's spine to stimulate respiratory activity if necessary. The nurse must be available immediately if the newborn develops distress.

INITIATION OF FIRST FEEDING The timing of the first feeding varies depending on whether the newborn is to be breastfed or formula-fed and whether there were any complications during pregnancy or birth, such as maternal diabetes or intrauterine growth restriction. The nurse should encourage mothers who choose to breastfeed their newborns to put the baby to the breast during the newborn's first period of reactivity. This practice should be encouraged because successful, long-term breastfeeding during infancy appears to be related to beginning such feedings in the first few hours of life. Sleep–wake states affect feeding behavior and need to be considered when evaluating the newborn's sucking ability.

Formula-fed newborns usually begin the first feedings by 5 hours of age, during the second period of reactivity when they awaken and appear hungry. Signs indicating newborn readiness for the first feeding are licking of the lips, placing a hand in or near the mouth, active bowel sounds, absence of abdominal distention, and a lusty cry that quiets with rooting and sucking behaviors when a stimulus is placed near the lips. Observing the earlier, more subtle cues that the baby is ready to nurse provides an opportunity to teach the parents to recognize these cues and respond before the baby is frustrated and crying.

SAFETY ALERT Newborns with respiratory distress should not be fed orally because of an increased risk of aspiration.

FACILITATION OF PARENT–NEWBORN ATTACHMENT To facilitate parent–newborn attachment, eye-to-eye contact between the parents and their newborn is extremely important during the early hours after birth, when the newborn is in the first period of reactivity. The newborn is alert during this time, the eyes are wide open, and the baby often makes direct eye contact with human faces within optimal range for visual acuity. It is theorized that this eye contact (*en face*) is an important foundation of establishing attachment in human relationships (Cassidy, Jones, & Shaver, 2013). Parents who cannot be with their newborns in this first period because of maternal or neonatal distress may need reassurance that the bonding process can proceed normally as soon as both mother and baby are stable.

Another situation that can facilitate attachment is the interactive bath. While bathing their newborn for the first time, parents attend closely to their baby's behavior. The bath is also an opportune time for the nurse to educate patients about normal variations in the newborn, and to allow parents to gain confidence handling and interacting with the newborn.

Care of the Newborn Following Transition

Once a healthy newborn has demonstrated successful adaptation to extrauterine life, the neonate needs appropriate observations for the first 6–12 hours after birth and the remainder of his or her stay in the birthing facility.

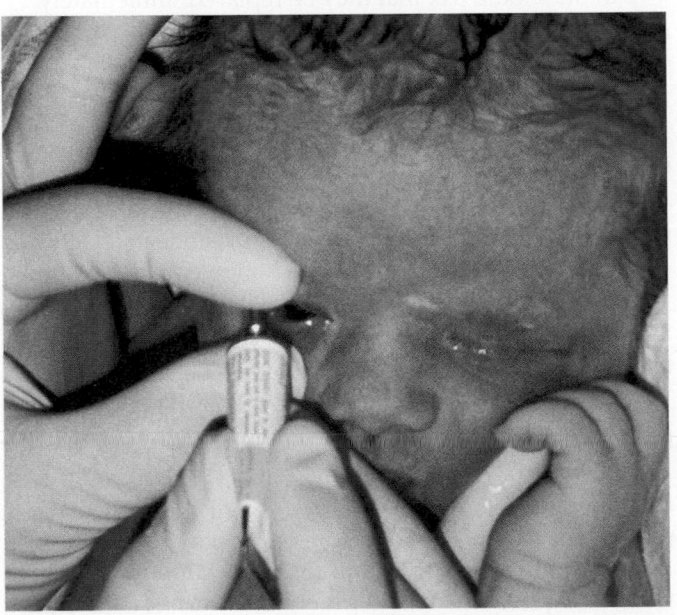

Figure 33–87 ≫ Ophthalmic ointment. Retract the lower eyelid outward to instill a 1-cm-(0.25-in.)-long strand of ointment from a single-dose tube along the lower conjunctival surface. *Make sure that the tip of the tube does not touch the eye.*

MAINTENANCE OF CARDIOPULMONARY FUNC-TION The nurse assesses vital signs every 4–8 hours or more, depending on the newborn's status. The nurse places the newborn on the back (supine) for sleeping and keeps a bulb syringe within easy reach should the baby need oral–nasal suctioning. If the newborn has respiratory difficulty, the nurse clears the airway. Vigorous fingertip stroking of the baby's spine will frequently stimulate respiratory activity. A cardiorespiratory monitor may be used on newborns who are not being observed at all times and are at risk for decreased respiratory or cardiac function. Indicators of risk are pallor, cyanosis, ruddy color, apnea, and other signs of instability. Changes in skin color may indicate the need for closer assessment of temperature, cardiopulmonary status, hematocrit, glucose, and bilirubin levels.

PROMOTION OF ADEQUATE HYDRATION AND NUTRITION The nurse records caloric and fluid intake and enhances adequate hydration by maintaining an NTE and offering early and frequent feedings. Early feedings promote gastric emptying and increase peristalsis, thereby decreasing the potential for hyperbilirubinemia by decreasing the amount of time fecal material is in contact with the enzyme beta-glucuronidase in the small intestine. This enzyme frees the bilirubin from the feces, allowing it to be reabsorbed into the vascular system.

The nurse records voiding and stooling patterns. The first voiding and the first passage of stool should occur within 24-48 hours. If they do not occur, the nurse continues the normal observation routine while assessing for abdominal distention, bowel sounds, hydration, fluid intake, and temperature stability.

The nurse weighs the newborn at the same time each day for accurate comparisons. The newborn must be kept warm during the weighing. A weight loss of up to 10% for term newborns is considered to be within normal limits during the first week of life. This weight loss is the result of limited intake, loss of excess extracellular fluid, and passage of meconium. Parents should be told about the expected weight loss, the reason for it, and the expectations for regaining the birth weight. Birth weight is usually regained by 2 weeks if feedings are adequate.

Excessive handling can cause an increase in the newborn's metabolic rate and caloric use and also cause fatigue. The nurse should be alert to the newborn's subtle cues of fatigue, including a decrease in muscle tension and activity in the extremities and neck as well as loss of eye contact, which may be manifested by fluttering or closure of the eyelids. The nurse quickly ceases stimulation when signs of fatigue appear. The nurse demonstrates to parents the need to be aware of newborn cues and to wait for periods of alertness for contact and stimulation.

The nurse also assesses the woman's comfort and latching-on techniques if breastfeeding. If the woman is not breastfeeding, the nurse assesses the mother's bottle-feeding techniques.

PROMOTION OF SKIN INTEGRITY Newborn skin care, including bathing, is important for the health and appearance of the individual newborn and for infection control within the nursery. Ongoing skin care involves cleansing the buttock and perianal areas with fresh water and cotton or a mild soap and water during diaper changes. If commercial baby wipes are used, those without alcohol should be selected. Perfume-free and latex-free wipes are also available.

The nurse should assess the umbilical cord for signs of bleeding or infection. Removal of the cord clamp within 24–48 hours of birth reduces the chance of tension injury to the area. Keeping the umbilical stump clean and dry can reduce the chance for infection. Many types of routine cord care are practiced, including the use of triple dye, an antimicrobial agent (e.g., bacitracin), or application of 70% alcohol to the cord stump. These practices are largely based on tradition rather than current research findings. The skin absorption and toxicity of triple-dye agents in newborns have not been carefully studied. Studies have shown that alcohol used alone is not effective in preventing umbilical cord colonization and infection (omphalitis) (AAP & ACOG, 2012). Folding the diaper down to avoid covering the cord stump can prevent contamination of the area and promote drying. The nurse is responsible for cord care per agency policy. It is also the nurse's responsibility to instruct parents in caring for the cord and observing for signs and symptoms of infection after discharge, such as foul smell, redness and drainage, localized heat and tenderness, or bleeding.

PROMOTION OF SAFETY Safety of the newborn is paramount. It is essential for the nurse and other caregivers to verify the identity of the newborn by comparing the numbers and names on the identification bracelets of the mother and newborn before giving a baby to a parent (AAP & ACOG, 2012).

The nurse should teach parents the following measures to prevent abduction and provide for safety:

- Parents should check that identification bands are in place as they care for their baby; if the bands are missing, parents should ask that they be replaced immediately.
- Parents should allow only individuals with proper birthing-unit picture identification to bring and/or remove the baby from the room. If parents do not know the staff person, they should call the nurse for assistance.
- Parents should report the presence of any suspicious individuals on the birthing unit.
- Parents should never leave their baby alone in their room. If they walk in the halls or take a shower, parents should have a family member watch the baby or should return the baby to the nursery.
- A parent who is feeling weak, faint, or unsteady should not lift the baby. Instead, the parent should call for assistance.
- Parents should always keep an eye and a hand on the baby when the newborn is out of the crib.
- Parents should ask visitors to leave if they have a cold, diarrhea, discharge from sores, or a contagious disease. Newborns need protection from infection even though they do possess some immunity.

PREVENTION OF COMPLICATIONS Newborns are at continued risk for the complications of hemorrhage, late-onset cardiac symptoms, and infection. Pallor may be an early sign of hemorrhage and must be reported to the healthcare provider. The newborn with pallor is placed on a cardiorespiratory monitor to permit continuous assessment. Several newborn conditions put newborns at risk for hemorrhage. Cyanosis that is not relieved by oxygen administration requires emergency intervention, may indicate a congenital cardiac condition or shock, and requires ongoing assessment.

Infection in the nursery is best prevented by requiring that all personnel who have direct contact with newborns scrub for 2–3 minutes from the fingertips up to and including the elbows at the beginning of each shift. Each caregiver's hands must also be washed with soap and rubbed vigorously for 15 seconds before and after contact with every newborn and after touching any soiled surface, such as the floor or one's hair or face. Parents are instructed to practice appropriate hand hygiene before touching the baby. They are also instructed that anyone holding the baby should practice good hand hygiene, even after the family returns home. In some clinical settings family members are asked to wear gowns (preferably disposable) over their street clothes during their contact with newborns. These are good opportunities for the nurse to reinforce the efficacy of hand hygiene in preventing the spread of infection.

Jaundice in newborns is caused by the accumulation of the pigment bilirubin in the skin. Jaundice occurs in most newborns. Most jaundice is benign, but because of the potential toxicity of bilirubin, newborns must be monitored to identify those who might develop severe hyperbilirubinemia and, in rare cases, acute bilirubin encephalopathy or kernicterus (AAP & ACOG, 2012). Current recommendations include obtaining a total serum bilirubin level in any neonate who is visibly jaundiced in the first 24 hours of life and obtaining either a serum or transcutaneous bilirubin level before discharge. Nomograms for evaluating risk factors based on bilirubin levels and age of the neonate are available.

CIRCUMCISION **Circumcision** is a surgical procedure in which the prepuce, an epithelial layer covering the penis, is separated from the glans penis and excised. This procedure permits exposure of the glans for easier cleaning. Controversy exists over the need to perform circumcisions.

Originally a religious rite practiced by Jews and Muslims, circumcision has gained widespread cultural acceptance in the United States but is much less common in Europe. Many parents choose circumcision because they want their male child to have a physical appearance similar to that of his father or the majority of other boys; some feel that it is expected by society. Another commonly cited reason for circumcising newborn males is to prevent the need for anesthesia, hospitalization, pain, and trauma if the procedure is needed later in life (AAP & ACOG, 2012). Failure to circumcise is a risk factor related to penile cancer in later life. During the prenatal period, the nurse ensures that parents have clear and current information regarding the risks and benefits of circumcision and supports their decision regarding the choice to circumcise.

As in the past, recommendations regarding circumcision have varied. The 1999 AAP policy statement was reaffirmed in 2005 and does not recommend routine circumcision, but it does acknowledge that medical indications for circumcision still exist (AAP & ACOG, 2012). The policy recommends that analgesia be used during circumcision to decrease procedural pain (AAP & ACOG, 2012); the dorsal penile nerve block and subcutaneous ring block are the most effective options (Cloherty et al., 2012). If a circumcision is to be performed, it should be done using the least painful method. Studies show that using oral sucrose for painful procedures can be effective in reducing pain for newborns and should be used with other nonpharmacologic measures to enhance its effectiveness (AAP & ACOG, 2012).

Circumcision should not be performed if the newborn is premature or compromised, has a known bleeding problem, or is born with a genitourinary defect, such as hypospadias or epispadias, which may necessitate use of the foreskin in future surgical repairs.

The nurse plays an essential role in providing parents with current information regarding the medical, social, and psychologic aspects of newborn circumcision. A well-informed nurse can allay parents' anxiety by sharing information and allowing them to express their concerns. In order for parents to make a truly informed decision, they must be knowledgeable about the potential risks and outcomes of circumcision. Hemorrhage, infection, difficulty in voiding, separation of the edges of the circumcision, discomfort, and restlessness are early potential problems. Later, there is a risk that the glans and urethral meatus may become irritated and inflamed from contact with the ammonia from urine. Ulcerations and progressive stenosis may develop. Adhesions, entrapment of the penis, and damage to the urethra are all potential complications of circumcision that could require surgical correction (AAP & ACOG, 2012).

The parents of a male newborn who will not be circumcised require information from the nurse about good hygiene practices. The nurse tells the parents that the foreskin and glans are two similar layers of cells that separate from each other. The separation process begins prenatally and is normally completed between 3 and 5 years of age. In the process of separation, sterile sloughed cells build up between the layers. This buildup looks similar to the smegma that is secreted after puberty, and it is harmless. Occasionally during the daily bath, the parent can gently test for retraction. If retraction has occurred, daily gentle washing of the glans with soap and water is sufficient to maintain adequate cleanliness. The parents should later teach the child to incorporate this practice into his daily self-care activities. Most uncircumcised males have no difficulty doing so.

If circumcision is desired, the procedure is performed when the newborn is well stabilized and has received his initial physical examination by a healthcare provider. The parents may also choose to have the circumcision done after discharge. However, parents need to be advised that if the baby is older than 1 month, the current practice is to hospitalize him for the procedure.

Before a circumcision, the nurse ensures that the physician has explained the procedure, determines whether the parents have any further questions about the procedure, and verifies that the circumcision permit is signed. As with any surgical procedure, the neonate's identification band should be checked to verify his identity before the procedure begins. The nurse gathers the equipment and prepares the newborn

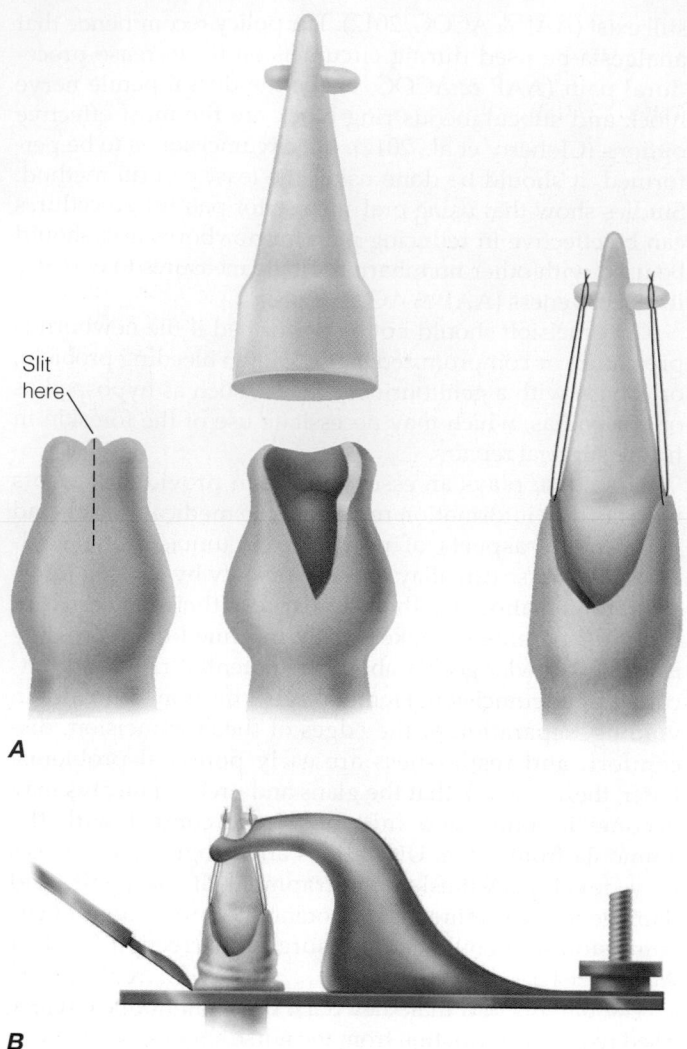

A

B

Figure 33–88 ≫ Circumcision using a circumcision clamp. *A,* The prepuce is drawn over the cone and *B,* the clamp is applied. Pressure is maintained for 3–4 minutes, and then excess prepuce is cut away.

Slit here

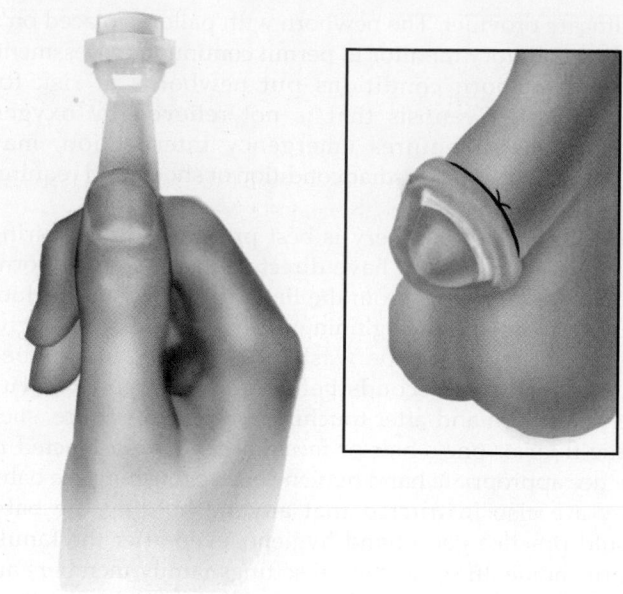

Figure 33–89 ≫ Circumcision using the Plastibell. The bell is fitted over the glans. A suture is tied around the bell's rim, and the excess prepuce is cut away. The plastic rim remains in place for 3–4 days until healing occurs. The bell may be allowed to fall off; it is removed if still in place after 8 days.

by removing the diaper and placing him on a padded circumcision board or some other type of restraint, but with only the legs restrained. These restraint measures, along with the application of warm blankets to the upper body, increase the newborn's comfort during the procedure. In Jewish circumcision ceremonies, the newborn is held by the father or godfather and is given wine before the procedure.

Various devices (Gomco clamp, Plastibell, and Mogen clamp) are used for circumcision (**Figures 33–88 ≫** and **33–89 ≫**), and all produce a small amount of bleeding. Therefore, the nurse should make special note of neonates with a family history of bleeding disorders or with mothers who took anticoagulants, including aspirin, prenatally. During the procedure, the nurse assesses the newborn's response. One important consideration is pain experienced by the newborn. A dorsal penile nerve block or ring block using 1% lidocaine without epinephrine or similar anesthetic significantly minimizes the pain and shifts in behavioral patterns, such as crying, irritability, and erratic sleep cycles, that are associated with circumcision. Other studies

are investigating the use of topical anesthetic applied 60–90 minutes before prepuce removal, acetaminophen, and cryo-analgesia. Studies indicate that a combination of methods is most effective in reducing pain during circumcision (AAP & ACOG, 2012). As indicated in Evidence-Based Practice: Breastfeeding to Control Procedural Pain in Newborns, a common method used to control pain associated with circumcision offers an opportunity for the mother to provide comfort for her newborn while diminishing anxiety related to concern about the procedure.

Following the circumcision, the newborn should be held and comforted by a family member or the nurse. The nurse must be alert to any behavioral cues that these measures are overstimulating the newborn instead of comforting him. Such cues include turning away of the head, increased generalized body movement, skin color changes, hyperalertness, and hiccoughing.

Ideally, the circumcision should be assessed every 30 minutes for at least 2 hours following the procedure. It is important to observe for the first voiding after a circumcision in order to evaluate for urinary obstruction related to penile injury and/or edema. Petroleum ointment and gauze may be applied to the site immediately following the procedure to help prevent bleeding and can be used to protect the healing tissue afterward.

The nurse must also teach family members how to assess for unusual bleeding, how to respond if unusual bleeding is present, and how to care for the newly circumcised penis. Parents of babies circumcised with a method other than the Plastibell should receive the following information:

- Clean the site with warm water with each diaper change.
- Apply petroleum ointment for the next few diaper changes to help prevent further bleeding.

Evidence-Based Practice
Breastfeeding to Control Procedural Pain in Newborns

Problem

What nonpharmacologic methods can help reduce the pain associated with common neonatal procedures?

Evidence

Assessment and management of pain are important issues in neonatal care. Most newborns will experience a venipuncture or heel lance for blood sampling during their hospital stay. Although healthcare providers agree that newborns are capable of responding to painful stimuli, most providers do not administer medication to control the short-term pain associated with these common procedures. A Cochrane systematic review investigated the use of breastfeeding—specifically, the oral administration of breast milk—to control the pain associated with common procedures (Harrison et al., 2016). Multiple systematic reviews with this quantity of randomized trials represent the strongest level of evidence for nursing practice.

Newborns who were feeding during heelsticks or venipuncture procedures demonstrated fewer physiologic and behavioral signs of pain. Actual feeding at the breast was associated with a reduction in heart rate change, percentage time crying, duration of crying, and improvement in validated neonatal pain measures. Breastfeeding led to significantly lower increases in heart rate and decreased crying time compared to those who were swaddled. All groups that were fed during the procedure—whether it was breast milk from the mother or expressed breast milk—had better pain control than babies who were swaddled, positioned, or given a pacifier without being held.

Implications

It does not appear that any of these measures completely eliminated the pain of routine procedures. In addition, these studies were focused on healthy newborns undergoing minimally invasive, singular painful procedures. The effectiveness of either breast milk for repeated painful procedures was not studied. With regard to preterm or sick newborns, there is insufficient evidence to support the safety of breast milk or sucrose as a routine, repeated comfort measure. For preterm and sick full-term newborns who are subjected to repeated painful procedures during hospitalization, the ideal analgesic has not yet been identified.

Newborns undergoing single painful procedures, such as venipuncture or heelstick, should be breastfed by the mother during the procedure if at all possible. If not, the baby can be fed expressed breast milk with a syringe, a bottle, or by dipping a pacifier in the solution. Holding the baby while doing so achieves the best pain control.

Critical Thinking Application

1. What are the challenges with breastfeeding to control procedural pain in newborns?
2. How could we measure the influence of breastfeeding on newborn pain during procedures?

- If bleeding does occur, apply light pressure with a sterile gauze pad to stop the bleeding within a short time. If this is not effective, contact the physician immediately, or take the baby to the caregiver's office.

- The glans normally has granulation tissue (a yellowish film) on it during healing. Continued application of a petroleum ointment (or ointment suggested by the healthcare provider) can help protect the granulation tissue that forms as the glans heals.

- Report to the care provider any signs or symptoms of infection, such as increasing swelling, pus drainage, and cessation of urination.

- When diapering, ensure that the diaper is not loose enough to cause rubbing with movement and is not tight enough to cause pain.

- If the newborn's care provider recommends oral analgesics, follow instructions for proper measuring and administration.

If the Plastibell is used, parents should receive information about normal appearance and how to observe for infection. The parents are informed that the Plastibell should fall off within 8 days. If it remains on after 8 days, they should consult with their physician. No ointments or creams should be used while the bell remains, but application of petroleum ointment may protect granulation tissue afterward.

STRENGTHENING PARENT–NEWBORN ATTACHMENT   The nurse encourages parent–newborn attachment by involving all family members with the new member of the family. The nurse can discuss waking activities, such as talking with the baby while making eye contact, holding the baby in an upright position (sitting or standing), gently bending the baby back and forth while grasping under the knees and supporting the head and back with the other hand, or gently rubbing the baby's hands and feet. Quieting activities may include swaddling or bundling the baby to increase a sense of security; using slow, calming movements; and talking softly, singing, or humming to the baby. See Focus on Integrative Health: Baby Massage.

When fostering parent–newborn attachment, it is important to be sensitive to the cultural beliefs and values of the family. The nurse must also be aware of cultural variations in newborn care (see Focus on Diversity and Culture:

Focus on Integrative Health
Baby Massage

Massage is a common child care practice in many parts of the world, especially Africa and Asia, that has recently gained attention in the United States. The nurse can teach parents to use massage as a method to facilitate the bonding process and to reduce the stress and pain associated with teething, constipation, inoculations, and colic. Massage not only induces relaxation for the baby, it also provides a calming and "feel-good" interaction for the parents that fosters the development of warm, positive relationships.

Focus on Diversity and Culture
Islamic Birth Traditions

At the birth of a child, Muslim families may follow one or more of several Islamic practices, a few of which are described here.

- The pregnant woman may choose to have only women attending at the birth of the baby. Note that Islam allows male providers to care for pregnant women. The father may attend the birth; Islam does not prohibit it.

- The father or an elder will speak the first words the newborn hears by whispering into the child's ear. These words are the *Adhan*, or *adhaan*, a call to prayer performed five times a day. By these words, the newborn is welcomed to a prayerful life, to Islam, and to the Muslim community.

- Within the child's first seven days, the parents may choose to circumcise the child, often doing so before leaving the hospital. Also during this first week, the parents will give the child a Muslim name.

Sources: Muslim Birth Rights. (2009). Retrieved from http://www.bbc.co.uk/religion/religions/islam/ritesrituals/birth.shtml; Huda. (2017). Common Practices of Islamic Birth Rights. Retrieved from https://www.thoughtco.com/islamic-birth-rites-2004500

Islamic Birth Traditions), complimenting the baby, and using good luck charms.

>> Go to **Pearson MyLab Nursing and eText** to see Chart 18: Promoting Attachment.

Prepare Family for Discharge

Although the adjustment to parenting is a normal process, going home presents a critical transition for the family. The parents become the primary caregivers for the newborn and must provide a nurturing environment in which the emotional and physical needs of the newborn can be met. Nursing interventions focus on promoting health and preventing possible problems.

PARENT TEACHING Nearly every contact with the parents presents an opportunity for sharing information that can facilitate their sense of competence in newborn care. To meet the parents' need for information, the nurse who is responsible for the care of the mother and newborn should assume the primary responsibility for parent education. The nurse should teach the family all necessary caregiving methods before discharge. A checklist may be helpful to determine whether the teaching has been completed and to verify the parents' knowledge on leaving the birthing unit (**Figure 33–90 >>**). The nurse needs to review all areas for understanding by the mother and father, without rushing, and then take the time to resolve all of their queries. Any concerns of the parents or nurse are noted. Unless their care methods are harmful to the newborn, the parents' methods of giving care should be reinforced rather than contradicted.

Caring for newborns in the hospital setting means that the nurse will have contact with patients from a wide variety of ethnic, religious, and cultural backgrounds. The nurse needs to recognize and respect the many good ways of providing safe care and must be sensitive to the cultural beliefs and values of the family. Although it may not be possible to be conversant with all cultures, the nurse can demonstrate

Parent Teaching Checklist

Check off each item once parents understand your instructions ✓

General Baby Care

Caring for skin

Caring for cord

Caring for circumcision and genital area

What to do if baby is sick

Using a thermometer

Using a bulb syringe

Burping baby

Comforting baby

Positioning baby

Breastfeeding

Waiting for milk to come in

Understanding let-down reflex

Positioning baby for feeding

Getting baby to latch on

When to breastfeed

How long to breastfeed

Removing baby from nipple

Understanding supply and demand

Supplementing

Comfort measures for sore nipples

Comfort measures for engorgement

Using a breast pump

Breastfeeding after returning to work

Bottle-feeding

Choosing formula

Mixing formula

Feeding baby from a bottle

Cleaning bottles

Safety

Placing baby to sleep on back

Preventing shaken baby syndrome

Using a car seat

Managing pets

Figure 33–90 >> A parent teaching checklist is completed by the time of discharge.

cultural sensitivity with both colleagues and patients as follows (Spector, 2017):

- Show respect for the inherent dignity of every human being, whatever the individual's age, gender, or religion.
- Accept the rights of individuals to choose their care provider, participate in care, and refuse care.
- Acknowledge personal biases, and prevent them from interfering with the delivery of quality care to individuals of other cultures.
- Recognize cultural issues, and interact with patients from other cultures in culturally sensitive ways.
- Incorporate the patient's cultural preferences, health beliefs and behaviors, and traditional practices into the plan of care.
- Develop appropriate educational materials that address the language and cultural beliefs of the patient.
- Access culturally appropriate resources to deliver care to patients from other cultures.
- Assist patients to access high-quality care within a dominant culture.

Parents may be familiar with handling and caring for babies, or this may be their first time interacting with a newborn. If they are new parents, the sensitive nurse gently teaches them by example and provides instructions geared to their needs and previous knowledge about the various aspects of newborn care.

The length of stay in the birthing unit for mother and baby after birth is often 72 hours or less. The challenge for the nurse is to use every opportunity to teach, guide, and support individual parents, fostering their capabilities and confidence in caring for their newborn. Including mother–baby care and home care instruction on the night shift assists with education needs for early-discharge parents.

The nurse observes how parents interact with their newborn during feeding and caregiving activities. Even during a short stay, the nurse will have opportunities to provide information and observe whether the parents are comfortable with changing the diapers of, wrapping, handling, and feeding their newborn. Do both parents get involved in the newborn's care? Is the mother depending on someone else to help her at home? Does the mother give reasons (e.g., "I'm too tired," "My stitches hurt," or "I'll learn later") for not wanting to be involved in her baby's care? As the family provides care, the nurse can enhance parental confidence by giving them positive feedback. If the parents encounter problems, the nurse can express confidence in their abilities to master the new skills or information, suggest alternatives, and serve as a role model. All of these factors need to be considered when evaluating the educational needs of the parents. In addition to the learning needs of parents, cultural factors must also be considered when providing patient education. As noted in Focus on Diversity and Culture: Examples of Cultural Beliefs and Practices Regarding Baby Care, parents from different cultures have differing views on subjects such as umbilical cord care, parent–newborn contact, feeding, circumcision, and health and illness.

Several methods may be used to teach families about newborn care. Daily newborn care videos and classes are nonthreatening ways to convey general information. Individual instruction is helpful to answer specific questions or to clarify an item that may have been confusing in class. Currently, many birthing centers have 24-hour educational video channels or videos to be viewed in the mother's room on a variety of postpartum and newborn care issues.

One-to-one teaching while the nurse is in the mother's room is the most effective educational method. Individual instruction is helpful both to answer specific questions and to clarify something that the parents may have found confusing in the educational video. With shorter stays, most teaching unfortunately tends to focus on newborn feeding and immediate physical care needs of the mothers, with limited anticipatory guidance provided in other areas.

>> Go to **Pearson MyLab Nursing and eText** to see Chart 19: What to Tell Parents About Newborn Care.

GENERAL INSTRUCTIONS FOR NEWBORN CARE   One of the first concerns of anyone who has not had the experience of picking up a baby is how to do it correctly. The newborn is easily picked up by sliding one hand under the neck and shoulders and the other hand under the buttocks or between the newborn's legs and then gently lifting upward. This technique provides security and support for the head, which the baby is unable to support until 3 or 4 months of age.

The nurse can be an excellent role model for families in the area of safety. Safety topics include proper positioning of the newborn on the back to sleep and correct use of the bulb syringe (discussed shortly). The baby should never be left alone anywhere but in the crib. The mother is reminded that while she and her newborn are together in the birthing unit, she should never leave her baby alone, both for security reasons and because newborns spit up frequently during the first day or two after birth.

Demonstrating a bath, cord care, and temperature assessment is the best way for the nurse to provide information on these topics to parents. Parents should be told to call their healthcare provider if redness, foul odor, bright-red bleeding, or greenish-yellow drainage occurs at the cord site or if the area remains unhealed 2–3 days after the cord stump has sloughed off. No single method of umbilical cord care (topical antimicrobials [triple dye, iodophor ointment, or hexachlorophene powder] or alcohol) has been proven to be superior in preventing colonization and disease (AAP & ACOG, 2012). The use of sterile water or air drying results in umbilical cords separating more quickly than those treated with alcohol (Fraser, 2014).

NASAL AND ORAL SUCTIONING   As mentioned, most newborns are obligatory nose breathers for the first months of life. They generally maintain air passage patency by coughing or sneezing. During the first few days of life, however, the newborn has increased mucus, and gentle suctioning with a bulb syringe may be indicated. The nurse can demonstrate the use of the bulb syringe in the mouth and nose and have the parents do a return demonstration. The parents should repeat this demonstration of suctioning and cleansing the bulb before discharge so that they feel confident in performing the procedure. Care should be taken to apply only gentle suction in order to prevent nasal bleeding.

Focus on Diversity and Culture
Examples of Cultural Beliefs and Practices Regarding Baby Care*

Umbilical Cord

- Individuals of Latin American, Filipino, and Haitian cultural background may use an abdominal binder or bellyband to protect against dirt, injury, and umbilical hernia. They may also apply oils to the stump of the cord or tape metal to the umbilicus to ward off evil spirits (Purnell, 2014).
- Individuals of northern European ancestry may expect a sterile cutting of the cord at birth. They may allow the stump to air dry and discard the cord once it falls off.
- Some Latin American parents cauterize the stump with a candle flame, hot coal, or burning stick.

Parent–Newborn Contact

- Individuals of Asian ancestry may pick up the baby as soon as it cries, or they may carry the baby at all times.
- Individuals of several native North American nations, notably the Navajos, may use cradle boards so that the baby can be with family even during work and feel secure (Woodring & Andrews, 2012).
- The Muslim father traditionally calls praise to Allah in the newborn's right ear and cleans the baby after birth (Purnell, 2014).

Feeding

- Some women of Asian heritage may breastfeed their babies for the first 1–2 years of life. Many Cambodian refugees practice breastfeeding on demand without restriction or, if formula feeding, provide a "comfort bottle" in between feedings.
- Individuals of Iranian heritage may breastfeed female babies longer than male babies. Many Muslim women will not breastfeed in public.
- Some individuals of African ancestry may wean their babies after they begin to walk.

- Some Asians, Haitian, Hispanics, Eastern Europeans, and Native Americans may delay breastfeeding because they believe colostrum is "bad."
- Haitian mothers may believe that "strong emotions" spoil breast milk.

Circumcision

- Individuals of Muslim and Jewish ancestry practice circumcision as a religious ritual (Purnell, 2014).
- Many natives of Africa and Australia practice circumcision as a puberty rite.
- Native Americans and individuals of Asian and Latin American cultures rarely perform circumcision.
- As of 2015, an estimated 38.7% of males worldwide were circumcised (Morris et al., 2016).

Health and Illness

- Some individuals with Latin American cultural backgrounds may believe that touching the face or head of a baby when admiring it will ward off the "evil eye." They may also neglect to cut the baby's nails to avoid nearsightedness and, instead, put mittens on the baby's hands to prevent scratching. They also may believe that fat babies are healthy (Woodring & Andrews, 2012).
- Some individuals of Asian heritage may not allow anyone to touch the baby's head without asking permission.
- Some Orthodox Jews believe that saying the baby's name before the formal naming ceremony will harm the baby.
- Some Asians and Haitians delay naming their babies until after confinement month (Purnell, 2014).
- Some individuals of Vietnamese ancestry believe that cutting a baby's hair or nails will cause illness.

Note: This information is meant only to provide examples of the behaviors that may be found within certain cultures. Not all members of a culture practice the behaviors described.

To suction the newborn, the bulb syringe is compressed before the tip is placed in the nostril. The nurse or parent must take care not to occlude the passageway. The bulb is permitted to reexpand slowly by releasing the compression on the bulb. The bulb syringe is removed from the nostril, and drainage is then compressed out of the bulb and onto a tissue. The bulb syringe may also be used in the mouth if the newborn is spitting up and unable to handle the excess secretions. The bulb is compressed, the tip of the bulb syringe is placed approximately 2.5 cm (1 in.) to one side of the newborn's mouth, and compression is released. This draws up the excess secretions. The procedure is repeated on the other side of the mouth. The roof of the mouth and the back of the throat are avoided, because suction in these areas might stimulate the gag reflex. The bulb syringe should be washed in warm, soapy water and rinsed in warm water daily and as needed after use. Rinsing with a half-strength white vinegar solution followed by clear water may help to extend the useful life of the bulb syringe by inhibiting bacterial growth. A bulb syringe should always be kept near the newborn. New parents and nurses who are inexperienced with babies may fear that

the baby will choke and are relieved to know how to take action if such an event occurs. They should be advised to turn the newborn's head to the side or hold the newborn with his or her head down as soon as there is any indication of gagging or vomiting and to use the bulb syringe as needed.

Some newborns may have transient edema of the nasal mucosa following suctioning of the airway after birth. The nurse can demonstrate the use of normal saline to loosen secretions and instruct parents in the gentle and moderate use of the bulb syringe to avoid further irritation of the mucous membranes. If parents will be using humidifiers at home, they should be instructed to follow the manufacturer's cleaning instructions carefully so that molds, spores, and bacteria from a dirty humidifier do not enter the baby's environment.

SWADDLING THE NEWBORN Swaddling (wrapping) helps the newborn maintain body temperature, provides a feeling of closeness and security, and may be effective in quieting a crying baby by having the newborn's hands near his or her mouth to allow sucking (Young et al., 2013). A

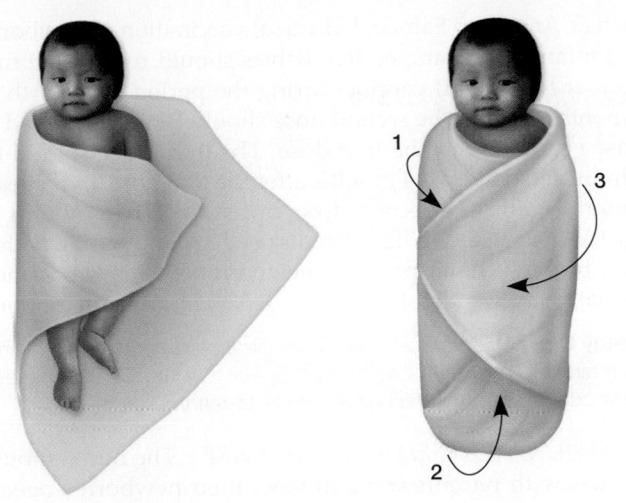

Figure 33–91 》 Steps in wrapping a baby.

blanket is placed on the crib (or secure surface) in the shape of a diamond. The top corner of the blanket is folded down slightly, and the newborn's body is placed with the head at the upper edge of the blanket. The right corner of the blanket is wrapped around the newborn and tucked under the left side (not too tightly—the newborn needs a little room to move and to allow for hands to get to the mouth). The bottom corner is then pulled up to the chest, and the left corner is wrapped around the baby's right side (**Figure 33–91 》**). The nurse can show this wrapping technique to new parents so that they will feel more skilled in handling their baby.

SLEEP AND ACTIVITY The National Institute of Child Health and Human Development and the AAP recommend that healthy term newborns be placed on their backs to sleep (**Figure 33–92 》**). Parents are taught the importance of

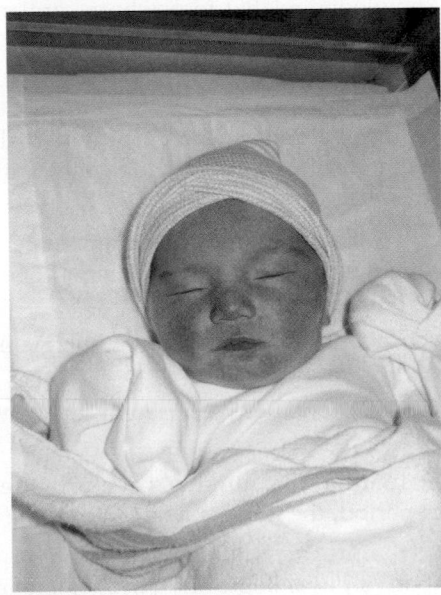

Source: Michele Davidson.

Figure 33–92 》 Babies should be placed on their backs when sleeping.

following "Safe to Sleep Guidelines" to reduce the incidence of sudden infant death syndrome (SIDS) (Healthy Children, 2015a). Though neonates may need to be placed on their sides initially because of copious or thick secretions, placing them on their backs in the newborn period serves to educate parents regarding safe sleep positioning. Studies indicate that parents position their babies in the same positions they observe in the hospital setting, so the nurse must demonstrate this behavior to reduce the risk of SIDS. If exceptions are warranted, these should be explained to families so that they do not misinterpret what they observe. The placement of babies in a prone position during wakeful play sessions ("tummy time") should be encouraged as well (AAP & ACOG, 2012). See the exemplar on Sudden Infant Death Syndrome, in the module on Oxygenation, for more information.

》Stay Current: Visit the Safe to Sleep website at https://www. nichd.nih.gov/sts/Pages/default.aspx to learn current recommendations for safe sleeping.

Perhaps nothing is more individual to each baby than the sleep–activity cycle. It is important for the nurse to recognize the individual variations of each newborn and to assist parents as they develop sensitivity to their baby's communication signals and rhythms of activity and sleep.

CAR SAFETY CONSIDERATIONS Half of the children killed or injured in automobile crashes could have been protected by the use of federally approved car seats. Newborns must go home from the birthing unit in a car seat adapted to fit them. Babies should never be placed in the front seat of a car equipped with a passenger-side airbag. The car seat should be positioned to face the rear of the car until the baby is 2 years old or until the child reaches the maximum height and weight for the seat (Healthy Children, 2015b). The nurse needs to ensure that all parents are knowledgeable about the proper installation and benefits of using a child safety seat. The nurse can encourage parents to have their safety seats checked by local groups trained specifically for that purpose. The Seat Check Initiative provides locations and information about child safety seats.

》Stay Current: Visit http://www.safercar.gov/parents/index.htm to learn how to install car seats properly and about occupant protection laws in each state.

NEWBORN SCREENING AND IMMUNIZATION PROGRAMS Before the newborn and mother are discharged from the birthing unit, the nurse informs the parents about the newborn screening tests and tells them when to return to the birthing center or clinic if further tests are needed. Some of the disorders that can be identified from a few drops of blood obtained by a heelstick are cystic fibrosis (see the exemplar on Cystic Fibrosis in the module on Oxygenation), galactosemia, congenital adrenal hyperplasia, congenital hypothyroidism, maple syrup urine disease, PKU, sickle cell trait (see the exemplar on Sickle Cell Disease in the module on Cellular Regulation), biotinidase deficiency, and hemoglobinopathies.

Early discharge has affected both the timing of newborn metabolic screening tests and the acquisition of subsequent immunization. Early newborn discharge increases the risk for a delayed or even missed diagnosis of PKU and congenital hypothyroidism because of decreased sensitivity of screening before 24 hours of age. Newborns should be retested by 2 weeks of age if the first test was done before 24 hours of age. A second test for PKU is required in most states, usually between 1 week and 1 month of age, to minimize the chance of a child with PKU going undetected.

New technology is quickly increasing the number of metabolic and other disorders that can be detected in the newborn period. The March of Dimes (2012) recommends newborn screening tests for 31 health conditions. In most states, newborn screening programs lead to the detection of several conditions before symptoms develop. While all states require screening for more than 50 congenital conditions, each state decides on the number and type of conditions (CDC, 2014b).

Hearing loss is found in 1 to 3 per 1000 babies in the normal newborn population (CDC, 2015c). Hearing screenings before discharge are now conducted in all 50 states. The recommended initial newborn hearing screening should be accomplished before discharge from the birthing unit with appropriate follow-up if the newborn fails to pass the initial screen in all hospitals providing obstetric services (**Figure 33–93 》》**).

Sometimes, newborns fail to pass these tests for reasons other than hearing loss. Amniotic fluid in the ear canals is a frequent cause of suboptimal test results. In these cases, babies are retested in a week or two. The current goal is to screen all babies by 1 month of age, confirm hearing loss with audiologic examination by 3 months of age, and treat with comprehensive early intervention services (CDC, 2015c). Typically, screening programs use a two-stage screening approach (autoacoustic emissions [OAE] repeated twice, OAE followed by auditory brain stem response [ABR], or automated ABR repeated twice). Families need to be educated about appropriate interpretation of screening test results and appropriate steps for follow-up (Healthy Children, 2015c).

Immunization programs against the hepatitis B virus during the newborn period and infancy are in place in many U.S. states, in at least 20 countries, and in high-incidence areas such as American Samoa. Universal vaccination of newborns and infants is recommended. Babies should receive the first dose of hepatitis B vaccine during the period from birth to 2 months of age. The second dose should be administered at least 1 month after the first dose. The third dose should be administered at least 4 months after the first dose and at least 2 months after the second dose, but not before 6 months of age (AAP & ACOG, 2012). Parents need to be advised whether their birthing center provides newborn hepatitis vaccination so that an adequate follow-up program can be set in motion.

》》Stay Current: Find up-to-date immunization schedules for children from birth to 6 years in English and Spanish at the CDC website at www.cdc.gov/vaccines/schedules/easy-to-read/child.html

COMMUNITY-BASED NURSING CARE The nurse should discuss with parents ways to meet their newborn's needs, ensure safety, and appreciate the newborn's unique characteristics and behaviors. By assisting parents in establishing links with their community-based healthcare provider, the nurse can get the new family off to a good start.

Key topics for parent education include:

- Knowing signs of illness and when to call the pediatrician
- Contact information for the pediatrician and nursery unit
- How to reach the pediatrician after hours
- Follow-up care after discharge
- Use of OTC medications and safety
- Importance of routine well-baby visits.

Some institutions have initiated postpartum and/or newborn follow-up home visits, especially for newborns discharged before 48 hours after birth. The follow-up home examination should be within 48 hours of discharge (AAP & ACOG, 2012) when the family is unable to visit their primary care physician within that time period. The home visit focuses on normal newborn care, assessment for hyperbilirubinemia (jaundice), extreme weight loss, feeding problems, and knowledge related to newborn care and feeding within the family unit.

Evaluation

When evaluating the nursing care provided during the period immediately after birth, the nurse may anticipate the following outcomes:

- The newborn's adaptation to extrauterine life is successful, as demonstrated by all vital signs being within acceptable parameters.
- The newborn's physiologic and psychologic integrity is supported.
- Positive interactions between parent and newborn are supported.

When evaluating the nursing care provided during the newborn period, the nurse may anticipate the following outcomes:

- The newborn's physiologic and psychologic integrity is supported by maintaining stable vital signs and interactions based on normal newborn behaviors.
- The newborn feeding pattern has been satisfactorily established.

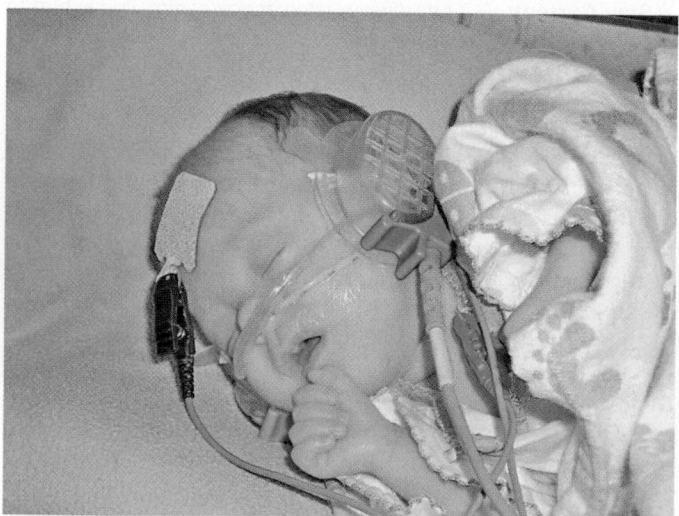

Source: Vanessa Howell, RN, MSN.

Figure 33–93 》》 Newborn hearing screen.

- The parents express understanding of the bonding process and display attachment behaviors.

When evaluating the nursing care provided in preparation for discharge, the nurse may anticipate the following outcomes:

- The parents demonstrate safe techniques in caring for their newborn.

- Parents verbalize developmentally appropriate behavioral expectations of their newborn and knowledge of community-based newborn follow-up care.

Conducting additional care evaluation determines if further care is needed based on newborn outcomes. If the outcomes are not met, the nurse may choose to continue or revise the plan of care for optimal outcome attainment. Continuation, revision, or discontinuation of a plan of care is decided through the collaboration of all members of the healthcare team.

As noted in the Nursing Care Plan: A Small-for-Gestational-Age Newborn, focused assessments include weight, thermoregulation, perfusion, and metabolism. Because these concepts are closely interrelated, an alteration in one may lead to alterations in others. Accurate assessment and identification of priority diagnoses allows for prompt intervention and improved patient outcomes.

Nursing Care Plan
A Small-for-Gestational-Age Newborn

Ellen, a term baby, was born 8 hours ago weighing 2500 g at 40 weeks of gestation. Two hours after birth, Ellen's temperature was 37.1°C (98.8°F) under the radiant warmer. She was swaddled and placed in an open crib. One hour later, Ellen is returned to the radiant warmer with a falling temperature reading of 36.1°C (97°F). Acrocyanosis has also been detected. The glucose level is 35 mg/dL. The nurse monitors the newborn for signs of hypothermia and hypoglycemia.

ASSESSMENT

Subjective: Alert and active.

Objective: 40 weeks of gestation; birth weight, 2500 g; length, 48.3 cm (19 in.); head circumference, 30 cm (11.8 in.); chest circumference, 28 cm (11 in.); temperature, 36.1°C (97°F) axillary; pulse, 140 beats/min; respirations, 45 breaths/min; vigorous cry, alert, and wide-eyed; dry skin; thin, meconium-stained umbilical cord; glucose, 35 mg/dL; and tremors.

DIAGNOSES

- *Hypothermia* related to decrease in subcutaneous fat tissue and increased body surface exposure to environment

- *Imbalanced Nutrition: Less Than Body Requirements* related to increased glucose consumption secondary to metabolic effects of hypothermia and poor hepatic glycogen stores

- *Risk for Injury* related to hypoglycemia secondary to the metabolic effects of hypothermia and poor hepatic glycogen stores

(NANDA-I © 2014)

PLANNING

- The newborn will maintain stable body temperature within normal range of 36.5°–37.4°C (97.7°–99.4°F) in an open crib.

- The newborn will not exhibit signs of acrocyanosis, mottling, or lethargy.

- The newborn will maintain a glucose level above 40 mg/dL.

- The newborn's weight will remain stable.

- The newborn will not exhibit any unusual jitteriness or tremors.

IMPLEMENTATION

- Monitor axillary temperature every 4 hours and prn.

- Monitor pulse and respirations every 4 hours and prn.

- Assess skin color and temperature every 15–30 minutes in presence of color change.

- Place newborn skin-to-skin with mother for mild hypothermia if the baby is stable and the parent is willing. If ineffective, place newborn under radiant warmer if temperature falls below 36.5°C (97.7°F).

- Place newborn in incubator if temperature is unstable.

- Initiate frequent feeding as tolerated (10 mL/kg is a general guideline for formula feeding).

- Initiate early feedings.

- Monitor glucose levels every 4 hours.

- Monitor for signs of hypoglycemia.

- Encourage on-demand feeding at least every 3–4 hours.

- Offer supplemental feedings or additional glucose.

- Maintain a neutral thermal environment.

EVALUATION

- The newborn's temperature remains between 36.5° and 37.4°C (97.7° and 99.4°F) in an open crib.

- The skin is pink in color, with no signs of acrocyanosis or mottling.

- The glucose level remains above 45 mg/dL.

- The newborn's weight is stabilized.

- No signs of jitteriness or tremors are present.

CRITICAL THINKING

1. What can the nurse do to prevent heat loss through convection when preparing the newborn for the open crib?

2. What measure can the nurse take to reduce heat loss through evaporation and conduction? How many calories can a SGA newborn lose through radiation?

3. Parents of an SGA newborn ask the nurse when they should expect their baby to catch up in weight to normal-growth newborns. What is the nurse's best response?

REVIEW Newborn Care

RELATE Link the Concepts and Exemplars

Linking the exemplar of newborn care with the concept of stress and coping:

1. What stressors does a newborn place on the family?

2. What assessment findings might you anticipate in a family that is not coping appropriately with the stress brought on by caring for their newborn? What actions might the nurse take to improve coping strategies?

Linking the exemplar of newborn care with the concept of immunity:

3. What recommendations would you make to the parents during discharge teaching related to their newborn's immune system?

4. While planning for discharge from the hospital, the mother of a newborn asks you, "What vaccinations does my baby need first?" How would you respond to this question?

READY Go to Volume 3: Clinical Nursing Skills

REFER Go to Pearson MyLab Nursing and eText

- Additional review materials
- Chart 14: Fetal and Neonatal Circulation
- Chart 15: Potential Birth Injuries
- Chart 16: Congenital Anomalies: Identification and Care in the Newborn Period
- Chart 17: Comparison of Cephalohematoma and Caput Succedaneum
- Chart 18: Promoting Attachment
- Chart 19: What to Tell Parents About Newborn Care

REFLECT Apply Your Knowledge

Maria and Carlos Ramirez are preparing to take their newborn daughter home. They have three other daughters at home, ages 7 years, 3 years, and 2 years. Mrs. Ramirez tells you that the middle child was very jealous when she brought the 2-year-old home from the hospital and is worried about how the children will respond to this new baby.

1. Mrs. Ramirez says she would like to breastfeed the baby, but wonders if that will increase the sibling rivalry among her other children. How would you respond to this concern?

2. What strategies might you recommend to Mrs. Ramirez to reduce sibling rivalry when introducing the new baby to the family?

3. Mr. Ramirez shares with you, while Mrs. Ramirez is out of the room, that he had really hoped this new baby would be a boy. What assessment questions might you ask of this father?

» Exemplar 33.E Prematurity

Exemplar Learning Outcomes

33.E Summarize care of premature newborns.

- Describe the physiology and risk factors of the premature newborn.
- Summarize alterations found in premature newborns.
- Describe the nursing process in assessing the premature newborn and implementing culturally competent care to the baby and the family.

Exemplar Key Terms

Apnea of prematurity, *2413*
Minimal enteral nutrition, *2412*
Preterm newborn, *2408*

Overview

A **preterm newborn** is a baby born at less than 37 completed weeks of gestation (ACOG & Society for Maternal-Fetal Medicine [SMFM], 2013, reaffirmed 2015; Spong, 2013). The incidence of all preterm births in the United States is approximately 10% (CDC, 2015d). With the help of modern technology, neonates are surviving at younger gestational ages, but not without significant morbidity. The rise in multiple birth rates has markedly influenced overall rates of low-birth-weight neonates. **Figure 33–94 »** shows a comparison of a premature neonate, a low-birth-weight neonate, and a full-term neonate.

The Preterm Newborn

The major problem of the preterm newborn is the variable immaturity of all systems. The degree of immaturity depends on the length of gestation. The preterm newborn

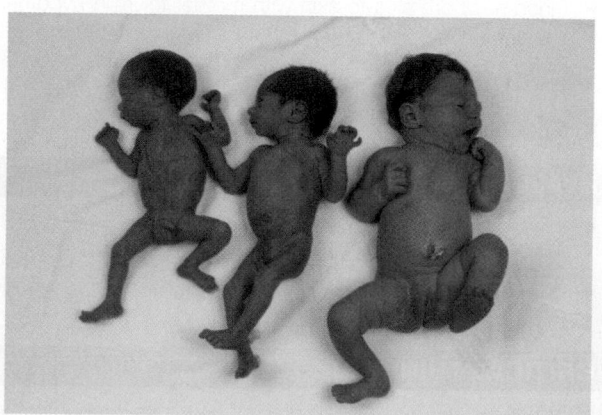

Figure 33–94 » *From left to right:* A 4-week-old neonate who was born 9 weeks premature, a 2-week-old neonate who weighed 1200 g at birth, and a full-term neonate, 2 days old, who weighed 3730 g at birth.

must traverse the same complex, interconnected pathways from intrauterine to extrauterine life as the term newborn. Because of immaturity, however, the premature newborn is ill equipped to make this transition smoothly. Maintenance of the preterm newborn falls within narrow physiologic parameters.

Respiratory and Cardiac Physiology

The preterm newborn is at risk for respiratory problems because the lungs are not fully mature and not fully ready to take over the process of oxygen and carbon dioxide exchange without assistance. Critical factors in the development of respiratory distress include the following:

- ***The preterm neonate is unable to produce adequate amounts of surfactant.*** Inadequate surfactant lessens compliance (ability of the lung to fill with air easily), thereby increasing the inspiratory pressure needed to expand the lungs with air. The collapsed (or atelectatic) alveoli will not facilitate an exchange of oxygen and carbon dioxide. As a result, the neonate becomes hypoxic, pulmonary blood flow is inefficient, and the preterm newborn's available energy is depleted.

- ***The muscular coat of pulmonary blood vessels is incompletely developed.*** As a result, the pulmonary arterioles do not constrict well in response to decreased oxygen levels. This lowered pulmonary vascular resistance leads to left-to-right shunting of blood through the ductus arteriosus, which increases the blood flow back into the lungs.

- ***The ductus arteriosus of the preterm neonate, who is more susceptible to hypoxia, may respond to increasing oxygen and prostaglandin E levels by remaining open rather than by vasoconstriction, which is how the ductus responds in the term neonate.*** A patent ductus increases the blood volume to the lungs, causing pulmonary congestion, increased respiratory effort, carbon dioxide retention, and bounding femoral pulses.

Thermoregulation

Heat loss is a major problem in premature newborns. Two factors limiting heat production are the availability of glycogen in the liver and the amount of brown fat available for heat production. Both of these limiting factors appear in the third trimester. In the cold-stressed baby, norepinephrine is released, which in turn stimulates the metabolism of brown fat for heat production. As a complicating factor, the hypoxic newborn cannot increase oxygen consumption in response to cold stress because of the already limited reserves; as a result, the hypoxic newborn becomes progressively colder. Preterm neonates have smaller muscle mass and diminished muscular activity, rendering them unable to shiver and further limiting heat production.

There are five physiologic and anatomic factors that increase heat loss in the preterm neonate.

1. ***The preterm newborn has a higher ratio of body surface to body weight.*** This means that the baby's ability to produce heat (based on body weight) is much less than the potential for losing heat (based on surface area). The loss of heat in a preterm neonate weighing 1500 g is five times greater per unit of body weight than that of an adult.

2. ***The preterm newborn has very little subcutaneous fat, which is the human body's insulation.*** Without adequate insulation, heat is easily conducted from the core of the body (warmer temperature) to the surface of the body (cooler temperature). Heat is lost from the body as the blood vessels, which lie close to the skin surface in the preterm neonate, transport blood from the body core to the subcutaneous tissues.

3. ***The preterm newborn has thinner, more permeable skin than the term neonate.*** This increased permeability contributes to a greater insensible water loss as well as to heat loss.

4. ***The posture of the preterm newborn influences heat loss.*** Flexion of the extremities decreases the amount of surface area exposed to the environment. Extension increases the surface area exposed to the environment and thus increases heat loss. The gestational age of the neonate influences the amount of flexion, from completely hypotonic and extended at 28 weeks to stronger flexion at 35 weeks and full flexion of all extremities at term (see Resting posture in Figure 33–69.

5. ***The premature newborn has a decreased ability to vasoconstrict superficial blood vessels and conserve heat in the body core.*** This lack of vasoconstriction allows heat to leave the premature neonate's body at a fast rate, thus leading to cold stress.

Thermoregulation is discussed more completely in the module on Thermoregulation. The essential point regarding thermoregulation of the premature neonate, however, is this: Gestational age is directly proportional to the ability to maintain thermoregulation; thus, the more preterm the newborn, the less able the neonate is to maintain heat balance.

The nurse can do much to prevent heat loss by providing a neutral thermal environment. This is one of the most important considerations in nursing management of the preterm neonate (see Maintain a Neutral Thermal Environment section later in this exemplar). Cold stress, with its accompanying severe complications, can be prevented.

Gastrointestinal Physiology

The basic structure of the gastrointestinal (GI) tract is formed early in gestation. The maturation of the digestive and absorptive process is more variable, however, and occurs later in gestation. As a result of GI immaturity, the preterm newborn has the following ingestion, digestive, and absorption problems:

- A marked danger of aspiration and its associated complications because of the premature neonate's poorly developed gag reflex, incompetent esophageal cardiac sphincter, and poor sucking and swallowing reflexes. The ability to coordinate sucking, swallow, and breathing is not established until 32–34 weeks' gestation.

- Difficulty in meeting high caloric and fluid needs for growth because of small stomach capacity.

- Limited ability to convert certain essential amino acids to nonessential amino acids. Some amino acids, such as histidine, taurine, and cysteine, are essential to the preterm neonate but not to the term neonate.

- Inability to handle the increased osmolarity of formula protein because of kidney immaturity. The preterm neonate requires a higher concentration of whey protein than of casein.

- Difficulty absorbing saturated fats because of decreased bile salts and pancreatic lipase. Severe illness of the newborn may also prevent intake of adequate nutrients.

- Initial difficulty with lactose digestion because processes may not be fully functional during the first few days of a preterm neonate's life. The preterm newborn can digest and absorb most simple sugars.

- Deficiency of calcium and phosphorus may exist because two thirds of these minerals are deposited in the last trimester. This can lead to rickets and significant bone demineralization.

- Increased basal metabolic rate and increased oxygen requirements caused by fatigue associated with sucking.

- Feeding intolerance and necrotizing enterocolitis (NEC) as a result of diminished blood flow and tissue perfusion to the intestinal tract because of prolonged hypoxia and hypoxemia at birth.

Renal Physiology

The kidneys of the premature neonate are immature compared with those of the full-term neonate, posing clinical problems in the management of fluid and electrolyte balance. Specific renal characteristics of the preterm neonate include the following:

- The glomerular filtration rate (GFR) is lower because of decreased renal blood flow. The GFR is directly related to lower gestational age, so the more preterm the newborn, the lower the GFR. The GFR is also decreased in the presence of diseases or conditions that decrease renal blood flow and perfusion, such as severe respiratory distress, hypotension, and asphyxia. Anuria and oliguria may also be observed.

- The preterm neonate's kidneys are limited in their ability to concentrate urine or to excrete excess amounts of fluid. This means that if excess fluid is administered, the neonate is at risk for fluid retention and overhydration. If too little fluid is administered, the neonate will become dehydrated because of the inability to retain adequate fluid.

- The kidneys of the preterm neonate begin excreting glucose (glycosuria) at a lower serum glucose level than those of the term newborn. Glycosuria with hyperglycemia can lead to osmotic diuresis and polyuria.

- The buffering capacity of the kidney is reduced, predisposing the neonate to metabolic acidosis. Bicarbonate is excreted at a lower serum level, and acid is excreted more slowly. Therefore, after periods of hypoxia or insult, the preterm neonate's kidneys require a longer time to excrete the lactic acid that accumulates. Sodium bicarbonate is frequently required to treat metabolic acidosis in the premature neonate.

- The immaturity of the renal system affects the preterm neonate's ability to excrete drugs. Because excretion time is longer, many drugs are given over longer intervals (i.e., every 24 hours instead of every 12 hours). Urine output must be carefully monitored when the neonate is receiving nephrotoxic drugs, such as gentamicin and vancomycin. If urine output is poor, drugs can become toxic much more quickly in the neonate than in the adult.

Immunologic Physiology

The preterm neonate is at much greater risk for infection than the term neonate. This increased susceptibility may be the result of an infection acquired in utero, which may have precipitated preterm labor and birth. However, all preterm neonates have immature specific and nonspecific immunity.

In utero, the fetus receives passive immunity against a variety of infections from maternal IgG immunoglobulins, which cross the placenta. Because most of this immunity is acquired in the last trimester of pregnancy, the premature neonate has few antibodies at birth, and these antibodies provide less protection and become depleted earlier than in a full-term neonate. The limited number of antibodies in the preterm neonate may be a contributing factor in the higher incidence of recurrent infection during the first year of life as well as in the immediate neonatal period.

The other immunoglobulin that is significant for the preterm neonate is secretory IgA, which does not cross the placenta but is found in breast milk at significant concentrations. The secretory IgA in breast milk provides immunity to the mucosal surfaces of the neonate's GI tract, protecting the baby from enteric infections such as those caused by *Escherichia coli* and *Shigella*.

Another altered defense against infection in the preterm neonate is the skin surface. In very small neonates, the skin is easily excoriated, and this factor, coupled with many invasive procedures, places the neonate at great risk for health-care-associated infections. It is vital to use good hand hygiene in the care of these neonates in order to prevent unnecessary infection.

SAFETY ALERT The sudden onset of apnea and bradycardia, coupled with metabolic acidosis in an otherwise healthy, growing premature neonate, may be suggestive of bacterial sepsis, especially if an invasive device, such as a central line or endotracheal tube, is in place.

Neurologic Physiology

The general shape of the brain is formed during the first 6 weeks of gestation. Between the second and fourth months of gestation, the brain's total complement of neurons proliferates. These neurons migrate to specific sites throughout the central nervous system, and nerve impulse pathways organize. The final step in neurologic development is the covering of these nerves with myelin, which begins in the second trimester of gestation and continues into adult life (Scheibel, 2012).

The period of most rapid brain growth and development occurs during the third trimester of pregnancy; therefore, the closer to term a neonate is born, the better the neurologic prognosis. A common interruption of neurologic development in the preterm neonate is caused by intraventricular hemorrhage and intracranial hemorrhage. Hydrocephalus may develop as a consequence of an intraventricular hemorrhage caused by the obstruction at the cerebral aqueduct.

Reactivity and Behavioral States

The neonate's response to extrauterine life is characterized by two periods of reactivity. The preterm neonate's periods of reactivity, however, are delayed. In the very ill neonate, these periods of reactivity may not be observed at all, because the neonate may be hypotonic and unreactive for several days after birth.

As the preterm newborn grows and the baby's condition stabilizes, identifying behavioral states and traits unique to each baby becomes increasingly possible. In general, stable preterm neonates do not demonstrate the same behavioral states as term neonates. Preterm neonates tend to be more disorganized in their sleep–wake cycles and are unable to attend as well to the human face and objects in the environment. Neurologically, their responses (sucking, muscle tone, and states of arousal) are weaker than those of full-term neonates.

By observing each neonate's patterns of behavior and responses, especially the sleep–wake states, the parents and nurse can plan nursing care around the times when the neonate is alert and best able to attend. In addition, the more knowledge parents have about the meaning of their newborn's responses and behaviors, the better prepared they will be to meet their newborn's needs and to form a positive attachment with their child. (See the Promote Developmentally Supportive Care section later in this exemplar.)

Nutritional and Fluid Requirements

Beginning feedings as soon as possible is extremely valuable in maintaining normal metabolism and lowering the possibility of such complications as hypoglycemia, hyperbilirubinemia, and azotemia. However, the preterm neonate is at risk for complications that may develop because of immaturity of the digestive system. Advancement of feedings should occur only as the neonate demonstrates tolerance of enteral feedings. Clinical signs of feeding intolerance or illness dictate discontinuing or holding the advancement of feedings.

Nutritional Requirements

Oral (enteral) caloric intake necessary for growth in a healthy preterm newborn is 95–130 kcal/kg per day (Blackburn, 2013). In addition to these relatively high caloric needs, the preterm neonate requires more protein than the full-term neonate. To meet these needs, many institutions use breast milk or special preterm formulas.

Whether breast milk or formula is used, feeding regimens are established on the basis of the neonate's weight and estimated stomach capacity. Initial formula feedings are gradually increased as the neonate tolerates them. It may be necessary to supplement oral feedings with parenteral fluids to maintain adequate hydration and caloric intake until the baby is on full oral feedings. Preterm neonates who cannot tolerate any oral (enteral) feedings are given nutrition by total parenteral nutrition (TPN).

In addition to a higher calorie and protein formula, preterm neonates should receive supplemental multivitamins, including vitamins A, D, and E, as well as iron and trace minerals. A diet high in polyunsaturated fats, which preterm neonates tolerate best, increases the requirement for vitamin E. Preterm neonates who are fed iron-fortified formulas have higher red cell hemolysis and lower vitamin E concentrations and thus require additional vitamin E. Preterm formulas also need to contain medium-chain triglycerides and additional amino acids, such as cysteine, as well as calcium, phosphorus, and vitamin D supplements to increase mineralization of bones. Rickets and significant bone demineralization have been documented in very-low-birth-weight neonates and otherwise healthy preterm neonates.

Nutritional intake is considered to be adequate when there is consistent weight gain of 20–30 g/day. Initially, no weight gain may be noted for several days, but total weight loss should not exceed 15% of the total birth weight or more than 1–2% per day. Some institutions add the criteria of head circumference growth and increase in body length of 1 cm (0.4 in.) per week once the newborn is stable.

Methods of Feeding

The preterm newborn is fed by various methods, depending on the baby's gestational age, health and physical condition, and neurologic status. The three most common oral feeding methods are bottle, breast, and gavage. In some cases, total parenteral nutrition is used.

BOTTLE FEEDING Preterm neonates who have a coordinated and rhythmic suck–swallow–breathing pattern are usually between 32 and 34 weeks of postconceptual age and may be fed by bottle. Oral readiness to feed is best described by the following engagement and hunger cues: bringing hands to mouth, being alert, exhibiting fussiness, sucking on fingers or pacifier, exhibiting rooting behavior, and showing relaxed facial expression and good tone (Newland, L'Huillier, & Petrey, 2013).

Those premature neonates who root when their cheek is stroked and actively search for the nipple are neurodevelopmentally ready to initiate oral feeding (**Figure 33–95 »**). To

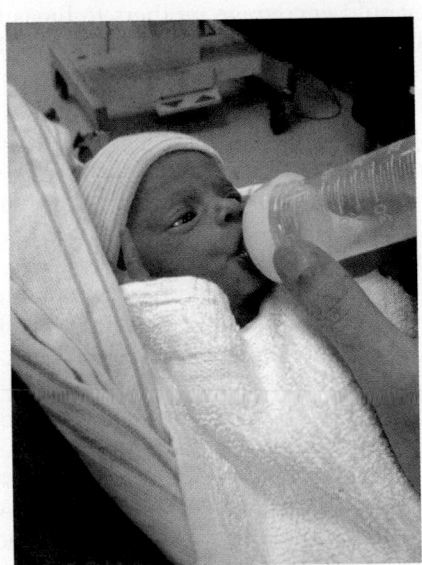

Source: Carol Harrigan, RN, MSN, NNP-BC.

Figure 33–95 » Mother bottle feeding her premature newborn with expressed breast milk.

avoid excessive expenditure of energy, a soft, yellow, single-hole nipple is generally used (milk flow is less rapid). The neonate is fed in a semisitting position and burped gently after each 0.5–1 oz. The feeding should take no longer than 30 minutes (nippling requires more energy than other methods). Premature neonates who are progressing from gavage feedings to bottle feeding should start with one session of bottle feeding a day and have the number of times per day a bottle is given slowly increase until the baby tolerates all feedings from a bottle.

In assessing the premature neonate's readiness for feeding, the nurse assesses the neonate's ability to suck. Sucking may be affected by age, asphyxia, sepsis, intraventricular hemorrhage, or other neurologic insult. Before initiating nipple feeding, the nurse observes for signs of stress, such as tachypnea (>60 respirations/min), respiratory distress, or hypothermia, which may increase the risk of aspiration. During the feeding, the nurse observes the neonate for signs of feeding difficulty (tachypnea, cyanosis, bradycardia, lethargy, or uncoordinated suck and swallow). Difficulty in bottle feeding is often associated with a milk bolus that is too large for the neonate's oral cavity, which can lead to aspiration. Demand feeding protocols, based on the neonate's hunger cues, should be considered for a growing premature neonate only when there is sufficient caloric intake to promote consistent weight gain (Newland et al., 2013).

Breastfeeding

Mothers who wish to breastfeed their preterm neonates are given the opportunity to put the baby to the breast as soon as the baby has demonstrated a coordinated suck and swallow reflex, is showing consistent weight gain, and can control body temperature outside of the incubator, regardless of weight. Preterm neonates tolerate breastfeeding with higher transcutaneous oxygen pressures and better maintenance of body temperature than during bottle feeding. Besides breast milk's many benefits for the neonate, breastfeeding allows the mother to contribute actively to the baby's well-being. The nurse should encourage mothers to breastfeed if they choose to do so. It is important for the nurse to be aware of both the advantages of breastfeeding and the possible disadvantages of breast milk as the sole source of food for the preterm neonate. Even if the neonate cannot be put to the breast, mothers can pump breast milk, which can be given via bottle or gavage. Use of the double-pumping system produces higher levels of prolactin than are obtained using sequential pumping of the breasts.

By initiating skin-to-skin holding of premature neonates in the early intensive care phase, mothers can significantly increase milk volume, thereby overcoming lactation problems (Lucas & Smith, 2015). The neonate is placed at the mother's breast. It has been suggested that the football hold is a convenient position for breastfeeding preterm babies. Feeding may take up to 45 minutes, and babies should be burped as they alternate breasts. The length of feeding time is monitored so that the preterm neonate does not burn too many calories.

The nurse should coordinate a flexible feeding schedule so that babies can nurse during alert times and be allowed to set their own pace. Feedings should be on demand, but a maximum number of hours between feedings should be set.

A similar regimen should be used for the baby who is progressing from gavage feeding to breastfeeding. The mother begins with one feeding at the breast and then gradually increases the number of times during the day that the baby breastfeeds. When breastfeeding is not possible because the neonate is too small or too weak to suck at the breast, an option for the mother may be to express her breast milk into a cup. The milk touches the neonate's lips and is lapped by the protruding motions of the tongue.

SAFETY ALERT For an otherwise healthy, growing premature neonate who is receiving total enteral intake and who has started to experience apnea and bradycardia, one differential diagnosis to think about is reflux rather than sepsis, although sepsis may need to be ruled out.

Gavage Feeding

The gavage feeding method is used with preterm neonates (32–34 weeks of gestation) who lack or have a poorly coordinated suck-and-swallow reflex or who are ill and ventilator dependent. Gavage feeding may be used as an adjunct to nipple feeding if the neonate tires easily. It may also be used as an alternative if a neonate is losing weight because of the energy expenditure required for nippling.

Gavage feedings are administered by either the nasogastric or orogastric route and by intermittent bolus or continuous drip method. Bolus feedings may be preferred, because these are thought to be more like normal feedings than the continuous feeding method and may enhance the release of certain GI hormones necessary for development of gastrointestinal tissues (Dawson et al., 2012). Currently, no conclusive studies support one method over the other. In common practice, bolus feedings are usually initiated, but if intolerance occurs, then the feedings are changed to continuous.

Early initiation of **minimal enteral nutrition** via gavage is now advocated as a supplement to parenteral nutrition. Minimal enteral nutrition refers to small-volume feedings of formula or human milk (usually <24 mL/kg per day), which are designed to "prime" the premature neonate's intestinal tract, thereby stimulating many of its hormonal and enzymatic functions (AAP & ACOG, 2012). Benefits of early feeding (as early as within the first 24–72 hours of life) include the following (Kenner & Lott, 2014):

- No increased incidence of NEC
- Fewer days on total parenteral nutrition, thereby decreasing the incidence of cholestatic jaundice
- Increased weight gain
- Increased muscle maturation of the GI function, which can lead to improved feeding tolerance
- Lower risk of osteopenia
- Possible decrease in the total number of hospital days in the neonatal intensive care unit (NICU).

SAFETY ALERT Orogastric gavage catheter placement is preferable to nasogastric, because most neonates are obligatory nose breathers. If nasogastric is used, a #5 French catheter should be used to minimize airway obstruction.

Total Parenteral Nutrition

Total parenteral nutrition is used in situations that do not allow the neonate to be fed through the GI tract. This method provides complete nutrition to the neonate intravenously and uses hyperalimentation to provide calories, vitamins, minerals, protein, and glucose, and uses intra-lipids to provide essential fatty acids.

Fluid Requirements

The calculation of fluid requirements must take into account the neonate's weight and postnatal age. Recommendations for fluid therapy in the preterm neonate are approximately 80–100 mL/kg per day for the first day, 100–120 mL/kg per day for the second day, and 120–150 mL/kg per day by the third day of life. These amounts may be increased up to 200 mL/kg per day if the baby is very small, receiving phototherapy, or under a radiant warmer because of the increased insensible water losses. Fluid losses can be minimized through the use of heat shields and added humidification in the incubator. Daily weights (and, sometimes, twice-a-day weights) are the best indicator of fluid status in the preterm neonate. The expected weight loss during the first 3–5 days of life in a preterm neonate is 15–20% of birth weight. Premature newborns being treated for complications such as respiratory distress syndrome or patent ductus arteriosus may be on diuretics that can influence their fluid requirements.

Long-term Needs

The care of preterm neonates and their families does not stop on discharge from the nursery. Follow-up care is extremely important: Many developmental problems are not noted until an infant is older and begins to demonstrate motor delays or sensory disability.

Within the first year of life, low-birth-weight preterm babies face higher mortality rates than term babies. Causes of death include sudden infant death syndrome (SIDS)—which occurs about five times more frequently in the preterm baby than the term baby—respiratory infections, and neurologic defects. (See the exemplar on Sudden Infant Death Syndrome, in the module on Oxygenation.) Morbidity is also much higher among preterm babies, those weighing less than 1500 g being at the highest risk for long-term complications.

The most common long-term needs observed in preterm neonates include the following:

- *Retinopathy of prematurity (ROP).* Premature newborns are particularly susceptible to characteristic retinal changes, known as ROP, which can result in visual impairment. The premature newborn's retina does not have all of the blood vessels the term newborn's has. As the blood vessels fill in, they may grow abnormally with the development of fibrous tissue that can contract and scar, resulting in retinal detachment. The disease is now viewed as multifactorial in origin. Increased survival of very-low-birth-weight babies may be the most important factor in the increased incidence of ROP. The acute stages of ROP may be treated with laser photocoagulation and cryotherapy. Most acute changes with ROP regress spontaneously with no long-term visual impairment.

- *Bronchopulmonary dysplasia (BPD).* Long-term lung disease is a result of damage to the alveolar epithelium secondary to positive-pressure ventilator therapy and a high oxygen concentration. These babies have long-term dependence on oxygen therapy and an increased incidence of respiratory infection during their first few years of life.

- *Speech defects.* The most frequently observed speech defects involve delayed development of receptive and expressive ability that may persist into the school-age years.

- *Neurologic defects.* The most common neurologic defects include cerebral palsy (CP), hydrocephalus, seizure disorders, lower IQ, and learning disabilities. (See the exemplar on Cerebral Palsy in the module on Development.) In the absence of major neurologic defects, the socioeconomic climate and family support systems are extremely important influences on the child's eventual school performance. Families should be reminded that risk does not equal injury, injury does not equal damage, and description of damage does not allow a precise prediction about recovery or outcome.

- *Auditory defects.* Preterm babies have a 1–4% incidence of moderate to profound hearing loss and should have a formal audiologic exam before discharge and at 3–6 months (corrected age). Tests currently used to measure hearing functions of the newborn are the evoked otoacoustic emissions or the automated auditory brain response test. Any baby with repeated abnormal results should be referred to speech-and-language specialists.

When assessing the baby's abilities and disabilities, parents must understand that developmental progress must be evaluated on the basis of chronologic age from the expected date of birth, not from the actual date of birth (corrected age). In addition, the parents need the consistent support of healthcare professionals in the long-term management of their child. Many new and ongoing concerns arise as the former premature neonate grows and develops; the goal is to promote the highest quality of life possible.

Many hospitals and NICUs provide referrals for parents of premature babies to local child health service coordination and early intervention service programs. Early intervention services for newborns, infants, and toddlers are mandated under Part C of the Individuals with Disabilities in Education Act. Nurses working with these families, either in the NICU or hospital setting or in a pediatric setting, should be aware of their agency's referral process or know about services available in their area.

Alterations of Prematurity

The goals of medical and nursing care are to meet the preterm neonate's growth and development needs and to anticipate and manage the complications associated with prematurity. The most common alterations associated with prematurity are as follows:

1. *Apnea of prematurity.* **Apnea of prematurity** refers to cessation of breathing for 20 seconds or longer, or for less than 20 seconds when associated with cyanosis, pallor, and bradycardia. Apnea is a common problem

in the preterm neonate less than 36 weeks' gestation, presenting between day 2 and day 7 of life. The etiology of apnea is multifactorial, but it is thought to be primarily a result of neuronal immaturity. This factor contributes to the preterm neonate's irregular breathing patterns. Other causes of apnea are obstructive apnea and gastroesophageal reflux. Obstructive apnea can occur when cessation of airflow is associated with blockage of the upper airway (resulting from a small airway diameter, increased pharyngeal secretions, or altered body alignment and positioning). Gastroesophageal reflux is defined as a movement of gastric contents into the lower esophagus caused by poor esophageal sphincter tone, in turn causing laryngospasm, which leads to bradycardia and apnea. Apnea of prematurity is then a diagnosis of exclusion.

2. **Patent ductus arteriosus (PDA).** The ductus arteriosus fails to close because of decreased pulmonary arteriole musculature and hypoxemia. Symptomatic PDA is often seen around the time when premature neonates are recovering from respiratory distress syndrome. PDA often prolongs the course of illness in a preterm newborn and leads to chronic pulmonary dysfunction.

SAFETY ALERT A growing premature neonate who is showing clinical signs of worsening respiratory status (i.e., increased oxygen needs or increased ventilatory settings), acidosis, and hypotension may be exhibiting signs and symptoms of a PDA.

---

3. **Respiratory distress syndrome.** Respiratory distress results from inadequate surfactant production.
4. **Intraventricular hemorrhage.** Intraventricular hemorrhage is the most common type of intracranial hemorrhage in small preterm neonates, especially those weighing less than 1500 g or of those less than 34 weeks of gestation. Up to 34 weeks, the preterm neonate's brain ventricles are lined by the germinal matrix, which is highly susceptible to hypoxic events, such as respiratory distress, birth trauma, and birth asphyxia. The germinal matrix is highly vascular, and these blood vessels rupture in the presence of hypoxia.
5. **Anemia of prematurity.** The preterm neonate is at risk for anemia because of the rapid rate of growth required, shorter red blood cell life, excessive blood sampling, decreased iron stores, and deficiency of vitamin E. The hemoglobin usually reaches its lowest level by 3–12 weeks and remains low for 3–6 months.

SAFETY ALERT An extremely premature, low-birth-weight neonate who presents with a sudden drop in hemoglobin along with the onset of severe metabolic acidosis, a "waxy" color, and hypotension may have experienced an intracranial hemorrhage.

NURSING PROCESS

Subtle signs and symptoms can indicate a change in a newborn's condition that may require rapid interventions to prevent lifelong complications. Nurses who want to care for premature neonates must obtain postgraduation specialized education offered by the hospital.

Assessment

The nurse needs to assess the physical characteristics and gestational age of the preterm newborn accurately. This allows the healthcare team to anticipate the special needs and problems of the baby.

Determining gestational age in preterm newborns requires knowledge and experience in administering gestational assessment tools. The tool used should be specific, reliable, and valid.

Physical characteristics vary greatly depending on gestational age, but the following characteristics are frequently present:

- **Color** is usually pink or ruddy but may show acrocyanosis. (Cyanosis, jaundice, and pallor are abnormal and should be noted.)
- **Skin** is reddened and translucent, blood vessels are readily apparent, and there is little subcutaneous fat.
- **Lanugo** is plentiful and widely distributed.
- **Head size** appears large in relation to the body.
- **Skull bones** are pliable; fontanel is smooth and flat.
- **Ears** have minimal cartilage and are pliable, folded over.
- **Nails** are soft and short.
- **Testes** may not be descended and scrotum nonrugated.
- **Clitoris and labia minora** are prominent.
- **Resting position** is flaccid, frog-like.
- **Cry** is weak and feeble.
- **Reflexes** (sucking, swallowing, and gag) are poor.
- **Activity** consists of jerky, generalized movements. (Seizure activity is abnormal.)

Diagnosis

Nursing diagnoses that may apply to the preterm newborn include the following:

- *Impaired Gas Exchange* related to immature pulmonary vasculature and inadequate surfactant production
- *Ineffective Breathing Pattern* related to immature central nervous system
- *Risk for Decreased Cardiac Tissue Perfusion* related to hypotension related to decreased tissue perfusion secondary to PDA
- *Risk for Ineffective Peripheral Tissue Perfusion* related to anemia of prematurity
- *Imbalanced Nutrition Less than Body Requirements* related to weak suck-and-swallow reflexes and decreased ability to absorb nutrients
- *Ineffective Thermoregulation* related to hypothermia secondary to decreased glycogen and brown fat stores
- *Deficient Fluid Volume* related to high insensible water losses and inability of kidneys to concentrate urine
- *Compromised Family Coping* related to anger or guilt at having given birth to a premature baby.

(NANDA-I © 2014)

Planning

Important goals of nursing care for the premature neonate often include the following:

- The neonate's oxygenation and normal breathing patterns will be promoted.
- The neonate's weight gain and normal growth will be promoted.
- The neonate's developmental needs will be supported.
- The neonate's parents will be educated to provide care when discharged.
- The nurse will support the neonate's parents and suggest strategies to reduce parental anxiety.

Implementation

Priorities for care of the premature neonate are many. Maintenance of respiratory function, a neutral thermal environment, fluid and electrolyte status, and adequate nutrition are essential to giving the neonate the greatest chance for healthy growth and development. Prevention of infection and of fatigue during feeding is also important, as are promoting parent–newborn attachment and developmentally supportive care and preparing for home care (**Figure 33–96 》**).

Maintain Respiratory Function

Premature newborns are at increased risk for respiratory obstruction because their bronchi and trachea are so narrow that mucus can obstruct the airway. The nurse must maintain patency through judicious suctioning, but only on an as-needed basis.

Positioning can also affect respiratory function. If the baby is in the supine position, the nurse should slightly elevate the head to maintain the airway, being careful to avoid hyperextension of the neck, which may cause the trachea to collapse. Also, because the newborn has weak neck muscles and cannot control head movement, place a small roll under the newborn's shoulders to maintain this head position. The prone position splints the chest wall and decreases the amount of respiratory effort used to move the chest wall, facilitating chest expansion and improving air entry and oxygenation. Weak or absent cough or gag reflexes increase the chance of aspiration in the premature newborn. The nurse should ensure that the newborn's position facilitates drainage of mucus or regurgitated formula.

The nurse monitors heart and respiratory rates with cardiorespiratory monitors and observes the newborn to identify alterations in cardiopulmonary status. Signs of respiratory distress include the following:

- Cyanosis (serious sign when generalized)
- Tachypnea (sustained respiratory rate >60 breaths/min after first 4 hours of life)
- Retractions
- Expiratory grunting
- Nasal flaring
- Apneic episodes
- Presence of rales or rhonchi on auscultation
- Diminished air entry.

If respiratory distress occurs, the nurse administers oxygen per physician or nurse practitioner orders to relieve hypoxemia. If hypoxemia is not treated immediately, it may result in PDA or metabolic acidosis. If oxygen is administered to the newborn, the nurse monitors the oxygen concentration with a pulse oximeter and blood gas analysis. Periodic arterial blood gas sampling to monitor oxygen concentration in the baby's blood is essential because hyperoxemia may lead to ROP and other complications.

The nurse also needs to consider respiratory function before and during feedings. To prevent aspiration and increased energy expenditure and oxygen consumption, the nurse must ensure that the newborn's gag and suck reflexes are intact before starting oral feedings.

Maintain a Neutral Thermal Environment

A neutral thermal environment minimizes the oxygen consumption required to maintain a normal core temperature; it also prevents cold stress and facilitates growth by decreasing the calories needed to maintain body temperature. The preterm newborn's small brown fat stores and immature central nervous system provide poor temperature control. A small premature neonate (> 1200 g) can lose 80 kcal/kg per day through radiation of body heat. To minimize heat loss and temperature instability for preterm and low-birth-weight newborns, the nurse should do the following:

- Monitor ambient temperature of the room where the newborn is kept.
- Allow skin-to-skin contact (*kangaroo care*) between the parents and newborn to maintain warmth and foster security.
- Warm and humidify oxygen to minimize evaporative heat loss and decrease oxygen consumption.
- Place the baby in a double-walled incubator, or use a Plexiglas heat shield over small preterm neonates in single-walled incubators, to avoid radiative heat losses. Some institutions use radiant warmers and plastic wrap

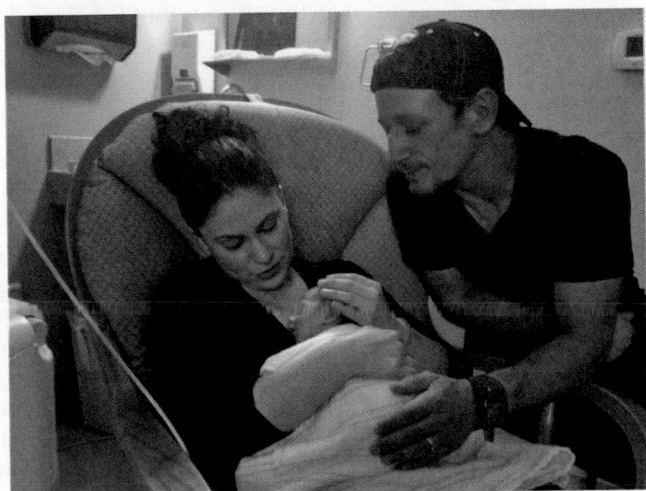

Source: Carol Harrigan, RN, MSN, NNP-BC.

Figure 33–96 》 Family bonding occurs when parents have opportunities to spend time with their premature newborn.

over the baby and pipe in humidity (swamping). Do not use Plexiglas shields on radiant warmer beds, however, because they block the infrared heat.

- Avoid placing the baby on cold surfaces, such as metal treatment tables and cold x-ray plates (conductive heat loss). Pad cold surfaces with diapers, and use radiant warmers during procedures. Place the preterm newborn on prewarmed mattresses, and warm hands before handling the baby to prevent heat transfer via conduction.

- Use warmed ambient humidity. Humidity can decrease insensible and transdermal water loss, especially in very-low-birth-weight newborns (Lund et al., 2013).

- Keep the newborn's skin dry (evaporative heat loss), and place a cap on the baby's head. The head makes up 25% of the total body size.

- Keep radiant warmers, incubators, and cribs away from windows or cold external walls (radiative heat loss) and out of drafts, which cause convection heat loss (conductive heat loss occurs when the newborn touches a cooler surface).

- Open incubator portholes and doors only when necessary, and use plastic sleeves on portholes to decrease convective heat loss.

- Use a skin probe to monitor the baby's skin temperature. Correlate ambient temperatures with the skin probe in the incubator using the servocontrol rather than the manual mode. The temperature should be 36°–37°C (96.8°–98.6°F). Temperature fluctuations indicate hypothermia or hyperthermia. Be careful not to place skin temperature probes over bony prominences; areas of brown fat; poorly vasoreactive areas, such as extremities; or excoriated areas.

- Warm formula or stored breast milk before feeding.

- Use a reflector patch over the skin temperature probe when using a radiant warmer bed so that the probe does not sense the higher infrared temperature as the baby's skin temperature and, therefore, decrease the heater output.

Once preterm newborns are medically stable, they can be clothed with a double-thickness cap, cotton shirt, and diaper and, if possible, swaddled in a blanket. The nurse begins the process of weaning to a crib when the premature newborn is medically stable, does not require assisted ventilation, weighs approximately 1500–2000 g (depending on facility policy), has had 5 days of consistent weight gain, and is taking oral feedings, and when apnea and bradycardia episodes have stabilized. The nurse should be familiar with the individual institution's protocol for weaning preterm babies to a crib.

Maintain Fluid and Electrolyte Status

The nurse maintains hydration by providing adequate fluid intake based on the newborn's weight, gestational age, chronologic age, and volume of sensible and insensible water losses. Adequate fluid intake should compensate for increased insensible losses and the amount needed for renal excretion of metabolic products. Insensible water losses can be minimized by providing high ambient humidity, humidifying

oxygen, using heat shields, covering the skin with plastic wrap, and placing the newborn in a double-walled incubator.

The nurse evaluates the hydration status of the baby by assessing and recording signs of dehydration. Signs of dehydration include the following:

- Sunken fontanel
- Loss of weight
- Poor skin turgor (skin returns to position slowly when squeezed gently)
- Dry oral mucous membranes
- Decreased urine output
- Increased specific gravity (> 1.013).

The nurse must also identify signs of overhydration by observing the newborn for edema or excessive weight gain and by comparing urine output with fluid intake.

The nurse weighs the preterm newborn at least once daily at the same time each day. *Weight change is one of the most sensitive indicators of fluid balance.* Weighing diapers is also important for accurate input and output measurement (1 mL = 1 g). A comparison of intake and output measurements over an 8- or 24-hour period provides important information about renal function and fluid balance. Assessment of patterns, and whether they show a net gain or loss over several days, is also essential to fluid management. In addition, the nurse monitors blood serum levels and pH to evaluate for electrolyte imbalances.

Accurate hourly intake calculations are needed when administering intravenous (IV) fluids. Because the preterm newborn is unable to excrete excess fluid, it is essential for the nurse to maintain the correct amount of IV fluid to prevent overload. Accuracy can be ensured by using neonatal or pediatric infusion pumps. To prevent electrolyte imbalance and dehydration, the nurse takes care to give the correct IV solutions as well as the correct volumes and concentrations of formulas. Urine-specific gravity and pH are obtained periodically. Urine osmolality provides an indication of hydration, although this factor must be correlated with other assessments (e.g., serum sodium). Hydration is considered to be adequate when the urine output is 1–3 mL/kg per hour.

Provide Adequate Nutrition and Prevent Fatigue During Feeding

The preterm newborn's feeding abilities and health status determine the feeding method. Both nipple and gavage methods are initially supplemented with IV therapy until oral intake is sufficient to support growth (110–130 kcal/kg per day). Early, small-volume enteral feedings, called *minimal enteral nutrition via gavage*, have proven to be beneficial for the very-low-birth-weight newborn (see Gavage Feeding earlier in this exemplar). GI priming with these small-volume feedings is not intended to contribute to the total nutritional intake but, rather, to enhance gut metabolism. Trophic feedings may also help encourage earlier advancement to full feedings, thereby decreasing the development of necrotizing enterocolitis and the complications of parenteral nutrition. Formula or breast milk (with or without fortifiers to increase caloric content) is incorporated into the feedings slowly. This is done to avoid overtaxing the digestive capacity of the preterm newborn. The nurse should carefully watch for any signs of feeding intolerance, including the following:

- Increasing gastric residuals
- Abdominal distention (measured routinely before feedings) with visible bowel loops
- Guaiac-positive stools (occult blood in stools)
- Lactose in stools (reducing substance in the stools)
- Vomiting
- Diarrhea
- Water-loss stools.

Before each feeding, the nurse measures abdominal girth and auscultates the abdomen to determine the presence and quality of bowel sounds. Such assessments permit early detection of abdominal distention, visible bowel loops, and decreased peristaltic activity, which may indicate necrotizing enterocolitis or paralytic ileus. The nurse also checks for residual formula in the stomach before feeding when the newborn is fed by gavage. This procedure also can be performed when the nipple-fed newborn presents with abdominal distention. The presence of increasing residual formula is an indication of intolerance to the type or amount of feeding or to the increase in amount of feeding.

SAFETY ALERT Residual feeding may indicate early necrotizing enterocolitis and should be called to the attention of the healthcare provider.

Preterm newborns who are ill or who fatigue easily with nipple feedings are usually fed by gavage. The neonate is essentially passive with these methods, thus conserving energy and calories. As the baby matures, gavage feedings are replaced with nipple (breast or formula) feedings to assist in strengthening the sucking reflex and in meeting the newborn's oral and emotional needs. While their nutrition may come from gavage feedings, nonnutritive sucking is important to the preterm newborn's development and should be encouraged. Signs that indicate readiness for oral feedings include a strong gag reflex, presence of nonnutritive sucking, and rooting behavior. Both low-birth-weight and preterm newborns nipple-feed more effectively in a quiet state. The nurse establishes a gradual nipple-feeding program, such as one nipple feeding per day, then one nipple feeding per shift, and then a nipple feeding every other feeding. The nurse should weigh the baby daily, because a small weight loss often occurs when nipple feedings are started. After feedings, the nurse places the baby on the right side (with support to maintain this position) or on the abdomen. These positions facilitate gastric emptying and decrease the chance of aspiration if regurgitation occurs. Gastroesophageal reflux is not uncommon in preterm newborns. Long-term gavage feeding may create nipple aversion that will require developmental occupational therapy interventions.

The nurse involves the parents in feeding their preterm baby. This is essential to the development of attachment between parents and baby. In addition, it increases parental knowledge about the care of their baby and helps them cope with the situation.

Prevent Infection

The nurse is responsible for minimizing the preterm newborn's exposure to pathogenic organisms. An immature immune system as well as thin and permeable skin make the preterm newborn susceptible to infection. Invasive procedures, techniques such as umbilical catheterization and mechanical ventilation, and prolonged hospitalization also place the neonate at greater risk for infection.

The practice of strict hand hygiene and use of separate equipment for each neonate help minimize the preterm newborn's exposure to infectious agents. Most nurseries have adopted the Centers for Disease Control and Prevention standard precautions of isolating every baby and the Joint Commission requirement that staff members have short-trimmed nails and no artificial nails. Staff members are required to complete a 2- to 3-minute scrub using an antibacterial solution, which inhibits growth of gram-positive cocci and gram-negative rod organisms. Other specific nursing interventions include limiting visitors, requiring visitors to wash their hands, maintaining strict aseptic practices when changing IV tubing and solutions (IV solutions and tubing should be changed every 24 hours or per agency protocols), administering parenteral fluids, and assisting with sterile procedures. Incubators and radiant warmers should be changed weekly. The nurse prevents pressure-area breakdown by changing the baby's position regularly, doing ROM exercises, and using water-bed pillows or an air mattress. To avoid skin tears, a protective, transparent covering can be applied over vulnerable joints; however, this method is used sparingly (Blackburn, 2013). Chemical skin preps and tape may cause skin trauma and should be avoided as much as possible.

If infection (sepsis) occurs in the preterm newborn, the nurse may be the first to identify its subtle clinical signs, such as lethargy and increased episodes of apnea and bradycardia. The nurse informs the healthcare provider of the findings immediately and implements the treatment plan per clinician orders in the presence of infection.

Promote Attachment

In some cases, preterm newborns are separated from their parents for prolonged periods after illness or complications that are detected in the first few hours or days following birth. This interrupts the bonding process, necessitating intervention to ensure successful attachment.

Nurses need to take measures to promote positive parental feelings toward the preterm newborn. They can give photographs of the baby to parents to take home. Photographs also may be given to the mother if she is in a different hospital or, if in the same hospital, is too ill to come to the nursery and visit. By placing the newborn's first name on the incubator as soon as it is known, nurses help the parents feel that their baby is a unique and special individual. A number of other interventions promote the bonding process, including the following:

- Give parents a weekly card with the baby's footprint, weight, and length.
- Give parents the telephone number of the nursery or intensive care unit and the names of staff members so that they have access to information about their baby at any time of the day or night.
- Encourage visits from siblings and grandparents.

Early involvement in the care of and decisions about their newborn provides the parents with realistic expectations for their baby. The individual personality characteristics of the newborn and the parents influence the bonding and contribute to the interactive process for the family. By observing each baby's patterns of behavior and responses, especially sleep–wake states, the nurse can teach parents the optimal times for interacting with their babies. The parents and nurse can plan nursing care around the times when the baby is alert and best able to attend.

Parents need education to develop caregiving skills and to understand the premature baby's behavioral characteristics. The more knowledge parents have about the meaning of their baby's responses, behaviors, and cues for interaction, the better they will be able to meet their newborn's needs and form a positive attachment with their child. For parents who cannot stay with their preterm baby, the nurse should encourage their daily participation (if possible) as well as early and frequent visits. The nurse should provide opportunities for parents to touch, hold, talk to, and care for the baby. Skin-to-skin holding (kangaroo care) helps parents feel close to their small newborn (**Figure 33–97 》》**). Kangaroo care has been shown to improve sleep periods and parents' perception of their caregiving ability (Ludington-Hoe, 2013).

Some parents will progress easily to touching and cuddling their newborn; however, others will not. Parents need to know that their feelings are normal and that the progression of acquaintanceship can be slow. Rooming-in can provide another opportunity for the stable preterm newborn and family to get acquainted; it offers both privacy and readily available help.

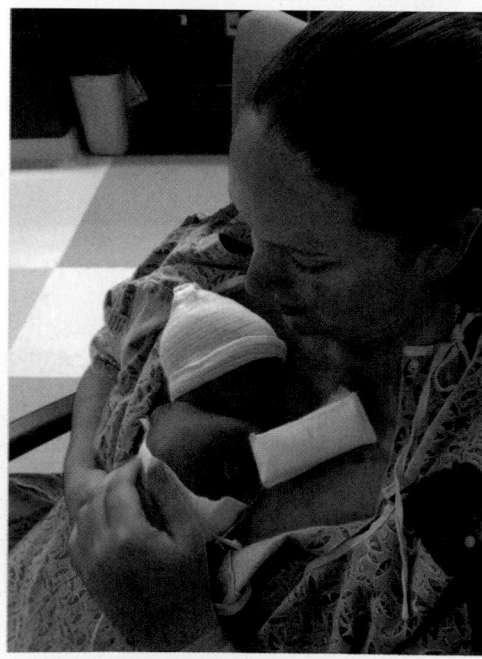

Source: Carol Harrigan, RN, MSN, NNP-BC.

Figure 33–97 》 Kangaroo (skin-to-skin) care facilitates closeness and attachment between mother and her premature newborn.

Promote Developmentally Supportive Care

Prolonged separation and the NICU environment necessitate individualized baby sensory stimulation programs. Developmentally supportive care (DSC) interventions include music therapy, light touch, massage, and vestibular stimulation (Westrup, 2014). The nurse plays a key role in determining the appropriate type and amount of visual, tactile, and auditory stimulation.

Some preterm newborns are not developmentally able to deal with more than one sensory input at a time. To ensure that the DSC interventions help the promotion of developmental support while simultaneously not inducing stress to the preterm newborn, a tool for assessing the behavior of preterm babies following provision of a DSC intervention in the NICU was developed (D'Souza, Kumar, & Lewis, 2014). This tool is used to assess the preterm newborn's behavior using two scales: autonomic/visceral system (color, respiration, visceral, and neurophysiologic responses) and the state and attention-interaction system (state regulation, auditory stimulus, and alertness). The preterm baby's behavioral reactions to stimulation are observed, and developmental interventions are then based on reducing detrimental environmental stimuli to the lowest possible level and providing appropriate opportunities for development (Blackburn, 2013).

Providing developmentally supportive, family-centered care improves the outcomes of the critically ill newborn. With this in mind, specially designed NICUs with the single-room care concept are being developed to minimize lighting and noise as well as to provide privacy for the parents of the convalescing newborn (White, Smith, & Shepley, 2013).

The NICU environment contains many detrimental stimuli that the nurse can help reduce. Simple actions that nurses can take include the following:

- If possible, replace alarms with lights to lower noise levels.
- Silence alarms quickly.
- Keep conversations away from newborns' bedsides.
- Use dimmer switches to shield newborns' eyes from bright lights.
- Place blankets over the top portion of each incubator.

Nursing care should also be planned to decrease the number of times the baby is disturbed. Signs (e.g., "Quiet Please") can be placed near the bedside to allow the baby some periods of uninterrupted sleep (Blackburn, 2013).

Some other suggested developmentally supportive interventions include the following:

- Facilitate handling by using containment measures when turning or moving the neonate or doing procedures such as suctioning. Use the hands to hold the neonate's arms and legs flexed close to the midline of the body. This helps stabilize the newborn's motor and physiologic subsystems during stressful activities.
- Touch the preemie gently, and avoid sudden postural changes.
- Promote self-consoling and soothing activities, such as placing blanket rolls or approved manufactured devices next to the neonate's sides and against the feet to provide

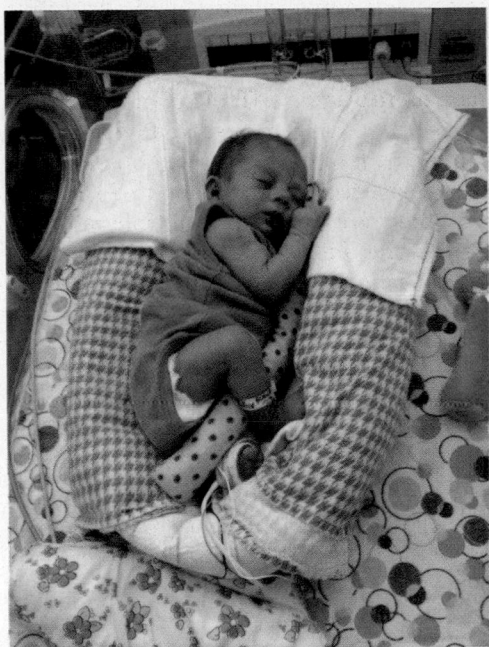

Source: Carol Harrigan, RN, MSN, NNP BC.

Figure 33–98 ❯❯ A 3-week-old, 31 weeks' gestational age baby is nested and developmentally positioned. Hand-to-mouth behavior facilitates self-consoling and soothing activities.

"nesting." Swaddle the preemie to maintain extremities in a flexed position while ensuring that the hands can reach the face. This permits the newborn to do hand-to-mouth activities, which can be consoling (**Figure 33–98** ❯❯).

- Simulate the kinesthetic advantages of the intrauterine environment by using sheepskin and approved water beds. Water bed and pillow use has been reported to improve sleep and decrease motor activity as well as lead to more mature motor behavior, fewer state changes, and a decreased heart rate.

- Provide opportunities for nonnutritive sucking with a pacifier (**Figure 33–99** ❯❯). This improves transcutaneous oxygen saturation; decreases body movements; improves sleep, especially after feedings; and increases weight gain.

- Provide objects for the preemie to grasp (e.g., a piece of blanket, oxygen tubing, or a finger) during caregiving. Grasping may comfort the baby.

The nurse teaches the parents how to read behavioral cues to help them move at their baby's own pace when providing stimulation. Parents are ideally equipped to meet the baby's need for stimulation. Stroking, rocking, cuddling, quiet singing, and talking to the baby can all be integral parts of the baby's care. Visual stimulation in the form of *en face* interaction with caregivers and mobiles is also important (see Figure 33–58).

Kangaroo (skin-to-skin) care is becoming more prevalent in NICUs across the United States (see Figure 33–97). It was first practiced in Bogota, Colombia, in the early 1980s because of fear about the spread of infection by sharing incubators. Skin-to-skin care is defined as the practice of holding newborns skin-to-skin against their parents. The newborn is

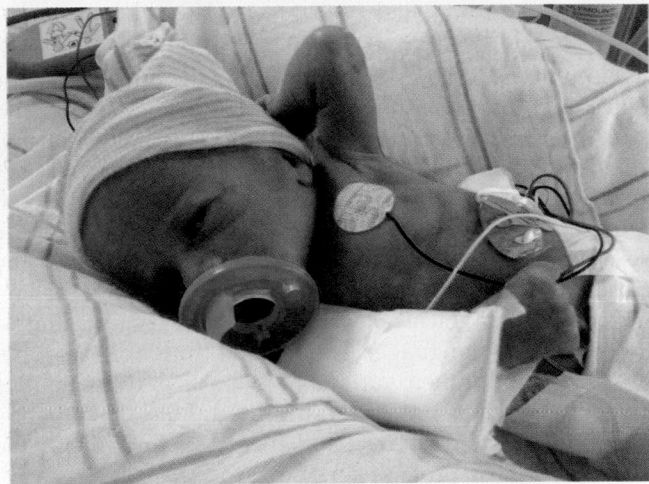

Source: Carol Harrigan, RN, MSN, NNP-BC.

Figure 33–99 ❯❯ Nonnutritive sucking on a pacifier has a calming effect on the preterm newborn and also facilitates readiness to bottle-feed.

usually naked, except for a diaper, and is placed on his or her parent's bare chest. They are then both covered with a blanket. Benefits of skin-to-skin care as a developmental intervention include the following (Ludington-Hoe, 2013):

- Improved oxygenation, as evidenced by an increase in oxygen saturation levels
- Enhanced temperature regulation
- Decline in the episodes of apnea and bradycardia
- Increased periods of quiet sleep
- Stabilization of vital signs
- Positive interaction between parent and baby, which enhances attachment and bonding
- Increased growth parameters
- Early discharge.

Skin-to-skin care may be limited because of staff uneasiness when moving the neonate while attached to multiple IV lines, monitor leads, and a ventilator. The confines of the nursery may be another limiting factor.

Music therapy as a noninvasive auditory stimulus has been shown to be advantageous in full-term newborns but has not been well studied in the premature neonate (Loewy et al., 2012). The music used in NICUs primarily includes lullabies and soft acoustical pieces that are pleasant, soothing, and calming. Such music has been shown to affect newborn physiologic responses, such as improving oxygenation and increasing weight gain. It also has behavioral effects, leading to enhanced parental bonding and increased intervals of nonnutritive sucking periods. Language development is also enhanced if the music is live and sung by the mother or another woman, which is preferential to the newborn. However, the overall noise level in the NICU needs to be considered before including any extra auditory stimulation, including music therapy (Kassity-Krich & Jones, 2014).

Massage and *gentle touch* have been practiced for many centuries. The types of stimulation include massage with stroking, gentle touch without stroking, and therapeutic touch or "hands-on" containment. Practitioners report such physiologic benefits as stimulating blood and lymphatic flow, promoting weight gain in premature newborns, and regulating sleep patterns (Smith, 2012). Many emotional and behavioral benefits are also cited by practitioners. Classes are available to teach parents how to perform massage on their babies. Massage demonstrates compassion while increasing the parent's empathy and understanding of the baby. It helps parents learn to interpret their baby's behavioral cues, such as facial expression, various crying patterns, and other body language. At the same time, it helps newborns learn about their various body parts and boundaries and feel how those integrate into the whole. Therapeutic touch reduces motor activity and energy expenditure by the newborn and also promotes comfort.

For ways to help new parents with a compromised newborn, see Patient Teaching: Parent Support.

Prepare for Home Care

Parents are often anxious when their premature newborn is transferred out of the NICU or is discharged home. Parents of preterm babies should receive the same postpartum teaching as any parent taking a new baby home. In preparing for discharge, the nurse encourages the parents to spend time caring directly for their baby. This familiarizes them with their baby's behavior patterns and helps them establish realistic expectations about the baby. Some hospitals have a special room near the nursery where parents can spend the night with their baby before discharge.

Discharge instruction includes breastfeeding and formula-feeding techniques, formula preparation, and vitamin administration. If the mother wishes to breastfeed, the nurse teaches her to pump her breasts to keep the milk flowing and provide milk even before discharge. The nurse gives information on bathing, diapering, hygiene, and normal elimination patterns and prepares the parents to expect changes in the color of the baby's stool, number of bowel

movements, and timing of elimination when the baby is switched from formula-feeding to breastfeeding. This information can prevent unnecessary concern by the parents. The nurse also discusses normal growth and development patterns, reflexes, and activity for preterm newborns. In these discussions, the nurse should emphasize ways to promote bonding behaviors and deal with newborn crying. Caring for the preemie with complications, preventing infections, recognizing signs of a sick baby, and the need for continued medical follow-up are other key issues.

Families with preterm newborns usually do not need to be referred to community agencies, such as visiting nurse assistance. However, referral may be necessary if the preemie has severe congenital abnormalities, feeding problems, or complications with infections or respiratory problems, or if the parents seem unable to cope with an at-risk baby. Parents of preterm babies can benefit from meeting with others in a similar situation to share common experiences and concerns. Nurses should refer parents to support groups sponsored by the hospital or by others in the community and make connections for parents with early education intervention centers.

Preterm and low-birth-weight babies are at greater risk of increased morbidity from vaccine-preventable diseases (AAP & ACOG, 2012). The optimal timing to initiate hepatitis B therapy in preterm newborns weighing less than 2000 g whose mothers are hepatitis B surface antigen negative has not been determined. Preterm newborns who weigh less than 2000 g and are medically stable and thriving do show consistently high rates of seroconversion following the first dose of hepatitis B vaccine, even when the first dose is given as early as 1 month after birth (AAP & ACOG, 2012). The medically stable preterm baby and low-birth-weight baby should receive full doses of diphtheria, tetanus, acellular pertussis, *Haemophilus influenzae* type b, poliovirus, and pneumococcal conjugate vaccines at a chronologic age consistent with the schedule recommended for full-term babies (AAP & ACOG, 2012). The influenza vaccine should be administered at 6 months of age before the beginning of and during the influenza season. Palivizumab for respiratory syncytial virus (RSV) should be administered during the local RSV season and before hospital discharge to preterm newborns born at less than 35 weeks of gestation as well as to those with bronchopulmonary dysplasia or congenital heart disease (AAP & ACOG, 2012). Immunoprophylaxis should be continued on a monthly basis until the local RSV season ends.

Evaluation

Expected outcomes of nursing care include the following:

- The preterm newborn is free of respiratory distress and establishes effective respiratory function.
- The preterm newborn gains weight and shows no signs of fatigue or aspiration during feedings.
- The preterm newborn demonstrates a serial head circumference growth rate of 1 cm (0.4 in.) per week.
- The parents are able to verbalize their feelings of anger and guilt about the birth of a preterm baby and show attachment behavior, such as frequent visits and growing confidence in their participatory care activities.

Patient Teaching
Parent Support

Although birth is often a highly anticipated and exciting experience, this event does not always result in the delivery of the healthy baby parents anticipate. When parents realize their newborn is not the "perfect" child they hoped for, both mothers and fathers experience an acute grief reaction (Valizadeh, Zamanzadeh, & Rahiminia, 2013). Whether related to prematurity or congenital anomaly, the birth of a seriously compromised baby may cause parents to experience anticipatory grief before an actual loss occurs. It is important to note that mothers and fathers may express grief in different ways. Women are more likely to openly express emotions and reactions associated with grief, while men may suppress their feelings because of their supportive and protective role (Valizadeh et al., 2013). Because nurses often participate in end-of-life care for critically ill babies and their families, they must be acutely aware of these differences and equipped to offer appropriate support measures. For more information, see the module on Grief and Loss.

Conducting additional care evaluation determines if further care is needed based on newborn outcomes. If the outcomes are not being met, the nurse may choose to continue or revise the plan of care for optimal outcome attainment.

Continuation, revision, or discontinuation of a plan of care is decided through collaboration of all members of the healthcare team.

Nursing Care Plan
A Premature Newborn

Baby Boy Johnson was born 12 weeks early at 28 weeks of gestation to Dennis and Alaina Johnson. He is their first child. The NICU nurse received the baby from the obstetrician after he was delivered vaginally. Apgar scoring was 5 at 1 minute, 5 at 5 minutes, and 4 at 10 minutes. He had a weak cry and was dusky and floppy, with an initial heart rate of greater than 100 beats/min. During resuscitation, the nurse provided blow-by oxygen. When his oxygenation status not only failed to improve but dropped, indicating that resuscitation was not effective, the nurse practitioner inserted an oral endotracheal tube, and oxygen was administered by bagging. He was transported to the NICU in a warm isolette where he was admitted, placed on a ventilator, and had an umbilical artery catheter placed.

His parents come to see him when his mother is moved from the labor area to her room on the postpartum unit. Their first question to the nurse is "Is he okay?" Their next question is "When will he be able to come home?" The nurse encourages his parents to touch him and talk to him before they leave the nursery.

ASSESSMENT

- Vital signs 36°C (96.7°F) axillary; pulse 172 beats/min; respiration 68/min; BP 42/24 mmHg
- Endotracheal tube taped in place to ventilator set to deliver 30 breaths/minute, with 4 mmHg of positive end-expiratory pressure
- Color pink with acrocyanosis
- Soft murmur audible in left midaxillary area
- Hypoactive bowel sounds in all quadrants
- Has not voided or stooled yet

DIAGNOSES

- *Ineffective Airway Clearance secondary to prematurity*
- *Attachment, Risk for Impaired*
- *Body Temperature: Imbalanced, Risk for*
- *Gas Exchange, Impaired*

(NANDA-I © 2014)

PLANNING

- The newborn will maintain adequate gas exchange to meet tissue requirements.
- The newborn will maintain a clear airway to promote oxygenation.
- The parents will bond with the newborn and recognize the characteristics of their baby.
- The newborn will receive adequate nutrition and fluid to promote growth.

IMPLEMENTATION

- Suction endotracheal tube as needed when secretions are heard in endotracheal tube.
- Monitor arterial blood gas studies to determine adequate gas exchange.
- Assist with surfactant administration as ordered to reduce alveolar collapse on expiration.
- Monitor daily weights.
- Monitor urine output and kidney function by testing urine for pH and specific gravity.
- Encourage parents to visit as often as possible, and point out the newborn's characteristics to help parents focus on the baby instead of the medical equipment.
- Assist parents to hold their baby, and offer the option of skin-to-skin (kangaroo) care to promote attachment.

- Monitor cardiorespiratory and oxygen saturation on a continuous basis. Change pulse oximeter location frequently (at least every 2 hours) to reduce the risk of altered skin integrity.
- Avoid use of tape to reduce altered skin integrity.
- Promote development by offering a pacifier for the newborn to suck on.
- Provide periods of reduced stimulation to promote rest and comfort.
- Maintain neonate in a neutral thermal environment, either on a radiant warmer or a heated isolette, until he is able to maintain a normal temperature independently.
- Monitor vital signs at a minimum of every 4 hours.

EVALUATION

After administration of surfactant, Baby Boy Johnson is extubated, placed on CPAP for 2 days, and then weaned to nasal cannula. Feedings are initiated via continuous gavage feedings. Once feedings are tolerated, he is changed to every-3-hour feedings. His murmur is diagnosed as a patent ductus arteriosus (PDA), and indomethacin is administered, which successfully closes the PDA.

He begins to have occasional apneic episodes and is placed on caffeine every 12 hours.

Within 4 weeks, he is showing steady weight gain and is moved to the low-risk NICU. His parents begin participating more in providing care, such as bathing and feeding him, and he is discharged at 12 weeks of age.

CRITICAL THINKING

1. How would you respond to the parents when they ask when the baby is likely to come home?

2. How can you maintain the neonate's temperature while he is being held by his parents?

3. If the neonate weighs 900 g, what are his fluid and caloric needs per day?

REVIEW Prematurity

RELATE Link the Concepts and Exemplars

Linking the exemplar of prematurity to the concept of grief and loss:

1. What factors might induce feelings of loss for the parents of a premature newborn, even if the newborn is doing well?

2. What nursing interventions would you implement to help the parents who are feeling grief and loss over the birth of their premature newborn?

Linking the exemplar of prematurity with the concept of development:

3. What developmental needs does a premature newborn have?

4. What nursing care would you provide the premature newborn in order to promote development?

READY Go to Volume 3: Clinical Nursing Skills

REFER Go to Pearson MyLab Nursing and eText

- Additional review materials

REFLECT Apply Your Knowledge

Jessica Marshall, 15 years old, delivers a baby girl at 32 weeks of gestation. Jessica sees her baby briefly in the delivery room before the newborn is transported to the NICU. Jessica names the baby Shamika, after her best friend. On the way from the labor and delivery recovery room, the nurse brings Jessica to the nursery to see the baby, who is under an oxygen hood with an IV through her umbilicus and cardiac monitor leads on her chest. When Jessica sees her baby, she begins to cry and says, "She's so small and looks so sick. It's all my fault!" The nurse caring for Shamika points out the baby's beautiful curly hair, long fingers, and aquiline nose. Jessica stops crying and says, "Oh, you're right. Look how beautiful she is—and so perfect." Shamika's nurse takes Jessica to her new room, gives her some information about premature babies to read, and encourages her to come back to visit Shamika as soon as she feels up to it.

1. When assigned to care for Shamika, what nursing diagnoses would you consider to be the greatest priority regarding this family?

2. How would you help Jessica bond with her premature newborn?

3. What risks does this premature newborn face as the result of being born to an adolescent mother?

References

Abu-Ouf, N. M., & Jan, M. M. (2015). The impact of maternal iron deficiency and iron deficiency anemia on child's health. *Saudi Medical Journal, 36*(2), 146–149. Retrieved from https://www.ncbi.nlm.nih.gov/pmc/articles/PMC4375689

Agency for Toxic Substance and Disease Registry (ATSDR). (2013). *Safeguarding communities from chemical exposure.* Retrieved from http://www.atsdr.cdc.gov/docs/apha-atsdr_book.pdf

AIDS.gov. (2015). *Pregnancy & childbirth.* Retrieved from https://www.aids.gov/hiv-aids-basics/prevention/reduce-your-risk/pregnancy-and-childbirth

Alan Guttmacher Institute (AGI). (2016). *American teens sexual and reproductive health.* Retrieved from https://www.guttmacher.org/fact-sheet/american-teens-sexual-and-reproductive-health

Alayed, N., Kezouh, A., Oddy, L., & Abenhaim, H. A. (2014). Sickle-cell disease and pregnancy outcomes: Population-based study on 8.8 million births. *Journal of Perinatal Medicine, 42*(4), 487–492.

Alio, A. P., Lewis, C. A., Scarborough, K., Harris, K., & Fiscella, K. (2013). A community perspective on the role of fathers during pregnancy: A qualitative study. *BMC Pregnancy and Childbirth, 13*(60), 1–11.

Al-Sayed, E. M., & Ibrahim, K. S. (2014). Second-hand tobacco smoke in children. *Toxicology and Industrial Health, 30*(7), 635–644.

American Academy of Pediatrics (AAP). (2004). AAP Subcommittee on Hyperbilirubinemia. Clinical Practice Guideline: Management of hyperbilirubinemia in the newborn infant 35 or more weeks of gestation. *Pediatrics, 114*, 297.

American Academy of Pediatrics (AAP). (2016a). *Erythromycin ointment.* Retrieved from http://www.healthychildren.org

American Academy of Pediatrics (AAP). (2016b). *Infant food and feeding.* Retrieved from https://www.aap.org/en-us/advocacy-and-policy/aap-health-initiatives/HALF-Implementation-Guide/Age-Specific-Content/Pages/Infant-Food-and-Feeding.aspx

American Academy of Pediatrics (AAP) & American College of Obstetricians and Gynecologists (ACOG). (2012). *Guidelines for perinatal care* (7th ed.). Elk Grove Village, IL: Author.

American Association of Colleges of Nursing. (2016). *Interdisciplinary education and practice.* Retrieved from http://www.aacn.nche.edu/publications/position/interdisciplinary-education-and-practice

American College of Obstetricians & Gynecologists (ACOG) (2009, reaffirmed 2013). *Intrapartum fetal heart rate monitoring: Nomenclature, interpretation, and general management principles.* (ACOG Practice Bulletin No. 106.) Washington, DC: ACOG.

American College of Obstetricians & Gynecologists (ACOG). (2012a). *Timing of umbilical cord clamping after birth.* (ACOG Committee Opinion No. 543.) *Obstetrics and Gynecology, 120*(6), 1522–1526. doi:10.1097/01.AOG.0000423817.47165.48.

American College of Obstetricians and Gynecologists (ACOG). (2012b). *Umbilical cord blood gas and acid base analysis.* (ACOG Committee Opinion No. 348.) Washington, DC: Author.

American College of Obstetricians and Gynecologists (ACOG). (2013a). Weight gain during pregnancy. (Committee Opinion No. 548.) Washington, DC: Author.

American College of Obstetricians and Gynecologists (ACOG). (2013b). *Oral health care during pregnancy and throughout the lifespan.* (Committee Opinion No. 569.) Washington, DC: Author.

American College of Obstetricians and Gynecologists (ACOG). (2013c). *Definition of term pregnancy.* (ACOG Committee Opinion No. 579.) Washington, DC: Author.

American College of Obstetricians and Gynecologists (ACOG). (2013d). *Gestational diabetes mellitus.* (ACOG Practice Bulletin No. 137.) Washington, DC: Author

American College of Obstetricians and Gynecologists (ACOG). (2013e). *Obesity in pregnancy.* (Committee Opinion No. 549.) Washington, DC: Author.

American College of Obstetricians and Gynecologists (ACOG). (2013f). *Induction of labor.* (ACOG Practice Bulletin No. 107.) Washington, DC: Author.

American College of Obstetricians and Gynecologists (ACOG). (2013g). *Non–medically indicated early-term deliveries.* (Committee Opinion No. 561.) Washington, DC: Author.

American College of Obstetricians and Gynecologists (ACOG). (2014). *Neural tube defects.* (ACOG Practice Bulletin No. 44.) Washington, DC: Author.

American College of Obstetricians and Gynecologists (ACOG). (2015a). *Nausea and vomiting in pregnancy.* (ACOG Practice Bulletin No. 153.) Washington, DC: Author.

American College of Obstetricians and Gynecologists (ACOG). (2015b). *Anemia in pregnancy.* (ACOG Practice Bulletin No. 95.) Washington, DC: Author.

American College of Obstetricians and Gynecologists (ACOG). (2015c). *Vaginal birth after previous cesarean delivery.* (Practice Bulletin No. 115.) Washington, DC: Author.

American College of Obstetricians and Gynecologists (ACOG). (2015d). *Screening for prenatal depression.* (Committee Opinion No. 630.) Washington, DC: Author.

American College of Obstetricians and Gynecologists (ACOG). (2016a). *Prenatal diagnostic testing for genetic disorders.* (Practice Bulletin No. 162.) Washington, DC: Author.

American College of Obstetricians and Gynecologists (ACOG). (2016b). *Premature rupture of membranes.* (Practice Bulletin No. 172.) Washington, DC: ACOG.

American College of Obstetricians and Gynecologist (ACOG). (2016c). *Optimizing postpartum care.* (Committee Opinion No. 666.) Washington, DC: Author.

American College of Obstetricians and Gynecologists (ACOG) & Society for Maternal-Fetal Medicine (SMFM). (2013, reaffirmed 2015.) *Definition of term pregnancy.* (Committee Opinion No. 579). Retrieved from http://www.acog.org/Resources-And-

Publications/Committee-Opinions/Committee-on-Obstetric-Practice/Definition-of-Term-Pregnancy

American Diabetes Association (ADA). (2014). Position statement: Standards of medical care in diabetes—2014. *Diabetes Care, 37*(Supp. 1), S81–S90.

Anderson, B. A., & Stone, S. (2013). Best practices in midwifery: Using the evidence to implement change. New York, NY: Springer.

Andrews, M.M., & Boyle, J. S. (2016). *Transcultural Concepts in Nursing Care* (7th ed.). Philadelphia, PA: Wolters Kluwer.

Angelini, D. J., & Lafontaine, D. (2013). *Obstetric triage and emergency care protocols.* New York, NY: Springer.

Apgar, V. (1966, August). The newborn (Apgar) scoring system, reflections and advice. *Pediatric Clinics of North America, 13,* 645.

Ara, F., Ara, B., Kaker, P., & Aslam, M. (2015). Childbirth: Comparison of complications between lithotomy and squatting positions during labor. *Professional Medical Journal, 22*(4), 390–394.

Assuncao, S., Camos, J. A., Bonini, D., Ibidi, S. M., Ruano, R., & Zugaib, M. (2012). Low Apgar scores at 5 minutes in a low-risk population: Maternal and obstetrical factors and postnatal outcome. *Revista da Associacao Medica Brasileira, 58*(5), 587–593. Retrieved from http://www.scielo.br/scielo.php?script=sci_arttext&pid=S0104-42302012000500017

Attanasio, L. B., Hardeman, R. R., Kozhimannil, K. B., & Kjerulff, K. H. (2017). Prenatal attitudes toward vaginal delivery and actual delivery mode: Variation by race/ethnicity and socioeconomic status. *Birth.* doi: 10.1111/birt.12305

Baggerly, C. A., Cuomo, R. E., French, C. B., Garland, C. F., Gorham, E. D., Grant, W. B., ... Wunsch, A. (2015). Sunlight and vitamin D: Necessary for public health. *Journal of the American College of Nutrition, 34*(4), 359–365.

Bagwell, G. A. (2014). Hematologic system. In C. Kenner & J. W. Lott (Eds.), *Comprehensive neonatal nursing care* (5th ed., pp. 334–375). New York, NY: Springer.

Ballard, J. L., Khoury, J. C., Wedig, K., Wang, L., Eilers-Walsmann, B. L., & Lipp, R. (1991). New Ballard Score, expanded to include extremely premature infants. *Journal of Pediatrics, 119*(3), 417–423.

Ballogh, V. (2015). The consequences of maternal obesity. *International Journal of Childbirth Education, 30*(1), 54–58.

Barron, M. L. (2014). Antenatal care. In K. R. Simpson & P. A. Creehan (Eds.), *AWHONN's perinatal nursing* (4th ed., pp. 89–121). Philadelphia, PA: Lippincott Williams & Wilkins.

Bhutani, V. K., Johnson, L., & Sivieri, E. M. (1999). Predictive ability of a predischarge hour-specific serum bilirubin for subsequent significant hyperbilirubinemia in healthy term and near-term newborns. *Pediatrics, 103,* 6–14.

Bishop, E. H. (1964). Pelvic scoring for elective inductions. *Obstetrics & Gynecology, 24,* 266.

Blackburn, S. T. (2013). *Maternal, fetal, & neonatal physiology: A clinical perspective* (4th ed.). St. Louis, MO: Saunders.

Blair, P. S. (2015). Co-sleeping and suffocation. *Forensic Science, Medicine, and Pathology, 11*(2), 1–2.

Borca, G., Bina, M., Keller, P. S., Gilbert, L. R., & Begotti, T. (2015). Internet use and developmental tasks: Adolescents' point of view. *Computers in Human Behavior, 52,* 49–58.

Born, A. (2012). Relationship violence and teenage parents. *Journal of Infant, Child, & Adolescent Psychotherapy, 11*(4), 368–375.

Bradshaw, E. A., Cuzzi, S., Kiernan, S. C., Nagel, N., Becker, J. A., & Martin, G. R. (2012). Feasibility of implementing pulse oximetry screening for congenital heart disease in a community hospital. *Journal of Perinatology, 32*(9), 710–715.

Brazelton, T. B. (1984). *Neonatal behavioral assessment scale* (2nd ed.). London, England: Heinemann.

Brazelton, T. B., & Nugent, J. K. (1995). *The neonatal behavioral assessment scale* (3rd ed.). London, England: MacKeith.

Brincat, C., Crosby, E., McLeod, A., & Fenner, D. E. (2015). Experiences during the first four years of a postpartum perineal clinic in the USA. *International Journal of Gynecology & Obstetrics, 128*(1), 68–71.

Caldwell, W. E., & Moloy, H. C. (1933). Anatomical variations in the female pelvis and their effect on labor with a suggested classification [Historical article]. *American Journal of Obstetrics and Gynecology, 26,* 479–505.

Callahan, I., & Caughley, A. (2013). *Blueprint in obstetrics & gynecology.* Philadelphia, PA: Lippincott Williams & Wilkins.

Cao, C., & O'Brien, K. O. (2013). Pregnancy and iron homeostasis: An update. *Nutrition Reviews, 71*(1), 35–51.

Carlson, S. E., Colombo, J., Gajewski, B. J., Gustafson, K. M., Mundy, D., Yeast, J., ... Shaddy, D. J. (2013). DHA supplementation and pregnancy outcomes. *The American Journal of Clinical Nutrition, 97*(4), 808–815.

Carmoney, P. (2014). Pica and pregnancy: A global view. *International Journal of Childbirth Education, 29*(3), 29–32.

Carolan, M. (2013). Maternal age ≥ 45 years and maternal and perinatal outcomes: A review of the evidence. *Midwifery, 29*(5), 479–489.

Cassidy, J., Jones, J. D., & Shaver, P. R. (2013). Contributions of attachment theory and research: A framework for future research, translation, and policy. *Development and Psychopathology, 25*(4 pt 2), 1415–1434. Retrieved from https://www.ncbi.nlm.nih.gov/pmc/articles/PMC4085672

Castle, P. (2012). Collaboration in open adoption: The birth mother's experience. *Australian Journal of Adoption, 6*(1), 1–9.

Caudle, P. W. (2014). Reproductive tract structure and function. In R. G. Jordan, J. L. Engstrom, J. A. Marfell, & C. L. Farley (Eds.), *Prenatal and postnatal care: A woman-centered approach.* Ames, IA: Wiley Blackwell.

Cavaliere, T. A. & Sansoucie, D. A. (2014). Assessment of the newborn and infant. In C. Kenner & J. W. Lott (Eds.), *Comprehensive neonatal nursing care* (5th ed., pp. 71–112). New York, NY: Springer.

Center for American Progress. (2015). *The adoption option.* Retrieved from http://www.americanprogress.org/issues/women/report/2010/10/18/8460/the-adoption-option

Centers for Disease Control (CDC). (2013). *Global tuberculosis 2013.* Retrieved from http://www.cdc.gov/tb/topic/globaltb/default.htm

Centers for Disease Control and Prevention (CDC). (2014a). *Guidelines for vaccinating pregnant women.* Retrieved from http://www.cdc.gov/VACCINes/pubs/preg-guide.htm

Centers for Disease Control and Prevention (CDC). (2014b). *Newborn screening quality assurance program.* Retrieved from http://www.cdc.gov/labstandards/nsqap.html

Centers for Disease Control and Prevention (CDC). (2015a). *Folic acid: Recommendations.* Retrieved from http://www.cdc.gov/ncbddd/folicacid/recommendations.html

Centers for Disease Control and Prevention (CDC). (2015b). *Births: Final data for 2014. National Vital Statistics Reports, 64*(10). Retrieved from https://www.cdc.gov/nchs/data/nvsr/nvsr64/nvsr64_12.pdf

Centers for Disease Control and Prevention (CDC). (2015c) *Hearing loss in newborn: Screening and diagnosis.* Retrieved from http://www.cdc.gov/ncbddd/hearingloss/screening.html

Centers for Disease Control and Prevention (CDC). (2015d). *Preterm birth.* http://www.cdc.gov/reproductivehealth/maternalinfanthealth/pretermbirth.htm

Centers for Disease Control and Prevention. (CDC). (2016). *Teen pregnancy in the United States.* Retrieved from http://www.cdc.gov/teenpregnancy/about

Cheng, Y. (2014). Normal labor and delivery. *Medscape.* Retrieved from http://emedicine.medscape.com/article/260036-overview

Cherry, A., & Dillon, M. (2014). International handbook of adolescent pregnancy: Medical, psychosocial, and public health responses. New York, NY: Springer.

Child Welfare Information Gateway. (2013a). *Grounds for involuntary termination of parental rights.* Retrieved from http://www.childwelfare.gov/systemwide/laws_policies/statutes/groundtermin.cfm

Child Welfare Information Gateway. (2013b). *Infant safe haven laws.* Retrieved from https://www.childwelfare.gov/pubPDFs/safehaven.pdf

Chou, C. (2017). Traditional postpartum practices and rituals: A qualitative systematic review. Ci. Lee-Dennis, K. Fung, S. Grigoriadis, G. Erlick-Robinson, S. Romans & L. Ross (Editors). *Embryo Project Encyclopedia.* Retrieved from https://embryo.asu.edu/.

Cloherty, J. P., Eichenwald, E. C., Hansen, A. R., & Stark, A. R. (2012). *Manual for neonatal care* (7th ed.). Philadelphia, PA: Lippincott Williams & Wilkins.

Creasy, R. K., Resnik, R., Iams, J. D., Lockwood, C. J., Moore, T. R., & Greene, M. F. (2014) *Creasy and Resnik's maternal-fetal medicine: Principles and practice* (7th ed.). St. Louis, MO: Elsevier.

Cunningham, F. G., Leveno, K. J., Bloom, S. L., Spong, C. Y., Dashe, G. S., Hoffman, B. L., ... Sheffield, G. S. (2014). *Williams obstetrics* (24th ed.). New York, NY: McGraw-Hill.

Dalfen, A. (2014). When baby brings the blues: Solutions for postpartum depression. New York, NY: Collins.

Davidson, M. R. (2013). Fast facts for the antepartum and postpartum nurse: An orientation in a nutshell. New York, NY: Springer.

Davidson, M., London, M., & Ladewig, P. (2017). *Olds' maternal–newborn nursing & women's health across the lifespan* (10th ed.). Hoboken, NJ: Pearson.

Dawson, J. A., Summan, R., Badawi, N., & Foster, J. P. (2012). Push versus gravity for intermittent bolus gavage tube feeding of premature and low birth weight infants. *Cochrane Database of Systematic Reviews, 11,* 1–17. doi:10.1002/14651858.CD005249.pub2

DeGroot, J. M., & Vik, T. A. (2017). Disenfranchised grief following a traumatic birth. *Journal of Loss and Trauma, 22*(4), 346–356.

Diab, Y., & Luchtman-Jones, L. (2015). The blood and hematopoietic system. In R. J. Martin, A. A. Fanaroff, & M. C. Walsh (Eds.), *Fanaroff & Martin's neonatal-perinatal medicine* (10th ed., pp. 1294–1343). St. Louis, MO: Elsevier Mosby.

D'Souza, S. R. B., Kumar, V., & Lewis, L. E. (2014). Development of a tool for assessing preterm infants. *Nursing and Midwifery Research Journal, 10*(3), 91–99.

Duff, P. (2014). Maternal and fetal infectious disorders. In R. K. Creasy & R. Resnik (Eds.), *Maternal-fetal medicine: Principles and practice* (7th ed., pp. 802–851). Philadelphia, PA: Saunders.

Ellis, C. R., & Schnoes, C. J. (2012). Pica. *Medscape.* Retrieved from http://emedicine.medscape.com/article/914765-overview#a1

Fantasia, H. C. (2014). A new pharmacologic treatment for nausea and vomiting of pregnancy. *Nursing for Women's Health, 18*(1), 73–77.

Field, T. (2012). Infant behavior and development. *Prenatal Exercise Research, 35*(3), 397–407.

Fontaine, K. L. (2014). *Contemporary and alternative therapies for nursing practice* (4th ed.). Upper Saddle River, NJ: Pearson.

Fraser, D. (2014). Newborn adaptations to extrauterine life. In K. R. Simpson & P. A. Creehan, *Perinatal nursing* (4th ed.). Philadelphia, PA: Lippincott Williams & Wilkins.

Freeman, R. K., Garite, T. J., Nageotte, M. P., & Miller, L. A. (2012). *Fetal heart rate monitoring* (4th ed.). Philadelphia, PA: Lippincott Williams & Wilkins.

Gabbe, S. G., Niebyl, J. R., Galan, H. Eric, R. M., & Jauniaux, E. R. M. (2012). *Normal and problem pregnancies* (6th ed.). Philadelphia, PA: Churchill Livingstone.

Gardner, S. L, Goldson, E. & Hernandez, J. A. (2016). The neonate and the environment: Impact on development. In S. L. Gardner, B. S. Carter, M. Enzman-Hines, & J. A. Hernandez (Eds.), *Merenstein & Gardner's handbook of neonatal intensive care* (8th ed., pp. 262–314). St. Louis, MO: Mosby.

Gavin, L., Warner, L., O'Neil, M. E., Duong, L. M., Marshall, C., Hastings, P. A., … Barfield, W. (2013). Vital signs: Repeat births among teens—United States, 2007–2010. *Morbidity and Mortality Weekly Report*, 62(13), 249–255. Retrieved from http://www.cdc.gov/mmwr/preview/mmwrhtml/mm6213a4.htm?s_cid=mm6213a4_w

Ghorashi, Z., Ashori, V., Aminzadeh, F., & Mokhtari, M. (2014). The effects of oral fluid intake an hour before cesarean section on regurgitation incidence. *Iranian Journal of Nurse Midwifery Research*, 19(4), 439–442.

Goer, H., & Romano, A. (2012). *Optimal care in childbirth: The case for a physiologic approach.* Seattle, WA: Classic Day.

Goetz, E., & Hokanson, J. (2011). *Pulse oximetry screening for congenital heart disease: Toolkit.* Retrieved from http://www.wisconsinshine.org/handouts/Pulse-Oximetry-Toolkit.pdf

Goldberg, A. E. (2015). Cervical ripening. *E-medicine.* Retrieved from http://emedicine.medscape.com/article/263311-overview#a6

Gomella, T. L. (Ed.). (2013). *Neonatology: management, procedures, on-call problems, diseases, and drugs* (7th ed.). New York, NY: McGraw-Hill Education.

Goodwin, M. (2015). Abdomen assessment. In E. P. Tapero & M. E. Honeyfield (Eds.), *Physical assessment of the newborn* (5th ed., pp. 111–120). Petaluma, CA: NICU Ink.

Gordon, M. C. (2012). Maternal physiology. In S. G. Gabbe, J. R. Niebyl, J. L. Simpson, M. B. Landon, H. L. Galan, E. R. M. Jauniaux, & D. A. Driscoll (Eds.), *Obstetrics: Normal and problem pregnancies* (6th ed.). Philadelphia, PA: Churchill Livingstone.

Greene, D. N., Schmidt, R. L., Kamer, S. M., & Grenache, D. G. (2013). Limitations in qualitative point of care hCG tests for detecting early pregnancy. *Clinica Chimica Acta, 415*, 317–321.

Groll, C. G. (2012). Fast facts for the L&D nurse: Labor and delivery orientation in a nutshell. New York, NY: Springer.

Gruneberg, F., & Crozier, K. (2015). Delayed cord clamping in the compromised baby. *British Journal of Midwifery 23*(2), 102–108.

Gurber, S., Bielinski-Blattmann, D., Lemola, S., Jaussi, C., von Wyl, A., Surbek, D., … Stadlmayr, W. (2012). Maternal mental health in the first 3 weeks postpartum: The impact of caregiver support and the subjective experience of childbirth—A longitudinal path model. *Journal of Psychosomatic Obstetrics and Gynaecology, 33*(4), 176–184.

Gurley, E. S., Halder, A. K., Streatfield, P. K., Sazzad, H. M., Huda, T. M., Hossain, M. J., & Luby, S. P. (2012). Estimating the burden of maternal and neonatal deaths associated with jaundice in Bangladesh: Possible role of hepatitis E infection. *American Journal of Public Health, 102*(12), 2248–2254.

Gurol-Urganci, I., Cromwell, D., Edozien, L., Mahmood, T., Adams, E., Richmond, D. H.… van der Meulen, J. (2013). Third- and fourth-degree perineal tears among primiparous women in England between 2000 and 2012: Time trends and risk factors. *British Journal of Obstetrics and Gynecology, 120*(12), 1534–1547. doi:10.1111/1471-0528.12363

Haines, T. M., Hildingsson, I., Pallant, J. F., & Rubertsson, C. (2013). The role of women's attitudinal profiles in satisfaction with the quality of their antepartal and intra-partum care. *Journal of Obstetric, Gynecologic, and Neonatal Nursing, 42*(4), 428–441. Retrieved from http://www.ncbi.nlm.nih.gov/pubmed/23773005

Hamel, M. S., & Hughes, B. L. (2016). Zika infection in pregnancy. *Contemporary OB/GYN, 61*(8), 16–42.

Hamilton, E. F., & Warrick, P. A. (2013). New perspectives in electronic fetal surveillance. *Journal of Perinatal Medicine, 41*(1), 83–92.

Haran, C., van Driel, M., Mitchell, B. L., & Brodribb, W. E. (2014). Clinical guidelines for postpartum women and infants in primary care—a systematic review. *BMC Pregnancy Childbirth, 14*(51).

Hardy, W., D'Agata, A., & McGrath, J. M. (2016). The infant at risk. In S. Mattson & J. E. Smith (Eds.), *Core curriculum for maternal-newborn nursing* (5th ed., pp. 363–416). St. Louis, MO: Saunders.

Harris, R., & Ayers, S. (2012). What makes labour and birth traumatic? A survey of intrapartum hot spots. *Psychology & Health, 27*(10), 1166–1177.

Harrison, D., Reszel, J., Bueno, M., Sampson, M., Shah, V., Taddio, A., … Turner, L. (2016). Breastfeeding for procedural pain in infants beyond the neonatal period. *Cochrane Database of Systematic Reviews, 2016*(10):CD011248.

Harvey, C. J., & Dildy, G. A. (2013). Obstetric hemorrhage. In N. H. Troiano, C. J. Harvey, & B. F. Chez (Eds.), *AWHONN's high-risk & critical care obstetrics* (3rd ed., pp. 246–273). Philadelphia, PA: Lippincott.

Healthy Children (2015a). *Sleep position: Why back is best.* Retrieved from http://www.healthychildren.org/English/ages-stages/baby/sleep/Pages/Sleep-Position-Why-Back-is-Best.aspx

Healthy Children. (2015b). *Car seats: Information for families 2014.* Retrieved from http://www.healthychildren.org/English/news/Pages/AAP-Updates-Recommendations-on-Car-Seats.aspx

Healthy Children. (2015c). *Purpose of newborn hearing screening.* Retrieved from http://www.healthychildren.org/English/ages-stages/baby/Pages/Purpose-of-Newborn-Hearing-Screening.aspx

Herdman, T. H. & Kamitsuru, S. (Eds.). *Nursing Diagnoses—Definitions and Classification 2015–2017.* Copyright © 2014, 1994–2014 NANDA International. Used by arrangement with John Wiley & Sons, Inc. Companion website: www.wiley.com/go/nursing-diagnoses.

Herrman, J. W., & Nandakumar, R. (2012). Development of a survey to assess adolescent perceptions of teen parenting. *Journal of Nursing Measurement, 20*(1), 3–20.

Hillman, N. H., Kallapur, S. G., & Jobe, A. H. (2012). Physiology of transition from intrauterine to extrauterine life. *Clinics of Perinatology, 39*, 769–783.

Hofmeyr, G. J., Gülmezoglu, A. M., & Pileggi, C. (2013). Vaginal misoprostol for cervical ripening and induction of labour. *Cochrane Database of Systematic Reviews, 2013*(1):CD000941.

Hoshiyama, E., Muento, T., Histake, I., Watanabe, H., Noryuki, I., & Kolchi, H. (2012). Postpartum migraines: A long-term prospective study. *Internal Medicine, 51*(22), 3119–3123.

Huda. (2017). Common practices of Islamic birth rights. Retrieved from https://www.thoughtco.com/islamic-birth-rites-2004500

Human Milk Banking Association of North America. (2011). *Best practice for expressing, storing and handling human milk in hospitals, homes and child care settings.* Raleigh, NC: Author.

Ingraham, N., Wingo, E., Foster, D. G., & Roberts, S. (2017). Best practices for LGBTQ inclusion and exclusion in reproductive health research. *Contraception, 96*(4), 299.

Institute of Medicine. (2009). *Weight gain during pregnancy: Reexamining the guidelines.* Washington, DC: National Academies Press. ©2009 National Academy of Sciences. Retrieved from http://www.nationalacademies.org/hmd/~/media/Files/Report%20Files/2009/Weight-Gain-During-Pregnancy-Reexamining-the-Guidelines/Report%20Brief%20-%20Weight%20Gain%20During%20Pregnancy.pdf

Institute of Medicine (IOM). (2010). *Dietary reference intakes (DRIs): Recommended dietary allowances and adequate intakes, vitamins and elements.* Washington, DC: Food and Nutrition Board, Institute of Medicine, National Academies.

James, D. C. (2014). Postpartum care. In K. R. Simpson & P. A. Creehan (Eds.), *Perinatal nursing* (4th ed., p. 530). Philadelphia, PA: Lippincott Williams & Wilkins.

Janke, J. (2014). Newborn nutrition. In K. R. Simpson & P. A. Creehan (Eds.), *Perinatal nursing* (4th ed., pp. 626–661). Philadelphia, PA: Lippincott Williams & Wilkins.

Jazayeri, A. (2012). Macrosomia. *E-medicine.* Retrieved from http://emedicine.medscape.com/article/262679-overview

Jazayeri, A. (2014). Premature rupture of membranes. *eMedicine.* Retrieved from http://emedicine.medscape.com/article/261137-overview#aw2aab6b3

Jessop, D. C., Craig, L., & Ayers, S. (2014). Applying Leventhal's self-regulatory model to pregnancy: Evidence that pregnancy-related beliefs and emotional responses are associated with maternal health outcomes. *Journal of Health Psychology, 19*(9), 1091–1102.

Johnson, P. (2015). Head, eyes, ears, nose, mouth, and neck assessment. In E. P. Tapero & M. E. Honeyfield (Eds.), *Physical assessment of the newborn* (5th ed.). Petaluma, CA: NICU Ink.

Kann, L., Kinchen, S., Shanklin, S. L., Flint, K. H., Hawkins, J., Harris, W. A., Lowry, R., … Zaza, S. (2014). Youth risk behavior surveillance—United States, 2013. *MMWR Surveillance Summaries, 63*(4), 1–172.

Kassity-Krich, N. A., & Jones, J. E. (2014). Complementary and integrative therapies. In C. Kenner & J. W. Lott (Eds.), *Comprehensive neonatal nursing care* (5th ed., pp. 773–782). New York, NY: Springer.

Katz, B. (2012). New focus of family-centered maternity care. *International Journal of Childbirth Education, 27*(3), 99–102.

Kenner, C., & Lott, J. W. (2014). *Comprehensive neonatal care: An interdisciplinary approach* (5th ed.). St. Louis, MO: Saunders/Elsevier.

Kenny, L. C., Lavender, T., McNamee, R., O'Neill, S. M., Mills, T., & Khashan, A. S. (2013). Advanced maternal age and adverse pregnancy outcome: Evidence from a large contemporary cohort. *PLoS One, 8*(2): e56583. doi:10.1371/journal.pone.0056583

Kim, S. (2017). Sanhujori: Korea's traditional postnatal care culture. *International Journal of Childbirth Education, 32*(3).

Kimberly, D. G., Niebyl, J. R., & Johnson, T. R. B. (2012). Preconception and prenatal care: Part of the continuum. In S. G. Gabbe, J. R. Niebyl, J. L. Simpson, M. B. Landon, H. L. Galan, E. R. M. Jauniaux, & D. A. Driscoll (Eds.), *Obstetrics: Normal and problem pregnancies* (6th ed.) Philadelphia, PA: Elsevier Saunders.

King, T. K., Brucker, M. C., Kriebs, J. M., Fahey, J. O., Gegor, C. L., & Varney, H. (2013). *Varney's midwifery* (5th ed.). Burlington, MA: Jones & Bartlett Learning.

Kovac, J. R., Addai, J., Smith, R. P., Coward, R. M., Lamb, D. J., & Lipshultz, L. I. (2013). The effects of advanced paternal age on fertility. *Asian Journal of Andrology, 15*(6), 723–728.

Ladewig, P. A., London, M. L., & Davidson, M. R. (2017). *Contemporary maternal-newborn nursing care* (9th ed. pp. 528–570). Hoboken, NJ: Pearson.

Lauderdale, J. (2012). Transcultural perspectives in childbearing. In M. M. Andrews & J. S. Boyle (Eds.), *Transcultural concepts in nursing care* (6th ed., pp. 91–122). Philadelphia, PA: Wolters Kluwer/ Lippincott Williams & Wilkins.

Lauwers, J., & Swisher, A. (2016). *Counseling the nursing mother: A lactation consultant's guide* (6th ed.). Burlington, MA: Jones & Bartlett Learning.

Leeman, L. M., & Rogers, R. G. (2012). Sex after childbirth: Postpartum sexual function. *Obstetrics & Gynecology, 119*(3), 647–655. doi:10.1097/ AOG.0b013e3182479611

Lehtonen, L. (2015). Assessment and optimization of neurobehavioral development in preterm infant. In R. J. Martin, A. A. Fanaroff, & M. C. Walsh (Eds.), *Fanaroff & Martin's neonatal-perinatal medicine* (10th ed., pp. 1001–1017). St. Louis, MO: Elsevier Mosby.

Lloreda-Garcia, J. M. (2017). Religion, spirituality and folk medicine: Superstition in a neonatal unit. *Journal of Religion & Health, 56*: 2276. doi.org/10.1007/ s10943-017-0408-y

Loewy, J., Steward, K., Dassler, A., Telsey, A., & Homel, P. (2012). The effects of music therapy on vital signs, feedings, and sleep in premature infants. *Pediatrics, 131*, 902. doi:10.1542/peds.2012-1367

London, M. L., Ladewig, P. A., Davidson, M. R., Ball, J. W., Bindler, R. C., & Cowen, K. J., (2017). *Maternal & Child Nursing Care.* (5th ed.). Hoboken, NJ: Pearson.

Lucas, R. F., & Smith, R. L. (2015). When is it safe to initiate breastfeeding for preterm infants? *Advances in Neonatal Care, 15*(2), 134–141.

Ludington-Hoe, S. M. (2013). Kangaroo care as a neonatal therapy. *NAINR, 13*(2), 73–75.

Lund, C. H., Brandon, D., Holden, A. C., Kuller, J., & Hill, C. M. (2013). *Neonatal skin care: Evidence-based clinical practice guidelines* (3rd ed.). Washington, DC, AWHONN.

Lunze, K., & Hamer, D. H. (2012). Thermal protection of the newborn in resource limited environments. *Journal of Perinatology, 32*(5), 317–324.

Lyndon, A., Lee, H. C., Gilbert, W. M., Gould, J. B., & Lee, K. A. (2012). Maternal morbidity during childbirth hospitalization in California. *Journal of Maternal–Fetal & Neonatal Medicine, 12*, 2529–2535.

MacKenzie, A. P., Stephenson, C. D., & Funai, E. F. (2016). Perinatal assessment of gestational age and estimated date of delivery. *UpToDate.* Retrieved from http://www.uptodate.com/contents/prenatal-assessment-of-gestational-age-and-estimated-date-of-delivery

Magann, E., & Ross, M. G. (2014). *Assessment of amniotic fluid volume. UpToDate.* Retrieved from http://www.uptodate.com/contents/assessment-of-amniotic-fluid-volume

Malhotra, N., Shah, P. K., Kumar, P., & Acharya, P. (2014). *Ultrasound in obstetrics & gynecology* (4th ed.). New Delhi, India: Jaypee Brothers Medical Publishers.

Malm, M. C., Lindgren, H., Rubertsson, C., Hildingsson, I., & Radestad, I. (2014). Development of a tool to evaluate fetal movements in full-term pregnancy. *Sexual & Reproductive Healthcare, 5*(1), 31–35.

March of Dimes (MOD). (2012). *Newborn screening.* Retrieved from http://www.marchofdimes.org/ baby/newborn-screening-tests-for-your-baby.aspx

March of Dimes (MOD). (2016). *Pregnancy after age 35.* Retrieved from http://www.marchofdimes.org/ pregnancy-after-age-35.aspx

Marcewicz, L. (2014, January 27). Late vitamin K deficiency bleeding in infants: Are we seeing a re-emergence? *Medscape.* Retrieved from http://www.medscape.com/viewarticle/819509

Martin, J. A., Hamilton, B. E., Osterman, M. J. K., Curtin, S. C., & Matthews, T. J. (2015). Births: Final data for 2013. *National Vital Statistics Reports, 64*(1), 1–65.

Mayo Clinic. (2016). *Infant and toddler health.* Retrieved from http://www.mayoclinic.org/healthy-lifestyle/ infant-and-toddler-health/basics/newborn-health/ hlv-20049400

McGrath, J. M., & Vittner, D. (2015). Behavioral assessment. In E. P. Tappero & M. E. Honeyfield (Eds.), *Physical assessment in the newborn* (5th ed., pp. 193–219). Petaluma, CA: NICU Ink.

MedlinePlus. (2012). *Quadruple screen test.* Retrieved from http://www.nlm.nih.gov/medlineplus/ency/ article/007311.htm

Menihan, C. A., & Kopel, A. (2014). *Point-of-care assessment in pregnancy and women's health: Electronic fetal monitoring and sonography.* Philadelphia, PA: Lippincott Williams, & Wilkins.

Mercer, R. T. (1995). *Becoming a mother.* New York, NY: Springer.

Mercer, R. T. (2004). Becoming a mother versus maternal role attainment. *Journal of Nursing Scholarship, 36*(3), 226–232.

Messerlian, G. M., Farina, A., & Palomaki, G. E. (2016). First trimester combined test and integrated test for screening for Down syndrome and trisomy 18. *UpToDate.* Retrieved from http://www.uptodate.com/contents/first-trimester-combined-test-and-integrated-tests-for-screening-for-down-syndrome-and-trisomy-18

Micali, N., Stavola, B. D., Santos-Silva, I., Steenweg-de Graaff, J., Jansen, P. W., Jaddoe, V. W., … Tiemeier, H. (2012). Perinatal outcomes and gestational weight gain in women with eating disorders: A population-based cohort study. *British Journal of Obstetrics and Gynecology, 119*(12), 1493–1502.

Miguelez, J., De Lourdes Brizot, M., Liao, A. W., De Carvalho, M., H., B., & Zugaib, M. (2012). Second-trimester soft markers: Relation to first-trimester nuchal translucency and unaffected pregnancies. *Ultrasound in Obstetrics & Gynecology, 39*, 274–278. doi:10.1002/uog.9024

Miller, L., Miller, D., & Tucker, S. M. (2013). *Mosby's pocket guide to fetal monitoring: A multidisciplinary approach* (7th ed.). St. Louis, MO: Mosby.

Modarres, M., Afrasiabi, S., Rahnama, P., & Montazeri, A. (2012). Prevalence and risk factors of childbirth-related post-traumatic stress symptoms. *BMC Pregnancy and Childbirth.* Retrieved from http:// bmcpregnancychildbirth.biomedcentral.com/articles/10.1186/1471-2393-12-88

Moore, E. R., Anderson, G. C., Bergman, N., & Dowswell, T. (2012). Early skin-to-skin contact for mothers and their healthy newborn infants. *Cochrane Database of Systematic Reviews, 2012,* CD003519. doi:10.1002/14651858.CD003519.pub3

Moore, K. L., Persaud, T. V. N., & Torchia, M. G. (2016). *The developing human: Clinically oriented embryology* (10th ed.). Philadelphia, PA: Saunders.

Morris, B. J., Wamai, R. G., Henenberg, E. B., Tobian, A. A. R., Klausner, J. D., Bannerjee, J., & Hankins, C. A. (2016). Estimation of country-specific and global prevalence of male circumcision. *Population Health Metrics, 14*(4). Retrieved from https://www.ncbi.nlm.nih.gov/pmc/articles/PMC4772313

Muchowski, K. E. (2014). Evaluation and treatment of neonatal hyperbilirubinemia. *American Family Physician, 89*(11), 873–878.

Muslim Birth Rights. (2009). Retrieved from http:// www.bbc.co.uk/religion/religions/islam/ritesrituals/birth.shtml

National Center for Complementary and Integrative Health (NCCIH). (2012). *Ginger.* https://nccih.nih. gov/health/ginger

Neis, R. (2017). The Reproduction of species: Humans, animals and species nonconformity in early Rabbinic science. *Jewish Studies Quarterly, 24*(4), 289–317.

Newland, L., L'Huillier, M. W., & Petrey B. (2013). Implementation of cue based feeding in a level III NICU. *Neonatal Network, 32*(2), 132–137.

Niebyl, J. R., & Simpson, J. L. (2012). Drugs and environmental agents in pregnancy and lactation: Embryology, teratology, epidemiology. In S. G. Gabbe, J. R. Niebyl, J. L. Simpson, M. B. Landon, H. L. Galan, E. R. M. Jauniaux, & D. A. Driscoll (Eds.), *Obstetrics: Normal and problem pregnancies* (6th ed.). Philadelphia, PA: Elsevier Saunders.

Nili, F., McLeod, L., O'Connell, C., Sutton, E., & McMillan, D. (2013). Maternal and neonatal outcomes in pregnancies complicated by systemic lupus erythematosus: A population-based study. *Journal of Obstetrics and Gynaecology Canada, 35*(4), 323–328. Retrieved from http://www.ncbi.nlm.nih.gov/pubmed/23660039

Nugent, J. K. (2013). The competent newborn and the Neonatal Behavioral Assessment Scale: T. Berry Brazelton's legacy. *Journal of Child and Adolescent Psychiatric Nursing, 26,* 173–179.

Ogburn, J. A., Espey, E., Pierce-Bulger, M., Waxman, A., Allee, L., Haffner, W. H., & Howe, J. (2012). Midwives and obstetrician-gynecologists collaborating for Native American women's health. *Obstetrics & Gynecology Clinics of North America, 39*(3), 359–366. doi:10.1016/j.ogc.2012.05.004

Oken, E., Kleinman, K. P., Rich-Edwards, J., & Gillman, M. W. (2003). A nearly continuous measure of birth weight for gestational age using a United States national reference. *BMC Pediatrics, 3,* 6. Retrieved from http://www.biomedcentral.com/1471-2431/3/6c 2003 Oken et al.; licensee BioMed Central Ltd.

O'Neill, E., & Thorp, J. (2012). Antepartum evaluation of the fetus and fetal well-being. *Clinical Obstetrics and Gynecology, 55*(3), 722–730.

Onoye, J. M., Shafer, L. A., Goebert, D. A., Morland, L. A., Matsu, C. R., & Hamagami, F. (2013). Changes in PTSD symptomatology and mental health during pregnancy and postpartum. *Archives of Women's Mental Health, 16*(6), 453–463.

Osborne, K., & Hanson, L. (2014). Labor down or bear down: A strategy to translate 2nd-stage labor evidence to perinatal practice. *Journal of Perinatal & Neonatal Nursing, 28*(2), 117–126.

Papadakis, M., McPhee, S., & Rabow, M. W. (2014). *Current medical diagnosis and treatment 2015.* Boston, MA: McGraw-Hill.

Pessel, C., & Tsai, M. C. (2013). The normal puerperium. In A. H. DeChemey, L. Nathan, N, & A. S. Roman (Eds.), *Current diagnosis & treatment: Obstetrics & gynecology* (11th ed., pp. 190–213). New York, NY: McGraw-Hill.

Phend, C. (2013). New form of misoprostol speeds up labor. *Medpage Today.* Retrieved from http://www.medpagetoday.com/meetingcoverage/ smfm/37406

Posner, G., Black, A., & Jones, G. (2013). *Oxorn-Foote labor and birth* (6th ed.). Philadelphia, PA: McGraw-Hill.

Powrie, R., Greene, M., & Camann, V. (2012). *De Swiet's medical disorders in obstetric practice* (5th ed.). New York, NY: John Wiley & Sons.

Purnell, L. D. (2014). *Guide to culturally competent health care* (3rd ed.). Philadelphia, PA: F. A. Davis.

Resnik, R. (2013). Electronic fetal monitoring: The debate goes on. *Obstetrics & Gynecology, 121*(5), 917–918.

Riordan, J. (2016). The biological specificity of breast-milk. In K. Wambach & and J. Riordan (Eds.), *Breastfeeding and human lactation* (5th ed. pp. 121–169). Boston, MA: Jones & Bartlett.

Robinson, J. N. (2015). Approach to episiotomy. *UpToDate*. Retrieved from http://www.uptodate.com/contents/approach-to-episiotomy?source=machineLearning&search=episiotomy&selectedTitle=1%7E52&sectionRank=1&anchor=H19#H19

Romm, A. J. (2011). *The natural pregnancy book: Herbs, nutrition, and other holistic choices.* New York, NY: Crown Publishing.

Rosenberg, A. A. (2013). The neonate. In S. G. Gabbe, J. R. Niebyl, & J. L. Simpson (Eds.). *Obstetrics: Normal and problem pregnancies* (6th ed., pp. 523–565). Philadelphia, PA: Churchill Livingstone/Elsevier.

Roy-Burne, P. B. (2016). Postpartum blues and unipolar depression: Epidemiology, clinical features, assessment, and diagnosis. *UpToDate*. Retrieved from http://www.uptodate.com/contents/postpartum-unipolar-major-depression-epidemiology-clinical-features-assessment-and-diagnosis

Rubin, R. (1984). *Maternal identity and the maternal experience.* New York, NY: Springer.

Sadler, T. W. (2015). *Langman's medical embryology* (13th ed.). Philadelphia, PA: Lippincott Williams & Wilkins.

Sahota, D. S., Leung, W. C., To, W. K., Chan, W. P., Lau, T. K., & Leung, T. Y. (2012). Quality assurance of nuchal translucency for prenatal fetal Down syndrome screening. *Journal of Maternal–Fetal & Neonatal Medicine, 25*(7), 1039–1043. doi:10.3109/14767058.2011.614658

Scheibel, A. B. (2012). Embryological development of the human brain. *New Horizons for Learning.* Retrieved from http://education.jhu.edu/PD/newhorizons/Neurosciences/articles/Embryological%20Development%20of%20the%20Human%20Brain

Sears, R. W., & Sears, J. M. (2016). *Ask Dr. Sears: Dad and baby bonding.* Retrieved from http://www.askdrsears.com/topics/pregnancy-childbirth/tenth-month-post-partum/bonding-with-your-newborn/dad-baby

Sedgh, G., Lawrence, B., Bankole, A., Eilers, M. A., Singh, S. (2015). Adolescent pregnancy, birth, and abortion rates across countries: Level and recent trends. *Journal of Adolescent Health, 56*(2), 223–230.

Shatken, S., Greenough, K., & McPherson, C. (2012). Epidural fever and its implications for mothers and neonates: Taking the heat. *Journal of Midwifery and Women's Health, 57*(1), 82–85. doi:10.1111/j.1542-2011.00105.x

Short, M. W., & Domagalski, J. E. (2014). Iron deficiency anemia: Evaluation and management. *American Family Physician, 87*(2), 98–104.

Sibai, B. M. (2012). Etiology and management of postpartum hypertension-preeclampsia. *American Journal of Obstetrics and Gynecology, 206*(6), 470–475. doi:10.1016/j.ajog.2011.09.002

Silverman, R. A. (2012). *Neonatal pustular melanosis.* Retrieved from http://emedicine.medscape.com/article/909753-overview

Simpson, K. R., & Creehan, P. A. (2013). *AWHONN's perinatal nursing* (4th ed.) Philadelphia, PA: Lippincott Williams & Wilkins.

Smith, J. R. (2012). Comforting touch in the very preterm hospitalized infant: An integrative review. *Advances in Neonatal Care, 12*(6), 349–365.

Snijder, C. A., Brand, T., Jaddoe, V., Hofman, A., Mackenbach, J. P., Steegers, E. P., & Burdorf, A. (2012). Physically demanding work, fetal growth and the risk of adverse birth outcomes: The Generation R study. *Occupational Environmental Medicine, 69*, 543–550.

Society for Maternal-Fetal Medicine. (2012). *Hi-risk pregnancy care, research, and education for over 35 years.* Retrieved from https://www.smfm.org/attached-files/SMFMMonograph3.1.pdf

Solan, T. D., & Lindow, S. W. (2014). Mercury exposure in pregnancy: A review. *Journal of Perinatal Medicine, 42*(6), 725–729.

Sonek, J., Molina, F., Hiett, A. K., & Glover, M. (2012). Prefrontal space ratio: Comparison between trisomy 21 and euploid fetuses in the second trimester. *Ultrasound in Obstetrics & Gynecology, 40*(3), 293–296. doi:10.1002/uog.11120

Sosa, M. E. (2014). Bleeding in pregnancy. In K. R. Simpson & P. A. Creehan (Eds.), *AWHONN's perinatal nursing* (4th ed., pp. 143–162). Philadelphia, PA: Lippincott Williams & Wilkins.

Spector, R. E. (2017). *Cultural diversity in health and illness* (9th ed.). Hoboken, NJ: Pearson Education.

Spong, C. Y. (2013). Defining "term" pregnancy: Recommendations from the defining "term" pregnancy workgroup. *JAMA, 309*, 2445–2446.

Stranges, E., Wier, L. M., & Elixhauser, A. (2012). *Complicating conditions of vaginal deliveries and cesarean sections, 2009* (Healthcare Cost and Utilization Project Statistical Brief No. 131). Rockville, MD: Agency for Healthcare Research and Quality.

Strauss, R. A. (2015). *Transverse fetal lie.* Retrieved from www.uptodate.com/contents/topic.do?topicKey=OBGYN/4447

Thompson, J. L., Kuller, J. A., & Rhee, E. H. (2012). Antenatal surveillance of fetal growth restriction. *Obstetrics and Gynecology Survey, 67*(9), 554–565.

Thorp, J. M., & Laughton, S. K. (2014). Clinical aspects of normal and abnormal labor. In R. K. Creasy & R. Resnik (Eds.), *Maternal-fetal medicine: Principles and practice* (7th ed., pp. 673–706). Philadelphia, PA: Saunders.

Tiran, D. (2012). Ginger to reduce nausea and vomiting during pregnancy: Evidence of effectiveness is not the same as proof of safety. *Complementary Therapies in Clinical Practice, 18*, 22–25.

Torvie, A. J., Callegari, L. S., Schiff, M. A., & Debiec, K. E. (2015). Labor and delivery outcomes among young adolescents. *American Journal of Obstetrics and Gynecology, 213*(1), 95.e1–95.e8.

Treister-Goltzman, Y., Peleg, R., & Biderman, A. (2015). Anemia among Muslim Bedouin and Jewish women of childbearing age in Southern Israel. *Annals of Hematology, 94*(11), 1777–1784.

Turnbull, V., & Petty, J. (2013). Evidence-based thermal care of the low birthweight neonates: Part one. *Nursing of Children & Young People, 25*(2), 18–22.

U.S. Department of Agriculture. (2016). *Supplemental Nutrition Assistance Program (SNAP).* Retrieved from http://www.fns.usda.gov/snap/supplemental-nutrition-assistance-program-snap

U.S. Department of Health and Human Services. (2015). *Recommended uniform screening panel.* Retrieved from http://www.hrsa.gov/advisorycommittees/mchbadvisory/heritabledisorders/recommendedpanel/index.html

U.S. Food and Drug Administration (FDA). (2013). *Food safety for moms-to-be: At-a-glance.* Retrieved from http://www.fda.gov/Food/FoodborneIllnessContaminants/PeopleAtRisk/ucm081819.htm

U.S. Food and Drug Administration (FDA). (2014). *Pregnancy and lactation labeling (drugs) final rule.* Retrieved from http://www.fda.gov/Drugs/DevelopmentApprovalProcess/DevelopmentResources/Labeling/ucm093307.htm

U.S. Preventive Services Task Force. (2014). *Final recommendation statement: Sexually transmitted Infections: Behavioral counseling.* Retrieved from https://www.uspreventiveservicestaskforce.org/Page/Document/RecommendationStatementFinal/sexually-transmitted-infections-behavioral-counseling1

Valizadeh, L., Zamanzadeh, V., & Rahiminia, E. (2013). Comparison of anticipatory grief reaction between fathers and mothers of premature infants in neonatal intensive care unit. *Scandinavian Journal of Caring Sciences, 27*, 921–926.

Van Woudenberg, C. D., Wills, C. A., & Rubarth, L. B. (2012). Newborn transition to extrauterine life. *Neonatal Network, 31*(5), 317–322.

Vargo, L. (2014). Newborn physical assessment. In K. R. Simpson & P. A. Creehan (Eds.), *Perinatal nursing* (4th ed., pp. 597–625). Philadelphia, PA: Lippincott Williams & Wilkins.

Ventura, S. J., Hamilton, B. E., & Mathews, T. J. (2014). National and state patterns of teen births in the United States, 1940–2013. *National Vital Statistics Reports, 63*(4), 1–34.

Walker, M. (2016). Breast pumps and other technologies. In K. Wambach and J. Riordan (Eds.), *Breastfeeding and human lactation* (5th ed., pp. 419–466). Boston, MA: Jones & Bartlett.

Westrup, B. (2014). Family-centered developmentally supportive care. *American Academy of Pediatrics NeoReviews, 15*(8). Retrieved from http://neoreviews.aappublications.org/content/15/8/e325

White, R. D., Smith, J. A., & Shepley, M. M. (2013). Recommended standards for newborn ICU design (8th ed.). *Journal of Perinatology, 33*(1), 2–12.

Wilson, B. A., Shannon, M. T., & Shields, K. M. (2017). *Pearson nurse's drug guide 2017.* Hoboken, NJ: Pearson.

Witt, C. (2015). Skin assessment. In E. P. Tappero & M. E. Honeyfield (Eds.), *Physical assessment of the newborn* (5th ed., pp. 45–60). Petaluma, CA: NICU Ink.

Wolfberg, A. (2016). The evolution of prenatal testing: How NIPT is changing the landscape in fetal aneuploidy screening. *Medical Laboratory Observer, 48*(1): 18.

Woodring, B. C., & Andrews, M. M. (2012). Transcultural perspectives in the nursing care of children and adolescents. In M. M. Andrews & J. S. Boyle (Eds.), *Transcultural concepts in nursing care* (6th ed., pp. 123–156). Philadelphia, PA: Lippincott.

World Health Organization (WHO). (2015). The global numbers and costs of additionally needed and unnecessary cesarean sections performed per year: Overuse as a barrier to universal coverage (World Health Report, Background Paper No. 30). Retrieved from http://www.who.int/healthsystems/topics/financing/healthreport/30C-sectioncosts.pdf

Yarrington, C., Valente, A. M., & Economy, K. (2015). Cardiovascular management in pregnancy: Antithrombotic agents and antiplatelet agents. *Circulation, 132*(14), 1354–1364.

Yogev, Y., Hiersch, L., Maresky, L., Wasserberg, N., Wiznitzer, A., & Melamde, N. (2014). Third and fourth degree perineal tears—The risk of recurrence in subsequent pregnancies. *Journal of Maternal–Fetal & Neonatal Medicine, 27*(2), 177–181. doi:10.3109/14767058.2013.806902

Young, J., Gore, R., Gorman, B., & Watson, K. (2013). Wrapping and swaddling infants: Child health nurses' knowledge, attitudes, and practice. *Neonatal, Paediatric & Child Health Nursing, 16*(3), 2–11.

Zaja, O., Tiljak, M., Stefanovic, J., & Zvonko, J. (2014). Correlation of UGT1A1 TATA-box polymorphism and jaundice in breastfed newborns: Early presentation of Gilbert's syndrome. *Journal of Maternal, Fetal, and Neonatal Medicine, 27*(8), 844–850.

Zerwekh, J., & Garneau, A. Z. (2014). *Nursing today: Transition and trends* (8th ed.). Philadelphia, PA: Saunders.

Part IV
Nursing Domain

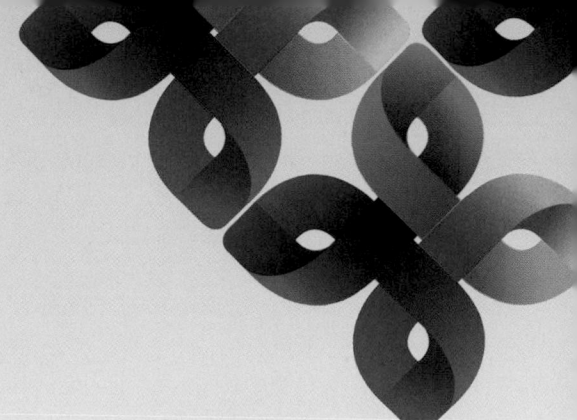

Part IV consists of modules that define and outline principles of nursing care, including assessment, clinical decision making, and communication. Each module presents a concept that directly relates to professional nursing and its impact on patient health and well-being and selected principles or topics of that concept presented as exemplars. In the concept of clinical decision making, for example, the exemplars include the nursing process, the nursing plan of care, and prioritizing care. Each module addresses the impact of that concept and selected exemplars on the care of individuals across the lifespan, inclusive of cultural, gender, and developmental considerations.

Module 34
Assessment

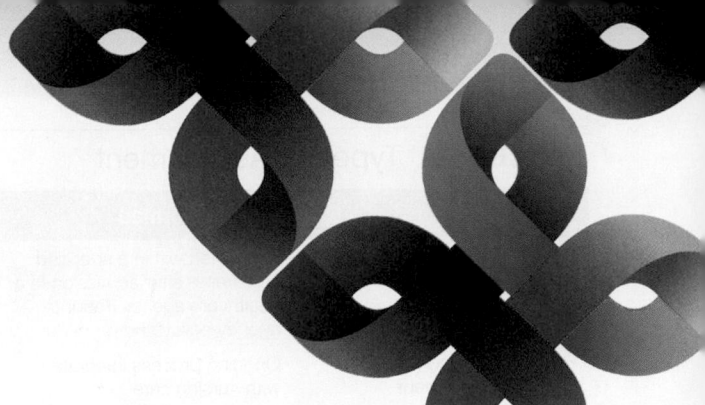

Module Outline and Learning Outcomes

The Concept of Assessment

Types and Sources of Data

34.1 Analyze the types and sources of data collected during a nursing assessment.

Collecting Data

34.2 Analyze the principal methods used to collect data during a nursing assessment.

Organizing Data

34.3 Analyze various methods of organizing assessment data.

Validating Data

34.4 Analyze the need for validating data collected during the nursing assessment.

Interpreting Data

34.5 Analyze the factors used when interpreting data from a nursing assessment.

Concepts Related to Assessment

34.6 Outline the relationship between assessment and other concepts.

Holistic Health Assessment Across the Lifespan

34.7 Differentiate considerations related to the assessment of patients throughout the lifespan.

» The Concept of Assessment

Concept Key Terms

Assessment, **2429**	Flatness, **2442**	Neutral question, **2434**	Palpation, **2439**	Signs, **2430**
Auscultation, **2442**	Holistic health, **2447**	Nondirective	Percussion, **2441**	Subjective
Clinical database, **2430**	Hydrocephalus, **2452**	interview, **2432**	Pitch, **2442**	data, **2430**
Closed questions, **2434**	Hyperresonance, **2442**	Objective	Pleximeter, **2442**	Symptoms, **2430**
Communication, **2446**	Inspection, **2439**	data, **2430**	Plexor, **2442**	Tympany, **2442**
Directive interview, **2432**	Intensity, **2442**	Open-ended	Quality, **2442**	Undernutrition, **2452**
Dullness, **2442**	Interview, **2432**	questions, **2434**	Rapport, **2432**	Validation, **2445**
Duration, **2442**	Leading question, **2434**	Overnutrition, **2451**	Resonance, **2442**	

Health **assessment** is a systematic method of collecting data about a patient for the purpose of determining the patient's current and ongoing health status, predicting risks to health, and identifying health-promoting activities (D'Amico & Barbarito, 2015). The focus of an assessment includes the problems presented by the patient and relevant physical, social, cultural, environmental, and emotional factors that affect the overall well-being of the patient. Data gathered about the patient's health status include wellness behaviors, illness and injury signs and symptoms, patient strengths and weaknesses, health history, and risk factors.

Use of effective communication techniques and critical thinking skills help the nurse gather the detailed, complete, relevant data needed to formulate a patient's plan of care. Health assessment includes the interview and physical assessment, which must be documented and interpreted. All future patient care is directed by the interpretation of findings from data collected throughout the assessment process.

Four different types of assessments are used: initial (or baseline) assessment, problem-focused (or system-specific) assessment, emergency assessment, and ongoing reassessment (see **Table 34–1 »**).

Types and Sources of Data

Data collection is the process of gathering information about a patient's health status. It must be both systematic and continuous to prevent the omission of significant data and to reflect a patient's changing health status. Data can be constant or variable. Constant data is information that does not

TABLE 34–1 Types of Assessment

Type	Time Performed	Purpose	Example
Initial (or baseline) assessment	Performed within a specified time frame after admission to a healthcare agency (Refer to agency policy and procedure)	■ To establish a baseline for problem identification, reference, and future comparison	■ Nursing admission assessment
Problem-focused (or system-specific) assessment	Ongoing process integrated with nursing care	■ To determine the status of a specific problem identified in an earlier assessment	■ Hourly assessment of patient's fluid intake and urinary output in an intensive care unit (ICU) ■ Assessment of patient's ability to perform self-care while assisting a patient to bathe
Emergency assessment	During any physiologic or psychologic crisis	■ To identify life-threatening problems ■ To identify new or overlooked critical problems	■ Rapid assessment of open airway, breathing status, and circulation during a cardiac arrest ■ Assessment of suicidal tendencies or potential for violence
Ongoing reassessment	Minutes to months after initial assessment	■ To compare the patient's current status to baseline data previously obtained	■ Reassessment of a patient's functional health patterns in a home care or outpatient setting, or change-of-shift assessments in an acute or long-term care facility

change over time, such as race or blood type. Variable data can change quickly, frequently, or rarely, and include data such as blood pressure, age, and level of pain.

A **clinical database** includes the nursing health history, physical assessment, primary care provider's history and physical examination, results of laboratory and diagnostic tests, and material contributed by other health personnel.

Patient data should include past history as well as current problems. For example, a previous allergic reaction to penicillin is a vital piece of historical data. Past surgical procedures, complementary or integrative health approaches that the patient has used, and chronic diseases are also examples of historical data. Current data relate to present circumstances, such as pain, nausea, sleep patterns, and religious practices. To ensure accuracy, both the patient and the nurse must participate actively in the data collection process.

Types of Data

Subjective data, also referred to as **symptoms**, are feelings or perceptions that can be described or verified only by the patient. Itching, pain, and feelings of anxiety are examples of subjective data. Subjective data include the patient's sensations (e.g., numbness, cold, tingling), feelings, values, beliefs, attitudes, and perception of personal health status and life situation.

Objective data, also referred to as **signs**, are detectable by an observer or can be measured or tested against an accepted standard. They can be seen, heard, felt, or smelled, and they are obtained by observation or physical examination. Examples of objective data include a discoloration of the skin and a blood pressure reading. During the physical examination, the nurse obtains objective data to validate subjective data and to complete the assessment phase of the nursing process.

Sources of Data

Sources of data are primary or secondary. The patient is the primary source of data. Family members or other support people, other healthcare professionals, records and reports, laboratory and diagnostic analyses, and relevant literature are secondary or indirect sources. In fact, all sources other than the patient are considered secondary sources. (Blood pressure measurements obtained by using an external cuff and manometer may be considered secondary or indirect data because they do not directly measure the pressure within the arteries.) All data from secondary sources should be validated if possible.

Patient

The best source of data is usually the patient, unless the patient is too ill, young, or confused to communicate clearly. The patient can provide subjective data that no one else can offer. Most often, primary data refer to statements made by the patient but also include the objective data that the nurse can obtain directly from the patient, such as gender. Some patients cannot or do not wish to provide accurate data. These include young children and patients who are confused, afraid, embarrassed, or distrustful or who do not speak the nurse's language (D'Amico & Barbarito, 2015).

Support People

Family members, friends, and caregivers who know the patient well often can supplement or verify information provided by the patient. They may convey information about the patient's response to illness, the stresses the patient was experiencing before the illness, family attitudes on illness and health, and the patient's home environment.

Support people are an especially important source of data for a patient who is very young, unconscious, or confused. In some cases—a patient who is physically or emotionally abused, for example—the individual giving information may wish to remain anonymous. Before eliciting data from support people, the nurse should ensure that the patient, if mentally able, approves the gathering of such input. The nurse should also indicate on the nursing history that the data were obtained from a support person.

Information supplied by family members, significant others, or other healthcare professionals is considered subjective if it is not based on fact. If a patient's daughter says, "Dad is very confused today," that is secondary subjective data because it is an interpretation of the patient's behavior by the daughter. The nurse should attempt to verify the reported confusion by interviewing the patient directly. However, if the daughter says, "Dad said he thought it was the year 1941 today," that may be considered secondary objective data because the daughter heard her father state this directly.

The presence or absence of support people in a patient's life can itself be a significant assessment finding. A young child who is brought in for a clinic visit by foster parents will require a different combination of assessment tools than a child who is brought in by his or her own parent. Similarly, an older patient who lives alone and is suspected of having dementia will require an assessment that differs from that of a healthy older patient who lives an active life with his or her spouse.

Patient Records

Patient records include information documented by various healthcare professionals. Patient records also contain data regarding the patient's occupation, religion, and marital status. By reviewing such records before interviewing the patient, the nurse can avoid asking questions for which answers have already been supplied. Repeated questioning can be stressful and annoying to patients and may cause concern about the lack of communication among health professionals. Types of patient records include medical records, records of therapies, and laboratory records.

Medical records (e.g., medical history, physical examinations, operative reports, progress notes, discharge summaries, consultations with specialists) provide information about a patient's present and past health, illness, and injury patterns. These records also can provide the nurse with information about the patient's coping behaviors, health practices, and allergies.

Records of therapies provided by other health professionals, such as social workers, nutritionists, dietitians, or physical therapists, help the nurse obtain relevant data not expressed by the patient. For example, a social service agency's report on a patient's living conditions or a home healthcare agency's report on a patient's self-care abilities can inform the nurse's assessment of the patient.

Laboratory records are another source of pertinent health information. For example, the determination of blood glucose level allows healthcare professionals to monitor the administration of oral hypoglycemic medications. Any laboratory data about a patient must be compared to the agency or performing laboratory's norms for that particular test, taking into account the patient's age, gender, and other significant patient data.

≫ Go to **Pearson MyLab Nursing and eText** to access Appendix B for descriptions of diagnostic studies and their normal values.

The nurse must always consider the information in patient records in light of the present situation. For example, if the most recent medical record is 10 years old, the patient's health practices and coping behaviors are likely to have changed. Older patients may have numerous previous records. These can be useful to understanding the patient's health history, especially if the patient's memory is impaired.

Healthcare Professionals

Because assessment is an ongoing process, verbal reports from other healthcare professionals serve as potential sources of information about a patient's health. Nurses, social workers, primary care providers, and physiotherapists, for example, may have information from either previous or current contact with the patient. Sharing of information among professionals is especially important to ensure continuity of care when patients are transferred to and from home and healthcare agencies.

Literature

Nursing and related literature, such as professional journals and reference texts, can provide additional information to assist the nurse in developing or interpreting an assessment. The nurse may review literature to gather additional information on one or more of the following:

- Standards or norms against which to compare findings (e.g., height and weight tables, normal developmental tasks for an age group)
- Cultural and social health practices
- Spiritual beliefs
- Assessment data needed for specific patient conditions
- Nursing interventions and evaluation criteria relevant to a patient's health problems
- Medical diagnoses, treatments, and prognoses
- Current methodologies and research findings.

Collecting Data

The principal methods used to collect data are observing, interviewing, and examining. Observation occurs whenever the nurse is in contact with the patient or support people. Interviewing is used mainly when the nurse is taking the nursing health history. Examining is the major method used in the physical health assessment.

In reality, the nurse uses all three methods simultaneously. For example, during the patient interview the nurse observes, listens, asks questions, and mentally retains information to explore in the physical examination. These topics are covered further in the module on Communication.

Observing

Observation has two aspects: (a) noticing the data and (b) selecting, organizing, and interpreting the data (**Table 34-2** ≫). A nurse who observes that a patient's face is flushed must relate that observation to findings such as body temperature, activity, environmental temperature, and blood pressure. The nurse often needs to focus on specific data to avoid being overwhelmed by a multitude of data. Observing, therefore, involves distinguishing data in a meaningful manner. For example, nurses caring for newborns learn to ignore the usual sounds of machines in the nursery but respond quickly to an infant's cry or movement. Errors can occur in selecting, organizing, and interpreting data. For example, a nurse might not notice certain signs, either

TABLE 34–2 Using the Senses to Observe Patient Data

Sense	Example of Patient Data
Vision	Overall appearance (e.g., body size, general weight, posture, grooming); signs of distress or discomfort; facial and body gestures; skin color and lesions; abnormalities of movement; nonverbal demeanor (e.g., signs of anger or anxiety); religious or cultural artifacts (e.g., books, icons, candles, beads)
Smell	Body or breath odors
Hearing	Lung and heart sounds; bowel sounds; ability to communicate; language spoken; ability to initiate conversation; ability to respond when spoken to; orientation to time, person, and place; thoughts and feelings about self, others, and health status
Touch	Skin temperature and moisture; muscle strength (e.g., hand grip); pulse rate, rhythm, and volume; palpatory lesions (e.g., lumps, masses, nodules)

because they are unexpected or because they do not conform to preconceptions about a patient's health.

The experienced nurse is often able to attend to an intervention (e.g., give a bed bath or monitor an intravenous infusion) and at the same time make important observations (e.g., note a change in respiratory status or skin color). The beginning student must learn to make observations and complete tasks simultaneously.

Interviewing

An **interview** is a planned communication or a conversation with a purpose. Interviews may be used to get or give information, identify problems of mutual concern, evaluate change, teach, and provide support, counseling, or therapy.

One example of the interview is the nursing health history, which is a part of the nursing admission assessment. See **Box 34–1 》** for the components of a nursing health history.

Nurses use two approaches to interviewing: directive and nondirective. The **directive interview** is highly structured and elicits specific information. The nurse establishes the purpose of the interview and controls the interview—at least at the outset. The patient responds to questions but may have limited opportunity to ask questions or discuss concerns. Nurses frequently use directive interviews to gather and to give information when time is limited (e.g., in an emergency situation).

During a **nondirective interview**, or rapport-building interview, the nurse allows the patient to control the purpose, subject matter, and pacing. **Rapport** is an understanding between two or more people.

A combination of directive and nondirective approaches is usually appropriate during the information-gathering interview. The nurse begins by determining areas of concern for the patient. If, for example, a patient expresses worry about surgery, the nurse pauses to explore the patient's worry and to provide support. Simply noting the worry, without dealing with it, can leave the impression that the nurse does not care about the patient's concerns or dismisses them as unimportant.

Planning the Interview

Before beginning an interview, the nurse reviews available information (for example, the operative report), information about the current illness, or literature about the patient's health problem. The nurse also reviews the agency's data collection form to identify which data must be collected and which data are within the nurse's discretion to collect based on the specific patient. If a form is not available, most nurses prepare an interview guide to help them remember areas of information and determine what questions to ask. The guide includes a list of topics and subtopics rather than a series of questions.

Both nurses and patients should be comfortable in order to encourage an effective interview by balancing several factors. Each interview is influenced by time, place, seating arrangement or distance, and language.

Time

If possible, the nurse plans interviews with patients when the patient is physically comfortable and free of pain, and when interruptions by friends, family, and other health professionals are minimal. The nurse should schedule interviews with patients in their homes at a time selected by the patient.

Place

A well-lighted, well-ventilated room that is relatively free of noise, movements, and distractions encourages communication. A place where others cannot overhear or see the patient is essential.

Seating Arrangement

The nurse who stands and looks down at a patient who is in bed or in a chair risks intimidating the patient. When a patient is in bed, the nurse can sit at a 45-degree angle to the bed. This position is less formal than sitting behind a table or standing at the foot of the bed. During an initial admission interview, a patient who is in bed may feel less confronted if an overbed table is placed between the patient and the nurse. A seating arrangement with the nurse behind a desk and the patient seated across creates a formal setting that suggests a business meeting between a superior and a subordinate. In contrast, a seating arrangement in which the parties sit on two chairs placed at right angles to a desk or table or a few feet apart, with no table between, creates a less formal atmosphere, and the nurse and patient tend to feel on equal terms (**Figure 34–1 》**). In groups, a horseshoe or circular chair arrangement can avoid a superior or head-of-the-table position.

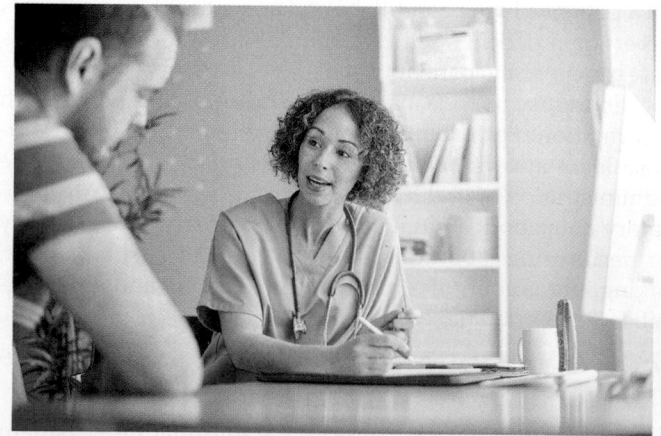

Source: Sturti/E+/Getty Images.

Figure 34–1 》 A seating arrangement in which the nurse and patient sit on two chairs placed at right angles to a desk puts them on equal terms.

Box 34-1
Components of a Nursing Health History

Biographical Data

The patient's name, address, age, sex, marital status, occupation, religious preference, healthcare financing, and usual source of medical care.

Chief Complaint or Reason for Visit

The chief complaint is the answer given to the question "What is troubling you?" or "Can you tell me the reason you came to the hospital or clinic today?" It should be recorded in the patient's own words.

History of Present Illness

- When the symptoms started
- Whether the onset of symptoms was sudden or gradual
- How often the problem occurs
- Exact location of the distress
- Character of the complaint (e.g., intensity of pain or quality of sputum, emesis, or discharge)
- Activity in which the patient was involved when the problem occurred
- Phenomena or symptoms associated with the chief complaint
- Factors that aggravate or alleviate the problem

Past History

- **Childhood illnesses**, such as chickenpox, mumps, measles, rubella (German measles), rubeola (red measles), streptococcal infections, scarlet fever, rheumatic fever, and other significant illnesses
- **Childhood immunizations** and the date of the last tetanus shot
- **Allergies** to drugs, animals, insects, or other environmental agents; the type of reaction that occurs; and how the reaction is treated
- **Accidents and injuries:** how, when, and where the incident occurred, type of injury, treatment received, and any complications
- **Hospitalization for serious illnesses:** reasons for the hospitalization, dates, surgery performed, course of recovery, and any complications
- **Medications and supplements:** all currently used prescription and over-the-counter medications, such as aspirin, nasal spray, vitamins, or laxatives
- **Complementary and integrative health approaches:** use of Chinese herbs, chiropractic medicine, acupuncture, or any traditional forms of treatment associated with cultural heritage or spiritual beliefs

Family History of Illness

To ascertain risk factors for certain diseases, the ages of siblings, parents, and grandparents and their current state of health or, if they are deceased, the cause of death are obtained. Particular attention should be given to disorders such as heart disease, cancer, diabetes, hypertension, obesity, allergies, arthritis, tuberculosis, bleeding, alcoholism, and any mental health disorders.

Lifestyle

- **Personal habits:** the amount, frequency, and duration of use of tobacco, alcohol, coffee, cola, tea, and illicit or recreational drugs
- **Diet:** description of a typical diet on a normal day or any special diet, number of meals and snacks per day, who cooks and shops for food, ethnically distinct food patterns, and food allergies
- **Sleep/rest patterns:** usual daily sleep–wake times, difficulties sleeping, and remedies used for difficulties
- **Activities of daily living (ADLs):** any difficulties experienced in the basic activities of eating, grooming, dressing, elimination, and locomotion
- **Instrumental ADLs (iADLs):** any difficulties experienced in food preparation, shopping, transportation, housekeeping, laundry, and ability to use the telephone, handle finances, and manage medications
- **Recreation/hobbies:** exercise activity and tolerance, hobbies and other interests, and vacations

Social Data

- **Family relationships/friendships:** the patient's support system in times of stress or need, what effect the patient's illness has on the family, and whether any family problems are affecting the patient
- **Ethnic affiliation:** health customs and beliefs; cultural practices that may affect healthcare and recovery
- **Educational history:** data about the patient's highest level of education attained and any past difficulties with learning
- **Occupational history:** current employment status, the number of days missed from work because of illness, any history of accidents on the job, any occupational hazards with a potential for future disease or accident, the patient's need to change jobs because of past illness, the employment status of spouses or partners and the way child care is handled, and the patient's overall satisfaction with the work
- **Economic status:** information about how the patient is paying for medical care (including what kind of medical and hospitalization coverage the patient has) and whether the patient's illness presents financial concerns
- **Home and neighborhood conditions:** home safety measures and adjustments in physical facilities that may be required to help the patient manage a physical disability, activity intolerance, and ADLs; the availability of neighborhood and community services to meet the patient's needs

Psychologic Data

- **Major stressors** experienced and the patient's perception of them
- **Usual coping pattern** with a serious problem or a high level of stress
- **Communication style**, or the ability to verbalize appropriate emotion; nonverbal communication—such as eye movements, gestures, use of touch, and posture; interactions with support people; and the congruence of nonverbal behavior and verbal expression

Patterns of Healthcare

Patterns of healthcare are all healthcare resources the patient is currently using and has used in the past. These include the primary care provider, specialists (e.g., ophthalmologist or gynecologist), dentist, traditional healers or folk practitioners (e.g., herbalist or *curandero*), health clinic, or health center; whether the patient considers the care being provided adequate; and whether access to healthcare is a problem.

Distance

The distance between the nurse and patient should be neither too small nor too great, because people feel uncomfortable when talking to someone who is too close or too far away. Most people in Western cultures feel comfortable maintaining a distance of 2–3 feet during an interview. Some patients require more or less personal space, depending on their cultural and personal needs.

Language

Failure to communicate in a language the patient can understand is a form of discrimination. The nurse must convert complicated medical terminology into common English usage. Interpreters or translators are needed if the patient and the nurse do not speak the same language or dialect (a variation in a language spoken in a particular geographic region). Translating medical terminology is a specialized skill because not all individuals who are fluent in the conversational form of a language are familiar with anatomic or other health terms. Interpreters, however, may make judgments about precise wording but also about subtle meanings that require additional explanation or clarification according to the specific language and ethnicity. Interpreters may also edit the original source to make the meaning clearer or more culturally appropriate.

If giving written documents to a patient, the nurse must determine whether the patient can read them, or if a translator is required. Live translation is preferred, because the patient can then ask questions for clarification. Services such as the commercial LanguageLine Solutions are available 24 hours a day in over 200 languages for a fee. Many large agencies have their own on-call translator services for the languages or dialects commonly spoken in their area.

SAFETY ALERT Check your healthcare institution's policies about offering language translation services. Nurses might be required to offer professional translators, rather than asking family members to translate for the patient. The concern is that family members may insert their own advice or alter information to reduce anxiety in the patient. Using patient visitors and agency nonprofessional staff should be avoided for reasons of confidentiality. It is important to remember that some patients may be more comfortable with an interviewer or translator who is of the same gender as the patient.

Even among patients who speak English, there may be differences in understanding terminology. Patients from different parts of the country may have strong accents, and teen patients and patients who are less well educated may ascribe different meanings to words. For example, "cool" may imply something good to one patient and something not warm to another. For some teens and young adults, the term "sick" means something very good. The nurse must always confirm accurate understandings.

Types of Interview Questions

Questions are often classified as closed or open ended, and neutral or leading. **Closed questions**, used in the directive interview, are restrictive and generally require only "yes" or "no" or short factual answers giving specific information. Closed questions often begin with "when," "where," "who," "what," "do (did, does)," or "is (are, was)." Examples of closed questions are "What medication did you take?" "Are you having pain now? Show me where it is." "How old are you?" "When did you fall?" The highly stressed individual and the individual who has difficulty communicating will find closed questions easier to answer than open-ended questions.

Open-ended questions, associated with the nondirective interview, invite patients to discover and explore, elaborate, clarify, or illustrate their thoughts or feelings. An open-ended question specifies only the broad topic to be discussed and invites answers longer than one or two words. Such questions give patients the freedom to divulge only the information that they are ready to disclose. The open-ended question is useful at the beginning of an interview or to change topics and to elicit attitudes.

Open-ended questions may begin with "what" or "how." Examples of open-ended questions are "How have you been feeling lately?" "What brought you to the hospital?" "How did you feel in that situation?" "Would you describe more about how you relate to your child?" "What would you like to talk about today?"

Nurses often find it necessary to use a combination of closed and open-ended questions throughout an interview to accomplish the goals of the interview and obtain needed information. See **Box 34–2 》** for advantages and disadvantages of open-ended and closed questions.

A **neutral question** is a question that the patient can answer without direction or pressure from the nurse, is open ended, and is used in nondirective interviews. Examples are "How do you feel about that?" and "Why do you think you had the operation?" A **leading question**, by contrast, is usually closed, used in a directive interview, and thus directs the patient's answer. Examples are "You're stressed about surgery tomorrow, aren't you?" "You will take your medicine, won't you?" The leading question gives the patient less opportunity to decide whether the answer is true or not. Leading questions create problems if the patient, in an effort to please the nurse, gives inaccurate responses. This can result in inaccurate data, which can negatively affect nursing care.

Stages of an Interview

An interview has three major stages: the opening or introduction, the body or development, and the closing (Stewart & Cash, 2014).

The Opening

The opening can be the most important part of an interview because it sets the tone for the remainder of the interview. What the nurse says, how the nurse says it, and the attitude the nurse projects to the patient can make a huge difference in the patient's attitude. The purposes of the opening are to establish rapport and orient the interviewee.

Establishing rapport is a process of creating goodwill and trust. It can begin with a greeting ("Good morning, Mr. Johnson") or a self-introduction ("Good morning. I'm Taylor James, a nursing student") accompanied by nonverbal gestures such as a smile, a handshake, and a friendly manner. The nurse must be careful not to overdo this stage; too much superficial talk can arouse anxiety and may appear insincere.

Box 34–2
Selected Advantages and Disadvantages of Open-Ended and Closed Questions

OPEN-ENDED QUESTIONS

Advantages	Disadvantages
They develop trust.	They take more time.
They let the patient do the talking.	Patients may give only brief answers.
The nurse is able to listen and observe.	Valuable information may be withheld.
They are easy for the patient to answer.	They can result in more information than necessary.
They reveal what the patient thinks is important.	Responses may be difficult to document.
They may reveal the patient's lack of knowledge.	The nurse requires skill in controlling an open-ended interview.
They can provide information the nurse may not ask for.	There may be language barriers if the nurse and patient don't have the same first language.

CLOSED QUESTIONS

Advantages	Disadvantages
Questions and answers can be controlled more effectively.	They may provide too little information and require follow-up questions.
They require less effort from the patient.	They may not reveal how the patient feels.
They may be less threatening because they do not require explanations or justifications.	They do not allow the patient to volunteer possibly valuable information.
They take less time.	They may inhibit communication and convey lack of interest by the nurse.
Information can be asked for sooner than it would be volunteered.	The nurse may dominate the interview with questions.
Responses are easily documented.	

In orientation, the nurse explains the purpose and nature of the interview, for example, what information is needed, how long it will take, and what is expected of the patient. The nurse tells the patient how the information will be used and usually states that the patient has the right not to provide information.

The following is an example of an interview introduction:

Step 1—Establish rapport:

Nurse: Hello, Ms. Goodwin, I'm Letisha Fellows. I'm a nursing student, and I'll be assisting with your care here today.

Patient: Hi. Are you a student from the college?

Nurse: Yes, I'm in my final year. Are you familiar with the campus?

Patient: Oh, yes! I'm an avid basketball fan. My nephew graduated from there, and I often attend basketball games with him.

Nurse: That's great! Sounds like fun.

Patient: Yes, I enjoy it very much.

Step 2—Orientation

Nurse: May I sit down with you for about 10 minutes to talk about how I can help you while you're here?

Patient: All right. What do you want to know?

Nurse: To help plan your care after your operation, I'd like to get some information about your usual daily activities and what you expect here in the hospital. I'll take notes while we talk to get the important points

and have them available to the other staff who will also look after you.

Patient: OK. That's all right with me.

Nurse: If there is anything you don't want to talk about, please feel free to say so. Everything you tell me will be confidential and will be shared only with others who have the legal right to know it.

Patient: Sure, that will be fine.

The Body

In the body of the interview, the patient communicates what he or she thinks, feels, knows, and perceives in response to questions from the nurse. Effective development of the interview demands that the nurse use communication techniques that make both parties feel comfortable and serve the purpose of the interview. For communicating during an interview, follow these guidelines:

- Listen attentively, using all your senses, and speak slowly and clearly.
- Use language the patient understands, and clarify points that are not understood.
- Plan questions to follow a logical sequence.
- Ask only one question at a time. Multiple questions limit the patient to one choice and may confuse the patient.
- Acknowledge the patient's right to look at things the way they appear to him or her and not the way they appear to the nurse or someone else.

- Do not impose your own values on the patient.
- Avoid giving personal viewpoints or advice, such as saying, "If I were you. . . ."
- Nonverbally convey respect, concern, interest, and acceptance.
- Be aware of the patient's and your own body language.
- Be conscious of the patient's and your own voice inflection, tone, and affect.
- Sit down to talk with the patient (be at an even level).
- Use and accept silence to help the patient search for more thoughts or to organize them.
- Use eye contact and be calm, unhurried, and sympathetic.

The Closing

The nurse terminates the interview when the necessary information has been obtained. In some cases, however, a patient terminates the interview. For example, the patient may decide not to give any more information or may be unable to offer more information for some other reason—fatigue, for example. The closing is important for maintaining the rapport and trust and for facilitating future interactions. The following techniques are commonly used to close an interview:

1. *Offer to answer questions.* "Do you have any questions?" or "I would be glad to answer any questions you have." Be sure to allow time for the individual to answer, or the offer will be regarded as insincere.
2. *Conclude by saying.* "Well, that's all I need to know for now" or "Well, those are all the questions I have for now." Preceding a remark with the word "well" generally signals that the end of the interaction is near.
3. *Thank the patient.* "Thank you for your time and help. The questions you have answered will be helpful in planning your nursing care." You may also shake the patient's hand.
4. *Express concern for the patient's welfare and future.* "Take care of yourself. I hope all goes well for you."
5. *Plan for the next meeting,* if there is to be one, or state what will happen next. Include the day, time, place, topic, and purpose: "Let's get together again here on the fifteenth at 9:00 a.m. to see how you are managing then." Or "Ms. Cho, I will be responsible for giving you care three mornings per week while you are here. I will be in to see you each Monday, Tuesday, and Wednesday between eight o'clock and noon. At those times, we can adjust your care as needed."
6. *Provide a summary to verify accuracy and agreement.* Summarizing serves several purposes, such as helping to terminate the interview, reassuring the patient that the nurse has listened, checking the accuracy of the nurse's perceptions, clearing the way for new ideas, and helping the patient to note progress and a forward direction: "Let's review what we have just covered in this interview." Summaries are particularly helpful for patients who are anxious or who have difficulty staying with the topic: "Well, it seems to me that you are especially worried about your hospitalization and chest pain because your father died of a

heart attack 5 years ago. Is that correct? . . . I'll discuss this with you again tomorrow, and we'll decide what plans need to be made to help you."

Clinical Example A

Martha Whitman is a 59-year-old recently retired elementary school teacher who complains of continued acute back pain. The findings from the physical assessment are all within normal limits. Ms. Whitman states that the pain started 2 weeks ago and has been getting worse, with only temporary relief with the use of aspirin. Before referring this patient for diagnostic studies, the nurse asks about any activities or events associated with the onset of the pain. Ms. Whitman reveals that she had enthusiastically taken up a new hobby of quilting about 3 weeks ago. She has been sitting and working with an embroidery hoop almost every day for an hour or two. In addition, she proudly adds that her garden "has never looked better—not a weed in sight!"

Critical Thinking Questions

1. How does the additional interview information assist the nurse in interpretation of Ms. Whitman's back pain?
2. What recommendations could the nurse make to prevent further straining the muscles of Ms. Whitman's back?
3. What timetable should the nurse give Ms. Whitman to expect decreased symptoms? What is the plan if this target date is not met?

Examining

The physical examination or physical assessment is a systematic data collection method that uses observation (i.e., the senses of sight, hearing, smell, and touch) to detect health problems. To conduct the examination, the nurse uses techniques of inspection, auscultation, palpation, and percussion.

The purposes of a physical examination include the following:

- To obtain baseline data about the patient's functional abilities
- To supplement, confirm, or refute data obtained in the nursing history
- To obtain data that will help establish nursing diagnoses and plans of care
- To evaluate the physiologic outcomes of healthcare and thus the progress of a patient in relation to health problems
- To make clinical judgments about a patient's health status
- To identify areas for health promotion and disease prevention.

A physical examination can be any of three types: (1) an initial assessment (e.g., when a patient is admitted to a healthcare agency), (2) a system-specific examination (e.g., the cardiovascular system), or (3) an examination of a body area (e.g., the lungs, when difficulty with breathing is observed). Most physical examinations begin by taking the patient's vital signs. **Table 34–3 »** lists normal vital signs across the lifespan.

Physical examinations typically reveal normal and abnormal findings. The nurse must analyze both types of findings and make critical decisions about their meaning and importance. For example, when the patient is being admitted with

TABLE 34–3 Normal Vital Sign Ranges Across the Lifespan[a]

	Pulse (per minute)[b]	Respirations (per minute)[b]	Temperature (°C)[c]	Blood Pressure (mmHg)[d] Systolic	Diastolic
Newborn	100–205 (awake) 90–160 (asleep)	30–80	Normal range: 36.5–37.5	At birth: 50–70[e] At day 10: 90	At birth: 30–45[e] At day 10: 50
Infant	100–180 (awake) 80–160 (asleep)	30–60	Normal range (axillary): 36.5–37.5	Age 1 Boys: 80–89 Girls: 83–90	Age 1 Boys: 34–39 Girls: 38–42
Toddler	98–140 (awake) 80–120 (asleep)	20–40	Normal range: 36–38.5 Extreme range: 35–40	Age 2 Boys: 84–92 Girls: 85–91	Age 2 Boys: 39–44 Girls: 43–47
Preschooler	98–140 (awake) 80–120 (asleep)	22–34	Normal range: 36–38.5 Extreme range: 35–40	Age 4 Boys: 88–97 Girls: 88–94	Age 4 Boys: 47–52 Girls: 50–54
School age	70–120 (awake) 50–90 (asleep)	15–25	Normal range: 36–38.5 Extreme range: 35–40	Age 9 Boys: 95–104 Girls: 96–103	Age 9 Boys: 57–62 Girls: 58–61
Adolescent	50–90	12–20	Normal range: 36–38.5 Extreme range: 35–40	Age 15 Boys: 109–117 Girls: 107–113	Age 15 Boys: 61–66 Girls: 64–67
Adult	60–100	12–20	Normal range: 36–38.5 Extreme range: 35–40	Less than 120	Less than 80
Older adult	60–100	15–20	Normal range: 36–38.5 Extreme range: 35–40	Less than 120	Less than 80

Notes:
a. There is a wide variety of "normal" at each stage of the lifespan, and vital signs are dynamic. While these ranges provide a general sense of the norm, it is important for the nurse to determine what "normal" is for each patient and to base further considerations on those parameters and the context of the patient presentation.
b. The ranges for pulse and respiration change dramatically from birth through adolescence, and then remain fairly stable throughout the rest of life.
c. The first set of numbers in each cell is the usual range of temperature; the second set shows extremes of normal temperature for when the weather is very cold, when it is early in the morning, or during exercise.
d. Data from American Heart Association (AHA). (2015). *Understanding blood pressure readings*. Retrieved from http://www.heart.org/HEARTORG/Conditions/HighBloodPressure/AboutHighBloodPressure/Understanding-Blood-Pressure-Readings_UCM_301764_Article.jsp
   Note that blood pressure readings for children are determined using the child's height percentile. The blood pressure values presented here are the 50th percentile for the child's age, sex, and height, which are considered the midpoint of the normal range. A reading above the 95th percentile indicates hypertension. To see the pediatric blood pressure tables, visit http://www.nhlbi.nih.gov/health-pro/guidelines/current/hypertension-pediatric-jnc-4/blood-pressure-tables.htm
e. Blood pressure is usually monitored before age 3 only if the patient has cardiac issues.

a diagnosis of appendicitis, the presence of pain in the right lower quadrant would be an expected initial finding, while a later absence of pain in that same location might indicate that the appendix has ruptured.

When findings are different than anticipated, the nurse must make decisions about their importance and what to do with the information. If unsure about the significance of a finding or to whom it should be reported, the nurse should consult with a more experienced nurse regarding the best course of action to follow.

A complete physical examination starts at the head and proceeds in a systematic manner downward (head-to-toe assessment), by body systems (neurologic system, respiratory system, and so forth), or by a combination of the two organizing principles. As shown in **Box 34–3** 》, Assessment of an Adolescent Woman, the physical examination starts with the upper part of the body before proceeding to a review of body systems.

Whichever approach is used, the nurse must adapt the examination according to the age of the individual, the severity of the illness, the preferences of the nurse and patient, the environment for the examination, and the agency's policies and procedures. Regardless of the procedure used, the patient's energy level and time constraints need to be considered. The physical assessment is conducted in a systematic and efficient manner with the fewest position changes for the patient.

Frequently, nurses assess a specific body area, instead of the entire body. These specific assessments are made in relation to patient complaints, the nurse's observations, the patient's presenting problem, available nursing interventions, and medical therapies. Examples of these situations and assessments are provided in **Table 34–4** 》.

Nurses use national guidelines and evidence-based practice while performing health assessments. For example, when screening for cancer, the nurse should keep in mind

Box 34–3
Assessment of an Adolescent Woman

General Health State (*present weight—gain or loss, reason for gain or loss, amount of time for gain or loss; fatigue, malaise, weakness, sweats, night sweats, chills*):

Skin (*history of skin disease, pigment or color change, change in mole, excessive dryness or moisture, pruritus, excessive bruising, rash or lesion*):

Hair (*recent loss or change in texture*):

Nails (*change in color, shape, brittleness*):

Head (*unusual headaches, frequency of headaches, head injury, dizziness, syncope or vertigo*):

Eyes (*difficulty or change in vision, decreased acuity, blurring, blind spots, eye pain, diplopia, redness or swelling, watering or discharge, glaucoma or cataracts*):

Ears (*earaches, infections, discharge and its characteristics, tinnitus or vertigo*):

Nose and Sinuses (*discharge and its characteristics, frequent or severe colds, sinus pain, nasal obstruction, nosebleeds, seasonal allergies, change in sense of smell*):

Mouth and Throat (*mouth pain, sore throat, bleeding gums, toothache, lesions in mouth, tongue, or throat, dysphagia, hoarseness, tonsillectomy, alteration in taste*):

Neck (*pain, limitation of motion, lumps or swelling, enlarged or tender lymph nodes, goiter*):

Neurologic System (*history of seizure disorder, syncopal episodes, CVA, motor function or coordination disorders/abnormalities, paresthesia, mood change, depression, memory disorder, history of mental health disorders*):

Endocrine System (*history of diabetes or insulin resistance, history of thyroid disease, intolerance to heat or cold*):

Breast and Axilla (*pain, lump, tenderness, swelling, rash, nipple discharge, any breast surgery*):

Respiratory System (*History of lung disease, smoking, chest pain with breathing, wheezing, shortness of breath, cough—productive or nonproductive. Sputum—color and amount. Hemoptysis, toxin or pollution exposure*):

Cardiac System (*history of cardiac disease, MI, atherosclerosis, arteriosclerosis, chest pain, angina*):

Peripheral Vascular System (*coldness, numbness, tingling, swelling of legs/ankles, discoloration of hands/feet, varicose veins, intermittent claudication, thrombophlebitis or ulcers*):

Hematologic System (*bleeding tendency of skin or mucous membranes, excessive bruising, swelling of lymph nodes, blood transfusion and any reactions, exposure to toxic agents or radiation*):

Gastrointestinal System (*appetite, food intolerance, dysphagia, heartburn, indigestion, pain [with eating or other], pyrosis, nausea, vomiting, history of abdominal disease, gastric ulcers, flatulence, bowel movement frequency, change in stool [color, consistency], diarrhea, constipation, hemorrhoids, rectal bleeding*):

Musculoskeletal System (*history of arthritis, joint pain, stiffness, swelling, deformity, limitation of motion, pain, cramps, or weakness*):

Urinary System (*recent change, frequency, urgency, nocturia, dysuria, polyuria, oliguria, hesitancy or straining, urine color, narrowed stream, incontinence; history of urinary disease; pain in flank, groin, suprapubic region or low back*):

Female Genital System (*menstrual history, age of first menses, last menstrual cycle, frequency of cycles, premenstrual pain, vaginal itching, discharge, premenopausal symptoms, age at menopause, postmenopausal bleeding*):

Sexual Health (*presently involved in relationship involving intercourse or other sexual activity, aspects of sex satisfactory, use of contraceptive, is relationship monogamous, history of STD*):

Source: From *Physical Examination and Health Assessment* by Carolyn Jarvis. Copyright © 2015 by Elsevier Health Sciences.

TABLE 34–4 Nursing Assessments Addressing Selected Patient Situations

Situation	Physical Assessment
Patient complains of abdominal pain.	Inspect, auscultate, and palpate the abdomen; assess vital signs.
Patient is admitted with a head injury.	Assess level of consciousness using the Glasgow Coma Scale (discussed in the module on Intracranial Regulation); assess pupils for reaction to light and accommodation; assess vital signs.
Nurse prepares to administer a cardiotonic drug to a patient.	Assess apical pulse, compare with baseline data and clinical standards for continued administration.
Patient has just had a cast applied to the lower leg.	Assess peripheral perfusion of toes, capillary refill, pedal pulse if accessible, and vital signs.
Patient's fluid intake is minimal.	Assess skin turgor, fluid intake and output, and vital signs.
Patient's spouse reports that the patient with limited mobility is "not making sense."	Assess vital signs. Check patient's body for signs that indicate fall or injury. Assess pupils for reactions to light and accommodation.
Patient is curled up in a fetal position, holding his head between his hands.	Assess the vital signs, including the possibility of pain or withdrawal. Palpate the forehead to check for elevated temperature.
Patient is throwing items around his hospital room.	Make contact with patient to calm him down before taking vital signs.
Patient receiving a blood transfusion reports "itchy skin."	Stop transfusion. Take vital signs and inspect the chest skin for signs of rash.
Parents report their child is unresponsive.	Assess the child's A, B, Cs (airway, breathing, circulation). Intervene as needed.

the American Cancer Society's guidelines (2017) for early detection. These guidelines include methods for early identification of breast, colorectal, cervical, endometrial, lung, and prostate cancers.

>> **Stay Current:** Visit the American Cancer Society website at www. cancer.org/healthy/findcancerearly/cancerscreeningguidelines/american-cancer-society-guidelines-for-the-early-detection-of-cancer to see their guidelines for early detection of cancer.

Preparing the Patient

Most patients need an explanation of the physical examination process. Often patients are anxious about what the nurse will find. The nurse provides reassurance by explaining each step of the examination. The nurse should explain when and where the examination will take place, why it is important, and what will happen, while ensuring the patient assents to each stage of the examination, an important component of informed consent. The nurse should inform the patient that all information gathered and documented during the assessment is kept confidential in accordance with the Health Insurance Portability and Accountability Act (HIPAA). Only healthcare providers who have a legitimate need to know the patient's information will have access to it. That may include health insurance companies in addition to clinicians.

Health examinations are usually painless; however, it is important to determine in advance any positions contraindicated for a particular patient. For example, patients having difficulty breathing may experience increased difficulty when lying in a supine position. The nurse assists the patient as needed to undress and put on a gown. Patients should empty their bladders before the examination. Doing so helps them feel more relaxed and facilitates palpation of the abdomen and pubic area. If a urinalysis is required, the urine should be collected in a container for that purpose.

Preparing the Environment

It is important to prepare the environment before starting the assessment. The time for the physical assessment should be convenient to both the patient and the nurse. The environment should be well lighted and the equipment organized for efficient use. A patient who is physically relaxed will usually experience little discomfort. The room should be warm enough to be comfortable for the patient.

Providing privacy is important. Most people are embarrassed if their bodies are exposed or if others can overhear or view them during the assessment. Culture, age, and gender of both the patient and the nurse influence how comfortable the patient will be and what special arrangements may be needed. For example, if the patient and nurse are of different genders, the nurse should ask if it is acceptable to perform the physical examination or if a nurse of the same gender is preferred. Family and friends should not be present unless the patient asks for someone.

Positioning

During the physical examination, the patient may need to maintain several positions. The nurse must consider the patient's ability to assume each position before asking him or her to do so. The patient's physical condition, energy level, and age should also be taken into consideration. Some positions are embarrassing or uncomfortable and therefore should not be maintained for extended periods. By organizing the assessment so that several body areas can be assessed in one position, the nurse can minimize the number of position changes needed and maximize the patient's comfort during the assessment (see **Table 34–5 >>**).

Methods of Examining

Four primary techniques are used in the physical examination: inspection, palpation, percussion, and auscultation. Each requires practice to develop expertise.

Inspection

Inspection is visual examination, or assessment using the sense of sight. The process should be deliberate, purposeful, and systematic. The nurse inspects with the naked eye and with a lighted instrument such as an otoscope (used to view the ear). In addition to visual observations, olfactory (smell) and auditory (hearing) cues are noted. Nurses frequently use visual inspection to assess moisture, color, and texture of body surfaces, as well as shape, position, size, color, and symmetry of the body. Lighting must be sufficient for the nurse to see clearly; either natural or artificial light can be used. When using the auditory senses it is important to have a quiet environment. Observation can be combined with the other assessment techniques.

Palpation

Palpation is the examination of the body using the sense of touch. The pads of the fingers are used because their concentration of nerve endings makes them highly sensitive to tactile discrimination. Palpation is used to determine the following characteristics:

- Texture (e.g., of the hair)
- Temperature (e.g., of a skin area)
- Moisture
- Vibration (e.g., of a joint)
- Swelling
- Rigidity or spasticity
- Crepitation
- Location, position, size, consistency, and mobility of organs, lumps, or masses
- Distention (e.g., of the urinary bladder)
- Amplitude of pulses
- The presence of tenderness or pain.

There are two types of palpation: light and deep. Light (superficial) palpation should always precede deep palpation because heavy pressure on the fingertips can dull the sense of touch. For light palpation, the nurse extends the dominant hand's fingers parallel to the skin surface and presses gently while moving the hand in a circle (see **Figure 34–2 >>**). With light palpation, the skin is slightly depressed. If it is necessary to determine the details of a mass, the nurse presses lightly several times rather than holding the pressure. See **Table 34–6 >>** for the characteristics of masses.

Deep palpation is done with one hand or with two hands (bimanually). In deep bimanual palpation, the nurse extends

TABLE 34–5 Patient Positions and Body Areas Assessed

Position	Description	Areas Assessed	Cautions
Dorsal recumbent	Back-lying position with knees flexed and hips externally rotated; small pillow under the head; soles of feet on the surface	Female genitals, rectum, and female reproductive tract	May be contraindicated for patients who have cardiopulmonary problems.
Supine (horizontal recumbent)	Back-lying position with legs extended; with or without pillow under the head	Head, neck, axillae, anterior thorax, lungs, breasts, heart, vital signs, abdomen, extremities, peripheral pulses	Tolerated poorly by patients with cardiovascular and respiratory problems.
Sitting	A seated position, back unsupported and legs hanging freely	Head, neck, posterior and anterior thorax, lungs, breasts, axillae, heart, vital signs, upper and lower extremities, reflexes	Older adults and weak patients may require support.
Lithotomy	Back-lying position with feet supported in stirrups; the hips should be in line with the edge of the table	Female genitals, rectum, and female reproductive tract	May be uncomfortable and tiring for older adults and embarrassing for most patients.
Sims	Side-lying position with lowermost arm behind the body, uppermost leg flexed at hip and knee, upper arm flexed at shoulder and elbow	Rectum, vagina	Difficult for older adults and people with limited joint movement.
Prone	Lies on abdomen with head turned to the side, with or without a small pillow	Posterior thorax, hip joint movement	Often not tolerated by older adults and people with cardiovascular, neuromuscular, and respiratory problems.

the dominant hand as for light palpation, then places the finger pads of the nondominant hand on the dorsal surface of the distal interphalangeal joints of the middle three fingers of the dominant hand (**Figure 34–3 >>**). The top hand applies pressure while the lower hand remains relaxed to perceive the tactile sensations. For deep palpation using one hand, the finger pads of the dominant hand press over the area to

be palpated. Often the other hand is used to support a mass or organ from below (**Figure 34–4 >>**). Deep palpation is usually not done during a routine examination and requires significant practitioner skill. It is performed with extreme caution because pressure can damage internal organs. Deep palpation is usually not indicated in patients who have acute abdominal pain or pain that is not yet diagnosed.

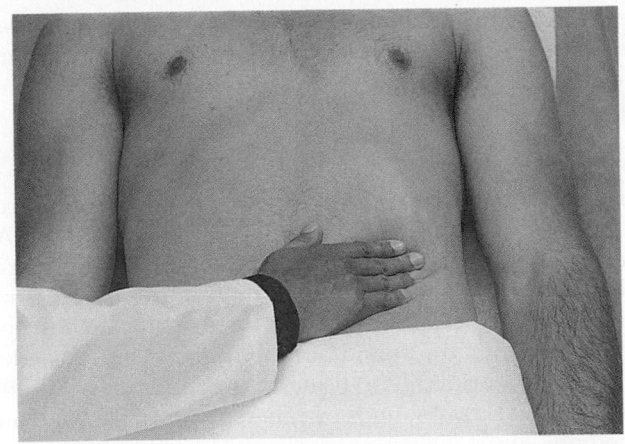

Figure 34–2 》 The position of the hand for light palpation.

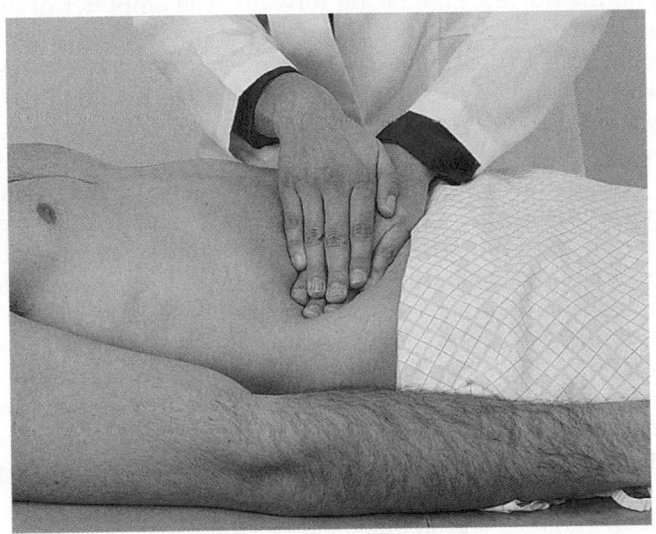

Figure 34–3 》 The position of the hands for deep bimanual palpation.

TABLE 34–6 Characteristics of Masses

Characteristic	Descriptors
Location	Site on the body, dorsal/ventral surface
Size	Length and width in centimeters
Shape	Oval, round, elongated, irregular
Consistency	Soft, firm, hard
Surface	Smooth, nodular
Mobility	Fixed, mobile
Pulsatility	Present or absent
Tenderness	Degree of tenderness to palpation

To test skin temperature, the nurse should use the dorsal aspect (back) of the hand and fingers where the skin is thinnest. To test for vibration, the nurse should use the base of the fingers (metacarpophalangeal joints) or ulnar surface of the hand. General guidelines for palpation include the following:

- The nurse's hands should be clean and warm, and the fingernails should be short.
- Palpation technique should be slow and systematic.
- Areas of tenderness should be palpated last.

The effectiveness of palpation depends largely on the patient's level of relaxation. The nurse can assist a patient to relax by (a) gowning and/or draping the patient appropriately, (b) positioning the patient comfortably, and (c) ensuring that the nurse's own hands are warm before beginning. During palpation, the nurse should be sensitive to the patient's verbal and nonverbal communications indicating discomfort.

Percussion

Percussion is the act of striking the body surface to elicit sounds that can be heard or vibrations that can be felt. There are two types of percussion: direct and indirect. In *direct percussion*, the nurse strikes the area to be percussed directly with the pads of two, three, or four fingers or with the pad of the middle finger. The strikes are rapid, and the movement is from the wrist (see **Figure 34–5 》**).

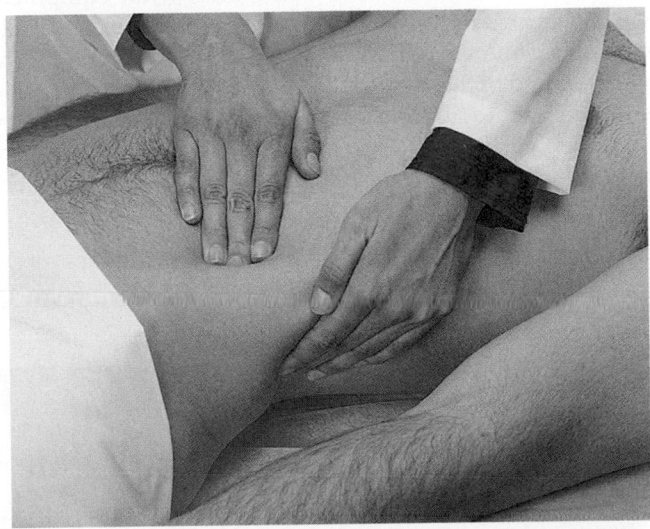

Figure 34–4 》 Deep palpation using the lower hand to support the body while the upper hand palpates the organ.

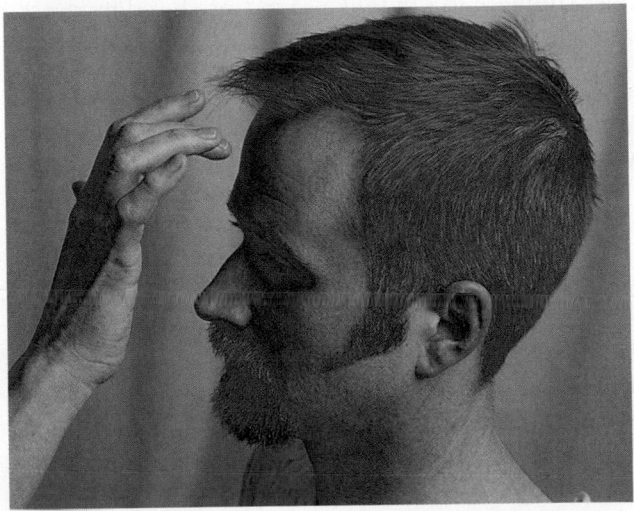

Figure 34–5 》 Direct percussion, in which one hand is used to strike the surface of the body.

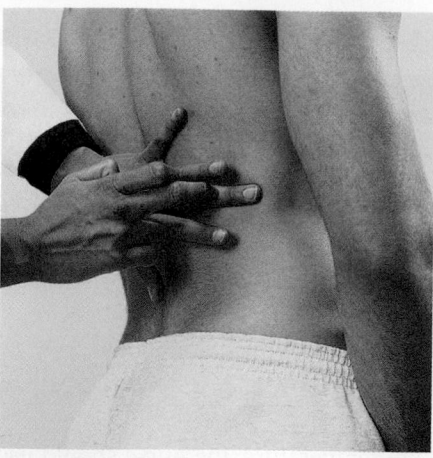

Figure 34–6 » Indirect percussion, in which the finger of one hand taps the finger of the other hand.

Indirect percussion refers to the striking of an object (e.g., a finger) held against the body area to be examined. In this technique, the middle finger of the nondominant hand, referred to as the **pleximeter**, is placed firmly on the patient's skin. Only the distal phalanx and joint of this finger should be in contact with the skin. Using the tip of the flexed middle finger of the other hand, called the **plexor**, the nurse strikes the pleximeter, usually at the distal interphalangeal joint (see **Figure 34–6 »**). Some nurses may find a point between the distal and proximal joints to be a more comfortable pleximeter point. The motion comes from the wrist; the forearm remains stationary. The angle between the plexor and the pleximeter should be 90 degrees, and the blows must be firm, rapid, and short to obtain a clear sound.

Percussion is used to determine the size and shape of internal organs by establishing their borders. It indicates whether tissue is fluid filled, air filled, or solid. Percussion elicits five types of sound: flatness, dullness, resonance, hyperresonance, and tympany. **Flatness** is an extremely dull sound produced by very dense tissue, such as muscle or bone. **Dullness** is a thudlike sound produced by dense tissue such as the liver, spleen, or heart. **Resonance** is a hollow sound, such as that produced by lungs filled with air. **Hyperresonance** is not produced in the healthy body. It is described as booming that can be heard over an emphysematous lung. **Tympany** is a musical or drumlike sound produced from an air-filled stomach. On a continuum, flatness reflects the most dense tissue (the least amount of air) and tympany the least dense tissue (the greatest amount of air). A percussion sound is described according to its intensity, pitch, duration, and quality (see **Table 34–7 »**).

Auscultation

Auscultation is the process of listening to sounds produced within the body. Auscultation may be direct or indirect. An example of *direct auscultation* is the use of the unaided ear to listen to a respiratory wheeze or the grating of a moving joint. *Indirect auscultation* refers to the use of a stethoscope, which transmits the sounds to the nurse's ears. A stethoscope is used primarily to listen to sounds from within the body, such as bowel sounds or valve sounds of the heart and blood pressure.

The stethoscope tubing should be 30–35 cm (12–14 in.) long, with an internal diameter of about 0.3 cm (1/8 in.). The earpieces of the stethoscope should fit comfortably into the nurse's ears, facing forward. The amplifier of the stethoscope is placed firmly but lightly against the patient's skin. If the patient has excessive body hair, it may be necessary to dampen the hairs with a moist cloth so that they will lie flat against the skin and not interfere with clear sound transmission.

Auscultated sounds are described according to their pitch, intensity, duration, and quality. The **pitch** is the frequency of the vibrations (the number of vibrations per second). Low-pitched sounds, such as some heart sounds, have fewer vibrations per second than high-pitched sounds, such as bronchial sounds. The **intensity** (amplitude) refers to the loudness or softness of a sound. Some body sounds are loud, such as bronchial sounds heard from the trachea; others are soft, such as normal breath sounds heard in the lungs. The **duration** of a sound is its length (long or short). The **quality** of sound is a subjective description of a sound, such as whistling, gurgling, or snapping.

Equipment

The physical examination requires use of common healthcare tools such as the stethoscope, penlight, gloves, or water-soluble lubricant. The nurse determines what equipment will be required for the specific examination to be performed and collects the supplies in advance to avoid extending the time required of the patient. The nurse should warm up cold equipment that will touch the patient's skin. All equipment should be cleaned after each use according to the recommendations for each instrument. **Table 34–8 »** describes some of the most commonly used tools.

TABLE 34–7 Percussion Sounds and Tones

Sound	Intensity	Pitch	Duration	Quality	Example of Location
Flatness	Soft	High	Short	Extremely dull	Muscle, bone
Dullness	Medium	Medium	Moderate	Thudlike	Liver, heart
Resonance	Loud	Low	Long	Hollow	Normal lung
Hyperresonance	Very loud	Very low	Very long	Booming	Emphysematous lung
Tympany	Loud	High (distinguished mainly by musical timbre)	Moderate	Musical	Stomach filled with gas (air)

TABLE 34–8 Tools Used for a Health Examination

Supplies		Purpose
Stethoscope		To listen to heart sounds
Sphygmomanometer		To take blood pressure readings
Oximeter		To determine oxygen saturation concentration of circulating blood
Flashlight or penlight		To assist viewing of the pharynx and cervix or to determine the reactions of the pupils of the eye
Nasal speculum		To permit visualization of the lower and middle turbinates; usually, a penlight is used for illumination
Ophthalmoscope		A lighted instrument to visualize the interior of the eye
Otoscope		A lighted instrument to visualize the eardrum and external auditory canal (a nasal speculum may be attached to the otoscope to inspect the nasal cavities)
Percussion (reflex) hammer		An instrument with a rubber head to test reflexes
Tuning fork		A two-pronged metal instrument used to test hearing acuity and vibratory sense
Vaginal speculum		To assess the cervix and the vagina
Cotton applicators		To obtain specimens

(continued on next page)

TABLE 34–8 Tools Used for a Health Examination *(continued)*

Supplies		Purpose
Gloves		To protect the nurse and the patient
Lubricant		To ease insertion of instruments (e.g., vaginal speculum)
Tongue blades (depressors)		To depress the tongue during assessment of the mouth and pharynx

Source: Stethoscope & Sphygmomanometer by London Robert/Pearson Education, Inc.; Oximeter by Juan R. Velasco/Shutterstock.

Clinical Example B

Clara and Roberto Galvez carry their screaming 7-year-old son John-nie into the emergency department. They tell the triage nurse that Johnnie woke up before dawn complaining that his stomach hurt. He then vomited, and when touched, he felt very hot and sweaty. He now holds both hands tightly on his abdomen and cannot be consoled.

The nurse conducts a physical examination that reveals the following: symmetrical abdomen, bowel sounds in all quadrants, tender to palpation in the lower quadrants, guarding. Johnnie has an oral temperature of 101.5°F, pulse of 122 bpm, and respiratory rate of 24/min.

Critical Thinking Questions

1. Classify the findings as objective or subjective data.
2. Prepare a narrative nursing note from the data.
3. What factors must be considered in conducting the comprehensive health assessment of Johnnie Galvez? What additional information might prove useful in the assessment? How would you gather that information?
4. Before developing a nursing diagnosis, what must the nurse do?

Organizing Data

Collected data must be recorded at the time of collection or shortly thereafter. Data are recorded in written or digital formats that organize assessment data systematically. Most schools of nursing and healthcare agencies have developed their own structured assessment formats. Many of these are based on selected nursing models or frameworks. The format may be modified according to the patient's physical status, such as one focused on musculoskeletal data for orthopedic patients. One example of a format used to document findings from an assessment uses the mnemonic **OLD CART & ICE**. For example, for a patient with a cough that is keeping her awake at night, the findings might look like:

Onset: 10 days ago
Location: Tickle begins in throat
Duration: Daily; coughing fits become worse at night
Characteristics: Painful to cough; can't catch breath. Clear mucus coughed up
Aggravating factors: Worse at night when lying in bed
Relieving factors: Hot liquids, steamy showers
Treatment: Acetaminophen and expectorant

Impact on ADLs: Not had a good night of sleep for over a week; asked other family members to shop and clean
Coping strategies: Afternoon naps
Emotional response: Since the patient has not become better over time, she worries her condition is much more serious than usual cough.

See the exemplar on Documentation in the module on Communication for more detailed information on recording data.

Maslow's Hierarchy of Needs

Maslow's hierarchy of needs can be used to organize data (see the module on Clinical Decision Making and the module on Stress and Coping for more information about Maslow's hierarchy). Such data clusters would pertaining to the following:

- Physiological needs (survival needs)
- Safety and security needs
- Love and belonging needs
- Self-esteem needs
- Self-actualization needs.

Developmental Theories

Several physical, psychosocial, cognitive, and moral developmental theories may be used by the nurse in specific situations (see the module on Development). Examples include the following:

- Havighurst's age periods and developmental tasks
- Freud's five stages of development
- Erikson's eight stages of development
- Piaget's phases of cognitive development
- Kohlberg's stages of moral development.

Functional Health Patterns and Body Systems

Assessment data can be organized according to one of several models. Most nursing programs develop their own framework for nursing assessment data based on these models. One example is to use 11 functional health patterns to organize the data by patterns (Gordon, 2014):

1. Health perception–health management pattern
2. Nutritional-metabolic pattern
3. Elimination pattern
4. Activity-exercise pattern
5. Sleep-rest pattern
6. Cognitive-perceptual pattern
7. Self-perception/self-concept pattern
8. Role-relationship pattern
9. Sexuality-reproductive pattern
10. Coping/stress-tolerance pattern
11. Value-belief pattern.

Assessment data may also be organized by body systems (see the exemplar on the Nursing Process in the module on Clinical Decision Making), such as:

1. Immune system
2. Respiratory system
3. Cardiovascular system
4. Nervous system
5. Musculoskeletal system
6. Gastrointestinal system
7. Genitourinary system
8. Reproductive system.

Once data have been organized, they are validated.

Validating Data

The information gathered during the assessment phase must be complete, factual, and accurate because the nursing diagnoses and interventions are based on this information. **Validation** is the act of double-checking or verifying data to confirm that they are accurate and factual. Validating data helps the nurse do the following:

- Ensure that assessment information is complete.
- Ensure that objective and related subjective data agree.
- Obtain additional information that may have been overlooked.
- Differentiate between cues and inferences.
- Avoid jumping to conclusions and focusing in the wrong direction to identify problems.

To collect data accurately, nurses need to be aware of their own biases, values, and beliefs and to separate fact from inference, interpretation, and assumption. For example, a nurse seeing a man holding his arm to his chest might assume that he is experiencing chest pain when in fact it is his hand that hurts.

Not all data require validation. For example, height, weight, birth date, and most laboratory studies that can be measured with an accurate scale can be accepted as factual. As a rule, the nurse validates data when discrepancies arise between data obtained in the nursing interview (subjective data) and the physical examination (objective data) or when the patient's statements differ at different times in the assessment. Failure to validate can lead to an inaccurate or incomplete nursing assessment and could compromise patient safety. Guidelines for validating data are shown in

TABLE 34–9 Validating Assessment Data

Guideline	Example
Compare subjective and objective data to verify the patient's statements with observations made.	Patient's perception of "feeling hot" needs to be compared with measurement of the body temperature.
Clarify any ambiguous or vague statements.	*Patient:* "I've felt sick off and on for 6 weeks." *Nurse:* "Describe what your sickness is like. Tell me what you mean by 'off and on.'"
Be sure assessment data consist of cues and not inferences.	*Observation:* Dry skin and reduced tissue turgor. *Inference:* Dehydration. *Action:* Collect additional data that are needed to make the inference in the diagnosing phase. For example, determine the patient's fluid intake, amount and appearance of urine, and blood pressure.
Double-check data that are extremely abnormal.	*Observation:* A resting pulse of 30 beats per minute or a blood pressure of 210/95 mmHg. *Action:* Repeat the measurement. Use another piece of equipment as needed to confirm abnormalities, or ask someone else to collect the same data.
Determine the presence of factors that may interfere with accurate measurement.	A crying infant will have an abnormal respiratory rate and will need quieting before accurate assessment can be made.
Use references (textbooks, journals, research reports) to explain phenomena.	A nurse considers tiny purple or bluish black swollen areas under the tongue of an older patient to be abnormal until the nurse reads about physical changes of aging. Such varicosities are common.

Table 34–9 ≫. Once data have been collected, organized, and validated, they can be analyzed to determine priorities for patient care.

Interpreting Data

Interpreting findings requires making determinations about all of the data collected in the health assessment process. The nurse must determine the following:

- Whether the findings fall within normal and expected ranges in relation to the patient's age, gender, and race
- The significance of the findings in relation to the patient's health status and immediate and long-range health-related needs.

Interpretation of findings is influenced by the ability to obtain, recall, and apply knowledge; to communicate effectively; and to take into account family history and dynamics. Other relevant influences include developmental, psychologic and environmental, cultural and diversity, and environmental factors.

Knowledge

Nurses obtain, recall, and apply knowledge from physical and social sciences, nursing theory, and all areas of research that affect current nursing practice. That knowledge includes human anatomy and physiology, growth and development across the lifespan, and characteristics specific to gender and race. Knowledge also reflects health-related and healthcare trends in groups and populations, such as the increased incidence of risk factors or actual illnesses in certain groups or populations. For example, in the United States one trend is the increased incidence of obesity in children and adults.

Nurses must be able to access and use reliable resources when interpreting findings. Resources include research; scientific literature; and charts, scales, and graphs to indicate ranges of norms and expectations about physical and psychologic development. Examples of the latter include Denver Developmental scores, mental status examinations, weight, body mass index, and growth charts prepared by centers for health statistics (D'Amico & Barbarito, 2015). In addition, the nurse must be able to communicate effectively, to think critically, to recognize and act on patient cues, to incorporate a holistic perspective, and to determine the significance of data in meeting immediate and long-term patient needs. The nurse must be able to recognize situations that require immediate attention, initiate care, and seek appropriate assistance.

Expectations about interpretation of findings change as the nurse gains skills and experience in nursing practice and with advanced practice education. A nursing student is expected to recall and apply knowledge to discriminate between normal and abnormal findings and use resources to understand the findings in relation to wellness or illness for a particular patient. For example, consider the findings from the assessment of Julie Connor, a 12-year-old girl: asymmetrical shoulders and elevated right scapula on inspection of the posterior thorax, and right lateral curvature of the thoracic spine on palpation of vertebrae. Normally, scapulae should be symmetrical and the vertebrae should be aligned. The findings are interpreted as a deviation from the normal. They do not, however, give sufficient information for the purposes of making nursing diagnoses. The nurse must collect more data to make diagnoses and design a plan of care for Julie.

The nurse gains confidence and ability to discriminate between normal and abnormal findings through experience and continuing education. With such experience, the nurse will learn to recognize patterns that predispose individuals to illness or are indicative of specific illnesses, and implement and evaluate appropriate nursing care.

Clinical Example C

James Long is a 46-year-old African American man: height 5'9", weight 220 lb, BP 156/94 mmHg. His mother died at age 62 from cerebrovascular accident (stroke), and his father died at age 42 from myocardial infarction (heart attack). Using knowledge of normal ranges of findings for vital signs, height, and weight, the nurse interprets Mr. Long's BP and weight results as abnormal findings: They indicate that he has high blood pressure and is obese. The nurse applies knowledge of trends associated with health problems to interpret the significance of the findings for this patient. The nurse knows that hypertension occurs more frequently in African American males than in Caucasians. Hypertension, obesity, and a family history of coronary artery disease increase the risk of acquiring both hypertension and its associated complications. By combining knowledge of risk factors and complications with the findings themselves, the nurse working with Mr. Long can develop a plan of care. The nurse

can collaborate with other healthcare professionals to address Mr. Long's need to reduce his weight and lower his blood pressure.

Critical Thinking Questions

1. What nursing diagnoses would be appropriate?
2. What patient outcomes would you plan for Mr. Long?
3. What resources are available in your community to assist you with intervening or advocating for patients such as Mr. Long?

Communication

Effective communication is essential to the assessment process. **Communication** refers to the exchange of information, feelings, thoughts, and ideas. Verbal techniques, such as open-ended or closed questions, statements, clarification, and rephrasing, are just a few of the techniques used to gather information. The communication techniques must incorporate regard for the individual in relation to the purposes of the data collection, the patient's age, and the patient's level of anxiety. In addition, the nurse must use techniques that accommodate language differences or difficulties, cultural influences, cognitive ability, affect, demeanor, and special needs.Communication is discussed in greater detail in the module on Communication.

Developmental Factors

The patient's developmental level affects the health assessment. Sources of information may vary depending on the patient's age and ability to communicate his or her symptoms. For patients with disabilities, findings must be interpreted according to the assessed developmental level, not the patient's age. Parents or guardians are the primary sources for information about children and patients with disabilities or impairments that affect their ability to communicate. The developmental level of the patient also influences the approach to assessment, including the words and terminology. For example, assessment of a pregnant adolescent would be different from assessment of a 38-year-old woman who is pregnant for the third time. Such differences are highlighted in the module on Development.

Psychologic and Emotional Factors

Psychologic and emotional factors affect physiologic health and must be considered as predisposing or contributing factors when interpreting findings from a health assessment. For example, anxiety triggers an autonomic response, resulting in increased pulse and blood pressure. Conversely, physical problems can affect emotional health, as when childhood obesity leads to problems with self-esteem and affects socialization and development. Psychologic problems such as anxiety and depression may interfere with the patient's ability to fully participate in health assessment. Grieving may limit a patient's ability to carry out required health practices or recognize health problems. See the module on Stress and Coping for more examples of how psychologic and emotional factors play a role in health.

SAFETY ALERT A simple statement such as, "I am required by law to ask you, are you safe at home? Do you feel safe in your relationship?" may be sufficient to ascertain whether or not the patient is at risk at home or in his primary relationship. The U.S.

Preventive Services Task Force (2013) recommends that question be asked of women of childbearing age and older or vulnerable adults. Similarly, consistent with the Joint Commission's National Patient Safety Goals, suicide screening at admission may be necessary or recommended for many patients. The question, "Do you have or have you had any thought of harming yourself or others? If so, do you have a plan?" provides the opportunity to begin assessing the patient's risk for harming self or others (The Joint Commission, 2016). A third type of screening, for depression, is recommended for routine use, but especially for pregnant and postpartum women (Siu et al., 2016).

Family History and Dynamics

The nurse must consider family history of illness or health problems when conducting a health assessment and interpreting findings. Individuals with a family history of some illnesses are considered at high risk for contracting those diseases. For example, having a first-degree relative (mother, sister, or daughter) with breast cancer about doubles a woman's risk of developing breast cancer herself (American Cancer Society, 2016). The nurse must recognize that family dynamics may influence one's approach to healthcare. In some families, health-related decisions are not made independently, but rather are made by the family leader or arrived at by group consensus. Circumstances within families can affect both physical and emotional health and must be considered as part of any health assessment. For example, children of people with alcoholism are not only at risk for alcoholism, but are also at risk for emotional issues not encountered by other children. Therefore, the nurse must view and interpret unexpected physical or emotional behaviors in relation to the alcoholic family situation. The module on Family considers the concept of Family in a more complete manner.

Cultural Factors

The nurse must consider cultural factors when collecting data and interpreting findings. Culture affects language, expression, emotional and physical well-being, and health practices. Findings regarding physical and emotional health must be interpreted in relation to the cultural norms for the patient. For example, many Asian cultures would not consider lack of eye contact during the interview as a lack of ability to interact, depression, or a problem with attention. The nurse must take care to provide clear explanations of abnormal findings, illnesses, and treatments because views of illness, causality, and treatment may be influenced by a patient's culture. Refer to the module on Culture and Diversity for more information on cultural considerations.

Environmental Factors

Internal and external environmental factors affect health assessment and interpretation of findings. The nurse must always consider data in relation to norms and expectation for age, race, and gender and in relation to factors affecting the individual patient.

Data from the comprehensive health assessment provide clues about the patient's internal environment, including emotional state, response to medication and treatment, and physiologic or anatomic alterations that influence findings and interpretations.

External environmental factors can also affect health, health assessment, and interpretation of findings. External factors may include any of the following:

- Inhaled toxins such as smoke, chemicals, and fumes
- Irritants that can be inhaled, ingested, or absorbed through the skin
- Noise, light, and motion
- Objects or substances encountered in the home, school, or workplace, such as animal dander or dust.

For more information about the external environmental factors themselves, consult the module on Safety. To become knowledgeable about nurses' exciting roles in making changes in the current environment, refer to the exemplar on Environmental Quality in the module on Advocacy.

Concepts Related to Assessment

Nursing care always begins with assessment. Nursing care depends on a strong knowledge base and the application of critical thinking. Regardless of the clinical setting, the role of the nurse is multifaceted. Each situation requires the nurse to use the nursing process, starting with strong assessment skills.

In the biophysical realm, thorough nursing assessment (including the fifth vital sign of pain) allows the nurse to identify an individual's problems with acid–base balance, cellular regulation, comfort, digestion, elimination, and fluids and electrolytes. Illness and injury will leave evidence that can be discovered through assessment.

In the psychosocial realm, a similarly thorough nursing assessment can point out a patient's difficulties with trauma, addiction, cognition, grief and loss, mood and affect, and stress and coping. At the same time, an assessment of the patient's strengths in the areas of family and spirituality can be a good foundation on which to build better health and wellness. The Concepts Related to Assessment feature lists some, but not all, of the concepts that are integral to assessment. They are listed in alphabetical order.

Holistic Health Assessment Across the Lifespan

Nursing assessment skills help the nurse interpret how the complex interactions of heredity, environment, and physiologic, cognitive, and psychologic development affect an individual at a particular time. By developing an image of what is usual or expected of children and adults of various ages, the nurse has a basis for a comparison with the norm. This knowledge and an understanding of individual variations provide a foundation for holistic health assessments across the lifespan.

Holistic health can best be defined as a clinical mindset that considers more than the physiologic health status of a patient. Holistic health includes all factors that affect the patient's physical and emotional well-being. With a holistic approach, the nurse recognizes that developmental, psychologic, emotional, family, cultural, and environmental factors combine to affect immediate and long-term actual and potential health goals, problems, and plans.

Concepts Related to
Assessment

CONCEPT	RELATIONSHIP TO ASSESSMENT	NURSING IMPLICATIONS
Legal Issues	Clinical trial enrollment opportunity → assessment of level of knowledge about risk-benefit ratio → informed consent	■ Nurse offers time and resources to answer questions about research study involvement.
Oxygenation	If assessment shows ↓ O_2, prioritize interventions to ↑ O_2	■ Decrease oxygen workload by having patient rest; administer O_2 by nasal cannula if needed.
Perfusion	If assessment shows ↓ blood flow to a limb, prioritize intervention to ↑ blood flow	■ Check for clothes restricting circulation. Use physical movement and exercise to keep fit.
Professional Behaviors	Professional approach ↑ knowledgeable assessment ↑ patient confidence	■ A professional approach helps build confidence and rapport with the patient, making it more likely that the patient will be honest and cooperative during the assessment.
Thermoregulation	If assessment shows ↑ temperature, discover cause of fever	■ Increase fluids and give antipyretic medications.
Safety	If assessment of home environment shows ↑ hazards, intervene to ↓ injury risk	■ Before discharge, scan home environments for obstacles that might cause a patient to slip or fall.
Sensory Perception	If assessment of preschooler shows ↓ visual acuity → assistance device to ↑ vision	■ Refer to optometrist to measure for eyeglasses prescription.
Tissue Integrity and Mobility	If older patient in wheelchair → constant sitting → assess skin → stage 2 pressure ulcer	■ Move patient to positions that do not cause pressure on area of breakdown. Continue to ↑ padding of seat.

A comprehensive assessment includes information about physical, cognitive, and emotional growth and development, including both subjective and objective data. When conducting health assessments, the nurse must be able to obtain accurate data and interpret findings in relation to expectations and predicted norms and ranges for patients at various stages of physical and emotional development. Knowledge of anatomic and physiologic changes as well as theoretical information about cognitive, psychoanalytical, and psychosocial events and expectations at each stage of human development is invaluable for the nurse. Further information about growth and development can be found in the module on Development.

Physical growth and development change across the lifespan. Stages from infancy through adolescence are marked by spurts of rapid growth and development. Health assessment includes the use of clinical growth charts to compare individual patient measurements of height and weight (and head circumference in infants) against expected normal values for age and gender. Additional indicators for normal growth and development throughout these stages include eating, sleeping, elimination, and activity patterns. Neurologic and sensory functions are assessed by monitoring development of speech and language, muscular growth, strength and coordination, and tactile sensibility.

Puberty is a period of rapid physiologic growth and development. Puberty occurs between the ages of 10 and 14 years in girls and is marked by menarche, breast development, axillary and pubic hair growth, and a spurt in height.

In boys, puberty occurs between the ages of 12 and 16 years and is characterized by a spurt in height, development of the penis and testicles, and body hair growth (axillae, chest, facial), including pubic hair. Young adulthood is the stage marked by completed growth in physical and mental structures. Physical development continues to be assessed by comparing individual findings to clinical growth charts and by assessing eating, sleeping, and activity patterns.

Middle age, occurring between the ages of 45 and 60 years, is another period in which dramatic changes in physical development occur. Primary changes are related to hormonal changes in both men and women, resulting in menopause in women. During middle age, changes occur in all systems; these include decreases in basal metabolic rate, muscle size, nerve conduction, lung capacity, glomerular filtration, and cardiac output. The middle-aged patient experiences increased adipose tissue deposit and skeletal changes leading to decreases in height, as well as changes in tactile sensibility, vision, and hearing. The physical changes continue into the stage of older adulthood. Middle-aged and older adults are at risk for obesity and associated health problems. Health assessment includes use of the BMI measurement to assess weight and risk for disease. Assessment also includes evaluation of the ability to carry out ADLs and regular testing of vision and hearing.

The leading causes of death throughout the lifespan are outlined in **Table 34–10 》**.

In addition to expectations about physical growth and development, there are expectations about cognitive, psychosocial, and emotional development across the lifespan. For

TABLE 34–10 Leading Causes of Death Throughout the Lifespan

Age Range	Leading Causes of Death and Number of Deaths in 2014 (Rounded to Nearest Hundred)
Birth–age 4 years	■ Conditions originating in the perinatal period (short gestation, maternal pregnancy complications, placenta/cord/membranes): 6800 ■ Congenital anomalies: 5100 ■ Unintentional injuries: 2400 ■ Sudden infant death syndrome (SIDS): 1500
Age 5–9 years	■ Unintentional injuries: 700 ■ Cancer: 400 ■ Congenital abnormalities: 200 ■ Heart and acute/chronic lung diseases: 200 ■ Homicide: 100
Age 10–24 years	■ Unintentional injuries: 12,600 ■ Suicide: 5500 ■ Homicide: 4300 ■ Cancer: 2000 ■ Heart and acute/chronic lung diseases: 1600
Age 25–64 years	■ Cancer: 175,000 ■ Heart and acute/chronic lung diseases: 153,700 ■ Unintentional injuries: 72,000 ■ Suicide: 29,600 ■ Liver disease: 24,700 ■ Diabetes mellitus: 22,100 ■ Cerebrovascular: 19,400
Age 65 and older	■ Heart and acute/chronic lung diseases: 659,300 ■ Cancer: 413,900 ■ Unintentional injuries: 48,300 ■ Cerebrovascular disease: 113,300 ■ Alzheimer disease: 92,600 ■ Diabetes mellitus: 54,200

Source: Data from Centers for Disease Control and Prevention, *10 Leading Causes of Death by Age Group, United States—2014*, retrieved from http://www.cdc.gov/injury/wisqars/pdf/leading_causes_of_death_by_age_group_2014-a.pdf

TABLE 34–11 Instruments to Assess Growth and Development in Infants and Children

Instrument	Description
Ages & Stages Questionnaire (ASQ)	The ASQ is a parent questionnaire that covers developmental areas of communication, gross motor, fine motor, problem solving, and personal-social in children.
Battelle Developmental Inventory	This inventory tests developmental domains of cognition, motor, self-help, language, and social skills in children from birth through 8 years of age.
Brigance Screens	These screens assess speech–language, motor, readiness, and general knowledge at younger ages and also reading and math. Used from 21 to 90 months of age.
Child Development Inventory	Scales used to measure social, self-help, gross motor, fine motor, expressive language, language comprehension, letters, numbers, and general development in children from 15 months to 6 years of age.
Denver II	Screening test administered to well children between birth and 6 years of age. It is designed to test 20 simple tasks and items in four sectors: personal-social, fine motor adaptive, language, and gross motor.
Hassles and Uplifts Scale	Scale used to measure adult attitudes about daily situations defined as "hassles" and "uplifts." It focuses on evaluation of positive and negative events in daily life rather than on life events.
Life Experiences Survey	This self-administered questionnaire reviews life-changing events of a given year. Ratings are used to evaluate the level of stress an individual is experiencing.
McCarthy Scale of Children's Abilities	The McCarthy scale evaluates the general intelligence level of children age 2½–8½ years. The scale identifies strengths and weaknesses in verbal, perceptual-performance, quantitative, memory, motor, and general cognitive skills.
Pediatric Symptom Checklist	Checklist of short statements used to identify conduct behaviors and behaviors associated with depression, anxiety, and adjustment in children age 4–16 years. Item patterns determine the need for behavioral or mental health referrals.
Stanford-Binet Intelligence Scale: Fourth Edition	The Stanford-Binet test measures general intelligence. The areas of verbal reasoning, quantitative reasoning, abstract/visual reasoning, and short-term memory can be tested from age 2 to 23 years.
Wechsler Preschool and Primary Scale of Intelligence—Revised (WPPSI-R)	The WPPSI-R is a standardized test of language and perception for children age 4½–6 years.

example, attachment is an essential element in infant development. Attachment refers to the tie between the infant and caregivers that promotes physical and psychosocial well-being. Assessment of attachment includes observing caregivers for eye contact, apparent interest in the child, talking or cooing to the child, response to infant needs, and communication.

Children are expected to develop language and cognitive abilities that enable them to learn and become independent over time. Young adults are expected to develop relationships with others and to become productive members of society. Maturity and aging lead individuals to contribute to the well-being of communities and their families and often to adapt to change and loss. Developmental milestones and crises occur in all stages of development and must be noted during assessment. A variety of instruments and scales can be used to identify developmental delays, behavioral patterns, and responses that indicate potential or actual problems with emotional, cognitive, and psychosocial development and adaptation in children and adults. **Table 34–11** » includes a list and description of some of the instruments available to measure aspects of growth and development.

Assessment of Infants, Children, and Adolescents

Children are not "little adults." Significant differences exist among infants, children, adolescents, and adults. These differences include variations in physiology, development, and cognition that must be incorporated into the nursing assessment. For instance, the head-to-toe approach to physical assessment is useful in many situations and with different types of patients, but it may not work with young children. Adults and adolescents will usually sit on an examination table, wear a paper gown, and follow the nurse's instructions. However, infants and toddlers often refuse to sit still or cooperate.

Furthermore, young children do not have the cognitive or verbal ability to describe symptoms or comply with complex instructions. The nurse must possess strong assessment skills to overcome the communication and situational challenges involved in pediatric physical assessment.

In assessing children, it may be helpful to conduct the nutrition history portion before the physical assessment in order to establish rapport and make the child more comfortable with the process. Rapport is essential, especially when assessing an adolescent. Infants and younger children need a caregiver present to assist with the assessment and to answer questions (**Figure 34–7 》**). Adolescents may be more comfortable having privacy during an assessment. The nurse may discuss the assessment arrangement with the adolescent and caregiver separately to allow the adolescent to give an unpressured answer. A caregiver can be interviewed separately if appropriate.

The parameters of the physical assessment in children include anthropometric measurements and clinical observations appropriate for each child's age. Determination of developmental milestones provides critical information and is part of a complete assessment. Developmental milestones are covered in the module on Development.

Anthropometric measurements in children should be obtained using equipment appropriate for the pediatric population. Recumbent length and weight measurements are needed for infants and young children. An infant's or toddler's weight should be measured without the child wearing a diaper. Older children can have their height and weight measured while standing. Skinfold measurements should be done using calipers calibrated to 0.2 mm because small changes in measurement can cause changes in assessment classification. The World Health Organization (WHO)

recommends weight for height as the standard in measuring children because skinfold and circumference measurements are prone to errors that could result in misclassification of nutritional health. Head circumference is a measurement unique to the assessment of growth in children at or under 3 years of age. Beyond age 3, head circumference is not a valid tool for assessing growth and nutritional status.

Anthropometric measurements have age-specific references established by the Centers for Disease Control and Prevention and WHO. In children under 20 years of age, references are described using charts with age-specific percentiles for height, weight, body mass index (BMI), and, for children under 36 months, head circumference. Percentiles are used to assess growth rate and health. Percentile charts are derived from the distribution of data from population studies and are age- and gender-specific descriptions of anthropometric measurements. The charts may change as new data are incorporated. For example, breastfed infants normally grow at a slightly slower rate than do formula-fed babies, and newer infant growth charts are more representative of the population-matched prevalence of breastfed infants compared to charts published before 2000.

Infants, children, and adolescents can be compared to their age-matched peers to determine their individual percentile within the population. A best use of percentile charts is in monitoring individual growth over time. Normally, children will remain within a narrow percentile range for each measurement over the course of childhood. For example, a child assessed sequentially in the 25th percentile for height (length) for age may have a small frame and parents with small stature and may not be at risk for poor nutritional health. However, a child sequentially in the 50th percentile for height for age who drops to the 25th percentile may be at risk for undernutrition. A significant drop or increase in percentile category is cause for further investigation to assess for undernutrition or overnutrition. Overweight and obesity (overnutrition) in children is defined as a BMI for age greater than the 85th percentile and the 95th percentile, respectively. Undernutrition is defined as a BMI for age less than the 5th percentile. Separate growth references exist for children with some chronic diseases and for knee–height estimates of stature. See the module on Nutrition for more information on overnutrition and undernutrition.

Children are physically different from adults. Each concept in the individual domain (Modules 1–33) discusses lifespan differences that can be anticipated when conducting the physical examination.

The nurse should use a caring, supportive, yet firm approach with children. Whenever possible, play should be incorporated into the assessment process. It is helpful to allow children to touch and manipulate equipment. Adhesive bandages or empty syringes can be provided for play-acting with dolls. The nurse should encourage children to talk about their fears and concerns. Painful procedures should not be performed while a child is seated on a parent's lap. Children need to know they are safe from painful experiences when they are with their parents.

When a child is ill, parents experience increased stress that results from interrupted sleep, concern for the child's well-being, and frustration at the inability to understand what is hurting or bothering their child. Each of these factors

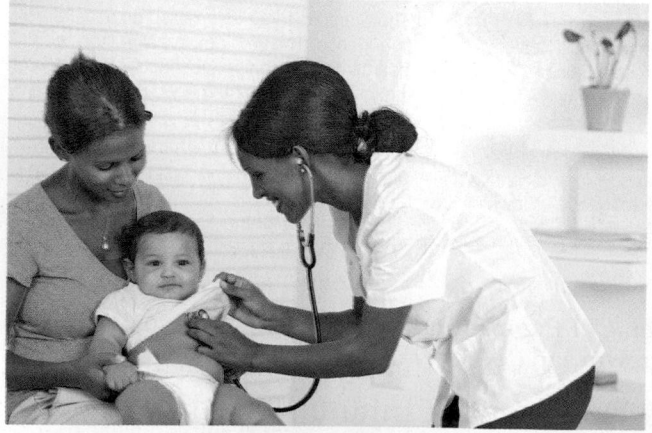

Source: Ruslan Dashinsky/E+/Getty Images.

Figure 34–7 》 This mother holds her baby while the nurse performs an examination.

may affect a parent's ability to recall information or to follow complex instructions. The nurse can help parents by providing them with written instructions as appropriate and encouraging patients and families to journal about their experiences or keep a notebook with information and details about the child's illness and treatment, including nutrition and activity levels. The nurse should consider parental stress levels when developing care plans.

The basic components of a health history are the same whether the nurse works with children or adults. However, a number of variations must be incorporated into a pediatric health history. It is essential for the nurse to determine the relationship between the child who seeks healthcare and the adult who presents with the child. State law determines which individuals can legally consent to medical treatment of a minor child. Federal privacy laws limit access to protected health information. One must never assume legal or family ties between children and the adults who accompany them. Nannies, babysitters, friends, siblings, and stepparents often transport children to healthcare appointments. Asking directly about the relationships is the easiest way to ensure compliance with the legal and ethical concerns regarding the medical treatment of children.

Many children are nonverbal or have limited language ability; therefore, the nurse depends on parents and guardians for health history information. This can limit the specificity of the history information. However, it is important to ask preschoolers and older children about their chief complaint and symptoms even though the information they provide may not be as detailed as the information provided by their parents or guardians.

Prior to the health interview, the nurse should determine whether the parent is stressed or distracted. Many parents of ill children are sleep deprived because of their child's altered sleep patterns. Sleep deprivation can result in altered recall, limited ability to follow complex questions, and diminished ability to remember verbal instructions. The presence of other children can be distracting, especially if the children are loud, active, or irritable. The nurse can distract energetic or fussy children with books, crayons, or toys.

The nurse should listen carefully to the parent or primary caregiver and use open-ended questions to elicit health information. Parents know their children better than anyone else. They are able to detect subtle differences in their child's behavior. It is essential to pay special attention to the chief complaints that parents describe. A thorough physical assessment is then conducted based on the issues and concerns raised in the health history.

The nurse should call the child by his or her name and use words that the child understands. For example, most preadolescents are not familiar with the word *abdomen*, but most children have used the word *tummy* or *belly* from infancy (**Figure 34–8 》**). Instead of asking "Does your head hurt?" the nurse should ask the child to touch the head where it hurts. It is necessary to be patient. Children often pause between words or repeat phrases when they are excited or nervous.

The nurse should give children who are at least 10 years old the option of being examined without their parents or other accompanying adult present. The patient is the child, not the parent. The nurse's legal and ethical responsibility is

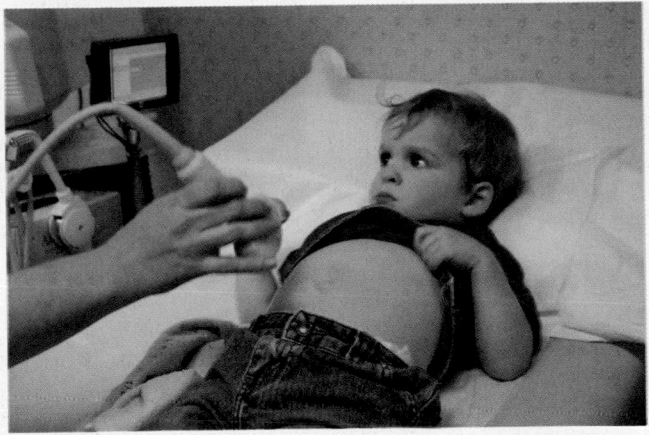

Source: Jessica Lewis/Moment/Getty Images.

Figure 34–8 》 This toddler knows that his belly hurts, but he would not understand if the nurse asked him if his abdomen hurt.

to the child first. The nurse must respect the confidentiality of the information provided by older children and be aware of state and federal laws regarding parental notification and mandatory reporting. The parent and the child should be told what the nurse can and cannot keep confidential. For example, statements such as "What you and I talk about will be between the two of us, unless you tell me that you are thinking about harming yourself or someone else, or if you tell me that someone is hurting you" help establish rapport and boundaries to the nurse–child and nurse–parent relationship. If a nurse is required to report health interview information to others (e.g., public health departments or child protective service agents), the nurse should always inform the child of the need to share the information with others prior to actually doing so. Failure to do so can jeopardize the rapport between nurse and child. Additional tips for effective assessment of pediatric patients are given in **Box 34–4 》**.

Assessment of Newborns

The assessment of newborns is covered in Module 33, Reproduction, in the exemplar on Newborn Care.

Assessment of Infants

Frequent assessments during the first year provide opportunities to monitor the infant's rate of growth and development as well as to compare the infant with the norm for age. Height, weight, and head circumference measurements are plotted on an appropriate growth chart at each assessment. The three measurements should fall within two standard deviations of each other. More importantly, each measurement should follow the expected rate of growth, following the same percentile throughout infancy.

Accurate assessment combining information obtained by history, physical assessment, and knowledgeable observation allows early identification of common problems that may easily be resolved with early intervention. Often basic parent education and support remedy problems that, if left untreated, could later result in significant health problems or disturbed parent–child interactions.

Overnutrition and undernutrition are identified by weight that crosses percentiles. In **overnutrition**, the rate of

Box 34–4
Tips for Effective Assessment of the Pediatric Patient

- Protect the modesty and privacy of children, just as you would for adults. Use standard precautions to examine children, just as you would for adults.
- Explain procedures and techniques in words that children can understand.
- Remember that young children are more comfortable and compliant when they sit on their parents' laps. However, avoid this location when performing painful activities.
- Establish rapport with the parent and child before initiating any physical examination.
- Begin with the least threatening examinations; a flexible approach to assessment is essential.
- Perform painful or invasive procedures at the end of the assessment.
- Encourage young children to take deep breaths by having them blow bubbles or blow out the light on the otoscope.
- Allow children to touch equipment (**Figure 34–9 ≫**). Use playful language to talk about examinations, such as asking children if they have elephants in their ears, before examining the tympanic membrane.
- Use toys, for example, finger puppets, as distractions.
- Use standard precautions.

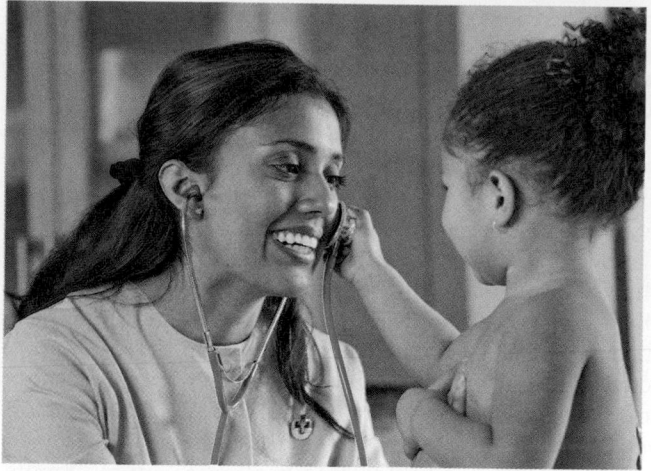

Source: Ariel Skelley/Blend Images/Getty Images.

Figure 34–9 ≫ A nurse allows her young patient to play with her stethoscope before using it to assess the child's heart.

weight gain is accelerated; in **undernutrition** the rate of weight gain diminishes. Overnutrition may occur when caregivers do not learn to read infants' cues but instead assume that every cry signals hunger. Cultural beliefs that a plump baby is a healthy baby may also lead parents and other caregivers to overfeed infants.

Undernutrition may be caused by inadequate caloric intake. This may result from lack of knowledge of normal infant feeding, a lack of financial resources to obtain formula, or inappropriate mixing of formula. Some quiet or passive infants do not demand feedings, and parents or caregivers may misinterpret this passivity as lack of hunger.

Head growth that crosses percentiles requires evaluation, because it may indicate **hydrocephalus** (enlargement of the head caused by inadequate drainage of cerebrospinal fluid). Early diagnosis and intervention for rapid head growth prevent or diminish serious neurologic effects.

Parents and caregivers generally enjoy relaying infants' new developmental milestones and can accurately describe infants' abilities. An infant who seems to be lagging behind on milestones may not be receiving appropriate stimulation. Assessment of caregivers' expectations and knowledge of infant development may reveal a knowledge deficit. Suggesting specific activities for caregivers to do with their infants may be the only intervention required. Infants who continue to lag significantly behind and are not achieving normal milestones require evaluation.

Healthy attachment is observed as a caregiver holds an infant close in a manner that encourages eye contact (the *en face* position). The caregiver looks at the infant, smiles, talks, and interacts with the infant. The infant responds by fixing on the caregiver's face, smiling, and cooing. The caregiver stays close to the infant, providing support and reassurance during examinations or procedures.

Failure to engage the infant through eye contact, talking, or a smile limits available opportunities for the caregiver to receive positive feedback from the infant. The infant, in turn, finds efforts to engage the parent frustrating, resulting in decreased attempts to interact. A negative pattern is quickly established, requiring more extensive intervention the longer it persists.

Assessment of Toddlers

Although the rate of growth of toddlers decreases, it proceeds in an expected manner. Height and weight continue to follow a percentile, although slight variations are often seen. Assessing caloric intake by obtaining a 24-hour recall provides clues to inappropriate feeding patterns. Toddlers generally feed themselves and begin to interact with the family at meals. A favorite food one week may be refused the next, causing frustration and confusion in caregivers. Concern for the toddler's health may precipitate a power struggle as parents try to force the toddler to eat. Poor weight gain may result as the toddler exerts a newfound independence by refusing to eat. Excessive weight gain occurs when caregivers use food to quiet or bribe their toddlers. Discussing appropriate eating expectations and weight gain helps parents resolve eating problems.

Because the young toddler is unlikely to cooperate, a health history is often the best way to assess development. Older toddlers are more willing to play with developmental testing materials or explore the environment while in proximity to a caregiver, enabling direct observations of development. Because toddlers might not speak in a strange or threatening environment, language assessment can be difficult. Listening to the child talk in a playroom or waiting room increases the probability of assessing the toddler's language.

The toddler wanders a short distance from a caregiver to explore, returning periodically to "touch base." After receiving reassurance and encouragement, the child is ready for further exploration. Exploration provides learning opportunities but also places the toddler at risk for accidental injury or poisoning.

Toddlers have frequent tantrums, usually in response to unwanted limits or frustration. An attitude of calm understanding limits the duration of tantrums and keeps tantrums from becoming power struggles or attention-getting behavior.

Toddlers quickly turn to caregivers for comfort or when confronted with a stranger. Observing the adult–child interaction and listening to how the adult speaks to the child provide information about the quality of the relationship.

Continuous clinging of a toddler to a caregiver in a nonthreatening situation is unusual. Failure of the child to look to a caregiver for comfort and support may indicate that trust did not develop during infancy. Inappropriate caregiver expectations, such as expecting a toddler to sit quietly in a chair, may interfere with the normal progression of the toddler's development. Caregiver inattention to the child's activities and failure to set limits result in the child's inability to develop self-control.

Assessment of Preschoolers

Preschoolers are generally pleasant, cooperative, and talkative. They are often less anxious if their caregiver is in view but do not need to return to the caregiver for comfort except in threatening situations. Talking with preschoolers about favorite activities allows the nurse to assess language ability, cognitive ability, and development. The nurse evaluates the child's use of language to express thoughts, sentence structure, and vocabulary. It may be possible to identify the ability to concentrate, magical thinking, and reality imitation as the child relays play activities. Lack of appropriate environmental stimulation may become evident, and the nurse may need to educate caregivers about age-appropriate activities for their children.

Preschoolers' slowed rate of growth is often of concern to caregivers. The nurse can allay anxiety by showing the preschooler's growth chart and discussing eating expectations.

A clinging, frightened preschooler in a nonthreatening situation may indicate a child who lacks a trusting relationship with his or her immediate caregivers. Lack of communication between caregiver and child limits the child's ability to learn appropriate social interaction and to practice language skills.

Children who do not exhibit appropriate achievement of developmental milestones should receive screenings and, if indicated, appropriate interventions. Periodic health assessments are necessary to ensure child well-being and to discuss child development with parents. Table 7–4: Health Screenings and Immunization Guidelines Across the Lifespan in Module 7 on Health, Wellness, Illness, and Injury provides a detailed listing of interventions recommended for newborns and infants, toddlers, and preschoolers. Depending on the results of the examination, additional screenings or referrals to agencies that conduct developmental screenings may be warranted.

Assessment of School-Age Children

The slow, steady growth and changing body proportions of school-age children can make them appear thin and gangly.

Assessing children's intake of nutrients and calories and reviewing their growth charts reassure parents that their children are not too thin. By educating parents to evaluate objectively their children's diets during the early school-age years, the nurse can help relieve family stress resulting from parents pushing children to eat and can help reinforce healthy eating habits that prevent obesity. Older school-age children have an increase in appetite as they enter the prepubertal growth spurt. During the growth spurt, height and weight increase and may normally cross percentiles.

School-age children are eager to talk about their hobbies, friends, school, and accomplishments. Increasing neurologic maturity allows them to master activities requiring gross and fine motor control, such as sports, dancing, playing a musical instrument, artistic pursuits, or building things. School-age children enjoy showing off newly acquired skills, and families display pride in their children's accomplishments.

School-age children frequently sort and classify collections of rocks, sports cards, dolls, coins, stamps, or almost anything. They are industrious in school, feeling pride in their accomplishments as they master difficult concepts and skills. Families provide positive feedback and encouragement to their children and speak of their children's successes with pride.

Adult family members and school-age children communicate openly, with adults setting appropriate and much-needed limits. Although peer relationships are becoming more important, the family remains the major influence during most of the school-age years. As children approach adolescence, the relationship with family may become strained as the children are drawn closer to peer groups and seek greater independence.

Children who lack hobbies or cannot think of any accomplishments may be environmentally deprived. Caregivers who are unable to think of anything positive to say about their children or who speak of them as a burden are likely to have a disturbed parent–child relationship. Children who lack encouragement and positive reinforcement at home for their achievements are at risk for gang recruitment. Gangs provide the "family" support children lack at home, increasing children's risk for violence, drug use, and illegal activity.

Problems in school may evolve at this time, and caregivers and children may have conflicts over grades and study time. The nurse can encourage the caregiver to help the child set a consistent place and time for homework. Caregivers should also be encouraged to communicate actively with the child's teacher. Teachers, adults, family members, and healthcare providers may identify learning disabilities at this time by careful observation.

Table 7–4: Health Screenings and Immunization Guidelines Across the Lifespan in Module 7 on Health, Wellness, Illness, and Injury provides a detailed listing of interventions recommended for school-age children.

Assessment of Adolescents

Parents and caregivers rarely express concern that their adolescents are not eating. The pubertal growth spurt requires adolescents to increase their caloric intake dramatically, causing parents concern that the adolescent eats constantly but never seems full. Despite this, adolescents (particularly women) are at risk for developing eating disorders. Information about eating disorders is included in the module on Self.

Adolescents often communicate better with peers and adults outside of the family than with family members. Assessing adolescents with their parents and then one-on-one affords a more complete picture of the adolescent–parent relationship and provides adolescents with an opportunity to express themselves and discuss concerns freely.

Most adolescents are able to hold an adult conversation and are often happy to discuss school, friends, activities, and plans for the future. They tend to be anxious about their bodies and the rapid changes that they are experiencing. Often adolescents are unsure if what is happening to them is normal, and they frequently express somatic complaints.

As adolescents become more independent, adult family members become anxious over their evolving lack of control. Parents may be uncomfortable with adolescents' sexuality, rebellious dress and hairstyles, and developing values that may differ from those of the parents. Communication between parents and adolescents is often challenging at this stage.

Severely restricting the activities and freedom of adolescents inhibits their ability to progress toward independence. Adolescents who lack social contacts and spend much time alone may be depressed and at high risk for suicide. Acting out and risk-taking behaviors place adolescents at risk for serious injury from accidents or drug or alcohol use. Alliance with gangs places adolescents at risk for violence and participation in illegal activities.

Table 7–4, Recommended Health Promotion Activities from Birth to Adolescence, in the module on Health, Wellness, Illness, and Injury provides a detailed listing of interventions recommended for the newborn period through adolescence.

Assessment of Pregnant Women

Prenatal care is important to ensure the health of both the developing fetus and the mother. Briefly, the changes that need to be assessed for comparison with normal expectations result from hormonal influences, the growing fetus, and the mother's physiologic and psychologic adaptation to the fact of being with child (**Figure 34–10 》**). Every system in the pregnant woman's body must adapt to support a new life and, at the same time, maintain the mother's body functions within normal limits.

The system changes include those in the reproductive system, including the uterus, cervix, ovaries, and vagina. Changes also happen in the breast, to prepare for possible lactation. The respiratory and cardiovascular systems change dramatically. Both need to support two individuals. The volume of air breathed increases 30 to 40%. Cardiac output peaks at 25 to 30 weeks' gestation at one third to one half above pre-pregnant levels.

Both the gastrointestinal system and the urinary tract prepare to provide digestion, absorption, and elimination for two individuals, instead of one. Both the musculoskeletal and central nervous systems alter their functioning only slightly to support the pregnancy. Finally, the mother's metabolism

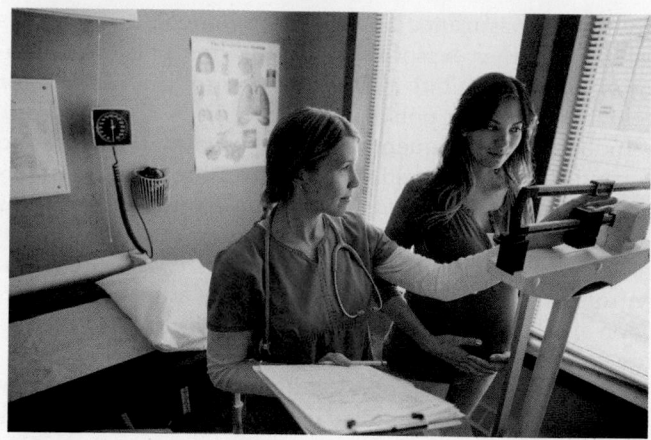

Source: Hero Images/Getty Images.

Figure 34–10 》 Prenatal checkups include a weigh-in to ensure that the mother is gaining weight appropriately.

accelerates to support the additional demands of the fetus, and the necessary preparation for labor and lactation.

The nine months of changes thoroughly affect the mother's life. Nursing assessment and education activities track the changes over time, comparing them to normal adaptations. For more in-depth details about how the mother, fetus, and obstetric-gynecologic team ensure a healthy pregnancy, see the four Assessment features in the module on Reproduction: Initial Prenatal Assessment, Subsequent Prenatal Assessment, Intrapartum Assessment during childbirth, and Postpartum Assessment after childbirth. See the module on Mood and Affect for an overview of assessment and nursing considerations related to preventing, identifying, and intervening in peripartum depression.

Assessment of Young Adults

Young adults tend to be busy, productive, and healthy. At their maximum physical potential, young adults actively pursue sports and physical fitness activities. They refine their creative talents and enjoy activities with peers.

Young adults form intimate partnerships with others in mature, cooperative relationships. Traditionally, such intimate relationships involved marriage. Increasingly, these relationships are formed and maintained without a formal marriage or between two people of the same sex. Developmentally, the important concept is the formation of the mature, intimate relationship.

People who want to have children in the 21st century have many more choices than their own parents and grandparents had: Surrogate motherhood, artificial insemination, in vitro fertilization, and other technologic innovations make it possible for couples in a variety of situations to choose to become parents. Deciding not to have children and delaying having children are increasingly accepted, as are the decisions of single women to have children and single men to adopt children.

Young adults have chosen an occupation, established their values, and adopted a lifestyle. Career advancement, a quest for financial stability, and emotional investment characterize the young adult years.

The young adult without a steady job may lack direction and self-confidence. Marital discord may trigger feelings of failure and insecurity. Failing to achieve intimacy may place the young adult at risk for depression, alcoholism, or drug abuse.

Table 7–5, Recommended Health Promotion Activities for Adults, in the module on Health, Wellness, Illness, and Injury provides a detailed listing of interventions recommended for young adults.

Assessment of Middle-aged Adults

Typically, the adult in the middle years of life is satisfied with past accomplishments and involved in activities outside the family. Healthy adjustment to the physical changes of aging includes developing appropriate leisure activities in preparation for an active retirement. Good financial planning during the middle adult years helps ensure financial security during retirement.

The middle adult years signal the end of childbearing and, most often, the end of childrearing. Individuals adjust to never having had children or to children leaving home. Couples may renew their relationships or find they have little in common and perhaps separate. Some women choose to delay childbearing until their late 30s or early 40s, after establishing their careers. They begin their childrearing years as many of their peers are completing this phase of life. Older mothers must make the transition from career women to mothers, even if they continue their careers.

The dissatisfied middle-aged adult is unhappy with the past and expresses little or no hope for the future. Sedentary and isolated, the individual complains about life, avoids involvement, and fails to plan appropriately for retirement.

Table 7–5, Recommended Health Promotion Activities for Adults, in the module on Health, Wellness, Illness, and Injury provides a detailed listing of interventions recommended for middle-aged adults.

Assessment of Older Adults

A comprehensive assessment is essential to understanding the health needs of the older adult. A comprehensive geriatric assessment should be carried out in the following circumstances:

1. Yearly for the older adult with complex health needs during the annual visit for routine health maintenance with the primary healthcare provider
2. After any abrupt change in physical, social, or psychologic function
3. When the older adult is hospitalized for acute illness or injury
4. When nursing home placement or a change in living status is being considered
5. When the older patient or the patient's family members would like a second opinion regarding an intervention or treatment protocol recommended by the primary care provider.

Because of the particular needs of older adult patients and the frequent need to work with healthcare providers in several disciplines, the nurse must be not only knowledgeable in the content area of gerontology and geriatrics, but

also educated regarding the issues of team dynamics. Essential skills in team dynamics include the following:

- An awareness of the roles and contributions of all team members
- Excellent communication skills in order to share information
- Conflict resolution skills
- The ability to see that multiple disciplines can provide information critical to solving the problems of the older patient.

Despite variations in instruments, structure of the interprofessional team, and methods employed, several strategies make the evaluation process more effective. These include the development of a close-knit interprofessional team with minimal redundancy in the assessments performed, the use of carefully designed questionnaires that reliable older patients or their caregivers can complete beforehand, and the effective use of assessment forms that are incorporated into computer databases (Kane et al., 2018).

The nurse can incorporate holistic assessment techniques and standardized instruments into routine evaluations (see **Table 34–12 》》** for a list of instruments used to assess older adults). In addition, the nurse is in an ideal position to advocate for older patients who would benefit from holistic assessment and to urge patients to seek the services of specialized geriatric assessment teams if these seem warranted.

》》 Stay Current: A set of more than 30 issues of Try This: Best Practices in Nursing Care to Older Adults is available from the Hartford Institute for Geriatric Nursing (2017), at the New York University College of Nursing. The general assessment series includes information on the purpose of the clinical measurement, the best tool, the target population, validity and reliability, strengths and limitations, and follow-up suggestions. It is available online at https://consultgeri.org/tools/try-this-series. Another set of geriatric assessment tools in 11 categories is available from the Iowa Geriatric Education Center (2017) at the University of Iowa. It is available online at https://igec.uiowa.edu/.

The three underlying principles of comprehensive geriatric assessment are as follows:

1. Physical, psychologic, and socioeconomic factors interact in complex ways to influence the health and functional status of the older individual.
2. Comprehensive evaluation of an older patient's health status requires an assessment in each of these domains. The coordinated efforts of various healthcare professionals are needed to carry out the assessment.
3. Functional abilities should be a central focus of the comprehensive evaluation. Other more traditional measures of health such as medical diagnosis, nursing diagnosis, physical examination results, and laboratory findings form the basic foundation of the assessment in order to determine overall health, well-being, and the need for social services (Kane et al., 2018).

The interrelationships among the physical, social, and psychologic aspects of aging and perhaps illness present a challenge to the nurse when beginning the geriatric evaluation. The nurse is often charged with the responsibility of

TABLE 34–12 Instruments for Evaluation of Older Adults

Instrument	Focus	Measurement	Uses
Tilburg or Groningen Frailty Indicators	Loss of resources causes inability to respond to physical or psychologic stress	Either professional or self-report of functioning in four domains: physical, cognitive, social, psychologic	Vulnerability to future poor health outcomes; to predict disability, healthcare use, and quality of life
World Health Organization Quality of Life questionnaire (WHOQOL-BREF)	Individual's perceptions of culture and value systems, and personal goals, standards, and concerns	Brief version is 26 items measuring four domains: physical health, psychologic health, social relationships, and environment	Can be used for people with intact cognitive functioning as well as mild-to-moderate dementia
Short Portable Mental Status	Mental process of knowing and understanding	Ten questions, can adjust for educational level	Assess cognitive functioning; can be repeated to check if decline in cognition
Mini–Mental State Examination (MMSE)	This brief, quantitative measure of cognitive status in adults can be used to screen for cognitive impairment, to estimate the severity of cognitive impairment at a given point in time, to follow the course of cognitive changes in an individual over time, and to document an individual's response to treatment. It is used frequently to track cognitive changes in patients with dementia	Eleven questions that assess areas such as orientation, recall, attention, and language	Assess cognitive functioning; can be repeated to check if decline in cognition
Katz's ADL Scale	Ability to independently bathe, dress, toilet, transfer, be continent, feed	Six yes/no questions, one for each functional area	Rate performance of independent activity
Instrumental Activities of Daily Living (iADLs)	Completion of complex activities; need for support services	Measures eight complex activities needed for independent functioning, assessing how much assistance is required, if any	If patient is not able to perform iADLs, assistance will be needed. If caregiver support is inadequate, a change in living situation might be indicated
Geriatric Depression Scale	Low mood accompanied by low self-esteem and loss of interest or pleasure in normally enjoyable activities	Short form has 15 yes/no questions, completion in 5 minutes; original form had 30 questions	Used to evaluate depression, which can exist alone or accompany dementia, as well as major illnesses: recent stroke, coronary artery bypass graft, or myocardial infarct. Older adult abuse can also cause depression
Barthel Index of Activities of Daily Living	Evaluates if disability is present, estimates its extent, determines when support needed	Can ask information of patient or relatives; can assess improvement over time	Assesses adequate functioning in mobility and daily self-care tasks
Palliative Performance Scale	Progression of disease, symptom management, prognosis, and timing of hospice referral	Scores are given in 10-point increments, ranging from 0 (death) to 100 (full or normal, no disease)	Response to palliative care services. Five categories of function are scored; lower scores indicate greater functional impairment
Get-Up-and-Go Test	Combination of gait and balance to produce mobility	Patient stands up from seated position in chair, walks short distance, turns around, returns to sitting in chair; can be timed or not	Patient's performance is scored on 5-point scale; higher score indicates greater gait and balance problems as well as an increased risk of falling
Kayser-Jones Brief Oral Health Status Examination (BOHSE)	Rates condition of patient's oral health from 0 (normal) to 2 (problematic)	Ten-item exam identifies oral health problems, using a pen light, tongue depressor, and gauze	Assesses need for referral
Clock Drawing Test (CDT)	Assessment of cognitive decline. If found, medications and management techniques can be used	Patient is asked to draw clock face with a specific time. Score for drawing closed circle, 12 correct numbers in correct positions, with hands pointed accurately	Often given with MMSE. The CDT detects impairments in executive function, while MMSE assesses orientation, memory, and language functions. Useful for detecting dementia in early stages
Zarit Burden Interview	Patient's care needs effect on daily life of caregiver	22 items that describe personal strain and role strain on 5-point scale	Used by aging agencies to rate caregiver stress
Braden Scale	Determines an individual's risk for developing pressure ulcers	Level of severity of six indicators: sensory perception, moisture, activity, mobility, nutrition, and friction or shear	Commonly used with older adults who have medical or cognitive impairments, on admission and on regular basis
Berg Balance Test or Single Leg Stance Test	To check for risk of falls; to monitor progress in physical therapy treatment	Choice of 14 tasks range from standing up from a sitting position, to standing on one foot	Clinical balance assessment; rated effective by 70% of physiotherapists
Fullmer SPICES	Conditions that warrant further assessment for fall risk	Checks for six conditions: Sleep disorders, Problems with eating and feeding, Incontinence, Confusion, Evidence of falls, and Skin breakdown	Used on admission to prompt fall risk precautions if needed
Mini–Nutritional Assessment (MNA)	Malnutrition and risk of developing malnutrition	Six questions on food intake, weight loss, mobility, psychologic stress or acute disease, presence of dementia or depression, and BMI	Suggested use: quarterly for institutionalized older adults and yearly for normally nourished community-dwelling older adults

obtaining the patient's past health history and history of the present illness.

Evaluation of the Assessment Environment

Before the assessment visit, clear instructions should be provided to the patient and family about parking arrangements and the registration process. To make the older patient and family comfortable, environmental modifications should be made, if possible. Environmental modifications may include adequate lighting, decreased background noise, comfortable seating for the older patient and family, easily accessible restrooms, examination tables that can be raised or lowered to assist patients with disabilities, and availability of water or juice for patient use. Patient comfort will ease communication and improve the data collection process.

Accuracy of the Health History

The more information that the patient and family can organize ahead of time, the more accurate and efficient the assessment will be. Many clinics mail an information packet in advance of the visit so that the older patient can come prepared. This packet might include the following:

1. A past medical history form. This form can be completed at home and is helpful for patients with complicated medical histories. The dates of hospitalizations, operations, serious injuries or accidents, procedures, and illnesses can be ascertained beforehand to save time during the assessment appointment. The form would also include any history of adverse drug effects or allergies.
2. Instructions to bring in all prescription and over-the-counter medications and herbal products/vitamins/mineral supplements for review by the nurse.
3. Instructions to bring any medical records, laboratory or x-ray reports, electrocardiograms, reports of vaccination, and other pertinent health records that the patient or family may possess.
4. Instructions to write down and bring the names of all healthcare providers involved with the patient's healthcare, including primary care providers, specialists, and alternative medicine practitioners (e.g., acupuncturists, massage therapists, chiropractors).
5. Instructions to bring hearing aids, eyeglasses, and any assistive devices (canes, walkers, and so on).

Patience is a virtue when obtaining a history from an older adult, because often the individual's thought and verbal processes are slower than those of younger patients. The patient should be allowed adequate time to answer questions and report information (Kane et al., 2018).

SAFETY ALERT When an older patient who has been asked to bring all medications to a geriatric evaluation session arrives carrying a large bag of medication bottles, the nurse knows that the first notation on the problem list is likely to be "at risk for adverse drug reaction related to polypharmacy."

The history should include emphasis on the following:

- Review of acute and chronic medical problems
- Medications

- Disease prevention and health maintenance review: vaccinations, PPD (tuberculosis), cancer screenings. (Table 7–5: Health Screenings and Immunization Guidelines Across the Lifespan in the module on Health, Wellness, Illness and Injury provides a detailed listing of interventions recommended for older adults.)
- Functional status (activities of daily living)
- Social supports (family, spiritual affiliations, caregiver stress, safety of living environment)
- Finances
- Driving status and safety record
- Review of symptoms (patient/family perception of memory, dentition, taste, smell, nutrition, hearing, vision, falls, fractures, bowel and bladder function).

Often, a standardized form is used to guide and direct the process of obtaining a health history. The nurse should be aware of potential difficulties in obtaining health histories from older patients, including the following:

- ***Communication difficulties.*** Decreased hearing or vision and decreased mental processing and response times have an effect on accurate and successful communication.
- ***Underreporting of symptoms.*** Fear of being labeled as a complainer, fear of institutionalization, and fear of serious illness and death can influence symptom reporting.
- ***Vague or nonspecific complaints.*** These may be associated with cognitive impairment, drug or alcohol use or abuse, or atypical presentation of disease.
- ***Multiple complaints.*** Associated "masked" depression, presence of multiple chronic illnesses, and social isolation are often an older adult's cry for help.
- ***Lack of time.*** New patients scheduled for a geriatric assessment should have at least a 1-hour appointment with the gerontologic nurse. Shorter appointments will result in a hurried interview with missed information (Kane et al., 2018).

Social History

Holistic evaluation is not complete without an assessment of the patient's social support system. Many frail older adults receive support and supervision from family members and significant others to compensate for functional disabilities.

Key elements of the social history include the following:

- Past occupation and retirement status
- Family history (helpful when constructing a family genogram)
- Present and former marital status, including quality of the relationship(s)
- Identification of family members, with designation of level of involvement and place of residence
- Current living arrangements
- Family dynamics
- Family and caregiver expectations
- Economic status, including adequacy of health insurance
- Social activities and hobbies

- Mode of transportation
- Community involvement and support
- Religious involvement and spirituality.

Older individuals who exhibit symptoms of sadness or social isolation, who question their existence, who feel they are being punished by God, or who ask about availability of religious or spiritual counseling should be asked if they would like help with their spiritual concerns. Religion and spirituality can be a great source of hope and strength in times of need and crisis. Many healthcare facilities and community agencies have access to religious and spiritual counselors. They can connect older patients and their families with such assistance, especially in the absence of an ongoing relationship with a priest, minister, rabbi, or spiritual counselor.

If an assessment team includes a social worker, the nurse may collaborate with him or her closely to identify and address social problems. Older patients with inadequate health insurance can often be helped by accessing community services, free hospital services, hardship funds established for indigent patients by major drug companies, and referrals to community-based free clinics. This information is helpful to the nurse working with older patients in many settings. It is crucial for patients admitted to long-term care facilities, those expressing feelings of severe loneliness, or those who do not have a close relationship with another individual.

Functional Evaluation

A key part of the evaluation of the older adult patient is the assessment or systematic evaluation of the patient's level of function and self-care. Ongoing research supports the need for regular assessment of the older adult's risk for falls regardless of setting. By properly evaluating older adults and targeting risk factors for falls and functional decline, the nurse can promote greater independence and safety in older patients. Areas to target include self-care abilities, cognition, nutrition and feeding, continence, mobility, sleep, and skin care. A home visit or comprehensive questions about the patient's home environment can provide useful information about fall risks, other safety issues, and the patient's ability to function in that environment (see Skills 15.2 and 15.5 in Volume 3).

Lifestyle and Health Considerations

Well-adjusted older adults maintain an active lifestyle and involvement with others and often do not appear their age (**Figure 34–11 》**). Lifestyle changes occur in response to declining physical abilities and retirement. Participation in activities that promote the older adult's sense of self-worth and usefulness also provides opportunities for developing new friendships with others of similar abilities and interests. Intellectual function is maintained through continued intellectual pursuits. Content with their life review, well-adjusted older adults often enjoy their retirement years and accept death as the inevitable end of a productive life. The older adult who has not successfully resolved developmental crises may feel that life has been unfair. Despair and hopelessness may be evident in the individual's lack of activity and bitter complaining.

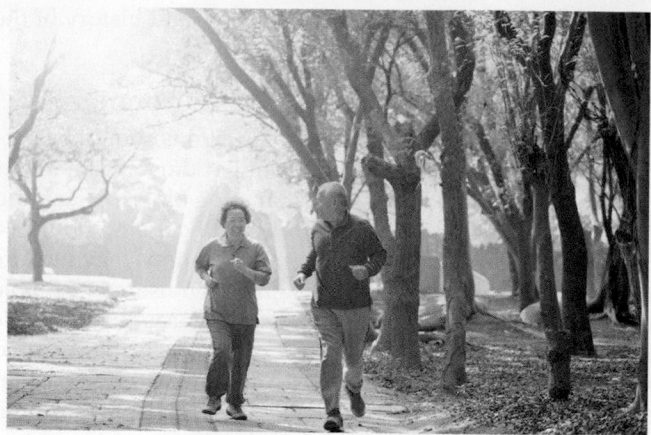

Source: Tom Wang/Shutterstock.

Figure 34–11 》 Well-adjusted older adults often enjoy their retirement.

Minimum Data Set

Assessment of an older patient for appropriate placement in a nursing home or within a long-term care system is done using the Minimum Data Set (MDS). The MDS is a comprehensive standardized multidisciplinary assessment used throughout the United States. The Omnibus Budget Reconciliation Act of 1987 (OBRA 87) mandated assessment of all residents of facilities funded by Medicare or Medicaid using the MDS. It is also completed on all residents admitted to Veterans Administration Community Living Centers (Saliba et al., 2012). The MDS is used for validating the need for long-term care, reimbursement, ongoing assessment of clinical problems, and assessment of and need to alter the current plan of care.

The MDS consists of a core set of screening, clinical, and functional measures:

- ***Resident Assessment Protocols (RAPs)*** are structured, problem-oriented guidelines that identify unique and relevant information about an older patient. This information is needed for formulating an individualized nursing care plan.

- ***Resident Utilization Guidelines (RUGs)*** determine the reimbursement the skilled nursing facility will receive for providing care to the older patient. Factors considered include the need for supportive therapy (physical, occupational, and/or speech), self-care ability of the older patient, and the need for special treatments such as feeding tubes or skin care.

- ***Resident Assessment Instrument (RAI)*** identifies medical problems and describes each older patient's functional ability in a comprehensive and standardized format. This information helps to formulate the plan of care and to evaluate progress toward goals, indicating when changes in the care plan are needed.

Categories of data gathered for the MDS include the following:

- Patient demographics and background
- Cognitive function
- Communication and hearing

- Mood and behavior patterns
- Psychosocial well-being
- Physical function and ADLs
- Bowel and bladder continence
- Diagnosed diseases
- Health conditions (weight, falls, and so on)
- Oral nutritional status
- Oral and dental status
- Skin condition
- Activity pursuits
- Medications

- Need for special services
- Discharge potential.

Certain information gathered for the MDS, such as data indicating functional decline or a poorly managed chronic disease, may trigger the need for further assessment using the RAPs. For instance, if information gathered for the MDS indicates that the nursing home resident has fallen, a RAP is triggered and indicates the need for direct gait assessment, medication review, and physical/occupational therapy evaluation.

Table 7–5, Recommended Health Promotion Activities for Adults, in the module on Health, Wellness, Illness, and Injury provides a detailed listing of interventions recommended for older adults.

REVIEW The Concept of Assessment

RELATE Link the Concepts

Linking the concept of assessment with the concept of caring interventions:

1. You are assigned to care for a patient who has been receiving tube feedings via a nasogastric tube that has been in place for several days. Prior to administering the first tube feeding of the shift, what assessments would you perform?

2. Would the assessment performed be an initial assessment or a problem-focused assessment? Explain your answer.

Linking the concept of assessment with the concept of clinical decision making:

3. You are assigned care of a 46-year-old man admitted for status asthmaticus. His condition has stabilized and discharge is planned for tomorrow. When you enter his room for the first time, you find that he is short of breath and he requests that you hand him his inhaler, which the physician ordered to be kept at the bedside for self-administration as needed. What will you do first? Which important assessment is needed? How would you handle a possible change in already-set discharge plans?

4. What critical thinking would you apply to the above situation?

Linking the concept of assessment with the concept of communication:

5. When collecting information for a health history, what strategies would you use when communicating with an older adult who has a hearing loss?

6. You are collecting information from the mother of a 3-year-old for a health history. The mother does not speak any English, but the 3-year-old does speak English. What communication strategies would you employ? What if the child was 9 years old and enrolled in third grade? Would those different characteristics cause you to change your communication strategy?

Linking the concept of assessment with the concept of legal issues:

7. You admit an adolescent to the adolescent unit of a local hospital and begin collecting data when you begin to suspect that the adolescent may be abusing substances. With an understanding of your legal obligation to the adolescent, as well as your knowledge that the parents want to help their child, how would you handle your suspicions if the parents are in the room with the child?

8. You are assessing an older adult and discover bruises that you suspect may be the result of abuse. The patient's son is in the room during the examination. What is the best legally appropriate action for you to take? What will you do if that initial approach does not clarify the situation?

READY Go to Volume 3: Clinical Nursing Skills

- Read Chapter 1 for general assessment skills, vital signs, and physical assessment.
- See Chapter 9 for skills related to assistive devices.
- See Chapter 10 for skills related to healthy eating habits.
- And see the skills in the Safety chapter for assessing for abuse, fall prevention, seizure precautions, environmental safety, fire safety, and preventing thermal and electrical injuries.

REFER Go to Pearson MyLab Nursing and eText

- Additional review materials

REFLECT Apply Your Knowledge

The nurse conducted a health history interview with Martha Washburn, a 67-year-old woman. The following are excerpts from the health history.

"Mrs. Washburn, I am going to ask you a lot of questions before your physical. I need to have correct responses, and I have to tell you, there will be a lot of them if we are to get to the root of your problem. I will use the information to develop a plan of care."

"What are you here for? Did someone come with you? I see on your chart that you have some problems with urination. Are you incontinent? How long have you had the problem?"

The nurse included the following questions: "What is your economic status? Do you go to church? What do you do when you are ill?"

"We need information about your family, so let's start with your parents. Are they alive? Do you have siblings?"

The nurse completed a review of symptoms and prepared the patient for the physical examination by showing her into a room and telling her to get undressed.

1. Critique the nurse's actions in the initial interview phase of the case study.

2. Identify the types of information the nurse was seeking in asking those questions.

3. Create alternative approaches and questioning techniques for the interview in the case study.

4. Describe your preparation for an interview of Mrs. Washburn.

References

American Cancer Society (2016). *Breast cancer risk factors you cannot change.* Retrieved from https://www.cancer.org/cancer/breast-cancer/risk-and-prevention/breast-cancer-risk-factors-you-cannot-change.html

American Cancer Society. (2017). *American Cancer Society guidelines for early detection of cancer.* Retrieved from http://www.cancer.org/healthy/findcancerearly/cancerscreeningguidelines/american-cancer-society-guidelines-for-the-early-detection-of-cancer

American Heart Association (AHA). (2015). *Understanding blood pressure readings.* Retrieved from http://www.heart.org/HEARTORG/Conditions/HighBloodPressure/AboutHighBloodPressure/Understanding-Blood-Pressure-Readings_UCM_301764_Article.jsp

Centers for Disease Control and Prevention. (2014). *10 Leading Causes of Death by Age Group, United States—2014.* Retrieved from http://www.cdc.gov/injury/wisqars/pdf/leading_causes_of_death_by_age_group_2014-a.pdf

D'Amico, D., & Barbarito, C. (2015). *Health & physical assessment in nursing* (3rd ed.). Upper Saddle River, NJ: Pearson Education.

Gordon, M. (2014). *Manual of nursing diagnosis* (13th ed.). Burlington, MA: Jones & Bartlett.

Hartford Institute for Geriatric Nursing. (2017). Try this: Series. Retrieved from https://consultgeri.org/tools/try-this-series

Iowa Geriatric Education Center, University of Iowa. (2017). *Geriatric assessment tools.* Retrieved from https://igec.uiowa.edu/.

Kane, R., Ouslander, J., Resnick, B. , & Malone, M. L. (2018). *Essentials of clinical geriatrics* (8th ed.). New York, NY: McGraw-Hill Professional.

Romero, A. (2011). *Health history and screening of an adolescent or young adult client.* Grand Canyon University. Retrieved from http://www.academia.edu/7722688/Health_History_and_Screening_of_an_Adolescent_or_Young_Adult_Client

Saliba, D., Jones, M., Streim, J., Ouslander, J., Berlowitz, D., & Buchanan, J. (2012). Overview of significant changes in the Minimum Data Set for nursing homes version 3.0. *Journal of the American Medical Directors Association, 13*(7), 595–601. doi:10.1016/j.jamda.2012.06.001

Stewart, C. J., & Cash, W. B., Jr. (2014). *Interviewing: Principles and practices* (14th ed.). New York, NY: McGraw-Hill.

Siu, A. L., the U.S. Preventive Services Task (USPSTF), Bibbins-Domingo, K., Grossman, D. C., Baumann, L. C., Davidson, K. W., . . . Pignone, M. P. (2016). Screening for depression in adults: U.S. Preventive Services Task Force Recommendation Statement. *Journal of the American Medical Association, 315*(4), 380–387.

The Joint Commission. (2016). *Sentinel event alert: Detecting and treating suicide ideation in all settings.* Retrieved from https://www.jointcommission.org/assets/1/18/SEA_56_Suicide.pdf

U.S. Preventive Services Task Force. (2013). *Intimate partner violence and abuse of elderly and vulnerable adults: Screening.* Retrieved from http://www.uspreventiveservicestaskforce.org/Page/Document/UpdateSummaryFinal/intimate-partner-violence-and-abuse-of-elderly-and-vulnerable-adults-screening

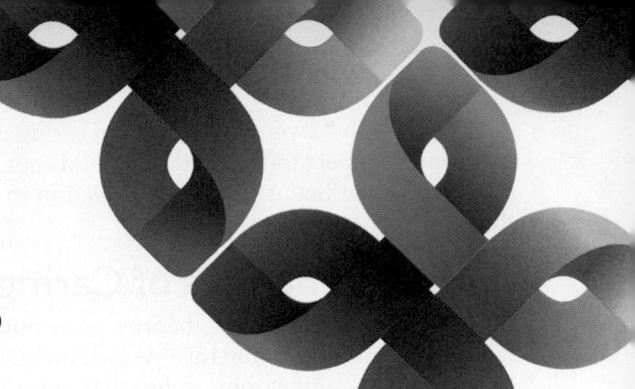

Module 35
Caring Interventions

Module Outline and Learning Outcomes

The Concept of Caring Interventions

Nursing Theories of Caring

35.1 Outline nursing theories that bridge the gap between theory and practice.

Concepts Related to Caring Interventions

35.2 Outline the relationship between caring interventions and other concepts.

Knowledge and Caring

35.3 Differentiate the four types of knowledge used in nursing.

Caring Encounters and Holistic Nursing

35.4 Analyze holistic nursing as it relates to caring interventions.

Lifespan Considerations

35.5 Differentiate caring interventions appropriate for patients at different stages throughout the lifespan.

Caring for the Caregiver: Self-Care in Nursing

35.6 Analyze the importance of nurses caring for themselves.

» The Concept of Caring Interventions

Concept Key Terms

Aesthetic knowing, **2464**	Caring practice, **2461**	Competence, **2467**	Empowerment, **2467**	Personal knowing, **2464**
Caring, **2461**	Compassion, **2467**	Empirical knowing, **2464**	Ethical knowing, **2465**	Presencing, **2466**

Caring is generally defined as ability "to feel interest or concern" (Merriam-Webster Online Dictionary, 2016), but in the context of the nursing profession, caring goes well beyond this simple explanation. Caring has been described as encompassing various intentions and actions. Brunton and Beaman (2000) identified the following caring behaviors: "In rank order [they] were appreciating the patient as a human being, showing respect for the patient, being sensitive to the patient, talking with the patient, treating patient information confidentially, treating the patient as an individual, encouraging the patient to call with problems, being honest with the patient, and listening attentively to the patient" (p. 451).

Caring is a concept that forms an integral part of nursing theory. That said, the concept of caring is not limited to the realm of academia. Research based on in-depth interviews of practicing nurses revealed that engaging in **caring practice** is an essential element in providing quality nursing care (Burhans & Alligood, 2010). One nurse participant who was chosen as representative of the initial sample described her experience of quality nursing: "If you have a person that's actually caring and compassionate and concerned about the welfare of that individual, it'll take you farther than if you are an expert clinician" (p. 1694).

To take it one step further, a currently accepted position within the field describes "nursing as situated caring" (Jarrin, 2012, p. 4); in other words, caring can only be understood in the context of the environment. Not only are physical time, space, and location relevant, but the nurse's level of development, the situation's specific circumstances, and both the nurse's and patient's value systems surrounding illness and healing are also central in affecting how caring is manifested. Depending on the perspective, nursing can be viewed as "technical actions and physical behavior . . . [or] caring thought, feeling, and intention behind the action" (p. 4), with the ideal being an amalgamation of the two. Although both elements form the foundation of nursing, "without caring our work would merely be tasks that could be performed by machines" (pp. 4–5).

Milton Mayeroff, author of the classic 1971 book *On Caring*, argued that at the heart of caring is "helping the other grow" (Mayeroff, 1990, p. 2). Mayeroff maintained that caring facilitates growth both in the person who exhibits caring and in the recipient, be it a person or thing, such as a concept, cause, or community. Under his framework, caring is not a finite action but rather a process that encourages self-actualization in the caregiver as well as development of the person receiving care. Central to Mayeroff's concept of caring is that the caregiver must respect the individuality and separateness of the other by not inflicting a specific direction in the growth of the other.

Nursing Theories of Caring

The various nursing caring theories grew out of humanism, which the American Humanist Association (2016) defines as "a progressive philosophy of life that, without theism and other supernatural beliefs, affirms our ability and responsibility to lead ethical lives of personal fulfillment that aspire to the greater good of humanity." Although each caring theory underscores different aspects and perspectives, all agree that caring is "the essence of nursing and a central and unifying feature" (Blais, 2015).

Bridging the gap between theory and practice has been an ongoing issue in nursing. Research has revealed that patients are clear on what constitutes a good nurse: Caring behaviors such as honesty, sincerity, the willingness to listen to others, and the perspective that the patient is a person and not just an illness are of central importance to patient satisfaction (Van der Elst et al., 2012). The question then is how to take the various theoretical perspectives on caring and translate them into practice (Swanson, 2012).

Tonges and Ray (2011) described how University of North Carolina Hospitals (UNCH) developed a successful nursing care delivery model known as the Professional Practice Model (PPM). The PPM is "one approach to actualizing caring theory across a healthcare organization by systematically incorporating interventions that link nursing actions, caring processes, and expectations" (p. 374). The PPM "translated caring theory into specific caring behaviors and incorporated them in practice" (p. 375). One example was the implementation of a "no passing zone" in which a "No Passing" sign was posted in hallways as a reminder that if a patient's call light was flashing, any nurse passing by the light was obligated to check in with the patient, even if that nurse was not assigned to that specific patient. "This practice is designed to convey the availability of the entire staff to *do for* all patients on the unit" (p. 377). Providing high-quality care and a climate accepting of innovations in caring depends on the development of concrete strategies that allow nurses to link theoretical concepts to their on-the-job duties (Tonges et al., 2015).

Although caring theories have been designed with the nurse–patient relationship in mind, the basic tenets of caring can and also should be applied to the nurse–nurse relationship. Intense levels of stress caused by staff shortages and high-needs patients underscore the importance of nurses supporting each other. When nurses are supportive of each other, they not only are able to solve problems that arise from challenging situations, but they also "are inspired to care by being cared for themselves" (Longo, 2011, p. 8). Inappropriate behaviors, such as bullying, are being scrutinized in healthcare because of the potential negative impact on patient care and safety and worker well-being and satisfaction. These behaviors will not be supported in environments with empowering initiatives that recognize the skills and knowledge that nurses contribute to patient care (Longo, 2013).

Leininger's Theory of Culture Care Diversity and Universality

In the mid-1980s, Madeleine Leininger revolutionized nursing and transformed the concept of caring with the development of a new discipline called transcultural nursing, currently referred to as the theory of Culture Care Diversity and Universality (George, 2011). In an early publication she said that "nurses often labeled, avoided or talked down to the cultural strangers when they did not understand their behavior and needs" (Leininger, 1989, p. 7). Her study of anthropology provided much insight as to how culture played a crucial role in providing nursing care in order to maintain or encourage health.

In order for nurses to provide the highest quality of care to culturally diverse patients, Leininger presents three modes of action:

- Culture care preservation and/or maintenance involves caregivers performing actions and making choices that help patients retain their specific cultural values and beliefs.

- Culture care accommodation and/or negotiation refer to caregivers' efforts to assist patients in adapting to or working with others to achieve the best possible care.

- Culture care repatterning and/or restructuring describes caregiver interventions that support patients in evaluating and changing their approaches to promote improved health outcomes (Leininger & McFarland, 2006).

Roach's Theory of Caring as the Human Mode of Being

Sister M. Simone Roach's philosophical theory declares caring to be a core element of how humans operate, as well as an expression of interconnectedness: "Caring, as the human mode of being, is caring from the heart; caring from the core of one's being; caring as a response to one's experience of connectedness" (Roach, 1997, p. 16).

Although Roach's theory views humans as caring entities, it also maintains that caring within the context of nursing is distinct in that the specific traits of nurses are all grounded in caring. She has labeled these attributes the six Cs of caring: compassion, competence, confidence, conscience, commitment, and comportment. Refer to **Box 35-1 》** for further explanation of each trait.

Boykin and Schoenhofer's Nursing as Caring Theory

In 1993, Anne Boykin and Savina O. Schoenhofer proposed their nursing theory of caring, which maintains that caring is a crucial element of being human, as well as an ongoing process rather than a goal to be achieved (George, 2011). They argue that nurses must be willing to accept that caring is never static; it continually changes and evolves throughout the span of their lives. At the heart of it all, nursing is caring. Boykin and Schoenhofer (2001) state that "being caring, that is, living one's commitment to this value 'important-in-itself' (Roach, 1984), fuels the nurse's growing in caring and enables the nurse in turn to nurture others in their living and growing in caring" (p. 19). Self-awareness is also essential to being a

Box 35–1
The Six Cs of Caring in Nursing

Compassion. Awareness of one's relationship to others, sharing their joys, sorrows, pain, and accomplishments. Participation in the experience of another.

Competence. Having the knowledge, judgment, skills, energy, experience, and motivation to respond adequately to others within the demands of professional responsibilities.

Confidence. The quality that fosters trusting relationships. Comfort with self, patient, and family.

Conscience. Morals, ethics, and an informed sense of right and wrong. Awareness of personal responsibility.

Commitment. Convergence between one's desires and obligations and the deliberate choice to act in accordance with them.

Comportment. Appropriate demeanor, dress, and language that are in harmony with a caring presence. Presenting oneself as someone who respects others and in turn demands respect.

Source: Adapted from Roach, M. S. (2002). *Caring, the human mode of being: A blueprint for the health professions* (2nd ed.). Ottawa, ON: CHA Press. Reprinted with permission.

---

caring and effective nurse. Patients respond positively to their caregiver's authenticity, which encourages their own growth.

Watson's Theory of Human Care

Jean Watson's theory of human care has evolved as a result of her intense interest, varied education, and extensive experience with nursing, philosophy, and metaphysics (Watson, 1999). At the crux of her theory is the assumption that genuine caring relationships have a positive impact on a patient's health and can facilitate the healing process, putting caring at the core of nursing. Equally important is the preservation of the patient's dignity and a respect for all people's inevitable interconnectedness (George, 2011).

Also key to Watson's theory of human care is that caring is considered transpersonal; in other words, both the nurse and the patient seek out meaning and a sense of connectedness. Furthermore, Watson (1999) maintained that caring involves addressing not just the mind and the body, but also the spirit: "The value of human care and caring involves a higher sense of spirit of self. Caring calls for a philosophy of moral commitment toward protecting human dignity and preserving humanity" (p. 31).

When Watson first developed her theory, she identified what she referred to as the 10 carative factors that needed to exist within a nurse–patient caring relationship. She later updated those characteristics and renamed them the 10 clinical caritas processes. These include the process of practicing loving kindness and equanimity within the context of providing care; being authentically present with the patient; being present to and supportive of patients' expression of feelings—both positive and negative; and creating a healing environment at all levels (George, 2011).

Benner and Wrubel's Theory of Caring

Patricia Benner and Judith Wrubel's contribution to caring theories is grounded in their book *The Primacy of Caring: Stress and Coping in Health and Illness* (1989), which places caring at the heart of providing quality service to patients and their families. In 2001, they further clarified their perspective as not focusing on nurse caregiving as much as on how care informs stress and coping responses: "Our main goal is to examine the phenomenon of care and caring practices to the experience of health and illness, not the caregiving of nurses" (p. 172). They describe a nurse's intent to care as only one factor in how caring is delivered and received. In other words, caring does not happen in a vacuum; it is dependent on other factors, such as the context of the situation, the physical environment, the nurse's training and experience, and the patient's unique capacities and perspectives (see Focus on Diversity and Culture) (Benner & Wrubel, 2001).

Focus on Diversity and Culture
Cultural Competence in Nursing

Cultural competence not only is imperative for nurses at the bedside but also relates to being a member of an influential global nursing community. There are many excellent cultural guides available detailing the healthcare concerns of various ethnicities; each new nurse should own one and refer to it frequently. Often, an overview to cultural care on ethnic groups commonly served by a hospital is provided in new graduate orientation. Below are some common areas of concern when providing care to someone from a different culture (Spector, 2017; Andrews & Boyle, 2016).

- Culture and religion can have an influence on how patients express pain and the meaning they attach to it. For instance, some cultures view pain as penance for a past wrongdoing or as a test of faith. Others see acknowledgment of pain and/or requests for pain relief as a sign of weakness.

- Certain cultures observe specific practices or rituals related to death and dying and may resist exploring the best options for end-of-life care.

- Families in some cultures approach healthcare decisions as a team as opposed to leaving the final decision of treatment to the individual in question.

- All distinctive practices of a specific culture or religion are not homogeneous within the same group, making it crucial that nurses be sensitive to such issues but also not make sweeping generalizations about an entire group of people. For example, younger members of a family may be less strict in their adherence to some cultural or religious practices than their grandparents or parents.

The Transcultural Nursing Society (Douglas et al., 2011), along with the Expert Panel for Global Nursing and Health of the American Academy of Nursing, has developed the Standards for Practice for culturally competent nursing care. These standards are broad-reaching, encompassing individual nursing care as well as actions by healthcare systems and governments. They address such concerns as social justice, knowledge of cultures; culturally competent practice; cultural competence in healthcare systems and organizations; patient advocacy and empowerment; a multicultural workforce; cross-cultural communication and leadership; and evidence-based practice and research (Douglas et al., 2011).

>> Stay Current: For additional information on nursing and other cultures, visit the website of the Transcultural Nursing Society at http://www.tcns.org/.

Concepts Related to Caring Interventions

The caring interventions are fundamental to the entire nursing process. Caring—both for self and for others—is the essence of nursing. Self-care includes recognizing and tending to the nurse's own physiologic and psychosocial needs, as well as seeking out activities that promote professional development. For the nurse, the negative impact of alterations in physical and mental health can extend to patient care, in terms of both the decision-making process and the actual care the nurse provides.

The relationship between caring interventions and professionalism carries important implications for nurses. In work environments where nurse shortages and poor working conditions exist, nurses have reported that quality of care suffers (Kutney-Lee et al., 2013). Furthermore, "improved work environments and reduced ratios of patients to nurses were associated with increased care quality and patient satisfaction," whereas patient satisfaction is much lower in institutions where many nurses feel burned out and dissatisfied with their work conditions (Aiken et al., 2012).

Caring is directly linked to ethics, because it "can be considered a commitment to attending to and becoming enthusiastically involved in the patient's needs" (Lachman, 2012, p. 114). Caring nurses are more inclined to hold high ethical standards, which unfortunately can lead to internal conflict, also referred to as moral distress. Moral distress is a phenomenon that encompasses many issues, such as a nurse knowing the right action to take, but being constrained from taking it; when nurses perceive less time available to give to their patients; when a leadership style is in conflict with providing better patient care; and when only inadequate consultative services are available to patients (de Veer et al., 2013).

Cultural influences affect coping styles, which, in turn, affect both care and self-care practices. For example, most Western cultures are considered to be individualist, which includes placing a high value on facing personal challenges individually and autonomously. In the context of an individualist culture, members from other cultures may be less likely to seek social support when managing stressful situations (Goh et al., 2015). As a result, when faced with a stressor, seeking social support may be viewed as unfavorable or even as a sign of weakness.

Cultural influences also inform the grieving process. Western expectations of autonomy may lead some providers to discount the importance of the family unit during times of grief but may also lead some patients to hesitate to ask family members for help or support. Similarly, individuals from different cultures may observe different rituals during the end of life. Nurses and other healthcare providers assess and facilitate the needs of all patients to observe cultural or traditional practices. Some, but not all, of the concepts integral to caring are shown in the Concepts Related to Caring Interventions feature. They are presented in alphabetical order.

Knowledge and Caring

In the context of nursing, researcher Barbara Carper (1978) outlined four types of knowledge, which she also refers to as knowledge patterns (p. 13): empirical, aesthetic, personal,

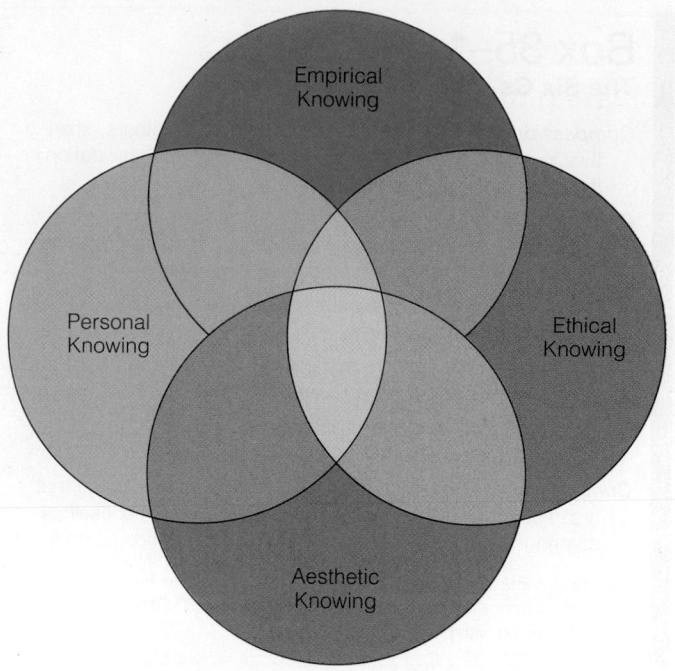

Figure 35–1 ⟩⟩ The four ways of knowing.

and ethical (see **Figure 35–1** ⟩⟩). Important to note is that they do not exist independently, but rather they overlap and interact with each other. With a greater awareness of what knowledge encompasses, nurses are able to more efficiently draw on the full scope of their understanding so as to provide the highest quality care possible.

Empirical Knowing

The first type of knowledge Carper (1978) identified is empirical, which she also referred to "the science of nursing" (p. 14). **Empirical knowing** is twofold in that it is based in facts and observations relevant to nursing, as well as the analyses and theories that attempt to explain them. Nurses can develop this pattern of knowing through ongoing academic education and increasing their skills at operating from a place of objectivity when making observations.

Aesthetic Knowing

The next type of knowledge, **aesthetic knowing**, is also referred to as "the art of nursing" (Carper, 1978, p. 14). In contrast to the objective nature of empirical knowing, aesthetic knowing is subjective and relates to the specific personal style the nurse possesses when delivering care. Key elements of this pattern of knowing are empathy (p. 17), holistic thinking, compassion, and sensitivity (Berman, Snyder, & Frandsen, 2016). Development of this type of knowing involves the nurse's commitment to increasing her awareness and respect regarding other people's unique perspectives and experiences.

Personal Knowing

Carper (1978) identified **personal knowing** as another pattern of knowledge within nursing, referring to the nurse's ongoing self-exploration and self-actualization. Developing this pattern of knowing involves "the nurse in the therapeutic use of

Concepts Related to
Caring Interventions

CONCEPT	RELATIONSHIP TO CARING INTERVENTIONS	NURSING IMPLICATIONS
Culture and Diversity	Western cultural influences → autonomous coping highly valued → sense of weakness associated with seeking social support → tendency to avoid asking for help when needed → ineffective self-care	■ Recognize cultural impact on beliefs about seeking help. ■ Assess personal beliefs regarding the value of social support. ■ Identify trusted sources of support and use resources as needed.
Ethics	Conflict between providing the best possible care for the patient could clash with the family's wishes or the constraining factors of the institution → leads nurse to experience moral distress → ↑ feelings of stress → ↑ risk for burnout	■ Share ethical concerns with supervisor and healthcare team and build supportive networks on the job. ■ Attend workshops on moral distress to increase coping strategies. ■ Identify common causes of moral distress among nursing peers.
Grief and Loss	Western cultural influences assume personal autonomy and involvement in end-of-life decisions and care → disregard for non-Western patient/family preferences regarding end-of-life preferences → impaired patient/family/provider communication → increased grief and unhappiness by patient and family during stressful life event	■ If patients/family from a non-Western culture reject such concepts as palliative care/hospice, advance directives, or organ donation, be respectful of these decisions. ■ Use chaplains and translators (if needed) to ensure that patient/family wishes regarding death and associated practices are fully understood by nurses and assistive personnel. ■ Accommodate patient/family wishes as much as possible to alleviate patient and family stress. ■ Demonstrate respect in all interactions with the patient/family.
Professionalism	Inadequate self-care → decreased level of physical and psychosocial wellness → decreased quality of work performance and weakened affiliation with profession of nursing → decreased level of demonstrated professionalism toward patients, peers, and other members of the healthcare team	■ Assess self-wellness and recognize when limitations are being exceeded. ■ Be aware of warning signs that may signal burnout. ■ Recognize areas of self-care that are unhealthy and identify solutions that promote wellness.
Safety	Lack of knowledge regarding patient culture → incomplete nursing assessment and miscommunication → poor patient outcomes and dissatisfaction with healthcare providers and facility	■ Use chaplains and translators (if needed) to ensure that information is accurately transmitted to patient and family. ■ Actively seek information about the patient's stated cultural and religious preferences. ■ Ensure that patient teaching is delivered using a culturally sensitive method that enhances understanding and supports decision making. ■ Safeguard against inserting racial or cultural stereotypes, biases, and prejudices that may affect patient care and safety.
Stress and Coping	Impaired coping → absence of self-care → stress, anxiety, or mild depression → errors in patient care	■ Identify and acknowledge stressors. ■ Evaluate the efficacy of personal coping methods. ■ Develop healthy, effective coping methods.

self [which] rejects approaching the patient–client as an object and strives instead to actualize an authentic personal relationship between two persons" (p. 19). In order to do this, the nurse must be willing to critically reflect on his own thoughts, emotions, and actions in a professional context.

Ethical Knowing

The last form of knowledge pattern is **ethical knowing**, which Carper (1978) calls the "moral component" (p. 20). She clarified that this type of knowing is more extensive than the

ethical codes by which nurses are expected to abide; it also encompasses "all voluntary actions that are deliberate and subject to the judgment of right and wrong" (p. 20). Sometimes nurses grapple with situations in which values and beliefs prove to be incompatible. To develop this pattern of knowledge, nurses must be aware of and fully understand the current codes of ethics outlined for nurses, in addition to the values held by the institution in which they work. Furthermore, they should possess "an understanding of different philosophical positions regarding what is good, what ought to be desired, what is right; of different ethical frameworks devised for dealing with the complexities of moral judgments; and of various orientations to the notion of obligation" (p. 20).

Clinical Example A

Mr. Bahdoon Osman, a 57-year-old man from Somalia, immigrated to Minnesota 5 years ago with his wife, son, and three daughters. Three days ago, he was rushed to the hospital for breathing and swallowing difficulties, the cause of which was a large tumor. Following emergent surgical resection of the tumor, Mr. Osman was diagnosed with stage IV esophageal cancer. The family is adamant that Mr. Osman not be informed of his terminal diagnosis, because Somali culture believes it is cruel to do so. The patient's physician has presented his treatment options.

The charge nurse instructed Mr. Osman's nurse, Joanne Williams, to speak only to the patient's son about Mr. Osman's care and not to his wife, explaining that according to Somali traditions, the father speaks for the family when outside the home. When the father is unable to do so, another adult man in the family, often the son, takes on the responsibility. The nurse finds this instruction challenging, especially seeing the obvious pain the patient's wife is in watching her husband suffer. The son tells Joanne that it is important that they reposition Mr. Osman's bed "so that it faces Mecca." Because Joanne does not understand the son's request, she asks Mr. Osman's wife for further explanation. His wife avoids Joanne's gaze and does not answer. The son firmly explains to Joanne that his mother does not have a say in the matter and repeats the request. Frustrated and upset at the lack of respect for Mr. Osman's wife, Joanne curtly responds by saying it is impossible to move the bed and leaves the room.

Critical Thinking Questions

1. Did Joanne demonstrate caring? If so, how?
2. How could have Joanne dealt with the Osman family differently?
3. What strategies could Joanne have employed to address culturally specific healthcare issues for the family?

Caring Encounters and Holistic Nursing

The healthcare field is moving from its traditional focus on disease management to a more holistic patient-focused approach to care. The American Holistic Nurses Association (AHNA) (2016a) defines holistic nursing as "all nursing practice that has healing the whole person as its goal." It is a philosophy and attitude that facilitates healing by recognizing the intertwined relationships among the "body, mind, emotion, spirit, social/cultural, relationship, context, and environment." Nurses practicing the holistic approach seek to develop a bond with the patient to create a more personal and supportive environment. Complementing traditional treatments with alternative therapies, such as reiki, meditation, biofeedback, and journaling, is also an important part of holistic nursing (Dossey & Keegan, 2012). The goal is to go beyond addressing the illness in order to help patients achieve balance in their lives. In this respect, it places the nurse in the role of health educator and emphasizes the patient's personal responsibility in maintaining health.

This approach to nursing has become more relevant in the face of the nation's changing demographics. Increasingly, the general population is turning to complementary and integrative health practices, formerly known as "alternative" medicine, to address health issues. *Complementary* is a term that

Focus on Integrative Health
How "Alternative" Is Complementary and Integrative Health in Nursing Today?

A growing number of adults and children in the United States have used healthcare approaches developed outside of Western, or conventional, medicine (NCCIH, 2016b). True alternative medicine is uncommon, because most people in the United States who use nonmainstream approaches use them along with conventional treatments (NCCIH, 2016b).

Integrative healthcare involves combining conventional and complementary approaches together in a coordinated way. NIH-affiliated researchers are currently exploring the potential benefits of integrative health in a variety of situations. Some of these include pain management for military personnel and veterans, using mindfulness meditation and self-hypnosis; relief of symptoms in cancer patients and survivors, using acupuncture and meditation; and programs to promote healthy behaviors using yoga and meditation- and mindfulness-based approaches (NCCIH, 2016b).

refers to a nonmainstream medical therapy or product used together with conventional medical practice, while the term *integrative* refers to a nonmainstream practice combined with conventional medicine. The latest figures from the National Health Interview Survey indicate that 32.2% of adults and almost 12% of children had made use of complementary health approaches in 2012 (National Center for Complementary and Integrative Health [NCCIH], 2016a). See the Focus on Integrative Health feature for more information.

Nurses must educate themselves on complementary health approaches and understand that not all alternative therapies work for all people, and some may even be harmful. Holistic understanding of the patient is required to advise patients on appropriate therapeutic interventions and treatments. Understanding the patient's context is of great importance when deciding on care strategies. For example, recommending costly supplements that can only be found in a few select specialty shops for an older adult who lives alone with limited mobility and income would prove problematic.

Nursing Presence

Presencing is a nursing concept developed by Rosemarie Rizzo Parse that involves the interpersonal arts of perception and communication. Through presencing, the nurse immerses himself in an interaction with the patient that helps the patient define her health choices. It is the patient, then, who has the authority to make decisions about her health. The nurse acts as a guide through his presence, not in the sense that the nurse tends to the patient, but rather by being open, receptive, and available at all levels without judging or labeling. The nurse's thinking flows with the patient's, and the value systems of the patient direct outcomes, not those of the nurse. Parse described presencing as "face-to-face discussions, silent immersions, and lingering presence" (as cited in George, 2011, p. 493). In this sort of interaction, the nurse lets the other lead, which could involve dialoguing, simply being there (even if silently), and leaving a lasting memory of the interaction in the patient's mind.

Another important nursing concept in this regard is *intentionality*, which refers to a nurse working in conjunction with those involved in the situation at hand as a cooperative force rather than attempting to impose her will. It is a philosophical mindset that surrenders the idea of directing outcomes and setting goals; instead, the nurse allows resistance to dissolve and a course of action to unfold (Watson, 2002). This perspective of "intentionality seeks to access the universal, life-spirit energy via manifesting one's deep intentional focus on a specific mental object of attention and awareness . . . [thus inviting] spirit-energy to enter into one's life and work, and into the caring-healing processes and outcomes" (p. 14).

Empowerment

Empowerment is a process whereby the patient develops the autonomy to identify her own health needs in lieu of being instructed how to do so (Berman et al., 2016). George (2011) said, "The basic element of empowerment is taking action to generate positive results at both the individual and the organizational level" (p. 199). Nurses, having established personal relationships of mutual respect, trust, and confidence with their patients, are in a unique position to empower them, thus increasing their independence. Nurses can facilitate empowerment by instructing patients on how they should perform certain functions, and in cases where a patient's abilities are hindered, provide only the amount of assistance that is absolutely necessary. In addition, nurses can provide information and resources to patients and their families, explain what they can expect beyond their hospital stay, and give voice to their concerns and desires to administrators and others providing care.

Compassion

When describing the ideal nurse, **compassion** is a must, but debate exists within the nursing community about how to precisely define this quality. It is not uncommon for the terms *compassion* or *compassionate care* to be used interchangeably with other characteristics such as caring, sympathy, and empathy, highlighting the subjective nature of the concept (Bramley & Matiti, 2014). Compassion is not something a nurse can learn through academic study, but only through the willingness to become intimately involved with the patient's experience. This often involves providing comfort to the patient—anything from validating the patient's experience through attentive listening and eye contact to holding the patient's hand in moments of pain, from adjusting the patient's position in bed to gently providing a warm sponge bath (see **Figure 35–2 》**). Another aspect of expressing compassion involves respecting the patient's spiritual beliefs or lack thereof, regardless of the nurse's personal opinions and values. Although nurses frequently cite time constraints as a barrier to compassion, research has shown that even brief interactions with patients can convey compassion, and that patients see compassion as closely aligned to the broader concept of conveying care within nursing practice (Bramley & Matiti, 2014).

Competence

Similar to Roach's (2002) description of competence, Takase and Teraoka (2011) define **competence** "as the ability of a

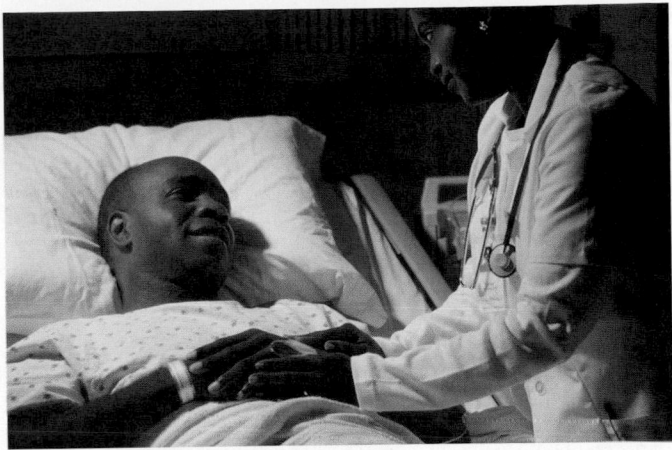

Source: Juan Silva Productions/Getty Images.

Figure 35–2 》 This nurse is using touch and presence to help comfort her patient.

nurse to effectively demonstrate a set of attributes, such as personal characteristics, professional attitude, values, knowledge, and skills, and to fulfill his/her professional responsibility through their practice. A competent person must possess these attributes, have the motivation and ability to use them, and must effectively use them to provide safe, effective, and professional nursing care to his/her patient" (p. 398). They outline specific attributes inherent in competence, including cognitive ability, participating in professional development, having an awareness of ethical and legal practices, guaranteeing quality and safety in care, and building relationships with patients and fellow nurses. Competence and compassion must coexist or patient care inevitably suffers. Competence without compassion can be, at best, off-putting and, at worst, impersonal and insensitive. Compassion in the absence of competence, however, presents real threats to patients' safety and health.

The classic theory regarding the development of nursing competence is Benner's (1982) novice-to-expert research on the lengthy process of nursing skills acquisition. Benner and Wrubel (1989) extended the thesis begun in the novice-to-expert work that caring is central to human expertise, to curing, and to healing. One of the unique goals of the latter publication was to distinguish the nursing perspective from purely psychologic, physiologic, or biomedical views (Benner & Wrubel, 1989).

Clinical Example B

Mrs. Julie Briggs is a 29-year-old woman who has undergone a left-breast lumpectomy, which also involved removing cancerous lymph nodes. As a result, she has been admitted to the hospital for a brief recovery period. The first postoperative day, Mrs. Briggs's nurse, Tomas Crespo, overhears an argument between the patient and her father, who is pressuring his daughter to have a double mastectomy as a preventive course of treatment because the patient's mother lost her life to breast cancer at age 36. Mrs. Briggs tells her father that she and her husband hope to conceive a child within the next year and she desperately wants to experience the bonding experience of breastfeeding. As he listens, Tomas is reminded of his wife's difficulty in breastfeeding and thinks the patient shouldn't place so much importance on it. After the patient's father leaves, Tomas enters the room and finds Mrs. Briggs crying. He pulls up a chair and asks her if she wants to talk. Mrs. Briggs says she's fine and collects herself. Tomas squeezes her hand and informs her that he is willing to listen, but she shakes her head no. While changing the patient's dressing, he allows a few minutes to pass before providing her with tips on how she can tend to her sutures when she is discharged in a couple of days, adding that he can also instruct her husband when he comes in later that evening. Upon completing Mrs. Briggs' care, Tomas tells her that there are support groups for young breast cancer survivors like her and promises to bring the information to her before the end of his shift.

Critical Thinking Questions

1. Did Tomas demonstrate presencing, empowerment, compassion, and competence in his interactions with Mrs. Briggs? If so, provide specific examples.
2. Could Tomas have approached the patient's dilemma differently? If so, how?

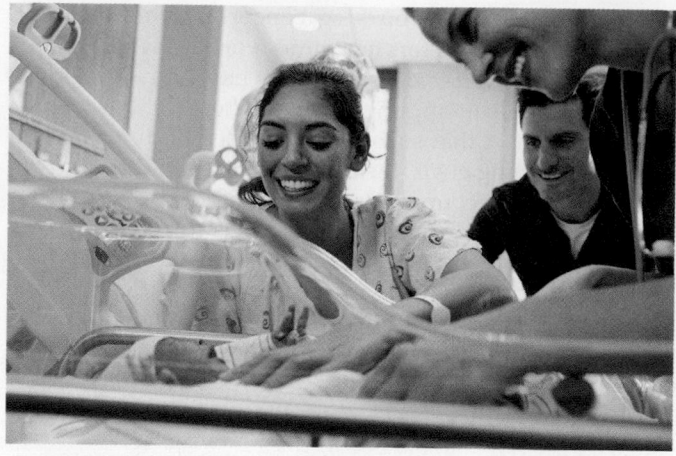

Source: Monkeybusinessimages/iStock/Getty Images.

Figure 35–3 》 Having the parents nearby when providing care for infants is soothing.

Lifespan Considerations

There are often some overarching themes that influence nurses as they provide caring interventions to patients of all ages. Obviously, one of the most important factors to consider, which is essential to all patient interactions and teaching, is the patient's developmental level. Developmental characteristics across the lifespan are discussed thoroughly in the module on Development. The presence of developmental delays and physical impairments will influence interactions with these patients and may require nurses to adjust delivery of their caring interventions to achieve optimal outcomes. Many areas can be impacted by developmental factors. Cultural and religious diversity, the presence of pain, the stress of a medical issue or emergency, the unfamiliar environment of the hospital or healthcare facility, and the context of the medical issue (e.g., accidents, chronic illnesses, the possibility of death, and associated psychologic issues such as grief and loss) all influence patient communication.

Furthermore, even though they may be performing caring interventions with only one patient, nurses often find that they are teaching and educating family members and caregivers at the same time. Thus, nurses find themselves accommodating a full range of developmental, psychologic, and sociocultural issues for several people when providing caring interventions. With the addition of family members and caregivers, caregiving becomes increasingly complicated and nuanced.

Caring Interventions for Infants

Nurses interacting with very young infants will likely find that as long as the environment is comfortable and a parent or caregiver present, infants will not object too much to being handled during caring interventions (see **Figure 35–3 》》**). Infants are fascinated by faces, and as they age they prefer faces that they know and recognize (Mash, Bornstein, & Arterberry, 2013). Babies are programmed to inherently provide important information—how they like to be treated, talked to, held, and comforted (American Academy of Pediatrics, 2016a). Aside from assessing developmental milestones and physical issues, nurses caring for infants must consider any pain or discomfort caused by interventions. Healthcare providers now know that infants experience

pain, and interventions such as sucking (with or without sucrose) or pain medications, depending on the procedure, are necessary (Stevens et al., 2014). Often in these cases, nurses must act as an advocate for the infant to receive pain-relieving interventions during routine procedures such as heelsticks and circumcision (Carter, 2013).

Other areas being assessed with parents and caregivers include whether infants, especially preterm infants, are thriving and gaining weight (American Academy of Pediatrics, 2016a); whether parents in vulnerable or underserved populations who are enrolled in early intervention or parenting programs are adequately caring for the child (Benzies et al., 2013); whether bonding seems to be taking place between infant and caregiver (American Academy of Pediatrics, 2016b); and the emotional and mental health of the mother and/or caregiver (Leis et al., 2014), with especial attention given to detection of postpartum depression (O'Hara & McCabe, 2013).

During the toddler years, physical growth and motor development will slow, but toddlers experience tremendous intellectual, social, and emotional changes. At this stage, parents may become concerned regarding speech and language development, temperament and personality traits such as shyness or aggression, and social isolation that may indicate autism (American Academy of Pediatrics, 2016c; Autism Speaks, 2016). Caring interventions will be affected by the toddlers' self-directed behavior and innate suspicion of strangers. Parents and caregivers will be necessary in providing care during this time.

Caring Interventions for Children

Children during the preschool and school years still need a parent or caregiver present during procedures. If a child has been exposed to uncomfortable medical procedures, he or she may be leery of or cry during caring interventions. Children at this stage become capable of developing psychic pain that the nurse may have to address. Some of the global issues facing children at this stage are stress, anger, conflict, and bullying; natural and human-caused disasters, such as terrorism and school shootings; poverty and uncertain housing; deployed parents and frequent moves (for children of military personnel); and emotional needs and emerging mental health problems (American Academy of Pediatrics, 2016d).

Caring Interventions for Adolescents

Adolescents may still need parents or caregivers present during times of medical challenge, such as surgery or an accident, but in general, they can handle medical procedures by themselves. They will also prefer privacy when interacting with healthcare providers. Nurses will find that adolescents will be more forthcoming with sensitive information regarding sexual practices and alcohol or drug use if questioned separately from their parents. Issues of concern with teens and parents include puberty; social development and relationships with peers, especially romantic attachments; gender identity; academic pressures; sexual, physical, and emotional abuse; and potential hazardous activities such as drunk driving and contact sports (American Academy of Pediatrics, 2016e). Parental relationship issues such as absent mothers or fathers, blended families with stepparents, or the presence of adopted/fostered children in the family may surge to the forefront during teen/family interactions with the provider (American Academy of Pediatrics, 2016f). The nurse may find that these issues, rather than a procedure or exam, become paramount during patient interactions.

Caring Interventions for Pregnant Women

Regardless of the caring intervention between the provider and pregnant woman, the nurse should keep in mind that he or she is always dealing with a dyad: the mother and the baby. Obviously, the expectant mother will assess every caring intervention in regard to its effect on the baby. Nurses must be sensitive to this concern and include this information in any patient teaching, especially regarding procedures, such as chorionic villus sampling to detect congenital abnormalities, that can present a genuine risk to the fetus (Mayo Clinic, 2016).

Nurses will also assess for signs of maternal alcohol or drug abuse and intimate partner violence (IPV). Pregnancy adds stress to interpersonal relationships and increases the incidence of IPV. The presence of partner alcohol misuse, jealousy, and suspicion of infidelity has been associated with psychologic and physical IPV victimization in the prenatal and postpartum periods (Hellmuth et al., 2013) and can lead to child abuse.

Research has indicated that the quality, rather than quantity, of prenatal care is more important to pregnant women (see **Figure 35–4** ⟫). Under ideal situations, prenatal care represents an opportunity for health promotion and illness prevention, screening and assessment, information sharing, continuity of care, non-medicalization of pregnancy, and women-centeredness (Sword et al., 2012). Pregnant women, especially those from vulnerable populations, form opinions regarding the quality of care based on access, physical setting, and staff and care provider characteristics. However, they rank as most important interpersonal care processes such as respectful attitude, emotional support, approachable interaction style, and taking time (Sword et al., 2012). The

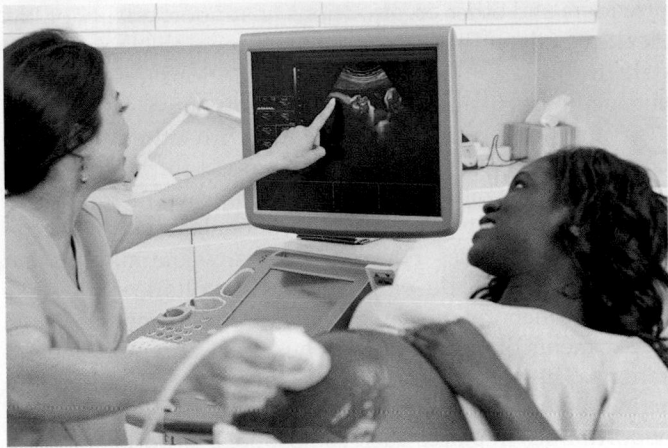

Source: Monkeybusinessimages/iStock/Getty Images.

Figure 35–4 ⟫ Having a good rapport with patients is important for nurses in an obstetrics practice.

meaningful relationship characterized by trust that exists between a woman and her prenatal care provider has been a recurrent theme in research. Nurses must respect this relationship in all interactions.

Caring Interventions for Adults

Perhaps the biggest obstacle clinicians face with adults is actually getting them to access healthcare. Lack of time and financial resources are large issues, as well as lack of health insurance coverage and lack of specialty providers in rural and less populated areas.

Many young and middle-aged adults can operate computers, although the abundance of poor-quality health information can complicate nurse–patient interventions and interactions. Nurses are encouraged to become aware of reliable internet sites for healthcare information and steer patients to them (Johns Hopkins Medicine, 2016). Another care issue is adults' increased reliance on retail clinics (e.g., drugstore chain walk-in clinics) for both acute and primary care. Although research has found that retail clinics handle new, simple medical conditions adequately, subsequent follow-up care is not as comprehensive as it would be with a primary care provider (Reid et al., 2013).

Finally, many young adults do not connect with the healthcare system for primary care. A large care gap emerges as young adults transition from pediatric care, monitored by parents, into autonomous primary care. The primary concern is that many young adults neglect getting care for chronic childhood conditions such as asthma and diabetes (American College of Physicians, 2016). In all caring interventions and interactions with adults, nurses can emphasize the importance of having a medical home and routinely monitoring and treating chronic conditions.

Caring Interventions for Older Adults

The term *active aging* refers to the fact that many older adults are aging independently or with limited assistance from friends, work associates, neighbors, and family members. Many older adults do not have chronic illnesses or cognitive decline and primarily seek interaction with care providers and other organizations to support quality of life. Healthy active older adults will seek complete and up-to-date information on caring interventions and will be engaged participants in their healthcare. Active older adults also seek opportunities to engage with others and live healthy, purposeful lives. Many may do so through interacting with organizations that work to improve the quality of life for older adults by creating vocational, social, and recreational opportunities. For example, many communities and organizations have developed extensive volunteer networks through collaborations among local Departments of Aging, Departments of Social Services, hospitals, and other organizations. These volunteer networks may recruit retired and active older adults to participate in meaningful volunteer opportunities in places such as hospitals, airports, libraries, and schools.

On the other hand, some older adults will develop physical and functional limitations and need to manage chronic medical conditions and comorbidities as they age. One of the largest issues elders face is securing care from providers, such as geriatricians, who can integrate all the findings from specialists into a comprehensive overview. There is a shortage of physicians and nurse providers of geriatric care in the United States because of factors such as limited payment, difficulty securing reimbursement from Medicare, and lower annual pay than other specialties (see **Figure 35–5** ≫) (AARP, 2016).

Nurses providing care to older adults should be mindful of negative attitudes that inhibit patient interactions: ageism, which is prejudice or discrimination based on age, and elderspeak, a type of simplified speech, characterized by shorter sentences and words, used when talking to older adults (Hanson, 2014). Research has shown that the primary factor causing negative nursing attitudes is lack of knowledge about gerontology and the aging process (Liu, Norman, & While, 2015). Other contributing factors are self-aging anxiety, commitment to nursing, and negative attitudes toward healthcare resources allocation among older people (Liu et al., 2015). Nurses can address these factors by continuing their education and by paying careful attention to patient–nurse interactions.

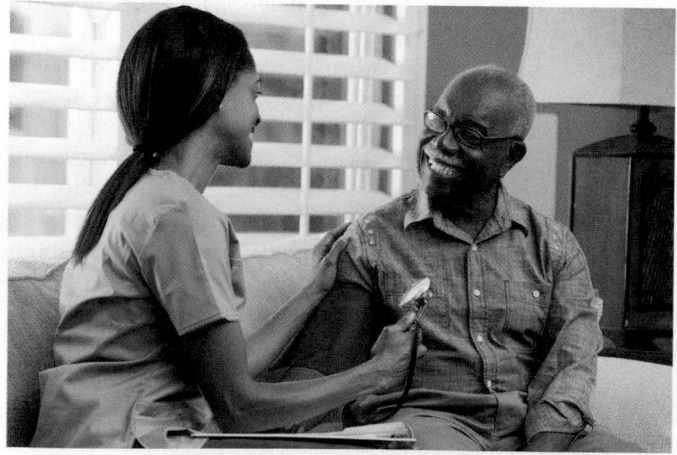

Source: Monkey Business Images Ltd/Monkey Business/Getty Images.

Figure 35–5 ≫ A home health nurse visits an older adult and provides palliative care.

Caring for the Caregiver: Self-Care in Nursing

Self-care is of vital importance in nursing and should not be treated as peripheral to patient care. George (2011) describes self-care as the activities an individual performs independently to ensure personal well-being and good health. Examples of such activities include a balanced diet, regular exercise, adequate rest and sleep, recreational activities, and meditation and/or prayer.

Self-care is particularly relevant to the nursing profession because nurses tend to overlook their own well-being while focusing on the health of others. According to the National Institute for Occupational Safety and Health (2016), "cases of nonfatal occupational injury and illness among healthcare workers are among the highest of any industry sector" (para. 3). Complicating the issue, healthcare is the fastest-growing sector of the U.S. economy, employing over 18 million workers, with women representing nearly 80% of the healthcare work force (National Institute for Occupational Safety and Health, 2015). Healthcare workers face a wide range of hazards on the job, including exposure to emerging pathogens, needlestick injuries, back injuries, latex allergy, violence, and stress.

In addition, the pressures of work, family, school, and community commitments experienced by nurses often lead to exhaustion, burnout, and stress with potentially debilitating effects on the quality of care delivered to patients. One study looking at nurses in the United States and Europe found that a substantial proportion of nurses in every country reported quality-of-care deficits, high nurse burnout, job dissatisfaction, and intention to leave their current positions (Aiken et al., 2012). The study concluded that modification of organizational behaviors toward nurses, improvement of the hospital work environment, and better nurse staffing would help retain a qualified and committed nurse workforce, improve hospital care safety and quality, and result in improved patient outcomes (Aiken et al., 2012).

Self-care for nurses encompasses more than just being physically fit and healthy. The practices that lead to increased well-being also build self-esteem, which in turn helps individuals problem-solve critically and face challenges more efficiently. Taking a self-esteem questionnaire helps individuals increase self-awareness by putting them in touch with their feelings and emotions; only through self-awareness can an individual begin to change those aspects that lower self-esteem. There are a number of self-esteem instruments available for use on the internet and at college counseling services. Worthy of note is the connection between self-awareness and self-control. A lack of self-awareness can contribute to decreased emotional control (Faguy, 2012), which could be problematic for nurses and the patients receiving their care.

AHNA (2016b) has maintained that holistic nursing practice requires the integration of self-care and personal development activities into one's life. Holistic nurses engage in self-assessment, self-care, and personal development, aware of being instruments of healing. Holistic nurses value themselves and mobilize the necessary resources to care for themselves, striving to achieve harmony and balance in their own lives and assisting others to do the same.

Evidence-Based Practice
Recognizing and Preventing Burnout in New Nurse Graduates

Problem

Nurses often function in high-pressure, short-staffed situations and are subject to rotating schedules and extended shifts. Despite the challenges associated with functioning in such an intense work environment, nurses tend to ignore feelings of fatigue, exhaustion, depression, and job dissatisfaction, believing that their colleagues must be feeling the same way. Consequently, many push self-care to the bottom of their list of priorities, ignoring even their most basic needs in order to meet job demands. This cycle leads to burnout.

The effects of nursing burnout take not only a personal emotional and physical toll, but they also adversely impact quality of care and patient satisfaction and lead to high turnover rates, contributing to the nursing shortage, which inevitably leads to even more burnout (Aiken et al., 2012; Chau et al., 2015). Much research has validated the relationship between poor patient outcomes, including 30-day inpatient mortality and failure-to-rescue rates, and factors such as nursing staffing levels, skill mix of baccalaureate-prepared registered nurses, and the overall nurse practice environment (Aiken et al., 2012; Chau et al., 2015).

Evidence

Most researchers have agreed that burnout consists of three components: emotional exhaustion, cynicism, and diminished personal efficacy, with emotional exhaustion and cynicism being considered the core elements of burnout (Spence Laschinger & Fida, 2014). Similar to other helping professions, the prevalence of burnout in nursing is particularly high because of the high emotional and physical demands of the work. Nursing burnout overall has been associated with heavy workloads, inadequate staffing levels, job dissatisfaction, absenteeism, turnover, depression, and career dissatisfaction (Ahola et al., 2014).

Alarmingly, new graduate nurses have the highest risk of experiencing burnout, with as many as 66% of new graduates experiencing severe burnout, primarily related to negative workplace conditions (Pineau Stam et al., 2015; Spence Laschinger & Fida, 2014). Moreover, approximately 17.5% of new nurses leave their first job within 1 year of starting their jobs (Kovner et al., 2014). Many factors causing burnout in recent graduates mirrored the concerns of experienced nurses. New-graduate burnout has been significantly related to lack of supervisor support, unmanageable workloads, absenteeism and turnover intentions, lower organizational commitment, and depression (Ahola et al., 2014).

A significant factor, usually considered to be part of the unfavorable working environment, is bullying or horizontal violence. Typically, nursing peers, physicians, or patient families were the main sources of bullying; some 29.5% of U.S. nurse graduates in one study had considered leaving the nursing profession because of bullying (Vogelpohl et al., 2013). Education of staff and authentic leadership committed to extinguishing horizontal violence are imperative for identifying and correcting negative behaviors in the workplace (Rush et al., 2014; Spence Laschinger, Wong, & Grau, 2012; Vogelpohl et al., 2013).

The personal and workplace resources can prevent new-graduate burnout. Research has shown that psychologic capital, structural empowerment, and perceived staffing adequacy were significant independent predictors of job satisfaction in recent graduates (Pineau Stam et al., 2015). Managers should ensure that empowerment structures are in place to support new graduate nurses' job satisfaction. Interventions that specifically support nurse graduates include orientation processes and ongoing management support that build psychologic capital in new graduate nurses and create positive perceptions of the workplace, thus enhancing job satisfaction (Pineau Stam et al., 2015).

Some of the essential components of successful programs for transitioning nurse graduates into the workplace have been identified. Formal new graduate transition programs have resulted in good retention and improved competency. Evidence has suggested that new graduate education should focus on practical skill development; preceptors should receive a level of formal training; formal support, including respectful feedback to improve confidence and competence in practice, should be available at least through the difficult 6- to 9-month post-hire period; opportunities for connection with their peers should be provided; and organizations should strive to ensure that clinical units operate with healthy work environments (for example, by allocating patient responsibilities commensurate with the new nurse's beginning skill set) (Phillips, Esterman, & Kenny, 2015; Rush et al., 2013).

Implications

Because burnout is detrimental to both the nurse and the patient, it is crucial that nurses recognize the signs and symptoms of this phenomenon. The Maslach Burnout Inventory (Maslach & Jackson, 1981) is the most widely used tool for measuring burnout (Poghosyan, Aiken, & Sloane, 2009). This questionnaire, which is designed to identify burnout, groups symptoms into three categories:

- **Emotional exhaustion.** This is one of the earliest signs of burnout and can cause headaches, insomnia, indigestion, and weight fluctuations. It may manifest itself as feelings of dread about going to work. Examples include uncontrollable crying, queasiness, and/or headaches during the nurse's commute.

- **Personal accomplishment.** Overworked nurses tend to feel that patients, supervisors, and hospital administrators do not appreciate their efforts. This can lead to underperformance, which is an adaptive response to stress.

- **Depersonalization.** When a nurse no longer feels compassion for some of her patients, it could cause insensitive behavior when providing care.

New graduate nurses experiencing any of these symptoms should seek the advice of colleagues and supervisors on how to overcome burnout. Strategies include physical exercise, talking it through, reducing patient load, learning to say "no" to extra assignments and committee appointments, switching shifts, and even changing jobs. Burnout is a sign that something must change. Nurses who choose to ignore it will discover that the symptoms and negative consequences of those symptoms will only worsen.

Critical Thinking Application

1. How can a nurse differentiate between the typical stress experienced by all healthcare professionals and burnout?

2. A nurse is experiencing symptoms of burnout and has approached her supervisor for support and guidance. The supervisor tells her it is simply a part of working as a caregiver and to "push through it." What steps can this nurse take to cope and improve her situation?

3. A nurse observes one of his colleagues being brusque with patients (e.g., lack of eye contact, not providing direct answers, cutting off patients when speaking). When he questions his coworker, she says that she doesn't want to get too emotionally involved with her patients and is just maintaining a healthy distance between them. He knows that she is also going through a difficult divorce and custody battle. What should he do?

Maslow's Hierarchy of Needs

Psychologist Abraham Maslow (1943, 1968) identified five levels of needs, the lower of which must be fulfilled before an individual can move to the next level and eventually achieve self-actualization, the highest level. For an illustration of Maslow's human needs hierarchy and a discussion of his work and its implication for the nursing care of patients, refer to the module on Stress and Coping.

Physiologic Needs

Physiologic needs are also referred to as survival needs and include the necessities of food, water, air, sleep, and shelter. For example, the extended work hours and rotating shifts common to the nursing profession make it challenging to maintain a regular eating schedule and sleep routine and to participate in regular physical activity. A lack of physical activity has been associated with high rates of lower back pain and other physical ailments reported by healthcare professionals (Sung, 2013).

Physiologic needs can be satisfied in healthy and unhealthy ways. Nurses practice self-care when they make healthy choices regarding food (e.g., by choosing fruit as a snack between meals), drinks (i.e., by drinking water instead of soft drinks), and sleep. Managing a sleep schedule can be particularly challenging, especially for nurses whose families operate on different schedules than the nurse. Physical recreational activities also help nurses cope with limited sleep while enhancing their fitness level. For more information, see the exemplars on Physical Fitness and Exercise and Normal Sleep–Rest Patterns in the module on Health, Wellness, Illness, and Injury.

Safety

Needs at this level have both physical and psychologic aspects, which include bodily safety, financial security, and personal health. The American Nurses Association's (ANA) *2011 Health and Safety Survey* (2013) reported that stress and overwork (74%) and musculoskeletal injury (62%) top the list of nurses' concerns; in addition, 34% of nurses reported concerns about physical assault by their patients, representing a 25% increase from the previous survey in 2001. Moreover, the ANA (2014) has recognized that nurse fatigue contributes to workplace errors and poor patient outcomes and has urged a stronger focus to prevent this problem. The ANA (2014) has endorsed some of the following recommendations:

- Involve nurses in the design of work schedules and use a regular and predictable schedule so nurses can plan for work and personal responsibilities.
- Limit work weeks to 40 hours within 7 days and work shifts to 12 hours.
- Eliminate the use of mandatory overtime as a "staffing solution."
- Promote frequent, uninterrupted rest breaks during work shifts.
- Enact official policy that confers RNs the right to accept or reject a work assignment based on preventing risks from fatigue. The policy should include conditions that a rejected assignment does not constitute patient abandonment, and that RNs should not experience adverse consequences in retaliation for such a decision.

Work–family conflict among nurses also has a negative effect on job satisfaction (Rantanen et al., 2013). When the quality of a nurse's personal and family life suffers, so does job performance, which directly impacts patient satisfaction and service quality.

Belonging and Love

According to Maslow, when the lower physical needs are met, an individual is in a position to address higher psychologic needs. The sense of love and belonging that comes from relationships with family, friends, and colleagues is particularly important to nurses, who depend on solid support networks to help them talk through and cope with pressures of work. Venting is a healthy way to unload stress, but it is vital that nurses maintain patient confidentiality at all times, even when venting to other nurses.

Unfortunately, new nurses may find their desire and efforts to fit in at work thwarted by a culture of bullying that is prevalent in the nursing profession. "Nurses eat their young" (Townsend, 2012) is an old, familiar refrain, and there is evidence to support it: As mentioned in the Evidence-Based Practice feature in this module, newly graduated nurses have significantly higher resignation rates in their first year of practice (Gaffney et al., 2012). Victims of bullying experience distress, anxiety, feelings of isolation, and depression, and they subsequently show an increased use of sick time. New graduates are particularly vulnerable because they often lack confidence in their skills and thus crave acceptance and positive feedback from their peers. In addition to adversely affecting job performance and satisfaction, bullying leads to increased absenteeism and staff turnover, therefore risking patient safety by interfering with teamwork, collaboration, and communication.

Clinical Example C

Mrs. Oden, the charge nurse on a medical–surgical unit, assigns extra patients to Celia Hammond, a new graduate nurse, in order to cover for a colleague who left unexpectedly to tend to a family emergency. Mr. Stephen Suskind, a 57-year-old man recovering from knee surgery, is among Celia's patients. In the early afternoon, Mr. Suskind falls while attempting to make his way to the bathroom unassisted. The sound of the fall and his subsequent cry prompt Celia to rush into his room. As Celia helps Mr. Suskind to stand, Mrs. Oden appears in the doorway and criticizes Celia harshly for having neglected her patient, as well as for attempting to move him after his fall. The commotion attracts the attention of other nurses on the floor, who stand behind Mrs. Oden, observing Celia as she is being chastised. Afterward, Celia discusses the incident with an experienced colleague who has worked at the hospital for more than a decade. When Celia complains about having been publicly humiliated, her colleague advises her to "suck it up" and closes the conversation by warning her that "no one likes a whiner."

Critical Thinking Questions

1. What should Celia do next?
2. How have Mrs. Oden, Celia's nurse colleague, and others reinforced a culture of bullying?
3. What actions might the nursing supervisor take to address incidents such as this one?

Self-esteem

Needs at this particular level include feelings of confidence, independence, competence, respect, and achievement. In nursing, a caregiver's self-esteem is based on how he/she is viewed by others. Nurses strive to be seen as competent and proficient and value the respect of peers. It is important for new nurses to realize that nursing proficiency comes through hands-on practice. Skills are improved and mastered over time; thus, new nurses should not compare themselves to more experienced colleagues by being overly self-critical. Instead, they should maintain a positive mindset and be open to learning. Knowledgeable, sympathetic preceptors can enhance the skills acquisition of new nurses during their orientation to a hospital or other healthcare facility.

A mentor can also play an important role in encouraging a new nurse's self-esteem needs by supporting the new nurse's skill development and sharing experiences. Many healthcare institutions have mentoring programs where new nurses are paired with established colleagues who serve to teach, counsel, aid, and encourage them. In cases where mentoring programs have not been institutionalized, new nurses can still reach out to experienced colleagues and build a mentoring relationship with someone whose style and behavior they admire (Sullivan, 2013).

Self-actualization

After meeting the lower-level needs, an individual can then strive to develop her maximum potential and fully realize her abilities and qualities. Part of self-actualization for nurses is the need to make time for themselves. This crucial aspect of self-care includes pursuing activities that bring joy and stimulate creativity. Artistic pursuits, such as writing, playing a musical instrument, and dancing, can serve as important outlets for self-expression. Hobbies are important to personal well-being, because they offer a healthy distraction from the pressures of work and encourage personal development. Taking a break to do nothing in particular is also an effective way to relax and reenergize.

Choosing Wellness

Wellness is a state of well-being involving sound nutrition, regular physical fitness, stable emotional health, self-responsibility, dynamic personal and professional growth, and preventive healthcare. Currently, nurses are promoting patient wellness through the *Healthy People 2020* program, which builds on efforts dating back to 1979 when the Surgeon General issued the original *Healthy People* report (Berman et al., 2016). (See the exemplars on Physical Fitness and Exercise and Normal Sleep-Rest Patterns in the module on Health, Wellness, and Illness for specifics.) Nurses would do well to adopt the same healthy principles in their own lives.

Avoiding Unhealthy Behaviors

In addition to adapting healthy behaviors, self-care is also about avoiding unhealthy ones. Smoking, abusing alcohol and drugs, and misusing medications are all destructive lifestyle choices that impact a nurse's personal and professional life.

An estimated 10–15% of all nurses may be impaired by or in recovery from some form of drug or alcohol addiction (Thomas & Siela, 2011). However, only a small percentage of the employed nursing population has been identified with substance use problems in the United States and its territories (Monroe et al., 2013). Approximately 71% of impaired nurses do enroll in substance abuse monitoring programs, which are viewed as less punitive than disciplinary programs run by state boards. The prevalence of nurses identified with a substance use problem requiring an intervention and treatment is lower than the prevalence of those receiving substance abuse treatment in the general population (0.51% vs. 1.0%) (Monroe et al., 2013).

Another major concern is the alcohol- or substance-impaired student nurse who increases risks to consumers by unsafe practice. Nursing students are at risk for alcohol and substance use for various reasons: lack of addiction/alcohol education; stress/anxiety from nursing program expectations; unhealthy habits, social isolation, and individual influences; peer influence/the college experience; and ineffective and unenforced campus policies (Nair et al., 2016). There has been little recent research about the numbers of nursing students with alcohol- and substance-use issues, but statistics presumably are in line with those of the general college population regarding to frequency of use and substance preference. One identified issue has been inconsistency among national and state healthcare organizations, clinical agencies, and colleges and universities regarding educational/professional policies addressing impaired nursing students (McCulloh Nair et al., 2015).

Nurses with a substance abuse problem are in a unique position given their access to drugs in the workplace. Further, beyond the harm they do to themselves, substance-abusing nurses may also inadvertently harm patients in their care. Fellow nurses are usually required to report impaired colleagues to management, and it is therefore vital that they recognize the telltale signs of substance abuse. Nurses with a drug or alcohol problem may exhibit one or more of the manifestations described in the module on Addiction (e.g., mood swings, tremors, slurred speech, or unsteady gait), as well as any of the following: discrepancies in documentation of controlled substances; volunteering to medicate coworkers' patients; wearing long sleeves in hot weather; committing frequent errors in care, particularly medication errors; arriving to work early or staying late; and coming in when not scheduled to work.

Workplace risk factors for substance use among nurses include the following (Bettinardi-Angres, Pickett, & Patrick, 2012):

- Easy access, role strain, and enabling behaviors by peers
- Seeing drugs as an acceptable means of coping with life's problems
- Developing an overarching faith in the ability of drugs to promote healing
- Rationalizing drug use on the basis of needing to continue working
- Feeling invulnerable to illnesses
- Developing a permissive attitude toward self-diagnosing
- Self-treating physical pain or stress.

Fellow nurses can help by making abusers aware of the issue and encouraging them to seek assistance options, such as counseling and treatment programs. Before reporting a colleague to management, a nurse may wish to give the fellow nurse the opportunity to self-report. Administrators tend to look more favorably on nurses who admit to their substance abuse problems (Cadiz et al., 2015). Nurses should especially keep an eye out for colleagues who have experienced a recent stressful life event, such as an accident or a divorce, because these experiences tend to increase the likelihood of resorting to some form of substance abuse to cope with the situation (Thomas & Siela, 2011).

Addiction is considered to be an illness. Nurses experiencing substance abuse should be referred to treatment, not punished. The majority of states have alternative-to-discipline programs (ADPs) affiliated with or recognized by their state boards of nursing. Increasingly, professional associations such as state nurses' associations are providing resources to help nurses recover from alcohol and drug addiction.

>> Stay Current: For more information about nurses and substance abuse, visit https://www.ncsbn.org/substance-use-in-nursing.htm.

Choosing Healthy Behaviors

A healthy lifestyle is particularly important to nurses for two main reasons: (1) They must maintain strong immune systems in order to work with people who are ill and (2) they should act as role models so as to maintain credibility when advising others about healthy choices. Balance and moderation are the keys to a healthy lifestyle, and this is especially true with respect to nutrition and exercise.

Because personal physical, mental, and emotional health is integral to successful nursing practice, the ANA has published a book on the subject, *Self-care and You: Caring for the Caregiver* (Richards, Sheen, & Mazzer, 2014). Suggestions include the following: Maintain a regular eating schedule; eat balanced, nutritious foods throughout the day; exercise at least three times a week (e.g., take a walk, work out, participate in sports); set aside time for rest and relaxation; seek the company of supportive people; do something enjoyable every day (e.g., play a musical instrument, cook, read, watch TV); avoid tobacco, alcohol, and drugs; maintain an optimistic attitude; set limits with others; and prioritize tasks (Richards et al., 2014).

Maintaining a regular eating schedule is a challenge in a profession where rotating shifts and unexpected events are the norm. Nonetheless, nurses need to make time to address their nutritional needs and not wait until the effects of hunger and thirst (pangs, dizziness, seeing spots, and so on) are felt. Nurses can accomplish this by planning ahead and making sure that healthy snacks and fresh water are on hand to consume at predetermined moments of the work shift. Nurses with physically demanding tasks often make the mistake of thinking they are getting enough physical exercise at work; however, standing for long periods of time, lifting patients, and performing other tasks that require physical exertion are not likely to build muscle tone or contribute to cardiovascular fitness (see **Figure 35–6 >>**) (Richards et al., 2014).

Self-awareness is the key to effective self-care. It involves self-discovery and leads to personal insights. For instance, a self-aware individual is able to identify personal strengths and weaknesses and is conscious of the assumptions, beliefs, values, and prejudices that can impair judgment. Through self-awareness, a nurse gains greater understanding of others, as well as increased respect and empathy for them (Sergeant

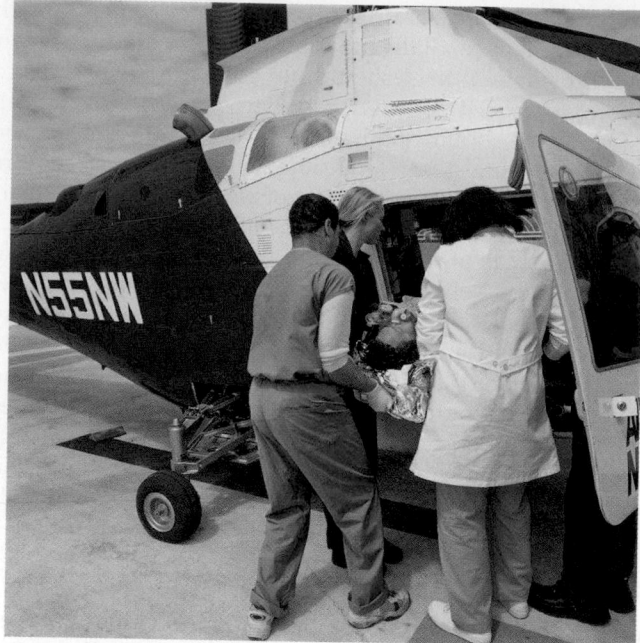

Source: Chad Baker/Jason Reed/Ryan McVay/Photodisc/Getty Images.

Figure 35–6 >> Many nursing tasks are physically demanding. Nurses should incorporate regular exercise into their schedules to build muscle tone and fitness.

& Laws-Chapman, 2012). Koren and Papamiditriou (2013) suggested that nurses take time to reflect and think about questions such as why they chose to go into nursing and what motivates them to go in to work every day.

In addition, nurses should take advantage of the support services available to them. At some healthcare facilities, nurses come together for weekly support groups to discuss their cases, providing a venue for them to reflect on their work and receive the benefit of their peers' experiences. Hospital chaplains are also available to listen to and support nurses (Koren & Papamiditriou, 2013). For problems such as addiction and depression or health promotion activities such as engaging in a wellness program, nurses may be able to turn to employee assistance programs that are part of their employee benefits (Claxton et al., 2013).

Several professional associations, such as AHNA and state nursing organizations, provide programs and additional resources to help nurses cope with the stressors and pressures of their everyday lives. Online services, such as community forums, offer nurses a safe space where they can vent freely to others who understand the issues they face. Nurses must remember to respect patient privacy and confidentiality during group discussions or in online forums.

REVIEW The Concept of Caring Interventions

RELATE Link the Concepts

Linking the concept of caring interventions with the concept of health, wellness, and illness:

1. Apply theories of caring to discuss how the benefits of self-care (improved physical fitness, overall health, self-esteem, and self-actualization) impact patient care.

2. Explain the relationship between self-care and wellness. Is the absence of illness a requirement for wellness? Why or why not?

Linking the concept of caring interventions with the concept of comfort:

3. In the psychosocial realm, how would an absence of genuine caring impact the nursing care for a patient who is receiving end-of-life care?

4. Describe the application of presencing when caring for the family members of a patient who is receiving end-of-life care.

Linking the concept of caring interventions with the concept of communication:

5. From the patient's perspective, how might inadequate self-care affect facets of the nurse's nonverbal communication, such as personal appearance and facial expression?

6. How does confidence, identified by Roach as a caring trait, impact the quality of communication between the nurse and the patient?

READY Go to Volume 3: Clinical Nursing Skills

All of *Volume 3: Clinical Nursing Skills* is devoted to individual caring interventions. The book is conveniently indexed to facilitate quick access to the step-by-step nursing skills. Often, nursing skills take place within the context of a nursing assessment, monitoring vital signs, or administering medications. Here are some links to performing these foundation skills:

- SKILL 1.1   Appearance and Mental Status: Assessing
- SKILL 1.5   Blood Pressure: Newborn, Infant, Child, Adult, Obtaining
- SKILL 1.9   Temperature, Newborn, Infant, Child, Adult, Obtaining
- SKILL 1.22   Neurologic Status: Assessing
- SKILL 2.11   Medications: Preparing and Administering

Finally, keep in mind that many hospitals and healthcare facilities maintain protocols and procedure guidelines for nurses and educational handouts for patients on the facility's intranet, or internal computer network. Nurses should be able to access these documents from computer workstations within the facility.

REFER Go to Pearson MyLab Nursing and eText

- Additional review materials

REFLECT Apply Your Knowledge

Ms. Ann Mah, a 26-year-old single woman, was admitted to the hospital following an automobile crash. She lost consciousness at the wheel while driving home from the gym by herself. Since her admission, she has been diagnosed with a neck injury, and a neurologic workup revealed she has epilepsy. Her nurse, Michael Robbins, is monitoring her blood pressure and assessing her for side effects related to her newly prescribed anticonvulsant medication, valproate (Depakote).

When Michael enters the room, he finds Ms. Mah gazing out the window. When he asks how she is doing, she responds with a curt "Fine." As he goes through his list of questions, she answers with just one or two words. He senses that she is a very private person, so he avoids asking her personal questions. Later in the day, he asks his mentor for advice on the case, who tells him to be patient and allow the patient time to open up. His mentor also informs him that some patients diagnosed with chronic illness may experience the diagnosis as a loss of their ideal selves and have difficulty accepting the diagnosis at first.

After his next assessment, Michael decides to spend an extra 5 minutes with Ms. Mah. He sits by her bedside quietly, observing her out of the corner of his eye as he pretends to review her file. Suddenly, she blurts out:

"I hate this! My life was perfect. I was promoted to regional director of sales last week. I drove around all over the city and I had a great social life. Now you tell me I'm epileptic. What are they going to say at work?"

Michael responds, "I hear your concern that the diagnosis of epilepsy may interfere with your life and work. And you're right, epilepsy does require adjustments. But you are the same woman you were before the accident. Except that now you know that the woman who was promoted to regional sales director has epilepsy. Tell me what else you're concerned about."

Ms. Mah looks away. "With this stupid medicine, I can't keep any food down!"

"I know that's frustrating, but it is important that we try to prevent another seizure, especially because of your neck injury. The idea is to gradually reduce the dosage to lessen the side effects as much as possible while still controlling the seizures. Does that make sense?"

"Yes, but I really don't want to take medication the rest of my life, especially not this stuff."

Michael nods his head to show that he's listening and answers, "I understand that. Let's do this: I'll email the attending provider who is managing your care and ask her to come around and discuss the medication with you. Would that be all right?"

Ms. Mah turns her head to look at Michael. "Yes. Thank you."

Michael says, "I know you're concerned about work and returning to your social life. How about we come up with a plan for how you might begin to manage your epilepsy after you leave here?"

Ms. Mah replies, "I'd like that. I spoke with my sister yesterday. She told me there are other ways to treat epilepsy. She mentioned acupuncture."

"I've heard that, too. Let's look into it and talk about some more ideas the next time I see you. Deal?"

Michael stretches out his hand and after a few seconds Ms. Mah takes it and they shake on it.

At his next assessment, Michael finds Ms. Mah reading information from an epilepsy website off a tablet.

"How are you today, Ms. Mah?" Michael asks.

"Fine. Today, I'll be asking the questions," Ms. Mah says.

1. Which caring theories are relevant to this case?

2. Which holistic approaches did Michael employ?

3. How did Michael's self-care aid him in caring for Ms. Mah?

References

AARP. (2016). *Where are the doctors you'll need?* Retrieved from http://www.aarp.org/health/conditions-treatments/info-2016/geriatrician-geriatric-doctor-physician.html

Ahola, K., Hakanen, J., Perhoniemi, R., & Mutanen, P. (2014). Relationship between burnout and depressive symptoms: A study using the person-centred approach. *Burnout Research, 1*(1), 29–37. doi:http://dx.doi.org/10.1016/j.burn.2014.03.003

Aiken, L. H., Sermeus, W., Van den Heede, K., Sloane, D. M., Busse, R., McKee, M., . . . Kutney-Lee, A. (2012). Patient safety, satisfaction, and quality of hospital care: Cross sectional surveys of nurses and patients in 12 countries in Europe and the United States. *BMJ, 344*. doi:10.1136/bmj.e1717. Published by BMJ Publishing Group Ltd, © 2012.

American Academy of Pediatrics. (2016a). *Ages and stages.* Retrieved from https://www.healthychildren.org/english/ages-stages/pages/default.aspx

American Academy of Pediatrics. (2016b). *Emotional and social development: Birth to 3 months.* Retrieved from https://www.healthychildren.org/English/ages-stages/baby/Pages/Emotional-and-Social-Development-Birth-to-3-Months.aspx

American Academy of Pediatrics. (2016c). *Social development: 2 year olds.* Retrieved from https://www.healthychildren.org/English/ages-stages/toddler/Pages/Social-Development-2-Year-Olds.aspx

American Academy of Pediatrics. (2016d). *Emotional wellness.* Retrieved from https://www.healthychildren.org/english/healthy-living/emotional-wellness/pages/default.aspx

American Academy of Pediatrics. (2016e). *Teen.* Retrieved from https://www.healthychildren.org/English/ages-stages/teen/Pages/default.aspx

American Academy of Pediatrics. (2016f). *Family dynamics.* Retrieved from https://www.healthychildren.org/english/family-life/family-dynamics/pages/default.aspx

American College of Physicians. (2016). *ACP Pediatric to Adult Care Transitions Initiative: About this project.* Retrieved from https://www.acponline.org/clinical-information/high-value-care/resources-for-clinicians/pediatric-to-adult-care-transitions-initiative/about

American Holistic Nurses Association (AHNA). (2016a). *What is holistic nursing?* Retrieved from http://www.ahna.org/About-Us/What-is-Holistic-Nursing

American Holistic Nurses Association (AHNA). (2016b). *What is self care?* Retrieved from http://www.ahna.org/Membership/Member-Advantage/What-is-self-care

American Humanist Association. (2016). *What is humanism?* Retrieved from http://americanhumanist.org/Humanism

American Nurses Association (ANA). (2013). *2011 Health and Safety Survey.* Retrieved from http://www.nursingworld.org/MainMenuCategories/WorkplaceSafety/SafeNeedles/2011-HealthSafety-Survey.html

American Nurses Association. (2014). *How to cope with stress on the job.* Retrieved from http://nursingworld.org/MainMenuCategories/Career-Center/Resources/How-to-Cope-with-Stress-on-the-Job.html

Andrews, M. M., & Boyle, J. S. (2016). *Transcultural concepts in nursing care* (7th ed.). Philadelphia, PA: Wolters Kluwer.

Autism Speaks. (2016). *Early intervention.* Retrieved from https://www.autismspeaks.org/family-services/tool-kits/100-day-kit/early-intervention

Benner, P. E. (1982). From novice to expert. *American Journal of Nursing, 82*(3), 402–407.

Benner, P. E., & Wrubel, J. (1989). *The primacy of caring: Stress and coping in health and illness.* Reading, MA: Addison-Wesley/Addison Wesley Longman.

Benner, P., & Wrubel, J. (2001). Response to: Edwards, S. D. (2001). Benner and Wrubel on caring in nursing. *Journal of Advanced Nursing, 33*(2), 167–171. Published by John Wiley & Sons, Inc., © 2001.

Benzies, K. M., Magill-Evans, J. E., Hayden, K. A., & Ballantyne, M. (2013). Key components of early intervention programs for preterm infants and their parents: A systematic review and meta-analysis. *BMC Pregnancy and Childbirth, 13*(1), 1–15. doi:10.1186/1471-2393-13-s1-s10

Berman, A., Snyder, S. J., & Frandsen, G. (2016). Pain management. In *Kozier and Erb's fundamentals of nursing: Concepts, process, and practice* (10th ed.). Hoboken, NJ: Pearson Education.

Bettinardi-Angres, K., Pickett, J., & Patrick, D. (2012). Substance use disorders and accessing alternative-to-discipline programs. *Journal of Nursing Regulation, 3*(2), 16–23.

Blais, K. (2015). *Professional nursing practice: Concepts and perspectives.* Upper Saddle River, NJ: Pearson.

Boykin, A., & Schoenhofer, S. O. (2001). *Nursing as caring: A model for transforming practice.* Sudbury, MA: Jones & Bartlett.

Bramley, L., & Matiti, M. (2014). How does it really feel to be in my shoes? Patients' experiences of compassion within nursing care and their perceptions of developing compassionate nurses. *Journal of Clinical Nursing, 23*(19–20), 2790–2799. doi:10.1111/jocn.12537

Brunton, B., & Beaman, M. (2000). Nurse practitioners' perceptions of their caring behaviors. *Journal of the American Academy of Nurse Practitioners, 12*(11), 451–456.

Burhans, L. M., & Alligood, M. R. (2010). Quality nursing care in the words of nurses. *Journal of Advanced Nursing, 66*(8), 1689–1697.

Cadiz, D. M., O'Neill, C., Schroeder, S., & Gelatt, V. (2015). Online education for nurse supervisors managing nurses enrolled in alternative-to-discipline programs. *Journal of Nursing Regulation, 6*(1), 25–32. doi:10.1016/s2155-8256(15)30006-5

Carper, B. (1978). Fundamental patterns of knowing in nursing. *Advances in Nursing Science 1*(1), 13–23.

Carter, B. (2013). *Child and infant pain: Principles of nursing care and management.* New York, NY: Springer.

Chau, J. P. C., Lo, S. H. S., Choi, K. C., Chan, E. L. S., McHugh, M. D., Tong, D. W. K., . . . Lee, D. T. F. (2015). A longitudinal examination of the association between nurse staffing levels, the practice environment and nurse-sensitive patient outcomes in hospitals. *BMC Health Services Research, 15*(1), 1–8. doi:10.1186/s12913-015-1198-0

Claxton, G., Rae, M., Panchal, N., Damico, A., Whitmore, H., Bostick, N., & Kenward, K. (2013). Health benefits in 2013: Moderate premium increases in employer-sponsored plans. *Health Affairs, 32*(9), 1667–1676. doi:10.1377/hlthaff.2013.0644

de Veer, A. J. E., Francke, A. L., Struijs, A., & Willems, D. L. (2013). Determinants of moral distress in daily nursing practice: A cross sectional correlational questionnaire survey. *International Journal of Nursing Studies, 50*(1), 100–108. doi:http://dx.doi.org/10.1016/j.ijnurstu.2012.08.017

Dossey, B. M., & Keegan, L. (2012). *Holistic nursing* (6th ed.). Burlington, MA: Jones & Bartlett.

Douglas, M. K., Pierce, J. U., Rosenkoetter, M., Pacquiao, D., Callister, L. C., Hattar-Pollara, M., . . . Purnell, L. (2011). Standards of practice for culturally competent nursing care: 2011 update. *Journal of Transcultural Nursing, 22*(4), 317.

Faguy, K. (2012). Emotional intelligence in healthcare. *Journal of the American Society of Radiologic Technologists, 83*(3), 237–253.

Gaffney, D. A., DeMarco, R. F., Hofmeyer, A., Vessey, J. A., & Budin, W. C. (2012). Making things right: Nurses' experiences with workplace bullying—A grounded theory. *Nursing Research and Practice.* Retrieved from http://www.hindawi.com/journals/nrp/2012/243210_doi:10.1155/2012/243210.

George, J. B. (Ed.). (2011). *Nursing theories: The base for professional nursing practice.* Upper Saddle River, NJ: Pearson Education.

Goh, Y.-S., Lee, A., Chan, S. W.-C., & Chan, M. F. (2015). Profiling nurses' job satisfaction, acculturation, work environment, stress, cultural values and coping abilities: A cluster analysis. *International Journal of Nursing Practice, 21*(4), 443-452. doi:10.1111/ijn.12318

Hanson, R. M. (2014). Is elderly care affected by nurse attitudes? A systematic review. *British Journal of Nursing, 23*(4), 225–229.

Hellmuth, J. C., Gordon, K. C., Stuart, G. L., & Moore, T. M. (2013). Risk factors for intimate partner violence during pregnancy and postpartum. *Archives of Women's Mental Health, 16*(1), 19–27. doi:10.1007/s00737-012-0309-8

Jarrin, O. F. (2012). The integrality of situated caring in nursing and the environment. *Advances in Nursing Science, 3*(1), 14–24. doi:10.1097/ANS.0b013e3182433b89. Published by Lippincott Williams and Wilkins, © 2012.

Johns Hopkins Medicine. (2016). *Finding reliable health information online.* Retrieved from http://www.hopkinsmedicine.org/johns_hopkins_bayview/patient_visitor_amenities/community_health_library/finding_reliable_health_information_online.html

Koren, M. E., & Papamiditriou, C. (2013). Spirituality of staff nurses: Application of modeling and role modeling theory. *Holistic Nurse Practitioner, 27*(1), 37–44.

Kovner, C. T., Brewer, C. S., Fatehi, F., & Jun, J. (2014). What does nurse turnover rate mean and what is the rate? *Policy, Politics, & Nursing Practice, 15*(3-4), 64–71. doi:10.1177/1527154414547953

Kutney-Lee, A., Wu, E. S., Sloane, D. M., & Aiken, L. H. (2013). Changes in hospital nurse work environments and nurse job outcomes: An analysis of panel data. *International Journal of Nursing Studies, 50*(2), 195–201. doi:10.1016/j.ijnurstu.2012.07.014

Lachman, V. D. (2012). Applying the ethics of care to your nursing practice. *MedSurg Nursing, 21*(2), 112–116. Published by MedSurg Nursing, © 2012.

Leininger, M. M. (1989). Transcultural nurse specialists and generalists: New practitioners in nursing. *Journal of Transcultural Nursing, 1*(1), 4–16. Published by Sage Publications, © 1989.

Leininger, M. M., & McFarland, M. R. (2006). *Culture care diversity and universality: A worldwide nursing theory.* Sudbury, MA: Jones & Bartlett.

Leis, J. A., Heron, J., Stuart, E. A., & Mendelson, T. (2014). Associations between maternal mental health and child emotional and behavioral problems: Does prenatal mental health matter? *Journal of Abnormal Child Psychology, 42*(1), 161–171. doi:10.1007/s10802-013-9766-4

Liu, Y.-E., Norman, I. J., & While, A. E. (2015). Nurses' attitudes towards older people and working with older patients: An explanatory model. *Journal of Nursing Management, 23*(8), 965-973. doi:10.1111/jonm.12242

Longo, J. (2011). Acts of caring: Nurses caring for nurses. *Holistic Nursing Practice,* 8–16.

Longo, J. (2013). Bullying and the older nurse. *Journal of Nursing Management, 21*(7), 950–955. doi:10.1111/jonm.12173

Mash, C., Bornstein, M. H., & Arterberry, M. E. (2013). Brain dynamics in young infants' recognition of faces. *Neuroreport, 24*(7), 359–363. doi:10.1097/WNR.0b013e32835f6828

Maslach, C., & Jackson, S. E. (1981). The measurement of experienced burnout. *Journal of Occupational Behaviour, 2*(2), 99–113.

Maslow, A. (1943). A theory of human motivation. *Psychological Review, 50*(4), 370–396.

Maslow, A. H. (1968). *Toward a psychology of being* (2nd ed.). New York, NY: Van Nostrand Reinhold.

Mayeroff, M. (1990). *On caring.* New York, NY: HarperCollins.

Mayo Clinic. (2016). *Chorionic villus sampling: Risks.* Retrieved from http://www.mayoclinic.org/tests-procedures/chorionic-villus-sampling/basics/risks/prc-20013566

McCulloh Nair, J., Nemeth, L. S., Sommers, M., & Newman, S. (2015). Substance abuse policy among nursing students: A scoping review. *Journal of Addictions Nursing, 26*(4), 166–174. doi:10.1097/jan.0000000000000094

Merriam-Webster Dictionary. (2016). Retrieved from http://www.merriam-webster.com/dictionary

Monroe, T. B., Kenaga, H., Dietrich, M. S., Carter, M. A., & Cowan, R. L. (2013). The prevalence of employed nurses identified or enrolled in substance use monitoring programs. *Nursing Research, 62*(1), 10–15. doi:10.1097/NNR.0b013e31826ba3ca

Nair, J. M., Nemeth, L. S., Sommers, M., Newman, S., & Amella, E. (2016). Alcohol use, misuse, and abuse among nursing students: A photovoice study. *Journal of Addictions Nursing, 27*(1), 12–23. doi:10.1097/jan.0000000000000107

National Center for Complementary and Integrative Health. (2016a). *What complementary and integrative approaches do Americans use? Key findings from the 2012 National Health Interview Survey.* Retrieved from https://nccih.nih.gov/research/statistics/NHIS/2012/key-findings

National Center for Complementary and Integrative Health. (2016b). *Complementary, alternative, or integrative health: What's in a name?* Retrieved from https://nccih.nih.gov/health/integrative-health

National Institute for Occupational Safety and Health. (2015). *Healthcare workers.* Retrieved from http://www.cdc.gov/niosh/topics/healthcare/

National Institute for Occupational Safety and Health. (2016). *NIOSH safety and health topics: Healthcare.* Retrieved from https://www.osha.gov/SLTC/healthcarefacilities/

O'Hara, M. W., & McCabe, J. E. (2013). Postpartum depression: Current status and future directions. *Annual Review of Clinical Psychology, 9*(1), 379–407. doi:10.1146/annurev-clinpsy-050212-185612

Phillips, C., Esterman, A., & Kenny, A. (2015). The theory of organisational socialisation and its potential for improving transition experiences for new graduate nurses. *Nurse Education Today, 35*(1), 118–124. doi:http://dx.doi.org/10.1016/j.nedt.2014.07.011

Pineau Stam, L. M., Spence Laschinger, H. K., Regan, S., & Wong, C. A. (2015). The influence of personal and workplace resources on new graduate nurses' job satisfaction. *Journal of Nursing Management, 23*(2), 190–199. doi:10.1111/jonm.12113

Poghosyan, L., Aiken, L. H., & Sloane, D. M. (2009). Factor structure of the Maslach Burnout Inventory: An analysis of data from large scale cross-sectional surveys of nurses from eight countries. *International Journal of Nursing Studies, 46*(7), 894–902.

Rantanen, J., Kinnunen, U., Mauno, S., & Tement, S. (2013). Patterns of conflict and enrichment in work-family balance: A three-dimensional typology. *Work and Stress, 27*(2), 141–163. doi:10.1080/02678373.2013.791074

Reid, R. O., Ashwood, J. S., Friedberg, M. W., Weber, E. S., Setodji, C. M., & Mehrotra, A. (2013). Retail clinic visits and receipt of primary care. *Journal of General Internal Medicine, 28*(4), 504–512. doi:10.1007/s11606-012-2243-x

Richards, K., Sheen, E., & Mazzer, M. C. (2014). *Self-care and you: Caring for the caregiver.* Silver Spring, MD: American Nurses Association.

Roach, M. S. (1984). *Caring: The human mode of being, implications for nursing, a monograph.* Toronto, ON: Faculty of Nursing, University of Toronto.

Roach, M. S. (Ed.). (1997). *Caring from the heart: The convergence of caring and spirituality.* Mahwah, NJ: Paulist Press.

Roach, M. S. (2002). *Caring, the human mode of being: A blueprint for the health professions* (2nd ed.). Ottawa, ON: CHA Press. Reprinted with permission.

Rush, K. L., Adamack, M., Gordon, J., & Janke, R. (2014). New graduate nurse transition programs: Relationships with bullying and access to support. *Contemporary Nurse, 48*(2), 219–228. doi:10.1080/10376178.2014.11081944

Rush, K. L., Adamack, M., Gordon, J., Lilly, M., & Janke, R. (2013). Best practices of formal new graduate nurse transition programs: An integrative review. *International Journal of Nursing Studies, 50*(3), 345–356. doi:10.1016/j.ijnurstu.2012.06.009

Sergeant, J., & Laws-Chapman, C. (2012). Creating a positive workplace culture. *Nursing Management, 18*(9), 14–19. doi:10.7748/nm2012.02.18.9.14.c8889

Spector, R. E. (2017). *Cultural diversity in health and illness* (9th ed.). Hoboken, NJ: Pearson Education.

Spence Laschinger, H. K., & Fida, R. (2014). New nurses burnout and workplace well being: The influence of authentic leadership and psychological capital. *Burnout Research, 1*(1), 19–28. doi:http://dx.doi.org/10.1016/j.burn.2014.03.002

Spence Laschinger, H. K., Wong, C. A., & Grau, A. L. (2012). The influence of authentic leadership on newly graduated nurses' experiences of workplace bullying, burnout and retention outcomes: A cross-sectional study. *International Journal of Nursing Studies, 49*(10), 1266–1276. doi:http://dx.doi.org/10.1016/j.ijnurstu.2012.05.012

Stevens, B. J., Gibbins, S., Yamada, J., Dionne, K., Lee, G., Johnston, C., & Taddio, A. (2014). The Premature Infant Pain Profile—Revised (PIPP-R): Initial validation and feasibility. *Clinical Journal of Pain, 30*(3), 238–243. doi:10.1097/AJP.0b013e3182906aed

Sullivan, E. J. (2013). *Becoming influential: A guide for nurses.* Upper Saddle River, NJ: Pearson Education.

Sung, P. S. (2013). Disability and back muscle fatigability changes following two therapeutic exercise interventions in participants with recurrent low back pain. *Medical Science Monitor, 19*, 40–48. doi:10.12659/MSM.883735

Swanson, K. M. (2012). What is known about caring in nursing science. In M. C. Smith, M. C. Turkel & Z. R. Wolf (Eds.), *Caring in nursing classics: An essential resource* (pp. 59–99). New York, NY: Springer.

Sword, W., Heaman, M. I., Brooks, S., Tough, S., Janssen, P. A., Young, D., . . . Hutton, E. (2012). Women's and care providers' perspectives of quality prenatal care: A qualitative descriptive study. *BMC Pregnancy and Childbirth, 12*(1), 1–18. doi:10.1186/1471-2393-1229

Takase, M., & Teraoka, S. (2011). Development of the holistic nursing competence scale. *Nursing and Health Sciences, 13*, 396–403.

Thomas, C. M., & Siela, D. (2011). The impaired nurse: Would you know what to do if you suspected substance abuse? *American Nurse Today, 6*(8). Retrieved from http://www.americannursetoday.com/article.aspx?id=8114&fid=8078

Tonges, M., & Ray, J. (2011). Translating caring theory into practice: The Carolina care model. *Journal of Nursing Administration, 41*(9), 374–381. Published by Lippincott Williams and Wilkins, © 2011.

Tonges, M., Ray, J. D., Overman, A. S., & Willis, B. (2015). Creating a culture of rapid change adoption: Implementing an innovations unit. *Journal of Nursing Administration, 45*(7/8), 384–390. doi:10.1097/nna.0000000000000219

Townsend, T. (2012). Break the bullying cycle. *American Nurse Today, 8*(1) 12–15.

Van der Elst, E., Dierckx de Casterlé, B., & Gastmans, C. (2012). Elderly patients' and residents' perceptions of "the good nurse": A literature review. *Journal of Medical Ethics, 38*, 93–97. doi:10.1136/medethics-2011-100046

Vogelpohl, D. A., Rice, S. K., Edwards, M. E., & Bork, C. E. (2013). New graduate nurses' perception of the workplace: Have they experienced bullying? *Journal of Professional Nursing, 29*(6), 414–422. doi:http://dx.doi.org/10.1016/j.profnurs.2012.10.008

Watson, J. (1999). *Nursing: Human science and human care: A theory of nursing.* Sudbury, MA: Jones & Bartlett.

Watson, J. (2002). Intentionality and caring-healing consciousness: A practice of transpersonal nursing. *Holistic Nurse Practitioner, 16*(4), 12–19.

Module 36
Clinical Decision Making

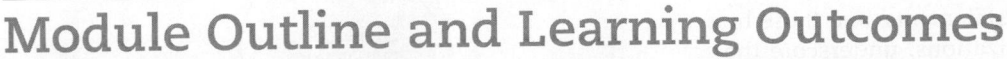

Module Outline and Learning Outcomes

The Concept of Clinical Decision Making

Critical Thinking

36.1 Analyze the use of critical thinking skills in nursing.

Clinical Decision Making

36.2 Analyze the components of clinical decision making.

Clinical Judgment

36.3 Outline the components of clinical judgment.

Lifespan Considerations

36.4 Differentiate considerations related to clinical decision making about patients throughout the lifespan.

Concepts Related to Clinical Decision Making

36.5 Outline the relationship between clinical decision making and other concepts.

Clinical Decision Making Exemplars

Exemplar 36.A The Nursing Process

36.A Analyze the nursing process as it relates to clinical decision making.

Exemplar 36.B The Nursing Plan of Care

36.B Analyze nursing plans of care as they relate to clinical decision making.

Exemplar 36.C Prioritizing Care

36.C Analyze prioritizing care as it relates to clinical decision making.

≫ The Concept of Clinical Decision Making

Concept Key Terms

Clinical decision making, **2479**	Clinical reasoning, **2483**	Deductive reasoning, **2483**	Inquiry, **2482**	Reflection, **2483**
Clinical judgment, **2482**	Creativity, **2481**	Inductive reasoning, **2483**	Intellect, **2480**	Salient cue, **2481**
	Critical thinking, **2480**		Intuition, **2484**	

Clinical decision making is a process nurses use in the clinical setting to evaluate and select the best actions to meet desired goals. Nurses use clinical decision making whenever choices are available, even when they evaluate a situation and decide not to act. In some cases, decisions are required in situations that have neither clear answers nor standard procedures and when conflicting forces add to the complexity. At other times, decisions are routine. For example, a nurse is assigned five patients:

- A patient with a 1-day-old abdominal surgical site
- A patient who was admitted in sickle cell crisis
- A patient with an arm wound infected with MRSA who is in contact isolation
- A patient who has been crying all night
- A patient who is already up and walking down the hall of the unit.

Clinical decision making applies across the continuum of nursing care, from direct patient care at the bedside to professional behaviors and accountability inherent in the profession of nursing. The nurse must evaluate each patient's needs and preferences as well as time-constraining activities (e.g., medication administration) to make appropriate decisions for each patient (see Exemplar 36.C on Prioritizing Care for further information). To make these decisions, the nurse must use critical thinking to choose among alternatives that support the best patient outcomes for all five patients.

Critical Thinking

Patient outcomes improve when the nurse uses critical thinking. Failure to employ critical thinking results in wasted time and energy, poor-quality patient outcomes, frustration, and anxiety (Elder & Paul, 2013). The American

Association of Colleges of Nursing's (2008) *The Essentials of Baccalaureate Education for Professional Nursing Practice* defines **critical thinking** as "All or part of the process of questioning, analysis, synthesis, interpretation, inference, inductive and deductive reasoning, intuition, application, and creativity." The Accreditation Commission for Education in Nursing speaks of critical thinking as "the deliberate nonlinear process of collecting, interpreting, analyzing, drawing conclusions about, presenting, and evaluating information that is both factually and belief based" (Benner, Hughes, & Sutphen, 2008). These statements, and those by other professional nursing organizations, underscore the importance of today's nurses being able to make meaningful observations, solve problems, and decide on a course of action. To do so, nurses must be able to process both previously learned and newly acquired information about their patients, the work environment, and resources at hand or in the community as well as applicable evidence related to care of the patient; the nurse must then be able to prioritize this information quickly and efficiently.

Nurses use critical thinking skills in a variety of ways. Because nurses manage patient care and human responses holistically, they must draw meaningful information from other disciplines in order to understand the meaning of patient data and plan effective interventions. This can be challenging because nurses work in rapidly changing situations. Routine actions are not always adequate to deal with the situation at hand. Familiarity with the routine for giving medications, for example, does not help the nurse in a situation with a patient who is frightened of injections or does not wish to take a medication. When unexpected situations arise, critical thinking enables the nurse to recognize the situation, respond quickly, and adapt interventions to meet specific patient needs. Nurses must use critical thinking, for example, to decide if observations should be reported to the primary care provider immediately or if those observations can wait to be reported after morning rounds. The skills and abilities necessary to develop critical thinking include intellect, creativity, inquiry, reasoning, reflection, and intuition (**Figure 36–1 »**). Critical thinking also requires maintaining an attitude that promotes critical thinking and working in an environment that encourages this skill (**Table 36–1 »**).

SAFETY ALERT A cross-sectional review of 2699 patient medical records from hospitals found that 76.8% of patient-related adverse events were attributable to nursing. Patients had an average of 15.3% risk of experiencing an adverse event. Of those patients who experienced adverse events attributed to nursing, 30% experienced at least two adverse events (D'Amour et al., 2014). In a time of economic restraint with healthcare reimbursement linked to patient satisfaction, adverse healthcare events are costly for institutions, pose a risk to patient safety, and diminish patient confidence in healthcare institutions and in nursing (D'Amour et al., 2014).

Intellect

Intellect is defined as the ability to think, understand, and reason. Building on clinical knowledge and skills expands the knowledge base nurses use for reasoning, analyzing, and predicting patient outcomes. Intellect helps to differentiate facts from opinions, approach situations objectively,

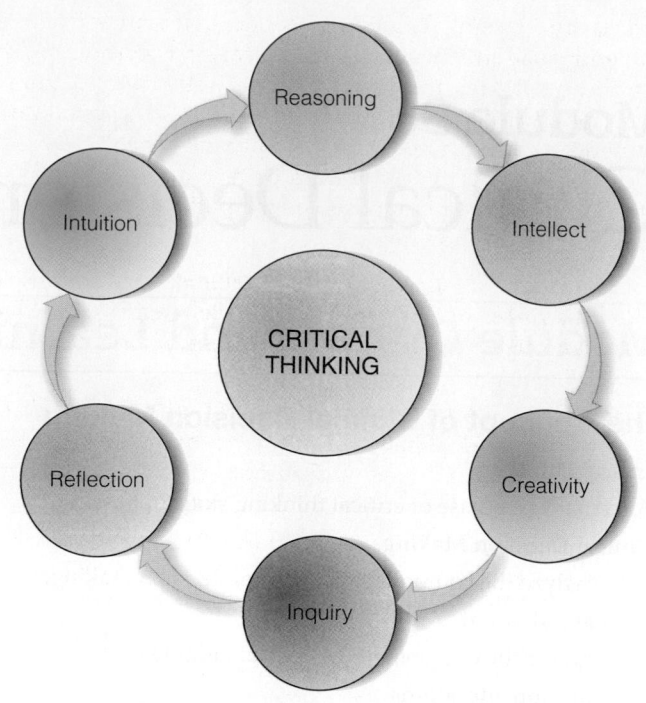

Figure 36–1 » Critical thinking skills are essential for making clinical decisions.

TABLE 36–1 Common Attitudes of Critical Thinkers

Attitudes	Examples
Independence	■ Does own thinking, objectively and honestly. ■ Is open minded about different methods used to reach same goal. ■ Looks for the facts; not easily swayed by opinions.
Fair-mindedness	■ Has neutral judgments without bias. ■ Considers opposing views to understand all aspects before making decisions. ■ Is open to new ideas and ways of doing things.
Aware of self-limits	■ Knows limits of intellect and experience. ■ Seeks new knowledge or skills in current evidence. ■ Expresses a willingness to self-reflect on own beliefs and ideas.
Integrity	■ Challenges own ideas and methods of doing nursing care. ■ Evaluates inconsistencies within own nursing practice. ■ Chooses the right thing to do over the popular thing to do.
Perseverance	■ Has stick-with-it motivation to find the best solution for quality patient outcomes. ■ Is patient with processes.
Confidence	■ Knows that he knows what he knows. ■ Trusts the skills and abilities of intellect, creativity, inquiry, reasoning, reflection, and intuition.

and clarify concepts. Thinking becomes an intentional action to identify **salient cues** within a clinical situation. *Salient,* or significant, means the leading, most noticeable, or most important, and *cue* refers to significant data that informs and influences conclusions about the patient's health status. Salient cues can cluster to form a pattern that can be translated into a nursing diagnosis for the patient. A salient cue does one of the following:

- *Indicates a negative or positive change in a patient's health status or pattern.* For example, the patient states, "I have been experiencing shortness of breath when climbing stairs."

- *Varies from norms of the patient population.* The patient's pattern may vary from norms of the general society. For example, an adult patient may consider a pattern of eating two small meals a day to be normal.

- *Indicates a developmental delay.* The nurse must be aware of the normal patterns and changes that occur as the person grows and develops. For example, by age 9 months an infant is usually able to sit alone without support. The infant who has not accomplished this task requires further assessment for possible developmental delays.

Once salient cues are recognized, they can be clustered to determine whether any patterns are present. The nurse can then interpret the pattern and take appropriate action. Awareness of cues and their significance can be valuable in making clinical decisions essential to nursing care for ever-changing conditions and reordering of priorities to meet patient needs (Burbach & Thompson, 2014). This dynamic method of thinking evolves over time, very much in the way that nurses advance through the stages of skill acquisition as they gain experience in clinical care. New nurses need to write down the assessment data and search the data for abnormal cues to help cluster significant cues that can be translated into a nursing diagnosis. See **Figure 36–2 ≫** for an example of cues and clustering of data.

Continuous learning is necessary for nurses to remain current with the best evidence for quality patient outcomes (see the feature on Evidence-Based Practice for further information). Many states now require that for licensure renewal, nurses complete continuing education credits to demonstrate up-to-date and current knowledge in patient care.

Creativity

Creativity is an outlet for the imagination that allows a nurse to take what can be seen in the mind and make it tangible. **Creativity** means finding unique solutions to unique problems when traditional interventions are not effective; for example, finding just the right way to connect with a patient who does not want to talk about her diabetes or finding interventions that best help a patient meet a goal so he can be discharged from the hospital.

A modification to an old adage, "No one size fits all" describes the importance of individualizing nursing care for each patient. When an attempt to help a patient is not successful, the nurse changes tactics and asks the question,

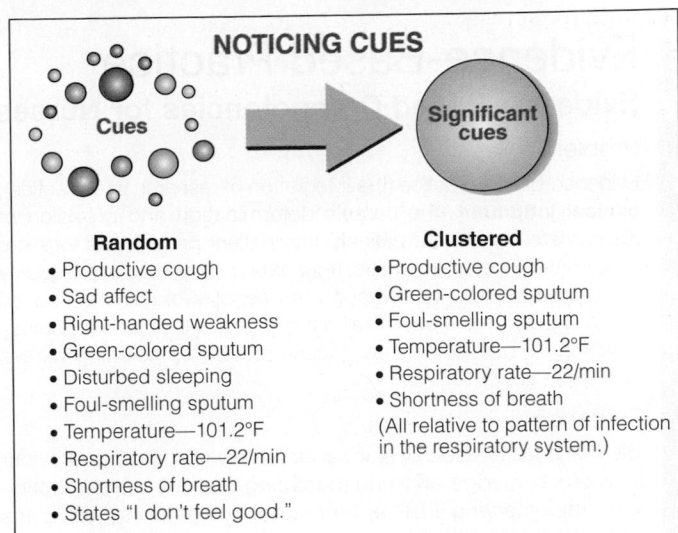

Figure 36–2 ≫ Random cues are not similar to each other, whereas significant cues that relate to each other can be clustered to form a pattern.

"What other approach might help this patient to succeed?" The ability to look for alternatives by "thinking outside the box" is necessary because the need for creative problem solving occurs every day. Some examples of opportunities for nurse creativity are:

- Helping a patient who is dehydrated to drink more liquids by mouth

- Helping a patient newly diagnosed with diabetes learn appropriate foods for controlling blood glucose levels

- Finding alternatives for an IV tubing label when a traditional label is not available

- Finding something to write vital signs on when paper, laptop, or computer are not at hand

- Using tape and tongue blades to make a toy house for a young child.

Sometimes the best way to find a good alternative is to increase the number of options available. This is where creativity and reality meet in much the same way creativity is used to figure out how many words can be spelled using the letters in "nursing care." Initially, you may have minimal success, but after more thought, you will begin to "see" more possibilities and spell more words from these few letters. Nurses can promote creative problem solving if they begin with asking "What if we . . . ?"

Creative thinkers must have knowledge of the problem. They must assess the problems before them and use their knowledge (intellect) of both underlying facts and, in this case, principles of development that apply to this situation (see Clinical Example A). The nurse knows the anatomy and physiology of respiratory function and is aware of the purpose of incentive spirometry. The nurse also understands pediatric growth and development. In trying to assist the child, the nurse builds on this knowledge and comes up with a creative solution.

Evidence-Based Practice
Evidence-Based Competencies for Nurses

Problem

Evidence-based practice (the integration of research into practice), **clinical judgment** (the nurse's determination and provision of appropriate care to the patient), and patient preferences together ensure the use of scientific rigor when providing high-quality healthcare to patients. Although the benefits of evidence-based practice (EBP) have been well established, a lack of consistency exists in its use among healthcare providers, including nurses (Melnyk et al., 2014).

Evidence

Clinicians fail to use EBP for several reasons, including provider lack of knowledge and understanding and the misperception that implementing EBP is time-consuming. These clinicians often follow traditional practices rather than evidence-based practices, because that's the way it's always been done, even when traditional practices have been proven to be harmful (Makic et al., 2013). Furthermore, many healthcare organizations fail to support EBP, and academic institutions continue to teach only traditional nursing methods. In order to begin implementing evidence-based practices, nurses must become proficient in critiquing current evidence, evaluating current practices, developing strategies to implement practice changes, and evaluating the outcomes related to changes in practice (Makic et al., 2013). To help combat clinicians' reluctance to implement evidence-based practices, the National Institutes of Health (NIH) has developed two programs: NIH Dissemination and Implementation (D&I) grants and the Improvement Science Research Network (Stevens, 2013).

Implications

Evidence-based practice has been an integral part of healthcare for at least a generation. Professional nursing and medicine strives to use this patient-centered practice methodology because it relies on the clinician's appraisal of the best evidence appropriate for the population the clinician serves. Furthermore, the added dimension of patient preference empowers the patient in healthcare decision making and allows the patient to be an active participant in his or her care as opposed to being the recipient of the traditional paternalistic physicians' orders or nursing interventions.

The National League of Nursing (NLN), the American Association of Critical-Care Nurses (AACN), and the Quality and Safety Education for Nurses (QSEN) have undertaken efforts to advance implementation of EBP among nurses at both the national and international levels (Melnyk et al., 2014). Research by Melnyk et al. (2014) supports both organizational and individual strategies for integrating EBP competencies into nursing practice, nursing research, organizational policies, management, and education.

Critical Thinking Application

1. How well do you understand EBP? Are you familiar with a healthcare institution or a healthcare provider that uses EBP? How does their use of EBP affect patient satisfaction and outcomes?

2. In your own words, describe how EBP affects the care patients receive.

3. How will you integrate evidence-based care into clinical decision making in your professional nursing practice?

Clinical Example A

A pediatric home health nurse is caring for Tyesha, a 9-year-old girl who has ineffective respirations following abdominal surgery. The primary care provider has ordered incentive spirometry (a treatment device that promotes alveolar expansion). Tyesha is frightened by the equipment and tires quickly during the treatments. The nurse offers her a bottle of bubbles and a blowing wand. Tyesha is delighted with blowing bubbles. The nurse knows that the respiratory effort in blowing bubbles will promote alveolar expansion and suggests that she blow bubbles between incentive spirometry treatments.

Critical Thinking Questions

1. What questions might the nurse ask of Tyesha to isolate the reasons the incentive spirometry device frightens her?
2. How might the nurse explain the purpose of the incentive spirometry device to Tyesha in a way that would make her less frightened of it?
3. Why is blowing bubbles an effective form of treatment for Tyesha? How much does it depend on Tyesha understanding the therapeutic component of what she is doing?
4. If Tyesha didn't want to blow bubbles, what might an effective alternative be that could fulfill the same purpose?
5. If an older, teenaged child didn't want to use the incentive spirometry device, what might be an effective alternative for a child of that age?
6. How might the nurse measure the positive effect of Tyesha's blowing bubbles?

Inquiry

Inquiry, a form of research, is defined as a search for knowledge or facts. When a nurse uses inquiry, he or she examines objective information to gain clarification and find solutions to problems. Inquiry differs from query in that a query is simply a question that requires an answer. Critical thinking requires nurses to use inquiry to examine both the situation at hand and their own nursing practice: "Why do we always need to apply the dressing this way?" "How can I help a patient who is on a salt-free diet avoid problems with her serum potassium levels?" "Why do we always need to put gloves on when we give injections?" "What would happen if we helped the patient exercise more than twice a day?" "Is there something else we can try when a patient is having trouble swallowing?" Nurses continuously use inquiry in the clinical setting. Nurses are inquisitive decision makers who ask questions about physician orders they do not understand, seek more information about an alternative therapy, or wonder if there is a better way of accomplishing an outcome for a patient. Nurses make changes in their practice based on new information, evidence, or innovative ways of doing things better. Clinical inquiry can resolve clinical problems and issues to promote improved patient outcomes.

Reasoning

To be able to walk into a patient's room and immediately observe significant data, come to a conclusion about the patient, and begin appropriate actions takes clinical reasoning by an experienced nurse. To be objective, the nurse needs to focus on salient cues and not be influenced by personal beliefs, biases, or assumptions that can result in errors, as illustrated by this statement made by a nurse: "The patient's a man, so I didn't think he was really in enough pain for an injection of morphine."

To help determine if decisions are reasonable, nurses use one of two forms of logical reasoning. In **deductive reasoning**, the nurse works from the "top down" by starting with general ideas, observations, or principles and analyzing them to develop specific predictions (Polit & Beck, 2017). For example, based on prior knowledge, the nurse knows that older adults have increased susceptibility to infection (general). Using deduction, the nurse can predict that when an 88-year-old man arrives at the emergency department with a 2-day complaint of increased sputum production, decreased appetite, productive cough, low energy, and complaints of chest pain when coughing, he has pneumonia (specific). Ask these questions: "What is the general idea?" and "What cues observed support it?" and, finally, "Do the significant cues make sense? Are they logical?"

Inductive reasoning involves working from the "bottom up." The nurse observes specific behaviors or symptoms and develops a general conclusion by putting significant, specific cues together (Polit & Beck, 2017). For example, the nurse has observed the following specific symptoms in patients diagnosed with pneumonia: increased sputum production, poor appetite and fluid intake, productive cough, little energy, and complaints of chest pain with coughing. Using inductive reasoning, the nurse concludes that the presence of these same signs and symptoms in other patients strongly indicates they may also have pneumonia. Ask these questions: "What are the significant cues observed?" and "What is the conclusion from the cues (the end result)?" And again, "Does the conclusion make sense? Is it logical?"

During the process of reasoning, the nurse needs to determine if patient information is a fact, an inference, a judgment, or an opinion, as described in **Table 36–2 »**. Evaluating the credibility of information sources is an important step in critical thinking. Unfortunately, nurses cannot always assume that all the things they read or hear are facts. The nurse may need to ascertain the accuracy of information by reviewing the evidence (e.g., conducting a literature search), checking other documents (e.g., facility procedures), or talking with other informants (e.g., supervising nurse).

Clinical reasoning, the use of careful reasoning in the clinical setting to improve patient care, is a learned skill that novice nurses must practice. Clinical reasoning requires critical thinking and the ability to reflect on previous situations and decisions and evaluate their effectiveness. With effort and time, new nurses learn critical thinking and integrate it into daily routines. Here are a few actions new nurses can take to improve their clinical reasoning:

1. On entering a patient's room, look around and observe the patient, any other people in the room, where they are positioned in the room, and what they are doing. Observe what items, smells, and sounds are present and what actions are taking place. This is similar to doing a 60-second safety check, a 3-minute brief assessment, or a 5-minute general survey of the patient. Careful use of the senses can help the nurse collect important cues.

2. Common cues nurses learn to recognize include facial expressions, patient activity, degree of respiratory effort, smell of cigarette smoke, complaints made by the patient, bed safety (e.g., rails up or down, bed low and locked, call bell within reach), patient affect, colors (e.g., red indicating bleeding, yellow indicating infection). These common cues can provide meaningful information quickly and help the nurse determine which cues are salient and if they form a pattern. Clusters of information may bring attention to a problem or issue the patient is having (e.g., presence of infection) or that is in the patient's immediate environment (e.g., visitors preventing appropriate rest). The nurse can then determine the best course of action and intervene as appropriate (Koharchik et al., 2015).

3. The nurse can evaluate previous actions and turn those actions into experiences that can be drawn upon in the future. The new nurse may ask him- or herself questions about a situation in order to analyze and learn from the experience. For example, "How well did that work?" "How did the patient respond?" "What could be done better next time?"

4. Build awareness of faulty reasoning, an occurrence that may cause new nurses to make mistakes in reasoning. Types of faulty reasoning are outlined in **Table 36–3 »**.

Reflection

Reflection is the action of retrospectively making sense of occurrences, experiences, situations, or decisions and consequently learning from them. It is the process of figuring out what worked or did not work, what could have

TABLE 36–2 Differentiating Types of Statements

Statement	Description	Example
Facts	Can be verified through investigation	Blood pressure is affected by blood volume.
Inferences	Conclusions drawn from facts; going beyond facts to make a statement about something not currently known	If blood volume is decreased (e.g., in hemorrhagic shock), the blood pressure will drop.
Judgments	Evaluation of facts or information that reflect values or other criteria; a type of opinion	It is harmful to the patient's health if the blood pressure drops too low.
Opinions	Beliefs formed over time; may include judgments that may fit facts or be in error	Nursing intervention can assist in maintaining the patient's blood pressure within normal limits.

TABLE 36–3 Types of Faulty Reasoning

Type of Faulty Reasoning	Action	Example
Bandwagon	Doing something because everyone else is doing it	Changing a patient's dressing without indicating date and time new dressing is applied because the dressing removed did not have this information.
Cause-and-effect fallacy	Linking something that happens to something that occurs before it happens	Thinking that the patient's nasogastric (NG) tube was draining fine until the nurse cleaned up the patient's bedside table; therefore, the nurse interfered with the NG tube drainage setup when cleaning up the bedside table.
Circular reasoning	Supporting an opinion by restating it using different words	Saying that a new dressing is very popular to use because a lot of nurses like using it. (The terms *popular* and *like using it* are saying the same thing.)
Either–or fallacy	Assuming that a problem has only two solutions	Thinking that the only way to help a patient with a headache is either with medication or a cold cloth on the head. (This ignores other interventions that may be helpful such as dimming the lights, decreasing noise, or giving the patient something to eat.)
Overgeneralizations	Coming to a conclusion when there is not enough evidence to do so	Concluding that a postoperative patient eats all of his meals based on the observation that he ate 100% of his last meal.
Using emotions instead of words	Reporting feelings about a situation rather than the facts	Saying the patient is an angry old man instead of saying that the older patient is anxious about being in the hospital.

been done differently to achieve better outcomes, what was done well, what necessary resources were available, and so on (Bulman & Schutz, 2013). To reflect on an experience, nurses need to learn to observe the significant factors of an experience that need to be included in reflective thinking. See **Box 36–1** ⟩⟩ for an example of guided reflection.

Evidence shows that debriefing, or reflective thinking after a simulated scenario, encourages reflective learning, a process that can help transfer book knowledge to practice application in complex situations (Decker et al., 2013). Reflective thinking can change a situation that is obscure, uncertain, and disturbing into one that is clear, understandable, and settled. For example, a nurse might be assigned to a patient who is anxious about going for surgery. The nurse can use guided reflection to help the patient "see" the surgical experience with better clarity, which may result in less anxiety for the patient.

Intuition

At times, nurses may experience what they call a "gut reaction" or a "feeling that something is wrong" when working with patients. Even though this awareness seems abstract and mysterious, it may be part of the nurse's reasoning and analysis of the constant data the nurse receives through the senses below a level of conscious awareness. In their article "How Expert Nurses Use Intuition," Benner and Tanner (1987) conclude that **intuition** is the use of nursing knowledge, experience, and expertise for understanding without the conscious use of reasoning. Many argue that intuition is a valuable cognitive skill in clinical decision making among professional expert nurses (Green, 2012; Pearson, 2013).

Intuition is a process. The data that are continuously received through senses are not always recognized consciously. Patterns and similarities of patterns are clustered and analyzed. Comparisons are made between a current patient's significant patterns and past patients' patterns

in response to similar situations. If the mind recognizes that a new pattern is similar to an old pattern, this recognition may bring the information to a level of cognitive awareness, making it available for the nurse to use in determining a course of action. Although the intuitive method of problem solving is gaining recognition as part of nursing practice, it is not recommended for new nurses or nursing students because they usually lack the knowledge base and clinical experience on which to make a valid judgment.

Courses are available to build critical thinking skills for nurses. For example, the National Council of State Boards of Nursing (NCSBN) has a continuing education course called "Sharpening Critical Thinking Skills."

Critical thinking remains the cornerstone of nursing care and patient intervention. As nursing continues to evolve, so too do the methods of thinking that influence those interventions that directly affect patient care. Benner (2015) emphasizes shifting from critical thinking alone to multiple thinking methods that expand the nurse's understanding and include understanding the patient's experience, the family's experience, and also the nurse's experience. Benner reasons that the complexity of illness and its effect on the patient and all elements of his being beyond that of being a patient are too broad and far-reaching to be explained by a single theory. Benner recommends multiple methods of thinking in addition to critical thinking, including practical reasoning, in which decisions for actions are determined in part by the actions that provide the best outcome for the patient.

Clinical Decision Making

Nurses make many decisions every day:

- "Which patient should I see first?"
- "When can I teach my patient with congestive heart failure about a no-salt diet?"

Box 36–1
Guided Reflection

This activity illustrates how one new nurse reflected on a situation he encountered during a clinical day that caused him to think about what happened and how he responded. Learning to organize thinking about patient care and professional nursing practice is an acquired skill. Reflecting on thinking processes supports recognizing the "lessons learned" for personal improvement in clinical judgment.

Task	Guided Reflection	New Nurse Response
Understanding the background of situation	1. Briefly describe what happened and what emotions you experienced during the situation. 2. What previous personal experience with a similar situation helped guide you through the situation?	1. "I was so busy giving my patient his bath that I forgot to give him a scheduled medication." 2. "I have worked as an unlicensed assistive personnel (UAP) in the past; I know that baths have to be given around other interventions that the patient has scheduled during the day."
Observing	3. What did you initially notice about the situation? 4. As time passed, what did you then notice?	3. "I started bathing the patient about 0850. I thought I had enough time to finish it, change his dressing, and then give him his medication that was scheduled to be given at 0930." 4. "The patient needed more time than I thought to bathe. When I checked my watch, it was already 1003, and the medication was late."
Interpreting	5. What further information about the situation did you decide you needed, and how did you get it?	5. "I should have remembered that some patients, particularly older adults, need more time to do things. I could have started the bath earlier, or I could have given the patient his medication first, and then helped him with his bath."
Responding	6. What was your nursing response to the situation? What interventions did you do? 7. Describe stresses you experienced as you responded to the situation.	6. "I had to tell the charge nurse what had happened. I then had to give the medication late." 7. "It stressed me out that I made a medication error. I felt stupid and was so embarrassed."
Reflecting	8. How did the situation end, and what emotion did you feel when the situation was over? 9. What might you do differently if this situation happens again? 10. What was your "take-away" from the experience?	8. "The patient received the medication 37 minutes late, so my actions didn't negatively impact the patient, but I could have kicked myself for this." 9. "I need to plan my work around medication administration times when I help a patient with morning care—or any intervention." 10. "Keep an eye on the clock and give priority to interventions and activities I need to do at specific times—work the other interventions around the timed ones."

Source: Based on Tanner, C. (2006). Thinking like a nurse: A research-based model of clinical judgment in nursing. *Journal of Nursing Education, 45*(6), 204–210. Retrieved from http://www.mccc.edu/nursing/documents/Thinking_Like_A_Nurse_Tanner.pdf.

- "How long should I wait before doing a bladder scan on my patient who hasn't voided since the indwelling catheter was removed?"

- "When's the best time for me to watch the video on that new dressing?"

- "Where can I find more linen for the UAPs to finish patient morning care?"

Wouldn't it be nice if there was a book to show nurses how to guarantee all clinical decisions they make would be 100% "successful"?

Good decisions come from careful consideration of resources; potential alternatives and their potential outcomes; the nurse's expertise, knowledge, skills, and clinical judgment; and the preferences of the patient. Typically, nurses make decisions during the process of solving problems. Types of decisions include:

- *Value decisions,* such as decisions regarding patient confidentiality

- *Time management decisions,* such as taking clean linens to a patient's room when taking medication to be administered

- *Scheduling decisions,* such as bathing a patient before visiting hours

- *Priority decisions* about which interventions are most urgent and which can be delegated.

Nurses also assist patients in making decisions. When a patient is trying to make a decision about what course of treatment to follow, the nurse may need to provide information or resources the patient can use in making a decision (see the Lifespan Considerations section). Nurses also make decisions in their professional lives. For example, nurses must decide whether to work in a hospital or community setting, whether to join a professional association, and whether to carry professional liability insurance.

The constantly changing healthcare environment requires strong clinical decision-making skills. New technology, expanding roles for nurses in healthcare systems, the complexity of patients entering the healthcare system, and the expanding body of knowledge and skills all add to the complexity of clinical decision making.

When nurses do not have enough clinical experience or nursing knowledge, skills, or imagination to make decisions, they can turn to available guidelines for help. Decision trees and protocols can assist in decision making for many aspects of nursing and nursing subspecialties. For example, many facilities have an emergency protocol for starting a patient on low-flow oxygen when the patient meets listed criteria. Sometimes when cycling through the alternatives, one alternative will just be exactly what is needed and may be chosen for use without further consideration of other alternatives. Many models for decision making are available, each suggesting steps in how to use cognitive processes to choose among alternatives. The following common steps are used in making decisions:

1. Identify the situation or problem: What decision needs to be made?
2. List all possible alternatives and information about the situation (i.e., risks, consequences).
3. Compare pros and cons of each alternative or solution and evaluate all of them.
4. Select the best option or alternative to try in a given environment.
5. Put the alternative into action.
6. Evaluate the success of using the alternative or the best option (Decision Making Confidence, 2013).

As nurses apply critical thinking to challenges in the workplace, they typically must choose among possible alternatives, engage in problem solving, use the nursing process, employ the scientific method, and sometimes engage in trial and error.

SAFETY ALERT The Texas Board of Nursing (n.d.) recommends the following six questions as part of a decision-making model and a tool for clinical judgment in order to ensure patient safety:

1. Is the activity consistent with your state's Nurse Practice Act?
2. Is the activity appropriately authorized by a valid order or protocol, and is it in accordance with established policies and procedures?
3. Is the act supported by either research reported in nursing- and health-related literature or in scope-of-practice statements by national nursing organizations?
4. Do you possess the required knowledge and have you demonstrated the competency required to carry out this activity safely?
5. Would a reasonable and prudent nurse perform this activity in this setting?
6. Are you prepared to assume accountability for the provision of safe care and the outcome of care rendered?

Choosing Among Alternatives

Many clinical situations present possible alternatives that must be considered prior to taking action. In clinical situations, alternatives may be selected from a range of nursing interventions or patient care strategies. Often priorities for care suggest or even determine the alternative chosen, but not always. For example, pain may be treated with oral or injectable medications as needed (prn) or on a schedule, or without any pharmacologic intervention by using nursing measures to support the patient's comfort. In all cases, the nurse analyzes the alternatives to ensure that there is an objective rationale for choosing one alternative over another. For example, for the patient with kidney stone pain, common nursing measures may not provide strong enough relief, and oral medication may take effect too slowly, so an intravenous narcotic might be the best choice. The nurse must consider the possibilities of adverse consequences due to a decision. This is also part of the decision-making process. If the intravenous narcotic is selected, should safety measures such as a narcotic antidote and supplemental oxygen be in place? Think about the following questions when choosing between alternatives in decision making:

1. Is there always just "one best" alternative?	Finding the "one best" alternative is very time consuming and may result in unnecessary delay.
2. Can consideration always be given to every alternative?	The list of alternatives could be quite lengthy, so limit the list to the top five options for serious consideration.
3. Is there always time to gather all the information about alternatives and consequences and then to think about them one at a time?	Is there ever enough time?

The nurse recognizes significant cues that form patterns and then uses intellect, intuition, and reasoning to quickly make decisions and choose a plan of action based on past experiences. Experienced nurses will recognize more patterns and possess a greater wealth of knowledge, enabling them to come to decisions quickly. Regardless of experience, all nurses cycle through alternatives until they find an appropriate choice based on their past experience, knowledge, and skills. At this point, the nurse mentally rehearses the choice and, if the alternative looks like it will work, selects a course of action. Every decision-making process helps nurses improve their decision-making skills and adds to their clinical experience.

Problem Solving

Problem solving is the norm rather than the exception for routine nursing responsibilities today. Nurses become skilled problem solvers in order to manage obstacles and maintain an unencumbered flow of care as they manage their workday. Sometimes patients are scheduled to be in two places at one time for various diagnostic tests, or perhaps a patient received the wrong diet tray and needs a different diet meal, or a patient needs a medication that has yet to arrive from the pharmacy department. Sometimes the problem itself is the number of problems that must be addressed in a short amount of time. Because some patients have complex health issues, their care is equally complex and involve problems that are not always easy to "fix." Some problems may occur repeatedly—for example, the nurse may realize that the pharmacy has been late delivering medications for several days. Nurses must be alert to recurrent problems and new problems and find the time to step in and correct the cycle (see the module on Quality Improvement for more information).

When problems arise, nurses use decision making as part of the problem-solving process. In problem solving, the nurse obtains information that clarifies the nature of the problem and identifies possible solutions. The nurse then carefully evaluates the possible solutions and chooses the best one to implement. After implementing the solution, the nurse monitors the situation over time to ensure the initial and continued effectiveness of the solution. The other possible solutions are held in reserve in the event that the first solution is not effective. The nurse may also encounter a similar problem in a different patient situation where another solution is found to be the most effective. Therefore, problem solving for one situation contributes to the nurse's body of knowledge for problem solving in similar situations. Commonly used approaches to problem solving include the nursing process, trial and error, intuition, and the scientific method.

The Nursing Process

The nursing process includes five phases that organize the problem-solving process (see Exemplar 36.A on the Nursing Process for more information). Nurses make clinical decisions using critical thinking during every phase of the nursing process. Experienced nurses also use their experiences, knowledge, skills, and current nursing research evidence to make decisions. As nursing students' knowledge, skills, and attitudes progress, they will be able to make better decisions faster using the nursing process as a decision-making tool. Clinical Example B outlines the five phases of the nursing process as they related to problem solving:

Clinical Example B

1. *Assessment:* Gathering information to determine the problem
   The nurse admits a 4-year-old patient, Austin Gates, who is suspected of having asthma. The patient has a history of frequent colds and has an allergy to grasses. His dad smokes three packs of cigarettes a day. Austin's mother tells the nurse that Austin has been playing with the neighbor's cats for the past few days. The nurse determines it is important to assess Austin for shortness of breath, respiratory effort, use of accessory muscles, lung sounds, vital signs, oxygen saturation, and the results of lab studies, including a complete blood count (CBC) and chest x-ray. With the help of Austin's mother, the nurse collects other data that may be relevant, such as the patient's past medical history, developmental behaviors, and activity level.

2. *Nursing Diagnosis:* Stating the specific problem to solve
   Based on the assessment data obtained, the nurse caring for Austin determines that his main complaint is difficulty in breathing secondary to airway obstruction. The obstruction is caused by both narrowing of airways and increased mucus production, evidenced by audible wheezing and adventitious lung sounds. The patient is anxious secondary to his shortness of breath and being in a strange environment. The patient has an elevated WBC and an increased respiratory rate. The nurse must decide which of these symptoms are top priorities for nursing care.

3. *Planning:* Stating how to know when the problem is resolved
   During the planning phase, the nurse caring for Austin decides that an important priority would be to monitor his wheezing, which indicates patency of airways. The goal might be "Austin's lung sounds will be clear bilaterally."

4. *Implementation:* Giving solutions to resolve the problem
   Interventions to help Austin meet his goal might be:

   - Assess lung sounds every 4 hours
   - Maintain supplemental oxygen via nasal cannula as ordered by physician
   - Administer medication prescribed by provider
   - Encourage oral (PO) fluids.

5. *Evaluation:* Evaluating if the problem has been resolved
   Nursing staff has documented "For the past 12 hours, Austin's lung sounds have been free from wheezes and are now clear."

Critical Thinking Questions

1. What interventions must the nurse address immediately in caring for Austin?
2. What interventions can be delayed?
3. What actions should the nurse anticipate related to Austin's presentation?

Trial and Error

One way to solve problems is through trial and error—trying out a solution, seeing if it works, and, if it does not, reflecting on why and making another, different attempt. Trial and error is an option only when time and safety allow multiple opportunities to select the correct solution. This problem-solving process is not an option when an error may result in harm to the patient. Trial and error may be more useful in situations related to patient comfort or preference. Two trial-and-error examples are when determining how far to raise the head of the bed for the patient to be comfortable enough to eat, or trying different methods to communicate with a patient who has a hearing impairment. The trial-and-error process is primarily used to solve problems; it may not result in the best solution, but it may reveal a workable solution. The use of trial and error requires creativity and patience, two qualities essential to nursing.

Intuition

Intuition is an unconscious awareness of a potentially compromising or dangerous situation. Intuition is an aspect of critical thinking. It is also relevant to problem solving. With practice, solving problems using rules and anticipatory thinking transforms into the ability to use thinking processes, knowledge, and intuition almost unconsciously.

The Scientific Method

The scientific method of problem solving is a formalized, logical, systematic investigative approach that is most successful when working in a controlled situation. Health professionals, often working with individuals in uncontrolled situations, require a modified approach to the scientific method for solving problems. For example, unlike experiments with animals, the effects of diet on health are complicated by a patient's genetic variations, lifestyle, and personal preferences.

Many aspects of nursing practice involve clinical decision making. Any time a patient's condition changes, those caring for the patient must decide how to respond. Decisions are usually made by problem solving or by choosing among alternatives. Some actions are performed routinely, such as measuring vital signs at the beginning of the shift or introducing oneself when meeting a new patient. Other actions require careful consideration, critical thinking, problem solving, and decision making in order to provide the highest quality nursing care and assure the safety of patients and staff. See Clinical Example C for an example of clinical decision making.

Clinical Example C

Anna Nadine, 64 years old, is admitted to the medical unit at a local healthcare facility with a medical diagnosis of pulmonary edema secondary to left-sided heart failure. Ms. Nadine has a history of type 2 diabetes requiring insulin injections, hypertension, and early-stage chronic renal failure. She is married, has no children, and lives with her husband in a high-rise apartment building that has a functioning elevator. Initial vital signs are T_O 99.2°F, P 90 bpm, R 24/min, and BP 136/86 mmHg. Oxygen saturation (O_2 Sat) is 91% on room air. Ms. Nadine is 5'2" and weighs 168 pounds. She has the following physician orders:

■ Vital signs, including oxygen saturation every 1 hour × 3, then every 2 hours × 3, then every 4 hours
■ Give oxygen at 2 LPM via nasal cannula
■ Chest x-ray
■ Electrocardiogram (ECG)
■ Lab work: CBC with differential, electrolytes, urinalysis (voided)
■ ABGs on oxygen
■ Daily weights
■ No-added-salt regular diet
■ Accu-Chek before meals and at bedtime, with sliding scale—cover with regular insulin

   200 or less = 0 coverage
   201–250 = 2 units subcutaneous injection
   251–300 = 4 units subcutaneous injection
   301–350 = 6 units subcutaneous injection
   351–400 = 8 units subcutaneous injection
   401 and higher = 10 units subcutaneous injection and call physician

■ Activity—out of bed to chair with assistance
■ Intake and output every 12 hours
■ D_5 ½ NS with 10 mEq potassium chloride (KCl) at 50 mL/hr
■ Lasix 40 mg IV STAT, then Lasix 20 mg PO daily (am)
■ Digoxin 0.125 mg PO daily (am)
■ Clonidine 0.1 mg PO BID.

Within 12 hours of admission, Ms. Nadine's weight is 160 pounds, and she is breathing more comfortably with breath sounds mostly clear with some fine crackles in the bases. Vital signs are T_O 99.2°F, P 78 bpm, R 18/min, BP 118/80 mmHg, and O_2 Sat 97% on 2 LPM via nasal cannula.

The next day when you return to the unit and are again assigned to her care, you receive a report from the previous shift that Ms. Nadine has been confused and disoriented for the past 2 hours. Her blood sugar when last checked 30 minutes ago was within normal limits. Her husband has been notified and plans to come in and sit with her today, but he has not yet arrived.

Critical Thinking Questions

1. What assessment information do you need to obtain?
2. What are the top three priority nursing actions for Ms. Nadine at this time?
3. What factors could be contributing to Ms. Nadine's confusion?
4. How important is it to gather additional assessment data prior to implementing any interventions for Ms. Nadine?
5. What discussion might you want to have with Mr. Nadine when he arrives?
6. Use critical thinking to determine what physician orders you would anticipate receiving for Ms. Nadine.

Clinical Judgment

The end product of the complex process that is clinical decision making is clinical judgment, the nurse's determination and provision of appropriate care to the patient. In other words, clinical judgment combines critical thinking abilities, evaluative decision making, and nursing experience to determine appropriate responses to a patient's complex and often layered situation to achieve the best patient outcomes (Thompson et al., 2013). Clinical judgment can be used in emergency situations and also for long-term planning of care.

This dynamic cognitive process brings all the elements of critical thinking and clinical decision making together in making clinical judgments about patient care through the application of nursing knowledge, skills, and attitudes. New nurses may find this skill difficult and slow to use, whereas experienced nurses will be faster and will be able to use their intuition for clinical judgment. The National League for Nursing (2016) lists nursing judgment as a competency for graduates of nursing programs. The National Council of State Boards of Nursing (2016) has models available for states to use in revising their scopes of nursing practice that relate to the accountability for clinical judgments. According to NANDA International (NANDA-I) (2016), a nursing diagnosis is a clinical judgment about an individual or family's situation or their response to a health concern or life process. Three nurse researchers have given the nursing profession important clinical research evidence related to clinical judgment: Patricia Benner, whose skill acquisition model describes five levels of clinical competence; Christine Tanner, whose clinical judgment model supports "thinking like a nurse;" and Kathie Lasater, who promotes the use of a clinical judgment rubric.

Benner's Skill Acquisition Model

The ability to make clinical judgments improves as nurses gain experience and build on their critical thinking and decision-making skills. A study in the late 1970s compared the performance of senior nursing students, new nurses, and experienced nurses over a 3-year period of time. The results of this study demonstrated distinct differences in clinical performance at these varying levels of nursing education and nursing experience (Benner, Tanner, & Chesla, 2009). Benner adapted these findings to the Dreyfus Model of Skill Acquisition and organized the evidence from the study into five levels of proficiency a nurse progresses through as he or she gains additional clinical experience (Benner, 2011). These levels are novice, advanced beginner, competent, proficient, and expert (see **Figure 36–3 》**).

The different levels of competence reflect four progressive changes in thinking processes:

1. Moving from not having nursing experiences on which to relate to having concrete clinical experiences to relate to new situations that require critical thinking
2. Progressing from following steps in a specific sequential order to customizing and adapting actions using nursing experience and intuition
3. Moving from taking in many significant cues and trying to make sense of all of them to identifying significant cues and clustering them to form patterns
4. Progressing from being an observant bystander to being an active participant.

Each level builds on the previous level as critical thinking skills are mastered and decision making becomes routine for the nurse. Experience further expands this process as the nurse gains confidence in his or her nursing skills.

Tanner's Clinical Judgment Model

Clinical judgment does not always include standard decision making or require all the skills of critical thinking. Tanner's "thinking like a nurse" approach in her clinical judgment model emphasizes the importance of elements the nurse uses in cognitive processing: different types of knowledge (e.g., textbook, transferred, on-the-job, abstract), length of nursing experience, values, morals, intuition, and knowing the patient (i.e., being familiar with expected patterns of responses to a medical condition or knowing the individual patient) (Tanner, 2006). Another element that influences clinical judgment is the culture of the work environment, including group norms and expectations of work routines. The Tanner model includes four features: noticing, interpreting, responding, and reflecting (**Table 36–4 》**).

Nursing education teaches fundamental nursing knowledge, skills, and attitudes that lay the foundation for expected high-level performance from students. Nursing education, both didactic and clinical, promotes safe and quality nursing performance. Nursing programs teach students to develop knowledge of their patients in order to care

Expert
- Many years experienced
- Intuitive practitioner
- Highly developed cognitive abilities

Proficient
- Can see the whole picture
- Formulates own rules for actions by analyzing significant cues

Competent
- After 2–3 years experience
- Intentional planning of care
- Still not able to see bigger picture from significant cues

Advanced beginner
- Typically new graduates
- Have limited nursing experience
- Beginning to recognize significant cues from internal cognitive processing

Novice
- Beginners without nursing experience
- Do actions by following rules
- Limited ability to act independent of being told what to, when to, and how to do nursing actions

Source: Data from Benner, P. (2011). From novice to expert. *Current Nursing.* Retrieved from http://currentnursing.com/nursing_theory/Patricia_Benner_From_Novice_to_Expert.html.

Figure 36–3 》 Benner's five levels of clinical competence from nursing student to graduate to professional.

TABLE 36–4 Features of the Tanner Clinical Judgment Model

Feature	Description
Noticing	■ Having a sense of what is happening in the patient situation
	■ May include recognition of or absence of expected significant cues from the patient's response to illness or a medical condition
	■ Includes influences of the nurse's own health beliefs about patient situations and expectations of the work culture for patient care
Interpreting	■ Using logical reasoning to gain understanding about a situation and determine appropriate actions
Responding	■ Includes analyzing a situation and choosing the best course of action
	■ Includes intuitive "knowing" from past similar experiences
	■ Includes using past similar experiences to "make sense" of a present clinical situation
	■ Includes responsive actions by the nurse
Reflecting	■ Using cognitive processes to review a clinical situation
	■ Considering appropriateness of assessment data obtained in the situation, actions taken, and positive and negative outcomes for patient
	■ Making mental response adjustments for similar future situations
	■ Learning from actions (done or not done)

Note. Based on Alfaro-Lefevre, R. (2017). *Critical thinking, clinical reasoning, and clinical judgment.* Philadelphia, PA: Elsevier; Gerdeman, J. L., Lux, K., & Jacko, J. (2013). Using concept mapping to build clinical judgment skills. *Nurse Education in Practice, 13*(1), 11–17; Tanner, C. (2006). Thinking like a nurse: A research-based model of clinical judgment in nursing. *Journal of Nursing Education, 45*(6), 204–210. Retrieved from http://www.mccc.edu/nursing/documents/Thinking_Like_A_Nurse_Tanner.pdf.

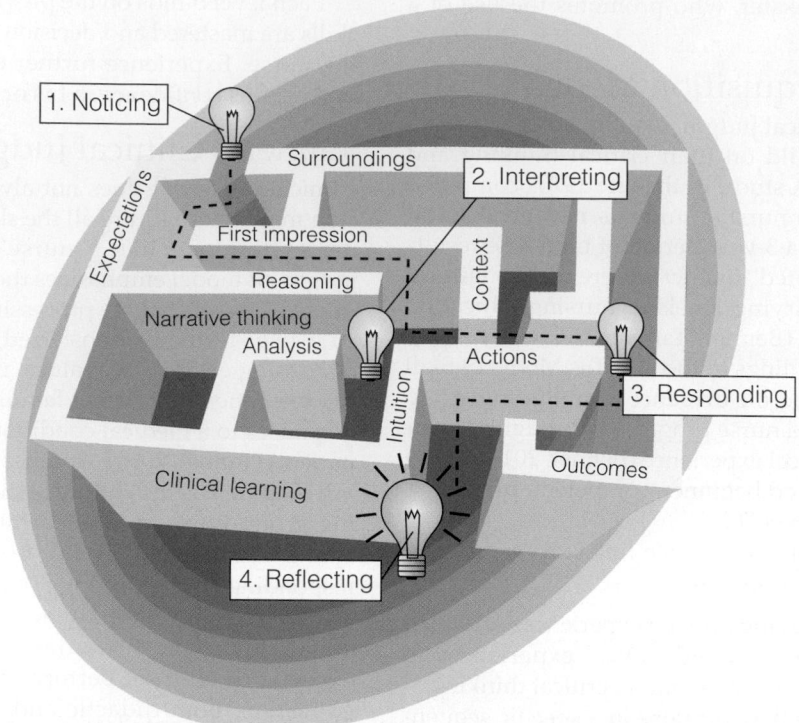

1. Noticing

Surroundings

2. Interpreting

Expectations

First impression

Context

Reasoning

Narrative thinking

Analysis

Actions

Intuition

3. Responding

Clinical learning

Outcomes

4. Reflecting

Source: Based on Tanner, C. (2006). Thinking like a nurse: A research-based model of clinical judgment in nursing. *Journal of Nursing Education,* 45(6), 204–210. Retrieved from http://jxzy.smu.edu.cn/jkpg/UploadFiles/file/TF_0692810354_thinking%20like%20a%20nurse.pdf.

Figure 36–4 》》 Tanner's clinical judgment model includes four major sequential cognitive steps: (1) noticing, (2) interpreting, (3) responding, and (4) reflecting.

for them responsibly and to develop a sense of their patients' situations in which they will need to intervene. Reflecting on clinical situations and learning from them help students build experiences they can use for future reference. In other words, "thinking like a nurse" begins with learning as a nursing student (Tanner, 2006). See **Figure 36–4 》》** for a diagram of these sequential cognitive steps.

Lasater's Clinical Judgment Rubric

Lasater developed the clinical judgment rubric to measure and evaluate clinical judgment using simulation (Bussard, 2015). Tanner's clinical judgment model served as the foundation for the rubric (see Figure 36–4). The rubric serves as a guide for learners to know the specific characteristics needed to reach quality levels of clinical judgment performance (**Figure 36–5 》》**). The rubric has been used successfully while observing learners in a simulation environment.

The rubric uses the four aspects of the Tanner model: noticing, interpreting, responding, and reflecting. Lasater developed additional dimensions for each of these aspects to describe associated behaviors and actions for each (see Figure 36–5, the vertical axis): for example, prioritizing data is an essential behavior of *interpreting* information. Lasater proposes measuring the four aspects of Tanner's model in a progressive developmental order: beginning, developing, accomplished, and exemplary (see Figure 36–5, the horizontal axis). The table provides descriptors and behavioral dimensions for each performance level. Students can use the rubric to measure their progress in

using clinical judgment. The rubric clearly defines characteristics for clinical judgment levels and dimensions (Bussard, 2015).

Focus on Integrative Health
Holistic Care and Autonomous Decision Making

Western medicine has long supported paternalistic management of healthcare decision making, often relegating most patients to a passive state in decisions about their health. Brophy (2014) writes that while all providers acknowledge a patient's right to self-determination, patient autonomy has been limited in traditional Western medicine. The integration of complementary medicine and holistic care into the U.S. healthcare system has altered patient healthcare decision making by supporting patient autonomy and the holistic relationship between the patient and the holistic-care provider.

Self-governance is the foundation of holistic care and autonomous decision making. Patients grounded in traditional paternalistic healthcare management will find that holistic providers spend time educating, building patient knowledge, and probing to ensure patient understanding in order to enable the patient to make the best decisions for his or her health. Holistic decision-making models are based on biopsychosocial, patient-centered, informed, and shared decision making, and evidence-based patient choice decision-making models in which patient–provider interactions focus on the whole person, not the disease.

	Progressive Development			
Dimensions	**Beginning**	**Developing**	**Accomplished**	**Exemplary**
Noticing • Focus on significant cues • Recognize differences • Look for cues				
Interpreting • Prioritize data • Make sense of data				
Responding • Calm and confident • Clear communication • Do planned actions • Skill abilities				
Reflecting • Evaluate/analyze self • Desire to be better				

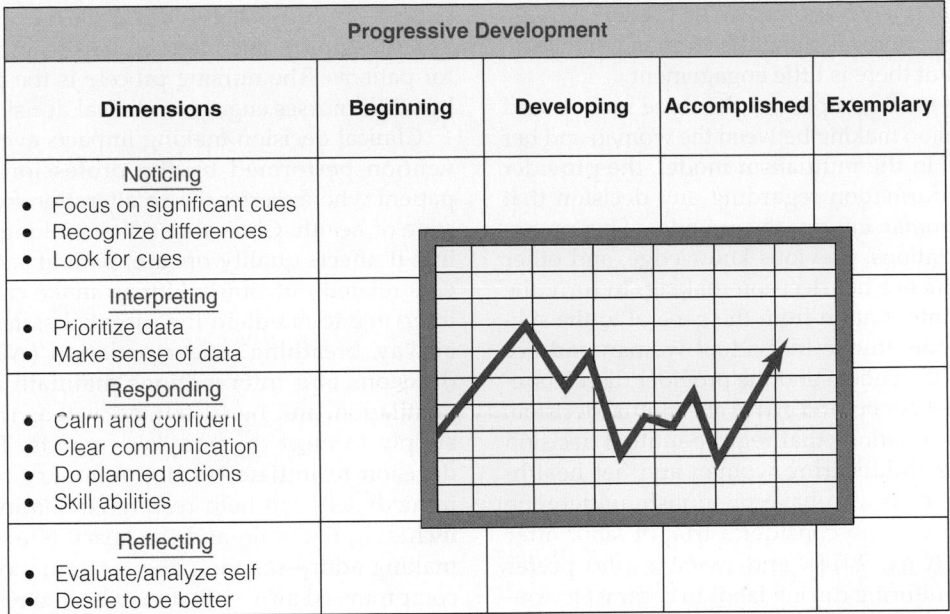

Source: Bussard, M. (2015). The nature of clinical judgment development in reflective journals. *Journal of Nursing Education,* 54(8), 451–454. doi:10.3928/01484834-20150717-05.

Figure 36–5 》 Lasater used the dimensions from Tanner's clinical judgment model and created developmental levels of clinical judgment for her rubric.

Lifespan Considerations

Clinical Decision Making Involving Children

Parents often make decisions about the healthcare of their children. Growing children can participate in those decisions in developmentally appropriate ways. As children mature and develop, they gain decision-making ability and an understanding of the consequences of their decisions. They are able to contribute to decisions about their health; however, healthcare providers must carefully evaluate and follow an established process if the child is involved in making his or her health-care decisions (Michaud et al., 2015). Children's ability to reason and think critically about themselves and their situation develops gradually. At each stage, nurses should be aware of the way children think and should be sensitive to how the child can be involved in healthcare decisions at each developmental stage:

- Infants progress from reflexive behavior to simple, repetitive behavior and then to imitative behaviors, learning the concepts of cause and effect and object permanence. Infants are not involved in healthcare decision making, but they need to be comforted and feel secure throughout the entire healthcare process, including during waiting periods.

- Toddlers and preschoolers are egocentric and engage in magical thinking. They cannot reason out the implications of care, but they need explanations in language they can understand. Play therapy and use of dolls and toys can help children in this age group understand healthcare in a manner appropriate to their developmental stage. Toddlers and preschoolers can sometimes be given options (e.g., "Do you want your dressing changed before breakfast or after?").

- School-age children tend to be concrete thinkers. They benefit from simple, direct explanations; hands-on exploration of equipment and materials; and helping the care provider as appropriate during procedures. Involving these children in care can increase cooperation and decrease anxiety.

- Adolescents are able to think abstractly and are able to participate in healthcare decisions. Adolescent involvement in clinical decision making is complex and, when possible, should involve the patient's assent to a procedure, though parental consent is still required. In some instances, an adolescent may provide assent as well as possess autonomous decision-making ability for clinical care. In such cases, the adolescent is also afforded both confidentiality and the ability to provide consent for procedures (Michaud et al., 2015). Healthcare providers, and if required, attorneys, must evaluate the adolescent and determine that he or she is competent and capable of making informed decisions.

Clinical Decision Making Involving Pregnant Women

Three decision-making models prevail in the health of the pregnant woman: paternalism, consumerism, and mutualism (Cox, 2014). Paternalism assumes that the provider, because of education and experience, knows best and will make the best decisions for the woman and the fetus. This assumption is based on the further assumption that the provider will make the best decision because of the need for a positive reputation among present and future patients.

The consumerism model takes a hands-off approach to decision making on the part of the clinician. In this model, the woman or her insurance provider pays for a service. The provider gives the woman what he or she believes is the best information based on science and research. There is a transfer of essential information, enabling the woman to make an informed decision, but there is little engagement.

Mutualism is the most complex of the three models and involves shared decision making between the woman and her healthcare provider. In the mutualism model, the provider gives the woman information regarding any decision that must be made. The woman informs the provider of her preferences, values, expectations, previous knowledge, and other factors that may influence her decision making. In turn, the provider molds the information from the general to the specific as it relates to the unique individual woman and her pregnancy. Together, the patient and the provider discuss scenarios and options, deliberate, and arrive at a mutual decision.

Two examples of situations that require mutual decision making between the childbearing woman and her healthcare provider are women who have previously undergone cesarean section but wish to consider a trial of labor after cesarean (TOLAC) (Cox, 2014), and women who prefer intermittent fetal monitoring during labor in contrast to constant fetal monitoring that requires bedrest. In these cases, as in others, women should be informed of risks, benefits, evidence, possible occurrences, and support measures (Hersh, Megregian, & Emeis, 2014). Mutualism and shared decision making provides the best model for managing these and other issues related to pregnancy, labor, and delivery.

For the childbearing woman, pregnancy, labor, and delivery can be intense times. Women value the input of providers; yet, some women have described providers as inadequate, insensitive, and coercive. Childbearing women expect providers who are both knowledgeable and sensitive and who value their patients' input in decision making about their bodies, their lives, and the lives of their unborn children.

Clinical Decision Making Involving Older Adults

All adult patients should be involved in clinical decision making and planning their nursing care; however, older adults with impaired cognition related to disease processes such as Alzheimer disease present a challenge. The nurse should allow these patients as much control and input as possible, keeping discussions simple, direct, and easy to understand. Older adults with impairments usually are unable to perform multiple tasks or to think of more than one step at a time. The nurse must be willing to calmly repeat instructions as necessary. Presenting and discussing issues in basic terms helps maintain the older adult's respect and dignity and allows older adults to participate in their care for as long and as much as possible. If the older adult is unable to perform self-care activities such as bathing or health-related activities such as dressing changes, the nurse should seek appropriate alternative methods for assisting the patient with these tasks.

Concepts Related to Clinical Decision Making

Clinical decision making is a complex process in which nurses observe and gather data, interpret that data through the use of salient cues, and identify patterns that provide critical information. Nurses analyze cues and patterns and determine patients' priority needs. Nurses also evaluate alternatives to provide appropriate interventions to support best outcomes for patients. The nursing process is the professional process by which nurses engage in clinical decision making.

Clinical decision making impacts every action and intervention performed by the professional nurse for every patient who experiences an alteration from his or her usual state of health. Clinical decision making is integral to nursing: it affects quality of care, patient satisfaction, cost, and care-related outcomes. Nurses make critical decisions and intervene to maintain the essential states necessary for life: airway, breathing, and circulation (ABC). Rapid clinical decisions and interventions maintain a patient's airway, ventilation, and perfusion, as well as the patient's oxygen supply to meet the body's demands. The nurse's clinical decision to initiate cardiopulmonary resuscitation (CPR) immediately can help restore circulation to major organs, including the brain and the heart. Nurses' critical decision making addresses the patient's actual or potential risk for compromised airway that may lead to respiratory arrest and alteration in the body's acid–base balance.

The nurse uses a vast body of knowledge in deciding appropriate interventions to resolve dehydration for the patient with fever in order to restore the patient to a state of normal hydration and to minimize the patient's electrolyte imbalance. However, the nurse's decisions and interventions must also reflect caution to avoid causing fluid overload that may exacerbate heart failure, compromise circulatory perfusion, and lead to respiratory failure.

The nurse caring for patients with neurologic deficits makes clinical decisions that reduce environmental stimuli with the potential to increase the patient's intracranial pressure. The nurse makes clinical decisions that avoid overwhelming the patient's sensory perceptions.

Nursing clinical decision making is integral to the postoperative patient, as the nurse's decision-making capability leads to interventions that assist patients who required surgical intervention for an inflammatory process, who undergo an orthopedic procedure related to mobility or orthopedic function, or have alteration in cellular regulation such as breast or colorectal cancer. The nurse uses knowledge and clinical decision making to perform interventions to decrease pain and promote patient comfort while continually assessing the patient and noting any postoperative alterations, including fever, a possible sign of infection; urinary retention after removal of an indwelling urinary catheter; or gastric alterations, a possible sign of digestive system complications that may compromise the patient's nutritional status. All hospitalized patients have increased risk of infection. Nurses' clinical decisions about a patient's already compromised immunity or recent surgery can alter the patient's risk of exposure to infection. Nurses' clinical decisions and interventions in the postoperative patient include interventions to promote tissue integrity and wound healing at the surgical site.

Almost every patient–nurse encounter requires a clinical decision that draws on the nurse's academic knowledge and work experience. Patients who benefit from nurses' sound decision-making ability experience satisfaction with quality nursing care. The Concepts Related to Clinical Decision Making feature links some, but not all, of the concepts integral to clinical decision making. They are presented in alphabetical order.

Concepts Related to
Clinical Decision Making

CONCEPT	RELATIONSHIP TO CLINICAL DECISION MAKING	NURSING IMPLICATIONS
Accountability	Standards of care set benchmarks for nursing performance expectations, including evidence of competent and effective clinical decision making that reflects professional behavior.	■ Nurses are responsible for the clinical decisions and judgments they make to support desired patient outcomes.
Cognition	The nurse assesses the cognitive ability of the patient and determines the severity of cognitive impairment. Based on this assessment, the nurse decides on the most effective way to communicate and to teach the patient.	■ Nurses are knowledgeable about the progression of cognitive impairment. Based on the patient's history and the nurse's assessment, the nurse decides on those interventions that have been found to be effective means of communicating and teaching patients who are cognitively impaired. The nurse creatively employs those methods.
Collaboration	The nurse's assessment determines the patient's post-discharge needs, which may include the need for subacute care; visiting nurse services for wound care, vital sign monitoring, teaching, and safety assessment; and the need for home physical therapy.	■ Nurses participate in a collaborative team approach when caring for patients. ■ Nurses refer patients to social services and case management to provide services outside of the hospital while continuing certain interventions for goal attainment.
Communication	Priorities of patient care need to be communicated to achieve continuity of care. Passing on correct information about patient status helps nurses on the next shift make competent decisions about patient care.	■ Nurses use the patient's plan of care, written or electronic, to communicate priority goals of the patient; document treatments, interventions and outcomes, and teaching; and record their work.
Safety	All clinical decisions, actions, and intervention on the part of the nurse must protect patients from harm. Clinical decision making and nursing actions and interventions must protect the nurse and nursing colleagues from harm.	■ Protecting patients from harm, or nonmaleficence, is one of the ethical foundations of nursing care. ■ Behaviors that endanger the nurse, nursing colleagues, and staff increase the risk of serious injury, loss of staff members due to injury, and possible health repercussions such as needlesticks and back injuries.
Thermoregulation	Patients with thermoregulatory dysfunction require immediate interventions to begin cooling and minimize organ and brain injury in cases of hyperthermia and immediate warming for patients with hypothermia to minimize tissue injury, loss of limb, or in cases of extreme exposure, death.	■ The nurse is knowledgeable about the need for immediate interventions and the necessary precautions in treating patients with exposure and thermoregulatory disorders. This knowledge, in combination with patient assessment, helps the nurse make appropriate decisions about the independent actions the nurse will take.

Focus on Diversity and Culture
Double Minority and Patient–Provider Relationships

Shared clinical decision making, the combination of clinical expertise and patient values and preferences, is an important part of the patient–provider relationship. Patients who belong to more than one minority group, for example patients who identify as lesbian, gay, bisexual, or transgender (LGBT), and also identify with an ethnic or cultural minority, are at risk for suboptimal shared decision making (DeMeester et al., 2016; Peek et al., 2016), which often results in poor clinical outcomes (Harvey & Housel, 2014). Patients describe healthcare providers' lack of knowledge regarding gender identity, cultural barriers, and distrust as factors that contribute to stigmatization and discrimination in the healthcare system. DeMeester et al. (2016) provide an extensive list of components for both patients and providers to assist in overcoming barriers to shared decision making for double-minority individuals. Peek and colleagues (2016) developed a model that depicts how race, gender identity, and other factors influence shared decision making. Shared decision making can help break down barriers between providers and patients to help increase trust and improve clinical outcomes.

REVIEW The Concept of Clinical Decision Making

RELATE Link the Concepts

Linking the concept of clinical decision making with the concept of legal issues:

1. What legal actions may occur if the nurse fails to make prudent clinical decisions? Explain your answer.

2. What role regarding sound clinical decision making in patient care is expected of the licensed registered nurse?

3. What role regarding sound clinical decision making in the workplace does the employer expect of the nurse?

Linking the concept of clinical decision making with the concept of evidence-based practice:

4. The nurse with strong critical thinking maintains an evidenced-based practice by _____.

5. A nurse reads a peer-reviewed article that recommends changing currently accepted practice. What critical thinking will the nurse perform before accepting the article's recommendations?

Linking the concept of clinical decision making with the concept of ethics:

6. What ethical obligation does the nurse hold toward the patient related to clinical decision making?

7. What ethical obligation does the nurse hold toward the hiring facility related to clinical decision making?

REFER Go to Pearson MyLab Nursing and eText

REFLECT Apply Your Knowledge

The nurse is caring for a patient who was admitted 3 days ago with acute abdominal pain. Following extensive diagnostic testing, the patient has received a medical diagnosis of stomach cancer, with suspected metastasis to the liver and pancreas. The oncologist has informed the patient that there are several options related to treatment. Option 1 is to surgically remove as much of the tumor as possible, followed by chemotherapy and radiation therapy. This is the most aggressive approach with the best odds for survival, but the oncologist tells the patient that with the amount of metastasis that has already occurred, the odds for survival are still not very good (less than 10%). The second option is to do nothing, allowing the patient to remain as comfortable as possible (palliative care) until death, which will likely occur in 3–6 months. The third option is the moderate option and involves chemotherapy to slow cancer growth, which may prolong the patient's life but will result in side effects (e.g., hair loss, vomiting, weakness) that will likely impact the patient's quality of life. After the oncologist leaves the room, the patient looks to the nurse and asks, "What do you think I should do? What would you do if you were me?"

1. What actions by the nurse would be most appropriate for this patient?

2. What ethical, legal, and moral duties guide the nurse when responding to this patient's questions?

3. How would you respond to each of the patient's questions?

≫ Exemplar 36.A The Nursing Process

Exemplar Learning Outcomes

36.A Analyze the nursing process as it relates to clinical decision making.

- Describe the assessment phase of the nursing process.
- Describe the diagnosis phase of the nursing process.
- Describe the planning phase of the nursing process.
- Describe the implementation phase of the nursing process.
- Describe the evaluation phase of the nursing process.
- Differentiate the use of the nursing process in caring for patients across the lifespan.

Exemplar Key Terms

Assessment, 2497
Cognitive skills, 2514
Collaborative interventions, 2511
Defining characteristics, 2502
Dependent interventions, 2511
Diagnostic label, 2501
Etiology, 2502
Evaluation, 2509
Evaluation statement, 2517
Goal, 2507
Health promotion diagnosis, 2501
Implementation, 2511
Independent interventions, 2511
Interpersonal skills, 2515
Modifiers, 2502
NANDA-I, 2500
Nursing diagnosis, 2500
Nursing process, 2494
Outcome, 2507
Planning, 2507
Problem-focused diagnosis, 2502
Risk factors, 2501
Risk nursing diagnosis, 2502
SMART, 2509
Syndrome diagnosis, 2502
Technical skills, 2515

Overview

The **nursing process** is used to identify a patient's health status and actual or potential healthcare problems or needs, to establish plans to meet the identified needs, to deliver specific nursing interventions to meet those needs, and to evaluate the success of those interventions. The patient may be an individual, a family, or a group.

The nursing process gained legitimacy in clinical practice in 1973 when the phases of the nursing process were included in the American Nurses Association (ANA) *Standards of Nursing Practice*. The standards of practice within the

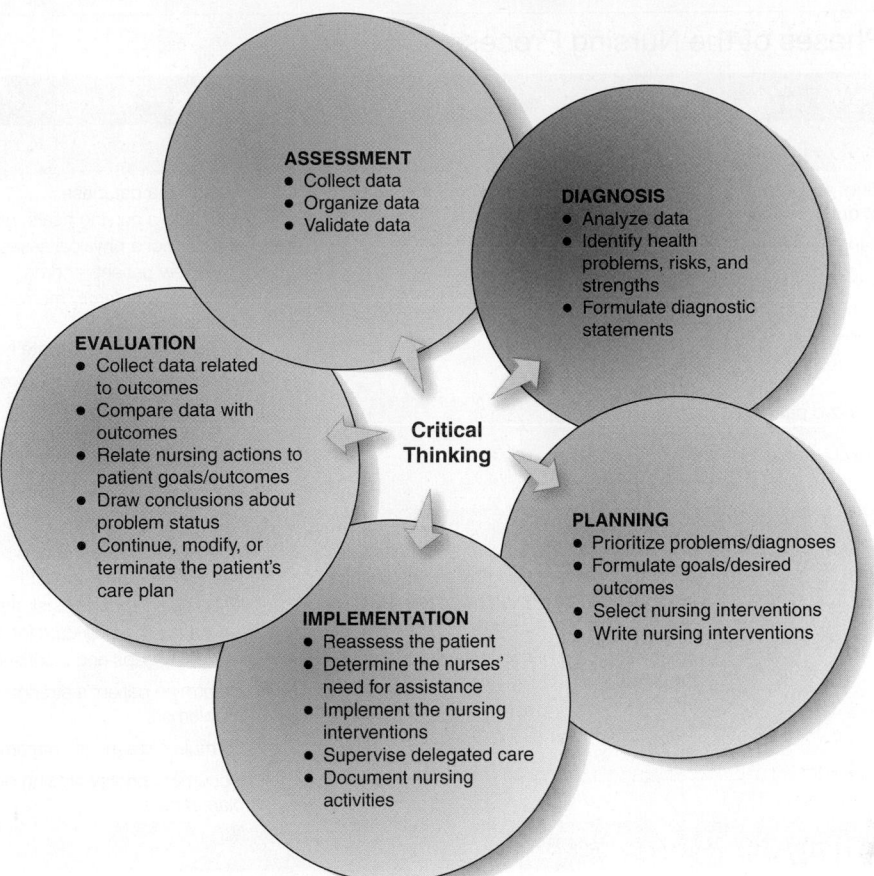

Figure 36–6 》 The nursing process in action.

most current *Scope and Standards of Nursing Practice* include five phases of the nursing process: assessment, diagnosis, planning, implementation, and evaluation (American Nurses Association, 2010a). Outcome or outcome identification is sometimes included as another phase of the nursing process; however, in this text, outcomes are used to evaluate the patient's response to the plan of care. Virtually every state has since revised its nurse practice acts to reflect the nursing process. See **Figure 36–6 》** for an illustration of the nursing process.

A few general characteristics of the nursing process complement its ease to organize the flow of nursing care and produce an individualized plan of care for all patients across the lifespan. The nursing process is a *dynamic* rather than static plan that can adapt to changes in the patient's status. The nursing process is *patient-centered.* The nurse organizes the plan of care according to a patient's need to achieve goals and outcomes.

Health is more than the absence of disease: it incorporates physical, spiritual, and emotional well-being. The nurse takes a holistic view of the patient and collects data related to the biological, psychologic, psychosocial, socioeconomic, and spiritual aspects of the patient. In other words, a holistic view sees the patient as the whole person rather than just the illness.

The nursing process is an adaptation of problem solving used by those involved with patient care. For example, physicians use the medical model, which focuses on physiologic

systems and the disease process. The nursing process is directed toward a patient's responses to the disease process and to the effects of the disease process, interventions, and therapies that interrupt the patient's standard of functioning in various aspects of his or her life. The nursing process assists the patient in restoring both physical health and general well-being within the limits of the patient's health condition.

Decision making is involved in every phase of the nursing process. Nurses can be very creative in making decisions to facilitate the individualized plan of care for each patient. The nursing process is interpersonal and *collaborative;* it requires the nurse to communicate directly and consistently with patients and families to meet their needs. The nursing process also requires that nurses collaborate with other members of the healthcare team in a joint effort to provide quality patient care. The universal characteristics of the nursing process make it an amenable framework for nursing care in all types of healthcare settings and with patients of all age groups, ethnicities, religions, cultures, genders, and sexual orientations.

An overview of the five phases of the nursing process is given in **Table 36–5 》**. The phases of the nursing process are not separate entities—they are interrelated and they overlap. For example, assessment, which may be considered the first phase of the nursing process, is also carried out during the implementation and evaluation phases. For instance, while administering medications (implementation), the

TABLE 36–5 The Phases of the Nursing Process

Phase and Description	Purpose	Activities
Assessment		
Collecting, organizing, validating, and documenting patient's assessment data Begin noting significant cues and how they may be clustering.	To establish a database about the patient's response to health concerns or illness and the ability to manage healthcare needs.	■ Establish a database: — Obtain a nursing health history. — Conduct a physical assessment. — Review patient records. — Speak with family members and significant support persons. — Speak with appropriate health professionals. ■ Update data to keep it current.
Look for significant cue clusters and patterns.		■ Organize data.
Seek more assessment data to clarify cue clusters and patterns.		■ Validate data. ■ Communicate/document data.
Nursing Diagnosis		
Analyzing and synthesizing data	To identify patient strengths and health problems that can be prevented or resolved by collaborative and nursing interventions. To develop a list of nursing and collaborative problems.	■ Interpret and analyze data: — Compare data against standards. — Cluster or group data (generate tentative hypotheses). — Identify gaps and inconsistencies. ■ Determine patient's strengths, risks, diagnoses, and problems. ■ Formulate diagnostic statements. ■ Document priority nursing diagnoses on the nursing plan of care.
Planning		
Determining how to prevent, reduce, or resolve the identified priority patient problems; how to support patient strengths; and how to implement nursing interventions in an organized, individualized, and goal-directed manner	To develop an individualized plan of care that specifies patient goals/desired outcomes, and related priority nursing interventions.	■ Set priorities and goals/outcomes in collaboration with patient. ■ Write goals/desired outcomes. ■ Select nursing strategies/interventions. ■ Consult other health professionals. ■ Write nursing interventions and nursing plan of care. ■ Communicate plan of care to relevant healthcare providers.
Implementation		
Carrying out (or delegating) and then documenting the planned nursing interventions	To assist the patient to meet desired goals/outcomes; promote wellness; prevent illness and disease; restore health; and facilitate coping with altered functioning.	■ Reassess the patient to update the database to keep it current. ■ Determine the nurse's need for assistance. ■ Perform planned priority nursing interventions. ■ Communicate what nursing actions were implemented: — Document care and patient responses to care. — Give verbal reports as necessary.
Evaluation		
Measuring the degree to which goals/outcomes have been achieved and identifying factors that positively or negatively influence goal achievement	To determine whether to continue, modify, or terminate the plan of care.	■ Collaborate with patient and collect data related to desired outcomes. ■ Judge whether goals/outcomes have been achieved. ■ Relate nursing actions to patient outcomes. ■ Make decisions about problem status. ■ Review and modify the plan of care as indicated or terminate it. ■ Document achievement of outcomes and modification of the plan of care.

nurse assesses the patient to determine the patient's continued need for the medication, response to the medication, and potential side effects of the medication.

SAFETY ALERT New nurses are often afraid to ask for help as they try to work independently. Undertaking a task better completed by more than one person is dangerous for the nurse and for the patient. Patient safety supersedes the desire to "do it all." Before undertaking any physical activity involving a patient, assess the safety risk to you and to the patient. Follow hospital guidelines for moving and transferring patients. Use assistive devices if available and ask for help from physical therapists, UAPs, and nursing colleagues. Although family members may be present and willing, they should not take part in transferring and moving patients. Remember, patient safety comes first.

Each phase of the nursing process affects the others. For example, if inadequate data are obtained during assessment, the nursing diagnoses will be incomplete or incorrect; inaccuracy will also be reflected in the planning, implementation, and evaluation phases. Because the nursing process is an organizing tool that guides the nurse's approach to patient care and decision making, the process always begins with accurate data collection.

Assessment

Assessment is the systematic and continuous collection of data about a patient for the purpose of determining the patient's current and ongoing health status, predicting the patient's health risks, and identifying appropriate health-promoting activities. Assessment is a continuous process carried out during all phases of the nursing process. For example, in the evaluation phase, the nurse assesses the outcomes of the nursing interventions and evaluates goal achievement. All phases of the nursing process depend on the accurate and complete collection of assessment data.

A nursing assessment focuses on a patient's responses to a health problem. It includes subjective data obtained from the patient or family about the patient's needs, health condition, health practices, values, health history, and lifestyle. It also includes objective data obtained through assessment and physical examination of the patient. Available sources, including the patient's medical record or office visit records, are used to assist the nurse in developing a database that includes the patient's past medical history and previous current health status (see the module on Assessment for further information).

Assessment data can be organized according to one of several models. Most nursing programs develop their own framework for nursing assessment data based on these models. One example is Gordon's 11 functional health patterns to organize the data (Gordon, 2010):

1. Health perception–health management pattern
2. Nutritional-metabolic pattern
3. Elimination pattern
4. Activity-exercise pattern
5. Sleep-rest pattern
6. Cognitive-perceptual pattern
7. Self-perception/self-concept pattern
8. Role-relationship pattern
9. Sexuality-reproductive pattern
10. Coping/stress-tolerance pattern
11. Value-belief pattern.

Another example is Roy's adaptation model, which states that the goal of nursing is to promote adaptation in each of four adaptive modes:

1. Physiologic
2. Self-concept
3. Role function
4. Interdependence (Roy, 2008).

Roy separates the assessment portion of the nursing process into two phases: assessment of behavior and assessment of stimuli. Behaviors include subjective and objective behaviors (i.e., symptoms and signs, respectively) as well as adaptive and ineffective behaviors (i.e., does the behavior promote health or not). Stimuli include focal, contextual, and residual stimuli. The focal stimulus is what the patient is most focused on and is often the origin of the "related to" phrase of the nursing diagnosis. Contextual stimuli are all the factors that contribute to the patient's interpretation of the focal stimulus, including environment, background, culture, and so on. Residual stimuli are factors that do not have a clear effect on the situation. Once the relationship between the factors is clear, then the stimulus is categorized as a focal or contextual stimulus.

Another common way to organize assessment data is by body systems:

1. Immune system
2. Respiratory system
3. Cardiovascular system
4. Nervous system
5. Musculoskeletal system
6. Gastrointestinal system
7. Genitourinary system
8. Reproductive system.

Figure 36–7 》 provides an example of how data might be organized according to a systems assessment or complete assessment (using the Case Study featuring Amanda Aquilini).

After data have been collected, it is validated (see the module on Assessment) and analyzed. Analysis involves three steps:

1. Comparing data against standards (to identify significant cues)
2. Clustering cues (to generate tentative hypotheses)
3. Identifying gaps and inconsistencies.

Experienced nurses perform these activities continuously rather than sequentially as data clusters around current health problems that require interventions. For this reason, nurses should think critically about what to assess.

When gathering and clustering assessment data for children, the nurse will need to include the parents as a major source of subjective data as well as asking the child about his or her feelings. Assessment of the family's needs related to the child's illness (e.g., does lack of insurance present a barrier to accessing services or paying for prescriptions?) is also necessary. See the Lifespan Considerations section for more detail on using the nursing process with children.

ADMISSION DATA

Date 4-16-17 Time 3:15p.m Primary Language English

Arrived Via: ☐ Wheelchair ☐ Stretcher ☑ Ambulatory

From: ☐ Admitting ☐ ER ☑ Home ☐ Nursing Home ☐ Other

Admitting M.D. R. Katz Time Notified 5 p.m.

ORIENTATION TO UNIT

	YES	NO		YES	NO
Arm Band Correct	☑	☐	Visiting Hours	☑	☐
Allergy Band	☑	☐	Smoking Policy	☑	☐
Telephone	☑	☐	TV, Lights, Bed Controls,		
Electrical Policy	☑	☐	Call Lights, Side Rails	☑	☐
Educational Material	☑	☐	Nurses Station	☑	☐
(TV Brochure)	☑	☐			

Family M.D. R. Katz

Weight 125 lb Height 5ft. 2in. BP:R — L 122/80

Temp. 103F Pulse 92, weak Resp. 28, shallow

Source Providing Information ☑ Patient ☐ Other

Unable to Obtain History ☐

Reason for Admission (Onset, Duration, Pt.'s Perception) ("Chest cold" X2 weeks S.O.B on exertion. "Lung pain, fever," "Dr. says I have pneumonia.")"

ALLERGIES & REACTIONS

Drugs Penicillin

Food/Other

Signs & Symptoms rash, nausea

Blood Reaction ☐ Yes ☑ No Dyes/Shellfish ☐ Yes ☑ No

MEDICATIONS

Current Meds	Dose/Freq.	Last Dose
Synthroid	0.1 mg. daily	4-16, 8 a.m.

Disposition of Meds: ☑ Home ☐ Pharmacy ☐ Safe *At Bedside

MEDICAL HISTORY

☑ No Major Problems ☐ Gastro

☐ Cardiac ☐ Arthritis

☐ Hyper/Hypotension ☐ Stroke

☐ Diabetes ☐ Seizures

☐ Cancer ☐ Glaucoma

☐ Respiratory ☑ Other Childbirth-2000

Surgery/Procedures	Date
Appendectomy	1985
Partial thyroidectomy	2000

SPECIAL ASSISTIVE DEVICES

☐ Wheelchair ☐ Contacts ☐ Venous ☐ Dentures

☐ Braces ☐ Hearing Aid Access ☐ Partial

☐ Cane/Crutches ☐ Prosthesis Device ☐ Upper

☐ Walker ☐ Glasses ☐ Epidural Catheter ☐ Lower

☐ Other None

VALUABLES

Patient informed Hospital not responsible for personal belongings.

Valuables Disposition: ☐ Patient ☐ Safe ☐ Given to

Patient/SO Signature None

PSYCHOSOCIAL HISTORY

Recent Stress None

Coping Mechanism Not assessed because of fatigue

Support System Husband, coworkers, friends

Calm: ☑ Yes ☐ No

Anxious: ☐ Yes ☐ No Facial muscles tense; trembling

Religion Catholic, Would want Last Rites

Tobacco Use: ☐ Yes ☑ No

Alcohol Use: ☐ Yes ☑ No

Drug Use: ☐ Yes ☑ No

NEUROLOGICAL

Oriented: ☑ Person ☑ Place ☑ Time ☐ Confused ☐ Sedated
☐ Alert ☐ Restless ☑ Lethargic ☐ Comatose

Pupils: ☑ Equal ☐ Unequal ☑ Reactive ☐ Sluggish
☐ Other 3mm.

Extremity Strength: ☑ Equal ☐ Unequal

Speech: ☑ Clear ☐ Slurred ☐ Other

MUSCULO-SKELETAL

Normal ROM of Extremities ☑ Yes ☐ No

☑ Weakness ☐ Paralysis ☐ Contractures ☐ Joint Swelling ☑ Pain
☐ Other ↓ related to fatigue when coughing

RESPIRATORY

Pattern: ☐ Even ☐ Uneven ☑ Shallow ☑ Dyspnea
☑ Other diminished breath sounds

Breathing Sounds: ☐ Clear ☑ Other inspiratory crackles

Secretions: ☐ None ☑ Other pink, thick sputum

Cough: ☐ None ☑ Productive ☐ Nonproductive

CARDIOVASCULAR

Pulses: Apical Rate 92-W ☑ Reg. ☐ Irregular ☐ Pacemaker
S = Strong W = Weak A = Absent D = Doppler

Radial R 92 L ___ Pedal R ___ L ___

Edema: ☑ Absent ☐ Present Site

Perfusion: ☐ Warm ☐ Dry ☑ Diaphoretic ☐ Cool (Hot)

GASTROINTESTINAL

Oral Mucosa ☐ Normal ☑ Other pale and dry

Bowel Sounds: ☑ Normal ☐ Other Abd. soft

Wt. Change: ☐ ☑ N/V Stool Frequency/Character 1/day; soft

Last B/M 4-15-07 ☐ Ostomy (type)

Equip.

GENITOURINARY

Urine: Last Voided This morning

☐ Normal ☐ Anuria ☐ Hematuria ☐ Dysuri ☐ Incontinent

☑ Other ↓ amount & frequency since ill

☐ Catheter (type) Other

LMP 4-1-07 ☐ Vaginal/Penile Discharge

Other

SELF CARE

Need Assist with: ☐ Ambulating ☐ Elimination
☐ Meals ☑ Hygiene ☐ Dressing
While fatigued

Amanda Aquilini [F, age 28]
#4637651

**� NORTH BROWARD HOSPITAL DISTRICT
NURSING ADMINISTRATION ASSESSMENT**

Figure 36–7 》 Assessment for Amanda Aquilini.

NUTRITION

General Appearance: ☑ Well Nourished ☐ Emaciated
☐ Other _____

Appetite: ☐ Good ☐ Fair ☑ Poor -x2 days
Diet _Liquid_ Meal Pattern _3/day_
☐ Feeds Self ☐ Assist ☐ Total Feed

SKIN ASSESSMENT

Color: ☐ Normal ☐ Flushed ☑ Pale ☐ Dusky ☐ Cyanotic
☐ Jaundiced ☑ Other _Cheeks flushed, hot_
General Description _Surgical scars:_
RLQ abdomen; anterior neck
_____
_____
_____
Note Cultures Obtained _____
_____
_____

PRESSURE SORE ™AT RISK SCREENING CRITERIA

OVERALL SKIN CONDITION
Grade
0	Turgor (elasticity adequate, skin warm and moist)
✓ 1	Poor turgor, skin cold & dry
2	Areas mottled, red or denuded
3	Existing skin ulcer/lesions

BOWEL AND BLADDER CONTROL
Grade
✓ 0	Always able to ask for bedpan
1	Incontinence of urine
2	Incontinence of feces
3	Totally incontinent Confined to bed

REHABILITATIVE STATE
Grade
0	Fully ambulatory
✓ 1	Ambulated with assistance
2	Chair to bed ambulation only
3	Confined to bed
4	Immobile in bed

NUTRITIONAL STATE
Grade
0	Eats all
✓ 1	Eats very little
2	Refuses food often
3	Tube feeding
4	Intravenous feeding

MENTAL STATE
Grade
✓ 0	Alert and clear
1	Confused
2	Disoriented/senile
3	Stuporous
4	Unconcious

CHRONIC DISEASE STATUS
(i.e. COPD, ASCVD. Peripheral Vascular Disease, Diabetes, or Renal Disease, Cancer, Motor or Sensory Deficits, Elderly, Other)
Grade
✓ 0	Absent
1	One Present
2	Two Present
3	Three or more Present

TOTAL _____ Refer to Skin Care Protocol

FALLS SCREENING

If one or more of the following are checked institute fall precautions/plan of care
☐ History of Falls ☐ Unsteady Gait ☐ Confusion/Disorientation ☐ Dizziness

If two or more of the following are checked institute fall precautions/plan of care
☐ Age over 80
☐ Impaired vision
☐ Multiple Diagnoses
☐ Inability to understand or follow directions
☐ Utilizes cane, walker, w/c
☐ Impaired hearing
☐ Sleeplessness
☐ Urgency/frequency in elimination
☐ Medication/Sedative /Diuretic etc.

NURSE SIGNATURE/TITLE	DATE	TIME
Mary Medina, RN	_4-16-17_	_3:30pm_
NURSE SIGNATURE/TITLE	DATE	TIME

EDUCATION/DISCHARGE PLANNING

1. What do you know about your present illness? _"Dr. says I have pneumonia." "I will have an I.V."_
2. What information do you want or need about your illness? _____
3. Would you like family/SO involved in your care? _Husband, Michael_
4. How long do you expect to be in the hospital? _"1-2 days"_
5. What concerns do you have about leaving the hospital? _____

CHECK APPROPRIATE BOX

Will patient need post discharge assistance with ADLs/physical functioning? ☐ Yes ☑ No ☐ Unknown
Does patient have family capable of and willing to provide assistance post discharge?
☑ Yes ☐ No ☐ Unknown ☐ No family
Is assistance needed beyond that which family can provide?
☐ Yes ☑ No ☐ Unknown
Previous admission in the last six months?
☐ Yes ☑ No ☐ Unknown
Patient lives with _Husband and 1 child_
Planned discharge to _Home_
Comments: _Fatigue and anxiety may have interfered with learning. Re-teach anything covered at admission, later._
_____

Social Services Notified ☐ Yes ☑ No

NARRATIVE NOTES

S--c/o sharp chest pain when coughing and dyspnea on exertion. States unable to carry out regular daily exercise for past week. Coughing relieved "if I sit up and sit still." Nausea associated with coughing. Having occasional "chills." Occasionally becomes frightened, stating, "I can't breathe." Well groomed but "too tired to put on make-up." O--Chest expansion < 3cm, no nasal flaring or use of accessory muscles. Breath sounds and insp. crackles in Ⓡ upper and lower chest. Assesses own supports as "good" (eg, relationship c̄ husband). Is "worried" about daughter. States husband will be out of town until tomorrow. Left 3-year-old daughter with neighbor. Concerned too about her work (is attorney). "I'll never get caught up." Had water at noon—no food today. Agrees to save urine for 24 hr. specimen. IV D₅W LR 1000 mL started in Ⓡ arm, 100 mL/hr. Slow capillary refill. Keeping head of bed↑ to facilitate breathing.

✸✸ **NORTH BROWARD HOSPITAL DISTRICT**
NURSING ADMINISTRATION ASSESSMENT

Figure 36–7 》》 Assessment for Amanda Aquilini. *(continued)*

Case Study >> Part 1

Amanda Aquilini, a 28-year-old married attorney with one child, was admitted to the medical unit of the local hospital with a medical diagnosis of pneumonia throughout her right lung. She has been assigned to Nurse Mary Medina, RN. After Mrs. Aquilini is oriented to her room by the UAP, Nurse Medina does her admission assessment (see **Figure 36–8 >>**).

During the interview, Nurse Medina learns that Mrs. Aquilini has had a "chest cold" for 2 weeks and has been experiencing shortness of breath when she tries to cook dinner or clean the house. Even putting her child to bed makes her short of breath. Mrs. Aquilini reports that for the past few days, she has not felt like eating very much and is only drinking a couple of glasses of tea every day. She states she has had a productive cough with a medium amount of thick, foul-smelling, pink sputum. Mrs. Aquilini tells Nurse Medina that she hasn't felt like going to work; she just feels tired all the time. She states she doesn't smoke and only drinks a glass of wine occasionally. Mrs. Aquilini likes to work out in the yard or go for a walk three or four times a week but lately has not had the energy to do these things. She currently takes levothyroxine 0.1 mg daily, and her last hospitalization was for the delivery of her child 3 years ago. Mrs. Aquilini states she is allergic to penicillin but not to foods, latex, or iodine.

On physical examination, Mrs. Aquilini is 62 in. (157 cm) tall and weighs 125 lbs. (56.7 kg). Vital signs: T_O 103°F (39.4°C); P 92 bpm; R 28/min; blood pressure 122/80 mmHg, and oxygen saturation (O_2 Sat) 95% on room air. Nurse Medina observes that Mrs. Aquilini's skin is dry, her cheeks are flushed, and she is experiencing chills. Auscultation reveals inspiratory rhonchi with diminished breath sounds in the right lung. Respirations are shallow. Her oral mucous membranes are pale and dry and her skin turgor when tented is >3 seconds. She speaks in short sentences. Peripheral pulses are weak and equal bilateral in all four extremities.

Clinical Reasoning Questions Level I

1. Which assessment data are salient cues?
2. Do these cues form any clusters? What are they?

Clinical Reasoning Questions Level II

3. Are there any other questions you would ask Mrs. Aquilini to further clarify her health status?
4. Which cluster of significant cues would be the priority? Why?

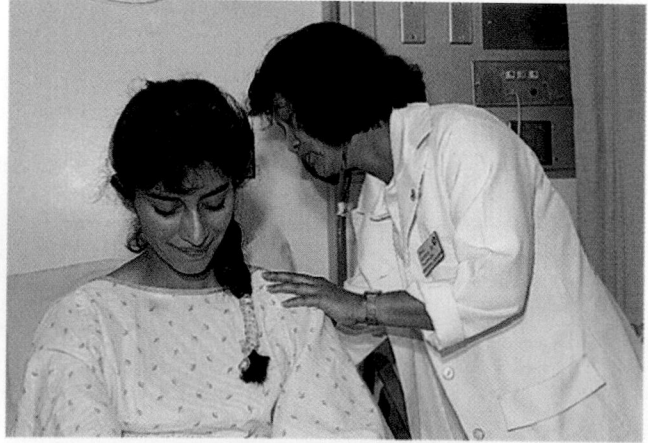

Figure 36–8 >> Assessment: Mrs. Aquilini's admission assessment reveals the following: temperature 103°F (39.4°C); pulse 92 bpm; respirations 28/min; and blood pressure 122/80 mmHg. Nurse Medina observes that Mrs. Aquilini's skin is dry, her cheeks are flushed, and she is experiencing chills. Auscultation reveals inspiratory crackles with diminished breath sounds in the right lung.

Diagnosis

In the diagnosis phase of the nursing process, nurses use critical thinking skills to cluster the assessment data and identify problems. Diagnosis is a pivotal step in the nursing process. Assessment activities preceding this phase are directed toward formulating a nursing diagnosis, and the care-planning activities following this phase are based on the nursing diagnoses.

Nursing diagnoses are developed and periodically updated by **NANDA-I** (formerly the North American Nursing Diagnosis Association). In 1990, NANDA-I adopted an official working definition of **nursing diagnosis**, "a clinical judgment concerning a human response to health conditions/life processes, or a vulnerability for that response, by an individual, family, group or community. A nursing diagnosis provides the basis for selection of nursing interventions to achieve outcomes for which the nurse has accountability" (NANDA-I, 2013). This definition implies the following:

- Registered nurses are responsible for making nursing diagnoses, even though other nursing personnel may contribute data to the process of diagnosing and may implement specified nursing care. In the *Standards of Professional Nursing Practice*, Standard 2 addresses the fact that registered nurses determine the diagnoses or issues from analysis of the assessment data (American Nurses Association, 2010a). The Joint Commission embraces ANA's *Nursing: Scope and Standards of Practice* and therefore requires evidence of nursing diagnoses in patients' medical records.

- The domains of nursing diagnoses include only those health states that nurses are educated and licensed to treat within their scope of practice (see the module on Legal Issues for further information). For example, nurses can diagnose and treat *Deficient Knowledge, Ineffective Coping*, or *Imbalanced Nutrition*, all of which are the human responses to the medical diagnosis of diabetes mellitus.

- A nursing diagnosis is a judgment made only after thorough, systematic assessment and data collection.

- Nursing diagnoses describe a continuum of health states: deviations from health, presence of risk factors, and areas of enhanced personal growth.

The current organization of nursing diagnoses is called Taxonomy II (NANDA-I, 2014). Taxonomy II has three levels: domains, classes, and nursing diagnoses. The diagnoses are coded according to seven axes that reflect elements of a patient's response addressed in the diagnosis: diagnostic focus, subject, judgment, location, age, time, and status.

>> **Stay Current:** For more information about NANDA-I-approved nursing diagnoses, refer to the NANDA-I website (www.nanda.org) and see Appendix A.

To identify nursing diagnoses effectively and then create and complete a nursing plan of care, the nurse must be familiar with:

- Common terms used with nursing diagnoses
- The difference between a nursing diagnosis and a medical diagnosis

- Types of nursing diagnoses
- Components of a nursing diagnosis.

Common Terms

A diagnosis is a statement or conclusion regarding the nature of a phenomenon. The standardized NANDA-I names for the nursing diagnoses are called **diagnostic labels**. The patient's problem statement is called a nursing diagnosis, and it includes the diagnostic label plus the etiology (causal relationship between a problem and its related or risk factors). **Risk factors** are factors that cause a patient to be vulnerable to developing a health problem. The term *diagnosing* refers to the reasoning process the nurse uses to formulate the nursing diagnosis.

Nursing diagnoses are developed using a multiaxial system. Axes are categories that address components of the diagnostic process. There are seven axes: the focus of the diagnosis, the subject of the diagnosis (patient, family, and so on), nursing judgment (impaired, inefficient, ineffective, and so on), locations (cardiac, pulmonary, leg, and so on), age (child, adult, adolescent, and so on), time (chronic, acute, intermittent, constant, and so on), and status of the diagnosis (problem-focused, risk, or health promotion).

Axis 1, the focus of the diagnosis, is the "principal element or the fundamental and essential part, the root, of the nursing diagnosis" (NANDA-I, 2014, p. 93). In the diagnosis *Compromised Family Coping*, coping is the principal element. Axis 2, the subject, may be explicit or implicit. For example, in the nursing diagnosis *Compromised Family Coping*, the subject, "family," comes from Axis 2. In the nursing diagnosis, *Ineffective Airway Clearance*, the subject, the patient, is implied. Axis 3 consists of modifiers that give meaning to the focus of the diagnosis. In the diagnosis *Compromised Family Coping*, the judgment is compromised (Axis 3). Other judgments in nursing diagnoses include complicated, decreased, delayed, ineffective, insufficient, and several other modifiers and descriptors.

Axis 4 provides a description, location, system, or function affected by the focus. In some cases, the location may not be a part of the body—for example, bed, wheelchair, or crutches. In the diagnosis *Ineffective Airway Clearance*, "airway" stems from Axis 4: airway is the location of the focus. Axis 5, age, represents the categorical age of the subject based on World Health Organization (WHO) definitions. Ages are categorized as fetus, neonate, infant, child, adolescent, and adult. For example, a nursing diagnosis that categorizes the age of the subject could be *Ineffective Infant Feeding Pattern*. By convention, an older adult is defined as an individual age 65 or older. Older adult is not defined by WHO (NANDA-I, 2014).

Axis 6 describes time as it relates to the nursing diagnosis. Time may be episodic, for example, perioperative, the time before and after surgery; it may be situational and relate to a set of circumstances, for example labor and delivery; or it may be intermittent or periodic. Time can also be acute, lasting less than 3 months, or chronic, lasting more than 3 months. In the diagnosis *Ineffective Coping Related to Chronic Back Pain*, the subject has endured back pain for at least 3 months. Other time-related terms include continuous and intermittent.

Axis 7, the status of a diagnosis, determines an actual or current health problem (a problem-focused diagnosis), a future problem (a risk diagnosis), or a desire to improve health and well-being (a **health promotion diagnosis**).

Nurses develop diagnoses by determining the focus (Axis 1) and adding a judgment (Axis 3). There are times when Axes 1 and 3 are combined—for example, *Nausea* or *Fatigue*. After determining the focus and the judgment, the subject is added. However, this is not necessary if the subject is an individual. Additional axes are then used to provide further detail and clarity.

Nursing Diagnosis Versus Medical Diagnosis

A nursing diagnosis is a statement of nursing judgment and refers to a condition that nurses, by virtue of their education, experience, and expertise, are licensed to treat. Nursing diagnoses describe the human response or a patient's physical, sociocultural, psychologic, and spiritual responses to an illness or a health condition. A medical diagnosis is made by a licensed provider such as a physician, advanced practice nurse, or physician assistant. Medical diagnoses refer to disease processes—specific pathophysiologic responses that are fairly uniform from one patient to another. Clinical Example D shows how these responses can vary among individuals:

Clinical Example D

Seventy-year-old Mary Cain and 20-year-old Kristi Vidan both have rheumatoid arthritis. Their disease processes are much the same. X-ray studies show that in both patients, the extent of inflammation and the number of joints involved are similar, and both patients experience almost constant pain. Mrs. Cain views her condition as part of the aging process and is responding with acceptance. Ms. Vidan, however, is responding with anger and hostility because she views her disease as a threat to her personal identity, role performance, and self-esteem.

Critical Thinking Questions

1. What barrier to effective pain management could Ms. Cain's acceptance of her rheumatoid arthritis possibly present?
2. How might the nurse separate the issue of personal identity for Ms. Vidan from her rheumatoid arthritis?
3. What are three issues of role performance that might be foremost in Ms. Vidan's mind when she thinks about her rheumatoid arthritis?
4. What aspects of rheumatoid arthritis mark it as an "old person's disease"?
5. How might the nurse help shift Ms. Vidan's concept of self-esteem from dwelling on her having rheumatoid arthritis to focusing on her effectively managing it?
6. Why might a results-based approach to the problem of rheumatoid arthritis be effective for helping Ms. Vidan manage the disease?

A patient's medical diagnosis remains the same for as long as the disease process is present, but nursing diagnoses change as the patient's responses change. Ms. Vidan's response to her illness may change over time to become more similar to those of Ms. Cain.

Types of Nursing Diagnoses

The current types of nursing diagnoses are problem-focused diagnoses (also referred to as actual diagnoses), risk diagnoses, health promotion diagnoses, and syndrome diagnoses (NANDA-I, 2014):

1. A **problem-focused diagnosis** is a patient problem that is present at the time of the nursing assessment. Examples are *Ineffective Breathing Pattern*, *Acute Pain*, and *Anxiety*. A problem-focused nursing diagnosis is based on a cluster of associated assessment data.

2. A **risk nursing diagnosis** is a clinical judgment that a problem does not exist, but the presence of risk factors indicates that a problem is likely to develop unless the nurse intervenes. For example, all hospitalized individuals have some possibility of acquiring an infection; however, a patient with diabetes or a compromised immune system is at higher risk than others. Therefore, the nurse would use the *Risk for Infection* nursing diagnosis to describe the patient's health status. The risk diagnosis documents a patient's health status vulnerability for a single diagnosis or his or her risk for a syndrome diagnosis.

3. A **health promotion diagnosis** reflects a patient's readiness to improve an aspect of health. For example, if a patient expresses the desire to improve eating habits, an appropriate diagnosis would be *Readiness for Enhanced Nutrition*. Similarly, if a woman expresses the desire to improve her health in order to prepare for pregnancy, *Readiness for Enhanced Childbearing Process* would be an appropriate health promotion nursing diagnosis. Health promotion diagnoses reflect patient awareness of well-being and the desire to maintain or enhance this state.

4. A **syndrome diagnosis** recognizes a cluster of individual nursing diagnoses that occur simultaneously and may result in the best patient outcomes if addressed concurrently (NANDA-I, 2016). Syndrome diagnoses may be problem-focused or risk diagnoses. For example, *Risk for Disuse Syndrome* may be assigned to patients who are bedridden. The cluster of diagnoses associated with disuse syndrome include *Impaired Physical Mobility*, *Risk for Impaired Tissue Integrity*, *Risk for Activity Intolerance*, *Risk for Constipation*, *Risk for Infection*, *Risk for Injury*, *Risk for Powerlessness*, and *Impaired Gas Exchange*.

Components of a Nursing Diagnosis

A nursing diagnosis has three components, and each component serves a specific purpose:

1. The **diagnostic label** ("What is the focus or subject of the problem?")
2. The **etiology** ("Where did it come from?" "What is it related to?")
3. The **defining characteristics** ("What does it look like?").

The Diagnostic Label

A NANDA-I diagnostic label describes the patient's response to a health problem for which nursing care is given. The diagnostic label describes the patient's health status clearly and concisely in a few words such as Infection, Nausea, or Urinary Incontinence. The diagnostic label identifies the topic that directs the formation of a patient goal

and desired outcomes. It may also suggest some nursing interventions.

To be clinically useful, diagnostic labels need to be specific; when the word *specify* follows the label, the nurse states the area in which the problem occurs. The only nursing diagnosis in the 2015–2017 list of NANDA-I diagnoses that requires specification is *Decisional Conflict*. For example, a family that is trying to decide whether to remove a feeding tube for an elderly parent at the end of life may receive the nursing diagnosis *Decisional Conflict* (removing feeding tube).

Modifiers, Axis 3, reflect nursing judgment, intensify the focus of the diagnosis, and give it specific meaning. For example, commonly used modifiers include

- *Deficient:* inadequate in amount, quality, or degree; not sufficient; incomplete
- *Impaired:* made worse, weakened, damaged, reduced, deteriorated
- *Decreased:* lesser in size, amount, or degree
- *Ineffective:* not producing the desired effect
- *Compromised:* to make vulnerable to threat.

Each diagnostic label approved by NANDA-I carries a definition that clarifies its meaning. For example, the definition of the diagnostic label *Activity Intolerance* is given in **Table 36–6 》》**.

The Etiology (Related Factors and Risk Factors)

The etiology component of a nursing diagnosis identifies one or more probable causes of the health problem, thereby giving a direction to the required nursing care and enabling the nurse to individualize the patient's care. Table 36–6 demonstrates the probable causes of *Activity Intolerance* that may include sedentary lifestyle, generalized weakness, and other factors. Differentiating among probable causes in the nursing diagnosis is essential because the cause of each problem may require different nursing interventions. **Table 36–7 》》** provides an example of patients with the nursing diagnosis of *Constipation* who have different etiologies; therefore, they require different interventions.

TABLE 36–6 Example of the Components of a Nursing Diagnosis

Diagnostic Label and Definition	Related Factors	Defining Characteristics
Activity Intolerance: Insufficient physiologic or psychologic energy to endure or complete required or desired daily activities	Bedrest or immobility Generalized weakness Imbalance between oxygen supply/demand Sedentary lifestyle	Verbal report of fatigue or weakness Abnormal heart rate or blood pressure response to activity Electrocardiographic changes reflecting arrhythmias or ischemia Exertional discomfort or dyspnea

Source: From NANDA-I. (2014). *NANDA nursing diagnoses: Definitions and classification 2015–2017.* Chichester, UK: Wiley-Blackwell. Adapted with permission.

TABLE 36–7 Example of a Nursing Diagnosis with Different Etiologies

Diagnostic Label (Problem)	Patient	Etiology
Constipation	Al Martinez	Long-term laxative use
	Jerry Wong	Inactivity and insufficient fluid intake
	Tanya Brown	Depression
	Caitlin Shea	Change in eating pattern

The Defining Characteristics

Defining characteristics refer to the cluster of signs and symptoms that indicate the presence of a particular diagnostic label. For actual nursing diagnoses, the defining characteristics are the patient's signs and symptoms. For risk nursing diagnoses, subjective and objective signs are not present. Thus, the factors that cause the patient to be more vulnerable to the problem are the etiology of a risk nursing diagnosis. Characteristics can be listed separately according to whether they are subjective or objective in nature. For example, the problem-focused diagnostic label *Fear* includes the following defining characteristics:

- Report of apprehension, being scared, having increased tension
- Diminished learning ability, unable to solve problems
- Diarrhea, vomiting, dry mouth, increase in pulse rate.

The risk diagnostic label *Risk for Falls* includes the following defining characteristics:

- Having a history of falling, using a cane to walk
- Lack of gate on the stairs, lack of parental supervision
- Tranquilizer use, anemia, visual difficulties.

Developing a Nursing Diagnosis

The skills and abilities of critical thinking discussed at the beginning of this module are used by nurses to analyze and apply reasoning to formulate nursing diagnoses. Data can be compared to standards, which are accepted measures, rules, or norms. For example, growth and development charts, normal ranges for laboratory values, or acceptable ranges for vital signs can provide standards against which to compare patient data when looking for norms. See **Table 36–8 ⟫** for some examples of how patient cues can compare with standards/norms.

An experienced nurse may enter a patient's room and immediately observe significant data and draw conclusions about the patient. As a result of attaining knowledge, skill, and expertise in the practice setting, the expert nurse may seem to perform these mental processes automatically. Novice nurses, however, need guidelines to understand and formulate nursing diagnoses (see the Critical Thinking section at the beginning of this module for further information).

Skillful assessment minimizes gaps and inconsistencies in data collection; however, data analysis should include a final check to ensure that assessment data are complete and current. Do the data make sense? For example, a nurse may learn from the nursing history that the patient reports not having seen a physician in 15 years, yet during the physical health examination he states, "My doctor takes my blood pressure every year." All inconsistencies must be clarified before a valid pattern can be established. See **Table 36–9 ⟫** for some examples of formulating nursing diagnoses based on patient cues.

After grouping and clustering the data, the nurse and patient together identify problems that support problem-focused and risk diagnoses, and if appropriate, health promotion diagnoses. This is primarily a decision-making process. In addition, the nurse determines whether the patient's problem is a nursing diagnosis, medical diagnosis, or collaborative problem. **Figure 36–9 ⟫** is a decision tree diagram that can help nurses make decisions about what kind of diagnosis is appropriate.

At this stage, the nurse and patient also establish the patient's strengths, resources, and abilities to cope. Most individuals have a clearer perception of their problems or weaknesses than of their strengths and assets, which they often take for granted. By taking an inventory of strengths,

TABLE 36–8 Examples of Patient Cues Compared to Standards/Norms

Cues from Patient	Standard/Norm	Interpretation of Cues
Height is 5 ft., 2 in. Woman with small frame Weighs 240 lb	Height and weight tables indicate that the "ideal" weight for a woman 5 ft., 2 in. with a small frame is 108–121 lb.	Deviation from population norms
Child is 17 months old. Parents state child has not yet attempted to speak. Child laughs aloud and makes cooing sounds.	Children usually speak their first word by 10–12 months of age.	Developmental delay
States, "I'm just not hungry these days." Ate only 15% of food on breakfast tray. Has lost 30 lb in past 3 months.	Patient usually eats three balanced meals per day. Adults typically maintain stable weight.	Changes in patient's usual health status
Mrs. Stuart reports that lately her husband angers easily. "Yesterday he even yelled at the dog." "He just seems so tense."	Mr. Stuart is usually relaxed and easygoing. He is friendly and kind to animals.	Changes in patient's usual behavior

TABLE 36–9 Examples of Formulating Nursing Diagnoses from Patient Cues

Patient Cue Clusters	Tentative Identification of Problems	Formulated Diagnostic Statements
"No appetite" since congestion Has not eaten today Last fluids at noon today Nauseated ×2 days	*Imbalanced Nutrition: Less Than Body Requirements*	*Imbalanced Nutrition: Less Than Body Requirements* related to decreased appetite and nausea (secondary to disease process)
Last fluids at noon today Oral temp 39.4°C (103°F) Skin hot and pale, cheeks flushed Mucous membranes dry Poor skin turgor Decreased urinary frequency and amount ×2 days	*Deficient Fluid Volume*	*Deficient Fluid Volume* related to intake insufficient to replace fluid loss secondary to fever, diaphoresis, anorexia
Difficulty sleeping because of cough "Can't breathe lying down"	*Disturbed Sleep Pattern*	*Disturbed Sleep Pattern* related to cough, pain, orthopnea, fever, and diaphoresis
States, "I feel weak" Short of breath on exertion *Cues from cognitive/perceptual pattern:* Responsive but fatigued "I can think OK, just weak." *Cues from cardiovascular pattern:* Radial pulses weak, regular; pulse rate 92 bpm	*Activity Intolerance*	*Activity Intolerance* related to general weakness, imbalance between oxygen supply/demand
Husband out of town; will be back tomorrow afternoon Child with neighbor until husband returns	*Interrupted Family Processes* related to mother's illness and temporary unavailability of father to provide child care	*Interrupted Family Processes* related to mother's illness and temporary unavailability of father to provide child care
Skin hot, pale, and moist Respirations shallow; chest expansion slight Cough productive of small amounts of thick pale pink sputum Inspiratory crackles auscultated throughout right upper and lower lungs Diminished breath sounds on right side	*Ineffective Airway Clearance* related to disease process	*Ineffective Airway Clearance* related to viscous secretions and shallow chest expansion secondary to pain, fluid volume deficit, and fatigue

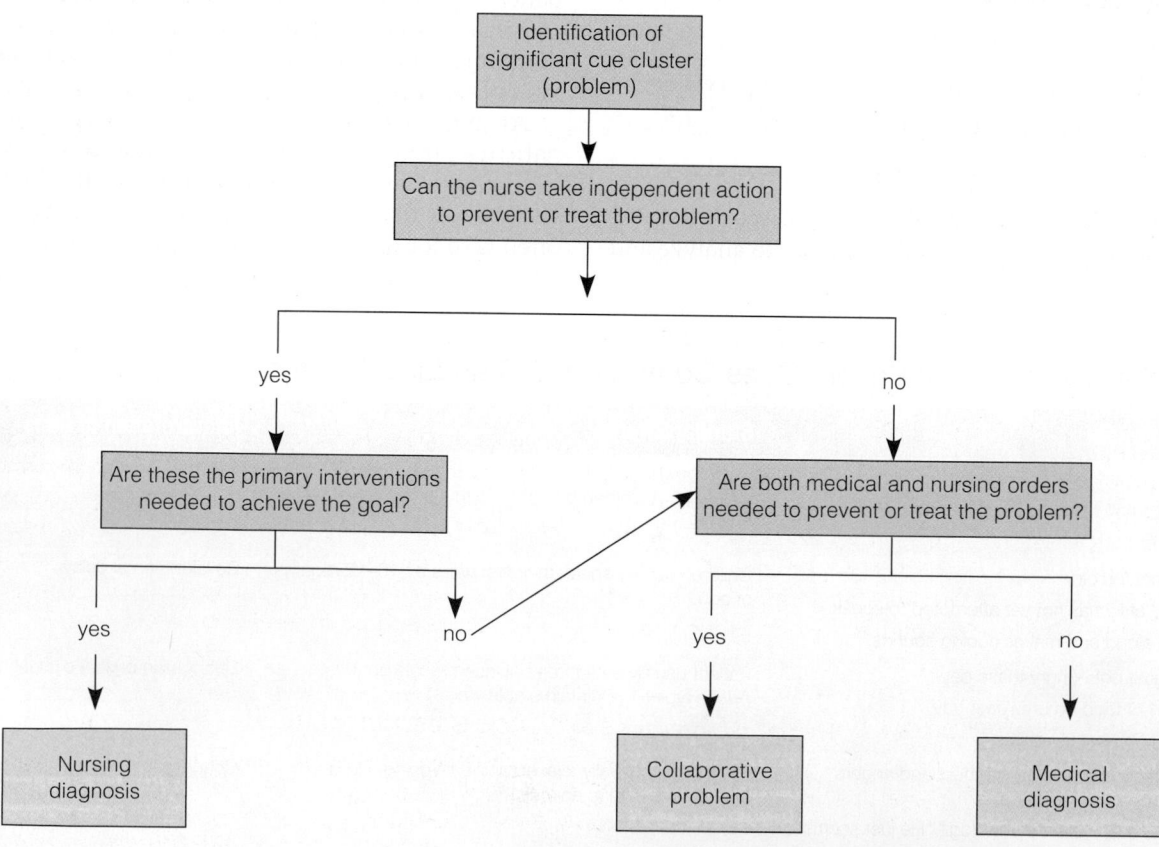

Figure 36–9 ▶ Decision tree for differentiating among nursing diagnoses, collaborative problems, and medical diagnoses.

TABLE 36–10 Examples of Two-Part Nursing Diagnosis Statements

Problem	Related to	Etiology
Constipation	related to	prolonged laxative use
Anxiety	related to	threat to physiologic integrity: possible cancer diagnosis

the patient can develop a more well-rounded self-concept and self-image. Strengths can be an aid to mobilizing health and regenerative processes. A patient's strength might include weight that is within the normal range for age and height, a strength that may enable the patient to recuperate from surgery faster and with fewer complications. Another patient's strength might be the absence of allergies or a non-smoking history.

A patient's strengths can be found in the nursing assessment record (health, home life, education, recreation, exercise, work, family and friends, religious beliefs, and sense of humor, for example), the health examination, and the patient's records.

Writing a Nursing Diagnosis Statement

Most nursing diagnoses are written as two-part or three-part statements.

Basic Two-Part Statement

The basic two-part statement includes the following:

1. *Problem (P):* NANDA-I label ("What's the problem?")
2. *Etiology (E):* related to . . . ("What's causing the problem?")

The two parts are joined by the words *related to* merely to imply a relationship. Some examples of two-part nursing diagnoses are shown in **Table 36–10 》**.

Basic Three-Part Statement

The basic three-part nursing diagnosis statement is called the PES format and includes the following:

1. *Problem (P):* NANDA-I label ("What's the problem?")
2. *Etiology (E):* related to . . . ("What's causing the problem?")
3. *Signs and symptoms (S):* defining characteristics of problem ("What's it look like?")

Actual nursing diagnoses can be documented by using a three-part statement (see **Table 36–11 》》**) because the signs and symptoms have been identified. This format cannot be used for risk diagnoses because the patient does not have signs and symptoms of the diagnosis. The PES format is especially recommended for beginner nurses

because the signs and symptoms validate why the diagnosis was chosen and make the problem statement more descriptive.

Basic One-Part Statement

Some diagnostic statements, such as health promotion diagnoses and syndrome nursing diagnoses, consist of a NANDA-I label only. As the diagnostic labels are refined, they tend to become more specific so that nursing interventions can be derived from the label itself. Therefore, an etiology may not be needed. For example, adding an etiology to the label *Rape-Trauma Syndrome* does not make the label any more descriptive or useful.

NANDA-I has specified that any new health promotion diagnoses will be developed as one-part statements beginning with the words *Readiness for Enhanced* followed by the desired higher level of wellness (for example, *Readiness for Enhanced Parenting*). Currently, the NANDA-I list includes several health promotion diagnoses. Some of these are *Spiritual Well-Being, Breastfeeding, Coping,* and *Sleep*. These are usually accepted as one-part statements but may be made more explicit by adding a descriptor, for example, *Readiness for Enhanced Communication* (English-speaking class). See **Table 36–12 》** for general guidelines for writing all of the nursing diagnostic statements.

Common Variations

Common variations of the basic one-, two-, and three-part statements include the following:

1. Writing *unknown etiology* when the defining characteristics are present but the nurse does not know the cause or contributing factors. An example is *Acute Confusion* related to unknown etiology.
2. Using the phrase *complex factors* when there are too many etiologic factors or when they are too complex to state in a brief phrase. The actual causes of chronic low self-esteem, for instance, may be long term and complex, as in the following nursing diagnosis: *Chronic Low Self-Esteem* related to complex factors.
3. Using *secondary to* divides the etiology into two parts, thereby making the statement more descriptive and useful. The part following *secondary to* is often a pathophysiologic or disease process or a medical diagnosis, as in *Risk for Impaired Skin Integrity* related to decreased peripheral circulation secondary to diabetes.
4. Adding a second part to the general response or NANDA-I label to make it more precise. For example, the diagnosis *Impaired Skin Integrity* does not indicate the location of the problem. To make this label more specific, the nurse can add a descriptor as follows: *Impaired Skin Integrity* (left lateral ankle) related to decreased peripheral circulation.

TABLE 36–11 Example of a Three-Part Nursing Diagnosis Statement

Problem	Related to	Etiology	As Manifested by	Signs and Symptoms
Situational Low Self-Esteem	related to (r/t)	feelings of rejection by husband	as manifested by (amb)	hypersensitivity to criticism; states, "I don't know if I can manage by myself," and rejects positive feedback

TABLE 36–12 Guidelines for Writing a Nursing Diagnostic Statement

Guideline	Correct Statement	Incorrect or Ambiguous Statement
1. State in terms of a problem, not a need.	*Deficient Fluid Volume* (problem) related to fever	Fluid Replacement (need) related to fever
2. Word the statement so that it is legally advisable.	*Impaired Skin Integrity* related to immobility (legally acceptable)	*Impaired Skin Integrity* related to improper positioning (implies legal liability)
3. Use nonjudgmental statements.	*Spiritual Distress* related to inability to attend church services secondary to immobility (nonjudgmental)	*Spiritual Distress* related to strict rules necessitating church attendance (judgmental)
4. Make sure that both elements of the statement do not say the same thing.	*Risk for Impaired Skin Integrity* related to immobility	*Impaired Skin Integrity* related to ulceration of sacral area (response and probable cause are the same)
5. Be sure that cause and effect are correctly stated (i.e., the etiology causes the problem or puts the patient at risk for the problem).	*Acute Pain:* Severe headache related to fear of addiction to narcotics	*Acute Pain* related to severe headache
6. Word the diagnosis specifically and precisely to provide direction for planning nursing interventions.	*Impaired Oral Mucous Membrane* related to decreased salivation secondary to radiation of neck (specific)	*Impaired Oral Mucous Membrane* related to noxious agent (vague)
7. Use nursing terminology rather than medical terminology to describe the patient's response.	*Ineffective Airway Clearance* related to accumulation of secretions in lungs (nursing terminology)	*Risk for Pneumonia* (medical terminology)
8. Use nursing terminology rather than medical terminology to describe the probable cause of the patient's response.	*Ineffective Airway Clearance* related to accumulation of secretions in lungs (nursing terminology)	*Ineffective Airway Clearance* related to emphysema (medical terminology)

Avoiding Errors in Diagnostic Statements

It is important that nurses make nursing diagnoses with a high level of accuracy. Nurses can avoid some common errors of reasoning by recognizing them and applying appropriate critical thinking skills. Errors can occur at any point in the diagnostic process: data collection, data interpretation, and data clustering. Nurses can do the following to minimize diagnostic errors:

- **Verify.** Hypothesize possible explanations of the data, but realize that all diagnoses are only tentative until they are verified. Begin and end the diagnostic process by talking with the patient and family. When collecting health data, ask patients to describe both the problem and the factors they believe to be the cause of the problem. At the end of the process, ask patients to confirm the accuracy and relevance of the nursing diagnoses.

- **Build a good knowledge base and acquire clinical experience.** Nurses must apply knowledge from many different areas to recognize significant cues and patterns and generate hypotheses about the assessment data. Principles from chemistry, anatomy, and pharmacology, psychology, and sociology, among other disciplines, help the nurse understand patient data in a different way.

- **Have a working knowledge of what is normal.** Nurses need to know the population norms for vital signs, laboratory tests, speech development, breath sounds, and other indicators. In addition, nurses must determine what is usual for a particular patient, taking into account age, physical makeup, lifestyle, culture, and the patient's own perception of her normal status. For example, the generally accepted normal blood pressure for adults is in the range of 110/60 to 140/80 mmHg. However, a nurse might obtain a reading of 90/50 that is normal for a particular patient. The nurse should compare actual findings to the patient's baseline when possible.

- **Consult resources.** Both novices and experienced nurses should consult appropriate resources whenever in doubt about a diagnosis. Professional literature, nursing colleagues, and other professionals are appropriate resources. The nurse should use a nursing diagnosis handbook to determine whether the patient's signs and symptoms truly fit the definition of the NANDA-I label chosen.

- **Base diagnoses on patterns—that is, on behavior over time—rather than on an isolated incident.** For example, even though the patient is concerned today about needing to leave her child with a neighbor, it is likely that this concern will be resolved without intervention by the next day. Therefore, the nurse should not diagnose *Interrupted Family Processes*.

- **Improve critical thinking skills.** Critical thinking skills help nurses increase awareness of patients' problems and also help nurses avoid errors in thinking, such as overgeneralizing, stereotyping, and making unwarranted assumptions about patients.

Case Study » Part 2

Nurse Medina wants to use the assessment data she obtained during the admission assessment of Mrs. Aquilini to identify the priority nursing diagnosis. First, she makes a list of all of the assessment data and then separates the significant cues that form clusters. Some of the significant cues came from Mrs. Aquilini's recent history at home, but others came from physical findings Nurse Medina obtained:

- "Chest cold" for 2 weeks
- Shortness of breath with activity
- Lung sounds—inspiratory crackles with diminished breath sounds in right lung

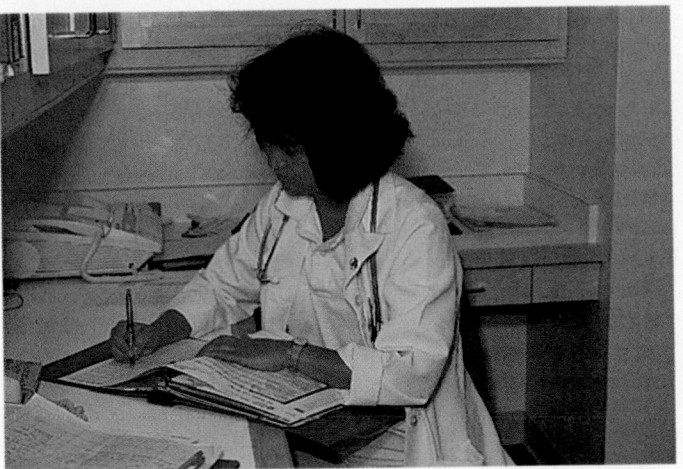

Figure 36–10 》 Diagnosis: After analysis, Nurse Medina formulates a nursing diagnosis: *Ineffective Airway Clearance* related to accumulated mucus obstructing airways (secondary to pneumonia).

- Drinking fluids less
- Feels tired all the time; no energy to do home activities or go to work
- Does not smoke
- T$_O$ 103°F (34.4°C), P 92 bpm, R 28/min, BP 122/80 mmHg, and O$_2$ Sat 95% on room air
- Productive cough with thick, foul-smelling green sputum
- Speaks in short sentences.

Based on the above assessment cluster and the fact that Mrs. Aquilini has a medical diagnosis of pneumonia, Nurse Medina feels confident that the priority nursing diagnosis would involve Mrs. Aquilini's response to the infection in her right lung. There are many NANDA-I nursing diagnoses related to the respiratory system. Nurse Medina decides the definition of the *Ineffective Airway Clearance* nursing diagnosis best fits Mrs. Aquilini's signs and symptoms. So the diagnostic statement for the top priority nursing diagnosis for Mrs. Aquilini is *Ineffective Airway Clearance* related to accumulated mucus obstructing airways (secondary to pneumonia) (**Figure 36–10 》**).

Clinical Reasoning Questions Level I

1. How do the assessment data support the nursing diagnosis made by Nurse Medina?
2. Can you identify the different components in this two-part diagnostic statement?

Clinical Reasoning Questions Level II

3. What might be the second and third priority nursing diagnoses for this patient?
4. What other assessment data could you hypothesize might be a potential problem for Mrs. Aquilini because of her medical diagnosis of pneumonia?

Planning

The **planning** phase is a deliberate, systematic phase of the nursing process during which the nurse refers to the patient's assessment data and nursing diagnoses for direction in formulating patient goals. Goals are different from outcomes, although many times these words are used to mean the same thing; the difference is outlined in **Box 36–2 》**.

Box 36–2
The Difference Between a Goal and an Outcome

Goals are observable patient responses; what the nurse hopes to achieve through nursing actions. Goals are developed in the planning phase of the nursing process. They are broad statements about something the patient strives to achieve and indicate progress toward desired patient behaviors or actions. Goals are what nurses and patients want to happen. They are individualized and specific for each patient. Goals are the responses to nursing interventions.

Outcomes are used to evaluate the patient's response to the plan of care. Desired outcomes are specific, observable criteria used to evaluate whether goals have been met. Desired outcomes are identified during the planning phase: during the evaluation phase, the nurse determines if outcomes have or have not been met. Outcomes are the end results of nursing actions—both desirable and undesirable. Outcomes indicate the effectiveness of nursing actions. The Nursing Outcomes Classification (NOC) identifies 490 standardized and classified patient outcomes that can be used to describe patient status in response to nursing actions (University of Iowa, College of Nursing, 2013). For example:

Nursing diagnosis: Ineffective Airway Clearance related to poor cough effort

Goal: Patient will demonstrate an effective cough by 1400 this afternoon.

Desired outcome: Patient maintains a clear airway during the postoperative period.

The terms *goal* and *desired outcome* are often used interchangeably. Sometimes the word "or" is used between them, "goals or outcomes," and sometimes they are written "goals/outcomes." In this text, goals are developed in the planning phase of the nursing process and desired outcomes are used to evaluate the patient's response to the plan of care.

The goals become the basis for the nursing interventions that are developed to prevent, reduce, eliminate, or improve the nursing diagnosis situation. For the plan to be effective, it is important for the patient and support persons (if applicable) to participate in the development of the plan: Nurses do not plan for the patient, but encourage the patient to participate actively to the extent possible. In a home setting, the patient's family members and caregivers are the ones who implement the plan of care; thus, its effectiveness depends largely on them.

When the nurse and patient identify a goal for every nursing diagnosis together, it helps support the nurse–patient relationship. This partnership achieves these other purposes as well:

1. Provides direction for selecting nursing interventions. Ideas for interventions come more easily if the goal clearly and specifically states what the patient is to achieve.
2. Serves as criteria for evaluating patient progress. Although developed in the planning phase of the nursing process, goals serve as the criteria for determining

the effectiveness of nursing interventions and patient progress for desired outcomes in the evaluation phase.

3. Enables closure of the nursing diagnosis situation when the patient and nurse determine the goal has been achieved.

4. Helps motivate the patient and nurse by providing a sense of achievement. As goals are met, both patient and nurse can see that their efforts have been worthwhile. This provides motivation to continue following the plan, especially when difficult lifestyle changes need to be made by the patient.

5. Supports a therapeutic nurse–patient relationship. Any time the nurse and patient are able to move forward together in the patient's plan of care, the patient gains trust in the nurse, further increasing the likelihood of the plan's success.

Long-Term and Short-Term Goals

Goals are customized to individual patients, which means they take varying amounts of time to achieve. Because of differences in time, goals are categorized as either short term or long term, depending on the time frames necessary to achieve them.

Short-term goals are useful for patients who require healthcare for a short time. In an acute care setting, much of the nurse's time is spent on the patient's immediate needs, so most goals are short term and can be achieved by the patient in a range of a few hours to a few days. Examples of short-term goals are:

- Patient will raise her right arm to shoulder height 4 days from today, January 23.

- Patient will identify five salty foods to avoid while on a salt-free diet by tomorrow, May 7.

- Patient will demonstrate how to change his leg dressing before discharge.

- Patient will use a cane to walk 20 feet down the hallway by April 22.

Long-term goals are often used for patients who live at home and have chronic health problems and for patients in nursing homes, extended care facilities, and rehabilitation centers. However, patients in acute care settings also need long-term goals to guide planning for their discharge to long-term care agencies or home care, especially in a managed-care environment. Long-term goals can be achieved by the patient in a range of 1 week to several months. Examples of long-term goals are:

- Patient will regain full use of her right arm 6 weeks from today, June 6.

- Patient will be able to discuss five effective coping strategies for dealing with stressful situations that he has used over a 6-month period of time from today, September 25.

- Patient will eat at least 60% of all meals by the end of 3 weeks from today, June 1.

- Patient will participate in two weekly group activities by sitting quietly and listening attentively by 3 months from today, May 13.

Developing a Goal

Goals are derived from the patient's nursing diagnoses—primarily from the diagnostic label. Each nursing diagnosis has one goal for the patient to achieve. When developing goals, the nurse should ask the following questions:

1. What about the nursing diagnosis needs to be changed for or by the patient?

2. Is there a healthy response to correct a problem stated in the nursing diagnosis that the patient can achieve as a goal?

3. How will the patient look or behave if the healthy response as a goal is achieved? (What will be seen, heard, measured, palpated, smelled, or otherwise observed through the senses?)

4. What action must the patient do and how well must the patient do it to demonstrate problem resolution or achievement of the goal?

For example, the nursing diagnosis is:

Deficient Fluid Volume related to diarrhea and inadequate intake secondary to nausea

The *diagnostic label* is "Deficient Fluid Volume."	This is the problem.
Related to is "diarrhea and inadequate intake."	This is the source of the problem.
Secondary to "nausea"	This is the origin of the "related to" factors.

The goal for this nursing diagnosis might be "Patient's intake and output of fluids will be balanced during his hospitalization." The patient's goal reflects maintaining a fluid balance during the time interval he is losing fluids through diarrhea. The goal of fluid balance is the opposite of the nursing diagnostic label *Deficient Fluid Volume*.

Writing a Goal

Goals have specific characteristics that should be included when writing them to fulfill their purpose in the planning phase of the nursing process. Setting a goal helps to identify desired change in a patient's situation and define the focus of nursing interventions. Common characteristics of goals include being:

- Patient centered (not about nurse activities)

- Specific and concise single actions

- A single goal for each nursing diagnosis

- Directional for nursing interventions

- Measurable

- Quantifiable

- Attainable for an individual patient

- Realistic to an individual patient

- Relevant to an individual patient

- Time limited.

All goals are patient centered in that the patient is always the subject, as indicated by beginning the goal with the words "The patient will" much of the time. Sometimes these three words are omitted in goals because it is assumed that the subject is the patient unless indicated otherwise. A quick and user-friendly format to follow to write a goal statement is the acronym **SMART** (College of Nurses of Ontario, 2014), which stands for:

Specific single action

Measurable

Attainable (achievable)

Relevant

Time limited.

Specific Single Action

The goal includes a clearly stated, single action for the patient to do that can be observed directly or indirectly. Any additional information defining how the action is to be done is included in this part of the statement. These are sometimes called *qualifiers* of the action. Information provided about the action is detailed so that other nurses following the nursing plan of care will be able to understand what the patient is to achieve to reach the goal.

Here are some examples of specific single actions for goals. The patient will:

- Walk 20 feet down the hall using a walker.
- Demonstrate giving herself an insulin injection using aseptic technique.
- Identify six foods to avoid that are high in salt content.
- State the purpose of his new medication, nitroglycerin, and when and how to take it.

Measurable

The goal includes a specific, measurable observation or result that is quantifiable. Any nurse observing the patient attempting the single action of the goal will be able to recognize when the patient reaches the goal. In the following examples, the first column does not provide specific measurements or quantities that all nurses would define the same, whereas the second column does. The patient will:

Poorly Written Quantified Measure	Correctly Written Quantified Measure
Go for a walk (need to know distance for goal to be reached).	Walk 20 feet down the hall using a walker.
Understand how to give insulin (understanding doesn't mean being able to do it).	Demonstrate giving herself an insulin injection using aseptic technique.
State foods not to eat (quantify how many and what kind so the understanding is consistent).	Identify six foods to avoid that are high in salt content.
Know about nitroglycerin (need to be specific about what to know).	State the purpose of his new medication, nitroglycerin, and when and how to take it.

Nurses must be aware that some phrases can lead to disagreements about whether the outcome was met. Avoid statements that start with *enable, facilitate, allow, let, permit,* or similar verbs followed by the word *patient.* These verbs indicate what the nurse hopes to accomplish, not what the patient will do.

Attainable (Achievable)

The goal is appropriate for the individual patient. The single action to be measured is realistic and one that the patient can complete based on the patient's physical, emotional, and psychologic capabilities and limitations (e.g., finances, equipment, family support, and social services). For example:

- Walking a mile would not be achievable for an end-stage COPD patient (20 feet might be more realistic).
- A 2-year-old would not be able to give her own insulin.
- A 24-year-old could identify foods high in salt content.
- A 68-year-old could discuss nitroglycerin.

Relevant

The goal is applicable to the individual patient. The attainable single action to be measured has a purpose that has been customized for the patient based on the needs of the patient. For example, typically:

- A patient on bedrest would not need a goal about walking.
- A nondiabetic patient does not need to know about insulin injections.
- An ordinary teenager does not need to watch his salt intake.
- A 22-year-old patient without angina does not need to know about nitroglycerin.

Time Limited

The goal has a specific time frame and deadline for the goal to be achieved. During this time period, the nurse evaluates the patient's progress in achieving the goal. **Evaluation** is a planned activity in which patients and healthcare professionals examine the patient's progress. Evaluation may serve as motivation for the patient to continue working to achieve the goal. The time frame is specific to date and hours, days, weeks, or months. For example:

- 3/2 at 0800
- In two months, starting 6/2
- Four hours from 1330
- 6/24 in the morning.

Putting all the SMART components together in the examples above results in the following appropriate goals:

- The patient will walk 20 feet down the hall using a walker by 3/3 at 0800.
- The patient will demonstrate giving herself an insulin injection using aseptic technique by discharge.
- The patient will identify six foods to avoid that are high in salt content in 4 hours from 1330.
- The patient will state the purpose of his new medication, nitroglycerin, and when and how to take it by discharge.

See **Table 36–13** ›› for examples of goals written in SMART format.

TABLE 36–13 SMART Format

Specific, Single Action	**M**easurable (Quantifiable, Determines How Often)	**A**ppropriate for Patient	**R**ealistic and Attainable for Patient	**T**ime Frame for Patient to Reach Goal
Patient will drink	2500 mL of fluids daily	Ask yourself "Is this goal appropriate for this specific patient?"	Ask yourself "Is this goal realistic and attainable for this specific patient?"	by _____ time, date
Patient will administer	correct insulin dose using aseptic technique			by day of discharge
Patient will list	three hazards of smoking			by _____ time, date
Patient will walk	30 feet down the hall with his cane			by day of discharge
Patient's right ankle will measure	less than 10 inches in circumference			in 48 hours from _____ time, date
Patient will identify	five foods that are allowed on a low-salt diet			by _____ time, date

The nurse writes the goal statement in the format of sub-ject, verb, goal and time limit. The *subject* in the goal state-ment is the patient. The *verb* is the specific action the patient is to perform that can be observed. The goal is the patient and nurse's intended achievement, and the time limit deter-mines by when the goal should be accomplished. Examples of action verbs include:

Apply	Discuss	Select
Change	Drink	Sit
Demonstrate	Explain	State
Describe	Inject	Verbalize
Differentiate	Prepare	Walk

Make sure the patient considers the goals important and valuable. Patients are motivated if goals are associated with personal meaning. The nurse should assess the patient's motivation to achieve goals or make behavioral changes. Some patients may know what they wish to accomplish with regard to their health problem; others may not be aware of their possible health goals. The nurse must actively listen to the patient to determine the patient's personal values and goals in relation to their current health concerns. Patients are usually motivated and expend the necessary energy to reach goals they consider important.

Case Study >> Part 3

Nurse Medina has formulated this diagnostic statement to be the top priority for Mrs. Aquilini based on the assessment cluster of significant cues: *Ineffective Airway Clearance* related to accumulated mucus obstructing airways (secondary to pneumonia). She is now ready to collaborate with Mrs. Aquilini to establish a goal. The following reason-ing is part of this discussion:

- Mrs. Aquilini hasn't been drinking much lately, so her mucus is thick and hard to expel.
- She has inspiratory rhonchi with diminished breath sounds in the right lung, which indicate partial obstructions from the thickened mucus in her airways.
- Because Mrs. Aquilini has increased mucus production from the infection in her lungs, she is experiencing impairment in gas exchange, which results in her intolerance to activities and short-ness of breath.

- Because she is breathing faster, she is using more energy to breathe.
- Mrs. Aquilini is experiencing general fatigue as her body fights the lung infection.

Nurse Medina helps Mrs. Aquilini understand that many of her problems are a result of the amount and type of mucus in her airways from the lung infection. Nurse Medina further explains the importance of liquefying the mucus so Mrs. Aquilini can cough more effectively and help clear her airways. Together they decide on a goal: "The patient will drink 3000 mL of fluids daily by 8/12." Both are satisfied that Mrs. Aquilini can reach this goal within the time frame. Now that the goal has been identified, they begin thinking about interventions that can help Mrs. Aquilini reach her goal (**Figure 36–11 >>**).

Clinical Reasoning Questions Level I

1. What role did the critical thinking skill of reasoning play in the discussion between Nurse Medina and Mrs. Aquilini?
2. Can you identify the different components of the SMART for-mat in the goal they created together?

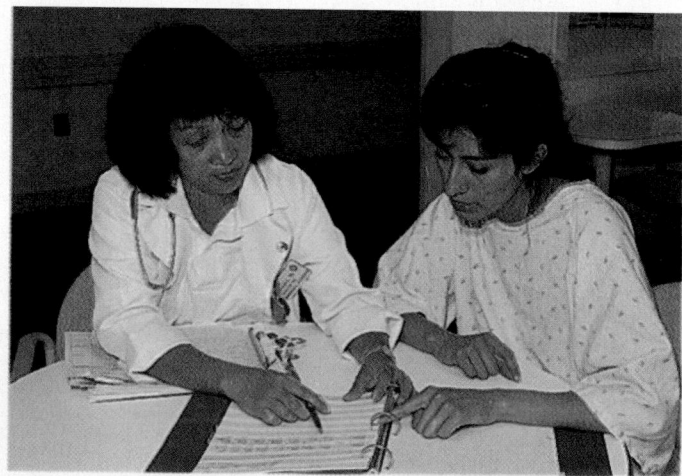

Figure 36–11 >> Planning: Nurse Medina and Mrs. Aquilini col-laborate to establish goals (e.g., restore effective breathing pat-tern and lung ventilation); set outcome criteria (e.g., have a symmetrical respiratory excursion of at least 4 cm); and develop a care plan that includes, but is not limited to, coughing and deep breathing exercises q3h, fluid intake of 3000 mL daily, and daily postural drainage.

Clinical Reasoning Questions Level II

3. Why does Nurse Medina include Mrs. Aquilini in deciding what the goal will be instead of just letting her know she needs to drink more every day?

4. If Mrs. Aquilini did not feel she could drink 3000 mL of fluids daily, what other goal would you suggest based on the information provided in the case study?

Implementation

Implementation is the action phase of the nursing process. In this phase, nurses take all the data acquired in the first three phases of the nursing process and determine interventions that would be most appropriate to help the patient reach the goal stated in the planning phase. Interventions provide data that will be used during the evaluation phase to determine patient outcomes. Implementation is a two-step process. The first step is identifying the best priority interventions for an individual patient, and the second step is the implementation of these interventions.

Nursing Interventions

Interventions include nursing actions, delegation of tasks, and documentation completed to help the patient achieve his or her goal based on the nursing diagnosis. These actions are listed in priority order (see Exemplar 36.C on Prioritizing Care within this module for further information). Nursing interventions focus on:

- Assessing to observe for changes in the patient's status
- Preventing complications
- Reducing risk factors
- Treating through teaching and providing physical care
- Improving health through health promotion and achieving higher levels of wellness.

Correct identification of the etiology during the assessment and nursing diagnosis phases provides the framework for choosing successful nursing interventions. For example, the diagnostic label *Activity Intolerance* may have several etiologies: pain, weakness, sedentary lifestyle, anxiety, or cardiac arrhythmias. Interventions will vary according to the cause of the problem. Sometimes nursing actions treat the patient's response to a disease, illness, or medical condition. Interventions for risk nursing diagnoses focus on measures to reduce the patient's risk factors found in the etiology of the risk nursing diagnosis. **Table 36–14** >> shows examples of typical nursing interventions based on the nursing diagnosis and its etiology.

Types of Nursing Interventions

Nursing interventions include both direct and indirect care. Direct care is an intervention performed through interaction with the patient. Indirect care is an intervention performed away from, but on behalf of, the patient. Attending an interprofessional meeting and managing the care environment are two examples of indirect care. A taxonomy of nursing interventions referred to as the Nursing Interventions Classification (NIC) Taxonomy, developed by the Iowa Intervention Project, can be used to describe the interventions that nurses perform. It includes seven domains and 30 classes of interventions (see the module on Informatics for further information). Nursing interventions are classified as independent, or nurse initiated; dependent, or physician initiated; and collaborative, or involving other providers (e.g., physical therapist) involved in the patient's treatments.

Independent interventions are those activities that nurses are licensed to do within their scope of practice; in other words, areas of healthcare that are unique to nursing and separate and distinct from medical management. These interventions include physical care, ongoing assessment, emotional support and comfort, teaching, counseling, environmental management, and making referrals to other healthcare professionals. For example, most patients with a nursing diagnosis of pain have medical orders for analgesics, but many independent nursing interventions also can alleviate pain (e.g., guided imagery or teaching a patient to "splint" an incision using a pillow). Recall that many nursing diagnoses are patient problems that can be treated primarily by independent nursing interventions. In performing an autonomous activity, the nurse determines that the patient requires certain nursing interventions. The nurse either carries these out or delegates them to other nursing personnel, and is accountable or responsible for the decision and the actions (see the module on Accountability for further information). An example of an independent action is planning and providing special mouth care for a patient after diagnosing impaired oral mucous membranes.

Collaborative interventions encompass **dependent interventions** employed by the nurse under a physician's orders, under supervision, or according to specified routines

TABLE 36–14 Examples of Typical Nursing Interventions Based on Nursing Diagnosis and Etiology

Type of Nursing Diagnosis	Etiology	Nursing Interventions
Problem focused	*Acute Pain* related to surgical site	■ Assess pain level using a pain rating scale of 0–10 at frequent intervals. ■ Give ketorolac 15 mg IV every 6 hours prn pain × 5 days.
Risk	*Risk for Falls* related to use of walker	■ Assess ability to move when using the walker. ■ Keep area from bed to bathroom free from clutter.
Health promotion	*Readiness for Enhanced Parenting* related to newborn in the home	■ Assess parents' feelings of impact of having a newborn in the home. ■ Discuss infant stimulation techniques with both parents.

and protocols, as well as actions the nurse carries out in collaboration with other healthcare team members, such as physical therapists, social workers, dietitians, and physicians. Collaborative nursing activities reflect the overlapping responsibilities of, and cooperative relationships among, healthcare personnel and demonstrate the benefits of multidisciplinary patient care. For example, the physician might order physical therapy to teach the patient crutch-walking. The nurse would be responsible for informing the physical therapy department and for coordinating the patient's care to include the physical therapy sessions. When the patient returns to the nursing unit, the nurse would assist with crutch-walking and collaborate with the physical therapist to evaluate the patient's progress.

Healthcare providers' prescriptions commonly direct nurses to provide medications, IV therapy, diagnostic tests, diet, and activity for patients. The nurse is responsible for assessing the need for, explaining, and administering medical orders. Nursing interventions should be written to customize the medical order based on the individual patient. For example, instead of writing "Administer NSAID as ordered" as an intervention, the nurse can write "Give ketorolac 15 mg IV every 6 hours prn pain × 5 days as prescribed by physician."

The amount of time the nurse spends in an independent versus a collaborative or dependent role varies according to the clinical area, type of facility, and specific position of the nurse.

Considerations When Selecting Interventions

Usually several potential interventions can be identified for each nursing goal. The nurse's task is to select those that are most likely to achieve the desired patient outcomes. There is also a need to prioritize potential interventions and include the patient's input. Weighing the pros and cons of each intervention can help the nurse make these decisions. For example, "Provide accurate information about diabetes" as an intervention could result in any one of the following patient responses:

- Increased anxiety
- Decreased anxiety
- Wish to talk with the primary care provider
- Desire to leave the hospital
- Relaxation.

Determining the pros and cons of each intervention requires nursing knowledge and experience. For example, the nurse's experience may suggest that providing information the night before the patient's surgery may increase the patient's worry and tension, whereas maintaining the usual rituals before sleep is more effective. The nurse might then consider providing the information several days before surgery. See examples of priority nursing interventions for the patient in **Table 36–15 》**.

The following guidelines can help the nurse choose the most appropriate priority nursing interventions to support patients in reaching their goal. Interventions need to be:

- Safe and appropriate for the individual patient's age, health, and condition (see the Lifespan Considerations feature).
- Achievable with the resources available. For example, a home care nurse might wish to include an intervention for an older adult patient to "check blood glucose daily," but in order for that to occur the patient must have intact sight, cognition, and memory to carry this out independently, or daily visits from a home care nurse must be available and affordable.
- Congruent with the patient's values, beliefs, and culture (see Focus on Diversity and Culture).
- Congruent with other therapies (e.g., if the patient is not permitted food, the strategy of an evening snack must be deferred until health permits).

TABLE 36–15 Examples of Priority Nursing Interventions

Nursing Interventions	Rationale
Nursing Diagnosis: *Ineffective Airway Clearance* related to viscous secretions and shallow chest expansion secondary to pneumonia	
Monitor respiratory status q4h: rate, depth, effort, skin color, mucous membranes, lung sounds, amount and color of sputum, and sensorium.	To identify progress toward or away from goal (i.e., pallor, cyanosis, lethargy, and drowsiness).
Monitor vital signs q4h: temperature, pulse, respiratory rate, blood pressure, and oxygen saturation.	To identify changes in vital signs, which may indicate changes in the patient's condition.
Administer oxygen at 2 LPM via nasal cannula as prescribed by physician.	Supplemental oxygen makes more oxygen available to the cells, which reduces the work of breathing.
Maintain in Fowler or semi-Fowler position.	Gravity allows for fuller lung expansion by decreasing pressure of abdomen on diaphragm.
Administer prescribed antibiotic to maintain therapeutic blood level.	Resolves infection by bactericidal effect.
Administer prescribed expectorant.	Helps loosen secretions so they can be coughed up and expelled.
Administer prescribed analgesic.	Controls pleuritic pain, enabling patient to increase thoracic expansion.
Encourage fluids by mouth (except when contraindicated by medical conditions such as cardiovascular or renal problems).	Helps liquefy the mucus, making it easier to cough up and expel.
Instruct in breathing and coughing techniques. Remind patient to perform, and assist as needed q2–3h.	To enable patient to cough up secretions.

Focus on Diversity and Culture
Cultural Considerations for Nursing Interventions

Patients will have their own cultural beliefs and values that need to be taken into consideration when selecting interventions. For example, patients who have strict dietary practices, such as not eating meat, will require advanced planning if their health problem requires dietary restrictions. Similarly, cultures that require daily care to be given by an individual of the same gender may require the nursing staff to reassign nurses to accommodate this request. In addition, patients who have strong religious beliefs may benefit from interventions related to prayer and meditation, whereas these same interventions would not be helpful for patients who do not have religious beliefs. Each step of the nursing process is important for providing culturally competent care. The assessment phase should be used to identify cultural practices through observation and interview questions. The diagnosis phase can be used to list nursing diagnoses that relate to cultural factors, such as *Spiritual Distress* or *Readiness for Enhanced Religiosity*. The planning and implementation phases should consider the patient's normal cultural practices and incorporate them into the plan of care. The patient has a greater chance of meeting goals and having positive outcomes if the interventions the nurse selects are consistent with the patient's values, beliefs, and practices.

- Based on current best nursing research evidence (see the module on Evidence-Based Practice for further information).
- Within established standards of care as determined by state laws, professional associations (e.g., ANA), and the policies of the facility. Many agencies have policies to guide the activities of health professionals and to safeguard patients. For example, there may be policies for visiting hours and procedures to follow for the patient who has had a cardiac arrest.

Writing a Nursing Intervention

After choosing the best priority nursing interventions, the nurse writes them in the patient's nursing plan of care. Interventions are dated when they are written and then reviewed regularly. Common characteristics of nursing interventions include that they:

- Are patient centered
- Have a specific and concise single action
- Include detailed information about the action (i.e., when, how, time, and where)
- Are realistic for the individual patient
- Are relevant to helping patient reach goal set in planning phase

Only the top 3–5 priority interventions are usually listed for each nursing diagnosis (instead of the 6–10 that could be listed). Nursing students often include a rationale for each selected intervention as they are learning about nursing actions expected with patient conditions and diseases. The following table shows examples of poorly and correctly written interventions:

Poorly Written Intervention	Correctly Written Intervention
Tell the patient about insulin.	Explain to the patient the actions of insulin.
Assess edema of left ankle daily.	Measure and record patient's left ankle circumference daily at 0800.
Apply dressing to left leg.	Change spiral dressing to left leg every shift as needed.
Give pain medication as needed.	Give acetaminophen 325 mg/oxycodone 5 mg 1 tablet PO 30 minutes prior to going to physical therapy and every 6 hours prn per physician order.

The Process of Implementation

Implementation refers to doing the actions in the interventions. The process of implementation commonly includes the following:

- Preassessment of the patient
- Determining the nurse's need for assistance
- Implementing the nursing interventions
- Supervising any delegated care
- Documenting nursing actions.

Preassessment of the Patient

Just before implementing an intervention, the nurse must reassess the patient to make sure the intervention is still needed and appropriate because the patient's condition may have changed. For example, a patient has a nursing diagnosis of *Disturbed Sleep Pattern* related to anxiety and unfamiliar surroundings. During rounds, the nurse discovers that the patient is sleeping; the nurse decides to defer the back massage intervention that had been planned as a relaxation strategy.

New data may indicate a need to change the priorities of care or the nursing activities. For example, a nurse begins to teach a patient who has diabetes how to give himself insulin injections. Shortly after beginning the teaching, the nurse realizes that the patient is not concentrating on the lesson. Subsequent discussion reveals that he is worried about his eyesight and fears he is going blind. Realizing that the patient's level of stress is interfering with his learning, the nurse ends the lesson and arranges for a primary care provider to examine the patient's eyes. The nurse also provides supportive communication to help alleviate the patient's stress.

Determining the Nurse's Need for Assistance

When implementing some nursing interventions, the nurse may require assistance for one or more of the following reasons:

- The nurse is unable to implement the nursing activity safely or efficiently alone (e.g., ambulating a patient who is obese and needs assistance).
- Assistance would reduce stress on the patient (e.g., turning an individual who experiences acute pain when moved).

- The nurse lacks the knowledge or skills to implement a particular nursing activity (e.g., a nurse who is not familiar with a particular type of orthopedic traction equipment needs assistance the first time turning the patient).

Implementing Nursing Interventions

Before beginning implementation, explain to the patient what interventions will be done, what sensations to expect, what the patient is expected to do, and the purpose of the intervention. For many nursing activities, it is important to ensure the patient's privacy by closing doors, pulling curtains, or draping the patient. The number and types of direct nursing interventions are almost unlimited and include coordination of patient care. Interventions involve scheduling patient contacts with other healthcare providers (e.g., laboratory and x-ray technicians, physical and respiratory therapists) and serving as a liaison among the members of the healthcare team. When implementing interventions, nurses should follow these guidelines:

- *Base nursing interventions on scientific knowledge, nursing research evidence, and professional standards of care.* The nurse must be aware of the scientific rationale as well as possible side effects or complications of all interventions. For example, a patient prefers to take an oral medication after meals; however, this medication is not absorbed well in the presence of food. Therefore, the nurse will need to explain why this preference cannot be honored.

- *Clearly understand the interventions to be implemented and question any that are not understood.* The nurse is responsible for intelligent implementation of physician-ordered interventions in the nursing plan of care. This requires knowledge of each intervention, its purpose in the patient's plan of care, any contraindications (e.g., allergies), and any changes in the patient's condition that may affect the order.

- *Adapt activities to the individual patient.* A patient's beliefs, values, age (chronologic and developmental), health status, and environment are factors that can affect the success of a nursing action. For example, the nurse determines that a patient chokes when swallowing pills, so she consults with the physician to change the order to a liquid form of the medication.

- *Implement safe care.* For example, when changing a sterile dressing, the nurse practices sterile technique to prevent infection; when giving a medication, the nurse follows the six rights of safe medication administration.

- *Provide teaching, support, and comfort.* The nurse should always explain the purpose of interventions, what the patient will experience, and how the patient can participate. The patient must have sufficient knowledge to agree to the plan of care and to be able to assume responsibility for as much self-care as possible.

- *Respect the patient's ethnic background and cultural preferences.* The nurse must always view the patient as a whole and give consideration to the patient's preferences. For example, whenever possible, the nurse honors the patient's expressed preference that interventions be planned for times that fit with the patient's usual schedule of visitors, work, sleep, eating, prayer, or meditation.

- *Respect the dignity of the patient and enhance the patient's self-esteem* by providing privacy and encouraging patients to make their own decisions as appropriate.

- *Encourage patients to participate actively in implementing nursing interventions.* Active participation enhances the patient's sense of independence and control. However, patients vary in the degree of participation they desire. Some want total involvement in their care, whereas others prefer little involvement. The amount of active involvement may be related to the severity of the illness; the patient's culture; or the patient's fear, understanding of the illness, and understanding of the intervention.

Delegation

Delegating patient care and assigning tasks are important responsibilities for registered nurses because healthcare facilities use licensed practical nurses and many unlicensed assistive personnel (UAP). To delegate appropriately, the nurse must match the needs of the patient and family with the scope of practice of the available caregivers. The RN remains responsible for making sure delegated tasks are carried out properly.

Other caregivers may be required to communicate their activities to the nurse by documenting them on the patient's medical record, reporting verbally, filling in a written form, or placing an entry in the patient's electronic medical record. The nurse validates and responds to any adverse findings or patient responses. This may involve modifying the nursing plan of care. For example, UAP may perform tasks such as measuring intake and output, but the RN is still responsible for analyzing data, planning care, and evaluating outcomes (see the module on Managing Care for further information).

Documentation

After carrying out the nursing activities, the nurse completes the implementation phase by recording the interventions performed and patient responses in the nursing progress notes. Nursing actions are communicated verbally, in writing, or by electronic entry. When a patient's health is changing rapidly, the charge nurse and/or the physician may want to be kept up to date with verbal reports. Nurses also report patient status to nursing colleagues at change of shift (see the module on Communication for further information).

Skills Necessary for Implementation

To implement the nursing plan of care successfully, nurses need several kinds of skills: cognitive (knowledge), interpersonal (attitudes), and technical (skills). Although these skills are distinct from one another, nurses use them in various combinations and with different emphasis depending on the activity. For instance, when inserting a urinary catheter, the nurse needs cognitive knowledge of the principles and steps of the procedure, interpersonal skills to inform and reassure the patient, and technical skill in draping the patient and manipulating the equipment.

Cognitive skills include problem solving, decision making, critical thinking, and creativity. They are crucial to safe, intelligent nursing care.

Interpersonal skills are the verbal and nonverbal communication methods nurses use when interacting with the patient or family. The effectiveness of a nursing action often depends largely on the nurse's ability to use therapeutic communication. A nurse also needs interpersonal skills to work effectively with others as a member of a healthcare team (see the module on Communication for further information). Interpersonal skills are necessary for all nursing activities and reflect knowledge, attitudes, feelings, interest, and appreciation of the patient's cultural values and lifestyle as well as the cultural and ethnic differences among fellow healthcare professionals.

Technical skills are purposeful, "hands-on" skills such as manipulating equipment; giving injections; bandaging; and moving, lifting, and repositioning patients. These skills are also called procedural or psychomotor skills. Technical skills require knowledge and, frequently, manual dexterity. The number of technical skills expected of a nurse has greatly increased in recent years because of the advances in the use of technology, especially in acute care hospitals.

Relationship to Other Nursing Process Phases

The first three phases of the nursing process—assessment, nursing diagnosis, and goal planning—provide the basis for the nursing actions performed during the implementation of interventions phase. In turn, the implementation phase provides the actual nursing activities and patient responses that are examined in the final phase, the evaluation phase. Using data acquired during assessment, the nurse can individualize the care given during the implementation phase.

While implementing nursing care, the nurse continues to reassess the patient at every contact, gathering data about the patient's responses to the nursing actions and about any new problems that may develop. Some routine nursing activities present new assessment data for the nurse making observations. For example, while bathing an older adult patient, the nurse observes a reddened area on the patient's sacrum. Or, when emptying a urinary catheter bag, the nurse measures 200 mL of foul-smelling, cloudy, brown urine.

Case Study >> Part 4

The goal for Mrs. Aquilini is "The patient will drink 3000 mL of fluids daily by 8/12." Nurse Medina and Mrs. Aquilini are now discussing interventions that will help Mrs. Aquilini reach her goal. Here is the list of potential interventions they have come up with:

- Perform postural drainage daily.
- Record daily weights.
- Have Mrs. Aquilini's favorite beverages available so she can drink them frequently.
- Do coughing and deep breathing exercises every 2 hours.
- Have Mrs. Aquilini's favorite snacks readily available.
- Encourage Mrs. Aquilini to drink a variety of beverages so she does not get bored with water.
- Keep a tally of how much Mrs. Aquilini is drinking and urinating each shift.
- Assess sputum for consistency, color, amount, and odor.

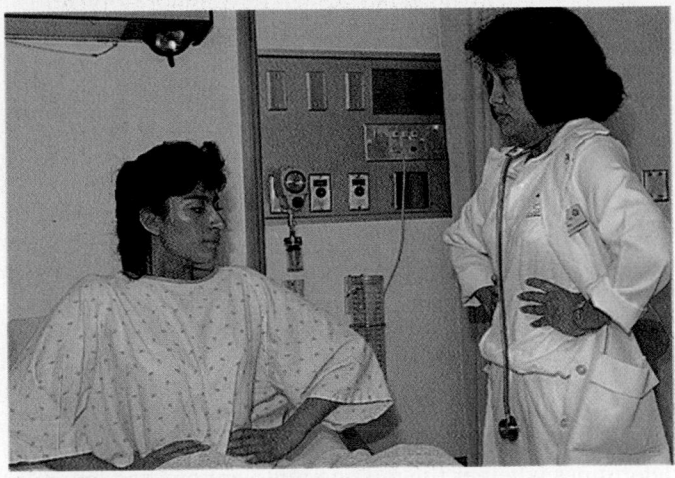

Figure 36–12 >> Implementation: Mrs. Aquilini agrees to practice deep breathing exercises q3h during the day. In addition, she verbalizes awareness of the need to increase her fluid intake and to plan her morning activities to accommodate postural drainage.

Nurse Medina explains to Mrs. Aquilini that they need to select the top four priorities from this list to add to her plan of care (**Figure 36–12 >>**). She further explains the importance of assessment to measure progress toward reaching the goal. Together, they decide these are the top four priorities:

- Measure intake and output every shift.
- Have Mrs. Aquilini's favorite beverages available so she can drink them frequently.
- Do coughing and deep breathing exercises every 3 hours.
- Perform postural drainage daily.

Clinical Reasoning Questions Level I
1. What is the importance of conducting an assessment before performing any interventions?
2. Would you have selected other interventions for Mrs. Aquilini? If so, what are they and why would you have selected them?

Clinical Reasoning Questions Level II
3. Which of the interventions listed are independent interventions nurses can do without physician orders?
4. Why do you think assessment of the sputum for consistency, color, amount, and odor was not selected as an intervention specific to helping Mrs. Aquilini reach her goal?

Evaluation

After implementing nursing care, the nurse evaluates the desired outcomes. In this context, evaluation is a planned, ongoing, purposeful activity in which patients and healthcare professionals determine (a) the patient's progress toward achievement of goals/outcomes and (b) the effectiveness of the nursing plan of care. On the basis of this evaluation, the plan of care is continued, modified, or terminated. As in all phases of the nursing process, patients and support persons are encouraged to participate as much as possible.

Evaluation continues until the patient achieves the health goals or is discharged from nursing care. Evaluation conducted during or immediately after implementation of a nursing action enables the nurse to make on-the-spot modifications to an intervention. Evaluation performed at specified intervals (e.g., once a week for the home care patient) shows the extent of progress toward goal achievement and enables the nurse to correct any deficiencies and modify the care plan as needed. Evaluation at discharge includes the status of goal achievement and the patient's self-care abilities with regard to follow-up care. Most facilities have a special discharge record for this evaluation.

Through evaluation, nurses demonstrate responsibility and accountability for their actions, indicate interest in the results of the nursing activities, and demonstrate a desire not to perpetuate ineffective actions but to adopt more effective interventions. During the evaluation process, the nurse determines whether the nursing interventions had any relation to the patient achieving his or her outcomes. It should never be assumed that a nursing action was the cause of or the only factor in meeting, partially meeting, or not meeting a goal.

Clinical Example E

Ruth Horowitz, a patient with obesity, needed to lose 14 kg (30 lb). When the nurse and Mrs. Horowitz drew up a plan of care, one goal was "Lose 1.4 kg (3 lb) in 4 weeks." A nursing intervention listed in the plan of care was "Explain how to plan and prepare a 1200-calorie diet." Four weeks later, Mrs. Horowitz weighed herself and had lost 1.8 kg (4 lb). The goal had been met—in fact, exceeded. It is easy to assume that the nursing intervention was highly effective. However, it is important to collect more data before drawing that conclusion. On questioning Mrs. Horowitz, the nurse might find any of the following: (a) She planned a 1200-calorie diet and prepared and ate the food; (b) she planned a 1200-calorie diet but did not prepare the correct food; or (c) she did not understand how to plan a 1200-calorie diet so she did not bother with it.

If the first possibility is found to be true, the nurse can safely judge that the nursing intervention "Explain how to plan and prepare a 1200-calorie diet" was effective in helping Mrs. Horowitz lose weight. However, if the nurse learns that either the second or third possibility actually happened, then it must be assumed that the nursing strategy did not affect the outcome. The next step for the nurse is to collect data about what Mrs. Horowitz actually did to lose weight. It is important to establish the relationship (or lack thereof) of the nursing actions to the patient responses.

Critical Thinking Questions

1. How might a nurse explain how to plan and prepare a 1200-calorie diet?
2. If a SMART goal is specific, measurable, attainable, realistic, and time-limited, then how do these criteria apply to the statement that "Ruth Horowitz, a patient with obesity, needs to lose 14 kg (30 lb)"?
3. If Ruth did not prepare the correct food, should the goal be explained more practically, revised, or abandoned?
4. What questions should the nurse ask to determine how Ruth lost weight if she did not follow her diet plan?
5. If Ruth did not understand how to plan and prepare the 1200-calorie diet, what should the nurse do first to determine how to better explain the practical steps involved?
6. What are potential indications that the problem might be Ruth's attitude and not her intellectual understanding of the practical issues involved in the 1200-calorie diet?

Drawing Conclusions

The nurse uses judgment about goal achievement to determine whether the plan of care was effective in resolving, reducing, or preventing the nursing diagnosis. When goals have been met, the nurse can draw one of the following conclusions about the status of the patient's problem:

- The actual problem stated in the nursing diagnosis has been resolved, or the potential problem is being prevented and the risk factors no longer exist. In these instances, the nurse documents that the goals have been met and discontinues the care for the problem.

- The risk problem stated in the nursing diagnosis is being prevented, but the risk factors are still present. In this case, the nurse keeps the problem on the plan of care.

- The actual problem still exists even though some goals are being met. For example, a desired goal on a patient's care plan is "Will drink 3000 mL of fluid daily." Even though the data may show this goal has been achieved, other data, for example the presence of dry oral mucous membranes, may indicate that the patient is still experiencing deficient fluid volume. Therefore, the nursing interventions must be continued even though this one goal was met.

When goals have been partially met or when goals have not been met, two conclusions can be drawn:

- The plan of care needs to be revised, since the problem is only partially resolved. The revisions may need to occur during the assessment, nursing diagnosis, planning, or implementation phase.
  OR

- The plan of care does not need revision because the patient merely needs more time to achieve the previously established goal(s). To make this decision, the nurse must assess why the goals are being only partially achieved, including whether the evaluation was conducted too soon.

Developing an Evaluation

The nurse collects data so that conclusions can be drawn about whether goals have been met. It is usually necessary to collect both objective and subjective data. Some data may require interpretation. Examples of objective data that may require interpretation are the degree of tissue turgor of a dehydrated patient or the degree of restlessness of a patient with pain. Examples of subjective data that may need interpretation include complaints of nausea or pain by the patient. When interpreting subjective data, the nurse must rely on either (a) the patient's statements (e.g., "My pain is worse now than it was after breakfast") or (b) objective indicators of the subjective data, even though these indicators may require further interpretation (e.g., decreased restlessness, decreased pulse and respiratory rates, and relaxed facial muscles as indicators of pain relief). Data must be recorded concisely and accurately to facilitate the next part of the evaluation process.

If the goal has been written following the guidelines given in this module, it will be relatively simple to determine whether a goal has been met. Both the nurse and patient play an active role in comparing the patient's actual responses with the desired outcomes. Did the patient drink 3000 mL of fluid in 24 hours? Did the patient walk unassisted the specified distance per day? When determining whether a goal has been achieved, the nurse can draw one of three possible conclusions:

1. The goal was met; that is, the patient's response is the same as the desired outcome.
2. The goal was partially met; that is, either a short-term goal was achieved but the long-term goal was not, or the desired outcome was only partially attained.
3. The goal was not met; that is, the patient did not achieve the goal within the time frame.

Writing an Evaluation

After determining whether a goal has been met, the nurse writes an evaluation statement (either on the care plan or in the nurse's notes). An **evaluation statement** consists of the following information:

- Date and time evaluation was done
- A conclusion statement about whether the goal was met, partially met, or not met
- A supporting statement giving the results of how the patient did or did not achieve the goal.

Here are examples of evaluation statements:

Date and Time of Evaluation	Conclusion Statement	Supporting Statement
12/3, 1345	Goal met.	Patient walked with cane 20 feet down hallway.
9/22, 0900	Goal partially met.	Patient is able to identify three foods instead of five foods high in sugar content.
5/14, 1030	Goal not met.	Patient did not change the dressing on his right arm using aseptic technique.

Continuing, Modifying, or Terminating the Nursing Plan of Care

After drawing conclusions about the status of the patient's problems, the nurse modifies the plan of care as needed. Depending on the facility, modifications may be made by drawing a line through portions of the plan of care or writing "discontinued," "goal met," or "problem resolved" and the date and time.

Whether or not goals were met, a number of decisions need to be made about continuing, modifying, or terminating nursing care for each problem. See **Table 36–16 »** for a checklist to use when reviewing a care plan. Although the checklist uses a closed, yes-or-no format, its only intent is to identify areas that require the nurse's further examination.

TABLE 36–16 Evaluation Checklist

Phase of Nursing Process	Checklist
Assessment	_____ Are data complete, accurate, and validated?
	_____ Do new data require changes in the care plan?
Diagnosis	_____ Are nursing diagnoses relevant and accurate?
	_____ Are nursing diagnoses supported by the data?
	_____ Has problem status changed (i.e., potential, actual, risk)?
	_____ Are the diagnoses stated clearly and in the correct format?
	_____ Have any nursing diagnoses been resolved?
Planning	**Desired Outcomes**
	_____ Do new nursing diagnoses require new goals?
	_____ Are goals realistic?
	_____ Was enough time allowed for goal achievement?
	_____ Do the goals address all aspects of the problem?
	_____ Does the patient still concur with the goals?
	_____ Have patient priorities changed?
	Nursing Interventions
	_____ Do nursing interventions need to be written for new nursing diagnoses or new goals?
	_____ Do the nursing interventions seem to be related to the stated goals?
	_____ Is there a rationale to justify each nursing diagnosis?
	_____ Are the nursing interventions clear, specific, and detailed?
	_____ Are new resources available?
	_____ Do the nursing interventions address all aspects of the patient's goals?
	_____ Were the nursing interventions actually carried out?
Implementation	_____ Was patient input obtained at each step of the nursing process?
	_____ Were goals and nursing interventions acceptable to the patient?
	_____ Did the caregivers have the knowledge and skill to perform the interventions correctly?
	_____ Were explanations given to the patient prior to implementing?

Before making modifications, the nurse must determine whether the plan as a whole was not completely effective. This requires a review of the entire plan of care and a critique of each step of the nursing process involved in its development.

Assessment

Incomplete or incorrect data influence all subsequent steps of the nursing process and plan of care. If data are incomplete, the nurse needs to reassess the patient and record the new data. In some instances, new data may indicate the need for new nursing diagnoses, new goals, and new nursing interventions.

Nursing Diagnosis

If the data were incomplete, new nursing diagnostic statements may be required. If the data were complete, the nurse needs to analyze whether the problems were identified correctly and whether the nursing diagnoses were relevant to the information collected. After making judgments about problem status, the nurse revises or adds new nursing diagnoses as needed to reflect current patient data.

Revising Patient Goals

If a nursing diagnosis was inaccurate, the goal statement(s) will need revision. If the nursing diagnosis was appropriate, the nurse then checks whether the goal was realistic and attainable. Unrealistic goals require correction. The nurse should also determine whether priorities have changed and whether the patient still agrees with the priorities. For example, the time frame for a specific amount of weight loss was possibly too short and should be extended. Goals must also be written for any new nursing diagnoses.

Selecting New Nursing Interventions

The nurse investigates whether the nursing interventions were appropriate for goal achievement and whether the priority nursing interventions were selected. Even when diagnoses and goals were appropriate, the nursing interventions selected may not have been the best ones to achieve the goal. New nursing interventions may reflect changes in the amount of nursing care the patient needs, scheduling changes, or rearranging nursing actions to group similar activities or to permit longer rest or activity periods for the patient. For example, for a patient who wishes to stop smoking, many potential interventions exist. If medication was prescribed but the patient is still smoking, a behavioral intervention such as group counseling may need to be added. If new nursing diagnoses have been written, then new nursing interventions will also be necessary.

Method of Implementation

Even if all sections of the plan of care appear to be satisfactory, the manner in which the plan was implemented may have interfered with goal achievement. Before selecting new interventions, the nurse should confirm whether the original interventions were carried out. Other personnel may not have carried them out, either because the interventions were unclear or because they were unreasonable in terms of external constraints such as money, staff, time, and equipment.

After making the necessary modifications to the plan of care, the nurse implements the modified plan and begins the nursing process cycle again. Refer to **Table 36–17 》》** to see how the plan for the patient in the plan of care throughout

this exemplar was modified after evaluation of goal achievement and review of the nursing process. Additions to the care plan are shown in italics. As well as evaluating the patient's response to the nursing plan of care, nurses also evaluate nursing care (see the module on Quality Improvement for further information).

Relationship to Other Nursing Process Phases

Successful evaluation depends on the effectiveness of the phases that precede it. Assessment data must be accurate and complete so that the nurse can formulate appropriate nursing diagnoses and desired goals. The goals must be stated concretely to be useful for evaluating patient responses. And finally, without the implementing phase in which the plan is put into action, there would be nothing to evaluate.

The evaluation phase includes assessment. As previously stated, assessment (data collection) is ongoing and continuous at every patient contact. However, data are collected for different purposes at different points in the nursing process. During the assessment phase, the nurse collects data for the purpose of making diagnoses. During the evaluation phase, the nurse collects data for the purpose of comparing it to the goal developed in the planning phase and making decisions about the effectiveness of the nursing care.

Case Study 》 Part 5

It is 8/12 and time for Nurse Medina and Mrs. Aquilini to evaluate whether or not Mrs. Aquilini has reached her goal. The first day her intake was 3100 mL and output was 2600 mL; the second day her intake was 3050 mL and output was 2825 mL. Mrs. Aquilini is pleased that she was able to increase her intake of fluids to at least 3000 mL daily. Nurse Medina was happy that Mrs. Aquilini has reached her goal that supports the outcome "to restore an effective breathing pattern." The goal statement was "Goal met. Patient has consumed at least 3000 mL of liquids daily by 8/12." (See **Figure 36–13 》》**.)

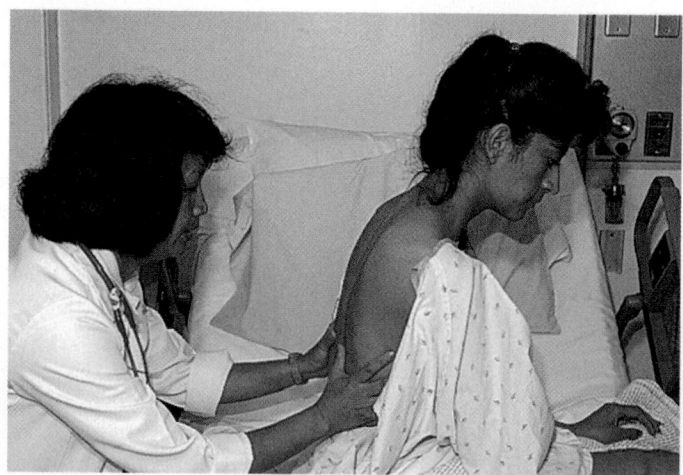

Figure 36–13 》》 Evaluation: Upon assessment of respiratory excursion, Nurse Medina detects failure of the patient to achieve maximum ventilation. She and Mrs. Aquilini reevaluate the care plan and modify it to increase coughing and deep breathing exercises to q2h.

TABLE 36–17 Example of Evaluation of Outcomes and Goals with Notes about Nursing Interventions

Desired Outcomes	Goal Statements	Nursing Interventions	Note about Nursing Interventions
Nursing Diagnosis: _Ineffective Airway Clearance_ related to viscous secretions and shallow chest expansion secondary to deficient fluid volume, pain, and fatigue			
Respiratory status: gas exchange as evidenced by the following:			_Retain nursing interventions to continue to identify progress. Goal status indicates problem not resolved._
▪ Absence of pallor and cyanosis (skin and mucous membranes)	Partially met. Skin and mucous membranes not cyanotic, but still pale.	Monitor respiratory status q4h: rate, depth, effort, skin color, mucous membranes, amount and color of sputum.	
▪ Use of correct breathing/ coughing technique after instruction	Partially met. Uses correct technique when pain well controlled by narcotic analgesics.	Monitor results of blood gases, chest x-ray studies, pulse oximetry, and incentive spirometer volume as available.	
▪ Productive cough	Met. Cough productive of moderate amounts of thick, yellow, pink-tinged sputum.	Monitor level of consciousness.	
▪ Symmetric chest excursion of at least 4 cm	Not met. Chest excursion 3 cm.	Auscultate lungs q4h.	
▪ Lungs clear to auscultation within 48–72 hours	Not met. Scattered inspiratory crackles auscultated throughout right anterior and posterior chest.	Monitor vital signs q4h: TPR, BP, pulse oximetry.	
▪ Respirations 12–22/min; pulse <100 bpm	Partially met. Respirations 26/min, pulse 96 bpm.	Instruct in breathing and coughing techniques. Remind to perform and assist q3h. _Support and encourage. (4/17/17, JW)_	_Does not need to be reinstructed because patient demonstrates correct techniques. May still need support and encouragement because of fatigue and pain of breathing._
▪ Inhaling normal volume of air on incentive spirometer	Not met. Tidal volume only 350 mL. _(Evaluated 4/17/17, JW)_	Administer prescribed expectorant; schedule for maximum effectiveness. Maintain Fowler or semi-Fowler position. Administer prescribed analgesics. Notify primary care provider if pain not relieved. Administer oxygen by nasal cannula as prescribed. Provide portable oxygen if patient goes off unit (e.g., for x-ray examination). Assist with postural drainage daily at 0930. _On 4/17, teach to continue PRN at home. (4/17/17, JW)_ Administer prescribed antibiotic to maintain constant blood level. Observe for rash and GI or other side effects.	_As soon as patient is hydrated and fever is controlled, she will probably be discharged to self-care at home._

In this plan of care, additions to the care plan are shown in _italics_.

Clinical Reasoning Questions Level I

1. Can you identify the different components in the goal statement?
2. How important is it for Nurse Medina to give Mrs. Aquilini positive feedback on reaching her goal?

Clinical Reasoning Questions Level II

3. If Mrs. Aquilini was not able to reach her goal, what would be Nurse Medina's next action?
4. Once a goal has been met successfully by the patient, what happens to this nursing diagnosis in the plan of care?

Lifespan Considerations

Applying the Nursing Process to Children

Assessment of a child is complex and can vary significantly depending on the child's chronologic age and developmental stage. Neonates and infants are not able to verbalize their complaints; therefore, collecting "subjective" data relies heavily on parents and caregivers; objective data are based on nursing observations, child–caregiver interactions, and physical assessment. Nevertheless, assessment of the child is a continuous process of collecting and developing a database of information. The nurse analyzes the data and develops accurate nursing diagnoses.

Data analysis supports a nursing diagnosis or diagnoses addressing the child's health-focused problem. Nursing diagnoses may also address risk problems that require interventions in order to decrease the risk of the child or family developing an actual problem. Furthermore, nurses must become familiar with the defining characteristics of diagnoses that address parenting, role conflict, and family processes and observe for cues that accurately support these diagnoses.

After developing nursing diagnoses, the nurse identifies a priority outcome that will be used to evaluate the pediatric patient's plan of care. A priority outcome states that (a) a healthcare problem does not exist and therefore health promotion is stressed; (b) a risk for health dysfunction is present that requires intervention to decrease or eliminate development of an actual problem; (c) an actual health-focused problem is present that requires interventions; or (d) the nurse identifies an outcome that addresses the child and the family's healthcare goals.

In addition to identifying an outcome to evaluate the plan of care, the nurse, the patient, and when applicable, the patient's family develop a plan with patient goals that will evaluate the patient's response to nursing interventions. Once the nurse develops patient- or family-focused goals, the next step is to develop and implement planned interventions and assess feedback by observation or by communication with patient, family, and other providers in order to determine the effectiveness of the interventions. The nurse ensures the child's physical and emotional safety and comfort while nurses or other providers perform interventions.

In the final step of the nursing process, the nurse evaluates data to determine that previously established goals and outcomes have been met and that nursing interventions were appropriate to the child's needs. If the goals have not been met, have been partially met, or have been met because of interventions not included in the plan of care, the nurse considers altering the plan of care, its goals, and its interventions.

Expected outcomes are not reviewed only during the child's hospitalization and at discharge but also at follow-up appointments with the child's pediatrician to evaluate for complete resolution of the actual health problem and, if applicable, the risk problem. School nurses and healthcare providers in daycare centers should also review expected outcomes for children with chronic diseases such as asthma, cystic fibrosis, diabetes, and other chronic diseases.

Clinical Example F

A 4-year-old girl is admitted following emergency surgery for a ruptured appendix. She is awake and alert, but refuses to talk. Her parents have had little sleep for over 24 hours and are extremely anxious.

- Gathering assessment data in this situation requires the nurse to be sensitive to the parents' needs for rest and assurance; at the same time, the nurse must collect information to compile an adequate database that can be used to make appropriate nursing care decisions. Assessment will be problem focused, monitoring the condition of the child as she recovers from surgery and being alert to potential problems.
- Objective data collected include vital signs; level of and response to pain (often called the fifth vital sign); bleeding or discharge from the incision; mobility; integrity of dressings, intravenous lines, catheters, nasogastric tubes, or other medical devices; and affect.
- Since children are a part of families, assessment will include observation of family dynamics and questions that could lead to care of the family system.

Critical Thinking Questions

1. What are the nursing priorities for the 4-year-old child?
2. What are the patient-centered outcomes for the child?
3. What might be an effective method of getting the patient to talk?
4. List three strategies that you would use to allay the parents' anxiety.
5. What objective data about the patient's parents is important for you to assess in relation to her care?

Applying the Nursing Process to Older Adults

Older adults make up the greater portion of all hospital admissions. As the older adult population increases, so does the cultural diversity of this segment of the population (U.S. Department of Health and Human Services, n.d.). Nurses are challenged to provide culturally sensitive care to the older population without cultural or age-related bias and assumptions.

In addition to acute care facilities, older adults function and seek care in various community settings. Nurses are involved in the care of older adults in patients' homes, nursing homes, adult daycare facilities, assisted-living communities, and various categories of subacute care facilities.

Assessment of the older adult in the acute-care or community setting may be complex because of factors related to physical health, cognition, and functionality. However, the nurse should not assume that all older adults have poor memory or impaired functionality; that they all experience depression, social isolation, or financial hardship; or that all older adults are dependent individuals.

The older adult has the potential for a complex and lengthy assessment database as the nurse attempts to organize information that spans a lifetime. For the older adult who may have visual and auditory impairment, assistive devices such as glasses and hearing aids should be used in order to engage in conversation with the nurse and to respond to questions appropriately. Some older adults may respond to questions with slower but accurate answers. The nurse allows the patient time to respond and does not rush the patient or fill in answers based on assumptions about older adults. Some older adult patients may have less than adequate recall due to cognitive dysfunction, medication, or illness. Patients with previous admissions to an institution should have an established database of health-related information that is supplemented and updated with each new admission. Assessment of the older adult should include up-to-date assessment of each patient's strengths, limitations, and means of social support, factors that may change over short periods of time due to illness, change in functionality, and death of spouse or friends.

The nurse must be aware that changes in an older adult's mental status, often reported by family members or caregivers, may indicate an underlying illness. In many cases, older adults do not present with typical signs and symptoms associated with infections or other healthcare problems. An acute change in mental status of the older adult is a cue for a high level of suspicion for a focused health problem and the need for thorough assessment.

The nurse determines the patient's diagnosis or diagnoses based on subjective data and observations from family members and caregivers and from objective data, including observations, physical and cognitive exams, and test results. The nurse then identifies a priority outcome related to the patient's diagnosis and identifies short- and long-term goals that will be used to evaluate nursing interventions. Outcomes and goals for the older adult must be realistic, individualized and within the realm of the patient's capability. As much as possible, older adult patients should be included when determining goals and interventions related to their care. Although care for every patient is individualized, common goals in caring for older adults revolve around learning needs related to chronic illnesses and medication regimens, safety concerns related to mobility and polypharmacy, and in some cases issues of physical and emotional safety related to caregiver mistreatment or socioeconomic well-being.

Once the nurse develops patient goals, the next step is to develop and implement planned interventions and assess feedback by observation or by communication in order to determine the effectiveness of the interventions. The nurse must take into consideration certain factors that prove challenging when developing interventions for some older adults, including the need for additional time, the patient's level of education and health literacy, the need to interact or teach the patient during the time of day the he or she has the most energy, and the need to use everyday language. The nurse may consider using multiple teaching modes and creativity when educating older adults.

In the final step of the nursing process, the nurse evaluates data to determine that previously established outcomes have been met and that nursing interventions were appropriate to the patient's goals. If the goals have not been met, have been partially met, or have been met because of interventions not included in the plan, the nurse considers altering the plan of care.

Expected outcomes are reviewed during the patient's hospitalization and at discharge. Outcomes should also be evaluated as patients return to the community, because health maintenance minimizes patient readmission. Although many older adults have chronic illnesses and actual health problems, nurses should not focus on these alone. Risk diagnoses are significant to the health of older adults, some of whom are vulnerable to additional healthcare, social, and socioeconomic problems.

Healthcare providers often associate health promotion with children and young adults; however, many older adults at various functional levels express the desire to maintain their level of health, improve their health status and functionality, and prevent disease. For older adults who express interest in improving their health status and in preventive care, health promotion diagnoses and interventions should be included in each patient's plan of care.

REVIEW The Nursing Process

RELATE Link the Concepts and Exemplars

Linking the exemplar of the nursing process with the concept of communication:

1. How does the nurse communicate the use of the nursing process when documenting?

2. The nurse is caring for a patient with postoperative pain and administers an analgesic 10 minutes before the end of the shift. How does the nurse communicate the need for evaluation of effectiveness of pain management to the oncoming shift?

Linking the exemplar of the nursing process with the concept of legal issues:

3. How does use of the nursing process in providing and documenting care reduce the nurse's risk of malpractice claims?

4. What legal obligations does the nurse have related to use of the nursing process?

REFER Go to Pearson MyLab Nursing and eText

- Additional review materials

REFLECT Apply Your Knowledge

Dr. Danilo Ocampo is a 74-year-old retired pathologist. He lives in his home with Lydia, his wife of 51 years. Their only child, a son, was killed at age 22 in an automobile crash. Dr. Ocampo was born and raised in the Philippines and came to the United States when he was 23. He is the last living member of his immediate family. He has a few nephews and nieces in the Philippines, but no relatives live nearby.

Dr. Ocampo's health has been declining for the past few years. He has a medical history that includes hypertension, myocardial infarction, angina, and heart failure. Because of these cardiovascular disorders, he takes multiple medications, including metoprolol; lisinopril; spironolactone; furosemide off and on; K^+ when taking furosemide; aspirin; isosorbide dinitrate; and nitroglycerin. He understands the pharmaceutical properties of the medications. At times, he is doubtful of the quality of healthcare he receives because of all the medications he has been prescribed. He often does not believe the medications are helpful because he experiences many side effects, and he has been readmitted to the hospital multiple times. He usually feels better after a few days in the hospital but typically checks himself out of the hospital before his physicians are ready to discharge him.

Because Lydia has dementia, most of Dr. Ocampo's time and energy are spent managing their household and taking care of her. He has been resistant to outside help, believing he can care for her better than anyone else does. He maintains a consistent schedule, and he and his wife get along quite well. Although at one time in their lives they were very socially active, at this point, they rarely go out.

Dr. Ocampo has become increasingly short of breath and is very fatigued. He notices his legs have become edematous. He goes to the neighborhood drugstore to use the "self-serve" blood pressure machine and finds his blood pressure to be 152/106 mmHg. He is resistant to the idea of seeing his physician or going to the emergency department for fear of being admitted. Instead, he increases the dose of furosemide and lisinopril by 1 tablet per day and tries to get a bit more rest. A week later when his symptoms fail to improve and seem to worsen slightly, Dr. Ocampo visits his healthcare provider's office and reports his symptoms and increase in medication dosages.

1. What are the priorities of care for Dr. Ocampo?

2. What data would you collect from Dr. Ocampo on initial examination?

3. Develop a nursing plan of care for this patient.

>> Exemplar 36.B
The Nursing Plan of Care

Exemplar Learning Outcomes

36.B Analyze nursing plans of care as they relate to clinical decision making.

- Define the nursing plan of care.
- Describe the column plan type of nursing care plan.
- Describe the concept map type of nursing care plan.
- Describe the standardized plan type of nursing care plan.
- Describe the clinical pathway type of nursing care plan.

Exemplar Key Terms

Clinical pathway, 2528
Column plan, 2524
Concept map, 2524
Nursing plan of care, 2522
Standardized plan, 2525

Overview

A **nursing plan of care** is a written or electronic guideline that organizes information about an individual patient or family's care. One plan may include several nursing diagnoses for a single patient. It is important to prioritize nursing diagnoses and to list only three to five nursing diagnoses; this helps the nurse focus on nursing care that provides the best patient outcomes. The RN initiates the plan when the patient is admitted to the facility. The plan of care is then constantly updated throughout the patient's stay in response to changes in the patient's condition and evaluations of goal achievement. Keeping the plan of care current is necessary to ensure appropriate, individualized care for the patient. When the patient is discharged from the facility, the plan is included as part of a patient's permanent record of the care

received and care the patient should have received (see the module on Communication for further information).

Although formats differ from facility to facility, the plan of care is often organized using the five phases of the nursing process (see **Figure 36–14 >>**). Whether written or electronic, plans have the following purposes:

- Provide individualized patient-centered care to meet the unique needs of each patient.
- Provide for continuity of care through communication with nursing staff and other healthcare providers involved with the care of the patient.
- Inform the nurse about which specific observations or actions need to be documented in the nurse's progress notes about the patient's care.

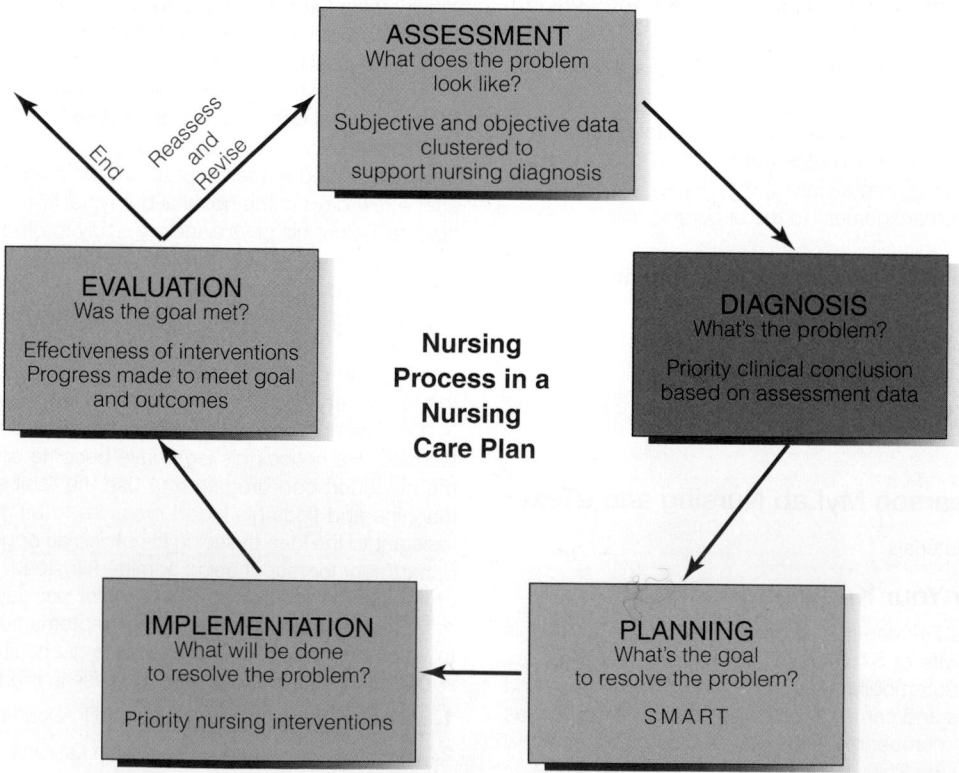

ASSESSMENT
What does the problem look like?
Subjective and objective data clustered to support nursing diagnosis

DIAGNOSIS
What's the problem?
Priority clinical conclusion based on assessment data

PLANNING
What's the goal to resolve the problem?
SMART

IMPLEMENTATION
What will be done to resolve the problem?
Priority nursing interventions

EVALUATION
Was the goal met?
Effectiveness of interventions Progress made to meet goal and outcomes

End   Reassess and Revise

Nursing Process in a Nursing Care Plan

Figure 36–14 >> Using the nursing process in a nursing plan of care.

- Provide health insurance companies documented proof for reimbursement amount to pay for services rendered to the patient.
- Provide the nurse with a guide when assigning nursing staff to care for each patient.

Accessibility

Nursing plans of care need to be readily accessible to all healthcare team members involved with the care of the patient. Availability of the plan supports communication with others for better continuity of care. The plan of care may be kept at the bedside but is more commonly kept within the medical record. In most institutions, the nursing plan of care is part of the electronic medical record that requires specific information about the patient's plan of care. The electronic medical record is accessible to all staff with appropriate access to the patient's record on all units and departments to which the patient may be transferred. The electronic medical record provides the healthcare team with information about the patient, such as demographic data, routines of daily care (i.e., bathing, nutrition), diagnostic studies, social history, oxygen therapy, monitoring needs, medications and IV fluids, and surgical drains.

Guidelines

The nurse should follow the guidelines in **Table 36–18 »** when writing nursing plans of care. Note that the guidelines include specificity and customization.

Clinical Example G

Marlene Fisher is a 52-year-old woman whose husband of 35 years died 5 weeks ago after a long battle with lung cancer. She says that she has come to the clinic today because she does not sleep more than 3 hours at night and feels tired all the time. She tells the nurse that she has lost about 15 pounds since her husband died because she is too tired to fix anything to eat.

Mrs. Fisher has two sons, both of whom attended the funeral, but they have not contacted Mrs. Fisher since then. One lives on the other side of town, and the other lives out of state.

For more than 40 years, Mrs. Fisher attended her place of worship every time the doors were opened for an activity. She also enjoyed singing in the choir. For the past couple of weeks, she has not been able to attend any activities because she doesn't understand why her husband had to die, and she feels disconnected from her place of worship. She stopped singing at home because she says she "doesn't feel the music anymore." Mrs. Fisher says she stays at home every night now to avoid seeing people that are "smiling and happy" when she feels so lost and alone.

Clinical Reasoning Questions Level I
1. What are the significant assessment data for Mrs. Fisher?
2. What related clusters do the significant assessment data form?

Clinical Reasoning Questions Level II
3. What are the top three priority nursing diagnoses from the clustered assessment data?
4. What goal would be appropriate for each of the three nursing diagnoses?
5. What are the top three priority nursing interventions to support Mrs. Fisher reaching her goals?

TABLE 36–18 Guidelines for Writing a Nursing Plan of Care

Guideline	Description
Date and sign the plan.	The date the plan is written is essential for evaluation, review, and future planning. The nurse's signature or login demonstrates accountability since the effectiveness of nursing actions can be evaluated.
Use category headings: "Assessment," "Nursing Diagnoses," "Goals/Desired Outcomes," "Nursing Interventions," and "Evaluation."	Headings may vary slightly with different facilities but are relative to the nursing process phases.
Use approved abbreviations and key words rather than complete sentences to communicate ideas unless facility policy dictates otherwise.	For example, write "Turn/reposition q2h" rather than "Turn and reposition the patient every two hours." Or, write "Clean wound c– H_2O_2 bid" rather than "Clean the patient's wound with hydrogen peroxide twice a day, morning and evening." (See the module on Communication for more information.)
Be specific, short, and concise.	Because nurses are now working shifts of different lengths (e.g., 12- or 8-hour shifts), the nurse must be specific about the timing of an intervention. An intervention reading "Change incisional dressing q shift," could mean either twice in 24 hours, or three times in 24 hours, depending on the length of the facility's shifts.
Refer to facility resources, such as procedure books, rather than including all of the steps on a written plan.	For example, write "See unit procedure book for tracheostomy care" or attach a standard nursing plan about such procedures as preoperative or postoperative care,
Customize the plan to include patient's choices, such as preferences about the times of care and the methods used.	This reinforces the patient's individuality and sense of control. For example, the written nursing intervention might read "Provide partial bath in the evening per patient's preference."
Ensure that the nursing plan incorporates preventive and health maintenance aspects as well as restorative ones.	For example, carrying out the intervention "Provide active assistance ROM (range-of-motion) exercises to affected limbs q2h" prevents joint contractures and maintains muscle strength and joint mobility.
Ensure that the plan contains interventions for ongoing assessment of the patient.	For example, "Inspect incision q8h."
Include collaborative activities in the plan.	For example, the nurse may write interventions to ask a nutritionist or physical therapist about specific aspects of the patient's care.
Include plans for the patient's discharge and health teaching needs.	The nurse begins discharge planning as soon as the patient has been admitted, often consulting and making arrangements with a community health nurse, social worker, and other community agencies to supply patient services, needed equipment, and supplies.

Written nursing plans of care are used in facilities that do not have electronic medical records. Plans can be kept in a separate notebook or with the patient's medical record. Similar to the electronic medical record, written plans of care support communication and continuity of care when patients are transferred from one unit to another or from one facility to another. The plan of care becomes a part of the patient's permanent record upon the patient's discharge from the facility. Each facility decides the format used for the plan of care. Facilities customize the following common types of plans of care for their patients: column plan, concept map, standardized plan, and clinical pathway.

Column Plan

Nursing students learn to develop patients' plans of care and to organize the patients' data from patients assigned to them for learning activities. As a result, care plans developed by students usually are lengthier and more detailed than plans of care used by experienced nurses. Students may be required to give a rationale, or reason, for selecting a particular nursing intervention as a priority. Students may also be required to cite research evidence from literature to support their stated rationale and to develop evidence-based practice habits.

The **column plan** of care uses columns to categorize data for each phase of the nursing process. This type of care plan may include four columns: (a) nursing diagnoses, (b) goals/desired outcomes, (c) nursing interventions, and (d) evaluation. Some agencies use a three-column plan in which evaluation is done in the goals column or in the nurses' notes; other agencies use a five-column plan that adds a column for assessment data preceding the nursing diagnosis column. **Figure 36–15 >>** shows a five-column framework for a nursing care plan for the patient in Clinical Example G, Mrs. Fisher.

Concept Map

A **concept map** is a visual representation of a nursing plan of care in a patterned diagram with data and ideas. Various shapes and colors are used to show relationships and connections in combination with lines or arrows. Concept maps are creative, conceptual images of concrete critical thinking. The visual image enhances clinical reasoning by "showing" how nursing diagnoses, goals, interventions, and evaluations relate to each other in a logical pattern. Concept maps can take many different forms and encompass various categories of data according to the creator's interpretation of the patient or health condition. They are an offshoot of mind maps or cognitive maps. A concept map can be a visual guide for analyzing relationships among clinical data to help prioritize meeting patient needs.

The concept map is another way of depicting the nursing plan of care. Concept maps can help nursing students view the patient and his or her problems holistically rather than as a single problem or medical diagnosis. Students are often asked to complete concept maps as a method of learning and demonstrating the links among disease processes, laboratory data, medications, signs and symptoms, risk factors, and other relevant data.

There are many different ways to make a concept map. Post-It notes are useful because they already come in a variety of colors and shapes; they also make it easy to move data around until the concept map is finished. Colored pencils or markers and paper cut into various shapes can be used as well. Software programs are available for creating electronic concept maps, and many websites offer free concept mapping programs.

Hints when making a concept map:

- Follow the sequence of the nursing process phases; always begin with assessment data collection and cluster significant related data to determine nursing diagnoses (see the exemplar on the Nursing Process for further information).

- Keep it simple. The more lines cross each other, the more difficult it is to follow the connections among data.

Assessment	Nursing Diagnosis	Plan	Implementation	Evaluation
• Doesn't understand why her husband died • Stopped attending place of worship because feels disconnected from it • Stopped singing in the choir	*Spiritual Distress*	Patient will meet with religious adviser by 4/12.	• Establish therapeutic relationship with patient. • Assist patient to cope with lifestyle changes. • Assist patient in finding a reason for living. • Discuss visit with religious adviser. • Encourage patient to talk about her feelings.	4/12 Goal ongoing–patient has appointment with religious adviser on 4/13.
• Not sleeping well • States she "feels so lost" • Lost 15 pounds • Not eating well	*Ineffective Coping*	Patient will eat three meals a day by 4/8.	• Assess for risk of hurting self or others. • Refer patient to counseling. • Discuss sleep promotion behaviors. • Have dietitian discuss cooking for one with patient.	4/8 Goal met–patient has eaten three meals a day × 4 days.
• No contact with sons since husband's death • Husband died 5 weeks ago • Avoids people • Stays at home every night	*Social Isolation*	Patient will phone each son by 4/10.	• Discuss promotion of social contacts. • Assist patient in developing a support system. • Support patient in reconnecting with sons. • Encourage outside activity–like walking.	4/10 Goal not met–patient has spoken with only one of her sons.

Figure 36–15 >> Five-column nursing plan of care for situational distress.

- Many nursing programs have developed a concept map format for nursing students to follow, but the nurse can still use creativity to individualize patient concept maps.
- Avoid becoming caught up in the artistic expression. Do not spend hours matching colors and shapes and coordinating patterns while developing a concept map: it is a visual representation of important concepts focused on nursing care for best patient outcomes.

Many approaches can be used to build a concept map. Here is an example that is basic and can be expanded if more data are being used:

1. Develop a legend for the concept map by assigning shapes and colors for each nursing process phase and one for other categories of patient information: demographics, outcomes, lab results, risk factors, or medications.
2. Put the shape with the patient's initials, age, gender, and priority medical diagnosis in the middle of the paper to illustrate the patient-centered nature of nursing care.
3. Look at the assessment data, subjective and objective, and then gather and sort the significant clusters. Each piece of significant data goes on one assessment shape. Place the clustered groups around the patient shape.
4. Determine the priority nursing diagnoses that are relative to each of the clusters and place one nursing diagnosis with each of them. Draw connecting lines from each shape with assessment data to the nursing diagnosis for which it is relative.
5. Determine one appropriate goal for each nursing diagnosis cluster and add its shape to the side of the nursing diagnosis cluster. Select priority nursing interventions and label them as independent, dependent, or collaborative for each goal. Write separate interventions on their designated shape and arrange them on the outer side of the nursing diagnosis. Draw connecting lines from each shape with an intervention to the nursing diagnosis for which it is relative.
6. Evaluate whether the goal was met, not met, or partially met, and place the evaluation shape on the side of the nursing diagnosis cluster. It can be located under the goal shape or on the opposite side.
7. The concept map is now complete. **Figure 36–16 »** uses the data for Mrs. Fisher from Clinical Example G to build a concept map.

Standardized Plan

A **standardized plan** of care specifies the nursing care for groups of patients with common needs (e.g., all patients with myocardial infarction). These plans can be developed by a standardized care committee composed of facility staff that use both medical and nursing research evidence (see the module on Evidence-Based Practice for more information). Facilities may also purchase standardized plans to complement their policies and procedures. A preprinted plan is time efficient for nurses compared to generating a single plan for a common set of interventions for patients with the same condition. Once the nursing assessment is completed, the standardized plan of care that is appropriate for the patient is selected, and the nurse adds or deletes information on the generalized care plan to individualize it to the unique needs of a particular patient.

A standardized plan of care frequently includes checklists, blank lines, or empty spaces to allow the nurse to individualize goals and nursing interventions. Standardized plans of care should not be confused with standards of care. Although the two have some similarities, they have important differences.

SAFETY ALERT Nurses must remember that standards of care are not the same as a standardized plan of care. Standards of care are nursing actions for patients that describe achievable nursing care. They define the interventions for which nurses are held accountable. Standards of care are developed by individual healthcare facilities for nurses working in the facility. National organizations and agencies, such as the ANA, the Joint Commission, and State Boards of Nursing, also set standards of nursing practice for nurse accountability (see the module on Accountability for further information). A standardized plan of care provides general nursing care for specific medical diseases or conditions. If the nurse determines that following any part of a standardized plan of care would jeopardize a patient's safety or health outcomes, the nurse is responsible for taking appropriate action to ensure the health and safety of the patient by altering or deleting that section of the plan of care.

Standardized care plans are usually categorized according to specific age groups, patient problems, and specialty categories. Standardized plans follow the nursing process phases so nurses are familiar with their format. Regardless of whether plans of care are handwritten, computerized, or standardized, nursing care must be individualized to fit the unique needs of each patient. In practice, a plan of care usually consists of both preprinted and nurse-created sections. The nurse uses standardized care plans for predictable, commonly occurring problems and creates an individual plan for unusual circumstances or problems that require special attention and are unique to the individual patient's needs.

For example, a standardized care plan for "patients with a medical diagnosis of pneumonia" would probably include a nursing diagnosis of *Deficient Fluid Volume* and direct the nurse to assess the patient's hydration status. On a respiratory or medical unit this would be a common nursing diagnosis; therefore, the patient's nurse would be able to obtain a standardized plan directing care commonly needed by patients with deficient fluid volume (see **Figure 36–17 »**). However, the nursing diagnosis *Interrupted Family Processes* would not be common to all patients with pneumonia, although it would be needed for a mother with three small children at home. Therefore, the goals and nursing interventions for that diagnosis for that patient would need to be created by the nurse.

SAFETY ALERT Documentation should always be clear, timely, and dated. Nursing documentation, handwritten or electronic, is the primary source of communication between the nurse and other members of the healthcare team. Documentation records nursing assessment, clinical problems, patient and family education, patient response to interventions, and patients' plan of care. Whereas documentation provides the most accurate and complete account of patient care, nursing documentation records nurses' work as well as patient outcomes. In addition, nursing documentation is the primary source for credentialing, accreditation, research, reimbursement, and legal affairs (American Nurses Association, 2010b).

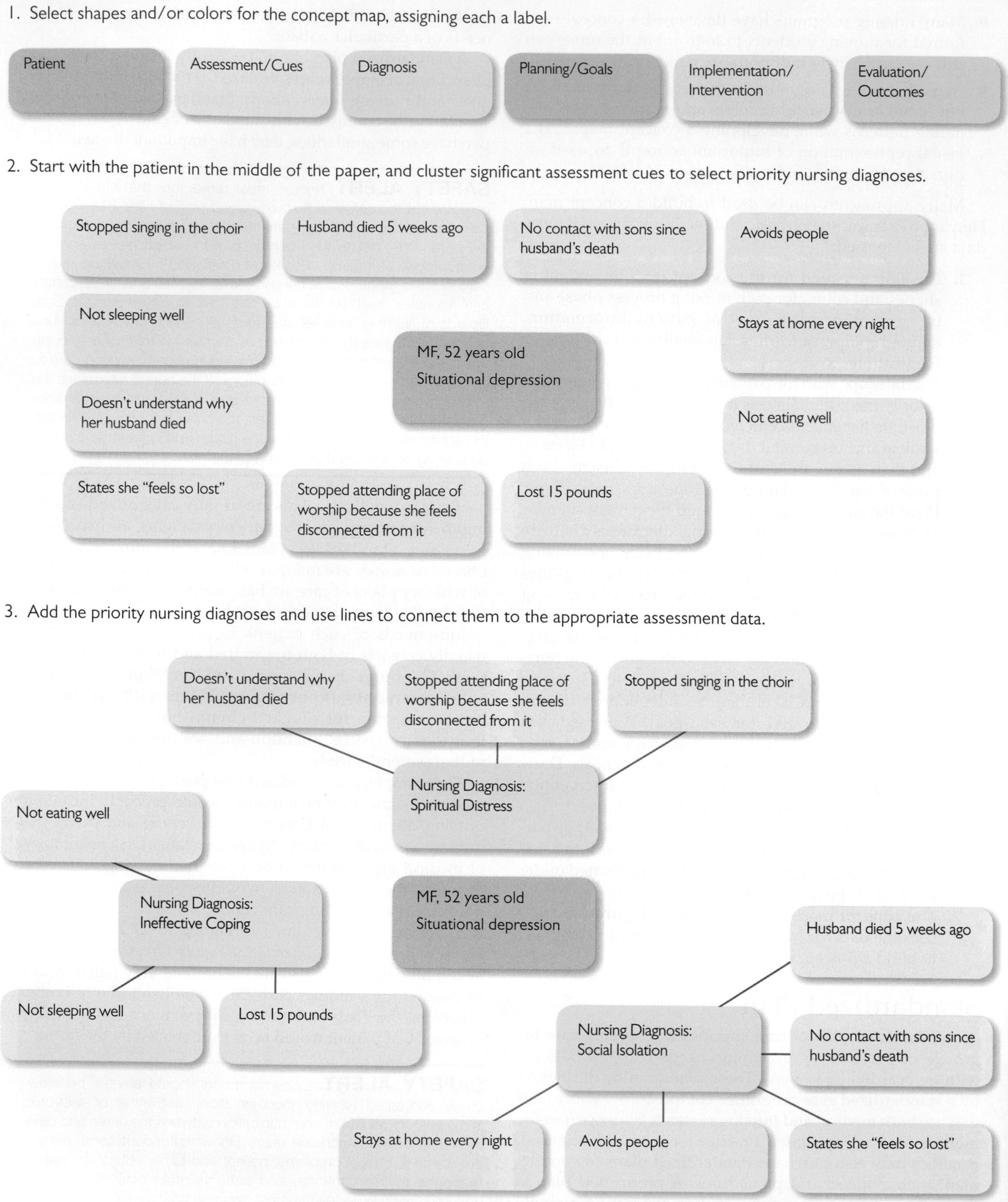

1. Select shapes and/or colors for the concept map, assigning each a label.
Patient
Assessment/Cues
Diagnosis
Planning/Goals
Implementation/ Intervention
Evaluation/ Outcomes
2. Start with the patient in the middle of the paper, and cluster significant assessment cues to select priority nursing diagnoses.
Stopped singing in the choir
Husband died 5 weeks ago
No contact with sons since husband's death
Avoids people
Not sleeping well
MF, 52 years old
Situational depression
Stays at home every night
Doesn't understand why her husband died
Not eating well
States she "feels so lost"
Stopped attending place of worship because she feels disconnected from it
Lost 15 pounds
3. Add the priority nursing diagnoses and use lines to connect them to the appropriate assessment data.
Doesn't understand why her husband died
Stopped attending place of worship because she feels disconnected from it
Stopped singing in the choir
Nursing Diagnosis: Spiritual Distress
Not eating well
Nursing Diagnosis: Ineffective Coping
MF, 52 years old
Situational depression
Husband died 5 weeks ago
Not sleeping well
Lost 15 pounds
Nursing Diagnosis: Social Isolation
No contact with sons since husband's death
Stays at home every night
Avoids people
States she "feels so lost"

Figure 36–16 » Steps for building a concept map.

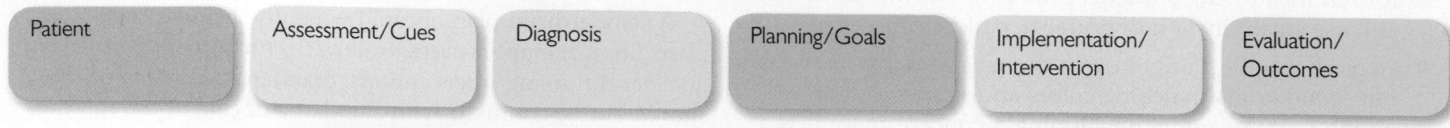

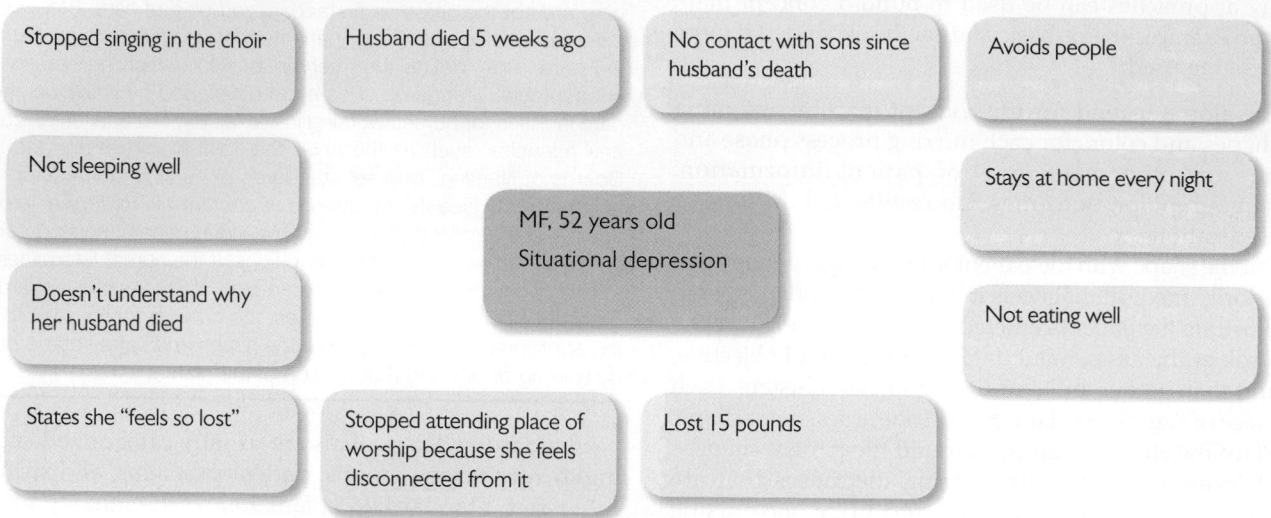

4. Select one or more measurable goals for the patient to work toward that will help the patient resolve the nursing diagnosis.

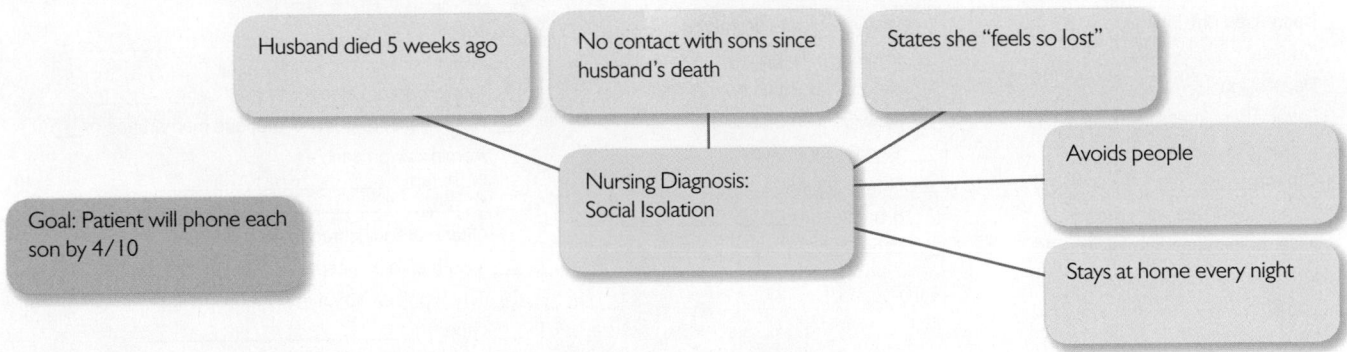

5. For each nursing diagnosis and corresponding goal(s), determine interventions that will help the patient meet the agreed upon goal(s).

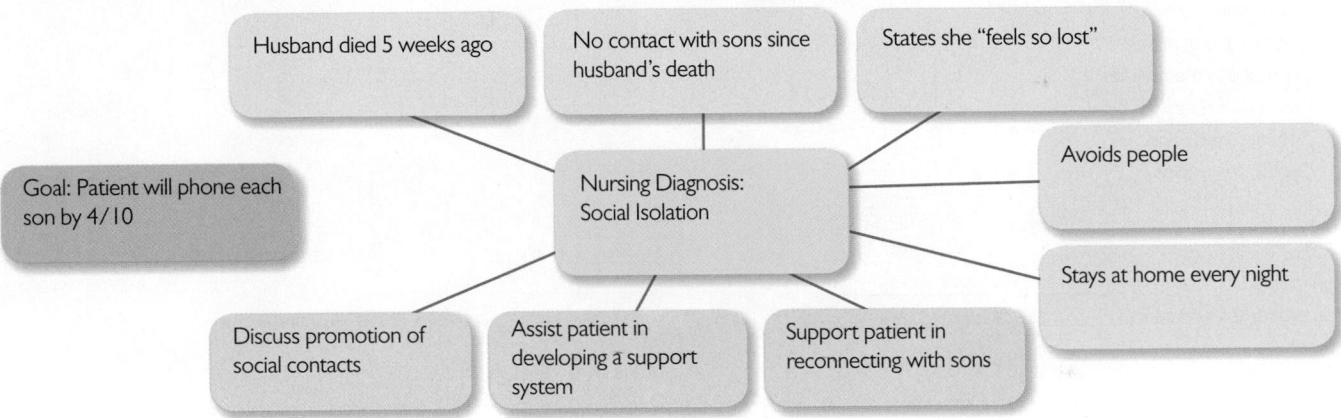

6. At the next healthcare interaction, evaluate whether or not the patient has met the goals (outcomes) and, if not, why.

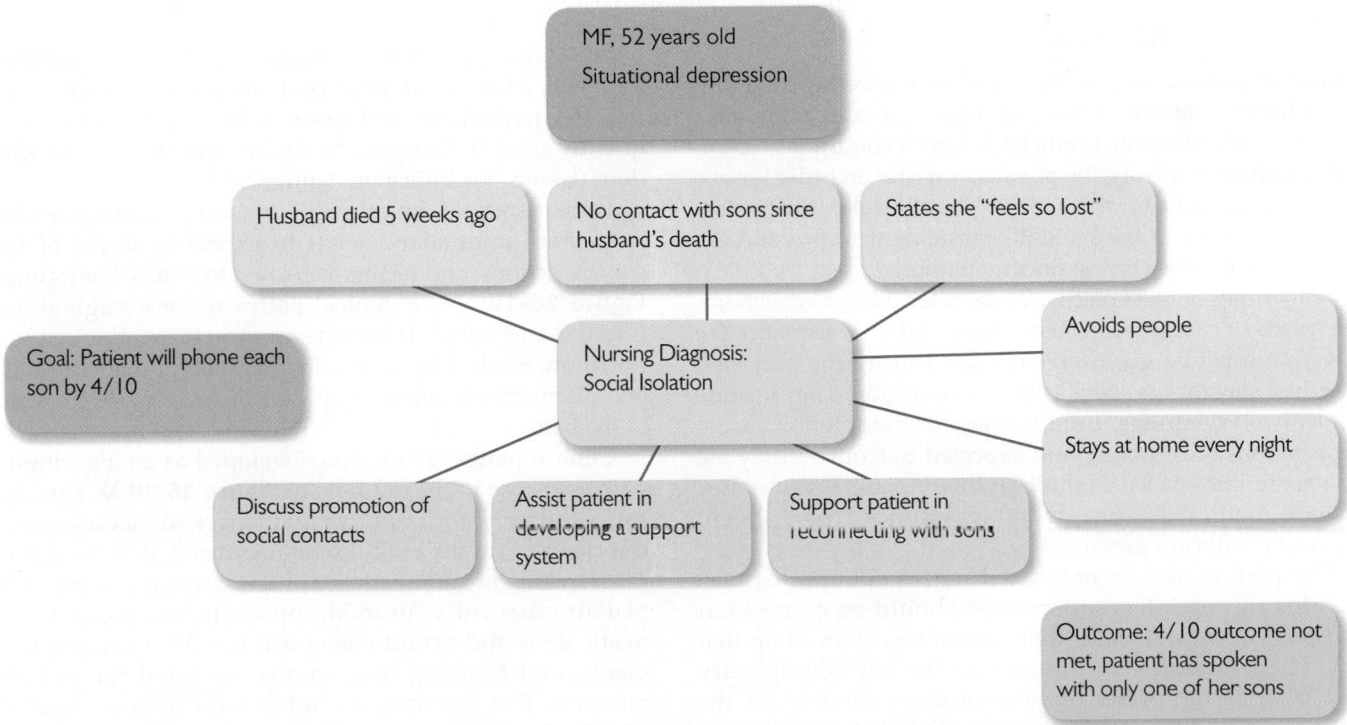

7. Repeat steps 4 – 6 for the nursing diagnoses of Ineffective Coping and Spiritual Distress. Arrange all the information into clusters with connecting lines, and complete a concept map on your own.

Figure 36–16 ⟩⟩ Steps for building a concept map. *(continued)*

Etiology	Desired Outcomes	Nursing Interventions (Identify Frequency)
___ Decreased oral intake	___ Urinary output >30 mL/hr	___ Monitor I&O q___ hr
___ Nausea	___ Urine specific gravity 1.005–1.025	___ Weight daily
___ Depression	___ Serum Na$^+$ within normal limits	___ Monitor serum electrolyte levels x_____
___ Fatigue, weakness	___ Mucous membranes moist	___ Assess skin turgor and mucous membranes q ___
___ Difficulty swallowing	___ Skin turgor elastic	___ Administer prescribed
___ Other: _____	___ No weight loss	IV therapy _____
___ Excess fluid loss	___ 8-hr intake = _____	_____
___ Fever or increased metabolic rate	___ Other: _____	___ Offer oral liquids frequently
___ Diaphoresis		___ Mouth care as needed
___ Vomiting		___ Teach patient about importance of fluid intake
___ Diarrhea		___ Other: _____
___ Burns		
___ Other: _____		
Defining Characteristics		
___ Insufficient intake		
___ Negative balance of I&O		
___ Dry mucous membranes		
___ Poor skin turgor		
___ Concentrated urine		
___ Rapid, weak pulse		
___ Lowered BP		
___ Weight loss		

Plan initiated by: _____ Date: _____

Plan/outcomes evaluated: _____ Date: _____

Patient: _____

Figure 36–17 》 Example of a standardized plan of care for *Deficient Fluid Volume*.

Clinical Pathway

A **clinical pathway** is a standardized, evidence-based, multidisciplinary plan that outlines the expected care required for patients with common, predictable health conditions. To initiate a clinical pathway, the physician writes an order for one that is appropriate for the patient. The clinical pathway documents are part of the patient's permanent record and are integrated into the clinical documentation.

Sometimes clinical pathways are referred to as collaborative plans or case management plans, and they sequence the care that must be given on each day during the projected length of stay for the specific type of condition. They include clinical interventions, time frames for completion, usual expectations of response, and expected outcomes. They are also sometimes called multidisciplinary plans because they include medical treatments to be performed by different types of healthcare providers.

The plan is usually organized with a column for each day, listing the interventions that should be carried out and the patient outcomes that should be achieved on that day. There are as many columns on the multidisciplinary care plan as the preset number of days allowed for the patient's diagnosis-related group (DRG). Clinical pathways do not include detailed nursing activities because they are multidisciplinary in nature. Because all patients are unique, each patient's care will be customized to meet his or her specific needs while keeping the guidelines in mind. Clinical pathways minimize variance in treatment plans in order to reduce cost, increase efficiency, and improve patient care outcomes. Clinical pathways are frequently used in Canada, Australia, and the United Kingdom (Centre for Policy on Aging, 2014).

Patient-specific clinical pathways are given to patients to help them understand what to expect in terms of time frames, actions, and results as related to DRGs. For example, **Figure 36–18** 》 is a clinical pathway for a vaginal birth (mother and baby). It includes information about activity, nutrition, medications, treatments, patient teaching, tests, and discharge planning for specific times from delivery time of the baby.

Clinical pathways may be developed as an algorithm or path as shown in the example of **Figure 36–19** 》. This clinical pathway is for pediatric patients with asthma and is directed toward the multidisciplinary team. It includes separate assessment and treatment progressive guidelines for the pediatric patient with mild, moderate, severe, and near-death signs and symptoms of asthma. Medications, treatments, and teaching instructions are listed for pediatric patients. The pathway includes information about the assessment, pretreatment, and treatment of these patients, and steps to be taken if the patient has not improved. Pathways like this one are designed to improve the quality of care and outcomes as well as to standardize care provided across clinical disciplines.

	MOTHER		NEWBORN	
	24 HOURS	**48 HOURS**	**24 HOURS**	**48 HOURS**
Activity	■ Up with assistance as needed, progress to up by self ■ Shower ■ Self-care with assistance ■ Baby care with assistance	■ Total self-care ■ Baby care by self with assistance as needed ■ Vaginal exercises	(To be done by nursing staff)	(To be done by nursing staff)
Nutrition	■ Regular diet as tolerated	■ Regular diet	■ Scheduled breastfeeding; minimum 6 feeds in 24 hours ■ Scheduled bottle feeding; minimum 6 feedings in 24 hours (each 15–30 mL)	■ Scheduled breastfeeding on cue; minimum 8 feeds in 24 hours ■ Scheduled bottle feeding; minimum 6 feedings in 24 hours (each 30–60 mL)
Medications	■ Pain medications as needed ■ Routine medications	■ Laxative as needed ■ Routine medications	■ Sucrose orally prior to procedures	■ Sucrose orally prior to procedures
Treatments	■ Routine vital signs and assessment ■ Comfort measures for perineum/episiotomy/hemorrhoids ■ Monitoring for signs of complications (e.g., excessive bleeding, difficulty urinating, constipation)	■ Routine vital signs and assessments ■ Sitz bath as needed ■ Comfort measures continued as needed ■ Monitoring for signs of complications continued	■ Routine vital signs and assessment ■ Vitamin K injection and erythromycin ointment to eyes at birth ■ Examination by physician ■ Baby care, height, weight ■ Circumcision if requested	■ Routine vital signs and assessment ■ Continued baby care, weight ■ Infant hearing screening ■ Circumcision care as needed
Patient Teaching	■ Discussion about self-care and newborn care ■ Review learning materials provided ■ Discussion about breastfeeding ■ Discussion about newborn feeding, safety, cord site care, comfort, bathing, sleeping, activity	■ Continue learning about at-home care for self and newborn ■ Continue learning about at-home newborn feeding needs	None	None
Tests	■ Procedures and diagnostic tests as needed	■ Procedures and diagnostic tests as needed	■ Newborn screening as needed before discharge	■ Newborn screening as needed before discharge
Discharge Planning	■ At-home care of self and newborn ■ Discussion about community resources available ■ Discussion about birth certificate, newborn's name, and health coverage	■ Continue at-home care of self and newborn discussions ■ Follow-up appointment for self scheduled	■ Appointment for newborn screening if needed	■ Follow-up appointment for baby scheduled before discharge

Figure 36–18 》 Clinical pathway for mother and baby (vaginal birth).

Focus on Diversity and Culture
Planning Care with Culture

The nurse develops the patient's plan of care with respect to the patient and family's sociocultural background, including the family's structure and organization, religious values, cultural beliefs, and the way in which culture and ethnicity relate to roles within the family. A patient's plan of care must address the role of family and family function within a specific culture, because after discharge, the family will be involved in the daily care of the patient. Nurses should employ effective communication, a holistic patient perspective, and respectful cultural care when caring for patients of varied cultures. Both in the hospital and at home, dietary recommendations should, as much as possible, fall within the patient's cultural dietary habits; it may be necessary to consult a dietitian for assistance with regard to dietary changes and recommendations. The nurse should note the patient's religious observances that may require fasting and the manner in which this practice can affect the patient's medication regimen and health. Religious practices may also influence the gender of the nurse who is able to care for the patient during hospitalization. This should also be taken into consideration if the patient is discharged to home with an order for visiting nurse services. In addition, patients who receive skilled nursing and other health-related therapies at home may benefit from having healthcare personnel who speak the same language or who share or have superior understanding of the patient's culture.

Sources: Based on Agency for Healthcare Research and Quality (2013); Re-engineered discharge to diverse populations. Retrieved from http://www.ahrq.gov/professionals/systems/hospital/red/toolkit/redtool4.html; Giger (2013); *Transcultural nursing: Assessment and intervention* (6th ed.). St. Louis, MO: Elsevier; Lors, Cooks, & Tluczek (2016). A proposed model of person-, family-, and culture-centered nursing care. *Nursing Outlook.* Retrieved from http://www.nursingoutlook.org/article/S0029-6554(16)30001-X/pdf.

EMERGENCY DEPARTMENT: PROTOCOL FOR ASSESSMENT AND TREATMENT OF PEDIATRIC ASTHMA

	ASSESSMENT	SYMPTOMS PRIOR TO TREATMENT	INTERVENTIONS AND THERAPIES	NEXT STEPS IF NOT IMPROVED
MILD ASTHMA	■ May be agitated ■ Can lie down ■ Nocturnal cough ■ Exertional dyspnea ■ Plays quietly ■ Can talk ■ Increased use of β-agonist ■ Good response to β-agonist	■ O_2 saturation >95% ■ Increased respiratory rate ■ Moderate wheeze-end expiratory Respiratory rates: Age Normal rate <2 months <60/min 2–12 months <50/min 1–5 years <40/min 6–8 years <30/min	■ O_2 to achieve $SaO_2 \geq 95\%$ ■ β-agonist—nebulizer, up to 3 doses in first hour ■ Oral systemic corticosteroids	
MODERATE ASTHMA	■ Agitated ■ Prefers sitting ■ Shorter cry ■ Difficulty feeding ■ Increased work of breathing ■ Some difficulty talking ■ Partial relief with β-agonist ■ β-agonist needed >q4h	■ SaO_2 92–95% room air ■ Increased resp rate ■ Increased heart rate ■ Wheezing throughout inhalation and exhalation Pulse rates Age Normal rate 2–12 months <160 bpm 1–2 years <120 bpm 2–8 years <110 bpm	■ O_2 to achieve $SaO_2 \geq 95\%$ ■ β-agonist and anticholinergic—nebulizer, up to 3 doses in first hour or continuous treatment for 1 hour ■ Systemic corticosteroids	**ADMIT**
SEVERE ASTHMA	■ Very agitated ■ Sits upright ■ Stops feeding ■ Marked limitation in talking ■ Dyspnea at rest ■ Grunting	■ SaO_2 < 92% ■ Labored respirations ■ Persistent tachycardia ■ Breath sounds are decreased ■ Wheezing throughout inhalation and exhalation	■ 100% O_2 ■ Continuous β-agonist and anticholinergics ■ Systemic corticosteroids ■ Systemic magnesium sulfate	**ADMIT TO ICU or TERTIARY CARE**
NEAR DEATH	■ Exhausted ■ Drowsy ■ Diaphoretic ■ Cyanotic ■ Apnea ■ Unable to talk ■ Use of accessory muscles to breath ■ Suprasternal retractions	■ SaO_2 < 80% ■ Decreased respiratory effort ■ Falling heart rate ■ Paradoxical thoracoabdominal movement ■ Silent chest	■ Cardiac monitoring ■ Oximetry, ABGs ■ Chest x-ray ■ Frequent reassessment ■ Medical supervision until clear signs of improvement ■ Consider alternative drugs: IV β-agonist Inhalation anesthetics Aminophylline Epinephrine	**RAPID SEQUENCE INTUBATION**

Figure 36–19 》 Clinical pathway for pediatric asthma for multidisciplinary team.

REVIEW The Nursing Plan of Care

RELATE Link the Concepts and Exemplars

Linking the exemplar of the nursing plan of care with the concept of communication:

1. What information in the nursing plan of care is communicated to members of other disciplines who are taking care of the same patient?

Linking the exemplar of the nursing plan of care with the concept of managing care:

2. How can using a standardized plan of care influence the cost of patient care?

Linking the exemplar of the nursing plan of care with the concept of professional behaviors:

3. Why is use of a nursing plan of care considered a professional behavior?

REFER Go to Pearson MyLab Nursing and eText

■ Additional review materials

REFLECT Apply Your Knowledge

Devon Bynum, an 11-year-old, is admitted to the hospital in sickle cell crisis. This is the first time he has been admitted to a hospital. He states he hurts all over and rates his pain as 7 out of 10. Devon has been in the emergency department all night and last received morphine 2 mg IV at 0400 for his pain. He is receiving oxygen at 2 liters per minute (LPM) via nasal cannula. He has an IV of D5 ½NS running at 83 mL/hr. His mom, who has been with him throughout the night, is anxious for her son to feel better. His latest vital signs are T 99.3° F; P 122 bpm; R 22/min; BP 100/64 mmHg; and oxygen saturation 93% on oxygen at 2 LPM. He says he is tired and just wants to go to sleep. Devon's mom tells the nurse that she doesn't know how she will be able to pay the hospital bills. She shares that she is a single parent with two other children at home.

1. What type of nursing plan of care would you use for Devon? Why?
2. Would you include his mom's concern about finances in his plan of care? How?
3. What other healthcare discipline(s) would you expect to include in Devon's plan of care?

» Exemplar 36.C Prioritizing Care

Exemplar Learning Outcomes

36.C Analyze prioritizing care as it relates to clinical decision making.

- Describe the need for nurses to prioritize care.
- Describe methods or identifying what to prioritize.
- Describe various processes of categorizing priorities.
- Outline factors to consider when prioritizing care.
- Summarize pitfalls of prioritization.

Exemplar Key Terms

ABC, *2533*
ABCD, *2533*
Effectiveness, *2532*
Efficiency, *2532*
Pitfall, *2538*
Pop-ups, *2538*
Prioritizing care, *2531*
Priority, *2531*
Resources, *2537*
Time constraints, *2534*
Time priority, *2534*
Triage, *2535*
Urgency factor, *2534*

Overview

The term **priority** refers to using judgment to discern which among competing problems should be addressed immediately. **Prioritizing care** is a process that helps nurses manage time and establish an order for completing responsibilities and care interventions for a single patient or for a group of patients. The ability to set priorities is a critical thinking skill that can optimize a nurse's time and productivity by categorizing responsibilities and care interventions in an order based on significance and urgency. Time is a constant factor in prioritizing care: nurses have only a limited amount of time to make clinical judgments about which interventions to perform and when to do them, whether for one patient or for several patients. Without some forethought and planning, a nurse may work for hours and yet accomplish very little. Nurses must learn to use time and energy wisely in today's busy healthcare settings.

A nurse's workload includes many objectives that need to be completed during each shift. Time management is an important skill that helps the nurse ensure that necessary activities are completed. Nurses can use a variety of approaches to accomplish nursing responsibilities and interventions. Unfortunately, some of these approaches may result in interventions being done poorly, incompletely, late, or not at all.

For example, some nurses simply plow into their work. They complete tasks as they go from patient to patient in no particular order, keeping busy by doing activities to meet patients' needs. They may start at one room and simply work their way down the hallway doing things for their patients. This strategy raises a number of questions. What about the nursing interventions with time constraints, such as medication administration? Are all nursing interventions equally important? Do all nursing interventions impact patients equally?

Sometimes nurses choose to work on the easiest tasks first, postponing the more challenging, complex tasks for a later time, but they may find themselves rushing to finish the complex tasks during that inevitable "crunch" time. The nurse may decide he or she does not have time to perform an important intervention and leave it undone. A nurse working at a hurried pace experiences an increased stress level, which interferes with clear thinking, clinical judgment, and decision making. As time to complete actions decreases, working at a hurried, task-oriented pace often negatively impacts both the quality of professional performance and the quality of patient care.

Many new nurses have difficulty prioritizing patient care, yet they are afraid to ask questions to get the help they need. New nurses often benefit from adequate orientation and preceptorship that include discussions about delegation, but they also benefit from having a mentor to address issues such as workflow and prioritizing patient care. As new nurses gain confidence, experience, and competency, they develop the ability to distinguish routine tasks from individualized care, they learn to advocate for their patients, and they develop their workflow based on prioritizing patient care (Veerapen & Purkis, 2014).

In contrast to less productive methods of completing activities, nurses can learn to prioritize their actions according to the importance of tasks and interventions and the appropriate timing for accomplishing them. As a result, interventions that have a high priority will be completed early. Just like learning any new skill, learning to prioritize care will take practice. When developing this skill, nurses have the advantage of being able to transfer other skills they have learned in nursing: assessment, critical thinking, clinical judgment, decision making, planning, implementation, and ongoing evaluation (see the Critical Thinking section earlier in this module for more information).

Identifying What to Prioritize

Nursing strives for quality productivity and patient satisfaction. Three factors can influence patient satisfaction with nursing care: availability of nursing staff to care for patients, the amount of time it takes nursing staff to meet patients' needs, and the quality of the care provided. **Effectiveness** (doing the right things) and **efficiency** (doing things right) are two qualities that impact patient perception of nursing care. Nurses employ effectiveness and efficiency by using the strategies of setting priorities, managing time, and delegating to staff. To support these qualities, nurses need to limit distractions and interruptions. Patients may perceive the nurses' distractions and interruptions as signs of inefficiency and conclude that the actions nurses perform are simply tasks instead of individualized, personal care. When providing patient-centered care, treat all patients with respect, dignity, and necessary attention.

Assessment

"Look before you leap" reflects the need to have accurate information prior to taking action. Setting priorities for nursing care always begins with assessment. Assessment includes observing and asking questions to gather the information necessary for decision making. Helpful assessment data include the following:

- Observing for cues about pace and emotions of staff already working on the unit (e.g., are they relaxed or stressed?).

- After receiving information from the previous nurse in shift report, conducting one's own assessment by making a quick safety check of patients.

- Becoming aware of any patients who have an unstable status, a risk of change in their condition, or who require closer observation.

- Asking if there are any complexities to patient problems.

- Asking about any special safety concerns for the patients (e.g., high risk for falls).

- Making note of routine responsibilities and interventions that have time constraints (e.g., physician rounds at 0900, medication administration at 1000 and 1200, nursing meeting at 1330).

- Knowing how many and what level of nursing staff are available for delegation of tasks to help with patient care. Delegation is the transfer of responsibility and authority for completing an activity to a qualified individual (see the module on Managing Care for additional information), although accountability for the task remains with the nurse.

- Noting the presence (and absence) of necessary resources on the unit (e.g., linen, supplies, and nourishments).

- Asking about patient preferences to take into consideration when providing care.

Airway, breathing, and circulation are vital for life. If a safety risk or physiologic deterioration threatens any one of these functions, the situation may quickly become life threatening without prompt assessment and intervention. Nurses must be able to assess and prioritize threats to these functions as they arise (see **Box 36–3 ≫**).

The Nursing Process

Since the 1950s, the nursing process has been used as a method of organizing nursing care of patients, and this process was made mandatory when it was codified by the ANA in 1973. The steps in the nursing process provide the framework nurses use to determine priorities when working with a single patient or a group of patients (see the exemplar on the Nursing Process for further information).

The National Council of State Boards of Nursing (NCSBN) provides models for states to use when revising their nurse practice acts and nursing administrative rules. The sections covering the scope and standards of nursing practice list the steps of the nursing process that develop a nursing plan of care. These sections also support accountability for clinical judgments, decision making, critical thinking, and competence of interventions in the course of nursing practice (prioritizing care and performing interventions) (NCSBN, 2016). See **Box 36–4 ≫** for two examples of state rules about prioritization of care.

Maslow's Hierarchy of Needs

Maslow's hierarchy of needs is a well-known method of assessing and organizing patients' needs. This hierarchy of needs is typically displayed as a five-level triangle or set of steps (see the module on Stress and Coping for further information). Beginning at the bottom, the levels of need progress from the most basic physiologic needs to more complex psychologic and social needs at the top. The most basic needs include food, air, water, shelter, elimination, and sleep (Cherry, 2015).

According to Maslow, these needs motivate behavior. The first four needs—physiologic, safety, social, and esteem—are sometimes called "deficiency needs" and indicate the patient is experiencing deprivation of one or more of those four needs. Needs on the lower levels must be met before an individual can move to higher levels. The last need, self-actualization, is called a "being need" and does not result from a deficiency, but rather indicates a desire for growth as an individual (Cherry, 2015).

Maslow ranked his hierarchy of needs with essential needs on the first (bottom) level and lowest needs on the last (top) level. Nurses can use Maslow's hierarchy as they establish priorities of patient care. For example, ineffective breathing pattern, a physiologic need, takes priority over body image disturbance, a self-esteem need.

The nursing process and Maslow's hierarchy of needs can be used to guide the nurse in thinking critically about the order in which patient needs should be addressed. Nurses

Box 36–3
Priority Assessment of Safety Risks and Physiologic Deterioration

A nurse walks into a patient's room and finds the patient pulling out his tracheostomy tube. Another nurse walking down the hallway passes the visitors' waiting room and finds a child patient climbing up a high metal file cabinet. A third nurse finds her patient unresponsive, not breathing, and without a pulse. These situations involve safety and physiologic deterioration; all require prompt assessment for the potential to become life threatening. Removal of the tracheostomy tube could leave the patient without a patent airway; the child patient could cause the file cabinet to fall and possibly crush his head; and the patient who is unresponsive with no respirations or pulse could die within minutes. Nurses continuously assess patients in their environments to recognize harmful situations. If the patient is in danger, intervention becomes a priority.

The mnemonic **ABC** represents the essential functions of airway, breathing, and circulation. It provides a guideline for use when assessing a patient. An initial assessment of basic body functions necessary to sustain life precludes a more definitive assessment or any patient intervention (discussed in the module on Perfusion). The initial ABC assessment includes:

Airway: A patent airway so oxygen will have a pathway into the lungs for gas exchange and for carbon dioxide to be expelled from the body

Breathing: An effective breathing pattern and respiratory effort to take in enough oxygen to meet cellular demands for oxygen throughout the body

Circulation: An effective circulatory system to deliver oxygen throughout the body and exchange carbon dioxide and oxygen through the pulmonary circulatory network.

Nurses working in a variety of settings follow priority emergency protocols developed by the American Heart Association (2015) to standardize CPR. Since its development, the ABCs of CPR have been enhanced and altered by various specialty groups and professional organizations, adding more letters or changing the meaning of the letters; however, ABC is the universally accepted priority in managing life-threatening emergencies.

Another popular enhancement to the basic ABCs mnemonic is to add a D at the end, creating **ABCD** to help define other priority emergency assessments to complete. The meaning of D varies from one organization to another, but D may stand for:

- **D**efibrillation (use an automated external defibrillator for an absent pulse)
- **D**eficiency (assess for sensory or neurologic changes)
- **D**eadly bleeding (assess for massive hemorrhaging and shock)
- **D**isability (assess for spinal cord trauma and injury with movement or sensory deficits) (American College of Surgeons Committee on Trauma, 2017; Thim et al., 2012).

The few seconds taken by the nurse to assess for a patent airway, effective breathing pattern, and effective circulation system are essential. If life-threatening problems are found on assessment, the nurse intervenes with appropriate nursing actions. When initiated immediately, these interventions can positively affect patient outcomes by preventing complications, resolving a deteriorating condition, or saving a life.

Assessment of airway, breathing, and circulation can be done very quickly by observing the patient. Is the patient awake? Moving? Talking? Responding? If there is no problem with airway, breathing, or circulation, a nurse can move on to a more holistic assessment to identify other patient needs. Assessment may include lung sounds, heart sounds, sensorium, emotional status, and psychologic status.

Box 36–4
Examples of Board of Nursing Rules Addressing Prioritization of Care

OHIO Board of Nursing

4723-4-07 Standards for Applying the Nursing Process as a Registered Nurse

(3) Planning

The registered nurse shall, in an accurate and timely manner:
- a. Develop, establish, maintain, or modify the nursing plan of care consistent with current nursing science, including the nursing diagnosis, desired patient outcomes or goals, and nursing interventions; and
- b. Communicate the nursing plan of care and all modifications of the plan to members of the healthcare team;

(d) Implementation:

The registered nurse shall, in an accurate and timely manner implement the current nursing plan of care which may include:
- a. Executing the nursing regimen;
- b. Implementing the current valid order authorized by an individual who is authorized to practice in this state and is acting within the course of the individual's professional practice;
- c. Providing nursing care commensurate with the documented education, knowledge, skills, and abilities of the registered nurse;
- d. Assisting and collaborating with other healthcare providers in the care of the patient;
- e. Delegating nursing tasks, including medication administration, only in accordance with Chapter 4723-13, 4723-23, 4723-26, or 4723-27 of the Administrative Code.

Source: From LAWriter, 2014.

Tennessee Board of Nursing

1000-01-.14 Standards of Nursing Competence

(1) (a). 2. Establish critical paths and teaching plans based on individual patient's plans of care after prioritizing need upon completion of a comprehensive assessment.

Source: From Tennessee Board of Nursing, 2015. Published by Department of Health Services.

can then use their clinical judgment to make decisions about ranking patient needs as low, medium, and high priorities.

Low Priority

Problems that typically can be resolved easily with minimal interventions and do not cause significant dysfunction are included in the low-priority category. For example, responding to a patient's request for a midafternoon snack could be delegated to unlicensed assistive personnel.

Medium Priority

These are problems that may result in unhealthy physical or emotional consequences but that are not life threatening. For example, the nurse could ask a patient who exhibits spiritual distress by saying, "God has forgotten about me" if she would like to have a hospital chaplain come visit.

High Priority

This category includes life-threatening problems of airway, breathing, and circulation, or conditions that have a potential to become life threatening within a short amount of time (Tunlind, Granstrom, & Engstrom, 2015). An example of a high-priority intervention is frequent monitoring for unexpected changes in the vital signs and drainage for a patient who has just had a chest tube inserted. See **Table 36–19** »» for examples of nursing diagnoses for patients experiencing low-, medium-, and high-priority circumstances.

SAFETY ALERT A survey of perioperative nurses indicated that priority safety issues exist for surgical patients despite increased efforts to reduce surgery-related errors. Perioperative nurses identified wrong site, procedure, and patient issues; medication errors; and pressure injuries from poor positioning, among several other types of errors in surgical cases (Steelman, Graling, & Perkhounkova, 2013). Patient safety is the responsibility of the entire healthcare team. As advocates for patients, nurses should voice their concerns and question and clarify any situation that may compromise patient safety.

TABLE 36–19 Examples of NANDA-I Nursing Diagnoses for Patients Experiencing Low-, Medium-, and High-Priority Circumstances

Low Priority	Medium Priority	High Priority
Readiness for Enhanced Self-Concept	Anxiety	Ineffective Airway Clearance
Fatigue	Diarrhea	Impaired Gas Exchange
Ineffective Health Maintenance	Acute Confusion	Impaired Spontaneous Ventilation
Disturbed Body Image	Disturbed Sleep Pattern	Ineffective Breathing Pattern
Deficient Knowledge	Impaired Bed Mobility	Risk for Bleeding
Powerlessness	Ineffective Coping	Decreased Cardiac Output
Interrupted Family Processes	Self-Care Deficit	Risk for Ineffective Cerebral Tissue Perfusion

Categorizing Priorities

Nurses must set priorities for nursing activities and interventions using assessment data with consideration of the category of the intervention: low, medium, or high priority. In addition, nurses must consider other priorities, including time constraints and the significance of the activities and interventions on patient outcomes. The urgency factor model will help nurses learn how to rank priorities based on time imperatives and severity of patient needs.

Time Constraints

When setting priorities, it is important to remember that some nursing interventions have **time constraints**, or deadlines for completion. One common intervention bound by time constraints is the administration of scheduled medications. Setting priorities for patient care includes planning the day in advance and determining which direct- and indirect-care activities must be completed at expected times (Antinaho et al., 2015). Essential activities not performed by the nurse may result in negative consequences for patients.

The Urgency Factor

Organizing times to provide nursing care is influenced by the urgency factor. The word *urgency* reflects the need to act. **Time priority** means a time constraint is present when completing actions. The **urgency factor** is a way to illustrate how much time can safely lapse before a patient's health status is compromised. Do all nursing interventions require an immediate action? Can some actions be performed within a short amount of time and others be delayed for a longer period without negative consequences for the patient?

Changes in the patient's condition, deterioration of status, or the complexities of a patient's condition can impact the urgency of performing interventions and the order in which the nurse performs those interventions. The urgency factor comprises four levels. These levels progress from not urgent (a low time priority) to high urgency (the highest time priority). The nurse can use the levels of the urgency factor to assist in setting patient-care priorities. By using the levels of urgency, the nurse can identify interventions that need to be completed and the order in which they should be accomplished. See **Figure 36–20** »» and the following sections for a diagram and discussion of the urgency levels when setting time priorities.

Nonacute

Interventions with a low urgency factor may be termed *nonacute*. A delay in providing these interventions would not negatively impact patient outcomes. Interventions at this level do not take priority. For example, at the beginning of a shift, the nurse could discuss with a patient scheduling a later time to teach him about changing a dressing.

Acute

Acute interventions are often considered medium priority: There is a low potential for the patient's condition to become life threatening if these interventions are not accomplished within a short amount of time. Typically, these are actions that nurses are expected to complete to meet identified patient needs. Interventions at this level can be scheduled

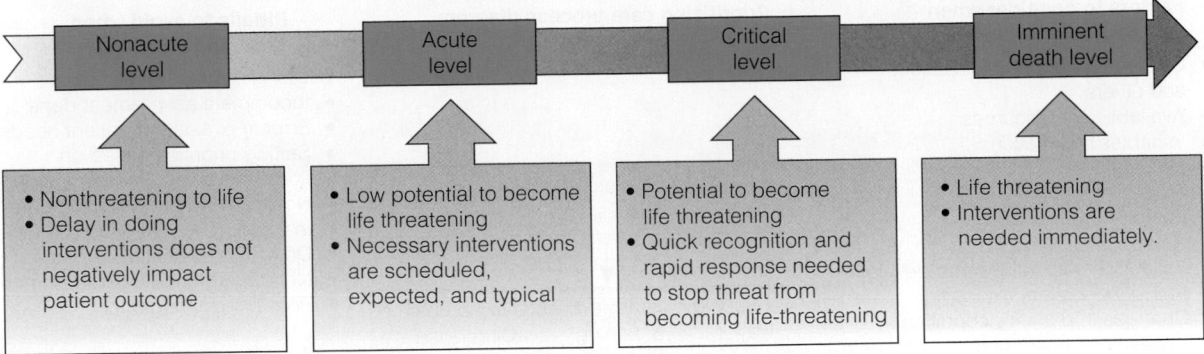

Figure 36–20 》 Urgency factor levels for setting time priorities.

during the shift when time constraints of higher priority interventions allow. For example, a nurse can schedule with unlicensed assistive personnel to turn and reposition a patient with impaired bed mobility every 2 hours to prevent skin breakdown.

Critical

This level is considered medium-high urgency: There is an urgent need for the nurse to respond quickly to high-priority physical or psychologic problems within a short amount of time because the potential exists for a patient's condition to become more serious and even life threatening if interventions are delayed. Quick recognition and a rapid response time are necessary to prevent further exacerbation of the patient's problem. For example, a patient develops shortness of breath and air hunger. If the patient does not receive high-flow supplemental oxygen, the patient may develop impaired gas exchange problems that may progress to severe hypoxemia and become life threatening.

Imminent Death

The highest urgency factor is *imminent death*. The time to take action to prevent threat to life takes priority over everything else. When the patient's airway is obstructed, the patient stops breathing, or the patient's heart becomes ineffective in pumping blood through the circulatory system, immediate intervention is necessary to try to save the patient's life. The nurse must act now, STAT, to prevent further deterioration and threat to life.

Of course, there are countless possible life-threatening situations. For example, a patient on suicide precautions is holding a knife against his neck and is threatening to kill himself. Immediate actions must be taken to try and prevent him from harming, and possibly killing, himself. Nurses are always on alert for situations that could result in death for patients. Many of the more common situations, including medication errors, patient identification errors, and other safety issues, are identified in the National Patient Safety Goals (see the module on Safety for additional information).

Ranking Activities

Learning to set priorities is the key to organizing patient care and efficiently using time to provide valued care. Setting priorities leads to providing efficient and effective patient care and can increase patient satisfaction (Papastavrou et al.,

2014). Nurses can set priorities by thinking in terms of these categories: "must do," "should do," and "nice to do."

Priority 1 or Must Do

These activities carry the highest priority for completion, take priority over other interventions, and must be done. For example, suctioning secretions from a tracheostomy tube to keep a patient's airway patent is a *must do* priority.

Priority 2 or Should Do

These activities should be done, but are not essential. These interventions can be accomplished once *must do* activities have been completed or covered. For example, restocking dressing supplies in the room of a patient who needs frequent dressing changes is a *should do* priority.

Priority 3 or Nice to Do

These activities are important to complete, but only after priority 1 and 2 actions have been completed. These actions can be done when time is available, but they are not essential. Nurses should also use their judgment to determine which "should do" and "nice to do" actions may be delegated to unlicensed assistive personnel.

Other category names for level of urgency can be used to rank priorities. See **Table 36–20 》** for examples of category names.

Triage

In emergency departments, emergency situations, and prehospital care, the process of identifying priorities for implementing care is called **triage**. Triage allows nurses and other healthcare staff to set priorities based on the severity and

TABLE 36–20 Examples of Common Names for Priority Categories

Priority 1	Priority 2	Priority 3
Need to do	Try to do	May not do
Vital to do	Important to do	May not do
Must do	Should do	Nice to do
High priority	Medium priority	Low priority
Most important	Less important	Least important

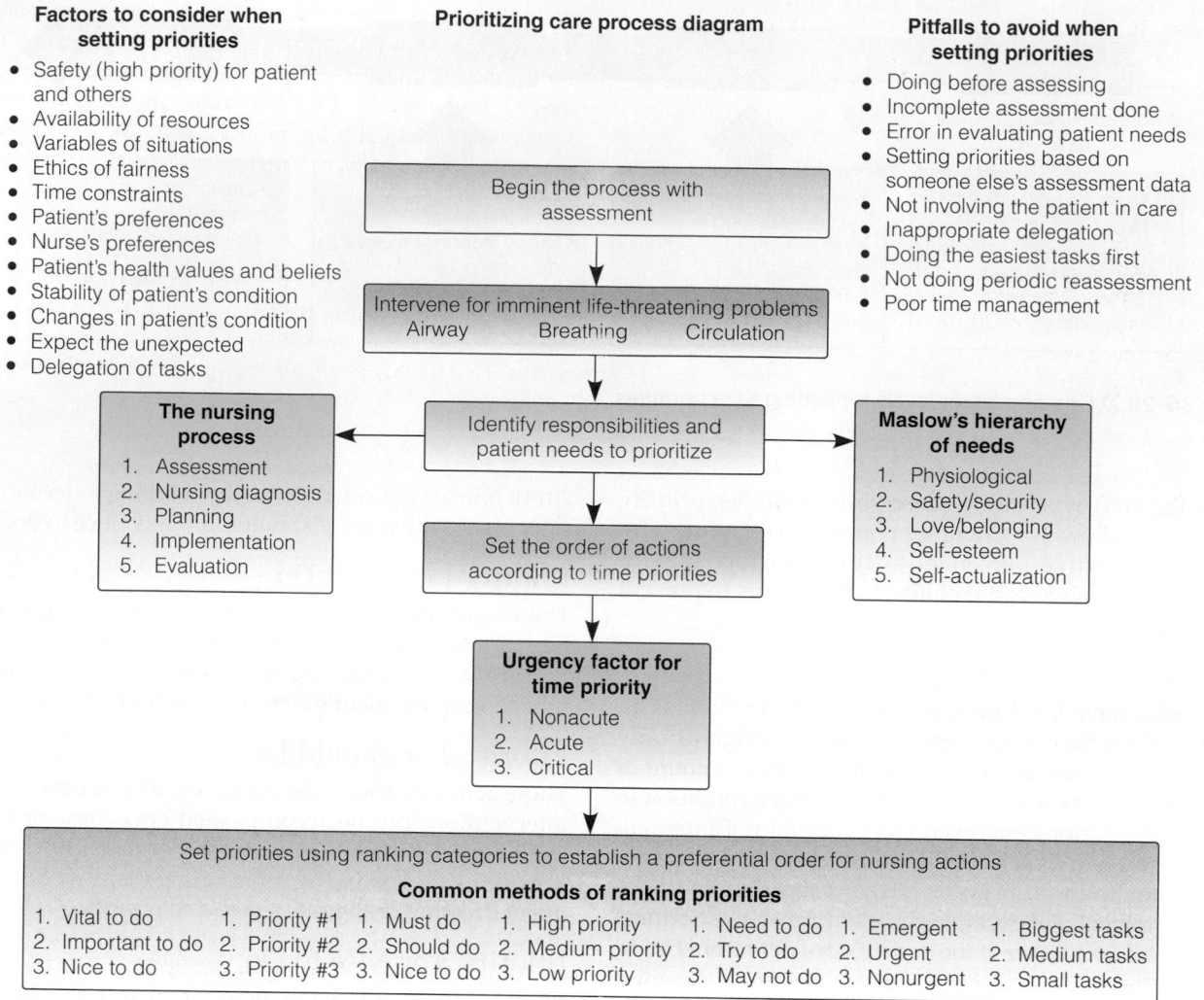

Factors to consider when setting priorities

- Safety (high priority) for patient and others
- Availability of resources
- Variables of situations
- Ethics of fairness
- Time constraints
- Patient's preferences
- Nurse's preferences
- Patient's health values and beliefs
- Stability of patient's condition
- Changes in patient's condition
- Expect the unexpected
- Delegation of tasks

Prioritizing care process diagram

Begin the process with assessment

Intervene for imminent life-threatening problems
Airway   Breathing   Circulation

Identify responsibilities and patient needs to prioritize

Set the order of actions according to time priorities

Pitfalls to avoid when setting priorities

- Doing before assessing
- Incomplete assessment done
- Error in evaluating patient needs
- Setting priorities based on someone else's assessment data
- Not involving the patient in care
- Inappropriate delegation
- Doing the easiest tasks first
- Not doing periodic reassessment
- Poor time management

The nursing process
1. Assessment
2. Nursing diagnosis
3. Planning
4. Implementation
5. Evaluation

Maslow's hierarchy of needs
1. Physiological
2. Safety/security
3. Love/belonging
4. Self-esteem
5. Self-actualization

Urgency factor for time priority
1. Nonacute
2. Acute
3. Critical

Set priorities using ranking categories to establish a preferential order for nursing actions

Common methods of ranking priorities

1. Vital to do	1. Priority #1	1. Must do	1. High priority	1. Need to do	1. Emergent	1. Biggest tasks
2. Important to do	2. Priority #2	2. Should do	2. Medium priority	2. Try to do	2. Urgent	2. Medium tasks
3. Nice to do	3. Priority #3	3. Nice to do	3. Low priority	3. May not do	3. Nonurgent	3. Small tasks

Figure 36–21 》 Prioritizing care process diagram.

urgency of a patient's illness, injury, and condition (see the module on Healthcare Systems for additional information). Common categories used to set priorities are discussed next.

Emergent (or Immediate)

This category is for life-threatening issues that require prompt treatment and care. Stabilization of the patient's condition is critical. For example, a trauma patient with a blood pressure of 88/56 mmHg and pulse of 108 bpm is emergent.

Urgent (or Delayed)

This category is for serious health conditions in which a delay of treatment and care would not result in life-threatening situations. For example, a patient who complains about having a productive cough for the past 4 days is urgent.

Nonurgent (or Minor)

Patients in this category have minor issues that do not require prompt care. Many of these patients can ambulate and are stable in their conditions. For example, a patient with a splinter in his foot that needs to be removed is nonurgent. Some emergency departments use satellite divisions for patients with nonurgent issues. This allows the main

emergency department to manage patients with emergent and urgent health problems with immediacy while decreasing wait times for nonurgent patients.

See **Figure 36–21 》** for a diagram of the prioritization of care process.

Factors to Consider When Prioritizing Care

Prioritization means more than just making decisions about which interventions to do first, second, third, and so forth. The assumption that nurses accomplish all of the things they want or need to do for all of their patients regardless of what order they do them in is no longer true. In some situations, nurses cannot get everything done within an allotted period of time. When nurses experience demands on their services that exceed the time available, they must be able to set priorities of care. Because of this, prioritization sometimes means the most important interventions get done, activities of lesser priority *may* get done, and the least important actions *may not get done at all* because there is insufficient time to complete them.

Prioritizing care in and of itself does not result in nurses being more productive in a given time period. Interventions take the same amount of time to complete regardless of the order in which they are done. Multitasking and learning to perform certain actions faster may improve effectiveness and efficiency but should never compromise patient safety.

Ethics

A holistic approach to nursing means caring for the physical, psychologic, spiritual, cultural, emotional, and developmental needs of patients. Often, patients have many more needs than nurses are able to meet. The principle of *justice* guides nurses in making decisions about setting priorities (see the module on Ethics). Nurses show *fairness* in treating individuals as equals. The difference among patients is the urgency of their needs; for example, a life-threatening situation will take priority over a psychosocial problem. Decisions are sometimes based on consideration of which actions will result in the best outcomes for the patient (Lachman, 2012).

Safety

Protecting patients and providing them with a safe environment is another aspect of justice. Safety in doing no harm to patients is a professional behavior (see the module on Professional Behaviors for further information). The Institute of Medicine (2011) published a document that emphasized the need to improve safety for patients that led to the National Patient Safety Goals developed by the Joint Commission. For example, safely administering medications to patients is a high priority (see the module on Safety for additional information).

Nurses can be fair in their allocation of time, attention, and skills to ensure patient safety. Unrealistic demands on nurses' physical and emotional abilities may result in nurses minimizing what they can do for their patients and may lead to feelings of dissatisfaction and exhaustion. Nurses' desire to help patients requires an environment that supports the delivery of quality care.

Availability of Resources

Resources are assets that help nurses meet patient needs. Problems arise when necessary resources are not available in the required quantity. Rationing or making decisions about which patients will receive the available resources may require prioritization. For example, a linen cart that has not been replenished leaves everyone without enough towels, washcloths, and gowns for patients. A nurse's creativity and resourcefulness can be valuable in finding solutions, such as borrowing the needed linen from another nursing unit and replenishing it when new linen arrives on the unit.

Nurses should use their time and resources efficiently and minimize activities that detract from patient care. Nurse managers should be made aware of situations that potentially compromise patient care, such as lack of sufficient resources. For example, in the scenario above, the nurse may suggest borrowing linen from another unit to the nurse manager, who then facilitates that arrangement and delegates assistive or supportive personnel to deliver the linen.

Time Management

Time priorities are determined by the urgency of completing interventions for patients. As nurses become proficient,

they develop a sense of how long it takes to complete certain interventions for patients, a skill that helps nurses better manage their time. Part of developing good time management is taking into account specific considerations, such as patient health preferences, changes in patient's condition, unexpected occurrences, and appropriate delegation of tasks.

Multiple Patients

Nurses generally take care of more than one patient at a time. Nurses can identify and plan interventions for all patients based on assessments of assigned individual patient needs, changes in patient status, and complexity of patient problems. Setting priorities is determined by the significance of the interventions for each of the individual patients. Time constraints such as medication administration for multiple patients requires more organization and focus from the nurse in order to complete medication administration within an allotted time frame. The pathophysiology of the individual patients would also require consideration when setting priorities among the assigned patients.

Patient Preferences

Patients are unique individuals who grow and develop as a result of genetic and environmental factors. Although patients share many similarities, such as the need for oxygen, they differ in terms of cultural rituals, spiritual practices, and routines of daily living. Some of these practices have time constraints, such as praying at specific times of day.

Health practices and beliefs of patients may conflict with some physicians' orders. Helping a patient maintain cultural or religious practices without compromising the patient's treatment plan sometimes requires extra effort on the part the nursing staff. The goal is to strive for a win–win situation by honoring the patient's wishes as much as possible and completing nursing interventions as needed. Working together for a mutually beneficial solution strengthens the patient–nurse relationship.

Prioritizing activities for the day can be done with most patients. The patient's individual preferences and expectations of care can help set time priorities. For example, some patients may prefer to have a shower in the evening instead of the morning. The patient can plan individual activities around nursing actions that are scheduled at certain times. For example, if the patient knows he needs to get medications at 1000 and 1400, he could schedule his walk down the hall at 1100. Activities the patient considers as priorities may differ from those ranked as priorities by the nurse. By assessing for patient preferences, nurses can help strengthen patient participation in and support for the plan of care. Such actions may result in improved patient outcomes, a positive experience for the patient, and greater patient satisfaction.

Change in Patient Condition

Patients need to be monitored continuously for changing circumstances. Assessing patients at 1200 and reporting on them at 1900 without reassessing them means 7 hours have elapsed in which one or more patients have likely experienced a change of status without reassessment by the nurse.

Such infrequent assessments may result in the nurse receiving the shift report receiving inaccurate or incomplete data about the patient.

Nurses depend on other nurses to let them know of problems and changes in their patients. Assessment is an ongoing process to recognize changes and provide appropriate interventions early. When a patient's condition changes or becomes unstable, the earlier it is discovered and addressed, the more quickly nurses and the healthcare team can intervene and prevent further deterioration. A change in patient status may require reevaluating priorities and changing the planned order of interventions. Revising priorities is especially important when planning care for multiple patients.

The Unexpected

Things do not always go as planned. Nurses could plan their workday more efficiently if they could depend on the initial schedule set at the beginning of the shift and follow that plan throughout the day. However, on most days, nurses encounter unexpected events, or **pop-ups**, that require their time and attention and take them away from their plan for the day. For example, a new admission to the unit, a patient whose blood pressure is dropping, or a patient complaining of shortness of breath all take precedence over interventions such as teaching a patient about food choices for a low-salt diet, changing a dressing for a surgical patient, or any number of other nursing interventions. Pop-ups can challenge the time management and organizational skills of the most experienced nurses.

Nurse Self-Care

A nurse's plan for a quick 15-minute break and a 30-minute meal break at the beginning of a shift may sound simple. However, when it is time for nurses to take a break, they often are busy with their patients or other responsibilities; because breaks are not considered a priority, they do not always happen. "I'll go when I finish this" may be a never-ending refrain.

A short time away for self-care can provide quality time to refresh, reenergize, and take care of body functions (drink some water, eat some food, go to the restroom, or do some stretching). A few quiet minutes can help break up the intensity of the work environment and relieve stress for nurses (American Holistic Nurses Association, n.d.).

Delegation

Delegating tasks to other nursing staff, such as LPNs and UAPs, can improve time management. Registered nurses must be aware of the legal responsibilities involved in delegating a task. The task must be within the scope of practice for the nursing staff member to whom the task has been delegated. The nurse who delegates the task must evaluate the task upon its completion (Yoon, Kim, & Shin, 2016). See the exemplar on Delegation in the module on Managing Care for more information.

Delegation between the RN and UAPs requires mutual trust and demonstrates the RN's confidence in staff members' abilities to assist in patient care. New RNs often do not delegate tasks because of fear of negative occurrences for which they will be responsible. Also, they are often unsure of which tasks may be delegated to UAPs, and they have yet to develop the skills to determine trustworthiness in UAP staff members (Ekstrom & Idvall, 2013; Yoon et al., 2016). Furthermore, novice nurses often fail to see themselves as leaders and fear being perceived as assertive by UAPs (Ekstrom & Idvall, 2013). Role-playing during orientation and preceptorship and discussions with a mentor may help the new nurse recognize when it is appropriate to delegate lower-level priorities to UAPs and that leadership is an inherent role of registered nurses.

Pitfalls of Prioritization

Nurses should learn to avoid pitfalls when prioritizing care. A **pitfall** is an unforeseen situation that often harbors consequences for nurses and can result in patient harm. Although nurses may not know all of the possible pitfalls, there are some pitfalls they can learn to recognize and avoid. When nurses follow ethical practices, use available resources, know the health concerns of their patients, have a sense about patient priorities, prioritize care appropriately, and use questions from clinical decision-making models, they can avoid many pitfalls. Common pitfalls are described in the following sections.

Prioritizing Without Assessment

Nurses need as much information as they can gather about their assigned patients, especially when they are assigned more than one patient. When providing care to multiple patients, nurses must consider interventions for all patients separately and set priorities. Without assessment, the first step in the prioritization process, nurses may forget important interventions or provide interventions based on old data. Patients may sustain severe consequences as a result.

Incomplete Assessment

Part of knowing how to do an assessment is learning what information is required to set priorities for patient care. Accurate and timely information about patient status, resources, available nursing staff, time constraints, and complexity of interventions is needed to prioritize care. If any of these are not assessed first, nurses will fail to include important and necessary information when setting priorities.

Relying Solely on Another's Assessment

Obtaining assessment data from another nurse, such as during shift report, can provide insight and give a picture of a patient's status during the previous shift. However, using only this information to set priorities, without also performing one's own assessment, may negatively affect patient outcomes.

Failing to Do Periodic Reassessments

Reassessment allows the nurse to adjust the time and order of actions to support completing interventions and activities on time and in order of importance. Sometimes the unexpected happens, taking the nurse in another direction and interrupting planned activities. Examples of these situations include a change in a patient's condition, arrival of a new patient who needs to be admitted to the unit, and a request from a relative or visitor to speak with the nurse. Periodic reassessments give the nurse a sense of the time available to perform actions, determine which actions still need to be done, and when to perform these actions throughout the shift.

Box 36–5
Time Management Suggestions

At home, the night before your shift:

1. Make a list of scheduled medication administration times (i.e., 0730, 0800, 1000, 1200, 1400, and 1600).
2. Under each time, list expected patient interventions that will happen close to the times (i.e., meals, safety checks, IV checks, pain management checks, physician rounds, AM care, and documentation). This is the blueprint to follow for managing your time.
3. If you know of any procedures you may need to do the next day, review and visualize how to do them so you will be prepared and not use time the next day to refresh how to perform the procedure (e.g., giving an IV piggyback medication, inserting an indwelling urinary catheter).

At the beginning of your shift:

1. Eat something before arriving; arrive early to put your things away.
2. Listen to the change-of-shift report to get a sense of how your day may go (acuity of patients assigned, problems you may have, patients who may require more time, and so on).

3. Add any time constraint activities to your blueprint (e.g., a meeting you need to attend).
4. Make safety check rounds on your patients to assess for additional information.
5. Begin setting priorities for patient care. Remember to include the urgency factor for time priorities. Delegate tasks to nursing staff working with you as appropriate. Remember to perform actions you've designated as priorities or difficult actions early and check them off of your to-do list.
6. Become more aware of time by checking your watch every couple of hours to get a sense of where you are with completing your activities.
7. Keep a notepad handy in a pocket to make notes about everything you do or want to remember later. This will increase your accuracy and relieve you from relying on memory. These notes will be useful for documentation time or for change of shift (Froedge, 2013).
8. Reprioritize your time as needed when pop-ups or unplanned events occur.
9. Check your progress in completing your to-do list throughout the shift. Reprioritize activities as needed.
10. Celebrate your success as you complete priority interventions.

Poor Time Management

Time management can be difficult for nurses to master, especially for those who do not check their watches every couple of hours to sense where they are in terms of accomplishing patient-care activities. Nurses may find that some actions have taken longer than expected to complete, while others have taken less time. Some actions have time constraints that may not be altered. Proficient time management ensures that priority tasks are accomplished in a timely manner and that the nurse remains productive during the shift. See **Box 36–5** 》 for suggestions on managing time.

SAFETY ALERT Nurses are aware of healthcare organizations' policies and procedures related to quality nursing care, patient safety, and general institutional safety guidelines, three essential factors in prioritizing patient care. However, a recent study found inconsistency between nurses' knowledge of policies and procedures regarding safety, and compliance with quality and safety indicators and safety implementation. The researchers state that factors such as improving nurse-to-patient ratio, increasing nurses' participation in clinical decision making, and promoting champions for nursing units, among other recommendations, may help close this gap (Alam & Alabdulaali, 2016). These factors may also help nurses avoid pitfalls that occur because of short staffing or, in some cases, lack of participation in nursing governance.

Patient care is individualized even when addressing routine tasks. When working with children and with older adults, more time may be needed for discussions, answering questions, and teaching, based on the patient's developmental stage and cognitive ability. In addition, during the course of the work shift, the nurse can expect to encounter family members and caregivers, in person and by phone, who will also require time as they present questions about

the state of the patient's health. Nurses often forget to include these occurrences when considering their plan for the day. By recognizing that interactions with patients and families will take time away from tasks, the nurse is able to plan the workday with consideration for such encounters. Patients and families must perceive that the nurse is fully engaged in responding to their needs: they should not feel rushed or hurried. Both patients and families recognize meaningful encounters and nursing attention as signs of quality care.

Not Involving Patients in Their Care

Nurses assess and determine patient needs when setting priorities. Nurses are also accountable for planning and carrying out interventions, but it is a mistake not to include the patient in planning his or her care. Patients have preferences in how they do things, when they want things to happen, and what they want to do. Preferences may be a result of culture, family influences, spirituality, or heritage. Asking patients about their needs is a way to recognize their individuality and deliver patient-centered nursing care. Observing patient behaviors can also provide the nurse with cues about time and order of patients' preferences.

Inappropriate Delegation

Nurses must follow certain rules when delegating tasks to others (see the module on Managing Care for further information). Other nursing staff, LPNs, and UAPs can assist in completing tasks for patients if the tasks are within the scope of practice found in their state's nurse practice act. Transferring responsibility for a task to an LPN or UAP does not remove accountability for the outcome from the registered nurse. Inappropriate delegation may result in the RN having to repeat an intervention or may even result in harm to the patient. Inappropriate delegation can have immediate ramifications for patient care.

Doing the Easiest Tasks First

Setting priorities means determining those actions that are more important than others and ordering actions based on their priority. Nurses become competent in the process of prioritizing through practice. Completing important, necessary, and sometimes complicated nursing tasks and interventions before easier, less complicated ones makes good, professional common sense. Positive patient outcomes occur when nurses provide intentionally planned care services to meet patients' needs.

REVIEW Prioritizing Care

RELATE Link the Concepts and Exemplars

Linking the exemplar of prioritizing care with the concept of clinical decision making:

1. What are some commonalities between these two nursing processes?

Linking the exemplar of prioritizing care with the concept of safety:

2. Why is safety a high priority for patients who have *Risk for . . .* nursing diagnoses?

Linking the exemplar of prioritizing care with the concept of professionalism:

3. What aspects of setting priorities for care are professional behaviors for nurses?

Linking the exemplar of prioritizing care with the concept of managing care:

4. Name some ways setting priorities for care contributes to improved management of care.

REFER Go to Pearson MyLab Nursing and eText

- Additional review materials

REFLECT Apply Your Knowledge

You have been assigned to take care of Mr. J. Rodriguez, a 48-year-old male patient, during clinical from 0645 to 1300. This patient was admitted to the medical unit yesterday with bilateral pneumonia. He has a history of shortness of breath and exertional dyspnea for the past week. He states he has had a productive cough for the past 4 days, with green, foul-smelling thick sputum. He complains of chest pain when he has to cough. His appetite is diminished and he is not drinking very much because he says he is too tired. He also states he was not able to go to work the 2 days before he was admitted to the hospital. Mr. Rodriguez lives with his wife and four children. His wife speaks very little English. His last set of vital signs were temperature 102.2°F (39°C), pulse 98 bpm, respirations 22/min; blood pressure 134/86 mmHg. He is friendly, quiet, and wants to get better. He is in no distress at this time.

Physician orders include:

- IV D_5 1/2NS with 20 mEq KCl at 100 mL/hr
- Rocephin 1 gram IV piggyback every 12 hours
- I&O every shift
- Vital signs every 4 hours, including pulse oximetry
- Out of bed to chair with assistance
- Regular diet, encourage fluids
- Use an incentive spirometer 10 times every hour while awake
- Oxygen via nasal cannula at 2 LPM oxygen.

Nursing interventions include:

- Assisting with bath and morning care as needed
- Changing bed linens on patient's bed
- Administering medications at 0800, 1000, 1200
- Assisting with breakfast as needed at 0800
- Assisting with lunch as needed at 1230
- Doing a 60-second patient safety check every 2 hours
- Doing a complete assessment on the patient early morning
- Reassessing the patient's condition every 4 hours
- Doing vital signs at 0800 and 1200
- Assisting the patient with incentive spirometry during morning hours
- Encouraging the patient to drink fluids
- Checking for new physician orders
- Checking for diagnostic test results
- Listening to report from previous shift nurse
- Assisting patient in menu selection for tomorrow's meals
- Teaching the patient how to splint his chest with a pillow when he needs to cough to prevent chest muscles from hurting with coughing
- Documenting in patient's electronic medical record throughout the day
- Checking the patient's IV every 4 hours
- Providing fresh ice water in the patient's water pitcher
- Measuring and tallying the I&O for the patient during the shift
- Assisting the patient to get up to the chair in the morning and again in the afternoon.

List any additional interventions you would want to do with this patient:

1.

2.

3.

Decide the priority of each of the above nursing interventions, both those listed and your own. Indicate your priority choice beside each one by writing a "1" for a high priority, a "2" for a medium priority, and a "3" for a low priority. Now decide which actions can be delegated to a UAP to assist in completing them all. Write a "D" beside the interventions that can be appropriately delegated to a UAP.

References

Agency for Healthcare Quality and Research (2013). *Re-engineered discharge to diverse populations.* Retrieved from http://www.ahrq.gov/professionals/systems/hospital/red/toolkit/redtool4.html

Alam, A. Y., & Alabdulaali, M. K. (2016). Awareness to implementation on select quality and patient safety indicators among nursing staff. *Journal of Community and Public Health Nursing, 2*(1), 1–5.

Alfaro-Lefevre, R. (2017). *Critical thinking, clinical reasoning, and clinical judgment.* Philadelphia, PA: Elsevier.

American Association of Colleges of Nursing. (2008). *The essentials of baccalaureate education for professional nursing practice.* Retrieved from http://www.aacn.nche.edu/education-resources/baccessentials08.pdf

American College of Surgeons Committee on Trauma. (2017). *Advanced trauma life support* (10th ed.). Chicago, IL: American College of Surgeons.

American Heart Association. (2015). *2015 American Heart Association guidelines for CPR and ECC.* Retrieved from https://eccguidelines.heart.org/index.php/circulation/cpr-ecc-guidelines-2/

American Holistic Nurses Association. (n.d.). *Holistic stress management for nurses.* Retrieved from http://www.ahna.org/Resources/Stress-Management

American Nurses Association. (2010a). *Nursing: Scope and standards of practice.* Retrieved from http://www.nursesbooks.org/ebooks/download/NursingScopeStandards.pdf

American Nurses Association. (2010b). *Principles for nursing documentation.* Retrieved from http://www.nursingworld.org/MainMenuCategories/ThePracticeofProfessionalNursing/NursingStandards/ANAPrinciples/PrinciplesforDocumentation.pdf

Antinaho, T., Kivinen, T., Turunen, H., & Partanen, P. (2015). Nurses' working time use—how value adding it is? *Journal of Nursing Management, 23*(8), 1094–1105. doi:10.1111/jonm.12258

Benner, P. (2011). From novice to expert. *Current Nursing.* Retrieved from http://currentnursing.com/nursing_theory/Patricia_Benner_From_Novice_to_Expert.html

Benner, P. (2015). Curricular and pedagogical implications for the Carnegie Study, educating nurses: A call for radical transformation. *Asian Nursing Research (Korean Society of Nursing Science), 9*(1), 1–6. doi:10.1016/j.anr.2015.02.001

Benner, P., Hughes, R. G., & Sutphen, M. (2008). Clinical reasoning, decisionmaking, and action: Thinking critically and clinically. In R. G. Hughes (Ed.), *Patient safety and quality: An evidence-based handbook for nurses* (Chap. 6). Rockville, MD: Agency for Healthcare Research and Quality. Retrieved from http://www.ncbi.nlm.nih.gov/books/NBK2643

Benner, P., & Tanner, C. (1987). How expert nurses use intuition. *American Journal of Nursing, 87*(1), 23–31.

Benner, P., Tanner, C., & Chesla, C. (2009). *Expertise in nursing practice: Caring, clinical judgment and ethics* (2nd ed.). New York, NY: Springer.

Brophy, E. (2014). Healthcare decision-making, CM, and the law. *Advances in Integrative Medicine, 1*(1), 40–43.

Bulman, C., & Schutz, S. (2013). *Reflective practice in nursing* (5th ed.). Oxford, UK: Wiley-Blackwell.

Burbach, B. E., & Thompson, S. A. (2014). Cue recognition by undergraduate nursing students: an integrative review. *Journal of Nursing Education, 53*(9 Suppl), S73–81. doi:10.3928/01484834-20140806-07

Bussard, M. (2015). The nature of clinical judgment development in reflective journals. *Journal of Nursing Education, 54*(8), 451–454. doi:10.3928/01484834-20150717-05

Centre for Policy on Aging. (2014). *The effectiveness of care pathways in health and social care.* Retrieved from www.ageuk.org.uk/.../CPA-Effectiveness_of_care_pathways.pdf

Cherry, K. (2015). *Hierarchy of needs: The five levels of Maslow's hierarchy of needs.* Retrieved from http://psychology.about.com/od/theoriesofpersonality/a/hierarchyneeds.htm

College of Nurses of Ontario. (2014). *Developing SMART learning goals.* Retrieved from http://www.cno.org/Global/docs/qa/DevelopingSMARTGoals.pdf

Cox, K. J. (2014). Counseling women with a previous cesarean birth: Toward a shared decision-making partnership. *Journal of Midwifery & Women's Health, 59*(3), 237–245. doi:10.1111/jmwh.12177

D'Amour, D., Dubois, C. A., Tchouaket, E., Clarke, S., & Blais, R. (2014). The occurrence of adverse events potentially attributable to nursing care in medical units: Cross sectional record review. *International Journal of Nursing Studies, 51*(6), 882–891. doi:10.1016/j.ijnurstu.2013.10.017

Decision Making Confidence. (2013). *Definitions: Definition of decision making.* Retrieved from http://www.decision-making-confidence.com/decision-strategies.html

Decker, S., Fey, M., Sideras, S., Caballero, S., Rockstraw, L., Boese, T., . . . Borum, J. C. (2013). Standards of best practice: Simulation standard VI: The debriefing process. *Clinical Simulation in Nursing, 9*(6), S26–S29.

DeMeester, R. H., Lopez, F. Y., Moore, J. E., Cook, S. C., & Chin, M. H. (2016). A model of organizational context and shared decision making: Application to LGBT racial and ethnic minority patients. *Journal of General Internal Medicine, 31*(6), 651–662. doi:10.1007/s11606-016-3608-3

Elder, L., & Paul, R. (2013). Becoming a critic of your thinking, *Critical Thinking Community, Foundation of Critical Thinking.* Retrieved from http://www.criticalthinking.org/pages/becoming-a-crit-of-your-thinking/478

Ekstrom, L., & Idvall, E. (2015). Being a team leader: Newly registered nurses relate their experiences. *Journal of Nursing Management, 23*(1), 75–86. doi:10.1111/jonm.12085

Froedge, Wendy L. (2013). *How to make the most of your nursing minutes.* Retrieved from http://www.americannursetoday.com/how-to-make-the-most-of-your-nursing-minutes/

Gerdeman, J. L., Lux, K., & Jacko, J. (2013). Using concept mapping to build clinical judgment skills. *Nurse Education in Practice, 13*(1), 11–17.

Giger, J. N. (2013). *Transcultural nursing: Assessment and intervention* (6th ed.). St. Louis, MO: Elsevier.

Gordon, M. (2010). *Manual of nursing diagnoses* (12th ed.). Boston, MA: Jones & Bartlett.

Green, C. (2012). Nursing intuition: A valid form of knowledge. *Nursing Philosophy, 13*(2), 98–111. doi:10.1111/j.1466-769X.2011.00507.x

Harvey, V. L., & Housel, T. H. (2014). *Healthcare disparities and the LGBT population.* Plymouth, UK: Lexington Books.

Herdman, T. H. & Kamitsuru, S. (Eds). *Nursing Diagnoses—Definitions and Classification 2015–2017.* Copyright © 2014, 1994–2014 NANDA International. Used by arrangement with John Wiley & Sons, Inc. Companion website: www.wiley.com/go/nursingdiagnoses.

Hersh, S., Megregian, M., & Emeis, C. (2014). Intermittent auscultation of the fetal heart rate during labor: An opportunity for shared decision making. *Journal of Midwifery & Women's Health, 59*(3), 344–349. doi:10.1111/jmwh.12178

Institute of Medicine. (2011, January 26). *The future of nursing: Focus on education.* Retrieved from http://www.iom.edu/Reports/2010/The-Future-of-Nursing-Leading-Change-Advancing-Health/Report-Brief-Education.aspx

Koharchik, L., Caputi, L., Robb, M., & Culleiton, A. L. (2015). Fostering clinical reasoning in nursing students. *American Journal of Nursing, 115*(1), 58–61. doi:10.1097/01.NAJ.0000459638.68657.9b

Lachman, V. (2012). Applying the ethics of care to your nursing practice. *MedSurg Nursing, 21*(2), 113–115.

LAWriter. (2014). *Ohio Administrative Code 4723-4-07: Standards for applying the nursing process as a registered nurse.* Retrieved from http://codes.ohio.gov/oac/4723-4-07v1

Lors, M., Cooks, N., & Tluczek, A. (2016). A proposed model of person-, family-, and culture-centered nursing care. *Nursing Outlook.* Retrieved from http://www.nursingoutlook.org/article/S0029-6554(16)30001-X/pdf

Makic, M. B. F., Martin, S. A., Burns, S., Philbrick, D., & Rauen, C. (2013). Putting evidence into nursing practice: Four traditional practices not supported by the evidence. *Critical Care Nurse, 33*(2), 28–43.

Melnyk, B. M., Gallagher-Ford, L., Long, L. E., & Fineout-Overholt, E. (2014). The establishment of evidence-based practice competencies for practicing registered nurses and advanced practice nurses in real-world clinical settings: Proficiencies to improve healthcare quality, reliability, patient outcomes, and costs. *Worldviews Evidence-Based Nursing, 11*(1), 5–15. doi:10.1111/wvn.12021

Michaud, P. A., Blum, R. W., Benaroyo, L., Zermatten, J., & Baltag, V. (2015). Assessing an adolescent's capacity for autonomous decision-making in clinical care. *Journal of Adolescent Health, 57*(4), 361–366. doi:10.1016/j.jadohealth.2015.06.012

NANDA-I. (2013). *Glossary of terms: Nursing diagnoses.* Retrieved from http://www.nanda.org/DiagnosisDevelopment/DiagnosisSubmission/PreparingYourSubmission/GlossaryofTerms.aspx

NANDA-I. (2016). *NANDA-I nursing diagnosis resources.* Retrieved from http://kb.nanda.org/article/AA-00266/38/English-/Frequently-Asked-Questions/Nursing-Diagnosis/Nursing-Diagnosis-vs.-Medical-Diagnosis/What-is-the-difference-between-a-medical-diagnosis-and-a-nursing-diagnosis-.html

National Council of State Boards of Nursing (NCSBN). (2016). *Nurse practice act, rules & regulations.* Retrieved from https://www.ncsbn.org/nurse-practice-act.htm

National League for Nursing. (2016). *NLN competencies for graduates of nursing programs.* Retrieved from http://www.nln.org/professional-development-programs/competencies-for-nursing-education/nln-competencies-for-graduates-of-nursing-programs

Papastavrou, E., Andreou, P., Tsangari, H., & Merkouris, A. (2014). Linking patient satisfaction with nursing care: The case of care rationing—a correlational study. *BioMed Central Nursing, 13*, 26. doi:10.1186/1472-6955-13-26

Pearson, H. (2013). Science and intuition: Do both have a place in clinical decision making? *British Journal of Nursing, 22*(4), 212–215. doi:10.12968/bjon.2013.22.4.212

Peek, M. E., Lopez, F. Y., Williams, S., Xu, L. J., McNulty, M. C., Acree, M. E., & Schneider, J. A. (2016). Development of a conceptual framework for understanding shared decision making among African-American LGBT patients and their clinicians. *Journal of General Internal Medicine, 31*(6), 677–687. doi:10.1007/s11606-016-3616-3

Polit, D. F., & Beck, C. T. (2017). *Nursing research: Generating and assessing evidence for nursing practice* (10th ed.). Philadelphia, PA: Wolters Kluwer.

Roy, C. (2008). *The Roy adaptation model* (3rd ed.). Upper Saddle River, NJ: Prentice Hall.

Steelman, V. M., Graling, P. R., & Perkhounkova, Y. (2013). Priority patient safety issues identified by perioperative nurses. *Association of periOperative Registered Nurses Journal, 97*(4), 402–418. doi:10.1016/j.aorn.2012.06.016

Stevens, K. (2013). The impact of evidence-based practice in nursing and the next big ideas. *OJIN: The Online Journal of Issues in Nursing, 18*(2), Manuscript 4.

Tanner, C. (2006). Thinking like a nurse: A research-based model of clinical judgment in nursing. *Journal of Nursing Education, 45*(6), 204–210. Retrieved from http://www.mccc.edu/nursing/documents/Thinking_Like_A_Nurse_Tanner.pdf

Tennessee Board of Nursing. (2015). *Rules of the Tennessee board of nursing.* Retrieved from http://share.tn.gov/sos/rules/1000/1000.htm

Texas Board of Nursing. (n.d.). *Six-step decision-making model for determining nursing scope of practice.* Retrieved from https://www.bon.texas.gov/pdfs/publication_pdfs/dectree.pdf

Thim, T., Krarup, N. H., Grove, E. L., Rohde, C. V., & Lofgren, B. (2012). Initial assessment and treatment with the airway, breathing, circulation, disability, exposure (ABCDE) approach. *International Journal of General Medicine, 5*, 117–121. doi:10.2147/IJGM.S28478

Thompson, C., Aitken, L., Doran, D., & Dowding, D. (2013). An agenda for clinical decision making and judgment in nursing research and education. *International Journal of Nursing Studies, 50*(12), 1720–1726. doi:10.1016/j.ijnurstu.2013.05.003

Tunlind, A., Granstrom, J., & Engstrom, A. (2015). Nursing care in a high-technological environment: Experiences of critical care nurses. *Intensive and Critical Care Nursing, 31*(2), 116–123. doi:10.1016/j.iccn.2014.07.005

University of Iowa, College of Nursing. (2013). *Overview: Nursing Outcomes Classification (NOC).* Retrieved from http://www.nursing.uiowa.edu/cncce/nursing-outcomes-classification-overview

U.S. Department of Health and Human Services, Administration for Community Living. (n.d.). *Administration on ageing.* Retrieved from http://www.aoa.acl.gov/AoA_Programs/Tools_Resources/diversity.aspx

Veerapen, K., & Purkis, M. E. (2014). Implications of early workplace experiences on continuing interprofessional education for physicians and nurses. *Journal of Interprofessional Care, 28*(3), 218–225. doi:10.3109/13561820.2014.884552

Yoon, J., Kim, M., & Shin, J. (2016). Confidence in delegation and leadership of registered nurses in long-term-care hospitals. *Journal of Nursing Management, 24*(5), 676–685. doi:10.1111/jonm.12372

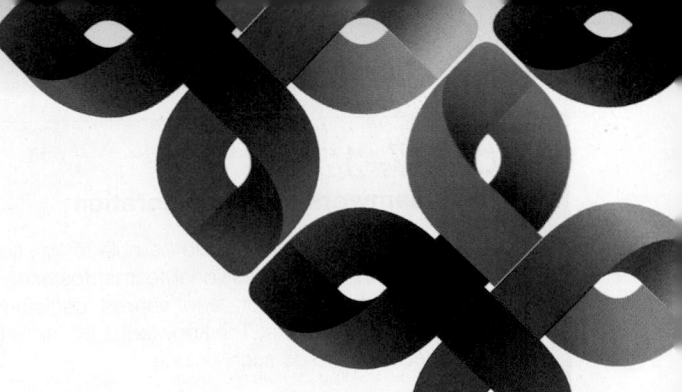

Module 37
Collaboration

Module Outline and Learning Outcomes

The Concept of Collaboration

The Nurse as Collaborator

37.1 Describe the nurse's role as a collaborative member of the healthcare team.

Concepts Related to Collaboration

37.2 Describe the relationship between collaboration and selected other concepts and implications for nursing care.

Competencies Basic to Collaboration

37.3 Identify competencies necessary for successful collaboration.

Interprofessional Collaborative Practice

37.4 Summarize the benefits and nature of interprofessional collaborative practice.

Conflict Prevention and Management

37.5 Analyze aspects of conflict prevention and management.

Incivility in the Workplace

37.6 Describe the effects of incivility in the workplace.

≫ The Concept of Collaboration

Concept Key Terms

The nature of healthcare today is so complex that it is impossible for any single provider or professional to provide high-quality patient care without working with others. The best care is delivered in a collaborative environment with all members of the healthcare team working to improve patient health outcomes. **Collaboration** is defined as two or more individuals working toward a common goal by combining their skills, knowledge, and resources while avoiding duplication of effort. In a healthcare environment, the common goal of each collaborative team is to improve patient outcomes, whether the patient is an individual, a group, or a community.

The American Nurses Association (ANA) Standards of Professional Nursing Practice recognize collaboration as a key component of nursing practice. Standard 10 of the ANA Standards of Professional Nursing Practice outlines specific competencies related to the nurse's role in collaboration (ANA, 2015) (**Box 37–1 ≫**). Cronenwett and coworkers (2007), as part of the QSEN (Quality and Safety Education for Nurses) project, identified six competencies necessary to improve the quality and safety of the patient care environment. Teamwork

and collaboration were identified as two of the major competencies necessary for achieving quality patient care. Virginia Henderson (1991), one of the pioneers of professional nursing, defined collaborative care as "a partnership relationship between doctors, nurses, and other healthcare providers with patients and their families" (p. 44). Mutual respect and a true sharing of both power and control are essential elements. Ideally, collaboration becomes a dynamic, interactive process in which patients (individuals, groups, or communities) work together with physicians, nurses, and other healthcare providers to meet their health objectives.

There has been an increased emphasis in the nursing community on the value of interprofessional collaboration and practice as a means to improve patient outcomes (National League for Nursing [NLN], 2015). The term **interprofessional** usually refers to professionals from various disciplines, whereas the term **interdisciplinary** is often used to denote that paraprofessionals or others (such as patients or family members) are also included. For the purposes of this module, we use the term *interprofessional* to refer to professionals from various disciplines along with support

Box 37–1
QSEN: Teamwork and Collaboration

According to QSEN, nurses should be able to function effectively within nursing and interprofessional teams, fostering open communication, mutual respect, and shared decision making to achieve quality patient care. The knowledge (K), skills (S), and attitudes (A) necessary to do such include:

- **(K)** Describe one's personal strengths, limitations, and values in functioning as a member of a team. **(S)** Demonstrate an awareness of personal strengths and limitations; initiate a plan for self-development as a team member and, act with integrity, consistency and respect for differing views. **(A)** Acknowledge your potential to be a contributing team member while appreciating the importance of collaboration.
- **(K)** Describe the scope of practice and roles of other health team members, the strategies for identifying and managing overlaps in team member roles, and recognize the contributions of other team members in helping patients and families to achieve goals. This can be achieved by **(S)** functioning within your scope of practice, assuming the role of team member or leader as appropriate, requesting help when needed, clarifying roles, and integrating the contributions of others in a **(A)** respectful manner.
- **(K)** Analyze differences in communication style and understand the impact of your own communication style on others by **(S)** communicating with and soliciting input from team members, and initiating actions to resolve conflict by **(A)** actively participating in the resolution process.
- **(K)** Describe the impact of team functioning on patient safety and quality care and explain how levels of authority have the potential to affect teamwork. **(S)** Follow best practice to minimize risks associated with handoffs and **(A)** acknowledge that care transition is risky.
- **(K)** Identify system barriers and facilitators of effective team functioning and examine strategies for improving systems to support team performance by **(S)** participating in designing systems that support teamwork and **(A)** valuing the influence of system solutions in achieving effective team functioning.

Source: Based on Cronenwett, L., Sherwood, G., Barnsteiner, J., Disch, J., Johnson, J., Mitchell, P., & Warren, J. (2007). Quality and safety education for nurses. *Nursing Outlook, 55*(3), 122–131.

staff, the patient, and family members—anyone who is working together for the benefit of the patient.

Successful collaboration requires that nurses develop skills in communication and teamwork, value the roles and responsibilities of other team members, and work to establish a climate of mutual respect. Successful interprofessional education and practice depends on healthcare professionals working in teams so as to provide safe, quality care (NLN, 2016).

The Nurse as Collaborator

Collaboration may occur between nurses, between healthcare providers and patients, and between healthcare providers from different professional backgrounds (**Figure 37–1 》**). According to the ANA (2015), collaborative interprofessional teams recognize each individual profession's value

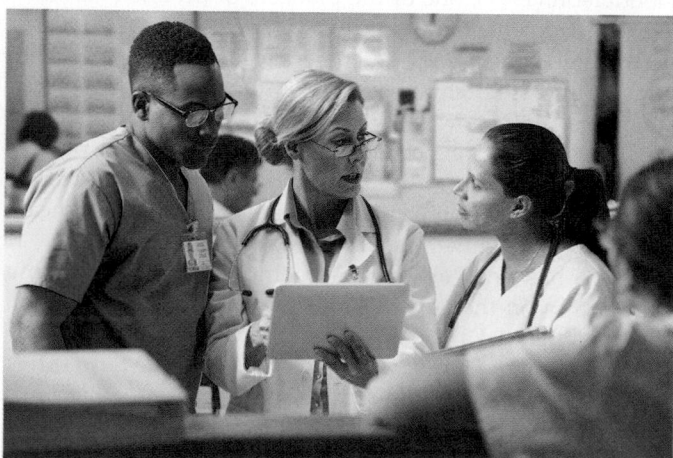

Source: Jose Luis Pelaez Inc./Blend Images/Getty Images.

Figure 37–1 》 The healthcare team works together to communicate concerns and mutually problem solve.

and contributions in an atmosphere of mutual trust and respect through open discussion and shared decision making (p. 8). In addition to collaborating with other professionals to provide individual patient care, nurses may also be involved in collaborating to develop community initiatives, write or revise legislation, or conduct health-related research. **Table 37–1 》** lists a number of professionals who may serve as members of an interprofessional healthcare team and their respective roles.

To fulfill a collaborative role, nurses need to assume accountability and increased authority in their practice areas. Continuing education in role exploration, communication, group work, and other areas helps members of the healthcare team understand the collaborative nature of their roles, specific contributions of each professional member, and the importance of working together. Each professional needs to understand how an integrated delivery system centers on the patient's healthcare needs rather than on the particular care given by any one group. **Box 37–2 》** describes selected aspects of the nurse's role as a collaborator.

Concepts Related to Collaboration

Effective collaboration affects healthcare positively on every level. At the organizational level, collaboration leads to increased efficiency and greater cost effectiveness. For patients, collaboration among members of the healthcare team promotes safety, resulting in decreased morbidity and mortality rates. Patients who are involved in the collaborative process report an increased sense of autonomy, which leads to greater overall satisfaction with care. Nurses who effectively collaborate report an increased sense of perceived autonomy and professionalism, along with greater job satisfaction. Some, but not all, of the concepts that are integral to collaboration are shown in the Concepts Related to Collaboration feature. They are presented in alphabetical order.

TABLE 37–1 Collaborative Members of the Healthcare Team

Healthcare Professional	Role
Nurse	The role of the nurse varies with the needs of the patient, the nurse's credentials, and the type of employment setting. A registered nurse (RN) assesses a patient's health status, identifies health problems, and develops and coordinates care. A licensed vocational nurse (LVN), in some states known as a licensed practical nurse (LPN), provides direct patient care under the direction of a registered nurse, physician, or other licensed practitioner. A Nurse Practitioner (NP) has a graduate degree and is qualified to treat certain medical conditions.
Unlicensed assistive personnel	Unlicensed assistive personnel (UAP) are healthcare staff who assume delegated aspects of basic patient care. These tasks include bathing, assisting with feeding, and collecting specimens. UAP titles include certified nurse assistants, hospital attendants, nurse technicians, patient care technicians, and orderlies. Some of these categories of provider may have standardized education and job duties (e.g., certified nurse assistants), while others do not. The parameters regarding nurse delegation to UAP are delineated by the state Boards of Nursing and statutes contained in state administrative codes.
Complementary healthcare providers	Non-mainstream practice used along with conventional medicine is considered as complementary. Examples of complementary practice groups include: chiropractors, herbalists, acupuncturists, massage therapists, reflexologists, holistic health healers, and other healthcare providers. These professionals, when used in conjunction with providers of allopathic or Western medicine, are considered to be complementary providers.
Case manager	The case manager's role is to ensure that patients receive fiscally sound, appropriate care in the best setting. This role is often filled by the member of the healthcare team who is most involved in the patient's care. Depending on the nature of the patient's concerns, the case manager may be a nurse, a social worker, or any other member of the healthcare team.
Dentist	Dentists diagnose and treat dental problems. Dentists are also actively involved in preventive measures to maintain healthy oral structures (e.g., teeth and gums). Many hospitals, especially long-term care facilities, have dentists on staff.
Dietitian or nutritionist	A dietitian, often a registered dietitian (RD), has special knowledge about the diets required to maintain health and to treat disease. Dietitians in hospitals generally are concerned with therapeutic diets, may design special diets to meet the nutritional needs of individual patients, and supervise the preparation of meals to ensure that patients receive the proper diet.
	A nutritionist is an individual who has special knowledge about nutrition and food. The nutritionist in a community setting recommends healthy diets and gives broad advisory services about the purchase and preparation of foods. Community nutritionists often function at the primary preventive level. They promote health and prevent disease, for example, by advising families about balanced diets for growing children and pregnant women.
Information technology expert	In healthcare organizations, an information technology (IT) expert offers knowledge and expertise in the ever-expanding field of computer science in application to health and health systems. The IT expert's knowledge base includes installing and repairing computer hardware, maintaining databases, and educating users about the use of computer applications, such as electronic health records (EHRs), and communication processes such as telemedicine.
Occupational therapist	An occupational therapist (OT) assists patients with impaired function to gain the skills to perform activities of daily living. For example, an occupational therapist might teach a man with severe arthritis in his arms and hands how to adjust his kitchen utensils so that he can continue to cook. The occupational therapist teaches skills that are therapeutic and at the same time provide some fulfillment. For example, weaving is a recreational activity but also exercises the arthritic man's arms and hands. Occupational therapists also perform developmental assessments and provide therapy for patients of all ages during recovery from or adaptation to a variety of alterations, including traumatic injuries, medical conditions that affect cognition, congenital disorders, and alterations related to prematurity.
Paramedical technologist	Laboratory technologists, radiologic technologists, and nuclear medicine technologists are just three kinds of paramedical technologists in the expanding field of medical technology. *Paramedical* means having some connection with medicine. Laboratory technologists, for example, examine specimens such as urine, feces, blood, and discharges from wounds to provide exact information that facilitates the medical diagnosis and the prescription of a therapeutic regimen.
Pharmacist	A pharmacist prepares and dispenses medications in hospital and community settings. The role of the pharmacist in monitoring and evaluating the actions and effects of medications on patients is becoming increasingly prominent. A clinical pharmacist is a specialist who guides physicians in prescribing medications.
Physical therapist	The licensed physical therapist (PT) assists patients with musculoskeletal problems. Physical therapists treat movement dysfunctions by means of heat, water, exercise, massage, and electric current. The physical therapist's functions include assessing patient mobility and strength, providing therapeutic measures (e.g., exercises and heat applications to improve mobility and strength), and teaching new skills (e.g., how to walk with an artificial leg). Physical therapists work in hospitals, offices, and in patients' homes.
Physician	The physician is responsible for medical diagnosis and for determining the therapy required by an individual who has a disease or injury. The physician's role has traditionally been the treatment of disease and trauma (injury); however, many physicians are now including health promotion and disease prevention in their practice. Some physicians are general practitioners (also known as primary care or family practitioners); others are specialists, such as dermatologists, neurologists, oncologists, orthopedists, pediatricians, psychiatrists, radiologists, or surgeons—to name a few.
Physician assistant	Physician assistants (PAs) perform certain tasks under the direction of a physician. They diagnose and treat certain diseases, conditions, and injuries. In many states, nurses are not legally permitted to follow a PA's orders unless the orders are cosigned by a physician.
Respiratory therapist	A respiratory therapist is skilled in therapeutic measures used in the care of patients with respiratory problems. These therapists are knowledgeable about oxygen therapy devices, intermittent positive pressure breathing respirators, artificial mechanical ventilators, and accessory devices used in inhalation therapy. Respiratory therapists administer many of the pulmonary function tests.
Social worker	A social worker counsels patients and their support people regarding problems, such as finances, marital difficulties, and adoption of children. It is not unusual for health problems to produce problems in day-to-day living and vice versa. For example, an older woman who lives alone and has a stroke resulting in impaired walking may find it impossible to continue to live in her third-floor apartment. Finding a more suitable living arrangement can be the responsibility of the social worker if the patient has no support network in place.

Box 37–2
The Nurse as a Collaborator

With Patients

- Acknowledges, supports, and encourages patients' active involvement in healthcare decisions.
- Encourages patient autonomy and equal position with other members of the healthcare team.
- Helps patients set mutually agreed-on goals and objectives for healthcare.
- Provides patients with consultation in a collaborative fashion.

With Peers

- Shares personal expertise with other nurses and elicits the expertise of others to ensure high-quality patient care.
- Develops a sense of trust and mutual respect with peers who value each member's unique contributions.

With Other Healthcare Professionals

- Recognizes the contribution that each member of the interprofessional team can make by virtue of his or her expertise.
- Listens to each individual's viewpoints.

- Shares healthcare responsibilities with other members of the team in order to explore care options, set realistic and attainable goals, and make decisions about the plan of care with patients and their families.
- Participates in collaborative interprofessional research to increase knowledge of a clinical problem or situation.

With Professional Nursing Organizations

- Seeks opportunities to collaborate with and within professional organizations.
- Serves on committees in state (or provincial), national, and international nursing organizations or specialty groups.
- Supports professional organizations in political action to create solutions for professional and healthcare concerns.

With Legislators

- Offers expert opinions on legislative initiatives related to healthcare.
- Collaborates with other healthcare providers and consumers on healthcare legislation in order to best serve the needs of the public.

Competencies Basic to Collaboration

Key features necessary for collaboration include mutual respect, trust, effective communication skills, giving and receiving feedback, decision making, and conflict management (Masters, 2013).

Communication Skills

Collaborating to solve complex problems requires effective communication skills. This is supported by the fact that miscommunication among providers has been identified as one of the most frequent root causes of sentinel events (unintended events that cause serious physical or psychologic injury or death) (The Joint Commission, 2012). The typical

Concepts Related to
Collaboration

CONCEPT	RELATIONSHIP TO COLLABORATION	NURSING IMPLICATIONS
Health Policy	↑ job satisfaction	▪ Acknowledgment by senior leader to support new approaches in workforce development and innovations that improve job working environments and increase job satisfaction.
Healthcare Systems	↑ collaboration among healthcare team members → ↓ duplication of patient services and ↓ healthcare costs	▪ Support and promote collaboration among healthcare team members. ▪ Apply principles of effective collaboration, including principles that facilitate clear communication. ▪ Be aware of the patient's plan of care, including ordered tests and diagnostics, and question apparent duplications using a polite, professional approach.
Professionalism	↑ nurse–physician collaboration → ↑ perceived professional autonomy → ↑ nursing professionalism	▪ Recognize the impact of collaboration on job satisfaction in nursing. ▪ Effectively apply principles of collaboration to promote collaborative nurse–physician relationships.
Quality Improvement	↑ situational awareness ↑ teamwork among healthcare team members	▪ Effectively identify threats to patient safety through open communication, identification of purpose and skill, and established plan of action.
Safety	↑ collaboration among healthcare team members → ↓ patient morbidity and ↓ patient mortality rates	▪ Support and promote collaboration among healthcare team members. ▪ Support the scheduling of interprofessional team meetings and attend all scheduled meetings. ▪ Educate healthcare team members about the safety-related benefits of collaboration.

patient environment is fraught with interruptions, distractions, conflicting goals, anxieties, and stressors that often hamper the best intentions. Even the most well-intended fundamental statement can be misinterpreted or misunderstood and compound the problem (Ruben, 2016).

True collaboration requires skilled communication and mutual respect in order to achieve desired patient outcomes. Expert collaborators hold themselves and each other accountable for serving as patient advocates, acting as skilled negotiators, and acting to resolve conflict. Instead of focusing on distinctions among members, each team must keep firmly in mind its common purpose, that of meeting the needs of the patient.

Each member of the healthcare team should be sensitive to differences among communication styles and the effects that her own style has on successful collaboration (see the module on Communication for information about communication styles). Team-centered communication, as opposed to status-based communication, demonstrates appreciation for member contributions. Team-centered approaches focus on the "we" — the work "we will do for this patient" — versus one-sided commands such as "give this, do that" statements that do not invite dialogue and do not promote collaboration. Effective communication can occur only if every team member is committed to understanding each member's professional role and appreciating each member as an individual. Team-centered communication focuses on shared responsibilities (Matzke et al., 2014). Identifying and preventing any potential cultural or language barriers also is critical to ensuring successful collaboration (see Focus on Diversity and Culture).

For all patients, communication is a key component (or competency) of effective nursing care and a means for promoting nurse–patient collaboration. Miscommunication among healthcare providers can lead to serious consequences. A lack of collaboration skills can impede safe practice. Acknowledging alternative perspectives, articulating one's own viewpoint, and engaging in mutual give and take are necessary qualities for effective collaboration. Using an attentive style of communication that encompasses active listening versus a dominant, take-charge, or contentious and argumentative style helps to remove the barriers that impede effective communication and collaboration.

Mutual Respect and Trust

Mutual respect occurs when two or more individuals show or feel honor or esteem toward one another. Trust occurs when an individual is confident in the actions of another individual. Both mutual respect and trust imply a shared process and outcome. They must be expressed both verbally and nonverbally. Sometimes professionals may *verbalize* respect or trust of others but *demonstrate* a lack of trust and respect through their actions. The healthcare system itself has not always created an environment that promotes respect or trust of the various healthcare providers. Although progress has been made toward creating more trusting relationships, past attitudes may continue to impede efforts toward collaborative practice (see the Evidence-Based Practice feature). Magnet hospitals are an example of successful efforts by healthcare organizations to foster respect among professionals. Placing the head of the nursing department (previously known as the director of nursing) on an equal managerial level with the chief of physicians (usually called the chief medical officer) has been found to improve mutual respect between physicians and nurses, thereby improving their relationships.

Decision Making

Collaboration involves shared responsibility for the outcome. To create a solution, the team must follow each step of the decision-making process, beginning with a clear definition of the problem (see the module on Clinical Decision Making). Team decision making must be directed at the objectives of the specific effort. Demonstration of mutual respect and timely, effective feedback facilitate the decision-making process.

Sound decision making regarding patient care requires that the healthcare team focus on the patient's priority needs and organize interventions accordingly. The discipline best able to address the patient's needs is identified, given priority in planning, and held responsible for providing its interventions in a timely manner. For example, when social needs (such as loss of a home or job) interfere with the patient's ability to respond to therapy, the team may agree that the social worker needs to intervene to help the patient resolve his social needs before starting therapy. Nurses, by the nature of their holistic practice, are often able to help the team identify priorities and areas requiring further attention. Ideally, the collaborative team will ensure that the patient is part of the decision-making process, even if the patient is not able to be present. Decision-making processes are discussed in greater detail in the module on Clinical Decision Making.

Focus on Diversity and Culture
Collaboration and the Dangers of Language

Ineffective management of cultural language barriers can impede collaboration and negatively impact medical and nursing diagnoses, as well as patient outcomes (Garcia & Duckett, 2009). Nurses should use evidence-based practice interventions that have been shown to be the most effective for culturally diverse populations. Universal guidelines for implementing culturally competent care require that nurses have an awareness of the patient's values, learning preferences, and behavior and work to include culturally appropriate verbal and nonverbal communication skills when working with patients. Nonverbal communication skills include an understanding of the patient's perceptions of space, silence, touch, modesty, and preference for provider gender. Acting as a true advocate, the nurse must do everything possible to ensure competent, quality care, including the use of an interpreter and selective print media appropriate for the patient's cultural values and age (Douglas et al., 2014). In addition, providing culturally competent care is a priority of The Joint Commission (2016), which recommends that hospitals provide staff training on the cultural health beliefs and practices and, in doing so, support systems that allow for effective communication and cultural competence.

See the module on Culture and Diversity for more information on providing culturally competent care.

Evidence-Based Practice
Overcoming Barriers: The Benefits of Nurse–Physician Collaboration

Problem

Despite research-based evidence that supports the benefits of effective collaboration between nurses and physicians, barriers to this process—several of which relate to the relationship between the nurse and the physician—remain intact.

Evidence

A review of the literature from 2009 to 2015 indicates that barriers in nurse–physician communication discourage collaboration (Fewster-Thuente, 2015). Reported obstructive behaviors are hierarchical and/or patriarchal nurse–physician relationships and misperceptions about how collaboration should occur. A culture of safety for patients depends on collaborative communication. Although nursing education programs have promoted a shift in the nurse's perception of the nurse–physician relationship from subservient–superior to collegial, some physicians at present view this collegial relationship as undermining their leadership and authority (Schneider, 2012).

Despite the barriers to nurse–physician collaboration, research strongly supports this practice. Interprofessional collaboration between physicians and nurses is linked to decreased patient morbidity and mortality (Schneider, 2012). Along with enhancing overall patient safety, benefits of effective collaboration between physicians and nurses also include a decreased risk for medication-related errors and improved cost containment (Nair et al., 2012).

Implications

Overcoming the barriers to effective collaboration is imperative. Some suggestions for promoting change are employing interprofessional rounding on patients during which each health team member has an opportunity to share pertinent information and suggestions for patient care; interprofessional simulations, and inter- and intraprofessional coursework. For the benefit of the patient, the healthcare system, and the professionals caring for the patient, nurses should support and promote the development of collaborative relationships with physicians, as well as with all other members of the healthcare team.

Critical Thinking Application

Development of a collaborative relationship requires mutual trust and respect, demonstrated efficacy with conflict resolution, clear methods of communication, and professionalism during all negotiation processes (Schneider, 2012). The common goal of providing the best care possible for the patient should be the starting point of all discussions and remain as the focal point throughout patient care. The expertise of each collaborator needs to be shared and appreciated; the physician or advanced practice nurse for the diagnostic information, the nurse for the patient- and family-specific knowledge, and the allied health team members (e.g., PT, OT, social work) for their skill and capability in condition-specific treatment and follow-up (Fewster-Thuente, 2015).

Clinical Example A

Bill Hainsley, 67 years old, will be transferring from the acute care hospital to a nearby rehabilitation facility following his knee replacement. Although Mr. Hainsley believes that he is perfectly capable of managing his rehabilitation at home, his wife is concerned about her ability to help him navigate their two-story house, which has only a small half-bath on the first floor. Mr. Hainsley is worried about the cost of going to a rehabilitation facility and is not sure how much, if any, of this will be covered by his insurance because he is retired. The RN case manager has decided to schedule a meeting with the Hainsleys that also includes the physical therapist and social worker. The nurse would like for the physical therapist to provide Mr. Hainsley and his wife with a description of the anticipated exercise protocol as well as some idea of the expected time frame for physical improvement and safe return to home. The nurse has included the social worker for help in addressing Mr. Hainsley's concern about what his insurance might cover, what Medicare will cover, and any anticipated out-of-pocket costs. The nurse acts as a facilitator in ensuring that all of Mr. and Mrs. Hainsley's fears are addressed before they make a decision about discharge. In addition, the nurse documents in the chart that the meeting occurred, who was involved, and the final decision by the patient about his discharge.

Critical Thinking Questions

1. Is there anyone else that the RN case manager should have included in this collaborative meeting with the patient and, if so, who and for what reason?
2. What other approach might the nurse case manager have used if the physical therapist and social worker were not available?
3. What approach can be used if Mr. Hainsley chooses to go home rather than to a rehabilitation facility?

Interprofessional Collaborative Practice

Many healthcare professionals believe that an interprofessional, collaborative framework can manage costs, enhance quality, and increase patient satisfaction with care. Interprofessional collaborative practice models attempt to achieve the following objectives:

- Provide patient-directed and patient-centered care using an interprofessional, integrated, participative framework.
- Enhance continuity of care across the continuum of health, from wellness and prevention through acute illness to recovery or rehabilitation.
- Improve patient and family satisfaction with care.
- Provide high-quality, cost-effective, evidence-based care that improves patient outcomes.
- Promote mutual respect, communication, and understanding between the patient and members of the healthcare team.
- Provide opportunities to address and resolve system-related issues and problems.
- Develop interdependent relationships and understanding among providers and patients.

Benefits of Interprofessional Collaboration

According to the World Health Organization (WHO), collaborative practice involves healthcare providers from a variety of disciplines working in tandem with patients, families, caregivers, and communities to provide the best possible quality of care. Collaboration has system-wide effects. WHO has linked interprofessional collaboration with a number of improved patient outcomes ranging from infectious disease to chronic disease as well as patient safety indicators such as complications, error rates, patient length of stay, and mortality (WHO, 2010).

A collaborative approach to healthcare ideally benefits patients, professionals, and the healthcare delivery system. Because care becomes patient centered and, most important, patient directed, patients are empowered as informed consumers and actively collaborate with the healthcare team in the decision-making process. When patients are empowered to participate actively and professionals share mutually set goals with patients, quality of care improves and everyone—including the organization and healthcare system—ultimately benefits. When quality improves, adherence to therapeutic regimens increases, lengths of stay decrease, and overall costs to the system decline. Sound application of collaborative strategies leads to decreased patient morbidity and mortality rates (Schneider, 2012). When professional interdependence develops among healthcare providers, collegial relationships emerge and overall job satisfaction increases.

The Process of Interprofessional Collaboration

A continuum of collaboration, as illustrated in **Figure 37–2 》**, reflects the following levels of communication and action, beginning with parallel communication and progressing toward co-management and referral:

- *Parallel communication* occurs when each professional communicates with the patient independently and asks the same or similar questions.

- *Parallel functioning* occurs when communication may be more coordinated, but each professional has separate interventions and a separate plan of care.

- *Information exchange* involves planned communication, but decision making is unilateral, involving little, if any, collegiality.

- *Coordination* and *consultation* represent midrange levels of collaboration seeking to maximize the efficiency of resources.

- *Co-management* and *referral* represent the upper levels of collaboration, where providers retain responsibility and accountability for their own aspects of care and patients are directed to other providers when the problem is beyond the initial provider's expertise.

Characteristics of effective interprofessional collaboration include the following:

1. Common purpose and goals identified at the outset
2. Clinical competence of each provider
3. Interpersonal competence
4. Humor
5. Trust
6. Valuing and respecting diverse, complementary knowledge.

Processes associated with these characteristics include recurring interactions that develop connections and, therefore, mutual respect and trust among the healthcare professionals. Interpersonal skills and respect for the competence of all collaborators are essential to achieving greater health outcomes for patients.

Interprofessional collaboration has positive psychosocial and professional effects as well. Both patients and nurses perceive a greater sense of autonomy when collaborative strategies are applied (Schneider, 2012). Within the context of workplace roles, autonomy refers to the ability of a professional to employ appropriate interventions as they relate to the quality and safety of patient care (Bularzik et al., 2013). For nurses, practicing autonomously means being authorized to provide nursing care that falls within the professional scope of practice as defined by existing regulatory boards, professional organizations, and institutional rules (Weston, 2008, 2010) while grounded in informedness, voluntariness, consent, and rationality (ANA, 2015). The ability to fully enact one's professional role contributes to career satisfaction, career retention, decreased absenteeism, and decreased turnover (Bularzik et al., 2013).

Interprofessional Settings

Interprofessional teams and collaborations can occur in any setting in which healthcare is provided, not just within a hospital. Examples of interprofessional settings outside the hospital environment include:

- *Skilled nursing, rehabilitation, and long-term care facilities:* Patients admitted to these facilities often require care from multiple disciplines, including nursing; medical (physician, nurse practitioner, specialist); physical, occupational, speech/language, or respiratory therapy; social services; and mental health or psychiatric services.

- *Schools and educational settings:* Children with special needs, children who are medically fragile, and children with acute or chronic conditions may require long- or short-term interprofessional care from nurses, teachers, school administrators or counselors, mental health specialists,

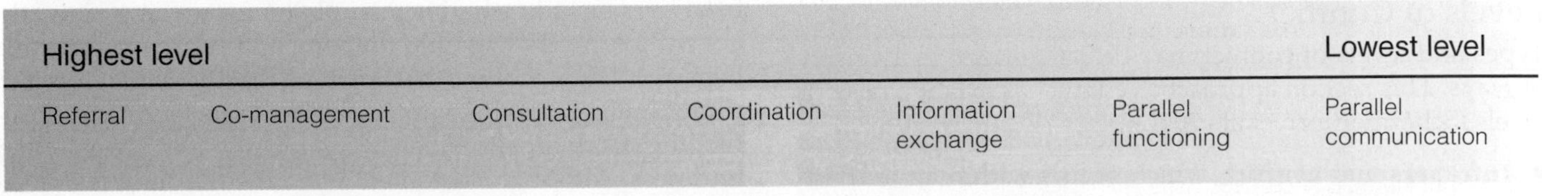

Highest level						Lowest level
Referral	Co-management	Consultation	Coordination	Information exchange	Parallel functioning	Parallel communication

Figure 37–2 》 Continuum of collaboration.

physical therapists, occupational therapists, speech/language therapists, physicians, and others.

■ ***Assertive community treatment (ACT):*** ACT provides mental health and support services in the community for individuals with serious mental illness, such as schizophrenia or bipolar disorder, to promote optimal functioning at home and within the community. Professionals participating in an individual patient's care team may include psychiatrists, psychologists, social workers, pharmacists, advanced practice nurses, employment counselors, and peer support specialists.

■ ***Elder care centers and services:*** Programs such as Programs of All-Inclusive Care for the Elderly (PACE) offers services for older adults on an inpatient or outpatient basis as appropriate. Services may include medically necessary services, respite care for caregivers, transportation to medical and social services appointment, and mental healthcare. Collaborative team members may include physicians, nurses, nutritionists, therapists, social workers, and mental health professionals, among others.

Conflict Prevention and Management

Conflict occurs when diverse interests about significant issues or concerns among individuals, groups, or organizations prevents progressive problem solving or when emotional opposition creates discord and stifles effective communication (Schermerhorn et al., 2012; Waite & McKinney, 2014). Conflict is a normal part of the work environment. Worldwide, nurses compose up to 80% of the healthcare workforce and deliver 90% of all healthcare services (International Council of Nurses, 2012). Considering the number of individuals with whom they must collaborate to provide care, conflict should be anticipated (Waite & McKinney, 2014). Responses to conflict depend on the nurse's leadership skills for effecting positive outcomes within the work environment. Conflict (both between individuals and within an organization) can never be eliminated; however, it can be managed, and it takes both skill and competence in order to be successful.

Types of Conflict

Conflicts can take place between individual nurses, between nurses and patients or family members, between nurses and other members of the healthcare team, within a unit, or within a department. Conflicts can be interunit and interdepartmental, can affect the entire organization, or can even occur between multiple organizations, between or within teams or units, or between an organization and the community.

Levels of Conflict

Types and levels of conflict may be categorized in a variety of ways. This section approaches conflict as existing on four levels (Schermerhorn et al., 2012):

■ **Intrapersonal conflict**, which occurs within an individual, is stress or tension that results from real or perceived pressure generated by incompatible expectations or goals. This may occur when an individual is expected to do something that produces both desirable and undesirable consequences. For example, intrapersonal conflict may occur when a nurse must choose either to accept an employment position that interferes with fulfilling family-related responsibilities or to prioritize family responsibilities while remaining unemployed and without an income (Schermerhorn et al., 2012).

■ **Interpersonal conflict** occurs between two or more individuals. It can arise from differences in goals or personalities, competition, or concern about territory, control, or loss. Interpersonal conflict may occur in the workplace when one staff member misunderstands the roles or responsibility of another. For example, a nurse may believe that someone from another discipline is not doing his or her job because the individual is neglecting to perform an activity that is really the responsibility of the nurse. Other interpersonal conflicts can arise as the result of bullying, when a member of the team belittles another or attempts to coerce others into behaving in ways that cause frustration, guilt, or other types of conflict.

■ **Intergroup conflict** occurs between teams that are in competition or opposition to one another. In some cases, the groups are competing for rewards or scarce resources. The groups may also be emotionally opposed to each other (Schermerhorn et al., 2012). One example of this level of conflict is the debate that is occurring between physician groups who want to bring nurse practitioners under the control of the medical board, whereas nurses feel strongly that nurse practitioners should remain under the control of the board of nursing.

■ **Interorganizational conflict** is most commonly considered to involve competition between two organizations that exist within one market (Schermerhorn et al., 2012). For example, hospitals within the same community may demonstrate interorganizational conflict, with different institutions advertising superior care for a subset of patients; or, colleges of nursing may compete for qualified applicants for program admission.

Covert and Overt Conflict

At any level, conflict may be overt or covert. Both approaches may be associated with benefits, as well as with negative consequences. In **overt conflict**, the individuals or group members who are in conflict address the conflict openly. Overt conflict is obvious, at least to most individuals, and thus coping with it is usually easier. Generally speaking, it is easier to arrive at an agreement that conflict is present and easier to arrive at a description of the conflict.

In **covert conflict**, the conflict is not discussed openly. It may be avoided or ignored. Covert conflict may be exhibited in reactive, repressive, and avoidant behaviors. Reactive behaviors include whining, complaining, agreeing with others without really listening to them, and passive-aggressive behavior. Gossip is another form of reactive behavior, and rumor mills are common in workplaces in which covert conflict thrives. Repressive behaviors include absenteeism and tardiness. Although sustained avoidance usually is associated with negative outcomes, it is worth noting that avoidance may be an effective method of temporarily managing conflict. Avoidance may be appropriate when emotions are flaring and the individual or individuals involved would benefit from taking time to regain composure before discussing the issues at the foundation of the conflict (Schermerhorn et al., 2012). However, sustained tactics of covert conflict result in increased stress, distress, and confusion about how to address the conflict. Acknowledging covert conflict is not easy, and everyone involved will have different perceptions of the conflict because it operates below the surface.

Causes of Conflict

To resolve conflict effectively, nurses must understand its cause. Some conflicts have more than one cause. Typical causes of conflict among individuals and among groups include the following: miscommunication, inaccurate information, mistrust, ambiguous role expectations, ineffective leadership, and resistance to change.

Within the healthcare setting, researchers have identified role boundary issues and accountability as two primary sources of conflict (Brown et al., 2011). Conflicts arising from role boundary issues include a lack of understanding of the value of all team members, including those outside the disciplines of nursing and medicine, relative to the care of the patient. Role boundaries also create conflicts with regard to awareness of which tasks each team member was authorized to perform. In the realm of accountability, conflict arises particularly when healthcare team members did not hold themselves accountable for their actions (Brown et al., 2011).

The Nurse–Physician Relationship

The nurse–physician relationship should be the strongest collaboration that nurses have in order to meet the needs of their patients. Unfortunately, it sometimes is not. This may be due to a lack of confidence on the part of the nurse, an attempt to save face, fear of repercussion, deference to the physician, or an attempt to preserve a patriarchal nurse–physician relationship (Matzke et al., 2014). Both nurses and physicians can contribute to inadequacies in this relationship. When conflict does occur, it often becomes a barrier to effective patient care. Cooperation and collaboration are also integral to the success of this relationship.

The Nurse–Patient Relationship

The close nature of the nurse–patient relationship allows little room for conflict between patient and nurse. Despite this, conflicts with patients or with family members or caregivers can arise. Causes of conflict in this relationship can include lack of knowledge on the part of the patient or family member; poor coping skills on the part of the patient or family member; fear or anxiety resulting in the patient or family member expressing frustration; and failure of the nurse to assess or meet patient needs or promote the therapeutic relationship. Whatever the cause, any conflict between the nurse and patient or family member can become a barrier to effective care.

Nurse–nurse and nurse–coworker conflicts also occur. When not managed properly, these may rise to the level of workplace bullying or incivility. Strategies for preventing and managing conflict (including workplace bullying and incivility) are outlined in the sections that follow.

Clinical Example B

Josiah Elliot, 72 years old, is admitted to the hospital with medical diagnoses of congestive heart failure, chronic renal failure, hypertension, and benign prostatic hypertrophy. The nurse admits him and develops his plan of nursing care, including the nursing diagnoses of *Excess Fluid Volume, Urinary Retention, Impaired Gas Exchange,* and *Anxiety* related to hypoxia. Three days later Mr. Elliot has lost 18 pounds and is breathing more easily. He also denies feeling anxious and reports, "I'm relaxed now that I can breathe!" The nursing diagnoses of *Excess Fluid Volume, Impaired Gas Exchange,* and *Anxiety* are all marked as resolved. During morning rounds, the nurse provides the physician with an update on the patient's condition and questions the need to continue administering the large doses of diuretics that were ordered when the patient was admitted. The physician agrees and reduces the dosage of the medications. The physician raises concerns about the patient's nutritional status and suitability for discharge to home. After some discussion, the physician and nurse agree to consult with a dietitian and a social worker for further evaluation of the patient's care.

Critical Thinking Questions

1. Describe the impact of the team's collaborative approach on Mr. Elliot's outcomes.
2. How might Mr. Elliot's care have differed if the team had not collaborated?
3. What further collaboration is indicated in providing care for Mr. Elliot?

Developing Conflict Competence

Caring for individuals requires groups of professionals working together in interprofessional settings. Resolving conflict requires increased cognitive, emotional, and behavioral skills, confidence, and competence. Purposeful development of these skills is also known as **conflict competence** (Waite & McKinney, 2014). Communication is key for both preventing and resolving conflict. Five different communication styles have been identified in the literature and have been repeatedly tested using the Thomas-Kilmann Conflict Mode Instrument (TKI). Those styles include:

1. *Competing:* An assertive, power-oriented approach; competing can be seen as self-centered or as defending one's position on behalf of the patient.
2. *Collaborating:* A cooperative approach; gaining insight to the perspectives of others can lead to creative problem-solving.
3. *Compromising:* An approach in which both parties are partially satisfied; compromising, at the very least, addresses rather than avoids the issue.
4. *Avoiding:* Seen as uncooperative or a preference to avoid addressing the conflict; however, avoidance can be a helpful approach when more information is needed or when the issue just is not worth risking further conflict or a loss of opportunity or consideration.
5. *Accommodating:* An attempt to satisfy the concerns of others while neglecting the self; accommodation works best when one individual or group is less interested in the issue than the other.

The ability to move among styles, depending on the situation at hand, is a skill that takes practice and awareness of self in order to develop one's conflict competence (Thomas & Kilmann, 1974).

Interprofessional communication has been identified by The Interprofessional Education Collaborative (IPEC) as one of its four core competencies as a framework for collaboration and practice (along with values & ethics, roles & responsibilities, and teams & teamwork) (NLN, 2015).

Communication can be status-based or team-centered. Status-based communication is, as the term implies, based on a hierarchy, typically the physician "giving orders" as the team captain. This type of communication focuses on the needs/desires of one individual (the physician) and/or the more powerful team member using forceful language to convey or reaffirm status. This approach does not lend itself to dialogue. Team-centered communication emphasizes shared problem-solving. Rather than the "I want" or "You need to do x" with the status-based approach, the team-centered approach invokes "How can we solve x" as a common strategy. Practice using "we" statements such as "Mr. X is concerned about. . . . What are your thoughts on this?" or "How can we work together to help him?" Statements such as these reflect shared responsibility and encourage open discussions (Matzke et al., 2014).

Using a relational approach helps individuals understand their own responses to conflict. The fundamental components of a therapeutic relationship—demonstrating respect, being self-aware, maintaining boundaries within the professional team, being empathetic, accepting individuality, and promoting equality among team members—are vital in communication. These qualities lay the groundwork for approaching communication about patient problems as one would in a relationship, moving from individual or "I" statements to "how best can we" type conversations that invite openness in dialogue. Using a relational approach can improve care coordination, which can, in turn, lead to better clinical outcomes (Gerardi, 2015a).

Preventing Conflict

Clear communication is essential to prevent misunderstandings that can lead to conflicts. Understanding and recognizing causes of conflict can assist individuals and organizations to develop strategies to prevent conflict. Nurses must be able to identify potential issues that can act as barriers to conflict resolution or increase the likelihood that a situation will turn into a conflict. First and foremost, nurses need to recognize their own tension or stress level in the workplace. **Mindsight** is a term that describes being self-aware of one's triggers to stress that can result in conflict, and purposefully "retraining" the brain to respond differently. Improving one's self-awareness is salient to growing as a leader and being able to redirect the typical response and course of action in a given situation. Taking steps to decrease or manage stress levels helps to reduce the likelihood of initiating conflict (see Focus on Integrative Health: Stress Reduction). Other strategies that help prevent conflict include the following (Greenberg, 2011; Porter-O'Grady & Malloch, 2013):

- Address issues as they arise.
- Avoid destructive criticism, including harsh words, threats, and generalized condemnation of behaviors or performance.

- Treat others with respect, which will decrease defensiveness.
- Avoid arguments. Sometimes people do need to vent, and as long as it is done appropriately and in a private place, it may be helpful in decreasing tension.
- Actively listen to each other.
- Consider the other individual's point of view, including cultural beliefs and values.

For individuals who are in leadership roles, strategies to promote conflict prevention include the following (Greenberg, 2011; Porter-O'Grady & Malloch, 2013):

- Allocate resources fairly, including fair distribution of workload balance and intensity when assigning patient care.
- Clearly define role expectations for all team members.
- Encourage staff to provide feedback and identify potential concerns without the threat of punitive action.
- Acknowledge team members' accomplishments and achievements, as well as significant life events.

Responding to Conflict

Not everyone responds to conflict in the same way, and individuals vary in how they respond to it in different circumstances. Often, interactions may be unpredictable and the accompanying behaviors unpredictable. In turn, one's response to such behaviors can trigger an unreasonable or inappropriate retort. Typical responses might be avoidance, minimizing, or prematurely "fixing" the problem but not the root cause. Such responses can set up barriers and prevent successful engagement and problem solving (Gerardi, 2015b).

When conflict occurs, each individual involved has a personal perspective of the issue and conflict. The nurse who can recognize the types of responses to conflict will be better equipped to predict and manage it. To respond effectively to conflict, the nurse should apply the following guidelines:

- Demonstrate honesty, trustworthiness, and respect.
- State the issue objectively and provide a factual basis for the concern.
- Avoid emotion-based discussions.
- Be open to hearing all individuals' viewpoints and avoid passing judgment.

Focus on Integrative Health
Stress Reduction

Integrative health approaches can have a positive impact for stress reduction. Knowing oneself and what is likely to trigger a reaction or a response to stress can be tempered by using integrative approaches, such as progressive relaxation, meditation, guided imagery, breathing exercises, aerobic exercise, and meditative movement therapies, including yoga and t'ai chi. Any method selected requires practice to improve adherence to health-promoting behaviors and lifestyle modifications. In the stressful world of nursing, early adoption of one or more of these approaches is encouraged in order to successfully deal with day-to-day events (Cramer et al., 2014).

- Allow all individuals involved to express their concerns without interruption.
- Apply active listening techniques.
- Focus on identifying solutions as opposed to exacerbating the problem.
- Throughout the process of conflict resolution, recognize that the delivery of safe, effective patient care is the central concern.

Managing Conflict Within the Healthcare Team

The common assumption about conflict is that it is destructive, and it certainly can be. However, when effectively managed, conflict can bring to light issues that need to be addressed and result in beneficial outcomes for individuals, groups, and organizations (Schermerhorn et al., 2012).

Nurses tend to resort to positions of avoidance, compromise, or accommodation rather than address an issue or deal with conflict. Such approaches, over time, can lead to resentment, which can further lead to ambivalence about one's job. Anticipating that conflict will occur and being prepared to deal with and manage conflict constructively is a leadership skill. Learning to manage and/or resolve conflict successfully is essential for professional growth. Although often viewed as being negative, conflict can actually be an impetus for better communication, stronger team relationships, and healthy changes. Nurses need to be able to competently and confidently address difficult situations in a constructive manner and in a safe space where all parties feel that they can have conversations about perceptions or misperceptions without fear of retribution. Successfully addressing conflict requires self-awareness for knowing how one responds in stressful situations. Self-inventory tools help to provide understanding of how one reacts to situations that trigger conflict. Self-awareness is key to therapeutic and respectful relationships. Personal inventories such as the Thomas-Kilmann Conflict Mode Instrument (Thomas & Kilmann, 1974), StrengthsFinder (Rath, 2007), and Emotional Intelligence Inventory (Stein & Book, 2000), to name but a few, help to increase personal awareness about personal reflexive responses that might hamper rather than help in stressful situations. Understanding one's own responses is important to reflect and learn how to change one's behavior from a reactionary stance to a relatable and intentional approach (Gerardi, 2015a; Waite & McKinney, 2014). At an organizational level, agency administrations need to promote programs that go beyond assertiveness training, conflict management, and collaborative processes. Agencies must engage employees in institution-wide programs that emphasize respect, acknowledge communication for the sake of patient safety, use nondisciplinary approaches to resolve issues, and model language and tactics that reduce tension and remove the barriers that impede resolution. Examples of these types of programs include Crucial Conversations, Crew Resource Management, TeamSTEPPS, and The Exchange (Rosenstein, Dinklin, & Munro, 2014).

Managing Conflict with Patients and Families

When conflict occurs with patients or their families, in addition to the strategies already presented, setting limits can be an effective way to manage expressions of negative behaviors.

For example, nurses set limits when a patient becomes loud or profane by providing instructions such as "I can see you are upset and I want to help you, but I will not tolerate abusive language." Setting limits can help anxious patients monitor their own behaviors and keep the nurse from being interrupted too frequently.

Patients or families should never be allowed to demonstrate anger inappropriately. When this occurs, the nurse needs to set reasonable limits that are based on an assessment of the situation. Anger and inappropriate behavior may stem from a number of causes, such as pain, medications, fear and anxiety, psychosis, and dysfunctional communication. Cultural differences must also be considered. Language barriers may result in misunderstandings, frustrations, and unmet needs, and some patients may display anger as a result. Further, some cultures consider it appropriate to be very emotional while others do not. In the long term, active listening and clear communication are critical to prevent and manage conflict. Although empathy and consideration are key components of the nurse's role, abusive behavior is never acceptable. Tolerance of verbal or physical acts of aggression may lead to escalation of these behaviors. To promote safety for both the healthcare provider and the patient, inappropriate demonstrations of anger, including hostile verbal or physical behaviors, should be reported immediately to the team leader or charge nurse.

Incivility in the Workplace

Incivility or disruptive behavior in the workplace can play out in many forms, including aggression, bullying, and violence. Studies on incivility indicate that such negativity can lead to adverse organizational outcomes, including decreased job satisfaction leading to absenteeism; loss of productivity; staff turnover; patient errors with the potential for adverse outcomes; and the associated costs of turnover or legal fees to resolve staff or patient issues. Although numbers vary, the financial burden is estimated to be more than $23 billion to cover the costs of uncivil workplace behaviors and associated outcomes (Lachman, 2015; Laschinger et al., 2014). The problem is more widespread than reports indicate, partly because individuals may not report out of fear of retribution, lack of knowledge of the reporting process, or an assumption that the behavior is acceptable. Other factors that discourage reporting of incivility in the workplace include the failure of administration to support or respond to previous reports and the overall lack of awareness on the part of the individual or the staff as a result of the normalization of the activity.

Aggressive or hostile behavior can lead to conflict. Aggressive behavior by even a single individual in the workplace can increase the anxiety of many others. The first response toward a hostile staff member should be to communicate control to that staff member and to insert calm into the situation. When the nurse manager or team leader is the one who is hostile, the situation carries greater complexity and requires assistance from higher level management. Regardless of who is exhibiting aggression or hostility, someone should gain control and try to move the aggressor to a private place. Demonstrations of open conflict with hostility should not take place in patient or public areas. If the suggestion to move to a private area does not work and the situation continues to escalate, simply walking away may help set some boundaries. This allows time for all parties to take a breath, calm down, and revisit the situation at a more appropriate time.

Workplace Bullying

Workplace bullying is a long-term behavior lasting a minimum of 6 months and plays out in the form of verbal attacks, refusal to help or assist others, speaking negatively or taunting. When not effectively managed or controlled, workplace bullying can escalate to physical threats (Lachman, 2015). **Verbal abuse** in professional settings is defined as malicious, repeated, harmful mistreatment of an individual with whom one works, regardless of whether that individual is an equal, a superior, or a subordinate. Verbal abuse occurs in healthcare settings between patients and staff, nurses and other nurses, physicians and nurses, and all other staff relationships.

Horizontal violence (HV) is a term used to describe aggressive acts committed against a nurse by one or more nursing colleagues (Longo & Sherman, 2007; Purpora & Blegen, 2012). Behaviors that reflect HV may include verbal acts, such as gossiping about and speaking sarcastically to the nurse who is the target, unkind or even antagonistic interactions, divisive behavior, sarcasm, and condescending or patronizing behavior (Lachman, 2015).

In any form, workplace bullying yields serious negative consequences. Victims of bullying experience adverse emotional effects, including depression, anxiety, and a sense of isolation (Murray, 2008, 2009). In healthcare organizations, research suggests that bullying is linked to increased rates of employee absenteeism and work-related injuries as well as decreased productivity (Felblinger, 2008; Longo & Sherman, 2007; Murray, 2008). It can impact patient safety and quality of care.

Incivility and disruptive behaviors violate the ANA *Code of Ethics for Nurses* (2015). Provision 1.5 of the code speaks to collegial relationships with others and the nurse's obligation to create a culture of civility and kindness. Provision 6 addresses the nurse's responsibility for creating a culture of excellence (ANA, 2015; Lachman, O'Connor Swanson, & Winland-Brown, 2015). In addition, within the Core Competencies for Interprofessional Collaborative Practice is the values/ethics competency stipulating that healthcare team members must place the interests of patients and populations at the center of care (Interprofessional Education Collaborative Expert Panel, 2011).

Maintaining a Culture of Excellence

Nurses have an obligation to create and maintain a culture of excellence, and within that is the obligation to report bullying. Nurses should recognize workplace bullying, be aware of its effects, and follow organizational policies and procedures with regard to reporting the behavior. Reports of bullying should include details such as the date, time, and description of events, as well as identification of any witnesses. Ideally, individuals in leadership positions within the organization will address the issue in such a manner that the bullying stops. The nurse should be aware of organizations that may be available to provide assistance

Box 37–3
Prevention of Workplace Bullying Among Nurses

- Educate team members about bullying behaviors and their adverse effects.
- Develop codes of conduct that clearly outline unacceptable behaviors.
- Promote a "zero-tolerance" attitude toward bullying.
- Encourage nurses to report bullying without fear of punishment or negative consequences.
- Offer the option of reporting bullying behaviors or recommendations for improvement of anti-bullying policies through use of comment or suggestion boxes.
- Assure nurses that reports of bullying will be taken seriously and thoroughly addressed, including through mandatory investigations of all allegations of bullying.
- Train leadership and management personnel to work collaboratively to prevent, identify, and address bullying behaviors.
- Create an environment in which courtesy and respect are valued.

Sources: Based *on* Lowenstein, L. F. (2013). Bullying in nursing and ways of dealing with it. *Nursing Times, 109*(11), 22–25; Broome, B. S., & Williams-Evans, S. (2011). Bullying in a caring profession: Reasons, results, and recommendations. *Journal of Psychosocial Nursing and Mental Health Services, 49*, 30–35; Cleary, M., Hunt, G. E., Walter, G., & Robertson, M. (2009). Dealing with bullying in the workplace: Toward zero tolerance. *Journal of Psychosocial Nursing and Mental Health Services, 47*, 34–41; and Mackintosh, J., Wuest, J., Gray, M. M., & Cronkhite, M. (2010). Workplace bullying in health care affects the meaning of work. *Qualitative Health Research, 20*, 1128–1141.

in case of bullying, including the appropriate state nursing association, the American Nurses Association, and the Department of Justice (Murray, 2009). Empowered nurses have access to information, support, and resources and work in environments whose leaders are committed to providing opportunities to learn and grow, all in an effort to minimize or greatly reduce workplace incivility (Laschinger et al., 2014). See **Box 37–3** ≫ for an overview of guidelines for prevention of bullying among nurses in the workplace. **Box 37–4** ≫ outlines the standards set by the American Association of Critical Care Nurses for establishing a healthy workplace. By following these standards, nurses and healthcare agencies can work to establish a culture of excellence.

Clinical Example C

Dee Johnston has worked in pediatric intensive care for the past year. She decides to leave her current position because she feels that her coworkers don't value the knowledge and skill that she has gained over time. Coworkers still make off-the-cuff remarks such as "She's just the newbie on the block" or "Wait until she has a really sick baby to deal with." Dee begins to feel nervous at the thought of just going to work and is afraid she is going to make a mistake. She decides to leave and accept a position as a staff nurse in the pediatric ICU at another facility. Within 3 weeks of orientation, her preceptor quickly recognizes her expertise and feels that additional orientation is unnecessary. She begins to gain more self-confidence and enjoys going to her job once again.

Critical Thinking Questions

1. How is Dee interpreting her coworkers' behavior?
2. Why might they be making such comments about Dee?
3. Do you think that leaving was the right thing for Dee to do? Why or why not?

Box 37–4
AACN Standards for Healthy Work Environments

The American Association of Critical Care Nurses (AACN, 2016) has worked diligently to promote healthcare environments that focus on meeting the needs of patients, families, nurses, and other healthcare professionals. As part of this work, the AACN has identified six essential standards based on evidence-based principles of professional performance. The six standards with sample critical elements include:

1. *Skilled communication*, with the expectation that individuals advance collaborative relationships, improve communication styles, establish zero-tolerance policies to protect against disrespectful behavior in the workplace, maintain accountability for words and actions, and encourage a focus on finding solutions and achievable outcomes.
2. *True collaboration*, wherein team members have access to interprofessional education opportunities, have high levels of integrity, and demonstrate competence in their roles.

3. *Effective decision making*, which ensures that nurses participate in all levels of decision making, that team members share fact-based information, and that effective processes are in place to objectively evaluate the results of decisions.
4. *Appropriate staffing* based on the professional obligation for nurses to provide high-level quality care and that organizations adopt technologies that increase the effectiveness of care.
5. *Meaningful recognition*, which acknowledges that team members should be recognized for the value they bring to the organization.
6. *Authentic leadership*, whereby leaders fully embrace and sustain a healthy work environment that promotes professional advancement.

Source: Based on AACN Standards for Establishing and Sustaining Healthy Work Environments. (2016). *A Journey to Excellence. 2nd ed. Executive Summary.* Aliso Viejo, CA:AACN, 1–9.

REVIEW The Concept of Collaboration

RELATE Link the Concepts

Linking the concept of collaboration with the concept of communication:

1. How does the nurse's communication skills affect his or her ability to collaborate?
2. How does communication style affect the process of collaboration? Give some examples.

Linking the concept of collaboration with the concept of oxygenation:

3. How would the care of a patient with chronic obstructive pulmonary disease (COPD) benefit from a nurse who collaborates well with other members of the healthcare team?
4. In caring for the patient with COPD, what aspects of care would require collaboration?

Linking the concept of collaboration with the concept of stress and coping:

5. How do different levels of stress affect both the occurrence of conflict and the management of conflict that arises?
6. How can an understanding of different individuals' coping mechanisms improve the ability to manage conflict?

REFER Go to Pearson MyLab Nursing and eText

■ Additional review materials

REFLECT Apply Your Knowledge

Abigail Lessarian, a 32-year-old patient, delivered her first baby prematurely at 32 weeks' gestation. Her infant son, Garrett, was apneic at birth and required a brief period of tracheal intubation and mechanical ventilation. Immediately after his delivery, Garrett was admitted to the neonatal intensive care unit (NICU) for treatment of neonatal respiratory distress syndrome (RDS). By day 3, Garrett had made excellent progress; he was extubated and oxygen administration was implemented via nasal cannula with continuous positive airway pressure (CPAP). By day 14 in the NICU, Garrett was breathing effectively enough to maintain his oxygen saturation at >98% on room air with CPAP via nasal cannula; however, he experienced intermittent apneic spells with bradycardia until day 22. Garrett also was diagnosed with an atrial septal defect (ASD), which his surgeon recommended monitoring in hopes that the ASD would resolve without requiring surgical treatment. He received gavage feedings via a nasogastric tube.

By day 30 in the NICU, Garrett had experienced no apneic spells for 7 days. On day 32, Garrett's gavage tube was removed, and he successfully transitioned to bottle feeding over a period of several days. On day 43, Garrett began transitioning to breastfeeding; despite having difficulty with sucking, his progress was slow but steady. By day 46, Garrett's neonatologist (pediatrician specializing in neonatal care) cleared him for discharge to home.

Prior to Garrett's discharge, his mother and father are scheduled to complete an infant CPR course. They also will receive teaching about the use of a home apnea monitor. During discussion of the numerous topics about which Garrett's parents will receive instruction, Garrett's mother states, "I don't know if I can handle much more. I feel so overwhelmed." When she becomes tearful, her husband puts his arm around her and says, "We'll do whatever it takes to help him get healthy. I can't believe I was concerned about whether or not he'd like playing baseball or football. Now, that seems so silly. I just want him to survive."

1. Identify three nursing diagnoses that are appropriate for inclusion in Garrett's nursing plan of care.
2. Identify three nursing diagnoses that are appropriate for inclusion in the nursing plan of care for Garrett's parents.
3. During preliminary discharge planning, Garrett's interprofessional team's recommendations include home visits by a nurse, occupational therapist, and social worker. What roles might each of these professionals serve in the care of Garrett and his family?
4. What other professionals might be beneficial to the care of Garrett and his parents in the home setting?

References

AACN Standards for Establishing and Sustaining Healthy Work Environments. (2016). *A Journey to Excellence.* 2nd ed. Executive Summary. Aliso Viejo, CA:AACN, 1–9.

American Nurses Association (ANA). (2015). *Code of ethics for nurses with interpretive statements.* Silver Spring, MD: Author.

Brown, J., Lewis, L., Ellis, K., Stewart, M., Freeman, T. R., & Kasperski, J. M. (2011). Conflict on interprofessional primary health care teams—Can it be resolved? *Journal of Interprofessional Care, 25,* 4–10.

Bularzik, A. M. H., Tullai, O., McGuinness, S., & Leibold Sieloff, C. (2013). Nurse's perceptions of their group goal attainment capability and professional autonomy: a pilot study. *Journal of Nursing Management, 21,* 581–590.

Cramer, H., Lauche, R., Moebus, S., Michalsen, A., Langhorst, J., Dobos, G., & Paul, A. (2014). Predictors of health behavior change after an integrative medicine inpatient program. *International Journal of Behavioral Medicine, 21,* 775–783.

Cronenwett, L., Sherwood, G., Barnsteiner, J., Disch, J., Johnson, J., Mitchell, P., & Warren, J. (2007). Quality and safety education for nurses. *Nursing Outlook, 55*(3), 122–131.

Douglas, M. K., Rosenkoetter, M., Pacquiao, D. F., Callister, L. C., Hattar-Pollara, M., & Fewster-Thuente, L. (2015). Working together toward a common goal: A grounded theory of nurse-physician collaboration. *MEDSURG Nursing, 24*(5), 356–362.

Felblinger, D. (2008). Incivility and bullying in the workplace and nurses' shame responses. *Journal of Obstetric, Gynecologic, and Neonatal Nursing, 37*(2), 234–242.

Fewster-Thuente, L. (2015). Working together toward a common goal: A grounded theory of nurse-physician collaboration. *MEDSURG Nursing, 24*(5), 356–362. Retrieved from https://www.ncbi.nlm.nih.gov/pubmed/26665873

Garcia, C., & Duckett, L. (2009). No te entiendo y tu no me entiendes: Language barriers among immigrant Latino adolescents seeking health care. *Journal of Cultural Diversity, 16*(3), 120–126.

Gerardi, D. (2015a). Perspectives on Leadership. Conflict engagement: a relational approach. *American Journal of Nursing, 115*(7), 56–60.

Gerardi, D. (2015b). Perspectives on Leadership. Conflict engagement: workplace dynamics. *American Journal of Nursing, 115*(4), 62–65.

Greenberg, J. (2011). *Behavior in organizations.* Upper Saddle River, NJ: Prentice Hall.

Henderson, V. A. (1991). *The nature of nursing: Reflections after 25 years.* New York, NY: National League for Nursing.

International Council of Nurses. (2012). *Reforming primary health care: A nursing perspective.* Geneva, Switzerland: Author.

Interprofessional Education Collaborative Expert Panel. (2011). *Core competencies for interprofessional collaborative practice: Report of an expert panel.* Washington, D.C.: Interprofessional Education Collaborative.

Lachman, V. D. (2015). Ethical issues in the disruptive behaviors of incivility, bullying, and horizontal/lateral violence. *Urologic Nursing, 35*(1), 39–42.

Lachman, V. D., O'Connor Swanson, E., & Winland-Brown, J. (2015). The new "code of ethics for nurses with interpretative statements" (2015): Practical clinical application, part II. *MEDSURG Nursing, 24*(5), 363–367.

Laschinger, H. K. S., Cummings, G. G., Wong, C. A., & Grau, A. L. (2014). Resonant leadership and workplace empowerment: The value of positive organizational cultures in reducing workplace incivility. *Nursing Economic$, 32*(1), 5–15.

Longo, J., & Sherman, R. O. (2007). Leveling horizontal violence. *Nursing Management, 38*(3), 34–37, 50, 51.

Masters, K. (2013). *Role development in professional nursing practice* (3rd ed.). Sudbury, MA: Jones & Bartlett.

Matzke, B., Houston, S., Fischer, U., & Bradshaw, M. J. (2014). Using a team-centered approach to evaluate effectiveness of nurse-physician communications. *Journal of Obstetric, Gynecological, and Neonatal Nursing, 43*(6), 684–694.

Murray, J. S. (2008). No more nurse abuse: Let's stop paying the emotional, physical, and financial costs of workplace abuse. *American Nurse Today, 3*(7), 17–19.

Murray, J. S. (2009). Workplace bullying in nursing: A problem that can't be ignored. *MedSurg Nursing, 18*(5), 273–276.

Nair, D. M., Fitzpatrick, J. J., McNulty, R., Click, E. R., & Glembocki, M. M. (2012). Frequency of nurse–physician collaborative behaviors in an acute care hospital. *Journal of Interprofessional Care, 26*(2), 115–120.

National League for Nursing (NLN). (2015). *NLN Vision Series: Transforming nursing education; leading the call to reform. Interprofessional Collaboration in Education and Practice: A living document from the National League for Nursing.* NLN Board of Governors.

National League for Nursing (NLN). (2016). *Vision for interprofessional collaboration in education and practice.* Retrieved from http://www.nln.org/docs/default-source/default-document-library/ipe-ipp-vision.pdf?sfvrsn=14

Porter-O'Grady, T., & Malloch, K. (2013). *Leadership in nursing practice: Changing the landscape of health care.* Burlington, MA: Jones & Bartlett.

Purpora, C., & Blegen, M. A. (2012). Horizontal violence and the quality and safety of patient care: A conceptual model. *Nursing Research and Practice, 2012,* 306948–306952.

Rath, T. (2007). *StrengthsFinder 2.0.* New York, NY: Gallup Press.

Rosenstein, A. H., Dinklin, S. P., & Munro, J. (2014). Conflict resolution: Unlocking the key to success. *Nursing Management, 45*(10), 34–39.

Ruben, B. D. (2016). Communication theory and health communication practice can be described by the axiom: The more things change, the more they stay the same. *Health Communication, 31*(11), 1–11.

Schermerhorn, J. R., Osborn, R. N., Hunt, J. G., & Uhl-Bien, M. (2012). *Organizational behavior* (12th ed.). New York, NY: John Wiley & Sons.

Schneider, M. A. (2012). Nurse–physician collaboration: Its time has come. *Nursing, 42*(7), 50–53.

Stein, S. J., & Book, H. E. (2000). *The EQ edge: Emotional intelligence and your success.* Toronto, Canada: Stoddart.

The Joint Commission. (2012). *Sentinel event data—Root causes by event type.* Retrieved from http://www.jointcommission.org/Sentinel_Event_Statistics/

The Joint Commission. (2016). *Advancing effective communication, cultural competence, and patient- and family-centered care: A roadmap for hospitals.* Oakbrook Terrace, IL: Author.

Thomas, K. W., & Kilmann, R. H. (1974). *Thomas-Kilmann Conflict Mode Instrument.* Palo Alto, CA: Consulting Psychologists Press.

Waite, R., & McKinney, N. S. (2014). Enhancing conflict competency. *Association of Black Nursing Faculty Journal, 25*(4), 123–128.

Weston, M. J. (2008). Defining control over nursing practice and autonomy. *Journal of Nursing Administration, 38,* 404–408.

Weston, M. J. (2010). Strategies for enhancing autonomy and control over nursing practice. *Online Journal of Issues in Nursing, 15*(1).

World Health Organization (WHO). (2010). *Framework for action on interprofessional education and collaborative practice.* Geneva, Switzerland: Author.

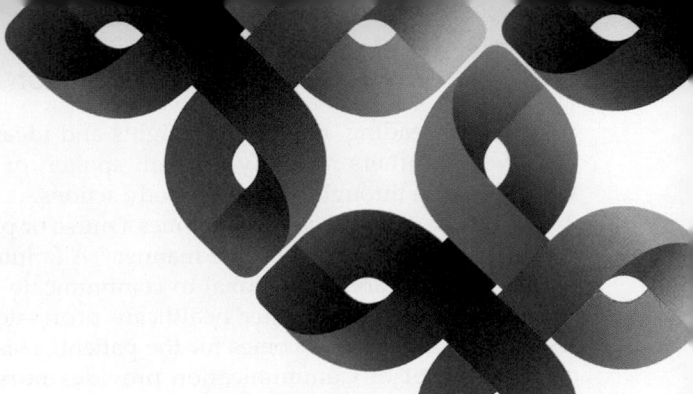

Module 38
Communication

Module Outline and Learning Outcomes

The Concept of Communication

The Communication Process

38.1 Analyze the process of communication.

Modes of Communication

38.2 Differentiate the various forms of communication.

Concepts Related to Communication

38.3 Outline the relationship between communication and other concepts.

Factors Influencing the Communication Process

38.4 Analyze the factors that influence the communication process.

Barriers to Communication

38.5 Analyze barriers to effective communication.

Types of Communicators

38.6 Analyze the various types of communicators.

Assertive Communication

38.7 Summarize the attributes of a nurse who uses assertive communication.

Lifespan Considerations

38.8 Differentiate considerations related to communication throughout the lifespan.

Nursing Practice

38.9 Analyze the nursing process as it relates to a patient with impaired verbal communication.

Communication Exemplars

Exemplar 38.A Groups and Group Communication

38.A Analyze groups and group communication.

Exemplar 38.B Therapeutic Communication

38.B Analyze the interactive process of therapeutic communication.

Exemplar 38.C Documentation

38.C Analyze documentation as it relates to communication.

Exemplar 38.D Reporting

38.D Analyze reporting as it relates to communication.

≫ The Concept of Communication

Concept Key Terms

Nursing involves interactions between nurses and patients, nurses and other health professionals, and nurses and the community. The process of human interaction occurs through communication: verbal and nonverbal, written and unwritten, planned and unplanned. Communication between individuals conveys thoughts, ideas, feelings, and information. To be effective in their interactions, nurses must be proficient in their verbal and written communication skills. They must be aware of what their words and body language say to others. Nurses also must demonstrate competency in computer and electronic communication skills.

The term *communication* has various meanings, depending on the context in which it is used. For example, communication can be the interchange of information, thoughts, or ideas between two or more individuals. This kind of communication uses methods such as talking and listening or writing and reading. However, thoughts and ideas can be conveyed to others not only through spoken or written words but also through gestures or body actions.

In healthcare professions, sometimes a nurse or physician is said to be lacking in "bedside manner." A failure on the part of a healthcare professional to communicate successfully with a patient or other healthcare professional can result in poor health outcomes for the patient. This section on the concept of Communication provides nurses with essential information they need in order to communicate successfully with patients, peers, and other healthcare professionals. For the purposes of this text, **communication** is any means of exchanging information or feelings between two or more individuals. Communication is a basic component of human relationships, including nursing.

The *intent* of any communication is to elicit a response. Thus, communication is a process that has two main purposes: to influence others to respond and to obtain information. Communication can be described as helpful or unhelpful. Positive or effective communication encourages a sharing of information, thoughts, or feelings between two or more individuals. Negative or ineffective communication hinders or blocks the transfer of information and feelings. In nursing, any form or failure of communication that prevents the sharing of information and feelings can have negative consequences for the patient.

Therapeutic as opposed to social communication is essential for the establishment of a healthy nurse–patient relationship. Nurses who communicate therapeutically are better able to collect assessment data, develop care plans in collaboration with patients, initiate interventions, evaluate outcomes of interventions, initiate changes that promote health, and prevent legal problems associated with nursing practice. This communication process depends on nurses having established trusting relationships with patients and caregivers.

The Communication Process

Face-to-face communication involves a sender, a message, a receiver, and a response, or feedback (**Figure 38–1 »**). In its simplest form, communication is a two-party process involving the sending and the receiving of a message. Because the intent of communication is to elicit a response, the process is ongoing: The receiver of the message then becomes the sender of a response, and the original sender in turn becomes the receiver.

During any communication interaction, communication is also occurring on an intrapersonal level—that is, an individual's thoughts are a form of communication. Intrapersonal communication, also called *self-talk*, describes the thoughts or communication individuals keep to themselves. Each individual will be thinking his or her own thoughts before, during, and after sending a message and while receiving a message from the other party. This intrapersonal communication occurs constantly and can interfere with an individual's ability to hear a message as the sender intended (**Figure 38–2 »**).

Sender

The **sender**, an individual or group who wishes to convey a message to another, can be considered the *source-encoder*. This term suggests that the person or group sending the message must have an idea or reason for communicating (source) and must put that idea or reason into a form that can be transmitted. **Encoding** involves the

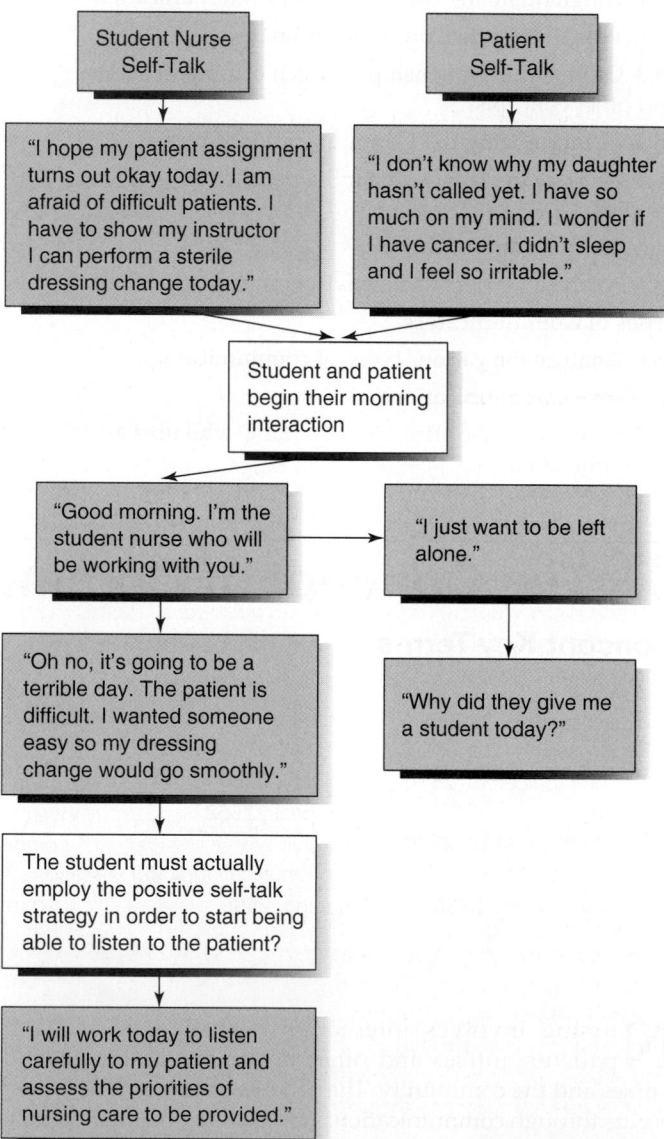

Figure 38–2 » Improving student nurse self-talk. The nurse's self-talk is shown in pink. The patient's self-talk is shown in purple. The verbal communication is shown in orange. Commentary is shown in white.

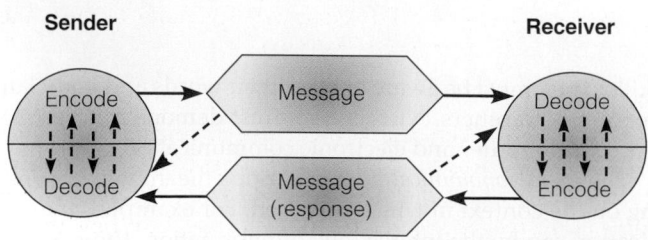

Figure 38–1 » The communication process. The dashed arrows indicate intrapersonal communication (self-talk). The solid lines indicate interpersonal communication.

selection of specific signs or symbols (codes) to transmit the message, such as which language and words to use, how to arrange the words, and what medium to use, which may involve tone of voice and gestures in oral communication. For example, if the receiver speaks English, the sender usually selects English words. If the message is "Mr. Johnson, you have to wait another hour for your pain medication," the tone of voice selected and a shake of the head can reinforce the message. Nurses must not only deal with dialects and foreign languages, but they must also cope with two language levels: the patient's and their own.

Message

The next component of the communication process is the **message** itself—the words actually spoken or written, the body language that accompanies the words, and how the words are transmitted. The medium used to convey the message is the **channel**, and it can target any of the receiver's senses. The channel must be appropriate for the message, and it should help make the intent of the message clearer. In some instances, for example, talking face to face with an individual may be more effective than telephoning or writing a message. Using recorded messages or communicating by radio or television may be more appropriate for large audiences. Written communication is often appropriate for long explanations or for a communication that needs to be preserved. The nonverbal channel of touch is often highly effective in establishing a bond or connection with the receiver. Some of the most effective communications use more than one sensory channel—for example, the nurse may combine the use of therapeutic touch with her verbal message.

Receiver

The **receiver**, the third component of the communication process, is the listener, who must listen, observe, and attend. This person is the *decoder*, who must perceive what the sender intended (interpretation). Perception entails using all of the senses to receive verbal and nonverbal messages. To *decode* means to relate the message perceived to the receiver's storehouse of knowledge and experience and to sort out the meaning of the message. Whether the receiver accurately decodes the message according to the sender's intent depends largely on their similarities in knowledge, experiences, and sociocultural background. If the meaning of the decoded message matches the intent of the sender, then the communication has been effective.

Ineffective communication occurs when the sender's message is misinterpreted by the receiver. For example, if a nurse preparing to feed a patient who requires assistance glances repeatedly at the clock, the patient may interpret this behavior as indicating that the nurse is in a hurry, which may make the patient feel rushed and like a burden. It is important for nurses to consider the unintended messages their behavior may be sending.

Response

The **response**, the fourth component of the communication process, is the message that the receiver returns to the sender. It is also called **feedback**. A response can be either verbal, nonverbal, or both. A nod of the head or a yawn is an example of a nonverbal response. Either way, feedback allows the sender to validate that the intended message has been received and correctly understood and, if not, then it provides the sender an opportunity to correct or reword a message. In the case of Mr. Johnson, who was told that he would have to wait an hour for his pain medication, the receiver may appear irritated and say, "Well, the nurse on the other shift gives me my pain medication early if I need it." The sender then knows the message was interpreted accurately. However, now the original sender becomes the receiver, who is required to decode and respond.

Modes of Communication

Communication is generally carried out in two different modes: verbal and nonverbal. **Verbal communication** uses the spoken or written word; **nonverbal communication** uses other forms, such as gestures, facial expressions, and touch. Although both kinds of communication occur concurrently, the majority of communication is nonverbal. Learning about nonverbal communication helps the nurse develop effective communication patterns and relationships with patients. A mode of communication that has evolved with technology is **electronic communication**. Email is perhaps the most common form of electronic communication, although social networking and text messaging are used frequently outside the workplace. It is important for the nurse to know when it is appropriate and not appropriate to use email and other forms of electronic communication to communicate with patients.

Verbal Communication

Because individuals choose the words they use, verbal communication is largely a conscious and purposeful activity. Words and phrasing used vary among individuals according to culture, socioeconomic background, age, and education. An abundance of words can be used to form messages. In addition, a wide variety of feelings can be conveyed when people talk. As a result, countless possibilities exist for the way ideas and information can be exchanged.

When choosing what words to say or write, the nurse needs to consider pace and intonation, simplicity, clarity and brevity, timing and relevance, adaptability, credibility, and humor.

Pace and Intonation

The manner of speech, as in the pace or rhythm and intonation, will affect the feeling and impact of the message. The intonation can express enthusiasm, joy, sadness, anger, or amusement. The pace of speech may indicate interest, anxiety, boredom, or fear. For example, speaking slowly and softly may help calm an excited patient.

Simplicity

Simplicity of speech refers to the use of commonly understood words, brevity, and completeness. Words such as *vasoconstriction* or *cholecystectomy* are meaningful to the nurse and may be easy for the nurse to use, but they are not meaningful to patients who have no background in healthcare. Nurses need to learn to select understandable terms that are appropriate for the developmental stage, knowledge, culture, and education of the patient. For example, instead of saying to a patient, "The nurses will be catheterizing you tomorrow for a urine analysis," it may be better to say, "Tomorrow we need to get a sample of your urine, so we will collect it by putting a small tube into your bladder." The latter statement is simpler and therefore easier to understand. It is more likely to convey to the patient why the procedure is needed and whether it will be uncomfortable.

Clarity and Brevity

The most effective type of message is one that is direct and simple. *Clarity* is saying precisely what is meant, and *brevity* is using the fewest words necessary. Using clarity and brevity results in a message that is simple and clear. An aspect of this is **congruent communication**, in which the nurse's behavior or nonverbal communication is congruent (consistent) with the words spoken. When the nurse tells the patient, "I am interested in hearing what you have to say," the nurse should use nonverbal behavior that includes facing the patient, making eye contact (if culturally appropriate), and leaning forward. The goal is to communicate clearly so that all aspects of a situation or circumstance are understood. To ensure clarity in communication, the nurse also needs to speak slowly and enunciate carefully. Note that careful enunciation does not require speaking loudly. Speaking loudly to a patient, even if the patient is hard of hearing, especially in a quiet setting, may be experienced by the patient as patronizing or aggressive. This can undermine the nurse–patient relationship.

Timing and Relevance

The nurse needs to be aware of both relevance and timing when communicating with patients. No matter how clearly or simply words are stated or written, the timing needs to be appropriate to ensure that the words are heard and understood. Moreover, the message needs to relate to the person who is the receiver or to the person's interests. This requires the nurse to be sensitive to the patient's needs and concerns. For example, a patient whose current focus is her fear of cancer may not hear the nurse's explanations about the upcoming gallbladder surgery. In this situation, the nurse should first encourage the patient to express her concerns and then deal with those concerns. The necessary explanations can be provided after the patient's primary fears have been addressed or at another time when the patient is able to listen.

Adaptability

Nurses must alter spoken messages in response to behavioral cues from the patient. This adjustment is referred to as *adaptability*. Nurses carefully consider and individualize what they say and how they say it. This requires both astute assessment and sensitivity. For example, suppose that a nurse who usually smiles, appears cheerful, and greets a patient with an enthusiastic "Hi, Mrs. Brown!" notices that the patient is not smiling and appears distressed. In this situation, the nurse should modify her tone of speech and express concern via her facial expressions while moving toward the patient.

Credibility

Credibility is the quality of being truthful, trustworthy, and reliable. Credibility is essential to effective communication. Nurses foster credibility by being consistent, dependable, and honest. Nurses need to be knowledgeable about the topic being discussed and to have accurate information. Nurses should convey confidence and certainty in what they are saying, while being able to acknowledge their limitations (e.g., "I don't know the answer to that, but I will find out").

Humor

Humor can be a positive and powerful tool in the nurse–patient relationship, but it must be used with care. Humor can be used to help patients adjust to difficult and painful situations. The physical act of laughter can provide an emotional and physical release, reducing tension by providing a different perspective and promoting a sense of well-being. However, in using humor, it is important to consider the patient's perception of what is considered funny. Timing is also important. For instance, inappropriate use of humor can serve to minimize patient concerns or anxieties. Although humor and laughter can help reduce stress and anxiety, the feelings of the patient should guide the nurse's use of humor (Tremayne, 2014).

Nonverbal Communication

Nonverbal communication is sometimes called *body language*. It includes gestures, body movements, use of touch, and physical appearance, including adornment. Nonverbal communication often conveys more about what an individual is feeling than what the person actually says, because nonverbal behavior is controlled less consciously than verbal behavior (**Figure 38–3 》**). Nonverbal communication can either reinforce or contradict what is said verbally. For example, if a nurse says to a patient, "I'd be happy to sit here and talk to you for a while," yet glances at the door every few seconds, the nurse's actions contradict the verbal message. The patient is more likely to believe the nonverbal behavior, which conveys "I am very busy and need to leave." By contrast, when the nurse enters the patient's room and finds the patient crying, if the nurse pulls a chair close to the bed and says quietly, "I can see how upset you are, tell me what is bothering you," the nurse conveys the

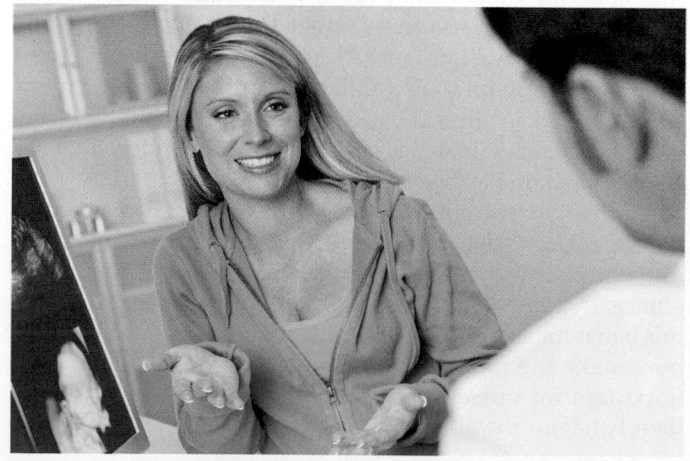

Source: Asiseeit/E+/Getty Images.

Figure 38–3 》 Nonverbal communication sometimes conveys meaning more effectively than words. This patient is clearly receptive to the healthcare provider's message.

message that the nurse cares and has the time and willingness to listen to the patient.

Observing and interpreting a patient's nonverbal behavior is an essential skill that nurses must develop. The efficient observation of nonverbal behavior requires a systematic assessment of the individual's overall physical appearance, posture, gait, facial expressions, and gestures.

Patients who have altered thought processes, such as patients with schizophrenia or dementia, may experience times when expressing themselves verbally is difficult or impossible. During these times, the nurse needs to be able to interpret the feeling or emotion that the patient is expressing nonverbally. An attentive nurse who clarifies observations very often portrays caring and acceptance to the patient. This can be a beginning for establishing a trusting relationship between the nurse and the patient, even for patients who have difficulty communicating appropriately.

Patients who are on the autism spectrum will likely have difficulty understanding nonverbal communication. Many individuals with autism find eye contact difficult, so they avoid it when communicating. When a nurse is speaking to a patient with autism, the nurse's communications should be direct and specific. The nurse should select words carefully, keeping in mind that the patient may not understand any nonverbal messages that may be communicated along with the words. It is critical for nurses to assess patients' communication abilities and communicate in ways that are most likely to result in successful communication with the patient.

Nonverbal communication varies widely among cultures. Even for behaviors such as smiling and handshaking, cultures differ. For example, many people feel that smiling and handshaking are an integral part of an interaction and essential to establishing trust. The same behavior might be perceived by others as insolent and frivolous. Refer to the module on Culture and Diversity for more information on cultural differences.

The nurse cannot always be sure of the correct interpretation of feelings that have been expressed nonverbally. The same feeling can be expressed nonverbally in more than one way, even within the same cultural group. For example, anger may be communicated by aggressive or excessive body motion, or it may be communicated by frozen stillness. In some cultures, a smile may be used to conceal anger. Therefore, the interpretation of such observations requires validation with the patient. For example, the nurse might say, "You look as though you have been crying. Is something upsetting you?"

Personal Appearance

Clothing and accessories can be sources of information about an individual. Although choice of apparel is highly personal, it may convey social and financial status, culture, religion, group association, and self-concept (**Figure 38–4 》**). Charms and amulets may be worn for decorative or for health protection purposes. When the symbolic meaning of an object is unfamiliar, the nurse can inquire about the object's significance. This may foster rapport with the patient and help the nurse gain a better understanding of the patient's beliefs.

How an individual dresses is often an indicator of how the person feels. Someone who is ill may not have the energy or the desire to maintain his normal level of grooming. When

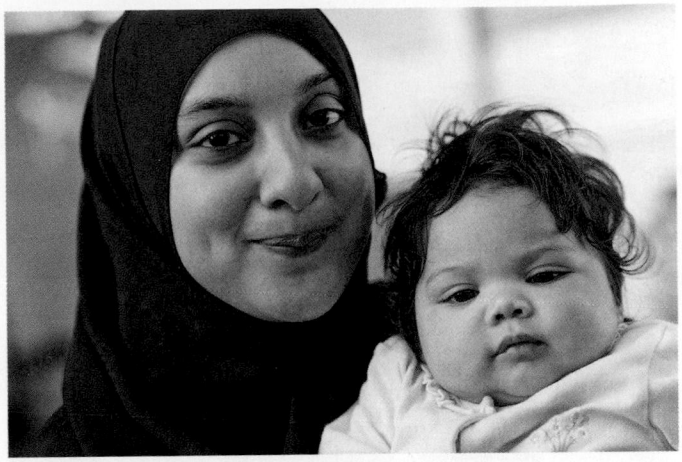

Source: Yuri Arcurs/E+/Getty Images.

Figure 38–4 》 Women who are Muslims may wear a headscarf as part of their hijab (proper clothing) to preserve their modesty. Muslim women may wear the hijab to reflect their devotion to God or as a means to express their Muslim identity. Not all Muslim women wear headscarves; many choose not to veil. In many American families who practice Islam, it is the woman's choice whether to wear a hijab (Arabs in America, n.d.).

someone known for immaculate grooming becomes lax about appearance, the nurse may suspect a loss of self-esteem, depression, or a physical illness. The nurse must validate these observed nonverbal data by asking the patient about them. For acutely ill patients in hospital or home care settings, a change in grooming habits or a desire to take a shower and dress may signal that the patient is feeling better.

Posture and Gait

The ways in which individuals walk and carry themselves are often reliable indicators of self-concept, current mood, and health. Erect posture and an active, purposeful stride suggest a feeling of well-being. Slouched posture and a slow, shuffling gait suggest depression or physical discomfort. Tense posture and a rapid, determined gait suggest anxiety or anger. The posture of individuals when they are sitting or lying can also indicate feelings or mood. Again, the nurse clarifies the meaning of the observed behavior by describing to the patient what the nurse sees and then asking what it means or whether the nurse's interpretation is correct. For example, "You look like it really hurts you to move. I'm wondering how your pain is and if you might need something to make you more comfortable?"

Facial Expression

No part of the body is as expressive as the face (see **Figure 38–5 》**). Feelings of surprise, fear, anger, disgust, happiness, and sadness can be conveyed by facial expressions. Although the face may express the person's genuine emotions, it is also possible to control these muscles so the emotion expressed does not reflect what the person is feeling. When the message is not clear, it is important to get feedback to be sure of the intent of the expression. No single expression can be interpreted accurately without considering other reinforcing physical cues, the setting in which the expression

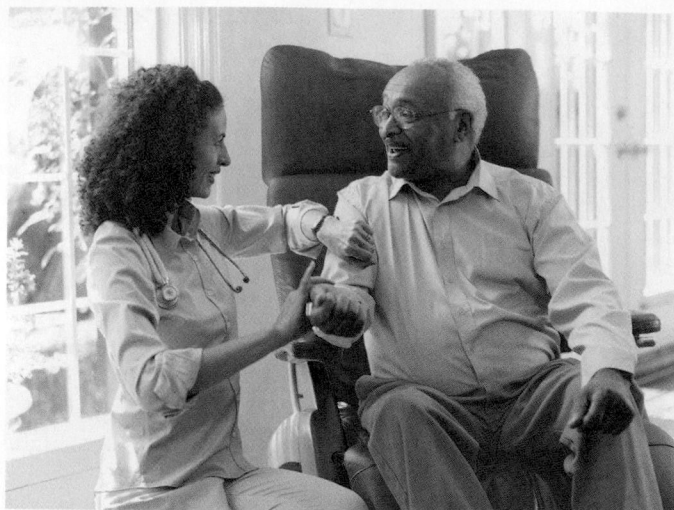

Source: Fuse/Corbis/Getty Images.

Figure 38–5 》 The nurse's facial expression communicates warmth and caring.

occurs, the expression of others in the same setting, and the cultural background of the patient.

Nurses need to be aware of their own expressions and what they are communicating to others. Patients are quick to notice a nurse's facial expression, particularly when the patient feels unsure or uncomfortable. The patient who questions the nurse about a feared diagnostic result will watch whether the nurse maintains eye contact or looks away when answering. The patient who has had disfiguring surgery will examine the nurse's face for signs of disgust. It is impossible to control all facial expressions, but the nurse must learn to control expressions of feelings such as fear or disgust in some circumstances.

Eye contact is another essential element of facial communication. In many cultures, mutual eye contact acknowledges recognition of the other person and a willingness to maintain communication. (See the module on Culture and Diversity.) In other cultures, direct eye contact is considered impolite. Often an individual initiates contact with another person with a glance, capturing the person's attention prior to communicating. However, a patient who averts his eyes may be signaling embarrassment or that the patient views the nature of the contact as threatening.

Gestures

Hand and body gestures may emphasize and clarify the spoken word, or they may occur without words to indicate a particular feeling or to give a sign. A father awaiting information about his daughter in surgery may wring his hands, tap his foot, pick at his nails, or pace back and forth. A gesture may indicate the size or shape of an object. Some gestures, such as waving goodbye or motioning to someone to have a seat, have relatively universal meanings. Other gestures, however, are culture specific. The Anglo American gesture meaning "shoo" or "go away" means "come here" or "come back" in some Asian cultures. In the Hmong culture, it is considered rude to point at something with your toe.

For individuals with special communication problems, such as those with hearing impairments, the hands are central

to communication. Many individuals who are deaf learn sign language, in which the hands are used along with facial expressions and other body language to form expressions with accepted meanings. Similarly, individuals who are unable to reply verbally may be able to communicate using their hands. For example, the patient who is intubated may be able to raise an index finger once for "yes" and twice for "no." Other signals can often be devised by the patient and the nurse to denote various meanings.

Electronic Communication

Nurses are increasingly using electronic communication media such as email, social media, and text messaging to communicate with patients, other nurses, other departments in their employment setting, and resources outside the employment setting. It is important for nurses to follow their agency's guidelines for the use of electronic communication and to understand the advantages and disadvantages of these media.

Advantages

Electronic communication has many advantages. As Kern and colleagues (2013) note, among organizations adopting electronic communication, researchers discovered that "changing clinical workflows to allow documentation into structured fields had a large effect on accuracy of electronic reporting, enabling corrections of rates of recommended care."

The use of email between providers and patients is becoming increasingly popular. The advantages of one-to-one email communication between nurses and patients are numerous, from email's instantaneous nature to the fact that email addresses tend to change less frequently than residential addresses. Additional benefits of email include increased efficiency, strengthened patient–provider communications, and informed decision making. Mass emailing provides still more benefits to healthcare providers, including the ability to automatically send condition-specific and stage-specific messages related to patients' diagnoses. Some healthcare facilities provide information to their patients on how to reach specified staff members by email. This improves communication and continuity of patient care.

Social networks such as Facebook and Twitter are less commonly used in healthcare, but they represent an important opportunity for the distribution of less critical health information. Nurses can use social networks to connect with colleagues worldwide for continuous learning through organizations such as the American Nurses Association. Posts on hospital Facebook and Twitter pages can provide followers with helpful information about community events such as health fairs or reminders about influenza vaccinations. During natural disasters, emergency management personnel and healthcare facilities may use social media as an additional method for sharing critically important information (such as evacuation orders and the location of shelters or medical care facilities).

Text messaging is another new frontier in electronic communication for healthcare providers, and it offers the benefits of convenience, ubiquity, immediacy, monitoring of symptoms, dissemination of emergency alerts, and multimedia capability. In communicating with patients, text messaging has been useful for disseminating public service announcements. Between nurses and other healthcare providers, text messaging can provide a convenient and low-cost means of electronic communication.

Disadvantages

The primary disadvantage of electronic communications media is the risk to patient confidentiality. The Health Insurance Portability and Accountability Act (HIPAA) requires organizations to apply "reasonable and appropriate safeguards" when emailing protected health information (PHI). Each healthcare agency needs to have an email encryption system to ensure security. An agency may use its own system or outsource an encryption service. Other disadvantages of email include problems incorporating electronic communications with patients into the electronic medical record and dangers that can arise if a provider overlooks a critical email communication from a patient.

Another disadvantage is one of socioeconomics. Not everyone has a computer or a cell phone capable of accessing the internet. And even if internet access is possible, not everyone has the necessary computer skills. Email and social media may enhance communication with some patients, but others will not have access to it at all. Alternative forms of communication will be needed for patients who have limited access to or limited abilities with using the internet.

The major drawbacks of text messaging in a healthcare context are related to its strengths of ubiquity and instantaneousness. Nurses who constantly receive work-related text messages may check their messages at inappropriate times or even use their devices for personal messages while at work. This can prove to be a barrier to effective communications with patients.

When Not to Use Electronic Communications Media

In certain situations, the use of electronic communication should be avoided:

- When the information is urgent and the patient's health could be in jeopardy if the patient doesn't read the message immediately
- When the information is highly confidential (e.g., HIV status, mental health, chemical dependency)
- When lab data are abnormal. If the information is likely to be confusing and could prompt many questions, it is better to either see or telephone the patient.

Other Guidelines

Agencies usually develop standards and guidelines for the use of electronic media in healthcare. It is important for nurses to know their employer's guidelines regarding the use of electronic media to communicate with patients. In the case of email, the patient is asked to sign an email consent form. This form provides information about the risks of email and authorizes the health agency to communicate with the patient at a specified email address. The website of the National Council of State Boards of Nursing also provides guidance to nurses on the use of social and electronic media in healthcare.

The nurse should indicate in the subject line that the email is confidential. It may also be prudent to include a disclaimer in the email stating that the message is to be read only by the person to whom it is addressed and that no one else is authorized to read the message. In addition, the disclaimer should state that if the email is sent to anyone else by mistake, the recipient should contact the sender.

Information sent to a patient via email is considered part of the patient's medical record. Therefore, a copy of the email needs to be put in the patient's chart. Emails, like other documentation in the patient's record, may be used as evidence during litigation. Rules for written communication (see the next section) also apply to email communication.

Email is another form of communication that can enhance effective relationships with patients. It is not, however, a substitute for effective in-person communication. The nurse needs to use professional judgment about what form(s) of communication will best meet the patient's health needs.

Written Communication

Written communication can be considered a form of verbal communication. Examples of forms of written communication include notes, letters, email messages, and text messages. Written communication has some limitations. For example, it lacks the nonverbal cues that accompany verbal communication. For example, you may receive a text message from a friend that says, "GET OUT OF HERE!!" Without an understanding of context, this message could be interpreted as shock and disbelief at something you told your friend, or anger and the wish for you to vacate the friend's life, or a request to be left alone. Only by hearing tone of voice and seeing body language can context be relayed. As a result, rules for written communication differ from rules for other forms of communicating.

Nurses have many requirements as well as opportunities for written communication. The most common form of written communication in nursing is the notes nurses make in the medical record about a patient's status, which are discussed in Exemplar 38.C on documentation. Nurses also write discharge instructions for patients and their families, memos to nursing colleagues and other healthcare professionals, and patient educational materials. Nurse-managers write employee evaluations, policies and procedures, and other communications to administrators, colleagues, and nursing staff. An important consideration in written communication is that decoding often occurs when the writer is not present and may occur long after the document is written. Therefore, clarity is important because it may not be possible to ask questions or process areas of confusion.

Characteristics of Effective Written Communication

In addition to simplicity, brevity, clarity, relevance, credibility, and humor (characteristics of effective oral communication), written communication must contain the following:

1. ***Appropriate language and terminology.*** Language and terminology must be appropriate for the developmental age, education and reading level, and culture of the reader. Health education materials written for children should be different from materials written for adults. For individuals whose primary language is not English, it may be more effective to have written materials translated into their primary language by a professional translator. Extensive use of illustrations can also aid in communication. Appropriate lay terminology may be substituted for medical terminology; for example, *high blood pressure* may be used instead of *hypertension*. National standards for culturally and linguistically appropriate services in health and healthcare (CLAS) are listed in **Box 38–1 》**.

》 **Stay Current:** For more information regarding the CLAS standards, go to https://www.thinkculturalhealth.hhs.gov/pdfs/EnhancedCLASStandardsBlueprint.pdf.

2. ***Correct grammar, spelling, and punctuation.*** The use of correct grammar, spelling, and punctuation provides clarity for the reader. Misspelled words, misplaced punctuation, and incorrect grammar can change the intended meaning, cause confusion, and undermine the reader's confidence in the sender.

3. ***Logical organization.*** Written materials are well organized when they are logical and easy for readers to follow. Simple and foundational information is usually provided first, followed by more complex information. Using examples can also assist readers.

4. ***Appropriate use and citation of resources.*** Information taken from other sources must always be credited to the original source. Failure to reference work taken from another writer is called plagiarism, is considered unethical, and may violate copyright laws. Various styles of referencing are in use, including the Modern

---

Box 38–1

National Standards for Culturally and Linguistically Appropriate Services in Health and Health Care (CLAS)

Standard 1: Provide effective, equitable, understandable, and respectful quality care and services that are responsive to diverse cultural health beliefs and practices, preferred languages, health literacy, and other communication needs.

Standard 2: Advance and sustain organizational governance and leadership that promotes CLAS and health equity through policy, practices, and allocated resources.

Standard 3: Recruit, promote, and support a culturally and linguistically diverse governance, leadership, and workforce that are responsive to the population in the service area.

Standard 4: Educate and train governance, leadership, and workforce in culturally and linguistically appropriate policies and practices on an ongoing basis.

Standard 5: Offer language assistance to individuals who have limited English proficiency and/or other communication needs, at no cost to them, to facilitate timely access to all health care and services.

Standard 6: Inform all individuals of the availability of language assistance services clearly and in their preferred language, verbally and in writing.

Standard 7: Ensure the competence of individuals providing language assistance, recognizing that the use of untrained individuals and/or minors as interpreters should be avoided.

Standard 8: Provide easy-to-understand print and multimedia materials and signage in the languages commonly used by the populations in the service area.

Standard 9: Establish culturally and linguistically appropriate goals, policies, and management accountability, and infuse them throughout the organization's planning and operations.

Standard 10: Conduct ongoing assessments of the organization's CLAS-related activities and integrate CLAS-related measures into measurement and continuous quality improvement activities.

Standard 11: Collect and maintain accurate and reliable demographic data to monitor and evaluate the impact of CLAS on health equity and outcomes and to inform service delivery.

Standard 12: Conduct regular assessments of community health assets and needs and use the results to plan and implement services that respond to the cultural and linguistic diversity of populations in the service area.

Standard 13: Partner with the community to design, implement, and evaluate policies, practices, and services to ensure cultural and linguistic appropriateness.

Standard 14: Create conflict and grievance resolution processes that are culturally and linguistically appropriate to identify, prevent, and resolve conflicts or complaints.

Standard 15: Communicate the organization's progress in implementing and sustaining CLAS to all stakeholders, constituents, and the general public.

Source: Based on Office of Minority Health. (2013). *National standards for culturally and linguistically appropriate services in health and health care: A blueprint for advancing and sustaining CLAS policy and practice.* Retrieved from https://www.thinkculturalhealth.hhs.gov/pdfs/EnhancedCLASStandardsBlueprint.pdf; Jacobs, C. G. (2012). *National standards for culturally and linguistically appropriate services in healthcare: Ensuring quality health care for all.* Retrieved from http://www.diversity-connection.org/diversityconnection/leadership-conferences/2012%20Conf%20Docs/Enchancing_Health_Care_with_CLAS.pdf; The National CLAS Standards. (2013). Retrieved from http://www.hdassoc.org/wp-content/uploads/2013/03/CLAS_handout-pdf_april-24.pdf.

Language Association (MLA), American Medical Association (AMA), and the American Psychological Association (APA) styles. Another benefit of citing references is that readers who want additional information can turn to the references listed.

Concepts Related to Communication

Communication is a concept that relates to every healthcare concept and is used in every healthcare setting. Communication is the cornerstone of patient care, and nurses, along with all healthcare providers, must be mindful of their communication techniques when providing care, regardless of setting. Communication binds healthcare workers, patients, and institutions together and is the means through which nurses provide both hospital-based and community-based care. Nurses should keep in mind the patient's needs and limitations and always take care to use technical terms and medical terminology judiciously during communication (Kourkouta & Papathanasiou, 2014). Listening is an essential component in nursing communication, and it is the foundation of responsible nursing practice. When listening, nurses should assess both the verbal and nonverbal statements of the patient. By being attentive to unspoken needs, nurses can enhance nursing diagnoses and the quality of care.

One of the most important components of providing effective communication in real-world nursing practice is tailoring communication efforts to the particular situation of the patient. Patients will vary dramatically in their ability to communicate and listen effectively at the time of treatment. Physiologic illness, cognitive impairment, substance abuse, mental illness, the emotional context of the healthcare encounter, and linguistic and cultural differences are all factors that can affect a patient's ability to communicate with the healthcare team. In all cases, the nurse is responsible for ensuring successful communication and for advocating for patients who are unable to advocate for themselves. The Concepts Related to Communication feature provides examples of some of the many concepts integral to communication. They are presented in alphabetical order.

Factors Influencing the Communication Process

Many factors influence the communication process. Some of these are development, gender, sociocultural characteristics, values and perceptions, personal space, territoriality, roles and relationships, environment, congruence, and attitudes.

Development

As individuals grow and develop, language and communication skills develop through various stages. It is important for the nurse to understand the developmental processes related to speech, language, and communication skills. Knowledge of the patient's developmental stage enables the nurse to select appropriate communication strategies. For example, when communicating with infants and toddlers whose language skills are not well developed, the nurse may rely more on the child's nonverbal communications to assess comfort and pain. The nurse may hold the child and use touch to provide comfort and demonstrate caring. For older children, the nurse may use pictures as an adjunct to verbal language to communicate. For adolescents and adults, the nurse is more able to rely on verbal language for communication. With older adults, physical changes associated with the aging process may affect communication. For example, it may be more effective to use visual communication methods for patients who have hearing impairments or aural communication methods for patients who have visual impairments. Also, intellectual processes develop across the lifespan as individuals acquire knowledge and experience. The knowledge and experiences that individuals have will influence their understanding and acceptance of transmitted information and feelings. The Lifespan Considerations section discusses some aspects of communicating with children as they grow from infancy to adolescence.

Gender

From an early age, females and males may exhibit differences in language development and communication tendencies. Examples often cited include the tendency of females to make requests and males to make demands, of males to address issues more directly and females to be more active listeners, often using statements that encourage a response. **Active listening**, also known as *attentive* or *mindful listening*, involves fully concentrating on both the content and emotion of a person's message, rather than just passively hearing the words a person says. (For more information on this topic, see Exemplar 38.B: Therapeutic Communication.) Although it has long been believed that these perceived differences result from psychosocial development, more recent research indicates that language development proceeds differently in girls than boys, indicating that both neuronal factors and psychosocial factors influence language and communication differences (Kaushanskaja, Gross, & Buac, 2013).

When working with patients or colleagues, nurses should be aware that men and women might interpret the same communication differently. Thus, nurses should always work to assess the ways in which a patient's or colleague's communication is gendered. Maintaining an understanding of the ways in which people communicate differently because of their socialization allows the nurse to respond accordingly.

An emerging area of awareness in healthcare communities is communicating with transgender individuals and individuals who identify as nonbinary or gender noncomforming (identifying as neither male nor female). In everyone, gender identity (how one sees oneself), gender expression (the outward expression of an individual's sense of maleness or femaleness), biological sex (one's anatomy), and sexual attraction (to whom one is sexually attracted) are distinct, and each element of identity can be well-defined or ambiguous. Transgender individuals who have not had sex reassignment surgery have a gender identity that may not align with their biological sex, and therefore, their name or appearance may not "match" their stated (or legal) sex. The nurse should always use a patient's preferred name and pronoun (whether "he," "she," "them," or something else) and guard the patient's privacy. By protecting the privacy and personal expression of transgender and nonbinary individuals and treating them with respect, nurses can reduce undue stress, promote the therapeutic

Concepts Related to
Communication

CONCEPT	RELATIONSHIP TO COMMUNICATION	NURSING IMPLICATIONS
Advocacy	Communication among nurses, patients, and physicians is a key component of effective healthcare. In addition to communication with patients, nurses directly or indirectly influence physician–patient communications.	▪ Assess what the healthcare provider has told the patient regarding the patient's condition. ▪ Encourage the patient to clarify the understanding with the healthcare provider. ▪ Help the patient identify and access high-quality sources of healthcare information. ▪ Always advocate for the best interests of the patient and the patient's expressed wishes.
Comfort	Pain → communication ability. Impaired communication may ↓ ability to report pain.	▪ Take patient's report of pain levels seriously. ▪ Assess for nonverbal signs of pain such as wincing and guarding. ▪ Communicate equally with patients across the lifespan. ▪ Use a pain management scale such as a numeric rating scale or the FACES pain rating scale that is appropriate for the patient's age and ability to communicate. ▪ Investigate palliative care options for patients at the end of life.
Grief and Loss	Grief or loss can adversely affect the way in which an individual communicates. Not only does the person experiencing the loss have trouble communicating needs to others, but others often do not know how to communicate their condolences to those who have experienced a loss. Cultural differences can exacerbate communication issues.	▪ Determine the effects of the loss on the patient. If the patient is grieving the loss of a primary caregiver or a spouse who provided financially for the patient, the patient may have a number of immediate needs. ▪ Consider the stages of grief when communicating with patients. ▪ Consider the cultural background of the patient and family related to expressions of grief and loss.
Intracranial Regulation	Impaired intracranial regulation → impaired communication. Traumatic brain injury → difficulty with word finding, sentence formation, and expression. Patients with severe increased intracranial pressure may enter a coma state.	▪ Recognize the communication difficulties caused by traumatic brain injuries early and respond appropriately. ▪ Help the patient with cognitive and/or physical limitations find an appropriate therapist to help them regain lost abilities. ▪ If patients have difficulty expressing their thoughts, calmly help them find ways of communicating.
Mood and Affect	A diagnosis of mental illness ↑ likelihood patient will experience discrimination/stigma, may ↑ reluctance to trust healthcare personnel. In addition, healthcare providers may miss signs that these patients are suffering from these disorders.	▪ Be aware that people of all ages suffer from mental and psychiatric disorders. ▪ Do not assume that someone does not have one of these conditions because of their physical appearance. ▪ Screen patients for depression or other psychiatric illness by asking open-ended questions with empathy. ▪ Research medical records for histories of mental illness and cognitive issues and shape communication appropriately. ▪ Be consistent and predictable in your nursing practice and communication.
Oxygenation	Decreased O_2 → hypoxemia → decreased level of consciousness (LOC) → decreased ability to communicate verbally (due to shortness of breath and LOC) and nonverbally (due to decreased LOC).	▪ Position patient in Fowler or semi-Fowler position as indicated to promote ease of breathing. ▪ Administer medications and supplemental oxygen as ordered. ▪ Consider other methods of communication for the patient (e.g., a tablet, a family member).
Safety	Impaired communication ↑ risk for illness and injury.	▪ Create a supportive environment that promotes communication and safety. ▪ Introduce opportunities for the patient to communicate needs and concerns. ▪ Be tactful and avoid abrupt, offensive, and accusatory statements. ▪ Maintain a nonthreatening approach and validate cooperation. ▪ Listen to the concerns of other members of the healthcare team. ▪ Apologize when needed. ▪ Agree when possible. ▪ Encourage the team to follow national standards.

relationship, and help these individuals feel safe in healthcare contexts (Booth, 2014).

Sociocultural Characteristics

Culture, education, and economic level can influence communication. Nonverbal communication characteristics such as body language, eye contact, and touch are influenced by cultural beliefs about appropriate communication behavior. Some cultures may believe that direct eye contact is disrespectful, whereas other cultures believe that direct eye contact shows trustworthiness. In some cultures touch would be appropriate to communicate caring and concern, but in other cultures physical touch would be offensive. Verbal communication may be difficult for the receiver whose primary language is not that of the sender. More information about the influence of culture on communication can be found in the module on Culture and Diversity.

An individual's level of education may affect the extent of that individual's vocabulary or ability to read written communication. Economic level may affect an individual's ability to access written or electronic communication, including email and the internet.

Values and Perceptions

Values are the standards that influence behavior, and **perceptions** are the personal views of an event. Because each person has unique personality traits, values, and life experiences, each will perceive and interpret messages and experiences differently. For example, if a nurse draws the curtains around a crying woman and leaves her alone, the woman may interpret this as either "The nurse thinks that I will upset others and that I shouldn't cry" or "The nurse respects my need to be alone." It is important for the nurse to be aware of a patient's values and to validate or correct perceptions to avoid creating barriers in the nurse–patient relationship.

Personal Space

Personal space is the distance individuals prefer to keep between themselves and others during interactions. **Proxemics** is the study of distance between individuals who are interacting. Many living in North America use definite distances in various interpersonal relationships, along with specific voice tones and body language. Communication thus alters in accordance with four distances in this culture, each with a close and a far phase (Samovar et al., 2016):

1. *Intimate:* touching to $1\frac{1}{2}$ feet
2. *Personal:* $1\frac{1}{2}$–4 feet
3. *Social:* 4–12 feet
4. *Public:* 12–15 feet

Intimate distance communication is characterized by body contact, heightened sensations of body heat and smell, and vocalizations that are low. Vision is intense, restricted to a small body part, and may be distorted. Nurses frequently use intimate distance. Examples include cuddling a baby, positioning a patient, observing an incision, and giving an injection. It is a natural protective instinct for individuals to maintain a certain amount of space immediately around them. That amount varies with individuals and cultures. When someone who wants to communicate moves too close,

the receiver automatically steps back a pace or two. In their therapeutic roles, nurses often are required to violate this personal space. However, it is important for the nurse to know when this will occur and to inform the patient in advance.

Personal distance is less overwhelming than intimate distance. At personal distance, voice tones are moderate, and body heat and smell are less noticeable. Physical contact such as a handshake or touching a shoulder is possible. Because more of the individual is experienced at a personal distance, nonverbal behaviors such as body stance or full facial expressions are seen with less distortion. Much communication between nurses and patients occurs at this distance. Examples include when the nurse is sitting with a patient, giving medications, or establishing an intravenous infusion. Communication at a close personal distance can convey involvement by facilitating the sharing of thoughts and feelings. On the other hand, it can also create tension if the distance encroaches on the other person's personal space (**Figure 38–6 »**). At the outer extreme of 4 feet, however, less involvement is conveyed. Bantering and some social conversations usually take place at this distance.

Social distance is characterized by a clear visual perception of the whole person. Body heat and odor are imperceptible, eye contact is increased, and vocalizations are loud enough to be overheard by others. Communication is therefore more formal and is limited to seeing and hearing. The person is protected and out of reach of touch or personal sharing of thoughts or feelings. Social distance allows more activity and movement back and forth. It is expedient for communicating with several individuals at the same time or within a short time. Examples include when the nurse makes rounds or waves a greeting to someone. Social distance is important in accomplishing the business of the day; however, it is frequently misused. For example, the nurse who stands in the doorway and asks a patient, "How are you today?" will receive a more noncommittal reply than the nurse who moves to a personal distance to make the same inquiry.

Public distance requires loud, clear vocalizations with careful enunciation. Although the faces and forms of people

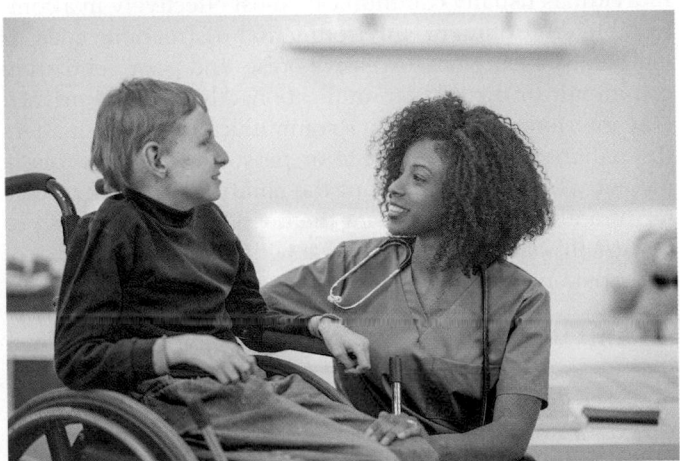

Source: Fat Camera/E+/Getty Images.

Figure 38–6 » Personal space influences communication in social and professional interactions. Encroachment into another individual's personal space may create tension.

are visible at public distance, individuality is lost. Instead, the perception is of the group of people or the community.

Territoriality

Territoriality is a concept of the space and things that an individual considers as belonging to the self. Territories marked off by individuals may be visible to others. For example, patients in a hospital often consider their territory as bounded by the curtains around the bed unit or by the walls of a private room. All healthcare workers must recognize this human tendency to claim territory. Patients often feel the need to defend their territory when it is invaded by others. For example, when a nurse removes a chair to use at another bed, the nurse has inadvertently violated the territoriality of the patient whose chair was removed. The nurse needs to obtain permission from the patient to remove, rearrange, or borrow objects in the patient's hospital area.

Roles and Relationships

The roles and the relationships between sender and receiver affect the communication process. Roles such as nursing student and instructor, patient and primary care provider, or parent and child affect content and responses in the communication process. Choice of words, sentence structure, message content and channel, body language, and tone of voice vary considerably from role to role. In addition, the specific relationship between the communicators is significant. The nurse who is meeting with a patient for the first time communicates differently from the nurse who has previously developed a relationship with that patient. The nurse may choose a more informal or comfortable stance when communicating with patients or colleagues and a more formal stance when communicating with physicians or administrators. The length of the relationship may also affect communication. For example, the nurse may use more formal language and stance when meeting a patient or colleague for the first time and a more relaxed posture when interacting with those whom the nurse has an established relationship.

Environment

Individuals usually communicate most effectively in a comfortable environment. Environmental distractions such as temperature extremes, excessive noise, and poor ventilation can impair or distort communication. Also, lack of privacy may interfere with a patient's communication about matters the patient considers private or personal. For example, a patient who is worried about the ability of his wife to care for him after discharge from the hospital may not wish to discuss this concern with a nurse within hearing distance of other patients, staff, or his wife.

Congruence

Patients more readily trust the nurse when they perceive the nurse's communication as congruent. This also helps prevent miscommunication. Congruence between verbal and nonverbal expression is easily observed by both the nurse and patient. Nurses are taught to assess patients, but patients are often just as adept at reading a nurse's expression or body language. If there is any incongruence, the true meaning is usually conveyed by the sender's body language. For example, when teaching a patient how to care for a colostomy, the

nurse might say, "You won't have any problem with this." However, if the nurse looks worried or disgusted while saying this, the patient is less likely to trust the nurse's words.

Nurses must strive to improve their nonverbal communication skills. One strategy is to refrain from indiscriminate use of nonverbal gestures, such as the overuse of smiling or nodding the head, because this can cause the patient to doubt the nurse's sincerity. Another strategy is to convey a relaxed attitude, rather than a distressed attitude. Being relaxed makes it easier for patients to feel at ease around the nurse.

Interpersonal Attitudes

Attitudes convey beliefs, thoughts, and feelings about people and events. Attitudes are communicated convincingly and rapidly to others. Attitudes such as caring, warmth, respect, and acceptance facilitate communication, whereas condescension, lack of interest, and coldness inhibit communication.

Kourkouta and Papathanasiou (2014) found that effective nursing communication is significantly related to patient satisfaction. When nurses communicate (both verbally and nonverbally) warmth, positivity, energy, and capability, patients express greater satisfaction with both competence and interpersonal care. Caring involves giving feelings, thoughts, skill, and knowledge. It requires psychologic energy and poses the risk of gaining little in return; yet by caring, both nurses and patients usually reap the benefits of greater communication and understanding.

Respect, an attitude that emphasizes the other person's worth and individuality, and *civility*, the use of courtesy in communication, are two qualities that promote effective communication. Respect conveys that the person's hopes and feelings are special and unique, even though they are similar to those of others in many ways. Being too different can be isolating and threatening. The use of civility shows respect to the individual with whom the nurse is communicating.

Healthcare providers may unknowingly show disrespect or incivility by using speech that they believe shows caring but that the patient perceives as demeaning or patronizing. This can happen in settings that provide healthcare to older adults and/or individuals with obvious physical or mental disabilities. **Elderspeak** is a style of speech similar to baby talk that sends the message to older adults that they are dependent and incompetent. It does not communicate respect. Many healthcare providers are not aware that they use elderspeak or that it can have negative meanings to the patient. The characteristics of elderspeak include use of inappropriate terms of endearment (such as "honey" or "dear"), plural pronouns (e.g., "Are we having a good day?"), tag questions, and slow, loud speech. Tag questions are short statements followed by a mini-question, such as "You feel better now, don't you?" Tag questions and other types of elderspeak should not be used with any age group. Alternative strategies to elderspeak include:

- Instead of using diminutives or terms of endearment, refer to and call the patient by full name (e.g., Ms. Applewhite) or preferred name.

- Instead of using inappropriate plural pronouns such as "we," always speak to the patient by using "you."

- Avoid tagging questions with words that would cause the patient to think that you are leading him or her to answer in a certain way. Instead, ask the question directly.

- Avoid the use of baby talk, as this is demeaning to the patient. Always address patients as the adults that they are.

Acceptance emphasizes neither approval nor disapproval. The nurse willingly receives the patient's honest feelings. An accepting attitude allows patients to express personal feelings freely and to be themselves. The nurse may need to restrict acceptance in situations in which patients' behaviors are harmful to themselves or to others. Helping the patient find appropriate behaviors for feelings is often part of patient teaching.

Barriers to Communication

Just as there are characteristics of effective communication, there are identified barriers to effective communication. Nurses need to be cognizant of these barriers and avoid them. Nurses also need to recognize the barriers when they occur and change to more effective means of communication. Failing to listen, improperly decoding the patient's intended message, and placing the nurse's needs above the patient's needs are major barriers to communication. Additional barriers to effective communication are given in **Table 38–1 》**.

TABLE 38–1 Barriers to Communication

Technique	Description	Examples
Stereotyping	Offering generalized and oversimplified beliefs about groups of individuals that are based on experiences too limited to be valid. These responses categorize patients and negate their uniqueness as individuals.	"Two-year-olds are brats." "Women are complainers." "Men don't cry." "Most people don't have any pain after this type of surgery."
Agreeing and disagreeing	Similar to judgmental responses, agreeing and disagreeing imply that the patient is either right or wrong and that the nurse is in a position to judge this. These responses deter patients from thinking through their position and may cause a patient to become defensive.	*Patient:* "I don't think Dr. Broad is a very good doctor. He doesn't seem interested in his patients." *Nurse:* "Dr. Broad is head of the department of surgery and is an excellent surgeon."
Being defensive	Attempting to protect an individual or healthcare service from negative comments. These responses prevent the patient from expressing true concerns. The nurse is saying, "You have no right to complain." Defensive responses protect the nurse from admitting weaknesses in the healthcare services, including personal weaknesses.	*Patient:* "Those night nurses must just sit around and talk all night. They didn't answer my light for over an hour." *Nurse:* "I'll have you know we literally run around on nights. You're not the only patient, you know."
Challenging	Giving a response that makes patients prove their statement or point of view. These responses indicate that the nurse is failing to consider the patient's feelings, making the patient feel it necessary to defend a position.	*Patient:* "I felt nauseated after that red pill." *Nurse:* "Surely you don't think I gave you the wrong pill?" *Patient:* "I feel as if I am dying." *Nurse:* "How can you feel that way when your pulse is 60?" *Patient:* "I believe my husband doesn't love me." *Nurse:* "You can't say that. Why, he visits you every day."
Probing	Asking for information chiefly out of curiosity rather than with the intent to assist the patient. These responses are considered prying and violate the patient's privacy. Asking "why" is often probing and places the patient in a defensive position.	*Nurse:* "Tell me about how you were sexually abused when you were a teenager." *Patient:* "I didn't ask the doctor about that when he was here." *Nurse:* "Why didn't you?"
Testing	Asking questions that make the patient admit to something. These responses permit the patient only limited answers and often meet the nurse's need rather than the patient's.	"Who do you think you are?" (forces the individual to admit to a lower status) "Do you think I am not busy?" (forces the patient to admit that the nurse really is busy)
Rejecting	Refusing to discuss certain topics with the patient. These responses often make patients feel that the nurse is rejecting not only their communication but also the patients themselves.	"I don't want to discuss that. Let's talk about. . . ." "Let's discuss other areas of interest to you rather than the two problems you keep mentioning." "I can't talk now. I'm on my way for coffee break."
Changing topics and subjects	Directing the communication into areas of self-interest rather than considering the patient's concerns is often a self-protective response to a topic that causes the nurse anxiety. These responses imply that what the nurse considers important will be discussed and that patients should not discuss certain topics.	*Patient:* "I'm separated from my wife. Do you think I can start sleeping with other women?" *Nurse:* "I see that you're 36 and that you like gardening. I bet you're looking forward to summer."
Unwarranted or false reassurance	Using clichés or comforting statements of advice as a means to reassure the patient. These responses block the fears, feelings, and other thoughts of the patient.	"You'll feel better soon." "I'm sure everything will turn out all right." "Don't worry."
Passing judgment	Giving opinions and approving or disapproving responses, moralizing, or imposing one's own values. These responses imply that the patient must think as the nurse thinks, fostering patient dependence.	"That's good (bad)." "You shouldn't do that." "That's not good enough." "What you did was wrong (right)."
Giving common advice	Telling the patient what to do. These responses deny the patient's right to be an equal partner. Note that giving expert advice that is appropriate for the patient's individual situation rather than common advice is therapeutic.	*Patient:* "Should I move from my home to a nursing home?" *Nurse:* "If I were you, I'd go to a nursing home where you'll get your meals cooked for you."

Types of Communicators

Different individuals have different ways or styles of communicating. Gender, culture, personality type, and degree of confidence can all play a role in how a nurse communicates with others. Communication is complex and requires that the nurse use a thoughtful process to communicate effectively. Communication style is something that is used daily in both the work and home environments but often is not viewed as important until there is a problem with it.

Individuals tend to express themselves in various ways. **Aggressive communicators** are those who tend to focus on their own needs and become impatient when these needs are not met. **Passive communicators** are those who focus on the needs of others. They often deny themselves any sort of power, which causes them to become frustrated. **Assertive communicators** are those who declare and affirm their opinions. In doing this, however, they respect the rights of others to communicate in the same fashion. The assertive communicator strikes a balance between the aggressive communicator and the passive communicator. It is the assertive communicator who has the most productive communication with others. **Table 38–2 》** compares and contrasts the three styles of communicating.

Individuals who use assertive communication express themselves effectively and stand up for their beliefs while respecting the rights of others (Mayo Clinic, 2014). Assertive communicators are honest, direct, and appropriate while being open to ideas and showing concern for the needs of others. They advocate for their patients. Assertive communication promotes patient safety by minimizing miscommunication with colleagues. Failure to communicate can result in negative patient outcomes.

An important characteristic of assertive communication includes the use of "I" statements versus "you" statements. The "you" statement places blame and puts the listener in a defensive position. On the other hand, the "I" statement encourages discussion. For example, a nurse who states "I am concerned about . . ." to a physician will gain the attention of the physician while also giving the message of the importance of working together for the benefit of the patient. Once the nurse has the physician's attention, it is important for the nurse to be clear, concise, organized, and fully informed when presenting the patient concern.

The passive, submissive communication style often causes rights violations. Individuals who use this style meet the demands and requests of others without regard to their own feelings and needs, as they believe their own feelings are not important. Some experts believe that individuals who use submissive behaviors or communication styles are insecure and try to maintain their self-esteem by avoiding conflict (e.g., negative criticism and disagreement from others).

Individuals who use aggressive communication assert their legitimate rights and options with little regard or respect for others. Aggressive communication is often perceived as a personal attack by the recipient because aggressive communication humiliates, dominates, controls, or embarrasses the recipient. By lowering the other person's self-esteem, the person using aggressive communication may feel superior, which helps increase the aggressive communicator's self-esteem. Aggressive communication takes several different forms, which can include screaming, sarcasm, rudeness, belittling jokes, and direct personal insults.

A nurse's approach to communication can have far-reaching impact on the quality of patient care delivered. Consider the following case study.

Clinical Example A

You are a nurse who is caring for Shannon Collins, a 41-year-old woman. Mrs. Collins has a standing order for vital signs every 2 hours because her temperature was elevated on admission to the facility. Since admission, Mrs. Collins's temperature has normalized, and her vital signs have consistently been within normal limits. She tells you that she isn't sleeping well because the nurses keep coming in and waking her every 2 hours and it takes her almost an hour to fall back to sleep. As a result, she is sleeping in 1-hour intervals and feels extremely sleep deprived. You approach the physician and request that the order be changed to every 4 hours during the day with 6 hours of uninterrupted sleep from midnight to 6:00 a.m. The physician responds by saying, "If she wants to sleep, she'll have to wait until she goes home. I want vital signs every 2 hours as ordered."

Critical Thinking Questions

1. Which type of communication style will best serve the needs of the patient? Provide a rationale for your response.
2. What type of response will the nurse have using an aggressive communication style?
3. What type of response will the nurse have using a passive communication style?
4. What type of response will the nurse have using an assertive communication style?

Assertive Communication

The goal of all true professionals is to achieve a mutual respect for boundaries in order to promote the best outcome for everyone involved. Assertive communication allows the

TABLE 38–2 Aggressive, Passive, and Assertive Styles

Aggressive Individuals	Passive Individuals	Assertive Individuals
■ Have loud, heated arguments	■ Conceal their feelings	■ Express their feelings without being nasty or overbearing
■ Are physically violent	■ Deny anger	■ Acknowledge emotions
■ Blame others	■ Feel that no one has the right to express anger	■ Stay open to discussion
■ Use name-calling and verbal insults	■ Avoid arguments	■ Express themselves while giving others that same opportunity
■ Walk out of arguments prior to their resolution	■ Are noncommittal	■ Use "I" statements to defuse arguments
■ Are demanding		■ Provide reasons and ask for the same in return

The Concept of Communication

nurse to express all ideas in a direct and nonconfrontational manner that promotes the rights of the nurse or the patient while respecting the rights of others to have a different outlook. Assertive communication does not use name-calling, is not judgmental, and does not blame others. It increases the likelihood of creating a win–win result in which both parties walk away feeling that their point of view was heard and understood while reaching a conclusion satisfactory to them both.

Characteristics of assertive communicators include freedom to express themselves, awareness of their own rights, and self-control over strong emotions such as anger, fear, or frustration. Assertive communicators are professional and serve as the best advocate for the patient. Assertive communicators express their opinions but are open to listening to others' points of view. They do not use sarcasm, biting comebacks, or passive-aggressive wounding to promote their superiority. Assertive communicators use body language that is relaxed and open to the words of others. They use a tone of voice that is well modulated with appropriate inflection and avoid raising their voice, whispering, or using aggressive overtones.

An assertive individual receives feedback from others with a willingness to consider both the positive and negative perspectives of the evaluator. Although assertive individuals may not believe everything that is said, they will listen to another individual's opinion without becoming defensive or angry and without attacking the speaker. Seeking clarification is appropriate to be sure that the perception of the message is the same as what the sender intended.

Some individuals may have more trouble accepting positive feedback and will dismiss it or negate it when offered. The assertive individual simply says "Thank you" and considers the value of the positive feedback for later application to similar situations.

Benefits of Assertive Communication

Assertiveness is an effective and professional communication style because it is based on mutual respect. An assertive style improves communication and reduces stress by de-escalating conflict, improving outcomes, and reducing the likelihood of angry encounters.

Techniques for Assertive Communication

Because no one technique works in every situation, the nurse must have an arsenal of strategies to use when faced with a situation requiring assertive communication. These techniques include the following:

- *"I" statements.* Assertive communicators voice their own feelings and wishes based on sound evidence without placing blame or raising the defenses of the individual to whom they are speaking. For example, "I have assessed that Patient A is. . . ."

- *Fogging.* Finding some area, no matter how small, on which both parties agree and building from there is a technique that assertive communicators use. In the example of the sleep-deprived patient described previously, both the nurse and the physician can agree that they want to maintain patient safety through careful monitoring of the patient's condition. This gives them a starting point

from which to reach consensus where both can feel patient care has been optimized.

- *Negative assertion.* An assertive communicator can agree with criticism without becoming upset or angry, thus moving the focus of the communication toward the desired goal. This can be particularly important to the nurse when receiving feedback related to the quality of the care the nurse delivers. For example, when the evaluator says, "Although you are very caring, I would like to see you improve your decision-making ability," the nurse may respond, "I could use improvement in my decision-making ability, but I believe the quality of the care I deliver is excellent." This prevents an ongoing debate about something that both parties agree on and allows the communication to move forward regarding the more important topic.

- *Repetition.* When being met with resistance to a request, repeating the request can be useful. However, each time the request is repeated, the power of the words is diminished. This strategy is effective only if the nurse has power within the relationship. For example, suppose the nurse calls the pharmacy to request a newly ordered medication that is to be given within the hour. The pharmacist explains that the pharmacy is very busy, cannot fill the prescription right now, and will not be able to deliver it to the unit for 3–4 hours. The nurse repeats, "I must give this medication within the hour" or "The patient needs the medication within the hour." The effectiveness of this approach may improve if the nurse attempts to find a compromise. The nurse might say, "I need to administer this medication within the hour," to which the pharmacy responds, "I'm sorry, I can't have it to the floor that quickly." The nurse then responds, "The patient needs that medication within the hour. What if I come to the pharmacy so you don't have to deliver it?" This allows for the nurse and the pharmacy to collaborate to reach a mutually effective solution to the problem through compromise.

- *Confidence.* Confidence is essential to assertive communication. A choppy or weak tone of voice implies uncertainty. The nurse should maintain an air of confidence in order to help others see their needs and wants as having merit.

- *Managing nonverbal communication.* Getting too close to the other individual, wagging a finger in someone's face, or glaring at the other person can all counteract assertive words. By maintaining open, assertive body language and keeping a neutral voice, the nurse promotes shared decision making and compromise.

- *Thinking before speaking.* Consider both the choice of words and the tone of voice before speaking. This helps the nurse avoid saying something she will later regret or that will reduce the effectiveness of her communication style.

- *Avoiding apologizing whenever possible.* This is particularly important for women, who have a tendency to say "I'm sorry" even when there is no call for an apology. A woman may say, "I'm sorry, I didn't hear you," or "I'm sorry to bother you, but. . . ." An unnecessary apology immediately places the communicator in a somewhat submissive position. Apologies should be given only when warranted.

■ *Performing a post-conversation evaluation.* Assertive communicators can continue to improve their skills by reviewing what was said and how the communication might have been handled differently to improve the final outcome. This should be done even when the communication interaction was successful because evaluation of what went well, in contrast to what did not, helps the nurse improve assertive communication skills.

Although some individuals may not prefer or feel comfortable with assertive communication, it is possible for all nurses to become assertive communicators and reach more positive outcomes through practice, self-evaluation, and ongoing efforts to improve their communication approach.

Lifespan Considerations

The ability to communicate is directly related to the development of thought processes, the presence of intact sensory and motor systems, and the extent and nature of an individual's opportunities to practice communication skills. As individuals grow and mature, their communication abilities change markedly.

Communicating with Infants

Infants communicate nonverbally, often in response to bodily sensations rather than in a conscious effort to be expressive. Infants' perceptions are related to sensory stimuli. For example, a gentle voice is soothing, whereas tension and anger displayed around an infant create distress. According to research (Rependa, 2012), infants use two types of nonverbal cues: engagement and disengagement cues. Each type of cue may be expressed in a subtle or direct manner. Disengagement cues include crawling away, crying, or lip compression. Engagement cues include smiling, babbling, and opening hands. Nurses can familiarize themselves with the expressive but nonverbal messages of infants to more effectively communicate with their youngest patients.

Communicating with Toddlers and Preschoolers

As they grow and develop toddlers and young children gain skills in both expressive (i.e., telling others what they feel, think, want, care about) and receptive (hearing and understanding what others are communicating to them) language. Toddlers need time to complete verbalizing their thoughts without interruption. Adults should provide simple responses to questions and straightforward, one-step directions because toddlers have short attention spans. Around the age of 4, children begin to follow two- and three-step directions and become more able to express feelings and sensations. For children at this age, drawing pictures or using pictures and photos to communicate can be helpful in a variety of settings.

Communicating with School-age Children

In interactions with school-age children, it is important to give them opportunities to be expressive, listen openly, and respond honestly, using words and concepts they understand. Talk to children at their eye level to help decrease any feelings of intimidation. Children have the ability to express themselves and take part in their healthcare, so if the child is present, include the child in the conversation. Several techniques are helpful when communicating with children. Play, the universal language, allows children to use other symbols, not just words, to express themselves. Drawing, painting, and other art forms can be used even by nonverbal children. Storytelling, in which the nurse and child take turns adding to a story or putting words to pictures, can help the child safely express emotions and feelings. Word games that pose hypothetical situations or put the child in control, such as "What if . . . ?" "If you could . . . ," or "If a genie came and gave you a wish . . ." can help a child feel more powerful or explore ideas about how to manage an illness. Reading books with a theme similar to the child's condition or problem and then discussing the meaning, characters, and feelings generated by the book can help the nurse communicate with the child about the condition and the child's experiences with it. Movies or videos can also be used in this way. Older children can use writing to reflect on their situation, develop meaning, and gain a sense of control.

Communicating with Adolescents

Adolescents have the ability to think abstractly and make decisions about their own healthcare. Adolescents are focused on the development of effective communication skills and feel a strong need to share thoughts, facts, and feelings with others (Koutoukidis, Stainton, & Hughson, 2013). It takes time to build rapport with adolescents. Nurses working with adolescents should use active listening and project a nonjudgmental attitude and nonreactive behaviors, even when an adolescent makes disturbing comments. Adolescents are very sensitive to feelings of judgment, so it is essential to remain open minded when communicating with them. Adolescents prefer expectations to be clearly explained, and they appreciate when praise is given.

Communicating with Adults

Young adults and middle-aged adults are at the peak of their communication abilities. They are fully grown/developed, and many have either completed their education or are earning advanced degrees. However, there is a wide range of communication abilities among adults based on cognitive ability, education levels, socioeconomic levels, exposure to professional and work environments, and health literacy. Young adults may still display some adolescent patterns of communication. And at the upper end of middle age, some adults may begin to have physical and cognitive problems usually seen in older adults. Nurses should identify any barriers to communication with adults and plan accordingly.

Communicating with Pregnant Women

Optimal pregnancy outcomes depend on clear communication, effective decision making, and teamwork (Zote, 2014). Effective therapeutic communication is essential to patient safety, creates a climate of confidence, and strongly affects the patient's comfort with the process of pregnancy and birth. Nurses can promote the patient's self-expression by establishing a therapeutic relationship, making the family feel welcome, and being nonjudgmental. Keys to communication during pregnancy include determining the cultural values of the family about birth, engaging in shared decision making, and listening to the patient as well as providing support. Refer to the module on Reproduction for more information on communicating with pregnant women.

Communicating with Older Adults

Older adults may have physical or cognitive problems that necessitate nursing interventions to improve communication. Some of the common problems include sensory deficits; cognitive impairment; neurologic deficits from strokes or other neurologic conditions; and psychosocial problems, such as depression. Recognizing specific needs and obtaining appropriate resources for patients can greatly increase their socialization and quality of life. Nurses can use a number of different interventions to improve communication in patients with these special needs. For example, nurses can ensure that the patient is using assistive devices, glasses, and hearing aids, and that these are in good working order. Nurses can also use communications aids, such as paper and pencil, communication boards, tablets or computers, or pictures, when possible. Referral to appropriate services and resources, such as speech therapy, may provide further support for the older adult who experiences communication difficulties.

To communicate effectively with older adults, the nurse should keep environmental distractions to a minimum. The nurse should seek to speak in short, simple sentences, one subject at a time, and reinforce or repeat what is said when necessary. In communicating effectively with older adults, the nurse must avoid elderspeak and should always face the patient when speaking; coming up behind someone may be frightening. Include family and friends in conversation. When verbal expression and nonverbal expression are incongruent, believe the nonverbal: clarification of this and careful attention to the patient's feelings will help promote a feeling of caring and acceptance. Find out what has been important and what has meaning to the patient, and try to maintain these things as much as possible. Simple things such as bedtime rituals become more important, especially in a hospital or extended-care setting.

NURSING PROCESS

Communication is an integral part of the nursing process. The nurse uses communication skills in each phase of the nursing process. Communication skills take on greater importance when the nurse is caring for a patient with sensory, language, developmental, or cognitive deficits. Timing also has a bearing on communication and patient care. See the Evidence-Based Practice feature for information on how nurses view timing related to providing nursing care.

Assessment

Assessment strategies related to communication include evaluating the patient's communication style and appraising any language or communication barriers. Remember that cultural values and practices may influence when and how a patient speaks. Obviously, language varies according to age and development. For example, with children,

the nurse observes sounds, gestures, facial expressions, and vocabulary.

Throughout the process of collecting data, the nurse uses communication skills to increase nurse–patient rapport, put the patient at ease when discussing personal matters, and interpret the patient's nonverbal communication, and to assess for and overcome barriers to communication as outlined below. Exemplar 38.B discusses the role of therapeutic communication in creating a helping relationship with the patient.

Language Deficits

The nurse determines whether the patient speaks another language or has an impairment that affects his or her ability to communicate verbally. When assessing for the need for an interpreter, remember that some patients who use English as a second language may have language skills that are inadequate to meet their needs in a healthcare environment.

Sensory Deficits

The abilities to hear, see, feel, and smell are important adjuncts to communication. A hearing impairment can significantly alter the message a patient receives; vision impairment may affect a patient's ability to observe nonverbal behavior, such as a smile or a gesture; and inability to feel and smell can impair the patient's ability to report injuries or detect smoke from a fire. If a patient appears to have severe hearing impairments, the nurse should follow these steps:

- Look for a medical alert bracelet, necklace, or tag indicating hearing loss.
- Determine whether the patient wears a functioning hearing aid.
- Observe whether the patient is attempting to see your face to read lips.
- Observe whether the patient is attempting to use hands to communicate with sign language.
- Evaluate feedback to validate that effective communication is taking place.

See the feature on Communicating with Patients Who Have a Visual or Hearing Deficit in the module on Sensory Perception for more information.

Cognitive Impairments

Any disorder that impairs cognitive functioning (e.g., cerebrovascular disease, dementia, and brain tumors or injuries) may affect a patient's ability to use and understand language. These patients may develop total loss of speech, impaired articulation, or the inability to find or name words. They may experience difficulty understanding others or tracking conversations, which may manifest through withdrawal, frustration, or changing the subject. Certain medications such as sedatives, antidepressants, and neuroleptics may also impair speech, causing the patient to use incomplete sentences or to slur words. Older adults are particularly likely to have cognitive impairments that may interfere with communication.

The nurse assesses whether these patients respond when asked a question and, if they do, assesses the following:

- Is the patient's speech fluent or hesitant?
- Does the patient use words correctly?

- Can the patient comprehend instructions as evidenced by following directions?
- Can the patient repeat words or phrases?

In addition, the nurse assesses the patient's ability to understand written words:

- Can the patient follow written directions?
- Can the patient respond correctly by pointing to a written word?
- Can the patient read aloud?
- Can the patient recognize words or letters even if unable to read whole sentences?

The nurse uses large, clearly written words when trying to establish abilities in this area.

SAFETY ALERT When the patient is unconscious, the nurse looks for any indication that suggests the patient has some ability to comprehend and communicate (e.g., tries to arouse the patient verbally and through touch). Ask a closed question such as "Can you hear me?" and watch for a nonverbal response such as a nod of the head for yes or a shake for no, or ask for a hand squeeze or blink of the eye: once for yes or twice for no. Because damage to the spinal cord may preclude movement, attempts to determine comprehension must be specific to the needs of the individual patient.

Other Impairments

Structural deficits of the oral and nasal cavities and respiratory system can alter an individual's ability to speak clearly and spontaneously. Examples include cleft palate, artificial airways such as an endotracheal tube or tracheostomy, and laryngectomy (removal of the larynx). Extreme dyspnea (shortness of breath) can also impair speech patterns.

If verbal impairment is combined with paralysis of the upper extremities that impairs the patient's ability to write, the nurse should determine whether the patient is able to point, nod, shrug, blink, or squeeze a hand. Any of these could be used to devise a simple communication system.

Style of Communication

In assessing communication style, the nurse considers both verbal and nonverbal communication. In addition to physical barriers, some psychologic illnesses (e.g., depression or psychosis) influence the patient's ability to communicate. The patient may demonstrate constant verbalization of the same words or phrases, a loose association of ideas, a flight of ideas (a continuous flow of rapid speech that switches from topic to topic), or other indicators of barriers posed by psychologic processes.

Verbal Communication

When assessing verbal communication, the nurse focuses on three areas: the content of the patient's message, the themes, and the emotions the patient verbalizes. In addition, the nurse considers the following:

- Whether the patient's communication pattern is slow, rapid, quiet, spontaneous, hesitant, evasive, and so on
- The patient's vocabulary, particularly any changes from the vocabulary normally used (for example, someone

who normally never swears may indicate increased stress or illness by an uncharacteristic use of profanity)

- The presence of hostility, aggression, assertiveness, reticence, hesitance, anxiety, or loquaciousness (incessant verbalization) in communication
- Difficulties with verbal communication, such as slurring, stuttering, inability to pronounce a particular sound, lack of clarity in enunciation, inability to speak in sentences, loose association of ideas, flight of ideas, or the inability to find or name words or identify objects
- The refusal or inability to speak.

SAFETY ALERT Changes in the patient's ability to put words together into sentences or to properly name an item or struggling to find the right word for common objects may be an indication of neurologic impairment. Assessment of the patient's communication ability, especially after any type of head trauma, is an important tool for detecting alterations in the patient's condition.

Diagnosis

Impaired Verbal Communication may be used as a nursing diagnosis when an individual experiences "a decreased, delayed, or absent ability to receive, process, transmit, and/or use a system of symbols" (NANDA-I, 2014). Communication problems may be *receptive* (e.g., difficulty hearing) or *expressive* (e.g., difficulty speaking).

A nursing diagnosis of *Impaired Verbal Communication* may not be useful when an individual's communication problems are caused by a psychiatric illness or acute anxiety or emotional distress. In those instances, a diagnosis of *Fear* or *Anxiety* may be more appropriate. Impaired verbal communication has implications for the patient in a number of areas, including patient self-esteem and social isolation.

Planning

When a nursing diagnosis related to impaired verbal communication has been made, the nurse and patient determine outcomes and begin planning ways to promote effective communication. Establishing communication with the patient may require creativity or technology. New devices are being developed, ranging from thought-activated computers that verbalize for the patient to devices that can be operated with a stylus in the mouth to verbalize needs.

Specific goals for nursing interventions will depend on the stated etiology and may include the following:

- The patient will have an effective means for communicating needs.
- The patient's ability to perceive messages accurately will be maximized.
- The patient will be provided with resources as needed to optimize the ability to communicate.

Implementation

Nursing interventions to facilitate communication with patients who have problems with speech or language include manipulating the environment, providing support,

Evidence-Based Practice
The Role of Time in Caring for the Patient with Complex Communication Needs

Problem

Effective nurse–patient communication is an essential aspect of healthcare. As Kourkouta and Papathanasiou (2014) note, "Good communication between nurses and patients is essential for the successful outcome of individualized nursing care of each patient." Unfortunately, time to communicate is often limited and subject to the workload demands of the nurse. Especially in the current era of healthcare institutions cutting costs and staff to stretch their limited resources, nurses are faced with more time pressure, a development that has been shown to undercut the quality of care for all patients (Ball et al., 2013). Little is currently known about how nurses manage the "lack of time" when caring for patients with developmental disabilities and those with complex communication needs. These groups tend to communicate at slower rates and a more concrete level, which can further undermine the communication process.

Evidence

Hemsley, Balandin, and Worrall (2012) investigated nurses' expressed concepts of "time" in stories about communicating with patients with developmental disabilities. They interviewed 15 nurses from two large hospitals about barriers to and strategies for successful communication with patients who have developmental disabilities.

The nurses identified "time" as both a barrier and a facilitator to a successful communication process. Time was a barrier when related to avoiding direct communication. It was also used as a means to avoid direct communication with patients and instead communicate with family members or other paid caregivers on behalf of the patient. Nurses viewed time positively when related to valuing communication, investing extra time, and the application of a range of adaptive communication strategies that established successful communication.

Implications

Time is perceived as both an enemy and a friend for the improvement of communication. Nurses who perceive that communication takes too long may avoid the communication process and miss opportunities to improve it. Those who take the time to communicate apply a wide range of strategies in order to achieve successful communication with patients.

Critical Thinking Application

1. What resources can the nurse use to communicate with patients with complex communication needs in the hospital setting?
2. What resources might the nurse use to communicate with these patients once they are discharged into the community?

---

employing measures to enhance communication, and educating the patient and support person.

Manipulate the Environment

A quiet environment with limited distractions provides the best setting for communication and increases the possibility of effective communication. Sufficient light helps in conveying nonverbal messages, which is especially important if visual or auditory acuity is impaired. Initially, the nurse needs to provide a calm, relaxed environment, which will help reduce any anxiety the patient may have. Any factor that affects communication can create feelings of frustration, anxiety, depression, or hostility in a patient. Communication normally contributes to a patient's sense of security and feelings of not being alone, so communication problems may cause some patients to feel isolated and confused. To reduce feelings of isolation, the nurse should acknowledge and praise the patient's attempts at communication.

Provide Support

The nurse should convey encouragement to the patient and provide nonverbal reassurance, perhaps by touch if appropriate. If the nurse does not understand a patient's communication, it is critical to let the patient know so that the patient can provide clarification with other words or through some other means of communication. When speaking with a patient who has difficulty understanding, check frequently to determine what the patient has heard and understood. Using open-ended questions will assist in obtaining accurate information about the effectiveness of communication.

Clinical Example B

You are providing care to Maria Perez, a 52-year-old Latina patient who has limited English skills. As part of the discharge teaching for this patient, you are teaching her about dietary changes that are necessary for managing Crohn disease. You ask Ms. Perez, "Do you understand what to eat?" She nods her head yes. You realize that the question did not elicit an answer that sufficiently confirms that Ms. Perez understood. You ask a follow-up question: "What do you think will be good for you to eat when you go home?" At the same time, your body language (e.g., gestures, posture, facial expression, and eye contact) conveys acceptance and approval. When Ms. Perez begins to explain what foods she should avoid, you are confident that you communicated the information to Ms. Perez successfully.

Critical Thinking Questions

1. What resources are available for teaching patients whose primary language is not English?
2. How does culture affect communication?
3. How does body language affect the communication process?

Employ Measures to Enhance Communication

To enhance communication, the nurse first determines how the patient can best receive messages: by listening, by looking, through touch, or through an interpreter. Ways to help communication include keeping words simple and concrete and discussing topics of interest to the patient. The use of alternative communication strategies, such as word boards, pictures, paper and pencil, or an iPad or other tablet may be helpful.

Avoid Potential Cultural Barriers to Communication

The nurse should remember several items when communicating with a patient whose primary language is not English. Avoid the use of slang, buzzwords, and medical terminology when possible. Show the patient respect by speaking clearly, directly, and at a normal pace. Avoid words that may impede the communication process, such as words that are slurred and those that have several syllables. Speak at a speed that does not overload the patient and allows the patient to follow the conversation. However, avoid speaking too slowly, because this may cause the nurse to lose the patient's attention. Use open-ended questions and rephrase them as necessary to obtain accurate information.

When using nonverbal communication with these patients, select gestures with care. This form of nonverbal communication underscores both words and actions and can be used to clarify meaning; however, gestures may have different meanings for different cultures. Therefore, the nurse must validate words and gestures with each patient on an individual basis.

If language is a barrier, the use of an interpreter may be necessary. In 2000, the federal Office for Civil Rights (OCR) of the Department of Health and Human Services mandated that any healthcare providers and agencies that receive federal funds must communicate effectively with patients, family members, and visitors who are deaf or hard-of-hearing and must take steps to provide meaningful access to their programs for persons who have limited English proficiency (LEP). Failure to do so is considered discrimination. ORC makes "information, resources, and tools available to healthcare organizations that assist people with limited English proficiency and people who are deaf or hard of hearing" (OCR, 2016).

Because the use of family members as interpreters can raise confidentiality and privacy issues, the nurse should enlist the aid of bilingual staff members to communicate information effectively. Most healthcare institutions have a list of bilingual staff members who can be used as personal interpreters, medical interpreters, or both. When working with an interpreter, the nurse must remember to always speak directly to the patient and not to the interpreter.

The nurse who is culturally competent will be appreciated by the patient. The following strategies can be used when caring for patients from a different culture:

1. Use the proper form of address for the patient's culture.
2. Know how individuals in the patient's culture greet one another. This may include the use of handshake, embraces, or kissing the cheeks. In some cultures, physical contact is prohibited.
3. Be aware of what a smile means in the patient's culture. A smile may indicate friendliness or be considered taboo. Also be aware of what eye contact means; in some cultures, it indicates respect, whereas in others, it may indicate aggression or be considered impolite.
4. Remember that not all gestures have a universal meaning.

While similarities may enhance the therapeutic relationship, differences can serve as topics for open discussion. Having an open and ongoing conversation between all parties will promote understanding.

Evaluation

Evaluation is useful for both patient and nurse communication. Evaluation of nurse communication is discussed in greater detail in Exemplar 38.B on therapeutic communication.

To establish whether patient outcomes have been met in relation to communication, listen actively and observe nonverbal cues. The overall patient outcome for individuals with impaired verbal communication is to reduce or resolve the factors impairing the communication. Examples of statements indicating outcome achievement include "Using a picture board effectively to indicate needs" or "The patient stated, 'I listened more closely to my daughter yesterday and found out how she feels about our divorce.'"

Examples of outcomes of care for the patient with impaired communication include the following:

- The patient communicates that needs are being met.
- The patient perceives the message accurately, as evidenced by appropriate verbal and/or nonverbal responses.
- The patient communicates effectively, using the patient's dominant language, a translator/interpreter, sign language, a word board or picture board, and/or a computer.
- The patient has regained maximum communication abilities.
- The patient expresses minimal fear, anxiety, frustration, and depression.
- The patient uses resources appropriately.

Nursing Practice

Communication is a critical skill for nursing. It is the process by which humans meet their survival needs, build relationships, and experience emotions. In nursing, communication is a dynamic process used to gather assessment data, to teach, to collaborate with other healthcare professionals, to advocate for patients, to express caring, and to provide comfort. It is an integral part of the helping relationship.

Four specific types of communication are explored in the exemplars of this module. Each of these is essential to successful nursing practice. Group communication is becoming ever more important in the process of making decisions in the current healthcare system. Therapeutic communication is an essential tool for developing the nurse–patient helping relationship. Documentation is the primary form of written communication used by nurses in all aspects of healthcare. Finally, reporting through handoff communication is the process of nurse-to-nurse communication that ensures continuity of care for the patient from one shift change or visit to another.

REVIEW The Concept of Communication

RELATE Link the Concepts

Linking the concept of communication with the concept of culture and diversity:

1. How can misunderstanding the patient's culture act as a barrier to communication when the nurse's culture differs from that of the patient?

2. The nurse is studying a culture different from the one in which the nurse was raised. What aspects of the culture would the nurse wish to learn about in order to understand how that culture's communication style may differ?

Linking the concept of communication with the concept of professional behaviors:

3. How do the nurse's communication skills affect the perceptions of others (both patients and other members of the healthcare team) regarding the nurse's professionalism?

4. A patient asks the nurse a question. Although the nurse is very knowledgeable about the subject, the nurse stumbles over words while answering the patient, repeatedly starts sentences over again, uses words such as "ahh" and "umm" a number of times, and gives the impression of weighing each word carefully. What impact will this delivery have on the patient's perception of the nurse's professionalism and knowledge of the subject matter being explained?

Linking the concept of communication with the concept of immunity:

5. How can a nurse's communication skills produce positive and negative patient teaching outcomes for patients with systemic lupus erythematosus?

6. Discuss some of the difficulties in communicating about a condition such as HIV/AIDS, which carries a social stigma. How can a nurse most effectively provide communication and allow the patient to express him- or herself?

REFER Go to Pearson MyLab Nursing and eText

■ Additional review materials

REFLECT Apply Your Knowledge

Madeline McCormick, 24 years old, is an RN who has worked in the local acute care hospital on the medical floor for the past 3 years. Last night her boyfriend proposed. She accepted and is so thrilled she can't wait to show her new diamond ring to all of her coworkers and tell them the good news. She arrives at work early to share the good news and they all congratulate her and shower her with questions about her ideas for the wedding.

You are a student nurse assigned to Ms. McCormick's floor today. As you walk by one of the patients' rooms you hear Ms. McCormick, who is providing a.m. care to a patient, talking to the patient and telling her all about how her boyfriend proposed, her wedding plans, and how happy she is.

1. Is it appropriate for Ms. McCormick to share her good news with her coworkers? Why or why not?

2. Is it appropriate for Ms. McCormick to share her news with her patient? Why or why not?

3. How does Ms. McCormick's excitement over her engagement affect the nurse–patient communication process?

» Exemplar 38.A
Groups and Group Communication

Exemplar Learning Outcomes

38.A Analyze groups and group communication.

■ Describe the types, functions, levels of formality, and characteristics of effective groups.

■ Outline the aspects of group dynamics.

■ List group problems that nurses should recognize and avoid.

■ Describe types and functions of healthcare groups.

Exemplar Key Terms

Apathy, 2581
Cohesiveness, 2580
Creativity techniques, 2580
Decision trees, 2580

Overview

A **group** is defined by Adams and Galanes (2014) as "three or more individuals who have a common purpose, interact with each other, influence each other, and are interdependent" (p. 11). Nurses participate in groups on a regular basis and may function as either a leader or a participant depending on the nature of the group and the nurse's qualifications. Group processes, called *group dynamics*, determine how groups function. For group work to be accomplished and goals to be achieved, group dynamics must be effective.

The changing healthcare system presents challenges for healthcare professionals if they are to be actively involved in decisions about policy and practice. Such decisions are made by groups of individuals at all levels of society: think tanks, advocacy groups, professional groups, and politicians at local, regional, state, national, and international levels. These challenges provide opportunities for nurses to participate as active members of the various decision-making groups. To be effective members of these groups, nurses must be knowledgeable about the dynamics of group interaction.

Groups

Groups exist to help individuals achieve goals that might be unattainable through individual effort alone. By pooling the ideas and expertise of several individuals, groups often can solve problems more effectively than one person acting alone (see the Concept of Collaboration). Information can be disseminated to groups more quickly and with more consistency than to individuals. In addition, groups often take greater risks than do individuals because group members support each other in decision making. Just as group members share responsibilities for the group's actions, they also share the consequences of those actions.

In the clinical setting, nurses work in groups as they collaborate with other nurses, other healthcare professionals, patients, and family members when planning and providing care. Nurses also work in groups in professional and specialty organizations and civic and community groups. Within these organizations, nurses promote the goals of nursing on professional, civic, and political levels. Group skills are therefore important for nurses in all settings.

Types of Groups

Groups are classified as either primary or secondary, according to their structure and type of interaction. A **primary group** is a small, intimate group in which the relationships among members are personal, spontaneous, sentimental, cooperative, and inclusive. Examples are the family, a play group of children, informal work groups, and friendship groups. Members of a primary group communicate with each other largely in face-to-face interactions and develop a strong sense of unity, or "oneness." What belongs to one person is often seen as belonging to the group. For example, a success achieved by one member is shared by all and is seen as a success of the group.

Primary groups set standards of behavior for their members. They also support and sustain each member in stressful situations that the member would otherwise not be able to withstand. In particular, the role of the primary group, particularly the family, in healthcare is increasingly recognized. Most individuals turn to their primary group for help and support when they have health problems. For this reason, healthcare providers and organizations expand their focus to include the family.

A **secondary group** is generally larger, more impersonal, and less sentimental than a primary group. Examples are professional associations, task groups, ad hoc committees, political parties, and business groups. Members view these groups simply as a means of getting things done. Interactions do not necessarily occur in face-to-face contact and do not require that the members know each other personally. Expectations of members are formally administered through impersonal controls and external restraints. Once the goals of the group are achieved or change, the interaction is discontinued.

Functions of Groups

Two classic studies outline the functioning of groups. Sampson and Marthas (1990) describe eight functions of groups: socialization, support, task completion, camaraderie, information, normative function, empowerment, and governance. Stewart, Manz, and Sims (1999) describe two ways of categorizing groups: functional perspectives and interpersonal perspectives. Any one group generally can have more than one function, and it may fulfill different functions for different group members. For example, for one member, a group may provide support; for another, it may provide information.

Levels of Group Formality

The three levels of groups are **formal**, **semiformal**, and **informal**. Traditional features of each type of group are shown in **Box 38–2 》**.

Characteristics of Effective Groups

To be effective, a group must achieve three main functions:

1. Accomplish its goals.
2. Maintain its cohesion.
3. Develop and modify its structure to improve its effectiveness.

Many factors can promote or inhibit a group's ability to achieve these functions. These include atmosphere, ability to set goals, and intergroup communication (**Figure 38–7 》**). These and other factors are compared in **Table 38–3 》**.

Group Communications

Group Dynamics

Group dynamics, which are also known as group processes, are related to how the group functions, communicates, sets goals, and achieves objectives. Every group has its own characteristics and ways of functioning. Five aspects of group dynamics are commitment, decision-making ability, member behavior, cohesiveness, and power.

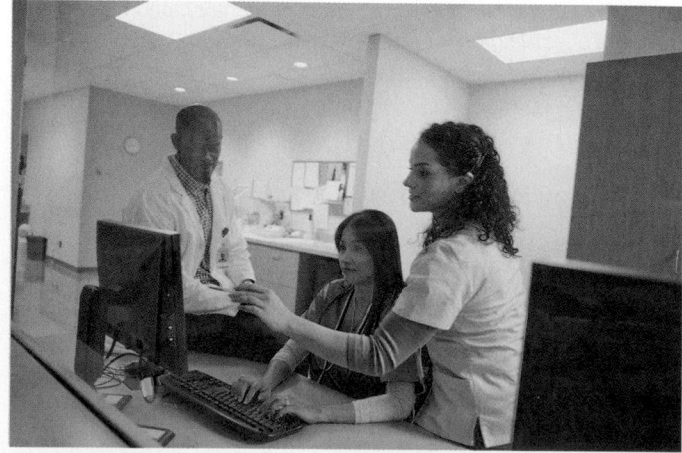

Source: Hero Images/Getty Images.

Figure 38–7 》 A healthcare team gathers to discuss issues affecting a patient's care.

Box 38–2
Characteristics of Formal, Semiformal, and Informal Groups

Formal Groups	Semiformal Groups	Informal Groups
■ Authority is imposed from above.	■ The structure is formal.	■ The group is not bound by any set of written rules or regulations.
■ Leadership selection is assigned from above and made by an authoritative and often arbitrary order or decree.	■ The hierarchy is carefully delineated.	■ Usually governed by a set of unwritten laws and a strong code of ethics.
■ Managers are symbols of power and authority.	■ Membership is voluntary but selective.	■ The group is purely functional and has easily recognized basic objectives.
■ The goals of the formal group are normally imposed at a much higher level than the direct leadership of the group.	■ Prestige and status are often accrued from membership.	■ Rotational leadership is common. The group recognizes that only rarely are all leadership characteristics found in one person.
■ Management is endangered by its aloofness from the members of the work group.	■ Structured, deliberate activities absorb a large part of the group's meeting time.	■ The group assigns duties to the members best qualified for certain functions. For example, the person who is recognized as outgoing and sociable will be assigned responsibilities for planning parties.
■ Behavioral norms (expected standards of behavior), regulations, and rules are usually superimposed. The larger the turnover rate of members, the greater the structuring of rules.	■ Objectives and goals are rigid; change is not recognized as desirable.	■ Judgments about the group's leader are made quickly and surely. Leaders are replaced when they make one or more mistakes or do not get the job done.
■ Membership in the group is only partly voluntary.	■ In many cases, the leader has direct control over the choice of a successor.	■ The group is an ideal testing ground for new leadership techniques, but there is no guarantee that such techniques can be transferred effectively to a large, formal organization.
■ Rigidity of purpose is often a necessity for protection of the formal group in the pursuit of its objectives.	■ The day-to-day operating standards and methods (group norms) are negotiable. Because most people become bored at quibbling about norms, someone can often "railroad" acceptance of a list of norms that person desires.	■ Behavioral norms are developed either by group effort or by the leader and adopted by the group.
■ Interactions within the group as a whole are limited, but informal subgroups often are formed.		■ Deviance by one member from the group's behavioral norms is more threatening to the perpetuation of small, informal groups than to large, formal, heterogeneous groups. Conformity and group solidarity are important for the protection and preservation of small groups.
		■ Group norms are enforced by sanctions (punishments) imposed by the group on those who violate a norm. Different values are placed on norms in accordance with the values of the leader. One leader may regard the action as a gross violation, whereas another leader may find it quite acceptable.
		■ Interpersonal interactions are spontaneous.

Commitment

The members of effective groups are committed to the goals and output of the group. Because groups demand time and attention, members must give up some autonomy and self-interest. Inevitably, conflicts arise between the interests of individual group members and those of the group as a whole. However, members who are committed to the group feel close to each other and willingly work for the achievement of the group's goals and objectives. Indications of group commitment include:

- Members feel a strong sense of belonging.
- Members enjoy each other.
- Members seek each other for counsel and support.
- Members support each other in difficulty.
- Members value the contributions of other members.
- Members are motivated by working in the group and want to do their tasks well.

- Members express good feelings openly and identify positive contributions.
- Members feel that the goals of the group are achievable and important.

Decision-making Methods

The ability to make sound decisions is essential to effective group functioning. Effective decisions are made when the following occur: when the group listens to all the ideas of its members and members feel satisfied with their participation; when the group atmosphere is positive; when the group uses time efficiently by focusing the discussion on the decision to be made; and when members feel committed to the decision and responsible for its implementation.

Huber (2014) describes several methods by which groups can make decisions: trial and error, pilot projects, creativity techniques, decision trees, scenario planning, and worst-case scenario. **Trial and error** techniques are the most haphazard: in these situations, a solution that seems viable is

TABLE 38–3 Comparative Features of Effective and Ineffective Groups

Factor	Effective Groups	Ineffective Groups
Atmosphere	Informal, comfortable, and relaxed. It is a working atmosphere in which individuals demonstrate their interest and involvement.	Obviously tense. Signs of boredom may appear.
Goal setting	Goals, tasks, and objectives are clarified, understood, and modified so that members of the group can commit themselves to cooperatively structured goals.	Unclear, misunderstood, or imposed goals may be accepted by members. The goals are competitively structured.
Leadership and member participation	Shift from time to time, depending on the circumstances. Different members assume leadership at various times, because of their knowledge or experience.	Delegated and based on authority. The chairperson may dominate the group, or the members may defer unduly. Members' participation is unequal, with high-authority members dominating.
Goal emphasis	All three functions of groups are emphasized: goal accomplishment, internal maintenance, and developmental change.	One or more functions may not be emphasized.
Communication	Open and two-way. Ideas and feelings are encouraged, both about the problem and about the group's operation.	Closed or one-way. Only the production of ideas is encouraged. Feelings are ignored or taboo. Members may be tentative or reluctant to be open and may have "hidden agendas" (personal goals at cross purposes with group goals).
Decision making	By consensus, although various decision-making procedures appropriate to the situation may be instituted.	By the higher authority in the group, with minimal involvement by members or an inflexible style is imposed.
Cohesion	Facilitated through high levels of inclusion, trust, liking, and support.	Either ignored or used as a means of controlling members, thus promoting rigid conformity.
Conflict tolerance	High. The reasons for disagreements or conflicts are carefully examined, and the group seeks to resolve them. The group accepts unresolvable basic disagreements.	Low. Attempts may be made to ignore, deny, avoid, suppress, or override controversy by premature group action. The group may choose to live with conflict rather than attempt to resolve it.
Power	Determined by the members' abilities and the information they possess. Power is shared. The issue is how to get the job done.	Determined by position in the group. Obedience to authority is strong. The issue is who controls.
Problem solving	High. Constructive criticism is frequent, frank, relatively comfortable, and oriented toward removing an obstacle to problem solving.	Low. Criticism may be destructive, taking the form of either overt or covert personal attacks. It prevents the group from getting the job done.
Self-evaluation of the group	Frequent. All members participate in evaluation and decisions about how to improve the group's functioning.	Minimal. What little evaluation there is may be done by the highest authority in the group rather than by the membership as a whole.
Creativity	Encouraged. There is room within the group for members to become self-actualized and interpersonally effective.	Discouraged. People are afraid of appearing foolish if they put forth a creative thought.

Sources: Data from Homestead Schools. (2016). *Section 10: Characteristics of effective and ineffective teams.* Retrieved from http://www.homesteadschools.com/lcsw/courses/TeamBuilding/Section10.htm; Arnold, E. C., & Boggs, K. U. (2013). *Interpersonal relationships: Professional communication skills for nurses* (6th ed.). St. Louis, MO: Elsevier Saunders; and Eventus. (2017). *Effective vs. ineffective teams.* Retrieved from http://www.eventus.co.uk/effective-vs-ineffective-teams/.

simply attempted. Managers and groups who use these techniques typically are seen as poor problem solvers, especially in a healthcare context. Evidence-based practice protocols have replaced trial and error as the standard in the nursing profession.

Pilot projects make use of limited trials to determine problems with problem-solving alternatives. Pilot project strategies may resemble research projects and may be linked to quality improvement initiatives. **Creativity techniques** such as brainstorming sessions use the creative potential of the group to generate a large number of possible options quickly. A **decision tree** is a graphic model that visually represents the choices, outcomes, and risks to be anticipated. A decision tree helps groups visualize the results of a series of branching options and helps streamline decision making by clearly spelling out alternative options as decisions lead to subsequent options.

Scenario planning is a group process strategy that encourages members of a group to create hypothetical or "possible future" situation. Scenario planning is most applicable to fluid and changing environments. Participants are encouraged to ask themselves, "What if?" Group members imagine pathways, forces in play, turning points, and deep behavioral undercurrents. Scenario planning helps illuminate early warning signs, create opportunities, and ensure against risks.

Worst-case scenario is a technique designed to help groups make decisions that involve risk. The worst-case outcome is outlined for each alternative, and then the scenario with the comparatively best outcome is selected as the preferred outcome. This technique helps ensure that the "least of all evils" is selected.

Member Behavior

The degree of input by members into goal setting, decision making, problem solving, and group evaluation is related to the group structure and leadership style, but members are responsible for their own behavior and participation. Each member participates in a wide range of roles (assigned or assumed functions) during group interactions. Individuals may perform different roles during interactions in the same group or may vary roles in different groups. Various roles have been identified. These include *information givers*, who provide factual information; *information seekers*, who seek factual information about tasks at hand; and *opinion givers*, who care more about values and beliefs than facts.

Cohesiveness

Groups that have cohesiveness possess certain characteristics. One characteristic is a group spirit. This is a sense of having a common purpose. **Cohesiveness** is the attachment that members feel toward each other, the group, or the task. Members of groups that have a high level of cohesiveness feel greater satisfaction with the group. Groups that lack cohesiveness are unstable and are more prone to disintegration.

SAFETY ALERT Effective group communication is essential for the patient's safety because the patient's care is overseen by an interdependent healthcare team. Team members must coordinate their efforts to ensure that medications are given in the correct dose at the correct time, that necessary education is provided, and that all interventions are implemented correctly. Poor group atmosphere, goal setting, leadership, goal emphasis, and all the other elements of group cohesion have a direct and cumulative impact on patient outcomes and safety.

Power

Patterns of behavior in groups are greatly influenced by the force of power. Power can be defined as the ability to influence another person in some way or the ability to do something, whether it is to decide the fate of a nation or to decide that a certain change in policy or practice is necessary. For example, a new member of a group may be more influenced by the group member who asked her to enter into membership than by other members. Similarly, group members may afford power to those group members who most closely share their interests.

Many individuals have a negative concept of power, likening it to control, domination, and even coercion of others by muscle and clout. However, power can be viewed as a vital, positive force that moves people toward the attainment of individual or group goals. The overall purpose of power is to encourage cooperation and collaboration in accomplishing a task.

Group Problems

In addition to conflict, problems that can occur in groups include monopolizing, groupthink, scapegoating, silence and apathy, and transference and countertransference. The nurse needs to be able to recognize and avoid these behaviors when working in collaborative groups because these behaviors function as barriers to successful group work.

Monopolizing

Monopolizing is the domination of a discussion by one member of a group. Because most group meetings have time restraints, monopolizing seriously deprives other individuals of their chance to participate. A sense of resentment among members then develops, and ultimately some members may direct their frustration and anger toward the group leader, whom they expect to do something to stop the monopolizer's behavior.

Monopolizing behavior may be motivated by anxiety or a need for attention, recognition, and approval. Often, compulsive talkers are unaware of their behavior and its effect on others and need help to recognize their behavior and its consequences.

Strategies for dealing with monopolizing include the following:

- *Interrupt simply, directly, and supportively.* This strategy is an initial attempt to get the individual to hear others.

- *Reflect the member's behavior.* This strategy is an attempt to help the individual become aware of the monopolizing behavior.

- *Reflect the group's feelings.* This strategy is an attempt to help the individual member become aware of the effects of his behavior on others.

- *Confront the person and/or the group.* This strategy can be directed toward the individual or toward the group to help members realize their own responsibility for the problem.

Groupthink

Groupthink is a type of decision making characterized by a group's failure to critically examine its own processes and practices. Groupthink may also occur when members of a group fail to recognize and respond to change. It may occur in highly cohesive groups when group members do not want to disagree or criticize the majority of the group's thinking for fear of being considered disloyal. For example, the administrators of a local urgent care center, failing to recognize that the staff is struggling to communicate with their many Latino patients, refuse to hire Spanish-speaking staff or engage the services of a full-time interpreter. Symptoms of groupthink include the group overestimating its power and morality, the group becoming closed minded, and group members experiencing pressure to conform.

Scapegoating

A **scapegoat** is an individual who has been selected to take the blame for another individual or for a group. Individuals and groups who engage in scapegoating minimize their own feelings of ineptitude by focusing on the weakness of others. For leaders to deal with scapegoating, they must be alert to its development and be prepared to accept anger when they confront individuals who are scapegoating. Scapegoating is a grossly unprofessional behavior that has no place within the profession of nursing, which emphasizes responsibility and accountability.

Silence and Apathy

Nonparticipation or **apathy** (lack of interest or enthusiasm) of one or more group members is sometimes best handled without intervention. Sometimes such silences are not a reflection of something in the immediate group setting but rather of some past experience. For example, after expressing an idea previously, this person may have been told "That was a stupid thing to say." Having been hurt once in a group, such individuals feel insecure about their views and are reluctant to express themselves again in groups. Continued nonparticipation or apathy, however, needs to be dealt with by the leader after a careful assessment of whether the apathy is a reflection of leadership style, task issues, or interpersonal conflicts.

Transference and Countertransference

Transference in the group setting is defined as the transfer of feelings that were originally evoked by one's parents or significant others to individuals in the present setting. An example is a group member who acts toward the leader as the member would act toward a parent. In addition, members of a group can transfer to others in the group personal feelings of love, guilt, or hate.

When leaders respond to group members because of reactions from earlier relationships, they are engaging in *countertransference*. For example, if a group member reminds a leader of a teacher who was menacing and demanding, the leader is likely to react with anxiety and may become unreasonably fearful. It is therefore important that group members and leaders recognize the possibility of overreaction because of countertransference and that it is not an unusual reaction among nurses who are highly involved in helping others.

Healthcare Groups

Much of a nurse's professional life is spent in a wide variety of groups. As a participant in a group, the nurse may be required to fulfill different roles as member or leader, teacher or learner, adviser or advisee. Common types of healthcare groups include committees or teams, task forces, teaching groups, self-help groups, therapy groups, and work-related social support groups. These various types of groups exhibit similarities and differences, as do the roles of nurses participating in them.

Committees or Teams

Committees are those groups that are relatively stable or those that are brought together in a formal manner. These are the most common type of work-related group. They usually have a specific purpose that is part of their organizational structure, and they typically meet at defined intervals. Examples are policy committees, quality improvement committees, healthcare planning committees, nursing organization committees, and governmental affairs committees. Committees may also be referred to as teams, such as nursing care teams or wound care teams. Teams are groups with a small number of consistent individuals who are committed to a relevant shared purpose. Groups have performance goals, complementary and overlapping skills, and a common approach to their work.

The leader of a committee or team must be accepted by the members as an appropriate leader and, therefore, should be an expert in the area of the committee's focus. The leader's role is to identify the specific task, clarify communication, and assist in expressing opinions and offering solutions. Within a single organization, committee or team members are generally selected on the basis of their individual functional roles and employment status rather than their personal characteristics. If a committee or team is composed of representatives from multiple organizations, the members are generally assigned by the member organizations. Committee members may reflect diverse expertise in order to assist the committee in achieving its purpose. In some cases, membership might be designated by rule or law. For example, membership in county child fatality review teams typically is designated by law and includes representatives of local hospitals, emergency medical systems, law enforcement, community health nurses, and so forth. Additional member positions, often called "at-large" positions, may be designated to enable local committees to add members from organizations whose membership would be helpful but who are not on the list of those designated by rule or law. Regardless of the type of committee or team, members are accountable for the group's results or outcomes.

Task Forces

Task forces or ad hoc committees are work groups that usually have a defined task that is limited in duration. In other words, the task force is brought together to perform a specific activity, such as preparation for a visit by The Joint Commission or Nurse Week. When the activity has been accomplished, the task force is dissolved. Task forces and ad hoc committees function in the same way as committees or work teams. The difference is in the duration of their work.

Teaching Groups

The major purpose of a teaching group is to impart information to the participants. Examples of teaching groups include group continuing education and patient healthcare groups. Numerous subjects are often handled using a group teaching format: childbirth techniques, exercise for older adults, and instructions to family members about follow-up care for discharged patients. A nurse who leads a group in which the primary purpose is to teach or learn must be skilled in the teaching–learning process discussed in the module on Teaching and Learning.

Self-Help Groups

A **self-help group** is a group of individuals who come together to face a common problem or difficulty. These groups are based on the helper-therapy principle: Those who help are helped most. A central belief of the self-help movement is that individuals who experience a particular social or health problem have an understanding of the condition that those without it do not. Twelve-step groups such as Alcoholics Anonymous (AA) are self-help groups. Other support groups may consist of individuals who have specialized knowledge to help individuals who have the problem or who have experienced it.

Therapy Groups

Therapy groups are composed of individuals coming together to receive psychotherapy through which they work toward self-understanding, more satisfactory ways of relating or handling stress, and changing patterns of behavior around health. Members are referred to as patients, participants, or, in some settings, clients. They are selected by health professionals based on the pattern of personalities, behaviors, needs, and identification of group therapy as the treatment of choice. The number of sessions or the termination date is usually mutually determined by the therapist and members. Therapy groups are characterized by different approaches to psychotherapy—for example, interpersonal groups, existential groups, cognitive–behavioral groups, and psychodrama.

Work-related Social Support Groups

Many nurses, especially hospice, emergency, and critical care nurses, experience high levels of vocational stress. Social support groups can help reduce stress if they provide various types of support to buffer the stress. Group members who know about the work of others can encourage and challenge members to be more creative and enthusiastic about their work. For example, a nurse may help another group member consider alternative strategies for intervention. Members also can share the joys of success and the frustration of failure through active listening without giving advice or making judgments. This type of social support is best provided outside the work-related support group.

REVIEW   Groups and Group Communication

RELATE Link the Concepts and Exemplars

Linking the exemplar of groups and group communication with the concept of addiction:

1. How do individuals work in groups and use group communication when dealing with addiction?

2. What are some group communication types that may be useful when working with addicts in a group setting?

Linking the exemplar of groups and group communication with the concept of family:

3. How can families use group communication techniques to increase communication?

4. How might communication within a family be affected as a result of health alterations?

REFER Go to Pearson MyLab Nursing and eText

- Additional review materials

REFLECT Apply Your Knowledge

As a substance abuse nurse, you are responsible for leading daily meetings for a group of people who have addiction challenges. You have been asked to lead your first meeting now that you have finished your 6-week preceptorship and are now taking your own patient assignments on the unit. You are nervous about running a group independently. You begin to plan your session and want your mentor's input on whether you are planning a session that will be effective for the participants.

1. What type of meeting should you plan for this group?
2. What type of group problems might occur during the session?
3. After the session you feel that the group is ineffective. What characteristics would lead you to believe that this group is ineffective?

» Exemplar 38.B
Therapeutic Communication

Exemplar Learning Outcomes

38.B Analyze the interactive process of therapeutic communication.

- Summarize the various techniques used by nurses to support patients.
- Outline the phases of the therapeutic relationship.
- Explain ways that nurses can develop therapeutic relationships with patients.

- Differentiate considerations related to therapeutic communication throughout the lifespan.

Exemplar Key Terms

Physical attending, *2585*
Therapeutic communication, *2583*
Therapeutic relationship, *2583*

Overview

Therapeutic communication is an interactive process between the nurse and the patient. It is an integral part of the **therapeutic relationship**, which is the caring relationship between a nurse and a patient that is based on mutual trust and respect, sensitivity, and nurturing. Therapeutic communication helps the patient overcome temporary stress, get along with other people, adjust to situations that cannot be changed, and overcome any psychologic blocks that may stand in the way of self-realizations. Therapeutic communication promotes understanding and can help establish a constructive relationship between the nurse and the patient. Unlike the social relationship, which might not have a specific purpose or direction, the nurse establishes a therapeutic relationship with the purpose of helping the patient achieve health goals.

In therapeutic communication, the nurse responds not only to the content (words and thoughts) of a patient's verbal message but also to feelings the patient expresses and to nonverbal cues. It is important for the nurse to understand how the patient perceives a situation and feels about it before responding. Sometimes an individual can convey a thought in words that contradict the individual's emotions; that is, the patient's words and feelings are incongruent. For example, a patient might say, "I am glad he has left me; he was very cruel." However, the nurse observes that the patient has tears in her eyes as she says this. To respond to the patient's *words*, the nurse might simply rephrase, saying, "You are pleased that he has left you." To respond to the patient's *feelings*, the nurse would need to acknowledge the tears in the patient's eyes, saying, for example, "You seem saddened by all this." Such a response helps the patient focus on her feelings. In some instances, the nurse may need to know more about the patient and her resources for coping with these feelings.

Sometimes patients need time to deal with their feelings, especially before coping with certain activities such as learning new skills or planning for the future. This is most evident in hospitals when patients learn that they have a terminal illness. Some patients require hours, days, or even weeks before they are ready to start other tasks. Some need time to themselves, others need someone to listen, others need assistance identifying and verbalizing feelings, and others need assistance in identifying alternatives for future courses of action. However, while the nurse should help the patient explore alternatives, the nurse should not participate in the patient's decision making.

Therapeutic Communication Techniques

Therapeutic communication is intended to help patients reach an understanding about their condition or treatment while encouraging them to express feelings and ideas. Therapeutic communication is rooted in acceptance of the patient's point of view. Nontherapeutic communication, on the other hand, interferes with the nurse–patient relationship by putting barriers in the way of open communication (Evesham, 2016).

Therapeutic communication relies on active listening and continuous confirmation that both the nurse and the patient are being understood. In therapeutic communication, nurses take time to answer questions and encourage patients to satisfy their curiosity. In therapeutic communication, the nurse focuses on the most important issues and summarizes important points of communication to ensure that the patient understands the nurse and that the nurse understands the patient. Nontherapeutic communication detracts from patient care and includes behaviors such as asking irrelevant personal questions, sharing unnecessary

personal information of your own, or showing disapproval. False reassurance and sympathy are also aspects of nontherapeutic communication.

The nurse can employ a number of different communication techniques to support patients as they deal with their feelings related to their health and healthcare. The nurse must embrace these techniques and adapt them to each situation to improve communication with patients. However, no one technique will guarantee a successful encounter with all patients. Each situation is unique. The nurse should use a holistic approach to communicating with patients in each situation that is presented.

Empathizing

Active listening (described in depth later in the exemplar) is a skill that nursing students are taught throughout their education. Merely listening, however, is not enough. The nurse must have an empathetic understanding of the situation and offer appropriate feedback to the patient. *Empathy* is best described as a process in which individuals are able to put themselves in someone else's situation. By using empathy, the nurse is able to embrace the attitudes of each patient in each encounter.

To be able to empathize with patients, the nurse must be able to understand and acknowledge the ideas that the patient is expressing or that the patient feels are important to the situation. The nurse must also accept and respect the patient's feelings as valid for the patient, whatever those feelings may be, even if the nurse would not feel the same way in similar circumstances. Using empathy allows the nurse to connect with patients, and it also validates the importance of the patient's message to the nurse.

The term *empathy* is often mistakenly used to mean *sympathy*. Empathy, however, contains no elements of condolence, agreement, or pity. Empathy focuses on the patient's feelings, not the nurse's feelings. Nurses who sympathize rather than empathize assume that there is a parallel between their own feelings and the patient's feelings. This perceived similarity can make professional judgment and objectivity difficult. The nurse who empathizes can interpret the patient's feelings and does not insert his own feelings into the patient's current situation. The process of establishing empathetic understanding has four phases:

1. ***Identification.*** This phase involves the relaxation of conscious control. In this phase, the nurse is able to contemplate the patient and the patient's experiences.
2. ***Incorporation.*** In this phase, the nurse considers the patient's experiences and feelings rather than his own experiences.
3. ***Reverberation.*** This phase involves an interplay of the patient's internalized feeling with the nurse's own experiences or fantasies. The nurse is fully absorbed in the patient's identity but is able to experience himself separately.
4. ***Detachment.*** In this phase, the nurse withdraws from subjective involvement with the patient and resumes his own identity. The nurse uses the insight that was gained from the reverberation phase, along with reason and objectivity, to offer meaningful and useful responses to the patient.

Empathizing with patients who are troubled can have some stressful consequences for nurses. Problems can arise at any phase of the process, and when a nurse fails to cope with one of the four phases of achieving empathy, obstacles occur in terms of the nurse–patient relationship. The nurse should not identify too closely with the patient, because this can lead to sympathy rather than empathy.

Active Listening

Active listening, also called *attentive* or *mindful listening*, involves listening with multiple senses, in contrast to listening passively with just the ear. It is probably the most important technique in therapeutic communication and is the basis of all other techniques. Active listening requires energy and concentration. It is more than being quiet while the other individual talks—it involves paying attention to the total message, both verbal and nonverbal, and noting whether these communications are congruent. Active listening means absorbing both the content and the feeling the individual is conveying, without selectivity. The nurse does not select or listen solely to what she wants to hear; also, the nurse focuses not on her own needs but on the patient's needs. Active listening conveys an attitude of caring and interest, thereby encouraging the patient to talk (**Figure 38–8 》**).

Active listening also involves listening for key themes in the communication. The nurse must be careful not to react quickly to the message. The speaker should not be interrupted, and the nurse should take time to think about the message before responding. As a listener, the nurse also should ask questions either to obtain additional information or clarification and to ensure that the nurse fully understands the message.

Nurses need to be aware of their own biases. A message that reflects values or beliefs that differ from the nurse's should not be discredited for that reason. The patient, who is the sender, should decide when to close the conversation, and the nurse should listen for the signal that the patient is ready to do so. When the nurse closes the conversation, the patient may assume that the nurse considers the message unimportant.

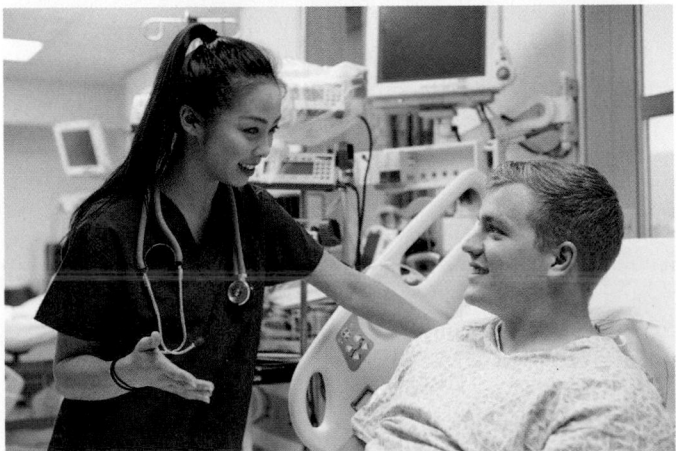

Source: Cathy Yeulet/123RF.com.

Figure 38–8 》 The nurse conveys active listening through a posture of involvement.

Box 38–3
Blocks to Active Listening

- *Rehearsing:* When the nurse is busy planning what to say next in the conversation
- *Being concerned with oneself:* When the nurse focuses on the nurse's own intelligence, competence, feelings, or accomplishments instead of focusing on the patient
- *Assuming:* When the nurse makes assumptions about what the patient is really trying to convey in the conversation
- *Judging:* When the nurse frames messages in the context of the nurse's own judgment about whether what the patient is saying is right or wrong, mature or immature, calm or anxious, sensible or paranoid, or depressed or simply quiet
- *Identifying:* When the nurse focuses on the nurse's own experiences, beliefs, or feelings; this may occur when what the patient communicates triggers memories or concerns from the nurse's own personal experiences
- *Getting off track:* When the nurse changes the subject or makes light of what the patient is expressing because the nurse is uncomfortable, bored, or tired
- *Filtering:* When the nurse tunes out certain topics in the conversation or hears only certain items that the patient is saying; this may occur because of anxiety on the part of the nurse.

There are some specific blocks to listening that may prevent the nurse from actually hearing what the patient says. This may convey a message to patients that what they have to say is not important (**Box 38–3 》**).

In summary, active listening is a highly developed skill that can be learned with practice. A nurse can listen actively and attentively to patients in various ways. Common responses that indicate active listening include nodding the head, uttering "uh huh" or "mmm," repeating the words that the patient has used, or saying "I see what you mean." Each nurse has characteristic ways of responding, and the nurse must take care not to sound insincere or patronizing.

Physical Attending

Physical attending is defined as the manner of being present to another or being with another. Listening, in a frame of reference, is what an individual does while attending. Five specific ways to convey physical attending, which in turn conveys involvement, include the following:

- *Look at the other person when speaking.* This position says, "I am available to you."
- *Adopt an open posture.* The nondefensive position is one in which neither arms nor legs are crossed. It conveys that the individual wishes to encourage the passage of communication, as the open door of a home or an office does.
- *Lean toward the person.* Individuals move naturally toward one another when they want to say or hear something—by moving to the front of a class, by moving a chair nearer a friend, or by leaning across a table with arms propped in front. The nurse conveys involvement by leaning forward, closer to the patient.
- *Maintain good eye contact.* Mutual eye contact, preferably at the same level, recognizes the other individual and

denotes willingness to maintain communication. Eye contact neither glares at nor stares down another but is natural.

- ***Try to be relatively relaxed.*** Total relaxation is not feasible when the nurse is listening with intensity, but the nurse can show relaxation by taking time when responding, allowing pauses as needed, balancing periods of tension with relaxation, and using gestures that are natural.

These five attending postures need to be adapted to the specific needs and cultural practices of patients in a given situation. For example, leaning forward may not be appropriate at the beginning of an interview. It may be reserved until a closer relationship grows between the nurse and the patient. The same applies to eye contact, which is generally uninterrupted when the communicators are very involved in the interaction, but which may be uncomfortable for or viewed as inappropriate by some patients.

Therapeutic communication techniques facilitate communication and focus on the patient's concerns. **Table 38–4** lists some common therapeutic communication techniques, with descriptions of the techniques and examples of their use. Touch can also be used as a part of therapeutic communication, but nurses are advised to use it with caution and intention (Anderson et al., 2016). As stated earlier, people from different cultures may view the use of touch differently. In addition, patients with a history of physical or sexual abuse and trauma and patients with certain mental illnesses, such as some personality disorders, may misinterpret the use of touch (Potter & Moller, 2016).

Using Silence

Nurses often feel that they must respond to each statement that is made by a patient. This, however, is not necessary.

The use of *silence* can be therapeutic and goes beyond active listening. The nurse who uses silence may sit or walk quietly with the patient. The goal is to provide a therapeutic purpose, such as:

- Encouraging the patient to communicate with the nurse
- Allowing the patient time to think about what has been said or to make connections
- Allowing the patient the necessary time to collect personal thoughts
- Allowing the patient time to consider possible alternatives.

The nurse who uses silence while remaining interested in what the patient is communicating maintains an open posture or a questioning look, which will encourage the patient to use the time effectively.

Silence is an effective communication technique only when it is used appropriately and purposefully for therapeutic communication. When an uncomfortable silence occurs, the nurse should break the silence and then analyze it. It is important not to allow the patient to become anxious or resistive. The nurse who is silent out of discomfort or a lack of knowledge or skill on how to communicate effectively should seek guidance from someone more experienced in order to analyze the personal and professional areas that are in need of growth.

Reflecting

In a 2013 article, Smith and Zsohar provide a number of other patient teaching techniques that can augment general therapeutic communication skills. One therapeutic teaching skill is the ability to assess a patient for individualized teaching. This requires the nurses to assess the patient's education

TABLE 38–4 Therapeutic Communication Techniques

Technique	Description	Examples
Using silence	Accepting pauses or silences that may extend for several seconds or minutes without interjecting any verbal response.	Sitting quietly (or walking with the patient) and waiting attentively until the patient is able to put thoughts and feelings into words.
Providing general leads	Using statements or questions that (a) encourage the patient to verbalize, (b) choose a topic of conversation, and (c) facilitate continued verbalization.	"Tell me how it is for you." "Perhaps you would like to talk about. . . ." "How might it help to discuss your feelings?" "Where would you like to begin?" "And then what?"
Being specific and tentative	Making statements that are specific rather than general and tentative rather than absolute.	"Rate your pain on a scale of 0 to 10" (specific statement) versus "Are you in pain?" (general statement) "You seem unconcerned about your diabetes" (tentative statement) versus "You don't care about your diabetes and you never will" (absolute statement)
Using open-ended questions	Asking broad questions that lead or invite the patient to explore (elaborate, clarify, describe, compare, or illustrate) thoughts or feelings. Open-ended questions specify only the topic to be discussed and invite answers that are longer than one or two words.	"I'd like to hear more about that." "Tell me about. . . ." "How have you been feeling lately?" "What brought you to the hospital?" "What is your opinion?" "You said you were frightened yesterday. How do you feel now?"
Sharing observations	The nurse openly informs the patient of the assessment and observations, especially those involving unconscious patient behavior.	"You are shaking." "You are biting your nails."

TABLE 38–4 Therapeutic Communication Techniques *(continued)*

Technique	Description	Examples
Restating or paraphrasing	Actively listening for the patient's basic message and then repeating those thoughts and/or feelings in similar words. This conveys that the nurse has listened and understood the patient's basic message and also offers patients a clearer idea of what they have said.	*Patient:* "I couldn't manage to eat any dinner last night—not even the dessert." *Nurse:* "You had difficulty eating yesterday?" *Patient:* "Yes, I was very upset after my family left." *Patient:* "I have trouble talking to strangers." *Nurse:* "You find it difficult talking to people you do not know?"
Seeking clarification	A method of making the patient's broad overall meaning of the message more understandable. It is used when paraphrasing is difficult or when the communication is rambling or garbled. To clarify the message, the nurse can restate the basic message or confess confusion and ask the patient to repeat or restate the message. Nurses can also clarify their own message with statements.	"I'm puzzled." "I'm not sure I understand that." "Would you please say that again?" "Would you tell me more?" "I meant this rather than that." "I'm sorry that wasn't very clear. Let me try to explain another way."
Perception checking or seeking consensual validation	A method similar to clarifying that verifies the meaning of specific words rather than the overall meaning of a message.	*Patient:* "My husband never gives me any presents." *Nurse:* "You mean he has never given you a present for your birthday or Christmas?" *Patient:* "Well—not never. He does get me something for my birthday and Christmas, but he never thinks of giving me anything at any other time."
Offering self	Suggesting one's presence, interest, or wish to understand the patient without making any demands or attaching conditions that the patient must comply with to receive the nurse's attention.	"I'll stay with you until your daughter arrives." "We can sit here quietly for a while. We don't need to talk unless you would like to." "I'll help you dress to go home if you'd like."
Giving information	Providing, in a simple and direct manner, specific factual information the patient may or may not request. When information is not known, the nurse states this and indicates who has it or when the nurse will obtain it.	"Your surgery is scheduled for 11 a.m. tomorrow." "You will feel a pulling sensation when the tube is removed from your abdomen." "I do not know the answer to that, but I will find out from Ms. King, the nurse in charge."
Acknowledging	Giving recognition, in a nonjudgmental way, of a change in behavior, an effort the patient has made, or a contribution to a communication. Acknowledgment may be with or without understanding, verbal or nonverbal.	"You trimmed your beard and mustache and washed your hair." "I notice you keep squinting your eyes." "You walked twice as far today with your walker."
Clarifying time or sequence	Helping the patient clarify an event, situation, or happening in relationship to time.	*Patient:* "I vomited this morning." *Nurse:* "Was that after breakfast?" *Patient:* "I feel like I have been asleep for weeks." *Nurse:* "You had your operation Monday, and today is Tuesday."
Presenting reality	Helping the patient differentiate the real from the unreal.	"The doorbell sound came from the program on television." "I see shadows from the window coverings." "Your magazine is here in the drawer. It has not been stolen."
Focusing	Helping the patient expand on and develop a topic of importance. It is important for the nurse to wait until the patient finishes stating the main concerns before attempting to focus. The focus may be an idea or a feeling; however, the nurse often emphasizes a feeling to help the patient recognize an emotion disguised behind words.	*Patient:* "My wife says she will look after me, but I don't think she can, what with the children to take care of. They're always after her about something—clothes, homework, what's for dinner that night." *Nurse:* "Sounds like you are worried about how well she can manage."
Reflecting	Directing ideas, feelings, questions, or content back to patients to enable them to explore their own ideas and feelings about a situation.	*Patient:* "What can I do?" *Nurse:* "What do you think would be helpful?" *Patient:* "Do you think I should tell my husband?" *Nurse:* "You seem unsure about telling your husband."
Summarizing and planning	Stating the main points of a discussion to clarify the relevant points discussed. This technique is useful at the end of an interview or to review a health teaching session. It often acts as an introduction to future care planning.	"During the past half hour we have talked about . . ." "Tomorrow afternoon we may explore this further." "In a few days I'll review with you what you have learned about the actions and effects of your insulin." "Tomorrow, I will look at your feeling journal."
Exploring	Investigating a patient's feeling related to a subject or idea.	"Would you describe your experience with that in more depth?" "Tell me more about your childhood."

and developmental level and also to determine what motivates the specific patient. Nurses can optimize the learning environment by turning off distractions and shutting the door, as well as sitting with the patient to create "space" for learning. Nurses should use effective teaching strategies such as demonstrating, involving the learner in the education process, and using videos for educational purposes. Nurses should confirm that their teaching efforts are understood. Nurses should ask themselves "Does my teaching reach the patient?" to help determine whether the patient is able to put the teaching into practice.

When nurses use reflection in the communication process, they are actively acknowledging what they have heard or seen from patients. *Reflecting* is what takes place when the nurse repeats the patient's verbal or nonverbal messages for the patient's benefit.

Reflecting Content

By reflecting the content of the message that the nurse receives from the patient, the nurse is essentially repeating the patient's statement. This allows the patient the opportunity to both hear and reflect on what she has told the nurse in the course of the conversation.

The technique of content reflecting is often misused or overused in the mental health environment. Overuse of this technique causes it to lose effectiveness. The nurse should use this technique judiciously.

Clinical Example C

Jason Smith is a 48-year-old man who has been admitted to the hospital with the diagnosis of acute inferior myocardial infarction. He says to the nurse, "I can't believe I had a heart attack. Those are for old people! I still feel young, but I guess I have to slow down." The nurse, using reflection, asks Mr. Smith, "Do you feel that you can no longer lead an active life because you have had a heart attack?" The nurse's statement will encourage Mr. Smith to continue sharing thoughts and explain why he believes this to be true. This will allow the nurse to correct any misunderstanding that he has about the recovery process after an MI.

Critical Thinking Questions

1. What physical attending communication techniques could be used in this interaction, and how might they impact the patient's communication?
2. How might the nurse use acknowledging in this encounter? What impact do you think it would have on this interaction?
3. What other communication techniques could the nurse use, and how might those impact the interaction with Mr. Smith?

Reflecting Feelings

In using the technique of *reflecting feelings*, the nurse verbalizes the feelings that are implied in the patient's comment. The nurse should respect that patients have the right to their own opinions and feelings even when the nurse personally disagrees with these. Some examples of reflecting feelings are as follows:

- "Sounds like you're really angry at your sister."
- "You're feeling anxious about being discharged from the hospital later today."

By reflecting feelings, the nurse attempts to identify any latent or connotative meanings that can either clarify or distort the content that is communicated. Reflection of feelings is useful because it will encourage the patient to make additional, clarifying comments in the conversation.

Imparting Information

In *imparting information*, the nurse is helping the patient by supplying additional data for consideration. This encourages further clarification because it is based on new or additional input. Some examples of statements that impart information are as follows:

- "Group therapy will be held on Wednesday afternoon from 3:30 until 5:00."
- "I am a mental-health nursing student."

Note that it is inappropriate to withhold information from a patient when the patient asks an information-seeking question. The nurse must be mindful not to cross the line between giving information and giving the patient advice. Also, the nurse should not give information as a way of avoiding conflict. Nurses who give patients personal or social information are moving outside of the realm of therapeutic communication. Information that the nurse must share with the patient includes the nurse's name, title, and position. New nurses must be cautioned to resist the temptation to divulge inappropriate information to patients.

The patient's participation in the decision-making process begins with the patient taking in and understanding information regarding his own condition. The ultimate goal of sharing essential information with the patient is to provide effective education that empowers the patient. Empowered patients are more likely to achieve a positive mental health and physical health outcome. They are also less likely to be admitted for inpatient therapy or be readmitted after discharge.

Additional examples of therapeutic techniques, annotated with the techniques used by the nurse, are provided in **Box 38–4 »**.

Avoiding Self-disclosure

Patients have been known to ask personal questions of nurses who are caring for them. This may include inquiring about the nurse's marital status, where the nurse lives, what religion the nurse practices, or information about personal issues. The best methods for deflecting requests for self-disclosure, outlined by Auvil and Silver in their classic 1984 study, include the following:

- *Using honesty:* "I don't feel comfortable sharing my address with you."
- *Using benign curiosity:* "Why are you asking me this today?"
- *Using refocusing:* "You were talking about how your mother treats you. Why are you changing the topic? You were saying. . . ."
- *Using interpretation:* "I notice that every time you talk about your sister, you change the subject and ask me a question." (pause)
- *Seeking clarification:* "You keep asking me where I live. I wonder if you have any concerns about me today?"

Box 38–4
Additional Examples of Therapeutic Communication

Example 1

Jeff Mastin, a 49-year-old man, is at the dermatologist's office having a basal cell carcinoma removed from his temple. Mr. Mastin teaches history and coaches baseball at the local high school. The procedure requires only a local anesthetic. Mr. Mastin's wife sits in a chair in the corner during the procedure. Dr. Keisha Thompson, the dermatologist, is conducting the procedure assisted by two nurses, Sheila Webber and Karl Kline. Ms. Webber's son is on the baseball team, and much of the conversation during the procedure revolves around baseball.

As Dr. Thompson finishes the procedure, Mr. Kline begins giving discharge instructions.

"You need to keep the bandage dry and intact for 48 hours. It's also important to minimize movement for 48 hours." **<giving information>**

"His baseball bag is in the trunk of the car, and he's planning on dropping me off at the house and going on to practice this afternoon." Ms. Mastin says.

"I understand you don't want to miss practice," Ms. Webber says, **<acknowledging>** "but the reason for limiting movement for 48 hours is because strenuous activity increases the risk of bleeding." **<being specific>**

Example 2

Junot Martinez, a 62-year-old man, is a professor of anthropology at the local college, and he was admitted to the hospital yesterday to have a noncancerous astrocytic brain tumor removed. Mr. Martinez just regained consciousness after being under anesthesia for many hours, and he is disoriented, asking disjointed questions of family, friends, and members of healthcare team. Clark Karabell, the nurse on duty, checks on Mr. Martinez during the period of his greatest confusion. Mr. Martinez has been mumbling for quite a few hours but eventually he poses a question to Mr. Karabell, "I feel like I've been asleep forever. How long have I been here?"

"You were admitted to the hospital yesterday morning, Mr. Martinez," Karabell responds. "That was Thursday morning, and now it is 4 p.m. on Friday." **<clarifying time>**

"Which one of you people stole my wallet?" Martinez asks, agitated.

"No one stole your wallet, Mr. Martinez," Karabell responds. "Your wife has your wallet, and she is downstairs at the food court right now." **<presenting reality>**

"Well, I guess nobody is looking out for me, then," Martinez says, looking downcast.

"Would you like me to stay with you until she returns?" Karabell asks. **<offering self>**

Example 3

Shuka Mansoori, a 50-year-old woman, is being released from the hospital following a heart attack. She is in a room with her husband, Blake, and seems withdrawn and moody despite being described normally as a sociable person. Francine Muhly, the nurse on duty, provides patient teaching on post–heart attack lifestyle changes when Ms. Mansoori unexpectedly asks, "Am I going to be okay?"

Ms. Muhly responds, "What specifically are you worried about, Ms. Mansoori?" **<seeking clarification, using open-ended questions>**

"I'm worried that I won't be able to play with the grandkids. I'm worried that I'm going to die," she says.

"So you're worried that you won't be able to do the things you enjoy and that you might have another heart attack?" Ms. Muhly summarizes. **<restating>**

"Yes," Ms. Mansoori says.

"I understand your concerns. However, if we work together to make a few simple changes to your diet, exercise routine, and smoking habit," Ms. Muhly says, "your overall health will improve. This will help reduce your risk of additional cardiovascular problems." **<planning>**

Example 4

Shen Liao, an 8-year-old boy, is admitted to the emergency department with significant bruising on his body. He is accompanied by his mother, Anya, and his 3-year-old sister, Laura. When asked how he received the bruises, Shen is silent, but his mother provides the explanation that he fell down a flight of stairs while playing with his younger sister.

Dave Musharraf, the nurse, is suspicious that the patient may have received the injuries through abuse, because most of the bruises are concentrated on the patient's back and forearms. He asks Shen and his mother, "Could you tell me more about the accident?" **<using open-ended questions, exploring>**

"Well," Mrs. Liao says, "he was at the top of the stairs and . . . tripped over a playground ball."

Musharraf turns to Shen and says "Shen, I'd like to hear your explanation. Could you tell me how the accident happened?" Musharraf then sits quietly while waiting for Shen to respond. **<using silence>**

"My dad hit me," Shen says quietly, looking away as his mother recoils.

"Thank you for telling me that, Shen," **<acknowledging>** responds Musharraf. "Can you tell me exactly what happened?" **<exploring>**

- **Responding with feedback and limit setting:** "I'm uncomfortable when you ask me who pays my tuition for school. Talking about my finances isn't part of our agreement to work together." Adding something like "The last time we met, you were deciding whether you were going to call your sister on the phone . . ." helps restructure the situation.

These communication techniques should be used within the context of the therapeutic relationship.

Therapeutic communication revolves around the needs of the patient. It is not appropriate for the nurse to talk to the patient about her experiences, such as what she did last night or her thoughts on a given subject. This wastes time that could be spent on learning about the patient's needs, thoughts, concerns, or problems. The nurse should always maintain a patient focus during communication.

Clarifying

Even when the nurse has listened carefully and thoughtfully to the patient, there may be a need to clarify information. *Clarifying* is an attempt to understand the basic nature of a patient's statement.

- "I'm confused about what is upsetting you. Could you go over that again, please?"

- "You say you're feeling anxious now. What's that like for you?"

Asking the patient to give an example allows the patient to clarify the meaning of the communication and helps the nurse understand the intended message. Clarification may be needed because of the language that the patient employs, such as slang used by adolescent patients, or when the nurse is not certain of adequate interpretation of what the patient is trying to convey.

Clinical Example D

The nurse is caring for Sara Kim, a 36-year-old woman who was recently diagnosed with breast cancer. The physician has informed Ms. Kim that her chance of full recovery is excellent and has recommended a course of treatment to include removal of the involved breast followed by chemotherapy. While the nurse is providing preoperative instructions, Ms. Kim says, "I'll sign the consent form, but I'll be dead before the surgery date." The nurse is not sure whether Ms. Kim is fearful of dying from cancer or whether this may be a statement of suicidal ideation. The nurse seeks clarification by asking, "Why do you think you'll be dead before the date for surgery arrives?"

Critical Thinking Questions

1. What would be an appropriate next step if Ms. Kim clarifies that she is considering suicide?
2. What would be an appropriate next step if Ms. Kim clarifies that she believes she will die from the cancer before the surgery can take place?
3. What is another therapeutic communication tactic that the nurse could have used instead of clarifying? How might the outcome have been changed with the use of a different technique?

Paraphrasing

By *paraphrasing*, the nurse restates in her own words what the patient has said. Some examples of paraphrasing statements are as follows:

- "In other words, you're tired of being treated like a child."
- "I hear you saying that when people compliment you, you feel embarrassed and if they knew the real you, they would not provide such praise."

The nurse is able to test her understanding of what the patient is trying to communicate through paraphrasing. Paraphrasing is reflective in nature as it lets the patient know what the nurse heard and how the nurse understands what is being discussed. It is also an opportunity for the patient to clarify the content of the message or the feelings behind it.

Checking Perceptions

Nurses can *check perceptions* by sharing how they perceived and heard the information. Once the nurse's perceptions have been shared, it is important to ask the patient to verify the perception, by using statements such as the following:

- "Let me know if this is how you see it, too."
- "I get the feeling that you're uncomfortable when we're silent. Does that seem right?"

The effective use of perception checking conveys that the nurse wants to understand what the patient is communicating.

It gives the patient the opportunity to correct inaccurate perceptions that the nurse may have. Essentially, *checking perceptions* allows the nurse to avoid actions that are based on false assumptions about the patient.

Questioning

Questioning is a very direct way of speaking that the nurse can use when communicating with a patient. This technique is quite useful when the nurse is seeking specific information. If the nurse is trying to engage in meaningful dialogue with a patient, questions should be limited, because they can affect the nature and the ranges of responses from the patient.

Open-ended questions can be used to elicit more information than closed questions. An *open-ended question* allows the nurse to focus the topic while allowing the patient freedom with responses. Examples of this include the following:

- "How did you feel when your brother said that to you?"
- "What's your opinion about . . . ?"

Closed questions should be used sparingly because they typically limit the patient's responses to "yes" or "no." Closed questions also limit therapeutic exploration. This type of question can be useful, however, for the patient who may have disorganized thinking. Closed questions can be used to guide these patients.

Questions that ask "why" are typically less helpful than open-ended questions. These questions tend to be hard to answer, in part because they require a higher level of insight on the part of the patient, and they rarely lead to the nurse having a clearer understanding of the current situation. Other types of closed questions, such as "who," "what," "when," and "how," can be useful if the nurse uses them wisely.

Nurses must be careful when questioning not to steer the patient to answer questions in a certain way. For example, "You don't exercise in excess, do you?" may suggest that the patient answer this question with a "no." Refer to the module on Assessment for more information on using open-ended and closed questions.

Structuring

The nurse can use a technique known as *structuring* in an attempt to create order or establish guidelines for patients. This helps patients become aware of their problems and the order in which they should deal with them. Examples of structuring statements are as follows:

- "You've mentioned that you want to improve your relationships with your husband, your son, and your boss. Let's put them in order of importance."
- "No, I won't be giving you advice, but we can discuss some solutions to these issues together."

The nurse can use structuring when a patient introduces a number of issues in a brief period and doesn't know where to begin. This technique can also be used to define the parameters of the nurse–patient relationship in terms of how the nurse will participate with the patient to facilitate the problem-solving process.

Pinpointing

The nurse can use a technique known as *pinpointing* to call attention to specific statements and relationships. For example, when the nurse points out inconsistencies among statements or similarities and differences in points of view, feelings, or actions, the nurse is engaging in pinpointing. This can also be used to determine differences between what an individual says and what one does. Examples of pinpointing statements include the following:

- "So, you and your husband aren't in agreement about how many children you want."
- "You say you're happy, but you're frowning."

Linking

When using the technique known as *linking*, the nurse responds to the patient in a way that ties together events, experiences, feelings, or people. Nurses often use linking to connect past experience with current behaviors that the patient is exhibiting. The nurse can also use linking when there is tension between two individuals during times of stress. Examples of statements that use linking include the following:

- "You felt depressed after the death of both of your parents."
- "So, the arguments didn't really begin until after you lost your job."

Giving Feedback

In using *feedback*, the nurse shares reactions to the patient's statements or behaviors. This technique can help a patient become aware of how their own actions and behaviors can affect others. The nurse who responds with feedback may engage in therapeutic self-disclosure because it allows the nurse to offer constructive information regarding how the patient's words or actions have affected the nurse as a communication partner. Total self-disclosure, however, is inappropriate in the nurse–patient relationship and should be avoided. This can place a burden of interdependence on the patient and may limit the time and energy the nurse has available to work on the patient's concerns. The use of reciprocal self-disclosure is more appropriate in friend and colleague relationships than in nurse–patient relationships.

Effective feedback should have three distinct qualities. It should be *immediate*, meaning that it is given as soon as possible; it should be *honest*, meaning that it provides a true reaction; and it should be *supportive*, meaning that it is provided in a way that is tolerable to comprehend and never hurtful or disrespectful to the patient. Examples of effective feedback statements include the following:

- "When you cross your arms while speaking, I feel your apprehension."
- "Sometimes when you look down while we are talking, I think you're angry."

Feedback should always be provided to the patient in a nonthreatening manner. Threatening feedback may increase the patient's defensiveness. The more defensive the patient is when engaging in therapeutic communication, the less able the patient is to hear and understand the feedback that the nurse is providing. Patients often feel offended if they perceive the nurse to be rejecting them. Feedback that is nontherapeutic, meaning that it is harsh, hurtful, cruel, or rejecting of the patient, will create an unnecessary boundary between the patient and the nurse. The nurse should take great care to prevent the patient from feeling personally rejected as a result of feedback from the nurse. **Table 38–5 »** lists strategies and rationales that the nurse can use for giving helpful, nonthreatening feedback.

Feedback goes both ways. Patients usually want to accomplish several items during their interactions with the

TABLE 38–5 Giving Helpful, Nonthreatening Feedback

Strategy	Rationale
Focus the feedback on behavior.	Feedback should relate to what the patient actually does rather than how the nurse imagines the patient to be.
Focus the feedback on observations.	Feedback should relate to what the nurse actually sees or hears the patient do. When inferences are used rather than observations, the nurse is drawing conclusions or making assumptions.
Focus the feedback on description.	Description reports what actually occurred rather than evaluating it in terms of good or bad, right or wrong.
Focus feedback on "more or less" rather than "either/or" descriptions of behaviors.	"More or less" descriptions stress quantity rather than quality (which may be value laden).
Focus feedback on here-and-now behavior rather than there-and-then behavior.	The most meaningful feedback from the nurse is given as soon as it is appropriate to do so.
Focus feedback on sharing of information and ideas.	Sharing of ideas and information helps the patient make decisions about the patient's own well-being. In contrast, by giving advice, the nurse takes away the patient's freedom to be self-determining.
Focus feedback on exploration of alternatives.	Focusing on a variety of alternatives for accomplishing a particular goal for the patient prevents premature acceptance of answers or solutions that may not be appropriate.
Focus feedback on its value to the patient.	Feedback should serve the patient's needs, not the needs of the nurse.
Limit feedback to the appropriate amount of information.	Overload of information will decrease the effectiveness of feedback for the patient.
Limit feedback to the appropriate time and place.	For feedback to be effective, it must be presented at the appropriate time.
Focus feedback on what is said rather than why it is said.	Focusing on why the patient has said something or done something moves away from observations and toward patient motive or intent. Motive or intent can only be assumed and, unless verified, such an assumption is counterproductive.

Box 38–5
Reflecting on Feedback from Patients

Input can be both positive and negative. Input can be received from a wide variety of individuals, including classmates, instructors, and patients. Input can allow the nurse to become more aware of "blind spots," that is, those characteristics about the self that are ignored, denied, or defended. Self-deception can interfere with the nurse's ability to relate and to communicate. Strategies to increase self-awareness include:

- Think about recent interactions with patients and how those patients responded to you.
- Identify the positive/negative elements in these interactions.
- Try to determine what the patients were telling you about yourself in the interactions. Ask these questions: What characteristics do you possess that enable patients to openly express their thoughts and feelings? What characteristics do you possess that prevent patients from openly expressing their thoughts and feelings?
- Discuss the interactions and your interpretations of them with an instructor, mentor, or preceptor.
- Ask for feedback on your behavior from others.

nurse. They want to express themselves, and they want to express information about their perception of the nurse. The nurse should be open and receptive when receiving cues from the patient, either solicited or unsolicited, because these can be useful in a more meaningful working relationship. **Box 38–5 »** provides strategies to help nurses reflect on feedback from patients.

Confronting

Used in a constructive way, confrontation can lead to productive change. *Confronting* is defined as the deliberate invitation to examine some aspect of personal behavior. Typically, confronting is used when there is a discrepancy or incongruence between what an individual says and what that individual does. It can also be used when expected behavior differs from actual behavior, such as when a patient who is prescribed a liquid diet asks family members to sneak in food from a restaurant. Confrontation requires careful attention to nonverbal communication and to both verbal and nonverbal discrepancies between messages.

The two basic types of confrontation are informational and interpretive. Each type can be directed toward the patient's resources and limitations. An *informational confrontation* describes the visible behavior of another individual (e.g., "You look sad and say you're 'not as smart as your brother and a sister,' yet you are the only one who made the honor roll"). *Interpretive confirmation* expresses thoughts and feelings about behavior and draws inferences (e.g., "Ever since Emily and Frank criticized the way you conducted the assembly, you haven't spoken to them. It looks like you're feeling angry").

Six skills can be used in incorporating constructive confrontations:

1. Use personal statements with the words *I, my,* and *me.*
2. Use relationship statements that express thoughts and feelings about the patient in the present.

3. Use statements that describe visible patient behaviors. This is known as behavior descriptions.
4. Use the description of personal feelings in which you specify the feeling by name.
5. Use responses that are aimed at understanding. Examples of these include paraphrasing and perception checking.
6. Use constructive feedback skills.

Summarizing

Summarizing is a technique that the nurse can use to highlight the main ideas that are expressed during interactions. It is used to convey the nurse's understanding to the patient, and it allows both nurse and patient to benefit from a review of the main ideas of a conversation. Summarizing can also be useful when the nurse wants to focus the patient's thinking and to aid in conscious learning.

In certain instances, summarizing is particularly appropriate. The nurse may want to use this technique in the first few minutes of patient interaction, because it is useful to review what occurred during previous interactions. This helps the patient recall items that were discussed and gives the patient an opportunity to see how the nurse synthesized the information from previous encounters. Summarizing also keeps all participants directed toward a common goal.

Processing

The nurse can also use a technique known as processing. *Processing* is a complex and sophisticated technique used to direct attention to the interpersonal dynamics of the nurse–patient relationship in terms of content, feelings, and behaviors that have been expressed. This is an advanced skill. Processing is most useful and meaningful when therapeutic intimacy has been achieved.

Clinical Example E

The nurse is preparing to conduct a home visit to Emily Bardinovich, an 86-year-old woman who has lived in an assisted living apartment for the past 5 years. Mrs. Bardinovich was recently discharged back to her apartment following an exacerbation of COPD. The nurse has cared for Mrs. Bardinovich for many years and knows her as a friendly, outgoing woman with a great sense of humor who loves to tease people. Today, the nurse finds Mrs. Bardinovich very quiet and reserved with little to say. The nurse comments, "You're very quiet today; you haven't teased me at all," to which Mrs. Bardinovich responds, "I'm just not in the teasing mood." The nurse has used processing to help the patient begin to talk about how she feels. This will allow the nurse to perform a more in-depth assessment of the patient's mood and thoughts.

Critical Thinking Questions

1. What therapeutic communication strategies could the nurse use to respond to the patient's statement, "I'm just not in the teasing mood?"
2. What are some potential outcomes if the nurse does not ask Mrs. Bardinovich why she is being so quiet?
3. Describe how the outcome might differ if the nurse uses linking instead of processing in this situation.

Common Mistakes

Nurses often make mistakes when it comes to therapeutic communication. It can be difficult for the nurse to both empathize and communicate with patients when the nurse is feeling uncomfortable with the situation. In addition to the barriers to communication discussed earlier and outlined in Table 38–1, some common mistakes the nurse should take care to avoid include the following:

- **Giving advice.** This carries the message that the patient is not capable of solving problems.
- **Minimizing or discounting feelings.** Attempts at reassurance often minimize and discount what the patient is feeling.
- **Deflecting.** Changing the subject or making jokes in an attempt to move the conversation to something that is less painful is not considered a positive shift because it gives the patient the message that the nurse does not know how to cope with the patient's experience.
- **Interrogating.** Asking a series of questions implies that the nurse is more interested in gaining information than in listening to what the patient has to say.
- **Sparring.** Debating or disagreeing with the patient sets up an adversarial dynamic and prevents the nurse from listening to what the patient is trying to communicate.

Clinical Example F

Anita Alvarez, a nurse, is providing care to Mark Walton, a 27-year-old man who has just been diagnosed with irritable bowel syndrome (IBS). Anita is teaching Mr. Walton about the dietary changes that he will need to make to manage his condition. Anita asks a series of questions quickly, changing the subject rapidly and not allowing Mr. Walton to provide answers or ask clarifying questions. During the session, she reads directly off a computer screen. When Mr. Walton does get a chance to ask questions, Anita takes several seconds to respond because she is busy looking at her phone. She focuses on herself for several minutes when Mr. Walton asks one question about her work. When Mr. Walton leaves, Anita says, "Everything's going to be all right" as she slams the door.

Critical Thinking Questions
1. Which mistakes or barriers to communication did Anita engage in?
2. What could Anita have done better or differently to ensure that Mr. Walton retained the information and to promote the therapeutic relationship?

The Therapeutic Relationship

Nurse–patient relationships are referred to by some as interpersonal relationships, by others as therapeutic relationships, and by still others as helping relationships. Helping is a growth-facilitating process that strives to achieve two basic goals (Egan, 2013):

1. Help patients manage their problems of living more effectively and develop unused or underused opportunities more fully.
2. Help patients become better at helping themselves in their everyday lives.

A therapeutic relationship may develop over weeks of working with a patient or within minutes. The keys to a therapeutic relationship are the development of trust and acceptance between the nurse and the patient and an underlying belief that the nurse cares about and wants to help the patient.

The therapeutic relationship is influenced by the personal and professional characteristics of the nurse and the patient. Age, sex, appearance, diagnosis, education, values, ethnic and cultural background, personality, expectations, and setting can all affect the development of the nurse–patient relationship. Consideration of all of these factors, combined with good communication skills and sincere interest in the patient's welfare, enables the nurse to create a therapeutic relationship. A therapeutic relationship:

- Is an intellectual and emotional bond between the nurse and the patient and is focused on the patient.
- Respects the patient as an individual, including the following:
  (a) Maximizing the patient's abilities to participate in decision making and treatments
  (b) Considering the patient's ethnic background and cultural practices
  (c) Considering family relationships and values.
- Respects patient confidentiality.
- Focuses on the patient's well-being.
- Is based on mutual trust, respect, and acceptance.

Phases of the Therapeutic Relationship

The therapeutic relationship process can be described in terms of four sequential phases: the preinteraction phase, introductory phase, working (maintaining) phase, and termination phase. Each phase is characterized by identifiable tasks and skills, and the relationship must progress through the stages in succession because each builds on the one before. The nurse can identify the progress of a relationship by understanding these phases.

Preinteraction Phase

The preinteraction phase is similar to the planning stage before an interview. In most situations, the nurse has information about the patient before the first face-to-face meeting. This information may include the patient's name, address, age, medical history, and/or social history. Planning for the initial visit may generate some anxious feelings in the nurse. If the nurse recognizes these feelings and identifies specific information to be discussed, positive outcomes can evolve.

Introductory Phase

The introductory phase, also referred to as the orientation phase or the pretherapeutic phase, sets the tone for the rest of the relationship. During this initial encounter, the patient and the nurse closely observe each other, and each forms judgments about the other's behavior. The goal of the nurse in this phase is to develop trust and security within the nurse–patient relationship (Boyd, 2014).

During the initial parts of the introductory phase, the patient may display some resistive behaviors. *Resistive behaviors* are those that inhibit involvement, cooperation, or change. These behaviors may arise from the patient's difficulty in acknowledging the need for help, fear of exposing and facing feelings, anxiety about the discomfort involved in changing problem-causing behavior patterns, and fear or anxiety in response to the nurse's approach, which may, in the patient's opinion, be inappropriate.

The nurse can overcome a patient's resistive behaviors by conveying a caring attitude, genuine interest in the patient, and competence. This will help the nurse foster the development of trust in the relationship. *Trust* can be described as a reliance on someone without doubt or question, or the belief that the other individual is capable of assisting in times of distress and in all likelihood will do so. To trust another individual involves risk; patients become vulnerable when they share thoughts, feelings, and attitudes with the nurse. Trust, however, enables the patient to express thoughts and feelings openly.

By the end of the introductory phase, patients should begin to do the following:

- Develop trust in the nurse.
- View the nurse as a competent professional capable of helping.
- View the nurse as honest, open, and concerned about the patient's welfare.
- Believe the nurse will try to understand and respect the patient's cultural values and beliefs.
- Believe the nurse will respect patient confidentiality.
- Feel comfortable talking with the nurse about feelings and other sensitive issues.
- Understand the purpose of the relationship and the respective roles of the patient and nurse.
- Feel like an active participant in developing a mutually agreeable plan of care.

Clinical Example G

While working in an ambulatory care setting, the nurse is asked by the physician to talk with a 24-year-old female patient named Raissa Kunin to explain the need for phlebotomy secondary to Ms. Kunin's diagnosis of polycythemia. Ms. Kunin's hemoglobin is 17.4 mg/dL; it has been steadily increasing since 1 year ago, when it was 16.2 mg/dL. The nurse enters the room and says, "Hello, Ms. Kunin, my name is Mikela Mathews. I'm a registered nurse working for Dr. Shah. He asked me to speak with you about the need to remove blood to lower your hemoglobin." Ms. Kunin says, "I'm just not sure I want to do that, but I'll call you after I have time to think about it." The nurse responds by stating, "You have every right to make a decision in your own best interest. What if I just give you some information while you're here so you can make your decision based on all the details. I can explain the risks of polycythemia, the process of removing blood, and answer any questions you may have." The nurse attempts to overcome resistance behavior by allowing the patient to maintain control. This also promotes a trusting relationship with the patient.

Critical Thinking Questions

1. How would you respond if the patient answered, "No, thank you. That's not necessary. I can look it up on the internet"?
2. If the patient agrees to listen to the nurse, what phase of the relationship will they be in once the nurse begins teaching?
3. What other types of resistive behaviors might you encounter, and how would you attempt to overcome them?

Working Phase

The working phase has two major stages: exploring and understanding thoughts and feelings, and facilitating and taking action. In this phase, the nurse helps the patient explore thoughts, feelings, and actions and plan a program of action to meet preestablished goals.

The nurse must have the following skills for this phase of the therapeutic relationship:

- *Empathetic listening and responding.* As discussed previously, the nurse must listen attentively and respond in ways that indicate that the nurse acknowledges the patient's concerns and feelings as important. Nonverbal behaviors indicating empathy include moderate head nodding, a steady gaze, moderate gesturing, and little activity or body movement.
- *Respect.* The nurse must show respect for the patient's willingness to be available, a desire to work with the patient, and a manner that conveys that the nurse takes the patient's point of view seriously.
- *Genuineness.* The nurse exudes genuine care for the patient by maintaining professional behaviors that promote the therapeutic helping relationship. Egan (2013) has outlined five behaviors that are components of genuineness: not taking refuge or overemphasizing the role of counselor, being spontaneous, being nondefensive, being consistent, and being capable of appropriate self-disclosure.
- *Concreteness.* The nurse must encourage the patient to be concrete and specific rather than to speak in generalities. When the patient says, "My blood pressure has been very unstable," the nurse narrows the topic to the specific by replying, "Show me your blood pressure log for the past 2 weeks."
- *Reflecting, paraphrasing, clarifying, and confronting.* These skills, as described earlier, assist nurses in making sure they understand the patient's messages and feelings and help the patient to identify discrepancies that inhibit the patient's self-understanding or exploration of specific areas and ideas.

During this first stage of the working phase, the intensity of interaction increases, and the patient may express or demonstrate feelings such as anger, shame, or self-consciousness. If the nurse is skilled in this stage and the patient is willing to pursue self-exploration, the outcome is a beginning understanding on the part of the patient about behavior and feelings.

Patients with dementia or cognitive impairments may not move between phases of the nurse–patient relationship in the same way as patients with normal cognitive function. Nurses working with these patients often find a need to reintroduce themselves at each meeting.

Termination Phase

The termination phase of the relationship is often expected to be difficult and filled with ambivalence. However, if the relationship has evolved effectively though the previous phases, the patient generally has a positive outlook and feels able to handle problems independently. On the other hand, because caring attitudes have developed, it is natural to expect some feelings of loss, and each individual in the relationship needs to develop a way of saying good-bye.

Many methods can be used to terminate relationships. Summarizing or reviewing the process can produce a sense of accomplishment. This may include sharing reminiscences of how things were at the beginning of the relationship and comparing them to how they are now. It is also helpful for both the nurse and the patient to express their feelings about termination openly and honestly. Thus, termination discussions need to start in advance of the termination interview. This allows time for the patient to adjust to independence. In some situations, referrals are necessary, or it may be appropriate to offer an occasional standby meeting to give support as needed. Follow-up phone calls or emails are other interventions that can ease the patient's transition to independence.

Developing Therapeutic Relationships

Whatever the practice setting, the nurse develops a therapeutic relationship in which to establish mutual goals (outcomes) with the patient or, if the patient is unable to participate, with support people. Although special training in counseling techniques is advantageous, there are many ways of helping patients that do not require special training:

- *Listen actively.* Active listening allows the nurse to gather pertinent information about the patient's physical and emotional health, and it also conveys that the nurse is fully interested in what the patient has to say.

- *Help identify what the person is feeling.* Patients who are troubled are often unable to identify or label their feelings and consequently have difficulty working them out or talking about them. Responses such as "You seem angry about your diagnosis" or "You sound as if you've been lonely since your wife died" can help patients recognize what they are feeling and talk about it.

- *Put yourself in the other person's shoes (i.e., empathize).* Communicate to the patient in a way that shows an understanding of the patient's feelings and the behavior and experience underlying these feelings.

- *Be honest.* In an effective relationship, the nurse honestly recognizes any lack of knowledge by saying "I don't know the answer to that right now;" can openly discuss the nurse's own discomfort by saying, for example, "I feel uncomfortable about this discussion;" and can also admit tactfully that problems do exist, for instance, when a patient says "I'm a mess, aren't I?"

- *Be genuine and credible.* Patients will sense whether you are truly concerned.

- *Use your ingenuity.* Consider all of the available actions when handling problems. Whatever course is chosen needs to further the achievement of the patient's goals (outcomes), be compatible with the patient's value system, and offer the probability of success.

- *Be aware of cultural differences that may affect meaning and understanding.* To facilitate nurse–patient interactions, recognize the language(s) and/or dialect(s) the patient uses. Provide a bilingual interpreter as needed for patients with limited English language ability.

- *Maintain patient confidentiality.* To maintain the patient's right to privacy, share information only with other healthcare professionals as needed for effective care and treatment.

- *Know your role and your limitations.* Clarify functions and roles, specifically what is expected of the patient, the nurse, and the primary care provider. Every individual has unique strengths and problems. When you feel unable to handle some of the patient's problems, you should inform the patient of this and refer the patient to the appropriate health professional.

Lifespan Considerations
Communicating with Children and Families

In caring for pediatric patients, the nurse should implement interventions that will establish an effective nurse–child–family relationship. The nurse must provide an appropriate environment that will foster nurse–child–family communication and ensure confidentiality while doing so. The techniques the nurse uses to develop this relationship are similar to the techniques that the nurse uses with an individual patient, tailoring communication techniques to the needs of both the child and the family (**Figure 38–9 》**).

The nurse can use any of several communication techniques with children. These include accepting, active listening, broad openings, clarifying, collaborating, exploring, focusing, giving recognition, observation, offering self, placing an event in time or sequence, reflection, restating or paraphrasing, summarizing, and validating perceptions. The nursing implications for each technique are explored in **Table 38–6 》**.

Establishing Rapport with Children

First and foremost, the nurse must establish rapport with the child to set the stage for a productive therapeutic relationship. All patients, including children, will be more responsive to

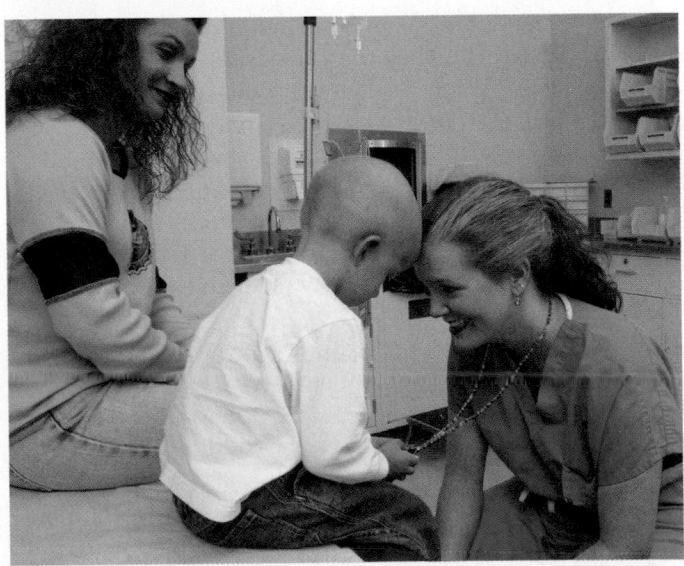

Figure 38–9 》 Taking time to listen to the child and family members is important for establishing trust and developing rapport.

TABLE 38–6 Nursing Implications of Using Therapeutic Communication Techniques with Children

Communication Technique	Nursing Implications
Accepting	By conveying acceptance, the nurse respects the child's emotions and allows the child to cry when in pain or lets the child know that crying is okay.
Active listening	The nurse involves the child in the discussion and encourages the child to communicate his point of view. It is important to face the child and parents when speaking. This conveys to the family that the nurse is listening and understands what is being said.
Broad openings	This includes using open-ended questions that allow the child to choose the topic for discussion.
Clarifying	By asking the child to clarify or elaborate on what is being expressed, the nurse communicates understanding.
Collaborating	The nurse suggests collaboration with the child and family and then assists them through the problem-solving process.
Exploring	This helps the child to organize their thoughts and focus on the current issue. It will also encourage the child to discuss the issue in more detail.
Focusing	This guides the direction of the conversation. It is useful with small children who may wish to discuss a variety of topics.
Giving recognition	This identifies observed behaviors and indicates an interest in the child.
Observation	This is particularly important with the behavioral aspect of communication. The nurse acknowledges behaviors that indicate the child's thoughts and feelings.
Offering self	This indicates that the nurse is available and willing to listen to the child.
Placing the event in time or sequence	The goal of this technique is to help the child and the nurse understand the order of events.
Reflection	This indicates that the nurse is interested in the discussion and also validates the child's concerns.
Restating or paraphrasing	This acknowledges to the child that the nurse is listening. It also validates appropriate interpretation of what the child is communicating.
Summarizing	This highlights the key facts of the conversation and also provides an opportunity to consider direction for future discussions. It can also provide closure. Summarizing can occur at varying points in the communication process.
Validating perceptions	This is when the nurse shares conclusions that have been drawn as a result of the discussions with the child. It provides an opportunity for the child to confirm or deny interpretations that the nurse has made throughout the process.

the nurse who makes an effort to help the patient feel that they are important in an interaction. The following guidelines can be used by the nurse to establish rapport with a child and encourage the sharing of information and feelings:

- *Position yourself on the same eye level as the child.* This suggests to the child that the nurse cares about and respects the child.

- *Show interest in what the child is doing.* This displays that the nurse is interested and encourages security.

- *Agree with the child when it is appropriate.* It may be appropriate for the nurse to share feelings. An example of this is telling the child, "I don't like the taste of that medicine either, but sometimes I have to take it when I am sick—but then I drink something that I like." Sharing experiences with the child offers encouragement to the child and family.

- *Compliment the child.* Examples include "You are really strong" or "You picked really nice colors for that picture." Complimentary statements by the nurse may reduce anxiety while conferring status on the child.

- *Use a calm tone of voice and language that is developmentally appropriate.* It is important to talk and share information with children that is on an appropriate level of comprehension.

- *Pace the discussion or procedure so that the child does not feel rushed.* Feeling rushed will increase the child's anxiety.

- *Explain concepts in terms the child can understand.* This is especially important for preschool-age children, who have a limited concept of time. For example, stating "Your mother will be back after lunch" is appropriate for this age level because it provides a concrete time frame that the child can understand.

- *Include the child in the discussion of care if developmentally appropriate.* This is particularly important for adolescents, because they have the cognitive ability to participate in abstract conversation and to comprehend some medical terminology.

- *Listen more than you talk, and avoid distractions.* This shows the child that the nurse is interested in what the child has to say.

Establishing Trust with Children and Families

Trust is critical to an effective nurse–child–family relationship. Strategies to establish trust with children and families include following through on promises made to the child and family, respecting confidentiality, and being truthful, even when the truth is not what they want to hear.

If a child asks whether a procedure is painful, answer truthfully, but follow with positive words. For example, if a child asks if his "shot" is going to hurt, you might reply, "Yes, most people say that a shot hurts, but it will hurt only for a moment, and then it will be over. Your mother can hold your hand while I give you the shot if that will make you feel better." By following difficult information with a positive rationale or comforting statement, the nurse can maintain credibility while still providing compassionate care.

Communicating with Pregnant Women

Whether a pregnancy is planned or unplanned, the patient is likely to experience stress and emotional distress. Therapeutic communication with pregnant women is especially important because the woman's emotional and physical health—as well as the health of the child—is at stake during pregnancy (Goodtherapy.org, 2016). Sources of emotional distress during pregnancy include worries about the health of the child, independent mental health issues such as anxiety and depression, strained romantic partnerships, financial issues, and physical challenges. Physical health issues include fetal development, physical strain on the mother, proper nutrition, and many others outlined in the Reproduction module.

Keys to communicating with pregnant women are relating medical information clearly and listening for patient questions and concerns. Nurses should use active listening techniques to be attentive to the patient's verbal and nonverbal communication. Silence can be a powerful tool to allow the patient to express herself fully so the nurse can address her concern. Making observations fills a similar role in that it allows the patient to communicate without the need for lengthy questioning. For example, the nurse can make observations such as "You look tired" to solicit communication by the patient. Using therapeutic communication techniques can help clarify patient concerns and protect the health of both mother and child.

Communicating with Older Adults and Their Families

Most older adults respond well to the therapeutic communication strategies outlined above. However, many older adults suffer from conditions that make communication difficult and require the nurse to adjust the therapeutic communication strategy (Potter et al., 2013). Approximately half of older adults suffer from hearing loss, and many also suffer from vision loss. These sensory impairments require the nurse to select communication techniques specifically tailored to the needs of the individual

older adult. For example, a nurse can change the environmental conditions of the individual with hearing loss to promote effective communication. Many of the difficulties in communicating effectively with older adults arise when the nurse and patient fail to establish a reliable nurse–patient communication system. The nurse can overcome communication impairments of all kinds by researching assistive communication devices and involving the patient's family in the communication process.

Establishing a reliable communication system with an older adult requires the nurse to continuously reevaluate the patient's communication needs. For instance, for a patient with a cognitive impairment such as dementia, the nurse can use simple, concrete sentences, ask one question at a time, allow time for the patient to reflect, be an active listener, and include family in conversation to ease the burden on the patient. For patients who are visually impaired, nurses can check for use of glasses, identify themselves when coming into contact with the patient, speak in a normal tone of voice, seldom use gestures, and employ fonts of readable size in printed materials. If the patient seems to not understand the nurse's questions or teaching, the nurse can reevaluate whether she can take any specific steps to change the communication pattern, such as moving to a different room or involving another member of the healthcare team. To communicate most effectively with the older patient, nurses should acquaint themselves with the patient's family and friends to learn about relevant health concerns and favorite conversational topics.

Conclusion

Whether teaching, advocating, assessing, planning, documenting, or intervening, the nurse requires strong communication skills. The ability to communicate effectively plays a large role in the nurse's ability to deliver the highest quality of care to patients. Whether communicating with patients, other members of the healthcare team, distraught family members, or peers, nurses need to be understood and understand the messages they receive. Strong verbal and written communication skills are required of the effective nurse, who must also monitor nonverbal communication to maintain consistency in the messages sent to others.

REVIEW Therapeutic Communication

RELATE Link the Concepts and Exemplars

Linking the exemplar of therapeutic communication with the concept of advocacy:

1. How do strong therapeutic communication skills contribute to the nurse's role as a patient advocate?

2. How do strong therapeutic communication skills contribute to the nurse's ability to work within groups to advocate for patients?

Linking the exemplar of therapeutic communication with the concept of teaching and learning:

3. The nurse is preparing to teach a patient who is newly diagnosed with diabetes about self-care. Describe the four phases of the therapeutic relationship as it applies to the patient-teaching plan.

4. While teaching the patient with diabetes, the nurse accidentally creates a barrier to the therapeutic relationship by misspeaking. What should the nurse do next?

REFER Go to Pearson MyLab Nursing and eText

■ Additional review materials

REFLECT Apply Your Knowledge

Zainah Kattan is a newly licensed nurse working at the Neighborhood Hospital. She is assigned the care of Lydia Ocampo, a 70-year-old woman who was born and raised in the Philippines, who has been diagnosed with Alzheimer disease. Ms. Ocampo was admitted with a fractured hip following a fall at home that occurred when she was wandering around her house late one

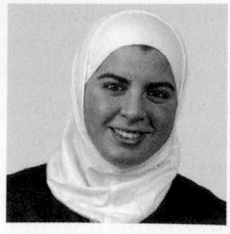 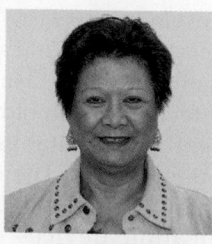

night. Ms. Ocampo was assigned a different nurse yesterday, but Danilo Ocampo, her husband, complained to the nurse manager when he came to visit and found her restrained and yelling for help with an untouched breakfast tray in front of her. Mr. Ocampo requested that a different nurse be assigned to his wife's care from now on. Ms. Kattan is happy to act as her primary nurse. She develops rapport with Mr. Ocampo and gets satisfaction from caring for his wife by helping her to feel more comfortable.

1. When communicating with a patient diagnosed with later-stage Alzheimer disease, what strategies will the nurse employ?
2. Why does the development of rapport with Mr. Ocampo improve the patient's ability to meet expected outcomes?
3. Mr. Ocampo complains to Ms. Kattan about the poor care provided to his wife by the other nurse, Bobby Schofield. How should Ms. Kattan respond to this statement?

≫ Exemplar 38.C
Documentation

Exemplar Learning Outcomes

38.C Analyze documentation as it relates to communication.

- Outline the legal and ethical considerations of documentation.
- Summarize the purposes of patient records.
- Outline various types of documentation systems.
- Summarize the documentation of nursing activities.
- Describe facility-specific documentation.
- Outline general guidelines for recording documentation.

Exemplar Key Terms

Assessment, 2602
Chart, 2598
Charting, 2598
Charting by exception (CBE), 2603
Discussion, 2598
Documenting, 2598
Evaluation, 2602

Flow sheet, 2602
Focus charting, 2602
Interventions, 2602
Narrative charting, 2600
Objective data, 2602
Patient record, 2598
PIE documentation model, 2602
Plan of care, 2602
Problem-oriented medical record (POMR), 2601
Problem-oriented record (POR), 2601
Record, 2598
Recording, 2598
Report, 2598
Revision, 2602
SOAP, 2601
SOAPIER, 2602
Source-oriented record, 2600
Subjective data, 2602
Variance, 2605

Overview

Effective communication among healthcare professionals is vital to the quality of patient care. Generally, healthcare personnel communicate through discussion, reports, and records. A **discussion** is an informal oral consideration of a subject by two or more healthcare personnel to identify a problem or establish strategies to resolve a problem. A **report** is oral, written, or electronic communication intended to convey information to others. For instance, nurses always report on patients at the end of a hospital work shift. A **record** may be handwritten or electronic. The process of making an entry on a patient record is called **recording**, **charting**, or **documenting**.

A clinical record, also called a **chart** or **patient record**, is a formal, legal document that provides evidence of a patient's care. Although healthcare organizations use different systems and forms for documentation, all patient records include similar information.

Each healthcare organization has policies about recording and reporting patient data, and each nurse is accountable for following the organization's standards. Agencies also indicate which nursing assessments and interventions can be recorded by RNs and which can be charted by unlicensed personnel. In addition, The Joint Commission requires patient record documentation to be timely, complete, accurate, confidential, and specific to the patient.

The need for documentation to be specific to the patient goes beyond simply ensuring that the individual patient's information is entered correctly in the healthcare record. Complete, accurate, and specific patient information includes entering relevant, objective information about cultural and other considerations that will help other members of the healthcare team who work with the patient to provide culturally appropriate, respectful care.

Ethical and Legal Considerations

The American Nurses Association (ANA) Code of Ethics (2015) states, "[T]he nurse has a duty to maintain confidentiality of all patient information" (p. 9). The patient's record is legally protected as a private record of the patient's care.

Access to the patient's record is restricted to healthcare professionals involved in giving care to that patient. The institution or agency is the rightful owner of the patient's record. This does not, however, exclude the patient's rights to the same records. See the module on Ethics and the module on Legal Issues for more information.

On April 14, 2003, changes were made to the Health Insurance Portability and Accountability Act (HIPAA) regulations to maintain the privacy and confidentiality of protected health information (PHI). PHI is identifiable health information that is transmitted or maintained in any form or medium, including verbal discussions, electronic communications with or about patients, and written communications.

For purposes of education and research, most agencies allow student and graduate healthcare professionals access to patient records. The records are used in patient conferences, clinics, rounds, patient studies, and written papers. The student or graduate is bound by a strict ethical code and legal responsibility to hold all information in confidence. Both students and practicing nurses have the responsibility to protect the patient's privacy by not using a name or any statements that may identify the patient in their worksheets, notes for class, or any notations they make that could potentially leave the facility's premises. Most facilities provide shredders or other receptacles for discarding material that contains PHI.

Ensuring Confidentiality of Electronic Records

Because of the increased use of computerized patient records, healthcare agencies have developed policies and procedures to ensure the privacy and confidentiality of patient information stored electronically. In addition, the Security Rule of HIPAA governs the security of electronic forms of protected health information and defines sanctions and fines for hospitals, clinics, and providers who violate this security. Some suggestions for ensuring the confidentiality and security of electronic records include:

1. A personal password is required to enter and sign off computer files. Do not share this password with anyone, including other healthcare team members, and do not display passwords in the computer area. Use only agency computers that have security functions built into the system for transmission of PHI.
2. After logging on, never leave a computer terminal unattended. Sign out of the computer before leaving it unattended to prevent unintended access to patient information.
3. Do not leave patient PHI displayed on the monitor where others may see it.
4. Shred all unneeded computer-generated worksheets.
5. Know the facility's policy and procedure for correcting an entry error.
6. Follow agency procedures for documenting sensitive material, such as a diagnosis of a sexually transmitted infection.
7. Information technology personnel must install a firewall to protect the server from unauthorized access.

Purposes of Patient Records

Patient records are kept for a number of purposes:

- **Communication.** The patient record serves as the vehicle by which different healthcare professionals who interact with a patient communicate with each other. This prevents fragmentation, repetition, and delays in patient care.
- **Planning patient care.** Each healthcare professional uses data from the patient's record to plan care for that patient. A primary care provider, for example, may order a specific antibiotic after establishing that the patient's temperature is steadily rising and that laboratory tests reveal the presence of a certain microorganism. The nurse uses baseline and ongoing data to evaluate the effectiveness of the nursing care plan.
- **Auditing health agencies.** An audit is a review of patient records for quality assurance purposes (see the module on Quality Improvement). Accrediting agencies such as The Joint Commission may review patient records to determine whether a particular health agency is meeting required standards.
- **Research.** The information contained in a record can be a valuable source of data for research. The treatment plans for a number of patients with the same health problems can yield information helpful in treating other patients.
- **Education.** Students in health disciplines often use patient records as educational tools. A record can frequently provide a comprehensive view of the patient, the illness, effective treatment strategies, and factors that affect the outcome of the illness.
- **Reimbursement.** Documentation helps a facility receive reimbursement from the federal government. For a facility to obtain payment through Medicare, for example, the patient's clinical record must contain the correct diagnosis-related group (DRG) codes and reveal that the appropriate care has been given. Codable diagnoses, such as DRGs, are supported by accurate and thorough recordings of a patient's care by nurses. Accurate coding not only facilitates reimbursement from the federal government but also facilitates reimbursement from insurance companies and other third-party payers. If additional care, treatment, or length of stay becomes necessary for the patient's welfare, thorough documentation will help justify these needs.
- **Legal documentation.** The patient's record is a legal document and usually is admissible in court as evidence. In some jurisdictions, however, the record is considered inadmissible as evidence when the patient objects, because information the patient gives to the physician is confidential.
- **Healthcare analysis.** Information from records may assist healthcare planners to identify agency needs, such as overused and underused hospital services. Records can be used to establish the costs of various services and to identify those services that cost the agency money and those that generate revenue.

Documentation Systems

A number of documentation systems are in current use. The most common are the source-oriented record; the problem-oriented medical record; the problems, interventions, evaluation (PIE) model; focus charting; charting by exception (CBE); and electronic documentation. In the American Recovery and Reinvestment Act (ARRA) of 2009, the federal government mandated that all healthcare facilities move to electronic medical records from paper records. Electronic records are the fastest growing type and are quickly replacing or augmenting the other methods of documentation.

Source-oriented Record

The traditional patient record is a **source-oriented record**. Each individual or department makes notations in a separate section or sections of the patient's chart. For example, the admissions department has an admission sheet; the physician has a physician's order sheet, a physician's history sheet, and progress notes; nurses use the nurses' notes; and other departments or personnel have their own records. In this type of record, information about a particular problem is distributed throughout the record. For example, if a patient had left hemiplegia (paralysis of the left side of the body), data about this problem might be found in the physician's history sheet, on the physician's order sheet, in the nurses' notes, in the physical therapist's record, and in the social service record. **Table 38–7 »** lists the components of a source-oriented record.

Source-oriented records may be compiled by narrative charting. **Narrative charting** consists of written notes that include routine care, normal findings, and patient problems

TABLE 38–7 Components of the Source-oriented Record

Form	Information
Admission (face) sheet	■ Legal name, birth date, age, gender ■ Identification number ■ Address ■ Marital status; closest relatives or individual to notify in case of emergency ■ Date, time, and admitting diagnosis ■ Food or drug allergies ■ Name of admitting (attending) physician ■ Insurance information ■ Any assigned DRGs
Initial nursing assessment	■ Findings from the initial nursing history and physical health assessment
Graphic record	■ Body temperature ■ Pulse rate ■ Respiratory rate ■ Blood pressure ■ Daily weight · ■ Special measurements such as fluid intake and output and oxygen saturation
Daily care record	■ Activity ■ Diet ■ Bathing ■ Elimination records
Special flow sheets	■ Examples: fluid balance record, skin assessment
Medication record	■ Name, dosage, route, time, date of regularly administered medications ■ Name or initials of individual administering the medication
Nurses' notes	■ Pertinent assessment of patient ■ Specific nursing care, including teaching and patient's responses ■ Patient's complaints and how patient is coping
Medical history and physical examination	■ Past and family medical history ■ Present medical problems ■ Differential or current diagnoses ■ Findings of physical examination by the primary care provider
Physician's order sheet	■ Medical prescriptions for medications, treatments, and so on
Physician's progress notes	■ Medical observations, treatments, patient progress, and so on
Consultation records	■ Reports by medical and clinical specialists
Diagnostic reports	■ Examples: laboratory reports, x-ray reports, CT scan reports
Consultation reports	■ Examples: physical therapy, respiratory therapy
Patient discharge plan and referral summary	■ Started on admission and completed on discharge ■ Includes nursing problems, general information, and referral data

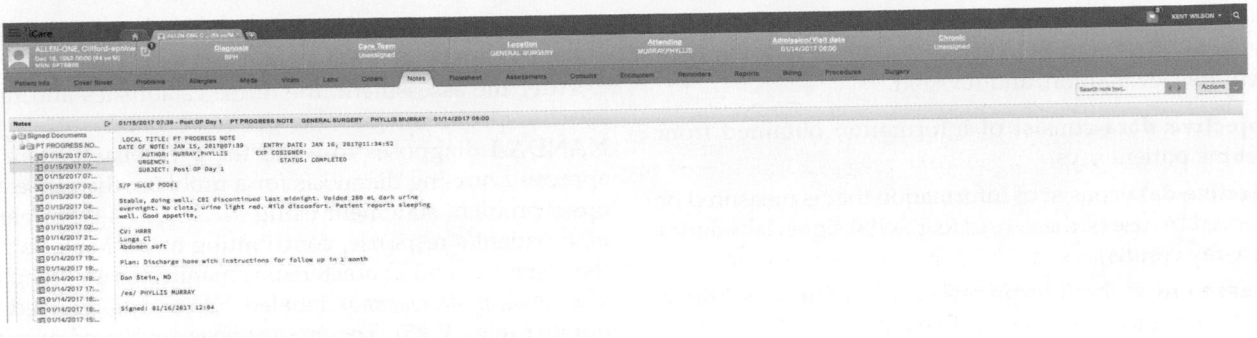

Source: RealEHRprep with iCare. Copyright © 2017 by iCare.

Figure 38–10 》 A narrative note in an electronic health record (EHR).

(Figure 38–10 》). There is no right or wrong order to the information, although chronologic order is frequently used. Although narrative charting is a traditional part of the source-oriented record, few institutions today use only narrative charting. It is being replaced by systems such as charting by exception and focus charting (discussed below). Many agencies combine narrative charting with another system. For example, an agency using a charting-by-exception system may use narrative charting only when describing abnormal findings. However, narrative charting is expedient in emergency situations. When using narrative charting, nurses must ensure the information is organized in a clear, coherent manner. Using the nursing process as a framework is one way to do this.

Source-oriented records are convenient because (a) care providers from each discipline can easily locate the forms on which to record data and (b) it is easy to trace the information specific to one's discipline. The disadvantage is that information about a particular patient problem is scattered throughout the chart, making it difficult to find chronologic information on a patient's problems and progress. This can lead to decreased communication among the healthcare team, an incomplete picture of the patient's care, and a lack of coordination of care (International Federation of Health Information Management Associations [IFHIMA], 2014).

Problem-oriented Medical Record

The **problem-oriented medical record (POMR)**, or **problem-oriented record (POR)**, was established by Lawrence Weed in the 1960s. In a POMR, data are arranged according to the problems the patient has rather than according to the source of the information. Members of the healthcare team contribute to the problem list, plan of care, and progress notes. Plans for each active or potential problem are created, and progress notes are recorded for each problem.

The advantages of POMRs are that they encourage collaboration, and that the problem list in the front of the chart alerts caregivers to the patient's needs, making it easier to track the status of each problem. The disadvantages of a POMR are that caregivers differ in their ability to use the required charting format, constant vigilance is required to maintain an up-to-date problem list, and it is somewhat inefficient because assessments and interventions that apply to more than one problem must be repeated.

The POMR has four basic components: database, problem list, plan of care, and progress notes. In addition, flow sheets and discharge notes are added to the record as needed.

Database

The database of a POMR consists of all information known about the patient when the patient first enters the healthcare agency. It includes the nursing assessment, the physician's history, social and family data, and the results of the physical examination and baseline diagnostic tests. Data are constantly updated as the patient's health status changes.

Problem List

The problem list is derived from the database. It is usually kept at the front of the chart and serves as an index to the numbered entries in the progress notes. Problems are listed in the order in which they are identified, and the list is continually updated as new problems are identified and others resolved. All caregivers may contribute to the problem list, which includes the patient's physiologic, psychologic, social, cultural, spiritual, developmental, and environmental needs. Primary care providers write problems as medical diagnoses, surgical procedures, or symptoms; nurses write problems as nursing diagnoses.

As the patient's condition changes or more data are obtained, problems may need to be redefined. When a problem is resolved, a line is drawn through it and the number is not used again for that patient.

Plan of Care

In the POMR method, the initial list of orders or plan of care is made with reference to the active problems. Care plans are generated by the individual who lists the problems. Physicians write physician's orders or medical care plans; nurses write nursing orders or nursing care plans. The written plan in the record is listed under each problem in the progress notes and is not isolated as a separate list of orders.

Progress Notes

A progress note in the POMR is a chart entry made by any of the healthcare professionals who are involved in a patient's care, who all use the same type of sheet for notes. Progress notes are numbered to correspond to the problems on the problem list and may be lettered for the type of data. The SOAP format is frequently used. **SOAP** is an acronym for subjective data, objective data, assessment, and planning.

Over the years, the SOAP format has been modified; the acronyms *SOAPIE* and **SOAPIER** refer to formats that add interventions, evaluation, and revision.

Subjective data consist of information obtained from what the patient says.

Objective data consist of information that is measured or observed by use of the senses (e.g., vital signs, laboratory and x-ray results).

Assessment is the interpretation or conclusions drawn about the subjective and objective data.

Plan of care is designed to resolve the stated problem. The initial plan is written by the individual who enters the problem into the record. All subsequent plans, including revisions, are entered into the progress notes.

Interventions refer to the specific interventions that have actually been performed by the caregiver.

Evaluation includes patient responses to nursing interventions and medical treatments. This is primarily reassessment data.

Revision reflects care plan modifications suggested by the evaluation. Changes may be made in desired outcomes, interventions, or target dates.

An example of a nursing progress note using SOAPIER is shown in **Figure 38–11 》**.

PIE Model

The **PIE documentation model** groups information into three categories. **PIE** is an acronym for

Problems,

Interventions

Evaluation of nursing care.

This system consists of a patient care assessment flow sheet and progress notes. The **flow sheet** uses specific assessment criteria in a particular format, such as human needs or functional health patterns. The time parameters for a flow sheet can vary from minutes to months. In a hospital intensive care unit, for example, a patient's blood pressure may be monitored by the minute, whereas in an ambulatory clinic a patient's blood glucose level may be recorded once a month.

After the assessment, the nurse establishes and records specific problems on the progress notes, often using NANDA-I diagnoses to word the problem. If there is no approved nursing diagnosis for a problem, the nurse develops a problem statement using NANDA-I's three-part format: patient's response, contributing or probable causes of the response, and characteristics manifested by the patient. The *problem statement* is labeled "P" and is referred to by number (e.g., P #5). The *interventions* employed to manage the problem are labeled "I" and are numbered according to the problem (e.g., I #5). The *evaluation* of the effectiveness of the interventions is labeled "E" and is numbered according to the problem (e.g., E #5).

The PIE system eliminates the traditional care plan and incorporates an ongoing care plan into the progress notes. Therefore, the nurse does not have to create and update a separate plan. One of the disadvantages to PIE is that the nurse must review all nursing notes before giving care to determine which problems are current and which interventions were effective.

Focus Charting

Focus charting is intended to make the patient and the patient's concerns and strengths the focus of care. Three columns for recording are usually used: date and time, focus, and progress notes. The *focus* may be a condition, nursing diagnosis, behavior, sign or symptom, acute change in the patient's condition, or patient strength. The progress notes are organized into (D) data, (A) action, and (R) response, referred to as DAR. The *data* category reflects the assessment phase of the nursing process and consists of observations of patient status and behaviors, including data from flow sheets (e.g., vital signs, pupil reactivity). The nurse records both subjective and objective data in this section.

The *action* category reflects planning and implementation and includes immediate and future nursing actions. It may also include any changes to the plan of care. The *response* category reflects the evaluation phase of the nursing process

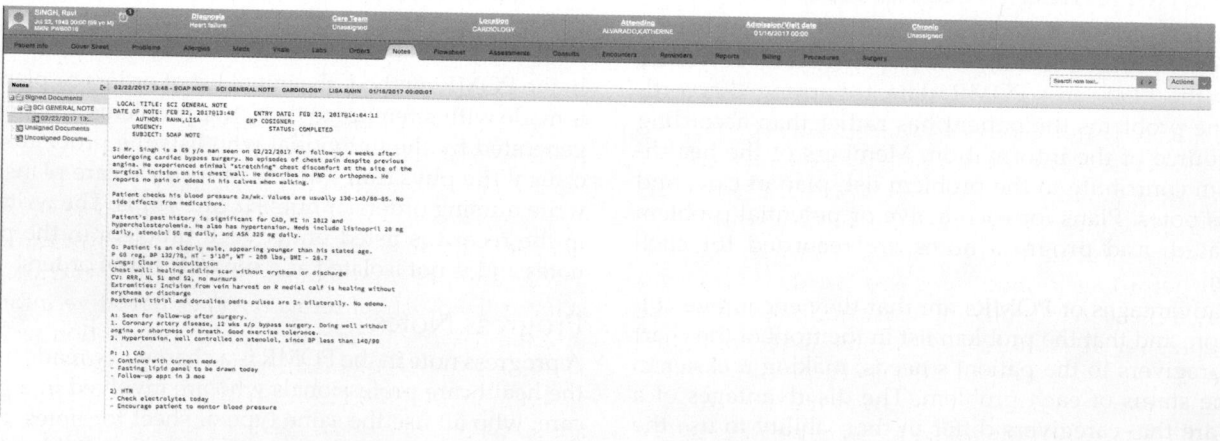

Source: From RealEHRprep with iCare. Copyright © 2017 by iCare.

Figure 38–11 》 An example of a nursing progress note using SOAPIER in an EHR.

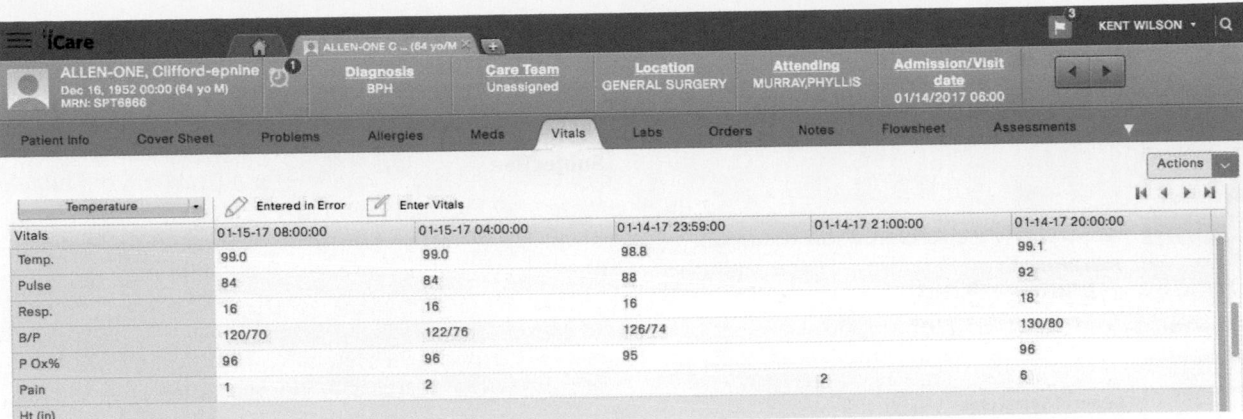

Figure 38–12 》》 A sample vital signs graphic record in an EHR.

and describes the patient's response to any nursing and medical care.

The focus charting system provides a holistic perspective of the patient and the patient's needs. It also provides a nursing process framework for the progress notes (DAR). The three components do not need to be recorded in order, and each note does not need to have all three categories. Flow sheets and checklists are frequently used on the patient's chart to record routine nursing tasks and assessment data.

Charting by Exception

Charting by exception (CBE) is a documentation system in which only abnormal or significant findings or exceptions to norms are recorded. CBE incorporates three key elements (Guido, 2013):

1. **Flow sheets.** Examples of flow sheets include a graphic record (**Figure 38–12 》》**), fluid balance record, daily nursing assessments record (**Figure 38–13 》》**), patient teaching record, patient discharge record, and skin assessment record.

2. **Standards of nursing care.** Documentation by reference to the agency's printed standards of nursing practice eliminates much of the repetitive charting of routine care. An agency using CBE must develop its own specific standards of nursing practice that identify the minimum criteria for patient care regardless of clinical area. Some units may also have unit-specific standards unique to the type of patient. For example, "The nurse must ensure that the unconscious patient has oral care at least every 4 hours." Documentation of care according to these specified standards involves only a check mark in the routine standards box on the graphic record. If not all of the standards are implemented, an asterisk on the flow sheet is made with reference to the nurses' notes. All exceptions to the standards are fully described in narrative form on the nurses' notes.

3. **Bedside access to chart forms.** In the CBE system, all flow sheets are kept at the patient's bedside to allow immediate recording and to eliminate the need to transcribe data from the nurse's worksheet to the permanent record.

The advantages to this system are the elimination of lengthy, repetitive notes and that it makes changes in the patient's condition more obvious. Inherent in CBE is the presumption that the nurse did assess the patient and determined what responses were normal and abnormal. Many nurses believe in the saying "not charted, not done" and subsequently may feel uncomfortable with the CBE documentation system. One suggestion is to write N/A on flow sheets where the items are not applicable and to not leave blank spaces. This would then avoid the possible misinterpretation that the assessment or intervention was not completed by the nurse.

Electronic Documentation

Computerized clinical record systems are the fastest growing sector in the field of documentation. Electronic health record (EHR) or electronic medical record (EMR) systems provide an efficient way to manage the huge volume of information required in contemporary healthcare. Nurses use computer databases to store the patient data, add new data, create and revise care plans, and document patient progress. Some institutions provide a computer terminal at each patient's bedside, such as a Computer on Wheels (COW) or a small handheld device for the nurse to carry; these technologies enable the nurse to document care immediately after providing it.

Computers and related electronic devices make care planning and documentation relatively easy. To record nursing actions and patient responses, the nurse either chooses from standardized lists of terms or types narrative information into the device. Automated speech-recognition technology allows nurses to enter data by voice for conversion to written documentation. However, according to HIPAA, if the spoken word is used to create or address protected health information, the nurse must be alert and aware of others who might hear the dictation and take care to protect the privacy of the patient's information. An expanding role in

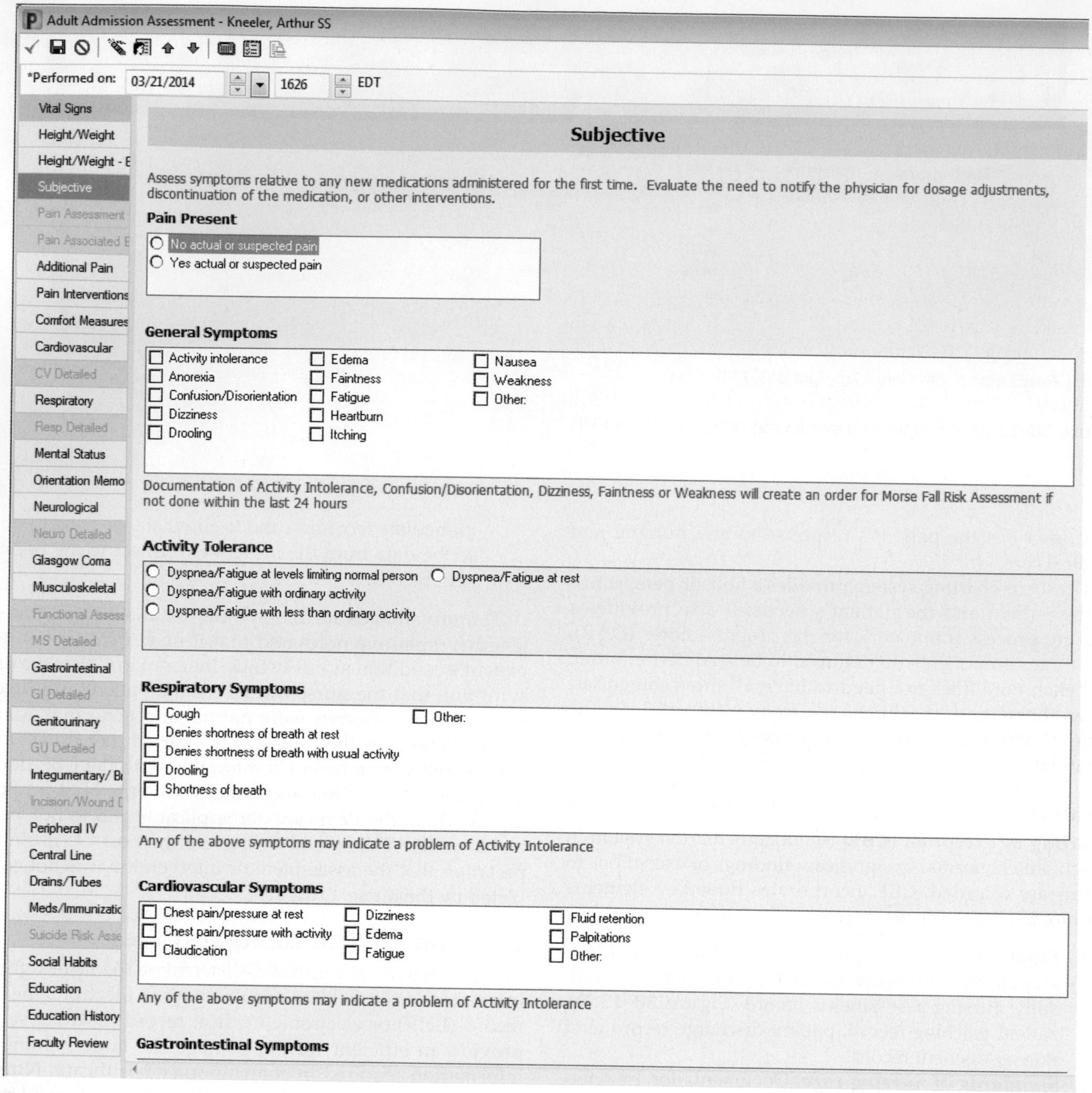
Adult Admission Assessment - Kneeler, Arthur SS

*Performed on: 03/21/2014 1626 EDT

Vital Signs
Height/Weight
Height/Weight - E
Subjective
Pain Assessment
Pain Associated E
Additional Pain
Pain Interventions
Comfort Measures
Cardiovascular
CV Detailed
Respiratory
Resp Detailed
Mental Status
Orientation Memo
Neurological
Neuro Detailed
Glasgow Coma
Musculoskeletal
Functional Assess
MS Detailed
Gastrointestinal
GI Detailed
Genitourinary
GU Detailed
Integumentary/ Br
Incision/Wound D
Peripheral IV
Central Line
Drains/Tubes
Meds/Immunizatic
Suicide Risk Asse
Social Habits
Education
Education History
Faculty Review

Subjective

Assess symptoms relative to any new medications administered for the first time. Evaluate the need to notify the physician for dosage adjustments, discontinuation of the medication, or other interventions.

Pain Present

- No actual or suspected pain
- Yes actual or suspected pain

General Symptoms

- Activity intolerance
- Anorexia
- Confusion/Disorientation
- Dizziness
- Drooling
- Edema
- Faintness
- Fatigue
- Heartburn
- Itching
- Nausea
- Weakness
- Other:

Documentation of Activity Intolerance, Confusion/Disorientation, Dizziness, Faintness or Weakness will create an order for Morse Fall Risk Assessment if not done within the last 24 hours

Activity Tolerance

- Dyspnea/Fatigue at levels limiting normal person
- Dyspnea/Fatigue with ordinary activity
- Dyspnea/Fatigue with less than ordinary activity
- Dyspnea/Fatigue at rest

Respiratory Symptoms

- Cough
- Denies shortness of breath at rest
- Denies shortness of breath with usual activity
- Drooling
- Shortness of breath
- Other:

Any of the above symptoms may indicate a problem of Activity Intolerance

Cardiovascular Symptoms

- Chest pain/pressure at rest
- Chest pain/pressure with activity
- Claudication
- Dizziness
- Edema
- Fatigue
- Fluid retention
- Palpitations
- Other:

Any of the above symptoms may indicate a problem of Activity Intolerance

Gastrointestinal Symptoms

Source: Neehr Perfect® networked educational EHR featuring WorldVistA, courtesy of Archetype Innovations, LLC 2010.

Figure 38–13 ›› Sample of a portion of a daily nursing CBE assessment form in an EHR.

healthcare is that of the "medical scribe," who is a paraprofessional trained to enter physician assessment data and medical orders directly into the EMR on behalf of the provider and accordingly free the physician to focus more attention on the patient than the computer.

EHRs make it possible to transmit information from one care setting to another. The nursing Minimum Data Set (MDS) is an effort to establish standards for collecting standardized, essential nursing data for inclusion in computer databases.

EMRs contain the standard medical and clinical data gathered in one provider's office. EHRs go beyond data collected at the individual healthcare provider's office and over time compile a comprehensive patient history (Office of the National Coordinator for Health Information Technology, 2014). EHR data can be created, managed, and consulted by healthcare staff within the same agency as well as across any number of healthcare organizations. EMRs and EHRs are more useful than paper records by most measures. In particular, electronic records can track data over time, identify patients who are due for particular procedures, monitor patients' vaccination schedules, and improve patient safety.

Documentation systems called electronic medication administration records (eMARs) are specifically used to keep track of patient medication information (Techopedia, 2016). eMARs use barcodes and a handheld scanner to send and fill prescriptions. Medication dosages, number of refills, types of medications, medication classifications, refill history, prescription status, and tracking information are all included in the eMAR. These records accelerate the prescribing process, and their quality assurance tools and audit tracking features enhance available information and severely limit the possibility of a medication error.

Case Management

The case management model emphasizes high-quality, cost-effective care delivered within an established length of stay. This model uses an interprofessional approach to planning and documenting patient care using *critical pathways*. These forms identify the outcomes that certain groups of patients are expected to achieve on each day of care, along with the interventions necessary for each day. **Figure 38–14 》** illustrates part of a critical pathway for a patient with a total hip replacement.

Along with critical pathways, the case management model incorporates graphics and flow sheets. Progress notes typically use some type of charting by exception. For example, if goals are met, no further charting is required. A goal that is not met is called a **variance**. A variance is a deviation from what is planned on the critical pathway, that is, an unexpected occurrence that affects the planned care or the patient's responses to care. When a variance occurs, the nurse writes a note documenting the unexpected event, the cause, and actions taken to correct the situation or justify the actions taken.

The case management model promotes collaboration and teamwork among caregivers, helps to decrease length of stay, and makes efficient use of time. Because care is goal focused, the quality of care may improve. However, critical pathways work best for patients with one or two diagnoses and few individualized needs. Patients with multiple diagnoses (e.g., a patient with a hip fracture, pneumonia, diabetes, and pressure sore) or those with an unpredictable course of symptoms (e.g., a patient with seizures) are difficult to document on a critical path.

Documenting Nursing Activities

The patient record should describe the patient's ongoing status and reflect the full range of the nursing process. Regardless of the records system used in an agency, nurses document evidence of the nursing process on a variety of forms throughout the clinical record (**Table 38–8 》**).

Admission Nursing Assessment

A comprehensive admission assessment, also referred to as an initial database, nursing history, or nursing assessment, is completed when the patient is admitted to the nursing unit. These forms can be organized according to health patterns, body systems, functional abilities, health problems and risks, nursing model, or type of healthcare setting (e.g., labor and delivery, pediatrics, mental health). The nurse generally records ongoing assessments or reassessments on flow sheets or on nursing progress notes.

Nursing Care Plans

The Joint Commission requires that the clinical record include evidence of patient assessments, nursing diagnoses and/or patient needs, nursing interventions, patient outcomes, and evidence of a current nursing care plan. Depending on the records system being used, the nursing care plan may be separate from the patient's chart, recorded in progress notes and other forms in the patient record, or incorporated into an interprofessional plan of care. See the module on Clinical Decision Making for information on types of nursing care plans and strategies for their development and use.

Flow Sheets

A flow sheet enables the nurse to record nursing data quickly and concisely and provides an easy-to-read record of the patient's condition over time.

CRITICAL PATHWAY: TOTAL HIP REPLACEMENT

	DOS/Day 1	Days 2–3
Pain Management	Outcome: • Verbalizes comfort or tolerance of pain Circle: V NV Variance:	Outcome: • Verbalizes comfort with pain control measures Circle: V NV Variance:
Respiratory	Outcomes: • Breath sounds clear to auscultation • Achieves 50% of volume goal on incentive spirometer Circle: V NV Variance:	Outcomes: • Breath sounds clear to auscultation • Achieves 100% of volume goal on incentive spirometer Circle: V NV Variance:

Key: V = Variance	NV = No Variance
Signature:	Initials:
Signature:	Initials:

Figure 38–14 》 Excerpt from a critical pathway documentation form.

TABLE 38–8 Documentation for the Nursing Process

Step	Documentation Forms
Assessment	Initial assessment form, various flow sheets
Nursing diagnosis	Nursing care plan, critical pathway, progress notes, problem list
Planning	Nursing care plan, critical pathway
Implementation	Progress notes, flow sheets
Evaluation	Progress notes

Note: All steps are recorded on discharge/referral summaries.

- *Graphic record.* This record typically indicates body temperature, pulse, respiratory rate, blood pressure, weight, and, in some agencies, other significant clinical data such as admission or postoperative day, bowel movements, appetite, and activity.
- *Intake and output (I&O) record.* All routes of fluid intake and all routes of fluid loss or output are measured and recorded on this form. Frequently this I&O form permits the recording of a daily weight and percentage of meal consumption.
- *Medication administration record.* Medication flow sheets usually include designated areas for the date of the medication order, the expiration date, the medication name and dose, the frequency of administration and route, and the nurse's signature. Some records also include a place to document the patient's allergies.
- *Skin assessment record.* A skin or wound assessment is often recorded on a flow sheet. These records may include categories related to stage of skin injury, drainage, odor, culture information, and treatments.

Progress Notes

Progress notes made by nurses provide information about the progress a patient is making toward desired outcomes. Therefore, in addition to assessment and reassessment data, progress notes include information about patient problems and nursing interventions and evaluation of these interventions. The format used depends on the documentation system in place in the institution.

Nursing Discharge/Referral Summaries

A discharge note and referral summary are completed when the patient is being discharged and transferred to another institution or to a home setting where a visit by a community health nurse is required. Many institutions provide forms for these summaries. Some records combine the discharge plan, including instructions for care, and the final progress note. Many are designed with checklists to facilitate data recording.

If the discharge plan is given directly to the patient and family, it is imperative that instructions be written in terms that can be readily understood. For example, medications, treatments, and activities should be written in layman's terms, and use of medical abbreviations (such as tid) should be avoided.

If a patient is transferred within the facility or from a long-term facility to a hospital, a report needs to accompany the patient to ensure continuity of care in the new area. It should include all components of the discharge instructions but also describe the condition of the patient prior to transfer. Any teaching or patient instruction that has been done should also be described and recorded.

If the patient is being transferred to another institution or to a home setting where a visit by a home health nurse is required, the discharge note takes the form of a referral summary. Regardless of format, discharge and referral summaries usually include some or all of the following:

- Description of patient's physical, mental, and emotional status at discharge or transfer
- Resolved health problems

- Unresolved continuing health problems and continuing care needs; may include a review-of-systems checklist that considers integumentary, respiratory, cardiovascular, neurologic, musculoskeletal, gastrointestinal, elimination, and reproductive problems
- Treatments that are to be continued (e.g., wound care, oxygen therapy)
- Current medications
- Restrictions that relate to (a) activity such as lifting, stair climbing, walking, driving, work; (b) diet; and (c) bathing, such as sponge bath, tub, or shower
- Functional/self-care abilities in terms of vision, hearing, speech, mobility with or without aids, meal preparation and eating, preparation and administration of medications, and so on
- Comfort level
- Support networks, including family, significant others, religious adviser, community self-help groups, home care and other community agencies available, and so on
- Patient education provided in relation to disease process, activities and exercise, special diet, medications, specialized care or treatments, follow-up appointments, and so on
- Discharge destination (e.g., home, nursing home) and mode of discharge (e.g., walking, wheelchair, ambulance)
- Referral services (e.g., social worker, home health nurse).

Facility-specific Documentation

Documentation systems and requirements vary by facility. The documentation required in an acute care setting, as discussed in the early part of this exemplar, is different from the documentation required by long-term care, home care, or other care delivery sites such as outpatient clinics.

Long-term Care Documentation

Long-term facilities usually provide two types of care: skilled or intermediate. Patients needing skilled care require more extensive nursing care and specialized nursing skills. In contrast, an intermediate-care focus is appropriate for patients who usually have chronic illnesses and may only need assistance with activities of daily living (such as bathing and dressing).

Requirements for documentation systems in long-term care settings are based on professional standards, federal and state regulations, and the policies of the healthcare agency. Laws influencing the kind and frequency of documentation required are found through the Health Care Financing Administration (HCFA), a branch of the U.S. Department of Health and Human Services, and the Omnibus Budget Reconciliation Act (OBRA) of 1987. The OBRA law, for example, requires that (a) a comprehensive assessment (the Minimum Data Set [MDS] for Resident Assessment and Care Screening) be performed within 4 days of a patient's admission to a long-term care facility, (b) a formulated plan of care must be completed within 7 days of admission, and (c) the assessment and care screening process must be reviewed every 3 months. Documentation must also comply with requirements set by Medicare and Medicaid. These requirements vary with the level of service provided and other factors. For example, Medicare provides little reimbursement for services provided in long-term care facilities except for services that require skilled care such as chemotherapy, tube feedings, and ventilators. For these patients, the nurse must provide daily documentation to verify the need for service and reimbursement.

Nurses need to familiarize themselves with regulations influencing the kind and frequency of documentation required in long-term care facilities. Usually the nurse completes a nursing care *summary* at least once a week for patients requiring skilled care and every 2 weeks for patients who require intermediate care. Summaries should address specific problems noted in the care plan; mental status; ADLs; hydration and nutrition status; safety measures needed; medications and other treatments; preventive measures; and any behavior modifications or assistive devices needed.

Home Care Documentation

In 1985, the HCFA mandated that home health agencies standardize their documentation methods to meet requirements for Medicare and Medicaid and other third-party disbursements. Two records are required: (1) a home health certification and plan of treatment form and (2) a medical update and patient information form. The nurse assigned to the home care patient usually completes the forms, which must be signed by both the nurse and the attending physician. Information in a home care medical record often includes reports to third-party payers, a list of medications, an interprofessional plan of care, referral and intake forms, and patient assessments.

Parts of the medical record remain in the patient's home, whereas other parts are transferred to the office (Potter et al., 2013). Duplication of medical records or use of a continuous EMR is necessary for the relevant information to be available in all necessary locations. Some home health agencies provide nurses with laptop computers, tablets, or smartphones to make records available in multiple locations. This allows the nurse to add new patient information to records at the agency without traveling to the office. Electronic records enable the entire healthcare team to have the information necessary to provide consistent and safe care.

General Guidelines for Recording

Because a patient's medical record is a legal document and may be used to provide evidence in court, many factors are considered in recording. Healthcare personnel must not only maintain the confidentiality of the patient's record but also meet legal standards in the process of recording.

Date and Time

Document the date and time of each recording. This is essential not only for legal reasons but also for patient safety. Record the time in the conventional manner (e.g., 9:00 a.m. or 3:15 p.m.) or according to the 24-hour clock (military clock), which avoids confusion about whether a time was a.m. or p.m.

Timing

Follow the agency's policy about the frequency of documenting, but adjust the frequency as a patient's condition indicates; for example, a patient whose blood pressure is changing requires more frequent documentation than a patient whose blood pressure is stable. As a rule, documenting should be done as soon as possible after an assessment or intervention. No recording should be done *before* providing nursing care.

Accepted Terminology

Use only commonly accepted abbreviations, symbols, and terms as specified by the agency. Many abbreviations are standard and used universally; others are used only in certain geographic areas. Many healthcare facilities supply an approved list of abbreviations and symbols to prevent confusion. A large number of healthcare facilities are now moving away from the use of any abbreviations. When in doubt about whether to use an abbreviation, write the term in full until certain about the abbreviation. **Table 38–9** ⟫ lists some common abbreviations used in healthcare.

In 2004, The Joint Commission developed National Patient Safety Goals to reduce communication errors. These goals are required to be implemented by all organizations accredited by The Joint Commission. As a result, accredited organizations must develop a "Do Not Use" list of abbreviations, acronyms, and symbols. These lists must include those banned by The Joint Commission.

⟫ **Stay Current:** Keep up with The Joint Commission's "Do Not Use" list by visiting its website at http://www.jointcommission.org/facts_about_do_not_use_list/.

Correct Spelling

Correct spelling is essential for accuracy in recording. If unsure how to spell a word, the nurse should look it up. Two decidedly different medications may have similar spellings with serious patient safety considerations, such as Fosamax and Flomax.

Signature

Each recording on the nursing notes is signed by the nurse documenting it. The signature includes the name and title, for example, "Susan J. Green, RN" or "S. J. Green, RN." With computerized charting, each nurse has her own code, which allows the person who entered the documentation to be identified.

The following title abbreviations are often used, but nurses need to follow agency policy about how to sign their names:

RN	registered nurse
LVN	licensed vocational nurse
LPN	licensed practical nurse
NA	nursing assistant
CNA	certified nursing assistant
MA	medical assistant
NS	nursing student
PCA	patient care associate
PCNA	patient care nursing assistant
SN	student nurse
NP	nurse practitioner
APRN	advanced practice registered nurse

TABLE 38–9 Commonly Used Abbreviations

Abbreviation	Term	Abbreviation	Term
Abd	Abdomen	meds	Medications
ABO	The main blood group system	mL, ml	Milliliter
ac	Before meals	mod	Moderate
ad lib	As desired	neg	Negative
ADL	Activities of daily living	Ø	None
Adm	Admitted or admission	#	Number or pounds
a.m.	Morning	NPO, NBM	Nothing by mouth
amb	Ambulatory	NS, N/S	Normal saline
amt	Amount	OD	Right eye or overdose
approx	Approximately	OOB	Out of bed
bid, BID	Twice daily	OS	Left eye
bm, BM	Bowel movement	pc	After meals
BP	Blood pressure	PE, PX	Physical examination
BRP	Bathroom privileges	per	By or through
c̄	With	p.m.	Afternoon
C	Celsius (centigrade)	po	By mouth
CBC	Complete blood count	postop	Postoperatively
c/o	Complains of	preop	Preoperatively
DAT	Diet as tolerated	prep	Preparation
drsg	Dressing	prn, PRN	When necessary
Dx	Diagnosis	qid, QID	Four times a day
ECG	Electrocardiogram	(R)	Right
F	Fahrenheit	s̄	Without
fld	Fluid	stat	At once, immediately
GI	Gastrointestinal	tid, TID	Three times a day
gtt	Drop	TO	Telephone order
h, hr	Hour	TPR	Temperature, pulse, respirations
H_2O	Water	VO	Verbal order
I&O	Intake and output	VS	Vital signs
IV	Intravenous	WNL	Within normal limits
(L)	Left	wt	Weight
LMP	Last menstrual period		

*Institutions may elect to include some of these abbreviations on their "Do Not Use" list. Check the agency's policy.

Accuracy

Before making an entry, the nurse should ensure they are in the correct chart or electronic record. Notations on records must be accurate and correct. Accurate notations consist of facts or objective observations rather than opinions or interpretations. It is more accurate, for example, to write that the patient "refused medication" (fact) than to write that the patient "was uncooperative" (opinion or a judgment), or to record that a patient "was crying" (observation) rather than that the patient "was depressed" (interpretation). Similarly, when a patient expresses worry about a diagnosis or problem, this should be quoted directly on the record: "Stated: 'I'm worried about my leg.'" When describing something, avoid general words, such as *large*, *good*, or *normal*, which can be interpreted in different ways. For example, chart specific data such as "2 cm × 3 cm bruise" rather than "large bruise."

Follow agency policies regarding documenting errors and recording the correct information. The original entry must remain visible.

Sequence

Document events in the order in which they occur; for example, record assessments, then the nursing interventions, and then the patient's responses. Update as needed or according to agency protocols.

Box 38–6
Dos and Don'ts of Documentation

DO

- Chart a change in a patient's condition **and** show that follow-up actions were taken.
- Read the nurses' notes prior to care to determine whether there has been a change in the patient's condition.
- Be timely. A late entry is better than no entry; however, the longer the period of time between actual care and charting, the greater the risk for recording inaccurate information or omitting necessary information.
- Use objective, specific, and factual descriptions.
- Correct charting errors in the manner specified by agency policy.
- Chart all teaching.
- Record the patient's actual words by putting quote marks around the words.
- Chart the patient's response to interventions.
- Review your notes. Are they clear? Do they reflect what you want to say?

DON'T

- Chart in advance of the event (e.g., procedure, medication).
- Use vague terms (e.g., "appears to be comfortable," "had a good night").
- Chart for someone else.
- Use "patient" instead of the patient's name.
- Alter a record even if requested by a superior or a physician.
- Record assumptions or words reflecting bias (e.g., "complainer," "disagreeable").

Appropriateness

Record only information that pertains to the patient's health problems and care. Any other personal information that the patient conveys is inappropriate for the record. Recording irrelevant information may be considered an invasion of the patient's privacy and/or libelous. For example, a patient's disclosure that she is recently divorced would *not* be recorded on her medical record unless it had a direct bearing on her health problem.

Completeness

Not all data that a nurse obtains about a patient can be recorded. However, the information that is recorded needs to be complete and helpful to the patient and healthcare professionals.

Nurses' notes need to reflect the nursing process. The nurse should record all assessments, dependent and independent nursing interventions, patient problems, patient comments and responses to interventions and tests, progress toward goals, and communication with other members of the health team.

SAFETY ALERT Do not assume that the individual who is reading your charting will know that a common intervention (e.g., turning) has occurred because you believe it to be an "obvious" component of care.

Care that is *omitted* because of the patient's condition or refusal of treatment must also be recorded. Document what was omitted, why it was omitted, and who was notified.

Conciseness

Recordings need to be brief as well as complete to save time in communication. The patient's name and the word *patient* are omitted. For example, write, "Perspiring profusely. Respirations shallow, 28/min." End each thought or sentence with a period.

Legal Prudence

Accurate, complete documentation should give legal protection to the nurse, the patient's other caregivers, the healthcare facility, and the patient. Admissible in court as a legal document, the clinical record provides proof of the quality of care given to a patient. Documentation is usually viewed by juries and attorneys as the best evidence of what really happened to the patient.

For the best legal protection, the nurse should not only adhere to professional standards of nursing care but also follow agency policy and procedures for intervention and documentation in all situations, especially high-risk situations (**Box 38–6** »).

REVIEW Documentation

RELATE Link the Concepts and Exemplars

Linking the exemplar of documentation with the concept of legal issues:

1. How does proper documentation reduce the risk of lawsuits?
2. What components of nursing care must be included in the nurse's documentation to meet legal requirements?

Linking the exemplar of documentation with the concept of quality improvement:

3. How is nursing documentation used to assess the quality of nursing care delivered?
4. How can incomplete documentation result in a negative evaluation of the quality of nursing care delivered?

REFER Go to Pearson MyLab Nursing and eText

- Additional review materials

REFLECT Apply Your Knowledge

Zainah Kattan is a 23-year-old nurse from a small, rural community. Zainah graduated from nursing school a few months ago and took a job working on a general medical–surgical inpatient unit at Neighborhood Hospital. Her goal is to eventually work in an adult intensive care unit. She recently received a sign-on bonus and looks forward to buying her first new car.

Zainah has a busy week because of increased patient loads. She has seven to eight patients of her own, and she has trouble managing her charting with all the patient care she has to do. She ends up staying up to

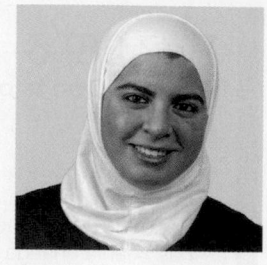

2 hours after each shift to get the charting done. Zainah's manager, Pat, talks with her about this and reviews the importance of point-of-care charting. The feedback he gives Zainah is generally positive.

1. Why is Zainah's manager trying to improve her point-of-care charting?
2. What are the potential drawbacks of waiting until the end of the shift to document care?
3. What strategies might you suggest to Zainah to help her improve point-of-care charting during a busy shift?

≫ Exemplar 38.D
Reporting

Exemplar Learning Outcomes

38.D Analyze reporting as it relates to communication.

- Explain the purposes of reporting.
- Describe the handoff report.
- Outline the SBAR technique of communication.
- Describe the process of telephone communication.
- Summarize the care plan conference.

Exemplar Key Terms

Change-of-shift report, *2611*
Handoff, *2610*
Handoff communication, *2610*
Reporting, *2610*
SBAR, *2611*
SHARE, *2610*

Overview

The purpose of **reporting** is to communicate specific information to an individual or group of individuals. A report, whether oral or written, should be concise, including pertinent information but no extraneous detail. In addition to change-of-shift reports and telephone reports, reporting can also include the sharing of information or ideas with colleagues and other health professionals about some aspect of a patient's care. Examples include the care plan conference and nursing rounds.

Note that the national CLAS standards (Office of Minority Health, 2013) have implications on reporting mechanisms in that agencies must consider culturally and linguistically appropriate services at all levels of communication throughout the agency. For example, consider a healthcare agency located in an urban area serving English-speaking, Spanish-speaking, and Arabic-speaking patients. As the agency employs more native Spanish and Arabic speakers to meet the needs of its patients, the agency must have policies and procedures in place to ensure that nurses and other healthcare providers who engage in reporting both in person (e.g., handoff reports) or through electronic means are able to communicate successfully with each other. Agencies must also ensure that communication and reporting mechanisms include opportunities for nurses and other providers to report pertinent cultural information about patients' healthcare and cultural needs.

Handoff Communication

Ineffective communication is the primary cause of sentinel events, which are serious, unexpected events (Popovich, 2016).

As a result, hospitals are required to implement a standardized approach to "handing off" communication. **Handoff** is defined as "the transfer of information (along with authority and responsibility) during transitions in care across the continuum. It includes an opportunity to ask questions, clarify, and confirm" (Agency for Healthcare Research and Quality [AHRQ], 2014). Hospital handoffs occur at many times, including but not limited to when a patient is transferred between units, at the change of shift, and at discharge (AHRQ, 2015). The **handoff communication** is a verbal or written exchange of information that encompasses the nursing care that has been provided along with all members of the healthcare team who have cared for the patient during the relevant time period (AHRQ, 2014).

The handoff process involves two groups, the senders and the receivers. The senders are the caregivers who are transmitting patient information and releasing care; the receivers are the caregivers who are accepting the patient and the patient's information.

The **SHARE** method can be used to accomplish a successful handoff:

Standardize critical content.

Hardwire within your system.

Allow opportunity to ask questions.

Reinforce quality and measurement.

Educate and coach.

The Joint Commission (2012) provides several items that can be helpful in the handoff communication process. The goal of the new Hand-off Communications Targeted Solutions Tool (TST) is "to assist health care organizations with the process of passing necessary and critical information about a patient from one caregiver to the next, or from one team of caregivers to another, to prevent miscommunication-related errors" (The Joint Commission, 2012).

>> **Stay Current:** For more information regarding the handoff communication process, visit the following website: https://www.aorn.org/guidelines/clinical-resources/tool-kits/patient-hand-off-tool-kit.

Change-of-Shift Report

A **change-of-shift report** is a type of handoff communication given to all nurses on the next shift. Its purpose is to provide continuity of care for patients by providing the new caregivers with a quick summary of patient needs and details of care to be given.

Change-of-shift reports may be written or given orally, either in a face-to-face exchange or by audio recording. The face-to-face report permits the listener to ask questions during the report; written and audio-recorded reports are often briefer and less time consuming. Reports are sometimes given at the bedside, and patients as well as nurses may participate in the exchange of information. A thorough change-of-shift report:

- Follows a particular order (e.g., follow room numbers in a hospital).
- Provides basic identifying information for each patient (e.g., name, room number, bed designation).
- For new patients, provides the reason for admission or medical diagnosis (or diagnoses), surgery (date), diagnostic tests, and therapies in the past 24 hours.
- Includes significant changes in the patient's condition and present information in order (i.e., assessment, nursing diagnoses, interventions, outcomes, and evaluation). For example, "Mr. Ronald Oakes said he had an aching pain in his left calf at 1400 hours. Inspection revealed no other signs. Calf pain is related to altered blood circulation. Rest and elevation of his legs on a footstool for 30 minutes provided relief."
- Provides exact information, such as "Ms. Jessie Jones received morphine 6 mg IV at 1500 hours," not "Ms. Jessie Jones received some morphine during the evening."
- Reports patients' need for special emotional support. For example, a patient who has just learned that his biopsy results revealed malignancy and who is now scheduled for a laryngectomy needs time to discuss his feelings before preoperative teaching is begun.
- Includes current nurse-prescribed and primary care provider–prescribed orders.
- Provides a summary of newly admitted patients, including diagnosis, age, general condition, plan of therapy, and significant information about the patient's support people.
- Reports on patients who have been transferred or discharged from the unit.
- Clearly states priorities of care and care that is due after the shift begins. For example, in a 7 a.m. report, the nurse might say, "Mr. Li's vital signs are due at 0730, and his IV bag will need to be replaced by 0800." This information is best given at the end of that patient's report because the receiver's memory is best for the first and last information given.

- Is concise. Don't elaborate on background data or routine care (e.g., do not report "Vital signs at 0800 and 1150" when that is the unit standard). Do not report coming and going of visitors unless there is a problem or concern or visitors are involved in teaching and care. Social support and visits are the norm.

SBAR

The SBAR technique, which was developed by the U.S. Navy, provides a framework for safe, efficient communication between members of the healthcare team. SBAR stands for:

Situation

Background

Assessment

Recommendation.

The tool provides an easy way to develop team cohesion and create a culture of patient safety (Institute for Healthcare Improvement, 2016). In the Situation step, the nurse provides a concise statement of the problem. In the Background step, the nurse relates information relevant to the situation. In the Assessment step, the nurse provides an analysis and consideration of options. And in the Recommendation step, the nurse provides a recommendation based on the relevant evidence. Using the SBAR technique during handoffs, transfers, and shift changes will reduce miscommunications that have the potential to cause patient harm, including those surrounding cultural considerations in patient care, as seen in the clinical example below. Improving communication skills among team members overall, and specifically in critical clinical situations, will help the nurse manager and the team improve patient safety and, in turn, team satisfaction.

Clinical Example H

Thomas Fullerton is a nurse in the postoperative recovery wing of a hospital. He is monitoring the vital signs of Mrs. Hussein, a 41-year-old woman who is recovering from a percutaneous endoscopic gastrostomy (PEG) placement earlier today. Thomas notices that Mrs. Hussein is having increasing dyspnea and complaining of chest pain, so he decides to alert the patient's physician. Thomas provides the information in SBAR format. He calls the physician and states the situation: "Mrs. Hussein is experiencing dyspnea and complaining of chest pain." Then, he provides background: "Mrs. Hussein had a PEG placement today, and a few hours ago she started complaining of chest pain. Her pulse is 122 and her blood pressure is 129 over 53. She is short of breath and restless." Then, Thomas provides his assessment: "I think she may be having a cardiac event or a pulmonary embolism." And finally, his recommendation: "I recommend that you see the patient as soon as possible and that we start her on O_2 stat." See a condensed version of Thomas's SBAR report in **Table 38–10** >>.

Critical Thinking Questions

1. Would you have provided any information that Thomas did not? Why or why not?
2. Is the SBAR an appropriate format in which to convey this information? Can you think of any mistakes that Thomas avoided by using SBAR?
3. Explain why this phone call between Thomas and the physician is a kind of hand-off event.

TABLE 38–10 Example of an SBAR Report

Phase	Action
Situation	Provide description of the patient's dyspnea and chest pain.
Background	Provide an explanation that the patient had a PEG placement this morning and that relatively recently she began complaining of chest pain.
Assessment	Provide an assessment that the patient is most likely having a cardiac event or pulmonary embolism.
Recommendation	Provide a recommendation that the physician see the patient immediately and that the patient be started on an O_2 stat.

Sources: Based on Safer Healthcare. (2016). *Why is SBAR communication so critical?* Retrieved from http://www.saferhealthcare.com/sbar/what-is-sbar/; Massachusetts Department of Higher Education. (2016). *Communication and documentation.* Retrieved from http://www.mass.edu/mcncps/orientation/m1Documentation.asp; Missouri Department of Health & Senior Services. (2017). *Best practice: Physician relationships.* Retrieved from http://health.mo.gov/seniors/hcbs/pdf/physiciannursetrack.pdf.

》》 Stay Current: Learn more about the SBAR technique by visiting the website of the Institute for Healthcare Improvement to read the article titled "SBAR Technique for Communication: A Situational Briefing Model": http://www.ihi.org/resources/pages/tools/sbartechniqueforcommunicationasituationalbriefingmodel.aspx.

SAFETY ALERT Employing effective communication techniques is essential throughout the nursing process, but communication may be most critical during reporting situations. If nurses do not receive adequate information from patients, provide the healthcare team with relevant details, and communicate effectively in groups, the patient's health may be jeopardized. Reporting techniques such as SBAR and handoff protocols are standardized techniques that streamline reporting safety.

Telephone Communication

Telephone Reports

Healthcare professionals frequently report about a patient by telephone. For example, a nurse informs the primary care provider about a change in a patient's condition, a radiologist reports the results of an x-ray study, or a nurse reports to a nurse on another unit about a transferred patient.

The nurse receiving a telephone report should document the date and time, note the name of the individual giving the information and subject of the information received, and then sign the notation. The individual receiving the information should repeat it back to the sender to ensure accuracy.

When giving a telephone report to a primary care provider, the nurse must be concise and accurate. Telephone reports usually include the patient's name and medical diagnosis, changes in nursing assessment, vital signs related to baseline vital signs, significant laboratory data, and related nursing interventions. The nurse should have the patient's chart ready in case the primary care provider requires further information.

After reporting, the nurse should document the date, time, and content of the call.

Telephone Orders

Physicians may order a therapy (e.g., a medication) for a patient by telephone. Most agencies have specific policies about telephone orders. Many agencies allow only registered nurses to take telephone orders. The increased use of electronic records and communications is reducing the use of telephone orders, as electronic transmission of orders allows for greater accuracy.

While the primary care provider gives the order, the nurse should *write* the complete order down and *read* it back to the primary care provider to ensure accuracy. Question the primary care provider about any order that is ambiguous, unusual (e.g., an abnormally high dosage of a medication), or contraindicated by the patient's condition. Then transcribe the order onto the physician's order sheet, indicating it as a verbal order (VO) or telephone order (TO). Once transcribed onto the physician's order sheet, the order must be countersigned by the primary care provider within a time period described by agency policy. Many acute care hospitals require that this be done within 24 hours. Guidelines for telephone and verbal orders include:

1. Know the state nursing board's position on who can give and accept verbal and phone orders.
2. Know the agency's policy regarding phone orders.
3. Ask the prescriber to speak slowly and clearly.
4. Ask the prescriber to spell the name of the medication if you are not familiar with it.
5. Question the drug, dosage, or changes if they seem inappropriate for the patient.
6. Write down the order or enter it into the computer on the physician's order form.
7. Read the order back to the prescriber. Use words instead of abbreviations.
8. Have the prescriber verbally acknowledge the read-back.
9. Record the date and time and indicate it was a telephone order.
10. Sign your name and credentials.
11. Transcribe the order.
12. Follow agency protocol to have the prescriber sign the telephone order.

Also:

- When writing a dosage, always put a number before the decimal point, such as 0.5.
- Write out units, i.e., 20 Units versus 20 U.
- Never follow a voice-mail order. Call the prescriber, write the order down, and read it back for confirmation.

Care Plan Conference

Care plan conferences allow for collaborative reporting among the healthcare professionals who provide care to the patient. They are most often used for patients who have complex care needs. During the conference, the patient's healthcare providers discuss possible solutions to certain problems of the patient, such as an inability to cope with an event or lack of progress toward goal attainment. The care plan conference allows each member of the healthcare team an opportunity to offer an opinion in order to reach a solution to the problem. The choice of healthcare professionals who are invited to attend the conference is based on the needs of the patient. Family members are an important part of the care plan conference, especially for patients who are unable to advocate for themselves. Other professionals may be invited. For example, a social worker may be present to discuss support for the family of a burned child or a pharmacist may be present at a conference when the patient requires multiple medications.

Care plan conferences are most effective when there is a climate of respect—that is, nonjudgmental acceptance of others even though their values, opinions, and beliefs may seem different. Interprofessional collaboration is discussed further in the module on Collaboration. The nurse needs to accept and respect each individual's contributions, listening with an open mind to what others are saying even when there is disagreement.

REVIEW Reporting

RELATE Link the Concepts and Exemplars

Linking the exemplar of reporting with the concept of legal issues:

1. What are the legal obligations of a nurse who is providing change-of-shift reporting to the oncoming nurse?

2. How can the nurse ensure that all legal obligations have been met when accepting telephone orders from the primary provider?

Linking the exemplar of reporting with the concept of safety:

3. How does handoff communication contribute to patient safety?

4. In providing a telephone report to a primary care provider because of a patient's sudden change in condition, what information should be included to maintain the safe care of the patient?

REFER Go to Pearson MyLab Nursing and eText

■ Additional review materials

REFLECT Apply Your Knowledge

Marjorie Newman, a 64-year-old woman, was admitted to the coronary care unit (CCU) with a diagnosis of acute anterior myocardial infarction. Her condition has remained stable, and she is to be transferred to the telemetry unit tomorrow or sooner if the CCU bed is required for an acutely ill patient. The nurse assigned to her care is called to the monitors by the monitor technician because Ms. Newman has suddenly begun having frequent premature ventricular contractions (PVCs). When the nurse enters Ms. Newman's room, she assesses the patient and finds her to be short of breath, experiencing severe left-sided chest pain radiating to the left arm, and very diaphoretic. Vital signs are T_O 98.6°F; P 108 bpm and irregular; R 28/min; and BP 92/44 mmHg. The nurse analyzes Ms. Newman's rhythm strip and finds elevated ST segments, tachycardia, with 10–14 PVCs per minute. A coworker agrees to stay with Ms. Newman and monitor her condition while the nurse assigned to Ms. Newman's care calls the primary care provider.

1. What information would the nurse report to the primary care provider when calling to notify of the change in the patient's condition?

2. Why did the nurse have a coworker stay with the patient while calling the primary care provider?

3. How should the nurse report Ms. Newman's condition in the SBAR portion of the handoff report?

References

Adams, K., & Galanes, G. J. (2014). *Communicating in groups: Applications and skills* (9th ed.). Boston, MA: McGraw-Hill Education.

Agency for Healthcare Research and Quality (AHRQ). (2014). *Pocket Guide: TeamSTEPPS.* Rockville, MD. Retrieved from http://www.ahrq.gov/professionals/education/curriculum-tools/teamstepps/instructor/essentials/pocketguide.html

Agency for Healthcare Research and Quality (AHRQ). (2015). *Handoffs and signouts.* Retrieved from https://psnet.ahrq.gov/primers/primer/9/handoffs-and-signouts

American Nurses Association (ANA). (2015). *Code of ethics for nurses with interpretive statements.* Silver Spring, MD: Author.

Anderson, J. G., Friesen, M. A., Fabian, J., Swengros, D., Herbst, A., & Mangione, L. (2016). Examination of the perceptions of registered nurses regarding the use of healing touch in the acute care setting. *Journal of Holistic Nursing, 34*(2), 167–176. doi:10.1177/0898010115592744

Andrews, M. M., & Boyle, J. S. (2016). *Transcultural concepts in nursing care,* 7th ed. Philadelphia: Wolters Kluwer, p. 22.

Arabs in America. (n.d.). What is the hijab and why do women wear it? Retrieved from http://arabsinamerica.unc.edu/

Arnold, E. C., & Boggs, K. U. (2013). *Interpersonal relationships: Professional communication skills for nurses* (6th ed.). St. Louis, MO: Elsevier Saunders.

Auvil, C. A., & Silver, B. W. (1984). Therapist self-disclosure: When is it appropriate? *Perspectives in Psychiatric Care, 22*(2), 57–61. Published by Wiley Periodicals, Inc., © 1984.

Ball, J. E., Murrells, T., Rafferty, A. M., Morrow, E., & Griffiths, P. (2013). "Care left undone" during nursing shifts: Associations with workload and perceived quality of care. *BMJ Quality and Safety,* doi:10.1136/bmjqs-2012-001767

Booth, J. (2014). *Viewpoint: Treating transgender patients with respect.* Retrieved from http://www.americannursetoday.com/viewpoint-treating-transgender-patients-respect/

Boyd, M. A. (2014). *Psychiatric nursing: Contemporary practice.* Philadelphia, PA: Lippincott Williams & Wilkins.

Egan, G. (2013). *The skilled helper: A problem-management approach to helping* (10th ed.). Pacific Grove, CA: Brooks/Cole. Published by Cengage Learning, © 2013.

Eventus. (2017). *Effective vs. ineffective teams.* Retrieved from http://www.eventus.co.uk/effective-vs-ineffective-teams/

Evesham, F. (2016). Therapeutic and non therapeutic communication. Retrieved from http://www.livestrong.com/article/188795-therapeutic-and-non-therapeutic-communication/

Goodtherapy.org. (2016). *Therapy and counseling for pregnancy.* Retrieved from http://www.goodtherapy.org/learn-about-therapy/issues/pregnancy-and-birthing

Guido, G. W. (2013). *Legal and ethical issues in nursing* (6th ed.). Upper Saddle River, NJ: Prentice Hall.

Hemsley, B., Balandin, S., & Worrall, L. (2012). Nursing the patient with complex communication needs: Time as a barrier and a facilitator to successful communication in hospital. *Journal of Advanced Nursing, 68*(1), 116–126.

Herdman, T. H. & Kamitsuru, S. (Eds) *Nursing Diagnoses—Definitions and Classification 2015–2017.* Copyright © 2014, 1994–2014 NANDA International. Used by arrangement with John Wiley & Sons, Inc. Companion website: www.wiley.com/go/nursingdiagnoses.

Homestead Schools. (2016). *Section 10: Characteristics of effective and ineffective teams.* Retrieved from http://www.homesteadschools.com/lcsw/courses/TeamBuilding/Section10.htm

Huber, D. (2014). *Leadership and nursing care management* (5th ed.). St. Louis, MO: Elsevier Saunders.

Institute for Healthcare Improvement. (2016). *SBAR technique for communication: A situational briefing model.* Retrieved from http://www.ihi.org/resources/pages/tools/sbartechniqueforcommunicationasituationalbriefingmodel.aspx

International Federation of Health Information Management Associations (IFHIMA). (2014). *Education module for health record practice.* Retrieved from https://ifhima.files.wordpress.com/2014/08/module1the-health-record.pdf

Jacobs, C. G. (2012). *National standards for culturally and linguistically appropriate services in healthcare:*

Ensuring quality health care for all. Retrieved from http://www.diversityconnection.org/diversityconnection/leadership-conferences/2012%20Conf%20 Docs/Enchancing_Health_Care_with_CLAS.pdf

Kaushankaja, M., Gross, M., & Buac, M. (2013). Gender differences in child word learning. *Learning and Individual Differences, 27*, 82–89.

Kern, L. M., Malhotra, S., Barron, Y., Quaresimo, J., Dhopeshwarkar, R., Pichardo, M., . . . Kaushal, R. (2013). Accuracy of electronically reported "Meaningful Use" clinical quality measures. *Annuals of Internal Medicine, 158*, 77–83. Published by American College of Physicians, © 2013.

Kourkouta, L., & Papathanasiou, I. V. (2014). Communication in nursing practice. *Materia Sociomedica, 26*(1), 65–67. Retrieved from http://www.ncbi.nlm.nih.gov/pmc/articles/PMC3990376/. Published by AVICENA, © 2014.

Koutoukidis, G., Stainton, K., & Hughson, J. (2013). *Tabbner's nursing care* (6th ed.). Melbourne, Australia: Elsevier.

Lambda Legal. (2016). *Creating equal access to quality healthcare for transgender patients.* Retrieved from http://www.lambdalegal.org/sites/default/files/publications/downloads/fs_20160525_transgender-affirming-hospital-policies.pdf

Management Sciences for Health. (2016). *Non-verbal communication.* Retrieved from http://erc.msh.org/mainpage.cfm?file=4.6.0.htm&module=provider&language=English

Massachusetts Department of Higher Education. (2016). *Communication and documentation.* Retrieved from http://www.mass.edu/mcncps/orientation/m1Documentation.asp

Mayo Clinic. (2014). *Being assertive: Reduce stress, communicate better.* Retrieved from http://www.mayoclinic.com/health/assertive/SR00042

Missouri Department of Health & Senior Services. (2017). *Best practice: Physician relationships.* Retrieved from http://health.mo.gov/seniors/hcbs/pdf/physiciannursetrack.pdf

Office for Civil Rights (OCR). (2016). *Effective communication in hospitals.* Retrieved from http://www.hhs.gov/civil-rights/for-individuals/special-topics/hospitals-effective-communication/

Office of Minority Health. (2013). *National standards for culturally and linguistically appropriate services in health and health care: A blueprint for advancing and sustaining CLAS policy and practice.* Retrieved from https://www.thinkculturalhealth.hhs.gov/pdfs/EnhancedCLASStandardsBlueprint.pdf

Office of the National Coordinator for Health Information Technology. (2014). *Benefits of EHRs.* Retrieved from https://www.healthit.gov/providers-professionals/electronic-medical-records-emr

Popovich, D. (2016). Cultivating safety in handoff communication. *Medscape.* Retrieved from http://www.medscape.com/viewarticle/746070

Potter, M. L., & Moller, M. D. (2016). *Psychiatric-mental health nursing: From suffering to hope.* Hoboken, NJ: Pearson Education.

Potter, P. A., Perry, A. G., Stockert, P., & Hall, A. (2017). *Fundamentals of nursing* (9th ed.). Philadelphia, PA: Elsevier Health Sciences.

Reeves, L. (2016). *How to use good communication skills for cross-cultural diversity.* Chron.com. Retrieved from http://work.chron.com/use-good-communication-skills-crosscultural-diversity-8317.html

Rependa, S. (2012). *Baby talk: Nonverbal infant communication.* Retrieved from http://trauma.blog.yorku.ca/2012/05/baby-talk-nonverbal-infant-communication/

Safer Healthcare. (2016). *Why is SBAR communication so critical?* Retrieved from http://www.saferhealthcare.com/sbar/what-is-sbar/

Samovar, L. A., Porter, R. E., McDaniel, E. R., & Roy, C. S. (2016). *Communication between cultures.* Boston, MA: Cengage Learning.

Sampson, E. E., & Marthas, M. S. (1990). *Group process for the health professions* (3rd ed.). Albany, NY: Delmar.

Smith, J. A., & Zsohar, H. (2013). Patient-education tips for new nurses. *Nursing2013.* Retrieved from http://www.nursingcenter.com/journalarticle?Article_ID=1603879

Stewart, G. L., Manz, C. C., & Sims, H. P. (1999). *Team work and group dynamics.* New York, NY: Wiley.

Techopedia. (2016). *What are Electronic Medication Administration Records (eMAR)?* Retrieved from https://www.techopedia.com/definition/25658/electronic-medication-administration-records-emar

The Joint Commission. (2012). *Improving transitions of care: Hand-off communication.* Retrieved from http://www.centerfortransforminghealthcare.org/projects/detail.aspx?Project=1

The National CLAS Standards. (2013). Retrieved from http://www.hdassoc.org/wp-content/uploads/2013/03/CLAS_handout-pdf_april-24.pdf

Tremayne, P. (2014). Using humour to enhance the nurse-patient relationship. *Nursing Standard, 28*(30), 37–40. Retrieved from http://journals.rcni.com/doi/pdfplus/10.7748/ns2014.03.28.30.37.e8412

Vermont Department of Health. (n.d.). *Cultural differences in non-verbal communication.* Retrieved from http://healthvermont.gov/family/toolkit/tools%5CF-6%20Cultural%20Differences%20in%20Nonverbal%20Communic.pdf

Zote, H. L. Z. (2014). *Therapeutic communication during pregnancy and labour.* Retrieved from http://www.slideshare.net/helenlr98/therapeutic-communication-labour

Module 39
Managing Care

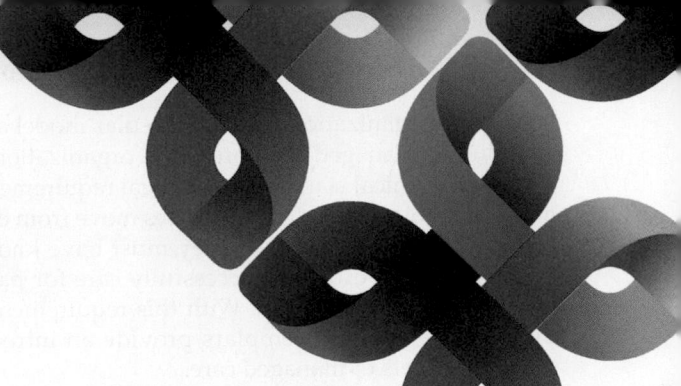

Module Outline and Learning Outcomes

The Concept of Managing Care

Managed Care and Care Delivery Models

39.1 Analyze frameworks for delivering care.

Concepts Related to Managing Care

39.2 Outline the relationship between managing care and other concepts.

Managing Care Exemplars

Exemplar 39.A Case Management

39.A Analyze case management as it relates to managing care.

Exemplar 39.B Cost-Effective Care

39.B Analyze cost-effective care as it relates to managing care.

Exemplar 39.C Delegation

39.C Analyze delegation as it relates to managing care.

Exemplar 39.D Leadership and Management

39.D Analyze leadership and management as they relate to managing care.

❯❯ The Concept of Managing Care

Concept Key Terms

Case management, **2616**	Functional method, **2617**	Patient-focused care, **2616**	Shared governance, **2617**
Case method, **2617**	Licensed practical nurses (LPNs), **2618**	Primary nursing, **2618**	Team nursing, **2618**
Differentiated practice, **2617**	Managed care, **2615**	Registered nurses (RNs), **2618**	Unlicensed assistive personnel (UAP), **2618**

Managed care is a healthcare delivery system that focuses on decreasing costs and improving outcomes for groups of patients. In this type of system, care is carefully planned from the initial contact with the patient through conclusion of the patient's specific health problem. Although exact methods used to manage care differ depending on the delivery model used, the overarching goals of lower costs and better outcomes remain constant.

Managed care is an important topic in modern nursing practice, because it shapes numerous aspects of the healthcare system. As payers search for ways to better contain rising costs, they continue to develop new incentives and standards, which in turn create trends in healthcare. Some of these trends have positive consequences, like an increased focus on preventive care. Others have the potential to create negative consequences, such as increases in hospital readmission following early release.

Within the managed care system, nurses may be involved in a variety of processes aimed at promoting high-quality care for patients while maintaining cost effectiveness. Delegation is one such process; by distributing routine tasks to other staff members, nurses are able to devote more time to skills unique to or required of the registered nurse role. Care coordination and case management are other examples. Care coordination is a collaborative effort in which an interprofessional team provides cohesive care as a patient proceeds from hospitalization to recovery and health maintenance. The case manager coordinates and facilitates patient use of healthcare services in the long term. These processes eliminate redundancy and promote consistency, therefore lowering costs and improving quality. Successful delegation, care coordination, and case management depend on the ability of nursing leaders and managers to inspire staff, monitor patients, and adhere to organizational requirements. As a result, nurses' interpersonal skills are at the heart of good managed care.

Understanding the basics behind managed care is important for nurses as they move through their careers, no matter their level of leadership or managerial responsibility. Each healthcare organization uses a particular model and understanding of managed care, and each organization layers its own goals, ethical standards, and legal requirements into its model of choice. Therefore, as nurses move from one organization or setting to another, they must have knowledge of these models in order to successfully care for patients and mature in their profession. With this requirement in mind, this module and its exemplars provide an introduction to the many facets of managed care.

Managed Care and Care Delivery Models

In managed care, healthcare providers and agencies work together to provide care that uses limited clinical resources wisely and effectively. Managed care strives to decrease unnecessary costs and increase patient satisfaction, in part by promoting health and delivering preventive services. Health maintenance organizations (HMOs) and preferred provider organizations (PPOs) are two examples of provider systems that are committed to managed care.

From the nurse's perspective, managing care is a learned process that requires strong communication, assessment, planning, and implementation skills (Leonard & Miller, 2012). The nurse's ability to apply these skills has important implications for direct patient care, coordination of care, and cost containment. For example, by scheduling the dietitian to meet with a patient at a different time than the physical therapist, the nurse makes sure that neither professional wastes time (and money) waiting for the other to finish seeing the same patient. This also may prevent the patient from becoming overtired by seeing too many providers within a short period. In addition to the skills mentioned above, effective managed care requires the abilities to prioritize, identify clinical pathways, and create concept maps and care plans. Information about these topics can be found in the module on Clinical Decision Making. The nurse must also understand patients' rights and advance directives and must be committed to quality improvement. The Advance Directives exemplar in the Legal Issues module, the Patient Rights exemplar in the Ethics module, and the Quality Improvement module include useful information on these topics.

From an organizational perspective, managed care has been embraced as a model for healthcare reform, but some people question the application of a business approach to something as personal and important as healthcare. Despite these concerns, many organizations have effectively combined managed care principles with a number of delivery models. As described in the following sections, each of these models requires nurses to draw upon their skills in different ways as they seek to promote patient well-being while controlling the costs of care.

Case Management

Case management is the coordination of patient care over time using the combination of health and social services necessary to meet the individual patient's needs. Case management is a fundamental element of many managed care systems. Case management offers intensive services, so it is most effectively and efficiently used for patients with multiple or complex chronic health problems (**Figure 39–1 》**). For

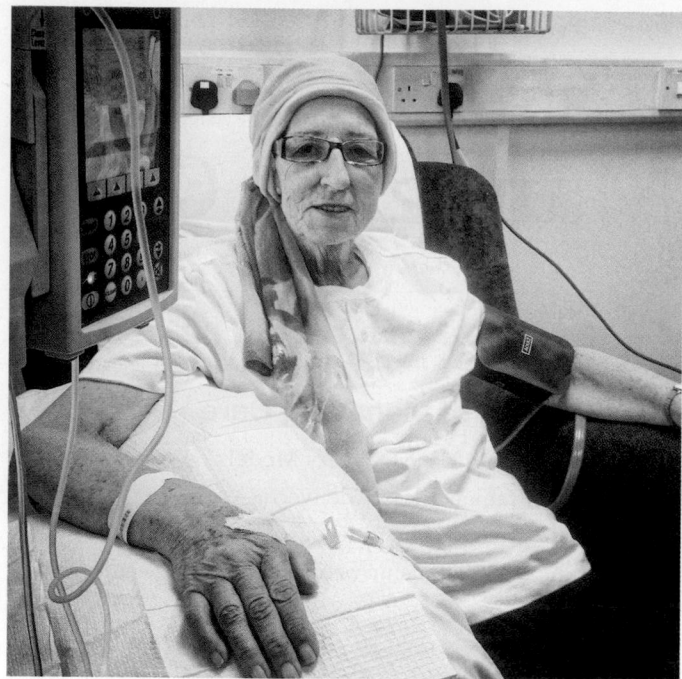

Source: Carole Gomez/Vetta/Getty Images.

Figure 39–1 》 Case management usually focuses on ongoing care of patients with chronic conditions or long-lasting problems, such as this patient who is receiving chemotherapy for cancer.

example, a patient with chronic obstructive pulmonary disease (COPD) who has just had hip replacement surgery would benefit from case management beginning at admission and continuing at the rehabilitation center or the skilled nursing facility to which he is discharged from the hospital.

Generally, case management involves interprofessional teams that collectively assume responsibility for planning and assessing the needs of groups of patients. These teams are also responsible for coordinating, implementing, and evaluating patient care from preadmission through discharge or transfer and recuperation. Each team is led by a case manager who is a nurse, social worker, or other appropriate professional. In some areas of the United States, case managers are referred to as discharge planners. These individuals may work for a patient's healthcare provider (e.g., clinic, hospital, or long-term care facility), insurance company, or perhaps even the patient's employer.

Patient-Focused Care

Patient-focused care is a delivery model that organizes healthcare around the expressed physical and emotional needs of the patient. This model incorporates concepts of patient- and family-centered care. Indeed, with this approach, patients and their families are considered integral components of the healthcare decision-making process.

In patient-focused care, the nurse takes time to learn about the patient's lifestyle, habits, and family. This includes being sensitive to diverse religious or cultural preferences. These preferences can impact diet, activity, and health practices, thus affecting patient adherence to the care regimen.

After gathering the necessary information about the patient's way of life, the nurse works with the patient to develop a plan of care that addresses both health and personal needs. As part of this plan, the nurse helps the patient acquire the knowledge and skills necessary to manage his or her health condition and make informed choices. The patient-focused model is based on the idea that care should be personalized and coordinated and that it should enable the patient to live as independent and fulfilling a life as possible (Health Foundation, 2014).

SAFETY ALERT With patient-focused care, the nurse should seek to honor the patient's preferences to the greatest degree possible. Still, the nurse has a duty to "do no harm." At no point should the nurse agree to a request that will potentially jeopardize the patient's well-being. Instead, the nurse should carefully and nonjudgmentally inform the patient of the risks associated with the requested practice or intervention.

Differentiated Practice

Differentiated practice is a system in which each nurse's educational preparation and skill sets are evaluated to determine how best to use the nurse. Thus, differentiated practice models consist of specific job descriptions for nurses according to their education or training—for example, LVN, ADN, BSN RN, MSN RN, and APN.

To establish a differentiated practice system, a healthcare organization must first identify the nursing competencies required by the patients it serves. The organization must also delineate the roles of licensed nursing personnel versus those of unlicensed assistive personnel (UAP). Such delineation enables nurses (as well as delegates) to assume roles and responsibilities appropriate to their level of experience, capability, and education. Differentiation maximizes the time and skill of individual staff members to help ensure that high-quality care is provided at an affordable cost.

Shared Governance

The **shared governance** model is used in concert with other models of care delivery. In this organizational model, members of the nursing staff participate with administrative personnel in making, implementing, and evaluating patient care policies. The focus of the shared governance model is to encourage nurses' participation in decision making at all levels of the organization.

With shared governance, individuals take part in decision making either at their own request or as part of their job role criteria. Typically, nurses participate by serving as members of decision-making groups, such as committees and task forces. The decisions made by these groups may address employment conditions, cost effectiveness, long-range planning, productivity, and wages and benefits. The underlying principle of shared governance is that employees are more committed to organizational goals if they provide planning and decision-making input.

Case Method

The **case method**, also referred to as *total care*, is one of the earliest nursing models. It is a patient-centered method in which one nurse is assigned to, and is responsible for, the

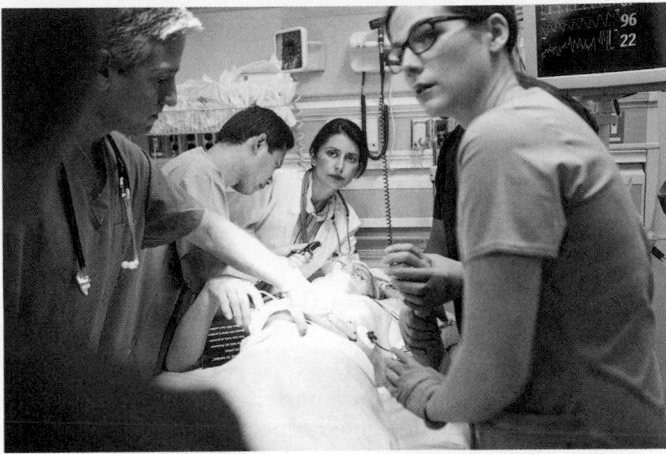

Source: Monkey Business Images/iStock/Getty Images.

Figure 39–2 》 The case method is often used in emergency departments.

comprehensive care of a group of patients during an 8- or 12-hour shift. For each patient, the nurse assesses needs, makes nursing plans, formulates nursing diagnoses, implements all care activities, and evaluates the effectiveness of care.

In the case method, a patient has consistent contact with one nurse during a shift but may have different nurses on other shifts. Considered to be the precursor of primary nursing (described later in the Concept), the case method continues to be used in a variety of practice settings, including emergency, acute, and intensive care units (**Figure 39–2 》》**).

SAFETY ALERT Information gaps often develop when patients are transferred from one facility to another, such as when a patient moves from the hospital to a rehabilitation facility. They may also occur during nursing shift changes. Communication breakdown during the transfer or shift-change process can result in life-threatening situations for the patient. To help prevent such situations, be sure to carefully and completely document all care provided to the patient, as well as to verbally communicate with a patient's new nursing staff whenever possible.

Functional Method

The **functional method** focuses on the jobs to be completed as part of patient care (e.g., bed making and temperature measurement). In this task-oriented approach, personnel with less educational preparation than the professional nurse (e.g., UAP) perform aspects of care with less complex requirements. The method is based on a production and efficiency model that gives authority and responsibility to the person assigning the work (e.g., the head nurse). Clearly defined job descriptions, procedures, policies, and lines of communication are required.

The functional approach to nursing is economical and efficient, and it permits centralized direction and control. Its disadvantages include fragmentation of care and the possibility that nonquantifiable aspects of care, such as meeting the patient's emotional needs, may be overlooked.

Team Nursing

Team nursing is the delivery of individualized nursing care to a group of patients by a team led by a professional nurse. A nursing team consists of the following members:

- **Registered nurses (RNs)**, who are specially licensed and trained to deliver direct patient care, including patient assessment, identification of health problems, and development and coordination of care
- **Licensed practical nurses (LPNs)**, who provide direct patient care under the direction of an RN, physician, or other licensed practitioner
- **Unlicensed assistive personnel (UAP)**, or healthcare staff, who assume delegated aspects of basic patient care such as bathing, assisting with feeding, and collecting specimens. UAP include certified nurse assistants (CNAs), hospital attendants, nurse technicians, and orderlies.

In team nursing, the RN retains responsibility and authority for patient care but delegates appropriate tasks to the other team members. Proponents of this model believe that the team approach increases the efficiency of the RN. Opponents believe that care of patients with acute illnesses requires greater attention from the professional nurse and allows little room for delegation.

Primary Nursing

Primary nursing is a delivery model in which one nurse is responsible for overseeing the total care of a number of patients 24 hours a day, 7 days a week, even if the nurse does not deliver all of the care personally. It is a method of providing comprehensive, individualized, and consistent care (**Figure 39–3 »**).

Primary nursing uses the nurse's technical knowledge and management skills. The primary nurse assesses and prioritizes each patient's needs, identifies nursing diagnoses, develops a plan of care with the patient, and evaluates the effectiveness of care (see the module on Clinical Decision Making). Associates provide some care, but the primary nurse coordinates it and communicates information about the patient's health to other nurses and health professionals.

Evidence-Based Practice
Nursing Ratio, Patient Outcomes, and Cost Effectiveness

Problem

The nursing ratio (i.e., the number of patients assigned to one nurse) in inpatient settings has long been thought to impact patient outcomes. The true impact of this ratio is difficult to quantify, however, because the nursing ratio is one of several components that can affect patient care. Addressing issues associated with the nursing ratio has the potential to influence the cost of care, which is a concern for organizations that adhere to the principles of managed care.

Evidence

Using objective measures such as the number of patients per nurse or the number of nursing hours per patient day, researchers have attempted to measure the impact of nursing ratios on patient outcomes. According to Mitchell (2012), higher nurse-to-patient ratios (assignment of fewer patients to one nurse) are linked with decreases in mortality, failure to rescue (failure to recognize and respond to a patient who is deteriorating), and specific adverse events among surgical patients. They are also associated with shorter lengths of stay and fewer complications. Lasater and McHugh (2016) further found that higher nursing ratios were associated with lower rates of hospital readmission following joint replacement surgery.

Kang, Kim, and Lee (2016) considered the way both the nursing ratio and the nonnursing responsibilities of nurses (e.g., housekeeping, patient transport, and food delivery) impact patient care. Their research revealed that the incidence of adverse patient events such as falls, healthcare-associated infections, and medication errors increased as nursing ratios decreased and nonnursing responsibilities increased. Roche et al. (2014) also explored the role nonnursing responsibilities play in provision of patient care. Their research suggests that increasing delegation of nonnursing responsibilities to UAP leads to improved quality of care, fewer incomplete tasks, and fewer delays in task completion.

Implications

Adverse events are detrimental to patients and increase the financial burden placed on the healthcare system. Research strongly suggests that higher nursing ratios reduce the likelihood of such events, though Shekelle (2013) points out there has not been a formal evaluation of adverse outcomes within a single organization following a ratio increase.

Increasing nursing ratios may mean increasing staff size, which has the potential to raise healthcare costs. However, research by Martsolf et al. (2014) suggests that increasing the nursing ratio by adding RNs results in a reduction of adverse event costs significant enough to offset the cost of additional staff. Pursuing delegation as a means of improving care also has the potential to increase costs if it involves hiring UAP, but as with RNs, decreases in adverse event costs may compensate for increases in UAP staffing costs.

Finding the right ratio of nurses to patients and the right mix of licensed and unlicensed staff has important implications for both patient care and healthcare costs. The ideal blend will vary from organization to organization, and it is affected by the care delivery model used. Evidence suggests that organizations committed to managed care stand to benefit from determining their ideal balance in both of these areas.

Critical Thinking Application

1. Evaluate how the loss of three licensed staff members from your unit might affect patient outcomes on the unit.

2. In the event that these staff members cannot be replaced, how would you, as the unit's director, prepare the remaining licensed and unlicensed personnel to prevent the most common adverse events that result from reductions in nursing staff?

3. In the event that these staff members cannot be replaced, what case management approach would you use to ensure that patients on your unit are adequately cared for and that their health is not jeopardized?

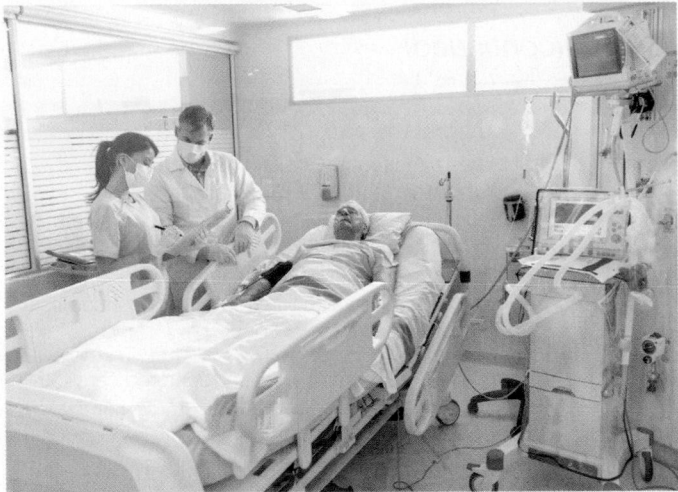

Source: Andresr/E+/Getty Images.

Figure 39–3 ≫ The primary nursing model is often used in ICUs.

Primary nursing encompasses all aspects of the professional role, including teaching, advocacy, decision making, and continuity of care. The primary nurse is the first-line manager of the patient's care, with all accountabilities and responsibilities inherent in that role.

Concepts Related to Managing Care

Managed care is designed to provide cost-effective, high-quality care for groups of patients from the time of their initial contact with the health system through the conclusion of their health problem. Managed care relies on collaboration among the patient, the patient's family, and healthcare pro-

viders. Care coordination and case management are significant components of managed care.

Communication is a key concept in managed care, and it encompasses both communication within the healthcare team and communication between the care team and the patient. Clear communication among nurses, doctors, and other care providers ensures continuity in patient care, improving the patient's perception and experience of care and eliminating costly duplications. Communication among team members and patients creates a relationship based in trust and helps patients be informed and active participants in the care they receive.

To provide high-quality, effective care, the nurse must have a clear understanding of the best ways to manage personal time and patient time, as well as the best ways to work with the schedules of other professionals on the care team. Flexibility and patience are key to effective time management, as is a clear understanding of a patient's care priorities. These skills are learned through practice and lead to more efficient clinical decision making. They are discussed in more detail in the module on Clinical Decision Making. In addition, when making clinical decisions, nurses must be aware of the types of care that will be most beneficial for patients and advocate for that care when necessary.

Nurses maintain high ethical standards as they work with other members of the healthcare team to ensure that the care provided is cost effective yet meets the patient's needs and does no harm. The nurse must also assume the role of teacher in managed care in order to educate the patient and family about the patient's acute and ongoing healthcare needs after discharge. This teaching role is especially important because it helps the patient maintain health and reduce or avoid the costs associated with an acute exacerbation or recurrence of disease or injury.

Some, but not all, of the concepts integral to managing care are shown in the Concepts Related to Managing Care chart. They are presented in alphabetical order.

Concepts Related to
Managing Care

CONCEPT	RELATIONSHIP TO MANAGING CARE	NURSING IMPLICATIONS
Advocacy	Nurses advocate to protect the rights of patients and defend patients from harm. Vulnerable populations depend on nurses to speak up for them as decisions about availability of healthcare services and resources are made.	■ Nurses work in a variety of healthcare settings with heterogeneous populations that need advocates to protect their rights. Nurse advocates empower and educate patients while managing their care.
Clinical Decision Making	Making decisions about patient care begins with analyzing assessment data to identify priorities of actions for best patient outcomes. Having a plan of care helps the nurse manage care by preventing duplication of services and communicating patient goals to other healthcare professionals.	■ Prioritizing care is a process nurses use to manage time and to establish an order for completing responsibilities and care interventions for a patient or group of patients. Competing priorities for care may mean initiating some interventions at a later time.

(continued on next page)

Concepts Related to Managing Care (continued)

CONCEPT	RELATIONSHIP TO MANAGING CARE	NURSING IMPLICATIONS
Communication	Communication among members of the collaborative team of healthcare providers is essential to ensure continuity of patient care. It also eliminates redundancy in testing and procedures. Therapeutic communication helps the patient learn about his or her condition and the care process.	■ Nurses direct communication within the collaborative team. They facilitate patient interactions with team members and coordinate care activities. In addition, they familiarize patients with their conditions and any necessary procedures. They also listen to patient concerns and answer patient questions.
Ethics	The ethical principles of altruism, autonomy, human dignity, integrity, and social justice influence decisions made in dispersing services and resources throughout healthcare systems.	■ Nurses need to provide patient-centered care to all patients in accordance with the common ethical nursing values of being truthful, promoting good, maintaining fairness, and doing no harm.
Healthcare Systems	Delivering and managing healthcare includes coordinating services and allocating resources as a means of meeting multiple patient needs and keeping costs in check. There is a need to close the gap between financial reimbursement and advances in medical interventions.	■ Nurses work with federal, state, and local guidelines in private and public healthcare settings to provide preventive, acute, chronic, and palliative care to patients. Adaptability, flexibility, and creativity are attributes nurses use to achieve good patient outcomes.
Teaching and Learning	Educating patients about their condition and health management is essential for enabling them to maintain health and avoid future complications. Mentoring staff members with less experience and familiarizing them with the components of managed care helps improve care delivery.	■ Nurses are primarily responsible for patient teaching; as such, they lay groundwork essential for keeping patients healthy and reducing the costs of care. Nurses also play an important role in helping other staff members develop their skills, particularly when tasks are delegated to less experienced staff members.

REVIEW The Concept of Managing Care

RELATE Link the Concepts

Linking the concept of managing care with the concept of communication:

1. How does the nurse's ability to communicate effectively contribute to managing the patient's care?

2. Describe a situation in which conflict management may be necessary when managing care for a patient who requires the services of several departments within a hospital.

Linking the concept of managing care with the concept of collaboration:

Mr. Montoya, a 54-year-old man, is to be discharged from an acute care facility after removal of a metastatic brain tumor. He will receive chemotherapy intrathecally as well as intravenously. The unit clerk has scheduled follow-up appointments with Mr. Montoya's surgeon, family provider, oncologist, and neurologist as well as with the infusion therapy department. The physician has provided referrals for consultation with a dietitian, social services, and home nursing care.

3. How can the nurse prioritize care to meet Mr. Montoya's needs while also ensuring that all of the services provided (e.g., predischarge nutritional screening, social services interview, and home nursing assessment to determine home care needs) fulfill the nurse's responsibilities to prepare Mr. Montoya for discharge?

4. What is the nurse's role in managing Mr. Montoya's care and collaborating with the other members of the healthcare team?

REFER Go to Pearson MyLab Nursing and eText

■ Additional review materials

REFLECT Apply Your Knowledge

John Seitz is the nursing director at a skilled nursing facility (SNF). He has received multiple complaints from patients and their families that care provided in one of the facility's units is inconsistent. For example, sometimes residents' trays are brought to the room but no one helps the residents eat. Similarly, beds often go unchanged, and baths are not always provided as requested by the residents.

1. Evaluate what type of nursing model may work best in an SNF.

2. Plan how you, as the nursing director, would ensure that the appropriate model is implemented by the facility's team members.

3. What tools would you design and apply to evaluate the effectiveness of the new plan?

>> Exemplar 39.A Case Management

Exemplar Learning Outcome

39.A Analyze case management as it relates to managing care.

- Describe the purpose of case management and the role of the case manager.
- Identify key elements of case management.
- Explain the need for critical pathways in the case management process.

Exemplar Key Terms

Care management model, 2621
Care map, 2623
Case management, 2621
Critical pathway, 2621
Patient-centered medical home (PCMH), 2621

Overview

Case management describes a range of models for integrating healthcare services for individuals or groups. Generally, case management involves multidisciplinary teams that assume collaborative responsibility for assessing needs, planning and coordinating, implementing, and evaluating care for groups of patients from preadmission to discharge or transfer and recuperation. A case manager may be a nurse, social worker, or other appropriate professional. In some areas of the United States, case managers may be referred to as discharge planners. Key responsibilities of case managers include:

- Assessing patients and their homes and communities
- Coordinating and planning patient care
- Collaborating with other health professionals
- Monitoring patients' progress
- Evaluating patient outcomes

The **care management model** focuses on the needs of the integrated delivery system. It has many similarities to case management in that it also includes planning, assessment, and coordination of health services. However, this model focuses on populations instead of individual patients. The population of interest might be all people in a specific region, the members of a managed care plan, or a group of individuals who share a particular health characteristic, such as diabetes. The goal of the care management model is to integrate a continuum of clinical services. Care management is concerned not only with medical care but also with health promotion, disease prevention, cost control, and use of resources. Case management is often used within the care management model. Typical tools used to facilitate care management are critical pathways, disease management programs, and benchmarking.

Case management may be used as a cost containment strategy in managed care. Both case management and managed care systems often use critical pathways to track patient progress. A **critical pathway** is a standardized plan that helps track care provided to patients with similar, predictable medical conditions. Critical pathways are also called critical paths, clinical pathways, interprofessional plans, anticipated recovery plans, interprofessional action plans, or action plans.

The Nurse as Case Manager

As previously mentioned, case management takes a variety of forms within the U.S. healthcare system. For instance, with the **patient-centered medical home (PCMH)** model, a patient's primary care provider works with the patient and family to develop a personalized plan that addresses the patient's physical and mental health needs across the lifespan. In this model, the provider's office serves as a "home base" from which the patient can access comprehensive preventive, acute, and chronic care services in a manner specific to his or her needs, values, and cultural and linguistic preferences (Patient-Centered Primary Care Collaborative, n.d.). Of course, provider-based case management also occurs in other settings. For example, hospital-based case managers plan and coordinate pre- and postdischarge care for patients with chronic or complex conditions, while community-based case managers work with patients in their homes to ensure they receive adequate ongoing care. In addition, many insurance companies and even some large employers have case managers on staff in an effort to control costs while obtaining better health outcomes.

Regardless of the exact setting, a high percentage of case manager positions are filled by registered nurses. Ideally, nursing case managers have advanced degrees and considerable clinical experience in nursing. These qualifications are crucial in that nurse case managers coordinate all aspects of care, advocate for patients at each stage of care, and plan an overall strategy to address each patient's problems. In an acute care setting, the case manager typically has a caseload of 10 to 15 patients and follows the patients' progress through the system from admission to discharge, accounting for variances from expected progress. Nursing case managers on a patient care unit may coordinate, communicate, collaborate, problem solve, and facilitate patient care for a group of patients and supervise the direct care that other nurses and UAP provide.

Clinical decision making and critical thinking skills are crucial to the development and execution of a well-coordinated care plan. The nurse assesses the patient's needs holistically to ensure that those needs are met and that the patient's independence and quality of life are maximized. The nurse also explores available resources to assist the patient with achieving or maintaining homeostasis and independence, including determining what materials or equipment (such as oxygen or assistive devices) the patient may need.

Actual and potential problems should be identified during care plan development. The nurse is responsible for identifying potential coordination challenges and ensuring that those challenges are addressed during the development phase. For example, challenges may arise related to a patient's religious practices, cultural beliefs and practices, or use of complementary approaches. The nurse assesses for any potential conflicts and works with the patient and the healthcare team to resolve them to ensure the provision of safe, appropriate care and the best possible outcomes for the patient.

The nurse must also ensure that planned care follows standard protocols or critical pathways and evidence-based guidelines. After evaluating the patient's care needs, the nurse organizes the required components of care and develops the nursing care plan in consultation with the patient. The care plan then serves as the nurse's framework for care coordination.

The nurse case manager initiates consultation with the interprofessional care team, recognizes the needs for referral, and obtains necessary orders. As consultations and referrals are implemented, the case manager updates the critical pathway and informs the other members of the interprofessional team. On an ongoing basis, the nurse communicates with patients, family members, and members of the healthcare team to ensure that the plan is executed and continues to meet the patient's needs. It is critical that the nurse coordinator monitor the plan execution and follow up with the patient, family, and team members when adjustments are needed. When necessary, the nurse revises the care plan. Changes in a patient's condition and plans to discharge or transfer the patient are automatic flags that the plan must be updated. The nurse is responsible for documenting the original care plan and any modifications.

Key Elements of Case Management

Nursing case management organizes patient care by major diagnoses or *diagnosis-related groups* (DRGs). DRGs allow nurses to work toward predetermined patient outcomes within specific time frames and resource allocations.

Nursing case management requires the following:

- Collaboration of all members of the healthcare team
- Identification of expected patient outcomes within specific time frames
- Use of principles of continuous quality improvement (CQI) and variance analysis
- Promotion of professional practice
- Promotion of cost-effective care

Research suggests that case management has been particularly successful in disability management, especially when applied to helping injured employees to return to work (Gardner et al., 2010). Likewise, home care and ambulatory settings lend themselves to case management. Patient involvement and participation are key to successful case management (Summers, 2012).

To initiate case management, specific patient diagnoses that represent high-volume, high-cost, and high-risk cases are selected. High-volume cases are those that occur frequently, such as total hip replacements on an orthopedic floor. High-risk cases include patients or case types who have complications, stay in a critical care unit longer than 2 days, or require ventilatory support. Patients also may be selected because they are being treated by a physician who supports case management. Whatever patient population is selected, baseline data must be collected and analyzed. These data provide the information necessary to measure the effectiveness of case management. Essential baseline data include length of stay, cost of care, and complication information.

Five elements are essential to successful implementation of case management:

1. Support by key members of the organization (administrators, physicians, nurses)
2. A qualified nurse case manager
3. Collaborative practice teams
4. A quality management system
5. Established critical pathways (see next section)

When a specific patient population is selected to be "case managed," a collaborative practice team is established. The team, which includes clinical experts from appropriate disciplines (e.g., nursing, medicine, physical therapy) needed for the selected patient population, defines the expected outcomes of care for that population. Based on expected patient outcomes, each member of the team, using that member's discipline's contribution, helps determine appropriate interventions within a specified time frame.

In case management, all professionals are equal members of the team; thus, one group does not determine interventions for other disciplines. All members of the collaborative practice team agree on the final draft of the critical pathways, take ownership of patient outcomes, and accept responsibility and accountability for the interventions and patient outcomes associated with their discipline. The emphasis must be on managing patient outcomes and building consensus among team members. Outcomes must be specified in measurable terms.

Clinical Example A

Martha Ellison is an RN with 10 years of experience and a master's degree in nursing. She is the case manager on the orthopedic unit of the city hospital. She is currently managing 10 patients on the unit: four with injuries that resulted from car crashes; two older adults, each with a fractured hip; and four adolescent patients who required placement of pins and traction to stabilize fractures. Ms. Ellison compares each patient's progress to the critical pathway for that patient and makes recommendations to the physician managing their care related to meeting specific needs.

One of the patients in Ms. Ellison's care is a 22-year-old man who experienced significant head injuries and multiple fractures as a result of a motor vehicle crash. Ms. Ellison works with the hospital physical therapy department to optimize his mobility and range of motion in order to prepare him for rehabilitation. She collaborates with a rehabilitation center that will continue his care following discharge. Ms. Ellison also collaborates with the neurologist and family care providers to ensure that the patient's other needs are met and he is able to be discharged as soon as possible.

Critical Thinking Questions

1. Identify the different individuals and organizations with whom Ms. Ellison is collaborating. Explain why collaboration is essential to meeting a patient's needs.
2. What is the purpose of a critical pathway? What are some other names for a critical pathway?
3. In the care of patients with orthopedic injuries, explain how case management for the older adult patient might differ from that needed for the younger adult patient.

Critical Pathways

Successful case management relies on critical pathways to guide care. The term *critical pathway*, also called a **care map**, clinical pathway, or critical path, refers to the expected outcomes and care strategies developed through collaboration by the healthcare team. Again, the interprofessional team must reach consensus regarding patient care and determine specific, measurable outcomes.

Critical pathways provide direction for managing the care of a specific patient during a specified time period. Critical pathways are useful because they accommodate the unique characteristics of the patient and the patient's condition while making use of the predictable characteristics of the course of the patient's disease or injury. Critical pathways use resources appropriate to the care needed, thereby reducing cost and length of stay. Critical pathways are used in every setting where healthcare is delivered.

A critical path quickly orients the nurse to the outcomes that should be achieved for the patient for that day. Nursing diagnoses identify the outcomes needed. If patient outcomes are not achieved, the case manager is notified and the situation is analyzed to determine how to modify the critical pathway.

Altering time frames or interventions is categorized as a variance, and the case manager tracks all variances. After a time, the appropriate collaborative practice teams analyze the variances, note trends, and decide how to manage them. Teams may then revise the critical pathway or decide to gather additional data before making changes.

Some features are included on all critical paths. These include the specific medical diagnosis, the expected length of stay, patient identification data, appropriate time frames (in days, hours, minutes, or visits) for interventions, and patient outcomes. Interventions are presented in modality groups (medications, nursing activity, and so on). The critical path must include a means to identify variances easily and to determine whether outcomes are met.

≫ **Stay Current:** Clinical pathways vary according to patient needs, agency protocols, and current best practices for care. Examples of clinical pathways can be found at the website of the Children's Hospital of Philadelphia: http://www.chop.edu/pathways#.V5JSfc-v6uM8 and at the University Health System, San Antonio, Texas: http://www.universityhealthsystem.com/services/pharmacy/clinical-pathways-guidelines

Case Management Across the Lifespan

Case management can yield positive results for patients of all ages and with any number of health concerns. However, some patients are more likely to benefit from case management than others. Prominent examples of such patients include at-risk pregnant women; children with congenital conditions or other special needs; children, adolescents, and adults with behavioral, intellectual, or mental health problems; and older adults who have chronic conditions or are approaching the end of life.

At-Risk Pregnant Women

Maternity case managers specialize in working with women who have one or more health-related, social, or economic factors in their lives that place them at increased risk for problems during pregnancy or childbirth. For example, a woman might benefit from maternity case management if she has a chronic disease, uses drugs or alcohol, is experiencing mental illness, lives in extreme poverty, and/or is involved in an abusive relationship. In such cases, the maternity case manager can help promote the health of mother and infant alike by ensuring receipt of adequate prenatal care and referring the patient to various community and government services as appropriate. The case manager also plays a critical role in educating the woman about topics such as obtaining proper nutrition and exercise during pregnancy; recognizing perinatal mood disorders; avoiding fetal exposure to alcohol, tobacco, and drugs; understanding the benefits of breastfeeding; and reducing the risk of maternal–fetal disease transmission at birth.

Children with Special Needs

Many children sustain physical and/or mental disability as a result of premature delivery, congenital disease, birth injury, childhood illness, or some other cause. Case managers are a valuable resource for these children and their families, not only at the time of the initial diagnosis or injury, but for months and sometimes years afterward.

For those children whose conditions can be remedied by surgical and other means (e.g., those with correctable heart or musculoskeletal defects), case managers help plan and coordinate the medical procedures required to correct the problem. They also arrange for the child and family to receive other services necessary to support their well-being throughout the entire treatment period, such as physical and occupational therapy, psychologic counseling, pharmacotherapy, and in-home nursing care.

For children whose conditions will persist for the rest of their life, case managers perform a similar set of actions. However, in addition to coordinating medical care and connecting patients and their families with available support services, they also work to ensure that the child receives adequate educational and other accommodations throughout childhood. Frequently, this requires the case manager to engage in advocacy efforts on behalf of these patients.

Patients with Behavioral, Intellectual, or Mental Health Problems

Patients of all ages may be affected by behavioral, intellectual, or mental health problems that limit their ability to participate in school, obtain or retain a job, engage in self-care, live independently in the community, or engage in any number of other activities of daily living. After working with these individuals to determine their unique limitations, case managers can help each patient formulate a set of realistic goals and expectations, then connect the patient with any number of resources necessary for meeting these goals. Examples include (but are not limited to) individual and/or group counseling; vocational training and structured workshops; nutritional services; disability advocacy organizations; group homes; housekeeping services; home care aides; transportation services; assistive technology; and resources for ensuring adherence with pharmacologic and other therapeutic regimens.

Older Adults

Case management is often a critical component of care for older adult patients. One reason is that many older adults experience multiple and/or chronic health conditions that require ongoing care and coordination. For patients like these, case management helps promote continuity of care, prevent duplication of services, and ensure that patients are not receiving therapies that counteract or otherwise work against one another. In this way, case management helps promote better patient outcomes while simultaneously fostering more efficient, cost-effective use of healthcare resources.

Case management is also an increasingly common aspect of end-of-life care for many older adults (as well as patients of any age who are affected by terminal illness). By working closely with these individuals and their families, case managers help ensure that their patients are able to achieve death with dignity. This means that patients are empowered to choose which treatments they wish to receive without feeling pressured to undergo potentially painful and/or expensive treatments that may only minimally extend their lifespan, yet they are not automatically precluded from receiving these treatments if they so choose. It also means that patients are able to die in the place of their choosing and/or in the presence of loved ones. Often, the case manager's first step in ensuring a patient's wishes are met is to simply speak honestly with the patient about his or her health and impending mortality—something that many healthcare providers and family members are reluctant to do. From this foundation of honesty and understanding, the case manager and patient can together explore options for many end-of-life decisions, including choices related to hospice, palliative care, financial affairs, advance directives, power of attorney, and other medical and legal concerns. The case manager can also help the patient and family arrange for grief counseling and other forms of emotional and spiritual support (Fink-Samnick, 2016; Meyer, 2012).

REVIEW Case Management

RELATE Link the Concepts and Exemplars

Linking the exemplar of case management with the concept of perfusion:

1. A neonate born with a severe congenital heart defect will require numerous open heart surgeries and regular follow-up with cardiology and pediatrics. The parents, who carry comprehensive medical insurance, will require assistance paying for medical bills because the cost of care is expected to exceed the child's lifetime maximum coverage within a few years. How might this family benefit from case management? What specifically would the case manager do for this family?

Linking the exemplar of case management with the concept of oxygenation:

2. The nurse is caring for two patients. One patient has pneumonia that is resolving with IV antibiotics; the other patient has had asthma for many years. Which patient would benefit most from case management? Explain your answer.

3. The nurse is caring for a patient with a chronic alteration in oxygenation requiring many different medications, frequent physician visits, and a history of two to three hospital admissions per year. How might case management help this patient?

REFER Go to Pearson MyLab Nursing and eText

- Additional review materials

REFLECT Apply Your Knowledge

Curt Ranier is a 42-year-old man who sustained a right femur fracture during a motor vehicle crash. Following surgical repair of his femur fracture, he is admitted to the orthopedic unit. Mr. Ranier's surgery and anesthesia were uneventful, and he is stable and alert. His medical history includes type 2 diabetes, which he manages through his diet. He also has a prior history of deep vein thrombosis (DVT) in his left leg. During his admission to the orthopedic unit, Mr. Ranier expressed his motivation to heal and go home; however, he states that he is concerned about caring for himself outside the hospital setting, as he lives alone and has no relatives nearby.

1. Considering Mr. Ranier's current condition and medical history, which nursing diagnoses (both actual and risk) should be included in his nursing plan of care?

2. How would Mr. Ranier benefit from case management? In addition to nursing, describe several other professional disciplines that should collaborate in Mr. Ranier's care.

3. Describe the benefits of using a critical pathway to guide Mr. Ranier's care. In addition to Mr. Ranier's medical diagnosis and patient identification data, identify three categories that would be included in Mr. Ranier's critical pathway.

>> Exemplar 39.B
Cost-Effective Care

Exemplar Learning Outcomes

39.B Analyze cost-effective care as it relates to managing care.

- Summarize payments sources in the United States.
- Describe the international perspective of healthcare.
- Outline factors influencing the provision of healthcare.
- Describe cost-containment strategies.
- Summarize the economics of nursing.

Exemplar Key Terms

Diagnosis-related groups (DRGs), *2628*
Mandatory health insurance, *2625*
Multi-payer systems, *2626*
Private insurance, *2625*
Prospective payment system (PPS), *2628*
Public insurance, *2625*
Single-payer systems, *2626*
Socialized insurance, *2625*
Socialized medicine, *2625*
Voluntary insurance, *2626*

Overview

Despite efforts to control costs, healthcare spending grew at an average annual rate of 4.6% during the period from 1960 to 2010. However, that rate slowed considerably between 2010 and 2013, dropping to 1.1% average annual growth (Council of Economic Advisers, 2014). In 2013, the Secretary of Health and Human Services, Kathleen Sebelius, commented on the change as follows:

> For years, health care costs have been rising faster than inflation, driving up the cost of health care and making it less affordable for families and businesses. But now, the good news about the slowing growth of health care spending nationwide is being increasingly recognized by independent analysts. . . . According to an analysis conducted by *USA Today* (2013), "health care spending last year rose at one of the lowest rates in a half-century." Further, health care providers and analysts found that "cost-saving measures under the health care law appear to be keeping medical prices flat."

Employers, legislators, insurers, and healthcare providers continue to collaborate in efforts to resolve issues surrounding how to best finance healthcare costs. Among these efforts, the United States has implemented several cost-containment strategies, including health promotion and illness prevention activities; managed care systems, including care coordination; and alternative insurance delivery systems.

Payment Sources in the United States

Payment for healthcare services in the United States may come from one or more of several sources. For example, an older patient may have Medicare and supplemental healthcare coverage purchased from a private insurance company; if this combination does not cover all costs, the patient may have to cover the remaining amount with his or her own money. Insurance is often classified as **public insurance** (insurance financed by the government) or **private insurance** (insurance provided by private or publicly owned companies such as Blue Cross Blue Shield, Kaiser Permanente, or Aetna). Many insurance plans, public or private, include a per-visit or per-prescription copayment and a deductible. Medical payment sources in the United States are discussed in greater detail in the module on Health Policy.

The International Perspective

A society's widely held values and attitudes (e.g., toward the government's role in private lives) influence the development of its healthcare systems and policies. Most developed countries outside of the United States have similar values with regard to healthcare; the United States is unique in its emphasis on self-reliance, self-determination, and limited government involvement. **Table 39–1 >>** contrasts U.S. values in relation to healthcare with those of other countries.

Each country has its own unique healthcare system, but these systems can be broadly divided into four categories based on the organization and financing of healthcare:

- The first category is **socialized medicine**, in which the state owns and controls healthcare services. Examples of socialized medicine are seen in the United Kingdom, Sweden, and Denmark, where physicians derive virtually all of their income from the government and have employment contracts with the state.

- The second category is **socialized insurance**, in which all medically necessary services are covered by the government (including physician care, hospital services, and to some extent, prescription drugs), but these services are delivered by a blend of private and public providers. Canada, France, and Australia have this form of healthcare system.

- **Mandatory health insurance** is the third category and is found in Germany and Japan. These nations have large, nonprofit health insurance organizations called "sickness funds." The sickness funds are usually organized around large employers or work-based associations. Government-sponsored programs cover citizens who are not part of a sickness fund. Everyone belongs to one of these two types of plans, thus ensuring universality of coverage.

TABLE 39–1 Comparison of Healthcare Values in the United States and Other Developed Countries

United States	Other Developed Countries
Pluralism and choice	Universality
Self-reliance	Shared responsibility
Emphasis on individual freedom	Acceptance of the role of government
Federalism	Centralization
Free enterprise	Equity
Fear of rationing	Acceptance of system constraints

Sources: Based on National Research Council & Institute of Medicine. (2013). Policies and social values. In S. H. Woolf and L. Aron (Eds.), *U.S. health in international perspectives.* Washington, DC: National Academies Press. Retrieved from http://www.ncbi.nlm.nih.gov/books/NBK154493/; Oberlander, J., & White, J. (2009). Public attitudes toward healthcare spending aren't the problem; Prices are. *Health Affairs, 28*(5), 1285–1293. doi:10.1377/hlthaff.28.5.1285; O'Mahony, J. (2012). *U.S. view of health care at odds with Europe.* Retrieved from http://www.marketwatch.com/story/us-view-of-health-care-at-odds-with-europe-2012-08-02.

- Finally, **voluntary insurance** provides no guarantee of universality because coverage may be expensive and difficult to purchase. The United States currently has this type of system, under which millions of Americans lack coverage due to financial and other constraints (see Focus on Diversity and Culture: Health Insurance and Socioeconomic Status). A major goal of the Patient Protection and Affordable Care Act, signed into law in March 2010 and often referred to as the ACA or "Obamacare," was to reduce the difficulties associated with securing voluntary insurance in the United States. Under the ACA, the majority of individuals who did not have health insurance through their employer or a government program were required to purchase coverage or pay a financial penalty. To make such coverage more accessible and affordable,

the ACA established subsidies for some Americans and called for the establishment of health insurance exchanges in all 50 states. Thus, the ACA attempted to move the United States toward a mandatory insurance system while still allowing people to opt out as long as they are willing to pay the associated penalty.

Note that both socialized medicine and socialized insurance are considered **single-payer systems**, because payment for all services ultimately comes from one source (i.e., the national government). In contrast, the mandatory and voluntary insurance systems are both considered **multi-payer systems** in that reimbursement is provided by a combination of sources (Ridic, Gleason, & Ridic, 2012).

Regardless of their exact form, healthcare systems throughout the world are in crisis. Most countries, regardless of their level of funding for healthcare, have run out of ways to finance their expenditures through taxation or other existing channels. They realize that costs must be contained in the future. Furthermore, there is concern in western European nations, Canada, and Australia about the increased sophistication and resulting expectations of their emerging middle classes.

Factors Influencing the Provision of Healthcare

A number of factors influence provision of and access to healthcare, regardless of the types of coverage available. Within the United States, economic factors including supply and demand and the inability to account for the actual costs of critical services (e.g., nursing services) are important influences on the provision of healthcare.

Supply and Demand

In the 1980s, an imbalance in supply and demand emerged as the cost of medical care began increasing faster than the

Focus on Diversity and Culture
Health Insurance and Socioeconomic Status

Health insurance is a major determinant of access to care—and in the United States, health insurance coverage is strongly tied to socioeconomic status.

Despite progress made in the numbers of insured individuals as a result of ACA, tens of millions of Americans continue to lack even basic healthcare coverage, and low-income families and minority groups continue to be disproportionately affected. For example, in 2014:

- More than 80% of uninsured Americans came from families in which at least one member worked.

- More than 50% of uninsured Americans came from low-income households, defined as those with a combined family income below 200% of the poverty level. (In 2014, the federal poverty level for a family of three was $19,055.)

- People of color accounted for over half of the nation's uninsured, even though they made up only 40% of the overall U.S. population. Uninsured rates were especially high among Hispanic Americans (20.9%) and non-Hispanic Black Americans (12.7%) as compared to White Americans, who had an uninsured rate of 9.1% (Kaiser Family Foundation, 2015).

A variety of socioeconomic factors place low-income and minority individuals at elevated risk for health problems—and lack of insurance only increases this risk. In fact, research indicates that about 27% of uninsured adults went without needed healthcare in 2014 because they couldn't afford the cost. Furthermore, even when they aren't sick, the uninsured are less likely to receive preventive care. As a result of this care deficit, uninsured Americans are more likely to experience catastrophic illness and less likely to afford treatment when they can no longer postpone it. The resulting increases in resource-intensive and uncompensated care drive up costs across the entire healthcare system (Kaiser Family Foundation, 2015).

These statistics also underline the importance of containing costs within nursing units and throughout care organizations as a means of improving the affordability of care. Making care more affordable for patients with low socioeconomic status will improve health and reduce suffering. It will also save money in the long run by eliminating costly complications associated with conditions that are preventable or more easily treated in the early stages.

gross national product. During this time, consumers came to expect that any and all services, regardless of cost, should be available and paid for by third-party payers. As a result, the price of insurance coverage in the private sector skyrocketed, creating further imbalance.

Today, many employers cannot or will not provide the same level of healthcare coverage to employees as in years past. Most employers now require their employees to pay a greater portion of the cost of insurance in the form of increased premiums. Others do not provide health insurance coverage at all. These changes diminish the ability of all consumers to afford care, yet many Americans continue to expect care on demand. From a healthcare economics standpoint, this has created a situation in which healthcare cannot be supplied at the level demanded by the public (Health Resources and Services Administration, 2013; Hoffman, 2013).

When there is an imbalance in supply and demand, rationing of healthcare may result. No country can afford to provide unlimited amounts of medical services to everyone, so each nation must decide how to ration, or limit access to, healthcare services. This can happen in two ways. The first is by having the government set limits. In this approach, the cost of services is kept low, and people wait for availability. This type of rationing is used in several industrialized countries, including Great Britain and Canada. Scarce services are kept at a reasonable cost but are allocated according to particular criteria, such as age or a waiting list. Even in these countries, however, individuals who can pay for more services have access to more services. In the United States, only Oregon has suggested such an approach. The Oregon legislature enacted a program to limit access to expensive procedures, such as transplantation, and then increase Medicaid eligibility to a larger number of low-income people. The second approach to healthcare rationing is to ration by ability to pay. This approach limits demand for more expensive procedures by offering them only to those who are willing and able to pay out of pocket or who have sufficient health insurance coverage (Hoffman, 2013).

There are important differences between these two rationing methods. One major difference involves the freedom of individuals to choose the amount and type of healthcare they use and to select who should deliver it. Freedom of choice is a traditional value of healthcare consumers in the United States. Under a system of strict government rationing, a patient cannot purchase a particular healthcare service unless it is made available to everyone by the government. Conversely, under the ability to pay method, a patient can theoretically purchase any healthcare service as long as he or she can afford it. For those who cannot afford a particular service, however, that service is not an option, no matter how great the individual's need.

SAFETY ALERT Under federal law, patients who are experiencing a true medical emergency cannot be denied treatment, regardless of their ability to pay. Specifically, the Emergency Medical Treatment and Labor Act (EMTALA) of 1986 requires all Medicare-participating hospitals that offer emergency services to examine and stabilize any patient who presents for an emergency medical condition, even if that patient cannot pay for services. Once the patient is stabilized, however, EMTALA protections no longer apply, and the patient may be transferred or discharged at the hospital's discretion.

Separate Billing for Nursing Services

Within the United States, bills submitted to third-party payers and consumers from healthcare organizations (e.g., hospitals) continue to bundle nursing services with flat daily charges (e.g., the cost of the room and housekeeping). The specific cost of nursing has neither been separated out nor given a dollar value. This bundling has hindered nurses' ability to receive payment from third-party payers. Many nursing leaders think that in order for nursing to be a profession, nursing services must be accounted for separately by healthcare institutions.

Several developments within the nursing profession have provided ways of quantifying nursing care. Some of the better-known projects have resulted in nursing diagnoses that can be used to categorize nursing interventions; these include the NANDA International (NANDA-I) diagnoses, the Nursing Interventions Classification (NIC), and the Nursing Outcomes Classification (NOC). The recent development of payment codes for care coordination is another example of such developments. Proponents of these systems argue that quantifying nursing care will help control costs by ensuring that patients pay only for the exact level of nursing care they require. Quantification of care will also provide useful data that allow facilities and providers to better track the cost effectiveness of various nursing actions, as well as allocate nursing resources in the most efficient way possible (Rutherford, 2012).

Cost-Containment Strategies

Over the past few decades, a number of strategies have been developed in an attempt to contain healthcare costs. Some of the most prominent cost-containment strategies are competition, price controls, and alternative insurance delivery systems. Managed care, health promotion and illness prevention, alternative care providers, and vertically integrated health service organizations are also popular. In addition, since its enactment in 2010, the ACA has put several cost-containment strategies in place. Various measures aimed at controlling the costs of care are discussed in the sections that follow.

Competition

During the 1970s, regulations in the United States were changed to permit competition among organizations that deliver healthcare and provide insurance. Currently, little reduction in costs appears to be attributable to competition. Competition has, however, led to the establishment and expanded use of walk-in clinics, urgent care clinics, and alternative healthcare providers (such as advanced practice registered nurses), all of which offer additional care choices for patients.

Price Controls

Price controls for healthcare services have been established in various ways. Freezes on physicians' fees have been imposed at various times for short periods and, as mentioned previously, many states limit reimbursement to physicians and hospitals for services provided to Medicaid patients.

The passage of the Tax Equity and Fiscal Responsibility Act (TEFRA) in 1982 brought about a dramatic restructuring of healthcare delivery in the United States. Through this act, the federal government changed the payment method for

Medicare from a retrospective system to a prospective one. In a retrospective payment system, billing is determined after services are rendered; in a **prospective payment system (PPS)**, billing is determined before the patient is ever admitted to the hospital. By making Medicare payments prospective, TEFRA limits the amount of Medicare reimbursements paid to hospitals. Limits are set using a system of **diagnosis-related groups (DRGs)**, by which hospitals are paid a predetermined amount for patients with a specific diagnosis. For example, a hospital that admits a patient with a diagnosis of myocardial infarction is reimbursed for a specific dollar amount, regardless of the cost of services, the length of stay, or the acuity or complexity of the patient's illness. DRG rates are set in advance of the year during which they apply and are considered to be fixed unless major, uncontrollable events occur.

Unfortunately, this type of PPS may result in healthcare agencies choosing to withhold borderline necessary tests and procedures and shorten hospital stays, thus avoiding the expenditures a prolonged stay generates. Doing so allows hospitals to keep their costs at or below the amount they are allowed to bill Medicare. Notable effects of these practices include the earlier discharge of patients, decreased admissions, increased outpatient services (both type and number), and increased focus on the costs of care. Earlier discharge of patients has led to expanded home care services and increased use of technology and specialists.

Another means of reducing healthcare costs is the development of group self-insurance plans. These plans are created for a designated group, such as employees in a large company, a group of companies, or a union. The designated group then assumes all or part of the costs of healthcare for its members. Group plans can often provide coverage at a lower cost than insurance companies because they are exempt from certain taxes and fees.

Cost-containment strategies such as PPS and group self-insurance plans have driven several trends in healthcare delivery. These include increased emphasis on preventive care to reduce the incidence of illnesses, provision of treatment in noninstitutional settings such as clinics or patients' homes, and use of best practices as documented in protocols and guidelines. These strategies focus on avoiding hospital and institutional placement unless absolutely necessary and ensuring that all care provided is scientifically based.

Vertically Integrated Health Services Organizations

Yet another cost-containment practice that has become increasingly common in recent decades is the establishment of *vertically integrated health services organizations*, or networks of hospitals, clinics, and individual providers that offer a broad range of care and support services to patients across the entire wellness spectrum. By integrating the provision of hospital care, ambulatory care, outpatient surgery, and home health services, these systems allow patients to receive the precise level of care they need in the most cost-effective way possible.

Two trends have contributed to the rise of vertically integrated health services organizations: the change in payment structures and the development of medical technology. As insurers became more concerned about the rising costs of healthcare during the 1970s, hospitals began to integrate horizontally to form multiple-hospital systems. By coordinating services within each system, hospitals were able to avoid duplication of services as well as underuse of expensive equipment at multiple sites.

The move to vertical integration began several years later as a result of TEFRA's creation of fixed Medicare payments based on DRGs. This legislation prompted hospitals to begin monitoring discharge practices and lengths of stay. Hospitals soon realized that patients could be discharged earlier to other suitable settings, such as nursing homes, rehabilitation centers, and their own homes. Earlier discharges were more cost effective. At the same time, hospitals realized it would be advantageous for them to own or contract with agencies that provide other levels of care. This vertical integration allowed hospitals to reduce inpatient costs and receive additional Medicare revenues.

Advances in medical technology have also contributed to the move from traditional inpatient hospitalization to outpatient settings. The length of hospital stay for many surgeries, such as cholecystectomies, hernia repairs, and some orthopedic surgeries, was once several days. New technologies now permit these surgeries to be performed on an outpatient or ambulatory surgery basis at less expense.

The goal of vertical integration is to create a "seamless" system of patient care in which movement from service to service is coordinated and well organized. Such a system improves outcomes and quality of care while increasing patient satisfaction and providing better cost control through more efficient use of resources. If a vertically integrated system is efficient, it can decrease transaction costs and allow greater accountability.

Cost Containment and the ACA

The ACA legally compelled healthcare organizations to adopt various cost-containment measures aimed at improving the quality of care provided, redesigning healthcare delivery systems, determining appropriate payment for services provided, modernizing the financial systems used to pay for services, and eliminating fraud and abuse. For example, the law established payment penalties as an incentive to prevent hospital readmissions and healthcare-associated conditions such as pressure injuries and infections. The ACA also called for provision of coordinated care by healthcare teams rather than individual providers and mandated reduction of medically unnecessary services that may be detrimental to a patient's health.

Nursing Economics

Quality of care and cost trade-offs in hospitals have dominated the literature for the past decade. Both consumers and healthcare professionals have expressed concerns about diminished quality of care resulting from cost constraints, early discharge, periodic nursing shortages, and increased use of UAP.

Determining the precise cost of services is a major challenge for nursing. What are the exact costs of high-quality nursing care? How many nursing care hours are required for each DRG? What is the best skill mix—that is, ratio of RNs to LPNs to UAP—on each hospital unit? Since 1983, many studies have sought to determine the actual costs and cost effectiveness of nursing care. Researchers have investigated such topics as the impact of nurse–physician collaboration;

new cost-effective interventions; the cost benefits of primary nursing, nurse practitioners, and nurse-midwives; and the cost effectiveness of home care. The quality of the nursing care of the future relies on ongoing research in the area of economics, as well as nurses' awareness of economic issues during the course of their daily practice.

Nursing Shortages

One factor that must be considered when discussing the economics of nursing in the United States is the impact of nursing shortages. One measure commonly used to gauge whether a shortage exists is the *nursing vacancy rate*, or the percentage of unfilled nursing positions for which an organization is recruiting.

When shortages occur, employers are forced to compete for the same available pool of nurses, which means they must increase wages in order to hire and retain staff. As employers fill positions and more nurses enter the workforce as a result of other factors, employers begin to slow the rate at which they increase wages. These shortage-linked salary fluctuations contribute to the challenge of determining the actual costs of nursing.

Trends in healthcare during the past 20 years have further contributed to the complexity of the problem. Because of the shift toward decreased lengths of stay, patients are often sent home "sicker and quicker." Many services that were historically provided in the hospital are now routinely done in a skilled nursing facility, an outpatient facility, or the patient's home. The ratio of nurses to non-nurses providing direct nursing care has also decreased in recent years. Some of this reduction is due to hospitals replacing portions of their nursing staff with UAP as a cost-containment measure. Another factor is increased demand for nurses to work in new roles; for example, nurses may leave the bedside to provide utilization and case management services for cost-containment companies. These staff reductions have left some nurses feeling disillusioned and doubtful of their ability to provide quality healthcare, prompting them to leave the profession altogether.

Ending the cycle of nursing shortages will require adjustments in the approaches used by employers and nurses alike. New opportunities and new roles for nurses may attract more people into the profession. However, as RNs increasingly perform more highly valued functions, administrators in healthcare organizations will need to respect and compensate them accordingly.

Cost-conscious Nursing Practice

All nurses must understand the costs associated with healthcare and the ways in which these costs impact nursing practice. Because the nursing staff is the largest professional group in a hospital, it is the most expensive. However, the nursing staff does not produce revenue, because nursing services are included as part of patients' room and board charges. As a result, it is incumbent on nurse managers to be mindful of employment and nonsalary expenses and to engage their staff in looking for ways to minimize expenditures at the unit level without negatively impacting patient care (Sherman, 2012a).

This level of financial accountability is relatively new to the nursing profession and comes at a time when nursing must compete for limited resources with other departments in the healthcare organization. Consider the following: Whether nurses work in a hospital, a school, home healthcare, or another setting, they are increasingly required to participate in strategies to make care more cost effective. Initially, this may sound intimidating. However, it is critical to understand that many evidence-based nursing interventions that nurses perform daily contribute to the goal of better cost containment. For example, hand washing to reduce the risk of healthcare-associated infections reduces costs, because these infections increase expenses for both individual patients and the healthcare setting. Similarly, nursing efforts to promote safety and improve quality also promote cost-conscious nursing practice.

Although cost containment is an essential component of nursing practice, it does not negate the essential roles of nursing. Nurses in all settings must continue to advocate for care that meets the standards of best practice while trying to find new ways to contain costs.

REVIEW Cost-Effective Care

RELATE Link the Concepts and Exemplars

Linking the exemplar of cost-effective care with the concept of health, wellness, and illness:

1. Explain how health promotion activities reduce the cost of care.

2. You are caring for an adolescent patient who admits to smoking "a couple" of cigarettes per week. What impact would helping this patient quit smoking have on the lifetime cost of his healthcare?

Linking the exemplar of cost-effective care with the concept of infection:

3. How does the cost of a healthcare-acquired infection impact the cost of a patient's admission?

4. How does the cost of reducing the risk of healthcare-acquired infections compare to the cost of treating a patient who contracts a healthcare-acquired infection?

REFER Go to Pearson MyLab Nursing and eText

- Additional review materials

REFLECT Apply Your Knowledge

A group of nurses works on an oncology unit with 30 beds, including a 6-bed bone marrow transplant unit. Each nurse is usually assigned four or five patients, depending on acuity levels. Only nurses with advanced training are allowed to administer chemotherapy, so it is not uncommon to have one nurse assigned to be a medication nurse when many others on the same shift have not yet attended or completed the chemotherapy certification course.

1. What actions could you, as a staff nurse on this unit, take to reduce the cost of providing care to these patients?

2. The hospital is considering replacing its 10-year-old x-ray machine with a newer model that uses less radiation and is completely digital, thereby eliminating the need for film cartridges and making it easier for radiologists to read x-rays from computers in their offices or homes. However, the cost of the machine is very high. You are asked to join the committee that will make the decision about whether to purchase this equipment. What are the pros and cons of buying this new radiology equipment?

» Exemplar 39.C
Delegation

Exemplar Learning Outcomes

39.C Analyze delegation as it relates to managing care.

- Summarize the principles of delegation.
- Describe the benefits of delegation.
- Outline the delegation process.
- Outline factors affecting delegation.
- Describe how liability affects delegation.

Exemplar Key Terms

Assignment, 2630
Delegate, 2630
Delegation, 2630
Delegator, 2630
Overdelegation, 2636
Reverse delegation, 2636
Underdelegation, 2636

Overview

Nurses play a major role in healthcare, and the United States continues to experience a nursing shortage secondary to increases in lifespan, the number of older adults requiring medical care, and the need for nursing care in nonhospital environments. As a result, registered nurses must dedicate increasingly larger portions of their time to the performance of highly skilled tasks. This often leaves them with little time to complete the less complex interventions required for attainment of successful patient outcomes. In order for such tasks to be accomplished, RNs frequently rely on the process of delegation.

In general terms, **delegation** is the transference of responsibility and authority for an activity to a competent individual. The **delegate** is the individual who assumes responsibility for the actual performance of the task or procedure. The **delegator** is the individual who assigns the task and retains accountability for the outcome. Delegation is a tool that allows the delegator to devote more time to tasks that cannot be delegated. It also enhances the skills and abilities of the delegate, which builds self-esteem, promotes morale, and enhances teamwork and attainment of the organization's goals.

Within the field of nursing, delegation refers to indirect care, meaning the intended outcome is achieved through the work of someone supervised by the nurse. It involves defining the task, determining who can perform the task, describing the expectation, seeking agreement, monitoring performance, and providing feedback to the delegate regarding performance.

Delegation is often confused with work allocation or assignment. Although the two concepts are related, they are not the same. **Assignment** refers to a skill or task that is a fundamental part of an individual's job that the individual is expected to accomplish on a regular basis (NCSBN, 2016). Asking an individual to perform a task that is a part of her regular responsibilities and job description is not delegating. In *delegation*, the nurse asks another individual to perform a task or skill that is not part of the individual's regular assigned work. In delegating, the nurse transfers the *responsibility* for completing the task to the delegate, but not the *accountability* for the task. Accountability remains with the nurse (NCSBN, 2016). Delegation is not easy. Complications may arise due to a number of factors, including variations in titles and

terminology, lack of training, issues of accountability and responsibility, and the nurse's discomfort with the delegation process. Still, today's emphasis on "doing more with less" means it is more critical than ever before that nurses master the skill of delegation. Once nurses learn how to delegate, they extend their ability to accomplish more by using others' help. Guidelines for successful delegation are listed in **Box 39-1** » and described in detail throughout this exemplar.

Principles of Delegation

Registered nurses increasingly delegate components of nursing care to other healthcare workers, including fellow RNs, licensed practical nurses (LPNs), licensed vocational nurses (LVNs), and UAP. An RN who delegates a task to another healthcare worker is accountable for selecting an appropriately skilled caregiver and for continually evaluating the care provided to the patient by that caregiver.

Delegating to Other Nurses

Registered nurses frequently delegate tasks to other RNs. For example, a charge nurse is engaging in delegation when she makes assignments for a shift. A nurse may also opt to delegate certain care activities for a patient to another nurse, as long as the second nurse is free and can accept the additional responsibility. For instance, an RN may assign a float RN to an unstable patient with a high temperature and high

Box 39-1
Guidelines for Successful Delegation

1. Follow your state's nurse practice act and your facility's policies and procedures when delegating.
2. Delegate only tasks for which you have both accountability and responsibility.
3. Follow state regulations, job descriptions, and agency policies when delegating.
4. Follow the delegation process and key behaviors for delegating.
5. Only accept delegation when you have a clear understanding of the task, time frame, reporting requirements, and other expectations.
6. Confront your fears about delegation; recognize which fears are realistic and which are not.

blood pressure. Caring for an unstable patient is within the RN scope of practice, so the RN who accepts the assignment will be responsible for completing the patient's care safely, ethically, and completely.

In addition, it may be appropriate for an RN to delegate specific interventions to an LPN or LVN. In these cases, the RN remains responsible for ensuring that the LPN or LVN completes the interventions both correctly and appropriately.

When delegating to other nurses of any type, the RN must use critical thinking and professional judgment. He or she must also follow the widely accepted *Five Rights of Delegation:*

1. *Right task:* The delegator must ensure that the task is one that can be delegated according to the agency's policies and procedures and is appropriate for the specific patient.

2. *Right circumstances:* The delegator must determine that the task addresses the patient's needs and contributes to a desired outcome, and that adequate supervision is available.

3. *Right person:* The delegator must assign the task to a delegate who has the necessary skills and experience. Moreover, the task must be within that individual's scope of practice.

4. *Right direction:* The delegator must provide a clear, concise description of the task, along with its objectives, limits, and expectations. This material may be communicated orally or in written format. The delegator must also verify that the delegate understands the information that has been communicated.

5. *Right supervision:* The delegator must monitor and evaluate the delegate's performance. This includes providing feedback and intervening if necessary (ANA & National Council of State Boards of Nursing [NCSBN], 2006; Yoost & Crawford, 2016).

Delegating to Unlicensed Assistive Personnel

UAP, who function as "nurse extenders," are identified by a variety of titles, including certified nursing aides/assistants (CNAs), home health aides (HHAs), medical technicians, orderlies, and surgical technicians. Each category and the individuals within it have diverse levels of training and experience. Even though UAP lack licensure, nurses may delegate to them as appropriate because they are employees of the healthcare provider. (Conversely, nurses may not delegate to family members or friends of patients even if these individuals provide personal care to the patients, because these individuals do not work for the healthcare provider.)

It is not possible to generate an exhaustive list of exactly which actions are acceptable for delegation to UAP. Remember, each state's nurse practice act defines what acts may or may not be delegated to UAP within that state. Still, some general examples of tasks that may and may not be delegated are provided in **Box 39–2 》**.

SAFETY ALERT Care of unstable patients should *never* be delegated to an LPN, LVN, or UAP. If an RN must delegate all or part of the care of an unstable patient, these tasks must be delegated to another RN as appropriate.

> ## Box 39–2
> ### Examples of Tasks That May and May Not Be Delegated to UAP
>
> **TASKS THAT MAY BE DELEGATED TO UAP**
> - Taking vital signs
> - Measuring and recording intake and output (I/O)
> - Patient transfers and ambulation
> - Postmortem care
> - Bathing
> - Feeding
> - Gastrostomy feedings in established systems
> - Attending to safety
> - Weighing
> - Suctioning chronic tracheostomies
>
> **TASKS THAT MAY NOT BE DELEGATED TO UAP**
> - Assessment
> - Interpreting data
> - Making a nursing diagnosis
> - Creating a nursing care plan
> - Evaluating care effectiveness
> - Care of invasive lines
> - Administering parenteral medications
> - Inserting nasogastric (NG) tubes
> - Patient education
> - Performing triage
> - Giving telephone advice

Principles guiding the nurse's decision to delegate help ensure the safety and quality of outcomes. These principles include the Five Rights of Delegation, along with those listed in **Box 39–3 》**. Note that even if a task is one that may be delegated legally, the individual nurse must still determine whether the task can be delegated to a particular UAP for a specific patient. Note also that UAP may not delegate tasks to another person.

Once a nurse has made the decision to delegate, he or she must communicate clearly to the UAP. The nurse must also verify that the UAP understands:

- The specific tasks to be done for each patient;
- When each task is to be done;
- The expected outcomes for each task, including parameters outside of which the unlicensed person must immediately report to the nurse (and any action that must urgently be taken);
- Who is available to serve as a resource if needed; and
- When and in what format (written or verbal) a task report will be completed.

As noted in Box 39–3, a specific task that can be delegated to one UAP may be inappropriate for a different UAP, depending on each person's experience, training, and individual skill set. Also, a task that is appropriate for a UAP to perform with one patient may be inappropriate with a different patient, or even with the same patient under altered circumstances. For example, taking routine vital signs may be delegated to the UAP for a patient who is in stable condition, but it would not be delegated for the same patient if he became unstable.

Box 39–3
Principles Used by the Nurse to Determine Delegation to Unlicensed Assistive Personnel

1. The nurse must assess the individual patient before delegating tasks.
2. The patient must be medically stable or in a chronic condition and not fragile.
3. The task must be considered routine for this patient.
4. The task must not require a substantial amount of scientific knowledge or technical skill.
5. The task must be considered safe for this patient.
6. The task must have a predictable outcome.
7. The nurse must know and understand the agency's procedures and policies about delegation.
8. The nurse must know the scope of practice and the customary knowledge, skills, and job description for each discipline represented on the healthcare team.
9. The nurse must be aware of individual variations in work abilities and training. Each individual UAP has different experiences and may or may not be capable of performing the task to be delegated.
10. The nurse, when unsure about a UAP's ability to perform a task, must observe while the UAP performs the task or must demonstrate the task to the UAP and get a return demonstration before allowing the UAP to perform it independently.
11. The nurse must clarify reporting expectations to ensure the task is accomplished.
12. The nurse must create an atmosphere that fosters communication, teaching, and learning. For example, the nurse should encourage the UAP to ask questions, listen carefully to concerns, and make use of every opportunity to teach.

Certain tasks should never be delegated by the RN. For example, discipline of other employees, highly technical tasks, and complex patient care tasks that require specific levels of licensure, certification, or training should not be delegated. Also, any situation that involves confidentiality or controversy should not be delegated to others.

SAFETY ALERT Each healthcare provider, licensed or unlicensed, is responsible for his or her own actions. Anyone who feels unqualified to perform a delegated task must decline to perform it until he or she receives appropriate training and is assessed for competency.

Delegation Versus Dumping

Nurses should delegate because it allows them to make better use of their time. They should not delegate in order to dump an undesirable task on someone else or to reward a productive employee with more work. Sometimes, a nurse may fear that he is "dumping" on another staff member by delegating routine care; in such cases, however, the nurse needs to maintain perspective on what tasks he can complete in a timely fashion and what tasks could be performed effectively by the delegate. Delegation should always be practiced in a way that provides the greatest benefit to the patient, makes the best use of the time of all staff members, and provides delegates with opportunities for growth.

Benefits of Delegation

The proper delegation of duties can benefit the nurse, the delegate, the manager, and the organization.

Benefits to the Nurse

By delegating some tasks to UAP, nurses are able to devote more time to those tasks that cannot be delegated, such as complex patient care. For example, a nurse has three central line dressing changes and two patients who require daily weights to be completed before the shift ends in 1 hour. The nurse may delegate the task of obtaining the patients' daily weights to a UAP and complete the central line dressing changes herself. In this example delegation improves patient care in that all the necessary tasks are done but the nurse is not rushed to complete more complex tasks. By alleviating task overload, delegation also increases nurses' job satisfaction and improves an organization's employee retention rate.

Benefits to the Delegate

Delegation allows delegates to gain new skills and abilities that can help them advance within a given organization or in their overall careers. In addition, delegation often brings with it trust and support, thereby helping build the self-esteem and confidence of the delegate. Subsequently, job satisfaction and motivation are enhanced as individuals feel stimulated by new challenges, morale improves, and a sense of pride and belonging develops, as does greater awareness of responsibility. Individuals feel more appreciated and learn to appreciate the roles and responsibilities of others, increasing cooperation and enhancing teamwork. Most delegates also feel a strong sense of internal satisfaction from knowing that their contributions assisted in the achievement of desired patient outcomes.

Benefits to the Manager

Delegation yields several benefits for the nurse manager. First, if nurses are delegating appropriately to UAP, the manager's unit will function better. Also, managers who themselves appropriately delegate tasks to staff members are able to devote more time to management functions that cannot be delegated. With the additional time gained through delegation, these managers have increased opportunity to develop new skills and abilities that facilitate career advancement.

Benefits to the Organization

As teamwork improves, the organization benefits by achieving its goals more efficiently. As efficiency increases, the quality of care and patient satisfaction improve. Employee overtime and absences decrease. Productivity increases, and the organization's financial position may improve.

The Delegation Process

Nurses may delegate only those tasks for which they have responsibility and authority. These include routine tasks, tasks for which the nurse does not have time, and tasks that have moved down in priority. Whenever a nurse opts to transfer authority for one or more of these tasks, he or she must engage in the delegation process. According to the

NCSBN (2012), this process consists of four distinct steps that should be followed for every situation involving delegation:

1. Assessment and planning
2. Communication
3. Surveillance and supervision
4. Evaluation and feedback

Each of these steps is described in detail in the following sections.

Assessment and Planning

Assessment and planning combine to form the critical first step in the delegation process. Prior to the actual delegation of any task, the nurse needs to consider the following questions:

- Is the task within the scope of the nurse's practice?
- Have the patient's needs been assessed?
- Is the nurse competent to make delegation decisions?
- Is the task consistent with the recommended criteria for delegation? (See Box 39–3 for a list of these criteria.)
- Does the delegate have the appropriate training, skills, and knowledge to perform the task safely, using current standards of practice?
- Are organizational policies, procedures, or protocols available for the task?
- Is adequate supervision available?

If the answer to each of these questions is "yes," then the nurse may continue to the next step in the delegation process (NCSBN, 2012).

Communication

The second step in delegation is to communicate with the delegate regarding expectations for the task. Appropriate communication goes both ways: from the delegator to the delegate, and from the delegate to the delegator. Specifically, the delegator must allow enough time to clearly describe the task and expectations for completing it, answer the delegate's questions, address any situations that must be reported to the delegate, and inform the delegate of the nurse's own availability in the event the delegate has further questions or needs assistance. Some behaviors that can assist in the accomplishment of these tasks are described in **Box 39–4 》**. The delegator must also consider any cultural factors that might affect the delegation process, as described in the Focus on Diversity and Culture feature.

The delegate also has certain responsibilities. In particular, the delegate needs to communicate understanding of the task, inform the delegator if she has never performed the task before, request training if needed, and describe what communication and action should be undertaken in an emergency situation. Both the delegator and the delegate should also have a clear understanding of how the delegated task will be documented in the nursing record (NCSBN, 2016).

Surveillance and Supervision

Surveillance is necessary to validate that the delegated task or function is being delivered in compliance with agency

Box 39–4
Key Behaviors When Delegating Tasks

When delegating a task to another staff member, the nurse should:

- Describe the task using "I" statements (e.g., "I would like …") and appropriate nonverbal behaviors (e.g., open body language, face-to-face positioning, and eye contact). The delegate needs to know what is expected, when the task should be completed, and also where and how (if appropriate). More experienced delegates may be able to define for themselves the where and how. The nurse must decide whether written reports are necessary or if brief oral reports are sufficient. If written reports are required, the nurse should indicate whether tables, charts, or other graphics are necessary. The nurse should be specific about reporting times. In patient care tasks, it is also important to determine who has responsibility and authority to chart certain tasks: UAP can enter vital signs, but if they observe changes in patient status, the RN must investigate and chart his or her assessment.
- Describe the importance of the task to the organization, the delegator, the patient, and the delegate.
- Clearly describe the expected outcome and the timeline for completion. Here, the nurse must also establish how closely the assignment will be supervised.
- Identify any constraints on completing the task or any conditions that could change. For example, the nurse may ask an assistant to feed a patient as long as the patient is not having difficulty swallowing; should the patient begin to demonstrate dysphagia, then the nurse will take over feeding activities.
- Have the delegate repeat back the task and specific directions. The nurse should further validate the delegate's understanding of the task and its expectations by eliciting questions and providing feedback.

policies and procedures and current standards of practice. Surveillance also validates that the delegate is working within his scope of practice. The amount of supervision required depends on the nature of the task, the delegate's experience, and the patient's needs. It is critical that the delegating nurse try to find a balance between too much and too little surveillance. The delegator should remain accessible because her support will build the delegate's confidence, reassure the delegate of her interest, and negate any concerns that she is dumping undesirable tasks; however, monitoring a delegate too closely may convey distrust.

In some instances, surveillance may reveal that the delegate needs closer supervision or assistance with the delegated task. For example, the delegator may notice subtle changes in the patient's signs and symptoms or observe that the delegate is having difficulty completing a particular activity. When situations such as these occur, the delegating nurse should intervene as appropriate, whether this involves providing the delegate with further guidance in task performance or opting to reassume responsibility and personally complete the task (NCSBN, 2016).

Evaluation and Feedback

Although often overlooked, evaluation and feedback are critical final elements of the delegation process. When engaging in evaluation, the delegator must compare the

Focus on Diversity and Culture
Transcultural Delegation

Just like patients, the members of a healthcare team often come from a variety of cultural backgrounds. Therefore, the nurse must take cultural phenomena into account when delegating to other nurses and UAP. These phenomena fall into six broad categories:

- **Communication:** Different cultures interpret certain elements of verbal and nonverbal communication in different ways. These include such things as eye contact, posture, volume, gesticulation, touch, and passive versus assertive wording.

- **Space:** Staff members' cultural backgrounds often influence their preferred zone of interpersonal space. For example, people from some cultures prefer to communicate at close distance, whereas people from other cultures view physical closeness as uncomfortable, rude, or intrusive.

- **Social organization:** Cultures vary in the level of importance they place on close social relationships. Thus, depending on cultural background, some staff members may desire higher levels of social support while carrying out delegated tasks.

- **Time:** A culture may be past, present, or future oriented. Staff members' orientation toward time can affect their attitudes toward such things as scheduling and short- versus long-range goals.

- **Environmental control:** Staff from cultures with an internal locus of control tend to focus on planning and acting proactively, whereas staff from cultures with an external locus of control are more likely to focus on overcoming obstacles and dealing with events as they arise.

- **Biological variations:** A person's background may influence certain physical characteristics (e.g., size, disease susceptibility), as well as his or her attitude toward particular biological conditions and variations.

Cultural variations should be considered when developing the plan for how a task will be explained, completed, reported, and evaluated. Consideration of such factors will help facilitate the best possible outcomes for patients, staff, and the healthcare organization as a whole.

Sources: Based on Kelly, P., & Tazbir, J. (2014). *Essentials of nursing leadership and management* (3rd ed.). Clifton Park, NY: Delmar-Cengage Learning; Poole, V. L., Davidhizar, R. E., & Giger, J. N. (1995). Delegating to a transcultural team. *Nursing Management 26*(8), 33–34; Yoost, B. L., & Crawford, L. R. (2016). *Fundamentals of nursing: Active learning for collaborative practice.* St. Louis, MO: Elsevier.

delegate's performance against appropriate policies, procedures, and standards of practice. The delegator must also determine whether the delegate's actions contributed to achievement of the agreed-upon objectives. Specific questions that can help the nurse evaluate the effectiveness of delegation include the following:

- Was the delegated task performed appropriately and successfully?

- Was the desired outcome achieved in a satisfactory manner?

- Was communication between the delegator and delegate both timely and effective?

- Which aspects of the task and/or the delegation process went well? Which aspects did not proceed so smoothly?

- Did any problems arise? If so, how were they addressed?

- Could the patient's need(s) be met in a more effective way?

- Should any adjustments be made to the patient's overall plan of care in light of the delegated task or activity?

If problem areas are identified, the nurse should promptly and quietly investigate the problem and explain any concerns to the delegate. An opportunity for feedback from the delegate must be given. The nurse should then instruct the delegate on how to prevent similar problems in the future. Note, however, that giving praise and recognition for a job well done is equally important (NCSBN, 2016).

The following Clinical Example explores how a school nurse would use this overall process when delegating the task of medication administration.

Clinical Example B

Lisa Ford is a school nurse for a suburban school district. She has responsibility for three school buildings, including a middle school, a high school, and a magnet school that offers a Spanish-English immersion program for elementary students as well as four classrooms of 4- and 5-year-old children with various special needs. Lisa's management responsibilities include providing health services for 1500 students, 80 faculty members, and 25 staff members, as well as supervising two unlicensed school health aides and three special education health aides. The logistics of managing multiple school sites means that Lisa must delegate many daily tasks, including medication administration, to the school-based health aides.

Nancy Andrews is an unlicensed health aide at the middle school. This is her first year as a health aide, and she has a limited background in healthcare. The nurse practice act in this state allows for delegation of medication administration in the school setting. Lisa is responsible for training Nancy to safely administer medication to students, documenting the training, evaluating Nancy's performance, and providing ongoing supervision. Part of Nancy's training will include a discussion of those medication-related decisions that must be made by a registered nurse.

To delegate medication administration to Nancy, Lisa must do all of the following:

- Understand the state nurse practice act and its applicability to the school setting.

- Implement school district policies related to health services and medication administration.

- Develop and implement an appropriate training program.

- Limit opportunities for error and decrease liability by ensuring that unlicensed health aides are appropriately trained to handle delegated tasks.

- Maintain documentation related to training and observation of medication administration by unlicensed staff.

- Audit medication administration records to ensure accuracy and completeness.

- Conduct several "drop-in" visits during the school year in order to track the competency of health aides.

- If necessary, report any medication errors to administration, and follow up with focused training and closer supervision.

- Provide constructive feedback and address any concerns.
- Acknowledge the effectiveness of the unlicensed health aide's efforts.

Critical Thinking Questions

1. If you were a school nurse, what would you include in your training of unlicensed health aides for medication administration?
2. Other than medication administration, what duties typically needed at a school could be delegated to the unlicensed personnel? What duties could not be delegated?
3. How would you respond if a task that you delegated to an unlicensed health aide was completed incorrectly and resulted in harm to a child?

Factors Affecting Delegation

A number of factors may affect delegation, including organizational culture, assignment patterns, and the personal qualities of the participants. Resource availability, such as having sufficient staff to whom the nurse may delegate tasks, also impacts delegation.

Assignment Patterns

Three assignment patterns affect delegation: unit-based assignment, pairing, and partnering. The unit-based approach assigns assistive personnel such as UAP to serve everyone on the unit by working from a task list. Limited planning between the RNs and support staff is a feature of unit-based assignment patterns; consequently, there is no sense of teamwork. With this type of assignment, RNs frequently ask for assistance as needed. Their requests are made in a vacuum; that is, none of the nurses are aware of the demands being placed on the UAP by others, thus placing the UAP in the position of managing conflicting requests. Not surprisingly, this approach does not lend itself to effective delegation and causes dissatisfaction among both RNs and support staff.

A more effective means of delegation is pairing, or the assignment of an RN, LPN, and/or UAP to work together as a team for a shift. Pairs are not scheduled to work together consistently; therefore, the team's composition varies from day to day. Pairs are able to plan care; team members identify priorities and plan each patient's individual outcomes for the shift. Pairing increases satisfaction among team members and facilitates delegation.

Partnering is the best assignment pattern. It is the consistent scheduling of a set team, such as an RN, LPN, and/or nursing assistant, who always work together. This consistency creates healthy interpersonal relationships and increases trust. Each partner is able to anticipate the others' needs and expectations. Partnering is the ideal approach to delegation and increases employee satisfaction and, in turn, patient satisfaction (Potter et al., 2017; Weydt, 2010).

Delegate Understanding, Acceptance, and Communication

Delegates are responsible for making sure they fully understand a task before accepting it. Before accepting the task, the delegate must evaluate whether she has the skills and abilities to complete it. If the delegate does not possess the necessary skills and abilities, she must inform the delegator. The delegate must also discuss with the delegator whether or not there is sufficient time to complete the task.

If the delegate does not have the necessary skills or abilities but the delegator is willing to train the delegate to complete the task, the delegate may accept the task provided there is time for sufficient training and questions before the task must be completed.

By accepting delegation, the delegate accepts full responsibility for the outcome of the task. Note that the delegate has the option to negotiate to perform only those parts of the task for which the delegate has been trained.

Once the delegate and delegator have agreed on the nature of the assignment and their roles and responsibilities, they should clarify the time frame and other expectations of the task as well as how the delegate is to report the outcome of the task and what kind of assistance and feedback the delegate can expect from the delegator. The delegate should keep the delegator informed of progress and report any concerns or unexpected events. Finally, the delegate should complete the assignment as agreed and report the task as completed in a timely manner. This fosters trust between delegator and delegate and builds the delegate's reputation for dependability and credibility.

Obstacles to Delegation

Delegation can yield many benefits, but it also has barriers that can potentially endanger patients and/or lead to unsuccessful outcomes. For example, when a patient does not receive ambulation because nursing staff fails to follow through on this important activity, the patient may be at increased risk for falls, pneumonia, and development of deep vein thromboses and pressure ulcers.

Some barriers to delegation are environmental, whereas others are the result of the delegator's or delegate's beliefs or inexperience, as described in the sections that follow.

A Nonsupportive Environment

Some environments simply do not support delegation. For example, the culture of an organization may, through rigid chains of command and autocratic leadership styles, restrict delegation. In this type of organizational culture, the norm is to do all work oneself because other staff members are not viewed as capable or skilled. These types of environments promote an atmosphere of distrust, as well as poor tolerance for mistakes.

A lack of resources can also inhibit delegation. For example, there may not be adequate staff to whom a nurse can delegate certain responsibilities. Consider the example of a sole RN in a skilled nursing facility. If the state's nurse practice act defines a particular task as one that only an RN can perform, then there is no one within the facility to whom the nurse can delegate that task.

Financial constraints also can interfere with delegation. For instance, if one member of a department must attend the annual conference in a nursing specialty area but the organization will pay only the manager's travel and conference expenses, then the manager cannot delegate the task of attending the conference to anyone else.

Educational resources may be another limiting factor. Others can learn how to do a task, but only if the proper equipment and a trainer are available.

Time resources can limit the ability to delegate as well. For example, suppose it is Friday, the schedule needs to be posted on Monday, and the nurse manager in charge of scheduling must leave town because of an unexpected family emergency. If no one on staff has been trained to develop the schedule, the schedule will not be posted or will be developed by someone who has not been trained to create it, thus leaving the unit open to the many problems that can result from poor scheduling.

Delegator Insecurity

Delegators often feel insecure about delegation, because they remain accountable for the tasks involved. Some delegators see delegates as competition. In reality, the success of a delegate reflects well on the delegate and on the delegator. Some delegators fear being blamed or being liable if a delegate makes a mistake. By following the delegation process and adhering to the Five Rights of Delegation, the delegator minimizes the risks of liability and the responsibility for any mistakes shifts to the delegate.

Beyond these fears, additional barriers to delegation on the part of the delegator include inadequate organizational skills, such as poor time management, and inexperience with delegation.

An Unwilling Delegate

Inexperience and fear of failure can motivate a potential delegate to refuse a delegated task. Delegates who lack confidence or experience need a great deal of reassurance and support. Furthermore, the delegator needs to equip this type of delegate to be able to handle the task. If the delegator follows the delegation process and the five rights of delegation, then the delegate should not fail.

The delegator can help boost the delegate's confidence by building on simple tasks. The delegate also needs to be reminded that everyone was inexperienced at one time. Another common concern for many delegates is how mistakes will be handled. Thus, when describing a task, the delegator should provide clear guidelines for handling problems—guidelines that adhere to organizational policies. The delegator also needs to ensure availability for any delegate needs.

Other delegate-related barriers to successful delegation include individuals who avoid responsibility or are too dependent on others. Success breeds success; therefore, it is important to engage the delegate in a simple task that guarantees success and to recognize the delegate's accomplishment when the task is finished.

Ineffective Delegation

When the delegation process is not followed or barriers remain unresolved, delegation is often ineffective. Ineffective delegation can also result from unnecessary duplication, underdelegation, reverse delegation, and overdelegation.

Unnecessary Duplication

If staff are duplicating the work of others, related tasks may have been given to too many people. To avoid unnecessary duplication, associated tasks should be delegated to as few people as possible. This allows each delegate to complete her assignment without spending time negotiating with others about which task should be done by which person. This also simplifies reporting for both the delegate and the delegator. If multiple people are involved in the delegation, then a team meeting should be held to develop a plan of who will be performing which tasks. This will both enhance teamwork and minimize duplication.

To further prevent duplication of work, the nurse should consider the following questions:

- How often do staff members duplicate an activity that someone else has recently performed?
- Why does this duplication occur, and is it necessary?
- What needs to be done to prevent this duplication?

Underdelegation

Underdelegation is a situation in which efforts at delegation fail because of one or more of the following factors:

- The delegator fails to transfer full authority to the delegate.
- The delegator takes back responsibility for certain aspects of a delegated task.
- The delegator fails to appropriately equip and direct the delegate.

As a result, the delegate is unable to complete the task, and the delegator must resume responsibility for its completion. The following Clinical Example describes a scenario in which underdelegation has occurred.

Clinical Example C

After completing Nancy's training (see the prior Clinical Example), Lisa gives Nancy the authority to begin administering medications to the students in her school. During the first week of classes, Nancy tries to "speed up" the medication administration process by setting out all of the noon medications in individual, unlabeled cups for the students. The cups are rearranged by students trying to find their medications, and Nancy cannot identify which meds belong to which students. Lisa is called back to the school to administer the correct medications, students are late to class, and Nancy is frustrated that she couldn't handle the task.

Critical Thinking Questions

1. Which of the four steps of the delegation process did Lisa fail to follow?
2. Which step or steps did Nancy fail to follow?
3. What should Lisa do to prevent this situation from happening again?

Reverse Delegation

In **reverse delegation**, someone with a lower rank delegates a task to someone with more authority. For example, say a nurse practitioner in a burn unit arrives on the unit to find several patients whose dressing changes have not been completed due to a code situation earlier in the morning. An LPN asks the nurse practitioner to complete a few dressing changes to help the staff before physician rounds begin. If the nurse practitioner agrees to the LPN's request, then reverse delegation has taken place.

Overdelegation

Overdelegation occurs when the delegator loses control of a situation by providing the delegate with too much authority or too much responsibility. This places the delegator in a risky position, increasing the potential for liability.

Liability and Delegation

Fear of liability often keeps nurses from delegating. State nurse practice acts determine the legal parameters for practice, professional associations set practice standards, and organizational policy and job descriptions define delegation appropriate to the specific work setting. Adherence to these rules should protect nurses from liability, but several additional guidelines can provide extra peace of mind when delegating. Perhaps the most useful guidelines for nurses to remember are the Five Rights of Delegation, as identified by the ANA and NCSBN in 2005 and described earlier in this exemplar. In addition, the ANA and NCSBN (2006) have issued a joint statement on delegation to explain both the profession's practice guidelines and the legal requirements for delegation. **Figure 39–4 》** shows a decision tree for delegation from the joint statement.

One situation that may present a challenge is when staff members receive written or verbal orders from a physician's office nurse. The same legal guidelines for the nurse giving the orders apply to the staff receiving them. If the nurse calling from the physician's office has a license that allows prescribing privileges, such as a nurse practitioner license, then the staff can accept appropriate orders from the physician's nurse. Otherwise, the orders must also be verified by the prescribing physician. The staff members put their own licenses in jeopardy if they do not obtain verification from the physician when necessary.

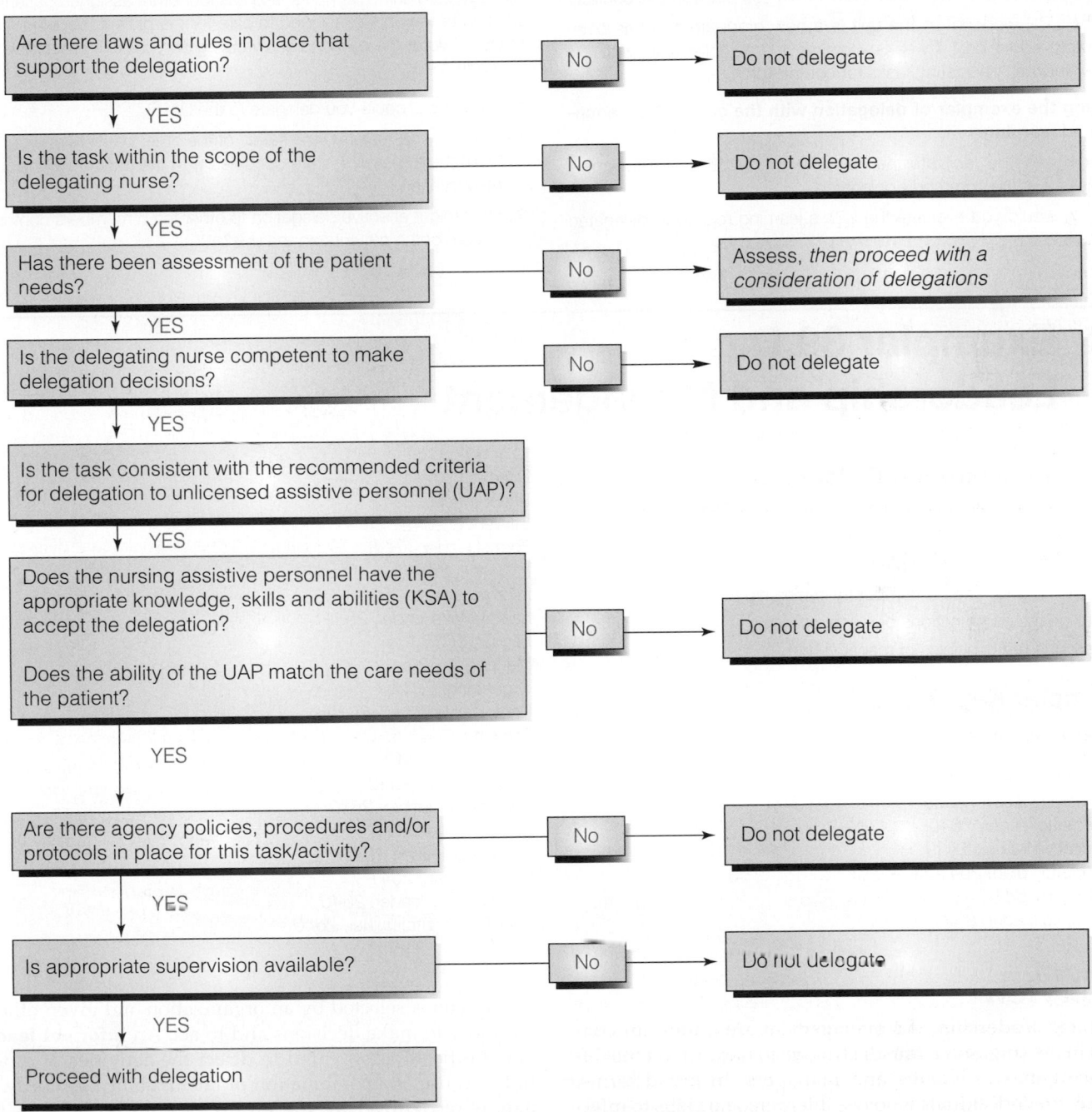

Source: Adapted from "Appendix B NCSBN, Decision Tree For Delegation To Nursing Assistive Personnel" from Joint Statement on Delegation by the American Nurses Association (ANA) and the National Council of State Boards of Nursing (NCSBN). Used by permission of the National Council of State Boards of Nursing (NCSBN).

Figure 39–4 》 Decision tree for delegation to unlicensed assistive personnel.

REVIEW Delegation

RELATE Link the Concepts and Exemplars

You are an RN working on a medical unit with two other RNs, an LPN, and two UAP. You receive a call informing you that two patients (both of whom are assigned to your care) must be transferred to another unit in order to make room for two patients who are to be admitted as soon as the rooms are ready.

Linking the exemplar of delegation with the concept of collaboration:

1. You delegate collection of one patient's possessions in preparation for transfer to one of the UAP, who says, "Why are you dumping this work on me? You do it." How would you manage this conflict?

2. The LPN working on the unit is a new graduate and has been employed for only 4 weeks. How would you collaborate with this nurse when delegating tasks for completion?

Linking the exemplar of delegation with the concept of teaching and learning:

3. How can you facilitate the new LPN's education in performing tasks that are commonly delegated?

4. How would you evaluate the LPN's learning related to delegated tasks?

REFER Go to Pearson MyLab Nursing and eText

- Additional review materials

REFLECT Apply Your Knowledge

You are working the night shift on a medical unit and have been assigned charge nurse responsibilities. You are working with four RNs, one LPN, and two UAP. A patient becomes pulseless and is not breathing, and the nurse assigned to the patient's care calls a code. The nurse is occupied at this patient's bedside for 1.5 hours until the resuscitation effort is completed and the patient is transferred to the intensive care unit. This nurse also has four other assigned patients. In addition to the nurse assigned to care for the patient requiring resuscitation, two of the other nurses working on your unit are assisting in the code.

1. What tasks could you delegate to the UAP?

2. How will you maintain the safety of the other patients on your unit while the three nurses are occupied with the patient who requires resuscitation?

3. How might effective delegation to other team members contribute to care of the patients on the unit?

≫ Exemplar 39.D
Leadership and Management

Exemplar Learning Outcomes

39.D Analyze leadership and management as they relate to managing care.

- Differentiate managers from leaders.
- Outline classic and contemporary leadership theories.
- Outline the four functions of management.
- Describe the principles of management.

Exemplar Key Terms

Accountability, 2642
Authoritarian leader, 2639
Autocratic leader, 2639
Bureaucratic leader, 2639
Charismatic leader, 2640
Consultative leader, 2639
Contingency plan, 2641
Controlling, 2641
Democratic leader, 2639

Directing, 2641
Effectiveness, 2642
Efficiency, 2642
Formal leader, 2638
Influence, 2640
Informal leader, 2638
Laissez-faire leader, 2639
Leader, 2638
Manager, 2639
Organizing, 2641
Participative leader, 2639
Planning, 2641
Productivity, 2642
Responsibility, 2642
Servant leadership, 2640
Shared leadership, 2640
Situational leader, 2640
Strategic plan, 2641
Transactional leader, 2640
Transformational leader, 2640

Overview

Although leadership and management are important concepts in nursing, some nurses struggle to understand the difference between leaders and managers. In broad terms, **leaders** are individuals who use interpersonal skills to influence others to accomplish specific goals. Leaders tend to be productive and persuasive and exhibit initiative and confidence, and they play a significant role in organizational success. Leadership may be formal or informal. A **formal leader** is one who is selected by an organization and given official authority to make decisions and to act. An **informal leader** is not officially appointed to direct the activities of others but, because of a combination of talent, ability, seniority, or age, is recognized by the group as a leader. Within the healthcare environment, formal and informal nurse leaders alike often participate in and guide teams that assess effectiveness of care, implement evidence-based practice, and construct process improvement strategies.

In contrast to leadership, management is always formal. **Managers** are individuals who hold an official position within an organization and are essential to the organization's success. Managers go by a variety of titles, including (but not limited to) *manager, director, supervisor,* and *administrator*. Nurse managers may manage units, departments, or entire facilities. On any given day, they must balance the needs of patients, professional staff, nonprofessional staff, contractors, the organization, and themselves. In order to meet the needs of these groups, nurse managers require a body of knowledge and skills distinct from those used in general nursing practice. Unfortunately, a gap often exists between what managers know and what managers need to know. New managers tend to apply skills learned through experiences with former supervisors rather than through formal management training. Increasing the number of nurses who hold BSN and MSN degrees could help close this gap.

All nurses manage and lead—at least in a practical sense. Whether through example, delegation, or the authority of their position, they formally and informally direct the work of professional and nonprofessional staff in order to achieve desired outcomes in patient care. As a result, all nurses should seek to build their leadership and management skills, no matter their current position or career aspirations.

Leadership Theories

Because leadership is a learned process, being an effective leader requires an understanding of the needs, goals, and rewards that motivate people. It also requires knowledge of leadership skills and of the group's activities as well as possession of the interpersonal skills necessary to influence others.

When learning leadership skills, it is helpful to be familiar with leadership theories. These theories describe the traits, behaviors, motivations, and choices leaders use to influence others. Classic leadership theories focus on what leaders are (trait theories), what leaders do (behavioral theories), and how leaders adapt their style according to the situation (contingency theories). Contemporary theories look at the emotions and relationships involved in leadership, as well as the importance of empowerment and shared responsibility. In practice, good leaders combine components of classical and contemporary theories into their daily interactions with others, and no single theory or type of theory adequately describes all of the components of leadership.

Classic Leadership Theories

Most classic leadership theories are classified as trait based or behavior based. Trait theories of leadership hold that successful leaders possess specific traits and abilities, including good judgment, decisiveness, knowledge, adaptability, integrity, tact, self-confidence, and cooperativeness. These theories have traditionally posited that leader traits and abilities are something an individual is born with, not something that is learned or acquired. In contrast, behavioral theorists believe that through education, training, and life experiences, leaders develop a particular leadership style. According to this point of view, an individual's leadership style can be described as autocratic, democratic, laissez-faire, or bureaucratic.

An **autocratic leader**, also called an **authoritarian leader**, makes decisions for the group based on the belief that individuals are externally motivated (in other words, they desire rewards from others) and are incapable of independent decision making. Similar to a dictator, the autocratic leader determines policies and gives orders and directions to the group. Under this leadership style, the group may feel secure because procedures are well defined and activities are predictable. Productivity may also be high. Under the autocratic leader, however, the group's needs for creativity, autonomy, and self-motivation are not met, and there is little or no openness and trust between the leader and group members. Although group members are often dissatisfied with this leadership style, there are times when an autocratic style is the most effective. For instance, when urgent decisions must be made (e.g., in the case of a cardiac arrest, unit fire, or terrorist attack), one individual must assume responsibility without being challenged by other team members. Similarly, when group members are unable or do not wish to participate in making a decision, the authoritarian style solves the problem and enables the group to move on. This style can also be effective when a project must be completed quickly and efficiently.

Unlike an autocratic leader, a **democratic leader** (also called a **participative** or **consultative leader**) encourages group discussion and decision making. This type of leader acts as a catalyst or facilitator, actively guiding the group toward its goals. Group productivity and satisfaction are high as group members contribute to the work effort. The democratic leader assumes that individuals are internally motivated (in other words, they desire personal satisfaction), are capable of making decisions, and value independence. Democratic leaders typically provide constructive feedback, offer information, make suggestions, and ask questions to gain information or help group members grow. This leadership style demands that the leader have faith in the group's ability to accomplish its goals. Although democratic leadership has been shown to be less efficient and more cumbersome than authoritarian leadership, it allows self-motivation and creativity among group members. It also calls for a great deal of cooperation and coordination. This leadership style can be extremely effective in the healthcare setting.

The **laissez-faire leader** recognizes the group's need for autonomy and self-regulation. This leader takes a hands-off approach, being less directive and more permissive than other types of leaders. The laissez-faire leader assumes that the group is internally motivated. However, under a laissez-faire leader, group members may work at cross purposes because of a lack of cooperation and coordination. A laissez-faire style is most effective for groups whose members have both personal and professional maturity, so that once the group has made a decision, the members are committed to it and have the required expertise to implement it. Individual group members then perform tasks in their area of expertise while the leader acts as a resource person.

Finally, the **bureaucratic leader** relies on the organization's rules, policies, and procedures to direct the group's work efforts. Group members are usually dissatisfied with a bureaucratic leader's inflexibility and impersonal relations with them.

In addition to trait and behavioral theories, contingency theories account for a third category of classic leadership theories. These theories propose yet another type of leader: the **situational leader**, who adapts his or her leadership style to the situation. According to contingency theorists, a situational leader is flexible in task and relationship behaviors, considers staff members' abilities, knows the nature of the task to be done, and is sensitive to the context or environment in which the task takes place. A task-oriented situational leader focuses on activities that encourage group productivity and getting necessary work done. A relationship-oriented situational leader focuses on interpersonal relationships and meeting group members' needs. Regardless of orientation, situational leaders adapt their leadership style to the readiness and willingness of the individual or group to perform the assigned task.

Contemporary Leadership Theories

Contemporary leadership theories break leaders into three groups: charismatic leaders, transactional leaders, and transformational leaders. They also consider the ideas of shared leadership, shared governance, and servant leadership.

A **charismatic leader** is rare and is characterized by the ability to cultivate an emotional relationship with group members. The charming personality of the leader evokes strong feelings of commitment in the group, and these feelings extend to both the leader and the leader's cause and beliefs. The followers of a charismatic leader often overcome extreme hardship to achieve the group's goals because of their faith in the leader.

The **transactional leader** has a relationship with group members based on an exchange for some resource valued by the members. These incentives are used to promote loyalty and performance. For example, in order to ensure adequate staffing on the night shift, a nurse manager might entice a staff nurse to work the night shift in exchange for a weekend shift off. The transactional leader focuses on the day-to-day tasks of achieving organizational goals and understanding and meeting the needs of the group.

In contrast, a **transformational leader** fosters creativity, risk taking, commitment, and collaboration by empowering the group to share in the organization's vision. The leader inspires others with a clear, attractive, and attainable goal and enlists them in reaching it. Through shared values, honesty, trust, and continual learning, the transformational leader empowers the group. This empowerment facilitates independence, individual growth, and change. Given these characteristics, it is not surprising that the Institute of Medicine (IOM) recommends use of a transformational model of nursing leadership. According to the IOM (2010), this model empowers nurses to lead efforts for change in a complex healthcare environment. For more information on the traits required by transformational nursing leaders, see **Box 39–5 》**.

Shared leadership is centered around the idea that a professional workforce is made up of many leaders. No one individual is believed to have knowledge or ability beyond that of other members of the work group. Appropriate leadership is thought to emerge in relation to the challenges that confront the work group. Examples of shared leadership in nursing include self-directed work teams, co-leadership, and shared governance. As described in the concept of

---

Box 39–5
Transformational Leadership in Nursing

Transformational leadership in nursing requires effective leaders who are compassionate and dedicated to their team, their patients, and the nursing profession. Research indicates that these leaders possess certain personal characteristics. Most notably, they are:

- Committed to excellence
- Trustworthy
- Accessible
- Empathetic and caring
- Committed to staff development
- Optimistic and positive
- Knowledgeable about nursing and leadership
- Aware of their own strengths and weaknesses
- Committed to lifelong learning

Evidence also reveals that effective nursing leaders possess a passion for nursing; good communication and crisis management skills; a clear vision and strategic focus for their team; a sense of responsibility to staff and patients; a strong moral compass; and high levels of common sense. Effective nursing leaders frequently call on these traits and skills as they strive to respect patients and team members, mentor staff, direct patient care, and build personal connections with their fellow employees.

Sources: Based on Anonson, J., Walker, M. E., Arries, E., Maposa, S., Telford, P., & Berry, L. (2014). Qualities of exemplary nurse leaders: Perspectives of frontline nurses. *Journal of Nursing Management, 22*(1), 127–136. doi:10.111/jonm.12092; Guyton, N. (2012). Nine principles of successful nursing leadership. *American Nurse Today, 7*(8). Retrieved from https://americannurseto-day.com/nine-principles-of-successful-nursing-leadership/; Sherman, R. (2012b). What followers want in their nurse leaders. *American Nurse Today, 7*(9). Retrieved from http://www.medscape.com/viewarticle/771912_2.

Managing Care, shared governance is a method that aims to distribute decision making among a group of people.

Finally, **servant leadership** is rooted in the belief that the most effective leaders are those who are motivated primarily by a desire to serve, rather than a desire to lead. According to this theory, by placing others' needs before their own, servant leaders inspire their followers to grow and become more self-directed. As a result of this personal growth, the followers themselves feel more empowered to act in the best interests of both the organization and the people around them. Servant leadership's emphasis on service, caring, and compassion make it an especially good fit for the healthcare environment and nursing in particular. Use of this leadership model cultivates not only stronger staff relationships, but also stronger nurse–patient relationships. Furthermore, effective servant leadership enhances the quality of care, promotes nurses' personal and professional development, increases nurses' job satisfaction, and helps empower nurses and patients alike to achieve better health outcomes (Huber, 2014; McCann, Graves, & Cox, 2014; Stanley, 2017).

No matter the theory or theories used, an effective leader must have *vision*—or a mental image of a possible and desirable future state—and must be able to transform this vision into a realistic future goal that others can understand. In doing this, leaders often rely on **influence**, or an informal strategy for gaining cooperation through persuasion and communication rather than authority. As part of influencing others, leaders act as positive role models, demonstrating caring toward coworkers and patients. Leadership may also be humanistic, or characterized by an emphasis on individuals' dignity and worth. As this suggests, being a good leader takes thought, care, insight, commitment, and energy.

Clinical Example D

Lauren Chavoen works in a hospital where senior management believes it is essential to engage nursing staff in planning, implementing, and evaluating patient care policies. Lauren realizes that she is not yet ready to assume a management position, but she understands that senior management's beliefs offer her a chance to develop some leadership and management skills through participation in policy development.

Critical Thinking Questions

1. How should Lauren convince her manager that her participation would benefit not only herself but her unit also?
2. Evaluate what skills Lauren will need to be successful on the committee she joins.

Management Functions

Management and leadership are closely tied to each other, although the functions associated with management tend to be more clearly defined than those associated with leadership. These functions were first described by French industrialist Henri Fayol in 1916 as *planning, organizing, directing,* and *controlling.* Though a century has passed, the fundamental functions identified by Fayol remain relevant for nurse managers today.

Planning

Planning is a four-stage process that involves the following:

1. Establishing objectives (goals).
2. Evaluating the present situation and predicting future trends and events.
3. Formulating a planning statement (means).
4. Converting the plan into an action statement.

Planning is important on both organizational and personal levels. It is an individual or group process that addresses the questions of what, why, where, when, how, and by whom. Decision making and problem solving are inherent in planning.

Organization-level plans, such as plans for organizational structure and staffing or operational budgets, evolve from the mission, philosophy, and goals of the organization. Within larger organizational plans, the nurse manager develops specific goals and objectives for his or her area of responsibility.

Planning is either strategic or contingent. A **strategic plan** defines the overall purpose and desired results of an organization and describes how those results will be achieved. A **contingency plan**, on the other hand, helps an organization prepare for unplanned events and determine in advance how it will respond to them. The strategic planning process uses continual assessment, planning, and evaluation to guide the future. Its purpose is creating an image of the desired future and designing ways to make that future a reality. For example, a nurse manager might be charged

with developing a plan to add a time-saving device to commonly used equipment. The manager must present the plan persuasively and develop operational strategies for implementation, such as acquiring the device and training staff in its use.

The contingency planning process requires the nurse manager to identify and manage unplanned and unexpected events that interfere with the quality of care and service delivered to patients. Contingency planning may be done *reactively*, in response to a crisis, or *proactively*, in anticipation of problems or in response to opportunities. Proactive planning is always preferable. Examples of problems that require contingency planning include the following:

- Two registered nurses call in sick for the 12-hour night shift.
- The manager of a specialty unit receives a call for an admission, but all of the unit's beds are taken.
- The manager of a pediatric oncology clinic discovers that a patient's sibling exposed several other immunocompromised patients to chickenpox.

Organizing

Organizing is the process of coordinating the work to be done. Formally, it involves identifying the work of the organization, dividing the labor, developing the chain of command, and assigning authority. Organizing is an ongoing process that systematically reviews the use of human and material resources. In healthcare, the mission, formal organizational structure, delivery systems, job descriptions, skill mix, and staffing patterns form the basis for organizing.

Directing

Directing is the process of getting the organization's work done. A manager's ability to direct is related to his or her power, authority, and leadership style. The manager's communication abilities, motivational techniques, and delegation skills are also important.

In today's healthcare organizations, professional staff members are autonomous, requiring guidance rather than direction. Thus, a manager is more likely to sell an idea, proposal, or new project to staff members than to tell them what to do. The manager coaches and counsels to achieve the organization's objectives. In fact, it may be the nurse who assumes the traditional directing role when working with unlicensed personnel.

Controlling

Controlling involves comparing actual results with projected results, similar to the evaluation step in the nursing process. Controlling includes establishing performance standards; determining how to measure performance; and creating the tools that permit consistent measurement, performance evaluation, and provision of feedback. The efficient manager constantly attempts to improve productivity by incorporating techniques of quality management, evaluating outcomes and performance, and instituting change as necessary.

Today, managers share many control functions with staff. In organizations that use a formal quality improvement process, such as continuous quality improvement (CQI), staff members participate in and lead the CQI teams. Organizations are also increasingly using peer review as a means of controlling the quality of care and service. Peer review is the evaluation of results by team members of similar skills and competence to those who produced the work. This process is educational, not judgmental or punitive. Peer review is a means for team members to hold each other accountable for the care and service they provide to patients.

Planning, organizing, directing, and controlling reflect a systematic, proactive approach to management. This approach is used widely in all types of organizations, including healthcare.

SAFETY ALERT Improving patient safety is an important function of the nurse manager. In doing so, the nurse manager must identify errors in patient care and help staff learn from those errors. When using errors as a teaching tool, it is essential that the manager do so without singling out the staff member or members who committed the error or attaching blame to those individuals.

Principles of Management

In addition to understanding managerial functions, nurse managers must have knowledge of the basic principles of management, including authority, accountability, and responsibility. As discussed in prior exemplars, *authority* is the right to direct other individuals and their activities. It is an integral component of managing. Authority is conveyed through leadership actions. It is largely determined by the situation and is always associated with responsibility and accountability. Managers must accept the authority granted to them.

Accountability is the ability and willingness to assume responsibility for one's actions and to accept the consequences of one's behavior. Accountability can be viewed as hierarchic, starting at the individual level, then the institutional or professional level, and finally the societal level. At the individual or patient level, accountability is reflected in the nurse's ethical integrity. At the institutional level, it is reflected in the statement of philosophy and objectives of the nursing department and in nursing audits. At the professional level, it is reflected in standards of practice developed by national or provincial nursing associations. At the societal level, it is reflected in legislated nurse practice acts.

Responsibility is an obligation to meet objectives and perform tasks. Managers are responsible for resources, employee performance, team building, and conflict resolution. They are also responsible for the way the team manages its time.

Managing Resources

One of managers' greatest responsibilities is their accountability for human, fiscal (financial), and material resources. Budgeting and determining variances between actual and budgeted expenses are crucial skills for managers. For more information about the allocation of resources, see the module on Healthcare Systems.

Enhancing Employee Performance

Managers help employees develop their skills by identifying appropriate learning opportunities, facilitating attendance at professional workshops and conventions, and encouraging achievement of advanced education, such as higher degrees or certifications. The nurse manager who empowers other nurses by providing information, support, resources, and opportunities will have team members who are more committed to the institution, more effective in their roles, and more confident in their abilities. These nurses are also better able to meet their own goals and to help the institution achieve its goals.

Building and Managing Teams

The manager is responsible for building and managing the work team. A manager who is familiar with the group process will be able to lead the group in a manner that promotes its development into an effective work team.

The term *group process* is used to summarize how a group works together to complete tasks. One of the elements of the group process is ensuring that all team members understand the team's purpose and their own individual roles, as well as those of other team members. Another element is helping each team member feel that his or her contributions are recognized by the manager and other team members. Yet another way that nurse managers can promote more effective group processes is through recognition and appreciation of the differences among staff members, as described in the Focus on Diversity and Culture.

Good communication within the team is also important. Effective communication promotes good personal relationships among team members and fosters a common understanding of the team's purpose, barriers faced, and opportunities for improvement. A healthcare team often consists of nurses, physicians, therapists, and unlicensed personnel who have different training and backgrounds. These individuals do not share the same vocabularies or medical knowledge, which can hamper communication. On teams such as these, it is particularly important for the nurse manager to facilitate good communication.

Evaluating the group's work is another responsibility of the manager. Effectiveness, efficiency, and productivity are three frequently used outcome measures. In healthcare, **effectiveness** entails providing services based on scientific knowledge to all patients who could benefit and refraining from providing services to those not likely to benefit (i.e., avoiding overuse and underuse). **Efficiency** is avoiding waste, in particular waste of the equipment, supplies, ideas, and energy used to provide nursing services. Finally, **productivity** is a performance measure of both the effectiveness and efficiency of nursing care. Productivity is frequently measured by the amount of nursing resources used per patient or in terms of required versus actual hours of care provided.

Managing Conflict

Nurse managers are frequently in a position to manage conflict between individuals and among groups or teams. Conflicts may arise from differing values, philosophies, or personalities. In healthcare, conflict can also arise as a result of competition for resources.

A nurse can use any of the available methods for managing conflict, each of which has its advantages and disadvantages. (See the module on Collaboration.) New nurse managers

Focus on Diversity and Culture
Embracing Staff Diversity

Today's nursing workforce is increasingly diverse, not only in terms of culture and ethnicity, but also in terms of age, experience, education, gender, religion, and many other factors. Increased diversity is beneficial, because it means America's nurses are better equipped than ever before to address the needs of a rapidly changing population. However, if not properly addressed and embraced, diversity among staff members can also serve as a potential impediment to communication, teamwork, and effective group processes.

Nurse managers play a key role in harnessing the benefits of a diverse workforce. First and foremost, they are responsible for enforcing legal and organizational requirements that prohibit workplace discrimination and harassment, as well as for ensuring that members of their staff do not engage in other forms of prejudicial behavior toward patients or one another. Perhaps more importantly, nurse managers can and should promote the celebration of diversity among their employees. Strategies for recognizing staff diversity and promoting inclusiveness include (but are not limited to) the following:

- Offering foreign language training to staff members
- Conducting educational sessions about communication preferences and/or healthcare practices among different cultures
- Using inclusive, nonbiased terminology when interacting with patients and staff
- Allowing staff members to discuss how their personal beliefs affect their feelings about different cultures
- Inviting staff members from different ethnic and religious groups to discuss how they might address specific scenarios in light of their culture
- Recognizing holidays celebrated by staff members from different backgrounds
- Selecting staff mentors and other unit leaders who place high value on cultivating a culturally diverse staff
- Not forcing employees from diverse backgrounds to conform to the behavior of the prevailing culture
- Encouraging open, honest, and respectful communication among staff

Measures such as these promote an environment of learning, cooperation, and personal growth in which all employees feel valued. This, in turn, contributes to more effective patient care.

Sources: Based on Clipper, B. (2012). *The nurse manager's guide to an intergenerational workforce.* Indianapolis, IN: Sigma Theta Tau International; Patrick, H. A., & Kumar, V. R. (2012). Managing workplace diversity: Issues and challenges. *SAGE Open* (April–June), 1–15. doi:10.1177/2158244012444615; Yoder-Wise, P. S. (2015). *Leading and managing in nursing* (6th ed.). St. Louis, MO: Elsevier Mosby.

may require training to become proficient in the use of these methods.

Managing Time

The effective nurse manager uses time effectively and assists others to do the same. Many factors inhibit good use of time, such as personal task preferences, emergencies or crises, and unrealistic demands from others. Strategies that the manager—and all nurses—can rely on in order to use time efficiently include setting goals and arranging priorities, with urgent tasks prioritized first; delegating tasks when possible; learning to ask for help when necessary; using regular schedules to avoid interruptions and limit time spent on activities; and striving to achieve balance (Froedge, 2013).

REVIEW Leadership and Management

RELATE Link the Concepts and Exemplars

Linking the exemplar of leadership and management with the concept of quality improvement:

1. What impacts might shared leadership and shared governance have on the quality improvement process?

Linking the exemplar of leadership and management with the concept of communication:

2. What is the nurse manager's role in improving communication at the time of patient hand-offs to promote patient safety?

3. Can an individual with poor communication skills act as a competent leader? Why or why not?

REFER Go to Pearson MyLab Nursing and eText

- Additional review materials

REFLECT Apply Your Knowledge

Taylor Bradakis graduated two years ago and worked in labor and delivery after graduation. He recently was transferred to the neonatal ICU. Martha Rivaldo is a staff nurse on Taylor's new unit; she has been in the ICU for 13 years and has a reputation for being an exceptionally skilled and competent nurse. She also has a reputation for being critical and unkind to new nurses on the unit. Taylor has yet to have an unpleasant encounter with Martha, but he has overheard her complaining to her friends about younger staff members and about the way the unit is managed. Several nurses confide in Taylor that they have complained about Martha to the nurse manager, but the nurse manager never does anything about her behavior. Instead, the nurse manager simply says, "How do you suggest correcting this issue?"

1. Is Martha a leader? Explain your answer.

2. Why might the nurse manager ask for staff nurses' input when they report problems with Martha?

3. If you were the ICU nurse manager and you had received several complaints about Martha's behavior, how would you respond?

4. What is Taylor's best course of action when he overhears complaints from both Martha and the other nurses on the unit?

References

American Nurses Association (ANA) & National Council of State Boards of Nursing (NCSBN). (2006). *Joint statement on delegation.* Retrieved from https://www.ncsbn.org/Joint_statement.pdf

Council of Economic Advisers. (2014). *Recent trends in health care costs.* Retrieved from https://www.whitehouse.gov/sites/default/files/docs/recent_trends_in_health_care_costs_9.24.14.pdf

Fink-Samnick, E. (2016). The evolution of end-of-life care: Ethical implications for case management. *Professional Case Management, 21*(4), 180–192.

Froedge, W. L. (2013). How to make the most of your nursing minutes. *American Nurse Today, 8*(10). Retrieved from http://www.medscape.com/viewarticle/813735_1

Gardner, B. T., Pransky, G., Shaw, W. S., Hong, Q. N., & Loisel, P. (2010). Researcher perspectives on competencies of return-to-work coordinators. *Disability & Rehabilitation, 32*(1), 72–78.

Health Foundation. (2014). *Person-centred care made simple: What everyone should know about person-centred care.* Retrieved from http://www.health.org.uk/sites/default/files/PersonCentredCareMadeSimple.pdf

Health Resources and Services Administration. (2013). *Projecting the supply and demand for primary care practitioners through 2020—In brief.* Retrieved from http://bhpr.hrsa.gov/healthworkforce/supplydemand/usworkforce/primarycare/primarycarebrief.pdf

Hoffman, B. (2013, January 18). Health care rationing is nothing new [excerpt]. *Scientific American.* Retrieved from http://www.scientificamerican.com/article.cfm?id=health-care-rationing-is

Huber, D. L. (2014). *Leadership and nursing care management* (5th ed.). St. Louis, MO: Elsevier Saunders.

Institute of Medicine (IOM). (2010). *The future of nursing: Leading change and advancing health.* Washington, DC: National Academies Press.

Kaiser Family Foundation. (2015). *Key facts about the uninsured population.* Retrieved from http://kff.org/uninsured/fact-sheet/key-facts-about-the-uninsured-population/

Kang, J., Kim, C., & Lee, S. (2016). Nurse-perceived patient adverse events depend on nursing workload.

Osong Public Health and Research Perspectives, 7(1), 56–62. doi:10.1016/j.phrp.2015.10.015.

Lasater, K. B., & McHugh, M. D. (2016). Nurse staffing and the work environment linked to readmissions among older adults following elective total hip and knee replacement. *International Journal for Quality in Health Care, 28*(2), 253–258. doi:10.1093/intqhc/mzw007.

Leonard, M., & Miller, R. (2012). *Nursing case management: Review and resource manual* (4th ed.). Silver Spring, MD: American Nurses Credentialing Center.

Martsolf, G. R., Auerbach, D., Benevent, R., Stocks, C., Jiang, H. J., Pearson, M. L., … Gibson, T. B. (2014). Examining the value of inpatient nursing staffing: An assessment of quality and patient care costs. *Medical Care, 52*(11), 982–988. doi:10.1097/MLR.0000000000000248.

McCann, J. T., Graves, D., & Cox, L. (2014). Servant leadership, employee satisfaction, and organizational performance in rural community hospitals. *International Journal of Business and Management, 9*(10), 28–38.

Meyer, S. (2012). Care management role in end-of-life discussions. *Care Management Journals, 13*(4), 180–183.

Mitchell, P. H. (2012). *Nurse staffing—A summary of current research, opinion, and policy.* Pullman, WA: William D. Ruckelshaus Center, Washington State University. Retrieved from http://www.ruckelshauscenter.wsu.edu/projects/documents/NurseStaffingfinal.pdf

National Council of State Boards of Nursing (NCSBN). (2012). *The four steps of the delegation process.* Retrieved from https://www.ncsbn.org/Communication-DelegationProces.pdf

National Council of State Boards of Nursing (NCSBN). (2016). National Guidelines for Nursing Delegation. *Journal of Nursing Regulation, 7*(1), 5–14.

Patient-Centered Primary Care Collaborative. (n.d.). *Defining the medical home: A patient-centered philosophy that drives primary care excellence.* Retrieved from https://www.pcpcc.org/about/medical-home

Potter, P. A., Perry, A. G., Stockert, P. A., & Hall, A. M. (2017). *Fundamentals of nursing* (9th ed.). St. Louis, MO: Elsevier.

Ridic, G., Gleason, S., & Ridic, O. (2012). Comparisons of health care systems in the United States, Germany and Canada. *Materia Sociomedica 24*(2), 112–120. doi:10.5455/msm.2012.24.112-120

Roche, M. A., Duffield, C., Friedman, S., Dimitrelis, S., & Rowbotham, S. (2016). Regulated and unregulated nurses in acute hospital setting: Tasks performed, delayed or not complete. *Journal of Clinical Nursing, 25*(1–2), 153–162. doi:10.111/jocn.13118.

Rutherford, M. M. (2012). Nursing is the room rate. *Nursing Economics 30*(4), 193–206.

Sebelius, K. (2013). Good news on health care spending. *HealthCare.gov.* Retrieved from http://www.healthcare.gov/blog/2013/03/health-care-spending.html

Shekelle, P. G. (2013). Nurse-patient ratios as a patient safety strategy: A systematic review. *Annals of Internal Medicine, 158*(5, Pt. 2): 404–409. doi:10.7326/0003-4819-158-5-20130305100007.

Sherman, R. (2012a). The business of caring: What every nurse should know about cutting costs. *American Nurse Today, 7*(11). Retrieved from https://americannursetoday.com/the-business-ofcaring-what-every-nurse-should-know-about-cutting-costs/

Sherman, R. (2012b). What followers want in their nurse leaders. *American Nurse Today, 7*(9). Retrieved from http://www.medscape.com/viewarticle/771912_2

Stanley, D. (2017). Leadership theories and styles. In D. Stanley (Ed.), *Clinical leadership in nursing and healthcare: Values into action* (2nd ed.). Chichester, UK: Wiley.

Summers, N. (2012). *Fundamentals of case management practice: Skills for the human services* (4th ed.). Belmont, CA: Brooks/Cole.

USA Today. (2013). Healthcare spending is transferred out of ICU—Dennis Cauchon.

Weydt, A. (2010). Developing delegation skills. *Online Journal of Issues in Nursing, 15*(2). Retrieved from http://www.nursingworld.org/MainMenu-Categories/ANAMarketplace/ANAPeriodicals/OJIN/TableofContents/Vol152010/No2May2010/DelegationSkills.html

Yoost, B. L., & Crawford, L. R. (2016). *Fundamentals of nursing: Active learning for collaborative practice.* St. Louis, MO: Elsevier.

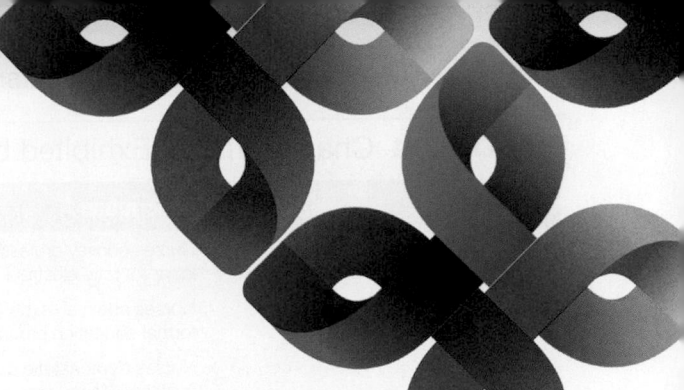

Module 40
Professionalism

Module Outline and Learning Outcomes

The Concept of Professionalism

Components of Professionalism in Nursing

40.1 Analyze the components of professionalism within the practice of nursing.

Concepts Related to Professionalism

40.2 Outline the relationship between professionalism and other concepts.

Unprofessional Behaviors

40.3 Analyze the components of unprofessional behaviors.

Professionalism Exemplars

Exemplar 40.A Commitment to Profession

40.A Analyze commitment to profession as it relates to professionalism.

Exemplar 40.B Work Ethic

40.B Analyze work ethic as it relates to professionalism.

≫ The Concept of Professionalism

Concept Key Terms

Abuse of power, **2650**	Formation, **2647**
Compassion, **2648**	Integrity, **2648**

Nurses hold the public's trust. In Gallup's annual survey of professions released on December 6, 2015, 80% of Americans called nurses' honesty and ethical standards either high or very high (Gallup, 2015). Nurses have topped Gallup's honesty and ethics ranking survey every year but one since being added to the list in 1999 (the exception being 2001, when the list included firefighters), and nursing continues to be the most well respected of 11 professions (Riffkin, 2014). At a time when the field of healthcare is in turmoil, this is a remarkable accomplishment.

Nurses are visible and present across the continuum of healthcare services, advocating for and caring for patients through the many facets of health promotion, education, maintenance, and restoration. Nurses may be found in diverse healthcare settings, including acute hospital settings, clinics, public health departments, private practice, hospice centers, birthing centers, schools, pharmacies, and doctors' offices. Nursing care extends beyond the confines of institutions and facilities. It is given in parish ministries, on military bases and in mobile field hospitals, at children's camps, at community health fairs, at motor vehicle crashes by emergency flight nurses, at places of employment in corporate health clinics, and in patients' homes. Nurse educators and researchers practice in colleges and universities and in clinical settings, and there are school nurses in schools

and colleges. Nurses are accessible 24 hours a day in the acute setting and may also be available via telehealth lines. Given that they interact so often with the community in health and wellness, in sickness, at work, at school, or at recreation sites, is it any wonder that nurses have secured trust in the community?

The first step in fostering trust is to be present and engaged in a professional manner. How then does the nursing profession, with such a large and varied practice arena, define professional behaviors for nurses?

Components of Professionalism in Nursing

Upon receiving their licenses, members of the nursing profession commit to a fundamental social contract that sets rules to guide the professional conduct of licensed registered nurses (American Nurses Association [ANA], 2016). Nurses, however, do not become professionals just by receiving a license. According to Dinmohammadi, Peyrovi, and Mehrdad (2013), nurses learn the complexities of professionalism over the course of years of engagement with comprehensive educational programs, competent role models, and field experiences. As nurses pass through the stages of "learning, interaction, development, and adaptation," they gradually

TABLE 40–1 Characteristics Exhibited by Professional Nurses

Characteristic	Description
Professional Behaviors	Nurses convey professionalism by adhering to dress codes, maintaining calm demeanors, refraining from inappropriate electronic media use, and demonstrating a strong work ethic.
Teaching and Learning	Nurses attain an expert level of nursing practice by actively engaging with both on-the-job learning opportunities and formal education programs.
Competence	Nurses demonstrate competence through rigorous application of universally accepted standards of care and evidence-based practice.
Collaboration	By working respectfully and communicating fluently with other members of the healthcare team, nurses display professional collaboration skills.
Advocacy	Nurses are accountable for advocating for patient safety and needs at all times and in all settings. Nurses act to reduce risk and improve patient outcomes.
Caring Interventions	By exemplifying a positive attitude and demonstrating compassion and cultural awareness for patients' needs, nurses provide a crucial aspect of patient care.
Ethics	By adhering to accepted nursing standards and considering the ethical implications of their actions, nurses protect patients and the healthcare team and demonstrate integrity.

learn to respond to novel situations with independent and creative applications of their nursing training. A brief overview of the characteristics of professionalism in nursing is presented in **Table 40–1 》**.

As the nursing profession expands to include the dynamic roles of case managers, nurse educators, and clinical nurse specialists, it is essential for nurses to educate the public to keep the image of nursing professionalism current (Hoeve, Jansen, & Roodbol, 2014). As the public and the healthcare team arrive at a coherent understanding of nursing as a healthcare profession in its own right, nurses gain incentive to perform to the best of their professional ability.

Professional Behaviors

One key component of professionalism is the nurse's commitment to behaving professionally by looking and acting like a professional, acting autonomously, and demonstrating a commitment to nursing. As a member of the profession of nursing, the individual nurse is always being observed and judged as a representative of that profession, even when off duty. How a nurse dresses, behaves, and communicates sets the stage for the development of trust or mistrust. Most healthcare employers provide employees with guidance and expectations for proper attire and conduct. Although most facilities have specific policies, those of one healthcare facility might not be relevant in another facility, and best practices are constantly being revised in light of new findings on patient safety, public perception, and shifting cultural attitudes. However, there are commonly accepted guidelines about dress, professional demeanor, and electronic media use (see **Table 40–2 》**).

Appearance also affects how others within the medical community see the nurse (**Figure 40–1 》**). Appearance is a form of nonverbal communication that evokes a response from others. Imagine a nurse talking on a cell phone while approaching a physician or other healthcare provider to question the validity of an order. Will the colleague have enough confidence in the nurse to accept the expressed concern and change the decision regarding the patient's plan of care?

Behavioral factors also play a large role in the nurse's self-identification and public presentation as a professional. In the past, nurses have been seen as accessories to doctors, but as nursing knowledge and practices have developed, nurses increasingly act autonomously in delivering care and prescribing nursing treatments (Hunt, 2015). As nursing continues to be increasingly recognized as an independent profession, patients and other members of the healthcare team alike will prize nurses' commitment to their profession and autonomy in performing their work.

An essential quality in acting with professionalism is demonstrating a strong work ethic. Nurses who go above and beyond to provide exemplary care, resolve conflicts, and collaborate respectfully with patients and the healthcare team will inevitably be seen as professionals.

Teaching and Learning

For generations, the on-the-job work of becoming a nurse has been considered a process of socialization. The old model of socialization carries with it a long history of

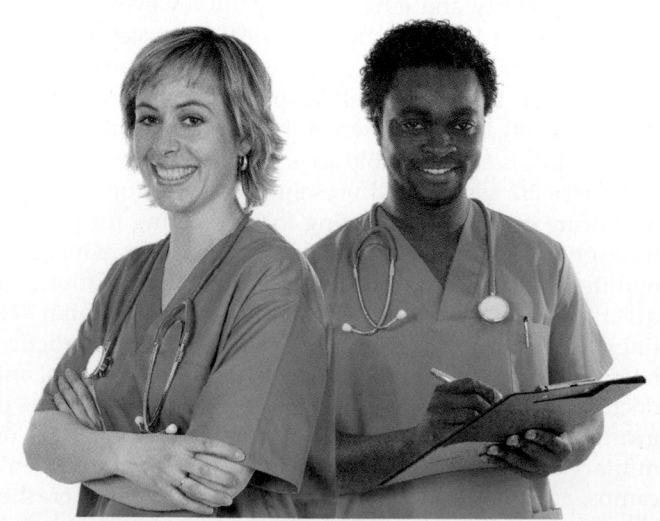

Source: Gelpi/Shutterstock.

Figure 40–1 》 A professional appearance supports the nurse's credibility.

TABLE 40–2 Common Guidelines for Professional Attire, Demeanor, and Electronic Media Use

Guidelines	Rationale
Professional Dress	
No excessive jewelry, long fingernails or artificial nails, or chewing gum	Avoidance of items that may harbor pathogens and threaten patient safety
Hair secured away from contact with the individual receiving care	Prevents contamination of sterile fields and spread of bacteria
Personal cleanliness, avoiding strong odors and perfumes	Prevents patient discomfort and annoyance
	Instills patient confidence and trust
	Shows respect for needs of allergic or nauseated patients
Clean uniform or clothing	Promotes good sanitation
	Builds patient trust
No visible body modifications or unusual ear piercings	Prevents patient discomfort
No tattoos visible on parts of the body not covered by scrubs	Shows respect for patients who find tattoos offensive
Professional Demeanor	
Avoid loud talking	Respect patients' need for rest
Maintain a positive attitude and instill hope	Encourages and shows respect for patients and families
Maintain a clean, uncluttered workstation	Shows respect for peers
Avoid taking personal calls at work	Keeps focus on patient care
Do not discuss personal problems with patients	Maintains professional boundaries
Never breach patient confidentiality	Avoids violation of HIPAA
Avoid gossiping with and bullying coworkers	Maintains and promotes civility and patient safety
Do not complain to patients or family members	Maintains professional boundaries
Do not use illegal substances	Shows respect for self and patient safety
Electronic Media Use	
Do not use personal cell phones to document patients	Prevents the sharing of photos, videos, and sound recordings that may violate HIPAA
Do not share patient information over social media	Avoids the violation of HIPAA
	Ensures that patient information cannot be shared or retrieved from servers later, even after the nurse removes the offending content from social media

subservient, dependent female roles, the acceptance of dominant behaviors for males, and a hierarchical structure in healthcare organizations. As an alternative to the socialization model of becoming a nurse, Benner et al. (2010) have formulated the concept of **formation**, a process that facilitates the transformation of an individual from a layperson to a professional nurse. Formation is an evolutionary process that requires the acquisition of lifelong learning, experience, technical expertise, and interdependent professional collaboration. The resulting integration of the nurse's thoughts, feelings, behavior, education, experience, and ethical behavior contributes to the formation of a professional nurse through the progressive stages of novice, advanced beginner, competent, proficient, and finally expert. Transformation can occur only with personal commitment to self, individuals, the community, organizations, society, and the profession. More information on the formation model can be found in the module on Accountability.

Continuously gaining knowledge is central to providing high-quality care and maintaining patient safety. Nursing students are required to learn the information the entry-level practicing nurse needs, but learning does not stop at graduation. Once licensed, nurses are expected to maintain and update their knowledge base throughout their career by engaging in continuing education programs and maintaining their licensure. Healthcare is changing constantly as new drugs enter the market, new treatments and technology are introduced, and ongoing research confirms or calls into question the effectiveness of past information. If nurses do not participate in continuing education, their knowledge base quickly becomes obsolete, and their practice may even endanger patients. Each state's board of nursing outlines requirements for nurses to participate in classes designed to help maintain and improve their knowledge (ANA, 2010). Many nurses also choose to pursue advanced degrees in nursing and other healthcare fields. See the module on Teaching and Learning for more information on the nurse as a student.

Accountability

A key component in nursing professionalism is accountability to expected standards of care. Organizations such as The Joint Commission, the ANA, and the National League for Nursing (NLN) define standards of care against which nurses' performance is measured (Davis, 2014). A nurse's competence, or ability to perform the job correctly, is the practical measure of accountability. The expectation of competence begins when the student enrolls in a nursing program and continues throughout nursing practice, whether the nurse is caring for patients, managing a department, or acting in an advanced practice role. The nurse must learn how to operate new equipment before it is put into general use; maintain an evidence-based practice that is current on the latest findings; and seek help from peers, mentors, and instructors to learn new skills and techniques. Each nurse is responsible for pinpointing his or her own areas of strength and weakness. Once an area of incompetence has been identified, the nurse should seek opportunities to gain competence in that area. This self-examination is a necessary ingredient in the formation of a truly professional nurse.

Nursing is defined as a profession in part because nurses are guided and assisted by professional organizations. In addition to the state boards of nursing and the National Council of State Boards of Nursing (NCSBN), which license nurses and define the standards of safe conduct, nurses can join a large number of professional organizations that promote information sharing, community building, and problem solving within the nursing profession. Nurses can join these organizations as a way of continuing their education and keeping up-to-date on the most recent developments in nursing practice. The module on Health Policy fully describes the professional organizations that govern and differentiate the profession of nursing.

Collaboration

How to work as a member of the team is discussed in detail in the module on Collaboration. Skill in working as a team member contributes to others' opinions of the nurse as a professional and improves the quality of care delivered to the patient.

Clinical Example A

Caroline Nava is a 28-year-old nursing student who is enrolled in her final clinical rotation and due to graduate in 2 months. She is working on a surgical unit managing care for five individuals. After completing her charting, she leaves the nursing unit 2 hours late. She returns home, exhausted from a particularly busy clinical day. Just as she sits down to enjoy some relaxation time, she remembers that she failed to obtain information from the chart of a new postoperative patient. Earlier today, her instructor asked Caroline to report back to her about this individual's laboratory results by the end of the day. The patient returned to the unit late from postanesthesia care, as Caroline was about to leave.

Caroline begins to panic and is uncertain what to do. Suddenly, she remembers that her friend Joan McIntyre, another student, is in clinical on the same unit until late that evening. Caroline calls Joan and asks her for a favor. She explains to Joan that she is in a bind and has to call her nursing instructor with the information as soon as possible. Caroline asks Joan to take a picture with her cell phone of the laboratory results in the patient's chart and send her the picture. Joan is glad to be able to help her friend and successfully sends the information to Caroline. Caroline is able to contact her instructor with the necessary information about her patient.

Critical Thinking Questions

1. Do you think Caroline handled the situation ethically? Support your answer.
2. If you were Joan, what would you have done in this situation?

Advocacy

Advocacy, the practice of expressing and defending patients' needs, is an essential component of professional nursing practice. The ANA Code of Ethics for Nurses emphasizes patient advocacy as a key concern (see the module on Ethics for more information). A nurse may be a patient advocate by conveying a patient's wishes to members of the healthcare team, by communicating with the patient's family, or simply by encouraging the patient to express his or her wishes. Patient advocacy is essential for patients in vulnerable populations, such as patients with disabilities or mental health diagnoses. Promotion of an organizational culture that is conducive to patient advocacy is of central importance to the development of a professionalism rooted in advocacy (Choi, 2015). See the module on Advocacy for more information.

Caring Interventions

The caring interventions of attitude and compassion are key to nursing professionalism. *Attitude* is a mental state involving values, beliefs, feelings, and mood. Each individual's attitude affects the individual and all others who are nearby. Professional behavior for the nurse includes maintaining a positive attitude while working with patients, their family members, and other healthcare professionals. A nurse with a positive attitude refrains from complaining and expresses an optimistic outlook. The Via Christi Health System survey revealed that nurses themselves view a positive attitude as an essential component of professionalism (Via Christi Regional Medical Center, 2003). Attitude is discussed in more detail in the exemplar on Work Ethic in this module.

Compassion is an awareness of and concern about other individuals' suffering. Nurses demonstrate compassion when they recognize a patient's need and respond appropriately to meet that need. In showing compassion, the nurse treats the patient as a unique and special individual and not as a number or a diagnosis. The nurse further demonstrates compassion by advocating in the community and communicating with politicians to develop laws that protect and promote the health of individuals and families. See the module on Caring Interventions for more information on compassion and attitude.

Ethics

As professionals, nurses adhere to the ANA Code of Ethics for Nurses, as well as evaluate the potential for any ethical conflicts between one's own ethical code and one's work as a nurse. Nurses who successfully engage in consistently ethical behavior demonstrate **integrity**, or adherence to a strict moral or ethical code. For nurses, integrity involves consistent behaviors based on the internalization of the values, ethics, and best practices of the profession of nursing. Nurses demonstrate integrity by accepting feedback (positive or negative) as a tool for improving their delivery of patient care, by maintaining accountability for their actions and freely admitting when they make mistakes, and by following their state's nurse practice act and never working outside their scope of practice.

Concepts Related to Professionalism

Professionalism is a central component of all effective nursing actions. Being professionally engaged enables nurses to make accurate assessments, perform caring interventions, collaborate, make clinical decisions expediently, and teach with compassion and care. How the concepts of accountability, collaboration, advocacy, and ethics relate to professionalism are outlined elsewhere in this module. Communication and application of culturally respectful, caring interventions through the nursing process are key elements valued by nursing students and nurses, especially in contrast to other members of the healthcare team (Delunas & Rouse, 2014). The profession of nursing is based in teamwork and respectful communication with patients as well as colleagues, and nurses must be fluent communicators to attain expert status.

Nurses' success within the discipline is predicated on a careful adherence to codes of ethics in all healthcare settings for all patients. According to Kangasniemi et al. (2013), the role of professional nurses is to incorporate ethical values of patient safety into decision making for nurses at every level of a healthcare organization or system, so that nurses in all roles consider ethical values when administering care.

Professional nurses are above all accountable to deliver the highest standard of care, which include as a crucial component caring interventions. Horsburgh and Ross (2013) found that nursing programs should prepare students for the necessity of delivering safe, culturally competent, and compassionate care despite busy schedules, an intervention that can be aided in practice by nurses' membership in nursing organizations and ongoing education programs. Some, but not all, of the concepts integral to Professionalism are outlined in the Concepts Related to Professionalism feature. The concepts are in alphabetical order.

Concepts Related to
Professionalism

CONCEPT	RELATIONSHIP TO PROFESSIONALISM	NURSING IMPLICATIONS
Caring Interventions	Professional behaviors help nurses provide caring interventions to patients and themselves.	■ Practicing theories of caring contributes to comprehensive patient care. ■ Emphasizing caring facilitates patients' empowerment. ■ Engaging in self-care contributes to holistic personal and professional wellness.
Clinical Decision Making	Nurses who engage in professional behaviors are better able to provide high-quality, evidence-based nursing care at all stages of the nursing process.	■ Use careful reasoning during assessment to ensure accurate and timely assessment while providing maximum comfort to the patient. ■ Use clinical decision making to determine priorities for care to ensure the best outcomes for the patient. ■ Use clinical decision making to determine the timing and order of interventions to promote patient trust and comfort.
Communication	Professional behaviors promote reliability and accountability for information and the methods by which it is conveyed.	■ Establish trust and rapport with patients and team members. ■ Ensure accurate and complete documentation and reporting, decreasing risks to patient safety.
Culture and Diversity	Professional standards of nursing require the nurse to work toward cultural competency and refrain from imposing the nurse's own values on the patient.	■ Assess patient and family cultural needs and practices. ■ Ensure that care provided incorporates patient and family cultural needs and practices whenever doing so will not cause injury to the patient. ■ Support the patient and family in maintaining cultural practices and rituals in outpatient, inpatient, and home care settings.
Healthcare Systems		■ By participating in primary prevention using evidence-based standards and professional guidelines, the nurse can help promote the health of the individual and the larger community. ■ By assessing the patient's insurance status and ability to access healthcare, the nurse can assist the patient in finding affordable and practical ways to meet healthcare needs.
Safety	Professional behaviors ensure that nurses follow safety guidelines and the principles of evidence-based practice.	■ Maintaining current knowledge of evidence-based practice facilitates patient safety. ■ Administering interventions according to knowledge of best practices across the lifespan promotes optimal health outcomes. ■ Maintaining a sense of one's own physical limits and boundaries promotes nurse and healthcare team safety.

Unprofessional Behaviors

Unprofessional behaviors undermine an individual nurse's credibility and negatively affect group morale, and they may affect patient outcomes.

Types of Unprofessional Behaviors

Unprofessional behaviors come in many forms, but they all make members of the healthcare team and patients feel uncomfortable, hurt, intimidated, threatened, or targeted in ways that interfere with the provision of high-quality patient care (Stringfellow, 2016). Some examples of unprofessional behaviors include the following:

- Belittling someone's opinion or using patronizing language
- Delivering negative or disparaging nonverbal messages
- Engaging in constant criticism, scapegoating, and fault-finding
- Engaging in elitism about experience, education, or practice area
- Undermining someone's activities or causing unnecessary disruptions
- Having emotional outbursts
- Being reluctant to answer questions
- Pitting staff members against one another and propagating rumors

Unprofessional behaviors such as breach of confidentiality, as defined by state nurse practice acts, are discussed in the module on Legal Issues. Other unprofessional behaviors, such as substance abuse and discrimination, are discussed in other modules. Unprofessional behaviors such as excessive absenteeism and tardiness are discussed in the exemplar on Work Ethic in this module.

It is important to recognize that the work environment sometimes carries over to social events, such as unit parties, company picnics, and informal gatherings. The rules of professionalism and the pitfalls of unprofessional behavior extend to these types of situations as well.

Abuses of Power

Any discussion of unprofessional behavior must include a discussion about abuses of power. An **abuse of power** is any attempt to use one's position or authority to shame, control, demean, humiliate, or denigrate another individual in order to gain emotional, psychologic, or physical advantage over that individual. In any professional environment, including the nursing profession, abuses of power such as sexual harassment, improper use of authority, bullying, and intimidation must be addressed immediately and appropriately.

SAFETY ALERT Acting with professionalism is not merely a matter of ensuring group cohesion and mutual respect. Behaving professionally is essential to healthcare workers' ability to ensure patient safety. According to the Agency for Healthcare Research and Quality (2014), 77% of healthcare staff report witnessing physicians engaging in disruptive behavior, and 65% report nurses engaging in these communication patterns. Most healthcare staff also believe that disruptive actions increase the potential for medical error and preventable deaths. Disruptive behaviors have been tied to nurses' workplace

dissatisfaction in addition to sentinel events in the operating room. There is no standard healthcare definition of disruptive behavior, but it is commonly defined as any behavior that shows disrespect for others or impedes the delivery of patient care.

Bullying

Evidence of bullying, lateral violence (violence directed toward peers), and incivility in the healthcare environment has been well documented in nursing research for over three decades. These behaviors are commonplace because of widespread tolerance within the healthcare arena. Furthermore, the long history of a hierarchical or tiered power structure perpetuates the dominance and empowerment of unprofessional individuals. The Joint Commission has identified "behaviors that undermine a culture of safety" in healthcare (such as bullying and incivility) as being among the leading causes of sentinel events (Wyatt, 2013). The Joint Commission calls for zero tolerance of intimidation and bullying in the workplace and recommends that healthcare facilities implement policies to stop such bullying. See the Evidence-Based Practice feature for more information.

Sexual Harassment

According to the Equal Employment Opportunity Commission (EEOC), the definition of sexual harassment is "unwelcome sexual advances, requests for sexual favors, and other verbal or physical conduct of a sexual nature" (Code of Federal Regulations, 2009). Because sexual harassment violates the harassed person's rights, it is a form of discrimination. The law against sexual discrimination in 1987 was held to apply to all federally funded educational and employment institutions. According to the 2009 Code of Federal Relations, sexual harassment occurs in any of the following circumstances (Code of Federal Regulations, 2009):

- An individual's employment is conditional on compliance with sexual requests or tolerance of sexual behavior, regardless of whether that condition is explicitly stated or simply implied.
- Employment decisions that affect the individual, such as promotion, are based on whether that individual consents to a sexual request or tolerates sexual behavior. (Whether the individual consents to or rejects the sexual request or behavior is irrelevant; it is sexual harassment in either event.)
- Sexual conduct interferes with an individual's performance on the job or creates an "intimidating, hostile, or offensive working environment."

The victim or violator may be either male or female in any of these cases, and it is not necessary for the victim and violator to be of the opposite sex.

To handle any sexual harassment they may encounter in the workplace, nurses must develop their assertiveness skills to be able to say no when necessary. They must also familiarize themselves with the sexual harassment policy and procedures at the institution that employs them. They must know the procedure for reporting sexual harassment (including to whom they should report incidents), the investigative process, and how their confidentiality will be protected and to what extent.

When providing patient care, nurses must use caution to avoid having patients misinterpret nursing behaviors as

Evidence-Based Practice
Bullying and Disruptive Behavior in the Workplace

Problem

Bullying and disruptive behaviors in the healthcare environment are top causes of sentinel events, and recent evidence links behaviors that undermine a culture of safety directly to medical errors (Wyatt, 2013).

Evidence

Over the past several decades, the phenomenon of disruptive behavior in the healthcare environment has been referred to as *lateral violence, incivility*, and a variety of other names. The existence of disruptive behavior is well documented in nursing research. Walrafen, Brewer, and Mulvenon (2012) describe disruptive behaviors as overly aggressive behaviors such as yelling, verbally dismissive and demeaning remarks, and the use of denigrating terms. Covert and overt actions are defined as verbal outbursts and physical threats as well as passive reluctance or refusal to answer questions, failure to return phone calls or pages, use of condescending language or voice intonation, and impatience with questions. A quantitative review of the literature on nursing violence that analyzed data from 136 articles gathered from 160 samples of 151,347 nurses revealed an exposure rate of 66.9% for nonphysical violence (Spector, Zhou, & Che, 2014). Even gossip, which might seem benign on the surface, is a frequent form of bullying in the workplace. Students and novice nurses are particularly vulnerable to bullying because of their lack of experience and power. In a study of 147 novice nurses, Berry et al. (2012) found that 72.6% of respondents reported a bullying event in the previous month. Workplace productivity was negatively affected by bullying, which reduced the novice nurses' ability to handle the cognitive demands of their workload.

Implications

The Institute of Medicine (2010) has challenged nurses to lead the way to changing and improving quality, efficiency, and safety in the healthcare environment. Nurses must possess and use good communication and conflict resolution skills to address bullying in the workplace and transform the healthcare environment in which they practice. The continued training of point-of-care nurses in assertiveness and leadership skill is necessary to effect a change.

Critical Thinking Application

Bullying is a threat to patient safety and the emotional well-being of nurses. What measures might a student or novice nurse use to address bullying by more experienced nurses in the healthcare setting? Describe a situation in which you may have observed or experienced incivility. Write down practical comments you would feel comfortable making to address the behavior in real time.

---

sexual harassment. For example, in lifting a patient's breast to bathe the chest or to place leads when performing an electrocardiogram, it is best to use the back of the hand rather than the palm of the hand. It is also important to explain the procedure and seek the patient's permission. In this way, the nurse can reduce the possibility that the action will be misinterpreted as sexual harassment and can avoid responses by the patient that might tend toward sexual harassment of the nurse.

Improper Use of Authority

Improper use of authority is widespread and has no place in the practice of nursing. Some nurses who, through use of their professional skills, have acquired administrative titles remove "Registered Nurse" from their title or name badge, perhaps to disassociate themselves from nursing's professional code of ethics. Once separated from the codes of ethical behaviors expected of nurses, bullies in administrative positions adopt a corporate rather than a professional demeanor and attitude. Such administrators serve their careers and no longer the priorities of patient-centered care. They can be identified by their attitude of arrogance, control, and acceptance of the hierarchical power structure that oppresses and is condescending to the voice of nursing at the point of care.

A nursing manager may use intimidation to show favoritism and to foster subordinate compliance, bias, and group pressure to exclude employees toward whom the manager has a less favorable attitude or who challenge the manager. Nurses in authority who emphasize principles over personality and who focus on patient safety can extinguish these negative behaviors and encourage nurses at the point of care. Nurses can facilitate effective leadership by becoming active in nursing leadership organizations such as the American Organization of Nurse Executives (AONE) and the ANA Leadership Institute following licensure and by lifelong learning within the discipline to promote professionalism and support the larger nursing community. Transformational leadership, which is discussed in the exemplar on Management and Leadership Principles in the module on Managing Care, is recommended as the leadership style for facilitating progress and innovation in nursing.

Clinical Example B

Mary Reynolds, who is a nurse of the baby-boomer generation, disagrees with Ashley Maloney, a new graduate, about how Ms. Maloney handled a situation with a patient's family. You overhear Ms. Reynolds telling a friend of hers that she hopes that Ms. Maloney never takes care of her or her family. Later, while you are on break, Ms. Reynolds repeats to you her story about Ms. Maloney. She informs you that Ms. Maloney "ignored the family" sitting at the bedside and that the family complained to Ms. Reynolds. She apologized for Ms. Maloney and told the family, "She is a problem. Thanks for telling me. I will take care of it for you." The family rewards Ms. Reynolds by writing a supportive note to the nurse manager about her and also detailing their perception of how Ms. Maloney dealt with their family.

Critical Thinking Questions

1. Using your knowledge of formation of professional behavior and bullying, how might you respond to Ms. Reynolds?
2. Using what you have learned about communication, frame a respectful confrontation of Ms. Reynolds.
3. If you were the nurse manager, how would you handle this situation while applying a provision of the ANA Code of Ethics?

Intimidation

Intimidation is bullying, threatening, or forcing someone who is physically or emotionally weaker to do something (or refrain from doing something) in order to avoid retribution. It is never appropriate for a nurse to threaten someone, whether a coworker, a patient, a patient's family member, or anyone else. Intimidation can be subtle, such as standing close to another individual with a hostile look on one's face, or it can be overt, such as telling someone to do something or that person will be "sorry." Even nurses with the best of intentions may not realize that they are using intimidation when they say things like "If you don't take your medicine [or go to physical therapy, or follow the treatment plan], you're only going to get worse." Even though what the nurse says may be true, this approach is intimidating and lacks professionalism.

REVIEW   The Concept of Professionalism

RELATE Link the Concepts

Linking the concept of professionalism with the concept of addiction:

1. What impact does a nurse's use of addictive substances (legal or illegal) have on the practice of nursing?

2. What is your professional responsibility when a nurse on your unit appears to be under the influence of a substance?

Linking the concept of professionalism with the concept of clinical decision making:

3. How do professional behaviors result from effective clinical decision making? How do competent clinical decisions stem from professional behaviors?

4. What conclusions would you draw, or have you drawn, about a nurse's ability to make clinical decisions on the basis of the nurse's professional or nonprofessional behaviors?

REFER Go to Pearson MyLab Nursing and eText

- Additional review material

REFLECT Apply Your Knowledge

Cheryl Goodwin is a nurse executive who is widely respected for her rapport with nurse educators. She is the dean of a nursing college and is a doctoral-prepared nurse who maintains a small private practice. She is active in state organizations and willing to help both faculty and students. A hospital administrator calls Ms. Goodwin in for a private meeting. In the course of the meeting, Ms. Goodwin is told that a faculty member in the nursing college has committed an act of abuse and neglect toward a patient in the hospital. The Chief Nurse Executive (CNE) of the hospital, who is also at the meeting, informs Ms. Goodwin that the faculty member is no longer permitted to practice at that hospital.

Upon questioning the faculty member involved, Ms. Goodwin discovers that the individual did in fact commit the offenses willfully, as reported by the CNE. Ms. Goodwin informs this faculty member that his actions created dire consequences for the patient involved and that his position at the college is terminated. He had been on probation for bullying and maltreatment of students before this incident.

The college administration permits the nursing faculty member to resign his position. He then begins a campaign to attack Ms. Goodwin, accusing her of making a number of false accusations. Friends rally around the dismissed employee, who has taught at the college for a number of years. He has been known for covering for and doing favors for other faculty members for extra cash, such as picking up an extra clinical day, and for granting favors to the faculty members who reported to him. As a senior faculty member, he also coordinated clinical rotations and scheduling.

Ms. Goodwin is not at liberty to discuss the incident that led to this faculty member's resignation. The other faculty members at the college are not aware of the consequences suffered by the hospital patient and family. The hospital has requested that the situation remain confidential, as the family has not been notified of the abuse. Faculty members who have known Ms. Goodwin for many years begin questioning her motives and labeling her as "sick." They talk behind her back and do not invite her to nursing functions that she has always attended. They bully any faculty member who associates with her. Ms. Goodwin acquires another position and leaves a position that she loved.

1. How would you describe the behaviors and actions of the faculty members in the scenario?

2. What recourse does Ms. Goodwin have?

3. Why do you suppose the faculty members who had a prior satisfactory relationship with Ms. Goodwin did not support her? Do you believe they did the right thing? How and why might they have handled the situation differently?

≫ Exemplar 40.A
Commitment to Profession

Exemplar Learning Outcomes

40.A Analyze commitment to profession as it relates to professionalism.

- Describe factors associated with professional commitment.
- Describe types of commitment.
- Outline the stages of the commitment process.
- Discuss ways to manage stress associated with commitment to a profession.

Exemplar Key Terms

Affective commitment, *2653*
Burnout, *2654*
Commitment, *2653*
Continuance commitment, *2654*
Normative commitment, *2654*
Organizational commitment, *2653*

Overview

Many experienced nurses view nursing as a vocation or calling. It is not a job or what they *do*; it is a part of who they *are*. They have made a commitment to their profession, incorporating the ethics and expectations of nursing into every aspect of their lives, whether at home, work, or play. This commitment is in essence a duty to the individual who is at the center of nursing care. Over time, some nurses may confuse professional commitment with organizational or corporate commitment.

Merriam-Webster's Online Dictionary (n.d.) defines **commitment** as "the state or an instance of being obligated or emotionally impelled." To understand the term *commitment* as it is applied to the profession of nursing, one must first look at the concept of organizational commitment. The most widely accepted definition of **organizational commitment** is that it is the relative strength of an individual's relationship to and sense of belonging to an organization. Although organizational commitment and professional commitment may intersect, it is important for nurses to distinguish between the two. Experienced nurses can cite many instances in which nursing ethics and corporate goals collide. The business of healthcare and the provision of care to the patient are not always the same issue. The nursing profession holds the trust of the community and individuals in our society. With this trust comes the moral responsibility of nurses to address the needs of patients and to advocate for safe care within the business of healthcare.

The IOM (2010) calls for nurses to step up and lead the transformation of healthcare and to protect a caring model within the business model of healthcare. It is essential for the safety and well-being of all individuals in our society that nurses be actively involved in health policy and the financial decisions that affect the delivery of care. The nurse's commitment must be synonymous with professional commitment, even when it may be at odds with organizational commitment.

Factors of Professional Commitment

Factors associated with professional commitment include the following:

1. A strong belief in and acceptance of the profession's code, role, goals, values, and morals.
2. A willingness to exert considerable personal effort on behalf of the profession.
3. A strong desire to maintain membership in the profession.
4. A pattern of behaviors congruent with the nurses' professional code of ethics.

As was discussed earlier, nursing education concerns not only teaching students how to think like nurses and perform nursing tasks but also is charged with the acculturation and formation of professional behaviors in students and novice nurses. This process begins when the student enters the first nursing class. Many of the policies and rules associated with a nursing program are intended to prepare the student for entry into the profession of nursing. The student who violates or ignores school policy is in danger of becoming the nurse who ignores practice and agency policy. For example, tardiness in coming to clinicals may result in significant consequences for the offender. Time and attendance are critical in nursing, as patients depend on the nurse for their safety. Especially during a nursing shortage, the nurse who is chronically late for work or excessively absent is subject to disciplinary action that could include suspension and termination. With frequent staff shortages, it is even more important for managers to be able to rely on staff members to be on the job when scheduled. Chronic lateness and frequent absenteeism place a greater burden on colleagues, compromise patient care, and lead to conflict among staff.

The values and goals of professional nursing are clearly delineated by standards of nursing practice, codes of ethics, nurse practice acts, national patient safety goals, accrediting agencies, and many other such resources. Entering the nursing profession is not just taking a job. It is assuming the obligation to protect, advance, and promote the health of self, individuals, and groups in the community, and it involves many role expectations not inherent in occupations that are just jobs.

Most students can easily identify with the willingness to exert considerable effort on behalf of the profession. Nursing programs have high standards of admission, and many programs receive far more applications than they have openings available. In times of economic recession, this imbalance is even more evident as displaced workers seek job security in the healthcare professions that have staff shortages. Nursing education is a rigorous program of study requiring considerable time and effort to prepare for entry into a demanding yet rewarding profession. The applicants who are accepted into nursing programs tend to be those who have demonstrated the ability to expend such time and effort to achieve their goals.

Students also can identify with the strong desire to maintain membership in the profession. Most students have already made sacrifices while taking related general education and science courses in preparation for the nursing major. The sacrifices required during nursing courses are even greater, as the number of hours required per credit earned increases when hours spent in lab and clinical are added. Most students who are accepted into a nursing program have a strong desire to complete the program, especially as their time in the program increases.

After graduation, the commitment to maintain membership in the nursing profession is demonstrated by membership in professional organizations and on various committees and by contributing to community organizations seeking input on laws related to healthcare and health promotion. Nurses must always maintain current knowledge related to changes in healthcare and the profession of nursing to keep their nursing practice up to date and therefore keep their patients safe.

Commitment to the profession of nursing is an obligation to behave in accordance with accepted codes of nursing professional practice. Many facilities that employ nurses require drug screenings and criminal background checks to assist them in the selection of individuals with high moral standards and to protect the populations that they serve.

Types of Commitment

Three types of commitment describe the psychologic link between an individual and the decision to continue in a profession: affective, normative, and continuance. **Affective commitment** is an attachment to a profession and includes

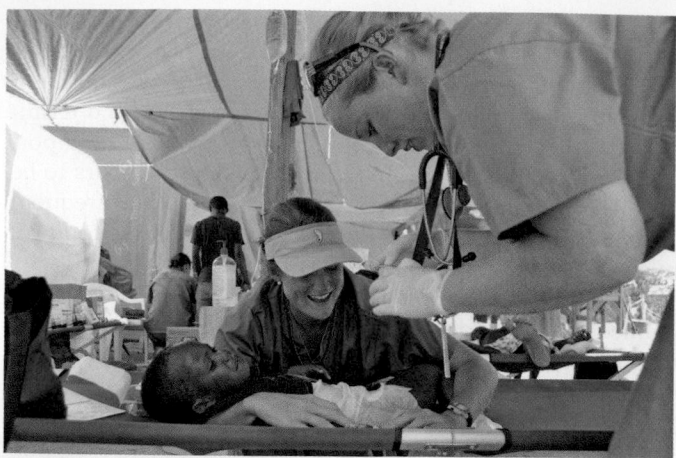

Source: Charlotte Observer/Tribune News Service/Getty Images.

Figure 40–2 ≫ Affective commitment leads nurses and other healthcare professionals to volunteer their services to help in disasters, such as the January 2010 earthquake in Haiti. Here, Tiffany Young, a pediatric nurse from North Carolina (center), holds a child with cholera who is receiving treatment.

identification with and involvement in the profession. Affective commitment develops when involvement in a profession produces a satisfying experience. The student or nurse who has a strong desire to continue in the profession, who is involved in keeping up with current information, and who becomes involved with profession-specific organizations and service activities demonstrates affective commitment (**Figure 40–2 ≫**). This individual is in school or working as a nurse because of a desire to be a nurse.

Normative commitment is a feeling of obligation to continue in the profession. Normative commitment develops as a result of having received benefits or having had positive experiences through engagement in the profession. The nurse who enters the field or remains in it because personal or family experiences with illness have created a desire to work in the healthcare field exemplifies normative commitment.

Continuance commitment, or the awareness of costs associated with leaving the profession, develops when negative consequences of leaving, such as loss of income, are seen as reasons to remain. Individuals who experience this type of commitment do not manifest the same ties to the profession as do those who are motivated by affective or normative commitment. In general, such individuals are not inclined to promote their profession. These students and nurses are in the field for the money and job security.

Stages of Commitment Development

The commitment to a profession develops in stages. The first stage is the *exploratory stage*, in which individuals explore the positive aspects of the profession. An example of this stage is the excitement of nursing students during the first weeks of their program as they model their new uniforms and ransack their lab kits. Commitment that begins as exploration leads to a positive orientation toward the profession.

The second stage is the *testing stage*, during which individuals discover negative elements of the profession. In this stage, individuals start to assess their willingness and ability

to deal with those negative elements. Some nursing students never get beyond this stage and drop out of school or change majors, deciding that the sacrifices are not worth the effort or that they are not suited to the nursing profession.

The third stage is the *passionate stage* of commitment, which begins as the individual synthesizes the positive and negative elements from the first two stages. Students in this stage not only are willing to commit to the profession but also are willing to contribute to its well-being. These students are the ones who become involved in student nursing associations, serve as class officers, or volunteer for activities not associated with a grade.

The fourth stage is the *quiet-and-bored stage* of commitment, in which students settle into the humdrum routines of the nursing program. This stage often occurs during the middle or late middle of the nursing program, as students begin to become more comfortable in their role and feel less anxiety about their performance.

The *integrated stage* is the final stage of commitment. Individuals who reach this stage have integrated both positive and negative elements of the profession into a more flexible, complex, and enduring form of commitment. They act out their commitment as a matter of habit. These students are in the final stages of their nursing program and are beginning to see themselves as nurses, eager to take the NCLEX-RN® and begin employment. As new graduates, they will once again proceed through the stages of commitment while transitioning from being nursing students to being registered nurses.

Managing Stress

Part of a commitment to any profession is learning how to manage the stress associated with that profession. Although most nurses find healthy ways to cope with the physical and emotional demands of the profession, these demands do create stress that can be difficult to manage. Nurses in some situations are overcome and develop **burnout**, which is similar to the exhaustion stage of the general adaptation syndrome (see the module on Stress and Coping) and should be understood as a complex syndrome of behaviors. In extreme cases, burnout may cause affected nurses to abandon the nursing profession altogether. The signs that a nurse has succumbed to burnout include feelings of helplessness and hopelessness, a negative attitude and self-concept, and physical and emotional exhaustion.

The use of healthy stress management techniques can help nurses prevent burnout. The first step is to recognize their stress and how they respond to stress. Some common responses to stress are angry outbursts, fatigue, feelings of being overwhelmed, physical illness, and increases in coffee drinking, smoking, or the use of alcohol or other mood-enhancing substances. After the nurses learn to recognize their stress and how they personally react to it, they must identify the trigger situations that tend to provoke the most pronounced stress reactions in them. Going through this recognition process will help nurses choose the stress reduction techniques that are best for them, which include the following:

- To reduce tension, engage in quiet activities that are personally meaningful (such as reading, listening to music, soaking in a tub, or meditating) as a daily relaxation program.

- To direct energy outward, establish and follow a regular exercise program.

- To overcome a feeling of powerlessness in relationships with others, learn techniques to increase assertiveness and develop the ability to say no.

- Turn errors and failures into constructive learning experiences by learning to accept such missteps as a part of life. By recognizing that most people do the best they can but do not always succeed, nurses learn to open up about their feelings with colleagues, ask for help, and reciprocate by supporting colleagues in their times of need.

- By recognizing that no situation is perfect and that certain limitations always exist, nurses learn to accept what cannot be changed; acceptance can decrease negative responses to stress.

- To improve organizational policies and procedures that may generate stress, nurses may get involved in efforts toward constructive change.

- To constructively handle the feelings and anxieties of working in a high-stress setting, nurses may develop collegial support groups.

- To address workplace issues, nurses may participate in professional organizations.

- To help clarify their problems and reactions to those problems, nurses may seek counseling.

Few professions are as demanding as nursing, which imposes unusual work schedule requirements, heavy demands on time and energy, and great responsibility. The work that nurses do often involves life and death, and nurses must face that possibility every day. Although the work of nursing can be highly satisfying and meaningful for many nurses as they help patients survive trauma and cope with problems to improve their lives, sustained professional commitment is necessary to avoid potential burnout.

REVIEW Commitment to Profession

RELATE Link the Concepts and Exemplars

Linking the exemplar of commitment to profession with the concept of development:

1. How might nurses in different life stages commit themselves to the profession of nursing in different ways?

2. Describe the impact of the nurse's moral development, according to Kohlberg's theory, on commitment to the profession of nursing.

Linking the exemplar of commitment to profession with the concept of collaboration:

3. How is nurses' commitment to profession demonstrated by their ability and willingness to collaborate with others?

4. A nurse working on a medical unit is approached by a newly graduated licensed practical nurse who asks for help in improving her skill in initiating an IV catheter. How would nurses with different levels of commitment to the profession respond to this request?

REFER Go to Pearson MyLab Nursing and eText

- Additional review material

REFLECT Apply Your Knowledge

Andrea Kamara is a nurse working on a very busy and often understaffed oncology unit. Two patients have died within the past week. They were both well known to the staff because each had been admitted several times with complications of their disease and treatment. The staff members who were working all cried, first for one patient and then, a few days later, for the other. Today, one of Ms. Kamara's assigned patients required cardiopulmonary resuscitation and was sent to the ICU, another developed septicemia and required many diagnostic tests and procedures, and a third was given bad news about her prognosis and was tearful and frightened. At the end of the day, Ms. Kamara felt that she had not done her best job because she was so busy. She wished she could have spent more time with each of her assigned patients, caring more for their emotional needs.

1. How will Ms. Kamara's commitment to the profession of nursing affect how she responds to her feelings of inadequacy and grief?

2. If Ms. Kamara is fully committed to nursing, how will she resolve her feelings about the quality of the care she delivers?

3. If Ms. Kamara has a continuance commitment to nursing, how will she respond to the shift she just worked and her feelings?

≫ Exemplar 40.B Work Ethic

Exemplar Learning Outcomes

40.B Analyze work ethic as it relates to professionalism.

- Describe the relationship of attendance and punctuality to work ethic.
- Outline the importance of reliability and accountability for the professional nurse.
- Describe the influence of attitude and enthusiasm on the work environment.
- Summarize generational differences in work ethic.

Exemplar Key Terms

Arrogance, *2657*
Corrective action, *2656*
Dismissal, *2656*
Generational cohort, *2657*
Insubordination, *2657*
Optimism, *2657*
Pessimism, *2657*
Punctual, *2656*
Work ethic, *2656*

Overview

A majority of employers identify a "strong work ethic" as the most important characteristic of a good employee. A belief in the importance and moral worth of work constitutes a **work ethic**. Because they place a high value on hard work and diligence, people with strong work ethics tend to stay focused on the job and leave their personal problems at home. Because they value doing the work right the first time, they take a thorough approach to tasks and apply themselves fully to what they do. People with strong work ethics assume responsibility for any mistakes they do make, fixing the mistakes if they can and willingly accepting the consequences of their actions. They know what management expects of them, and they exercise self-discipline and self-control to meet these expectations. They are proactive, taking the initiative and approaching work tasks positively and enthusiastically.

Nursing students may develop a better grasp of the expectations of the nursing profession by examining the components of a strong work ethic and, through developing a strong work ethic themselves, demonstrating a commitment to their job and to their employer.

Attendance and Punctuality

Attendance is a fundamental requirement to demonstrate commitment to a job. To perform the duties of a job requires showing up for work every day. A key component of attendance is being on time, or **punctual**.

Other employees are required to take on more than their usual workloads to cover for employees who do not come to work. An employee may have a legitimate reason for being absent, but even so, frequent absences increase stress for other employees and decrease productivity. Funding shortages force many healthcare agencies to employ no more employees than are absolutely required. Accordingly, all employees have full workloads that, even under the best of circumstances, require their full commitment and the best of their ability. If employees have to take on some or all of an absent employee's work, this increases the burden for everyone. Accordingly, every nurse (and nursing student) has the responsibility to be at work and to arrive on time.

Employees who arrive late for work create delays and other inconveniences for their coworkers. A nurse's failure to be punctual might force the rescheduling of a patient's procedure and could delay that patient's (or another's) diagnosis, treatment, surgery, or discharge from the hospital. That nurse might be late in delivering needed supplies and filing paperwork by its appointed deadline, forcing other people to work overtime to compensate for the delays. Nurses must report to work on time because of the interconnected nature of professional healthcare roles. Being "on time" does not mean arriving at the parking lot at the time work is scheduled to begin; "on time" means that at the start of a nurse's shift, that nurse is already at work and in place, ready to begin.

It is inevitable for almost everyone to occasionally miss work or arrive late. However, habitual poor attendance and lack of punctuality are performance issues and may be grounds for steps to overcome the problem (**corrective action**) or even terminate employment (**dismissal**).

Professional commitment, then, dictates that nursing students must arrive on time for work every day and be ready to work immediately when the shift starts. To assist with this, nursing students should anticipate potential emergencies, such as a child being sick or a car being in the shop, and set up contingency plans to prepare for them.

A component of forming a good work ethic for nurses is taking steps to protect their own health and safety, such as by getting enough rest, avoiding unnecessary risks, and taking preventive measures such as receiving flu shots.

Another part of maintaining a good work ethic is avoiding excessively long or unscheduled breaks. This involves trying to allow some extra time at the end of every shift in case they are held over. Above all, nurses must never rush out the door the minute the shift ends if that might mean leaving a patient, coworker, visitor, or guest hanging. Staying long enough to complete work or to hand it off properly to the individual who follows is every nurse's (and nursing student's) responsibility. Doing so facilitates a smooth transition between shifts and ensures that work in progress is not left for other people to finish.

Reliability and Accountability

Professionalism involves the essential factors of reliability and accountability. From a systems perspective, each nurse must complete the duties of the job appropriately so that others who depend on the nurse can complete their own work. Part of reliability and accountability is following through on commitments—for example, honoring agreements to trade shifts or taking on additional work when someone is absent. Honoring commitments helps the team function properly and builds trust and team cohesion (**Figure 40-3 》**). It is also important to take responsibility for the consequences of one's actions. Professionals do not blame others for their mistakes but instead hold themselves personally accountable.

Professional nurses should refuse work assignments only when the nurse is not qualified or is not prepared to perform the assignment. In either case, the nurse should discuss the situation immediately with the supervisor. Otherwise, the nurse should be ready to complete all assigned tasks,

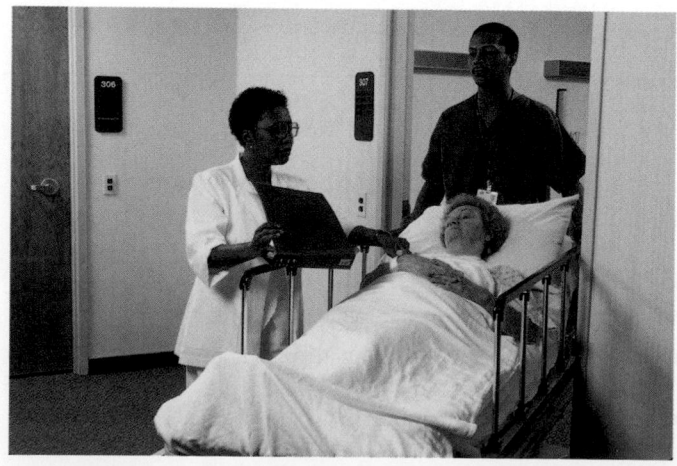

Figure 40-3 》 Nurses are responsible for completing their duties so that other people can complete their own work.

especially because refusal to do so may be regarded as **insubordination** (defiance of authority) and grounds for dismissal.

Nurses act professionally when they avoid judging patients or forcing their own personal beliefs onto patients. When a nurse feels a conflict between an assigned task and the nurse's religious beliefs, morals, or values, it is the nurse's responsibility to bring this conflict to the supervisor's attention and discuss it reasonably. Many employers will allow a nurse to opt out of participation in activities to which the nurse has moral objections, but the nurse should anticipate such conflicts and report them to the employer at the earliest opportunity. For more information, refer to the module on Accountability.

Attitude and Enthusiasm

A positive attitude—an essential professional characteristic for nurses—involves a sense of **optimism**, or a feeling that things will turn out for the best. Professional nurses are typically optimistic, but unfortunately, a negative attitude is a way of life for some people. This negativity expresses itself as **pessimism**, or the belief that the current situation is always bad and may become worse. Pessimists complain about everything and tend to be dissatisfied with what they have. Pessimists do not convey enthusiasm about their work. They rarely smile and often appear unhappy, which, whether the pessimist consciously intends it or not, may spread negativity to their coworkers, undermining morale, teamwork, and cooperative spirit. Pessimism is a dangerous attitude that nurses must guard against, because it erodes trust and confidence. Instead, nurses should convey optimism and enthusiasm about their work, especially to patients and their families. A commitment to positivity contributes to a more pleasant, collegial, and productive work environment.

Arrogance is another negative attitude that can damage a nurse's professionalism. **Arrogance**, or excessive pride and a feeling of superiority, can be an extremely dangerous characteristic in the nurse, as it can lead to a false belief that the nurse is always right and does not need input from others. For example, when the unit begins using a new IV infusion pump, the arrogant nurse does not bother attending the in-service, believing that it is possible to "figure things out" independently. Accurate self-assessment of strengths and weaknesses, as well as acceptance of feedback from others, promotes both safety and growth and is therefore an essential ability for the nurse.

Generational Differences in Work Ethic

Discussions about cultural diversity often focus on differing ethnic, national, or religious perspectives. Studies, including an international research project by Papastavrou et al. (2012), have traced the key differences in cross-cultural perceptions of nursing professionalism (see the module on Culture and Diversity for more information). But at this moment in the United States, the major cultural divide currently impacting nurses' work ethic is the generational gap.

For the first time in American history, four generations of people are working shoulder to shoulder. Research has shown that generation membership is a key variable in determining behavior (Hendricks & Cope, 2012). Different generations hold different ideals, values, traits, goals, and characteristics, which play a significant role in how employees of one generation relate to those of other generations. These differences can be seen in communication styles, expectations, work styles, values and norms, attitudes about work and life, comfort with technology, views regarding loyalty and authority, and acceptance of change.

The term **generational cohort** refers to people born in the same general time span who share key life experiences, including historical events, public heroes, pastimes, and early work experiences. These common life experiences create cohesiveness in perspectives and attitudes and lead generational cohorts to develop distinct values and workforce patterns. Differences between generations (sometimes called a *generation gap*) can have negative effects in the workplace, causing conflicts and interpersonal tension. Learning to create collegial relationships with people from different generations is a critical skill for nurses who work in multigenerational teams.

While the literature sometimes disagrees on specific years or generational names, there is consistent agreement on the characteristics of each generational cohort. An understanding of the historical influences on each generation, their common life experiences, and the workforce the members entered when first employed is necessary to understand their attitudes and values related to work (see **Table 40–3 》》**).

Different generational styles can lead to workplace conflict. Older nurses may experience considerable conflict over younger nurses' behaviors and may describe younger nurses as arrogant, lacking in commitment, and having a "slacker" attitude. Younger nurses may see themselves as self-reliant rather than arrogant. Older nurses may be dismayed and struggle with a perceived lack of professionalism among their younger colleagues, evidenced by younger nurses' dress, hair styles, piercings, and tattoos. Younger nurses may be disillusioned by older nurses' perceived unwillingness to become technologically competent.

While differences between generations are not new, two significant changes over the past 60 years have forced the current generations in the workforce into more intense interaction. First, the nature of the work itself has shifted. In traditional bureaucratic structures, interactions between generations followed hierarchical lines. People from younger generations traditionally held entry-level positions and reported to people of the older generation in more senior positions. As a result, younger employees took direction from and followed the rules of people who were older. With the advent of continuous quality improvement and shared governance structures, individuals from various "levels" of the organization are now equal members of a team. This arrangement has increased the interaction of employees from different generations.

Second, the transformation from the industrial age to the information age has altered the interactions between people of differing generations. Historically, the most senior members of an organization offered the most reliable information and knowledge. Young nurses relied on their more senior colleagues for instruction and advice when confronted with an unusual diagnosis or a complex patient situation. With

TABLE 40–3 Description of Four Generations in the American Workforce

NOTE: Generational trends exist and everyone is, to some extent, shaped by things that happened in their particular generation; however, nurses should approach each colleague as an individual and should not stereotype based on generation.

Generational Cohort and Their Historical Influences	Life Experiences	Workforce Entered	Work Ethic
Veterans: Born 1925–1944			
Great Depression World War II	News came from newspapers and radio. Long-distance phone calls were rare and expensive. Shopping was mostly done at locally owned stores. Movies were seen only in theaters. Attitude toward children: They should be "seen and not heard."	End of Depression and war Economic prosperity Emergence of middle class Able to thrive in a nice home on a single income Large, bureaucratic organizations Rules, policies, and procedures plainly outlined	Sacrifice and hard work are rewarded. Seniority is important to advance career. Value loyalty. Respect authority. Like working in teams with designated leaders. Prefer personal forms of communication.
Baby Boomers: Born 1945–1960			
Introduction of television Humans landed on the moon Assassination of President Kennedy Assassination of Dr. Martin Luther King, Jr. Civil rights movement Summer of Love Vietnam War Woodstock Watergate	Grew up in a healthy, flourishing economy. Watched variety shows, movies, and sitcoms in their own home. News became more visual and dramatic. Raised in two-parent households in which father worked and mother was home caretaker. Were members of smaller families.	Emphasis was on freedom to be yourself—the "me" generation. Heroes were those who questioned the status quo. People in positions of power were not to be trusted. Raised to be independent, critical thinkers. Many female college graduates went on to become secretaries, nurses, or teachers because of the perception that these were primarily female professions.	Are workaholics. Embrace sense of professionalism. Self-worth closely tied to work ethic. Question authority. Status quo can be transformed by working together. Desire financial prosperity but long to make a significant contribution with their experience and expertise.
Generation X: Born 1961–1980			
Rising divorce rates Microwaves Video games Computers Space shuttle *Challenger* disaster Numerous scandals involving high-profile public figures Operation Desert Storm	Lived in two-career households. Many raised in single-parent homes. "Latch key" generation; learned to manage on their own, becoming adept, clever, and resourceful. Allowed to be equal participants in family discussions.	Dramatic downsizing, reengineering, and layoffs seen. Hierarchical structures had begun to flatten, eliminating promotion opportunities for younger workers. Large cohort of baby boomers remained in workforce, filling limited managerial positions. Assume responsibility to keep themselves employable by constantly updating their skills.	Seek challenges. Are self-directed. Expect instant access to information. Desire employment in which they can create balance in work and personal life. Prefer managers to be mentors and coaches. Desire more control over their own schedule.
Millennials (Generation Y): Born 1981–2000			
Established infrastructure (child care, preschool, after-school care) to assist dual-career parents Global generation Internet School shootings Terrorist attack of September 11, 2001 Wars in Afghanistan and Iraq Obama presidency	Mostly children of baby boomers born to older mothers. Life highly structured and scheduled. Parents heavily involved in their upbringing, often chaperoning or coaching extracurricular activities. Accept multiculturalism. Raised enmeshed in digital technology. Mass consumption of pop culture but via the internet.	Economic downturn Drying up of job opportunities in many industries. Belief that education is the key to success. Resurgence of heroism and patriotism. Diversity a given. Renewed sense of interest in contributing to collective good. Volunteering for community service. Joining organizations in record numbers.	Collaborative, open-minded, achievement-oriented. Expectation of daily feedback, high maintenance. Potential to become the highest-producing workforce in history. Personal smart devices a necessity for daily life.

the advent of the information age, young nurses are not as reliant on their older peers, since they can easily access information from around the world on their computers and smartphones. Computerization has not only broken the dependence of younger generations on more senior generations for information, it has also resulted in the unprecedented situation in which the youngest individuals in the workforce are the most expert at a critical skill. Instead of younger nurses turning to their older colleagues for advice, older nurses often depend on their younger peers for guidance in using new technologies.

Members of each generation typically operate as if their own values and expectations are universal. For example, veteran nurses who entered the workforce when success occurred through long-term employment with one organization assume that the same approach will ensure achievement today. They see their younger colleagues' frequent job changes or working as independent agents as unreliability or a lack of commitment. Younger nurses may assume that their older peers who have remained in one place of employment have done so because of failure to take advantage of opportunities. Also, having grown up in a world in which their voice and contributions are expected, younger nurses are often misunderstood when they advise their more senior colleagues who were taught to respect and listen to their elders. An older nurse may see the voiced criticisms of a novice nurse at a staff meeting as disrespectful and therefore discount the younger nurse. From the younger nurse's perspective, speaking up even with limited experience is contributing to the unit.

Learning to develop collegial relationships with people from different generations is a critical skill for nurses who work in multigenerational teams. Working with nurses from different generations offers the opportunity to explore new and different ways of thinking. Rather than focusing on what is "wrong" with another generation, nurses should look for ways to capitalize on each generation's strengths. Nurses of the veteran generation value hard work and respect authority, baby boomers value teamwork, Generation X nurses value self-reliance, and millennial nurses value achievement. In the workplace, a veteran nurse might say, "Do it because I say so," and a baby-boomer nurse might say, "Let's get together and reach a consensus about how to do it." The Generation X staff nurses might say they will do it themselves, and the millennial nurses might not care who does it as long as the work gets done.

Veteran nurses should be valued for the wisdom and organizational history they bring to nursing teams. When technology fails, veteran nurses can assist a unit to quickly shift back to the traditional ways of assessing and caring for patients. Baby boomers should be valued for their clinical and organizational experience and should be used to coach and mentor younger nurses. Generation X nurses should be valued for their innovative ideas and creative approaches to unit issues and problems. They can be important in helping organizations design new approaches to nursing care delivery. Millennial nurses should be valued for their understanding of technology and insights into how it can be used in practice. They can also serve as technology coaches for members of older generational cohorts.

Appreciation of the unique strengths of each generation can decrease interpersonal tension and facilitate personal growth. Nurses who learn to acknowledge and appreciate their colleagues from different backgrounds, including generational backgrounds, have a distinct advantage. Successful teamwork is increasingly required for job satisfaction and the ability to positively affect patient outcomes. This teamwork requirement is reflected in the recent introduction of relationship-based nursing care delivery systems such as the primary nursing model, as discussed in the module on Healthcare Systems. All too frequently, intergenerational interactions lead to conflicts due to lack of appreciation or understanding, or simply to misinterpretation of other perspectives.

Particular attention should be paid to engaging the perspective of younger nurses, as the youngest generation is always at a distinct disadvantage. The existing organizational structure is based on strategies that were used successfully in the past rather than having been designed for the future. Because of their longevity, older generations often dominate in the powerful leadership positions and are more influential when changes are made. These nurses update processes and rewards in a way that makes sense from their generational perspective, often not recognizing that younger nurses might not hold the same perspective and might have a valuable perspective of their own. Incorporating younger nurses' values of participation, access to information, and balance into nursing operations is important. Older nurses need to learn to welcome input from their younger colleagues, encouraging them to use their fresh viewpoints to identify where opportunities exist. Younger nurses need to be taught and learn to value the experience and expertise of more senior nurses who have a wealth of lived experiences to share.

The best teams use the contributions of each generation's skill set and strengths. The hardworking, loyal veterans; the idealist, passionate baby boomers; the techno-literate, adaptable Generation Xers; and the young, optimistic millennials can come together in a powerful network of nurses with a remarkable ability to support each other and maximize each nurse's contribution to patient care (**Figure 40–4 ≫**).

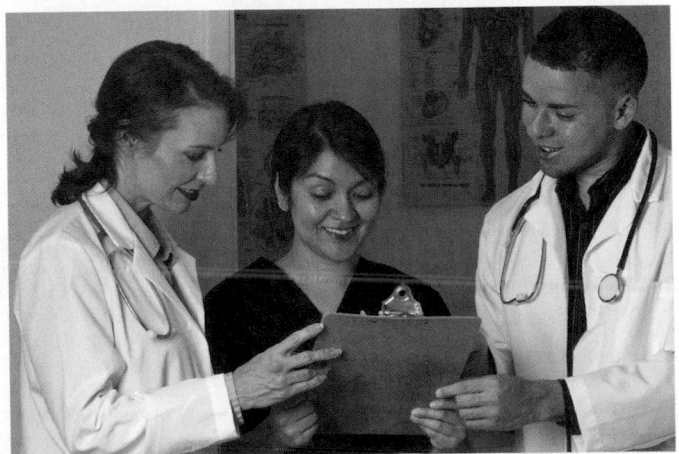

Source: JHDT Productions/Fotolia.

Figure 40–4 ≫ The best nursing teams use the contributions of each generation's strengths.

REVIEW Work Ethic

RELATE Link the Concepts and Exemplars

Linking the exemplar of work ethic with the concept of collaboration:

1. How does the work ethic of the individual nurse affect collaboration?

2. How might nurses from different generations respond to a rude and confrontational physician?

Linking the exemplar of work ethic with the concept of teaching and learning:

3. How does the nurse's generational work ethic affect how the nurse teaches patients?

4. How does the nurse's generational work ethic affect learning style?

REFER Go to Pearson MyLab Nursing and eText

- Additional review material

REFLECT Apply Your Knowledge

How would you respond in each of the following situations?

1. You were out with friends until very late last night and were scheduled to report for work this morning at 7 a.m. You arrive on time, but you know that your coworkers won't get there for another half hour. You have just enough time for a quick run to the corner coffee shop before your coworkers arrive.

2. You promised your coworkers that you would work the day shift on Thanksgiving so they could be home with their families. Two days before the holiday, an old friend from out of town calls to say that he would like you to be his guest for lunch on Thanksgiving Day.

3. You have an appointment with your supervisor next week to review the results of your annual performance evaluation. You overhear one of your teammates telling another individual that she gave you a low score on your 360-degree feedback evaluation because you refused to trade shifts with her over the Easter weekend.

4. Your shift ends in 30 minutes, and you have about 30 minutes of work left to do, but you have not been able to take your afternoon break yet.

5. One of your neighbors is admitted to the unit where you work. A member of your family calls to tell you that he has heard a rumor that the neighbor has a communicable disease. Because you work on the unit and have access to patient records, your family member asks you to find out whether the rumor is true.

6. A new piece of equipment has been installed in your department, but you missed the in-service session in which everyone was trained in how to operate it. Today a procedure is to be done using this equipment, and it is your responsibility to use it.

7. A coworker invites you to a party. When you arrive, you notice three other people you work with complaining about low wages and telling a group of strangers that one of the surgeons at your hospital made a mistake in surgery last week and lied to the patient's family to try to cover it up.

References

Agency for Healthcare Research and Quality. (2014). *Disruptive and unprofessional behavior*. Retrieved from https://psnet.ahrq.gov/primers/primer/15/disruptive-and-unprofessional-behavior

American Nurses Association (ANA). (2010). Standard 8: Education. In *Nursing: Scope and standards of practice*. Washington, DC: Author.

American Nurses Association (ANA). (2016). *Bill of Rights FAQs*. Retrieved from http://nursingworld.org/DocumentVault/NursingPractice/FAQs.aspx

Benner, P., Sutphen, M., Leonard, V., & Day, L. (2010). *Educating nurses: A call for radical transformation*. San Francisco, CA: Jossey-Bass.

Berry, P. A., Gillespie, G. L., Gates, D., & Schafer, J. (2012). Novice nurse productivity following workplace bullying. *Journal of Nursing Scholarship, 44*(1), 80–87.

Choi, P. P. (2015). Patient advocacy: The role of the nurse. *Nursing Standard, 29*(41), 52–58.

Code of Federal Regulations. (2009). Title 29—Labor: Section 1604-11—Sexual harassment. Retrieved from https://www.gpo.gov/fdsys/pkg/CFR-2009-title29-vol4/pdf/CFR-2009-title29-vol4-sec1604-11.pdf. Published by U.S. Government Publishing Office.

Davis, C. (2014). The importance of professional standards. *Nursing Made Incredibly Easy! 12*(5), 4.

Delunas, L. R. & Rouse, S. (2014). Nursing and medical student attitudes about communication and collaboration before and after an interprofessional education experience. *Nursing Education Perspectives, 35*(2), 100–105.

Dinmohammadi, M., Peyrovi, H., & Mehrdad, N. (2013). Concept analysis of professional socialization in nursing. *Nursing Forum, 48*(1), 26–34.

Gallup. (2015). *Honesty/ethics in professions*. Retrieved from http://www.gallup.com/poll/1654/honesty-ethics-professions.aspx

Hendricks, J. M. & Cope, V. C. (2012). Generational diversity: What nurse managers need to know. *Journal of Advanced Nursing, 69*(3), 717–725.

Hoeve, Y. T., Jansen, G., & Roodbol, P. (2014). The nursing profession: Public image, self-concept and professional identity. A discussion paper. *Journal of Advanced Nursing, 70*(2), 295–309.

Horsburgh, D. & Ross, J. (2013). Care and compassion: The experiences of newly qualified staff nurses. *Journal of Clinical Nursing, 22*(7–8), 1124–1132.

Hunt, D. D. (2015). *The nurse professional: Leveraging your education for transition into practice*. New York, NY: Springer.

Institute of Medicine. (2010). *The future of nursing: Leading change, advancing health*. Retrieved from https://www.nationalacademies.org/hmd/~/media/Files/Report%20Files/2010/The-Future-of-Nursing/Future%20of%20Nursing%202010%20Recommendations.pdf

Kangasniemi, M., Vaismoradi, M., Jasper, M., & Turunen, H. (2013). Ethical issues in patient safety: Implications for nursing management. *Nursing Ethics, 20*(8), 904–916.

By permission. From *Merriam-Webster's Online Dictionary* (n.d.) (11th ed.). Commitment. Retrieved from www.merriam-webster.com/dictionary/commitment

Papastavrou, E., Efstathiou, G., Tsangari, H., Suhonen, R., Leino-Kilpi, H., Patiraki, E., . . . Merkouris, A. (2012). A cross-cultural study of the concept of caring through behaviours: Patients' and nurses' perspectives in six different EU countries. *Journal of Advanced Nursing, 68*(5), 1026–1037.

Riffkin, R. (2014). *Americans rate nurses highest on honesty, ethical standards*. Retrieved from http://www.gallup.com/poll/180260/americans-rate-nurses-highest-honesty-ethical-standards.aspx

Spector, P. E., Zhou, Z. E., & Che, X. X. (2014). Nurse exposure to physical and nonphysical violence, bullying, and sexual harassment: A quantitative review. *International Journal of Nursing Studies, 51*(1), 72–84.

Stringfellow, S. (2016). Promoting professional behavior. *Vanderbilt University Medical Center*. Retrieved from http://www.mc.vanderbilt.edu/root/vumc.php?site=nurse-wellness&doc=40086

Via Christi Regional Medical Center. (2003). *Survey on professionalism*. Retrieved from www.via-christi.org/workfiles/Professionalism%20in%20Nursing.ppt

Walrafen, N., Brewer, K., & Mulvenon, C. (2012). Sadly caught up in the moment: An exploration of horizontal violence. *Nursing Economics, 30*(1), 6–12, 49.

Wyatt, R. M. (2013). *Revisiting disruptive and inappropriate behavior: Five years after standards introduced*. Retrieved from http://www.jointcommission.org/jc_physician_blog/revisiting_disruptive_and_inappropriate_behavior/

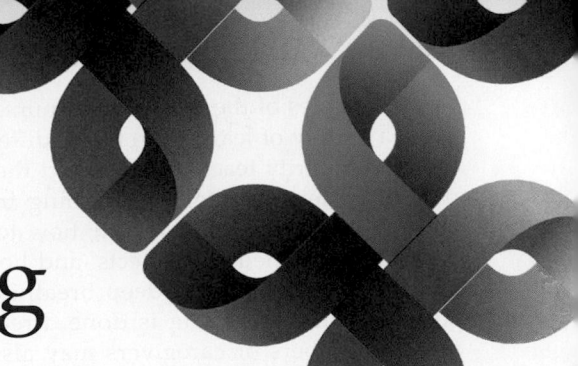

Module 41
Teaching and Learning

Module Outline and Learning Outcomes

≫ The Concept of Teaching and Learning

Concept Key Terms

Adherence, **2664**	Compliance, **2664**	Feedback, **2666**	Modeling, **2665**	Social learning theory, **2665**
Adult learning theory, **2665**	Constructivist theory, **2665**	Learning, **2661**	Observational learning, **2665**	Teaching, **2661**
Behaviorist theory, **2665**	E-health, **2671**	Learning need, **2664**	Positive reinforcement, **2665**	Theory of multiple intelligences, **2665**
Cognitive theory, **2665**	Emotional intelligence, **2665**	Mentors, **2662**		

Teaching is a system of activities designed to produce learning. **Learning** is a change in human disposition or capability that persists and cannot be solely accounted for by growth. Broadly speaking, learning is represented by a change in behavior; in other words, the learner is able to apply or demonstrate what is learned. Some additional attributes of learning are described in **Box 41–1 ≫**.

Box 41–1
Attributes of Learning

Learning is:

- An experience that occurs within the learner
- The discovery of the personal meaning and relevance of ideas
- A consequence of experience
- A collaborative and cooperative process
- An evolutionary process that builds on past learning and experiences
- A process that is both intellectual and emotional

The teaching–learning process involves dynamic interaction between teacher and learner. Each participant in the process communicates information, emotions, perceptions, and attitudes to the other person. Because nurses constantly gather information from and provide information to patients and other individuals, they require a clear understanding of the roles of teacher and learner alike.

This concept takes an in-depth look at the teaching–learning process and the nurse's responsibility as a patient and family educator. In doing so, it examines major domains and theories of learning as well as factors that affect an individual's ability to learn. The concept concludes with a discussion of ways in which nurses can use their knowledge of the teaching–learning process to design more successful patient and family education activities.

Nurses as Teachers and Learners
Nurses as Teachers

The American Nurses Association (ANA) Standards of Practice for Registered Nurses (2010) identify teaching as one of the many roles of the professional nurse. Although nurses teach a variety of learners in many different settings, most nurses primarily teach patients and their families. Examples of patient and family teaching include instruction about how to perform self-care; how to take medications and recognize their side effects; and how to perform prescribed treatments (e.g., deep breathing and coughing). Although most teaching is done directly with patients, family members or caregivers may also be instructed in care of the patient. This is especially important for those patients who have difficulty performing self-care. For example, parents who need to give medication to their children must be instructed in the proper administration of that medication. Patients with diabetes who have visual impairments may need assistance when administering insulin or when assessing their feet and lower extremities for skin breakdown. When teaching patients about diet, it is important to include the person who purchases and prepares the food.

In addition to teaching patients and their families, nurses teach professional colleagues and other healthcare personnel in academic settings such as vocational schools, colleges, and universities, as well as in healthcare facilities such as hospitals or nursing homes. Teaching occurs through a variety of formal and informal encounters, including mentoring, continuing education classes, and clinical experiences for nursing students. **Box 41–2 》** describes the mentoring relationship among nurses.

A number of factors affect the ways in which nurses teach patients and others in the healthcare system. Federal and state regulations influence what content should be taught and indicate what documentation is required of nursing schools, certifying agencies, and agencies employing and training nurses and other healthcare professionals. Nurses who provide patient education do so for individuals who vary in age, cultural and socioeconomic background, primary language, and previous knowledge and experience. Information is constantly changing as new research becomes available. Today's resources are numerous and readily available through the internet. These factors combine to make providing patients with accurate, current information a challenge for nurses.

Nurses as Learners

The field of nursing requires that its members be not only teachers, but also learners. Before entering the profession, all aspiring nurses must complete formal education programs that teach them effective beginning nursing skills. Furthermore, because changes occur quickly and often in healthcare, nurses must continue learning to keep their knowledge current. The ANA Standards of Professional Performance recognize this (Standard 8, Education), and each state's board of nursing outlines continuing education requirements designed to increase nurses' knowledge and skill (ANA, 2010).

To help nurses maintain their licenses and ensure quality of care, many employers provide continuing education programs at the work site, although some nurses may need to travel to specialized centers to gain advanced skills. In addition, many nurses return to school to obtain advanced degrees in nursing and other health-related disciplines.

Concepts Related to Teaching and Learning

The concepts of development, communication, health, wellness, and illness are directly related to the concepts of teaching and learning. Nurses must understand various theories of psychosocial development and basic principles of

Box 41–2
Mentoring

Mentoring is an important career development tool for nurses in any setting or specialty. **Mentors** are experienced nurses who coach, advise, and support the personal and professional growth of a less-experienced or novice mentee or protégé in a professional relationship by discussing mutual goals and providing accountability (Hnatiuk, 2012). Fortunately, modern technology provides more opportunities for mentoring via the internet and other rapid communication methods when the protégé is not physically in the same location as the mentor.

Often, the mentor relationship is one of teacher–learner. The mentor instructs the protégé in her expected role, introduces the protégé to individuals important to the achievement of her goals, helps the protégé evaluate new ideas, and challenges the protégé to advance her professional practice. Mentor programs are important for both student nurses and newly graduated nurses when transitioning from the role of a student into the role of a professional nurse. Mentoring is also important for professional development in nursing administration and nursing education and when nurses enter a new position (Hnatiuk, 2012; McCallum, Lamont, & Kerr, 2016; Rush et al., 2012).

Nurse mentor programs also benefit the nursing profession as a whole. Transitioning to practice can affect a new nurse's job satisfaction, job retention, and stress levels, as well as patient safety (National Council of State Boards of Nursing [NCSBN], 2016; Spector et al., 2015). Hospitals with an evidence-based, structured transition-to-practice program have higher job satisfaction, retention, and competency levels. They also have decreased stress and patient care errors among new graduate nurses compared to hospitals without transition-to-practice programs (Spector et al., 2015).

The mentoring relationship requires work and time from both the mentor and protégé. Some mentoring relationships have negative effects, including power struggles, intimidation, and loyalty issues. Nurses should recognize their individual strengths and encourage excellence in one another rather than feeling intimidated by each other. Employees must feel safe in their workplace, and a commitment to improving intrapersonal and interpersonal communication among nurses should provide a safe learning environment and encourage growth. Mindful creation of collaborative work environments is an essential task of nurse leaders (Warshawsky, Havens, & Knafl, 2012). Such environments help nurses unite and support each other, which helps ensure safety and excellence in nursing practice.

communication to create effective teaching plans and transmit information appropriate to each patient's level of understanding. Combining psychologic theories such as Erik Erikson's stages of psychosocial development, Jean Piaget's phases of cognitive development, and John B. Watson's behaviorism theory will provide direction and explanations for a fundamental understanding of mental, emotional, and social development during the lifespan. Similarly, cultural competency has become increasingly relevant for nurses providing teaching and therapeutic communication to diverse populations and in diverse settings. Educational materials and care plans must be patient specific and written after all aspects of a patient's cultural, mental, and physical status are assessed.

Knowledge of basic principles of teaching and learning is crucial because nurses empower individuals to lead healthier lives. Teaching and promoting general health principles such as good nutrition practices, illness and infection prevention, and safety measures are among the primary roles and responsibilities of nurses as patient advocates and, in some cases, professional educators of colleagues. Education empowers individuals to be active participants in their healthcare and promotes individual recovery, self-control, and personal responsibility for health and well-being. Some, but not all, of the concepts that are integral to teaching and learning are outlined in the Concepts Related to Teaching and Learning feature. They are presented in alphabetical order.

Concepts Related to
Teaching and Learning

CONCEPT	RELATIONSHIP TO TEACHING AND LEARNING	NURSING IMPLICATIONS
Communication	Teaching and learning processes require nurses and patients alike to engage in verbal, nonverbal, and written communication.	■ Use various elements of verbal communication—including pace, intonation, clarity, credibility, timing, relevance, and humor—in ways that are appropriate and help promote desired learning outcomes. ■ Effectively employ different elements of nonverbal communication, including posture, appearance, facial expressions, and gestures. ■ Create, distribute, and recommend written communication items (e.g., handouts, computer programs, mobile device apps) that are reflective of patients' literacy levels.
Culture and Diversity	Understanding and appreciating cultural diversity will encourage and promote trusting, interactive communication in patient care and interprofessional relationships.	■ Evaluate personal attitudes and beliefs regarding cultural diversity. ■ Recognize and consider patients' cultural background when planning care. ■ Coordinate interprofessional participation for resources such as interpreters or social and faith-based services to meet patients' culture-specific needs.
Development	As children develop, their learning abilities become more complex. As adults age, their vision, hearing, and motor function may become impaired. They may also experience declines in cognitive functioning.	■ Assess patient's age and developmental stage. ■ Use teaching methods appropriate to the patient's age and level of development. ■ Be aware that age does not always indicate specific developmental characteristics.
Health, Wellness, Illness, and Injury	Knowledge empowers individuals to make lifestyle choices that promote health and may prevent illness and injury.	■ Educate patients to be effective healthcare consumers. ■ Reinforce healthy patient behaviors. ■ Guide patients in problem solving health-related issues.
Nutrition	Understanding basic nutritional requirements and food preparation guidelines can help individuals promote health, prevent illness, and manage existing disease processes.	■ Promote the importance of a balanced diet for disease prevention. ■ Provide information and teaching on specific diets related to disease management. ■ Provide referrals to a nutritionist or dietitian.
Safety	Knowledge of safe practices can help both patients and healthcare personnel avoid accidents and injury.	■ Assess patient's level of safety and risk for injury related to the environment. ■ Evaluate safety risks related to patient's cognitive and/or physical development. ■ Provide information about and teach basic safety precautions.

The Art of Teaching

Teaching is a system of activities intentionally designed to produce specific learning. It is a goal-directed activity that results in improved learning for the learner. Teaching is more than giving information; the art of teaching lies in creating a learning environment that helps the learner cultivate knowledge, skills, and an internal desire to change some aspect of his or her life. Just as care plans are patient specific, teaching plans should also be specific to each learner. This means the nurse must carefully evaluate and consider the learning capabilities and preferences of each individual, remembering that even people within the same cultural or social group will have their own distinct learning styles.

Nurses should also recognize when patients misinterpret health teaching, or when the patient's health education needs are beyond the nurse's scope of practice or specialty knowledge base. Quality teaching requires knowledge, an understanding of the learning process, good judgment, and a sense of intuition. Most importantly, it encourages learners to be actively involved and accountable in the learning process. For a more complete description of the characteristics of effective teaching, refer to **Box 41–3** »».

SAFETY ALERT Safe, effective teaching relies on the nurse's knowledge of the subject matter. Inaccurate or incomplete knowledge may result in the patient receiving incorrect information about a condition or treatment and may compromise the patient's safety.

The relationship between teacher and learner is essentially one of trust and respect. The learner trusts that the teacher has the knowledge and skill to teach, and the teacher respects the learner's ability to attain the recognized goals. Once a nurse starts to instruct a patient or other learner, it is important that the teaching process continue until the participants achieve the mutually agreed-upon learning goals, change the goals, or decide that the goals cannot be met.

As teachers, nurses must understand a number of learning theories. By understanding how people learn and the factors that impact learning, nurses can develop more successful teaching plans for individual patients and their families, as well as for various groups of learners.

Aspects of Learning

Individuals have a variety of learning needs. A **learning need** is a desire or requirement to know something that is currently unknown to the learner. Learning needs may include new knowledge or information, a new or different skill or physical ability, a new behavior, or a need to change an old behavior.

One important aspect of learning is compliance, or the individual's desire to learn and to act on that learning. In the healthcare context, **compliance** refers to the extent to which an individual's behavior coincides with medical or health advice. Compliance is best illustrated when the individual accepts the need to learn, then follows through with appropriate actions that reflect the learning. For example, a patient who is diagnosed with diabetes would be compliant if he willingly learned about the recommended special diet, then followed that diet. However, many people view the term *compliance* negatively because it implies the learner is submissive, and submission conflicts with the learner's right to make his or her own healthcare decisions. At the same time, some professionals are too quick to label a patient as noncompliant. It is important to determine why a patient is not following a recommended course of action before applying this label. For example, a patient may have intended to comply with a prescription regimen but was unable to do so because he could not afford the cost of the medications.

A related aspect of learning described in healthcare literature is **adherence**, or attachment to a prescribed regimen. Modern healthcare promotes and encourages patients to be committed, active participants in maintaining personal health and wellness. According to Maningat, Gordon, and Breslow (2013), "Compliance suggests that the patient is passively following the physician's orders, while adherence acknowledges that the patient is part of the decision-making process" (p. 2). Adherence identifies the level of a patient's behavioral patterns in response to mutually agreed-upon healthcare providers' teaching and treatment recommendations (Centers for Disease Control and Prevention [CDC], 2013). When evaluating responses and results of treatment plans, nurses may use the terms *adherence* and *compliance* interchangeably. Although both terms convey the same general concept, adherence has more positive connotations and emphasizes the collaborative nature of the patient–provider relationship (van den Bemt, Zwikker, & van den Ende, 2012). The term *adherence* also recognizes that factors other than patient willingness to comply (e.g., financial considerations) may affect the treatment process.

Learning Theories

A number of different theories can help nurses understand the ways in which people learn. Adult learning theory, behaviorist theory, cognitive theory, social learning theory, and

---

Box 41–3
Characteristics of Effective Teaching

Effective Teaching

- Holds the learner's interest.
- Involves the learner in the learning process, and creates a partnership between the learner and the teacher.
- Fosters a positive self-concept in the learner such that he or she believes that learning is possible and probable.
- Is appropriate for the learner's age, condition, and abilities.
- Sets realistic goals directed at helping learners meet their objectives.
- Supports the learner with optimistic, positive reinforcement and feedback.
- Uses accurate and current evidence-based information from reliable sources.
- Uses several methods of teaching to accommodate a variety of learning styles, and provides learning opportunities through hearing, seeing, and doing.
- Uses methods to evaluate learning.
- Is cost effective (i.e., the cost of the nurse's time spent teaching is less than the cost of treating health problems that occur when patients do not follow recommended treatments, fail to take medications correctly, or do not adapt their lifestyle to changing health needs).

TABLE 41–1 Major Learning Theories and Their Implications for the Teaching Process

Learning Theory	Summary	Implications for Teaching
Adult learning theory	Adult learners differ from child learners in fundamental ways. In particular, adults: ■ Need to know why they should learn something. ■ Prefer that others treat them as capable of self-direction. ■ Have accumulated life experiences that can enhance their current learning. ■ Are often ready to learn what they must know in order to take care of themselves.	When providing teaching to adult patients or caregivers, communicate how and/or why information is important and useful. Respect the learner as an independent, competent adult. Identify previous experiences and help the learner scaffold or incorporate new information with previous experiences.
Behaviorist theory	Learning occurs when an individual's response to a stimulus is either positively or negatively reinforced. It is possible to change an individual's behavior by either altering the stimulus condition or altering what happens after the individual responds to the stimulus. Providing **positive reinforcement**, or a pleasant experience such as praise and encouragement, is especially useful in fostering repetition of an action.	Provide praise or encouragement with each attempt or at each phase of the learning process. Allow sufficient time for the learner to practice new skills (e.g., return demonstrations). Consider environmental influences that affect the learning process.
Cognitive theory	Learning involves three mental processes that can occur sequentially or simultaneously: (1) acquiring information, (2) processing the information, and (3) using the information. An individual's capacity to learn is shaped by his or her developmental level as well as by the social, emotional, and physical contexts in which learning takes place. Learning occurs across three primary domains: the cognitive (or "thinking") domain, the affective (or "feeling") domain, and the psychomotor (or "skill") domain.	Develop appropriate strategies to meet each learner's unique learning style and preferences. Assess each learner's developmental stage and emotional readiness to learn, then adapt teaching strategies to the learner's level. Select behavioral objectives and teaching strategies that encompass the cognitive, affective, and psychomotor domains of learning.
Constructivist theory	Learning is a developmental process constructed from individual experiences. Knowledge acquisition is the ongoing assimilation and accommodation of new experiences and interpretations. Cooperative learning and problem-solving in collaboration with others promote learning.	Acknowledge the importance of and build on the learner's prior learning experiences. Encourage the learner to engage with the nurse and others during the learning process.
Social learning theory	Learning primarily results from instruction and **observational learning**, or the process of acquiring new skills or altering old behaviors by watching other people. This process focuses on imitation and **modeling**. The cognitive aspect of social learning theory suggests that an individual's beliefs, perceptions, and cognitive competencies influence the way in which the individual interacts with the environment.	By modeling how to perform skills (such as changing a wound dressing) and asking for repeat demonstrations until the patient can perform the skill satisfactorily, the nurse provides an opportunity for imitation and modeling.

Sources: Data from Bloom, B. S. (Ed.). (1956). *Taxonomy of education objectives. Book 1: Cognitive domain.* New York, NY: Longman; Bruner, J. (1966). *Toward a theory of instruction.* Cambridge, MA: Harvard University Press; Candela, L. (2012). From teaching to learning: Theoretical foundations. In *Teaching in nursing: A guide for faculty* (4th ed., pp. 202–243). St. Louis, MO: Elsevier Saunders; Knowles, M. S., Holton, E. F., & Swanson, R. A. (2005). *The adult learner* (6th ed.). Burlington, MA: Elsevier Butterworth-Heinemann (original work published 1973).

humanistic learning theory are among the theories most commonly used by nurses when teaching individuals and groups of learners. Additional concepts that the nurse should keep in mind when formulating teaching plans include the theories of categorization and constructivism. **Table 41–1 》** provides a brief description of these theories and highlights some ways nurses can apply each theory in the teaching process.

In addition to the learning theories discussed in the table, nurses should understand the **theory of multiple intelligences**. This theory was presented by researcher Howard Gardner and is based on observations of the ways in which stroke damage can impact one area of the brain while leaving other areas of mental functioning intact. Initially, Gardner (1983) cited seven intelligences:

1. Linguistic
2. Musical/rhythmic (music)
3. Logical/mathematical
4. Spatial (visual)
5. Kinesthetic/movement (body)
6. Personal
7. Symbols as intellectual strengths or ways of knowing

Gardner has since added an eighth intelligence, naturalist intelligence, which is associated with recognition of environmental elements and patterns (Candela, 2012).

Gardner's work is one of several theories that challenge the notion that intelligence is static and is solely based on the learner's intelligence quotient, or IQ, which is a score derived from standardized tests. Another important theory that disputes the concept of IQ was put forth by researcher Daniel Goleman. Goleman (1995) proposed that **emotional intelligence**—or EQ—is as relevant to learning and success as IQ, or even more so. EQ measures individuals' abilities to differentiate between their own thoughts and feelings, recognize the thoughts and feelings of others, and show discernment when using emotions to influence decisions.

It is important for nurses to understand the focus and limitations of the various learning theories, as well as Gardner's and Goleman's theories. Intelligence levels are unique and specific to every person, and individuals can exhibit one or more intelligences at higher operant levels than the others. By knowing the various theories, the nurse can select the most appropriate theory or theories when developing a teaching plan for a specific patient.

Clinical Example A

Patrick Johnson is a 60-year-old man who owns a small business. Mr. Johnson underwent coronary bypass surgery (CABG) 3 days ago after experiencing a myocardial infarction at his retail store. He is scheduled for hospital discharge within the next 48 hours. The nurse responsible for Mr. Johnson's care and discharge planning notes that the healthcare provider has ordered several new medications, as well as dietary restrictions and follow-up appointments.

Mr. Johnson is used to working 7 days per week. He lives with his 56-year-old wife, who occasionally helps at the store but also works as a part-time substitute teacher. The Johnsons have two grown children who are married and reside out of state. Mr. Johnson states that he is very worried that his business (and therefore his income) will decline due to his recent health problems and potential lifestyle changes.

Critical Thinking Questions

1. Discuss the impact of Mr. Johnson's recent health impairment and stated concerns on his ability to "learn," and apply information based on the cognitive and psychomotor domains of learning. What factors might hinder Mr. Johnson's ability to learn? Do any real and/or potential factors exist to promote his learning?

2. Is teaching a priority of care for Mr. Johnson at this time? Why or why not?

Factors Affecting Learning

Many factors can facilitate or inhibit a patient's ability to learn, including stress level, effects of medication, fatigue, or pain. The nurse should be aware of these factors, particularly when available teaching time is limited.

Factors That Facilitate Learning

A number of factors promote learning. Although these factors are common to all people, how they promote learning in the individual learner will vary. What motivates one individual to learn, for example, may not motivate another individual at all.

- **Motivation:** Motivation to learn is personal and affects how much an individual learns. It can also influence the rate of learning. Motivation must be identified and experienced by the patient—the nurse's recognition of a need is not sufficient to motivate a patient, although the nurse can help the patient identify and embrace the need. Furthermore, the nurse can help persuade support people that a need exists by providing information and/or reminding the patient how his behaviors affect the people around him. For example, a man who has smoked for 20 years may not embrace the need to quit for the benefit of his own health. However, if the nurse provides patient education that includes the dangers of secondhand smoke, especially to young children, the man may recognize the need to quit smoking for the benefit of a child or grandchild.

- **Readiness:** Readiness to learn refers to an individual's demonstration of behaviors or cues that reflect her motivation to learn at a specific time. Readiness reflects not only the desire or willingness to learn, but also the ability to learn. The nurse's role is often to encourage the development of readiness. For example, a patient may want to learn self-care during a dressing change, but if the patient is experiencing pain or discomfort, she may not be able to

learn. In this case, the nurse can provide pain medication to make the patient more comfortable and ready to learn.

- **Active Involvement:** When a learner is actively involved in the process of learning, learning becomes more meaningful. If the learner actively participates in planning and discussion, he will learn more quickly and retain more information. Active learning promotes critical thinking, enabling learners to solve problems more effectively. Patients who are actively involved in learning about their healthcare may be more able to apply that learning to their own situation. For example, patients who are actively involved in learning about their therapeutic diets may be more able to apply the principles being taught to their cultural food preferences and usual eating habits. Passive learning, such as listening to a lecture or watching a film, does not foster optimal learning.

- **Relevance:** Patients learn more quickly and retain more information when what they are learning is personally relevant to them. It also helps when they can connect the new knowledge to things they already know or have experienced. For example, if a patient is diagnosed with hypertension, is overweight, and has symptoms of headaches and fatigue, he is more likely to understand the need to lose weight if he remembers having more energy when he weighed less. The nurse needs to validate the relevance of learning with the patient throughout the learning process.

- **Feedback:** Feedback is information regarding an individual's performance in relation to a desired goal. To be effective, feedback must be meaningful to the learner. Nurses can provide either positive or negative feedback when teaching patients. Positive feedback or reinforcement may include praise, positively worded corrections, and gently worded suggestions of alternative methods, all of which encourage patients to continue engaging in a desired behavior. In contrast, negative feedback, including ridicule, anger, or sarcasm, can lead people to withdraw from learning. Such feedback, viewed as a type of punishment, may cause the patient to avoid the teacher in order to avoid punishment.

- **Nonjudgmental Support:** People learn best when they believe they are accepted and will not be judged. The individual who expects to be judged as a "poor" or "good" patient will not learn as well as the individual who feels no such threat. Once learners have succeeded in accomplishing a task or understanding a concept, they gain self-confidence in their ability to learn. This confidence reduces their anxiety about failure and can motivate greater learning.

For example, when a nurse cares for a patient who did not graduate from high school, she should independently assess the patient's ability to learn and not make a judgment about the patient's ability based on education level. Completing high school is an indication of the patient's level of formal education, not an indication of the patient's intellect or ability to learn. The patient may be highly intelligent and self-taught, but the nurse will not know this unless she begins by assessing the patient's ability to learn.

- **Information That Proceeds from Simple to Complex:** Learning is facilitated by material that is logically organized and proceeds from the simple to the complex. Such organization enables the learner to comprehend new information, assimilate it with previous learning, and form new understandings. Of course, *simple* and *complex* are relative terms, depending on the level at which a person is learning. What is simple for one person may be complex for another.

- **Repetition:** Repetition of key concepts and facts facilitates retention of newly learned material. Similarly, practicing psychomotor skills (particularly with feedback from the nurse) improves an individual's performance of those skills and facilitates their transfer to other settings.

- **Timing:** People retain information and psychomotor skills best when there is a short time interval between learning and using what they have learned; the longer the time interval, the easier it is for people to forget new skills and information. For example, a patient who is only shown literature and videos about administering insulin but is not permitted to administer his own insulin until discharge from the hospital is unlikely to remember what he learned. However, giving his own injections while in the hospital (and with feedback from the nurse) enhances the patient's learning.

- **Environment:** An optimal learning environment facilitates learning by reducing distractions and providing physical and psychologic comfort. It has adequate lighting that is free from glare, a comfortable room temperature, and good ventilation. Most students know what it is like to try to learn in a hot, stuffy room; the consequent drowsiness interferes with concentration. Noise can also distract the student and interfere with listening and thinking. To facilitate learning in a hospital setting, nurses should choose a time when no visitors are present and interruptions are unlikely.

  In some situations, privacy during the learning process is essential. For example, when a patient is learning to change a colostomy bag, the presence of others can be embarrassing and thus interfere with learning. However, when a patient is particularly anxious, having a support person present may give the patient confidence.

Clinical Example B

Angela Simpson, a 22-year-old woman, recently gave birth to her first child, and she is eager to learn how to safely care for her newborn. Angela believes that babies should sleep on their stomachs (prone position), and she has grown up observing family members, including her own mother, use this position with her younger siblings at naps and bedtime. As Angela's nurse, you know that evidence-based research discourages this tradition, because stomach sleeping is linked to an increased risk for sudden infant death syndrome (SIDS). You also note that Angela is currently staying with her mother (the baby's grandmother), who is actively involved in caring for her grandchildren.

Critical Thinking Questions

When developing a plan for teaching infant care to this mother:

1. What essential information would you want Ms. Simpson to learn?
2. How could you assess Ms. Simpson's motivation to apply this information?
3. In what setting would Ms. Simpson be most likely to learn and retain the information?

Factors That Inhibit Learning

Many factors can inhibit patient learning. Some of the most common barriers to learning are described in **Table 41–2 》**. Several of these barriers are described below:

- **Emotions:** Emotions such as fear, anger, and depression can impede learning. Similarly, high levels of anxiety can result in agitation and an inability to focus or concentrate, thereby also inhibiting learning. Patients or families who are experiencing extreme emotional states may not hear spoken words or may retain only part of the communication. However, emotional responses such as fear and anxiety decrease with information that relieves uncertainty. In some cases, patients (and perhaps even families) who are extremely distraught may be prescribed medications in order to reduce their anxiety and put them in an emotional state in which learning can occur.

- **Physiologic Events:** Physiologic events such as critical illness, pain, or sensory deficits inhibit learning. Because the patient cannot concentrate and apply energy to learning, the learning process itself is impaired. For this reason, the nurse should try to reduce the patient's physiologic barriers to learning as much as possible before teaching. For patients who are experiencing a physiologic event, analgesics and rest before teaching may be helpful.

- **Cultural Aspects:** Cultural barriers to learning arise when the patient's language, beliefs, or values are different from those of the healthcare team. The most obvious barrier is language: A patient who does not understand the nurse's language may learn very little. Another impediment to learning is differences between the values held by the patient and those held by the healthcare team. Western medicine also may conflict with a patient's cultural healing beliefs and practices. To be effective, nurses must be culturally competent; otherwise, patients may be partially or totally noncompliant with recommended treatments.

- **Psychomotor Ability:** Nurses should be aware of patients' psychomotor ability when planning teaching. Psychomotor skills can be affected by health. For example, an older patient who has severe osteoarthritis of the hands may not be able to wrap a bandage. The following physical abilities are especially important for learning psychomotor skills:

  - **Muscle strength.** Patients must possess the strength necessary to carry out a new skill. For example, an older patient who cannot rise from a chair because of insufficient leg and muscle strength cannot be expected to learn to lift herself out of a bathtub.

  - **Motor coordination.** Gross motor coordination is required for movements such as walking, whereas fine motor coordination is needed for tasks like eating with utensils. For example, a patient who has advanced amyotrophic lateral sclerosis involving the lower limbs will probably be unable to use a walker.

  - **Energy.** Patients need energy for most psychomotor skills—and learning these skills requires even more energy. People who are ill or older often have limited energy resources. Therefore, nurses should schedule the teaching and practice of new skills for times when patients' energy levels are at their peak.

TABLE 41–2 Barriers to Learning

Barrier	Explanation	Nursing Implications
Acute illness	Patient requires all resources and energy to cope with illness.	Defer teaching until patient is less ill.
Pain	Pain decreases the ability to concentrate.	Conduct pain assessment before teaching.
Prognosis	Patient can be preoccupied with illness and unable to concentrate on new information.	Defer teaching to a better time.
Biorhythms	Mental and physical performances have a circadian rhythm.	Adapt time of teaching to suit patient's circadian rhythms. For example, plan a teaching session during the part of the day when the patient is most alert.
Emotions (e.g., anxiety, denial, depression, or grief)	Emotions require energy and distract from learning.	Deal with emotions and possible misinformation prior to providing patient teaching.
Language	Patient may not be fluent in the nurse's language.	Obtain the services of an interpreter or nurse with appropriate language skills.
Older adults	Vision, hearing, and motor control can be impaired in older adults.	Consider possible sensory and motor deficits, and adapt the teaching plan as needed.
Children	Children have a shorter attention span and different vocabulary than adult patients.	Plan shorter and more active learning episodes.
Culture/religion	A patient's culture and/or religion may place restrictions on certain types of knowledge (e.g., birth control information).	Assess the patient's cultural and/or religious needs when planning learning activities.
Physical disability	Visual, hearing, sensory, or motor impairments may interfere with a patient's ability to learn.	Plan teaching activities appropriate to the learner's physical abilities. For example, provide audio learning tools for a patient who is blind or large-print materials for a patient whose vision is impaired.
Mental disability	Impaired cognitive ability may affect a patient's capacity for learning.	Assess patient's capacity for learning. Plan teaching activities to complement the patient's ability while also planning more complex learning for the patient's caregivers.

- **Sensory acuity.** Sight is vital to the learning and completion of many psychomotor tasks, such as walking with crutches, changing a dressing, or drawing a medication into a syringe. Thus, patients who have a visual impairment often need the assistance of a support person to carry out such tasks.

Clinical Example C

Margaret Kim, a 36-year-old woman, is being transferred from the hospital to a long-term care facility to recover following a motor vehicle crash. Ms. Kim sustained multiple fractures resulting in partial paralysis on her right side. She and the nurse planned a learning session at 1:00 p.m. to discuss wound care and medications for post-hospitalization treatment and care. At 1:00 p.m., the nurse comes to Ms. Kim's room with supplies and handouts to help Ms. Kim learn. The nurse finds Ms. Kim crying.

Critical Thinking Questions

1. What actions should the nurse take at this time?
2. Can learning take place? Why or why not?
3. Discuss strategies that the nurse could use to enhance Ms. Kim's readiness to learn.

Lifespan Considerations

As individuals progress from infancy to older adulthood, their capacity to learn changes in many different ways. To ensure that their efforts to educate patients are as successful as possible, nurses must carefully assess each patient's level of development before creating a teaching plan. Generally speaking, patients within certain age groups tend to be at similar levels of development, and they often face similar physical, cognitive, and psychosocial factors that impact learning. A comprehensive discussion of these levels and factors and how they affect the nursing process (including patient teaching efforts) is provided in the module on Development. In addition, the following sections highlight some of the most important points to keep in mind when planning and delivering teaching to patients at various stages throughout the lifespan.

Teaching Children

Children are constantly developing new cognitive and motor skills and becoming increasingly purposeful when interacting with their environment. Therefore, when developing a teaching plan for a pediatric patient, the nurse must first assess the child's level of development. Teaching plans for patients in this age group typically focus on primary healthcare, health promotion, and illness/injury prevention. In most cases, the teaching plan should be directed toward the parent or primary caregiver; however, the nurse must include the child in the teaching and provide basic instructions at the child's level of understanding.

To ensure successful outcomes, seek to establish trust by addressing the child by name. Be sure all teaching interventions are implemented in a safe environment using a calm approach, and take care to address any concerns or fears of the child or parent/caregiver. Allow time for questions and practice if the teaching involves patient or caregiver performance of a skill or task. When appropriate, use props to demonstrate treatment procedures

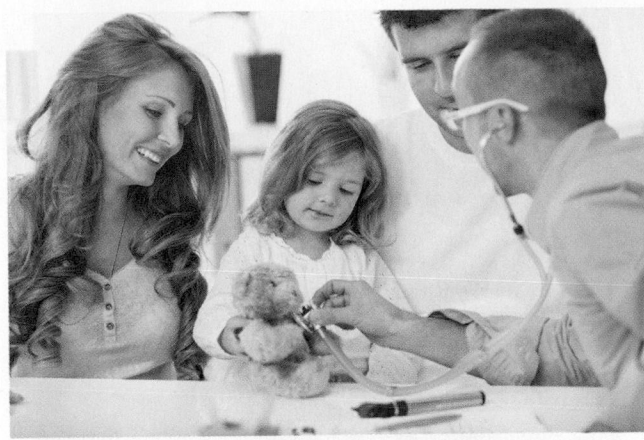

Source: Vgajic/iStock/Getty Images.

Figure 41–1 ≫ This preschooler is holding a teddy bear that the nurse "examined" first to show the child what to expect.

(**Figure 41–1 ≫**). Always provide feedback, praise, and encouragement; evaluate the effectiveness of the teaching/learning experience; reinforce teaching as needed; and document the intervention (Ball et al., 2017). See the Patient Teaching feature for tools to use when teaching children.

Teaching Adolescents

Adolescents experience many cognitive, moral, and physical changes as part of the transition from childhood to adulthood. Interpersonal communication, development of trusting relationships, and increased independence are of primary importance to patients in this age group. Health alterations can deeply affect personal identity, including feelings of well-being and perceptions of body image, and may carry long-term effects.

Before constructing a teaching plan for an adolescent patient, assess the patient's level of development and independence from parents and caregivers. During the teaching session, acknowledge and show respect for the patient's fears and feelings, and strive to provide a calm environment. Involving adolescents in the teaching effort facilitates a trusting relationship between the nurse and the patient and is essential for successful teaching. Teaching and health promotion for adolescent patients should focus on safety, consequences, and personal responsibility due to environmental influences that may involve peer pressure and risk-taking behavior. As with younger patients, allow time for questions and practice if teaching involves performance of a skill or task, and provide feedback, praise, and encouragement. Always evaluate the effectiveness of the learning and teaching, reinforce teaching as needed, and document the intervention (**Figure 41–3 ≫**).

Teaching Adults

An individual's critical thinking skills, cognitive development, and learning styles or preferences are influenced by personal experience and may change over a lifetime. Accordingly, before teaching, the nurse must seek to determine the adult patient's unique learning preferences, even if the nurse has worked with the patient in the past. In addition,

Patient Teaching
Tools for Teaching Children

- **Visits.** Have children visit the hospital and treatment rooms so they can see people dressed in uniforms, scrub suits, and protective gear.
- **Dress-up.** Have children touch and dress up in the clothing they will see and wear (**Figure 41–2 ≫**).
- **Coloring books.** Use coloring books to prepare children for treatments, surgery, or hospitalization. These books should show what the rooms, people, and equipment will look like.
- **Storybooks.** Storybooks describe how the child will feel, what will be done, and what the place will look like. Parents can read these stories to children several times before the experience. Younger children like this repetition.
- **Dolls.** To give children a sense of mastery of their situation, have them practice procedures that they will later experience on dolls or teddy bears. Custom dolls are often available for inserting tubes and giving injections.
- **Puppet play.** Puppets can be used in role-play situations to provide information and show the child what an experience will be like. Use of puppets can help the child express emotions.
- **Health fairs.** Health fairs can educate children about their bodies and ways to stay healthy. Fairs can focus on high-risk problems children face, such as accident prevention, poison control, and other topics identified in the community as a concern.

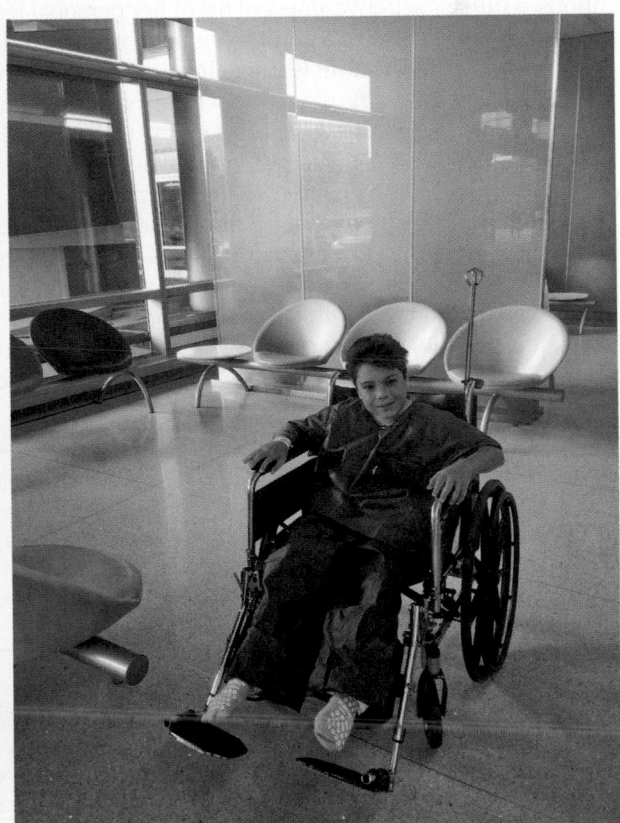

Source: Courtesy of Kelly Block.

Figure 41–2 ≫ Aiden, age 11, visited the hospital in preparation for upcoming surgery. While there, he got to have a wrist band, try on a hospital gown, and use a wheelchair.

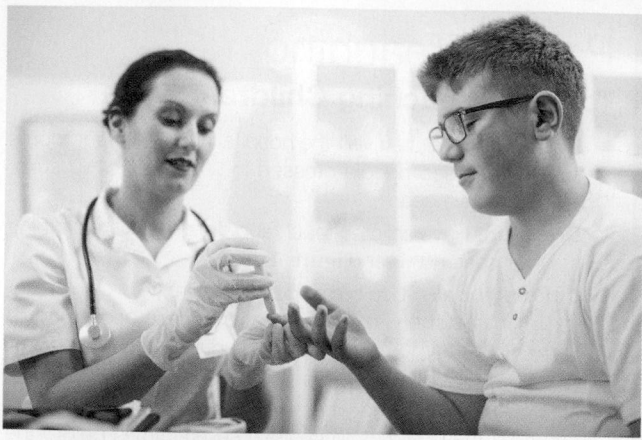

Source: Jovanmandic/iStock/Getty Images.

Figure 41–3 》》 An adolescent with diabetes is learning how to check his blood sugar. The nurse will next provide an opportunity for the patient to try it on his own.

gathering subjective and objective data regarding the patient's personal demands, responsibilities, educational level, cultural influences, and motivation to learn is essential to setting realistic teaching goals and preparing the patient for success.

Because teaching is one of the most critical nursing interventions, a nurse's self-awareness of his or her personal learning style may be helpful when developing individualized patient teaching plans. Adult learners have a "need to know," so it is important for the nurse to allow time for questions and practice if teaching involves return demonstrations of skills or tasks **(Figure 41–4 》》)**. Providing feedback, reassurance, and support promotes a positive learning experience.

Nurses should also emphasize and promote the importance of positive health practices and actively involve patients in their care during patient teaching. However, it is imperative for nurses to remember that adult patients are responsible for their behaviors, and nurses cannot control responses or change patients' habits. Providing knowledge and awareness are the primary goals.

SAFETY ALERT Patient teaching documents are often written above the reading level of the average adult, increasing the potential for negative patient outcomes. Many formulas are available for assessing the reading level of written material, and most word processing programs have a feature that calculates readability. Materials should target a fifth- or sixth-grade level.

Teaching Older Adults

Teaching for older patients primarily focuses on health promotion, disease management, and illness/injury prevention. Many older adults have chronic illnesses that require various medications and therapies, so teaching with regard to these treatments is essential for symptom control and prevention **(Figure 41–5 》》)**. Teaching plans for older adults commonly center on nutrition, physical activity, personal safety, medications, and the need for follow-up healthcare appointments (Bastable, 2014).

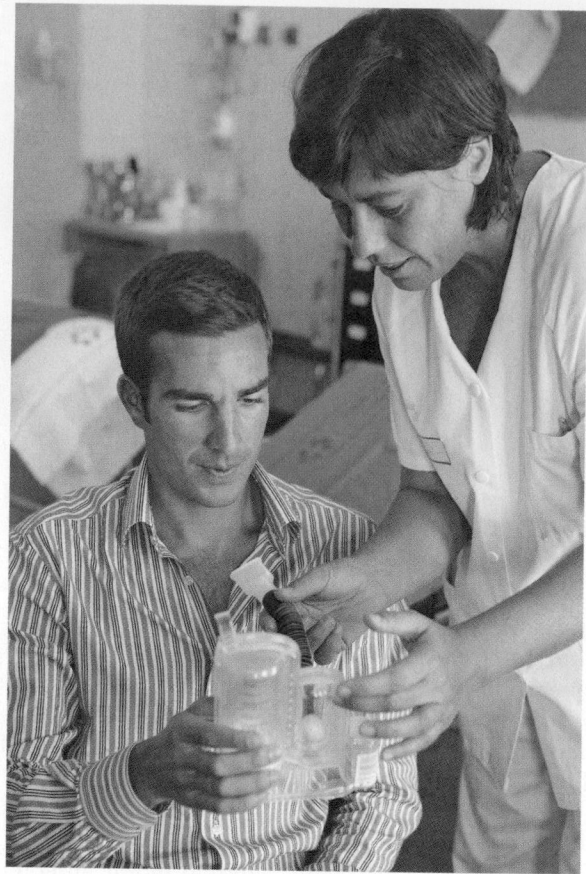

Source: Javier Larrea/age fotostock/Alamy Stock Photo.

Figure 41–4 》》 When teaching adult patients, make sure to answer all their questions so that they understand the need for and benefit from the treatment.

When teaching older adults, nurses must address aging factors that influence comprehension and develop teaching plans that ensure maximal learning can take place. Sensory alterations (especially hearing, vision, and touch), energy level, physical abilities, cultural influences, memory, response time, and stress can all affect an older adult's ability to learn and/or retain information, and they may be significant factors in nonadherence with treatment regimens. Older adults also have past experiences, insight, and knowledge that affect their current attitudes toward healthcare teaching. The nurse should respect older patients and use these past experiences, knowledge, and skills to help them learn.

To maximize learning and establish trust, the nurse must include older adults when developing a teaching plan and setting goals. Moreover, to achieve outcomes specific to older adults, the nurse should allow adequate time for processing information, provide repetition, and include significant others or primary caregivers as necessary. Teaching handouts that are written at a fifth- to sixth-grade reading level and use large (e.g., at least 14-point font) black print on matte paper are practical and effective tools. As with all age groups, the nurse should use a calm approach; create a peaceful environment; allow time for questions and practice if teaching a skill or task; and provide feedback and encouragement. The nurse must also

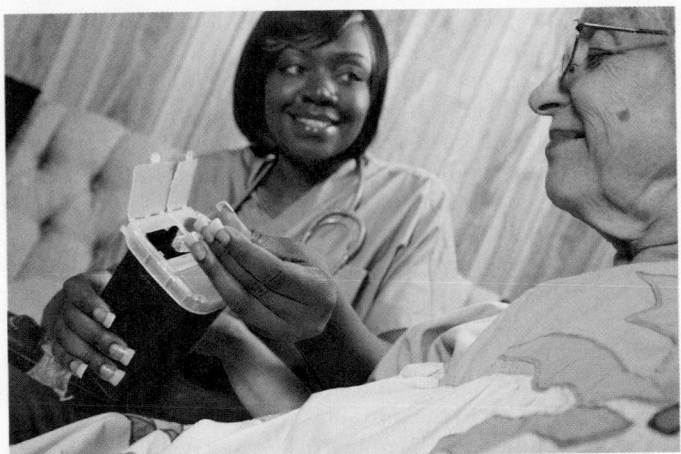

Source: Fstop123/E+/Getty Images.

Figure 41–5 》 A home healthcare nurse demonstrates for an older patient how to properly dispose of unused medication.

evaluate the effectiveness of the teaching and learning, reinforce teaching as needed, and document the intervention (Osborn et al., 2013).

Teaching Patients with Special Needs

The term *special needs* encompasses not only patients with physical, cognitive, and/or developmental impairments, but also patients facing social and environmental issues that affect their health and well-being. When working with a special needs patient, the nurse should perform a complete assessment of the individual's home environment, support systems, and unique level of development prior to any teaching efforts. Later, during teaching, the nurse may need to stress the importance of interprofessional interventions from therapists or medical social workers to ensure that all of the patient's health and wellness needs are met.

Clinical Example D

Lily is an active 5-year-old girl who fell off a swing at the playground, fracturing her left clavicle for the second time in 18 months. The physician tells Lily's mother that CT scans reveal the need for minor surgical correction that will require a 2-day hospital stay. As the nurse prepares to teach both Lily and her mother about the upcoming procedure, Lily begins tearfully asking for her favorite doll "so my booboo can feel better." Lily's mother also verbalizes concern about what her daughter's postsurgical care may require. She is a single working mother with minimal support and another daughter—an 11-year old who she thinks may be too young to stay home with her little sister. She further explains that she cannot afford to take much time off from work.

Critical Thinking Questions
1. What priority actions should the nurse take at this time?
2. Can learning take place? Why or why not?
3. What strategies could the nurse use to enhance Lily's learning and calm her fears?
4. Discuss strategies that the nurse could use to teach and provide reassurance to Lily's mother and address her concerns.

Technology, Health Information, and Patient Teaching

Technology has dramatically transformed many aspects of healthcare, including the ways in which patients and healthcare providers obtain and use health information.

Patients and Online Health Information

The internet in particular has changed the way that patients search for information about medical conditions and treatments on their own. In addition, technology-based tools offer nurses new and innovative methods for working with patients. These tools are part of the **e-health** movement, which focuses on making healthcare resources more accessible to patients by transferring them to electronic media (World Health Organization, 2013a).

The Pew Research Center reports that 87% of American adults use the internet and 72% seek health information online (Pew Research Center, 2014). Many published articles, clinical studies, and scholarly journal publications are available online and through health-related applications. Unfortunately, many websites contain unreliable, questionable, and biased information. Healthcare providers must review online sources carefully to identify those that are reliable. They must also teach patients how to discern trustworthy information from false or potentially dangerous health advice. The following points may be helpful for both nurses and patients who are searching for health information on the internet:

- Consider the author's credentials and whether or not the information is on a personal website or a site sponsored by an organization.
- Review any "About Us," "Philosophy," or "Background" links on the page.
- Look for citations or references documented with footnotes and working links to other sources of information.
- Check the publication or posting date on the page.

Authors with credentials from known and respected universities or organizations are preferable to authors with unknown or questionable credentials. However, information provided on a blog or personal website should be questioned, even if the author appears credible.

Organizational websites should be carefully vetted as well. In general, websites associated with reputable organizations such as the Mayo Clinic, the Cleveland Clinic, or the American Heart Association are reliable, whereas sites associated with private companies promoting medical products should be viewed cautiously. Reputable sites will often acknowledge that the information they provide is not a substitute for professional advice and will encourage individuals to follow up with their healthcare providers. In addition, .gov, and .edu domains are generally reliable sources of health information. The domain .org is generally reserved for nonprofit organizations. The information from nonprofit professional organizations, such as the American Academy of Allergy, Asthma, and Immunology, and nonprofit advocacy organizations, such as the Alzheimer's Association and the National Parkinson

Foundation, is usually helpful and reliable, but caution patients to vet information from sites that are less well known.

Citations and references should be reliable and of high quality. Journal articles, research studies, and documents from the National Institutes of Health (NIH) and the Centers for Disease Control and Prevention (CDC) are examples of quality references; popular nonscientific or "wiki" websites are not. References should be current unless they are classic or foundational studies in a particular field or area of medicine. In general, information published in the past 4 to 5 years can be considered current (HealthIT.gov, 2013). The publication or posting date on the page itself should also be current. (See the Stay Current feature for more about identifying current, reliable web-based health information.)

>> **Stay Current:** The Health on the Net Code of Conduct (HONcode) was established by the Health on the Net Foundation to accredit health related websites for reliability (Health on the Net Foundation, 2016). It has become an important resource for validating ethical, internet-based information. Any health or medical website intended for patients, health professionals, or the general public can request a review in order to receive the HONcode certification of reliability. Once approved, the HONcode logo can be publicly displayed on the website to indicate its credibility. For further information see: Health on the Net Foundation, http://www.hon.ch/HONcode/Patients/Visitor/visitor.html

Incorporating Technology in Patient Teaching

In addition to helping patients become more informed consumers of web-based health information, nurses can use a variety of technologies when teaching patients. The type of technology used will depend on the particular health topic; the resources available; and patients' comfort with, preferences about, and willingness to use technology.

One of the most basic—and simplest—forms of technology in patient teaching is directing patients to specific health-related websites. Before doing so, the nurse must carefully vet websites to ensure that the information is reputable, accurate, and easy to understand. For example, a patient with chronic obstructive pulmonary disease (COPD) might benefit from information and resources available on the American Lung Association's website.

In addition, some hospitals and clinics have e-health portals that enable nurses to print educational information personalized for each patient based on condition and age. These resources may be particularly useful for patients who are not tech-savvy or who prefer to keep printed information on hand. If patients show interest in accessing this information on their own and the portal is structured for patient access, the nurse can also provide information to the patient about logging on to the portal from a home computer.

Some facilities also have smart TVs that enable patients to watch videos and use health learning applications. Some of these applications may be downloadable to patients' tablets or mobile phones, enabling patients to work through them at their own pace or revisit them at a later time. The applications may also include tutorials and quizzes that can help reinforce patient learning.

More individualized uses of technology may also be used in patient teaching. For example, webcams allow the nurse to video chat with patients at remote locations. This may be particularly useful when working with patients who are homebound. It can also be effective for observing patients performing self-care tasks in the home.

Use of e-health interventions may be especially helpful with the adolescent population, which is acclimated to obtaining and sharing information online. A review of five randomized controlled trials that examined the use of e-health with youth patients with depression or anxiety found that online cognitive–behavioral therapy (CBT) interventions may be helpful in reducing levels of acuity when offered with supervision in school and clinical settings (O'Dea, Calear, & Perry, 2015). E-health interventions for use with adolescents with other disorders, such as diabetes, are also being investigated.

REVIEW The Concept of Teaching and Learning

RELATE Link the Concepts

Linking the concept of teaching and learning with the concept of communication:

1. How does the quality of a nurse's communication skills impact his or her ability to teach?

2. How does the ability to communicate with people who speak a different language impact the teaching process?

Linking the concept of teaching and learning with the concept of advocacy:

3. How does the role of the nurse as teacher combine with the role of the nurse as advocate?

4. A nurse teaches a patient newly diagnosed with diabetes how to provide self-care to reduce the risk of complications. How does teaching this patient serve the nurse's advocacy role?

REFER Go to Pearson MyLab Nursing and eText

- Additional review materials

REFLECT Apply Your Knowledge

Samuel Jordan is a 33-year-old man who has worked as a nurse on the medical unit of a local acute care facility for the past 4 years. He has 9 years of nursing experience, having worked at another facility for 5 years before accepting this position. The unit is usually staffed with registered nurses (RNs), nursing assistants, and licensed practical nurses, along with a clinical secretary who transcribes orders, answers the phone, and obtains supplies. Throughout the course of an average day, Samuel interacts with many different members of the healthcare team.

1. What teaching opportunities is Samuel likely to encounter on a normal workday?

2. What teaching opportunities might Samuel encounter on his days off?

3. How does teaching impact Samuel's self-evaluation of his work performance?

>> Exemplar 41.A
Patient/Consumer Education

Exemplar Learning Outcomes

41.A Analyze patient/consumer education as it relates to teaching and learning.

- Differentiate environments where nurses teach.
- Outline the steps of developing a teaching plan.
- Summarize the aspects of identifying learning needs.
- List special teaching strategies.

Exemplar Key Terms

Anticipatory guidance, *2684*
Anticipatory problem solving, *2685*
Health literacy, *2677*
Return demonstration, *2674*
Teach-back method, *2686*

Overview

Providing patient education is a major aspect of nursing practice and an important independent nursing function. A variety of sources support this idea, beginning as early as 1992 with the American Hospital Association's passage of *A Patient's Bill of Rights*, which recognizes education as a right of all patients. The Joint Commission (TJC) followed suit in 1993 when it first established standards for patient education; TJC has continued to expand its standards over the years and emphasizes the importance of ensuring patient understanding of the material taught (Bastable, 2014). In 2010, the U.S. Department of Health and Human Services initiated *Healthy People 2020,* which promotes education that improves individuals' ability to make informed health choices. In addition, state nurse practice acts include teaching as a function of nursing and a legal and professional responsibility.

Although nurses play a key role in educating patients, patients are not passive recipients of information. In fact, many patients are taking an increasingly active role in all aspects of their health.

Good patient education efforts recognize the patient's role as consumer. Accordingly, education should help patients take a more active role in their health by providing them with information about methods for reducing health risk factors, increasing their level of wellness, and taking protective measures. **Box 41–4 >>** lists specific areas of health teaching that address these areas.

This exemplar takes a closer look at the steps nurses can take to provide teaching that promotes patient health and empowers patients as consumers. It begins with a discussion of the different environments in which nurses may engage in teaching. It also discusses methods for developing specific, individualized patient teaching plans. In addition, it looks at methods for identifying patient learning needs and implementing teaching plans. Finally, the exemplar explores methods for evaluating teaching and learning.

Teaching Environments

Nurses teach patients in many different settings, including hospitals, primary care clinics, urgent care centers, their homes, and assisted living and long-term care facilities.

Box 41–4
Common Topics for Patient Education

Health Promotion

- Human growth and development
- Fertility control
- Hygiene
- Nutrition
- Exercise
- Stress management
- Lifestyle modification
- Resources within the community

Illness/Injury Prevention

- Health screening (e.g., blood glucose levels, blood pressure, blood cholesterol, Pap tests, mammograms, vision and hearing tests, routine physical examinations)
- Reducing health risk factors (e.g., lowering cholesterol levels)
- Specific protective health measures (e.g., immunizations, use of condoms, use of sunscreen, use of medication, umbilical cord care)
- First aid
- Safety (e.g., proper use of seat belts, helmets, walkers)

Health Restoration

- Information about tests, diagnoses, treatment, and medications
- Self-care skills or skills needed to care for a family member
- Resources within the healthcare setting and the community

Adaptation to Altered Health and Function

- Lifestyle adaptations
- Problem-solving skills
- Adaptation to changing health status
- Strategies to deal with current problems (e.g., home IV skills, medications, diet, activity limits, prostheses)
- Strategies to deal with future problems (e.g., fear of pain with terminal cancer, future surgeries, or treatments)
- Information about available treatments and likely outcomes
- Referrals to other healthcare facilities or services
- Facilitation of strong self-image
- Grief and bereavement counseling

TABLE 41–3 Comparison of the Teaching Process and the Nursing Process

Step	Teaching Process	Nursing Process
1	Collect data; analyze patient's learning strengths and deficits.	Collect data; analyze patient's strengths and deficits.
2	Make educational diagnoses.	Make nursing diagnoses.
3	Prepare teaching plan: ■ Write learning outcomes. ■ Select content and time frame. ■ Select teaching strategies.	Plan nursing goals/desired outcomes and select appropriate interventions.
4	Implement teaching plan.	Implement nursing strategies.
5	Evaluate patient learning based on achievement of learning outcomes.	Evaluate patient outcomes based on achievement of goal criteria.

Nurses may also teach large and small groups of learners in community health education programs.

Teaching Individual Patients

When teaching individual patients and their families, the nurse is in a position to promote healthy lifestyles through the application of health knowledge, the change process, learning theories, and nursing and teaching processes. As with nursing interventions, patient education opportunities should be tailored to needs identified via consultation with patients and their families. In fact, the teaching process shares many similarities with the nursing process, including assessment of needs, planning, implementation, and evaluation. See **Table 41–3** >> for a more detailed comparison of the teaching and nursing processes.

Nurses may teach individual patients in one-to-one teaching episodes. For example, the nurse may teach about wound care while changing a patient's dressing or may teach about diet, exercise, and other lifestyle behaviors that minimize the risk of heart attack when caring for a patient who has a cardiac problem. The nurse may also be involved in teaching family members or other support people who are caring for a patient. For instance, nurses who work in obstetric and pediatric areas regularly teach parents (and sometimes grandparents) how to care for children.

Because of the current trend toward shorter hospital stays, nurses often face time constraints on patient education. Accordingly, nurses must take care to provide education that will ensure the patient's safe transition from one level of care to another, then make appropriate plans for follow-up education in the patient's home if necessary. Discharge plans must include information about what the patient has been taught before transfer or discharge, as well as what the patient still must learn to perform self-care in the home or other residence.

When educating patients, the nurse must ensure that the environment is conducive to learning. In addition, both the patient and the nurse must be adequately prepared for the teaching session. The following is a list of recommendations nurses should keep in mind when preparing the environment, the patient, and themselves for teaching:

■ Provide a calm environment to decrease distractions.

■ Take time in teaching. Observe the patient for signs or feelings of being overwhelmed, confused, and/or anxious.

■ Adapt your teaching plan to reflect the patient's reactions. For example, if the patient seems confused, avoid

moving on to more information. Determine where the patient became confused and address the issue until understanding occurs before moving to new information.

■ Remember that instructions may need to be repeated several times, depending on the patient's level of anxiety and stress.

■ Evaluate the patient's (or support person's) ability to perform a skill through **return demonstration**. Having the patient (or support person) demonstrate how they would perform the skill in response to a "what if" situation allows that individual to exhibit mastery of the skill.

Teaching in the Community

Nurses are often involved in community health education programs. Such teaching activities may be voluntary as part of the nurse's involvement in an organization (e.g., the American Red Cross, Planned Parenthood), or they may be part of the nurse's job responsibilities. Nurses work in a variety of community settings, including local health departments, schools, and colleges and universities. Community teaching activities may be aimed at large groups of people who have an interest in some aspect of health; examples include nutrition classes, cardiopulmonary resuscitation (CPR) or cardiac risk factor reduction classes, and bicycle or swimming safety programs. Community education programs also can be designed for small groups or individual learners, as is often the case with childbirth classes or family planning classes.

Clinical Example E

When providing teaching to groups, it is essential to tailor the teaching to the members of each group. Consider the following example: During fall sports season, three athletes at a local high school develop staph infections. When deciding how to best provide education related to this situation, the school nurse identifies several groups who have a stake in the health and well-being of student athletes: (1) the athletes themselves, (2) their parents and immediate family members, (3) the coaches, and (4) the teachers and other staff at the school.

The nurse recognizes that providing each group with only a handout will be insufficient. Instead, she decides to work with the school's athletic director and physical trainer to develop a teaching session for the coaches that reinforces individual hygiene and also provides local and state regulations related to preventing staph infections. She further plans to demonstrate how to properly clean equipment such as wrestling mats.

In collaboration with the trainer, the nurse also develops and schedules a teaching session for the athletes themselves. Recognizing the importance of peer influence in this group, the nurse obtains parental permission for one of the athletes who acquired a staph infection to come speak to the others about what it was like and to help her persuade the other students to take steps to avoid infection.

Critical Thinking Questions

1. What are the primary takeaways from the teaching sessions for each stakeholder group?
2. How would the teaching methods used in the session for the coaches differ from those used in the session for athletes?
3. Discuss strategies that the nurse could use to promote individual hygiene among student athletes.

Developing a Teaching Plan

Before creating a teaching plan, the nurse must assess the needs of the patient or group. For individual patients (and their families), the nurse should consider the patient's health history, physical and psychosocial assessment, and available support systems (e.g., caregivers or access to transportation). The nurse should also note various factors that influence the learning process, such as readiness and motivation to learn, reading and comprehension level, and mobility.

Using the Health History

Several elements of a patient's health history can provide clues about the patient's learning needs. These elements include age and developmental level; the patient's understanding and perceptions of the health problem; the patient's

health beliefs and practices; cultural factors; economic factors; the patient's learning style; and the patient's support systems. Some examples of interview questions that help elicit this information are provided in **Box 41–5 》**.

Note that the same elements that affect an individual patient's learning needs also affect the needs of individuals in communities. For example, consider a nurse who is planning a teaching session on health promotion for individuals with high blood pressure. This session will be presented to residents at an independent living facility. Although the teaching plan for the group will be different from that for a single patient, the plan should still consider factors such as the residents' primary language, age and developmental level, and economic situation (e.g., access to transportation, health insurance coverage). The following sections take a closer look at these and other elements that influence patients' learning needs.

Age and Developmental Level

Age generally provides information about a patient's developmental status that may indicate the need for distinctive health teaching content and teaching approaches. Posing simple questions to school-age children and adolescents can elicit information on what they know. Observing young children at play also provides information about motor and intellectual development as well as relationships with other children. For older adults, conversation and questioning may reveal slow recall or limited psychomotor skills, sensory

Box 41–5
Interview Questions That Help Reveal Patient Learning Needs

Questions About the Primary Health Problem

- Tell me what you know about your current health problem. What do you think caused it?
- What concerns do you have about your health problem?
- How has the problem affected what you can or cannot do during your usual activities (e.g., work, recreation, shopping, and housework)?
- What do you or did you do at home to relieve the problem? How helpful was it?
- Have the treatments you have started helped your problem? If so, how?
- What, if any, difficulties have the treatments caused you (e.g., inconvenience, cost, discomfort)?
- Tell me about the tests (surgery, treatments) you are going to have.

Questions About Health Beliefs

- How would you describe your health generally?
- What things do you usually do to keep healthy?
- What health problems do you think you may be at risk for because of family history, age, diet, occupation, inadequate exercise, or other habits, such as smoking?
- What changes would you be willing to make to decrease your risk for these problems or to improve your health?

Questions About Cultural Factors

- What language do you use most often when speaking and writing?
- Are you seeking the advice of another health practitioner?

- Do you use herbs or other medications or treatments commonly used by members of your cultural group? If so, does your current primary care provider know about these?
- Has your primary care provider given you any advice or treatments that conflict with values or beliefs you consider important?
- When a conflict arose, what did you do?

Questions About Learning Style

- Note the patient's age and developmental level.
- What level of education have you achieved?
- Do you like to read?
- Where do you usually obtain health information (e.g., primary care provider, nurse, magazines, books, internet, or pharmacist)?
- How do you best learn new things?
  - By reading about them?
  - By talking about them?
  - By watching a movie or demonstration?
  - By using a computer?
  - By listening to a teacher?
  - By first being shown how something works, then doing it yourself?
  - On your own or in a group?

Questions About Support Systems

- Would you like a family member or friend to help you learn about the things you must do to take care of yourself?
- Who do you think would be interested in learning with you?

deficits, and learning difficulties. (See the section on Life-span Considerations for additional information.)

Understanding of the Health Problem

Patients' perceptions of their current health problems and concerns may indicate deficient knowledge or misinformation. In addition, discussion of the problem's effects on the patient's usual activities can alert the nurse to other areas that require instruction. For example, individuals who cannot manage self-care at home often need information about community resources and services.

Health information can be difficult to obtain prior to providing teaching in a group setting. Whenever possible, the nurse should try to assess participants' health perceptions in advance. Some strategies for doing so include the following:

- Circulating brief surveys
- Surveying staff at the setting where teaching will be provided
- Conducting brief surveys as patients arrive for the teaching session

For instance, in the staph example mentioned earlier, the school nurse might ask the coaches to circulate surveys to athletes at the beginning of practice a week before the session. An alternative might be to hold a brief question-and-answer session with team captains to get a sense of athletes' general habits, practices, and attitudes toward hygiene.

Health Beliefs and Practices

A patient's health beliefs and practices are important to consider in any teaching plan. The health belief model described in the module on Health, Wellness, and Illness provides a predictor of preventive health behavior. However, even if a nurse is convinced that a particular patient's health beliefs should be changed, doing so may not be possible because so many factors are involved in patient health beliefs.

Cultural Factors

Many cultural groups have their own beliefs and practices, some of which are related to diet, health, illness, and lifestyle. The cultural practices and values held by patients will affect their learning needs. For example, a patient may understand the healthcare information being taught, but she may not use any of this information if she believes in following the practices of her culture of origin.

Economic Factors

Economic factors can also affect learning. For example, a patient who cannot afford to obtain a new sterile syringe for each insulin injection may find it difficult to learn to administer insulin when the nurse teaches that a new syringe should be used every time. In a group setting, nurses may be teaching individuals who have limited access to transportation, who lack health insurance, or who are dependent on others for their financial security. Nurses must take these factors into account when planning education sessions in the community.

Learning Styles

Considerable research exists with regard to learning styles. In general, this research indicates that the best way to learn varies with the individual. Some individuals are visual learners and learn best by watching. Others do not visualize an activity well but learn best by actually manipulating equipment and discovering how it works. Many individuals learn best from reading information presented in an orderly fashion. Still others learn best in groups where they can relate to other people. For some, stressing the thinking part of a skill and its logic will promote learning. For other people, stressing the feeling part or interpersonal aspect motivates and promotes learning.

The nurse seldom has the time or skills to assess each learner, identify his or her particular learning style, then adapt teaching accordingly. What the nurse can do, however, is ask patients how they have learned information best in the past or how they like to learn. Many people know what helps them learn, and the nurse can use this information to plan the teaching. Using a variety of teaching techniques and varying activities during teaching are good ways to match learners with learning styles. One technique will be most effective for some patients, whereas other techniques will be suited to patients with different learning styles.

It is particularly important to use a variety of teaching techniques when providing education in community settings. The nurse can combine videos, whiteboards, and opportunities to practice demonstrations to ensure the highest rate of retention among group members. PowerPoint presentations can also be helpful. Some learners may benefit from receiving a copy of the plan or agenda of the session in advance so they can follow along with the presentation.

Support Systems

When compiling the health history, the nurse must explore the patient's support systems to determine the extent to which other people may enhance learning and offer support. In many cases, family members or close friends can help patients perform required skills at home and maintain necessary lifestyle changes.

Using the Physical Examination

When working with individual patients, the general survey part of the physical examination provides useful clues to the patient's learning needs, including those related to mental status, energy level, and nutritional status. Other parts of the physical examination reveal data about the patient's physical capacity to learn and to perform self-care activities. For example, visual ability, hearing ability, and muscle coordination affect the selection of content and approaches to teaching.

Determining Readiness to Learn

Patients who are ready to learn often behave differently from those who are not. A patient who is ready may search out information, for example, by asking questions, reading books or articles, talking to others, and generally showing interest. The individual who is not ready to learn is more likely to avoid the subject or situation. In addition, the unready patient may change the subject when it is brought up by the nurse. For example, if the nurse says, "I was wondering about a good time to show you how to change your dressing," a patient who is not ready to learn might respond "Oh, my wife will take care of everything." Using cues from the patient can result in teaching moments (small chunks of time in which the patient is receptive to information). Always observe the patient's reaction during a teaching moment because it may lead into a longer period of receptiveness.

When assessing a patient's readiness to learn, the nurse should consider the following characteristics:

- **Physical readiness.** Is the patient able to focus on things other than physical status, or are pain, fatigue, and immobility consuming all of the patient's time and energy?

- **Emotional readiness.** Is the patient emotionally ready to learn self-care activities? Patients who are extremely anxious, depressed, or grieving over their health status are not ready.

- **Cognitive readiness.** Can the patient think clearly at this point? Are the effects of anesthesia and analgesia altering the patient's level of consciousness?

Nurses can promote readiness to learn by providing physical and emotional support during the critical stage of recovery. As the patient stabilizes physically and emotionally, the nurse can then provide actual opportunities to learn.

In group settings, when attendance is voluntary, patients are more likely to be ready to learn new information. When attendance is compulsory, such as in a school setting or an inpatient treatment facility, patient readiness to learn may vary considerably. In these instances, it is especially important that nurses be able to manage problem behaviors, such as monopolizing. (See the module on Communication for more information.)

Assessing Motivation

Motivation relates to whether the patient wants to learn, and it is usually greatest when the patient is ready, the learning need is recognized, and the information being offered is meaningful to the patient. Assessment of motivation, however, may be difficult. Nurses should be alert for information that indicates a readiness for change, such as a patient saying, "I'm really ready to lose weight this time." On the other hand, nonverbal behaviors such as lack of interest, wandering attention, and missed appointments can indicate decreased motivation to learn.

Nurses can use the following strategies, as appropriate, to increase patient motivation in both individual and group settings:

- Relate the learning to something the patient values and help the patient see the relevance of the learning.

- Help the patient make the learning situation pleasant and nonthreatening.

- Encourage self-direction and independence.

- Demonstrate a positive attitude about the patient's ability to learn.

- Offer continuing support and encouragement as the patient attempts to learn (i.e., positive reinforcement).

- Create a learning situation in which the patient is likely to succeed. (Succeeding in small tasks motivates the patient to continue learning.)

- Assist the patient in identifying the benefits of changing behavior.

Box 41–6
Populations Most Likely to Experience Limited Health Literacy

- Adults older than 65 years of age
- Recent refugees and immigrants
- Individuals with less than a high school degree or GED
- Individuals with incomes at or below the poverty level
- Nonnative speakers of English (USDHHS, n.d.)

Assessing Health Literacy

Literacy and *health literacy* are two closely related ideas. Literacy is a comprehensive measurement of an individual's mathematical, reading, writing, and language skills. A patient's literacy level affects her ability to understand and use information. **Health literacy** refers to the individual's ability to use literacy skills as a means of obtaining, understanding, and applying health information (CDC, 2015). Essentially, health literacy allows the patient to make sense of health information and use that information to make sound decisions about healthcare. The nurse must assess a patient's health literacy to create an effective teaching plan.

Health literacy is important because it impacts patient outcomes. Typically, patients with higher levels of health literacy have better outcomes. For example, patients with higher health literacy are more likely to read a prescription label accurately and take the correct number of pills at the correct times of day. Patients with low health literacy, on the other hand, are more likely to experience adverse events and hospitalization. Research suggests that more than 50% of North Americans do not possess the skills needed to learn about and manage their health adequately (Hadden, 2015; Manafo & Wong, 2012). **Box 41–6 >>** lists the groups at the greatest risk of low health literacy. The Focus on Diversity and Culture feature goes into further detail about health literacy in immigrant populations.

The large percentage of people with low health literacy is particularly worrisome in light of the increased availability of health information online. In order to address this concern, U.S. government health agencies have developed programs and initiatives designed to educate individuals and promote national and global health. In 2010, the U.S. Department of Health and Human Services (USDHHS) released the *National Action Plan to Improve Health Literacy*. This plan is intended to help meet the goals and objectives outlined by *Healthy People 2020* (USDHHS, 2010). The CDC also developed a website for individuals, organizations, and healthcare providers that aims to improve health literacy and public health (CDC, 2016). This site is simply titled *Health Literacy* and can be accessed at http://www.cdc.gov/healthliteracy/.

Clinical Example F

David Rodriquez is a 28-year-old man who had an emergency appendectomy yesterday. He is to be discharged home later today. During discharge teaching, the nurse provides Mr. Rodriquez with handouts relating to wound care, medications, activity restrictions, and follow-up appointments. The nurse knows the handouts will fit Mr. Rodriquez's learning style because he said he likes to read; in fact, the nurse observed Mr. Rodriquez reading a couple of times this morning.

Critical Thinking Questions

1. Should the nurse have used the handouts as a learning tool? Why or why not?
2. What strategies might patients use to avoid embarrassment by having to admit they cannot read English?
3. What strategies might a nurse use to help a patient who cannot read English learn about self-care?

Nurses play a major role in improving health literacy. An important first step for nurses is assessing a patient's general literacy. (See the Patient Teaching feature for information about patient behaviors that suggest a literacy problem.) Once a patient's literacy level has been determined, the nurse should adjust written materials to the patient's level. In general, educational materials should be written at a fifth- or sixth-grade reading level. Materials should use the active voice rather than the passive voice and be written in second person (*you*) rather than third person (*the patient*). Priority information should appear first and be repeated several times. Sentences should be short and use easy, common one- or two-syllable words. For example, the word *use* should take the place of *utilize*, and the word *give* should be used rather than *administer*. Larger type size (14- to 16-point font)

should be used, and important words should be boldfaced for emphasis. Simple pictures, drawings, or cartoons should also be used if appropriate.

SAFETY ALERT Individuals with low reading skills may struggle not only with health teaching but with giving accurate informed consent for treatment. When working with these patients, review all components of the procedure and the consent document carefully, allowing time for the patient to ask questions.

Individuals with good reading skills are unlikely to be offended by simple reading material; in fact, they may prefer easy-to-read information. However, even the simplest written directions will not be helpful to a patient with low or no reading skills. When working with these patients, the nurse should use multiple teaching methods, including pictures, role playing, and hands-on practice. The nurse can also read important information to the patient, taking care to emphasize key points in simple terms. It may also be helpful to associate new information with information the patient already knows or associates with his job or lifestyle.

Regardless of a patient's health literacy level, it is generally a good idea for the nurse to limit the amount of information presented in a single teaching session. Instead of one long session that provides a great deal of information, it is often better to provide more frequent sessions that focus on one or two major points. All teaching should involve the patient and use repetition to reinforce the information presented. Finally, the nurse should obtain feedback during the session by asking the patient specific questions about the information presented or asking the patient to repeat what was learned in her own words.

SAFETY ALERT Highly technical language and nursing jargon are confusing to patients—even those with higher levels of health literacy. Confusing instructions may be ignored, placing the patient's health at risk. Verbal and written teaching must use simple, clear language that is readily understood by laypersons.

Focus on Diversity and Culture
Health Literacy in Immigrant Populations

Immigrants tend to have lower health literacy than non-immigrants. Low health literacy is more responsible for a perceived lower quality of care in immigrants than many other factors, including education, income, and health insurance coverage (Calvo, 2016). Public initiatives intended to improve health literacy do not always reach immigrants. This may be the result of economic status, language and other social barriers, or both. In addition, the combination of low health literacy and limited English proficiency cause immigrants to be at high risk for poor health (Sentell & Braun, 2012). For the same reasons, health promotion and disease prevention services are often underused by immigrant populations as well (World Health Organization, 2013b).

Interventions that have been found effective for improving health literacy and access to services in immigrant populations include the use of informational pictograms and signs translated into multiple languages. Translated signs in particular are useful not only for helping patients learn, but also for creating feelings of inclusion and belonging at the facility where they are used.

The use of cultural mediators may also be successful in improving health literacy and quality of care for immigrant patients. Cultural mediators are individuals with an understanding of patients' native cultures and that culture's view of health, wellness, and medical interventions (World Health Organization, 2013b). The cultural mediator may also be versed in the migrant experience and may speak the patients' native language.

A key to improving immigrants' health literacy and access to healthcare initiatives is engaging these groups in the planning and implementation of strategies. The effectiveness of these strategies should regularly be evaluated by immigrant patients, cultural mediators, and healthcare providers.

Patient Teaching
Identifying Low Literacy Behaviors in Patients

Patients often will not admit to having difficulty reading because of the embarrassment it brings them, and many people at the lowest reading levels report that they "read well." A nurse who suspects a patient has difficulty reading may ask the patient tactful questions, such as "Would you like me to go over it with you?"

It can be difficult to assess a patient's health literacy skills because the shame and stigma associated with limited literacy are major barriers. The following patient behaviors may cause a nurse to suspect a literacy problem:

- A pattern of nonadherence
- Insistence that they already know the information
- Reliance on friends or family members to read the document aloud
- A pattern of excuses for not reading the instructions (e.g., claiming that glasses are broken)

Identifying Learning Needs

Nursing diagnoses for patients with learning needs can be designated in two ways: as the patient's primary concern or problem, or as the etiology of a nursing diagnosis associated with the patient's response to health alterations or dysfunction.

Learning Need as the Diagnostic Label

NANDA International (NANDA-I) is charged with providing evidence-based diagnosis terminology and guidance to the nursing community to assist in providing consistent, evidence-based care across all settings in which nurses care for patients. NANDA-I's diagnostic labels list includes *Deficient Knowledge*, which is an appropriate diagnosis whenever a patient's learning need is the primary concern because the patient lacks knowledge related to a specific healthcare issue or topic (NANDA-I © 2014).

Whenever the nursing diagnosis label *Deficient Knowledge* is used, either the patient is seeking health information or the nurse has identified a learning need. The area of deficiency should always be included in the diagnosis. The following examples both use the NANDA-I label *Deficient Knowledge* as the primary concern:

- *Deficient Knowledge* of low-calorie diet related to inexperience with newly ordered therapy.
- *Deficient Knowledge* of home safety hazards related to denial of declining health and living alone.

  (NANDA-I © 2014)

When working with patients who have a knowledge deficit, the nurse should provide information that has the potential to change the patient's behavior rather than focus on the behaviors caused by the patient's lack of knowledge.

A second nursing diagnosis label that may apply when a learning need is the primary concern is *Readiness for Enhanced Knowledge*. When this diagnostic label is used, the patient is seeking information. Note that the patient may or may not have an altered response or dysfunction at the time of the diagnosis; he or she may simply be seeking information to improve health or prevent illness. This diagnosis is especially appropriate for patients attending community health education programs. The following example uses the NANDA-I label *Readiness for Enhanced Knowledge* as the primary concern:

- *Readiness for Enhanced Knowledge* related to desire to improve health behaviors and decrease risk of heart disease.

This diagnosis may be appropriate for the patient who has identified a personal health risk for a cardiac condition and wants to minimize that risk through exercise.

Noncompliance is a third nursing diagnosis label that may be appropriate when a learning need is the primary concern. This label recognizes that the individual or caregiver may not always be able to follow the treatment or care plan as agreed (NANDA-I © 2014). The *Noncompliance* diagnostic label generally is used when patients have intent to comply but barriers affect their compliance. Factors that influence a patient's compliance with health teaching include understanding or comprehension of the teaching, any negative side effects of the treatment, financial inability to carry out the treatment plan, language barriers, or poor teaching on the part of the healthcare team. *Noncompliance* should *not* be used for patients who are unable to follow instructions (e.g., because of cognitive disability) or for patients who make an informed decision to refuse or not follow the medical treatment (Wilkinson, 2013).

Deficient Knowledge as the Etiology

Another way to deal with patients' identified learning needs is to include deficient knowledge as the etiology, or second part, of the diagnosis statement.

Examples include the following:

- *Risk for Impaired Parenting* related to deficient knowledge of skills required for infant care and feeding.
- *Risk for Infection* related to deficient knowledge of sexually transmitted infections and their prevention.
- *Anxiety* related to deficient knowledge of bone marrow aspiration.

  (NANDA-I © 2014)

Other nursing diagnoses in which a knowledge deficit can be the etiology include the following:

- *Injury, Risk for*
- *Breastfeeding, Ineffective*
- *Coping, Ineffective*
- *Health Maintenance, Ineffective.*

  (NANDA-I © 2014)

Note also that most nursing diagnoses approved by NANDA-I imply a teaching–learning need. For example, the nursing diagnosis *Constipation* suggests the need for a review of bowel hygiene practices, including diet, hydration, and exercise/activity.

Establishing the Teaching Plan

When developing a teaching plan, the nurse should follow a series of steps, each of which is described in the following sections. Involving the patient in each step promotes the formation of a meaningful plan and stimulates patient motivation. In fact, patients who help develop the teaching plan are more likely to achieve the desired outcomes.

Determining Teaching Priorities

The first step in creating a teaching plan is to rank the patient's learning needs according to priority. The patient and the nurse should do this together, with the patient's priorities always being considered. Once a patient's priorities have been addressed, the patient is generally more motivated to concentrate on other identified learning needs. For example, a man who wants to know all about coronary artery disease may not be ready to learn how to change his lifestyle until he meets his own need to learn more about the disease. Nurses can also use theoretical frameworks, such as Maslow's hierarchy of needs, to establish priorities.

Setting Learning Outcomes

Once a patient's learning needs have been prioritized, the patient and nurse should work together to determine the desired learning outcomes. Learning outcomes are essentially the same as desired outcomes for other nursing diagnoses. In fact, they are written in the same way. Like patient outcomes, good learning outcomes:

- *State the patient (learner) behavior or performance, not the nurse behavior.* For example, an appropriate learning outcome would be "Identify personal risk factors for heart disease" (patient behavior), *not* "Teach the patient about cardiac risk factors" (nurse behavior).

- *Reflect an observable, measurable activity.* Performance of this activity may be visible (e.g., walking) or invisible (e.g., adding a column of figures). However, the nurse must be able to evaluate whether an unobservable activity has been mastered from some performance that represents the activity. For example, the performance of an outcome might be written as "Selects low-fat foods from a menu" (observable), *not* as "Understands low-fat diet" (unobservable). Examples of measurable verbs that can be used in learning outcomes are shown in **Box 41–7 》**. Avoid using words such as *knows, understands, believes,* and *appreciates* because they are neither observable nor measurable.

- *May add conditions or modifiers as required to clarify what, where, when, or how the behavior will be performed.* Examples include "Demonstrates four-point crutch gait *correctly*" (condition), "Administers own insulin *independently* (condition) as taught," or "States *three* (condition) factors that affect blood sugar level."

- *Include criteria specifying the time by which learning should have occurred.* For example, "The patient will state three things that affect blood sugar level *by the end of the second diabetes class.*"

Learning outcomes can reflect the learner's command of simple to complex concepts. For example, the learning outcome "The patient will list cardiac risk factors" is a low-level knowledge outcome that simply requires the learner to identify all cardiac risk factors; it does not suggest application of the knowledge to the learner's own behaviors. In comparison, the learning outcome "The patient will list personal cardiac risk factors" requires that the learner not only know cardiac risk factors in general, but also know his own behaviors that place him at risk for cardiac disease.

When writing learning outcomes, the nurse must be specific about what behaviors and knowledge (cognitive, psychomotor, and affective) learners must have to positively influence their health state. In most cases, a patient's learning needs are more complex than simple acquisition of knowledge and include the application of that knowledge to oneself.

Choosing Content

The content of a teaching plan—or what is to be taught—is determined by the identified learning outcomes. For example, the learning outcome "Identify appropriate sites for insulin injection" requires that the teaching plan include content about the body sites suitable for insulin injections.

When choosing content, nurses can select among many sources of information, including books, nursing journals, the internet, and other nurses and primary care providers. Whatever sources the nurse chooses, the content should be:

- Accurate
- Current
- Based on learning outcomes
- Adjusted for the learner's age, culture, and ability
- Consistent with information the nurse is teaching
- Selected with consideration of how much time and what resources are available for teaching

Selecting Teaching Strategies

The method of teaching that the nurse chooses should be suited to the individual and to the material to be learned. For example, a patient who cannot read needs material presented in other ways; discussion is usually not the best strategy for teaching a patient how to give an injection; and a nurse who uses group discussion for teaching should be a competent group leader. As stated earlier, some people are visually oriented and learn best through seeing; others learn best through hearing and having a skill explained to them. **Table 41–4 》** lists some teaching strategies the nurse may find useful.

Organizing Learning Experiences

To save nurses time in constructing their own teaching guides, some health agencies have developed guides for teaching sessions that nurses commonly give. These guides standardize content and teaching methods and make it easier for the nurse to plan and implement patient teaching. Standardized teaching plans also ensure consistency of

Box 41–7
Examples of Verbs for Writing Learning Outcomes

Cognitive Domain	Affective Domain	Psychomotor Domain
Compares	Accepts	Assembles
Describes	Attends	Calculates
Evaluates	Chooses	Changes
Explains	Discusses	Demonstrates
Identifies	Displays	Measures
Labels	Initiates	Moves
Lists	Joins	Organizes
Names	Participates	Shows
Plans	Shares	Performs
Selects	Uses	
States		
Writes		

TABLE 41–4 Selected Teaching Strategies

Strategy	Major Type of Learning	Characteristics
Explanation or description (e.g., lecture)	Cognitive	Teacher controls content and pace.
		Learner is passive and therefore retains less information than when actively participating.
		Feedback is determined by teacher.
		May be given to individual or group.
One-to-one discussion	Affective, cognitive	Encourages participation by learner.
		Permits reinforcement and repetition at learner's level.
		Permits introduction of sensitive subjects.
Answering questions	Cognitive	Teacher controls most of content and pace.
		Learner may need to overcome cultural perception that asking questions is impolite and may embarrass the teacher.
		Can be used with individuals and groups.
		Teacher sometimes needs to confirm whether question has been answered by asking learner, for example, "Does that answer your question?"
Demonstration	Psychomotor	Often used with explanation.
		Can be used with individuals and small or large groups.
		Does not permit use of equipment by learner; learner is passive.
Discovery	Cognitive, affective	Teacher guides problem-solving situation.
		Learner is active participant; therefore, retention of information is high.
Group discussions	Affective, cognitive	Learner can obtain assistance from supportive group.
		Group members learn from one another.
		Teacher needs to keep the discussion focused and prevent monopolization by one or two learners.
Practice	Psychomotor	Allows repetition and immediate feedback.
		Permits hands-on experience.
Printed and audiovisual materials	Cognitive	Includes use of books, pamphlets, films, programmed instruction, and computer learning.
		Learners can proceed at their own speed.
		Nurse can act as resource person and need not be present during learning.
		Potentially ineffective if materials are written at too high a reading level.
		If English is the patient's second language, nurse should select materials that use the patient's preferred language (e.g., Spanish).
Role playing	Affective, cognitive	Permits expression of attitudes, values, and emotions.
		Can assist in development of communication skills.
		Involves active participation by learner.
		Teacher must create supportive, safe environment for learners to minimize anxiety.
Modeling	Affective, psychomotor	Nurse sets example by attitude, psychomotor skill.
Computer-assisted learning programs	All types of learning	Learner is active.
		Learner controls pace.
		Provides immediate reinforcement and review.
		Can be used with individuals or groups.

content for the learner, thereby decreasing the risk of confusion if different practices are taught. For example, when teaching infant bathing, the nurse on the unit should be consistent about which soaps are appropriate for the infant's bath and distinguish those that are not.

Whether the nurse is implementing a plan devised by another person or developing an individualized teaching plan, the following guidelines can help the nurse sequence the learning experience:

- Start with something the learner is concerned about; for example, before learning how to administer insulin to himself, an adolescent patient may want to know how to adjust his lifestyle and yet still play football.

Evidence-Based Practice

Finding Teaching Strategies That Help Patients Understand, Apply, and Retain Information

Problem

Patient teaching is a professional obligation of nurses, but determining the most effective teaching strategy or strategies for each patient is challenging. The selected strategy must be appropriate for the patient's health literacy level and readiness to learn. It should help patients understand, apply, and retain the necessary information. With the many teaching methods available to nurses, identifying the ideal strategy for these outcomes can be difficult.

Evidence

A number of studies have been conducted to assess the effectiveness of various teaching methods on different patient populations. Ackerman et al. (2017) looked at patients' perceptions of understanding associated with various teaching methods. They looked specifically at information delivered to osteoarthritis patients age 55 and under via group-based programs, online resources, telephone helplines, mailed information, social media, and mobile applications. Patients rated understanding and accessibility of these methods on a scale from 1.0 (ineffective/inaccessible) to 10.0 (highly effective/highly accessible). Social media was rated as the least effective and least accessible method (with scores of 2.0 in each category). Mailed information and online programs were rated the most effective and most accessible (with effectiveness scores of 8.0 and 7.0 respectively for effectiveness and 10.0 and 9.0 respectively for accessibility).

Park et al. (2016) compared the application of information by patients exposed to two different teaching methods. Their research focused on patients' at-home bowel preparation for colonoscopy as assessed by the providers conducting the scope. Participants were divided into two groups: one group received traditional instruction about bowel preparation from a care provider while the other received instruction via video. Providers reported that 78.5% of traditional teaching patients exhibited good bowel preparation compared to 91.6% of video patients. As a result, colonoscopies for patients in the video group were of shorter duration than those of the traditional group; however, polyp detection among the two groups was not significantly different (19.0% in the traditional group and 19.2% in the video group).

White et al. (2013) addressed retention of information by patients exposed to the teach-back method for teaching self-care. (The teach-back method is explained in greater depth later in this exemplar.) The researchers examined the impact of this method on exacerbations and readmissions of patients with heart failure. Although the researchers did not find a strong relationship between the use of the teach-back model and readmission rates, the model was found to be effective in patient education: most patients were able to recall 75% of the information during their hospitalization (84.4%) and at 7 days after discharge (77.1%).

Implications

Although each of these studies assesses different components of effectiveness, they all suggest teaching methods involving visual media improve patient understanding, application, and retention of material. The types of visual media available to nurses vary widely, and the type selected by the nurse will be based on patient health literacy levels and readiness to learn. Visual media may be used alone or in combination with verbal teaching. One type of visual media may also be used to reinforce information taught via another type of visual media—for example, providing a patient with a written set of instructions after a teach-back session.

Critical Thinking Application

1. Discuss the ways in which visual media might be used differently to teach pediatric patients and adolescents about leukemia.

2. How do patient goals dictate the way in which visual media are used for patient teaching? Consider two diabetic patients, one who is learning to administer insulin and one who is struggling to stay active and lose weight. Assume both patients have similar health literacy and readiness to learn.

3. Is visual media appropriate for a patient who is visually impaired? In what ways could visual media be adapted for teaching this patient?

- Discover what the learner knows, then proceed to the unknown. This gives the learner confidence. Sometimes you will not know the patient's knowledge or skill base and will need to elicit this information either by asking questions or by having the patient fill out a form in advance of the session.

- Address early any area that is causing the patient anxiety. A high level of anxiety can impair concentration in other areas. For example, a woman who is highly anxious about her fear of needles breaking off in her skin may not be able to learn how to self-administer insulin injections until her fear is resolved.

- Teach the basics before proceeding to the variations or adjustments (i.e., proceed from simple to complex). It is confusing to learners to have to consider possible adjustments and variations before they master the basic con-

cepts. For example, when teaching a female patient how to insert a retention catheter, it is best to teach the basic procedure before teaching any adjustments that might be needed if the catheter stops draining after insertion.

- Schedule time for review of content and questions the patient may have to clarify information.

- If the patient does not have any questions, you can help introduce questions by saying, "A few frequently asked questions are. . . ."

Showing Flexibility

The nurse needs to be flexible in implementing any teaching plan because the plan may need to be revised. For example, the patient may tire sooner than anticipated or be faced with too much information too quickly, the patient's needs may change, or external factors may intervene. For instance, say the nurse and the patient plan to change the patient's dressing at 10 a.m., but when the time comes, the patient wants to observe the nurse once more before actually doing it himself. In this case, the nurse alters the teaching plan and discusses any desired information, provides another demonstration, and defers teaching the psychomotor skill until the next day.

It is also important for nurses to use teaching techniques that enhance learning and reduce or eliminate any barriers to learning, such as pain or fatigue. Many nurses find that they teach while performing nursing care (e.g., giving medication). Remember to document this informal teaching also.

Implementing the Teaching Plan

Knowledge alone is not enough to motivate individuals to change their behaviors. Rather, evidence indicates that patients are more likely to adopt new behaviors and follow their treatment plan when they are actively engaged in their care (Blazeck et al., 2016). The Institute of Medicine's (IOM) 2012 report *Best Care at Lower Cost* also recommends that patients be "fully engaged participants at all levels" of their care.

Thus, when implementing a teaching plan, the nurse must actively seek ways to get the patient interested and involved in not just the teaching process, but the entire care process. This requires that the nurse reflect on the changes required as part of the care plan, the stages of the change process, the patient's willingness and perceived need to change, and any barriers to the change process. When the patient is ready to change his or her health behavior, the nurse can begin implementing the teaching plan. In doing so, the nurse may find it useful to keep the following guidelines in mind:

- Rapport between teacher and learner is essential. A relationship that is both accepting and constructive will best assist learning. The nurse should know the learner and the previously described factors that affect learning before planning and delivering the teaching.

- The teacher who uses the patient's previous learning in the present situation encourages the patient and facilitates learning new skills. For instance, an individual who already knows how to cook can use this knowledge when learning to prepare food for a special diet.

- The optimal time for each session depends largely on the learner. Whenever possible, ask the patient for help to choose the best time (e.g., when the patient feels most rested or when no other activities are scheduled). Be alert for patient cues that indicate a readiness to learn. For example, if a patient asks you why he needs a certain medication, the question provides an opportunity to explain the reason for the medication, signs to watch for, and whether follow-up laboratory work is needed.

- The nurse teacher must be able to communicate clearly and concisely. The words used in the teaching session need to have the same meaning to the patient as to the teacher. For instance, a patient who is taught not to put water on an area of skin may think a wet washcloth is permissible for washing the area. In effect, the nurse needs to explain that no water or moisture should touch the area.

- Using a layperson's vocabulary enhances communication. Often nurses use terms and abbreviations that have meaning to other health professionals but make little sense to patients. Even words such as *urine* or *feces* may be unfamiliar to some patients, and abbreviations such as ICU (intensive care unit) or PACU (postanesthesia care unit) are often misunderstood.

- The pace of each teaching session affects patient learning. Nurses should be sensitive to any signs that the pace is too fast or too slow. A patient who appears confused or does not comprehend material when questioned may be finding the pace too fast. When the patient appears bored and loses interest, the pace may be too slow, the learning period may be too long, or the patient may be tired.

- The environment can detract from or assist learning. For example, noise or interruptions usually interfere with concentration, whereas a comfortable environment promotes learning. If possible, the patient should be out of bed for learning activities. Most people associate their bed with rest and sleep, not with learning. Placing the patient in a position and location associated with activity or learning may influence the amount of learning that takes place. For instance, a patient who is shown a video while in bed may be more likely to become drowsy during instruction than a patient who is sitting in a bedside chair.

- Teaching aids can foster learning and help focus a learner's attention. To ensure the transfer of learning, the nurse should use the type of supplies or equipment the patient will eventually use. Before the teaching session, the nurse needs to assemble all equipment and visual aids and ensure that all audiovisual equipment is functioning effectively.

- Teaching that involves a number of the learner's senses often enhances learning. For instance, when teaching about changing a surgical dressing, the nurse can tell the patient about the procedure (hearing), show how to change the dressing (sight), and show how to manipulate the equipment (touch).

- Learning is more effective when the learners discover the content for themselves. Ways to increase learning include stimulating motivation and self-direction by, for example, providing specific, realistic, achievable outcomes; giving feedback; and helping the learner derive satisfaction from learning. The nurse may also enhance self-directed independent learning by encouraging the patient to explore sources of information. If certain activities do not assist the learner in attaining identified outcomes, these activities need to be reassessed; perhaps other activities can replace them. For instance, explanation alone may not be able to teach a patient to handle a syringe; actually handling the syringe may be more effective.

- Repetition reinforces learning. Summarizing content, rephrasing (using other words), and approaching the material from another point of view are ways of repeating and clarifying content. For instance, after discussing the kinds of foods that can be included in a diet, the nurse can describe the foods again, but in the context of the three meals eaten during one day.

- It is helpful to employ "organizers" to introduce the material to be learned. Advanced organizers provide a means of connecting unknown material to known material and generating logical relationships. For example, the following statement could be an advanced organizer: "You understand how urine flows down a catheter from the bladder. Now I will show you how to inject fluid so that it flows up the catheter into the bladder." The details that follow are then seen within a framework that adds meaning.

- The anticipated behavioral changes that indicate learning has taken place must always be within the context of the patient's lifestyle and resources. For example, it would be unreasonable to expect a woman to soak in a tub of hot water two times a day if she did not have a bathtub or had to heat water on a stove.

Special Teaching Strategies

One-to-one discussion is the most common method of teaching used by nurses. However, nurses can choose from a number of special teaching strategies, including anticipatory guidance, patient contracting, group teaching, technology-assisted instruction, discovery/problem solving, behavior modification, the teach-back method, and transcultural teaching. Any strategy the nurse selects must be appropriate for the learner and the learning objectives.

Anticipatory Guidance

Anticipatory guidance has been primarily associated with health promotion activities in pediatrics. In this context, nurses use anticipatory guidance to provide parents with information about developmental changes they can expect their child or children to exhibit as they grow and develop. However, anticipatory guidance can be used any time during the lifespan with the same focus: health promotion. For example, the nurse may provide anticipatory guidance to a family whose mother has Alzheimer disease to help them recognize safety concerns as the disease progresses. Anticipatory guidance may be provided to both individuals and groups. Nurses should consider several factors before providing anticipatory guidance, including the patient's age, developmental stage, health status, and health literacy level. See **Box 41–8** ⟫ for suggested anticipatory guidance topics.

Anticipatory guidance provided by healthcare professionals can help patients prevent health alterations or complications. Nurses can expect to use anticipatory guidance in the form of patient teaching in various settings, including:

- Prenatal visits
- Well-child/adolescent visits
- Annual medical/dental visits
- Community programs such as health screenings, health fairs, and safety programs.

Because the time for each visit is limited, nurses should build on a patient's current knowledge and care practices and start with a topic in which the patient expresses interest. Nursing using anticipatory guidance should reinforce what the patient and family are doing well and clear up any poorly understood concepts.

Box 41–8
Topics for Anticipatory Guidance

Children and Parents
- Growth and development
- Nutrition
- Mental health issues
- Risks of secondhand smoke
- Sleep safety and patterns
- Sunscreen use
- Automobile and bicycle safety
- Family and peer stress and relationships
- Disease and injury/accident prevention

Adults
- Injury prevention strategies for mechanical equipment
- UVA/UVB protection
- Responsible sexual behaviors
- Alcohol and drug use

Older Adults
- Fall prevention
- Medication use and side effects
- Age-related nutritional needs
- Safe driving evaluations
- Advance directives

Nurses rely on resources in the community to enhance the guidance provided. For example, Bright Futures provides information for anticipatory guidance regarding children. State and local Safe Kids coalitions help inform families about injury prevention strategies. Schools provide health and safety programs throughout the year. Nurses need to be aware of the types of programs available in the community to reinforce concepts.

⟫ **Stay Current:** Visit Bright Futures at www.brightfutures.org and Safe Kids at www.safekids.org to enhance your teaching strategies for children.

Patient Contracting

Learning contracts are mutually developed verbal or written agreements between the teacher and the learner. They are an increasingly popular, effective teaching strategy to encourage independence and control over personal health management and wellness. Essential elements include what the learner will learn, information resources and the way in which learning will be accomplished, and rewards for consistent contract adherence and goal achievement (Bastable & McLees, 2016). Use of a learning contract allows for freedom, mutual respect, and mutual responsibility.

The following is an example of a patient contract:

I, Kirsten Hugo, will exercise strenuously for 20 minutes three times per week for a period of 2 weeks and will then buy myself six yellow roses.

Kirsten Hugo
A. Tucker RN
July 30, 2017

Group Teaching

Group instruction is economical, and it provides members with an opportunity to share with and learn from others. A small group allows for discussion in which everyone can participate. A large group often necessitates a lecture technique or use of films, videos, slides, or role-playing by teachers.

All members involved in a particular group should have a common need (e.g., prenatal health or preoperative instruction). Sociocultural factors also should be considered when a group is being formed.

Technology-Assisted Instruction

Technology-assisted instruction (TAI) is increasingly popular. Initially, the primary use of computer educational methods was for cognitive learning of facts. Now, however, computers and other electronic devices (e.g., smartphones and tablets) can also be used to teach the following:

- Application of information (e.g., answering questions after reading information about a health subject)
- Psychomotor skills (e.g., filling a syringe on the computer screen to the correct dosage line)
- Complex problem-solving skills (e.g., responding to questions based on a patient situation)

TAI can also be used in various other ways. For example:

- Individual healthcare professionals or patients may use an electronic device for teaching/learning.
- Families or small groups of three to five patients may gather around one electronic device and take turns running a program and answering questions together.
- Large groups may view a display of a computer's monitor that is projected onto an overhead screen, while a teacher or a learner uses a keyboard or other device to change the display.
- Individuals or small groups may use computers or other electronic devices through shared network platforms or through websites.

Individuals using an electronic device are able to set the pace that meets their particular learning needs. Small groups are less able to do this, and large groups progress through the program at a pace that may be too slow for some learners and too fast for others. It is therefore helpful to group learners of similar needs and abilities together.

Whether using an electronic device alone or in large groups, learners read and view informational material, answer questions, and receive immediate feedback. The correct answer is usually indicated by the use of colors, flashing signs, or written praise. When the learner selects an incorrect answer, the program may respond with an explanation of why that was not the best answer and encouragement to try again. Many programs ask learners whether they want to review material on which the question and answer were based. Some programs feature simulated situations that allow learners to manipulate objects on the screen to learn psychomotor skills. When used to teach such skills, TAI must be followed up with practice on actual equipment supervised by the teacher.

Some patients may have a negative attitude about electronic devices that creates a barrier to learning. The nurse can help these patients by explaining how the device helps meet their needs. Matching a program or website to the patient's individual health circumstances may encourage the use of electronic devices. Providing a resource list of free available community sites for training and access may also help. For patients who use the internet, it is important for the nurse to teach the patient how to evaluate whether the site is a relevant, credible source for health information. In addition, it is important to recognize that some individuals still do not embrace technology. This may be due to a number of factors, including affordability, access, and literacy level.

Most media catalogs, professional journals, and healthcare libraries contain information about computer software programs and mobile device applications available to the nurse for patient education. The media specialist or librarian in a healthcare facility or college is an excellent resource to help locate appropriate programs. Technological educational material is also available for patients with different language needs, for patients with special visual needs, and for patients at various growth and development levels.

Discovery/Problem Solving

In using the discovery/problem-solving technique, the nurse presents some initial information, then asks the learner a question or presents a situation related to the information. The learner applies the new information to the situation and decides what to do. Learners can work alone or in groups. This technique is well suited to family learning. The teacher guides the learners through the thinking process necessary to reach the best solution to the question or the best action to take in the situation. This may also be referred to as **anticipatory problem solving**. For example, the nurse educator might present information on diabetes and glucose management. Then the nurse might ask the learners how they think their insulin and/or diet should be adjusted if their morning glucose reading is too low. In this way, patients learn what critical components they need to consider to reach the best solution to the problem.

Behavior Modification

The basic assumptions of the behavior modification system are (a) that human behaviors are learned and can be selectively strengthened, weakened, eliminated, or replaced; and (b) that an individual's behavior is under conscious control. Under this system, desirable behavior is rewarded and undesirable behavior is ignored. The patient's response is the key to behavior change. For example, patients who are trying to quit smoking are not criticized when they smoke, but they are praised or rewarded when they go without a cigarette for a certain period of time. For some people, a learning contract is combined with behavior modification and includes the following pertinent features:

- Positive reinforcement (e.g., praise) is used.
- The patient participates in the development of the learning plan.
- Undesirable behavior is ignored, not criticized.
- The expectation of the patient and the nurse is that the task will be mastered (i.e., the behavior will change).

Teach-Back Method

With the **teach-back method**, the nurse provides teaching on a particular topic, then asks the patient to describe the main points from that teaching using his or her own words. This method is similar to return demonstration, except it requires the patient to show understanding through verbal communication instead of through actual physical performance of a task (Agency for Healthcare Research and Quality [AHRQ], 2015).

In order to successfully employ the teach-back method, the nurse should keep several points in mind. First and foremost, the nurse must provide all information in plain language that the patient can understand. The nurse should also pause periodically throughout the teaching session to check that the patient understands and remembers the material delivered so far. If the nurse asks for certain information but the patient cannot provide it or restates the information incorrectly, the nurse must clarify the areas of confusion before moving on to the next topic in the teaching session. Once the nurse has addressed all of the teaching topics, he or she should once again ask the patient to explain major points not only from the most recent part of the session, but also from earlier portions. To help increase and reinforce patient understanding throughout the session, the nurse may supplement the teach-back method with use of handouts and/or return demonstration (AHRQ, 2015).

Although the teach-back method seems simple on its surface, it requires a great deal of preparation on the part of the nurse. Not only must the nurse plan the teaching session and select language and educational materials appropriate for each patient, but he or she must also anticipate which topics are most likely to elicit confusion and necessitate further follow-up. The nurse must also practice use of this method so that it does not seem awkward or off-putting to patients or unnecessarily extend the length of the teaching session. Finally, the nurse should remember that the teach-back method is not a test of the patient's knowledge or learning capacity, but rather of how well the nurse explained the information (AHRQ, 2015).

Transcultural Teaching

Nurses and patients from different cultural and ethnic backgrounds have additional barriers to overcome in the teaching–learning process. These barriers include language and communication problems, differing concepts of time, conflicting cultural healing practices, beliefs that may positively or negatively influence compliance with health teaching, and unique high-risk or high-frequency health problems that can be addressed with health promotion instruction. Nurses should consider the following guidelines when teaching patients from various ethnic backgrounds:

- Obtain teaching materials, pamphlets, and instructions in languages used by patients. Nurses who are unable to read the foreign language material for themselves can have a translator read the material to them. The nurse can then evaluate the quality of the information and update it with the translator's help as needed.

- Use visual aids, such as pictures, charts, or diagrams, to communicate meaning. Audiovisual material may be helpful if the English is spoken clearly and slowly. Even if

understanding the verbal message is a problem for the patient, seeing a skill or procedure may be helpful. In some instances, a translator can be asked to clarify the video. Alternatively, the video may be available in several languages, and the nurse can request the necessary version from the company.

- Use concrete rather than abstract words. Use simple language (short sentences, short words) and present only one idea at a time.

- Allow time for questions. This helps the patient mentally separate one idea or skill from another.

- Avoid the use of medical terminology or healthcare language, such as "taking your vital signs" or "apical pulse." Rather, nurses should say they are going to take a blood pressure reading or listen to the patient's heart.

- If understanding the patient's pronunciation is a problem, validate brief information in writing. For example, during assessments, write down numbers, words, or phrases and have the patient read them to verify accuracy.

- Use humor very cautiously. Meaning can change in the translation process.

- Do not use slang words or colloquialisms. These may be interpreted literally.

- Do not assume that a patient who nods, uses eye contact, or smiles is indicating an understanding of what is being taught. These responses may simply be the patient's way of indicating respect. The patient may feel that asking the nurse questions or stating a lack of understanding is inappropriate because it might embarrass the nurse or cause the nurse to "lose face."

- Invite and encourage questions during teaching. Let patients know they are urged to ask questions and be involved in making information clearer. When asking questions to evaluate patient understanding, avoid asking negative questions. These can be interpreted differently by people for whom English is a second language. "Do you understand how far you can bend your hip after surgery?" is better than the negative question "You don't understand how far you can bend your hip after surgery, do you?" With particularly difficult information or skills teaching, the nurse might say, "Most people have some trouble with this. May I please help you go through this one more time?" In some cultures, expressing a need is not appropriate, and expressing confusion or asking to be shown something again is considered rude.

- When explaining procedures or functioning related to personal areas of the body, it may be appropriate to have a nurse of the same sex do the teaching. Because of modesty concerns in many cultures and beliefs about what is considered appropriate and inappropriate male–female interaction, it is wise to have a female nurse teach a female patient about personal care, birth control, sexually transmitted infections, and other potentially sensitive areas. If a translator is needed during explanation of procedures or teaching, the translator should also be female.

- Include the family in planning and teaching. This promotes trust and mutual respect. Identify the authoritative family member and incorporate that person into the planning and teaching to promote compliance and support of health teaching. In some cultures, the male head of household is the critical family member to include in health teaching; in other cultures, it is the eldest female member.

- Consider the patient's time orientation. The patient may be more oriented to the present than the nurse. Cultures with a predominant orientation to the present include the Mexican American, Navajo Native American, Appalachian, Eskimo, and Filipino American cultures. Preventing future problems may be less significant for these patients than for others, so teaching prevention may be more difficult. For example, teaching a patient why and when to take medications may be more difficult if the patient is oriented to the present. In such instances, the nurse can emphasize preventing short-term problems rather than long-term problems. Failure to keep clinic appointments or to arrive on time is common in patients who have a present-time orientation. The nurse can help by accommodating these patients when they arrive for their appointment.

Schedules may be very flexible in present-oriented societies, with sleeping and eating patterns varying greatly. Teaching patients to take medications at bedtime or with a meal does not necessarily mean that these activities will occur at the same time each day. For this reason, the nurse should assess the patient's daily routine before teaching the patient to pair a treatment or medication with an event the nurse assumes occurs at the same time every day. When teaching a patient when to take medication, the nurse should determine whether a clock or watch is available to the patient and whether the patient can tell time.

- Identify cultural health practices and beliefs. Noncompliance with health teaching may be related to conflict with folk medicine beliefs. Noncompliance may also be related to lack of understanding or fatalism, a belief system in which life events are held to be predestined or fixed in advance and the individual is powerless to change them. Provide an opportunity for patients to explain their views and rationale for not adhering to the treatment plan or why it did not work.

The nurse should treat the patient's cultural healing beliefs with respect and try to identify whether any are in agreement or in conflict with what is being taught. The nurse can then focus on the ones in agreement to promote the integration of new learning with the familiar health practices. The goal is to arrive at a mutually agreeable plan: Decide which instructions must be followed for patient safety, then negotiate less crucial folk healing practices. See the Focus on Diversity and Culture feature for information specific to teaching Hispanic patients.

Evaluating Teaching and Learning

Evaluation is both an ongoing and a final process in which the patient, the nurse, and often the patient's support people determine what has been learned.

Focus on Diversity and Culture
Teaching Hispanic Patients

Hispanic patients are a diverse and growing population with special teaching considerations. One key consideration is language. Use of interpreters is helpful for overcoming this issue, as is use of written material in the patient's native language. In addition to these techniques, the "teach-back" method is also particularly helpful. This method can be time consuming, but it has been shown to result in better understanding and adherence in Hispanic patients (Juckett, 2013).

In addition, the nurse's observance of the Hispanic cultural values of *simpatía* (kindness), *personalismo* (friendliness), and *respeto* (respect) are essential for building trust with Hispanic patients and enhancing learning (Juckett, 2013). *Simpatía* can be defined as politeness and avoidance of conflict. For example, a nurse who compliments a patient on the health maintenance practices he observes rather than criticizing him for those he does not observe is exhibiting *simpatía*. *Personalismo* is a personal connection between two people. A nurse who asks a patient about his family is showing *personalismo*. *Personalismo* is similar to the phenomenon of connectedness that was found to be important for providing culturally competent care for Hispanic patients (Sobel & Sawin, 2016). *Respeto* is concern for the individual and respect for age and experience. By calling the patient "Señor" rather than using his first name, the nurse demonstrates *respeto*.

Evaluating Learning

The process of evaluating learning is the same as evaluating patient achievement of desired outcomes for other nursing diagnoses. Learning is measured against the predetermined learning outcomes selected in the planning phase of the teaching process. Thus, the outcomes serve not only to direct the teaching plan but also to provide outcome criteria for evaluation. For example, the outcome "Selects foods that are low in carbohydrates" can be evaluated by asking the patient to name such foods or to select low-carbohydrate foods from a list.

The best method for evaluating learning depends on the type of learning. For cognitive learning, the patient should be able to demonstrate acquisition of knowledge. Examples of evaluation tools for cognitive learning include the following:

- Direct observation of behavior (e.g., observing the patient demonstrate use of a blood pressure monitor)
- Written measurements (e.g., tests)
- Oral questioning (e.g., asking the patient to restate information or correct verbal responses to questions)
- Patient reports and self-monitoring. These can be useful during follow-up phone calls and home visits. Evaluating individual self-paced learning, as might occur with computer-assisted instruction, often incorporates self-monitoring.

The acquisition of psychomotor skills is best evaluated by observing how well the patient carries out a procedure, such as self-administration of insulin.

Affective learning is more difficult to evaluate. Whether attitudes or values have been learned may be inferred by listening to the patient's responses to questions, noting how the patient speaks about relevant subjects, and observing patient behavior that expresses feelings and values. For example, have parents learned to value health sufficiently to have their children immunized? Do patients who state that they value health actually use condoms every time they have sex with a new partner?

Following evaluation, the nurse may find it necessary to modify or repeat the teaching plan if the objectives have not been met or have been met only partially. Follow-up teaching in the home or by phone may be needed for the patient discharged from a health facility.

Behavior change does not always take place immediately after learning. Often individuals accept change intellectually first and then change their behavior only periodically (for example, a patient who knows that she must lose weight may diet and exercise off and on). If the new behavior is to replace the old behavior, it must emerge gradually; otherwise, the old behavior may prevail. The nurse can assist patients with behavior change by allowing for patient vacillation and by providing encouragement.

Evaluating the Learning Experience

It is important for nurses to evaluate their own teaching and the content of the teaching program, just as they evaluate the effectiveness of nursing interventions for other nursing diagnoses. Evaluation should include a consideration of all factors—the timing, the teaching strategies, the amount of information, whether the teaching was helpful, and so on. The nurse may note, for example, that the patient was overwhelmed with too much information, was bored, or was motivated to learn more. The patient should also evaluate the learning experience by providing feedback on what information, materials, approaches, and other elements were helpful, interesting, or confusing. To gather such information, the nurse might provide patients with a feedback questionnaire or perhaps even video learning sessions to see which aspects of the session seem to be most and least effective.

The nurse should not feel ineffective as a teacher if the patient forgets some of what is taught. Forgetting is normal and should be expected. Having the patient write down information, repeating it during teaching, giving handouts on the information, and having the patient be active in the learning process all promote retention.

Documenting

Documentation of the teaching process is essential because it provides a legal record that the teaching took place and communicates the teaching to other health professionals. If teaching is not documented, legally it did not occur.

It is also important to document the responses of the patient and support people to teaching activities. What did the patient or support person say or do to indicate that learning occurred? Has the patient demonstrated mastery of a skill or the acquisition of knowledge? The nurse records this in the patient's chart as evidence of learning. The following is a sample of documentation charting:

SAMPLE DOCUMENTATION

11/8/2017 1130 Learning to use glucometer to check own capillary blood glucose levels. Noted a slight hesitation with each step. Demonstrated correct technique. Stated "feeling more comfortable" each time she does it but still "needs to stop and think about the process." Will continue to monitor patient's progress. *C. Brown RN*

Many agencies have multiple-copy patient teaching forms that include the medical and nursing diagnoses, the treatment plan, and the patient education. After the teaching session is completed, the patient and the nurse sign the form, and a copy of the form is given to the patient as a record of teaching and as reinforcement of the content taught. A second copy of the completed and signed form is placed in the patient's chart. The parts of the teaching process that should be documented in the patient's chart include the following:

- Diagnosed learning needs
- Learning outcomes
- Topics taught
- Patient outcomes
- Need for additional teaching
- Resources provided.

The written teaching plan that the nurse uses as a resource to guide future teaching sessions might also include these elements:

- Actual information and skills taught
- Teaching strategies used
- Time framework and content for each class
- Teaching outcomes and methods of evaluation.

Nursing Care Plan
A Patient Who Requires Teaching About Wound Care

Kevin McArthur is a 22-year-old male college student who received a laceration on his leg while playing in an intramural hockey game. During the game, Kevin became entangled with another player. He fell as a result of the encounter and landed on the other player's skate blade.

Kevin indicates that the injury occurred two nights ago and that it is no longer bleeding. He tells you that he does not think the wound is a "big deal," but came to the health center today at his roommate's insistence. He also admits to you that he is a little embarrassed that his "clumsiness" has resulted in this injury.

Nursing Care Plan (continued)

ASSESSMENT	DIAGNOSES	PLANNING
Kevin is alert and oriented. He tells you he lives in a dormitory on campus and confirms that he is able to understand, read, and write English. He seems distracted, bored, and uninterested in performing wound self-care. You check his vitals and make the following assessments: T_O 38.7°C (101.6°F); P 66 beats/min; R 17/min; BP 115/74 mmHg. Kevin's weight is 85 kg (187.4 lb) and within normal limits for his height. Physical examination reveals a 7-cm (2.5-in) laceration on the left lower anterior leg. There is redness and minor swelling around the laceration. You also note the presence of serous exudate.	■ *Impaired Skin Integrity* ■ *Risk for Infection* related to alteration in skin integrity ■ *Deficient Knowledge* of care of sutured wound related to lack of prior experience (NANDA-I © 2014)	■ The patient will describe normal wound healing. ■ The patient will identify three main signs and symptoms of infection. ■ The patient will identify supplies needed for wound care. ■ The patient will correctly perform a return demonstration of wound cleansing and bandaging. ■ The patient will describe appropriate action if questions or complications arise. ■ The patient will identify date, time, and location of follow-up appointment for suture removal.

IMPLEMENTATION

- Assist the healthcare provider with cleansing, suturing, and dressing the wound as ordered.
- Describe normal wound healing and provide written and visual instructions of the signs and symptoms of local infection and complications, including increased redness, swelling, purulent drainage, and pain at wound site. Discuss the symptoms of systemic infection, including fever and malaise.
- Identify and provide wound care supplies such as bandaging material (e.g., gauze wrap, nonadhesive pads, adhesive tape) and cleansing solution as prescribed by provider (e.g., mild soap and water, antimicrobial solution, triple-antibiotic ointment).

- Demonstrate wound cleansing and bandaging on the patient's wound. Remove wound dressings and have the patient perform return demonstration. Provide a written handout describing the procedure.
- Instruct on appropriate actions and follow-up if questions or complications occur Provide written instructions listing available resources, clinic contact information, and treatment plan. Include the date, time, and location of next follow-up appointment in 10 days in written instructions.

EVALUATION

At the 10-day follow-up appointment, Kevin reports that he has forgotten to clean the wound and change the dressing "a few times." The dressing on his leg is clearly several days old and was haphazardly applied. His wound shows signs of local infection, including thick yellow discharge, redness, and swelling. Kevin's temperature is also elevated. The healthcare provider diagnoses Kevin with an abscess. His stitches are removed and the wound is drained. Kevin is prescribed a 2-week course of antibiotics. He is also advised to soak the infected area with warm towels three times per day to aid the healing process.

CRITICAL THINKING

1. Discuss Kevin's readiness to learn at his initial appointment and describe indicators of his level of readiness. How might the nurse enhance his readiness to learn?

2. What are the priority learning outcomes for Kevin at his follow-up appointment? Which teaching methods might improve his compliance with the treatment regimen?

3. How would you handle the situation if Kevin continues to show a lack of interest in self–wound care in spite of the changes to your teaching methods?

REVIEW Patient/Consumer Education

RELATE Link the Concepts and Exemplars

Linking the exemplar of patient/consumer education with the concept of development:

1. How does the concept of development impact teaching and learning?

2. How should the nurse incorporate characteristics of each developmental stage when choosing teaching strategies?

Linking the exemplar of patient/consumer education with the concept of culture and diversity:

3. What aspects of culture should be considered before developing a teaching plan for a patient?

4. How should the nurse address teaching and learning when a patient's health beliefs and values differ from his or her own?

Linking the exemplar of patient/consumer education with the concept of cognition:

5. How should the nurse address teaching and learning for a patient with altered cognition?

6. How does the concept of cognition impact the nurse's teaching plan and the patient's learning?

REFER Go to Pearson MyLab Nursing and eText

- Additional review materials

REFLECT Apply Your Knowledge

Mrs. Yorty is a 59-year-old female bank vice president who is heavily relied on by her boss and coworkers. Three days ago, she was admitted to the hospital with complaints of shortness of breath and mild chest pain. A diagnostic evaluation indicates that she has significant coronary artery disease but has not yet had a heart attack. Her primary care provider has indicated that Mrs. Yorty will need to make significant lifestyle changes to reduce her heart attack risk.

As her nurse, you have been asked to teach Mrs. Yorty about her disease process, diet, exercise, and stress reduction. As you begin teaching Mrs. Yorty, you note that she is very pleasant and frequently nods her head, but she also seems preoccupied and is easily distracted.

1. How would you evaluate Mrs. Yorty's readiness to learn?

2. Of what benefit would a learning needs assessment be since Mrs. Yorty is obviously a well-educated patient?

3. You recognize that you have a great deal of information to deliver to Mrs. Yorty, and you are concerned that you will not be able to teach it all. What can you do to help Mrs. Yorty and still accomplish the learning outcomes?

4. How will you know if your teaching is effective?

5. How might your teaching differ if you were teaching Mrs. Yorty at home rather than in a hospital or acute care setting?

References

Ackerman, I. N., Bucknill, A., Pate, R. S., Broughton, N. S., Rogers, C., Cavka, B., … Brand, C. A. (2017). Preferences for disease-related education and support among younger people with hip or knee osteoarthritis. *Arthritis Care & Research, 69*(4), 499–508. doi:10.1002/acr.22950

Agency for Healthcare Research and Quality (AHRQ). (2015). *Health literacy universal precautions toolkit, 2nd edition: Use the teach-back method.* Retrieved from http://www.ahrq.gov/professionals/quality-patient-safety/quality-resources/tools/literacy-toolkit/healthlittoolkit2-tool5.html.

American Nurses Association (ANA). (2010). Standard 8: Education. In *Nursing: Scope and standards of practice.* Washington, DC: Author.

Ball, J. W., Bindler, R. C., Cowen, K., & Shaw, M. (2017). *Principles of pediatric nursing: Caring for children* (7th ed.). Hoboken, NJ: Pearson Education.

Bastable, S. B. (2014). *Nurse as educator: Principles of teaching and learning for nursing practice* (4th ed.). Burlington, MA: Jones & Bartlett Learning.

Bastable, S. B., & McLees, E. P. (2016). Behavioral objectives and teaching plans. In *Essentials of patient education* (2nd ed., pp. 347–376). Burlington, MA: Jones & Bartlett Learning.

Blazeck, A. M., Katrancha, E., Drahnak, D., Sowko, L. A., & Faett, B. (2016). Using interactive video-based teaching to improve nursing students' ability to provide patient-centered discharge teaching. *Journal of Nursing Education, 55*(5), 296–299. http://dx.doi.org/10.3928/01484834-20160414-11

Calvo, R. (2016). Health literacy and quality of care among Latino immigrants in the United States. *Health Social Work, 41*(1), e44–e51.

Candela, L. (2012). From teaching to learning: Theoretical foundations. In *Teaching in nursing: A guide for faculty* (4th ed., pp. 202–243). St. Louis, MO: Elsevier Saunders.

Centers for Disease Control and Prevention (CDC). (2013). *Medication adherence* [Educational standard PowerPoint]. Retrieved from https://www.cdc.gov/primarycare/materials/medication/docs/medication-adherence-01ccd.pdf

Centers for Disease Control and Prevention (CDC). (2015). *Learn about health literacy.* Retrieved from http://www.cdc.gov/healthliteracy/learn/

Centers for Disease Control and Prevention (CDC). (2016). *Health literacy.* Retrieved from http://www.cdc.gov/healthliteracy/

Gardner, H. (1983). *Frames of mind: Theory of multiple intelligences.* New York, NY: Basic Books.

Goleman, D. (1995). *Emotional intelligence.* New York, NY: Bantam Books.

Hadden, K. B. (2015). Health literacy training for health professions students. *Patient education and counseling, 98,* 918–920. Retrieved from http://dx.doi.org/10.1016/j.pec.2015.03.016

HealthIT.gov. (2013). *e-health: Find quality resources.* Retrieved from https://www.healthit.gov/patients-families/find-quality-resources

Health on the Net Foundation. (2016). *The commitment to reliable health and medical information on the internet.* Retrieved from http://www.hon.ch/HONcode/Patients/Visitor/visitor.html

Herdman, T. H. & Kamitsuru, S. (Eds). *Nursing Diagnoses—Definitions and Classification 2015–2017.* Copyright © 2014, 1994–2014 NANDA International. Used by arrangement with John Wiley & Sons, Inc. Companion website: www.wiley.com/go/nursingdiagnoses.

Hnatiuk, C. N. (2012). Mentoring nurses toward success. *Minority Nurse, Summer 2012,* 43–45. Retrieved from http://minoritynurse.com/mentoring-nurses-toward-success/

Institute of Medicine. (2012). *Best care at lower cost: The path to continuously learning health care in America.* Retrieved from http://www.nationalacademies.org/hmd/~/media/Files/Report%20Files/2012/Best-Care/Best%20Care%20at%20Lower%20Cost_Recs.pdf

Juckett, G. (2013). Caring for Latino patients. *American Family Physician, 87*(1), 48–54. Retrieved from http://www.aafp.org/afp/2013/0101/p48.html.

Manafo, E., & Wong, S. (2012). Health literacy programs for older adults: A systematic literature review. *Health Education Research, 27*(6), 947–960. http://dx.doi.org/10.1093/her/cys067

Maningat, P., Gordon, B. R., & Breslow, J. L. (2013). How do we improve patient compliance and adherence to long-term statin therapy? *Current Atherosclerosis Reports, 15*(291), 2–8. Retrieved from http://link.springer.com/article/10.1007/s11883-012-0291-7

McCallum, J., Lamont, D., & Kerr, E. L. (2016). First year undergraduate nursing students and nursing mentors: An evaluation of their experience of specialist areas as their hub practice learning environment. *Nurse Education in Practice, 16*(1), 182–187. Retrieved from http://dx.doi.org/10.1016/j.nepr.2015.06.005

National Council of State Boards of Nursing [NCSBN]. (2016). *Transition to practice.* Retrieved from https://www.ncsbn.org/transition-to-practice.htm

O'Dea, B., Calear, A. L., & Perry, Y. (2015). Is e-health the answer to gaps in adolescent mental health service provision? *Current Opinions in Psychiatry 28*(4), 336–42.

Osborn, K. S., Wraa, C. E., Watson, A. B., & Holleran, R. (2013). *Medical-surgical nursing: Preparation for practice.* Upper Saddle River, NJ: Pearson.

Park, J. S., Kim, M. S., Kim, H., Kim, S. I., Shin, C. H., Lee, H. J., … Moon, S. (2016). A randomized controlled trial of an educational video to improve quality of bowel preparation for colonoscopy. *BMC Gastroenterology, 16*(1), 64. doi:10.1186/s12876-016-0476-6

Pew Research Center. (2014). *Health fact sheet.* Retrieved from http://www.pewinternet.org/fact-sheets/health-fact-sheet/

Rush, K. L., Adamack, M., Gordon, J., Lily, M., & Janke, R. (2012). Best practices of formal new graduate nurse transition programs: An integrative review. *International Journal of Nursing Studies, 50,* 345–356. Retrieved from http://dx.doi.org/10.1016/j.ijnurstu.2012.06.009

Sentell, T. & Braun, K. (2012). Low health literacy, limited English proficiency, and health status in Asians, Latinos, and other racial/ethnic groups in California. *Journal of Health Communication, 17*(Suppl 3), 82–99.

Sobel, L. L., & Sawin, E. M. (2016). Guiding the process of culturally competent care with Hispanic patients: A grounded theory study. *Journal of Transcultural Nursing, 27*(3), 226–232.

Spector, N., Blegan, M. A., Silvestre, J., Barnsteiner, J., Lynn, M. R., Ulrich, B., … Alexander, M. (2015). Transition to practice study in hospital settings. *Journal of Nursing Regulation 5*(4), 24–38.

U.S. Department of Health and Human Services (USDHHS). (n.d.). Quick guide to health literacy. Retrieved from https://health.gov/communication/literacy/quickguide/factsbasic.htm

U.S. Department of Health and Human Services (USDHHS), Office of Disease Prevention and Health Promotion. (2010). *National action plan to improve health literacy*. Washington, DC: Author.

Retrieved from http://www.health.gov/communication/hlactionplan/pdf/Health_Literacy_Action_Plan.pdf

Van den Bemt, B. J.., Zwikker, H. E., & van den Ende, C. H. (2012). Medication adherence in patients with rheumatoid arthritis: A critical appraisal of the existing literature. *Expert Review of Clinical Immunology, 8*(4), 337–351. doi:10.1586/eci.12.23

Warshawsky, N. E., Havens, D. S., & Knafl, G. (2012). The influence of interpersonal relationships on nurse managers' work engagement and proactive work behavior. *Journal of Nursing Administration, 42*(9), 418–425. Retrieved from http://dx.doi.org/10.1097/NNA.0b013e3182668129

White, M., Garbez, R., Carroll, M., Brinker, E., & Howie-Esquivel, J. (2013). Is "teach-back" associated with knowledge retention and hospital readmission in hospitalized heart failure patients? *Journal of Cardiovascular Nursing, 28*(2), 137–146. doi:10.1097/JCN.0b013e31824987bd

Wilkinson, J. M. (2013). *Nursing diagnosis handbook with NIC interventions and NOC outcomes* (10th ed.). Upper Saddle River, NJ: Prentice Hall Health.

World Health Organization. (2013a). *E-health*. Retrieved from http://www.who.int/trade/glossary/story021/en

World Health Organization. (2013b). *Health literacy: The solid facts*. Retrieved from www.euro.who.int/__data/assets/pdf_file/…/e96854.pdf

References 2001

Part V
Healthcare Domain

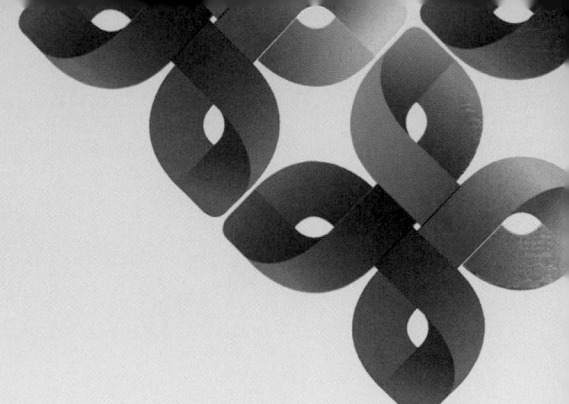

Part V consists of modules that outline and define principles related to the healthcare domain, including accountability, ethics, and quality improvement. Each module presents a concept that relates directly to professional nursing, its relationship to healthcare systems and policies, and how nursing within the healthcare system impacts patient health and well-being. Selected principles or topics of each concept are presented as exemplars. The exemplars in the module on Accountability, for example, cover Competence and Professional Development. Each module addresses the effect of that concept and the selected exemplars on the care of individuals across the lifespan, inclusive of their culture, their gender, and their developmental status.

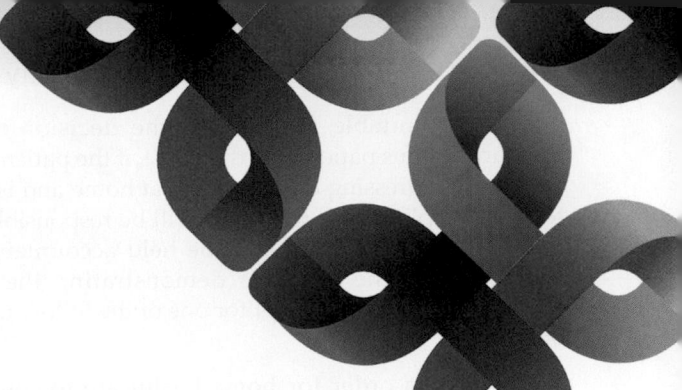

Module 42
Accountability

Module Outline and Learning Outcomes

The Concept of Accountability

Components of Accountability

42.1 Analyze how the nursing profession promotes accountability.

Concepts Related to Accountability

42.2 Outline the relationship between accountability and other concepts.

Socialization to Nursing

42.3 Analyze the process of socialization to nursing.

Factors Influencing Nursing Practice and Accountability

42.4 Differentiate factors that influence nursing practice and accountability.

Accountability Exemplars

Exemplar 42.A Competence

42.A Analyze competence as it relates to accountability.

Exemplar 42.B Professional Development

42.B Analyze professional development as it relates to accountability.

» The Concept of Accountability

Concept Key Terms

Accountability, **2695**
Autonomy, **2697**
Consumer, **2701**

Governance, **2697**
Patient Self-Determination Act (PSDA), **2702**

Responsibility, **2695**
Socialization, **2699**
Standards of care, **2695**

Standards of practice, **2695**
Telecommunication, **2702**

Telehealth, **2702**
Telenursing, **2702**

Accountability and *responsibility* are words that are often used interchangeably. However, they have some important distinctions. **Accountability** involves being answerable for the outcomes of a task or assignment. Nurses are accountable for their own actions and behaviors, but they may also be accountable for the actions of others, such as subordinates or trainees. **Responsibility** is the specific obligation associated with the performance of duties of a particular role, and it belongs to the individual performing the duties. Nurses are responsible for performing their assigned tasks reliably, dependably, and to the best of their abilities. Nurses' sense of accountability guides their performance, which ultimately determines patient outcomes.

Accountability in nursing cannot be achieved without clear definitions of what is an accepted standard of care. **Standards of care**, also known as **standards of practice**, are professional standards or guidelines used to determine what a nurse should or should not do. These standards are established by organizations such as The Joint Commission, the American Nurses Association (ANA), and the National League for Nursing (NLN). They describe the responsibilities for which nurses are accountable, thereby setting a

desirable and achievable benchmark against which the performance and care standards of individual nurses may be measured (Davis, 2014). For example, a standard of practice/care for medication administration set forth by The Joint Commission is to require two patient identifiers prior to giving the prescribed dose. A nurse who chooses not to meet this requirement is failing to practice at the minimum standard acceptable to the profession and will be held accountable to the patient and the facility for which he or she works.

As another example, suppose a nurse has a patient who will need continued wound care for his left foot after discharge to home. The patient has said that he thinks he understands the procedure for changing his dressing and has promised to call if he needs any further teaching. The nurse knows that the standards of care dictate asking the patient to demonstrate how to change the dressing so that the nurse can evaluate the patient's understanding and ability to care for himself. The nurse must decide whether to allow the patient to go home without seeing him perform the dressing change or whether discharge needs to be delayed until the patient can demonstrate his understanding. In this scenario, the nurse is responsible for upholding the standards of care and is accountable for making the decision regarding discharge of this patient. Furthermore, if the patient does not perform the dressing care properly at home and is readmitted for complications, the nurse will be responsible for that particular outcome and may be held accountable. As an alternative to the patient's demonstrating the dressing change, the nurse could opt for one of the following courses of action:

- Request an order for home healthcare to continue the teaching and follow up until the patient is comfortable on his own.

- Teach a family member to perform the dressing change in case the patient is not feeling well enough to do it on his own.

- Arrange for the patient to travel to an outpatient nursing facility for daily dressing changes.

Regardless of the chosen method, the nurse is accountable at discharge for ensuring that the patient can get his wound dressed as often as the order advises. The patient must rely on the nurse's judgment for the most favorable outcome.

》》 Stay Current: To learn more about your state's board of nursing and standards of practice, visit the National Council of State Boards of Nursing website at https://www.ncsbn.org/nurse-practice-act.htm.

Unfortunately, the term *accountability* often carries a negative connotation. When an error is made, the question "Who is accountable?" often translates into "Who is to blame?" The implication is that someone has failed. The negative image of accountability is what the public tends to see, especially since the release of *To Err Is Human* (1999), a landmark report by the Institute of Medicine (IOM). In the years since that report, healthcare organizations have worked hard to regain the public's trust. Organizations such as The Joint Commission, NLN, and ANA have revised and created standards for nurses to follow independently and jointly to ensure delivery of the safest, most competent care possible. More recently, the Robert Wood Johnson Foundation sponsored Quality and Safety Education for Nurses (Cronenwett, Sherwood, & Gelmon, 2009; QSEN, 2014), an initiative to improve quality and safety in prelicensure nursing programs. This initiative endorsed the idea that quality and safety education must become core competencies embedded in all programs that prepare nurses for basic practice. Indeed, according to QSEN (2014), the six competencies critical to the nursing role are patient-centered care, teamwork and collaboration, evidence-based practice, quality improvement, safety, and informatics.

》》 Stay Current: To learn more about the QSEN competencies, visit the QSEN Institute website at http://qsen.org/.

Research supports the importance of accountability in preventing errors as well as after making them (Flynn et al., 2012). However, if nurses practice in a positive and supportive environment and celebrate accountability for their successes as well as their errors, the culture of the profession will remain positive. Thus, focusing on and honoring successes are as important as examining and correcting errors.

Components of Accountability

Nursing as a profession embraces and promotes personal and professional accountability. Aspects of the profession that promote accountability include:

- The requirement to successfully complete exhaustive, specialized training to acquire the body of knowledge necessary for performance of the role;

- The direction of the professional individual toward service, whether in a community or an organizational capacity;

- Allegiance to a code of ethics;

- The autonomy of the role; and

- Membership in a professional organization.

These factors are described in greater detail in the sections that follow.

Specialized Education

Specialized education is an important aspect of professional status. Today, entry into registered nursing in the United States is open to any individual who successfully earns either a hospital diploma or an associate's, bachelor's, master's, or doctorate degree in nursing and subsequently passes the National Council Licensure Examination, or NCLEX. Fewer than 70 hospitals around the country still offer diploma programs, so the vast majority of new RNs hold either an associate's or bachelor's degree (NLN, 2014; Salsberg, 2015). The ANA recommends a bachelor's degree to enter professional practice, and many magnet hospitals and academic health centers require that their RNs have at least a bachelor's degree. Thus, many associate's degree RNs later opt to pursue their bachelor's degree, typically through participation in an RN-to-BSN program that builds on their existing knowledge and skill set. Similarly, many bachelor's degree RNs go on to earn a master's or doctorate degree in order to further advance in their careers (American Association of Colleges of Nursing, 2015).

Body of Knowledge

As a profession, nursing has a well-defined body of knowledge and expertise that is always expanding. This knowledge base is the product of various conceptual nursing frameworks that direct practice, education, and ongoing research. The nursing profession continues to grow and develop its body of knowledge over time, maintaining an evidence-based practice based on current research that promotes accountability for safe nursing practice (see the Evidence-Based Practice feature).

Service Orientation

A service orientation means that nursing, unlike some occupations, is not primarily driven by considerations of profit. Rather, nursing emphasizes service to others as a matter of tradition and as a basis for accountability. Rules, policies, and codes of ethics guide and shape this tradition of service. Nursing has been and continues to be an integral component of the system for delivering healthcare.

Evidence-Based Practice
Leadership Interventions to Establish Evidence-Based Practice

Problem

What is the impact of leadership facilitation strategies on nurses' beliefs about the importance and frequency of using evidence in their daily practice? How can nursing leaders encourage nurses to adopt evidence-based practice (EBP) methods?

Evidence

In one study by Hauck, Winsett, and Kuric (2013), a 429-bed non-teaching, faith-based hospital located in a moderate-sized city in the Midwest conducted a prospective descriptive comparative study that involved three surveys. The Evidence-Based Practice Beliefs Scale, the Implementation Scale, and the Organizational Culture and Readiness for System-Wide Integration Survey measured change before and after facilitation of strategies for EBP enculturation. They found that the hospital's nursing leadership facilitated infrastructure development in three major areas: incorporating EBP outcomes in the strategic plan; supporting mentors; and advocating for resources for education and outcome dissemination. Following interventions in these areas, nurses' total group scores regarding their belief in the value of EBP improved significantly. Hauck et al. (2013) concluded that the most successful strategies for changing nurses' perceptions of EBP and organizational readiness were EBP education and establishing internal opportunities to disseminate findings. They also noted that transformational nursing leadership drives organizational change and provides vision, human and financial resources, and time that empowers nurses to include evidence in practice.

Several years later, another study (Guerrero et al., 2016) used semistructured interviews and surveys to identify the approaches used by leaders of addiction treatment centers when implementing EBP methods in their facilities. In their study, Guerrero et al. (2016)

determined that the top strategies for encouraging staff to use EBP techniques involved the "recruitment and selection of staff members receptive to change, offering support and requesting feedback during the implementation process, and offering in-vivo and hands-on training." Leadership behaviors that encouraged EBP techniques included being proactive to implementation needs, supportive to staff members, knowledgeable to guide the implementation process, and willing to address ongoing barriers to EBP implementation.

Implications

Because of the continual nursing shortage, healthcare facilities must recruit and retain competent nursing staff, as well as effectively implement evidence-based changes in the practice environment. Studies such as those by Hauck et al. (2013) and Guerrero et al. (2016) provide insight as to the most effective methods for making EBP part of an organization's nursing culture. In doing so, they also highlight strategies that can be used to improve nursing practice and prevent errors—thereby contributing to higher-quality patient care, better nursing retention, and lower costs.

Critical Thinking Application

1. In the study by Hauck et al. (2013), nurses were encouraged to search for evidence to support their daily practice. How have you been encouraged to use evidence-based research findings as a nursing student?

2. Although not discussed in these particular studies, from the authors' findings, what role could nursing education programs take in assisting with EBP implementation in acute care nursing units where student nurses are practicing?

Code of Ethics

Another important part of the nursing tradition is respect for the inherent worth and dignity of all people. To preserve this value, professionals in the nursing field must do what is considered right, even if doing so means they incur a personal cost. In other words, nurses must strive to maintain their integrity.

As the needs and values of society change, so do its ethical codes. To promote accountability in the use of ethical behaviors, the nursing profession has developed its own codes of ethics specific to the aims of nursing and the problems that nurses typically face. These codes are discussed in detail in the module on Ethics.

Autonomy

Generally speaking, **autonomy** means independence or freedom; thus, a profession is autonomous if it is able to regulate itself and set standards of practice for its own members. One of the purposes of a professional association is to give its members autonomy. Professional status for nursing hinges to a large degree on the nursing profession's ability to function autonomously in how it formulates nursing policy and controls its own activity. Professional autonomy involves legal authority; a professional group is autonomous only if it possesses the legal authority to define its goals and responsibilities in how it delivers its services, describe its particular functions and roles, and

determine its scope of practice. With respect to the autonomy of the nursing profession, state Boards of Nursing (detailed in the module on Legal Issues) hold this legal authority.

Autonomy for nurses on an individual level means professional responsibility, accountability for their actions, and the freedom to do their jobs as necessary while at work. Nurses at all levels of practice take accountability for their actions when they advocate for their own autonomy and for that of their nurse colleagues.

Professional Organization

Professions are different from occupations in that they operate under the umbrella of a professional organization. This organizational structure provides **governance**, which establishes and maintains social, political, and economic arrangements that give professionals the means to control their professional affairs, including their practice, self-discipline, and working conditions. The module on Health Policy fully describes the professional organizations that govern and differentiate the profession of nursing.

Concepts Related to Accountability

Because accountability is a key aspect of professional nursing, it affects all areas of nursing practice. On a basic level, nurses are answerable for ensuring that patients' essential health and

Concepts Related to
Accountability

CONCEPT	RELATIONSHIP TO ACCOUNTABILITY	NURSING IMPLICATIONS
Comfort	The nurse is accountable for assessing the patient's level of comfort and providing effective interventions to promote or maintain patient comfort.	■ Assess patient's reported level of comfort at least once per shift, or more often as indicated by patient's condition. ■ Document patient's comfort level and any nursing interventions provided.
Evidence-Based Practice	The nurse is accountable for practice within an EBP environment and for implementing evidence in his or her own practice.	■ Develop a clinical question using the format described in the EBP Concept. ■ Conduct a literature search for current evidence. ■ Select appropriate nursing interventions based on evidence from the literature search.
Health, Wellness, Illness, and Injury	The nurse is accountable for assessing the patient's current level of health and wellness, then providing teaching, interventions, and referrals aimed at preserving and/or promoting health and preventing illness.	■ Assess patient's current overall health, including biophysical, cognitive, psychologic, and spiritual components. ■ Provide teaching on general health promotion and illness prevention measures beneficial to all individuals (e.g., regular exercise, immunizations), as well as measures specific to the patient's risk factors and lifestyle (e.g., smoking cessation, heart-healthy diet). ■ Refer patients to counselors, clergy, dietitians, physical therapists, support groups, and other outside resources as appropriate.
Safety	The nurse is accountable for keeping patients safe within the healthcare environment, as well as for teaching patients ways to reduce the risk of illness and injury in their daily lives.	■ Identify and address safety hazards in the immediate healthcare environment. ■ Assess patients' risk for various types of injury outside the healthcare environment. ■ As appropriate, teach patients about actions that can reduce their risk of injury (e.g., helmet use when bicycling, proper use of child safety restraints).
Teaching and Learning	The nurse is accountable for patient education concerning all aspects of care. The nurse is accountable for staying up to date with the latest evidence for best practices. The nurse is accountable for providing current and accurate teaching to subordinates, especially nursing leaders who are mentoring nursing students.	■ Assess patient and family learning needs. ■ Assess readiness for learning. ■ Design and implement appropriate educational interventions. ■ Read current journal articles and attend workshops or seminars that provide up-to-date information about procedures, medications, and other standards of practice.
Trauma	Patients may present with signs or symptoms of trauma, and/or they may be at risk for abuse or violence. The nurse is accountable for taking action to prevent further harm; in some circumstances, the nurse may also have a legal duty to report.	■ Assess for signs of prior physical, emotional, or sexual abuse as part of the admission process. ■ Assess for both risk of abuse and suicide risk as part of the admission process. ■ Be aware of warning signs of abuse or suicide that may be demonstrated or verbalized by patients.

wellness needs are addressed. This means the nurse is accountable for providing information about measures that protect and promote patients' physical health, such as preventive screenings, recommended immunizations, smoking cessation, adequate exercise, and a healthy diet. It also means that nurses must address the cognitive, psychologic, and spiritual dimensions of health, examples of which include teaching patients about stress management and making referrals to counselors, clergy, and similar resources as needed.

Beyond issues of health and wellness, nurses are also accountable for certain physical outcomes of patient care. These vary depending on setting, the patient's condition, state nurse practice acts, and healthcare providers' orders. Still, there are some things for which nurses are nearly always answerable. For example, in the hospital setting, nurses are typically accountable for ensuring that patients receive appropriate fluids and nutrition, have an environment that permits adequate rest and sleep, maintain appropriate oxygenation levels, and receive assistance with elimination if necessary. Similarly, all nurses are accountable for promoting patient safety. This encompasses not just maintaining a safe physical environment within the healthcare setting, but also teaching patients about ways to reduce their risk of injury in various aspects of their daily lives. Helping patients maintain comfort (or at least achieve a manageable level of pain) is a related concern. Indeed, encouraging patients to give voice to any needs and providing appropriate comfort interventions are major accountability roles for nurses in their own right, and they also help promote a safer care environment.

Yet another key area of nursing accountability relates to trauma. Per both legal requirements and the ethical standards of the profession, nurses have a duty to report certain types of trauma to the proper authorities. This includes known and suspected abuse of children and the elderly, as well as certain categories of violence-related injuries (e.g., gunshot wounds); exact requirements vary from state to state. Nurses must also continually remain aware of the potential for abuse of any vulnerable child or adult with whom they come into contact during their practice. Nurses are further accountable for preventing patients from engaging in self-directed violence, which means they must routinely assess patients for factors that may indicate an increased risk of self-harm, suicide, and suicidal intent.

Because teaching is a critical nursing function, it too is an important area of accountability—and one that extends to all patient care areas. As previously mentioned, nurses must provide patients with broad-based information about health, illness, and safety, but they are also accountable for educating patients about tests, procedures, diagnoses, treatments, and other self-care measures specific to their condition. In order to provide such teaching, nurses must first assess each patient's learning style and readiness to learn. Nurses are also accountable for their own ongoing education and professional development. This encompasses not just meeting state and institutional continuing education requirements, but also taking steps to apply what they have learned via evidence-based practice.

The Concepts Related to Accountability feature links some, but not all, of the concepts integral to accountability. They are presented in alphabetical order.

Case Study » Part 1

Jen Sturges is a new RN on the medical unit in a 245-bed hospital. During the evening shift, Jen starts her rounds with her five patients. One of her patients is a 45-year-old woman named Kathryn Miller, who has been admitted with a GI diagnosis and also has a history of back pain. During Jen's assessment of her pain level, Ms. Miller says she is "doing just fine," although she seems very anxious. As Jen reviews Ms. Miller's vital signs, which the CNA had recently taken, she notes a blood pressure much higher than usual. Jen comments that one of the symptoms of pain is elevated blood pressure. Ms. Miller describes trying to overrule her body by ignoring its signals and by having a dialogue between the "body me" and the "real me." Ms. Miller also states, "If I refuse to pay attention to my body, my pain will go away."

Jen realizes that Ms. Miller, although actually in pain, might not be allowing herself to pay attention. Jen asks Ms. Miller if she has discussed pain management with her primary healthcare provider. Ms. Miller laughs: "My doctor tries to have me take narcotics, but I worry about those types of meds." As she speaks, Ms. Miller's hands are gripping the bed sheets and she is shaking. She says, "The pain is my enemy, and I don't talk to my enemies."

Jen knows that ignoring the body's signals of pain can cause serious consequences; for example, the pain could intensify and the patient's blood pressure could rise significantly. Jen also realizes that Ms. Miller needs to get appropriate treatment for her pain. After her assessment, Jen discusses her concerns about Ms. Miller with the unit charge nurse, including Ms. Miller's need for pain management and comfort.

Clinical Reasoning Questions Level I

1. Why is it important for Jen to complete her patient's assessment before leaving the room?
2. What further symptoms does Jen observe while she speaks with her patient?
3. What information should Jen share with the charge nurse to assist in meeting her patient's needs?

Clinical Reasoning Questions Level II

4. With what staff should Jen and the charge nurse plan to collaborate to find a better method for managing Ms. Miller's pain?
5. When a patient refuses pain management, why should the nurse pursue other solutions rather than simply acquiescing?

Socialization to Nursing

As previously mentioned, the members of a profession—and not outsiders—determine the standards of education and practice for that profession. Entering a profession is therefore similar to entering a new society, so it involves a complete socialization process far more extensive than what most nonprofessional occupations require. Socialization into a profession supports accountability because it has consequences for the nurse by instilling critical values and providing opportunities for interactions that support and promote accountability.

Socialization is the process by which individuals learn to become members of groups and society as well as learn the social rules defining the relationships into which they will enter. In a traditional sense, socialization involves learning how to behave, feel, and see the world in your chosen role as others do in that same role (Hardy & Conway, 1988). Professional socialization is a more complex process. Dinmohammadi et al. (2013) conducted a meta-analysis to clarify the process of professional socialization and to identify its attributes, antecedents, and consequences in nursing. They argue that professional socialization is a complex process with four critical attributes: learning, interaction, development, and adaptation. Comprehensive educational programs, competent faculty and role models, and adequate field experiences were found to be the antecedents of these attributes. Additional research by Price (2009) further underscores the need for mentors and peers in nursing.

Interaction with fellow students is a powerful driver for professional socialization among nursing students (Fettig & Friesen, 2014; Houghton, 2014). Through this interaction, students naturally and collectively set norms for and determine

Box 42–1
National Student Nurses Association Code of Academic and Clinical Conduct

Preamble

Students of nursing have a responsibility to society in learning the academic theory and clinical skills needed to provide nursing care. The clinical setting presents unique challenges and responsibilities while caring for human beings in a variety of healthcare environments.

The Code of Academic and Clinical Conduct is based on an understanding that to practice nursing as a student is an agreement to uphold the trust that society has placed in us. The statements of the code provide guidance for the nursing student in the personal development of an ethical foundation and need not be limited strictly to the academic or clinical environment but can assist in the holistic development of the individual.

A Code for Nursing Students

As students are involved in the clinical and academic environments we believe that ethical principles are a necessary guide to professional development. Therefore within these environments we:

1. Advocate for the rights of all clients.
2. Maintain client confidentiality.
3. Take appropriate action to ensure the safety of clients, self, and others.
4. Provide care for the client in a timely, compassionate and professional manner.
5. Communicate client care in a truthful, timely and accurate manner.
6. Actively promote the highest level of moral and ethical principles and accept responsibility for our actions.
7. Promote excellence in nursing by encouraging lifelong learning and professional development.

8. Treat others with respect and promote an environment that respects human rights, values, and choice of cultural and spiritual beliefs.
9. Collaborate in every reasonable manner with the academic faculty and clinical staff to ensure the highest quality of client care.
10. Use every opportunity to improve faculty and clinical staff understanding of the learning needs of nursing students.
11. Encourage faculty, clinical staff, and peers to mentor nursing students.
12. Refrain from performing any technique or procedure for which the student has not been adequately trained.
13. Refrain from any deliberate action or omission of care in the academic or clinical setting that creates unnecessary risk of injury to the client, self, or others.
14. Assist the staff nurse or preceptor in ensuring that there is full disclosure and that proper authorization is obtained from clients regarding any form of treatment or research.
15. Abstain from the use of alcoholic beverages or any substances in the academic and clinical setting that impair judgment.
16. Strive to achieve and maintain an optimal level of personal health.
17. Support access to treatment and rehabilitation for students who are experiencing impairments related to substance abuse and mental or physical health issues.
18. Uphold school policies and regulations related to academic and clinical performance, reserving the right to challenge and critique rules and regulations as per school grievance policy.

Note: This code was adopted by the NSNA House of Delegates, Nashville, Tennessee, on April 6, 2001. Reprinted with permission.

---

the direction of their scholastic efforts. They develop perspectives about the situations in which they are involved, the goals they are trying to achieve, and the kinds of activities and behaviors that are appropriate for nurses, and they establish a set of practices in keeping with all of these things. Students become bound together by feelings of mutual cooperation, support, and solidarity that continue after they graduate and enter the world of professional nursing.

Nursing education aids students in the development of individual professional values by helping them clarify and internalize these values. The nursing code of ethics (described in the module on Ethics), standards of nursing practice (described in the exemplar on Professional Development in this module), and the legal system itself (described in the module on Legal Issues) define specific values all professional nurses should share. The National Student Nurses Association (NSNA) also adopted a code of academic and clinical conduct in 2001 (**Box 42–1 »**) that is an integral part of ethical practice (NSNA, 2013). This code addresses students' responsibility in the academic environment and to society at large as they learn clinical skills in nursing care.

Case Study » Part 2

Jen Sturges meets with the charge nurse, Melinda Menendez, and briefly but clearly discusses her concerns about Ms. Miller's pain management and the objective signs she noted during her shift. Ms.

Menendez asks Jen what she thinks is going on with Ms. Miller. Jen tells her that this is her first experience with a patient who has a history of pain but does not want to use any pain medications and ignores her apparent pain.

Ms. Menendez is concerned that Ms. Miller would be unable to participate in her care and other daily activities if she has uncontrolled pain during hospitalization. She asks Jen to join her while she speaks with Ms. Miller. After a few minutes of discussion, it becomes clear that Ms. Miller is afraid of the potential for narcotic abuse. It also appears that uncertainty about the meaning of her body's pain signals worries Ms. Miller about the safety of her physical activities at home and in the hospital. Ms. Menendez gently holds Ms. Miller's hand and tells her how important it is for her to take part in care activities and to allow the staff to manage pain and keep her as comfortable as possible. "To help you with this care," Ms. Menendez says, "I would like our social worker and clinical pharmacist to see you about your pain and other needs while you are here." Ms. Miller agrees with this plan.

Clinical Reasoning Question Level I

1. As the charge nurse, Ms. Menendez took an active role in further assessment of the patient's needs and communicated with Ms. Miller in a truthful and calm manner. Of what aspect of the ethical principles listed in the Code for Nursing Students is this an example?

Clinical Reasoning Question Level II

2. If Jen had waited to collaborate with Ms. Menendez, would this have prevented further care and appropriate patient outcomes? Explain your answer.

Factors Influencing Nursing Practice and Accountability

Various factors influence nursing as a profession, and because of the integral part nursing plays in the healthcare system as a whole, these factors typically also influence the entire healthcare system. Essentially, what affects the healthcare system will affect nursing as a profession, and the reverse is also true. Some of the most important factors affecting nursing practice include economics, consumer demand, science and technology, information availability and telecommunications, legislation, demographics, and the current nursing shortage.

Economics

In recent years, changes in public and private health insurance programs, particularly Medicare, have affected the demand for nursing care. Multiple and ongoing changes in the American healthcare system present challenges to both nurses and the organizations in which they practice. For many years, the healthcare industry has been shifting its emphasis from inpatient to outpatient care with preadmission testing, increased outpatient same-day surgery, posthospitalization rehabilitation, home healthcare, health maintenance, physical fitness programs, and community health education programs. As a result, while acute care remains the primary nursing practice area, more nurses are being employed in community-based health settings, such as home health agencies, hospices, and community clinics.

Focus on Integrative Health
Integrative Health and Accountable Care Organizations

According to the Centers for Medicare and Medicaid Services (CMS), accountable care organizations (ACOs) are groups of doctors, hospitals, and other healthcare providers that come together voluntarily to give coordinated high-quality care to their Medicare patients. The goal of an ACO is ensuring that patients, especially the chronically ill, get the right care at the right time, while avoiding unnecessary duplication of services and preventing medical errors (CMS, 2015). The linkage of healthcare institutions through ACOs ensures that healthcare providers in all phases of a patient's care are accountable to the core goal: ensuring the patient's health.

Integrative health techniques have a unique ability to serve the three-part aim of ACOs: improving the health of the population, enhancing the patient experience of care, and reducing the per capita cost of care. Integrative health strategies focus on the whole person, not just the disease, and emphasize preventive care, thus improving the health of the population. Surveys reveal that they increase patient satisfaction, thus enhancing the experience of care. Furthermore, these strategies reduce the overall cost of healthcare compared with traditional therapies alone, thus reducing the per capita cost of care (CHP Group, 2014). In fact, Davis et al. (2013) have found that "the inclusion of integrative health providers in new delivery systems such as accountable care organizations could help slow growth in national healthcare spending," providing an enticing salve to rising healthcare costs.

These changes affect nursing education, nursing research, and nursing practice, particularly with regard to the nurse's competence to practice within these settings.

As with acute care environments, the field of outpatient care has developed specialty areas to meet patient needs. For example, there are now outpatient facilities dedicated to such things as oncology symptom management, ostomy care, diabetes management, and palliative care for terminally ill patients. Various models of integrative care have also arisen in an attempt to better control rising healthcare costs, as described in the Focus on Integrative Health feature.

Consumer Demand

A **consumer** is any person or group that uses a service or commodity; thus, a consumer might be an individual, a group of individuals, or even an entire community. Because everyone has healthcare needs, the consumers of nursing services are the general public. Consumer needs are a driver for any market or service. For example, the drive for integrative healthcare services is motivated by more than the need to consolidate and lower the costs of healthcare; it is also motivated by consumer interest in the use of complementary health approaches. In a 2012 survey, nearly 18% of adults reported using a nonvitamin, nonmineral dietary supplement (Clark et al., 2015). Another factor affecting consumer use of the healthcare system is that today's healthcare consumers are more knowledgeable and vocal about their needs, in part due to the increasing amount of information available on the internet.

Science and Technology

Advances in science and technology greatly affect nursing practice, competence, and accountability. For example, recent progress in the field of molecular genetics has made it possible to identify individuals who are at elevated risk for a variety of hereditary diseases. However, the testing of healthy children for diseases that would develop only in adulthood raises many important ethical, legal, and social questions. These questions are further amplified by the fact that genetic testing is now available outside the traditional healthcare system, often without the mediation of physicians, nurses, or other healthcare professionals. Nurses therefore need to expand their knowledge base and technical skills as they adapt to meet new patient needs emerging out of the expanded use of technology.

Science and technology have affected other areas of nursing practice as well. Healthcare practitioners in most settings are now expected to learn how to use technologic advances such as sophisticated computerized equipment to monitor or treat patients. They are also expected to be able to use online Electronic Health Report Systems (CMS, 2016). In both acute inpatient settings and primary care practices, healthcare practitioners have integrated electronic health records (EHRs) successfully and have reported increased efficiency in retrieving medical records, storing patient information, and coordinating care and general office operations (Goldberg et al., 2012).

Technologic innovations have also had dramatic effects on nurses' clinical training. Simulation-based training activities are increasingly common, and they have been shown to improve clinical decision making and have an overall positive impact on student learning and patient safety (Lafond & Van Hulle Vincent, 2013; Secomb, Mckenna, & Smith, 2012; Spooner, Hurst, & Khadra, 2012). As technologies continue to change, nursing education must also continue to evolve so that nurses have the knowledge and experience necessary to provide safe, effective care.

Information Availability and Telecommunications

Increased use of the internet has dramatically affected healthcare, particularly as more patients become well informed about their health concerns. With easy access to the internet at home and on mobile devices, ever-greater numbers of patients and caregivers are searching the web for answers to their health questions. For instance, by 2012, 81% of American adults used the internet, 72% searched the web for health information, and 45% reported owning and using smartphones. Furthermore, many Americans regularly logged on to online forums surrounding their particular concerns (Fox, 2013).

As the internet has evolved, so have various forms of **telecommunication**, or the means by which information is transferred from one site to another via cable, radio, and other systems. Today, videoconferencing, telepractice, telerehabilitation, and virtual visits all allow individuals and/or groups in two or more locations to communicate by simultaneous two-way video and audio transmissions. It is now even possible to monitor critical care patients in an ICU in a different city or rural area and to manage patient care from another part of the world. Education has also been enhanced

by web-based distance learning. Technology-delivered education has been shown to augment existing curricula by increasing students' access to clinical experts in specialty areas, thus supporting more efficient use of faculty resources (American Telemedicine Association [ATA], 2012). As the use of **telehealth**, the provision of long-distance healthcare through the use of technology such as videoconferencing, computers, or telephones, continues to grow, **telenursing**, the provision of care via telecommunication systems, will also continue to expand.

Legislation

Changes in health legislation affect not just the nursing profession, but also consumers. The **Patient Self-Determination Act (PSDA)**, for example, requires that all competent adults be informed in writing upon admission to a healthcare institution about their rights to accept or refuse medical care and to use advance directives (American Bar Association, 2017). In many institutions, nurses are responsible for ensuring compliance with this law, as well as with similar regulatory requirements. In this way, legislative and other regulatory changes can directly affect the nurse's role in supporting patients and their families.

The Current Nursing Shortage

The present nursing shortage involves multiple new factors (**Box 42–2 >>**) that did not contribute to previous nursing shortages. For example, even though registered nurses make up the largest group of healthcare providers, fewer nurses are entering the workforce now, and certain geographic

---

Box 42–2
Factors Contributing to the Nursing Shortage

Nursing School Enrollment Not Growing Fast Enough

■ There was a 2.6% increase in entry-level BSNs in 2013, but this was not sufficient to meet demand.
■ With changes in access to healthcare, more Americans may soon require nursing services.

Aging Nurse Workforce

■ According to a 2015 study conducted by the National Council of State Boards of Nursing (2015) and the Forum of State Nursing Workforce Centers, 50% of the RN workforce is age 50 or older. Furthermore, the U.S. Department of Health and Human Services, Health Resources and Services Administration (2014) predicts that in the next 10 to 15 years, more than 1 million RNs will reach retirement age and begin to withdraw from the workforce.
■ New graduates are entering the workforce at an older age and will have fewer years to work.

Shortage of Nursing Faculty

■ U.S. nursing schools turned away more than 79,659 qualified applicants in 2012 due to budget constraints and insufficient faculty and clinical sites.
■ There is a 12% shortfall in the number of nurse educators needed.

Changing Demographics

■ The number of individuals in the U.S. population age 65 and older is expected to double between 2000 and 2030.
■ The ratio of potential caregivers to older adults will decrease by 40% between 2010 and 2030.

Increased Demand for Nurses

■ Because of the increased acuity of hospital patients, demand for skilled and specialized nurses is rising.
■ Shorter hospital stays mean that more nurses are needed to care for patients in long-term care and community settings.

Workplace Issues

■ Inadequate wages and low nurse recruitment contribute to staffing shortages.
■ Staffing shortages, including insufficient support staff, result in excessive workloads and greater reliance on overtime.
■ Long hours and task overload cause high nurse turnover and vacancy rates, with many experienced nurses leaving the profession altogether.

Sources: Data from American Association of Colleges of Nursing (AACN). (2014). *Nursing shortage fact sheet.* Retrieved from http://www.aacn.nche.edu/media-relations/NrsgShortageFS.pdf; Cox, P., Willis, K., & Coustasse, A. (2014, March). *The American epidemic: The U.S. nursing shortage and turnover problem.* Paper presented at BHAA 2014, Chicago, IL; U.S. Department of Health and Human Services, Health Resources and Services Administration. (2014). *The future of the nursing workforce: National and state-level projections, 2012–2025.* Retrieved from http://bhpr.hrsa.gov/healthworkforce/supplydemand/nursing/workforceprojections/nursingprojections.pdf.

areas are experiencing acute nursing shortages. Simply put, demand for nurses exceeds supply, especially in specialized areas such as critical care, and this situation is only expected to get worse (AACN, 2014).

Healthcare systems, policy makers, nursing educators, and professional organizations must work together to fix the nursing shortage problem. Some recommended actions for addressing this problem include the following:

- Giving nursing students the means to enter and progress through educational programs more rapidly and efficiently
- Stepping up efforts to recruit young people early in the course of their education (e.g., in middle and high school)
- Providing greater scheduling flexibility, better rewards for experienced nurses who serve as mentors, more adequate staffing, and increased salaries to improve nurses' work environment
- Increasing funding for nursing education

Case Study » Part 3

Lisa Rossi, the social worker, meets with Ms. Miller and learns that she is a single mother with a long history of back pain who appears dejected about the amount of time and effort she puts into being a mom. "I am not a person who gives in to things easily," Ms. Miller said. "That's why I think it is so unfair. Why me? There are so many things I should be able to do. And if I don't ignore my pain, it ruins so much in my life. I have been suffering through many snowboarding and camping trips with my children, but I don't want them to know that."

Ms. Rossi allows time for Ms. Miller to discuss her concerns and then briefly teaches her how to do slow yoga-type breathing to help her anxiety. After Ms. Miller practices the slower breathing, Ms. Rossi asks her whether she is ready to meet with the clinical pharmacist who will work with her to find the best options for pain management both while she is in the hospital and after discharge. Ms. Miller agrees to the plan.

The information from the social worker helps Dan Kramer, the clinical pharmacist, plan appropriate interventions for Ms. Miller. Dr. Kramer is able to meet with Ms. Miller that evening, and afterward he discusses the medication plan with Jen Sturges and Ms. Menendez. The next day, after a few doses of IV morphine and some oral narcotics, Ms. Miller is able to relax and take part in care activities. By the time the doctor discusses discharge plans with her, Ms. Miller describes how she had learned to recognize the pain not so much as an enemy, but rather as a signal to move or to calm down. She also learns that medication is not an enemy if it helps her with her daily life. In addition, she mentions that working with an occupational therapist has helped her understand how to calculate and plan all of her daily activities, physical and otherwise, to ensure her ability to participate in her usual social and occupational roles.

Clinical Reasoning Questions Level I

1. What role did technology play in the patient's care plan?
2. What information would you expect the social worker to share with Jen Sturges?

Clinical Reasoning Questions Level II

3. What role did the social worker take with Ms. Miller? How did the social worker's interview and discussion help with the patient's care and further activity?
4. Why was it important for the pharmacist to meet with the patient and then discuss the plans with Jen Sturges and Ms. Menendez?

REVIEW The Concept of Accountability

RELATE Link the Concepts

Linking the concept of accountability with the concept of legal issues:

1. What is the nurse's legal obligation to the patient related to accountability, and how is it regulated?
2. A nurse makes a medication error that results in harm to the patient. The nurse demonstrates accountability by immediately informing the physician and nursing supervisor when the error is recognized. How does the nurse's proper demonstration of accountability affect the nurse's legal responsibility?

Linking the concept of accountability with the concept of comfort:

3. What is the nurse's role in assessment and appropriate interventions to ensure comfort for the patient?
4. How does lack of patient comfort impede the patient's taking part in care plans and activities?

Linking the concept of accountability with the concept of ethics:

5. How does the nursing code of ethics reflect the expectation that the nurse is accountable when providing patient care?
6. A nurse believes that the physician has written orders that may endanger the patient. The nurse consults the physician, who refuses to alter the orders. What is the nurse's ethical obligation to the patient in order to demonstrate accountability?

REFER Go to Pearson MyLab Nursing and eText

- Additional review materials
- Additional case study

Reflect Apply Your Knowledge

Frank Epworth is a 78-year-old man who presents to the emergency department complaining of nausea, vomiting, and severe pain in his left side and back, just below his ribs. Mr. Epworth states that these symptoms began suddenly. He also mentions that he is having difficulty passing urine; despite increased urge and several attempts to "go," he last urinated two hours ago, and at that time, he noted small amounts of blood in his urine. Based on these symptoms, the patient's reported medical history, and the physical examination, the physician suspects that Mr. Epworth has urolithiasis, or kidney stones. Imaging studies confirm the diagnosis. The physician has requested a urology consult. She has also ordered additional urinalysis and blood testing to learn more about Mr. Epworth's condition, but the results are still pending. In the meantime, you are the RN charged with Mr. Epworth's care.

As you review Mr. Epworth's chart, you note that the physician has authorized administration of Dilaudid 1–4 mg IV prn for pain management. The physician has also ordered you to push IV fluids at a rate of 500 mL/hour in hopes of helping Mr. Epworth pass the stone. Mr. Epworth's urine must also be collected, measured, and strained so that any stone fragments can be analyzed to determine their composition. After consulting the chart, you perform a brief nursing assessment during which Mr. Epworth rates his pain as 8 on a scale of 0 to 10. Therefore, after starting IV fluids as ordered, you administer 1 mg of Dilaudid. You also task the LPN involved in Mr. Epworth's care with urine collection responsibilities and helping Mr. Epworth remain as comfortable as possible.

1. Half an hour later, you speak with the LPN. He notes that Mr. Epworth passed 30 mL of urine about 5 minutes ago, which he noted in the patient's chart. He also states that he disposed of the urine without straining it for stones. As the RN, are you accountable for the LPN's error? Why or why not?

2. An hour after the initial administration of Dilaudid, you reassess Mr. Epworth's pain level. He says that the medication didn't seem to provide any relief, so you administer another 3 mg of Dilaudid per the doctor's order. Will you be accountable if this additional dose fails to control Mr. Epworth's pain? Why or why not?

3. Shortly after starting Mr. Epworth's IV, you recall reading recent clinical guidance advising that large fluid pushes are rarely effective in facilitating stone passage. In this scenario, how might the standards of nursing accountability affect your subsequent course of action?

» Exemplar 42.A
Competence

Exemplar Learning Outcomes

42.A Analyze competence as it relates to accountability.

- Describe the areas of competence.
- Explain the importance of lifelong competence for nurses.

Exemplar Key Terms

Caring for the dying, *2705*
Competence, *2704*
Health promotion, *2704*
Health restoration, *2704*
Illness prevention, *2704*
Wellness, *2704*

Overview

Competence is defined as possessing the knowledge and skills necessary to perform one's job appropriately and safely (Makely, 2012). In the past, nurses were considered able to do their job if they could simply provide care and comfort. Today, nurses are held to a higher standard of competence. Each nurse is expected to achieve and maintain competence within four main areas: health promotion, illness prevention, health restoration, and caring for the dying.

Areas of Competence

A variety of knowledge bases and professional skills are involved in the four major areas described below. Within each area, nurses are expected to achieve and demonstrate competence in the application of the nursing process, as well as in those skills necessary to provide safe and appropriate care.

Health and Wellness Promotion

According to the World Health Organization (WHO, 2017), health is a complete state of physical, mental, and social well-being and not just the absence of disease. Thus, **health promotion** can be defined as a process that enables individuals and communities to increase their control over the determinants of well-being, thereby improving their overall health (Dawson & Grill, 2012). Similarly, **wellness** can be described as a state of being in which individuals engage in activities and behaviors that enhance their quality of life and maximize their personal potential, including their physical fitness and emotional health (Lerner et al., 2013). Both patients who are healthy and patients who are ill may benefit from wellness-related nursing services. This process of health promotion may involve such things as improving nutrition and physical fitness, preventing drug and alcohol misuse, restricting smoking, preventing accidents and injury in the home and workplace, and other health-enhancing activities at the individual, community, and workplace levels. Educating patients is an especially important element of health and wellness promotion. See the Module on Teaching and Learning for information on the nurse's role in providing patient teaching.

SAFETY ALERT When engaging in health and wellness promotion activities, nurses may encourage regular exercise, a key intervention that can significantly reduce the risk of many common conditions. Exercise comes with its own set of risks for injury, though, and some medical conditions require restricting physical activity, so the nurse should work with the patient to develop an appropriate exercise plan that aligns with the patient's specific needs.

Illness Prevention

Nurses engage in **illness prevention** in every setting in which they work. Illness prevention programs in community settings are designed to maintain optimal health by preventing disease. Some examples of community-level illness prevention include immunization programs, prenatal and infant care programs, and programs aimed at stopping the spread of sexually transmitted infections. These programs are frequently facilitated by nurses working in school settings, hospital outreach programs, and local health departments.

Within clinical settings, nurses engage in illness prevention in a variety of ways, such as by observing equipment sterilization precautions and engaging in patient teaching. These and other methods of illness prevention are discussed throughout Parts I, II, and III of this text.

Health Restoration

Ill patients are the focus of **health restoration**, which extends from early detection of disease through the process of helping patients during the recovery period. Critical nursing competencies in the area of health restoration include providing direct care; conducting assessments; patient teaching about recovery activities; and assisting patients with achieving optimal functional level of physical, cognitive, psychologic, and spiritual health.

Caring for the Dying

Caring for the dying involves helping terminally ill patients of all ages live as comfortably as possible until death, as well as helping these patients' support individuals cope with death. Nurses care for the dying in a variety of settings, including homes, hospitals, and extended care facilities. The End-of-Life Care exemplar in the module on Comfort provides more information on caring for the dying.

Promoting Lifelong Competence

Nurses gain competence gradually throughout nursing school until they reach a level at which they are judged safe and skillful enough to function as newly graduated nurses. Nurses continue to build competence throughout their career, with expertise coming from experience, gaining new knowledge, and improving their performance of skills.

Maintaining and increasing competence in nursing require the nurse to continue learning. Professional development and continuing education opportunities come in a variety of forms, including seminars offered by colleges and professional organizations, professional and peer-reviewed journals, hospital- or employer-sponsored classes on new equipment or procedures, and formal and informal discussions with peers and other members of the healthcare team. All nurses must assess their own level of knowledge and identify areas in which they need additional knowledge in order to provide appropriate patient care.

Even the most competent nurses sometimes encounter situations that make them question how best to respond. Luckily, nurses can collaborate with each other and with others on the interprofessional team, sharing opinions, ideas, and information. Although collaboration is helpful and even critical, each nurse is nevertheless accountable for his or her own choices and must weigh all information and choose the best course of action. The nurse who recognizes that there will always be a need to collaborate with others maintains a safe practice.

Various models have been developed in an attempt to explain the process by which nurses attain competence. One classic model is that developed by Benner (2001), which describes five levels of proficiency in nursing: novice, advanced beginner, competent, proficient, and expert (**Box 42–3 》》**). Benner's model proposes that experience is essential for the development of professional expertise—and this idea has significant implications for teaching and learning.

SAFETY ALERT As nurses pass through Benner's stages of nursing expertise, they gain not only knowledge and fluency, but also a more intuitive sense of patient safety. By the expert level, medication

---

Box 42–3
Benner's Stages of Nursing Expertise

Stage I: Novice

No experience (e.g., a nursing student). Performance is limited, inflexible, and governed by context-free rules and regulations rather than experience.

Stage II: Advanced Beginner

Demonstrates marginally acceptable performance.

Recognizes the meaningful aspects of a real situation. Has experienced enough real situations to make judgments about them.

Stage III: Competent

Has 2 or 3 years of experience. Demonstrates organizational and planning abilities. Differentiates important factors from less important aspects of care. Coordinates multiple complex care demands.

Stage IV: Proficient

Has 3 to 5 years of experience. Perceives situations as wholes rather than in terms of parts as in Stage II. Uses maxims as guides for what to consider in a situation. Has holistic understanding of the client, which improves decision making. Focuses on long-term goals.

Stage V: Expert

Performance is fluid, flexible, and highly proficient; no longer requires rules, guidelines, or maxims to connect an understanding of the situation to appropriate action. Demonstrates highly skilled intuitive and analytic ability in new situations. Is inclined to take a certain action because "it felt right."

Source: Benner, P. (2001). *From novice to expert: Excellence and power in clinical nursing practice, commemorative edition* (1st ed.). Upper Saddle River, NJ: Pearson Education. Reprinted and electronically reproduced by permission of Pearson Education, Inc., New York, NY.

---

doses and sterilization procedures that once required careful training and memorization become easy to perform. Even at the expert level, however, nurses must double-check their actions to ensure that patients' safety needs are always being met.

Regardless of their exact level of proficiency, all nurses must hold themselves accountable by frequently weighing and assessing their own competence. This includes competence not just in applying nursing knowledge and carrying out clinical skills, but also in recognizing and dealing with various cultural issues that may arise. (See the Focus on Diversity and Culture feature for more information.) Furthermore, in all situations, nurses should understand that it is more honorable to say "I don't know" or ask "Would you help me?" than to say "I'm not sure but I think this is right" or "I'll figure it out as I go along." In fact, the first rule of competence in providing patient care is to ask for help whenever there is uncertainty about the safety of any given action. By doing so, nurses both invite opportunities to increase their own level of competence and hold themselves accountable for providing the highest quality of patient care.

Focus on Diversity and Culture
Teaching Cultural Competence

Adequate healthcare is a universal human right, so it is essential that nurses gain the skills necessary to communicate cross-culturally in this era of increasing diversity. According to Jeffreys (2015), "culturally congruent" healthcare refers to healthcare that is customized to fit with the patient's cultural values. Nurses must learn to practice culturally congruent healthcare by actively seeking to expand their level of cultural competence. This means embracing a "broader, more inclusive worldview that appreciates various forms of diversity and [considers] various philosophies and approaches to learning" (Jeffreys, 2015). Healthcare organizations and schools of nursing must also seek to provide current and future nurses with cultural competence training. But what, exactly, should this sort of teaching entail?

Many researchers have considered this question, with varying results. Still, several broad recommendations have emerged. For instance, Raman (2015) highlights multiple studies suggesting that cultural competence training is most effective when delivered by a diverse team of nurse educators who have engaged in thorough self-assessment of their own cultural knowledge and limitations. Raman also recommends that these educators have significant experience working among individuals who are "ethnically and culturally different from themselves." Similarly, Truong, Paradies, and Priest (2014) point out several studies recommending that healthcare organizations evaluate their own strengths and weaknesses, along with the unique needs of their patients, prior to developing in-house cultural competence training programs. Evidence from several studies also indicates that such programs are most effective when they "connect cultural competency to professional values rather than legal or organizational requirements, fostering a safe and respectful learning environment, cultivating cultural humility, and avoiding stereotypes throughout the training" (University of Wisconsin Population Health Institute, 2015). This last point is echoed by George, Thornicroft, and Dogra (2015), who emphasize the value of cultural competence training programs that are driven by clinical need rather than political concerns and that avoid assuming that all members of a particular cultural group are homogeneous in terms of their beliefs and practices.

REVIEW Competence

RELATE Link the Concepts and Exemplars

Linking the exemplar on competence with the concept of legal issues:

1. What is the nurse's legal obligation to society and the profession to maintain competence?

2. How can nurses who lack competence in one area of nursing strengthen their knowledge and skills?

Linking the exemplar on competence with the concept of ethics:

3. What is the nurse's ethical obligation related to competence?

4. How does the nursing code of ethics address the issue of competence?

REFER Go to Pearson MyLab Nursing and eText

- Additional review materials

REFLECT Apply Your Knowledge

Tyree Campbell has worked in the labor and delivery unit of a large metropolitan hospital since graduating from nursing school 8 years ago. A new private hospital recently opened in town, and the census on Ms. Campbell's unit has been significantly lower. Tonight, Ms. Campbell reports to work and learns that more nurses are scheduled to work than there are patients. The decision has been made to float the excess staff to other units, and Ms. Campbell is asked to float to the neonatal intensive care unit (NICU). Her heart sinks, and she begins to feel the early signs of panic as she thinks, "How can I work in the NICU? I don't have any experience working there!"

1. What is Ms. Campbell's responsibility in this situation?

2. Can Ms. Campbell agree to float to the NICU if she is not competent to care for the patients on this unit? Explain your answer.

3. What should Ms. Campbell say to the nursing supervisor who has given her this assignment?

» Exemplar 42.B
Professional Development

Exemplar Learning Outcomes

42.B Analyze professional development as it relates to accountability.

- Analyze the history of nursing.
- Explain the effects of women's status, religion, war, and societal attitudes on nursing.
- List nursing leaders who made notable contributions to the profession.
- Differentiate the components of contemporary nursing practice.
- Differentiate expanded careers for nurses.

Exemplar Key Terms

Authority, 2710
Chain of command, 2710
Line authority, 2710
Organizational chart, 2711
Responsibility, 2710
Staff authority, 2710
Standards of Practice, 2710
Standards of Professional Performance, 2710

Overview

Professional development takes on different meanings in the many different areas of nursing. The term may be associated with advanced education, an increase in experience or seniority, involvement or membership in an organization that governs the profession, or continuing education classes or offerings. Professional development encompasses all of these activities.

Nursing today is very different from nursing as it was practiced years ago, and it is expected to continue changing. To understand nursing in the present as well as prepare for the future, nursing students must understand not only past events but also contemporary nursing practice and its sociologic and historical influences.

Historical Perspectives

Over the centuries, societal needs and influences have brought about dramatic changes in nursing. From its beginnings, nursing has struggled for autonomy and professionalization—a struggle that continues in the present. A renewed interest in nursing history has in recent decades produced a growing body of literature on the subject. The following sections touch on only selected aspects of influential events in nursing practice. Themes that recur throughout this history of nursing include issues related to women's roles and status, religious values, war, societal attitudes, and visionary nursing leadership. Many of these factors continue to influence nursing in the present.

Women's Roles and Status

The female roles of wife, mother, daughter, and sister have traditionally included the care and nurturing of others. Women have cared for infants and children from the beginning of time, and nursing could legitimately be said to have its roots in "the home." Additionally, women, who in general occupied a subservient and dependent role, were frequently called on to care for others in the community who were ill. Most often, this care involved the promotion of physical maintenance and comfort. Humanistic caring, nurturing, comforting, and supporting have thus always been components of the traditional nursing role.

Religion

Religion has also played a significant role in the development of nursing. Although many of the world's religions emphasize benevolence, Western nursing in particular has been influenced by the Judeo-Christian commandment to "love thy neighbor as thyself" and Christ's parable of the Good Samaritan. Throughout its history, nursing has also drawn on other religious values such as self-denial, devotion to duty and hard work, and the idea of a spiritual calling. In the early history of nursing, religious organizations supported or provided nursing care. Examples include the Daughters of Charity of Vincent de Paul in France, who provided psychiatric nursing care as early as the 17th century. Deaconess groups also provided nursing care, most notably when Theodore Fliedner reinstituted the Order of Deaconesses in Kaiserswerth, Germany, in 1836 and opened a small hospital and training school there. This school is where Florence Nightingale received her training in nurs-

ing. Religion continues to influence nursing, albeit in different ways. Most notably, today's nurses are increasingly seeking ways to honor patients' religious beliefs in their practice (Sayles, 2016).

War

Throughout history, wars have demanded nurses to care for the wounded. Several orders of knights—including the Knights of Saint John of Jerusalem (also known as the Knights Hospitalers), the Teutonic Knights, and the Knights of Saint Lazarus—were formed during the Crusades to provide nursing care to their sick and injured comrades. Eventually, these groups began to provide care to others as well. For example, because the group's original members were themselves lepers, the Knights of Saint Lazarus chose to dedicate themselves to the care of individuals with leprosy, syphilis, and chronic skin conditions. These orders also built hospitals, the organization and management of which set a standard for hospital administration throughout Europe at that time.

Centuries later, the inadequacy of the care given to soldiers during the Crimean War (1854–1856) led to a public outcry in Great Britain. Florence Nightingale played a well-known role in addressing this problem when Sir Sidney Herbert of the British War Department asked her to recruit a contingent of female nurses to care for the sick and injured in the Crimea. Nightingale and her nurses set up practices that transformed sanitation standards for military hospitals, such as hand washing and laundering clothing. Through efforts like these, Nightingale and her nurses helped decrease the mortality rate in the Barrack Hospital in Turkey from 42% to a remarkable 2% (Donahue, 1996, p. 197).

Shortly after Nightingale's work in the Crimea, several Americans made notable contributions during the U.S. Civil War (1861–1865). Although not technically nurses, Harriet Tubman and Sojourner Truth provided care and safety to slaves fleeing to the North on the Underground Railroad. Meanwhile on the battlefields, Mother Biekerdyke and Clara Barton provided care to injured and dying soldiers. Dorothea Dix became the Union Army's superintendent of female nurses. In this role, she was responsible for recruiting nurses and supervising the care provided by all women nurses working in army hospitals during the Civil War.

American, British, and French women all rushed to volunteer their nursing services when World War I broke out in the 1910s. These nurses had to endure harsh environments and treat unprecedented injuries. World War I also brought progress in other areas of healthcare, particularly in the surgical field. Other examples of war-related advances included more effective use of anesthetic agents, infection control, blood typing, and prosthetics.

Approximately 90% of the 11,000 American military women stationed in Southeast Asia during the Vietnam War were nurses. Most of these women volunteered to go to Vietnam immediately following graduation from nursing school, making them the youngest group of medical personnel ever to serve in wartime (Vietnam Women's Memorial Foundation, n.d.).

Today, U.S. military nurses serve individuals and populations worldwide during times of war and peace. For example,

Army nurses responded to and helped to develop protocols for the Ebola crisis in Africa and the United States. Their work continues to influence the health and safety of active service men and women, the nation's veterans, and civilians at home and abroad (Military Health System Communications Office, 2015).

Societal Attitudes

Over the years, professional nursing has been significantly influenced by societal attitudes concerning nurses and nursing. For example, nurses lacked organization, education, or social status prior to the mid-1800s because of the pervasive attitude that a woman's place was in the home. During this time, it was not respectable for women to pursue careers. Most hospital-based nurses of the era were poorly educated, and some were even incarcerated criminals. Charles Dickens' novel *Martin Chuzzlewit* (1896) reflected society's attitudes about nursing during this period; in that book, Sairey Gamp's "care" for the sick included neglect, theft, and physical abuse (Donahue, 1996, p. 192). This character's portrayal did much to influence the negative image of nurses.

In the latter part of the nineteenth century, thanks largely to Florence Nightingale's efforts during the Crimean War, a contrasting image of the nurse as *guardian angel* or *angel of mercy* arose in the popular imagination. Nightingale brought new respectability to the nursing profession, changing the image of nurses from cruel and exploitive to noble, compassionate, moral, religious, dedicated, and self-sacrificing.

As the nursing profession developed during the twentieth century, so did the efforts of nurses to take more active steps to improve the image of nursing. For example, during the early 1990s, the Tri-Council for Nursing (which consists of the American Association of Colleges of Nursing, the ANA, the American Organization of Nurse Executives, and the NLN) initiated a national effort titled Nurses of America, which focused on elevating nursing's professional image. In 2002, the Johnson & Johnson corporation launched the Campaign for Nursing's Future, which promoted nursing as a positive career choice and a trusted profession. In 2010, the Institute of Medicine (IOM) and the Robert Wood Johnson Foundation (RWJF) launched the Initiative on the Future of Nursing, which focused on identifying solutions of nursing care that not only addressed many of the issues facing the profession, but also transformed the way Americans receive healthcare. This initiative was based on the belief that nurses are a linchpin for health reform and will be vital in implementing systemic changes in the delivery of care (IOM, 2010).

Nursing Leaders

Leaders such as Florence Nightingale, Clara Barton, Lillian Wald, Lavinia Dock, Margaret Sanger, and Mary Breckinridge made notable contributions to both nursing's history and women's history, and their skills at influencing others and bringing about change make them potent models for political nurse activists today. Contemporary nursing leaders have also played important roles in the profession. For example, Virginia Henderson created a modern worldwide definition of nursing, and Martha Rogers made important theoretical contributions.

Florence Nightingale (1820–1910)

Florence Nightingale's contributions to nursing are well documented. During the Crimean War, she made such great strides in improving standards of care for war casualties that her efforts earned her the title "Lady with the Lamp." She also became an accomplished political nurse—the first nurse, in fact, to exert political pressure on government—in her zeal to reform hospitals and produce and implement public health policies. Her greatest achievements, however, were her contributions to nursing education and her pioneering work *Notes on Nursing: What It Is, and What It Is Not* (1859/1969), which established Nightingale as nursing's first scientist–theorist.

Clara Barton (1812–1912)

A schoolteacher who volunteered as a nurse during the American Civil War, Clara Barton was given the responsibility of organizing the nursing services. She established the American Red Cross and in 1882 persuaded Congress to ratify the Treaty of Geneva (the first Geneva Convention), which linked the American Red Cross with the International Red Cross to perform humanitarian efforts in times of peace.

Linda Richards (1841–1930)

Linda Richards graduated from the New England Hospital for Women and Children in 1873, thereby becoming America's first trained nurse. Richards did pioneering work in psychiatric and industrial nursing, and the practices of nurse's notes, doctor's orders, and nurses wearing uniforms all originated with her (ANA, 2016a).

Mary Mahoney (1845–1926)

In 1879, Mary Mahoney graduated from the New England Hospital for Women and Children to become the first African American professional nurse. Mahoney promoted equal opportunities and worked constantly for African Americans to be accepted in nursing (Donahue, 1996, p. 271). The ANA (2016b) gives the Mary Mahoney Award biennially to recognize significant contributions, whether by individual nurses or groups of nurses, to the advancement of racial integration in nursing.

Lillian Wald (1867–1940)

Lillian Wald is considered the founder of public health nursing. Wald and Mary Brewster were the first to offer trained nursing services to the poor in the New York slums. They provided nursing and social services as well as organized educational and cultural activities. Wald pushed for school nursing as an adjunct to visiting nursing soon after founding the Henry Street Settlement.

Lavinia Dock (1858–1956)

A friend of Lillian Wald and a feminist, prolific writer, political activist, and suffragist, Lavinia L. Dock campaigned both for the passage of the 19th Amendment securing women's right to vote, but also for legislation to make the profession of nursing autonomous by allowing nurses, not physicians, to control it. Dock, assisted by Mary Adelaide Nutting and Isabel Hampton Robb, founded the American Society of Superintendents of Training Schools for Nurses of the

United States and Canada in 1893; this was a precursor to the current National League for Nursing.

Margaret Sanger (1879–1966)

A public health nurse in New York, Margaret Higgins Sanger had a lasting impact on women's healthcare and reproductive rights. She was imprisoned for opening America's first birth control information clinic and is considered the founder of Planned Parenthood. Sanger brought attention to the large number of unwanted pregnancies among the working poor and pushed for this issue to be addressed.

Mary Breckinridge (1881–1965)

In 1918, immediately following the end of World War I, Mary Breckinridge worked with the American Committee for Devastated France to distribute food, clothing, and supplies to rural villages and care for sick children. After returning to the United States in 1921, Breckenridge acted on her plans to provide healthcare to the people of rural America, establishing the Frontier Nursing Service (FNS) in 1925 with two other nurses in Leslie County, Kentucky. Within the FNS, Breckinridge started one of the first midwifery training schools in the United States.

Contemporary Nursing Practice

Examining the definitions of nursing, who receives nursing services, the settings for nursing practice, nurse practice acts, and current standards for clinical nursing can help cultivate a deeper understanding of contemporary nursing practice.

Definitions of Nursing

Almost 150 years ago, Florence Nightingale defined nursing as "the act of utilizing the environment of the patient to assist him in his recovery" (Nightingale, 1859/1969). She considered a clean, well-ventilated, and quiet environment to be essential for patient recovery. Nightingale raised the status of nursing through education and is often considered the first nurse theorist. Thanks to her efforts, nurses were no longer untrained housekeepers but professional individuals formally educated in the care of the sick.

Virginia Henderson was one of the first modern nurses to define nursing. In her words, "The unique function of the nurse is to assist the individual, sick or well, in the performance of those activities contributing to health or its recovery (or to peaceful death) that he would perform unaided if he had the necessary strength, will, or knowledge, and to do this in such a way as to help him gain independence as rapidly as possible" (Henderson, 1966, p. 3). Henderson described nursing in relation to the patient and the patient's environment, just as Nightingale did, but unlike Nightingale, Henderson saw the nurse as concerned with both healthy and ill individuals. She acknowledged that nurses interact with patients even when it might not be possible for them to recover and promoted the role of the nurse as both teacher and advocate.

In 1952, Hildegard Peplau published her landmark *Interpersonal Relations in Nursing*, which described and emphasized the importance of the nurse–patient relationship as a therapeutic process. Her pioneering work on nurse–patient relations and on anxiety led to her being widely consider as the founder of modern psychiatric nursing.

In the latter half of the 1900s, a number of nurse theorists developed definitions of nursing. These theoretical definitions are important because they go beyond simplistic common definitions to describe not only what nursing is, but also the interrelationship among nurses, nursing, the patient, the environment, and the intended patient outcome. Certain themes are common to many of these definitions; for example, most theoretical definitions view nursing as:

- Caring
- An art
- A science
- Patient centered
- Holistic
- Adaptive
- Concerned with health promotion, health maintenance, and health restoration
- A helping profession

Professional nursing associations have also scrutinized the nursing profession and contributed their own definitions of nursing. In 1973, the ANA described nursing practice as "direct, goal oriented, and adaptable to the needs of the individual, the family, and community during health and illness" (p. 2), but the organization changed its definition of nursing in 1980 to this: "Nursing is the diagnosis and treatment of human responses to actual or potential health problems" (p. 9). Later, in 1995, the ANA recognized the contribution that the science of caring had made to nursing philosophy and practice. Its current definition of professional nursing is therefore much broader than earlier definitions: "Nursing is the protection, promotion, and optimization of health and abilities, preventions of illness and injury, alleviation of suffering through the diagnosis and treatment of human response, and advocacy in the care of individuals, families, communities, and populations" (ANA, 2003, p. 6).

Settings for Nursing

The many and varied settings for nursing practice include acute care hospitals, community agencies, ambulatory clinics, long-term care facilities, health maintenance organizations (HMOs), nursing practice centers, and patients' homes (see **Figure 42–1 》**).

Depending on the setting, nurses may have different degrees of autonomy and responsibility. They may provide direct care, or they may teach patients and support individuals. They may also serve as advocates and agents of change, helping determine the health policies that affect consumers in hospitals and in the community.

Nurse Practice Acts

Nurse practice acts are legal acts that regulate the practice of nursing in the United States and Canada. Each state in the United States and each province in Canada has its own nurse practice act. Although their content differs from jurisdiction to jurisdiction, the common purpose of all nurse practice acts is to protect the public. Nurses are responsible for knowing how their state's nurse practice act governs

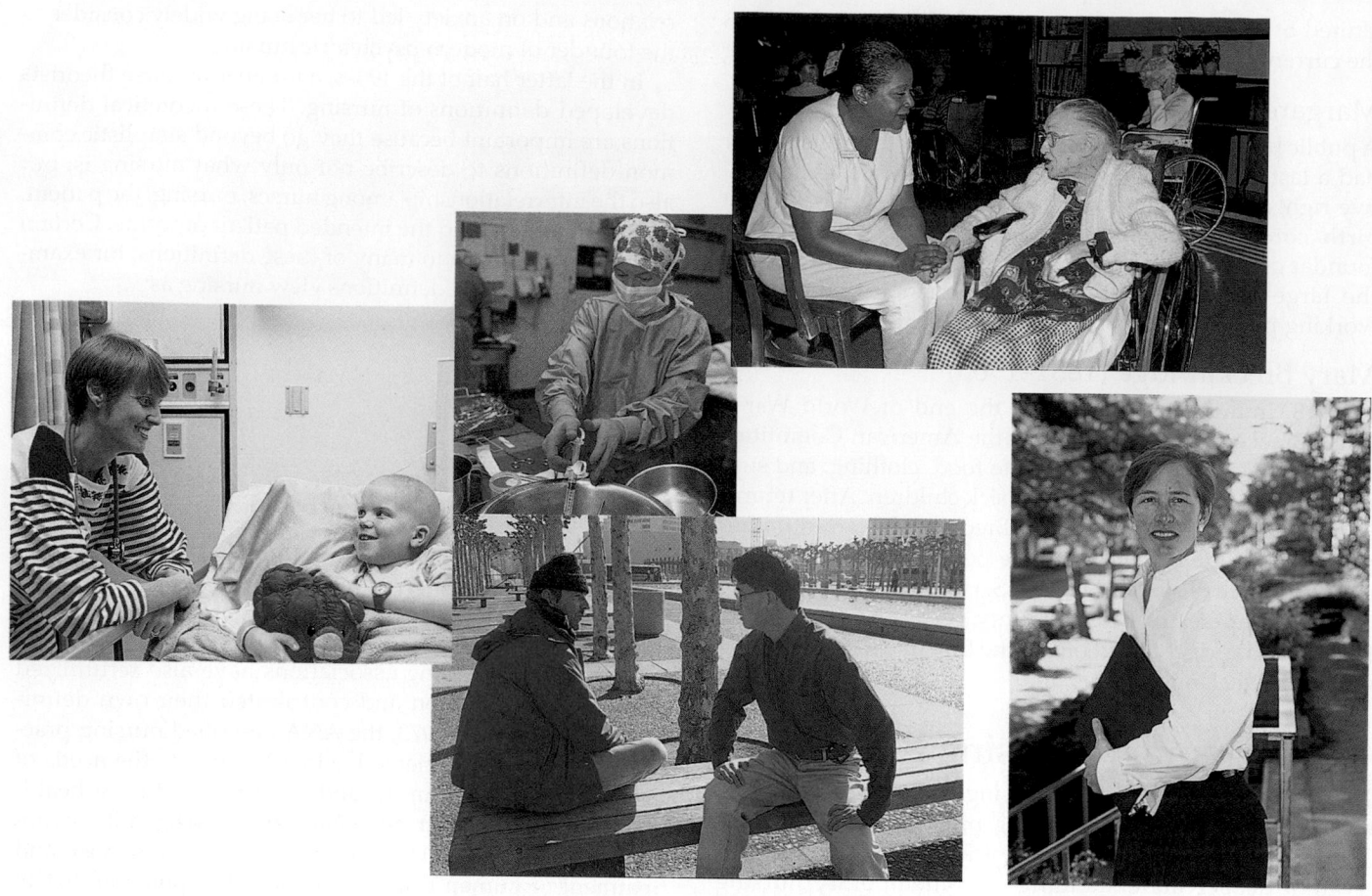

Figure 42–1 》 Nurses practice in a variety of settings. Clockwise from left: pediatric nursing, operating room nurse, geriatric nursing, home nursing, and community nursing.

their practice. The module on Legal Issues discusses nurse practice acts in detail.

Standards of Nursing Practice

A professional organization's major functions include establishing and implementing standards of practice. The ANA's **Standards of Practice**, for example, are intended to describe the responsibilities for which American nurses are accountable. The ANA uses the nursing process as a foundation to develop generic standards of nursing practice that apply regardless of area of specialization. Similarly, the ANA uses its **Standards of Professional Performance** to describe the expected behavior of professional nurses. Professional performance standards refer to enhancing general practice, ensuring appropriate education level, and maintaining collegiality with peers and collaboration with the entire care team. Because of the increasing use of the internet and social networking sites such as Facebook and Twitter, in 2011 the ANA published principles for social networking in nursing. In addition to the ANA, specialty nursing organizations have developed standards of nursing practice specific to their areas of specialization. Each province or territory in Canada also establishes its own standards of practice for nurses.

Competent nurses use the nursing process—that is, the steps of assessment, diagnosis, planning, implementation, and, ultimately, evaluation—in their nursing practice. A

professional nurse also integrates ethics in all areas of practice and considers appropriate use of resources while functioning in relevant leadership roles (ANA, 2015).

Chain of Command

The **chain of command** is the hierarchy within an organization. The authority and responsibility of the individuals in the organization depend on their position in the chain of command. **Authority** is the power to command other individuals and direct their activities; **responsibility** is being accountable for meeting personal or organizational objectives and performing required tasks.

Line authority is the power to direct the activities of subordinates within the organization. In **Figure 42–2 》**, examples of line authority include the relationships among the chief nurse executive, the nurse manager, and the staff nurse. **Staff authority** is the power to provide advice and support to employees or departments but not to assign tasks. In Figure 42–2, staff authority is illustrated by the relationship between the acute care nurse practitioner and the nurse manager. Neither is responsible for the work of the other; rather, they collaborate to optimize care in the unit for which the nurse manager is responsible.

A chain of command provides structure, so employees understand how to perform their tasks and how to manage supervisory relationships within the organization. It also

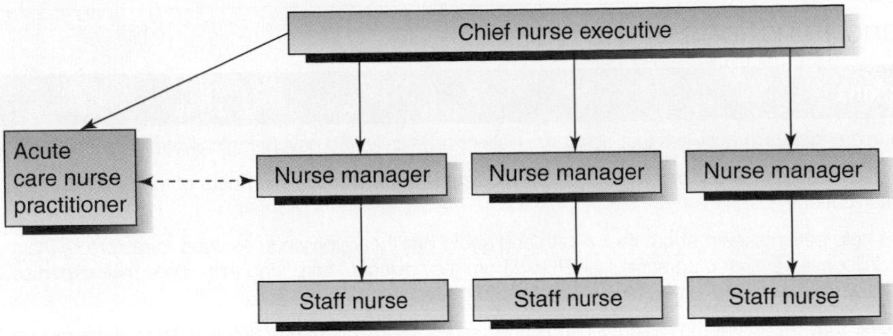

Figure 42–2 》 Organizational chart showing chain of command in a nursing unit.

provides a structure for reporting issues that need management's attention. Any nurse who identifies such an issue should follow the organization's chain of command. For example, in a hospital, a problem is usually first reported to the charge nurse, then to the unit manager. If the problem is still not resolved, the nurse may approach someone in middle or upper management.

The student nurse should always follow the chain of command, and the nursing instructor acts as the first link in that chain. When a problem arises, whether in the clinical area or the classroom, the student should first discuss the problem with the instructor. If the instructor is unable to resolve the issue to the student's satisfaction, the student should then approach the program director. Failure to follow the chain of command is considered unprofessional and slows the resolution process. In some organizations, failure to follow the chain of command may result in disciplinary action.

In traditional organizations, an **organizational chart** depicts the formal hierarchical structure and related responsibilities of the individuals or positions that are depicted on the chart. However, organizations also have informal structures that are not reflected in a chart. For instance, nurses who function as leaders but do not have a formal title in the hierarchy would not appear in the organizational chart. Similarly, managers who have strong personalities or other characteristics may have more actual power than other managers with the same formal level of authority, but these differences are not shown in the chart.

The traditional hierarchical structure is not the only model used in healthcare settings. Many organizations have moved toward a shared governance model that flattens the organizational chart as appropriate participants (such as nursing staff, pharmacy staff, and medical staff) share ownership of patient care issues and outcomes (Charland, 2015).

Roles and Functions of the Nurse

When they provide patients with care, nurses perform a number of roles, often simultaneously. The nurse, for example, may not only provide physical care, but also act as a counselor to teach the patient aspects of that care. The needs of the patient and the aspects of the patient's environment at a particular time determine which roles a nurse will be required to fulfill. These roles, briefly outlined in **Table 42–1 》**, are discussed throughout this text.

As the nursing profession has grown in autonomy through professional organizations, nursing leaders and managers have seen a need for a number of expanded roles in the nursing profession. Some of these roles, such as that of the nurse-midwife, have come about partly as a response to needs expressed by patients. Others, such as that of the nurse educator, have resulted primarily from the profession's desire to continue to improve, educate, and renew its own members.

Expanded Career Roles for Nurses

Expanded career roles that allow greater independence and autonomy are available to many nurses. Such roles include nurse practitioner, clinical nurse specialist, nurse-midwife, nurse educator, and nurse anesthetist. Although exact requirements for these roles are defined in each state's nurse practice act, they almost universally reflect the standards below.

Nurse Practitioner

The basic requirements for becoming a nurse practitioner are advanced education (master's degree or higher), graduation from a nurse practitioner program, and American Nurses Credentialing Center (ANCC) certification in a particular area. These areas include adult nurse practitioner, family nurse practitioner, school nurse practitioner, pediatric nurse practitioner, and gerontology nurse practitioner. Nurse practitioners must hold both an RN license and a nurse practitioner license in order to practice. Nurse practitioners usually provide primary ambulatory care as well as care for patients with nonemergency acute or chronic illness, and they are employed in healthcare agencies or in community-based settings.

Clinical Nurse Specialist

A clinical nurse specialist is a nurse who possesses an advanced degree (master's or higher) with emphasis on a specialized area of practice, such as gerontology or oncology. To become a clinical nurse specialist, the nurse must hold RN licensure and pass a certification exam administered by the ANCC. Most states then require the nurse to obtain separate licensure as a clinical nurse specialist. Depending on their specialty and job setting, clinical nurse specialists provide direct patient care, educate others, consult, conduct research, and manage care.

TABLE 42–1 Roles and Functions of the Nurse

Nursing Role	Functions
Caregiver	The nurse engages in activities that assist the patient physically and psychologically while preserving the patient's dignity.
Communicator	The nurse identifies patient problems and communicates these to other members of the healthcare team. (See the module on Communication.)
Teacher	Nurses help patients learn about their health and about healthcare procedures used to restore or maintain their health. Nurses also teach unlicensed assistive personnel (UAP) to whom they delegate care, and they share their expertise with other nurses and healthcare professionals. (See the module on Teaching and Learning.)
Patient advocate	The nurse may represent the patient's needs and wishes to other health professionals, such as relaying the patient's wishes for information to the physician. The nurse also assists patients in exercising their rights and helps them speak up for themselves.
Counselor	Nurses counsel healthy individuals with normal adjustment difficulties and focus on helping these individuals develop new attitudes, feelings, and behaviors by encouraging them to look at alternative behaviors, recognize the choices, and develop a sense of control. Nurses counsel ill patients in how to develop more healthy and self-protective behaviors and how to recognize and respond to triggers, signs, and symptoms in a timely manner.
Change agent	Nurses assist patients to make modifications in their behavior. Nurses also often act to make changes in a system, such as clinical care, if it is not helping a patient return to health. Nurses are continually dealing with changes in the healthcare system. Technologic changes, changes in the age of the patient population, and changes in medications are just a few that nurses deal with daily.
Leader	A leader influences others to work together to accomplish a specific goal. The leader role can be employed at different levels: individual patient, family, groups of patients, colleagues, or the community. Effective leadership is a learned skill requiring an understanding of the needs and goals that motivate individuals, the knowledge to apply the leadership skills, and the interpersonal skills to influence others. (Leadership is discussed further in the module on Professional Behaviors.)
Manager	The nurse manages the nursing care of individuals, families, and communities. The nurse manager also delegates nursing activities to ancillary workers and other nurses, as well as supervises and evaluates their performance. Managing requires knowledge about organizational structure and dynamics, authority and accountability, leadership, change theory, advocacy, delegation, and supervision and evaluation. (See the module on Collaboration for more information.)
Case manager	Nurse case managers work with the multidisciplinary healthcare team to measure the effectiveness of the case management plan and to monitor outcomes. Each agency or unit specifies the role of the nurse case manager. In some institutions, the case manager works with primary or staff nurses to oversee the care of a specific caseload. In other agencies, the case manager is the primary nurse or provides some level of direct care to the patient and family. Insurance companies have also developed a number of roles for nurse case managers, and responsibilities may vary from managing acute hospitalizations to managing high-cost patients or case types. Regardless of the setting, case managers help ensure that care is oriented to the patient while also controlling costs. (See the module on Managing Care for more information.)
Research consumer	Nurses often use research to improve patient care. In a clinical area, nurses need to (a) have some awareness of the process and language of research, (b) be sensitive to issues related to protecting the rights of human subjects, (c) participate in the identification of significant researchable problems, and (d) be a discriminating consumer of research findings.

Nurse Anesthetist

Nurse anesthetists administer general anesthetics for surgery under the supervision of a physician prepared in anesthesiology, as well as carry out preoperative and postoperative patient assessments. A nurse may qualify to be a nurse anesthetist after completing advanced education (master's degree or higher) in an accredited program in anesthesiology. Nurses who obtain this degree and already hold RN licensure may then sit for a certification examination offered by the National Board on Certification and Recertification of Nurse Anesthetists (NBCRNA). Nurses who pass this exam earn the title of Certified Registered Nurse Anesthetist (CRNA). Maintenance of the CRNA credential requires nurses to meet certain continuing education requirements set by the NBCRNA. Some states also require that CRNAs obtain separate licensure beyond that of a registered nurse.

Nurse-Midwife

Nurse-midwives provide prenatal and postnatal care and manage deliveries in normal pregnancies. They practice in association with a healthcare agency, which enables them to quickly obtain medical services should complications occur. Nurse-midwives may also conduct routine Papanicolaou tests, family planning counseling, and routine breast examinations. To become a nurse-midwife, a registered nurse must complete an accredited graduate program in midwifery, earning a master's degree or higher. The nurse must then pass a certification exam offered by the American College of Nurse-Midwives. In many states, specialized licensure is also required.

Nurse Researcher

The role of the nurse researcher is to investigate problems in nursing and to discover solutions that may improve nursing care and refine and expand nursing knowledge. Academic institutions, teaching hospitals, and research centers, such as the National Institute for Nursing Research in Bethesda, Maryland, all employ nurse researchers. Nurse researchers typically have advanced education at the doctoral level.

Nurse Administrator

A nurse administrator manages patient care, including delivery of nursing services. He or she may have a middle management position, such as head nurse or supervisor, or a more senior management position, such as director of nursing services. The nurse administrator's functions include budgeting, staffing, and planning programs. To prepare for their role, nurse administrators complete at least a baccalaureate degree in nursing and frequently a master's or doctoral degree as well.

Nurse Educator

The nurse educator usually has a baccalaureate degree or more advanced preparation and frequently has expertise in a particular area of practice. Nurse educators work in nursing programs, at educational institutions, or in hospital staff education programs. They are responsible for classroom, skills laboratory, and often clinical teaching.

Nurse Entrepreneur

A nurse entrepreneur is someone who manages a health-related business and typically has an advanced degree. The nurse entrepreneur's business may involve education, consultation, or research.

Clinical Nurse Leader

The American Association of Colleges of Nursing (AACN) developed the role of clinical nurse leader to address the challenges of providing high-quality healthcare in the current environment (Wilson et al., 2013). Quality improvement and use of evidence-based solutions are hallmarks of this role. Clinical nurse leaders must hold a master's degree and have completed specialized coursework in areas such as pathophysiology, clinical assessment, finance management, epidemiology, and pharmacology. They must also pass a certification examination offered by the Commission on Nurse Certification.

REVIEW Professional Development

RELATE Link the Concepts and Exemplars

Linking the exemplar on professional development with the concept of legal issues:

1. What role does the nurse's continued professional development play in meeting the legal requirements for the profession?

2. What nursing regulations require continued professional development?

Linking the exemplar on professional development with the concept of ethics:

3. Can the nurse meet the ethical responsibilities of the profession without belonging to a professional organization? Explain.

4. How does the nursing code of ethics address the issue of professional development?

REFER Go to Pearson MyLab Nursing and eText

■ Additional review materials

REFLECT Apply Your Knowledge

Francois Guardiene graduated from nursing school 4 years ago and accepted a position working in the coronary care unit (CCU) of a large metropolitan hospital. He was required to attend 6 weeks of hospital orientation and a 3-month class for CCU nurses. He worked under the supervision of a preceptor for an additional 3 months. During his first year of practice, Francois checked with more experienced nurses frequently, but with time, he began to have more confidence in his competence and established a more autonomous practice. Over the past 2 years, he has noticed that some individuals seek to collaborate with him, and he considers himself a good CCU nurse.

1. Has Mr. Guardiene satisfied the need for professional development? Explain your answer.

2. What obligations does Mr. Guardiene have to continue developing his professional practice?

3. How would a nurse's hospital orientation differ if the position involved an area less specialized than the CCU?

References

American Association of Colleges of Nursing (AACN). (2014). *Nursing shortage fact sheet*. Retrieved from http://www.aacn.nche.edu/media-relations/NrsgShortageFS.pdf

American Association of Colleges of Nursing (AACN). (2015). *Degree completion programs for registered nurses: RN to master's degree and RN to baccalaureate programs*. Retrieved from http://www.aacn.nche.edu/media-relations/fact-sheets/degree-completion-programs

American Bar Association. (2017). *Law for older Americans*. Retrieved from https://www.americanbar.org/groups/public_education/resources/law_issues_for_consumers/patient_self_determination_act.html

American Nurses Association (ANA). (1973). *Standards of nursing practice*. Kansas City, MO: Author.

American Nurses Association (ANA). (1980). *Nursing: A social policy statement*. Kansas City, MO: Author.

American Nurses Association (ANA). (2003). *Nursing's social policy statement*. Washington, DC: American Nurses Publishing.

American Nurses Association (ANA). (2015). *Nursing: Scope and Standards of Practice* (3rd ed.). Retrieved from http://www.nursesbooks.org/Homepage/Hot-off-the-Press/Nursing-Scope-and-Standards-3rd-Ed.aspx.

American Nurses Association (ANA). (2016a). *ANA hall of fame*. Retrieved from http://nursingworld.org/FunctionalMenuCategories/AboutANA/Honoring-Nurses/NationalAwardsProgram/HallofFame/19761982/richla5574.html

American Nurses Association (ANA). (2016b). *ANA hall of fame*. Retrieved from http://www.ana.org/hof/mahome.htm

American Telemedicine Association (ATA). (2012). *What is telemedicine?* Retrieved from http://www.americantelemed.org/learn/what-is-telemedicine

Benner, P. (2001). *From novice to expert: Excellence and power in clinical nursing practice* (commemorative ed.). Upper Saddle River, NJ: Pearson Education. Reprinted and electronically reproduced by permission of Pearson Education, Inc., New York, NY.

Centers for Medicare and Medicaid Services (CMS). (2015). *Accountable care organizations*. Retrieved from https://www.cms.gov/Medicare/Medicare-Fee-for-Service-Payment/ACO/index.html?redirect=/ACO/

Centers for Medicare and Medicaid Services (CMS). (2016). *EHR incentive programs*. Retrieved from https://www.cms.gov/Regulations-and-Guidance/Legislation/EHRIncentivePrograms/index.html?redirect=/ehrincentiveprograms

Charland, B. (2015). *Organizational context, shared governance structure and outcomes in veterans affairs hospitals*. Retrieved from http://digitalcommons.uri.edu/oa_diss/344/

CHP Group. (2014). *Complementary and alternative medicine (CAM) in accountable care organizations*. Retrieved from http://www.chpgroup.com/wp-content/uploads/2014/12/CHP-WP_CAM-in-ACOs_12.12.2014.pdf

Clark, T. C., Black, L. I., Stussman, B. J., Barnes, P. M., & Nahin, R. L. (2015). Trends in the use of complementary health approaches among adults: United States, 2002–2012. *National Health Statistics Report,*

79. Retrieved from http://www.cdc.gov/nchs/data/nhsr/nhsr079.pdf

Cronenwett, L., Sherwood, G., & Gelmon, S. B. (2009). Improving quality and safety education: The QSEN learning collaborative. *Nursing Outlook, 57*, 304–312.

Davis, C. (2014). *The importance of professional standards.* Retrieved from http://journals.lww.com/nursingmadeincrediblyeasy/Fulltext/2014/09000/The_importance_of_professional_standards.1.aspx

Davis, M. A., Martin, B. I., Coulter, I. D., & Weeks, W. B. (2013). US spending on complementary and alternative medicine during 2002–08 plateaued, suggesting role in reformed health system. *Health Affairs, 32*(1), 45–52. Published by Project HOPE: The People-to-People Health Foundation, Inc., © 2013.

Dawson, A., & Grill, K. (2012). Health promotion: Conceptual and ethical issues. *Public Health Ethics, 5*(2), 101–103.

Dinmohammadi, M., Peyrovi, H., & Mehrdad, N. (2013). Concept analysis of professional socialization in nursing. *Nursing Forum, 48*(1). Retrieved from http://onlinelibrary.wiley.com/doi/10.1111/nuf.12006/pdf

Donahue, M. P. (1996). *Nursing: The finest art. An illustrated history* (2nd ed.). St. Louis, MO: Mosby.

Fettig, K. J., & Friesen, P. K. (2014). Socialization of nontraditional nursing students. *Creative Nursing, 20*(2), 95–105.

Flynn, L., Liang, Y., Dickson, G. L., Xie, M., & Suh, D. (2012). Nurses' practice environments, error interception practices, and inpatient medication errors. *Journal of Nursing Scholarship, 44*(2), 180–186.

Fox, S. (2013). *Pew internet: Health.* Retrieved from http://pewinternet.org/Commentary/2011/November/Pew-internet-Health.aspx

George, R. E., Thornicroft, G., & Dogra, N. (2015). Exploration of cultural competency training in UK healthcare settings: A critical interpretive review of the literature. *Diversity and Equality in Health and Care, 12*(3), 104–115.

Goldberg, D. G., Kuzel, A. J., Feng, L. B., DeShazo, J. P., & Love, L. E. (2012). EHRs in primary care practices: Benefits, challenges, and successful strategies. *American Journal of Managed Care, 18*(2), e48–e54.

Guerrero, E. G., Padwa, H., Fenwick, K., Harris, L. M., & Aarons, G. A. (2016). Identifying and ranking implicit leadership strategies to promote evidence-based practice implementation in addiction health services. *Implementation Science, 11*(1), 1.

Hardy, M. E., & Conway, M. E. (1988). *Role theory: Perspectives for health professionals* (2nd ed.). Norwalk, CT: Appleton & Lange.

Hauck, S., Winsett, R. P., & Kuric, J. (2013). Leadership facilitation strategies to establish evidence-based practice in an acute care hospital.

Journal of Advanced. Nursing 69(3), 664–674. doi:10.1111/j.1365-2648.2012. 06053.x

Henderson, V. (1966). *The nature of nursing: A definition and its implications for practice, research, and education.* New York, NY: Macmillan.

Houghton, C. E. (2014). "Newcomer adaptation": A lens through which to understand how nursing students fit in with the real world of practice. *Journal of Clinical Nursing, 23*(15–16), 2367–2375.

Institute of Medicine. (1999). *To err is human.* Washington, DC: National Academies Press.

Institute of Medicine. (2010). *The future of nursing: Leading change, advancing health.* Washington, DC: Author. Retrieved from http://www.iom.edu/Reports/2010/The-Future-of-Nursing-Leading-Change-Advancing-Health.aspx

Jeffreys, M. R. (2015). *Teaching cultural competence in nursing and healthcare: Inquiry, action, and innovation.* New York, NY: Springer.

Lafond, C. M., & Van Hulle Vincent, C. (2013). A critique of the National League for Nursing/Jeffries simulation framework. *Journal of Advanced Nursing, 69*(2), 465–480.

Lerner, D., Rodday, A. M., Cohen, J. T., & Rogers, W. H. (2013). A systematic review of the evidence concerning the economic impact of employee-focuses health promotion and wellness programs. *Journal of Occupational and Environmental Medicine, 55*(2), 209–222.

Makely, S. (2012). *Professionalism in health: A primer for career success* (4th ed.). Upper Saddle River, NJ: Prentice Hall.

Military Health System Communications Office. (2015). *Military public health nurses stabilize, protect communities worldwide.* Retrieved from http://www.health.mil/News/Articles/2015/06/04/Military-Public-Health-Nurses-Stabilize-Protect-Communities-Worldwide

National Council of State Boards of Nursing. (2015). *National nursing workforce study.* Retrieved from https://www.ncsbn.org/workforce.htm

National League for Nursing. (2014). *Number of basic RN programs, total and by program type: 2005 to 2014.* Retrieved from http://www.nln.org/docs/default-source/newsroom/nursing-education-statistics/number-of-basic-rn-programs-total-and-by-program-type-2005-to-2014.pdf

National Student Nurses Association. (2013). *Code of ethics.* Retrieved from http://www.nsna.org/Portals/0/Skins/NSNA/pdf/Pieces_Appendix_B.pdf

National Student Nurses Association House of Delegates. (2001). *The code of academic and clinical conduct.* Nashville, TN: Author.

Nightingale, F. (1969). *Notes on nursing: What it is, and what it is not.* New York, NY: Dover. (Original work published 1859)

Peplau, H. (1952). *Interpersonal relations in nursing: A conceptual frame of reference for psychodynamic nursing.* New York, NY: Putnam.

Price, S. L. (2009). Becoming a nurse: A meta-study of early professional socialization and career choice in nursing. *Journal of Advanced Nursing, 65*(1), 11–19.

Quality and Safety Education for Nurses Institute. (2014). *Prelicensure KSAs.* Retrieved from http://qsen.org/competencies/pre-licensure-ksas/

Raman, J. (2015). Improved health and wellness outcomes in ethnically/culturally diverse patients through enhanced cultural competency in nurse educators. *Online Journal of Cultural Competence in Nursing and Healthcare, 5*(1), 104–117.

Salsberg, E. (2015). Recent trends in the nursing pipeline: US educated BSNs continue to increase. *Health Affairs Blog.* Retrieved from http://healthaffairs.org/blog/2015/04/09/recent-trends-in-the-nursing-pipeline-us-educated-bsns-continue-to-increase/

Sayles, N. (2016). Religion in nursing. *Nursing School Hub.* Retrieved from http://www.nursingschool-hub.com/religion-in-nursing/

Secomb, J., Mckenna, L., & Smith, C. (2012). The effectiveness of simulation activities on the cognitive abilities of undergraduate third-year nursing students: A randomised control trial. *Journal of Clinical Nursing, 21*(23/24), 3475–3484.

Spooner, N., Hurst, S., & Khadra, M. (2012). Medical simulation technology: Educational overview, industry leaders, and what's missing. *Hospital Topics, 90*(3), 57–64.

U.S. Department of Health and Human Services, Health Resources and Services Administration. (2014). *The future of the nursing workforce: National- and state-level projections, 2012–2025.* Retrieved from http://bhpr.hrsa.gov/healthworkforce/supplydemand/nursing/workforceprojections/nursingprojections.pdf

Truong, M., Paradies, Y., & Priest, N. (2014). Interventions to improve cultural competency in healthcare: A systematic review of reviews. *BMC Health Services Research, 14*(99).

University of Wisconsin Population Health Institute. (2015*). Cultural competence training for healthcare professionals.* Retrieved from http://whatworks-forhealth.wisc.edu/program.php?t1=22&t2=17&t3=28&id=47.

Vietnam Women's Memorial Foundation. (n.d.). *During the Vietnam era… .* Retrieved from http://www.vietnamwomensmemorial.org/pages/frames/vwmp.html

Wilson, L., Orff, S., Gerry, T., Shirley, B. R., Tabor, D., Caiazzo, K., & Rouleau, D. (2013). Evolution of an innovative role: The clinical nurse leader. *Journal of Nursing Management, 21*, 175–181.

World Health Organization (WHO). (2017). Frequently asked questions. Retrieved from http://www.who.int/suggestions/faq/en/

Module 43
Advocacy

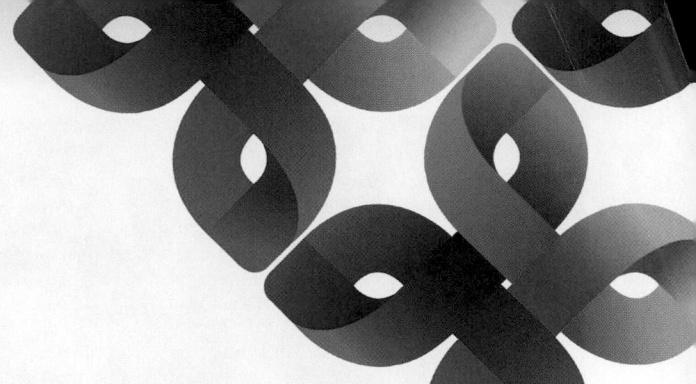

Module Outline and Learning Outcomes

The Concept of Advocacy

The Advocate's Role

43.1 Analyze the role of the advocate in the practice of nursing.

Advocacy Interventions

43.2 Summarize advocacy interventions used by nurses.

Concepts Related to Advocacy

43.3 Outline the relationship between advocacy and other concepts.

Unethical or Unsafe Practice or Unprofessional Conduct

43.4 Describe the nurse's role in reporting unprofessional activities.

Advocacy Exemplar

Exemplar 43.A Environmental Quality

43.A Analyze the health indicator of environmental quality as it relates to advocacy.

» The Concept of Advocacy

Concept Key Terms

Advocacy, **2715**
Patient advocacy, **2715**

Advocacy is a concept integral to both the American Nurses Association Code of Ethics for Nurses with Interpretive Statements (see the module on Ethics) and the International Council of Nurses' Code of Ethics for Nurses. **Advocacy** is generally defined as the act or process of supporting, defending, or assisting in another's cause. **Patient advocacy** can be defined as a process or strategy for acting on behalf of others (including patients, families, groups, or communities) to help them obtain services and rights that they might not otherwise receive but that they need to advance their well-being (Hanks, 2013; Jansson et al., 2014). Patient advocacy is a primary nursing role. The nurse may demonstrate advocacy by communicating the patient's needs to other health professionals; by facilitating, clarifying, or mediating communication between the patient and the primary care provider (PCP); or by assisting patients to exercise their right to receive care that is consistent with their circumstances, values, beliefs, and preferences. Successful advocacy results in positive outcomes for patients. It also provides nurses with a sense of professional satisfaction, having met a duty to provide individualized, culturally sensitive, patient-centered care.

Nurses are ethically obligated to act as advocates for all patients, but particularly for those who cannot advocate for themselves. Advocacy can occur at any level, in any setting, from the bedside to the healthcare provider's office, from advocating for the individual patient to advocating for an entire population through advocacy for changes in public policies and services.

Successful advocacy requires a balanced approach. It may not be possible to act on every patient request. Skilled nurse-advocates are able to explain the rationale for care limitations to the patient in plain language and also manage their own ability to cope with disappointing outcomes to prevent frustration and burnout.

Learning the patient advocate role begins during the nursing education experience. With time, the nurse will gain proficiency in this role and incorporate advocacy activities into daily professional practice.

The Advocate's Role

Navigating the healthcare system is a challenge for any patient. Advances in healthcare knowledge, technology, and system complexity have progressed exponentially in the 21st century. The result is that patients are rapidly moved through diagnosis and treatment in both inpatient and outpatient healthcare settings, often with little time for thoughts about self-determination or consideration of quality-of-life decisions. In addition, disparities in access

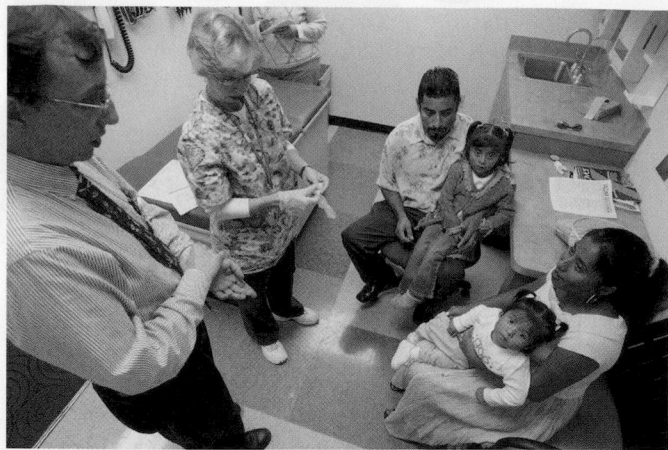

Source: Gene J. Puskar/AP Images.

Figure 43–1 》 At this clinic in Pittsburgh, Pennsylvania, patients not only receive healthcare, but also are helped to find a place to take English lessons, the closest Hispanic grocery store, and anything else they might need.

and quality of healthcare, particularly for underserved ethnic minority and socioeconomically disadvantaged populations or those with poor literacy, are apparent in the U.S. healthcare system. These patients have additional difficulty navigating the system, and they lack the resources to make quality decisions about their care. Even patients who are competent in terms of English literacy, and/or who have advanced education, may have issues with healthcare literacy and a need for information provided in plain language. All of these patients, as well as their families and support systems, need assistance and empathy to help them manage information about their diagnosis, determine the best course through their treatment plan, and penetrate the layers of bureaucracy to access the required resources (**Figure 43–1 》**).

As an advocate, the nurse provides patients with much of the information they need to make informed healthcare decisions and supports patients' right to decide. Ideally, medical treatment decision making is shared between the patient and the PCP. When the patient makes decisions other than what is recommended by the PCP, the nurse can help mediate further conversation between the two and ensure that the patient is making an informed decision. The nurse advocates for the patient's right to make autonomous choices, even when those choices are incongruent with the nurse's own beliefs and values. The nurse-advocate must be careful to remain objective and respect the patient's choices without conveying approval or disapproval.

Attributes of the Nurse-Advocate

Although patient advocacy is considered to be an essential nursing function, supported and reinforced in contemporary nursing codes of conduct (American Nurses Association Scope and Standards of Nursing Practice [ANA, 2010]; ANA Code of Ethics for Nurses with Interpretive Statements [ANA, 2015]; and International Council of Nurses

Code of Ethics for Nurses [ICN, 2012]), perspectives on how to approach patient advocacy and the boundaries of advocate roles are open to discourse. Questions have been raised historically (Hyland, 2002; Schwartz, 2002), and continue to appear in current nursing and healthcare literature (Cole, Wellard, & Mummery, 2014), regarding the definition of patient advocacy and whether advocacy means supporting any healthcare decision the patient might make, regardless of its rationality or the extent of the resources available. Additional questions include the potential for advocacy to interfere with autonomous decision making, as well as whether nurses are the only healthcare professionals with a duty to safeguard patients' right to decide. Hyland's (2002) seminal discussion on advocacy asked the question, "Do nurses, in fact, have any right to assume a unique position as a patient advocate among a multitude of health professionals?" (p. 472). Bu and Jezewski's mid-range theory of patient advocacy (2007) has become the "gold standard" from the nursing point of view. This theory acknowledges the importance of patient advocacy as an essential nursing role and provides a clear definition. According to the authors, "patient advocacy is viewed as a process or strategy consisting of a series of specific actions for preserving, representing and/or safeguarding patients' rights, best interests and values in the healthcare system" (p. 104).

The overall goal of patient advocacy is to create an environment in which patients can exercise their right to decide, and in which those rights can be protected, regardless of the environment or setting. Patient advocacy is complicated, because of the complexity of healthcare and legal systems, and also because healthcare decision making is dependent on multiple patient-specific factors. Therefore, the nurse's actions to advocate for any patient must be individualized and depend on the clinical and situational context (Bu & Jezewski, 2007). Within each individual context, three broad core attributes of advocacy form the foundation for action:

1. Safeguarding patients' autonomy
2. Acting on behalf of patients
3. Championing social justice in the provision of healthcare (Bu & Jezewski, 2007).

Safeguarding Patients' Autonomy

Safeguarding patients' autonomy is the first core attribute. It requires respecting and promoting each patient's right to self-determination, except in those situations when the patient is incompetent to decide or does not wish to be involved in decision making (see the Focus on Diversity feature on Patient Autonomy). Safeguarding the autonomy of a patient includes specific actions that both respect and promote the patient's ability to make healthcare decisions. For the patient to be able to exercise autonomy, two assumptions must be made. First is that the patient holds primary responsibility for her own health and decision making. Second is that the patient is legally competent to make healthcare decisions. The patient will likely need information to reach an informed decision; however, for this core attribute to apply, the patient's competency to decide cannot be in question (Bu & Jezewski, 2007). Examples of effective nursing actions that safeguard patients' autonomy include (Bu & Jezewski, 2007):

- Encouraging patients to share and document their goals, preferences, values, and beliefs
- Supporting patient values and choices even when they conflict with those of individual healthcare providers
- Providing patients with sufficient, timely information for making informed decisions about healthcare, assuring a match between patients' health information literacy and the information provided.

Acting on Behalf of Patients

The second core attribute consists of acting on behalf of patients. When patients are unable to act on their own behalf, or do not wish to represent themselves in the decision-making process, a series of advocacy actions can both preserve and represent the patient's values, benefits, and rights. Examples of situations in which this core attribute applies includes periods during which patients are under anesthesia/sedation or when patients make a conscious choice to have an advocate act on their behalf. Acting on behalf of patients differs from safeguarding patient autonomy, and the two do not conflict because the nurse is advocating for patients who are in very different circumstances (Bu & Jezewski, 2007). If a patient lacks decision-making capacity (e.g., the patient with advanced dementia or the unconscious patient), is legally incompetent, or is a minor, a designated healthcare surrogate or legal guardian is usually appointed to act on behalf of the patient (see the module on Legal Issues for more information).

Focus on Diversity and Culture
Patient Autonomy

Patient control over health decisions is a Western view that is not necessarily accepted in other cultures. In other societies, such as the Hmong population, health decisions may be made by the head of the family, a member of the community, or a religious leader. Some Hmong families make their healthcare decisions depending on how they classify their illness based on symptoms (for example, whether the cause is physical or spiritual) and their beliefs about the effectiveness of Western or traditional treatment for the problem. Religious leaders are then called on to decide how to treat spiritual health problems (Lor et al., 2016). In traditional Vietnamese families, husbands make decisions beyond the home, but wives make family healthcare decisions as a part of caring for the home and children (Centers for Disease Control and Prevention [CDC], 2012). The nurse must respect the patient's and family's views and honor their traditions regarding healthcare decision making. Even within the United States, a variety of American cultures and traditions may practice healthcare customs that are unfamiliar to the nurse. In American cultures such as Appalachia, fatalistic beliefs are common and affect the likelihood that people will receive preventive care. For example, some Appalachian women are less likely to complete a full HPV vaccine series, and therefore have higher rates of cervical cancer (Vanderpool et al., 2015). The ethics of advocacy require that the nurse honor the patient's and family's values, preferences, expressed needs, and right to self-determination.

Examples of advocacy interventions in which the nurse acts on behalf of patients include (Bu & Jezewski, 2007):

- Monitoring the quality and safety of healthcare delivered to the patient
- Taking action to intervene if the nurse has information that a treatment or intervention may violate the patient's wishes, directives, or best interests, when appropriate
- Expressing patients' wishes when patients cannot do so for themselves (e.g., during procedures requiring anesthesia/sedation)
- Ensuring that patients who are incompetent to make autonomous decisions have appropriate legal representation (e.g., power of attorney, guardianship).

Championing Social Justice in Healthcare

Championing social justice in the provision of healthcare is the third core attribute of advocacy. This attribute is based on the ethics of justice (see the module on Ethics). Whereas the first two core attributes represent nursing advocacy at the microsocial level (i.e., working with individual patients), this core attribute represents nursing advocacy at the macrosocial level. This attribute calls for nurses to become social activists by becoming involved in matters of health, education, and welfare related to the patients they serve in their organizations, community, or the larger society (Bu & Jezewski, 2007). This attribute could be actualized at the committee level in the nurse's organization, or the nurse might become active in her professional association, for example by serving on a legislative committee. Examples of advocacy actions related to championing social justice in healthcare include (Bu & Jezewski, 2007):

- Helping individual patients achieve healthcare goals by mobilizing resources available in the agency and/or community
- Acting on behalf of patients at policy and legislative levels, both within the agency and at the local, state, or federal level or by advocating to eliminate disparities in any area of healthcare.

Empowering the Patient

The patient–healthcare professional relationship has historically been characterized as paternalistic, with the physician or provider generally guiding decision making. However, the cultural ethic in Western healthcare is moving toward empowering patients to make informed decisions (Barr et al., 2015). The advancement of patient empowerment is beneficial for patients, health professionals, and the healthcare system. Patient empowerment has formally taken hold across Europe and is defined as a "process that helps [patients] gain control over their own lives and increases their capacity to act on issues that they themselves define as important" (European Patients Forum [EPF], 2016). The EPF identifies five aspects of empowerment:

1. Self-efficacy
2. Self-awareness
3. Confidence
4. Coping skills
5. Health literacy.

The idea of patient partnership and empowerment is seen as a way to reduce healthcare costs. By engaging patients, diagnosis is reached more quickly, and unnecessary treatment can be avoided (Richards et al., 2013). Strategies to promote empowerment (Elwyn et al., 2012; Vanderpool et al., 2015) include:

- A thorough and sensitive explanation about available options that provides patients with the opportunity to ask questions
- Always addressing the potential benefits and risks when explaining options to patients
- Eliciting the patient's concerns, ideas, and expectations.

These strategies help ensure that patients have the information they need and are especially applicable to nursing because the nurse often has more opportunity to be present with patients when they need time, conversation, and empathy. There are additional ways for nurses to foster patient empowerment. One way is by assisting patients to cultivate responsibility for their own health. Reminding patients that they are at the center of their own care may help them regain a sense of control. Educating patients about responsible and safe avenues for support can also promote patient empowerment; for example, an online support group for adolescents with cancer operated by a hospital may assist in promoting patient empowerment through social media. Using these strategies to empower patients to navigate healthcare decision making will help build a nurse–patient relationship of mutual respect, trust, and confidence.

Collaborating with Other Healthcare Providers

Given the complexity of healthcare systems, collaborating with other providers on the healthcare team as a way to advocate for the patient's needs has developed on a global scale. In its seminal report a *Framework for Action on Interprofessional Education and Collaborative Practice*, the World Health Organization (2010) reported on the countless benefits of collaborative practice, including greater collaborative decision making with patients. The Interprofessional Education Collaborative Expert Panel (2011) defines the concept of interprofessionality as "the process by which professionals reflect on and develop ways of practicing that provide an integrated and cohesive answer to the needs of the patient/population . . . [I]t involves continuous interaction and knowledge sharing between professionals . . . to solve or explore a variety of . . . care issues all while seeking to optimize the patient's participation" (D'amour & Oandasan, 2005, p. 8). Interagency and interprofessional collaborations as described in the module on Collaboration are essential to making healthcare services work for patients. In some cases, collaboration with advocacy programs can result in additional avenues of instructional, emotional, and financial support for patients. For example, the National Alliance on Mental Illness (NAMI) (www.nami.org) comprises hundreds of local affiliates and state organizations. NAMI provides support for individuals with mental illness and their families, including education, awareness, and advocacy to promote solutions for the nation's mental health crisis and advances for mental health research (NAMI, 2016).

Advocacy Programs

The federal government encourages states to develop advocacy programs to serve as a resource regarding the rights of those with mental illness or disability. Each state designates an agency or group to advocate for the rights of those with mental illness or disability and to investigate reported incidents involving neglect and abuse of these vulnerable patients in public or private mental health treatment settings, research facilities, and nursing homes. For example, Disability Rights North Carolina (www.disabilityrightsnc.org) is a federally mandated nonprofit organization charged with protecting the rights of children and adults with disabilities living in North Carolina (NC). Another example, Disability Rights Ohio (www.disabilityrightohio.org), a nonprofit corporation, is a federally mandated Protection and Advisory System for Individuals with Mental Illness (PAIMI).

The U.S. military has been faced with a number of health policy challenges, and subsequently has instituted advocacy measures for veterans and active duty personnel. Military personnel are at high risk for developing mental health conditions, one of which is posttraumatic stress disorder (PTSD). Those at risk for PTSD include individuals who have experienced deployment for long periods of time associated with extreme combat conditions. The Department of Defense developed baseline mental health standards military personnel must meet prior to deployment, and also post-deployment assessment screening standards, so persons at risk can be referred for treatment (Murray & Chaffee, 2014). Nurses working with military personnel, veterans, or others at risk for PTSD should be aware of these standards, as well as other related standards, benefits, and interventions available to these patients.

Professional and Public Advocacy

Professional nursing organizations advocate at the state and national levels for the profession of nursing, for its members, and for those who benefit from the services nurses provide. Professional organizations include the American Nurses Association (ANA) and are discussed in the module on Health Policy. As advocates, nurses are in a position to promote and effect change. They need to understand the ethical issues in nursing and healthcare and to have an understanding of state and federal laws and regulations affecting nursing practice and the health of society.

Nurses may advocate as individuals speaking on their own behalf, or they may be asked to speak as a representative of their professional association. There are multiple and varied opportunities to speak publicly for the health, welfare, and safety of patients, to take steps to protect patient rights, to inform the public about issues and concerns by writing articles for the popular press, to lobby state legislators or congressional representatives on behalf of better healthcare for all people, and to run for political office. Gains made by nursing in developing and improving health policy at the organizational, institutional, and governmental levels help to achieve better healthcare for the public.

Advocating for Children and Families

To be an effective advocate for children and families, the nurse must be aware of the child's and family's needs, the family's resources, and the available healthcare options. The nurse should ensure that the family has adequate information about treatment options and that information is provided a level matched with their health literacy and appropriate to the child's level of understanding. Treatment options should be in accord with the family's values and resources. Collaboration with other members of the healthcare team is essential, particularly if the family situation is complex, the healthcare issue has significant consequences, or the family's resources are minimal. If the nurse has the best information about these factors from the child/family point of view, communicating this information to the PCP and any other member of the healthcare team who will be helping to facilitate the child's care is essential. The nurse can then play an important role in assisting the family and the child to make informed decisions and to act in the child's best interests. As an advocate for the child and family, the nurse must also intervene to prevent any potential or real harm during planning or treatment and must follow through in whatever way is most appropriate and matched to the situation.

Ensuring that the policies and resources of healthcare organizations meet the psychosocial needs of children and their families is also a part of nursing's role. For example, membership on a committee that develops policies or evidence-based practice guidelines, or a team planning modernization of the healthcare facility design, allows the nurse to contribute knowledge of the developmental and psychosocial needs of children that can help ensure that the organization addresses the needs of children and families (**Figure 43–2 »**).

Table 43–1 » lists some examples of how nurses can advocate for children and families in their community.

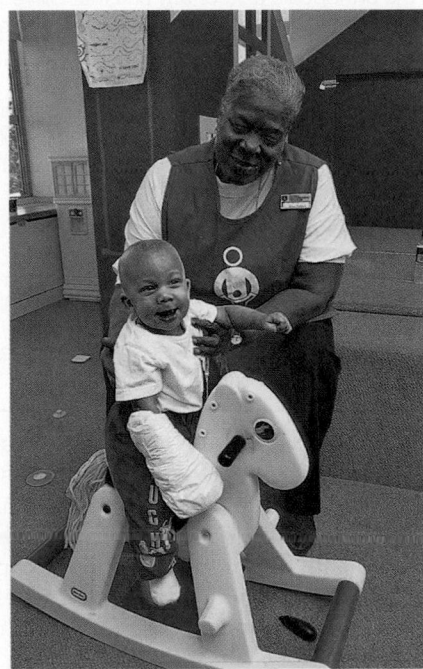

Figure 43–2 » Nurses must be aware of the needs of pediatric patients for play time and advocate for children to have play time as well as rest time and appropriate nutrition. Here, a volunteer grandmother plays with a young boy to provide stimulation and nurturing during his lengthy hospitalization.

TABLE 43–1 Advocating for Children and Families

Health Need Example	Nurse Advocacy Actions
Members of the community need information about places to obtain immunizations.	■ Make a list of agencies that provide immunizations, including those with low-cost immunizations through the Vaccines for Children program. ■ Obtain financial assistance from a local foundation to print your findings. ■ Make copies available in child care centers and other community agencies.
A local homeless shelter has little in the way of self-care amenities for the patients.	■ Obtain donations of hotel lotions, soaps, and shampoos from classmates and faculty that can be given to the shelter. ■ Visit several local hotels and ask whether they will each donate a box of small toiletries for the residents. ■ Encourage volunteers to provide haircuts and styling, or obtain donations to provide this service.
Your state has a law protecting the rights of any woman to bring her unwanted newborn baby to certain sites for the purpose of giving up her child without legal recriminations. Because many women do not know about the law, babies are abandoned in unsafe locations.	■ Find a local newspaper reporter who is willing to write an article about the law. ■ Run off copies of the article to distribute. ■ Make posters with necessary information for several community sites and the emergency department.

Source: Ball, J. W., Bindler, R. C., & Cowen, K. J. (2014). *Child health nursing: Partnering with children & families* (3rd ed., p. 336, Table 8–3: Advocating for Children and Families). Upper Saddle River, NJ: Prentice Hall. Reprinted and electronically reproduced by permission of Pearson Education, Inc., New York, NY.

Advocating for Vulnerable Populations

Vulnerable populations generally include groups who are at greater risk for disease, disability, and reduced lifespan because of a lack of resources, risk factors, or a combination. These groups often include the socioeconomically disadvantaged, such as low-income seniors, younger persons with either physical or mental health–related disabilities, and individuals of limited English proficiency. Many older individuals in vulnerable groups are considered "dual eligible," in that they are enrolled in both Medicare and Medicaid programs. These individuals—who consist of the sickest and poorest patients, with higher rates of diabetes, pulmonary disease, stroke, mental health disorders, and Alzheimer disease—must navigate both government programs to access the services they need. In its most recent report on vulnerable populations, the American Hospital Association reported that approximately 9.2 million individuals were classified in this highly vulnerable "dual eligible" category. New care coordination models have developed to help vulnerable older adults receive home-based care and improve care coordination, and they ensure integration of cultural competency and care equity standards (American Hospital Association, 2011).

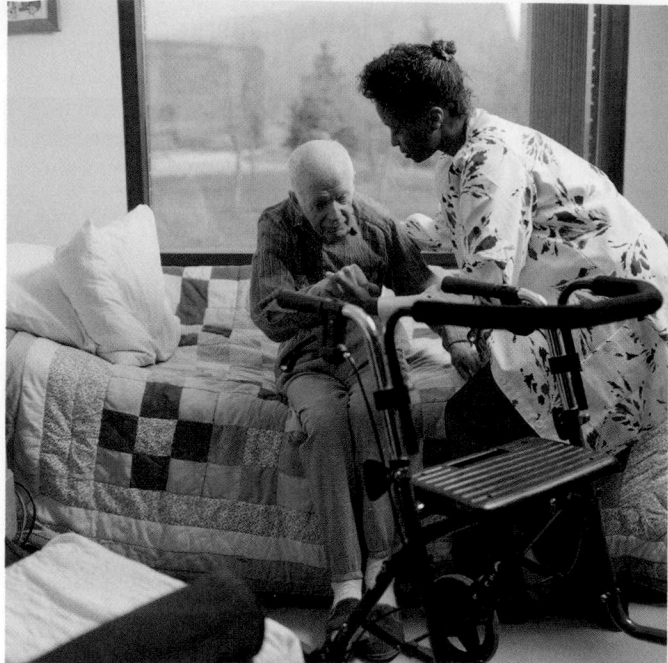

Source: Stockbyte/Getty Images.

Figure 43–3 》 Patients in long-term care facilities are often unable to advocate for themselves. Nurses should advocate for these individuals in many areas, including effective pain control.

An additional category of vulnerable populations is patients who serve as research subjects. The National Institutes of Health established vulnerable research subjects categories in 2005 that are currently in effect. These include pregnant women, human fetuses and neonates, prisoners, and children (National Institutes of Health, 2005). Nurses are strong advocates for all of these vulnerable populations, both those in in their care and those who are the subjects of healthcare research.

In the twenty-first century there is a need for new energy and political activism to ensure that the needs and the rights of individuals representing vulnerable populations are not overlooked. Advances in science, technology, and evidence-based practice continue to revolutionize how nurses practice (**Figure 43–3 》》**), and nurses must continue to advocate for fair and equitable access to high-quality care for all patients in a variety of settings, including acute care, free clinics, and primary care and specialty practices.

Clinical Example A

Lois Potter is a 78-year-old woman with a number of medical conditions, including type 2 diabetes mellitus. She is seen regularly in a community-based primary care clinic. The nurse practitioner has just talked with Mrs. Potter about the fact that her lab values indicate she needs to switch from the oral antidiabetic medication she has been taking to insulin injections. Mrs. Potter knew this was a possibility, but she is distressed about glucose monitoring and self-injection. Mrs. Potter is on a very limited income and is insured by Medicare and a supplemental policy. The RN working alongside the nurse practitioner teaches her self-injection in the office, but Mrs. Potter's return demonstration is worrisome.

Critical Thinking Questions

1. What information should the nurse communicate to the health-care team regarding Mrs. Potter's injection competency?

Which team members should be a part of this collaborative conversation?
2. What options does the nurse have for advocating that Mrs. Potter receive follow-up home care until she is comfortable with self-injection?
3. How can the nurse advocate for the patient in a way that maintains Mrs. Potter's dignity?

Two federal laws ensure the rights of individuals with disabilities. The Patient Self-Determination Act (PSDA) was enacted in 1991 to require healthcare institutions to inform patients of their healthcare decision-making rights, and the institution's policies regarding recognition of advance directives. This law provided general protection rights to all patients, including those with disabilities (see the module on Legal Issues for more information about the PSDA). However, the Americans with Disabilities Act (ADA), first enacted in 1990, is a civil rights law that ensures people with disabilities have the same rights as everyone else. It prohibits discrimination against individuals by providing federal protection to those with physical and/or mental health disabilities, in areas of public life such as employment, schools, transportation, and both public and private places open to the general public. Amendments to the law made significant changes to the definition of "disability" and became effective January 1, 2009 (ADA National Network, n.d.).

Clinical Example B

Ms. Marina Smith is an RN with 20 years of clinical experience. While caring for a patient on the orthopedic unit, Ms. Smith injures her back and is no longer able to work on a clinical nursing unit. During a visit to her PCP for follow-up care, Ms. Smith explains that although she is currently on medical leave, she is no longer able to function as a staff nurse on the orthopedic unit, or any unit that will require lifting or moving more than 20 pounds. She is uncertain what next steps her career can take, and she is very concerned. She reports that she applied for a position at a different hospital, but did not get an interview when the agency discovered she had physical limitations. She has not yet had a conversation about her predicament with her supervisor, so she does not know if options are open to her at her existing workplace.

Critical Thinking Questions

1. What would you say to Ms. Smith at this time?
2. If you were Ms. Smith's nurse, what would be the most appropriate way to advocate on her behalf? Explain your answer.
3. With whom on the healthcare team would you collaborate to be sure Ms. Smith gets the care she needs?

Nurses should be aware of the rights of two categories of individuals with disabilities: the physically disabled and those with cognitive disabilities. The prevalence of individuals with disabilities is staggering, and it crosses the lifespan. Seventy percent of students in public schools who are either secluded or physically restrained have disabilities, and 60% of individuals in jail have some type of mental disability. In addition, these individuals are socioeconomically disadvantaged: 48% have a personal annual income of $15,000 or less (American Civil Liberties Union, 2016).

Individuals with mental health issues are particularly vulnerable to abuse and neglect, either in their communities or in mental health settings that provide substandard care. The nurse's role is to advocate for the disabled person's physical, sexual, and emotional safety, both in the community setting, during institutionalization, or during a short-stay admission or outpatient visit. Their rights include (Disability Rights of Ohio, 2016):

- Personal rights, including the right to safety with people they know, including family, staff, and strangers.
- The right to be respected and treated with dignity.
- The right to have or not have a sexual relationship, including the right to permit or deny another person's touch.
- The right to control their money and possessions, including items such as cigarettes and clothing.
- The right to treatment in a place that respects their freedom and includes a current, written treatment plan that the patient participated in creating.
- The right to refuse or accept a suggested medication. In most states, psychiatric facilities cannot force patients to take medication except in an emergency.
- The right to exercise these rights without punishment, withholding of treatment, loss of privileges, or physical/emotional abuse.
- The right to a living space that provides reasonable protection from harm, including physical or emotional abuse and the use of overmedication or excessive restraint.

Clinical Example C

Mr. William Johnson is a 53-year-old patient being seen in the outpatient clinic for treatment of an acute exacerbation of chronic bronchitis related to his chronic obstructive pulmonary disease (COPD). He is also being treated for schizophrenia. He takes the medication he receives from the clinic because he wants his symptoms to remain under control, but he doesn't like the side effects. He has been a smoker for 40 years and has no intention of stopping. He is currently living with several other men in a housing project, and he has an entry-level job at a local fast food restaurant. Mr. Johnson has been disciplined by his generally understanding employer several times for behavior issues, but during his examination he tells you he fears being sent back to the mental health facility. On his last admission, the night staff who had previously treated him well during past admissions had been replaced by two new "orderlies" (psychiatric technicians). When the nurse was on another unit, one of them restrained him in his bed when he refused to share his cigarettes with him.

Critical Thinking Questions

1. How is this action by the psychiatric technician a violation of Mr. Johnson's rights?
2. What is the nurse's next step in advocating for Mr. Johnson?
3. Is this an example of advocacy at the level of the individual patient, at the community/policy level, or both?

Although laws protect basic healthcare rights and those of the disabled, miscommunication among providers and patients, and medical error, may still occur. Even when the letter of the law is followed, the spirit of the law may not be satisfied, particularly when working with patients with disabilities. For example, even if a patient reads and signs an informed consent document, comprehension of the information may be incomplete or absent. Nurses are often in a position to ensure that the procedures for procuring informed consent conform to both the letter and spirit of the law, particularly in the matter of patients with mental disabilities severe enough that capacity is questionable or incompetency

has been determined. In these cases, the patient's guardian, or individual with durable power of attorney, should be present and engaged in the informed consent process on the patient's behalf. Note that the nurse may not legally serve in that role; to do so would be considered a conflict of interest and could result in consequences for both the nurse and the organization. However, nurses are uniquely sensitive to the complex biopsychosocial issues involved in coping with disabilities, and they are in a position to advocate for these patients as they navigate the healthcare system. If the nurse discovers that the patient is not competent to make healthcare decisions, and no durable power of attorney is on record, the nurse should contact the PCP and may also need to work with social services to ensure that the appropriate next steps occur.

Advocacy Interventions

Novice nurses need to understand the organization in which they work, appreciate the legal implications of their actions, and carefully think through options before advocating on behalf of patients. In addition, it is essential that nurses anticipate patients' advocacy needs. Even a quick assessment can reveal the extent of the patient's understanding of their health problem, their plan of care, their health literacy, support system, and coping ability *in that moment*. Then the nurse can plan initial advocacy interventions accordingly. It is always necessary to safeguard the patient, but action must be taken in context. In designing and conducting advocacy interventions, it is important to do the following:

- Assess the patient's ability to cooperate and to make decisions.
- Assess the reliability of information provided *by the patient*, with regard to health history and family situation, especially if the patient exhibits impairment of cognitive function or mental instability. When necessary, engage family members as partners, or if appropriate, ensure the presence of the guardian or person with durable power of attorney.

Specific advocacy interventions may include:

- Educating patients and their families about their legal rights regarding informed decision making
- Ensuring patients have a voice in their care and are intentionally engaged in shared decision making by all providers involved in their care
- Ensuring that patients have the necessary information to give informed consent
- Monitoring patients' care to safeguard patient rights
- Evaluating organizational policies and procedures to ensure protection of patient rights
- Intervening if other healthcare professionals provide care that does not consider the patient's stated preferences and values or does not engage the patient in the decision, if the patient is competent to decide.

Concepts Related to Advocacy

Nurses must take many other concepts into consideration when advocating for their patients. Examples include ethics, legal issues, professional behaviors, culture and diversity, and healthcare systems.

Concepts Related to
Advocacy

CONCEPT	RELATIONSHIP TO ADVOCACY	NURSING IMPLICATIONS
Cellular Regulation	↑ advocacy → ↑ awareness of individual and global needs, as well as ↑ funding for research and treatment needs	■ Nurses ensure access to treatments and services, that holistic needs are met, and that patients do not face discrimination based on their health issue. ■ Nurses advocate, nationally or locally, for cancer research funding or for community cancer patient-friendly services.
Culture and Diversity	By advocating for patients' cultural and religious preferences, nurses ↑ patient satisfaction with care, promote the therapeutic relationship.	■ The nurse should practice culturally competent care by respecting the unique patient values and advocating for patient's rights to culturally competent care provided by healthcare organization, systems, and providers. ■ Nursing advocates should respect the patient's diversity and promote equity of care.
Ethics	Ethics → advocacy, ↑ patient safety and autonomy	■ The nurse's primary commitment is to the patient. The patient should trust that the nurse will act on behalf of the patient's best interests. ■ Nurses have an obligation to intervene when ethical dilemmas arise. The nurse should call ethical dilemmas to the attention of the PCP, the healthcare team, and the organization's ethics committee, as necessary and appropriate. ■ The nurse protects the patient's right to make choices about care and to refuse treatment.
Healthcare Systems	Vulnerable patients experience ↑ barriers to access and ↑ challenges and discrimination.	■ The nurse should support the patient by advocating for their right to access and receive equitable care in the healthcare system.
Legal Issues	Nurses who advocate ↑ patient safety and autonomy ↓ risk for negligence or error, ↑ trust in the profession.	■ The nurse-advocate should uphold the rights of the patient in any situation and also monitor the care provided by other professionals caring for patients. The nurse has an obligation to report any unethical or illegal behavior by another nurse, healthcare provider, or other staff member.
Mobility	Advocacy is necessary to improve patient and caregiver understanding, ↓ risk for further injury or immobility, ↑ patient and caregiver quality of life.	■ Nurses ensure patients have access to appropriate care, mobility devices, and live in mobility-restricted safe environments. ■ Nurses may advocate at the national, state, or community level for patients with mobility limitations, e.g., for research funding, or to ensure public place accessibility.
Professional Behaviors	By acting professionally, nurses ↑ their credibility, thereby ↑ opportunities and chances for successful advocacy.	■ The nurse should continuously advocate for the patient as a component of the professional scope of practice. ■ The nurse-advocate should act in accordance with professional and ethical standards.

As stated earlier, the nurse's role as an advocate is based in nursing codes of ethics, a system of principles or standards that governs nursing behaviors and relationships, guiding right conduct. Ethics and morals are related—morals are the principles on which judgments about right or wrong are based from a personal point of view. The role of the advocate is to uphold nursing's ethical principles.

Legal issues encompass the rights, the responsibilities, and scope of nursing practice as expressed in national standards of care, state practice acts, and associated rules (regulations). All patients have the right to expect safe, effective, competent nursing practice.

Patients have the right to exercise their individual cultural beliefs and values and to have their unique health needs met. Nurses who advocate for culturally competent care, both in specific individual situations and in everyday practice, help ensure that patients' cultural beliefs, values, and needs are respected. In turn, this increases patient satisfaction with care and promotes the therapeutic relationship.

Access to healthcare remains challenging to millions of Americans. In many rural settings, for example, access to specialty care and quality mental healthcare is limited. Nurses who work in areas or with patient populations with limited access can advocate for their patient or region by seeking ways to collaborate with other agencies, advocating for increased funding from their local legislators, and advocating for affordable alternatives, such as telemedicine, as ways to improve and promote patient access to healthcare.

The nurse's duty to advocate on behalf of patients requires careful collaboration in the form of clear and continuous communication with the patient, family members, and other healthcare professionals on the decision-making team. It is important to remember to balance the role and duty of advocacy "watchdog" with an attitude of teamwork when it comes to working alongside other professionals on the healthcare team. For example, a busy consulting physician may engage a patient in a one-on-one discussion about a treatment option and obtain written informed consent, unaware that the patient was recently medicated with an opioid drug to manage pain and is having difficulty both concentrating and remembering. The nurse's role would be to inform the physician and together with the physician decide whether a family member of the patient's choice should be present for a rescheduled conversation, wait until such time as the effects of the opioid did not affect decision making, or both. Regardless, a time for the physician to repeat the conversation should be scheduled, and the consent form signed again. The nurse would document the facts in the patient's record. The duty of advocacy is then fulfilled, the patient's rights safeguarded, and a collaborative nurse–physician relationship established or advanced.

Patients with alterations in cellular regulation, especially any type of cancer, need strong advocates. At the microsocial level, nurses help ensure that patients have access to necessary treatments and services and that patients' holistic needs are met. For example, nurses working with children with cancer advocate that patients have access to playtime and help their parents find ways to continue their schooling. At the macrosocial level, nurses may find themselves advocating through professional organizations for increased funding or may advocate at their agency level for play areas that can accommodate pets.

Patients with alterations in mobility, particularly those who depend on the use of mobility assistive equipment, also need strong advocates. At the microsocial level, nurses ensure that patients have access to the equipment and devices they need, and accompanying treatments, services, and personnel who can assist them with activities of daily living, if necessary. Nurses can advocate for affiliate home healthcare agencies to ensure that the patient's home environment is safe relative to their mobility limitations. At the macrosocial level, nurses may advocate through their professional associations to increase funding for

research and care for mobility-related health issues, or work with community organizations to ensure accessibility to public places is accommodated. The Concepts Related to Advocacy feature links some, but not all, of the concepts integral to advocacy. They are presented in alphabetical order.

Unethical or Unsafe Practice or Unprofessional Conduct

Nurses have a legal responsibility to intervene on behalf of any patient if they have reason to believe that another professional is engaging in practice that is unethical, unsafe, substandard, or unprofessional. State nurse practice acts include sections regulating the actions of the nurse in this regard, as well as reporting requirements. However, if the professional in question is not a nurse, the nurse should still intervene to safeguard the patient. The nurse who needs to intervene to protect a patient will follow established reporting procedures for her agency or facility, but the first step is to notify the nurse's own direct supervisor— the person to whom the nurse reports directly. That individual can be essential in assisting the nurse who discovered the breach of conduct and in facilitating the reporting procedure. That person is also the nurse's resource if immediate assistance is needed to stop an unsafe practice before harm is done to the patient.

Common examples of unethical or unsafe conduct that require nurses to advocate with one another or on behalf of a patient include boundary violations and nurses or team members working under the influence of drugs or alcohol. Boundary violations, such as engaging in an inappropriate relationship with a patient or coercing or restraining a patient to benefit the professional in some way (as in Clinical Example B in this module), are included in the category of ethical issues that may be addressed by a state board of nursing. Both state nurse practice acts and the ANA Code of Ethics require nurses to report unethical nurse behaviors, including boundary violations.

Impairment of a coworker or team member is the most commonly encountered situation that combines unethical, unsafe, and unprofessional conduct. Impairment to practice may be the effect of a substance—legal, illegal, prescription, or over-the-counter. Impairment to practice safely may also result from extreme emotional distress (e.g., a nurse who returns to work too soon following the death of a close family member). Because impairment has the potential to interfere with safe clinical practice, the nurse who observes or suspects impairment in any other health professional, nurse or non-nurse, is obligated to immediately report to a supervisor (ANA, 2010). For more information, including warning signs that indicate impairment, please see the section on Impaired Nurses in the module on Addiction.

A growing concern in healthcare regulation is the violation of a patient's privacy related to the inappropriate use of social and electronic media by healthcare providers. Nurses must consider confidentiality and privacy laws, patients' rights to be treated with dignity and respect, and trust as a foundation for nurse–patient relationships. Whether or not a post was an unintentional or nonmalicious act, posting confidential information about patients, including any health-related facts, conversations, or photographs, constitutes a breach of privacy. Such action may subject a nurse to disciplinary action by both the employing institution and the state board of nursing. In addition, the nurse may be subject to civil and criminal penalties. In response to alarm about this increasingly widespread practice, the National Council of State Boards of Nursing published its seminal White Paper on the use of social media (National Council of State Boards of Nursing, 2011). It is important that nurses work with their colleagues to keep one another attuned to the inappropriateness of using social media in this way, advocate for patient privacy and protection, and if aware, report infractions.

REVIEW The Concept of Advocacy

RELATE Link the Concepts

Linking the concept of advocacy with the concept of culture and diversity:

1. Consider each of the groups included within the description of vulnerable populations, and provide examples of how the nurse can advocate for each.

2. Why might patients with values and beliefs that differ from the mainstream population require greater efforts with regard to advocacy?

Linking the concept of advocacy with the concept of ethics:

3. How does the ANA Code of Ethics with Interpretive Statements (ANA, 2015) address advocacy? Under what circumstances might a nurse experience conflict of interest when advocating for a patient? Is the nurse the sole healthcare provider taking on the advocacy role; i.e., how do nurses balance the unique contributions of the profession with the team approach?

4. Differentiate between the nurse's role of advocate for individuals who are temporarily unable to speak for themselves (e.g., persons under anesthesia) versus the role of advocate for those who are competent to speak for themselves but, for whatever reason, do not.

Linking the concept of advocacy with the concept of legal issues:

5. What is the nurse's advocacy role when caring for a patient who is not competent to make healthcare decisions? Provide examples of other members of the healthcare team or organization who could be helpful in ensuring that the patient's advocacy needs are met.

6. How does the nurse practice act in your state address reporting of unethical or unsafe practice, or boundary violations (e.g., posting patient healthcare information on social media). Is the reporting requirement for licensees (i.e., nurses), employers, or both?

REFER Go to Pearson MyLab Nursing and eText

- Additional review materials

REFLECT Apply Your Knowledge

Heather Adams is a neighbor in your apartment building. On weekends, the two of you sometimes get together for morning coffee. Last weekend, Ms. Adams shared a concern that has been troubling her for a few weeks. She is 31 years old and unmarried, and she lives alone. Her father is deceased, and her mother, who was diagnosed with Alzheimer disease several years ago, is now a resident in a long-term care facility for people with cognitive impairments. Ms. Adams is estranged from her only brother. When she was in her early 20s, Ms. Adams was hospitalized and treated for depression. Her fear is that, should she become incapacitated again with depression, the brother whom she actively dislikes and with whom she does not get along will make treatment decisions as her next of kin.

You have decided to invite Ms. Adams for coffee. Because Ms. Adams seems to be an individual who would benefit from a healthcare power of attorney, your intent is to have a conversation with her about her choices.

1. On what basis do you act as an advocate for Ms. Adams (i.e., as a neighbor/friend, or as her nurse)?

2. Would it be ethical for you to serve as the surrogate decision maker? Explain your answer.

3. In your discussion with Ms. Adams, should you encourage her to see an attorney? Explain your answer.

» Exemplar 43.A Environmental Quality

Exemplar Learning Outcomes

43.A Analyze the health indicator of environmental quality as it relates to advocacy.

- Outline the components of environmental quality.
- Summarize the major impacts of environmental quality on public health.

- Describe community responses to alterations in environmental quality.
- Explain the nurse's role in advocating for patients affected by environmental quality.

Exemplar Key Terms

Environmental health hazards, *2724*
Environmental quality, *2724*

Overview

Environmental quality is one of the 12 leading health indicators published in *Healthy People 2020*. Its effect on health status is direct. For example, premature death, cancer, and long-term damage to respiratory and cardiovascular systems are all linked to poor air quality (Office of Disease Prevention and Health Promotion [ODPHP], 2016). **Environmental health hazards** include natural or human-made substances, states, or events that affect the natural environment, produce negative effects on the human ecosphere, and adversely affect health. Air and water pollution are the two most common environmental health issues, and the data regarding exposure is staggering. *Healthy People 2020* reports that approximately 127 million people in the United States live in counties where air pollution exceeds national air quality standards, and 88 million nonsmokers are exposed to secondhand smoke annually (ODPHP, 2016). These issues and many others affect the health of citizens in the United States and globally; the actions of nurse-advocates focused on environmental quality can have profound effects.

Classification of Environmental Hazards

Healthy People 2020 and the CDC categorize environmental quality and its determinants differently; together, these classifications provide an overview of the breadth of environmental factors that affect the nation's health. These lists are provided in **Table 43–2 》**.

The two most common environmental health hazards are air and water pollution (CDC, 2016b). A key factor in air pollution is the level of ground-level ozone, which is a component of smog. Ground-level ozone is often responsible for increases in emergency department visits and hospitalizations for individuals with health problems associated with diminished lung function, such as asthma and chronic obstructive lung disease. Individuals at higher risk are those who live in geographic areas where ground-level ozone is most likely to form at greater levels; contributing factors include heat, concentrations of precursor chemicals, methane emissions, wildfire emissions, and air stagnation (CDC, 2016b). Individuals at higher risk within high-ozone geographic areas include those with diminished lung function, but who are also socioeconomically disadvantaged (e.g., may be without air conditioning during times of high ground-level ozone), the elderly, children, or those with comorbidities.

Water pollution is also a concern. Water supplies may be contaminated with either natural or human-made substances. Contaminants in the public drinking-water supply that can cause health hazards include, but are not limited to, arsenic, nitrate, radium, uranium, and disinfection by-products (CDC, 2016b). Water pollution includes contamination of water supplies for public use (e.g., drinking water, bathing water) but also includes contamination of water resources, such as the pollution of rivers, lakes, and oceans. Contaminants, garbage, and oil spills are common pollutants of resources that can impact environmental quality over time.

Other environmental hazards include ionizing radiation, a variety of other chemicals such as lead and cadmium (ODPHP, 2016), and noise pollution.

The Effects of Environmental Quality on Public Health

A number of public health problems can be linked to exposure to environmental hazards, including asthma, birth defects, heat stress illness, poor reproductive and birth outcomes, lead poisoning, heart disease, cancer, carbon monoxide poisoning, and developmental disabilities. Three of the most common health effects related to environmental hazards, and their associated environmental links, are shown in **Table 43–3 》**.

TABLE 43–2 Determinants of Environmental Quality

Healthy People 2020 Determinants of Environmental Quality[1]	CDC Environmental Hazards and Health Effects[2]
■ Improving air and water quality	■ Air Pollution and Respiratory Health
■ Decreasing mental health stresses	■ Asthma
■ Strengthening the social fabric of a community	■ Carbon Monoxide
■ Providing fair access to employment opportunities, education, and resources	■ Clean Water for Health
	■ Climate and Public Health
■ Increasing options for physical activity and healthful diets	■ Health Studies, which includes epidemiologic investigations in response to outbreaks believed to have environmental causes, and responding to natural/technologic disasters
■ Decreasing injuries and accidents	■ Radiation Studies, which includes information about both ionizing and nonionizing radiation

[1] Based on HealthyPeople.gov. (2016). *Environmental quality.* Retrieved from https://www.healthypeople.gov/2020/leading-health-indicators/2020-lhi-topics/Environmental-Quality/determinants.
[2] Adapted from Centers for Disease Control and Prevention (CDC). (2016a). *National Center for Environmental Health.* Retrieved from http://www.cdc.gov/nceh/default.htm.

TABLE 43–3 Selected Health Effects and Related Environmental Hazards

Common Health Problems	Related Environmental Hazards
Asthma	■ Exposure to allergens and triggers, including tobacco smoke, dust mites, furry pets, mold, certain chemicals, and the particulate matter in outdoor air pollution ■ Particulate matter, which includes dust, dirt, soot, and smoke ■ When these pollutants from vehicles, power plants, factories, and other sources come in contact with heat and sunlight, ground-level ozone forms, putting individuals with asthma who spend time outside at greater risk
Birth defects	■ Environmental exposures to substances such as ionizing radiation, some endocrine-disrupting chemicals (e.g., polychlorinated biphenyls, or PCBs), dioxins, and pesticides have been linked to defects of the nervous system and developmental problems ■ Disinfection by-products in drinking water (e.g., trihalomethanes, or TMHs) may increase risk for brain and spinal cord, urinary tract, and heart birth defects ■ Living near hazardous waste has been linked to birth defects such as spina bifida, cleft lip/palate, gastroschisis, Down syndrome, and others ■ More data are needed to make clear connections between environmental exposures and birth defects
Cancer	■ Exposure to ionizing radiation ■ Exposure to some industrial chemicals ■ Environmental tobacco smoke (secondhand smoke) ■ It may take up to 40 years of environmental exposure for a cancer to develop

Source: From Centers for Disease Control and Prevention (CDC). (2016c). *National Environmental Public Health Tracking Network.* Retrieved from http://ephtracking.cdc.gov/showHome.action.

Community Responses to Environmental Issues

A community's citizens are directly affected by local, national, and global environmental issues. One way for citizens to respond is to be empowered to make positive change and become active regarding one or more environmental issues that affect them directly. Communities can serve as activists locally in municipalities, or join larger communities to make a larger impact. For example, the Natural Resources Defense Council (NRDC) is a global group of more than 2 million online activists, including scientists, lawyers, and policy advocates, who work to safeguard air, water, and natural systems. The NRDC identifies six ways to keep water clean, including (1) looking at how water flows across outdoor surfaces and into storm drains; (2) advising against flushing nondegradable products in a toilet or (3) a sink; (4) disposing of pet waste appropriately; (5) regular car maintenance, to reduce leaking of oil, coolant, and antifreeze; and (6) reporting polluters by contacting local environmental groups, such as the Clean Water Network or Waterkeeper Alliance (NRDC, 2016). These are steps that are possible for nurses working with community activist groups to actualize.

Advocating for Patients Affected by Their Environment

Nurses can intervene on behalf of patients affected by environmental quality in a number of ways across a variety of care settings. Nurses working in emergency departments, acute care, and primary care see the effects of environmental quality when they work with patients who experience health conditions affected by, or caused by, environmental hazards (**Figure 43–4 》**). For example, nurses may care for individuals with asthma or COPD who are admitted with exacerbations during periods of poor air quality. Community/public health nurses are also well positioned to serve as advocates. For example, underserved patients who live in substandard housing may have children at risk for lead poisoning from old peeling paint or old plumbing. Nurses can educate

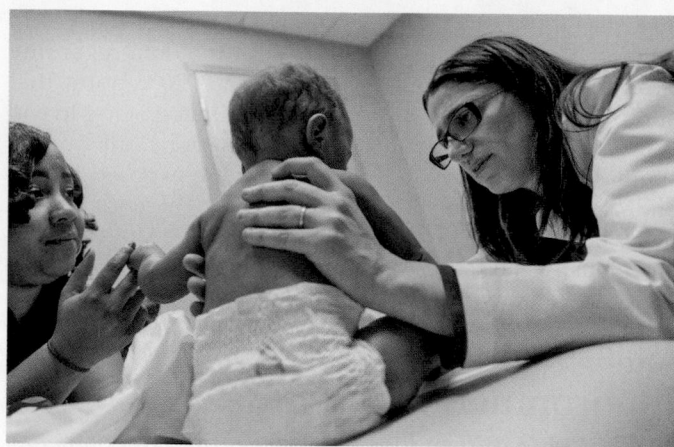

Source: ZUMA Press Inc/Alamy Stock Photo.

Figure 43–4 》 Dr. Hanna-Attisha of Flint, Michigan, knew that an investigation of the water quality in Flint showed that it contained dangerous amounts of lead. She decided to conduct her own analysis using hospital records. She found that the number of Flint children with elevated levels of lead had doubled and tripled in some areas since Flint had switched to a new water source 2 years earlier. Dr. Hanna-Attisha was so alarmed that she chose to hold a press conference rather than go through the months-long process of publishing her findings in a medical journal. She said she and her team had "an ethical, moral, professional responsibility to alert our community about this crisis."

patients about environmental hazards and strategies to safeguard themselves, or develop programs to educate the larger community. Nurses can act locally at the municipal, state, or national level to lobby government officials for change—for example, if community industries are known to be noncompliant with air pollution standards. Professional nursing associations generally identify legislative agendas focusing on state or federal legislation, depending on the scope of the association; as members, nurses can become involved on legislative committees and assist by providing data, or testimony, to support measures that safeguard the environment.

REVIEW Environmental Quality

RELATE Link the Concepts and Exemplars

Linking the exemplar of environmental quality with the concept of ethics:

1. Consider the air pollution exemplar, and how different vulnerable populations, for example children with asthma, might be affected by living in areas prone to high summertime ground-level ozone measurements. What is the nurse's ethical responsibility to advocate for environmental quality that improves the health of vulnerable populations? Provide examples of how nurses could advocate for environmental quality improvement.

Linking the exemplar of environmental quality with the concept of healthcare systems:

2. Why might patients who experience health problems made worse by environmental hazards (e.g., lung disease, heart disease), and

also represent vulnerable populations (e.g., socioeconomically disadvantaged or the elderly), experience barriers to access to healthcare treatment for environmentally related health issues? Consider the Flint, Michigan, water crisis as an exemplar. Why might these patients require greater advocacy?

Linking the exemplar of environmental quality with the concept of legal issues:

3. What is the nurse's role when advocating for the mother of a child with asthma who is living in substandard housing in poor condition with a leak in the roof?

4. What is the nurse's advocacy role when a patient presents with a health problem related to an unsafe work environment, such as constant exposure to toxic fumes?

5. What advantage does professional nursing hold when advocating, as a group, for environmental health and safety?

6. When nurses testify for an environmental quality issue, how do they represent themselves—as an individual, or as a member of the profession?

REFLECT Apply Your Knowledge

Jonathan Baker comes to the emergency department (ED) where you work complaining of difficulty breathing and shortness of breath. He has no other symptoms of upper respiratory disease, no history of chronic lung disease, and otherwise is in good health. As a part of your assessment you ask him about his living conditions, and he tells you that he lives in a subdivision very near the river that has flooded twice during the spring rainy season. The last flood was significant,

and several weeks later, Jonathan and his wife are still working at cleaning up the aftermath. You ask him if he has noticed any musty, earthy smell or foul odor in the house, and he states that he has. He knows that there has been mold growth in the basement and first floor, but he has not had the time to deal with it or to call his insurance company.

You determine that Mr. Baker's respiratory problem is likely due to mold, and you immediately notify the PCP so the diagnosis can be confirmed and his condition appropriately treated.

1. What are your next steps advocating for Mr. Baker's health?

2. Is there any other role in which you might advocate for the health and well-being of other flood victims in your city/region?

References

ADA National Network. (n.d.). *What is the Americans with Disabilities Act (ADA)?* Retrieved from https://adata.org/learn-about-ada

American Civil Liberties Union. (2016). *Disability rights*. Retrieved from https://www.aclu.org/issues/disability-rights#current

American Hospital Association 2011 Committee on Research. (2011). *Caring for vulnerable populations.* Chicago: American Hospital Association. Retrieved from http://www.aha.org/research/cor/content/caring_vulnerable_populations_report.pdf

American Nurses Association (ANA). (2010). *Professional standards*. Retrieved from http://www.nursingworld.org/MainMenuCategories/ThePracticeofProfessionalNursing/NursingStandards

American Nurses Association (ANA). (2015). *Code of ethics for nurses and interpretive statements.* Silver Spring, MD: Author.

Ball, J. W., Bindler, R. C., & Cowen, K. J. (2014). *Child health nursing: Partnering with children & families* (3rd ed.). Upper Saddle River, NJ: Prentice Hall. Reprinted and electronically reproduced by permission of Pearson Education, Inc., New York, NY.

Barr, P. J., Scholl, I., Bravo, P., Faber, M. J., Elwyn, G., & McAllister, M. (2015). Assessment of patient empowerment—A systematic review of measures. *PLoS One 10*(5): e126553. Doi:101371/journal.pone.0126553

Bu, X., & Jezewski, M. A. (2007). Developing a mid-range theory of patient advocacy through concept analysis. *Journal of Advanced Nursing, 57*(1), 101–110. Published by John Wiley and Sons, © 2007.

Centers for Disease Control and Prevention (CDC). (2012). Chapter 2: Overview of Vietnamese culture. In *Promoting cultural sensitivity: A practical guide for tuberculosis programs that provide services to persons from Vietnam.* Retrieved from http://www.cdc.gov/tb/publications/guidestoolkits/ethnographicguides/vietnam/

Centers for Disease Control and Prevention (CDC). (2016a). *National Center for Environmental Health.* Retrieved from http://www.cdc.gov/nceh/default.htm

Centers for Disease Control and Prevention (CDC). (2016b). *Climate and health: Climate effects on health—air pollution.* Retrieved from http://www.cdc.gov/climateandhealth/effects/air_pollution.htm

Centers for Disease Control and Prevention (CDC). (2016c). National environmental public health tracking network. Retrieved from http://

ephtracking.cdc.gov/showHome.action http://www.cdc.gov/tb/publications/guidestoolkits/ethnographicguides/vietnam/

Cole, C., Wellard, S., & Mummery, J. (2014). Problematising autonomy and ethics in nursing. *Nursing Ethics, 21*(5), 576–582.

D'amour, D., & Oandasan, I. (2005). Interprofessionality as the field of Interprofessional practice and Interprofessional education: An emerging concept. *Journal of Interprofessional Care.* Supplement 1: 8–20. Published by John Wiley & Sons, Inc. ©2005.

Disability Rights of Ohio. (2016). *Abuse and neglect: awareness and reporting for individuals labeled as mentally ill.* Retrieved from http://www.disability-rightsohio.org/abuse-neglect-mi

Elwyn, G., Frosch, D., Thomson, R., Joseph-Williams, N., Lloyd, A., Kinnersley, P., ... Barry, M. (2012). Shared decision making: A model for clinical practice. *Journal of General Internal Medicine, 27*(10), 1361–1367. doi:10.1007/s1 1606-012-2077-6

European Patients Forum [EPF]. (2016). *Patient empowerment campaign.* Retrieved from http://www.eu-patient.eu/campaign/PatientsprescribE/

Hanks, R. G. (2013). Social advocacy: A call for nursing action. *Pastoral Psychology, 62,* 163–173. doi:10.1007/s11089-011-0404-1

HealthyPeople.gov. (2016). *Environmental quality.* Retrieved from https://www.healthypeople.gov/2020/leading-health-indicators/2020-lhi-topics/Environmental-Quality/determinants

Hyland, D. (2002). An exploration of the relationship between patient autonomy and patient advocacy: Implications for nursing practice. *Nursing Ethics, 9*(5), 472–482. Published by Sage Publications (US), © 2002.

International Council of Nurses (ICN). (2012). *The ICN code of ethics for nurses.* Retrieved from http://www.icn.ch/images/stories/documents/about/icncode_english.pdf

Interprofessional Education Collaborative Expert Panel. (2011). *Core competencies for interprofessional collaborative practice: Report of an expert panel.* Washington, DC: Interprofessional Education Collaborative.

Jansson, B. S., Nyamathi, A., Duan, L., Kaplan, C., Heidemann, G., & Ananias, D. (2015). Validation of the patient advocacy engagement scale for health professionals. *Research in Nursing and Health, 38*(2), 162–172.

Lor, M., Xiong, P., Park, L., Schwei, R. J., & Jacobs, E. A. (2016, March 3). Western or traditional

healers? Understanding decision making in the Hmong population. *Western Journal of Nursing Research.* Advance online publication. doi:10.1177/0193945916636484

Murray, J. S., & Chaffee, M. W. (2014). The United States military health system: Policy challenges in wartime and peacetime. In D. J. Mason, J. K. Leavitt, & M. W. Chaffee (Eds.), *Policy & politics in nursing and health care* (6th ed., revised reprint, pp. 176–181). St. Louis, MO: Elsevier Saunders.

National Alliance on Mental Illness. (2016). *About NAMI.* Retrieved from https://www.nami.org/About-NAMI

National Council of State Boards of Nursing (2011). *White paper: A nurse's guide to the use of social media.* Retrieved from https://www.ncsbn.org/Social_Media.pdf

National Institutes of Health, Office of Extramural Research. (2005). *Research involving vulnerable populations.* Retrieved from http://grants.nih.gov/grants/policy/hs/populations.htm

Natural Resource Defense Council (NRDC). (2016). *6 ways you can help keep our water clean.* Retrieved from https://www.nrdc.org/stories/6-ways-you-can-help-keep-our-water-clean?gclid=CK_8y7_SicwCFQEJaQod_JgBuw

Office of Disease Prevention and Health Promotion (ODPHP). (2016). Healthy People 2020: Environmental quality. Retrieved from https://www.healthypeople.gov/2020/leading-health-indicators/2020-lhi-topics/Environmental-Quality

Richards, T., Montori, V. M., Godlee, F., Lapsley, P., & Paul, D. (2013). Let the patient revolution begin. Patients can improve healthcare: it's time to take partnership seriously. *BMJ, 346,* f2614. doi:http://dx.doi.org.proxy.lib.ohio-state.edu/10.1136/bmj.f2614

Schwartz, L. (2002). Is there an advocate in the house? The role of health care professionals in patient advocacy. *Journal of Medical Ethics, 28,* 37–40.

Vanderpool, R. C., Dressler, E. V., Stradtman, L. R., & Crosby, R. A. (2015). Fatalistic beliefs and completion of the HPV vaccination series among a sample of young Appalachian Kentucky women. *Journal of Rural Health, 31*(2), 199–205. doi:10.1111/jrh12102

World Health Organization. (2010). *Framework for action on interprofessional education and collaborative practice.* Geneva, Switzerland: WHO Press. (WHO/HRH/HPN/10.3). Retrieved from http://apps.who.int/iris/bitstream/10665/70185/1/WHO_HRH_HPN_10.3_eng.pdf?ua=1

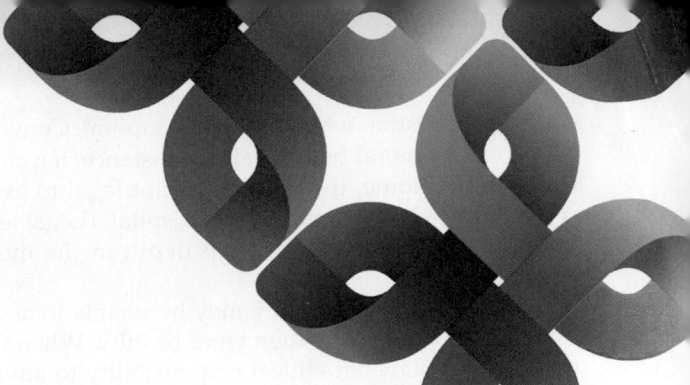

Module 44
Ethics

Module Outline and Learning Outcomes

The Concept of Ethics

Values

44.1 Analyze the relationship between values and ethics in nursing.

Concepts Related to Ethics

44.2 Outline the relationship between ethics and other concepts.

Nursing Codes of Ethics

44.3 Differentiate the various codes of ethics used in nursing.

Principles and Practices of Ethical Decision Making

44.4 Analyze the principles of ethical decision making.

Strategies to Enhance Ethical Decisions and Practice

44.5 Summarize strategies to enhance ethical decisions in practice.

Ethics Exemplars

Exemplar 44.A Morality

44.A Analyze morality as it relates to ethics.

Exemplar 44.B Ethical Dilemmas

44.B Analyze dilemmas related to ethics.

Exemplar 44.C Patient Rights

44.C Analyze patient rights as they relate to ethics.

» The Concept of Ethics

Concept Key Terms

Advocate, **2730**	Beneficence, **2736**	Integrity, **2730**	Nonmaleficence, **2736**	Values clarification, **2730**
Altruism, **2730**	Code of ethics, **2734**	Justice, **2736**	Social justice, **2730**	Veracity, **2736**
Autonomy, **2730**	Ethics, **2729**	Morality, **2729**	Values, **2730**	
Belief, **2730**	Human dignity, **2730**			

Ethics, as applied in professional nursing, is defined as a system of moral principles or standards governing behaviors and relationships that is based on professional nursing beliefs and values. More broadly defined, ethics refers to the standards of right and wrong that influence human behavior, usually in terms of rights, obligations, benefits to society, fairness, or specific virtues. Ethical standards are based on the values of the group that holds to those standards, whether the group consists of individuals of the same religion, people from the same community, or individuals who share the same profession. Within the field of nursing, some of the most important ethical standards relate to the rights of patients and their families, such as the rights to privacy and self-determination.

The term *ethics* also refers to the study and development of the ethical standards of an individual, community, or profession. Nurses should constantly examine their personal ethical standards and understand how their personal ethics and morals compare to the ethical standards of the nursing profession.

Morality (or morals) is similar to ethics, and many people use the terms interchangeably. However, **morality** usually refers to private, personal standards of what is right and wrong in conduct, character, and attitude. Sometimes the first clue to the moral nature of a situation is the awareness of feelings such as guilt, hope, or shame. Another indicator is the tendency to respond to the situation with words such as *ought, should, right, wrong, good,* and *bad.* Moral issues are concerned with important social values and norms; they are not about trivial things.

Just as nurses should be able to distinguish between ethics and morality, they should be able to distinguish between morality and law. Laws reflect the moral values of a society and offer guidance in determining what is moral; however, an action can be legal but not moral. For example, an order for full resuscitation of a dying patient is legal, but one could still question whether the act is moral. Conversely, an action can be moral but illegal. For instance, if a child stops breathing at home, it is moral but not legal to exceed the speed limit when driving to the hospital. (Legal aspects of nursing practice are covered in depth in the module on Legal Issues.)

When people are ill, they may be unable to assert their rights as they would if they were healthy. When this happens, nurses have an ethical responsibility to advocate on behalf of the patient based on what the patient would want. An **advocate** is a person who expresses and defends the cause of another person. Therefore, the nurse advocates for the patient's best interest on the basis of the patient's values, not on the basis of the nurse's own ethical or moral values. Nursing advocacy takes many forms and is discussed in detail in the module on Advocacy. However, to function successfully in his or her capacity as an advocate for patients, each nurse needs an understanding of ethical issues in nursing and healthcare.

Values

Values provide the foundation on which an individual's or group's ethical standards are built. Guido (2014) defines **values** as "personal beliefs about the truths and worth of thoughts, objects, or behavior" (p. 32). A **belief** is an interpretation or conclusion that one accepts as true. Values can reflect both beliefs that are based on a particular tenet (doctrine) or body of tenets accepted by a group of individuals and beliefs that are based on a pattern of mental views established by cumulative prior experience. For example, many traditional Jewish beliefs are based on the tenets found in the Jewish Torah, but individual Jews may hold other or additional beliefs based on their own experiences. Personal values are developed through individual observation and experience and may be heavily influenced by social traditions and the cultural, ethnic, and religious norms experienced within a person's family and associated groups.

Nurses acquire professional values through socialization into the nursing profession by nursing school faculty and other nurses, through clinical and life experiences, and by following established professional codes of ethics. As part of this socialization, nurses develop insight into their own values and how their values influence their actions. One of the most helpful ways for nurses to develop such insight is through **values clarification** (Johnstone, 2012a). Through this process of consciously identifying, examining, and developing individual values, nurses gain the ability to choose actions on the basis of deliberately adopted values.

Values clarification is important to both nurses and patients in supporting the provision of patient-centered care, because it helps nurses learn how to identify patients' values and distinguish patients' values from their own (Yoost & Crawford, 2016). Values clarification is not a once-in-a-lifetime activity but an ongoing process of examining what one's values are and how these values inform or affect one's decisions and actions. Nursing students and professional nurses alike need to have a clear sense of their values specific to life, death, health, and illness. Values clarification

exercises and real-life experience in carrying out treatment plans that contradict or challenge their beliefs about patients' best interests will assist nurses at all levels to develop expertise in responding to ethical issues.

Values Essential for the Professional Nurse

Although each nurse ultimately has his or her own unique set of personal values, certain core values are shared by all members of the nursing profession. Nurses typically acquire these values through the process of socialization to the profession. According to the American Association of Colleges of Nursing (AACN, 2008), five values that are essential for all professional nurses are altruism, autonomy, human dignity, integrity, and social justice:

- **Altruism** is concern for the welfare and well-being of others. In practice, altruism is reflected in the nurse's concern for the welfare of patients, other nurses, and other healthcare providers.

- **Autonomy** is the right to self-determination. Professional practice reflects autonomy when the nurse respects patients' rights to make decisions about their healthcare.

- **Human dignity** refers to the inherent worth and uniqueness of individuals and populations. The nurse who values and respects all patients and colleagues shows respect for human dignity.

- **Integrity** is acting in accordance with an appropriate code of ethics and accepted standards of practice. Integrity is reflected in professional practice when the nurse is honest and provides care based on an ethical framework that is accepted within the profession (e.g., the American Nurses Association Code of Ethics).

- **Social justice** refers to the upholding of justice, or what is fair, on a social scale. Nurses act in accordance with social justice by treating all patients equally without regard to economic status, ethnicity, age, gender, religion, citizenship, disability, or sexual orientation.

Some professional behaviors associated with these five essential values are outlined in **Box 44–1 》**.

Clarifying Patients' Values

To plan effective care, nurses must also identify patients' values, because these values often influence and relate to particular health problems. For example, a patient with failing eyesight will probably place a high value on the ability to see, whereas a patient with chronic pain will likely place high value on comfort. When patients hold unclear or conflicting values that are detrimental to their health, the nurse should use values clarification as an intervention. Some behaviors that may indicate the need for clarification of a patient's health values are listed in **Table 44–1 》**.

Nurses can help patients clarify their values through the use of the following seven-step process:

1. ***List alternatives.*** First, make sure the patient is aware of all alternative actions. A good way to start this conversation is by asking, "Are you considering other courses of action? If so, tell me about them."

Box 44–1
Professional Behaviors Associated with Core Nursing Values

Nurses embody the core values of their profession whenever they do the following:

- Demonstrate the professional standards of moral, ethical, and legal conduct.
- Assume accountability for personal and professional behaviors.
- Promote the image of nursing by modeling the values and articulating the knowledge, skills, and attitudes of the nursing profession.
- Demonstrate professionalism—including attention to appearance, demeanor, and respect for self and others—and professional boundaries with patients and families as well as among fellow caregivers.
- Demonstrate an appreciation of the history of and contemporary issues in nursing and their impact on current nursing practice.
- Reflect on their own beliefs and values as they relate to professional practice.

- Identify personal, professional, and environmental risks that impact personal and professional choices and behaviors.
- Inform the healthcare team of any personal biases on difficult healthcare decisions that may impact their ability to provide care.
- Recognize the impact of attitudes, values, and expectations on the care of the very young, frail older adults, and other vulnerable populations.
- Protect patient privacy and the confidentiality of patient records and other privileged communications.
- Access interprofessional and intraprofessional resources to resolve ethical and other practice dilemmas.
- Act to prevent unsafe, illegal, or unethical care practices.
- Articulate the value of pursuing practice excellence, lifelong learning, and professional engagement to foster professional growth and development.
- Recognize the relationship between personal health, self-renewal, and the ability to deliver sustained quality care.

Source: American Association of Colleges of Nursing. (2008). *The essentials of baccalaureate education for professional nursing practice* (p. 29). Washington, DC: Author. Used with permission.

---

2. ***Examine possible consequences of choices.*** Next, make sure the patient has thought about the potential results of each possible course of action. Some questions to aid in this effort include "What do you think you will gain from doing that?" and "What benefits do you foresee from doing that?"

3. ***Freely choose a course of action.*** To determine whether a patient chose freely, pose questions such as "Did you have any say in that decision?" or "Did you have a choice?"

4. ***Feel good about the choice.*** To determine how the patient views the choice, ask, "How do you feel about this decision (or action)?" Because some patients may not feel satisfied with their decision, a more sensitive question might be "Some people feel good after a decision is made, while others feel bad. How do you feel?"

5. ***Affirm the choice.*** Ask the patient, "How will you discuss this choice with others (family, friends, and so on)?"

6. ***Act on the choice.*** Find out whether the patient is prepared to act on the decision by asking for specifics about his or her plan of action.

7. ***Act with a pattern.*** To determine whether the patient consistently behaves in a certain way, ask, "How many times have you done that before?" or "Would you act that way again?"

When implementing this clarification process, the nurse should help the patient think each question through, but the nurse should not impose his or her personal values on the patient. In fact, the nurse should rarely, if ever, offer an opinion, even when the patient asks for it—and then only with great care or when the nurse is an expert in the content area. Each person's situation is different, and what the nurse would choose in his or her own life might not be relevant to the patient's circumstances. If the patient asks the nurse, "What would you have done in my situation?" the nurse should redirect the question back to the patient rather than answering from the nurse's personal viewpoint.

Concepts Related to Ethics

Ethical patient care encompasses more than managing difficult care decisions or facing the moral issues surrounding a patient. Ethical care also involves appropriate completion of common care tasks, including pain control; providing adequate patient teaching; demonstrating respect for patients from diverse backgrounds; advocating for the rights of all patients, regardless of their level of development or cognition; ensuring confidentiality; advocating for patients' safety; and supporting patients' right to self-determination.

TABLE 44–1 Patient Behaviors That May Indicate Unclear Values

Behavior	Example
Ignoring a health professional's advice	A patient with heart disease who values hard work ignores advice to exercise regularly.
Inconsistent communication or behavior	A pregnant woman says she wants a healthy baby but continues to drink alcohol and smoke tobacco.
Numerous admissions to a health agency for the same problem	A man with obesity repeatedly seeks help for back pain but does not lose weight.
Confusion or uncertainty about which course of action to take	A woman wants to obtain a job so she can meet her financial obligations but also wants to stay at home to care for her ailing husband.

Concepts Related to
Ethics

CONCEPT	RELATIONSHIP TO ETHICS	NURSING IMPLICATIONS
Advocacy	Nurses must ensure patients receive sufficient information on which to base consent for care and related treatment. Nurses must also provide an environment that allows patients to make their own care decisions, as appropriate.	■ Make sure medical staff clearly discuss all interventions with the patient and provide information sufficient to ensure informed consent. ■ Discuss the plan of care with the patient and allow self-determination as appropriate (e.g., allow the patient to choose which medication dosage to try first). ■ Recognize the patient's right to refuse treatment and procedures.
Cognition and Development	Patients with developmental limitations or disorders that affect their cognitive function may not be able to understand the implications of a situation or may make important decisions on their own without adequate support. Nurses have a duty to advocate on behalf of these patients, not only to help preserve their rights to autonomy, dignity, and respect, but also to help ensure that they do not become victims of abuse.	■ Understand state laws regarding the determination of incapacity and state and federal laws protecting the rights of disabled individuals. ■ Assume that patients have the capacity to make their own decisions unless there is clear evidence or documentation otherwise. ■ Understand the concept of guardianship, including when patients should be under the care of a guardian, as well as what limitations are placed on the guardian role. ■ Advocate for patients with limited cognition or intellectual ability when their rights appear to be in jeopardy or when others make decisions that may not be in their best interest.
Comfort	Chronic pain is a common problem in the United States, but many affected individuals lack access to healthcare resources that can help them adequately control their pain. Other people with chronic pain consume excessive amounts of healthcare resources, causing shortages of these resources for other patients. Both sides of this situation raise ethical issues related to resource allocation, social justice, and what constitutes an acceptable outcome of care for patients with chronic pain. The nurse also has an ethical obligation to collaborate with the patient and care team to manage the patient's pain in a way that minimizes the likelihood of medication abuse.	■ Become educated about chronic pain. ■ Engage with patients to develop a deeper understanding of the duration and severity of their pain. ■ Refer patients to pain management specialists as appropriate. ■ Help patients develop realistic expectations about the degree to which their pain can be alleviated. ■ Ask for support from supervisors or peers when advocating for appropriate patient care. ■ Recognize and set aside personal assumptions or biases surrounding narcotic use. ■ Educate patients about and monitor for signs of painkiller abuse or addiction.
Communication	Nurses are obligated to ensure the confidentiality of patient information during all care and in all care areas.	■ Ensure that access to patient information, such as online charting, is made available only to appropriate staff members. ■ Do not discuss a particular patient's situation with individuals who do not require this information as part of their job. ■ Observe all laws and institutional policies related to the confidentiality of patient information. ■ Inform the patient of policies and procedures that ensure confidentiality.
Legal Issues	The Health Insurance Portability and Accountability Act (HIPAA) sets forth specific guidelines nurses must follow to protect patient information. Thus, preserving patient confidentiality is both an ethical duty and a legal obligation. Nurses also help to protect patients' right to self-determination by ensuring that advance directives are in place and followed correctly.	■ Understand what constitutes "protected health information" under HIPAA's Privacy Rule. ■ Take appropriate measures to preserve the confidentiality of protected health information. ■ Discuss different types of advance directives with patients before surgery and other procedures that carry a degree of risk. ■ When patients are incapacitated, ensure that any advance directives are followed correctly and in the manner the patient intended.

Concepts Related to (continued)

CONCEPT	RELATIONSHIP TO ETHICS	NURSING IMPLICATIONS
Teaching and Learning	Because they are now sent home earlier than in years past, patients often require detailed instructions regarding critical aspects of their own care. The nurse has a professional obligation and an ethical duty to provide this teaching and to ensure that the patient understands the teaching and can properly carry out any self-care tasks.	■ Assess the patient's learning needs and abilities at the time of the initial encounter (whether in the ED, operative unit, acute care unit, clinic, or home). ■ Plan teaching interventions for the patient using appropriate methods and materials. ■ Recognize and set aside personal assumptions and values about the best ways to receive care information. ■ Follow up to ensure that the patient understands the teaching and that the teaching furthers the patient's sense of autonomy and self-determination.

American society is increasingly diverse, and this diversity has ethical implications for nursing practice. In particular, nurses have a responsibility to show respect to all of their patients, regardless of gender, race, ethnicity, religion, disability, sexual orientation, or any other personal characteristic. This obligation is clearly stated in the American Nurses Association's *Code of Ethics for Nurses with Interpretive Statements* (ANA, 2015a), which declares that nurses must respect the inherent dignity and rights of all patients, provide nursing services without bias or prejudice, work to eliminate disparities in care, and consider each patient's "culture, value systems, religious or spiritual beliefs, lifestyle, social support system, sexual orientation or gender expression, and primary language" when creating a plan of care (p. 1). In addition, ethical standards require that nurses neither project their own cultural preferences onto their patients nor view patients' cultural beliefs as inferior to or less valid than their own. For additional discussion of the intersection between diversity and nursing ethics, see the Focus on Diversity and Culture feature.

Of course, nurses have a responsibility to advocate for all patients, not just those who differ in terms of culture, cognition, or development. Part of the advocate role involves making sure that each patient's right to confidentiality is preserved. This requires the nurse to observe all laws and institutional policies meant to protect patient information. Ensuring confidentiality also means that the nurse must exercise good professional judgment when communicating with others, including the patient's family and other members of the healthcare team. Similarly, nurses must advocate for every patient's right to self-determination, including the right to establish advance directives and have them carried out according to the patient's wishes. Some, but not all, of the concepts integral to ethics are outlined in the Concepts Related to Ethics feature. They are listed in alphabetical order.

Focus on Diversity and Culture
Religion, Ethics, and Nursing Practice

For many people, including many nurses, the concepts of religion and ethics are intimately intertwined. For example, an individual's religion often informs his or her beliefs about social justice, end-of-life issues, the nature of suffering, and the very meaning of human existence, to list just a few topics. When nurses encounter patients whose religious beliefs differ from their own, ethical conflicts may arise. Nurses can help to minimize the likelihood of such conflicts by keeping several principles in mind:

■ First, nurses should seek to identify any ethical common ground that exists between themselves and their patients. Despite the significant differences that exist between the world's many religions, most belief systems place some value on helping the less fortunate, taking responsibility for one's actions, and treating others as you wish to be treated, among other things. In many situations in which an ethical conflict initially seems to exist, the nurse and patient can reach a shared understanding of which course of action is most ethical by looking at the situation through the lens of these common beliefs.

■ Nurses should also recognize that not every person adheres to all of the beliefs typically associated with the person's religious background. For example, although official Roman Catholic teaching forbids the use of birth control and sets specific guidelines regarding end-of-life care, many Catholics find it morally and ethically acceptable to disregard these teachings. A thorough assessment of each patient's unique belief system can help the nurse to avoid assuming that religion-based ethical conflicts exist when they do not.

■ Above all, nurses must remember that they have an ethical obligation to respect the patient's beliefs and right to autonomy throughout the care process. The nurse should honor the patient's beliefs and decisions unless the patient's choices will cause the nurse to act in a way that violates his or her own deeply held beliefs. In such cases, the nurse should seek guidance from supervisors, ethics committees, and other resources as appropriate.

Case Study » Part 1

June D'Angelo, a 49-year-old woman of Italian descent, presents to the emergency department (ED) late at night complaining of a severe migraine headache. Her vital signs show that her blood pressure is elevated at 210/104 mmHg. The ED physician discusses her history and finds that Ms. D'Angelo has been in the ED five times in the past year for the same problem. Ms. D'Angelo was prescribed a daily blood pressure medication by her primary physician 3 weeks earlier; however, she says she is not taking the medication and has not even filled the prescription but instead has decided to take daily walks to manage her blood pressure.

The ED physician asks Ms. D'Angelo how recently her headaches began and how long each one typically lasts. Ms. D'Angelo sighs and said that her migraines mostly never end and have gotten worse in the past 24 hours. When the physician leaves the bedside to call Ms. D'Angelo's healthcare provider, he gives orders to the nurse for IV blood pressure medication for Ms. D'Angelo. As the nurse prepares to provide the IV medication, Ms. D'Angelo says, "I'll take this medication, because I know it will make the pain go away. But I'm not taking that daily medication." The nurse then speaks with Ms. D'Angelo to complete a brief nursing assessment to determine why Ms. D'Angelo is reluctant to take daily blood pressure medication. Findings from the assessment indicate that Ms. D'Angelo relies on the ED to manage her pain and does not follow her primary healthcare provider's instructions, and that she feels exercise should be enough to manage her high blood pressure.

Critical Thinking Questions

1. What ethical issue is the nurse facing as she assesses this patient with frequent ED admissions?
2. What topics should be included in patient teaching for Ms. D'Angelo?
3. What further information should the nurse assess before planning patient teaching?
4. How can the nurse assist Ms. D'Angelo in planning how to manage her symptoms better?
5. Who should be involved in this patient's discharge planning and self-care? Explain.

Nursing Codes of Ethics

Ethical standards and behaviors are at the core of nursing practice. As a result, the nursing profession has developed formal codes of ethics to guide nurses in their work with patients and other healthcare professionals. A **code of ethics** is both a general guide for a profession's membership and a social contract with the public that that the profession serves.

The Nightingale Pledge is considered the first code of nursing ethics used in the United States. Written in 1893 by Lystra Gretter, principal of the Farrand Training School for Nurses in Detroit, and patterned after the Hippocratic Oath for medicine, the Nightingale Pledge was named in honor of Florence Nightingale. The Nightingale Pledge is still used at many nursing schools' graduation ceremonies. It reads as follows:

> I solemnly pledge myself before God and in the presence of this assembly to pass my life in purity and to practice my profession faithfully. I will abstain from whatever is deleterious and mischievous, and will not take or knowingly administer any harmful drug. I will do all in my power to elevate the standard of my profession, and will hold in confidence all personal matters committed to my keeping, and all family affairs coming to my knowledge in the practice of my profession. With loyalty will I endeavor to aid the physician in his work and devote myself to the welfare of those committed to my care (Gretter, 1910).

Over the years, the Nightingale Pledge was modernized, then largely replaced by longer, more comprehensive codes of ethics. Today, the nursing profession depends primarily on two major codes of ethics: the International Council of Nurses (ICN) *Code of Ethics* and the American Nurses Association (ANA) *Code of Ethics for Nurses*. These codes were initially adopted in the early 1950s and have undergone changes to reflect social and technologic change. The ICN code was most recently updated in 2012. The current version is presented in **Box 44–2 »**.

The latest version of the ANA *Code of Ethics for Nurses with Interpretive Statements* was released in 2015, after a four-year period of input and revision (ANA, 2015b). Within the United States, this code serves as a statement of nurses' ethical obligations and duties, as the profession's nonnegotiable ethical standard, and as the nursing profession's statement of commitment to society. All nurses should regularly refer to the ANA *Code of Ethics* to direct how they perform their duties in daily practice. The nine provisions of the ANA *Code of Ethics* appear in **Box 44–3 »**.

Using codes of ethics in everyday practice requires seeking knowledge and understanding of the patient's needs and preferences (whether the patient is a single individual, a family, a group, a community, or a population) as well as self-awareness on the part of the nurse. The following questions can help nurses apply Provision 2 to ethical problems (Kangasniemi & Haho, 2012; Lachman, 2012):

- What do I know about this patient's situation?
- What do I know about the patient's values and moral preferences?
- What assumptions am I making that require more data to clarify?
- What are my own feelings (and values) about the situation? How might they be influencing how I view and respond to the situation?
- Are my own values in conflict with those of the patient?
- What else do I need to know about this case, and where can I obtain this information?
- What can I never know about this case?
- Given my primary obligation to the patient, what should I do to be ethical?

SAFETY ALERT Although nurses have a duty to protect all research participants, they must pay special attention to research involving vulnerable populations, such as children, pregnant women, prisoners, older adults, and people with cognitive impairments. Because members of these groups often have limited autonomy, they are especially vulnerable to coercion, undue influence, and abuse.

Box 44–2
The ICN Code of Ethics

1. Nurses and people
   - The nurse's primary professional responsibility is to people requiring nursing care.
   - In providing care, the nurse promotes an environment in which the human rights, values, customs and spiritual beliefs of the individual, family and community are respected.
   - The nurse ensures that the individual receives accurate, sufficient and timely information in a culturally appropriate manner on which to base consent for care and related treatment.
   - The nurse holds in confidence personal information and uses judgement in sharing this information.
   - The nurse shares with society the responsibility for initiating and supporting action to meet the health and social needs of the public, in particular those of vulnerable populations.
   - The nurse advocates for equity and social justice in resource allocation, access to health care and other social and economic services.
   - The nurse demonstrates professional values such as respectfulness, responsiveness, compassion, trustworthiness and integrity.

2. Nurses and practice
   - The nurse carries personal responsibility and accountability for nursing practice, and for maintaining competence by continual learning.
   - The nurse maintains a standard of personal health such that the ability to provide care is not compromised.
   - The nurse uses judgement regarding individual competence when accepting and delegating responsibility.
   - The nurse at all times maintains standards of personal conduct which reflect well on the profession and enhance its image and public confidence.
   - The nurse, in providing care, ensures that use of technology and scientific advances is compatible with the safety, dignity and rights of people.
   - The nurse strives to foster and maintain a practice culture promoting ethical behaviour and open dialogue.

3. Nurses and the profession
   - The nurse assumes the major role in determining and implementing acceptable standards of clinical nursing practice, management, research and education.
   - The nurse is active in developing a core of research-based professional knowledge that supports evidence-based practice.
   - The nurse is active in developing and sustaining a core of professional values.
   - The nurse, acting through the professional organisation, participates in creating a positive practice environment and maintaining safe, equitable social and economic working conditions in nursing.
   - The nurse practices to sustain and protect the natural environment and is aware of its consequences on health.
   - The nurse contributes to an ethical organisational environment and challenges unethical practices and settings.

4. Nurses and co-workers
   - The nurse sustains a collaborative and respectful relationship with co-workers in nursing and other fields.
   - The nurse takes appropriate action to safeguard individuals, families and communities when their health is endangered by a co-worker or any other person.
   - The nurse takes appropriate action to support and guide co-workers to advance ethical conduct.

Source: From International Council of Nurses. (2012). *The ICN Code of Ethics for Nurses.* Retrieved from http://www.icn.ch/images/stories/documents/about/icncode_english.pdf. Used by permission of International Council of Nurses.

Box 44–3
The Provisions of the Code of Ethics for Nurses

Provision 1. The nurse practices with compassion and respect for the inherent dignity, worth, and unique attributes of every person.

Provision 2. The nurse's primary commitment is to the patient, whether an individual, family, group, community, or population.

Provision 3. The nurse promotes, advocates for, and protects the rights, health, and safety of the patient.

Provision 4. The nurse has authority, accountability, and responsibility for nursing practice; makes decisions; and takes action consistent with the obligation to promote health and to provide optimal care.

Provision 5. The nurse owes the same duties to self as to others, including the responsibility to promote health and safety, preserve wholeness of character and integrity, maintain competence, and continue personal and professional growth.

Provision 6. The nurse, through individual and collective effort, establishes, maintains, and improves the ethical environment of the work setting and conditions of employment that are conducive to safe, quality health care.

Provision 7. The nurse, in all roles and settings, advances the profession through research and scholarly inquiry, professional standards development, and the generation of both nursing and health policy.

Provision 8. The nurse collaborates with other health professionals and the public to protect human rights, promote health diplomacy, and reduce health disparities.

Provision 9. The profession of nursing, collectively through its professional organizations, must articulate nursing values, maintain the integrity of the profession, and integrate principles of social justice into nursing and health policy.

Source: From American Nursing Association. (2015a). *Code of Ethics for Nurses and Interpretive Statements.* Silver Spring, MD: Author, page v. Retrieved from http://nursingworld.org/DocumentVault/Ethics-1/Code-of-Ethics-for-Nurses.html.

Case Study >> Part 2

After June D'Angelo receives her IV hypertension medication, she tells both her nurse and the physician that she feels much better, "just like last time." The ED physician asks the nurse to stay by the bedside as he tells Ms. D'Angelo about his phone conversation with her primary healthcare provider. During the call, the physician learned about Ms. D'Angelo's tendency to miss appointments with her primary provider and her failure to fill prescriptions. The ED physician suggests that the best way for Ms. D'Angelo to avoid further ED visits is for her to collaborate with her primary provider to control her hypertension and headaches. The nurse then asks Ms. D'Angelo what barriers are preventing her from trusting and collaborating with her provider. Ms. D'Angelo says that her main worry is that her blood pressure will be so high that she will miss work and need to see the physician too many times. The physician tells Ms. D'Angelo that he wants her to take responsibility for her own well-being, then asks a clinical nurse specialist to meet with Ms. D'Angelo to prepare an outpatient blood pressure management plan. Before Ms. D'Angelo is discharged from the ED, she is given a calendar listing her next two outpatient appointments and a prescription for a new blood pressure medication.

Critical Thinking Questions

1. Why was it important for the nurse to ask Ms. D'Angelo about barriers to outpatient care management?
2. How did the discussion at Ms. D'Angelo's bedside maximize her well-being?
3. How did the nurse and clinical nurse specialist assist the patient's need for autonomy?
4. Analyze how the bedside discussion was an example of collaborative practice in which nurses function effectively in cooperation with other healthcare professionals.

Principles and Practices of Ethical Decision Making

An individual's personal, community, and professional values ultimately inform his or her decision-making processes. In turn, each profession has its own set of values or principles that shape how its members approach ethical decisions. For professional nurses, the four primary principles that shape ethical decision making are autonomy, beneficence, justice, and veracity.

Autonomy

Autonomy is the right to self-determination. Individuals have "inward autonomy" if they have the ability to make choices; they have "outward autonomy" if their choices are not limited or imposed by others. In the context of nursing, autonomy means that patients have the right to determine their own care. The nurse honors this principle by respecting the patient's decisions even if those decisions are in conflict with what the nurse believes is in the patient's best interest. In a healthcare setting, the principle of autonomy is violated, for example, when a nurse disregards patients' subjective accounts of their symptoms (e.g., pain). Furthermore, respect for autonomy means that no

individual should be treated as an impersonal source of knowledge or training.

Beneficence

Beneficence requires that "the actions one takes should promote good; it is the basic obligation to assist others" (Guido, 2014, p. 36). For nurses, this obligation extends to include the related principle of **nonmaleficence**, which requires that nurses do no harm and instead safeguard their patients. Intentional harm is clearly not in keeping with this principle, but there can also be risk of harm in performing nursing interventions that are intended for good. Nonmaleficence does *not* mean that the nurse performs only actions that carry no risk to the patient. After all, many actions, such as administering medications, carry some degree of risk. In most cases, the risk of harm is weighed against the potential for benefit. Also, before the action is taken, the patient is given information about the potential benefits and risks, and the patient decides whether to accept the treatment. Consider the example of administering pain medication to a patient after an operation. The risks of discomfort from the injection and side effects from the medication are typically outweighed by the goal of relieving the patient's suffering. Unintentional harm occurs when a risk could not have been anticipated. For instance, while catching a patient who is falling, a nurse might grip the patient tightly enough to cause bruises to the patient's arm.

Justice

Nurses must uphold the principle of justice in their practice. Here, **justice** means treating all patients fairly and in accordance with honor, standards, or law. This principle most commonly arises when decisions about the allocation of scarce resources must be made. For example, suppose that a nurse who is making home visits finds one patient tearful and depressed. The nurse knows that she could help this patient by staying for 30 more minutes to talk. However, that would take time from the nurse's next patient, who has diabetes and needs a great deal of teaching and observation. The nurse must weigh the facts carefully in order to divide her time justly among her patients.

Veracity

Individuals who always tell the truth reflect the principle of **veracity** (Guido, 2014, p. 37). Veracity can be a particularly challenging principle for the nurse, who may be faced with providing a patient with complete information about his or her illness even though family members or significant others want the information withheld. Veracity is the principle that underlies the need for healthcare providers to give patients complete information before obtaining informed consent for any procedure. Veracity is also one of several principles behind timely and accurate documentation of nursing interventions.

Applying the Principles

The ultimate goal of the ethical reasoning process should be to arrive at a decision that is in the patient's best interest and

The nurse has an obligation to:

- Maximize the patient's well-being.
- Balance the patient's need for autonomy with family members' responsibilities for the patient's well-being.
- Support each family member and enhance the family support system.
- Carry out hospital, clinic, or agency policies.
- Protect other patients' well-being.
- Protect his or her own standards of care.

at the same time preserves the integrity of all individuals involved. Nurses have ethical obligations to their patients, to themselves, to the agency that employs them, and to primary care providers. Therefore, nurses must weigh competing factors when making ethical decisions. Responsible ethical decision making is rational and systematic. It should be based on the ethical principles and codes described throughout this module and not on emotions, intuition, fixed policies, or precedent (i.e., an earlier similar occurrence). **Box 44–4** ≫ provides some examples of the obligations nurses must take into account.

Although the nurse's input is important, several individuals are usually involved in ethical decision making. Frequently, the patient, family, and other members of the healthcare team all work together in reaching a decision (see **Figure 44–1** ≫). Sometimes families will seek help from a spiritual advisor, such as a minister, priest, imam, rabbi, or other trusted individual. Therefore, collaboration, communication, and compromise are important skills that contribute not only to successful nursing practice, but also to a more ethical practice environment. Stress management is another valuable skill for the professional nurse. In many

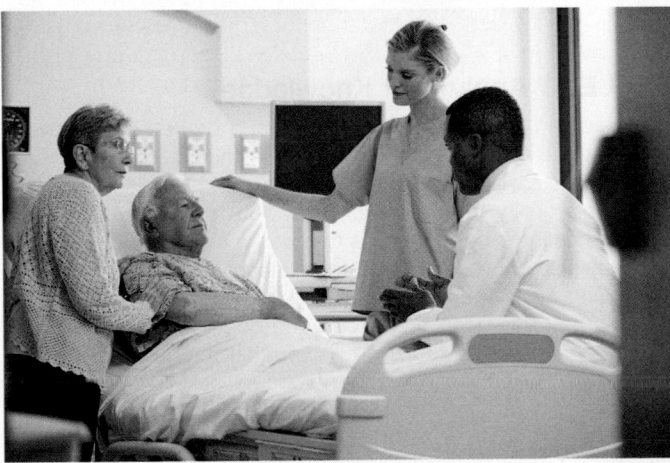

Source: Monkey business images/iStock/Getty Images.

Figure 44–1 ≫ When there is a need for ethical decisions with regard to patient advocacy, the patient, family, and healthcare team contribute to the final outcome.

cases, the nurse may feel torn among his or her obligations to patient, family, and employer. Also, what is in the patient's best interest might be contrary to the nurse's personal belief system. To help control their stress levels and allow for expression of their feelings, nurses who work in settings in which ethical issues frequently arise should establish support systems such as team conferences and use of counseling professionals.

Of course, many nursing problems are not moral or ethical problems at all; they are simply questions of good nursing practice. Therefore, an important first step in ethical decision making is to determine whether a moral dilemma actually exists. Generally speaking, a moral dilemma is said to exist when the following criteria are satisfied:

- A difficult choice exists between actions that conflict with the needs of one or more individuals.
- There are moral principles or frameworks that can be used to provide some justification for one or more of the actions.
- The choice is guided by a process of weighing reasons.
- The decision is freely and consciously chosen.
- The choice is affected by personal feelings and by the particular context of the situation.

When these conditions are met, the nurse should proceed with the ethical reasoning process. When they are not, the nurse should refer to professional standards of practice for guidance in determining the appropriate course of action.

Strategies to Enhance Ethical Decisions and Practice

Even when nurses do their best to adhere to the principles of their profession and engage in sound decision making, they still occasionally encounter organizational and social constraints that can hinder the ethical practice of nursing and create moral distress. Several strategies can help them overcome these hurdles. In particular, nurses can do the following:

- Become aware of their own values and the ethical aspects of nursing.
- Be familiar with the nursing codes of ethics.
- Seek continuing education opportunities to stay knowledgeable about ethical issues in nursing.
- Respect the values, opinions, and responsibilities of other healthcare professionals that may be different from their own.
- Participate in or establish ethics rounds. Ethics rounds use hypothetical or real cases that focus on the ethical dimensions of patient care rather than clinical diagnosis and treatment.
- Serve on institutional ethics committees.
- Strive for collaborative practice in which nurses function effectively in cooperation with other healthcare professionals.

One resource that is available to help nurses maintain current, evidence-based ethical practice is the National Guideline Clearinghouse (NGC). Maintained by the Agency for Healthcare Research and Quality (AHRQ) within the Department of Health and Human Services, the NGC provides an index to more than 2000 guidelines for evidence-based practice on a number of health issues, including ethical issues. For example, the Hartford Institute of Geriatric Nursing has developed a number of evidence-based nursing protocols for working with older patients. These protocols address topics such as advance directives, working with older adults with dementia, and discussing sexual health with older adults (NGC, 2017). Guidelines criteria were revised in 2013, and the Advanced Search page on the NGC website allows users to easily locate any of the nearly 500 guidelines that satisfy these new criteria.

>> **Stay Current:** Visit the National Guideline Clearinghouse online at www.guideline.gov

Ethical dilemmas can occur in the normal provision of care. The frequency of ethical dilemmas was reported as being negatively correlated with the level of nursing skills (Dekeyser Ganz & Berkovitz, 2012). In effect, this study found that the less experienced nurses are, the more likely they are to encounter ethical dilemmas. Thus, for many nurses, seeking advice from a mentor or a more experienced peer is a strategy that can facilitate effective solutions and approaches to perceived ethical challenges.

Another strategy that hospitals and other organizations have used to enhance ethical decision making is to implement a multidisciplinary ethics committee. In fact, the ethical standards of The Joint Commission (2013a) mandate that healthcare institutions provide ethics committees or similar structures to write guidelines and policies and to provide education, counseling, and support on ethical issues. These multidisciplinary committees, which include nurses, physicians, and hospital administrators, can be asked to review a case and provide guidance to a competent patient, to an incompetent patient's family, or to healthcare providers. Ethics committees provide a forum in which diverse views can be expressed, support is provided for caregivers, and the institution's legal risks can be reduced. (For additional information on this topic, see the module on Quality Improvement.)

Case Study >> Part 3

Reread Parts 1 and 2 of the case study. Before the end of the shift, another staff member in the ED asks the nurse to pick up the phone. As soon as she says hello, a woman asks her, "Did June D'Angelo come to your department earlier today?" The nurse immediately realizes that this situation will become a HIPAA issue if she does not manage it carefully and correctly. She asks the woman, "Who is calling, please?" The woman groans loudly and says, "This is Mrs. Jones. I am June's supervisor where she works, and I need to know if she was there today." The nurse answers, "Mrs. Jones, I am sorry, but due to privacy rules, we cannot discuss any patient information or names on the phone and cannot confirm whether any patient was or was not in our department." Mrs. Jones becomes upset and states, "Then how can I know what is going on? June missed her shift today!" The nurse remains calm and replies, "My best suggestion is that you contact your employee directly yourself." At that point, Mrs. Jones hangs up.

Critical Thinking Questions

1. How did the nurse realize that this was a possible HIPAA issue?
2. What privacy and confidentiality rules and ethical guidelines was the nurse following?
3. Do you think the nurse managed the call correctly?

REVIEW   The Concept of Ethics

RELATE Link the Concepts

Linking the concept of ethics with the concept of addiction:

1. How does substance abuse affect people's ability to make ethical decisions based on their personal values and beliefs?
2. What parts of the ANA *Code of Ethics for Nurses* address impaired nurses?

Linking the concept of ethics with the concept of reproduction:

3. What are your personal beliefs regarding fertility treatments? How would you feel about a patient who has conceived multiple fetuses through fertility treatments and now wants to have selective reduction to reduce the number of fetuses she will carry to term?
4. As a nurse, what are your responsibilities to a teenager who is seeking information on birth control methods?

REFER Go to Pearson MyLab Nursing and eText

■ Additional review materials

REFLECT Apply Your Knowledge

Keith Morgan, a 46-year-old man, fell and broke his leg several weeks ago. He is now receiving home healthcare. You are a home health nurse case manager, and you go to Mr. Morgan's home to assess his ability to ambulate. When you arrive, Mr. Morgan is alert and oriented but continues to report a high pain level. During your assessment, he tells you that Tylenol just isn't effective in controlling his pain. When you ask him about the effect of the narcotic that has been prescribed and documented as given by his primary nurse, Mr. Morgan tells you that the nurse told him all he needed was Tylenol and that he has not taken any other pain medication.

1. How should you respond to Mr. Morgan?
2. What is your legal responsibility in this scenario? What is your ethical responsibility? What actions do you need to take?

>> Exemplar 44.A
Morality

Exemplar Learning Outcomes

44.A Analyze morality as it relates to ethics.

- Explain the development of morality.
- Explain how moral theories can be used as a framework for examining ethical dilemmas.
- List three types of moral theories.
- Summarize moral principles.

Exemplar Key Terms

Accountability, *2740*
Consequence-based (teleologic) theories, *2739*
Cultural relativism, *2741*
Fidelity, *2740*
Moral development, *2740*
Moral principles, *2740*
Moral rules, *2740*
Principles-based (deontologic) theories, *2739*
Relationship-based (caring) theories, *2739*
Responsibility, *2740*
Utilitarianism, *2739*
Utility, *2739*

Overview

Morality typically refers to an individual's private standards of what is right and wrong, not only in terms of conduct, but also in terms of character and attitude. When the members of a group share many of these standards, morals may serve as the basis for the group's ethics, that is, its system of standards governing behaviors and relationships. Morals also help shape the laws of a society, although some actions may be legal but not moral, while others may be moral but illegal.

Just as people tend to confuse morality and ethics, they also tend to wrongly conflate morality and spirituality. Certainly, an individual's spiritual and/or religious beliefs may shape his or her ideas regarding right and wrong. For example, a person may be morally opposed to blood transfusions, sterilization, abortion, contraception, or any number of medical interventions because his or her religion forbids these things. However, people need not hold any spiritual beliefs whatsoever to cultivate a clear sense of morality. (For more information, refer to the module on Spirituality.)

Theories of Morality and Moral Development

Because morality intersects with so many of humankind's "big questions" about life and death, it has long been a topic of philosophical interest and debate. Much of this interest has revolved around the theoretical basis of morality, while some of it has focused on formulating a clearer picture of the process by which a person's moral standards emerge.

Moral Frameworks

Moral theories provide different frameworks through which nurses can view and clarify patient care situations. Nurses can use moral theories in developing explanations for their ethical decisions and actions and in discussing problem situations with others. Three types of moral theories are widely used, and they can be differentiated by their emphasis on (a) consequences, (b) principles and duties, or (c) relationships:

- **Consequence-based (teleologic) theories** look to the outcomes of an action in judging whether that action is right or wrong; these theories generally focus on issues of fairness. **Utilitarianism**, one form of consequentialist theory, views a moral act as one that brings the most good and the least harm for the greatest number of people; this is called the principle of **utility**. A utilitarian approach is often used in making decisions about the funding and delivery of healthcare.

- **Principles-based (deontologic) theories** involve logical and formal processes and emphasize individual rights, duties, and obligations. With these theories, the morality of an action is determined not by its consequences, but by whether the action is done according to an impartial, objective principle. For example, following the rule "Do not lie," a nurse might believe that he or she should tell the truth to a dying patient, even though the family has given instructions not to do so. There are many deontologic theories; each justifies the rules of acceptable behavior differently.

- **Relationship-based (caring) theories** stress courage, generosity, commitment, and the need to nurture and maintain relationships. Unlike consequence-based and principles-based theories, which frame problems in terms of justice (fairness) and formal reasoning, relationship-based theories judge actions according to a perspective of caring and responsibility. Whereas principles-based theories stress individual rights, relationship-based theories promote the common good or the welfare of the group.

A moral framework guides moral decisions, but it does not determine the outcome. For example, imagine a situation in which a frail older patient has made it clear that he does not want further surgery but his family and surgeon insist otherwise. Three nurses have decided that they will not help with preparations for surgery and that they will work through proper channels to try to prevent it. Using consequence-based reasoning, Nurse A thinks, "Surgery will cause the patient more suffering. He probably will not survive it anyway, and his family may even feel guilty later." Using principles-based reasoning, Nurse B thinks, "This violates the principle of autonomy. The patient has a right to decide what happens to his own body." Using relationship-based reasoning, Nurse C thinks, "My relationship with this patient commits me to protecting him and meeting his needs, and I feel such compassion for him. I must try to help the family understand that he needs their support." Each of these different perspectives is based on the individual nurse's moral framework.

Moral Development

Ethical decisions require individuals to think and reason. Reasoning is a cognitive function and is, therefore, developmental. **Moral development** is the process of learning to tell the difference between right and wrong and of learning what ought and ought not to be done. This process is complex, beginning in childhood and continuing throughout life.

Theories of moral development attempt to answer questions such as "How does an individual become moral?" and "What factors influence the way an individual behaves in a situation involving a question of morals?" Two well-known theorists of moral development are Lawrence Kohlberg and Carol Gilligan. Kohlberg's theory emphasizes rights and formal reasoning; Gilligan's theory emphasizes care and responsibility, although it points out that individuals use the concepts of both theorists in their moral reasoning. (For a full discussion of these two theories, see the module on Development.)

Moral Principles of Professional Nursing

Moral principles are statements about broad, general, philosophical concepts such as autonomy and justice. They provide the foundation for **moral rules**, which are specific prescriptions for actions. For example, the rule "People should not lie" is based on the moral principle of respect for individuals (autonomy). Principles are useful in ethical discussions because even if individuals disagree about which action is right in a situation, they may be able to agree on the principles that apply. Such an agreement can serve as the basis for a solution that is acceptable to all parties. For example, most individuals would agree to the principle that nurses are obligated to respect their patients, even if they disagree about whether the nurse should deceive a particular patient about his or her prognosis.

Like many professions, nursing is shaped by a set of guiding moral principles that shape how their members act. For nurses, the most important moral principles are autonomy, nonmaleficence, beneficence, justice, fidelity, veracity, responsibility, and accountability. Autonomy, beneficence, nonmaleficence, justice, and veracity were discussed earlier in this module.

Fidelity

Fidelity means being faithful to agreements and promises. By virtue of their standing as professional caregivers, nurses have responsibilities to patients, employers, government, and society, as well as to themselves. Nurses often make promises such as "I'll be right back with your pain medication" or "I'll find out for you." Patients take such promises seriously, and so should nurses, because doing so is central to the principle of fidelity.

Accountability and Responsibility

Nurses must also have professional accountability and responsibility. **Accountability** involves being answerable for the outcomes of a task or assignment. Nurses are accountable for their own actions and behaviors, but they may also be accountable for the actions of others, such as subordinates or trainees. **Responsibility** is the specific obligation associated with the performance of duties of a particular role, and it belongs to the individual performing the duties. Thus, the ethical nurse is able to explain the rationale behind every action and recognizes the standards to which he or she will be held. (For more information, see the module on Accountability.)

NURSING PROCESS

Morality shapes the profession of nursing in many different ways. Not only do certain moral principles drive nursing theory, practice, and decision making, but they also serve as the foundation for the professional codes of ethics described earlier in this module. Nonetheless, unethical or immoral behavior still occurs among nurses. Although only a very few individuals in the profession exhibit this behavior, all nurses must be able to identify, discourage, and report it. In fact, failure to report certain forms of immoral behavior by another healthcare professional is a violation of the ANA *Code of Ethics for Nurses* and the nurse–patient relationship.

SAFETY ALERT Nurses have both an ethical and a legal responsibility to report certain forms of abuse to the appropriate authorities. Depending on the state in which a nurse practices, mandatory reporting laws may include known and/or suspected child abuse and neglect; elder abuse and neglect; and/or domestic violence. Nurses must also take action to ensure the safety of suspected victims of abuse and neglect.

To guard against questionable and unethical practices, nurses must have a thorough understanding of their own morality and what constitutes right and wrong for them as individuals. They must also have a thorough understanding of their professional code of ethics and be able to identify when the ethics of another professional or agency are contrary to the *Code of Ethics for Nurses*. Furthermore, nurses must recognize that they will encounter patients at various stages of moral development, patients with questionable or confusing morals, and patients who are immoral. Nursing ethics and professional codes of conduct require nurses to deliver high-quality, professional care to all patients, regardless of the patients' morality. This can sometimes challenge even the most professional, experienced nurse. Examples of such challenges include the following:

- A patient with HIV is transferred to the critical care unit (CCU) of a hospital from the prison infirmary. The patient is paraplegic with no ability to move his legs. He is serving a life sentence in prison for repeated child molestation and rape.

- A young woman comes to the local free health clinic with her boyfriend to get a pregnancy test. The test is positive. The boyfriend immediately starts talking to her about how she'll have to get an abortion.

- An older woman is brought to the emergency department by a friend who came to visit and found the woman lying in her own feces. She is weak and dehydrated. The friend says that the woman lives with her son and his wife.

To care for patients such as these, nurses must have an awareness of their own morality and ethics, a thorough understanding of the requirements they must follow under the professional code of ethics, and an understanding of the reporting requirements in their state and the procedures they must follow in their place of employment. Although a nurse's own personal beliefs, morality, and bias will influence how the nurse manages each situation, the nurse must ultimately remember his or her moral duty to provide the best possible care, no matter what the patient's morality or immorality may be. (See the Focus on Diversity and Culture feature for additional information.) The following sections take a closer look at how this duty comes into play during all stages of the nursing process.

Assessment

As with any patient, assessment of the patient who is immoral or who is exposed to immorality that involves abuse or mistreatment includes a nursing history and physical examination. Patients who are immoral may not be able or willing to participate in a trusting nurse–patient relationship and may not respond to attempts at therapeutic communication. In interviewing these patients, the nurse should maintain a calm, nonjudgmental manner and should ask open-ended questions in a matter-of-fact tone.

Diagnosis

Nursing diagnoses for an individual with moral dilemmas or distress or a patient with a family member or significant other with questionable morals will vary. For example, appropriate diagnoses in the scenarios mentioned earlier may include the following:

- The prisoner transferred to the CCU will have a number of diagnoses appropriate to his medical condition. In addition, the following nursing diagnoses may be appropriate:

  Health Behavior, Risk Prone

  Moral Distress

  Noncompliance

  Social Isolation.

  (NANDA-I © 2014)

- The young woman who has just found out she is pregnant may be diagnosed with the following:

  Self-Esteem, Situational Low, Risk for

  Resilience, Impaired.

  (NANDA-I © 2014)

- The older woman who was brought to the emergency department by a friend may be diagnosed with the following:

  Family Processes, Interrupted

  Powerlessness

  Self-Esteem, Chronic Low

  Social Isolation

  Post-Trauma Syndrome.

  (NANDA-I © 2014)

Focus on Diversity and Culture
Cultural Relativism

Cultural relativism is the idea that people's morals are deeply rooted in the beliefs and behaviors of their particular culture. According to this principle, even though a person's moral principles may conflict with our own, we should not automatically assume that these principles are indefensible or incorrect, because they likely make sense when viewed through the lens of that person's culture (Butts & Rich, 2013; Ellis & Hartley, 2012).

Cultural relativism was first popularized by anthropologists and other social researchers who wanted to describe and compare cultures in a systematic manner that was free from bias. This concept has become increasingly widespread throughout the field of nursing as theorists and practitioners alike place greater emphasis on cross-cultural care. Nursing's embrace of this concept has helped to bring about a care environment in which many patients feel more autonomous, more respected, and more valued. However, cultural relativism also creates moral and ethical dilemmas for the nurse.

Consider, for example, the practice of female genital mutilation (FGM), sometimes also known as "female circumcision." Although FGM involves physical mutilation of underage girls, some African and Middle Eastern cultures view it as morally acceptable and an important rite of passage into adulthood. Most Western cultures, however—as well as the United Nations and the World Health Organization (WHO)—regard FGM as a clear violation of the rights to autonomy, consent, and freedom from harm. Cultural practices that raise similar concerns include child marriage and severe limitations on the rights of females. When nurses encounter situations like these, they must carefully evaluate what course of action will produce greater benefit and/or lesser harm to the patient. In some cases, as in the case of FGM, the nurse's duty to preserve the patient's rights to self-determination, consent, and freedom from harm far outweigh the nurse's duty to honor the cultural preferences of the patient and the patient's family. The nurse may also be legally required to act in a certain way. Because situations like these are fraught with potential moral, ethical, and legal implications, it is always wise for the nurse to seek the counsel of a mentor or supervisor before deciding on an appropriate course of action.

Planning

Individuals with moral dilemmas or distress may find it difficult to participate in the planning process; they may even show disdain for it. The nurse may try to obtain cooperation by capitalizing on needs the patient presents during the assessment. For example, the nurse might say, "You said you didn't want to be in pain anymore, so we need to run these tests to find out what is causing your pain so that we can treat it," or "I know you don't like the food here, but remember we discussed that to feel better, you have to get appropriate nutrition." Although outcomes for these patients will vary widely, a few frequently appropriate outcomes include the following:

- The patient will participate appropriately as able in the therapeutic regimen.
- The patient will refrain from causing disruptions that affect other patients and staff.
- The patient will be appropriately supervised during caring interventions, diagnostic procedures, and other

activities. For example, a security staff member or member of law enforcement will be present during caring interventions for a patient with a history of assault.

Implementation

Caring for individuals with moral dilemmas or distress can be challenging, unpleasant, and time consuming. Interventions

that may be appropriate when working with these patients could include any of the following:

- Following procedures that ensure the safety of staff working with the patient and adding precautions or procedures as necessary to ensure safety of other patients and staff. Refer to the Safety Alert for additional information.

Nursing Care Plan
A Patient Presenting Morality Issues

Michael Dunham is a 50-year-old man with HIV who is also paraplegic. Mr. Dunham is admitted to the critical care unit (CCU) of the local hospital from the prison infirmary, where he has been for more than a month.

ASSESSMENT

Mr.Dunham has a history of IV drug use and having sexual relations with female sex workers. He is admitted to the critical care unit of the local hospital from the prison infirmary, where he has been for more than a month. He is on oxygen by cannula. He is restrained to his bed. Almost every time members of the nursing staff work with him, he tries to spit on them in an effort to "give" them his disease. Upon arrival, the prison transport unit informs the head nurse that Mr. Dunham is serving a life sentence for molesting children and that he used his disability to trick preteen girls into coming close enough for him to handcuff them to his wheelchair so they could not escape his sexual abuse. Before releasing them, he would threaten to kill their parents if the girls told anyone what happened.

Upon physical examination, the nurses working with Mr. Dunham find the following:

- Temperature 37.9°C oral (100.2°F), P 104 beats/min, R 32/min, BP 102/60 mmHg
- Oxygen saturation 84%; breath sounds reveal coarse crackles in the left lower base
- Mild cyanosis of nail beds and mucous membranes
- Use of accessory muscles to breathe with intercostal and suprasternal retractions
- Flaccid paralysis of lower extremities since the patient was 8 years old
- ECG shows 2–3 premature ventricular contractions per minute
- HIV positive with CD4 T-cell count of 64; CBC showed WBC of 9.8, elevated lymphocyte and low segs
- Chest x-ray shows characteristic appearance of *Pneumocystis jirovecii*

DIAGNOSES

- *Moral Distress*
- *Social Interaction, Impaired*
- *Social Isolation*
- *Gas Exchange, Impaired*
- *Health Behavior, Risk-Prone*

(NANDA-I © 2014)

PLANNING

- The patient will participate appropriately as able in the therapeutic regimen.
- The patient will refrain from causing disruptions that affect other patients and staff.
- The patient will be appropriately supervised during caring interventions, diagnostic procedures, and other activities.
- Nursing staff will take appropriate precautions to prevent the spread of HIV.

IMPLEMENTATION

- A correctional officer or member of the hospital security staff will be present during any intervention in which removing the restraints is necessary.
- Nurses will provide care in groups of two or more.
- The patient will be offered counseling and a referral to the hospital chaplain.

- The nurses caring for the patient will share their concerns with their supervisor or mentor.
- The patient will be consulted and asked to give permission for all treatments and therapies.
- Additional interventions will be used as warranted by medical condition and ordered by the attending physician.

EVALUATION

Mr. Dunham's condition continued to deteriorate, and he was placed on a mechanical ventilator. As it became increasingly difficult to meet his oxygenation needs, he was given paralytics. Mr. Dunham ultimately died of cardiorespiratory failure.

CRITICAL THINKING

1. Does a nurse who is assigned to care for this patient have the option of requesting a different assignment on the basis of his or her feelings of revulsion, disgust, or anger at the patient's past history and behavior? Why or why not?

2. What interventions would be the most difficult for you to provide this patient? Explain your answer.

3. How would your moral beliefs regarding this patient's history and behavior affect your nursing care of the patient? Is it appropriate to reduce the quality of care you provide as a result? Explain your answer.

SAFETY ALERT When working with patients who are potentially dangerous, the nurse can help to ensure both personal safety and the safety of others by staying between the patient and the door and by notifying security to be present as necessary. Other appropriate measures may include restraining the patient, providing additional staff for interventions and procedures, and transporting the patient during times when hallways and other areas have the fewest people around.

- Encouraging patients to make informed decisions without pressure from others. In the earlier example of the young woman who learned that she was pregnant, her boyfriend was attempting to influence her decision. Although patients are free to seek advice from whomever they wish, the nurse must ensure that the patient makes a treatment decision free from coercion.

- Referring patients to spiritual leaders or mental health professionals as necessary. Consulting with these individuals may assist patients in the ethical decision-making process.

Evaluation

Treatment options that challenge individual morality and ethics, such as abortion and organ transplantation, often leave patients and family members second-guessing decisions after they have been made. Evaluation of patients who are faced with decisions that poses a challenge to their morality or of patients who lack morality should be based on the question "Is the patient satisfied that the best possible decision was made?" Nurses who work with patients in these situations should support autonomy; provide a listening, nonjudgmental ear; and continue to support the patient's decision after the conclusion of treatment.

REVIEW Morality

RELATE Link the Concepts and Exemplars

Linking the exemplar of morality with the concept of development:

A mother brings her 13-year-old daughter to the gynecologist's office for the girl's first pelvic examination. The daughter is autistic and has a spoken vocabulary of fewer than 500 words. The mother tells the nurse that she wants to talk to the physician about getting her daughter's tubes tied or some other procedure that will keep her daughter from getting pregnant if anyone molests her.

1. How does the daughter's developmental level interfere with her ability to make autonomous decisions?

2. What ethical responsibilities do you have to the daughter in this situation?

Linking the exemplar of morality with the concept of comfort:

3. What moral or ethical issues are involved in patients' advance directives and do-not-resuscitate orders?

4. What are your feelings about the morality of do-not-resuscitate orders? How would you keep these feelings from influencing your discussions with a patient about do-not-resuscitate orders? Would your feelings change if the patient were a child or adolescent?

REFER Go to Pearson MyLab Nursing and eText

- Additional review materials

REFLECT Apply Your Knowledge

The nurse on the day shift at an inpatient rehabilitation center is making her morning rounds when she finds a young woman awake and crying in her bed. The woman has bruises on her wrists and forearms that were not there when the nurse last saw the patient the previous afternoon. When the nurse asks the patient what happened, the patient responds only by shaking her head, and she pulls away when the nurse reaches out to comfort her. The nurse checks the visitor logs and confirms that the patient had no visitors the night before.

1. What are the priorities of care for the patient at this moment?

2. What steps should the nurse take to try to determine what happened to this patient?

3. How should the nurse document her findings, and with whom should the nurse share these findings?

4. Does the nurse have an obligation to report these findings? If so, to whom must she report them?

>> Exemplar 44.B
Ethical Dilemmas

Exemplar Learning Outcomes

44.B Analyze dilemmas related to ethics.

- Propose solutions to ethical dilemmas based on an individual's problem and ethical principles.

- Analyze conflicts among nursing loyalties and obligations to patients, families, the multiprofessional team, and outside organizations.

- Critique the bioethical dilemmas that may arise during the care of patients and families.

- Explore the nurse's role in supporting patients' rights to information and counseling when making genetic testing decisions.

- Analyze the challenges and dilemmas patients and their families face when managing end-of-life care choices, advance directives, euthanasia, and the withdrawal of life support.

- Differentiate considerations related to ethical dilemmas for patients across the lifespan.

Exemplar Key Terms

Active euthanasia, *2749*
Assisted suicide, *2749*
Bioethical dilemma, *2746*
Ethical dilemma, *2744*
Euthanasia, *2749*
Withdrawing or withholding life-sustaining therapy (WWLST), *2749*

Overview

An **ethical dilemma** exists when two or more rights, values, obligations, or responsibilities come into conflict. Conflict may arise between the nurse's personal values and those of another individual or the organization. Conflict may also develop between the nurse's principles and the need to achieve a desired outcome. Conflict may occur between two or more individuals or groups to whom the nurse has an obligation, such as the patient, a colleague, the nursing profession, the nurse's employer, or society (Dekeyser Ganz & Berkovitz, 2012; Lachman, 2012).

A number of factors contribute to ethical dilemmas. Rapidly changing technology and conflicting societal and cultural values are among the most important factors today. Technology pervades most aspects of our lives, and today's nurses have grown up in a tech-driven society. The result is new ethical concerns that didn't exist 10—or even 5—years ago. Social change is also altering the way in which patients and nurses approach routine aspects of the healthcare experience. Nurses must be prepared to handle dilemmas related to these key drivers of change.

Other factors that contribute to ethical dilemmas include the development of conflicting loyalties and obligations among nurses. Competing allegiances to patients, families, colleagues, employers, and self can make it difficult for the nurse to determine the most ethical course of action. In addition, increasing pressure to contain healthcare costs at the organizational level may result in situations that give rise to ethical dilemmas.

No matter the contributing factors, the nurse must recognize ethical dilemmas and take appropriate action. Some dilemmas affect the care patients receive, and the nurse must be prepared to inform the patient and other staff members of these issues. Other dilemmas may involve an individual's nursing practice. When such issues arise, the nurse must act in a manner consistent with the ANA *Code of Ethics for Nurses*. No matter the dilemma a nurse faces, recognizing and managing ethical challenges—and evaluating the outcomes of interventions taken—promote ethical practice.

Factors Contributing to Ethical Dilemmas

Ethical dilemmas arise in many situations and touch many areas of nursing practice. In spite of the diverse nature of these dilemmas, they often start with common contributing factors. Technologic change, social change, and conflicting loyalties are three such factors.

Technologic Changes

Technologic change creates new ethical dilemmas that did not previously exist. From the nursing perspective, there are two areas of technology that must be considered: medical technology and communications technology.

Medical technology has been changing nursing practice throughout the twentieth and twenty-first centuries as new treatments and devices revolutionize healthcare. Some devices, such as monitors, respirators, and feeding tubes, have been around for 50 to 100 years or more, but as they have become more sophisticated, they have presented more occasions for ethical dilemmas. For example, the decision of whether to provide life-sustaining measures to an 800-gram premature infant would not exist without modern technology.

Devices are not the only medical technology to radically change the healthcare landscape. For example, organ transplantation is another procedure that has experienced great advances and is also subject to ongoing ethical debate. These debates focus on both the donor and the recipient and concern the definitions of donor death in relation to organ viability and the proper procedure for selecting recipients on the basis of age, health factors, and time on the waiting list.

Communications technology is also of critical importance to nurses. Cell phones, tablets, and other "smart" devices have made people and organizations more connected. They have also changed the nature of what people share with one another. The downside of this connectedness is that it can be difficult to separate what it is appropriate to share from what is inappropriate to share and when it is appropriate to do so. For example, an excited student nurse may snap a picture of herself and her preceptor on the first day of clinical education in the emergency department (ED). If she posts the photo to her social media page, the confidentiality of any patients in the background has been compromised. In addition, taking the photograph and posting it during the time designated for clinical education is ethically questionable, as it takes the student's attention away from learning and from providing high-quality patient care.

In this situation, the student nurse also opens herself up to questions that may present an ethical dilemma. Suppose a friend's father was admitted to the ED that day and the friend saw the picture. The friend may ask the student nurse whether she saw his father, what his father's condition is, and whether his father is still in the ED. The student nurse is faced with the ethical dilemma of answering her friend's questions or maintaining his father's privacy.

SAFETY ALERT Photos or comments posted to social media may be impossible to remove from the internet, even if you have deleted them from your social media accounts. Before posting anything that could negatively affect a patient or your career, consider the potential repercussions.

Patients now have unprecedented access to medical information through their smart devices. Patients can search for information about their symptoms or condition and find numerous sources within seconds. Unfortunately, not all health information available on the internet is up to date, accurate, or trustworthy. This can create ethical issues for nurses. For instance, during a patient interview, a nurse may learn that a patient is treating her condition using a remedy she found online. The remedy is unlikely to cause harm to the patient but is also unlikely to provide any benefit. The nurse feels uncomfortable addressing the issue for fear of upsetting the patient. The nurse must decide whether it is ethically responsible to allow the patient to continue with a remedy that he knows will not do her any good. Often, situations such as these can be avoided if nurses proactively direct patients to reliable online sources of health information.

Medical and communications technology converge in some areas of nursing. Electronic health records (EHRs) are one example of this convergence. EHRs offer patients ready access to their own medical records via their devices and allow providers to quickly get a comprehensive view of a patient's history and care. In some organizations, care providers access EHRs on in-room computers or using tablet devices provided by the organization for that purpose. These records, although useful, present their own set of ethical dilemmas. For example, suppose a nurse knows that her brother is a patient at the clinic where she works. She suspects that he is ill, but when she asks him about it, he brushes her off. She can review his EHR via the clinic's system, but from a professional standpoint, she should not do so unless she is providing care to him at the clinic, a situation that in itself presents an ethical dilemma. Other issues may arise if a nurse fails to log out of an EHR access device before taking a break or notices that another nurse has failed to log out. In addition, it may be tempting for nurses to use devices designated for EHR access for unauthorized personal purposes.

Social Changes

Social beliefs and ideas are constantly changing, in part because of the advances brought about by new technology. The increasing interconnectedness of people around the globe contributes to the pace at which these ideas are spread. These changes bring with them a variety of ethical dilemmas for all members of society. They have a particularly big impact on healthcare providers because they often affect how people choose to live and maintain their health.

One particularly important change relates to the way in which people define life. Some believe that life should be allowed to end naturally; others believe that everything possible should be done to preserve life. Modern medical technology has made it possible to preserve or extend life for individuals who are terminally ill or in a vegetative state. These patients may survive for weeks or months with medical assistance. This assistance is expensive and draws on scarce clinical resources. Patients or their families may feel strongly about maintaining life via this technology even if healthcare providers do not consider it appropriate. Conversely, the patient or family may be strongly opposed to such treatments even if care providers think that they are necessary. The nurse must be prepared to provide care in either of these scenarios. In addition, the nurse may be called on to participate in difficult conversations about these topics with patients, their families, and other healthcare providers.

Closely related to this is the issue of quality of life. Although life can be prolonged or maintained, it may not include the freedoms and experiences that are considered important by many people. For example, suppose a 14-year-old cancer patient has been given 2 months to live. A new treatment may extend his life an additional 2 months but is likely to be very painful. The patient and his family must weigh whether length of life or quality of life is more important to them. Another potentially complicating issue here is the patient's age; his parents may be in favor of the treatment while the patient himself may be against it. Unless the care is being provided in a state that recognizes the decision-making capabilities of mature minors, the patient cannot make this decision for himself. (See the module on Legal Issues for more information about mature minors and minor consent.) This situation can be particularly challenging for the nurse who has strong personal opinions about the issues.

The way in which individuals define and pursue wellness is changing, too. One way this is evidenced is in the adoption of nontraditional diets. For instance, gluten-free diets (in which only foods that do not contain gluten protein are consumed) have become much more popular. Some individuals adopt these diets because of celiac disease or gluten intolerance. For others, the diets are a conscious choice based on personal beliefs about health. Issues may arise, however, if patients' nutritional needs are not being met.

Complementary health approaches are also becoming increasingly popular. These include natural products—such as herbs and vitamins—and dietary supplements that contain these products. They also include mind and body practices such as yoga, meditation, and chiropractic manipulation. Some other complementary health approaches include traditional medicines, homeopathy, and naturopathy (National Center for Complementary and Integrative Health, n.d.). A number of complementary practices can be integrated into traditional healthcare in ways that benefit the patient. For example, incorporating massage therapy into treatment for a cancer patient may improve comfort and reduce stress. Ethical dilemmas arise, however, when a patient relies on a complementary treatment that either is ineffective or has potential to harm the patient.

Another social change is the increasing public support of the use of medical marijuana—either whole, unprocessed plants or their extracts—to treat diseases or symptoms (National Institutes of Health [NIH], 2017a). Research suggests that the chemicals in marijuana can be useful for treating a variety of illnesses. Legal use of medical marijuana is regulated on the state level; the federal government does not recognize or approve medical use of the drug. Medical marijuana has the potential to create ethical dilemmas for the nurse. For example, the nurse may believe that it is a useful and appropriate treatment for a patient's condition, but the patient may be adamantly opposed to consumption of the drug. The converse may also occur: The nurse is opposed, but the patient is in favor.

Conflicting Loyalties and Obligations

Because of their unique position in the healthcare system, nurses experience conflicts among their loyalties and obligations to patients, families, primary care providers, employing institutions, and licensing bodies. Patient needs may conflict with institutional policies, primary care provider preferences, needs of the patient's family, or even state or federal laws.

According to the ANA *Code of Ethics for Nurses* (ANA, 2015a), the nurse's primary commitment is to the patient. As part of that commitment, the nurse must engage the patient in care planning. In planning care with patients, it is not always easy to determine which actions best serve the patient's needs. For instance, the nurse may be aware that medical marijuana has been shown to be effective for a patient's condition. The patient has not responded to mainstream therapies, but medical marijuana is not legal in the state where the nurse and patient live. Although legal issues are involved, the nurse must determine whether, ethically, the patient should be made aware of this potentially effective alternative.

When planning and caring for a patient, the nurse must also consider the patient's family relationships. The nurse also has an obligation to the patient's family as well as the patient; however, it is important to remember that the nurse's first loyalty always lies with the patient. This is particularly important should conflicts arise between the patient and the family about care. Suppose a patient with necrotizing fasciitis of the foot has been presented with several care options by her physician, including amputation. The patient wants to pursue amputation, but her spouse would prefer that she receive a different treatment. The nurse may help the patient and her spouse reach an understanding but is ultimately obligated to ensure that the patient's wishes are met.

The nurse may also have loyalties to colleagues and the healthcare organization. For example, suppose a hospital denies a $2 per hour cost-of-living raise for the nursing staff. The staff as a whole chooses to strike, but each individual nurse must decide whether to honor the picket lines during the strike. The nurse may experience conflicting feelings about the need to support coworkers in their efforts to improve working conditions, the need to show loyalty to the organization, and the need to ensure that patients receive care and are not abandoned.

Ethical Dilemmas in Patient Care

Specific ethical issues related to human life or health often develop in the course of caring for patients. These issues are referred to as **bioethical dilemmas**. Bioethical dilemmas arise during the care of patients and families and often emerge from a combination of causative factors. HIV/AIDS, genetic testing, organ transplantation, and end-of-life decisions all present their own unique ethical dilemmas.

HIV and AIDS

HIV is a virus that attacks the immune system and eventually leads to AIDS. It is spread through contact with bodily fluids, including blood, breast milk, rectal fluids, semen, and vaginal fluids. Because contact with these fluids is often associated with sexual behavior and illicit drug use, HIV/AIDS bears a social stigma (De Bruyn, 2012). According to an ANA position statement on risk and responsibility in nursing, the nurse cannot set aside the moral obligation to care for the patient infected with HIV/AIDS unless the risk associated with providing that care exceeds the responsibility (ANA, 2015c). More information can be found in the exemplar on HIV/AIDS in the module on Immunity.

There is no safe or effective cure for HIV/AIDS, which means that an individual who contracts the virus will have it for life. However, antiretroviral therapy (ART) can effectively control HIV. Before the introduction of ART in the 1990s, HIV infection progressed to AIDS over the course of a few years; with ART, patients with HIV who receive early treatment can have close to a normal life expectancy (Centers for Disease Control and Prevention [CDC], 2016). Use of ART can also reduce the patient's risk of transmitting HIV.

Although ART is an important treatment that has changed the course of HIV infection for many patients, the combination of drugs involved is expensive. Private health insurance, Medicare, or Medicaid covers a portion of costs, but patients are responsible for deductibles and copayments, which may be costly. For patients without insurance, Medicare, or Medicaid coverage, the cost associated with ART may be prohibitive. This reality presents a number of ethical dilemmas, including whether it is ethical to allow a patient to endure a controllable condition because of inability to pay. Programs such as the Ryan White HIV/AIDS Program and the Health Center Program attempt to address these issues by providing care and medication to individuals who could not otherwise afford it. The Health Center Program in particular serves individuals in minority and traditionally underserved communities, which tend to have higher HIV infection rates (AIDS.gov, 2014, 2015).

Patients have a duty to inform past and future sexual partners about their infection status. These conversations are difficult and have the potential to be confrontational; as a result, patients may avoid having them. The extended life expectancy and lowered risk of transmission associated with ART may help patients feel justified in this decision. Such a choice presents an ethical dilemma for the nurse. The nurse has an obligation to the patient to maintain his or her privacy, but the patient's partners also have a right to know they are at risk, to get testing, and to receive treatment if necessary (CDC, 2016).

Other ethical issues related to HIV/AIDS center on testing for HIV status and the presence of AIDS in healthcare professionals and patients. Questions arise about whether testing of all providers and patients should be mandatory or voluntary and whether test results should be released to insurance companies, sexual partners, and caregivers. As with all ethical dilemmas, each possibility has positive and negative implications for specific individuals.

Genetic Testing

Patients with genetic risk factors for chronic illness must make difficult decisions about genetic testing and test findings. For example, a patient with a family history of Huntington disease must decide whether to have predictive testing for the condition. If the test indicates that she will develop the condition, she must make decisions about the type of care she wants to receive in the future and whether to share information about her condition with others who may be affected by her diagnosis. Genetic testing can also present dilemmas for pregnant patients. If prenatal test results indicate a genetic condition, the patient must decide whether to undergo an elective abortion or deliver a child who may require medical and social support throughout his or her life.

Working with individuals who are seeking information about genetic testing for themselves or for their children is a new and interesting ethical challenge for nurses. The increasing prominence of genetics in the media has contributed to growing awareness among families and patients about inherited conditions (**Figure 44–2 》**). As a result, patients are asking more questions of the nurses who care for them. The nursing code of ethics supports patients' rights to information and counseling in making genetic testing decisions. To provide the best information, nurses should know the legal requirements of their state related to genetic testing. For example, nurses should know whether their state requires parental consent for a minor to seek genetic testing and counseling.

It is important that nurses understand the limitations of genetic testing and explain them to patients in an unbiased manner. Genetic tests typically provide information about the nature of the condition a patient has or may be

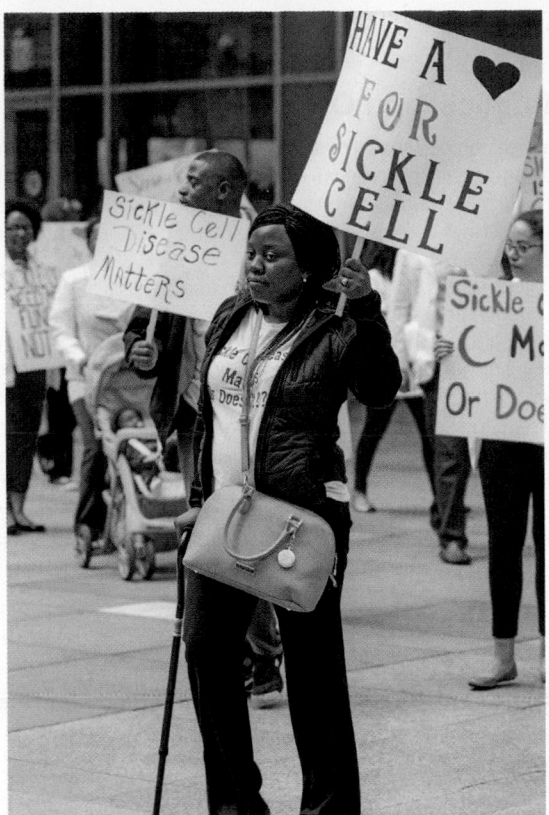

Source: 400tmax/iStock/Getty Images.

Figure 44–2 》 The "Have a Heart for Sickle Cell" campaign promotes the importance of genetic testing to help prospective parents determine their children's risk for having the disease.

at risk for developing. They do not, however, provide information about the severity of the condition or about the age or timing of occurrence (Centre for Genetics Education, 2016). Understanding these limitations can complicate the ethical dilemmas genetic testing presents to patients, including the decision about whether or not to be tested. For this reason, organizations that provide genetic testing also offer genetic counseling.

Genetic counseling may not be available to patients who use direct-to-consumer genetic tests rather than physician-ordered genetic tests. Direct-to-consumer tests are purchased by individual patients, who collect a genetic sample at home and mail the sample to the laboratory that sells the test. Results are sent to the consumer by mail or email. Some companies that provide these tests connect patients to counselors or physicians who can explain the results; some do not (NIH, 2017b). This scenario may present nurses with a number of dilemmas. For example, patients may misinterpret their results and pursue treatment based on this misunderstanding. The nurse must decide whether to intervene and must be prepared to provide accurate information, support, and referrals as part of the intervention process.

Organ Transplantation

Organ transplantation is a sensitive issue in terms of both organ donation and organ allocation. In general, organs are

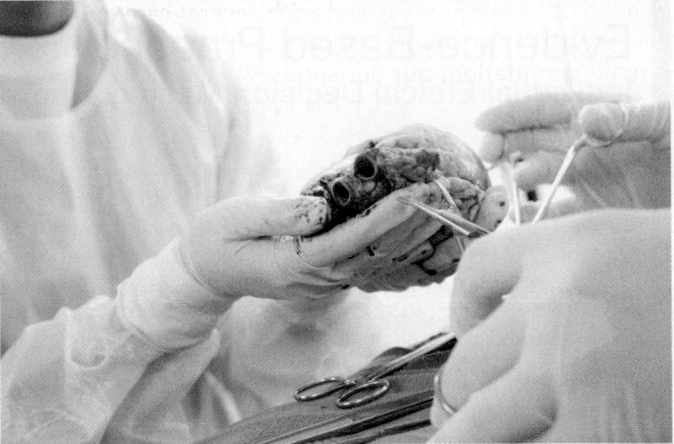

Source: Fstop123/iStock/Getty Images.

Figure 44–3 》 Organ transplantation programs use formulas that balance utility, justice, and respect for persons to determine which patients receive organs.

procured from patients who are brain dead but whose hearts are still beating, though some organs may be recovered after circulatory death has occurred (McKeown, Bonser, & Kellum, 2012). Under the Uniform Anatomical Gift Act (UAGA), patients may elect to donate their organs after their death. Life support systems may be used around the time of death to maximize procurement of donor organs. According to provisions in the act, the need to use life support under UAGA overrides patient desires related to such measures in an advance directive. Although the intent of this provision is to prevent organ failure following brain death, it creates a clear ethical dilemma for healthcare providers, who may have to balance a patient's wish to donate her organs and her wish not to be placed on life support. Educating patients and their families about these issues when discussing organ donation and advance directives may reduce the occurrence of these dilemmas.

Ethical issues also surround the allocation of donated organs, in part because there are many more patients in need of organs than there are organs available (**Figure 44–3 》》**). Typically, beyond the more clear-cut issues of tissue or blood type compatibility, geography, and organ size and the more ambiguous issue of medical urgency (United Network for Organ Sharing, 2015), organ transplantation programs use formulas that balance utility, justice, and respect for persons to determine which patients receive which organs and when they receive them. Utility weighs the good the transplant will do against the harm it may do. Justice explores whether distribution of the organ is fair. Respect for persons looks at the autonomy of the patients in decision making (Organ Procurement and Transplantation Network [OPTN], 2015). These concepts are abstract, often in conflict with one another, and difficult to apply to individual human lives. Suppose, for example, that two patients are in need of a liver but only one liver is available. One patient is a 60-year-old alcoholic with cirrhosis of the liver; the other is a 20-year-old with a hereditary condition who will die soon without a new liver. The 60-year-old is a brilliant scientist who conducts lifesaving research. The 20-year-old is young, with decades

Evidence-Based Practice
Individual Ethical Decision Making, Knowledge of Ethics, and Organizational Support

Problem

Nurses are faced with ethical dilemmas every day, and these dilemmas often must be resolved quickly. Research suggests that nurses may feel vulnerable both before and after dealing with ethically volatile situations. In some cases, nurses do not feel sufficiently competent in their knowledge of ethics to be comfortable with their role in the decision-making process; in other cases, nurses do not feel that they receive adequate organizational support.

Evidence

Numminen et al. (2015) explored newly graduated nurses' perception of ethics in the organizations in which they worked. In general, these nurses had a positive perception of the ethical climate; however, these positive perceptions were primarily reserved for patients, physicians, and fellow nurses. The organization itself and nurse managers were viewed less favorably. The nurses with the most positive perceptions of the ethical environment were those who self-identified as feeling very competent in their understanding of ethics.

Kim, Seo, and Kim (2016) assessed intensive care, medical–surgical, emergency, and oncology nurses on specific areas of difficulty in ethical decision making. Among the most significant difficulties, nurses identified a lack of education regarding ethics, a lack of organizational support for ethical decision making, and struggles to provide evidence-based care. However, the nurses' desire for organizational ethical support varied from department to department.

Jansen and Hanssen (2016) conducted a similar survey with psychiatric nurses. Their research suggested that nurses often felt squeezed between their own ethical values and the values of the organization as a whole. Nurses indicated that they often found themselves in the role of negotiator between the various stakeholder groups, which contributed to feelings of burnout and moral distress.

Implications

Nurses need organizational support in order to manage ethical dilemmas and cope with their role in the process. Kim et al. (2016) identify ethical counseling as a means of preventing fatigue in nurses' personal and professional lives. They also suggest that unit-specific in-house training be provided to improve nurses' feelings of ethical competence and aid in the development of practical solutions to ethical problems.

Poikkeus et al. (2016) suggest that nurse leaders take a greater role in orienting nurses to the ethical procedures and practices on their units and facilitate multiprofessional discussions on ethics. They also support continuing ethics education for nurses.

Finally, Chooljian et al. (2016) encourage organizational ethics committees to serve in a supportive role for nurses. Typically, these committees are involved with nurses' ethical issues only when a dispute arises that requires committee attention. The researchers believe that organizations as a whole and nurses in particular could benefit from guidance and reassurance from the ethics committee throughout the decision-making process, even when the dilemmas involved do not require committee attention.

Critical Thinking Application

1. What conclusions can you draw about the way in which nurses build an ethical support network according to the research of Numminen et al.? In what ways do you think this type of support network is beneficial to nurses? In what way might it be detrimental to nurses?

2. In their research, Jansen and Hanssen describe that nurses feel squeezed between personal and organizational ethics. What does this suggest about the practicality of organizational ethics in clinical situations?

3. How would the increased involvement by organizational ethics committees suggested by Chooljian et al. improve the ethical climate of the organization? How would it help nurses avoid fatigue and burnout associated with ethical decision making?

---

full of potential ahead. Determining which patient receives the organ is an ethical dilemma that is only somewhat simplified by the use of an allocation formula based on the principles of utility, justice, and respect for persons.

>> **Stay Current:** For more information on how donor kidneys from deceased individuals are allocated for transplant, visit the website of the United Network for Organ Sharing (UNOS) at https://www.unos.org/transplantation/matching-organs/

End-of-life Issues

Advances in medical technology and the increasing population of older adults have expanded the ethical dilemmas faced by older adults and the healthcare professionals who work with them. Some of the most frequent and disturbing ethical dilemmas for nurses involve death and dying. Euthanasia, assisted suicide, termination of life-sustaining treatment, and withdrawing or withholding of food and fluids are among these dilemmas.

In spite of increasing interest in and the urgent need for high-quality end-of-life care, there is no exact definition of the "end of life" interval or consensus about what constitutes end-of-life care (Izumi et al., 2012). Current definitions of end-of-life care tend to be based on the time until death and the stage of illness. These definitions are problematic because the time frames involved are not always predictable, which puts patients at risk of being left without adequate end-of-life care (Izumi et al., 2012). Nurses who see a patient's life as a whole are better suited to understand the patient's condition and guide the patient and family through preparation for end of life (Watts, 2013).

Advance Directives

Many of the ethical dilemmas surrounding end-of-life care can be resolved if patients complete advance directives and ensure that they are available to healthcare providers. Advance directives are legal documents representing a patient's end-of-life decisions; they may include how patients want medical decisions to be made or whom they would like to make those decisions (Phillips, 2014). Advance directives instruct caregivers about patients' treatment preferences and provide an ongoing voice for patients when they no longer have the capacity to make or communicate decisions. An advance directive may provide instructions regarding do-not-resuscitate (DNR) orders, the withholding of emergency measures to sustain life, the termination of life-sustaining measures, or any combination thereof. Nurses working with a patient who is experiencing a life-threatening event or who is approaching the end of life should make sure they understand the patient's advance directive as well as their employer's policies and procedures regarding advance directives. See the module on Legal Issues and the exemplar on End-of-Life Care in the module on Comfort for more information about advance directives.

Euthanasia and Assisted Suicide

Euthanasia, a Greek word meaning "good death," is sometimes referred to in the popular press as "mercy killing." **Active euthanasia** involves taking direct action to bring about a patient's death, with or without patient consent (Johnstone, 2012b). An example of this is the administration of a lethal dose of medication to end the patient's suffering. Regardless of the caregiver's intent, active euthanasia is forbidden by law and can result in criminal charges against the individual who brings about the patient's death.

A variation of active euthanasia is **assisted suicide** (sometimes called "right to die"), in which patients are given the means to kill themselves if they request it. The ethics and morality of assisted suicide have been debated in the United States for a long time. For years, only Oregon, which passed the Death with Dignity Act in 1997, allowed physicians to provide lethal medications to qualifying patients who requested assistance (Drum, 2016). In January 2006, the U.S. Supreme Court upheld Oregon's assisted suicide regulations. After this decision, Washington (2008), Montana (2009), Vermont (2013), and California (2016) passed similar legislation. Several other countries also have assisted suicide laws in place.

Right-to-die legislation is still controversial in our society, and opposition to it by some cultural, religious, and other groups makes it an ethical issue that many nurses will be confronted with during their careers. The ANA's position statement on assisted suicide (ANA, 2013) states that performing active euthanasia and participating in assisted suicide violate the ANA *Code of Ethics for Nurses*. Nurses should understand the assisted suicide laws in their state so that they can adequately answer patients' questions; in doing so, they must be able to balance facts and patient concerns against their own personal biases and the ethics of their profession.

Withdrawing or Withholding Life-sustaining Therapy

Withdrawing or withholding life-sustaining therapy (WWLST) involves the withdrawal of extraordinary means of life support. It includes removing a ventilator, making no special attempts to revive a patient, and allowing the patient to die of the underlying medical condition (e.g., aspiration pneumonia). WWLST is a complex process that can take several days to complete. During that time, nurses must be prepared to manage the process, the complex emotions experienced by the patient's family, and their own feelings about the process (Stacy, 2012).

Antibiotics, organ transplants, and technologic advances such as ventilators can prolong life but do not necessarily restore health. Patients may specify that they wish to have life-sustaining measures terminated; they may also include these wishes in advance directives or appoint a healthcare surrogate to make these decisions on their behalf. Even when WWLST is in accordance with the patient's wishes, it is often troubling for healthcare professionals to withdraw treatment. Nurses must understand that a decision to withdraw treatment is not a decision to withdraw care. As primary caregivers, nurses must ensure that sensitive care and comfort measures (palliative care) are given as the patient's illness progresses after withdrawal of treatment. When the patient is at home, nurses may provide this type of education and support through hospice services (see the module on Comfort for more information on hospice and end-of-life care).

Because withdrawal of treatment is difficult for families, it is very important that they fully understand the patient's treatment (Stacy, 2012). Families may misunderstand which treatments are life sustaining and which are palliative, and they may be confused when certain treatments are withdrawn while others are maintained. Keeping patients and families informed about the process is an ongoing concern, and it is important to keep in mind that family members need time to ask questions and discuss the situation. It is also essential for patients and families to understand that they can reevaluate and change their decision if they wish.

Withdrawing or Withholding Nutrition and Fluids

It is generally accepted that providing nutrition and fluids is part of ordinary nursing practice and, therefore, a moral duty. However, for patients who are dying or who are unconscious and not expected to improve, provision of nutrition and fluids is considered a medical intervention rather than a comfort measure (Danis, 2015).

During the dying process, patients exhibit decreased oral intake, progressive fluid deficits, and progressive accumulation of drugs. These changes can worsen existing symptoms or create new ones; these, in turn, lead to further declines in oral intake. Research consistently suggests that, when this occurs, it is more harmful to administer nutrition and fluids to the patient than it is to withhold them (Danis, 2015). As a result, nurses in this situation are morally obligated to withhold nutrition and fluids—or any treatment.

The nurse must also honor competent and informed patients' refusal of nutrition and fluids, referred to as voluntary cessation of intake. The ANA *Code of Ethics for Nurses* (2015a) supports this position through the nurse's role as a patient advocate and through the moral principle of autonomy. Some religions oppose voluntary cessation on the grounds that it involves a decision that will lead to patient death; however, some groups consider voluntary cessation preferable to euthanasia or assisted suicide (Danis, 2015).

Families may view provision of nutrition and hydration as important care and comfort measures and may strongly oppose withdrawal or withholding. This can create ethical dilemmas for the nurse. The nurse must be prepared to explain the withdrawal and withholding process to the family and why doing so is important. In addition, nurses should be familiar with the laws in their state pertaining to voluntary cessation.

Clinical Example A

Conner Wolfe is a 14-year-old patient with cancer who is refusing chemotherapy after becoming very ill and weak after his first round of chemo. His oncologist has made it very clear that Conner has a 90% chance of being cured if he undergoes chemotherapy followed by radiation and an equal chance that he will die without it. Although Conner and his family do not follow any specific spiritual or cultural traditions, they believe in using "natural medicine" for curing illness. Conner is adamant that he does not want any more chemotherapy. His parents state that he was in "better health" before the first chemo treatment and that is proof that the chemo is bad for him. When asked what the parents intend to do if Conner's cancer metastasizes, the Wolfes say they will discuss that with Conner in the unlikely event that it occurs.

Critical Thinking Questions

1. What ethical dilemmas can you identify in this situation?
2. What is the nurse's responsibility regarding addressing these dilemmas?
3. What, if any, action should the hospital take regarding Conner's treatment? Why?

Ethical Issues in Nursing Practice

Ethics in nursing is not limited to bioethical dilemmas; it also includes nursing practice and the nurse's identity as a moral agent. This identity is shaped by contextual and organizational forces that impact the role, obligations, and duties of the nurse. These forces include corporate healthcare values and hierarchies and the growing demand for healthcare (Edmonson, 2015).

Some everyday ethical challenges identified by nurses were categorized in a classic publication by Varcoe et al. (2004), who posited that nurses work as the "in-betweens." Specifically, nurses are caught in between various other players involved in healthcare, including healthcare providers and the patient, and the patient and the family. Nurses are also caught between family members, between staff members, between managers, and between other colleagues. Within these relationships, nurses must constantly balance their loyalties.

Conflicts also arise from traditional power structures in healthcare. For example, nurses have expressed concern about being intimidated or dismissed by physicians when the nurses report observations that are not congruent with the proposed medical treatment plan. They have also voiced anxiety about being ignored by senior medical staff when they report concerns related to physician behavior or by administrators when they express concern over corporate values. In some cases, nurses may be threatened with job and license loss over such reports and concerns.

Additional conflicts arise as a result of staffing shortages and other situations in which the organization functions inefficiently (Iglesias & De Bengoa Vallejo, 2012). When faced with inefficiencies, nurses must balance their limited time with the care that must be provided. In these situations, patient teaching, counseling, and support suffer as the nurse's focus moves to performance of physical tasks and functions.

The behavior of nurses is shaped by their organizational and professional roles and the settings in which they work. Their responses to ethical dilemmas are inseparable from the scenarios in which those dilemmas arise (Johansen & O'Brien, 2015). Therefore, clinical experiences are important for helping nurses develop ethical behaviors. In addition, supportive colleagues, educators, and approachable and responsible managers are important resources for ethical practice. In fact, nurses have reported that having the opportunity to discuss ethical concerns is both personally and professionally sustaining (Johnstone, 2012a).

Focus on Diversity and Culture
Variations in Autonomy and Information Sharing

In providing ethical care to patients, it is important to understand the key role that culture plays in healthcare and the ways in which different cultures view autonomy and information sharing. For example, in the United States, autonomous individual decision making is highly valued; as a result, respect for patient autonomy is central to healthcare in this country. Autonomy is not a universal cultural value, however, and some patients from Chinese, Korean, and Hispanic backgrounds may prefer to involve family members or tribal or spiritual leaders in their decision-making process (Segal & Hodges, 2012). For example, in the Hmong culture, the clan leader may make the decision regarding whether or not an individual has surgery (Carteret, 2012).

It is also common for U.S. healthcare providers to disclose all information about a patient's condition to the patient, including whether the condition is life threatening. In some other cultures, it is common to withhold information about terminal prognoses from patients. The rationale for this approach is that it enables the patient to maintain hope. Some patients from Central and South America, the Middle East, and Eastern Europe may prefer this approach. Chinese, Taiwanese, and Japanese patients may also subscribe to this ideology (Segal & Hodges, 2012).

In addition, cultural beliefs may require healthcare providers to carefully choose their language when disclosing information to patients and families. In some cultures, discussing the specifics of a patient's condition is seen as impolite and disrespectful; some groups may even consider it dangerous. For example, the Navajo culture traditionally believes that speaking about something can result in that thing taking place. Thus, discussing death can make it occur. The underlying concern for this and other cultures with similar belief structures is that patients may become depressed, anxious, or hopeless as a result of a poor prognosis, and this can hasten their physical decline (Segal & Hodges, 2012). Nurses working with patients from cultures with these belief structures should seek guidance on strategies for imparting negative information. Elders, spiritual leaders, and colleagues from these cultures may be the most appropriate sources of reliable information.

Nurses may fear ethical or even legal repercussions related to information sharing or withholding from patients with diverse cultural backgrounds. It is important for the nurse to develop a relationship with the patient and family and work with them to determine the best means of sharing essential information based on their beliefs and values (Segal & Hodges, 2012).

Workplace Issues

A number of workplace issues outside of the bioethical realm affect nurses. Many of them are the result of financial constraints, personnel issues, and other organizational challenges. Two of the most common ethical dilemmas stemming from these factors involve limited resources and short staffing.

Allocation of Limited Health Resources

As healthcare costs continue to rise and more stringent cost containment strategies are implemented, allocation of limited supplies of healthcare goods and services has become an especially urgent issue. Examples of the goods and services affected include organs suitable for transplantation, artificial joints, and specialist services. The moral principle of autonomy cannot be applied if a patient cannot obtain the treatment he or she chooses. In these situations, healthcare providers may use the principle of justice by attempting to choose what is most fair to all. Nurses, other healthcare professionals, legislators, and patients must continue to look for ways to balance economics and care in the allocation of health resources. For more information on resource allocation in healthcare, see the modules on Managing Care and Healthcare Systems.

Short Staffing

Because of a nationwide shortage of nurses, nursing care is becoming a limited health resource. Short staffing is a critical concern because a number of studies link staffing levels to safe patient care (AACN, 2014). Unfortunately, some facilities continue to staff nursing units with fewer registered nurses and more unlicensed caregivers. When this occurs, staffing may not be adequate to ensure patient safety or allow nurses to provide an appropriate level of care. California is the only state that has enacted legislation mandating specific nurse-to-patient ratios in hospitals and other healthcare settings (Schultz, 2013). Unfortunately, this is not the simple solution that it might seem. The need to maintain adequate staffing levels could force changes elsewhere in the organization that are detrimental to patient care. For example, the need to maintain adequate staffing may force an ED to limit the number of patients it can accept at one time. As a result, patients in need of emergency care might be turned away when that limit is reached.

Clinical Example B

The director of nursing is having difficulty staffing all the units adequately. Two units have already been closed. The director can either spread the available staff around the facility and keep the remaining units open, but with fewer nurses than is really safe, or close more units. The director needs to consider the welfare of the institution, the nursing staff, and the patients.

Critical Thinking Questions

1. How would you assess the ethical aspects of this issue?
2. What actions would you take? Why?
3. How does the ANA *Code of Ethics* inform the possible actions?

Working with Patients and Families

Working with patients and families is both rewarding and challenging. Clear communication and good clinical decision-making skills help the nurse develop positive relationships with these individuals. Ethical challenges may still arise, however; they include ensuring patient autonomy and maintaining patient privacy and confidentiality.

Patient Autonomy

Respect for patient autonomy is fundamental to nursing ethics, and nurses must recognize and defend the right of each patient to make his or her own decisions about healthcare. However, situations often arise in which patient autonomy is at risk. This risk may come in the form of a well-meaning family member who disagrees with the patient's decision or a physician or other healthcare provider who either fails to hear the patient's concerns or disagrees with the patient's request or decision (Rasmussen, 2012). In these situations, the nurse is ethically obligated to advocate for the patient's right to make his or her own decision.

Patient Privacy and Confidentiality

In keeping with the principle of autonomy, nurses are obligated to respect patients' privacy and confidentiality. Privacy is both a legal and an ethical mandate. The Health Insurance Portability and Accountability Act of 1996 (HIPAA) includes standards that protect the confidentiality, integrity, and availability of data and standards defining appropriate disclosures of identifiable health information and patient rights protection (see the module on Legal Issues).

Patients must be able to trust that nurses will reveal details about their history and care only when appropriate and will communicate only the information necessary to provide for their healthcare. Computerized patient records make sensitive data accessible to more people and make issues of confidentiality more complex and more important. Nurses should help develop and follow security measures and policies that ensure that patient data are used appropriately (see the modules on Informatics and Communication).

Academic Dishonesty

Ethical dilemmas are not just the concern of practicing nurses and are not limited to the workplace or to patient interactions; nursing students may find themselves facing ethical dilemmas in the classroom. Academic dishonesty is an important example of an ethical dilemma faced by nursing students. Examples of academic dishonesty include cheating, plagiarism, and failure to follow academic policies, such as the requirement to return examinations after test review sessions (Olafsen et al., 2013).

Academic dishonesty affects student nurses in two primary ways. First, there is the temptation for the student nurse to personally engage in academic dishonesty. Busy schedules and the need to maintain grades at a certain level can make dishonesty appealing; however, engaging in dishonesty negatively affects learning and personal growth and, in turn, the student's future nursing practice. Second, student nurses may witness or be aware of friends engaging in academic dishonesty. In these situations, balancing friendship and ethics can be difficult.

The way student nurses approach academic dishonesty is important to their development of personal ethics. In personal ethics, the individual makes decisions on the basis of his or her values and best interests (Lachman, 2012). The individual is accountable for the consequences of his or her actions. This is in contrast to a professional ethical dilemma, in which the decision reflects the autonomy of the patient and the nurse is accountable to the patient's values and best interests. In spite of the differences between personal and professional ethics, personal ethics contribute to professional ethics. With increased experience and exposure on both personal and professional levels, students become better able to identify conflicting values and variables that affect the practicing nurse. See the clinical example that follows and **Box 44–5 》**.

Clinical Example C

Elizabeth, a first-year nursing student, has obtained a copy of the first examination given last year in Nursing 110 from Jasmine, her assigned "Big Sister" from the second-year class. Jasmine emphasized that questions on nursing examinations are particularly hard to answer because they require application of information, not just recall. Elizabeth informs her selected study group that she has the exam and is willing to share it to help them focus their study time. You are a member of Elizabeth's study group.

Critical Thinking Questions

1. Will you participate? Why or why not?
2. Will you report Elizabeth to your instructor? Why or why not?
3. What ethical principle is involved in your decision process?
4. What conflicting values are involved in this scenario?
5. What additional information might help you make your decision? What difference does it make if you learn that Jasmine did not turn in the exam after a test review session?
6. What school policies are involved? What aspects of the ANA *Code of Ethics* apply?

Box 44–5
An Exercise in Ethical Decision Making

When ethical dilemmas arise, the individual often has the choice of multiple courses of action. To determine the best course of action, you must consider the pros and cons of each and the consequences that may result. This can be difficult to do, especially for individuals who are new to the concept of ethical decision making.

For this exercise, refer to the clinical example of Elizabeth and Jasmine. Then build your ethical decision-making skills by answering the following questions:

1. ***Identify a range of actions with potential outcomes.***
   What are the pros? What are the cons?
   If you choose to participate in the study group and then inform the instructor?
   If you choose to participate and not tell the instructor?
   If you choose not to participate and not tell the instructor?
   If you choose not to participate and to tell the instructor?

2. ***Decide on a course of action and carry it out.***
   What are you going to decide?
   On what do you base your decision?
   What does your decision tell others about you and your values?
   Does your decision predict future decisions/actions?

3. ***Evaluate/reevaluate the consequences of your decision/action.***
   What tools would you use to evaluate your decision/action after the fact?
   How would you determine what effect your decision/action had on others?

Coping with Ethical Dilemmas

Ethical dilemmas occur frequently in everyday clinical practice. They require decision and action on the part of the nurse, and they have important implications for compassionate, high-quality patient care (Epstein & Turner, 2015).

Nurses may be blindsided by ethical dilemmas and wonder why they did not recognize the potential for these dilemmas before they arose. Several ethical decision-making models have been proposed to assist nurses in these situations; however, these models may not always consider the underlying values of both the practitioner and the patient involved in the dilemma (Crowley & Gottlieb, 2012). The primary risk management model below is an example. It was designed to assist clinical staff in managing ethical decisions, and it includes the following:

- ***Resource accumulation.*** Acquisition of the requisite resources and skills before the occurrence of a stressor.
- ***Time.*** Engagement in "free time" activities to relieve pressure and anxiety in order to better perceive the subtle cues that alert the practitioner to potential ethical dilemmas.
- ***Education.*** Development of primary risk management skills through education and didactic training.
- ***Organization and planning.*** Enhancement of organization and planning through teaching and modeling.
- ***Peer support and consultation.*** Reliance on the practitioner's professional network, consisting of peers, supervisors, and colleagues, as a resource for primary prevention of ethical challenges (Crowley & Gottlieb, 2012, pp. 67–68).

Lifespan Considerations

When caring for patients at all stages of life, nurses may be faced with ethical dilemmas. Often, these dilemmas are specific to certain population groups; other times, they are related to bioethical issues common to patients of all ages. Regardless of the patient's age, the nurse must be prepared to handle these dilemmas in an ethically responsible manner.

Ethical Dilemmas Related to Infants and Children

Ethical dilemmas commonly arise in working with the pediatric population. This is in part because pediatric patients cannot make their own decisions. Parents or guardians have the authority to make healthcare decisions for their children. Dilemmas arise when parents and children do not agree on whether to go forward with a recommended treatment. In most cases, the nurse and other members of the healthcare team who have developed a therapeutic alliance with the child and family may be able to help the family reach a joint decision by providing additional information and opportunity to discuss their concerns calmly and openly.

In some cases, the healthcare team may need to seek guidance from the organization's ethics committee related to parental decision making for a minor child. For example, when there is a potential conflict of interest—such as suspected child abuse and neglect—other measures may be necessary to provide appropriate care for the pediatric patient. In some cases, these measures may include obtaining a court order stating that the child is able to make his or her own decisions or assigning care decisions for the child to an individual or entity other than the parent, such as the Department of Child Services.

In addition to these concerns, the bioethical issues discussed previously in this exemplar can take on different aspects when applied to the pediatric population. WWLST decisions can be especially difficult when the patient is an infant, child, or adolescent. In discussing the withdrawal or withholding of medical treatment for pediatric patients with their parents, it is critical to provide complete, clear information about the child's condition, prognosis, degree of pain and suffering, and potential for good quality of life (Larcher et al., 2015).

When facing these situations, healthcare providers must follow the requirements of the Child Abuse and Treatment Act of 1984, which deemed withholding of medically indicated treatment as child abuse except in cases in which providing care is futile, that is, cases in which the treatments will not provide any clear clinical benefit (Ball, Bindler, & Cowen, 2017). Although it is rare for parents to refuse a medically indicated treatment that may benefit their child, the decision can be exceedingly difficult when the proposed treatment itself carries a high degree of risk, such as an organ transplantation or major surgery.

There are particular issues involving children as organ transplant recipients. For instance, the Organ Transplant and Procurement Network (OPTN) prefers to allocate organs from child donors—rather than adult donors—to child recipients. This is due to the difference in size between child and adult organs and the fact that children often respond better to organs from child donors (OPTN, n.d.). OPTN also encourages the use of special considerations in allocating organs that gives pediatric patients priority in some situations. These include the prudential lifespan account, in which the unique quality of life benefits enjoyed by child recipients is considered; the fair innings principle, in which the ability to maximize the recipient's lifespan is considered; and the maximin principle, in which giving priority to the most disadvantaged individual or group is considered (OPTN, 2014). Taken together, these concepts present ethical dilemmas that affect both child and adult patients in need of organ transplantation.

Ethical Dilemmas Related to Adolescents

Ethical dilemmas involving the adolescent population tend to focus on issues of consent and confidentiality. Parents or guardians must consent to medical treatment for adolescents under the age of 18 unless the adolescent has been emancipated, resides in a state that recognizes mature minors, or is seeking specific types of treatment recognized by state law, such as birth control, prenatal care, and diagnosis and treatment of sexually transmitted infections. Minors may also be able to give consent for mental health counseling and substance abuse treatment

(American Civil Liberties Union of Ohio, 2014; Goodwin et al., 2012).

Adolescent patients seeking care may wish to be examined without their parents being present; they may also prefer that their treatment remain confidential. Nurses should inform adolescent patients about mandatory reporting of imminent danger, evidence of abuse, and communicable diseases to the proper authorities (American Academy of Family Physicians [AAFP], 2016). Nurses should also notify adolescent patients that if the patient is covered under a parent's insurance, billing statements provided to that parent may include information about care. In addition, EHRs for minors are typically set up with parents as proxy. As a result, parents can read the information contained in the EHR unless the system is designed to restrict proxy access to confidential information (American College of Obstetricians and Gynecologists [ACOG], 2014).

Nurses must be aware of state statutes related to adolescent care and confidentiality as well as their ethical obligations to their adolescent patients. Nurses may encourage adolescent patients to involve their parents or guardians in care decisions related to sexual or mental health, but they must respect adolescent patients' right to autonomy in decision making. Failure to do so may give rise to patient concerns over confidentiality and result in patient refusal of treatment. For additional information, see the module on Legal Issues.

Ethical Dilemmas Related to Pregnant Women

Ethical issues related to pregnancy often focus on the delicate balance of maternal rights and fetal rights. For example, if a pregnant woman is in an accident that leaves her brain dead, it can be difficult to determine whether her life should be artificially sustained in order to deliver the child or whether life-sustaining technology should be discontinued. Two highly publicized cases occurred in 2014 and 2015. In one, the hospital attempted to keep the woman's body on life support against her wishes and those of her family (Goodwyn, 2014). In the other, the hospital and family collaborated to keep the woman's body alive for nearly 2 months, and her baby was born via cesarean section (Izadi, 2015). While the cases differed in many ways, they were similar in that the families and care providers faced a dilemma with no clear ethical or legal solution.

Ethical issues can also arise in situations in which the mother's life is in danger. This may occur as a result of complications of pregnancy that threaten the mother's life or as a result of medical conditions unrelated to pregnancy, such as cancer. In these situations, the woman, family, and healthcare providers are faced with the difficult question of whether the mother's life or the child's life takes priority. In these situations, personal opinions about abortion and the medical necessity of treatments that could harm the fetus complicate the decision-making process.

Fetal protection laws enacted by some states have complicated the ethics of healthcare during pregnancy. The intent of these laws is to protect mothers and fetuses from individuals who abuse them; however, broad interpretation of these laws has led to questions about the mother's right to accept or decline certain tests and treatments during pregnancy (Graham, 2014). Fetal protection laws are discussed further in the module on Legal Issues.

The discussion of maternal and fetal rights often stirs up complex emotions and strong opinions about the ethics and morality of pregnant patient care. Nurses should understand their state laws and organizational policies on these topics. They should also understand their rights and responsibilities related to conscientious objection (Lachman, 2014). For more information on this topic, see the module on Legal Issues.

Ethical Dilemmas Related to Older Adults

End-of-life issues are common sources of ethical dilemmas for nurses working with the older adult population. These may include issues associated with advance directives, assisted suicide, withdrawal or withholding of life sustaining treatment, and withdrawal or withholding of nutrition and fluids.

Issues related to autonomy, competency, and decision making also commonly arise in the older adult population. Some older adults experience age-related cognitive impairments or untreated depression that may affect the decisions they make related to healthcare. In addition, family members or caregivers may have strong opinions about what the patient should or should not do and may question the patient's ability to make healthcare decisions (Seamen & Erlen, 2013). The combination of these factors can place the nurse in a difficult position. If the patient is competent to make her own medical decisions, the nurse must respect her autonomy in decision making. However, the nurse must consider the factors that may be at work and the risks and benefits associated with a treatment. In addition, the nurse must be prepared to face anger, disappointment, and questions from the patient's family. When these situations arise, it may be useful for the nurse to facilitate a discussion between the major stakeholders—including the physician, patient, and family—to ensure that everyone understands what the treatment entails and what its risks and benefits are and to help the patient reach a decision that affirms her autonomy while being acceptable to the other parties involved (Seamen & Erlen, 2013).

Consent can also present issues with older adult patients who have been hospitalized. Typically, when patients are admitted to the hospital, they sign a blanket consent for treatment. By signing this form, the patient gives implicit consent for routine care. However, the patient can refuse or question any individual treatment. For example, the patient may refuse to allow the nurse to draw blood or administer a medication. When these situations arise, the nurse must respect the patient's autonomy, even if the nurse disagrees with the patient's decision. In many cases, these dilemmas can be worked through if the nurse explains the procedure and its purpose to the patient and asks about his or her reasons for refusing it (Seamen & Erlen, 2013).

SAFETY ALERT Forcing or coercing a patient to have a procedure that the patient has refused is unlawful and can result in legal consequences for the nurse.

REVIEW Ethical Dilemmas

RELATE Link the Concepts and Exemplars

Linking the exemplar of ethical dilemmas with the concept of legal issues:

1. What are your beliefs about advance directive planning for any patient who has a chronic illness, such as a cardiac illness, diabetes, or renal failure, regardless of the patient's age?

2. What is the nurse's role in discussing future care plans, such as end-of-life care, with chronically ill patients?

Linking the exemplar of ethical dilemmas with the concept of comfort:

3. What are your beliefs about ensuring comfort for patients with chronic pain?

4. Assess your understanding of pain management options to ensure comfort. What are your beliefs about the use of high-level narcotics for patients?

REFER Go to Pearson MyLab Nursing and eText

- Additional review materials

REFLECT Apply Your Knowledge

David Lewis is a 50-year-old man who is recovering from a stroke at a rehabilitation facility. He is medically stable and able to participate fully in his therapies. However, he has requested DNR (do-not-resuscitate) status. He reasons that if he has another stroke or cardiac arrest, he could lose much more cognitive and motor function, and if he were resuscitated after such an event, it would place too heavy a burden of care on his family. Day after day, he and his family ask about the DNR order. The nurses working with Mr. Lewis repeatedly ask the attending physician for an order, and the physician continues to respond that Mr. Lewis does not need a DNR order—he is stable. Finally, the primary nurse goes to the facility's ethics committee to discuss the problem. This results in another physician reviewing the chart, speaking with the patient and family, and entering the DNR order.

1. What ethical dilemma did the primary nurse working with Mr. Lewis face?

2. What principles did the primary nurse follow in going to the ethics council?

3. How do you feel about DNR orders? Why?

4. In what ways did the nurses working with Mr. Lewis advocate on his behalf? How is the nurse's role as an advocate related to nursing ethics?

≫ Exemplar 44.C
Patient Rights

Exemplar Learning Outcomes

44.C Analyze patient rights as they relate to ethics.

- Examine the rights of patients in the healthcare system.
- Analyze support systems that exist for patients who feel that their rights have been violated by a healthcare agency or provider.
- Compare the contents of different documents or laws that address patient rights.
- Differentiate considerations related to patient rights across the lifespan.

Exemplar Key Terms

Patient responsibilities, *2757*
Patient rights, *2755*

Overview

All patients have rights when it comes to the healthcare they receive. Popularly called **patient rights**, these represent the fundamental care owed to patients by healthcare providers and the government (WHO, 2016). Some of these rights are guaranteed by federal law, such as the right to informed consent mandated in the Patient Self-Determination Act (see the module on Legal Issues). Other rights are governed by state laws. In addition, healthcare organizations often have a patient bill of rights, which details the rights the organization promises to uphold for its patients.

The importance of patient rights is evident in the American Nurses Association's Standards of Practice and Code of Ethics and the accreditation standards for various types of healthcare agencies set by The Joint Commission. The Joint Commission also encourages patients to become more informed about their rights and more involved in their care through the Speak Up program (The Joint Commission, 2013b). The essential points of this program are outlined in **Box 44–6 ≫**.

Nurses should be aware of national and state laws pertaining to patient rights, as well as their employer's policies and procedures. Nurses should also be knowledgeable about the standards enacted by professional nursing bodies in an effort to protect patient rights and ensure nurse compliance with applicable laws.

Beyond laws, policies, and standards, nurses should understand their role in protecting patient rights. In addition, nurses should introduce patients to their patient rights and responsibilities and encourage patients to engage as partners with their healthcare providers. Methods of doing so will vary depending on the patient's age and condition, but it is an important component of the nurse's role as a patient advocate.

Protecting Patients' Rights

In spite of the legal requirement and ethical duty to protect patient rights, many patients still experience violations of these rights as they navigate the healthcare system. Some of the most common violations involve confidentiality, privacy, informed consent, and nondiscrimination. Less commonly, violations may involve treatment that does not respect the

---

Box 44–6
Patient Rights from The Joint Commission's Speak Up Campaign

Know Your Rights

- You have the right to be informed about the care you will receive.
- You have the right to get important information about your care in your preferred language.
- You have the right to get information in a manner that meets your needs, if you have vision, speech, hearing or mental impairments.
- You have the right to make decisions about your care.
- You have the right to refuse care.
- You have the right to know the names of the caregivers who treat you.
- You have the right to safe care.
- You have the right to have your pain addressed.
- You have the right to care that is free from discrimination. This means you should not be treated differently because of age, race, ethnicity, religion, culture, language, physical or mental disability, socioeconomic status, sex, sexual orientation, or gender identity or expression.
- You have the right to know when something goes wrong with your care.
- You have the right to get a list of all your current medications.
- You have the right to be listened to.
- You have the right to be treated with courtesy and respect.
- You have the right to have a personal representative, also called an advocate, with you during your care. Your advocate is a family member or friend of your choice.

Source: From The Joint Commission. (2013b). *Speak up: Know your rights.* Retrieved from http://www.jointcommission.org/assets/1/6/Know_Your_Rights_brochure.pdf.

---

dignity of the patient or that jeopardizes the patient's healthcare outcomes (Cohen & Ezer, 2013).

To protect patient rights, nurses must follow requirements related to informed consent. They must also be aware of the patient protection systems in place within their organizations and their state. In addition, they must recognize the importance of patient bills of rights and patient responsibilities in patient care.

Informed Consent

To ensure patient rights, the nurse must first identify the appropriate individual to provide informed consent for the patient (e.g., patient, parent, legal guardian). Also, it is vital to provide written materials in the patient's spoken language. The nurse needs to understand and describe components of informed consent and how to participate in obtaining informed consent.

When obtaining informed consent, the nurse must understand how to verify that the patient comprehends and consents to care and procedures. In addition, the nurse must discuss various treatment options and decisions with the patient. Similarly, the nurse must educate patients and staff about patients' rights and responsibilities (e.g., ethical/legal issues) and know how to evaluate patient and staff understanding of patients' rights.

SAFETY ALERT When discussing informed consent with patients, the nurse should explain to the patient his or her right to refuse a treatment or procedure.

Organizational and State Protections

Individual patients who feel that their rights are in danger or have been violated have a number of options. Many healthcare organizations have patient advocates who help patients navigate the organizational system and intervene when necessary to ensure that the patient's rights are respected. This type of advocacy is particularly important for patients who require long-term care. In addition, many states have offices designated by the governor or secretary of health to assist patients with issues related to patient rights in long-term care.

The state department of health may also be able to help with patient rights issues. Nursing homes, homes for frail older adults, and licensed facilities for people with disabilities are regulated at the state level, and violations committed by these agencies may be reported for investigation (Hicks et al., 2012). Legislatures in many states have also passed declarations of patients' rights that must be followed by nursing homes and other agencies that provide medical care and housing for patients.

Patient Bills of Rights

The first patient bill of rights was drafted by the American Hospital Association during the 1970s; since then, a number of different groups have created their own patient bills of rights (American Cancer Society, 2016). For example, in 1998, the U.S. Advisory Commission on Consumer Protection and Quality in the Health Care Industry adopted a bill of rights. This bill included, among other things, provisions about information disclosure, provider and plan choice, access to emergency services, participation in treatment decisions, nondiscrimination, and confidentiality. It also included information about filing complaints and appeals (President's Advisory Commission on Consumer Protection and Quality in Healthcare, 1998). The bill was intended to protect all consumers and was adopted by the federal government for employees covered under their insurance plans. A summary of this bill of rights is provided in **Box 44–7 》**.

The 1998 bill of rights served as the inspiration for a number of other patient bills of rights. Hospitals, patient organizations, government agencies, and insurance plans are among the different groups that have created patient bills of rights. Patient bills of rights have also been developed for hospice patients and patients with mental illness. Although these bills of rights differ from one another to some degree, most discuss privacy and confidentiality, nondiscrimination, language preferences, and patient involvement in treatment decisions.

Box 44–7

A Summary of the Bill of Rights of the U.S. Advisory Commission on Consumer Protection and Quality in the Health Care Industry

- *Information disclosure.* You have the right to accurate and easily understood information about your health plan, healthcare professionals, and healthcare facilities. If you speak another language, have a physical or mental disability, or just don't understand something, help should be provided so you can make informed healthcare decisions.

- *Choice of providers and plans.* You have the right to a choice of healthcare providers who can give you high-quality healthcare when you need it.

- *Access to emergency services.* If you have severe pain, an injury, or sudden illness that makes you believe that your health is in serious danger, you have the right to be screened and stabilized using emergency services. These services should be provided whenever and wherever you need them, without the need to wait for authorization and without any financial penalty.

- *Participation in treatment decisions.* You have the right to know your treatment options and to take part in decisions about your care. Parents, guardians, family members, or others who you select can represent you if you cannot make your own decisions.

- *Respect and nondiscrimination.* You have a right to considerate, respectful care from your physicians, health plan representatives, and other healthcare providers that does not discriminate against you.

- *Confidentiality of health information.* You have the right to talk privately with healthcare providers and to have your healthcare information protected. You also have the right to read and copy your own medical records. You have the right to ask that your physician change your record if it is not accurate, relevant, or complete.

- *Complaints and appeals.* You have the right to a fair, fast, and objective review of any complaint you have against your health plan, physicians, hospitals, or other healthcare personnel. This includes complaints about waiting times, operating hours, the actions of healthcare personnel, and the adequacy of healthcare facilities.

Source: Based on President's Advisory Commission on Consumer Protection and Quality in the Health Care Industry. (1998). Consumer bill of rights and responsibilities: Executive summary. *Agency for Healthcare Research and Quality.* Retrieved from http://archive.ahrq.gov/hcqual/cborr/exsumm.html.

Passage of the Affordable Care Act in 2010 was accompanied by a new patient bill of rights. This bill differs in content from other bills of rights in that it specifically addresses patient protections related to health insurance coverage. Areas discussed in this patient bill of rights include coverage for individuals with preexisting conditions, free preventive care, elimination of dollar limits, accountability for rate increases, and provider choice (HealthCare.gov, n.d.). The Affordable Care Act may be replaced in the coming years. Nurses should stay abreast of changes in healthcare laws and the way in which they affect patients.

Patient Responsibilities

In addition to patient bills of rights, some organizations now publish lists of **patient responsibilities**. These lists emphasize that healthcare is a partnership between the patient and caregivers, that other patients have the right to be comfortable, and that there are consequences when patients do not comply with treatment plans. Common patient responsibilities include the following:

- Tell your healthcare team how you feel.
- Provide information about your health, past illnesses, and use of medications.
- Report accurate and complete information about your health to your healthcare team.
- Ask your healthcare team whether you need to change your medications before a procedure or test.
- Answer questions asked by your healthcare team.
- Cooperate with your healthcare team.
- Listen to instructions, read written material given to you, and ask questions if you do not understand something.
- Be considerate of the staff and other patients by limiting visitors, following smoking regulations, and using the telephone and television so as not to disturb others.
- Provide information about your health insurance, and work with the hospital to arrange for payment if needed.
- Recognize the effects of your lifestyle on your health, and work with your hospital team to change your lifestyle as necessary.
- Follow the treatment plan recommended by your healthcare team.
- Accept the consequences if you fail to comply with instructions given to you.

Patient responsibilities lists are intended to encourage patients to take a more active role in their care and promote consideration of others within the healthcare environment. They are not intended to be a list of rules that patients must follow. In introducing patients to these responsibilities, it is important for nurses to make sure patients understand this difference.

Lifespan Considerations

At different points in the lifespan, patients experience different needs and concerns related to patient rights. In addition, some organizations have patient bills of rights that are specific to patients at different points in the lifespan. The nurse must ensure that the specific rights of these patients are respected.

Patient Rights Pertaining to Infants and Children

When working with pediatric patients, nurses are responsible for protecting the rights of both patients and their families. To support nurses in these efforts, the Association for the Care of Children's Health (ACCH) has developed the pediatric bill of rights, which outlines the need for family-centered care that provides developmentally appropriate psychosocial support. The Society of Pediatric Nurses (SPN) encourages hospitals and children's units across the country to adopt some version of this bill of rights (Mott, 2014). In doing so, the SPN hopes to better prepare families to understand the care that is being provided to their child and to create more positive healthcare experiences for pediatric patients and their loved ones.

A central theme in the pediatric bill of rights is allowing patients and families to remain together whenever possible during treatments and hospital stays. In some cases, this includes making arrangements for a family member to remain with the child overnight. Other supportive measures include allowing the child to have toys or clothes from home when possible and providing children with opportunities to play and engage in activities related to their personal interests. The goal of all these measures is to make patients and families comfortable and to maintain a sense of normalcy rather than emphasizing the child's illness (Mott, 2014).

The pediatric bill of rights includes many of the same provisions as other patient bills of rights with relation to privacy, information sharing, and respect for the individual. The primary difference is the focus on age-appropriate and developmentally appropriate applications of these concepts. Another difference is the application of these concepts to the family as a whole rather than to the patient as an individual.

Patient Rights Pertaining to Adolescents

Adolescent patients are also covered under the pediatric bill of rights. An important difference in caring for adolescents rather than young children is the role of family. As children reach adolescence, they may engage in behaviors or have care needs that they are embarrassed or worried about sharing with their families. In these situations, it is essential that nurses understand the state laws related to confidential care for adolescents and are prepared for the ethical dilemmas involved in providing this kind of care. (See the module on Legal Issues and the exemplar on Ethical Dilemmas in this module for more information.)

The pediatric bill of rights includes a privacy provision that is useful for working with adolescent patients. It states that patients have the right for their privacy to be honored as long as it is safe for the patient (Mott, 2014). Though the right of privacy must be honored, the American Academy of Family Physicians encourages healthcare providers to make a reasonable effort to encourage adolescents to involve their family in their healthcare (AAFP, 2016). This encouragement should be provided in a supportive manner with the clear understanding that involving parents or guardians in the decision-making process is not essential for the patient to receive care.

Another important consideration in caring for adolescent patients is their inclusion in nonconfidential healthcare decisions. For example, a teenage patient being treated for leukemia may have strong opinions about the types of treatment he would like to receive, even though his parents serve as his decision-making proxy. Adolescent patients have a right to have their opinion heard and considered by healthcare providers and family members (Dikema, 2014). The nurse must facilitate conversations with family and other healthcare providers in these situations. See the Ethical Dilemmas exemplar in this module for more information on this topic.

Patient Rights Pertaining to Pregnant Women

Many pregnant patients may not be fully aware of their rights in regard to making healthcare decisions on behalf of themselves and their children and so may not exercise their rights. As a result, a major rights-related issue that nurses face with this population involves informing patients of their rights. Rights specific to the pregnant patient include the right to prenatal care, the right to choose a physician or midwife, and the right to give birth in the setting of her choice (see Focus on Diversity and Culture feature). In addition, the pregnant patient has the right to move freely during labor, to deliver in the position of her choice, and to have uninterrupted contact with her newborn provided that neither mother nor child experience a medical condition that prevents this (Childbirth Connection, 2006).

Focus on Diversity and Culture
Diversity in Labor and Delivery

A pregnant patient has the right to receive labor and delivery care in accordance with her cultural background (Childbirth Connection, 2006). For example, patients from African cultures may choose to have their mothers or respected female elders in the delivery room rather than the child's father. Middle Eastern patients may prefer to walk or remain otherwise mobile during the labor process and to squat during delivery. Chinese, Japanese, Vietnamese, and Korean patients may remain silent during the birthing process because of the traditional belief that crying out takes energy away from laboring. Patients from East Indian cultures may have the child's father or grandfather whisper traditional prayers to the infant immediately following birth (HealthCare Chaplaincy, 2013).

If these actions do not jeopardize the mother or the child, the nurse must respect the mother's wishes for culturally based practices. The nurse should also advocate with other healthcare providers for the patient's right to engage in these practices (Kang, 2014).

A number of issues can develop that endanger a pregnant patient's rights. For example, the patient's right to prenatal care depends on the patient's access to care. As a result, patients without health insurance or in underserved communities may not be able to exercise this right. In addition, labor and delivery rights may be affected by organizational or unit regulations that limit patient movement, by healthcare providers who are unaware of the various rights of the pregnant patient, or by medical emergencies that necessitate that certain protocols be followed. The nurse should work with the patient and other providers to protect the patient's rights to the extent possible in a given situation.

Patient Rights Pertaining to Older Adults

One of the biggest patient rights issues for older patients involves long-term care provided in nursing homes and in skilled nursing facilities. Federal law requires that nursing homes protect and promote the rights of each resident. These include the rights of nondiscrimination, respect, freedom from abuse and neglect, and freedom from physical restraints. In addition, residents must be informed about fees and services in writing before admission, be allowed to manage their money as they see fit, be allowed to keep personal property in their rooms, and be able to see the healthcare provider of their choice. Visitors must be allowed during reasonable hours, and necessary social services must be provided to residents. Residents must be able to file complaints without fear of reprisals and cannot be transferred or discharged unfairly (Medicare.gov, n.d.). Recently the Centers for Medicare and Medicaid Services (CMS) issued a rule that bars nursing homes that receive federal funding from requiring that residents resolve disputes in arbitration instead of in court, making it easier for residents of nursing homes and their families to sue if necessary for claims such as elder abuse, sexual harassment, and wrongful death (CMS, 2016).

The rights of older patients may also be endangered in hospital settings, particularly if friends or family members are concerned about the patients' capacity for making their own medical decisions. In addition, the rights of patients who are no longer able to speak or make decisions for themselves may be at risk if the patients do not have advance directives in place. These issues are discussed in greater detail in the module on Legal Issues and in the exemplar on Ethical Dilemmas in this module.

REVIEW Patient Rights

RELATE Link the Concepts and Exemplars

Linking the exemplar of patient rights with the concept of healthcare systems:

1. Patients have the right to emergency care without bias. What are your beliefs about patients who use emergency care in place of primary care?

2. What are your beliefs about patient privacy when emergent or critical care is needed and the patient cannot provide approval for his or her own care?

Linking the exemplar of patient rights with the concept of addiction:

3. Patients with persistent admissions for alcohol withdrawal therapy due to alcohol addiction need support to make the decision to get over this addiction. What are your beliefs about alcohol addiction and the nursing role in assisting a patient with these issues?

4. When adults who have had an extensive history of back pain with several narcotics taken each day need surgery, they often require a higher level of narcotics postoperatively. What is the nurse's role in supporting this type of patient in appropriate pain management?

REFER Go to Pearson MyLab Nursing and eText

■ Additional review materials

REFLECT Apply Your Knowledge

James Casper is a 75-year-old widower who was admitted to the ED after a hit-and-run accident. Upon arrival, he was intubated, a chest tube was inserted, and he was rushed into surgery to repair damage to his spleen. After surgery, he was taken to the trauma unit to recover.

Mr. Casper has been on the trauma unit for 3 days now. He is awake and alert but still reports that he is experiencing pain. He has become increasingly agitated during his time on the unit. He has also complained repeatedly about nurses' "constant poking and prodding" of him. He has refused to see his daughter on several occasions when she has come to visit him.

Today, Candace Jones, the nurse assigned to Mr. Casper, has come to perform a venipuncture to get a blood sample for lab testing. Mr. Casper refuses to allow her to draw the blood. At first, he simply refuses to give her his arm; then, he began to yell at Ms. Jones and verbally berate her.

1. Upon admission into the ED, Mr. Casper signed a general consent for care form. Does this form supersede his right to refuse the venipuncture? Why or why not?

2. What is Ms. Jones' best means of proceeding in this situation without violating Mr. Casper's rights?

3. In what way has Mr. Casper violated his patient responsibilities in this scenario?

References

AIDS.gov. (2014). *U.S. statistics*. Retrieved from https://www.aids.gov/hiv-aids-basics/hiv-aids-101/statistics/

AIDS.gov. (2015). *Addressing the cost of care*. Retrieved from https://www.aids.gov/hiv-aids-basics/just-diagnosed-with-hiv-aids/find-care-and-treatment/addressing-cost-barriers/

American Academy of Family Physicians (AAFP). (2016). *Adolescent health care, confidentiality*. Retrieved from http://www.aafp.org/about/policies/all/adolescent-confidentiality.html

American Association of Colleges of Nursing (AACN). (2008). *The essentials of baccalaureate education for professional nursing practice*. Washington, DC: Author. Used with permission.

American Association of Colleges of Nursing (AACN). (2014). *Nursing shortage fact sheet*. Retrieved from http://www.aacn.nche.edu/media/FactSheets/NursingShortage.htm

American Cancer Society. (2016). *Patient's bill of rights*. Retrieved from http://www.cancer.org/treatment/findingandpayingfortreatment/understandingfinancialandlegalmatters/patients-bill-of-rights

American Civil Liberties Union of Ohio. (2014). *Your health and the law: A guide for teens*. Retrieved from http://www.acluohio.org/wp-content/uploads/2014/06/TeenHealthGuide.pdf

American College of Obstetricians and Gynecologists (ACOG). (2014). Committee opinion: Adolescent confidentiality and electronic health records. *Committee on Adolescent Health Care, Number 599.* Retrieved from http://www.acog.org/Resources-And-Publications/Committee-Opinions/Committee-on-Adolescent-Health-Care/Adolescent-Confidentiality-and-Electronic-Health-Records

American Nurses Association (ANA). (2013). *Position statements: Euthanasia, assisted suicide, and aid in dying*. Retrieved from http://www.nursingworld.org/MainMenuCategories/EthicsStandards/Ethics-Position-Statements/Euthanasia-Assisted-Suicide-and-Aid-in-Dying.pdf

American Nurses Association (ANA). (2015a). *Code of ethics for nurses with interpretive statements*. Retrieved from http://nursingworld.org/DocumentVault/Ethics-1/Code-of-Ethics-for-Nurses.html

American Nurses Association (ANA). (2015b). The year of ethics commences with first revision of code since 2001. Retrieved from http://nursingworld.org/FunctionalMenuCategories/MediaResources/PressReleases/2015-NR/The-Year-of-Ethics-Commences-with-First-Revision-of-Code-since-2001.html

American Nurses Association (ANA). (2015c). *Position statement: Risk and responsibility in providing nursing care*. Retrieved from http://www.nursingworld.org/MainMenuCategories/EthicsStandards/Ethics-Position-Statements/Risk-and-Responsibility-in-Providing-Nursing-Care.html/RiskandResponsibilityPositionStatement2015.pdf

Ball, J. W., Bindler, R. C., Cowen, K., & Shaw, M. (2017). *Principles of pediatric nursing: Caring for children* (7th ed.). Hoboken, NJ: Pearson Education.

Butts, J. B., & Rich, K. L. (2013). *Nursing ethics: Across the curriculum and into practice* (3rd ed.). Burlington, MA: Jones & Bartlett.

Carteret, M. (2012). *Providing healthcare to Hmong patients and families*. Retrieved from http://www.dimensionsofculture.com/2012/01/providing-healthcare-to-hmong-patients-and-families/

Centers for Disease Control and Protection (CDC). (2016). Today's HIV/AIDS epidemic. *CDC Fact Sheet*. Retrieved from https://www.cdc.gov/nchhstp/newsroom/docs/factsheets/todaysepidemic-508.pdf

Centers for Medicare and Medicaid Services. (2016). *Reform of requirements for long-term care facilities*. Retrieved from https://s3.amazonaws.com/public-inspection.federalregister.gov/2016-23503.pdf

Centre for Genetics Education. (2016). *Fact sheet 19: Ethical issues in human genetics and genomics*. Retrieved from http://www.genetics.edu.au/Publications-and-Resources/Genetics-Fact-Sheets/FactSheetELSI

Childbirth Connection. (2006). *The rights of childbearing women*. Retrieved from http://www.nationalpartnership.org/research-library/maternal-health/the-rights-of-childbearing-women.pdf

Chooljian, D. M., Hallenbeck, J., Ezeji-Okoye, S. C., Sebesta, R., Iqbal, H., & Kuschner, W. G. (2016). Emotional support for health care professionals: A therapeutic role for the hospital ethics committee. *Journal of Social Work in End of Life and Palliative Care, 12*(3), 277–288. doi:10.1080/15524256.2016.1200519

Cohen, J., & Ezer, T. (2013). Human rights in patient care: A theoretical and practical framework. *Health and Human Rights Journal, 15*(2). Retrieved from https://www.hhrjournal.org/2013/12/human-rights-in-patient-care-a-theoretical-and-practical-framework/

Crowley, J. D., & Gottlieb, M. C. (2012). Objects in the mirror are closer than they appear: A primary prevention model for ethical decision making. *Professional Psychology: Research and Practice, 43*(1), 65–72.

Danis, M. (2015). *Stopping artificial nutrition and hydration at the end of life*. Retrieved from http://www.uptodate.com/contents/stopping-artificial-nutrition-and-hydration-at-the-end-of-life

De Bruyn, M. (2012). HIV, unwanted pregnancy and abortion—Where is the human rights approach? *Reproductive Health Matters, 20*(Suppl. 39), 70–79.

Dekeyser Ganz, F., & Berkovitz, K. (2012). Surgical nurses' perceptions of ethical dilemmas, moral distress and quality of care. *Journal of Advanced Nursing 68*(7), 1516–1525. doi:10.1111/j.1365-2648.2011.05897.x

Dikema, D. S. (2014). *Parental decision making*. Retrieved from https://depts.washington.edu/bioethx/topics/parent.html

Drum, K. (2016, January/February). My right to die. *Mother Jones*. Retrieved from http://www.motherjones.com/politics/2016/01/assisted-suicide-legalization-california-kevin-drum

Edmonson, C. (2015). Strengthening moral courage among nurse leaders. *Online Journal of Issues in Nursing, 20*(2). Retrieved from http://www.nursingworld.org/MainMenuCategories/ANAMarketplace/ANAPeriodicals/OJIN/TableofContents/Vol-20-2015/No2-May-2015/Articles-Previous-Topics/Strengthening-Moral-Courage.html

Ellis, J. R., & Hartley, C. L. (2012). *Nursing in today's world: Trends, issues and management* (10th ed.). Philadelphia: Wolters Kluwer Health/Lippincott Williams & Wilkins.

Epstein, B., & Turner, M. (2015). The nursing code of ethics: Its value, its history. *Online Journal of Issues in Nursing, 20*(2). doi:10.3912/OJIN.Vol20No02Man04

Goodwin, K. D., Taylor, M. M., Brown, E. C., Winscott, M., Scanlon, M., Hodge, J. G., Jr., … England, B. (2012). Protecting adolescents' right to seek treatment for sexually transmitted diseases without parental consent: The Arizona experience with Senate Bill 1309. *Public Health Reports, 127*, 253–258.

Goodwyn, W. (2014). *The strange case of Marlise Munoz and John Peter Smith Hospital*. Retrieved from http://www.npr.org/sections/health-shots/2014/01/28/267759687/the-strange-case-of-marlise-munoz-and-john-peter-smith-hospital

Graham, R. (2014, February 16). For pregnant women, two sets of rights in one body. *Boston Globe.* Retrieved from https://www.bostonglobe.com/ideas/2014/02/16/for-pregnant-women-two-sets-rights-one-body/5Pd6zntIViRBZ9QxhiQgFJ/story.html

Gretter, L. (1910). Florence Nightingale pledge: Autograph manuscript dated 1893. *American Journal of Nursing, 10*(4), 271. Published by Wolters Kluwer Health.

Guido, G. W. (2014). *Legal and ethical issues in nursing* (6th ed.). Upper Saddle River, NJ: Prentice Hall.

HealthCare Chaplaincy. (2013). *Handbook of patients' spiritual and cultural values for health care professionals.* Retrieved from http://www.healthcarechaplaincy.org/userimages/Cultural%20Sensitivity%20handbook%20from%20Health-Care%20Chaplaincy%20%20(3-12%202013).pdf

HealthCare.gov. (n.d.). *Health coverage rights and protections.* Retrieved from https://www.healthcare.gov/health-care-law-protections/

Hicks, E., Sims-Gould, J., Byrne, K., Khan, K. M., & Stolee, P. (2012). "She was a little bit unrealistic": Choice in healthcare decision making for older people. *Journal of Aging Studies, 26,* 140–148.

Herdman, T. H. & Kamitsuru, S. (Eds) *Nursing Diagnoses—Definitions and Classification 2015–2017.* Copyright © 2014, 1994–2014 NANDA International. Used by arrangement with John Wiley & Sons, Inc. Companion website: www.wiley.com/go/nursingdiagnoses.

Iglesias, M. E., & De Bengoa Vallejo, R. B. (2012). Conflict resolution styles in the nursing profession. *Contemporary Nurse, 43*(1), 73–80.

International Council of Nurses. (2012). *The ICN code of ethics for nurses.* Retrieved from http://www.icn.ch/images/stories/documents/about/icncode_english.pdf

Izadi, E. (2015, May 1). Woman delivers baby 54 days after being declared brain dead. *Washington Post.* Retrieved from https://www.washingtonpost.com/news/morning-mix/wp/2015/05/01/a-brain-dead-woman-was-kept-alive-for-54-days-to-deliver-her-baby/

Izumi, S., Nagae, H., Sakurai, C., & Imamura, E. (2012). Defining end-of-life care from perspectives of nursing ethics. *Nursing Ethics, 19*(5), 608–618.

Jansen, T. L., & Hanssen, I. (2016). Patient participation: Causing moral stress in psychiatric nursing? *Scandinavian Journal of Caring Science,* epub ahead of print. doi:10.1111/scs.12358

Johansen, M. L., & O'Brien, J. L. (2015). Decision making in nursing practice: A concept analysis. *Nursing Forum, 51*(1), 40. doi:10.1111/nuf.12119

Johnstone, M. (2012a). Workplace ethics and respect for colleagues. *Australian Nursing Journal, 20*(2), 31.

Johnstone, M. (2012b). Ethics. *Australian Nursing Journal, 20*(4), 43.

Kang, H-K. (2014). Influence of culture and community perceptions on birth and perinatal care of immigrant women: doulas' perspective. *The Journal of Perinatal Education, 23*(1):25–32.

Kangasniemi, M., & Haho, A. (2012). Human love—The inner essence of nursing ethics according to Estrid Rodhe: A study using the approach of history of ideas. *Scandinavian Journal of Caring Science, 26,* 803–810.

Kim, S., Seo, M., & Kim, D. R. (2016). Unmet needs for clinical ethics support services in nurse: Based on focus group interviews. *Nursing Ethics.* doi:10.1177/0969733016654312

Lachman, V. D. (2012). Applying the ethics of care to your nursing practice. *MEDSURG Nursing, 21*(2), 112–115.

Lachman, V. D. (2014). Conscientious objection in nursing: Definition and criteria for acceptance. *MEDSURG Nursing, 23*(3), 196–198. Retrieved from http://www.nursingworld.org/MainMenuCategories/EthicsStandards/Resources/Conscientious-Objection-in-Nursing.pdf

Larcher, V., Craig, F., Bhogal, K., Wilkinson, D., & Brierley, J. (2015). Making decisions to limit treatment in life-limiting and life-threatening conditions in children: a framework for practice. *Archives of Disease in Childhood, 100*(2), s1–s23.

McKeown, D. W., Bonser, R. S., & Kellum, J. A. (2012). Management of the heart-beating brain-dead organ donor. *British Journal of Anaesthesia, 108.* doi:10.1093/bja/aer351

Medicare.gov. (n.d.). *What are your rights in a skilled nursing facility?* Retrieved from https://www.medicare.gov/what-medicare-covers/part-a/rights-in-snf.html

Mott, S. (2014). The pediatric bill of rights. *Journal of Pediatric Nursing, 29*(6), 709. doi:10.1016/j.pedn.2014.08.008

National Center for Complementary and Integrative Health. (n.d.) *Complementary, alternative, or integrative health: What's in a name?* Retrieved from https://nccih.nih.gov/health/integrative-health

National Guideline Clearinghouse (NGC). (2017). Nursing. *Agency for Healthcare Research and Quality.* Retrieved from https://www.guideline.gov/search?f_Clinical_Specialty=Nursing&fLockTerm=Nursing

National Institutes of Health (NIH). (2017a). DrugFacts: What is medical marijuana? *National Institute on Drug Abuse.* Retrieved from https://www.drugabuse.gov/publications/drugfacts/marijuana-medicine

National Institutes of Health (NIH). (2017b). What is direct-to-consumer genetic testing? *Genetics Home Reference.* Retrieved from https://ghr.nlm.nih.gov/primer/testing/directtoconsumer

Numminen, O., Leino-Kilpi, H., Isoaho, H., & Meretoja, R. (2015). Ethical climate and nurse competence—newly graduated nurses' perceptions. *Nursing Ethics, 22*(8), 845–859. doi:10.1177/0969733014557137

Olafsen, L., Schraw, G., Nadelson, L., Nadelson, S., & Kehrwald, N. (2013). Exploring the judgment–action gap: College students and academic dishonesty. *Ethics & Behavior, 23*(2), 148–162.

Organ Procurement and Transplantation Network (OPTN). (2014). *Ethical principles of pediatric organ allocation.* Retrieved from https://optn.transplant.hrsa.gov/resources/ethics/ethical-principles-of-pediatric-organ-allocation/

Organ Procurement and Transplantation Network (OPTN). (2015). *Ethical principles in the allocation of human organs.* Retrieved from https://optn.transplant.hrsa.gov/resources/ethics/ethical-principles-in-the-allocation-of-human-organs/

Organ Procurement and Transplantation Network (OPTN). (n.d.). *How organ allocation works.* Retrieved from https://optn.transplant.hrsa.gov/learn/about-transplantation/how-organ-allocation-works/

Phillips, E. (2014). *How to help patients prepare for end-of-life decisions.* Retrieved from http://www.advisorperspectives.com/articles/2014/03/18/how-to-help-patients-prepare-for-end-of-life-decisions

Poikkeus, T., Suhonen, R., Katajisto, J., & Leino-Kilpi, H. (2016). Organisational and individual support for nurses' ethical competence: A cross-sectional survey. *Nursing Ethics,* epub ahead of print. pii:0969733016642627

President's Advisory Commission on Consumer Protection and Quality in the Health Care Industry. (1998). Consumer bill of rights and responsibilities: Executive summary. *Agency for Healthcare Research and Quality.* Retrieved from http://archive.ahrq.gov/hcqual/cborr/exsumm.html

Rasmussen, L. M. (2012). Patient advocacy in clinical ethics consultation. *American Journal of Bioethics, 12*(8), 1–9.

Schultz, D. (2013). Nurses fighting state by state for minimum staffing laws. *Kaiser Health News.* Retrieved from http://www.kaiserhealthnews.org/Stories/2013/April/24/nurse-staffing-laws.aspx

Seamen, J. B., & Erlen, J. A. (2013). "Everyday ethics" in the care of hospitalized older adults. *Orthopaedic Nursing, 32*(5), 286–289. Retrieved from http://www.nursingcenter.com/journalarticle?Article_ID=1601851

Segal, B., & Hodges, M. (2012, March–April). Care across cultures: Does every patient need to know? *Health Progress.* Retrieved from http://oregon.providence.org/~/media/files/providence%20or%20migrated%20pdfs/patients%20toolkit/care%20across%20cultures%20%20does%20every%20patient%20need%20to%20know.pdf

Stacy, K. M. (2012). Withdrawal of life-sustaining treatment: A case study. *Critical Care Nurse, 32*(3), 14–23. Retrieved from http://www.aacn.org/wd/cetests/media/c1232.pdf

The Joint Commission. (2013a). *Ethics committee.* Retrieved from http://www.jcrinc.com/Ethics-Framework/Organizational-Ethics-Statements/Ethics-Committee

The Joint Commission. (2013b). *Speak up: Know your rights.* Retrieved from http://www.jointcommission.org/assets/1/6/Know_Your_Rights_brochure.pdf

United Network for Organ Sharing. (2015). *How organs are matched.* Retrieved from https://www.unos.org/transplantation/matching-organs

Varcoe, C., Doane, G., Pauly, B., Rodney, P., Storch, J. L., Mahoney, K., … Starsomski, R. (2004). Ethical practice in nursing: Working the in-betweens. *Journal of Advanced Nursing, 45*(3), 316–325.

Watts, T. (2013). End-of-life care pathways and nursing: A literature review. *Journal of Nursing Management, 21,* 47–57.

World Health Organization (WHO). (2016). *Patients' rights.* Retrieved from http://www.who.int/genomics/public/patientrights/en/

Yoost, B. L., & Crawford, L. R. (2016). *Fundamentals of nursing: Active learning for collaborative practice.* St. Louis, MO: Elsevier.

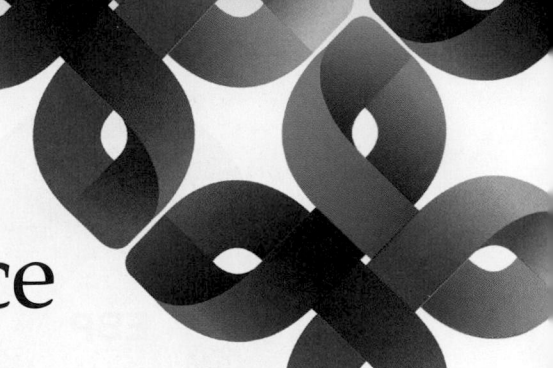

Module 45
Evidence-Based Practice

Module Outline and Learning Outcomes

The Concept of Evidence-Based Practice

Overview of Evidence-Based Practice

45.1 Summarize the evolution of evidence-based practice.

Concepts Related to Evidence-Based Practice

45.2 Outline the relationship between evidence-based practice and other concepts.

Nursing Clinical Research

45.3 Summarize the fundamentals of research methodology.

Developing Evidence-Based Practice

45.4 Analyze the four steps of developing evidence-based practice.

Lifespan Considerations

45.5 Differentiate considerations related to evidence-based practice throughout the lifespan.

Strategies to Implement Evidence-Based Practice

45.6 Outline activities used to implement evidence-based practice.

≫ The Concept of Evidence-Based Practice

Concept Key Terms

Background questions, 2766	Evidence-based practice (EBP), 2761	Institutional review boards (IRBs), 2765	PICOT, 2767	Research, 2761
Evidence, 2761	Foreground questions, 2766	Nursing clinical research, 2764	Qualitative research, 2764	Research participants, 2765
Evidence-based nursing, 2761	Informed consent, 2765	Nursing research, 2764	Quantitative research, 2764	Translational research, 2762

The Institute of Medicine's (IOM) 2000 publication *To Err Is Human* established the high cost of medical errors, including the cost in terms of human life. The IOM's 2001 publication *Crossing the Quality Chasm: A New Health System for the 21st Century* addressed the failure of the healthcare delivery system to consistently provide high-quality healthcare to all people. Evidence-based practice is one response to intensifying public and professional demands for safety and high quality improvement in health care. Goals of evidence-based practice include using the best evidence to reduce inappropriate variations in healthcare and to facilitate the standardization of safe, effective healthcare practices (Stevens, 2013).

Overview of Evidence-Based Practice

Evidence-based practice (EBP) is used to form a bridge between **research** (a formal, systematic way of answering a question or approaching a problem) and nursing practice. **Evidence** can be defined as clinical knowledge, expert opinion, or information resulting from research. Although there are many definitions of EBP, they generally include three components: (a) the best evidence from the most current research available, (b) the nurse's clinical expertise, and (c) the patient's preferences, which reflect values, needs, interests, and choices (see a **Figure 45–1 ≫**). By integrating the three components of EBP into the clinical decision-making process, nurses can individualize patient care and provide best practice for patient-centered care.

Although different professional organizations and healthcare agencies vary slightly in their definitions, most agree that **evidence-based nursing** seeks, considers, and synthesizes the combination of the best available research evidence, the nurse's own clinical experience, and each patient's cultural values and personal preferences to provide individualized, optimal nursing care appropriate for the patient at the point of care (Sigma Theta Tau International, 2002; American Association of Nurse Anesthetists, n.d.; UNC Health Sciences Library, 2016).

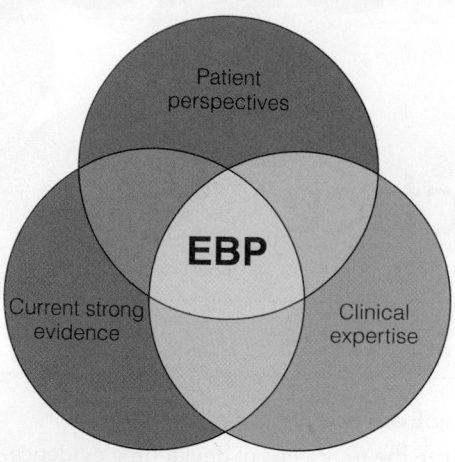

Figure 45–1 >> These three components provide the framework for evidence-based practice that nurses use to provide optimized individual clinical care to patients.

Implementing research evidence is not a new concept (**Box 45–1 >>**). However, a reordering of priorities in the medical field led to an emphasis on practice-oriented research. In the early 1970s, Dr. Archie Cochrane, a British epidemiologist who is generally credited with developing EBP, campaigned among healthcare providers to use evidence when making healthcare decisions. Professional nursing organizations saw the wisdom in this idea and encouraged nursing research in the development of best nursing practice based on current best knowledge. In 1996, Dr. David Sackett and colleagues provided the following commonly accepted definition of EBP: "The conscientious, explicit and judicious use of current best evidence in making decisions about the care of the individual patient. It means integrating individual clinical expertise with the best available external clinical evidence from systematic research" (Sackett et al., 1996, p. 71).

Translational research is a systematic approach of converting research knowledge into applications of healthcare for improved patient outcomes. The translation of scientific evidence into practical applications allows for enhanced human health, particularly when information flows back and forth between researchers and clinicians, allowing for further investigation of diseases and their effects on humans. The National Institutes of Health supports translational research through the Clinical and Translational Science Awards Consortium. The Centers for Disease Control and Prevention has translational centers around the country. Educational institutions are partnering with communities to do translational projects.

Translational research has clear benefits for the development of EBP across nursing and the various disciplines involved in healthcare systems. In particular, translational research may speed the process from discovery to application. However, this potential benefit also carries risks. Researchers have expressed concerns that rapid translation may lead to the introduction of applications and technologies that have not been sufficiently evaluated from ethical and social perspectives (Ostergren et al., 2014).

Box 45–1
Florence Nightingale

Florence Nightingale introduced to nursing the importance of collecting data through the process of observation to help make decisions about the health status of an individual (see **Figure 45–2 >>**). As Nightingale (1859/1946) explained:

> The most important practical lesson that can be given to nurses is to teach them what to observe—how to observe—what symptoms indicate improvement—what the reverse—which are of importance—which are of none—which are the evidence of neglect—and of what kind of neglect. All of this ought to make part, and an essential part, of the training of every nurse. (p. 59)

Observation continues to be one of the most powerful tools in nursing practice. Nurses employ physical assessment, including observation, as a way to gain immediate information about a patient's health status. EBP extends the nurse's realm of information to incorporate research—the data observed and recorded by others—to improve patient outcomes.

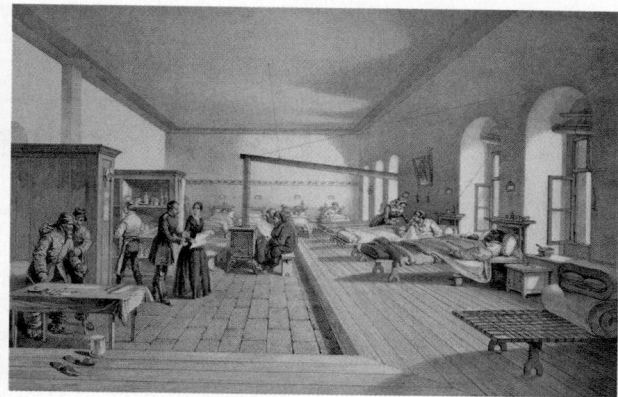

Source: Universal Images Group/Getty Images.

Figure 45–2 >> A ward of the hospital at Scutari where Florence Nightingale worked, from an 1856 lithograph by William Simpson. In the 1800s, Nightingale changed her concepts of disease prevention and promotion of health when she observed patients with and without the advantage of sanitation measures during their care. She concluded that patients situated in well-ventilated rooms and treated with clean equipment and supplies, such as fresh linens and dressings, healed faster and had fewer complications. Washing hands resulted in a decrease in patient deaths. This is an example of an early informal randomized controlled trial that provided objective evidence to support a change in best practice for nurses to improve patient outcomes.

Concepts Related to Evidence-Based Practice

EBP has widespread implications for all areas of nursing, because it informs nursing procedures during the day-to-day care of patients. From simple tasks, such as the use of standard hand hygiene procedures to prevent infection and turning patients every 2 hours to prevent pressure injuries,

Concepts Related to
Evidence-Based Practice

CONCEPT	RELATIONSHIP TO EVIDENCE-BASED PRACTICE	NURSING IMPLICATIONS
Accountability	Best practice standards of care, responsibility, and scope of nursing practice reflect EBP.	■ Nurses are responsible for providing best current nursing care to their patients.
Clinical Decision Making	EBP provides scientific support for nurses in clinical thinking processes, making decisions, and using clinical judgment.	■ As problem solvers, nurses depend on current best practice to deliver high-quality care throughout the individual patient's nursing plan of care.
Health, Wellness, and Illness	Routine habits, including sleep patterns, hygiene practices, and exercise, impact an individual's current and future state of health and wellness.	■ Nurses are responsible for educating patients about evidence-based self-care practices that promote health and wellness and that reduce the risk for illness.
Legal Issues	The evidence that supports EBP includes clinical knowledge, expert opinion, and information resulting from research. Evidence serves as an essential component of the foundation for professional nursing's scope and standards of practice.	■ Conduct that deviates from professional standards of practice constitutes malpractice.
Professional Behaviors	As a credible professional discipline, nursing has a responsibility to use EBP.	■ Best evidence needs to be integrated with the nurse's clinical experience and patient preferences.
Quality Improvement	Improving nursing care is a continuous process using current evidence to deliver safe and effective interventions resulting in best patient outcomes.	■ Improvement of the "Why?" "When?" and "What?" of nursing care is a dynamic process that can lead to changes in how nursing care is provided.

to more complex tasks such as administering medications, monitoring for adverse effects, and preparing patients for surgery, EBP is intimately associated with all nursing standards of care and nursing procedures. Part of the reason that EBP is so important is that it assists nurses in examining the *why* behind existing processes and procedures, encouraging nurses to advocate for patients by asking questions such as the following:

■ Is this the best practice method available to support positive patient outcomes?

■ Is there evidence supporting an improvement?

With the abundance of research available today, nurses are challenged to continuously evaluate and change their nursing practices based on current evidence. At the same time, as healthcare team members, nurses face the challenge of cost containment in managing care. Factors that influence decisions about potential interventions include availability of resources and requirements regarding reimbursement for services as stipulated by payment sources. Nurses must use best evidence related to finance and economics to develop a cost-conscious nursing practice (see the module on Managing Care for additional information).

Patients' participation in decisions about care is based on their individual influences and preferences, including health beliefs, culture, spirituality, and traditions (see the modules on Culture and Diversity and Spirituality for more information). For example, patients can agree to a treatment such as supplemental oxygen, refuse a treatment such as a blood transfusion, ask for a second opinion from a specialist

physician, and establish advance directives to ensure that they will be treated according to their preferences. Patients also may choose to incorporate integrative medicine into the plan of care (see Focus on Integrative Health). Many patients have access to resources that provide them with medical knowledge and clinical information through technology, including television and the internet, which can increase awareness of their condition and possible care options. Patients need to be a part of the process, and their preferences should be taken into consideration in clinical decisions about their care (see the module on Clinical Decision Making for further information). The Concepts Related to Evidence-based Practice feature outlines some, but not all, of the concepts that are integral to EBP. They are listed in alphabetical order.

Nursing Clinical Research

Nurses actively collaborate with other healthcare disciplines to provide high-quality patient care. They help patients navigate the healthcare environment and assume many roles, such as provider of care, advocate, teacher, and researcher (refer to the module on Accountability for additional information). Nurses help to ensure open and effective communication and continuity among all members of the healthcare team and patients and their families. Nurses who are actively involved in EBP access and use evidence from a variety of sources and disciplines to help guide their clinical practice and improve patient care. By using EBP, nurses also ensure the credibility of their profession and provide accountability for nursing care (**Box 45–2 »**).

Focus on Integrative Health
The Evidence for Integrative Medicine

As explained by the Academy of Integrative Health and Medicine (AIHM, n.d.), the term *alternative medicine* was replaced by *complementary and alternative medicine (CAM)*. CAM embodied the various philosophical approaches to healing that extended beyond conventional treatments and could be used either independently or in addition to traditional medical care (AIHM, n.d.). More recently, the term *integrative medicine* has replaced CAM. Integrative medicine combines the principles of CAM with conventional medical approaches. Integrative medicine, which emphasizes interprofessional collaboration among members of the healthcare team, has been successfully used in the treatment of individuals with a wide variety of conditions, including chronic pain, gastrointestinal disorders, stress, depression, and anxiety (AIHM, n.d.). Primary goals of integrative medicine include establishing best practices for promoting health and healing by way of combining evidence-based therapies with holistic approaches to healthcare (AIHM, n.d.). A study of 29 integrative medicine centers and programs across the United States found that integrative lifestyle change programs are particularly beneficial for individuals who experience chronic illness (Horrigan et al., 2012). Likewise, for individuals with depression, research has indicated that integrative interventions, such as hypnotherapy and meditation, are of benefit (Horrigan et al., 2012). Furthermore, research evidence suggests that integrative prevention strategies such as eliminating toxins from home and work environments and regular exercise are beneficial to all individuals (Horrigan et al., 2012).

Box 45–2
An Example of Using EBP to Inform Practice

Traditionally, the hypoxic drive theory has held that patients with chronically elevated blood carbon dioxide levels, such as occurs with chronic obstructive pulmonary disease (COPD), may experience respiratory failure if exposed to high levels of supplemental oxygen. The hypoxic drive theory is based on the premise that, for individuals with an abnormally high level of carbon dioxide in the blood (a condition known as hypercarbia), a high level of carbon dioxide in the air no longer serves as a stimulus for breathing. Rather, according to this theory, when chronic hypercarbia is present, the stimulus for breathing is a low level of oxygen in the air (hypoxia), and administering supplemental oxygen to a patient with chronic hypercarbia may cause respiratory depression and respiratory failure (Jerath et al., 2015).

Despite research suggesting that patients with chronic hypercarbia generally do not depend on hypoxia as a stimulus for breathing (Kim et al., 2008), the hypoxic drive theory continues to influence clinical practice (Makic et al., 2013). However, Global Initiative for Chronic Obstructive Lung Disease (GOLD) guidelines, which are based on current evidence, recommend supplemental oxygen administration for patients who demonstrate a PaO_2 of ≤55 mmHg and an oxygen saturation of ≤88%, with or without the presence of hypercarbia that has been confirmed twice in a period of 3 weeks (GOLD, 2015).

Because evidence is a product of research, being familiar with the research process helps nurses to select and evaluate practices for best patient outcomes. In a very broad definition, *research* is obtaining information and objective facts to advance knowledge about a specific topic. **Nursing research** is the use of a systematic and strict scientific process to analyze phenomena of interest to all areas of nursing, including practice, education, and administration (Nieswiadomy, 2012). **Nursing clinical research** seeks answers to questions that will ultimately improve patient care, such as the following:

- What are the links between diet and the development of diabetes and cardiovascular disease?
- Is a new drug or medical device more effective than one already on the market?
- Do patients who undergo surgery at one medical center have a higher complication rate than those who are treated at another?
- Are patients satisfied with their care during hospitalization?

Familiarity with research methodology is becoming increasingly important to nursing practice. The ability to weigh the scientific merit of a research study is key to understanding the interpretation and implications of the research findings. Not all research findings have equal validity. One factor that influences the validity of a research study is the type of methodology that is used. The various methodologies used in clinical research include quantitative research and qualitative research.

Quantitative research uses precise measurement to collect data and analyze it statistically for a summary and a description of the resulting findings or to test relationships among variables. An example of a quantitative question is "Are there differences in skin breakdown between premature infants who are bathed with plain water and those who are bathed with bacteriostatic soap?"

Qualitative research investigates a question through narrative data that explores the subjective experiences of human beings and can provide nursing with a better understanding of the patient's perspective. Goals of qualitative research include the identification of patterns and themes. An example of a qualitative question is "What is the nature of coping and adjustment after a radical mastectomy?"

Today's nurses have a wealth of nursing research available that uses the scientific method to obtain evidence (**Box 45–3 »**). Using this method limits subjective

Box 45–3
General Elements of the Scientific Method

- A question is asked about a phenomenon.
- A literature review is done to identify past research findings on the phenomenon.
- A hypothesis is proposed.
- A study, or experiment, is planned and executed.
- Data are collected, organized, and evaluated.
- A conclusion about the phenomenon is presented.

influences and bias and enhances the validity and reliability of the data.

Funding

Funding from many sources is available to nurses who are interested in doing research to advance nursing science and generate evidence that supports improved patient care (American Nurses Association [ANA], n.d.). This funding ranges from small research grants from local professional nursing chapters to larger grants awarded by state or national nursing organization foundations. Corporations, state agencies, and federal organizations also support nursing research grants. Awards are given in all areas of nursing, including gerontology, quality of life, health disparities, disease prevention, and nursing practice specialties. Examples of sources of awards and grants are Sigma Theta Tau International Honor Society of Nursing, Agency for Healthcare Research and Quality, National Institute of Nursing Research, National Council of State Boards of Nursing, Robert Wood Johnson Foundation, and the American Cancer Society.

Participants

All research studies require participants. Because each study targets a specific population (e.g., women older than 65 years with a history of hypertension), researchers develop a list of criteria, which normally includes factors such as age, weight, gender, medical history, type and present stage of a disease, and present medications taken. These qualifiers can be categorized as inclusion (acceptable) or exclusion (not acceptable) criteria. Inclusion and exclusion criteria are used to guide selection of participants that represent the target population while also ensuring protection of potential participants' physical safety and psychosocial well-being. Vulnerable populations that are subject to strict legal and ethical considerations include human fetuses, neonates, children, prisoners, educationally disadvantaged individuals, and individuals who are cognitively impaired (U.S. Department of Health and Human Services [HHS], 2016a). Even for individuals who are legally capable of consenting to participation in a research study, in some cases, safety concerns may prohibit participating. For example, particularly with medication-related research, individuals with certain medical diagnoses may be excluded from participating because of potential health risks. **Research participants** are defined as volunteers for a specific study project who meet all the inclusion criteria, have been informed of all aspects of the study, and have given informed consent.

Ethical and Legal Issues

Ethical principles used by nurses to protect patients receiving care are also used to protect participants in clinical research studies (see the module on Ethics for further information). Ethical principles are at the core of such questions as "Did the researchers maintain the participants' confidentiality?" and "Did the participants experience physical harm or psychologic distress as a result of participating in the study?" **Institutional review boards (IRBs)** review research protocols and ensure that such protocols adhere to ethical standards. As established by the 1979 landmark publication *The Belmont Report*, research must adhere to three main ethical principles: respect for persons, beneficence, and justice (HHS, 2016b).

Respect for persons comprises acknowledging and protecting the autonomy of all individuals, including individuals whose capacity to exercise autonomy is diminished because of disability, illness, circumstances that restrict liberty, or immaturity (HHS, 2016b). Researchers must ensure that the volunteers are participating freely in a study, without coercion and after receiving full disclosure about the study and the potential risks involved. *Beneficence* requires that researchers protect participants from physical injury, psychologic harm, economic insult, and exploitation during or as a result of the study. It also addresses the requirement that the study be conducted for the benefit of others. *Justice* requires the fair treatment of all participants, including the right of participants to expect their personal information to be maintained under strict confidentiality and the protection of participant anonymity. The Health Insurance Portability and Accountability Act (HIPAA) includes a Privacy Rule, which creates a national standard for the disclosure of private health information.

Legal practices related to research studies include following criminal, civil, and tort laws. Study volunteers have a legal right to full disclosure of the study's purpose, required procedures, length, expectations, risks, and possible benefits before consenting to participate. **Informed consent** includes the right to receive this information as well as the right of participants to withdraw from the study at any time. Participants must give informed consent, usually in written form, before the study begins (refer to the module on Legal Issues for further information).

Implications for Nursing Practice

The nursing profession includes both nurse clinicians and nurse researchers who are working to determine best evidence. Nursing clinical research is important to provide best evidence for EBP, to support nursing as a separate professional discipline, and to define current best practice standards of nursing care.

Providing Best Evidence for EBP

Best practices in nursing have continuously evolved as a result of research. In today's healthcare environment, it is especially crucial to participate in EBP. Practice based on the reasoning "we do it that way because we've always done it that way" is inadequate and fails to consider the research evidence supporting new and improved nursing practices. Integrating EBP is necessary to meet the current standards of high quality in nursing performance.

Supporting Nursing as a Professional Discipline

Simply stated, nurses want to be in control of nursing. Nursing history reflects its growth as a professional discipline and efforts to gain recognition as a profession in the eyes of the general public and in the eyes of members of the other healthcare professions.

The criteria for nursing to be recognized as a profession continue to evolve. They currently include the following:

1. Specialized education requirements
2. A body of well-defined knowledge and expertise
3. Conducting ongoing research

4. An orientation toward service to others
5. Following a code of ethics
6. Having autonomy as a profession
7. Professional organization (see the modules on Professional Behaviors and Accountability for additional information)

Note that the first two items in this list—specialized education requirements and a body of well-defined knowledge and expertise—both depend, in part, on nursing research.

Defining Current Best Practice Standards of Nursing Care

EBP supports changes in the responsibilities of nurses, including clinical decision making and clinical judgment, and the level and extent of nurses' accountability. Standards of nursing care are defined by the ANA, the National League for Nursing (NLN), and The Joint Commission (see the module on Accountability for more information about standards of nursing care). These organizations periodically update these standards to reflect current best evidence. Rights, responsibilities, and scopes of nursing practice are legally defined by state nurse practice acts from each state's Board of Nursing (see the modules on Professional Behaviors and Legal Issues for additional information).

In addition to the standards set by professional organizations and state boards, each healthcare facility sets performance expectations for nursing care in its policies and procedures, in accordance with the state's nursing scope of practice. To protect themselves from liability, nurses need to follow policies and procedures as written. When practice evidence supporting better patient outcomes is discovered, the nurse becomes an advocate of that best evidence. Each facility has a process to follow in suggesting changes in policies and procedures; it may be a quality improvement committee, a policies and procedures committee, or a nursing unit's chain of command. There is room for any change that benefits staff and patients, and it is incumbent on nurses, as professionals, to advocate for changes that benefit their patients.

Developing Evidence-Based Practice

EBP is a combination of the knowledge that is generated from the clinician's experience, the research evidence, and the preferences of the patient. Nurses must commit to expanding the implementation of EBP within the nursing profession. Through such efforts, nurses continue their quest for the provision of safe, effective, high-quality patient care.

Step 1: Develop a Clinical Question

Formulating the clinical question is the first step in engaging in EBP (see **Figure 45–3 》》**). Clinical questions are generated in many ways but are usually encountered during patient care. A clinical question may be knowledge-based (a background question) or practice-based (a foreground question). The type of question developed helps determine how and where to search for an answer. **Background questions** are general questions that seek more information about a topic,

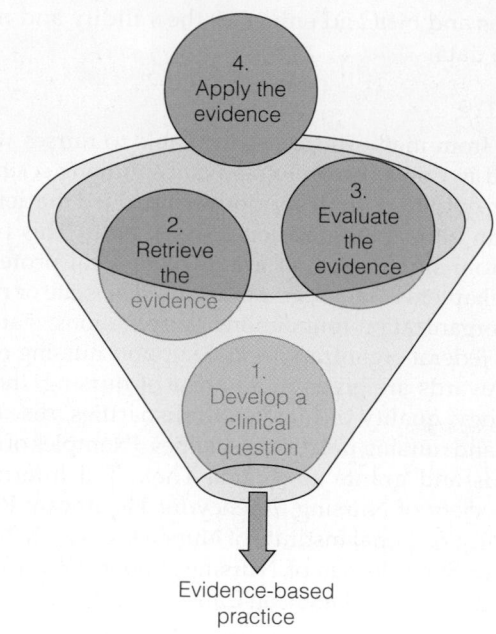

Figure 45–3 》》 The four steps in developing evidence-based practice funnel together to produce best nursing practice for safe, effective, high-quality patient care.

such as diseases or medications. These questions serve to fill gaps in knowledge about a specific topic and take the form "What is . . ." or "What does. . . . " The following are examples of background questions:

- Who is at risk for hypoglycemia?
- What are the side effects of a specific diuretic?

Answers to these questions can be found in textbooks, medical dictionaries, drug handbooks, and other educational materials.

Foreground questions are narrower in focus and are about a specific clinical issue. They are useful for finding nursing interventions that improve patient outcomes; in other words, they identify useful information about direct patient care. The following are examples of foreground questions:

- How does using an incentive spirometer (or not using one) affect the length of stay for a surgical patient?
- How does using a cooling blanket compare to using antipyretic medication as treatment for a patient with a high temperature?

Answers to these questions can be found in the studies conducted to elicit evidence. Types of research studies include the following:

- ***Meta-analysis.*** A group of studies on a given topic are examined, and their results are combined and analyzed as if they were from one large study.
- ***Case study.*** A case study is specific to one individual, issue, or event.
- ***Cohort study.*** A longitudinal study follows two groups and measures the outcomes of an exposure group with those of a nonexposure group.

TABLE 45–1 PICOT

PICOT	Definition	Factors to Consider	Examples
Population or **P**roblem of interest	What is the common factor in the group of patients? Alternatively, what is the problem that will be addressed?	Characteristic(s) common to patients in the group.	A specific age, gender, health problem, or medication taken by all group members
Intervention	What will be done to the patients?	Activity shows the difference in the patient before and after the intervention.	A treatment, medication, therapy, test, or new routine of care
Comparison group or comparing interventions	What is the difference (alternative) in the intervention being used when comparing two groups?	1. Can contrast an experimental group that receives an intervention with a control group that does not receive the intervention. 2. Can contrast an experimental group that receives the intervention of interest with a comparison group that receives a different intervention. 3. Can help establish a relationship, or the lack of a relationship, between an intervention and a predicted outcome.	1. Comparing two ways of doing something to find the best way. 2. Identifying the effect of taking medication A by comparing one group receiving medication A with a group receiving a placebo.
Outcome or desired effects	1. In response to the intervention, what is the desired effect for the patient? 2. In relationship to a selected problem, what is the desired improvement?	1. Desired effects of an intervention can be proved or disproved. 2. Improved outcomes can result from an intervention.	1. The desired effect is to minimize or eliminate a specific symptom. 2. An improved outcome is to reduce the time needed to accomplish a task.
Time frame (optional)	1. How long will the study last? 2. How long will it take to achieve the desired outcome?	Extent of time needed to study the impact of an intervention on a group may be brief or extended.	1. A brief time could be the first 12 hours after taking a medication. 2. An extended time could be 6 months following a treatment regimen.

- ***Case-control study.*** Individuals with and without a specific condition are compared to identify predictive variables.
- ***Randomized controlled trial (RCT).*** This is the strongest type of study in terms of validity. RCTs are designed to illustrate a cause-and-effect relationship by using a control group (participants who do not receive an intervention) and an experimental group (participants who do receive an intervention) (Duke University Medical Center Library, 2016).

Another consideration is determining the type of question that is of interest. This information helps to further narrow the clinical question. Types of questions are as follows:

- ***Diagnosis.*** How to select and interpret diagnostic tests; accuracy, safety, cost effectiveness
- ***Therapy.*** How to select treatments that do more good than harm to patients and lead to the best outcomes
- ***Etiology.*** How to identify causes of a condition or disease

- ***Prognosis.*** How to predict a clinical course over time and possible complications related to a condition or disease process.

Clinicians commonly use the mnemonic PICOT (or, alternatively, PICO) to define and formulate a clinical question that will contribute to EBP. **PICOT** represents the elements of a clinical question (Nieswiadomy, 2012; University of Wisconsin–Madison, 2016):

Population (of patients) or **P**roblem of interest
Intervention, prognostic factor, or type of exposure
Comparison of interventions or main alternative to the intervention (including no intervention)
Outcome (desired effect)
Time frame (optional)

Both research studies and EBP projects use PICOT questions. PICOT develops foreground questions that apply EBP to clinical situations and problems (**Table 45–1 》**).

Table 45–2 》 shows an example of the following clinical question in PICOT format: Among postoperative orthopedic patients, does hourly rounding increase patient satisfaction ratings related to nursing care?

TABLE 45–2 Example of Clinical Question in PICOT Format

Population	**I**ntervention	**C**omparison	**O**utcome	**T**ime
Postoperative orthopedic patients	Scheduled hourly rounding on a selected group of patients	No intervention/ patients who are not subject to the hourly rounding protocol	Increased patient satisfaction ratings	Four weeks of implementation and data collection

Case Study ›› Part 1

Brent Calloway is the new nurse educator for a local hospital's medical–surgical unit. During the past few months, he has observed a high number of incident reports related to nursing procedures. He wonders whether there is something he can do to lower this number and improve patient safety in the unit. One of his responsibilities is to organize a continuing education program for the annual review of competencies for the nurses. In past years, the nurses have had a mandatory meeting annually in which competencies were presented and demonstrated by the nurse educator while the nurses sat and watched. Brent is curious whether there is another, better approach to emphasize patient safety when the nurses review knowledge and skills for patient care.

Brent is aware that the staff development department uses computer technology for simulation scenarios during orientation for new nurses, and he wonders whether he could use that learning approach for continuing education programs in his division. He has helped with simulations in past employment and thinks that using this teaching strategy could support better patient safety. He questions whether changing the method of training could decrease the number of safety reports and improve patient outcomes.

Brent formulates the following PICOT elements:

P: Nursing staff

I: Simulation-based safety education

C: No intervention

O: Decreased incidence of procedural errors

T: 12 weeks for implementation of intervention and data collection

On the basis of the identified PICOT elements, Brent formulates the following clinical question: "Among nursing staff, what is the effect of simulation-based safety education on the incidence of procedural errors?"

Before developing the EBP project, Brent plans to search for current research evidence related to the use of simulation-based education to promote safe nursing practice.

Clinical Reasoning Questions Level I

1. How does an EBP project differ from a research study? How would Brent's project development change if he were planning a research study instead of an EBP project?
2. What role did Brent's experience with computer-based simulation play in development of his clinical question?
3. Using the same PICOT elements, what are some other potential versions of the clinical question?
4. In Brent's clinical question, why is the target population stated as "nursing staff" instead of "medical–surgical patients"?

Clinical Reasoning Questions Level II

5. How important is it for Brent to have the support of his manager to be motivated to explore the potential of finding a better method of providing continuing education?
6. What is the value of nurses being inquisitive about the way things are done in their nursing practice?
7. Refer to the exemplar on Competence in the module on Accountability: What role does experiential learning play in the development of clinical expertise for nurses?

Step 2: Retrieve the Evidence

Looking for clinical evidence from research sources usually includes a review of the pertinent literature. When doing a literature review for evidence, nurses look for scientific elements in the journal article, including the abstract, or

TABLE 45–3 Order of Sections Typically Found in a Professional Research Article

Section	Function
Title	Gives the main topic of the research study.
Abstract	Provides a summary of the entire content of the journal article.
Introduction	Presents the question, or focus, of the investigative study; includes background of older research on same hypothesis.
Methods	Describes in detail all the aspects and methods of the study.
Results of study	Reports statistical data; may be in the form of charts or tables.
Conclusion	Summarizes and interprets the results of the study and statistical data in relation to the hypothesis; evaluates the findings of the study.
References	Lists the resources available for additional information.

summary of the article; an overview of the study conducted, including its methodology; a written conclusion based on the results of the study; and relevant references. The order of sections typically found in a professional research article is shown in **Table 45–3** ››.

Nursing databases and resource links can yield a list of evidence articles related to the question at hand (**Table 45–4** ››). Many databases have a tutorial available. Some databases offer only abstracts; others offer the full text of the article. All sources and sites should be judged on their degree of credibility. Research resources can be found in various ways. One is to use a review-of-literature article that presents studies relative to a topic and ends with an evaluative statement, or recommendation, regarding the studies described. Another way is to use a primary resource, which is the original published article. Secondary resources, when

TABLE 45–4 Common Nursing Research Links

Name	Internet Website
Cochrane Review Database	http://www.cochrane.org
PubMed or MEDLINE Database (OVID) (includes international nursing index)	http://pubmed.gov
EBSCO Database a. DynaMed b. Cumulative Index to Nursing and Allied Health Literature (CINAHL) c. PsycINFO	a. ebscohost.com (through libraries and other institutions) b. mynursingkit.com (access EBSCO through Pearson Publishing, My Nursing Kit, My Search Lab)
Books and Articles Database	http://www.sciencedirect.com (Elsevier Publishing)
Agency for Healthcare Research and Quality (AHRQ)	http://www.ahrq.gov/about/nursing/ http://guideline.gov http://www.qualitymeasures.ahrq.gov
Evidence-Based Nursing BMJ journals (Evidence-Based Nursing, 2012)	http://ebn.bmj.com
Evidence-Based Practice Network (Evidence-Based Practice Network, 2012)	http://www.nursingcenter.com/ evidencebasedpracticenetwork/ (Lippincott Publishing)

Box 45–4
Nursing Journals

Examples of Research Journals in Nursing

Evidence-Based Nursing
Journal of Nursing Scholarship
Applied Nursing Research
International Journal of Nursing Studies
Nursing Research
Research in Nursing and Health
Scholarly Inquiry for Nursing Practice

Examples of Clinical and Specialty Nursing Journals That Publish Research

American Journal of Nursing
Journal of Emergency Nursing
Journal of Gerontologic Nursing
Journal of Nursing Administration
Journal of Nursing Education
Journal of Obstetric, Gynecologic and Neonatal Nursing
Journal of Pediatric Nursing
Journal of the American Psychiatric Nursing Association
MedSurg Nursing

Focus on Diversity and Culture
Pharmacology and Genetics

Two fields of study in particular—pharmacogenetics and pharmacogenomics—represent an intersection of research, genetics, and pharmacology (U.S. National Library of Medicine, Genetics Home Reference [GHR], 2016). Pharmacogenetics emphasizes application of the research process to study the genetic basis for unexpected drug responses demonstrated by individuals (Patil, 2015). Inherited differences, particularly those related to ethnicity and race, are key considerations to pharmacogenetics researchers. For example, pharmacogenetics is used to investigate why beta-1 blocker medications have limited efficacy when used to treat congestive heart failure among some individuals who are of African American heritage (Ortega & Meyers, 2014).

By comparison, pharmacogenomics takes a broader approach to exploring the link between genetics and pharmacology. By combining pharmacology with the study of genes and their functions (GHR, 2016), pharmacogenomics focuses on examining a multitude of genes that may influence the pharmacologic response (Patil, 2015). Both pharmacogenetics and pharmacogenomics have important implications for the development of medications that will more effectively treat health problems among a culturally diverse population.

one author is writing about the original work of another author, can also be helpful. Focusing on the most recently published materials can help narrow the number of evidence resources.

The nurse who has difficulty accessing electronic databases from work or home should make use of local reference librarians and other available resources. Many libraries, particularly at colleges and universities, have access to nursing journals both online and in print (**Box 45–4 ≫**). The nurse who cannot get support from employers and colleagues may want to do more networking with local chapters of professional organizations such as the ANA.

The Agency for Healthcare Research and Quality (AHRQ) funds 13 Evidence-Based Practice Centers (EPCs). Through their efforts, these centers improve the quality and effectiveness of healthcare by reviewing all relevant scientific literature, synthesizing the evidence, and helping to translate the evidence-based research findings so they are more readily available to clinicians who are at the bedside providing care (AHRQ, 2015).

≫ Stay Current: For more information on the 13 Evidence-Based Practice Centers, go to http://www.ahrq.gov/research/findings/evidence-based-reports/overview/index.html

Case Study ≫ Part 2

Recently, Brent Calloway read an article in his staff development journal about a research study that suggested that the use of simulation enhanced nursing competence and benefited patient safety. He wonders whether his unit could experience similar results. In the article, the nurses participating in the study reported high levels of satisfaction related to the use of simulation in a safety-controlled environment to support their learning. The results of the study also suggested that the incidence of nursing errors decreased by 30% following several sessions of simulation training.

By searching multiple databases, Brent finds several current, peer-reviewed resources, including research studies that suggest that there is a correlation between simulation-based safety training and a decreased incidence of nursing-related errors in patient care. Brent is excited about exploring the impact of implementing simulation-based education to improve nursing practice in his unit and, ultimately, to promote patient safety and improve patient outcomes.

Clinical Reasoning Questions Level I
1. Which search terms would be appropriate for Brent to use when searching an online database for scholarly resources related to his topic?
2. When seeking current scholarly resources, what limits should Brent place on the publication dates?

Clinical Reasoning Questions Level II
3. What are peer-reviewed resources? What is the rationale for Brent's inclusion of only peer-reviewed resources in the research review?
4. If Brent decided to search authoritative websites for information, what criteria would be most appropriate for use in the selection of the authoritative websites?

Step 3: Evaluate the Evidence

Evidence that is gathered must be critically appraised for validity (the degree to which the study measured what it intended to measure), reliability (the ability to produce consistent results with each use), and usefulness in applying the evidence in clinical practice. Nurses must be able to critique research articles to identify the strengths and weaknesses of the studies and their resulting evidence. By doing this, nurses can discard materials that do not meet the standards for application in patient care. Appraising clinical significance answers the question "Is the comparison difference significant enough to change nursing practice?" In other words, does the study yield

Hierarchy of Research						
Least powerful evidence	**Somewhat stronger evidence**	**More compelling evidence comes from research studies**				**Gold standard**
Opinions of reviewers that are based on their experience and knowledge	Opinions that come from well-known experts and respected authorities	Non-experimental studies: correlational, descriptive, qualitative	Quasi-experimental studies: time series, matched case-controls	Individual experimental studies	Meta-analysis of controlled studies	Large randomized controlled studies and meta-analyses of controlled studies

Figure 45–4 》 Hierarchy of research.

information that is reliable and useful enough to warrant a change in practice? Unfortunately, it is sometimes difficult to know which evidence yields best nursing practice patient care.

Measure the significance of the information gathered by rating the strength of the evidence to determine its validity and its relevance to a given clinical situation (Oncology Nursing Society, 2012). Rating the strength of evidence helps to identify best choices to support greater effectiveness and positive outcomes in specific clinical situations. To categorize scientific data, various companies and organizations use different methods to illustrate the hierarchy or levels of evidence. Assigning levels of evidence can help nurses identify the strongest evidence available for use as best practice. There is general agreement that the highest level of research (research that is considered the most reliable and valid) includes large randomized controlled studies and meta-analyses of controlled studies (**Figure 45–4 》**). Following this hierarchy, nurses can rate evidence strengths, compare the results, choose the strongest ones, and apply them to patient care for best results.

Many professional nursing organizations have developed guidelines to provide their members with evidence-based information they can use in the caring interventions of their nursing specialty. For example, the Institute for Emergency Nursing Research (IENR), which was launched by the Emergency Nurses Association (ENA, n.d.a), publishes Clinical Practice Guidelines (CPGs). Based on a comprehensive literature review and analysis, CPGs rate the strength of evidence and provide recommendation levels for practice: high, moderate, weak, and not recommended for practice (ENA, n.d.b).

Another example of rating the strength of evidence is called Putting Evidence into Practice (PEP) used by the Oncology Nursing Society. PEP helps identify and qualify evidence-based interventions for patient care and teaching. The stoplight is used as an analogy to demonstrate the following categories of evidence strength:

Green light: Strong evidence supports interventions that are likely to be effective and helpful.

Yellow light: Not enough evidence is available to determine the effectiveness of the interventions as harmful or helpful.

Red light: Strong evidence indicates that interventions are likely to be ineffective or possibly harmful (Oncology Nursing Society, 2012).

As nursing clinical research grows, so too does the amount of new published materials on nursing. Strategies that nurses can use to stay abreast of current information include participating in research committees, continuing education programs, and listservs or newsletters. Participation with other nurses in a research or journal club is an excellent way to maximize critical evaluation of current articles related to specific interests.

Case Study 》 Part 3

When Brent Calloway discussed with the vice president of his division the use of evidence to make decisions about changing training methods to improve patient safety, she agreed that it was a good idea and was very excited about it. Brent has organized a team to help him explore the topic of using simulation for experiential learning, which could positively affect patient safety outcomes. The team includes a nurse from the staff development department who is familiar with using simulation training; two staff nurses and one nurse manager from the medical–surgical division, who would be directly affected by any changes that might be implemented; and a nurse from the quality improvement division, who has experience in developing EBP.

At the first meeting, Brent explains the group's objective. He gives each member a copy of the journal article he had previously read, and he discusses his plan for the medical–surgical division. The group members decide on a course of action after discussing several possible ways to proceed. They decide to use the PICOT question Brent developed. Members of the team are asked to do a literature search for research evidence, critically appraise the evidence they find, and bring the highest-rated evidence to the next meeting for further evaluation by the team. The team will then evaluate the EBP outcomes and decide whether to change the current practice based on any new evidence found. Everyone is very enthusiastic, and they want to do all they can to help with this project.

Clinical Reasoning Questions Level I

1. Why would careful selection of members for this project team be important for the success of the project?
2. How would each team member evaluate the research evidence?
3. In the context of research findings, what is the difference between reliability and validity?

4. What other participants might Brent have asked to be on the project team to help during this EBP process?
5. What is the value of having all team members achieve consensus regarding the clinical question?

Step 4: Apply the Evidence

Once the evidence related to the clinical question has been collected and evaluated, the nurse is ready to integrate the best evidence with the nurse's own clinical experience and the patient's personal preferences. But that process in itself is not sufficient; once the nurse (or division or healthcare team) implements the change in practice, the change needs to be evaluated for its impact on patient outcomes. This process begins at implementation, with monitoring the process to make sure the change is replicated as intended. Is it being done correctly? Does it yield the intended results? Were there any unexpected results? What areas need improvement? The nurse analyzes the data collected and decides to accept, reject, or modify the change for clinical practice. If the change shows benefits to the patient, the facility, through committee work, can choose to modify policies and procedures to reflect the new practice. The change then becomes a part of the nursing routine until it is fully integrated into the standards of care.

Individual nurses can follow this process to identify the best evidence for specific clinical questions they may have about delivering care to patients assigned to them. They can evaluate and change their routines of care to maximize positive patient outcomes, such as reducing the length of stay or promoting cost effectiveness. However, the EBP process does not end with the individual nurse. After evaluation and satisfaction with patient outcomes, nurses should expand the "EBP loop" by sharing the findings with other colleagues. The results can be disseminated in a variety of ways, both informally at the agency level and, more important, formally through presentations at national conferences and by submission of articles for publication in professional journals.

Many medical facilities and professional organizations are providing more support for EBP and the dissemination of best evidence patient care outcomes. An evidence committee may be available to facilitate the evaluation of evidence. Pilot trials may be used on one nursing unit and then rolled out to the whole facility.

If this development process sounds familiar, it is probably because the steps are very similar to those of the nursing process of assessment, diagnosis, planning, implementing, and evaluation. Where the nursing process seeks to address the patient's holistic needs, the process of EBP deals with a specific clinical question that may be researched in an attempt to improve patient outcomes related to the clinical question.

The explosion of informatics in healthcare has also generated a need for a common language that individuals can use to access and share information. This common language allows nurses to code information to track nursing care processes and revise as necessary. Information technology involves more than providing or improving access to information; it also involves developing new ways for nurses to share information on best practice. Listservs, social media groups, blogs, and videoconferencing are just a few of the ways in which information may be shared through technology.

EBP is a continuing process because new evidence replaces older evidence; healthcare is not a static system; and over time, nurses advance their clinical expertise. What is known today may be changed tomorrow as science progresses. EBP gives a framework and set of tools that nurses can use systematically to improve as clinicians, using the best of its three components: patient preferences, clinical nursing experience, and current evidence (see Figure 45–3).

Case Study » Part 4

Evidence found by Brent Calloway's group demonstrated that simulation was an effective method of learning for nurses, as shown by several study outcomes brought before the group for discussion. The study outcomes the group included:

- Decreased time required to implement interventions
- Improved organization and completion of simulated tasks
- Improved infection control
- Improved communication skills that supported quick, efficient actions
- Increasing ability of nurses to anticipate needed patient interventions

These results were very exciting to the team and reinforced the value of how changes in the delivery of continuing education can achieve a positive impact on patient safety.

After reflecting on all the evidence, the group decided on an educational plan for the nurses using a simulation teaching strategy. The medical–surgical division would be able to use the simulation unit in staff development for nurse competence. The two nurses and nurse manager would answer questions from nursing staff and would serve as the division champions for simulation. The nurse with additional training in EBP would continue to serve as a resource to staff.

In addition, Brent developed a schedule to visit all units in the division to discuss simulation, and the group posted flyers in the staff break rooms about simulation. The vice-president of the medical–surgical division remained supportive of this EBP change process.

Two months after the first nurse competence simulation training was completed, Brent and the team reviewed safety reports related to nursing procedures. Initial results showed a 73% reduction in the number of safety problems. The nurses in the division reported an increased awareness of safety for patients because of the hands-on simulation training they had received. An increase in patient safety was demonstrated that supported better patient outcomes. As a result, other divisions in the hospital are interested in hearing more information about how the EBP change could enhance learning outcomes and positively affect patient safety in their divisions. A potential rollout for the whole hospital is on the agenda for discussion at the next quarterly management meeting.

Clinical Reasoning Questions Level I

1. Why was work done in advance to let the nurses know of an upcoming change in how things were being done?
2. What steps did Brent's team use to develop and implement the changes they sought?
3. Who ultimately benefited most from the EBP change in training? How?

Clinical Reasoning Questions Level II

4. For the EBP change in training to be successful, how important is "buy-in" from the nurses? From management? From the facility, as a whole, to support a general culture of EBP?

5. How could the project team integrate best evidence with nursing expertise and patient preferences in changing to an EBP method of training for the nurses?

6. In addition to improved patient safety outcomes, what benefits might result from implementation of EBP in this situation for the nurses? The facility?

Lifespan Considerations

Without exception, nurses must work within their scope of practice and adhere to federal, state, and local laws that govern their practice. Similarly, all patient care should be reflective of EBP. Although nursing care is tailored for individual patients according to a multitude of factors (for example, the patient's health, weight, age, allergies, culture, and personal preferences), the degree to which nursing practice is based on evidence should not vary. Any intervention either is based on current evidence or is not.

Healthy People 2020 provides an excellent source of national health objectives, which serve to highlight areas in which EBP is needed as well as the availability of evidence-based resources. The following sections provide an overview of selected *Healthy People 2020* objectives and resources related to caring for individuals throughout the lifespan.

Evidence-Based Practice in Care of Infants

Healthy People 2020 (HHS, 2016c) objectives include reducing the rate of fetal, neonatal, and infant deaths, including deaths resulting from birth defects and sudden unexpected infant deaths (SUIDs). Evidence-based resources related to newborns and infants address topics such as screening protocols for phenylketonuria and sickle cell disease (HHS, 2016d).

Evidence-Based Practice in Care of Children

Healthy People 2020 objectives include reducing child mortality rates as well as decreasing the incidence of transmission of preventable diseases among children. Increasing access to a *medical home*—which is a model of care that promotes physician-led, patient-centered, coordinated health services—for children with special needs is also an objective (HHS, 2016c). Evidence-based resources related to the care of children address topics including vaccination programs, obesity prevention, and screening for visual impairment among children between the ages of 1 and 5 years (HHS, 2016d).

Evidence-Based Practice in Care of Adolescents

For adolescents, *Healthy People 2020* objectives include reducing the mortality rate among this population as well as increasing the proportion of adolescents with special healthcare needs who receive patient care within a comprehensive, coordinated, family-centered system (HHS, 2016c). Evidence-based resources related to adolescent care address topics including vaccination programs, obesity prevention, and reduction of secondhand smoke exposure (HHS, 2016d).

Evidence-Based Practice in Care of Pregnant Women

For pregnant women, *Healthy People 2020* objectives include reducing mortality rates among this population, reducing the rate of pregnancy-related complications, and reducing the occurrence of cesarean births among women who are at low risk for complications (HHS, 2016c). Evidence-based resources address topics including preventing excessive alcohol consumption among pregnant women, educating mothers about breastfeeding, and screening for illnesses such as hepatitis B and bacterial vaginosis (HHS, 2016d).

Evidence-Based Practice in Care of Adults

Healthy People 2020 objectives address numerous issues related to the care of adults, including genomics and global health (HHS, 2016a). Targeting health promotion from a genomic standpoint allows for more accurate risk prediction, diagnosis, and treatment of a variety of health alterations, such as heart disease, stroke, cancer, diabetes, and Alzheimer disease (HHS, 2016e). Goals associated with the promotion of global health include protecting the health of the national population as well as limiting the international transmission of infectious diseases during travel (HHS, 2016f). Evidence-based resources related to global health and genomics are emerging.

Evidence-Based Practice in Care of Older Adults

For older adults, *Healthy People 2020* objectives address topics including increasing the number of individuals who are up to date on basic preventive care and decreasing the incidence of health alterations such as pressure ulcers and fall-related injuries (HHS, 2016e). Evidence-based resources discuss topics including screening for illnesses such as breast cancer and colorectal cancer (HHS, 2016f).

Strategies to Implement Evidence-Based Practice

Some basic activities can provide a foundation for implementing EBP. These strategies can spark the necessary stimulus to engage in behaviors that encourage best practice. Participating in EBP contributes to the knowledge of nursing and patient care in today's healthcare systems and delivery of high-quality nursing care for best outcomes.

- Assess yourself to determine how much of your current nursing practice is evidence-based. Make a list of actions you do in a clinical day. Beside each action, make a note whether it is evidence-based, the routine everyone follows, or a shortcut or whether you perform the action that way because that is how you learned it.

- Assess the obstacles that inhibit you from using EBP more frequently. These may include internal factors, such as beliefs or misconceptions, or external factors, such as lack of management support (**Box 45–5 》**).

- Practice raising questions about current clinical practices and problem solving.

- Acquire more information to correct your misperceptions of EBP.

- If you only have limited time, focus on evidence from high-yield sources—those that are current, are known for their high quality, and have content applicable to patient care.

- Go to www.guideline.gov (AHRQ) for free resource compilations of evidence reviews and practice guidelines published by a variety of groups on a wide range of topics, such as hearing screening, learning disorders, screening, treatment, and prognosis.

- Use the internet when doing searches to cut down the time needed to find good evidence choices.

- Learn how to do a critical appraisal of evidence to determine the best evidence.

- Build your awareness of how and why things are done to identify how much EBP is being used.

- Identify others interested in searching for evidence and evaluating it for collaborative opportunities such as a journal club.

- Volunteer to participate on a professional nursing practice committee.

- Participate in a research project to be a part of an EBP process.

>> **Stay Current:** AHRQ sponsors evidence reports and technology assessments through systematic reviews for health literacy interventions and outcomes from their Evidence-Based Practice Centers. Search for reports of interest to you at http://www.ahrq.gov/research/findings/evidence-based-reports/search.html.

Box 45–5
Barriers to Evidence-Based Practice

A barrier is anything that makes it difficult to progress or succeed in achieving an objective. Even though EBP can provide nurses with the satisfaction of knowing that they have given best evidence-based care to their patients to promote high positive outcomes, some typical barriers challenge nurses in implementing EBP in their daily practice. Some common barriers nurses confront in using EBP are the following:

- Work schedule and workload demands
- Patient preferences that might conflict with best practice care
- Lack of access to technology to find evidence when needed
- Limited knowledge in skills for finding and evaluating evidence
- Lack of experience and confidence in developing strategies to promote evidence-based care
- Lack of support from supervisors or agency personnel
- Lack of access to continuing education programs (e.g., due to lack of time, lack of funding, distance from program site)
- Attitudes of individual nurses (including lack of confidence in using EBP, misperceptions about EBP, lack of motivation in integrating EBP into routines of patient care, and failure to understand the value of EBP)
- Resistance to change from traditional patient care routines.

By learning the skills of EBP and gaining confidence in it, nurses are in the best position to overcome such barriers.

REVIEW   The Concept of Evidence-Based Practice

RELATE Link the Concepts

Linking the concept of evidence-based practice with the concept of cellular regulation:

1. While caring for a pediatric patient with severe stomatitis secondary to chemotherapy, the nurse is concerned because the patient's mouth ulcers are not responding to current treatment. How can the nurse ensure that he is using current EBP?

2. The nurse learns of a new treatment that has had great results with treatment-resistant stomatitis. What should the nurse do next?

Linking the concept of evidence-based practice with the concept of advocacy:

3. How can the nurse best advocate for a patient who is considering becoming a participant in a clinical trial?

4. The nurse is caring for a patient who is involved in a clinical research study. The patient says to the nurse, "I don't want to be a part of this study any longer. How do I get out of it?" What would be the nurse's therapeutic response to this patient?

REFER Go to Pearson MyLab Nursing and eText

- Additional review materials

REFLECT Apply Your Knowledge

You are caring for a patient with severe persistent asthma who requires daily doses of inhaled corticosteroids, with frequent use of oral steroids during periods of exacerbation. The patient has been invited to join a research study to determine the effects of a new medication for patients with severe persistent asthma. The lead researcher has provided the patient with the necessary information for informed consent. The patient has asked for time to think about it and discuss it with his spouse. When you enter the room, the patient asks, "What if I agree to participate and the medication doesn't work? Will that mean my asthma will get worse? Does that increase my chances of dying from an asthma attack?"

1. How can you best respond to the patient's questions?

2. How can you best advocate for this patient?

3. What are your ethical obligations to help this patient?

References

Academy of Integrative Health & Medicine (AIHM). (n.d.). *What is integrative medicine?* Retrieved from https://www.aihm.org/about/what-is-integrative-medicine/

Agency for Healthcare Research and Quality (AHRQ). (2015). *Evidence-based practice centers (EPC) program overview.* Retrieved from http://www.ahrq.gov/research/findings/evidence-based-reports/overview/index.html

American Association of Nurse Anesthetists. (n.d.) Evidence-based Practice. Available at http://www.aana.com/resources2/professionalpractice/Pages/Evidence-Based-Practice.aspx

American Nurses Association (ANA). (n.d.). *Opportunities for research funding.* Retrieved from http://nursingworld.org/research-toolkit/Research-Funding

Duke University Medical Center Library. (2016). *Introduction to evidence-based practice: Type of study.* Retrieved from http://guides.mclibrary.duke.edu/c.php?g=158201&p=1036068

Emergency Nurses Association (ENA). (n.d.a). *Practice & research.* Retrieved from http://www.ena.org/practice-research/Pages/about.aspx

Emergency Nurses Association (ENA). (n.d.b). *Clinical practice guidelines (CPGs).* Retrieved from https://www.ena.org/practice-research/research/CPG/Pages/Default.aspx

Evidence-Based Nursing. (2012). *About evidence-based nursing.* Retrieved from http://ebn.bmj.com/site/about/

Evidence-Based Practice Network. (2012). *Understanding evidence-based practice.* Retrieved http://www.nursingcenter.com/evidencebasedpracticenetwork/Home/Tools-Resources/Collections/UnderstandingEvidenceBasedPractice.aspx

Global Initiative for Chronic Obstructive Lung Disease (GOLD). (2015). *Global strategy for the diagnosis, management and prevention of COPD.* Retrieved from http://www.goldcopd.it/materiale/2015/GOLD_Report_2015.pdf

Horrigan, B., Lewis, S., Abrams, D. I., & Pechura, C. (2012). Integrative medicine in America: How integrative medicine is being practiced in clinical centers across the United States. *Global Advances in Health and Medicine, 1*(3), 18–94.

Institute of Medicine (IOM). (2000). *To err is human: Building a safer health system.* Washington, DC: National Academy Press.

Institute of Medicine (IOM). (2001). *Crossing the quality chasm: A new health system for the 21st century.* Committee on Quality of Health Care in America, Institute of Medicine. Washington DC: National Academies Press.

Jerath, R., Crawford, M. W., Barnes, V. A., & Harden, K. (2015). Widespread depolarization during expiration: A source of respiratory drive? *Medical Hypotheses, 84*(1), 31–37.

Kim, V., Benditt, J. O., Wise, R. A., & Sharafkhaneh, A. (2008). Oxygen therapy in chronic obstructive pulmonary disease. *Proceedings of the American Thoracic Society, 5*(4), 513–518.

Makic, M. B. F., Martin, S. A., Burns, S., Philbrick, D., & Rauen, C. (2013). Putting evidence into nursing practice: Four traditional practices not supported by the evidence. *Critical Care Nurse, 33*(2), 28–42.

Nieswiadomy, R. M. (2012). *Foundations of nursing research* (6th ed.). Upper Saddle River, NJ: Pearson Education.

Nightingale, F. (1946). *Notes on nursing: What it is and what it is not* (p. 59). Facsimile of the first edition printed in London, 1859, and reproduced by Edward Stern, Philadelphia, PA. (Original work published 1859). Published by Harrison.

Oncology Nursing Society. (2012). *Evidence-based practice resource area: Levels of evidence.* Retrieved from http://www.ons.org/Research/EBPRA/Process/Critique/Levels

Ortega, V. E., & Meyers, D. A. (2014). Pharmacogenetics: Implications of race and ethnicity on defining genetic profiles for personalized medicine. *Journal of Allergy and Clinical Immunology, 133*(1), 16–26.

Ostergren, J. E., Hammer, R. R., Dingel, M. J., Koenig, B. A., & McCormick, J. B. (2014). Challenges in translational research: The views of addiction scientists. *PLoS One, 9*(4), e93482.

Patil, J. (2015). Pharmacogenetics and pharmacogenomics: A brief introduction. *Journal of Pharmacovigilance, 3*, e139.

Sackett, D. L., Rosenberg, W. M., Gray, J. A., Haynes, R. B., & Richardson, W. S. (1996). Evidence based medicine: What it is and what it isn't [Editorial]. *BMJ, 312*, 71–72.

Sigma Theta Tau International. (2002). *Evidence-based nursing position statement.* Retrieved from http://www.nursingsociety.org/why-stti/about-stti/position-statements-and-resource-papers/evidence-based-nursing-position-statement

Stevens, K. (2013). The impact of evidence-based practice in nursing and the next big ideas. *OJIN: The Online Journal of Issues in Nursing, 18*(2).

UNC Health Sciences Library. (2016). Evidence-based Nursing Introduction. Available at http://guides.lib.unc.edu/c.php?g=8362&p=43029.

University of Wisconsin-Madison—Health Sciences, Ebling Library. (2016). *Nursing resources: PICO-clinical question.* Retrieved from http://research-guides.ebling.library.wisc.edu/nursing?p=1953396

U.S. Department of Health and Human Services (HHS), National Institutes of Health. (2016a). *Research involving human subjects.* Retrieved from https://humansubjects.nih.gov/

U.S. Department of Health and Human Services (HHS), Office for Human Research Protections (OHRP). (2016b). *The Belmont report.* Retrieved from http://www.hhs.gov/ohrp/regulations-and-policy/belmont-report/#xrespect

U.S. Department of Health and Human Services (HHS), Office of Disease Prevention and Health Promotion. (2016c). *Healthy people 2020 topics and objectives: Maternal, infant, and child health.* Retrieved from https://www.healthypeople.gov/2020/topics-objectives/topic/maternal-infant-and-child-health/objectives

U.S. Department of Health and Human Services, Office of Disease Prevention and Health Promotion. (2016d). *Healthy people 2020 interventions and resources: Maternal, infant, and child health.* Retrieved from https://www.healthypeople.gov/2020/topics-objectives/topic/maternal-infant-and-child-health/ebrs

U.S. Department of Health and Human Services (HHS), Office of Disease Prevention and Health Promotion. (2016e). *Healthy people 2020 topics and objectives: Older adults.* Retrieved from https://www.healthypeople.gov/2020/topics-objectives/topic/older-adults/objectives

U.S. Department of Health and Human Services, Office of Disease Prevention and Health Promotion. (2016f). *Healthy people 2020 interventions and resources: Older adults.* Retrieved from https://www.healthypeople.gov/2020/topics-objectives/topic/older-adults/ebrs

U.S. National Library of Medicine, Genetics Home Reference. (2016). *What is pharmacogenomics?* Retrieved from https://ghr.nlm.nih.gov/primer/genomicresearch/pharmacogenomics

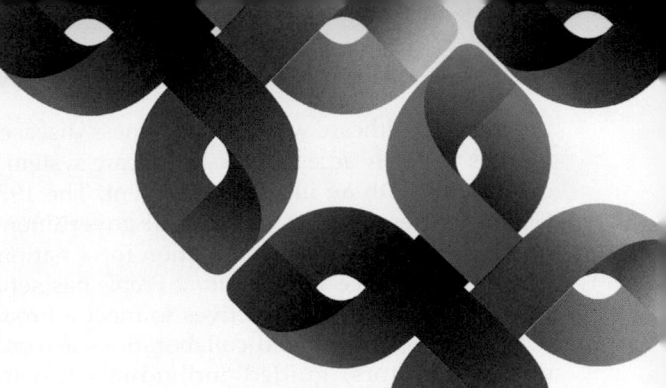

Module 46
Healthcare Systems

Module Outline and Learning Outcomes

The Concept of Healthcare Systems

Types of Healthcare Services and Settings

46.1 Differentiate the three levels of preventive healthcare systems.

Factors Affecting Delivery of Healthcare

46.2 Outline the factors affecting delivery of healthcare.

Frameworks for Providing Care

46.3 Differentiate the three common models of healthcare.

Access to Healthcare

46.4 Outline the factors that limit access to healthcare.

Nursing Care Delivery Systems

46.5 Differentiate the three models of nursing care delivery most frequently used.

Concepts Related to Healthcare Systems

46.6 Outline the relationship between healthcare systems and other concepts.

Resource Allocation

46.7 Explain the issues with allocation of resources and the nurse's role in decision making.

Healthcare Systems Exemplar

Exemplar 46.A Emergency Preparedness

46.A Analyze emergency preparedness as it relates to healthcare systems.

» The Concept of Healthcare Systems

Concept Key Terms

Case management, **2778**	Managed care, **2778**	Primary prevention, **2775**	Team nursing, **2782**	Uninsured, **2779**
Functional nursing, **2782**	Patient-focused care, **2779**	Resource allocation, **2784**	Tertiary prevention, **2775**	Unlicensed assistive personnel (UAP), **2782**
Health literacy, **2778**	Primary nursing, **2782**	Secondary prevention, **2775**	Underinsured, **2779**	
Health promotion, **2776**				

The concept of healthcare systems relates to the methods of healthcare delivery and management, including financing and coordination of services. Particularly in the past two decades, new cost-containment strategies and advances in technology—both informatics and medical technology—have combined to significantly change healthcare systems in the United States.

Nurses must have a solid understanding of the different types of healthcare settings and frameworks used to provide care. Some agencies use a combination of models, and each agency has its own specific policies and procedures. Nurses must understand that the concept of healthcare systems impacts all other concepts. Nurses must know the requirements of the agency in which they practice.

In addition, nurses must understand the barriers patients face to accessing healthcare, the issues they themselves face when resources are insufficient to meet patients' needs, and their agency's and community's expectations for them when a disaster occurs.

Types of Healthcare Services and Settings

Healthcare delivery can be classified by the type of services offered. Today's healthcare systems tend to be oriented toward prevention. A **primary prevention** service focuses on health promotion and illness prevention. **Secondary prevention** services include the diagnosis and treatment of disease. **Tertiary prevention** consists of the restoration of health following an illness or accident and includes rehabilitation and palliative services.

Primary Prevention

Primary prevention attempts to avoid development of disease as much as possible and promotes healthy living. Until the 1980s, healthcare was actually illness/disease care. Individuals typically accessed the healthcare system only when confronted with an illness or accident. The 1979 Surgeon General's Report from the federal government's *Healthy People* program laid the foundation for a national prevention agenda. Since 1979, *Healthy People* has set and monitored national health objectives to meet a broad range of health needs, encouraged collaborations across communities and sectors, guided individuals toward making informed health decisions, and measured the impact of prevention activities. *Healthy People 2020* sets a number of goals and identifies a number of leading health indicators (discussed in the module on Health, Wellness, Illness, and Injury), which, if addressed, should result in an increase in the quality and length of life and the eradication of health disparities.

Healthy People 2020 includes new initiatives that address health issues that came to the forefront of healthcare in the previous 10 years, such as dementias (including Alzheimer disease); healthcare-associated infections; early and middle childhood health; and lesbian, gay, bisexual, and transgender health (Office of Disease Prevention and Health Promotion [ODPHP], 2017a). Work has begun collecting data for *Healthy People 2030*, and the Office of Disease Prevention and Health Promotion seeks public feedback on their efforts (ODPHP, 2017b).

>> **Stay Current:** For the full list of *Healthy People 2020* topics and objectives, visit www.healthypeople.gov/2020/topicsobjectives2020/default.aspx. To keep abreast of or even participate in the development of the *Healthy People 2030*, you can subscribe to the Healthy People listserv, and follow @GoHealthyPeople on Twitter.

Health promotion is another tool used to improve individuals' health. The World Health Organization (1998) defines **health promotion** as the process of enabling people to increase control over and to improve their health. While the primary purpose of health promotion is to improve an individual's quality of life, there are additional benefits. For example, preventing disease and using health promotion techniques to improve health are more cost effective than treating illness and disease; therefore, both approaches help to reduce healthcare expenses.

The nurse has an integral role in health promotion. The nurse's aim should be to teach patients how to remain healthy, thus preserving wellness. The overarching goal is to ensure that patients understand the importance of setting health goals for themselves and their children and that patients are able to assess, implement, and evaluate the goals, and modify them as their health needs change. Some examples of how nurses participate in health promotion include providing health education at every opportunity; evaluating and screening patients to identify prevention opportunities such as immunizations; and promoting wellness in the community by organizing and participating in community events such as health fairs.

Examples of current health promotion topics, identified both by *Healthy People 2020* and by individual states and communities, are childhood obesity and nutrition, physical activity across the lifespan, dental/oral health, tobacco use and smoking cessation, and health screening recommendations.

By implementing health promotion strategies, the nurse has an opportunity to step out of the secondary prevention area and into the primary prevention area. This shift increases nurses' satisfaction because they have an opportunity to contribute to the health of all patients—not just those who are ill but also those whose overall health status is free of illness, such as smokers who are disease free.

Secondary Prevention

Secondary prevention activities are aimed at early disease detection and treatment to prevent the progression of the disease and its associated symptoms. Screening is a means of early detection of diseases such as hypertension and vision or hearing problems. Screenings may be provided by primary healthcare providers and through health fairs. They may be offered to the general population or focused on groups at high risk.

Tertiary Prevention

Tertiary prevention involves restoring function and decreasing disease-related complications of an already established disease. When restoration to the previous level of functioning is not possible, care is focused on controlling symptoms and promoting the highest quality of life. Tertiary prevention includes rehabilitation and palliative care.

The three levels of prevention are summarized in **Table 46–1 >>**.

Healthcare Settings

Primary care is delivered in a variety of settings, including physicians' offices, hospital-based clinics, community health centers, and public health service locations (**Figure 46–1 >>**). Primary care should not be confused with primary prevention described in the previous section. Community health centers and public health organizations frequently offer health promotion activities at locations such as churches, shopping malls, and community cultural events.

In the context of managed care, the primary care setting is often the point of entry and the location of gatekeeping for all other care. Primary care involves the provision of health maintenance services such as routine physicals, immunizations, treatment of common acute illnesses, and support for psychosocial needs.

Secondary care is typically delivered in a hospital, outpatient surgical center, or specialist's office. The most cost-effective, efficient place of service should be selected as the optimal place of service. For example, a dermatologist may remove an adult's uncomplicated basal cell carcinoma in the office. In this instance, the office setting is the most appropriate, cost-effective place of service because removal of this type of lesion involves only a minor surgical procedure under local anesthesia.

Tertiary care that involves complicated diagnostic or therapeutic procedures may be provided in a place of service such as a hospital, a rehabilitation center, or an extended care facility. Wherever a patient receives tertiary care, the nurse, as the patient's advocate, will coordinate the patient's care and treatment and ensure the patient's compliance with treatment.

TABLE 46–1 Levels of Prevention

Level and Description	Examples
Primary Prevention	
Take action to prevent disease in generally healthy people and populations. Give people tools that empower them to improve their own health through positive actions such as smoking cessation and eating well.	■ Educate individuals, families, and populations on topics such as the importance of nutrition, exercise, dental hygiene, prenatal care, immunization, and smoking cessation. ■ Educate employers and employees about occupational safety as well as avoidance of occupational hazards. ■ Improve environmental sanitation and provide adequate housing and nutrition (e.g., removing lead from housing units, making fresh produce available in areas designated as food deserts).
Secondary Prevention	
Detect and then treat identified injuries and diseases early so that they can be cured or their associated symptoms and complications can be prevented or limited.	■ Perform risk assessments for healthy people who have risk factors for specific diseases such as coronary artery disease and diabetes; then work with each patient to develop and implement a risk reduction plan. ■ Encourage regular dental, vision, and medical screening examinations for children and adults (primary care providers should follow guidelines such as *Healthy People 2020* or the recommendations of the U.S. Preventive Services Task Force when evaluating patients' screening needs). ■ Teach patients to perform self-screening examinations such as testicular examinations and mole checks for possible melanoma. ■ In all settings, develop and implement care plans to treat patients' illnesses and injuries (e.g., administer medication and treatment regimens) and prevent complications (e.g., turn, position, and exercise patients to prevent pressure ulcers and deep venous thromboses); ensure adequate rest, food intake, and fluid intake to promote healing and promote fecal and urinary elimination.
Tertiary Prevention	
Begins after a condition is treated and stabilized or recognized as incurable. Includes the restoration of function and decrease of complications of an established disease. If restoration to the previous level of function is not possible, care focuses on controlling symptoms and promoting the highest quality of life possible. Rehabilitation and palliative care are included in tertiary prevention.	■ Refer a patient with a new urostomy to an RN ostomy management specialist to learn how to care for and improve life with an ostomy. ■ Refer a patient with diabetes to a registered dietitian for education on how diet can affect the complications of diabetes. ■ Refer individuals with severe or chronic pain to a pain specialist to manage pain with an appropriate medication regimen and/or alternative treatment methods. ■ Refer individuals with mobility issues to physical therapy or rehabilitation services to promote mobility and prevent falls and other mobility-related complications.

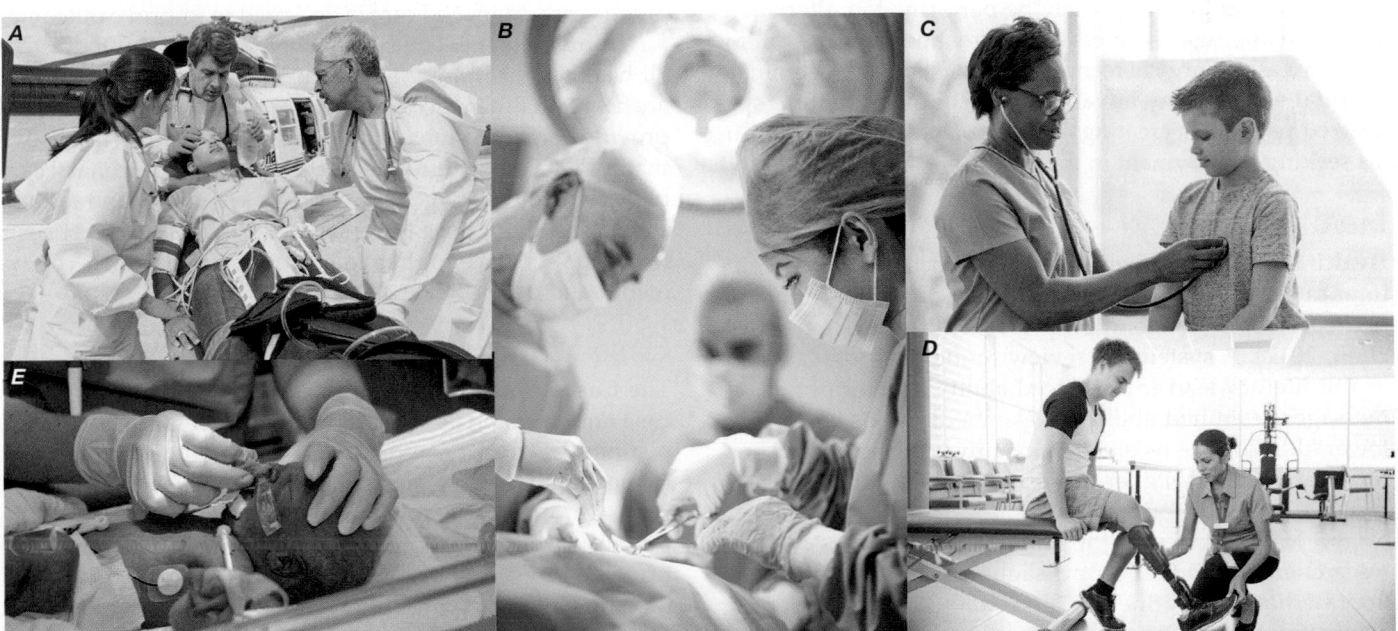

Source: **A,** Sturti/iStock/Getty Images. **B,** Comstock/Stockbyte/Getty Images. **C,** Johnny Greig/E+/Getty Images. **D,** FatCamera/E+/Getty Images. **E,** Pelicankate/iStock/Getty Images.

Figure 46–1 》 Nurses practice in many healthcare settings. Clockwise from top left: **A,** a nurse in the emergency department with a patient coming in from a medical flight; **B,** a surgical nurse in the OR; **C,** a nurse in a pediatrician's office; **D,** a nurse working in a rehabilitation hospital; **E,** and a nurse in the neonatal intensive care unit. Other settings where nurses work include schools, public health departments, patient's homes, prisons, insurance companies, colleges and universities, and publishing companies.

Factors Affecting Delivery of Healthcare

A number of factors affect the ability of the nurse to deliver patient care, regardless of the competency or proficiency of the nurse or the level of care or the setting in which care is being delivered. These include changing demographics, advances in technology, and levels of health literacy of patients in the community.

Changing Demographics

By the mid-21st century, the United States will be more racially and ethnically diverse, as well as much older, according to projections released by the U.S. Census Bureau (2014). Life expectancy is also expected to increase among all groups. The other major change that will impact healthcare delivery systems is drivers of mortality. Whereas the rates of smoking have decreased among those age 25–44, the rates of obesity have dramatically increased between 1980 and 2008, doubling for adults and tripling for children. This will lead to increases in obesity-related conditions such as adverse lipid concentrations, type 2 diabetes, and hypertension.

Advances in Technology

Scientific knowledge related to healthcare continues to increase rapidly, leading to ever more sophisticated technology. Information management systems have been created and are continually being refined. Such systems support bedside charting, barcoding for medication administration, and use of online evidenced-based guidelines to provide appropriate care. Advances in laparoscopic surgical techniques have resulted in fewer hospitalizations for some surgeries because they can safely be performed at alternative sites such as surgical centers. Other treatments such as minimally invasive surgical techniques may shorten or eliminate hospital stays. Many advances in technology require specialized personnel, creating new opportunities for individuals seeking employment in the healthcare sector.

Health Literacy

Health literacy is defined the as the capacity to obtain, communicate, process, and understand basic health information and services to make appropriate health decisions (Koh et al., 2012). A systematic review found that low levels of health literacy lead to a reduced ability to interpret health messages, a limited ability to take medications correctly, a lower likelihood of receiving preventive care, increased hospitalizations, and higher use of emergency care (Berkman et al., 2011). In the only population-level survey conducted by the National Center for Educational Statistics in 2003, researchers found that only a slight majority of adults had intermediate health literacy skills and 36% had a basic or below basic level. Despite this, our healthcare systems function as if all patients have literacy skills (Koh et al., 2012). For many tasks in the healthcare systems, patients must employ print literacy (writing and reading), oral literacy (listening and speaking) and numeracy (using and understanding numbers such as medication dosages).

Healthcare illiteracy and ineffective communication place patients at risk for poor health outcomes. According to the National Institutes of Health (2013), African Americans, Hispanics, Native Americans, and Asian Pacific Islanders, representing about 25% of the U.S. population, continue to experience health disparities, including shorter life expectancy and higher rates of diabetes, cancer, heart disease, stroke, substance abuse, infant mortality, and low birth weight. Providing health education programs for these populations is one of the key strategies for overcoming this health disparity.

Health literacy also involves policies and strategies at the organizational level. Agencies that strive to be health-literate organizations continuously work to improve verbal interactions, improve written communications, link to support systems, and engage patients and caregivers as partners in care and improvement efforts. Technology also plays a role. Many agencies offer virtual patient portals and websites that provide an array of evidence-based information and resources ranging from topics such as how to prepare a child for surgery to tips on how to care for loved ones with chronic illnesses.

Frameworks for Providing Care

In the United States, the three common models of healthcare are managed care, case management, and patient-focused care. Sometimes the frameworks overlap (e.g., services may be coordinated through a case management model to patients whose health insurance plan uses a managed care model).

Managed Care

Managed care, discussed in detail in the module on Managing Care, is a method of delivering cost-effective and high-quality care. Managed care is designed to improve outcomes for groups of patients; its framework can be adapted across all healthcare settings. The primary managed care models are health maintenance organizations (HMOs) and preferred provider organizations (PPOs). HMOs are more restrictive than PPOs and require that a patient select a primary care physician who manages the patient's secondary and tertiary services. Although a PPO is less restrictive, the direct costs to the patient are higher (e.g., higher premiums, copayments, and deductibles).

Case Management

The Case Management Society of America (2012) defines **case management** as "a collaborative process of assessment, planning, facilitation and advocacy for options and services to meet an individual's and family's comprehensive health needs through communication and available resources to promote quality, cost-effective outcomes." Multidisciplinary teams led by a case manager are at the heart of successful case management. Case management is essential when a patient has multiple care needs and requires the services of multiple providers. The goal of case management is to reach and then maintain the individual's optimal level of health, quality of life, and activities of daily living (ADLs) by ensuring that the individual's healthcare needs are met. The case manager may be a nurse, a social worker, or another healthcare team member. Case management enables patients to experience continuity of care, regardless of the location at which the care is provided. This activity on behalf of a patient may be limited to a hospitalization or may occur across settings for patients receiving care in the community and/or at home.

Patient-focused Care

Patient-focused care is a delivery model that organizes healthcare around the expressed physical and emotional needs of the patient. Patient-focused care is generally understood to be an approach that considers patients and their families to be integral to decisions regarding healthcare delivery.

Access to Healthcare

For most Americans who have healthcare coverage through an employer, high-quality healthcare is available without a long wait and at a reasonable cost. However, such healthcare is often beyond the reach of the many Americans who work for small employers, the unemployed and underemployed, the self-employed, the poor, and members of underserved minorities. These groups face many challenges to accessing healthcare and, as a result, often have poorer health outcomes—in some cases worse than those of residents of developing countries. A 2011 report from the Agency for Healthcare Research and Quality (AHRQ, 2011), titled *National Healthcare Disparities Report*, confirms that people of racial and ethnic minority groups and those of low socioeconomic status have disproportionately more access problems than others. Inadequate access to healthcare has a large impact on society. For example, a failure to receive immunizations against or early treatment of contagious diseases can result in community outbreaks. The healthcare reform acts signed into law by President Obama in early 2010 were designed to remedy some of the disparities in access to health insurance coverage and other related problems.

Uninsured individuals are those without any type of healthcare coverage. Uninsured individuals do not qualify for public health insurance programs, such as Medicaid, and cannot buy health insurance, usually because they work for employers who do not offer health insurance coverage. Uninsured patients also include those who cannot afford to purchase insurance through their employer because the insurance premiums are too expensive. During recent decades, even individuals who were self-employed had difficulty purchasing health insurance privately, either because the premiums were unaffordable or because they were denied coverage because of preexisting conditions. One of the most popular provisions of the Affordable Care Act was that it prevented insurance companies from denying coverage based on preexisting conditions, even for those who with employer-based insurance. **Underinsured** individuals have healthcare coverage that is insufficient to meet their needs. Examples include the child who is covered under a parent's company policy, but the policy does not include immunizations, and the patient with a chronic illness whose insurance does not include coverage for medications. Continued healthcare reform may resolve these gaps in coverage.

Access to healthcare means having "the timely use of personal health services to achieve the best health outcomes" as documented in the Institute of Medicine's 1993 report titled *Access to Healthcare in America*, a document that is still widely cited today. As noted in the report and more recently quoted in *Healthy People 2020*, accessing healthcare requires three discrete steps:

1. Gaining entry into the healthcare system
2. Getting access to sites of care where the patient can receive needed services
3. Finding providers with whom the patient can communicate, develop a trusting relationship, and have individual needs met.

Lack of Health Insurance

In 2013, the rate of uninsured non-elderly had dropped to 16.7%, and it continued to drop over the next 3 years. As of January 2017, some 28 million people were enrolled through the ACA Marketplace (12.2 million) or Medicaid expansion (over 16 million) (Centers for Medicare & Medicaid Services, 2017; Macpac, 2017; Mangan, 2016). Many of these newly insured had gone without insurance for long periods of time. The largest gains in coverage were seen among poor and low-income individuals and people of color. Hispanic and Black populations had the largest declines in uninsured rates. Despite these improvements, there are still people who do not have health insurance.

The primary reason individuals are uninsured is that they cannot afford to be insured. Some 3 million poor uninsured adults earn too much money to qualify for Medicaid. People who are uninsured may delay treatment or opt not to receive it because they must choose to pay either for medical care or for basic necessities such as food and housing. Most uninsured individuals do not receive healthcare services for free or at a reduced charge and are often billed at a higher rate. In 2014, one third of uninsured adults had medical debts sufficient to put them at risk of bankruptcy (Henry J. Kaiser Family Foundation, 2015).

Children with health insurance are more likely to stay healthy and do well in school, setting them on a course for better health and better opportunities throughout their childhood and teens. Children with healthcare coverage receive preventive care; are treated for sickness and injuries when they occur; are immunized against childhood diseases; are seen for well-child visits required for participation in school and sports; and receive treatment for recurring illnesses such as ear infections. Well children are more likely to attend school regularly and have an easier time focusing on their schoolwork (Insure Kids Now, 2013).

The Affordable Care Act affected children favorably because it prevented insurance companies from denying coverage for preexisting conditions and from dropping insured individuals or their dependents because of the onset of serious illness (Henry J. Kaiser Family Foundation, 2013).

SAFETY ALERT In 1986, Congress enacted the Emergency Medical Treatment and Active Labor Act (EMTALA) to ensure public access to emergency services regardless of ability to pay. Prior to the enactment of this law, providers of emergency services often refused to treat patients who were uninsured and who could not afford to pay for services. Under Section 1867 of the Social Security Act, Medicare-participating hospitals that offer emergency service must provide a medical screening examination (MSE) when a patient asks for examination for or treatment of an emergency medical condition (EMC), including active labor. The law requires that this service be provided regardless of an individual's ability to pay. Hospitals must also provide stabilizing treatment for patients with EMCs. If unable to stabilize a patient or if the patient requests it, the emergency care provider must arrange for an appropriate transfer (EMTALA, 2011).

Lack of a Usual Source of Care

According to the AHRQ (2011), individuals with a *usual source of care* (i.e., a facility where the individual regularly receives care) experience improved health outcomes, fewer health disparities, and lower costs. A usual source of care is sometimes referred to as a *medical home* or *healthcare home*.

If a patient has a primary care provider (i.e., a physician or nurse from whom the patient regularly receives care), trust and communication between the patient and provider are improved, resulting in the likelihood that the care provided to the patient will be appropriate and of high quality (AHRQ, 2011). A primary care provider who learns about the diverse needs of patients over time is better able to meet those needs. Despite this fact, over 40 million Americans do not receive regular care from a primary care provider.

The United States Department of Health & Human Services (USDHHS), the American Academy of Pediatrics, and the American Medical Association developed national guidelines for preventive health services for infants, children, and adolescents (**Box 46–1 》**). These guidelines are supported by the National Association of Pediatric Nurse Associates and Practitioners (NAPNAP).

Children and families are better served when they have a usual source of healthcare that allows parents to forge an ongoing relationship and a high comfort level with their provider and increases the likelihood that they will seek healthcare for their children. Providers are able to give comprehensive, family-centered treatment because of their knowledge of the child and family, including the family's dynamics, possible risks, and need for protection. One source of such treatment is the patient-centered medical home, which is not a location but a standards-based approach to providing primary care in which the healthcare facility forges a partnership with the patient and the patient's family (**Box 46–2 》**).

Box 46–1
National Guidelines for Health Promotion

- *Bright Futures*, American Academy of Pediatrics (original editions by Maternal and Child Health Bureau, Health Resources and Services Administration, USDHHS)
- *Put Prevention Into Practice*, Agency for Healthcare Research and Quality
- *Guide to Clinical Preventive Services*, U.S. Preventive Services Task Force
- *Guidelines for Adolescent Preventive Services*, American Medical Association

Box 46–2
Six Principles of a Patient-centered Medical Home

The most standard definition of a patient-centered medical home is provided in the *Joint Principles of the Patient-Centered Medical Home*, adopted by the American Academy of Family Physicians, American Academy of Pediatrics, American College of Physicians, and the American Osteopathic Association in 2007. This groundbreaking concept is still in use and was quoted by Andrea Bachrach et al. (2011) in *Pediatric Medical Homes: Laying the Foundation of a Promising Model of Care*.

This joint statement defines medical homes as both "an approach to providing comprehensive primary care for children, youth and adults" and "a healthcare setting that facilitates partnerships between individual patients, and their personal physicians, and when appropriate, the patient's family." It lists seven principles that characterize medical homes. Six are listed below; the seventh (omitted here) addresses appropriate payment to medical home providers.

1. *Personal physician.* Each patient develops an ongoing relationship with a personal physician who provides comprehensive medical care from the initial visit onward.
2. *Physician-directed medical practice.* The patient's personal physician leads a healthcare team that works together and accepts responsibility for the ongoing care of the patient.
3. *Whole person orientation.* The personal physician, who is responsible not only for providing and overseeing medical care to the patient but also for ensuring that all healthcare needs are met, prevents fragmentation of care by arranging for and following up on care provided by other qualified professionals, such as specialists, and ensuring that the patient returns to the medical care home.
4. *Coordinated and integrated care.* Care must be coordinated and/or integrated across all elements of the complex healthcare system and the patient's community, and it must be provided in a way that meets the patient's cultural and linguistic needs. Coordination and integration are facilitated by using strategies such as such as electronic health records and health information exchanges.
5. *Quality and safety.* Quality and safety are critical elements of the medical home.
6. *Access to care.* Access to care is facilitated by systems such as open scheduling; expanded hours; and improved means of communication among patients, their personal physician or nurse practitioner, and practice staff.

Perceptions of Need

Perceived need often affects an individual's decision to access the healthcare system. Patients may not always be able to assess their own need for care. However, when they believe they need care for illness and injury and are unable to obtain it, they perceive that care is difficult to access. These perceived difficulties include delays in getting care as soon as it is wanted.

Clinical Example A

A nurse working for a large insurance company as a telephone triage nurse receives a call late at night from a member reporting that her 4-year-old daughter woke with ear pain that has not responded to acetaminophen administered by mouth 15 minutes ago. The mother reports that the child is crying in pain and requests authorization to go to the hospital emergency department. The nurse provides strategies to treat the child's pain and explains that oral analgesics require 45–60 minutes to begin taking effect. The nurse offers to make an appointment with the primary care provider in the morning. When the mother states that the child must be seen immediately, the nurse suggests that the mother take the child to a 24-hour urgent care center. The mother declines, insisting that the child be treated immediately at the emergency department.

Critical Thinking Questions

1. Does this nurse have the right to inform parents they cannot take the child to the emergency department because this is not an emergency?
2. How does the mother's perception of need affect her response?
3. What else might the nurse do to help the parent more accurately perceive the child's healthcare needs?

Uneven Distribution of Services

The distribution of healthcare services in the United States is problematic because it is uneven. Many geographic areas and populations are medically underserved. Rural areas come to mind as areas that are likely to lack medical resources; however, suburban and urban areas may also be underserved because of poverty as well as cultural and linguistic barriers to healthcare access. Another factor that causes a community or population to be underserved is a shortage of primary care professionals such as primary care physicians, nurse practitioners, nurses, and physician assistants. Availability varies from region to region, from state to state, and even within cities themselves, where the poorest communities may be underserved.

This uneven distribution is seen across professions in the healthcare field. There are 3.1 million registered nurses in the United States and the District of Columbia. Except for California and Texas, the states with the highest number are found in the eastern half of the U.S. The same pattern holds for nurse practitioners, who numbered 153,092 in 2016. Family medicine practitioners are only slightly more evenly distributed. There are no states that have enough primary care providers to meet their needs. The desirable ratio of primary care physician to population is 1 to 3000, assuming the needs of the population are average (Henry J. Kaiser Family Foundation, 2016). Uneven distribution is aggravated by the increasing number of healthcare providers who specialize. This shift to specialization decreases the number of primary care providers who are available at any given time. Specialization can be advantageous, given the complexity of healthcare today, but it is also disadvantageous because it may increase fragmentation of care and costs. Increased specialization is a factor that increases the need for care management.

Solutions

The United States has addressed and continues to address the problem of the uninsured and the underinsured in many ways. Although controversial, the most far-reaching recent solution has been the Affordable Care Act, which was created to ensure that all U.S. citizens have access to affordable, quality care and to curb the growth of healthcare costs. The ACA will likely be changed significantly in the coming years.

>> **Stay Current:** Keep abreast of the changes in healthcare and insurance laws by visiting the U.S. Department of Health & Human Services at https://www.hhs.gov/healthcare/about-the-aca/index.html and Medicaid.gov at https://www.medicaid.gov/affordable-care-act.

Other older programs include the following:

- Medicare for older adults
- Medicaid, which assists people with lower incomes and older adults who require services not covered by Medicare, such as nursing homes, as well as some people with disabilities.
- CHIP, which assists with coverage for children whose families earn too much to qualify for Medicaid coverage but too little to afford private health insurance.

Local health departments and community health centers are sources of care for individuals without health insurance or who have gaps in their coverage. Community health centers offer primary and preventive care to millions of Americans for free or at a low cost. Anyone may obtain care from these clinics regardless of income. The cost of care is determined by using a sliding scale that is based on an individual's income (HealthCare.gov, 2013). The ACA increased the funding so Medicaid pay to physicians is increased for 2 years and the availability in many states has risen by 8% (Blumenthal et al., 2015). In addition, the ACA has funded the National Health Service Corps for physicians and refunded the Nurse Service Corps for nurses to support education and loan repayment.

As illustrated in the clinical example above, a patient's perceived need for healthcare services can be a barrier to access. It may cause patients to seek care that is unnecessary or care that is necessary but provided at an inappropriate and often more expensive place of service than needed. The nurse can change the patient's perception of need (thereby promoting appropriate and timely healthcare) by managing patient care; teaching adults about self-care and the care of their children; and teaching them when and how to access appropriate care.

Implementation of a team approach to healthcare favorably affects the availability of primary care. As physicians are teamed with nurses and nurse practitioners who manage those aspects of patient care that do not require a physician's expertise, physicians will have more time available to devote to those elements of care requiring their knowledge and skills.

Clinical Example B

Helena Alvarez is a pregnant, 19-year-old woman, who arrives at the emergency department of a small rural hospital with severe cramping pains and bleeding. She has no health insurance. No maternity services are available at this hospital, and no obstetricians are available in the community. There is a tertiary care facility about 100 miles away.

Critical Thinking Questions

1. How would you determine what options are available for providing care for Ms. Alvarez?
2. As a nurse, what are your obligations to Ms. Alvarez?

Nursing Care Delivery Systems

Three models of nursing care delivery are frequently used where patient care is provided. These are functional nursing, team nursing, and primary nursing.

Functional Nursing

Functional nursing is a task-oriented approach to care delivery. Although it is not used routinely, it may be implemented when systems are stressed by factors such as inadequate staffing resulting from nursing shortages or significant weather events such as major snowstorms. In this approach, the head nurse delegates tasks to team members who complete these specific tasks rather than caring for specific patients. For example, one nurse is responsible for delivering medications and changing dressings while another performs administrative functions such as monitoring orders and communicating with physicians and other departments to arrange for services. Functional nursing is an efficient approach because it enables the nursing team to complete many tasks in a short time. **Unlicensed assistive personnel (UAP)** are a critical component of functional nursing. They are paraprofessionals who are unlicensed but may be certified. The primary role of the UAP is to assist patients with ADLs and provide other types of basic care. UAPs act under the direction of licensed professionals such as registered nurses who delegate activities to them. When UAPs assist patients with activities such as feeding, bathing, and ambulating, registered nurses are able to focus on performing more complex tasks.

Because fewer nurses are needed, functional nursing is cost effective. However, depersonalization and fragmentation of care may result because there is limited opportunity for team members to view the patient holistically. Nurses often become dissatisfied with their role in patient care because it is limited to tasks. Patients also may be dissatisfied because they cannot identify "their nurse," that is, one individual who is responsible for their care.

Team Nursing

Team nursing is the delivery model most frequently used today. It is a means of providing individualized care to patients that was developed in response to the fragmentation of care inherent in the functional model. The registered nurse who serves as the team leader is accountable for the care provided to the patients assigned to the team. The team leader retains responsibility and authority for the patients' overall well-being but delegates some tasks to UAPs. Team members are assigned tasks based on their ability to perform them. While this model frees the professional nurse to attend to more complex patient care tasks, frequent changes in assignments may lead to a lack of continuity of care for patients. A modification to the team nursing concept is pod nursing. In pod nursing, larger units are broken down into smaller pods and teams of nurses and UAPs work together in closer geographical areas where they have closer access to supplies to keep them closer to their patients. This model maintains smaller teams with greater degrees of partnership (Friese et al., 2014).

Primary Nursing

In the **primary nursing** model, one nurse has 24/7 authority and responsibility for the care of an assigned group of patients. The primary nurse (PN) cares for the assigned patients during her shift from the time of admission through discharge. Primary care nursing is a relationship-based model of care. The PN is responsible for assessing patients, developing care plans, and providing direct care. When the PN is absent, an associate nurse will provide care under the guidance of the care plan developed by the PN. In this model, UAPs are actively involved in providing direct patient care and are assigned tasks by the PN or associate nurse in the PN's absence.

Concepts Related to Healthcare Systems

Healthcare systems refers to the broad array of people, institutions, and resources that provide care to people locally, within a state, across the nation, and internationally. Care is provided at many different places of service, and the nurse must be prepared to function in each. Each of these components of the healthcare system faces its own ethical dilemmas, legal issues, managed care issues, and clinical decision-making challenges. These challenges are particularly acute in a time of disaster, when concise, accurate, and timely communication becomes even more important. For example, nurses will face ethical and legal issues associated with the provision of care in mass casualty events (MCEs) (e.g., who will not receive care, who will receive care, and when and where care will care be provided). They will also be challenged as they decide what care to provide to the patients they are caring for during a disaster (e.g., when has sufficient care been provided to permit the patient to be transported, and how does one safely provide care when resources are strained?). Communication among the various emergency team members must be concise, accurate, and timely during an MCE. Nurses must use their knowledge to foster better communication. The Concepts Related to Healthcare Systems feature lists some, but not all, of the concepts integral to healthcare systems. They are listed in alphabetical order.

Resource Allocation

For more than two decades, the escalating cost of healthcare in the United States has been a concern. Gaining control over increasing healthcare expenditures has been a goal of both the government and private entities. Many factors are responsible for the increasing cost of healthcare. These include increased longevity, increases in the prevalence of chronic diseases such as diabetes, continued medical advances (which may result in more accurate diagnoses and better treatment but are often more expensive than existing methods), technologic advances, consumer demand, and defensive medicine (ordering a test or procedure to avoid litigation). Inappropriate healthcare treatment choices by consumers have also contributed to increased healthcare costs. As discussed in the module on Managing Care, employees have enjoyed the benefits of employer-negotiated

Concepts Related to
Healthcare Systems

CONCEPT	RELATIONSHIP TO HEALTHCARE SYSTEMS	NURSING IMPLICATIONS
Communication	Because of the uncertainties, confusion, and sheer demands of an emergency, communications may be fragmented and difficult. Yet an emergency is the very time when clear, effective communication is critical.	■ You will immediately identify and communicate important information to the individuals in charge. ■ You will continually communicate information with others on the team to which you are assigned. ■ You will ensure that documentation regarding patient condition, treatments completed, and so on, is maintained and transported with the patient to ensure a smooth transition in care and to prevent harm to the patient. ■ You will use tools for communication (e.g., SBAR) that result in concise exchanges of critical information.
Ethics	A nurse who is in the midst of a disaster faces many ethical dilemmas. Perhaps the first is whether to provide care (i.e., "show up"). The nurse, who is trained to provide the best care possible to any assigned patient, may be challenged by decisions made for the greater good, such as not providing care to individuals who are unlikely to survive and keeping care for others very basic to preserve available resources.	■ Develop an individual disaster plan for yourself and your family so that it will be easier to make a decision to participate during a disaster or not. ■ Familiarize yourself with the disaster preparedness plans of your employer and community, which will facilitate a decision and, by virtue of having a plan in place, will make it easier to respond. ■ Participate in disaster drills, which will enable you to understand the requirements of participation and make a quicker decision about participation. ■ Obtain CERT (Community Emergency Response Team) Training. ■ Never exceed your professional scope of practice, because doing so may result in loss of your license and subject you to personal liability for negligence or malpractice. ■ Ensure that you understand the Code of Ethics and Standards of Practice of the American Nurses Association (ANA) and how they relate to emergency situations.
Legal Issues	Despite the good intentions of nurse volunteers, they must understand that state and federal law may not provide legal protection if the nurse is practicing outside of the jurisdiction where the nurse is licensed.	■ If you plan to respond to disasters, then volunteer with a disaster registry, such as federal disaster medical assistance teams nationally or locally with the American Red Cross. Doing so will provide you with the proper credentialing and training necessary to respond to a disaster, and your participation will be less problematic because you are part of an organized system. ■ Know your state's laws regarding emergency response, and ensure that you adhere to the requirements of your state licensing board.
Managing Care	Care coordination will be required to ensure that the needs of disaster victims are met. The leader of the disaster team will work with all present to ensure that the medical emergency response is effective.	■ Know the disaster plans for your employer and be prepared to follow them. ■ When you report to the disaster team, immediately go to the command center to receive your assignment rather than beginning care where you stand. ■ You may need to delegate care to other individuals; ensure that, despite the emergency, you follow the principles of delegation (e.g., confirm that the delegate has been trained to perform the procedure, understands the procedure, completes the procedure, and reports back).
Perioperative Care	One of the outcomes of triage will be determining which patients will need to go to the OR now or which ones can be stabilized and sent to the OR later.	■ Know the disaster plans for your employer and be prepared to follow them. ■ The nurse will need to assist with quickly preparing patients for the OR, while ensuring that all critical safety procedures are done such as timeouts, site marking, and appropriate patient identification. ■ The nurse will use tools for communications such as SBAR to ensure a safe and complete handoff.

insurance plans but, as patients, have been insulated from and are often unaware of the cost of care, resulting in uninformed decisions about the type and amount of healthcare needed. Mass advertising by pharmaceutical manufacturers and specialty treatment centers directed at consumers has also contributed to inappropriate treatment choices being made by the public.

As healthcare expenditures have increased, the need for **resource allocation**, the distribution of resources among competing groups of people or programs, has been recognized. When resources are being allocated, three levels of decision making must be considered:

Level 1: Allocating resources to healthcare versus other social needs

Level 2: Allocating resources within the healthcare sector

Level 3: Allocating resources among individual patients (AHC).

Clinical Example C

An 8-year-old boy with a chronic blood disorder requires weekly blood transfusions. The hospital struggles to maintain enough of his rare blood type. The 8-year-old arrives at the emergency department at the same time as another patient who is bleeding profusely and has the same blood type. There is enough blood for only one of these patients.

Critical Thinking Questions

1. Which patient should receive the blood? Why?
2. What models or methods should be used to make the decision? Who should be responsible for making the decision?

Examples of Resource Allocation

Rationing is one means of allocating healthcare resources. Rationing is a method used by individuals, insurance companies, and the government to prevent increases in the cost of healthcare or to reduce the cost of healthcare. Individuals ration when they decide to provide self-care for an illness or injury rather than seeking care from a healthcare provider. Methods used by insurance companies to ration healthcare resources include limiting the number of healthcare providers that patients can choose and denying coverage for services (e.g., services deemed to be experimental or those that are not supported by scientific evidence that prove their efficacy). The government also rations healthcare resources, such as inclusion of the coverage gap in Medicare Plan D (known as the "donut hole") that sometimes forces beneficiaries to purchase fewer prescriptions (Torrey, 2012).

The Organ Procurement and Transplantation Network

One of the best-known systems of allocating certain healthcare resources is the Organ Procurement and Transplantation Network (OPTN). In the United States, on average 92 people receive a donated organ each day (USDHHS, 2017a). There are currently almost 120,000 people awaiting organ transplantation, and 75,000 are on the active waiting list. Unfortunately, there simply are not enough donated organs to meet the demand for transplants. The OPTN, a contracted service of the USDHHS, maintains the only national patient waiting list for organ transplantation. Multiple factors determine

who receives a donor organ. A few of the factors are blood and tissue type, medical urgency, organ size, time on the waiting list, and the geographic distance between the donor and the recipient (USDHHS, 2017b).

》Stay Current: More information on organ donation, including statistics updated daily and how to register as a donor, can be found at http://optn.transplant.hrsa.gov.

H1N1 Vaccine Distribution

During 2009, there was an outbreak of H1N1 influenza. Initially an inadequate supply of vaccine was available, but as H1N1 began to spread, the Centers for Disease Control and Prevention (CDC) realized that guidelines had to be developed and implemented to ensure that the most vulnerable individuals had first access to the vaccine. As more vaccine became available, the CDC (2009) rationed its distribution by considering factors such as the amount of vaccine being requested by local health departments, the speed at which the vaccine was becoming available, and the need to ensure availability for not only the community but also active-duty military personnel.

Once the vaccine arrived in local communities, further decisions were made about who could receive it if the supply was insufficient to meet the demand. Many local health departments screened potential recipients and initially administered the vaccine only to individuals with risk factors for H1N1, such as small children and adults with diagnosed respiratory disease (**Figure 46–2 》》**). Later, when sufficient quantities of the vaccine became available, healthcare providers were able to administer the vaccine to anyone who asked for it.

Nurses and Allocation of Resources

The role of the nurse in the allocation of resources is a collaborative one. Nurses are the largest group of health professionals, and as part of the interprofessional healthcare team, the nurse participates in allocating healthcare resources. Thus, nurses develop a significant understanding of how appropriate allocation and misallocation of healthcare resources can affect patient needs and outcomes. Nurses must be aware of and participate in discussions that affect

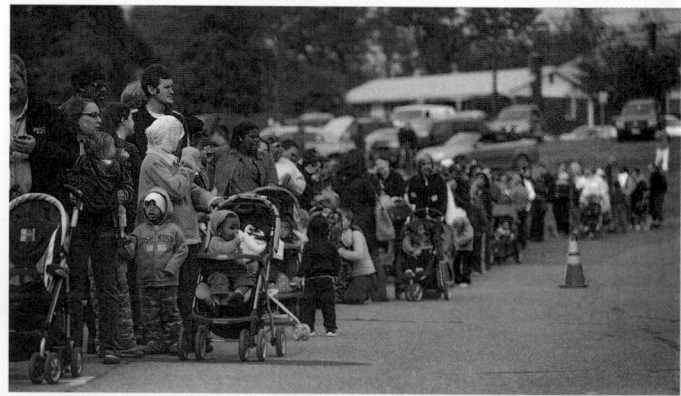

Source: Tim Sloan/Staff/Getty Images.

Figure 46–2 》 Hundreds of county residents wait in a long line for the H1N1 vaccination shot at a clinic held by the Montgomery County Health and Human Services on October 14, 2009, at the Dennis Avenue County Health Center in Silver Spring, Maryland.

the allocation of healthcare resources in the workplace, in their communities, and at the federal level. Nurses are uniquely placed to advocate on behalf of patients when allocation of resources is being considered in their communities. They may advocate by talking with local legislators, writing to politicians, and engaging in discussions in their neighborhoods and social groups. As working professionals, nurses have the opportunity to participate in national discussions about resources through a number of professional organizations, such as the American Nurses Association.

REVIEW The Concept of Healthcare Systems

RELATE Link the Concepts

Linking the concept of healthcare systems with the concept of oxygenation:

You are a registered nurse leading a team that includes LPNs and UAPs on a critical care unit of a hospital. You are planning care for a patient on a mechanical ventilator.

1. What aspects of this patient's care may be delegated to UAPs?

2. What factors related to the delivery of healthcare may affect your ability to provide care for this patient, and how?

Linking the concept of healthcare systems with the concept of clinical decision making:

You are a registered nurse working in the emergency department (ED) of a rural hospital. Harvesting season has brought large numbers of Spanish-speaking families to the community. Almost all of the men and many of the women are migrant workers. A mother who speaks limited English brings her 5-year-old son to the ED. She says he has been vomiting for 2 days. He has a fever of 102 degrees. She says he does not have a regular healthcare provider. He is not enrolled in any type of health insurance plan.

3. What factors will affect your ability to plan care for the child?

4. Which model of nursing care delivery would most benefit the child and his mother? Why?

Linking the concept of healthcare systems with the concept of reproduction:

5. What resources in your community are available to uninsured pregnant women?

6. Are the risks to the fetus any greater or any different when the pregnant mother is uninsured? Explain.

Linking the concept of healthcare systems with the concept of ethics?

7. What provisions of the ANA Code of Ethics address resource allocation?

8. What ethical considerations do you as an individual value that might affect how you would determine resource allocation?

REFER Go to Pearson MyLab Nursing and eText

- Additional review materials

REFLECT Apply Your Knowledge

Juan Santiago, 41 years old, makes an appointment with a healthcare provider he has never seen before for an annual physical examination. During the nurse's initial assessment, the patient explains that he has never had a complete physical because he has always been healthy and hasn't had health insurance. After his recent college graduation, he accepted a new job that offered full healthcare benefits, so he decided it was time to take care of his health. Although he appears anxious about what will happen during the exam, he does not ask any questions and avoids making eye contact with the nurse.

During the collection of his health history, Mr. Santiago reports smoking approximately 20 cigarettes per day, drinking 2–3 alcoholic beverages per week, and, until recently, working as a landscaper, a very physically demanding job. He describes the physical requirements of his new job as "a little bit of walking but mostly desk work."

During the physical examination the nurse notes a wound the size of a quarter on the anterior aspect of Mr. Santiago's left foot. It is erythematous and warm to the touch, and a small amount of purulent drainage seeps from the side of the wound. Mr. Santiago reports that the wound has been there for more than 6 weeks. He has applied over-the-counter antibiotic cream daily but it still has not healed. The nurse asks Mr. Santiago about his weight; he admits losing about 10 pounds in the past month but denies changing his diet.

1. Describe primary, secondary, and tertiary care requirements for this patient.

2. What referrals to other healthcare providers might be appropriate to assist in the treatment plan for this patient?

3. What type of assessment of health literacy would the nurse conduct with this patient before providing written information?

4. What factors will influence care delivery to this patient? How will that alter the nurse's approach to providing care for this patient?

» Exemplar 46.A
Emergency Preparedness

Exemplar Learning Outcomes

46.A Analyze emergency preparedness as it relates to healthcare systems.

- Describe the four phases of emergency management.
- Outline the organizations responsible for emergency management and response.

- Summarize the process of triage.
- Describe the safety zones used in site-specific disaster response.
- Summarize the methods used for handling bioterrorism disasters.
- Analyze the importance of collaboration during disaster response.
- Explain the role of nurses in emergency management and response.

Exemplar Key Terms

Overview

An **emergency** is a sudden, often unforeseen event that threatens health or safety. A public emergency necessitating assistance from outside the affected community is a **disaster**. Disasters have three things in common: little or no warning before the event; available personnel and emergency services that are overwhelmed initially; and a serious threat to life, public health, and the environment. Infectious diseases may accompany disasters or can become disasters themselves. A **pandemic** is an infection that spreads rapidly around the world.

Emergency preparedness is the act of making plans to prevent, respond to, and recover from emergencies. The CDC recommends an *all-hazards* approach to emergency preparedness. This approach provides for general preparation, including training that can be applied in a wide variety of emergency situations. The impact on health and the healthcare system is similar regardless of the nature of the disaster. **Surge capacity** refers to a community's ability to rapidly meet the increased demand for qualified personnel and resources, including healthcare resources, in the event of a disaster.

The Four Phases of Emergency Management

Emergency management consists of four phases: mitigation, preparedness, response, and recovery.

Mitigation

The **mitigation** phase, which takes place both before and after an emergency occurs, consists of identifying potential hazards, taking action to reduce the likelihood of their occurrence, and minimizing the effects of those that cannot be prevented. An example of mitigation in an individual's disaster plan would be the purchase of flood insurance by someone living in a flood zone. Implementation of warning systems for tornadoes and tsunamis are examples of mitigation by local, state, or regional agencies. Installation of a warning system prior to an occurrence of a disaster is an example of excellent disaster planning. Installation after an event is an example of using lessons learned from a disaster to reduce the effect of future occurrences. Both examples are mitigation.

Preparedness

The **preparedness** phase takes place before an emergency occurs. Risks are assessed and plans are developed to address them. Plans are designed to save lives and to assist first response and rescue teams that are often overwhelmed by the initial demands of an emergency. Emergency plans are developed at the federal, regional, state, and local levels. The Federal Emergency Management Agency (FEMA), the Department of Homeland Security, and the CDC identify national threats, create plans at the national level, and coordinate planning efforts among many people, agencies, and levels of government. They provide guidance for the development of plans in local communities. For communities, the most critical task performed during the preparedness phase is the development of an emergency operations plan. These plans often include multiple components that address each of the many hazards and natural disasters that the community may face. They include identifying, organizing, and training emergency personnel; stockpiling equipment and supplies; implementing communication and warning systems; establishing emergency operations centers; and implementing response and evacuation plans.

Ideally, the agencies that participate in the emergency plan's development will also be involved in emergency response efforts and, therefore, will understand the risks the community may face and the responses that will be required. When agencies prepare for emergencies in advance and continually update their plans over time, their preparedness efforts will be more effective and result in better outcomes for the community.

During the preparedness phase, individual nurses must gain an understanding of their expected roles in an emergency and prepare for them. Because nurses will be required to allocate scarce resources and supplies and make unbelievably difficult patient care decisions, they must understand the ethics associated with such choices. The ANA is a good source of information to guide nurses' understanding of their roles and possible consequences. Public health nurses have a specific role to play in this phase. They plan ahead of time in their communities to assess the region for populations at risk for access and functional needs during a disaster and develop care plans to address those needs. They also conduct training drills and evaluate operational plans and work with local stakeholders (Association of Public Health Nurses [APHN], 2014).

Nurses also must be aware of their employer's response plans and have a sense of how their state and local community will operate during an emergency. Nurses who choose to become disaster volunteers should register with an agency such as the American Red Cross to ensure they are properly trained and recognized as part of an organized system (ANA, 2016).

During the preparedness phase, nurses must also develop an emergency plan for themselves and their immediate families. When this plan is complete, nurses can be confident that their families are prepared to weather an emergency in relative safety. With this assurance, nurses who choose to assist in a disaster or who are required to remain at the hospital during a disaster will be able to leave their families without delay and remain available until no longer needed. FEMA and the Red Cross are two organizations that provide detailed information to assist individuals with the development of personal emergency plans. It is important for everyone to develop a plan for themselves and their families. They must ensure that not only the adults but also the children know what to do in an emergency. Plans should address the basic emergency needs of any disaster. They should also include instructions for specific disasters, such as tornadoes, that may occur in the individual's location. Everyone should assemble a disaster kit that can be used in place or taken if evacuation is necessary. Escape routes for disasters that could occur within the home itself (e.g., gas leaks and fires) or for disasters that would require mass evacuation (e.g., floods and hurricanes) should be determined. Meeting places should be designated—someplace inside or outside the home where the family can unite. Family members should be provided contact information in case they are separated during a disaster. Someone outside of the immediate area should be identified as a central contact if family members are unable to reach each other locally. It is very important to shut off utilities as directed by emergency authorities or when forced to leave home. Insurance, medical, financial, and other vital records should be duplicated and stored in an off-site, safe location. Special needs such as medications, medical equipment, and so forth, should be considered and availability planned for. Family members should be trained in first aid, including CPR. Review and update of the emergency plan on a regular basis are critical because someday one's life may depend on it.

>> **Stay Current:** Visit www.ready.gov/are-you-ready-guide for FEMA's *Are You Ready? Guide—An In-Depth Guide to Citizen Preparedness.*

Despite a community's best preparedness efforts, there will be instances when a variety of factors result in failure to meet community needs. The evacuation of New Orleans in advance of hurricane Katrina and the efforts to provide shelter immediately following Katrina are stunning examples of how preparedness efforts can fail (see **Figure 46–3 >>**).

Emergency Response

The third phase, **emergency response**, is the implementation of emergency preparedness plans. These plans provide a means for responders to save lives, prevent additional property damage, and meet basic human needs. As soon as possible, disaster victims are triaged and given appropriate treatment. Other emergency activities include search and rescue operations, opening shelters to house survivors, and repairing utility infrastructure (**Figure 46–4 >>**).

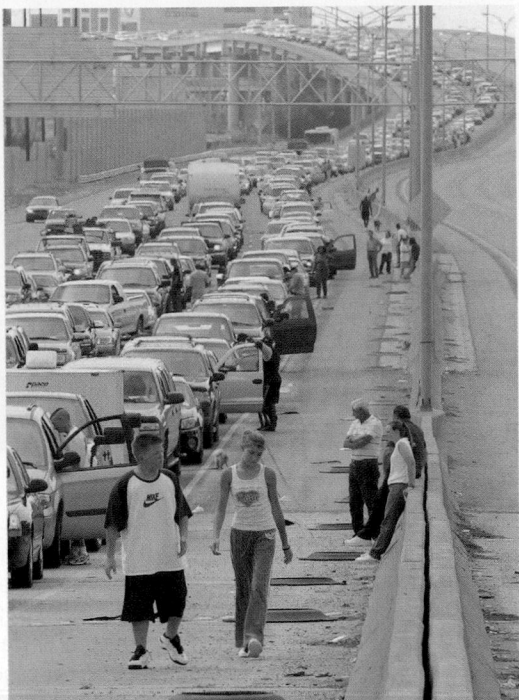

Source: Rick Wilking/Reuters/Alamy Stock Photo.

Figure 46–3 >> Authorities in New Orleans ordered hundreds of thousands of residents to flee on Sunday, August 28, 2005, as Hurricane Katrina strengthened into a rare, top-ranked storm and barreled toward the vulnerable U.S. Gulf Coast city. Those who had vehicles were caught in traffic jams for hours.

The emergency response plan is followed during and immediately after the emergency, simultaneously with the community's assessment of the disaster's immediate effects. Community agencies such as local law enforcement, paramedics, and emergency department personnel, as well as local governmental staff employed in the disaster response unit, are responsible for implementing the overall plan and its components. Public health nurses are part of this response effort. They ensure that logistics are in place to support community care during the crisis and provide ongoing response planning during the incidence (APHN, 2014). Federal, state, and other outside resources support local efforts by providing first aid and other emergency medical assistance and by establishing or restoring communication and transportation. Public health nurses use population-based triage to assess communicable disease outbreak impact and needed response, assessing the probability of infectious diseases and addressing them, and identifying and providing support to individuals with mental health problems.

During the preparedness phase, nurses must become familiar with the emergency plans of their employers and communities. They must also familiarize themselves with the ANA's positions on nurses' emergency and disaster responsibilities. During the emergency response phase, nurses will put this information to use. The responsibility of nurses during an emergency, like that of other first

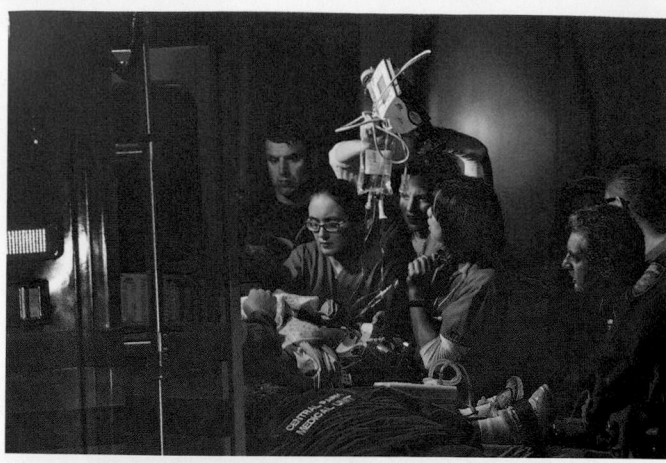

Source: John Minchillo/AP Images.

Figure 46–4 》 Medical workers assist a patient into an ambulance during an evacuation of New York University's Langone Medical Center, Monday, October 29, 2012. The New York City hospital moved out more than 200 patients, including 20 infants from the NICU, after its backup generator failed when the power was knocked out by Hurricane Sandy.

responders, is to do the greatest good for the greatest number of casualties. During an emergency, nurses will be asked to perform the fundamentals of nursing practice but will do so in a very stressful environment under extraordinary circumstances. They will be working under intense time constraints and must care for each victim quickly, then move on to the next one. They should not use their time to provide care that will be of minimal or questionable benefit. Nurses must observe both the physical and mental status of victims and ensure appropriate triage and treatment. Advanced practice nurses who have received training in emergency and trauma care will have significantly greater responsibilities than nurses with less training. During the crisis, nurses should be constantly aware of their defined scope of practice and must not exceed it even when circumstances would seem to dictate otherwise.

Recovery

The **recovery** phase takes place after the emergency and is designed to restore the community to normal balance (restoration) or create a new, safer normal by updating the community's preparedness plan to address lessons learned during the emergency (mitigation). The recovery phase includes the reconstitution of government operations and services, if necessary, and includes the provision of public assistance by the private and public sectors. Other elements of the recovery phase may include rebuilding, reemployment, and the repair of essential infrastructure. During the recovery phase, each community must reassess risks and update plans to ensure that newly identified risks are addressed. Because of their education and experience, nurses are well qualified to participate in risk assessment

and planning at the local, state, and national levels following a disaster. Nurses are also perfect candidates to educate their patients and communities about disaster preparation. In particular, public health nurses conduct rapid ongoing needs assessments at intervals to determine health and critical resource capacity after a natural disaster and work with community stakeholders to plan for any long-term health concerns following an incident. They also participate in the reconstruction of critical services and evaluate the long-term impact of the disaster consequences on the community (APHN, 2014).

Responsibility for Emergency Management and Response

State divisions of emergency management act as the **local emergency management agency (LEMA)** for each state. This is a governmental agency with expertise in public safety, emergency medical services, and management. The U.S. Department of Homeland Security has created federal guidelines called the National Incident Management System (NIMS) that local governments must follow during an emergency or disaster. Local governments have the primary responsibility for emergency management and response. In the event of an emergency, first responders such as local fire departments and emergency medical technicians will be challenged to meet the needs of the public because of the sheer volume of assistance they will be asked to provide. In situations like this, citizen volunteers often act as extensions of the first responders. For this reason, it is beneficial for a community to develop a corps of trained citizens to provide such support.

In recognition of this, FEMA has developed the **Community Emergency Response Team (CERT) program** to prepare interested community members. Participants gain an understanding of their responsibility for preparing for a disaster so they will be ready to safely assist themselves, their families, and their neighbors. The CERT program provides citizens with facts about what to expect following a major disaster in terms of immediate services; alerts citizens to their responsibility for mitigation and preparedness; trains citizens in needed lifesaving skills with an emphasis on decision-making skills, rescuer safety, and doing the greatest good for the most people; and organizing teams that act as an extension of first responder services, offering immediate help to victims until professional services are on site (U.S. Department of Homeland Security, 2016).

The CDC manages the Clinician Outreach Communication Activity (COCA) program to ensure that clinicians have up-to-date information. COCA is designed to provide two-way communication between clinicians and the CDC about emerging health threats such as pandemics, natural disasters, and terrorism. COCA keeps a list of emergency preparedness and training resources offered by federal agencies and COCA partners.

》 Stay Current: Visit www.bt.cdc.gov/coca/training.asp for COCA's list of conferences and training opportunities and to sign up for e-mail updates from COCA.

Nursing Competencies for Emergency Response

Nurses represent the largest pool of healthcare professionals and, for this reason, are called on to assist in mass casualty events (MCEs). Training in preparation for, recognition of, and response to MCEs will be beneficial to the nurse, the nurse's family, the nurse's employer, and the community. Some of the ways in which nurses have received training regarding MCEs include reading professional journal articles, participating in mock disaster drills, volunteering in community services, obtaining CERT certification, and actual nursing during an MCE. Emergency preparedness is a necessity, regardless of the nurse's educational preparation, area of expertise, or practice setting (Whitty & Burnett, 2012).

In 2003, the International Nursing Coalition for Mass Casualty Education (INCMCE) (2003) published educational competencies for registered nurses to facilitate their response to MCEs, with a strong recommendation that these core competencies be included in initial nursing education programs (**Box 46–3 》**).

The National Nurse Emergency Preparedness Initiative is a highly interactive, web-based course that provides emergency preparedness training for nurses working in hospitals/acute care, schools, public health, ambulatory care, hospice/palliative care, long-term care, occupational health, and home health settings. This training focuses on providing opportunities for dynamic and interactive application of both theory and practice through scenario-based learning.

》 Stay Current: Visit the National Nurse Emergency Preparedness Initiative website at http://nnepi.gwnursing.org to sign up for its interactive learning module that teaches nurses about a critical thinking framework that can be applied during disasters.

Emergency Plans

Individuals and agencies that respond to MCEs are expected to act within the framework of emergency plans that were prepared in advance. Most agencies are mandated by law to develop plans that dictate the roles and responsibilities of all individuals who will respond during emergencies, disasters, and MCEs. Individual healthcare agencies such as hospitals, health departments, and residential facilities for older adults and people with disabilities will create emergency plans that prescribe the roles and responsibilities of their own employees. All nurses not only must familiarize themselves with the policies and procedures of the agency that employs them, but also must create an individual emergency plan for themselves and their families.

Triage

The process of **triage** involves prioritizing patients for treatment based on severity of illness or injury and in light of the supplies and resources available. The objective of triage is to ensure early assessment of patients and prioritize care based on severity of symptoms. Nurses perform triage every day in emergency departments. During a mass casualty event (more than 100 victims), the demand on nurses' knowledge and skills will be even greater. Mass casualties call for the implementation of **reverse triage**, in which the most severely injured or ill victims who require the greatest resources are treated last to allow the greatest number of victims to receive medical attention. A simple color classification system (START) is used to prioritize adult patients (see **Figure 46–5 》**). A separate algorithm, Jump START, has been developed for pediatric victims (**Figure 46–6 》**). It is recommended that emergency medical personnel be assigned to triage. This frees physicians and nurses to provide needed care.

Site-specific Disaster Zones

When a site-specific disaster occurs, access to the site of contamination is limited and safety zones are established. Examples of such disasters are the release of weapons, such as bombs, and toxic chemical leaks due to tanker car derailment. The designated safety zones should be located uphill, upwind, and upstream from the site of the disaster. The configuration of each zone will vary based on the site of the occurrence. Topography, weather, and the physical layout (buildings, roads, and so on) will play an important role in designating the zones. The initial site of the incident is considered the hot zone. Only personnel with appropriate protective equipment are allowed in the hot zone. **Box 46–4 》** provides more information on zone breakdown.

Bioterrorism

Bioterrorism is the deliberate release of viruses, bacteria, or other microbes as weapons. The U.S. public health system and primary healthcare providers must be prepared to respond to and treat the diseases caused by these agents,

---

Box 46–3
Categories of Educational Competencies for Registered Nurses Responding to Mass Casualty Incidents

Core Competencies

1. Critical thinking
2. Assessment
3. Technical skills
4. Communication

Core Knowledge Areas

1. Health promotion, risk reduction, and disease prevention
2. Healthcare systems and policies
3. Illness and disease management
4. Information and healthcare technologies
5. Ethics
6. Human diversity

Professional Role Development

1. A description of nursing roles during MCEs
2. Identification of the most appropriate or most likely healthcare role for oneself during an MCE

Source: Based on Nursing Emergency Preparedness Education Coalition. (2003). Retrieved from http://www.nursing.vanderbilt.edu/incmce/overview. html.

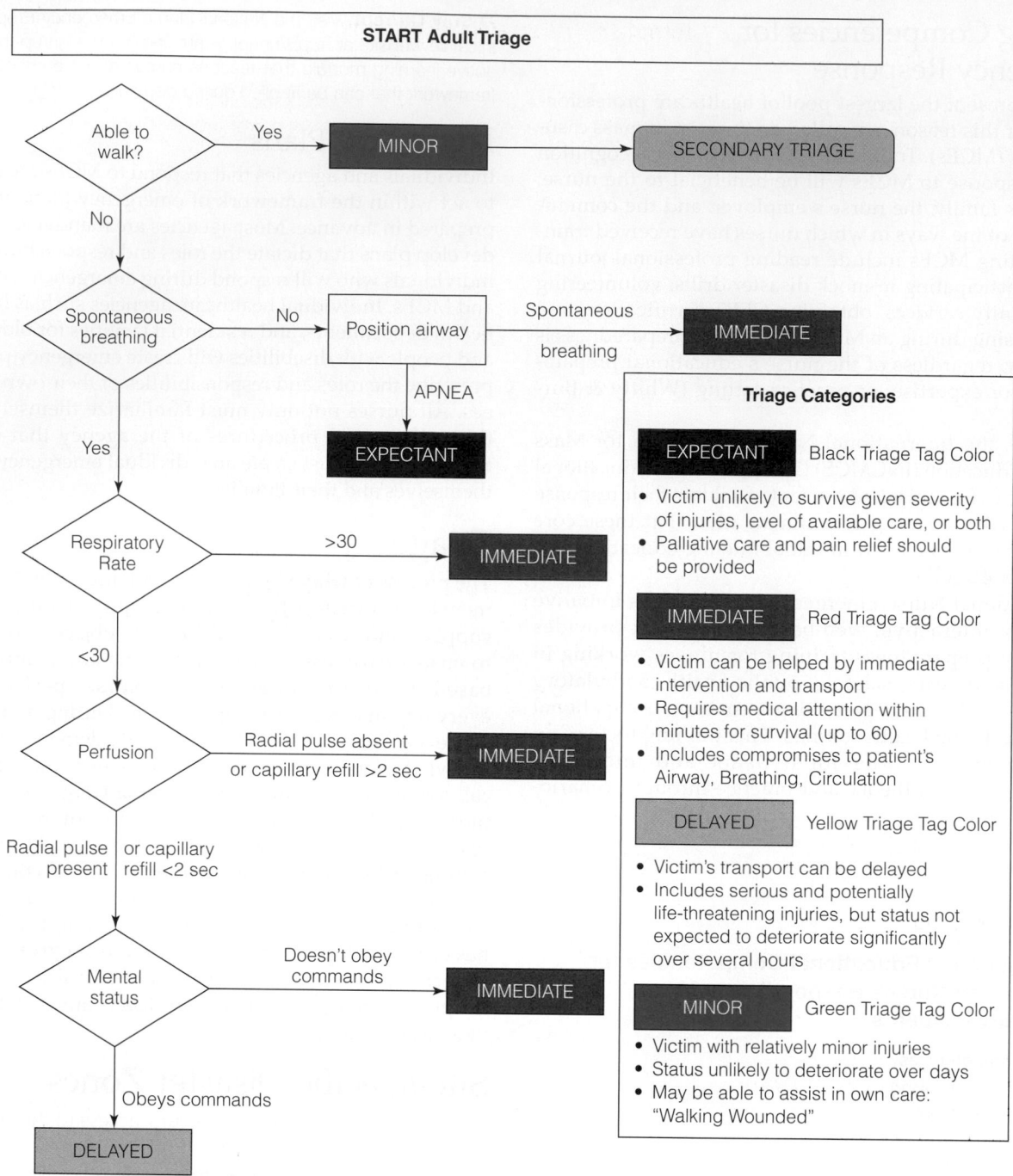

Figure 46–5 ▶ START adult triage algorithm.

many of which are rarely seen in the United States. The CDC has assigned the highest priority to biological agents that can be easily disseminated or transmitted from individual to individual; cause a high mortality rate; have a significant impact on public health; cause public panic; and disrupt society and government. The primary agents identified by the CDC as potential bioterrorist threats are anthrax (*Bacillus anthracis*), botulism (*Clostridium botulinum* toxin), plague (*Yersinia pestis*), smallpox (variola major), tularemia (*Francisella tularensis*), and viral hemorrhagic fevers (filoviruses [e.g., Ebola and Marburg] and arenavirsuses [e.g., Lassa and Machupo]) (CDC, 2013).

Nurses must be aware of the early signs and symptoms of these diseases as well as the methods of transmitting them. See **Table 46–2 ▶**.

Immediate treatment for the primary biological agents used in terrorism is limited. Inhalation of anthrax has been effectively treated with ciprofloxacin 400 mg administered intravenously every 12 hours. There are no effective therapies for treating patients infected by most of the other viruses that could be used in a bioterrorism attack. For some viruses, a vaccine could be created to stimulate the body's immune system such that the individual may be protected from infection if exposed to the virus at a later date.

JumpSTART Pediatric MCI Triage

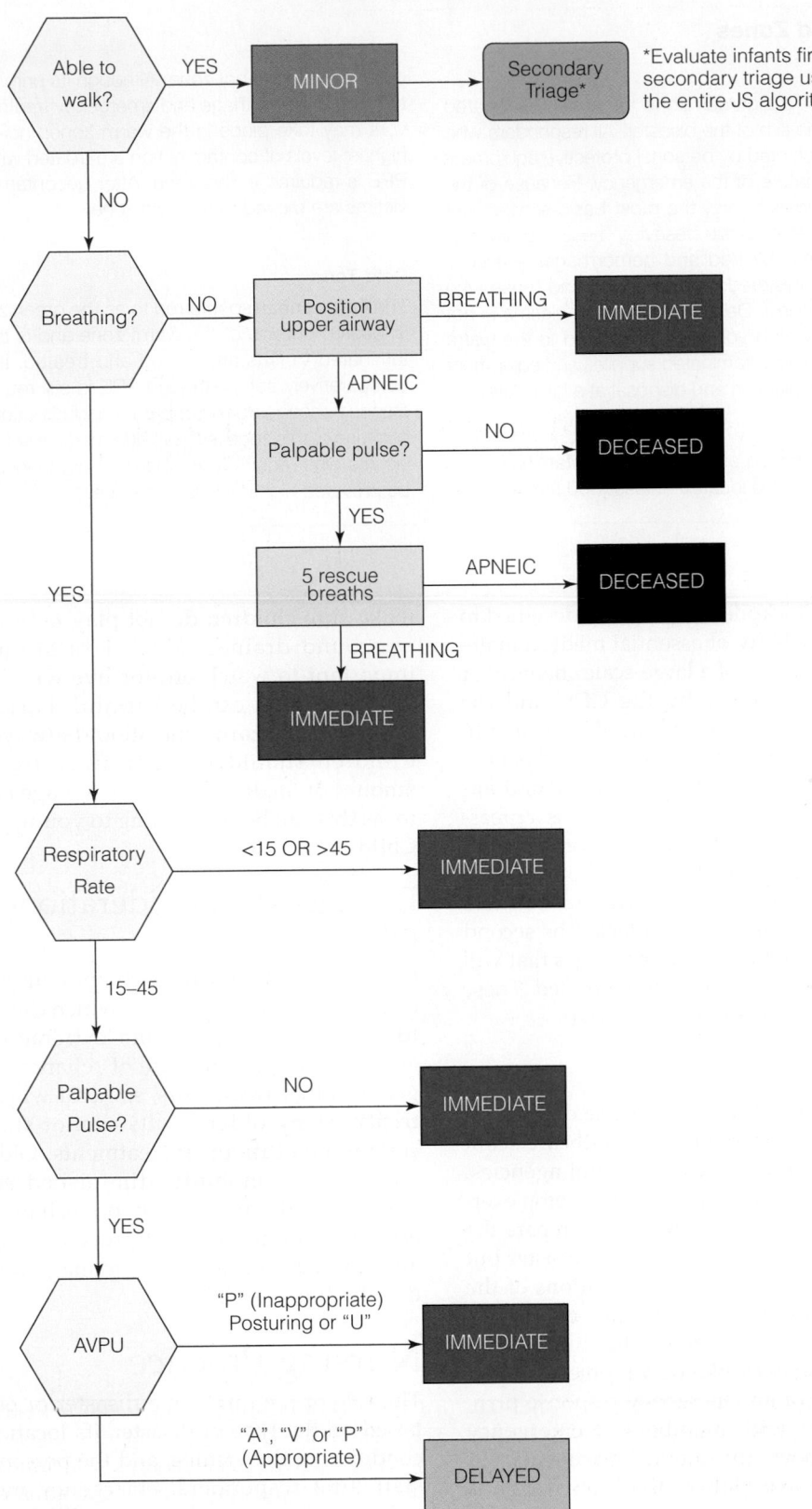

Figure 46–6 》 JumpSTART algorithm for pediatric victims.

Box 46–4
Hot, Warm, and Cold Zones

Hot Zone

The **hot zone** is the most dangerous zone because it is located immediately adjacent to the site of the disaster. All responders who enter the area must be protected by personal protective equipment (PPE) appropriate to the nature of the emergency. Because of the dangers inherent in this location, only the most basic services are performed: Victims are located; basic lifesaving measures are provided (e.g., airways are established and hemorrhages are controlled); antidotes are administered; and the dead and those who cannot be saved are identified. Decontamination of victims is not performed in the hot zone. Survivors are transported to the warm zone for decontamination. All contaminated supplies and equipment are left in the hot zone for collection and disposal at a later date.

Warm Zone

The **warm zone** (also referred to as the yellow, contamination, or contamination reduction zone) is located at least 300 feet from the outer edge of the hot zone. Although its primary purpose is decontamination, rapid triage and emergency treatment to stabilize survivors may take place in the warm zone. Individuals who have the highest levels of contamination are treated with the highest priority. PPE is required in this zone. After decontamination is completed, victims are moved to the cold zone.

Cold Zone

The **cold zone**, also referred to as the green zone or support zone, is located outside of the warm zone and is the site where decontaminated victims are triaged and treated. It is considered to be comparatively safe, although PPE is still required in case circumstances change (for example, if wind direction shifts). The primary purpose of this zone is to provide medical services and to transport victims who require more than first aid to locations where they will be provided higher levels of service.

The Strategic National Stockpile is a program designed to ensure the immediate availability of essential medical materials to a community in the event of a large-scale chemical or biological attack. Managed jointly by the CDC and the Department of Homeland Security, it consists of large quantities of antibiotics; vaccines; and medical, surgical, and patient support supplies such as bandages, IV equipment, and airway supplies. The first component of the stockpile is a preassembled "push package" designed to meet the community's needs in the case of an undetermined biological or chemical threat. The push packages are stored in locations that will permit delivery within 12 hours after an attack. The second component is vendor-managed inventory packages that will be shipped once the threat has been clearly identified. These packages are designed to arrive within 24–36 hours.

Collaboration

Emergency preparedness and disaster response depend on the collaboration of an interprofessional healthcare team involving local, state, and federal governmental agencies. Interprofessional training and participation in tabletop exercises, simulations, and mock incidents not only prepare the team members to assume their roles in case of disaster but also provide opportunities for frequent evaluations of the plan. These evaluations lead to a more effective emergency plan and facilitate communications across the interprofessional team that is responsible for the development, implementation, and evaluation of an emergency response plan. Nurses often have contact with members of emergency medical services (EMS) in both emergency departments and disaster situations. A brief overview of the EMS system is presented in **Box 46–5 »**.

Lifespan Considerations

Emergency Considerations for Children

After a disaster such as a tornado or hurricane, it is important to keep children safe. Parents need to be aware to make sure children do not play in or around floodwaters or around drainage ditches or storm drains. It is also important to watch out for live wires or other sources of electricity that can be harmful. Portable generators can pose safety hazards and should always be used outdoors. Children should be kept away from them. Limit the amount of media and news coverage children are exposed to, as this can be frightening to younger children (HealthyChildren.org, 2015).

Emergency Considerations for Older Adults

Older adults are particularly vulnerable to disasters. They often have chronic diseases, which can worsen quickly due to lack of food, water, and extreme heat or cold. Older adults have a greater rate of reliance on medication, oxygen, or other treatments, some of which will require electricity. Many older adults cannot survive long without certain medications or treatments. Older adults may also have limited mobility, diminished sensory awareness, inadequate thermoregulation mechanisms, and social and economic limitations that prevent adequate preparedness and limited their ability to manage during and/or after a disaster hits (CDC, 2016).

Nursing Practice

The role of the nurse in a disaster or emergency will vary based on the type of disaster, its location, the number and condition of the victims, and the personnel (e.g., command staff, first responders, emergency medical technicians, police) and supplies that are available at the time it occurs. Nurses may be called on to perform triage of patients, to perform first aid, or to stabilize patients in preparation for transfer for more advanced care.

Initially, the nurse must decide whether to assist during the disaster or not. This decision will be based on individual safety, family safety and needs, and the greater needs of the

TABLE 46–2 Biological Pathogens of Highest Concern for Bioterrorism Attacks

Pathogen	Cause	Symptoms	Transmission
Anthrax	*Bacillus anthracis*, a spore-forming bacterium Three types: ■ Cutaneous ■ Respiratory ■ Gastrointestinal	■ Cutaneous: The first symptom is a small sore that becomes a blister, then progresses to a skin ulcer with a black spot in the center. All lesions are painless. ■ Respiratory: *Initially:* sore throat, mild fever and muscle aches. *Later:* respiratory symptoms, e.g., cough, chest discomfort, shortness of breath, tiredness and achy muscles. ■ Gastrointestinal: Nausea, loss of appetite, bloody diarrhea, and fever followed by bad stomach pain.	■ Cutaneous: direct skin contact with spores; often result from handling products, such as wool, from infected animals ■ Respiratory: inhalation of aerosolized spores (rare unless weaponized) ■ Gastrointestinal: eating undercooked meat or dairy products from infected animals (rare)
Botulism	*Clostridium botulinum* toxin	Foodborne botulism symptoms: ■ Usually develop within 12–36 hours after exposure. ■ May include visual effects, e.g., double vision; neurologic symptoms, including slurred speech, dysphagia, and muscle weakness that begins in the shoulders and descends through the body to the calves; and paralysis of the breathing muscles, which, if left untreated, may result in death.	■ Foodborne: individual ingests preformed toxin. ■ Infant: Occurs in small number of infants who harbor *C. botulinum* in their intestinal tract. ■ Wound botulism: Occurs when existing wounds are infected with the toxins of *C. botulinum.*
Plague	*Yersinia pestis*, a bacterium	■ Pneumonic plague develops within 1–6 days of exposure. ■ Fever, weakness, rapidly developing pneumonia with dyspnea, chest pain, cough, and sometimes bloody or watery sputum	■ An old mnemonic is "The fleas and lice on rats and mice cause plague." ■ Bubonic plague is transmitted via an infected flea bite or exposure of broken skin to infected material. ■ Pneumonic plague is of particular interest as a biological weapon because it can be released via weaponized aerosol. It can also be transmitted from individual to individual.
Viral hemorrhagic fevers (VHF)	Several distinct families of zoonotic viruses that reside in an animal reservoir host (e.g., rodent) or arthropod vector (e.g., ticks and mosquitos)	Signs and symptoms, which develop after a 5- to 10-day incubation period, vary by the type of VHF. Early signs and symptoms often include marked fever, fatigue, dizziness, myalgia, weakness, exhaustion, and a rash on the trunk. Severe cases may be accompanied by bleeding under the skin, in internal organs, or from body orifices such as the mouth, eyes, or ears. Patients rarely die from this blood loss. Severe cases may cause shock, nervous system breakdowns, coma, delirium, and seizures. Renal failure may occur in some types of VHF.	■ VHFs are most commonly spread by exposure to an animal reservoir host or arthropod vector. Humans are not natural reservoirs for VHFs; however, some VHFs can be transmitted from individual to individual after an initial human has been infected.
Smallpox	Variola virus	■ During the incubation period (from 7 to 17 days), an infected individual has no symptoms and is not contagious. ■ Prodromal phase (2–4 days) symptoms include a fever of 101°–104°F, head and body aches, and possibly vomiting. This phase may be contagious. ■ The early rash phase is the most contagious period. The rash first appears as spots on the tongue and in the mouth, which then progress into sores that break open, allowing large amounts of the virus to spread into the mouth and throat. The disease is highly contagious during this phase. Within 24 hours the rash, which begins on the face, spreads down and across the entire body. By the third day of the rash, raised bumps develop. By the fourth day of the rash, the bumps fill with thick, opaque fluid and have a depression in the center that resembles a belly button—a distinguishing characteristic of smallpox. Fever increases again. ■ Pustular rash (duration of 5 days): Pustular bumps develop (they feel like BBs under the skin), then form a crust and scab over. The scabs fall off, leaving pitted scars. The individual is contagious until all the scabs have fallen off.	■ Direct and fairly long face-to-face exposure is usually necessary under normal circumstances; however, weaponized smallpox can be spread by aerosol. ■ Direct contact with body fluids or contaminated items such as clothing or bed linen could spread the disease. ■ Humans are the only natural host of variola.
Tularemia	*Francisella tularensis*	■ Sudden fever, chills, headache, diarrhea, muscle aches, joint pain, dry cough, and progressive weakness ■ If *F. tularensis* was used as a biological weapon and made airborne for exposure by inhalation, the infected people would experience severe respiratory illness, including life-threatening pneumonia and systemic infection.	Spread by bacterium found in animals (especially rodents, rabbits, and hares). Means of spread include: ■ Being bitten by infected ticks, deerflies, other insects ■ Handling infected animal carcasses and skins ■ Eating or drinking contaminated food or water ■ Inhaling *F. tularensis.*

Source: Based on Centers for Disease Control and Prevention. (2013). *Bioterrorism agents: Emergency.* Retrieved from http://emergency.cdc.gov/agent/agentlist.asp.

Box 46–5
The Emergency Medical Services System

The emergency medical services (EMS) system is a network of resources that provides emergency care and transportation, that is, prehospital care, to victims of illness, injury, or disaster. EMS personnel, who must be trained and licensed, work under the auspices of a medical director, usually a hospital-based physician, who is consulted as needed. There are four levels of EMS professionals.

EMRs and EMTs provide basic life support:

- *Emergency medical responders (EMRs)* provide initial emergency care, including assessment, opening airways, ventilating, controlling bleeding, performing CPR, stabilizing the spine and injured limbs, assisting with childbirth, and aiding other EMS personnel.
- *Emergency medical technicians (EMTs)* do everything EMRs do, but have received additional training and certification. This permits them to assist patients with prescribed medications and give aspirins, NSAIDs, oral glucose, and other medications when indicated.

AEMTs and paramedics are qualified to provide advanced life support:

- *Advanced emergency medical technicians (AEMTs)* have received advanced emergency training so they may start and administer IV fluids; give medications; and assess the need for and provide advanced airway procedures.
- *Paramedics* receive the most training and are qualified to do more in-depth assessments of patients, including the assessment of abnormal heart rhythms, and to perform some invasive procedures.

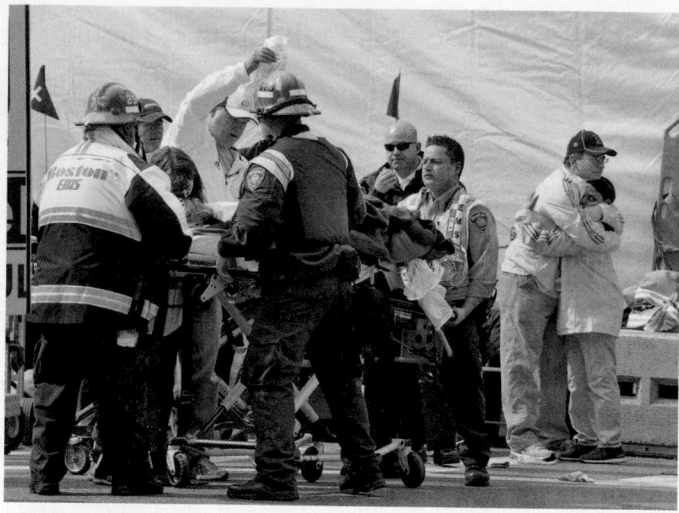

Source: Elise Amendola/AP Images.

Figure 46–7 ⟫ EMS personnel and volunteer nurses helped care for hundreds of victims of the Boston Marathon bombings on April 15, 2013.

community at large. Nurses are never expected to jeopardize their own safety or the safety of their families or other rescuers by responding to a disaster. Nurses must also consider whether they have the appropriate skills to respond—that is, whether the skills of the nurse are adequate for the job or whether the job would be better left to individuals with advanced training in disaster response.

If the decision is made to participate, the nurse will follow the emergency preparedness plans created by the employing agency or within the community. The nurse must operate within the defined nursing scope of practice despite the temptation to step outside of those bounds when faced with critical care needs outside the nurse's scope of practice.

Individuals who choose to provide care during disasters must be aware of the ethics of doing so and the personal risk that may be involved. The American Nurses Association provides guidance in this area and is working hard to ensure that nurses who work within the framework suggested by ANA are protected from risks associated with providing care.

The injuries experienced during a disaster are specifically related to the type of disaster. For example, nurses working where an earthquake has occurred will treat multiple crush injuries. During the Boston Marathon on April 15, 2013, two explosions occurred. Nurses who had volunteered to provide medical services during the marathon suddenly found themselves in the unexpected position of caring for mass casualties who had sustained fractures, head trauma, severe abdominal injuries, and amputations (**Figure 46–7 ⟫**).

Nurses should assist their communities not only by providing emergency care during a disaster but also by becoming leaders as their communities prepare for potential disasters by creating or revising emergency preparedness and contingency plans.

REVIEW Emergency Preparedness

RELATE Link the Concepts and Exemplars

Linking the exemplar of emergency preparedness with the concept of professional behaviors:

1. What is the nurse's professional duty in a time of disaster?

Linking the exemplar of emergency preparedness with the concept of managing care:

2. Uninsured Americans are the most vulnerable in the event of a pandemic event. How is early recognition related to access to care?

Linking the exemplar of emergency preparedness with the concept of ethics:

3. What ethical considerations are involved when allocating scarce resources, such as medication, equipment, and healthcare personnel, during a disaster?

REFER Go to Pearson MyLab Nursing and eText

- Additional review materials

REFLECT Apply Your Knowledge

Ed Jones is a 75-year-old retired cabinet maker who makes small toys in the basement of his home, located on the banks of the Deep River. He is independent and a widower. His primary care physician has prescribed antihypertensive medications and monitors his blood pressure regularly. When a week of heavy rainstorms flooded Mr. Jones's neighborhood, his home sustained much water damage and most of his equipment and wood were ruined. Mr. Jones waded through waist-deep water to reach a rescue boat rather than waiting for it to pick him up. The EMTs who triage him decide to transfer him to the nearest emergency department.

You are the nurse assessing Mr. Jones. You observe that he has multiple cuts on his hands that are a result of woodworking and an ulcer on his right foot. Mr. Jones reports that the ulcer developed after a tool fell on his foot. He adds that he has not sought medical treatment for it. His physical assessment findings reveal: T 100.7°F PO; P 96 beats/min, R 20/min, and BP 178/100 mmHg; his skin is cool and dry with multiple lesions on both hands and a stage II ulcer on his right dorsal foot with yellow-green exudate. His pain rated as 2 on a 0–10 scale with 10 being the worst pain there could be. His lungs are clear, and his heart rate is regular. No edema is noted.

1. What actions did Mr. Jones take that probably exacerbated his skin lesions?

2. What additional information is needed so that you can form nursing diagnoses for Mr. Jones?

3. What nursing diagnoses do you believe would be appropriate?

References

Agency for Healthcare Research and Quality (AHRQ). (2011). *National healthcare disparities report*. Retrieved from http://www.ahrq.gov/research/findings/nhqrdr/nhdr11/nhdr11.pdf

American Nurses Association (ANA). (2016, May). *Disaster preparedness and response*. Retrieved from http://nursingworld.org/MainMenuCategories/HealthcareandPolicyIssues/DPR.aspx

Association of Public Health Nurses (APHN). (2014). *The role of the public health nurse in disaster preparedness, response, and recovery*. Retrieved from http://www.achne.org/files/public/APHN_RoleOfPHNinDisasterPRR_FINALJan14.pdf

Bachrach, A., Isakson, E., Seth, D., & Brellochs, C. (2011, October). *Pediatric medical homes: Laying the foundation of a promising model of care*. Retrieved from http://www.nccp.org/publications/pdf/text_1041.pdf. Published by National Center for Children in Poverty, © 2011.

Berkman, N. D., Sheridan, S. L., Donahue, K. E., Halpern, D. J., & Crotty, K. (2011). Low health literacy and health outcomes: an updated systematic review. *Annals of Internal Medicine*, 155(2), 97–107.

Blumenthal, D., Abrams, M., & Nuzum, R. (2015). The Affordable Care Act at 5 years. *New England Journal of Medicine*, 372(25), 2451–2458.

Case Management Society of America. (2012). *What is a case manager?* Retrieved from http://www.cmsa.org/Home/CMSA/Whatisacasemanager/tabid/224/default.aspx

Centers for Disease Control and Prevention (CDC.) (2009). *H1N1 flu allocation and distribution Q&A*. Retrieved from http://www.cdc.gov/H1N1flu/vaccination/statelocal/centralized_distribution_qa.htm

Centers for Disease Control and Prevention (CDC). (2013). *Bioterrorism agents: Emergency*. Retrieved from http://www.bt.cdc.gov/agent/agentlist-category.asp

Centers for Disease Control and Prevention (CDC) (2016). *CDC's disaster planning goal: Protect vulnerable older adults*. Retrieved from [0]http://www.cdc.gov/aging/pdf/disaster_planning_goal.pdf

Centers for Medicare & Medicaid Services. (2017). *Health insurance marketplaces 2017 open enrollment period final enrollment report: November 1, 2016–January 31, 2017*. Retrieved from https://www.cms.gov/Newsroom/MediaReleaseDatabase/Fact-sheets/2017-Fact-Sheet-items/2017-03-15.html

Emergency Medical Treatment and Active Labor Act (EMTALA). (2011). *Frequently asked questions on EMTALA*. Retrieved from http://www.emtala.com/faq.html

Friese, C. R., Grunawalt, M. J. C., Bhullar, S., Bihlmeyer, M. K., Chang, R., & Wood, M. W. (2014). Pod nursing on a medical/surgical unit: implementation and outcomes evaluation. *Journal of Nursing Administration*, 44(4), 207.

HealthCare.Gov. (2013). *Community health centers*. Retrieved from http://www.healthcare.gov/using-insurance/low-cost-care/community-health-centers

Healthy Children. (2016). *Keeping children safe in Sandy's wake*. Retrieved from https://www.healthychildren.org/English/safety-prevention/at-home/Pages/Keeping-Children-Safe-in-Sandys-Wake.aspx

Henry J. Kaiser Family Foundation. (2013). *Key facts about healthcare reform*. Retrieved from http://kff.org/health-reform/fact-sheet/summary-of-the-affordable-care-act/

Henry J. Kaiser Family Foundation. (2015). *Key facts about the uninsured*. Retrieved from http://kff.org/uninsured/fact-sheet/key-facts-about-the-uninsured-population/

Henry J. Kaiser Family Foundation. (2016). *State health facts*. Retrieved from http://kff.org/state-category/providers-service-use/

Institute of Medicine. (1993). *Access to healthcare in America*. Washington, DC: National Academies Press.

Insure Kids Now. (2013). *Questions and answers: Why is healthcare so important?* Retrieved from http://www.insurekidsnow.gov/qa

International Nursing Coalition for Mass Casualty Education (INCMCE). (2003, August). *Educational competencies for registered nurses related to mass casualty incidents*. Retrieved from http://www.aacn.nche.edu/leading-initiatives/education resources/INCMCECompetencies.pdf

Koh, H. K., Berwick, D. M., Clancy, C. M., Baur, C., Brach, C., Harris, L. M., & Zerhusen, E. G. (2012). New federal policy initiatives to boost health literacy can help the nation move beyond the cycle of costly "crisis care." *Health Affairs*, 31(2), 434–443.

Macpac. (2017). *Medicaid enrollment changes following the ACA*. Retrieved from https://www.macpac.gov/subtopic/medicaid-enrollment-changes-following-the-aca/

Mangan, D. (2016). Record number of Obamacare sign-ups on HealthCare.gov for 2017 health insurance coverage. Retrieved from http://www.cnbc.com/2016/12/21/record-number-of-obamacare-signups-on-healthcaregov-for-2017-health-insurance-coverage.html

National Institutes of Health. (2013). *Health disparities*. Retrieved from http://report.nih.gov/NIHfactsheets/ViewFactSheet.aspx?csid=124

Office of Disease Prevention and Health Promotion (ODPHP). (2017a). *Healthy People 2020*. Retrieved from https://www.healthypeople.gov/2020/topics-objectives

Office of Disease Prevention and Health Promotion (ODPHP). (2017b). *Development of national health promotion and disease prevention objectives for 2030*. Retrieved from https://www.healthypeople.gov/2020/About-Healthy-People/Development-Healthy-People-2030

Torrey, T. (2012, April). *What is healthcare rationing? From denial of care to healthcare reform, rationing is a consideration*. Retrieved from http://patients.about.com/od/patientempowermentissues/a/rationing.htm

U.S. Census Bureau. (2014). 2014 national population projections. *Population projections*. Retrieved from https://www.census.gov/population/projections/data/national/2014.html

U.S. Department of Health and Human Services (USDHHS). (2017a). About donation. *Organ Procurement and Transplantation Network (OPTN)*. Retrieved from https://optn.transplant.hrsa.gov/learn/about-donation/

U.S. Department of Health and Human Services (USDHHS). (2017b). How organ allocation works. *Organ Procurement and Transplantation Network (OPTN)*. Retrieved from https://optn.transplant.hrsa.gov/learn/about-transplantation/how-organ-allocation-works/

U.S. Department of Homeland Security. (2016). *Community emergency response teams. FEMA*. Retrieved from https://www.fema.gov/community-emergency-response-teams

Whitty, B., & Burnett, M. (2012). From our readers: Are you prepared for a mass casualty event? *American Nurse Today*, 7(4). Retrieved from http://www.nursingworld.org/MainMenuCategories/Policy-Advocacy/Positions-and-Resolutions/Issue-Briefs/Disaster-Preparedness.pdf

World Health Organization. (1998). *Health promotion glossary*. Retrieved from http://whqlibdoc.who.int/hq/1998/WHO_HPR_HEP_98.1.pdf.

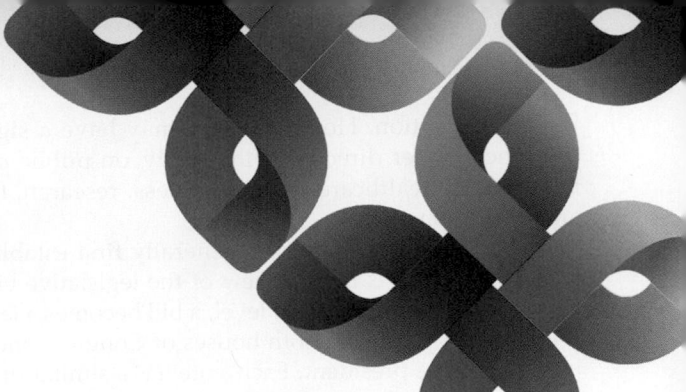

Module 47
Health Policy

Module Outline and Learning Outcomes

The Concept of Health Policy

Overview of Health Policy

47.1 Describe health policy, as an entity and as a process.

Developing Health Policies

47.2 Summarize the process of developing health policies.

Concepts Related to Health Policy

47.3 Outline the relationship between health policy and other concepts.

Federal, State, Local, and International Agencies

47.4 Outline the agencies or organizations involved in oversight or influence of health policy.

Accrediting Bodies

47.5 Analyze the role of accrediting organizations in the advancement of health policy.

Professional Associations

47.6 Analyze professional organizations' influences on health policy.

Healthcare Funding

47.7 Analyze types of health insurance and the health policies that regulate reimbursement.

>> The Concept of Health Policy

Concept Key Terms

Accreditation, **2801**	Copayment, **2804**	Health policy, **2797**	Point-of-service (POS) plan, **2805**	Primary care provider (PCP), **2805**
Children's Health Insurance Program (CHIP), **2806**	Domestic partner, **2804**	Indemnity, **2805**	Preferred-provider organization (PPO), **2805**	Regulation, **2797**
	Executive branch agency, **2798**	Law, **2797**		
Consumer-driven healthcare plan (CDHP), **2805**	Health maintenance organization (HMO), **2805**	Medicaid, **2805**		
		Medicare, **2805**		
		Medigap policy, **2805**		

Health policies drive the availability, safety, and quality of the healthcare provided in the United States. A poorly constructed policy or the absence of a needed policy can have a significant negative impact on the health and well-being of individuals or whole populations. Professional nurses must understand how healthcare policy affects patients, their own practice, and the organizations in which they work. Every day, nurses see the public's healthcare needs and can envision how new or revised health policies could improve the quality and safety of healthcare. Nurses can influence change by working with public officials at the local, community, state, and national levels as representatives of their professional association or as individual citizens.

Overview of Health Policy

The term **health policy** refers to actions taken by government bodies and other societal actors to attain specific health-related goals. Health policies include laws, regulations, government agency guidelines, position statements, resolutions, judicial decrees, and budget priorities.

Public health policy is established in **law** (statute) and **regulation** (rules) at the federal or state levels and is therefore enforceable by the government agency responsible for implementing the policy. Public health policy is subject to influence by nongovernmental healthcare organizations and health professions associations, education accreditation agencies, and private citizens. Public health policies have powerful effects on healthcare delivery systems, the health and well-being of U.S. citizens, and professional nursing issues ranging from scope of practice and safe staffing to nursing education funding and universal access to health insurance.

Private agencies may also develop health policy. Policies generated by private associations representing the interests of healthcare organizations, health professions, or health professions education associations are not established in law or regulation. However, they may have a significant influence, either directly or indirectly, on public policy in the areas of healthcare practice, access, research, funding, and education.

Public healthcare policy is generally first established in law. Lawmaking is the purview of the legislative branch of government. On the federal level, a bill becomes a law when it is passed by votes in both houses of Congress and signed into law by the president. Each state has a similar procedure for passing state laws, which are signed into law by the governor. Presidential vetoes, executive orders, and judicial interpretations of law also have the force of law; courts may determine the outcome of health policy if laws are vague or controversial (Milstead, 2016).

Once a law has been passed, an **executive branch agency** of the federal or state government is responsible for administering it. The Centers for Disease Control and Prevention (CDC), for example, is an executive branch agency authorized to implement laws to protect the public against exposure and spread of highly communicable disease (CDC, 2014). State executive branch agencies include state health departments and state Boards of Nursing. A state health department may have jurisdiction over local health departments and boards of health, sanitarians, and vital statistics, among other responsibilities. Boards of Nursing are authorized to implement the nurse practice act in their state, and license or discipline license holders to protect the public.

Laws provide broad mandates and are written somewhat generally to provide flexibility and so they can withstand the test of time. Therefore, the laws that create public health policy and the laws that create executive branch agencies also give the administering executive branch agencies the authority to write regulations. Regulations provide the detail that describes how the executive branch agency will carry out the law. A regulation must always refer directly to the law it seeks to amplify, and an agency cannot write rules that exceed its statutory authority; the original intent of the legislature that created the law must be honored (**Figure 47–1 》**).

Developing Health Policies

Public healthcare policies are the product of both government processes and political forces. The process often begins when legislators or leaders in executive branch health agencies commit to solve a problem or bridge a gap in services. Sometimes constituents bring problems or gaps to their legislators' attention. In other cases, special interest groups, such as health professions associations, raise awareness and begin to lobby for a new health policy. Some initial questions precede construction of a bill's first draft, such as the following:

■ What population of citizens will benefit? Is it large or small? Is it underserved and economically disadvantaged?

■ What is the anticipated cost of implementing the policy? Do the benefits outweigh the cost of implementation?

■ Who are the stakeholders? Is there support for the policy? If not, what issues are in question?

■ Is there a body of scientific evidence to support the efficacy of the policy? Are there similar models in other states that have been successful?

The four major stages in policymaking are agenda setting, government response, implementation, and evaluation. In each stage, formal and informal relationships develop between stakeholders both inside and outside of government. Those serving in government positions can include legislators, bureaucrats such as regulatory officials, the president's or governor's staff, or the courts. Stakeholders outside government can include interested citizens who may or may not be constituents of specific legislators, institutions, and professional associations or other special interest groups.

How resources are allocated, and to whom, is determined within a political framework. Influence, negotiation, bargaining, and compromise are all part of this process, which is not necessarily logical or linear (Milstead, 2016). For example, interested parties may resist certain provisions in a bill midway through the process, which may lead to a revision of the political agenda. An example of developing a health policy is described in **Box 47–1 》**.

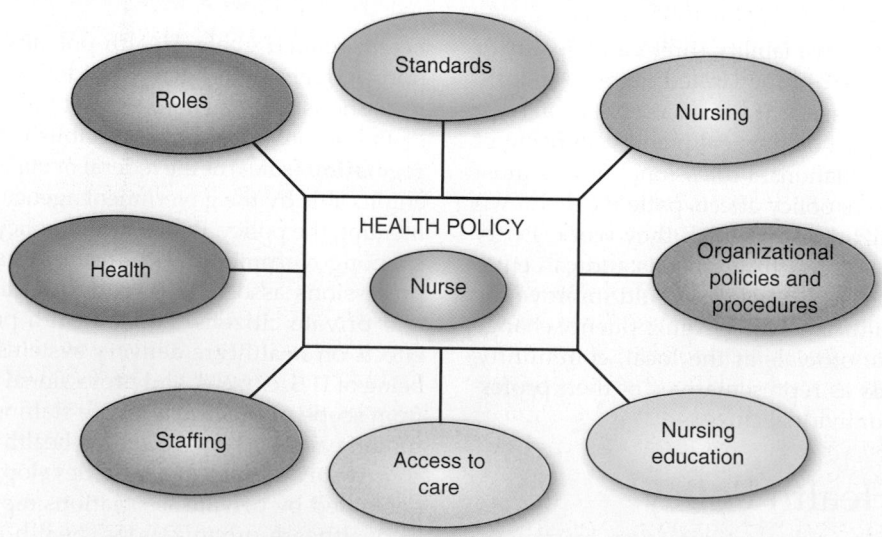

Figure 47–1 》 Why is health policy relevant to nurses?

Box 47–1
Developing an Evidence-informed Health Policy: An Example

Evidence-based practice models provide processes to address clinical problems and improve healthcare outcomes. The same processes can be used to address health policy problems. For example, opioid and heroin abuse is a significant public health problem that has reached epidemic proportions in the United States. A specific issue is that individuals who overdose on opioids are often in respiratory and cardiac arrest when EMS arrives. EMS personnel administer naloxone (Narcan) onsite, but the time between the cardiopulmonary arrest and naloxone administration may be too long to ensure a positive outcome for the individual. The literature demonstrates:

1. Individuals with an opioid addiction are at particularly high risk for overdose immediately post-rehabilitation, when their tolerance has been reduced.
2. Individuals who are most likely to be in the vicinity of the person who is overdosing are family or close friends, who may or may not have emergency medical training, supplies, or equipment.

3. The safety profile on naloxone suggests that it is about as safe for laypeople to administer as is epinephrine during anaphylaxis.

Using an evidence-informed health policy process, policymakers and stakeholders would examine the external evidence (including scientific evidence that naloxone is safe for administration by non-healthcare personnel), combine the evidence with their issue expertise (discussions with and testimony from stakeholders, professional experts, and so on), and combine that with lawmaker and stakeholder values and ethics (e.g., the value of making lifesaving naloxone available to those in a position to administer naloxone when it will be most effective: family and friends of individuals addicted to opioids) (Loversidge, 2016). This process can help to inform the dialogue necessary for the drafting of lifesaving legislation that will permit family and friends of persons addicted to opioids to have a dose of naloxone on hand, the training to administer the drug, and the education to understand the importance of follow-up by calling EMS.

Concepts Related to Health Policy

A number of concepts in the Healthcare Domain relate to health policy. These include accountability, advocacy, ethics, healthcare systems, legal issues, quality improvement, and safety. A few of these integral to health policy are discussed in the Concepts Related to Health Policy feature. They are presented in alphabetical order.

Federal, State, Local, and International Agencies

Agencies with the authority to affect the health of citizens exist at the federal, state, local, and international levels. Their missions and scope of authority differ. Some have a broad scope of responsibility; others have very specific responsibilities. Some have extensive regulatory authority; others receive authority to enact programs from their parent departments.

Federal Agencies

Healthcare policies with direct effects on the nation's health are administered through the U.S. Department of Health and Human Services (HHS) and the agencies it oversees. Other federal departments also administer policies that affect the nation's health. For example, the U.S. Department of Labor oversees policies that affect worker safety; these policies are administered through the Occupational Safety and Health Administration. The U.S. Environmental Protection Agency (2015) is responsible for protecting the environment; this also affects the nation's health.

Department of Health and Human Services

The HHS is the principal federal health agency. It has 11 operating divisions: Administration for Children and Families (ACF), Administration for Community Living (ACL), Agency for Healthcare Research and Quality (AHRQ), Agency for Toxic Substances and Disease Registry (ATSDR), Centers for Disease Control and Prevention (CDC), Centers for Medicare & Medicaid Services (CMS), Food and Drug Administration (FDA), Health Resources and Services Administration (HRSA), Indian Health Service (IHS), National Institutes of Health (NIH), and Substance Abuse and Mental Health Services Administration (SAMHSA).

HHS is a powerful agency that administers more grant dollars than all other federal agencies combined (HHS, 2017). The 2017 HHS budget of $1.150 trillion was allocated to fund more than 300 divisions and programs. Examples of HHS programs include those that improve maternal and infant health, protect mental health, promote better nutrition and physical activity, and prevent and manage the impact of infectious and chronic diseases and conditions (HHS, 2017).

>> **Stay Current:** To learn more about the programs and services of the U.S. Department of Health and Human Services, go to http://www.hhs.gov/programs/index.html.

Occupational Safety and Health Administration

The Occupational Safety and Health Administration (OSHA), an agency of the U.S. Department of Labor, is tasked with ensuring the health and safety of Americans in the workplace. The OSHA legislation covers most private sector employers and their workers plus some employers and workers in the public sector. Part of OSHA's mission is to provide assistance to employers, who are responsible for providing a safe workplace and for reducing or eliminating workplace hazards. OSHA standards address a wide variety

Concepts Related to
Health Policy

CONCEPT	RELATIONSHIP TO HEALTH POLICY	NURSING IMPLICATIONS
Healthcare Systems	Access to healthcare is directly related to insurability. The Affordable Care Act changed the profile of insurability for millions of previously uninsured adults and children who would otherwise have been unable to afford healthcare insurance. Public health policies direct coding, billing, and reimbursement for care, which in turn may affect how care is provided and documented.	■ Nurses may find that insured individuals use primary care services more often. Continuity of care may improve for them, especially for individuals with chronic conditions. ■ Health policies related to managed care may have a variety of impacts on patients' healthcare. For example, one patient's health insurance plan may cover brand name prescription medication with a small copayment. A patient on another plan might have a much higher copayment for a brand name prescription; the nurse may need to work with the prescribing provider to ensure that the patient receives a prescription for the more cost-effective generic medication.
Legal Issues	The U.S. Constitution grants states the authority to govern selected professions such as nursing, medicine, and pharmacy. Authority to enforce the laws, known as practice acts, is granted by law, usually to Boards of Nursing, or in some states, to an "umbrella board" that includes a division responsible for oversight of nursing.	■ Current licensure is required for practice as a nurse. Nurses are held accountable for knowing the legal nursing scope of practice in their state and what actions could place their licensure status in jeopardy, as well as all regulations that accompany the nurse practice act. State Boards of Nursing also have authority to write regulations to amplify the practice act. Regulations typically address standards of safe and competent practice, delegation, and continuing education requirements.
Quality Improvement	Some public health policies are enacted to advance science, translate science to practice, and support national health imperatives. The Agency for Healthcare Research and Quality (AHRQ), an agency of the Public Health Service in the U.S. Department of HHS, determines standards of healthcare quality by using a system of quality indicators. If providers are not meeting those standards. AHRQ provides training for health professionals.	■ Nurses are accountable for competent, safe patient care. Part of that responsibility is becoming engaged in organizational quality improvement and quality management projects at the unit level or the organization committee level. Joint Commission–accredited hospitals typically use AHRQ quality indicators specific to their setting, which can provide helpful means to reach The Joint Commission National Patient Safety Goals and other quality improvement objectives.

of hazards in industrial and healthcare workplaces (**Figure 47–2 》**). One example is the availability of emergency eye-wash stations (U.S. Department of Labor, n.d.).

》 Stay Current: Go to www.osha.gov for the latest information from the Occupational Safety and Health Administration.

State Health Agencies

Each state mandates its own health policies and regulations in accord with federal policies and regulations. Each state has its own division or department of health and human services, with a scope of responsibility determined by that state. These departments generally report to the state's governor and are part of the executive branch of state government. State health departments enforce regulation of county health departments and may license or register healthcare facilities such as hospitals and long-term care facilities, child care centers, clinical laboratories, and other service providers such as

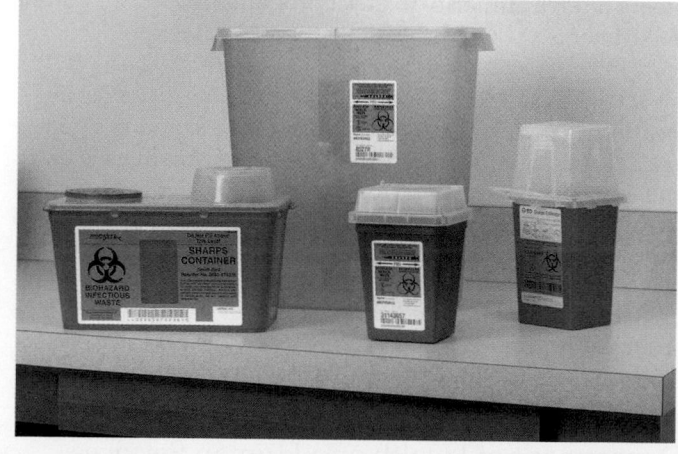

Figure 47–2 》 OSHA regulations require use of sharps containers for discarding used needles.

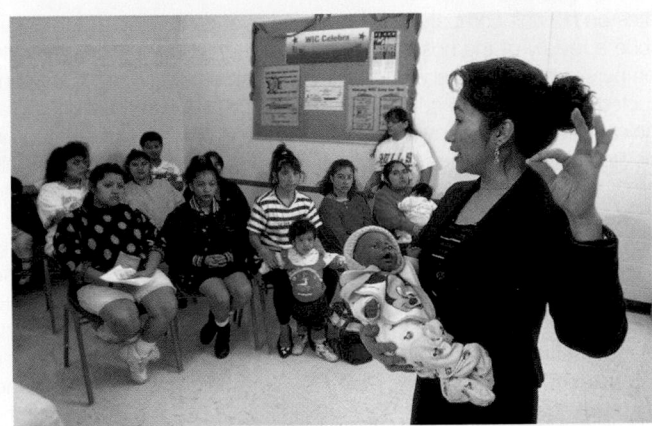

Source: A. Ramey/PhotoEdit Inc.

Figure 47–3 >> An instructor uses a doll to demonstrate breast-feeding techniques to a group of women in a WIC program.

portable x-ray suppliers. The departments may also be responsible for overseeing the planning and construction of medical facilities and for receiving and resolving complaints about the facilities they regulate. They are often responsible for tracking state health data and statistics; maintaining birth, death, marriage, and divorce records; and enforcing state-wide health laws, such as smoking bans.

State offices of emergency medical services (OEMSs) may be structurally connected to a larger state department, such as a state department of public safety. OEMSs are usually responsible for establishing training and certification standards for EMS personnel, accrediting training programs, overseeing the state's trauma system, and/or licensing medical transportation services. By ensuring that local emergency medical services (EMS) systems comply with the applicable regulations, OEMSs provide citizens access to high-quality emergency medical care.

Local Health Departments

At the county or municipal level, local departments of health administer health policies and offer many vital services to their communities. In counties that surround cities with large populations, both county and city health departments may exist, often with a division of responsibility. For example, the county health department may be responsible for regulating health issues with widespread effects, such as sanitation, retail food establishment safety, and waste disposal. City health departments may provide clinical, environmental, health promotion, and population-based services such as free clinics, sexual health, HIV/AIDs testing, and TB and dental clinics. City health departments are often responsible for developing and enforcing city-wide health codes and for disease monitoring.

Local departments of health may oversee child care center sanitation and food safety and typically offer community-wide disease and injury prevention programs, which may be federally supported or arise in response to local issues. Such programs include injury prevention campaigns, lead poisoning prevention efforts, and making safety equipment such as smoke detectors, children's bicycle helmets, and infant car seats available to families at no cost. Local social

services departments are typically responsible for administering Medicaid, the Child Health Insurance Program, and the Women, Infants, and Children (WIC) supplemental nutrition program, which provides food assistance to pregnant women and children under age 5 who are at risk for malnutrition (**Figure 47–3 >>**).

Clinical Example A

Richard Taylor is a 46-year-old man who works as an assistant to social workers in a residential homeless shelter in an underserved area of the city. An increasing number of shelter residents have been showing symptoms of active tuberculosis (TB). Social workers have been sending these individuals to the free clinic associated with the shelter for treatment. Now Mr. Taylor and his coworkers have become concerned about their own risk, even though they have taken measures to quickly identify residents at risk and work appropriately with them. Mr. Taylor finds that his city health department does not conduct TB screening, so he seeks screening at a local drugstore with a nurse-managed clinic. He tests positive for TB.

Critical Thinking Questions

1. What information should the nurse practitioner have at hand to assist Mr. Taylor to access low-cost or free treatment?
2. What recommendations could the nurse make to Mr. Taylor to advocate for improved TB risk exposure prevention for employees and residents at the homeless shelter?

International Health Agencies

International health organizations fall into three groups, depending on their funding sources and location: multilateral organizations, bilateral organizations, and nongovernmental organizations (NGOs). All the major multilateral organizations are part of the United Nations (UN). The premier international health organization is the World Health Organization (WHO), which is an intergovernmental agency related to the UN and is the only international health organization with legal authority. Bilateral agencies are governmental agencies with a home in a single country, such as the U.S. Agency for International Development. They provide aid to developing countries. NGOs, also known as private voluntary organizations (PVOs), are independent of any government. More than 130 health-related NGOs based in the United States were reported in 2013; of these, 20 were faith-based (Moss, 2014). An example is Project Hope, which provides essential medicine and supplies, volunteers, medical training, and disaster response. International health organizations typically provide support services and establish guiding policy.

Accrediting Bodies

Accreditation is a process of gaining recognition through a peer review process that evaluates the quality of an organization on the basis of the standards and criteria of the accreditation organization. Reputable accreditation organizations establish standards using a rigorous process based on evidence. Whereas state or federal licensing or certification is governmental, accreditation is private and voluntary; but achieving accreditation certifies that the organization meets quality criteria and is competent to provide the services or programs it offers. Accredited organizations must be reevaluated at intervals specified by the accrediting body. To achieve reaccreditation, an organization must provide evidence that it has continuously evaluated its own performance, has acted to correct deficiencies and continuously improved its performance, and continues to meet the accreditation standards.

The accreditation body conducts an on-site survey to validate the organization's self-assessment and performance and to determine whether the organization meets the required standards. This occurs at the initial accreditation visit and during periodic reaccreditation visits. Benefits of accreditation and the nurse's role in the process depend on the type of accreditation.

The Joint Commission

The Joint Commission is an independent, nonprofit organization that sets standards for and accredits healthcare provider organizations, such as ambulatory care centers, behavioral healthcare providers, hospitals, and long-term care facilities. Its standards address key functions for each type of organization it accredits—for example, infection prevention and control, provision of care, treatment and services, medical management, environment of care, and performance improvement (The Joint Commission, 2016). Healthcare organizations are highly motivated to achieve Joint Commission accreditation, which brings not only greater consumer trust and respectability, but also credibility with private third-party payers, and helps organizations meet qualifications for Medicare and Medicaid reimbursement.

Although The Joint Commission is an independent, nongovernmental organization, its work significantly influences national quality and safety standards and the advancement of healthcare policy. For example, since 2003, The Joint Commission has identified annual National Patient Safety Goals (NPSGs) (see the module on Safety) to help accredited organizations address specific patient safety concerns (The Joint Commission, 2015). The Joint Commission also has requirements for reporting sentinel events (see the module on Quality Improvement). The NPSGs and the Sentinel Event reporting system provide benchmarks for quality improvement processes in healthcare organizations across the country.

A nurse's role in The Joint Commission accreditation process may include helping to develop, revise, or facilitate use of policies and procedures for nursing practice that are current and evidence-based. The nurse may also participate in an organization's self-review activities. Nurses, especially those in management positions, may also be part of meetings with the accreditation survey team; survey teams are often interested in speaking with the healthcare providers who are most involved in maintaining standards at the point of care.

>> **Stay Current:** Go to www.jointcommission.org for the latest information from The Joint Commission.

Clinical Example B

Darren Langdon is a 34-year-old staff RN on a medical–surgical unit in a hospital classified by The Joint Commission as a Critical Access Hospital. The nursing department has been preparing for a Joint Commission reaccreditation survey visit. Unrelated to the visit, Darren's unit has been concerned about the rate of catheter-associated urinary tract infections (CAUTI). Darren has taken the lead in gathering data about the CAUTI

rates on his unit compared to other units over the past 6 months, has done a review of the hospital's policies and procedures, has talked to the nurses on his unit about how they implement these, and has conducted a review of the current literature on CAUTI. Having learned that the current hospital policy is outdated in comparison to what he found in the literature, Darren has been encouraged by the nurse manager, his fellow staff members, and nursing leadership to draft a new policy to present to the hospital's policy and procedure committee.

The Joint Commission survey visitors come to Darren's unit during a reaccreditation survey visit. They have noticed the data on the CAUTI rates and are asking the nurse manager and staff to respond to questions about possible causes and actions. Darren's nurse manager asks him to meet with her and the visitors to discuss the unit's process and plan to address the CAUTI rates, at both the unit and organizational levels.

Critical Thinking Questions

1. What should Darren be aware of with regard to the National Patient Safety Goals? Is there a National Patient Safety Goal related to CAUTI?
2. How should Darren explain to the survey visitors the process he used to address the CAUTI problem on his unit?

Nursing Education Program Accreditation

Although nursing program accreditation is considered voluntary, most graduate nursing programs and many RN-to-BSN programs require applicants to graduate from an accredited prelicensure/BSN program as a criterion for admission. The Commission on Collegiate Nursing Education (CCNE), an autonomous arm of the American Association of Colleges of Nursing (AACN), accredits baccalaureate and graduate education programs. The Accreditation Commission for Education in Nursing (ACEN) accredits all types of nursing education programs (clinical doctorate, master's degree, baccalaureate degree, associate degree, diploma, and practical nursing education programs). The National League for Nursing Commission for Nursing Education Accreditation (NLN CNEA) was established in 2013. In the spring of 2016, the NLN CNEA issued standards of accreditation for practical nursing/vocational nursing, diploma, associate, bachelor, master's, and clinical doctorate degree programs. CNEA is an autonomous accreditation division of NLN (NLN, 2016a).

Many accrediting organizations belong to the Association of Specialized and Professional Accreditors (ASPA). The ASPA Code of Good Practice for Accrediting Bodies, which has been adopted by CCNE, states that accrediting organizations focus on educational quality, "not narrow interests, or political action" (AACN, 2016a). By conforming to this ethical principal and focusing on education quality, nursing education accreditation commissions also work toward improving the quality of nursing education and healthcare by influencing educators and the membership of their parent or affiliate organizations. AACN, the national voice for baccalaureate and graduate nursing education, has a Government Affairs division that oversees its federal policy agenda. AACN's policy agenda focuses on expanding federal funding streams to support nursing education; supporting higher education policy priorities that affect affordability, access, transparency, and diversity; and advancing federal initiatives relevant to nursing education (AACN, 2016b).

Professional Associations

Nursing associations exist to serve their specialized membership and advance the nursing profession. Professional nursing associations define standards of practice and professional behaviors, establish codes of ethics for their members, support nursing research, and participate in policy development at a level commensurate with the scope of their membership. Some associations are state branches of the national association representing all registered nurses; others serve one of the many specialized memberships.

International Council of Nurses

The International Council of Nurses (ICN), which represents more than 16 million nurses worldwide, is the world's oldest organization for health professionals. It is a federation of more than 130 national nurses' associations with the mission to "represent nursing worldwide, advancing the profession and influencing health policy" (ICN, 2015). The ICN addressed a number of key issues for nursing at the 69th World Health Assembly in Geneva, Switzerland. These included the ICN's commitment to work with world government leaders to implement an action plan to address violence as the first point of care for elder abuse and intimate partner violence and in conflict, post-conflict, and humanitarian settings. Another issue identified was the need to remove regulatory barriers on nursing scopes of practice to strengthen primary healthcare systems as a key to improving elder well-being (ICN, 2016).

Sigma Theta Tau International

Sigma Theta Tau International (STTI) is an international nursing organization with more than 135,000 active members in 500 chapters in 90 countries around the globe. It was founded in the United States in 1922 and incorporated as an international organization in 1985. Its mission is "advancing world health and celebrating nursing excellence in scholarship, leadership, and service" (STTI, 2016). Membership is by invitation to baccalaureate and graduate nursing students who demonstrate excellence in scholarship and to nurse leaders who exhibit exceptional achievements in nursing. STTI's benefits to its members include leadership summits, funding and forums for disseminating research, continuing education opportunities, and career services. STTI's Global Health Policy Position Statement states that "the membership is engaged in education, clinical practice and leadership endeavors that inform health policy at local, national, and international levels" (STTI, n.d.). Other STTI Position Statements that have policy implications include topics such as international nurse migration, global health and nursing research priorities, and universal access to affordable, high-quality healthcare.

American Nurses Association

The American Nurses Association (ANA) represents the 3.6 million registered nurses in the United States through joint membership with its constituent and state nurses' associations and direct membership in ANA. Its mission statement is "Nurses advancing our profession to improve health for all" (ANA, n.d.). The ANA fosters high standards of nursing practice, promotes the rights of nurses in the workplace, projects a positive and realistic view of nursing, and lobbies Congress and federal regulatory agencies on healthcare issues affecting nurses and the health of Americans. There are constituent or state nurses' associations in each of the 50 states and in Guam, the Virgin Islands, and Washington, DC, as well as the Federal Nurses Association (ANA, 2016a). Membership for the Federal Nurses Association is open to registered nurses who are classified as active duty in the U.S. armed forces: Army, Navy, Air Force, or U.S. Public Health Service.

The ANA Membership Assembly and/or Board of Directors respond to current events related to the ANA's policy agenda by writing a position statement or resolution. ANA Position Statement topics include specific issues related to bloodborne and airborne diseases, consumer advocacy, drug and alcohol abuse, environmental health, and ethics and human rights. The ANA also writes issue briefs expressing the association's opinion on how federal or state laws or proposed federal rules, regulations, policies or guidelines affect nurses and patients (ANA, 2016b). In addition, the ANA publishes a number of documents that serve as guiding principles and standards for all RNs in the United States.

>> **Stay Current:** Go to www.nursingworld.org for more about the American Nurses Association.

National Student Nurses Association

The National Student Nurses Association (NSNA) is a nonprofit organization that mentors nursing students preparing for initial licensing as registered nurses. Students may be enrolled in associate, baccalaureate, diploma, and prelicensure (second-degree) graduate programs. NSNA is dedicated to fostering the professional development of these students by conveying "the standards, ethics, and skills students will need as responsible and accountable leaders and members of the profession" (NSNA, n.d.). NSNA membership provides opportunities for workshop participation, networking, scholarships, and career planning. NSNA also links interested members to the ANA Nursing Strategic Action Team (N-STAT program), which unites nurses across the nation who aspire to let lawmakers know their position on bills moving through Congress.

Specialty Practice Nursing Associations

Most nursing specialties are supported by a professional specialty practice association, which advances nursing practice in the affiliated specialty area and provides support to practitioners and their patients. The missions of the organizations include advocacy, education, provision of networking opportunities, and strengthening professional identities among members. Examples of specialty practice associations include the Academy of Medical-Surgical Nurses; the American Assisted Living Nurses Association; the American Association of Critical-Care Nurses; the Association of Pediatric Oncology Nurses; the Association of Women's Health, Obstetric, and Neonatal Nurses; the National Association of Orthopaedic Nurses; and the Oncology Nursing Society.

Several professional nursing associations exist to support and promote the interests of special nursing profession demographics. These include the Asian American/Pacific Islander Nurses Association, the American Assembly for Men in Nursing, the National Black Nurses Association, and the National Association of Hispanic Nurses.

Clinical Example C

Marsha Johnson, RN, BSN, graduated from a university college of nursing 10 years ago. Three years ago, she decided to continue her education and applied to an accredited certified registered nurse anesthetist (CRNA) program. She completed the program, passed the national certification exam, and was hired by a small-volume ambulatory surgery center. She competently delivers care and enjoys her advanced practice role. She works with an anesthesiologist but is the only CRNA on staff. She recently realized that as a nurse anesthetist, she has a limited number of professional contacts with other nurses employed at the center and that because the surgery center requires only one nurse anesthetist, she will not have many opportunities for interaction with peers or on-site educational opportunities specific to her role. She is starting to feel isolated.

Critical Thinking Questions

1. What professional association would you recommend to Ms. Johnson to fulfill her need for peers and CRNA-specific continuing education?
2. What networking and support is available from this association?
3. Where else could Ms. Johnson go for professional support?

National League for Nursing

The National League for Nursing (NLN), the first nursing organization in the United States, was founded in 1893 as the American Society of Superintendents of Training Schools for Nurses. The NLN's mission is "to promote excellence in nursing education to build a strong and diverse nursing workforce to advance the health of our nation and the global community" (NLN, 2016b). Its membership consists of nursing education programs, nursing faculty, and leaders in nursing education, both nurses and non-nurses. NLN nursing education program membership includes practical nursing, associate degree, baccalaureate, master's, and doctoral programs. Member services include professional development, research, student exam services, nurse educator certification, public policy, and networking (NLN, 2016c). The organization's public policy focuses on influencing policies affecting nursing workforce development, nursing education, and healthcare for underserved populations (NLN, 2015).

The American Association of Colleges of Nursing

The American Association of Colleges of Nursing (AACN) is "the national voice for America's baccalaureate and graduate nursing education" (AACN, 2016c). Its membership consists of 790 member schools of nursing, which includes baccalaureate, graduate, and postgraduate programs. AACN serves the school of nursing administrative staff, faculty, and students. It facilitates programs in instructional development, research, organizational leadership, faculty practice, and other services. AACN establishes *Essentials*, which are the standards for the education curricula of its member nursing programs. AACN's government relations team works to advance public policy related to nursing education, research, and practice. AACN has served as a leader in securing federal support for nursing education and research and has helped shape policy affecting nursing education programs and financial assistance for nursing students (AACN, 2016c).

Healthcare Funding

Perhaps the most important issue in health policy today is how healthcare is funded. Healthcare has historically been considered a market-based commodity in the United States. The sweeping social welfare legislation embodied in the Social Security Act of 1935 did not include healthcare coverage for all Americans. Blue Cross and Blue Shield, the earliest private insurance plans, were developed in the early 1930s and covered hospital and physician care. With the advent of private insurance, the political pressure to enact government-operated health insurance was diffused. No progress was made on this issue until 1965, when the federal government entered healthcare financing with Medicare and Medicaid (Pulcini & Hart, 2014).

Health insurance in the United States is available through private insurance companies and through government-funded programs for those who qualify. As part of the Affordable Care Act (ACA) passed by Congress in 2010, many individuals who did not qualify for Medicare or Medicaid and who would otherwise not have had access to health insurance gained improved access to health insurance coverage. Access to health insurance for individuals who do not qualify for Medicare or Medicaid or who do not have employer-based health insurance coverage varies from state to state and depends on policies enacted by state legislatures and Congress.

Private Healthcare System

Any health insurance not funded by government is private health insurance. Individuals purchase private health insurance plans to protect themselves from all or some of the medical, surgical, and preventive care expenses they would incur without coverage. The three basic private insurance plan types are employer-sponsored insurance, self-employment-based plans, and direct-purchase plans. There are also private insurance policies to supplement Medicare coverage.

Employment-sponsored insurance (ESI) is offered through one's employer or union. The percentage of adult Americans under 65 who subscribe to this type of health insurance fell from 69.7% in 2000 to 59.5% in 2011 (Robert Wood Johnson Foundation, 2013). Group health insurance is usually purchased by large employers that offer healthcare coverage to eligible company employees. ESI coverage may be extended to include the spouse, dependents, or domestic partner of the employee. A **domestic partner** is an unmarried partner of the same or opposite sex. Group coverage may also be purchased through voluntary and membership associations, such as professional and trade groups, bar associations, local chambers of commerce, and AARP. Benefits of group health insurance, especially when provided by large employers, may include lower premium costs (the amount of money paid for insurance coverage) and better coverage for eligible employees and their families. The employer may pay nothing toward the premium or may make partial or full payment; the employee is responsible for the premium amount not paid by the employer. The insured may also be responsible for additional costs such as deductibles, coinsurance, and copayments. Deductibles are commonly between $100 and $300 per individual and $500 to $2000 per family annually for medical care. A **copayment** is a set amount paid at the time of service (e.g., $20 for a primary-care physician office visit). Copayments for specialty care are usually higher than those for primary care. An out-of-pocket maximum protects the patient from catastrophic healthcare costs; if medical expenses reach a certain amount during a 12-month period, the plan covers all usual and customary fees for the remainder of the year.

Self-employment-based health insurance coverage is available only to individuals who are self-employed, and only the policyholder is covered by the plan. Individuals who are self-employed and have chronic health conditions often experience difficulty trying to purchase health insurance through private insurers.

An individual who needs private health insurance and is ineligible for group coverage purchases an individual policy. The individual purchasing an individual plan is responsible for paying the premium as well as copayments and deductibles. Individual health insurance policies are usually more expensive and coverage is more restricted than under group health coverage. A medical examination may be required to determine eligibility, and individuals with pre-existing medical conditions may find it difficult to find a company that will provide health insurance.

Types of Private Health Insurance Plans

Health insurance plans offered in the United States range from health maintenance organizations (HMOs), the most restrictive type, to indemnity plans (also known as "fee-for-service" plans), the least restrictive. Plans in the middle of the spectrum are point-of-service (POS) plans and preferred provider organizations (PPOs); both are considered managed-care plans and include features of both HMO and indemnity coverage. Usually, a greater selection of in-network providers is available in PPO and POS options than in HMOs.

Health maintenance organizations (HMOs) are insurance plans that limit coverage to care from physicians who contract with the specific HMO. Out-of-network care is not generally covered except in emergencies. HMOs may require that the person live or work in the service area. Participants must often select a **primary care provider (PCP)**, who serves as the gatekeeper to care and refers the patient to in-network hospitals and specialists when additional care is needed. HMOs typically provide a broad range of healthcare benefits; they often provide integrated care, covering preventive care and wellness.

A **preferred-provider organization (PPO)** does not require the insured to select a PCP. PPOs usually have larger networks of providers than HMOs and provide financial incentives that encourage insured persons to seek care from in-network providers. PPOs are less restrictive than HMOs but typically have higher copayments.

A **point-of-service (POS) plan** is a hybrid of an HMO and a PPO. Each time insured individuals seek healthcare, they decide which option—HMO or PPO—to use. Members pay less if they use in-network physicians, hospitals, and other healthcare providers. If they opt to use out-of-network providers, they pay higher copayments, coinsurance, and deductibles. The advantages of the POS plan are its flexibility and freedom of choice in comparison with a traditional HMO.

Indemnity plans allow the insured to self-select healthcare providers; that is, there is no network. These plans may use some managed-care techniques to control costs (e.g., preauthorization of MRIs).

The **consumer-driven healthcare plan (CDHP)** is a type of employer-sponsored coverage that combines a private insurance plan with a health savings account (HSA) or health reimbursement account (HRA). This type of plan typically has a higher deductible but lower monthly premiums. As part of the plan, the employer offers HSA or HRA accounts to all employees. Employees then save money in the HSA or HRA so that they can pay for deductibles and noncovered services. In some cases, the amount that goes into the HSA or HRA is provided by the employer as part of the employee benefits package.

Medigap Policy

A **Medigap policy** (i.e., Medicare supplemental insurance) is private health insurance designed to supplement Medicare coverage. These policies may pay copayments, coinsurance, deductibles, and "gaps" in Medicare coverage (i.e., noncovered health care costs). If an individual has a Medigap policy, Medicare will pay its share first; then the Medigap policy will pay its share. Medigap policies are required to comply with federal and state laws and must be transparent in stating they are "Medicare Supplement Insurance." State laws designate the letters by which these policies can identify themselves.

Federally Funded Public Healthcare

The Centers for Medicare and Medicaid Services (CMS) is the federal agency and public funding system responsible for administering Medicare, Medicaid, and the Children's Health Insurance Program (CHIP). Other public funding systems include the Veteran's Administration (VA); the Defense Health Program (TRICARE) for military personnel, their families, and military retirees; the Indian Health Service, which covers American Indians and Alaskan Natives; and the Federal Employees Health Benefits (FEHB) Program, which covers federal employees. Federally funded healthcare is subject to relevant federal legislation.

Medicare

Medicare is a federally funded health insurance program available to people age 65 or older who have worked in a Medicare-covered employment setting, younger people with disabilities, and people with end-stage renal disease or amyotrophic lateral sclerosis (ALS). Medicare covers 16% of Americans (Kaiser Family Foundation, 2012). Four types of coverage are available through Medicare (**Box 47-2 》》**).

Medicare does not cover all medical expenses. Excluded services include long-term care, routine dental and eye care, hearing aids and the exams for fitting them, and cosmetic surgery. People often purchase Medigap policies from private companies to supplement or fill in the gaps in their Medicare coverage.

》》 Stay Current: For additional information about CMS and its programs, visit http://www.cms.hhs.gov

Programs Financed at the Federal, State, and Local Levels

Medicaid

Medicaid was established in 1965 under Title 19 of the Social Security Act. It is available to certain lower-income individuals and families, the elderly, and people with disabilities who

Box 47–2
The Different Parts of Medicare

Medicare Part A (Hospital Insurance)

- Helps to cover inpatient care in hospitals.
- Helps to cover home healthcare and care in skilled nursing facilities and hospice.
- The covered individual must be age 65 or older, and either the individual or the individual's spouse must have been employed in a Medicare-covered employment setting and paid Medicare taxes for at least 10 years. Copayments, coinsurance, or deductibles may apply.

Medicare Part B (Medical Insurance)

- Helps to cover medically necessary services provided by physicians and other healthcare providers, outpatient care, home healthcare, and durable medical equipment.
- Coverage includes partial payment for office visits to physicians and other healthcare providers; outpatient services, including screening exams such as mammograms and colonoscopies; and preventive services such as flu shots.
- All individuals covered by Medicare Part B pay an annual deductible and a 20% copayment; the remaining covered costs are paid by Medicare.

Medicare Part C (Medicare Advantage Plans)

- A health coverage option run by private insurance companies approved by and under contract with Medicare.
- Includes all services covered under Parts A and B, usually includes Plan D prescription drug coverage, and may cover other services such as hearing and vision testing.
- Medicare pays the insurer for each individual enrolled in the plan. The insured must cover out-of-pocket expenses, including the Part B premium, an additional premium to the company providing the coverage, and applicable copayments.

Medicare Part D (Medicare Prescription Drug Coverage)

- A prescription drug option run by private insurance companies, such as HMOs and PPOs, approved by and under contract with Medicare.
- May help lower prescription drug costs and help protect against higher costs in the future.

Source: Data from Centers for Medicare and Medicaid Services. (2016). *Medicare and You 2016.* Retrieved from www.medicare.gov

meet the eligibility requirements. Medicaid is jointly funded and administered by states and the federal government. Each state sets its own guidelines regarding eligibility and covered services, which are then matched by federal funding. Federal mandates require coverage of certain services (e.g., hospitalization, physician services, laboratory services, radiology studies, preventive services, prenatal care, nursing home and home health services, and medically necessary transportation). The federal match enables states to ensure comprehensive health coverage for as many of their residents as possible (Pulcini & Hart, 2014). In 2014, the ACA changed the Medicaid eligibility requirements to allow more people to qualify. Also, the ACA offers additional community-based care programs as an alternative to nursing home care.

Supplemental Security Income

Supplemental Security Income (SSI) is a federal and state public assistance program funded by general taxes. SSI is designed to help aged, blind, and disabled people who have little or no income, including children who are blind and disabled. It provides cash for basic needs such as food, clothing, and housing.

Children's Health Insurance Program

Federal and matching state funding combine to provide the **Children's Health Insurance Program (CHIP)**, previously known as the State Child Health Insurance Program (SCHIP). CHIP provides health insurance coverage to children under the age of 19 whose families earn more than the Medicaid limits but cannot afford to purchase private healthcare coverage. Within broad federal guidelines, each state determines the design of its program, eligibility requirements, benefit packages, payment levels for coverage, and administrative and operating procedures. Federal requirements mandate that states include routine checkups, immunizations, dental and vision care, inpatient and outpatient hospital care, and laboratory and x-ray services in their benefits.

State-funded Healthcare

State governments may administer programs targeting specific public health priorities, which are funded by either states or localities, frequently in combination with federal grants. Examples include maternal and child health, smoking cessation, obesity prevention, HIV/AIDS, substance abuse, and environmental health. In addition, state governments have a degree of responsibility for oversight related to the regulation of health insurance, healthcare providers, and public health activities (Pulcini & Hart, 2014).

Local/County Level Healthcare

In many states, local and county governments may fund public health initiatives or programs. Some local governments fund indigent care by subsidizing and running public hospitals and clinics. Two examples are New York City's Health and Hospital's Corporation, and Chicago's Cook County Hospital. These hospitals, which serve individuals regardless of their ability to pay, also receive a large amount of operating money from Medicaid and Medicare. Therefore, health policy at the federal and local/county levels plays a part in shaping the funding models for these subsidized institutions.

The Affordable Care Act

From the beginning, the ACA met with controversy and troubled implementation (see the Focus on Diversity and

Focus on Diversity and Culture
Implementing the Affordable Care Act

To be fully effective, even a health policy crafted to address health-care disparities may need significant overhaul either in the original language or in the implementation by federal or state agencies. The first state to implement the ACA was California, a state with a very diverse population. A study found major issues associated with its early implementation. For instance, racial disparities in enrollment were found. At the end of the enrollment period in April 2014, the percentage of new White enrollees was 7.4% higher than that of Latinos, 14% higher than that of Asian-Pacific Islanders, and more than 12 times higher than that of African Americans.

Two factors were cited for this trend. The first was that Latinos and African Americans had internet access at less than half the rate of Whites. In addition, general website difficulties and failures on the Spanish language website were cited as issues. Also, the combination of language, fear of legal reprisal against undocumented immigrants, and unfamiliarity with both medical and insurance terms served as obstacles. Another issue the study established was that the e-verify system was set up for middle-class individuals with standard credit profiles and with access to the internet and email. The study also found that the process was not immigrant-friendly.

Despite its initial implementation difficulties, the ACA did improve access to healthcare. However, it did not make healthcare affordable for many Californians. For example, a seasonal construction worker said that his coverage minimum would have been $240 a month, with an additional premium to add his daughter. He simply did not have the money, so he did not apply (Alliance for a Just Society, 2015).

Source: Based on Alliance for a Just Society. (2015). *Report on Breaking Barriers (Obamacare) in California.* Retrieved from http://allianceforajustsociety.org/wp-content/uploads/2015/04/BBReport_CALIF.pdf

Culture feature). However, as of January 2017, more than 20 million previously uninsured individuals had gained health-care insurance coverage through the provisions of the Affordable Care Act (Greenberg, 2017; Levey, 2017). Between 2013 and 2014, the uninsured rate dropped from 16.2% to 12.1% (Kaiser Family Foundation, 2016). As with any government-funded program, ACA came with a tax burden. The taxpayers' share of U.S. health expenditures for 2013 has been estimated to be $1.877 trillion; this is an estimated 64.3% of national health expenditures in that year. This figure is projected to increase to $3.624 trillion in 2024 (Himmelstein & Woolhandler, 2016).

The ACA included a number of provisions that reformed the health insurance market. These included measures to ensure that consumers receive value for the cost of their premiums, restricts insurers from charging unreasonable health insurance premiums, and hold insurance companies accountable for unjustified premium increases. In addition, the ACA banned annual dollar limits on essential coverage such as hospitals, physician, and pharmacy benefits; required that children of the insured be covered until they turn 26 years old; required new health plans to cover certain evidence-based preventive services and eliminate cost sharing for those services; and made it possible for Americans with preexisting conditions to gain and keep their coverage. The ACA included many additional provisions that benefits the consumer and requires health insurers to provide fair, equitable coverage and transparency of information.

REVIEW The Concept of Health Policy

RELATE Link the Concepts

Linking the concept of health policy with the concept of ethics:

1. How does enacting evidence-based policies or legislation align with ethical standards of nursing?

2. Which federal law protects patient privacy?

Linking the concept of health policy with the concept of legal issues:

3. Explore the board of nursing website in your state, and find the section of law or rules related to the nurse's accountability for patient care and safety. What nursing actions or protective measures promote compliance with those sections of law or rule?

Linking the concept of health policy with the concept of safety:

4. Review The Joint Commission National Patient Safety Goals. Choose one that is relevant to a clinical area in which you have recently had experience. What nursing actions could you take to ensure that the NPSG is met?

REFER Go to Pearson MyLab Nursing and eText

■ Additional review materials

REFLECT Apply Your Knowledge

Emma Jones is a 29-year-old woman who works for a small manufacturing firm. The demand for the firm's product has grown. To keep pace with the orders, the manufacturer bought some used equipment and hired more people, but the used equipment is noisier and less efficient than newer models. Ms. Jones visits the ear, nose, and throat clinic with a chief complaint of persistent ringing in her ears. As she provides her history, she and the nurse realize that the ringing began a week after the additional equipment was put into use. The ear protection that is available has to be shared because of the influx of new employees. This means that Ms. Jones and the other employees must rotate wearing ear protection. The supervisor has not yet purchased additional ear protection, and employees lack ear protection for about one quarter of their work shift.

1. What is the employer's responsibility for protecting his employees' hearing health?

2. What options does an employee have if the employer does not fulfill this responsibility?

3. As the nurse at the clinic, what could you do to advocate for a safer workplace for Ms. Jones and her fellow employees?

References

American Association of Colleges of Nursing (AACN). (2016a). *ASPA code of good practice.* Retrieved from http://www.aacn.nche.edu/ccne-accreditation/why-accreditation/aspa.

American Association of Colleges of Nursing (AACN). (2016b). *2016 Federal policy agenda.* Retrieved from http://www.aacn.nche.edu/government-affairs/2016-Federal-Policy-Agenda.pdf

American Association of Colleges of Nursing (AACN). (2016c). *About AACN.* Retrieved from http://www.aacn.nche.edu/about-aacn

American Nurses Association (ANA). (2016a). Constituent and state nurses associations. Retrieved from http://nursingworld.org/FunctionalMenuCategories/AboutANA/WhoWeAre/CMA

American Nurses Association (ANA). (2016b). Policy & advocacy: Positions and resolutions. Retrieved from http://nursingworld.org/MainMenuCategories/Policy-Advocacy/Positions-and-Resolutions/default.aspx

American Nurses Association (ANA). (n.d.). *About ANA.* Retrieved from http://nursingworld.org/FunctionalMenuCategories/AboutANA

Centers for Disease Control and Prevention (CDC). (2014). Legal authorities for isolation and quarantine. Retrieved from http://www.cdc.gov/quarantine/aboutlawsregulationsquarantineisolation.html

Greenberg, J. (2017). Medicaid expansion drove health insurance coverage under health law, Rand Paul says. Retrieved from http://www.politifact.com/truth-o-meter/statements/2017/jan/15/rand-paul/medicaid-expansion-drove-health-insurance-coverage/

Himmelstein, D. U., & Woolhandler, S. (2016). The current and projected taxpayer shares of US health costs. *American Journal of Public Health, 106*(3), 449–452.

International Council of Nurses (ICN). (2015). *Who we are: Our mission, strategic intent, core values and priorities.* Retrieved from http://www.icn.ch/who-we-are/who-we-are/

International Council of Nurses (ICN). (2016). *International Council of Nurses addresses key issues for nursing at 69th World Health Assembly.* Retrieved from http://www.icn.ch/images/stories/documents/news/press_releases/2016_PR_24_WHA_2016.pdf

Kaiser Family Foundation. (2012). *The unemployed, a primer.* Retrieved from http://kaiserfamilyfoundation.files.wordpress.com/2013/01/7670-03.pdf

Kaiser Family Foundation. (2016). *Key facts about the uninsured population.* Retrieved from http://kff.org/uninsured/fact-sheet/key-facts-about-the-uninsured-population/

Levey, N. M. (2017). *Obamacare enrollment drops, to 12.2 million, as Congress debates repeal.* Retrieved from http://www.latimes.com/nation/nationnow/la-na-pol-obamacare-sign-up-20170315-story.html

Loversidge, J. M. (2016). An evidence-informed health policy model: adapting evidence-based practice for nursing education and regulation. *Journal of Nursing Regulation, 7*(2), 27–33.

Milstead, J. A. (2016). What is public policy? In J. A. Milstead (Ed.), *Health Policy & Politics: A Nurses Guide* (pp. 1–43). (5th ed.). Burlington, MA: Jones & Bartlett.

Moss, K. (2014). NGO engagement in U.S. global health efforts: U.S.-based NGOs receiving USG support through USAID. *Kaiser Family Foundation Report.* Retrieved from http://kff.org/report-section/us-ngos-in-global-health-report/

National League for Nursing (NLN). (2015). *Public policy agenda 2015–2016.* Retrieved from http://www.nln.org/docs/default-source/advocacy-public-policy/public-policy-brochure2015-2016.pdf?sfvrsn=0

National League for Nursing (NLN). (2016a). *FAQs: National League for Nursing Commission for Nursing Education Accreditation (CNEA)—general questions.* Retrieved from http://www.nln.org/accreditation-services/faqs.

Mission statement from National League for Nursing (NLN). (2016b). *About the NLN: Mission and goals.* Retrieved from http://www.nln.org/about/mission-goals. Used by permission of National League for Nursing.

National League for Nursing (NLN). (2016c). *Membership: Overview.* Retrieved from http://www.nln.org/membership.

National Student Nurses Association (NSNA). (n.d.). *About us.* Retrieved from http://www.nsna.org/AboutUs.aspx

Pulcini, J. A., & Hart, M. A. (2014). Financing healthcare in the United States. In D. J. Mason, J. K. Leavitt, & M. S. Chaffee (Eds.), *Policy & politics in nursing and healthcare* (6th ed., revised reprint, pp. 135–146). St. Louis, MO: Elsevier Saunders.

Robert Wood Johnson Foundation. (2013). *Number of Americans obtaining health insurance through an employer declines steadily since 2000.* Retrieved from http://www.rwjf.org/en/library/articles-and-news/2013/04/number-of-americans-obtaining-health-insurance-through-an-employ.html

Sigma Theta Tau International (STTI). (2016). *STTI organizational fact sheet.* Retrieved from http://www.nursingsociety.org/why-stti/about-stti/sigma-theta-tau-international-organizational-fact-sheet

Sigma Theta Tau International (STTI). (n.d.). *"Global" health policy position statement.* Retrieved from http://www.nursingsociety.org/docs/default-source/position-papers/stti-global-health-policy-position_final.pdf?sfvrsn=4

The Joint Commission. (2015). *Facts about the national patient safety goals.* Retrieved from https://www.jointcommission.org/facts_about_the_national_patient_safety_goals/

The Joint Commission. (2016). *About the Joint Commission.* Retrieved from https://www.jointcommission.org/about_us/about_the_joint_commission_main.aspx

U.S. Department of Health and Human Services (HHS). (2017). *HHS agencies & offices.* Retrieved from http://www.hhs.gov/about/agencies/hhs-agencies-and-offices/index.html#

U.S. Department of Labor. (n.d.). *OSHA: About OSHA.* Retrieved from https://www.osha.gov/about.html

U.S. Environmental Protection Agency. (2015). *Our mission and what we do.* Retrieved from https://www.epa.gov/aboutepa/our-mission-and-what-we-do

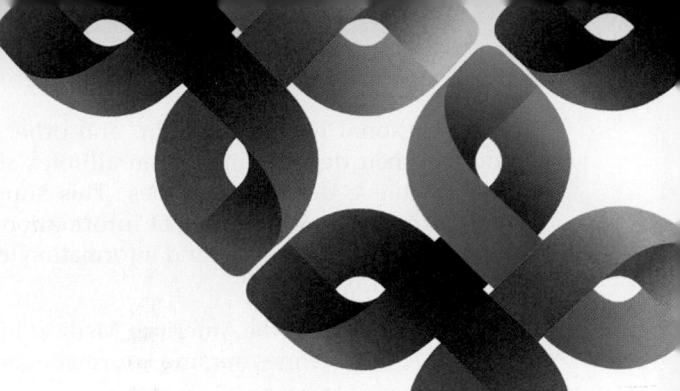

Module 48
Informatics

Module Outline and Learning Outcomes

The Concept of Informatics

Nursing Informatics

48.1 Analyze informatics as a key component of nursing practice.

Concepts Related to Informatics

48.2 Outline the relationship between informatics and other concepts.

Healthcare Information Systems

48.3 Explain the use of informatics in healthcare.

Computerized Medical Records

48.4 Analyze the uses of computerized medical records.

Telehealth

48.5 Analyze the use of informatics for telehealth.

Geographic Information Systems

48.6 Explain the use of geographic information systems.

Patient Education and E-Health

48.7 Analyze the use of the internet for patient education and e-health.

Ergonomic Considerations

48.8 Differentiate good ergonomics from poor ergonomics.

Informatics Exemplars

Exemplar 48.A Clinical Decision Support Systems

48.A Analyze clinical decision support systems as they relate to informatics.

Exemplar 48.B Individual Information at Point of Care

48.B Analyze individual information at point of care as it relates to informatics.

» The Concept of Informatics

Concept Key Terms

Biomedical informatics, **2809**	Computer vision syndrome, **2819**	Electronic health record (EHR), **2812**	Geographic information system (GIS), **2816**	Nursing informatics (NI), **2809**
Clinical decision support system, **2815**	Device integration, **2814**	Electronic medical record (EMR), **2812**	Health Level 7 (HL7), **2812**	Repetitive strain injury, **2819**
Clinical information system, **2811**	E-health, **2817**	Ergonomics, **2818**		Telehealth, **2815**

Today's healthcare professionals handle extraordinary amounts of information. At the bedside and in the examination room, nurses and other clinicians assess patients' health status and prioritize and provide care. Each action creates new data that must be recorded and used at different points of service from direct care to billing related to the cost of that care. In today's clinical environment, that information is created, stored, and accessed with the help of technology. **Biomedical informatics** is the "interdisciplinary science that deals with biomedical information, its structure, acquisition and use. Biomedical informatics is grounded in the principles of computer science, information science, cognitive science, social science, and engineering, as well as the clinical and basic sciences" (Vanderbilt University School of Medicine, 2013).

Nursing Informatics

The relationship between nursing and informatics is so critical that the American Nurses Association (ANA) recognized nursing informatics as a specialty in 1992, and the American Nurses Credentialing Center began offering board certification for nursing informatics in 1995. The ANA defines **nursing informatics (NI)** as

the specialty that integrates nursing science with multiple information management and analytical sciences to identify, define, manage, and communicate data, information, knowledge, and wisdom in nursing practice. NI supports nurses, consumers, patients, the

2809

interprofessional healthcare team, and other stakeholders in their decision-making in all roles and settings to achieve desired outcomes. This support is accomplished through the use of information structures, information processes, and information technology (ANA, 2015).

The nursing section of the American Medical Informatics Association (AMIA) defines nursing informatics as the

science and practice (that) integrates nursing, its information and knowledge, with information and communication technologies to promote the health of people, families, and communities worldwide (AMIA adapted from IMIA Special Interest Group on Nursing Informatics, 2016).

Even in the few practices that do not yet use electronic health records (EHRs), nurses use technology every day: Cardiac monitors, mechanical ventilators, and many blood pressure cuffs use computer technology, as do most telephone systems. Informatics is an everyday occurrence in the practice of nursing.

Informatics and Health Policy

Both professional organizations and government entities recognize and support the careful, purposeful implementation of informatics in healthcare environments. The Healthcare Information and Management Systems Society (HIMSS) works to improve healthcare quality, safety, and outcomes through improving the use of information technology (IT) and systems. HIMSS is a nonprofit organization with both individual and corporate members. The American Medical Informatics Association (AMIA) is another organization dedicated to the development and application of health informatics to support patient care and teaching. The Alliance for Nursing Informatics (ANI) works to support and advance the areas of informatics leadership, practice, education, policy, and research. It works closely with other organizations such as HIMSS and AIMIA. These groups promote the use of health IT and sponsor conferences as well as policy development. The Technology Informatics Guiding Educational Reform (TIGER) initiative focuses on integrating technology and informatics competencies into nursing education as well as practice. The TIGER initiative is currently integrated into the HIMSS network.

》Stay Current: For more information about the TIGER initiative, visit http://www.himss.org/professionaldevelopment/tiger-initiative.

The administrations of both President George W. Bush and President Barack Obama contributed to the use of informatics in the delivery of healthcare across the United States. Electronic medical documentation is thought to help reduce errors, reduce healthcare costs, and improve the quality of care delivered to patients. The Bush administration introduced a policy that, over the course of 10 years, would encourage the use of electronic documentation of the healthcare record. The Obama administration took this policy further with the introduction of the American Recovery and Reinvestment Act of 2009 (ARRA), which provided $27 billion worth of incentives to healthcare providers to promote the use of electronic medical records. Through the Health

Information Technology for Economic and Clinical Health Act (HITECH), the funding is directed toward EHRs. The Centers for Medicare and Medicaid Services (CMS) and the Office of the National Coordinator for Health Information Technology (ONC) are charged with the oversight of health information technology efforts. ONC is overseeing the achievement of meaningful use objectives, which are reported back to CMS to authorize financial reimbursement. Meaningful use is built on the five pillars of health outcomes (CMS, 2016):

- Improving care coordination
- Reducing health disparities among U.S. citizens, by improving the safety and quality of care
- Ensuring the security and privacy of protected medical information
- Engaging patients and their families in the patient's care
- Improving population and public health.

As of November 2016, approximately 605,000 eligible professionals and hospitals had signed up for the meaningful use incentive program (CMS, 2017).

Informatics and Service Delivery

Informatics has broad implications for service delivery. For example, addiction and overdoses of prescription opioids are an increasing problem in the United States. Reports of overdoses have increased more than threefold since the 1990s. In 2010, prescription medication overdose caused almost 17,000 deaths (Substance Abuse and Mental Health Services Administration, 2016). Efforts are being made to enhance tracking of prescriptions of opioids through electronic tracking at the state level. In addition, the Centers for Disease Control and Prevention (CDC) works with healthcare agencies to track prescriptions and emergency department visits for overdoses in an attempt to identify people who are or have been abusers (CDC, 2016). The ability to link computerized written orders with patient EHRs on regional and national levels can help identify and monitor individuals who are at risk, and make it easier to identify people who engage in "doctor shopping" to obtain narcotics for abuse or illegal sale. Tracking mechanisms can also help identify healthcare providers who write bogus opioid prescriptions and receive a financial kickback from sellers.

One of the often-cited benefits of EHRs is improved quality of care delivered to patients. As part of the meaningful use requirements, clinical quality measures must be reported (CMS, 2013a). An example of a large quality improvement project that can be facilitated with informatics is the Surgical Care Improvement Project (SCIP). The target population is all patients who are undergoing surgery, and the goal is to reduce surgical complications and improve surgical care. Hospitals started collecting data on certain quality indicators in July 2006. This is a collaborative project between The Joint Commission and CMS, and reimbursement for surgical procedures and hospital stays is tied to meeting SCIP measures (The Joint Commission, 2012). Informatics and the ability to retrieve information from patients' EHRs can help with such large-scale projects and also help facilities identify their own quality projects and areas for process improvement.

Concepts Related to Informatics

The use of informatics has created many new challenges for nurses. Patients have increasing access to a variety of health-related information, such as recommendations for diet and monitoring weight. Nurses must be attentive to ensure that their patients are getting good-quality information and using it appropriately. It is also important to recognize that some patients will be unable or unwilling to use electronic means to access health information. Nurses are in a good position to help patients find the most appropriate means of getting and using healthcare information.

Protecting health information is also important, and vigilance is necessary to protect patient information and to ensure that protected information is not released inadvertently. The rise of social media has created ethical challenges, especially when nurses and patients know each other socially from events or activities outside the workplace. Despite the great possibilities for improving patient care through quality improvement efforts and tracking patient use of medications, nurses must take care to use informatics within established guidelines consistent with the scope of nursing practice and professional, ethical, and legal requirements. Some, but not all, of the concepts integral to informatics are outlined in the Concepts Related to Informatics feature. They are presented in alphabetical order.

Healthcare Information Systems

The increasing use of technology by healthcare facilities requires that nurses have a basic knowledge of the types of information systems used, the purposes and abilities of these systems to support patient care, and the nurse's responsibilities related to using these systems.

In the days of paper charts, only one individual at a time could access a patient's chart and add information to it. A **clinical information system** allows multiple disciplines to simultaneously access the patient's chart and record data that can be viewed and analyzed by a number of healthcare providers in real time, providing the most accurate and current information about the patient so that the best decisions about the care of that patient can be made.

A clinical information system must give the nurse the ability to access patient information and provide data necessary to execute the nursing process of assessing, diagnosing, planning, implementing, and evaluating the care of the patient. When the system is used at the point of care, the nurse can immediately record patient information based on assessment of the patient's current condition. The nurse should also have access to diagnostic data (e.g., laboratory values), diagnoses, assessments, plans, and evaluations of the patient from the viewpoint of other healthcare professionals (e.g., physicians, physical therapists). Pharmacy information, such as medication, route, dose, and time, should be available in the patient's chart in real time. The chart should also include safety features, such as warnings for drug interactions or incorrect dosages. Most clinical information systems also contain clinical decision support, which is discussed later in this module. The system should also allow the nurse to print discharge instructions to review with the patient (Duke University, 2012; Locatelli et al., 2012).

Computerized Medical Records

On the surface, a computerized medical record may appear to be nothing more than a digital form of a patient's paper chart. Many systems start out that way. However, rapid technologic advances have transformed these static charts into dynamic systems.

Purpose

The purpose of a computerized medical record is to unify a patient's entire health history into one single source of information about the patient's health, including the patient's medical and surgical histories, diagnostic tests and treatments, medications, and therapies. It is meant to be multidisciplinary and multispecialty in nature. It is meant not to simply record the past but to aid clinicians in the patient's future healthcare, improve quality of care, lower costs of care, and facilitate research. It is meant to be portable, so that if a patient lives in New York but requires emergency care in Los Angeles, all of the patient's medical information is available to help the healthcare providers in Los Angeles make the best possible decisions about the care of the patient (Open Clinical, 2016). A survey of physicians found that 78% of physicians using EHRs reported that their use enhanced patient care overall; 81% indicated it helped them access a patient's chart remotely; and 65% stated it alerted them of a potential drug error (King et al., 2014).

To deliver the best quality of care, promote safety, and maintain efficiency, computerized health records should contain the following functionality (Open Clinical, 2016):

- *Patient support.* Patients should be able to access their health records. Patients can take a more active role in their care if they have the ability to track appointments and health maintenance, monitor their weight and laboratory results, and access educational materials related to their health condition.

- *Health information and data.* Important data, such as chronic and acute medical and psychiatric diagnoses, medications, allergies, and diagnostic tests, can help clinicians make rapid decisions if necessary.

- *Administrative processes.* The ability to manage schedules, insurance information, and inventory can help healthcare facilities focus on patient-centered care.

- *Results management.* Access to past and current diagnostic tests can help clinicians recognize changes in a patient's state of health faster.

- *Reporting.* Healthcare facilities can comply more easily with regulatory requests and help report disease surveillance and patient safety matters such as medical device recalls.

- *Secure electronic communication and connectivity.* Secure and accurate communication between medical providers at different facilities that are caring for the same patient help with continuity of care and timely diagnoses.

- *Order management.* Computerized physician order entry (CPOE) helps with accuracy and decreases times from order to treatment. CPOE should be available for pharmacy, laboratory, radiologic tests, and ancillary services such as physical and occupational therapy.

Concepts Related to
Informatics

CONCEPT	RELATIONSHIP TO INFORMATICS	NURSING IMPLICATIONS
Addiction	EHRs give healthcare providers, including nurses, access to the patient's entire health history, not just information from this particular encounter at this particular facility. Linking of EHR information may help identify individuals who are at risk for opioid addiction and who are engaged in obtaining these drugs illegally.	■ Assess appropriate use of addictive medications; many patients have legitimate need for prescription opioids. ■ Be alert for duplicate opioid prescriptions within a patient's record, especially from multiple providers.
Ethics	With social media, lines between patients and providers can be blurred.	■ Nurses must be aware that many employers monitor their employees' activity on social media; the legality of disciplinary action for a post showing the employee intoxicated and/or engaging in illegal activity or requiring employees to give employers their passwords is still being established. ■ Nurses must weigh the implications of "friending" patients that they care for (especially in areas with long-term interaction). ■ *Anticipate* how to handle patients who attempt to cross boundaries by using social media.
Legal Issues	It is necessary to keep protected health information confidential and to ensure that the information entered in a patient's health record is accurate.	■ Nurses must be aware of HIPAA and HITECH rules. Among the most critical activities: — Keep passwords private. — Do not leave screens containing protected health information unattended. — Access charts only of patients to whom you are assigned. — Always verify that you are charting on the correct patient's chart and that the information is recorded accurately.
Nutrition	Smartphone applications allow patients to determine and track the nutritional value of foods they eat.	■ Use of these applications may increase ease of tracking nutritional intake for the purposes of dietary recall and weight monitoring. ■ Anticipate that some patients may not have smartphones or may have minimal data plans that limit their ability to use this technology. Work with patients to establish other, convenient means to track dietary intake.
Quality Improvement	With many EHRs, quality metrics can be easily tracked for improvement within a department or hospital system. Tracking information to use for quality improvement initiatives requires users to understand how to use technology correctly. Nurses must be at the table as new systems are evaluated and put in place, and they must advocate to ensure that they will receive adequate training to implement the system safely and accurately.	■ Assess your own comfort and ability level related to use of electronic/computer equipment. Attend and pay attention in training sessions; seek follow-up help as necessary. ■ Be alert for the possibility for error; enter information accurately the first time.
Safety	EHRs can provide tools to improve patient safety such as reminders. Clinical Decision Support Systems are also used to ensure that appropriate protocols are used when patients meet certain criteria.	■ Nurses benefit from electronic reminders to assist them when they are busy to ensure that key assessments such as neurologic assessments in stroke patients are done in a timely manner. ■ Flags in the system alert nurses to complete screening tools such as falls risk or pressure ulcer screening. Healthcare providers can access evidence-based practice care bundles for patients who meet criteria for sepsis and other diagnoses.

- *Decision support.* The care of the patient can be enhanced through the use of a clinical decision support system. These systems can display best practice standards, notifications for preventive screenings, and alerts for drug interactions.

Terminology

A nurse will hear many different terms to describe a computerized medical record, and the list will probably continue to change. The two most commonly used terms are electronic medical records and EHRs.

Electronic medical records (EMRs) are similar to an electronic chart used in a clinician's office. Their focus is on diagnosis and treatment. They can help track information over time (e.g., weight, blood pressure, cholesterol readings) and identify when patients are due for routine preventive health maintenance such as vaccines and mammograms. A disadvantage of these systems is that most of them are designed to stay within a clinical setting and are not meant to travel beyond it. A patient who needs to see a specialist may need a paper printout of the EMR to take to the specialty appointment.

Electronic health records (EHRs) give a broader view of the patient's health. They are designed so that multiple clinicians from multiple disciplines (e.g., family practice, nursing, pharmacy, specialists) can all have simultaneous access to the patient's health information. This access provides patients with more comprehensive management of their health and is designed to improve the quality of care they receive. EHRs enhance communication with other clinicians, they provide easy access to patient information, they can provide automated formulary checks by health plans to avoid problems with prescriptions, and they can link to public health systems such as registries and communicable disease data banks (HealthIT.gov, n.d.a). One significant advantage is e-prescribing, in which healthcare providers can communicate directly with the pharmacy to order prescriptions. This can reduce errors, lower costs, and improve care (HealthIT.gov, n.d.b).

This text uses *EHR* when discussing documentation, as it is the broader, more encompassing term.

Components

Real-time documentation of patient data can help all clinicians care for the patient. The nurse should be given the tools to record assessments, nursing diagnoses, plans, interventions, and evaluations. The work that nurses have done in caring for the patient has traditionally been invisible to other disciplines, so the ability to carry the nursing process over into electronic records will help promote the work that nurses do in caring for the patient. *Uniform language* is the consistent use of the same terminology among providers, facilities, institutions, and organizations when describing all patient data, including that pertaining to assessment and treatment. Uniform language (discussed further in the exemplar on Clinical Decision Support Systems in this module) is vital for communicating to other nurses and health professionals the value that nurses provide in the care of the patient.

NANDA International (NANDA-I) has been involved in developing uniform language for nursing since the 1970s.

NANDA-I diagnoses are available in many electronic health systems (Meum, 2013). The Nursing Interventions Classifications (NIC) include both physiologic and psychologic interventions that nurses perform with patients and their families. Nurses use both NANDA-I and NIC to formulate care plans for the patient in the EHR (Meum, 2013). The Nursing Outcomes Classification (NOC) is designed to assess the outcomes of patients based on the nursing interventions performed. Both NIC and NOC have been approved for use in **Health Level 7 (HL7)** terminology, which provides a framework and composes standards "for the exchange, integration, sharing, and retrieval of electronic health information that supports clinical practice and the management, delivery and evaluation of health services" (Health Level Seven International, 2013).

Health Insurance Portability and Accountability Act of 1996

A major concern for both patients and healthcare providers is the protection of private health information. Private health information includes any details that could identify a particular patient, such as name, phone number, hospital medical record number, diagnosis, or Social Security number. The U.S. Department of Health and Human Services issued a set of privacy rules called the Health Insurance Portability and Accountability Act of 1996, commonly referred to as HIPAA. It set rules to limit who may have access to a patient's health information, whether that information is in written, oral, or electronic form. It also gives patients the right to view their own health records, make corrections to their records, and receive notification of how their information may be used or shared (e.g., for research or marketing purposes; U.S. Department of Health and Human Services, n.d.). The Health Insurance Technology for Economic and Clinical Health Act (HITECH) added more strength to the existing HIPAA protection of patients' medical information (Solove, 2013).

Nurses should use many of the same rules for protecting patient privacy that were practiced before the advent of electronic records. Information about a patient should not be discussed in public areas, such as hospital cafeterias or elevators. Any paper documents that may contain protected health information should be placed in designated shred bins. Newer considerations for nurses include not sharing passwords, not leaving a computer screen with protected health information unattended, and not posting any patient information on public social networks such as Facebook, Instagram, or Twitter (see **Box 48–1 》** and **Figure 48–1 》**). Commonsense habits related to confidentiality must be practiced. In the days of paper charts, it may have been possible to obtain unauthorized access to a neighbor's or celebrity's chart without being detected. Now it is very easy to ascertain electronically each time a patient's chart is accessed and by whom. A nurse who improperly accesses a patient's chart could face loss of employment and possible fine, loss of licensure, and/or legal action.

Despite the move to EHRs, medical fraud still occurs. The cost to Medicare and Medicaid is roughly $98 billion and the cost to the entire healthcare systems is around $272 billion per year. Fraud occurs through the charging of "false visits,"

Box 48–1
Social Media and the Workplace

In 2016, almost 2 billion people worldwide used some form of social media; Facebook had the largest share of users (Statista, 2016). In a study conducted in 2011, 87% of physicians surveyed reported personal use of social media, and 67% reported professional use (Federation of State Medical Boards, 2012). Social networking can pose several ethical dilemmas for healthcare providers. Some employers have demanded access to their employees' social media accounts or have monitored employees' activities. As of 2016, over a dozen states had made it illegal for employers to require employees to provide passwords or access to an employee's social media accounts, and several other states have legislation pending (Guerin, 2016).

The other challenge in the workplace is navigating the use of social media by providers. The National Council of State Boards of Nursing (NCSBN) has developed a set of media guidelines for nurses (NCSBN, 2014). They caution that inappropriate posts by nurses to social media can result in licensure and legal repercussions. Sharing any information at all about patients with your friends on social media is inappropriate and violates HIPAA and the Nursing Code of Ethics.

>> **Stay Current:** Visit the website of the National Council of State Boards of Nursing to view a video of guidelines for use of social media.

Many institutions have developed policies to guide staff and providers on whether or not they can "friend" patients on Facebook. Many providers do not "friend" patients on personal Facebook, as this generally is a less professional site and reserved for their friends and family (NPR, 2015). However, social media is a powerful tool and a great way to communicate with the millennial generation, so many institutions and provider practices set up institutional Facebook, Twitter, Instagram, Pinterest, and Google Plus sites where they can distribute general information to patients. They can provide educational videos on subjects such as diabetes, remind patients to get flu shots, or disseminate other important information (U.S. News, 2014).

Social media is not the only electronic tool presenting challenges for providers. Some hospitals and healthcare offices use emails and text messages to notify physicians about a patient's status (Baum, 2015). If this information is not encrypted and includes a patient's name or other identifying factors, it may be classified as a HIPAA violation. To mitigate this risk, employers now require the use of mobile security services that protect devices at both the device and application levels so that if a device is lost or stolen, access to the sensitive data can be disabled. Text messages can also be set to delete after having been read ("Text messaging apps for hospitals," n.d.).

---

overbilling for services, prescription fraud, and unnecessary ambulance transports. To combat this, CMS is enlisting patients to scrutinize their bills for charges that don't seem accurate. Nurses should educate patients about these scams and how to protect themselves (The Economist, 2014).

Quality Assurance

On the surface, the implementation of EHRs would seem likely to automatically improve the quality of patient care. It has the potential to do that, but an EHR is just a tool, and outcomes of care depend, in part, on how this tool is used.

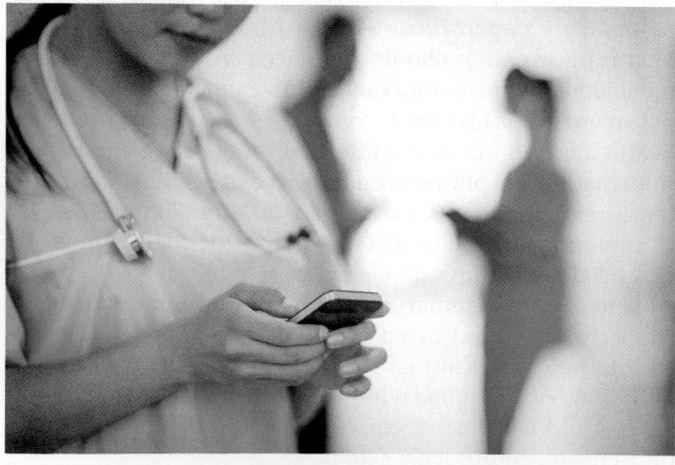

Source: Wavebreakmedia/iStock/Getty Images.

Figure 48–1 >> Do not post any information at all on any social media about any patient in your facility.

Accuracy

Recording accurate patient health information is vital, whether the nurse is using a paper or an electronic system. First encounters with an electronic charting system involve a learning curve that increases the chance of errors in recording data that will be left in a patient's chart. For example, someone who is new to the system may not know how to remove a blood pressure reading that was 225/124 because the arterial line transducer was on the floor or how to mark that reading as faulty data. In many charting systems, more than one chart may be open at the same time, so entering information on the wrong chart may be easy. An accidental click of a mouse on the wrong medication can cause the provider who is not paying attention to order or give the wrong medication. **Device integration**, which automatically enters patient vital signs into the EHR, is possible in some systems. This has increased in use and is found not only in intensive care units but also in telemetry, obstetrics, and even general care units. Device integration allows real-time accurate data to be recorded in the patient's chart directly from the device (e.g., a blood pressure monitor or cardiac monitor). It allows the nurse to more quickly analyze and interpret that data and make adjustments to the plan of care based on the most current information. In one study of ICU patients, 95% of vital signs were recorded at least once per hour, and clinicians validated most of the data within 15 minutes of its being recorded (Pizzi, 2013). As EHRs evolve, more departments are likely to use device integration.

Some EHR systems use templates and cut-and-paste functions designed to promote efficiency. For example, a pediatric clinic seeing 10 otherwise healthy children who have ear infections can use a template or cut/copy function to forward the information that is within normal limits and just focus on the infection, saving precious time that would otherwise be spent manually clicking boxes for negative or normal findings. However, overuse of these functions can result in inaccurate data being recorded in a patient's chart, risking future decisions about medical care based on faulty information. For example, if there has been a significant change in the patient's condition and a practitioner uses a "copy forward" function to duplicate the previous day's progress notes, then care of the patient can be seriously compromised. One study found that up to 20% of material in a patient's chart was the result of copy-and-paste (Stokes, 2013). A patient's medical record is only as valuable as the information that is entered in it, and nurses have a duty to ensure that they enter only timely and accurate information. Risk management, insurance companies, and regulatory bodies as well as other clinicians will be looking at the data in the patient's record, so it is imperative that nurses take the time to learn proper documentation within the electronic system that their employer adopts.

Critical Thinking

The fact that the EHR is merely a tool cannot be overemphasized. As with paper charting, the patient and not the record should have first priority in the nurse's attention. Although it may be difficult when electronic records are used, nurses must learn to focus their attention on the patient and not the computer. Employers should give nurses adequate training on the use of their electronic system and provide mentors to help decrease the stress of adding one more activity to the nurses' already busy workload (Goldberg et al., 2012).

Clinical decision support systems are a type of artificial intelligence that analyzes data and provides information about evidenced-based practices. These systems can help improve patient safety and quality of care. However, they cannot take the place of sound nursing judgment. The use of clinical decision support systems in nursing practice is described further in the exemplar on Clinical Decision Support Systems in this module.

Uniform Language

For greater efficiency, nurses should use uniform language in their documentation. Uniform nursing diagnoses, along with uniform descriptors of nursing interventions and outcomes, can help clarify care of the patient not only to other nurses, but to other disciplines as well. Some documentation within an electronic record may have only standardized descriptors available for the end user. The use of uniform language also aids nursing research (National Association of School Nurses, 2012).

Clinical Example A

Mary Wilson is a 19-year-old with a history of grand mal seizures. She takes two antiepileptic medications: phenytoin and topiramate. Her seizures are fairly well controlled, and she has an average of three seizures per year. Ms. Wilson is getting ready to go out of state to college and visits her primary care provider for a physical before she leaves. The office has just installed a new EHR system. Because of an early regional outbreak of influenza, the office is overbooked on appointments. The practitioner that Ms. Wilson usually sees is on vacation. The other practitioner rushes through Ms. Wilson's appointment and

does not take a thorough history or discuss medications that she is taking. Ms. Wilson presents as a healthy 19-year-old, so the practitioner uses the "copy and paste healthy adult" format for her chart.

Ms. Wilson goes out of state to school. After class one day, she decides to go for a run to relieve the stress of her classes. While she is on her run, she experiences a grand mal seizure. A motorist finds her unconscious in a postictal state and calls for emergency services. Ms. Wilson is transported to the hospital, which happens to be on the same EHR system as her primary care provider. She is still not conscious when she is examined, but she has identification with her name and birthdate on it. The emergency department staff looks at Ms. Wilson's EHR, but there is no mention of her seizure disorder. She is sent for emergency CT scans and an MRI of her brain.

Critical Thinking Questions

1. What mistakes did the provider at Ms. Wilson's primary care office make with her record?
2. How did the omission of information affect the care that Ms. Wilson received at the hospital?
3. What complications regarding health insurance might arise if she is at an out-of-state school?

Telehealth

Telehealth uses telecommunications technologies (e.g., videoconferencing, streaming media, store and forward imaging, and land-based and wireless communications) to allow patients access to care that they might not otherwise be able to obtain. The terms *telehealth* and *telemedicine* are often used interchangeably, but according to the Health Resources Administration, *telehealth* is much broader and can encompass health-related education, public health, and health administration (HealthIT.gov, n.d.b). Telehealth is not meant to replace all provider face-to-face visits, but it can be used to help manage patients with chronic physical and mental disorders, particularly those who live in rural areas where access to specialists is limited or requires travel. In many states, reimbursement for telehealth visits is the same as that for in-person visits. This makes telehealth an attractive and cost-effective option for both patients and providers (Pena & Sanders, 2016). Patients still must see a provider in person, and there are limits on the number of telehealth visits that insurance will pay for. However, not all states have agreed to pay for telehealth services in the same way; for example, Texas and Arizona are more restrictive in the reimbursement and use of telehealth services (Lagase, 2016).

Research on the effectiveness of telehealth has found evidence to support its use in patients with chronic conditions and with those receiving psychotherapy as part of behavioral health. In particular, improvement in outcomes such as mortality, quality of life, and reductions in admissions were seen in patients who were followed with chronic diseases (Landi, 2016).

Benefits of telehealth include:

- **Access to healthcare is increased.** Patients in rural areas can reduce the need to travel, and they receive access to specialists that may not be available in their community.

- **Health outcomes are improved.** Increased access to care can reduce complications and increase diagnostic and treatment options from specialists.

- **Healthcare costs can be reduced.** The expenses involved in frequent long-distance travel are reduced or eliminated, and home monitoring of chronic conditions can help reduce hospital admissions.

- **Telehealth may help with shortages of healthcare providers.** Many new graduates are not willing to move to rural communities. Telehealth can give patients access to primary care providers and specialists from other areas.

A 2016 survey by the American Telemedicine Association (ATA) found that approximately 15 million Americans had received some kind of medical care remotely in the past year. In addition, the ATA surveyed 280 healthcare executives and found that 72% of hospitals and 52% of physician groups use some kind of telemedicine program (Beck, 2016).

>> **Stay Current:** Visit the website of the American Telehealth Organization for updates on current policies, including the latest on CMS reimbursement and support for telehealth (http://www.americantelemed.org/home).

Barriers to Patient Participation

Some patients may be reluctant to use telehealth services because their insurance company may not cover the cost (California HealthCare Foundation, 2013a, b). Older adults who lack understanding of or experience with technology may be reluctant to use telehealth services. The lack of availability of broadband internet service throughout the country also limits participation. In addition, many patients are not aware that these services exist or that their healthcare provider is willing to participate in this type of interaction. On the provider side, reimbursement challenges still exist and vary from state to state. Obtaining a license to practice across state lines varies by state. Some offer a special telehealth license, and some allow providers to practice in bordering states (Center for Connected Health Policy, 2016).

Clinical Example B

Jack Anderson is an 85-year-old retired machinist. He has an eighth-grade education and lives on a fixed income in a rural community 100 miles from a major city. He has congestive heart failure (CHF) and takes a loop diuretic (furosemide) and digoxin for his condition, both of which he gets through a mail-order pharmacy. Mr. Anderson has Medicare but tries to limit his doctor visits because he doesn't like to drive to the city, and the cost of gas puts a strain on his monthly budget. His community has high-speed internet, but Mr. Anderson has not installed it because "he moved to the country to get away from everyone."

Critical Thinking Questions
1. Discuss several factors that would make Mr. Anderson an ideal candidate for telehealth.
2. When Mr. Anderson comes in for an appointment, what could the nurse say to encourage Mr. Anderson to participate in telehealth to manage his CHF?
3. If Mr. Anderson agrees to participate in telehealth, what should the practitioner assess in each of the telehealth sessions with Mr. Anderson?

Geographic Information Systems

A **geographic information system (GIS)** uses location to capture, manage, and analyze data. This technology has been used both inside and outside of healthcare. It relies on satellite imaging and the global positioning system (GPS) to capture geographic data. Those data are then managed and stored on a database. Healthcare policy makers, researchers, and public health professionals use GIS to understand a health problem, decide the best response to that problem, and plan ways to avoid the same or a similar problem or keep it from occurring again (HIT, 2015). GIS is being used to:

- **Identify health trends.** This combines individuals' health data from electronic records, data from wearables, and data from their environment to determine if there are clusters of cancer in an area or obesity related to certain areas or climates
- **Track the spread of infectious diseases.** Data is used to map where diseases are mostly likely to spread next and gain an understanding of vaccination rates
- **Use personal technology.** Data from wearable technologies has the ability to determine trends in heart rate and sleeping patterns of individuals and to determine if that varies in different geographic areas
- **Incorporate social media.** Through the use of social media, researchers are able to query posts or tweets for keywords such as *flu* or *influenza* to create a visual map of where the flu outbreaks are geographically located.

Public health nurses and administrators can use GIS to track where chronic disease programs should be placed, to monitor the effectiveness of these programs, to plan new treatment facilities, and to track acute health problems, among many other uses. GIS gives healthcare providers the tools to show where services are provided and where health services are needed. Gaps between available programs and the needs of the community can be identified easily (Miliard, 2014).

Patient Education and E-Health

Besides changing the ways in which healthcare providers handle and use information, informatics is changing the way patients view their health. Some studies have indicated that when patients have access to their EHRs, they feel more knowledgeable about their health and disease processes, are more engaged during visits with their primary care provider, and feel more empowered to participate in disease management and wellness activities (Woods et al., 2013). Smartphone technology offers many add-on utilities and applications. Individuals can read and monitor their blood pressure or track their blood glucose levels using smartphones. Many fitness training applications allow users to share their successes on social media sites. Other applications are available for tracking calories in certain food items, recording caloric intake for the day, and tracking weight loss.

Wearable technologies such as fitness bands (Fitbit, Garmin, Apple Watch) have become popular. Many people use them to track steps, count calories, track quality of sleep, and set fitness goals. As these devices become more sophisticated and more personalized, they will be able learn each individual's habits and give more personal advice (Ghose, 2015). As records and applications continue to evolve, this information may eventually become directly transferrable into a patient's EHR. However, the need to ensure that these devices and applications are without risk to patients and do not compromise their privacy presents a complicated challenge to government regulators (Hamel et al., 2014). Nurses need to understand a patient's level of e-health literacy as more people turn to online sources of health information and patient portals are increasingly being used for patient information (Park et al., 2016).

Online Consumer Medical Information

E-health uses electronic information that can be retrieved online or through a mobile device to improve a person's health or healthcare (U.S. Department of Health and Human Services, 2013). A survey found that 71% searched for information online. Of those searches, 60% searched for information about prescription drugs and 35% asked their physician to make a change by either adding a drug or discontinuing a drug. Another 57% searched for a diagnosis based on their symptoms and then proposed a diagnosis to their healthcare provider. The survey also found that nearly half of Americans go online to find reviews of healthcare providers. Despite the increased use of the internet to search for information, they still track key health factors on paper or in their heads as opposed to mobile devices (Wire, 2015). Another study found that when people have difficulty accessing health services, they turn to the internet and online resources to find health information more often than do those who have good access to healthcare.

Box 48–2 ≫ provides some information on evaluating health-related websites that is useful for both patients and nurses who want to stay current.

Box 48–2
Evaluating Web-based Health Information

When looking online for medical information, ask yourself the following questions:

- *Where does the information come from?* Reliable websites clearly indicate the source of the information. They often provide additional sources of information.
- *Who hosts the site?* Websites that end in *.gov* are government-sponsored; *.org* indicates a noncommercial sponsor; and *.edu* identifies an academic or university sponsor. These are usually reliable sources of information. Websites that end in *.com* indicate commercial sponsorship and may or may not provide accurate information.
- *What type of information is presented?* Is the information authored by a health professional or scientist? Is the information evidenced-based? Does it contain research information?
- *Is the information current?* Review dates should be clearly posted. The most current information should be used, as practices in some areas change rapidly.
- *Is the website trying to sell a product?* Websites that are promoting a product or supplement probably do not contain accurate information and should be avoided.
- *Is your privacy being protected?* Read the website's privacy policy. Do not provide personal information unless you are comfortable with how the website will handle that information.

Sources: Based on National Institutes of Health. (2014). Evaluating Web-based health resources. Retrieved from http://nccam.nih.gov/sites/nccam.nih.gov/files/D337.pdf; National Network of Libraries of Medicine. (2016). Evaluating health websites. Retrieved from https://nnlm.gov/professional-development/topics/health-websites.

Online Patient Medical Information

Many health facilities are using the internet to give patients access to and control over their own health records. Some of these sites are called *patient portals*. Online registration is required, and a user identification and password are needed for each visit. Through many of these portals, patients can schedule routine appointments and request prescription refills from their primary care office (**Figure 48–2 ≫**). Patients also can communicate electronically with their health provider, although some portals are not yet encrypted to allow secure transmission of protected health information. Hospitals are using the internet to schedule some radiology procedures such as mammograms online. Some EHRs allow patients to access parts of their health records. Information such as laboratory and pathology reports, medication records, and due dates for routine screenings and immunizations may be available. The use of these services leads to higher patient satisfaction and retention within the health system (Turley et al., 2012). However, with increased access comes a concern over security of the data. A 2015 survey conducted by the Pew Research Center found that people are sensitive about their personal health information and worry about the security of the data that might be accessible online through the patient portals (Pew Research Center, 2015).

Online Administrative Tools

Patient portals can also perform administrative functions. Patients are able to view and verify their demographic and insurance information. Many providers are placing their new patient paperwork online for patients to complete before their first appointment. Some systems send automated text or voice message reminders for upcoming appointments. Other systems may send automated messages to a group of patients, such as reminders for influenza vaccinations. The patient often has the ability to view any outstanding balances and make payments online.

Many hospitals are using the internet to have patients complete questionnaires about their treatment preferences. Patients can request the gender of the physician, the distance they are willing to travel, and a language accommodated other than English.

A major health insurance program is now allowing patients to price-shop the costs of surgical procedures or diagnostic tests such as MRIs. It also allows patients to see out-of-pocket costs for each health service and keeps track of the patient's contributions to deductibles for the year (Weisman, 2013).

Health insurance companies give providers online access to information about the patient's insurance coverage, including information on providers and hospitals in the insurance company's network. Providers often can see the dates of coverage and co-pays and deductibles paid to date, and in some cases, they can obtain instant online authorization of procedures such as MRIs.

Some websites allow patients to compare health professionals based on specialty, languages spoken, and clinical training. Hospitals and nursing homes can be compared based on quality measures and demographics (e.g., location, size). Websites vary: Some use only patients' ratings, and others use less subjective data.

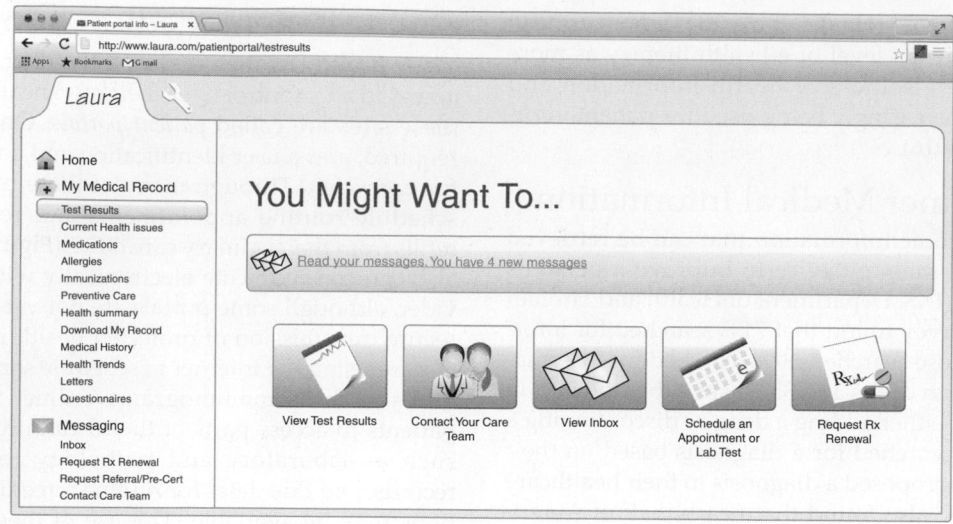

Figure 48-2 》 Patients can use their patient portal to send and receive messages, view test results, schedule an appointment, and order prescription refills.

Ergonomic Considerations

More and more individuals—patients and professionals—are using technology, often for hours a day. Use of technology can impact both work flow and body mechanics. The addition of computers in healthcare may seem innocent enough, but without proper planning and implementation, it can lead to serious injuries to the user. The risk of injury increases with professions that require pushing, pulling, frequent or heavy lifting, prolonged awkward positions, or repetitive, forceful, or prolonged exertion of the hands (U.S. Department of Labor, n.d.a).

Ergonomics is "the science of fitting workplace conditions and job demands to the capabilities of the working population"

(U.S. Department of Labor, n.d.a). Ergonomics examines the type of work being done, the tools being used, and the body mechanics of both the work and the tools, and then suggests the best way to do that work with those tools to limit overuse and harm (U.S. National Library of Medicine, 2016).

For working on a computer, the goal of ergonomics is to set up a workstation that allows a neutral body position (**Figure 48-3 》**). The head, neck, and torso should be in alignment. Shoulders and upper arms should be perpendicular to the floor and relaxed. The upper arms and elbows should be close to the body. Forearms, wrists, and hands should be straight and in line. When the worker is sitting, the thighs should be parallel to the floor and the feet should rest flat on

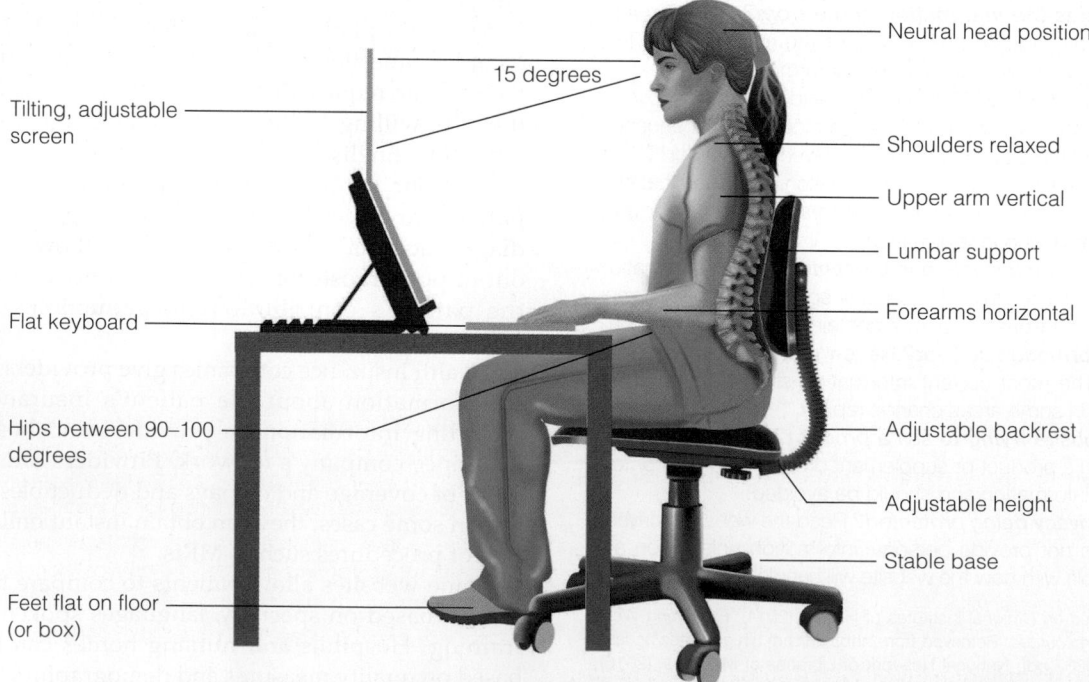

Neutral head position

15 degrees

Tilting, adjustable screen

Shoulders relaxed

Upper arm vertical

Lumbar support

Flat keyboard

Forearms horizontal

Hips between 90–100 degrees

Adjustable backrest

Adjustable height

Stable base

Feet flat on floor (or box)

Figure 48-3 》 Maintaining neutral position while working at a computer will help prevent the development of repetitive strain injuries.

the floor or be supported by a footrest (U.S. Department of Labor, n.d.a).

» Stay Current: A checklist that looks at each component of the computer system (keyboard, monitor, chair, and work surfaces) is available online at www.osha.gov/SLTC/etools/computerworkstations/checklist.html.

Workstations on wheels (WOWs) add requiring the user to pull or push them to different locations for use. The position of the monitor, keyboard, or mouse on the WOW can also lead to bad posture and injury. These carts should be as lightweight and maneuverable as possible. Ideally, the user should be able to tilt the screen at different angles, and workstation platforms should be adjustable to varying heights. See **Box 48–3 »** for ways to incorporate good ergonomics in computer use.

Improper workstation setup or improper body mechanics can lead to injury. Common complaints after prolonged computer use include fatigue or pain in the neck, shoulders, back, arms, wrists, and hands. Some of these symptoms can be alleviated by proper ergonomics or breaks from the computer when possible. Sometimes simple aches and pains can lead to more serious injuries that cause disability. The two most common injuries are repetitive strain injury (RSI) and computer vision syndrome (Princeton University, University Health Services, 2017).

Repetitive strain injury, or repetitive motion disorder, occurs when the limbs are subjected to repetitive use, awkward positions, or forced positions. These injuries can affect nerves, tendons, and muscles. Tendinitis is a common occurrence, but carpal tunnel syndrome is more serious and can lead to permanent disability if not treated. Symptoms of tendinitis include pain in the wrist, elbow, shoulder, or neck; numbness or tingling in the fingers; difficulty grasping objects; and a decrease in the size of the affected hand. Treatment should not be delayed and can include changes in posture, stretching, muscle strengthening, and rest. Rest is a key component; treatment and healing require time. Carpal tunnel syndrome is a more serious repetitive strain injury caused by repeated bending or use of the fingers or wrists that results in median nerve compression. Pain, numbness, and tingling in the palm of the hand and in the thumb and index fingers or the middle fingers are common symptoms. Surgery may be required if the injury is severe enough or does not respond to conservative treatment. If left untreated,

---

Box 48–3
Good Ergonomics for Computer Use

- Maintain good posture whether sitting or standing, aligning your ears, shoulders, and hips.
- Avoid overreaching. Keep the keyboard and mouse within easy reach.
- Keep your wrists in a straight position and your elbows at a slightly open angle.
- Position the monitor so that you can see the screen without tilting your neck up or down or turning your head.
- Use light force when typing on the keyboard.
- Customize font sizes and screen resolution to maximize comfort.
- Take frequent breaks. Eye breaks are important as well as stretching and moving around at regular intervals.
- Ensure proper lighting and reduce glare from the screen.

If you experience numbness, weakness, or pain, seek medical attention.

Sources: Based on University of California at Los Angeles. (2012). *Tips for computer users.* Retrieved April 20, 2013, from http://ergonomics.ucla.edu/homepage/office-ergonomics/tips-for-computer-users.html; Princeton University, University Health Services. (2017). *Ergonomics and computer use.* Retrieved from http://www.princeton.edu/uhs/healthy-living/hot-topics/ergonomics; University of Michigan Health Services. (2017). *Computer ergonomics: how to protect yourself from strain and pain.* Retrieved from https://www.uhs.umich.edu/computerergonomics.

---

carpal tunnel syndrome can lead to muscle wasting, decreased sensation, and permanent disability (Princeton University, University Health Services, 2017).

Computer vision syndrome, or eyestrain, is the most common sequela of computer use. Using the computer for more than 3 hours a day puts one at risk, so many individuals are affected. Symptoms include eye fatigue, headaches, blurred vision, dry eyes, and changes in color perception. If left untreated, computer vision syndrome can lead to a decrease in work efficiency, general fatigue, and increased myopia. It can be caused by monitor glare, monitor position (too close or incorrect angle), or quick eye movements while typing and looking at a source document. Correct monitor position, antiglare screen covers, correct lighting, and proper document placement can all help reduce the effects of computer vision syndrome. It is also important to take breaks and to blink (Princeton University, University Health Services, 2017).

REVIEW The Concept of Informatics

RELATE Link the Concepts

Linking the concept of informatics with the concept of legal issues:

1. Name three ways in which a nurse can keep protected health information secure.

2. What are some ramifications of looking up information in a local celebrity's chart if you are not taking care of that individual?

Linking the concept of informatics with the concept of addiction:

3. You are a nurse at a busy inner city emergency department. It is 3 a.m. on a Saturday when a patient comes in asking for a narcotic prescription. She reports that she usually gets her prescription from her primary care provider for ankle pain from an old injury, but she forgot to call during the week. Describe how an EHR can assist you in caring for this patient.

4. What type of questionnaire tools could be built into an EHR to assist with screening patients for chemical dependency?

REFER Go to Pearson MyLab Nursing and eText

- Additional review materials

REFLECT Apply Your Knowledge

Susan Johnson is a 45-year-old RN who works in a busy medical–surgical unit. Her hospital just installed an EHR system, and because of the layout of the unit, it was decided that the nurses would chart using workstations on wheels. Susan is excited about the new computerized system and has adapted to it quickly. She usually works three 12-hour shifts a week, but a few nurses are out on maternity leave, so she has been picking up extra hours. She has been noticing some tension and pain in her neck and shoulders, especially after her shifts.

1. What are some factors that may be contributing to the tension and pain in Susan's neck and shoulders?
2. What are some things that Susan could try to alleviate these symptoms?
3. What are some advantages to using WOWs for patient documentation?

» Exemplar 48.A
Clinical Decision Support Systems

Exemplar Learning Outcomes

48.A Analyze clinical decision support systems as they relate to informatics.

- Describe the role of uniform languages in clinical decision support systems.
- Describe the use of computers in nursing research.
- Describe the use of computers in nursing administration.

Exemplar Key Terms

Clinical decision support systems, *2820*
Dashboard, *2821*

Overview

Clinical decision support systems (CDSSs) are an important addition to EHRs. A CDSS can be a general system that is used as developed by the vendor, or it can be customized by the organization. A CDSS uses a knowledge base and programmed rules, protocols, and evidence-based guidelines to match against patient data in the EHR and deliver alerts or recommendations to the provider. A CDSS can improve patient care by through the reduction of medication errors, increase adherence to best practice protocols, and decreased costs. However, a CDSS can be challenging: If it is not set up correctly, too difficult to navigate, or creates too many alerts leading to alert fatigue, users will become frustrated, and this can impact patient care. Users also may become dependent on the system and not use their own critical thinking and judgment (Castillo & Kelemen, 2013).

Nurses' Use of Clinical Decision Support Systems

EHRs and CDSSs are designed to provide nurses with alerts, reminders, and recommendations to guide best practice and support clinical decision making. Piscotty and Kalisch (2014) conducted a literature review that examined nurses' use of these systems. They found four factors that impact the use of CDSSs: patient factors, nurse factors, technology design factors, and organizational factors. Nurses tended to use the guidelines more often early in their careers or when caring for unfamiliar patients. They also used the guidelines to back up their decisions. Technology design factors that supported use were limiting the number of reminders, strategic location of the workstations, administrative support for issues, ability to adapt the technology, and good ergonomics.

Barriers to use were heavy workload, poor interface, lack of trust in the information, and lack of reminder flexibility. Organizational support was necessary for adoption of use (Piscotty & Kalisch, 2014).

Using Research

The use of EHRs that contain clinical decision support systems should help promote best practices through nursing research and make it easier to use current nursing research at the point of care (Topaz et al., 2012). Research in the area of adoption of CDSS is helpful in understanding the barriers to using those best practices. A study by Khong et al. (2015) found that some nurses were resistant to using a CDSS and instead relied on their own "gut" instinct for how best to manage wound care or continued to conduct wound care as they had in the past.

Computers in Nursing Research

With the introduction of the EHR, computers will be available to nurses in all practice settings. Research environments will be no different. Conducting nursing research should be easier with the use of uniform language and the ability to query EHRs. The steps of the nursing research process should remain the same. Technology can assist nurses in many ways to gain additional information: The nurse can use the EHR to research the patient's medical history to determine if the patient has been prescribed a particular drug and what responses the patient experienced following administration. The nurse can use the internet to conduct a literature search to determine if there is more information on use of that drug in certain populations or to get additional information related to potential side effects. For a detailed discussion of nursing research, including a list of nursing research databases, see the module on Evidence-Based Practice.

Computers in Nursing Administration

Many EHRs give administrators tools to manage budgets, staffing, quality initiatives, and productivity information. The use of dashboards puts all of this information at the administrator's fingertips. A **dashboard** presents information about a healthcare facility's key performance indicators and displays the information in an easy-to-read format, often with charts or graphs. Some information can be displayed in real time. EHRs can create reports that track data over short-term periods (the past week) or long-term periods (the past year).

Human Resources

Human resource departments and payroll departments can benefit from computerization by tracking personnel within the healthcare system. Professional licenses and credentials expire and must be renewed. It would be a daunting task to keep track of this information manually for a large facility that employs thousands of healthcare professionals. A computerized system can monitor license expiration and when recredentialing of a provider is required. Mandatory hospital education, employee attendance, and performance reviews can all be tracked. When government regulatory agencies make their visits, all of this information is easier to obtain and review. Payroll systems are more accurate with a computerized system. Employees can have access to their available hours of vacation and sick time and may be able to view their paycheck online a few days before they are paid.

Medical Records Management

Much of medical records management revolves around finances. The process begins when a patient schedules an appointment or enters the system on an emergency basis. An informatics system can help schedule the appointment, verify insurance coverage and co-pay information, collect the patient's demographic information, and collect any outstanding payments or co-pays. If the patient is being admitted to the hospital, the system can help with obtaining insurance authorization and assigning a room and bed that have been marked clean and available by the system (and a roommate of the same gender if it is not a private room). The patients' condition can be coded for payment based on their ICD-10, CPT, or HCPCS code (HIMSS, 2016). ICD-10 codes replaced ICD-9 codes on October 1, 2015. The International Classification of Diseases (ICD) codes are used to report inpatient procedures and medical diagnosis (CMS, 2013b). Current procedural terminology (CPT) describes surgical, medical, and diagnostic services; hearing and vision services; occupational and physical therapy services; and transportation services (such as an ambulance; American Medical Association [AMA], 2013). The Healthcare Common Procedure Coding System (HCPCS) contains two levels. Level I is the CPT coding. Level II codes a wide array of services, such as durable medical equipment, outpatient chemotherapy drugs, medical supplies, orthotics, and prosthetics (American Academy of Professional Coders [AAPC], 2016).

Facilities Management

Another system that most nurses are unfamiliar with is materials management and supply chain. When a patient needs a surgical dressing changed, the nurse goes to the supply room and grabs a new dressing without much thought about how it got there. As in many areas of healthcare, the materials management and supply chain community pushed for standardization for efficiency and cost savings. The first standard is that each institution has a Global Location Number (GLN) instead of an account number to make location of the institution easier. The second standard is that each product used in a facility has a Global Trade Item Number (GTIN) instead of a custom item number. It is thought that these standards will help by reducing errors in shipments, streamlining recall processes, enabling facilities to negotiate better contract pricing, and improving the supplier's ability to meet contract requirements. Electronic systems, with or without barcode scanning, can help make equipment use and tracking more efficient and help reduce costs (GS1 Healthcare US Location Identification Workgroup, 2012). These systems also make it easier to keep track of supplies on hand and assist with ordering supplies or materials as they are used.

Budget and Finance

Before the patient's chart can be finalized and closed, it is reviewed to make sure all coding is correct so that proper information is sent to the billing department. Some facilities do their own billing; others hire separate companies for this. If a patient is receiving care in the hospital, there are usually two separate billing processes. One is professional billing, which covers fees for services provided by surgeons, radiologists, and anesthesiologists. The other is hospital billing, which covers room and board and supplies. Incorrect billing can result in the claim's being denied by a patient's insurance company. This denial could leave either the patient or the hospital responsible for the bill, so there is usually a process for billers to submit appeals or resolve claim denials. It is a very complicated system that can be made easier through an electronic administration system.

Reimbursement rates for procedures and diagnoses change regularly, and a computerized contract management system helps facilities track rates of reimbursement and real-time changes in policies for different health insurance plans. Pay-for-performance systems will drive areas of reimbursement such as chronic disease management and care for acute disease without causing unnecessary harm (Miliard, 2015).

Financial systems within healthcare facilities can benefit greatly from use of an electronic system. They are responsible for sharing information between billing systems, materials management, and staffing/human resources in order to determine the financial health of the facility. The data provided is crucial for making strategic decisions about a healthcare institution and in planning organizational budgets. Executives and managers can view financial information over both short- and long-term time frames and adjust their resources and fiscal planning appropriately.

Quality Assurance and Utilization Reviews

Computerized systems facilitate the tracking of patient outcomes. Unexpected or poor patient outcomes can be tracked by risk management (the legal department of a health system). Quality outcomes information can also be easily tracked. Outcome tracking helps identify faulty processes and assists in modifying policies and procedures to improve patient outcomes for a particular diagnosis or department within a health organization. Using CDSS and quality improvement efforts, health centers can build in best practice protocols to improve blood pressure management or

standardized risk assessment tools to improve patient care and outcomes (Miliard, 2015).

Accreditation

The availability of quality metrics will make it easier to meet and document the requirements of regulatory agencies. Agencies such as the Centers for Medicare and Medicaid Services and The Joint Commission implement policies that health facilities must follow in order to receive reimbursement by many health insurance plans. There are also smaller yet still important standards that must be maintained for certification, such as trauma status from the American College of Surgeons or stroke center status from The Joint Commission. EHRs simplify the data-gathering process when each of these agencies reviews a facility for accreditation.

REVIEW Clinical Decision Support Systems

RELATE Link the Concepts and Exemplars

Linking the exemplar of clinical decision support systems to the concept of cellular regulation:

1. Discuss how clinical decision support systems could improve outcomes for patients with cancer.

2. Name three cancer screening tools that could be built into an EHR.

3. Discuss the benefits of making reminders for cancer screening available to healthcare providers and to patients.

Linking the exemplar of clinical decision support systems to the concept of health policy:

4. You are working in the operating room, and your supervisor always requires that the employees in the department enter a higher level-of-diagnosis code on each trauma patient's chart. What are some ramifications?

5. What impact does a change in a federal or state health policy have on clinical decision support systems?

REFER Go to Pearson MyLab Nursing and eText

- Additional review materials

REFLECT Apply Your Knowledge

You are the nurse manager for an orthopedic unit that has just installed an EHR system with an administrative system. You have been short-staffed for several months.

1. How can an administrative system help get more nursing positions approved for your unit?

2. What other features of an administrative system do you think will have the greatest impact on your unit and why?

≫ Exemplar 48.B
Individual Information at Point of Care

Exemplar Learning Outcomes

48.B Analyze individual information at point of care as it relates to informatics.

- Summarize the advantages of point-of-care service delivery.
- Outline uses of computer-based patient records in community and hospital settings.

Exemplar Key Terms

Case managers, 2823
Point of care, 2822

Overview

Studies have proven that the more direct nursing care a patient receives, the better the quality and safety of the care that is delivered and the more satisfied both nurse and patient are with the care. Nurses have reported that charting is an activity that consumes much of their time and takes time away from the bedside. The ability to enter data into a

patient's chart while at the patient's bedside seems like a valid compromise. Most EHRs allow recording of vital signs, medication documentation, assessment notes, and responses to nursing intervention (**Figure 48–4 ≫**). One of the selling points of an EHR is that charting at point of care is possible and that it helps to increase efficiency. Interventions at **point of care** refers to interventions or testing that takes place

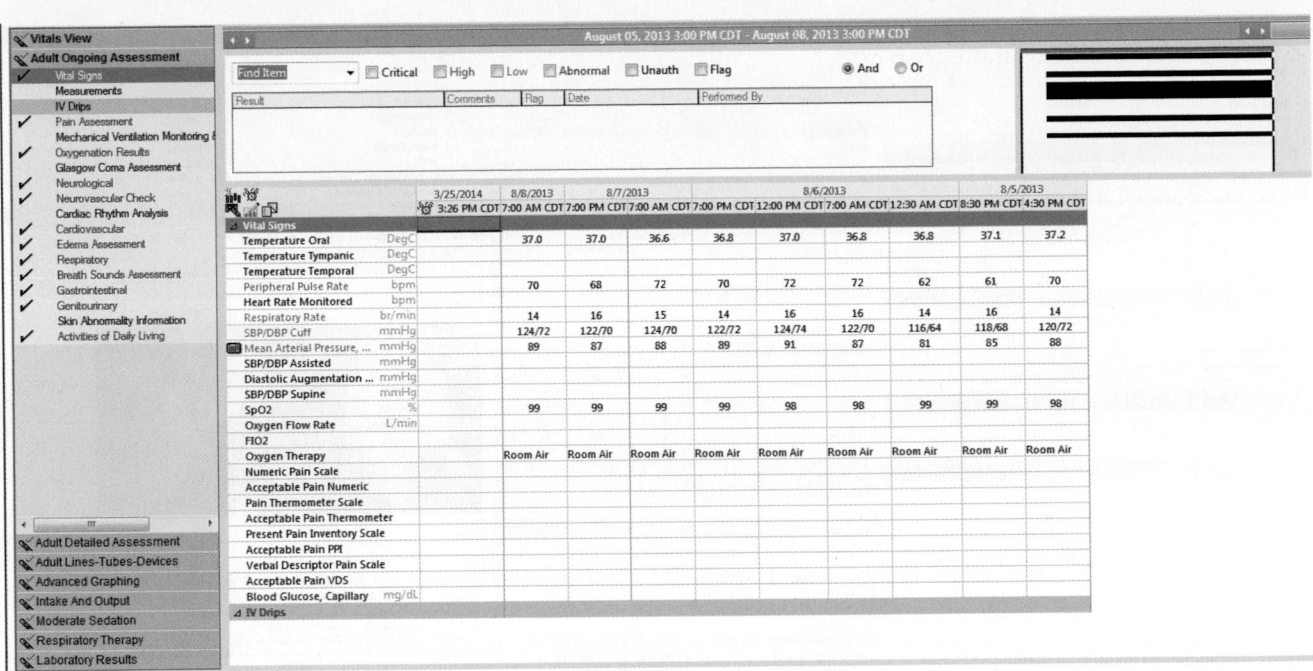

Figure 48–4 ≫ This EHR screen displays the patient's vital signs. They can be entered by the nurse (or anyone with security rights to do so) at the bedside, and they can be displayed wherever needed.

using transportable, portable, or handheld devices near the patient (ASC Quality Collaboration, 2013). This setup provides on-the-spot information about the patient rather than having to wait for the results from blood or urine samples sent to the laboratory.

Computer-based Patient Records

Although the EHR has the potential to forever change how healthcare is delivered in the United States, it is important to understand that, in many instances, the electronic record cannot and should not replace real-time (face-to-face or telephone) communication with peers, other health professionals, and especially the patient. An acute change in the patient's condition still requires a phone call to the physician. News of pathology reports that indicate cancer should still be delivered in person by the physician and not discovered by the patient online. As systems become more advanced and interfaces more integrated, nurses must not lose sight of the human element in the delivery of care.

Patient Monitoring and Computerized Diagnostics

Advances in electronic systems are changing monitoring and tracking of patient care. Many facilities now use systems that allow electronic transmission of information such as the weight from the scale on the bed, intravenous pump rates, barcode scanning of medications that are administered, vital sign information, barcode scanning of blood administration, and ventilator settings. Many departments within a hospital or other facility may enter data about the patient into the record so that all practitioners have the information easily available rather than having to flip through a paper chart. Some examples are the laboratory

and many radiologic exams, such as MRI and CT scans (**Figure 48–5 ≫**). With some systems, the radiologic image is available at the bedside in addition to the radiologist's report. The patient's medical administration record (MAR) also may be viewed by all providers involved in care of the patient (**Figure 48–6 ≫**).

Community and Home Health

More than 4 million people are admitted to or reside in nursing homes and skilled nursing facilities annually; another 1 million reside in assisted living communities (CDC, 2015). In 2013, nearly 5 million patients received some degree of home healthcare (Harris-Kojetin et al., 2016). Nurses are the main providers of this care to patients, many of whom are receiving home healthcare for a chronic disease such as diabetes or congestive heart failure. It is difficult sometimes to stay current with the management of complex medical issues that home healthcare nurses are facing. The incorporation of current evidence-based clinical practice guidelines into the EHR system that is used by the home healthcare agency can improve the quality of care that these patients receive.

Case Management

Case managers help manage the care of certain patient populations, including patients with chronic medical conditions, such as diabetes; patients recovering from acute conditions, such as those receiving joint replacement; and patients managing psychiatric disorders. EHRs can assist the case manager by allowing trending of patient progress, documentation of patient education, and observation of quality metrics to help decrease readmission rates for these populations. EHRs also allow improved coordination of care between providers because they are all working off of one chart.

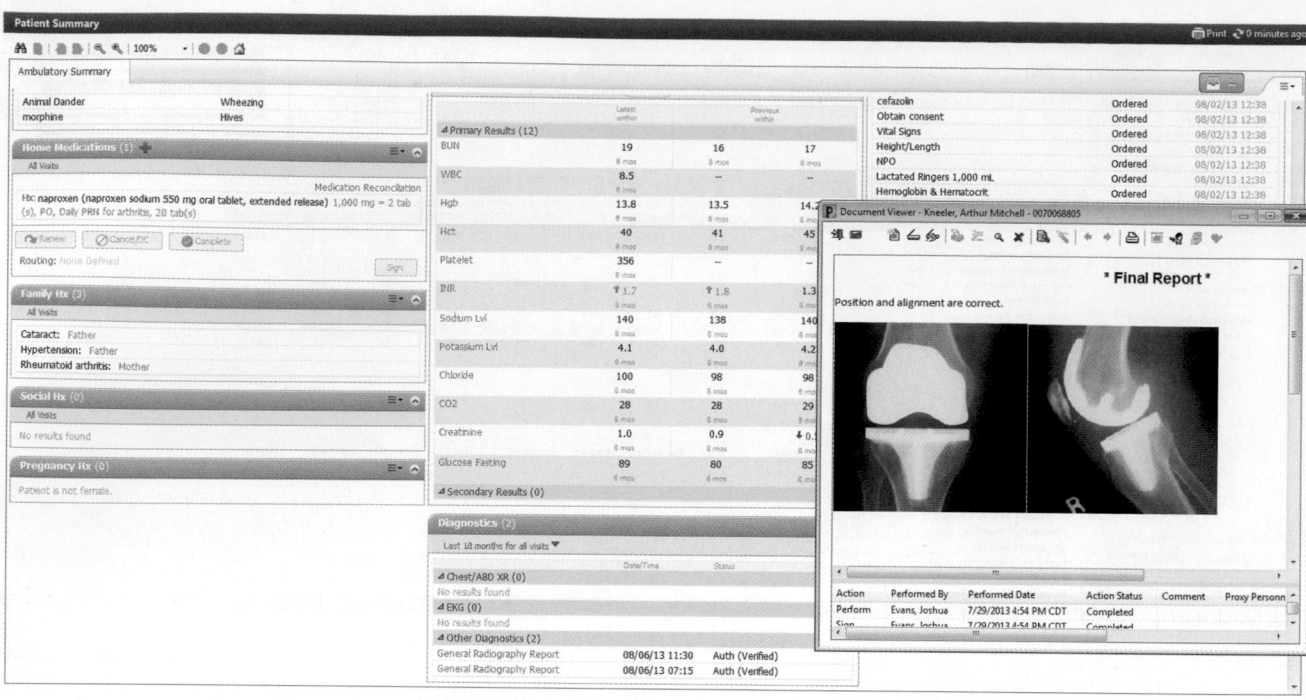

Figure 48–5 ≫ This EHR screen displays a summary view of all available laboratory results and diagnostic imaging for a particular patient. The information is reported from most summarized to most detailed so that the user gets the overview first and can then "drill down" to see the details.

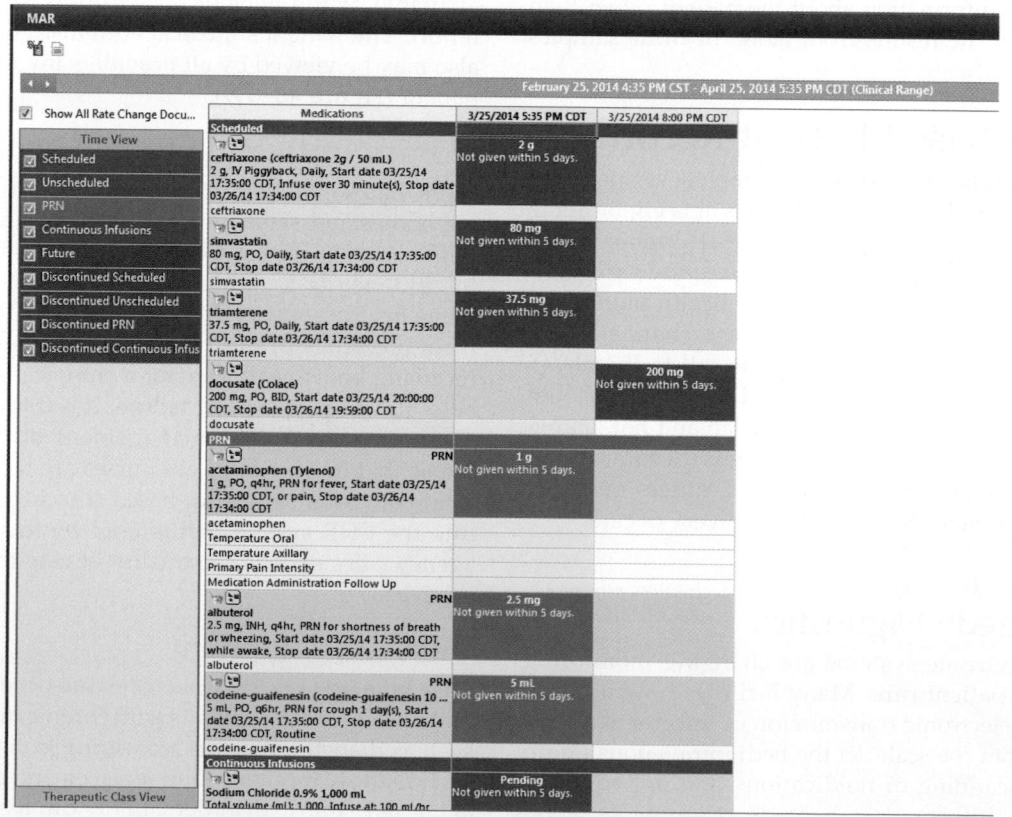

Figure 48–6 ≫ This EHR screen shows a medication administration record (MAR) for several regularly scheduled medications. The worksheet displays the next time the medications are scheduled to be administered.

Patient Education

Instructions for health conditions and procedures are available in most EHR systems. The patient's health problem can be identified through menus and educational information printed so that the nurse can review the information with the patient or the patient's family. Standardization of the record means that the patients will receive the same educational material whether they are being treated in the emergency department, on a surgical unit, or in a healthcare provider's office. The information contained within the educational material should be current and evidenced based, so that the task of patient education is more accurate and meaningful. Some material may provide links to websites for additional information. Many systems can print out or be linked to educational information in different languages as well (Agency for Healthcare Research and Quality, 2016; National Learning Consortium, 2012). Note that use of standardized printed material does not negate the nurse's responsibility to (a) assess the patient or family member's ability to read and understand the information, (b) review the information in person with the patient or family member, and (c) ensure that the patient or family member understands the information prior to discharge.

REVIEW Individual Information at Point of Care

RELATE Link the Concepts and Exemplars

Linking the exemplar of individual information at point of care with the concept of assessment:

1. Discuss the advantages of being able to document the assessment of your patient at the point of care with an electronic record rather than a centralized charting location.

2. Explain how point-of-care documentation of your patient assessment can be used as an opportunity for patient teaching.

Linking the exemplar of individual information at point of care with the concept of oxygenation:

3. What point-of-care information can you obtain from an electronic medical record about the patient's past and present oxygenation status that may influence immediate nursing interventions?

4. How might point-of-care recording of pulse oximeter values have an advantage over recording them from a centralized monitoring station in the intensive care unit?

REFER Go to Pearson MyLab Nursing and eText

■ Additional review materials

REFLECT Apply Your Knowledge

You are caring for an Albanian patient who just had his appendix removed. You log into your health system's electronic record to obtain discharge information. The patient and the family speak limited English. Albanian is not a language choice for appendectomy discharge instructions.

1. What are some options that you can use to try to educate the patient on taking care of his incision site?

2. How would you document your interventions in the electronic record?

References

Agency for Healthcare Research and Quality. (2016). *Practice facilitation handbook: Module 17. Electronic health records and meaningful use.* Retrieved from http://www.ahrq.gov/professionals/prevention-chronic-care/improve/system/pfhandbook/mod17.html

American Academy of Professional Coders. (2016). *What is HCPCS?* Retrieved from http://www.aapc.com/resources/medical-coding/hcpcs.aspx

American Medical Association. (2013). *CPT frequently asked questions.* Retrieved from http://www.ama-assn.org/ama/pub/physician-resources/solutions-managing-your-practice/coding-billing-insurance/cpt/frequently-asked-questions.page

American Nurses Association. (2015). *Nursing informatics: Scope and standards of practice.* (2nd ed.). Silver Spring, MD: Nursebooks.org

AMIA. (2016). *Nursing informatics.* Retrieved from https://www.amia.org/programs/working-groups/nursing-informatics. Used by permission of American Medical Informatics Association.

ASC Quality Collaboration. (2013). *Point of care devices toolkit.* Retrieved from http://www.ascquality.org/PointofCareDevicesToolkit.cfm

Baum, S. (2015). *Report: Emails, text messages helped hospital cut readmissions for congestive heart failure patients.* Retrieved from http://medcitynews.com/2015/04/philly-hospital-emails-text-messages-cut-readmissions-chronic-heart-failure-patients/

Beck, M. (2016). How telemedicine is transforming health care. *The Wall Street Journal.* Retrieved from http://www.wsj.com/articles/how-telemedicine-is-transforming-health-care-1466993402

California HealthCare Foundation. (2013a). *Brief highlights: Ways to promote the successful adoption of telehealth.* Retrieved from http://www.ihealthbeat.org/articles/2013/2/1/brief-highlights-ways-to-promote-the-successful-adoption-of-telehealth

California HealthCare Foundation. (2013b). *1.8 million patients will use telehealth tools by 2017, report says.* Retrieved from http://www.ihealthbeat.org/articles/2013/1/23/18-million-patients-will-use-telehealth-tools-by-2017-report-says.aspx?topic=telehealth

Castillo, R. S., & Kelemen, A. (2013). Considerations for a successful clinical decision support system. *Computers Informatics Nursing, 31*(7), 319–326.

Center for Connected Health Policy (2016). *State telehealth laws and Medicaid program policies.* Retrieved from http://cchpca.org/sites/default/files/resources/50%20STATE%20COMPLETE%20REPORT%20PASSWORD%20AUG%202016 1.pdf

Centers for Disease Control and Prevention. (2015). *Nursing homes and assisted living (long-term care facilities [LCTFs]).* Retrieved from https://www.cdc.gov/longtermcare/

Centers for Disease Control and Prevention. (2016). *State successes.* Retrieved from http://www.cdc.gov/drugoverdose/policy/successes.html

Centers for Medicare and Medicaid Services. (2013a). *Clinical quality measures (CQMs).* Retrieved from http://www.cms.gov/Regulations-and-Guidance/Legislation/EHRIncentivePrograms/Clinical-QualityMeasures.html

Centers for Medicare and Medicaid Services. (2013b). *ICD-10.* Retrieved from http://www.cms.gov/Medicare/Coding/ICD10/index.html?redirect=/icd10

Centers for Medicare and Medicaid Services. (2016). *Meaningful use.* Retrieved from http://www.cdc.gov/ehrmeaningfuluse/introduction.html. Published by U.S. Department of Health & Human Services.

Centers for Medicare and Medicaid Services. (2017). *Data and program reports.* Retrieved from https://www.cms.gov/regulations-and-guidance/legislation/ehrincentiveprograms/dataandreports.html

Duke University. (2012). *Health management information systems: Administrative, billing, and financial systems lecture A.* Retrieved from http://www.healthinformaticsforum.com/page/component-6-unit-9-lecture-a

Federation of State Medical Boards. (2012). *Model policy guidelines for the appropriate use of social media and social networking in medical practice.* Retrieved from http://www.fsmb.org/pdf/pub-social-media-guidelines.pdf

Ghose, T. (2015) 10,000 steps, new trackers go beyond the data dump. Retrieved from http://www.livescience.com/49380-fitness-trackers-analyze-data.html

Goldberg, D., Kuzel, A., Feng, L., DeShazo, J., & Love, L. (2012). EHRs in primary care practices: Benefits, challenges, and successful strategies. *American Journal of Managed Care, 18*(2), e48–e54

GS1 Healthcare US Location Identification Workgroup. (2012). *GLN roadmap: A collaborative industry implementation plan for U.S. healthcare.* Retrieved from http://www.gs1us.org/DesktopModules/Bring2mind/DMX/Download.aspx?Command=Core_Download&EntryId=535& PortalId=0&TabId=785

Guerin, L. (2016). *Can employers ask for passwords to my social media accounts?* Retrieved from http://www.nolo.com/legal-encyclopedia/can-employers-ask-passwords-my-social-media-accounts.html

Hamel, M. B., Cortez, N. G., Cohen, I. G., & Kesselheim, A. S. (2014). FDA regulation of mobile health technologies. *New England Journal of Medicine, 371*(4), 372–379.

Harris-Kojetin, L., Sengupta, M., Park-Lee, E., Valverde, R., Caffrey, C., Rome, V., & Lendon, J. (2016). Long-term care providers and services users in the United States: Data from the National Study of Long-Term Care Providers, 2013–2014. *Vital Health Statistics, 3*(38), x–xii, x–105.

Healthcare Information and Management Systems Society. (2016). *ICD-9 to ICD-10 transition.* Retrieved from http://www.himss.org/library/icd-10-transition

HealthIT.gov. (n.d.a). *Medical practice efficiencies and cost savings.* Retrieved from [0] https://www.healthit.gov/providers-professionals/medical-practice-efficiencies-cost-savings

HealthIT.gov. (n.d.b). *What is telehealth? How is it different from telemedicine?* Retrieved from https://www.healthit.gov/providers-professionals/faqs/what-telehealth-how-telehealth-different-telemedicine

Health Level Seven International. (2013). *About HL7.* Retrieved from http://www.hl7.org/about/index.cfm?ref=nav. Copyright © 2013 by Health Level Seven International.

HIT. (2015). 5 benefits of geographic information systems in healthcare. Retrieved from http://hitconsultant.net/2015/10/29/5-benefits-of-geographic-information-systems-in-healthcare/

Khong, P. C. B., Hoi, S. Y., Holroyd, E., & Wang, W. (2015). Nurses' clinical decision making on adopting a wound clinical decision support system. *Computers Informatics Nursing, 33*(7), 295–305.

King, J., Patel, V., Jamoom, E. W., & Furukawa, M. F. (2014). Clinical benefits of electronic health record use: National findings. *Health Services Research, 49*(1), 392–404. Retrieved from http://onlinelibrary.wiley.com/doi/10.1111/1475-6773.12135/abstract

Lagase, J. (2016). *Arkansas, Texas look to ease telehealth restrictions.* Retrieved from http://www.healthcareitnews.com/news/arkansas-texas-look-ease-telehealth-restrictions

Landi, H. (2016). *AHRQ Study: Teleheath use effective for remote monitoring, counseling of chronic disease patients.* Retrieved from http://www.healthcare-informatics.com/news-item/telemedicine/ahrq-study-telemedicine-use-effective-remote-monitoring-counseling-chronic

Locatelli, P., Restifo, N., Gastaldi, L., & Corso, M. (2012). *Healthcare information systems: Architectural models and governance.* Retrieved from http://cdn.intechopen.com/pdfs/37320/InTech-Health_care_information_systems_architectural_models_and_governance.pdf

Meum, T. (2013). "Lost in translation": The challenges of seamless integration in nursing practices.

International Journal of Medical Informatics, 82(5), e200–e208.

Miliard, M. (2014). *Mapping a new future for GIS.* Retrieved from http://www.healthcareitnews.com/news/mapping-new-future-gis

Miliard, M. (2015). *Clinical decision support system no longer just nice to have.* Retrieved from http://www.healthcareitnews.com/news/clinical-decision-support-no-longer-just-nice-have

National Association of School Nurses. (2012). *Standardized nursing languages.* Retrieved from http://www.nasn.org/Policy/Advocacy/PositionPapersandReports/NASNPositionStatementsFullView/tabid/462/ArticleId/48/Standardized-Nursing-Languages-Revised-June-2012-Standardized Nursing Languages

National Council of State Boards of Nursing. (2014). *Social media guidelines for nurses.* Retrieved from https://www.ncsbn.org/347.htm

National Learning Consortium. (2012). *Providing patients with patient-specific education resources.* Retrieved from https://www.healthit.gov/sites/default/files/providing_patients_with_patient-specific_education_resources.docx

NPR. (2015, August). *Why your doctor won't friend you on Facebook.* Retrieved from http://www.npr.org/sections/health-shots/2015/08/25/434604425/why-your-doctor-won-t-friend-you-on-facebook

Open Clinical. (2016). *Electronic medical records.* Retrieved from http://www.openclinical.org/emr.html

Park, H., Cormier, E., Gordon, G., & Baeg, J. H. (2016). Identifying health consumers' ehealth literacy to decrease disparities in accessing ehealth information. *Computers Informatics Nursing, 34*(2), 71–76, quiz 99.

Pena, K. D., & Sanders, K. A. (2016) *Bumps along the road: using telemedicine to treat chronic disease in rural communities.* Retrieved from http://www.healthcareitnews.com/blog/bumps-along-rural-road-using-telemedicine-treat-chronic-disease-rural-communities

Pew Research Center. (2015). *Scenario health information convenience and security.* Retrieved from http://www.pewinternet.org/2016/01/14/scenario-health-information-convenience-and-security/

Piscotty, R., & Kalisch, B. (2014). Nurses' use of clinical decision support: a literature review. *Computers Informatics Nursing, 32*(12), 562–568.

Pizzi, R. (2013). Stage 7 health system raises the bar. *Healthcare IT News.* Retrieved from http://www.healthcareitnews.com/news/mdi-boosts-quality-saves-time

Princeton University, University Health Services. (2017). *Ergonomics and computer use.* Retrieved from http://www.princeton.edu/uhs/healthy-living/hot-topics/ergonomics

Solove, D. J. (2013, April 4). HIPAA turns 10: Analyzing the past, present, and future impact. *Journal of AHIMA, 84*(4), 22–28. Retrieved from https://ssrn.com/abstract=2245022

Statista. (2016). *Number of social network users worldwide from 2010 to 2020 (in billions).* Retrieved from http://www.statista.com/statistics/278414/number-of-worldwide-social-network-users/

Stokes, T. (2013). *Copying common in electronic medical records.* Retrieved from http://www.reuters.com/article/2013/01/04/us-electronic-medical-records idUSBRE9030IJ20130104

Substance Abuse and Mental Health Services Administration. (2016). *Opioid overdose.* Retrieved from http://www.samhsa.gov/medication-assisted-treatment/treatment/opioid-overdose

"Text messaging apps for hospitals." (n.d.). *HIPAA Journal.* Retrieved from http://www.hipaajournal.com/text-messaging-apps-for-hospitals/

The Economist. (2014). *The $272 billion swindle.* Retrieved from http://www.economist.com/news/united-states/21603078-why-thieves-love-americas-health-care-system-272-billion-swindle

The Joint Commission. (2012). *Surgical care improvement project.* Retrieved from http://www.jointcommission.org/surgical_care_improvement_project/

Topaz, M., Radhakrishnan, K., Masterson-Creber, R., & Bowles, K. H. (2012). Putting evidence to work: Using standardized terminologies to incorporate clinical practice guidelines in homecare electronic health records. *Online Journal of Nursing Informatics, 16*(2). Retrieved from http://ojni.org/issues/?p=1694

Turley, M., Garrido, T., Lowenthal, A., & Zhou, Y. (2012). Association between personal health record enrollment and patient loyalty. *American Journal of Managed Care, 18*(7), e248–e253.

U.S. Department of Health and Human Services. (2013). *What is e-health?* Retrieved from http://www.health.gov/communication/ehealth/

U.S. Department of Health and Human Services. (n.d.). *Your rights under HIPAA.* Retrieved from www.hhs.gov/hipaa/for-individuals/guidance-materials-for-consumers/index.html

U.S. Department of Labor, Occupational Safety and Health Administration. (n.d.a). *Prevention of musculoskeletal disorders in the workplace: Ergonomics.* Retrieved from http://www.osha.gov/SLTC/ergonomics

U.S. Department of Labor, Occupational Safety and Health Administration. (n.d.b). *Computer workstations: Checklist.* Retrieved from http://www.osha.gov/SLTC/etools/computerworkstations/checklist.html

U.S. National Library of Medicine, National Institutes of Health. (2012). *MedlinePlus guide to healthy Web surfing.* Retrieved from http://www.nlm.nih.gov/medlineplus/healthywebsurfing.html

U.S. National Library of Medicine, National Institutes of Health. (2016). *Ergonomics.* Retrieved from http://www.nlm.nih.gov/medlineplus/ergonomics.html

U.S. News & World Report. (2014). Health care harnesses social media. Retrieved from https://www.usnews.com/news/articles/2014/06/05/health-care-harnesses-social-media

Vanderbilt University School of Medicine, Department of Biomedical Informatics. (2013). *Frequently asked questions.* Retrieved from https://medschool.vanderbilt.edu/dbmi/frequently-asked-questions

Weisman, R. (2013, January 27). New insurance tools will let patients discover costs. *The Boston Globe.*

Wire, K. (2015). *71% have searched for information online.* Retrieved from https://www.klick.com/health/news/blog/strategy/71-have-searched-for-health-information-online/

Woods, S., Schwartz, E., Tuepker, A., Press, N., Nazi, K., Turvey, C., & Nichol, W. (2013). Patient experiences with full electronic access to health records and clinical notes through the My HealtheVet Personal Health Record Pilot: Qualitative study. *Journal of Medical Internet Research, 15*(3), e65. doi:10.2196/jmir.org/2013/e65/

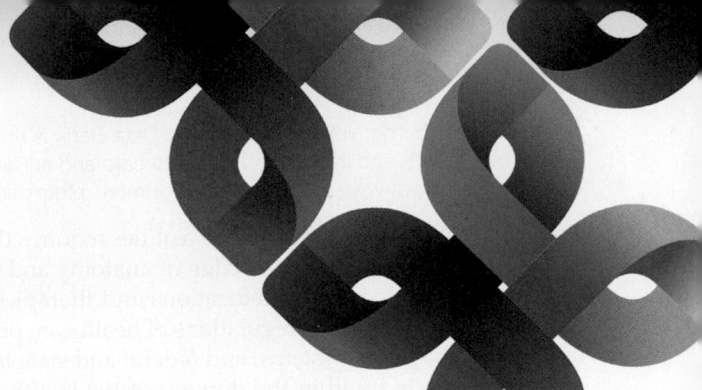

Module 49
Legal Issues

Module Outline and Learning Outcomes

The Concept of Legal Issues

Sources and Types of Laws

49.1 Analyze the sources of laws and types of laws.

Tort Law

49.2 Analyze tort law and its implication for nursing.

Concepts Related to Legal Issues

49.3 Outline the relationship between legal issues and other concepts.

Strategies to Prevent Incidents of Professional Negligence

49.4 Outline strategies to prevent incidents of professional negligence.

The Standard of Care

49.5 Analyze the impact of the standard of care on legal issues.

Selected Laws That Affect Nursing Practice

49.6 Outline laws that affect nursing practice.

Lifespan Considerations

49.7 Differentiate considerations related to legal issues throughout the lifespan.

Legal Issues Exemplars

Exemplar 49.A Nurse Practice Acts

49.A Analyze nurse practice acts as they relate to legal issues.

Exemplar 49.B Advance Directives

49.B Analyze advance directives as they relate to legal issues.

Exemplar 49.C Health Insurance Portability and Accountability Act

49.C Analyze HIPAA as it relates to legal issues.

Exemplar 49.D Mandatory Reporting

49.D Analyze mandatory reporting as it relates to legal issues.

Exemplar 49.E Risk Management

49.E Analyze risk management as it relates to legal issues.

» The Concept of Legal Issues

Concept Key Terms

Administrative laws, 2828	Competency, 2834	Expressed consent, 2834	Informed consent, 2833	Standards of care, 2831
Assault, 2831	Controlled Substances Act (CSA), 2835	False imprisonment, 2831	Law, 2828	Statute of limitations, 2830
Battery, 2831	Crime, 2829	Foreseeability, 2829	Liability, 2829	Statutory laws, 2828
Breach of duty, 2829	Criminal law, 2829	Good Samaritan laws, 2835	Malpractice, 2827	Tort, 2829
Causation, 2829	Damages, 2830	Implied consent, 2834	Negligence, 2829	Whistleblower, 2836
Civil law, 2829	Duty, 2829		Seven Rights, 2832	Whistleblowing, 2836

Legal issues in nursing encompass the rights, responsibilities, and scope of nursing practice as defined by state nurse practice acts and as legislated through criminal and civil laws. All patients have a privilege, demand, or claim by virtue of law or *right* (that which is proper or just) to expect competent nursing services. The nursing student must be equipped to provide safe nursing care consistent with legal requirements and to gain an awareness of ways to minimize the risks of errors due to accident, carelessness, system failures, or malpractice.

Malpractice is conduct that deviates from the standard of practice dictated by a profession. According to the 2012 Annual Report of the National Practitioner Data Bank, professional nurses were responsible for 6167 malpractice payments from 2003 to 2012. That is 4.2% of malpractice payments made during that time period (Health Resources and Services Administration [HRSA], 2014a). The number of nursing malpractice cases is associated with both the liability risks of nursing practice and an increasingly well-informed patient base.

>> Stay Current: The National Practitioner Data Bank is an excellent source of research and information on healthcare and nursing topics. Visit their website at www.npdb.hrsa.gov for more information.

Providing safe care in light of these realities requires the nurse to have more than just a knowledge of anatomy and physiology, pathophysiology, and medications and therapies. It also requires knowledge of the regulations of healthcare providers, institutions, payment systems, and federal and state laws that are interconnected within the domain of the healthcare system. Upon enrollment, the nursing student begins learning about laws and regulations that affect nursing practice. Legal and professional regulations address both nursing practice and the practices of healthcare organizations that serve as workplaces for nurses at all levels of practice. Many healthcare agency policies and procedures exist to ensure that relevant laws are followed (1) to promote patient safety and reduce the risk for errors resulting in adverse events and (2) to protect both healthcare staff and healthcare agencies as a whole. For example, policies regarding identifying and managing patient valuables help ensure that patients' belongings are cared for and respected and also act to prevent theft or accidental loss.

To provide safe, effective care and maintain personal protection from liability, nurses must be aware of the applicable regulations they must follow in every nursing encounter. Awareness begins with understanding general legal concepts and continues as the nursing student starts to learn about the laws and regulations that directly affect the daily activities of nursing.

Sources and Types of Laws

Guido (2014, p. 2) defines **law** as the "sum total of the rules and regulations by which a society is governed." Law is made at the federal, state, and local levels to reflect the ever-changing needs and expectations of a society. **Statutory laws** are made by the legislative branches of the government, including the U.S. Congress, state legislatures, and city and county governments. The U.S. Constitution grants the federal government power to make laws; the states have inherent power to act to maintain health, public order, safety, and welfare except where the Constitution restricts their ability to do so.

Nursing laws are examples of state statutory laws. Each state has a nurse practice act that contains the laws pertaining to nursing practice in that state. Nurse practice acts are discussed in detail in Exemplar 49.A. Other statutory laws that affect the practice of nursing include statutes of limitation, protection and reporting laws, natural death acts, and informed consent laws.

A legislative body, through statutory law, delegates the responsibility for the administration and enforcement of those laws to administrative agencies. Administrative agencies may be granted additional power to interpret those laws and enact policies or procedures by which those laws will be implemented and enforced. These policies or procedures are often referred to as **administrative laws**. State Boards of Nursing are examples of administrative agencies that are delegated the power to interpret and enforce law by the legislatures that govern them.

An overview of the sources of law is shown in **Figure 49–1 >>**. Selected categories of law that may affect nurses are shown in **Table 49–1 >>**.

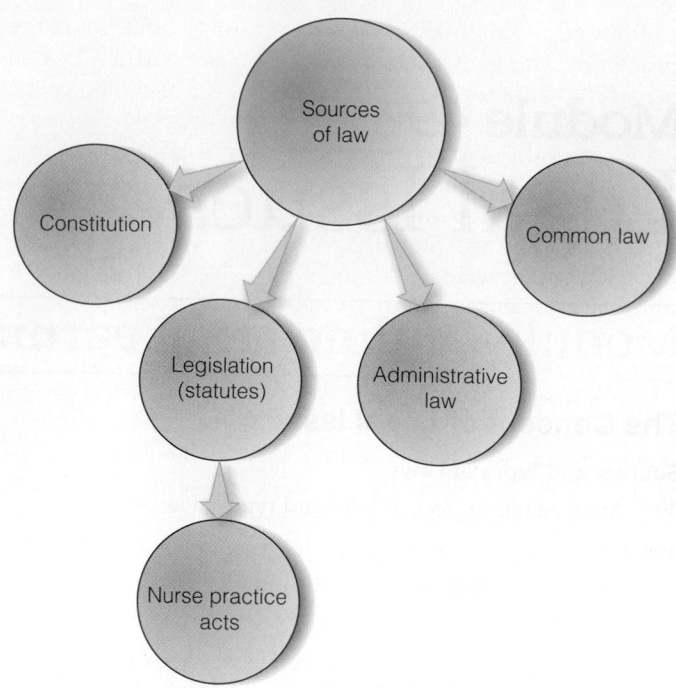

Figure 49–1 >> Overview of the sources of law.

TABLE 49–1 Selected Categories of Laws Affecting Nurses

Category	Examples
Constitutional	Due process
	Equal protection
Statutory (legislative)	Nurse practice acts
	Good Samaritan acts
	Child and adult abuse laws
	Advance directives
	Sexual harassment laws
	Americans with Disabilities Act
Criminal (public)	Homicide, manslaughter
	Theft
	Arson
	Active euthanasia
	Sexual assault
	Illegal possession of controlled drugs
Contracts (private/civil)	Nurse and patient
	Nurse and employer
	Nurse and insurance provider
	Patient and agency
Torts (private/civil)	Negligence/malpractice
	Libel and slander
	Invasion of privacy
	Assault and battery
	False imprisonment
	Abandonment

Both criminal and civil laws have implications for the practicing nurse. **Criminal law** defines conduct that is harmful to another individual or to society as a whole and that may be punishable by fines or imprisonment. A **crime** is an act prohibited by statute or by common-law principles. Crimes are considered to be committed against the state rather than the individual. Examples of crimes include homicide, theft, and manslaughter. Crimes are classified by severity, more serious crimes being classified as *felonies* and lesser offenses being termed *misdemeanors*. Criminal laws are enforced by law enforcement and government prosecutors.

Civil law deals with the rights and duties of private individuals or citizens and is most often enforced through lawsuits. A **tort** is a civil wrong committed against an individual or an individual's property. An individual who violates tort law may be sued and compensation awarded to those wrongfully injured by those violations. Torts may be intentional or unintentional.

Tort Law

Tort law defines and addresses unintentional and intentional actions or omissions that result in harm to another person or persons or harm to another's personal property. Unintentional torts discussed here include negligence and malpractice. Intentional torts include assault, battery, false imprisonment, and invasion of privacy.

Unintentional Torts

It is especially important for nurses and other healthcare providers to understand negligence and malpractice.

Negligence

Negligence is conduct that deviates from what a reasonable person would do in a particular circumstance. The "reasonable person" standard describes an individual in society who exercises average care, skill, and judgment in conduct as a comparative standard for determining liability. According to this standard, an individual who undertakes a particular activity is ordinarily considered to have the knowledge common to others who engage in that activity; for example, a motorist must know the rules of the road. A negligent act occurs when an individual damages the person or property of another without any intent to injure. This damage may be due to carelessness on the part of the individual who committed the act. For example, a motorist who is talking on a cell phone or otherwise not paying attention and causes an automobile crash by failing to stop at a stop sign may be considered negligent and would be liable for any damages to any person or property.

In a legal action to establish negligence, the injured party needs to prove that the other party had a *duty of reasonable care*, that the other party *did not maintain reasonable care*, and that the failure to maintain such reasonable care *caused* (resulted in) *injuries* to the aggrieved party. In the example of the automobile crash, all drivers have the duty to operate their vehicles safely and follow traffic laws. If a driver fails to do so and this failure results in injury to any other person or damage to property, that driver would meet all of the criteria to be held negligent and would therefore be accountable for paying damages to the injured party.

Malpractice

When discussing negligence, it is important to note that the standard of a "reasonable person" is different for individuals in specific professional occupations. If an individual engages in an activity that requires special skills, education, training, or licensure—such as piloting a plane or providing professional nursing care—the standard by which that person's conduct is measured is the conduct of a reasonably skilled, competent, and experienced individual who is a qualified member of the group that is authorized to engage in that activity (**Box 49–1 》》**). Should an individual fail to meet the standard of conduct for his or her profession, this failure may be considered an instance of *professional negligence*, also known as *malpractice*.

Malpractice includes acts and omissions committed by a professional in the course of performing his or her professional duties. Malpractice is one of the most important areas of the law for nurses, because any negligent act or omission, however unintentional, may rise to the standard of malpractice and may jeopardize the professional nurse's license and, more importantly, patient safety. It is also important to remember that anyone who performs the special skills associated with a particular profession, whether qualified or not, is held to the standards of conduct of those who are properly qualified to do so, because the public relies on the special expertise of those who engage in such activities. Thus, a nursing student is held to the same standard of conduct as an experienced, licensed professional nurse.

Elements of Professional Negligence or Malpractice

Five elements of professional negligence or malpractice are required to establish **liability**, which is defined as the state of being legally obliged and responsible:

- The patient must be owed a **duty**, a legally enforceable obligation to adhere to a particular standard of care (Guido, 2014). The formation of a provider–patient relationship is the basis for finding that the healthcare provider owes a duty to the patient. A nurse–patient relationship begins when the nurse accepts responsibility for providing nursing care to a patient (North Carolina Board of Nursing, 2012).

- A deviation from the standard of care owed to the patient, called a **breach of duty**, must occur by either commission or omission. For example, the nurse has a duty to correctly administer medication to a patient. Giving the patient the wrong dose of medication would be a breach of duty.

- The element of **foreseeability** (certain events may reasonably be expected to cause specific results) must be present. The nurse should know in advance, or reasonably anticipate, that damage or injury will probably ensue from acts or omissions.

- The injury must have resulted as a direct result of the professional's breach of duty, called **causation**. Typically, a patient cannot successfully make a claim for malpractice on acquiring a healthcare-associated infection. Only if the patient could show that a specific nurse did not follow the standard of aseptic technique would the standard of causation be met.

Box 49–1
Categories and Examples of Negligence That Result in Malpractice

Failure to Follow Standards of Care

Failure to:

- Perform a complete admission assessment or design a plan of care.
- Adhere to standardized protocols or institutional policies and procedures (e.g., using an improper injection site).
- Follow a physician's verbal or written orders, if appropriate.

Failure to Use Equipment in a Responsible Manner

Failure to:

- Follow the manufacturer's recommendations for operating the equipment.
- Check the equipment for safety prior to use.
- Place the equipment properly during treatment.

Failure to Communicate

Failure to:

- Notify a physician in a timely manner when conditions warrant it.
- Listen to a patient's complaints and act on them.
- Communicate effectively with a patient (e.g., providing inadequate or ineffective communication of discharge instructions).
- Seek clarification of orders for treatment when necessary.
- Discuss medication errors with team and patient.

Failure to Document

Failure to note in the patient's medical record:

- A patient's progress and response to treatment.
- A patient's injuries.
- Pertinent nursing assessment information (e.g., drug allergies).
- A physician's medical orders.
- Information about telephone conversations with physicians, including time, content of communication between nurse and physician, and actions taken.

Failure to Assess and Monitor

Failure to:

- Complete a shift assessment.
- Implement a plan of care.
- Observe a patient's ongoing progress.
- Interpret a patient's signs and symptoms.

Failure to Act as a Patient Advocate

Failure to:

- Question discharge orders when a patient's condition warrants it.
- Question incomplete or illegible medical orders.
- Provide a safe environment.

Sources: From Anselmi, K. K. (2012). Nurses' personal liability vs. employer's vicarious liability. *MEDSURG Nursing, 21*(1), 45–48; Reising, D. (2012). Make your nursing care malpractice-proof. *American Nurse Today, 7*(1), 24–28; Tzeng, H.-M., Yin, C. Y., & Schneider, T. E. (2013). Medication error–related issues in nursing practice. *MEDSURG Nursing, 22*(1), 13–16, 50.

- The plaintiff must demonstrate that some type of physical, financial, or emotional injury or harm resulted from the breach of owed duty. If the nurse gave the wrong medication but no harm occurred, the elements are not present for malpractice.

SAFETY ALERT Nurses administering medications must know why the patient is receiving the medication, the acceptable dosage range, possible adverse effects, toxicity levels, and contraindications.

The basic purpose of a malpractice lawsuit is to award damages sufficient to restore the plaintiff to his or her original position, as far as is financially possible. The amount of the **damages**, or compensation, for the plaintiff's loss or injury may include enough money to pay for the plaintiff's medical fees associated with the injury. If the plaintiff lost the ability to work as a result of the injury, damages could include compensation for lost wages as well as for medical fees. Punitive damages may be awarded if the nurse's misconduct is deemed malicious, willful, or wanton (Guido, 2014). Punitive damages are considered punishment for misconduct (Sleasman, 2013).

Related Doctrines

Several legal doctrines, or principles, are related to negligence and malpractice. One such doctrine is *respondeat superior* ("let the master answer"). A lawsuit for a negligent act or omission performed by a nurse generally will also name the nurse's employer. Employers may also be held liable for negligence if they fail to provide adequate human and material resources for nursing care, fail to properly educate nurses on the use of new equipment or procedures, or fail to orient nurses to the facility. Another doctrine is *res ipsa loquitur* ("the thing speaks for itself"). In some cases, the harm cannot be traced to a specific healthcare provider or standard but does not normally occur unless there has been some type of negligence. An example is harm that results when a surgical instrument is inadvertently left in a patient during surgery.

Statute of Limitations

There is a limit to the amount of time that can pass between recognition of harm and bringing a suit. This is referred to as the **statute of limitations**. The exact time limitation varies by type of suit and state, but plaintiffs typically have 1 to 2 years from the time that they knew of the injury or had reason to believe that an injury was sustained to file a malpractice lawsuit. Statutes of limitations applying to minors vary from state to state; some states identify specific variances such as extended time limits for specific types of injuries.

Intentional Torts

A number of intentional torts—actions taken by an individual with the intent to perform the action—have a bearing on nursing practice. The willful nature of these actions and the intent behind them separate intentional torts from negligence and malpractice.

Assault, Battery, and False Imprisonment

Assault is the action of creating an apprehension of offensive, insulting, or physically injurious touching. Assault can occur without an individual's actually being touched. Threatening a patient who refuses to agree with starting an intravenous line is assault. **Battery**, on the other hand, is defined as willful touching of another individual (or the individual's clothes or even something the individual is carrying) that is unwanted, embarrassing, or unwarranted, such as touching done without permission or giving an injection without a patient's consent. Even the simple act of ambulation requires the patient's consent. Forcing a patient to ambulate against his or her will may be considered battery (Guido, 2014).

Guido (2014) defines **false imprisonment** as the "unjustifiable detention of a person without legal warrant to confine the person." False imprisonment includes confining the patient to his or her room or restraining the patient to the bed with the intent to restrict or prevent the patient's freedom. Detaining a patient who wishes to leave against medical advice is generally considered false imprisonment.

Because **standards of care** (the skills and learning common to their profession, including the nursing process) prohibit nurses from forcing patients to participate in treatment or to engage in any action against the patient's will, assault, battery, and false imprisonment are actions that violate standards of care and may rise to the level of civil or criminal action against the nurse.

Invasion of Privacy

According to the Fourth Amendment to the U.S. Constitution, individuals have the right to privacy. Information concerning patients is confidential and may not be disclosed without authorization. The patient's right to privacy extends to use of the patient's name as well as photographic or videographic representations of the patient (e.g., the patient's picture may not be used without proper authorization). This right extends to control of the patient's personal belongings, personal space, and immediate territory. The nurse–patient relationship is based on trust. Searching a patient's room, touching personal belongings without first requesting permission, and entering a patient's room without knocking are behaviors that potentially violate this trust. Most healthcare agencies have policies and procedures that specify to whom and under what circumstances patient information can be released, and they have appropriate procedures for managing patient environments and personal property within the agency. Failure to follow these policies could lead to a claim of invasion of privacy.

Nurses are bound by the Privacy Rule of the Health Insurance Portability and Accountability Act (HIPAA) to protect the privacy of the patient's protected health information. This includes information related to mental and physical conditions, healthcare services provided, and payment for services rendered. It also includes name, address, birth date, and Social Security number (McGowan, 2012). HIPAA protections represent the minimum requirements for privacy. State law and professional codes may afford additional protections, in which case the more strict law is enforced. HIPAA and the Privacy Rule are discussed in more detail in Exemplar 49.C.

Concepts Related to Legal Issues

Safety and legal issues are closely connected. Ensuring patient safety and preventing care errors have important legal implications for nurses, as well as implications for the health of their patients. As many as 1 in 10 patients experience adverse events, such as falls and infections, during hospital stays; approximately 15% of these events involved medication errors (Tzeng, Yin, & Schneider, 2013). Prevention measures are essential for reducing these events; equally important is properly reporting any errors that do occur. Proper reporting can minimize the impact errors have on patients and help organizations and individuals gain valuable insight into the causes of errors. Unfortunately, nurses sometimes do not report errors. If uncovered later on, these errors and the subsequent failure to report could have professional and legal ramifications.

Issues of consent are important for all nurses but present special considerations in managing care. Nurse managers must adhere to legal requirements related to safety, communication, and many other areas; they must also ensure that other members of the care team follow these requirements. When requirements are not followed by team members, the nurse manager must identify and correct the situation. In addition, managers must ensure that patient care tasks are delegated appropriately to licensed and unlicensed staff and that these tasks are carried out correctly and completely according to state nurse practice acts and facility policy.

The Concepts Related to Legal Issues feature outlines some of the many ways in which legal issues intersect with other concepts. The concepts are presented in alphabetical order.

Strategies to Prevent Incidents of Professional Negligence

Situations may arise in nursing practice that can lead to reported negligence or malpractice cases. A continuing issue in nursing is medication errors, which must be clearly documented and discussed with the patient (Tzeng et al., 2013). Other situations in which problems may arise include communicating care concerns and key information about the patient's condition; ensuring that physicians' orders are clear; understanding how to use equipment in practice; and providing appropriate mentoring, assessment, and care plans for patients (Anselmi, 2012; Lipley, 2012).

Maintaining Patient Safety

Patients often fall accidentally, which sometimes results in injury. Some falls can be prevented through appropriate use of bed alarms, side rails, and other safety measures. If a nurse fails to take appropriate measures to prevent patient injury, that nurse may be held liable for malpractice if the patient falls and is injured as a direct result. Most hospitals and nursing homes have policies regarding the use of safety devices. The nurse needs to be familiar with these policies and needs to take the indicated precautions to prevent injuries (see the modules on Mobility and Safety).

SAFETY ALERT Assess every patient for fall potential. Document all nursing measures taken to protect the patient (e.g., "Instructed patient how to use the call light").

Concepts Related to
Legal Issues

CONCEPT	RELATIONSHIP TO LEGAL ISSUES	NURSING IMPLICATIONS
Cognition	Patients demonstrate the capacity to understand the benefits, risks, and alternatives for care. If this capacity exists, consent must be given voluntarily.	■ Provide information about procedures and conditions appropriate to the patient's cognitive level. ■ Work with the care team to assess the patient's capacity to give consent. ■ Assist the patient with consent forms and answer any questions the patient may have. ■ Work with the surrogate decision maker if the patient lacks the capacity to provide consent.
Comfort	Patients have the legal right to receive appropriate end-of-life (EOL) care. All hospitals receiving Medicare and Medicaid funds are legally responsible to provide advance directive information and support patients' advance directive needs.	■ Assess own assumptions or biases surrounding EOL care. ■ Assess self-understanding of appropriate EOL care options in your practice area. ■ Ask for support from supervisor or peers to assist in advocating for appropriate EOL care. ■ Anticipate further assessment of information patients and family members may need. ■ Be aware that advance directives (ADs) improve the EOL planning process by giving patients peace of mind and easing family conflict during health crises.
Communication	Nurses must ensure the privacy of all patient information during all care and in all care areas and must follow HIPAA regulations.	■ Ensure that patient information, such as online charting, is accessible only for appropriate use by appropriate staff members. ■ Discuss with your patients how you ensure privacy. ■ Ensure that patient care is discussed only with appropriate individuals and not outside the care unit.

In some instances, ignoring a patient's complaints can result in malpractice. This type of malpractice is termed *failure to observe and take appropriate action*. For example, the nurse who does not report a patient's complaint of acute abdominal pain is negligent and may be found liable for malpractice if the patient's appendix ruptures and the patient dies. If a nurse fails to take the blood pressure and pulse and to check the dressing of a patient who has just had cardiac surgery, the nurse is omitting important assessments. If the patient hemorrhages and resulting brain hypoxia renders the patient unable to return to his or her former occupation, the nurse may be held liable for injury and loss of wages.

Incorrect identification of patients is a problem, particularly in busy hospital units. Unfortunate occurrences, such as removal of a healthy gallbladder from the wrong patient, have resulted from nurses preparing the wrong patient for surgery. Cases of mistaken identity are costly and possibly very painful for the patient and render the nurse liable for malpractice.

Using Effective Communication

Nurses interact with patients and families during the provision of care. Poor communication skills may create a perception in the patient that the nurse is less than competent. Poor communication coupled with a negative outcome can increase the chance of a malpractice claim. Clear communication of directions and explanations and provision of effective patient education regarding the patient's healthcare requirements can help decrease the risk of bad outcomes (see the module on Teaching and Learning). Attentive listening

skills demonstrate the element of caring. Accurate documentation and reporting (see the module on Communication) provide a source of information that will either support or refute allegations of malpractice. Nursing documentation should be completed according to policy and should clearly depict the timeline of care, including assessments, interventions, the patient's response to interventions, and notification of information outside treatment protocol (e.g., abnormal lab values, changes in patient assessment). Remember that this document serves as the legal record of what occurred, so the nurse should document defensively, be inclusive, and not rely on their own or the patient's memories of the details of care.

Minimizing the Risk of Medication Errors

Administration of medications has been identified as a high-risk activity for error. Prevention of medication errors requires a systems approach involving all interprofessional healthcare personnel. Nurses need to strictly apply the **Seven Rights** of medication administration:

1. **Right assessment**
2. **Right drug**
3. **Right dose**
4. **Right patient**
5. **Right route**
6. **Right time**
7. **Right documentation.**

Strategies that integrate new technology, such as barcoding and electronic records, need to be evaluated for effectiveness in reducing errors.

Nothing can replace nursing judgment in preventing errors in administering medications. Unclear orders need to be clarified. Questions need to be answered. The nurse needs to have knowledge of each medication prior to administration. A culture of safety instead of blame will facilitate identification of errors and evaluation of causes and strategies to reduce errors.

Obtaining Professional Liability Insurance

Nurses, like physicians, should carry professional liability insurance to manage their personal financial risk. Occurrence-based coverage covers incidents that occurred during the time period the policy was in effect, regardless of whether the policy was still in effect when the claim was made. Claims-made policies provide coverage only if the incident occurred and the claim was reported during the active policy period. Policies should identify limits of liability, declarations, deductibles, exclusions, reservation of rights, covered injuries, defense costs, coverage conditions, and supplementary payments.

Policies may be individual, group, or employer sponsored. Individual coverage provides the broadest coverage to the policyholder. This type of policy covers the named policyholder on a 24-hour basis as long as his or her actions fall within the scope of practice. Employer-sponsored coverage provides the narrowest coverage for the individual nurse; the policy covers only actions performed during work as an employee of the institution. Nursing students are generally required to carry liability insurance for the duration of the education program, although some programs insure students under a broad institutional policy.

The Standard of Care

The applicable state nurse practice act and administrative rules form the basis of the standard of care to which each nurse is held. They define professional conduct and the scope of practice for the licensed nurse and identify activities for all levels of personnel providing nursing care. These laws are not static, and every nurse needs to be aware of any changes. The nurse's specific job description will contribute to defining the standard of care. Employers can limit but not expand the scope of practice, and the nurse is held to functioning within the scope of employment.

Although agency policies and procedures may seem to contain overwhelming amounts of information, they serve to define the standard of care. The prudent nurse reviews and implements the policies and procedures relevant to her or his practice. If there is a conflict between current practice and policy, the nurse should be proactive in resolving the conflict through quality improvement processes (see the module on Quality Improvement).

A primary source for defining the standard of care is the prevailing national nursing standards. These include the American Nurses Association (ANA) Standards of Practice as well as specialty practice standards appropriate to a nurse's practice (e.g., standards for critical care nurses).

Nurses who follow these standards will provide their patients with the best care possible and minimize the likelihood of committing any unintentional act that may rise to the level of malpractice.

Selected Laws That Affect Nursing Practice

In addition to tort laws, a number of other laws affect nursing practice. These include laws related to informed consent and competency, as well as laws regarding the Controlled Substance Act and the Good Samaritan Act. Because states have the freedom to enact additional legislation that may further define or restrict aspects addressed by federal law, all nurses should be aware of the laws that govern or affect nursing practice in their own states.

Informed Consent

Informed consent refers to the patient's legal and ethical rights to be informed of, and give or refuse permission for, any healthcare procedure or treatment. The healthcare provider has the duty to disclose information about proposed treatment in terms the patient can reasonably understand. The healthcare provider must also disclose information about available alternatives, the risks and benefits of each treatment option, and the patient's right to refuse treatment.

General guidelines regarding the information that should be provided to the patient include the following:

- The diagnosis or condition that requires treatment
- The purposes of the treatment
- What the patient can expect to feel or experience
- The intended benefits of the treatment
- Possible risks or negative outcomes of the treatment
- Advantages and disadvantages of possible alternatives to treatment (including no treatment).

To give informed consent voluntarily, the patient must not be coerced or pressured in any manner. For example, if the patient is motivated to consent by fear of disapproval on the part of a healthcare provider, such consent is not considered to be voluntary.

Patient understanding is an essential element of informed consent. Technical words and language barriers can inhibit understanding and, when a patient has a lower literacy level, may encourage a signature without discussion of its actual meaning. Therefore, cultural competence in managing patient care is critical (Agency for Healthcare Research & Quality [AHRQ], 2012). If a patient cannot read, the healthcare provider must read the consent form to the patient, and the patient must state an understanding before signing the form. If the patient and the healthcare provider do not speak the same language, a medical interpreter must be present. However, even with an interpreter, it is important to remember that errors in translation may occur. The nurse should also consider the patient's cultural and spiritual preferences when asking a patient to make decisions about a procedure or treatment. Some religions and some cultures have specific mores that affect healthcare, although patients may or may not follow those mores (Arritt, 2014).

The nurse should follow the employing agency's specific protocols regarding informed consent. Obtaining informed consent for specific medical and surgical treatments is the responsibility of the individual who will perform the procedure. Consent must be obtained for all procedures and treatments, including nursing care. However, this does not require written consent before each occurrence. Most nurses rely on **expressed consent** (an oral or written agreement) or **implied consent** based on a patient's action. The patient either verbally indicates participation in the care or nonverbally takes actions that are consistent with the care. For example, patients who position their bodies for an injection or cooperate with the taking of vital signs are expressing implied consent. While state laws provide for protection from liability for failure to obtain informed consent, nurses need to understand implied versus obtained consent (Cole, 2012).

Competency for Consent

Competency is a legal presumption applied to individuals when they become adults. Competency gives adults the right to negotiate certain legal activities, such as making a will or entering into a contract. In most states, an individual is considered to be competent at 18 years of age unless some evidence to the contrary persuades a court to declare that individual incompetent.

Adults who have been declared legally incompetent through a court order are provided a legal guardian. The legal guardian should give healthcare providers a copy of the court order giving him or her the authority to make healthcare decisions on the other adult's behalf. Examples of adults who may be legally incompetent include those who have sustained a debilitating brain injury as a result of a motor vehicle crash and those who have profound intellectual disability.

An adult may be rendered temporarily incompetent by narcotic medication or a serious fall or may gradually be rendered incompetent as a result of dementia. The nurse who has concerns about a patient's level of competency should alert the primary care provider. If the primary care provider determines that the patient is not competent for the purposes of informed consent, the provider will determine whether the emergency doctrine applies (see the Consent in an Emergency section below) or whether someone else can validly make healthcare decisions on the patient's behalf. State laws regarding consent for adults who are rendered temporarily incompetent vary. Courts generally presume continuing competency of adults unless the healthcare facility can show that the patient is unable to understand the consequences of his or her actions (Guido, 2014). All healthcare staff, including nurses, should be familiar with their state's laws and with the policies and procedures of their employing agency. Nurses should recognize the effect of issues related to competency on providing nursing care, because patients have the right to decline nursing care as well as medical procedures. The Focus on Diversity and Culture feature discusses how a patient's cognitive impairment may affect the process of obtaining informed consent.

Consent in an Emergency

In most states, the law assumes an individual's consent to medical treatment when the individual is in imminent danger of loss of life or limb and unable to give informed consent. In other words, the emergency doctrine assumes that the individual would reasonably consent to treatment if able to do so. This doctrine serves as a guiding principle that permits healthcare providers to perform potentially lifesaving procedures under circumstances that make it impossible or impractical to obtain consent. The emergency doctrine may not always apply. For example, it does not extend to allowing healthcare providers to implement a treatment or procedure to which the patient would not reasonably consent if the patient were able to do so. It also does not permit healthcare providers to provide a treatment or procedure that the patient previously refused. For example, if a patient has previously refused a procedure on religious grounds, healthcare providers may not implement the procedure if the patient becomes unconscious.

Child Participation in Healthcare Decisions

For a minor child (under age 18), a parent or guardian must give informed consent for medical treatment. Specific legal exceptions do exist, however, including situations in which the emergency doctrine applies, when the child is an *emancipated minor* (one who is no longer under parental control and manages his or her own financial affairs), when the child is a resident of a state that allows a *mature minor* to give valid consent (for example, 14- and 15-year-old adolescents who are able to understand treatment risks), when a court order to proceed with treatment exists, or when the law recognizes the minor as having the ability to consent to a specific treatment. In the majority of states, a minor who is the parent of a child may give informed consent for healthcare treatment of the child. Some states also permit teenagers of a certain age who are seeking certain types of care to do so without parental consent. Types of care that may not require

---

Focus on Diversity and Culture
Cognitive Impairment and Informed Consent

Cognitively impaired adult patients present special particular concerns when it comes to informed consent. The presence of cognitive impairment does not automatically preclude a patient from giving consent, although some patients who have been declared legally incompetent by a court will have a legal guardian who must give consent. In determining whether a patient without a legal guardian is able to give informed consent, the patient's capacity to understand the benefits, risks, and alternatives for care and to make and communicate a decision must be considered (Vanderbilt Kennedy Center, 2016). This capacity can change over time and may be affected by the nature and complexity of the decision involved; therefore, the patient's capacity should be assessed and documented for each treatment. If a patient does not have the capacity to consent or it is unclear whether the patient has the capacity, decision making should be delegated to a surrogate, following agency procedure. Consent is required for elective and therapeutic surgeries, diagnostic procedures, and procedures that involve sedation or anesthesia. Consent is not required for time-sensitive, lifesaving emergency procedures (Vanderbilt Kennedy Center, 2016).

Box 49–2
Overview of Minor Consent Laws

Contraceptive Services

Twenty-one states and the District of Columbia allow all minors (age 12 years and older) to consent to contraceptive services. Twenty-five states allow only certain categories of minors to consent to contraceptive services.

Sexually Transmitted Infections Services

All states and the District of Columbia allow all minors to consent to services for sexually transmitted infections.

Prenatal Care

Thirty-two states and the District of Columbia explicitly allow all minors to consent to prenatal care.

Adoption

Twenty-eight states and the District of Columbia allow all minor parents to choose to place their child for adoption.

Medical Care for a Child

Thirty states and the District of Columbia allow all minor parents to consent to medical care for their child. The remaining 20 states have no relevant explicit policy or case law.

Abortion

Two states and the District of Columbia explicitly allow all minors to consent to abortion services. Twenty-one states require that at least one parent consent to a minor's abortion, while 13 states require prior notification of at least one parent. State laws regarding abortion may change; be sure to know the laws in your state.

Sources: Data from Guttmacher Institute. (2016b). *An overview of minors' consent law.* Retrieved from http://www.guttmacher.org/statecenter/spibs/spib_OMCL.pdf; Guttmacher Institute. (2016c). *Minors' access to contraceptive services.* Retrieved from https://www.guttmacher.org/sites/default/files/state_policy_overview_files/spib_macs.pdf; National District Attorneys Association. (2013, January). *Minor consent to medical treatment laws.* Retrieved from http://www.ndaa.org/pdf/Minor%20Consent%20to%20Medical%20Treatment%20(2).pdf.

parental permission, depending on state law, include contraceptive services, prenatal care, mental health counseling, diagnosis and treatment of sexually transmitted infections, and treatment of substance abuse (American Civil Liberties Union [ACLU] of Ohio, 2014; Goodwin et al., 2012).

In some states, mature minors are permitted to give consent for treatment or to refuse treatment. In some cases, the minor must convince a judge that he or she is mature enough to make an independent judgment about consent for treatment. Nurses need to know the state and federal laws regarding consent as well as the agency's policies and procedures regarding informed consent (Brent, 2013). North Carolina law, for example, provides for all minors over the age of 12 to consent for contraceptive services, treatment of sexually transmitted infections, and prenatal care (Moore, 2015). For an overview of minor consent laws in the United States, see **Box 49–2** ⟫.

Clinical Example A

Marvin Martinice, a 15-year-old boy with acute myelocytic leukemia, has come out of his second remission with an acute onset of fever, joint pain, and petechiae. A bone marrow transplant is one of the few remaining therapeutic options. Although Marvin has agreed to

a transplantation if a suitable donor is found, he does not want to be resuscitated and placed on life-support equipment should he go into a cardiac arrest. Marvin has talked extensively with the hospital chaplain and social worker and feels comfortable with his decision. His parents want an all-out effort to sustain his life until a donor is located.

Critical Thinking Questions

1. In general, what happens when parents and children have conflicting opinions about treatment?
2. Assume you are a nurse involved in Marvin's care. What is your role, if any, in addressing the difference of opinion between Marvin and his parents regarding available treatment options?

Controlled Substances Act

The **Controlled Substances Act (CSA)** is a federal law that requires drugs to be classified on the basis of the substance's medical use, potential for abuse, and safety risks. The classifications are referred to as schedules and are numbered from I to V; Schedules I and II have the highest potential for abuse (**Table 49–2** ⟫). The CSA is enforced by the U.S. Drug Enforcement Agency, which regulates a closed system of distribution. This system provides for registration with unique identifiers for legitimate handlers of controlled substances and required record keeping that traces the flow of any drug from the time it is first imported or manufactured, through the distribution level, to the pharmacy or hospital that dispenses it, and then to the patient who receives it. Each state has its own requirements for prescribers. Nurses must abide by the rules and regulations of their state.

⟫ **Stay Current:** For more information about the Controlled Substance Act, visit the Office of Diversion Control's website at www.deadiversion.usdoj.gov/21cfr/21usc.

Good Samaritan Laws

Most states have **Good Samaritan laws** that encourage healthcare providers to help victims in an emergency. These laws are designed to protect the healthcare worker from potential liability when volunteering his or her skills outside of an employment contract (**Figure 49–2** ⟫). To be protected by Good Samaritan laws, a nurse must adhere to the standard of nurs-

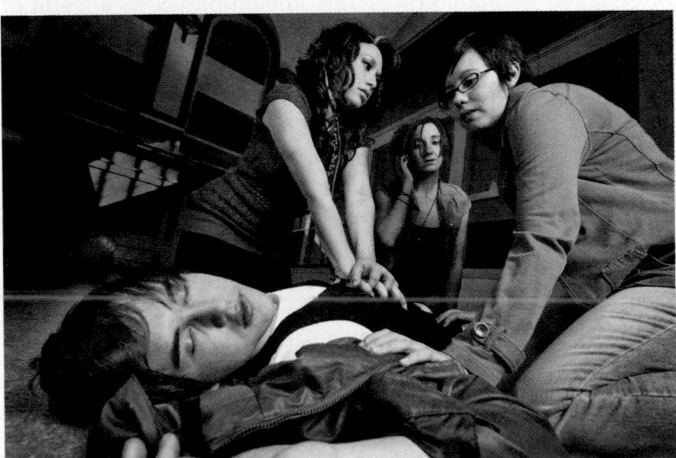

Source: Jsteck/E+/Getty Images.

Figure 49–2 ⟫ Good Samaritan laws protect healthcare workers from liability when they volunteer their services in an emergency.

TABLE 49–2 U.S. Drug Schedules and Examples

Drug Schedule	Dependency Potential			Examples	Therapeutic Use
	Abuse Potential	Physical Dependence	Psychologic Dependence		
I	Highest	High	High	Heroin, peyote, marijuana, MDMA ("ecstasy")	Medical use of marijuana/cannabis limited to specific states
II	High	High	High	Morphine, opium, cocaine, oxycodone, fentanyl, methadone, amphetamine, pentobarbital	Current accepted medical use in the United States with severe restrictions; prescription required
III	Moderate	Moderate	High	Tylenol with codeine, anabolic steroids, buprenorphine, ketamine	Current accepted medical use in the United States; prescription required
IV	Lower	Lower	Lower	Alprazolam, clonazepam, lorazepam, midazolam, diazepam	Current accepted medical use in the United State; prescription required
V	Lowest	Lowest	Lowest	Cough medicine containing codeine, ezogabine	Current accepted medical use in the United States; no prescription required

ing care during all volunteer activities. The nurse should provide only care that is consistent with his or her level of training and licensure. Once having made the decision to render emergency care, the nurse is responsible for following through by providing the necessary care or safely placing the victim in the care of someone who can provide the appropriate care (Howie, Howie, & McMullen, 2012). Before volunteering their skills, nurses should review the nurse practice act and the Good Samaritan law in the state in which they work.

Whistleblowing Laws

Whistleblowing is the disclosure of an employer's unsafe or illegal practices and/or polices by an employee (Guido, 2014). The employee who reports such practices or policies is called a **whistleblower**. The Whistleblower Protection Act of 1989 establishes certain protections for individuals who report gross misconduct on the part of their employers to federal authorities; additional protections may vary by state. To qualify for protection under the federal act, the employee must make every effort to resolve the issue via the employer's internal reporting procedures before going outside of the organization. In addition, an employee does not qualify for protection under the act unless the employer has threatened or engaged in retaliation against the employee as a result of the employee's complaint.

Simple error or misconduct on the part of the employer does not qualify under the Whistleblower Protection Act. Typically, the activity or policy in question must violate a state or federal law or rule, and the employer must be aware that the activity or policy is a violation. Examples include billing fraud, failure to maintain safety equipment, and chronic insufficient staffing. The employee making the complaint must give the employer written notice and an appropriate amount of time to correct the issue. To be considered a whistleblower, the employee must also make or threaten to make a report to the appropriate state or federal agency.

Whistleblower laws exist to prevent retaliation by the employer against reasonable, good-faith reporting of illegal, unethical, or unsafe conduct in order to provide a safe environment for patients. However, the nurse who makes a report outside of the employing agency should be prepared for the possibility of negative consequences. These may include personal consequences such as losing the support or friendship of coworkers. They may also include retaliatory or discriminatory actions, including dismissal, demotion, discipline, or intimidation. These actions are prohibited by the Occupational Safety and Health Act. To prevail in a discrimination claim, an employee must report discriminatory actions to the Occupational Safety and Health Administration (OSHA) before resigning from the place of employment.

Lifespan Considerations

Nurses should be aware of how legal issues may affect patients of different age groups and must understand their responsibilities for protecting their patients and themselves when these issues arise. No matter the age or condition of the patients with whom the nurse works, failure to keep up with changes in laws or regulations can endanger patients and place the nurse at risk for liability.

Legal Issues Pertaining to Infants and Children

Nurses are mandated reporters of child abuse or suspected child abuse, including physical, emotional, and sexual maltreatment. Although statutes related to reporting vary from state to state, nurses who fail to report abuse may face civil charges. Reports should be complete and accurate and should be made according to the policy of the organization for which the nurse works. In addition to reporting the abuse within the organizational framework, the nurse should personally report the abuse to the proper authorities. When abuse is reported, all pertinent information in the patient's medical record is required by law to be disclosed to the reporting agency. As such, reporting abuse or suspected abuse represents an exception to patient confidentiality rules (Merrick & Latzman, 2014).

Nurses should be aware of common signs of abuse in both infants and children. For example, bruising in infants can indicate physical abuse; vomiting, irritability, and lethargy may indicate head injury. Older children may exhibit unexplained injuries or bruises, injuries that do not match the explanations given, and untreated medical problems. Children and adolescents who report sexual abuse may exhibit no abnormal physical findings in an exam, though cultures may indicate the presence of sexually transmitted diseases (STDs). If the parent or guardian of a child is responsible for the abuse, health history and interview information provided by that individual may be vague or intentionally misleading (Herendeen et al., 2014).

Accurate reporting of abuse and suspected abuse is essential for protecting the child and safeguarding the nurse both professionally and personally. The nurse is required to report the facts or circumstances that led to the belief that abuse occurred but does not have the burden of proof. Reports must be made in good faith and without malicious intent. Most states allow reports to be made anonymously but may encourage the reporter to provide identifying and contact information to aid in the investigation. In most states, if the reporter's identity is known, it is not disclosed to the individual suspected of committing the abuse (Child Welfare Information Gateway, 2016). Mandatory reporting is discussed further in Exemplar 49.D.

>> **Stay Current:** Nurses should be familiar with the child abuse reporting statutes in their state. Search by state and topic at the U.S. Department of Health and Human Services' Child Welfare Information Gateway at https://www.childwelfare.gov/topics/systemwide/laws-policies/state/.

Legal Issues Pertaining to Adolescents

Confidentiality is a concern for some adolescents seeking care, particularly care related to contraception, sexual health, substance abuse, or mental health. Nurses should be familiar with federal and state laws related to adolescent confidentiality. Trust and honesty are essential. Nurses should ensure that patients understand that confidentiality will be maintained when possible but that confidentiality cannot be guaranteed in some circumstances. For example, if the patient is covered under a parent's or guardian's insurance, billing and benefits statements provided to the parent or guardian may include information about care. It is also important that patients understand that the authorities must be contacted if a patient is in imminent danger, if there is evidence of abuse, or if the patient has certain communicable diseases (American Academy of Family Physicians [AAFP], 2013).

Adolescent patients may wish to be examined or receive counseling separately from their parents. The nurse should make every effort to honor this request, though doing so may lead to confrontation with the parents. Understanding state statutes and organizational policy related to adolescent confidentially is essential when situations such as this arise.

The use of electronic health records (EHRs) presents additional concerns about confidentiality for adolescents. In general, child and adolescent EHRs are set up with parents or guardians as proxy. As a result, these individuals are able to view information contained in the EHR. Some EHR systems offer customizable modules that can be configured to restrict the proxy's access to confidential or sensitive information; some systems do not. Certain information gathered during general exams—such as social or sexual history—may be accessible to parents or guardians via the EHR unless it is included with the restricted information. If the system does not allow for customization to restrict information, patients should be informed that parents or guardians can access these records (American College of Obstetricians and Gynecologists [ACOG], 2014).

When providing confidential care to adolescents, the nurse should encourage adolescents to consider involving parents or guardians in their decision making. The nurse should make it clear that this is a suggestion and not a requirement for receiving care. Patients who feel pressured to involve parents or who fear that their confidentiality may be breached may refuse treatment and may not receive the care they need.

Legal Issues Pertaining to Pregnant Women

Legal rights of pregnant women in the United States have been a subject of debate for many years. Perhaps the most famous example of this surrounds the Supreme Court's 1973 ruling in *Roe v. Wade*. In this ruling, the court deemed it unconstitutional for states to outlaw abortion during the first trimester of pregnancy and placed restrictions on states' ability to regulate abortion during the second and third trimesters. Since the ruling, abortion has remained a contentious issue in the United States. Statutes related to abortion vary from state to state and include regulations related to gestational limits, insurance coverage for procedures, and mandated counseling (Guttmacher Institute, 2016a).

In addition to statutes related directly to abortion, a number of states have passed fetal protection laws. The intent of these laws is to protect both mothers and fetuses and punish individuals who harm them. In some cases, however, these laws have raised questions about a woman's right to refuse certain tests or treatments during pregnancy (Graham, 2014).

Abortion and fetal protection laws may create ethical or moral dilemmas for nurses. It is of the utmost importance that nurses know their state's statutes and their organization's policies on these matters. In addition, nurses should understand their rights of conscientious objection and their responsibilities in the event that they choose to be a conscientious objector. Conscientious objection is the refusal by the nurse to engage in a procedure because doing so would violate his or her moral or ethical principles (Lachman, 2014). Abortion, sterilization, and contraception are reproduction-related procedures that may give rise to conscientious objection. Currently, 45 states allow individual healthcare providers to refuse to participate in abortions, and 42 states allow institutions to refuse to provide them (Guttmacher Institute, 2016). Nurses who choose to be conscientious objectors should make their refusal known in advance of the procedure to allow for necessary staffing adjustments. If advance notice is not possible, the nurse is duty bound to remain with the patient until another nurse can take over the patient's care. Failure to do so may be considered patient abandonment (Lachman, 2014).

Legal Issues Pertaining to Older Adults

In many states, nurses are mandatory reporters of elder mistreatment, which encompasses elder abuse, neglect, and exploitation; Medicare requires that nursing facilities monitor patients for signs of mistreatment. Specific types of elder mistreatment include physical, emotional, verbal, and sexual abuse. They also include neglect and financial abuse. Signs of possible elder abuse include bruises, lacerations, fractures, open wounds, and untreated injuries in various stages of healing. Dehydration, malnutrition, and poor personal hygiene may signal elder neglect. Agitation, withdrawal, and sudden changes in behavior or financial situation may be indicative of other types of mistreatment (National Center on Elder Abuse [NCEA], n.d.). It is the nurse's responsibility to understand the reporting laws in his or her state and to report mistreatment or suspected mistreatment to the appropriate authorities. Failure to do so may result in civil or criminal penalties (Falk, Baigis, & Kopac, 2012). Even if state law does not identify them as mandatory reporters, it is advisable for nurses to report mistreatment or suspected mistreatment.

Screening and assessment are essential for identifying elder mistreatment. Patient interviews are commonly included in the assessment process, but age-related cognitive impairments can limit their effectiveness. Patients may also be hesitant to disclose mistreatment in an interview for fear that the abuse will worsen if they do so (Falk et al., 2012). Elder mistreatment can be a difficult topic to broach with patients and family members or care providers who may be involved in the mistreatment. In addition, some signs of elder mistreatment are similar to signs associated with normal age-related changes and conditions. To help nurses better address and identify elder mistreatment, many state and national resources exist. State Boards of Nursing and the National Center on Elder Abuse offer useful information on this topic.

>> **Stay Current:** The website of the National Center on Elder Abuse can be found at https://ncea.acl.gov.

End-of-life (EOL) care is another important consideration for nurses working with older adults. EOL encompasses both planning and delivery of care. When an advance directive (AD) exists, the nurse is bound to provide care in accordance with the patient's wishes and organizational policy. When no AD exists, patients with capacity to make EOL decisions for themselves may work with the nurse to determine the type of care they prefer (American Cancer Society, 2015). Advance directives are discussed in more detail in Exemplar 49.B. For more on EOL care, see the exemplar on End-of-Life Care in the module on Comfort.

REVIEW The Concept of Legal Issues

RELATE Link the Concepts

Linking the concept of legal issues with the concept of clinical decision making:

1. How does the nursing process support nurses in maintaining appropriate standards of care?

2. What type of consent is necessary for the nurse to take a patient's temperature and vital signs? For the patient to undergo an x-ray if a broken leg is suspected?

Linking the concept of legal issues with the concept of communication:

3. How does a change-of-shift report minimize the nurse's risk for professional negligence or malpractice?

4. What types of communication result in the best quality of patient care and are therefore most likely to prevent the nurse from being accused of malpractice?

REFER Go to Pearson MyLab Nursing and eText

- Additional review materials

REFLECT Apply Your Knowledge

Joanne Otunde, an RN coworker on your surgical unit, returned to work about 6 weeks ago following back surgery. Since her return, you have noticed that she is frequently and uncharacteristically late for work and has called in sick six times. Twice you have witnessed her treating a nurse's aide harshly. Ms. Glancy, a patient who is 2 days postoperative, puts her light on and tells you that she is in severe pain and that the pain medication she received did not have any effect on the pain level. She states, "It's the strangest thing. The pill never seems to work in the evenings the way it does in the daytime and at night." You report Ms. Glancy's pain to Joanne, who is her primary nurse. At the end of the shift, you and an oncoming nurse are doing the narcotic count and notice that Joanne has given six doses of the same narcotic during the shift and one dose is documented as having been given at 8 p.m. to a patient who had been discharged at 5 p.m.

1. What are your responsibilities? Should you take any action? If so, why? If not, why not?

2. What laws do you need to review? What policies?

>> Exemplar 49.A
Nurse Practice Acts

Exemplar Learning Outcomes

49.A Analyze nurse practice acts as they relate to legal issues.

- Explain how Boards of Nursing oversee licensure.
- Describe the National Council of State Boards of Nursing.
- Outline the Nurse Licensure Compact.
- Differentiate credentialing and certification.
- Explain the duties and responsibilities of nursing students.

Exemplar Key Terms

Certification, 2841
Credentialing, 2841
Mutual recognition model, 2840
Nolo contendere, 2840
Nurse practice act (NPA), 2839
Responsibility, 2841

Box 49–3
Anatomy of a Nurse Practice Act

Typically, the following components are addressed in an NPA. Each nursing student and practicing nurse should understand the NPA for the state in which she or he is working and how each component of the NPA affects practice. Components of an NPA include the following:

- Definition of nursing
- Requirements for licensure
- Penalty for practicing without a license
- Exemptions from licensure
- Licensure across jurisdictions.

Overview

The practice of nursing is regulated at the state level through a **nurse practice act (NPA)**. An NPA is a series of state statutes that define the scope of practice, standards for education programs, licensure requirements, and grounds for disciplinary actions. The law provides a framework for establishing nursing actions in the care of patients (**Box 49–3 »**). Laws set the boundaries for and maintain a standard of nursing practice (**Figure 49–3 »**). The nurse is held accountable to the specific standards for licensure and grounds for revocation in the state of employment. For the registered nurse (RN), the provisions of NPAs are quite similar from state to state. Greater variation exists in the scope of practice for the licensed practical nurse (LPN) and licensed vocational nurse (LVN).

Each state's NPA is enforced and administered by a state board of nursing (BON), though some states use other titles for this regulatory board. BONs were established some 100 years ago to standardize the education of nurses, establish standards for safe nursing practice, and issue licenses to protect the public from unprepared, unsafe practitioners. Over the years, BONs have expanded their scope. Programs for impaired nurses, remediation of practice issues, and participation in multistate licensure compacts are all part of BONs today. BONs also act as a forum for citizens to report and discuss concerns regarding nursing services they have received. In this way, BONs continue to work toward their goal of protecting the public health.

The state's NPA dictates the membership of the state's BON, which usually includes a mix of RNs, LPNs/LVNs, advanced practice registered nurses (APRNs), and consumers. The members of the BON are appointed according to the regulations in each state, with the exception of North Carolina. North Carolina is the only state in which licensed nurses serving on the board are elected by other licensed nurses and members of the public who serve are appointed.

Licensure

Licensure allows a nurse the legal privilege to practice nursing as defined in the state's NPA. Through the process of licensure, the BON ensures the provision of safe nursing care to the public. Typically, BONs oversee licensure through the following activities:

- Establishing and monitoring educational standards for nursing education programs
- Defining professional standards
- Examining and renewing the licenses of duly qualified applicants
- Investigating violations of the NPA
- Sanctioning (to the point of initiating prosecution against) those who violate the NPA
- Holding disciplinary hearings for possible suspension or revocation of a license
- Establishing and overseeing diversity programs in some states. The Focus on Diversity and Culture feature looks at efforts to increase diversity in the nursing workforce.

Focus on Diversity and Culture
Diversity and the Nursing Workforce

Since 2004, the Institute of Medicine (IOM) has emphasized the connection between a diverse nursing workforce and culturally competent nursing care. In particular, the IOM posits that diversity among nurses will improve access to care for minority patients and will result in greater patient satisfaction (American Association of Colleges of Nursing [AACN], 2016).

A diverse workforce begins by increasing the number of minority students enrolled in nursing programs. The AACN reports that the number of minority students in nursing programs has steadily increased since 2011, with nearly 30% of students at all levels representing minority populations. The number of male students in nursing programs has also increased; as of 2015, roughly 12% of nursing students were male (AACN, 2016).

Federal government involvement has been an important factor in these increases. Through the Nursing Workforce Diversity (NWD) program, the Health Resources and Services Administration (HRSA) is striving to increase educational opportunities for groups that are underrepresented in the registered nurse population (HRSA, 2014b). The program provides grants to schools of nursing that are committed to increasing the number of minority graduates. Recipient organizations can use funds for scholarships, stipends, and advanced education preparation. Between $14 million and $16 million in grants have been awarded through this program each year since 2006 (AACN, 2016).

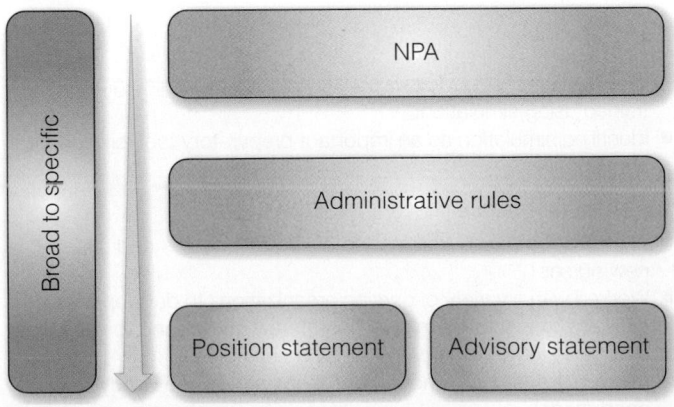

Figure 49–3 » Relationship among nurse practice acts, administrative rules, and position/advisory statements.

Each BON oversees the administration of a licensure examination that measures the competencies needed to perform safely and effectively as a newly licensed, entry-level nurse. The National Council of State Boards of Nursing (NCSBN) has developed two licensure examinations, the National Council Licensure Examination for Registered Nurses (NCLEX-RN®) and the National Council Licensure Examination for Practical Nurses (NCLEX-PN®), for state and territory BONs to implement as part of their requirements for licensure. The NCSBN also offers two additional examinations: the National Nurse Aide Assessment Program and the Medication Aide Certification Examination (NCSBN, 2016a).

Licenses are issued by the state or territory in which the applicant nurse wishes to practice. For licensed nurses at all levels of practice, the BON monitors compliance with state laws, including maintaining continued competency and annual renewal of licensure. To maintain the privilege to practice afforded by the license, the individual nurse is required to demonstrate awareness and application of standards of nursing care and meet his or her responsibilities to both patients and the healthcare system. The board is also responsible for taking action against nurses who have exhibited unsafe nursing practice or otherwise engaged in professional misconduct or who fail to meet requirements for licensure renewal.

Each BON details what charges of professional misconduct may result in the revocation or suspension of a nurse's license. Most BONs will take action against the nurse who is found guilty of charges that include the following:

- Giving false information or withholding material information from the board in procuring or attempting to procure a license to practice nursing.

- Being convicted of or pleading either guilty or *nolo contendere* to any crime that indicates the nurse is unfit or incompetent to practice or has deceived or defrauded the public. In pleading **nolo contendere**, the individual neither admits nor denies that he or she has committed the crime but agrees to a punishment (usually a fine or jail time) as if guilty. Usually, this type of plea is entered because it can-

not be used as an admission of guilt if a civil lawsuit is initiated following the conclusion of a criminal trial.

- Engaging in conduct that endangers the public health.

- Being unfit or incompetent to practice by reason of deliberate or negligent acts or omissions, regardless of whether actual injury to the patient is established.

- Engaging in conduct that deceives, defrauds, or harms the public in the course of professional activities or services.

National Council of State Boards of Nursing

The NCSBN provides leadership to advance regulatory excellence for public protection. The membership of the NCSBN includes BONs in the 50 states, the District of Columbia, and four U.S. territories (Guam, Virgin Islands, American Samoa, and the Northern Mariana Islands). Four states (California, Georgia, Louisiana, and West Virginia) have separate BONs for RNs and LPNs/LVNs.

The NCSBN offers a number of services that support member BONs. It is responsible for developing the licensure and assessment exams mentioned earlier. In addition, the NCSBN offers continuing education opportunities via its e-learning community.

The NCSBN also serves as an important source of data and research about nursing practice (**Box 49–4 》**). It maintains a central nursing database called Nursys that coordinates nurse licensure information for the United States. It also works with BONs to promote uniform regulation of nursing practice. The Nurse Licensure Compact is an important outcome of these activities.

》 Stay Current: Contact information for state Boards of Nursing and information about licensure and NCSBN research can be found at https://www.ncsbn.org/boards.htm.

Nurse Licensure Compact

The **mutual recognition model** of nurse licensure allows a nurse to have a single license that confers the privilege to practice in other states that are part of the Nurse Licensure

---

Box 49–4
NCSBN Research in 2015

National Nursing Workforce Survey

- Collected demographic and other information related to the supply of RNs and LPNs/VNs in the United States.
- Explored trends in the nursing workforce and compared them to trends in past years' surveys.
- Examined the impact that telehealth is having on nursing practice.

National Simulation Study

- Explored the role and outcomes of simulation training in nursing education.
- Used a three-phase approach to study the current use of simulation, to examine the impact of simulation in place of traditional

clinical hours, and to follow clinical practice of nursing graduates trained using simulation.
- Identified simulation as an important preparatory tool for student nurses.

Transition to Practice

- Explored the issues that lead to high attrition rates and stress in new nurses.
- Worked with a variety of nursing organizations to develop a standardized model to aid in retention of new nurses and to improve outcomes for patients cared for by these nurses.
- Designed e-learning modules to supplement the newly developed model.

Source: National Council of State Boards of Nursing (NCSBN). (2016c). *Recent Research.* Retrieved from https://www.ncsbn.org/recent-research.htm.

Box 49–5
Mutual Recognition Model

- Each state has to enter into an interstate compact, called the Nurse Licensure Compact (NLC), that allows nurses to practice in more than one state.
- Multistate licensure privilege means the nurse has the authority to practice nursing in another state that has signed an interstate compact. It is not an additional license.
- A nurse must have a license in his or her primary state of legal residency if that state is an NLC state.
- The states continue to have authority in determining licensure requirements and disciplinary actions.
- The nurse is held accountable for knowing and practicing the nursing practice laws and regulations in the state where the patient is located.
- Enactment does not change a state's nurse practice act.
- Complaints and/or violations are addressed by the home state (place of residence) and the remote state (place of practice).
- RNs and LPNs/LVNs are included in the interstate compact or NLC. Since 2002, there has been a separate APRN Compact. A state must be a member of the NLC for RNs and LPNs before entering into an APRN Compact. A state must adopt both compacts to cover LPNs/RNs and APRNs for mutual recognition.

Source: National Council of State Boards of Nursing (NCSBN). (2016b). *Nurse licensure compact: Information for new grads.* Retrieved from https://www.ncsbn.org/NLC_New_Grads.pdf.

Compact (**Box 49–5 》**). Monitoring the nurse's license and taking any needed disciplinary actions are the responsibilities of the state that issues the license. It is similar to the driver's license model: A single license to drive is issued in the individual's state of primary residency, but this license also gives the individual the privilege to drive in other Drivers' License Compact states.

SAFETY ALERT When practicing in a mutual recognition state, the nurse is held accountable for following the laws and rules of the state in which he or she is practicing or where the patient is located, not the state that issued the license.

To achieve mutual recognition, each state must enact legislation or regulations authorizing the Nurse Licensure Compact. States that enter the compact also adopt administrative rules and regulations for implementation of the compact. Twenty-five states are currently part of the compact.

》 Stay Current: For information on states participating in the compact, go to https://www.ncsbn.org/nurse-licensure-compact.htm.

Credentialing

Although a nursing license grants the legal privilege to practice, **credentialing** is the formal identification of professionals who meet predetermined standards of professional skill or competence. The federal government has used the term **certification** to define the credentialing process by which a nongovernmental agency or association recognizes the professional competence of an individual who has met certain predetermined qualifications specified by the agency or association. The American Nurses Credentialing Center (ANCC), a subsidiary of the ANA, provides credentialing programs to certify nurses in specialty practice areas, recognizes healthcare organizations for nursing excellence through the Magnet Recognition Program, and accredits providers of continuing nursing education and nursing specialty organizations.

Federal organizations, such as The Joint Commission and the Centers for Medicare and Medicaid Services, and federal guidelines affect the standards of care the nurse is held accountable for practicing. Individual healthcare agencies must implement policies, procedures, and job descriptions to ensure that the nurses they employ follow all applicable regulations and guidelines. The nurse needs to know the employing institution's policies and procedures and the specific job descriptions of the licensed and unlicensed nursing personnel. The purpose of knowing the standards of care is to protect both the patient and the nurse.

The impact of laws and standards on nurses is profound (**Figure 49–4 》**). The professional nurse is held accountable for many standards and statutes. Knowledge of the laws that regulate and affect nursing practice enables the nurse to practice within current legal principles and be aware of his or her legal obligations and responsibilities.

Nursing Students

Each NPA addresses the duties and responsibilities of nursing students in that state. Typically, this includes language that allows nursing students the privilege to practice nursing without a license while engaged in the clinical practicum of an approved nursing education program under the supervision of qualified faculty. Nursing students have the ultimate **responsibility** (accountability for their actions that includes the obligation to answer for an act done and to repair any injury one may have caused) for their own actions. Guidelines for clinical performance for nursing students include the following (Virginia Board of Nursing, 2012):

1. Provide safe nursing care.
2. Understand program and facility policies and procedures before undertaking any clinical assignment.
3. Demonstrate knowledge about the patient's condition, interventions, medications, and treatments.

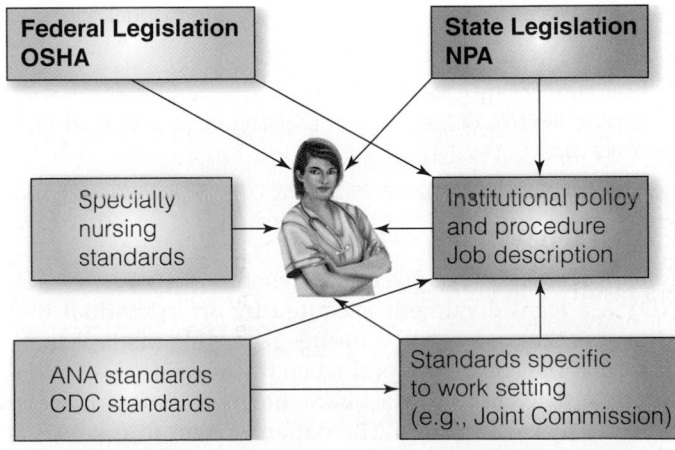

Figure 49–4 》 Impact of laws and standards on nurses.

4. Perform care only to the highest level of nursing knowledge; if you are unprepared for a clinical assignment, inform your instructor.

5. Seek help before beginning a procedure about which you are unsure; if the instructor is not readily available, allow the staff nurse to perform the intervention.

Nursing students are held accountable to the same standard of care as licensed nurses. Nursing faculty members are held accountable for appropriate assignment and supervision of students.

SAFETY ALERT Student nurses do not practice on a faculty member's license. The only individual who can legally practice on a license is the individual whose name appears on the license.

Standards of Practice

Nursing, as a profession, has a responsibility to self-regulate by defining the practice of nursing, researching and developing the practice, establishing standards of practice, and providing for the education and credentialing of nurses. The ANA, the largest professional nursing organization, has established Standards of Clinical Nursing Practice. These address both standards for nursing care and standards for professional performance. Standards of practice are also available for various nursing specialties, including pediatric nursing, nurse anesthesia practice, critical care nursing, and psychiatric nursing.

REVIEW Nurse Practice Acts

RELATE Link the Concepts and Exemplars

Linking the exemplar of nurse practice acts with the concept of addiction:

1. What resources does your state's board of nursing offer for nurses who are struggling with substance abuse?

2. What would you do if you realized that a nurse you were working with was under the influence of drugs or alcohol? Explain.

Linking the exemplar of nurse practice acts with the concept of accountability:

3. What does your state's Nurse Practice Act say about the accountability of nursing students? How is that different from what the NPA says about the accountability of registered nurses?

4. How does your state's board of nursing support or assist nurses in their professional development?

REFER Go to Pearson MyLab Nursing and eText

- Additional review materials

REFLECT Apply Your Knowledge

Sarah Coulton is a registered nurse who works with you in a primary care clinic. Her husband has been notified that his employer is transferring him to another state, and Sarah and her family will be moving in a couple of months.

1. Where will Sarah be able to find information on which states have mutual recognition with your state?

2. What steps might Sarah need to take if she learns that she is moving to a state that is not part of the Nurse Licensure Compact?

≫ Exemplar 49.B
Advance Directives

Exemplar Learning Outcomes

49.B Analyze advance directives as they relate to legal issues.

- Describe types of healthcare advance directives.
- Outline elements of advance directives.
- Explain the role of the nurse in assisting families with advance directives.

Exemplar Key Terms

Durable power of attorney for healthcare, 2843
Healthcare advance directive, 2842
Living will, 2843
Patient Self-Determination Act, 2842

Overview

A **healthcare advance directive** (sometimes referred to as an AD) is a legal document executed by an individual that expresses that individual's desires regarding medical treatment that may be used if and when the individual is no longer able to communicate his or her preferences directly (Ryan & Jezewski, 2012). The patient's right to use ADs is guaranteed in the Patient Self-Determination Act. The **Patient Self-Determination Act** is a federal law requiring

healthcare institutions that receive federal funding (but not individual healthcare providers) to do the following:

1. At the time of admission, give patients a written summary of:
   - Healthcare decision-making rights. (Each state has developed such a summary for hospitals, nursing homes, and home health agencies to use.)
   - The facility's policies with respect to recognizing ADs.

Focus on Diversity and Culture
Advance Directives

A majority of Americans feel that individuals have the right to direct what sort of medical treatment they receive at the end of life. Despite this widespread belief, fewer than one third of Americans have established ADs—and this percentage is even lower among people of color. As a result, members of minority groups are significantly less likely than White Americans to have their final wishes followed (Benson & Aldrich, 2012; Minority Nurse, 2013).

There are multiple reasons why people of color are less likely to have ADs than their White counterparts. For example, individuals who do not understand English and those who are non-native speakers may find it difficult, if not impossible, to understand AD forms and/or the terminology used by healthcare workers when discussing ADs. Still other individuals might not create ADs because of cultural beliefs, mistrust of the healthcare system, or inaccurate perceptions of how ADs actually work. Some Chinese patients, for instance, tend to view death as a taboo subject, and they may believe that planning for EOL care will doom them to dying in the near future. Similarly, some African American patients may view ADs as a sign that they've given up on God or abandoned hope for recovery. Some African Americans further believe that ADs are unnecessary because their family will make the right decisions for them, or they fear that they won't actually receive the care described in their ADs because of past instances of institutional racism in healthcare. In comparison, Latino patients may lack ADs because they are unfamiliar with the concept. Some members of Latino populations may also believe that hospice care is the same thing as nursing home care and thus violates their traditional cultural belief that sick and dying individuals be cared for in the home by family members (Minority Nurse, 2013). Yet other possible explanations for differences in AD use among minority groups include lower health literacy levels, physician bias, and reduced access to care (Fischer et al., 2012).

Nurses are in an ideal position to help people of color better understand the value of ADs and establish these documents as needed. One key step is to encourage patients to discuss EOL issues with their loved ones; here, the nurse should emphasize the importance of the discussion itself rather than the need to obtain a signed AD. To foster such discussions, nurses should approach the topic in a manner that is appropriate to each patient's cultural, religious, and personal preferences. This requires that nurses be knowledgeable about other cultures and try to consider the situation from their patients' point of view. It is often useful to frame ADs as positive devices that clarify what care measures an individual wants, rather than what measures he or she wishes to avoid. Patients may also find reassurance in the idea that ADs relieve their loved ones of the burden of making life-or-death decisions on their behalf. Nurses should be sure to explain any unclear or culturally sensitive terminology used in AD documents. In addition, nurses can further promote AD adoption by encouraging their employers and other healthcare organizations to use EOL planning documents that are simple to read and understand, as well as culturally and linguistically appropriate to various communities (Minority Nurse, 2013).

---

2. Ask patients whether they have an AD and document the AD's existence in the medical record. (It is up to the patient to provide a copy of the AD.)
3. Educate staff and community about ADs.
4. Ensure that the individuals know that the facility never discriminates on the basis of whether or not the individual has an AD.

Competent patients may execute ADs at any time. ADs are formal, written documents that typically outline the patient's desires regarding the following:

- Use or withholding of hydration and/or total parenteral nutrition
- Resuscitation or intubation in the event of a life-threatening emergency (Do-not-resuscitate and do-not-intubate orders are discussed in the exemplar on End-of-Life Care in the module on Comfort)
- The individual with the authority to make decisions on the patient's behalf in the event the patient is unable to do so (referred to as a healthcare surrogate).

Types of ADs include the living will and the durable power of attorney for healthcare. A **living will** provides specific instructions about what medical treatment the patient chooses to omit or refuse (e.g., ventilator support) in the event that the patient is unable to make such a decision. Through a **durable power of attorney for healthcare**, the patient may designate another individual (usually a family member, significant other, or close personal friend) as *healthcare surrogate* or *healthcare proxy* and give that individual power to make healthcare decisions on behalf of the patient if the patient is unable to do so. These may be combined into a single document or may be two separate documents. The Focus on Diversity and Culture feature looks at the use of ADs by various populations.

>> **Stay Current:** Information about advance directives can be found at the Health in Aging Organization website at https://www.nia.nih.gov/health/publication/end-life-helping-comfort-and-care/planning-end-life-care-decisions.

Clinical Example B

Gary Casper, a 65-year-old man, has been in the hospital several times in the past year with a deteriorating diagnosis. After Shondra Lewis, the patient's RN, completes her assessment of Mr. Casper's current condition and his concerns, she contacts the case management department for assistance with his concerns regarding his end-of-life care choices. Ms. Lewis tells the case manager that the patient's wife will not allow him to prepare an AD, which Mr. Casper wants to do, since he decided to be DNR on this current admission. The next day, the social worker meets with Mr. Casper separately from his wife to discuss his right for self-determination and how to prepare an AD form. Mr. Casper is relieved that he can complete the form in the hospital, but he is concerned that his wife will still be able to prevent this, as he does not want her to have a power of attorney for him. Plans are put in process for Mr. Casper to complete the advance directive with appropriate staff and another family member while the physician speaks with Mrs. Casper in a conference room.

Critical Thinking Questions

1. How did the staff support this patient's right to self-determination?
2. Did the physician violate the wife's right to be with her spouse in this case? Explain.
3. How can nursing staff further assist Mr. Casper in facing end-of-life care choices?
4. How can the staff support Mrs. Casper as she faces the end of her husband's life?

Elements of an Advance Directive

A broadly drafted AD usually gives an agent or surrogate decision maker authority to do the following:

- Consent to or refuse any medical treatment or diagnostic procedure relating to the individual's physical or mental health, including artificial nutrition and hydration.

- Hire or discharge medical providers, and authorize admission to medical and long-term care facilities.

- Consent to measures for comfort care and pain relief.

- Have access to all medical records.

- Take whatever measures are necessary to carry out wishes, including granting releases or waivers to medical facilities and seeking judicial remedies if problems arise.

Each state, through legislation, determines the specific requirements for healthcare ADs. In most states, ADs must be witnessed by two people and do not require review by an attorney. Many states require that a specific legislated form be used. The majority of states do not permit relatives, heirs, or primary care providers to serve as witnesses for ADs (Ryan & Jezewski, 2012). In some states, the patient has the option to limit the authority of the healthcare agent as desired. Nurses working with a patient who has an AD should ensure that they understand what the patient's AD includes and should know the laws in the state related to self-determination as well as the employing agency's policies and procedures for following ADs.

Figure 49–5 》》 shows an example of a healthcare AD that combines a living will declaration and a durable power of attorney for healthcare.

》》 Stay Current: Samples of state-specific forms can be obtained from the National Hospice and Palliative Care Organization at www.nhpco.org.

One popular AD is Five Wishes. This form was developed to simplify the process of drafting an AD and is specifically designed to address not only the healthcare aspects of EOL, but the emotional and spiritual issues as well (Aging with Dignity, 2015). The form addresses five areas:

1. The person who will make care decisions when the patient cannot
2. The kinds of medical treatment the patient does and does not want
3. The level of comfort the patient would prefer
4. The way the patient would prefer to be treated by others

5. The information the patient would like his or her loved ones to know.

Specific concerns in each of these areas is addressed via questions on the form. Patients circle or cross out answers or write one- or two-sentence responses to these questions (Aging with Dignity, 2015). Questions and responses are written in simple language that is easy for laypeople to understand.

Five Wishes is widely used, and 42 states currently accept the form as an AD. Patients 18 and older may use the form. It is available in 27 languages (Aging with Dignity, 2015). Five Wishes does not meet the technical requirements for an AD in Alabama, Indiana, Kansas, New Hampshire, Ohio, Oregon, Texas, and Utah. Patients living in these states who wish to use the Five Wishes AD must append it to the government-approved AD form required by their state.

Role of the Nurse

Patients and families often have difficulty making advance treatment decisions for EOL matters. The nurse should reassure them that if they make a decision and have an AD, they will have the option to change their decision. For example, the patient may have decided not to have ventilator support in the case of terminal illness, but when the situation occurs, the patient has the right to change his or her mind or take more time to make the decision.

SAFETY ALERT Nurses can assist patients and their families by instructing patients to provide a copy of their advance directives to their next of kin, primary healthcare providers, and any healthcare facility to which they are admitted, including emergency departments, rehabilitation facilities, and senior living centers.

The nurse needs to assess whether the patient and family have an accurate understanding of life-sustaining measures. Patients and families may misunderstand what actions may sustain life and base their decisions on these misconceptions. The nurse needs to incorporate teaching in this area and continue to be supportive of patients' decisions. The Evidence-Based Practice feature looks at additional aspects that may affect a patient's likelihood to have an AD.

For patients without an AD who no longer have capacity to make decisions, a surrogate may be selected. Nurses may be involved in assessing a patient's capacity, but selection of a surrogate is typically dictated by the state. Generally, the spouse is the first choice as surrogate, followed by an adult child, a parent, and an adult sibling. Decision making by the surrogate is generally governed by one of two criteria. The first is the substituted judgment standard. With this standard, the surrogate infers the choice the patient would make on the basis of past conversations with the patient or knowledge of the patient's beliefs and values. The second is the best interest standard. With this standard, the surrogate weighs the benefits and risks of treatment options and selects the one that he or she believes will be most beneficial for the patient.

POWER OF ATTORNEY FOR HEALTH CARE
(1) **DESIGNATION OF AGENT:** I designate the following individual as my agent to make health care decisions for me: _____

_____

(Name of individual you choose as agent)

_____

(address) (city) (state) (zip code)

_____

(home phone) (work phone)

OPTIONAL: If I revoke my agent's authority or if my agent is not willing, able, or reasonably available to make a health-care decision for me, I designate as my first alternate agent:

_____

(Name of individual you choose as first alternate agent)

_____

(address) (city) (state) (zip code)

_____

(home phone) (work phone)

OPTIONAL: If I revoke the authority of my agent and first alternate agent or if neither is willing, able, or reasonably available to make a health care decision for me, I designate as my second alternate agent:

_____

(Name of individual you choose as second alternate agent)

_____

(address) (city) (state) (zip code)

_____

(home phone) (work phone)

(2) **AGENT'S AUTHORITY:** My agent is authorized to make all health care decisions for me, including decisions to provide, withhold, or withdraw artificial nutrition and hydration, and all other forms of health care to keep me alive, **except** as I state here:

(3) **WHEN AGENT'S AUTHORITY BECOMES EFFECTIVE:** My agent's authority becomes effective when my primary physician determines that I am unable to make my own health care decisions unless I mark the following box. If I mark this box [ ], my agent's authority to make health care decisions for me takes effect immediately.

(4) **AGENT'S OBLIGATION:** My agent shall make health care decisions for me in accordance with this power of attorney for health care, any instructions I give below, and my other wishes to the extent known to my agent. To the extent my wishes are unknown, my agent shall make health care decisions for me in accordance with what my agent determines to be in my best interest. In determining my best interest, my agent shall consider my personal values to the extent known to my agent.

(5) **AGENT'S POSTDEATH AUTHORITY:** My agent is authorized to make anatomical gifts, authorize an autopsy, and direct disposition of my remains, except as I state here or elsewhere in this form:

INSTRUCTIONS FOR HEALTH CARE
Strike any wording you do not want.

(6) **END-OF-LIFE DECISIONS:** I direct that my health care providers and others involved in my care provide, withhold, or withdraw treatment in accordance with the choice I have marked below: **(Initial only one box)**
[ ] (a) **Choice NOT To Prolong Life**
I do not want my life to be prolonged if (1) I have an incurable and irreversible condition that will result in my death within a relatively short time, (2) I become unconscious and, to a reasonable degree of medical certainty, I will not regain consciousness, or (3) the likely risks and burdens of treatment would outweigh the expected benefits, **OR**
[ ] (b) **Choice To Prolong Life**
I want my life to be prolonged as long as possible within the limits of generally accepted health care standards.

(7) **RELIEF FROM PAIN:** Except as I state in the following space, I direct that treatment for alleviation of pain or discomfort should be provided at all times even if it hastens my death:

DONATION OF ORGANS AT DEATH
(8) Upon my death: (mark applicable box)
[ ] (a) I give any needed organs, tissues, or parts,
OR
[ ] (b) I give the following organs, tissues, or parts only: _____
[ ] (c) My gift is for the following purposes:
(strike any of the following you do not want)
(1) Transplant
(2) Therapy
(3) Research
(4) Education

(9) **EFFECT OF COPY:** A copy of this form has the same effect as the original.

(10) **SIGNATURE:** Sign and date the form here:

_____   _____
(date)   (sign your name)

_____   _____
(address)   (print your name)

_____   _____
(city)   (state)

(11) **WITNESSES:** This advance health care directive will not be valid for making health care decisions unless it is either: (1) signed by two (2) qualified adult witnesses who are personally known to you and who are present when you sign or acknowledge your signature; or (2) acknowledged before a notary public.

Figure 49–5 ≫ Sample advance healthcare directive.

Evidence-Based Practice
End-of-Life Care for Patients with Terminal Cancer

Problem

When working with patients diagnosed with terminal cancer, nurses must be prepared to discuss advance directives (ADs). If an AD does not exist, the nurse needs to understand the complex psychosocial and emotional issues the patient is experiencing and incorporate these into a compassionate, professional conversation about end-of-life (EOL) care. When doing so, the nurse should understand that patient wishes related to EOL are tied to a number of complex influences.

Evidence

Miljoković et al. (2015) surveyed adults with cancer about the existence of and attitudes toward do not resuscitate (DNR) and allow natural death (AND) orders. The researchers discovered that, although the patients surveyed were identified as terminal by their physicians, only 42% considered themselves terminally ill. In addition, only 50% of patients had a DNR or AND order in place. Patients were increasingly likely to create DNR or AND orders as their prognosis worsened and their survival time shortened. In addition, the researchers hypothesized that the concept of an AND order might be more acceptable than a DNR order for emotional reasons, but patients did not exhibit a statistically significant preference for one type of order over the other.

Crosby et al. (2016) explored the link between gender and DNR orders in patients with cancer. The researchers discovered that female patients were 1.3 times more likely to have DNR orders early in their illness than male patients. They also discovered that female physicians were 1.5 times more likely to write early DNR orders for their female patients than for their male patients. The researchers did not find a similar correlation in male patient–male physician pairs. Age at time of diagnosis, comorbid conditions, and disease progression were also found to be factors in the timing of DNR order creation.

Ahmed and colleagues (2015) looked specifically at DNR orders in patients with lung cancer. Their research revealed that, while patients at all disease stages typically received family support for creating DNR orders, patients' uncertainty about the extent of their disease and amount of time remaining were key factors in DNR order preparation. Most patients indicated that, even if they did not have a DNR order in place, they had considered the need for one; many had also sought advice about DNR orders from their physicians. A primary area of concern for patients without DNR orders was linked to hope; many patients felt that creating a DNR order was akin to giving up hope for long-term survival. Others indicated concern about the reversibility of DNR orders and the quality of care they would receive if healthcare providers knew they had a DNR in place.

Implications

Patients diagnosed with terminal cancer have differing views on ADs, and individual patient opinions related to ADs may be affected by prognosis, time remaining, gender, and feelings of hope. It is essential that the nurse not make assumptions about whether a patient has an AD; it is equally important that the nurse use tact and understanding when addressing this complex issue with a patient. In addition, the nurse should ensure that the patient understands the legal aspects of DNR orders, including the reversibility of orders and the process that must be undertaken to change a DNR order. The nurse should also make clear the healthcare providers' legal obligation to provide high-quality care even in the presence of a DNR order.

Critical Thinking Application

1. Why might a patient's perception of the terminal nature of a cancer diagnosis affect the patient's likelihood of having a DNR or AND order?

2. What reasons might explain the higher likelihood of female patients with cancer to have DNR orders earlier than male patients? Why is the female patient–female physician information important to consider?

3. Why is family support for creation of a DNR order important in working with a terminally ill patient with cancer? How can the nurse leverage this support?

REVIEW Advance Directives

RELATE Link the Concepts and Exemplars

Linking the exemplar of advance directives with the concept of cognition:

1. Why might it be advisable to discuss development of ADs with a patient who is in the early stages of Alzheimer disease?

2. How might a patient with schizophrenia benefit from an AD that includes instructions related to psychiatric care and treatment?

Linking the exemplar of advance directives with the concept of communication:

3. What communication strategies would you use to address the need to develop ADs with a patient? With the patient's family members?

4. What communication strategies would you use to help a family member understand that his mother is no longer able to make her own decisions and it is time to review and follow the ADs that she put in place?

REFER Go to Pearson MyLab Nursing and eText

- Additional review materials

REFLECT Apply Your Knowledge

Heather King is a 53-year-old woman who is hospitalized with a newly diagnosed malignant brain tumor. She has signed an AD that indicates she does not want any extraordinary measures to keep her alive if she has an incurable or irreversible condition that will result in her death within a relatively short period of time. The neurosurgeon has presented her with treatment options. Ms. King refuses treatment for the tumor, requesting only palliative care "until the time comes." Her husband speaks to the neurosurgeon outside of Ms. King's room, stating, "I want everything possible done! The children and I have discussed this, and we don't agree with not treating the tumor."

1. What should happen with Ms. King's treatment? Why?

2. How may the family's reaction affect implementation of the AD?

3. In what circumstances could the patient's family member refuse or consent to treatment for the patient?

4. What law, rule, or policy describes the nurse's responsibility?

>> Exemplar 49.C
Health Insurance Portability and Accountability Act

Exemplar Learning Outcomes

49.C Analyze the Health Insurance Portability and Accountability Act (HIPAA) as it relates to legal issues.

- Explain the purpose of HIPAA.
- Explain how the Privacy Rule covers protected health information.
- Differentiate privacy and confidentiality.

Exemplar Key Terms

Confidentiality, *2848*
Health Insurance Portability and Accountability Act (HIPAA), *2847*
Privacy, *2848*
Protected health information, *2847*

Overview

The **Health Insurance Portability and Accountability Act (HIPAA)** of 1996 was enacted by Congress to minimize the exclusion of preexisting conditions as a barrier to healthcare insurance, designate special rights for individuals who lose other health coverage, and eliminate medical underwriting in group plans. The act includes the Privacy Rule, which creates a national standard for the disclosure of private health information. This rule affects all healthcare providers as well as health insurance plan providers (McGowan, 2012).

Protected Health Information

The Privacy Rule protects all "individually identifiable health information" held or transmitted in any form or medium, whether electronic, paper, or oral. The rule calls this information **protected health information** and delineates it further to include information that identifies the individual (e.g., name, address, birth date, and Social Security number) or for which a reasonable basis exists to believe the information can be used to identify the individual as it relates to the following:

- The individual's past, present, or future physical or mental health or condition
- The provision of healthcare to the individual
- The past, present, or future payment for the provision of healthcare to the individual.

HIPAA also includes provisions for the protection of patients that address access to medical records, requires notice of privacy practices and opportunity for confidential communications, limits on use of medical information beyond the sharing among healthcare providers directly involved in providing care, and prohibition of the use of personal information for marketing.

In the event that a patient feels a healthcare plan or provider has violated his or her rights according to HIPAA, the individual may file a formal complaint either directly to the entity that committed the violation or to the office for Civil Rights of the U.S. Department of Health and Human Services. Information about how to file a complaint should be included in each entity's notice of privacy practices. Willful violation of the Privacy Rule can result in civil or criminal penalties for the individuals involved. In most cases, violations that are corrected within 30 days are not subject to civil penalties (American Medical Association [AMA], 2016).

Nurses must maintain an understanding of current law in order to protect the patient's privacy and to avoid civil punitive damage suits and possible criminal charges. Nurses should be familiar with the particular policies of their employers.

Clinical Example C

D'Alice Jones and Otis Harvey are RNs in the oncology unit at Mercy Hospital. They are standing behind the nurse's station having a whispered conversation about Sandy Wagner, a 60-year-old female patient with terminal cancer.

"She didn't do well with today's treatment. She's been vomiting at least twice an hour for the last three hours," D'Alice says.

"Poor Mrs. Wagner. I wish there was more we could do to make her feel better. But she's refused all pain and antinausea medication," Otis replies.

"I know. She told me today that she's about ready to give up on treatments and just let whatever happens happen," D'Alice responds.

Just then, D'Alice and Otis notice Mrs. Wagner's son standing a few feet from the nurses' station with a horrified look on his face. When he sees them looking at him, he quickly turns and walks away.

Critical Thinking Questions

1. Assuming that the patient's son overheard their conversation, are the two nurses in violation of the Privacy Rule? Why or why not?
2. What additional precautions could the nurses have taken to avoid their conversation being overheard?

In spite of the extensive efforts of the healthcare industry, the general population remains confused about their actual rights, and some healthcare workers remain unclear about what is and is not allowed under HIPAA (Bova, Drexler, & Sullivan-Bolyai, 2012; McGowan, 2012). Ultimately, maintaining the security of protected health information provides for the protection of the most vulnerable populations, and personnel in covered entities will need to continue to learn and implement the HIPAA standards.

SAFETY ALERT Disclosure of patient information is a breach of confidentiality that may subject a nurse to legal action. Disclosure of confidential information occurs when a patient's condition—for example, a diagnosis of HIV infection—is discussed inappropriately with any third party. In addition, privacy must be provided when calling individuals in for office visits and in all provision of care.

Privacy Versus Confidentiality

Privacy includes the right of individuals to keep their personal information from being disclosed. The individual decides when, where, and with whom to share his or her health information. **Confidentiality** refers to the assurance the patient has that private information will not be disclosed without his or her consent. Confidentiality applies both to the nature of the information the nurse obtains from the patient and to how the nurse treats patient information once it has been disclosed to the nurse (ANA, 2015):

- *Obtaining information.* Nurses should request and record only information pertinent to the health status of patients to whom they are assigned. If the nurse runs into a neighbor in the emergency department waiting room, for example, it would be inappropriate for the nurse to ask the neighbor, "What are you doing here?" This would inadvertently invite protected information that this nurse does not need for provision of healthcare.

- *Disclosing information.* Information obtained from the patient should be disclosed only to individuals who are directly involved in providing that patient's healthcare. Even the presence of the individual in the healthcare setting is protected information. It would be a breach of confidentiality, for example, for the nurse to go home and tell her family that a state senator or representative, the family's pastor, a neighbor, or anyone else was a patient. Protection of patient information, once disclosed, is one tenet of the nurse's responsibility as the patient's advocate, and challenges to patient privacy can include other members of the interprofessional team.

- *Advocating for confidentiality.* Nurses are professionally obligated not only to avoid participating in discussions of patients outside communications directly related to providing care but also to curb others from participation. Gossiping at work is common in many organizations, but it has no place in the healthcare setting. Celebrity status, notoriety, and an unusual medical

condition all add to the potential risks to confidentiality. If the nurse is in a coffee shop and hears another nurse or healthcare provider discussing a patient, the nurse is expected to redirect those professionals to maintain patient privacy.

In addition to the actions and behaviors described here, nurses should be familiar with the specific policies and procedures for protecting patient privacy and confidentiality for the healthcare agency in which they work.

Disclosure

A patient's protected health information can be disclosed under certain conditions without express permission from the patient. These disclosures include providing information to the patient, to other providers who are treating the patient, and to individuals involved in payment processing and other healthcare operations. Information must also be disclosed where required by law or court order, where necessary to protect public health, and when abuse or neglect are suspected. When such disclosure occurs, information should be limited to the minimum necessary for the situation. Providing information beyond what is required is a breach of the Privacy Rule. Informal patient permission may be sufficient for providing information to the patient's family, friends, or other individuals identified by the patient (McGowan, 2012). In general, when circumstances give the patient the opportunity to agree or object, the nurse should ask for the patient's permission to disclose information.

Incidental disclosure of patient information may occur in some circumstances. For example, conversations with patients or colleagues about patient care may be overheard by others. The Privacy Rule permits some incidental disclosure of this sort, provided that appropriate safeguards are in place. In this case, reasonable safeguards would include holding such conversations in private locations if possible; if this is not possible, the nurse should try to speak quietly (McGowan, 2012).

REVIEW Health Insurance Portability and Accountability Act

RELATE Link the Concepts and Exemplars

Linking the exemplar of Health Insurance Portability and Accountability Act with the concept of trauma:

1. When and how is it appropriate to break the confidentiality of patients who threaten harm to themselves or others?

2. What additional considerations are involved when it comes to protecting the confidentiality of victims of domestic violence? Of child abuse?

Linking the exemplar of Health Insurance Portability and Accountability Act with the concept of reproduction:

You are the nurse at a local high school. A 16-year-old student has been in the bathroom off and on all morning. She is very nauseated but has been adamant about staying at school. You sit down to talk with her and learn that she thinks she is pregnant. She says, "I don't know what to do. I don't want my parents to know."

3. What are your responsibilities to this patient regarding her privacy and confidentiality?

4. What are the laws in your state that relate to the ability of minors to make independent decisions regarding their own pregnancies?

REFER Go to Pearson MyLab Nursing and eText

- Additional review materials

REFLECT Apply Your Knowledge

Michael Nguyen is a nurse on the medical–surgical unit of a busy suburban hospital. Approximately 20 minutes ago, the nursing unit was notified that seven patients who were involved in a motor vehicle crash and are receiving treatment in the emergency department (ED) are expected to be admitted to the med–surg unit in varying conditions. Carole Fulton, another nurse working on the unit, has been liaising with the ED staff about the situation. Michael goes to answer a patient call bell. When he returns to the nursing desk, he overhears Carole on her cell phone saying, "Yes, that accident on Highway 40. Yeah, apparently it's really bad. I saw Reverend Mitchell downstairs. Yeah. No. His daughter was a passenger. OK. Bye." Carole hangs up the phone and puts it in her purse, saying, "My mom. She called to tell me she got home safely from work." Thirty minutes later, Michael receives a report on a patient named Elizabeth Mitchell who is being transported up from the ED.

1. What concerns might Michael have about the content of Carole's phone call with her mother? How might Carole have violated Ms. Mitchell's privacy or confidentiality?
2. If you had been Michael, what responsibility would you have to address your concerns?

» Exemplar 49.D
Mandatory Reporting

Exemplar Learning Outcomes

49.D Analyze mandatory reporting as it relates to legal issues.

- Describe the legalities of mandatory reporting.
- Outline situations that require mandatory reporting.
- Differentiate considerations related to mandatory reporting across the lifespan.

Exemplar Key Terms

Good faith immunity, *2849*
Mandatory reporting, *2849*

Overview

The term **mandatory reporting** refers to the legal requirement to report an act, event, or situation that is designated by state or local law as a reportable event (Katner, 2012). Disclosure statutes mandate the reporting of certain types of health information, and all states mandate the reporting of certain vital statistics, including births and deaths. Many states also require healthcare providers to report abortions and neonatal deaths. Federal and state laws mandate the reporting of communicable diseases, including venereal diseases. This exemplar discusses the nurse's responsibilities related to mandatory reporting as well as the types of acts, events, and situations that are reportable.

Legal Requirements for Mandatory Reporting

In most states, nurses are required to report abuse or suspected abuse, certain types of injuries and illness, and crimes involving minors. Nurses have a legal obligation to report conduct that is incompetent, unethical, and illegal. This may include reporting violence, abuse, or neglect toward patients or other nurses and extends to reporting conduct involving third parties, including family members and other healthcare providers. Each state's NPA includes requirements for reporting nurses who are in violation of the act.

As a general rule, when reporting situations involving patients, the nurse reports the required information through the administrative chain of the institution, beginning with the nurse's immediate supervisor and the primary healthcare provider. All information reported is documented in the patient record. When reporting nurses who are in violation of the NPA, the nurse may be required to report the relevant facts to both the institution and the state BON.

Regardless of the situation, the nurse is not required to conduct any type of investigation or otherwise confirm that the suspected act or incident has, in fact, occurred. The nurse is required only to have a good faith suspicion based on information disclosed by a patient, physical symptoms observed in a patient, or the nurse's personal observations of behavior on the part of a patient, colleague, or third party. The reporting nurse may be granted immunity from liability unless he or she knows that the report is false or acts with reckless disregard, without concern for the validity of the allegations made.

Good Faith Immunity

In every state, healthcare workers are protected from civil or criminal liabilities when they report suspected child abuse in good faith, even if the subsequent investigation does not make a determination of abuse. This is called **good faith immunity**. Good faith immunity also typically applies to reports of elder mistreatment, particular illnesses or injuries, and crimes involving minors.

When reporting incidents subject to good faith immunity, the nurse or healthcare provider may be required to disclose protected health information. This includes patient name, age, gender, race, residence, or present location as well as the nature and extent of the abuse, injury, or illness. Disclosure of this information under these circumstances is not considered a violation of the HIPAA Privacy Rule. Guidelines regarding disclosure of health information as a mandatory reporter are presented in **Box 49–6 »**.

SAFETY ALERT Good faith immunity applies only to required information that is reported to the appropriate agency or office. Information reported above and beyond that which is mandated may not be protected under good faith immunity.

Box 49–6
Guidelines Regarding Disclosure of Health Information

Depending on the setting, the nurse may be the only professional with firsthand information necessary for making an accurate report. General guidelines that nurses should follow regarding reporting health-related information include the following:

- Know the federal and state laws concerning duty to report.
- Report the required information to the appropriate governmental agency promptly.
- Comply with reporting laws in good faith.
- Follow agency policy carefully when making a report.
- Avoid a breach of confidentiality, and report only the information mandated.

Source: Based on Guido, G. W. (2014). *Legal and ethical issues in nursing* (6th ed.). Upper Saddle River, NJ: Pearson Education.

Mandatory Reporting of Abuse or Neglect of Minors and Older Adults

The circumstances in which a nurse must report child abuse vary among states. In most states, a report must be made when the nurse has reason to believe abuse has occurred because of things that are seen, heard, or observed in the work environment. In addition, nurses may be required to report knowledge or observation of a child being subjected to conditions that are likely to result in harm. Mandatory reporters must cite the facts or circumstances that led to their suspicions of abuse, but do not have the burden of proof (Child Welfare Information Gateway, 2016).

States also have specific laws pertaining to the mistreatment of adults and older adults (**Figure 49–6 》**). These laws may be similar to those that govern the abuse and neglect of children. For example, many states generally offer good

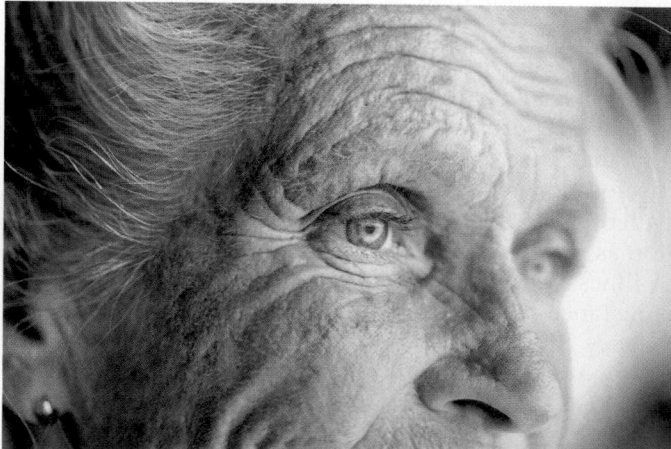

Source: Jodi Jacobson/E+/Getty Images.

Figure 49–6 》 Elder mistreatment includes physical, emotional, verbal, and sexual abuse and neglect.

faith immunity to individuals who report suspected abuse or neglect of an older adult or an adult with a disability. Nurses should know the laws of their individual states and their agency's policies for reporting suspected mistreatment of an adult or older adult (Daly, Klein, & Jogerst, 2012). Additional information on this topic can be found in the module on Trauma.

Mandatory Reporting of Certain Injuries and Illnesses

Primary healthcare providers are mandated to report certain types of injuries and illnesses to the appropriate authorities. Injuries and illnesses that typically fall under the reporting laws include the following:

- Bullet wounds, gunshot wounds, powder burns, or any other injuries arising or suspected of arising from the discharge of a gun or firearm
- Illnesses that appear to be caused by poisoning
- Injuries caused by, or appearing to be caused by, a knife or other sharp or pointed instrument if the physician or surgeon treating the individual suspects that a criminal act may have been involved
- Any wound, injury, or illness resulting in bodily harm as a result of a suspected criminal act or act of violence
- Infectious diseases, such as tuberculosis, HIV/AIDS, and *Escherichia coli* infection.

Most agencies have a policy and procedure in place for routine reporting of these injuries and illnesses. For example, injuries that are or appear to be due to violence are typically first seen in the emergency department; therefore, organizations typically designate the emergency department to report these injuries. A diagnosis of an infectious disease, on the other hand, may occur at any point in the healthcare interaction, so the nurse needs to be familiar with the agency policy for reporting infectious diseases and ensure that the report is made when warranted. As with abuse situations, good faith immunity typically applies.

Mandatory reporting of infectious conditions is a cornerstone of maintaining public health. Since 1878, the U.S. Public Health System has been collecting information on infectious conditions for the purpose of early identification and control of massive outbreaks, including, when necessary, instituting quarantines. High-profile diseases and threats of bioterrorism have brought renewed attention to this system of ongoing monitoring. The Centers for Disease Control and Prevention National Notifiable Diseases Surveillance System (NNDSS) has identified more than 50 infectious diseases in the United States that must be reported. Among these are anthrax, botulism, cholera, hepatitis, HIV infection, and syphilis.

Data are reported at the county level, with primary care providers reporting these diseases and conditions to local health departments. For diseases and conditions that must be reported within 24 hours, the initial report is made by telephone to the health department, and the written report is made within 7 days. Each county health department reports to the state's department of health, where data are managed and maintained. Data on many diseases and conditions are provided from the state level to the Centers for Disease Control and

Prevention, which publishes the *Morbidity and Mortality Weekly Report*. Although the law targets physician reporting, nurses need to be aware of the policies and procedures for reporting within their place of employment, especially nurses who are employed directly by their local health department.

>> **Stay Current:** Visit the National Diseases Surveillance System (NNDSS) website at https://wwwn.cdc.gov/nndss for more information. A complete list of the 2016 event codes of the NNDSS can be found at https://wwwn.cdc.gov/nndss/case-notification/related-documentation.html#event-code-lists.

Clinical Example D

Randy Wallace is a 6-year-old boy who is a first grader at Park Hills Elementary school, where Maya Anderson is the school nurse. One afternoon, Randy's teacher brings him to Miss Anderson's office because of an injury he sustained during recess. While tending to Randy's injury, Miss Anderson notices a number of bruises on Randy's arms in various states of healing. After dressing Randy's injury and sending him back out on the playground, Miss Anderson asks Randy's teacher about his bruises. Randy's teacher laughs and says, "Randy? He's my little daredevil. I can't turn my back on him for a second or I find him climbing up on desks, dancing across the radiator, or otherwise risking his life. His mom says he is the same way at home."

Critical Thinking Questions

1. Are Randy's injuries sufficient to produce good faith suspicion of child abuse? If not, what additional information might be necessary to produce good faith suspicion?
2. In what ways might the teacher's attitude about Randy's injuries suggest negligence by a mandatory reporter?

Mandatory Reporting of Nurses Who Are in Violation of the Nurse Practice Act

Not all instances of mandatory reporting by nurses involve patients; nurses must also report other nurses who are in violation of their state's NPA. Violations of the NPA and proper reporting procedures for violations are governed by the state BON. For example, North Carolina's General Statutes (NCGS § 90-171.47) mandate that any individual who has reasonable cause to suspect that a nurse is in violation of the NPA has the duty to report the relevant facts to the BON. BONs take these reports very seriously; as a result, their websites generally make reporting forms readily available. Employers typically use a different reporting form than that used by members of the general public.

The NPA spells out any formal action the board may take, and it usually requires clear and convincing evidence that the nurse has violated state nursing laws or rules. The nature of alleged violations varies widely, and cases are decided on their own merits. Many complaints are resolved through informal processes, though in some instances, a formal administrative hearing is held.

BONs are required to respect each nurse's right to due process. This ensures that the nurse is informed of any allegations regarding his or her practice, that the nurse has an opportunity to respond to and defend against the allegations, and that the matter is heard by a fair and impartial body.

REVIEW   Mandatory Reporting

RELATE Link the Concepts and Exemplars

Linking the exemplar of mandatory reporting with the concept of trauma:

1. Why do you think nurses and healthcare providers have a duty to report injuries sustained during or as a result of a criminal act?
2. Why do you think mandatory reporting laws include the requirement to report injuries resulting from the discharge of a firearm?

Linking the exemplar of mandatory reporting with the concept of infection:

3. How do requirements and procedures for reporting HIV infection in your state or agency differ from requirements and procedures for reporting anthrax?
4. How do requirements and procedures for reporting shigellosis in your state or agency differ from requirements and procedures for reporting meningococcal disease?

REFER Go to Pearson MyLab Nursing and eText

■ Additional review materials

REFLECT Apply Your Knowledge

Jenny Erickson, an 85-year-old woman who is a widow, came into the emergency department after she apparently fell at home. Her neighbor and friend, Elinor Jones, was waiting for Mrs. Erickson to go to lunch with her and tried calling her several times. After getting no response for more than an hour, Mrs. Jones called the police, who found Mrs. Erickson on the kitchen floor. During the ED assessment, the nurse, Lynn Gutierrez, noted multiple bruises on Mrs. Erickson's legs, her upper arms, and both sides of her rib cage. When she asked Mrs. Erickson about the bruises, Mrs. Erickson said that she has been "falling a lot." The bruises were in several different stages of healing and bruised colors.

When Lynn asked whether she lived alone, Mrs. Erickson began crying and shivering. Mrs. Jones heard her friend crying and asked to speak with the nurse. Lynn spoke with Mrs. Jones away from the ED bedside. "I don't mean to get anyone in trouble, but Jenny has been living with her daughter and son-in-law for the past two years. I'm worried that they are upset having her there." Lynn realized that Mrs. Jones might have information that could explain why Mrs. Erickson had so many bruises. "Has Mrs. Erickson complained at all? I mean, has her family hurt her?" Mrs. Jones nodded her head. "I think so. I've heard her son-in-law yelling at her before, and Jenny had a big bruise on her forehead a month ago right after that."

1. What does the nurse need to do next?
2. How can the ED staff support Mrs. Erickson and ensure her safety while she is in the ED?
3. How can the nursing staff further assist Mrs. Erickson with the possible abuse?
4. What report must be done for this patient, and by whom?

» Exemplar 49.E
Risk Management

Exemplar Learning Outcomes

49.E Analyze risk management as it relates to legal issues.

- Explain the concept of risk management.
- Outline strategies for risk management.
- Explain the use of incident reports.

Exemplar Key Terms

Discovery, 2854
Incident report, 2854
Risk management, 2852
Variances, 2854

Overview

Risk management focuses on limiting a healthcare agency's financial and legal risk associated with the delivery of care, particularly in terms of lawsuits, ideally before incidents occur. Risk management is a process that identifies, analyzes, and treats potential hazards within a setting for the purpose of identifying and rectifying the hazards, thus preventing harm. Nurses play an important role in risk management because they are responsible for both patient safety and high-quality care.

Risk management focuses on areas at high risk for incidents, such as overall patient safety, medication administration, assessment and communication of allergies, and falls. The use of equipment and technology—including assessment of the functioning of equipment prior to use—also falls under the risk management umbrella.

Strategies for Risk Management

A facility may have an individual or a team dedicated to risk management. In most cases, there will be a designated risk manager whose overall role is to collaborate with the interprofessional healthcare team to maintain a safe and effective healthcare environment and prevent or reduce financial and legal risk to the organization (Kable, Guest, & McLeod, 2012).

Healthcare organizations can use several strategies to minimize risk. One of the most basic strategies is protecting against financial risk by purchasing insurance or by self-insuring. Other strategies involve identifying the areas in which incidents commonly occur and implementing practices to minimize the likelihood of incidents in these areas. Data collection, incident report systems, and staff education related to risk and documentation are all important for identifying and protecting against these types of risks. Strategies related to three common incident areas—implementing physician's orders, providing competent nursing care, and reducing pediatric medical errors—are discussed later in this section.

No matter how well an organization manages risk, incidents do still occur. Organizations should develop an investigation and reporting protocol for incidents that have the potential to result in lawsuits. When such incidents occur, investigation should begin as soon as possible after the incident.

Risk management strategies, reporting systems, and investigation practices should be regularly monitored and updated as needed. In addition, information gathered by reporting systems and via investigation should be used to educate staff in preparation for future incidents. For more information on how to prevent risk, see the modules on Quality Improvement and Safety.

SAFETY ALERT In addition to patient safety, healthcare organizations must consider risks to nonpatient visitors. These include community members and patients' family and friends. The organization can be found liable for falls and other accidents that occur on its property and should have proper protocols and risk management strategies in place for these occurrences.

Implementing a Physician's Orders

Nurses can minimize risk by analyzing procedures and medications ordered by the physician. It is the nurse's responsibility to seek clarification of ambiguous or seemingly erroneous orders from the prescribing physician. Seeking clarification from any other source is unacceptable and is regarded as a departure from competent nursing practice.

If the order is neither ambiguous nor apparently erroneous, the nurse is responsible for implementing it. For example, if the physician orders oxygen to be administered at 4 L/min, the nurse must administer oxygen at that rate and not at 2 or 6 L/min. If the orders state that the patient is not to have solid food after a bowel resection, the nurse must ensure that no solid food is given to the patient.

There are several categories of orders that nurses must question to protect themselves legally:

- *Question any order a patient questions.* For example, if a patient who has been receiving an intramuscular injection tells the nurse that the physician changed the order from an injectable to an oral medication, the nurse must recheck the order before giving the medication.

- *Question any order if the patient's condition has changed.* The nurse is considered responsible for notifying the physician of any significant changes in the patient's condition, whether the physician requests notification or not. For example, if a patient who is receiving an intravenous infusion suddenly develops a rapid pulse, chest pain, and a cough, the nurse must notify the physician immediately and question continuance of the ordered rate of infusion. If a patient who is receiving morphine for pain develops severely depressed respirations, the nurse must withhold the medication and notify the physician.

- *Question and record verbal orders to avoid miscommunications.* In addition to recording the time, the date, the physician's name, and the orders, the nurse documents the circumstances that occasioned the call to the physician, reads the orders back to the physician, and documents that the physician confirmed the orders as the nurse read them back.

- *Question any order that is illegible, unclear, or incomplete.* Misinterpretation of the name of a drug or the amount of a dose, for example, can easily occur with handwritten orders. The nurse is responsible for ensuring that the order is interpreted the way it was intended and that it is a safe and appropriate order.

Providing Competent Nursing Care

Nurses further minimize and manage risk by providing competent patient care. Nurses need to provide care that is within the legal boundaries of their practice and within the boundaries of agency policies and procedures. Nurses therefore must be familiar with their various job descriptions, which may be different from agency to agency. Every nurse is responsible for ensuring that his or her education and experience are adequate to meet the responsibilities delineated in the job description. If the nurse feels that his or her knowledge is inadequate, the supervisor or manager should be alerted.

SAFETY ALERT Competent care also involves protecting patients from harm. Nurses need to anticipate sources of patient injury, educate patients about hazards, and implement measures to prevent injury.

Application of the nursing process is another essential aspect of providing safe and effective patient care. Patients need to be assessed and monitored appropriately and involved in care decisions. All assessments and care must be documented accurately. Effective communication can also protect the nurse from negligence claims. Nurses need to approach every patient with sincere concern and include the patient in conversations. In addition, nurses should always acknowledge when they do not know the answer to a patient's questions, tell the patient they will find the answer, and then follow through.

Methods of legal protection for nurses are summarized in **Box 49–7 》**.

Reducing Pediatric Medical Errors

Children are at a higher risk for medical errors than other patients and may also be more vulnerable to harm from errors because of their immature physiology (Tzeng et al., 2013). Reasons for increased medical errors among children include the following (Kaufman, Laschat, & Wappler, 2012; Tzeng et al., 2013):

- Medication dosage calculations for children are more complex than those for adults. Many medications are produced in adult concentrations that require dilution when given to a child, or the dosages need to be calculated based on weight or body surface area. This means that the optimal dose is based on mg/kg and divided by number of doses to be given a day. An additional problem is

---

Box 49–7
Guidelines for Legal Protection for Nurses

- Function within the scope of your education, job description, and nurse practice act.
- Follow the procedures and policies of the employing agency.
- Build and maintain good rapport with patients.
- Always check the identity of a patient to make sure it is the right patient.
- Observe and monitor the patient accurately. Communicate and record significant changes in the patient's condition to the physician.
- Promptly and accurately document all assessments and care given.
- Be alert when implementing nursing interventions, and give each task your full attention and skill.
- Perform procedures correctly and appropriately.
- Make sure the correct medications are given in the correct dose, by the right route, at the scheduled time, and to the right patient. Document the administration of the medication.
- When delegating nursing responsibilities, make sure that the individual who is delegated a task understands what to do and that the individual has the required knowledge and skill.
- Protect patients from injury.
- Report all incidents involving patients.
- Always check any order that a patient questions.
- Know your own strengths and weaknesses. Ask for assistance and supervision in situations for which you feel inadequately prepared.
- Maintain your clinical competence. For students, this demands study and practice before caring for patients. For graduate nurses, it means continued study to maintain and update clinical knowledge and skills.

---

that children often need suspensions or liquid preparations, adding to the dosage calculation complexity. Not only must the correct dose be calculated, but so must the amount of liquid preparation with that dose. Mistakes in mathematical calculations are one of the most common causes of medication errors.

- A misplaced decimal point in the medication dosage calculation can result in an overdose that can cause harm to the child or even death. This is particularly important for critically ill or injured children who do not have the reserves to deal with an overdose of medication.

- Many drug preparations require dilution to achieve the small dosage required by infants.

- Medications are sometimes prescribed that have not yet been approved by the FDA for use in children and for which pediatric standard dosage guidelines have not been established.

- Young children may be unable to communicate that they are having a reaction to the medication.

Another occasion of potential medical error involves families with limited English proficiency. There is a risk for errors in interpretation between the healthcare professional and the family member regarding care. For example, failure to obtain historical information about a drug allergy may lead to serious adverse effects. Even when a hospital interpreter is used, errors such as omitting instructions on dose, route, frequency, and duration of medications have potentially harmful clinical consequences (AHRQ, 2012).

Incident Reports

As part of risk management, each healthcare organization has an incident reporting system (Kable et al., 2012). Nurses participate in this process by completing the required forms when they are involved in an incident and by following policies and procedures.

An **incident report** is an agency record of an accident or incident that occurred within the agency. It is designed to collect adequate information to assist personnel in preventing future incidents or occurrences. Incident reports are also called variance reports or unusual occurrence reports. Examples of occurrences that would be reported include medication administration **variances** (e.g., wrong medication, wrong dose, wrong route, wrong time, or omissions) and a patient or visitor falling.

In some jurisdictions, incident reports may be used in discovery. **Discovery** is the legal process of obtaining information before a trial. Although most incidents do not result in lawsuits, a nurse completing an incident report should always fill out the report as though it is discoverable. No language regarding liability should be included. The report should completely and accurately document the facts without

assumptions, conclusions, or blame. The report should include the patient's account of the incident in direct quotes and should identify all witnesses to the incident. Incident reports generally include the following:

- Names and identifying information of any patients and healthcare personnel involved in the incident as well as information on witnesses (if any)
- The location, time, and date of the incident
- Equipment or medication involved (if medication, state the medication's name and dosage).

Although the event that prompted the incident report is noted in the patient's chart, there should be no entry in the patient's chart to indicate that an incident report was completed. For example, if the patient was given the wrong medication, the actual administration of the medication will be noted in the patient's chart. If the patient required any treatment as a result of the event, that also is noted in the patient's chart (Guido, 2014).

Nurses engage in risk management by following ANA standards of care and practice, by following their employing agency's policies and procedures, and by working collaboratively to ensure that patient safety is maintained at all times. Risk management is required of every nurse every day in the course of practicing nursing.

REVIEW Risk Management

RELATE Link the Concepts and Exemplars

Linking the exemplar of risk management with the concept of assessment:

1. How does a thorough assessment of a patient contribute to risk management?

2. Nurses are required to do their own assessment of a patient after receiving a report during shift change or patient transfer. How might failure to conduct this assessment or failure to do it in a timely manner affect the patient's risk for adverse outcomes?

Linking the exemplar of risk management with the concept of communication:

3. How does a change-of-shift report minimize the nurse's risk for professional negligence or malpractice?

4. How does accuracy in documentation contribute to risk management?

REFER Go to Pearson MyLab Nursing and eText

- Additional review materials

REFLECT Apply Your Knowledge

Three nurses were getting ready for the shift change report outside the room of an older adult patient. Kim Nelson whispered to the other

two nurses, "The doctor ordered the wrong dosage for Mr. Stivers. It took more than an hour to get in contact with her to clarify the order."

Randy Carson shook his head, knowing that this had become a common problem on their unit. "So, Kim, did she finally fix the order?"

Kim sighed and said, "Yes, but it didn't end there. Shortly after I gave Mr. Stivers the medication, he had difficulty breathing."

Pam Troy felt worried about this. She had been a nurse for only 2 years, but she knew that any problems when a medication is given are of critical concern. "Well, was it still the wrong dosage?"

Kim avoided looking at the other two nurses. "I need to get ready for report."

Randy was also concerned. "Wait, Kim. What happened?"

"Okay, so then I found out he's allergic to the medication I gave him."

Pam spoke up again. "Are you going to do an incident report?"

Kim shook her head. "No, I don't want to be sued or lose my job."

1. Is this case an example of nursing negligence? Explain.

2. What is the evidence that this issue may need an incident report?

3. What further information should the nurse seek before reporting an error?

4. Who else needs to know that there was a medication error with the patient?

References

Agency for Healthcare and Research Quality (AHRQ). (2012). Improving patient safety systems for patients with limited English proficiency: A guide for hospitals. *AHRQ Publication No. 12-0041.* Retrieved from http://www.ahrq.

gov/sites/default/files/publications/files/lepguide.pdf.

Aging with Dignity. (2015). *Five Wishes.* Retrieved from https://agingwithdignity.org/five-wishes/about-five-wishes.

Ahmed, N., Lobchuk, M., Hunter, M. W., Johnston, P., Nugent, Z., Sharma, A., ... Sisler, J. (2015). Perceptions and preferences of patients with terminal lung cancer and family caregivers about DNR. *Cureus, 7*(5). doi:10.7759/cureus.271

American Academy of Family Physicians (AAFP). (2013). *Adolescent health care, confidentiality.* Retrieved from http://www.aafp.org/about/policies/all/adolescent-confidentiality.html

American Association of Colleges of Nursing (AACN). (2016). *Policy brief: The changing landscape: Nursing student diversity on the rise.* Retrieved from http://www.aacn.nche.edu/government-affairs/Student-Diversity-FS.pdf

American Cancer Society. (2015). *Advance directives.* Retrieved from http://www.cancer.org/acs/groups/cid/documents/webcontent/002016-pdf.pdf

American Civil Liberties Union (ACLU) of Ohio. (2014). *Your health and the law: A guide for teens.* Retrieved from http://www.acluohio.org/wp-content/uploads/2014/06/TeenHealthGuide.pdf

American College of Obstetricians and Gynecologists (ACOG). (2014). Committee opinion: Adolescent confidentiality and electronic health records. *Committee on Adolescent Health Care, Number 599.* Retrieved from http://www.acog.org/Resources-And-Publications/Committee-Opinions/Committee-on-Adolescent-Health-Care/Adolescent-Confidentiality-and-Electronic-Health-Records

American Medical Association (AMA). (2016). *HIPAA violations and enforcement.* Retrieved from http://www.ama-assn.org/ama/pub/physician-resources/solutions-managing-your-practice/coding-billing-insurance/hipaahealth-insurance-portability-accountability-act/hipaa-violations-enforcement.page?

American Nurses Association (ANA). (2015). *American Nurses Association position statement on privacy and confidentiality.* Retrieved from http://www.nursingworld.org/DocumentVault/Position-Statements/Ethics-and-Human-Rights/Position-Statement-Privacy-and-Confidentiality.pdf

Anselmi, K. K. (2012). Nurses' personal liability vs. employer's vicarious liability. *MEDSURG Nursing, 21*(1), 45–48.

Arritt, T. (2014). Caring for patients of different religions. *Nursing Made Incredibly Easy!, 12*(6): 38-45. Retrieved from http://www.nursingcenter.com/cearticle?an=00152258-201411000-00008&JournalID=417221&Issue_ID=2603606

Benson, W. F., & Aldrich, N. (2012). Advance care planning: Ensuring your wishes are known and honored if you are unable to speak for yourself. *Critical Issue Brief, Centers for Disease Control and Prevention.* Retrieved from http://www.cdc.gov/aging/pdf/advanced-care-planning-critical-issue-brief.pdf

Bova, C., Drexler, D., & Sullivan-Bolyai, S. (2012). Reframing the influence of the Health Insurance Portability and Accountability Act on research. *Chest, 141*(3), 782–786.

Brent, N. J. (2013). *Who can give informed consent and what is the nurse's role in obtaining consent for treatment?* Retrieved from http://www.cphins.com/blog/post/who-can-give-informed-consent-and-what-is-the-nurses-role-in-obtaining-consent-for-treatment

Child Welfare Information Gateway. (2016). *Mandatory reporters of child abuse and neglect.* Washington, DC: U.S. Department of Health and Human Services, Children's Bureau.

Cole, C. A. (2012). Implied consent and nursing practice: Ethical or convenient? *Nursing Ethics, 19*(4), 550–557.

Crosby, M. A., Cheng, L., DeJesus, A. Y., Travis, E. L., & Rodriguez, M. A. (2016). Provider and patient gender influence on timing of do-not-resuscitate orders in hospitalized patients with cancer. *Journal of Palliative Medicine, 19*(7): 728–733. doi:10.1089/jpm.2015.0388

Daly, J. M., Klein, A. N., & Jogerst, G. J. (2012). Critical care nurses' perspectives on elder abuse. *Nursing in Critical Care, 17*(4), 172–179.

Falk, N. L., Baigis, J., & Kopac, C. (2012). Elder mistreatment and The Elder Justice Act. *OJIN: The Online Journal of Issues in Nursing, 17*(3). Retrieved from http://nursingworld.org/MainMenu-Categories/ANAMarketplace/ANAPeriodicals/OJIN/TableofContents/Vol-17-2012/No3-Sept-2012/Articles-Previous-Topics/Elder-Mistreatment-and-Elder-Justice-Act.html

Fischer, S. M., Sauaia, A., Min, S., & Kutner, J. (2012). Advance directive discussions: Lost in translation or lost opportunities? *Journal of Palliative Medicine, 15*(1): 86–92. doi:10.1089/jpm.2011.0328

Goodwin, K. D., Taylor, M. M., Brown, E. C., Winscott, M., Scanlon, M., Hodge, J. G., Jr., … England, B. (2012). Protecting adolescents' right to seek treatment for sexually transmitted diseases without parental consent: The Arizona experience with Senate Bill 1309. *Public Health Reports, 127*, 253–258.

Graham, R. (2014). *For pregnant women, two sets of rights in one body.* Retrieved from https://www.bostonglobe.com/ideas/2014/02/16/for-pregnant-women-two-sets-rights-one-body/5Pd6zntIViRBZ9QxhiQgFJ/story.html

Guido, G. W. (2014). *Legal and ethical issues in nursing* (6th ed.). Upper Saddle River, NJ: Pearson Education.

Guttmacher Institute. (2016a). *An overview of abortion laws.* Retrieved from https://www.guttmacher.org/state-policy/explore/overview-abortion-laws

Guttmacher Institute. (2016b). *An overview of minors' consent law.* Retrieved from http://www.guttmacher.org/statecenter/spibs/spib_OMCL.pdf

Guttmacher Institute. (2016c). *Minors' access to contraceptive services.* Retrieved from https://www.guttmacher.org/sites/default/files/state_policy_overview_files/spib_macs.pdf;

Health Resources and Services Administration of the U.S. Department of Health and Human Services (HRSA). (2014a). *National practitioner data bank: 2012 annual report.* Retrieved from http://www.npdb-hipdb.hrsa.gov/resources/annualRpt.jsp

Health Resources and Services Administration of the U.S. Department of Health and Human Services (HRSA). (2014b). *Nursing workforce diversity (NWD).* Retrieved from http://bhpr.hrsa.gov/nursing/grants/nwd.html

Herendeen, P. A., Blevins, R., Anson, E., & Smith, J. (2014). Barriers to and consequences of mandated reporting of child abuse by nurse practitioners. *Journal of Pediatric Health Care, 28(1):* e1–e7. doi:10.1016/j.pedhc.2013.06.004.

Howie, W. O., Howie, B. A., & McMullen, P. C. (2012). To assist or not assist: Good Samaritan considerations for nurse practitioners. *The Journal for Nurse Practitioners, 8*(9), 688–694. Retrieved from http://www.micnp.org/files/chapters/detroit/articles/JNP%20article%20for%20Metro%20Chapter%20Oct2012.pdf

Kable, A., Guest, M., & McLeod, M. (2012). Organizational risk management of resistance to care episodes in health facilities. *Journal of Advanced Nursing 68*(9), 1933–1943. doi:10.1111/j.1365-2648.2011.05874.x

Katner, D. R. (2012). Mandatory reporting of oral injuries indicating possible child abuse. *Journal of the American Dental Association, 143*(10), 1087–1092.

Kaufman, J., Laschat, M., & Wappler, F. (2012). Medication errors in pediatric emergencies: A systemic analysis. *Deutsches Arzteblatt International, 109*(38), 609–616. Retrieved from http://www.ncbi.nlm.nih.gov/pmc/articles/PMC3471264/

Lachman, V. D. (2014). Conscientious objection in nursing: Definition and criteria for acceptance. *MEDSURG Nursing, 23*(3), 196–198. Retrieved from http://www.nursingworld.org/MainMenu-Categories/EthicsStandards/Resources/Conscientious-Objection-in-Nursing.pdf

Lipley, N. (2012). Service failures put down to poor monitoring of patients. *Emergency Nurse, 20*(8), 5.

McGowan, C. (2012). Patients' confidentiality. *Critical Care Nurse, 32*(5), 61–64. Retrieved from http://www.aacn.org/wd/Cetests/media/C1252.pdf

Merrick, M. T., & Latzman, N. E. (2014). Child maltreatment: A public health overview and prevention considerations. *The Online Journal of Issues in Nursing, 19*(1). doi:10.3912/OJIN.VOL19No01Man02

Miljković, M. D., Emuron, D., Rhodes, L., Abraham, J., & Miller, K. (2015). "Allow natural death" versus "do not resuscitate": What do patients with advanced cancer choose? *Journal of Palliative Medicine, 18*(5), 457–460. doi:10.1089/jpm.2014.0369

Minority Nurse. (2013, March 30). *Making their wishes known.* Retrieved from http://minoritynurse.com/making-their-wishes-known/

Moore, J. D. (2015). *Consent to medical treatment for minor children: Overview of North Carolina law.* Retrieved from https://www.sog.unc.edu/sites/www.sog.unc.edu/files/course_materials/Consent%20to%20Medical%20Treatment%20for%20Minor%20Children_0.pdf

National Center on Elder Abuse (NCEA). (n.d.) *Types of abuse.* Retrieved from http://www.ncea.aoa.gov/FAQ/Type_Abuse/index.aspx

National Council of State Boards of Nursing (NCSBN). (2016a). *NCLEX & other exams.* Retrieved from https://www.ncsbn.org/NCLEX.htm

National Council of State Boards of Nursing (NCSBN). (2016b). *Nurse licensure compact: Information for new grads.* Retrieved from https://www.ncsbn.org/NLC_New_Grads.pdf

National Council of State Boards of Nursing (NCSBN). (2016c). *Recent research.* Retrieved from https://www.ncsbn.org/recent-research.htm

North Carolina Board of Nursing. (2012). *Nursing practice.* Retrieved from http://www.ncbon.com/content.aspx?id=34

Ryan, D., & Jezewski, M. A. (2012). Knowledge, attitudes, experiences, and confidence of nurses in completing advance directives: A systematic synthesis of three studies. *The Journal of Nursing Research, 20*(2), 131–140.

Sleasman, P. (2013). Damages. In *Federal practice manual for legal aid attorneys* (Chapter 9). Retrieved from http://federalpracticemanual.org/node/51

Tzeng, H. M., Yin, C. Y., & Schneider, T. E. (2013). Medication error–related issues in nursing practice. *MEDSURG Nursing, 22*(1), 13–16, 50.

Vanderbilt Kennedy Center. (2016). *Health care for adults with intellectual and developmental disabilities: Toolkit for primary care providers.* Retrieved from http://vkc.mc.vanderbilt.edu/etoolkit/general-issues/informed-consent/

Virginia Board of Nursing. (2012). *Guidance on clinical learning experiences.* Retrieved from https://www.dhp.virginia.gov/nursing/guidelines/90-21.doc

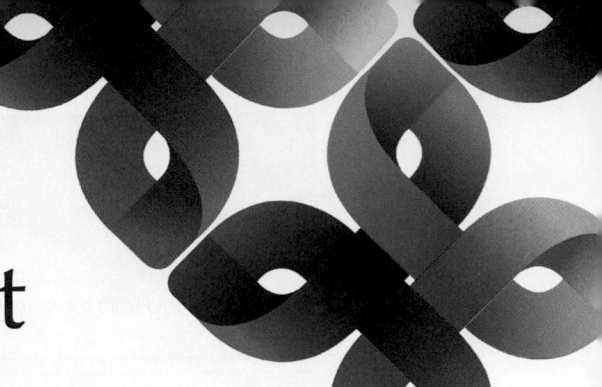

Module 50
Quality Improvement

Module Outline and Learning Outcomes

The Concept of Quality Improvement

Improving the Quality of Healthcare

50.1 Summarize the need for improving the quality of healthcare.

National Initiatives

50.2 Summarize federal, state, and local initiatives to improve healthcare.

Concepts Related to Quality Improvement

50.3 Outline the relationship between quality improvement and other concepts.

The Quality Improvement Process

50.4 Outline the quality improvement process.

Quality Management Programs

50.5 Differentiate commonly used quality management programs.

>> The Concept of Quality Improvement

Concept Key Terms

Affordable Care Act (ACA), **2858**	Continuous quality improvement (CQI), **2866**	Just culture, **2864**	Process standards, **2861**	Root cause analysis, **2862**
Audit, **2859**		Lean Six Sigma, **2867**	Quality, **2857**	Sentinel event, **2862**
Benchmarking, **2859**	External customers, **2866**	Outcome standards, **2861**	Quality assurance, **2865**	Six Sigma, **2867**
Blame-free environment, **2864**	Indicator, **2861**	Outcomes management, **2860**	Quality improvement, **2857**	Standards, **2861**
Breach of care, **2862**	Internal customers, **2866**	Peer review, **2859**	Quality management, **2857**	Structure standards, **2861**
Breach of duty, **2862**	Interprofessional assessment, **2860**	Performance improvement, **2859**	Retrospective audit, **2859**	Total quality management (TQM), **2866**
Concurrent audit, **2860**	Intraprofessional assessment, **2859**	Plan–Do–Study–Act (PDSA), **2866**	Risk management, **2862**	Utilization review, **2860**

The Institute of Medicine (IOM) (2001) has defined **quality** as "the degree to which health services for individuals and populations increase the likelihood of desired health outcomes and are consistent with current professional knowledge." In addition, high-quality care involves "providing patients with appropriate services in a technically competent manner, with good communication, shared decision making, and cultural sensitivity."

Improving the Quality of Healthcare

One way in which nurses can provide high-quality care is participating in quality improvement and quality management. **Quality improvement** consists of "systematic and continuous actions that lead to measurable improvement in healthcare services and the health status of targeted patient groups" (Health Resources and Services Administration [HRSA],

2011). **Quality management** includes evaluation of medical and nursing processes for quality and effectiveness compared to accepted standards in order to correct problems before they harm patients and to prevent errors in treatment. Quality management also aims to provide cost-effective care by preventing overuse, misuse, and underuse of medical resources.

In its report *To Err Is Human: Building a Safer Health System*, the IOM (2000) stated that medical errors account for approximately 98,000 deaths per year. Since the report's release, multiple studies have investigated the incidence of preventable medical errors. An updated study was conducted in 2011, and the estimated rates of medical errors were found to be closer to a range of 210,000–400,000 preventable deaths per year (James, 2013). This puts medical errors as the third leading cause of death. Medication errors alone are often studied, and a recent systematic review study found that overall medication error rates are occurring at a median rate of 19.6–25.6% (Keers et al., 2013).

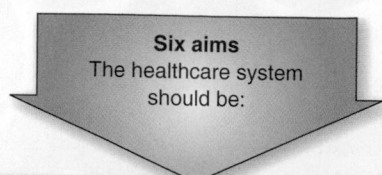

Six aims
The healthcare system should be:

Safe—avoiding injuries to patients from the care that is intended to help them

Effective—providing services based on scientific knowledge to all who could benefit and refraining from providing services to those not likely to benefit (avoiding underuse and overuse, respectively)

Patient-centered—providing care that is respectful of and responsive to individual patient preferences, needs and values and ensuring that patient values guide all clinical decisions

Timely—reducing wait time that may result in harmful delays for both those who receive and those who give care

Efficient—avoiding waste, including waste of equipment, supplies, ideas, and energy

Equitable—providing care that does not vary in quality because of personal characteristics such as gender, ethnicity, or geographic location

Figure 50–1 》 Six aims for improving the healthcare system.

In 2001, the IOM released a follow-up report entitled *Crossing the Quality Chasm: A New Health System for the 21st Century*. This report concluded that the current healthcare system was too disorganized to adequately care for individuals with multiple chronic illnesses. The report suggested that a new healthcare system should be developed that improves care, partly through the use of rapidly advancing technology. In an effort to improve the healthcare system, *Crossing the Quality Chasm* proposed six aims for improvement: The healthcare system should be safe, effective, patient-centered, timely, efficient, and equitable (**Figure 50–1 》**).

National Initiatives

Following the IOM reports, the healthcare industry began to embrace quality improvement. The need to improve patient safety and health outcomes and to implement changes to support these improvements was obvious to individuals working at every level of healthcare. State and federal governments have also contributed to initiatives aimed at improving the quality of healthcare.

Federal Initiatives

Governmental agencies such as the U.S. Department of Health and Human Services (USDHHS), physicians' groups such as the American Medical Association, and professional nursing organizations such as the American Nurses Association (ANA) have developed indicators of high-quality care and measures to document the quality of care. Three important efforts are the development of the National Database of

Nursing Quality Indicators (NDNQI), the publication of *Patient Safety and Quality: An Evidence-Based Handbook for Nurses*, and the development of National Patient Safety Goals by The Joint Commission. These programs and documents aim to collect and provide data that identify areas for improvement and encourage facilities to meet quality goals.

More recently, the Patient Protection and Affordable Care Act (PPACA), commonly known as the **Affordable Care Act (ACA)**, was passed by Congress and signed into law by President Barack Obama on March 23, 2010. This 906-page law, along with its thousands of pages of regulations, was enacted in an attempt to make healthcare affordable for all Americans. Some of these changes included expanding and reforming Medicaid and Medicare; incentives to reduce 30-day readmission rates; and incentives to reduce wasteful spending by healthcare facilities. Changes to the healthcare system that are detailed in the ACA began implementation in 2010 and may continue into 2020. However, healthcare laws are constantly changing, and the ACA may be changed significantly in the coming years.

》Stay Current: Keep abreast of the changes in healthcare and insurance laws by visiting the U.S. Department of Health & Human Services at https://www.hhs.gov/healthcare/about-the-aca/index.html and Medicaid.gov at https://www.medicaid.gov/affordable-care-act

To improve the health of the population, the USDHHS (2015) has developed the National Quality Strategy, which contains three broad aims:

- **Better Care:** Improve the overall quality by making healthcare more patient centered, reliable, accessible, and safe.
- **Healthy People/Healthy Communities:** Improve the health of the U.S. population by supporting proven interventions to address behavioral, social, and environmental determinants of health in addition to delivering higher-quality care.
- **Affordable Care:** Reduce the cost of quality healthcare for individuals, families, employers, and government.

To achieve these aims, the National Quality Strategy will focus on six priorities (**Box 50–1 》**).

State and Local Initiatives

Even with the advent of the ACA, states are partially responsible for providing state health insurance programs for low-income individuals and families. The ACA offers states the option of implementing a basic health program (BHP) for low-income adults and legal immigrants. Under the BHP, states contract with health plans and providers to provide at least the minimum essential benefits under the ACA, and the federal government helps to subsidize the program (Henry J. Kaiser Family Foundation, 2013).

Quality Initiatives

A review of the first 5 years of the ACA has found some improvements in the quality of healthcare, although it is too early to determine whether the trends will continue and whether the improvements are related to the new laws or to other initiatives that were already ongoing. Overall 30-day readmission rates for Medicare patients have declined by over 1%, and the incidence of hospital-acquired conditions is also showing a decline. Many healthcare organizations have signed up for bundled payment options, which should reduce costs, and early reports show a stabilization in healthcare expenditures (Blumenthal, Abrams, & Nuzum, 2015).

Concepts Related to Quality Improvement

Some ways in which healthcare quality can be improved include properly using advance directives, following privacy laws, and striving to reduce errors. Quality improvement uses a variety of methods to improve care, including the use of evidence-based practices and quality improvement methods adopted from industry. Quality management programs track overall patient progress on certain key indicators such as infection rates, fall rates, and incidence of pressure injuries to determine how well patients are cared for and what measures need to be taken to improve care on the unit. If new devices are used on the unit for the prevention of pressure injuries, they are tracked by the quality department to determine whether pressure injury rates decline. Patients' records are also used to track quality measures called core measures, and certain key measures are tracked to make sure patients are being discharged with the appropriate medications and follow-up for conditions such as stroke and myocardial infarction.

Safety culture is important to monitor, and many health systems use the Agency for Healthcare Quality and Research's (AHRQ) Patient Safety Culture Survey to monitor the safety culture to evaluate how staff perceive the environment and if they are comfortable reporting errors so improvements can be made. Patient-centered care is also an important area for safety. Including patients' preferences is an important area to support high-quality care. Selected concepts integral to quality improvement are outlined in the Concepts Related to Quality Improvement feature. They are presented in alphabetical order.

The Quality Improvement Process

Quality improvement is a continuous multistep, multilevel process that identifies areas for improvement based on performance and industry standards. Quality improvement involves analyzing current protocols of care and their associated outcomes, comparing those outcomes to the outcomes of leaders in high-quality care (**benchmarking**), identifying areas for improvement, researching factors that contribute to better outcomes, and implementing changes to improve outcomes. Patient outcomes must then be analyzed to determine the effectiveness of the changes and identify areas for further improvement. In addition, if a facility consistently provides a better quality of care than similar facilities do, the facility that is demonstrating excellence is responsible for documenting its methods to help improve care at other facilities. When quality improvement is directly linked to the performance of an individual, team, unit, or organization, it is called **performance improvement**.

Analysis of Current Protocols and Outcomes

To begin quality improvement, an individual, unit, or facility must understand its baseline performance records. Performance can be assessed on an intraprofessional level or an interprofessional level. In addition, it can focus on patient outcomes, cost effectiveness, resource utilization, or the integration of these aspects of care.

Intraprofessional Assessment

Intraprofessional assessment occurs within a group of individuals who have similar positions within a healthcare system, such as a group of nurses or a group of surgeons. Such an assessment is important for identifying areas of improvement at each level of care. Intraprofessional assessment includes peer reviews, audits, and outcomes management.

Peer Reviews

A **peer review** is used to professionally critique a colleague's work on the basis of predetermined standards. This allows nurses to assess other nurses in a safe, nonpunitive environment. Using this process, nurses are together able to analyze complicated cases and determine the standards by which they will collectively be held accountable. It also allows issues to be discussed by those with firsthand knowledge and produces recommendations that the nursing staff will understand and accept.

Audits

An **audit** is an examination of records to verify accuracy and proper use. An audit usually examines financial or medical records, and the audit can be for a single patient, a group of similar patients, an individual clinician, a unit, or a whole facility. If the audit is focused on one discipline (e.g., nursing), it is an intraprofessional assessment. If the audit is focused on multiple disciplines (e.g., both nurses and physicians), it becomes an interprofessional assessment.

In nursing, most audits are either retrospective or concurrent. A **retrospective audit** is performed after a patient's discharge. It compares care provided to one patient with care

Concepts Related to
Quality Improvement

CONCEPT	RELATIONSHIP TO QUALITY IMPROVEMENT	NURSING IMPLICATIONS
Ethics	Patients have the right to the best quality of care.	■ Anticipate the need to provide high-quality care to all individuals, regardless of race, gender, sexual orientation, or ability to pay for services. ■ Be aware of disparities in treatment among population groups; advocate for high-quality care for all individuals. ■ Consult with patients to determine their preferences for care; provide culturally competent care. ■ Be aware of patient preferences that are not ethical, such as refusal of lifesaving blood transfusions for a child.
Informatics	Electronic health records can be used at the point of care and can be easily transmitted to collaborating healthcare workers to improve continuity of care.	■ Accurately record a patient's medical history and results of diagnostic tests for current and future use and to share patient information with relevant healthcare providers. ■ Realize the importance of keeping all electronic and paper records up to date. ■ Provide education on the use of electronic records at the point of care. ■ Use informatics to identify areas for improvement, such as tracking healthcare-associated infections or identifying geographic locations that are without adequate healthcare resources.
Legal Issues	Consistently following federal and state laws will improve the quality of patient care.	■ Be alert to potential abusive situations; quality of care can be improved by preventing future abuse. ■ Be alert to behavior of healthcare workers (including one's self) that could increase risk of harm to patients or violate any patient's privacy; seek to counsel individuals performing reckless acts. ■ Anticipate asking patients or family members about legal documents such as living wills, healthcare proxy, preference for do not resuscitate (DNR) orders. ■ Avoid blaming healthcare workers for inadvertent mistakes that result in patient harm; instead, console the individual and provide education on how to avoid future errors. ■ Participate in efforts to improve laws and healthcare protocols and treatments.

provided to patients with similar conditions, and recommendations are made to change procedures if needed. A **concurrent audit** is performed while the patient is still undergoing care at the healthcare facility. It is used to evaluate the adequacy of the nursing care the patient is receiving and to determine whether desired outcomes are being met. This allows changes to be made, if needed, to prevent adverse events or improve the patient's care.

Outcomes Management

Outcomes management uses patient experiences to guide improvement in all areas of healthcare by providing a link between medical interventions and health outcomes and between health outcomes and cost of care. An outcomes management system implements evidence-based practices, guides case decision making, incorporates better and more efficient clinical management, and provides information to improve services (Hodges & Wotring, 2012). Outcomes management can be used both to discover areas for improvement and to analyze areas of excellence to determine factors that contribute to success or failure. In 2004, the National Institutes of Health (n.d.) began an outcomes management program called PROMIS (Patient Reported Outcomes Measurement

Information System) that collects information from patients to measure their health status in the areas of physical, mental, and social well-being. This program continues to provide clinicians with access to patient-reported information about the effectiveness of treatments and the symptoms that patients experience to help improve communication, manage chronic diseases, and design treatment plans.

Interprofessional Assessment

Patient care involves collaboration among providers in multiple disciplines. For example, a patient with obesity and type 2 diabetes who is recovering from bariatric surgery may require care from a surgeon, a physician, a nurse, and a dietitian. To collaborate effectively, these individuals must have efficient communication, coordination, and integration of care. An **interprofessional assessment** (or interdisciplinary assessment) involves more than one discipline such as nursing and physical therapy.

In addition to peer reviews, audits, and outcomes management, interprofessional assessments include utilization reviews. A **utilization review** analyzes the use of resources to identify areas of overuse, misuse, and underuse. This protects the facility from unnecessary and inappropriate use of resources. Utilization review is required by Medicaid for specific services and by The Joint Commission for facility accreditation. A utilization review may identify areas in which resources are being overused, such as urinary catheterization for incontinent patients who are ambulatory, or areas in which resources are lacking, such as inadequate staffing.

Clinical Example A

Ruth Davison is a 74-year-old woman who has been admitted to the same-day surgery center for elective right carpal tunnel repair (CTR). One hour before surgery, Mrs. Davison receives cefazolin (Ancef) 1 g IV as a prophylactic antibiotic. Anesthesia for the procedure consists of injection of local anesthetic at the surgical site with no administration of sedation.

After completion of the CTR, Mrs. Davison is stable, awake, and alert. She is monitored in the postanesthesia care unit (PACU) for 1 hour. Once she meets all discharge criteria, she is prepared for discharge to her home. Mrs. Davison's discharge instructions include keeping her surgical dressing in place for 2 days, after which time she may remove the dressing. She is further instructed to keep the dressing clean and dry while it is in place and to immediately report any drainage noted on the dressing. Mrs. Davison also is instructed to immediately report any redness, drainage, or swelling noted at her incision site following dressing removal. She is further advised that her sutures are absorbable and, thus, do not need to be removed. After verbalizing understanding of her discharge instructions and signing the discharge record, Mrs. Davison is transported to her home by her daughter.

The following morning, the same-day surgery center receives a phone call from Mrs. Davison, who reports that she has removed her dressing and now notes "a little" bleeding and redness at her incision site. After reviewing Mrs. Davison's discharge record, the nurse reminds Mrs. Davison that her instructions included leaving her dressing in place for 2 days. Mrs. Davison states that she does not recall being told to leave her dressing intact for 2 days and asks, "How was I supposed to be able to tell if the wound looked okay with the dressing covering it?" She further notes that she is concerned that her surgical wound may be infected.

Mrs. Davison is scheduled for a follow-up appointment with her surgeon that afternoon. At her follow-up appointment, Mrs. Davison's wound is evaluated and cleansed, and a dressing is reapplied. Her surgeon instructs Mrs. Davison to return to his office in 3 days, at which time her dressing will be removed and her wound will be reevaluated for signs and symptoms of infection.

As a result of Mrs. Davison's apparent misunderstanding of her discharge instructions and subsequent need for two additional appointments with her physician, an intraprofessional assessment is initiated. Two registered nurses who provided care to Mrs. Davison, two additional registered nurses, and the nurse manager review Mrs. Davison's case. They compare Mrs. Davison's case to the cases of patients of similar age, cultural background, and surgical procedure. The nurse manager also follows up with Mrs. Davison to hear her perspective on the care she received, her understanding of the discharge instructions, the symptoms she experienced, and her overall satisfaction with her care.

Critical Thinking Questions

1. Identify the portions of the intraprofessional assessment that reflect peer review, auditing, and outcomes management.
2. Why is it important to compare Mrs. Davison's care with care received by other patients who correctly followed discharge instructions?
3. Describe the impact that a patient's perspective can have on quality improvement.

Benchmarking

Benchmarking is a method that is used to compare the performance of an individual or organization to industry standards. **Standards** of care are based on established models of high-quality performance and may reflect the performance of industry leaders, scientific or clinical research, or recommendations of professional organizations such as the ANA. These standards are continually being updated, so nurses must use research and other reliable sources of information to stay up to date on current recommendations and standards.

The Donabedian model of quality improvement (originally developed by physician and researcher Avedis Donabedian) states that standards usually relate to three dimensions of high-quality care: structure, process, and outcome. **Structure standards** relate to material resources, human resources, and general organizational structure. They focus on the organization's capacity and systems for providing care. **Process standards** focus on the steps used to lead to a particular outcome. They are used to determine whether a set of steps exists and whether those steps are being followed. **Outcome standards** focus on the performance of a process, such as the number of bedridden patients who develop a pressure injury (Joint Commission Resources, 2012).

Benchmarking uses **indicators**, or statistics, that reflect the organization's performance in a specific area, to compare the quality of care within the organization to industry standards. Indicators must be measurable, objective, and sensitive to changes in performance. Indicators can include generic or specific standards of care as stated by the ANA, specialty organizations, or the organization or unit implementing quality improvement strategies.

For example, a nursing unit decides to evaluate the quality of the care provided to newly admitted patients. The unit determines that the indicators for the study will be a completed initial assessment within 1 hour of admission, a documented and accurate nursing plan of care by the end of the shift, and accurate implementation of physicians' orders. The indicators are then compared against each newly admitted patient's medical records to benchmark the frequency with which the indicators were met. The nurses on the unit will be informed if the study indicates that the nursing care provided does not comply with the standards for the unit.

Targeting Areas for Improvement

Once the current level of performance has been compared with industry standards, areas that need improvement can be identified. On the basis of the policies and procedures already in place, each healthcare facility will have different areas in need of improvement. These may reflect general practices such as use of a specific ointment for wounds or specific practices such as frequency of checking vital signs on older patients after pacemaker implantation. They may be identified on the basis of a bad outcome for one patient or a trend of poor outcomes for multiple patients. Some areas needing improvement are identified as a result of a required investigation after adverse events such as sentinel events and breach of care. Risk management can also be used to identify risk factors and develop associated protocols for reducing or preventing adverse events.

Sentinel Events

The Joint Commission (2013) has defined a **sentinel event** as "an unexpected occurrence involving death or serious physical or psychologic injury, or the risk thereof. Serious injury specifically includes loss of limb or function. The phrase 'the risk thereof' includes any process variation for which a recurrence would carry a significant chance of a serious adverse outcome." Sentinel events require immediate investigation and response. In an effort to continuously improve the safety and quality of healthcare provided to the public, The Joint Commission reviews a facility's response to sentinel events as part of its accreditation process. The goals of the sentinel event policy are to have a positive impact on patient care, prevent sentinel events, understand the factors that contributed to the event, increase the general knowledge about sentinel events, and maintain the confidence of the public in accredited organizations.

If a sentinel event occurs, accredited organizations are expected to respond appropriately, including conducting a credible **root cause analysis** (problem solving to identify the root cause of faults), developing a plan to reduce future risk of sentinel events, implementing improvements, and monitoring the effectiveness of improvements (The Joint Commission, 2013). In addition, The Joint Commission conducts reviews for a specific subset of sentinel events, including the following:

- Unanticipated death or major permanent loss not associated with the patient's original illness
- Invasive procedures on the wrong patient, at the wrong site, or with the wrong procedure
- Unintended retention of a foreign object in a patient after surgery
- Radiation overdose or delivery of radiation to the wrong body region
- Administration of an incompatible blood transfusion
- Abduction, rape, assault, homicide, or suicide of any patient or staff member while at the healthcare facility or suicide within 72 hours of discharge
- Unanticipated death of a full-term infant
- Discharge of an infant to the wrong family.

Breach of Care

A **breach of care** or **breach of duty** occurs when a nurse deviates from the standard of care. Guido (2014) states that this occurs when the nurse does something that should not have been done (e.g., gives the incorrect medication) or does not do something that should have been done (e.g., fails to administer a scheduled medication). Thirty years ago, malpractice suits involving nurses were rare; in recent years, they represented about 5% of the medical malpractice payment reports (HRSA, 2013). These suits are usually related to deficits in treatment and care management, assessment, monitoring, professional conduct, and medication administration (in order of frequency). An analysis of closed cases revealed nurses failing to identify a worsening pressure injury or failing to contact a physician for additional treatment in the assessment category. In the monitoring category, failure to monitor vital signs in postoperative patients was found. The medication administration category has seen a reduction in number of incidents, but those that have occurred are more severe (Nurses Service Organization, 2015).

Quality improvement efforts seek to determine weaknesses in procedures and processes as well as organizational issues that can affect nurses' ability to provide nursing care consistent with established professional standards of care. Nurses can reduce the risk of committing a breach of care by reporting problems to nursing supervisors, remaining current in their skills and education, basing all care on the nursing process model, and documenting care provided as well as the patient's response to interventions (Guido, 2014). Following these procedures reduces the risk of an adverse event and resulting malpractice suit.

Risk Management

Risk management is "the process by which vulnerabilities are identified and changes are made to minimize the consequences of adverse patient outcomes and liability" (Raso & Gulinello, 2010, p. 26). Risk management includes both proactive components to prevent adverse events and reactive components to minimize damage from adverse events. Risk assessment must occur daily, and all individuals must be dedicated to keeping patients safe from harm.

The risk management process identifies risks that may lead to patient or staff injury or financial loss; reviews systems that monitor risks, such as patient questionnaires or incident reports; analyzes the frequency, severity, and cause of past adverse events; analyzes new procedures with potential risk to patients; stays up to date on current laws pertaining to healthcare; and identifies the need for patient and staff education. Using this information, the risk management team can identify areas of risk and implement strategies to reduce risk as much as possible.

Because of their close contact with patients, nurses are perfectly positioned to analyze patient satisfaction, identify specific patient risks, and implement strategies at the bedside to reduce patient risk of an adverse event. Patient satisfaction is a key factor in risk management, because a dissatisfied patient presents a higher risk for liability than a satisfied patient. A nurse who becomes aware of patient dissatisfaction should take steps to communicate with the patient to clarify misunderstandings, advocate for the patient to receive better care, and notify a supervisor about potential problems. Personal care by a nurse and a nurse manager can calm a patient or the patient's family, identify problems before they become an emergency, and improve the quality of care. (For more information, see the exemplar on Risk Management in the module on Legal Issues.)

Clinical Example B

At an extended care facility, Reuben Meyers, an 84-year-old man with Alzheimer disease, was discovered to be missing from his bed at 2:15 a.m. A search resulted in finding Mr. Meyers lying in the street, the victim of a hit-and-run motor vehicle accident. He was unconscious when he was found, and a physical assessment identified a right hip injury, which later was revealed to be a fractured right hip. He also had a 2-inch-long open gash in the right temporal region of his head. After closure of his head wound and surgical repair of his hip, Mr. Meyers remained unconscious until his death 12 days later. An investigation found that security cameras had recorded Mr. Meyers wandering from the extended care facility at 1:30 a.m. Traffic cameras recorded the hit-and-run accident at 2:08 a.m.

Critical Thinking Questions

1. On the basis of the limited description of this sentinel event, what standards of nursing care may have been breached?
2. What potential legal ramifications may this event have for the nurses who were caring for Mr. Meyers and for the nursing home facility?
3. Develop a risk management program to identify risks for similar sentinel events, and propose strategies to improve the quality of care and reduce the risk of wandering outdoors for patients with Alzheimer disease.

Identifying Factors That Promote Better Outcomes

Identification of problem areas or adverse events demands intervention to improve patient safety. This involves a planning process that identifies the cause of adverse events through a root cause analysis and researches the literature for methods of improvement. Nurses can participate with a team of other clinicians to plan the changes needed to improve the quality of care. Organizations such as The Joint Commission identify patient safety goals every year for organizations to focus on. The 2017 goals include ensuring patients are identified safely (e.g., right patient; see the module on Safety), improving staff communication (see the module on Communication), using alarms safely, and preventing infections (see the module on Infection) (The Joint Commission, n.d.). Nursing has a role in impacting all of these goals to promote better patient outcomes. Additional factors that promote better outcomes are summarized next.

Root Cause Analysis

A root cause analysis is required by The Joint Commission for sentinel events and is recommended for any adverse event. The goals of the root cause analysis are to identify the reasons for failures or problems and to develop an action plan for improvement to decrease the likelihood of future adverse events. This analysis focuses on systems and processes, not on individual performance, and it analyzes both special causes (factors that cause variation beyond what is normal) and common causes (factors that occur because of normal variation in the system). The action plan should include identification of who is responsible for implementing and overseeing improvements, pilot testing to ensure the success of the changes, timelines for implementing changes, and strategies for measuring the effectiveness of changes (The Joint Commission, 2013).

Reducing Medication Errors

The National Coordinating Council for Medication Error Reporting and Prevention (n.d.) defines a medication error as "any preventable event that may cause or lead to inappropriate medication use or patient harm while the medication is in the control of the healthcare professional, patient, or consumer." An adverse drug event (ADE) is defined as harm experienced by a patient as a result of exposure to a medication. Not all ADEs are the result of a medication error, but about half of ADEs are preventable. One of the highest-risk drugs used in the inpatient setting is anticoagulant intravenous

Box 50–2
Methods to Reduce Medication Errors

Nurses can implement several methods to reduce medication errors, including the following:

- Double check the "seven rights" *every time* medication is administered: right assessment, right individual, right medication, right dose, right time, right route, and right documentation.
- Have a second nurse check the medication order.
- Check known allergies before administering medication to a patient.
- Avoid disruptions and distractions during medication administration duties.
- Verify tubing placement (e.g., IV, chest, NG) before administering drugs or nutrition.
- Document and understand the interactions among *all* medications a patient is taking, including over-the-counter medicines, herbal remedies, and nutritional supplements.
- Do not combine medications with the same active ingredient.
- Always check a child's weight before medication administration to ensure correct dosing.
- Consult with the prescriber of the patient's medication and possibly a pharmacist if unsure about a medication order.
- Maintain a current resource to reference for drugs that are not familiar.
- Provide thorough education to patients about the use of all medications.
- Conduct medication reconciliation at every transition in care.
- Use smart infusion pumps for intravenous medications.

heparin. The Institute for Safe Medication Practice (ISMP) maintains a list of high alert medications such as look-alike, sound-alike medications to assist clinicians with identifying medications that can either look similar or have similar names, but that have very different chemical properties that can cause harm to the patient if the medications are mixed up. Another group of high-alert medications are medications that can cause problems in older adults, such as benzodiazepines and oral antidiabetic agents (AHRQ, 2015b).

Several national- and facility-implemented interventions have been designed to decrease medication errors, including barcoding both patients' identification bands and medications, regulating similar names of drugs that may cause confusion, and using a computerized physician order entry system. Many other interventions specifically help nurses prevent medication errors (**Box 50–2 »**).

Staffing Practices in Nursing

Multiple studies have established a link between decreased nurse staffing and adverse patient outcomes. One consideration of nurse staffing is the nurse-to-patient ratio (quantity). One systematic review found that an increased number of nursing hours was associated with reduced inpatient mortality (Shekelle, 2013). Readmission rates are also improved with better staffing. A study of Medicare patients from California, New Jersey, and Pennsylvania found that readmission rates in patients with heart failure, pneumonia, and myocardial infarction increased when nursing workload increased (McHugh & Ma, 2013). Nursing skill is also a critical factor related to patient outcomes (quality). One

Box 50–3
Nursing-Sensitive Indicators

Nursing-sensitive indicators reflect the quantity and quality of nursing care in the areas of structure, process, and outcome (Jones, 2016; NDNQI, n.d.).

Structure	Process	Outcome
■ Nursing hours per patient day ■ Nursing turnover ■ RN education/certification ■ Nursing skill mix (RN, LPN/LVN, UAP, agency staff)	■ Pain assessment, intervention, reassessment (AIR) cycles completed ■ Peripheral intravenous infiltration rate ■ RN job satisfaction ■ RN Practice Environment Scale (PES)	■ Healthcare-associated infections (e.g., catheter-associated UTI, central line–associated bloodstream infections, ventilator-associated pneumonia) ■ Patient falls (with or without injury and injury level) ■ Pressure injury rate (community-, hospital-, or unit-acquired) ■ Psychiatric physical or sexual assault ■ Physical restraint prevalence ■ Patient satisfaction

study found that an increase in the ratio of LPN hours to total nursing hours was associated with an increase in mortality and sepsis in trauma patients (Glance et al., 2012). Nursing-sensitive indicators are measured by many healthcare systems as part of the NDNQI. The NDNQI was established by the ANA in 2007 to evaluate linkages between staffing and quality of care (Montalvo, 2007). The original database was managed by the University of Kansas; however, in 2014 the database was sold to Press Ganey, a leader in the industry of performance measurement, including patient care satisfaction (ANA, 2014). Currently Press Ganey has combined the NDNQI with patient experience and nurse engagement to provide nursing (Press Ganey, n.d.) and other leaders with a comprehensive set of quality data that allow them to gain insights into where there are areas that need improvement and where things are going well. The NDNQI indicators are listed in **Box 50–3 》**.

Resource Utilization

The value of healthcare can be increased by reducing costs while maintaining or improving the quality of care. This can be accomplished by implementing measures to reduce waste that may result from unnecessary or inefficient services, prices that are too high, excess administrative costs, missed prevention opportunities, and medical fraud (IOM, 2010). Examples of waste that are directly applicable to nurses include medical errors that result in prolonged inpatient days, scheduling an additional visit for patient education only, and lost time because of unorganized supplies, poorly maintained equipment, or inadequate documentation.

Blame-free Environment

According to the IOM's report *To Err Is Human* (2000), most errors in healthcare are a result of the healthcare system and not the fault of any single individual. If a clinician is afraid to report errors for fear of punishment or because reporting does not result in positive change, then problems within the system cannot be identified and addressed. Therefore, a key component in quality improvement is establishing a **blame-free environment** in which healthcare providers can report errors or near misses without the fear of punishment (AHRQ, 2012). This helps identify problems so corrections

can be made and future adverse events can be prevented. The Evidence-Based Practice feature discusses methods for reducing errors and increasing the reporting of errors.

Just Culture

One difficulty in establishing a blame-free environment is that whereas many errors are a result of the healthcare system, some errors are the result of personal mistakes and demand accountability. **Just culture** attempts to balance the blame-free environment with appropriate accountability by focusing on correcting problems that lead individuals to engage in unsafe behavior while maintaining individual accountability by establishing zero tolerance for reckless behavior (AHRQ, 2012). Just culture differentiates among human error, at-risk behavior, and reckless behavior, in contrast to the "no blame" approach of the blame-free environment. Just culture is based on the understanding that errors are often the result of system failures rather than human failures. It recognizes that an atmosphere of punishment impedes error prevention by promoting intimidation and secrecy rather than shared accountability. Just culture focuses on the system rather than the individual while still maintaining an environment of individual accountability for both front-line staff and leaders and managers. This is critical; when front-line staff fail to report safety errors because of a fear of suspension or termination, healthcare managers may develop an inaccurate understanding of the care provided by the organization. This hampers ongoing quality improvement efforts, further risking patient safety (Dekker & Breakey, 2016). Successfully establishing an environment of just culture requires that leadership encourage proactive system management as well as individual accountability. It also requires that employees consider themselves stakeholders and act to establish and maintain the just culture environment. Just culture does not, however, accept or tolerate gross misconduct (e.g., employees working under the influence of alcohol or narcotics) or conscious disregard of patient and staff safety.

In a just culture environment, each member has the responsibility to take action to prevent errors and also to respond to errors, recognizing that errors are more often the result of system failures than individual error, and that when individual

Evidence-Based Practice

Methods to Reduce Errors

Problem

The most effective way to identify and correct problems in health-care is by consistently reporting errors and potential errors/near misses so that they can be learned from. However, studies indicate that safety climate and safety culture and clinician willingness to report errors are linked (Weaver et al., 2013).

Evidence

One method to reduce medical errors is to eliminate barriers to error reporting. The primary reasons that healthcare workers do not report errors are the fear of being blamed and the fear of being punished (Gorini, Miglioretti, & Pravettoni, 2012). Other reasons include increased time associated with paperwork, a fear of lawsuits, self-perceptions of incompetence, embarrassment or guilt about the mistake, reluctance to incriminate other providers, lack of knowledge about what constitutes an error or how to report errors, and lack of feedback when errors are reported (Hartnell et al., 2012). In addition, many clinicians do not realize that near misses and errors that do not cause harm should also be reported.

Another method to reduce medical errors is to improve the nurses' work environment. The American Association of Critical Care Nurses (AACN) has established six standards for a healthy work environment: skilled communication, true collaboration, effective decision making, appropriate staffing, meaningful recognition, and authentic leadership (AACN, n.d.). In addition, fostering a safety culture can lead to decreased errors and increased reporting. A recent systematic review of interventions to promote safety cultures found that a combination of interventions such as patient safety rounds, implementation of best care practices, teamwork interventions, and continuous learning improves patient safety and quality (Weaver et al., 2013).

Implications

Eliminating barriers to error reporting and establishing a healthy work environment can lead to reduced errors and increased reporting of errors. However, changing from the current culture of blame to a safety culture will require time and dedication from the entire organization. As individuals on the front line of patient care, nurses play a critical role in the establishment of a safety culture by helping to identify problems and by working to implement changes to practice that will reduce errors. Education about a blame-free environment and taking personal responsibility to report errors are two ways in which nurses can contribute to quality improvement in healthcare.

Critical Thinking Application

1. Consider situations in which you, a fellow nurse, or a physician makes medication errors that do not result in patient harm. In which situations would you complete an error report? Why?

2. Identify personal barriers that would prevent you from reporting a medical error caused by the system, a coworker, or yourself.

3. Research the current error reporting systems in place at a local hospital, nursing home, and primary care clinic.

---

error does occur, it is more likely to be accidental than willful or neglectful. For example, if the hospital pharmacy dispenses the wrong medication or the wrong dosage or if the department in charge of stocking supplies for a unit fails to make an appropriate inventory and orders an inadequate amount of supplies, those errors may result from inadequate systems as much as from individual carelessness.

As more organizations begin to embrace just culture, front-line staff are likely to feel more support from management in critical areas, including staffing. From time to time, however, nurses and other front-line staff may find themselves in situations in which management is unresponsive to suggestions for improvement or reporting of critical shortages or potential for errors related to patient safety. In these cases, staff may find themselves in the awkward position of needing to report these problems outside the agency.

Personal Responsibility

All nurses must be involved in quality improvement. The nursing student demonstrates concern for quality by making a commitment never to perform an act that the student is uncertain how to perform, by showing accountability for his or her actions, and by admitting to errors if they occur. Each nurse, whether a nursing student or a practicing nurse, has the responsibility to know the policies and procedures in the facility where clinical training is performed and to follow them exactly. In addition, nurses are responsible for understanding how to report errors, including paperwork that should be completed and individuals to whom errors should be reported.

Implementation of New Protocols

When a problem has been identified and a plan has been put in place to improve the quality of care, that plan must be implemented. The most important step in implementing new procedures is educating nurses and other clinicians about the importance of the new process, the steps involved, and associated reporting procedures. Education can take place in large or small groups, as a self-study, or during orientation. Each individual must then take personal responsibility to implement the needed changes to improve the quality of care.

Evaluation of Efficacy of New Protocols

Finally, the implemented changes must be evaluated to assess their impact on patient care, patient outcomes, patient and clinician satisfaction, and resource utilization. Data related to the original problem must be collected and are then analyzed on the basis of the benchmark standards to determine whether standards are being met. This process is called **quality assurance**. If standards are not met, the quality improvement is continued with the goal of achieving the desired goals.

Quality Management Programs

The process of quality improvement is accomplished through use of a quality management program. A quality management program must include both information about current practices and outcomes and accountability for the individuals who oversee and perform patient care. Advances in technology are vital to quality management, because clinical information systems (see the module on Informatics) can be used to track patient outcomes and actions that led to patient harm. For example, data from a clinical information system can be used to track the occurrence of healthcare-associated infections, including the location of the infection (e.g., urinary system, respiratory system, skin), frequency of patient assessment, materials used to treat the patient, and other relevant factors. Changes in hand hygiene protocols, equipment and medical supplies used, wound care protocols, and patient placement can then be implemented to reduce the incidence of healthcare-associated infections. To be successful, these changes must then be accepted and used by the entire staff.

Healthcare organizations use different quality management programs depending on their clientele and specialty area. Commonly used quality management programs include total quality management, continuous quality improvement, Six Sigma, and Lean Six Sigma. Each of these programs includes a comprehensive quality management plan.

Comprehensive Quality Management

A quality management plan is used to help healthcare facilities integrate new programs, models, and technologies with the primary care services that are already in place. The plan should address needs of engagement (improving the experience of care), population health, and value (per capita costs). The plan should be comprehensive, looking at quality and safety in clinical, managerial, administrative, and facility-related aspects of the organization. It should design, implement, monitor, and improve methods to increase the quality of care in keeping with the organization's mission and core values. Most organizations will develop quality management plans that require cooperation between departments as well as unit-specific plans.

Quality management plans should be patient focused, collecting and evaluating data for improvement of patient outcomes, expectations, and satisfaction. Patient satisfaction surveys can be used to track the effectiveness of changes from the patient's perspective. Nurses often perform this follow-up through personal visits, forms, or phone calls. If any problems are noted, the nurse can then report back to the healthcare provider or nurse manager to help improve patient care.

Total Quality Management

Total quality management (TQM), a comprehensive management philosophy that was invented by Walter Shewhart and made famous by W. Edwards Deming, is used to improve quality and productivity by using data and statistics to improve systems processes. The hallmark of TQM is that it involves teamwork throughout the organization, involving all departments and employees and including both suppliers and customers. Its essential elements include communication, feedback, fact-based decision making, and a focus on continual improvement.

A system of quality improvement most often associated with TQM is Deming's **Plan–Do–Study–Act (PDSA, Figure 50–2 ≫)**, which was modified from Shewhart's Plan–Do–

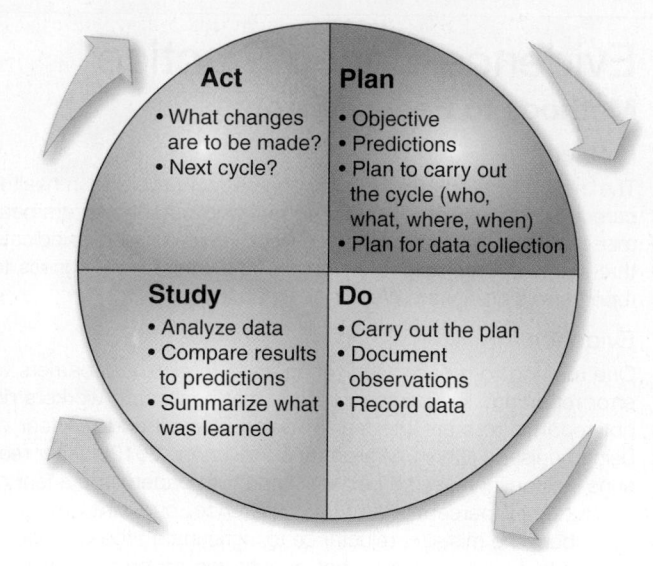

Figure 50–2 ≫ PDSA cycle.

Check–Act or Plan–Do–Check–Adjust (PDCA). During planning, individuals on the TQM team define the goal, collect data, and outline a strategy to reach the goal. In the Do phase, the plan is implemented on a small scale to determine whether it will be effective. This is followed by the Study phase, in which the outcomes of the Do phase are analyzed and compared to the expected outcomes. In the Act phase, the team must decide whether the goal was met, plan further changes, and decide whether the original goal is attainable based on the results of the previous interventions. If the goal was met, then the team must decide whether the changes should be implemented throughout the organization.

Continuous Quality Improvement

In healthcare, **continuous quality improvement (CQI)** is defined as "a structured organizational process for involving personnel in planning and executing a continuous flow of improvements to provide quality health care that meets or exceeds expectations" (Sollecito & Johnson, 2013, p. 4). CQI can be applied to a specific problem, development and implementation of policies and procedures, resource utilization, or implementation of evidence-based practices.

CQI is a customer-driven process. In healthcare, the customer can be internal or external to the system. **Internal customers** include employees of a healthcare organization, such as nurses, physicians, therapists, medical record staff, billing specialists, and other employees. **External customers** include the individuals who seek healthcare as well as their family members and significant others. External customers also include other individuals and entities with whom internal patients interact, such as insurance companies, managed care organizations, equipment or material suppliers, social service agencies, and law enforcement officials. Customer satisfaction is the end goal of CQI. CQI is also system focused, emphasizing system errors rather than individual errors. Therefore, CQI requires involvement by everyone with knowledge of the system, from senior management to individuals providing everyday care to patients (Sollecito & Johnson, 2013).

Clinical Example C

An unidentified middle-aged woman is transported to the emergency department (ED) by two law enforcement officers. The officers report that the individual was observed "wandering around on a highway" and that complaints were received from passing motorists about the woman's behavior. The officers also report that, upon their arrival, the woman was unable to provide any identification, nor was she verbally responsive to their questions. She did, however, willingly seat herself in their squad car upon request. The officers state that the woman is being transferred to the ED for evaluation, as they are uncertain about the etiology of her behaviors.

Lynne Bryten, RN, is the ED triage nurse. The unidentified woman, who is clutching a doll, appears to be awake and alert. She is clean and dressed appropriately, and her tennis shoes appear to be relatively new. Ms. Bryten attempts to perform an initial interview, but the woman does not respond to her questions. She permits Ms. Bryten to assess her vital signs, all of which are within normal limits. She exhibits no apparent indications of traumatic injury, and her pupils are equal and responsive to light. Although the woman is not verbally responsive to Ms. Bryten's questions, she appears to follow directions during the assessment. The woman is admitted to the ED as an unidentified patient. Ms. Bryten escorts the patient and the law enforcement officers into the ED and notifies the ED physician of their arrival.

Dr. Terrence Garvinner, the attending ED physician, receives Ms. Bryten's report. Upon entering the patient's room, he introduces himself and performs a brief patient assessment. The patient remains verbally unresponsive, but she follows Dr. Garvinner's directions. Afterward, Dr. Garvinner asks the law enforcement officers to speak with him privately. They accompany him to an empty ED room.

Dr. Garvinner informs the law enforcement officers that the patient does not appear to have any physical injury; rather, she may be developmentally delayed. He suggests that the officers check missing person reports and contact residential treatment centers to determine whether or not the patient may have wandered away from one of the local residential care centers. Dr. Garvinner questions the officers as to why they did not use this approach initially. One of the officers responds, "We have no way of knowing if she has a medical problem. That's why we brought her here. Plus, we have other calls coming in—we're swamped." Dr. Garvinner responds, "We have no way of identifying this woman. She appears to be a vulnerable adult who may be lost. We have a full waiting room, but we don't have staff available to serve as detectives. I believe you have an entire department dedicated to performing detective work."

Critical Thinking Questions

1. Identify the internal and external customers in this scenario.
2. Summarize the conflict between the law enforcement officers and the ED physician. Is either argument correct? Why or why not?
3. In the context of healthcare, how can conflict between internal and external customers affect the patient who is seeking treatment or in need of assistance?
4. What additional external customers may be helpful in identifying the patient and assisting with her safe return to her residence?
5. How might the process of quality management be applied to address and manage future situations such as the one described in the scenario?

Six Sigma

Six Sigma is a quality improvement program that was originally implemented by Motorola and General Electric to reduce variation within a process to produce a near-perfect product. Sigma is a Greek letter often used to measure deviation from a standard; to receive a sigma level of 6, only 3.4 products per million are allowed to be defective. In this system, a defect is defined as anything that could lead to patient dissatisfaction. Defects in healthcare could range from relatively minor problems such as providing the wrong size gown to a patient to major problems such as performing an amputation on the wrong limb. Six Sigma primarily uses the **DMAIC** system to improve outcomes (Mason, Nicolay, & Darzi, 2015):

Define the problem, determine a goal, and form a team to address the problem.

Measure: Obtain data related to the current process, the problem, and the desired goal.

Analyze: Look at the data to determine cause-and-effect relationships related to the problem.

Improve: Develop solutions to problems and implement those solutions.

Control: Implement measures to sustain positive changes and continuously monitor the process to ensure goals are being met.

Six Sigma may also use the DMADV methodology: Define, Measure, Analyze, Design, and Verify.

Six Sigma uses teams of individuals with intimate knowledge of the problem and training in Six Sigma principles. Master Black Belts are experts in Six Sigma who can assist in data calculations and function as a resource for the team. The team is led by a Black Belt with extensive knowledge of Six Sigma. Green Belts are team members with some experience with Six Sigma, and Yellow and White Belts are relatively new to the Six Sigma system. Six Sigma is most successful when the entire organization, including both administrators and clinicians, is involved in planning and implementing changes.

Multiple studies have illustrated the success of the Six Sigma system in healthcare. In one study, a 92.6% rate of hyponatremia for postoperative kidney transplantation patients was improved to a 92.2% rate of normal serum sodium levels after application of Six Sigma principles (Leaphart et al., 2012). In another study, implementation of Six Sigma principles decreased patient transfer times from general medical floors to a critical care area by almost 60%, resulting in increased customer satisfaction, improved utilization of resources, a decreased risk of adverse events, and better economic profit (Silich et al., 2012).

Lean Six Sigma

Lean Six Sigma combines the strategies of Six Sigma, described above, with the Lean system. The objective of the Lean system is to eliminate waste to maximize value. Waste is defined as anything that does not bring value to the customer. Therefore, Lean Six Sigma is a methodology used to reduce waste and provide consistency in the quality of care. It primarily uses the DMAIC system that is used in Six Sigma.

REVIEW The Concept of Quality Improvement

RELATE Link the Concepts

Linking the concept of quality improvement with the concept of collaboration:

1. How can the nurse use conflict management skills to resolve patient or family member dissatisfaction with care?

2. How does strong interprofessional team communication improve the outcomes of total quality management?

Linking the concept of quality improvement with the concept of managing care:

3. How does an effective quality improvement process reduce the cost of care?

4. How does proper care coordination improve the quality of care provided to patients?

REFER Go to Pearson MyLab Nursing and eText

■ Additional review materials

REFLECT Apply Your Knowledge

Jose Hernandez is a newly graduated nurse who has successfully passed the NCLEX-RN and has accepted a job working on a busy genitourinary unit in the local community hospital. During orientation, he is working the evening shift with a preceptor. On this particular evening, the unit has been very busy, and the charge nurse asks Jose's preceptor, Fred McFarlane, to take a few patients in addition to acting as a preceptor for Jose with his assigned patients. Fred agrees and instructs Jose to seek him out if he needs help or has any questions.

Quite by chance, Jose notices that Fred makes a medication error when he fails to administer an ordered medication at an appropriate time to one of Fred's assigned patients. Jose doesn't say anything because Fred acknowledges the error independently, but Jose isn't sure what to do at the end of the shift when he realizes that Fred is not going to fill out an incident report.

1. Should an incident report be filled out regarding Fred's late administration of a medication to the patient if no harm resulted? Explain the rationale for your answer.

2. Who is responsible for completing an incident report if one is required? Explain.

3. What is Jose's responsibility related to the error if he had no care responsibility related to the patient who received the medication later than ordered?

4. How would you handle this situation if you were Jose?

References

Agency for Healthcare Research and Quality (AHRQ). (2012). *Safety culture.* Retrieved from http://psnet.ahrq.gov/primer. aspx?primerID=5

Agency for Healthcare Research and Quality (AHRQ). (2015a). *2015 national healthcare quality and disparities report and 5th anniversary update on the national quality strategy.* Retrieved from http://www.ahrq.gov/research/findings/nhqrdr/nhqdr15/index.html

Agency for Healthcare Research and Quality (AHRQ). (2015b). *Medication errors.* Retrieved from https://psnet.ahrq.gov/primers/primer/23/medication-errors

American Nurses Association (ANA). (2014). NDNQI changes hands. *The American Nurse.* Retrieved from http://www.theamericannurse.org/2014/09/02/ndnqi-changes-hands/

American Association of Critical Care Nurses (AACN). (n.d.). *Is your work environment healthy?* Retrieved from https://www.aacn.org/nursing-excellence/healthy-work-environments

Blumenthal, D., Abrams, M., & Nuzum, R. (2015). The Affordable Care Act at 5 years. *New England Journal of Medicine, 372*(25), 2451–2458.

Dekker, S. W., & Breakey, H. (2016). "Just culture": Improving safety by achieving substantive, procedural and restorative justice. *Safety Science, 85,* 187–193.

Glance, L. G., Dick, A. W., Osler, T. M., Mukamel, D. B., Li, Y., & Stone, P. W. (2012). The association between nurse staffing and hospital outcomes in injured patients. *BMC Health Services Research, 12,* 247. doi:10.1186/1472-6963-12-247

Gorini, A., Miglioretti, M., & Pravettoni, G. (2012). A new perspective on blame culture: An experimental study. *Journal of Evaluation in Clinical Practice, 18*(3), 671–675. doi:10.1111/j.1365-2753.2012.01831.x

Guido, G. W. (2014). *Legal and ethical issues in nursing* (6th ed.). Hoboken, NJ: Pearson Education.

Hartnell, N., MacKinnon, N., Sketris, I., & Fleming, M. (2012). Identifying, understanding and overcoming barriers to medication error reporting in hospitals: a focus group study. *BMJ Quality & Safety, 21*(5), 361–368.

Health Resources and Services Administration (HRSA). (2011). *Quality improvement.* Retrieved from http://www.hrsa.gov/quality/toolbox/508pdfs/qualityimprovement.pdf

Health Resources and Services Administration (HRSA). (2013). *National Practitioner Data Bank: 2011 annual report.* Retrieved from http://www.npdb-hipdb.hrsa.gov/resources/reports/2011NPDBAnnualReport.pdf

Henry J. Kaiser Family Foundation. (2013). *Key facts about healthcare reform.* Retrieved from http://kff.org/health-reform/fact-sheet/summary-of-the-affordable-care-act/

Hodges, K., & Wotring, J. R. (2012). Outcomes management: Incorporating and sustaining processes critical to using outcome data to guide practical improvement. *Journal of Behavioral Health Services & Research, 39*(2), 130–143. doi:10.1007/s11414-011-9262-y

Institute of Medicine (IOM). (2000). *To err is human: Building a safer health system.* Washington, DC: National Academies Press.

Institute of Medicine (IOM). (2001). *Crossing the quality chasm: A new health system for the 21st century.* Washington, DC: National Academies Press.

Institute of Medicine (IOM). (2010). *The healthcare imperative: Lowering costs and improving outcomes.* Washington, DC: National Academies Press.

James, J. T. (2013). A new, evidence-based estimate of patient harms associated with hospital care. *Journal of Patient Safety, 9*(3), 122–128.

Joint Commission Resources. (2012). *Benchmarking in health care.* Oakbrook Terrace, IL: Author.

Jones, T. L. (2016). Outcome measurement in nursing: Imperatives, ideals, history, and challenges. *OJIN: The Online Journal of Issues in Nursing, 21*(2). Retrieved from http://www.nursingworld.org/MainMenuCategories/ANAMarketplace/ANAPeriodicals/OJIN/TableofContents/Vol-21-2016/No2-May-2016/Outcome-Measurement-in-Nursing.html

Keers, R. N., Williams, S. D., Cooke, J., & Ashcroft, D. M. (2013). Prevalence and nature of medication administration errors in health care settings: a systematic review of direct observational evidence. *Annals of Pharmacotherapy, 47*(2), 237–256.

Leaphart, C. L., Gonwa, T. A., Mai, M. L., Prendergast, M. B., Wadei, H. M., Tepass, J. J. III, & Taner, C. B. (2012). Formal quality improvement curriculum and DMAIC method results in interdisciplinary collaboration and process improvement in renal transplant patients. *Journal of Surgical Research, 177*(1), 7–13. doi:10.1016/j.jss.2012.03.017

Mason, S. E., Nicolay, C. R., & Darzi, A. (2015). The use of Lean and Six Sigma methodologies in surgery: a systematic review. *The Surgeon, 13*(2), 91–100. Published by Elsevier Inc., © 2014.

McHugh, M. D., & Ma, C. (2013). Hospital nursing and 30-day readmissions among Medicare patients with heart failure, acute myocardial infarction, and pneumonia. *Medical Care, 51*(1), 52.

Montalvo, I. (2007). The national database of nursing quality indicators (NDNQI). *The Online Journal of Issues in Nursing, 12*(3). Retrieved from http://www.nursingworld.org/MainMenuCategories/ANAMarketplace/ANAPeriodicals/OJIN/TableofContents/Volume122007/No3Sept07/NursingQualityIndicators.html

National Coordinating Council for Medication Error Reporting and Prevention. (n.d.). *About medication errors.* Retrieved from http://www.nccmerp.org/aboutMedErrors.html

National Database of Nursing Quality Indicators (NDNQI). (n.d.). *Nursing-sensitive indicators.* Retrieved from http://www.nursingquality.org/data.aspx

National Institutes of Health. (n.d.). *PROMIS overview.* Retrieved from http://www.nihpromis.org/about/overview

Nurses Service Organization. (2015). *CNA HealthPro Nurses Claims Study.* Retrieved from http://www.nso.com/Documents/pdfs/CNA%20NURSE%20EXEC%20SUMMARY%20101315.pdf

Press Ganey. (n.d.). Retrieved from http://www.pressganey.com/solutions/clinical-quality/nursing-quality

Raso, R., & Gulinello, C. (2010). Creating cultures of safety: Risk management challenges and strategies. *Nursing Management, 41*(12), 26–33. Published by Wolters Kluwer Health, Inc. doi:10.1097/01.NUMA.0000390459.88752.0c

Shekelle, P. G. (2013). Nurse–patient ratios as a patient safety strategy: a systematic review. *Annals of Internal Medicine, 158*(5 Part 2), 404–409.

Silich, S. J., Wetz, R. V., Riebling, N., Coleman, C., Khoueiry, G., Rafeh, N. A., ... Szerszen, A. (2012). Using Six Sigma methodology to reduce patient transfer times from floor to critical-care beds. *Journal for Healthcare Quality, 34*(1), 44–54. doi:10.1111/j.1945-1474.2011.00184.x

Sollecito, W. A., & Johnson, J. K. (2013). *McLaughlin and Kaluzny's continuous quality improvement in health care* (4th ed.). Burlington, MA: Jones & Bartlett.

The Joint Commission. (2013). *Sentinel event policy and procedures.* Retrieved from http://www.jointcommission.org/Sentinel_Event_Policy_and_Procedures

The Joint Commission. (n.d.). *2017 National patient safety goals.* Retrieved from https://www.jointcommission.org/assets/1/6/2017_NPSG_HAP_ER.pdf

U.S. Department of Health and Human Services (USDHHS). (2015). *2015 National Healthcare Quality and Disparities Report and 5th anniversary update on the National Quality Strategy.* Retrieved from https://www.ahrq.gov/research/findings/nhqrdr/nhqdr15/index.html

Weaver, S. J., Lubomksi, L. H., Wilson, R. F., Pfoh, E. R., Martinez, K. A., & Dy, S. M. (2013). Promoting a culture of safety as a patient safety strategy: a systematic review. *Annals of Internal Medicine, 158*(5 Part 2), 369–374.

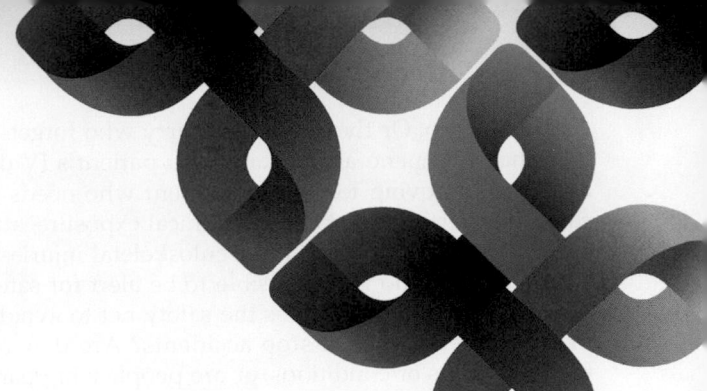

Module 51
Safety

Module Outline and Learning Outcomes

The Concept of Safety

Attributes of Safety

51.1 Analyze the attributes of safety.

Alterations to Safety

51.2 Differentiate common alterations of safety.

Concepts Related to Safety

51.3 Summarize the relationship between safety and other concepts.

Health Promotion

51.4 Explain the promotion of health safety.

Nursing Assessment

51.5 Differentiate common assessment data used to examine safety.

Independent Interventions

51.6 Explain independent interventions that can be implemented for the patient's safety.

Collaborative Efforts

51.7 Summarize collaborative efforts used by interprofessional teams and patients for safety in healthcare settings.

Safety Exemplars

Exemplar 51.A Health Promotion and Injury Prevention Across the Lifespan

51.A Analyze health promotion and injury prevention across the lifespan as they relate to safety.

Exemplar 51.B Patient Safety

51.B Analyze safety as it relates to patients in home care and healthcare settings.

Exemplar 51.C Nurse Safety

51.C Analyze safety as it relates to being a nurse.

» The Concept of Safety

Concept Key Terms

Attributes of safety, **2872**

National Patient
    Safety Goals
    (NPSGs), **2880**

Never event, **2872**

Quality, **2872**

Quality and Safety
    Education for Nurses
    (QSEN), **2880**

Safety, **2872**

Safety culture, **2880**

Standard
    precautions, **2877**

How important is the quality of safety in healthcare settings? Is it only essential in an acute healthcare facility? Or extended healthcare facility? What about healthcare at a community setting? Or in a patient's home? When quality and safety are not priorities in healthcare settings, safety records reflect increases in accidents, errors, injuries, and infections. Statistics about patients in healthcare settings reflect that every year, 1 of 25 patients acquires a healthcare-associated infection; a patient on Medicare has a 1 in 4 chance of experiencing harm, injury, or death when admitted to a hospital; and every day more than 1000 patients will die as a result of preventable harm or adverse events (Hospital Safety Score, 2015). Many of these adverse occurrences could have been prevented.

Is safety limited to patients, or does it also include the healthcare workforce? It is a safety issue when the patient is left in a tightly tied wrist restraint throughout the night shift without being checked and complains of tingling and numbness below the restraint. But what about the patient with congestive heart failure who is on a salt-free diet but who is being given packs of salt from staff? Don't accidents just happen sometimes? As in the example of an elderly patient who was told not to get out of bed without help, but who does, and then trips over a towel left on the floor, falls, and fractures a hip. Or the nurse in a hurry who forgets to perform hand hygiene after changing a patient's IV dressing and before moving to the next patient who needs a Foley catheter inserted. What about chemical exposure, attacks of violence, needlesticks, and musculoskeletal injuries nurses may receive? Who is responsible to be alert for safety hazards like these, and where is the safety net to avoid errors, prevent infections, and stop accidents? Are they all from faulty systems or conditions, or are people a big part of the problem, too?

Attributes of Safety

Unsafe situations related to the quality of safety can occur in healthcare facilities, homes of patients, and community settings. **Safety** refers to decreasing risks of dangers or hazards to prevent accidents, injuries, mistakes, and harm. **Quality** relates to the level of performance consistent with current evidence that increases efficiency and effectiveness for desired safety outcomes (Agency for Healthcare Research and Quality [AHRQ], 2013). It requires everyone in a healthcare facility to engage in safe behaviors and have awareness of surroundings to protect against unsafe situations and prevent safety hazards.

Attributes of safety are the qualities or properties of remaining safe. They are the precautions individuals take to be safe and prevent adverse occurrences. Examples of attributes or precautions healthcare facilities can implement to improve quality and safety include the following (Occupational Safety and Health Administration [OSHA], 2015):

1. Schedule hazard surveys and safety/health inspections in all areas.
2. Implement an effective hazard reporting system available to employees.
3. Investigate all safety incidents for root causes.
4. Perform job hazard analysis for all departments.
5. Keep safety, health rules, and work practices readily available.
6. Have applicable OSHA-mandated safety programs in place.
7. Make sure personal protective equipment (PPE) is being used effectively.
8. Ensure appropriate housekeeping is properly maintained.
9. Confirm the facility has disaster plans for internal and external emergency situations.
10. Analyze workplace injury/illness data.
11. Promote the performance of safety and health responsibilities through organizational policies.
12. Provide safety and health training for all levels of employees at least annually.

Active partnership between healthcare staff and patients is an effective way to maximize the quality of safety and minimize risks of hazards and errors resulting in accidents and injuries. Everyone positively or negatively impacts safety and quality in the healthcare environment, including patients. Nurses need to encourage patients to:

- Be assertive to actively speak up and ask questions about medications, therapies, tests, and procedures to know the "what" and "why" of these and anticipated results.

- Be knowledgeable about their condition or illness and have awareness of how to prevent complications while in a healthcare facility.

- Have a support person to assist in these areas and be vigilant about the safety of care for the patient.

- Practice safe behaviors such as washing hands appropriately, asking for help when needed, eating appropriate foods on their prescribed diet, and reporting any mistakes noticed to the nurse or another staff member.

Healthcare employees need to be competent in and willing to use a range of safety skills. They also need to have the ability to identify safety hazards, take responsibility for correcting them, and be part of the solution to prevent them from happening again. Quality improvement and risk management of health services within healthcare concentrate on identifying and making changes to improve quality and safety for everyone (see the module on Quality Improvement for more information).

Alterations to Safety

Nurses play a major role as safety gate keepers, but even still, sometimes tragic adverse events happen, assessments may be incomplete, or a step or two during a procedure may be skipped. Even unintentional mistakes may result in longer hospital stays, accidents, injuries, infections, functional decline, or death. **Figure 51–1 》** illustrates how sometimes decisions made may seem to make sense at the time, but later can negatively impact patient safety.

In some cases, catastrophic adverse events serve as motivators for prevention, spurring healthcare facilities, advocacy organizations, and even families to act to try to prevent tragic events from happening to others. Small safety initiatives may grow into national initiatives using public service announcements, social media, and other forms of media communication. This can help build awareness of how routine procedures can quickly become life-threatening safety hazards within healthcare facilities. An example of one such initiative is *CampaignZERO*. This initiative advocates for patient safety by providing patients and their family members free checklists to use when admitted to a healthcare facility to help remain safe until discharge. The checklists have items listed that support patient safety and quality of care to help prevent **Never Events**, which are preventable hazards that can result in injury or death and that should never happen to patients (CampaignZERO, 2014). A checklist may give information about a given topic, such as pressure injuries or falls, what to do to avoid complications, how to notice something is wrong, how to talk with the physician, when to notify a nurse for help, and how to ask appropriate questions. Never events are considered sentinel events by The Joint Commission. See the Concept of Quality Improvement for a discussion of sentinel events.

》 Stay Current: Visit the website of the Patient Safety Movement to see the checklists from CampaignZERO: http://patientsafety-movement.org.

Another national initiative from the CDC and the Safe Injection Practices Coalition began after an investigation was completed on multiple cases of hepatitis exposure. Evidence showed that the problem stemmed from basic infection

Three Nurses Making Decisions About a Patient's Safety

First: Read about Tammy, our patient.

Tammy Odom is a 6-year-old patient with a history of bronchial asthma. Tammy is 40 inches tall, weighs 42 pounds, and is allergic to peanuts. She was admitted through the emergency department at 0200 this morning with acute exacerbation/bronchitis. Tammy's mother, Mrs. Odom, told the nurse that Tammy had a cold a few days ago. She also said that Tammy had been at her friend's house spending the night. At approximately 1900, the friend's mother called her and told her that Tammy had to use her rescue inhaler and still was having a hard time breathing. At that time, she found out the friend's father smokes in the house. Mrs. Odom said the recent drop in temperature may also have contributed to Tammy's breathing problems and reported that Tammy is allergic to peanuts and shellfish.

The nurse making rounds before breakfast notes the following assessment data: temperature 99.2°F (o), pulse 112, respirations 26, blood pressure 112/52, O_2 saturation 95% on room air, minimal wheezing bilateral lower lobes, no retractions or use of accessory muscles for respirations, and speaking in whole sentences. Tammy tells the nurse about the bag of candy her friend gave her the night before. When looking at the candy, the nurse notes some peanut butter cups and explains to Tammy she should not eat them because of her allergy to peanuts. Tammy says she is saving those for her mother who likes them, but that she has not eaten any of them. The nurse notes an empty wrapper in the candy bag. An unlicensed assistive personnel (UAP) is assigned to help Tammy and her mother as needed.

Answer the following questions:

1. What else do you want to assess about Tammy's situation and physical condition?
2. What do you suspect as the trigger of her asthma exacerbation? Why?
3. What is your priority intervention at this time?

Second: Read about nurses A, B, and C.

Nurse A	Nurse B	Nurse C
The nurse thinks Tammy looks better now, safe in the hospital, so she thinks about her other patients that need her help.	The nurse thinks Tammy ate a peanut butter cup causing her asthma problem, so she takes the bag of candy away so she won't eat anymore of them.	The nurse thinks about what might be triggering Tammy's asthma and discusses this with her mother—her recent cold, the change in weather, the smoker's home, the peanut butter cups.
The nurse tells Tammy's mother to call her if Tammy needs anything.	The nurse thinks Tammy is safe now and just needs to rest, so busies herself caring for her other patients.	The nurse plans to keep close check on Tammy and asks other team members caring for her to keep an eye on her also.
Throughout the morning, Tammy had episodes of increased wheezing, dyspnea, and respirations, lasting about 10 minutes each time. She is having more distress, speaking in broken sentences, and working harder to breathe with increased wheezing in all lung fields in the afternoon. Vital signs are temperature 99.6 (o), pulse 118, respirations 34, blood pressure 118/62, and O_2 saturation 92% room air. While Tammy is trying to play a game with the UAP, her dyspnea worsens and her mother puts the call light on for help.		While checking on Tammy at 1000, the UAP was cleaning up Tammy's bedside table. The nurse observed Tammy was having trouble breathing and coughing. She heard Tammy tell the UAP that she smelled funny. The nurse smelled the UAP and smelled tobacco smoke on the clothing. She pulled the UAP outside the door and discovered the UAP was a smoker. The nurse determined every time the UAP had gone into Tammy's room during the morning, it was triggering Tammy's asthma and she would begin having more breathing difficulty. The UAP was unaware that the smoke smell would cause Tammy a breathing problem. The nurse immediately reassigned this UAP to another patient and had a nonsmoker UAP assigned to Tammy. Within an hour Tammy was breathing in a more relaxed way and resting comfortably with minimal wheezing heard.
The nurse walks in the room, and quickly notices the respiratory distress Tammy is having. She tells Tammy's mother she was sorry but thought Tammy was better because she hadn't heard from her. She tells Tammy's mother she needs to call the physician and leaves the room.	When the nurse finally gets to Tammy's room about 15 minutes later, she can't understand what happened and becomes very anxious because she thought she had taken care of the problem when she took the bag of candy away. She calls for help, gets the HOB up, starts Tammy on oxygen, and has someone call the physician.	

Answer the following questions:

4. At what point do you consider Tammy safe from respiratory distress from her asthma? Explain.
5. What was the faulty thinking from Nurse A? Nurse B?
6. Nurse C used reasoning based on significant cues to make a clinical judgment about what was triggering Tammy's respiratory distress. Can you follow her critical thinking process?
7. What should Nurse C say to the UAP with smoke in her clothing?
8. Can you identify eight mistakes in thinking or lack of knowledge in this scenario? How would they have been avoided?
9. What were the consequences for Tammy due to decisions by Nurse A and Nurse B?
10. What were the benefits for Tammy due to decisions by Nurse C?

Figure 51–1 》》 Three nurses making decisions about a patient's safety. This is a scenario looking at perspectives of three different nurses based on decisions they make about the same situation. Follow the directions and answer the questions.

control inconsistencies involving the unsafe medication administration practice of reusing syringes, which caused contamination of medication vials used on subsequent patients. The coalition developed an initiative called *One Needle, One Syringe at One Time*, whose goal is to eliminate adverse events resulting from unsafe injection practices. Since its inception, this initiative has notified more than 130,000 patients of potential exposure to hepatitis or HIV related to unsafe medication administration (One and Only Campaign, 2014).

>> Stay Current: Visit the One and Only website at http://www.oneandonlycampaign.org/ to learn more about this campaign.

Healthcare facilities can help decrease adverse events by using a three-pronged approach to quality and safety for everyone. The first prong is the organization's support for keeping quality in safety a priority by promoting a safety culture that encourages all employees to intentionally and actively make safe choices in what they do and how they do it as they keep a mind-set for quality of safe practice. A nonprofit organization, the Leapfrog Group, ranks the safety of hospitals around the country with letter grades (**Box 51–1 >>**).

The second prong is the involvement and sustainability of healthcare employees to consistently choose to follow health safety rules and standards for the environment, patient care, and be safety advocates for others. Healthcare employees are needed to responsibly maintain the safe environment and care within a facility. The last prong is encouragement given to patients to be actively engaged in every aspect of their care throughout their course of stay. They need to ask questions about the quality and safety of procedures done, medications administered, or other care provided to them.

Box 51–1
Hospital Safety Scores Reflecting Alterations to Safety

The Leapfrog Group uses the Hospital Safety Score to rank general acute care healthcare facilities on how safe they are for patients. This not-for-profit organization is composed of companies and private healthcare companies that want healthcare in the United States to be safe, have high quality, and be affordable by promoting transparency and value-based incentives to healthcare facilities. The 28 performance measures used in the scoring process are from AHRQ, CDC, Centers for Medicare and Medicaid Services (CMS), and the Leapfrog Hospital Survey.

These 28 measures are divided into two categories, process/structural measures and outcome measures. These safety scores are publicly reported through the annual Leapfrog Hospital Survey (Hospital Safety Score, 2015). Scores for more than 2500 acute care healthcare facilities throughout the United States are available. Consumers of healthcare are encouraged to consider safety when selecting a healthcare facility for procedures, surgeries, and hospitalizations, which can serve as an incentive for healthcare facilities to make safety more of a priority.

>> Stay Current: Visit http://www.hospitalsafetyscore.org/what-is-patient- to see the 28 measures and to find the safety score of your local hospital.

Concepts Related to Safety

Every area of nursing is related to safety. Many nursing actions, such as hand hygiene and patient identification validation, promote well-being and safety for patients and others. As partners in their own plans of care, patients can participate in safety behaviors such as infection control, fall precautions, and accident prevention. Nurses also ensure their own safety by following policies and procedures, by engaging in therapeutic communication that promotes patient self-esteem and reduces patient anxiety, and by using critical thinking to prioritize patient care. The Concepts Related to Safety feature links some, but not all, of the concepts integral to safety. They are presented in alphabetical order.

Health Promotion

In the United States, there is a collaborative effort of several federal agencies to improve the nation's health. Workplace promotion programs are offered to employees at many companies and organizations that include wellness programs about nutrition, smoking cessation, stress management, and safety. Individuals can select from a variety of wellness, exercise, weight management, and stress management programs available to meet their own needs (see the module on Health, Wellness, Illness, and Injury for more information). Health promotion practices are given in **Table 51–1 >>**.

>> Stay Current: Follow individual state laws on child passenger safety seats for infants and children at http://www.ghsa.org/html/stateinfo/laws/childsafety_laws.html.

Nursing Assessment

Patients admitted to healthcare facilities initially undergo a comprehensive nursing assessment, including observation, an interview, and a physical examination. As a proactive measure, this initial assessment includes specific age-appropriate questions and observations that focus on safety needs. All healthcare settings will have their own safety checklists based on recommendations of healthcare organizations such as The Joint Commission. Risk-based assessment data help to identify patients who may require special precautions to prevent harm and minimize consequences from debilitation or exacerbation of a preexisting risk while in healthcare settings. This assessment process can further be divided into three levels based on patient responses: low, medium, or high safety risk.

Observation and Patient Interview

During initial interviews with patients, nurses may use checklists quickly to identify physical, psychologic, and emotional areas to further explore for potential safety issues or health promotion needs. For example, if the patient is asked, "Have you ever noticed blood in your stool?" and the patient responds, "Yes," the nurse should then explore this with the patient. If the patient responds "Yes, sometimes" to the question, "Have you ever thought about hurting yourself?" the nurse takes this seriously and assesses the patient's current risk for suicide or self-harm.

In addition to gathering assessment data through the interview, nurses are constantly observing patients for age-appropriate assessment data such as communication

Concepts Related to
Safety

CONCEPT	RELATIONSHIP TO SAFETY	NURSING IMPLICATIONS
Accountability	■ Unsafe nursing practice, behaviors, and thinking could cause harm to patients and others, and if not addressed, will continue to occur.	■ Unsafe nursing practice should be reported and addressed. ■ Competency in providing quality safe nursing care develops when following standards of care.
Advocacy	■ Vulnerable populations may unintentionally make unsafe decisions about their healthcare. ■ Sometimes unethical, immoral, or illegal actions result in unsafe treatments and behaviors by professionals.	■ Nurses can support patients in making safe appropriate decisions by providing accurate and complete information using their primary language to help them understand the decision to be made. ■ Nurses can uphold the rights of patients, including the right to have quality safe treatment in a safe environment.
Assessment	■ Data are used to monitor for changes in conditions of patients. ■ Data can show numerical values indicating safe or unsafe parameters for patient's body systems.	■ Nurses continuously collect assessment data, interpret it, and intervene as appropriate for quality and safety of patient care. ■ Data can change, and nurses need to monitor these changes to help prevent unsafe physical, emotional, or psychologic conditions for patients.
Clinical Decision Making	■ Nurses consider safety (both the patient's safety and the safety of other healthcare workers) in all phases of the nursing process, and while prioritizing patient needs.	■ Assess patients for safety risks, factors that impact risks for falls, and ability to perform activities of daily living (ADLs) such as vision, hearing, mobility, and balance, and risk for or presence of abuse or neglect. ■ Provide patient teaching regarding safety measures as appropriate based on assessment and evaluation of interventions.
Evidence-Based Practice	■ Evidence supports that many errors occurring in the healthcare setting can be avoided with improved performance of healthcare workers. ■ Evidence supports that everyone in the healthcare environment, including patients, can improve quality and safety.	■ Nurses can form partnerships with patients to work together for quality and safety of care. ■ Evidence provides best practices for safety in nursing interventions. ■ Improvements in quality and safety of patient-centered care contribute to best patient outcomes.
Quality Improvement	■ Improving quality of care for all patients involves ensuring and considering the safety of patients at all times when providing nursing care.	■ Ensure a high quality of care in all interactions with patients. ■ Resolve any safety concerns in the patient's immediate bed area. ■ Ensure that the correct patient is receiving the correct type and amount of medication. ■ Follow safety and procedural guidelines for patient care.

and speech patterns, mobility, eye contact, general appearance, balance, and other data. Some assessment data observed may need to be explored with the patient verbally. Common safety risk assessment data from the patient or family member during the interview include:

- Ability to communicate
- Ability to provide self-care
- Cognitive ability
- Memory deficiencies
- Bowel and bladder elimination and control
- Susceptibility to falls or any other safety risks
- Visual or other sensory deficiencies
- Mobility deficiencies

- Use of assistive devices
- Presence of Foley catheter, PEG tube, colostomy, or tracheostomy
- Skin integrity
- Vulnerability to injury
- Nutritional status
- Developmental considerations.

Teaching patients protective measures to reduce their vulnerability for safety issues in a healthcare facility, home setting, or community setting can help keep patients engaged in their nursing plan of care. See the feature on Patient Teaching: Patient Practices That Promote Safety in Healthcare Settings.

TABLE 51-1 Health Promotion Practices

Practice	Actions
Be physically active at any age to achieve health benefits as abilities and conditions allow.	■ Make exercise a part of every day ■ Do effective exercising for long-term health benefits ■ Ongoing daily activity will increase energy ■ Physical activities can relieve stress
Use protection against injuries and accidents with appropriate safety gear and sports equipment; do activities in safe environments; choose appropriate activities to do; and follow rules for safety.	■ Use gear such as helmets, mouth guards, knee and elbow pads, skin guards, padding, and protective eyewear as appropriate ■ Use well-lit populated sidewalks, supportive shoes, and stay hydrated ■ Follow game rules and fair play ■ Avoid risk areas ■ Check with healthcare provider before beginning new physical activities
Be smoke-free and avoid secondhand smoke.	■ Participate in a cessation program ■ Avoid secondhand smoke areas ■ Health risks of respiratory and cardiovascular diseases are decreased
Motor vehicle safety.	■ Follow guidelines for infant/child car seats ■ Don't be distracted by talking on a cell phone or texting; stay focused ■ Wear safety seat belts ■ Follow laws and road rules ■ Avoid aggressive drivers ■ Avoid driving when tired or sleepy
Eat appropriate diet and drink suitable beverages in moderation.	■ Decrease portion sizes ■ Increase vegetable and fruit portions ■ Limit fats, sugar, and salt ■ Use low-fat dairy products
Include doing activities that are fun and relaxing.	■ Do hobbies that stretch the mind and body ■ Practice stress management techniques
Maintain healthy weight.	■ Minimize eating processed foods and fast foods ■ Eat an assortment of fruits, vegetables, and meats ■ Decrease obesity, currently found in all ages
Be smart about health promotion.	■ Increase knowledge through online courses, attending training programs, and learning from others ■ Become empowered to make healthy choices ■ Avoid risk behaviors that can develop into chronic diseases such as smoking, poor eating habits, lack of physical activity, high stress environments, and low air quality
Attend local health fairs; participate in health screenings for eyesight, hearing, bone density, blood pressure, and blood glucose, and other community health activities.	■ Periodic measurements can be used to look at health trends and changes in the body ■ Activity levels can show trends in mobility and flexibility
Allow time to de-stress.	■ Disconnect from emails and phones for short periods to reduce stress ■ Take a short walk around workplace or home settings
Monitor personal health status.	■ See a healthcare provider annually ■ Take medications as prescribed ■ Have immunizations recommended for specific age group
Allow for enough restful sleep.	■ Have bedtime rituals to prepare the body to sleep ■ Follow routines of sleep habits
Have protection against temperature variances while inside or outside.	■ Wear appropriate clothing ■ Use sunscreen to protect skin ■ Avoid long periods of time in temperature extremes ■ Control thermostats to maintain comfort ■ Use safe heating and cooling equipment ■ Use carbon monoxide alarms when inside of home

Source: Based on Rural Assistance Center. (2015). *Defining health promotion and disease prevention.* Retrieved from https://www.raconline.org/communityhealth/health-promotion/1/definition.

Patient Teaching

Patient Practices That Promote Safety in Healthcare Settings

Patients are at a higher risk for acquiring a healthcare-associated infection or injury because of the quality of safety in some healthcare settings. By following the steps below, patients can help make healthcare safer and help prevent healthcare-associated infections and injuries.

1. Have annual eye exams and update eyeglasses to maximize vision.
2. Exercise regularly to improve balance, joint mobility, and leg strength.
3. Eat a variety of nutrients and protein; drink adequate amount of water.
4. Follow directions for medications prescribed.
5. Wash hands appropriately as needed.
6. Know your body so that you notice changes in it.
7. Get vaccinations as prescribed for age group.
8. Use assistive walking aids as prescribed.
9. Maintain hygiene and self-care as able.
10. Recognize limitations of ability.

Source: From Centers for Disease Control and Prevention. (2013a). Patient safety: Ten things you can do to be a safe patient. *The National Institute for Occupational Safety and Health (NIOSH).* Retrieved from http://www.cdc.gov/Features/PatientSafety/.

Physical Examination

Nurses are continuously observing patients, monitoring for unsafe changes in conditions, and making decisions about appropriate responses. For example, a nurse walks into a patient's room and assesses a patient with diabetes who is confused, agitated, and has a respiratory rate of 28 with a sweet odor to the breath. The nurse notices several candy wrappers on the bedside table. Based on this assessment data, the nurse quickly has a glucometer check done and finds the patient's blood glucose reading to be consistently 308 after two checks. The patient has changed from a safe blood glucose level to an unsafe increased level outside of normal range for this patient. Intervention is required.

There are four acute changes in condition that nurses must investigate to determine appropriate interventions and urgency in responding to them:

- *Cognitive changes,* such as decreased level of consciousness, change in memory, change in mood, difficulty thinking, and acute confusion.

- *Physical changes,* such as changes in vital signs, change in oxygen saturation, change in skin color, change in appearance of an incision, onset of diaphoresis, seizure activity, and an onset of pain.

- *Functional changes,* such as respiratory distress, change in mobility, onset of slurred speech, weakness of an extremity, numbness of extremity, and acute function deficit.

- *Behavioral changes,* such as inappropriate movements, disorientation to time and place, hallucinating, depression, and wandering (American Medical Directors Association [AMDA], 2015).

For example, changes in sputum color from clear to yellow, consistency from watery to tenacious, and amount from small to copious will influence the quality and safety of the patient's airway, so intervention is needed. Another example would be the older adult who develops acute slurring of speech, inability to move an arm, drooling, and inability to talk coherently, and has facial drooping on one side of the face, indicating a neurologic situation that needs immediate intervention for the safety of the patient.

Independent Interventions

Everyone, including healthcare workers, patients, families, and visitors, must assertively perform safety behaviors to prevent injuries, accidents, infections, and errors in all healthcare environments. In all settings, policies and procedures such as standard precautions assist nurses and other healthcare providers in ensuring the safety of the environment.

Standard Precautions

Standard precautions incorporate those guidelines previously referred to as universal precautions and body substance isolation (BSI). Standard precautions include measures such as the use of proper hand hygiene, protective equipment, and safe injection practices and the effective management of potentially contaminated surfaces or equipment. The transfer of infectious agents between nurses and patients is a serious safety concern to be addressed (see the module on Infection for further information).

Latex Exposure

Latex precautions are of particular importance to nurses, because products containing latex are common in the healthcare industry. Latex gloves, blood pressure cuffs, IV tubes, bandages, syringes, and catheters are among some of the common devices found in medical settings that can contain latex. Exposure to latex can trigger a latex allergy, which can become a serious problem for nurses, patients, and others. Symptoms may begin as itching, burning, redness, and swelling of the hands and fingers when latex gloves are worn or contact with other latex equipment or supplies occurs. Symptoms may become more severe, leading to asthma or anaphylaxis. Over a period of time, exposure to latex can develop into occupational asthma (AHRQ, 2008).

A number of precautions can be employed to avoid latex exposure for both healthcare workers and patients. Hypoallergenic (and specifically latex-free) and powderless gloves are helpful in preventing exposure. Not all hypoallergenic gloves are latex-free, so this should be ensured if an allergy or sensitivity is indicated. The powder from gloves can absorb the latex and then spread it when the gloves are removed; this can then release the allergen into the air, potentially affecting those with a severe sensitivity. Hand washing after taking off gloves is extremely important in preventing exposure to others.

Chemical Exposure

Exposure to hazardous and toxic substances is of paramount concern in the healthcare environment. Many chemicals found in this setting can be dangerous, including cleaning

Evidence-Based Practice

The World Health Organization (WHO) Hand Hygiene and Control of the 2015 Ebola Outbreak

Problem

Hand hygiene among healthcare providers was highlighted during the 2014–2015 West African Ebola outbreak as a cost-effective safety practice in the prevention and control of healthcare-associated infections (HAIs). Ebola virus disease (EVD) is a serious and often fatal disease that is spread through person-to-person transmission. This latest outbreak involved multiple countries and included people living in cities as well as rural villages. The number of cases and deaths during this EVD outbreak was higher than that for all other EVD outbreaks in the past combined. The West Africa outbreak was declared a Public Health Emergency of International Concern by WHO (**Figure 51–2 》**).

Many materials and tools developed by the WHO were used in the response and recovery of the areas involved in this outbreak. The people in the communities of these countries were brought onboard by making hand hygiene resources available at public places such as banks, churches, and schools. Public service announcements were developed to inform people of the value of hand hygiene in controlling the transmission of this infectious disease.

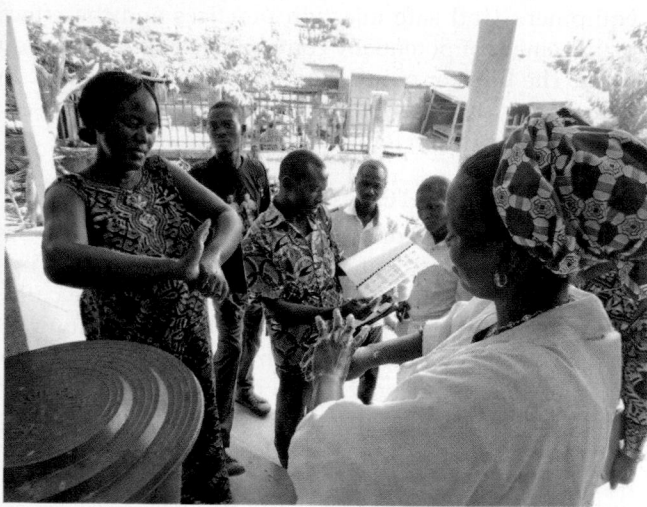

Source: Centers for Disease Control and Prevention (CDC).

Figure 51–2 》 Hand hygiene played an important role in controlling the 2015 Ebola outbreak. People had to be taught proper hand hygiene techniques that would help control this contagious disease.

Evidence

To reduce the spread of infection from pathogenic microorganisms and prevent HAIs, global initiatives from WHO are implemented. WHO works with different levels of development and cultural environments around the world promoting hand hygiene as an effective solution. In 2004, WHO developed *Guidelines on Hand Hygiene in Healthcare,* an assortment of evidence reviewed and organized into documents.

Two years later, WHO launched a *Clean Care Is Safer Care* campaign. In 2006–2008 these strategies were used during a 2-year field test pilot program across six WHO regions. The project was to collect data and test the data for the reliability, validity, and sustainability of the guidelines to improve safety. Evidence determined that there was:

- Improved hand hygiene compliance found in all professional categories
- Increased knowledge of the importance of hand hygiene in preventing HAIs
- An enhanced culture of safety in healthcare facilities
- Scientific evidence that supported WHO hand hygiene strategies as a successful model for preventing HAIs (WHO, 2015a).

Implications

When this outbreak ended, the major African countries involved declared support to continue addressing HAIs with preventive actions, including improved hand hygiene among healthcare providers. Improvements in hand hygiene compliance for healthcare providers will support continued sustainability and prevention of HAIs. Conversations and actions addressing safety of water, sanitation, and waste management will also lessen the incidence of HAIs.

To continue to improve patient safety and prevent HAIs, the WHO Guidelines and Toolkit are kept current through organized reviews of scientific data and published studies about HAIs around the world. For example, the WHO *Multimodel Hand Hygiene Improvement Strategy* tool is used to implement change in safety practices of hand hygiene. Cleaning hands at the right times and in the right way, actions of simple hand hygiene, can make the difference (WHO, 2015b).

Critical Thinking Application

1. To reinforce the importance of hand hygiene to others, what can nurses do? Who can they teach hand hygiene practices to in the healthcare setting?
2. How does hand hygiene compliance change the number of HAIs that occur in the healthcare setting? Who needs to participate in this safety prevention behavior?

Sources: World Health Organization. (2015a). *Clean care is safer care. Testing the WHO Guidelines on hand hygiene In healthcare in eight pilot sites worldwide.* Retrieved from http://www.who.int/gpsc/country_work/pilot_sites/introduction/en/; World Health Organization. (2015b). *Clean care is safer care. Hand hygiene in the control of Ebola and health system strengthening.* Retrieved from http://www.who.int/gpsc/hand-hygiene_ebola/en/; World Health Organization. (2015c). *Ebola virus disease.* Fact sheet no. 103. Retrieved from http://www.who.int/mediacentre/factsheets/fs103/en/#.

---

supplies, disinfectants, paints, and certain forms of air pollutants. To reduce hazardous exposures, healthcare facilities are using safer alternatives that are now available. Product solutions can not only be safe in the work environment, but also support a safer environment. One initiative to reduce environmental hazards for hospitals is *Go Green,* which advocates disposing of medical waste in an environmentally

friendly way following regulations developed by OSHA. Improved green safety products that are eco-friendly and reliable are now available (National Safety Council [NSC], 2014).

》 Stay Current: For more information on hospitals going green, visit http://www.healthcarebusinesstech.com/going-green-hospital/.

Collaborative Efforts

Many local organizations in addition to international, federal, and state agencies collaborate to support quality health, safety, and cost efficiency initiatives in healthcare. Collaborative community initiatives may be started by community members in response to a serious, community-wide health issue. They may start through state-funded or federally funded initiatives that begin in response to larger statewide or nationally recognized health issues and that provide funding at the community level to address these issues. Although national healthcare safety initiatives vary in approach, in general they support collaboration of government agencies, healthcare facilities, and people who work in healthcare to have safe healthy work environments and to provide patients safe quality care for best patient outcomes. **Table 51–2 »** lists a number of current safety initiatives.

Even with safety initiatives in place, injuries, accidents, and errors can still happen in healthcare facilities, homes, and

TABLE 51–2 Safety Initiatives

Organization	Intent	Contributions
AHRQ, U.S. Department of Health & Human Services	Produce evidence that supports healthcare safety, make it more available, have a higher quality, be equitable, and cost effective while reducing medical errors and improving patient safety.	■ *Patient Safety and Quality: An Evidence-Based Handbook for Nurses* (2008), developed with the Robert Wood Johnson Foundation. http://www.ncbi.nlm.nih.gov/books/NBK2651/ ■ For other AHRQ publications and products: http://www.ahrq.gov/research/publications/index.html
CDC	Engages in health research, surveillance, promotion, and response to promote and increase the health security of the United States.	■ A list of some of the CDC's numerous national health and safety initiatives, strategies, and plans of action that provide leadership to public health efforts across the United States can be found on their website, http://www.cdc.gov/stltpublichealth/strategy/index.html
Institute of Medicine (IOM)	Provides reliable evidence to the government and the private sector to support informed health decisions about assessment and improvement of healthcare systems and policies.	■ *To Err Is Human: Building a Safer Health System* (1999) http://iom.nationalacademies.org/~/media/Files/Report%20Files/1999/To-Err-is-Human/To%20Err%20is%20Human%201999%20report%20brief.pdf ■ *Crossing the Quality Chasm: A New Health System for the 21st Century* (2001) ■ *Keeping Patients Safe: Transforming the Work Environment of Nurses* (2004) ■ *Envisioning the Future of Health Professional Education* (2015) http://iom.nationalacademies.org/Reports/2015/Envisioning-the-Future-of-Health-Professional-Education.aspx ■ For more IOM studies and activities: http://iom.nationalacademies.org/~/media/Files/About%20the%20IOM/2015/CARR-20September%202015.pdf?la=en
The Joint Commission	Promotes quality and safety through accreditation and certification of healthcare facilities representing high quality, safety, and value for patients.	■ National Patient Safety Goals https://www.jointcommission.org/standards_information/npsgs.aspx ■ SpeakUp initiative http://www.jointcommission.org/speakup.aspx
The National Institute for Occupational Safety and Health (NIOSH)	A federal agency that provides evidence-supported recommendations on the prevention of worker injuries and illnesses to preserve human resources.	■ Develops and enforces workplace safety and health regulations http://www.cdc.gov/niosh/programs.html ■ Provides multiple training programs and educational publications/products http://www.cdc.gov/niosh/topics/safety.html
OSHA, U.S. Department of Labor	A national public health regulatory agency that protects workers against safety and health hazards in the work environments by enforcing compliance with health and safety standards.	■ Occupational Safety and Health Act (OSH Act), 1970 https://www.osha.gov/pls/oshaweb/owasrch.search_form?p_doc_type=oshact ■ Enforcement inspections https://www.osha.gov/oshstats/index.html ■ Worker, environmental and nuclear safety laws enforced https://www.osha.gov/law-regs.html ■ Worker's rights law https://www.osha.gov/workers/index.html
Quality and Safety Education for Nurses (QSEN)	Designed to prepare nursing students with knowledge, skills, and attitudes (KSAs) needed to improve quality of patient care and safety of providing healthcare using systems thinking.	■ Six core nursing competencies (using IOM healthcare clinician competencies) http://qsen.org/competencies/ ■ KSAs for undergraduate prelicensure nursing programs http://qsen.org/competencies/pre-licensure-ksas/ ■ KSAs for graduate education nursing programs http://qsen.org/competencies/graduate-ksas/
WHO	International authority to direct and coordinate health within the United Nations' system.	■ International preparedness, surveillance and response to health emergencies threatening human health security http://www.who.int/csr/alertresponse/en/ ■ Multiple WHO patient safety training programs and activities http://www.who.int/patientsafety/education/en/

communities. Initiatives, policies and mandates need to include the "people factor" to be successful. Everyone in healthcare wants to have a safe and healthy environment, and it takes everyone to make it happen by creating a culture of safety. A **safety culture** is a general feeling of shared attitudes, values, practices, and beliefs that result in behaviors and feelings of responsibility for safety in all daily routines (OSHA, 2015). Safety awareness is heightened throughout all areas.

Organizations and employees working together can build and maintain a safety culture, resulting in improved safety and quality of care for patients and fewer unsafe and unhealthy conditions for themselves. This means anyone can report unsafe conditions or behaviors and help find solutions to correct them.

A safety culture is a blame-free environment. With a focus on systems, individuals can report errors or near misses without fearing reprimand or punishment. Some healthcare facilities have created a "just culture" that looks not only at systems but also at how they may have contributed to an individual's unsafe action (see the module on Quality Improvement for further information). Everyone in a healthcare safety culture is aware of the importance of how they work and is determined to consistently do their work correctly and safely. They all are involved with the planning, implementation, and evaluation of initiatives for safety and health concerns, actively working together to find methods for quality improvement.

Some things healthcare facilities can do to support safety initiatives are to:

1. Make necessary resources available
2. Include all levels of employees in committees making decisions about initiatives
3. Celebrate improvements when quality programs are implemented
4. Do management walk-arounds to support staff
5. Offer periodic safety training
6. Share successes in improved patient outcomes and safety goals attained.

One way to measure the success of safety cultures is to use a validated survey. Two examples of these surveys are the AHRQ's *Patient Safety Culture Surveys* and the *Safety Attitudes Questionnaire* (AHRQ, 2014). For those who work in a safety culture environment, there can be improved job satisfaction for protecting patients and others from safety and health hazards. Safety hazards and health risks can also be minimized for the employees in this environment, resulting in a decrease in injuries, accidents, illnesses, and errors. Healthcare is about those who provide the care and those who receive the care; healthcare facilities need safety and health protection for everyone.

In 2005, the Robert Wood Johnson Foundation funded a group of distinguished nursing leaders and faculty to use the Institute of Medicine's healthcare clinician competencies from the *Crossing the Quality Chasm: A New Health System for the 21st Century* report to develop core nursing competencies. These nursing competencies, called **Quality and Safety Education for Nurses (QSEN)**, would better prepare nursing students with practical experience in providing safer more effective care. They were further defined with specific knowledge, skills, and attitudes (KSAs) necessary to provide better quality and safety in healthcare settings (see **Table 51–3 ⟫**) (QSEN, 2014a, 2014b, 2014c).

The Joint Commission began its **National Patient Safety Goals (NPSG)** program in 2002 to help accredited organizations deal with specific topics on patient safety. NPSGs are developed and revised by the Patient Safety Advisory Group (PSAG), which is a panel of nurses, physicians, pharmacists, risk managers, engineers, and other professionals who have expertise related to patient safety issues within healthcare organizations. PSAG determines topics for NPSGs by analyzing safety concerns and evaluating which ones will have the maximum impact and usefulness for the minimum cost. Input is also solicited from practitioners, provider organizations, purchasers, consumer groups, and others. NPSGs are updated annually. Each goal is accompanied by elements of performance that The Joint Commission identifies as necessary to meet the goal. For example, among the NPSGs required for hospital accreditation in 2016 is the *goal* that agencies identify patients correctly, which is accompanied by two *elements of performance*, which relate to (1) consistently using two methods of identifying the patient, and (2) ensuring that patients receiving blood transfusions are correctly identified prior to transfusion (The Joint Commission, 2016).

⟫ **Stay Current:** For the most current National Patient Safety Goals, go to the website of The Joint Commission: www.jointcommission.org.

TABLE 15–3 QSEN Nursing Competencies

QSEN Competency	Definition
Patient-Centered Care	Patients are partners in their care, and thus their perspectives, beliefs, and culture need to be taken into consideration during their care.
Quality Improvement	Adverse events must be monitored and reported so they can be tools for learning in similar situations in the future and catalysts for improvements in quality and safety.
Evidence-Based Practice	Medicine is evolving and changing every day, and thus current medical findings must be monitored for the possibility of improved care.
Teamwork and Collaboration	Because treatment sometimes involves multiple departments and 24-hour care, teamwork across departments and shifts is necessary for optimal care.
Informatics	As information technology becomes further integrated into medicine, nurses' input is an essential part of the design process.
Safety	Activities such as knowledge sharing and error reporting must be taken seriously to help improve safety.

Source: Based on QSEN Institute. (2014a). *Competencies*. Retrieved from http://qsen.org/competencies/. Reproduced with permission.

REVIEW The Concept of Safety

RELATE Link the Concepts

Linking the concept of safety with the concept of tissue integrity:

1. Describe safety precautions that can be taken to prevent skin breakdown.

2. The nurse is caring for a patient with third-degree burns over 50% of his body. Identify three nursing interventions that promote safety while also facilitating the patient's healing and providing comfort.

Linking the concept of safety with the concept of ethics:

3. Explain the ethical considerations in a scenario in which a patient has been given the wrong medication, but with no adverse effects. Discuss the patient's right to be informed about the mistake. How should the nurse who committed the error handle this situation?

4. A surgeon nearly performed the wrong surgery on a patient, but the mistake was caught before a surgical incision was made. The correct surgery was performed, but the surgeon has not reported the original error. Does this scenario require submitting a report? Describe the dilemma faced by the surgical team in this scenario.

5. Describe the ethical dilemma associated with the use of restraints and respect for a patient's autonomy. Under what circumstances are restraints indicated for use in a patient's care?

Linking the concept of safety with the concept of oxygenation:

6. What are some teaching points the nurse should discuss with a chronic obstructive pulmonary disease (COPD) patient who keeps changing his oxygen settings?

7. Describe safety considerations when beginning supplemental oxygen on an asthmatic patient.

Linking the concept of safety with the concept of cognition:

8. Contrast differences in etiology between acute confusion and chronic confusion.

9. Plan safety interventions for the patient with early signs of dementia.

Linking the concept of safety with the concept of caring interventions:

10. Explain why safety when doing invasive interventions such as inserting a Foley catheter is a priority.

11. Relate the safety reasons for using evidence-based instead of traditional methodology for performing caring interventions.

READY Go to Volume 3: Clinical Nursing Skills

- Safe Delegation headings are found at beginning of many of the skills
- Clinical Alert features about safety are found throughout many of the skills
- Safe Practice features are found throughout many of the skills
- Safety chapter includes Home Care Safety, Environmental Safety, and Immobilizers and Restraints

REFER Go to Pearson MyLab Nursing and eText

- Additional review materials

REFLECT Apply Your Knowledge

A 72-year-old patient is admitted to the hospital for treatment of severe dehydration secondary to advanced and untreated urinary tract infection. She is normally very independent and does not often like to ask for help, particularly when she needs to use the bathroom. The patient's nurse recognizes the patient's desire for independence, but also realizes that she is at a heightened risk for falling because of the infection and corresponding dehydration-related signs and symptoms, including weakness and dizziness. The nurse talks to the patient about the risk of falling, as well as the possible injuries that could occur if she were to fall. He does not want the patient to lose her sense of independence, so he rearranges the chairs in the room so she has a clear line from the bed to the bathroom. The nurse then discusses the need for the patient to wear socks and/or slippers with gripper bottoms when she walks to the bathroom to further prevent falling. Together the nurse and patient develop a plan of care that respects the patient's needs and also works to ensure her overall safety.

1. Describe three reasons why the patient's situation represents an advanced risk for falling.

2. Explain the nurse's approach to the situation described above. What communication and collaboration efforts does he employ?

3. Evaluate the nurse's recommendations for the patient. Are these recommendations appropriate? Why or why not?

4. Would the situation above be any different if the patient were 30 years old? If so, how? Explain your answer.

≫ Exemplar 51.A
Health Promotion and Injury Prevention Across the Lifespan

Exemplar Learning Outcomes

51.A Analyze health promotion and injury prevention across the lifespan as they relate to safety.

- Summarize the risks for injury, health promotion, and injury prevention in the perinatal period and for infants.
- Outline the risks for injury, health promotion, and injury prevention for toddlers and preschoolers.
- Contrast safety considerations in healthcare settings for patients across the lifespan.
- Summarize the risks for injury, health promotion, and injury prevention for young and middle-aged adults.
- Outline the risks for injury, health promotion, and injury prevention for older adults.
- Plan nursing interventions for health promotion and injury prevention for individuals with special needs.

Overview

Health promotion includes activities that increase well-being and enhance health, such as appropriate nutrition, oral health, physical activity, and mental health. To be more effective, nurses can build partnerships with families so healthcare visits include all family members present to participate in discussions about questions or health topics they may have, support family strengths, improve communication, and work together as a team. These family visits also provide opportunities for nurses to observe each family member; note family dynamics; assess nutrition, growth and development, mental and spiritual health; and promote injury prevention strategies for everyone.

Illness prevention strategies focus mainly on the prevention of disease. **Screening tests** are procedures used to detect the possible presence of health conditions before symptoms are apparent. Vision and hearing screening tests are frequently conducted when children begin attending school. Most screening tests are not diagnostic by themselves but are followed by further diagnostic tests if the screening result is positive. Once a screening test identifies the existence of a health condition, intervention can begin.

Health promotion and safety needs vary across the lifespan, with parents taking care of the needs of infants and young children, school-age children adolescents accepting more responsibility for their health, adults bearing complete responsibility for their health, and older adults often sharing responsibility with their adult children.

Safety in the Perinatal Period and for Infants

The Perinatal Period

A total of 23,595 fetal deaths at 20 weeks' gestation or more were reported in the United States in 2013. This translates to a mortality rate of 5.96 fetal deaths per 1000 live births. These numbers compared to the previous year show that there were more fetal deaths than infant deaths occurring in the United States. Fetal mortality rates were highest for teenagers, women aged 36 and over, unmarried women, and women with multiple pregnancies (CDC, 2015a). **Fetal mortality** is the intrauterine death of a fetus at any gestational age. The majority of fetal deaths occur early in pregnancy. The following risk factors for perinatal mortality (the time immediately before or just after birth) have been identified: maternal obesity, smoking during pregnancy, severe hypertension or diabetes, congenital anomalies, infections, placental and cord problems, and intrauterine growth retardation (CDC, 2015a).

Early and regular prenatal care can result in having a healthy pregnancy, which promotes a healthy birth. Some women will make changes in their health routines before they actually are pregnant to further promote a healthy pregnancy such as to stop smoking, attain a healthy weight,

and learn about familial health conditions. Genetic counseling can help people learn more about genetic health conditions and the chances of having a child with a gene-related condition. Prenatal care can help prevent complications and provide women information about things they can do to protect the fetus and ensure fetal health and development. The healthcare provider can monitor the mother's health and development of the fetus during the pregnancy. Some prenatal risks are controllable, such as cessation of smoking, drinking alcohol, or taking certain medications during pregnancy, and some are not, such as first-time pregnancy after the age of 35 or occurrence of a familial physical abnormality. Having prenatal care as soon as pregnancy is determined by a healthcare provider can help increase incidence of having a healthy baby. See the exemplar on Antepartum Care in the module on Reproduction for more information.

Infants

Birth defects are common occurrences in the United States. Nearly 120,000 babies are affected by birth defects each year. **Birth defects** are changes in physical structure present at birth that can affect many parts of the body, such as the heart, foot, or palate. Depending on the severity and location of the birth defect, expected lifespan may or may not be affected (CDC, 2015b). Examples of birth defects include congenital heart defects, Down syndrome, spina bifida, and lower limb reduction defects. Birth weight is a good predictor of the survival and healthy development of a newborn. Newborns are screened while still in the hospital for critical birth defects that cannot be seen, such as hearing loss, heart defects, hemoglobin disorders, hormonal insufficiency, cystic fibrosis, or inability to process certain nutrients. Types of screening and how many conditions to look for are determined by each state. See the exemplar on Newborn Care in the module on Reproduction for more information.

Congenital anomalies and short gestation continue to be common causes of mortality as the neonate, or newborn, matures into an infant. Sudden infant death syndrome (SIDS) is the leading cause of death among infants between 1 and 12 months (U.S. National Library of Medicine, 2015). Complications during delivery and unintentional injuries also can result in infant death, with the most common unintentional injuries resulting from suffocation, often as a result of co-sleeping (CDC, 2013b). See the exemplar on Sudden Infant Death Syndrome in the module on Oxygenation for more information.

Maltreatment of children, abuse or neglect, causes injuries or deaths each year. In 2012, 27% of victims were younger than 3 years, 20% were age 3–5 years, and children younger than 1 year had the highest rate of victimization, 21.9 per 1000 children. Of the child victims, 78% were victims of neglect; 18% of physical abuse; 9% of sexual abuse; and 11% of emotional and threatened abuse or lack of supervision. An estimated 1640 children died from child maltreatment, with 70% of those deaths occurring among children

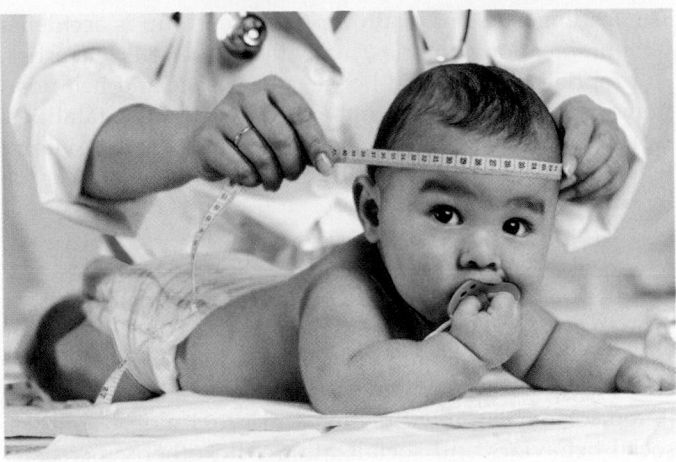

Source: ArtMarie/iStock/Getty Images.

Figure 51–3 》 An infant's head circumference is measured at every well-child visit.

younger than age 3 (CDC, 2014a). See the exemplar on Abuse in the module on Trauma for more information.

Because of their immature musculoskeletal systems and relative immobility, infants are also susceptible to a number of unintentional injuries. Falls accounted for nearly 50% of these injuries, and because of their soft heads, infants are particularly susceptible to traumatic brain injury. Another 14% were unintentionally struck by or against something, and an additional 7% of injuries were due to bites or stings (CDC, 2013b).

Nursing Implications

Newborns and infants are measured for growth and developmental trends at each visit to the healthcare provider. Measurements of their length, weight, and head circumference can be compared with weight gain and growth percentile ranges (**Figure 51–3 》》**). Observing the newborn and infant for developmental milestones such as lifting the head, smiling, rolling front to back, sitting without support, playing with toys, and imitating sounds readily provides assessment data for trending as the infant grows older. First-time parents may need more teaching and demonstrations of

---

Patient Teaching
When to Contact the Infant's Healthcare Provider

Encourage parents to call the healthcare provider any time they have a question. Teach parents to call the pediatrician's office for the following situations:

- Seizure activity
- Temperature of 100.4°F or above
- Skin change in color and presence of petechiae or skin rash
- Refusal to eat or drink
- Change in behavior or activity unusual for infant
- Vomiting
- Diarrhea
- Decreased urine
- Respiratory infection unusual for infant

Source: From Centers for Disease Control and Prevention (CDC). (2013c). *Leading causes of death reports, 1999–2010.* Retrieved from http://webappa.cdc.gov/sasweb/ncipc/leadcaus10_us.html.

---

newborn care to be comfortable and safe in caring for their new infant at home. See **Table 51–4 》》** for strategies for promoting infant safety. Teach parents when to contact the infant's healthcare provider as outlined in the Patient Teaching feature.

》》 Stay Current: The CDC provides information for current recommended immunization schedules for children aged 0 through 18 years old. http://www.cdc.gov/vaccines/schedules/downloads/child/0-18yrs-child-combined-schedule.pdf.

Safety for Toddlers and Preschoolers

Among all ages of children, unintentional injuries are the leading cause of death. Risks related to unintentional injury vary by age; for example, the toddler's mobility increases his risk for drowning in a swimming pool, whereas the infant is more likely to drown in the bathtub or a bucket, and

---

TABLE 51–4 Strategies for Promoting Infant Safety

Strategies for Injury Prevention	Strategies for Disease Prevention
■ Swaddle newborns so they feel secure; allow free movement of arms and hands	■ Other considerations: motor vehicle safety restraints, shaken baby syndrome, bed-sharing, drowning, suffocation, burns, falls, pet safety, fire safety, poisoning, and gun safety
■ Position infants on the back during sleep periods; put infants to sleep in warm clothing on a firm mattress in a crib or bassinet; do not place blankets, bumpers, pillows, or toys in the crib	■ Avoid secondhand smoke exposure
■ Position infant on the abdomen during supervised play periods	■ Reduce risks for sudden infant death syndrome
	■ Use proper hand hygiene before handling infant
■ Encourage appropriate toys such as crib mobile, soft toys, musical toys	■ Limit exposure to large crowds, especially in cold season
	■ Begin oral care by gently wiping gums with soft gauze 1–2 times a day
■ Create an environment that is infant-centered, allowing for learning, thinking, responding, and solving problems	■ Vaccinate infant with routine immunizations such as hepatitis B, DTP, *Haemophilus influenzae* type b, inactivated poliovirus, pneumococcus, influenza, and rotavirus
■ Know choking and CPR procedures for an infant	

Sources: Ball, J. W., Bindler, R. C., Cowen, K., & Shaw, M. (2017). *Principles of pediatric nursing: Caring for children* (7th ed.). Hoboken, NJ: Pearson Education.; CDC. (2014a). Violence prevention. *Child Maltreatment. Facts at a Glance.* Retrieved from http://www.cdc.gov/violenceprevention/pdf/childmaltreatment-facts-at-a-glance.pdf; CDC. (2015c). Ten leading causes of death and injury. *Injury Prevention & Control: Data & Statistics (WISQARS™).* Retrieved from http://www.cdc.gov/injury/wisqars/leadingcauses.html; National Institute of Child Health and Human Development. (2016). *Safe to sleep.* Retrieved from https://www.nichd.nih.gov/sts/Pages/default.aspx.

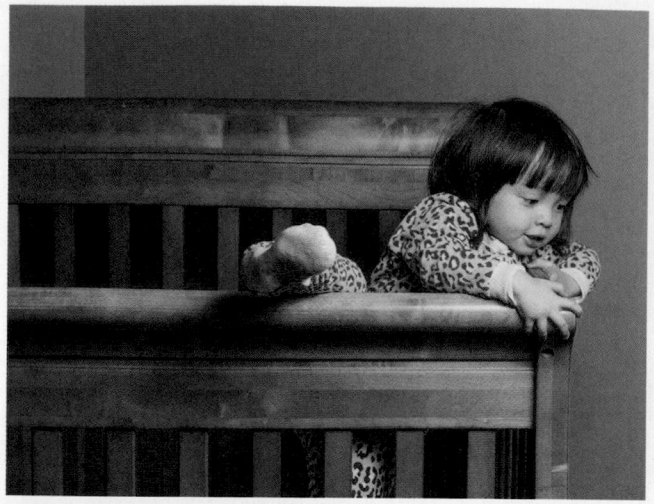

Source: Michael Pettigrew/Shutterstock.

Figure 51–4 》 Toddlers are vulnerable to accidents as they try out new skills and explore the world.

bicycle accidents are more common among school-age children. Note that the risk for ingesting chemicals or medications is highest among toddlers, preschoolers, and school-age children. Patient education for parents and caregivers of children in these age group includes keeping all medications and chemicals out of reach.

Toddlers

Toddlers begin walking, exploring the world around them, testing limits, and playing with anything in reach (**Figure 51–4 》**). Their small size and developing bones make them particularly vulnerable during motor vehicle crashes or when hit, pushed, or shaken. Drowning is of particular concern, particularly around swimming pools. The leading causes of death for this age group are accidents with unintentional injuries, and congenital malformations, deformations, and chromosomal abnormalities (CDC, 2015c). Toddlers also are at risk for injury or death due to fires or burns and suffocation. Another cause of death for young children occurs when they are left locked in parked motor vehicles.

SAFETY ALERT Even on a mild day (72°F), the temperature inside a closed car can escalate 30–40°F in an hour. Heat stroke may occur when the body temperature exceeds 104°F. Each year, an average of 38 children die in hot cars in the United States (Kids and Cars, 2016).

》 Stay Current: For a list of safety tips and strategies parents and caregivers can use to prevent children from being locked in vehicles, visit the Kids and Cars website at http://www.kidsandcars.org/heatstroke.html.

Preschoolers

Preschool-age children are more mobile and coordinated than toddlers, yet not fully aware of the dangers that surround them. Although the number of injuries and fatalities are reduced compared to toddlers, the most common causes of injury and fatality in preschoolers are generally the same.

The leading cause of death for this age group is accidents with unintentional injuries, many by motor vehicle crashes. Appropriate car seat and booster seat usage and belt positioning can reduce the numbers of injuries and fatalities. Approximately 14% of preschooler fatalities related to unintentional injuries are caused by fires or burns, and over 6% by suffocation (CDC, 2013c).

Nursing Implications

Toddlers and preschoolers continue to be measured for growth and developmental trends. Measurements of their standing height, weight, and BMI are done and compared with height and weight percentile ranges. Children are monitored for development of fine and gross motor abilities, social behaviors and socialization with others, increased skill in language development, and temperament. Observing the toddler and preschooler for developmental milestones such as walking, drinking from a cup, feeding self, kicking a ball, drawing lines on paper, stating name, and building a tower of blocks provides assessment data for trending as the child grows older. Screen children for anemia, number and condition of teeth, signs of possible abuse such as bruising, and skin or gait problems. Teaching parents about risk factors associated with these age groups can help reduce the incidence of unintentional injuries. See **Table 51–5 》** for strategies to teach parents for promoting safety for toddlers and preschoolers.

Safety for School-age Children and Adolescents

School-Age Children

Children age 5–10 are much more active than younger children and can play farther from home with less supervision. They are less dependent on their parents and move faster on foot and on bicycles, leading to more falls, accidents, and playground injuries. Unintentional injuries account for almost one third of deaths, of which more than 40% are caused by motor vehicle crashes. Nonfatal injuries mainly come from unintentional falls. In line with the increased activity of children this age, overexertion and bicycle accidents both accounted for 5% of injuries (CDC, 2013c).

Adolescents

Adolescents age 11–18 are exposed to a number of new risks. They are trying to develop their own identities apart from their parent(s), facing increasing peer pressure from all directions, receiving driver's licenses, and playing contact sports. They are most likely to start experimenting with drugs and alcohol in this age range. They are also experiencing emotional turmoil, leading to outward aggression and fighting, or internalizing and suicide. Now competing more seriously in sports and play, adolescents age 10–14 have the highest rate of injury during sports and play (**Figure 51–5 》**).

Most deaths for this age group are due to unintentional injury from motor vehicle crashes, poisoning (with 80% of these due to drug exposure of some kind), and drowning. Suicides, which do not qualify as unintentional but which are preventable, account for a small percentage of adolescent deaths. Other unintentional nonfatal injuries are from

TABLE 51–5 Strategies for Promoting Safety for Toddlers and Preschoolers

Strategies for Injury Prevention	Strategies for Disease Prevention
■ Help with food choices and eating patterns. Eat fewer fast foods and more fruits and vegetables	■ Avoid secondhand smoke exposure
■ Provide physical activities that use large muscle groups	■ Teach child to brush teeth; have scheduled dentist visits
■ Help child learn about what is right and wrong, and rules that guide behaviors	■ Encourage adequate sleep and rest
■ Discipline the child for undesirable behaviors	■ Teach child safety around strangers
■ Prevent air, water, or other toxic exposures	■ Be alert for electrical cords hanging down, water temperature higher than 120°F, sun exposure, and playing unsupervised
■ Prevent lead exposure in the home	■ Teach child about hand washing, calling for help using the telephone
■ Use appropriate harness straps or lap and shoulder belts for car safety	■ Vaccinate child with routine immunizations such as hepatitis B #3 in series and A, DTP, *Haemophilus influenzae* type b, inactivated poliovirus, pneumococcal, influenza, measles, mumps, rubella, varicella
■ Other considerations: falls, drowning, poisoning, burns, motor vehicle crashes, pedestrian accidents	■ Teach children about crossing streets, riding bicycles, playing in water safety, and avoiding fire hazards
	■ Know choking and CPR procedures for a child

Sources: Ball, J. W., Bindler, R. C., Cowen, K., & Shaw, M. (2017). *Principles of pediatric nursing: Caring for children* (7th ed.). Hoboken, NJ: Pearson Education.; CDC. (2014a). Violence prevention. *Child Maltreatment. Facts at a Glance.* Retrieved from http://www.cdc.gov/violenceprevention/pdf/childmaltreatment-facts-at-a-glance.pdf; CDC. (2015c). Ten leading causes of death and injury. *Injury Prevention & Control: Data & Statistics (WISQARS™).* Retrieved from http://www.cdc.gov/injury/wisqars/leadingcauses.html.

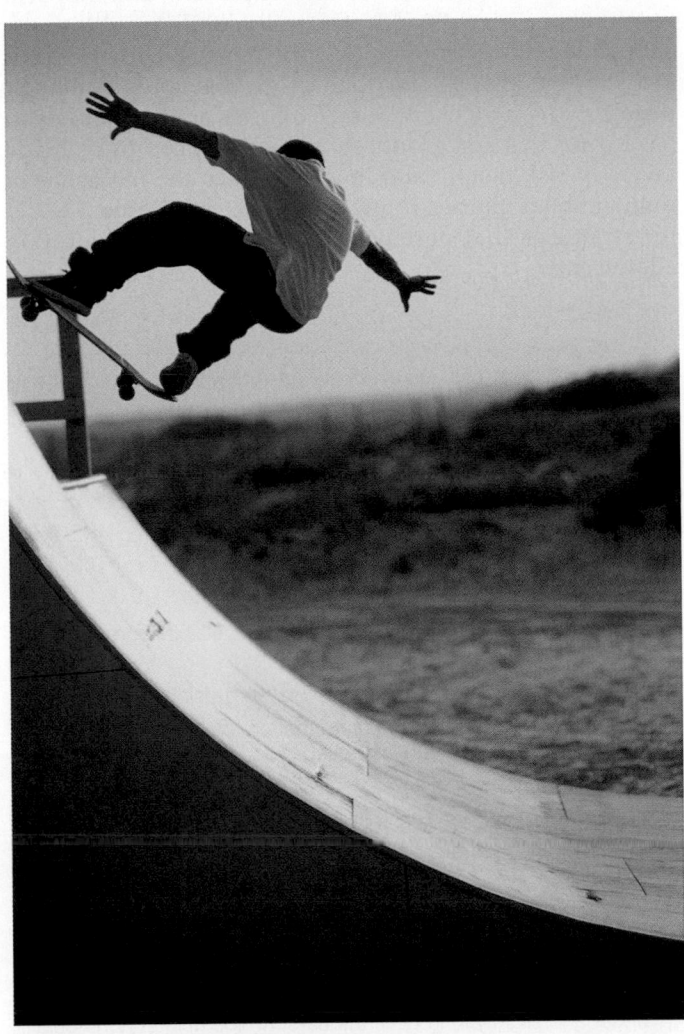

Source: Michael Krasowitz/Taxi/Getty Images.

Figure 51–5 >> This teenage skateboarder is at risk for fractures and head injury because he is not wearing protective equipment.

unintentionally being struck by or against something, unintentional falls, overexertion, and as a motor vehicle occupant (CDC, 2013c).

Nursing Implications

School-age children continue to have their height, weight, and BMI monitored. Their bodies are refining muscular strength and coordination. They need encouragement to establish good health habits for nutrition, physical activity, and mental health, and to avoid tobacco, alcohol, and drugs. Children are learning decision-making, problem-solving skills, and refining skills with sports such as eye-hand coordination, agility, and speed. Their deciduous teeth are being replaced by permanent teeth. They are increasingly more active in after-school activities such as sports and clubs.

Continue observation for developmental milestones such as independence in bathroom and dressing activities, reading, developing hobbies, playing musical instrument, writing well, skill at computer use, developing self-esteem more with feelings of self-worth related to physical appearance and social interactions, developing body image of self, having prepuberty changes (girls may begin to menstruate), common mental disorders such as anxiety, worrying, fears, stress, sleep disorders, depression, and building relationships outside of family. This observation provides assessment data for trending as the child grows older. Screen for blood pressure, bruising, repeated infections, changes in school performance or behavior, medications being taken, and any integrative therapies used.

Parents need to adapt discipline methods to actions such as withholding privileges and using time-out; spanking and yelling should be avoided. School-age children can be taught risk factors and how to help reduce the incidence of unintentional injuries, such as by wearing a helmet when riding a bicycle. See **Table 51–6 >>** for strategies for parents to promote safety for school-age children; also see the Patient Teaching feature on use of bicycle helmets.

TABLE 51–6 Strategies for Promoting Safety in School-Age Children

Strategies to Prevent Injury	Strategies to Prevent Disease
▪ Latchkey children who come home to an empty house after school need encouragement to remain safe, responsible, and have feelings of security ▪ Teach children about fire, firearms, water, and other safety hazards and what to do in emergencies ▪ Teach children about safety around interacting with strangers—accepting rides from them, chatting with them online, or talking with them on the phone ▪ Promote healthy sleep behaviors ▪ Use proper safety equipment to avoid sports injuries, especially from sports such as skateboarding, football, soccer, skiing, rollerblading, and motorcycle and ATV riding ▪ Teach children safe resources such as teachers, school counselors, and police or security ▪ Watch for signs of risky behaviors such as substance abuse, smoking, aggression and violence, eating disorders, and anxiety ▪ Other considerations: pedestrian or biking accidents, handling firearms unsupervised, burns from experiments with flames or toxic substances, assault from a stranger, and what to do when scared and alone in a public or private area	▪ Encourage independent food choices, including fruits and vegetables; suggest frequent snacks of nonfat and nonsugar choices ▪ Continue oral health with brushing, flossing, and dentist visits ▪ Teach children how to prevent diseases by washing their hands, avoiding respiratory infections, and avoiding causes of gastrointestinal illness ▪ Connect health with risk behaviors such as smoking, poor oral hygiene, low physical activity, having above-normal weight, and skin problems ▪ Limit television and video game time ▪ Continue with immunizations as needed

Sources: Ball, J. W., Bindler, R. C., Cowen, K., & Shaw, M. (2017). *Principles of pediatric nursing: Caring for children* (7th ed.). Hoboken, NJ: Pearson Education.; CDC. (2015c). Ten leading causes of death and injury. *Injury Prevention & Control: Data & Statistics (WISQARS™).* Retrieved from http://www.cdc.gov/injury/wisqars/leadingcauses.html; CDC. (2015d). *Influenza vaccination information for health care workers.* Retrieved from http://www.cdc.gov/flu/healthcareworkers.htm.

When caring for adolescents, continue to monitor height, weight, and BMI. Observing the adolescent for developmental milestones provides assessment data for trending as the individual grows older. Self-concept continues to evolve; body changes may lead to decisions about sexual behaviors. Older adolescents should be asked if they are having sexual intercourse and, if so, if they are using protection against pregnancy and sexually transmitted infections. Ask about confusion with sexuality, sexual practices, and gay, lesbian, or bisexual activities. Their relationships and friends are very important, and they will test limits of parents and engage in conflicts with them. School offers peer support and meaningful activities, but also causes stress, worry about grades, and violent or unsupportive school situations. Injuries are a major health hazard for this age group, so caregivers need to be made aware of risk factors and how to reduce the incidence of unintentional injuries to prevent them. See **Table 51–7 》** for strategies that parents can use to promote safety in adolescents.

Patient Teaching
Bicycle Safety

Children age 5–14 years have a high rate of nonfatal bicycle-related injuries. Helmets can reduce the number of head and brain injuries if worn correctly (**Figure 51–6 》**); unfortunately, they often are either not worn or worn incorrectly (too far back on the head) (CDC, 2015e).

Suggested interventions for reducing injuries and fatalities to bicyclists include:

▪ Wearing fluorescent clothing to be more visible from farther away

▪ Wearing retro-reflective clothing to be more visible at night

▪ Wearing age-appropriate helmets that are well maintained

▪ Adding lights on the bicycle or bicyclist such as front white lights and rear red lights

▪ Making sure the helmet is properly fitting; it should fit snugly all around with no spaces between the foam and the bicyclist's head

▪ Wearing helmet correctly: (1) the bottom of the pad inside the front of the helmet is one or two fingerwidths above the bicyclist's eyebrows, (2) the back of the helmet should not touch the top of the neck, (3) side straps should form a "V" shape under and slightly in front of the ears, (4) the chin strap should be centered under the bicyclist's chin and fit snugly, not moving in any direction.

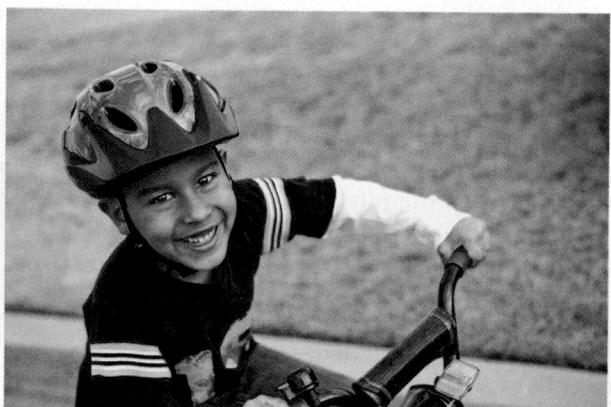

Source: Mari/E+/Getty Images.

Figure 51–6 》 Wearing an age-appropriate, well-fitting helmet helps reduce the risk of head and brain injuries.

TABLE 51–7 Strategies for Promoting Safety in Adolescents

Strategies to Prevent Injury	Strategies to Prevent Disease
■ Encourage consumption of nutritional foods to support immune system, physical activity, and metabolism ■ Encourage adequate sleep ■ Encourage regular physical activity ■ Avoid high noise levels such as when listening to music through earbuds or headphones ■ Encourage oral health behaviors; be alert for ulcers or unusual growths in mouth, self-induced vomiting with anorexia or bulimia which harms tooth enamel, chewing tobacco resulting in oral ulcers, cancers, and certain sports that are higher risk for injuries, such as hockey and football ■ Observe for signs of depression such as changes in behavior, school performance, sleep, and appetite; sadness; poor concentration; feelings of worthlessness; thoughts of death or suicide ■ Observe for signs of substance abuse such as changes in behavior, school performance, sleep, and appetite, lack of responsibility, inability to set goals, hopelessness, multiple accidents ■ Teach and encourage safe driving behaviors ■ Other considerations: safety with four-wheelers, boats, jet skis, farm machinery, tools, drowning, sun exposure, fires, firearms, hearing problems from loud music, abuse	■ Seek medical attention for acne and skin infections ■ Seek medical treatment for anemia, monitor dietary choices, encourage rest periods ■ Encourage use of appropriate safety equipment to avoid sports overuse injuries, teach safety for flexibility and muscular limitations ■ Discuss bowel and bladder patterns and recognition of constipation and diarrhea, teach dietary choices to avoid bowel problems, teach importance of fluid intake to support bowel habits ■ Discuss aseptic technique needed for body piercing and tattooing to avoid infection, discuss decision-making that has long-range impacts later in life ■ Discuss wellness habits to help prevent fatigue, such as healthy eating, exercise activity, amount of sleep, and emotional support ■ Use sunscreen to avoid sunburn and risk for later skin lesions ■ Discuss and provide information about sexually transmitted infections such as HIV, herpes, syphilis, gonorrhea, hepatitis A, and the viruses that cause warts and herpes that can be transmitted through unprotected intercourse or oral sex; provide options to protect adolescents against acquiring these diseases and conditions ■ Discuss physical and emotional complications of eating disorders such as anorexia and bulimia; obtain counseling if needed ■ Discuss safety and protection if being abused or bullied by another individual, observe for signs of abuse, provide information about strategies to remain calm and protect oneself from altercations, provide safe adults to go to when needing assistance ■ Observe for signs and symptoms of substance abuse and provide medical help as needed, monitor for any drug paraphernalia or drugs, discuss addiction and safety implications of certain drugs in the body ■ Stress importance of cessation of smoking and use of nicotine products to avoid addiction and chronic health conditions ■ Common immunizations recommended: TD if last one >10 years ago, second measles-mumps-rubella, meningococcal vaccine recommended, human papillomavirus vaccine (3-dose series), annual influenza vaccine

Sources: Ball, J. W., Bindler, R. C., Cowen, K., & Shaw, M. (2017). *Principles of pediatric nursing: Caring for children* (7th ed.). Hoboken, NJ: Pearson Education.; CDC. (2015b). Child health. *FastStats.* Retrieved from http://www.cdc.gov/nchs/fastats/child-health.htm; CDC. (2015c). Ten leading causes of death and injury. *Injury Prevention & Control: Data & Statistics (WISQARS™).* Retrieved from http://www.cdc.gov/injury/wisqars/leadingcauses.html.

Safety for Adults

Young Adults

Young adults, ages approximately 19–45, are generally striking out on their own, getting jobs, being educated, getting married, and having kids. However, this independent living means making their own choices and mistakes, some of which can lead to life-altering changes. Young adults die from unintentional injuries resulting from poisoning mostly by drugs, narcotics, medicines, or biological agents; motor vehicle crashes; malignant cancers; heart disease; suicide; and homicides (**Figure 51–7 »**) (CDC, 2013c). Sources of nonfatal injuries include unintentional falls, inadvertent overexertion, being accidentally struck by or against something, and unintentional cuts or piercing wounds. Overexertion can be a particular concern among recreational athletes, who may be at greater risk for dehydration, exposure-related illness, or sports-related injury.

Middle Adults

Middle adults, ages 46–65, are beginning to look toward retirement. Middle adults have started to slow down, probably becoming less active and developing some chronic health problems as the healing process slows. For the first time, unintentional injuries are not the leading cause of death. Instead, malignant cancers account for one third of deaths. Heart disease is the second leading cause of death, due to age and obesity. Unintentional injuries that result in

death are caused by poisoning, mostly from drugs, narcotics, medicines, or biological agents. A little over one quarter of fatalities are due to motor vehicle traffic and falls. Suicides in this age group represent a small percentage of deaths (CDC, 2013c). For the middle adults who experience injuries that do not end in fatality, the majority of these injuries are due to unintentional falls, and the others due to overexertion, accidental injury due to being hit by or against something, and motor vehicle crashes (CDC, 2013b).

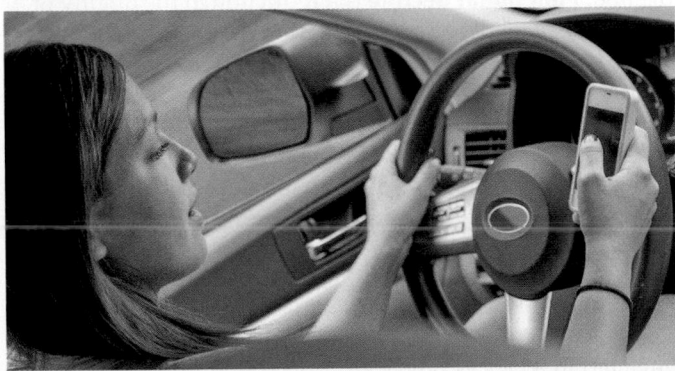

Source: Nycshooter/iStock/Getty Images.

Figure 51–7 » Individuals who text while driving are 23 times more likely to be in a crash than those who do not text while driving.

TABLE 51–8 Strategies for Promoting Safety in Adults

Strategies to Prevent Injury	Strategies to Prevent Disease
■ Do not be distracted when driving a motor vehicle, such as texting, talking on cell phone, eating, drinking, looking at a GPS device, or adjusting the radio	■ Do basic medical screening for conditions that may lead to chronic medical illness or disease
■ Do appropriate exercise activities, check with healthcare provider before beginning new physical activities	■ Have annual health checkups
■ Seek medical help if at-home care does not improve an injury	■ Maintain healthy weight by eating nutritious foods
■ Avoid stressing back when lifting or moving heavy objects	■ Practice health behaviors such as handwashing
■ Stay alert and use caution when using equipment and household appliances	■ Follow a prudent lifestyle and take medications as prescribed to control chronic conditions such as hypertension and diabetes
■ Stay alert and use caution to avoid tripping on objects and falling	■ Avoid exposure to infectious conditions such as crowds in cold season
■ Use ergonomic aids when using a computer	■ Use sunscreen to avoid sunburn and risk for later skin lesions
■ Use safety seat belt when driving or riding in a motor vehicle	■ Follow immunization guidelines appropriate for adults such as annual flu vaccine, Tdap every 10 years, shingles zoster vaccine, and pneumococcal vaccine
■ Keep a simple first aid kit at home and in motor vehicle in case of accidents	
■ Use integrative health therapies such as herbs, green tea, massages, and yoga to relax the body and mind	■ Omit lifestyle risks such as smoking, drinking alcohol, drug abuse, and unprotected sexual intercourse with many partners

Sources: CDC. (2013c). *Leading causes of death reports, 1999–2010.* Retrieved from http://webappa.cdc.gov/sasweb/ncipc/leadcaus10_us.html; CDC. (2013b). *Leading causes of nonfatal injury reports, 2001–2011.* Retrieved from http://webappa.cdc.gov/sasweb/ncipc/nfilead2001.html; CDC. (2015c). Ten leading causes of death and injury. *Injury Prevention & Control: Data & Statistics (WISQARS™).* Retrieved from http://www.cdc.gov/injury/wisqars/leadingcauses.html.

Strategies for promoting safety for adults are shown in **Table 51–8 》**.

》 Stay Current: The CDC provides information for current recommended immunization schedules for adults: http://www.cdc.gov/vaccines/schedules/downloads/adult/adult-schedule-easy-read.pdf.

Safety for Older Adults

About 65% of older adults retire by the time they turn 65. Of those still working past 65, more than a third work part time (Sightings, 2014). As older adults continue to age, living independently can become challenging for those experiencing chronic illnesses that impact cognition or mobility. Chronic diseases such as heart disease, malignant cancers, cerebrovascular illness (stroke), chronic respiratory disease, Alzheimer disease, and diabetes are common causes of fatality in this age group. The highest cause of death from unintentional injury is falls, then motor vehicle crashes, suffocation, poisoning, and fire (CDC, 2013c).

Older adults in assisted living facilities or living in their own homes need to take steps to actively prevent functional decline. **Functional decline** is a reduction in the quality of or ability for physical or cognitive function. It may only take a couple of days to begin to manifest through changes such as diminished ability to complete ADLs, impaired mobility, decreased musculoskeletal strength, and reduced physical endurance (Government of South Australia, 2016).

By reducing the risk of functional decline, nurses and independent older adults can help prevent complications of this condition, such as pressure injuries, delirium and depression, decreased mobility, loss of independence, and incontinence. Reducing functional decline may be helped by encouraging older adults to keep mobile, active, and engaged in ADLs as physically and cognitively able. Precautionary measures need to be implemented for the prevention of injury in the elderly with impaired mobility or altered cognitive function. Reorientation to the patient's room, how to get to a restroom, and how to call for help will also help reduce functional decline when in an assisted living facility.

Some communities have daycare centers with staff trained to work with older adults. Another community-based resource for the elderly is a senior center that offers a variety of activities for the elderly to participate in and socialize with others their age (**Figure 51–8 》**). There are also many federal, state, local, and private advocacy organizations dedicated to providing services for the elderly. Oral care remains important to prevent periodontal diseases such as oral and pharyngeal cancers. See the Patient Teaching feature for factors affecting oral health and **Table 51–9 》** for strategies to promote safety in older adults who live in the community.

Safety for Individuals with Special Needs

Safety is focused on the developmental level and physical capabilities of individuals. Strategies to prevent unintentional injuries can be adapted for those with special needs.

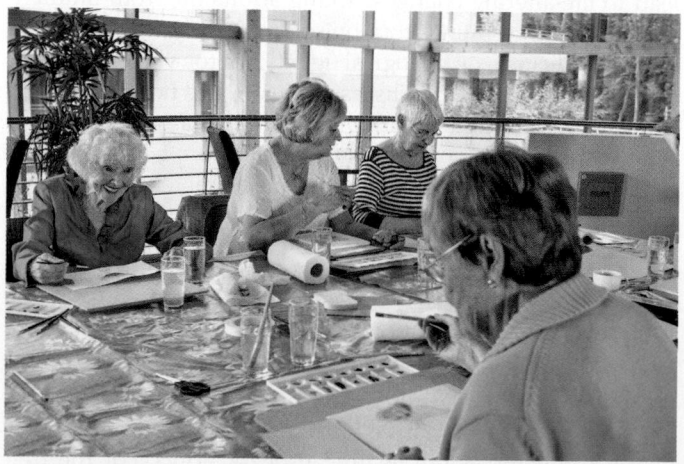

Source: Horsche/iStock/Getty Images.

Figure 51–8 》 Senior centers offer companionship and activities for older adults.

Patient Teaching

Oral Health for Older Adults

Older adults are at risk for poor oral health for a number of reasons. Approximately 25% of older adults no longer have their natural teeth, which may lead them to choose soft, easily chewed foods and avoid fresh fruits and vegetables (CDC, 2013d). Older adults face increasing severity of periodontal disease. Oral and pharyngeal cancers, primarily diagnosed in older adults, have poor prognoses. Those with the poorest oral health are those who are economically disadvantaged, do not have dental insurance, and are members of ethnic minorities. Those who are disabled, bedbound, homebound, or institutionalized have higher risk of poor oral health (CDC, 2013d).

Another factor that contributes to poor oral health is the high number of prescription and over-the-counter drugs older adults take that cause a dry mouth. Saliva contains antimicrobial components as well as minerals that help rebuild tooth enamel attacked by decay-causing bacteria, so when saliva production is decreased, the risk for oral disease is increased. There are also chronic neurologic or musculoskeletal conditions such as Alzheimer disease and stroke that limit the ability of older adults to perform oral health self-care.

Nurses should encourage older adults and/or those assisting them to:

- Periodically assess the mouth for changes in appearance, tenderness of gums, sensitivity of teeth, presence of saliva, cracked skin areas, ulcerations, or pain, and report anything unusual to their healthcare provider.
- Observe for bleeding gums when brushing natural teeth, red swollen gums, and chronic bad taste or bad breath, as these may indicate gum disease.
- Remember to stay hydrated to maintain good salivary flow. Dry mouth may occur as a side effect of certain medications prescribed.
- Notice if the corners of the mouth and the lips are dry and cracked. A lubricant can be applied as needed to prevent problems with skin integrity.
- Clean any dentures daily and rinse them after every meal. Ensure food particles and other debris are removed after each meal.
- Brush teeth every day, as able, and after every meal, or have assistance with oral care.
- Have oral hygiene materials available, such as toothbrushes, toothpaste, denture cleaning products, and mouthwash.
- Prevent aspiration with positioning and assistance as needed during mouth care.
- Schedule annual appointments with the dentist.

Source: From CDC. (2013d). *Oral health for older Americans. Adult oral health. Division of Oral Health.* Retrieved from http://www.cdc.gov/OralHealth/publications/factsheets/adult_oral_health/adult_older.htm.

Individuals with special needs refers to individuals with mental, emotional, or physical disabilities who may require special care or assistance to communicate, ambulate, perform self-care activities, or make decisions. Types of special needs include autism, Down syndrome, speech and language impairments, reading and learning disabilities, and cerebral palsy. Individuals with conditions that affect attention, memory, or communication, such as Alzheimer disease and ADHD, may also be included in this category.

Individuals with special needs require assistance or accommodation in all settings. For example, parents and care providers can create a safe home environment by using safety equipment, such as smoke alarms that signal with a light, handrails to prevent falls, and life jackets for water safety that are specially fitted to the individual. If the individual with special needs is a wanderer, family can talk with neighbors and ask for their help keeping watch and to contact them if they see the individual unsupervised. As appropriate, the individual with special needs can wear a bracelet or some other kind of identification. Special locks or alarms on exit doors may be necessary to alert caregivers that the individual is trying to leave the building.

TABLE 51–9 Strategies for Promoting Safety in Community-Dwelling Older Adults

Strategies to Prevent Injury	Strategies to Prevent Disease
■ Maintain mobility, activity, and function as tolerated and able to do	■ Schedule an annual comprehensive assessment of physical, cognitive, emotional, and functional status
■ Have safety supports in the home for mobility, such as handrails, shower seats, chairs with adjustable heights, adequate lighting, and low beds	■ Maintain appropriate body weight by eating a variety of fruits, vegetables, and proteins
■ Seek help when needed for household upkeep, yard maintenance, repair work, and so on	■ Drink adequate fluids to stay hydrated
■ Minimize clutter in the home	■ Exercise joints and muscles to maintain mobility and flexibility
■ Wear footwear with skid-resistant soles	■ Do assessment self-checks for changes to skin integrity, respiratory status, musculoskeletal movements, and routine body functions
■ Keep assistive devices such as canes, walkers, glasses, and hearing aids, close and accessible to use	■ Be actively engaged in health safety behaviors such as frequent hand washing
■ Know about prescribed medications and their side effects	■ Be aware of surroundings and alert for safety hazards to avoid
■ Be aware of physical limitations to avoid injuries and accidents	■ Avoid temperature extremes
■ Socialize with others for psychosocial healthiness as desired	

Sources: Administration on Aging (AoA). (2015). Administration for Community Living. *National organizations. Comprehensive national organizations.* Retrieved from http://www.aoa.acl.gov/AoA_Programs/Tools_Resources/national_organizations.aspx#; CDC. (2013e). *Falls among older adults: An overview.* Retrieved from http://www.cdc.gov/Homeand_RecreationalSafety/Falls/nursing.html; Office of Disease Prevention and Health Promotion (ODPHP). (2015a). *The Office of Disease Prevention and Health Promotion.* Retrieved from http://health.gov.

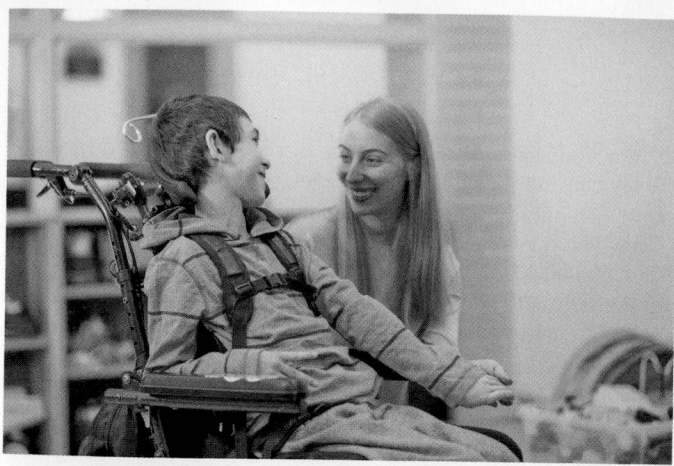

Source: FatCamera/E+/Getty Images.

Figure 51–9 》 Because of IDEA, all students are guaranteed a free and appropriate education. Here a boy with cerebral palsy works with his aide in the classroom.

In school systems, the Individuals with Disabilities Education Act (IDEA) mandates the provision of a free and appropriate public school education for individuals who have a disability that adversely affects academic performance or need special education and related services (**Figure 51–9 》**). During the school year 2012–2013, about 6.4 million children or about 13% of all public school students were receiving special education services (National Center for Education Statistics [NCES], 2015). Individuals with special needs may be bullied, teased, or harassed physically, verbally, or socially leading to feelings of low self-esteem, health problems, and depression. Individuals can learn how to protect themselves from bullying with instruction and by practicing behaviors at home. They can also learn safe people to go to while at school, such as the school counselor, teacher, or security guard.

Here are suggested questions to address for safety and injury prevention:

1. Can the individual move about, handle things, and explore?

2. Is there any safety equipment or modifications that are appropriate for the individual?
3. Does the individual have difficulty talking or understanding?
4. Does the individual have difficulty making decisions? (CDC, 2014b)

Individuals with special needs depend on others to help them have safety and security. Parents and other family members may need assistance to locate community resources to help provide appropriate care and respite care. Nurses can assess what needs the individual has that will require assistance from others and discuss resources with the family. Nurses can provide support and encouragement for the individuals and their families. Teaching is important to show family members how equipment, supplies, and procedures are used or performed. A team of caregivers may be essential to provide supervision and care. This also can provide a variety of relationships with caregivers and the special needs individual. Family members may need encouragement and support to accept respite care as a time of refreshing and reenergizing without feelings of guilt. Strategies for promoting safety for individuals with special needs are outlined in **Table 51–10 》**.

NURSING PROCESS

Individualized patient care includes appropriate developmental and chronologic health promotion and injury prevention considerations. Safety is often a priority. Nurses need to take into account safety hazards that may result in injuries associated with all age groups across the lifespan, such as accidental poisoning for small children or falls for older adults.

Assessment

Both objective and subjective data are used to assess the need for maintaining the current level of health or readiness to improve it:

■ ***Observation and patient interview.*** History of lifestyle risk behaviors, frequency of injuries from chronic conditions,

TABLE 51–10 Strategies for Promoting Safety for Individuals with Special Needs

Strategies to Prevent Injury	Strategies to Prevent Disease
■ Adapt safety restraints and seats in motor vehicles as appropriate to keep individual safe	■ Avoid secondhand smoke exposure
■ Advocate to have neighborhood audible crosswalk signals installed	■ Teach individual to brush teeth, have scheduled dentist visits
■ Have safety evacuation plans at home for fire, include flashing lights for hearing impaired, include special equipment as appropriate	■ Encourage adequate sleep and rest
■ Install soft surfaces in outside play areas	■ Teach individual safety around strangers
■ Match sports activities to individual's abilities	■ Maintain airway with suctioning as needed, or if able, effective coughing
■ Provide special equipment or protection for individuals needing assistive devices	■ Teach individual about hand washing and using a telephone to call for help
■ Match toys, games, and hobbies to individual's developmental level	■ Schedule routine immunizations for age group
■ Dress appropriately for the weather	■ Provide oxygen therapy as prescribed
■ Be alert for home safety issues: electrical outlets, electrical cords, climbing on furniture, hot water temperature; knowing where to find bathroom, bedroom, dining room	

Source: Center for Children with Special Needs (CCSN). (2015). Early intervention, childcare & schools>Safety tips>Playground safety for your child with special needs. *Seattle Children's Hospital Research Foundation.* Retrieved from http://cshcn.org/childcare-schools-community/safety-tips/playground-safety-for-your-child-with-special-needs; CDC. (2014a). Violence prevention. *Child Maltreatment. Facts at a Glance.* Retrieved from http://www.cdc.gov/violenceprevention/pdf/childmaltreatment-facts-at-a-glance.pdf; CDC. (2014b). *Keeping children with disabilities safe.* Retrieved from http://www.cdc.gov/ncbddd/disabilityandsafety/child-safety.html.

developmental challenges, sensory and motor deficits, change in sustainability of current health status, changes in family dynamics, ability to live independently, and so on

- **Physical examination.** Vital signs, heart and lung sounds, mobility, sensory and motor disabilities, changes due to lifestyle risk behaviors, cognition abilities, current injuries noted, and so on.

Diagnosis

There are many NANDA-I nursing diagnosis labels about promoting health and preventing injuries for all ages of patients. Promoting health can focus on psychologic, emotional, physical, spiritual health, and preventing injuries can address environmental conditions, the patient's current state of well-being, or the patient's homeostasis status. Here are a few common examples of safety and health promotion nursing diagnoses:

- *Protection, Ineffective*
- *Health Behavior, Risk-Prone*
- *Health Maintenance, Ineffective*
- *Self-Care, Readiness for Enhanced.*

(NANDA-I © 2014)

Planning

Goals for improved health reflect the nursing diagnosis label and include input from the patient, such as:

- The patient will assess his skin for lesions every month.
- The patient will verbalize three ways to be physically active each day.
- The patient will actively participate in a community-based smoking cessation program.
- The patient will be able to correctly demonstrate how to empty his colostomy bag by discharge.

Implementation

There are many nursing actions that help patients improve their health while in a healthcare setting (acute care facility, extended care facility, community facility, or home setting). There are many opportunities for nurses to teach patients about being more active in safe self-care behaviors to prevent injuries. All interventions need to be prioritized to best meet patient needs. Some intervention examples are:

- Demonstrate to patient how to use a mirror to assess for skin lesions on his back.
- Assist patient in finding a smoking cessation program in his community.
- Encourage patient to observe and then participate in emptying his colostomy bag.
- Collaborate with the physical therapist to teach patient appropriate physical exercises.

Evaluation

Expected outcomes may include the following:

- The patient is able to correctly empty his colostomy bag when needed.
- The patient attends a smoking cessation program in his community.
- The patient is able to verbalize how to assess for lesions on his back using a mirror.
- The patient is able to demonstrate three physical activities that can be done during the day.

The safety and health conditions of a patient can change quickly. Because of this, the nurse needs to continuously monitor the patient's health status by observing for cues indicating a difference between previous and current assessment data. Promoting safety and well-being for the patient needs to be a priority during every nurse–patient interaction.

REVIEW Health Promotion and Injury Prevention Across the Lifespan

RELATE Link the Concepts and Exemplars

Linking the exemplar on health promotion and injury prevention across the lifespan with the concept of culture and diversity:

1. Discuss how an individual's culture may impact his or her environmental exposures and lifestyle choices.
2. How might the nurse integrate cultural considerations in an assessment of an individual's safety throughout the lifespan?

Linking the exemplar of health promotion and injury prevention across the lifespan with the concept of communication:

3. Differentiate ways of teaching an adult, a school-age child, and a toddler about hand hygiene safety.
4. Contrast safety considerations when providing care to a primary English-speaking patient and to a patient who speaks English as a secondary language.

READY Go to Volume 3: Clinical Nursing Skills

REFER Go to Pearson MyLab Nursing and eText

- Additional review materials

REFLECT Apply Your Knowledge

An older adult patient was admitted to the hospital 3 days ago subsequent to a fall. She sustained a right hip fracture and a mild concussion. The patient had been outside gardening on an afternoon where the temperature reached a high of 92 degrees. When she stood up to walk in the house, she experienced vertigo and fell to the ground. After she recovers from surgical repair of her hip fracture, she will be transferred to a rehabilitation facility.

1. How might age-related physiologic changes have contributed to the patient's fall and subsequent injuries?
2. Why is the patient being transferred to a rehabilitation facility, as opposed to being discharged to her home?
3. Develop a nursing plan of care for the patient.

≫ Exemplar 51.B
Patient Safety

Exemplar Learning Outcomes

51.B Analyze safety as it relates to patients in home care and healthcare settings.

- Evaluate the quality of safety in home care settings.
- Write safety nursing interventions for patients in healthcare settings.
- Contrast lifespan considerations for safety in healthcare settings.
- Plan nursing interventions for quality, safety, and best patient outcomes.

Exemplar Key Terms

Adverse drug event (ADEs), 2893
Chemical restraints, 2895
Elder abuse, 2892
Handoff reporting, 2893
Healthcare-associated infections (HAIs), 2894
National Healthcare Safety Network, 2894
Never events, 2895
Physical restraints, 2895
Polypharmacy, 2893
Safety devices, 2895
SBAR, 2893
Seclusion, 2895
Sentinel events, 2895
Wrong-site surgery (WSS), 2895

Overview

Individualized patient care incorporates numerous developmental considerations. Patients who present with illness or injuries are assessed not only in terms of their developmental age group, but also about safety concerns for the age group. Nurses need to take into account common injuries and safety hazards associated with all age groups across the lifespan. These considerations for safety should take place in all healthcare settings; acute care facilities, extended care facilities, community settings, and home settings.

Safety in Home Care Settings

Home healthcare has become an established regulated program of care and services that older adults are using more now that they are living longer. A variety of medical, therapeutic, and nonmedical services, such as wound care, dietary counseling, physical therapy, skilled nursing services, occupational therapy, and homemaker services, are now available in private homes from healthcare professionals. Data show that 23.1% of noninstitutionalized older adults are in fair or poor health, so many need some level of assistance in the home. The home health industry is responding to these needs (CMS, 2015).

As the older adult population continues to grow, so does the suspected number of unreported elder abuse cases (National Center on Elder Abuse [NCEA], 2015). **Elder abuse** is defined as intentional actions by a family member, caregiver, or other that inflicts harm or puts the older adult at risk for harm, including failure to meet basic needs or protect the older adult from harm. In a national study, it was reported that approximately 90% of abusers were family members (NCEA, 2015).

Older adults over the age 65 with disabilities are more vulnerable to abuse that puts their health, safety, well-being, and ability to take care of themselves at risk. Another high-risk group for abuse is those with dementia. Victims of elder abuse and neglect have additional health conditions, such as digestive problems, depression, anxiety, chronic pain, and

heart problems. Many older adults on fixed incomes also experience financial exploitation with very damaging losses affecting their lifestyles and ability to take care of themselves (NCEA, 2015). See the exemplar on Abuse in the module on Trauma for further information.

≫ **Stay current:** Learn more about federal and state policies on elder abuse at https://ncea.acl.gov/index.html.

There are many environmental improvements that address safety risk measures in home settings. Best patient outcomes from these interventions could include that the patient remained unharmed, did not fall, was comfortable with room temperatures, remained accident free, and felt secure and safe. These improvements can be adapted to individual home settings. Examples of environmental safety improvements are:

1. Installing handrails along the walls
2. Installing grab bars in the bathroom, at toilet and tub/shower areas
3. Designing wider hallways and doorways for using walkers and wheelchairs
4. Installing easy-grip door handles, water faucets, and cabinets
5. Removing scatter rugs or adding nonslip padding underneath
6. Ensuring that a bell or way to call for help is easily accessible
7. Providing adequate lighting
8. Using raised toilet seats
9. Giving the patient the ability to control room temperatures for comfort
10. Ensuring that fire and disaster plans are available.

Older adults with one or more chronic illnesses may be taking medications that can increase risk for confusion or compromise mobility. Nurses working with patients from this population assess for risks to safety related to both prescribed and over-the-counter medications and supplements (see the Patient Teaching feature).

Patient Teaching
Promoting Medication Safety for Older Adults

Nurses can provide patient teaching to help older adults and their families know how to reduce the risk of harm related to medications and in particular from **polypharmacy**, which is using a large number of medications for one or more conditions. The following suggestions can help promote medication safety for older adults in a home setting:

1. Carry a list of medications to each appointment with a healthcare provider. Share the list with a family member.
2. Take medication as prescribed until it is finished, especially antibiotics, or discontinued under the direction of the healthcare provider. Do not skip doses of medication.
3. Use a pill organizer, or ask a family member or close neighbor for help filling pill compartments for each day of the week.
4. Keep emergency and contact phone numbers near the telephone.
5. Do not store multiple medications in a single container; this can make it difficult to identify individual medications.
6. If the patient has difficulty remembering to take medications, reading labels, hearing instructions, swallowing tablets or capsules, or opening medication bottles, encourage the patient to inform the pharmacist and all healthcare providers and to ask a family member or close neighbor for assistance as needed.
7. If the nursing assessment indicates that the patient needs regular assistance taking medications, work with the patient to come up with solutions that ensure the patient's safety, such as having a family member or a friend assist with medications.

Safety in Healthcare Settings

Because patient care can be very complicated in the healthcare setting, there is a need for coordination, flexibility, and adjustments made among the team of physicians, nurses, and other disciplines involved. Treatment protocols can be complicated and time sensitive; healthcare providers can modify their prescribed orders by changing them, adding new ones, or stopping old ones by the telephone, face-to-face, or in writing. Keeping quality and safety priorities for everyone is a continuous challenge.

Communication of patient information, called **handoff reporting**, between nursing units, between shifts, other departments, staff, and physicians is critical. Unfortunately, it is also a common cause of error if not all patient information is given, or if there is not enough time to give complete information and information about the patient is fragmented (The Joint Commission, 2013). To organize necessary patient information and standardize handoff communication, many healthcare facilities are using a communication tool called **SBAR**, which stands for:

Situation

Background

Assessment

Recommendations

For further information, go to the module on Communication, and see **Figure 51–10 》**.

For these reasons, and despite the best intentions of nurses and other providers, adverse events and medical errors occur frequently. Healthcare staff constantly strive to keep these adverse events to a minimum, targeting common clinical occurrences such as adverse drug events, falls, healthcare-associated infections (HAIs), improper use of restraints, and wrong-site surgery (WSS) (CDC, 2015f). Unfortunately, in some healthcare facilities safety may not be a high priority, leading to complacency and tolerance of low performance, which can contribute to poor quality and patterns of unsafe behaviors and uncaring attitudes.

Adverse Drug Events

Injuries that result from medication-related medical interventions are called **adverse drug events (ADEs)** (ODPHP, 2015b). They can occur anywhere throughout the medication administration process, starting when medications are pre-

SBAR Report		
Report given by:		Time :_____
Report received by:		Phone:_____
S	**Situation:** Patient name Age Location Code status Current vital signs and O_2 saturation Patient's current status	
B	**Background:** Admitting date and diagnosis Allergies Diagnostic tests pending Patient's physical/mental status Oxygen in use or not	
A	**Assessment:** Lungs, heart, neurologic status IV sites/fluids/rates Diet and intake/output Active precautions Isolation precautions Special care—tubes, wounds	
R	**Recommendations:** Suggestions for diagnostic tests Treatments Transfer to critical care Come to see patient	

Figure 51–10 》 Information included in an SBAR handoff report.

scribed and ending when patients receive them. ADEs can occur in a variety of healthcare settings such as acute care hospitals, outpatient clinics, physician offices, community offices, extended care facilities, and home care settings. They can involve professionals who prescribe, prepare, and administer medications, and patients who receive medications.

Approximately 1 of 3 inpatient hospital adverse events are due to ADEs, affecting about 2 million hospital stays per year by extending those hospital stays by 1.7 to 4.6 days. In outpatient settings, ADEs yearly cause more than 3.5 million physician office visits, approximately 1 million emergency department visits, and about 125,000 hospital admissions (ODPHP, 2015b). The majority of ADEs are preventable. High-alert medications, such as insulin, anticoagulants, and opioids, have the highest risk of causing harm and thus require special alertness to safety guidelines when administering them. Nurses can provide safe medication administration by following rights of medication administration, including:

1. **Right assessment**
2. **Right drug**
3. **Right dose**
4. **Right patient**
5. **Right route**
6. **Right time**
7. **Right documentation.**

By ensuring that the right assessment has been done and the right medication and the right dose are being given to the right patient at the right time and by the right route, the nurse acts to ensure quality and safety for the patient, protecting the patient against the possibility of adverse effects or an overdose. In addition, by correctly documenting when and how the medication was given (as well as which medication at what dose), the nurse prevents anyone else from accidentally duplicating administration of the medication order. Patient teaching to avoid medication errors is outlined in **Box 51–2 »**.

Falls

Falls are very common in healthcare facilities and homes and are a special risk for those age 65 and older. One third of older adults fall every year (National Patient Safety Foundation [NPSF], 2013). Falls among older adults result in 2 million

---

Box 51–2
Medication Teaching

Nurses can help prevent medication errors in a number of additional ways, including by engaging patients and discussing their medication with them. Medication teaching begins with assessment of current medications prescribed as well as patient's use of them and use of over-the-counter medications and supplements. Medication teaching includes:

- The name and function of each medication.
- When and how medication should be taken.
- Common side effects and how to address them.
- Adverse effects that should be reported to the provider.
- Drug interactions with other drugs, food, and diseases.

---

emergency department visits every year, making falls the most common cause of nonfatal injuries and the leading cause of injury death in older adults (CDC, 2013c). In nursing homes, 50–75% of residents fall each year, with an average of 2.6 falls per person per year (CDC, 2013f).

Falls can cause numerous injuries, including fractured bones, excessive bleeding, traumatic brain injury, and death. Patients who display memory impairment and muscle weakness, as well as those individuals who require assistive devices such as canes or walkers for ambulation, are especially at risk. Numerous prescription and over-the-counter medications also increase the risk of falls (CDC, 2013f).

In a clinical setting, numerous strategies can be implemented to reduce the risk of falls. Examples of nursing interventions that may be applicable to the care of the patient who is at risk for falling may include the following:

- Remove obstacles from walking paths, including patient rooms, corridors, and stairwells.

- Keep frequently used items within easy reach.

- Ensure that patient rooms are well lit.

- Make sure patients wear shoes with soles that provide adequate traction, as opposed to wearing slippers or going barefoot.

- Assess the patient's vision and make sure he is using any prescribed eyewear, because poor and blurry vision increases the risk of falling.

- Use side rails on patient beds to prevent falls while the patient is sleeping.

- Be aware of each patient's medication regimen, including side effects and interactions, because side effects such as dizziness or drowsiness can substantially increase the risk of a fall. Request that a physician or pharmacist review patient medications when necessary (CDC, 2013e).

Healthcare-associated Infections

Healthcare-associated infections (HAIs) are infections that occur while a patient is being treated for another condition. Approximately 5% of hospitalized patients contract an HAI during their hospital-stay (NPSF, 2013). Infections of this nature can be quite serious, because hospital patients are usually weaker or immunocompromised due to the injury or illness that hospitalized them in the first place. Common HAIs and pathogens that are commonly associated with HAIs are discussed in the module on Infection.

In 2011, the CDC prevalence survey based on a large sample of U.S. acute care hospitals showed that 1 in 25 hospital patients had at least one HAI. For the same year, there were approximately 722,000 HAIs in U.S. acute care hospitals. These HAIs resulted in an estimated 75,000 patient deaths during their hospital stay (CDC, 2015a).

The CDC HAI Progress Report for 2013 uses data reported to the CDC using the **National Healthcare Safety Network**. This is an annual report on progress at the national and state levels in preventing HAIs. On the national level, the report gave the following results between 2008 and 2013: (1) a 46% decrease in central line–associated bloodstream infections, (2) a 19% decrease in surgical-site infections related to the 10 select procedures tracked, (3) a 6% increase in catheter-associated urinary tract infections, (4) an 8% decrease in hospital-onset methicillin-resistant *Staphylococcus aureus* (MRSA) bacteremia, and (5) a 10% decrease in hospital *Clostridium difficile* infections (CDC, 2015f).

Patients can help prevent infection through becoming knowledgeable about their treatment and recovery plan, being proactive about blood sugar control, losing weight prior to surgery, and quitting smoking. Nurses are also vital in preventing HAIs and must take appropriate measures to ensure that they are not unknowingly spreading illness between patients. Among other safety measures, appropriate hand hygiene and disinfectant techniques are particularly important.

Safety Devices

Safety devices include a variety of physical restraints that are intended to partially or fully limit the patient's mobility. They are applied only when absolutely necessary to protect the patient from injuring self or others and only with a physician's order. Two other types of safety restraints are chemical restraints and seclusion.

Chemical restraints are pharmacologic agents, such as sedatives, hypnotics, neuroleptics, and antianxiety medications, that are administered to agitated patients to control unsafe physical movements and behaviors. **Seclusion** is confining a patient to a room involuntarily and preventing the patient from leaving. Typically, acute care units do not have space for a seclusion room, so this category is more appropriate for emergency departments and psychiatric units than acute care settings. Other devices that may be considered forms of restraints include wheelchairs with stationary lap trays, bed rails, and geri chairs. Generally, if the patient can release or remove the device without assistance, the device is not considered to be a restraint. Infant and child restraints include crib nets, elbow restraints, and mummy restraints.

Physical restraints are wrapped, buckled, or tied to a patient's arms, legs, or trunk of the body to limit or restrict movement. They cannot be used as a form of punishment, a convenience measure, or to prevent a patient from leaving a given setting. Regulations stipulate the following conditions for restraints: (1) a physician or other healthcare provider must order specific restraints, physical or chemical, to be applied to the patient, (2) the order for restraints cannot be a standing order or prn order, and (3) when there is an urgency to protect the patient and others, restraints can be applied and then the physician can be notified as soon as possible for an order. Legally, a competent patient who simply does not comply with his care cannot be restrained; this may be construed as assault and battery or false imprisonment.

Restraint alternatives and least restrictive forms of restraint must be tried first, and if they are unsuccessful, then chemical or physical restraints can be implemented as a last resort for the safety of the patient and others. There must be documented evidence of less restrictive measures that were tried but unsuccessful, including interventions to modify the patient's behavior or the environment. Some examples of restraint alternatives to help control the patient's behaviors and avoid restraints include:

- Having a family member or sitter stay with the patient
- Using bed or chair alarms

- Using distractions and diversional activities
- Using a calm voice and soothing tone
- Limiting the number of staff working with the patient
- Using de-escalation strategies
- Using portable electronic GPS sensors to locate patient
- Reorienting the confused patient
- Assessing/addressing problems causing agitation such as wanting to get up and go to the bathroom, or wanting some water to drink
- Offering therapeutic self and reassurance (ASHRM, 2015).

Although restraints are intended to protect the patient, their use also may result in injury or even death. Psychosocial effects are also a concern; adult patients may experience depression, as well as a sense of dehumanization, and pediatric patients may feel they are being punished. Whenever restraints are used, the nurse must follow strict guidelines to ensure the patient's safety. These guidelines include:

- Assessment is to be done at least every 2 hours and includes skin and circulation status, patient's response, and effect of restraints
- New verbal order is needed every 24 hours if there is not a written order
- Removal of restraints must be done periodically so patient can freely move body part, range-of-motion (ROM) exercises can be done, and patient can be repositioned
- Toileting, food, and fluids are offered periodically
- Evaluation to determine if continued restraint is needed, and restraints reapplied if needed
- Appropriate and complete documentation of the restraint intervention.

Commonly used restraints include limb, soft belt, safety strap, or vest immobilizers or mitt, elbow, or hand restraints (**Figure 51–11 》**). Limb restraints and mitts, which are typically made of cloth, may be used when limb immobilization is needed for therapeutic purposes—for example, to prevent dislodgement of an intravenous infusion device or removal of dressings. To ensure the safety of patients who are transported by wheelchair or gurney, soft belt restraints, safety strap body restraints, or vest restraints are used. Soft belt restraints and immobilizers may be used to protect patients who are confined to a chair or a bed. To protect confused patients or very small children from scratching and injuring their skin, mitt restraints, mittens, or hand restraints may be used.

Wrong-Site Surgery

Wrong-site surgery (WSS), or wrong-site, wrong-procedure, wrong-patient surgery, are errors that should not occur and are called **sentinel events** by The Joint Commission and **never events** by the National Quality Forum. *Wrong-site* refers to surgery performed on an incorrect body site or to surgery performed on the wrong side of the correct body site: for example, removing the right upper lung lobe instead of the left upper lung lobe, or removing the right side of the right upper lung lobe instead of removing the left side of

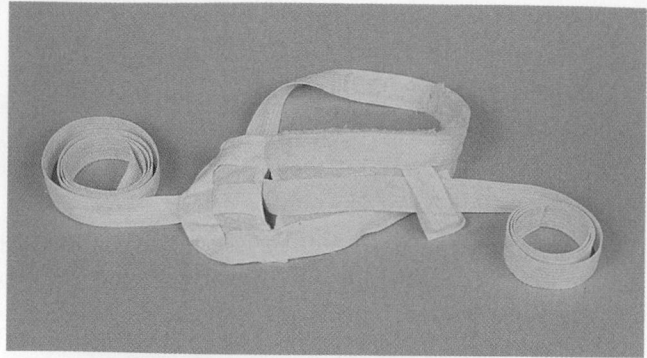

A

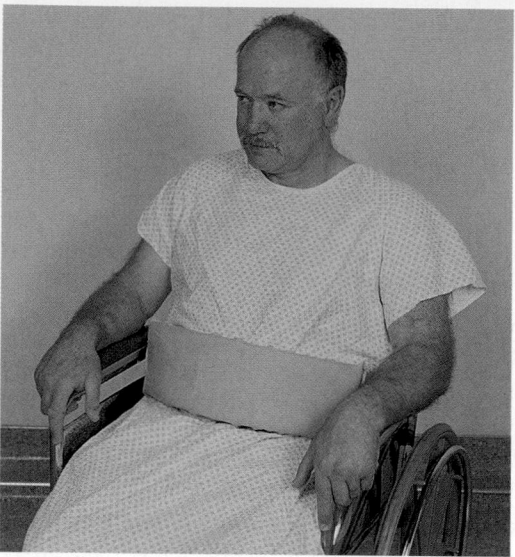

B

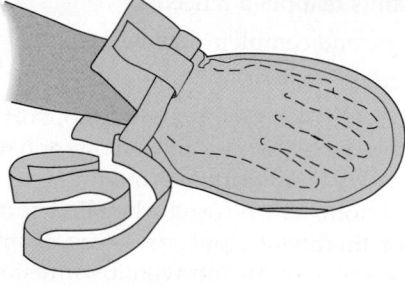

C

Figure 51–11 》 Various types of restraints. *A,* Limb restraint. *B,* Belt restraint. *C,* Mitt restraint.

the right upper lung lobe. *Wrong procedure* refers to the right patient undergoing an incorrect surgical procedure. *Wrong-patient surgery* refers to the patient undergoing a surgical procedure intended for another patient. WSSs are fairly rare and happen approximately 1 in every 112,000 surgical procedures, averaging one such error every 5–10 years in a given healthcare facility (AHRQ, 2015). Some factors are:

- Inadequate patient assessment
- Inadequate safety culture
- Communication failure
- Inadequate medical record review
- Multiple procedures on multiple parts of a patient performed during a single operation

- Failure to include the patient and family when identifying the correct operation site
- Failure to clearly mark the correct operation site
- Failure to recheck information before starting the operation.

WSS is a serious patient risk, because it subjects a patient to severe and unnecessary trauma. Surgery teams also feel the effects because they can be subjected to negative morale, insurers that will not pay for WSS, malpractice claims, and disciplinary actions by licensing boards. To prevent WSS, The Joint Commission developed a universal protocol that has been adopted by numerous medical and professional organizations. The universal protocol is outlined in the module on Perioperative Care (The Joint Commission, 2015).

Lifespan Considerations in Healthcare Settings

Healthcare facilities are strange environments, full of strange new sounds, people, equipment, and activity. Preparing for this experience can help reduce patient anxiety and promote patient comfort and satisfaction with care. In general, giving patients honest information at a level they can understand, answering any questions they may have, and providing them support and encouragement will help them be more at ease. The following sections present some common safety considerations for pediatric, pregnant, and geriatric patients.

Safety Considerations for Pediatric Patients

1. Very young children learn about their world by touching and playing with objects around them, so keep medications, sharp objects, and equipment out of reach.
2. Suggest parents bring in a few comfort items the child is familiar with, such as photos, a favorite blanket, or a favorite small toy.
3. Maintain the child's daily routines and habits as much as appropriate.
4. Suggest that parents help their child stay busy with age-appropriate activities they like to do.
5. Encourage parents to respect safety signs such as washing hands, keeping a security door closed, and not allowing the pediatric patient to run down the hallways or be out of their sight at any time.
6. Be aware when parents leave the child alone.
7. Remember that children and infants can move very quickly and fall from a crib or bed.
8. Communicate with children using language that is appropriate for their developmental level.
9. Infant and child patients must wear proper identification at all times.
10. Nurses should provide patient-centered care and also family-centered care to keep the patient and family engaged in how they can support the quality and safety of care.

Safety Considerations for Pregnant Patients

1. Patients need to continue to follow prenatal care guidelines as approved by their healthcare provider.
2. When patients have chronic conditions requiring treatment, such as asthma, diabetes, or heart problems, they should be more careful about managing these conditions. Their healthcare providers may change or stop certain medications or treatments during their pregnancy.
3. Patients need to know how medications, procedures, and treatments could affect their pregnancy or their child. Nurses can reinforce information provided by the patient's treating physician or provider.
4. Nurses can encourage pregnant patients to do safety behaviors and be especially careful to avoid risks of infection, injuries, and accidents.
5. Nurses can encourage pregnant patients to use their call button to ask for assistance to get out of bed or move about to prevent falls.

Safety considerations for the newborn include teaching the mother and other family members to never leave the baby alone in the mother's room, only give the baby to personnel with appropriate photo identification name badges, always use an infant crib when transporting the baby, always leave the baby on the postpartum unit, and never give interested strangers on the unit personal information about themselves or the baby.

Safety Considerations for Geriatric Patients

1. Encourage patients to have a family member or someone they trust to advocate for them while they are in the hospital.
2. Encourage patients to have someone bring their prescription and over-the-counter medications, herbs, and dietary supplements to the hospital to review and include in their admission information.
3. If a patient has any known allergies to medicines, materials, foods, soaps, and so on, this information needs to be posted in appropriate places such as on the medical record, the medication administration record, and as hospital policy dictates.
4. Emphasize to patients the importance of using the call button to ask for help getting up to the restroom or walking around the hallway.
5. Emphasize to patients the need to keep the bed in a low and locked position with upper side rails raised.
6. If a patient will be in the hospital for a few days, suggest that a family member bring in a few comfort items familiar to the patient, such as a bathrobe, photo, or favorite item.
7. Help patients and family members be comfortable with asking questions about care, diagnostic tests, or procedures for understanding.
8. Emphasize the importance of wearing an identification band while in the hospital and encourage patients to make sure it is checked before receiving medications or treatments.
9. Discuss routines of mealtimes, bathing, procedures, treatments, and other care with patients and, as appropriate, accommodate any cultural, spiritual, or personal rituals, habits, or activities patients would like to continue doing while in the hospital.
10. Communicate with patients in their language and at their developmental level for understanding. Provide orientation of day, place, and name to patients as needed.

NURSING PROCESS

Individualized patient care includes appropriate developmental and chronologic age-specific safety considerations. Safety is a common priority for many patients because of motor or sensory changes from acute or chronic conditions inhibiting functional abilities to protect themselves. For example, patients who have had strokes may not independently be able to reposition themselves to protect the integrity of their skin from breakdown, and children with cystic fibrosis may not be able to cough up and remove their secretions in order to protect their airways and keep them open for air exchange.

Assessment

Both objective and subjective data are used to assess the safety needs of patients:

- **Observation and patient interview.** History of falls, balance issues, medications that may cause orthostatic hypotension, chronic conditions, mobility deficits, sensory deficits, and so on

- **Physical examination.** Vital signs, ROM, skin assessment, hearing or visual difficulties, heart and lung sounds, tremors, impaired balance, and so on

Diagnosis

Because of the nature and large number of safety hazards in healthcare settings, there are many NANDA-I nursing diagnosis labels appropriate for patients focused on safety. Safety can include elements in the environment, the patient's situation, or the patient's homeostasis status. Here are a few examples:

- *Knowledge, Deficient*
- *Skin Integrity, Impaired*
- *Airway Clearance, Ineffective*
- *Thermoregulation, Ineffective*
- *Risk for Infection* from bleeding, falls, injury, poisoning, and suicide.

(NANDA-I © 2014)

Planning

Safety goals are decided on by the patient and the nurse and would reflect the nursing diagnosis label, such as:

- The patient will have clear breath sounds by discharge.
- The patient will be able to correctly demonstrate walking with a cane 25 feet by (date).
- The patient will remain free from infection, bleeding, falls, injury, poisoning, and suicide.
- The patient will verbalize three things to do to safely get up out of the bed and sit in the chair by (date).

Implementation

There are many nursing actions that can be done to keep patients safe while in a healthcare setting (acute care facility, extended care facility, community facility, or home setting).

There are many opportunities for nurses to teach patients about using safety behaviors to prevent accidents. All interventions need to be prioritized to best meet the safety needs for the patient. Some intervention examples are:

- Assess patient's feet for cracking and dryness and apply lotion after bathing time.
- Collaborate with the physical therapist to teach patient correct cane walking.
- Encourage the patient to use the incentive spirometer every hour while awake as tolerated.
- Staff will promptly respond when patient's call light is activated for assistance to get up to the restroom.

Evaluation

Expected outcomes may include the following:

- The patient has clear breath sounds at time of discharge.
- The patient is able to correctly demonstrate walking with a cane for 25 feet.
- The patient remains free from infection, bleeding, falls, injury, poisoning, suicide, and so on.
- The patient is able to verbalize three things to do to safely get up out of the bed and sit in the chair.

The nursing plan of care follows a sequence of actions that have a causal relationship. Clustering assessment data results in the identification of the nursing diagnosis; the nursing diagnosis informs goal setting; goals stimulate decisions regarding what interventions will help the patient reach the goal; and evaluation is completed to determine if the interventions were successful in supporting the goal to be obtained. If the goal is not reached, the whole process is reevaluated to determine if the goal and interventions were appropriate for the assessment data and nursing diagnosis. Changes in the goal or interventions may be necessary to individualize them for best patient outcomes.

REVIEW Patient Safety

RELATE Link the Concepts and Exemplars

Linking the exemplar of patient safety with the concept of perioperative care:

1. The nurse notices that the child patient waiting to go to surgery is drinking a glass of milk. What are the priority safety actions for the nurse? Why?

2. Immediate postoperative assessment of the patient postanesthesia would include which priority safety data?

Linking the exemplar of patient safety with the concept of mood and affect:

3. Sometimes patients who are in the manic phase of bipolar disorder are placed in seclusion for a period of time. What are the safety concerns of the staff for making this decision?

4. Is it a potential safety problem when a depressed patient begins putting her affairs in order? Why or why not?

Linking the exemplar of patient safety with the concept of acid–base balance:

5. When a diabetic patient has hyperglycemia, the blood pH goes down indicating metabolic acidosis. How will the body attempt to correct the metabolic acidosis and return to a pH within normal range?

6. When a patient overuses bicarbonate of soda for his indigestion problem, what safety problem might this cause for the patient's acid–base balance? What needs to be done to correct it?

READY Go to Volume 3: Clinical Nursing Skills

REFER Go to Pearson MyLab Nursing and eText

- Additional review materials

REFLECT Apply Your Knowledge

A 9-year-old patient is admitted for observation to the medical unit with closed head trauma after falling off his bicycle and hitting his head; he was not wearing his safety helmet. He is drowsy, crying at times, and complaining of a headache. He had two episodes of vomiting while in the emergency department. Last set of vital signs were T—98.8°F, P—102, R—16, B/P—108/72, O_2 saturation 96% room air. His pupils are slightly sluggish but PERRLA. His HOB is to be elevated 30 degrees. Phenytoin has been ordered 125 mg IV BID, and he can have acetaminophen 480 mg po every 6 hours prn headache.

He is currently NPO and to have neuro checks every 2 hours using the Glasgow Coma Scale.

1. What are priority safety considerations with this patient?
2. What might be the reason the patient is receiving phenytoin? What might be the reason he is NPO? What might be the reason his HOB is up 30 degrees?
3. What priority teaching should the nurse identify at this time to do when the patient is more alert and awake and the parents are present before discharge?

›› Exemplar 51.C
Nurse Safety

Exemplar Learning Outcomes

51.C Analyze safety as it relates to being a nurse.

- Outline the agencies that regulate workplace safety for nurses.
- Describe the etiology and prevalence of injuries to nurses.
- Summarize strategies to prevent injury in nursing practice.

Exemplar Key Terms

Compassion fatigue, *2903*
Job burnout, *2903*
National Institute for Occupational Safety and Health (NIOSH), *2899*
Nurse Practice Act (NPA), *2900*
Occupational Health Safety Network (OHSN), *2900*
Occupational Safety and Health Administration (OSHA), *2899*
Scoop method, *2902*
Workplace violence, *2902*

Overview

Workplace safety is a concern in most professions, but it is of particular concern to healthcare workers. In 2014, of the more than 18 million individuals working in healthcare occupations, registered nurses had the highest employment number, a total of 2.7 million (BLS, 2015a). All of these occupations face numerous risks on the job. Some of these risks include bloodborne pathogens, needlesticks, latex allergies, musculoskeletal injuries, mental stress, and violence from patients. Injury and illness within the healthcare sector represent the highest percentage of nonfatal occupational injuries in any sector, including both construction and agriculture—two industries known for work-related injuries (CDC, 2013g).

Safety in the workplace is critical to job satisfaction and employee retention rates. In nursing, protocols for safety promotion and injury prevention have become more prevalent over the years. These protocols are designed to protect members of the healthcare team and patients.

Regulation of Workplace Safety

The Occupational Safety and Health Act of 1970 created both the **Occupational Safety and Health Administration (OSHA)** and the **National Institute for Occupational Safety and Health (NIOSH)**. OSHA is part of the U.S. Department of Labor. It is a national public health agency to protect workers from safety hazards and health risks in the workplace. NIOSH is part of the U.S. Centers for Disease Control and Prevention in the U.S. Department of Health and Human Services. It is a U.S. federal agency that conducts research and produces evidence used to find solutions and interventions to protect the safety and health of workers (CDC, 2017).

Occupational Safety and Health Administration

OSHA enforces the guidelines presented in the OSHA Act of 1970, requiring its covered employees to report specific incidents and illnesses in a timely manner. OSHA developed standards, enforcement actions, compliance assistance, and cooperative programs to prevent injuries and illnesses. OSHA enforces the rights of workers to have a safe work environment. Workers can file a complaint about unsafe work conditions through their whistleblower program asking for an on-site inspection of the situation from OSHA and will be protected from employer retaliation (U.S. Department of Labor, 2017).

One of the primary functions of OSHA includes consulting with both employees and employers regarding prevention methods for the injuries and illnesses that are most prevalent in each particular work environment. For example, OSHA's involvement with those in the nursing sector includes preventive measures against needlesticks, bloodborne pathogens, and aggression from patients. Inspections of the workplace are conducted by OSHA employees to ensure that individuals are complying with standards. In the healthcare setting, for example, hand hygiene procedures could be monitored, or the use of gloves when working with patients, or the availability of puncture-resistant sharps containers.

National Institute for Occupational Safety and Health

According to the CDC (2014c), "the mission of NIOSH is to generate new knowledge in the field of occupational safety and health and to transfer that knowledge into practice for the betterment of workers." NIOSH conducts scientific research to provide advances in safety both in the workplace and for the population at large. In addition to research, NIOSH also develops recommendations for safety procedures, distributes information, provides training videos, and evaluates workplace health hazards.

Research conducted by NIOSH focuses on numerous topics relating to different sectors of the workforce. For example, NIOSH compiles research on the effects of stress in the workplace, which is particularly common in the healthcare community because of the nature of the work being performed. NIOSH can evaluate work environments for health hazards and recommend ways to reduce or eliminate them through its *Health Hazard Evaluation Program*.

Boards of Nursing

In order to protect the public's health and welfare from nurses who are not prepared or competent to provide safe nursing care, state governments used their police powers to enact laws to protect citizens and minimize harm of unsafe nursing practice. These laws are included in the **Nurse Practice Act (NPA)** of each state and authorized by the state's legislature. Each state has a Board of Nursing empowered to adopt, amend, or repeal rules and regulations as necessary. The guidelines in the NPA focus on safety parameters for nurses to provide safe and effective nursing care for public protection (NCSBN, 2012).

Boards of Nursing act to ensure safety by establishing academic requirements for nursing prelicensure programs, identifying standards for all areas from clinical learning experiences to faculty qualifications. Boards of Nursing also establish requirements for licensure, including taking the National Council Licensure Examination for Registered Nurse (NCLEX-RN) and continuing education requirements (NCSBN, 2015). Equally as important, Boards of Nursing establish procedures for reporting errors and violations made by licensed nurses and act to investigate such reports. Employers, coworkers, the public, healthcare facilities and others can send anonymous complaints to the Board of Nursing. Complaints about conduct include sexual misconduct, stealing, fraud, confidentiality issues, boundary violations, impairment while working, and drug diversion. Unsafe nurse practice includes inappropriate delegation, abandonment, neglect, exceeding scope of practice, and documentation issues (NCSBN, 2015).

》》 **Stay Current:** It is important for nurses to stay abreast of changes in the Nurse Practice Act in the state for which they work. Each state Board of Nursing will have this information. The NCSBN website has a list of all states at https://www.ncsbn.org/npa.htm.

Etiology of Injury and Illness

Injuries and illnesses in the workplace occur in almost every profession. Causes of workplace illness and injury vary by profession. The following categories make up the majority of workplace incidents resulting in fatalities: transportation accidents (41%), violence in the workplace (17%), trauma from objects and/or equipment (15%), falling or tripping (15%), exposure to dangerous environments or substances (9%), and explosions or fires (3%) (Bureau of Labor Statistics, 2013).

Prevalence

In 2012, a total of 4383 workers in the United States died from injuries sustained at work, an average of 12 deaths per day. There were an estimated 2.8 million work-related injuries treated in emergency departments, resulting in 140,000 hospitalizations. Reports from employers included nearly 3 million injuries and illnesses to private industry workers and 793,000 injuries to state and local government workers (CDC, 2015a). All occupational injuries and illnesses have social and economic implications for the workers and their families, with medical costs, differences in quality of lifestyle, pain and suffering. Employers and society also share the burden for consequences of occupational safety and health hazards in the workplace.

One in five reported nonfatal occupational injuries involved healthcare and social assistance workers in 2013. This was the highest number of this type of injury reported throughout all private industries. In 2011, healthcare workers experienced seven times the national rate of musculoskeletal disorders when compared to all other private workers (CDC, 2015a). Data collection is dependent on national surveillance systems to record new cases and provide information that can be used to reduce occupational hazards and health issues to prevent injuries, illnesses, and death among healthcare personnel. To enhance details of data collected, NIOSH and others began the **Occupational Health Safety Network (OHSN)** to track injuries by type, demographic location, occupation, and risk factors. The three injury types recorded are (1) patient handling and movement; (2) slips, trips, and falls; and (3) workplace violence.

Injury data was collected by OHSN over a 2-year span of time that ended in September 2014. The data, which came from 112 healthcare facilities located in 19 states with a collective workforce of 162,535 full-time employees, reported 10,680 injuries: 4674 from patient handling and movement; 3972 from slips, trips, and falls; and 2034 from workplace violence (CDC, 2015a). Of the 4674 injuries from patient handling and movement, 82% occurred when lifting devices were not being used. Of the 3972 injuries from falls, 89% occurred from same-level falls. Of the 2034 workplace violence injuries, 99% were physical assaults and 95% were committed by patients. These figures are included in the total number of occupational injuries in healthcare reported by the National Bureau of Labor Statistics (Gomaa et al., 2015) (**Figure 51–12** 》》).

Nurses accounted for 38% of the 10,680 reported injuries. Nurses and nursing assistants had the highest injury rates of all other occupations reported. Using the data collected and analyzed, OHSN was able to identify how lifting devices and training could help reduce patient handling and movement injuries. Guidelines were made available to help protect personnel from common preventable injuries that could be disabling. Between 2012 and 2014, the rate of workplace violence injuries nearly doubled for nurses and nursing assistants and increased for all other occupations. These injuries occurred mainly on inpatient adult units, although incident numbers in emergency departments, stand-alone acute care centers, and critical care units were elevated. High fall rates occurred on inpatient adult units as well as nonpatient maintenance areas.

In 2013, there were 66,910 occupational musculoskeletal disorder injuries reported in the healthcare and social assistance private sector. Almost 50% of these cases included patients in acute and nonacute settings. Of the acute care cases, 20% were nurse musculoskeletal disorder injuries (BLS, 2015b). Injuries to nurses include pinched nerve,

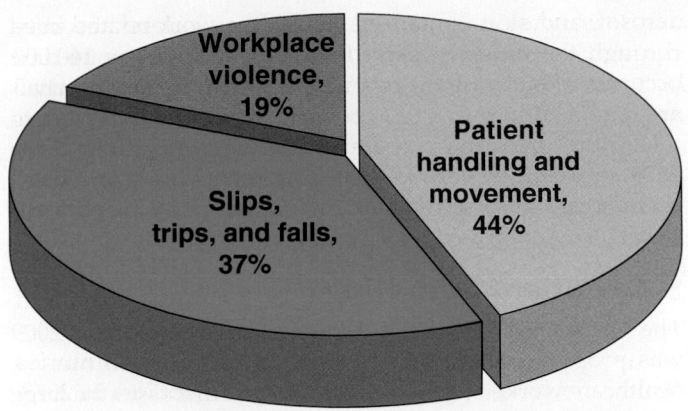

Source: Data from Gomaa, A. E., Tapp, L. C., Luckhaupt, S. E., Vanoli, K., Sarmiento, R. F., Raudabaugh, W. M., … Sprigg, S. M. (2015). Occupational traumatic injuries among workers in health care facilities—United States, 2012–2014. *Morbidity and Mortality Weekly Report (MMWR), 64*(15), 405–410.

Figure 51–12 》 Categories of 10,680 injuries reported by healthcare employees over a 2-year study.

herniated disk, meniscus tear, sprains, strains, tears, carpal or tarsal tunnel syndrome, and musculoskeletal system and connective tissue diseases. Nurses are at high risk for these injuries because of their work patterns, the increased acuity of patients, the need to keep patients mobilized, and the increase in obese patients. Increased resources such as training, lifting devices, and lift teams can potentially reduce the number of occupational injuries of healthcare workers. Healthcare facilities can establish and support a safety culture among their employees. Emphasis on occupational safety and health practices can promote a safer work environment and support patient safety. OHSN can help healthcare facilities identify hazards of safety and health and provide them with a variety of tools and materials to improve employee safety and health. These strategies can protect healthcare employees from injuries, accidents, and illnesses that could be disabling and life-changing.

Illness and Injury Prevention in Nursing Practice

Nurse safety from workplace-related health problems is important not only to nurses but also to the patients under their care. Nurses experience not only physical but also psychologic demands throughout their shifts. Pressures can come from workforce downsizing, working more hours, the work pace, increased acuity levels of patients, the escalating number of older patients, the complexity of the environment, extended workloads, an older nurse workforce, and potential for violence and chemical exposures. These factors can contribute to acute or long-term health problems from musculoskeletal injuries and disorders, infections, mental health changes, insufficient sleep patterns, and chronic exhaustion (AHRQ, 2008).

Work-related illnesses in nursing may arise from contact with contagious patients or from contact with bloodborne pathogens as the result of needlestick or sharps injuries.

Exposure to many illnesses can be minimized with simple measures such as hand hygiene and sanitization efforts.

There are many occupational hazards for nurses and other healthcare workers found in all healthcare settings, including acute care, extended-care, and community-based facilities and the home environment. In 2014, workplace illnesses accounted for 4.9% of the nearly 3.0 million injury and illness cases (BLS, 2015b). These hazards put healthcare workers at risk for a variety of safety concerns, including exposure to infectious diseases, such as blood and body fluid pathogens, and injuries or accidents. To create a safer work environment and prevent illness and injury in nursing practice, the focus needs to be on building an awareness of potential safety hazards and finding solutions to prevent them.

Nurses provide care for patients with diagnosed and sometimes undiagnosed infectious diseases such as influenza, norovirus, methicillin-resistant *Staphylococcus aureus* (MRSA), tuberculosis, and HIV (CDC, 2013g; Hospital Jobs Online [HJO] & Burgess, 2012). Vaccines are available to protect against some pathogens, and healthcare providers are encouraged to take advantage of employer-provided vaccination programs.

》 Stay Current: Visit http://www.cdc.gov/vaccines/adults/rec-vac/hcw.html for current CDC recommended vaccines and changes in immunizations for nurses and other healthcare workers.

The CDC has developed comprehensive infection control recommendations that include standard, contact, and airborne precautions for all settings of patient care. Healthcare facilities and organizations that provide home healthcare services have policies and procedures that address safety infection control measures. The CDC provides considerations when choosing personal protective equipment to protect against infectious exposures. Guidelines for preventing the transmission of infectious pathogens are available. The proper use of respirators by nurses and other healthcare workers is another preventive practice. Information about the proper cleaning and sterilization of equipment and procedures to do the cleaning and sterilization are available to help prevent the transmission of infections. Nurses can implement the following tips to avoid illness:

1. Keep Tdap (combination vaccine for tetanus, diphtheria, and pertussis) immunization current; get boosters every 10 years
2. Take advantage of annual influenza vaccinations
3. Get the hepatitis-B vaccination series and maintain positive titers for adequate immunity
4. Get the MMR (measles, mumps, and rubella combination) vaccine following CDC guidelines
5. Get the varicella (chickenpox) vaccine following CDC guidelines (CDC, 2014d)
6. Perform frequent and complete hand washing or hygiene
7. Don personal protective equipment (PPE) following CDC guidelines *every time*
8. If working with a patient in isolation, call for assistance as needed
9. Avoid touching the nose, eye areas, and mouth on one's own face
10. Provide own self-care to keep the immune system healthy: appropriate diet, sleep, relaxation, activity, and self-time

11. If beginning to feel sick at work, go home as soon as appropriate

12. If feeling sick at home, don't go to work; stay at home.

Nurses must be vigilant in the prevention of injuries and illness in their workplace environment, in their nursing practice, and for their own personal safety. Healthcare facilities have policies for preventing injuries and maintaining a safe work environment. Safe practice and protocols can be implemented to sustain a nurse's well-being when working with infectious (or potentially infectious) agents, needles, latex, chemical exposure, and patient handling.

Needlestick Injuries

Needlestick and sharps injuries are a large and growing problem in the healthcare industry. It is estimated that approximately 385,000 sharps-related incidents occur each year in hospitals across the country. The CDC believes that over half of all sharps injuries are not reported as required, including those that happen to physicians, laboratory personnel, and housekeeping staff. Sharps injuries are very serious and can result in numerous illnesses. The *STOP STICKS* campaign, initiated by NIOSH, works to raise awareness of the risks associated with bloodborne pathogens most commonly associated with sharps injuries, such as HIV and hepatitis B and C. Although this campaign was originally developed for emergency departments and operating rooms, the ideas extend to all other healthcare fields that use sharps. The *STOP STICKS* campaign provides resources for exposure prevention methods and equipment evaluations and the requirements for sharps disposal containers (CDC, 2013c).

Nurses incur most injuries from reported needlesticks (CDC, 2013h). When working with used or contaminated sharps, nurses should employ extra precautions so as to avoid unnecessary injuries. Needles that have been used are almost never recapped (unless this is necessary because of protocol) and are disposed of in an appropriate sharps container. Approved disposal containers should be present wherever sharps are being used and must be both puncture resistant and leakproof on the bottom and all sides. If sharps do need to be recapped, this should be done with the use of another device (such as a hemostat), or with the **scoop method**. In the scoop method, the cap is placed on a table or hard surface and the tip of the needle is guided into the cap; to ensure the cap is on tight, it can be pressed against a hard surface such as a table or wall. Nurses should *never* hold the cap in one hand while trying to guide the tip of the needle into the cap with the other—this method substantially increases the risk of a sharps-related injury. Needlestick and sharps injuries arise from a number of different situations, such as not implementing proper disposal techniques, failure to recap the needle, bumping into an uncapped and used needle, or contact with a used scalpel (CDC, 2013h).

>> Stay Current: Visit http://www.cdc.gov/niosh/stopsticks/ for more information on the STOPSTICKS campaign.

Chemical Exposure

Nurses can be exposed to a high level of chemicals used in sterilizing, pest control, volatile organic compounds such as formaldehyde, and pharmaceuticals such as antineoplastics. These products come in a variety of forms, including gas, aerosol, and skin contaminants, so they can be absorbed through the lungs or skin. Exposure may be a one-time occurrence, but it can also occur over time. Some chemicals are regulated in terms of exposure, requiring employees to take more precautionary measures when handling these substances. However, many common chemicals and compounds can cause both injury and illness if they are accidentally spilled or ignited (OSHA, 2015).

Safe Patient Handling

The Nurse and Healthcare Worker Protection Act of 2009 was proposed in an effort to prevent injuries to nurses, healthcare workers, and patients. The act discusses the large number of musculoskeletal disorders and injuries that affect nurses that are often the result of helping to move, lift, or reposition patients. The safe patient handling and injury prevention standard within the act requires the use of mechanical devices to lift or move patients, unless the use of these devices proves to be unsafe or is contraindicated for the patient for some reason. Using mechanical devices to help move patients aids in avoiding unnecessary musculoskeletal injuries for both nurses and other healthcare workers (**Figure 51–13 >>**). The act also establishes extensive training in safe patient handling methods for all nurses (Govtrack, 2015).

Effective and safe patient handling helps to promote patient safety as well as nurse safety. Patient handling can be done more safely by using height-adjustable electric beds, mobile mechanical and ceiling-mounted patient lifts, anti-friction devices, band transfer aids, and bed or chair repositioning. Another strategy is to have peer safety leaders available to help nursing staff make practice changes to improve safety.

Workplace Violence Protection

Workplace violence is defined by NIOSH as "any physical assault, threatening behavior or verbal abuse occurring in the work setting" (CDC, 2014e). Nurses and other healthcare workers are at particular risk of violence in the workplace. Violence can come from patients, their families, or visitors, because of inadequate workplace security, unrestricted movement by visitors around the healthcare facility, personal relationship altercations in the workplace, or a healthcare

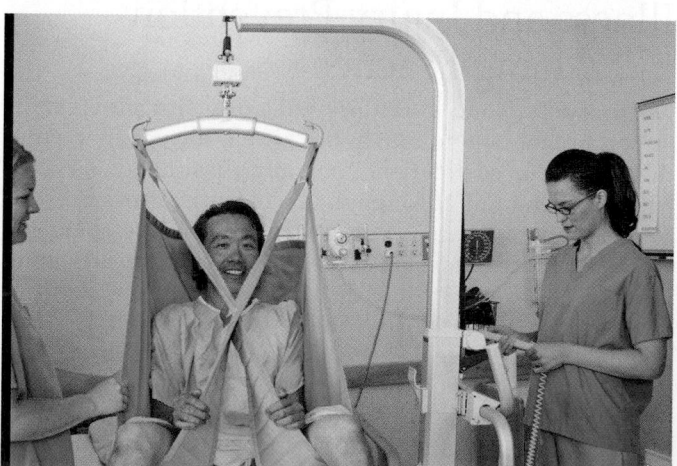

Source: Trish233/iStock/Getty Images.

Figure 51–13 >> Nurses using a floor-mounted mechanical lift to move a patient.

worker bullying another worker. Although routinely there are higher risks of injuries from assaults by patients or their families in an emergency department or mental health nursing unit, no department in a healthcare facility is immune from workplace violence. Potential injuries include nurses being scratched, hit, kicked, beat, bitten and sometimes threatened with weapons such as knives or guns.

Some strategies to prevent workplace violence are: keep hair tucked away, use breakaway lanyards, be aware of and note any change in surroundings, note verbal and nonverbal cues that signal increasing patient agitation or anger, note inappropriate abusive language or behaviors from coworkers, and note signs that someone may be acutely emotionally upset to the degree that he or she is unable to think clearly with a change in rational behaviors. Some healthcare facilities offer employees training in managing aggressive behaviors (**Figure 51–14 》**).

Many states have enacted legislation to address violence in the workplace by increasing punishments for those who attack nurses and by requiring employers to provide training on workplace violence. NIOSH collects data on reports of violence against nurses in order to aid in further prevention efforts and to develop training programs and new policies aimed at increasing safety measures for nurses and other healthcare workers (CDC, 2014e).

Mental Health Safety

Caring for others is a hallmark of the nursing profession. As a helping profession, nursing involves significant responsibility for the well-being of others on many levels in addition to working in a highly stressful environment. Prolonged response to the many nursing work stressors mentioned at the beginning of this exemplar can lead not only to fatigue and distress but also to physical, mental, and emotional depletion, often referred to as **job burnout** or **compassion fatigue**. Nurses who experience compassion fatigue also experience less satisfaction from their work and are less engaged with their patients. The quality of their performance and interactions is affected.

It is essential for nurses to take care of their own physical and emotional selves so they can be physically, mentally, and emotionally prepared to care for their patients. Nurses need to look at themselves and recognize where stressors are coming from and think about what they can do about them to reduce stress and strain. Taking care of their bodies will support having healthy immune systems to avoid frequent bouts of sickness and disease. Nurses need to develop balance with lifestyle activities such as work and play, relaxation and activity, exercise and rest/sleep, aloneness and socializing, hobbies and family, and self and others. They can renew their spiritual selves, have fun, and decompress by appropriately expressing their thoughts and feeling their emotions. There is a need to refresh support systems at work, at home, and with others. Nurses can reaffirm all the reasons they went into nursing to care for others and make a difference for them. They can learn to say "No" at appropriate times to avoid extra demands on time and sometimes remember that they have a sense of humor.

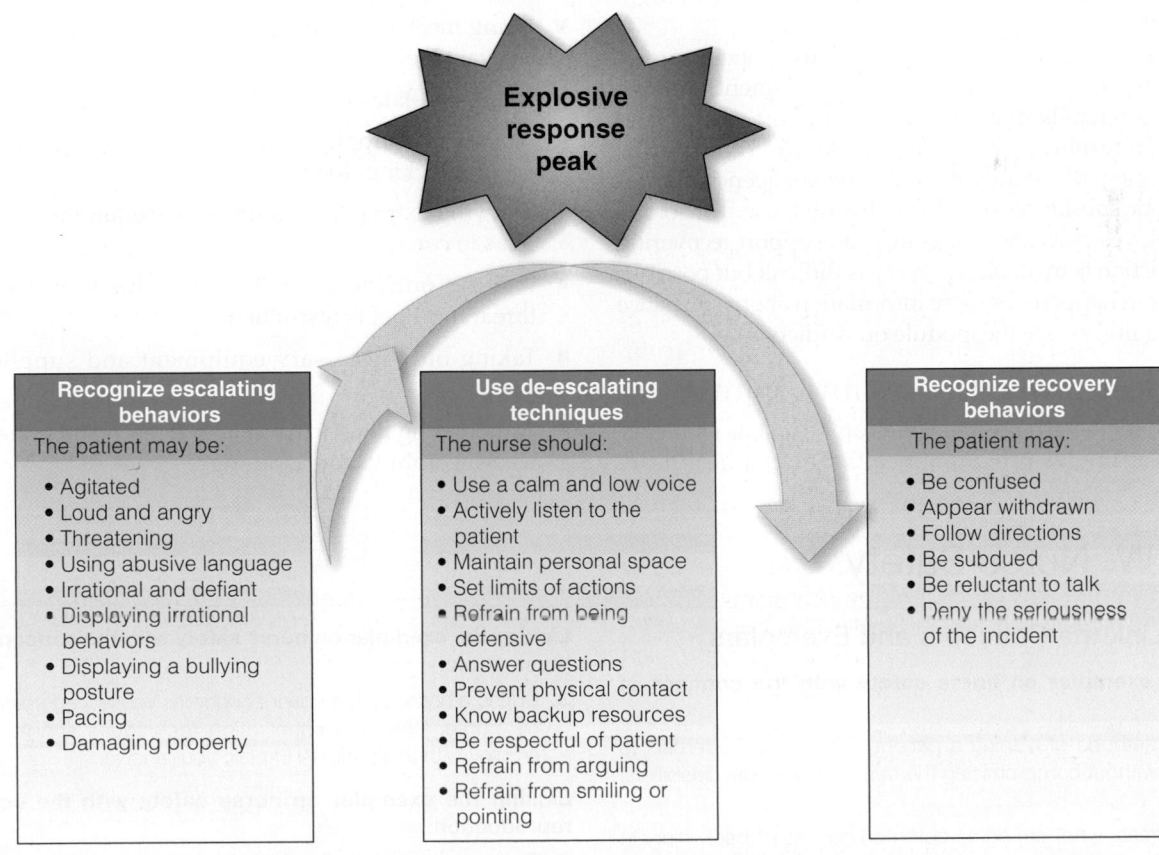

Figure 51–14 》 The process of de-escalating aggressive behaviors includes three stages: recognizing escalating behaviors, using de-escalating techniques, and recognizing recovery behaviors.

Healthcare facilities can and should take actions to support their nursing workforce. For example, they can invest in reduced nurse–patient ratios to lessen nurse work pressures. This would give nurses more time with patients and potentially improve patient outcomes and provide short periods of time for nurses to eat and refresh themselves. Workplace morale can be enhanced with appreciation and incentives for improvements made in patient safety and satisfaction. Debriefing teams can be developed to work with nurses and others after psychologically stressful situations occur. An employee assistance program can be started to help avoid compassion fatigue. When nurses are refreshed, recommitted to helping care for others, taking care of themselves, and physically and emotionally healthy, they will be able to withstand the challenges of nursing and once again enjoy helping their patients. They will again be able to provide safe, effective, and quality care for their patients.

Substance Abuse and Safety

In order for nurses to provide quality and safety for their patients, they must be able to withstand the many pressures of physical, mental, and emotional demands in the work environment and strains from their personal lives and families. Impaired nurses under the influence of alcohol or drugs will not be able to proficiently perform necessary procedures, make accurate decisions about their nursing responsibilities, or make necessary critical clinical judgments about patient care. Dysfunctional nurses in a clinical environment can mean more errors, injuries, and accidents. Patients needing their prn pain or sleep medications may remain in pain or unable to have restful sleep. This quickly becomes a high-priority safety hazard for patients and others.

Every board of nursing has substance abuse policies, procedures, and expectation guidelines about treatment, nursing license status, rehabilitation, peer nurse support groups, and conditions of returning to the nursing workforce. There may be legal involvement of federal drug enforcement agencies if controlled narcotic substances have been diverted, used, or sold to others. Employee assistance programs can support recovering nurses. Addiction is treatable, recovery is difficult but possible, and relapse can happen (for more information about substance abuse among nurses, see the module on Addiction).

Home Healthcare Nurses and Injuries

Providing home health nursing care can be just as challenging and rewarding as providing healthcare in a healthcare facility. Unfortunately, it also can have many of the same safety hazards—for example, bloodborne and infectious pathogens, needlesticks, latex, chemical exposure, and patient handling. In addition to these, home healthcare nurses also contend with hostile animals, unhygienic and dangerous surroundings, and road travel to patients' homes. OSHA has many materials on safety available for healthcare workers on their website (CDC, 2015g).

Safety measures for the home health nurse begin with an assessment of the patient's home and neighborhood to identify potential risks. This assessment can be a part of the discharge planning and patient/family education to help create a safe environment for everyone. Ongoing safety training for nurses should include personal protection maneuvers, prevention of infectious disease, needlestick safety, minimizing latex allergic reactions, avoiding chemical exposure, and prevention of musculoskeletal injuries.

Common steps to follow to maintain safety for the home health nurse include:

- Being aware of immediate surroundings
- Using a GPS system or detailed map to know address locations
- Making home visits during daylight hours as possible
- Parking the car in a lighted area with minimal shrubs close by
- Avoiding setting personal items or supply bags on carpeted floor
- Using mechanical devices to assist in lifting and moving as available
- Using non-latex gloves and hand sanitizer
- Not leaving supplies or personal belongings visible in the car and locking doors
- Carrying extra personal protective equipment (PPE) supplies in car
- Waiting outside door if unrestrained animal poses a threat until pet is restrained
- Taking only necessary equipment and supplies inside home
- Anticipating homes that may not be cooled or heated and wearing appropriate clothing.

REVIEW Nurse Safety

RELATE Link the Concepts and Exemplars

Linking the exemplar on nurse safety with the concept of mobility:

1. Describe methods of helping a patient with multiple sclerosis to reposition without compromising the nurse's own musculoskeletal health.

2. Among nurses, what are some common causes of back injury in the workplace? What are some methods for decreasing the incidence of these injuries?

Linking the exemplar on nurse safety with the concept of communication:

3. During a home visit, a patient becomes verbally aggressive toward his nurse. What communication techniques should the nurse employ with this patient? Explain your answer.

Linking the exemplar on nurse safety with the concept of reproduction:

4. The new parent is trying to hold her newborn while eating breakfast. What are some potential safety problems with this situation? What should the nurse do?

5. As the nurse is making rounds on her patients, she notices that a newborn is being carried by the mother taking a short walk down the hallway. Is this a safety concern? Why or why not?

READY Go to Volume 3: Clinical Nursing Skills

REFER Go to Pearson MyLab Nursing and eText

- Additional review materials

REFLECT Apply Your Knowledge

The nurse is inserting an intravenous (IV) access device into a patient's arm. The patient has advanced hepatitis C and has been admitted to the hospital because of hepatitis-induced liver failure. After inserting the IV device, the nurse places the needle portion on the patient's bed so he can quickly secure infusion tubing to the IV port. When the patient moves her arm, the needle falls to the floor. Upon retrieving the needle, the nurse accidentally punctures himself. Once the needle has punctured his skin, he immediately stops what he is doing and washes the injury site thoroughly with warm soapy water.

1. After cleansing the injury site, what should be the nurse's next action?

2. Could the nurse have done anything differently in this situation to avoid the injury? Explain your answer.

3. Explain the postexposure follow-up guidelines for individuals who sustain needlestick injuries.

References

Administration on Aging (AoA). (2015). Administration for Community Living. U.S. Department of Health and Human Services. *National organizations. Comprehensive national organizations.* Retrieved from http://www.aoa.acl.gov/AoA_Programs/Tools_Resources/national_organizations.aspx#

Agency for Healthcare Research and Quality (AHRQ). (2008). Classic. *Patient safety and quality: An evidence-based handbook for nurses.* Publication No. 08-0043. Chapter 39, Personal safety for nurses. R. G. Hughes (Ed.). Rockville (MD): Author. Retrieved from http://www.ncbi.nlm.nih.gov/books/NBK2651/

Agency for Healthcare Research and Quality (AHRQ). (2013). *Mission and vision.* Retrieved from http://www.ahrq.gov/news/newsroom/highlights/highlt12.html

Agency for Healthcare Research and Quality (AHRQ). (2014). *20 tips to help prevent medical errors. Patient fact sheet.* Retrieved from http://www.ahrq.gov/patients-consumers/care-planning/errors/20tips/index.html

Agency for Healthcare Research and Quality (AHRQ). (2015). PSNet Patient Safety Network. *Patient safety primer. Wrong-site, wrong-procedure, and wrong-patient surgery.* Retrieved from https://psnet.ahrq.gov/primers/primer/18/wrong-site-wrong-procedure-and-wrong-patient-surgery

American Medical Directors Association (AMDA). (2015). Acute change of condition. Frequently asked questions (FAQs) from acute change of condition in the long term care setting. *CPG News Organization.* Retrieved from http://www.cpgnews.org/ACC/askexperts.cfm

American Society for Healthcare Risk Management (ASHRM). (2015). *Welcome to the ASHRM Patient Safety Portal.* Retrieved from http://www.ashrm.org/resources/patient-safety-portal/index.dhtml

Ball, J. W., Bindler, R. C., Cowen, K., & Shaw, M. (2017). *Principles of pediatric nursing: Caring for children* (7th ed.). Hoboken, NJ: Pearson Education.

Bureau of Labor Statistics (BLS), U.S. Department of Labor. (2015a). *Injuries, illnesses, and fatalities.* Retrieved from http://www.bls.gov/opub/ted/2015/registered-nurses-have-highest-employment-in-healthcare-occupations-anesthesiologists-earn-the-most.htm

Bureau of Labor Statistics (BLS), U.S. Department of Labor. (2015b). *Employer-reported workplace injuries and illnesses—2015.* [News release]. Retrieved from http://www.bls.gov/news.release/pdf/osh.pdf

CampaignZERO. (2014). *CampaignZERO. Families for patient safety.* Retrieved from campaignzero.us9.list-manage.com/subcribe?u=fd735a6a4fd51b8f208ef5989&id=fb397e0a19

Center for Children with Special Needs (CCSN). (2015). Early intervention, childcare & schools>Safety tips>Playground safety for your child with special needs. *Seattle Children's Hospital Research Foundation.* Retrieved from http://cshcn.org/childcare-schools-community/safety-tips/playground-safety-for-your-child-with-special-needs/

Centers for Disease Control and Prevention (CDC). (2013a). Patient safety: Ten things you can do to be a safe patient. *The National Institute for Occupational Safety and Health (NIOSH).* Retrieved from http://www.cdc.gov/Features/PatientSafety/

Centers for Disease Control and Prevention (CDC). (2013b). *Leading causes of nonfatal injury reports, 2001–2011.* Retrieved from http://webappa.cdc.gov/sasweb/ncipc/nfilead2001.html

Centers for Disease Control and Prevention (CDC). (2013c). *Leading causes of death reports, 1999–2010.* Retrieved from http://webappa.cdc.gov/sasweb/ncipc/leadcaus10_us.html

Centers for Disease Control and Prevention (CDC). (2013d). *Oral health for older Americans. Adult oral health. Division of Oral Health.* Retrieved from http://www.cdc.gov/OralHealth/publications/factsheets/adult_oral_health/adult_older.htm

Centers for Disease Control and Prevention (CDC). (2013e). *Falls among older adults: An overview.* Retrieved from http://www.cdc.gov/Homeand_RecreationalSafety/Falls/nursing.html

Centers for Disease Control and Prevention (CDC). (2013f). *Falls in nursing homes.* Retrieved from http://www.cdc.gov/HomeandRecreational-Safety/Falls/adultfalls.html

Centers for Disease Control and Prevention (CDC). (2013g). *Healthcare workers.* Retrieved from http://www.cdc.gov/niosh/topics/healthcare

Centers for Disease Control and Prevention (CDC). (2013h). *Stop sticks campaign. The National Institute for Occupational Safety and Health (NIOSH).* Retrieved from http://www.cdc.gov/niosh/stopsticks/sharpsinjuries.html

Centers for Disease Control and Prevention (CDC). (2014a). Violence prevention. *Child Maltreatment. Facts at a Glance.* Retrieved from http://www.cdc.gov/violenceprevention/pdf/childmaltreatment-facts-at-a-glance.pdf

Centers for Disease Control and Prevention (CDC). (2014b). *Keeping children with disabilities safe.* Retrieved from http://www.cdc.gov/ncbddd/disabilityandsafety/child-safety.html

Centers for Disease Control and Prevention (CDC). NIOSH. (2014c). *Workplace safety & health topics.* Retrieved from http://www.cdc.gov/niosh/topics/healthcare/

Centers for Disease Control and Prevention (CDC). (2014d). *Vaccine information for adults. Recommended vaccines for healthcare workers.* Retrieved from http://www.cdc.gov/vaccines/adults/rec-vac/hcw.html

Centers for Disease Control and Prevention (CDC). (2014e). Occupational violence. training and education. *The National Institute for Occupational Safety and Health (NIOSH). Workplace Violence Prevention for Nurses.* CDC Course No. WB1865 NIOSH Pub. No. 2013-155. Retrieved from http://www.cdc.gov/niosh/topics/violence/training_nurses.html

Centers for Disease Control and Prevention (CDC). (2015a). Occupational traumatic injuries among workers in healthcare facilities—United States, 2012–2014. *Morbidity and Mortality Weekly Report, 64*(15), 405–410. Retrieved from http://www.cdc.gov/mmwr/preview/mmwrhtml/mm6415a2.htm

Centers for Disease Control and Prevention (CDC). (2015b). Child health. *FastStats.* Retrieved from http://www.cdc.gov/nchs/fastats/child-health.htm

Centers for Disease Control and Prevention (CDC). (2015c). Ten leading causes of death and injury. *Injury Prevention & Control: Data & Statistics (WISQARS™).* Retrieved from http://www.cdc.gov/injury/wisqars/leadingcauses.html

Centers for Disease Control and Prevention (CDC). (2015d). *Influenza vaccination information for health care workers.* Retrieved from http://www.cdc.gov/flu/healthcareworkers.htm

Centers for Disease Control and Prevention (CDC). (2015e). *Bicycle safety.* Retrieved from http://www.cdc.gov/motorvehiclesafety/bicycle/index.html

Centers for Disease Control and Prevention (CDC). (2015f). *Healthcare-associated infections (HAI). Data and statistics.* Retrieved from http://www.cdc.gov/HAI/surveillance/index.html

Centers for Disease Control and Prevention (CDC). (2015g). Caring for yourself while caring for others. Module 7: Tips for safely handling threatening behavior when providing homecare. NIOSH. Retrieved from https://www.cdc.gov/niosh/docs/2015-102/pdfs/homecare-module-7_2015-102.pdf

Centers for Disease Control and Prevention. (2017). The National Institute for Occupational Safety and Health (NIOSH). Retrieved from https://www.cdc.gov/niosh/index.htm

Centers for Medicare and Medicaid Services (CMS). (2015). *Welcome to the partnership for patients.* Retrieved from http://partnersshipforpatients.cms.gov

Gomaa, A. E., Tapp, L. C., Luckhaupt, S. E., Vanoli, K., Sarmiento, R. F., Raudabaugh, W. M., ... Sprigg, S. M. (2015). Occupational traumatic injuries among workers in health care facilities —United States, 2012–2014. *Morbidity and Mortality Weekly Report (MMWR), 64*(15), 405–410.

Government of South Australia. (2016). What is functional decline? *SA Health.* Retrieved from http://www.sahealth.sa.gov.au/wps/wcm/connect/public+content/sa+health+internet/clinical+resources/clinical+topics/older+people/care+of+older+people+toolkit/what+is+functional+decline+-+the+toolkit

Govtrack. (2015). H.R. 2480 (113th): Nurse and Healthcare Worker Protection Act of 2013. Retrieved from https://www.govtrack.us/congress/bills/113/hr2480

Herdman, T. H. & Kamitsuru, S. (Eds). *Nursing Diagnoses—Definitions and Classification 2015–2017.* Copyright © 2014, 1994–2014 NANDA International. Used by arrangement with John Wiley & Sons, Inc. Companion website: www.wiley.com/go/nursingdiagnoses.

Hospital Jobs Online (HJO) & Burgess, N. (2012). *Occupational hazards for nurses.* Retrieved from http://www.hospitaljobsonline.com/career-center/healthcare-careers/occupational-hazards-for-nurses.html

Hospital Safety Score. (2015). *What is patient safety? Errors, injuries, accidents, infections.* Retrieved from http://www.hospitalsafetyscore.org/what-is-patient-safety_m#errors

Kids and Cars. (2016). *Heat stroke.* Retrieved from http://www.kidsandcars.org/heatstroke.html

National Center for Education Statistics (NCES). (2015). *Children and youth with disabilities.* Retrieved from http://nces.ed.gov/programs/coe/indicator_cgg.asp

National Center on Elder Abuse (NCEA). (2015). *Statistics/data.* Retrieved from http://www.ncea.aoa.gov/library/data/

National Council of State Boards of Nursing. (2012). Nurse practice act, rules & regulations. *Nurse Practice Acts Guide and Govern Nursing Practice.* Retrieved from https://www.ncsbn.org/2012_JNR_NPA_Guide.pdf

National Institute of Child Health and Human Development. (2016). *Safe to sleep.* Retrieved from https://www.nichd.nih.gov/sts/Pages/default.aspx

National Patient Safety Foundation (NPSF). (2013). *Key facts about patient safety.* Retrieved from http://www.npsf.org/for-patients-consumers/patients-and-consumers-key-facts-about-patient-safety

National Safety Council (NSC). (2014). Going "green." *Safety + Health Magazine.* Retrieved from http://www.safetyandhealthmagazine.com/articles/9975-going-green

Occupational Safety and Health Administration (OSHA). (2015). *We can help. Creating a safety culture.* Retrieved from https://www.osha.gov/SLTC/etools/safetyhealth/mod4_factsheets_culture.html

Office of Disease Prevention and Health Promotion (ODPHP). (2015a). *The Office of Disease Prevention and Health Promotion.* Retrieved from http://health.gov

Office of Disease Prevention and Health Promotion (ODPHP). (2015b). Healthcare quality and patient safety. Prevent adverse drug events (ADEs). *National Action Plan for Adverse Drug Event Prevention.* Retrieved from http://health.gov/hcq/ade.asp

One and Only Campaign (OOOC). (2014). The One & Only Campaign. *Centers for Disease Control and Prevention and the Safe Injection Practices Coalition.* Retrieved from http://www.oneandonlycampaign.org/about/the-campaign

QSEN Institute. (2014a). *Competencies.* Retrieved from http://qsen.org/competencies/

QSEN Institute. (2014b). *Competencies. Pre-licensure KSAs.* Retrieved from http://qsen.org/competencies/pre-licensure-ksas/

QSEN Institute. (2014c). *Competencies. Graduate KSAs.* Retrieved from http://qsen.org/competencies/graduate-ksas/

Sightings, T. (2014). *On retirement, expert planning, ideas and advice. 12 baby boomer retirement trends.* Retrieved from http://money.usnews.com/money/blogs/on-retirement/2014/07/22/12-baby-boomer-retirement-trends

The Joint Commission. (2013). *SBAR—a powerful tool to help improve communication!* Retrieved from http://www.jointcommission.org/at_home_with_the_joint_commission/sbar_%E2%80%93_a_powerful_tool_to_help_improve_communication/default.aspx

The Joint Commission. (2015). *Our award-winning patient safety program. SpeakUp™.* Retrieved from http://www.jointcommission.org/speakup.aspx

The Joint Commission. (2016). *2016 Hospital National Patient Safety Goals.* Retrieved from http://www.jointcommission.org/asets/1/6/2016_NPSG_HAP_ER.pdf

U.S. Department of Labor. (2017). *Occupational Safety and Health Administration.* Retrieved from https://www.osha.gov

U.S. National Library of Medicine. (2015). *Sudden infant death syndrome.* Retrieved from https://www.nlm.nih.gov/medlineplus/suddeninfantdeathsyndrome.html

World Health Organization (WHO). (2015a). *Clean care is safer care. Testing the WHO Guidelines on hand hygiene in healthcare in eight pilot sites worldwide.* Retrieved from http://www.who.int/gpsc/country_work/pilot_sites/introduction/en/

World Health Organization (WHO). (2015b). *Clean care is safer care. Hand hygiene in the control of Ebola and health system strengthening.* Retrieved from http://www.who.int/gpsc/hand-hygiene_ebola/en/.

World Health Organization (WHO). (2015c). *Ebola virus disease. Fact sheet no. 103.* Retrieved from http://www.who.int/mediacentre/factsheets/fs103/en/#

Appendix A
NANDA-Approved Nursing Diagnoses 2015–2017

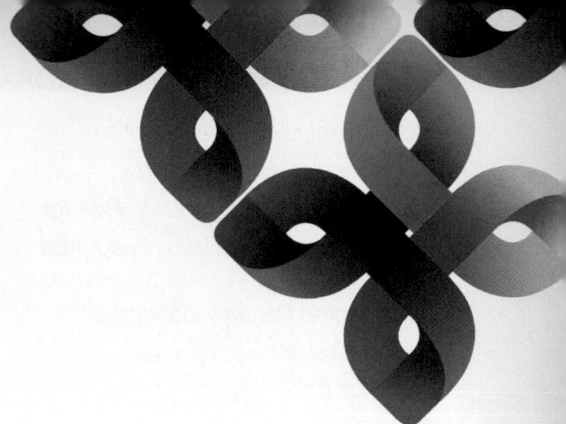

Activity, Deficient Diversional

Activity Intolerance

Activity Intolerance, Risk for

Activity Planning, Ineffective

Activity Planning, Risk for Ineffective

Adaptive Capacity: Intracranial, Decreased

Adverse Reaction to Iodinated Contrast Media, Risk for

Airway Clearance, Ineffective

Allergy Response, Risk for

Allergy Response, Latex

Allergy Response, Latex, Risk for

Anxiety

Anxiety, Death

Aspiration, Risk for

Attachment, Risk for Impaired

Bleeding, Risk for

Blood Glucose Level, Risk for Unstable

Body Image, Disturbed

Body Temperature: Imbalanced, Risk for

Bowel Incontinence

Breast Milk, Insufficient

Breastfeeding, Ineffective

Breastfeeding, Interrupted

Breastfeeding, Readiness for Enhanced

Breathing Pattern, Ineffective

Cardiac Output, Decreased

Cardiac Output, Decreased, Risk for

Cardiovascular Function, Impaired, Risk for

Caregiver Role Strain

Caregiver Role Strain, Risk for

Childbearing Process, Ineffective

Childbearing Process, Readiness for Enhanced

Childbearing Process, Risk for Ineffective

Chronic Pain Syndrome

Comfort, Impaired

Comfort, Readiness for Enhanced

Communication, Readiness for Enhanced

Communication: Verbal, Impaired

Confusion, Acute

Confusion, Chronic

Confusion, Risk for Acute

Constipation

Constipation, Perceived

Constipation, Risk for

Contamination

Contamination, Risk for

Coping: Community, Ineffective

Coping: Community, Readiness for Enhanced

Coping, Defensive

Coping: Family, Compromised

Coping: Family, Disabled

Coping: Family, Readiness for Enhanced

Coping: Readiness for Enhanced

Coping, Ineffective

Corneal Injury, Risk for

Decision Making, Readiness for Enhanced

Decisional Conflict (Specify)

Denial, Ineffective

Dentition, Impaired

Development: Delayed, Risk for

Diarrhea

Disuse Syndrome, Risk for

Dry Eye, Risk for

Dysreflexia, Autonomic

Dysreflexia, Autonomic, Risk for

Electrolyte Imbalance, Risk for

Emancipated Decision-Making, Impaired

Emancipated Decision-Making, Impaired, Risk for

Emancipated Decision-Making, Readiness for Enhanced

Emotional Control, Labile

Falls, Risk for

Family Processes, Dysfunctional

Family Processes, Interrupted

Family Processes, Readiness for Enhanced

Fatigue

Fear

Fluid Balance, Readiness for Enhanced

Fluid Volume: Deficient

Fluid Volume: Deficient, Risk for

Fluid Volume: Excess

Fluid Volume: Imbalanced, Risk for

Frail Elderly Syndrome

Frail Elderly Syndrome, Risk for

Functional Constipation, Chronic

Gas Exchange, Impaired

Gastrointestinal Motility, Risk for Dysfunctional

Gastrointestinal Motility, Dysfunctional

Grieving

Grieving, Complicated

Grieving, Risk for Complicated

Growth: Disproportionate, Risk for

Health: Community, Deficient

Health Behavior, Risk-Prone

Health Maintenance, Ineffective

Health Management, Family, Ineffective

Health Management, Ineffective

Health Management, Readiness for Enhanced

Home Maintenance, Impaired

Hope, Readiness for Enhanced

Hopelessness

Human Dignity, Risk for Compromised

Hyperthermia

Hypothermia

Hypothermia, Risk for

Impulse Control, Ineffective

Infant Behavior: Disorganized

Infant Behavior: Disorganized, Risk for

Infant Behavior: Organized, Readiness for Enhanced

Infant Feeding Pattern, Ineffective

Infection, Risk for

Injury, Risk for

Insomnia

Jaundice, Neonatal

Jaundice, Neonatal, Risk for

Knowledge, Deficient

Knowledge, Readiness for Enhanced

Labor Pain

Lifestyle, Sedentary

Liver Function, Risk for Impaired

Loneliness, Risk for

Maternal/Fetal Dyad, Risk for Disturbed

Memory, Impaired

Mobility: Bed, Impaired

Mobility: Physical, Impaired

Mobility: Wheelchair, Impaired

Mood Regulation, Impaired

Moral Distress

Nausea

Neglect, Unilateral

Neurovascular Dysfunction: Peripheral, Risk for

Noncompliance

Nutrition, Imbalanced: Less than Body Requirements

Nutrition, Readiness for Enhanced

Mucous Membrane: Oral, Impaired

Mucus Membrane: Oral, Impaired, Risk for

Obesity

Overweight

Overweight, Risk for

Pain, Acute

Pain, Chronic

Parenting, Impaired

Parenting, Readiness for Enhanced

Parenting, Risk for Impaired

Perfusion: Gastrointestinal, Risk for Ineffective

Perfusion: Renal, Risk for Ineffective

Perioperative Hypothermia, Risk for

Perioperative Positioning Injury, Risk for

Personal Identity: Disturbed

Personal Identity: Disturbed, Risk for

Poisoning, Risk for

Post-Trauma Syndrome

Post-Trauma Syndrome, Risk for

Power, Readiness for Enhanced

Powerlessness

Powerlessness, Risk for

Pressure Ulcer, Risk for

Protection, Ineffective

Rape-Trauma Syndrome

Relationship, Ineffective

Relationship, Risk for Ineffective

Relationship, Readiness for Enhanced

Religiosity, Impaired

Religiosity, Readiness for Enhanced

Religiosity, Risk for Impaired

Relocation Stress Syndrome

Relocation Stress Syndrome, Risk for

Resilience, Impaired

Resilience, Readiness for Enhanced

Resilience, Risk for Impaired

Role Conflict, Parental

Role Performance, Ineffective

Self-care, Readiness for Enhanced

Self-care Deficit: Bathing

Self-care Deficit: Dressing

Self-care Deficit: Feeding

Self-care Deficit: Toileting

Self-Concept, Readiness for Enhanced

Self-Esteem, Chronic Low

Self-Esteem, Chronic Low, Risk for

Self-Esteem, Situational Low

Self-Esteem, Situational Low, Risk for

Self-Mutilation

Self-Mutilation, Risk for

Self Neglect

Sexual Dysfunction

Sexuality Pattern, Ineffective

Shock, Risk for

Sitting, Impaired

Skin Integrity, Impaired

Skin Integrity, Risk for Impaired

Sleep Deprivation

Sleep Pattern, Disturbed

Sleep, Readiness for Enhanced

Social Interaction, Impaired

Social Isolation

Sorrow, Chronic

Spiritual Distress

Spiritual Distress, Risk for

Spiritual Well-Being, Readiness for Enhanced

Standing, Impaired

Sudden Infant Death Syndrome, Risk for

Stress Overload

Suffocation, Risk for

Suicide, Risk for

Surgical Recovery, Delayed

Surgical Recovery, Delayed, Risk for

Swallowing, Impaired

Thermal Injury, Risk for

Thermoregulation, Ineffective

Tissue Integrity, Impaired

Tissue Integrity, Impaired, Risk for

Tissue Perfusion: Cardiac, Risk for Decreased

Tissue Perfusion: Cerebral, Risk for Ineffective

Tissue Perfusion: Peripheral, Ineffective

Tissue Perfusion: Peripheral, Risk for Ineffective

Transfer Ability, Impaired

Trauma, Risk for

Trauma: Vascular, Risk for

Urinary Elimination, Impaired

Urinary Elimination, Readiness for Enhanced

Urinary Incontinence, Functional

Urinary Incontinence, Overflow

Urinary Incontinence, Reflex

Urinary Incontinence, Stress

Urinary Incontinence, Urge

Urinary Incontinence, Urge, Risk for

Urinary Retention

Urinary Tract Injury, Risk for

Ventilation: Spontaneous, Impaired

Ventilatory Weaning Response, Dysfunctional

Violence: Other-Directed, Risk for

Violence: Self-Directed, Risk for

Walking, Impaired

Wandering

Glossary

ABC The essential functions of airway, breathing, and circulation.

ABCD An enhancement of the **ABC** mnemonic, with the **D** representing one of four indicators depending on agency use: defibrillation, deficiency, deadly bleeding, or disability.

Abortion Loss of pregnancy before the fetus is viable outside the uterus. Also called *miscarriage*.

Absence seizures Also called petit mal seizures, absence seizures involve both hemispheres of the brain as well as deeper structures such as thalamus, basal ganglia, and upper brainstem. They are considered a type of generalized seizure.

Absorption The process of moving nutrients and fluid from the external environment of the gastrointestinal tract to the internal environment. May also refer to the intake of any specific nutrient.

Abstinence Voluntarily going without alcohol, drugs, or other pleasurable substances or activities.

Abuse of power An attempt by an individual to use his or her position or authority in a manner that shames, controls, demeans, humiliates, or denigrates another individual to gain emotional, psychologic, or physical advantage over that individual.

Accelerations A transient increase in the fetal heart rate normally caused by fetal movement.

Accommodation 1. The ability of the eye to adjust to variations in distance. 2. The process of a change whereby cognitive processes mature sufficiently to allow an individual to solve problems that were unsolvable before.

Accountability The ability and willingness of an individual to assume responsibility for his or her actions and to accept the consequences of his or her behavior.

Accreditation A peer review process that evaluates and certifies the quality of an organization.

Acculturation The process of adapting to the majority culture and accepting it as one's own.

Acid indigestion A condition in which an individual can taste the stomach acid when it flows back into the esophagus.

Acidosis The condition that results when hydrogen ion concentration increases above normal, causing the pH to drop below 7.35.

Acids Substances that release hydrogen ions in solution.

Acquaintance phase The first few days after a child's birth, when the new mother applies herself to the task of getting to know her baby.

Acquaintance rape A broad term used to describe a rape committed by an acquaintance or other familiar individual.

Acquired immunity Immunity developed after exposure to a pathogen.

Acquired immunodeficiency syndrome (AIDS) An immune system deficit induced by infection with the human immunodeficiency virus (HIV). AIDS is characterized by opportunistic infections.

Acrocyanosis A bluish discoloration of the hands and feet.

Acromegaly Excessive growth of bone from growth hormone hypersecretion.

Actinic keratosis An epidermal skin lesion directly related to chronic sun exposure and photodamage. Also called *senile keratosis* or *solar keratosis*.

Action potential The electrical activity produced by movement of ions across cell membranes that stimulates muscle contraction.

Active acquired immunity Antibodies formed in response to an illness or an immunization while a woman is pregnant.

Active euthanasia Actions to bring about a patient's death directly, with or without patient consent.

Active immunity Production of antibodies or development of immune lymphocytes against specific antigens.

Active listening Fully concentrating on both the content and emotion of a person's message, rather than just passively hearing the words a person says.

Active transport A method that requires additional energy (in the form of adenosine triphosphate) to move substances against the concentration gradient (from low concentration to high concentration).

Activities of daily living (ADLs) Activities used routinely in daily life, such as grooming, eating, bathing, and dressing.

Activity-exercise pattern An individual's routine of exercise, activity, leisure, and recreation, including activities of daily living that require energy expenditure.

Activity tolerance The type and amount of exercise or daily living activities that an individual is able to perform without experiencing adverse effects.

Actual loss A change in or unavailability of something or someone of value that can be recognized by others.

Acute coronary syndrome (ACS) Any condition that develops due to sudden, reduced blood flow to the heart.

Acute fatigue A sudden onset of physical and mental exhaustion or weariness, particularly after a period of mental or physical stress.

Acute illness An alteration in health or functioning characterized by severe symptoms of relatively short duration.

Acute infection An infection that appears suddenly and lasts for a short time.

Acute kidney injury (AKI) Proposed as a more accurate term for *acute renal failure*, AKI is defined as a sudden decline in kidney function that causes disturbances in fluid, electrolyte, and acid–base balances.

Acute lymphocytic leukemia (ALL) The most common type of leukemia in children and adolescents, marked by the proliferation of malignant cells that resemble immature lymphocytes.

Acute myeloid leukemia (AML) A disorder characterized by uncontrolled proliferation of myeloblasts and hyperplasia of the bone marrow and spleen.

Acute myocardial infarction (AMI) A life-threatening condition that occurs when blood flow to a portion of the cardiac muscle is blocked. If circulation to the affected myocardium is not promptly restored, loss of functional myocardium affects the heart's ability to maintain an effective cardiac output, ultimately leading to cardiogenic shock and death.

Acute pain Temporary, localized, and sudden pain that lasts for less than 6 months and has an identifiable cause, such as trauma, surgery, or inflammation.

Acute pancreatitis An inflammatory disorder that involves self-destruction of the pancreas by its own enzymes through autodigestion.

Acute postinfectious glomerulonephritis (APIGN) Inflammation of the glomerular capillary membrane that is most often seen in children as a response to a group A beta-hemolytic streptococcal infection of the skin or pharynx or as a result of infection by *Staphylococcus*, *Pneumococcus*, or Coxsackie virus.

Acute renal failure (ARF) A rapid decline in renal function with azotemia, fluid, and electrolyte imbalances. ARF may be reversed with prompt intervention.

Acute respiratory distress syndrome (ARDS) A disorder with rapid onset characterized by noncardiac pulmonary edema and progressive refractory hypoxemia. ARDS is a life-threatening emergency.

Acute retroviral syndrome (ARS) Primary human immunodeficiency virus infection.

Acute stress disorder A condition that may occur following an individual experiencing, learning of, or witnessing an extremely stressful event that involves the threat of death, actual or threatened serious injury, or actual or threatened physical or sexual violation.

Acute tubular necrosis (ATN) The destruction of tubular epithelial cells, which causes an abrupt and progressive decline of renal function.

Adaptation 1. The ability to handle the demands made by the environment. Also called *coping behavior*. 2. The return to normal functioning, even when homeostasis cannot be regained.

Adaptation phase The phase during a crisis in which the individual meets the challenges presented and uses his or her resources to successfully resolve the crisis.

Adaptive behavior Everyday skills, including conceptual skills, social skills, and practical skills.

Adaptive functioning The ability of an individual to meet the standards expected for his or her cultural group.

Adaptive mechanisms Methods the ego uses to fulfill the needs of the id in a socially acceptable manner. Also called *defense mechanisms*.

Addiction A psychologic or physical need for a substance (such as alcohol) or process (such as gambling) to the extent that the individual will risk negative consequences in an attempt to meet the need.

Addictive behaviors Compulsive, problematic patterns of action resulting in psychologic and/or physiologic dependence.

Addison disease A disorder that results from adrenal insufficiency, particularly a cortisol deficiency.

Adherence Commitment or attachment to a regimen. Also called *compliance*.

Adhesions Fibrous bands of scar tissue.

Adjustment disorder with depressed mood A maladaptive reaction to an identifiable psychosocial stressor or stressors that occurs within 3 months after the onset of the stressor and has persisted for no longer than 6 months. Also called *adjustment disorder* or *situational depression*.

Adjustment phase Initial phase experienced in response to crisis, characterized by disorganization and unsuccessful attempts to meet the crisis.

Adjustment reaction to depressed mood See Postpartum blues.

Administrative laws Responsibilities that may be interpreted and enforced by an agency that has been delegated the power of oversight by the governing legislation.

Adolescent family A family in which one or more parents are adolescents.

Advance healthcare directives Legal documents that allow an individual to plan for healthcare and/or financial affairs in the event of incapacity. Also called *advance directives* or *healthcare advance directives*.

Advocacy Protecting an individual by expressing and defending the individual's cause on his or her behalf.

Advocate An individual who expresses and defends the cause of another.

Aerobic exercise An activity during which the amount of oxygen taken into the body is greater than that used to perform the activity.

Aesthetic knowing The subjective elements and personal style a nurse uses when delivering care, including empathy, holistic thinking, compassion, and sensitivity.

Afebrile Without fever.

Affect The immediate and observable emotional expression of mood, which people communicate verbally and nonverbally; the outward manifestation of what the individual is feeling.

Affective commitment An attachment to a profession that includes identification with and involvement in the profession.

Affective domain The learning domain encompassing an individual's emotional response to tasks, including feelings, emotions, interests, attitudes, and appreciation. Also called the *feeling domain*.

Afterload The force that ventricles must overcome to eject their blood volume.

Afterpains Cramplike pains caused by intermittent contractions of the uterus that occur after childbirth.

Age-related macular degeneration (AMD) A gradual degeneration in the macular area of the retina that is the leading cause of blindness in people over age 65.

Ageism A deep and profound prejudice in American society against older adults.

Aggravated assault An unlawful attack by one individual on another for the purpose of inflicting severe or aggravated bodily injury. This type of assault usually is accompanied by the use of a weapon or by means likely to produce death or great bodily harm.

Aggression Any form of behavior directed toward the goal of harming or injuring another living being.

Aggressive behavior Behavior directed toward getting what one wants without considering the feelings of others.

Aggressive communicators Individuals who tend to focus on their own needs and become impatient when these needs are not met.

Agnosia The inability to recognize one or more objects that previously were familiar.

Agoraphobia A condition that is characterized by anxiety associated with two or more of the following situations: being in enclosed spaces, being in open spaces, using public transportation, being in a crowd or standing in a line of people, or being alone outside the home environment.

Agraphia The inability to write properly.

AIDS dementia complex The most common cause of mental status changes for patients with HIV infection. This dementia results from a direct effect of the virus on the brain and affects cognitive, motor, and behavioral functioning. Fluctuating memory loss, confusion, difficulty concentrating, lethargy, and diminished motor speed are typical manifestations.

Air trapping Decreased airflow with exhalation caused by edema of the air passages.

Airborne precautions Used for patients who are known to have or suspected of having serious illnesses transmitted by airborne droplet nuclei smaller than 5 microns, such as tuberculosis.

Airway clearance techniques Nonpharmacologic strategies for clearing the airway. Examples include coughing, huffing, and **chest physical therapy**.

Airway remodeling Structural changes of the airway caused by a disease, such as asthma, resulting in progressive or permanent loss of lung function.

Airway resistance The effort or force needed to move oxygen through the trachea to the lungs.

Akathisia Restlessness.

Alcohol dependence A primary, chronic disease characterized by use or abuse of alcohol; genetic, psychosocial, and environmental factors influence its development and manifestations. Also called *alcoholism*.

Alcohol poisoning A toxic condition that results from excessive consumption of large amounts of alcohol in a very short period of time.

Alcohol withdrawal delirium A medical emergency usually occurring 3–5 days following alcohol withdrawal and lasting 2–3 days. Characterized by paranoia, disorientation, delusions, visual hallucinations, elevated vital signs, vomiting, diarrhea, and diaphoresis. Also known as *delirium tremens (DTs)*.

Alcohol withdrawal syndrome Condition that typically begins about 6–8 hours after an individual with alcoholism takes his or her last drink. Early symptoms include irritability, anxiety, insomnia, tremors, sweating, and a mild tachycardia.

Alcoholic cirrhosis A progressive, irreversible liver disorder resulting from excessive consumption of alcohol. Also called *Laënnec cirrhosis*.

Alcoholism A primary, chronic disease characterized by use or abuse of alcohol; genetic, psychosocial, and environmental factors influence its development and manifestations. Also called *alcohol dependence*.

Alkalosis The condition that results when hydrogen ion concentration falls below normal and the pH level rises above 7.45.

Allen test A measurement of radial or ulnar artery patency; either the radial or ulnar artery is digitally compressed by the examiner after blood has been forced out of the hand by clenching it into a fist.

Allergen An environmental or exogenous antigen that provokes a hypersensitivity response.

Allergic contact dermatitis A cell-mediated or delayed hypersensitivity to a wide variety of allergens.

Allergy A hypersensitivity response to environmental or exogenous antigens.

Allogeneic blood transfusion A transfusion using blood that has been donated by the community.

Allogeneic bone marrow transplant A transplant using bone marrow from a matched donor.

Allografts Grafts between members of the same species who have different genotypes and HLA antigens. Human skin that has been harvested from cadavers is usually used. Also called *homograft*.

Alloimmunization The reaction of the immune system to donated tissue.

Allostasis Necessary changes that must occur to achieve the characteristic stability of homeostasis.

Allostatic load The physical cost of adaptation to physiologic or psychosocial stressors.

Alogia Limited or impoverished speech.

Alopecia Hair loss.

Alternative therapies (also referred to as *alternative medicine*) A term used to describe use of these diverse therapies *instead of* conventional therapies, including acupuncture; cultural practices related to food preparation or practices at specific times of the day or during the week.

Altruism A concern for the welfare and well-being of others.

Alveoli Terminal structures of the respiratory system where gas exchange occurs.

Alzheimer disease (AD) The most common kind of dementia, Alzheimer disease involves progressive dementia, memory loss, and the inability to care for one's self.

Ambulation The ability to walk from place to place independently with or without an assistive device.

Amblyopia Lazy eye; one eye has reduced vision even with no identifiable cause, and the reduced vision is not correctable by corrective lenses.

Amenorrhea The absence of menstruation.

Amniocentesis A procedure used to obtain amniotic fluid for genetic testing to determine fetal abnormalities or fetal lung maturity in the third trimester of pregnancy.

Amnion A thin protective membrane that contains amniotic fluid.

Amniotic fluid The liquid surrounding the fetus in utero. It absorbs shocks, permits fetal movement, and prevents heat loss.

Amphetamine A powerful stimulant that, when used improperly or abused, poses a severe health risk due to its devastating physical and neurologic consequences, including amphetamine-induced mental disorders.

Ampulla The outer third of the fallopian tube, where fertilization usually occurs.

Amyloid plaques Seen in Alzheimer disease and formed when groups of nerve cells degenerate and clump around the amyloid core in the spaces between the neurons in the brain. Amyloid plaques consist primarily of insoluble deposits of beta-amyloid, a protein fragment from a larger protein called amyloid precursor protein, mixed with other neurons and nonnerve cells.

Anaerobic exercise Activity in which the muscles cannot draw out enough oxygen from the bloodstream, and anaerobic pathways are used to provide additional energy for storing for a short time.

Anal stimulation The stimulation of the anus with the fingers, mouth, or sex toys for sexual pleasure.

Anaphylactic shock Shock resulting from a widespread hypersensitivity reaction. Also called *anaphylaxis*.

Anaphylaxis An acute systemic type I hypersensitivity (allergic) response that may result in shock and death. It occurs in highly sensitive persons following exposure to a specific antigen, usually through injection or ingestion.

Anaplasia The regression of a cell to an immature or undifferentiated cell type.

Anasarca Severe, generalized edema.

Andragogy The art and science of teaching adults.

Androgen A hormone that stimulates the development and maintenance of male sex characteristics.

Androgyny Flexibility in gender roles.

Anemia An abnormally low number of circulating red blood cells, low hemoglobin concentration, or both.

Anergic Unable to react to common antigens.

Anergy Fatigue and decreased energy associated with a depressive disorder. Also called *anergia*.

Anger A subjective sense of intense displeasure, irritation, or animosity.

Angina pectoris Chest pain resulting from reduced coronary blood flow caused by a temporary imbalance between myocardial blood supply and demand. Also called *angina*.

Angle-closure glaucoma A type of glaucoma that results from a narrowing of the anterior chamber angle due to corneal flattening or bulging of the iris into the anterior chamber. Also called *narrow-angle* or *closed-angle glaucoma*.

Anhedonia The inability to feel pleasure.

Animism Giving lifelike qualities to nonliving things.

Anion Ion that carries a negative charge.

Anomia Difficulty naming people and things.

Anorexia Loss of appetite.

Anorexia nervosa (AN) A potentially life-threatening disorder characterized by extreme perfectionism, weight fear, significant weight loss, body image disturbances, strenuous exercising, peculiar food-handling patterns, and reductions in heart rate, blood pressure, metabolic rate, and the production of estrogen or testosterone.

Anorgasmia Absence of orgasm.

Antagonism One of the six trait domains associated with personality disorders that is composed of manipulativeness, deceitfulness, callousness, hostility, grandiosity, and attention seeking.

Antepartum Time between conception and the onset of labor; usually used to describe the period during which a woman is pregnant.

Anthropometric measurements Measurements that can help identify individuals who are at risk for undernutrition or overnutrition. Specific measurements include height, length (in babies), weight, body mass index, waist-to-hip circumference, and skinfold thickness.

Antibodies Proteins that work against antigens.

Antibody-mediated (humoral) immune response Activation of B cells to produce antibodies to respond to antigens such as bacteria, bacterial toxins, and free viruses.

Anticipatory grief Grief experienced in advance of a loss, such as the wife who grieves before her ailing husband dies.

Anticipatory guidance Information about developmental changes that can be expected in the future. Including the recognition of the potential for a crisis and assistance with identifying potential methods for averting the crisis.

Anticipatory learning Learning necessary to effectively reach a desired outcome or in anticipation of a need for information that has not yet occurred.

Anticipatory loss A loss that is experienced before the loss actually occurs. For example, the gradual decline and eventual death of a family member who has Alzheimer disease.

Anticipatory problem solving Initial information is presented to a learner, who is then asked a question or presented with a situation related to the information. The learner applies the new information to the situation and decides what to do.

Antigen Foreign substance that triggers the immune response.

Antigen-antibody complex The complex formed by the binding of an antibody to an antigen.

Antigenic drift Describes small changes that occur continuously as a virus makes copies of itself.

Antigenic shift When two different strains of a virus infect the same cell and exchange genetic material to create a new subtype of the virus.

Antiretroviral therapies Pharmacologic therapies that stop or suppress the activity of a retrovirus, preventing further weakening of the immune system and thereby minimizing opportunistic infections.

Antiseptics Agents that inhibit the growth of some microorganisms.

Antisocial personality disorder (ASPD) One of several types of personality disorders defined by the DSM-5, it is characterized by a pattern of disregard for and violation of the rights of others.

Anuria The failure of the kidneys to produce urine, resulting in a total lack of urination or output of less than 100 mL/day in an adult.

Anxiety A stress response characterized by feelings of apprehension, dread, mental uneasiness, and a sense of helplessness in response to an actual or perceived threat to the well-being of oneself or others.

Anxious distress A combination of symptoms often associated with anxiety, including restlessness, impaired concentration due to worry, fear of something awful happening, and fear of losing control. Anxious distress often manifests in patients with depression and bipolar disorders and is associated with an increased risk for suicide.

Aortic stenosis Narrowing of the aortic valve that obstructs blood flow to systemic circulation.

Apathy A lack of interest or enthusiasm.

Apgar score A physical assessment of a newborn at 1 minute and 5 minutes after birth on a scale from 1 to 10 that includes heart rate, respiratory effort, muscle tone, reflex irritability, and skin color.

Aphakia Absence of the lens of the eye (e.g., after surgical removal of a cataract).

Aphasia Defective or absent language function.

Apical-radial pulse A comparison of the apical and radial pulses, which are normally identical. A pulse deficit can indicate certain cardiovascular disorders.

Aplastic anemia A disorder that results when the bone marrow fails to produce all three types of blood cells.

Apnea Absence of breathing.

Apnea of prematurity Absence of breathing for 20 seconds or longer, or for less than 20 seconds when associated with cyanosis, pallor, and

bradycardia. A common problem in a preterm infant of less than 36 weeks' gestation, usually presenting between day 2 and day 7 of life.

Appendectomy Surgical removal of the appendix.

Appendicitis Inflammation of the vermiform appendix.

Appendicular skeleton Pectoral girdles, upper limbs, pelvic girdle, and lower limbs.

Approach-coping The use of confrontation to change the stressor by taking direct action.

Approximated Term describing successful closure of a wound with little or no tissue loss.

Apraxia The inability to perform purposeful movements and use objects correctly.

Areflexia The loss of reflex function.

Areola Pigmented ring surrounding the nipple of the breast.

Arousal In the brain, arousal, or alertness, is regulated by the **reticular activation system**.

Arrhythmogenic tissue Tissue that affects the generation and conduction of electrical impulses in the heart.

Arrogance Excessive pride and a feeling of superiority.

Arrhythmogenic right ventricular dysplasia (ARVD) A condition that results when the body progressively replaces the muscle of the right ventricle with fatty and fibrous tissue.

Arterial blood gas (ABG) A laboratory test used to evaluate oxygen and carbon dioxide exchange and the acid–base balance within the blood.

Arterial blood pressure A measure of the pressure exerted by the blood as it flows through the arteries.

Arteriosclerosis An arterial disorder characterized by thickening, loss of elasticity, and calcification of arterial walls.

Arteriovenous (AV) fistula An artificial connection between a vein and an artery created for long-term vascular access.

Arthrodesis A procedure that permanently fuses two or more bones together at a joint using pins, plates, screws, and rods. Also called *joint fusion*.

Arthroplasty Total joint replacement.

Arthroscopy A surgical procedure in which a thin, lighted tube with a camera in one end is inserted into a joint in order to allow a surgeon to visualize joint structure more easily.

Artificial disc surgery Surgery to replace a herniated disc with an artificial disc in order to maintain flexibility of the spinal joint.

Artificial rupture of membranes A process of rupturing of the membranes by the certified nurse-midwife or physician using an instrument called an amniohook. Completed if spontaneous rupture of membranes does not occur.

ASA Physical Classification Scale A physical risk classification category that determines the type and dosage of sedation a patient can receive.

Ascites Excess fluid in the peritoneal cavity.

Asepsis The absence of disease-causing organisms.

Assault The action of creating an apprehension of offensive, insulting, or physically injurious touching.

Assertive behavior Behavior that consists of expressing one's wishes and opinions, or taking care of oneself, but not at the expense of others.

Assertive communicators Individuals who tend to declare and affirm their opinions. In doing this, however, they respect the rights of others to communicate in the same fashion.

Assertive community treatment (ACT) A therapeutic regimen for individuals with moderate to severe mental illness that provides patients with individually tailored services within their communities.

Assessment The systematic and continuous collection of data about a patient for the purpose of determining the patient's current and ongoing health status, predicting the patient's health risks, and identifying appropriate health-promoting activities.

Assignment The transfer of responsibility to accomplish a task, without the transfer of authority.

Assimilation 1. The process of adapting to and integrating characteristics of the dominant culture as one's own. 2. The process by which humans encounter and react to new situations by using the mechanisms they already possess.

Assisted suicide Self-administration of a lethal dose of medication provided by a physician or healthcare provider in order to intentionally end a patient's life with the goal of relieving pain and suffering.

Associative play A stage of play in which children play together or share tasks during play.

Astereognosis The inability to identify objects by touch.

Asthma A chronic inflammatory disease of the lungs characterized by recurrent episodes of wheezing, breathlessness, chest tightness, and coughing.

Asynclitism A condition that occurs when the sagittal suture is directed toward either the symphysis pubis or the sacral promontory and is felt to be misaligned.

Asystole Cardiac standstill.

Ataxia Lack of muscle coordination.

Atelectasis Collapse of lung tissue following obstruction of the bronchus or bronchioles.

Atherectomy A procedure to remove plaque from a lesion, specifically an **atheroma**.

Atheroma Complex lesion consisting of lipids, fibrous tissue, collagen, calcium, cellular debris, and capillaries. The formation of atheromas is the final stage of **atherosclerosis**.

Atherosclerosis A form of arteriosclerosis in which deposits of fat and fibrin obstruct and harden the arteries.

Atrial gallop (S$_4$) A heart sound produced by atrial contraction and ejection of blood into the ventricle during late diastole. Also called the *fourth heart sound*.

Atrial kick An extra bolus of blood delivered to the ventricles before they contract.

Atrial natriuretic factor (ANF) A peptide hormone released from cells in the atrium of the heart in response to excess blood volume and stretching of the atrial walls.

Atrial septal defect (ASD) An opening in the atrial septum that permits left-to-right shunting of blood.

Atrioventricular (AV) canal defect A combination of defects in the atrial and ventricular septa and portions of tricuspid and mitral valves. A complete AV canal defect allows blood to travel freely among all four chambers of the heart. Also called *endocardial cushion defect*.

Atrophy The wasting away or decrease in size of an organ, muscle, or tissue.

Attention deficit disorder (ADD) A variation in central nervous system processing characterized by developmentally inappropriate behaviors involving inattention.

Attention-deficit/hyperactivity disorder (ADHD) A variation in central nervous system processing characterized by developmentally inappropriate behaviors involving inattention, hyperactivity, and impulsivity.

Attention impairment A condition marked by an inability to process information and respond to such information appropriately; a patient with attention impairment will have poor concentration and be easily distracted.

Attentive listening The process of listening actively, using all the senses. Also called *mindful listening*.

Attributes of safety The quality or properties of remaining safe.

Audiologist A healthcare professional specializing in identifying, diagnosing, treating, and monitoring disorders of the auditory and vestibular portions of the ear.

Audit An examination of records to verify accuracy and proper use.

Auditory Of or relating to hearing.

Aura An olfactory or visual sensory sensation that may provide an early warning sign of a seizure.

Auscultation Listening to the sounds produced within the body. Auscultation can be direct using the unaided ear or indirect using a stethoscope or other listening device.

Authority 1. The power to command other individuals and direct their activities. 2. The right to act or to accomplish the task.

Autism spectrum disorders (ASDs) A developmental disorder in which individuals have persistent deficits in social communication and social interaction, and restricted, repetitive patterns of behavior, interest, or activities.

Autoantibodies Antibodies that react to the individual's own tissues.

Autocratic (authoritarian) leader A leader who makes decisions for the group based on the belief that individuals are externally motivated and are incapable of independent decision making.

Autografting A procedure performed in the surgical suite in which part of a patient's healthy skin is removed and used to effect permanent skin coverage over a wound area.

Autoimmune disorder/disease Failure of immune system to recognize itself, resulting in normal host tissue being targeted by immune defenses.

Autologous blood transfusion A blood transfusion using a patient's own blood.

Autologous bone marrow transplant Bone marrow transplant using a patient's own bone marrow.

Automatism A repetitive reaction that occurs automatically, without conscious thought. Examples include lip smacking, eyelid fluttering, aimless walking, picking at clothing, and swallowing.

Autonomic dysreflexia An abrupt onset of excessively high blood pressure as the result of an overactive autonomic nervous system. An exaggerated sympathetic response that occurs in patients with spinal cord injuries at or above the T6 level. Also called *autonomic hyperreflexia*.

Autonomy 1. The state of being independent and self-directed without outside control. 2. The right to make one's own decisions.

Autosomal chromosomes Genetic material found in a cell nucleus that determines physical characteristics (excluding gender) of the individual.

Autosome A single chromosome from any one of the 22 pairs of chromosomes not involved in sex determination (X or Y); humans have 22 pairs of autosomes.

Avascular necrosis The death of bone tissue due to lack of blood supply. Also called *osteonecrosis*.

Avian influenza Also known as "bird flu," it is a form of influenza that commonly infects birds. This virus has not yet demonstrated the ability to spread among humans; however, concerns are that it will mutate to allow person-to-person spread. This viral strain has a mortality rate of greater than 50% in people who have been infected due to close association with infected birds.

Avoidance-coping The use of both behaviors and cognitive processes to avoid a stressor.

Avoidant personality disorder (APD) One of several types of personality disorders recognized by the DSM-5, APD is characterized by a pattern of social withdrawal along with a sense of inadequacy, fear, and hypersensitivity to potential rejection or shame.

Avolition The inability to persist in goal-directed activities.

Awareness The ability to perceive environmental stimuli and body reactions and to respond appropriately through thought and action.

Axial loading The application of vertical force to the spinal column.

Axial skeleton Ribs, sternum, vertebral column, and skull.

Axon A nerve fiber.

Azotemia Increased levels of nitrogenous wastes in the blood.

B lymphocytes (B cells) Integral to specific immune response, they are activated and mature into either plasma cells, which secrete antibodies, or memory cells.

Babinski reflex The fanning and extension of the toes or flexion of the toes due to gentle stroking on the sole of the foot. Also called the *Babinski response*.

Bacilli Rod-shaped bacteria.

Background questions General questions asked of a patient that seek more information about a topic, such as diseases and medications.

Bacteremia The presence of bacteria in the blood.

Bacteria The most common category of infection-causing microorganisms.

Bactericidal agent Destroys bacteria.

Bacteriostatic agent Prevents the growth and reproduction of some bacteria.

Balanitis Inflammation of the glans.

Balloon tamponade The inflation of the balloon tip of a multiple-lumen nasogastric tube to control bleeding.

Barlow maneuver A procedure used to evaluate an infant for hip dislocation or instability in which the healthcare provider grasps and adducts the infant's thigh and then applies gentle downward pressure.

Barotrauma Lung injury caused by alveolar overdistention. Also called *volutrauma*.

Barrel chest An increase in the anteroposterior chest diameter resulting from air trapping and hyperinflation.

Basal cell carcinoma An epithelial tumor believed to originate either from the basal layer of the epidermis or from cells in the surrounding dermal structures. Also called *basal cell cancer*.

Basal metabolic rate (BMR) The amount of energy expended by the body at rest.

Base excess (BE) A calculated value also known as *buffer base capacity*. The BE measures substances that can accept or combine with hydrogen ions. It reflects the degree of acid–base imbalance by indicating the status of the body's total buffering capacity.

Baseline fetal heart rate The average fetal heart rate (FHR) rounded to increments of 5 bpm observed during a 10-minute period of monitoring. This excludes periodic or episodic changes, periods of marked variability, and segments of the baseline that differ by more than 25 bpm.

Baseline fetal heart rate variability Fluctuation in the FHR baseline of 2 cycles per minute or greater, with irregular amplitude and inconstant frequency.

Bases Substances that accept hydrogen ions in solution. Also called *alkalis*.

Basic needs The physical needs of an individual, such as eating, sleeping, resting, self-care, and physical stability.

Battery The willful touching of another individual, an individual's clothes, or even something the individual is carrying that is unwanted, embarrassing, or unwarranted.

Behavioral therapy A form of therapy in which patients learn techniques to modify or change maladaptive behaviors.

Behaviorist theory A theory that suggests that learning takes place when an individual's reaction to a stimulus is either positively or negatively reinforced.

Belief An interpretation or conclusion that one accepts as true.

Belief system The way in which a culture explains the mysteries of the universe and life.

Belt restraint Restraint used to ensure the safety of patients who are transported by wheelchair or gurney, or to protect patients confined to a bed or a chair. Also called *safety strap body restraint*.

Benchmarking A method used to compare the performance of an individual or organization to industry standards.

Beneficence The act of doing good or beneficial actions.

Benign Referring to a growth or tumor that does not endanger life or health and tends to not recur after treatment.

Benign prostatic hyperplasia (BPH) Nonmalignant enlargement of the prostate gland commonly seen in the aging man.

Bereavement The subjective response experienced by the surviving loved ones after the death of an individual with whom they have shared a significant relationship.

Bias The favoring of a group or individual over another.

Bidirectional influence Influences exerted between an individual and his or her family that may negatively affect the emotional health of the individual, the family, or both.

Bilevel ventilator (BiPAP) Mechanical ventilation that provides inspiratory positive airway pressure as well as airway support during expiration.

Biliary colic A severe, steady pain in the epigastric region or right upper quadrant of the abdomen.

Binge drinking The consumption of five or more drinks containing alcohol in a single session.

Binge eating The ingestion of huge amounts of food (about 3,500 kcal) within a short time (about 1 hour).

Binge eating disorder (BED) An eating disorder characterized by recurring episodes of binge eating, a sense of lack of control, and negative feelings about oneself, but without intervening periods of behavior such as self-induced vomiting, purging by laxatives, fasting, or prolonged exercise.

Binuclear family A postdivorce family in which the biologic children are members of two nuclear households—that of the father and that of the mother—and the children alternate between the two homes.

Bioethics The application of ethics to issues of human life or health (e.g., to decisions about abortion or euthanasia).

Bioethical dilemmas Ethical dilemmas of human life or health that arise in the care of patients and families; they often emerge from a combination of causative factors.

Biologic rhythm A cyclical event or function that consists of repeated occurrences and repeated, regular intervals between occurrences. Biologic rhythms can refer to both physical and psychologic patterns.

Biomedical informatics The interprofessional science that deals with biomedical information's structure, acquisition, and use.

Bioterrorism The deliberate release of viruses, bacteria, or other microbes as weapons.

Bipolar disorder A mood disorder characterized by alternating depression and elation, with periods of normal mood in between. Formerly called *manic–depressive disorder*.

Birthing room A single room in a hospital where a pregnant woman and her partner or other family members will stay for the labor, birth, recovery, and possibly the postpartum period.

Bisexual An individual who is attracted to members of both sexes.

Bisphosphonates Drugs used to treat osteoporosis that inhibit bone reabsorption by suppressing osteoclast activity.

Blackouts A form of amnesia about events that occurred during a drinking period. This is often seen in the early stages of alcoholism.

Bladder training Gradually increases the bladder capacity by increasing the intervals between voidings and resisting the urge to void.

Blame-free environment An environment in which healthcare providers can report errors or near misses without the fear of punishment.

Blended family A family formed after the death or divorce of a parent; may include stepparents on both sides, stepchildren, half-siblings.

Blepharism Spasms that cause the eye to blink continuously.

Blighted ovum One of the most common causes of miscarriage, it occurs when the egg has been fertilized and both the membrane and placenta have formed, but the embryo has not formed.

Blood flow The volume of blood transported in a vessel, in an organ, or throughout the entire circulation over a given period of time.

Blood pressure The force that blood exerts against the walls of the arteries as it is pumped from the heart.

Blood urea nitrogen (BUN) A measure of blood level of urea, the end product of protein metabolism.

Bloodborne pathogens Microorganisms carried in blood and body fluids that are capable of infecting other individuals with serious and difficult-to-treat viral infections.

Bloody show The pink-tinged secretions resulting from a small amount of blood loss from the exposed cervical capillaries during pregnancy.

Blunt trauma Trauma that occurs without any communication between the damaged tissues and the outside environment.

Body fluid Any fluid that is essential to homeostasis; water is the primary body fluid.

Body image The mental image of the physical self.

Body mass index (BMI) A method of comparing weight to height as an indirect measure of body fat.

Body substance isolation (BSI) System that employs generic infection control precautions for all patients, except those with the few airborne diseases.

Body surface area (BSA) The relationship between height and weight measured in square meters.

Body temperature The core or surface measurement of a patient's internal heat production and loss.

Bone marrow transplant The treatment of disease by infusing a patient with his or her own bone marrow or that of a healthy donor.

Borborygmus Hyperactive, high-pitched, tinkling, rushing, or growling bowel sounds heard in diarrhea or at the onset of bowel obstruction.

Borderline personality disorder (BPD) One of several personality disorders defined in the DSM-5, BPD is marked by unstable interpersonal relationships, self-image, affect, and impulsiveness.

Bouchard nodes Bony lumps in the middle joint of the digit.

Boundaries The invisible lines that define the amount and kind of contact allowable among members of a family and between the family and outside systems.

Boutonnière deformity A flexion deformity of the PIP joints with extension of the DIP joint.

Bowel incontinence The inability to voluntarily control the passage of fecal contents and intestinal gas through the anal sphincter. Also called *fecal incontinence.*

Brachytherapy Radiation treatment given by placing radioactive material directly in or near the target, which is often a tumor.

Bradycardia A heart rate in an adult of less than 60 bpm.

Bradydysrhythmia Abnormally slow rhythms.

Bradykinesia Slowed movements due to muscle rigidity.

Bradyphrenia Slowed thinking and a decreased ability to form thoughts, to plan, or to make decisions.

Bradypnea A respiratory rate of less than 10 breaths per minute in adults.

Brain death The cessation and irreversibility of all brain functions, including those of the brainstem.

Brainstem Contains the midbrain, pons, and medulla oblongata. Located between the cerebrum and spinal cord, the brainstem connects pathways between the higher and lower structures. Ten of the 12 pairs of cranial nerves originate in the brainstem.

Brainstorming A decision-making method in which group members meet and generate diverse ideas about the nature, cause, definition, or solution to a problem.

Braxton Hicks contractions Intermittent painless uterine contractions that may occur every 10–20 minutes and occur more frequently near the end of pregnancy.

Brazelton neonatal behavioral assessment scale A scale developed to assess a newborn's state changes, temperament, and individual behavioral patterns.

Breach of care See Breach of duty.

Breach of duty A deviation from the standard of care owed a patient. Also called *breach of care.*

Breakthrough pain A sudden flare or increase in pain despite comfort with or without baseline analgesia.

Breast Mammary gland.

Breast cancer The unregulated growth of abnormal cells in breast tissue.

Breathing exercises Techniques used to slow the breathing rate by focusing on taking regular and deep breaths from the diaphragm.

Brief psychotic disorder Rapid onset of at least one of the following psychotic symptoms: delusions, hallucinations, disorganized speech, or disorganized behavior. The episode lasts at least 1 day but less than 1 month, after which the person returns to the premorbid level of functioning.

Bronchial sounds Loud, high-pitched sounds heard over the trachea that are longer on exhalation than inhalation.

Bronchiectasis Chronic dilation of the bronchi and bronchioles.

Bronchiolitis A lower respiratory tract illness that occurs when an infecting agent (virus or bacterium) causes inflammation and obstruction of the small airways.

Bronchitis Inflammation of the mucous membranes of the bronchial tubes.

Bronchogenic carcinomas Tumors of the airway epithelium.

Bronchoscopy A procedure that allows direct visualization of the lungs by inserting a bronchoscope orally into the trachea and advancing it to the bronchi bifurcation.

Bronchovesicular sound The sound created as air moves within the bronchial tree.

Brown adipose tissue (BAT) A specific store of fat in newborn infants that appears dark brown due to enriched blood supply, dense cellular content, and abundant nerve endings.

Bruits Blowing sound sometimes heard due to restriction of blood flow through the vessels.

Buffers Substances that prevent major changes in pH by releasing hydrogen ions.

Bulimia nervosa (BN) A type of eating disorder characterized by an obsessive focus on weight and body size and cycles of binge eating followed by purging.

Bullying Any unwanted aggressive behavior committed against another who is not a sibling or dating partner.

Bureaucratic leader A leader who relies on the organization's rules, policies, and procedures to direct the group's work efforts.

Burn An injury resulting from exposure to heat, chemicals, radiation, or electric current.

Burn shock Hypovolemic shock resulting from the shift of a massive amount of fluid from the intracellular and intravascular compartments into the interstitium following burn injury. Also called *hypovolemic shock.*

Burnout A complex syndrome resulting from unmanaged stress that manifests as physical and emotional depletion, a negative attitude and self-concept, and feelings of helplessness and hopelessness.

Cachexia Physical wasting from weight loss and loss of muscle mass due to the rapid growth and reproduction of cancer cells and their need for increased nutrients.

Caffeine A stimulant that increases the heart rate and acts as a diuretic.

Calcium oxalate A chemical compound from which kidney stones may form.

Calcium phosphate A chemical compound from which kidney stones may form.

Calculi Renal stones.

Cancellous bone The spongy tissue of bone.

Cancer A family of complex diseases with manifestations that vary according to body system and type of tumor cells.

Cancer pain Pain that may result from the direct effects of the cancerous disease and its treatment, or it may be unrelated to the disease and its treatment in individuals with cancer.

Candidiasis A common, opportunistic fungal infection in patients with AIDS.

Cannabis sativa The plant source of marijuana.

Caput succedaneum A localized, easily identifiable, soft area of the scalp, generally resulting from a long and difficult labor or vacuum extraction.

Carbohydrate One of the three major macronutrients primarily derived from plant foods. These foods contain simple and complex sugars, and starches.

Carcinogen A substance that causes cancer.

Carcinogenesis The production or origin of cancer.

Cardiac arrest The cessation of heart function that precedes biologic death.

Cardiac cycle One contraction and relaxation of the heart; a single heartbeat.

Cardiac index The cardiac output adjusted for the patient's body size or body surface area (BSA).

Cardiac markers Proteins released from necrotic heart muscle.

Cardiac output (CO) The amount of blood pumped by the ventricles into the pulmonary and systemic circulations in 1 minute.

Cardiac rehabilitation A medically supervised program designed to aid people with their recovery from heart attacks, heart surgeries, and percutaneous coronary interventions.

Cardiac reserve The heart's ability to respond to the body's changing need for cardiac output.

Cardiac tamponade Compression of the heart caused by collected blood or fluid in the pericardium.

Cardinal ligament Major ligament of the uterus containing the uterine artery and vein.

Cardinal movements A series of changes in position that allow the fetus to move through the birth canal. Also called *mechanisms of labor.*

Cardiogenic shock Shock that occurs when the heart's pumping ability is compromised to the point that it cannot maintain cardiac output and adequate tissue perfusion.

Cardiomyopathy Disease that affects the heart muscle's ability to pump effectively. Primary abnormality of the heart muscle that affects its structural or functional characteristics.

Cardiopulmonary resuscitation (CPR) A mechanical attempt to maintain tissue perfusion and oxygenation using oral resuscitation and external cardiac compressions.

Care coordination The means by which a multidisciplinary team works with a patient to ensure that the care received across the healthcare continuum meets the patient's needs.

Care management model Planning, assessment, and coordination of health services to provide an integrated continuum of clinical services, including medical care, health promotion, disease prevention, costs, and use of resources.

Care map Expected outcomes and care strategies developed through collaboration by the healthcare team. Also called a *critical pathway.*

Caring To feel interest, concern, and respect for a patient while demonstrating sensitivity, sincerity, honesty, and patience.

Caring for the dying The act of helping patients live as comfortably as possible until death and helping the patient's support individuals cope with death.

Carpal spasm Involuntary contraction of the hand and fingers due to decreased calcium levels.

Carphologia Involuntary, repeated lint picking.

Carrier Human or animal reservoir of a specific infectious agent that usually does not manifest any clinical signs of the disease.

Cartilage A type of flexible connective tissue found throughout the body.

Case management (CM) The coordination of patient care over time using the combination of health and social services necessary to meet the individual patient's needs.

Case managers Individuals who help manage the care of certain patient populations, including patients with chronic medical conditions, such as diabetes; patients recovering from acute conditions, such as those receiving joint replacement; and patients managing psychiatric disorders.

Case method A patient-centered method of managing care in which one nurse is assigned to, and is responsible for, the comprehensive care of a group of patients during an 8- or 12-hour shift.

Caseation necrosis A process in which tissue infected with *Mycobacterium tuberculosis* dies and forms a cheeselike center in the infectious bacilli.

Cast A rigid device applied to immobilize injured bones and promote healing.

Catabolism The breakdown of body proteins.

Cataract An opacification (clouding) of lens of the eye due to a breakdown of proteins within the lens.

Catatonia Unresponsiveness to the environment or others.

Catatonic excitement Includes hyperactivity and bizarre behavior and is a positive symptom of schizophrenia.

Catatonic inhibition Involves decreased activity level; limited speech; minimal self-care; and, at times, a trancelike state. Catatonic inhibition is a negative symptom of schizophrenia.

Cation Ion that carries a positive charge.

Cauda equina syndrome (CES) A condition that occurs when the nerve roots of the cauda equine are compressed. It may result in permanent neurologic impairment, including urinary incontinence and paralysis.

Causation To make a successful claim for malpractice, an injury must have occurred as a direct consequence of a nurse's or other healthcare professional's breach of duty.

Cavitation Formation of a cavity or bubble.

Celiac disease A chronic immune-mediated disorder of the small intestine in which the absorption of nutrients, particularly fats, is impaired. Also known as celiac sprue or nontropical sprue.

Cell cycle The four phases of cell growth and development.

Cell-mediated (cellular) immune response Direct or indirect inactivation of antigen by lymphocytes.

Cellulitis An acute bacterial infection of the dermis and underlying connective tissue. Cellulitis is characterized by red or lilac, tender, warm, edematous skin that may have an ill-defined, nonelevated border.

Central nervous system (CNS) One of two principal parts of the neurologic system, the central nervous system consists of the brain and the spinal cord.

Central nervous system (CNS) depressants A type of drug that acts to slow brain function, decreasing levels of alertness and awareness. CNS depressants include barbiturates, benzodiazepines, paraldehyde, meprobamate, and chloral hydrate.

Central pain 1. A type of pain related to a lesion in the brain that may spontaneously produce high-frequency bursts of impulses that are perceived as pain. 2. A type of pain caused by damage to the central nervous system that may manifest in constant pain, pain paroxysms, evoked pain, or allodynia. Patients may describe their pain as "pins and needles," aching, or lacerating.

Centration Focusing only on one particular aspect of a situation or the ability to concentrate.

Cephalocaudal development Growth that proceeds in the direction from head to toe.

Cephalohematoma A collection of blood resulting from ruptured blood vessels between the surface of a cranial bone and the periosteal membrane. Also called an *entrapped hemorrhage*.

Cerebellum Located below the cerebrum and behind the brainstem, it coordinates stimuli from the cerebral cortex to provide precise timing for skeletal muscle coordination and smooth movements.

Cerebral palsy (CP) A group of chronic conditions affecting body movement, coordination, and posture that results from a nonprogressive abnormality of the immature brain.

Cerebral perfusion pressure (CPP) The pressure it takes for the heart to provide the brain with blood. It is calculated by finding the difference between arterial pressure and intracranial pressure. Normal CPP is 0–95 mmHg.

Cerebrum The largest portion of the brain, it is composed of gray matter and has two hemispheres divided into four regions or lobes.

Certification The credentialing process by which a nongovernmental agency or association recognizes the professional competence of an individual who has met the predetermined qualifications specified by the agency or association.

Cerumen Earwax.

Cervical cap A latex cup-shaped contraceptive device, used with spermicidal cream or jelly, that fits snugly over the cervix and is held in place by suction.

Cervical collar A device that stabilizes and maintains neutral alignment of the cervical spine; it is used with patients with potential or suspected cervical spine injury. Also called *C-collar*.

Cervical ripening The softening and effacing of the cervix.

Cervix The narrow neck of the uterus.

Cesarean birth The birth of an infant through an abdominal and uterine incision.

CFTR modulators A treatment for **cystic fibrosis** that attacks the cause of the problem—issues with the CFTR protein—rather than just CF's clinical manifestations.

Chain of command The hierarchy of authority and responsibility within an organization.

Chancre A painless ulceration formed during the first stage of syphilis.

Change-of-shift report A type of handoff communication given to all nurses on the next shift.

Channel A medium used to convey messages.

Charcot-Marie-Tooth disease The most common inherited form of **peripheral neuropathy,** it is characterized by a slowly progressive degeneration of the muscles of the foot, lower leg, hand, and forearm. Symptoms usually present between adolescence and young adulthood.

Charismatic leader A rare type of leader who is characterized by a strong, emotional relationship between the leader and the group members.

Chart A formal, legal document that provides evidence of a patient's care. Also called a *patient record* or a *clinical record*.

Charting The process of making an entry on a patient record. Also called *recording* or *documenting*.

Charting by exception (CBE) A documentation system in which only abnormal or significant findings or exceptions to norms are recorded.

CHCT A biopsy of thigh skeletal muscle tissue to determine sensitivity to caffeine and halothane.

Cheilosis Cracking of lips.

Chemical conjunctivitis An irritation of the conjunctiva by chemicals used to treat the eyes.

Chemical restraints Pharmacologic agents administered for the purpose of controlling hyperactive behavior in agitated patients.

Chemical thermogenesis The stimulation of heat production in the body through increased cellular metabolism. Also called *nonshivering thermogenesis* or *NST*.

Chemotaxis The movement of cells in response to a chemical stimulus.

Chemotherapy Cancer treatment involving the use of cytotoxic medications to decrease tumor size, adjunctive to surgery or radiation therapy; or to prevent or treat suspected metastases.

Chest physical therapy An **airway clearance technique** that involves clapping and **percussion**.

Chest x-ray Allows for two-dimensional visualization of the contents of the thoracic cavity.

Child abuse Any act or failure to act on the part of a parent or caretaker which results in the death, serious physical or emotional harm, sexual abuse, or exploitation of a child.

Child Health Insurance Program (CHIP) State and federal funded healthcare coverage for children under the age of 19 whose families earn more than the Medicaid limits but cannot afford to purchase private healthcare coverage.

Childhood traumatic grief A grief reaction that occurs when an important person in a child's life dies as the result of a traumatic event or circumstances the child views as traumatic.

Childfree family A family without children.

Chlamydia A group of sexually transmitted infections caused by *Chlamydia trachomatis*.

Chloasma Brownish pigmentation over the bridge of the nose and the cheeks during pregnancy and in some women who are taking oral contraceptives. Also called *melasma gravidarum* or *mask of pregnancy*.

Cholangitis Duct inflammation.

Cholecystitis Inflammation of the gallbladder.

Cholelithiasis The formation of stones (*calculi* or *gallstones*) in the gallbladder or biliary duct system.

Chromosomes Tightly coiled strands of DNA within the nucleus that contain genetic information.

Chronic bronchitis A disorder of excessive bronchial mucous secretion.

Chronic fatigue Profound fatigue of long duration that is not improved by rest.

Chronic fatigue syndrome A complex disorder in which the patient experiences unrelenting fatigue and associated symptoms that are not alleviated by substantial rest and that cannot be otherwise explained for a period of 6 months or longer. Also called *myalgic encephalomyelitis*.

Chronic illness An alteration in health or function that lasts for an extended period of time, usually 6 months or longer, and often for the duration of the individual's life.

Chronic infection An infection that develops slowly and persists for months or sometimes years.

Chronic intermittent colitis A recurrent form of ulcerative colitis characterized by insidious onset, few systemic manifestations, and attacks lasting 1–3 months that occur at intervals of months to years.

Chronic kidney disease A type of renal failure that progresses slowly with few symptoms until the kidneys are severely damaged and unable to meet the excretory needs of the body. Also called *chronic renal failure.*

Chronic lymphocytic leukemia (CLL) A disorder characterized by the proliferation and accumulation of small, abnormal, mature lymphocytes in the bone marrow, peripheral blood, and body tissues.

Chronic myeloid leukemia (CML) A disorder characterized by abnormal proliferation of all bone marrow elements.

Chronic obstructive pulmonary disease (COPD) A specific progressive disorder that slowly alters the structures of the respiratory system over time, irreversibly affecting lung function.

Chronic pain Prolonged pain, usually lasting longer than 6 months. It is not always associated with an identifiable cause and is often unresponsive to conventional medical treatment.

Chronic pancreatitis An irreversible process characterized by chronic inflammation, fibrosis, and gradual destruction of functional pancreatic tissue.

Chronic traumatic encephalopathy (CTE) A form of dementia associated with a history of multiple concussions.

Chronic renal failure See Chronic kidney disease.

Chronic venous insufficiency (CVI) A disorder of inadequate venous return over a prolonged period of time.

Chvostek sign Facial grimacing caused by repeated contractions of the facial muscle. A test used to check for hypocalcemia.

Circadian rhythms Regular fluctuations in the body's physiologic processes occurring in a 24-hour cycle.

Circumcision A surgical procedure in which the prepuce, an epithelial layer covering the penis, is separated from the glans penis and excised. This procedure permits exposure of the glans for easier cleaning.

Cirrhosis The end stage of chronic liver disease. It is a progressive, irreversible disorder, eventually leading to liver failure.

Civil law The area of law that deals with the rights and duties of private persons or citizens and is most often enforced through the awarding of damages or compensation.

CK-MB A subset of CK enzyme specific to cardiac muscle. Elevated CK-MB is an indicator of myocardial infarction. Also called *MB-bands.*

Clang Repetition of rhyming words without apparent meaning.

Classism The oppression of groups of people based on their socioeconomic status.

Clean A state of medical asepsis in which almost all microorganisms are absent.

Client An individual who engages the advice or services of another person who is qualified to provide this service.

Clinical database The full extent of information about a patient, including the nursing health history, physical assessment, primary care provider's history and physical examination, results of laboratory and diagnostic tests, and material contributed by other health personnel.

Clinical decision support system A system that analyzes data and provides information about evidence-based practices. These systems can help improve patient safety and quality of care when used with sound nursing and medical judgment.

Clinical information system A software-based system that allows multiple disciplines to simultaneously access the patient's chart and record data that can be viewed and analyzed by a number of healthcare providers in real time. These systems are designed to provide the most accurate and current information about the patient so that the best decisions concerning the care of that patient can be made.

Clinical pathway A standardized, evidence-based, multidisciplinary plan that outlines the expected care required for patients with common, predictable—usually medical—conditions.

Clonic phase Typically the second phase in a generalized or tonic–clonic seizure, characterized by alternating muscular contraction and relaxation.

Closed fracture A bone fracture in which the skin remains intact. Also called a *simple fracture.*

Closed questions Restrictive questions in an interview that require only a "yes" or "no" or short, specific answer.

Clotting Also known as **coagulation,** the process by which blood changes from liquid into a gel-like substance in order to stop bleeding from a damaged vessel.

Club drugs Substances popular among adolescents and young adults who frequent dance clubs and "raves." The most common is MDMA (methylenedioxymethamphetamine), better known as Ecstasy.

Coaching The process that encourages the development of individuals through personal interaction within an organization.

Coagulation Also known as **clotting,** the process by which blood changes from liquid into a gel-like substance for the purpose of forming a clot to stop bleeding from a damaged vessel.

Coagulation cascade A process that activates clotting factors, plasma proteins used in the formation of blood clots.

Coanalgesics Drugs that have analgesic properties, potentiate the effects of pain medications, relieve other discomforts, or reduce the side effects of analgesic drugs. Coanalgesics are especially effective at reducing neuropathic pain.

Coarctation of the aorta Narrowing or constriction in the descending aorta, often near the ductus arteriosus or left subclavian artery, which obstructs the systemic blood outflow.

Cobb angle A technique to estimate the degree of curvature of the spine using lines drawn from the vertebrae at the upper and lower limits of the curve that tilt most dramatically toward the apex of the curve.

Cocaine A powerful stimulant of natural origin that acts at the nerve terminals to prevent the reuptake of dopamine and norepinephrine, which in turn results in vasoconstriction, tachycardia, and hypertension.

Code of ethics A general guide for a profession's membership and a social contract with the public that it serves.

Codependence A cluster of maladaptive behaviors exhibited by significant others of a substance-abusing individual that serves to enable and protect the abuse at the expense of living a full and satisfying life.

Cognition The complex set of mental activities through which individuals acquire, process, store, retrieve, and apply information.

Cognitive appraisal The process of appraising, sorting, assessing, categorizing, evaluating, and framing the significance of an event or stressor with respect to an individual's own well-being.

Cognitive–behavioral therapy (CBT) The use of cognitive techniques and behavior modification to change detrimental beliefs and thought patterns.

Cognitive development The manner in which people learn to think, reason, and use language.

Cognitive domain The learning domain that includes the six intellectual abilities and thinking processes: knowing, comprehending, applying, analysis, synthesis, and evaluation. Also called the *thinking domain.*

Cognitive skills Intellectual skills or thought processes that include problem solving, decision making, critical thinking, and creativity.

Cognitive symptoms Cognitive symptoms of schizophrenia include deficits in memory, attention, language, visual-spatial awareness, social and emotional perception, and intellectual and executive function.

Cognitive theory A learning theory that recognizes the developmental level of learners and acknowledges the learner's motivation and environment. Also called *cognitivism.*

Coitus interruptus A method of contraception in which the man withdraws from the woman's vagina when he feels that ejaculation is impending.

Cold zone When a disaster occurs, this zone, located outside the warm zone, is where decontaminated victims are triaged and treated. Also called the *green zone* or the *support zone.*

Colectomy Surgical resection and removal of the colon.

Collaboration Two or more people working toward a common goal.

Collaborative intervention The actions a nurse carries out in collaboration with other healthcare team members, such as physical therapists, social workers, dietitians, and physicians.

Collagen A whitish protein substance that adds tensile strength to a wound.

Collateral channels Small blood vessels that develop to connect small arteries. Also called *collateral circulation*.

Colloid osmotic pressure A pulling force exerted by colloids that helps maintain the water content of blood by pulling water from the interstitial space into the vascular compartment. Also called *oncotic pressure*.

Colloids Substances such as large protein molecules that do not readily dissolve into true solutions.

Colon cancer Cancer of the third segment of the large bowel that may or may not include the anus.

Colonization The process by which strains of microorganisms become resident flora, capable of growing and multiplying.

Colorectal cancer Cancer of both the colon and rectum.

Colostomy A surgical opening into the colon.

Colostrum The initial milk that begins to be secreted during midpregnancy and that is immediately available to the baby at birth.

Column plan A nursing care plan that uses columns to categorize data for each phase of the nursing process. This type of care plan may include four columns: (1) nursing diagnoses, (2) goals/desired outcomes, (3) nursing interventions, and (4) evaluation. Some include only three columns.

Combined oral contraceptives (COCs) A safe, highly effective contraceptive pill combining estrogen and progestin. Also called *birth control pills*.

Comfort To ease the grief or trouble of others; to give hope.

Commitment The state or an instance of being obligated or emotionally impelled.

Communicable disease An illness that is transmitted directly from one person or animal to another by contact with body fluids, or that is indirectly transmitted by contact with contaminated objects or vectors.

Communication The exchange of information, feelings, thoughts, and ideals through verbal or other techniques.

Communication deviance Communication patterns that are distracting and confusing to listeners who are trying to share a common focus or meaning with a speaker. Communication deviance has been identified as a social-environmental trigger for schizophrenia symptoms.

Communicator style The manner in which an individual communicates; includes the way the individual interacts with others.

Community-based care Care that focuses on the political, social, institutional, and physical environments of the patient.

Community Emergency Response Team (CERT) program A Federal Emergency Management Agency–organized program that prepares participants to safely assist themselves, their families, and their neighbors in case of a disaster.

Comorbidity The presence of two or more disease processes.

Compartment syndrome A condition in which the tissue pressure in a muscle compartment exceeds the microvascular pressure, interrupting cellular perfusion.

Compassion An awareness of and concern for other individuals' suffering.

Competence Possessing the knowledge and skills necessary to perform one's job appropriately and safely.

Complementary health approaches (also referred to as alternative therapies) Any of the diverse array of practices, therapies, and supplements that are not considered part of conventional or traditional medicine that are used in addition to conventional treatments.

Complete spinal cord injury An injury that involves a total loss of all sensory and motor function below the level of the injury; usually the damage is irreversible.

Compliance 1. The relationship between the volume of the intracranial components and intracranial pressure. 2. The amount of distention or expansion the ventricles can achieve to increase stroke volume. 3. The extent to which an individual's behavior coincides with medical or health advice.

Complicated grief A form of grief in which the individual's strategies to cope with a loss are maladaptive. Also called *prolonged grief disorder (PGD)*.

Compression A condition that occurs when a vertical force is applied to the spinal column, such as occurs by falling and landing on the feet or buttocks or diving into shallow water.

Compromised host An individual who is at increased risk of infection.

Compulsion A repetitive behavior or mental activity used in response to obsessive thoughts that helps the individual lower his or her anxiety level.

Compulsivity One of the six trait domains associated with personality disorders that is distinguished by extreme inflexibility in a quest for perfection, in relation to both the individual's own actions and others' behaviors.

Computer vision syndrome The most common sequela of computer use. Symptoms include eye fatigue, headaches, blurred vision, dry eyes, and changes in color perception. Also called *eye strain*.

Concept map A visual representation of a nursing plan of care in a patterned diagram with data and ideas. Various shapes and colors are used to show relationships and connections in combination with lines or arrows.

Concrete thinking A type of thinking characterized by a focus on facts and details coupled with an inability to generalize or think abstractly.

Concurrent audit An evaluation of the adequacy of the nursing care a patient is receiving and a determination of whether desired outcomes are being met while the individual is still undergoing care at the healthcare facility.

Concussion Mild **traumatic brain injury**.

Condom A sheath of synthetic material that covers the penis to prevent conception or disease.

Conduction The process of heat transfer through physical contact of one surface with another surface.

Confabulation Making up information to fill memory gaps; used as a defensive mechanism to protect the person's attempt to protect self-esteem when confronted with memory loss.

Confidentiality The assurance the patient has that private information will not be disclosed without the patient's consent.

Conflict A situation that occurs when an agreement cannot be reached with regard to significant issues and concerns or when emotional opposition creates discord within an individual or among individuals, groups, or organizations.

Conflict competence Purposeful development of cognitive, behavioral, and emotional skills that assist individuals in preventing and reducing conflict.

Confusion An alteration in cognition that makes it difficult to think clearly, focus attention, or make decisions.

Confusion assessment method (CAM) A two-part test that differentiates between delirium and dementia. It is specifically designed to account for and control ageism.

Congenital cataracts A type of cataract that may appear in a child at birth or in childhood, usually in both eyes.

Congenital glaucoma A primary form of **glaucoma** caused by an abnormal development in the ocular drainage system that is sometimes diagnosed at birth but is usually diagnosed within the first year.

When diagnosed within the first year, it is often referred to as **infantile glaucoma**. When diagnosed after age 3, it may be referred to as **juvenile glaucoma**.

Congenital heart defect A defect of the heart or great vessels that is present at birth.

Congruent communication Communication in which the verbal and nonverbal aspects of the message match.

Conjugate vera The true conjugate, which extends from the middle of the sacral promontory to the middle of the pubic crest.

Conjunctiva The thin, transparent membrane that covers the anterior surface of the eye and lines the inner surfaces of the eyelids.

Conjunctivitis Inflammation of the conjunctiva. The most common eye disease, conjunctivitis is usually caused by a bacterial or viral infection.

Connective tissue Tissue made of fiber that forms the framework for support of the body's tissue and organs.

Consciousness A condition in which the individual is aware of self and environment and is able to respond appropriately to stimuli. Full consciousness requires both normal arousal and full cognition.

Consequence-based (teleologic) theories Theories that look to the outcomes (consequences) of an action in judging whether that action is right or wrong.

Conservation The concept that matter is not changed when its form is altered.

Consolidation Solidification of damaged cells and tissue during immune response to inflammation, specifically in the lungs.

Constant fever A condition that occurs when the body temperature fluctuates minimally but always remains above normal.

Constipation Fewer than three bowel movements per week or the difficult passage of stools.

Constructivism A collection of theories with the common thread of individuals actively constructing knowledge in order to solve realistic problems, often in collaboration with others.

Consumer An individual, a group of people, or a community that uses a service or commodity.

Consumer-driven healthcare plan (CDHP) A type of employer-sponsored coverage that combines a private insurance plan with a Health Savings Account (HSA) or Health Reimbursement Account (HRA).

Contact dermatitis An inflammation of the skin that occurs in response to direct contact with an allergen or irritant.

Contact precautions Used for patients who are known to have or suspected of having serious illnesses that are easily transmitted by direct contact with the patient or by contact with items in the environment, such as *Shigella*.

Contingency contracts A reinforcement process. Contingency contracts operate by "if–then" rules. If the patient performs a targeted response, such as abstinence from the addictive behavior (gambling, drug use, cutting, and so on), then the patient receives desired reinforcers.

Contingency planning The process of identifying and managing unplanned and unexpected events that interfere with getting work done efficiently, effectively, and in a timely manner.

Continuance commitment The awareness of costs associated with leaving a profession that inhibit an individual from leaving that profession. Considered the weakest type of commitment to a profession.

Continuous bladder irrigation (CBI) A method used to prevent the formation of blood clots.

Continuous positive airway pressure (CPAP) Mechanical ventilation that applies positive pressure to the airways of a patient who is breathing spontaneously. Breathing is patient triggered and pressure controlled. CPAP is used to help maintain open airways and alveoli, decreasing the work of breathing.

Continuous quality improvement (CQI) A structured organizational process for involving personnel in planning and executing a continu-ous flow of improvements to provide quality healthcare that meets or exceeds expectations.

Continuous renal replacement therapy (CRRT) A form of dialysis in which blood is continuously circulated through a highly porous hemofilter from artery to vein or vein to vein.

Contractility The inherent capability of the cardiac muscle fibers to shorten.

Contraction stress test (CST) A method of evaluating the respiratory function (oxygen and carbon dioxide exchange) of a placenta.

Contracture Permanent shortening of connective tissue.

Contralateral deficit Loss or impairment of sensorimotor functions on the side of the body opposite the side of the brain that is damaged by stroke.

Contrecoup injury This injury occurs when the brain strikes the side of the skull opposite to the side of impact.

Controlled Substance Act (CSA) A federal law that requires drugs to be classified based on the substance's medical use, potential for abuse, and safety risks.

Controlling The managerial process of comparing actual results with projected results, similar to the evaluation step in the nursing process. Controlling includes establishing performance standards, determining how to measure performance and creating the tools that will permit consistent measurement, evaluating performance, and providing feedback.

Convection The process of heat transfer through the fluid motion of air or water across the skin.

Convergence The medial rotation of the eyeballs so that each is directed toward the viewed object.

Co-occurring disorders Concurrent diagnosis of a substance use disorder and a psychiatric disorder. One disorder can precede and cause the other, such as the theorized relationship between alcoholism and depression.

Cooperative play The stage of play in which children work together to contribute to a unified whole, such as forming a sports team or dancing in an ensemble.

Copayment The set payment owed by an insured individual at the time a covered service is rendered.

Coping A dynamic process through which an individual applies cognitive and behavioral measures to handle internal and external demands that are perceived by the individual as exceeding available resources.

Cor pulmonale Right-sided heart failure.

Corneal abrasion Disruption of the superficial epithelium of the cornea.

Corneal reflex Closure of eyelids (blinking) due to corneal irritation.

Cornu The elongated portion of the uterus where the fallopian tubes enter.

Coronary artery bypass grafting (CABG) A procedure in which a section of a vein or artery is used to create a connection, or bypass, between the aorta and the blocked coronary artery beyond the obstruction.

Coronary artery disease (CAD) The most common type of heart disease, CAD is caused by impaired blood flow to the myocardium.

Coronary circulation A network of vessels that supply the heart muscle.

Corpus The upper triangular portion of the uterus. Also called the *uterine body*.

Corpus luteum A small yellow body that develops within a ruptured ovarian follicle.

Corrective action The steps taken to overcome a job performance problem.

Coryza Inflammation of the mucous membranes lining the nose, usually associated with nasal discharge.

Countershock phase The second part of an alarm reaction during which the sympathetic nervous system stimulation triggers the body's defenses.

Coup injury An injury that occurs when the brain strikes the same side of the skull as the side of impact.

Coup-contrecoup injury In this type of injury, the brain strikes the coup side, then bounces back and strikes the contrecoup side, resulting in contusions on both sides of the brain.

Couplet Two premature ventricular contractions in a row.

Couvade In some cultures, the man's observance of certain rituals and taboos to signify the transition to fatherhood.

Covert conflict Conflict that is avoided, ignored, or not discussed openly.

Crack A form of freebase cocaine that is made of baking soda, water, and cocaine mixed into a paste and microwaved to form a rock.

Crackles High-pitched popping sounds heard on inspiration due to fluid associated with or resulting from inflammation, or exudates, within the lung fields, or localized atelectasis.

Creatinine clearance A test that uses 24-hour urine and serum creatinine levels to determine the glomerular filtration rate; a sensitive indicator of renal function.

Creatine kinase (CK) An enzyme important for cellular function that is found principally in cardiac and skeletal muscle and the brain.

Creativity The ability to find or create a unique solution to a unique problem when traditional interventions are not effective.

Creativity techniques Strategies, such as brainstorming sessions, that use the creative potential of the group to generate a large number of possible options quickly.

Credentialing The formal identification of professionals who meet predetermined standards of professional skill or competence.

Credibility The quality of being truthful, trustworthy, and reliable.

Crepitation A grating or cracking sound.

Crime An act prohibited by statute or by common law principles.

Criminal law The area of law that deals with conduct that is harmful to another individual or to society as a whole and that may be punishable by fines or imprisonment.

Crisis An event or circumstance that overwhelms an individual's inherent ability to resolve, manage, or process the event or circumstance.

Crisis counseling A meeting that focuses on brief solutions, focused interventions, and supportive care during or after a crisis. It also considers the individual's physical vulnerability and degree of emotional stability.

Crisis intervention An emergent approach to care that is intended to assist patients with recognizing a crisis situation, and identifying and implementing an immediate, short-term solution.

Crisis intervention centers Organizations that provide telephone counseling for patients in crisis. Some organizations also provide consultation through email and online chatting.

Critical pathway Expected outcomes and care strategies developed through collaboration by the healthcare team. Also called a *case map*.

Critical thinking All or part of the process of questioning, analysis, synthesis, interpretation, inference, inductive and deductive reasoning, intuition, application, and creativity.

Crohn disease A chronic, relapsing inflammatory bowel disorder affecting the gastrointestinal tract. Also known as *regional enteritis*.

Cross-dressing Occurs when an individual of one gender (typically male) dresses in clothing specific to the opposite gender.

Crowning During birth, the appearance of the newborn's head or presenting fetal part at the vaginal orifice.

Crystalloids Salts that dissolve readily into true solutions.

Cultural deprivation A lack of culturally assistive, supportive, or facilitative acts.

Cultural groups Racial, ethnic, religious, or social groups with specific group behaviors and characteristics that are learned and shared, including language, customs, beliefs, and values.

Cultural humility The recognition that a healthcare provider's personal cultural values are not superior to the cultural values of others, thus preventing an abuse of power.

Cultural values Preferred ways of behaving or thinking that are sustained over time and used to govern a cultural group's actions and decisions.

Culture The patterns of behavior and thinking that people living in social groups learn, develop, and share.

Cultures Laboratory cultivations used to identify probable microorganisms by their characteristics, such as shape, growth patterns, and Gram-staining qualities.

Curling ulcers Acute ulcerations of the stomach or duodenum that form following a burn injury.

Cushing syndrome A disorder resulting from too much cortisol in the body. It can develop in individuals who take too much exogenous glucocorticosteroid for asthma or other disorders, or it can develop as a result of the overproduction of endogenous cortisol due to a pituitary or adrenal tumor.

Cyanosis Gray to blue or purple skin color caused by deoxygenated hemoglobin.

Cyber-bullying Aggression or bullying that occurs through the use of technology (e.g., social media, texting, or email).

Cycle of violence Violence that occurs with a patterned frequency, usually in three phases: initial tension due to communication failures, an abusive incident, and a honeymoon stage in which the aggressor may show love and affection. Cycle of violence may also refer to violence that spans multiple generations in a family.

Cyclothymic disorder A type of bipolar disorder characterized by chronic, fluctuating mood disturbances involving numerous periods of hypomanic symptoms and numerous periods of depressive symptoms.

Cystic fibrosis (CF) An inherited disorder that affects the secretory glands, particularly the glands that are responsible for secreting mucus, digestive enzymes, and sweat.

Cystic fibrosis transmembrane conductance regulator (CFTR) protein. A protein that is central to the movement of chloride into and out of the body cells.

Cystitis Inflammation of the urinary bladder.

Cystoscopy Endoscopy of the urinary tract. Also called *catheterization*.

Cytokines Proteins that carry messages for immune system function.

Damages Compensation sufficient to restore the plaintiff to his or her original position, so far as is financially possible.

Dashboard An interface that gathers, organizes, and displays a healthcare facility's key performance indicators in an easy-to-read format, often with charts or graphs.

Dashboard knee Tearing of the posterior cruciate ligament or any knee injury resulting from an individual's knee slamming into the dashboard or back of a seat during a motor vehicle collision.

Database A compilation of all information about a patient, including the nursing health history, physical assessment, primary care provider's history, physical examination, and test results.

Date rape A term used when dating violence takes the form of rape.

Dating violence A type of intimate partner abuse; this type occurs most often in relationships among youth.

Dawn phenomenon A rise in blood glucose between 4 a.m. and 8 a.m. that is not a response to hypoglycemia.

Dead space Areas of the lung that are ventilated but not perfused.

Death anxiety Worry or fear related to death or dying.

Debridement The process of removing painful or necrotic material, including all loose tissue, wound debris, and dead tissue, from a wound.

Decelerations The periodic decreases in fetal heart rate from the normal baseline.

Decerebrate posturing An abnormal posture adopted by an unconscious individual that indicates deteriorating brain function. It is characterized by an extended neck; clenched jaw; arms pronated, extended, and close to the sides; legs extended and feet plantar flexed.

Decibels (dB) Units of loudness.

Decision tree A graphic model that visually represents the choices, outcomes, and risks to be anticipated.

Declarative memory Memory that is related to people and facts, is consciously accessible, and can be verbally expressed.

Decode The process of relating the message perceived to the receiver's storehouse of knowledge and experience and sorting out the meaning of the message.

Decompensation Loss of effective compensation.

Decorticate posturing An abnormal posture adopted by an unconscious individual that indicates deteriorating brain function. It is characterized by the upper arms kept close to the sides; the elbows, wrists, and fingers flexed; the legs extended and internally rotated; and the feet plantar flexed.

Deductible A set annual cost for healthcare paid by an individual or family participating in a health insurance plan.

Deductive reasoning A "top-down" method of logical thinking that starts with a conclusion and analyzes the situation for valid, significant cues. One of two methods of logical thinking that are used to determine if decisions are reasonable.

Deep brain stimulation (DBS) A procedure in which a neurostimulator is implanted into the individual to send electrical signals to one of three brain regions—the subthalamic nucleus, the globus pallidus, or the thalamus—in order to reduce symptoms of Parkinson disease.

Deep venous thrombosis (DVT) A blood clot that forms along the intimal lining of a large vein, usually in a leg.

Defecation The expulsion of feces from the anus and rectum.

Defense mechanism See Adaptive mechanisms.

Defibrillation An emergency procedure that delivers an electrical shock to stop ventricular fibrillation and return to a rhythm that promotes cardiac output sufficient to sustain life.

Deficiency A term used to describe when intake of a nutrient is less than recommended.

Defining characteristics The cluster of signs and symptoms that indicate the presence of a particular diagnostic label.

Deformation The alteration of the spinal cord and soft tissues caused by abnormal movement.

Dehiscence An unintended separation of wound margins due to incomplete healing.

Dehydration A condition that occurs when a body does not take in as much water as it loses or lacks sufficient reserves to maintain proper function.

Delayed ejaculation Once called **male orgasmic disorder**, involves extreme difficulty ejaculating, despite the ability to maintain an erection for long periods (in some cases, an hour or more).

Delayed union The delayed healing of bones beyond the expected time period.

Delegate An individual who assumes responsibility for the actual performance of an assigned task or procedure.

Delegation The transfer of responsibility and authority for completing an activity to a qualified individual.

Delegator An individual who assigns a task to another individual to perform, but retains accountability for the outcome.

Delirium An acute cognitive disorder that affects functional independence.

Delirium tremens (DTs) A medical emergency usually occurring 3–5 days following alcohol withdrawal and lasting 2–3 days. Characterized by paranoia, disorientation, delusions, visual hallucinations, elevated vital signs, vomiting, diarrhea, and diaphoresis. Also known as *alcohol withdrawal delirium.*

Delusions False ideas or beliefs not based in reality.

Dementia The progressive, irreversible loss of cognitive function.

Democratic leader A leader who assumes that individuals are internally motivated, are capable of making decisions, and value independence. Democratic leaders typically provide constructive feedback, offer information, make suggestions, and ask questions to gain information or to help group members grow in their ability to make decisions.

Demography The study of population, including statistics about distribution by age and place of residence, mortality, and morbidity.

Demyelination A condition in which cells of the immune system, such as lymphocytes and macrophages, cross the blood–brain barrier and attack and destroy the myelin sheath.

Denominations Groups of members that adhere to the same practices and beliefs.

Dental caries Cavities.

Deoxyribonucleic acid (DNA) One of two types of nucleic acid made by cells, DNA contains the genetic instructions for the development and functioning of human beings.

Dependence A physiologic need for a substance that the patient cannot control, and which results in withdrawal symptoms if the substance is withheld.

Dependent intervention Activities carried out under a physician's orders or supervision, or according to specified routines or protocols.

Dependent personality disorder (DPD) One of several personality disorders defined in the DSM-5, it is marked by a pervasive, excessive, and unrealistic need to be cared for; fear of separation; lack of self-confidence; an inability to make decisions; and an inability to function independently.

Depersonalization A feeling of strangeness or unreality about the physical self.

Depolarization 1. The rapid inflow of sodium ions, causing an electrical change in which the inside of a cell becomes positive in relation to the outside. 2. The phase in which the heart contracts as a result of ion channel functions.

Depo-Provera A long-acting progesterone that provides highly effective birth control for 3 months when given as a single injection.

Depression A disorder characterized by a sad or despondent mood or loss of interest in usual activities.

Depressive disorder with peripartum onset See Postpartum depression.

Derealization A feeling of disconnection from an individual's own body or the environment.

Dermatome An area of skin innervated by the cutaneous branch of one spinal nerve.

Dermis The second layer of skin, which is made of a flexible connective tissue. It is richly supplied with blood cells, nerve fibers, and lymphatic vessels, as well as most of the hair follicles, sebaceous glands, and sweat glands.

Desaturated blood Blood that is low in oxygen as a result of oxygenated and deoxygenated blood mixing due to a congenital heart defect.

Desire phase The first phase of the sexual response cycle is the arousal of sexual interest by means of real or symbolic stimuli.

Detachment One of the six trait domains associated with personality disorders that is broken down into withdrawal, intimacy avoidance, anhedonia, and restricted affectivity.

Detrusor muscle The smooth muscle layers of the bladder wall, the detrusor muscle allows the bladder to expand as it fills with urine and contract as it releases urine during voiding.

Development An increase in the complexity and function of skill progression, the individual's capacity and skill to adapt to the environment. Related to growth.

Developmental disability Any of a variety of chronic conditions characterized by mental and/or physical impairment.

Developmental stage A level of achievement for a particular segment of an individual's life.

Developmental task A skill or behavior pattern learned during stages of development.

Device integration Real-time, accurate data is recorded in the patient's chart directly from a device (e.g., blood pressure monitor). Device integration allows the nurse to more quickly analyze and interpret that data and make adjustments to the plan of care based on the most current information.

Diabetes mellitus Group of chronic disorders of the endocrine pancreas, all categorized under a broad diagnostic label. The condition is characterized by inappropriate hyperglycemia caused by a relative or absolute deficiency of insulin or by a cellular resistance to the action of insulin. Also called *diabetes.*

Diabetic ketoacidosis (DKA) A form of metabolic acidosis that develops when there is an absolute deficiency of insulin and an increase in the insulin counterregulatory hormones. It may also be induced by stress in an individual with type 1 diabetes.

Diabetic nephropathy Disease of the kidneys in patients with diabetes that is characterized by the presence of albumin in the urine, hypertension, edema, and progressive renal insufficiency.

Diabetic neuropathy A disorder of the peripheral nerves and the autonomic nervous system in patients with diabetes, which manifests in one or more of the following: sensory and motor impairment, muscle weakness and pain, cranial nerve disorders, impaired vasomotor function, impaired gastrointestinal function, and impaired genitourinary function.

Diabetic retinopathy The collective name for the changes in the retina that occur in the person with diabetes. The retinal capillary structure undergoes alterations in blood flow, leading to retinal ischemia and a breakdown in the blood–retinal barrier.

Diagnosis-related groups (DRGs) A system of price control regulation that classifies patient illnesses based on diagnoses and pays hospitals a predetermined sum for each specific diagnosis regardless of the actual cost of services, the length of stay, or the acuity or complexity of the patient's illness.

Diagnostic label Standardized NANDA names for nursing diagnoses.

Diagonal conjugate Distance from the lower posterior border of the symphysis pubis to the sacral promontory.

Dialysate Dialysis solution.

Dialysis A process by which fluids and molecules pass through a semipermeable membrane from an area of higher solute concentration to one of lower solute concentration according to the rules of osmosis. Dialysis is used to remove excess fluid and metabolic waste products in renal failure.

Diaphragm A flexible disc that covers the cervix to prevent conception.

Diaphysis The shaft of a bone.

Diarrhea The passage of liquid feces and an increased frequency of defecation.

Diastasis recti abdominis A separation of the abdominal muscle.

Diastole The phase of ventricular relaxation between heartbeats.

Diastolic blood pressure The minimum pressure within the arteries during diastole.

Diathermy Treatment with heat generated by high-frequency electrical currents.

Diencephalon Area of the brain consisting of the thalamus (sometimes called the dorsal thalamus), hypothalamus, epithalamus, and subthalamus.

Diet recall Patient history of intake over a specified period of time.

Dietary Reference Intakes (DRIs) A standardized, recommended nutrient intake to support a healthy diet often provided by health organizations.

Differentiated practice A system in which each nurse's educational preparation and skill sets are evaluated and used to determine how he or she will be best used.

Differentiation A process occurring over many cell cycles that allows cells to specialize in certain tasks.

Diffuse axonal injury An injury that occurs because of a rotational deceleration that is dramatic enough to cause damage to the brain's white matter in the form of widespread disruption of axon fibers and myelin sheaths.

Diffusion The continual intermingling of molecules in liquids, gases, or solids brought about by the random movement of the molecules.

Digestion The conversion of food by means of its mechanical and chemical breakdown into absorbable substances in the gastrointestinal tract.

Digital rectal examination (DRE) An examination to detect for abnormalities in the rectum that can be detected through palpation.

Dihydrotestosterone (DHT) The androgen that mediates prostatic growth at all ages; formed in the prostate from testosterone.

Dilated cardiomyopathy The most common form of cardiomyopathy, it is characterized by the dilation of the heart chambers and impaired ventricular contraction.

Directing The managerial process of effectively motivating, communicating, and delegating tasks in order to complete an organization's work.

Directive interview A highly structured interview that elicits specific health information.

Dirty In medical asepsis, a term used to indicate that microorganisms are likely to be present.

Disaster An event that occurs with little or no warning in which available personnel and emergency services are initially overwhelmed and a serious threat to life, public health, and the environment is posed.

Discharge planning A plan of care that prepares the patient for discharge, including training in any necessary health skills.

Discipline A method of teaching children the rules for how to behave in society and what is expected in different circumstances.

Discoid lesions Raised, scaly, circular lesions with an erythematous rim.

Discovery The legal process of obtaining information before a trial.

Discrimination The differential treatment of individuals or groups, based on categories such as race, age, weight, gender, or social class, that occurs when an individual acts on prejudice and denies other people one or more of their fundamental rights.

Discussion An informal oral consideration of a subject by two or more healthcare personnel to identify a problem or establish strategies to resolve a problem.

Disease A detectable alteration in body function resulting from infection by microorganisms that causes a reduction of capacities or a shortening of the normal lifespan. Also called *pathogenesis.*

Disease surveillance Monitoring patterns of disease occurrence from cases of infections and communicable diseases reported by healthcare workers to state officials.

Diseases of adaptation Stress-related illnesses, such as peptic ulcers and hypertension.

Disenfranchised grief Grief that occurs when an individual is unable to acknowledge a loss to other persons. Also called *ambiguous loss.*

Disinfectants Agents that destroy pathogens other than spores.

Disinhibition One of the six trait domains associated with personality disorders that is noted for the presence of irresponsibility, impulsivity, and risk taking.

Disc Fluid-filled "shock absorber" that holds together and insulates the vertebrae. Also called *spinal disc.*

Discectomy The removal of all or part of the nucleus pulposus of an intervertebral disc.

Dismissal Termination of employment.

Disorganized behavior The inability to start or finish goal-oriented activities to a degree that it interferes with an individual's ability to lead a normal life.

Disorganized thinking Difficulty logically connecting thoughts, leading to garbled speech.

Dissatisfaction problems Issues that arise from unmet sexual needs and expectations.

Disseminated intravascular coagulation (DIC) A disruption of hemostasis characterized by widespread intravascular clotting and bleeding. It may be acute and life threatening, or it may be relatively mild.

Distracted driving The act of driving a motor vehicle while doing any activity that takes attention away from the road. Activities include texting, talking on the phone, eating, drinking, reading a map, talking to passengers, looking at a GPS, and adjusting the radio.

Distress A stress that is associated with inadequacy, insecurity, and loss.

Distributive shock Shock that results from widespread vasodilation and decreased peripheral resistance. Also called *vasogenic shock.*

Diuresis The production and excretion of abnormally large amounts of urine. Also called *polyuria.*

Diuretics Pharmacologic agents that increase urine formation and secretion.

Diversity The unique variations among and between individuals, variations that are informed by genetics and cultural background, but that are refined by experience and personal choice.

Diverticula Saclike projections of mucosa through the muscular layer of the wall of a canal or organ, e.g., the bladder wall, colon, or large intestine.

Documenting The process of making an entry on a patient record. Also called *recording* or *charting.*

Doll's eye reflex An oculomotor response in which the eyes move in opposite direction as head turns to the side. Also called the **oculocephalic reflex.**

Domestic partner An unmarried partner of the same or opposite sex.

Do-not-intubate (DNI) order Usually written by the physician for the patient who has a terminal illness or is near death, this order is usually based on the wishes of the patient and family that no lifesaving measures be provided once the patient stops breathing.

Do-not-resuscitate (DNR) order Usually written by the physician for the patient who has a terminal illness or is near death, this order is usually based on the wishes of the patient and family that no cardiopulmonary resuscitation be performed for respiratory or cardiac arrest. Also called a *no-code order.*

Dopamine A brain neurotransmitter that regulates voluntary movement, reward-seeking behavior, memory and learning, attention, sleep, affect, and many other functions.

Dormant Temporarily inactive but not dead.

Double-bind theory The theory that schizophrenia symptoms are partially an expression of contradictory family interactions.

Double depression A term used to describe a situation in which an individual experiences dysthymic disorder in combination with major depressive disorder.

Doula A paid caregiver who has typically received special training and may even be certified in caring for laboring women.

Down syndrome A developmental disorder that occurs when an individual is born with an extra full or partial chromosome. Down syndrome is associated with intellectual disability and a wide variety of physical impairments that can range from mild to severe.

Dramatic play The stage of play in which individuals use props to act out the drama of human life.

Dressler syndrome A symptom complex characterized by fever and chest pain that may develop days to weeks after an AMI. It is thought to be a hypersensitivity response to necrotic tissue or an autoimmune disorder.

Droplet nuclei Residue of evaporated droplets emitted by an infected host; can remain in the air for long periods of time.

Droplet precautions Used for patients who are known to have or suspected of having serious illnesses transmitted by particle droplets larger than 5 microns, such as pertussis or pneumonia.

Dual diagnosis Term used to refer to concurrent diagnoses of a psychiatric disorder and a substance use disorder.

Dubowitz tool A tool for assessing newborns that includes neuromuscular tone assessments, such as head lag, ventral suspension, and leg recoil.

Dullness A thudlike sound produced by dense tissue such as the liver, spleen, or heart.

Duodenal ulcer A peptic ulcer occurring in the duodenum.

Durable power of attorney A legal document that can delegate the authority to make health, financial, and/or legal decisions on an individual's behalf.

Durable power of attorney for healthcare A legal designation of another individual, usually a family member, significant other, or close personal friend, to make healthcare decisions on an individual's behalf.

Duration 1. The length of a sound. 2. The length of time from the beginning of a contraction to the completion of that same contraction.

Duty A legally enforceable obligation to conform to a particular standard of conduct that is owed to the patient.

Dwarfism Excessively short stature caused by insufficient growth hormone, typically resulting from a genetic abnormality.

Dysfunctional uterine bleeding (DUB) Vaginal bleeding that is usually painless but abnormal in amount, duration, or time of occurrence. Also called *abnormal uterine bleeding.*

Dysmenorrhea Painful menstruation.

Dyspareunia Painful intercourse.

Dysphagia Difficulty swallowing.

Dysplasia A loss of DNA control over differentiation occurring in response to adverse conditions.

Dyspnea Shortness of breath or difficulty breathing that is uncomfortable or painful; or when breathing is insufficient to meet oxygen demand.

Dysrhythmia Abnormal heart rate or rhythm. Also called *arrhythmia.*

Dysthymia A chronic depressive disorder with symptoms that are less severe than those of major depressive disorder. Also called *persistent depressive disorder* or *dysthymic disorder.*

Dystonia Severe muscle spasms, particularly of the back, neck, tongue, and face.

Dysuria Difficult or painful urination.

Early deceleration During birth, a condition that occurs when the fetal head is compressed and cerebral blood flow decreases, causing central vagal stimulation. Usually associated with the onset of uterine contractions.

Early (primary) postpartum hemorrhage Hemorrhage that occurs in the first 24 hours after childbirth.

Eating disorder A set of maladaptive responses to stress or anxiety characterized by obsessions with food and weight, often to the extent that daily functioning is impaired and physical and psychologic health are threatened.

Echolalia The compulsive parroting of a word or phrase just spoken by another.

Echopraxia The compulsive imitation of the movements of another.

Eclampsia A major complication of pregnancy characterized by hypertension, albuminuria, oliguria, tonic and clonic convulsions, and coma.

Ecologic theory A theory of development that emphasizes the presence of mutual interactions between the individual and all of life's settings.

Ecomap Visual representation of how the family unit interacts with the external community environment, including schools, religious institutions, occupational duties, and recreational pursuits.

Ectopic beats Impulses originating outside normal conduction pathways of the heart that interrupt the normal conduction sequence and may not initiate a normal muscle contraction.

Edema Swelling caused by excess fluid trapped in body tissue.

Effacement The drawing up of the internal os and the cervical canal into the uterine side walls.

Effectiveness In healthcare, effectiveness is providing services based on scientific knowledge to all who could benefit and refraining from providing services to those not likely to benefit.

Efficiency In healthcare, efficiency is avoiding waste of equipment, supplies, ideas, and energy.

Ego defense mechanisms Unconscious psychologic processes developed for the purpose of defending the personality. Also called *defense mechanisms*.

Egocentrism Ability to see things only from one's own point of view.

Ego-syntonic The perception that one's behaviors and beliefs are normal and any difficulties with other people are external to oneself.

E-health Electronic information that can be retrieved and transferred online or through a mobile device to improve a person's health or healthcare.

Ejection fraction The fraction or percentage of the diastolic volume that is ejected from the heart during systole.

Elasticity of the arterial wall An indicator of the health of an artery. A healthy, normal artery feels straight, smooth, soft, and pliable. Older adults often have inelastic arteries that feel twisted (tortuous) and irregular upon palpation.

Elder abuse The intentional physical, emotional, or sexual mistreatment or neglect of an individual 65 years of age or older.

Elderspeak A speech style similar to baby talk that communicates a message of dependence and incompetence to older adults.

Elective surgery Performed when surgical intervention is the preferred treatment for a condition that is not imminently life threatening (but may ultimately threaten life or well-being) or to improve the patient's life.

Electrocardiogram (ECG) A graphic record of the heart's activity.

Electrocardiography A diagnostic test of cardiac function.

Electroconvulsive therapy (ECT) A treatment procedure during which an electric current is passed through the brain. It is useful to patients with severe depression, acute mania, some psychotic conditions, and those who are acutely suicidal.

Electroencephalogram (EEG) Measures and records the brain's electrical activity.

Electrolyte A charged ion capable of conducting electricity.

Electromyogram A diagnostic technique that measures the electrical activity of the muscles at rest and during contraction.

Electronic communication Transmitting information though email, social networking, text messaging, and other electronic means.

Electronic fetal monitoring (EFM) The measurement and tracing of the fetal heart rate (FHR), which allows many characteristics of the FHR to be visually assessed.

Electronic health record (EHR) A health record system that is designed so that multiple clinicians from multiple disciplines (e.g., family practice, nursing, pharmacy, specialists) can all have simultaneous access to the patient's health information.

Electronic medical record (EMR) A system focused on diagnosis and treatment. EMRs track information over time (weight, blood pressure, cholesterol readings) and identify when patients are due for routine preventive health maintenance such as vaccines and mammograms.

Elimination The secretion and excretion of body wastes from the kidneys and intestines.

Embolus A particle or aggregate of blood, fat, or pathogens or a bubble of air that obstructs a blood vessel.

Embryo The early stage of development of the young of any organism. In humans the embryonic period is from about 2 to 8 weeks' gestation and is characterized by cellular differentiation and predominantly hyperplastic growth.

Embryonic membranes The amnion and chorion.

Emergency A sudden, often unforeseen event that threatens health or safety.

Emergency preparedness The act of making plans to prevent, respond to, and recover from emergencies.

Emergency response The implementation of emergency preparedness plans.

Emergency surgery Surgery that is performed immediately to preserve function or the life of the patient.

Emesis The act of vomiting; occurs when inspiratory muscles of the thorax (including the diaphragm) and abdomen contract, increasing intrathoracic and intra-abdominal pressures.

Emigration The movement of leukocytes through the blood vessel wall into affected tissue spaces in response to illness or injury.

Emotion-focused coping The regulation of emotional responses to distress when the stressor is perceived to be beyond the individual's control.

Emotional availability The quality of parent–child interactions, including parental sensitivity, structuring, and degree of intrusiveness and hostility.

Emotions Feeling responses to a wide variety of emotional stimuli.

Emphysema A progressive pulmonary disease characterized by destruction of the walls of the alveoli, with resulting enlargement of abnormal air spaces.

Empirical knowing The twofold understanding of facts and observations relevant to nursing, and of the analyses and theories that attempt to explain them. Also called the *science of nursing*.

Empyema Accumulation of purulent (infected) exudate in a space, for example, the pleural cavity or the gallbladder.

Enabling behavior Any action by an individual that consciously or unconsciously facilitates substance dependence.

Enamel A hard substance that encapsulates the crown, the uppermost part of the tooth.

Encapsulated Enclosed.

Encoding The selection of specific signs or symbols to transmit a message, such as which language and words to use, how to arrange the words, and what tone of voice and gestures to use.

Encopresis Abnormal elimination pattern characterized by recurrent soiling or passage of stool at inappropriate times.

Enculturation The process by which children learn culture from adults. Also called *cultural transmission*.

End-of-dose medication failure Pain experienced at the end of one dose of medication before the next dose is scheduled.

End of life The final weeks of life when death is imminent.

End-of-life care The nursing care provided to a patient who is dying or who is near death.

End-stage renal disease (ESRD) The final stage of chronic kidney disease, when the kidneys are unable to excrete metabolic wastes and regulate fluid and electrolyte balance adequately.

Endocardial cushion defect A combination of defects in the atrial and ventricular septa and portions of the tricuspid and mitral valves. A complete AV canal defect allows blood to travel freely among all four chambers of the heart. Also called *atrioventricular (AV) canal defect*.

Endocardial cushions Fetal growth centers for mitral and tricuspid valves and AV septum.

Endogenous Developing from within.

Endogenous insulin Insulin that is produced by an individual's own body.

Endogenous pyrogens Interleukins, interferons, and tumor necrosis factor released by macrophages in response to an infection.

Endometriosis A condition that occurs when endometrial tissue implants on organs outside the uterus, causing pain, fibrosis, and adhesions.

Endometrium The innermost mucosal layer of the uterus.

Endotoxins Found in the cell wall of gram-negative bacteria, endotoxins are released only when the cell is disrupted. They act as activators of many human regulatory systems, producing fever, inflammation, and potentially clotting, bleeding, or hypotension when released in large quantities.

Engagement The passing of the fetus into the pelvic inlet in preparation for birth.

Engrossment The characteristic sense of absorption, preoccupation, and interest in an infant demonstrated by fathers during early contact.

Enophthalmos Sunken appearance of the eyes.

Enteral nutrition Tube feeding used to meet calorie and protein requirements in patients who are unable to consume enough food on their own.

Entropion Inversion of the eyelid.

Enuresis Involuntary passing of urine in children after bladder control is achieved.

Environmental health hazards Factors that impede individual and community health and include natural or human-made substances, states, or events which affect the natural environment, produce negative effects on the human ecosphere, and adversely affect health.

Environmental quality One of the 12 leading health indicators identified by *Healthy People 2020*, environmental quality refers to the ability of the environment to promote and sustain individual and community health.

Enzymes Chemicals that induce a chemical reaction in order to assist in the breakdown of nutrients.

Eosinophil A type of leukocyte found in large numbers in the respiratory and gastrointestinal tracts. Eosinophils are thought to be responsible for protecting the body from parasitic worms. They also play a role in the hypersensitivity response by inactivating some of the inflammatory chemicals released during the inflammatory response.

Epidemic Widespread outbreak of infectious disease with many infected people.

Epidermis The surface or outermost part of the skin consisting of four to five layers of epithelial cells.

Epigenetic External influences or effects on gene expression.

Epilepsy A chronic disorder characterized by recurrent, unprovoked seizures secondary to a central nervous system disorder.

Epiphyseal plate Cartilage between the epiphysis and diaphysis found in the long bones of children.

Episiotomy A surgical incision of the perineal body to enlarge the outlet.

Epispadias Congenital abnormality in which the meatus is located on the upper side of the glans.

Epstein's pearls Small, glistening, white specks that feel hard to the touch on the hard palate and gum margins.

Erb-Duchenne paralysis Damage affecting the upper arm between the fifth and sixth cervical nerves, causing paralysis. Also called *Erb palsy*.

Erectile disorder Term used to describe **erectile dysfunction** when the cause of the disorder is unrelated to physical causes (for example, it results as a side effect of a substance or medication).

Erectile dysfunction (ED) The inability of a man to attain and maintain an erection sufficient to permit satisfactory sexual intercourse.

Ergonomics The science of fitting workplace conditions and job demands to the capabilities of the working population.

Erik Erikson A German-born psychologist and psychoanalyst who created a theory of development comprising eight stages or age-related tasks faced by an individual throughout the lifespan.

Erythema A reddening of the skin.

Erythema toxicum An eruption of lesions in the area surrounding a hair follicle that are firm, vary in size from 1 to 3 mm, and consist of a white or pale yellow papule or pustule with an erythematous base. Also called *newborn rash* or *flea bite dermatitis*.

Eschar Hard, leathery crust that covers a burn wound and harbors necrotic tissue.

Escharotomy Surgical removal of eschar from the torso or extremity to prevent circumferential constriction.

Essential nutrients The macro- and micronutrients needed for the body's survival.

Essential tremors Tremors that are not associated with another condition and may be genetic in origin.

Estimated date of birth (EDB) The approximated date of childbirth. Also called estimated date of delivery.

Estrogen The primary hormone responsible for female sex characteristics.

Ethical knowing Understanding and applying the ethical codes by which nurses are expected to abide, as well as upholding the various philosophical, cultural, and moral frameworks of the institution and of the patient. Also called the *moral component*.

Ethics The rules or principles that govern right or moral conduct.

Ethnic group Group of individuals who have common racial characteristics and share a cultural heritage.

Etiology A causal relationship between a problem and its related or risk factors.

Eupnea Breathing within the expected respiratory rates.

Eustachian tube Connects the middle ear with the nasopharynx to help equalize the pressure in the middle ear with the atmospheric pressure.

Eustress Good stress that is associated with accomplishment and victory.

Euthanasia From the Greek for *painless*, *easy*, *gentle*, or *good death*, now commonly used to signify a killing prompted by a humanitarian motive.

Euthymia Stable or normal mood.

Euthyroid A normal thyroid state.

Evaluation Reassessment of a patient following nursing or medical intervention or therapy.

Evaluation statement A written comment on the care plan or in the nurse's notes about progress following an evaluation. An evaluation statement must contain the date and time evaluation was done; a conclusion statement determining goal met, partially met, or not met; and a supporting statement giving the results of how the patient did or did not achieve the goal.

Evaporation The process of converting water to a vapor.

Evidence Clinical knowledge, expert opinion, or information resulting from research.

Evidence-based nursing An integration of the best evidence available, nursing expertise, and the values and preferences of the individuals, families, and communities who are served.

Evidence-based practice The application of research in areas that are of interest to nursing and in the actual practice of nursing.

Evisceration Protrusion of internal viscera through a surgical wound.

Exacerbation A reappearance of symptoms of a chronic illness. Also called a *flare*.

Excess More than is needed in order for the body to survive and remain productive.

Excitement phase This second phase of the sexual response cycle is marked by an increase in blood flow to various body parts, resulting in erection of the penis and clitoris and swelling of the labia, testes, and breasts.

Excoriation Area of loss of the superficial layers of the skin. Also called *denuded area*.

Executive function The mental skills involved in planning and executing complex tasks.

Exercise Physical activity that is planned, structured, and involves repetitive body movements; the goal is to improve or maintain one or more components of physical fitness.

Exercise addiction Excessive pattern of exercising regardless of physical injury, personal inconvenience, or disruption to other areas of life, including marital strain, interference with work, and lack of time for other activities.

Exercise intolerance Decreased ability to participate in activities using large skeletal muscles because of fatigue or dyspnea.

Exogenous Developing from outside sources.

Exogenous insulin Insulin from a source outside the body.

Exophthalmos Protruding eyes.

Exotoxins Soluble proteins that microorganisms secrete into surrounding tissue. Exotoxins are highly poisonous, causing cell death or dysfunction.

Expectorate To expel or spit out.

Expiration The act of exhaling air in respiration.

Expressed consent An oral or written agreement.

Expressive jargon Using unintelligible words with normal speech intonations as if truly communicating in words.

Expressive speech The ability to speak and be understood by others.

Extended family The relatives of nuclear families, such as grandparents, aunts, and uncles.

Extended kin network family A form of extended family in which two nuclear families of primary or unmarried kin live in proximity to each other and share a social support network, goods, and services.

External patients The individuals who seek healthcare as well as their family members and significant others; and other individuals and entities with whom internal patients interact, such as insurance companies, managed care organizations, equipment or material suppliers, social service agencies, and law enforcement officials.

External environmental stressors Triggers outside of an individual that demand change or disrupt homeostasis.

External locus of control The belief that an individual's health is controlled by forces outside of his or her control such as chance or fate.

Extracapsular extraction A surgical treatment for cataracts in which the anterior capsule, nucleus, and cortex of the lens are removed, leaving the posterior capsule intact.

Extracapsular hip fracture A hip fracture involving the trochanteric region between the neck and diaphysis of the femur.

Extracellular fluid (ECF) Fluid found outside the cells. It accounts for about one third of total body fluid and is subdivided into compartments. The two main compartments of ECF are intravascular and interstitial.

Extracorporeal shock wave lithotripsy (ESWL) A noninvasive technique for fragmenting kidney stones using shock waves generated outside the body.

Extrapulmonary tuberculosis Results when tuberculosis spreads through the blood and lymph system to other organs.

Extrapyramidal side effects (EPS) A particularly serious set of adverse reactions to antipsychotic drugs. EPS includes acute dystonia, akathisia, parkinsonism, and tardive dyskinesia.

Extubation The process of withdrawing a breathing tube on completion of anesthesia and the surgical case.

Exudate Material, such as fluid and cells, that has escaped from blood vessels during the inflammatory process and is deposited in tissue or on tissue surfaces.

Exudative macular degeneration A form of macular degeneration characterized by the formation of new, weak blood vessels in the potential space between the choroid and the retina. Also referred to as the wet form of macular degeneration.

Eye movement desensitization and reprocessing (EMDR) A form of psychotherapy that contains elements of a number of types of therapy, including cognitive–behavioral therapy and body-centered therapy.

Failure to thrive (FTT) 1. Inability to meet or maintain developmental milestones related to physical growth due to undernutrition. 2. A syndrome in which an infant falls below the fifth percentile for weight and height on a standard growth chart or is falling in percentiles on a growth chart.

Faith To believe in or be committed to something or someone.

Fallopian tubes Tubes that extend from the lateral angle of the uterus and terminate near the ovary. Also called *oviducts* and *uterine tubes*.

False imprisonment The unjustifiable detention of an individual without legal warrant to confine the person.

False pelvis The portion of the pelvis above the linea terminalis that supports the enlarged pregnant uterus.

Familial AD (FAD) One of the two basic types of Alzheimer disease, it has a strong inherited component and usually manifests before the age of 65. Also called *early-onset Alzheimer disease*.

Family Individuals who are joined together by marriage, blood, adoption, or residence in the same household.

Family burden The overall level of distress experienced by a family as a result of a family member's illness.

Family-centered care A model of healthcare service that is provided in partnership with the patient and family.

Family-centered nursing Nursing that considers the health of the family as a unit in addition to the health of individual family members.

Family cohesion The emotional bonding between family members.

Family communication Includes listening, speaking, self-disclosure, and tracking abilities of the family as a group.

Family coping mechanisms The behaviors families use to deal with stress or changes imposed from either within or without the family.

Family development The dynamics or changes a family experiences over time, including changes in relationships, communication patterns, roles, and interactions.

Family flexibility The amount of change in a family's leadership, role relationships, relationship rules, and ability to respond to stress.

Family recovery Family response to a member's mental illness.

Family support Support from family members as they care for other family members; for example, one sister relieves another to care for their aging mother over the weekend.

Family therapy A form of therapy in which the family system is treated as a unit and the focus is on family dynamics.

Fascial excision Excising a wound to the level of fascia. Also called *fasciectomy*.

Fasciculation An irregular movement or a twitch.

Fasciectomy Excising a wound to the level of fascia. Also called *fascial excision*.

Fat embolism syndrome (FES) Occurs when fat globules lodge in the pulmonary vascular bed or peripheral circulation.

Fatigue A condition characterized by a lack of energy and motivation that may or may not be accompanied by drowsiness.

Fear A sense of apprehension triggered by a perceived threat to safety or well-being, including a painful stimuli or dangerous event.

Febrile Having a fever.

Febrile seizures Generalized seizures that usually occur in children as the result of rapid temperature rise above 39°C (102°F), usually in association with an acute illness. No evidence of intracranial infection or other defined cause is found in relation.

Fecal impaction A mass or collection of hardened feces in the folds of the rectum.

Fecal incontinence The loss of voluntary ability to control fecal and gaseous discharges through the anal sphincter. Also called *bowel incontinence*.

Fecalith A hard mass of feces.

Feces Body wastes and undigested food eliminated from the bowel. Also called *stool*.

Feedback 1. The mechanisms by which some of the output of a system is returned to the system as input. 2. The response a receiver of a message gives to the message's sender.

Female orgasmic disorder The persistent delay or absence of orgasm following a phase of normal sexual excitement.

Female reproductive cycle (FRC) The monthly rhythmic changes in sexually mature women; composed of the ovarian cycle, during which ovulation occurs, and the uterine cycle, during which menstruation occurs.

Female sexual interest/arousal disorder Persistent decreased or absent sexual thoughts, interest in sexual activity, mental or physical feelings of arousal, and/or pleasurable sensation during sexual activity.

Fertility awareness-based methods Contraception based on an understanding of the changes that occur throughout a woman's ovulatory cycle. Also called *natural family planning*.

Fertilization The process by which a sperm fuses with an ovum to form a new diploid cell, or zygote.

Festination Rapid, small steps, as if an individual is trying to run.

Fetal alcohol spectrum disorder See Fetal alcohol syndrome (FAS).

Fetal alcohol syndrome (FAS) A developmental disorder that occurs when a developing fetus is exposed to ethyl alcohol. Fetal alcohol syndrome is associated with physical, intellectual, behavioral, and/or learning disabilities. Also called *fetal alcohol spectrum disorder*.

Fetal attitude The flexion or extension of the fetal body and extremities.

Fetal bradycardia A fetal heart rate of less than 110 bpm during a 10-minute period or longer.

Fetal demise Death of a fetus that occurs after 20 weeks' gestation. Also called a *stillbirth* or *intrauterine fetal death (IUFD)*.

Fetal heart rate (FHR) The number of times the fetal heart beats per minute; normal range is 120–160.

Fetal lie The relationship of the cephalocaudal axis, or spinal column, of the fetus to the cephalocaudal axis, or spinal column, of the woman. The fetus may be in a longitudinal or transverse lie.

Fetal movement record A noninvasive technique that enables the pregnant woman to monitor and record movements easily and without expense.

Fetal position The relationship of the landmark on the presenting fetal part to the front, sides, or back of the maternal pelvis.

Fetal presentation The body part of the fetus entering the pelvis in a single or multiple pregnancy.

Fetal tachycardia A fetal heart rate of 161 bpm or more during a 10-minute period of continuous monitoring.

Fetoscope An adaptation of a stethoscope that facilitates auscultation of the fetal heart rate.

Fetoscopy A technique for directly observing the fetus and obtaining a sample of fetal blood or skin.

Fetus The child in utero from about the seventh to ninth week of gestation until birth.

Fever A protective immune response to foreign antigens within the body that increases the cellular metabolic rate, thus increasing the body's temperature.

Fever of unknown origin A temperature above 100.9°F (38.3°C) that occurs on several occasions within a short time span, lasts for more than 3 weeks, and does not have a definitive cause after 1 week of clinical investigation.

Fever phobia Fear felt by caregivers about the harmful effects of a fever on a child, such as seizure, brain damage, and death.

Fever spike A temperature that rises to fever level rapidly, following a normal temperature, and then returns to normal within a few hours.

Fiber A polysaccharide that contributes to disease prevention, especially in the gastrointestinal tract and the cardiovascular system.

Fibrin Connective tissue.

Fibrin degradation products Potent anticoagulants.

Fibromyalgia A chronic disorder characterized by widespread musculoskeletal pain, fatigue, and multiple tender points.

Fidelity A moral principle that obligates an individual to be faithful to agreements and responsibilities one has undertaken.

Filtration A process whereby fluid and solutes move together across a membrane from a compartment with higher pressure to a compartment with lower pressure.

Filtration pressure The pressure in the compartment that results in the movement of the fluid and substances dissolved in fluid out of the compartment.

Fimbria A funnel-like enlargement of the fallopian tube with many fingerlike projections (fimbriae) reaching out to the ovary.

First heart sound (S_1) The heart sound produced by the closure of the AV valve; characterized by the syllable "lub."

Five P's neurovascular assessment An assessment checklist for pain, pulse, pallor, paralysis/paresis, and paresthesia.

Fixation The immobilization or inability of an individual to proceed to the next developmental stage because of anxiety.

Flaccidity Absence of muscle tone. Also called *hypotonia*.

Flashbacks The recurrence of images, sounds, smells, or feelings from a traumatic event; often triggered by daily events, such as a car backfiring on the street or the smell of a perpetrator's cologne.

Flat affect Minimal facial expression and movement, sometimes monotone speech patterns.

Flatness An extremely dull sound produced by very dense tissue, such as muscle or bone.

Flatulence The presence of excessive amounts of gas in the stomach or intestines.

Flatus Gas or air normally present in the stomach or intestines.

Flight of ideas Rapidly changing, fragmentary thoughts.

Flow sheet A specific assessment criteria in a particular format, such as human needs or functional health patterns.

Fluid resuscitation The administration of intravenous (IV) fluids to restore circulating blood volume during an acute period of increasing capillary permeability.

Fluid volume deficit (FVD) Substantial loss of both water and electrolytes in similar proportions from the extracellular fluid. Also called *hypovolemia*.

Fluid volume excess (FVE) Excessive fluid retained by the body. The retention of both water and sodium in similar proportions to normal extracellular fluid (ECF). Also called *hypervolemia*.

Fluoroscope A scope used to project visual examination images on a fluorescent screen.

Focal seizures Seizures that are caused by abnormal electrical activity in one hemisphere or in a specific area of the cerebral cortex, most often the temporal, frontal, or parietal lobes. The seizure may spread regionally, and the symptoms are related to the region of the cortex that is affected. Also known as *partial seizures*.

Focus charting Date and time, focus, and progress notes are recorded for a specific condition, nursing diagnosis, and behavior to make the patient and the patient's concerns and strengths the focus of care.

Folic acid A vitamin that is required for normal growth, reproduction, and lactation and that prevents the macrocytic, megaloblastic anemia of pregnancy.

Follicle-stimulating hormone (FSH) Hormone produced by the anterior pituitary during the first half of the menstrual cycle, stimulating development of the graafian follicle.

Fontanels The intersections of membranous spaces between the cranial bones of a fetus.

Food choice An individual's decision of what and how much to eat of a specific food. This decision can be influenced by a number of conscious and unconscious factors such as taste, preparation, smell, habits, convenience, availability, and cost.

Food insecurity Results when one or more members of a household must reduce their eating patterns due to a lack of money or lack of resources to access appropriate amounts and varieties of food.

Food security Results when all members of a household have sufficient resources to access appropriate amounts and varieties of food.

Foramen ovale An opening between the atria of the fetal heart.

Foraminotomy An enlargement of the opening between the disc and the facet joint to remove bony overgrowth.

Forced expiratory volume in 1 second (FEV$_1$) The amount of air that can be exhaled in 1 second as measured by a spirometer.

Forceps-assisted birth The use of forceps to assist the birth of a fetus by providing traction or by providing the means to rotate the fetal head to an occiput-anterior position. Also called an *instrumental delivery*, *operative delivery*, or *operative vaginal delivery*.

Forceps marks Reddened areas over the cheeks and jaws on an infant caused by a difficult forceps birth.

Foreground question Questions that are narrow in focus about a specific clinical issue.

Foreseeability The ability to foresee events that reasonably may be expected to cause specific results.

Formal group A group with formalized goals, designated management, and only partly voluntary membership.

Formal leader A leader who is selected by an organization and given official authority to make decisions and act.

Formation The process that facilitates the transformation of an individual from a layperson to a professional nurse.

Foster family A family consisting of one or more adults caring for one or more children from other families when the children can no longer live with their birth parents.

Fourth heart sound (S$_4$) A heart sound produced by atrial contraction and ejection of blood into the ventricle during late diastole. Also called *atrial gallop*.

Fracture A break in the continuity of a bone.

Fragile X syndrome A developmental disorder caused by a single recessive gene abnormality on the X chromosome. Fragile X syndrome is associated most notably with intellectual disability, often accompanied by ADHD and other behavioral problems.

Frank–Starling mechanism An increase in venous return increases ventricular filling and myocardial stretch, which increases the force of contraction.

Free-floating anxiety Excessive worry about everyday events; worry that is hard to control and the focus of which may shift from moment to moment.

Freezing A condition in which an individual feels like his or her feet are stuck to the floor.

Frequency The time between the beginning of one contraction and the beginning of the next contraction.

Friend support Support or assistance from nonfamily members, such as friends or coworkers, for a family during a time of illness or stress.

Frostbite An injury of the skin resulting from freezing.

Frustration An emotion that occurs when an individual is prevented from reaching a desired goal. Intense frustration may trigger violent aggressive tendencies resulting in assault or homicide.

Fulguration A procedure that destroys tissue with electrical current.

Full-thickness burn A burn that involves all layers of the skin, including the epidermis, the dermis, and the epidermal appendages.

Fulminant colitis An acute form of ulcerative colitis that involves the entire colon; manifestations include severe bloody diarrhea, acute abdominal pain, and fever.

Functional assessments Typically a combination of assessments that includes observations of child behavior, responses, and abilities. It is used to assess how a child functions on a daily basis in his or her environment and to determine if the child has any developmental delays or special needs.

Functional method A method of coordinating care that focuses on the jobs to be completed as part of patient care (e.g., bed making and temperature measurement). In this task-oriented approach, personnel with less educational preparation than the professional nurse (e.g., unlicensed assistive personnel) perform aspects of care with less complex requirements.

Functional nursing A task-oriented approach to care delivery used in situations of inadequate staffing or nursing shortages.

Functional strength The body's ability to perform work.

Fundus The rounded, uppermost portion of the uterus.

Fungi A type of microorganism capable of producing infection. Yeasts and molds are common types of fungi.

Galanin A neuropeptide that is released by neurons as they are injured or die. Often associated with Alzheimer disease, although the exact role galanin plays in the disease is unknown.

Gallstone ileus A large gallstone.

Gambling disorder An **addiction** to gambling characterized by gambling despite the risk of losing something of value (e.g., a home) and an inability to stop gambling.

Gamete Female or male germ cell; contains a haploid number of chromosomes.

Gametogenesis The process by which germ cells are produced.

Gastric lavage Irrigation of the stomach with large quantities of normal saline.

Gastric outlet obstruction Obstruction of the pyloric region of the stomach and duodenum that impairs gastric outflow; a potential complication of peptic ulcer disease.

Gastric ulcer A peptic ulcer that occurs in the stomach.

Gastrocolic reflex The increased peristalsis of the colon after food has entered the stomach.

Gastroesophageal reflux disease (GERD) A disease in which stomach contents flow back up into the esophagus.

Gate control theory Melzack and Wall's 1965 theory stating that the perception of pain is controlled by the overall activity of small-diameter (pain) fibers vs. large-diameter (heat, cold, mechanical) fibers.

Gender identity One's self-image as a female or male.

Gender-role behavior The outward expression of an individual's sense of maleness or femaleness as well as the expression of what is perceived as gender-appropriate behavior.

General adaptation syndrome (GAS) A three-stage chain of events in an individual's stress response.

Generalized anxiety disorder (GAD) A condition that occurs when an individual experiences intense tension and worry, even if no external stressors are present.

Generalized seizures The result of diffuse electrical activity that often begins in both hemispheres of the brain simultaneously, then spreads throughout the cortex into the brainstem. As a result, movements and spasms displayed by the patient are bilateral and symmetric.

Generational cohort Individuals born in the same general time span who share key life experiences, including historical events, public heroes, pastimes, and early work experiences.

Genital herpes A sexually transmitted infection caused by the herpes simplex virus.

Genital intercourse Penetration of the vagina by the penis. Also called *coitus*.

Genital warts A sexually transmitted infection caused by the human papillomavirus (HPV).

Genito-pelvic pain/penetration disorder Persistent or recurrent dyspareunia (pain) or fear of pain before or during vaginal penetration.

Genogram Visual representation of gender showing lines of birth descent through the generations.

Genotype The pattern of genes on chromosomes.

Geographic information system (GIS) A system that relies on satellite imaging and global positioning systems to capture, manage, and analyze geographical data.

Geragogy The process of stimulating and helping older adults to learn.

Geriatric failure to thrive (GFTT) A condition in which older patients experience a multidimensional decline in physical functioning that is characterized by weight loss of more than 5% of baseline body weight, decreased appetite, undernutrition, dehydration, depression, and cognitive and immune impairment.

Gestation Period of intrauterine development from conception through birth; pregnancy.

Gestational age assessment tools Methods to determine an infant's age at birth assessing external physical characteristics and neurologic or neuromuscular development.

Gestational diabetes mellitus (GDM) A carbohydrate intolerance of variable severity with onset or first recognition during pregnancy.

Gingiva The gum.

Gingivitis Red, swollen gingiva.

Glaucoma A condition characterized by optic neuropathy with gradual loss of peripheral vision and, usually, increased intraocular pressure of the eye.

Global evaluative dimension of the self The degree to which an individual likes him- or herself overall, as a whole being. Also called *global self-esteem*.

Global self The collective beliefs and images an individual holds about him- or herself.

Global self-esteem See Global evaluative dimension of the self.

Glomerular filtration rate (GFR) The rate at which fluid is filtered through the kidneys.

Glomerulonephritis Inflammation of the glomerular capillary membrane.

Glomerulus Found in the nephrons of the kidneys, a tuft of capillaries surrounded by the Bowman capsule.

Glucagon Produced by alpha cells, glucagon is a hormone that decreases glucose oxidation and promotes an increase in the blood glucose level by signaling the liver to release glucose from glycogen stores. In addition to stimulating the breakdown of glycogen in the liver, glucagon stimulates the formation of carbohydrates in the liver and the breakdown of lipids in both the liver and adipose tissue.

Gluconeogenesis The formation of glucose from fats and proteins.

Glucosuria The excretion of glucose in the urine.

Glycogenolysis The breakdown of liver glycogen.

Glycosuria The excretion of carbohydrates into the urine.

Goiter An enlarged thyroid gland

Gonadotropin-releasing hormone (GnRH) A hormone secreted by the hypothalamus that stimulates the anterior pituitary to secrete follicle-stimulating hormone and luteinizing hormone.

Gonorrhea A sexually transmitted infection caused by *Neisseria gonorrhoeae*.

Good-faith immunity Law or laws that protect healthcare workers from civil or criminal liabilities when they report suspected child abuse in good faith, even if the subsequent investigation does not make a determination of abuse.

Good Samaritan laws Specific laws designed to protect healthcare workers from potential liability when volunteering their skills outside of an employment contract.

Goodpasture syndrome A rare autoimmune disorder of unknown etiology that is characterized by formation of antibodies to the glomerular basement membrane.

Governance The establishment and maintenance of social, political, and economic arrangements by which professionals control their practice, their self-discipline, their working conditions, and their professional affairs.

Graafian follicle The ovarian cyst containing the ripe ovum, which secretes estrogens.

Grading A standardized method of judging a tumor's aggressiveness based on the level of differentiation and mitotic rate; where the least malignant cells are classified grade 1 and the most aggressive malignant cells are classified grade 4.

Graft-versus-host disease (GVHD) A series of immunologic reactions in response to transplanted cells.

Gram stain A diagnostic test conducted to identify infecting organisms in urine by shape and characteristic.

Granulation tissue Young connective tissue with new capillaries formed in the healing process.

Grasping reflex The closing and grasping of an infant's fingers in response to a finger placed in the palm of the infant's hand.

Graves disease An autoimmune disorder marked by an enlarged thyroid and signs of hyperthyroidism.

Grief The total psychologic, biological, and behavioral response to the emotional experience related to loss.

Group Three or more individuals who have a common purpose, interact with each other, influence each other, and are interdependent.

Group therapy A form of therapy that allows group members to help each other with psychologic, cognitive, behavioral, and spiritual dysfunctions through a process of change, aided by a professional group therapist.

Groupthink A type of decision making characterized by a group's failure to critically examine their own processes and practices or to recognize and respond to change.

Growth Physical change and increase in size.

Guillain-Barré syndrome (GBS) An acute inflammatory demyelinating disorder of the peripheral nervous system characterized by an acute onset of motor paralysis (usually ascending).

Gustatory Of or relating to taste.

Gynecomastia Abnormal enlargement of the breast(s) in men.

H₁ receptors Cellular histamine receptors that are present in the smooth muscle of the vascular system, the bronchial tree, and the digestive tract. Stimulation of these receptors results in itching, pain, edema, bronchoconstriction, and other characteristic symptoms of inflammation and allergy.

H1N1 influenza A form of the influenza virus that consists of avian genes, human genes, and genes from flu viruses typically found in pigs from Asia and Europe. Once mistakenly called *swine flu*, it can be spread through human-to-human transmission.

H₂ receptors Cellular histamine receptors present primarily in the stomach; their stimulation results in the secretion of large amounts of hydrochloric acid.

Habit training Attempts to keep patients dry by having them void at regular intervals.

Habituation The newborn's ability to process and respond to complex stimulations.

Hallucination The perception of seeing, hearing, or feeling something that is not present in reality.

Hallucinogen A type of drug that induces the same types of thoughts, perceptions, and feelings that occur in dreams. Hallucinogens include PCP, 3,4-MDMA, D-lysergic acid diethylamide (LSD), mescaline, dimethyltryptamine (DMT), and psilocin.

Hand restraints A device used to protect confused patients from scratching or injuring their skin, or dislodging intravenous access devices. Also called *mitt restraints.*

Handoff The transfer of information along with authority and responsibility during transitions in care across the continuum.

Handoff communication A verbal or written exchange of information. It encompasses the nursing team and all other members of the healthcare team who care for a patient at any given time.

Hardware The physical component of technology, including computers, keyboards, and display screens.

Harlequin sign A reddening of the skin on one side of an infant's body while the other side remains pale. Also called *clown color change.*

Hashimoto thyroiditis An autoimmune disorder in which antibodies destroy thyroid tissue.

Hassles Day-to-day tension/stressors.

Health A state of complete physical, mental, and social well-being.

Health beliefs Concepts about health that an individual believes are true, regardless of whether or not they are founded in fact.

Health Insurance Portability and Accountability Act (HIPAA) Legislation enacted by Congress to minimize the exclusion of preexisting conditions as a barrier to healthcare insurance, designate special rights for those who lose other health coverage, and eliminate medical underwriting in group plans. The act includes the Privacy Rule, which creates a national standard for of the disclosure of private health information.

Health Level Seven (HL7) A framework designed for the exchange, integration, sharing, and retrieval of electronic health information that supports clinical practice and the management, delivery, and evaluation of health services.

Health literacy The ability to read, understand, and act on health information, including such tasks as comprehending prescription labels, interpreting appointment slips, completing health insurance forms, and following instructions for diagnostic tests.

Health maintenance organization (HMO) The most restrictive type of private health insurance plan. HMO participants must select a primary care provider who provides basic medical services and, as the gatekeeper to care, refers the patient to in-network hospitals and specialists when additional care is needed.

Health policy The actions and decisions by government bodies and professional organizations that affect whether or not healthcare organizations and individuals working within the healthcare system can achieve their healthcare goals.

Health promotion A way of thinking and acting in order to increase individuals' overall health and well-being regardless of their health and illness status or age.

Health restoration Care focusing on the ill patient that extends from early detection of disease through helping the patient during the recovery period.

Healthcare advance directive Legal document that allows an individual to plan for healthcare and/or financial affairs in the event of incapacity. Also called *advance directive* or *advance healthcare directive.*

Healthcare-associated infection (HAI) Infections associated with the delivery of healthcare services in a facility such as a hospital or nursing home. Also called a *nosocomial infection.*

Healthcare disparity A difference in a measurement of access to or quality of healthcare services between an individual or group possessing a defined characteristic when other variables have been controlled, such as individual health choices, disease courses, and other variations from the normative measure.

Healthcare proxy An individual selected to speak to physicians and other healthcare providers on behalf of a patient to determine the best course of treatment.

Healthcare surrogate An individual selected to make medical decisions when someone is no longer able to make them for him- or herself.

Heart block A block in the normal electrical conduction of the heart.

Heart failure The inability of the heart to pump adequate blood to meet the metabolic demands of the body.

Heart murmur Harsh, blowing sounds caused by disruption of blood flow into the heart, between the chambers of the heart, or from the heart into the pulmonary or aortic systems.

Heartburn A burning sensation in the chest or throat. Also called *pyrosis.*

Heat balance When the amount of heat produced by the body equals the amount of heat lost.

Heat exhaustion Excessive heat exposure and dehydration that causes paleness, dizziness, nausea, vomiting, fainting, and a moderately increased temperature (38.3°–38.9°C [101°–102°F]).

Heat stroke A serious form of heat exhaustion that can be life threatening, generally caused by exercising in hot weather. Patients will have warm, flushed skin, often do not sweat, and have a temperature of 41°C (106°F) or higher. A patient may be also delirious, unconscious, or having seizures.

Heat transfer The four ways heat moves from one place or object to another place or object.

Heaving Lifting of the chest wall during contraction.

Heberden nodes Bony lumps on the end joint of a digit.

Helper T cells Play a vital role in normal immune system function, recognizing foreign antigens and infected cells and activating antibody-producing B cells. They are the primary cells infected by the human immunodeficiency virus.

HELPP syndrome A cluster of changes, including hemolysis, elevated liver enzymes, and low platelet count, sometimes associated with preeclampsia.

Hematochezia Bright blood in the stool.

Hematocrit The proportion of cells and plasma in blood. Also refers to the laboratory test that measures the hematocrit. This test can also be used to detect severe dehydration or overhydration.

Hematogenous spread Describes the spread of infection or disease through the blood.

Hematoma A localized collection of blood underneath the skin that may appear as a bruise.

Hematopoiesis Blood cell formation.

Hematuria The presence of blood in the urine.

Hemianopia The loss of half of the visual field of one or both eyes.

Hemiarthroplasty Hip replacement that involves replacement of the ball, the head, or the femur.

Hemiarthroscopy The surgical replacement of the femoral head with a smooth metal sphere.

Hemiparesis Weakness of the left or right half of the body.

Hemiplegia Paralysis of the left or right half of the body.

Hemispheres The two halves created by the division of the cerebrum by the deep fold.

Hemodialysis A process by which a patient's blood flows through vascular catheters, passes by the dialysate in an external machine, and then returns to the patient.

Hemodynamics The study of forces involved in blood circulation.

Hemoglobin The oxygen-carrying molecule within red blood cells; a laboratory test to measure the amount of hemoglobin.

Hemoglobinopathy A disorder of hemoglobin.

Hemolysis The destruction of red blood cells; releases hemoglobin into the circulation.

Hemolytic anemia A disorder that results from the premature destruction of red blood cells.

Hemoptysis Bloody sputum.

Hemorrhage Rapid or excessive bleeding.

Hemosiderosis The storage of excessive iron in tissues and organs.

Hemostasis The cessation of bleeding.

Hemotympanum Bleeding into or behind the tympanic membrane.

Hepatitis The inflammation of the liver triggered by a virus, alcohol, medications, toxins, autoimmune disorder, or other pathogens.

Here-and-now concept A concept used in group therapy that recognizes that only in the present moment of a group's experience can change be made.

Hernia A protrusion in the intestine through the inguinal wall or canal.

Herniated intervertebral disc A rupture of the cartilage surrounding the intervertebral disc with protrusion of the nucleus pulposus. Also called a *ruptured disc*, *slipped disc*, or *herniated nucleus pulposus*.

Heroin An illicit, central nervous system depressant narcotic that alters perception and produces euphoria.

Heterograft Skin used for transplantation that was obtained from an animal, usually a pig. Also called a *xenograft*.

Heterosexism The view that heterosexuality is the only correct sexual orientation.

Heterosexual An individual who is attracted to members of the opposite sex.

Highly active antiretroviral therapy (HAART) Effective treatment of AIDS that combines at least three medications to inhibit HIV replication.

Hip fracture A fracture of the femur at the head, neck, or trochanteric regions.

Hippocampus A small, curved body in the brain. Part of the limbic system, it plays a major role in memory formation.

Hirsutism An increased growth of coarse hair on the face and trunk.

Histamine A key chemical mediator of inflammation.

Histrionic personality disorder (HPD) One of several personality disorders defined in the DSM-5, it is characterized by a lifelong tendency for dramatic, egocentric, attention-seeking response patterns.

Hoarding compulsion An excessive collection and accumulation of objects, extreme cluttering of the living environment, accompanied by a lack of regard for the embarrassment of family member or others whose living is impacted.

Holistic health A clinical mindset that considers more than the physiologic health status of an individual.

Holosystolic Term used to describe the sounds heard during the entire phase of systole.

Holy day A day set aside for special religious observance.

Homan sign Pain in the calf when the foot is dorsiflexed.

Homeostasis The body's ability to maintain a state of physiologic balance in the presence of constantly changing conditions.

Homicide The killing of one individual by another; for legal purposes, this act is further specified by whether the act was intentional or due to negligence.

Homocysteine An amino acid that is a homologue of cysteine.

Homograft Grafts between members of the same species who have different genotypes and HLA antigens. Usually human skin that has been harvested from cadavers. Also called an *allograft*.

Homologous chromosomes The two paired chromosomes that are inherited, one from each parent.

Homophobia The fear, hatred, or mistrust of gays and lesbians often expressed in overt displays of discrimination.

Homosexual An individual who is attracted to members of the same sex.

Hope To expect or desire with confidence.

Horizontal violence (HV) Aggressive acts committed against a nurse by one or more nursing colleagues.

Hormone replacement therapy (HRT) Administration of hormones, usually estrogen and a progestin, to alleviate the symptoms of menopause.

Hormones Chemical messengers secreted by various glands that exert controlling effects on the cells of the body.

Hospice An organization that provides end-of-life care for patients either in their homes or in a hospital setting.

Hospice care The support and care for persons in the last phase of an incurable disease so that they may live as fully and comfortably as possible until their death.

Hot zone When a disaster occurs, the hot zone is the most dangerous zone because it is located immediately adjacent to the site of the disaster. All responders who enter the area must be protected by personal protective equipment.

Human chorionic gonadotropin (HCG) A hormone produced by the chorionic villi that is found in the urine of pregnant women. Also called *prolan*.

Human dignity The inherent worth and uniqueness of individuals and populations.

Human immunodeficiency virus (HIV) A primary immunodeficiency disorder that is spread primarily through sexual contact with an infected person. HIV is the virus that causes acquired immunodeficiency syndrome (AIDS).

Human leukocyte antigen (HLA) The major histocompatibility complex gene.

Humanistic learning theory A learning theory that focuses on the unique cognitive and affective qualities of a learner.

Humoral immune response Hyperreactive response of B cells characteristic of systemic lupus erythematosus (SLE).

Hunger The feeling that makes individuals think of food and encourages them to satisfy this feeling by eating.

Hyaluronic acid (HA) A lubricating substance in cartilage and joint synovial fluid.

Hydrocephalus A condition characterized by enlargement of the head caused by inadequate drainage of cerebrospinal fluid.

Hydronephrosis An accumulation of urine in the renal pelvis as a result of obstructed outflow.

Hydrostatic pressure The pressure a fluid exerts within a closed system on the walls of its container. The hydrostatic pressure of blood is the force blood exerts against the vascular walls (e.g., the artery walls). The principle involved in hydrostatic pressure is that fluids move from an area of greater pressure to an area of lesser pressure.

Hydroureter Distention of the ureter with urine.

Hyperalgesia Increased response to a pain stimulus because of peripheral sensitization.

Hypercalcemia Elevated blood levels of calcium.

Hypercapnia A condition marked by a PaCO$_2$ level above 45 mmHg. Also known as **hypercarbia**.

Hypercarbia See Hypercapnia.

Hyperchloremia Elevated chloride levels in the blood.

Hypercyanotic episode A potentially life-threatening episode of hypoxia. Also called a *tet episode*.

Hyperemia Increased blood flow to an area.

Hyperextension Forcible backward bending.

Hyperflexion Forcible forward bending.

Hyperglycemia Elevated glucose levels.

Hyperkalemia Elevated potassium levels in the blood.

Hypermagnesemia Elevated magnesium levels in the blood.

Hypernatremia Elevated sodium levels in the blood.

Hyperopia Farsightedness.

Hyperosmolar hyperglycemic state (HHS) A disorder characterized by a plasma osmolarity of 340 mOsm/L or greater, greatly elevated blood glucose levels, and altered levels of consciousness. It occurs in individuals who have type 2 diabetes mellitus.

Hyperphosphatemia Increased blood levels of phosphate.

Hyperplasia An increase in the number or density of normal cells.

Hyperresonance An abnormal, booming sound that can be heard over an emphysematous lung.

Hyperresponsiveness An exaggerated response, as with bronchoconstriction in asthma.

Hypersensitivity An overreaction of the immune system to an antigen or antigens.

Hypersomnia The inability to stay awake during the day, despite obtaining sufficient sleep at night.

Hypertension Excess pressure in the arterial portion of the circulatory system, specifically a systolic blood pressure of 140 mmHg or higher or a diastolic blood pressure of 90 mmHg or higher.

Hypertensive crisis A systolic blood pressure greater than 180 mmHg and diastolic blood pressure higher than 120 mmHg. Also called *malignant hypertension*.

Hypertensive encephalopathy A syndrome characterized by extremely high blood pressure, altered level of consciousness, increased intracranial pressure, papilledema, and seizures.

Hyperthermia A condition that occurs when a body produces more heat than is lost.

Hyperthermia blanket An electronically controlled blanket that provides a specified temperature

Hyperthermic A body temperature above 37.8°C (100°F).

Hyperthyroidism A disorder caused by excessive delivery of thyroid hormone to the peripheral tissues. Also called *thyrotoxicosis*.

Hypertonic Refers to solutions that have a higher osmolality than body fluids; 3% sodium chloride is a hypertonic solution.

Hypertonic dehydration Occurs when sodium loss is proportionately less than water loss. Also called *hypernatremic dehydration*.

Hypertrophic cardiomyopathy A disorder characterized by decreased compliance of the left ventricle and hypertrophy of the ventricular muscle mass.

Hypertrophic scar An overgrowth of dermal tissue that remains within the boundaries of the wound.

Hypertrophy An enlargement of glandular cells or muscles.

Hyperventilation Unusually fast respirations, or overbreathing causing an imbalance of oxygen and carbon dioxide.

Hypervolemia The excessive retention of both water and sodium in similar proportions to normal extracellular fluid (ECF). Also called *fluid volume excess*.

Hyphema Bleeding into the anterior chamber of the eye.

Hypoactive sexual desire disorder A deficiency in or absence of sexual fantasies and persistently low interest or a total lack of interest in sexual activity.

Hypocalcemia Decreased blood levels of calcium.

Hypocapnia A condition that results when PaCO$_2$ falls below 35 mmHg. Also called **hypocarbia**.

Hypocarbia See Hypocapnia.

Hypochloremia Decreased blood levels of chloride.

Hypodermis The layer of loose connective tissue and fat cells that lies below the dermis. Also called *subcutaneous tissue*.

Hypodermoclysis Fluid administered subcutaneously.

Hypoglycemia Diminished glucose levels.

Hypokalemia Decreased blood levels of potassium.

Hypomagnesemia Decreased blood levels of magnesium.

Hypomania A less extreme form of mania that is not severe enough to markedly impair functioning or require hospitalization.

Hyponatremia Decreased blood levels of sodium.

Hypoperfusion Decreased blood flow.

Hypophonia A lowered voice volume.

Hypophosphatemia Decreased blood levels of phosphate.

Hypoplastic left heart syndrome (HLHS) One of the most severe congenital heart defects, characterized by absence or stenosis of mitral and aortic valves, an abnormally small left ventricle, a small aorta, and aortic or mitral stenosis or atresia.

Hypotension A below-normal blood pressure reading between 85 and 110 mmHg.

Hypothalamic-pituitary axis In the brain, the HPA is responsible for the regulation of endocrine glands, and consequently, hormones.

Hypothermia A condition that occurs when a body loses more heat than it produces.

Hypothermic A body temperature below 36°C (97°F).

Hypothyroidism A disorder resulting when the thyroid gland produces an insufficient amount of thyroid hormone.

Hypotonic Refers to solutions that have a lower osmolality than body fluids, such as one half normal saline.

Hypotonic dehydration Occurs when fluid loss is characterized by a proportionately greater loss of sodium than water. Also called *hyponatremic dehydration*.

Hypoventilation An abnormally slow respiratory rate leads to inadequate oxygen delivery to the lungs as well as an increase in retention of carbon dioxide.

Hypovolemia Loss of both water and electrolytes in similar proportions from extracellular fluid. Also called *fluid volume deficit*.

Hypovolemic shock Shock caused by a decrease in intravascular volume of 15% or more.

Hypoxemia Decreased oxygen levels in the blood that result when PaO$_2$ falls below 80 mmHg.

Hypoxia Decreased delivery of oxygen to the tissues.

Iatrogenic Refers to a condition induced by the effects of treatment.

Iatrogenic infection A type of infection that results directly from diagnostic or therapeutic procedures.

Ideal body image A mental representation of what an individual believes his or her body should look like.

Ideal self How the individual thinks he or she should be or would prefer to be.

Idiopathic pain A type of pain that occurs unpredictably and is not associated with any known cause, making it difficult to treat.

Ileostomy A surgical opening made in the ileum of the small intestine.

Ileus A condition that causes a temporary cessation of the passage of material through the intestines, usually lasting 24–48 hours.

Illness A state in which an individual's physical, emotional, intellectual, social, developmental, or spiritual functioning is diminished.

Illness behavior A coping mechanism that includes the ways in which an individual describes, monitors, and interprets symptoms, and the individual's ability to take remedial action and use the healthcare system.

Illness prevention Healthcare focusing on maintaining optimal health by preventing disease through programs on immunizations, prenatal and infant care, and prevention of sexually transmitted infections.

Illusion A distorted perception of actual sensory stimuli.

Imagery A relaxation technique in which the patient focuses on pleasant images such as a beach or a garden to replace negative images such as pain and darkness. Also called *guided imagery*.

Imitation The process by which individuals copy or reproduce what they have observed.

Immobility A reduction in the amount and control of one's movement.

Immunity The body's natural or induced response to infection and the conditions associated with its response.

Immunization Introduces an antigen into the body, allowing immunity against a disease to develop naturally.

Immunocompetent Term used to describe patients who have an immune system that identifies antigens and effectively destroys or removes them.

Immunodeficiency A condition that develops when the immune system is incompetent or unable to respond effectively.

Immunoglobulin (Ig) A protein that functions as an antibody.

Immunosuppression Inability of the immune system to respond to an antigen. Occurs in response to disease or medications; may be intentional to prevent rejection of transplants or a side effect of some medications.

Implied consent Nonverbal consent indicated by a patient's cooperative actions.

Impotence Inability to achieve or maintain an erection.

Impulse conduction The transmission of an impulse along the nerve pathways to the spinal cord and directly to the brain.

Impulsiveness Acting without considering the consequences of one's behavior. Also called *impulsivity*.

In vitro fertilization A process in which a woman's eggs are collected from her ovaries, fertilized in the laboratory, and then placed into her uterus after normal embryo development has begun.

Incentive spirometry A breathing exercise using an incentive spirometer that helps patients breathe deeply to expand the lungs. This process can help patients clear mucus secretions and increase the amount of oxygen delivered to the bronchi and alveoli.

Incident pain A type of breakthrough pain that is predictable because it is precipitated by an event or activity such as coughing or changing position.

Incident report An agency record of an accident or incident occurring within the agency. This record is designed to collect adequate information to assist personnel in preventing future incidents or occurrences. Also called *variance reports* or *unusual occurrence reports*.

Incomplete spinal cord injury An injury that involves only a partial loss of sensory and motor function below the level of the injury.

Increased intracranial pressure (IICP) Sustained, elevated pressure (15 mmHg or higher in adults) in the cranial cavity.

Indemnity plan A type of health insurance program that allows the insured to self-select healthcare providers and has no predefined network.

Independent intervention The activities that nurses are licensed to do within their scope of practice; in other words, areas of healthcare that are unique to nursing and separate and distinct from medical management.

Indicator A statistic that reflects the organization's performance in a specific area.

Inductive reasoning A "bottom-up" method of logical thinking that starts with putting significant cues together in order to reach a conclusion. It is a method of logical thinking that is used to determine if decisions are reasonable.

Infantile glaucoma **Congenital glaucoma** diagnosed within the first year of life.

Infection An invasion of the body tissue by microorganisms with the potential to cause illness or disease.

Infectious disease Any communicable disease that is caused by microorganisms that are commonly transmitted from one person to another or from an animal to an individual.

Infertility A lack of conception despite unprotected sexual intercourse for at least 12 months.

Inflammation An adaptive response to what the body sees as harmful, such as an allergen, illness, or injury. Inflammation typically is characterized by pain, heat, redness, and swelling. Also called *inflammatory response*.

Inflammatory bowel disease (IBD) Chronic inflammation of the bowel common to a group of conditions that includes Crohn disease and ulcerative colitis.

Influenza A highly contagious viral respiratory disease characterized by coryza (inflammation of the mucous membranes lining the nose usually associated with nasal discharge), fever, cough, and systemic symptoms such as headache and malaise (vague feeling of physical discomfort).

Informal groups A type of group that functions with much less structure than a formal or semiformal group. Characteristics of informal groups include easily recognized, basic objectives; rotational leadership; and no set of written rules or regulations.

Informal leader A leader who is not officially appointed to direct the activities of others but, because of seniority, age, or special abilities, is recognized by the group as a leader and plays an important role in influencing colleagues, coworkers, or other group members to achieve the group's goals.

Informed consent 1. A patient's legal and ethical rights to be informed of and give permission for any healthcare procedure or treatment. 2. A study volunteer's legal right to be informed with full disclosure of the study's purpose, required procedures, length of the study, expectations, risks, and possible benefits before consenting to participate. Informed consent also includes the right to withdraw from the study at any time.

Infundibulopelvic ligament A ligament that suspends and supports the ovaries.

Inhalant A substance inhaled to produce euphoria. Categorized into three types: anesthetics, volatile nitrites, and organic solvents.

Injury An act or event that causes damage, harm, or loss to a body's functioning.

Input Information, material, or energy that enters a system.

Inquiry A search for knowledge or facts in order to gain clarification and find solutions to problems.

Insensible fluid loss Fluid loss that is not perceptible to the individual and cannot be measured.

Insomnia The inability to fall asleep or remain asleep.

Inspection A visual, auditory, and olfactory examination or assessment of a patient to note health condition.

Inspiration The act of inhaling air in respiration.

Instrumental aggression Aggression executed in the absence of emotional arousal.

Insubordination Defiance of authority, such as the refusal to complete a task as assigned.

Insulin A hormone that facilitates the uptake and use of glucose by cells and prevents an excessive breakdown of glycogen in the liver and muscle. In doing so, insulin acts to decrease blood glucose levels.

Insulin reaction Low blood glucose levels, or hypoglycemia. Also called *insulin shock*.

Integrative health The process of incorporating **complementary health approaches** into mainstream Western healthcare.

Integrity Adherence to a strict moral or ethical code.

Integumentary system The body's system that includes skin, hair, and nails and the sebaceous, sweat, and mammary glands.

Intellect The ability to learn and understand knowledge; the capacity for thinking and reasoning intelligently.

Intellectual disability Significant limitations in intellectual functioning and adaptive behavior prior to the age of 18. Previously called *mental retardation*.

Intellectual functioning General intelligence or mental capacity, including an individual's abilities to learn, use logic, and solve problems.

Intensity 1. The amplitude of a sound produced. 2. The strength of the contraction during acme, the peak of a uterine contraction during the birth process.

Interdisciplinary assessment An assessment that involves more than one discipline such as nursing and physical therapy. Also called *interprofessional assessment*.

Interdisciplinary team A team that seeks to achieve a common goal, though the team members are professionals with varied backgrounds. Also called *interprofessional team*.

Intergroup conflict Conflict that occurs between teams that are in competition or opposition to one another.

Intermittent claudication A cramping or aching pain in the calves of the legs, the thighs, and the buttocks that occurs with a predictable level of activity

Intermittent fever Occurs when body temperature alternates at regular intervals between periods of fever and periods of normal or subnormal temperatures.

Internal environment The physical, spiritual, cognitive, emotional, and psychologic well-being of an individual that depends on the satisfaction of these basic human needs.

Internal locus of control A belief that an individual can impact her or his own health and well-being.

Internet gaming disorder The persistent use of the internet to engage in games, often with other players, leading to clinically significant impairment or distress. May also be referred to as *internet gaming addiction*.

Interdisciplinary Referring to professionals or paraprofessionals from various disciplines.

Interorganizational conflict Usually conflict that occurs between two organizations that exist within one market.

Interpersonal conflict Conflict that occurs between two or more individuals due to differences, competition, or concern about territory, control, or loss.

Interpersonal violence Violence that occurs within relationships, between family members, intimate partners, acquaintances, or strangers that does not aim to further the goals of a formal group or cause.

Interprofessional Referring to professionals from multiple or various disciplines.

Interprofessional team A team that seeks to achieve a common goal, though the team members are professionals with varied backgrounds. Also called *interdisciplinary team*.

Intersex A general term used to describe a variety of conditions in which reproductive or sexual anatomy does not fit the typical definitions of male or female.

Interstitial fluid Accounts for approximately 75% of extracellular fluid; interstitial fluid surrounds the cells.

Intervention Activities conducted or attempts made by the nurse to influence a positive change in a patient's health status or behavior; a personalized confrontation that prevents an addict from denying the addiction problem and forces them to face the negative aspects of their behavior and enroll in treatment.

Intimacy A relationship that entails commitment, companionship, affective intimacy, social support, physical closeness, and mutuality.

Intimate distance Communication that is characterized by body contact, heightened sensations of body heat and smell, and vocalizations that are low.

Intimate partner violence (IPV) The act of inflicting sexual, emotional, or physical harm on a current or previous partner or spouse.

Intra-aortic balloon pump (IABP) Also called intra-aortic balloon counterpulsation, the IABP is a mechanical circulatory support device that may be used after cardiac surgery or to treat cardiogenic shock following AMI. The IABP temporarily supports cardiac function, allowing the heart to recover gradually by decreasing myocardial workload and oxygen demand and increasing perfusion of the coronary arteries.

Intracapsular hip fracture A hip fracture involving the head or neck of the femur.

Intracellular fluid (ICF) Fluid found within the body cells that contains solute vital to the metabolic processes of the cells. Also called *cellular fluid*.

Intracranial hypertension A sustained state of increased intracranial pressure that is potentially life threatening.

Intracranial regulation The processes that affect intracranial compensation and adaptive neurologic function.

Intractable seizures Seizures that continue to occur even with optimal medical management.

Intradiscal electrothermal therapy (IDET) The use of thermal energy to treat pain from a bulging spinal disc.

Intradisciplinary assessment An evaluation that occurs within a group of individuals with a similar position in the healthcare system, such as a group of nurses or a group of surgeons, to identify areas of improvement at each level of care.

Intradisciplinary team A team that seeks to achieve a common goal with team members from the same background.

Intergenerational family A family in which more than two generations live together.

Internal patients Employees of a healthcare organization, such as nurses, physicians, therapists, medical record staff, billing specialists, and other employees.

Intraocular pressure A force within the eye that causes tissue damage.

Intraoperative The phase of an operative process in which the surgical procedure actually takes place.

Intrapartum The time from the onset of true labor until the birth of the infant and expulsion of the placenta.

Intrapersonal conflict Conflict that occurs within an individual, arising from stress or tension that results from real or perceived pressure generated by incompatible expectations or goals

Intrauterine contraception (IUC) A safe, effective method of reversible contraception that is designed to be inserted into the uterus by a qualified healthcare provider and left in place for an extended period, providing continuous contraceptive protection.

Intrauterine device (IUD) A small plastic or metal form that is placed in the uterus to prevent implantation of a fertilized ovum.

Intrauterine fetal death (IUFD) Death of a fetus that occurs after 20 weeks' gestation. Often referred to as *stillbirth* or *fetal demise*.

Intrauterine pressure catheter (IUPC) A device that measures the pressure in the uterine cavity.

Intravascular fluid Accounts for approximately 20% of the extracellular fluid and is found within the vascular system. Also called *plasma*.

Intravenous pyelography (IVP) A diagnostic test used to evaluate the structure and excretory function of the kidneys, ureters, and bladder.

Introspection The personal exploration and evaluation of one's own thoughts, emotions, behaviors, and values incorporating both verbal and nonverbal feedback from others.

Intubation The process of inserting a breathing tube.

Intuition The use of nursing knowledge, experience, and expertise for understanding without the conscious use of reasoning.

Invasion Occurs when cancerous cells overtake adjacent tissues.

Involuntary admission The detention of a patient in a psychiatric or medical facility against the patient's will, normally reserved for cases in which the patient is a danger to himself or others.

Involution The rapid reduction in size of the uterus and the return of the uterus to a nonpregnant state.

Ions Electrically charged particles.

Iron deficiency anemia A disorder that results when the supply of iron in the body is insufficient for the formation of red blood cells.

Irritant contact dermatitis An inflammation of the skin from irritants; it is not a hypersensitivity response.

Ischemia Insufficient blood supply.

Ischemic Deprived of oxygen.

Ischial spines Prominences that arise near the junction of the ilium and ischium and jut into the pelvic cavity.

Isoelectric line A straight line on an electrocardiograph that indicates the absence of electrical activity.

Isokinetic exercises Resistive exercises that involve muscle contraction or tension against resistance; can be either isotonic or isometric.

Isolation Measures designed to prevent the spread of infection to health personnel, patients, and visitors.

Isometric exercises Static or sitting exercises in which muscles contract without moving the joint.

Isotonic A solution that has the same osmolality as body fluids. Normal saline, 0.9% sodium chloride, is an isotonic solution.

Isotonic dehydration A type of fluid imbalance that occurs when fluid loss is not balanced by intake and the losses of water and sodium are in proportion. Also called *isonatremic dehydration*.

Isotonic exercises Dynamic exercises in which the muscle shortens to produce muscle contractions and active movement.

Isotonic fluid volume deficit A type of fluid imbalance that occurs when electrolytes are lost along with fluid.

Isotonic imbalance A fluid imbalance that occurs when water and electrolytes are lost or gained in equal proportions, so that the osmolality of body fluids remains constant.

Isthmus That portion of the uterus between the internal cervical os and the endometrial cavity.

Jaundice A yellow pigmentation of body tissues caused by the presence of bile pigments.

Joint arthroplasty The reconstruction or replacement of a joint.

Joint custody Occurs when two parents who are not married have equal responsibility and legal rights for their shared children.

Joint fusion A procedure that permanently fuses two or more bones together at a joint using pins, plates, screws, and rods. Also called *arthrodesis*.

Joint irrigation A fluid injected into the joint to allow the surgeon to visualize joint structures more easily and to help remove debris and infection in the joint.

Joint resurfacing A procedure in which a little bone is removed at the articulating surface of the joint and a metal replacement is fitted over the end of the bone.

Just culture An attempt to balance the blame-free environment with appropriate accountability by focusing on correcting problems that lead individuals to engage in unsafe behavior while maintaining individual accountability by establishing zero tolerance for reckless behavior.

Justice Fairness.

Juvenile glaucoma **Congenital glaucoma** diagnosed after age 3.

Juvenile idiopathic arthritis (JIA) See Juvenile rheumatoid arthritis (JRA).

Juvenile macular degeneration A pediatric form of **age-related macular degeneration** that is inherited rather than acquired.

Juvenile rheumatoid arthritis (JRA) A chronic inflammatory autoimmune disease diagnosed in children that is characterized by joint inflammation resulting in decreased mobility, swelling, and pain.

Kaposi sarcoma (KS) Often the presenting symptom of AIDS, it remains the most common cancer associated with the disease. Kaposi sarcoma is caused by a virus called the Kaposi sarcoma–associated herpes virus, also known as human herpes virus 8.

Kardex A widely used, concise method of organizing and recording data about a patient, making information quickly accessible to all healthcare professionals.

Karyotype A pictorial analysis of chromosomes.

Kcalorie See Kilocalories.

Kegel exercises The act of tightening the perineal muscle in order to strengthen the pubococcygeus muscle and increase its elasticity.

Keloid A scar that extends beyond the boundaries of the original wound.

Keratin A fibrous, water-repellent protein that gives the epidermis its tough, protective quality.

Keratotic basal cell carcinoma A type of skin cancer.

Ketonuria The presence of ketones in the urine.

Ketosis An accumulation of ketone bodies produced during oxidation of fatty acids.

Kilocalories A term used to identify the energy-producing ability of nutrients. Also called *Kcalories* or *kcal*.

Kindling Long-term changes in brain neurotransmission that occur after repeated detoxifications.

Kinesthesia The ability to perceive movement and sense of position.

Kinesthetic A term referring to awareness of the position and movement of body parts.

Korotkoff sounds The series of sounds identified while taking a blood pressure using a stethoscope.

Korsakoff psychosis A condition typically seen in alcoholics that is characterized by intact intellectual functioning but an inability to retrieve long-term memory events or retain new information.

Kosher Acceptable to or prepared according to Jewish law.

Kussmaul respirations Deep, rapid respirations associated with compensatory mechanisms.

Kyphosis A convex curvature of the spine that may decrease mobility.

Labor induction The stimulation of uterine contractions before the spontaneous onset of labor, with or without ruptured fetal membranes, for the purpose of accomplishing birth.

Labyrinthitis Inflammation of the inner ear. Also called *otitis interna*.

Laceration Disruption of the brain tissue caused by the entrance of a foreign object such as a bullet, knife, or skull fragment.

Lactase deficiency An individual's inability to digest lactose because of a deficiency of lactase, the enzyme that breaks down lactose into monosaccharides. Also called *lactose intolerance*.

Lactation consultant A specially trained individual who provides breastfeeding support and care to mothers, infants, children, families, and communities.

Lacto-ovovegetarians Vegetarians who include milk, dairy products, and eggs in their diets.

Lactase deficiency Occurs when the body lacks that substance that triggers the chemical breakdown to metabolize lactose.

Lactose intolerance An individual's inability to digest lactose because of a deficiency of lactase, the enzyme that breaks down lactose into monosaccharides. Also called *lactose deficiency*.

Lactovegetarians Vegetarians who include dairy products but no eggs in their diets.

Laënnec cirrhosis A progressive, irreversible liver disorder resulting from excessive alcohol consumption. Also called *alcoholic cirrhosis*.

Laissez-faire leader A leader who recognizes a group's need for autonomy and self-regulation. The leader assumes a "hands-off" approach, being less directive and more permissive than other types of leaders.

Lamellar A type of bone that is stronger and more compact with better blood circulation compared to woven bone.

Laminectomy The surgical removal of the vertebral lamina.

Laminotomy The surgical removal of part of the vertebral lamina.

Lanugo A large quantity of fine hair found on some newborns.

Laparoscopic cholecystectomy Removal of the gallbladder using an endoscope.

Late deceleration A condition caused by uteroplacental insufficiency resulting from decreased blood flow and oxygen transfer to the fetus through the intervillous spaces during uterine contractions.

Late (secondary) postpartum hemorrhage Postpartum hemorrhage that occurs from 24 hours to 6 weeks after birth.

Law The sum total of the rules and regulations by which a society is governed.

Laxatives Medications that stimulate bowel activity and assist in fecal elimination.

Lead An insulated wire that connects an electrocardiograph to the electrodes attached to a patient.

Leader An individual with the ability to rule, guide, or inspire others to think or act as that individual recommends.

Leading question A closed question that gives the patient an opportunity to decide whether the answer is true or not.

Lean Six Sigma A methodology used to reduce waste and provide consistency in the quality of care.

Learned helplessness A sense of helplessness that nothing the individual does can change an aspect of a situation or stressor; often reinforced by repeated failures, learned helplessness is common in individuals with major depressive disorder.

Learning A change in human disposition or capability that persists and that cannot be solely accounted for by growth.

Learning disabilities Disorders that impair an individual's ability to receive and process information, causing reduced functioning in verbal, linguistic, reasoning, and academic skills; neurologic conditions in which the brain cannot receive or process information normally.

Learning need A desire or a requirement to know something that is presently unknown to the learner.

Lecithin/sphingomyelin (L/S) ratio The measurement of lecithin and sphingomyelin in order to determine the lung maturity of a fetus.

Leopold maneuvers A systematic way to evaluate the maternal abdomen.

Lesbian A woman who prefers relationships with other women.

Lesion An observable change in skin structure that may indicate disorders in other systems and organs.

Leukemia A group of chronic malignant disorders of white blood cells (WBCs) and WBC precursors.

Leukocytes The primary cells involved in both nonspecific and specific immune system responses. Also known as *white blood cells (WBCs)*.

Leukocytosis An increase in the number of leukocytes in the blood (above $10,000/mm^3$), in response to infection or inflammation.

Leukopenia A decrease in the number of circulating leukocytes.

Level of injury The vertical location of an injury along the spinal column.

Lewy bodies Abnormal aggregates of proteins, including alpha-synuclein.

Liability The state of being legally obliged and responsible.

Libido Sexual desire.

Licensed practical nurses (LPNs) Members of a nursing team who provide direct patient care under the direction of an RN, physician, or other licensed practitioner.

Lichenification The thickening of the skin.

Lifestyle An individual's general way of living, including living conditions and individual patterns of behavior that are influenced by sociocultural factors and personal characteristics.

Ligaments Connective tissue between bones to create joints.

Lightening The effects that occur when the fetus begins to settle into the pelvic inlet.

Limb restraints A device typically made of cloth that may be used when limb immobilization is needed for therapeutic purposes, for example, to prevent dislodgement of an intravenous infusion device.

Limbic system A set of structures located deep inside the brain; includes the hippocampus.

Limit setting Establishing clear and consistent rules or guidelines for child or patient behavior.

Line authority The power to direct the activities of subordinates within an organization.

Lipids The macronutrient that provides most of the body's energy at 9 kcal/g. There are three categories of lipids: triglycerides, phospholipids, and sterols. Also called *fats*.

Lipoatrophy Atrophy of subcutaneous tissues.

Lipodystrophy Excessive growth of subcutaneous tissue.

Lithiasis Stone formation.

Lithotripsy The preferred treatment for urinary calculi; uses sound or shock waves to crush a stone.

Living will A document that provides written directions about life-prolonging procedures to provide instructions when an individual can no longer communicate in a life-threatening situation.

Lobes Specialized cognitive regions in the hemispheres of the brain.

Local adaptation syndrome (LAS) A stress response that affects only one organ or body system.

Local emergency management agency (LEMA) A governmental agency with expertise in public safety, emergency medical services, and management.

Local infection Invasion by a microorganism that is limited to the specific part of the body where the microorganism remains.

Localized responses Common manifestations of type I hypersensitivity, they are typically atopic responses; that is, they have a strong genetic predisposition. Atopic reactions are the result of localized, rather than systemic, IgE-mediated responses to an allergen. They are prompted by contact of the allergen with IgE in the bronchial tree, nasal mucosa, and conjunctival tissues.

Lochia The discharge through which the uterus rids itself of the debris remaining after birth. The discharge should change appearance and contents as healing commences.

Lochia alba The final discharge as the uterus completes healing; composed primarily of leukocytes, decidual cells, epithelial cells, fat, cervical mucus, cholesterol crystals, and bacteria.

Lochia rubra The dark red initial discharge as the uterus eliminates epithelial cells, erythrocytes, leukocytes, shreds of decidua, and occasionally fetal meconium, lanugo, and vernix in the first 1–2 days following birth.

Lochia serosa A light pink discharge of serous exudate, shreds of degenerating decidua, erythrocytes, leukocytes, cervical mucus, and numerous microorganisms from the uterus 3–10 days following birth.

Locked-in syndrome A state of consciousness in which the patient is alert and fully aware of the environment and has intact cognitive abilities but is unable to communicate through speech or movement because of blocked efferent pathways from the brain. Motor paralysis affects all voluntary muscles, although the upper cranial nerves (I through IV) may remain intact, allowing the patient to communicate through eye movements and blinking.

Locus of control (LOC) The extent to which patients believes their health status is under their own or others' control.

Long-term memory The final process or destination for information to be stored indefinitely.

Longboard spinal immobilization A device that provides support and immobilization of the entire spine below the level of the neck, instituted for patients with a potential or suspected spinal cord injury from a motor vehicle collision.

Loose association An indication of disordered thinking characterized by the shifting of verbal ideas from one topic to another, with no apparent relationship between thoughts, and the person speaking being unaware that the topics are unconnected. Commonly seen in schizophrenia.

Lordosis A concave curvature of the spine that may decrease mobility.

Loss A situation in which someone or something that is valued becomes altered or no longer available.

Lower body obesity Identified by a waist-to-hip ratio of less than 0.8; more commonly seen in women. Also called *peripheral obesity*.

Lumpectomy Removal of a tumor and the surrounding margin of breast tissue followed by radiation therapy. Also called *segmental mastectomy* or *breast conservation surgery*.

Lung abscess A local area of necrosis and pus formation within the lung.

Lupus nephritis Inflammation of the kidneys resulting from systemic lupus erythematosus (SLE).

Luteinizing hormone (LH) Anterior pituitary hormone responsible for stimulating ovulation and for development of the corpus luteum.

Lymphadenopathy The enlargement of lymph nodes with or without tenderness. It may be caused by inflammation, infection, or malignancy of the nodes or the regions drained by the nodes.

Lymphangitis Inflammation of a lymph vessel.

Lymphedema Accumulation of fluid in the soft tissues of the arm caused by removal of lymph channels.

Lymphocytes The principal effector and regulator cells of specific immune responses to protect the body from microorganisms, foreign tissue, and cell mutations or alterations.

Lyse Disintegrate.

Maceration Tissues softened by prolonged wetting or soaking.

Macronutrients Essential nutrients needed by the body in large amounts to survive: carbohydrates, proteins, and fats.

Macrophages Large phagocytes that are important in the body's defense against chronic infections.

Macular degeneration A progressive disorder involving loss of central vision due to damage to the retina.

Magical thinking Believing that events occur because of one's thoughts or actions.

Major depressive disorder (MDD) A mood disorder characterized by loss of interest in life and unresponsiveness, moving from mild to severe, with severe symptoms lasting at least 2 weeks. Also called *unipolar depression*.

Major depressive episode Characterized by a change in several aspects of an individual's emotional state and functioning consistently over a period of 14 days or longer.

Major trauma A serious single-system injury (such as the amputation of a leg) or multiple-system injuries (simultaneous injuries such as a punctured lung, traumatic brain injury, and crushed bones in the arms and legs). Also called *multisystem trauma*.

Malabsorption A condition in which the intestinal mucosa is unable to absorb nutrients, resulting in nutrients being excreted in the stool.

Malaise Vague feeling of physical discomfort.

Maldigestion A condition in which there is inadequate preparation of chyme for absorption of nutrients; also can result in malabsorption.

Male hypoactive sexual desire disorder A deficiency in or absence of sexual fantasies and persistently low interest or a total lack of interest in sexual activity.

Male orgasmic disorder A condition that occurs when a man can maintain an erection for long periods, but has difficulty ejaculating.

Malignant Term used to refer to a cell or growth that, if not treated, will recur, continue to grow, and spread to other sites in the body, ending in death.

Malignant hyperthermia A musculoskeletal disorder resulting from an inherited cellular deficit that places the patient in a hypermetabolic state.

Malnutrition Health effects due to insufficient nutrient intake or stores. Also called *undernutrition*.

Malpractice Conduct deviating from the standard of practice dictated by a profession.

Malpresentation A condition that occurs when a fetus passes into the pelvic inlet with a breech or shoulder presentation. These presentations are associated with difficulties during labor.

Malunion The healing of bones in an anatomically incorrect position. Surgical correction may be needed.

Managed care A healthcare delivery system designed to provide cost-effective, high-quality care for groups of patients from the time of their initial contact with the health system through the conclusion of their health problem.

Manager An individual employed by an organization and granted the required authority, responsibility, accountability, and power to accomplish the organization's goals.

Mandatory health insurance Health insurance is provided by large, nonprofit health organizations centered around large employers or work-based associations or else is provided by government-sponsored programs. Everyone belongs to one of these two types of insurance plans, thus ensuring universal coverage.

Mandatory reporting A legal requirement to report an act, event, or situation that is designated by state or local law as a reportable event.

Mania An abnormal and persistently elevated, expansive, or irritable mood lasting at least 1 week, significantly impairing social or occupational functioning and generally requiring hospitalization.

Manipulation Controlling behavior used to exploit others for personal gain.

Margination The accumulation of leukocytes along the inner surface of blood vessels. Occurs as part of the inflammatory process.

Marital rape Rape that occurs when one spouse forces the other to have sex against his or her will.

Maslow's hierarchy of needs A concept proposed by Abraham Maslow in which he proposed the existence of levels of human needs that could be organized into five categories: physiologic, safety, love and belonging, esteem, and self-actualization.

Massage therapy The scientific manipulation of the soft tissues of the body for the purposes of promoting healing and wellness.

Massive transfusion A series of blood parcels, including packed red blood cells, fresh frozen plasma, cryo units, and platelet pheresis administered to a patient who has lost a substantial amount of blood.

Mast cells Leukocytes that detect foreign agents or injury and respond by releasing histamine, thereby activating the inflammatory process.

Masturbation The self-stimulation of one's genitals for sexual pleasure.

Maternal role attainment (MRA) The process by which a woman learns mothering behaviors and becomes comfortable with her identity as a mother.

Maturational crisis A crisis that occurs normally as an individual progresses through the life cycle.

Mature milk A white or slightly blue-tinged color milk that presents by 2 weeks postpartum and continues thereafter until lactation ceases.

McDonald sign A probable sign of pregnancy characterized by an ease in flexing the body of the uterus against the cervix.

Mean arterial pressure (MAP) The average pressure in the arterial circulation throughout the cardiac cycle.

Meaning-focused coping The use of revaluation to reduce the appraisal of a threat.

Meatus A body passage or opening.

Meconium The first fecal material passed by a newborn, normally within 8–24 hours after birth.

Medicaid A state-administered health insurance program available to certain lower-income individuals and families, older adults, and people with disabilities.

Medical asepsis All practices intended to confine a specific microorganism to a specific area, thus limiting the number, growth, and transmission of the microorganism.

Medicare A federally funded health insurance program available to people ages 65 or older, younger people with disabilities, and people with end-stage renal disease.

Medigap policy A private health insurance plan designed to supplement Medicare coverage. It may pay copayments, coinsurance, deductibles, and "gaps" in Medicare coverage (i.e., noncovered healthcare costs). Also called *Medicare supplemental insurance.*

Meditation The act of focusing one's thoughts or engaging in self-reflection or contemplation.

Meiosis A reductive division of sex cells, producing ova or sperm with a half set (haploid) of chromosomes.

Melanin A shield that protects the keratinocytes and the nerve endings in the dermis from the damaging effects of ultraviolet light.

Melanoma A type of malignant skin cancer.

Melasma gravidarum See Chloasma.

Mendelian inheritance Traits that are passed on by a single gene. Also called *single-gene inheritance.*

Meninges Three connective tissue membranes that cover, protect, and nourish the central nervous system.

Menometrorrhagia Irregular, excessive, prolonged menstruation.

Menopause The permanent cessation of menses.

Menorrhagia Excessive or prolonged menstruation that occurs at regular intervals.

Menstrual cycle The cyclic phases of menstruation that normally occur about every 28 days.

Menstruation The periodic shedding of the uterine lining in a woman of childbearing age who is not pregnant.

Mental health A state of well-being in which an individual is able to work productively, cope with change and adversity, engage in meaningful relationships, and realize his own potential.

Mental illness A condition that affects emotions, thinking, behavior, or any combination of the three; mental illness is characterized by symptoms that are severe enough to impair functioning.

Mental retardation See Intellectual disability.

Mentor A competent, experienced professional who develops a relationship with a novice for the purpose of providing advice, support, information, and feedback in order to encourage development of the individual.

Message Content that is actually said or written, the body language that accompanies the words, and how the words are transmitted.

Metabolic acidosis This bicarbonate deficit is characterized by a low pH (<7.35), low bicarbonate (<24 mEq/L), and $PaCO_2$ less than 38 mmHg. It may be caused by excess acid in the body or loss of bicarbonate from the body.

Metabolic alkalosis This bicarbonate excess is characterized by a high pH (>7.45), a high bicarbonate (>28 mEq/L), and $PaCO_2$ higher than 45 mmHg. It may be caused by loss of acid or excess bicarbonate in the body.

Metabolic syndrome A disorder characterized by the presence of three or more of the following: increased waist circumference, hypertension, elevated blood triglycerides and fasting blood glucose, and low HDL cholesterol.

Metabolism The complex process of biochemical reactions occurring in the body's cells necessary to produce energy, repair cells, and sustain life.

Metacognition The human ability to think about thinking.

Metaphysis The portion of the bone between the diaphysis and the epiphysis.

Metaplasia A change in the normal pattern of differentiation such that dividing cells differentiate into cell types not normally found at that location in the body.

Metastasis The process by which spreading of malignant neoplasms occurs; the transfer of disease from one organ or part to another.

Metrorrhagia Bleeding between menstrual periods.

Microalbuminuria An abnormally low level of albumin in the urine.

Micronutrients Essential nutrients needed by the body in small quantities, such as vitamins and minerals.

Microstaging The assessment of the level of invasion of a malignant melanoma and the maximum tumor thickness.

Micturition Releasing urine from the urinary bladder. Also called *voiding* or *urination.*

Middle ear effusion Results when negative pressure in the middle ear causes sterile serous fluid to move from the capillaries into the space.

Milia Exposed sebaceous glands that appear as raised white spots on the face, especially across the nose on infants within the first month after birth.

Miliary tuberculosis Results from hematogenous spread (through the blood) of the tuberculosis bacilli throughout the body.

Milieu therapy A therapeutic recovery environment that supports behavior changes, teaches new coping skills, and helps the patient move from addiction to sobriety.

Milliequivalent The chemical combining power of the ion, or the capacity of cations to combine with anions to form molecules.

Minerals Salts dissolved in water that carry electrical charge and work with other nutrients to maintain fluid balance throughout the body. Also called *electrolytes.*

Minimal enteral nutrition Small-volume feedings of formula or human milk (usually <24 mL · kg^{-1} · day^{-1}) designed to "prime" the premature infant's intestinal tract and stimulate many of its hormonal and enzymatic functions.

Minor trauma Trauma that affects a single part or system of the body and is usually treated in a physician's office or in a hospital's emergency department.

Miscarriage The loss of a fetus prior to 20 weeks' gestation. Also called a *spontaneous abortion.*

Mitigation A phase that takes place before and after an emergency that consists of identifying potential hazards, minimizing effects, and reducing the likelihood of their occurrence.

Mitosis The process of cell division.

Mitt restraints A device used to protect confused patients from scratching or injuring their skin or dislodging intravenous access devices. Also called *hand restraints.*

Modeling Observing the behavior of people who have successfully achieved a goal that they have set for themselves and, through observing, acquiring ideas for behavior and coping strategies.

Modified radical mastectomy The removal of the breast tissue and lymph nodes under the arm, leaving the chest wall muscles intact.

Molding The asymmetrical appearance of an infant's head caused by overlapping of the cranial bones during labor and birth.

Mongolian spots Macular areas of bluish-black or gray-blue pigmentation on the dorsal area and the buttocks; common in newborns of Asian, Hispanic, and African descent and in newborns of other dark-skinned races.

Monoamine oxidase inhibitor (MAOI) A drug that inhibits monoamine oxidase, an enzyme that terminates the actions of neurotransmitters such as dopamine, norepinephrine, epinephrine, and serotonin. These drugs are used to treat individuals who have not responded to typical treatments for depression.

Mononeuropathies Isolated peripheral neuropathies that affect a single nerve.

Monophasic A term used to describe rheumatoid arthritis when it occurs for a limited time and then improves.

Monopolizing The domination of a discussion by one member of a group.

Monosomy Absence of a chromosome.

Monro-Kellie hypothesis A hypothesis that states if the volume of any of the three intracranial components (the brain, cerebrospinal fluid, and blood) increases, the volume of the others must decrease to maintain normal pressures in the cranial cavity.

Mood An individual's internal, subjective, sustained emotional state.

Mood stabilizers Drugs used for treatment of bipolar disorder because they moderate extreme shifts in emotions between mania and depression.

Moral behavior The way in which an individual perceives and responds to society's requirements.

Moral development 1. The process of learning to tell the difference between right and wrong and of learning what ought and ought not to be done. 2. The pattern of change in moral behavior that occurs with age.

Moral principles Statements about broad, general, philosophical concepts such as autonomy and justice.

Moral rules Specific prescriptions for actions.

Morality Private, personal standards of what is right and wrong in conduct, character, and attitude; the requirements necessary for people to live together in society.

Morbid obesity A condition in which an individual weighs more than 200% of his or her ideal body weight or has a BMI >40 kg/m^2.

Morning sickness A term that refers to the nausea and vomiting that a woman may experience in early pregnancy. This lay term is sometimes used because these symptoms frequently occur in the early part of the day and disappear within a few hours.

Moro reflex In response to being lifted, then suddenly lowered or surprised by a loud noise, a newborn will straighten the arms and hands outward while the knees flex. Slowly, the arms return to the chest, as in an embrace. The fingers spread, forming a "C," and the newborn may cry.

Morpheaform basal cell carcinoma A type of skin cancer.

Morula Developmental stage of the fertilized ovum in which there is a solid mass of cells.

Mosaicism The expression of two cell lines, each with a different chromosomal number, in an individual.

Motility The process of moving food and fluid through the gastrointestinal tract from the mouth to the anus.

Motivation to learn The individual's personal desire and need to learn that affects how much and how fast the individual will learn.

Motor vehicle crash (MVC) The unintentional collision of one or more motor vehicles with another vehicle or object.

Mottling A lacy pattern of dilated blood vessels under the skin.

Mourning The behavioral process through which grief is eventually resolved or altered; it is often influenced by culture, spiritual beliefs, and custom.

Movement disorder A disorder associated with schizophrenia. There are two general forms: The first involves increased body movements that may appear agitated, repetitive, or purposeless. The second form involves catatonia, or unresponsiveness to the environment or others.

Movement technique A relaxation technique, such as yoga or tai chi, designed to improve strength, balance, and mental calmness.

Mucolytics Medications that help break up thick mucus secretions in the airways.

Multi-payer system Healthcare insurance coverage or payment system in which funds come from multiple sources.

Multiculturalism Characterized by many subcultures coexisting within a given society in which no one culture dominates.

Multidisciplinary team approach An approach to healthcare in which team members work together to deliver patient care, but a single team member—usually a physician—makes the treatment decisions.

Multifocal A term used to describe premature ventricular contractions (PVCs) that arise from different ectopic sites and appear distinct on the ECG.

Multigravida Term used to describe a woman who has been pregnant more than once.

Multipara Term used to describe a woman who has had more than one pregnancy in which the fetus was viable.

Multiple pregnancy More than one fetus in the uterus at the same time.

Multiple sclerosis (MS) A chronic demyelinating neurologic disease of the central nervous system associated with an abnormal immune response to an environmental factor.

Multiple trauma Trauma that involves serious single-system injury or multiple-system injuries. Also called *major trauma.*

Mural thrombi Blood clots in the heart wall.

Muscle relaxation A relaxation technique that involves consciously tightening and then relaxing each muscle progressively from either head to toe or toe to head.

Mutual recognition model A licensing system that allows a nurse to have a single license that confers the privilege to practice in other states that are part of the Nurse Licensure Compact.

Mutual respect A state in which two or more individuals show or feel honor or esteem toward one another.

Mycobacterium tuberculosis The bacteria that causes tuberculosis.

Mydriasis Abnormal or excessive dilation of the pupil of the eye, usually caused by a disease or drug.

Myelin The fatty, segmented wrappings that normally protect and insulate nerves. Also called *myelin sheath.*

Myelogram A diagnostic technique in which dye is injected into the spinal fluid and visualized by x-ray in order to identify areas of pressure on the spinal cord or nerves due to herniated discs.

Myocardial hypertrophy An increase in the size of muscle cells of the myocardium.

Myometrium The middle muscular layer of the uterus.

Myopia Nearsightedness.

MyPlate A nutrient intake guide from the U.S. Department of Agriculture that outlines suggested food intake by food groups.

Myringotomy A surgical incision of the tympanic membrane.

Myxedema The hypothyroid state with characteristic accumulation of nonpitting edema in the connective tissues throughout the body.

Myxedema coma A life-threatening complication of long-standing, untreated hypothyroidism, usually triggered by an acute illness or trauma.

Nägele rule A common method of determining the estimated date of birth using the first day of the last menstrual period, subtracting 3 months, and adding 7 days.

NANDA The acronym for North American Nursing Diagnosis Association.

Narcissism Self-centered behavior in which the individual feels entitled to special favors due to a mistaken perception that they are superior to others.

Narcissistic personality disorder (NPD) One of several personality disorders defined in the DSM-5, it is marked by in a pattern of grandiosity, difficulty regulating self-esteem, and the need for admiration and attention from others.

Narcolepsy A disorder characterized by daytime sleep attacks or excessive daytime sleepiness.

Narcotics See Opioids.

Narrative charting A traditional part of the source-oriented record. It consists of written notes that include routine care, normal findings, and patient problems.

National Institute for Occupational Safety and Health (NIOSH) An organization that focuses on generating new knowledge in the field of occupational safety and health and transferring that knowledge into practice for the betterment of workers.

National Patient Safety Goals (NPSGs) Formulated goals to assist accredited organizations with specific topics about patient safety.

Natural killer (NK) cells Large, granular cells found in the spleen, lymph nodes, bone marrow, and blood. NK cells provide immune surveillance and resistance to infection, and they play an important role in the destruction of early malignant cells.

Nature The genetic or hereditary capability of the individual.

Nausea A vague, but unpleasant, subjective sensation of sickness or queasiness.

Necrosis Dead tissue.

Negative affectivity One of the six trait domains associated with personality disorders that is distinguished by anxiousness, emotional lability, separation insecurity, depressive tendencies, perseveration, and suspicion.

Negative airflow room A room where airflow is controlled to prevent the air from circulating into the hallway or other rooms. Multiple fresh-air exchanges dilute the concentration of droplet nuclei in a negative airflow room. Also called *negative flow room.*

Negative feedback Output of a system that returns to the system as input and which inhibits system change.

Negative pressure ventilators A device that creates negative pressure externally to draw the chest outward and air into the lungs, mimicking spontaneous breathing.

Negative punishment The removal of a positive reward if an undesirable behavior occurs.

Negative symptom Loss or absence of a normal function seen in mentally healthy adults, such as the ability to care for one's self; commonly seen in schizophrenia.

Neglect syndrome A disorder of attention that can result from stroke, which is characterized by the inability to integrate and use perceptions from the affected side. Also called *unilateral neglect.*

Negligence Any conduct that deviates from what a reasonable person would do in a particular circumstance.

Neologisms Use of meaningless words that only have meaning to the individual using them.

Neonatal abstinence syndrome (NAS) A combination of neonatal signs and symptoms caused by withdrawal of gestational opioid exposure.

Neonatal anemia A disorder caused by blood loss, hemolysis, and impaired red blood cell production related to birth.

Neonatal mortality risk An infant's chance of death within the first 28 days of life.

Neonatal transition The first few hours after birth, in which a newborn's body systems adapt to extrauterine life.

Neonatology The field of medicine providing care for sick and premature infants.

Neoplasm A mass of new tissue that grows independently of its surrounding structures and has no physiologic purpose.

Nephrectomy Removal of a kidney.

Nephritis Inflammation of the kidneys.

Nephrolithiasis The formation of stones in the kidney.

Nephrolithotomy A procedure for removal of a staghorn calculus that invades the calyces and renal parenchyma.

Nephrotoxins Substances that damage nerves or nerve tissue.

Nerve block A chemical interruption of a nerve pathway, effected by injecting a local anesthetic into the nerve.

Networking The act of developing and maintaining relationships with others within and outside of the nursing profession and affiliated organizations to improve nursing practice, advance career goals, offer support, share information, and provide advice.

Neurofibrillary tangles Seen in patients with Alzheimer disease, they are thick, insoluble clots of protein inside the damaged brain cells or neurons.

Neurogenic bladder Interference with the normal mechanisms of urine elimination in which the patient does not perceive bladder fullness and is unable to control the urinary sphincters; usually the result of impaired neurologic function.

Neurogenic shock The result of an imbalance between parasympathetic and sympathetic stimulation of vascular smooth muscle.

Neuroleptic malignant syndrome (NMS) A potentially fatal condition caused by antipsychotic medications that block dopamine receptors. It is characterized by fever, rigidity, and increased prolactin levels.

Neuron The basic or specialized cell of the nervous system that carries electrical impulses throughout the body.

Neuropathic pain A type of pain experienced by people who have damaged or malfunctioning nerves.

Neurotransmitters Chemical messengers that carry information between neurons.

Neutral question An open-ended question the patient can answer without direction or pressure.

Neutral thermal environment (NTE) A specific environmental temperature range in which the rates of oxygen consumption and metabolism are minimal and the internal body temperature is maintained because of thermal balance.

Never events Preventable hazards that can result in injury or death, and that should never happen to patients.

Nevi Moles.

Nevus flammeus A capillary angioma directly below the epidermis. It is a nonelevated, sharply demarcated, red-to-purple area of dense capillaries. In infants of African descent, it may appear as a purple-black stain. Also called *port-wine stain.*

Nevus vasculosus A capillary hemangioma consisting of newly formed and enlarged capillaries in the dermal and subdermal layers. It is a raised, clearly delineated, dark red, rough-surfaced birthmark commonly found in the head region. Also called a *strawberry mark.*

New Ballard score Specific criteria designed for accurate assessment of the gestational age of newborns between 20 and 28 weeks of gestation and weighing less than 1500 g.

Newborn Infant from birth through the first 28 days of life.

Nicotine A highly addictive chemical that is found in tobacco and enters the body via the lungs (cigarettes, pipes, and cigars) and oral mucous membranes (chewing tobacco as well as smoking).

Nicotine replacement therapy (NRT) A pharmacologic therapy designed to relieve some of the physiologic effects of withdrawal, including cravings, for patients trying to quit smoking or using tobacco. NRT transdermal patches and gums are available over the counter; nicotine inhalers and nasal sprays are available by prescription only.

Nicotinic receptors Found in the hippocampus and involved with new sensory information and memory formation, they are thought to be impaired in patients with schizophrenia.

Nidation The cyclical preparation of the uterine lining by steroid hormones for implantation of the embryo.

Nociceptive pain A type of pain resulting from external stimuli on an uninjured, fully functional nervous system.

Nociceptors The nerve receptors for pain.

Nocturia Voiding two or more times at night.

Nocturnal emissions Orgasm and emission of semen during sleep. Also called *wet dreams.*

Nocturnal enuresis Involuntary urination at night after bladder control has been achieved. Also called *bed wetting.*

Nocturnal frequency The need for older adults to arise during the night to urinate.

Nodular basal cell carcinoma A type of skin cancer.

Noise-induced hearing loss (NIHL) A condition associated with prolonged exposure to sound of greater than or equal to 85 dB.

Nolo contendere A term used when an individual neither admits to nor denies committing a crime but agrees to a punishment as if guilty.

Nominal group technique (NGT) A process that alternates between individual work and group work. Individuals meet as a group, but they write their responses without any discussion.

Nondirective interview An unstructured interview in which the nurse allows the patient to control the purpose, subject matter, and pacing.

Nonexudative macular degeneration The most common form of macular degeneration, it is characterized by the accumulation of deposits beneath the pigment epithelium of the retina, causing the pigment epithelium to detach and interfere with the sensory function of the macula. Also referred to as the dry form of macular degeneration.

Noninvasive ventilation (NIV) Ventilator support using a tight-fitting face mask, thus avoiding intubation.

Nonmaleficence The duty to do no harm.

Non-Mendelian inheritance Traits that are passed on by the influence of multiple genes. Also called *multifactorial inheritance.*

Nonpenetrating injury Also called a close injury, this type of injury is associated with blunt-force injuries that do not result in the entrance of a foreign object into the body.

Nonshivering thermogenesis (NST) The stimulation of heat production in the body through increased cellular metabolism. Also called *chemical thermogenesis.*

Non-small-cell carcinoma Lung cancers other than small-cell carcinoma.

Nonstress test (NST) A widely used method of evaluating fetal status; may be used alone or as part of a more comprehensive diagnostic assessment called a biophysical profile.

Non-suicidal self-injury behaviors (NSSI) Intentional self-inflicted acts of harm to body tissue without the intent of suicide.

Nonunion Failure of the ends of a fracture to heal together after at least 3 months.

Nonverbal communication Transmitting information through gestures, facial expressions, or touch.

Normal sinus rhythm (NSR) The normal heart rhythm, in which impulses originate in the sinus node and travel through all normal conduction pathways without delay.

Normative commitment A feeling of obligation to continue in the profession due to benefits or positive experiences derived from the profession.

Normothermia Normal body temperature.

Nosocomial infections Infections that are associated with the delivery of healthcare services in a facility such as a hospital or nursing home. Also called *healthcare-associated infections (HAIs).*

NREM Sleep Non-rapid-eye-movement sleep occurs when activity in the *reticular activating system* is inhibited.

Nuclear family A family structure consisting of a husband and wife and their biological children.

Nucleation The formation of a crystal from a liquid.

Nucleotomy The surgical removal of a herniated disc.

Nulligravida Term used to describe a woman who has never been pregnant.

Nullipara Term used to describe a woman who has not given birth to a viable fetus.

Nurse practice act (NPA) State-level statutes that define and regulate nursing practices.

Nursing clinical research Research that seeks to answer questions that ultimately will improve patient care.

Nursing diagnosis A clinical judgment about individual, family, or community responses to actual and potential health problems/life processes.

Nursing ethics Ethical issues that occur in nursing practice.

Nursing informatics (NI) A specialty that integrates nursing science, computer science, and information science to manage and communicate data, information, knowledge, and wisdom in nursing practice.

Nursing plan of care A written or electronic guideline that organizes information about an individual patient's or family's care.

Nursing process The process used to identify a patient's health status and actual or potential healthcare problems or needs, to establish plans to meet the identified needs, to deliver specific nursing interventions to meet those needs, and to evaluate the success of those interventions.

Nursing research A systematic and strict scientific process that tests hypotheses about health-related illness and conditions and processes of nursing care practices.

Nursing transactional model The relationship among the nurse, the patient, and the environment in which they interact.

Nurture The effects of the environment on an individual's performance.

Nutrient density The ratio of good nutrients to calories a food contains.

Nutrients Substances found in food used by the body to promote growth, maintenance, and repair.

Nutrition The process by which the body ingests, absorbs, transports, uses, and eliminates nutrients in food.

Nutritional health The physical result of the balance between nutrient intake and nutritional requirements.

Nystagmus Involuntary rapid eye movement.

Obesity An excess of adipose tissue.

Object permanence The ability to understand that when something is out of sight it still exists.

Objective data Information that is detectable by an observer or can be measured or tested against an accepted standard. Also called *overt data* or *signs.*

Objective family burden Actual, identifiable family problems associated with the mental illness of a family member.

Obligatory losses Essential fluid losses required to maintain body functioning.

Observational learning The acquisition of new skills or the alteration of old behaviors simply by watching other children and adults.

Obsession A recurrent, unwanted, and often distressing thought or image that leads to feelings of fear and anxiety.

Obsessive-compulsive disorder (OCD) A disabling disorder characterized by obsessive thoughts and compulsive, repetitive behaviors that dominate an individual's life.

Obsessive–compulsive personality disorder (OCPD) One of several personality disorders defined in the DSM-5, it is marked by fear and anxiety concerning loss of control over situations, objects, or people.

Obstetric conjugate The distance from the middle of the sacral promontory to an area approximately 1 cm below the pubic crest.

Obstructive shock Shock caused by an obstruction in the heart or great vessels that either impedes venous return or prevents effective cardiac pumping action.

Occult blood Blood in stool that cannot be seen with the naked eye.

Occupational exposure Skin, eye, mucous membrane, or parenteral contact with blood or other potentially infectious materials that may result from the performance of an employee's duties.

Occupational Safety and Health Administration (OSHA) An organization that enforces the guidelines presented in the OSHA Act of 1970, requiring its covered employees to report specific incidents and illnesses in a timely manner.

Oculocephalic reflex An oculomotor response in which the eyes move in opposite direction as head turns to the side. Also called **doll's eye reflex.**

Olfactory Of or relating to smell.

Oligodendrocytes Cells that produce myelin.

Oligomenorrhea Light or infrequent menstruation and occurs when cycles are longer than 6–7 weeks. Usually related to hormonal imbalances such as those seen in polycystic ovary syndrome.

Oliguria The production of abnormally small amounts of urine by the kidney.

On–off effect A sudden lack of symptom control and unexpected dyskinesias appearing as drug effectiveness diminishes.

Oncogenes Genes that promote cell proliferation and are capable of triggering cancerous characteristics.

Oncology The study of cancer.

Oncotic pressure A pulling force exerted by colloids that helps maintain the water content of blood by pulling water from the interstitial space into the vascular compartment. Also called *colloid osmotic pressure.*

Online shopping addiction Excessive online shopping, often associated with overspending and aided by the internet, and characterized by compulsive and addictive forms of consumption and buying behavior.

Oogenesis The process that produces the female gamete, called an ovum (egg).

Open-angle glaucoma The most common form of glaucoma, it is a chronic, gradually progressive disease that typically affects both eyes.

Open-ended question A question that allows patients to discover, explore, elaborate, clarify, or illustrate their thoughts or feelings.

Open fracture A fracture in which the skin integrity is disrupted. Also called a *compound fracture.*

Open reduction and internal fixation (ORIF) The surgical insertion of nails, screws, plates, or pins to hold fractured bones in place.

Opiates A type of drug derived from natural or synthetic opiates that is used as a pain reliever. Opiates include morphine, meperidine, codeine, hydrocodone, and oxycodone.

Opioids Drugs that act on one or more of three opioid receptors: mu, delta, and kappa. They are controlled substances due to their potential for abuse. Also called *narcotics.*

Opportunistic infection An invasion of the body tissue by microorganisms appearing in an individual with immunodeficiency that would normally not affect an individual with an intact immune system.

Opportunistic pathogen A microorganism that causes disease only in susceptible individuals.

Optimism A feeling that things will turn out for the best.

Oral–genital sex Kissing, licking, or sucking of the genitals for sexual pleasure.

Orchiectomy Surgical removal of the testes.

Organizational chart A chart that depicts the formal hierarchical structure and related responsibilities within a traditional organization.

Organizational commitment The relative strength of an individual's relationship and sense of belonging to an organization.

Organizing The process of coordinating the work to be done. Formally, it involves identifying the work of the organization, dividing the labor, developing the chain of command, and assigning authority.

Orgasmic phase The phase of the sexual response cycle that is marked by the involuntary release of sexual tension accompanied by physiologic and psychologic release.

Orientation 1. A structured program of activities to help new employees adapt to their new workplace; it is geared toward helping newly employed nurses to be successful. 2. A newborn's ability to be alert to, follow, and fixate on appealing and attractive, complex visual stimuli. 3. A component of normal perception that includes four basic elements: person, place, time, and situation.

Orthopnea Difficulty breathing when supine.

Orthopneic position A body position with the head and arms supported on the overbed table to facilitate breathing.

Orthotic devices Orthopedic devices that may include splints or braces applied to reduce strain on a joint.

Ortolani maneuver A procedure used to evaluate an infant for developmental dysplastic hip.

Osmolality A measure of the concentration of solutes in body fluids. Osmolality is determined by the total solute concentration within a fluid compartment and is measured as parts of solute per kilogram of water.

Osmolar imbalance A fluid imbalance that involves the loss or gain of only water, so that the osmolality of the serum is altered.

Osmosis The movement of water across cell membranes, from a less concentrated solution to a more concentrated solution.

Osmotic pressure The power of a solution to draw water across a semipermeable membrane.

Ossification The development of bone.

Osteoarthritis (OA) The most common form of arthritis in older adults. It is caused by chronic degenerative changes in the cartilage and synovial membranes of the joints.

Osteoblasts Cells that form bone.

Osteoclasts Cells that resorb bone.

Osteocytes Cells that maintain bone matrix.

Osteodystrophy A complex bone disease process of chronic kidney disease in which chronic hyperparathyroidism causes increased resorption of bone.

Osteomyelitis Infection of the bone in a compound fracture.

Osteophytes Bony spurs that form as cartilage deteriorates.

Osteoporosis A metabolic bone disorder characterized by loss of bone mass, increased bone fragility, and increased risk of fractures.

Osteotomy 1. Surgical removal of a wedge of bones above or below a joint to realign the joint and shift weight away from the damaged potion of a joint. 2. An incision into or transection of the bone.

Otitis externa Inflammation of the ear canal. It is often called *swimmer's ear* because it is most frequently found in people who spend significant time in the water.

Otitis interna An inflammation of the inner ear. Also called *labyrinthitis*.

Otitis media Inflammation of the middle ear.

Otoscope A handheld instrument with a light and a cone-shaped attachment; known as an *ear speculum*.

Outcome The specific, observable criteria used to evaluate whether goals have been met and the effectiveness of nursing actions.

Outcome standards Standards that focus on the performance of a process, such as the number of bedridden patients who develop a pressure injury.

Outcomes management Management process that uses patient experiences to guide improvement in all areas of healthcare by providing a link between medical interventions and health outcomes and between health outcomes and the cost of care.

Output Energy, material, or information that a system gives out as a result of its processes.

Ovarian cycle The three cyclical phases of oogenesis that occur about every 28 days.

Ovarian ligaments Ligaments that anchor the lower pole of the ovary to the uterus.

Ovaries Female sex glands in which the ova are formed and in which estrogen and progesterone are produced. Normally, a woman has two ovaries.

Overdelegation A situation that occurs when a delegator loses control over a situation by providing a delegate with too much authority or too much responsibility. This places the delegator in a risky position, increasing the potential for liability.

Overnutrition Health effects caused by excessive or accelerated nutrient intake or stores, such as obesity, hypertension, hypercholesterolemia, or toxic levels of stored vitamins or minerals.

Overt conflict Conflict that is addressed openly and is generally obvious to the individuals involved.

Ovulation Normal process of discharging a mature ovum from an ovary approximately 14 days before the onset of menses.

Oxygenation The mechanism that facilitates or impairs the body's ability to supply oxygen to all cells of the body.

Pacemaker An external or implanted pulse generator used to provide an electrical stimulus to the heart when the heart fails to generate or conduct its own stimulus at a rate that maintains the cardiac output.

PaCO$_2$ A measure of the pressure exerted by dissolved carbon dioxide in the blood; it reflects the respiratory component of acid–base regulation and balance because it is regulated by the lungs.

Pain An unpleasant sensory and emotional experience associated with actual or potential tissue damage.

Pain threshold The point at which pain is initially perceived.

Pain tolerance The duration of time or intensity of pain an individual will endure before demonstrating pain responses.

Palliation Measures taken not to cure a disease, but to relieve disease-related symptoms and enhance the patient's quality of life. See also Palliative care.

Palliative care Nursing care that improves the quality of life of patients and their families facing life-threatening illness by preventing, assessing, and treating pain and other physical, psychosocial, and spiritual problems.

Palliative procedure A surgical or interventional cardiac catheterization procedure that does not create normal anatomic or hemodynamic results but allows adequate blood flow to oxygenate the tissues.

Pallidotomy A surgical technique for Parkinson disease in which the neurosurgeon locates the affected areas of the globus pallidus and destroys the involved tissue in order to improve tremors and mobility.

Palpation A method of assessment that involves touching the areas related to the body system to determine symmetry, equality of the size, shape, or condition of opposite sides of the body.

Pancreatitis Inflammation of the pancreas that occurs when pancreatic enzymes are released into the pancreas itself, causing autodigestion of pancreatic tissues.

Pandemic Widespread global outbreak of an infectious disease.

Panic disorder A sudden attack of terror, sometimes accompanied by a pounding heart, sweating, fainting, or dizziness.

Pannus An abnormal tissue layer that includes newly formed blood vessels. Pannus leads to scar tissue formation that immobilizes joints.

PaO$_2$ A measure of the pressure exerted by oxygen that is dissolved in the plasma.

Para Term used to describe a woman who has borne offspring who reached the age of viability.

Paracentesis Aspiration of fluid from the peritoneal cavity.

Parallel play A stage of play in which toddlers play side by side with similar objects, but do not play together.

Paranoia An extreme suspicion that others are "out to get you" and delusions that one is being followed and that others are trying to harm oneself; experienced by some individuals with psychosis.

Paranoid personality disorder (PPD) One of several personality disorders defined in the DSM-5, it is characterized by the inability to trust others, hypervigilance, pathologic jealousy, and prejudicial and judgmental tendencies.

Paraplegia Paralysis of all or part of the lower portion of the body.

Paraphimosis Condition in which the retracted foreskin becomes trapped over the glans and tightens on the penis, causing painful swelling.

Parasite One of the four categories of microorganisms, parasites live on other organisms.

Parasomnias Abnormal behaviors that may interfere with sleep and may occur during sleep.

Parenteral nutrition (PN) The intravenous administration of amino acids, often with added carbohydrates, fats, electrolytes, vitamins, and minerals.

Parenting The ongoing act of guiding children to learn acceptable behaviors, morals, and rituals of the family and of teaching them to become socially responsible, contributing members of society.

Paresis Weakness.

Paresthesia Sensation of prickling, tingling, or numbing.

Parkinson disease (PD) A degenerative disorder of the central nervous system resulting from the death of neurons that produce the brain neurotransmitter dopamine.

Parkinsonian gait Altered gait characterized by small, shuffling steps, as well as bradykinesia or festination.

Parkinsonism The motor symptoms of Parkinson disease: tremors, muscle rigidity, postural instability, and bradykinesia.

Paroxysmal Occurring in bursts with an abrupt onset and termination.

Paroxysmal nocturnal dyspnea A sudden episode of shortness of breath occurring at night during sleep.

Partial-thickness burns Burns that involve the entire dermis and the papillae of the dermis (superficial partial-thickness burns) or extend into the hair follicles (deep partial-thickness burns).

Passive acquired immunity A condition that occurs when a pregnant woman passes IgG antibodies to a fetus in utero.

Passive behavior Behavior that seeks to avoid conflict at any cost, even at the expense of one's own happiness.

Passive communicators Individuals who focus on the needs of others. They often deny themselves any sort of power, which causes them to become frustrated.

Passive immunity Temporary protection—provided by antibodies produced by other people or animals—against disease-producing antigens. Protection is gradually lost when these acquired antibodies are used up either by natural degradation or by combining with the antigen.

Patch testing A test used to identify allergens causing dermatitis. An adhesive patch with common allergens is placed on the back between the scapulae. The patch is generally removed after several days; if there is no reaction to a particular allergen, that allergen is eliminated as a possible cause of dermatitis.

Patent airway An airway that is open and free of obstruction.

Patent ductus arteriosus (PDA) A congenital connection between the great vessels that normally closes after birth, allowing blood from the right and left side of the heart to mix.

Pathogen A microorganism that causes disease.

Pathogenicity The ability to produce disease.

Pathologic fracture A fracture that results from disease that has weakened the bone.

Patient An individual who is waiting for or undergoing medical treatment and care.

Patient advocacy Process or strategy for acting on behalf of others, including patients, families, groups, or communities, to help them obtain services and rights that they might not otherwise receive but that they need to advance their well-being.

Patient-centered medical home A model of care in which a patient's primary care provider works with the patient and family to develop a personalized plan that addresses the patient's physical and mental health needs across the lifespan.

Patient-controlled analgesia (PCA) A pump with a control mechanism that allows the patient to self-manage pain.

Patient-focused care A delivery model that organizes healthcare around the expressed physical and emotional needs of the patient.

Patient Protection and Affordable Care Act (PPACA or ACA) A law enacted during the presidency of Barak Obama designed to increase access to and affordability of healthcare. Also called *Obamacare*.

Patient record A formal, legal document that provides evidence of a patient's care. Also called a *chart* or a *clinical record*.

Patient Self-Determination Act (PSDA) A federal law that requires every competent adult to be informed in writing on admission to a healthcare institution about his or her rights to accept or refuse medical care and to use advance directives.

Pauciarticular arthritis A form of juvenile rheumatoid arthritis that primarily affects the knees, ankles, and elbows; it occurs more frequently in females.

Peak expiratory flow rate (PEFR) A measurement used to monitor the ability of an individual to exhale a specific volume of air related to the individual's age, gender, height, and weight.

Pedagogy The study or science of teaching, specifically referring to children and adolescents.

Pedigree The graphic representation of a family tree, usually to trace genetic abnormalities.

Peer review A method to professionally critique a colleague's work based on predetermined standards.

Pelvic cavity Bony portion of the birth passage; a curved canal with a longer posterior than anterior wall.

Pelvic diaphragm Part of the pelvic floor, composed of deep fascia and the levator ani and the coccygeal muscles.

Pelvic floor exercises Isometric exercises to strengthen the pelvic floor muscles for increased support of the neighboring organs.

Pelvic inlet Upper border of the true pelvis.

Pelvic outlet Lower border of the true pelvis.

Pelvic tilt An exercise that helps prevent or reduce back strain as it strengthens abdominal muscles. Also called *pelvic rocking*.

Penetrating injury Also called an open injury, a penetrating injury causes an open wound with focal damage around the site of the injury. When referring to eye injuries specifically, in a penetrating injury, the layers of the eye spontaneously reapproximate after entry of a sharp-pointed object or small missile (e.g., a BB) into the globe.

Penetrating trauma Trauma that occurs when a foreign object enters the body, causing damage to body structures.

Penta screen Maternal screening that measures five indicators whose presence may suggest fetal complications: AFP, beta hCG, unconjugated estriol, inhibin A, and invasive trophoblast antigen.

Penumbra A band of minimally perfused cells that surrounds a central core of dead or dying cells.

Peplau, Hildegard A nursing theorist who is widely considered the mother of psychiatric nursing; she presented nursing as a therapeutic interpersonal process, rather than as a task-oriented process.

Peptic ulcer A break in the mucosal lining of the GI tract exposed to acid-pepsin secretions, including the esophagus, stomach, and duodenum.

Peptic ulcer disease (PUD) A break in the mucous lining of the GI tract where it comes in contact with gastric juice.

Perceived loss A loss that is experienced by one person but cannot be verified by others.

Perception Awareness and interpretation of stimuli; the ability of the individual to interpret the environment.

Percussion A method of tapping the chest or back to assess underlying structures. More forceful striking of the skin with cupped hands is sometimes called *clapping*.

Percutaneous coronary revascularization (PCR) Procedures are used to restore blood flow to the ischemic myocardium in patients with CAD.

Percutaneous transluminal coronary angioplasty (PTCA) A type of PCR (see above entry) in which a balloon-tipped catheter is threaded over the guidewire, with the balloon positioned across the area of narrowing.

Perforating injury A type of eye injury in which the layers of the eye do not spontaneously reapproximate after the entry of a sharp-pointed object or small missile (e.g., a BB) into the globe, which results in rupture of the globe and potential loss of ocular contents.

Perforation Rupture, as in the penetration of ulcer through mucosal wall.

Performance improvement Quality of care improvement is directly linked to the performance of an individual, team, unit, or organization.

Pericarditis Inflammation of the pericardial tissue surrounding the heart.

Pericardium A double layer of fibroserous membrane that encases and anchors the heart.

Perimenopause A period of hormonal change during which the body gradually transitions toward permanent infertility.

Perimetrium The outermost layer of the uterus.

Perinatal loss Death of a fetus or infant that occurs between the time of conception and the end of the newborn period 28 days after birth.

Perineal body The wedge-shaped mass of fibromuscular tissue between the lower part of the vagina and the anus.

Periodic breathing A breathing pattern characterized by pauses lasting 5–15 seconds.

Periodontal disease Gum disease.

Perioperative The three phases of a surgical procedure: the preoperative phase, intraoperative phase, and postoperative phase.

Perioperative nursing care Nursing care provided during any or all of the three phases of surgery: preoperative, intraoperative, and postoperative.

Peripartum cardiomyopathy A rare but serious dysfunction of the left ventricle that occurs in the last month of pregnancy or the first 5 months postpartum in a woman with no previous history of heart disease.

Peripheral nervous system (PNS) One of two principal parts of the neurologic system, the peripheral nervous system consists of the cranial nerves and the spinal nerves.

Peripheral neuropathy A condition that results when trauma or a disease process interferes with innervation of peripheral nerves.

Peripheral pulse A pulse located away from the heart, in the foot or the wrist.

Peripheral vascular disease (PVD) A disorder in which arteriosclerosis and atherosclerosis affect circulation to peripheral tissues, particularly the lower extremities.

Peripheral vascular resistance The opposing forces or impedance to blood flow as the arterial channels become more and more distant from the heart.

Peristalsis The process of wavelike muscular contractions that propels food and digestive products through the digestive tract.

Peritoneal dialysis The process by which dialysate is instilled into the abdominal cavity through a catheter, allowed to rest there while fluids and molecules exchange, and then removed through the catheter.

Peritonitis Inflammation and bacterial infection of the abdominal area.

Pernicious anemia A disorder that results from a failure to absorb dietary vitamin B_{12}.

Perseveration Use of the same words or phrases repetitively.

Persistent A term used to describe a disease or disorder (such as rheumatoid arthritis) that lasts for a period of 3–6 months or longer.

Persistent bacteriuria The reappearance of bacteria in urine due to a persistent source of infection causing repeated infection after the initial cure.

Persistent depressive disorder Chronic depression that affects an individual for the majority of most days for at least 2 years (1 year for children and adolescents). May be interrupted by periods of normal mood that do not exceed 2 months over the course of the 2 years. Also called *dysthymic disorder*.

Persistent vegetative state A permanent condition of complete unawareness of self and the environment and loss of all cognitive functions. Also called *irreversible coma*.

Personal distance Communication characterized by moderate voice tones, less noticeable body heat and smell. Physical contact such as a handshake or touching a shoulder is possible.

Personal identity The conscious sense of individuality and uniqueness that is continually evolving throughout life.

Personal knowing A nurse's commitment to ongoing, individual self-exploration and self-actualization.

Personal space The distance people prefer in interactions with others.

Personality The individual qualities, including habitual behavior patterns, that make an individual unique; the outward expression of the inner self.

Personality disorder (PD) Rigid, stereotyped behavioral patterns that deviate markedly from the norm of an individual's culture and persist throughout the person's life. Personality disorders are characterized by a lifelong maladaptive pattern of perceiving, thinking, and relating that impairs social or occupational functioning.

Personality traits The elements and patterns that make up an individual's personality.

Pessimism A feeling that a situation is always bad and may become worse.

pH A measurement of the hydrogen ion concentration of a solution.

Phagocytosis A process by which a foreign agent or target cell is engulfed, destroyed, and digested. Neutrophils and macrophages, known as phagocytes, are the primary cells involved in phagocytosis.

Phantom pain A confusing pain syndrome that occurs following surgical or traumatic amputation of a limb. The patient experiences pain in the missing body part even though there is complete mental awareness that the limb is gone. Also called *phantom limb syndrome*.

Phase of mutual regulation Time period during which a mother and her infant seek to determine the degree of control each partner in their relationship will exert. In this phase of adjustment, a balance is sought between the needs of the mother and the needs of the infant.

Phenotype The observable expression of genetic traits.

Philadelphia chromosome The balanced translocation of chromosome 22 to chromosome 9; associated with chronic myeloid leukemia.

Phimosis Tightness of the prepuce that prevents retraction of the foreskin.

Phobia An intense, persistent, irrational fear of a simple thing or social situation that compels the individual to avoid the stressor that elicits the fear.

Photophobia Sensitivity to light.

Physical activity Body movement produced by skeletal muscle contraction that increases energy expenditure.

Physical fitness The ability to carry out tasks with vigor and alertness and without fatigue, while still maintaining enough energy for other tasks.

Physical attending The conveyed act of being with another individual through physical posturing.

Physical restraint Any manual method, material, device, or equipment that is attached to the patient's body with the intention of limiting or restricting free movement of the patient's head, arms, legs, or body.

Physiologic anemia of infancy A type of anemia that occurs as a result of the normal, gradual drop in hemoglobin for the first 6–12 weeks of life.

Physiologic anemia of pregnancy Apparent anemia that results because during pregnancy the plasma volume increases more than the erythrocytes increase. Also called *pseudoanemia*.

Physiologic jaundice A yellow discoloration of the skin caused by accelerated destruction of fetal red blood cells, impaired conjugation of bilirubin, and increased bilirubin reabsorption from the intestinal tract.

Physiologic pain Experienced when an intact, properly functioning nervous system sends signals that tissues are damaged, requiring attention and proper care.

Physiologic tremors Tremors that occur normally as a result of physiologic exhaustion or emotional stress.

Pica The craving for and persistent eating of nonnutritive substances not ordinarily considered to be edible or nutritionally valuable, such as soil, clay, and soap.

PICOT A mnemonic method used by clinicians to define and formulate a clinical question driving the search for evidence-based practice. PICOT stands for Population of a group, Intervention or activity focus, Comparison group, Outcome(s) or desired effects, and Time frame.

Pigmented basal cell carcinoma A type of skin cancer.

Pill-rolling Rubbing of the thumb and fingers together accompanying other tremors.

Piloerection Goosebumps.

Pilot projects Limited trials to determine problems with problem-solving alternatives. Pilot project strategies may resemble research projects and may be linked to quality improvement initiatives.

Pitch The frequency of vibrations in a sound.

Pitfall A hidden trap that catches people unaware and undermines their plans.

Pitting edema Edema that retains indentation caused by pressure.

Placenta A flat, disc-shaped organ that is highly vascular and normally forms in the upper segment of the endometrium of the uterus; exchanges nutrients and gases between the fetus and the mother.

Placenta previa Occurs when the placenta partially or totally covers the mother's cervix; can result in severe bleeding before or during delivery.

Placental abruption A condition that occurs when the placenta detaches from the uterine wall before delivery. May or may not result in fetal demise, but a fetus's survival depends on the stage of development and prompt medical treatment.

Plan–do–study–act (PDSA) A system of quality improvement most often associated with total quality management.

Planning The four-stage managerial process that establishes objectives, evaluates the present situation in order to predict future trends and events, formulates a planning statement, and converts the plan into an action statement.

Plaque 1. An invisible soft film that adheres to the enamel surface of teeth. Consists of bacteria, saliva molecules, and remnants of epithelial cells and leukocytes. 2. Scar tissue on myelin sheath due to repeated attacks by the immune system.

Plateau phase A phase of the **sexual response cycle** during which individuals experience strong, prolonged sexual arousal. The plateau phase is typically maintained by physical stimulation.

Plasmapheresis Removal of a harmful component from plasma. Also called *plasma exchange therapy*.

Play therapist A therapist who designs and provides recreational activities to promote emotional and/or physical healing and wellness.

Pleural effusion Accumulation of excess fluid in the pleural cavity.

Pleural friction rub Associated with pleural inflammation, it occurs when inflamed pleural surfaces slide across one another. This low-pitched, crackling sound typically is present during both inspiration and expiration.

Pleural space The region between the visceral and parietal pleura.

Pleuritic pain Sharp localized chest pain that increases with breathing and coughing.

Pleuritis Local extension of an infection to involve the pleura.

Pleximeter The middle finger of the nondominant hand. Often used in indirect percussion techniques.

Plexor The middle finger of the dominant hand. Often used in indirect percussion techniques.

Pneumatic retinopexy A surgical procedure to correct retinal detachment in which air is injected into the vitreous cavity and the patient is positioned so that the air bubble pushes the detached portion of the retina into contact with the choroid.

Pneumocystis jirovecii **pneumonia** An opportunistic infection that is not pathogenic in those with intact immune systems.

Pneumomediastinum The presence of air in the mediastinum.

Pneumonia Inflammation of the lung parenchyma (the respiratory bronchioles and alveoli).

Pneumopericardium Air in the pericardial sac.

Pneumothorax A partial lung collapse due to air or gas collecting in the lung or in the pleural space that surrounds the lungs.

Point of care Interventions or testing that provides on-the-spot information about the patient rather than having to send blood or urine samples down to the laboratory and wait for results to be returned.

Point of maximal impulse (PMI) A pulse located at the apex of the heart. Also called the *apical pulse*.

Point-of-service (POS) plan An insurance plan that allows the insured to choose between a health maintenance organization or a preferred provider organization each time they seek healthcare.

Polyarticular arthritis A form of juvenile rheumatoid arthritis that involves many joints (five or more), particularly the small joints of the hands and fingers. It may also affect the hips, knees, feet, ankles, and neck.

Polycyclic Describes a periodically recurring course of rheumatoid arthritis.

Polycythemia An increase in the production of red blood cells.

Polydipsia Excessive thirst.

Polyneuropathies Bilateral sensory disorders; they are the most common types of neuropathy associated with diabetes.

Polyp A small vascular growth on the surface of any mucous membrane.

Polyphagia Excessive hunger.

Polysomnography (PSG) A recording of the biophysical changes that a patient experiences during sleep.

Polysubstance abuse The simultaneous use of many substances.

Polyuria The production of abnormally large amounts of urine. Also called *diuresis*.

Pop-ups Unexpected things or events occurring during the day that require time and attention in addition to the regular plan for the day.

Positive end-expiratory pressure (PEEP) Mechanical ventilation in which a positive pressure is maintained in the airways during exhalation and between breaths to help keep alveoli open.

Positive feedback Output of a system that returns to the system as input and which promotes system change.

Positive pressure ventilator A mechanical device that pushes air into the lungs through an invasive device such as an endotracheal tube or tracheostomy tube, rather than drawing air in by negative pressure.

Positive punishment The addition of a negative consequence if undesirable behavior occurs.

Positive reinforcement Giving rewards such as praise or encouragement for a learner's achievements.

Positive symptoms Excessive or added behaviors that are not normally seen in healthy adults, such as delusions; commonly seen in schizophrenia.

Postanesthesia care unit (PACU) Designated unit for postoperative recovery of patients who do not require intensive care following a surgical procedure with anesthesia.

Postcoital contraception A drug taken after intercourse to avoid pregnancy. Also called *Plan B* or the *morning after pill*.

Postconception age periods Period of time in embryonic/fetal development calculated from the time of fertilization of the ovum.

Postconcussion syndrome A series of concussion-like symptoms that occur 7–10 days after a concussion. Manifestations include nausea, headache, dizziness, fatigue, memory problems, difficulty concentrating, insomnia, light and noise sensitivity, and/or personality changes.

Postictal period A period immediately following seizure activity in which level of consciousness is decreased. The length of the postictal period varies.

Postmenopausal bleeding Bleeding that occurs after menopause has occurred; may be caused by endometrial polyps, endometrial hyperplasia, or uterine cancer.

Postoperative The third phase of an operative process in which recovery occurs.

Postpartal hemorrhage A loss of blood of greater than 500 mL following birth. The hemorrhage is classified as *early* if it occurs within the first 24 hours and *late* if it occurs after the first 24 hours.

Postpartum After childbirth.

Postpartum blues A maternal adjustment reaction occurring in the first few postpartum days, characterized by mild depression, tearfulness, anxiety, headache, and irritability. Also called *adjustment reaction to depressed mood*.

Postpartum depression A severe form of depression that affects new mothers, often beginning within 3 months of delivery but which may strike at any time during the first year after having a child. Also called *depressive disorder with peripartum onset*.

Postpartum endometritis (metritis) An inflammation of the endometrium portion of the uterine lining occurring anytime up to 6 weeks postpartum.

Postpartum psychosis Severe psychosis occurring within the first 3 months after birth that usually requires hospitalization.

Postterm labor Labor that occurs after 42 weeks' gestation.

Postterm newborn Any infant born after 42 weeks' gestation.

Postterm pregnancy Pregnancy that lasts beyond 42 weeks' gestation.

Posttraumatic stress disorder (PTSD) A trauma- and stressor-related disorder that can evolve after exposure to a traumatic or overwhelming event in which an individual's physical health was endangered.

Postural drainage The drainage by gravity of secretions from various lung segments.

PPD Tuberculin skin test. See Purified protein derivative.

Prader–Willi syndrome (PWS) A congenital disorder of the 15th chromosome that causes an unrelenting feeling of hunger, but also low muscle tone, short stature, incomplete sexual development, mild to severe mental retardation, and behavioral problems.

Prayer Human communication with divine and spiritual entities.

Preceptor An experienced nurse who provides knowledge and emotional support, as well as a clarification of role expectations, on a one-to-one basis.

Precipitating factor A practice, behavior, or environmental factor that gives rise to a specific incident of violence.

Predisposing factor A practice, behavior, or environmental factor that increases the potential of an individual's risk of violent victimization or perpetration of violence.

Preeclampsia An increase in blood pressure after 20 weeks of gestation accompanied by proteinuria. May also be accompanied by albuminuria and edema. Also called *toxemia of pregnancy.*

Preferred provider organization (PPO) A type of health insurance program that does not require its insureds to select a primary care provider. PPOs usually have larger networks of providers than health maintenance organizations (HMOs) and provide financial incentives that encourage insureds to seek care from in-network providers. They are less restrictive than HMOs but typically have higher copayments.

Prejudice A negative belief or preference that is generalized about a group that leads to prejudgment.

Preload The amount of cardiac muscle fiber tension, or stretch, that exists at the end of diastole.

Premature ejaculation Ejaculation that occurs consistently before or shortly after penetration; i.e., before both partners are able to achieve satisfaction.

Premature junctional contractions Heartbeats that occur before the next expected beat of the underlying rhythm.

Premature rupture of membranes (PROM) Spontaneous rupture of membranes and leakage of amniotic fluid before the onset of labor at any gestational age.

Premenstrual syndrome (PMS) A complex of manifestations (e.g., mood swings, breast tenderness, fatigue, irritability, food cravings, and depression) that occurs 3–14 days before menstruation and is relieved by the onset of menses.

Prenatal education Programs offered to expectant families, adolescents, women, or partners to provide education regarding the pregnancy, labor, and birth experience.

Preoperative The first phase of an operative process in which the patient is identified as a candidate for surgical intervention, assessed, and prepared for surgery.

Preorgasmic Never having had an orgasm.

Preparedness The phase that takes place before an emergency occurs during which risks are assessed and plans are developed to address them.

Preprocedure verification process A standardized process used to verify that the correct procedure is being implemented on the correct patient at the correct site, and that all items necessary for the procedure are available.

Presbycusis Age-related loss of the ability to hear high-frequency sounds; may occur because of cochlear hair cell degeneration or loss of auditory neurons in the organ of Corti.

Presbyopia Impaired near vision resulting from a loss of elasticity of the lens related to aging.

Presencing Being present with a patient and being open, receptive, and available at all levels without judging or labeling.

Presenting part The first part of the fetus to enter and settle in the pelvic inlet during fetal presentation.

Pressure injury Ischemic lesions of the skin and underlying tissue caused by external pressure that impairs the flow of blood and lymph.

Preterm infant An infant born at less than 37 completed weeks of gestation.

Preterm premature rupture of the membranes (PPROM) A condition that occurs when membranes rupture and amniotic fluid leaks from the vagina before 37 weeks of gestation.

Pretibial myxedema The bilateral formation of edematous, erythematous, and sometimes hyperpigmented plaques and nodules over the shins and dorsal surface of the feet. A characteristic sign of Graves disease.

Priapism Persistent, painful erection of the penis.

Primary appraisal The evaluation of an event or circumstance in terms of its potential to harm, benefit, threaten, or challenge the individual.

Primary care provider (PCP) A healthcare provider who provides basic medical service and acts as a gatekeeper to more specialized care, referring patients to in-network hospitals and specialists.

Primary group A small, intimate group in which the relationships among members are personal, spontaneous, sentimental, cooperative, and inclusive.

Primary hypertension A persistently elevated systemic blood pressure. Also called *essential hypertension.*

Primary immune response When an individual is exposed to an antigen, the B-lymphocyte system produces antibodies that react specifically with that antigen over the first 3 days.

Primary intention healing Healing that occurs where the tissue surfaces have been closed and there is minimal or no tissue loss. It is characterized by the formation of minimal granulation tissue and scarring. Also called *primary union* or *first intention healing.*

Primary nursing A model in which one nurse has 24/7 authority and responsibility for the care of an assigned group of patients.

Primary prevention Methods designed to focus on health promotion and illness prevention.

Primary sex characteristics The reproductive organs.

Primigravida A woman who is pregnant for the first time.

Primipara Term used to describe a woman who has given birth to her first child (past the point of viability), whether or not that child is living or was alive at birth.

Principles-based (deontologic) theories Theories that involve logical and formal processes and emphasize individual rights, duties, and obligations.

Prioritizing care A process that helps nurses manage time and establish an order for completing responsibilities and care interventions for a single patient or for a group of patients.

Priority Something given or meriting attention before competing alternatives.

Privacy The right of individuals to keep their personal information from being disclosed.

Private insurance Health insurance provided by private or publicly owned companies such as Blue Cross Blue Shield, Kaiser, or Aetna.

Probiotics Microorganisms that aid in digestion and help to protect the body from harmful bacteria.

Problem-focused coping Managing or altering a stressor, event, or circumstance in response to distress.

Problem, intervention, evaluation (PIE) An assessment system consisting of patient care flow sheets and progress notes.

Problem-oriented medical record (POMR) A recording system in which data are arranged according to the problems the patient has rather than the source of the information. Also called *problem-oriented record (POR)*.

Problem-oriented record (POR) See Problem-oriented medical record (POMR).

Procedural memory Recall of information that does not require conscious awareness and involves the memory of motor skills and procedures.

Process addictions Compulsive behaviors that serve to reduce anxiety such as workaholism, gambling, shopping, cutting, pornography, spending and indebtedness, internet surfing or gaming, eating disorders, and sexual addictions.

Process standards Standards that focus on the steps used to lead to a particular outcome. It is used to determine if a set of steps exists and if those steps are being followed.

Productivity The performance measure of both the effectiveness and efficiency of nursing care.

Profession An occupation that requires extensive education or a calling that requires special knowledge, skill, and preparation.

Professional behaviors Effective nursing actions based on ethical principles, clinical reasoning, and technical knowledge and expertise that form helping relationships.

Professional development Continued staff education, planned activities to enhance role performance, and defined goals to improve patient outcomes. Also called *staff development*.

Professional support Assistance provided by professionals in the community who exhibit a nonblaming and respectful attitude toward families and patients and who provide information and help locating community resources.

Professionalism Acting with the knowledge, skill, and preparation of a professional.

Professionalization The process of establishing qualifications, ethical guidelines, and a standardized knowledge base by which an occupation transforms itself into a profession.

Progesterone Hormone produced by the corpus luteum, adrenal cortex, and placenta whose function is to stimulate proliferation of the endometrium to facilitate growth of the embryo.

Projectile vomiting Vomiting in which emesis may be spewed up to 2–3 feet out of a baby's mouth. A major symptom of pyloric stenosis.

Prone Face-down.

Proprioception The body's sense of its position.

Proptosis Forward displacement of the eye.

Prospective payment system (PPS) A system in which hospitals determine the amount to be billed to the insurance company before the patient is ever admitted to the hospital.

Prostaglandins (PGs) Complex lipid compounds synthesized by many cells of the body.

Prostate specific antigen (PSA) A protein produced in the cells of the prostate gland.

Prostatectomy Surgical removal of part or all of the prostate gland.

Prostatitis An inflammation of the prostate gland.

Prostatodynia A condition in which the patient experiences the symptoms of prostatitis, but shows no evidence of inflammation or infection.

Protected health information Personal information or healthcare data that could identify an individual. This information is protected and defined by HIPAA's Privacy Rule.

Protective factor 1. A practice, behavior, or environmental factor that provides strength and assistance to children and families in dealing with crises and risk factors. 2. A practice, behavior, or environmental factor that decreases the potential of an individual to perpetuate violence or victimization.

Protein A macronutrient that contains nitrogen and is a critical component of all tissues in the human body, including muscle, bone, and blood.

Protein-calorie malnutrition Problem of patients with long-term deficiencies in caloric intake; characteristics include depressed visceral proteins (e.g., albumin), weight loss, and visible muscle and fat wasting.

Proteinuria Excess protein in urine.

Proxemics The study of distance between people in their interactions.

Proximodistal Growth that proceeds from the center of the body outward.

Proximodistal development Development that proceeds from the center of the body outward.

Pruritus Itching of the skin.

Pseudoaddiction A term applied to patients who display drug-seeking behaviors but differ from addicts in that they have true underlying pain for which they are seeking relief. These behaviors will generally stop when adequate pain control is achieved.

Pseudoexacerbation A temporary aggravation of symptoms that is directly related to a trigger and subsides as soon as the trigger is removed.

Pseudomenstruation Blood or whitish discharge may occasionally be observed on the diapers of female newborns caused by the withdrawal of maternal hormones.

Purified protein derivative (PPD) Used to screen for tuberculosis in a tuberculin test. A small amount of the PPD is injected and the body's response interpreted.

Purulent exudate A large quantity of cells and necrotic debris that form an opaque or milky discharge that is thicker than serous exudate. Also called *pus* or *suppuration*.

Pus The common name for *purulent exudate.*

Psychoanalytic theory A framework for personality development that emphasizes the presence of unconscious impulses and their influence on behaviors and the formation of self; developed by Sigmund Freud (1856–1939).

Psychogenic pain Pain that is experienced in the absence of any diagnosed physiologic cause or event.

Psychomotor domain The learning domain that includes fine motor skills. Also called the *skill domain.*

Psychomotor retardation A state in which thinking and body movements are noticeably slower than normal and speech is slowed or absent.

Psychosis A mental health condition characterized by delusions, hallucinations, illusions, disorganized behavior, and a difficulty relating to others. Also called *psychotic disorder.*

Psychosocial skills Skills that enable an individual in crisis to maintain relationships with family and friends throughout and after the crisis period.

Psychostimulants Stimulants that have a high potential for abuse. Psychostimulants include cocaine and amphetamines.

Psychoticism One of the six trait domains associated with personality disorders that is composed of eccentricity, cognitive and perceptual dysregulation, and unusual beliefs and experiences.

Ptosis Drooping of the eyelid.

Ptyalism Excessive, often bitter salivation.

Puberty The stage during which an individual reaches sexual maturity.

Pubis Pertaining to the pubes or pubic area.

Public distance Communication that requires loud, clear vocalizations with careful enunciation.

Public insurance Health insurance financed by the government.

Public self How the individual wishes to be perceived by others.

Puerperium That time immediately following childbirth during which physiologic changes that occurred during pregnancy begin to return to normal. Also called *postpartum period.*

Pulmonary atresia The absence of communication between the right ventricle and the pulmonary artery.

Pulmonary circulation Circulation through the right side of the heart, the pulmonary artery, the pulmonary capillaries, and the pulmonary vein.

Pulmonary edema An abnormal accumulation of fluid in the interstitial tissue and alveoli of the lung.

Pulmonary embolism (PE) The obstruction of blood flow in part of the pulmonary vascular system by an embolus. Also called *pulmonary thromboembolism.*

Pulmonary function test (PFT) A test designed to provide information about ventilation airflow, lung volume, and the capacity and diffusion of gas.

Pulmonary vascular resistance The force or resistance of the blood in the pulmonary circulation.

Pulse A wave of blood created by the contraction of the left ventricle of the heart.

Pulse oximetry A noninvasive method of assessing arterial blood oxygenation.

Pulse pressure The difference between the systolic and diastolic pressure.

Pulse rhythm The pattern of the beats and the intervals between the beats.

Punctual On time.

Punishment 1. Action taken to enforce rules when a child misbehaves. 2. Consequences that lead to a decrease in undesirable behavior.

Pupillary light reflex Reflex in which the pupil contracts in response to a bright light.

Purging Self-induced vomiting or misuse of laxatives, diuretics, or enemas.

Pursed-lipped breathing Exhaling through a narrow opening between the lips to prolong the expiratory phase in an effort to promote more alveolar emptying while maintaining open alveoli.

Pyelolithotomy An incision into and removal of a stone from the kidney pelvis.

Pyelonephritis Inflammation of the renal pelvis and parenchyma, the functional kidney tissue.

Pyloric stenosis A thickening of the pyloric muscle resulting in a narrowing of the pyloric sphincter between the stomach and small intestine.

Pyogenic bacteria Bacteria that produces purulent exudate or pus.

Pyorrhea Advanced periodontal disease.

Pyuria Cloudy or pus-filled urine.

Quadriplegia Complete loss of function of the upper and lower body, including the arms, trunk, legs, and pelvic organs. Also called *tetraplegia.*

Quadruple screen The most widely used test to screen for Down syndrome (trisomy 21), trisomy 18, and neural tube defects.

Qualifiers Words that have been added to some NANDA nursing diagnosis labels to give additional meaning to the diagnostic statement.

Qualitative research Investigates a question through narrative data from interviews, storytelling, and description of observation to provide a better understanding of the patient's perspective.

Quality 1. A subjective description of a sound, for example: whistling, gurgling, or snapping. 2. The degree to which health services for individuals and populations increase the likelihood of desired health outcomes and are consistent with current professional knowledge.

Quality and Safety Education for Nurses (QSEN) A program designed to identify and standardize the six core competencies or nursing: patient-centered care, teamwork and collaboration, evidence-based practice, quality improvement, safety, and informatics.

Quality assurance The process of collecting data related to a problem and then analyzing the data based on benchmark standards to determine if standards are being met.

Quality improvement The process of using systematic and continuous actions that lead to measurable improvement in healthcare services and the health status of targeted patient groups.

Quality management The evaluation of medical and nursing processes for quality and effectiveness compared to accepted standards in order to correct problems before they harm patients and to prevent errors in treatment.

Quantitative research Uses precise measurements for data collection and employs statistical analysis to provide specific and objective data about a topic.

Quickening The mother's perception of fetal movement.

Race A term used to describe socially defined populations that share genetically transmitted physical characteristics, such as skin color and bone structure.

Racism The oppression of a group of people based on their perceived race.

Radiation The process of heat transfer with no physical contact.

Radiation cataracts A type of cataract that may result from long-term exposure to radiation.

Radical mastectomy The removal of an entire affected breast, its underlying chest muscles, and the lymph nodes under the arms. Compare with Simple mastectomy.

Range of motion (ROM) The degree to which a joint can be moved; a measurement of flexion and extension.

Range-of-motion (ROM) exercises Exercises designed to take each joint through all possible movements to maintain flexibility and movement in the joint.

Rape Any penetration, no matter how slight, of the vagina or anus with any body part or object, or oral penetration by a sex organ of another person, without the consent of the victim.

Rape-trauma syndrome (RTS) A series of psychologic sequelae that many victims experience following rape in addition to physiologic sequelae.

Rapport An understanding between two or more people.

Readiness to learn The demonstration of behaviors or cues that reflect a learner's motivation to learn at a specific time.

Real self The perceived true self.

Reappraisal An individual's ongoing evaluation and reinterpretation of an event or circumstance, as well as continued evaluation of the efficacy of the coping strategies.

Receiver This is the third component of the communication process. The receiver is the listener, who listens, observes, and attends.

Receptive speech The ability to understand the spoken word.

Receptor A nerve cell that converts a stimulus to a nerve impulse. Most receptors are specific, that is, sensitive to only one type of stimulus.

Record A formal, legal document that provides evidence of a patient's care. Also called a *patient record* or a *clinical chart.*

Recording The process of making an entry on a patient record. Also called *charting* or *documenting.*

Recovery 1. Return to (or exceed) preillness levels of functioning. 2. A continued state of voluntary sobriety in which an individual maintains personal health and functions normally. 3. A phase of mental illness in which symptoms of the disorder are present but under control.

Recurrence A later recurrence of a disorder after recovery.

Red blood cells (RBCs) Blood cells shaped like biconcave discs that contain the hemoglobin required for oxygen transport to body tissues; the most common type of blood cell. Also called *erythrocytes.*

Reduction Surgical placement of a broken bone in the correct alignment.

Referred pain Pain that is perceived in an area distant from the site of the stimuli.

Reflection The action of making sense of occurrences, situations, or decisions by carefully considering the totality of the experience: what worked or did not work, what could have been done differently to achieve better outcomes, what was done well, what necessary resources were available, and so on.

Reflexes The rapid, involuntary, predictable motor responses to a stimulus.

Reflux A backward flow of acidic secretions into the lower esophagus.

Refraction The bending of light rays as they pass from one medium to another medium of different optical density.

Refractory hypoxemia The decrease of particle arterial oxygen despite administration of oxygen at high flow rates.

Refractory period A phase during which myocardial cells resist stimulation.

Refractory septic shock A persistently low mean arterial blood pressure despite vasopressor therapy and adequate fluid resuscitation.

Regeneration The replacement or renewal of destroyed tissue cells by cells that are identical or similar in structure and function.

Registered nurses (RNs) The members of a nursing team who are specially licensed and trained to deliver direct patient care, including patient assessment, identification of health problems, and development and coordination of care.

Regurgitation The backflow of blood into the atria during systole.

Rehabilitation A level of wellness in which symptoms of the condition are under control to the extent that the affected individual can engage in goal-directed activities.

Reinfection The development of a new infection with a different pathogen following successful treatment.

Reinforcement Consequences that lead to an increase in a particular behavior.

Relapse Return of an acute phase of illness after recovery.

Relapsing fever Short febrile periods of a few days are interspersed with periods of 1–2 days of normal temperature.

Relationship-based (caring) theories Theories that stress courage, generosity, commitment, and the need to nurture and maintain relationships.

Relaxation response A healthful physiologic state that can be elicited through deep relaxation breathing with emphasis on a prolonged exhalation phase.

Religion A set of doctrines accepted by a group of people who gather together regularly to worship that offers a means to relate to God or a higher power; an organized system of beliefs and practices.

REM sleep Rapid-eye-movement sleep that occurs during sleep about every 90 minutes and lasts 5–30 minutes. The brain is highly active in this phase, and most dreams will take place during REM sleep.

Remission 1. A period during a chronic illness in which the symptoms of the illness disappear. 2. A sustained recovery lasting 8 weeks or more.

Remittent fever A wide range of fluctuating temperatures (more than 2°C [3.6°F]), all of which are above normal and occur over a 24-hour period.

Remyelination Repair of the damaged myelin sheath by oligodendrocytes.

Renal colic Acute, severe flank pain on an affected side that develops when a stone obstructs the ureter, causing ureteral spasm.

Renal failure A condition in which the kidneys are unable to remove accumulated metabolites from the blood or produce urine, resulting in altered fluid, electrolyte, and acid–base balance.

Renal insufficiency Decrease in the kidneys' ability to conserve sodium and concentrate the urine.

Renin–angiotensin–aldosterone system System initiated by specialized receptors in the juxtaglomerular cells of the kidney nephrons that respond to changes in renal perfusion.

Repetitive strain injury A nerve, tendon, or muscle condition that occurs when the limbs are subjected to repetitive use, awkward positions, or forced positions. Also called *repetitive motion disorder*.

Repolarization The process that returns the cell to its resting, polarized state.

Report An oral, written, or electronic communication intended to convey information to others.

Research participants Volunteers for a specific study project that meet all the inclusion criteria, have been informed of all aspects of the study, and have signed informed consent.

Reservoir A source of microorganisms.

Residual urine Urine that remains in the bladder after voiding.

Resilience/resiliency The ability to function with healthy responses, even when experiencing significant stress or adversity; the personal patterns, behaviors, or processes that promote an individual's recovery from or adaptation to adversity.

Resolution phase The fourth and final phase of the sexual response cycle is marked by a return to an unaroused state.

Resonance A hollow sound, such as the sound produced by lungs filled with air.

Resource An asset that helps nurses meet patient needs.

Resource allocation The distribution of resources among competing groups of people or programs.

Respiration The act of inhaling (inspiration) and exhaling (expiration) air to transport oxygen to the alveoli so that oxygen may be exchanged for carbon dioxide, and the carbon dioxide expelled from the body.

Respiratory acidosis A condition that is caused by an excess of dissolved carbon dioxide, or carbonic acid. It is characterized by a pH of less than 7.35 and a $PaCO_2$ greater than 45 mmHg. It may be caused by hypoventilation.

Respiratory alkalosis A condition that results when pH rises above 7.45 and $PaCO_2$ falls below 35 mmHg. It is caused by hyperventilation (unusually fast respiration, or overbreathing), leading to a carbon dioxide deficit.

Respiratory depression A decrease in the depth and rate of breathing.

Respiratory syncytial virus (RSV) A highly contagious respiratory infection that affects almost all children before 2 years of age.

Response This is the fourth component of the communication process; it is the message that the receiver returns to the sender. Also called *feedback*.

Responsibility The specific accountability or liability associated with the performance of duties of a particular role.

Rest pain Cramping or aching pain in the calves of the legs, the thighs, and the buttocks that occurs while at rest.

Restless leg syndrome A neurologic sensorimotor disorder that is characterized by an overwhelming urge to move the legs when at rest.

Restraints Any devices or medications intended to protect the patient from injuring self or others through partially or fully limiting the patient's mobility.

Restrictive cardiomyopathy A disorder characterized by rigid ventricular walls that impair diastolic filling.

Reticular activating system Modulation of sleep–wake transitions that occurs when the reticular formation, a network of ascending nerves, relays information about alertness and arousal to the cerebral cortex and directs the brain's attention to sensory events.

Retinal detachment Separation of the retina or sensory portion of the eye from the choroid.

Retractions Visible sinking of the chest wall, or sunken areas seen between the ribs during inspiration.

Retrograde conduction Cardiac conduction against the normal flow or pattern.

Retrograde ejaculation Ejaculation that occurs with fluid traveling into the bladder instead of out through the urethra.

Retropulsion The tendency to topple backward when bumped or when rising, standing, or turning.

Retrospective audit An evaluation performed after a patient's discharge comparing the care provided to the patient with care provided to patients with similar conditions.

Reverse delegation A situation that occurs when someone with a lower rank delegates to someone with more authority.

Reverse triage A method in which the most severely injured or ill victims who require the greatest resources are treated last to allow the greatest number of victims to receive medical attention.

Revision surgery The replacement of an artificial joint after 10 years or more.

Reward deficiency syndrome The decreased ability to experience pleasure. Reward deficiency syndrome drives the person to seek external forms of gratification through the use of substances, pathologic gambling, or other high-risk behaviors.

Rh disease A rare condition where the mother is Rh negative while the child is Rh positive. If this condition arises, the mother's body will see the Rh-positive cells in the fetus as foreign, and will then produce antibodies to fight off the Rh-positive cells. May result in fetal demise in extreme cases.

Rheumatoid arthritis (RA) A chronic systemic autoimmune disease that causes inflammation of connective tissue, primarily in the joints.

Rhinorrhea Drainage of mucus from the nose. Commonly known as a runny nose.

Rhonchi A long, low-pitched sound that continues throughout inspiration suggesting a blockage of large airway passages.

Ribonucleic acid (RNA) One of two types of nucleic acid made by cells. Ribonucleic acid is made up of ribose rather than deoxyribose and contains information that has been copied from DNA (the other type of nucleic acid).

Rigidity Resistance to movement because of the involuntary contraction of all skeletal muscles.

Risk diagnosis A clinical judgment that a problem does not exist, but the presence of risk factors indicates a problem is likely to develop unless the nurse intervenes.

Risk factor A practice, behavior, or environmental factor that increases the potential of negative effects on an individual's health.

Risk management Preventive policies and processes that focus on limiting a healthcare agency's financial and legal risk associated with the delivery of care, particularly in terms of lawsuits.

Role A set of expectations about how an individual occupying one position behaves.

Role ambiguity Occurs when expectations are unclear and when people do not know how to perform their roles and/or are unable to predict the reactions of others to their behavior.

Role conflict Emotional conflict arising when competing demands are made on an individual in the fulfillment of his or her multiple social roles.

Role development Teaching and modeling the behaviors needed to successfully assume a particular role.

Role mastery Occurs when an individual's behaviors meet or exceed social expectations.

Role performance The demonstration of behaviors or actions associated with a given role.

Role strain The stress or strain experienced by an individual when incompatible behavior, expectations, or obligations are associated with a single social role.

Root cause analysis An evaluation required by the Joint Commission that is focused on identifying areas of improvement that would decrease the likelihood of future adverse events and to develop an action plan for improvement.

Rooting reflex In response to a light touch of a finger on an infant's cheek close to the mouth, the infant's head will rotate toward the stimulation and attempt to suck the finger.

Rotational injury An injury caused by lateral flexion or twisting of the head and neck.

Round ligaments The ligaments that hold the ovaries in place.

Rupture of membranes The rupturing of amniotic membranes before the onset of labor.

Sacral promontory A projection into the pelvic cavity on the anterior upper portion of the sacrum, which serves as a landmark for pelvic measurements.

Sarcopenia The process of atrophy due to age.

Safety Decreasing risks of dangers or hazards to prevent accidents, injuries, mistakes, and harm.

Safety culture A general feeling of shared attitudes, values, practices, and beliefs which result in behaviors and feelings of responsibility for safety in all daily routines.

Safety strap body restraint Restraints used to ensure the safety of patients who are transported by wheelchair or gurney, or to protect patients confined to a bed or a chair. Also called *belt restraint.*

Salient cue The leading, most noticeable, or most important information about a patient's health status.

Saline An isotonic solution of 0.9% sodium chloride.

Sanguineous exudate A large amount of red blood cells that form a bright or dark red discharge indicating new or old damage to capillaries. Also called *hemorrhagic exudate.*

Satiety The sensation of fullness and satisfaction that should inhibit eating until the next meal.

Saturated fat A triglyceride fat that contains all of the hydrogen ions it is capable of holding.

SBAR A method of reporting information about a patient in the following order: situation, background, assessment, and recommendation.

Scaling The rating of the severity of symptoms or problems.

Scapegoat An individual who has been selected to take the blame for another individual or for a group.

Scenario planning A group process strategy that encourages members of a group to create hypothetical or "possible future" situations.

Scheduled toileting Toileting at regular intervals.

Schemes Adaptive cognitive structures formed in response to environmental stimuli according to Jean Piaget's theory of cognitive development.

Schistocytes Fragmented red blood cells.

Schizoaffective disorder A psychotic disorder with features of both schizophrenia and mood disorders.

Schizoid personality disorder (SPD) One of several personality disorders defined in the DSM-5, it is characterized by a lifelong pattern of indifference to others, absence of humor, and social isolation.

Schizophrenia The most common psychotic disorder, schizophrenia is a combination of disordered thinking, perceptual disturbances, behavioral abnormalities, affective disruptions, and impaired social competency.

Schizophreniform disorder A disorder with rapid onset of psychotic symptoms, very similar to schizophrenia, lasting less than 6 months.

Schizotypal personality disorder One of several personality disorders defined in the DSM-5, it is characterized by a pattern of disturbed interpersonal relationships, thought patterns, appearance, and behavior.

Sciatica Lumbar back pain that radiates down the posterior leg to the ankle due to irritation or compression of all or part of the sciatic nerve.

Scleral buckling A surgical procedure to correct retinal detachment.

Scoliometer A diagnostic test used to measure a patient's rib hump when in the Adam position.

Scoliosis A lateral, or sideways, curvature of the spine.

Scoop method A safe method of recapping sharps in which the cap is placed on a needle or a hard surface and the needle is guided into the cap.

Seasonal affective disorder (SAD) A mood disorder typically characterized by depression during fall and winter and normal mood or hypomania during spring and summer.

Second heart sound (S$_2$) The heart sound produced by closure of the semilunar valves; characterized by the syllable "dub."

Second impact syndrome (SIS) A constellation of clinical manifestations that can occur when an individual receives a second concussion before the initial concussion is completely healed.

Secondary appraisal Evaluation of an individual's available coping resources and potential options for responding to an event or circumstance.

Secondary cataracts A type of cataract that may form after surgery to treat another eye disorder, such as glaucoma, or as an effect of medication or another primary disorder.

Secondary group A group that is larger, more impersonal, and less sentimental than a primary group.

Secondary hypertension Elevated blood pressure resulting from an identifiable underlying process.

Secondary immune response Subsequent encounters with an antigen following the primary immune response that result in triggering memory cells.

Secondary infertility The inability to conceive after one or more successful pregnancies, or the inability to sustain a pregnancy.

Secondary intention healing Healing that occurs when a wound's edges cannot or should not close. Repair time is typically longer, scarring is greater, and susceptibility to infection is greater.

Secondary prevention Methods that focus on the diagnosis and treatment of disease.

Secondary sex characteristics Bodily traits that develop over time and are influenced by a person's sex but not directly involved in reproduction.

Segmental mastectomy See *Lumpectomy*.

Seizures Periods of abnormal electrical discharges in the brain that cause involuntary movement, as well as behavior and sensory alterations.

Selective perception The process of filtering out unnecessary and distracting information in order to focus on what is important at any given moment.

Selective serotonin reuptake inhibitor (SSRI) A drug that selectively inhibits the reuptake of serotonin into nerve terminals; used mostly for depression.

Selectively permeable Refers to membranes separating body fluid compartments across which solutes can move with relative ease.

Self The entirety of an individual's being, including body, sensations, emotions, and thoughts, as well as a conscious awareness of one's own being.

Self-awareness The relationship between an individual's perception of himself or herself and others' perceptions of him or her.

Self-concept The personal perception of the self formed in response to interactions with others and the environment throughout the course of an individual's lifetime.

Self-efficacy The expectation that someone can produce a desired outcome.

Self-esteem One's judgment of one's own worth.

Self-help group A group of individuals who come together to face a common problem or difficulty.

Self-quieting ability The ability of newborns to use their own resources to quiet and comfort themselves.

Semen Sperm mixed with seminal fluid, ejaculated during sexual activity.

Semiformal group A group with formalized structure, delineated hierarchy, and voluntary, but selective, membership.

Sender An individual or group who wishes to convey a message to another; can be considered the *source-encoder*.

Sensate focus A mindfulness technique commonly employed as part of sex therapy.

Sensitization An increased reaction to pain over time, or a reduced threshold for reaction to painful stimuli.

Sensory memory The earliest stage of memory in which visual input and auditory information are retained for less than a few seconds.

Sensory perception The conscious organization and translation of external data or stimuli into meaningful information.

Sensory reception The process of receiving external stimuli or data. External stimuli are visual (sight), auditory (hearing), olfactory (smell), tactile (touch), and gustatory (taste).

Sentinel event An unexpected occurrence involving death or serious physical or psychologic injury, or the risk thereof.

Sepsis 1. A whole-body inflammatory process resulting in acute illness. 2. A state of infection.

Septal defect A congenital heart defect that connects the right and left side of the heart.

Septic shock Altered perfusion resulting from a systemic infection that manifests with hypotension, delayed capillary refill, and inadequate perfusion and oxygenation of vital body tissues. Also called *septicemia*.

Septicemia See Septic shock.

Serious mental illness Mental illness that is severe enough to impair daily functioning and the ability to achieve life goals.

Seroconversion Antibody response to a disease or vaccine.

Serosanguineous exudate A clear or blood-tinged discharge commonly seen in surgical incisions.

Serotonin syndrome A condition that may occur in individuals taking two or more medications that increase serotonin levels. Symptoms include hypertension or hypotension, agitation, shivering, changes in mental status, symptoms of gastrointestinal distress, restlessness, tremor, muscle rigidity, unreactive pupils, and tachypnea.

Serous exudate A watery, clear or straw-colored discharge that accompanies mild inflammation.

Serum bicarbonate (HCO$_3$) A value that reflects the renal regulation of acid–base balance. The normal HCO$_3$ value is 24–28 mEq/L.

Serum sickness A systemic type III hypersensitivity response, usually in response to a drug such as penicillin or a sulfonamide.

Servant leadership A theory of leadership rooted in the belief that the most effective leaders are those who are motivated primarily by a desire to serve, rather than a desire to lead.

Severe sepsis Sepsis associated with acute organ failure.

Seven rights of medication administration Right person, right assessment, right drug, right dose, right route, right time, right documentation.

Sex addiction Persistent, excessive sexual behaviors.

Sex chromosomes The 23rd pair of chromosomes found in a cell's nucleus; it determines an individual's gender.

Sexism When male values, beliefs, or activities are preferred over female ones.

Sexual abuse Any sexual act that is perpetrated against someone's will including rape, attempted sexual acts, unwanted sexual contact, voyeurism, and sexual harassment. Also called *sexual violence*.

Sexual aversion disorder A disorder characterized by severe distaste for sexual activity or the thought of sexual activity.

Sexual dysfunction Any persistent disturbance in an individual's sexual response.

Sexual health A state of physical, emotional, mental, and social well-being in relation to sexuality, not merely the absence of disease, dysfunction, or infirmity. Sexual health requires a positive and respectful approach to sexuality and sexual relationships.

Sexual orientation The sexual attraction of an individual to the same sex, the opposite sex, or both sexes.

Sexual self-concept How one values oneself as a sexual being.

Sexually transmitted infections (STIs) Infections transmitted by vaginal, oral, and anal intimate contact and intercourse.

SHARE A method of handoff reporting: Standardize critical content; hardwire within your system; allow opportunity to ask questions; reinforce quality and measurement; educate and coach.

Shared governance A method that aims to distribute decision making among a group of people.

Shared leadership The concept that a professional workplace is made up of many leaders.

Shared psychotic disorder A condition that results when an individual who is in a close relationship with another person who is delusional comes to share the delusional beliefs.

Shearing force A condition that results when one tissue layer slides over another.

Shock A clinical syndrome characterized by a systemic imbalance between oxygen supply and demand.

Shock phase The initial part of an alarm reaction during which the sympathetic nervous system is suppressed and an individual may experience manifestations such as hypotension, decreased body temperature, and decreased muscle tone.

Short bowel syndrome A condition in which the transit time of ingested foods and fluids is reduced and digestive processes are impaired because of a resection of significant portions of the small intestine.

Short-term memory Information held in the brain for immediate use; what an individual has in mind at a given moment.

Shunt A natural or artificially created tunnel or passage that allows blood to flow through an area.

Sickle cell anemia An inherited chronic hemolytic anemia, sickle cell anemia is the most common form of sickle cell disease.

Sickle cell crisis Severe episodes of fever and intense pain that are the hallmark of sickle cell disease. Also called *vaso-occlusive crisis*.

Sickle cell disease A hereditary hemoglobinopathy characterized by replacement of normal hemoglobin with abnormal hemoglobin S (Hgb S) in RBCs.

Sickle cell trait Carrying one copy of the defective sickle cell gene, which can be passed on to children but does not usually cause the illness.

Sickling A process in which red blood cells take on the characteristic sickle shape following deoxygenation in patients who have sickle cell disease.

Sick-role behavior A combination of illness behaviors, such as engaging in self-care and using the healthcare system, combined with dependent behaviors, such as avoiding usual responsibilities.

Signs See Objective data.

Simple assault An unlawful physical attack by one person upon another in which neither the offender displays a weapon, nor the victim suffers any obvious severe or aggravated bodily injury involving apparent broken bones, loss of teeth, possible internal injury, severe laceration, or loss of consciousness.

Simple mastectomy The removal of a complete breast only. Compare with Radical mastectomy.

Single-parent family A family in which only one parent resides in the home and is the primary caretaker and provider for the family.

Single-payer system Healthcare coverage arising from a single source, usually the government.

Situational crisis A crisis that involves an unexpected stressor or circumstance that occurs in the course of daily living.

Situational depression A maladaptive reaction to an identifiable psychosocial stressor or stressors that occurs within 3 months after the onset of the stressor and has persisted for no longer than 6 months. Also called *adjustment disorder with depressed mood*.

Situational leader A leader who is flexible in task and relationship behaviors, considers the staff members' abilities, knows the nature of the task to be done, and is sensitive to the context or environment in which the task takes place.

Six Sigma A quality improvement program originally implemented by Motorola and General Electric that focuses on reducing variation within a process to produce a near-perfect product.

Skin turgor The elasticity of skin.

Sleep An altered state of consciousness in which an individual's perception and reaction to the environment are decreased.

Sleep apnea A disorder characterized by frequent short breathing pauses during sleep.

Sleep architecture The basic organization of normal sleep.

Sleep hygiene Interventions used to promote quality sleep at night.

Sleep loss A duration of sleep shorter than the recommended 7–8 hours a night for an adult.

Small cell carcinoma A highly malignant cancer usually associated with the lung.

SMART An acronym to provide assistance in writing a patient-centered goal statement. SMART is Single action (choose a specific, single action to focus on), Measurable result (observable or measurable result), Attainable (level appropriate), Relevant (customized specifically for patient's needs), and Time-limited (specific time frame for goal to be completed).

SOAP An acronym for collective data in a progress note; it stands for subjective data, objective data, assessment, and planning.

SOAPIER Short for subjective data, objective data, assessment, plan of care, intervention, evaluation, and revision.

Sobriety A state of habitually refraining from using alcohol or drugs.

Social cognition The ability to process and apply social information accurately and effectively.

Social distance Communication characterized by a clear visual perception of the whole person. Body heat and odor are imperceptible, eye contact is increased, and vocalizations are loud enough to be overheard by others.

Social justice A framework in which to explore the complexities surrounding the variety of factors that impact diverse and vulnerable populations.

Social microcosm The concept that group members eventually behave in a therapy group the same way they behave with family and friends.

Social phobia A condition that is characterized by a pervasive, extreme fear of one or more social situations that may lead to scrutiny by others. Also called *social anxiety disorder*.

Socialization The process by which individuals learn to become members of groups and society and learn the social rules defining relationships into which they will enter.

Socialized insurance A system in which all medically necessary services are covered, including physician care, hospital services, and to some extent, prescription drugs.

Socialized medicine State government-owned and controlled healthcare services.

Solitary play A stage of play in which an infant still plays primarily alone, but enjoys the presence of others.

Solute Substance that dissolves in liquid.

Solvent The component of a solution that can dissolve a solute.

Somatic cells Cells that make up the tissue of the body, with a full complement (diploid) of chromosomes, as opposed to sex cells.

Somatic pain Pain arising from nerve receptors originating in the skin or close to the surface of the body.

Somatization The process by which psychologic distress is experienced and communicated in the form of somatic symptoms.

Somatostatin A substance, believed to be a neurotransmitter, that inhibits the production of both glucagon and insulin.

Somnology The study of sleep.

Somogyi phenomenon A combination of hypoglycemia during the night with a rebound, morning rise in blood glucose to hyperglycemic levels.

Source-oriented record Patient record in which each healthcare provider or department member makes notations in a separate section or sections of the patient's chart.

Spasticity Increased muscle tone, usually with some degree of weakness.

Specific defenses Immune system responses directed against identifiable bacteria, viruses, fungi, or other infectious agents.

Specific gravity An indicator of urine concentration that can be performed quickly and easily by nursing personnel.

Specific phobia An intense or extreme fear with regard to a particular object or situation.

Specific self-esteem How much one approves of a certain parts of oneself.

Spermatogenesis The process by which mature spermatozoa are formed.

Spermicide A cream, jelly, foam, vaginal film, or suppository that is inserted into the vagina before intercourse to destroy sperm and prevent conception.

Spinal cord A continuation of the medulla oblongata, it has the ability to transmit impulses to and from the brain via the ascending and descending pathways.

Spinal cord injury (SCI) Trauma to the spinal cord that results from excessive force to the spinal column.

Spinal cord stimulation (SCS) A form of therapy used with persistent pain that has not been controlled with less invasive therapies. SCS involves the insertion of an electrode (a single channel or multichannel device) adjacent to the spinal cord in the epidural space. The electrode(s) is attached to an impulse-generator (external or implanted) that sends electric impulses to the spinal cord to control pain.

Spinal fusion The insertion of a wedge-shaped piece of bone or bone chips between the vertebrae to stabilize them and reduce pain.

Spinal shock A condition that is characterized by spinal cord swelling, decreased blood flow and blood pressure, and complete loss of motor function, spinal reflexes, and autonomic function below the level of injury.

Spiritual distress A challenge to the spiritual well-being or to the belief system that provides strength, hope, and meaning to life; a feeling of being separated from interconnectedness with others or with a higher power.

Spiritual health The overall feeling of strength, hope, and fulfillment that encourages people to find life-sustaining and enriching opportunities.

Spiritual skills Skills that help an individual find meaning in and understand the personal significance of an unexpected event.

Spiritual support Assistance to patients and families in providing meaning and sustaining courage during difficult times.

Spiritual well-being A feeling of inner peace and of being generally alive, purposeful, and fulfilled; the feeling is rooted in spiritual values and/or specific religious beliefs.

Spirituality The part of being human that seeks meaningfulness through personal connection, which may include belief in or relationship with some higher power, creative force, driving being, or infinite source of energy.

Spirometry A means of measuring inhalation and exhalation, although the key measurements are forced expiratory volume over 1 second (FEV_1) and the ratio of FEV_1 to forced vital capacity (FEV_1/FVC). In other words, how much and how quickly an individual exhales air as measured by spirometry is an indicator of the degree of pulmonary function deficit.

Splint An easily adjustable device that stabilizes injuries, usually before swelling has subsided or after the reparative phase of healing.

Splitting 1. The inability to integrate contradictory experiences. 2. The inclination to perceive people or situations as one extreme or the other.

Spontaneous abortion The loss of a fetus prior to 20 weeks of gestation. Also called *miscarriage*.

Spontaneous rupture of membranes (SROM) The rupturing of membranes during the height of an intense contraction with a gush of fluid out of the vagina.

Sporadic AD One of the two basic types of Alzheimer disease, it shows no clear pattern of inheritance, although genetic factors may contribute to the disorder. Sporadic AD typically does not develop until after the age of 65. Also called *late-onset Alzheimer disease*.

Sprain A stretching or tearing of ligaments.

Sputum Mucus or mucopurulent matter expectorated from the lungs.

Squamous cell carcinoma A malignant tumor of the squamous epithelium of the skin or mucous membranes.

Staff authority The power to provide advice and support to employees or departments but not to assign tasks.

Staff development Continued staff education, planned activities to enhance role performance, and defined goals to improve patient outcomes. Also called *professional development*.

Stage of exhaustion Stage in which the body ceases to maintain its adaptation to a stressor; the stressor overwhelms the individual's ability to cope or mount a continued defense, resulting in the depletion of energy and resources.

Stage of resistance Stage in which the body attempts to move toward restoration of homeostasis while continuing to respond to the stressor.

Staghorn calculi A type of calculi associated with a urinary tract infection caused by urease-producing bacteria such as *Proteus*. These stones can grow to become very large, filling the renal pelvis and calyces. Also called *struvite calculi*.

Staging A system of classifying cancer according to the size of the tumor, involvement of lymph nodes, and metastasis to distant sites.

Standard precautions Safety guidelines, such as proper hand hygiene, use of proper protective equipment, safe injection practices, and effective management of potentially contaminated surfaces or equipment, that are designed to decrease the risk of transmitting unidentified pathogens. Also called *universal precautions* and *body substance isolation (BSI)*.

Standardized plan A nursing care plan that specifies the nursing care for groups of patients with common needs (e.g., all patients with myocardial infarction).

Standards Models of high-quality performance that may reflect the performance of industry leaders, scientific or clinical research, or recommendations of professional organizations such as the ANA.

Standards of care Guidelines used to determine what a nurse should or should not do, and may be defined as a benchmark of achievement based on a desired level of excellence.

Standards of practice A standardized description of the responsibilities for which nurses are responsible.

Standards of professional performance The behaviors expected in the professional nursing role by the American Nurses Association.

Station The location of the fetal presenting part in the maternal pelvis in relation to the ischial spine.

Status asthmaticus A severe, prolonged form of asthma that is difficult to treat.

Status epilepticus A continuous seizure that lasts for more than 30 minutes or a series of seizures during which time consciousness is not regained.

Statute of limitations The limit to the amount of time that can pass between recognition of harm and bringing a suit.

Statutory laws Laws made by any legislative branch of the government, including the U.S. Congress, state legislatures, and city and county governments.

Steatorrhea Fatty, frothy, foul-smelling stools caused by a decrease in pancreatic enzyme secretion.

Stem cell transplant The infusion of immature stem cells to replenish a patient's blood cell lines; used as an alternative to bone marrow transplantation.

Stenosis Narrowing of the valve, valve area, or great artery above the valve.

Stent A short, narrow tube inserted into the lumen of a vessel (e.g., artery) to relieve blockage.

Step-down therapy A gradual reduction in the dosage and number of drugs used in a therapeutic regimen.

Stepfamily Consists of a biological parent with children and a new spouse who may or may not have children.

Stereognosis The ability to perceive and understand an object through touch.

Stereotaxic thalamotomy An x-ray taken during neurosurgery to guide the insertion of a needle into a specific area of the brain.

Stereotyping The act of generalizing that all people in a group are the same.

Stereotypy Rigid and obsessive behavior.

Sterile field An area free of microorganisms.

Sterile technique Practices that keep an area or object free of all microorganisms. Also known as *surgical asepsis*.

Sterilization 1. A process that destroys all microorganisms, including spores and viruses. 2. An inclusive term that refers to surgical procedures that permanently prevent pregnancy.

Stigma A collection of negative attitudes and beliefs that lead people to fear, reject, avoid, and discriminate against people with mental illness.

Stillbirth Death of a fetus that occurs after 20 weeks of gestation. Also called *fetal demise* or *intrauterine fetal death (IUFD)*.

Stimulus The agent or act that stimulates a nerve receptor.

Stimulus-based stress model A model that defines stress as being a life event that requires change or adaptation on the part of the individual who is experiencing the life event.

Stoma An artificial opening in the abdominal wall; it may be permanent or temporary.

Stool Body wastes and undigested food eliminated from the bowel. Also called *feces*.

Strabismus Misalignment of the eyes.

Strain A stretching or tearing of a muscle or tendon.

Strategic planning The process of continual assessment, planning, and evaluation to guide future decisions and developments.

Stress The body's general, nonspecific response to the demands placed on it by a stressor.

Stress fracture A fracture that results from disease that has weakened the bone.

Stress mediators Hormonal triggers that are intended to promote adaptation through mechanisms such as triggering a necessary increase in heart rate and blood pressure when faced with physical danger.

Stress response Physiologic changes triggered by stress; includes activation of the neural, neuroendocrine, and endocrine systems, as well as activation of target organs.

Stressor An external influence that threatens to disrupt the equilibrium that is needed to maintain homeostasis.

Striae Whitish-silver stretch marks seen in obesity and during or after pregnancy.

Stridor A high-pitched sound within the trachea and larynx that suggests narrowing of the tracheal passage.

Stroke A condition in which neurologic deficits result from a sudden decrease in blood flow to a localized area of the brain. Also called *cerebrovascular accident* or *brain attack*.

Stroke volume (SV) The amount of blood pumped into the aorta with each contraction of the left ventricle that is measured by the difference between the end-diastolic volume and the end-systolic volume.

Structural-functional theory Focuses on family structure and function, examining family relationships and how they affect the functions of the family and relationships with other systems.

Structure standards Standards related to material resources, human resources, and general organizational structure.

Struvite calculi A type of calculi associated with a urinary tract infection caused by urease-producing bacteria such as *Proteus*. These stones can grow to become very large, filling the renal pelvis and calyces. Also called *staghorn stones*.

Subconjunctival hemorrhage Temporary, nonpathogenic hemorrhages that are caused by the changes in vascular tension or ocular pressure during birth.

Subculture groups Minority groups characterized by specific norms, beliefs, and values that coexist with a dominant culture.

Subcutaneous tissue The layer of loose connective tissue and fat cells that lies below the dermis. Also called *hypodermis*.

Subdermal implant Capsules implanted within the skin that slowly release medication, such as for contraception.

Subfertility Occurs when both partners of a couple have reduced fertility.

Subinvolution A slowing of the descent of the uterus during the postpregnancy healing process.

Subjective data Information that is apparent to only the patient affected and can be described or verified by only that patient. Also called *symptoms* or *covert data*.

Subjective family burden The psychologic distress of family members in relation to the objective family burden of having a family member with a mental illness.

Substance abuse The use of any chemical in a fashion inconsistent with medical or culturally defined social norms despite physical, psychologic, or social adverse effects.

Substance dependence A condition in which the patient can no longer control use of the substance, continues to use it despite adverse effects, and experiences withdrawal symptoms without continued use of the substance.

Subsystem A component of a larger system.

Sucking reflex Occurs in response to a finger or nipple inserted into an infant's mouth; the infant responds by beginning to rhythmically suck on the finger.

Suctioning Aspirating secretions through a catheter connected to a suction machine or wall suction outlet.

Sudden cardiac death (SCD) Unexpected death occurring within 1 hour of the onset of cardiovascular symptoms.

Sudden infant death syndrome (SIDS) The sudden death of an apparently healthy infant that remains unexplained after other possible causes have been ruled out through autopsy, death scene investigation, and review of the medical history.

Sudden unexpected death in epilepsy (SUDEP) Sudden and unexpected death in an individual diagnosed with epilepsy.

Suicidal ideation A case of an individual constantly considering, planning, or thinking about suicide.

Suicide An act of an individual inflicting self-harm resulting in death.

Suicide attempt An act of an individual inflicting self-harm with the intent to cause death that is not successful.

Sundowning A behavioral change commonly seen in patients with dementia, characterized by increased agitation, time disorientation, and wandering behaviors during afternoon and evening hours; it is accelerated on overcast days.

Superficial basal cell carcinoma A type of skin cancer.

Superficial burn A burn that involves only the epidermal layer of the skin.

Superficial thrombophlebitis A blood clot blocking one or more veins near the skin's surface.

Superimposed preeclampsia Occurs when a woman previously diagnosed with chronic hypertension develops hypertension-related end-organ dysfunction in pregnancy or worsening hypertension that is resistant to treatment.

Supersaturated urine A condition that results when the concentration of salt in the urine is very high.

Supine On the back.

Suppuration A large quantity of cells and necrotic debris that form an opaque or milky discharge that is thicker than serous exudate. Also called *pus* or *purulent exudate*.

Suprasystem An overarching system to which smaller systems or subsystems belong. For example, the family is the suprasystem of the individual.

Surface temperature Body temperature taken at the skin's surface that may rise or fall in response to the environment.

Surfactant Specialized cells that control surface tension and keep alveoli from collapsing and sticking to themselves.

Surge capacity A community's ability to rapidly meet the increased demand for qualified personnel and resources, including healthcare resources, in the event of a disaster.

Surgical asepsis Practices that keep an area or object free of all microorganisms. Also called *sterile technique*.

Surgical debridement The process of excising a wound to the level of fascia or sequentially removing thin slices of a burn wound to the level of viable tissue.

Sutures The membranous spaces between the cranial bones of a fetus.

Swan-neck deformity Caused by rheumatoid arthritis, it is characterized by hyperextension of the proximal interphalangeal joints with compensatory flexion of the distal interphalangeal joints.

Sweat test Typically administered twice, it measures the amount of salt in the baby's sweat and is most effective for a CF diagnosis; a high level of salt confirms the diagnosis.

Switching A term used in disorders of mood and affect to describe a new illness phase (manic or depressed) without recovery.

Symmetry Equality of the size, shape, or condition of opposite sides of the body.

Sympathetic tone A state of partial smooth muscle contraction around arteries and veins.

Symphysis pubis Fibrocartilaginous joint between the pelvic bones in the midline.

Symptom See Subjective data.

Synchronized cardioversion Delivery of direct electrical current synchronized with the patient's heart rhythm.

Synclitism A condition that occurs when the sagittal suture is midway between the symphysis pubis and the sacral promontory and is felt to be aligned.

Syncope Transient loss of consciousness and muscle tone after exercise or activity.

Syndrome diagnosis A cluster of nursing diagnoses that occur together and may result in best patient outcomes if addressed at the same time.

Synovectomy Excision of synovial membrane; this procedure is used as a treatment for rheumatoid arthritis.

Synovitis Inflammation of the synovial membrane lining the articular capsule of a joint.

Syphilis A complex systemic sexually transmitted infection caused by the spirochete *Treponema pallidum*.

System A set of interacting identifiable parts or components.

Systematized delusions A manifestation of schizophrenia characterized by an extensively developed central delusional theme from which conclusions are deduced.

Systemic arthritis A form of juvenile rheumatoid arthritis that characteristically is manifested by high fever, polyarthritis, and rheumatoid rash. Systemic arthritis also affects internal organs and joints.

Systemic circulation Circulation through the left side of the heart, the aorta and its branches, the capillaries that supply the brain and peripheral tissues, the systemic venous system, and the vena cava.

Systemic infection Occurs when an invading microorganism spreads and damages different parts of the body.

Systemic inflammatory response syndrome (SIRS) Describes the body's response to a critical illness that can result from an infectious or noninfectious cause precipitating a whole-body inflammatory process.

Systemic lupus erythematosus (SLE) A chronic, inflammatory connective tissue disease.

Systemic response Results because of a widespread antibody-antigen reaction. Systemic responses include anaphylaxis, urticaria, or angioedema.

Systemic vascular resistance The force or resistance of the blood in the body's blood vessels that helps return blood to the heart.

Systems theory The study of how a system operates, including how it interacts with other systems and how its components interact with each other within the system itself.

Systole The phase of ventricular contraction.

Systolic blood pressure The maximum pressure exerted within the arteries when the heart compresses.

T lymphocyte (T cells) A type of leukocyte that matures in the thymus gland and is integral to the specific immune response.

Tachycardia An excessively fast heart rate greater than 100 bpm in an adult.

Tachypnea A respiratory rate greater than 20 bpm in adults.

Tactile Of or relating to touch.

Tangential excision The sequential removal of thin slices of a burn wound to the level of viable tissue.

Tanner stages Stages of physical growth of the breasts and pubic hair in girls and the genitalia and pubic hair in boys.

Tardive dyskinesia A condition characterized by repetitive, involuntary body movement of varying severity that may not cease after medication cessation; includes unusual tongue and face movements such as lip smacking and wormlike motions of the tongue.

Tartar A visible, hard deposit of plaque and dead bacteria that forms at the gumlines. Also called *dental calculus*.

Tau A protein found in the neurons.

Teach-back method A patient teaching strategy in which the nurse provides information to a patient and asks the patient to restate the information to ensure that the patient understands it correctly.

Teaching A system of activities intended to produce learning.

Team Two or more individuals who agree to work in tandem to accomplish a common goal.

Team nursing The delivery of individualized nursing care to a group of patients by a team led by a professional nurse.

Telangiectatic nevi Pale pink or red spots frequently found on the eyelids, nose, lower occipital bone, and nape of the neck of young children. These areas have no clinical significance and usually fade by the second birthday. Also called *stork bites*.

Telecommunication The transmission of information from one site to another, using equipment to send information in the form of signs, signals, words, or pictures by cable, radio, or other systems.

Telehealth A system that employs the use of telecommunications technologies (e.g., videoconferencing, streaming media, real-time forwarding imaging, and land-based and wireless communications) to allow patients access to care that they might not otherwise be able to obtain. Also called *telemedicine* or *remote patient monitoring*.

Telenursing The provision of nursing care via **telecommunication**.

Temperament The combination of biological and physical characteristics that influence personality and behavior specific to each individual.

Tender points Tenderness that occurs in precise, localized areas, particularly in the neck, spine, shoulders, and hips.

Tendon Tissue that connects bones to muscles and carries the contractile forces from the muscle to the bone to cause movement.

Tendonitis Inflammation of a tendon.

Teratogen Any substance that adversely affects the normal growth and development of the fetus.

Terminal weaning The gradual withdrawal of mechanical ventilation when survival without assisted ventilation is not expected.

Territoriality A concept of the space and things that an individual considers as belonging to the self.

Tertiary intention healing Healing that occurs after closing a wound that has been left open for 3–5 days to allow edema or infection to resolve. Also called *delayed primary intention*.

Tertiary prevention Methods that focus on the restoration of health following an illness or accident and include rehabilitation and palliative services.

Testosterone The primary male sex hormone produced by the testes.

Tetany Tonic muscle spasms.

Tetralogy of Fallot A rare disease that consists of four defects: pulmonic stenosis, right ventricular hypertrophy, ventricular-septal defect, and an overriding aorta.

Tetraplegia Complete loss of function of the upper and lower body, including the arms, trunk, legs, and pelvic organs. Also called *quadriplegia*.

Thalassemia Inherited disorder of hemoglobin synthesis in which either the alpha or beta chains of the hemoglobin molecule are missing or defective.

Thelarche The beginning of breast development in females.

Therapeutic communication An interactive process between the nurse and the patient that helps the patient to overcome temporary stress, to get along with other people, to adjust to situations that cannot be altered, and to overcome any psychologic blocks that may stand in the way of self-realizations.

Therapeutic insemination The process of depositing semen at the cervical os or in the uterus by mechanical means.

Therapeutic relationship Nurse–patient relationship that is focused on helping patients manage problems and become better at helping themselves.

Thermoregulation The body process that balances heat production and heat loss to maintain the body's temperature.

Third heart sound (S₃) Heart sound that is sometimes heard after the second heart sound in children, young adults, and pregnant women during the third trimester. Also called a *ventricular gallop*.

Third spacing A shift of fluid from the vascular space into an area where it is not available to support normal physiologic processes.

Thoracentesis Needle insertion into the pleural space to remove fluid accumulation.

Thoracolumbar sacral orthosis (TLSO) A brace contoured to conform to the body and support the spine. Also called an *underarm brace* or *Boston brace*.

Thought blocking Speech stopped in midsentence as if the thought disappeared from the individual's head.

Thought disorders Disorders associated with schizophrenia that involve an abnormal way of thinking, such as disorganized thinking, sensory overload, thought blocking, neologisms, loose association, clang, and perseveration.

Threshold potential The point at which an action potential is capable of being generated.

Thrill A palpable vibration over the precordium or an artery.

Thromboemboli Emboli created by a blood clot.

Thrombophlebitis Sometimes called phlebitis, condition in which a blood clot forms and blocks one or more veins. Clots typically form in the legs but can form in the arms and neck in rare instances.

Throughput The process by which information, energy, or material that enters a system (input) is used by the system.

Thrush White patches that look like milk curds that adhere to the mucous membranes usually caused by an infected vaginal tract during birth, antibiotic use, or poor hand hygiene. Bleeding may occur if patches are removed.

Thyroid crisis See Thyroid storm.

Thyroid storm An extreme state of hyperthyroidism. Now extremely rare due to improved diagnosis and treatment methods. Also called *thyroid crisis*.

Thyroidectomy Surgical removal of all or part of the thyroid gland.

Thyroiditis Inflammation of the thyroid gland.

Thyrotoxicosis A disorder caused by excessive delivery of thyroid hormone to the peripheral tissues. Also called *hyperthyroidism*.

Tics Semi-involuntary movements that are sudden, repetitive, and non-rhythmic. They may involve muscle groups or vocalizations (motor or phonic).

Time constraints Deadlines for completion.

Time-out A preprocedure verification to ensure the correct procedure is being performed at the right site on the right patient.

Time priority A time constraint to complete an action.

Tine test Test in which a multiple-puncture device is used to introduce tuberculin into the skin.

Tinea pedis Fungal infection of the feet. Also called *athlete's foot*.

Tinnitus The perception of sound or noise in the ears without stimulus from the environment.

Token economies Formalized programs of contingency contracts.

Tolerance State in which a particular dose elicits a smaller response than it formerly did. With increased tolerance, the individual needs higher and higher doses to obtain the desired response.

Tone 1. The amount of tension or resistance to movement in a muscle. 2. The ability of vessels to constrict or dilate to maintain normal pressure.

Tonic–clonic seizures Alternating contraction (tonic phase) and relaxation (clonic phase) of muscles during seizure activity.

Tonic neck reflex In response to an infant's head being turned to one side while the infant lies on the back, the infant will extend the arm and leg on the side the infant faces while the opposite arm and leg will be flexed.

Tonic phase Initial phase of a generalized seizure, manifested by unconsciousness and continuous muscular contraction.

Tonicity The osmolality of a solution. Solutions may be termed *isotonic*, *hypertonic*, or *hypotonic*.

Torsades de pointes A type of ventricular tachycardia associated with a prolongation of the QT interval.

Tort A civil wrong committed against an individual or an individual's property.

Total anomalous pulmonary venous return The pulmonary veins empty into the right atrium or into veins leading to the right atrium, rather than into the left atrium.

Total lymphoid irradiation A procedure sometimes used in the treatment of rheumatoid arthritis; it decreases total lymphocyte levels.

Total quality management (TQM) A comprehensive management philosophy that improves quality and productivity by using data and statistics to improve system processes.

Toxic multinodular goiter A tumor characterized by small, discrete, independently functioning nodules in the thyroid gland tissue that secrete excessive amounts of thyroid hormone.

Toxoplasmosis Space-occupying lesions common in patients with AIDS that may cause headache, altered mental status, and neurologic deficits.

Trachoma A chronic conjunctivitis caused by *Chlamydia trachomatis*. It is a significant preventable cause of blindness worldwide.

Traction The application of a straightening or pulling force to return or maintain fractured bones in their normal anatomic position.

Traditional family An autonomous unit in which both parents reside in the home with their children, the mother assuming the nurturing role and the father providing the necessary economic resources.

Transactional leader A leader who has a relationship with followers based on an exchange of some resource valued by the follower.

Transcellular fluid One of the compartments where extracellular fluid is found. Examples of transcellular fluid are cerebrospinal, pericardial, pancreatic, pleural, intraocular, biliary, peritoneal, and synovial fluids.

Transcendence A person's recognition that there is something other or greater than the self and a seeking and valuing of that greater other, whether it is an ultimate being, force, or value.

Transcranial magnetic stimulation (TMS) A promising alternative therapy for individuals with schizophrenia that uses electromagnetic stimulus to affect brain activity in the cerebral cortex.

Transductive reasoning Connecting two events in a cause-and-effect relationship simply because they occur together in time.

Transection An injury that occurs when an individual is injured by a gunshot, stabbing, or similar force, which may partially or completely sever the spinal cord.

Transference The transfer of feelings that were originally evoked by one's parents or significant others to people in the present setting.

Transformational leader A leader who fosters creativity, risk taking, commitment, and collaboration by empowering a group to share in an organization's vision. The leader inspires others with a clear, attractive, and attainable goal and enlists them to participate in attaining the goal.

Transfusion reaction A type II or cytotoxic hypersensitivity reaction to blood of an incompatible type.

Transgender Gradations of human characteristics running from female to male; more commonly, an individual who expresses a gender identity different from that with which he or she was born.

Transient ischemic attack (TIA) A brief period of localized cerebral ischemia that causes neurologic deficits lasting for less than 24 hours. Also called a *mini-stroke*.

Transitional milk A light yellow milk that is more copious than colostrum and contains more fat, lactose, water-soluble vitamins, and calories; it usually presents between the second and fifth day following birth.

Transjugular intrahepatic portosystemic shunt (TIPS) An expandable metal stent inserted through a transcutaneous needle to channel blood from the portal vein into the hepatic vein, bypassing the cirrhotic liver.

Translational research A systematic approach of converting research knowledge into applications of healthcare for improved patient outcomes.

Transplacental immunity Passive immunity transferred from mother to infant.

Transposition of the great arteries (TGA) A congenital heart defect in which the pulmonary artery, the outflow tract for the left ventricle, and the aorta, the outflow tract for the right ventricle, are transposed.

Transsexual An individual who feels his or her sexual anatomy is not consistent with his or her gender identity.

Transurethral incision of the prostate (TUIP) Small incisions are made in the smooth muscle where the prostate is attached to the bladder in order to reduce pressure on the urethra.

Transurethral needle ablation (TUNA) A procedure that uses low-level radio-frequency through twin needles to burn away a region of the enlarged prostate in order to improve the flow of urine.

Transurethral resection of the prostate (TURP) A procedure that removes obstructing prostate tissue using the wire loop of a resectoscope and electrocautery inserted through the urethra.

Transverse diameter The largest diameter of the pelvic inlet; helps determine the shape of the inlet.

Trauma An injury to human tissues and organs resulting from the transfer of energy from an external environmental source, such as a motor vehicle, a fire, or a sharp object.

Traumatic brain injury (TBI) An injury resulting from an external physical force, such as a blow or jolt to the head, that causes displacement of the brain within the skull and disruption of normal brain function.

Traumatic cataracts A type of cataract that may result from an injury to the eye.

Tremors Rhythmic, involuntary movements or twitching of the extremities.

Triage The process of identifying priorities for implementing care.

Trial and error A group decision strategy in which the most viable solution is attempted.

Tricuspid atresia The absence of the tricuspid valve.

Tricyclic antidepressant (TCA) A class of drugs that inhibit the reuptake of both norepinephrine and serotonin into presynaptic nerve terminals. TCAs are primarily used in the pharmacotherapy of depression.

Triglycerides Substances converted from dietary fats and carbohydrates to store energy in fat cells.

Triplet Three premature ventricular contractions in a row.

Tripod position A position of sitting and leaning forward; often used by patients who are having difficulty breathing.

Trisomy An extra chromosome.

Trisomy 21 A condition that occurs when an individual born with Down syndrome has an additional full chromosome present.

Troponins Proteins released during a myocardial infarction that are sensitive indicators of myocardial damage.

Trousseau sign Spasmodic contraction of the hand and fingers in response to occlusion of the blood supply by a blood pressure cuff; caused by decreased blood calcium levels. A test used to check for hypocalcemia.

True pelvis The portion that lies below the linea terminalis; made up of the inlet, cavity, and outlet.

Truncus arteriosus A heart defect in which a single large vessel empties both ventricles and provides circulation for the pulmonary, systemic, and coronary circulations.

Trunk incurvation In response to stroking an infant's spine, the infant's pelvis will turn toward the stimulated side. Also called *Galant reflex*.

Tubal ligation A surgical procedure to clip, tie off, band, or plug the fallopian tubes to sterilize a female patient.

Tubercle A granulomatous lesion (a sealed-off colony of bacilli) formed from *Mycobacterium tuberculosis*.

Tuberculosis (TB) A chronic, recurrent infectious disease caused by *Mycobacterium tuberculosis*. TB usually affects the lungs, but any organ can be affected.

Tubular sound The sound air makes moving through a clear and functioning trachea.

Tumor lysis syndrome (TLS) A condition that occurs when tumor cells dissolve and release intracellular contents into circulation, causing hyperkalemia, hyperuricemia, and hyperphosphatemia.

Tumor marker A protein molecule detectable in serum or other body fluids that is used to highlight suspicious regions for follow-up.

TURP syndrome A condition that is characterized by hyponatremia, decreased hematocrit, hypertension, bradycardia, nausea, and confusion.

Two-career family A family in which both partners are employed by choice or necessity. A two-career family may or may not have children.

Tympanic membrane A thin, tense membrane that separates the middle ear from the external auditory canal, protecting the middle ear from the external environment.

Tympanocentesis A surgical incision of the tympanic membrane. Also called *myringotomy*.

Tympanogram A test that provides a graph of the middle ear's ability to transmit sound.

Tympanostomy tubes Pressuring-equalizing tubes inserted to provide the middle ear with ventilation and drainage during healing.

Tympany A musical or drumlike sound produced from an air-filled stomach.

Type 1 diabetes mellitus An absolute deficiency of insulin related to pancreatic beta cell destruction that results in severe hyperglycemia and diabetic ketoacidosis, among other symptoms.

Type 2 diabetes mellitus A relative deficiency of insulin, which may be related to insulin resistance and inadequate secretion of insulin to meet body needs. Both of these components are usually present at time of diagnosis.

Ulcer A break in the GI mucosa that develops when the mucosal barrier is unable to protect the mucosa from damage by hydrochloric acid and pepsin, the gastric digestive juices.

Ulcerative colitis A chronic inflammatory bowel disorder that affects the mucosa and submucosa of the colon and rectum.

Ultrafiltration Removal of excess body water using a hydrostatic pressure gradient.

Ultrasound A test using intermittent ultrasonic waves transmitted by an alternating current to a transducer and applied to the abdomen.

Unconscious mind The part of an individual's mental life of which he or she is unaware.

Underinsured Individuals whose healthcare coverage is insufficient to meet their needs.

Undernutrition Health effects due to insufficient or diminished nutrient intake or stores. Also known as *malnutrition*.

Unifocal When a ventricular impulse arises from one ectopic site.

Unilateral lobar pneumonia A pattern of pneumonia in which bacteria tend to be distributed evenly throughout one or more lobes of a single lung.

Uninsured Individuals who are without any type of healthcare coverage.

Unipolar depression A mood disorder characterized by loss of interest in life and unresponsiveness, moving from mild to severe, with severe symptoms lasting at least 2 weeks. Also called *major depressive disorder (MDD)*.

Universal precautions (UP) Safety guidelines, such as proper hand hygiene, use of proper protective equipment, safe injection practices, and effective management of potentially contaminated surfaces or equipment, that are designed to decrease the risk of transmitting

unidentified pathogens. Also called *standard precautions* and *body substance isolation (BSI)*.

Universal protocol Established guidelines for healthcare professionals to prevent errors during surgical procedures, including wrong-site surgery.

Unlicensed assistive personnel (UAP) Members of a nursing team who assume delegated aspects of basic patient care such as bathing, assisting with feeding, and collecting specimens. UAPs include certified nurse assistants, hospital attendants, nurse technicians, and orderlies.

Unresolved bacteriuria The presence of bacteria in urine that fails to resolve with treatment.

Unsaturated fat A triglyceride fat that does not contain all of the hydrogen ions it is capable of holding.

Upper body obesity Identified by a waist-to-hip ratio of greater than 1 in men or 0.8 in women. Also called *central obesity*.

Uremia Excessive amounts of urea in the blood.

Uremic fetor A urine-like breath odor often associated with a metallic taste in the mouth.

Uremic frost Crystallized deposits of urea on the skin.

Ureteral stent A thin catheter inserted into the ureter to provide for urine flow and ureteral support.

Ureterolithotomy An incision in the affected ureter to remove a calculus.

Ureteroplasty The surgical repair of a ureter.

Urgency The sudden, strong desire to void.

Urgency factor A way to illustrate how much time can safely lapse before doing interventions without compromising patient outcomes.

Uric acid stones Develop when the urine concentration of uric acid is high.

Urinary calculi Stones in the urinary tract.

Urinary drainage system Those organs required to drain urine from the kidneys, including the ureters, urinary bladder, and urethra.

Urinary frequency The need to urinate often, specifically more than four to six times a day.

Urinary hesitancy A delay and difficulty in initiating voiding; often associated with dysuria.

Urinary incontinence Involuntary urination due to the temporary or permanent inability of the external sphincter muscles to control the flow of urine from the bladder. Also called *involuntary urination*.

Urinary reflux Backward flow of urine.

Urinary retention The accumulation of urine in the bladder and inability of the bladder to empty itself, resulting in overdistention of the bladder.

Urinary stasis Stagnation of urinary flow.

Urination Releasing urine from the urinary bladder. Also called *voiding* or *micturition*.

Uroflowmetry A method of measuring urine flow rate.

Urolithiasis The formation of stones in the urinary tract.

Urticaria Patches of pale, itchy wheals in an erythematous area. Also known as *hives*.

Uterine atony The relaxation of uterine muscle tone.

Uterosacral ligaments Ligaments that provide support for the uterus and cervix at the level of the ischial spines.

Uterus The hollow muscular organ in which the fertilized ovum is implanted and in which the developing fetus is nourished until birth.

Utilitarianism A form of consequentialist theory that views a good act as one that brings the most good and the least harm for the greatest number of people. This is called the principle of utility.

Utility See Utilitarianism.

Utilization review An evaluation of the use of resources to identify areas of overuse, misuse, and underuse.

Uveitis Inflammation of the middle layer of the eye called the uvea.

Vaccine Suspensions of whole or fractionated bacteria or viruses that have been treated to make them nonpathogenic; introduced by immunization to provoke active immunity.

Vacuum extraction An obstetric procedure used by physicians and CNMs to assist the birth of a fetus by applying suction to the fetal head.

Vagina The muscular and membranous tube that connects the external genitals with the uterus.

Vaginal birth after cesarean (VBAC) An option for a mother to choose a trial of labor and vaginal birth after having a cesarean for a previous child, provided the previous cesarean was required due to a nonrecurring indication and the mother meets the guidelines established by the American College of Obstetricians and Gynecologists.

Vaginismus The involuntary spasm of the outer one third of the vaginal muscles, making penetration of the vagina painful and sometimes impossible.

Validation The act of verifying the accuracy and factuality of data.

Valsalva maneuver Forced exhalation against a closed glottis.

Values Personal beliefs about truth and the worth of behaviors or objects; standards that influence behavior.

Values clarification A process of consciously identifying, examining, and developing individual values that helps nurses gain the ability to choose actions on the basis of deliberately adopted values.

Variable decelerations A condition that occurs if the umbilical cord becomes compressed, reducing blood flow between the placenta and fetus. Fetal hypertension stimulates the baroreceptors in the aortic arch and carotid sinuses, slowing the fetal heart rate.

Variance 1. An unmet goal. 2. An incident or accident that affects a patient or a visitor in a healthcare facility.

Vasectomy A procedure to surgically sever the vas deferens on both sides of the scrotum to sterilize a male patient.

Vasogenic shock Shock that results from widespread vasodilation and decreased peripheral resistance. Also called *distributive shock*.

Vaso-occlusive crisis See Sickle cell crisis.

Vegan A type of vegetarian diet that excludes all animal and fish products, including dairy, meat, eggs, and honey.

Venous stasis The collection and stagnation of blood in the lower extremities.

Venous thrombectomy Surgical removal of a blood clot from the femoral vein to prevent pulmonary embolism or gangrene.

Venous thrombosis A condition in which a blood clot (thrombus) forms on the wall of a vein, accompanied by inflammation of the vein wall and some degree of obstructed venous blood flow. Also called *thrombophlebitis*.

Ventilation The exchange of oxygen and carbon dioxide.

Ventilation-perfusion (V-Q) The movement of oxygen across the alveolar–capillary membrane into a well-perfusing capillary.

Ventricular aneurysm An outpouching of the ventricular wall that does not contract during systole, causing stroke volume to decrease.

Ventricular bigeminy A premature ventricular contraction following each normal beat.

Ventricular gallop (S_3) Heart sound sometimes heard after the second heart sound in children, young adults, and pregnant women during the third trimester. Also called the *third heart sound.*

Ventricular septal defect (VSD) An opening in the ventricular septum that causes increased pulmonary blood flow.

Ventricular trigeminy A premature ventricular contraction every third beat.

Veracity A moral principle that holds that an individual should tell the truth and not lie.

Verbal abuse The use of berating, humiliating, ridiculing, blaming, or threatening language toward an individual.

Verbal communication Transmitting information through the spoken or written word.

Vernix caseosa A whitish, cheeselike substance that covers a fetus while in utero.

Vertical rotation The degree of rotation of the vertebrae.

Vertical transmission Perinatal transmission of an infection, such as the human immunodeficiency virus, from mother to infant.

Vertigo A sensation of whirling or rotation.

Very-low-calorie diets A program providing a protein-sparing modified fast (400–800 kcal/day or less) under close medical supervision.

Vesicoureteral reflux A condition in which urine moves from the bladder back toward the kidney. A common risk factor in children who develop pyelonephritis that may also be seen in adults whose bladder outflow is obstructed.

Vesicular sounds The soft and breezy sounds of air moving in and out of the lobes at the alveolar level.

Vestibulitis Pain of the outer portion of the vagina upon touch or attempted penetration.

Vibration A series of vigorous quiverings produced by hands that are placed flat against the patient's chest wall.

Violence The use of excessive force against other individuals or oneself, often resulting in physical or psychologic injuries or death.

Virchow triad Three factors associated with thrombophlebitis: stasis of blood, vessel damage, and increased blood coagulability.

Virions Virus particles unable to grow and reproduce outside a host.

Virulence The ability of a microorganism to produce disease.

Virus A type of microorganism that must enter living cells in order to reproduce.

Visceral Of or relating to any large organ in the body.

Visceral pain Pain arising from body organs. It is dull and poorly localized because of the low number of nociceptors.

Viscosupplementation A treatment for osteoarthritis of the knee that involves injecting lubricating substances directly into the knee.

Visual Of or relating to sight.

Vitamins Micronutrient compounds that are involved in regulating body functioning. Most vitamins, with the exceptions of vitamins D and K, cannot be manufactured within the body and must be consumed through dietary intake.

Vitiligo An autoimmune disorder that results in loss of melanin in patches of the face, hands, or groin.

Voiding Releasing urine from the urinary bladder. Also called *urination* or *micturition*.

Voiding cystourethrography Use of a contrast medium and x-rays to assess the bladder and urethra when filled and during voiding.

Volatile acid Acids eliminated from the body as a gas.

Volkmann contracture Impaired mobility of the arm and inability to extend the arm completely, which is a common complication of elbow fractures.

Voluntary admission The detention of a patient in a psychiatric or medical facility at the patient's request.

Voluntary insurance Healthcare insurance that provides no guarantee of universality because coverage may be expensive and difficult to purchase.

Vomiting The forceful expulsion of the contents of the upper gastrointestinal tract resulting from contraction of muscles in the gut and abdominal wall.

Vulnerability An individual's susceptibility to react to a specific stressor.

Vulnerability factors A practice, behavior, or environmental factor that increases the potential of an individual becoming a victim of violence.

Vulnerable populations Social groups with inadequate access to healthcare because they lack resources and are exposed to more risk factors.

Vulva The external female genitals.

Vulvodynia Constant, unremitting burning that is localized to the vulva with an acute onset.

Warm zone When a disaster occurs, this zone, located at least 300 feet from the outer edge of a hot zone, is where decontamination occurs and rapid triage and emergency treatment are given to stabilize victims. Also called the *yellow zone*, *contamination zone*, or *contamination reduction zone*.

Water An essential nutrient for the body's survival, it contributes to fluid balance and plays an important role in nerve and muscle functioning and in the transport of nutrients to all body systems.

Weaning 1. The process of removing ventilator support and reestablishing spontaneous, independent respirations. 2. The process of discontinuing breastfeeding and transitioning an infant to another feeding method.

Well-being A subjective perception of feeling well that can be described objectively and measured.

Wellness A state of well-being that encompasses self-responsibility, dynamic growth, nutrition, physical fitness, emotional health, preventive healthcare, and the whole being of the individual.

Wellness diagnosis A term that describes human responses to levels of wellness in an individual, family, or community that have a readiness for enhancement. For example, *Readiness for Enhanced Coping*.

Wernicke encephalopathy A condition typically seen in people with alcoholism that is characterized by ataxia (lack of coordination), abnormal eye movements, and confusion.

Wheezing A high-pitched whistling sound most often heard on expiration and caused by the narrowing of bronchi; wheezes can also be heard on inspiration.

Whiplash An injury that results from sudden impact to a motor vehicle that causes an individual's head and neck to be forcibly contorted, resulting in injury to the spine.

Whistleblower A nurse or other individual who goes outside of an organization for the public's best interest when the organization fails to follow procedures regarding safety and patient care.

Whistleblowing The act of going outside of an organization for the public's best interest when an organization fails to follow procedures regarding safety and patient care.

White blood cells (WBCs) See Leukocytes.

Withdrawing or withholding life-sustaining therapy (WWLST) The withdrawal of extraordinary means of life support, such as removing a ventilator or withholding special attempts to revive a patient, and allowing the patient to die of the underlying medical condition.

Work ethic A belief in the importance and moral worth of work.

Workplace bullying Malicious, repeated, harmful mistreatment of an individual with whom one works, regardless of whether that individual is an equal, a superior, or a subordinate.

Workplace violence Any physical assault, threatening behavior, or verbal abuse occurring in the workplace.

Worldview The way in which people in a culture perceive ideas and attitudes about the world, other people, and life in general.

Worst-case scenario Technique designed to help groups make decisions that involve risk. The worst-case outcome is outlined for each alternative, and then the scenario with the comparatively best outcome is selected as the preferred outcome. This technique helps ensure that the "least of all evils" is selected.

Wrong-site surgery (WSS) A surgical operation that is performed at the wrong location on a patient's body due to error.

Xenograft Skin used for transplantation that was obtained from an animal, usually a pig. Also called *heterograft*.

Xenophobia The fear or dislike of people different from one's self.

Xerostomia Dry mouth that occurs when an individual's supply of saliva is reduced.

Zollinger-Ellison syndrome A form of peptic ulcer disease caused by a gastrinoma, or gastrin-secreting tumor of the pancreas, stomach, or intestines.

Zygote A fertilized egg.

Combined Index

Special Features

FOCUS ON DIVERSITY AND CULTURE

FOCUS ON INTEGRATIVE HEALTH

MEDICATIONS